## Part 4

## RHYTHM AND CONDUCTION DISORDERS



## Part 5

## SYNCOPE, SUDDEN DEATH, AND CARDIOPULMONARY RESUSCITATION



## Part 6

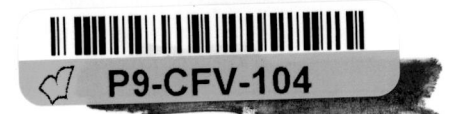

## CORONARY HEART DISEASE

# HURST'S
# THE HEART

## NOTICE

Medicine is an ever-changing science. As new research and clinical experience broaden our knowledge, changes in treatment and drug therapy are required. The authors and the publisher of this work have checked with sources believed to be reliable in their efforts to provide information that is complete and generally in accord with the standards accepted at the time of publication. However, in view of the possibility of human error or changes in medical sciences, neither the authors nor the publisher nor any other party who has been involved in the preparation or publication of this work warrants that the information contained herein is in every respect accurate or complete, and they disclaim all responsibility for any errors or omissions or for the results obtained from use of the information contained in this work. Readers are encouraged to confirm the information contained herein with other sources. For example and in particular, readers are advised to check the product information sheet included in the package of each drug they plan to administer to be certain that the information contained in this work is accurate and that changes have not been made in the recommended dose or in the contraindications for administration. This recommendation is of particular importance in connection with new or infrequently used drugs.

# HURST'S THE HEART

VOLUME 1

ELEVENTH EDITION


## Editors

### VALENTIN FUSTER, MD, PhD

Director, The Zena and Michael A. Wiener Cardiovascular Institute and The Marie-Josée and Henry R. Kravis Center for Cardiovascular Health
Richard Gorlin, MD/Heart Research Foundation, Professor of Cardiology, The Mount Sinai Medical Center and School of Medicine
New York, New York

### R. WAYNE ALEXANDER, MD, PhD

R. Bruce Logue Professor and Chair
Department of Medicine
Emory University School of Medicine
Atlanta, Georgia

### ROBERT A. O'ROURKE, MD

Charles Conrad Brown Distinguished Professor in Cardiovascular Disease
University of Texas Health Science Center at San Antonio
San Antonio, Texas

## Associate Editors

### ROBERT ROBERTS, MD

Professor of Medicine
President and CEO
University of Ottawa Heart Institute
Ottawa, Ontario, Canada

### SPENCER B. KING III, MD

Fuqua Chair of Interventional Cardiology
The Fuqua Heart Center at Piedmont Hospital
Co-Director, American Cardiovascular Research Institute
Clinical Professor of Medicine
Emory University School of Medicine
Atlanta, Georgia

### IRA S. NASH, MD

Associate Professor of Medicine
Mount Sinai School of Medicine
Associate Director, The Zena and Michael A. Wiener Cardiovascular Institute and The Marie-Josée and Henry R. Kravis Center for Cardiovascular Health
Mount Sinai Medical Center
New York, New York

### ERIC N. PRYSTOWSKY, MD

Director, Clinical Electrophysiology Laboratory
St. Vincent Hospital
Indianapolis, Indiana
Consulting Professor of Medicine
Duke University Medical Center
Durham, North Carolina



McGRAW-HILL
Medical Publishing Division

New York Chicago San Francisco Lisbon London Madrid Mexico City
Milan New Delhi San Juan Seoul Singapore Sydney Toronto

The McGraw-Hill Companies

Hurst's
THE HEART
Eleventh Edition



1234567890 DOWDOW 0987654

ISBN 0-07-142264-1 (Single vol. ed.)
0-07-142265-X (2-vol. set ed.)
0-07-143224-8 (Vol. 1)
0-07-143225-6 (Vol. 2)

This book was set in Times Roman by *The GTS Companies*/York, PA Campus.
The editors were Darlene B. Cooke, Marc Strauss, Marsha Loeb,
and Lester A. Sheinis.
The production supervisor was Richard C. Ruzycka.
The text designer was Marsha Cohen / Parallelogram Graphics.
The cover designer was Aimee Nordin.
The indexer was Alexandra Nickerson.
RR Donnelley was printer and binder.

This book is printed on acid-free paper.

**Library of Congress Cataloging-in-Publication Data**

Hurst's the heart / edited by Valentin Fuster ... [et al.].—11th ed.
p. ; cm.
Includes bibliographical references and index.
ISBN 0-07-142264-1 (single vol.)—ISBN 0-07-142265-X (2-vol. set)
1. Cardiovascular system—Diseases. 2. Heart—Diseases. I. Title: Heart.
II. Fuster, Valentin.
[DNLM: 1. Cardiovascular Diseases. WG 100 H9662 2004]
RC667.H88 2004
616.1—dc22

2003059615

# CONTENTS

## Part 3

## HEART FAILURE



## Part 4

## RHYTHM AND CONDUCTION DISORDERS



## Part 5

## SYNCOPE, SUDDEN DEATH, AND CARDIOPULMONARY RESUSCITATION



## Part 6

## CORONARY HEART DISEASE

## Part 11

## CARDIOMYOPATHY AND SPECIFIC HEART MUSCLE DISEASES



## Part 12

## PERICARDIAL DISEASES AND ENDOCARDITIS



## Part 13

## ANESTHESIA, SURGERY, AND THE HEART



## Part 14

## MISCELLANEOUS CONDITIONS AND CARDIOVASCULAR DISEASE



## Part 15

## DISEASES OF THE GREAT VESSELS AND PERIPHERAL VESSELS

# CONTRIBUTORS


### Fadi G. Akar, PhD
Post Doctoral Fellow
School of Medicine
Division of Cardiology
Johns Hopkins University
Baltimore, Maryland
Chapter 10

### Masood Akhtar, MD, FACC, FACP
Clinical Professor of Medicine
University of Wisconsin School of Medicine
Cardiology Department
Milwaukee Clinical Campus
Aurora Sinai Medical Center and St. Luke's Medical Center
Milwaukee, Wisconsin
Chapter 34

### R. Wayne Alexander, MD, PhD
R. Bruce Logue Professor and Chair
Department of Medicine
Emory University School of Medicine
Atlanta, Georgia
Chapters 7 and 52

### Suhail Allaqaband, MD
Clinical Assistant Professor
Department of Cardiology
University of Wisconsin Medical School–Milwaukee Clinical Campus
Consultant Interventional Cardiologist
Aurora Sinai Medical Center and St. Luke's Medical Center
Milwaukee, Wisconsin
Chapter 103

### Jeffrey L. Anderson, MD
Associate Chief of Cardiology
Professor of Internal Medicine
University of Utah School of Medicine
Salt Lake City, Utah
Chapter 81

### Juan Jose Badimon, PhD
Professor of Medicine
Director
Cardiovascular Biology Reserch Laboratory
Mount Sinai School of Medicine
New York, New York
Chapter 45

### Lina Badimon, PhD
Professor and Director
Cardiovascular Institute
High Council for Scientific Research
Director
Catalan Institute for Cardiovascular Sciences
Hospital de la Santa Creu I Sant Pau
Barcelona, Spain
Chapter 45

### James M. Bailey, MD
Department of Anesthesiology
North East Georgia Diagnostic Hospital
Gainesville, Georgia
Chapter 59

### Steven R. Bailey, MD
Professor of Medicine and Radiology,
Director
Interventional Cardiology
Director
Cardiac Catheterization Laboratory
University of Texas Health Science Center San Antonio
San Antonio, Texas
Chapter 68

### Tanvir K. Bajwa, MD
Associate Professor of Medicine
University of Wisconsin Medical School–Milwaukee Clinical Campus
Director
Cardiac Catheterization Laboratory
Director
Interventional Cardiology Fellowship
Aurora Sinai Medical Center and St. Luke's Medical Center
Milwaukee, Wisconsin
Chapter 103

### George L. Bakris, MD, FACP
Professor of Preventive Medicine and Internal Medicine
RUSH Medical College of RUSH University at RUSH-Presbyterian-St. Luke's Medical Center
Vice-Chairman
Department of Preventive Medicine
Director
Section of Clinical Research
Department of Preventive Medicine
Chicago, Illinois
Chapter 61

### Emelia J. Benjamin, MD, ScM
Clinical Associate Professor
Department of Medicine
Boston University School of Medicine
Boston, Massachusetts
Director
Echocardiography Laboratory
Framingham Heart Study
Framingham, Massachusetts
Staff Cardiologist
Boston Medical Center
Cardiology Department
Boston, Massachusetts
Chapter 2

### Daniel S. Berman, MD
Professor of Medicine
Department of Nuclear Cardiology
Director
Cardiac Imaging
Cedars-Sinai Medical Center
Los Angeles, California
Chapter 19

### Gerald J. Berry, MD
Associate Professor of Pathology
Director of Cardiac Pathology
Stanford University School of Medicine
Stanford University Medical Center
Stanford, California
Chapter 26

### Alan L. Bisno, MD

Professor of Medicine
Department of Medicine
University of Miami School of Medicine
Medical Service
VA Medical Center
Medical Service
Miami, Florida
Chapter 65

### Henry R. Black, MD

The Charles J. and Margaret Roberts
Professor of Preventive Medicine
Professor of Internal Medicine and
Pharmacology
Associate Dean for Research
RUSH Medical College of RUSH University
at RUSH-Presbyterian-St. Luke's
Medical Center
Chicago, Illinois
Chapter 61

### Daniel G. Blanchard, MD

Professor of Medicine
Department of Medicine (Cardiology)
University of California
San Diego School of Medicine
Director
Cardiac Noninvasive Laboratory
University of California San Diego Medical
Center
San Diego, California
Chapter 15

### Rob A. Bleasdale, MD

Lecturer
Wales Heart Institute
Heath Park, Cardiff, United Kingdom
Chapter 38

### Teresa Bohlmeyer, MD

Division of Cardiology
University of Colorado Health Sciences
Center
Denver, Colorado
Chapter 76

### Wendy M. Book, MD

Assistant Professor of Medicine
Emory University School of Medicine
Director
Emory Adult Congenital Program
Division of Cardiology
Emory Hospital
Atlanta, Georgia
Chapter 89

### Harisios Boudoulas, MD

Emeritus Professor of Medicine
Cardiology
Ohio State University College of Medicine
and Public Health
Columbus Ohio
Director
Clinical Research Center
Foundation of Biomedical Research
Academy of Athens
Athens, Greece
Chapter 40

### Kenneth L. Brigham, MD

Vice Chair for Research
Department of Medicine
Emory University School of Medicine
Atlanta, Georgia
Chapter 64

### Michael R. Bristow, MD, PhD

Division of Cardiology
University of Colorado Health Sciences
Center
Denver, Colorado
Chapter 76

### Bruce R. Brodie, MD

Clinical Professor of Medicine
University of North Carolina Teaching
Service
Moses H. Cone Heart and Vascular Center
Greensboro, North Carolina
Chapter 56

### Ramon Brugada, MD, FACC

Masonic Medical Research Laboratory
Molecular Genetics Department
Director
Molecular Genetics Program
Utica, New York
Chapter 72

### Allen P. Burke, MD

Adjunct Professor of Pathology
Georgetown University
Associate Chair
Department of Cardiovascular Pathology
Armed Forces Institute of Pathology
Washington, District of Columbia
Chapter 49

### Hugh Calkins, MD

Professor of Medicine
Divison of Cardiac Electrophysiology
John Hopkins School of Medicine
Johns Hopkins Hospital
Baltimore, Maryland
Chapter 30

### Louis R. Caplan, MD

Professor of Neurology
Harvard Medical School
Chief
Cerebrovascular Disease
Beth Israel Deaconess Medical Center
Boston, Massachusetts
Chapter 99

### Agustin Castellanos, MD, FACC, FAHA

Professor of Medicine
Director
Clinical Electrophysiology
Division of Cardiology
Jackson Memorial Medical Center
University of Miami School of Medicine
Miami, Florida
Chapter 13

### Simon Chakko, MD

Chief
Cardiology Section
University of Miami School of Medicine
Veterans Affairs Medical Center
Professor of Medicine
University of Miami School of Medicine
Miami, Florida
Chapter 65

### Nisha Chandra-Strobos, MD

Professor of Medicine
Johns Hopkins University School of
Medicine
Director
Coronary Care Unit
Johns Hopkins Bayview Medical Center
Baltimore, Maryland
Chapter 42

### Pamela Charney, MD, FACP
Clinical Professor of Medicine
Albert Einstein College of Medicine
New York, New York
Program Director
Internal Medicine Residency
Norwalk Hospital
Norwalk, Connecticut
Chapter 97

### Melvin D. Cheitlin, MD
Emeritus Professor of Medicine
University of California San Francisco
Former Chief of Cardiology
San Francisco General Hospital
Cardiology Service
San Francisco, California
Chapter 88

### James T. T. Chen, MD
Professor Emeritus of Radiology
Duke Medical Center
Durham, North Carolina
Chapter 14

### Domenico Cianflone, MD, FESC
Director Coronary Care Unit
San Raffaele University Hospital
Milan, Italy
Chapter 46

### Michael Clark, MD, FACC
Senior Vice President
Chief Medical Director
Swiss RE Life & Health
Medical Department
Armonk, New York
Chapter 105

### Stephen D. Clements Jr., MD
Professor of Medicine
Cardiology
Emory University School of Medicine
Atlanta, Georgia
Chapter 59

### Lynn Clemow, MD
Behavioral Cardiovascular Health and Hypertension Program
Columbia Presbyterian Medical Center
New York, New York
Chapter 107

### Stefano Coli, MD
Coronary Care Unit
San Raffaele University Hospital
Milan, Italy
Chapter 46

### Denton A. Cooley, MD
Clinical Professor of Surgery
University of Texas Medical School
Houston, Texas
Chapter 85

### Roberto Corti, MD
Consultant
Division of Cardiology
University Hospital
Zurich University
Zurich, Switzerland
Chapter 45

### Ralph B. D'Agostino, PhD
Professor of Mathematics
Statistics and Public Health
Mathematics and Statistics Department
Boston University
Boston, Massachusetts
Director of Data Management and Statistical Analysis
Framingham Heart Study
Framingham, Massachusetts
Chapter 2

### Karina W. Davidson, PhD
Behavioral Cardiovascular Health and Hypertension Program
Columbia Presbyterian Medical Center
New York, New York
Chapter 107

### John E. Deanfield, MB, FACC
Cardiothoracic Unit
Great Ormond Street Hospital for Children
Professor of Cardiology
Cardiac Unit
Institute of Child Health
London, United Kingdom
Chapter 74

### Louis J. Dell'Italia, MD
University of Alabama at Birmingham
Birmingham, Alabama
Chapter 67

### Anthony N. DeMaria, MD
Judith and Jack White Chair in Cardiology
Professor of Medicine
Chief
Division of Cardiology
University of California at San Diego
San Diego, California
Chapter 15

### Howard V. Dinh, MD
Cardiology Fellow
Division of Cardiology
David Geffen School of Medicine at UCLA
UCLA Medical Center
Los Angeles, California
Chapter 21

### Thomas F. Dodson, MD
Associate Professor of Surgery
Vice Chairman for Education
Program Director for General Surgery Residency Program
Emory University School of Medicine and the Emory Clinic
Atlanta, Georgia
Chapter 102

### John S. Douglas Jr., MD
Professor of Medicine
Emory University Hospital School of Medicine
Director of Interventional Cardiology
Emory University Hospital
Atlanta, Georgia
Chapters 17, 55, 57

### W. Lane Duvall, MD
Cardiovascular Fellow
Mount Sinai School of Medicine
The Zena and Michael A. Wiener Cardiovascular Institute and The Marie-Josée and Henry R. Kravis Center for Cardiovascular Health
Mount Sinai Medical Center
New York, New York
Chapter 54

### Victor J. Dzau, MD

Chairman
Department of Medicine
Brigham and Women's Hospital
Hershey Professor of the Practice and Theory of Medicine
Harvard University
Medical School
Boston, Massachusetts
Chapter 11

### Kim A. Eagle, MD

Albion Walter Hewlett Professor of Internal Medicine
Clinical Director
Cardiovascular Center
University of Michigan Health System
Ann Arbor, Michigan
Chapter 82

### William D. Edwards, MD

Professor of Pathology
Mayo Medical School and Mayo Graduate School of Medicine
Consultant in Anatomic Pathology
Mayo Clinic and Mayo Foundation
Rochester, Minnesota
Chapter 3

### Kenneth Ellenbogen, MD

Kontos Professor of Medicine
Director
Cardiac Electrophysiology and Pacemaker Laboratory
Medical College of Virginia at Virginia Commonwealth University
Richmond, Virginia
Chapter 32

### William J. Elliott, MD, PhD

Professor of Preventive Medicine
Internal Medicine and Pharmacology
RUSH Medical College of RUSH University at RUSH-Presbyterian-St. Luke's Medical Center
Chicago, Illinois
Chapter 61

### Domien J. Engelen, MD

Diakonessen Hospital
Utrecht, The Netherlands
Chapter 53

### Gregory Engle, MD

Chief Fellow
Cardiovascular Medicine
Cardiovascular Medicine Division
Stanford University School of Medicine
Stanford, California
Chapter 16

### Erling Falk, MD, PhD

Professor of Experimental Cardiovascular Pathology
Department of Cardiology
Aarhus University Hospital (Skejby)
Aarhus, Denmark
Chapter 44

### Michael E. Farkouh, MD

Associate Professor of Medicine
NYU School of Medicine
Director, Cardiac Care Unit
NYU Medical Center
New York, New York
Chapter 86

### Michael D. Faulx, MD

Cardiology Fellow
Case Western Reserve University
University Hospitals of Cleveland
Cleveland, Ohio
Chapter 80

### Zahi A. Fayad, PhD

Imaging Science Laboratories
Departments of Radiology and Medicine (Cardiology)
The Zena and Michael A. Wiener Cardiovascular Institute
The Marie-Josée and Henry R. Kravis Cardiovascular Health Center
Mount Sinai School of Medicine
New York, New York
Chapter 22

### Maksin A. Fedaru, MD

Research Fellow
Department of Internal Medicine/Cardiology
University of Michigan
Research Fellow
Division of Cardiovascular Medicine
University of Michigan Health System
Ann Arbor, Michigan
Chapter 50

### Gerald F. Fletcher, MD

Professor of Medicine
Mayo Clinic College of Medicine
Rochester, Minnesota
Director
Preventive Cardiology
Mayo Clinic
Jacksonville, Florida
Chapter 95

### Thomas R. Flipse, MD

Consultant
Cardiovascular Diseases and Internal Medicine
Mayo Clinic
Jacksonville, Florida
Chapter 95

### Richard I. Fogel, MD

The Heart Center of Indiana
The Care Group
Indianapolis, Indiana
Chapter 28

### Robert H. Franch, MD

Professor of Medicine
Emeritus (Cardiology)
Emeritus Staff Emory University Hospital
Egleston Children's Hospital
Grady Memorial Hospital
Department of Cardiology
Emory University Medical School
Atlanta, Georgia
Chapter 17

### Gary S. Francis, MD, FACC

Professor of Medicine and Director
Coronary Intensive Care Unit
Cleveland Clinic Lerner College of Medicine at Case Western Reserve University
Cleveland Clinic Foundation
Cardiology Department
Cleveland, Ohio
Chapter 24

### O. Howard Frazier, MD

Professor of Surgery
University of Texas Health Science Center
Clinical Professor, Department of Surgery
Baylor College of Medicine
St. Luke's Episcopal Hospital
Chief, Transplant Service
Director, Cardiovascular Surgical Research
Houston, Texas
Chapter 85

### Michael D. Freed, MD

Associate Professor of Pediatrics
Harvard Medical School
Senior Associate in Cardiology
Children's Hospital
Boston, Massachusetts
Chapter 73

### William T. Friedewald, MD

Clinical Professor
Departments of Medicine, Epidemiology, and Biostatistics
Columbia University School of Medicine
New York, New York
Chapter 105

### William H. Frishman, MD, MACP

Professor and Chair
Department of Medicine
New York Medical College
Westchester Medical Center
Valhalla, New York
Chapters 25 and 90

### Victor F. Froelicher, MD

Professor of Medicine
Director
ECG and Exercise Testing
Division of Cardiovascular Medicine
Stanford University School of Medicine
Palo Alto, California
Chapter 16

### David R. Fulton, MD

Associate Professor of Pediatrics
Harvard Medical School
Senior Associate in Cardiology
Chief
Cardiology Outpatient Services
Department of Cardiology
Children's Hospital at Boston
Boston, Massachusetts
Chapter 73

### Valentin Fuster, MD, PhD

Director, The Zena and Michael A. Wiener Cardiovascular Institute and The Marie-Josée and Henry R. Kravis Center for Cardiovascular Health
Richard Gorlin, MD/Heart Research Foundation, Professor of Cardiology, The Mount Sinai Medical Center and School of Medicine
New York, New York
Chapters 21, 22, 44, 45, 48, 54, 86

### William Gerin, MD

Behavioral Cardiovascular Health and Hypertension Program
Columbia Presbyterian Medical Center
New York, New York
Chapter 107

### Guido Germano, PhD

Professor of Medicine and Radiological Sciences
UCLA School of Medicine
Director
Artificial Intelligence Program
Cedars-Sinai Medical Center
Los Angeles, California
Chapter 19

### Gary Gerstenblith, MD

Johns Hopkins University School of Medicine
Department of Medicine
Division of Cardiology
Baltimore, Maryland
Chapter 96

### Edward M. Gilbert, MD

University of Utah Health Sciences Center
Salt Lake City, Utah
Chapter 76

### Anton P. Gorgels, MD, PhD

Associate Professor of Cardiology
Cardiovascular Research Institute Maastricht
University Maastricht
Cardiologist
University Hospital Maastricht
Department of Cardiology
Maastricht, The Netherlands
Chapter 53

### Kathy K. Griendling, PhD

Professor of Medicine
Division of Cardiology
Emory University School of Medicine
Atlanta, Georgia
Chapter 7

### Scott M. Grundy, MD, PhD

Center for Human Nutrition
University of Texas Southwestern Medical Center at Dallas
Dallas, Texas
Chapter 43

### Gary L. Grunkemeier, MD

Director
Medical Data Research Center
Providence Health Systems
Portland, Oregon
Chapter 70

### Patricia A. Gum, MD

Staff
Department of Cardiovascular Medicine
Cleveland Clinic Foundation
Cleveland, Ohio
Chapter 100

### Rory Hachamovitch, MD, MSc

Associate Professor of Medicine
Division of Cardiovascular Medicine
Keck School of Medicine
University of Southern California
Los Angeles, California
Chapter 19

### Robert J. Hall, MD

Director
Cardiac Education
St. Luke's Episcopal Hospital and Texas Heart Institute
Clinical Professor of Medicine
Baylor College of Medicine and University of Texas Medical School at Houston,
St. Luke's Episcopal Hospital
Houston, Texas
Chapter 85

### Jonathan L. Halperin, MD

Director of Clinical Sevices,
The Zena and Michael A. Wiener Cardiovascular Institute and
The Marie-Josée and Henry R. Kravis Center for Cardiovascular Health
Mount Sinai Medical Center
Robert and Harriet Heilbrenner Professor of Medicine
Mount Sinai School of Medicine
New York, New York
Chapter 98

### David G. Harrison, MD
Director
Division of Cardiology
Bernard Marcus Professor of Medicine
Emory University School of Medicine
Emory Clinic
Atlanta, Georgia
Chapter 7

### Sean Hayes, MD
Cedars-Sinai Medical Center
Los Angeles, California
Chapter 19

### Brian D. Hoit, MD
Professor of Medicine
Director
Echocardiography
Case Western Reserve University
Cleveland, Ohio
Chapters 78 and 80

### J. Willis Hurst, MD, MACP
Active Consultant to the Division of Cardiology
Candler Professor and Chairman
Department of Medicine Emeritus
Emory University School of Medicine
Atlanta, Georgia
Foreword

### Julia H. Indik, MD
Assistant Professor of Medicine
Section of Cardiology
Department of Internal Medicine
University of Arizona
Tucson, Arizona
Chapter 35

### Alberto Interian Jr., MD
Professor of Medicine
Associate Chief
Division of Cardiology
Director of Electrophysiology
University of Miami School of Medicine
Miami, Florida
Chapter 13

### Vinod K. S. Jayam, MD
Senior Clinical Fellow
Division of Cardiac Electrophysiology
Johns Hopkins Hospital
Johns Hopkins University
Baltimore, Maryland
Chapter 30

### Mark E. Josephson, MD
Chief
Cardiovascular Division
Director
Harvard Thorndike Electrophysiology Institute and Arrhythmia Services
Electrophysiology Institute
Beth Israel Deaconess Medical Center
Cardiology
Boston, Massachusetts
Chapter 41

### Ronald J. Kanter, MD
Associate Professor of Pediatrics
Director of Pediatric Electrophysiology
Department of Pediatrics
Duke University School of Medicine
Duke University Medical Center
Durham, North Carolina
Chapter 39

### Samir Kapadia, MD
Staff
Cardiovascular Medicine
Cleveland Clinic Foundation
Cleveland, Ohio
Chapter 100

### Joel A. Kaplan, MD
Executive Vice President
Chancellor, Health Sciences Center
Professor of Anesthesiology
University of Louisville
Department of Anesthesia
University of Louisville Hospital
Louisville, Kentucky
Chapter 83

### Marinka Kartalija, MD
Department of Medicine
University of Utah
Salt Lake City, Utah
Alaska Native Medical Center
Anchorage, Alaska
Chapter 81

### G. Neal Kay, MD
Professor of Medicine
Division of Cardiovascular Disease
University of Alabama at Birmingham
Birmingham, Alabama
Chapter 29

### Bradley B. Keller, MD
Professor of Pediatrics
University of Pittsburgh
Chief
Pediatric Cardiology
Children's Hospital of Pittsburgh
Pittsburgh, Pennsylvania
Chapter 8

### Richard E. Kerber, MD
Professor of Medicine
Department of Internal Medicine
University of Iowa
Staff Physician
Department of Internal Medicine
University of Iowa Hospitals and Clinics
Iowa City, Iowa
Chapter 37

### Morton J. Kern, MD
Professor
St. Louis University
Director
Catheterization Lab
St. Louis University Hospital
St. Louis, Missouri
Chapter 17

### Michael C. Kim, MD
Assistant Professor of Medicine
Mount Sinai School of Medicine
New York, New York
Chapter 48

### Spencer B. King III, MD
Fuqua Chair of Interventional Cardiology
The Fuqua Heart Center at Piedmont Hospital
Co-Director, American Cardiovascular Research Institute, Clinical Professor of Medicine
Emory University School of Medicine
Atlanta, Georgia
Chapters 17 and 55

### Annapoorna S. Kini, MD
Assistant Professor of Medicine
Mount Sinai School of Medicine
New York, New York
Chapter 48

## Timothy Knilans, MD

Associate Professor of Clinical Pediatrics
Department of Pediatrics
University of Cincinnati
Cincinnati Children's Hospital Medical Center
Division of Cardiology
Director
Clinical Cardiac Electrophysiology and Pacing
Cincinnati, Ohio
Chapter 39

## Mitchell W. Krucoff, MD, FACC, FCCP

Associate Professor of Medicine
Cardiology
Duke University Medical Center
Durham, North Carolina
Chapter 108

## Harlan Krumholz, MD, MSc

Professor of Medicine
Cardiology
Epidemiology and Public Health
Department of Internal Medicine
Yale University of Medicine
New Haven, Connecticut
Chapter 104

## Nils Kucher, MD

Venous Thromboembolism Research Group
Cardiovascular Division
Brigham and Women's Hospital
Harvard Medical School
Boston, Massachusetts
Chapter 63

## Edward G. Lakatta, MD

Professor of Medicine
Johns Hopkins School of Medicine
Johns Hopkins University
Adjunct Professor of Physiology
University of Maryland
School of Medicine
Baltimore, Maryland
Chapter 96

## Gaetano Antonio Lanza, MD, FESC

Institute of Cardiology
Universita Cattolica del Sacro Cuore
Roma, Italy
Chapter 46

## E. Clinton Lawrence, MD

Augustus J. McKelvey Professor of Medicine
Director
Andrew J. McKelvey Lung Transplantation Center
Medical Director of Lung Transplantation
Emory University School of Medicine
Emory University Hospital
Atlanta, Georgia
Chapter 64

## Megan C. Leary, MD

Instructor in Neurology
Harvard Medical School
Beth Israel Deaconess Medical Center
Boston, Massachusetts
Chapter 99

## Thierry H. LeJemtel, MD

Professor of Medicine
Department of Medicine
Albert Einstein College of Medicine
Montefiore Medical Center
Bronx, New York
Chapter 25

## Martin M. LeWinter, MD

Professor of Medicine and Molecular Physiology and Biophysics
University of Vermont College of Medicine
Director
Heart Failure Program
Fletcher Allen Health Care
Burlington, Vermont
Chapter 4

## Richard P. Lewis, MD

Professor Emeritus, Attending Physician
Cardiovascular Medicine
Ohio State University Hospitals
Columbus, Ohio
Chapter 40

## Richard Liebowitz, MD

Assistant Professor of Clinical Medicine
Duke University
Executive Medical Director
Center for Living
Duke University
Durham, North Carolina
Chapter 108

## Richard P. Lifton, MD

Chairman
Department of Genetics
Professor of Genetics
Internal Medicine and Molecular Biophysics and Biochemistry
Yale University School of Medicine
Associate Investigator
Howard Hughes Medical Institute
Yale University
New Haven, Connecticut
Chapter 9

## Bruce Whitney Lytle, MD

Department of Thoracic and Cardiovascular Surgery
The Cleveland Clinic Foundation
Cleveland, Ohio
Chapter 58

## John J. Mahmarian, MD

Professor of Medicine
Section of Cardiology
Department of Medicine
Baylor College of Medicine
Medical Director
Nuclear Cardiology Laboratory
Methodist DeBakey Heart Center
The Methodist Hospital
Houston, Texas
Chapter 20

## Joseph F. Malouf, MD

Consultant
Division of Cardiovascular Disease
Mayo Clinic
Rochester, Minnesota
Chapter 3

## Donna Mancini, MD

Associate Professor
Columbia University
New York, New York
Chapter 79

## Ali J. Marian, MD

Associate Professor
Baylor College of Medicine
Cardiologist
Baylor Heart Clinic
The Methodist Hospital
Houston, Texas
Chapter 72

## Daniel Mark, MD, MPH

Director
Outcomes Research
Duke Clinical Research Institute
Professor of Medicine
Department of Medicine
Duke University Medical Center
Durham, North Carolina
Chapter 108

## Roger R. Markwald, PhD

Professor and Chairman
Department of Cell Biology and Anatomy
Medical University of South Carolina
Charleston, South Carolina
Chapter 8

## David J. Maron, MD

Associate Professor of Medicine
Division of Cardiovascular Medicine
Vanderbilt University Medical Center
Nashville, Tennessee
Chapter 43

## Attilio Maseri, MD, FACC, FESC

Professor of Cardiology
Director Cardio-Thoracic and Vascular Department
San Raffaele University Hospital
Milan, Italy
Chapter 46

## Jay W. Mason, MD

Adjunct Professor of Medicine
University of Utah
Salt Lake City, Utah
Professor of Medicine
University of Kentucky
Lexington, Kentucky
Medical Director
Covenance Central Diagnostics
Reno, Nevada
Chapter 75

## Tahsin Masud, MD

Assistant Professor of Medicine
Renal Division
Emory University School of Medicine
Atlanta, Georgia
Chapter 94

## Hugh A. McAllister Jr., MD

Clinical Professor
Department of Pathology
Baylor College of Medicine
Clinical Professor
Department of Pathology
University of Texas Medical School
Houston, Texas
Chapter 85

## John H. McAnulty, MD

Professor of Medicine
Oregon Health and Science University
Portland, Oregon
Chapters 71 and 92

## William M. McDonald, MD

J.B. Fuqua Chair of Late-Life Depression
Associate Professor of Psychiatry and Behavioral Sciences
Emory University School of Medicine
Wesley Woods Geriatric Hospital
Atlanta, Georgia
Chapter 91

## Donogh F. McKeogh, MD

Assistant Professor
Division of Cardiology
Department of Medicine
Oregon Health and Science University
Portland, Oregon
Chapter 71

## Luisa Mestroni, MD

Associate Professor of Medicine
Department of Cardiology
Director, Molecular Genetics Program
University of Colorado Cardiovascular Institute
University of Colorado
Denver, Colorado
Chapter 76

## James Metcalfe, MD

Professor Emeritus of Medicine
Oregon Health Sciences University
School of Medicine
Portland, Oregon
Chapter 92

## Darryl Miller, MD

Cardiology Fellow
Case Western Reserve University
University Hospitals of Cleveland
Cleveland, Ohio
Chapter 78

## William E. Mitch, MD

Edward Randall Distinguished Chair in Internal Medicine
Chair of Medicine
Department of Medicine
University of Texas at Galveston
Galveston, Texas
Chapter 94

## Alexander Mittnacht, MD

Instructor
Anesthesiology
Clinical Assistant Attending
Department of Anesthesiology
Mount Sinai School of Medicine
New York, New York
Chapter 83

## Susan D. Moffatt, MD

Department of Cardiothoracic Surgery
Stanford University School of Medicine
Stanford, California
Chapter 26

## Douglas C. Morris, MD

J. Willis Hurst Professor of Medicine
Emory University School of Medicine
Vice Chairman of Medicine for Clinical Affairs
Emory Clinic
Atlanta, Georgia
Chapter 59

## Joseph B. Muhlestein, MD

Department of Cardiology
LDS Hospital
Salt Lake City, Utah
Chapter 81

## Debabrata Mukherjee, MD

Assistant Professor
Division of Cardiology
University of Michigan
Ann Arbor, Michigan
Chapter 82

## Dominique L. Musselman, MD, MS

Associate Professor
Department of Psychiatry and Behavioral Sciences
Emory University School of Medicine
Atlanta, Georgia
Chapter 91

## Robert J. Myerburg, MD

Lemberg Professor of Medicine and Physiology
Director
Division of Cardiology
Department of Medicine
American Heart Association Chair in Cardiovascular Research
University of Miami School of Medicine
Miami, Florida
Chapter 13

## Elizabeth G. Nabel, MD

Scientific Director
Clinical Research
National Heart, Lung, and Blood Institute
National Institute of Health
Bethesda, Maryland
Chapter 11

## Yoshifumi Naka, MD

Mechanical Circulatory Support Program
New York–Presbyterian Hospital
Chapter 50

## Ira S. Nash, MD

Associate Professor of Medicine
Mount Sinai School of Medicine
Associate Director
The Zena and Michael A. Wiener Cardiovascular Institute and The Marie-Josée and Henry R. Kravis Center for Cardiovascular Health
Mount Sinai Medical Center
New York, New York
Chapter 106

## Steven D. Nelson, MD

Associate Professor of Medicine
The Ohio State University
Director
Clinical Cardiac Electrophysiology
Division of Cardiology
Department of Internal Medicine
Columbus, Ohio
Chapter 40

## Charles B. Nemeroff, MD, PhD

Reunette W. Harris Professor and Chairman
Department of Psychiatry and Behavioral Sciences
Emory University School of Medicine
Atlanta, Georgia
Chapter 91

## Konstantin Nikolaou, MD

Department of Clinical Radiology
University of Munich
Grosshadern, Germany
Chapter 22

## Rick A. Nishimura, MD

Judd and Mary Morris Leighton Professor of Medicine
Mayo Clinic College of Medicine
Rochester, Minnesota
Chapter 77

## Steven E. Nissen, MD

Professor of Medicine
Cleveland Clinic Lerner College of Medicine
Medical Director
Cleveland Clinic CV Coordinating CTR
Cleveland, Ohio
Chapter 18

## R. Joe Noble, MD, FACC

Clinical Professor of Medicine
Indiana University School of Medicine
The Heart Center of Indiana
St. Vincent's Hospital
Indianapolis, Indiana
Chapter 33

## Peter A. O'Callaghan, MD

Consultant Electrophysiologist
Clinical Teacher
University of Wales College of Medicine
Consultant Electrophysiologist
Department of Cardiology
University Hospital of Wales
Heath Park, Cardiff, United Kingdom
Chapter 38

## Patrick O'Gara, MD

Associate Professor of Medicine
Harvard Medical School
Director, Clinical Cardiology
Vice Chairman, Clinical Affairs
Department of Medicine
Brigham and Women's Hospital
Boston, Massachusetts
Chapter 57

## Keith R. Oken, MD

Consultant
Cardiovascular Diseases
Mayo Clinic, Florida
Assistant Professor of Medicine
Mayo College of Medicine
Jacksonville, Florida
Chapter 95

## Jeffrey W. Olin, DO

Professor of Medicine
Mount Sinai Medical School of Medicine
Director, Vascular Medicine, The Zena and Michael A. Wiener Cardiovascular Institute and The Marie-Josée and Henry R. Kravis Center for Cardiovascular Health
Mount Sinai Medical Center
New York, New York
Chapter 98

## Steven R. Ommen, MD

Assistant Professor of Medicine
Mayo Clinic College of Medicine
Consultant
Division of Cardiovascular Disease and Internal Medicine
Department of Internal Medicine
Rochester, Minnesota
Chapter 77

## William W. O'Neill, MD, FACC

Corporate Chairman of Cardiology
William Beaumont Hospital System
Royal Oak and Troy, Michigan
Chapter 56

## LIONEL OPIE, MD, DPhil, FRCP

Director
Hatter Institute
Cape Heart Centre and Department of Medicine
University of Cape Town
Senior Consultant
Hypertension Clinic
Groote Schuur Hospital
Cape Town, South Africa
Chapter 90

## ROBERT A. O'ROURKE, MD

Charles Conrad Brown Distinguished Professor in Cardiovascular Disease
University of Texas Health Sciences Center
San Antonio, Texas
Chapters 12, 14, 51, 57, 68, 69, 84, 85

## GEORGE OSOL, PhD

Professor and Director of Research
Department of OB/GYN
University of Vermont College of Medicine
Burlington, Vermont
Chapter 4

## RICHARD L. PAGE, MD

Robert A. Bruce Professor
Head
Division of Cardiology
Department of Medicine
University of Washington School of Medicine
Seattle, Washington
Chapter 31

## EUGEN C. PALMA, MD

Assistant Professor of Medicine
Arrhythmia Service
Albert Einstein College of Medicine
Montefiore Medical Center
Bronx, New York
Chapter 36

## THOMAS A. PEARSON, MD, MPH, PhD, FACC

Albert D. Kaiser Professor and Chair
Community and Preventative Medicine
Professor of Medicine
University of Rochester School of Medicine and Dentistry
Attending Physician
Department of Medicine
Director
Preventative Cardiology Clinic
Co-Director
Stony Heart Program
University of Rochester Medical Center
Rochester, New York
Chapter 43

## THOMAS G. PICKERING, MD, DPhil

Director
Behavioral Cardiovascular Health and Hypertension Program
Columbia Presbyterian Hospital
New York, New York
Chapter 107

## SEAN P. PINNEY, MD

Instructor of Medicine
Department of Internal Medicine
Columbia University–College of Physicians and Surgeons
Attending Physician
Department of Medicine
Division of Circulatory Physiology
New York Presbyterian Hospital
New York, New York
Chapter 79

## DAVID J. PINSKY, MD, FACC

Division Chief
Cardiovascular Medicine
Professor
Cardiovascular Medicine
Scientific Director
Cardiovascular Center
Internal Medicine
Cardiology
University of Michigan
Ann Arbor, Michigan
Chapter 50

## DUANE S. PINTO, MD

Instructor of Medicine
Harvard Medical School
Program Director
Fellowship Training Program
Cardiovascular Division
Beth Israel Deaconess Medical Center
Boston, Massachusetts
Chapter 41

## VANCE J. PLUMB, MD

Professor of Medicine
Division of Cardiovascular Disease
Department of Medicine
University of Alabama at Birmingham
School of Medicine
Birmingham, Alabama
Chapter 29

## MICHAEL POON, MD

Associate Professor of Medicine (Cardiology)
Mount Sinai School of Medicine
Director of Clinical Cardiac MR/CT Imaging Program and Pulmonary Hypertension Program
Director of Cardiology
Cabrini Medical Center
New York, New York
Chapter 22

## CRAIG M. PRATT, MD

Professor of Medicine
Baylor College of Medicine
Director of Research
DeBakey Heart Center
Director, Coronary Care Unit
The Methodist Hospital
Houston, Texas
Chapter 52

## JOHN O. PRIOR, MD

David Geffen School of Medicine at UCLA
Visiting Associate Professor
Department of Molecular and Medical Pharmacology
University of California at Los Angeles
Los Angeles, California
Chapter 23

## Eric N. Prystowsky, MD

Director
Clinical Electrophysiology Laboratory
St. Vincent Hospital
Indianapolis, Indiana
Consulting Professor of Medicine
Duke University Medical Center
Durham, North Carolina
Chapters 28 and 33

## Shahbudin H. Rahimtoola, MB, FRCP, MACP, MACC, DSc(Hon),

Distinguished Professor
University of Southern California
G. C. Griffith Professor of Cardiology
Professor of Medicine
Keck School of Medicine
LAC and USC Medical Center
Los Angeles, California
Chapters 66, 67, 70, 71

## Elliot J. Rayfield, MD

Clinical Professor of Medicine
Attending Physician
Mount Sinai School of Medicine
New York, New York
Chapter 86

## David L. Reich, MD

Professor of Anesthesiology
Mount Sinai School of Medicine
Vice-Chair for Academic Affairs
Department of Anesthesia
Mount Sinai Medical Center
New York, New York
Chapter 83

## Robert W. Rho, MD

Assistant Professor of Medicine
University of Washington
School of Medicine
Seattle, Washington
Chapter 31

## Paul M. Ridker, MD

Eugene Braunwald Professor of Medicine
Harvard Medical School
Director
Center for Cardiovascular Disease
Prevention
Division of Preventive Medicine
Brigham and Women's Hospital
Boston, Massachusetts
Chapter 43

## Robert C. Robbins, MD

Associate Professor
Department of Cardiac Surgery
Stanford University
Stanford, California
Chapter 26

## Robert Roberts, MD

Professor of Medicine
President and CEO
University of Ottawa Heart Institute
Ottawa, Ontario, Canada
Chapters 5, 9, 52, 72

## William C. Roberts, MD

Director
Baylor Heart and Vascular Institute
Baylor University Medical Center
Dallas, Texas
Chapter 84

## Jose F. Roldan, MD

Resident
Department of Rheumatology
University of Texas Health
Science Center
San Antonio, Texas
Chapter 84

## Thom W. Rooke, MD

Professor of Medicine
Department of Internal Medicine
Division of Cardiovascular Diseases
Mayo Graduate School of Medical
Education
Rochester, Minnesota
Chapter 101

## Lewis J. Rubin, MD

Professor of Medicine
Pulmonary and Critical Care Medicine
University of California at San Diego
School of Medicine
La Jolla, California
Chapter 62

## Bruce Rudisch, MD

Resident in Psychiatry
Department of Psychiatry and Behavioral
Sciences
Emory University School of Medicine
Atlanta, Georgia
Chapter 91

## Jeremy N. Ruskin, MD

Director
Cardiac Arrhythmia Service
Massachusetts General Hospital
Associate Professor of Medicine
Harvard Medical School
Boston, Massachusetts
Chapter 38

## Thomas J. Ryan, MD

Professor of Medicine
Boston University School of Medicine
Senior Consultant in Cardiology and Chief
of Cardiology Emeritus
Boston University Medical Center
Boston, Massachusetts
Chapter 52

## Merle A. Sande, MD

Professor of Medicine
Department of Medicine
University of Utah School of Medicine
Salt Lake City, Utah
Chapter 81

## Stephen F. Schaal, MD

Professor of Medicine
Ohio State University
College of Medicine and Public Health
Columbus, Ohio
Chapter 40

## Melvin M. Scheinman, MD

Professor of Medicine
Shorenstein Chair in Cardiology
University of California at San Francisco
San Francisco, California
Chapter 36

## Heinrich R. Schelbert, MD, PhD

Geroge V. Taplin Professor
Division of Nuclear Medicine
Department of Molecular and Medical
Pharmacology
UCLA School of Medicine
Los Angeles, California
Chapter 23

### JOHN S. SCHROEDER, MD

Professor of Medicine
Department of Cardiology
Stanford University School of Medicine
Stanford Medical Center
Stanford, California
Chapter 26

### STEVEN P. SCHULMAN, MD

Associate Professor of Medicine
Director of Coronary Care Unit
Johns Hopkins University School of Medicine
Baltimore, Maryland
Chapter 96

### JAMES B. SEWARD, MD

Professor of Medicine and Pediatrics
Director
Echo Lab
Consultant
CV Diseases
Mayo Clinic
Rochester, Minnesota
Chapter 3

### PREDIMAN K. SHAH, MD

Shapell and Webb Chair and Director
Division of Cardiology and Atherosclerosis Research Center
Cedars Sinai Medical Center
Professor of Medicine
David Geffen School of Medicine at UCLA
Los Angeles, California
Chapter 44

### JAMES A. SHAVER, MD

Professor of Medicine
Cardiovascular Institute
University of Pittsburgh
Director of Cardiovascular Fellowship Program
University of Pittsburgh Medical Center
Presbyterian University Hospital
Pittsburgh, Pennsylvania
Chapter 12

### LESLEE J. SHAW, PhD

Associate Professor
Department of Medicine
Duke University
Durham, North Carolina
Director
Outcomes Research
Atlanta Cardiovascular Research Institute
Atlanta, Georgia
Chapter 19

### DOMENIC A. SICA, MD

Professor of Medicine and Pharmacology
Chairman
Section of Clinical Pharmacology and Hypertension
Division of Nephrology
Medical College of Virginia
Virginia Commonwealth University
Richmond, Virginia
Chapter 90

### MARK E. SILVERMAN, MD, MACP, FRCP, FACC

Professor of Medicine
Cardiology
Emory University School of Medicine
Chief of Cardiology
The Fuqua Heart Center
Piedmont Hospital
Atlanta, Georgia
Chapters 1 and 12

### ANDREW L. SMITH, MD

Associate Professor of Medicine
Emory University School of Medicine
Medical Director
Heart Failure and Transplantation
Division of Cardiology
Emory Hospital
Atlanta, Georgia
Chapter 89

### ROBERT B. SMITH III, MD

John E. Skandalakis Professor of Surgery Emeritus
Emory University School of Medicine
Medical Director
Emory University Hospital
Associate Chairman
Department of Surgery
Emory University School of Medicine
Atlanta, Georgia
Chapter 102

### EDMUND H. SONNENBLICK, MD, FACC

Edward J. Safra Professor of Medicine
Albert Einstein College of Medicine
Weiler Hospital/Montefiore Medical Center
Bronx, New York
Chapters 24 and 25

### ALBERT STARR, MD

Professor of Surgery
Oregon Health Sciences University
Director
Heart and Vascular Institute
Providence St. Vincent's Hospital
Portland, Oregon
Chapter 70

### LISA M. SULLIVAN, MD

Associate Professor of Biostatistics, Mathematics and Statistics
Assistant Dean for Undergraduate Education in Public Health
Boston University
Boston, Massachusetts
Chapter 2

### H. ROBERT SUPERKO, MD, FACC, FAHA, FACSM

Director
Cholesterol, Genetics and Heart Disease Institute
Portola Valley, California
Director
Advanced Cardiovascular Disease Prevention
Fuqua Heart Center/Piedmont Hospital
Atlanta, Georgia
Director of Research
Berkeley HeartLab, Inc.
Burlingame, California
Chapter 87

### PANAGIOTIS N. SYMBAS, MD

Professor of Cardiothoracic Surgery
Emory University School of Medicine
Emory Affiliated Hospitals
Atlanta, Georgia
Chapter 93

### A. JAMIL TAJIK, MD

Thomas J. Watson, Jr., Professor
Professor of Medicine and Pediatrics
Mayo Clinic
Consultant
Division of Cardiovascular Diseases
Mayo Clinic
Rochester, New York
Chapters 3 and 77

## W. H. Wilson Tang, MD

Assistant Professor of Cardiovascular Medicine
Cleveland Clinic Lerner College at Medicine at Case Western Reserve University
Staff Physician
Kaufman Center for Heart Failure
Department of Cardiovascular Medicine
Cleveland Clinic Foundation
Cleveland, Ohio
Chapter 24

## Victor F. Tapson, MD

Associate Professor of Medicine
Pulmonary and Critical Care Medicine
Duke University Medical Center
Durham, North Carolina
Chapter 63

## Thomas T. Terramani, MD

Vascular Surgery and Endovascular Therapy
San Diego, California
Chapter 102

## Gordon F. Tomaselli, MD

Professor of Medicine
Johns Hopkins School of Medicine
Johns Hopkins University
Baltimore, Maryland
Chapter 10

## Kent Ueland, MD

Professor Emeritus
Department of OB/GYN
Stanford University School of Medicine
Stanford, California
Chapter 92

## Ramachandran S. Vasan, MD

Clinical Associate Professor
Department of Medicine
Boston University School of Medicine
Boston, Massachusetts
Assistant Director
Echocardiography Laboratory
Framingham Heart Study
Framingham, Massachusetts
Chapter 2

## Pugazhendhi Vijayaraman, MD

Assistant Professor of Medicine
Medical College of Virginia
Virginia Commonwealth University
Co-Director
Cardiac Electrophysiology Section
McGuire Veterans Affairs Medical Center
Richmond, Virginia
Chapter 32

## Renu Virmani, MD

Chairman
Department of Cardiovascular Pathology
Armed Forces Institute of Pathology
Washington, District of Columbia
Chapter 49

## John H. K. Vogel, MD

Chairman
Cardiology
Santa Barbara Cottage Hospital
Santa Barbara, California
Chapter 108

## David A. Vorchheimer, MD

Assistant Professor of Medicine
Mount Sinai School of Medicine
Director
Coronary Care Unit
The Zena and Michael A. Wiener Cardiovascular Institute
Mount Sinai Medical Center
New York, New York
Chapter 54

## Albert Waldo, MD

Walter H. Pritchard Professor of Cardiology
Professor of Medicine
Professor of Biomedical Engineering
Case Western Reserve University
Cleveland, Ohio
Chapter 27

## Bruce F. Waller, MD

Clinical Professor of Medicine and Pathology
Indiana University School of Medicine
Director
Cardiovascular Pathology Registry
St. Vincent's Hospital
Cardiologist
The Care Group
Medical Director
The Care Group Laboratory
Indianapolis, Indiana
Chapter 47

## Richard A. Walsh, MD

John H. Hord Professor and Chairman
Department of Medicine
Case Western Reserve University
Physician-in-Chief
University Hospitals of Cleveland
Department of Medicine
Case Western University/University Hospitals of Cleveland
Cleveland, Ohio
Chapter 6

## Carole A. Warnes, MD, MRCP, FACC

Professor of Medicine
Mayo Medical School
Consultant in CV Diseases
Internal Medicine and Pediatric Cardiology
Mayo Clinic
Rochester, Minnesota
Chapter 74

## William S. Weintraub, MD

Professor of Medicine
Cardiology
Emory University School of Medicine
Director
Cardiovascular Epidemiology
Emory Healthcare
Atlanta, Georgia
Chapter 104

## Myron L. Weisfeldt, MD

Chair of Medicine
Johns Hopkins University School of Medicine
Johns Hopkins Hospital
Baltimore, Maryland
Chapter 42

## Hein J.J. Wellens, MD

Professor of Cardiology
University of Maastricht
Chairman
Department of Cardiology
University Hospital Maastricht
Maastricht, The Netherlands
Chapter 53

## Nanette K. Wenger, MD

Professor of Medicine
Cardiology
Emory University School of Medicine
Chief of Cardiology
Grady Memorial Hospital
Atlanta, Georgia
Chapter 60

## Paul W. Wennberg, MD

Associate Professor of Medicine
Department of Internal Medicine
Division of Cardiovascular Diseases
Mayo Graduate School of Medical Education
Rochester, Minnesota
Chapter 101

## Andy Wessels, PhD

Associate Professor
Department of Cell Biology and Anatomy
Medical University of South Carolina
Charleston, South Carolina
Chapter 8

## Andrew L. Wit, PhD

Professor of Pharmacology
College of Physicians and Surgeons of Columbia University
New York, New York
Chapter 27

## Charles F. Wooley, MD

Department of Cardiovascular Medicine
Ohio State University Medical Center
Columbus, Ohio
Chapter 1

## Raymond L. Woosley, MD, PhD

Vice President for Health Sciences
University of Arizona
College of Medicine
Tucson, Arizona
Chapter 35

## Jay S. Yadav, MD

Director
Vascular Intervention
Department of Cardiovascular Medicine
Cleveland Clinic Foundation
Department of Cardiology
Cleveland, Ohio
Chapter 100

# FOREWORD

The very personal story you are about to read is offered here at the request of the editors of the eleventh edition of *Hurst's The Heart.* They wanted a historical account of the conception, birth, and development of the book, *Hurst's The Heart.* I am honored to tell the story that, to a major degree, consumed many of my waking hours during several decades of my life.

There were two factors involved in the original creation of the book: the *mind-set* that was clearly present and the *trigger* that initiated the action.

The *mind-set* gradually evolved in the late forties and fifties. I completed my cardiology fellowship with Dr. Paul Dudley White at the Massachusetts General Hospital in Boston in 1949. His scholarly work inspired me to take care of people with heart disease, engage in clinical research, teach, and write. His book, *Heart Disease,* was my constant companion. I was pleased beyond description when he asked me to contribute a few pages on spatial vector electrocardiography to the fourth edition of his masterpiece.

I joined Dr. Bruce Logue in Dr. Paul Beeson's department of medicine at Emory University in Atlanta, Georgia, in 1950. Bruce was a walking encyclopedia, a remarkable clinician, a rapid decision maker, and the leading cardiologist in Atlanta. We worked side by side and wrote several articles together. I was beginning to appreciate that writing improved my teaching and that both improved my knowledge base, which in turn improved my diagnostic and therapeutic skills. My work with Dr. Robert Grant, who was also at Emory, in electrocardiography led me to write my first book, *Atlas of Spatial Vector Electocardiography*. I began work on the book when I was 29 years old; it was published by Blakiston, a division of the McGraw-Hill Company, 3 years later in 1952. This event showed me that I could put a book together. Bruce Logue had worked with Meakins at McGill and was asked to write the section on the heart in the new edition of *Meakins' Textbook of Medicine;* Bruce passed this task and opportunity along to me. I organized the section and wrote much of it but asked several people to write various chapters in the section. These events led me to conclude that the time was right for a multiauthored book on the heart, arteries, and veins. However, I was in my early thirties and realized not only that there were several good books on these subjects already available but also that I was perhaps a bit young to dream such a dream. I realized too that I did not have the resources required for such an endeavor. Meanwhile, I was asked to become chairman of the department of medicine at Emory in late 1956 and began work there in January 1957. This gave me more resources. By then, I was a few years older and had edited and written part of a small multiauthored book on cardiac resuscitation.

The *trigger* that stimulated me to act came in 1962. I invited the internationally famous Dr. Paul Wood to visit my department at Emory in 1962. His book *Diseases of the Heart and Circulation* had become a classic, along with White's *Heart Disease* and Friedberg's *Diseases of the Heart*. Wood's reputation preceded him. He was known to be uninhibited in making vitriolic remarks to others regarding their competence. He was said to be pedantic and intolerant of anything short of perfection. Despite this, he was considered a genius who rarely made a diagnostic error. I showed him patients with the most difficult problems and waited for his caustic attacks. The hospital auditorium was filled to capacity with house officers, clinical faculty, and practicing physicians. Like the expert swordsman who always hits the right spot, he never missed. Surprisingly, there were no caustic remarks. However, he seemed to be somewhat aloof and obviously frustrated. I asked him, in my own way, to state his problem, hoping that I might make his visit more pleasant. He answered, "I realize that I can't complete the next edition of my book *Diseases of the Heart and Circulation*. By the time I write the last chapter, the first chapter will be out of date." That was the *trigger*. I reasoned then and there that if Paul Wood could not write a single-authored book on the heart, no one could. As I walked and talked with him, he did not complain of chest discomfort. He died in London of a myocardial infarction about 2 weeks after visiting us.

Paul White had already decided not to write a fifth edition of his book, *Heart Disease*. Dr. Charles Friedberg's excellent book was the only remaining established complete treatise on the heart then available. I sensed that he too would have trouble continuing to write a single-authored book. This was obviously true, because cardiovascular research was beginning to bring many new insights to every area of cardiology and no single person could hope to master them all.

The book that was later titled *Hurst's The Heart* was conceived during Paul Wood's visit to Emory. I asked Dr. Logue to join me as co-editor and asked my colleagues Dr. Robert Schlant and Dr. Nanette Wenger to be assistant editors. I also asked Ruth Strange, who was my secretary for many years, to help us keep order. Ruth was unusually gifted and could have served as the chief operating officer of a modern company.

The editorial managers of the Blakiston Division of McGraw-Hill, which published my book on vector electrocardiography in 1952, expressed their interest in the creation of a complete treatise on the heart. This was the beginning of my long and pleasant relationship with the McGraw-Hill Company.

The goals for the book were established as follows: It would be a complete treatise on the heart, arteries, and veins. The Emory staff would write a large part of the book, but authors from elsewhere would be asked to contribute chapters as well. These latter authors would be chosen because they had taught their subjects through their writing and were considered to be experts in their fields. Most importantly, we chose authors with whom we agreed. We were delighted when no one turned down the invitation to write for the new book.

I have always believed that there are two types of reading. The *quick read* is used by physicians who wish to look up information that is needed immediately. Reading about the criteria required to diagnose hypertrophic cardiomyopathy is an example of the *quick read*. The *long read* is used when physicians want to understand certain aspects of a disease process. This type of reading is done in a more leisurely fashion without a feeling of urgency. Reading about and understanding the evolution of an atherosclerotic plaque is an example of the *long read*.

The book I planned would serve clinicians whose professional purpose in life was to take care of patients with heart disease but who also wanted to understand the etiology, pathology, and altered physiology of the disease that produced the clinical problems they identified in their patients. This book, I felt, had to be a rich source for a *quick read* and an excellent source for a *long read*.

In order to create a book, it is necessary to visualize the finished product before the first words are written. This initial step is fortunately relatively easy for me. I created a grid listing the *parts* of the book as well as the *chapters*, showing the authors' names and the dates on which their chapters were due. The grid was placed on the door of my office. It covered the door from top to bottom. I studied it many times each day and could, at a glance, follow the flow of the work in progress.

Dr. Logue and I spent several hours every Thursday morning for more than a year reviewing every sentence of every manuscript before it was sent to the publisher. The authors reviewed every sentence of every page of galley proof and I reviewed every sentence of the page proof before signing off on the project.

The naming of the book was an interesting experience. The choice of names was limited and most names had already been used by the creators of other books. Two gentlemen from McGraw-Hill came to Atlanta from New York to discuss the matter with Dr. Logue and me. The night we named the book was like a scene from an old movie. Dr. Logue and I were seated in a small room of an Atlanta hotel while the two gentlemen from McGraw-Hill walked the floor. We each tossed out names and they would shake their heads. I suggested the name *The Heart.* They stood still—stretched out their hands—changed their facial expressions, and said, "That's it—that's it!" The words *Arteries and Veins* were to be added in smaller print in order to emphasize the book's comprehensive nature.

The authors delivered their manuscripts to us on time and the first edition of *Hurst's The Heart* appeared in 1966.

Having lived with the book night and day for 4 years, we waited for the reactions of readers and book reviewers. We were more than pleased with their responses. The prompt worldwide acceptance of *The Heart* led to its translation into other languages. Eventually, it appeared in French, Spanish, Portuguese, Japanese, Chinese, and Greek editions.

Dr. Charles Friedberg congratulated me and stated how much he liked the book. He was a great man. As stated earlier, Dr. White had decided not to write the fifth edition of his book, but he was well pleased with the first edition of *Hurst's The Heart.* Dr. Paul Wood had died and Dr. Friedberg unfortunately died a few years later as the result of an automobile accident. In my mind's eye, I do remember that other books became available about the time *The Heart* was published. Luisada created a huge three-volume, multiauthored treatise on the heart and circulation, but, perhaps because of its great size, there was only one edition. Another new, multiauthored, comprehensive treatise on the heart was published before or after *The Heart* appeared, but it too did not reappear after the first edition. Accordingly, *Hurst's The Heart* stood alone for many years and I am happy to say gained a strong foothold throughout most of the world. Now, of course, the book *Hurst's The Heart* has many playmates, because most large publishing houses believe that they must have a heart book.

The second edition of *Hurst's The Heart* was published 4 years after the first. It was somewhat obese, but it too was well received. One reader said it was a bit heavy and that he had his first episode of angina while carrying it! I learned from the second edition the problem we would face in future editions—that is, to control the book's size. The problem was the antithesis of Paul Wood's problem. He realized that a single author could not master the details of the progress being generated in the world's many research laboratories. On the other hand, the multiple authors of *Hurst's The Heart* could, to some degree, do that. So, the authors of *Hurst's The Heart* needed to cover more pages, but chapters had to be shortened, references decreased in number, and many lovely sentences omitted.

Dr. Logue's workday became so crowded that he could not continue as coeditor after the third edition of *Hurst's The Heart,* and I became the sole editor-in-chief. Dr. Logue continued to provide valuable help as an associate editor through the sixth edition.

Ruth Strange died of leukemia in 1972. Thereafter, Carol Miller became responsible for keeping order, typing manuscripts, writing to authors, and so on. She too was a genius and a healthy perfectionist.

The book thrived through its childhood over the next few editions. After that, it entered and left the adolescent period and came to maturity in the sixth edition, which was published in 1986. It was at this time that I gave up the chairmanship of the department of medicine at Emory University. I had held that position for 30 years and was then 66 years old. I was asked to continue my teaching, patient care, clinical investigation, and writing. Although I enjoyed being chairman, I also relished the opportunity to relinquish the shackles of administrative work. I planned to complete the seventh edition of *Hurst's The Heart,* but I thought that after it was on the shelf, it would be wise to relinquish my role as editor-in-chief so that I could help the next editor-in-chief to make a smooth transition in his effort to create the eighth edition. I urged the selection of my friend and associate Dr. Robert Schlant to succeed me. I also asked that Dr. Wayne Alexander, who was at the time director of the division of cardiology at Emory, be added to the editorial staff.

McGraw-Hill officials honored me by naming the book *Hurst's The Heart* in deference to my role in the creation of the book and its nurturance to maturity.

As I close, may I offer a prediction? The future editors of *Hurst's The Heart,* and any other similar book, will find their task to be increasingly difficult for the following reason. When the first edition of *Hurst's The Heart* was created in the early sixties, there were only a few drugs and only a few procedures to consider. A consensus of opinion regarding their use was easy to achieve. With the plethora of new information generated by the explosion of research, there is now often legitimate disagreement as to what would be best for the patient. For example, there is a debate regarding the definition of proper diet and an argument about the value or harm that may result from the use of estrogens in postmenopausal women. Should the editors of a book insist on a single view, or should the physician reading the book be given various options from which to choose? I have no doubt that the smart editors now on the editorial board will address such problems and continue to create an excellent single-source book for all physicians who wish to learn more about the heart. But it will not be easy.

I am especially pleased to have the chance to thank once again all the individuals who helped me to create *Hurst's The Heart*. The dedicated workers of centuries ago set the stage for modern authors (see Chapter 1). They, in turn, passed the baton to the splendid authors who have contributed chapters to the present book and its earlier editions. I thank them all from every cardiac myocyte in my body.

Nelie, my wife, tolerated the transformation of our home into a library filled with manuscripts and books. She deserves much credit, because a stable, secure, and happy home is needed in order to remain focused on any creative act. So I say once again "No Nelie—no book."

Now, as I rush, with a smile of anticipation, to meet the students, house staff, and cardiology fellows at Emory University, please join me and the trainees as we search in the eleventh edition of *Hurst's The Heart* for answers to the questions we are certain to raise. Because of the competence of Fuster, Alexander, who is now chairman of the department of medicine at Emory University, O'Rourke, King, Roberts, Nash, Prystowsky, and numerous other splendid authors who spearheaded the creation of this edition of *Hurst's The Heart*—I can properly say, without timidity, "It is a great book."

J. Willis Hurst, MD, MACP
Emory University
Atlanta, Georgia

# PREFACE

The first edition of *The Heart,* published in 1966, was the first multiauthored and comprehensive textbook on cardiovascular disease. The history of the book and its subsequent development are elucidated by its editor J. Willis Hurst in his Foreword to this 11th edition (pages xxv to xxvii). This 11th edition of *Hurst's The Heart,* with 108 chapters written by outstanding and highly recognized experts in each of the examined fields, has several unique features that distinguish it from previous editions.

1. Each chapter of the 11th edition will be updated on an ongoing basis on the website, including the incorporation of "late breaking" clinical trials. Thus, the 11th edition of *Hurst's The Heart* and its continually evolving website will keep you abreast of the latest developments in cardiovascular medicine.
2. Forty percent of the chapters have been modified extensively, particularly those concerned with electrophysiology and with the diagnosis and treatment of acute coronary syndromes.

   Ten new chapters have been added spanning the latest exciting developments concerning the human genome and the genetic basis of many diseases, "high" and "low" risk coronary and noncoronary atherothrombotic plaques, evolving imaging technology for the assessment of coronary and noncoronary atherosclerotic disease and plaque characterization, and the most recent advances in the pathophysiology and treatment of pulmonary hypertension and heart failure. The many major advances in interventional cardiology are discussed in detail.
3. Three revised chapters focus on the new therapeutic challenges and socioeconomic issues affecting medicine in general and cardiovascular medicine in particular: a discussion of alternative and complementary medicine in the treatment of cardiovascular disease, the importance of behavioral modification as the basis of risk factor modification, and the cost-effectiveness of various noninvasive and interventional diagnostic methods and forms of treatment.
4. The ACC/AHA Clinical Practice Guidelines are emphasized throughout the text as well as in a special chapter concerning the use of Clinical Practice Guidelines. Each table utilizing ACC/AHA recommendations is clearly identified.
5. The 11th edition of *Hurst's The Heart* includes hundreds of new references including many that were still in press at the time of publication. The book has been shortened by reducing the number of references and eliminating duplication. The quality of the text paper, the illustrations, and the print size have been made more "reader friendly."

The editors are grateful to the outstanding group of authors who participated in the 11th edition of *Hurst's The Heart* for their extraordinary and timely contributions. As in the previous 10th edition, from the moment that the group of authors accepted to participate in this 11th edition of *Hurst's The Heart* to the moment of the book appearing on the shelves has only taken 15 months. Again, this is an absolute record for a textbook of this size and complexity. Such an approach represents the highest tribute and acknowledgment to our authors.

We thank J. Willis Hurst, the editor of the first seven editions and the author of the Foreword of this 11th edition for his continuous and enthusiastic support.

Finally we wish to thank our families for their support and for the many sacrifices they made to make this volume possible. We especially thank our wives for their strength, love, and support: Maria Fuster, Jane W. Alexander, Suzann O' Rourke, Donna Roberts, Gail King, Beth Nash, and Bonnie Prystowsky.

THE EDITORS
Valentin Fuster, MD, PhD
R. Wayne Alexander, MD, PhD
Robert A. O' Rourke, MD
Robert Roberts, MD
Spencer B. King III, MD
Ira S. Nash, MD
Eric N. Prystowsky, MD

# HURST'S

# THE HEART

PART ONE

# FOUNDATIONS OF CARDIOVASCULAR MEDICINE

CHAPTER 1

# A HISTORY OF THE HEART

Mark E. Silverman / Charles F. Wooley



> "The heart ... is the beginning of life; the sun of the microcosm ... for it is the heart by whose virtue and pulse the blood is moved, perfected, made apt to nourish, and is preserved from corruption and coagulation; it is the household divinity which, discharging its function, nourishes, cherishes, quickens the whole body, and is indeed the foundation of life, the source of all action." William Harvey, 1628 [1]

The history of the heart is a remarkable story, with origins in antiquity, centered initially on clinical observations and palpation of the pulse. The heart, thought at one time to be impervious to disease, was long a source of mystery and wonder. How best to describe this history? Most historians would agree that William Harvey's discovery of the circulation of blood in the early seventeenth century is a good place to start. Following Harvey, in a general sense, cardiology has followed the pathway of descriptive anatomy and pathology in the seventeenth and eighteenth centuries, auscultation and its correlations in the nineteenth century, an understanding of cardiac disease and its pathophysiology in the last half of the nineteenth and first half of the twentieth century, and major advances in the diagnosis and treatment of heart disease resulting from bacteriology, chemistry, surgery, molecular genetics, and vascular biology in the later twentieth century.[2–4] The clinical practice of cardiology, in which physicians identified themselves as heart specialists, originated in early-twentieth-century London with James Mackenzie. At that time, the examination of patients with instruments of precision, beginning with the blood pressure, chest x-ray, and electrocardiogram, transformed the entire field of medicine. Since the 1950s, the field of cardiology has splintered into multiple highly specialized disciplines and is increasingly laboratory-focused and less bedside-rooted. Many of the initial discoveries are recalled as eponyms attached to diseases or physical signs. As the number of investigators and institutions has grown exponentially and internationally, it is increasingly difficult to assign priority to contributions for which many are ultimately responsible. Taking all of these considerations into account, we have chosen to provide a condensed narrative by subject, selectively highlighting important events and key figures in the grand and complex story of cardiology written by our illustrious predecessors.[2–10]

## WILLIAM HARVEY AND THE CIRCULATION OF THE BLOOD

Early civilizations considered the heart to be a source of heat and believed that the blood vessels carried *pneuma*, the life-sustaining spirit of the vital organs. This concept was most fully elaborated by Claudius Galen (A.D. 130–200), whose erroneous teachings were entrenched for 1300 years, until Andreas Vesalius corrected his anatomy (1543) and William Harvey proposed that blood circulates due to the force of the heart (1616).[2]

The discovery of the circulation of blood by Harvey (Fig. 1-1) in London is often considered to mark the beginning of cardiology as well as the introduction of experimental observation. Starting in 1603, Harvey dissected the anatomy and observed the motion of the cardiac chambers and flow of blood in more than 80 species of animals. His experimental questions "to seek unbiased truth" can be summarized as follows:

1. How much blood is present and how long would its passage take?
2. What is the relationship of the motion of the auricle to the ventricle and which is the systolic and which the diastolic motion of the heart?
3. What is the propulsive force that distends the arteries?
4. How does blood travel from the right ventricle to the left side of the heart?
5. What purpose is served by the orientation of the cardiac valves?
6. What is the direction of the flow of blood in the veins and the arteries?

After many experiments and without the knowledge of the capillary circulation of the lungs, which was not known until 1661, Harvey stated: "It must of necessity be concluded that the blood is

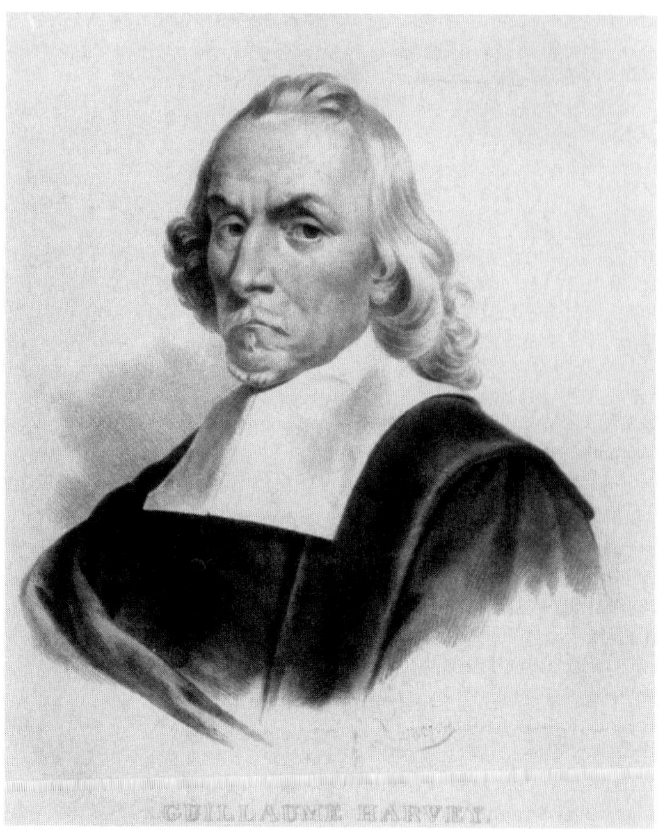


FIGURE 1-1 William Harvey. (Courtesy of the National Library of Medicine.)

driven into a circular motion and that it moves perpetually and that this is the action or function of the heart which the heart performs by means of its pulse." This concept was first presented in 1616 to the Royal College of Physicians, London, and published in 1628 as *Exercitatio Anatomica de Motu Cordis et Sanguinis in Animalibus.*[1] Though attacked, this revolutionary concept became accepted in Harvey's lifetime and remains the foundation for our understanding of the purpose of the heart.

## THE CARDIAC EXAMINATION

### The Arterial Pulse

Until the seventeenth century, the examination of the patient was primarily devoted to palpating and interpreting the pulse, which was thought to reveal the disease and predict the prognosis. Chinese acupuncture, for example, depended on analyzing the pulse in different sites, applying varying digital pressure to elicit more information, then timing the pulse according to the respiration of the physician. In the second century, Claudius Galen wrote 18 books on the arterial pulse, providing elaborate descriptions that influenced clinical practice into the eighteenth century.[2,3] The 1-min pulse watch, invented by Floyer in 1707, offered the first opportunity to make accurate observations about the heart rate; however, this did not become a routine part of medical practice until the mid-nineteenth century.[3] Since the nineteenth-century observations of Dominic Corrigan, the carotid arterial pulse has been linked to aortic valve disease and essential for timing the onset of systole at the bedside. Pulsus alternans was described by Ludwig Traube in 1872, and Adolf Kussmaul called attention to the paradoxical pulse in 1873, noting that the arterial pulse could transiently disappear on inspiration even though the heart sounds were still audible. Before electrocardiography, arterial recordings were applied to diagnose arrhythmias, as shown so well by James Mackenzie in his *The Study of the Pulse* (1902).[11]

### Percussion

In 1761, Leopold Auenbrugger, a Viennese physician, published a book proposing "percussion of the human thorax, whereby, according to the character of the particular sounds thence elicited, an opinion is formed of the internal state of that cavity."[2] He had observed his father, an innkeeper, use this technique to check wine levels in his casks. Although his discovery was ignored at that time, his work was translated and reintroduced by Jean-Nicolas Corvisart in nineteenth-century France, and percussion became an important addition to the examination.

### The Jugular Venous Pulse

Evaluation of the jugular venous waves began in mid-nineteenth-century France with Pierre-Carl Potain and was more fully realized in the 1870s by James Mackenzie, a general practitioner who sought to interpret arrhythmias by understanding arterial and venous waves. Using a kymographic sphygmometer and then an ink-writing polygraph of his invention, Mackenzie applied his intuitive skills to the interpretation of jugular waves, which he labeled "a, c, and v."[12] Thomas Lewis, a disciple of Mackenzie, later (1930) described the current technique of bedside assessment of jugular venous pressure.

### Auscultation

Auscultation of the chest was practiced by Hippocrates (460–370 B.C.), who applied his ear directly to the chest. The invention of the wooden monaural stethoscope (Greek: *stethos,* chest; *skopein,* to view or to see) by René Läennec in 1816 forever changed the examination by providing a relatively simple technique to listen to cardiovascular sounds and murmurs.[13–15] This technique spread to Europe and Great Britain—where it was promoted by Skoda, Stokes, Hope, and others—and to America, where Austin Flint became its champion. The stethoscope quickly became an indispensable tool for the clinical examination, and the nineteenth century became known as the "golden age of stethoscopy." Diagnoses based on percussion and auscultation were also subjected to the critical analysis of the autopsy by Läennec, Rokitansky, and Skoda, and murmurs were assigned to the underlying pathology. Symptoms not supported by auscultatory or autopsy findings were often thought to be functional or unreliable. The stethoscope evolved from a monaural to a binaural device in 1855, and zseparate heads were later developed for listening to different frequencies. Grading of systolic murmurs was introduced by Samuel Levine in 1933. The acoustic principles of cardiovascular sound became better understood in the 1940s through the work of Rappaport and Sprague, and correlations were made using auscultation, chest x-ray, phonocardiography, and cardiac catheterization by Paul Wood, Aubrey Leatham, and others between 1950 and 1975. In 1961, the physiologist Robert Rushmer proposed the acceleration-deceleration theory that is our current concept of the generation of normal and abnormal heart sounds. Auscultation has continued to be valuable in the assessment of the cardiovascular system, though it is less relied upon today, when bedside skills are decreasingly prized and taught.

## TECHNOLOGY AND THE HEART

### The Electrocardiogram

The Nobel Prize in 1924 was given to Willem Einthoven of the Netherlands "for his discovery of the mechanism of the electrocardiogram." The story begins with Galvani's 1786 discovery that animal tissue generated electricity.[16] In 1856, von Kölliker and Müller demonstrated that the heart also produced electricity. Augustus Waller, with a capillary electrometer device, was the first to show, in 1887, that cardiac electricity could be detected from the limbs, a crude recording that he called an "electrogram." Willem Einthoven, a physiologist in Utrecht, found the capillary electrometer too sluggish and invented (1902) the string galvanometer, which is still in use today. Initially weighing 600 lb and requiring five people to operate, the electrocardiograph eventually became lightweight, portable, and universally available (Table 1-1).[16]

With this far more sensitive equipment, the activation and sequence of stimulation of the human heart could now be recorded and measured and the anatomic basis for the conduction system confirmed. Disorders of the heartbeat and abnormalities in the activation of the human heart, heretofore unknown or inferred from pulse tracings or experimental observations, became new clinical currency: palpitations became premature atrial or ventricular beats and tachycardias and atrioventricular block could be understood. When electrocardiography was added to the chest x-ray and cardiac fluoroscopy in the early twentieth century, clinical cardiology became a field of its own, inextricably linked to technology. Those who interpreted the complicated tracings, known as cardiologists, became practitioners of this new specialty.[10] Beginning in the 1920s, the electrocardiogram would be considered a necessary confirmation for the clinical diagnoses of myocardial ischemia or infarction. Continuous bedside monitoring (1956) and the ambulatory detection of arrhythmias (1961) became commonplace in the 1960s; implanted loop recording appeared more recently. When exercise testing with electrocardiography was introduced—beginning with the two-step test in the 1940s, then stress testing in the 1960s, and nuclear and echo imaging in the 1970s—an entirely new diagnostic approach to patients with chest pain became available.

Electrophysiologic testing in humans began as an offshoot of basic catheterization laboratory investigations in the early pacemaker era. Catheter techniques were used to localize the His bundle by Sherlag and Damato (1967) and to identify accessory pathways. Programmed electrical stimulation of the heart, a technique introduced by Durrer and Wellens (1972), was designed to provoke arrhythmias, which could then be matched against antiarrhythmic drugs to see if

TABLE 1-1 Advances in Cardiac Diagnosis and Technology

**Ancient Times**

General inspection
Palpation of the pulse (Egypt, China, India)

**Eighteenth Century**

Physician's one minute pulse watch (1707)
Percussion of the chest (1761)

**Nineteenth Century**

Stethoscopic auscultation of the heart (1816)
Pleximeter (1826)
Kymographic recording of pulses (1847)
Sphygmograph for blood pressure measurement (1855, 1863)
Polygraphic recording of pulses (1883)
Chest x-ray (1895)
Fluoroscopy (1896)

**Twentieth Century**

**1900–1929**

Orthodiagraphy (1902)
Electrocardiogram (1902)
Auscultation of blood pressure (1905)
Phonocardiogram (1907, 1950s)
Electrocardiography for myocardial infarction (1920)
Leukocytosis in myocardial infarction (1916)
Vectorcardiography (1920)
Portable electrocardiogram (1928)
First cardiac catheterization (1929)
Precordial electrocardiography (1932)
Unipolar ECG leads (1932)

**1930–1959**

Bedside measurement of venous pressure (1930)
Cardiac output measurement (1870, 1930)
Circulation time (1931)
Angiography (1931, 1937)
Sedimentation rate for myocardial infarction (1933)
Development of cardiac catheterization (1941)
Augmented unipolar leads (1942)
Master's two-step exercise test (1942)
Scintillation scanner (1949, 1952)
Left heart catheterization (1950)
Image intensification (1953)
M-mode echocardiography (1954)
Serum glutamic oxaloacetic transaminase (1954)
Treadmill exercise testing (1956)
Cardiac monitoring (1956)
Selective coronary arteriography (1958)

**1960–1979**

Computerized electrocardiography (1961)
Ambulatory monitoring (1961)
Creatine phosphokinase (1965)
His bundle recording (1967)
Transfemoral catheterization (1967)
Contrast echocardiography (1968)
Swan-Ganz flotation catheter (1970)
Digoxin level (1971)
CT scanning (1971)
Electrophysiologic testing (1972)
Nuclear stress cardiology (1973)
2-D echocardiography (1974)
Doppler echocardiography (1975)
Positive emission tomography (1979)
Stress echocardiography (1979)
Ultrafast computed tomography (1979, 1990)

**1980–Present**

Signal-averaged electrocardiography (1981)
Doppler color-flow echocardiography (1982)
Magnetic resonance imaging of the heart (1984)
ST segment monitoring (1984)
Transesophageal echocardiography (1985)
Dobutamine stress echocardiography (1986)
Heart rate variability (1973, 1987)
Troponin T (1991)
Troponin I (1992)
B-type natriuretic peptide (1984)
Intracoronary ultrasound (1996)
3-D echocardiography (2003)

reinduction could be prevented. Mapping techniques, initially applied to the surface of the exposed heart for the localization and resection of accessory pathways (1968) and for the surgical excision of malignant ventricular arrhythmias, became an important next step. As catheter methods of ablation developed, first coupled with intracardiac electric shock of the atrioventricular node and then with radiofrequency current, ablation moved from the surgery suite into the laboratory setting, populated by a new subspecialty group—the electrophysiologists. More recently, understanding the biophysical and molecular determinants of the cardiac action potential, identification of the genes for specific channels, and investigations of the genetic and molecular mechanisms of heritable cardiac disorders, such as the long-QT syndromes, has elevated the indispensable electrocardiogram to a new level of importance.

## The Cardiac Catheter

The Nobel Prize in 1956 was awarded to André Cournand, Dickinson Richards, and Werner Forssmann "for their discoveries concerning heart catheterization and pathological changes in the circulatory system." If the electrocardiograph was a touchstone for the identification of the cardiologist at the dawn of the twentieth century, it was the cardiac catheter that completed the modern definition of cardiology. Many of the fundamentals of modern cardiovascular instrumentation and physiology originated in mid-nineteenth-century France. Claude Bernard in 1844 was the first to insert a catheter into the heart of animals in order to measure temperature and pressure.[7] In the 1860s, Etienne Jules Marey combined the kymographic instrumentation created by Carl Ludwig in Leipzig in 1847 with an air-filled manometer for the graphic registration of biological phenomena.[5] Marey's pulse writer—the sphygmograph—was used for recording the external pulsation of the heart and arteries and was a prototype for noninvasive devices in cardiology. Marey was also the first to record an electrogram of the heart in animals (1876) using the capillary electometer, and he pioneered the calibration and standardization of recording instruments. In the early 1860s, Auguste Chauveau, a veterinary physiologist, and Marey collaborated to develop a system of devices called sounds, forerunners of the modern cardiac catheter, which they used to catheterize the right heart and left ventricle of the horse.[5] They recorded true values of intracardiac pressure with superb tracings and correlated the intracardiac events with precision to show the relation of atrial and ventricular systole to the apex impulse. In 1870, Adolph Fick provided his oximetric formula to measure cardiac output.

Everything was in place for cardiac catheterization in the clinical arena; however, cardiac catheterization in humans remained an inconceivable risk for almost 70 years until Werner Forssmann, a 29-year-old surgical resident in Germany, performed a self-catheterization.[17,18] Forssmann was interested in discovering a method of injecting adrenaline in order to treat cardiac arrest. He passed a ureteral catheter into the right atrium, first on cadavers and then on himself, confirming its right atrial position on an x-ray (1929). The next year he attempted to image his heart using an iodide injection. However, he was reprimanded and did not experiment further. Catheterization began in earnest in the early 1940s in New York and London. André Cournand and Dickinson Richards at Bellevue, interested in respiratory physiology, developed and demonstrated the safety of complete right heart catheterization, for which they shared the Nobel Prize with Forssmann in 1956.[2,5,8]

The cardiac catheter was viewed initially as an instrument to measure pressure and cardiac output, sample blood contents, or deliver contrast agents for cardiovascular angiography. Brannon and Warren in Atlanta were the first to apply the catheter to diagnose heart disease—an atrial septal defect—in 1945. It was the impetus of cardiac surgery requiring an accurate diagnosis, initially for congenital heart and rheumatic mitral disease, that brought cardiac catheterization out of the physiology laboratory and to the forefront of clinical cardiology in the 1950s. Improved catheters and pressure manometers, automatic film changers, and the introduction of retrograde left heart catheterization by Henry Zimmerman (1950) and a percutaneous approach by Sven Seldinger (1953) advanced the technique, accompanying heart surgery into the era of valve replacement in the 1960s. Mason Sone's accidental injection of contrast directly into a right coronary artery (1958) was quickly recognized by him to be a serendipitous leap forward. The transfemoral approach by Judkins (1967) simplified selective coronary catheterization. Visualization of the coronary circulation ultimately led to the introduction of coronary bypass surgery by René Favoloro (1967) and angioplasty by Andreas Grüntzig (1977).[18,19] Since then, the versatile cardiac catheter has continued to evolve, carrying delivery systems or instruments ranging from ultrasound, balloons, and stents to defibrillators (Tables 1-1 and 1-2).

## Imaging of the Heart

Imaging of the heart can be traced to Leonardo da Vinci. His remarkable drawings of the heart provide two-dimensional representations of three-dimensional objects, and his knowledge of fluid dynamics interposed hydraulic technology into cardiac anatomy and function. His use of a glass cast to visualize the inside of the heart marks the beginning of medical imaging.

### RADIOGRAPHY

Modern imaging technology began with Konrad Röntgen's discovery of x-rays in 1895, for which he was awarded the Nobel Prize in Physics in 1901 "in recognition of the extraordinary services he has rendered by the discovery of the remarkable rays subsequently named after him."[20,21] Within a year, fluorescent screens were available to view and produce images on photographic film. These radiographic techniques were soon applied clinically to view the contents of the thorax and the cardiac pulsations. Contrast agents incorporating sodium iodide were necessary to visualize the organ cavities. Antonio Moniz in Lisbon (1931) and Castellanos in Cuba (1937) were the first to image the interior of the heart with intravenous angiograms.[2] It was not until the mid-twentieth century that electronic x-ray technology and the image intensifier provided the basis for enhanced viewing of dynamic events in real time (Table 1-1). Angiography became the essence of cardiovascular imaging for several decades after the mid-twentieth century, vital to the diagnosis and management of coronary disease during the 1960s, and it continues to play an important role.

### NUCLEAR CARDIOLOGY

Nuclear cardiology began with Herrman Blumgart, who injected radon to measure the circulation time in 1927; followed by G. Liljestrand, who determined normal blood volume in 1939; and Myron Prinzmetal, who monitored the transit of radiolabeled albumin through the heart in 1948.[5,22] Following World War II, radioactive isotopes and scintillation cameras became available for imaging purposes. The gamma camera of Hal Anger, a key development introduced in 1952, provided a high-resolution scanning capability that could visualize the cardiac chambers and assess function and shunting without moving the patient. Electrocardiographic gating greatly improved the analysis of wall motion and ejection fraction starting in

TABLE 1-2 Advances in Medical Therapy: 1900–Present

**Available in 1900**

Alcohol
Amyl nitrite (1867)
Atropine (1833, 1867)
Caffeine (1879)
Chloroform (1831)
Diet
Digitalis (1785)
Ether (1842)
Exercise
Leeches
Morphine (1821)
Nitroglycerine (1879)
Salicylic acid (1876)
Southey trochars
Spa therapy
Squill (seventeenth century)
Theobromine (1879)
Venesection
Veratrium viride (1859)

**1900–1949**

Adrenaline (1900)
Oxygen (1908)
Quinidine (1918)
Heparin (1918, 1935)
Mercurial diuretics (1920)
Magnesium (1935)
Dicoumarol (1941)
Rice diet (1944)
Cation exchange resins (1946)
Open chest defibrillation (1947)
Reserpine (1949)

**1950–1959**

Hexamethonium (1950)
Hydralazine (1951)
Procainamide (1951)
Ambulation post-MI (1952)
Carbonic anhydrase inhibitors (1952)
External cardiac pacing (1952)
Warfarin (1954)
Alpha methyl dopa (1955)
Closed chest defibrillation (1956)
Chlorothiazide (1957)
Streptokinase for MI (1958)
Guanethidine (1959)

**1960–1969**

Closed chest cardiac massage (1960)
Implantable pacemaker (1960)
AV synchronous pacemaker (1962)
Beta blockers (1962)
Coronary care units (1961)
Synchronized cardioversion (1962)
Intra-aortic balloon pump (1962)
Disopyramide (1963)
Lidocaine (1963)
Furosemide (1964)
Balloon atrial septostomy (Rashkind procedure, 1966)
Programmed electrophysiologic stimulation (1967)
Mobile ICU (1967)
Bretylium tosylate (1968)
Outpatient cardiac rehabilitation (1968)

**1970–1979**

Calcium channel blocking agents (1970)
Vasodilator therapy (1971)
Dopamine (1972)
Lithium battery pacemakers (1972)
Intravenous verapamil (1972)
Nitroprusside (1974)
Beta blockers for heart failure (1975)
Dobutamine (1975)
Coronary angioplasty (1977)
Amiodarone (1961, 1979)
Intracoronary thrombolysis (streptokinase) (1979)
Intravenous nitroglycerine

**1980–1989**

ACE inhibitors (1981)
Phosphodiesterase inhibitors (1980)
Propafenone (1980)
Automatic implanted defibrillator (1980)
Transmyocardial laser (1981)
Flecainide (1982)
Antitachycardia pacemaker (1982)
AV nodal ablation (1982)
Catheter ablation of Wolff-Parkinson-White (1984)
Coronary stents (1986)
Dual chamber pacing (1980)
Low-molecular weight heparin (1986)
Lovastatin (1986)
Intravenous thrombolysis (tPA) (1987)
Aspirin for acute coronary disease (1988)
Aspirin for primary prevention (1989)
Ticlopidine (1989)

**1990–Present**

Hirudin (lepirudin) (1991)
Angiotensin II receptor blocking agents (1992)
Directional atherectomy (1993)
$GII_b$–$III_a$ inhibitors (1993)
Carvedilol (1995)
Nesiritide (1996)
Biphasic cardioversion–defibrillation (1996)
Clopidogrel (1998)
Biventricular pacing (1998)
Dofetilide (1999)
Brachytherapy (2000)
Drug eluding stents (2001)

the early 1970s, as did single-photon emission computed tomography (SPECT) in the 1990s. Nuclear stress testing for ischemia was reported by Zaret and Strauss in 1973 using potassium 43 as the tracer. Redistribution studies, taking advantage of the properties of thallium 201 and technetium 99m, have improved the performance of the test, and pharmacologic stress testing with dipyridamole and adenosine has expanded their utilization.[5,22]

## ECHOCARDIOGRAPHY

Ultrasound imaging dates back to the production of sound waves from piezoelectric crystals in 1880 and the military use of sonar for the detection of reflected sound waves during World War II.[5] Cardiac ultrasound was introduced in Sweden by Inge Edler, who detected the anterior mitral leaflet by M-mode echo (1954). In the 1960s and 1970s, M-mode echo was developed into a powerful clinical technique by Harvey Feigenbaum and others, who also taught its interpretation to the first generation of echocardiographers. Since then, two-dimensional echo (1974), Doppler echo (1975), stress echo (1979), and both color-flow (1982) and transesophageal imaging (1985) have added to its success. Intraoperative transesophageal monitoring and the intrauterine diagnosis of congenital heart disease have become possible. Echocardiography has safely and brilliantly illuminated the heart.[20,21]

## TOMOGRAPHY AND MAGNETIC RESONANCE IMAGING

The three decades following the introduction of the gamma camera and ultrasound brought unbelievable largesse to the medical imaging field, including computed tomography (CT; 1963–1971), single-photon emission computed tomography (SPECT; 1963–1981), positron emission tomography (PET; 1975–1987), and magnetic resonance imaging (MRI; 1972–1981), each delivering its own exciting ability to look at the heart in a different way (Table 1-1). Each of these imaging techniques has initiated new clinical disciplines in cardiology and radiology that continue to the present. As with cardiac catheterization and angiography, industrial developments have provided the bases for each technological advance. The computer has been a major asset for all technologies.

## CORONARY ARTERY DISEASE

On July 21, 1768, William Heberden presented "Some Account of a Disorder of the Breast" to the Royal College of Physicians, London, in which he stated: "But there is a disorder of the breast marked with strong and peculiar symptoms, considerable for the kind of danger belonging to it, and not extremely rare. The seat of it, and sense of strangling and anxiety with which it is attended, may make it not improperly be called angina pectoris."[2,23] Heberden appropriated the term *angina* (from a Latin word meaning "strangling") because of its use in describing cases of sore throat, speculating that it was due to a cramp or an ulcer. Heberden's classic account is considered to mark the beginning of our appreciation of coronary artery disease. Edward Jenner and Caleb Parry were the first to suspect a coronary etiology. This was supported by their 1793 autopsy findings of ossified coronaries in their friend, the temperamental surgeon John Hunter, who suffered from angina, saying that his "life was in the hands of any rascal who should choose to annoy and tease me." Crediting Jenner, Parry published this coronary implication in 1799 in *Syncope Anginosa*. Allan Burns, in Scotland, likened the pain of angina pectoris to the discomfort brought about by walking with a tight ligature placed on a limb (1809), a prescient concept that remains current. Nevertheless, a coronary cause of angina pectoris was not readily accepted until the late nineteenth century for several reasons: (1) the heart was thought to be immune to disease; (2) autopsies showed other heart or aortic conditions or the cardiac scarring was interpreted as myocarditis; (3) the coronaries were not carefully dissected; (4) symptoms were intermittent, though coronary disease seemed fixed; and (5) coronary disease was found in asymptomatic patients and might be absent in patients with chest pain.[23] Additionally, Corvisart failed to mention angina in his influential 1806 textbook; Läennec and Flint attributed chest pain to neuralgia; Skoda, Hope, Stokes, and others—believing in the stethoscope and physical diagnosis—found little or nothing to corroborate a coronary cause in patients with chest pain. The term *arteriosclerosis*, derived from Greek roots, was coined by Johann Lobstein (1833). Key pathologic observations were made by Rudolf Virchow, who established the importance of thrombosis of arteries as a cause of disease (1846); Richard Quain, who associated the fatty degeneration of cardiac muscle with coronary obstruction (1850); Karl Weigert, who described the pathology of myocardial infarction and remarked on the importance of collateral vessels (1880); and Karl Huber, who suggested that atheroma could cut off the blood supply and lead to myocardial fibrosis (1882).[23] Adam Hammer was the first to report the premortem diagnosis of myocardial infarction (1878).

By the late nineteenth century, angina pectoris was linked with coronary artery disease by William Osler and others, although there was confusion between angina pectoris and myocardial infarction. The disease was thought to be uncommon at that time, when the average life expectancy was 40 years. Julius Cohnheim, an experimental pathologist, taught that coronary arteries were end arteries, noting that experimental ligation of a coronary artery resulted in ventricular fibrillation (1881). In 1901, Osler classified angina into several types, calling the anterior branch the "artery of sudden death." He agreed that coronary thrombosis was invariably fatal and later stated that "the tragedies of life are largely arterial." The concept that coronary thrombosis was always fatal was finally dispelled by James Herrick in his article entitled "Clinical Features of Sudden Obstruction of the Coronary Arteries" (1912).[25,26] He concluded "there is no inherent reason why the stoppage of a large branch of a coronary artery, or even of a main trunk, must of necessity cause sudden death." Herrick is credited as having been the first to grasp the variable course of myocardial infarction. Willem Einthoven's three-lead electrocardiogram, used by Herrick and Smith in 1918 to diagnose infarction experimentally and clinically by Pardee in 1920, provided clinical confirmation.[16] Precordial leads, introduced by Frank Wilson in the 1930s, supplemented the diagnosis. Other diagnostic aids included the elevated white cell count (1916), an increase in the sedimentation rate (1933), and the determination of transaminase (1954), creatine kinase (1965) and its isoenzymes (1972), and troponin (1991). Between 1920 and 1950, large series of patients—analyzed by John Parkinson and Evan Bedford in London, Samuel Levine and Paul Dudley White in Boston, Charles Friedberg in New York, and others—provided a broad understanding of the clinical, electrocardiographic, and laboratory findings of myocardial infarction and its prognosis and autopsy correlations.[9] By the 1930s, myocardial infarction was a familiar diagnosis which was felt to be increasing in frequency. The clinical and pathologic correlations of arteriosclerosis and thrombosis with angina and infarction were greatly strengthened by the 1940 postmortem coronary injection studies of Blumgart, Schlesinger, and Davis in Boston. As late as the 1970s, considerable argument still persisted about whether a coronary thrombosis was the initiating cause of infarction or occurred afterwards. This was resolved by the autoradiographic postmortem studies of Fulton in Glasgow (1976) and DeWood's coronary arteriographic studies of patients with acute infarction, which demonstrated that a thrombus was the primary event and indicated that the clot might subsequently lyse (1980). More recently, the "vulnerable plaque" hypothesis, evidenced by Michael Davies in London and Erling Falk in Denmark and New York and dating back to Constantinides' 1966 description of fissured plaques leading to thrombosis, has gained enthusiastic support. The role of inflammation as a primary or secondary event, supported by serum markers, has led many to believe that atherosclerosis is at least in part an inflammatory condition.

### Coronary Care and the Treatment of Coronary Disease

Before the development of the defibrillator and coronary care units, the mortality of infarction was commonly quoted to be 25 to 30 percent. Cardiac arrest was assumed to be irreversible. With the development of the external pacemaker by Paul Zoll (1952) and the defibrillator by William Kouwenhoven (1930s–1950s), used by Claude Beck (1947) and Zoll (1956), the rescue of victims of cardiac arrest became feasible. Beck dramatically stated that "The death factor in coronary artery disease is often small and reversible.... The heart wants to beat and often it needs only a second chance." His concept that "the heart is too good to die" instilled optimism into the care of coronary patients. The monitoring of patients in close proximity to skilled nursing personnel to treat ventricular arrhythmias and perform cardiopulmonary resuscitation was initiated in 1961 and then spread throughout the world. Since then, coronary care has gone through recognizable phases: resuscitation and the important role of the nurse, prevention of arrhythmias, hemodynamic catheter monitoring and treatment of pump failure, reduction of infarct size—first with beta blockers and now with thrombolytic therapy, and primary angioplasty. Clinical and electrocardiographic distinctions have been drawn between unstable angina (previously called preinfarction angina), an acute coronary event, nontransmural/non–Q wave infarction, and transmural infarction. The mortality of transmural infarction has fallen as low as 3 percent and the period of hospitalization has been progressively reduced from weeks to a few days for many patients.

Treatment of angina pectoris begins with the use of amyl nitrite by Lauder Brunton (1867) and nitroglycerine by William Murrell (1879). At one time or another before 1970, xanthine derivatives, sedatives, opiates, diet, prolonged rest, alcohol, long-acting nitrites, paravertebral alcohol injections, dorsal sympathectomy, induction of myxedema, instillation of talc or bone dust into the pericardium, denervation of the heart, radiation to the anterior chest, and carotid sinus pacing were in vogue. Beta-adrenergic blockade, first available in the early 1970s, greatly improved the management of angina, and trials in the 1980s showed that myocardial infarction can often be prevented by the regular use of beta blockade. Calcium channel blockers and nitroglycerine administered by paste and intravenously were introduced in the late 1970s (Table 1-2). Dicumarol became available in 1941, and starting in the 1950s, anticoagulation was strongly recommended by Paul Wood and others for myocardial infarction. Strict bed rest, often for weeks, was rigidly advised for heart attacks until 1952, when Levine and Lown suggested that an "armchair" approach was better. Aspirin has been as an important adjunct for acute infarction since 1988 and has been strongly recommended for primary prevention since 1989. Thrombolytic therapy for acute myocardial infarction, using small doses of intravenous streptokinase, was first tried in 1958 by Fletcher and Sherry and given as an intracoronary infusion by Boucek and Murphy in 1960 and Chazov in 1976.[27] Its current use, which has so radically changed our approach to acute infarction, began with the intracoronary infusion of streptokinase in 1979 by Rentrop and was extended with intravenous streptokinase in 1983 and intravenous tissue plasminogen activator (t-PA) in 1987. Large randomized studies confirmed their benefit, bringing a cooperative international approach to clinical trials. Percutaneous angioplasty for angina was conceived and developed by Andreas Grüntzig (1977), followed by the first stenting of coronary arteries by Sigwart and Puel (1986), primary angioplasty for acute infarction (1988), brachytherapy (2000), and drug-eluding stents (2001).[19] The benefit of angiotensin converting enzyme (ACE) inhibitors in the remodeling of myocardium was shown in the early 1990s. Potent platelet inhibition with GIIb-IIIa inhibitors became available in 1993 for acute coronary syndromes. The internally implanted automatic defibrillator, developed by Michel Mirowsky, was first used in a human in 1980. Although it was initially highly controversial, it is now in widespread use to prevent sudden cardiac death. Epidemiologic studies, especially those of Ancel Keys in Minnesota and the Framingham study, have emphasized primary and secondary prevention through the recognition and treatment of risk factors, especially smoking, hypertension, and hyperlipidemia, as essential to the management of patients with coronary disease or at high risk for future events. The role of the statin drugs, introduced during the past decade to prevent heart attack and stroke, has been especially promising.

## VALVULAR HEART DISEASE

Claudius Galen (A.D. 130–200) noted that "the general purpose of the valves is to prevent a reversal of flow." Valvular pathology was described in the seventeenth and eighteenth centuries; however, Läennec was the first to hear heart murmurs, calling them "blowing, sawing, filing, and rasping."[13] Originally, he attributed the noise to valvular disease, but he later decided that they were due to spasm or contraction of a cardiac chamber. James Hope in England was the first to classify valvular murmurs in *A Treatise on the Diseases of the Heart and Great Vessels,* originally published in 1832.[28] Hope found valvular disease much more likely to occur on the left side of the heart and showed how to separate murmurs of all four valves. He interpreted physical findings in early physiologic terms and provided detailed pathologic correlations. His description of mitral regurgitation was especially memorable: "When the valve is permanently open, admitting of regurgitation, the first sound is attended with a murmur. It may be rough (rasping), or smooth (bellows murmur), according to the nature of the contraction.... Its key is low, more like whispering Who."[29] Constriction of the mitral valve was recorded by John Mayow (1668) and Raymond Vieussens (1715); the latter also recognized that it could cause pulmonary congestion.[30] The presystolic murmur of mitral stenosis was heard by Bertin (1824), timed as both early diastolic and presystolic by Williams (1835), and placed on firmer grounds by Fauvel (1843) and Gairdner (1861). Aortic stenosis was first described pathologically by Rivière (1663), and Läennec pointed out that the aortic valve was subject to ossification (1819).[31] Corvisart showed an astute grasp of the natural history of aortic stenosis (1809), commenting:

> When it is considered how narrow the opening is, which these constrictions leave, it is difficult to conceive how such an organic derangement can continue for years. It is evident, if such an obstacle to the circulation were suddenly introduced into a healthy subject, death would immediately follow; but as these obstacles are slowly formed, the circulation is gradually impeded, and nature seems in some measure to be habituated to such a perversion of her laws.

Early descriptions of aortic regurgitation were by William Cowper (1706) and Raymond Vieussens (1715).[32] Morgagni recognized the hemodynamic consequences of aortic regurgitation (1761). In 1832, Dominic Corrigan provided his classic description of the arterial pulse and murmur of aortic regurgitation. Austin Flint added the presystolic murmur sometimes heard with severe aortic regurgitation (1862).[14] The etiology of valvular disease in the nineteenth and first half of the twentieth century revolved about the role of rheumatic fever. David Pitcairn was the first to suggest rheumatism of the heart (1788), and William Charles Wells described acute rheumatic fever with cardiac involvement in 1812.[9,33] The most important figure was Jean Baptiste-Bouillaud, who established that acute articular rheumatism was associated with inflammation of the endocardium, myocardium, and pericardium, leading to valvular deformities (1836). Called *Bouillaud's disease* by the French, it became well-known as "a disease that licks the joints but bites the heart."[9] Acceptance of the association between "rheumatism"—i.e., rheumatic fever—and subsequent valvular heart disease slowly took hold. By the late 1800s, treatment of rheumatic episodes with salicylic acid had been introduced. Over time, the link between the throat, heart, and rheumatic fever was clarified; the role of the *Streptococcus* was identified; and attention paid to environmental factors—poverty, overcrowding, and malnutrition. Antibiotic therapy and prophylaxis have contributed to the great decrease in rheumatic fever in the western world; however, a precise understanding of the causative factors of rheumatic heart disease is still lacking.

The story of valvular heart disease in the second half of the twentieth century overlaps with developments in cardiac catheterization, imaging technology, and cardiac surgery. Beginning with cardiac catheterization in the 1950s and supplemented by echocardiographic imaging in the 1970s, the severity of valvular disease could be more easily analyzed and its progression followed. Until the last 40 years, valvular murmurs continued to be ascribed to rheumatic heart disease, to the detriment of recognizing valvular heart disease of other etiologies. Our understanding of the etiology of valvular heart disease changed dramatically with the recognition of nonrheumatic causes of valvular disease.[34] The expanded list includes heritable and congenital causes (the floppy mitral valve with mitral valve prolapse, bicuspid aortic valve, the Marfan syndrome); inflammatory causes (immunologic disorders including rheumatic fever, acquired immunodeficiency syndrome, radiation, endocardial proliferative disorders, collagen diseases, and antiphospholipid syndrome); diseases or disorders of other organs (chronic renal failure, carcinoid heart disease); myocardial disease with valvular regurgitation; valvular disease in the aging population (calcific aortic stenosis, mitral annular calcification); valvular disease following interventions (valvuloplasty, valve reconstruction, and valve replacement); and valve disease related to diet drugs and physical agents.

## CONGENITAL HEART DISEASE

The first complete description of a congenital heart, with defects later known as tetralogy of Fallot, was given by Niels Stensen in Denmark (1672).[5] Early textbooks in cardiology by Jean-Baptiste Senac (1749) and Allan Burns (1809) included comments on cardiac malformations. Cyanotic heart disease is mentioned; however, its mechanism was debated because some patients with septal defects had cyanosis while others did not. John Farre in England was the first to use the word *clubbing* in 1814. An early, comprehensive book devoted to cyanotic and acyanotic congenital heart disease, *On Malformations, of the Human Heart,* was published in 1858 and 1866 by Thomas Bevill Peacock, a London physician with a special interest in pathology.[2] In his book, Peacock reviews the previous literature and provides detailed case studies, beautiful engravings of the pathology, personal insights, and an anatomic classification of more than 100 patients.

Following Peacock's book, advances in congenital heart disease were limited primarily to pathologic descriptions and summaries until the seminal work of the pathologist Maude Abbott. Beginning in 1908, with encouragement from William Osler, Maude Abbott catalogued the pathology collection at the Montreal General Hospital, compiling 1000 cases that were fully analyzed in her 1936 classic *Atlas of Congenital Heart Disease.*[5,35] Her meticulous work provided a new classification correlating the history, examination, and postmortem with illustrations; it became the foundation for the study of congenital heart disease.

The pivotal breakthrough came from Helen Taussig and Alfred Blalock at Johns Hopkins Hospital with their "blue baby operation." Taussig had observed that patients with cyanotic heart disease worsened and died when their ductus arteriosus closed. She suggested creating an artificial ductus to improve oxygenation.[36] Alfred Blalock, Chair of Surgery, ably assisted by Vivian Thomas, created a shunt from the subclavian to the pulmonary artery, which Blalock performed successfully in November 1944. This innovative operation, in which a blue baby was dramatically changed to a pink one—the Blalock-Taussig shunt—was highly publicized, and other shunt operations soon followed (Table 1-3). Taussig's *Congenital Malformations of the Heart,* a 1947 compendium of her vast knowledge of the subject with easy-to-understand schematics explaining the pathophysiology of the defect, became the bible of congenital heart disease. Many of her trainees, and those of Alexander Nadas and Robert Gross in Boston, would become future leaders in the field, extending their influence worldwide.

Studies in the 1950s correlated the clinical with the cardiac catheterization findings and led to a firmer basis for selecting patients who might benefit from the upcoming advances in congenital heart surgery. Natural history studies helped to clarify their prognosis.

In 1966, Rashkind introduced the balloon septostomy—the Rashkind procedure—a novel catheter therapeutic technique that launched the entire field of interventional cardiology and bought time for severely cyanotic infants with transposition of the great arteries.[5] In the 1980s, catheters were further adapted to dilate stenotic aortic and pulmonic valves and coarctation of the aorta. More recently, atrial and some ventricular septal defects and patent ductus arteriosus have been closed with transcatheter devices. On the near horizon are catheter techniques capable of restricting excessive pulmonary blood flow, inserting cardiac valves, and redirecting blood flow through stents.

Treatment with indomethacin to enable closure of a patent ductus in the premature infant (1976) and prostaglandin infusion to maintain ductal patency in duct-dependent circulations (1981) has profoundly changed the medical management of fragile newborns. Infants with severe congenital heart disease, such as pulmonary atresia and hypoplastic left hearts, can now be safely stabilized before surgery. Until the 1970s, confirmation of a complex clinical diagnosis, necessary for critical surgical decisions, required cardiac catheterization and angiography. In the late 1970s and 1980s, two-dimensional echo and color-flow Doppler technique and later MRI became available to provide an immediate diagnosis. With new medical and catheter management, the approach to many infants with congenital heart disease was radically changed. Improvements in operative techniques allowed innovative surgeons to operate earlier on smaller and sicker hearts while offering palliation or complete repair for congenital defects. During the last half of the twentieth century, our understanding of the etiology of congenital heart disease has been greatly furthered by genetic, biochemical, and environmental studies.

## BLOOD PRESSURE MEASUREMENT AND HYPERTENSION

In 1711, Reverend Stephen Hales, an English minister with an intense curiosity, cannulated the crural artery of a recumbent horse and found that the pulsation of the arterial blood rose to a height over 8 ft above the heart—the first measurement of arterial pressure.[36,37] His pioneering efforts stood alone until 1828, when Jean Poiseuille introduced a crude mercury manometer device to measure blood pressure.[39] Over the next 60 years, various sphygmomanometric methods were developed—notably by Ludwig (1847), Vierordt (1855), and Marey (1863)—to refine the precision of measuring arterial blood pressure. The inflatable arm cuff coupled to the sphygmograph, a device small enough to allow measurement outside the laboratory, was invented by Riva-Rocci (1896), who also noted the "white-coat effect" on blood pressure (see Chap. 12).[40] In 1901, Harvey Cushing visited Riva-Rocci and then instituted a new anesthesia record at Johns Hopkins Hospital to chart blood pressures during surgery. Not everyone was convinced. James Mackenzie in England, devoted to his polygraphic method of pulse recording, was skeptical that blood pressure measurement was necessary and complained in 1904 that it separated the physician from the patient. The 1905 discovery by Nicolai Korotkoff, a Russian military surgeon, that brachial arterial sounds can be auscultated when the Riva-Rocci cuff is deflated, marks the advent of modern blood

TABLE 1-3 Advances in Cardiovascular Surgery

| Nineteenth Century |
|---|
| Drainage of pericardial effusion (1810) |
| Surgical closure of stab wound of heart (1835) |
| Introduction of ether anesthesia (1842) |
| Removal of foreign body from heart (1873) |
| Surgical closure of stab wound of heart (1897) |
| **Twentieth Century** |
| **1900–1925** |
| End-to-end arterial anastomosis (1902) |
| Animal heart transplantation (1905) |
| Arterial patch graft (1910) |
| Coronary artery bypass in animal (1910) |
| Insufflation endotracheal anesthesia (1910) |
| Attempted external dilatation of aortic stenosis (1912) |
| Pericardial resection for constriction (1913) |
| Sympathectomy (1917) |
| Heparin anticoagulation (1918) |
| Mitral stenosis valvulotomy (1923) |
| Pulmonary embolectomy (1924) |
| Lumbar sympathectomy (1925) |
| Mitral stenosis dilatation by finger (1925) |
| **1926–1950** |
| Thyroidectomy for angina pectoris (1933) |
| Cardio-omentopexy (1930s) |
| Ligation of patent ductus arteriosus (1938) |
| Coarctation repair (1944) |
| Subclavian artery to pulmonary artery anastomosis for tetralogy of Fallot (Blalock-Taussig shunt, 1944) |
| Cardiac missile removal (WW II) |
| Side-to-side anastomosis of aorta to pulmonary artery for tetralogy of Fallot (Potts procedure, 1946) |
| Valvotomy for pulmonic stenosis (Brock procedure, 1947) |
| Closed mitral commissurotomy (1948) |
| Resection of infundibulum of right ventricle (1948) |
| Extracorporeal circulation (1949) |
| Atrial septostomy (Blalock-Hanlon procedure, 1949) |
| Internal mammary tunnel implant into myocardium (Vineberg, 1950) |
| Hypothermia (1950) |
| **1951–1975** |
| First prosthetic ball valve—into aorta for aortic regurgitation (1952) |
| Closure atrial septal defects (1950s) |
| Pulmonary artery banding (1953) |
| Extracorporeal circulation (1954) |
| Closure ventricular septal defect (1954) |
| Carotid endarterectomy (1954) |
| Aortic dissection repair (1955) |
| Potassium cardioplegia (1955) |
| Aortic valvotomy (1956, 1958) |
| Tetralogy of Fallot repair (1957) |
| Transection of ventricular septum for idiopathic hypertrophic subaortic stenosis (IHSS) (1957) |
| Ventricular aneurysectomy (1958) |
| Superior cava to pulmonary artery shunt (Glenn procedure, 1959) |
| Transposition of great vessels repair (Senning procedure, 1960) |
| Mitral ball and cage valve replacement (1960) |
| Excision of ventricular aneurysm (1961) |
| Aortic ball and cage valve (1961) |
| Intraaortic balloon pump (1962) |
| Homograft valve (1962) |
| Aorto-pulmonary window (Waterston procedure, 1963) |
| Left ventricular assist (1963) |
| Cardioplegia (1964) |
| Double outlet right ventricle repair (1964) |
| Internal mammary to coronary graft (1964) |
| Transposition of aorta intra-atrial baffle (Mustard procedure, 1965) |
| Cardiac transplantation (1966) |
| Coronary artery saphenous bypass (1964, 1967) |
| Pulmonary autograft for aortic valve disease (Ross procedure, 1966) |
| Wolff-Parkinson-White surgery (1967) |
| Truncus arteriosus repair (1968) |
| Extracardiac conduit (Rastelli procedure, 1969) |
| Tilting disc valve (1969) |
| Heart and lung transplant (1969) |
| Connection of right atrial appendage to pulmonary artery for tricuspid atresia (Fontan procedure, 1970) |
| Bioprosthetic valve (1970) |
| Annuloplasty ring (1971) |
| Bovine pericardial valve (1971) |
| Porcine valve (1975) |
| **1976–Present** |
| Arterial switch procedure for transposition of great vessels (1976) |
| Mitral valve repair (1977) |
| Tilting disc valve (1977) |
| Bi-leaflet hinged valve (1977) |
| Pericardial valve (1980) |
| Artificial heart (1982) |
| Cardiomyoplasty (1985) |
| Heart transplants in infants with hypoplastic left heart (1986) |
| Minimally invasive bypass surgery (1997) |
| Robotic surgery (2000) |

pressure recording (see Chap. 12). This eventually ensured its widespread adoption and successful use by the 1920s. In 1939, blood pressure recordings were first standardized by committees of the American Heart Association and the Cardiac Society of Great Britain and Ireland. Since then, blood pressure measurements have changed little except for the adoption of aneroid manometers and the recent hospital practice of automated blood pressure recordings, a backward step in the accuracy of the measurement.

Richard Bright was the first to associate kidney disease with hypertrophy of the heart, dropsy, and hardening of the arteries (1827).[39] In the 1870s, the studies of Frederick Mahomed in London established that elevated blood pressure could occur in the absence of nephritis and produce secondary kidney and arteriolar disease.[40] Secondary causes of hypertension became known, including pheochromocytoma (1922), Cushing's disease (1932), renal artery stenosis (1934), coarctation of the aorta (1938), and primary aldosteronism (1955). Although Robert Tigerstedt in Stockholm discovered a pressor substance in the renal cortex, which he named renin (1898), Goldblatt's experiments showing that renal artery stenosis caused hypertension (1934) eventually led to our understanding of renin, angiotensin, and aldosterone by Pickering, Page, Braun-Menendez, Laragh, and others.[41] In the mid- and late nineteenth century and early twentieth century, vasomotor, neurohormonal, and baroreceptor reflexes as well as genetic determinants of blood pressure became known. Whether or not there was a dividing line between normal and abnormal blood pressure was debated between Pickering and Platt in the late 1950s. In 1972, Pickering stated: "There is no dividing line. The relationship between arterial pressure and mortality is quantitative: the higher the pressure, the worse the prognosis."[33] Subsequent studies have supported this and lowered the level where treatment should begin, especially in diabetics and patients with known vascular disease.

Studies on hypertensive heart disease, defined initially as a systolic blood pressure greater than 160, date to 1913, when Janeway showed that patients with symptoms lived an average of 4 to 5 years. The asymptomatic state of most patients with hypertension (leading to its label as "the silent killer" in the 1970s), the lack of effective treatment, and a prevalent view that lowering the blood pressure would be deleterious to the kidney lulled most physicians into accepting the condition as not serious or just due to aging. In the 1970s, the Framingham studies showed hypertension to be a major contributing cause to stroke, heart attack, heart failure, and kidney failure. Other studies followed, indicating that treatment of severe, moderate, and even mild hypertension could reduce stroke and heart failure, though not heart attacks. Educational programs started by the National High Blood Pressure Education Program in 1972 urged physicians to treat blood pressure elevation, and outposts to measure blood pressure, utilizing grocery stores and fire stations, became common. The initial emphasis was on the treatment of diastolic hypertension; systolic hypertension was commonly attributed to aging and thought to be unimportant. More recently systolic hypertension and wide pulse pressure have been found to be more serious and to warrant treatment.

### Treatment of Hypertension

President Franklin Roosevelt's death in 1945 from severe hypertension and stroke called international attention to the consequences of hypertension and its inadequate treatment—he had been managed with diet, digitalis, and phenobarbital. Effective oral treatment became possible in 1949, first with reserpine then hydrochlorothiazide.[42] Lumbar sympathectomy (1925), the last resort for severe cases, was abandoned. Subsequently, beta-adrenergic blockers and calcium channel blockers as well as angiotensin converting enzyme (ACE) inhibitors and angiotensin blocking agents have brought antihypertensive relief to many, though controversy was sparked over the risk posed by short-acting calcium channel blockers (Table 1-2). Severe salt restriction, as practiced earlier with the Kempner rice diet, has taken a lesser role, while diet, exercise, and alcohol restriction are still considered important. Since 1973, recommendations published by the Joint National Committee on Detection, Evaluation, and Treatment of High Blood Pressure (JNC) have been very helpful; however, the majority of patients remain imperfectly controlled and many are not yet detected.

## HEART FAILURE

Medieval physicians commented upon suffocative catarrh, dyspnea, asthma, orthopnea, and dropsy, though failing to recognize a possible connection with the heart.[43] This was primarily due to the entrenched teaching of Galen that the purpose of the heart was to generate heat and distribute vital spirit, a view that persisted for 1500 years into the seventeenth century. Marcello Malpighi believed that dyspnea was caused by retarded circulation in the pulmonary vessels (1660s). Vieussens (1706) and Lancisi (1707) were the first to fault the heart as the direct cause of failure, a concept more fully elaborated by Albertini (1726).[43]

Initially, clinical observation was based on case reports describing signs and symptoms. In this setting, clinicians understood that valve obstruction, the most common cardiac problem at that time, caused dyspnea and fluid accumulation. Correlating the clinical with the autopsy findings of hypertrophy and dilatation of the heart was a particular puzzle for eighteenth-century physicians. Jean-Baptiste de Senac commented: "The volume of the heart can be contracted or it can dilate; this diminution and expansion present two illnesses that are not equally felt, but can be equally fearsome" (1749). Giovanni Morgagni was the first to understand that overload from valvular disease could elicit a compensatory hypertrophic response and dilatation, leading to failure (1761). At the beginning of the nineteenth century, Corvisart's distinction between the causes of hypertrophy and dilatation led to an appreciation of the beneficial effects of hypertrophy and the harmful effects of dilatation. The primary role of the myocardium versus valvular disease in the production of symptoms and a basis for prognosis followed, was lost, and was then rediscovered. Richard Bright's 1836 discovery of the relationship of cardiac hypertrophy and dropsy to shrunken kidneys introduced the kidneys as a cause of heart failure long before hypertension was known.[37] Toward the end of the nineteenth century, the beneficial role of hypertrophy was questioned by Schroetter (1876), Osler (1892), and others, who saw that it was harmful in its later stages. James Mackenzie, in his influential 1908 textbook *Diseases of the Heart,* stressed the functional role of the heart muscle and its reserve force, downplaying valvular disease as "an embarrassment to the heart muscle." He felt that it was exhaustion of the heart muscle that led to symptoms and signs of heart failure.[9] His insistence that "A heart is what a heart can do" was the beginning of a functional classification that redirected thinking toward physiology and away from just the presence of murmurs and arrhythmias. The definition of normal circulatory physiology was the precursor for an understanding of abnormal circulatory phenomena. In the late nineteenth and early twentieth centuries, the hemodynamic physiologists Otto Frank, Ernest Starling, and Carl Wiggers established the basic principles of cardiac function, pressure, and flow abnormalities in the failing heart. In the mid-twentieth century, studies by Sarnoff and others heightened our understanding of the performance of normal and abnormal heart muscle. The widespread application of cardiac catheterization, selective angiography, and imaging studies has resulted in more precise diagnostic criteria and hemodynamic information for differentiating ischemic heart disease, hypertensive heart disease, and dilated and hypertrophic forms of cardiomyopathies. *Congestive heart failure* was a term first used in the 1920s; however, a definition for heart failure based on its pathogenesis has been controversial. The primary debate initially centered over whether the elevated venous pressure was a primary or secondary event. Two opposing camps evolved: the first holding that "backward failure," or an upstream obstruction (aortic stenosis, for example) was the central factor, and the second championing "forward failure," in which myocardial dysfunction with low cardiac output was the problem. Over time, the rigid concepts embodied in "backward" and "forward failure," "right-sided" and "left-sided failure," have given way to definitions based on the cardiac output as the discriminator: "low-output" and "high-output failure." More recently "systolic heart failure" and "diastolic heart failure" have climbed to the top of the clinical lexicon. Cell biochemistry and biophysics have contributed to our understanding of the abnormalities in cardiac contraction, relaxation, and energetics, while molecular biology has helped to define the pathways responsible for alterations in growth.

### Treatment of Heart Failure

Clarification of the etiologic and contributing factors in heart failure has provided insights into a more directed rationale of treatment. In the late nineteenth and early twentieth centuries, heart failure was treated with venesection, digitalis, saline purges, a low-salt diet, mercurial cathartics, incision and drainage of edema (Southey tubes) or ascites, bromides, theophylline or urea for diuresis, and carbonic acid baths at a spa. By the 1930s, cathartics had been replaced by intramuscular mercurial injections to remove fluid. Thyroidectomy was advised in advanced cases. The introduction of potent oral diuretics, beginning with chlorothiazide (1957) and then furosemide (1964), brought miraculous relief to volume-overloaded cardiac patients, ending the common practice of twice-weekly "merc shots." The concept of afterload reduction with vasodilators by Cohn (1971) soon led to the use of nitroprusside (1974), ACE inhibitors (1981), and angiotensin receptor blockers (1992), which have greatly improved the quality of life and prognosis for patients with heart failure (Table-1-2). Beta-adrenergic blockers, initially thought to be absolutely contraindicated for heart failure, were shown to be otherwise in 1975 by Wagstein and are now a first-rank drug, along with carvedilol (1995). While digitalis is still used, its effect on mortality has been questioned; newer oral inotropic agents have consistently been found to worsen the prognosis. Biventricular pacing to resynchronize the ventricles, introduced in 2000, has shown early promise in selected patients. Cardiac transplantation has been a last resort for selected patients since the late 1960s. Cell therapy for cardiac repair, using transplanted skeletal myoblasts and bone marrow stem cells, is an exciting new approach (2002).

## CARDIAC SURGERY

The Nobel Prize in Physiology or Medicine in 1912 was given to Alexis Carrel, a French experimental surgeon working at the Rockefeller Institute, "in recognition of his work on vascular suture and the transplantation of blood vessels and organs." In addition to pioneering the anastomosis of vessels, Carrel also invented methods of preserving and transplanting vessels, organs, and limbs. His many contributions to the basic science of surgery provided the essential foundation and encouragement for the clinical surgeons who would eventually follow his bold path[5] (Table 1-3). A few attempts were made to repair cardiac wounds in the late nineteenth century and to remove pericardial adhesions or correct valvular disease in the first quarter of the twentieth century; however, the surgeon was constantly thwarted by the problems of correct diagnosis, cerebral oxygenation, pneumothorax, anesthesia, bleeding, clotting, infection, arrhythmias, blood pressure control, fluid, acid-base and electrolyte management, and so on.[44] Surgery was a "get in, get out, and pray for the best" proposition. As Comroe pointed out, 25 separate bodies of knowledge had to evolve to permit successful open-heart surgery.[45] Extracardiac surgery—ligation of a patent ductus by Gross (1938), repair of coarctation of the aorta by Craaford (1944), the Blalock-Taussig shunt (1944), and removal of intracardiac missile fragments by Harken during World War II—led the way.[44] Simple and quick intracardiac surgery, such as repair of an atrial septal defect, was successfully accomplished by Swan, Holmes-Sellars, and others using hypothermia in the 1950s, though the risk of ventricular fibrillation and air embolism presented a hazard. John Gibbons's development of extracorporeal circulation, work he and his wife initiated in the early 1930s, became the essential solution that would propel intracardiac surgery forward. In 1953, his pump-oxygenator was finally able to provide 45 min to repair an atrial septal defect.[47] With the relative leisure of cardiopulmonary bypass, the surgeon had time to operate more safely and explore new horizons. In the 1950s, mitral stenosis was the major hurdle, and mitral valvotomy was performed by Bailey, Harken, Brock, and others with increasing success.[33] Surgery for congenital defects was next. More complicated surgery, including aortic dissection repair (DeBakey, 1955), mechanical prosthetic valve replacement (Starr, 1960), cardiac transplantation (Barnard and Shumway, 1966), bioprosthetic valve replacement (1970), mitral valve repair (Carpentier, 1971), and repair of complex congenital heart disease followed as diagnostic and surgical techniques, artificial valves, and intensive postoperative care improved.[44,46] In 1910, the ingenious Alexis Carrel attempted the first experimental coronary bypass, fashioning an anastomosis between the descending aorta and the left coronary artery. Efforts to improve the coronary circulation using pericardial irritants (Beck, 1934), omental or pectoral grafts (O'Shaunessy, Beck, 1930s), internal mammary implants tunneled directly into the heart muscle (Vineberg, 1950), and coronary endarterectomy (Bailey, Longmire, 1956) were touted but provided inconsistent benefit. Garrett was the first to use an aortocoronary saphenous vein graft (1964); however, René Favoloro, working with Mason Sones at the Cleveland Clinic, deserves the credit for ushering in the era of coronary bypass surgery (1967).[48,49] Mortality rates from all cardiac surgery have progressively fallen to low levels, and the surgical benefit has been extended to sicker and older people. Cardiac transplantation has become almost routine, but attempts to manufacture an artificial heart have been disappointing. Minimally invasive cardiac surgery, avoiding cardiopulmonary bypass, has become feasible though not yet proven. Heart surgery has truly been one of the great success stories of the twentieth century.

## FINAL COMMENT

In the 1970 (second) edition of *The Heart,* Paul Dudley White (Fig. 1-2) wrote a chapter entitled "The Evolution of Our Knowledge of the Heart and Its Diseases," in which he concluded: "But the most important advance of all ... is emphasis on the prevention of the very diseases which we have prided ourselves on being so clever to diagnose and to treat, both medically and surgically. Heart disease before 80 is our fault, not God's or nature's will." Studies since then have shown a dramatic and continuing decline in the mortality from heart disease, and many people are living longer productive lives. This 11th edition of *The Heart*, 34 years later, documents many more advances in cardiology, including an emphasis on the prevention of heart disease. No doubt Dr. White would be pleased, but he would also point out that with all our knowledge and all our technology, we are not quite there yet.

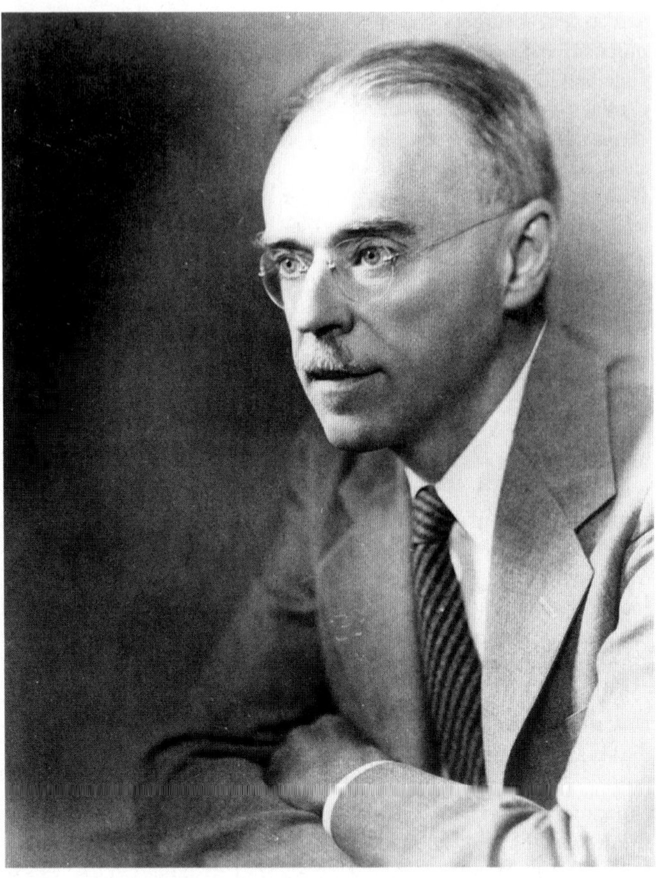

FIGURE 1-2 Paul Dudley White. (Courtesy of the National Library of Medicine.)

## References


1. Harvey W. *Anatomical Studies on the Motion of the Heart and Blood.* Leake CD, transl. Springfield, IL: Charles C Thomas; 1970.
2. Acierno LJ. *The History of Cardiology*. London: Parthenon; 1994.
3. Willius FA, Dry TJ. *A History of the Heart and the Circulation.* Philadelphia: Saunders; 1948.
4. Rolleston HD. *Cardiovascular Diseases since Harvey's Discovery: The Harveian Oration of 1928.* London: Cambridge University Press; 1928.
5. Bing RJ. *Cardiology: The Evolution of the Science and the Art.* Basel: Harwood; 1992.
6. Herrick JB. *A Short History of Cardiology*. Springfield, IL: Charles C Thomas; 1942.
7. Lee HSJ. *Dates in Cardiology*. New York: Parthenon; 2000.
8. Fishman AP, Dickinson WR. *Circulation of the Blood: Men and Ideas*. Bethesda, MD: American Physiological Society; 1982.
9. Fleming P. *A Short History of Cardiology*. Amsterdam: Rodopi; 1997.
10. Fye B. *American Cardiology: The History of a Specialty and Its College*. Baltimore: The Johns Hopkins University Press; 1996.
11. Mackenzie J. *The Study of the Pulse*. Edinburgh: Pentland; 1902.
12. Mackenzie J. The venous and liver pulses, and the arrhythmic contraction of the cardiac cavities. *J Pathol Bacteriol* 1894; 2:84–154.
13. Duffin JM. The cardiology of RTH Laënnec. *Med Hist* 1989; 33:42–71.
14. Hanna IR, Silverman ME. A history of cardiac auscultation and some of its contributors. *Am J Cardiol* 2002; 90:259–267.
15. McKusick VA. *Cardiovascular Sound in Health and Disease*. Baltimore: Williams & Wilkins; 1958.
16. Burch GE, DePasquale NP. *A History of Electrocardiography.* Chicago: Year Book; 1964.
17. Forssmann-Falck R. Werner Forssmann: A Pioneer of Cardiology. *Am J Cardiol* 1997; 79:651–660.
18. Mueller RL, Sanborn TA. The history of interventional cardiology: Cardiac catheterization, angioplasty, and related interventions. *Am Heart J* 1995; 129:146–172.
19. King SB. The development of interventional cardiology. *J Am Coll Cardiol* 1998; 31(suppl B):64B–88B.
20. Muir AL. Cardiac imaging 50 years on. *Br Heart J* 1987; 58:1–5.
21. Roelandt JRTC. Seeing the heart, the success story of cardiac imaging. *Eur Heart J* 2000; 21:1281–1288.
22. Zaret BL. A brief historical perspective on nuclear cardiology. In: Iskandrian AE, Verani MS, eds. *Nuclear Cardiac Imaging*. 3d ed. London: Oxford University Press; 2003:1–6.
23. Leibowitz JO. *The History of Coronary Heart Disease*. Berkeley, CA: University of California Press; 1970.
24. Rolleston H. The history of angina pectoris. *Glasgow Med J* 1937; 9:205–225.
25. Fye B. The delayed diagnosis of myocardial infarction: It took half a century! *Circulation* 1985; 72:262–271.
26. Herrick JB. Clinical features of sudden obstruction of the coronary arteries. *JAMA* 1912; 59:2015–2020.
27. Sherry S. The origin of thrombolytic therapy. *J Am Coll Cardiol* 1989; 14:1085–1092.
28. Flaxman N. The hope of cardiology: James Hope (1801–1841). *Bull Hist Med* 1938; 6:1–21.
29. VanderVeer JB. Mitral insufficiency: Historical and clinical aspects. *Am J Cardiol* 1958; 2:5–10.
30. Rolleston H. The history of mitral stenosis. *Br Heart J* 1941; 3:1–12.
31. Vaslef SN, Roberts WC. Early descriptions of aortic valve stenosis. *Am Heart J* 1993; 125:1465–1474.
32. Vaslef SN, Roberts WC. Early descriptions of aortic regurgitation. *Am Heart J* 1993; 125:1475–1483.
33. Silverman ME, Fleming PR, Hollman A, et al. *British Cardiology in the 20th Century*. London: Springer; 2000.
34. Boudoulas H, Vavuranakis M, Wooley CF. Valvular heart disease: The influence of changing etiology on nosology. *J Heart Valve Dis* 1994; 3:516–526.
35. Abbott ME. *Atlas of Congenital Heart Disease*. New York: American Heart Association; 1936.
36. Engle MA. Growth and development of state of the art care for people with congenital heart disease. *J Am Coll Cardiol* 1989; 13:1453–1457.
37. Naqvi NH, Blaufox MD. *Blood Pressure Measurement: An Illustrated History*. New York: Parthenon; 1998.
38. Dustan HP. History of clinical hypertension: From 1827 to 1970. In: Oparil S, Weber MA, eds. *Hypertension: A Companion to Brenner and Rector's The Kidney*. Philadelphia: Saunders; 2000: 1–4.
39. Ruskin A. *Classics in Arterial Hypertension*. Springfield, IL: Charles C Thomas; 1956.
40. Posten-Vinay N. *A Century of Arterial Hypertension: 1896–1996*. Chichester: Wiley; 1996.
41. Pickering G. Systemic arterial hypertension. In: Fishman AP, Richards DW, eds. *Circulation of the Blood: Men and Ideas*. Bethesda, MD: American Physiological Society; 1982: 487–541.
42. Piepho RW, Beal J. An overview of antihypertensive therapy in the 20th century. *J Clin Pharmacol* 2000; 40:967–977.
43. Jarcho S. *The Concept of Heart Failure from Avicenna to Albertini*. Cambridge, MA: Harvard University Press; 1980.
44. Shumacker HB Jr. *The Evolution of Cardiac Surgery*. Bloomington, IN: Indiana University Press; 1992.
45. Comroe JH. The heart and lungs. In: Comroe JH, ed. *Advances in American Medicine*. New York: Josiah Macey; 1976.
46. Johnson SL. *The History of Cardiac Surgery: 1896–1955*. Baltimore: Johns Hopkins Press; 1970.
47. Gibbon JH Jr. The development of the heart-lung apparatus. *Am J Surg* 1978; 135:608–619.
48. Brewer LA. Open heart surgery and myocardial revascularization. *Am J Surg* 1981; 141:618–631.
49. Favaloro RG. Landmarks in the development of coronary artery bypass surgery. *Circulation* 1998; 98:466–478.

C H A P T E R 2

# THE BURDEN OF INCREASING WORLDWIDE CARDIOVASCULAR DISEASE*

Ramachandran S. Vasan / Emelia J. Benjamin / Lisa M. Sullivan / Ralph B. D'Agostino



It is widely acknowledged that heart disease and stroke are the leading causes of death and disability in the United States and other developed countries.[1] What is less appreciated is that this holds true for the developing countries as well.[1,2] We are in the midst of a true global cardiovascular disease (CVD) epidemic.[3,4] CVD is responsible for about 30 percent of all deaths worldwide each year.[5] Of note, nearly 80 percent of these deaths occur in developing countries. Indeed, CVD is the leading cause of mortality in every region of the world with the sole exception of sub-Saharan Africa where infectious diseases are still the leading cause. It is anticipated that even in sub-Saharan Africa, CVD will be the leading cause of mortality within the next few years.

This chapter describes the current global burden of CVD and its risk factors, emphasizing the evolution of the CVD epidemic in developing countries and its contributory factors. Furthermore, the projected trends in the global burden of CVD over the next 2 decades is elucidated, and ongoing efforts by the world community [including the World Health Organization (WHO)] to combat and contain the current epidemic are outlined. The broad term *CVD* includes coronary heart disease [CHD, includes myocardial infarction (MI), angina, coronary insufficiency, and coronary death], cerebrovascular disease (includes stroke and transient ischemic attacks), peripheral vascular disease, congestive heart failure (CHF), hypertension, and valvular and congenital heart disease.

*This work was supported in part through NHLBI Contract NO1-HC-25195, NHLBI grant 1K24HL04334 (RS Vasan).

## THE WORLD IN TRANSITION: IMPLICATIONS FOR CARDIOVASCULAR DISEASE

### Demographic Transition

The last two centuries have witnessed major changes in the demographic characteristics of the human population.[6] This transformation (termed *demographic transition*) involved a progressive change from very high birth and infant mortality rates to low ones. This change was accompanied by a shift from low population growth rates through an intermediate phase of high growth rates, with a consequent major increase in total population. This then was followed by a reversal to low or zero growth rates. The demographic transition results in a conversion of the age distribution of the population from one with a preponderance of young to one with nearly equal representation of all age groups.

The demographic transition has been driven by the most dramatic improvements ever in the history of human health. Improvements in sanitation, nutrition, and infectious disease control and advances in perinatal care have resulted in lower infant and child mortality rates and an enhancement of overall life expectancy. The improvement in life expectancy began in Europe in the late nineteenth century and by the second half of the twentieth century had spread to the rest of the world. Life expectancy at birth has increased from a global average of 46 years in 1950 to 66 years in 1998.[7]

### Economic, Social, and Nutritional Transition

The developing countries have been undergoing rapid industrialization, urbanization, economic development, and market globalization over the last four decades.[2,8] As a consequence, standards of living have improved but with a detrimental shift toward inappropriate dietary patterns and a reduction in physical activities. The nutritional status of populations has been adversely influenced by the aforementioned changes, a phenomenon referred to as *nutritional transition*.[9,10]

Globalization has resulted in the expansion of the food economies from local to broad-based ones in which there is easy access to large amounts of unhealthy food products.[11] The shift in dietary patterns comprises a change in all three major food constituents (namely, fats, proteins, and carbohydrates).[12] Local diets that are traditionally rich in fiber and have a low fat content are being replaced by cheap energy-dense micronutrient-poor foods with a high content of saturated fats.[13] Vegetarian diets characterized by high intake of plant proteins have been substituted with nonvegetarian diets rich in animal proteins. Complex carbohydrates in diets have been supplanted by refined carbohydrates and sugars that have a high glycemic index.[12] The overall increased caloric consumption occurs in a milieu of reduced energy expenditure due to sedentary lifestyles, with the advent of motorized transport, and increased use of labor-saving home and office appliances. Additionally, leisure time physical activities have given way to physically undemanding pastimes including watching television.

These changes in dietary and lifestyle patterns foreshadow in both developing and newly developed countries an increasing burden of diet-related diseases—including obesity, dyslipidemia, diabetes mellitus, hypertension, and eventually CVD—and various forms of cancer. In essence, although referred to under the umbrella of noncommunicable disease, CVD is to some extent a *communicated* disease, spread by the forces of globalization.

### Epidemiologic Transition

The previously mentioned demographic, economic, and nutritional changes lead inexorably to major changes in the patterns of human diseases, a phenomenon referred to as *epidemiologic transition*.[6] Epidemiologic transition is characterized by a progressive shift from a predominance of nutritional deficiencies and infectious diseases to those categorized as degenerative (i.e., chronic diseases such as CVD, cancer, and diabetes).[6]

## CHALLENGES OF THE CARDIOVASCULAR DISEASE EPIDEMIC IN DEVELOPING COUNTRIES: DIFFERENCES FROM DEVELOPED COUNTRIES

While the determinants of the health transition in developing countries are similar to those in the developed countries, it is important to emphasize that the dynamics of health transition are different in the former.[2,14–16]

1. In developing countries the epidemic of CVD is occurring over a compressed time frame (in part related to the rapidity of globalization), whereas in developed countries it took decades for the CVD epidemic to establish itself. Such a compression of the time course of the epidemic requires a greater intensity of public health response.
2. Unfortunately, the transition that is fueling the CVD epidemic in developing countries occurs in settings of poverty and international debt: factors that restrict resources available for public health action. An accentuating factor is the easy access to low-cost cigarettes in developing countries early in the transition phase. Tobacco is a cash crop and the tobacco industry is a potential employer: factors that pose a major challenge to the governmental implementation of tobacco control.
3. Individual responses to the CVD epidemic in developing countries are restricted by low levels of education and limited personal resources to purchase drugs required for lowering elevated levels of CVD risk factors. An additional aggravating factor is that CVD afflicts individuals at an earlier age in developing countries, resulting in loss of economic productivity, often of the sole wage-earning member of the family.
4. Very often these countries face a dual burden of communicable and noncommunicable diseases, resulting in a competition for limited public health resources.
5. The global response to the ongoing epidemic is challenged by a paucity of epidemiologic data and the necessary infrastructure to define, characterize, and track the CVD epidemic in most developing countries.
6. The societal response to the CVD epidemic lags behind because of a lack of awareness and the popular belief that CVD is largely a disease of developed countries.
7. It is important to note that for several countries in Asia and Africa, increases in blood pressure and tobacco use preceded the impact of nutrition transition by decades. This has resulted in a differing CVD profile with higher levels of stroke but relatively low levels of CHD. These differing CVD patterns underscore an opportunity to implement strong CHD preventive programs focusing on nutrition and physical activity and aggressive control of blood pressure and tobacco use.

## MEASURING BURDEN OF DISEASE: GLOBAL BURDEN OF DISEASE PROJECT AND CONCEPT OF DISABILITY-ADJUSTED LIFE-YEAR

In 1993, the Harvard School of Public Health in collaboration with the World Bank and WHO commenced the Global Burden of Disease (GBD) Project.[17] The GBD project has generated the most comprehensive set of estimates of morbidity and mortality due to various disease conditions according to age, sex, and region. The investigators subdivided the world into 14 regions based on levels of child (<5 years) and adult (15 to 59 years) mortality for WHO member states (Fig. 2-1, Plate 1).[18]

The GBD project also introduced a new metric, disability-adjusted life-year (DALY), to quantify the burden of disease.[19] The DALY is a health gap measure that summates the potential years of life lost due to premature death and the years of "healthy" life lost in states of less than full health, broadly termed *disability*. A "premature" death is defined as a death that occurs before the age to which the person could have expected to survive if he or she was a member of a standardized model population with a life expectancy at birth equal to that of the world's longest-surviving population, Japan. Thus, one DALY can be thought of as 1 lost year of healthy life. The burden of disease is the gap between current health status of a population and an ideal situation where everyone lives into old age free of disease and disability.

WHO has undertaken an assessment of the GBD for the year 2000 (GBD 2000) with the specific objectives to quantify the burden of premature mortality and disability by age, sex, and WHO subregion for 135 major causes or groups of causes, to analyze the contribution of selected risk factors to this burden, and to develop various projection scenarios of the burden of disease over the next 30

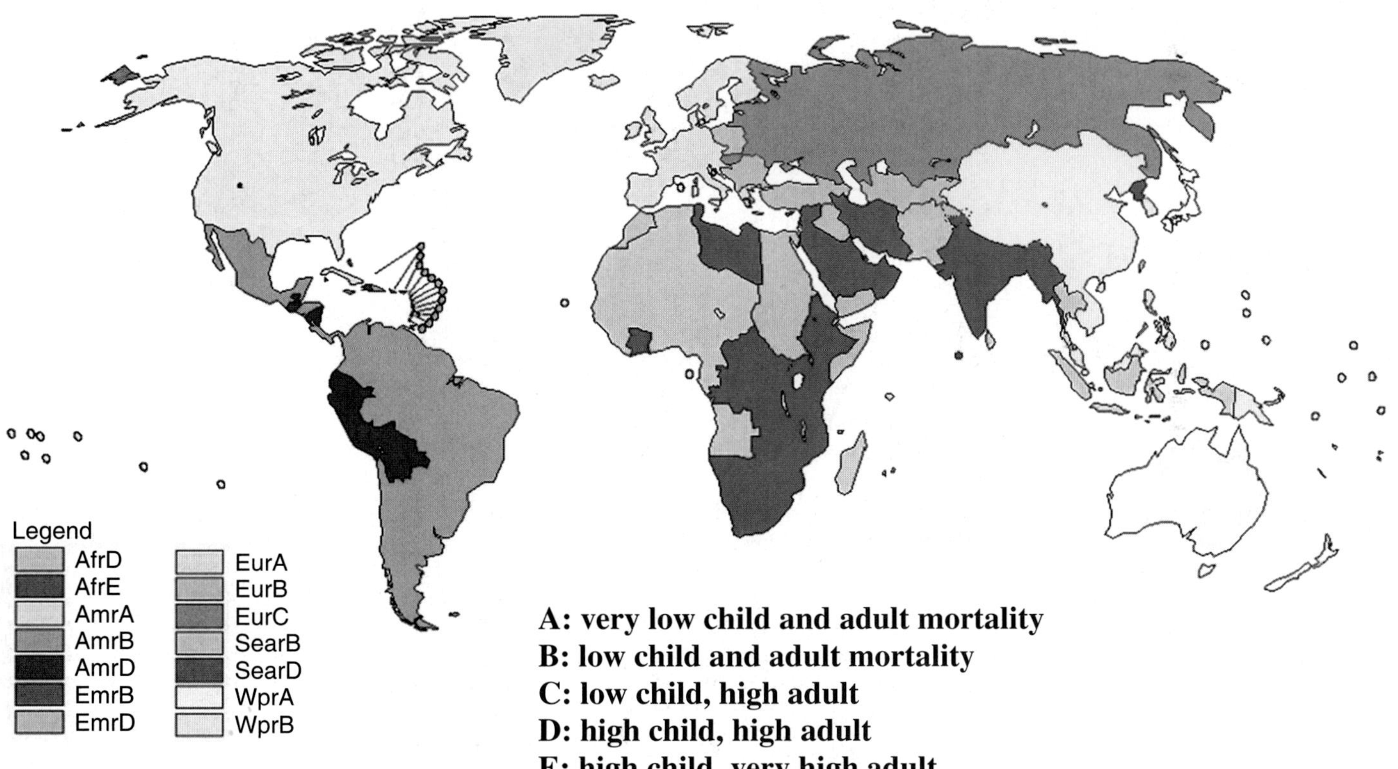


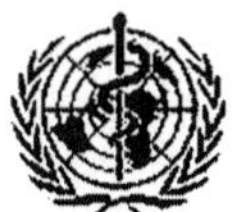

FIGURE 2-1 (Plate 1) World Health Organization (WHO) subregions for global burden of disease. For geographic disaggregation of the global burden of disease, the six WHO regions of the world have been further divided into 14 subregions, based on levels of child (under 5 years) and adult (15 to 59 years) mortality for WHO member states. The classification of WHO member states into the mortality strata were carried out using population estimates for 1999 (United Nations population division, 1998) and estimates of 5q0 and 45q15 based on WHO analyses of mortality rates for 1999. Five mortality strata were defined in terms of quintiles of the distribution of 5q0 and 45q15 (both sexes combined). Adult mortality 45q15 was regressed on 5q0 and the regression line used to divide countries with high child mortality into high adult mortality (stratum D) and very high adult mortality (stratum E). Stratum E includes the countries in Sub-Saharan Africa where HIV/AIDS has had a very substantial impact. (Adapted from Mathers CD, Stein C, Fat DM, et al. Global burden of disease 2000: Version 2 methods and results. Global program on evidence for health policy discussion Paper No. 50. World Health Organization, October 2002 From http://www.hoffmanpr.com/Press_Releases/Archived_Press_Releases/WHO/Cardio2002/CardioGraphs.ppt, used with permission.)

years.[20] Detailed tables for DALYs by subregion, cause, sex, and age group are available at the WHO website at http://www.who.int/evidence/bod.

## CARDIOVASCULAR DISEASES

### Global Burden

CVD is the leading cause of mortality worldwide; responsible for one-third of all deaths.[5] According to WHO estimates, 16.6 million people died of CVD in 2001 (Table 2-1). Developing countries contributed to 78 percent of CVD deaths. There is considerable variation in CVD mortality rates across countries (Fig. 2-2).[21] Potential reasons for such variation include differing stages of epidemiologic transition in various countries, varying environmental effects due to dissimilar burden of CVD risk factors, inherent genetic differences, and distinct early childhood programming influences.[14,22]

In terms of combined morbidity and mortality, CVD accounted for 145 million DALYs lost worldwide in 2001. Eighty-six percent of the DALYs lost due to CVD were in the developing world. Conversely, of total DALYs lost in developing countries, about 10 percent were due to CVD (Fig. 2-3).

### Global Trends in Mortality

The WHO projections indicate that a pattern of premature CVD mortality is likely to persist and may accentuate further in developing countries.[23] By 2010, CVD is projected to be the leading cause of death in developing countries. By 2020, WHO estimates there will be nearly 25 million CVD deaths worldwide.[17]

### Burden in the United States

Since 1900, CVD has been the leading cause of death in the United States every year (except for 1918).[24] In 2000, CVD accounted for 39 percent of all deaths. In fact, CVD claims more lives each year than

TABLE 2-1 Global Burden of CVD

| CVD | AFR | AMR | EUR | SEAR | WPR | EMR | World |
|---|---|---|---|---|---|---|---|
| | | | MORTALITY, THOUSANDS | | | | |
| CHD | 333 | 967 | 2423 | 1972 | 963 | 523 | 7181 |
| Cerebrovascular | 307 | 454 | 1479 | 1071 | 1926 | 218 | 5454 |
| HTN heart disease | 54 | 130 | 174 | 138 | 285 | 92 | 874 |
| Rheumatic | 29 | 111 | 34 | 132 | 108 | 24 | 338 |
| Inflammatory | 34 | 66 | 87 | 78 | 81 | 29 | 375 |
| Other CVD | 227 | 352 | 845 | 407 | 380 | 152 | 2363 |
| All CVDs | 985 | 1980 | 5042 | 3797 | 3745 | 1037 | 16585 |
| | | | TOTAL BURDEN, DALYS MILLIONS | | | | |
| CHD | 3.26 | 6.51 | 16.00 | 20.24 | 7.37 | 5.35 | 58.72 |
| Cerebrovascular | 3.32 | 4.06 | 10.44 | 9.95 | 15.74 | 2.36 | 45.87 |
| HTN heart disease | 0.56 | 1.01 | 1.18 | 1.46 | 2.27 | 0.83 | 7.31 |
| Rheumatic | 0.76 | 0.16 | 0.43 | 2.56 | 1.61 | 0.58 | 6.11 |
| Inflammatory | 0.77 | 0.84 | 1.20 | 1.57 | 0.82 | 0.46 | 5.67 |
| Other CVD | 2.69 | 2.57 | 4.88 | 5.75 | 2.70 | 2.20 | 20.79 |
| All CVDs | 11.36 | 15.14 | 34.14 | 41.53 | 30.51 | 11.79 | 144.47 |

Rheumatic heart disease includes symptomatic cases of congestive heart failure due to rheumatic heart disease. Hypertensive (HTN) heart disease includes symptomatic cases of congestive heart failure due to hypertensive heart disease. Ischemic heart disease includes acute myocardial infarction; definite and possible episodes of acute myocardial infarction according to MONICA study criteria; angina pectoris, cases of clinically diagnosed angina pectoris or definite angina pectoris according to Rose questionnaire. Congestive heart failure includes mild and greater (Killip scale k2–k4). Cerebrovascular disease includes first-ever stroke cases, first-ever stroke according to World Health Organization definition (includes subarachnoid hemorrhage but excludes transient ischemic attacks, subdural hematoma, and hemorrhage or infarction due to infection or tumor); long-term stroke survivors: persons who survive more than 28 days after first-ever stroke. Inflammatory heart diseases include myocarditis, symptomatic cases of congestive heart failure due to myocarditis; pericarditis, symptomatic cases of congestive heart failure due to pericarditis; endocarditis, symptomatic cases of congestive heart failure due to endocarditis. For detailed definition refer to: Mathers CD, Stein C, Fat DM, et al. *Global Burden of Disease 2000: Version 2 methods and results. Global Programme on Evidence for Health Policy Discussion Paper No. 50.* World Health Organization, October 2002.

ABBREVIATIONS: CVD = cardiovascular disease; CHD = coronary heart disease; AFR = Africa; AMR = America; EUR = Europe; SEAR = South East Asia Region; WPR = Western Pacific Region; EMR = Eastern Mediterranean Region; DALYs = disability-adjusted life-years.

SOURCE: http://www3.who.int/whosis/menu.cfm?path=evidence,burden,burden_estimates, burden_estimates_2001,burden_estimates_2. Accessed on May 5, 2003.

**Death Rates for Total Cardiovascular Disease, Coronary Heart Disease, Stroke and Total Deaths in Selected Countries (most recent year available)**

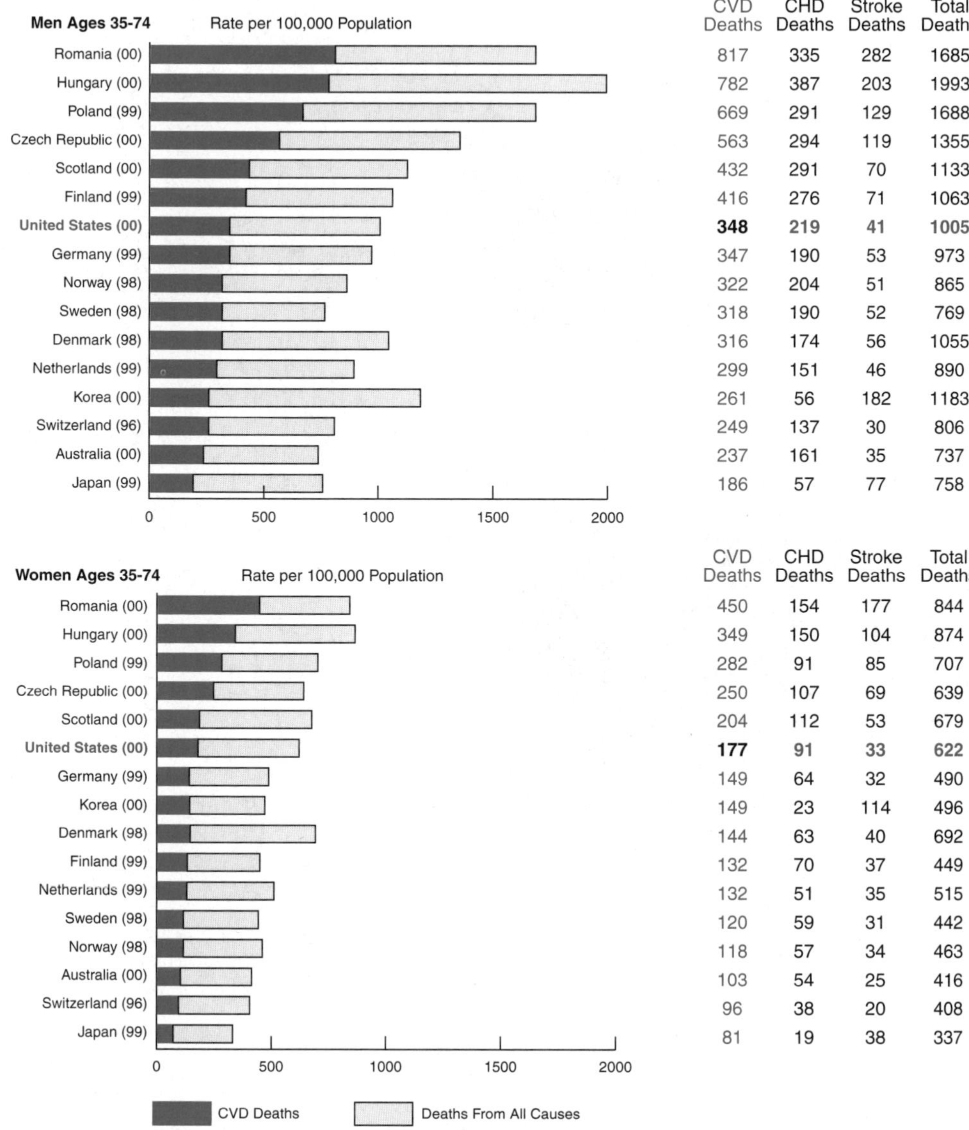


| Men Ages 35-74 | CVD Deaths | CHD Deaths | Stroke Deaths | Total Deaths |
|---|---|---|---|---|
| Romania (00) | 817 | 335 | 282 | 1685 |
| Hungary (00) | 782 | 387 | 203 | 1993 |
| Poland (99) | 669 | 291 | 129 | 1688 |
| Czech Republic (00) | 563 | 294 | 119 | 1355 |
| Scotland (00) | 432 | 291 | 70 | 1133 |
| Finland (99) | 416 | 276 | 71 | 1063 |
| **United States (00)** | **348** | **219** | **41** | **1005** |
| Germany (99) | 347 | 190 | 53 | 973 |
| Norway (98) | 322 | 204 | 51 | 865 |
| Sweden (98) | 318 | 190 | 52 | 769 |
| Denmark (98) | 316 | 174 | 56 | 1055 |
| Netherlands (99) | 299 | 151 | 46 | 890 |
| Korea (00) | 261 | 56 | 182 | 1183 |
| Switzerland (96) | 249 | 137 | 30 | 806 |
| Australia (00) | 237 | 161 | 35 | 737 |
| Japan (99) | 186 | 57 | 77 | 758 |

| Women Ages 35-74 | CVD Deaths | CHD Deaths | Stroke Deaths | Total Deaths |
|---|---|---|---|---|
| Romania (00) | 450 | 154 | 177 | 844 |
| Hungary (00) | 349 | 150 | 104 | 874 |
| Poland (99) | 282 | 91 | 85 | 707 |
| Czech Republic (00) | 250 | 107 | 69 | 639 |
| Scotland (00) | 204 | 112 | 53 | 679 |
| **United States (00)** | **177** | **91** | **33** | **622** |
| Germany (99) | 149 | 64 | 32 | 490 |
| Korea (00) | 149 | 23 | 114 | 496 |
| Denmark (98) | 144 | 63 | 40 | 692 |
| Finland (99) | 132 | 70 | 37 | 449 |
| Netherlands (99) | 132 | 51 | 35 | 515 |
| Sweden (98) | 120 | 59 | 31 | 442 |
| Norway (98) | 118 | 57 | 34 | 463 |
| Australia (00) | 103 | 54 | 25 | 416 |
| Switzerland (96) | 96 | 38 | 20 | 408 |
| Japan (99) | 81 | 19 | 38 | 337 |

Note: Rates adjusted to the European Standard population. ICO/10 codes are 100-199 for cardiovascular disease; 120-125 for coronary heart disease; and 160-169 for stroke. For better comparisons between countries, we have omitted not using ICD/10 mortality.

*Source: The World Health Organization Web page, www.who.int/whosis/ and NCHS.*

FIGURE 2-2 Heterogeneity in cardiovascular disease mortality rates across countries. (Reproduced with permission from American Heart Association World Wide Web Site, URL address: http://www.americanheart.org/downloadable/heart/1043250000063IntStats2003.pdf, International Cardiovascular Disease Statistics and Burden of CVD Risk Factors in the US © 2003, Copyright American Heart Association.)

the next 5 leading causes of death combined. According to the American Heart Association (AHA) estimates, approximately 2600 Americans die of CVD each day, an average of 1 death every 33 s.[24] The overall death rate per 100,000 from CVD in the United States was 343.1 in the year 2000. CVD death rates are higher for men than they are for women, and for blacks as compared to whites; in 2000, CVD death rates were 397.6 for white males versus 509.6 for black males, while among women, rates ranged from 285.8 for white females to 397.1 for black females. In the United States, there are marked regional disparities, with the southeast experiencing the highest CVD mortality rates. The pathogenesis of ethnic and regional disparities in CVD morbidity and mortality are multifactorial and will be discussed later in this chapter.

## INCIDENCE IN THE UNITED STATES

Data from the Framingham Heart Study, a predominantly Caucasian cohort followed from 1948 (original cohort) and 1971 (offspring cohort), provide estimates of CVD event rates. The average annual rates of first major CVD events increase with age, rising from 7 per 1000 men at ages 35 to 44 years to 68 per 1000 at ages 85 to 94 years (Table 2-2). For women, CVD rates comparable to men are achieved 10 years later in life, with the gender difference in rates narrowing with advancing age. CHD is the predominant cardiovascular event, comprising more than one-half of all CVD events in men and in women under age 75 (Table 2-3). The proportions of cardiovascular events due to CHD decline with age, due to the increasing proportions of stroke and CHF.

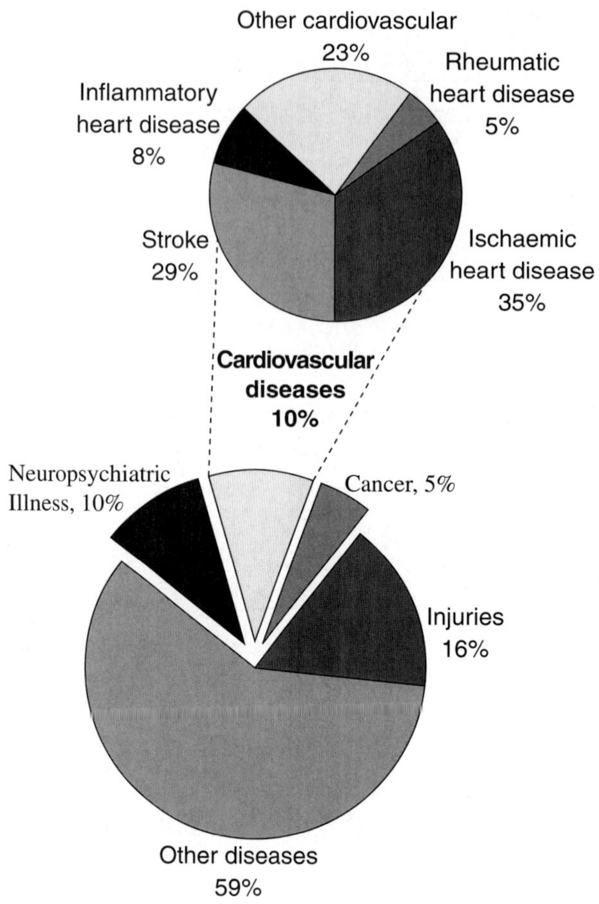


FIGURE 2-3 Disability-Adjusted Life-Years (DALYs) attributable to cardiovascular disease in developing countries. (From World Health Report 1999. Making a difference. Geneva: WHO; 1999. Available at http://www.who.int/ whr/, used with permission.)

TABLE 2-2 Incidence of Major Cardiovascular Events: Framingham Study, 44-Year Follow-Up of Cohort and 20-Year Follow-Up of Offspring Cohort*

| | Cardiovascular Disease, (All Types) | | Coronary Heart Disease | | Stroke & Transient Ischemic Attack | | Congestive Heart Failure | |
|---|---|---|---|---|---|---|---|---|
| Age, Yrs | Men | Women | Men | Women | Men | Women | Men | Women |
| 35–44 | 7 | 3 | 4 | 1 | † | † | † | † |
| 45–54 | 15 | 7 | 10 | 4 | 2 | 1 | 2 | 1 |
| 55–64 | 26 | 15 | 21 | 10 | 4 | 3 | 4 | 2 |
| 65–74 | 39 | 24 | 24 | 14 | 11 | 8 | 9 | 6 |
| 75–84 | 59 | 40 | 33 | 18 | 20 | 15 | 18 | 12 |
| 85–94 | 68 | 63 | 35 | 28 | 12 | 25 | 39 | 31 |
| 35–64‡ | 17 | 9 | 12 | 5 | 2 | 2 | 2 | 1 |
| 65–94‡ | 44 | 30 | 27 | 16 | 13 | 11 | 12 | 9 |

*Average annual incidence per 100 persons free of specified disease.
†Results are omitted when fewer than 5 individuals experience an event.
‡Age-adjusted rates.
Source: The Framingham Study.

TABLE 2-3 Percentage of First Cardiovascular Event by Type of Event: Framingham Study, 44-Year Follow-Up of Cohort and 20-Year Follow-Up of Offspring Cohort

| | Cardiovascular Disease (N) | | Coronary Heart Disease (%) | | Stroke & Transient Ischemic Attack (%) | | Congestive Heart Failure (%) | |
|---|---|---|---|---|---|---|---|---|
| Age, Yrs | Men | Women | Men | Women | Men | Women | Men | Women |
| 35–54 | 352 | 200 | 76.1 | 60.9 | 9.6 | 13.8 | 5.0 | 10.6 |
| 55–64 | 437 | 329 | 69.9 | 62.2 | 11.1 | 14.6 | 5.2 | 8.7 |
| 65–74 | 358 | 364 | 57.9 | 53.6 | 20.8 | 24.5 | 7.2 | 8.4 |
| 75–94 | 199 | 312 | 51.0 | 39.3 | 26.0 | 35.0 | 13.5 | 16.8 |

SOURCE: The Framingham Study.

## Mortality Trends in the United States

CVD mortality has declined in the United States progressively since about 1940, with sustained long-term declines since the mid-1960s (see Fig. 2-4).[25–27] CVD mortality decreased by just less than 1 percent per year in the 1950s and 1960s. The decline became steeper in the 1970s, with the rate falling 3 percent per year since then. Of note, while the initial rapid decrements in CVD mortality rates were consistent across racial groups, since mid-1980s, a divergence in CVD trends have been noted, with black males experiencing a slower decline as compared to white males.[27]

# CORONARY HEART DISEASE

## Risk Factors

Numerous epidemiologic investigations have characterized the risk factors for CHD. Age, male sex, elevated LDL cholesterol levels, low HDL cholesterol levels, diabetes mellitus, and smoking are key risk factors for CHD.[28–38] Risk scores have been developed that can aid the determination of CHD risk.[29,37,39,40] The Framingham risk score[37] is one of the most popular ones but requires recalibration

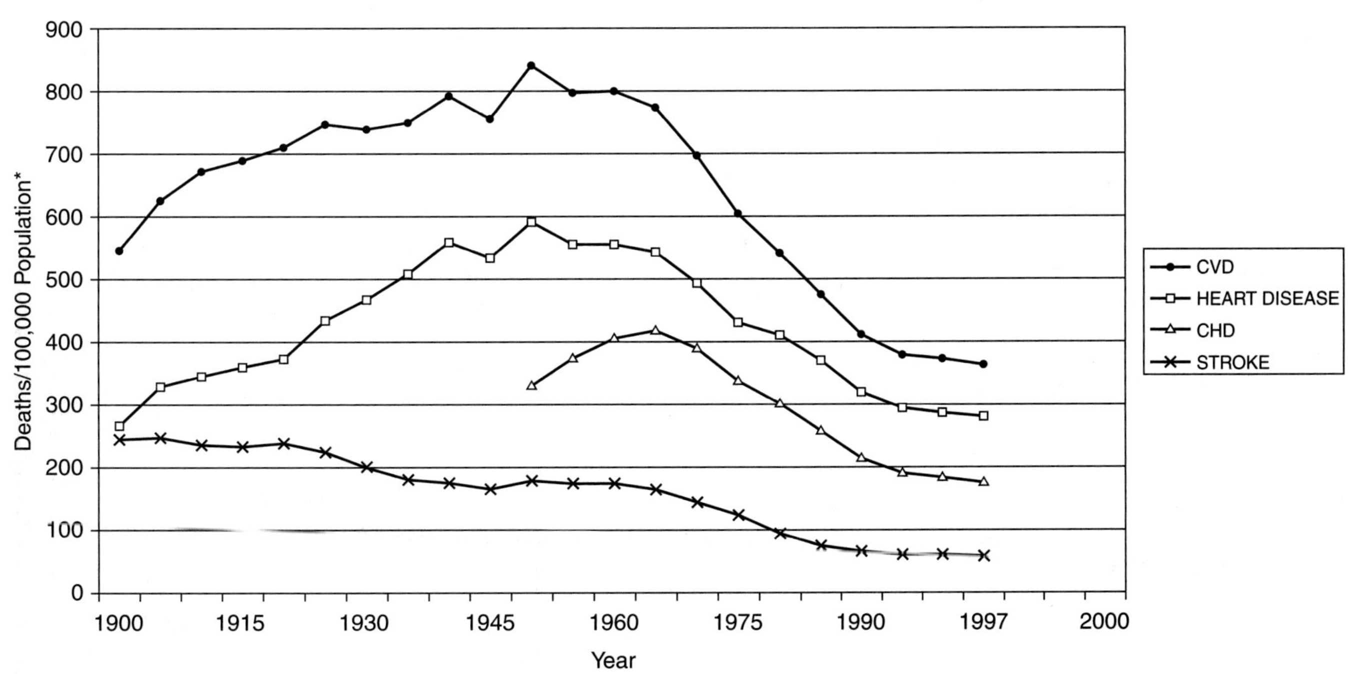


FIGURE 2-4 Decline in cardiovascular disease mortality in the United States. (From Achievements in Public Health, 1900–1999: Decline in deaths from heart disease and stroke—United States, 1900–1999. *MMWR Morb Mortal Wkly Rep* 1999;48:649, used with permission.)

TABLE 2-4 Global Incidence and Prevalence of CVD

| CVD | AFR | AMR | EUR | SEAR | WPR | EMR | World |
|---|---|---|---|---|---|---|---|
| **Annual Incidence in 2000, thousands** | | | | | | | |
| CHD* | 292 | 877 | 1932 | 1665 | 647 | 431 | 5844 |
| Cerebrovascular† | 271 | 292 | 1010 | 678 | 1436 | 167 | 3855 |
| **Point Prevalence in 2000, thousands** | | | | | | | |
| CHD‡ | 2739 | 5969 | 9945 | 12001 | 6985 | 2925 | 40,064 |
| Cerebrovascular§ | 1637 | 5299 | 11669 | 5752 | 13706 | 1391 | 39,455 |

*acute MI.
†strokes
‡includes angina
§first-ever stroke survivors
ABBREVIATIONS: CVD = cardiovascular disease; CHD = congestive heart disease; AFR = Africa; AMR = America; EUR = Europe; SEAR = South East Asia Region; WPR = Western Pacific Region; EMR = Eastern Mediterranean Region.
SOURCE: http://www3.who.int/whosis/menu.cfm?path=evidence,burden,burden_estimates,burden_estimates_2001,burden_estimates_2001_regi_on&language=English. Accessed on May 5, 2003.

when used to estimate absolute CHD risk in other populations. There is increasing awareness that obesity is a key risk factor that antedates and promotes several CHD risk factors. Obesity does not appear in many risk prediction tools because the risks are partly mediated through other risk factors.

## Global Burden

In 2001, CHD caused 7.2 million deaths worldwide and accounted for loss of 59 million DALYs (see Table 2-1). Each year there are about 5.8 million new CHD cases and about 40 million individuals with prevalent CHD are alive today (Table 2-4).

## Global Heterogeneity in Coronary Event Rates

Data collected from 35 populations that were part of the Monitoring Trends and Determinants in Cardiovascular Disease (MONICA) Project during the mid-1980s until the mid-1990s reveal substantial heterogeneity in coronary event rates (MI and coronary deaths) across countries.[41] Thus, the coronary event rate (per 100,000) in men varied 10-fold, being highest in Finland (835) and lowest in China (81). Likewise, an eightfold variation in coronary event rates was observed among women; the highest event rate was in the United Kingdom (265), while the lowest rates (35) were noted both in Spain and China. Potential reasons for such geographic variation have been noted in an earlier section.

## Global Trends in Mortality

The MONICA Project tracked coronary event rates, risk factors, and coronary care in predefined populations in 31 countries over a 10-year period from the mid-1980s to the mid-1990s.[41–43] On average, coronary event rates decreased from 23 (women) to 25 (men) percent, while CHD mortality rates reduced by 34 (women) to 42 (men) percent during the observation period.[44,45] The greatest decline in coronary event rates in men occurred in north European populations—namely, Finland, which had the highest levels at the beginning of the observation period, and Northern Sweden. Populations experiencing notable increases in coronary event rates were predominantly from central and Eastern Europe and Asia, although the general pattern of increases and decreases appeared to be less consistent in women.

In regions where coronary mortality rates were falling, it is estimated that improvements in survival contributed one third and change in heart attack rates accounted for two thirds, on average, of the total change in survival rates.[44,45] These data underscore the importance of both the prevention of heart disease and improved care of acute events in determining CHD mortality rates at the population level.

The decline in CHD mortality in developed countries is in sharp contrast to future projections for the developing countries. Between 1990 and 2020, CHD mortality is expected to increase by 120 percent in women and by 137 percent in men in developing countries. This represents a substantial increase compared with developed countries where CHD mortality is projected to increase by 29 percent in women and by 48 percent in men.[17]

## Burden in the United States

In the United States, an estimated 13 million people have CHD, about one-half of whom have acute MI and one-half have angina pectoris (Table 2-5).[2] For men, prevalence of MI is 1 percent at ages 35 to 44 years, and 16 percent at age 75 years and over. Corresponding figures for women are less than 1 percent and 13 percent, respectively.

**INCIDENCE IN THE UNITED STATES:** In the United States, CHD causes about 650,000 new and 450,000 recurrent MIs per year.[24] According to the AHA, the annual rates per 1000 population of new and recurrent heart attacks in non-black men are 26.3 for ages 65 to 74, and 53.6 for age 85 and older; corresponding rates in black men are16.3, and 40.8. For non-black women in the same age groups the heart attack rates are 7.8 and 24.2, respectively, while for black women the rates are 13.3 and 14.1, respectively.[24]

The incidence of CHD events in women lags behind that in men by 5 to 10 years. In premenopausal women, annual CHD event rates are less than 1 percent, but there is a two- to threefold increase after menopause. The average age of a person having a first heart attack is 65.8 years for men and 70.4 years for women. The first coronary presentation for women is more likely to be angina, whereas in men it is more likely to be a MI.

Unrecognized MIs are common, numbering at least one in three infarctions in the Framingham Study.[46–48] Half the unrecognized MIs are silent, and the rest are atypical so that neither the patient nor the physician entertains the possibility. More than one half of these people eventually develop some overt clinical manifestations of CHD and hence come under medical care. Angina is less frequent in individuals with unrecognized MI than it is in those with recognized

TABLE 2-5 Burden of CVD in the United States

| Group | CHD | | | MI | | | Stroke | | | CHF | | |
|---|---|---|---|---|---|---|---|---|---|---|---|---|
| | Prevalence | Incidence | Mortality | Prevalence | Incidence | Mortality | Prevalence | Incidence | Mortality | Prevalence | Incidence | Mortality |
| Total | 12,900,000 | 1,100,000 | 515,204 | 7,600,000 | 540,000 | 192,898 | 4,700,000 | 700,000 | 167,661 | 4,900,000 | 550,000 | 51,546 |
| Men (M) | 6,300,000 | 660,000 | 260,574 | 4,700,000 | 330,000 | 100,306 | 2,300,000 | 329,000 | 64,769 | 2,400,000 | — | 19,384 |
| Women (F) | 6,600,000 | 440,000 | 254,630 | 2,900,000 | 210,000 | 92,585 | 2,400,000 | 371,000 | 102,892 | 2,500,000 | — | 32,162 |
| White M | 6.9% | — | 230,951 | 5.2% | — | 89,383 | 2.2% | 267,160 | 54,938 | 2.3% | — | 17,440 |
| White F | 5.4% | — | 224,449 | 2.0% | — | 81,201 | 1.5% | 300,800 | 89,642 | 1.5% | — | 29,143 |
| Black M | 7.1% | 68,200 | 24,625 | 4.3% | — | 9,045 | 2.5% | 52,960 | 8,026 | 3.5% | — | 1,701 |
| Black F | 9.0% | 47,700 | 26,640 | 3.3% | — | 10,067 | 3.2% | 62,390 | 11,195 | 3.1% | — | 2,726 |
| Mexican American M | 7.2% | — | — | 4.1% | — | — | 2.3% | — | — | — | — | — |
| Mexican American F | 6.8% | — | — | 1.9% | — | — | 1.3% | — | — | — | — | — |

Total population data include children, and prevalence estimates are age-adjusted to Americans age 20 years and older. Incidence data refer to annual events.
ABBREVIATIONS: CHD = coronary heart disease; CHF = congestive heart failure; MI = myocardial infarction.
SOURCE: American Heart Association. Heart Disease and Stroke Statistics—2003 Update, Dallas, Texas: American Heart Association; 2002.[24]
http://www.americanheart.org/downloadable/heart/10461207852142003HDSStatsBook.pdf.

symptomatic MI, either before or after the infarction occurs. Despite the apparent mild nature of unrecognized MI, the risk of subsequent mortality is nearly the same as in patients with recognized infarction.[46–48] Men with diabetes and persons with hypertension of both sexes are particularly susceptible to silent or unrecognized MIs.[46–48]

### LIFETIME RISK OF CARDIOVASCULAR DISEASE IN THE UNITED STATES

The long-term risk of developing CHD in an individual is best described by the *lifetime risk* statistic (i.e., the probability that an individual will develop CHD over the course of his or her lifetime). Lifetime risk estimates are computed as cumulative incidence of the disease, usually for conveying to the general public the risk of experiencing a disease event from age 40 to 90 years. The lifetime risk of developing CHD after age 40 years is 49 percent in men and 32 percent in women. Even at age 70 years, the risk is 35 percent for men and 24 percent for women.[49]

### PROGNOSIS

In patients who survive the acute stage of an MI, the morbidity and mortality ranges from 1.5 to 15 times that of the general population, depending on the person's sex and clinical outcome. The rates of reinfarction, sudden death, angina pectoris, cardiac failure, and stroke are all substantial. The relative and absolute risks of these events are as great in women as in men after MI. Within 6 years following a recognized MI, 18 percent of men and 35 percent of women have a recurrent infarction, and 27 percent of men and 14 percent of women develop angina. About 22 percent of men and 46 percent of women are disabled with CHF; 8 percent of men and 11 percent of women will have a stroke. Sudden death will be experienced by 7 percent of men and 6 percent of women.

### MORTALITY IN THE UNITED STATES

CHD is the single leading cause of death in adults in the United States, accounting for 1 in 5 deaths.[24] About every 29 s an American will sustain a coronary event, and about every minute someone will die from one. There are about 515,000 coronary deaths every year (see Table 2-5).[24]

Age, gender, ethnicity, and geographic origin are key correlates of CHD mortality. CHD mortality increases with age, and CHD is also a prominent cause of death in adults at the peak of their productive lives. CHD is the leading cause of death in both men and women and in every racial or ethnic group (except Asian-American females). Overall, the CHD death rate is almost three times higher in men than it is in women at ages 25 to 34 years, but this ratio declines to 1.6 by ages 75 to 84 years. In 2000 the overall CHD death rate was 186.9 per 100,000 in the population. CHD death rates are higher in blacks (262.4 for black males and 187.5 for black females) compared to whites (238.0 for white males and 145.3 for white females). The CHD death rate is more than 50 percent higher in blacks than it is in whites at ages 25 to 34 years but this difference disappears by age 75 years. CHD mortality is not as high among the Asian and Hispanic population (rates ranging from 100 to 125, respectively) as it is among blacks and whites. There has been more than a 58 percent decline in the age-adjusted CHD death rate between the peak mortality rate reached in 1963 and that observed in 1997; the current decline is 2.7 percent per year.[26]

***Sudden Coronary Death*** In a substantial number of CHD deaths, the progression from inapparent clinical disease to death is swift. Sudden, unexpected, out-of-hospital coronary death that occurs too rapidly to allow arrival alive at the hospital accounts for one-half of all coronary fatalities. Age, gender, and time since MI are important determinants of sudden death. The proportion of coronary deaths that are sudden is lower in women than it is in men, and lower in elderly men than it is in the young.

## STROKE

### Risk Factors

Age, elevated blood pressure, smoking, diabetes mellitus, electrocardiographic left ventricular hypertrophy, and atrial fibrillation are the major risk factors for stroke.[32,50–53] A stroke risk score has been developed to estimate the risk of stroke using the experience of the Framingham cohort.[54]

### Global Burden

It is estimated that there are 5.5 million stroke deaths worldwide each year.[55] Strokes accounted for loss of 43.5 million DALYs worldwide in 2001 (see Table 2-1). Every year there are about 3.9 million new strokes and 39 million prevalent cases worldwide (see Table 2-2).

### Global Trends in Mortality

Stroke mortality has declined in the developed world over the last two decades. Data from the MONICA Study demonstrate a modest contribution of reduction in risk factors such as hypertension to the decline in stroke mortality in women, but not in men.[56]

Global mortality due to cerebrovascular disease in the next two decades will parallel the CHD trends noted in an earlier section, with a 124 percent increase in women and a 107 percent increase in men in the developing countries, compared to increments of 56 percent in women and 28 percent in men in developed countries.[17]

### Burden in the United States

Two percent of the U.S. adult population, 4.7 million people, has prevalent cerebrovascular disease (stroke or transient ischemic attack; see Table 2-5). More than 1 million of these individuals are limited in their usual activity. Prevalence rises from 2 percent in men at 45 to 54 years to 12.5 percent for men aged 75 and over, and from 1 to 10.7 percent in the corresponding age groups in women.[24]

#### INCIDENCE IN THE UNITED STATES

In the Framingham Study, the chance of having a stroke before age 70 was 5 percent for both sexes. Overall in the United States, the age-adjusted stroke incidence rates (per 100,000) for first-ever strokes are 167 for white males, 138 for white females, 323 for black males, and 260 for black females.[24] Thus, blacks have almost twice the risk of first-ever stroke as compared with whites. Overall, there are about 100,000 more women than men with prevalent stroke. This is because the average life expectancy for women is greater than for men, and the stroke rates are highest in the oldest age groups.[24]

The age-adjusted annual incidence rate (per 1000) has declined markedly for total stroke from 5.1 to 2.4, for thromboembolic stroke from 3.5 to 1.9, and for hemorrhagic stroke from 1.1 to 0.6 between 1970 and 1990.

#### TYPE OF STROKE

Of the incident stroke events in the United States, 88 percent are ischemic strokes, while 12 percent are hemorrhagic.[24] Among the

54 percent classified as definite thrombotic brain infarctions, 38 percent were classified as lacunar, with more than twice as many found in blacks as were found in whites.

#### DISABILITY FOLLOWING STROKE

The time course of functional recovery is strongly related to initial stroke severity. Of survivors of an initial event, 50 to 70 percent return to functional independence, but 15 to 30 percent become permanently dependent. Institutional care is required by 20 percent at 3 months after onset. Stroke attacks have become less severe in recent years.

#### MORTALITY IN THE UNITED STATES

Cerebrovascular disease is the third leading cause of death in the United States and is responsible for 167,000 deaths each year (see Table 2-5). On average, every 3.1 min someone in the United States dies of a stroke.[24] Stroke accounts for 7 percent of all deaths, and 44,000 of them occur in individuals younger than 75 years of age. The proportion of strokes that result in death within 1 year is about 22 percent in men and 25 percent in women; less if the stroke occurs before age 65 years. For men or women under age 65, however, only 50 percent survive past 8 years.

Age, ethnicity, and geographic region are principal determinants of stroke mortality. Overall, stroke mortality is higher in the elderly and in blacks. The 2000 overall death rate for stroke was 60.8. Death rates were 58.6 for white males and 87.1 for black males, and 57.8 for white females and 78.1 for black females. Under age 65, the mortality rate is 3 times greater in blacks than it is in whites, largely as a result of the higher prevalence and increased severity of hypertension in the former. Stroke death rates are lower in other ethnicities (40.0 for Hispanics, 39.7 for American Indians/Alaska Natives, and 52.4 for Asian/Pacific Islanders in 1999). Stroke death rates are higher in regions in Southeastern United States, referred to as the stroke belt.

#### MORTALITY TRENDS IN THE UNITED STATES

In the United States, the age-adjusted death rate for stroke has also declined by more than 50 percent over the last 4 decades, although the decline appears to have almost ended in the 1990s;[26,57] the rate of decline was 4 to 6 percent per year in the 1970s and early 1980s, but decreased to less than 1 percent per year between 1990 and 1996.[27] The overall decline in stroke mortality is remarkable because the population of older persons increased substantially during that time. There are data to suggest that the stroke belt is moving to more south-central and northwestern regions of the United States.[58]

## CONGESTIVE HEART FAILURE

### Risk Factors

Advancing age, MI, hypertension, diabetes mellitus, valvular heart disease, and obesity are key risk factors for CHF.[59–64] A clinical risk score has been formulated to estimate the risk of developing CHF, based on several of these risk factors.[65]

### Global Burden

CHF is clearly a major clinical and public health problem. The exact magnitude of the problem is difficult to assess because we lack broadly based population estimates of its prevalence, incidence, and mortality rates. It is estimated that there are nearly 23 million people with heart failure worldwide.[63,66]

### Global Trends in Mortality

It is estimated that the burden of CHF will increase over the next 2 decades in developed countries.[67] Despite a stable incidence rate, increasing prevalence may result due to a reduction in CHF mortality.[68]

### Burden in the United States

The AHA estimates that there are 4.7 million people in the United States who have CHF as of 2000, and that 550,000 new cases are reported each year (see Table 2-5).[24] CHF is reported to be the leading diagnosis for hospitalization of persons over age 65 years.

National estimates for the United States suggest that CHF afflicts 1.5 to 2 percent of the total population and as much as 6 to 10 percent of the elderly.[24] It is estimated that as many as 20 million additional persons have an asymptomatic impairment of cardiac function likely to become symptomatic over the course of 1 to 5 years. Prevalence estimates from the Framingham Study include both systolic and diastolic dysfunctional varieties but is confined mainly to those who are symptomatic. The population-based estimate from the Framingham Study indicates an increase in prevalence in men from 8 per 1000 at age 50 to 59 years to 66 per 1000 at age 80 to 89 years. In women the prevalence at these ages increases from 8 per 1000 to 79 per 1000. The prevalence of heart failure in blacks is reported to be higher than it is in whites.[24] The age-adjusted prevalence of heart failure in non-Hispanic whites is 2.3 percent in men and 1.5 percent in women. In non-Hispanic blacks, the age-adjusted prevalence is 3.5 percent in men and 3.1 percent in women. Blacks with CHF have a different spectrum of underlying cardiovascular disorders and risk factors; they have a higher prevalence of hypertension and electrocardiographic left ventricular hypertrophy but a lower prevalence of CHD and valvular disease.[69]

#### PREVALENCE OF DIASTOLIC VERSUS SYSTOLIC HEART FAILURE IN THE UNITED STATES

At present, epidemiologic population-based assessment of the prevalence of diastolic CHF uses the occurrence of clinically overt heart failure in persons with normal left ventricular systolic function for case ascertainment. Approximately 30 to 50 percent of patients with CHF are reported to have a normal or nearly normal left ventricular ejection fraction.[70] In the Framingham Study, women predominated in the diastolic CHF subgroup, with 65 percent of the heart failure occurring in association with a normal left ventricular ejection fraction. In men, 75 percent of the heart failure cases occurred in those with left ventricular systolic dysfunction.[71] The high prevalence and female preponderance in diastolic CHF have been corroborated by numerous other community-based investigations.[70]

#### INCIDENCE IN THE UNITED STATES

The Framingham Study reported that the incidence of CHF increased steeply with age, approximately doubling with each decade.[60] Between the ages of 35 to 64 and 65 to 94 years, the annual incidence rate in men increased from 3 per 1000 to 12 per 1000. In women, the corresponding rates were 2 and 9 per 1000. The higher rate in men at all ages is chiefly attributable to the greater vulnerability of men to CHD. Similar figures for the incidence of CHF have been reported by other cohort studies and investigations examining new cases in other geographic regions worldwide.[63]

#### LIFETIME RISK IN THE UNITED STATES

The Framingham Study reported that the lifetime risk of CHF is 21 percent in men and 20 percent in women.[72] Furthermore, lifetime risk of CHF, even in the absence of a myocardial infarction, is 11 percent in men and 15 percent in women.[72]

### MORTALITY OF HEART FAILURE IN THE UNITED STATES

The annual death rate for CHF was 18.7 per 1000 population in the year 2000. In population-based studies the survival rates of CHF patients are appalling. The overall population rate of expected life-years lost due to CHF is 6.7 years per 1000 in men, and 5.1 years per 1000 in women. Geographically, there is about a 10-fold range of reported mortality from CHF, the highest rates reported from the southern stroke belt. The age-adjusted death rates are 25 percent higher in men than they are in women, and 40 percent higher in blacks than they are in whites. The lower mortality in women may be related to a greater likelihood of a false-positive diagnosis of CHF, a lower probability of coronary disease as the basis of heart failure, a higher prevalence of intact left ventricular systolic function, and possibly a greater capacity of women to withstand cardiac pump failure.

In the Framingham Study a number of other conditions were associated with a poor survival experience in individuals with CHF. Advancing age was associated with increased mortality—27 percent per decade in men and 61 percent in women. Valvular heart disease increased the hazard by 68 percent in men, while in women diabetes mellitus imposed a 70 percent higher mortality rate. Additional prognostic factors associated with an adverse outcome include the presence of atrial fibrillation, renal dysfunction, underlying diabetes mellitus, a low body mass index, and a low systolic blood pressure. In the Framingham Study, diastolic CHF had an annual mortality rate of 8.7 percent compared to 18.9 percent for systolic CHF. Compared to age- and sex-matched controls, diastolic and systolic CHF were associated with hazard ratios for mortality of 4.1 and 4.3, respectively.

Data from several sources suggest that blacks with CHF have a worse prognosis relative to whites even after adjusting for multiple factors including socioeconomic status. Blacks with CHF also suffer more hospital readmissions compared to whites with this condition.[73]

## ATRIAL FIBRILLATION

### Risk Factors

The risk factors for atrial fibrillation include advancing age, gender, hypertension, diabetes, heart failure, MI, valvular heart disease, and increasing left atrial size.[74–76] In contrast to industrialized countries, in developing countries valvular heart disease appears to be the most common predisposing condition.[77,78] However, with the globalization of cardiovascular disease risk factors, hypertension and CHD are increasing in importance in developing countries.[78]

### Global Burden

The global burden of atrial fibrillation is unknown because most atrial fibrillation research has been conducted in North America and Western Europe.[79] Even within these geographic constraints, the reported studies have been from predominantly Caucasian cohorts.[79] Also, our ability to compare the epidemiology of atrial fibrillation in different countries and ethnicities has been limited by study design issues, such as differences in ages studied, case ascertainment, case definition (chronic versus paroxysmal; atrial flutter and atrial fibrillation), duration of follow-up, and frequency of electrocardiographic surveillance across studies.[79,80] For instance, the prevalence of atrial fibrillation in a community-based study of Japanese at least 40 years of age with a single-occasion electrocardiogram (ECG) was 1.3 percent;[81] the prevalence of chronic atrial fibrillation in Indo-Asians over 50 years retrospectively identified from a chart review of 6 general practices in England was 0.6 percent.[82] Higher prevalence rates have been described from U.S. cohort studies with routine surveillance of ECGs (see later and review[79] for country-specific data).

### Burden in the United States

Atrial fibrillation is the most common persistent arrhythmia, with an estimated prevalence in the United States of 2.3 million.[80] The prevalence increases significantly with advancing age, ranging from 0.1 percent in adults less than 55 years to 9.0 percent in people age 80 years or older.[80] The age-specific prevalence is higher in men than it is in women, but women constitute about one-half of atrial fibrillation cases because women in general enjoy a longer life span.[80] Several studies have suggested that black Americans may have a lower prevalence[80] and incidence than do whites,[75] for reasons that are incompletely understood. The prevalence also varies by the chronicity of atrial fibrillation studied; one study has reported that paroxysmal, chronic, and recent onset atrial fibrillation were 22.1 percent, 51.4 percent, and 26.4 percent of atrial fibrillation cases, respectively.[83]

Data from a number of sources suggest that the prevalence of atrial fibrillation is increasing,[84] and it is projected that 5.6 million Americans will have the condition by 2050.[80] The increasing prevalence is partly related to the aging of the population, but speculation also has centered on improved survival with established CVDs such as CHF and MI.

#### INCIDENCE IN THE UNITED STATES

In the Framingham Heart Study, the incidence of atrial fibrillation doubles for each successive decade of life and ranges from 3.1 for men 55 to 64 years and 38.0 for men 85 to 94 years per 1000 person-years; corresponding rates for women were 1.9 and 31.4 per 1000 person-years.[74] Similar incidence rates are reported from the Cardiovascular Health Study.[75]

#### LIFETIME RISK IN THE UNITED STATES

Based on data from the Framingham Study, the lifetime risk of atrial fibrillation is substantial; at age 40 the lifetime risk is about 26 percent for men and 23 percent for women and by 80 years it declines to only 23 percent and 21 percent, respectively.[85] Similar to CHF, the residual lifetime risk does not change substantially with increasing index age despite the decreasing life span, because of the rapidly rising incidence of atrial fibrillation with advancing age.[85]

#### RELATIONS TO STROKE AND CONGESTIVE HEART FAILURE

Atrial fibrillation has been demonstrated to be an independent risk factor for stroke[86] in virtually all settings and countries studied, with an annual stroke rate averaging about 5 percent in untreated patients. In Japan the adjusted risk ratio for stroke was 4.3 in women and 6.9 in men[81] Canadian male air force recruits with atrial fibrillation have an age-adjusted doubling of stroke risk in follow-up.[87] Data from the Framingham Heart Study suggest that while the relative risk of atrial fibrillation for stroke does not change substantively with advancing age (relative risk, RR, 3 to 5), the percentage of strokes attributable to atrial fibrillation increases markedly from 1.5 percent in subjects in their 50s to 24 percent in subjects 80 to 89 years, reflecting the higher prevalence of atrial fibrillation with advancing age.[86]

The relation between atrial fibrillation and heart failure is complex, because they share common risk factors and can each predispose to the other's development. Atrial fibrillation doubles to triples the risk of developing CHF, adjusting for the coexistent risk factors. In addition, in individuals with either atrial fibrillation or CHF, development of the other condition increases mortality.[88] Risk prediction models for stroke,[89] and stroke and death,[90] have been developed to help clinicians assess the prognosis of patients with atrial fibrillation.

#### MORTALITY IN THE UNITED STATES

Atrial fibrillation is associated with a 1.3- to twofold increased risk of death, even accounting for the frequently coexistent risk factors.[91,92] In contrast to many other cardiovascular conditions, data from several sources suggest that the age-adjusted mortality of atrial fibrillation has been increasing over time. For instance, one study analyzing death certificates noted that the age-standardized death rate (per 100,000) has increased from 27.6 in 1980 to 69.8 in 1998.[93]

## HYPERTENSION

### Definition

Numerous epidemiologic investigations have demonstrated that blood pressure is related to vascular mortality in continuous fashion.[32,34,94,95] Given the continuous relations of blood pressure to vascular risk, any definition of hypertension is somewhat arbitrary, and largely based on thresholds for which there is evidence that the benefits of lowering blood pressure outweigh potential risks of treatment. It is not surprising, therefore, that the definition of "high" blood pressure (hypertension) has been lowered in successive blood pressure guidelines over the past 35 years. Guidelines of the seventh Joint National Committee on prevention, detection, evaluation, and treatment of high blood pressure in the United States (JNC VII) and the WHO-International Society for Hypertension define hypertension as a systolic blood pressure of 140 mmHg or greater, or a diastolic blood pressure of 90 mmHg or greater, or the use of antihypertensive medication.[96,97] The JNC VII also has categorized blood pressure readings in the range of a systolic of 120 to 139 mmHg or a diastolic of 80 to 89 mmHg as "prehypertension."[97] An important reason for this change is to simplify the classification system of blood pressure and to emphasize the continuous risk of relations of blood pressure to vascular disease.

### Risk Factors

Advancing age, sedentary lifestyle, excess weight, increased dietary salt consumption, and reduced intake of potassium and increased alcohol consumption have been identified as risk factors for developing high blood pressure.[98] Family history of hypertension and African-American ancestry have also been observed to elevate the risk of developing high blood pressure.[98] Prehypertension is associated with increased risk of progression to hypertension, relative to those with optimal levels of blood pressure.[99]

### Global Burden

Hypertension is the most common CVD disorder, affecting about 20 percent of the adult population.[100] It is considered both as a disease condition and as one of the major risk factors for heart disease, stroke, and kidney disease. Worldwide an estimated 691 million people have high blood pressure.[101] About 15 to 37 percent of the adult population worldwide is afflicted with hypertension. In those older than 60 years of age, as many as one-half are hypertensive in some populations. In general, hypertension prevalence is higher in urban settings as compared with rural settings.

#### GLOBAL AWARENESS, TREATMENT, AND CONTROL OF HYPERTENSION

The detection and control of hypertension remains a challenge even in developed countries.[100,102–108] The detection rates in most developed countries vary from 32 to 64 percent, while in many developing countries the reported detection rates are substantially lower.[100,102–105,107,108] The control rates in those already being treated for hypertension varies from 13 to 29 percent.[100,102–105,107,108] However, in African countries, control rates were reported to be as low as 2 percent.[100] Data from the MONICA Study demonstrate small decreases in mean systolic blood pressures in most countries evaluated and in both sexes during the time period 1979 to 1996.[43]

### Burden in the United States

In the United States, 24 percent of the adult population, representing 43.2 million persons, have hypertension.[109] An additional 13 million adults classified as nonhypertensive report being told on one or more occasions that they have hypertension, so that the potential burden may be as high as 50 million (Table 2-6).[109] The age-adjusted prevalence varies with ethnicity, ranging from 22.6 percent in Mexican American populations, 23.3 percent in non-Hispanic white populations, to 32.4 percent in non-Hispanic black populations. A distinct geographic variation has also been noted, prevalence being greater in the southeastern United States.

The prevalence of hypertension in blacks in the United States is among the highest in the world. Compared with whites, blacks develop hypertension earlier in life and their average blood pressures are much higher. Within the African-American community, rates of hypertension vary substantially; those with the highest rates are more likely to be middle age or older, less educated, overweight or obese, physically inactive, and diabetic.

#### LIFETIME RISK IN THE UNITED STATES

The lifetime risk of hypertension reflects the probability that a person will develop high blood pressure during his or her lifetime and has been shown to be as high as 90 percent in middle-aged and elderly Framingham Study participants.[110]

#### AWARENESS, TREATMENT, AND CONTROL OF HYPERTENSION IN THE UNITED STATES

In the United States, 32.2 million, or 77 percent of Americans with hypertension, have inadequately controlled hypertension. Over two thirds of patients with hypertension were aware of their diagnosis (69 percent), and slightly more than one-half were taking prescribed medication (53 percent). About one-half of those taking medication (27 percent overall) have their blood pressure controlled at or below the 140/90 mmHg threshold. Thus, there are over 20 million Americans with hypertension who are treated and about 12 million with treated but uncontrolled hypertension.

Treatment rates and control vary by ethnicity, but the pattern that consistently emerges across ethnicities is one of lost opportunities for prevention. Only one-third of Mexican Americans with hypertension were treated (35 percent), and only 14 percent achieved control, in contrast to control rates of about 25 percent for both the non-Hispanic black and non-Hispanic white populations with hypertension. Those with uncontrolled high blood pressure who are not taking

TABLE 2-6 Burden of CVD Risk Factors in the US

| Risk Factor | Smoking | Physical Inactivity (%) | Excess Weight | | Hypertension | Dyslipidemia | | | Diabetes |
|---|---|---|---|---|---|---|---|---|---|
| | | | Overweight | Obesity | | Tc > 240 | LDL > 130 (%) | HDL < 40 (%) | |
| Total | 48,700,000 | — | 129,250,000 | 61,200,000 | 50,000,000 | 42,000,000 | — | — | 10,910,000 |
| Men(M) | 26,000,000 | — | 64,660,000 | 26,370,000 | 26.4% | 18,000,000 | 48.6 | 39.0 | 5,030,000 |
| Women (F) | 22,700,000 | — | 64,590,000 | 34,830,000 | 21.4% | 24,000,000 | 43.3 | 14.9 | 5,880,000 |
| White M | 25.8% | 32.5 | 67.4% | 27.3% | 25.2% | 18% | 49.6 | 40.5 | 5.4% |
| White F | 21.6% | 36.2 | 57.3% | 30.1% | 20.5% | 20% | 43.7 | 14.5 | 4.7% |
| Black M | 26.1% | 44.1 | 60.7% | 28.1% | 36.7% | 15% | 46.3 | 24.3 | 7.6% |
| Black F | 20.8% | 55.2 | 77.3% | 49.7% | 36.6% | 18% | 41.6 | 13.0 | 9.5% |
| Mexican American M | 24.1% | 48.9 | 74.7% | 28.9% | 24.2% | 18% | 43.6 | 40.1 | 8.1% |
| Mexican American F | 12.3% | 57.4 | 71.9% | 39.7% | 22.4% | 17% | 41.6 | 18.4 | 11.4% |

Other than for smoking and excess weight (that are crude), all prevalence data are age-adjusted to Americans age 20 and older.
SOURCE: American Heart Association. Heart Disease and Stroke Statistics—2003 Update. Dallas, Texas: American Heart Association 2002.[24]
http://www.americanheart.org/downloadable/heart/10461207852142003HDSStatsBook.pdf.

antihypertensive medication tend to be male, young, and have infrequent contact with a physician. Awareness, treatment, and control of hypertension have improved substantially since the 1976 to 1980 National Health and Nutrition Examination Survey (NHANES) but continue to be suboptimal, especially in Mexican Americans.

## Risks Associated with Hypertension

Worldwide, high blood pressure is estimated to cause 7.1 million deaths (see Table 2-1), about 13 percent of the global fatality total. Across WHO regions, research indicates that about 62 percent of strokes and 49 percent of heart attacks are caused by blood pressure levels exceeding optimal levels.[5] Every year 64.3 million DALYs (4.4 percent of total) are lost due to high blood pressure.

It is important to emphasize that while 10 to 30 percent of adults worldwide suffer from high blood pressure as currently defined, an additional 50 to 60 percent would improve their prognosis if they had levels in the healthy range.[5] Even small reductions in blood pressure for this "silent majority" would reduce their heart attack and stroke risk.[5] A meta-analysis of 61 prospective observational studies evaluated individual records from 958,074 participants (Prospective Studies Collaboration).[111] Based on 56,000 vascular deaths over a follow-up period of 12.7 million person-years, the report concluded that "usual" blood pressure is related to vascular mortality without evidence of a threshold down to 115/75 mmHg.[111] Across the entire blood pressure distribution, middle-aged persons (40 to 69 years) with a 20-mm higher systolic blood pressure (or a 10-mm higher diastolic blood pressure) experienced a twofold greater risk of death due to stroke or coronary disease. These data, the largest of their kind, strongly support the notion that a usual blood pressure of 115/75 mmHg would be "optimal" from a vascular risk standpoint.[111]

### RISKS IN THE UNITED STATES

In the United States, there is both ethnic and geographic variation in morbidity due to high blood pressure. Compared with hypertensive whites, blacks with high blood pressure have a 1.3 times greater rate of nonfatal stroke, a 1.8 times greater rate of fatal stroke, a 1.5 times greater rate of heart disease death, and a 4.2 times greater rate of end-stage kidney disease.[24] Death rates from stroke are higher in hypertensive individuals within the stroke belt than they are among those in other regions.[24]

# RHEUMATIC VALVULAR HEART DISEASE

## Global Burden

Acute rheumatic fever and subsequent rheumatic heart disease remain important cardiovascular problems in the tropical and subtropical developing countries of the Middle East, South America, Africa, and Asia, and there have been outbreaks in the United States in recent years. Although preventable, rheumatic fever occurs more frequently because of overcrowding and the mild and often clinically inapparent nature of streptococcal infections. The availability of penicillin to treat these infections, living conditions that are less crowded than formerly, and evolution of different milder strains of *Streptococcus* have made rheumatic fever uncommon in developed countries. The incidence, however, remains higher in subgroups such as Polynesians, Australian aborigines, Maoris in New Zealand, and within the United States among blacks, Puerto Ricans, Mexican Americans, and Native Americans. Rheumatic fever is rare before age 3, occurring most frequently between 5 and 15 years of age, when streptococcal infections are most frequent. During epidemics of streptococcal pharyngitis, the rheumatic fever attack rate may be 3 percent, whereas in endemic situations it is usually only 0.3 percent.

In developing countries, rheumatic fever is the most frequent cause of heart disease in the pediatric age group, accounting for 25 to 40 percent of all CVD and 33 to 50 percent of all hospital admissions. It is estimated that 12 million patients with rheumatic heart disease require further treatments to prevent disability and death due to rheumatic heart disease; of these, 8 million are children of school age.[21,24] More than 2 million require repeated hospital admissions and 400,000 die due to the illness every year. Another 1 million will need heart surgery in the next 5 to 20 years.[21,24]

### Burden in the United States

An estimated 1.8 million persons have rheumatic heart disease in the United States, more than 6 per 1000 persons.[24] In the United States, rheumatic fever accounted for about 3500 deaths in the year 2000; 70 percent were females. From 1990 to 2000, death rate due to rheumatic fever or rheumatic heart disease fell by 39 percent.[24]

## GLOBAL BURDEN OF CARDIOVASCULAR DISEASE RISK FACTORS

### Aging

The world population was 2.8 billion in 1955 and is 5.8 billion currently. It is estimated that the global population will increase by nearly 80 million people per year to reach a staggering 8 billion by the year 2025.[23] Life expectancy will increase from the current 68 years to about 73 years in 2025, representing a 50 percent improvement in life expectancy from that in 1950 (48 years). This will translate into a marked increase in the number of people aged over 65, from 390 million at present to 800 million by 2025.[112] The elderly segment will constitute over 10 percent of the total human population, and over two third of them will reside in developing countries.[23] In addition, the number of centenarians will increase markedly. For example, while there were only 200 centenarians in France in 1950, by the year 2050, the number is projected to reach 150,000—a 750-fold increase in 100 years.

The aging of the world population will have major implications for CVD morbidity and mortality. By 2025, more than 60 percent of all deaths will be among those over 65 years of ages, and more than 40 percent among over age 75 years.

### Smoking

#### GLOBAL BURDEN

It is estimated that there are about 1.15 billion smokers (250 million women) in the world today, and these individuals consume an average of 14 cigarettes each per day.[23] Of these, 300 million live in developed countries, while 800 million reside in developing countries. Overall, 47 percent of men and 12 percent of women in the world are current smokers. In developing countries, it is estimated that 48 percent of men and 7 percent of women smoke, while in developed countries, 42 percent of men and 24 percent of women are smokers. East-Asian countries account for a disproportionately high percentage (38 percent) of world smokers.[113] More than 60 percent of men in China are present smokers,[114] as are over 40 percent of men in India.[115]

#### GLOBAL TRENDS IN TOBACCO CONSUMPTION

Tobacco consumption fell between 1981 and 1991 in most developed countries.[116] In developed countries the decrease in smoking prevalence has been lowest among the least educated.

By contrast, consumption is increasing in developing countries by about 3.4 percent per annum, having risen dramatically in some countries in recent years. Data from the MONICA Study suggest that whereas smoking rates are declining in most of the male populations, rates in women are increasing.[43,117] Smoking is increasing at an alarming rate among young women, especially in Eastern Europe.[43,117,118] It is estimated that the number of individuals who smoke will increase by 500 million throughout the world in the next quarter century.

#### BURDEN IN THE UNITED STATES

For Americans age 18 and older, the current prevalence of cigarette smoking is 25.7 percent of men and 21.0 percent of women (see Table 2-6).[119] Native Americans have the highest smoking rates, while Asian Americans and Hispanic Americans have lower rates relative to whites. There are striking disparities by educational level, with individuals who have a 9 to 11 grade education having 3 times the prevalence of smoking (36.8 percent) as individuals with a college education (11.3 percent). Similarly, there is also marked geographic variation in smoking rates, with the highest rate in Kentucky (30.9 percent) and the lowest rate in Utah (13.3 percent). Adolescent smoking is a known precursor of adult smoking habits, and it is estimated that about 20 percent of twelfth graders in the United States currently smoke.

#### TRENDS IN TOBACCO CONSUMPTION IN THE UNITED STATES

In the United States, the prevalence of smoking rose steadily from the 1930s and reached a peak in 1964 when more than 40 percent of all adult Americans (60 percent of men) smoked. Since then smoking prevalence has declined markedly, decreasing to about 23 percent by 1997.[119]

#### HEALTH RISKS AND FUTURE TRENDS

Smokers of all ages have a two- to threefold elevated risk of dying prematurely compared to nonsmokers.[120–123] It has been estimated that between ages 35 to 69, smokers lose about 20 years of life expectancy relative to nonsmokers.[120] After age 70 years, smokers lose about 8 years of life relative to nonsmokers.[120] Smoking is an important CVD risk factor in both men and women, being particularly harmful in the latter after menopause and in those who use oral contraceptives. Prospective studies show that cigarette smoking causes about 30 percent of CVD deaths worldwide.[120,121,124] This is especially evident in populations with clustering of CVD risk factors (i.e., those with diets that are high in saturated fat with subsequent high blood cholesterol and high blood pressure). Smoking is responsible for 90 percent of all lung cancers and for 75 percent of chronic obstructive pulmonary disease.[120,121] It is estimated that tobacco kills 560 people every hour or 13,400 people per day. WHO estimates that tobacco was responsible for 10 percent of the total global mortality, and caused about 4.9 million deaths worldwide in 2000, or about 1 million more deaths than it did in 1990. Over 59 million DALYs (4.1 percent of total) were lost due to smoking in 2000. In the United States, from 1995 to 1999, an average of 442,400 individuals died each year from smoking-related illnesses. One third of these were CVD related.

Based on current smoking patterns and trends, smoking is expected to kill 10 million people annually worldwide by 2025—this is more than the total of deaths from malaria, maternal and major childhood conditions, and tuberculosis combined.[125] Of specific concern is that over 70 percent of these deaths will be occurring in developing countries. By 2020, smoking will cause about one in three of all adult deaths.

Health risks diminish with smoking cessation. According to WHO, 1 year after quitting, the risk of CHD decreases by 50 percent, and within 3 years, the relative risk of dying from CHD for an exsmoker approaches that of a long-time (lifetime) nonsmoker.[126]

#### RISKS ASSOCIATED WITH ENVIRONMENTAL TOBACCO EXPOSURE

The risk of death from CHD increases by up to 30 percent among those exposed to environmental tobacco smoke at home or work.[127]

It is estimated that about 35,000 nonsmokers die from CHD each year as a result of exposure to environmental tobacco smoke.[5]

### TOBACCO FREE INITIATIVE

WHO established the Tobacco Free Initiative in July 1998 to coordinate an improved global strategic response.[128] While the long-term mission of global tobacco control is to reduce smoking prevalence, the goals of the Tobacco Free Initiative are to (1) galvanize global support for evidence-based tobacco-control policies and actions; (2) to build new partnerships for action and strengthen existing ones; (3) to raise awareness of the need to address tobacco issues at all levels of society; and (4) to accelerate the implementation of national, regional, and global strategies.[128] Specific strategies for tobacco control include a ban on advertising and expansion of public health information; use of taxes and regulations to reduce consumption; promotion of cessation of tobacco use, the building of antitobacco coalitions.[128]

## Physical Inactivity

### SIGNIFICANCE

It is widely accepted that daily moderate-intensity physical activity helps lower blood pressure, reduce body fat, and improve glucose metabolism.[129] Indeed, physical activity is essential to maintain overall good health and is important in maintaining a healthy weight. Physical activity also reduces the risk of diabetes mellitus, hypertension, CVD, and all-cause mortality.[129]

### GLOBAL BURDEN AND TRENDS

WHO estimates that 60 percent of the world population is insufficiently physically active, a situation that is particularly striking among women and that undoubtedly has contributed to the increased prevalence of obesity and diabetes.[13,129] Physical inactivity is widespread in developed countries and is increasing in urban areas of developing countries, especially in poorer communities. This trend for physical inactivity is influenced by cultural patterns, local traditions, and the lack of civic organizations to promote the benefits of exercise. In developing countries that previously relied on walking or bicycling for transportation, there has been a progressive increase in the use of automobiles and motorized public transportation.

### BURDEN IN THE UNITED STATES AND TRENDS

According to national data in the United States, 38 percent of Americans age 18 or older indulge in no leisure-time physical activity, Sixty-two percent engaged in at least some physical activity, while only 23 percent performed light to moderate physical activity at least 5 times per week as per current AHA guidelines.[130] Physical inactivity is more common in women, elderly, blacks, and Hispanics (see Table 2-6) and among the less affluent.[24] The prevalence of physical inactivity is particularly high in rural areas in southern and western parts of the country. Physical inactivity among adolescents is a harbinger of continued inactivity during adulthood. It is estimated that only 70 percent of adolescent boys and 54 percent of girls engage in vigorous physical activity for 20 min 3 times per week. Of specific concern is that attendance at physical education classes fell from 41 percent in 1991 to 28 percent in 1997, in the Youth Risk Behavior Survey.[131]

### RISKS

Physical inactivity caused about 1.9 million deaths globally in 2000.[5] It is estimated that about 20 percent of cases of CHD, 15 percent of diabetes and some cancers, and 10 percent of strokes are attributable to physical inactivity.[5] The relative risk of CHD associated with physical inactivity ranges from 1.5 to 2.4, relative to people who do follow current minimum physical activity recommendations. This increase in risk associated with physical inactivity is comparable to that observed for high blood cholesterol, high blood pressure, or cigarette smoking.

### WHO PHYSICAL ACTIVITY INITIATIVE

WHO has begun formulating a Global Strategy on Diet, Physical Activity and Health, under a May 2002 mandate from the World Health Assembly.[13,129] This extensive, population-wide, prevention-based strategy will be developed over 2 years.

## Obesity

### DEFINITION

Overweight and obesity are currently defined by body mass index (BMI, calculated as weight in kilograms per height in meters$^2$). A BMI of 25.0 to 29.9 defines overweight, and a BMI ≥30.0 defines obesity.[132,133]

### GLOBAL BURDEN

Obesity is a disease condition that is highly prevalent in both developing and developed countries (Fig. 2-5). According to WHO data, an estimated 1 billion people across the world are now overweight or obese.[134,135] It is estimated that between 50 and 75 percent of the adults studied in the MONICA study were overweight or obese.[42] Low levels of education are associated with increased body mass index in the MONICA populations.[136] In the European Union, between 27 to 35 percent of adults are overweight, and from 7 to 12 percent are obese. The WHO estimates that about 18 million children under the age of 5 are overweight, and these children are at increased risk of developing adult obesity and related problems of dyslipidemia and hypertension in their teen years.[134,137,138]

### GLOBAL TRENDS IN PREVALENCE

Obesity rates have risen threefold or more in some parts of the Middle East, North America, Eastern Europe, the Pacific Islands, Australia, and China since 1980.[134,139] Data from the MONICA Study indicate that BMI increased in about half of the female populations and in two thirds of the male population.[43]

### BURDEN IN THE UNITED STATES

In the United States, 35 percent of United States adults were considered overweight (BMI 25.0 to 29.9 kg/m$^2$), and another 26 percent were considered obese (BMI ≥ 30.0 kg/m$^2$) in 1999. Hispanic men and Hispanic and black women were more likely to be overweight or obese than were their white counterparts.[140] Among non-Hispanic black women, more than one half of females over age 40 years were obese, and more than 80 percent were overweight. A socioeconomic gradient is evident, with excess weight being more common in those in a low social class and with the least education.[141]

### TRENDS IN PREVALENCE IN THE UNITED STATES

In the United States, the age-adjusted prevalence of overweight increased from 56 percent in National Health and Nutrition Examination Survey III (NHANES III) (1988 to 1994) to 65 percent in 1999 to 2000.[142,143] The prevalence of obesity (BMI ≥ 30.0) also increased during this period from 23 percent to 31 percent. Prevalence of extreme degrees of obesity (BMI ≥ 40.0) increased from 3 to 5 percent. Increases in obesity occurred for both men and women in all age groups and for all ethnicities.[142,143]

Based on data from the 1999 to 2000 NHANES, the prevalence of overweight in children ages 6 to 11 increased from 4.2 to 15.3 percent compared with data from 1963 to 1965. The prevalence of overweight in adolescents ages 12 to 19 increased from 4.6 to 15.5 percent.[144]

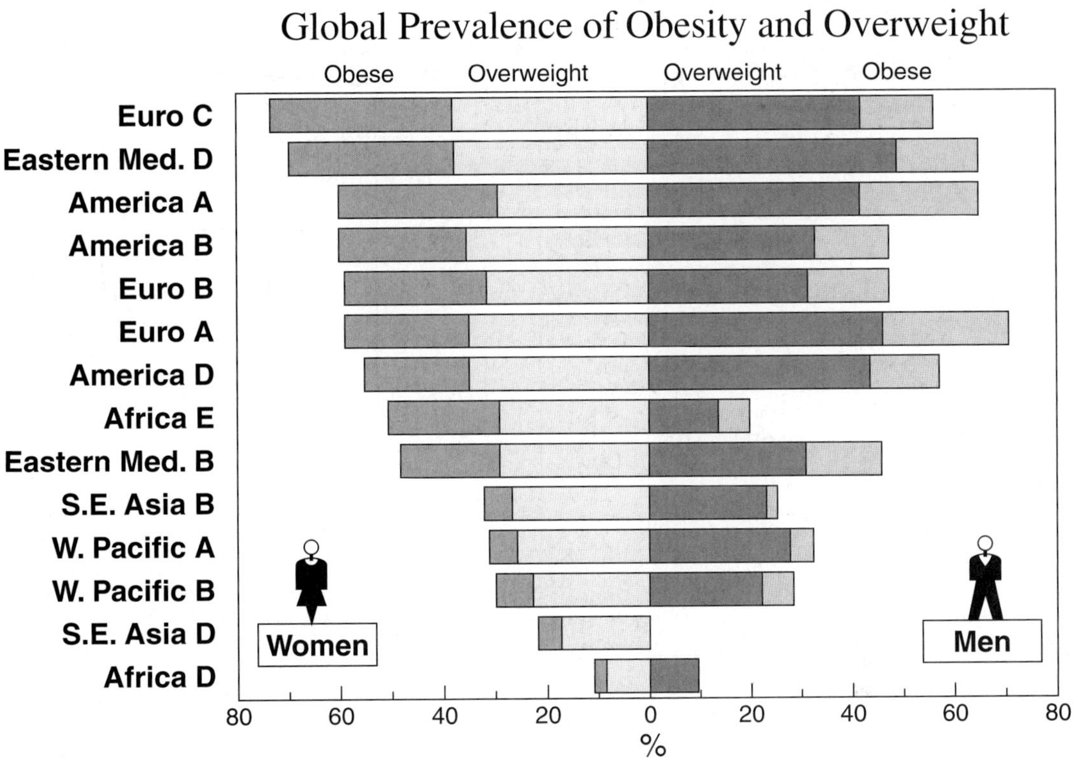

**HEALTH RISKS**

Obesity accounts for 60 percent of cases of diabetes mellitus, and 40 percent of cases of hypertension.[38] Conversely, weight loss significantly improves CVD risk factors including lipid profile,[98] blood pressure,[98,145] blood glucose,[146] and inflammatory markers.[147] In addition, obesity accounts for 20 percent of CHD and stroke in the community. It is also a major cause of mortality. About 500,000 people in North America and Western Europe die from obesity-related disease every year.[134] Obesity kills about 220,000 men and women annually in the United States and Canada, and about 320,000 men and women in 20 countries of Western Europe. It accounted for loss of 33 million DALYs (2.3 percent of total) in 2000.

Global Prevalence of Obesity and Overweight

FIGURE 2-5 Global burden of obesity. (From James PT, Leach R, Kalamara E, Shayeghi M. The worldwide obesity epidemic. *Obes Res* 2001;9(90004):228S, used with permission.)

## Dyslipidemia

**GLOBAL BURDEN AND TRENDS**

It is estimated that over 80 percent of the world population has suboptimal levels of serum cholesterol (i.e., in excess of 150 mg/dL). Excessive levels of serum cholesterol are estimated to cause 18 percent of global cerebrovascular disease (mostly nonfatal events) and 56 percent of global CHD. Overall this amounts to about 4.4 million deaths (7.9 percent of total; Fig. 2-6) and 40.4 million DALYs (2.8 percent of total). Data from the MONICA Study demonstrate small decreases in mean cholesterol levels of the populations studied between 1979 and 1996.[43]

**BURDEN AND TRENDS IN THE UNITED STATES**

In the United States, the age-adjusted mean cholesterol is 5.27 mmol/L (203 mg/dL).[148] An estimated 42 million Americans have serum cholesterol levels of 240 mg/dL or higher, an estimated 18 percent of the adult population (see Table 2-6). An estimated 105 million, or one half of the adult population, have serum cholesterol levels in excess of 200 mg/dL. Of note, about 10 percent of adolescents (ages 12 to 19 years) have total serum cholesterol levels exceeding 200 mg/dL. The overall prevalence of elevated serum cholesterol level is similar in men and women and comparable across ethnicities. However, beginning at age 50 years a higher proportion of women than men have total blood cholesterol of 200 mg/dL or higher. The mean level of low-density lipoprotein (LDL) cholesterol for American adults age 20 and older is 127 mg/dL. About 48 percent of men and 43 percent of adults have LDL cholesterol levels in excess of 130 mg/dL. Values of high-density lipoprotein (HDL) cholesterol of less than 40 mg/dL are considered low. About 40 percent of men and 15 percent of women have values below this threshold. The prevalence of a low HDL cholesterol value is slightly lower in black women relative to white and Hispanic females.

**TRENDS IN THE UNITED STATES**

Serial NHANES surveys I to III have demonstrated a sequential decrease in the percentage of individuals with elevated serum cholesterol levels. This observation is consistent across all ethnicities, both sexes, and in all educational strata. These data suggest a change in population determinants of serum cholesterol levels in the United States, such as the dietary content of saturated fats, despite the increase in the prevalence of overweight noted across the surveys. After NHANES III, decline in serum cholesterol levels has been limited. Between NHANES III and NHANES 1999–2000, the age-adjusted mean total cholesterol concentration decreased marginally from 5.31 mmol/L (205 mg/dL) in NHANES III to 5.27 mmol/L (203 mg/dL) in NHANES 1999 to 2000.[148]

**AWARENESS, TREATMENT, AND CONTROL IN THE UNITED STATES**

In the United States awareness, treatment, and control levels for hypercholesterolemia mirror the suboptimal patterns observed with hypertension. In the NHANES investigation between 1999 and 2000, among participants who had a total cholesterol concentration ≥5.2

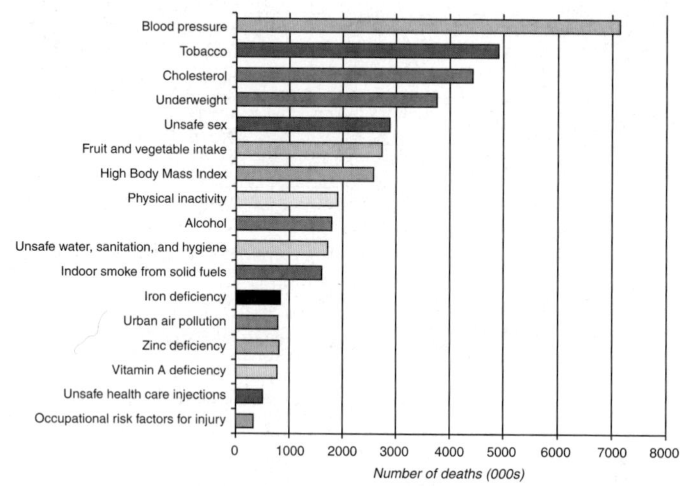


FIGURE 2-6 Contribution of select risk factors to global mortality. (From http://www.hoffmanpr.com/Press_Releases/ Archieved_Press_Releases/WHO/Cardio2002/CardioGraphs.ppt, used with permission.)

mmol/L (200 mg/dL) or who reported using cholesterol-lowering medications, 69.5 percent reported having had their cholesterol checked, 35.0 percent were aware that they had hypercholesterolemia, only 12.0 percent were being treated, and a meager 5.4 percent had a total cholesterol concentration < 5.2 mmol/L (200 mg/dL) after age adjustment.[148]

## Diabetes Mellitus

### GLOBAL BURDEN

An estimated 177 million people are affected by diabetes—the majority by type 2 diabetes.[149] Two-thirds of these individuals live in the developing world.[149] The top 10 countries, in terms of absolute numbers of individuals with the condition, are India, China, United States, Indonesia, Russia, Japan, United Arab Emirates, Pakistan, Brazil, and Italy. The overall prevalence is below 10 percent in people below age 65 years and between 10 to 20 percent in individuals beyond this age.[150]

### GLOBAL TRENDS

The prevalence of diabetes worldwide is increasing at an alarming rate. The prevalence of diabetes in adults globally was estimated to be 4.0 percent in 1995 and was projected to rise to 5.4 percent by the year 2025. The number of adults with diabetes in the world was 30 million in 1985 and is projected to rise from 135 million in 1995 to 300 million in 2025.[149,151] The proportional rise projected by 2025 is much larger in developing countries where a 170 percent increase (from 84 million to 228 million) is estimated, compared to a 42 percent increase in developed countries (from 51 million to 72 million). The highest increase is projected to occur in India and China. Indeed, the prevalence of diabetes in these 2 countries combined will rise from 45 million in 1995 to an estimated 95 million in 2025. The vast majority of people with diabetes in developing countries are likely to be between the ages of 45 and 64 years, while those in developed countries will be age 65 years or older. The main reasons for the rising epidemic of diabetes are population aging, unhealthy diets, increasing epidemics of obesity, and sedentary lifestyles.[149]

### BURDEN IN THE UNITED STATES

In the United States, it is estimated that about 16 million people have diabetes, but only about 10 million have been diagnosed. Approximately 798,000 new cases of diabetes are diagnosed annually.[152] The risk of diabetes for Hispanics and non-Hispanic blacks is about 1.5-fold to twice that for non-Hispanic whites. The median percentages with physician-diagnosed diabetes varies from 4.7 (women) to 5.4 (men) percent in whites, from 7.6 (men) to 9.5 (women) percent in non-Hispanic blacks, to 8 (men) to 11 (women) percent in Hispanics (see Table 2-6).

### TRENDS IN THE UNITED STATES

In the United States, the number of persons diagnosed with diabetes has increased sixfold, from 1.6 million in 1958 to 10 million in 1997.[152] The rise has been particularly striking in the last decade; the prevalence of diabetes rose from 4.9 percent in 1990 to 6.5 percent in 1998, an increase of 33.3 percent.[153] Of note, this increase preceded the introduction of the new diagnostic criteria that use a lower fasting blood sugar threshold. Increases in prevalence of diabetes have been observed in both sexes, all ages, all ethnic groups, all education levels, and in nearly all states. Type II diabetes is increasing in frequency in young people, including children and adolescents.[154] Similar numbers of people have impaired glucose tolerance. In the San Antonio Study, the incidence of diabetes has tripled in Hispanics and among whites between 1987 and 1996.[155]

### HEALTH RISKS

The number of deaths attributed to diabetes was previously estimated at just over 800,000 worldwide. However, it has long been known that the number of deaths related to diabetes is considerably underestimated. A more plausible figure is likely to be around 4 million deaths per year related to the presence of the disorder. This is about 9 percent of the global total mortality. Most deaths due to diabetes are premature. About 75 percent of the mortality among diabetic men and 57 percent among diabetic women are attributable to CVD. Among people with diabetes, CVD is 2 to 4 times more common; the risk of stroke is 2 to 4 times higher; and over 60 percent have high blood pressure.[152,156]

## Metabolic Syndrome

### DEFINITIONS

The metabolic syndrome has been defined by the Adult Treatment Panel (ATP) III as the presence of 3 or more of the following abnormalities: waist circumference greater than 102 cm (40 inches) in men and 88 cm (36 inches) in women; serum triglyceride level of at least 150 mg/dL (1.69 mmol/L); HDL cholesterol level <40 mg/dL (1.04 mmol/L) in men and 50 mg/dL (1.29 mmol/L) in women; blood pressure of at least 130/85 mmHg; or serum glucose level of at least 110 mg/dL (6.1 mmol/L).[157] WHO defines the *metabolic syndrome* as the presence of diabetes, impaired glucose tolerance, impaired fasting glucose, or insulin resistance plus two or more of the following abnormalities:

1. High blood pressure defined as a value ≥160/90 mmHg.
2. Hyperlipidemia identified by a triglyceride concentration ≥150 mg/dL (1.695 mmol/L) and/or HDL cholesterol <35 mg/dL (0.9 mmol/L) in men and <39 mg/dL (1.0 mmol/L) in women.
3. Central obesity characterized by a waist-to-hip ratio of >0.90 in men or >0.85 in women and/or BMI >30 kg/m$^2$.
4. Microalbuminuria denoted by a urinary albumin excretion rate ≥20 μg/min or an albumin-to-creatinine ratio ≥20 mg/g (see also Chap. 87).[158]

#### GLOBAL BURDEN

The prevalence of the metabolic syndrome varies from 10 to 25 percent based on the criteria used, the population investigated, and the age of the sample.[159–167] Prevalence increases with age and is much higher in individuals with diabetes mellitus.[165,168]

#### BURDEN IN THE UNITED STATES

It is estimated that there are 47 million Americans with the metabolic syndrome, with an overall age-adjusted prevalence of 24 percent.[168] Older age, postmenopausal status, higher BMI, high carbohydrate consumption, physical inactivity, and Mexican American ethnicity are key correlates of the metabolic syndrome.[165] Prevalence increases with age exceeding 40 percent in individuals over age 65 years.[168] Among different ethnicities, Mexican Americans have the highest age-adjusted prevalence of the metabolic syndrome (31.9 percent). The age-adjusted prevalence is similar for men (24.0 percent) and women (23.4 percent). However, among African Americans, women have about a 57 percent higher prevalence than do men, and among Mexican Americans, women have about a 26 percent higher prevalence than do men.[168]

#### RISKS

The presence of the metabolic syndrome is an ominous indicator of future CVD risk.[169–172] In a prospective study of Finnish men, the metabolic syndrome was associated with a threefold increased risk of CHD/CVD and twofold elevated mortality relative to individuals without the syndrome.[164]

### Inflammation

Inflammation is a fundamental component of atherosclerosis.[173] Plasma levels of several inflammatory markers have been used as a surrogate for vascular inflammation, including that in the atherosclerotic plaque. C-reactive protein (CRP) has emerged as a premier inflammatory marker. There is a paucity of data in the published literature regarding the distribution of CRP levels in developing countries.

#### DISTRIBUTION AND DETERMINANTS IN THE UNITED STATES

The distribution of CRP (using high sensitivity assays, hs-CRP) has been investigated in men in the NHANES 1999-2000 survey.[174] The median CRP concentrations were 1.6 mg/L for all men, 1.6 mg/L for white men, 1.7 mg/L for African-American men, 1.5 mg/L for Mexican-American men, and 1.8 mg/L for other men. Age, BMI, and smoking are other positive correlates of CRP.[174]

#### CARDIOVASCULAR DISEASE RISKS

Plasma levels of CRP are elevated in CHD patients.[173] Plasma CRP predicts a wide variety of CVD endpoints including CHD, peripheral vascular disease, and stroke. There is an increased risk of CHD, even at levels below those indicating acute inflammation in clinical practice.[175]

Assays for hs-CRP to assess cardiovascular risk are not yet used in routine clinical practice. On the basis of the available evidence, a Writing Group of the AHA recommended against screening of the entire adult population for hs-CRP as a public health measure.[176] The Writing Group concluded that it is reasonable to measure hs-CRP as an adjunct to the major risk factors to further assess absolute risk for coronary disease primary prevention.[176] The Group recommended that hs-CRP measurement appears to have its best utility when performed to detect enhanced absolute risk in persons in whom multiple risk factor scoring indicates an intermediate 10-year CHD risk (10 to 20 percent).[176] However, the benefits of this strategy or any treatment based on this strategy remain uncertain.[176]

### Homocysteine

#### DISTRIBUTION AND DETERMINANTS

Homocysteine is a sulfur-containing amino acid that is an intermediate product of the metabolism of methionine and cysteine. Plasma homocysteine levels show a strong inverse correlation both with dietary intake and with plasma levels of the vitamins folate, $B_6$, and $B_{12}$, all of which are essential cofactors in homocysteine metabolism.[177–181] A common polymorphism in the gene for methylenetetrahydrofolate reductase appears to influence the sensitivity of homocysteine levels to folic acid deficiency (see also Chap. 43).

In the NHANES III examination, plasma homocysteine levels varied according to age, sex, and ethnicity. The mean plasma homocysteine level was 21.5 percent higher in men than it was in women, 11.8 percent higher in non-Hispanic whites than it was in Mexican Americans, and 42 percent higher in persons 70 years or older as compared to individuals below the age of 30 years. Others have suggested that Asians may have higher plasma homocysteine levels compared to other ethnicities.[182]

#### CARDIOVASCULAR DISEASE RISKS

Rare homozygous defects of the key enzyme cystathionine-beta-synthase cause homocystinuria, which is associated with an up to 10-fold elevation of plasma homocysteine levels and with premature atherosclerosis, recurrent thromboses of coronary, cerebral, or peripheral arteries and venous thrombosis. Prospective studies and case control studies have shown that even moderately elevated levels of plasma homocysteine also increase the risk of both atherosclerosis of the coronary, cerebral, and peripheral arteries and of cardiovascular death. A meta-analysis calculated that each 5 μmol/L increase in the plasma homocysteine level increases the risk for CHD by about 15 to 25 percent.[183,184]

At present, there is insufficient evidence to recommend measuring homocysteine levels in the general population.[185] Homocysteine levels should be measured in patients with a history of premature coronary artery disease and/or stroke who do not have classical risk factors. It should also be determined in individuals with a history of venous thromboembolism.[185]

## GLOBAL BURDEN OF CARDIOVASCULAR DISEASE: GLOBAL RESPONSES TO THE EPIDEMIC

### Future Challenges and Opportunities

Organized efforts at CVD prevention began in high-income countries when the epidemic had peaked, and they have helped accelerate a secular downswing in CVD. The efforts in low- and middle-income countries are starting when the epidemic is still on its upswing. Strategies to control CVD internationally must be based on recognition of global similarities and differences. Principles of prevention must be based on the evidence gathered in high-income countries, but the interventions must be context-specific and resource sensitive.

#### GENERAL PRINCIPLES OF PRIMARY AND SECONDARY PREVENTION

1. Classical risk factors (i.e., smoking, dyslipidemia, elevated blood pressure, and hyperglycemia/diabetes mellitus) account for over 75 percent of CVD. For each of these variables, CVD risk operates across a continuum (Table 2-7, Fig. 2-7).[32–34,186] Indeed, CVD is rare when none of these risk factors are present.[35]
2. CVD risk factors are pathogenetically interrelated and frequently cluster in individuals. For instance, physical inactivity predisposes to the development of obesity, which further exacerbates tendencies toward sedentary lifestyle, and contributes to the development of a host of other risk factors.
3. Many more events arise from the "moderate" middle of the distribution than from the "high-risk" tail.[187] CVD risk is increased when risk factors coexist.[28,29] Consequently, a majority of CVD events occur in persons with modest levels of multiple risk factors rather than in those with a high level of a single risk factor.
4. "Comprehensive" or "absolute" CVD risk is the best guide for individual interventions, while "population-attributable risk" should guide mass interventions, maximizing benefits by bringing about modest distributional shifts.[187] Risk scores have been formulated to assess the absolute risk of developing CVD events.[29,37] It is important to note that while qualitatively the same set of risk factors determine CVD risks in different populations, there are quantitative differences in the relative importance of select risk factors, the relative risks associated with them, and the absolute risks.[36,50,53] Risk scores, therefore, have to be recalibrated based on CVD rates of the indigenous population.
5. CVD risk factors evolve in childhood and adolescence so that a synergistically complementary blend of cost-effective "population-wide" and "high-risk" interventions must extend to the pediatric age group too.
6. Epidemiologic principles dictate that compared with intensive individual treatment of high-risk patients, small improvements in the overall distribution of risk in a population will yield larger gains in disease reduction, when the underlying conditions that confer risk are widespread in the population (see Fig. 2-7).[187] Hence, at a population level primary prevention must be combined in children, and adults free of disease must be combined with secondary prevention in older adults.

#### IMPORTANCE OF PRIMORDIAL PREVENTION

An emerging concept in CVD prevention is a focus on primordial prevention, which proposes strategies to prevent the emergence of risk factors.[188] Primary and secondary prevention strategies intervene at the stage when atherosclerosis is established.[188] Attention to the prevention of the emergence of risk factors is critical, because secular trend data suggest both optimistic and pessimistic developments. For instance in the Minnesota Heart Study from 1980 through 1982 to 1995 through 1997 there were improvements in prevalence of hypertension, cigarette smoking, and dietary fat consumption. However, mirroring national data there was a plateau in lipid levels and less favorable trends in adiposity and physical activity.[189]

It must be emphasized that primordial prevention is not a theoretical objective. Work from several cohort studies suggest that maintenance of optimal risk factor status results in significantly decreased relative risk (RR 0.15 to 0.60) of CVD mortality and an average gain in life expectancy of 5.8 to 9.5 years.[35] Unfortunately, only 5 to 10 percent of individuals screened were in the low-risk subgroup defined as having a serum cholesterol level < 200 mg/dL (5.17 mmol/L), blood pressure ≤ 120/80, no diabetes or MI, or did not smoke cigarettes.[35,105] Furthermore, research increasingly demonstrates that the emergence of risk factors can be prevented. For instance, the Diabetes Prevention Program randomized individuals at risk for diabetes to a lifestyle (7 percent weight loss and 150 min physical activity per week), metformin, or placebo.[146] The incidence of diabetes was reduced to 58 percent by lifestyle intervention and 31 percent by medication—to prevent 1 case of diabetes over 3 years

TABLE 2-7 Global Burden of Suboptimal Blood Pressure and Serum Cholesterol

| | AFR | AMR | EUR | SEAR | WPR | EMR | World |
|---|---|---|---|---|---|---|---|
| Blood pressure | | | | | | | |
| Mean SBP, mmHg | 129–133 | 127–128 | 135–138 | 125–128 | 124–133 | 131–133 | 128 |
| % SBP > 115 | >70 | >70 | >80 | >60 | >60 | >70 | >70 |
| % CV burden due to suboptimal SBP | 50–58 | 44–53 | 51–66 | 44–55 | 53–56 | 55–58 | 50 |
| Cholesterol | | | | | | | |
| Mean, mmol/L | 4.8 | 5.1–5.3 | 5.1–6.0 | 4.7–5.1 | 4.6–5.2 | 5.0 | 5.0 |
| % >3.8 mmol/L (150 mg/dL) | >80 | >80 | >80 | >80 | >70 | >80 | >80 |
| % CV burden due to suboptimal cholesterol | 24 | 26–39 | 32–48 | 24–40 | 19–28 | 37–38 | 31 |

1 mmol/L = 38.7 mg/dL

ABBREVIATIONS: AFR = Africa; AMR = America; EUR = Europe; SEAR = Southeast Asia Region; WPR = Western Pacific Region; EMR = Eastern Mediterranean Region; SBP = systolic blood pressure; CV = cardiovascular.

SOURCE: http://www.hoffmanpr.com/Press_Releases/Archived_Press_Releases/WHO/Cardio2002/CardioGraphs.ppt.

only 7 persons would have to participate in the lifestyle-intervention program.[146] Similar approaches are advocated and efficacious for the prevention of hypertension.[98,190]

## GLOBAL EFFORTS FOR CVD PREVENTION

WHO and several international organizations have commenced a series of measures and investigations to stem the rising burden of global CVD. Several of these efforts are summarized in Table 2-8.[4,191–200]

The World Health Report (WHR) 2002 identifies 5 important risk factors for noncommunicable disease in the top 10 leading risks to health (Fig. 2-6).[5] These are raised blood pressure, raised cholesterol level, tobacco use, alcohol consumption, and overweight. The disease burden caused by these leading risk factors is global. In every region of the world, including the poorest, raised blood pressure, cholesterol, and tobacco use are causing serious disease and untimely deaths.[5]

The WHR 2002 underscores the fact that blood pressure alone causes about 50 percent of CVD worldwide (see Table 2-7).[5] Cholesterol causes about one third of CVD (see Table 2-7). Inactive lifestyles, tobacco use, and low fruit and vegetable intake account for 20 percent each. Overall, approximately 75 percent of CVD can be attributed to the established risks assessed in the report, far higher than the one third to one half commonly thought.[5] The CVD burden is about equally shared among men and women. A fundamental message of the WHR 2002 is that more than 50 percent of deaths and disability from CVD can be avoided by a combination of simple, cost-effective, national efforts and individual actions to reduce the major risk factors, such as high blood pressure, high cholesterol, obesity, and smoking.[5]

Because the causes of CVD are multifactorial, it follows that the response needs to be multifaceted and multi-institutional.[5] The evidence is overwhelming that prevention is possible when sustained actions are directed both at individuals and families, as well as the broader social, economic, and cultural determinants of CVD. The WHR 2002 also urges countries to adopt policies and programs to promote population-wide interventions such as reducing salt in processed foods, cutting dietary fat, encouraging exercise and higher consumption of fruits and vegetables, and limiting smoking. However, primary prevention must be complemented by secondary prevention.[5] Demographic and epidemiologic changes have steeply increased the need for long-term care of people of all ages suffering from CVD. Fortunately, large randomized clinical trials have established the efficacy of antiplatelet agents, beta-blockers, angiotensin-converting enzyme inhibitors, diuretics, and statins in the primary and secondary prevention of CVD.[94,145,201–207] Cost-effective pharmacologic treatments for risk factors such as high blood pressure, diabetes, and raised cholesterol levels have lifesaving impacts and should be routinely implemented at the primary health care level. The WHR 2002 shows that countries in all epidemiologic settings will achieve major additional reductions in the disease burden by treating people identified to be at risk. Dietary, physical activity, and smoking cessation programs should also be integral to the management of these diseases. Ensuring good health demands a "life course" approach to eating and physical activity that begins with prepregnancy, includes breast-feeding, and extends to old age.[5] WHO has also formulated the CVD-Risk Management Package, which is designed to select and target high-risk patients in different countries with varying availability of resources.[192]

A. Continuous Relations of BP and Cholesterol to CHD Risk

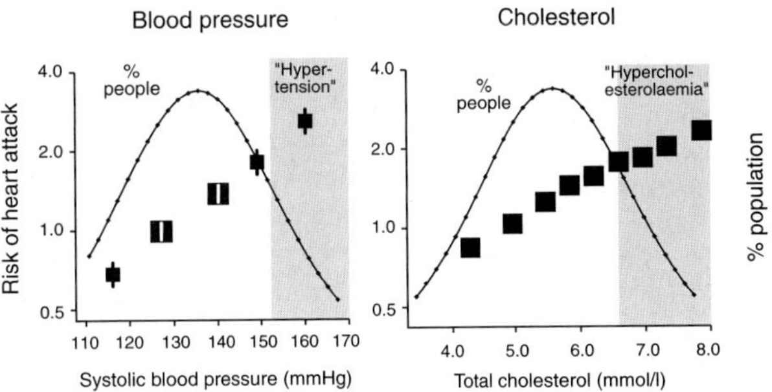


Population-based and High-Risk Strategies for CHD Prevention

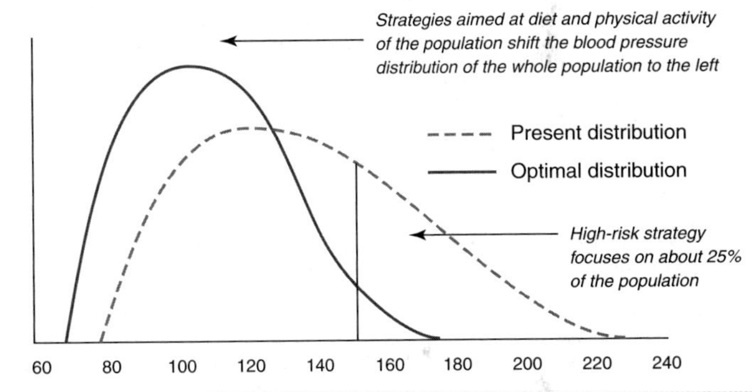


FIGURE 2-7 *A.* Risk factors and coronary heart disease risk. *B.* Complementary approaches to risk reduction. (From http://www.hoffmanpr.com/Press_Releases/Archived_Press_Releases/WHO/Cardio2002/CardioGraphs.ppt, used with permission.)

## CARDIOVASCULAR DISEASE PREVENTION IN THE UNITED STATES: CHALLENGE OF ETHNIC DISPARITIES

Numerous studies have unequivocally documented the existence of profound ethnic disparities in CVD care and outcome in the United States. Ethnic minorities, particularly African Americans, experience excess CVD morbidity and mortality and receive less diagnostic and therapeutic interventions than do their white counterparts.[27] For instance, since the 1980s CHD mortality has declined more slowly in black men and women than it did in their white counterparts. Disparities in cardiac testing and treatment have also been documented (see review in the Kaiser Family Foundation and American College of Cardiology Report).[208] From 1984 to 2001, 84 percent of the 81 studies reviewed observed ethnic disparities in care for at least one minority group.[208] African Americans have been the most intensively investigated minority group; the vast majority of studies find that African Americans are less likely to undergo diagnostic catheterization (odds ratios 0.23 to 0.85), percutaneous transluminal coronary angioplasty (odds ratios 0.20 to 0.87), coronary artery bypass graft

TABLE 2-8 **Global Efforts to Prevent CVD**

| Key Reports/Programs | Essential Features |
|---|---|
| The Institute of Medicine Report, 1998[191] | • U.S. National Academy of Sciences recommendations on the control of international cardiovascular disease (CVD).<br>• Research to fully determine the magnitude of CVD in developing countries, the development of targeted primary prevention strategies, reduction in tobacco use, control of hypertension, access to low-cost drugs, and the development of affordable clinical care algorithms.<br>• Build capacity to conduct research and development activities.<br>• Develop institutional frameworks that would facilitate CVD prevention and control. |
| World Heart Forum[195] | • International coalition to confront global cardiovascular issues (American Heart Association is founding member).<br>• Conduct research to better understand the epidemiology of CVD in various regions of the world and to more accurately track its toll in terms of death, disability, and health care costs.<br>• Development of prevention guidelines to identify common principles for lowering CVD risk, while at the same time providing flexibility to address regional differences (e.g., it is expected that, in some countries or regions of the world, tobacco use and hypertension may take precedence, whereas cholesterol reduction or weight control may be of primary importance in others).<br>• Development of programs to assist medical schools in establishing core curricula that focus on the prevention of CVD.<br>• Advocacy initiatives that address regional issues of tobacco, exercise, nutrition, and access to care. |
| CVD Research Initiative[194] | • Joint program of World Health Organization and the Global Forum for Health Research.<br>• Initiative has developed six multicenter collaborative research projects on capacity assessment, surveillance, community-based interventions, clinical management, and global information networks. |
| WHO Programs for Disease Surveillance (STEPS) | • Based on the concept that CVD surveillance systems need to be simple, focusing on a minimum number of risk factors that predict disease, before placing too much emphasis on costly disease registers that are difficult to sustain long-term.<br>• Step 1 gathers information on risk factors by questionnaires. This includes information on sociodemographic features, tobacco use, alcohol consumption, physical inactivity, and fruit/vegetable intake.<br>• Step 2 includes objective data by simple physical measurements needed to examine risk factors that are physiologic attributes of the human body. These are height, weight, and waist circumference (for obesity) and blood pressure.<br>• Step 3 carries the objective measurements of physiologic attributes one step further with the inclusion of blood samples for measuring lipid and glucose levels.<br>• STEPS is now being planned or implemented in 33 countries. |
| WHO Programs for CHOosing Interventions that are Cost-Effective (CHOICE) | • First-ever system of identifying and reporting cost-effective health interventions consistently across settings.<br>• These interventions can be implemented on an à la carte basis, depending on each country's individual circumstances.<br>• CHOICE options are contained in a new statistical database that is also a part of the World Health Report 2002. |
| INTER-HEART[194] | • Global case-control study that seeks to understand the importance of both traditional and emerging risk factors for acute myocardial infarction.<br>• Findings will be relevant for developing health policies that can be applied to different countries and ethnic groups. |
| CARMEN[193] | • The Pan American Health Organization (PAHO) is promoting CARMEN (Spanish acronym for: Actions for the Multifactorial Reduction of Noncommunicable Diseases) as a general framework for the prevention and control of noncommunicable diseases, particularly CVD, in the Americas by coordinating health promotion and disease prevention activities in communities and community health services.<br>• This model includes the identification of risk factors, regional surveillance using a common methodology, early detection of cases, delivery of comprehensive and long-term care, and more active participation of all members of the health team and the community.<br>• Management of hypertension and diabetes are particularly important in the model. |

(*Continued*)

TABLE 2-8 Continued

| | |
|---|---|
| CINDI[193] | • In Europe, the Countrywide Integrated Noncommunicable Diseases Intervention (CINDI) program aims to reduce modifiable risk factors, such as smoking and high blood pressure, by integrating health promotion and disease prevention; at present, 27 countries participate.<br>• Two other programs also aim to improve the quality of life of people with CVD: (1) The Helsingborg Declaration on stroke management. (2) The second program is a pilot project aimed at improving the education skills of general practitioners by showing them how to educate coronary heart disease patients about improving the quality of their lives, and how rehabilitation and secondary prevention can be improved. |
| Prevention of REcurrences of Myocardial Infarction and StrokE Study (PREMISE) | • The PREMISE is a jont WHO-Welcome trust program aimed at using community and health services-based interventions to prevent recurrences of CVD. |
| SHARE (200) | • Investigators at the McMaster University have just completed SHARE (Study of Health Assessment and Risk in Ethnic groups), in which atherosclerosis, clinical CVD, and traditional and emerging risk factors were measured in 997 randomly chosen individuals of 3 ethnic groups (South Asian, Chinese, and European Canadian).<br>• Preliminary data indicate marked differences in lipid profile, glucose abnormalities, coagulation parameters, and homocysteine levels between the 3 groups. Although within each ethnic group the degree of carotid atherosclerosis predicted clinical CVD, the relationship varied (steepest among South Asians, least steep among Chinese, intermediate among European Canadians). |

Adapted in part from the World Health Report 2000.[5]

(odds ratios 0.26 to 0.68), and thrombolytic therapy (odds ratios 0.51 to 0.76). The report concludes that these disparities persist after controlling for clinical and socioeconomic factors.[208]

The pathogenesis of ethnic disparities in CVD morbidity and mortality in the United States is highly complex, multifactorial, and likely due to a mix of patient, provider, health care systems, and societal issues. Skepticism has emerged that genetic "racial" differences will explain most ethnic disparities. Investigators have noted that race is a social construct as opposed to a meaningful genetic determination.[209] The increased burden of CVD risk factors experienced by ethnic minorities[210] undoubtedly contributes to ethnic disparities in CVD outcomes, but begs the question of why such profound inequalities in risk factor burden exist. Diminished access to health care, insurance, and ability to pay also contribute to worse treatment and control of CVD risk factors and less utilization of diagnostic and therapeutic interventions.[211] But undertreatment of CVD risk factors exists even when individuals have health insurance.[212] Yet another possible explanation is patient preference. The Institute of Medicine was charged by the U.S. Congress to examine the extent of ethnic disparities in health care. After reviewing the literature, the authors found that patient preference or treatment refusal is an unlikely explanation, because African Americans were only slightly more likely to reject recommended treatments (3 to 6 percent).[211] The Institute of Medicine report concluded that "some evidence suggests that bias, prejudice, and stereotyping on the part of health care providers may contribute to differences in care."[211] While the precise mix of factors causing the ethnic disparities remains unknown, consensus has emerged on the part of multiple organizations (American Heart Association, American College of Cardiology, and Kaiser Family Foundation)[27,208] and governmental agencies (The National Heart, Lung and Blood Institute and Centers for Disease Control and Prevention)[213] that to successfully decrease CVD morbidity and mortality in the twenty-first century ethnic disparities in CVD must be addressed with intensive research and programmatic efforts.

## CONCLUSIONS

CVD has no geographic, gender, or socioeconomic boundaries. The global burden of disease due to CVD is rising, principally due to a sharp rise in the developing countries that are experiencing rapid health transition. Contributory causes include the aging of the world population, lifestyle changes due to urbanization, progressive industrialization and burgeoning globalization, probable effects of fetal undernutrition on adult susceptibility to vascular disease, and possible gene–environment interactions influencing ethnic disparities. Altered diets and diminished physical activity are critical factors contributing to the acceleration of CVD epidemics, along with tobacco use. The prevalence of risk factors for CVD, however, varies across developing regions with consequent variations in the burden of CVD. The CVD epidemic in developing countries differs from that observed in developed countries in the last century by virtue of its rapidity, occurrence in a milieu of limited health care infrastructure, widespread poverty, and low levels of societal education. A global public health response must integrate policies and programs that effectively impact the multiple determinants of these diseases in a resource-sensitive and context-specific manner and provide protection over the life span through primordial, primary, and secondary prevention.

### References

1. Pearson TA. Cardiovascular disease in developing countries: Myths, realities, and opportunities. *Cardiovasc Drugs Ther* 1999;13(2): 95–104.
2. Chockalingam A, Balaguer-Vinto I (eds). *Impending Global Pandemic of Cardiovascular Diseases: Challenges and Opportunities for the Prevention and Control of Cardiovascular Diseases in Developing Countries and Economies in Transition.* World Heart Federation. Barcelona: Prous Science; 1999.

3. Murray CJL, Lopez AD. Mortality by cause for eight regions of the world: Global Burden of Disease Study. *Lancet* 1997;349(9061): 1269–1276.
4. Bonow RO, Smaha LA, Smith SC Jr, et al. World Heart Day 2002: The International Burden of Cardiovascular Disease: Responding to the Emerging Global Epidemic. *Circulation* 2002;106(13):1602–1605.
5. World Health Organization. The World Health Report 2002: Reducing risks, promoting healthy life. Geneva: WHO; 2002.
6. Omran AR. The epidemiologic transition: A key of the epidemiology of population change. *Millbank Memorial Fund Q* 1971;49:509–538.
7. Sen K, Bonita R. Global health status: Two steps forward, one step back. *Lancet* 2000;356:577–582.
8. Bloom DE, Williamson JG. Demographic transitions and economic miracles in emerging Asia. *World Bank Econ Rev* 1998;12(3):419–455.
9. Drewnowski A, Popkin BM. The nutrition transition: New trends in the global diet. *Nutr Rev* 1997;55(2):31–43.
10. Popkin BM, Popkin BM, Lu B, Zhai F. Understanding the nutrition transition: Measuring rapid dietary changes in transitional countries. *Public Health Nutr* 2002;5(6A):947–953.
11. Lang T. The public health impact of globalisation of food trade. In: Shetty PS, McPherson K (eds.). *Diet, Nutrition and Chronic Disease: Lessons From Contrasting Worlds.* Chichester, UK: Wiley; 1997:173–187.
12. Chopra M, Galbraith S, Darnton-Hill I. A global response to a global problem: The epidemic of overnutrition. *Bull World Health Organ* 2002;80(12):952–958.
13. Diet, nutrition and the prevention of chronic diseases: Report of a joint WHO/FAO expert consultation. WHO Technical Report Series 916. Geneva: WHO; 2002.
14. Reddy KS, Yusuf S. Emerging epidemic of cardiovascular disease in developing countries. *Circulation* 1998;97(6):596–601.
15. Janus ED, Postiglione A, Singh RB, Lewis B. The Modernization of Asia: Implications for Coronary Heart Disease. *Circulation* 1996; 94(11):2671.
16. Reddy KS. Cardiovascular diseases in the developing countries: Dimensions, determinants, dynamics and directions for public health action. *Public Health Nutr* 2002;5(1A):231–237.
17. Murray CJ, Lopez AD. The Global Burden of Disease: A Comprehensive Assessment of Mortality and Disability From Disease, Injuries and Risk Factors in 1990 and Projected to 2020. Cambridge, Mass: Harvard School of Public Health, 1996.
18. World Health Organization. *The World Health Report 2000: Health Systems: Improving Performance.* Geneva: WHO; 2000.
19. Murray CJ, Lopez AD. Global Health Statistics. Cambridge: Harvard University Press, 1996.
20. Murray CJ, Lopez AD, Mathers CD, Stein C. The Global Burden of Disease 2000 project: Aims, methods and data sources. GPE Discussion Paper No. 36, 2001. Geneva: WHO; 2001.
21. International Cardiovascular Disease Statistics. 2003. Dallas: Texas; American Heart Association. Available at http://www.americanheart.org/downloadable/heart/1043250000063IntStats2003.pdf, accessed May 2003.
22. Barker DJP. Fetal origins of coronary heart disease. *BMJ* 1995; 311(6998):171.
23. World Health Report 1999. Making a difference. Geneva: WHO; 1999.
24. American Heart Association. Heart Disease and Stroke Statistics—2003 Update. Dallas Texas: American Heart Association; 2002, 31.
25. Decline in Deaths From Heart Disease and Stroke—United States, 1900–1999. *JAMA* 1999;282(8):724.
26. Achievements in Public Health, 1900–1999: Decline in deaths from heart disease and stroke—United States, 1900–1999. *MMWR Morb Mortal Wkly Rep* 1999;48(30):649.
27. Cooper R, Cutler J, Desvigne-Nickens P, et al. Trends and disparities in coronary heart disease, stroke, and other cardiovascular diseases in the United States: Findings of the National Conference on Cardiovascular Disease Prevention. *Circulation* 2000;102(25):3137.
28. Grundy SM. Primary prevention of coronary heart disease: Integrating risk assessment with intervention. *Circulation* 1999;100(9):988–998.
29. Grundy SM, D'Agostino S, Mosca L, et al. Cardiovascular risk assessment based on US cohort studies: Findings from a National Heart, Lung, and Blood Institute Workshop. *Circulation* 2001;104(4):491.
30. Neaton JD, Wentworth D. Serum cholesterol, blood pressure, cigarette smoking, and death from coronary heart disease. Overall findings and differences by age for 316,099 white men. Multiple Risk Factor Intervention Trial Research Group. *Arch Intern Med*1992;152(1):56–64.
31. Tunstall-Pedoe H, Woodward M, Tavendale R, et al. Comparison of the prediction by 27 different factors of coronary heart disease and death in men and women of the Scottish heart health study: Cohort study. *BMJ* 1997;315(7110):722–729.
32. MacMahon S, Peto R, Cutler J, et al. Blood pressure, stroke, and coronary heart disease. Part 1, Prolonged differences in blood pressure: Prospective observational studies corrected for the regression dilution bias. *Lancet* 1990;335(8692):765–774.
33. Magnus P, Beaglehole R. The Real Contribution of the Major Risk Factors to the Coronary Epidemics: Time to End the "Only-50%" Myth. *Arch Intern Med* 2001;161(22):2657.
34. Stamler J, Stamler R, Neaton JD. Blood pressure, systolic and diastolic, and cardiovascular risks. US population data. *Arch Intern Med* 1993;153(5):598–615.
35. Stamler J, Stamler R, Neaton JD, et al. Low risk-factor profile and long-term cardiovascular and noncardiovascular mortality and life expectancy: Findings for 5 large cohorts of young adult and middle-aged men and women. *JAMA* 1999;282(21):2012.
36. van den Hoogen PC, Feskens EJ, Nagelkerke NJ, et al. The relation between blood pressure and mortality due to coronary heart disease among men in different parts of the world. Seven Countries Study Research Group. *N Engl J Med* 2000;342(1):1–8.
37. Wilson PW, D'Agostino RB, Levy D, et al. Prediction of coronary heart disease using risk factor categories. *Circulation* 1998;97(18):1837–1847.
38. Wilson PW, D'Agostino RB, Sullivan L, et al. Overweight and obesity as determinants of cardiovascular risk: the Framingham experience. *Arch Intern Med* 2002;162(16):1867–1872.
39. Durrington PN, Prais H. Methods for the prediction of coronary heart disease risk. *Heart* 2001;85(5):489–490.
40. Jones AF, Walker J, Jewkes C, et al. Comparative accuracy of cardiovascular risk prediction methods in primary care patients. *Heart* 2001; 85(1):37–43.
41. WHO MONICA Project Principal Investigators. Monitoring trends and determinants in cardiovascular disease: A major international collaboration. *J Clin Epidemiol* 1988;41:105–114.
42. Keil U, Kuulasmaa K. WHO MONICA Project: Risk factors. *Int J Epidemiol* 1989;18(3 suppl 1):S46–S55.
43. Evans A, Tolonen H, Hense HW, et al. Trends in coronary risk factors in the WHO MONICA Project. *Int J Epidemiol* 2001;30(90001):35S.
44. Kuulasmaa K, Tunstall-Pedoe H, Dobson A, et al. Estimation of contribution of changes in classic risk factors to trends in coronary-event rates across the WHO MONICA Project populations. *Lancet* 2000; 355:675–687.
45. Tunstall-Pedoe H, Vanuzzo D, Hobbs M, et al. Estimation of contribution of changes in coronary care to improving survival, event rates, and coronary heart disease mortality across the WHO MONICA Project populations. *Lancet* 2000;355:688–700.
46. Kannel WB, Abbott RD. Incidence and prognosis of unrecognized myocardial infarction. An update on the Framingham study. *N Engl J Med* 1984;311(18):1144–1147.
47. Sheifer SE, Manolio TA, Gersh BJ. Unrecognized myocardial infarction. *Ann Intern Med* 2001;135(9):801–811.
48. Sigurdsson E, Thorgeirsson G, Sigvaldason H, Sigfusson N. Unrecognized myocardial infarction: Epidemiology, clinical characteristics, and the prognostic role of angina pectoris. The Reykjavik Study. *Ann Intern Med* 1995;122(2):96–102.
49. Lloyd-Jones DM, Larson MG, Beiser A, Levy D. Lifetime risk of developing coronary heart disease. *Lancet* 1999;353(9147):89–92.
50. Cholesterol, diastolic blood pressure, and stroke: 13,000 strokes in 450,000 people in 45 prospective cohorts. Prospective studies collaboration. *Lancet* 1995;346(8991–8992):1647–1653.

51. Goldstein LB, Adams R, Becker K, et al. Primary prevention of ischemic stroke: A statement for healthcare professionals from the Stroke Council of the American Heart Association. *Stroke* 2001;32(1):280.
52. Jeerakathil TJ, Wolf PA. Prevention of strokes. *Curr Atheroscler Rep* 2001;3(4):321–327.
53. Stroke and Coronary Heart Disease Collaborative Research Group E. Blood pressure, cholesterol, and stroke in eastern Asia. *Lancet* 1998; 352(9143):1801–1807.
54. D'Agostino RB, Wolf PA, Belanger AJ, Kannel WB. Stroke risk profile: Adjustment for antihypertensive medication. The Framingham Study. *Stroke* 1994;25(1):40–43.
55. Kalache A, Aboderin I. Stroke: The global burden. *Health Policy Plan* 1995;10(1):1–21.
56. Tolonen H, Mahonen M, Asplund K, et al. Do trends in population levels of blood pressure and other cardiovascular risk factors explain trends in stroke event rates? Comparisons of 15 populations in 9 countries within the WHO MONICA Stroke Project. *Stroke* 2002;33(10):2367.
57. Gillum RF, Sempos CT. The end of the long-term decline in stroke mortality in the United States? *Stroke* 1997;28(8):1527.
58. Howard G, Howard VJ, Katholi C, et al. The decline in stroke mortality: An analysis of temporal patterns by gender, ethnicity, and geographic region. Paper presented at the National Conference on CVD Prevention, September 27–29, 1999. Bethesda, Md: 2003.
59. He J, Ogden LG, Bazzano LA, et al. Risk factors for congestive heart failure in US men and women: NHANES I Epidemiologic Follow-up Study. *Arch Intern Med* 2001;161(7):996.
60. Kannel WB, Ho K, Thom T. Changing epidemiological features of cardiac failure. *Br Heart J* 1994;72(2 suppl):S3–S9.
61. Kenchaiah S, Evans JC, Levy D, et al. Obesity and the risk of heart failure. *N Engl J Med* 2002;347:305–313.
62. Levy D, Larson MG, Vasan RS, et al. The progression from hypertension to congestive heart failure. *JAMA* 1996;275(20):1557–1562.
63. McMurray JJ, Stewart S. Epidemiology, aetiology, and prognosis of heart failure, *Heart* 2000;83(5):596–602.
64. Wilhelmsen L, Rosengren A, Eriksson H, Lappas G. Heart failure in the general population of men—morbidity, risk factors and prognosis. *J Intern Med* 2001;249(3):253–261.
65. Kannel WB, D'Agostino RB, Silbershatz H, et al. Profile for estimating risk of heart failure. *Arch Intern Med* 1999;159(11): 1197–1204.
66. McMurray JJ, Petrie MC, Murdoch DR, Davie AP. Clinical epidemiology of heart failure: Public and private health burden. *Eur Heart J* 1998;19(suppl P):9–16.
67. Bonneux L, Barendregt JJ, Meeter K, et al. Estimating clinical morbidity due to ischemic heart disease and congestive heart failure: The future rise of heart failure. *Am J Public Health* 1994;84(1):20–28.
68. Levy D, Kenchaiah S, Larson MG, et al. Long-term trends in the incidence of and survival with heart failure. *N Engl J Med* 2002;347(18): 1397.
69. Yancy CW. Heart failure in blacks: Etiologic and epidemiologic differences. *Curr Cardiol Rep* 2001;3(3):191–197.
70. Vasan RS, Benjamin EJ, Levy D. Prevalence, clinical features and prognosis of diastolic heart failure: An epidemiologic perspective. *J Am Coll Cardiol* 1995;26(7):1565–1574.
71. Vasan RS, Larson MG, Benjamin EJ, et al. Congestive heart failure in subjects with normal versus reduced left ventricular ejection fraction: Prevalence and mortality in a population-based cohort. *J Am Coll Cardiol* 1999;33(7):1948–1955.
72. Lloyd-Jones DM, Larson MG, Leip EP, et al. Lifetime risk for developing congestive heart failure: The Framingham Heart Study. *Circulation* 2002;106(24):3068–3072.
73. Senni M, Tribouilloy CM, Rodeheffer RJ, et al. Congestive heart failure in the community: A study of all incident cases in Olmsted County, Minnesota, in 1991. *Circulation* 1998;98(21):2282–2289.
74. Benjamin EJ, Levy D, Vaziri SM, et al. Independent risk factors for atrial fibrillation in a population-based cohort. The Framingham Heart Study. *JAMA* 1994;271(11):840–844.
75. Psaty BM, Manolio TA, Kuller LH, et al. Incidence of and risk factors for atrial fibrillation in older adults. *Circulation* 1997;96(7):2455.
76. Vaziri SM, Larson MG, Benjamin EJ, Levy D. Echocardiographic predictors of nonrheumatic atrial fibrillation. The Framingham Heart Study. *Circulation* 1994;89(2):724–730.
77. Chowdhury KS, Siddiqui MN. Etiological pattern of atrial fibrillation. *Mymensingh Med J* 2002;11(2):100–103.
78. Shatoor AS, Ahmed ME, Said MA, et al. Patterns of atrial fibrillation at a regional hospital in Saudi Arabia. *Ethn Dis* 1998;8(3): 360–366.
79. Ryder KM, Benjamin EJ. Epidemiology and significance of atrial fibrillation. *Am J Cardiol* 1999;84(9A):131R–138R.
80. Go AS, Hylek EM, Phillips KA, et al. Prevalence of diagnosed atrial fibrillation in adults: National implications for rhythm management and stroke prevention: The AnTicoagulation and Risk Factors in Atrial Fibrillation (ATRIA) Study. *JAMA* 2001;285(18):2370–2375.
81. Nakayama T, Date C, Yokoyama T, et al. A 15.5-Year Follow-up Study of Stroke in a Japanese Provincial City: The Shibata Study. *Stroke* 1997;28(1):45.
82. Lip GYH, Bawden L, Hodson R, et al. Atrial fibrillation amongst the Indo-Asian general practice population: The West Birmingham Atrial Fibrillation Project. *Intern Cardiol* 1998;65(2):187–192.
83. Levy S, Maarek M, Coumel P, et al. Characterization of different subsets of atrial fibrillation in general practice in France: The ALFA Study. *Circulation* 1999;99(23):3028.
84. Wolf PA, Benjamin EJ, Belanger AJ, et al. Secular trends in the prevalence of atrial fibrillation: The Framingham Study. *Am Heart J* 1996;131(4):790–795.
85. Wang TJ, Larson MG, Lloyd-Jones DM, et al. The lifetime risk of atrial fibrillation: The Framingham Heart Study. *Circulation* 2002;106: II–456.
86. Wolf PA, Abbott RD, Kannel WB. Atrial fibrillation as an independent risk factor for stroke: the Framingham Study. *Stroke* 1991;22(8): 983–988.
87. Krahn AD, Manfreda J, Tate RB, et al. The natural history of atrial fibrillation: Incidence, risk factors, and prognosis in the Manitoba Follow-Up Study. *Am J Med* 1995;98(5):476–484.
88. Wang TJ, Larson MG, Levy D, et al. The temporal relations of atrial fibrillation and congestive heart failure and their joint influence on mortality: The Framingham Heart Study. *Circulation* 2003;107(23):2920–2925.
89. Gage BF, Waterman AD, Shannon W, et al. Validation of clinical classification schemes for predicting stroke: Results from the National Registry of Atrial Fibrillation. *JAMA* 2001;285(22):2864.
90. Wang TJ, Massaro JM, D'Agostino RB, et al. A Risk profile for stroke or death in atrial fibrillation: The Framingham Heart Study. *J Am Coll Cardiol* 2002;39:86A.
91. Benjamin EJ, Wolf PA, D'Agostino RB, et al. Impact of atrial fibrillation on the risk of death: The Framingham Heart Study. *Circulation* 1998;98(10):946.
92. Stewart S, Hart CL, Hole DJ, McMurray JJV. A population-based study of the long-term risks associated with atrial fibrillation: 20-year follow-up of the Renfrew/Paisley study. *Am J Med* 2002;113(5):359–364.
93. Wattigney WA, Mensah GA, Croft JB. Increased atrial fibrillation mortality: United States, 1980–1998. *Am J Epidemiol* 2002;155(9):819.
94. Collins R, Peto R, MacMahon S, et al. Blood pressure, stroke, and coronary heart disease. Part 2, Short-term reductions in blood pressure: overview of randomised drug trials in their epidemiological context. *Lancet* 1990;335(8693):827–838.
95. Vasan RS, Larson MG, Leip EP, et al. Impact of high-normal blood pressure on the risk of cardiovascular disease. *N Engl J Med* 2001; 345(18):1291–1297.
96. 2003 World Health Organization (WHO)/International Society of Hypertension (ISH) statement on management of hypertension. *J Hypertens* 2003;21(11):1983 1992.
97. Chobanian AV, Bakris GL, Black HR, et al. The Seventh Report of the Joint National Committee on Prevention, Detection, Evaluation, and Treatment of High Blood Pressure: The JNC 7 Report. *JAMA* 2003; 289:2560–2571.
98. Whelton PK, He J, Appel LJ, et al. Primary prevention of hypertension: Clinical and public health advisory from The National High Blood Pressure Education Program. *JAMA* 2002;288(15):1882–1888.

99. Vasan RS, Larson MG, Leip EP, et al. Assessment of frequency of progression to hypertension in non-hypertensive participants in the Framingham Heart Study: A cohort study. *Lancet* 2001;358(9294):1682–1686.
100. Fuentes R, Ilmaniemi N, Laurikainen E, et al. Hypertension in developing economies: A review of population-based studies carried out from 1980 to 1998. *J Hypertens* 2000;18(5):521–529.
101. Mensah GA. The global burden of hypertension: Good news and bad news. *Cardiol Clin* 2002;20(2):181–185.
102. Gu D, Reynolds K, Wu X, et al. Prevalence, awareness, treatment, and control of hypertension in China *Hypertension* 2002;40(6):920.
103. Ibrahim MM, Rizk H, Appel LJ, et al. Hypertension prevalence, awareness, treatment, and control in Egypt: Results from the Egyptian National Hypertension Project (NHP). *Hypertension* 1995;26(6):886.
104. Primatesta P, Brookes M, Poulter NR. Improved hypertension management and control: Results from the Health Survey for England 1998. *Hypertension* 2001;38(4):827.
105. Resengren A, Dotevall A, Eriksson H, Wilhelmsen L. Optimal risk factors in the population: Prognosis, prevalence, and secular trends. Data from Goteborg population studies. *Eur Heart J* 2001;22(2):136–144.
106. Pan WH, Chang HY, Yeh WT, et al. Prevalence, awareness, treatment and control of hypertension in Taiwan: Results of Nutrition and Health Survey in Taiwan (NAHSIT) 1993–1996. *J Hum Hypertens* 2001; 15(11):793–798.
107. Wolf HK, Tuomilehto J, Kuulasmaa K, et al. Blood pressure levels in the 41 populations of the WHO MONICA Project. *J Hum Hypertens* 1997;11(11):733–742.
108. Wu Z, Yao C, Zhao D, et al. Sino-MONICA Project: A collaborative study on trends and determinants in cardiovascular diseases in China, Part I: Morbidity and mortality monitoring. *Circulation* 2001;103(3):462.
109. Burt VL, Whelton P, Roccella EJ, et al. Prevalence of hypertension in the US adult population: Results from the Third National Health and Nutrition Examination Survey,1988–1991. *Hypertension* 1995;25(3):305.
110. Vasan RS, Beiser A, Seshadri S, et al. Residual lifetime risk for developing hypertension in middle-aged women and men: The Framingham Heart Study. *JAMA* 2002;287(8):1003–1010.
111. Lewington S, Clarke R, Qizilbash, et al.—Prospective Studies Collaboration. Age-specific relevance of usual blood pressure to vascular mortality: a meta-analysis of individual data for one million adults in 61 prospective studies. *Lancet* 2002;360(9349):1903–1913.
112. Trends in aging—United States and worldwide. *MMWR Morb Mortal Wkly Rep* 2003;52(6):101–104, 106.
113. Jha P, Ranson MK, Nguyen SN, Yach D. Estimates of global and regional smoking prevalence in 1995, by age and sex. *Am J Public Health* 2002;92(6):1002.
114. Yang G, Fan L, Tan J, et al. Smoking in China: Findings of the 1996 National Prevalence Survey. *JAMA* 1999;282(13):1247.
115. Shimkhada R, Peabody JW. Tobacco control in India. *Bull World Health Organ* 2003;81(1):48–52.
116. Osler M, Prescott E, Gottschau A, et al. Trends in smoking prevalence in Danish adults, 1964–1994. The influence of gender, age, and education. *Scand J Soc Med* 1998;26(4):293–298.
117. Molarius A, Parsons RW, Dobson AJ, et al. Trends in cigarette smoking in 36 populations from the early 1980s to the mid-1990s: Findings from the WHO MONICA Project. *AM J Public Health* 2001;91(2):206.
118. Dobson AJ, Kuulasmaa K, Moltchanov V, et al. Changes in cigarette smoking among adults in 35 populations in the mid-1980s. *Tob Control* 1998;7(1):14.
119. Prevalence of current cigarette smoking among adults and changes in prevalence of current and some day smoking—United States, 1996–2001. *MMWR Morb Mortal Wkly Rep* 2003;52(14):303.
120. Peto R, Lopez AD, Boreham J, et al. Mortality from tobacco in developed countries: Indirect estimation from national vital statistics. *Lancet* 1992;339(8804):1268–1278.
121. Peto R, Lopez AD, Boreham J, et al. Mortality from smoking worldwide. *Br Med Bull* 1996;52(1):12.
122. Liu BQ, Peto R, Chen ZM, et al. Emerging tobacco hazards in China: 1. Retrospective proportional mortality study of one million deaths. *BMJ* 1998;317(7170):1411.
123. Niu SR, Yang GH, Chen ZM, et al. Emerging tobacco hazards in China: 2. Early mortality results from a prospective study. *BMJ* 1998; 317(7170):1423.
124. Yuan JM, Ross RK, Wang XL, et al. Morbidity and mortality in relation to cigarette smoking in Shanghai, China. A prospective male cohort study. *JAMA* 1996;275(21):1646–1650.
125. World development report 1993—Investing in health. New York: Oxford University Press for The World Bank; 1993.
126. Rosenberg L, Palmer JR, Shapiro S. Decline in the risk of myocardial infarction among women who stop smoking. *N Engl J Med* 1990; 322(4):213–217.
127. He J, Vupputuri S, Allen K, et al. Passive smoking and the risk of coronary heart disease—A meta-analysis of epidemiologic studies. *N Engl J Med* 1999;340(12):920.
128. Tobacco free initiative. 2003. Available at http://www5.who.int/tobacco/. Accessed May 2003.
129. WHO global strategy on diet, physical activity and health, 2003. Available at http://www.who.int/hpr/global.strategy.shtml. Accessed May 2003.
130. U.S. Department of Health and Human Services. *Physical Activity and Health: A Report of the Surgeon General.* Atlanta, GA: U.S. Department of Health and Human Services, Centers for Disease Control and Prevention, National Center for Chronic Disease Prevention and Health Promotion; 1996.
131. Physical activity trends—United States, 1990–1998. *MMWR Morb Mortal Wkly Rep* 2001;50(9):166–169.
132. Obesity: Preventing and managing the global epidemic. Report of a WHO Consultation on Obesity, Geneva, June 3–5, 1997. Geneva: World Health Organization; 1998.
133. *Clinical Guidelines on the Identification, Evaluation, and Treatment of Overweight and Obesity in Adults.* Bethesda, MD: National Institutes of Health; 1998. NIH Publication No. 98-4083.
134. Obesity: Preventing and managing the global epidemic. Report of a WHO Consultation on Obesity, Geneva, June 3–5, 1997. Geneva: World Health Organization; 1998.
135. James PT, Leach R, Kalamara E, Shayeghi M. The worldwide obesity epidemic. *Obes Res* 2001;9(90004):228S.
136. Molarius A, Seidell JC, Sans S, et al. Educational level, relative body weight, and changes in their association over 10 years: An international perspective from the WHO MONICA Project. *Am J Public Health* 2000;90(8):1260.
137. Ebbeling CB, Pawlak DB, Ludwig DS. Childhood obesity: Public-health crisis, common sense cure. *Lancet* 2002;360(9331):473–482.
138. Strauss RS, Pollack HA. Epidemic increase in childhood overweight, 1986–1998. *JAMA* 2001;286(22):2845–2848.
139. Torrance GM, Hooper MD, Reeder BA. Trends in overweight and obesity among adults in Canada (1970–1992): Evidence from national surveys using measured height and weight. *Int J Obes Relat Metab Disord* 2002;26(6):797–804.
140. McTigue KM, Garrett JM, Popkin BM. The natural history of the development of obesity in a cohort of young U.S. adults between 1981 and 1998. *Ann Intern Med* 2002;136(12):857–864.
141. Gordon-Larsen P, Adair LS, Popkin BM. The relationship of ethnicity, socioeconomic factors, and overweight in U.S. adolescents. *Obes Res* 2003;11(1):121.
142. Flegal KM, Carroll MD, Ogden CL, Johnson CL. Prevalence and trends in obesity among US adults, 1999–2000. *JAMA* 2002;288(14):1723.
143. Mokdad AH, Serdula MK, Dietz WH, et al. The continuing epidemic of obesity in the United States. *JAMA* 2000;284(13):1650–1651.
144. Ogden CL, Flegal KM, Carroll MD, Johnson CL. Prevalence and trends in overweight among US children and adolescents, 1999–2000. *JAMA* 2002;288(14):1728.
145. Ebrahim S, Smith GD. Systematic review of randomised controlled trials of multiple risk factor interventions for preventing coronary heart disease. *BMJ* 1997;314(7095):1666.
146. Diabetes Prevention Program Research Group. Reduction in the incidence of type 2 diabetes with lifestyle intervention or metformin. *N Engl J Med* 2002;346(6):393.

147. Esposito K, Pontillo A, Di Palo C, et al. Effect of weight loss and lifestyle changes on vascular inflammatory markers in obese women: A randomized trial. *JAMA* 2003;289(14):1799.
148. Ford ES, Mokdad AH, Giles WH, Mensah GA. Serum total cholesterol concentrations and awareness, treatment, and control of hypercholesterolemia among US adults. Findings from the National Health and Nutrition Examination Survey, 1999 to 2000. *Circulation* 2003; 107(17):2185–2189.
149. King H, Aubert RE, Herman WH. Global burden of diabetes, 1995–2025: Prevalence, numerical estimates, and projections. *Diabetes Care* 1998;21(9):1414–1431.
150. The DECODE Study Group. Age- and sex-specific prevalences of diabetes and impaired glucose regulation in 13 european cohorts. *Diabetes Care* 2003;26(1):61–69.
151. Amos AF, McCarty DJ, Zimmet P. The rising global burden of diabetes and its complications: Estimates and projections to the year 2010. *Diabetes Med* 1997;14(suppl 5):S1–85.
152. Diabetes Fact sheets. 2003. Available at http://www.cdc.gov/diabetes/pubs/factsheet.htm Accessed May 2003.
153. Harris MI, Flegal KM, Cowie CC, et al. Prevalence of diabetes, impaired fasting glucose, and impaired glucose tolerance in U.S. adults. The Third National Health and Nutrition Examination Survey, 1988–1994. *Diabetes Care* 1998;21(4):518.
154. Type 2 diabetes in children and adolescents. American Diabetes Association. *Diabetes Care* 2000;23(3):381.
155. Burke JP, Williams K, Gaskill SP, et al. Rapid rise in the incidence of type 2 diabetes from 1987 to 1996: Results from the San Antonio Heart Study. *Arch Intern Med* 1999;159(13):1450.
156. Asia Pacific Cohort Studies Collaboration. The effects of diabetes on the risks of major cardiovascular diseases and death in the Asia-Pacific region. *Diabetes Care* 2003;26(2):360–366.
157. Executive Summary of The Third Report of The National Cholesterol Education Program (NCEP) Expert Panel on Detection, Evaluation, and Treatment of High Blood Cholesterol in Adults (Adult Treatment Panel III). *JAMA* 2001;285(19):2486–2497.
158. Alberti KG, Zimmet PZ. Definition, diagnosis and classification of diabetes mellitus and its complications. Part 1: Diagnosis and classification of diabetes mellitus provisional report of a WHO consultation. *Diabetes Med* 1998;15(7):539–553.
159. Abdul-Rahim HF, Husseini A, Bjertness E, et al. The metabolic syndrome in the West Bank population: An urban-rural comparison. *Diabetes Care* 2001;24(2):275.
160. Alvarez Leon EE, Ribas BL, Serra ML. [Prevalence of the metabolic syndrome in the population of Canary Islands, Spain]. *Med Clin (Barcelona)* 2003;120(5):172–174.
161. Balkau B, Charles MA, Drivsholm T, et al. Frequency of the WHO metabolic syndrome in European cohorts, and an alternative definition of an insulin resistance syndrome. *Diabetes Metab* 2002;28(5): 364–376.
162. Ford ES, Giles WH. A comparison of the prevalence of the metabolic syndrome using two proposed definitions. *Diabetes Care* 2003;26(3): 575.
163. Jia WP, Xiang KS, Chen L, et al. Epidemiological study on obesity and its comorbidities in urban Chinese older than 20 years of age in Shanghai, China. *Obes Rev* 2002;3(3):157–165.
164. Lakka HM, Laaksonen DE, Lakka TA, et al. The metabolic syndrome and total and cardiovascular disease mortality in middle-aged men. *JAMA* 2002;288(21):2709.
165. Park YW, Zhu S, Palaniappan L, et al. The metabolic syndrome: Prevalence and associated risk factor findings in the US population from the Third National Health and Nutrition Examination Survey, 1988–1994. *Arch Intern Med* 2003;163(4):427.
166. Vanhala MJ, Kumpusalo EA, Pitkajarvi TK, Takala JK. Metabolic syndrome in a middle-aged Finnish population. *J Cardiovasc Risk* 1997;4(4):291–295.
167. Zimmet PZ, McCarty DJ, de Courten MP. The global epidemiology of non-insulin-dependent diabetes mellitus and the metabolic syndrome. *J Diabetes Complications* 1997;11(2):60–68.
168. Ford ES, Giles WH, Dietz WH. Prevalence of the metabolic syndrome among US adults: Findings from the Third National Health and Nutrition Examination Survey. *JAMA* 2002;287(3):356.
169. Trevisan M, Liu J, Bahsas FB, Menotti A. Syndrome X and mortality: A population-based study. Risk Factor and Life Expectancy Research Group. *AM J Epidemiol* 1998;148(10):958.
170. Isomaa B, Almgren P, Tuomi T, et al. Cardiovascular morbidity and mortality associated with the metabolic syndrome. *Diabetes Care* 2001;24(4):683.
171. Grundy SM. Obesity, metabolic syndrome, and coronary atherosclerosis. *Circulation* 2002;105(23):2696.
172. Resnick HE, Jones K, Ruotolo G, et al. Insulin resistance, the metabolic syndrome, and risk of incident cardiovascular disease in nondiabetic American Indians: The Strong Heart Study. *Diabetes Care* 2003;26(3):861.
173. Libby P, Ridker PM, Maseri A. Inflammation and atherosclerosis. *Circulation* 2002;105(9):1135.
174. Ford ES, Giles WH, Myers GL, Mannino DM. Population distribution of high-sensitivity C-reactive protein among US men: Findings from National Health and Nutrition Examination Survey, 1999–2000. *Clin Chem* 2003;49(4):686.
175. Ridker PM, Rifai N, Rose L, et al. Comparison of C-reactive protein and low-density lipoprotein cholesterol levels in the prediction of first cardiovascular events. *N Engl J Med* 2002;347(20):1557.
176. Pearson TA, Mensah GA, Alexander RW, et al. Markers of inflammation and cardiovascular disease: Application to clinical and public health practice. A statement for Healthcare Professionals from the Centers for Disease Control and Prevention and the American Heart Association. *Circulation* 2003;107(3):499.
177. Jacques PF, Bostom AG, Wilson PW, et al. Determinants of plasma total homocysteine concentration in the Framingham Offspring cohort. *Am J Clin Nutr* 2001;73(3):613–621.
178. Jacques PF, Rosenberg IH, Rogers G, et al. Serum total homocysteine concentrations in adolescent and adult Americans: Results from the third National Health and Nutrition Examination Survey. *Am J Clin Nutr* 1999;69(3):482–489.
179. Nygard O, Refsum H, Ueland PM, Vollset SE. Major lifestyle determinants of plasma total homocysteine distribution: the Hordaland Homocysteine Study. *Am J Clin Nutr* 1998;67(2):263.
180. Saw SM, Yuan JM, Ong CN, et al. Genetic, dietary, and other lifestyle determinants of plasma homocysteine concentrations in middle-aged and older Chinese men and women in Singapore. *Am J Clin Nutr* 2001;73(2):232.
181. Ganji V, Kafai MR. Demographic, health, lifestyle, and blood vitamin determinants of serum total homocysteine concentrations in the third National Health and Nutrition Examination Survey, 1988–1994. *Am J Clin Nutr* 2003;77(4):826.
182. Chandalia M, Abate N, Cabo-Chan AV Jr, et al. Hyperhomocysteinemia in Asian Indians living in the United States. *J Clin Endocrinol Metab* 2003;88(3):1089.
183. Homocysteine Studies Collaboration. Homocysteine and risk of ischemic heart disease and stroke: A meta-analysis. *JAMA* 2002; 288(16):2015.
184. Wald DS, Law M, Morris JK. Homocysteine and cardiovascular disease: Evidence on causality from a meta-analysis. *BMJ* 2002; 325(7374):1202.
185. Malinow MR, Bostom AG, Krauss RM. Homocysteine, diet, and cardiovascular diseases: A statement for healthcare professionals from the Nutrition Committee, American Heart Association. *Circulation* 1999; 99(1):178–182.
186. Beaglehole R, Saracci R, Panico S. Editorial—Cardiovascular diseases: Causes, surveillance and prevention. *Int J Epidemiol* 2001; 30(90001):1S.
187. Rose G. Sick individuals and sick populations. *Int J Epidemiol* 1985;14(1):32–38.
188. Benjamin EJ, Smith J, Cooper RS, et al. Task Force #1—magnitude of the prevention problem: Opportunities and challenges. *J Am Coll Cardiol* 2002;40(4):588–603.

189. Arnett DK, McGovern PG, Jacobs DR Jr, et al. Fifteen-year trends in cardiovascular risk factors (1980–1982 through 1995–1997): The Minnesota Heart Survey. *Am J Epidemiol* 2002;156(10):929.
190. Writing Group of the PREMIER Collaborative Research Group. Effects of comprehensive lifestyle modification on blood pressure control: Main results of the PREMIER clinical trial. *JAMA* 2003; 289(16):2083.
191. Howson CP, Reddy KS, Ryan TJ, Bale JR. *Control of Cardiovascular Diseases in Developing Countries. Research, Development and Institutional Strengthening.* Washington, DC: Institute of Medicine, National Academy Press; 1998.
192. Integrated management of cardiovascular risk: Report of a WHO meeting, Geneva, July 9–12 2002. Geneva: WHO; 2003.
193. Regional activities to the global CVD strategy. 2003. Available at http://www5.who.int/cardiovascular-diseases/main.cfm?p=0000000464. Accessed May 2003.
194. Research and global partnership initiatives. 2003. Available at http://www5.who.int/cardiovascular-diseases/main.cfm?p=0000000463. Accessed May 2003.
195. Bayes de Luna A. International cooperation in world cardiology: The role of the World Heart Federation. *Circulation* 1999;99(8):986.
196. Michaud CM, Murray CJL, Bloom BR. Burden of disease—Implications for future research. *JAMA* 2001;285(5):535.
197. Pearson TA, Smith SC Jr, Poole-Wilson P. Cardiovascular specialty societies and the emerging global burden of cardiovascular disease: A call to action. *Circulation* 1998;97(6):602–604.
198. Yusuf S, Reddy S, Ounpuu S, Anand S. Global burden of cardiovascular diseases: Part II: Variations in cardiovascular disease by specific ethnic groups and geographic regions and prevention strategies. *Circulation* 2001;104(23):2855–2864.
199. Yusuf S, Reddy S, Ounpuu S, Anand S. Global burden of cardiovascular diseases: Part I: General considerations, the epidemiologic transition, risk factors, and impact of urbanization. *Circulation* 2001; 104(22):2746–2753.
200. Anand SS, Yusuf S, Vuksan V, et al. Differences in risk factors, atherosclerosis, and cardiovascular disease between ethnic groups in Canada: The Study of Health Assessment and Risk in Ethnic groups (SHARE). *Lancet* 2000;356(9226):279–284.
201. Indications for ACE inhibitors in the early treatment of acute myocardial infarction: Systematic overview of individual data from 100,000 patients in randomized trials. *Circulation* 1998;97(22):2202.
202. Antithrombotic Trialists' Collaboration. Collaborative meta-analysis of randomised trials of antiplatelet therapy for prevention of death, myocardial infarction, and stroke in high risk patients. *BMJ* 2002; 324(7329):71.
203. Murray CJ, Lauer JA, Hutubessy RC, et al. Effectiveness and costs of interventions to lower systolic blood pressure and cholesterol: A global and regional analysis on reduction of cardiovascular-disease risk. *Lancet* 2003;361(9359):717–725.
204. Rodgers A, Lawes C, MacMahon S. Reducing the global burden of blood pressure-related cardiovascular disease. *J Hypertens Suppl* 2000;18(1):S3–S6.
205. Staessen JA, Wang JG, Thijs L. Cardiovascular protection and blood pressure reduction: A meta-analysis. *Lancet* 2001;358(9290): 1305–1315.
206. Gould AL, Rossouw JE, Santanello NC, et al. Cholesterol reduction yields clinical benefit: Impact of statin trials. *Circulation* 1998;97(10): 946.
207. LaRosa JC, He J, Vupputuri S. Effect of statins on risk of coronary disease: A meta-analysis of randomized controlled trials. *JAMA* 1999; 282(24):2340.
208. Racial/Ethnic differences in cardiac care. Henry J. Kaiser Family Foundation and the American College of Cardiology. Available at http://www.kff.org/content/2002-20021009c/6042v2.pdf. Accessed May 2003.
209. Cooper RS, Kaufman JS, Ward R. Race and genomics. *N Engl J Med* 2003;348(12):1166.
210. Winkleby MA, Kraemer HC, Ahn DK, Varady AN. Ethnic and socioeconomic differences in cardiovascular disease risk factors: Findings for women from the Third National Health and Nutrition Examination Survey, 1988–1994. *JAMA* 1998;280(4):356.
211. Institute of Medicine. Unequal treatment: Understanding racial and ethnic disparities in health. National Academy Press, 2002. Available at http://www.iom.edu/iom/iomhome.nsf/WFiles/Disparitieshcproviders8pgFINAL/$file/Disparitieshcproviders8pgFINAL.pdf Accessed on May 2003.
212. Hyman DJ, Pavlik VN. Characteristics of patients with uncontrolled hypertension in the United States. *N Engl J Med* 2001;345(7):479.
213. National Heart, Lung and Blood Institute Strategy for Addressing Health Disparities FY 2002–2006. National Heart, Lung, and Blood Institute, 2002. Available at http://www.nhlbi.nih.gov/resources/docs/plandisp.htm. Accessed May 2003.


## Web Sources

**American Heart Association**
http://www.americanheart.org/
Heart Disease and Stroke Facts 2003:
http://www.americanheart.org/downloadable/heart/10461207852142003HDSStatsBook.pdf
International statistics:
http://www.americanheart.org/downloadable/heart/1043250000063IntStats2003.pdf

**British Heart Foundation–Coronary Heart Disease Statistics**
http://www.bhf.org.uk/professionals/index.asp?secondlevel=519
This site includes European CVD statistics.

**(Canadian) Cardiovascular Disease Surveillance Online**
http://dsol_smed.hc.gc.ca/dsol_smed/cvd/index_e.html
Health Canada provides this site on CVD statistics for Canada. See also:

**Center for Disease Control**
http://www.cdc.gov/nchs/

**Changing Face of Heart Disease and Stroke in Canada, The**
http://www.hc-sc.gc.ca/hpb/lcdc/bcrdd/hdsc2000/index.html

**Centers for Disease Control (CDC)–Cardiovascular Health–International Information**
http://www.cdc.gov/cvh/library/international_resources.htm
This page includes links to CDC affiliated publications and international CVD projects.

**European Society of Cardiology**
http://www.escardio.org/

**Eurostat**
http://europa.eu.int/en/comm/eurostat/eurostat.html

**G8 Promoting Heart Health**
http://www.med.mun.ca/g8hearthealth/pages/enter.htm

**Global Cardiology Network**
http://www.globalcardiology.org/

**Global Cardiovascular Infobase**
http://cvdinfobase.ca/

**Global Health.gov–World Health Statistics**
http://www.globalhealth.gov/worldhealthstatistics.shtml

**Heart and Stroke Foundation of Canada**
http://www.heartandstroke.ca
This site includes Canadian CVD statistics.

**Institute for International Health–Global Burden of Disease**
http://www.iih.org/about/burden.html

**International Burden of Disease Network**
http://www.ibdn.net/

**International Task Force for Prevention of Coronary Disease**
http://www.chd-taskforce.de/

**LAC Health Accounts**
http://www.lachealthaccounts.org/en/webguide.php

***Morbidity and Mortality Weekly Report (MMWR)* International Bulletins**
http://www.cdc.gov/mmwr/international/world.html

**PAHO Pan American Health Organization**
http://www.paho.org/Project.asp?SEL=HD&LNG=ENG&CD=HTREN
**ProCOR Conference on Cardiovascular Health**
http://procor.org/
**UNICEF–Statistical Data**
http://www.unicef.org/statis/
**World Health Organization Web Site**
www.who.int/cardiovascular_diseases/en/
**World Health Organization Burden of Disease Web site**
www3.who.int/whosis/menu.cfm?path=evidence,burden
Detailed tables for DALYs subregion, cause, sex and age group are available at this website.
**World Health Organization (WHO) Publications–Cardiovascular Diseases**
http://www.who.int/cardiovascular_diseases/resources/publications/en/
This page includes links to WHO MONICA Project information.
**World Health report, 2002**
http://www.who.int/whr/en/
Supplementary data on:
http://www.hoffmanpr.com/Press_Releases/Archived_Press_Releases/WHO/Cardio2002/CardioGraphs.ppt
**World Federation of Public Health Associations**
http://www.apha.org/wfpha/about_wfpha.htm
**World Health Reports**
http://www.who.int/whr/previous/en/
**World Heart Federation–White Book**
http://www.worldheart.org/publications/intro.asp
This site gives information on how to order the White Book on Cardiovascular Diseases.
**World Heart Day (from World Heart Federation, WHO, UNESCO)**
http://www.worldheartday.com/index.asp
**United Nations Population Fund (UNFPA)**
http://www.unfpa.org/
**United Nations, Department of Economic and Social Affairs–Statistical Division**
http://unstats.un.org/unsd/methods/inter-natlinks/sd_intstat.htm

CHAPTER 3

# FUNCTIONAL ANATOMY OF THE HEART

Joseph F. Malouf / William D. Edwards / A. Jamil Tajik / James B. Seward



## BACKGROUND

The study of the heart and great vessels has come a long way since the days of Andreas Vesalius, the great sixteenth-century anatomist who recognized the impact of anatomy on the practice of medicine.[1] During the European Renaissance, the tomographic approach to the study of cardiac anatomy became popular because of its artistically based correlations. This is vividly depicted in the drawings of Leonardo da Vinci[2] (Fig. 3-1), who was called the first comparative anatomist since Aristotle (see Chap. 1). During the ensuing nearly four hundred years, however, interest in cardiac anatomy was very sporadic and limited to a few zealous and pioneering physicians, anatomists, and artists. The nineteenth century ushered in the era of anatomic dissection for the study of physiologic and pathophysiologic processes. Virchow in 1885 described the *inflow-outflow method of cardiac dissection,* which followed the direction of blood flow.[3] It was quick and simple and became the dissection method of choice. The works of Virchow and Osler paved the way to understanding the pathophysiologic basis of such diseases as pulmonary embolism, endocarditis, and heart failure.[4] Renewed interest in the study of cardiac anatomy and pathology was facilitated by the rise in autopsy rates in Europe and North America during the first half of the twentieth century.[5] Herrick described the clinical features of coronary thrombosis.[5] Later, Blumgart, Schlesinger, and Zoll advanced our understanding of coronary artery disease through elegant clinicopathologic correlations.[5]

These achievements notwithstanding, however, they were limited to postmortem examinations. The advent of cardiac surgery in the 1950s, followed by coronary angiography, was a major impetus for promoting the study of in vivo clinicopathologic anatomic correlations. While cardiac surgeons were quick to appreciate the importance of having a detailed understanding of cardiac anatomy, clinical cardiologists were more interested in pathophysiology. However, with the introduction of noninvasive imaging techniques [echocardiography, computed tomography (CT), magnetic resonance imaging (MRI), and single-photon-emission computed tomography (SPECT)] over the past two decades, the perception of cardiac anatomy and pathophysiology radically changed for all of medicine in general and cardiology in particular.

With increasing use of tomographic techniques in the diagnosis and management of cardiovascular diseases, there has been a corresponding decrease in the use of autopsy for anatomic correlations. The reasons for this decrease are complex and controversial and include an increased confidence in technology, lack of reimbursement for the cost of autopsy, and rescinding the mandate for autopsies for hospital accreditation.[4] Nonetheless, autopsy still uncovers unexpected processes in about 15 percent of cases and is an invaluable tool for quality assurance programs.

Today, at the beginning of the twenty-first century, there is a resurgence in the clinicopathologic correlative approach to cardiovascular morphology. In particular, the tomographic presentation of cardiac structure, which had remained dormant for over a century, has become relevant because the diagnostic techniques used today are tomographic in nature.[6] The specialties associated with cardiovascular diseases have been quick to embrace these newer anatomic presentations. Echocardiography was brought into the operating room, and with the advent of transesophageal echocardiography, the cardiologist became an indispensable member of the surgical team (see Chap. 15).[7,8] Because of increasingly more sophisticated cardiac surgical techniques coupled with closer interaction between the cardiac surgeon and the noninvasive cardiologist, there has been a growing demand for precise diagnostic tools with greater spatial and temporal resolution to guide the planning of surgical procedures and, therefore, to ensure their success.[7,8,8a,8b]

The interest in cardiac anatomy among cardiologists is by no means limited to those instances involved in imaging the heart. Over the past few years, there has been an explosion of interest in anatomically guided electrophysiologic mapping and ablation techniques,

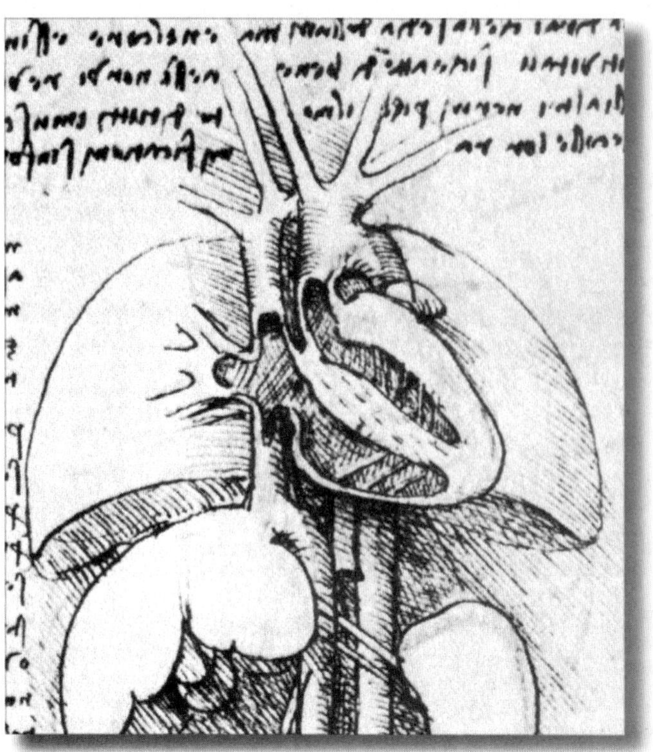

FIGURE 3-1 Four-chamber tomographic section of the heart as illustrated by Leonardo da Vinci. Note the thin-walled right ventricle and thick-walled left ventricle and detailed anatomic connections. (From O'Malley and Saunders,[2] with permission.)

which are increasingly guided by intracardiac ultrasound (see Chap. 36).[9–13] It has thus become feasible to accurately pinpoint the anatomic location of the source of many arrhythmias[9–13] (Figs. 3-2 and 3-3). By providing the electrophysiologist with a real-time visual "road map," the "search and destroy" mission during an ablation procedure will be made much easier and results, as well as complications, will be recognized immediately.[9–13] By providing a new window to the heart, real-time anatomic-electrophysiologic correlations

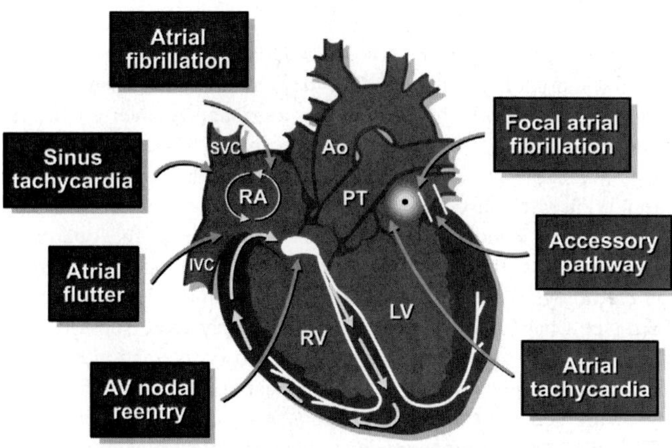


FIGURE 3-2 Anatomic considerations in the treatment of supraventricular arrhythmias. AV, atrioventricular; Ao, ascending aorta; IVC, inferior vena cava; LV, left ventricle; PT, pulmonary trunk; RA, right atrium; RV, right ventricle; SVC, superior vena cava. (Courtesy of Dr. Douglas L Packer, Mayo Clinic, Rochester, MN.)

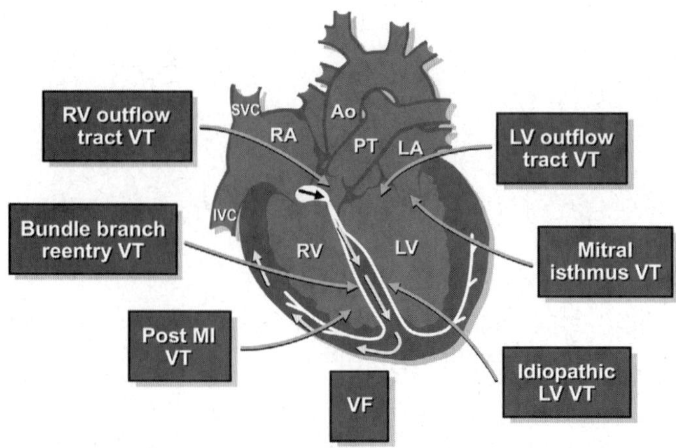


FIGURE 3-3 Anatomic considerations in the treatment of ventricular arrhythmias. LV, left ventricle; LA, left atrium; MI, myocardial infarction; VT, ventricular tachycardia; VF, ventricular fibrillation; other abbreviations as in Fig 3-2. (Courtesy of Dr. Douglas L Packer, Mayo Clinic, Rochester, MN.)

may also help to enhance our understanding of the mechanisms of propagation of various arrhythmias.

In this technologically driven era, a new appreciation of cardiac anatomy has emerged as the cornerstone for clinical cardiology. The purpose of this chapter is to describe the anatomy of the heart by principally using the tomographic format prevalent in current CT, MRI, and echocardiography, with special emphasis and focus on clinically relevant anatomic details. We will make only passing note of the next generation of imaging techniques. The intent is to emphasize the important anatomic features of various cardiovascular disease processes relative to diagnosis and management.[13a,13b]

## Orientation of the Heart within the Thorax

The body may be viewed in three standard anatomic planes: (1) frontal (coronal), (2) horizontal (transverse), and (3) sagittal, which are orthogonal to one another.[6,7] However, the three primary planes of the heart [short axis (transverse), four-chamber (frontal), and long-axis (sagittal)] do not correspond to the standard anatomic planes of the body[6,7] (Fig. 3-4, Plate 2). *Incorrect photographic or artistic orientation of surgical or autopsy specimens of the heart, presented out of context, can result in the display of two-dimensional images in nonanatomic positions and actually contribute to misconceptions regarding the position of the heart within the thorax*[6] (Fig. 3-5, Plate 3).

Thus, first, in describing the orientation of a specific organ such as the heart, one must take into account both the position of the heart and the position of adjacent structures such as the thoracic aorta and esophagus. In interpreting two-dimensional images, clinicians must avoid making correlations that yield impossible anatomy[6] (Fig. 3-6). Accurate anatomic diagnoses require close interdisciplinary interactions between cardiovascular pathologists, clinicians, radiologists, anesthesiologists, and surgeons and emphasize a critical need for teamwork and a "common language" in describing cardiac anatomy and pathology.

## Methods Used to Study Cardiac Anatomy

The two conventional approaches to the study of cardiac anatomy that have stood the test of time are (1) the inflow-outflow method (Fig. 3-7) and (2) the tomographic ventricular slice method[3,6] (Fig. 3-8, Plate 4). Although the inflow-outflow method readily demonstrates

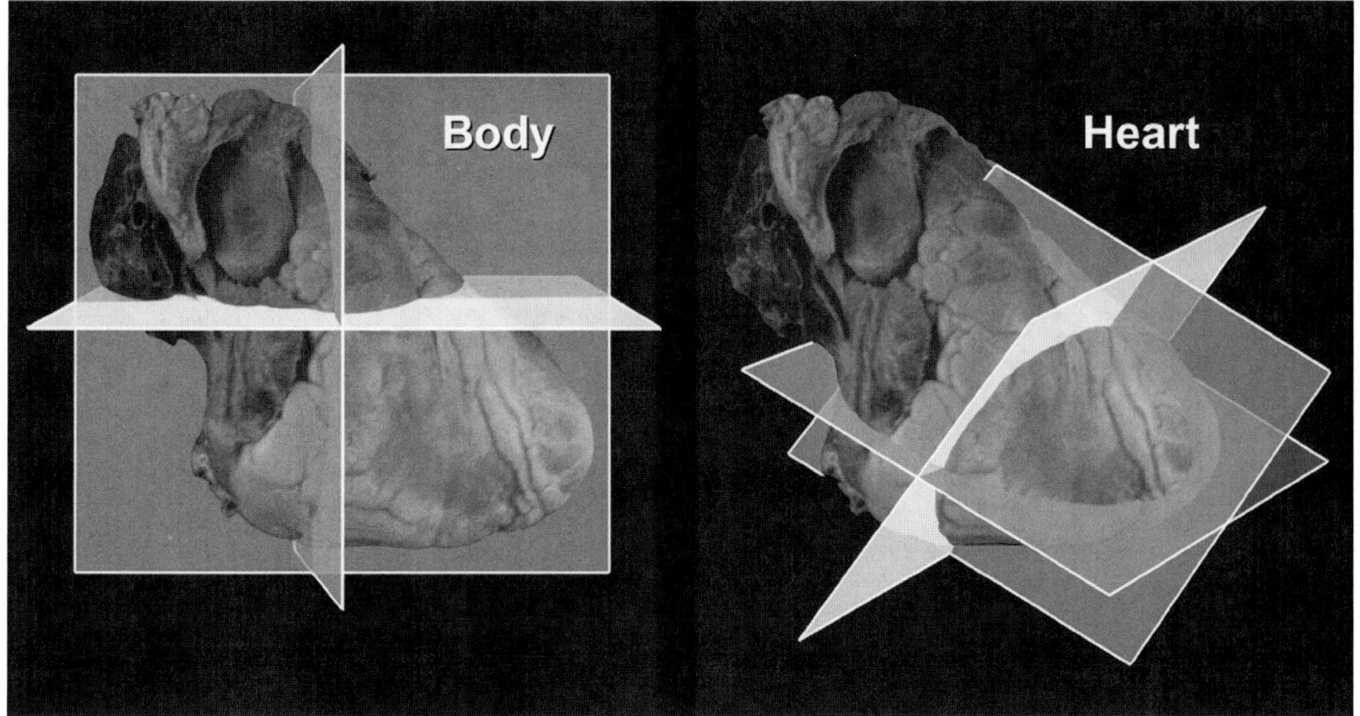


FIGURE 3-4 (Plate 2) The three primary planes of the body (*left*) and heart (*right*). Note that the planes of the body are aligned with vertical midline structures, such as the esophagus. In contrast, the major axis of the heart is oriented obliquely. Thus the heart's long and short axes do not lie in the same plane as the body's long and short axes. The body planes cut the heart obliquely and not in its primary planes. Conversely, the heart's primary planes cut the body obliquely.

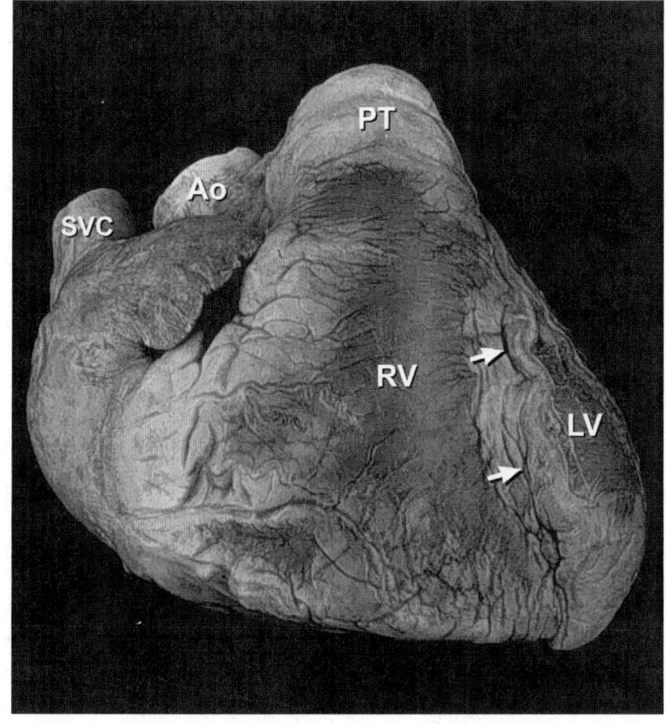


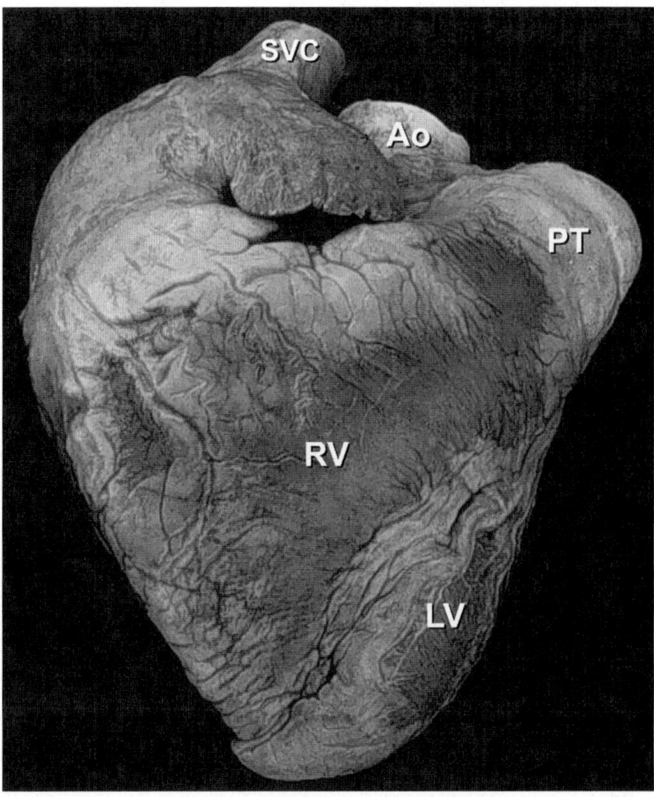


FIGURE 3-5 (Plate 3) *A*. Anterior view of the heart in its usual anatomic position with its apex directed from right to left. Arrows point to the anterior interventricular groove. *B*. Nonanatomic positioning of the normal heart with its apex directed downward, thereby resembling a "valentine." The position of the cardiac apex is normally leftward (levocardia) but may anomalously be rightward (dextrocardia) or midline and inferiorly (mesocardia). Ao, ascending aorta; LV, left ventricle; PT, pulmonary trunk; RV, right ventricle; SVC, superior vena cava.

disease processes in a given cardiac chamber or valve, it does not allow simultaneous visualization of the effects of that process on contiguous structures.[6] Furthermore, the inflow-outflow method does not correspond well to clinical tomographic imaging modalities except possibly cavitary angiography.[6] With the ventricular slice technique (see Fig. 3-8), the ventricles are "bread sliced" perpendicular to the plane of the ventricular septum. This technique is ideal for the evaluation of ischemic heart disease but may have to be carried basally, well beyond the papillary muscle tips.[6]

## TOMOGRAPHIC METHOD

Renaissance anatomists such as da Vinci used the *tomographic approach* principally because of its *artistic correlations*.[2] Modern anatomists and

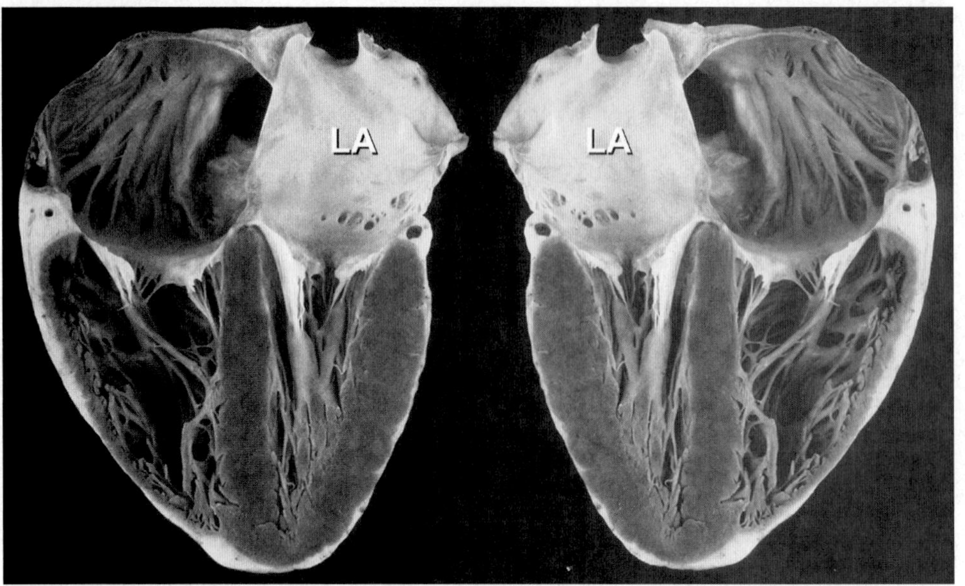

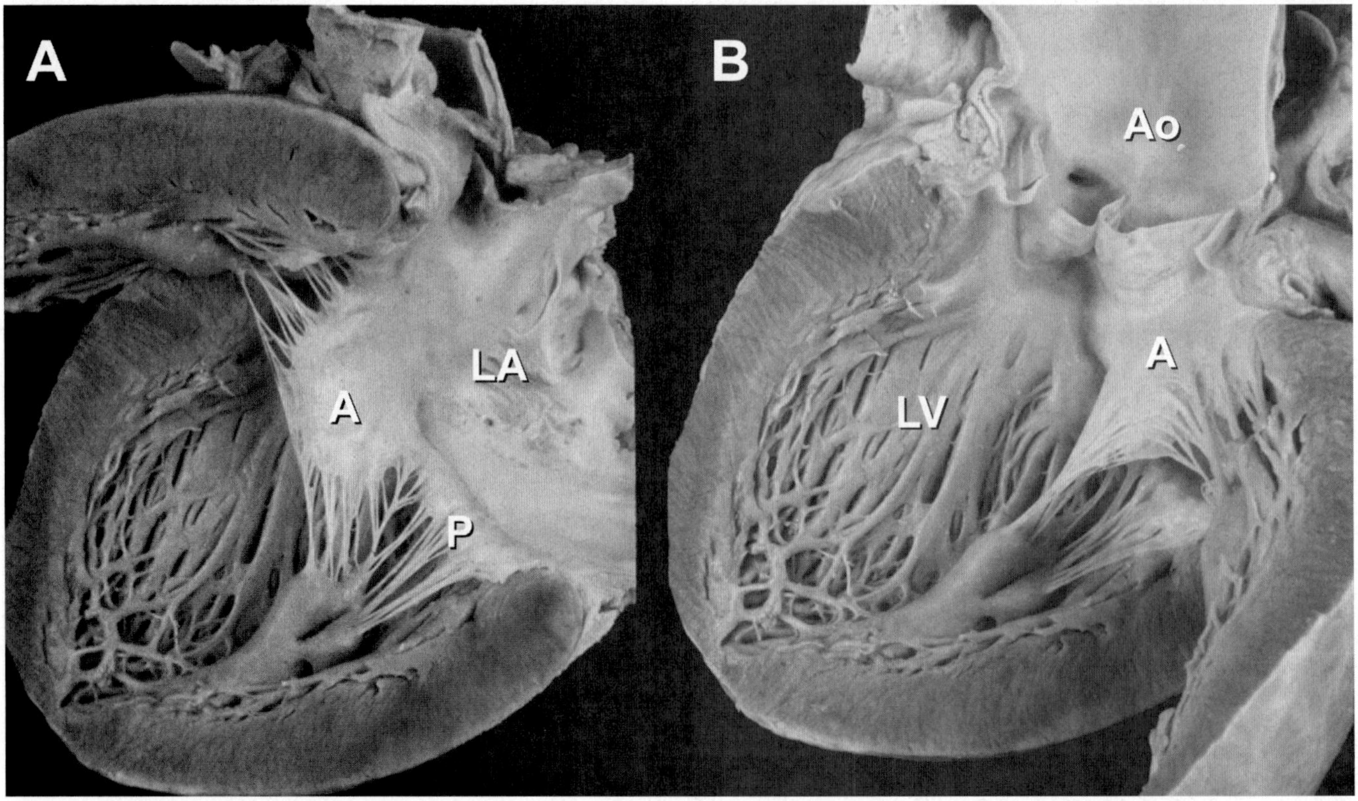

FIGURE 3-6 Apex-down four-chamber view of the heart (*left*) and mirror-image photograph (*right*). Mirror-image depiction (though commonly used in publications) to depict normal four-chamber, apex-up echocardiographic anatomic images does not correspond to normal anatomic reality. Obviously, three-dimensional anatomic correctness is essential for accurate clinicopathologic correlations. LA, left atrium.

FIGURE 3-7 Inflow-outflow method of cardiac dissection. *A*. Left ventricular inflow view. *B*. Left ventricular outflow view. A, anterior mitral leaflet; Ao, ascending aorta; LA, left atrium; LV, left ventricle; P, posterior mitral leaflet.

pathologists have resorted to this method because it correlates with conventional diagnostic tomographic-anatomic techniques. With this method, cardiac dissection involves bisecting the heart into two pieces using a single plane of section.[6] Anatomy contained within the depth of each section fosters a perception of three-dimensional anatomy. Commonly used planes bisect the heart perpendicular to the base-apex axis (*short-axis "transverse" views*) (Fig. 3-9, Plate 5) or parallel to it (*long-axis and four-chamber "frontal" views*)[6] (Fig. 3-10, Plate 6). Planes that bisect the heart parallel to the conventional body planes (frontal "coronal," transverse "short-axis," and sagittal "long-axis" views) (Fig. 3-11, Plate 7) replicate *body tomography*.[6,14]

The *short-axis tomographic planes*[6,7] of the heart (Fig. 3-12) are similar to the ventricular slice method but differ in two important respects. The "bread slicing" of the heart is continued to the base of the heart and

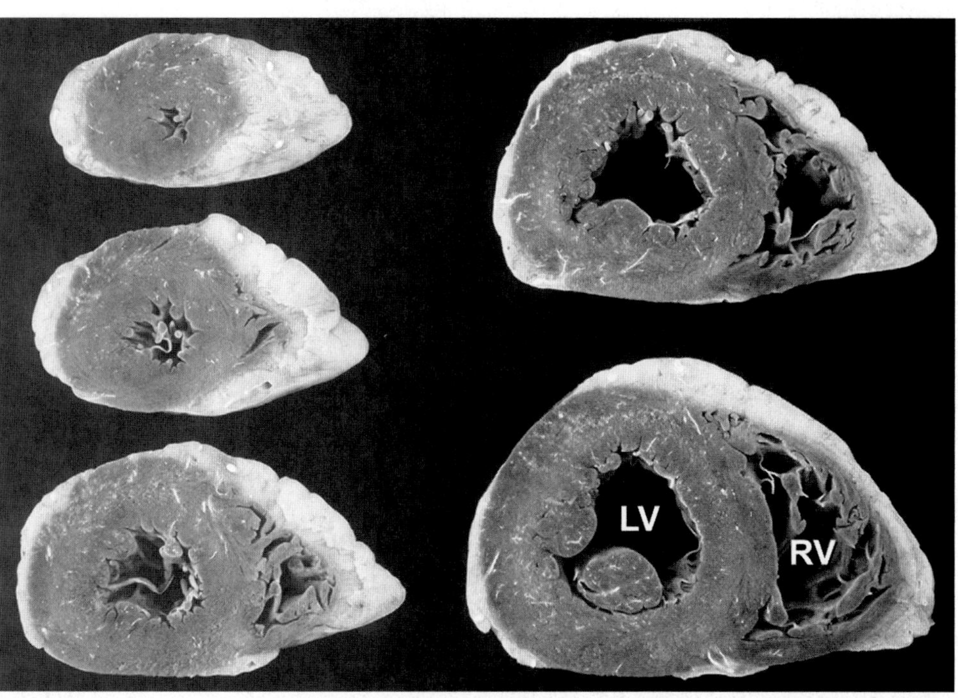


FIGURE 3-8 (Plate 4) Ventricular slice method of cardiac dissection. Display of five slices (LV, left ventricle; RV, right ventricle) viewed as though looking from the base of the heart toward the apex.

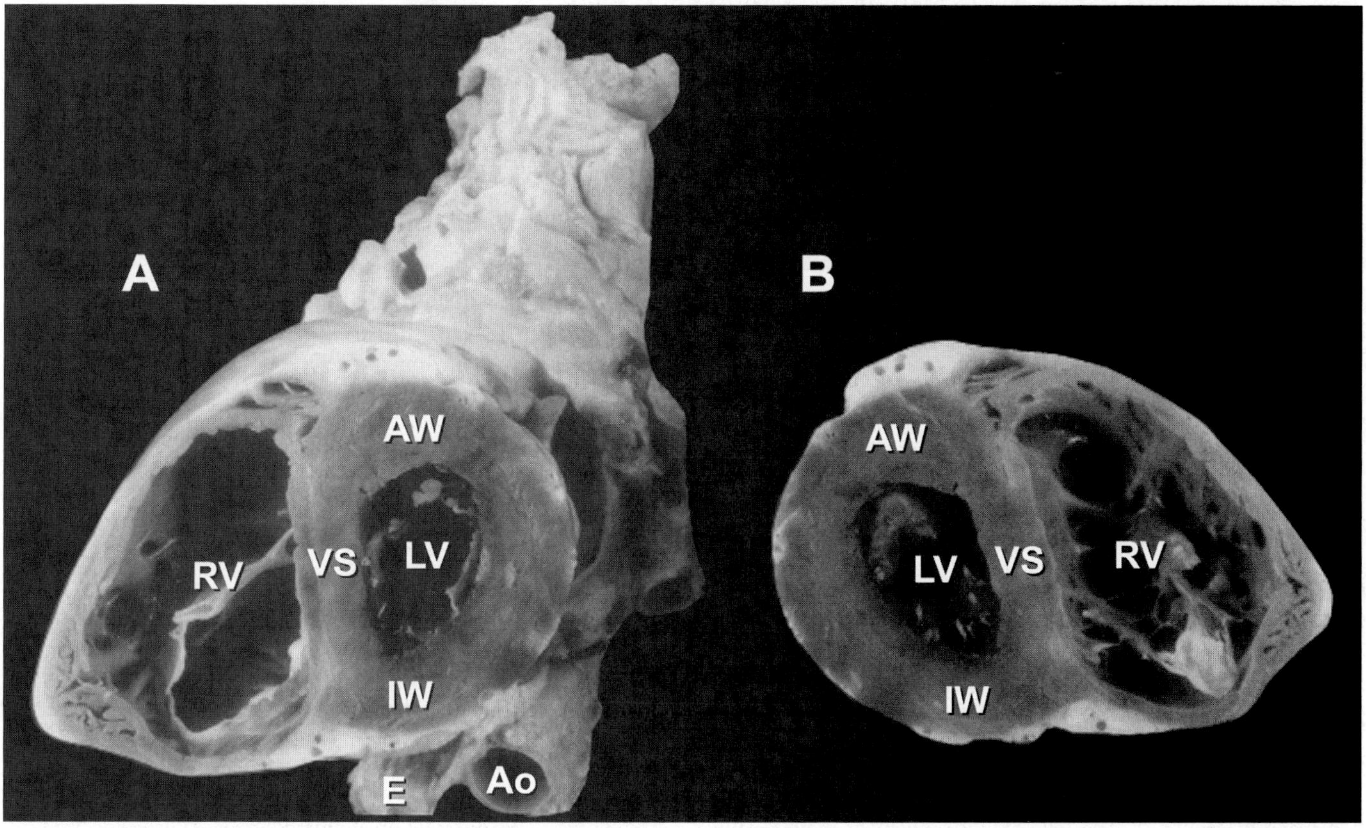

FIGURE 3-9 (Plate 5) Bisected cardiac specimen, viewed in the short axis. *A*. The specimen is viewed from the apex toward the base. The esophagus (E) is posterior and adjacent to both the thoracic aorta (Ao) and the inferior wall of the left ventricle (LV). The right ventricular (RV) cavity is to the left. *B*. The other half of the bisected specimen is viewed as though looking from the base toward the apex (comparable with Fig. 3-8). AW, anterior wall; IW, inferior wall; VS, ventricular septum.

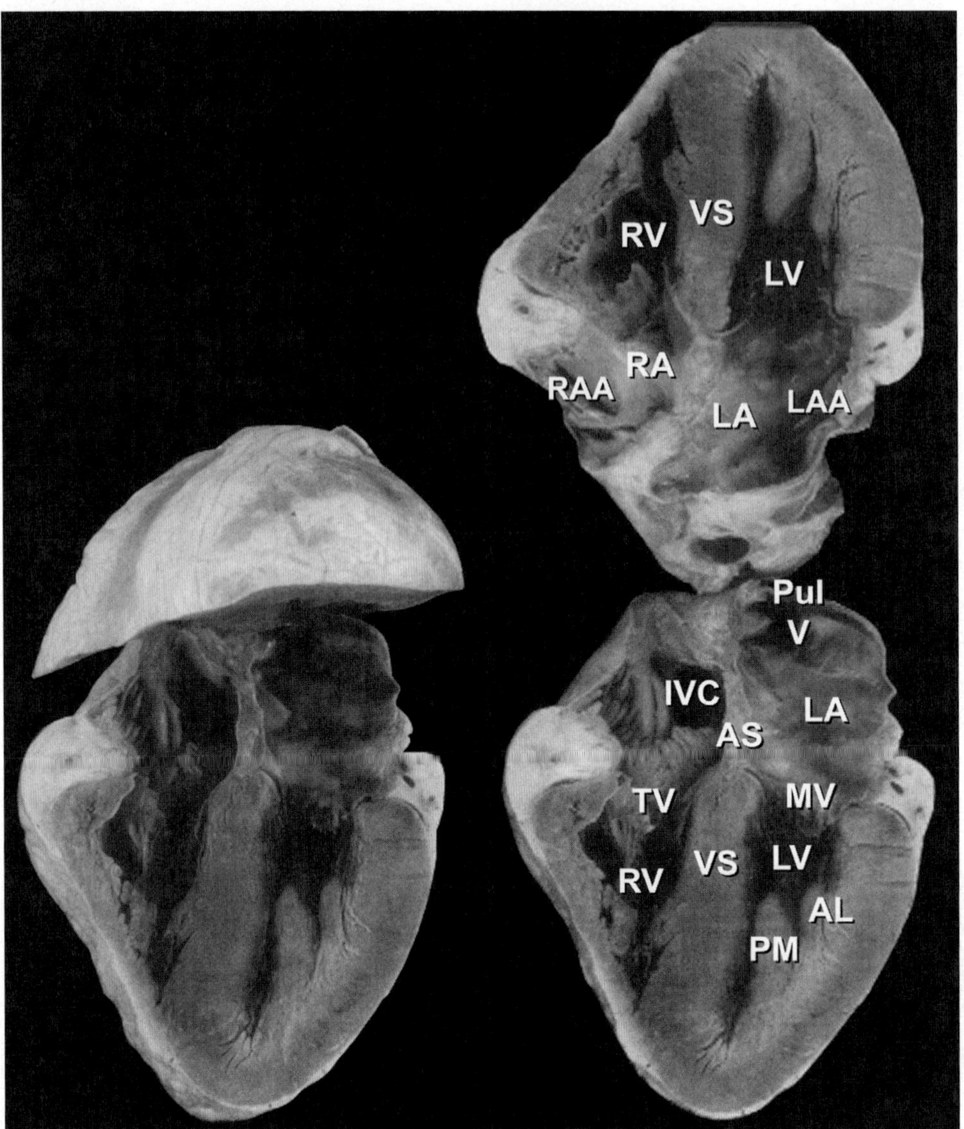


FIGURE 3-10 (Plate 6) Bisected cardiac specimen in the four-chamber view parallel to the base-apex axis of the heart. The bisected specimen (*left*) has been partially opened to show the relative relationship of the bisected halves. The two components of the bisected specimen (*right*) are opened completely. Note the positions of the pulmonary veins posteriorly and the positions of the atrial appendages at the atrioventricular groove. AL, anterolateral papillary muscle; AS, atrial septum; IVC, inferior vena cava; LA, left atrium; LAA, left atrial appendage; LV, left ventricle; MV, mitral valve; PM, posteromedial papillary muscle; PulV, pulmonary vein; RA, right atrium; RAA, right atrial appendage; RV, right ventricle; TV, tricuspid valve; VS, ventricular septum.

great vessels, and the slices are oriented as though the heart were being viewed from the apex toward the base rather than in the opposite direction, as has been the case with the ventricular slice technique. Photographs should correspond with diagnostic tomographic scans.

The *long-axis and four-chamber planes* are orthogonal to the short-axis planes. The four-chamber planes of cardiac dissection (Fig. 3-13) involve sectioning the heart along both lateral walls, from apex to base, such that both ventricles and both atria are included in the plane of section.[6,7] The long-axis two-chamber method (Fig. 3-14) involves bisecting the heart from the left ventricular apex through the mitral orifice and into the left atrium.[6,7] The long-axis plane can cut through both the left ventricular inflow tract (including the left atrium and mitral valve) and the left ventricular outflow tract (including the ventricular septum, anterior mitral leaflet, and ascending aorta) (Fig. 3-15). This plane also cuts obliquely through the right ventricular outflow tract.[6,7]

These three tomographic planes of the heart have been particularly useful in echocardiography. Serial sections within each plane produce a collage of anatomic slices (Fig. 3-16, Plate 8) that can be used for three-dimensional reconstruction, which is beyond the scope of this chapter (see Chap. 15). The tomographic planes of section can be tailored to the different imaging modalities. *Thus echocardiography and* SPECT *generally employ the primary planes of the* heart. *In contrast, CT and MRI use the primary planes of the* body. *The parasagittal or oblique planes of the body serve radionuclide angiography and left ventriculography.*[6] When the tomographic

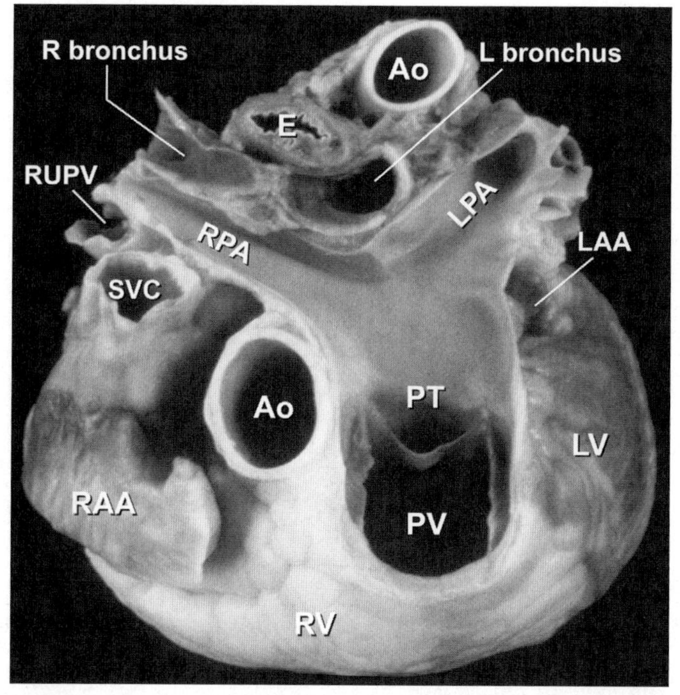


A

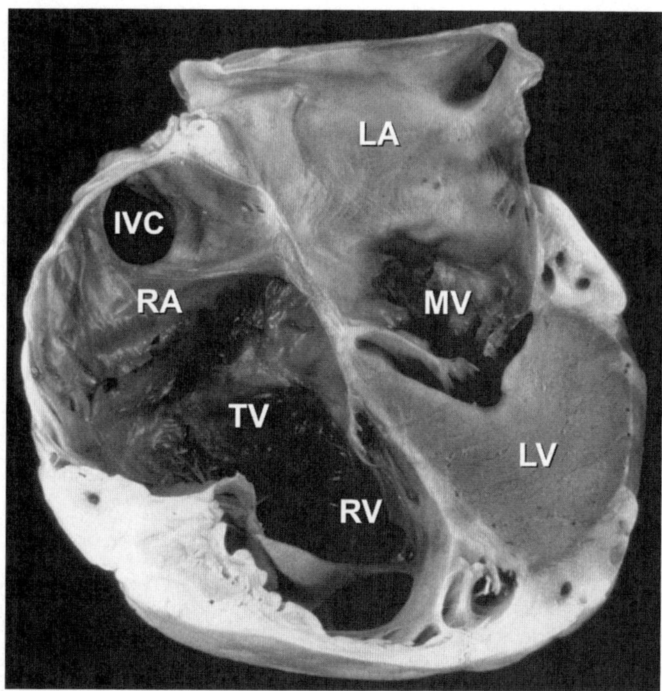


B

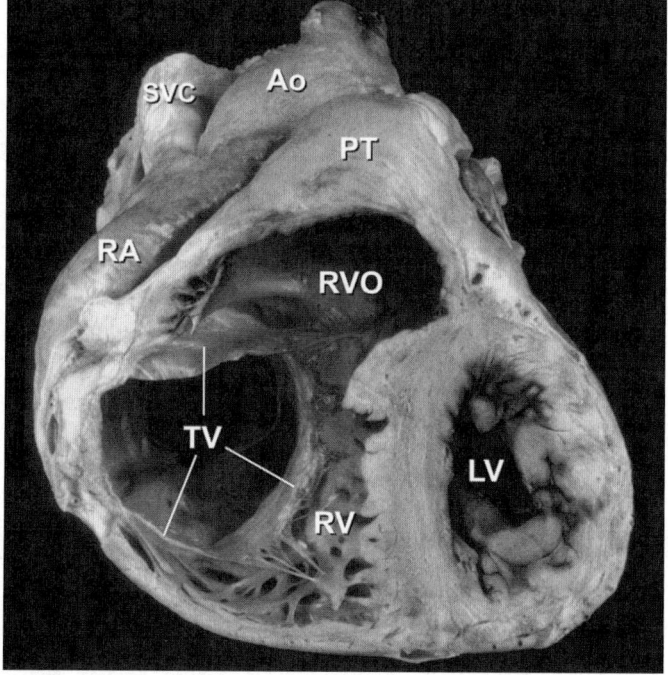

C

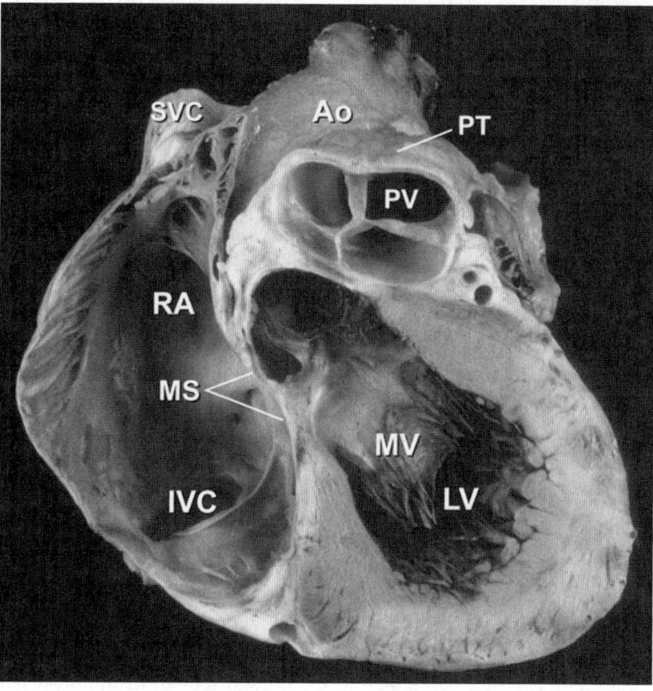


D

FIGURE 3-11 (Plate 7) Tomographic cardiac dissection along the body primary planes. *A, B.* Transverse sections (looking from head toward feet) at the level of the great vessels (*A*) or the cardiac chambers (*B*). The aortic arch travels over the left bronchus and the right pulmonary artery. *C, D.* Frontal sections (looking from anterior to posterior) through both ventricles (*C*) or left ventricle and right atrium (*D*). *E,F.* Parasagittal sections looking from right (*E*) to left (*F*). Ao, ascending aorta; CS, coronary sinus; E, esophagus; IA, innominate artery; IVC, inferior vena cava; LA, left atrium; LAA, left atrial appendage; LB, left bronchus; LCX, left circumflex coronary artery; LIV, left innominate vein; LLPV, left lower pulmonary vein; LPA, left pulmonary artery; LUPV, left upper pulmonary vein; LSA, left subclavian artery; LV, left ventricle; MS, membranous ventricular septum; MV, mitral valve; PS, pericardial sac; PT, pulmonary trunk; PV, pulmonary valve; RA, right atrium; RAA, right atrial appendage; RPA, right pulmonary artery; RUPV, right upper pulmonary vein; RV, right ventricle; RVO, right ventricular outflow; SVC, superior vena cava; TV, tricuspid valve.

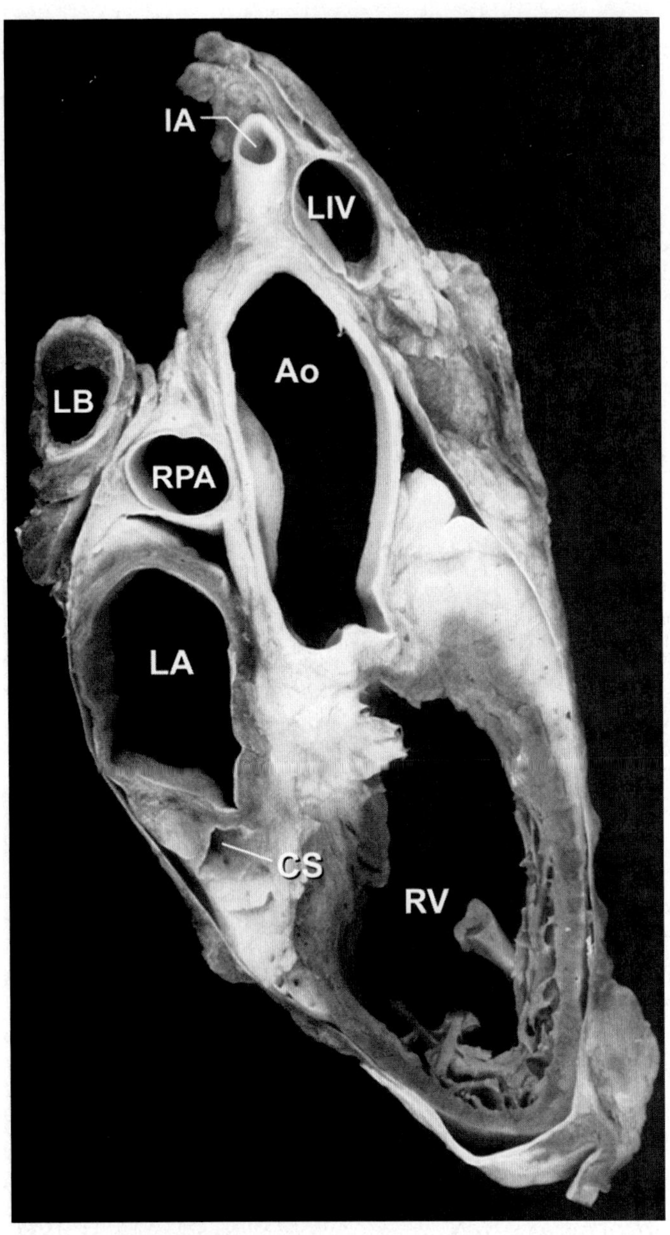


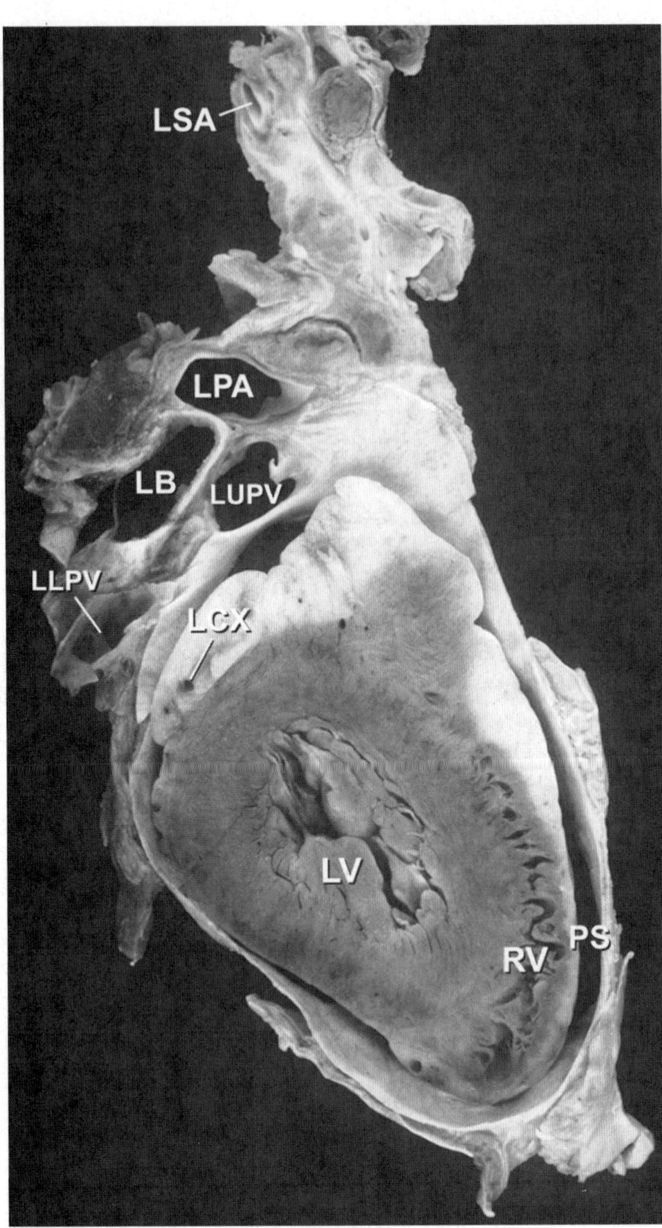


FIGURE 3-11 *(Continued)*

examination is not configured to the primary planes of the heart but rather to the planes of the body, the terms *short, long,* and *frontal* can be misleading (Figs. 3-17 and 3-18).

Pathologic lesions in both congenital and acquired heart diseases often involve contiguous chambers, valves, or vessels. The tomographic method is the optimal technique for demonstrating intracardiac relationships and is ideal for any disease that involves several cardiac chambers. The proliferation of noninvasive tomographic imaging techniques makes this method particularly ideal for clinicopathologic correlations. Limitations of tomographic dissection can be overcome by photography, computer imagery, and interestingly, the use of glue. After each tomographic section has been produced and photographed, the bisected specimens can be glued back together using any cyanoacrylate glue, such as Krazy Glue or Superglue, and resectioned along a different tomographic plane.[6] A step-by-step photographic documentation is necessary, since once the specimen has been glued and recut, the preceding tomographic plane of section will be available only in the photograph and not in the actual specimen.

## CORRELATIVE ANATOMY

This section provides an illustrated review of applied cardiac anatomy. The clinical significance of the anatomy described is highlighted in italics.

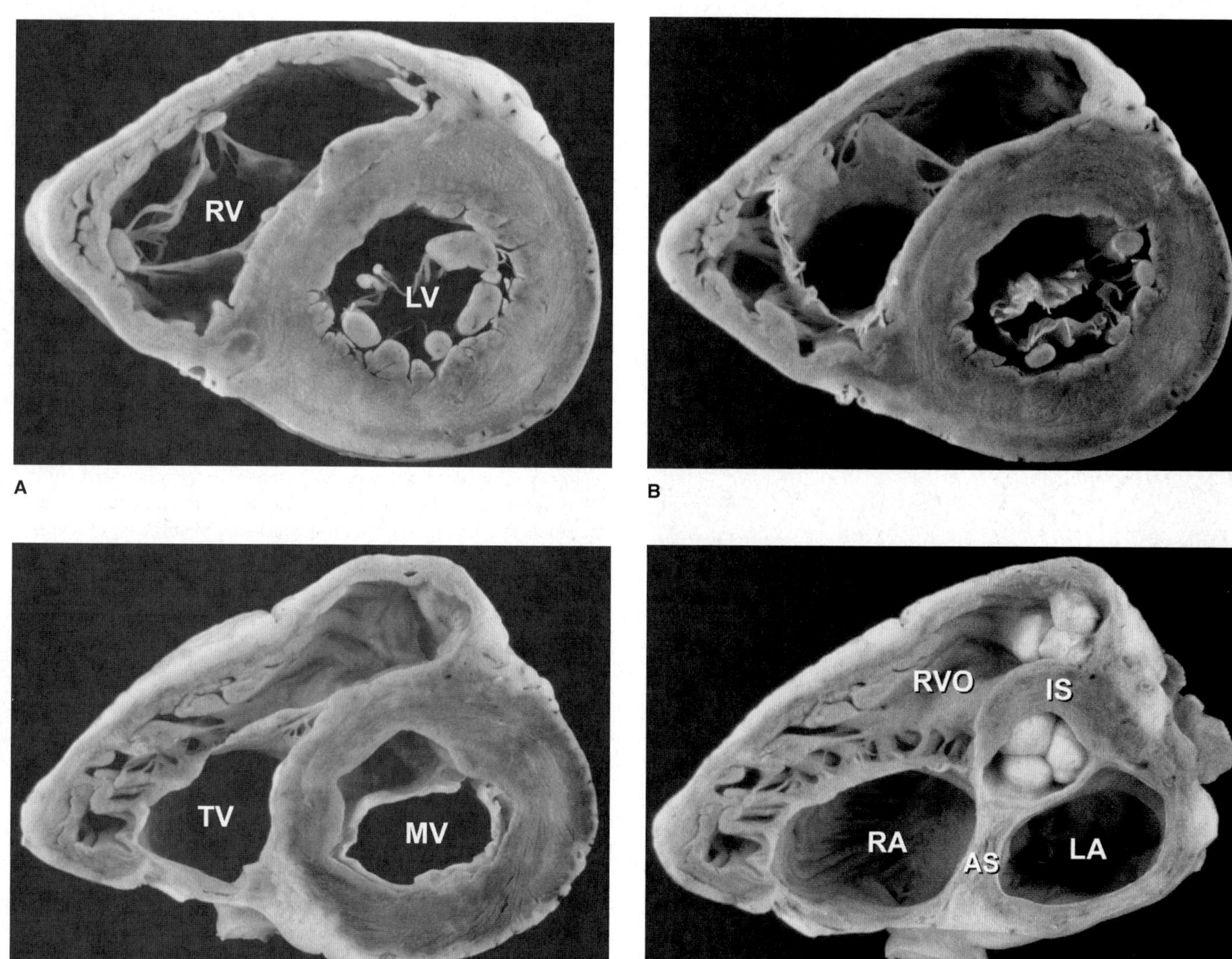


FIGURE 3-12 *A–D*. Tomographic cardiac dissections along the heart's primary short-axis plane. This method of tomographic dissection shows the crescentic right ventricle (RV) and circular left ventricle (LV). The atrioventricular valves are sectioned at the level of their papillary muscles (in *A*), chordae tendineae (in *B*), atrioventricular valve leaflets (in *C*), and their annuli and the semilunar valves (in *D*). The infundibulum septum (IS) separates the pulmonary and aortic valves. The atrial septum (AS) separates the tricuspid and mitral valves and abuts the posterior (noncoronary) cusp of the aortic valve. LA, left atrium; MV, mitral valve; RA, right atrium; RVO, right ventricular outflow; TV, tricuspid valve.

## Pericardium

The fibrous (parietal) pericardium is a resilient sac that envelops the heart and attaches onto the great vessels.[15] Almost the entire ascending aorta and main pulmonary artery and portions of both venae cavae and all four pulmonary veins are intrapericardial (Fig. 3-19). *These are important anatomic landmarks to remember in evaluating diseases of the pericardium. Given the intrapericardial location of the ascending aorta, diseases such as localized aortic wall hematoma, aortic dissection, or aortic rupture can produce a rapidly fatal hemopericardium. Because the sac is collagenous, with little elastic tissue, it cannot stretch acutely. In patients with total anomalous pulmonary venous connection, the confluence of pulmonary veins is intrapericardial. In contrast, the right and left pulmonary arteries and ductal artery (ductus arteriosus) are extrapericardial structures.*[16]

The serous pericardium forms the delicate inner lining of the fibrous pericardium as well as the outer lining of the heart and great vessels (visceral pericardium). Over the heart, it is referred to as the *epicardium,* and it contains the epicardial coronary arteries and veins, autonomic nerves, lymphatics, and a variable amount of adipose tissue. The junctions between the visceral and parietal pericardium lie along the great vessels and form the pericardial reflections. The reflections along the pulmonary veins and vena cavae are continuous and form a posterior midline cul-de-sac known as the *oblique sinus*. Behind the great arteries, the *transverse sinus* forms a tunnel-like passageway (Fig. 3-20). *After open-heart surgery, localized accumulation of blood within the oblique sinus can produce*

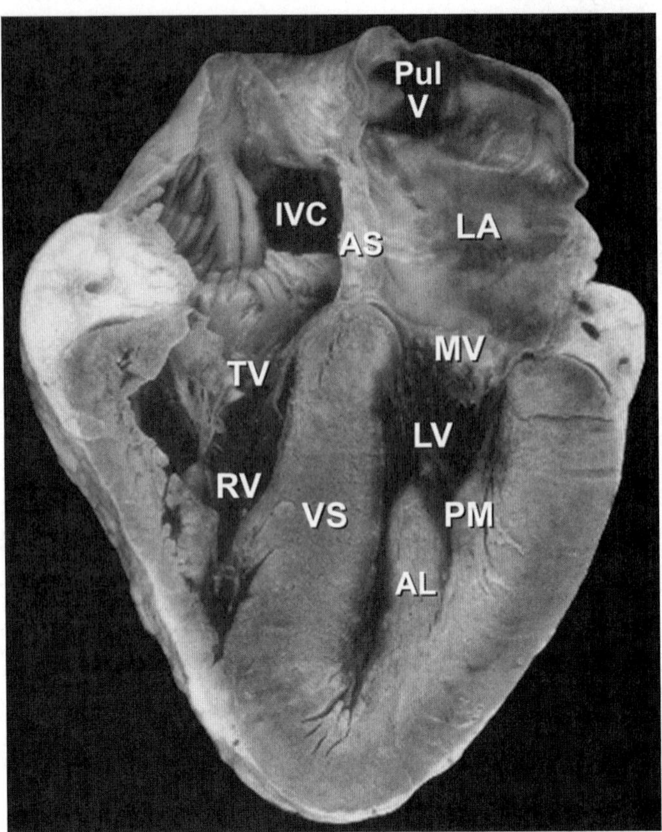


FIGURE 3-13 Tomographic cardiac dissection along the heart's primary four-chamber plane. The heart is viewed as though one were looking from the anterosuperior surface toward the posteroinferior surface. In the floor of the right atrium is the orifice of the inferior vena cava (IVC). The pulmonary veins (PulV) enter the posterior aspect of the left atrium. AL, anterolateral mitral papillary muscle; AS, atrial septum; LA, left atrium; LV, left ventricle; MV, mitral valve; PM, posteromedial mitral papillary muscle; RV, right ventricle; TV, tricuspid valve; VS, ventricular septum.

*isolated left atrial tamponade.*[16] *Similarly, a hematoma adjacent to the low-pressure right atrium can cause isolated right atrial tamponade* (see Chap. 80). With increasing age and with obesity, fat can accumulate within the parietal pericardium and epicardium.[16] *In imaging the heart, it is important not to misinterpret epicardial fat as an abnormal structure or a tumor.*

## Cardiac Skeleton

The four cardiac valves are anchored to their annuli, or valve rings. These fibrous rings, at the base of the heart, join to form the fibrous skeleton of the heart[16] (Fig. 3-21, Plate 9). The centrally located aortic valve forms the cornerstone of the cardiac skeleton, and its fibrous extensions abut each of the other three valves. The cardiac skeleton contains not only the four valve annuli but also the membranous septum and the aortic intervalvular, right, and left fibrous trigones. The fibrous trigones form the anatomic substrate for direct mitral-aortic continuity[16] (Fig. 3-21, Plate 9, and Fig. 3-22). The intervalvular fibrosa also forms part of the floor of the transverse sinus (see Figs. 3-22 and 3-23). *In patients with infective endocarditis of the mitral or aortic valves, infection may burrow through the intervalvular fibrosa and produce characteristic fistulas between the left ventricle and the adjacent left atrium, ascending aorta, or transverse sinus* (see Chap. 81).[17] The right fibrous trigone (Fig. 3-21, Plate 9), also known as the *central fibrous body*, welds together the aortic, mitral, and tricuspid valves and forms the largest and strongest component of the cardiac skeleton. It is through the right fibrous trigone that the atrioventricular (His) bundle passes. Otherwise, the fibrous cardiac skeleton serves to electrically isolate the atria from the ventricles. *Diseases or surgical alterations of one valve may affect the shape or angulation of adjacent valves (e.g., aortic valve replacement causing severe mitral regurgitation) and may affect the nearby coronary arteries or conduction tissue.*[17]

## Tricuspid Valve

The tricuspid valve is comprised of five components (i.e., annulus, leaflets, commissures, chordae tendineae, and papillary muscles). The anterior tricuspid leaflet is the largest and most mobile and forms an intracavitary curtain that partially separates the inflow and outflow tracts of the right ventricle (Fig. 3-23). The posterior leaflet is usually the smallest. The septal leaflet is the least mobile because of its many direct chordal attachments to the ventricular septum. A distensible fibroadipose annulus is unique to the tricuspid valve.[17] Consequently, dilatation of the right ventricle commonly produces circumferential tricuspid annular dilatation that results in variable degrees of tricuspid valve regurgitation (see Chap. 69).[16]

## Mitral Valve

The mitral apparatus is composed of the same five components as the tricuspid valve. Competent mitral valve function is a complex process that requires the proper interaction of all components, as well as adequate left atrial and left ventricular function. *Abnormalities of the mitral valve apparatus may involve any of these components or combinations thereof. The pattern of pathologic involvement often determines the feasibility of mitral valve repair (surgical or percutaneous)* (see Chaps. 67 and 68).[18] The mitral valve annulus forms a complete fibrous ring that is firmly anchored along the circumference of the anterior leaflet by the tough fibrous skeleton of the heart[17] (see Fig. 3-21, Plate 9). Therefore, dilatation of the mitral valve annulus primarily affects the posterior leaflet. *All current operative mitral valve repair techniques are based on this principle of asymmetric annular dilatation. Mitral valve annuloplasty reduces the mitral valve inlet area by reducing the circumference of the posterior leaflet.*[17] *This is the rationale for using a partial posterior annuloplasty ring.*

Unlike the other cardiac valves, the mitral valve has only two leaflets. The anterior leaflet is large and semicircular, and it partially separates the ventricular inflow and outflow tracts (see Fig. 3-23). However, unlike its right-sided counterpart, it also forms part of the outflow tract. *In patients with hypertrophic obstructive cardiomyopathy, the anterior mitral leaflet may be pulled toward the basal anterior septum by a Venturi effect, resulting in midsystolic outflow obstruction and mitral regurgitation.*[16] The posterior mitral leaflet is rectangular and is usually divided into three scallops. The middle scallop is the largest of the three in more than 90 percent of normal hearts. Occasionally, however, either the anterolateral or the posteromedial scallop is larger, and rarely there are accessory scallops[15,17] (Fig. 3-24, Plate 10). *Posterior mitral leaflet prolapse usually involves the middle scallop and may be associated with chordal rupture.* Both mitral leaflets are normally similar in area. The anterior leaflet is twice the height of the posterior leaflet but has half its annular length.[17] With advanced age, the mitral leaflets thicken somewhat, particularly along their closing edges.[15]

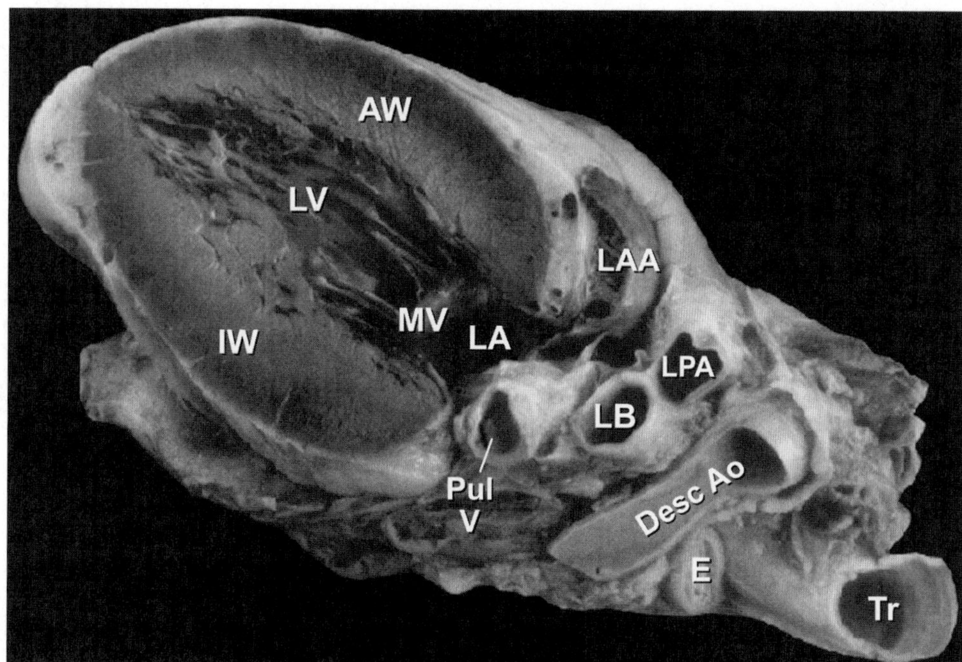


A

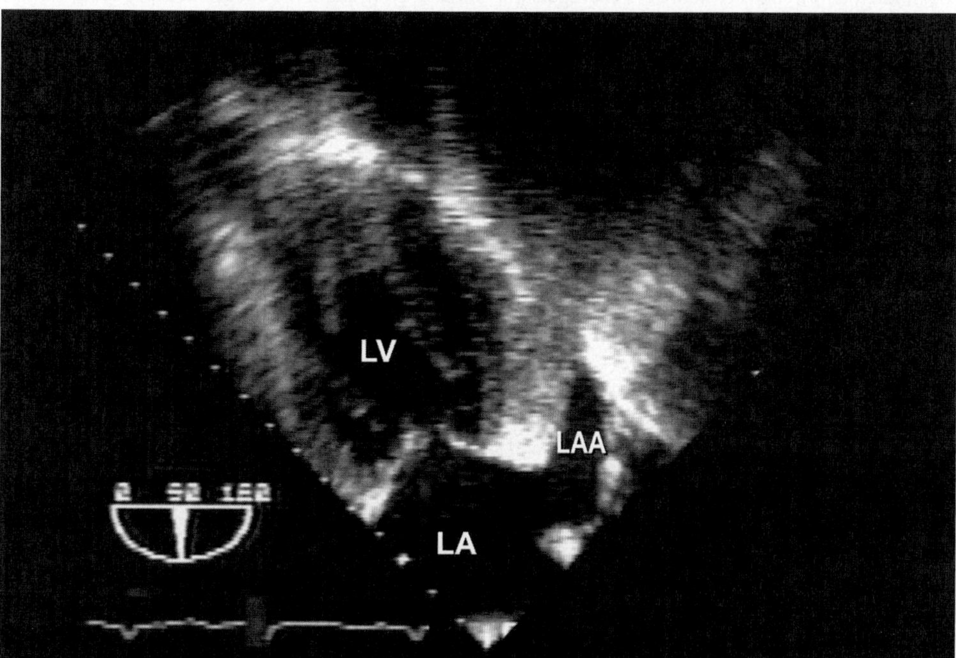


B

FIGURE 3-14 Tomographic cardiac dissection along the heart's primary long-axis plane. *A*. Tomographic section showing the left ventricle and left atrium. The mitral valve is also well demonstrated. The left atrial appendage is located anteriorly. The specimen is viewed as though one were looking from the tip of the left scapula toward the right nipple. *B*. Two-chamber transesophageal echocardiography (TEE) analogous to the two-chamber transthoracic echocardiography (TTE). AW, anterior wall; Desc Ao, descending thoracic aorta; E, esophagus; IW, inferior wall; LA, left atrium; LAA, left atrial appendage; LB, left bronchus; LPA, left pulmonary artery; LV, left ventricle; MV, mitral valve; PulV, pulmonary vein; Tr, trachea.

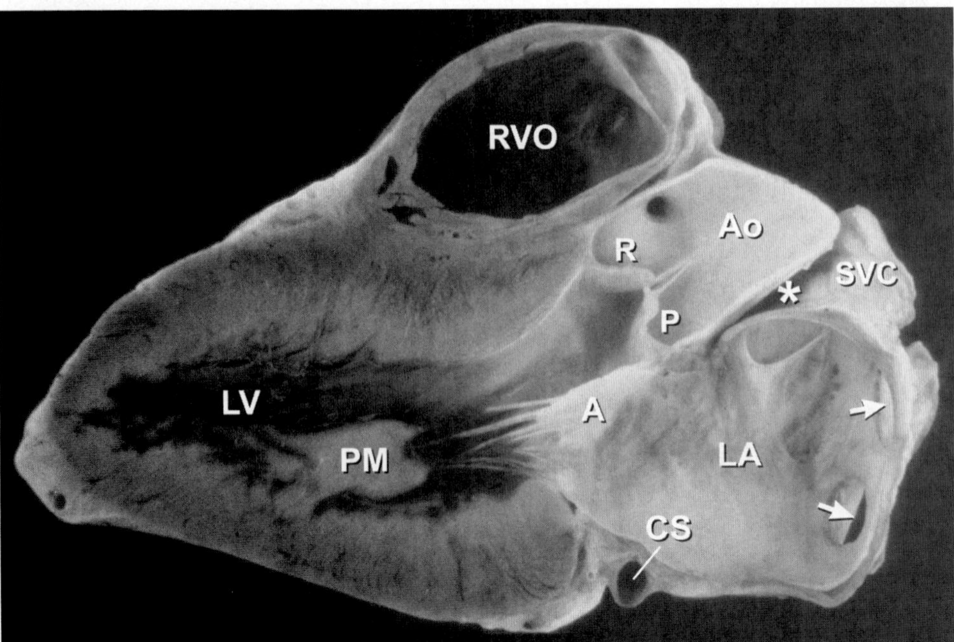


FIGURE 3-15 Left ventricular long-axis method of tomographic cardiac dissection (looking from left flank toward the midsternum). Continuity between mitral and aortic valves is clearly seen. The oblique sinus (*) abuts the wall of the left atrium. A, anterior mitral leaflet; Ao, ascending aorta; CS, coronary sinus; LA, left atrium; LV, left ventricle; P, posterior aortic cusp; PM, posteromedial mitral papillary muscle; R, right aortic cusp; RVO, right ventricular outflow; SVC, superior vena cava; arrows point to the right upper and lower pulmonary veins.

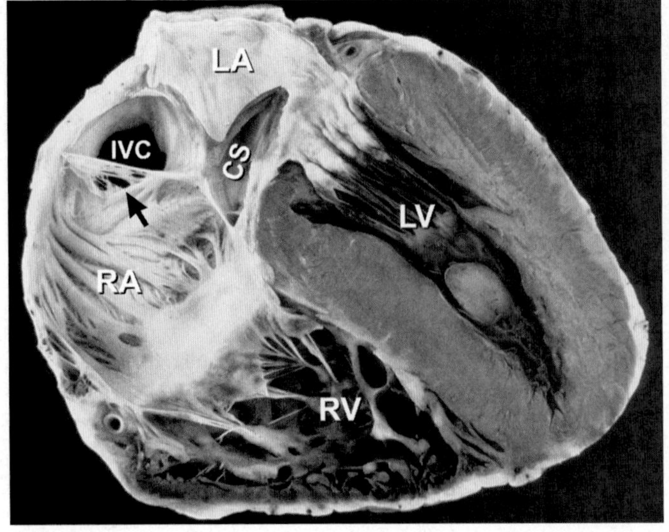


A

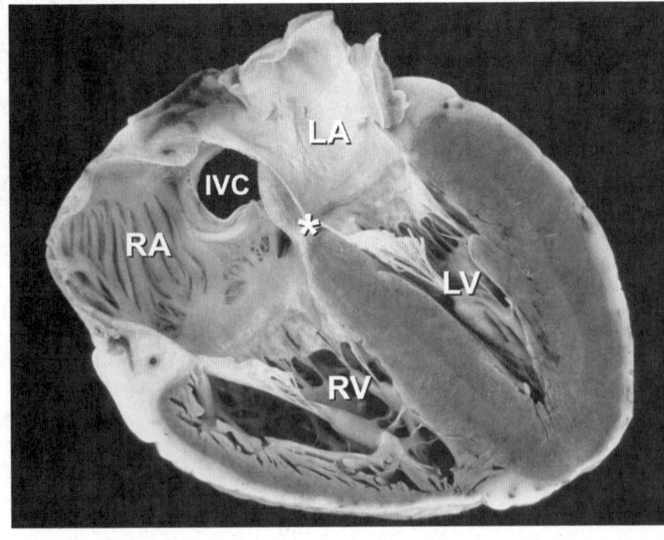


B

FIGURE 3-16 (Plate 8) Collage of four-chamber tomographic sections cutting from inferior wall to anterosuperior wall showing coronary sinus (*A*), internal cardiac crux (*) (*B*), and aortic valve (*C*). Ao, ascending aorta; CS, coronary sinus; IVC, inferior vena cava; LA, left atrium; LV, left ventricle; RA, right atrium; RV, right ventricle; arrow in *A* points to a fenestrated eustachian valve.

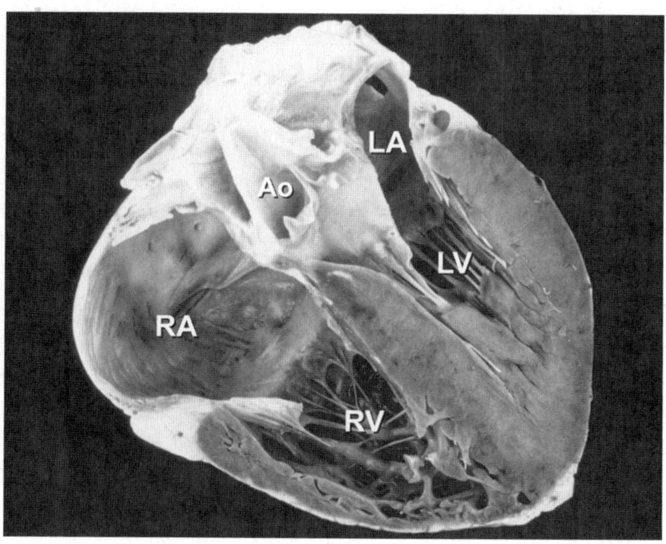


FIGURE 3-16 *(Continued)*

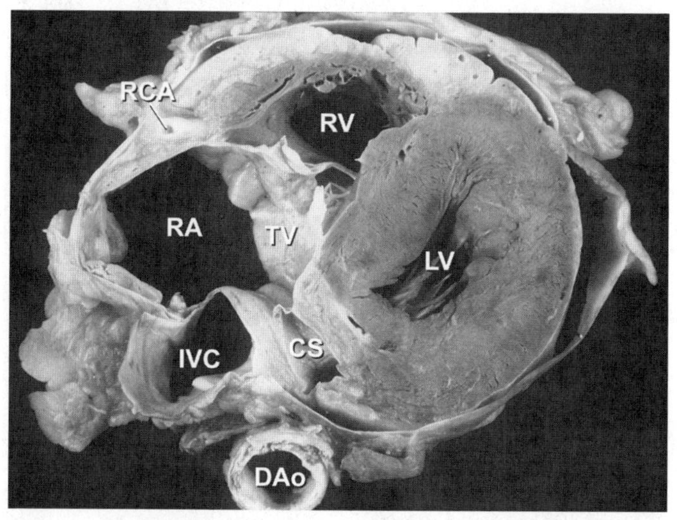


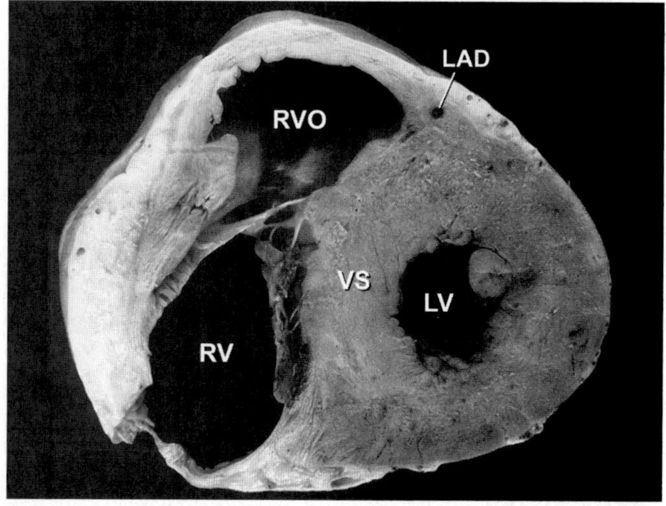


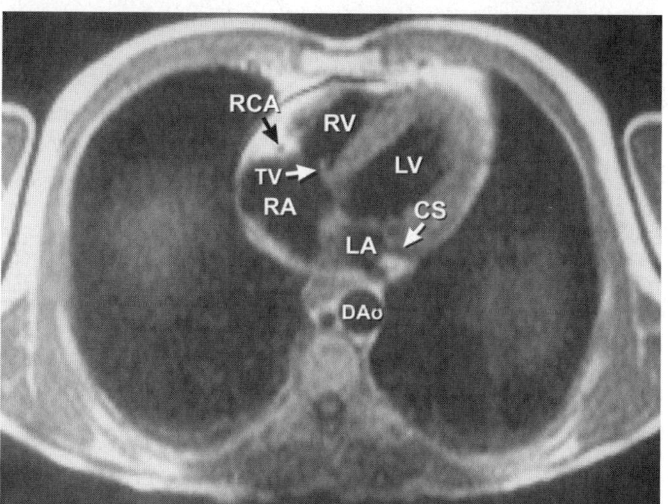


FIGURE 3-17 Tomographic sections of the heart in the transverse (*A*) and frontal (*B*) planes of the body. A tomographic section in the transverse plane of the body (*A*) results in an on-off axis four-chamber view of the heart. A tomographic section along the frontal plane of the body (*B*) results in an oblique short-axis view of the heart. *C*. MRI image corresponding to *A*. CS, coronary sinus; DAo, descending thoracic aorta; IVC, inferior vena cava; LA, left atrium; LAD, left anterior descending coronary artery; LV, left ventricle; RA, right atrium; RCA, right coronary artery; RV, right ventricle; RVO, right ventricular outflow; TV, tricuspid valve; VS, ventricular septum.

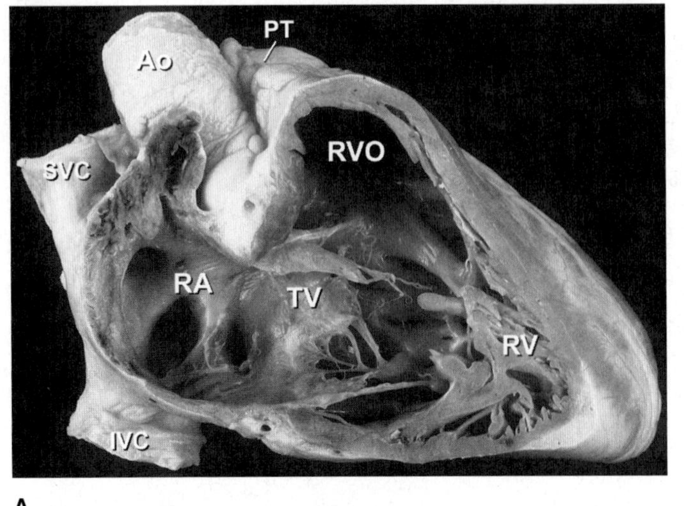


A

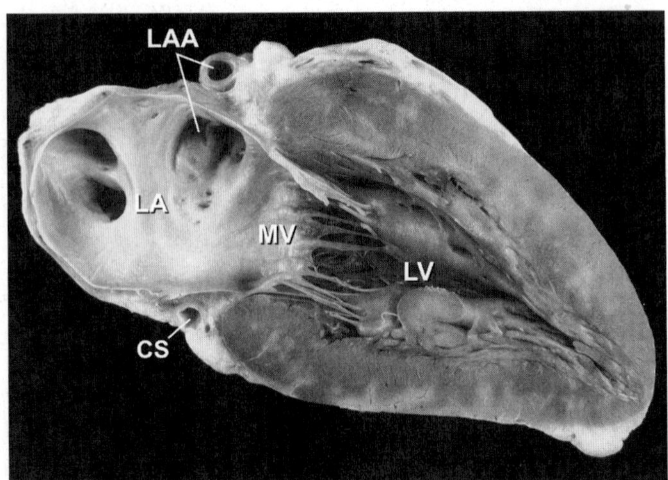


B

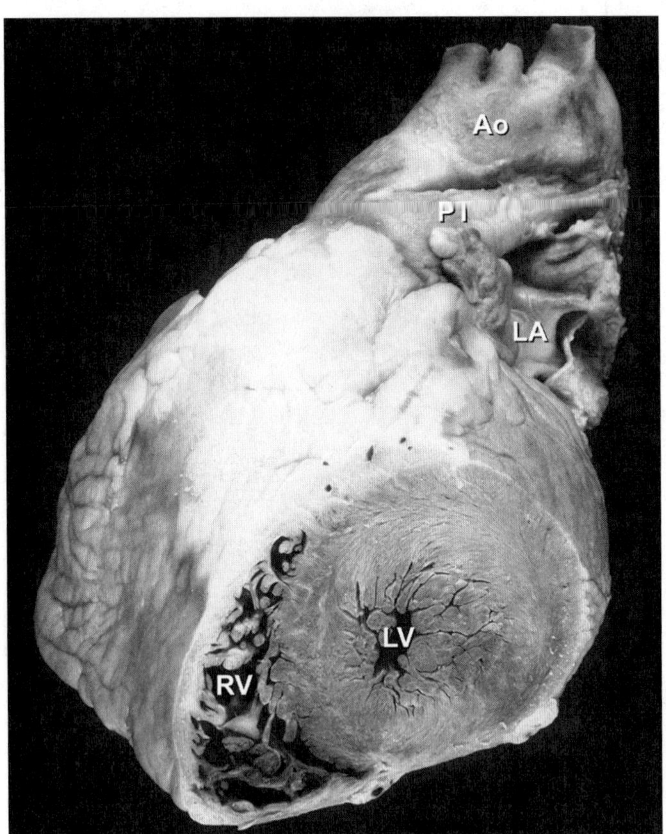


C

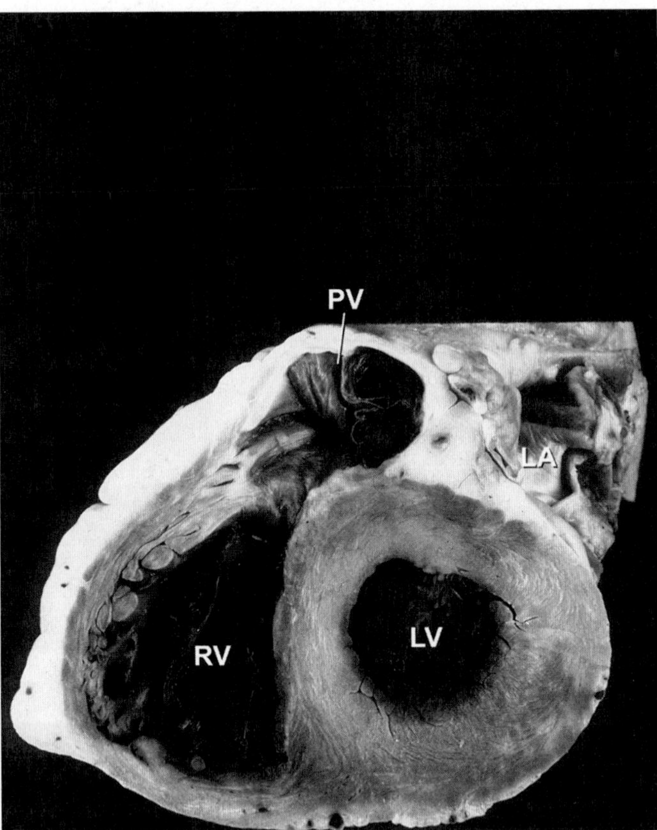


D

FIGURE 3-18 Oblique methods of tomographic cardiac dissection. *A, B.* Right anterior oblique sections, viewed from the right, are taken parallel to the ventricular and atrial septa, may include the right side of the heart (*A*) or the left side of the heart (*B*), and are similar to the two-chamber tomographic sections. *C,D.* Left anterior oblique sections, viewed from the apex toward the base, may be taken at various levels and are similar to the short-axis tomographic sections. Ao, aorta; CS, coronary sinus; IVC, inferior vena cava; LA, left atrium; LAA, left atrial appendage; LV, left ventricle; MV, mitral valve; PT, pulmonary trunk; PV, pulmonary valve; RA, right atrium; RV, right ventricle; RVO, right ventricular outflow; SVC, superior vena cava; TV, tricuspid valve.

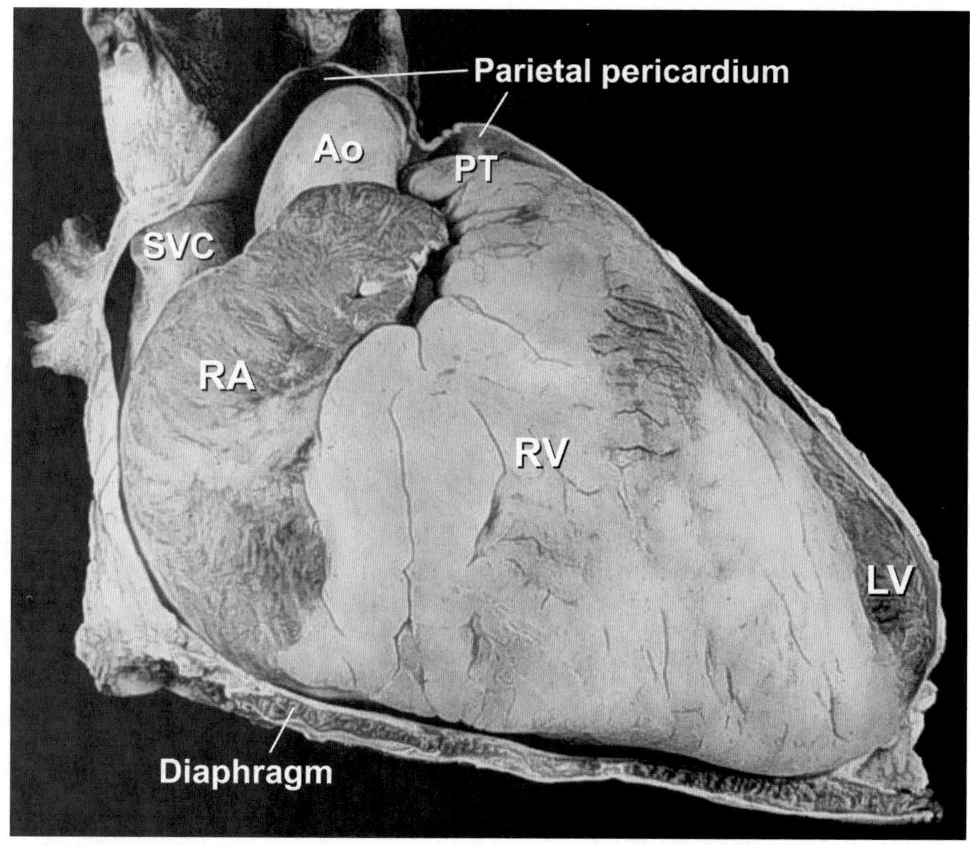


FIGURE 3-19 Anterior view of the heart. The anterior portion of the parietal pericardium has been removed, exposing the intrapericardial portions of the superior vena cava (SVC), ascending aorta (Ao), and pulmonary trunk (PT). LV, left ventricle; RA, right atrium; RV, right ventricle.

The commissures are cleftlike splits in the leaflet tissue that represent the sites of separation of the leaflets (Figs. 3-25 and 3-26*A*). Beneath the two mitral commissures lie the anterolateral and posteromedial papillary muscles, which arise from the left ventricular free wall (see Figs. 3-18*B* and 3-25). Commissural chords arise from each papillary muscle and extend in a fan-like array to insert into the free edge of both leaflets adjacent to the commissures (major commissures)[17] (see Figs. 3-24 and 3-26*A*, Plate 10) or into two adjacent scallops of the posterior leaflet (minor commissures) (see Figs. 3-24, Plate 10, and 3-25). *In contrast to congenital clefts, a true commissure is always associated with an underlying papillary muscle and an intervening array of chordae tendineae.*[17] The attachments of commissural chords precisely demarcate the commissure. *Because the commissural chords are seldom elongated, they serve as accurate reference points for determining the proper closing plane for the leaflets during surgical repair.*

The anterolateral papillary muscle is commonly single and usually has a dual blood supply from the left coronary circulation.[16] In contrast, the posteromedial papillary muscle usually has multiple heads and is most commonly supplied only by the right coronary artery.[16] Small left atrial branches supply the most basal aspects of the mitral leaflets.[17]

Papillary muscle contraction pulls the two leaflets toward one another and thereby promotes valve closure. The line of closure for either mitral leaflet is not its free edge but an ill-defined junction between a thin, clear zone and a thicker, rough zone[17] (see Fig. 3-26, Plate 11). The major chordae supporting a leaflet insert into its free edge and rough zone. The chordae tendineae anchor and support the leaflets and, by doing so, prevent leaflet prolapse during ventricular

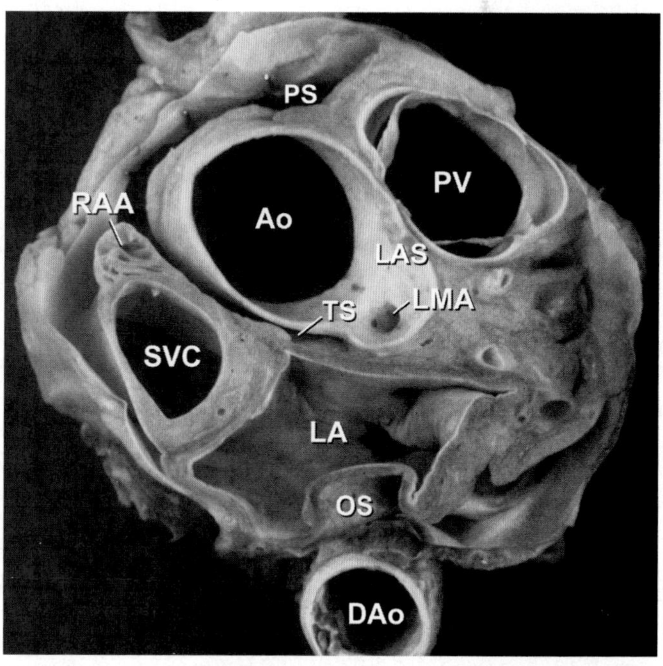


FIGURE 3-20 Tomographic section in the short-axis plane of the body, looking from apex toward the base, showing the oblique (OS) and transverse (TS) pericardial sinus. Ao, ascending aorta; DAo, descending thoracic aorta; LA, left atrium; LAS, left aortic sinus; LMA, left main coronary artery: PS, pericardial sac; PV, pulmonary valve; RAA, right atrial appendage; SVC, superior vena cava.

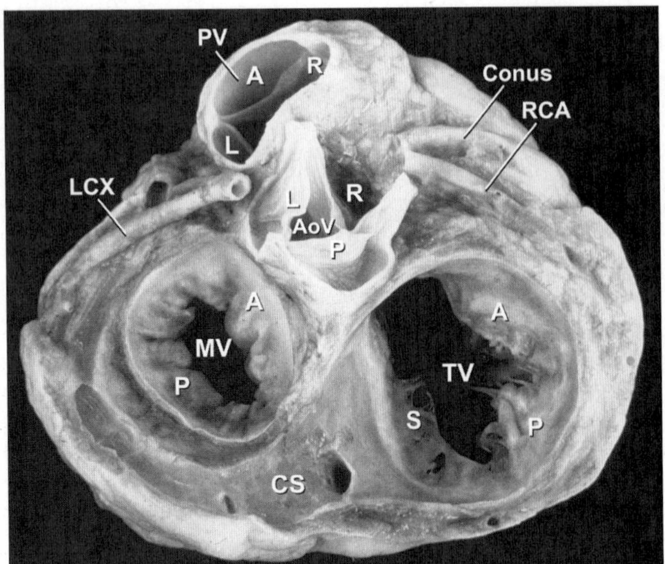


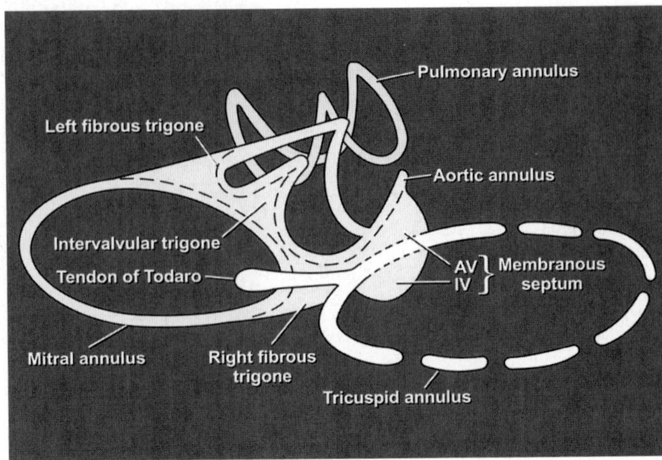


FIGURE 3-21 (Plate 9) Base of heart. *A*. Section through the base of the heart, looking from base toward apex, with the atria and great arteries removed, shows all four cardiac valves. *B*. A comparable schematic diagram of the fibrous cardiac skeleton. The centrally located aortic valve forms the cornerstone of the cardiac skeleton. Its fibrous extensions anchor and support the other three valves. *A*, anterior; AoV, aortic valve; AV, atrioventricular; CS, coronary sinus; IV, interventricular; L, left; LCX, left circumflex coronary artery; MV, mitral valve; P, posterior; PV, pulmonary valve; R, right; RCA, right coronary artery; S, septal; TV, tricuspid valve.

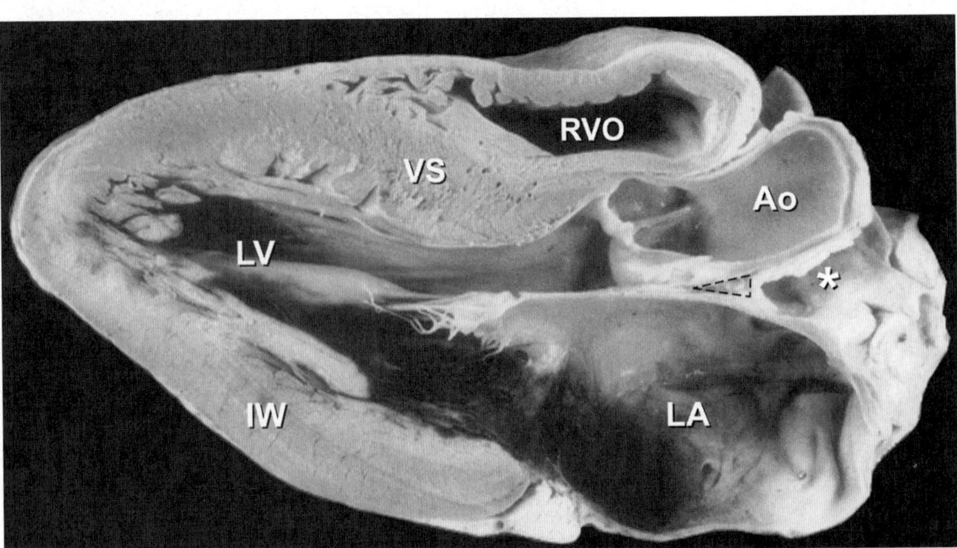


FIGURE 3-22 Long-axis section of the left ventricle. The intervalvular fibrosa (dashed triangle) lies between the anterior mitral leaflet and the posterior cusp of the aortic valve and abuts the floor of the transverse pericardial sinus (*). Ao, ascending aorta; IW, inferior wall; LA, left atrium; LV, left ventricle; RVO, right ventricular outflow; VS, ventricular septum.

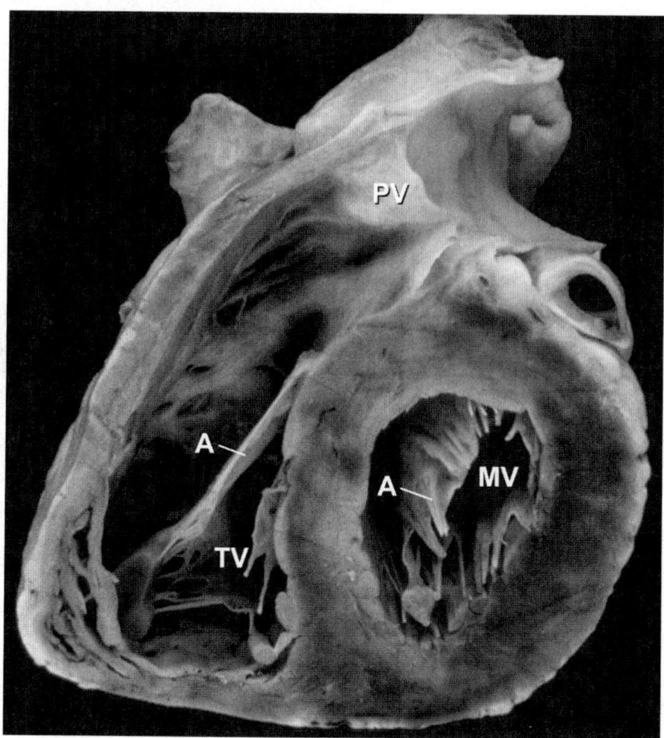


FIGURE 3-23 This oblique short-axis view of the heart shows the triangular-shaped tricuspid orifice (TV) and the elliptical mitral orifice (MV) at midleaflet level. The anterior tricuspid and anterior mitral leaflets (A) separate the inflow and outflow tracts of the right and left ventricles, respectively, and are parallel to one another. PV, pulmonary valve.

systole. Two particularly prominent rough zone chords, referred to as *strut chordae,* insert along each half of the ventricular surface of the anterior mitral leaflet and provide additional leaflet support.[17] They may contain cardiac muscle and tend to calcify with age. Unlike the tricuspid valve, *the normal mitral leaflets have no chordal insertions into the ventricular septum.*[16]

*The functional orifice of the mitral valve is defined by its narrowest diastolic cross-sectional area. This may be at the annulus when there is extensive annular calcification or close to the papillary muscle tips in patients with rheumatic mitral stenosis.*

*Mitral valve prolapse is characterized by thickened and redundant leaflets, annular dilatation (with or without calcium), and thickened and elongated chordae tendineae (with or without rupture). Prolapse of the posterior leaflet occurs more frequently than that of the anterior leaflet. Rheumatic involvement of the mitral valve causes chordal shortening and thickening without annular dilatation. Rheumatic mitral stenosis is produced by chordal and commissural fusion, often with calcification, whereas rheumatic mitral insufficiency results from scar retraction of leaflets and chords.*[15] *Chronic postinfarction mitral regurgitation is associated with left ventricular dilatation and scarring of a papillary muscle and its subjacent ventricular free wall. Acute postinfarction mitral regurgitation may be associated with partial or complete rupture of a papillary muscle, usually the posteromedial one.*

*Anatomically important structures during mitral valve surgery include the left circumflex coronary artery, which courses within the left atrioventricular groove near the anterolateral commissure, and the coronary sinus, which courses within the left atrioventricular groove adjacent to the annulus of the posterior mitral leaflet*[17] (see Fig. 3-21*A*, Plate 9).

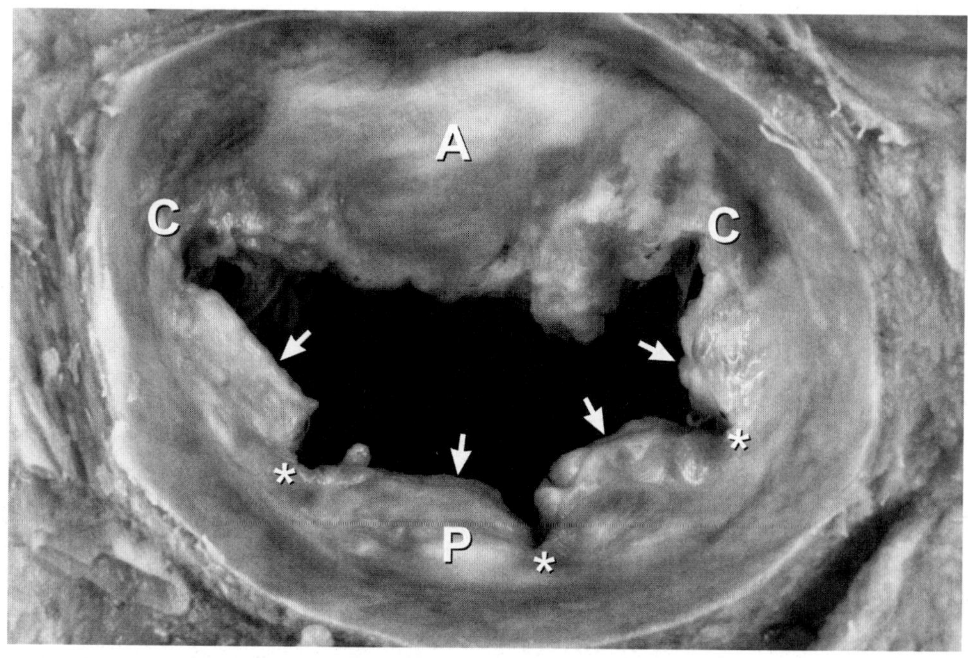


FIGURE 3-24 (Plate 10) Mitral valve, viewed from left atrial aspect. Minor commissures (*) divide the posterior leaflet into four scallops (arrows). A, anterior; C, major commissures; P, posterior.

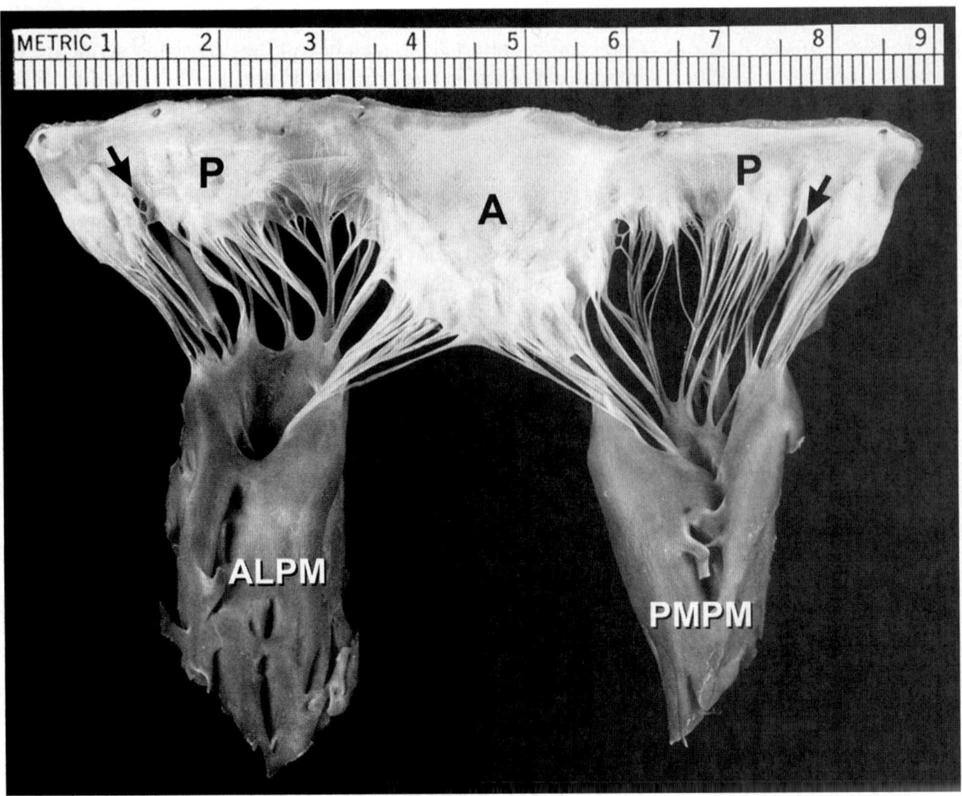


FIGURE 3-25 Gross anatomy of the mitral valve and papillary muscles–chordal apparatus, as demonstrated in an excised and unfolded valve. Each commissure overlies a papillary muscle. Arrows point to minor commissures. A, anterior leaflet; ALPM, anterolateral papillary muscle; P, posterior leaflet; PMPM, posteromedial papillary muscle.

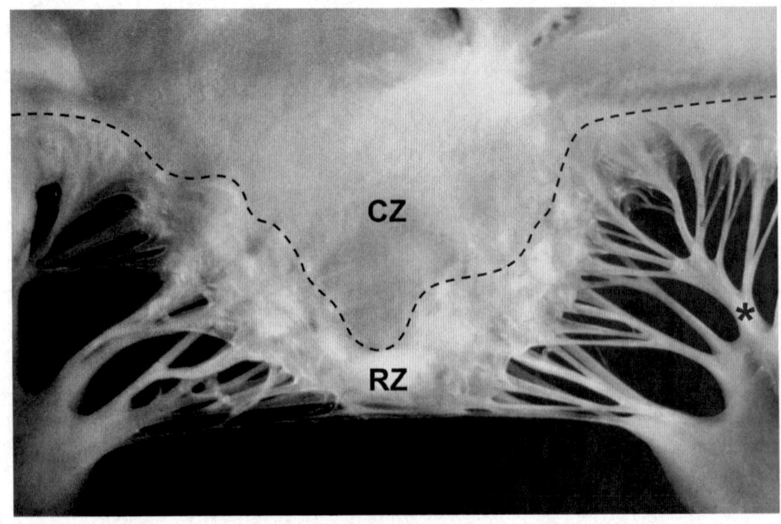


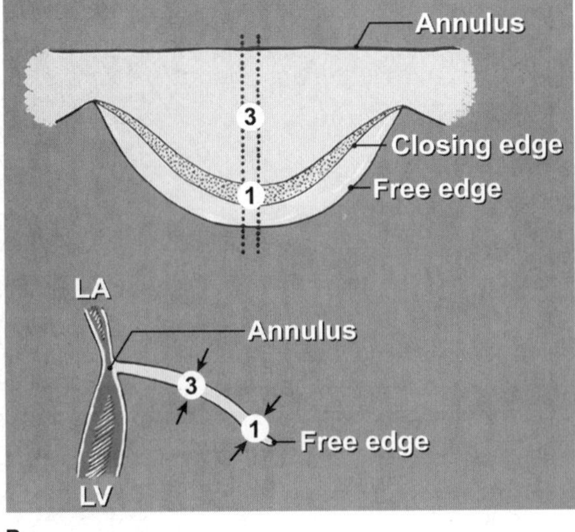


FIGURE 3-26 (Plate 11) Components of the mitral valve. *A*. Each leaflet has a large clear zone (CZ) and a smaller rough zone (RZ) between its free edge and closing edge (*dotted line*). A fanlike commissural chordae tendinea (*) connects the tip of the papillary muscle to the commissure. *B*. Schematic diagram of an open anterior mitral leaflet comparable to *A*. Section obtained along the dotted lines shows the relationship of the mitral annulus and free edge to the closing edge.

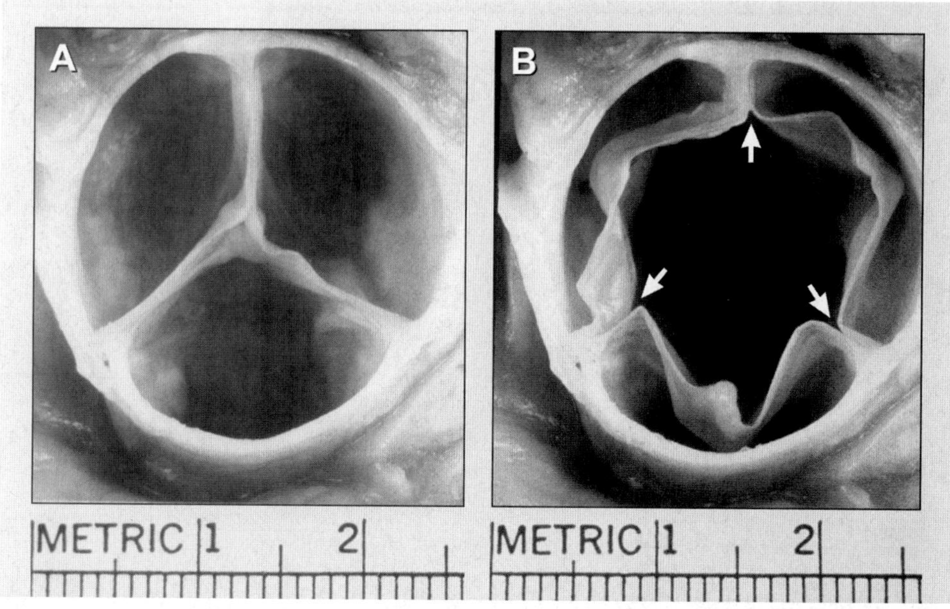


FIGURE 3-27 Each cusp of a semilunar valve is pocket-shaped. The aortic valve is viewed from above in simulated closed (*A*) and open (*B*) positions, showing the three commissures (arrows). Note that the length of the closing edge exceeds the straight-line distance between the commissures.

## Aortic Valve

The aortic valve, like the pulmonary valve, is composed of three components (i.e., annulus, cusps, and commissures). In contrast to the mitral and tricuspid valves, the two semilunar valves have no tensor apparatus (i.e., chordae tendineae or papillary muscles). The commissures form tall, peaked spaces between the attachments of adjacent cusps (Figs. 3-27 and 3-28) and attain the level of the aortic sinotubular junction, the ridge that separates the sinus and tubular portions of the ascending aorta (originally described by Leonardo da Vinci as the "supraortic ridge")[15] (see Fig. 3-28). The functional aortic valve orifice may be at the sinotubular junction or proximal to it.[17]

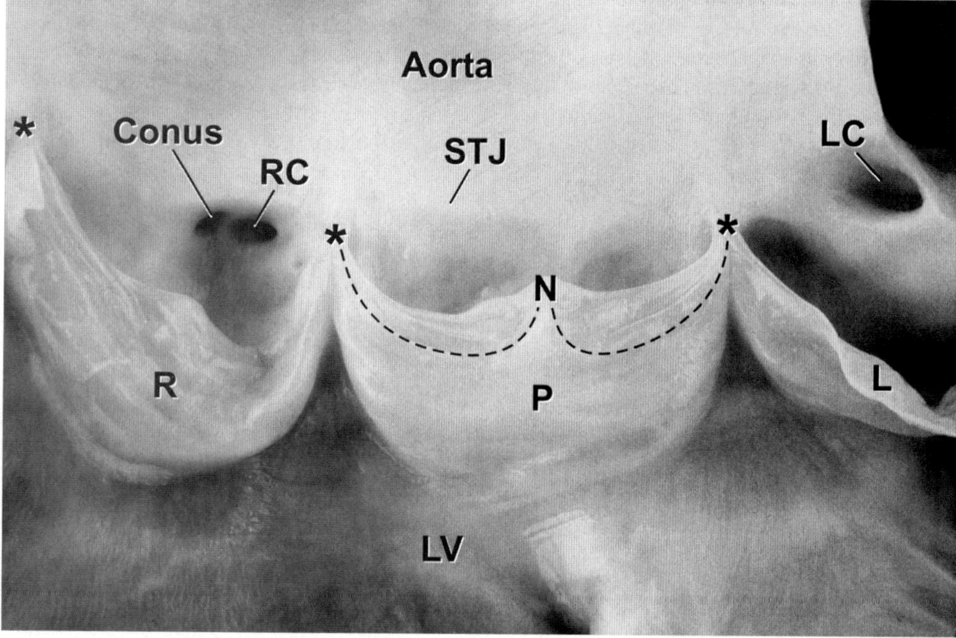


FIGURE 3-28 An opened aortic valve shows the right (R), left (L), and posterior (P) cusps. The dashed line marks the closing edge. Between the free and closing edges of each cusp are two lunular areas, representing the surfaces of apposition between adjacent cusps during valve closure. The commissures (*) attain the level of the aortic sinotubular junction (STJ). Conus, conus coronary ostium; LC, left coronary ostium; LV, left ventricle; N, nodule of Arantius; RC, right coronary ostium.

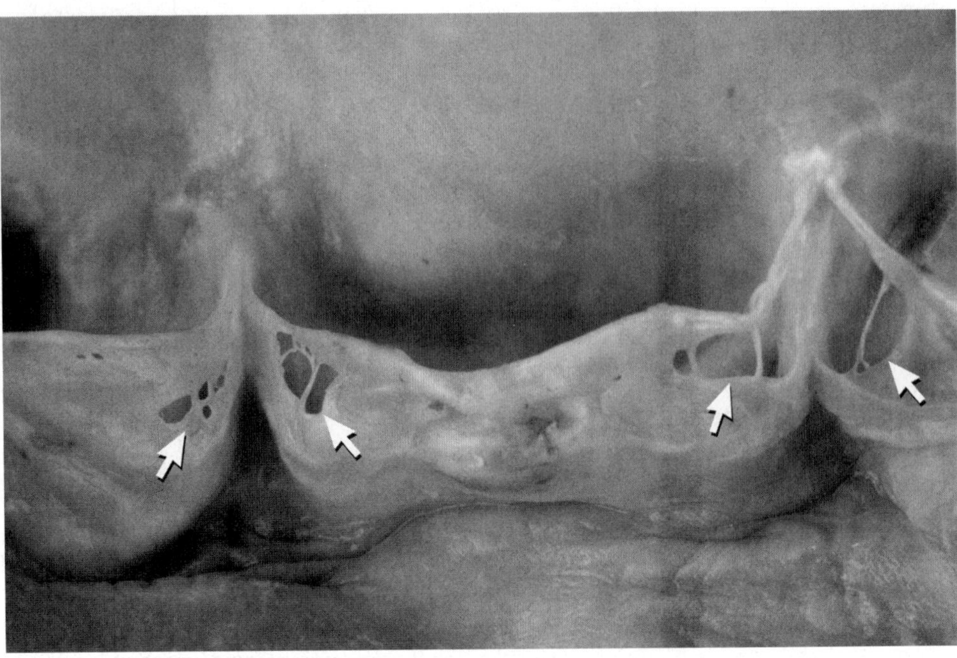

FIGURE 3-29 Aortic cusp fenestrations (arrows) occurring in the lunular regions near the commissures. This is a common age-related degenerative finding and normally accounts for little or no aortic valve regurgitation.

The three half moon–shaped (semilunar) aortic cusps form pocket-like tissue flaps that are avascular. In only about 10 percent of hearts are they truly equal in size. In two-thirds of hearts, either the right or posterior cusp is larger than the other two.[17] Just below the free edge of each cusp is a ridge-like closing edge (see Fig. 3-28). At the center of each cusp the closing edge meets the free edge and forms a small fibrous mound, the *nodule of Arantius*[15] (see Fig. 3-28). Between the free and closing edges, to each side of the nodule are two crescent-shaped areas known as the *lunulas*, which represent the sites of cusp apposition during valve closure.[15] Lunular fenestrations, near the commissures are common and increase in size and incidence with age[15] (Fig. 3-29). However, owing to their position distal to the closing edge, they rarely produce valvular incompetence.[17] When viewed from above, the linear distance along the closing edge of a cusp is much greater than the straight-line distance between its two commissures[15] (see Fig. 3-27). This extra length of cusp tissue is necessary for nonstenotic opening and nonregurgitant closure of the valve.[15] Normally, the diameter of the aortic annulus at the hinge points of the aortic valve is about equal to the diameter of the ascending aorta at the sinotubular junction.[8]

*These are important anatomic details in patients undergoing aortic valve repair. In hearts from adults with bicuspid valves and other congenital aortic valve disease, the annular diameter is usually enlarged. In contrast, patients with normal aortic cusps and central aortic regurgitation show enlargement at the level of the sinotubular junction.*[7] *A prebypass intraoperative transesophageal long-axis view of the left ventricular outflow tract is used to measure the aortic valve annular diameter prior to replacement by a homograft. In doing so, precious bypass time is saved while the homograft is being prepared.*[8] *Disease processes that produce commissural fusion such as rheumatic valvulitis or which decrease cusp mobility such as fibrosis or calcification may lead to aortic stenosis.*[15] *In contrast, those disorders that decrease cusp size, such as rheumatic valvulitis, or that cause aortic root dilatation may lead to aortic regurgitation.*[15] *Combinations of these processes may produce combined stenosis and regurgitation.*

The commissure between the right and posterior aortic cusps overlies the membranous septum (Fig. 3-30) and contacts the commissure between the anterior and septal leaflets of the tricuspid valve (see Fig. 3-40). The commissure between the right and left aortic cusps contacts its corresponding pulmonary commissure and overlies the infundibular septum (see Fig. 3-12*D*). The intervalvular fibrosa, at the commissure between the left and posterior aortic cusps, fuses the aortic valve to the anterior mitral leaflet.[15,17]

*During aortic valve replacement, the anterior mitral leaflet, left bundle branch, or coronary ostia may be injured inadvertently.*[17] *Annular abscesses due to infective endocarditis involving the aortic valve may burrow into adjacent structures and thereby produce endocarditis of the other valves; conduction disturbances with septal involvement; aortoatrial, aortopulmonary artery, or aortoventricular fistulas; pericarditis; or fatal hemopericardium.*[15]

## Pulmonary Valve

The pulmonary valve is virtually identical in design to the aortic valve.[17] The pulmonary artery sinuses are partially embedded within the muscle bundles of the right ventricular infundibulum, particularly adjacent to the right and left sinuses.[16,19] *In pulmonary valve atresia with an intact ventricular septum, hypertrophy of the muscle bundles and the narrow right ventricular outflow tract accentuate this relationship.*[19] Also, unlike the aortic valve, which is continuous with the mitral valve, the pulmonary and tricuspid valves are separated by infundibular muscle.[17]

## Age-Related Valve Changes

Several age-related changes in the cardiac valves may have clinical significance.[20] In normal hearts, the thickness of the aortic and mitral leaflets increases progressively with each decade, particularly along their closure margins.[20] Probably the most common clinical manifestation of these changes is aortic valve sclerosis, characterized by valve thickening without hemodynamic dysfunction.[20] However, age-related degenerative calcification of an otherwise anatomically normal-appearing aortic valve may result in progressive aortic stenosis.[20]

Age-related thickening along the nodule of Arantius and closing edges may be associated with the formation of whisker-like projections called *Lambl's excrescences*. These fine fibrous-like strands also can develop on the mitral valve.[17] *Lambl's excrescences can be detected by echocardiography and have been associated with cardioembolic stroke.*[21] *Larger clusters, having the appearance of a sea anemone, are considered to be either neoplastic or reactive and are known as* papillary fibroelastomas.[22]

The circumferences of all four cardiac valves increase with age in normal hearts. This is particularly evident in the semilunar valves.[20]

# THE COLOR PLATES

**WHO Regions for Global Burden of Disease**

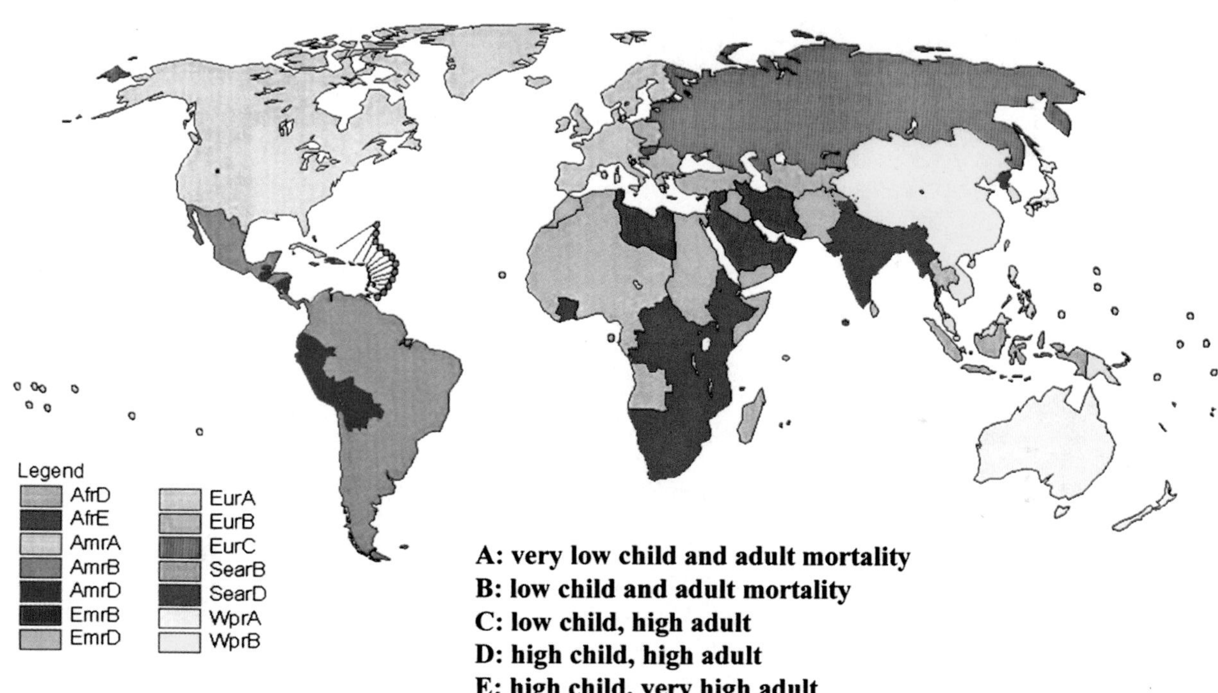


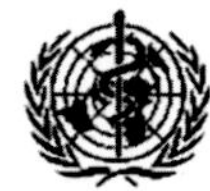

Plate 1 (FIGURE 2-1) World Health Organization (WHO) subregions for global burden of disease. For geographic disaggregation of the global burden of disease, the six WHO regions of the world have been further divided into 14 subregions, based on levels of child (under 5 years) and adult (15 to 59 years) mortality for WHO member states. The classification of WHO member states into the mortality strata were carried out using population estimates for 1999 (United Nations population division, 1998) and estimates of 5q0 and 45q15 based on WHO analyses of mortality rates for 1999. Five mortality strata were defined in terms of quintiles of the distribution of 5q0 and 45q15 (both sexes combined). Adult mortality 45q15 was regressed on 5q0 and the regression line used to divide countries with high child mortality into high adult mortality (stratum D) and very high adult mortality (stratum E). Stratum E includes the countries in Sub-Saharan Africa where HIV/AIDS has had a very substantial impact. (Adapted from Mathers CD, Stein C, Fat DM, et al. Global burden of disease 2000: Version 2 methods and results. Global program on evidence for health policy discussion Paper No. 50. World Health Organization, October 2002 From http://www.hoffmanpr.com/Press_Releases/Archived_Press_Releases/WHO/Cardio2002/CardioGraphs.ppt, used with permission.)

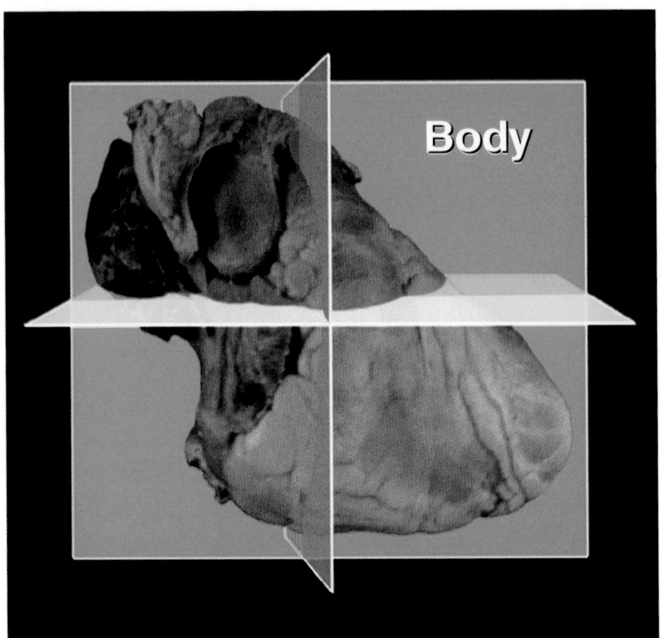


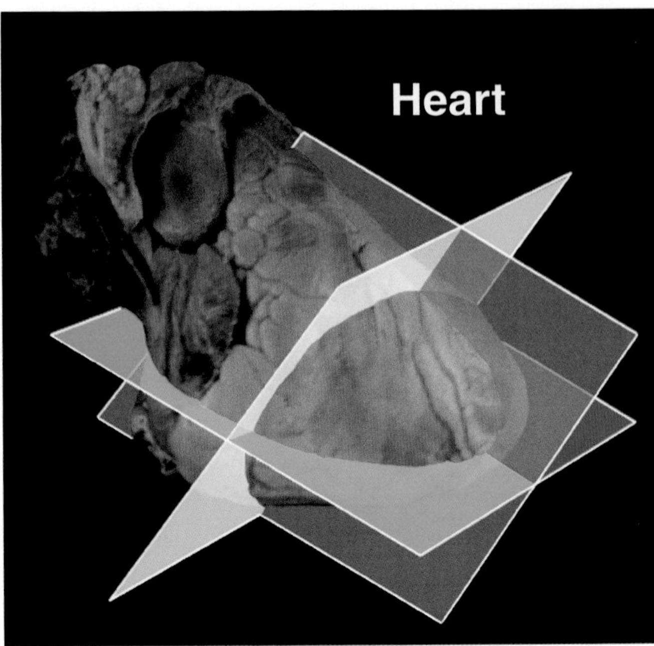


Plate 2 (FIGURE 3-4) The three primary planes of the body (*left*) and heart (*right*). Note that the planes of the body are aligned with vertical midline structures, such as the esophagus. In contrast, the major axis of the heart is oriented obliquely. Thus the heart's long and short axes do not lie in the same plane as the body's long and short axes. The body planes cut the heart obliquely and not in its primary planes. Conversely, the heart's primary planes cut the body obliquely.

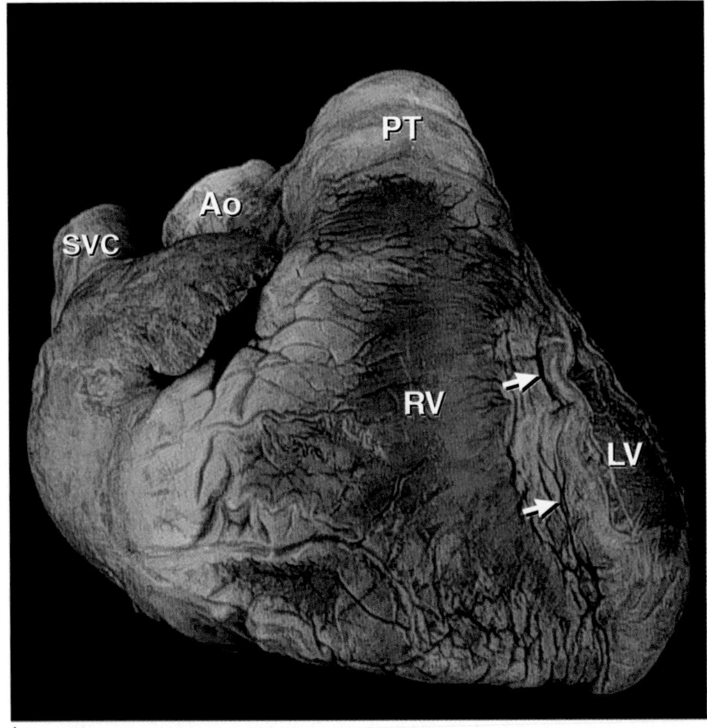


*A*

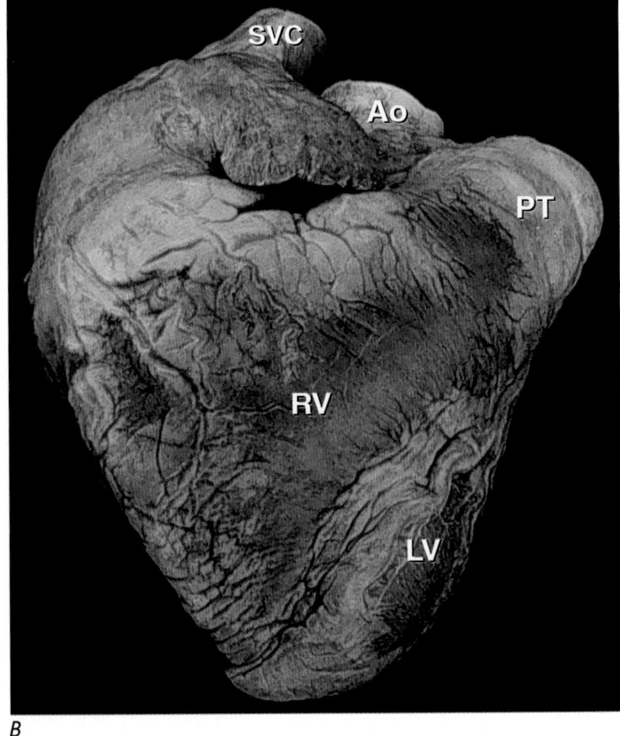


*B*

Plate 3 (FIGURE 3-5) *A*. Anterior view of the heart in its usual anatomic position with its apex directed from right to left. Arrows point to the anterior interventricular groove. *B*. Nonanatomic positioning of the normal heart with its apex directed downward, thereby resembling a "valentine." The position of the cardiac apex is normally leftward (levocardia) but may anomalously be rightward (dextrocardia) or midline and inferiorly (mesocardia). Ao, ascending aorta; LV, left ventricle; PT, pulmonary trunk; RV, right ventricle; SVC, superior vena cava.

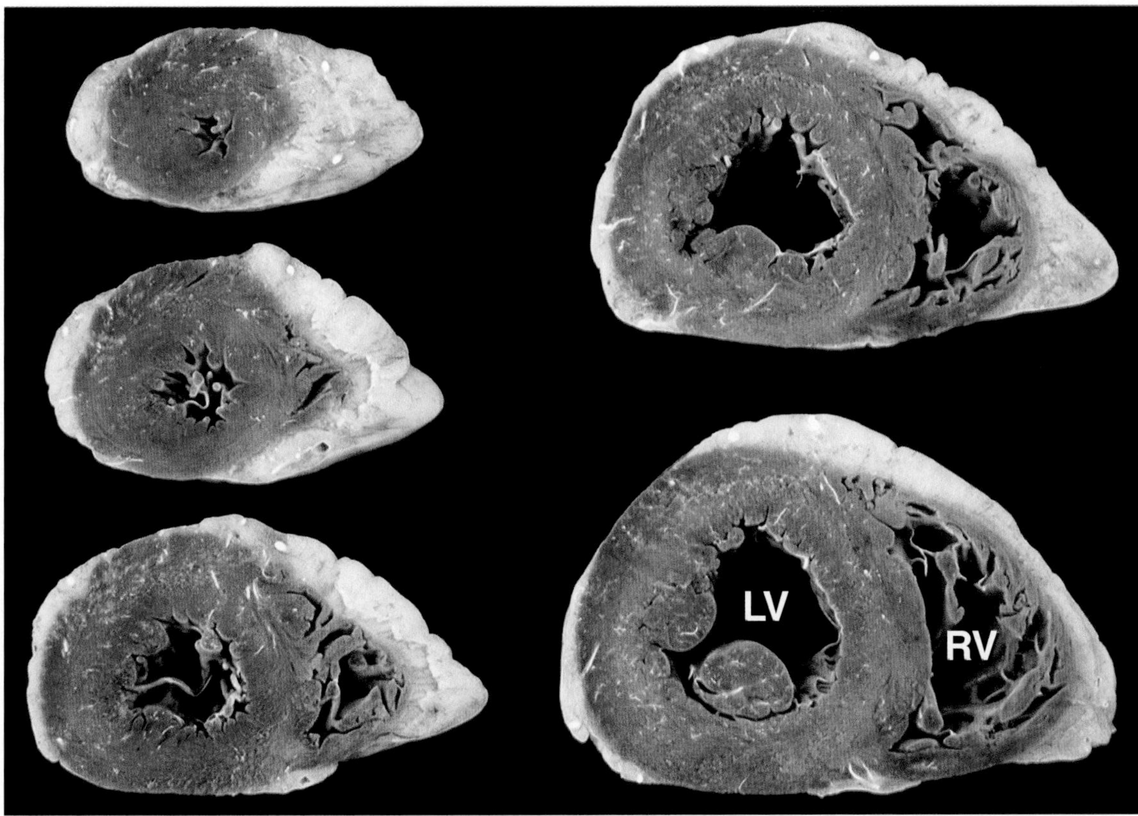


Plate 4 (FIGURE 3-8) Ventricular slice method of cardiac dissection. Display of five slices (LV, left ventricle; RV, right ventricle) viewed as though looking from the base of the heart toward the apex.

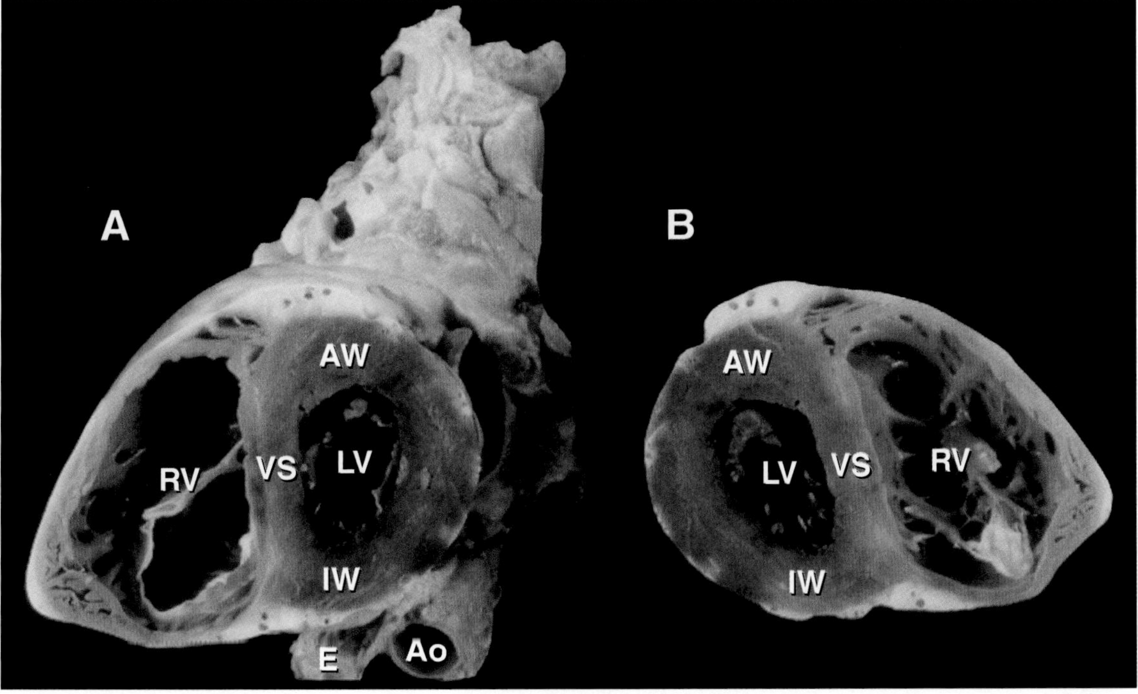


Plate 5 (FIGURE 3-9) Bisected cardiac specimen, viewed in the short axis. *A*. The specimen is viewed from the apex toward the base. The esophagus (E) is posterior and adjacent to both the thoracic aorta (Ao) and the inferior wall of the left ventricle (LV). The right ventricular (RV) cavity is to the left. *B*. The other half of the bisected specimen is viewed as though looking from the base toward the apex (comparable with Fig. 3-8). AW, anterior wall; IW, inferior wall; VS, ventricular septum.

Plate 6 (FIGURE 3-10) Bisected cardiac specimen in the four-chamber view parallel to the base-apex axis of the heart. The bisected specimen (*left*) has been partially opened to show the relative relationship of the bisected halves. The two components of the bisected specimen (*right*) are opened completely. Note the positions of the pulmonary veins posteriorly and the positions of the atrial appendages at the atrioventricular groove. AL, anterolateral papillary muscle; AS, atrial septum; IVC, inferior vena cava; LA, left atrium; LAA, left atrial appendage; LV, left ventricle; MV, mitral valve; PM, posteromedial papillary muscle; PulV, pulmonary vein; RA, right atrium; RAA, right atrial appendage; RV, right ventricle; TV, tricuspid valve; VS, ventricular septum.

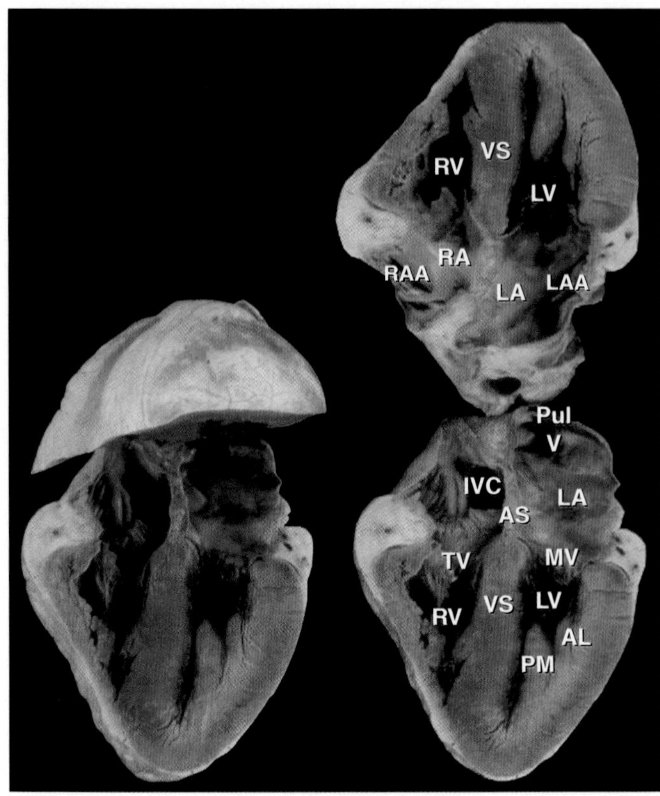


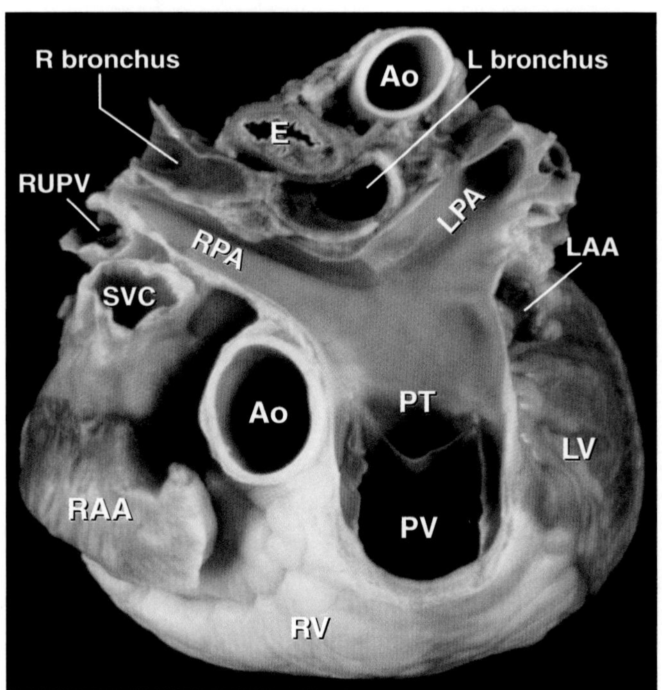


*A*

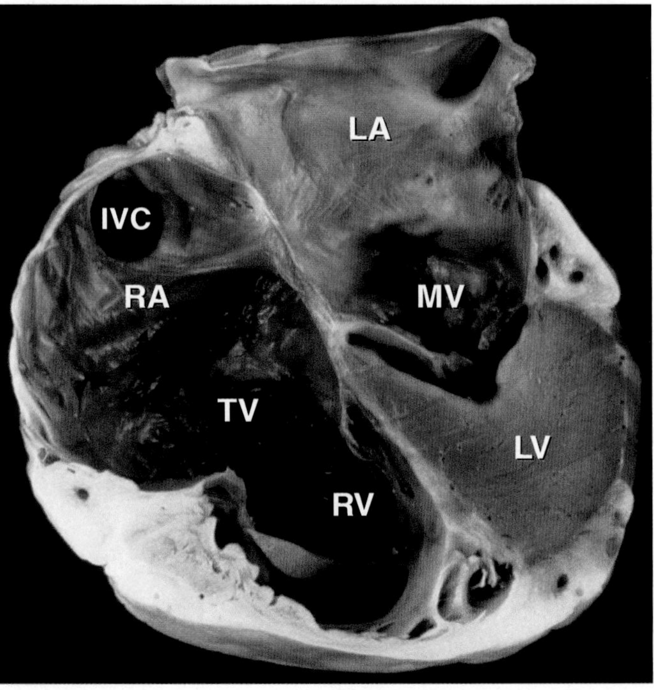


*B*

Plate 7 (FIGURE 3-11) Tomographic cardiac dissection along the body primary planes. *A*, *B*. Transverse sections (looking from head toward feet) at the level of the great vessels (*A*) or the cardiac chambers (*B*). The aortic arch travels over the left bronchus and the right pulmonary artery. *C*, *D*. Frontal sections (looking from anterior to posterior) through both ventricles (*C*) or left ventricle and right atrium (*D*). *E*,*F*. Parasagittal sections looking from right (*E*) to left (*F*). Ao, ascending aorta; CS, coronary sinus; E, esophagus; IA, innominate artery; IVC, inferior vena cava; LA, left atrium; LAA, left atrial appendage; LB, left bronchus; LCX, left circumflex coronary artery; LIV, left innominate vein; LLPV, left lower pulmonary vein; LPA, left pulmonary artery; LUPV, left upper pulmonary vein; LSA, left subclavian artery; LV, left ventricle; MS, membranous ventricular septum; MV, mitral valve; PS, pericardial sac; PT, pulmonary trunk; PV, pulmonary valve; RA, right atrium; RAA, right atrial appendage; RPA, right pulmonary artery; RUPV, right upper pulmonary vein; RV, right ventricle; RVO, right ventricular outflow; SVC, superior vena cava; TV, tricuspid valve.

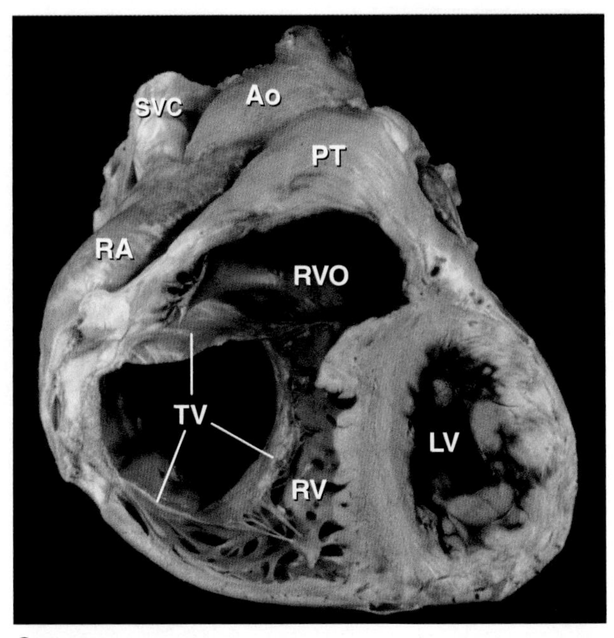
SVC
Ao
PT
RA
RVO
TV
RV
LV
C

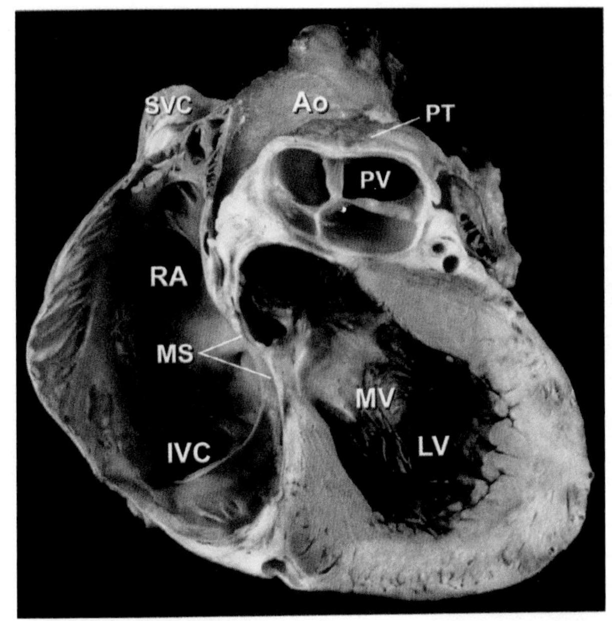
SVC
Ao
PT
PV
RA
MS
MV
IVC
LV
D

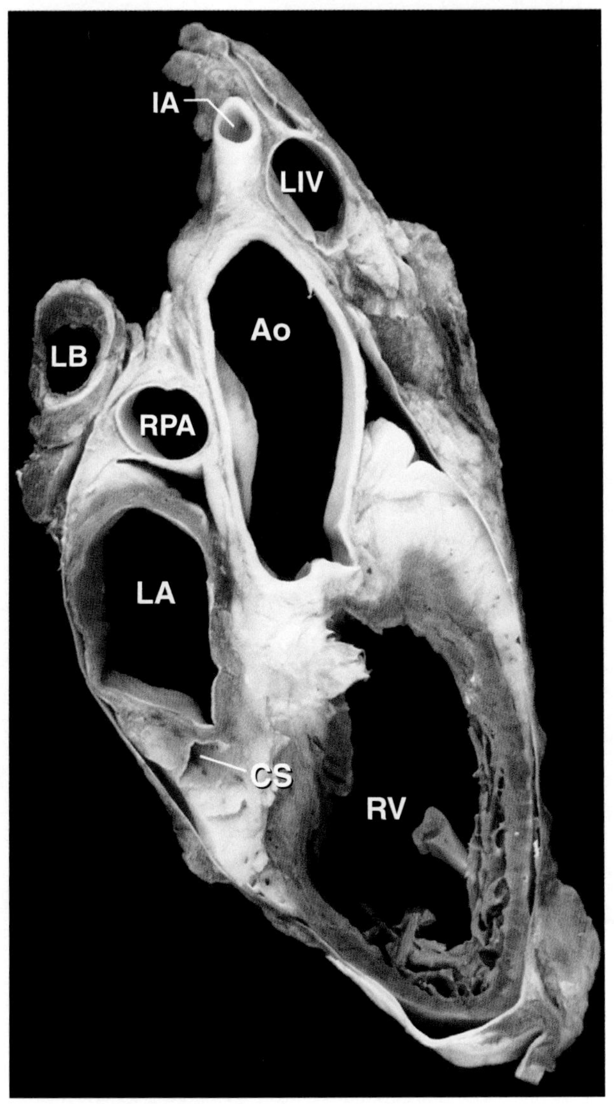
IA
LIV
Ao
LB
RPA
LA
CS
RV
E

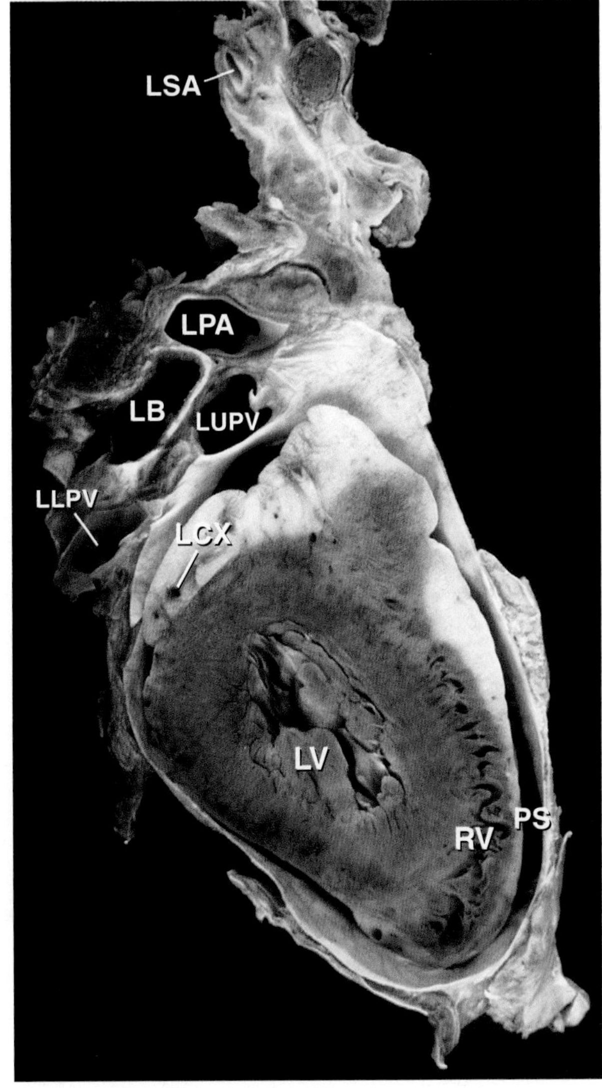
LSA
LPA
LB
LUPV
LLPV
LCX
LV
RV
PS
F

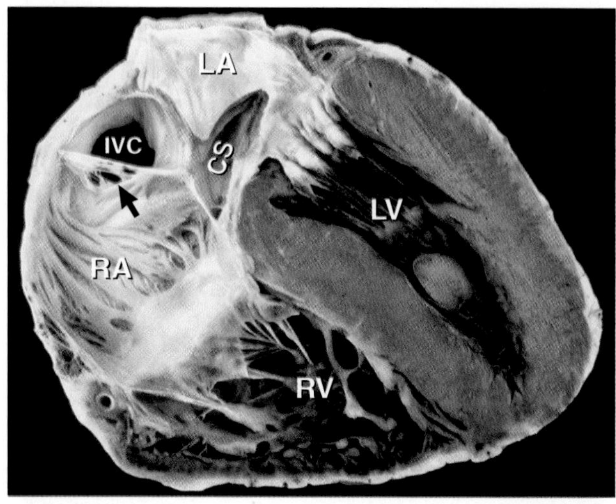


A

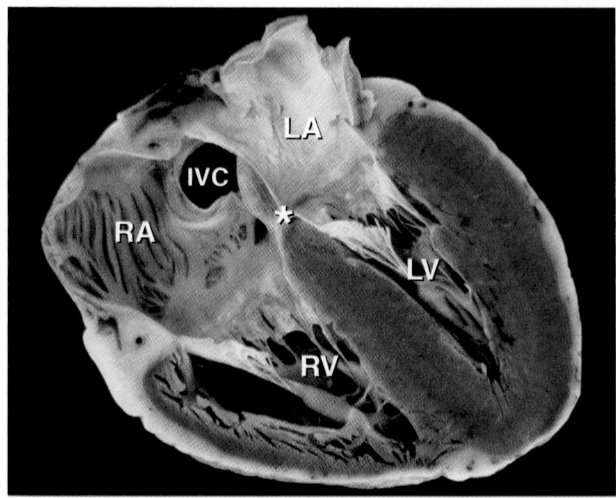


B

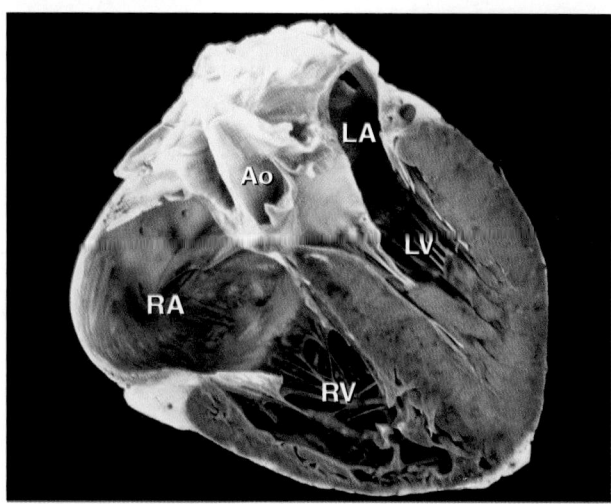

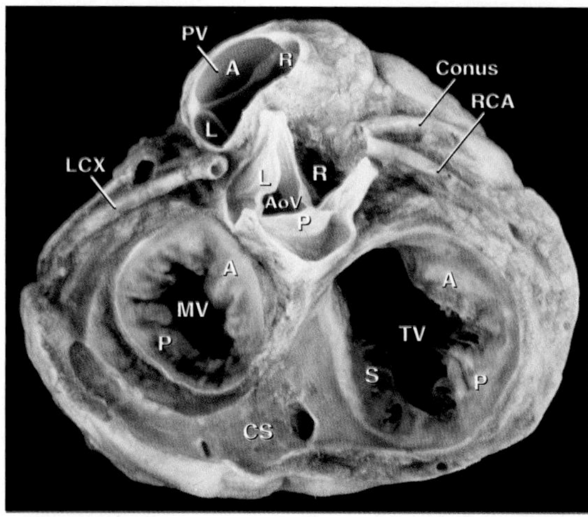


C

Plate 8 (FIGURE 3-16) Collage of four-chamber tomographic sections cutting from inferior wall to anterosuperior wall showing coronary sinus (*A*), internal cardiac crux (*) (*B*), and aortic valve (*C*). Ao, ascending aorta; CS, coronary sinus; IVC, inferior vena cava; LA, left atrium; LV, left ventricle; RA, right atrium; RV, right ventricle; arrow in *A* points to a fenestrated eustachian valve.

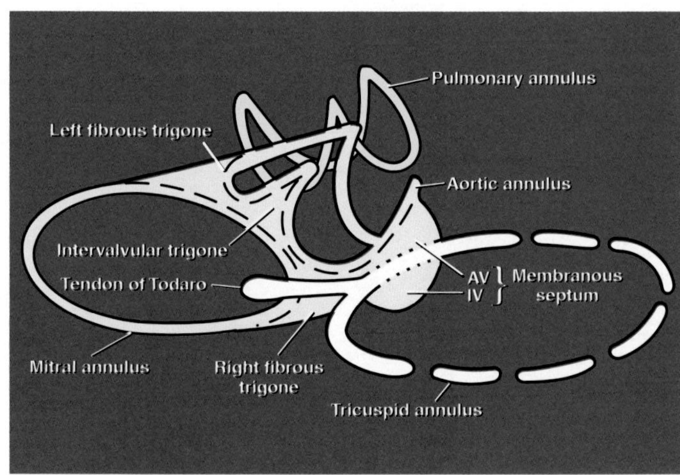


A B

Plate 9 (FIGURE 3-21) Base of heart. *A*. Section through the base of the heart, looking from base toward apex, with the atria and great arteries removed, shows all four cardiac valves. *B*. A comparable schematic diagram of the fibrous cardiac skeleton. The centrally located aortic valve forms the cornerstone of the cardiac skeleton. Its fibrous extensions anchor and support the other three valves. *A*, anterior; AoV, aortic valve; AV, atrioventricular; CS, coronary sinus; IV, interventricular; L, left; LCX, left circumflex coronary artery; MV, mitral valve; P, posterior; PV, pulmonary valve; R, right; RCA, right coronary artery; S, septal; TV, tricuspid valve.

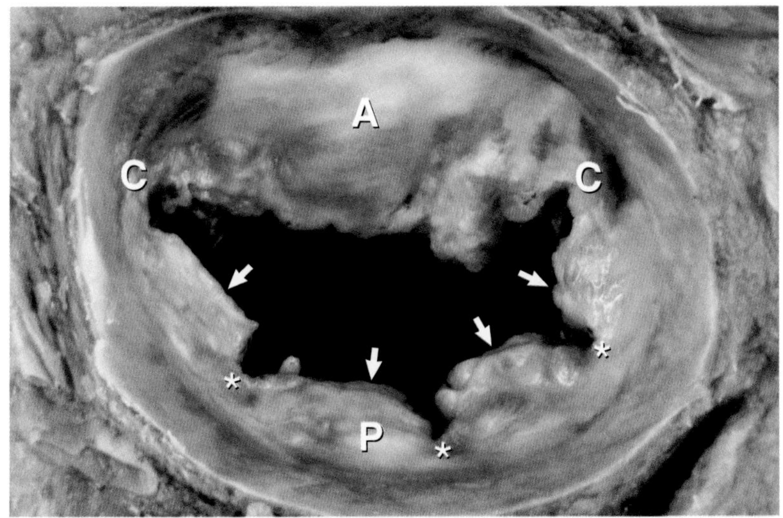


◀ Plate 10 (FIGURE 3-24) Mitral valve, viewed from left atrial aspect. Minor commissures (*) divide the posterior leaflet into four scallops (arrows). A, anterior; C, major commissures; P, posterior

▼ Plate 11 (FIGURE 3-26) Components of the mitral valve. *A*. Each leaflet has a large clear zone (CZ) and a smaller rough zone (RZ) between its free edge and closing edge (*dotted line*). A fanlike commissural chordae tendinea (*) connects the tip of the papillary muscle to the commissure. *B*. Schematic diagram of an open anterior mitral leaflet comparable to *A*. Section obtained along the dotted lines shows the relationship of the mitral annulus and free edge to the closing edge.

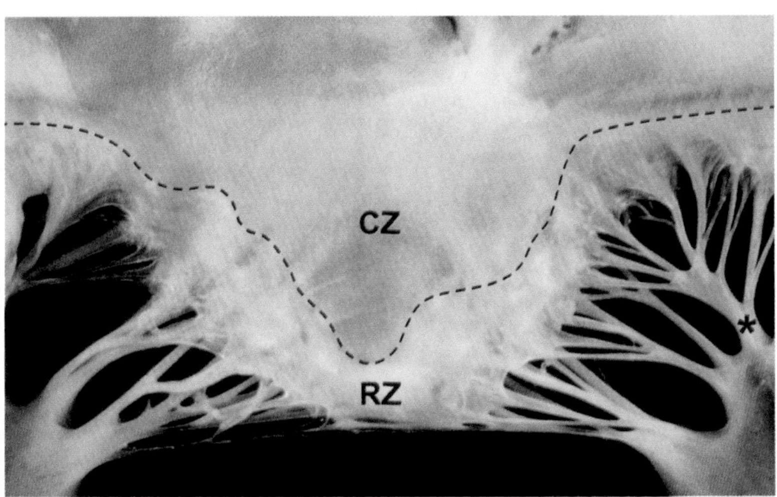


*A*

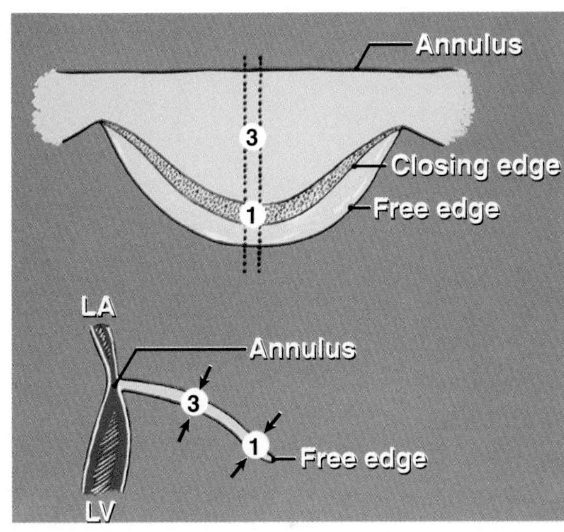


*B*

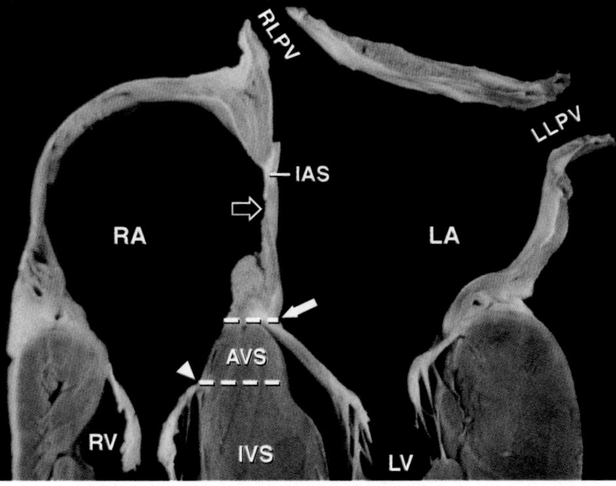


Plate 12 (FIGURE 3-34) Internal cardiac crux. Four-chamber slice of the heart shows the characteristic normal apical displacement of the tricuspid valve septal leaflet insertion (arrowhead) when compared with septal insertion of the mitral valve (solid arrow). This tomographic section also shows the interatrial septum (IAS), atrioventricular septum (AVS), and interventricular septum (IVS). Open arrow points to fossa ovalis. LA, left atrium; LLPV, left lower pulmonary vein; LV, left ventricle; RA, right atrium; RLPV, right lower pulmonary vein; RV, right ventricle.

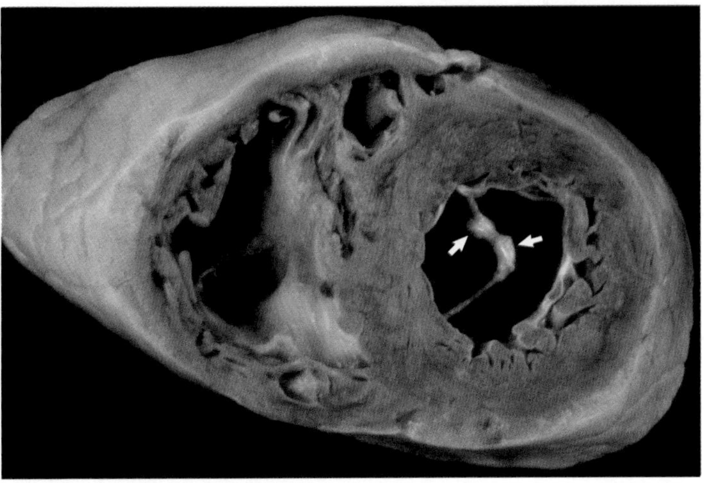

Plate 13 (FIGURE 3-36) Calcified left ventricular false tendon (arrows) seen in short-axis view.

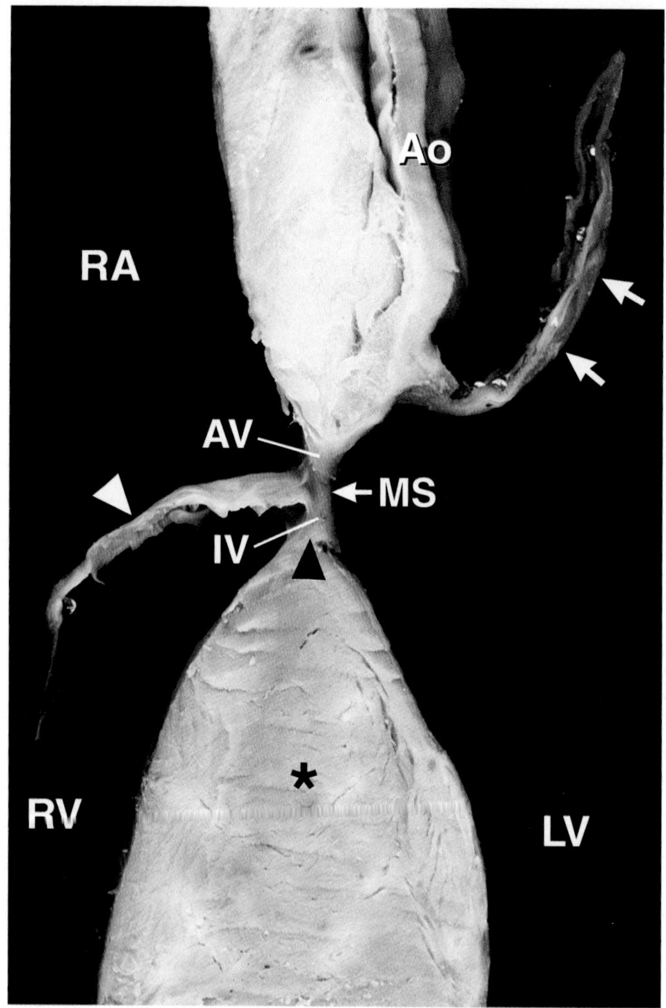


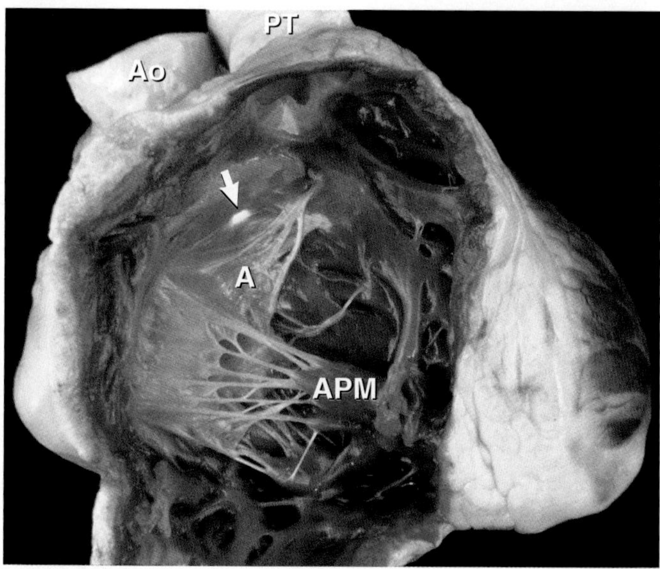


Plate 15 (FIGURE 3-40) A view of the right ventricle. Transilluminated membranous ventricular septum (arrow) in contact with the commissure between the anterior and septal leaflets of the tricuspid valve. A, anterior tricuspid leaflet; Ao, ascending aorta; APM, anterior tricuspid papillary muscle; PT, pulmonary trunk.

◀ Plate 14 (FIGURE 3-38) Four-chamber tomographic slice through the aortic root (Ao) and aortic valve (arrows) showing the small membranous (MS) and large muscular (*) portion of the ventricular septum. The membranous septum is divided into atrioventricular (AV) and interventricular (IV) components by the septal tricuspid leaflet (white arrowhead). Black arrowhead points to the expected location of the AV (His) bundle. LV, left ventricle; RA, right atrium; RV, right ventricle.

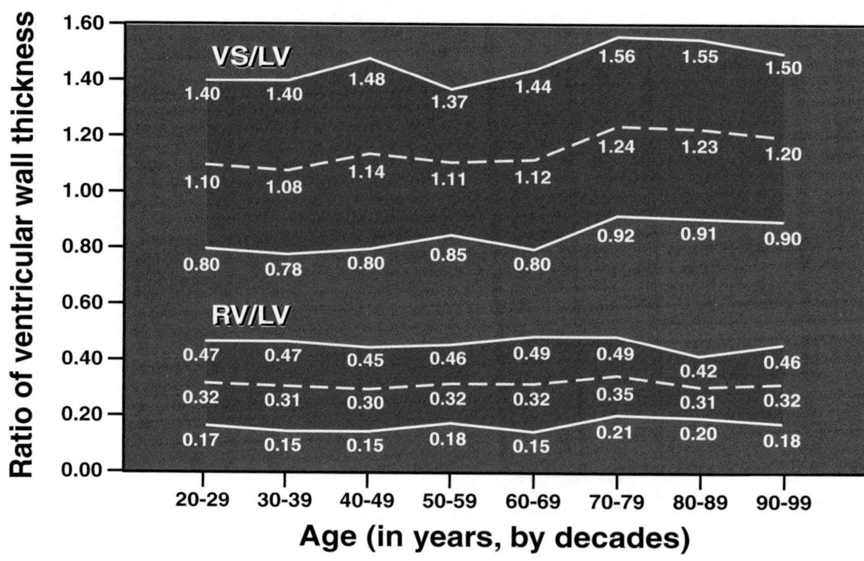


Plate 16 (FIGURE 3-41) Ratios of ventricular wall thicknesses (means ± 2 standard deviations) versus age. RV/LV, ratio of right to left ventricular wall thickness; VS/LV, ratio of ventricular septal to left ventricular free wall thickness. (From Kitzman DW et al. *Mayo Clin Proc* 1988; 63:137–146. Reproduced with permission of Mayo Foundation.)

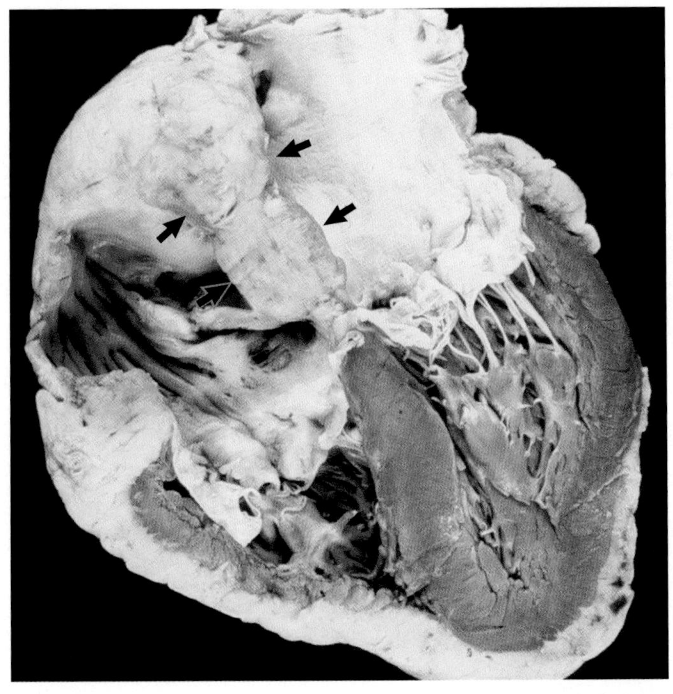

Plate 17 (FIGURE 3-45) Four-chamber slice through the heart showing lipomatous hypertrophy of the atrial septum (arrows).

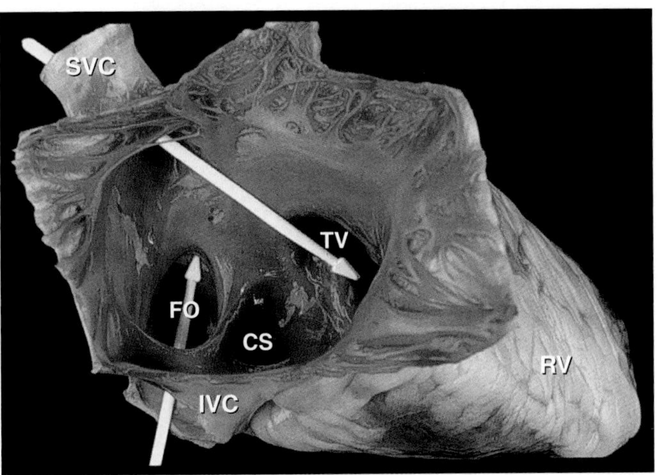


Plate 18 (FIGURE 3-47) Opened right atrium. Two arrow-shaped probes show that superior vena caval flow is directed toward the tricuspid orifice and inferior vena caval flow is directed toward the fossa ovalis (FO). CS, coronary sinus; IVC, inferior vena cava; RV, right ventricle; SVC, superior vena cava; TV, tricuspid valve.

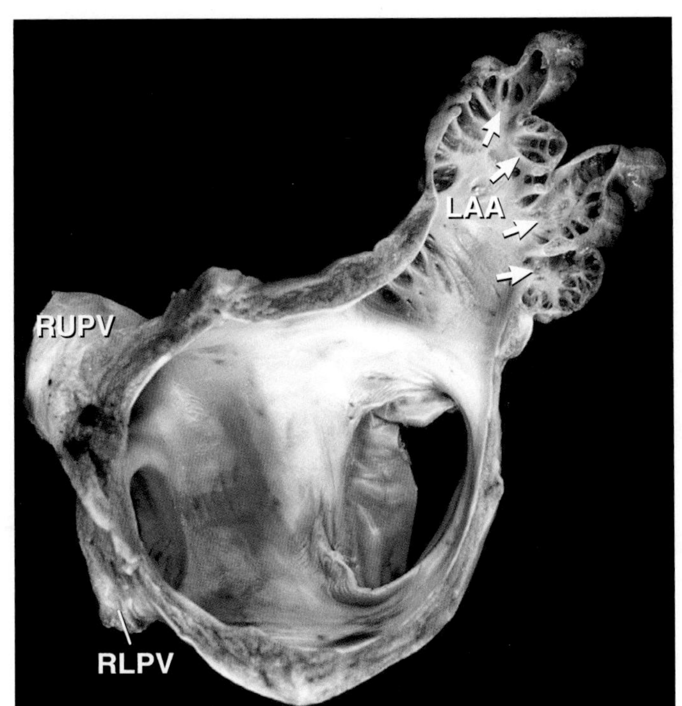


*A*

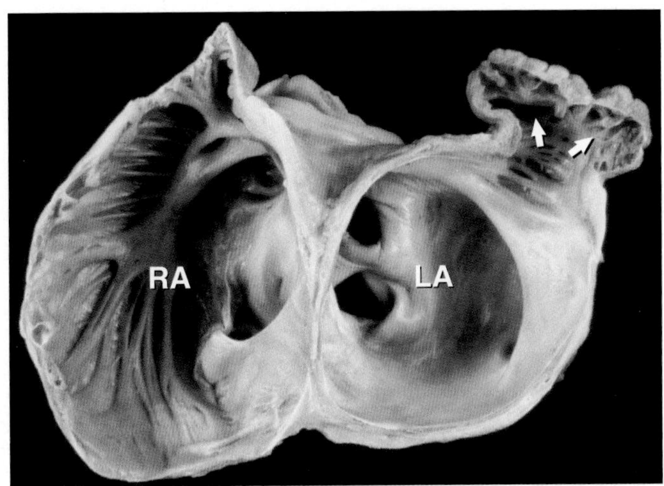


*B*

Plate 19 (FIGURE 3-49) Left atrial appendages (LAA). *A.* Left atrial free wall showing appendage with four lobes (arrows). *B.* Biatrial specimen demonstrating left atrial appendage with two lobes (arrows). LA, left atrium; RA, right atrium; RLPV, right lower pulmonary vein; RUPV, right upper pulmonary vein.

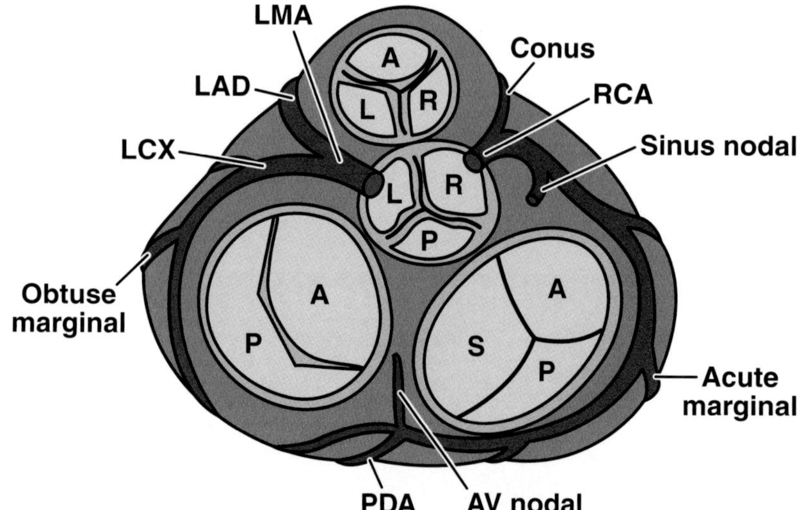


Plate 20 (FIGURE 3-50) Schematic diagram of coronary artery distribution viewed at the base of the heart. In this right-dominant system, the right coronary artery (RCA) gives rise to the posterior descending artery (PDA), and the left main coronary artery (LMA) gives rise to the left anterior descending (LAD) and left circumflex (LCX) branches. A, anterior; AV, atrioventricular; L, left; P, posterior; R, right; S, septal.

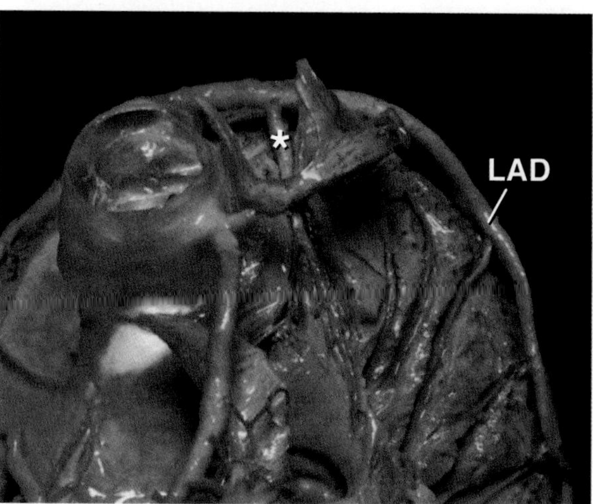


Plate 21 (FIGURE 3-53) Septal branches of the left anterior descending coronary artery (LAD);* points to the first septal perforator. (From McAlpine,[30] with permission.)

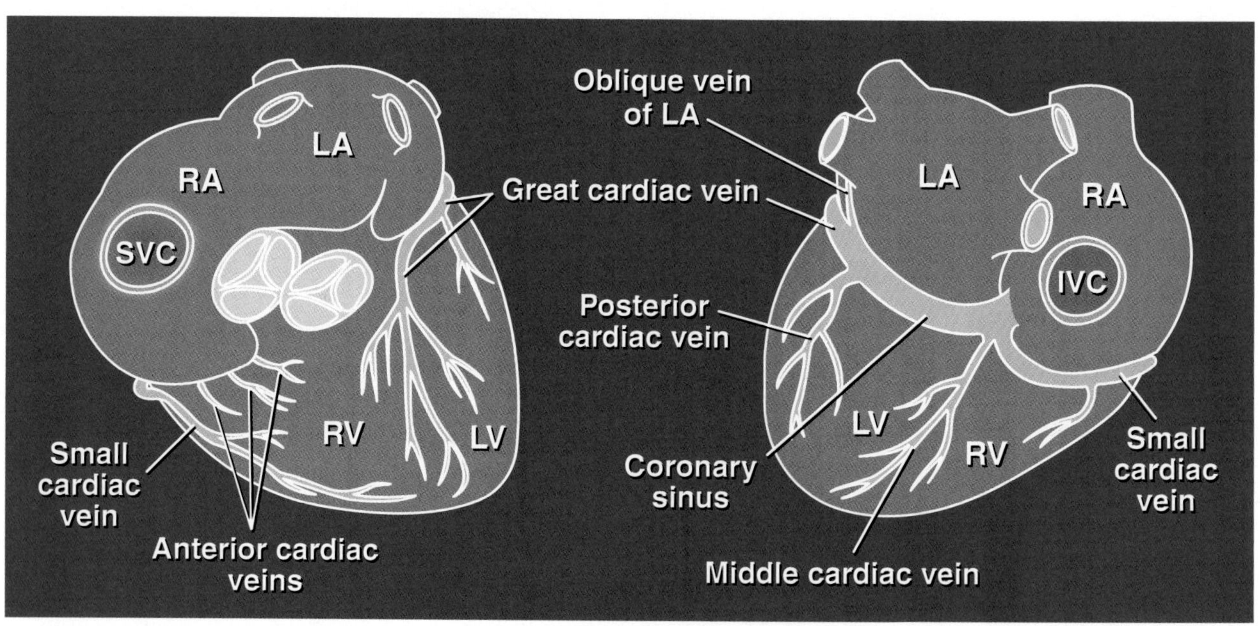


Plate 22 (FIGURE 3-55) Schematic diagram of the coronary venous circulation. IVC, inferior vena cava; LA, left atrium; LV, left ventricle; RA, right atrium; RV, right ventricle; SVC, superior vena cava.

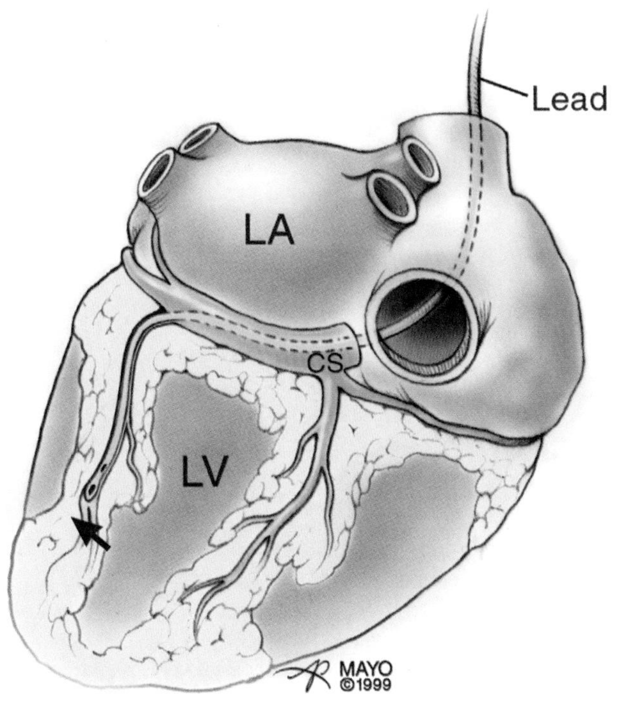


Plate 23 (FIGURE 3-56) Schematic diagram shows placement of the tip of a pacing/mapping catheter within a coronary vein (arrow) via the coronary sinus (CS). LA, left atrium; LV, left ventricle.

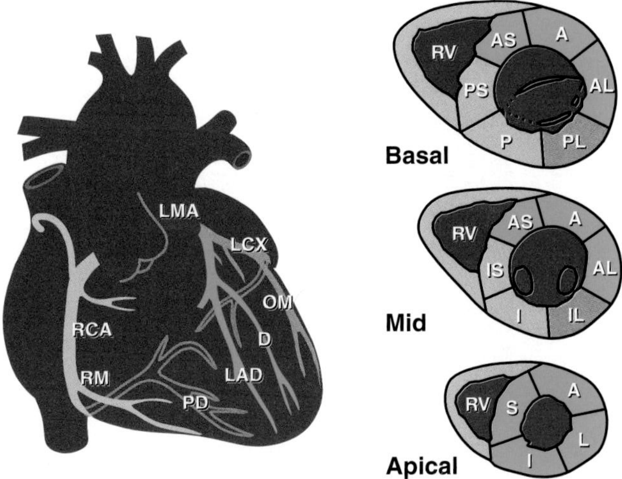


Plate 24 (FIGURE 3-60) Coronary distribution using a 16-segment model. D, diagonal branch of the left anterior descending coronary artery; LAD, left anterior descending coronary artery; LCX, left circumflex coronary artery; LMA, left main coronary artery; OM, obtuse marginal branch of the circumflex coronary artery; PD, posterior descending coronary artery; RCA, right coronary artery; RM, right marginal branch; other abbreviations as in Fig 3-58.

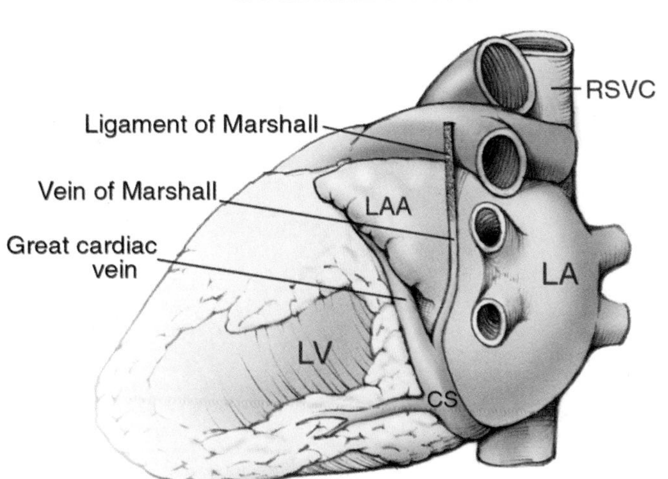


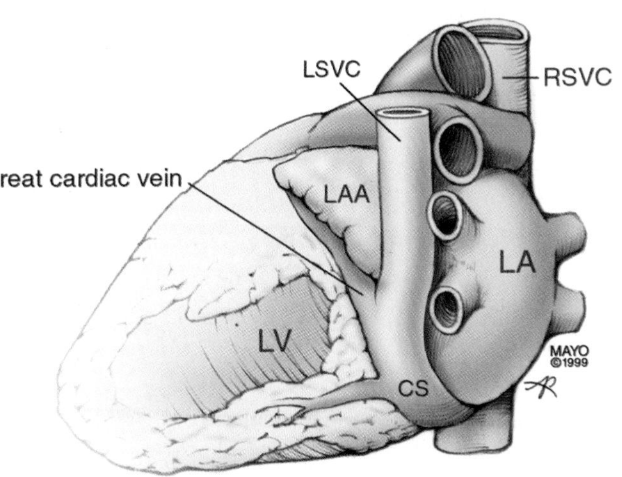


Plate 25 (FIGURE 3-64) Schematic diagrams showing the ligament/vein of Marshall in normal hearts (*left*) and persistent left superior vena cava (LSVC) (*right*). CS, coronary sinus; LA, left atrium; LAA, left atrial appendage; LV, left ventricle; RA, right atrium; RSVC, right superior vena cava.

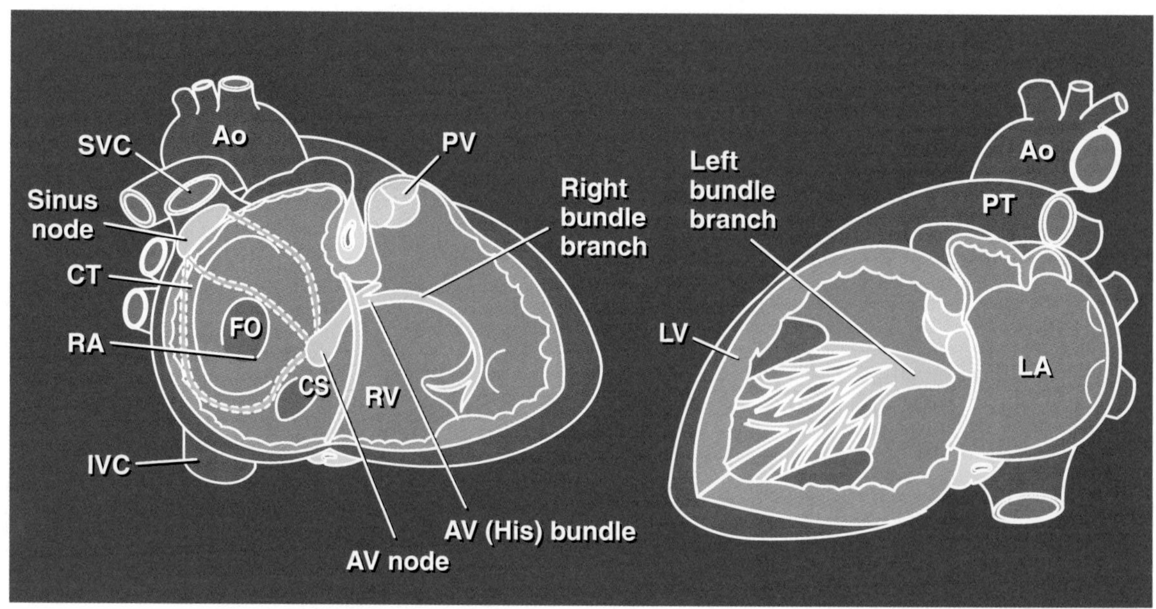


Plate 26 (FIGURE 3-67) Schematic diagram of the cardiac conduction system. The right side of the heart (*left*) showing the sinus node, atrioventricular (AV) node, AV (His) bundle, and right bundle branch. The left side of the heart (*right*) showing incomplete anatomic separation of the left bundle into antero and posterior fascicles. Ao, ascending aorta; AV, atrioventricular; CS, coronary sinus; CT, crista terminalis; FO, fossa ovalis; IVC, inferior vena cava; LA, left atrium; LV, left ventricle; PT, pulmonary trunk; PV, pulmonary valve; RA, right atrium; RV, right ventricle; SVC, superior vena cava.

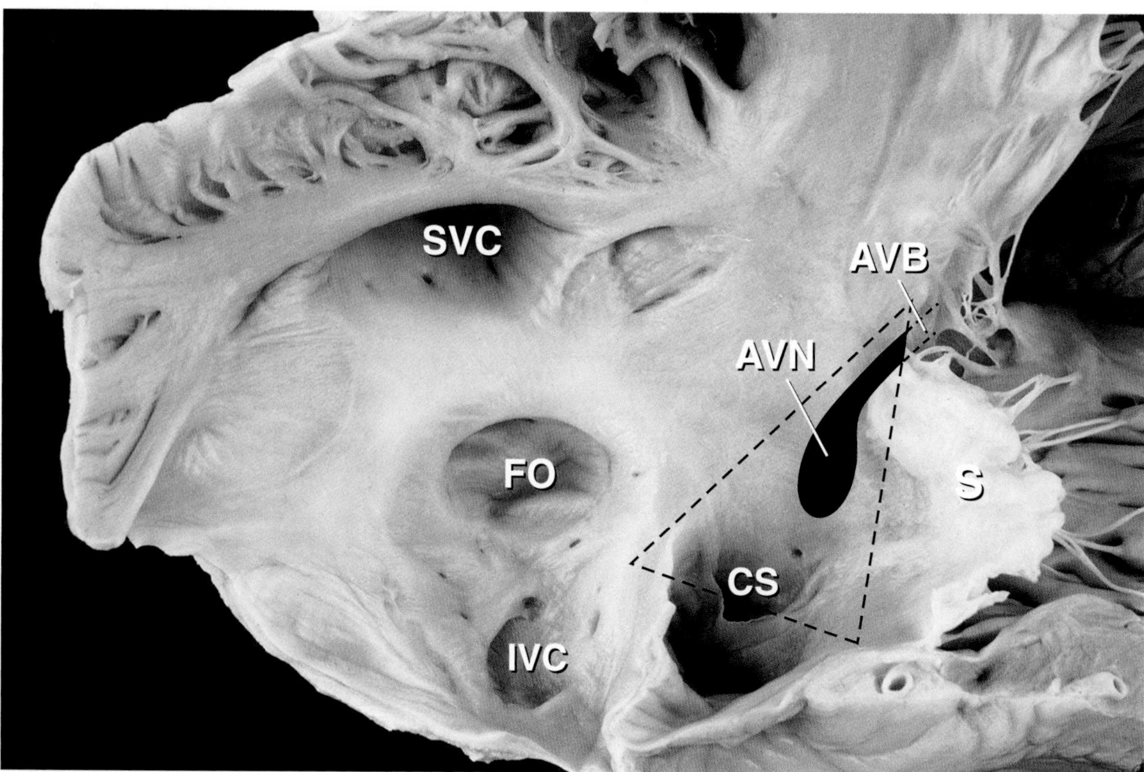


Plate 27 (FIGURE 3-68) The atrioventricular node (AVN) lies within the triangle of Koch (dashed triangle), and the AV (His) bundle (AVB) travels through the tricuspid annulus to rest along the summit of the ventricular septum. CS, coronary sinus; FO, fossa ovalis; IVC, inferior vena cava; S, septal leaflet of the tricuspid valve; SVC, superior vena cava.

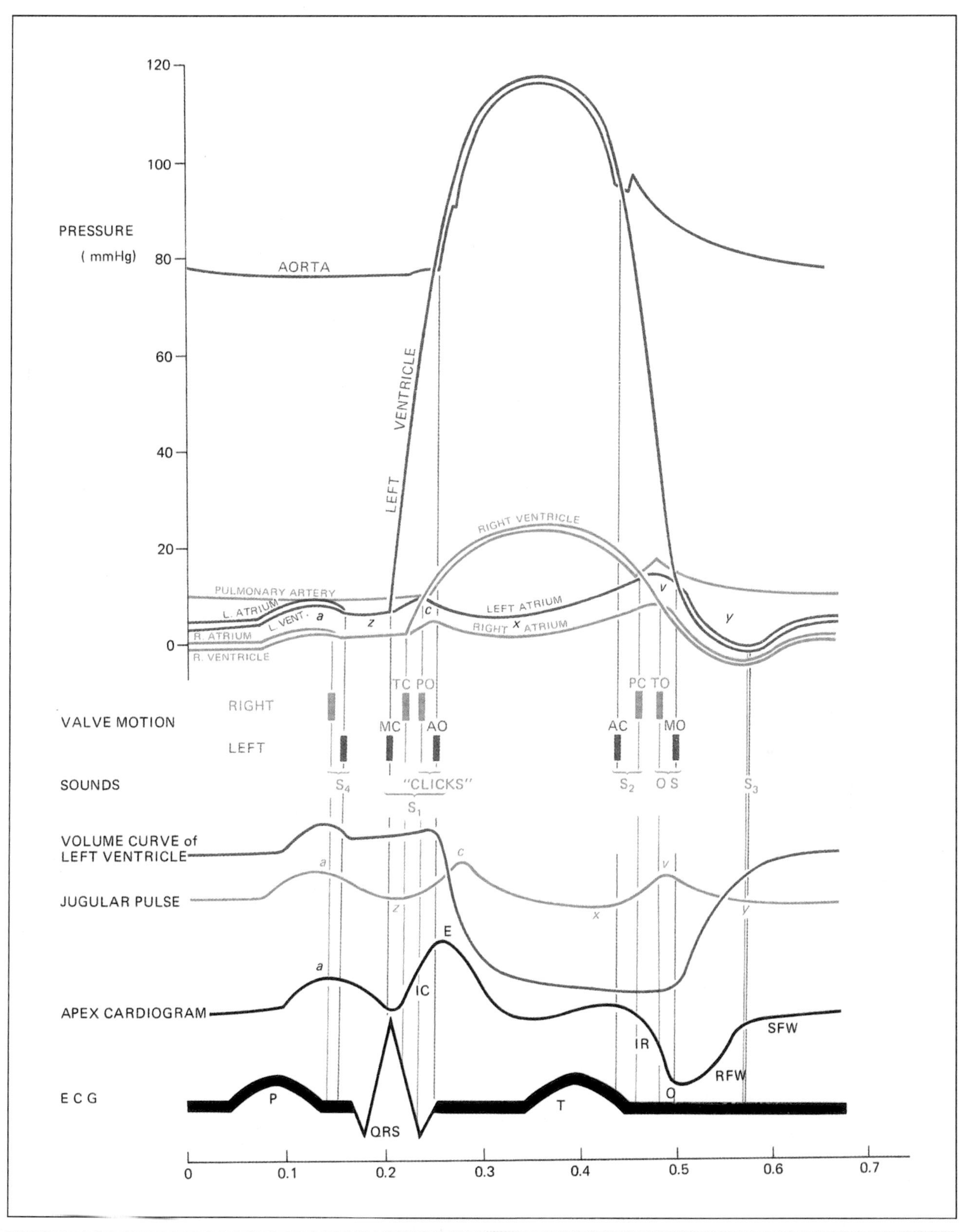


Plate 28 (FIGURE 4-1) Electrical and mechanical events during the cardiac cycle. Shown are pressure curves of great vessels and cardiac chambers, valvular events, timing of heart sounds, LV volume curve, jugular venous pulse wave, and electrocardiogram (ECG). MC and TC, mitral and tricuspid valve closure; PO and AO, pulmonic and aortic valve opening; AC and PC, aortic and pulmonic valve closure; TO and MO, tricuspid and mitral valve opening.

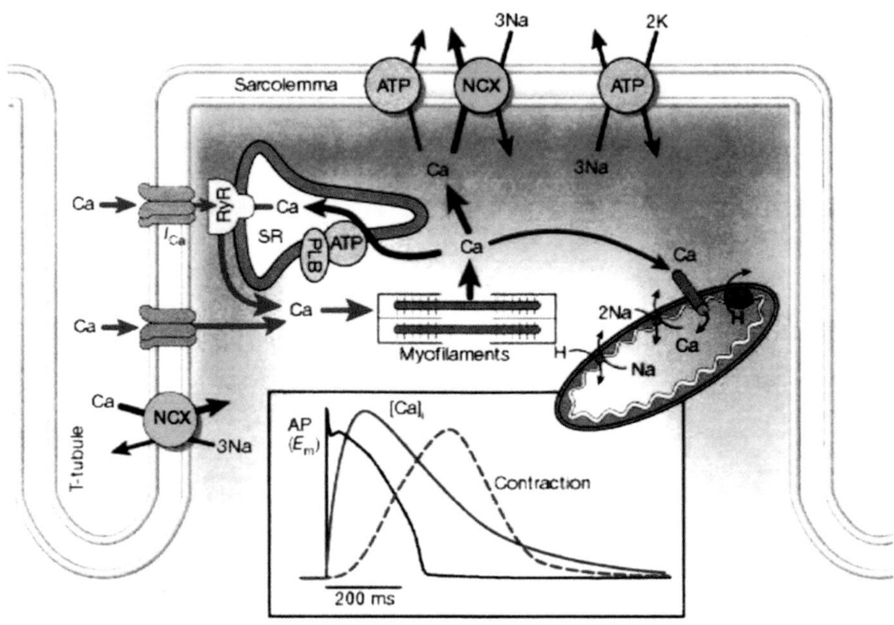


Plate 29 (FIGURE 4-3) Schematic diagram of the major cellular components involved in contraction of the myocyte, with emphasis on calcium transport mechanisms. SR, sarcoplasmic reticulum; RyR, ryanodine receptor; ATP, sarcolemmal and SR ATPase pumps, PLB, phospholamban; NCX, sodium-calcium exchanger. Mitochondrion shown lower right. Inset, time course of myocyte AP (action potential), intracellular calcium transient, force of contraction. (From Bers.[21] Reprinted with permission of the publisher.)

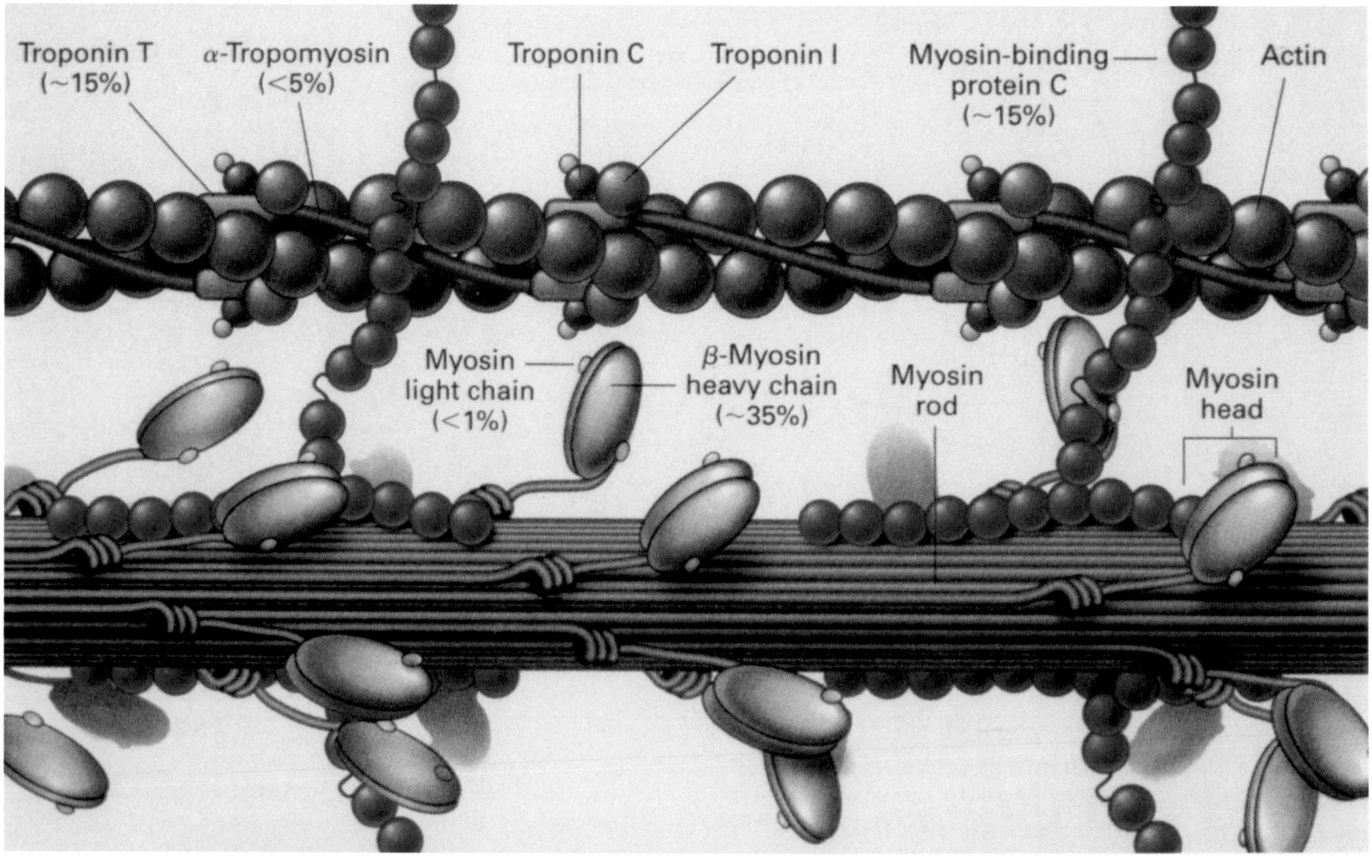

Plate 30 (FIGURE 4-8) Cartoon of sarcomeric proteins (titin not shown). (From Spirito P, Seidman CE, McKenna WJ, Maron BJ. The management of hypertrophic cardiomyopathy. *N Eng J Med* 1997; 336:775. Reprinted with permission of the publisher.)

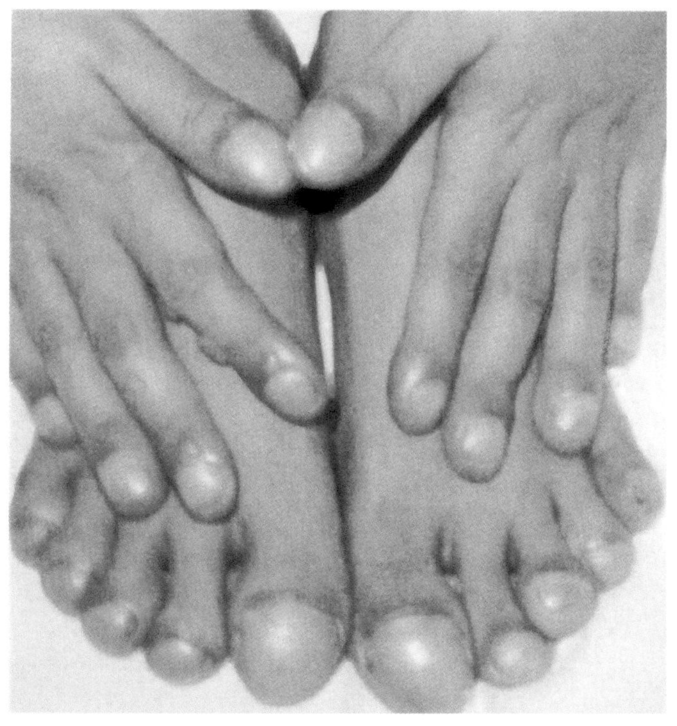

Plate 31 (FIGURE 12-1) *Symmetric cyanosis*. Equal cyanosis and clubbing of hands and feet due to transposition of the great vessels and a ventricular septal defect without patent ductus arteriosus.

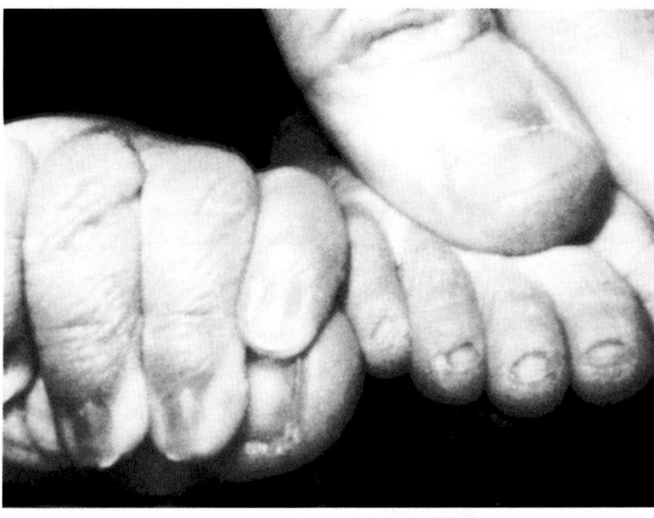

Plate 32 (FIGURE 12-2) *Differential cyanosis*. Clubbing of left hand (compare thumbs) and cyanosis of left hand and all toes due to patent ductus arteriosus with pulmonary hypertension and normally related great vessels. (Courtesy of Dr. Joseph K. Perloff, University of California, Los Angeles.)

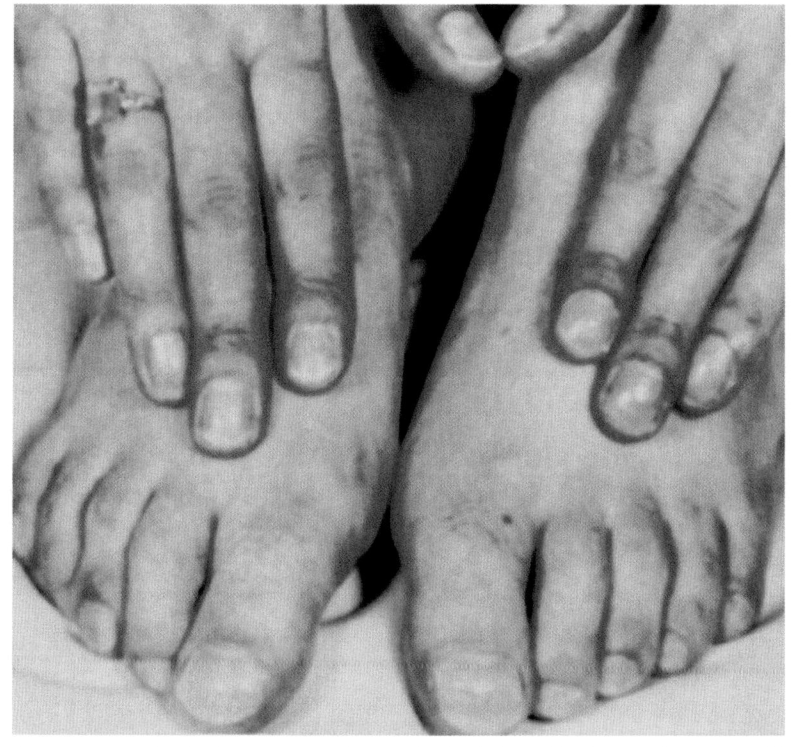

Plate 33 (FIGURE 12-3) *Differential cyanosis*. Cyanosis of fingers (*left*) greater than that of toes due to transposition of the great vessels with patent ductus arteriosus.

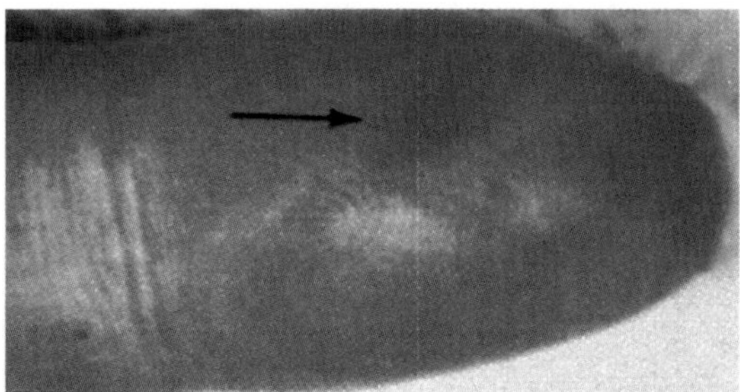

*A*

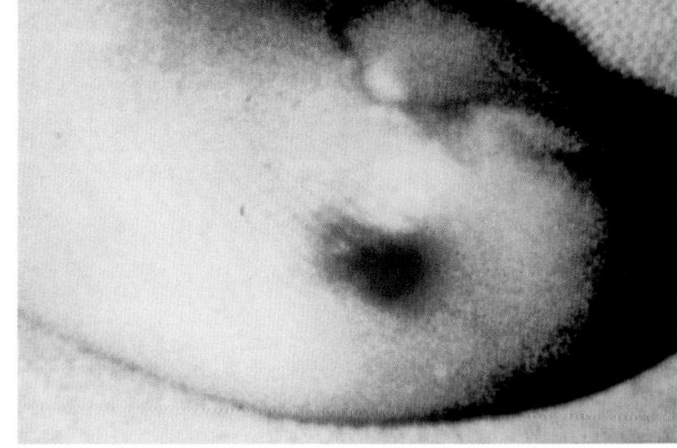

*B*

PLATE 34 (FIGURE 12-15) *Bacterial endocarditis: A.* Valvular infection associated with a tender, purplish nodule (Osler's node) in the finger pad (*arrow*). *B.* Osler's node from another patient.

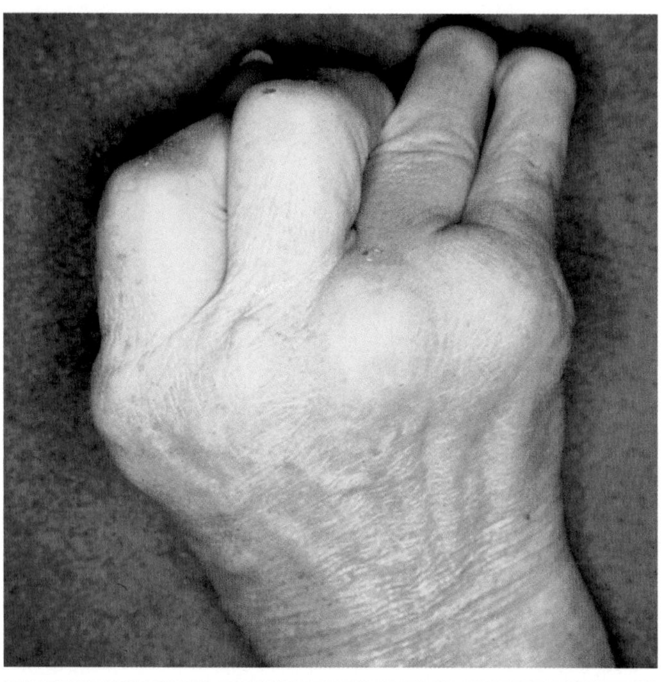

Plate 35 (FIGURE 12-22) *Rheumatoid arthritis:* with ulnar deviation of the fingers and flexion of the distal interphalangeal joints with hyperextension of the proximal interphalangeal joints.

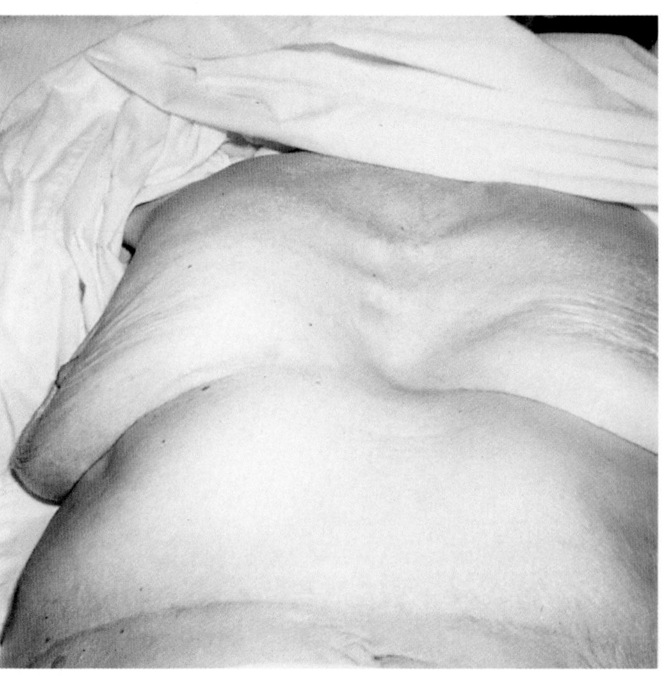

Plate 36 (FIGURE 12-25) Marked pectus excavatum.

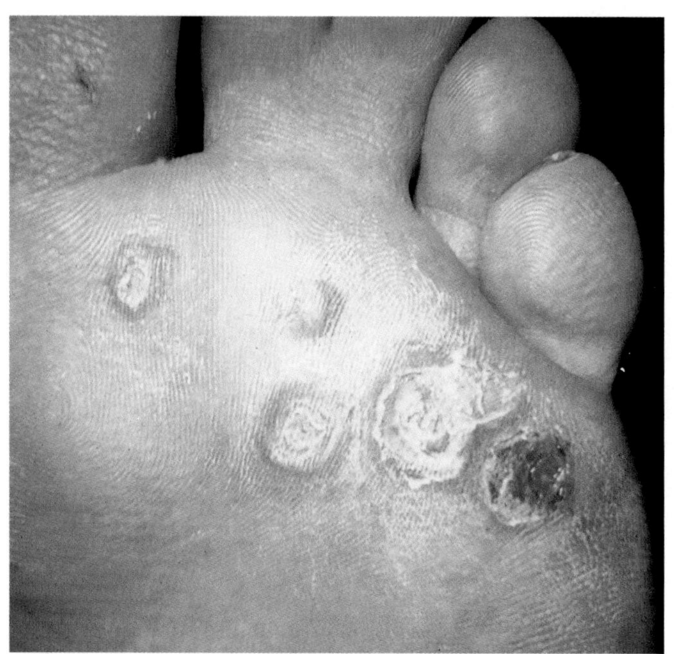

Plate 37 (FIGURE 12-27) *Hyperkeratotic lesions* encrusted on the soles of the feet in Reiter's syndrome.

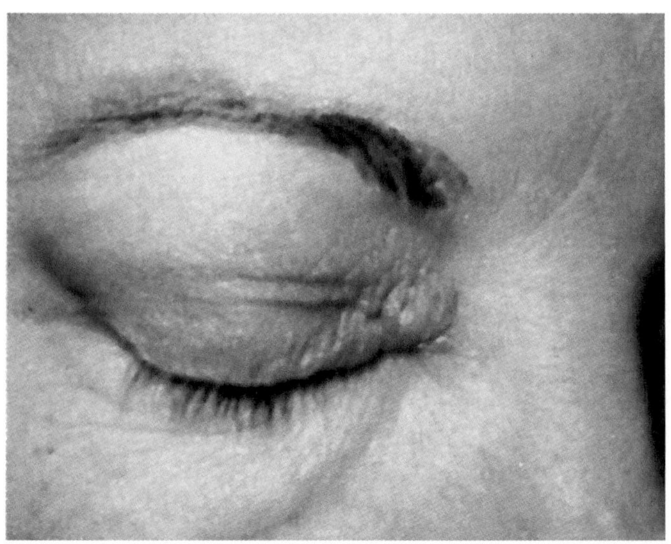

Plate 38 (FIGURE 12-29) *Dermatomyositis.* A violaceous hue and edema of upper eyelid may be associated with myocardial disease.

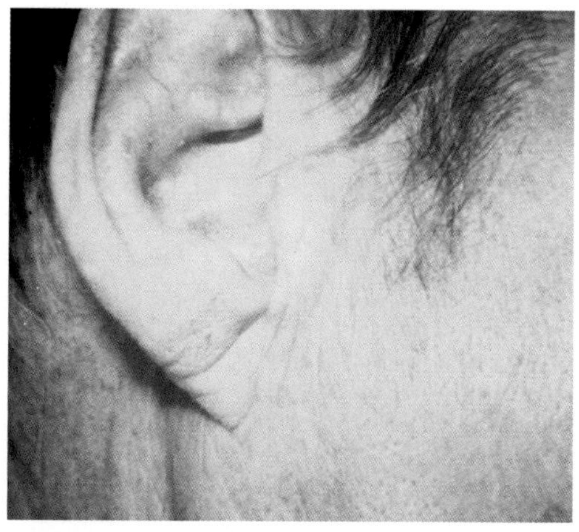

Plate 39 (FIGURE 12-32) Horizontal ear creases are often associated with the presence of extensive CAD.

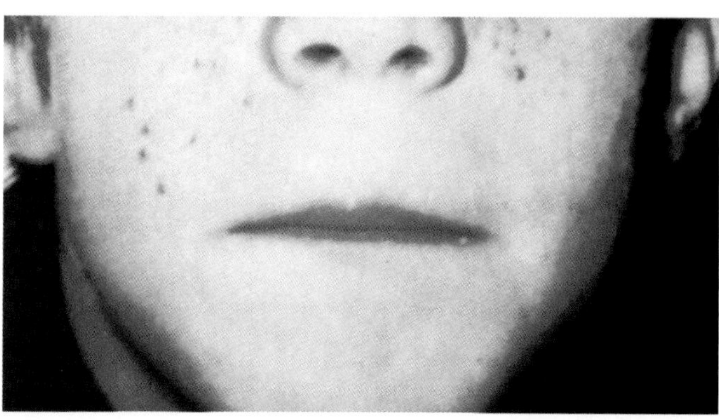

Plate 40 (FIGURE 12-35) Tuberous sclerosis. Adenoma sebaceum may be associated with rhabdomyomas of the myocardium.

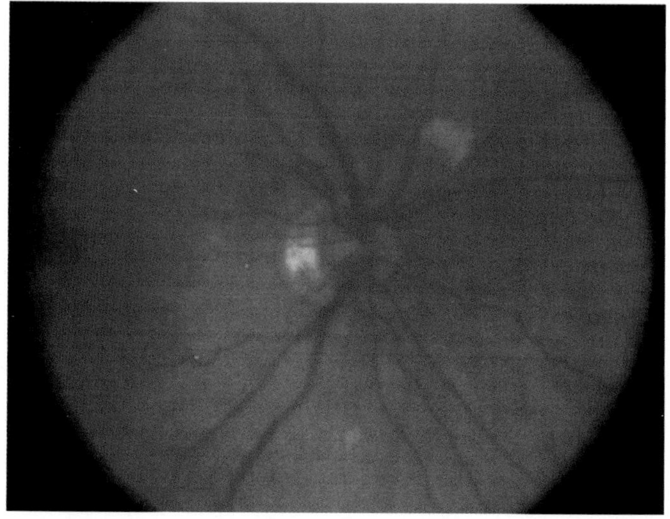

Plate 41 (FIGURE 12-42) Retinal cotton-wool spot. Cotton-wool spots are most frequently found close to the optic disk. Although they occur in acute uncontrolled systemic hypertension, the more common cause now, in younger patients, is infection with the human immunodeficiency virus (HIV). This normotensive 37-year-old man had no visual symptoms and no other retinopathy. There is a myopic crescent at the temporal disk edge, which is not abnormal. He died of complications related to the acquired immunodeficiency syndrome (AIDS) 2 years later.

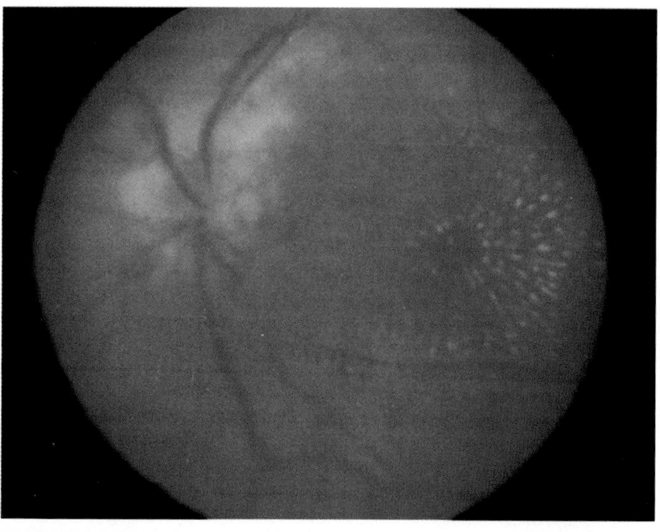

Plate 42 (FIGURE 12-43) Disk swelling and hard exudate in a macular "star" pattern. In this hypertensive patient with periarteritis nodosa, vascular leakage has led to the deposition of hard exudates around the fovea. The star pattern of the exudate is due to radial perifoveal connective tissue. Note also that the optic disk is edematous, with blurred margins, secondary to hypertension.

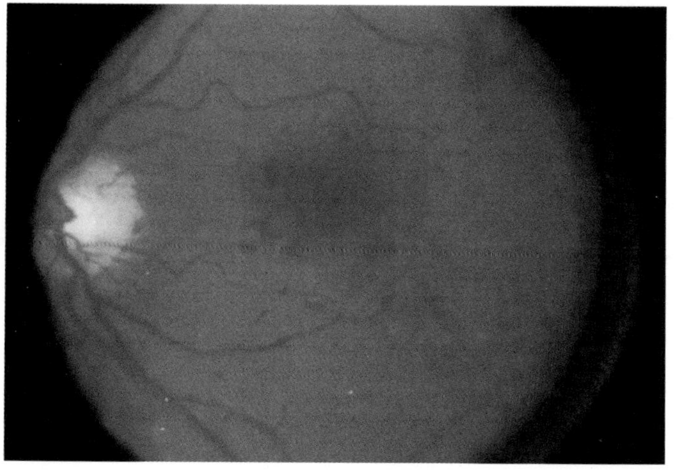

Plate 43 (FIGURE 12-44) Background diabetic retinopathy. Retinal microaneurysms, dot-and-blot hemorrhages, and a few fine upper temporal hard exudates are diagnostic of early diabetic retinopathy. The patient had no visual symptoms, but retinopathy of this magnitude can often be seen in patients with insulin-requiring diabetes of 15 or more years' duration.

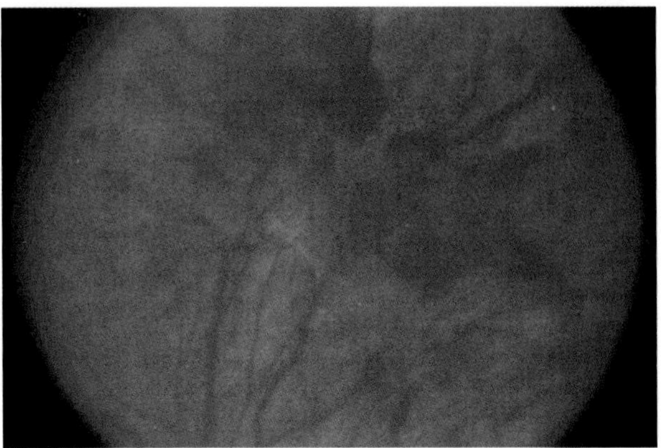

Plate 44 (FIGURE 12-45) Proliferative diabetic retinopathy with preretinal hemorrhage. When neovascularization develops, preretinal and vitreous hemorrhages are much more likely to occur. Easily visible neovascularization either in the periphery of the retina, as in this diabetic patient, or at the disk is an indication for immediate panretinal laser photocoagulation.

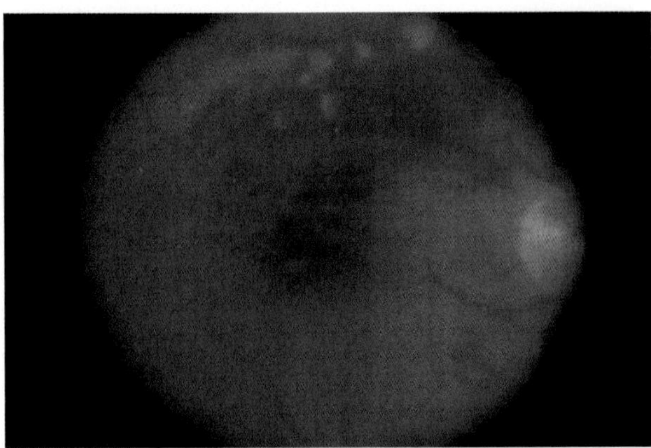

Plate 45 (FIGURE 12-47) Branch retinal vein obstruction. Thickening of the retinal arterial wall in diabetes and hypertension may compromise the lumen of the vein, where artery and vein share a common adventitial sheath at an arteriovenous crossing. The resulting obstruction produces hemorrhage retinopathy in the drainage area of the affected vein. Note how the flame-shaped pattern of blood outlines the arcuate pattern of the nerve fibers as they run toward the optic disk.

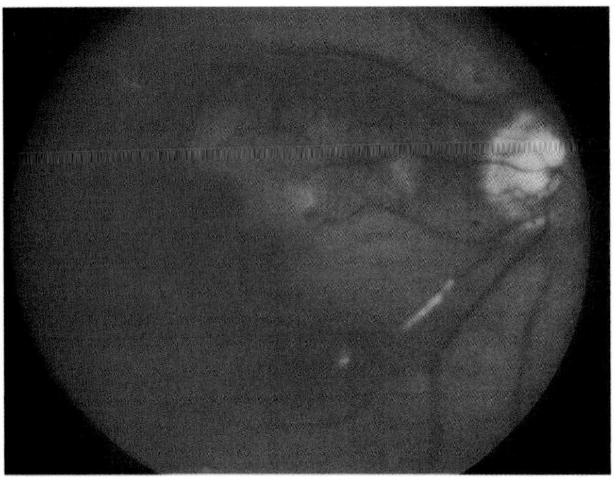

*A*

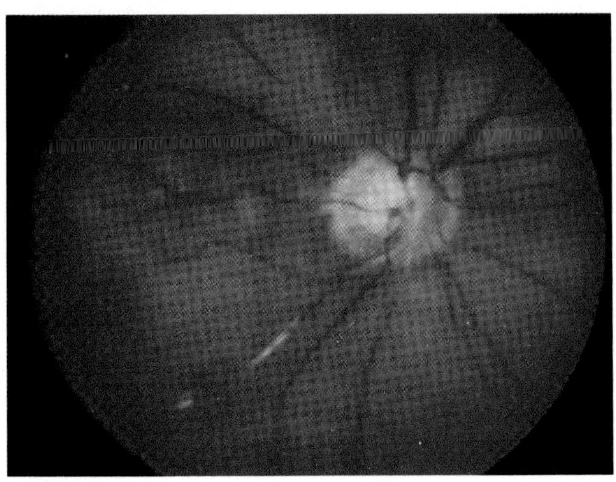

*B*

Plate 46 (FIGURE 12-48) Embolic retinal arterial obstruction (*A* and *B*). Cholesterol crystals may dislodge from the walls of the heart, aortic arch, or carotids. Carried into the retinal circulation as Hollenhorst plaques, they seldom obstruct the arterioles completely. Although amaurosis fugax is more common, the embolic burden may occasionally be so large as to produce retinal infarction. Note in the photograph of the macular area (*A*) that this patient's fovea remains red, while there is a pale, cloudy swelling nasal to it. This has produced a half "cherry-red" spot. With complete central retinal artery occlusion, the red foveal area is completely surrounded by pale swollen retina. Hollenhorst cholesterol plaques can be seen in both the upper and lower temporal retinal arteries. In *A*, the inferior temporal arteriole demonstrates "box-car" segmentation of the blood column, indicative of very slow flow.

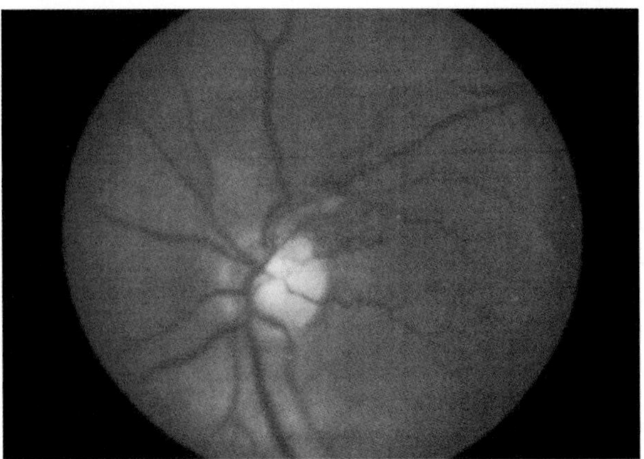

Plate 47 (FIGURE 12-49) Neovascularization after branch retinal vein obstruction. New vessels may develop late after obstruction of a branch of the central retinal vein. These most often serve to shunt flow around the obstructed vessel site and are thus not as exuberantly proliferative as those seen in diabetic retinopathy.

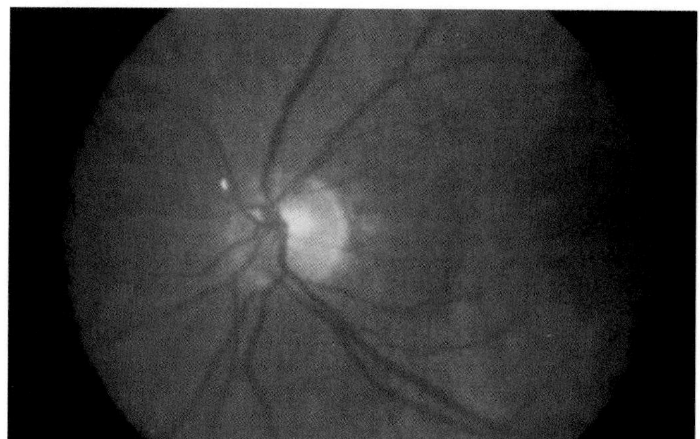

Plate 48 (FIGURE 12-51) Calcific retinal embolus associated with aortic valvular disease. Calcific aortic valvular disease and valve replacement surgery may give rise to retinal emboli. Like cholesterol emboli, these calcific flecks lodge at arterial bifurcations but seldom obstruct flow completely. They are white and glitter in the ophthalmoscope beam. Somewhat similar emboli may be seen after the intravenous injection of illicit drugs expanded with talc.

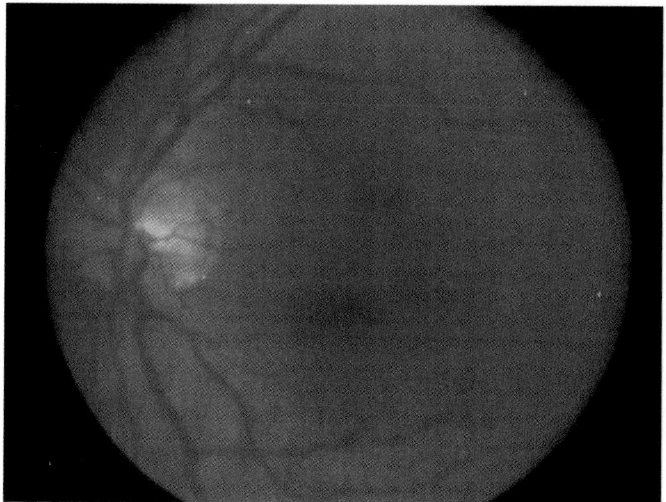

Plate 49 (FIGURE 12-52) Retinal hemorrhages, such as may occur after cardiac catheterization. They can be either symptomatic or asymptomatic, although the latter are more common. Presumably these are the result of embolic events. Note, in this recently catheterized patient, the two oval hemorrhages and a small area of cloudy swelling just inferior and temporal to the fovea.

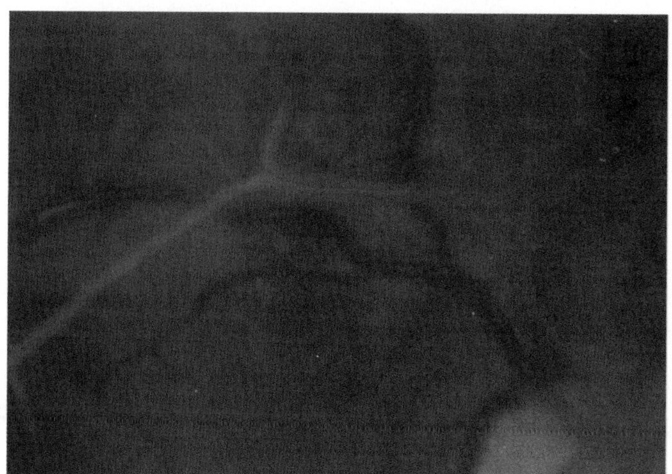

*A*

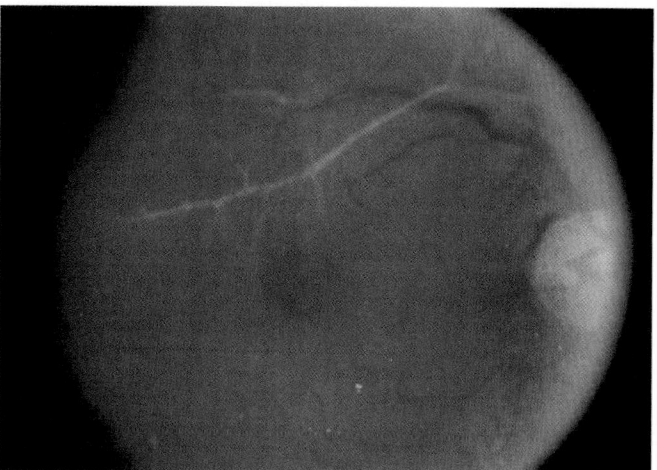

*B*

Plate 50 (FIGURE 12-54) *A.* Retinal arteriosclerosis. This 75-year-old hypertensive woman has marked arteriosclerosis of the upper temporal retinal arteriole and its branches. When the narrowed blood column can no longer be seen, the thickened wall produces the "silver wire" appearance seen here. Where the arteriole crosses its associated vein, the course of the vein is altered and its blood column cannot be seen. This venous "nicking" and "banking" is associated with impairment of outflow, and the affected veins become darker, larger, and more tortuous. *B.* Low-power view showing the silver-wire arteriole.

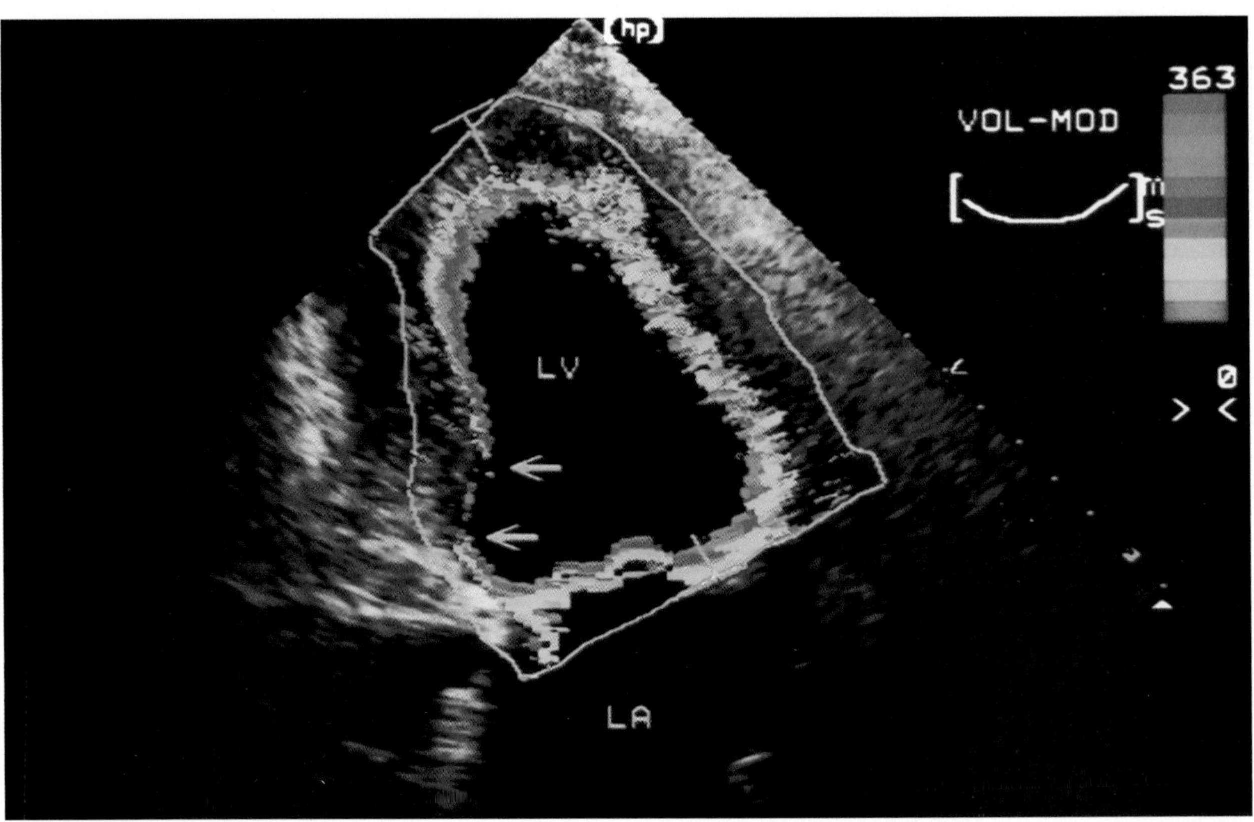


Plate 51 (FIGURE 15-23) Color kinesis image (apical two-chamber view) from a patient with an inferobasal infarction. Systolic motion in this area (*arrows*) is markedly diminished.

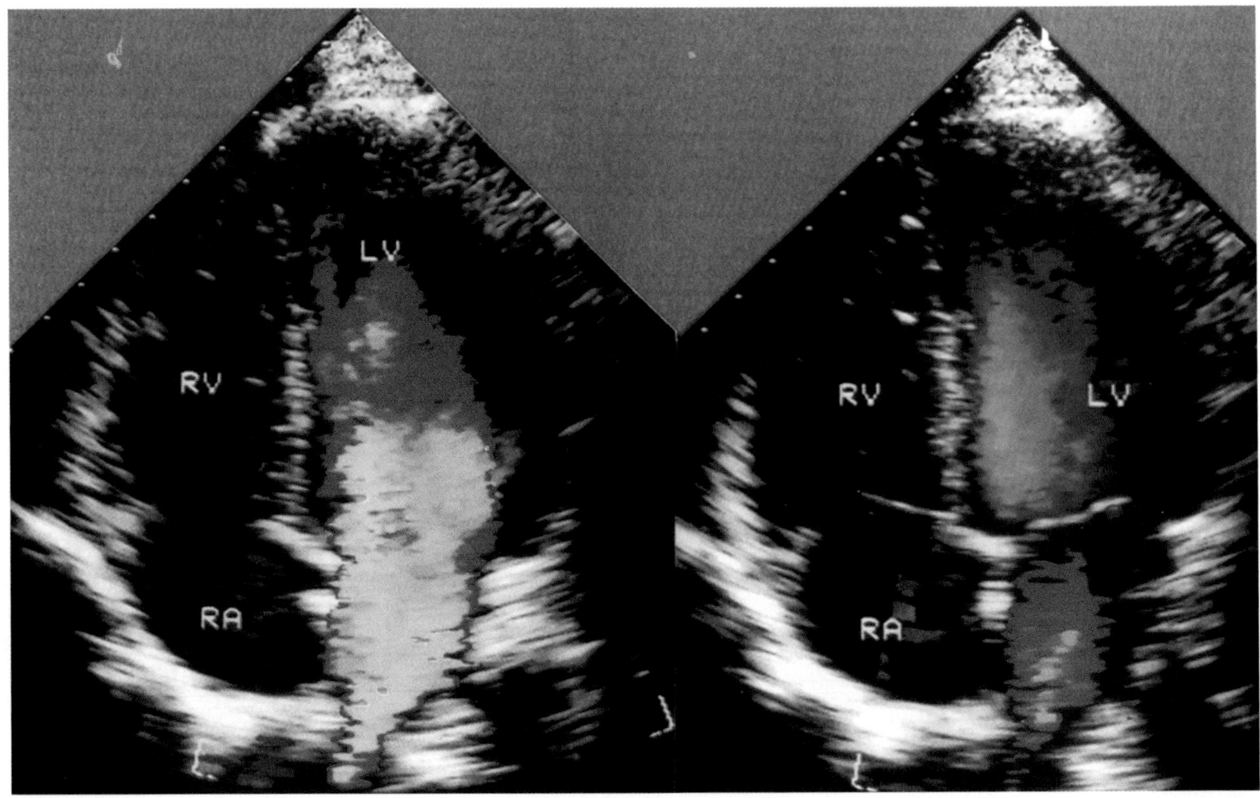


Plate 52 (FIGURE 15-30) Apical four-chamber images with color-flow Doppler during diastole and systole. Red flow indicates movement toward the transducer (diastolic filling); blue flow indicates movement away from the transducer (systolic ejection). LV = left ventricle; RA = right atrium; RV = right ventricle.

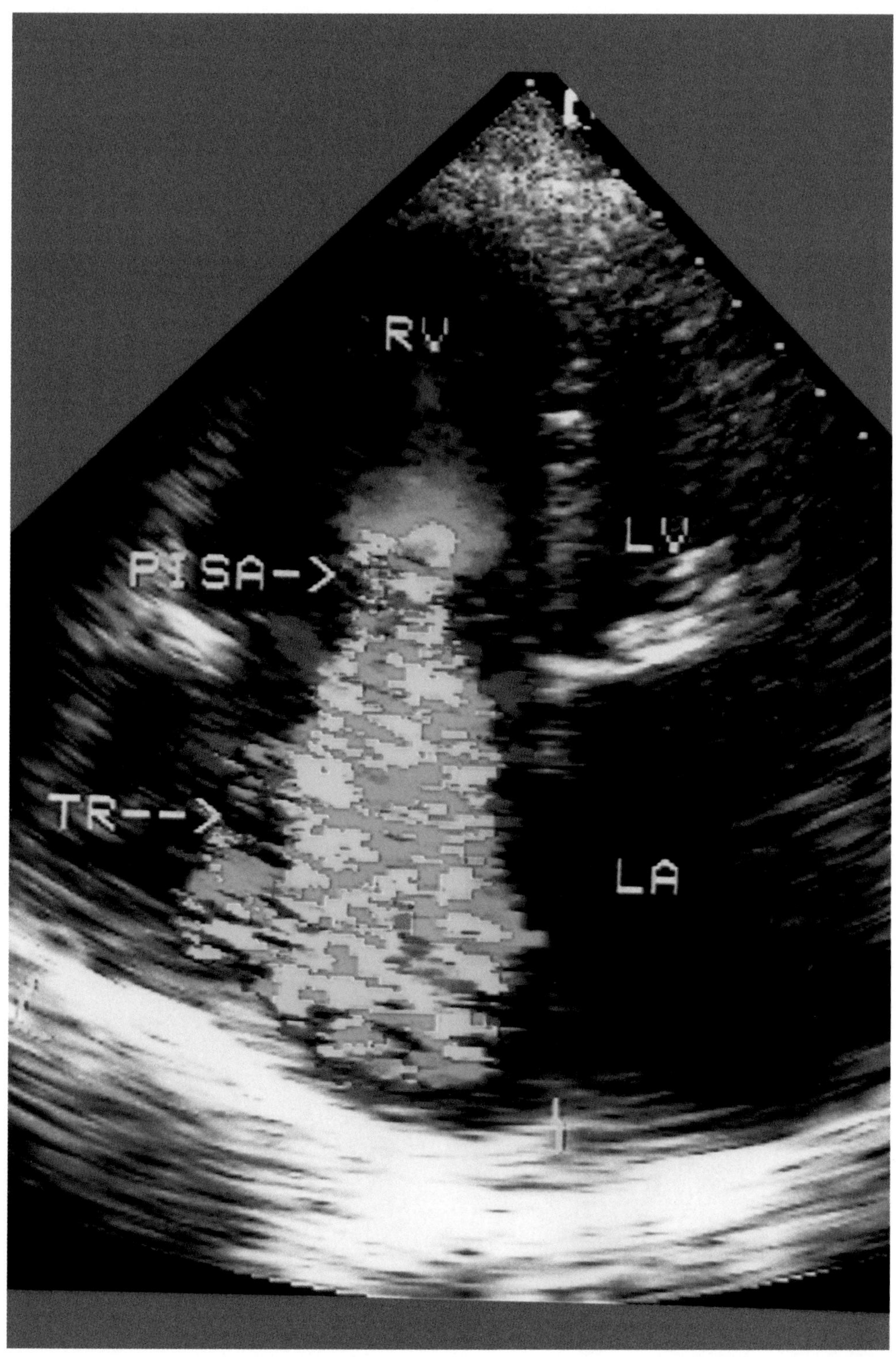


Plate 53 (FIGURE 15-31) Apical four-chamber view of severe tricuspid regurgitation. The Doppler color jet fills the right atrium (RA). PISA = proximal isovelocity surface area; LV = left ventricle; LA = left atrium; RV = right ventricle.

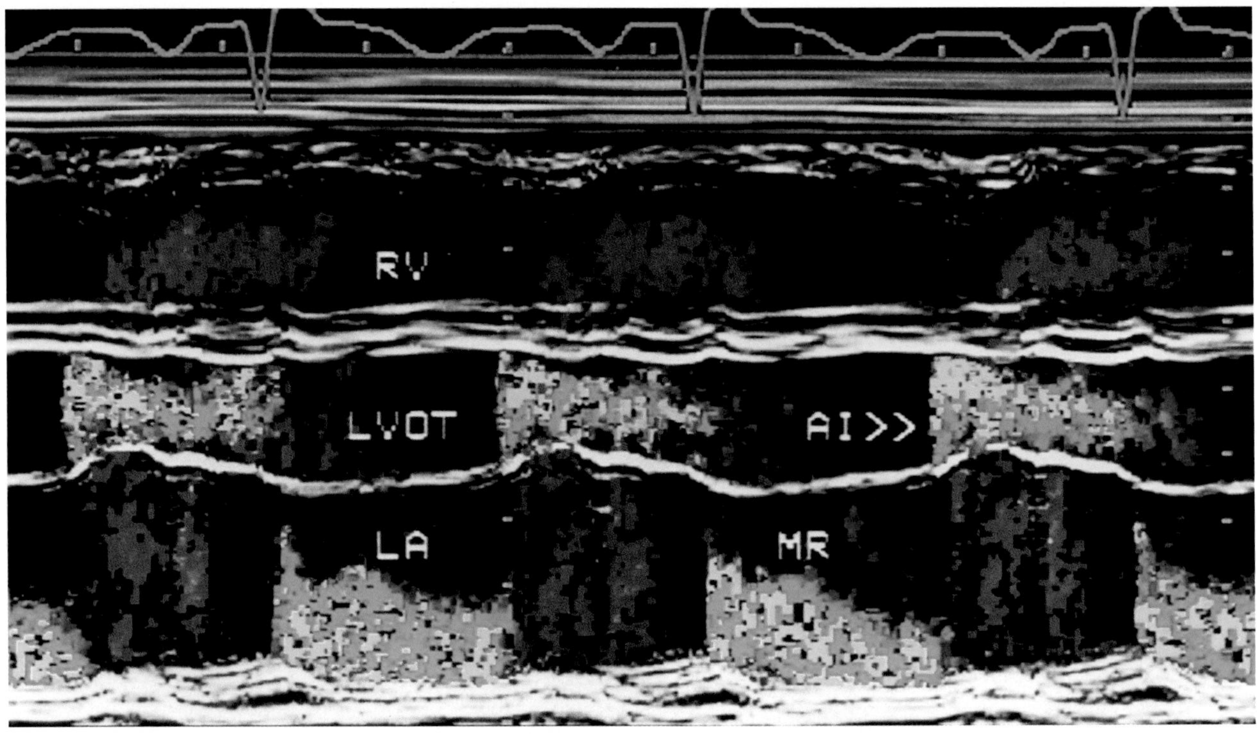


Plate 54 (FIGURE 15-32) Color-flow Doppler superimposed on an M-mode image. The transducer is in parasternal position and the cursor is directed through the left ventricular outflow tract (LVOT) and left atrium (LA). The patient under study has both aortic insufficiency (AI) and mitral regurgitation (MR). RV = right ventricle.

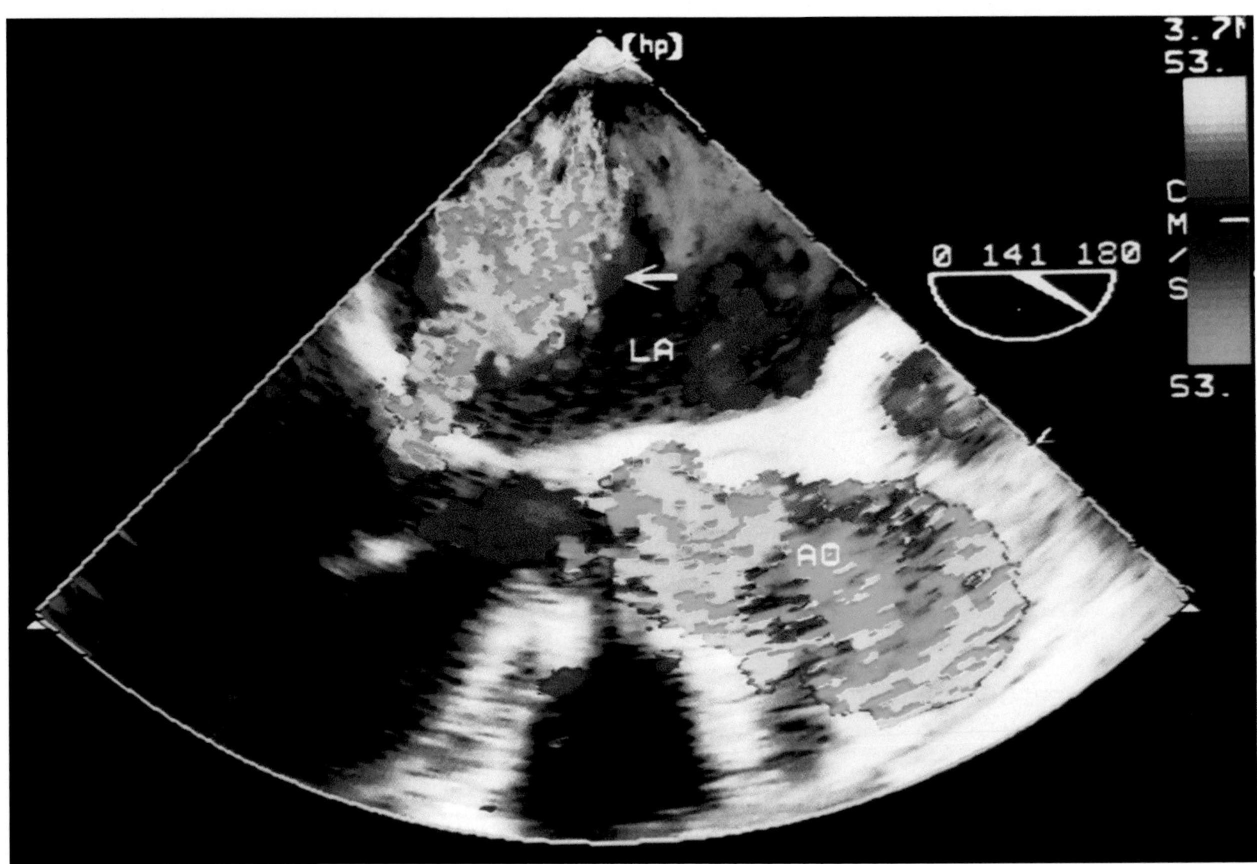


Plate 55 (FIGURE 15-49) Transesophageal echocardiography image (three-chamber plane) demonstrating a jet of mitral regurgitation (*arrow*) in the left atrium (LA). AO = aorta; LV = left ventricle.

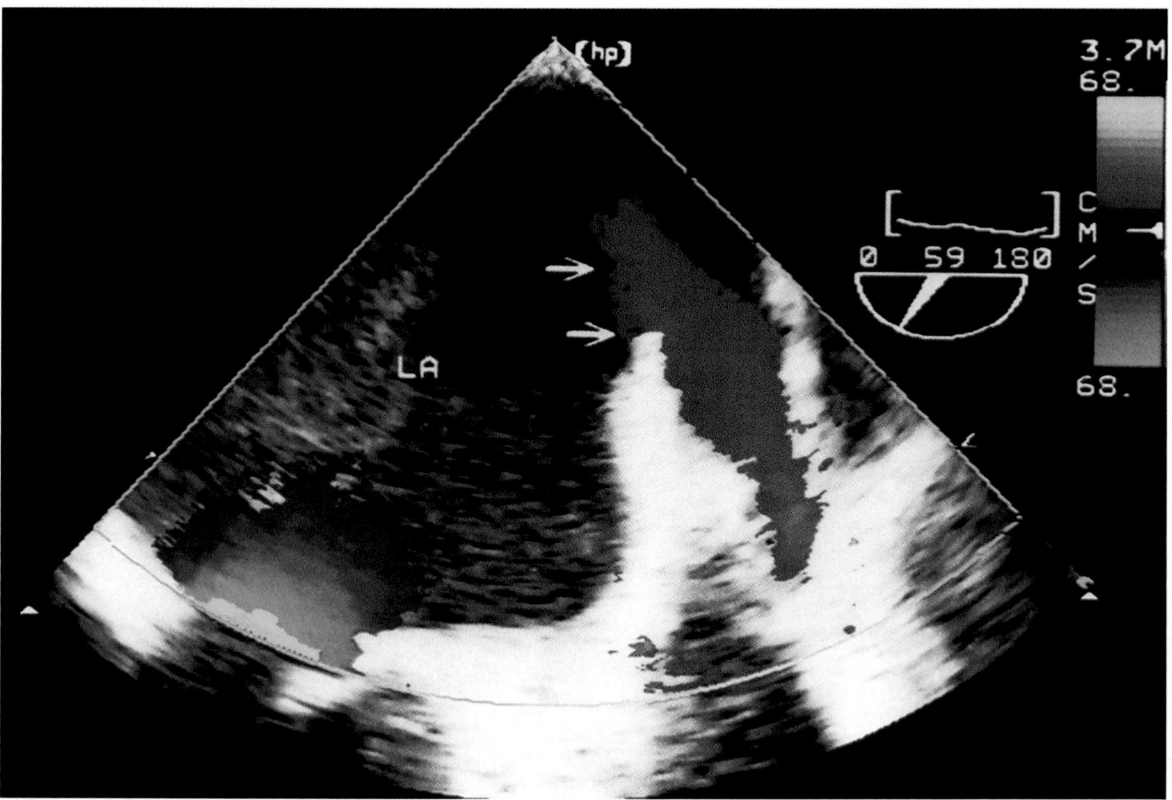


Plate 56 (FIGURE 15-50) Transesophageal echocardiography image of pulmonary venous flow (*arrows*) entering the left atrium (LA) during diastole.

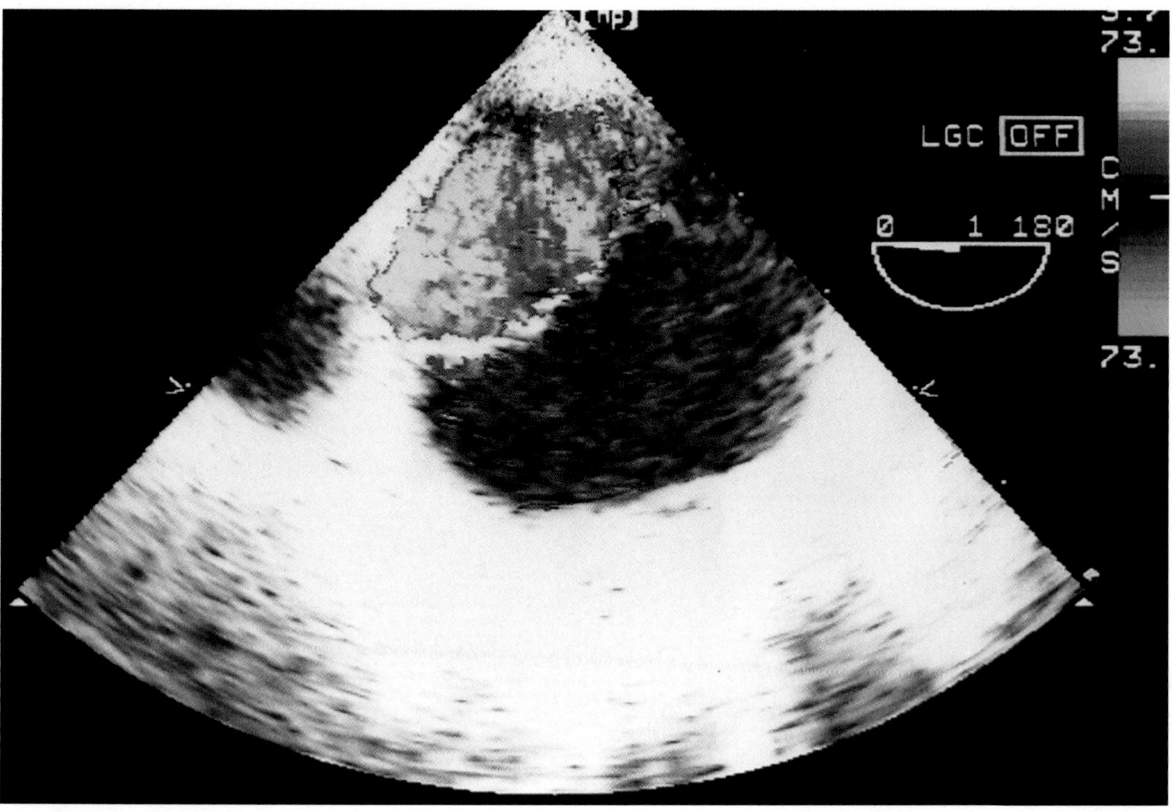


Plate 57 (FIGURE 15-51) Transverse TEE image of a descending aortic dissection. The true lumen is color-coded orange. The false lumen is mostly devoid of flow, but a small blue jet of communication between the two channels is present.

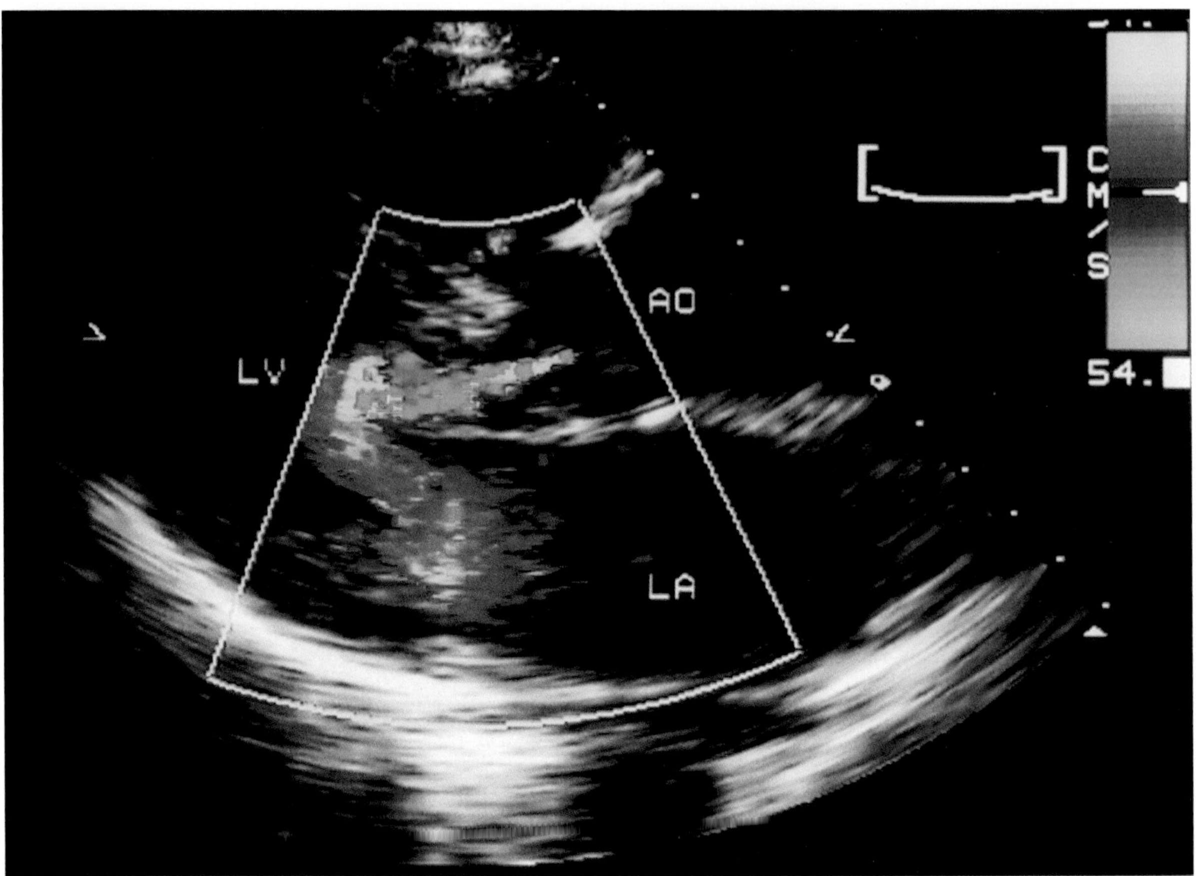


*A*

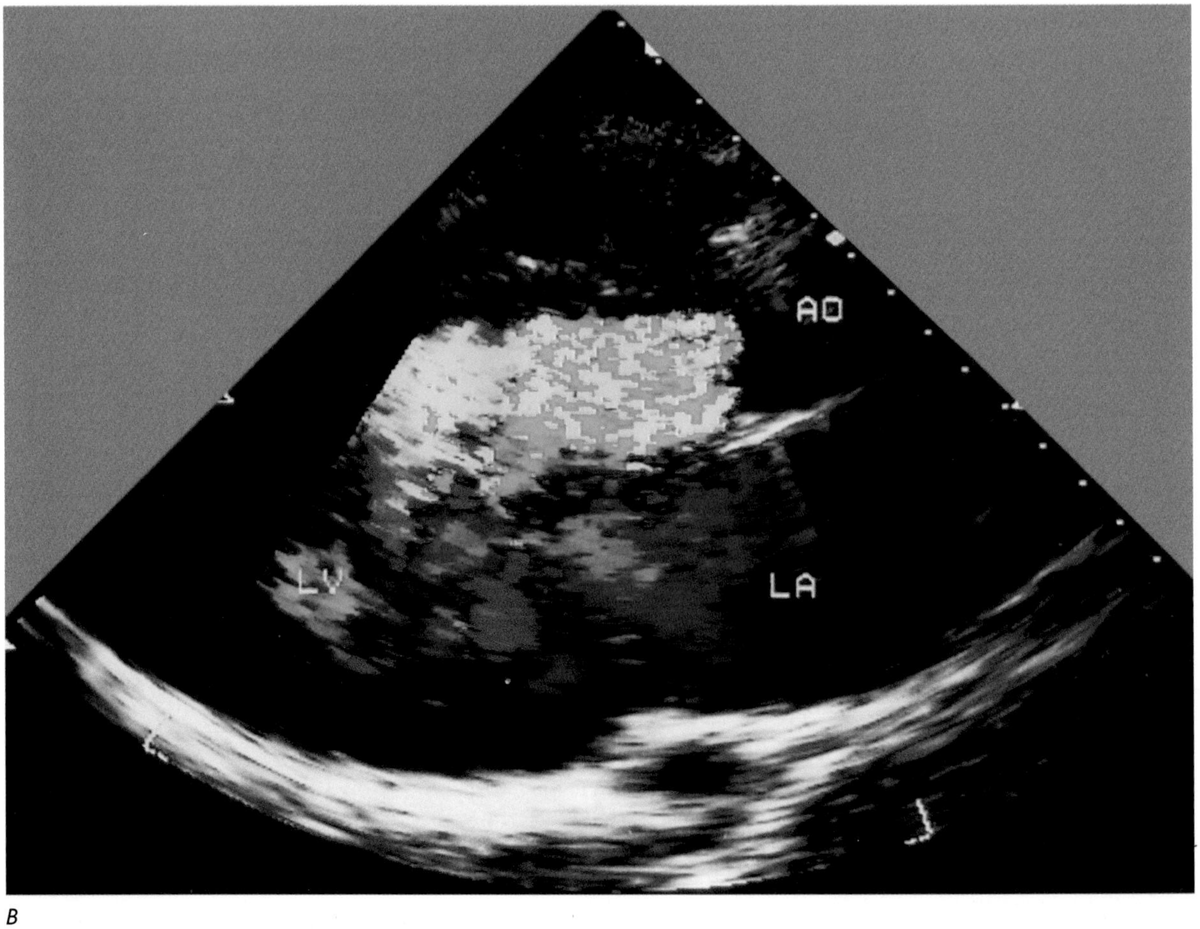

*B*

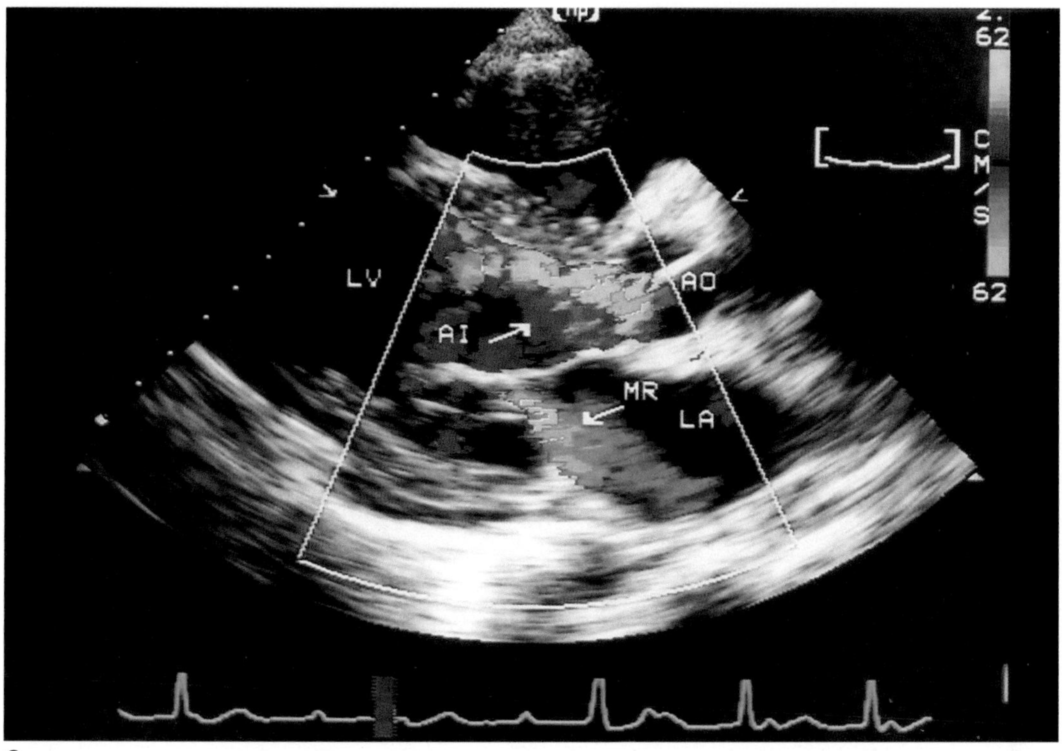


*C*

Plate 58 (FIGURE 15-64) *A.* Parasternal long-axis plane showing a multicolor jet (indicating turbulent flow) of aortic regurgitation in the left ventricular outflow tract. The jet is narrow in width, suggesting mild regurgitation. AO = aorta; LA = left atrium; LV = left ventricle. *B.* Parasternal long-axis plane with color-flow Doppler imaging. The aortic regurgitant (AR) color jet is as wide as the left ventricular outflow tract, suggesting severe AR. AO = aorta; LA = left atrium; LV = left ventricle. *C.* Parasternal long-axis image of acute severe aortic regurgitation (AI). The accompanying marked elevation of left ventricular (LV) diastolic pressure causes diastolic mitral regurgitation (MR). AO = aorta; LA = left atrium.

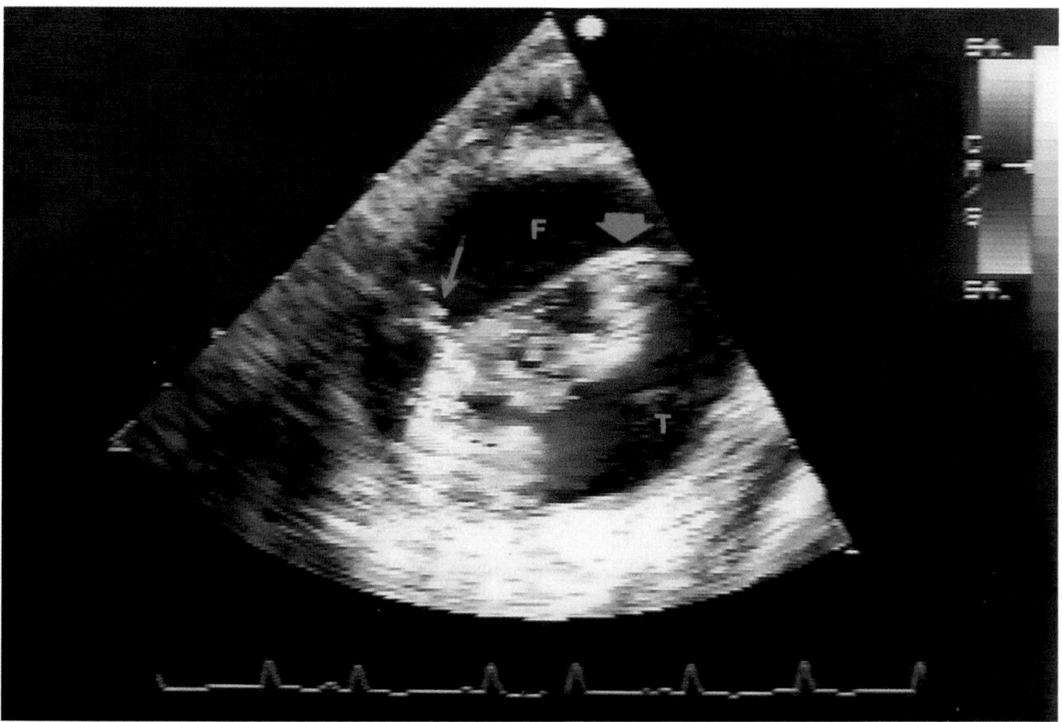


Plate 59 (FIGURE 15-69) Transverse TEE view of an aortic dissection. The false (F) and true (T) lumens are separated by an intimal flap (*large arrow*). The communication between the two channels is visible (*small arrow*).

Plate 60 (FIGURE 15-70B) TEE image of a ruptured sinus of Valsalva aneurysm. The upper image shows focal aneurysmal dilatation of the right coronary sinus with the appearance of a "windsock." Color Doppler (*lower image*) reveals a high-velocity flow jet from the aorta into the right ventricle. Agitated saline was injected intravenously to highlight right heart structures.

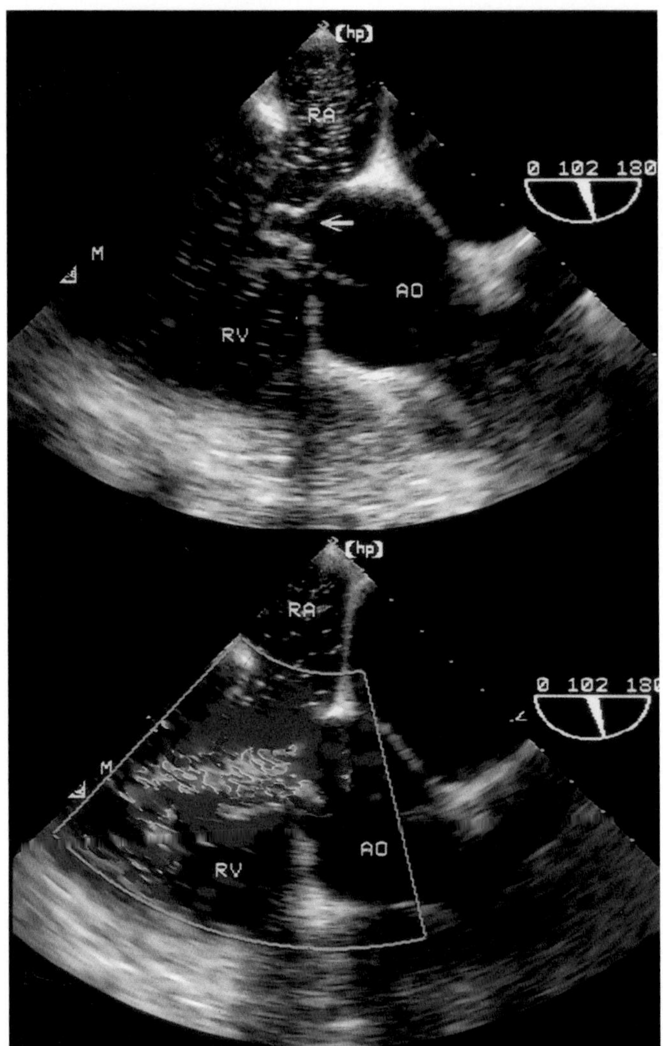


Plate 61 (FIGURE 15-71) Transverse TEE view of penetrating ulceration in the proximal portion of the descending aorta (A). The mouth of the ulcer crater is visible (*large arrowhead*), as is blood flow within the atheroma (*arrow*).

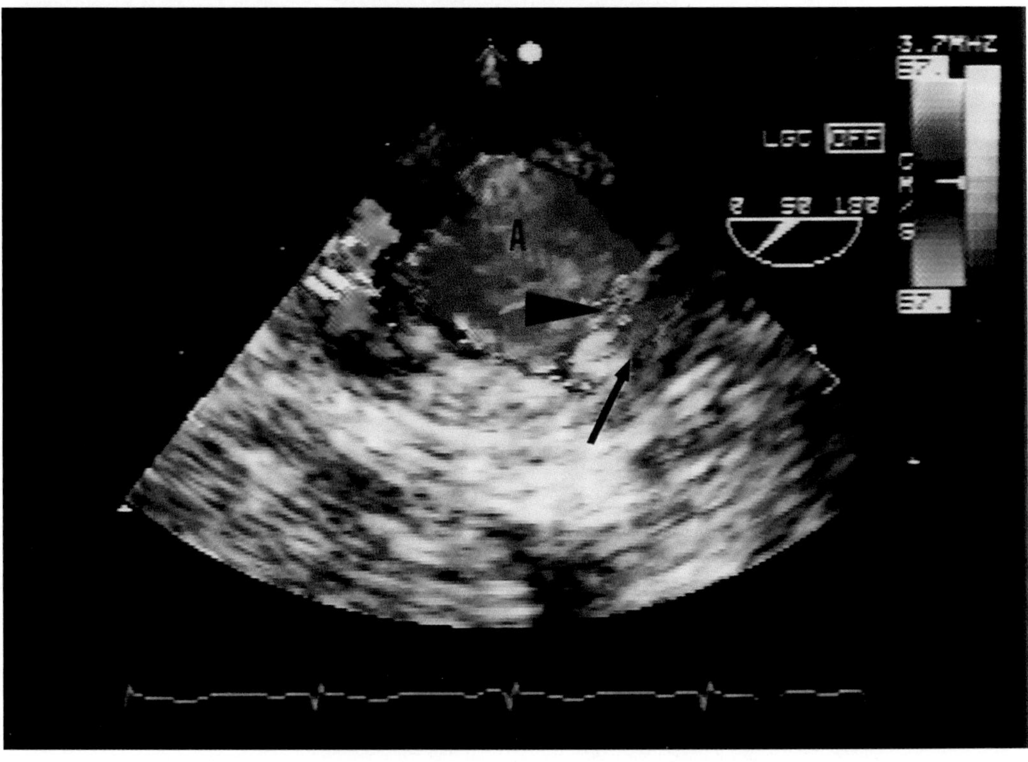

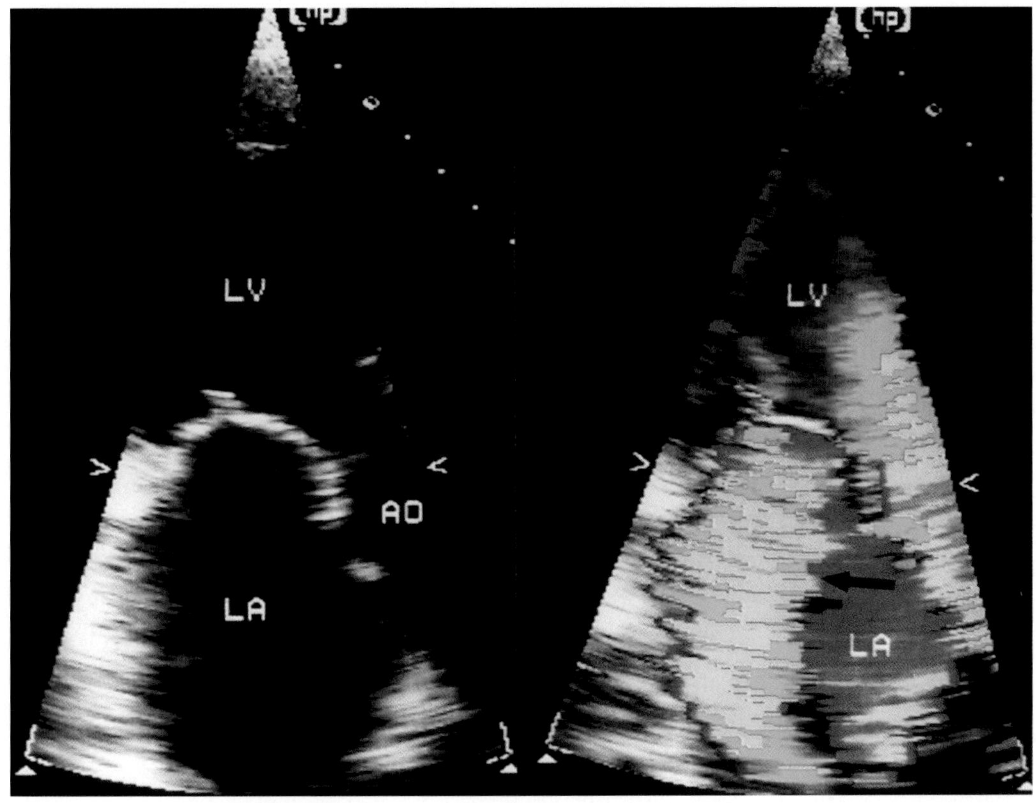


*A*

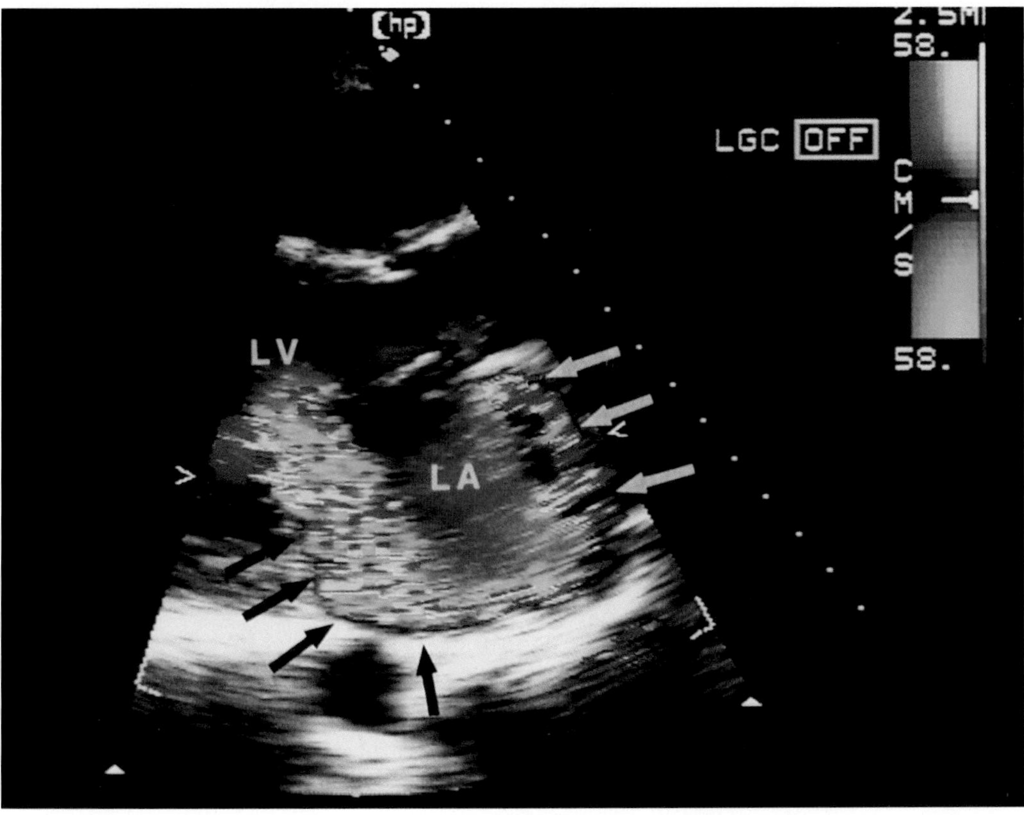


*B*

Plate 62 (FIGURE 15-77) *A.* Mitral regurgitation. *Left:* apical three-chamber plane. Right: same plane with color Doppler imaging. A large jet of mitral regurgitation (*arrow*) is present. AO = aorta; LA = left atrium; LV = left ventricle. *B.* Parasternal long-axis view from a patient with angiographically proved severe mitral regurgitation. The color Doppler jet in this case is directed posteriorly and eccentric (*black arrows*). The jet hugs the wall of the left atrium (LA) and wraps around all the way to the aortic root (*white arrows*). LV = left ventricle.

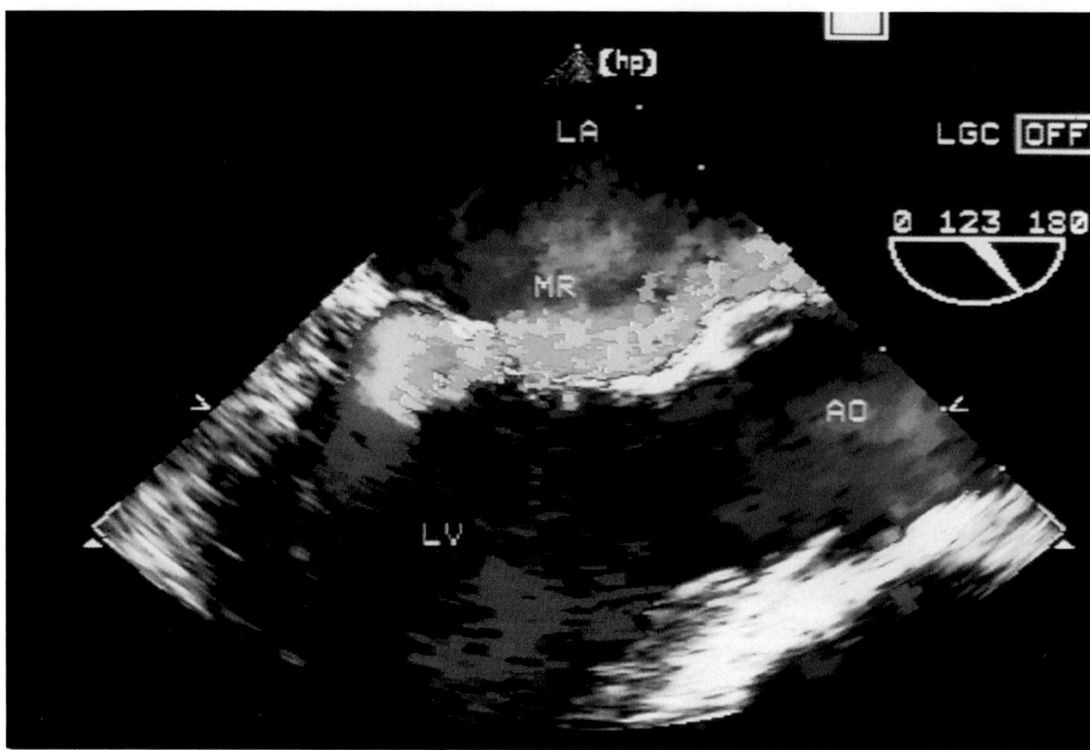


Plate 63 (FIGURE 15-78) TEE images from a case of severe mitral regurgitation secondary to a flail posterior mitral valve leaflet. *A.* abnormal coaptation and prolapse of the posterior leaflet is apparent. *B.* Color Doppler imaging demonstrates an eccentric jet of MR directed anteriorly toward the aortic root (AO). LA = left atrium; LV = left ventricle.

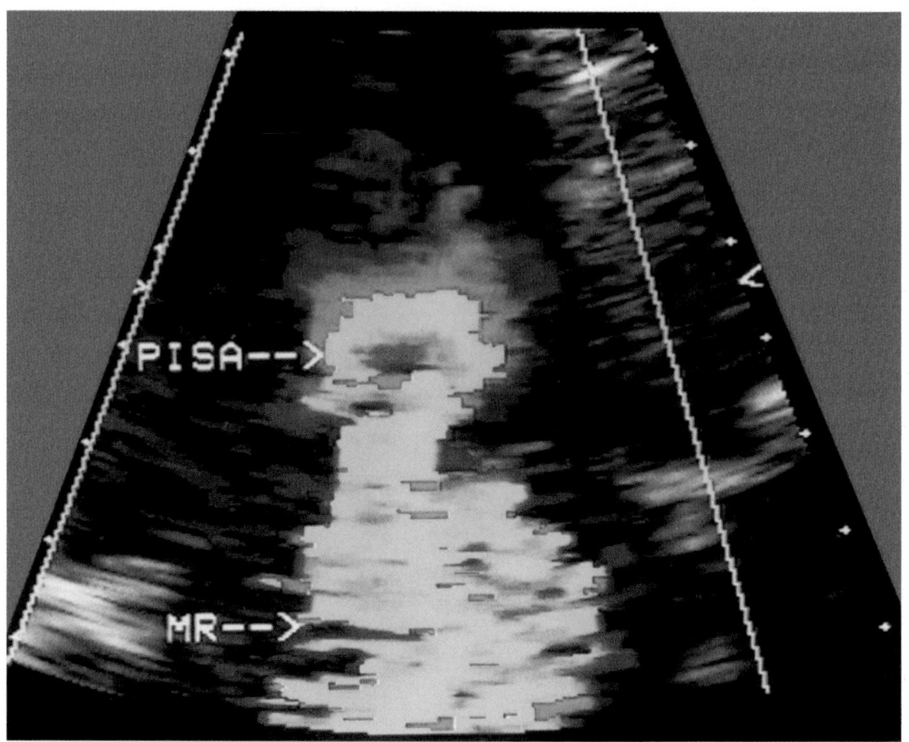


Plate 64 (FIGURE 15-80) *A.* Proximal isovelocity surface area (PISA). See text for details. Q = flow; FCR = flow convergence region; r = radius of isovelocity hemisphere; Vr = velocity of flow at distance r from the orifice. (From Bargiggia GS, Tronconi L, Sahn DJ, et al. A new method for quantitation of mitral regurgitation based on color flow Doppler imaging of flow convergence proximal to regurgitant orifice. *Circulation* 1991;84:1481–1489, with permission.) *B.* Magnified view (from the apical four-chamber plane) of mitral regurgitation (MR) demonstrating color Doppler flow convergence proximal to the mitral valve (PISA).

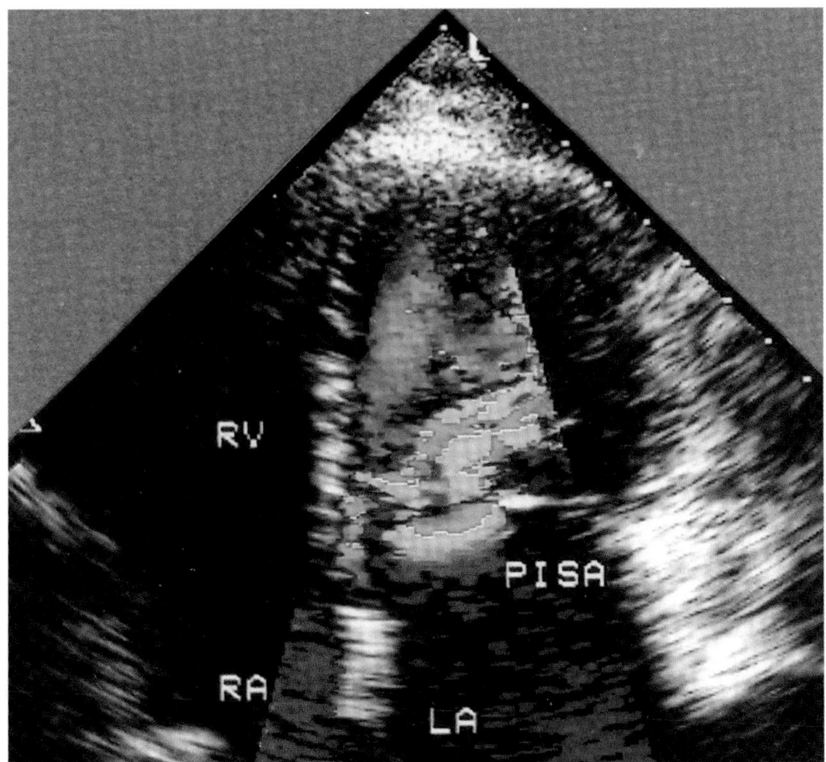


Plate 65 (FIGURE 15-81) Apical four-chamber plane in mitral stenosis. Color flow imaging in the mitral valve region shows flow convergence (PISA) proximal to the valve during diastole. LA = left atrium; RA = right atrium; RV = right ventricle.

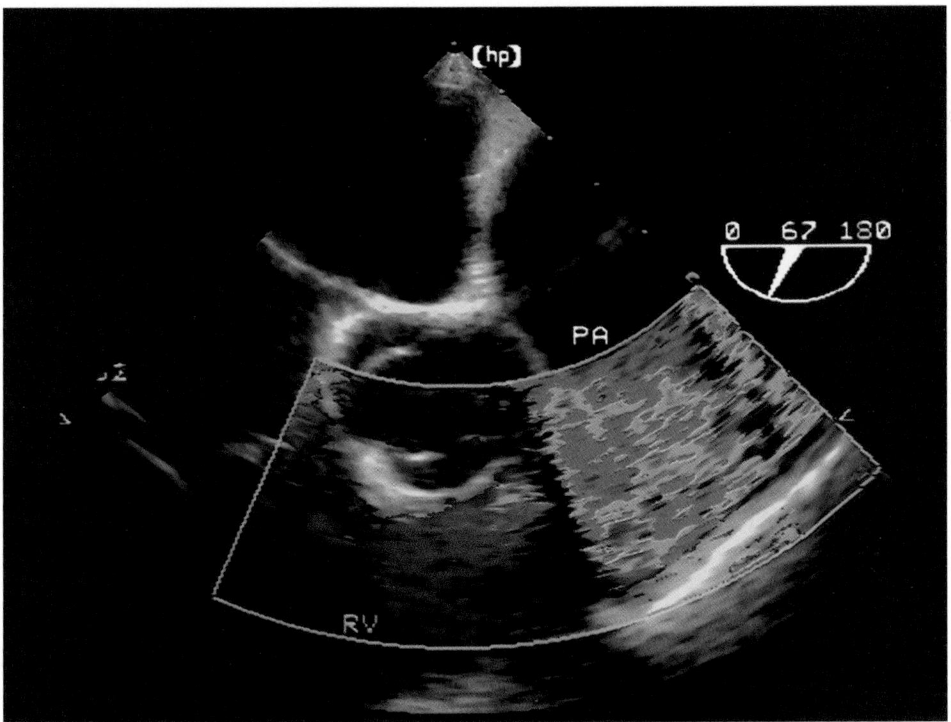


Plate 66 (FIGURE 15-85) *A.* Pulmonic stenosis. The pulmonic valve leaflet is thickened and echo-reflective, and does not open completely during systole (*arrow*). RA = right atrium; LA = left atrium; AO = aorta; PA = pulmonary artery; RV = right ventricle. *B.* Doppler interrogation reveals increased flow velocity (4 m/s) through the valve orifice. *C.* Transesophageal image of pulmonic stenosis. The valve leaflets exhibit doming during systole (arrow). *D.* TEE image with color Doppler, showing high-velocity, turbulent flow in the main pulmonary artery.

Plate 67 (FIGURE 15-102) Modified apical four-chamber image of a distal septal ventricular septal rupture. With 2D imaging (*left*), the distal septum is incompletely visualized. With color Doppler imaging, however, a high-velocity aliased color jet is seen in the right ventricle (RV). In addition, an area of flow convergence is seen on the left ventricular (LV) side of the rupture (*arrow*).

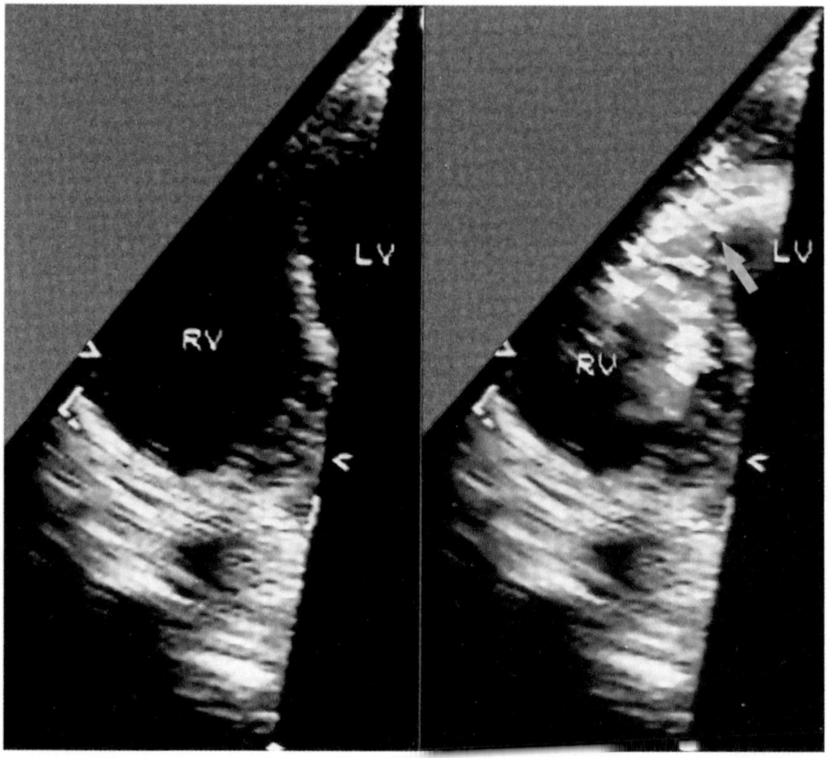


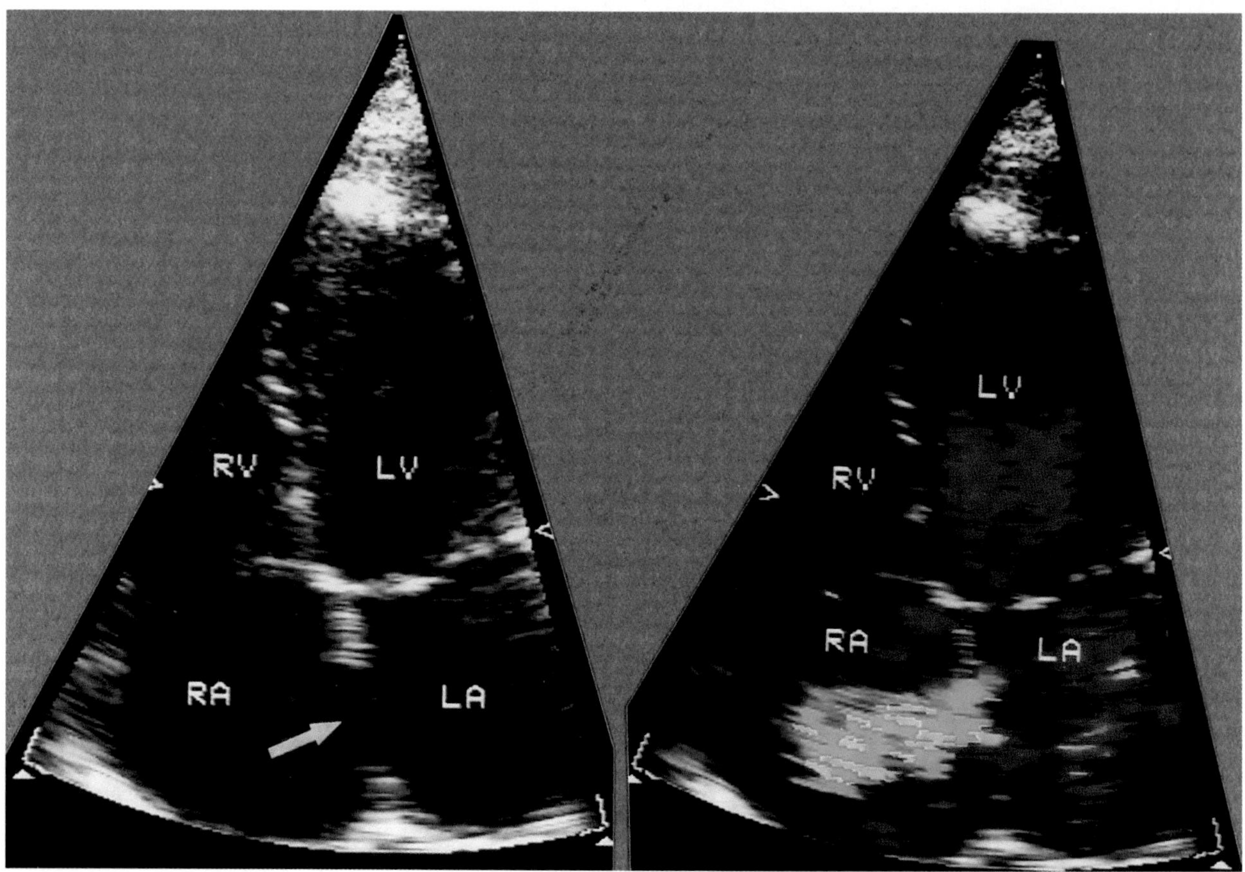


Plate 68 (FIGURE 15-110) *A*. Apical four-chamber view of an ostium secundum atrial septal defect (ASD). On the left, a defect in the mid atrial septum is apparent (*arrow*). On the right, there is color flow through the shunt. RV = right ventricle; RA = right atrium; LA = left atrium; LV = left ventricle. *B*. Apical four-chamber view of a large ostium primum atrial septal defect (as well as an inlet VSD) in a patient with Down's syndrome. RA = right atrium; LA = left atrium; LV = left ventricle; RV = right ventricle.

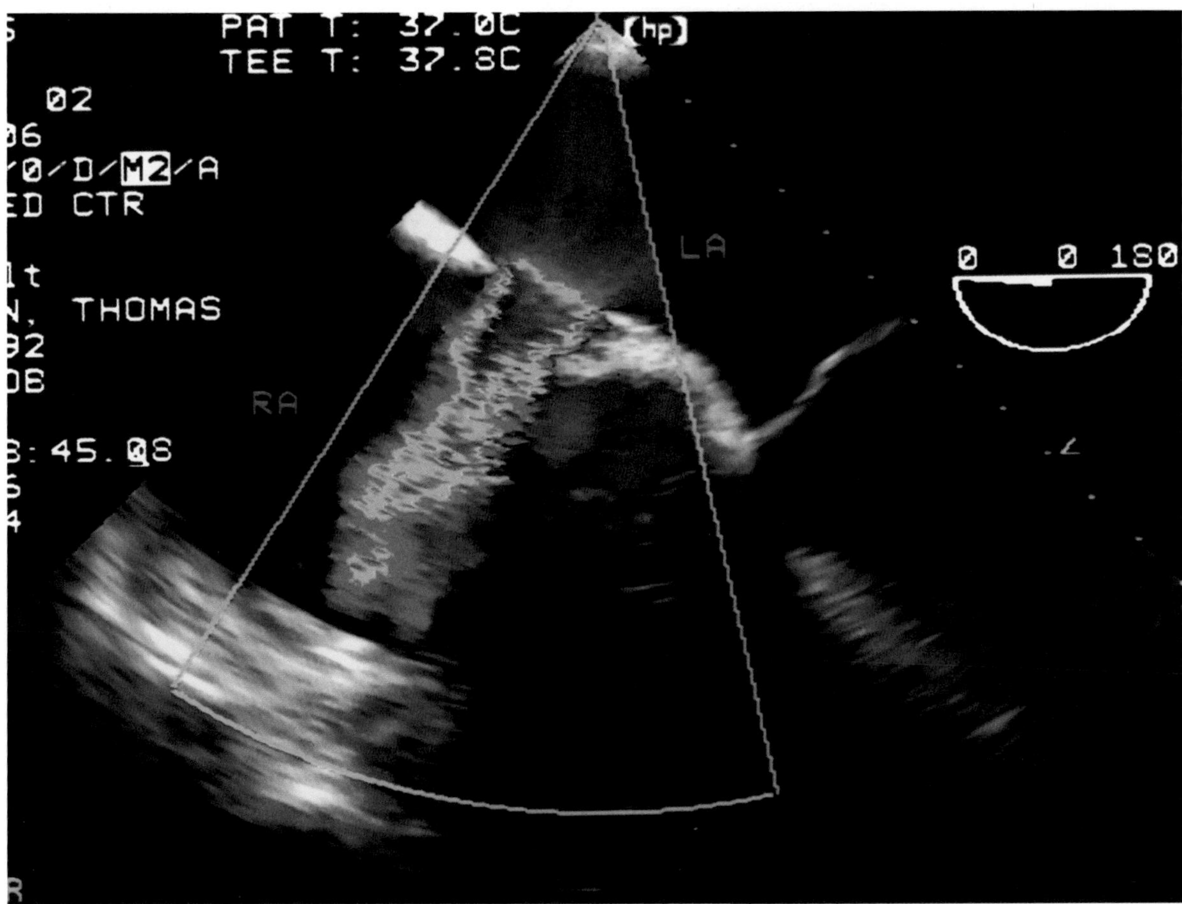


Plate 69 (FIGURE 15-111) *A*. Transesophageal image of a sinus venosus atrial septal defect (ASD) (longitudinal plane). The defect is present in the superior portion of the interatrial septum. RA = right atrium; LA = left atrium; ASD = atrial septal defect; PA = pulmonary artery. *B*. Transesophageal image of an ostium secundum ASD. Color-flow Doppler confirms a left to right shunt, and the size of the defect can be measured accurately.

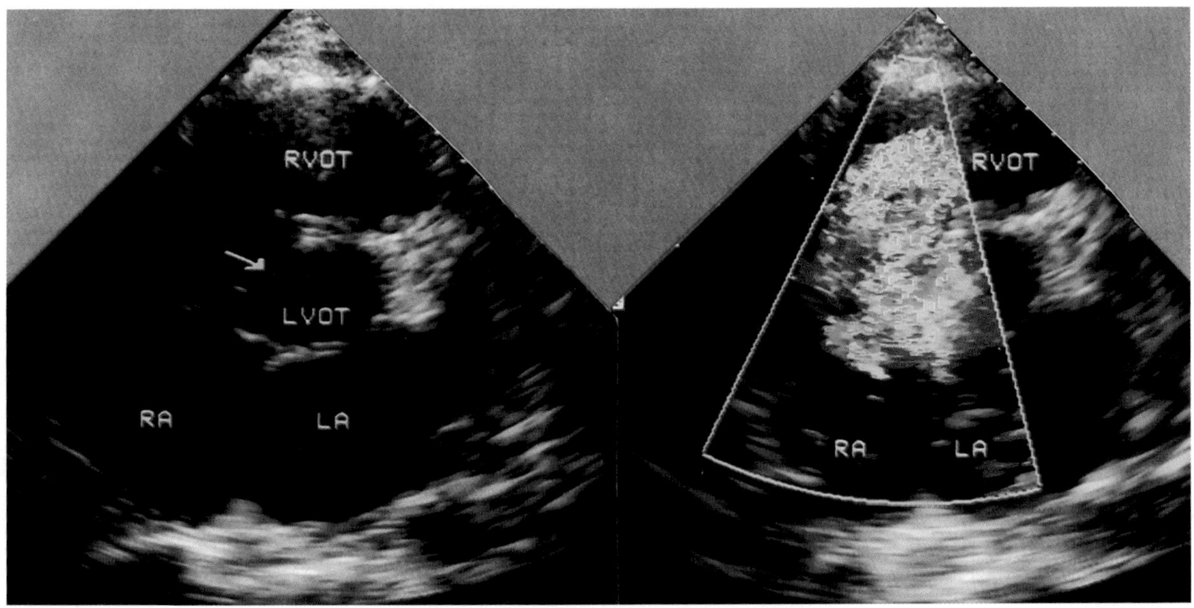


Plate 70 (FIGURE 15-114) Parasternal short-axis images of a large perimembranous ventricular septal defect (VSD) (*arrow*) without (*left*) and with (*right*) superimposed color flow Doppler. A large, turbulent color jet crosses the VSD during systole (*right*). RVOT = right ventricular outflow tract; RA = right atrium; LA = left atrium; LVOT = left ventricular outflow tract.

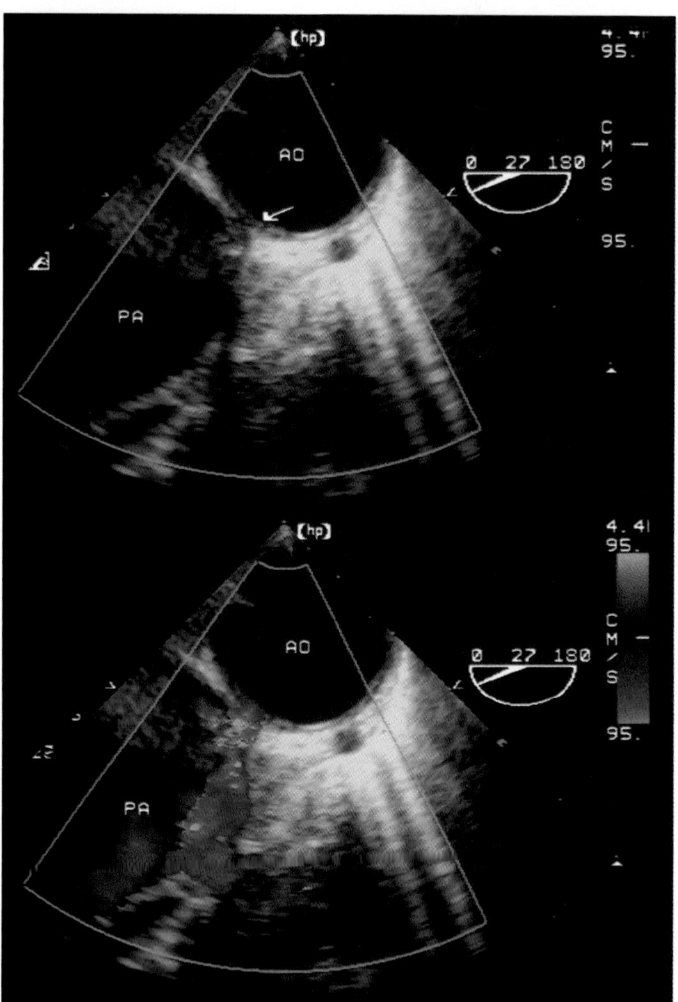


A

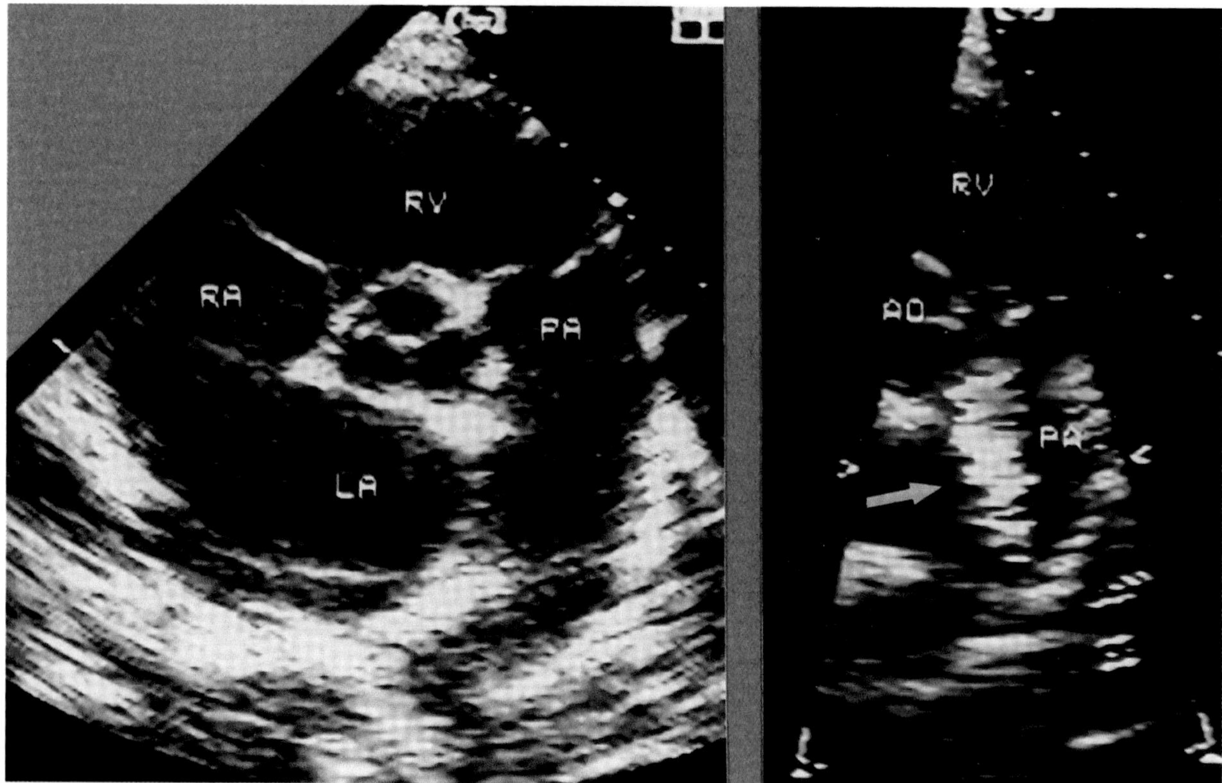


B

Plate 71 (FIGURE 15-115) *A*. Transesophageal image of a patent ductus arteriosus (PDA). The upper panel shows a small communication (arrow) between the aorta (AO) and pulmonary artery (PA), which is confirmed with color-flow Doppler imaging (lower panel). *B*. Parasternal short-axis images at the aortic valve level. On the left, the pulmonary artery (PA) is somewhat enlarged. On the right, color imaging reveals diastolic flow within the PA, consistent with a patent ductus arteriosus. RV = right ventricle; RA = right atrium; LA = left atrium; AO = aorta.

Plate 72 (FIGURE 15-121) *A*. Continuous-wave Doppler tracing of the descending aorta (from the suprasternal position) in aortic coarctation. Peak systolic velocity is 3.7 m/s, and there is persistent flow during diastole, suggesting severe coarctation. *B*. Suprasternal image of aortic coarctation. The descending aorta (DAo) is focally narrowed and tortuous, and turbulent (aliased) flow is present distal to the site of coarctation.

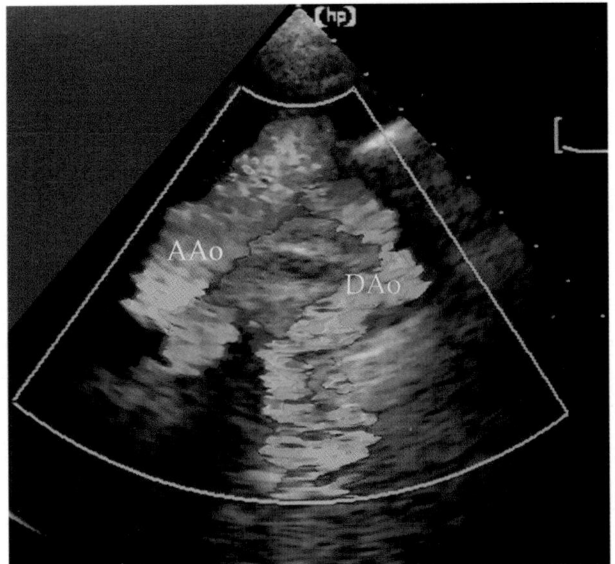


*A*

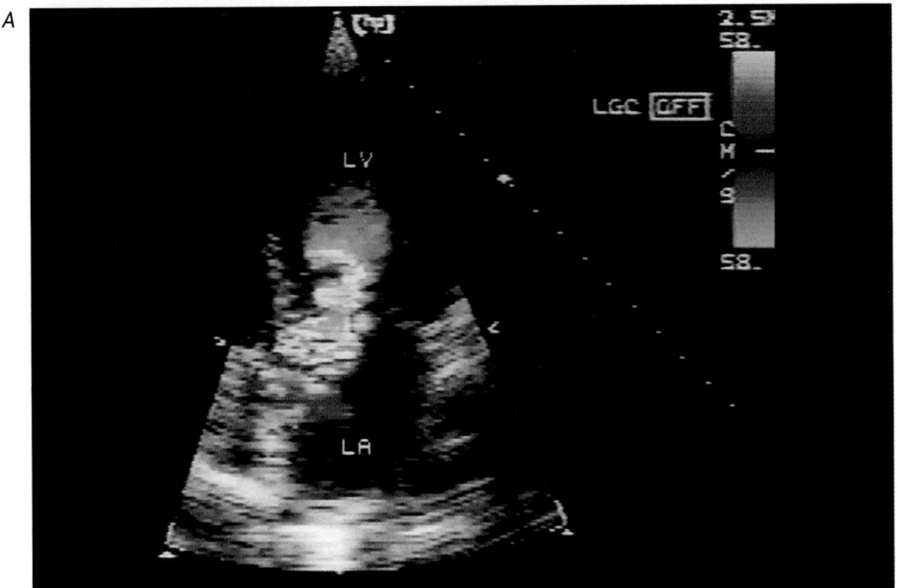


*B*

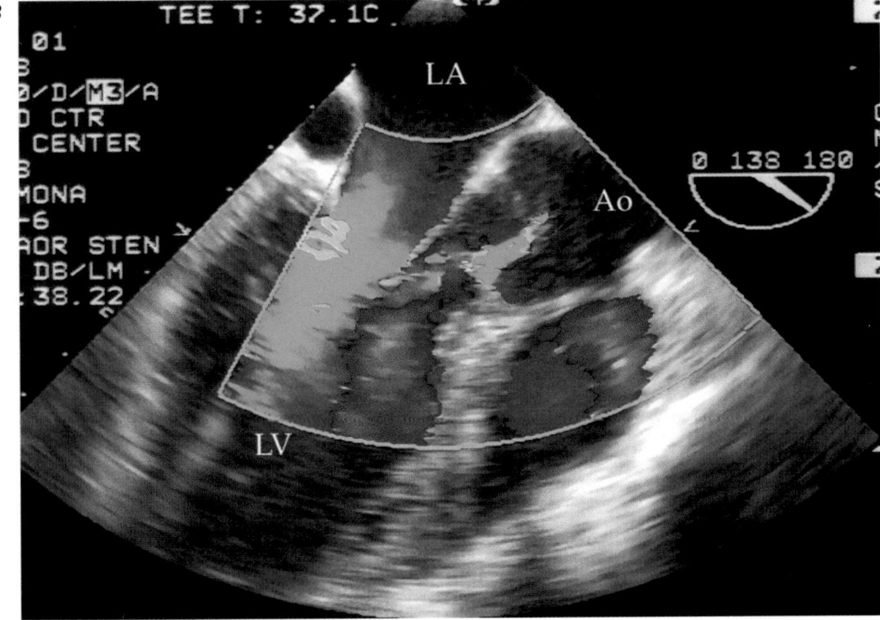


Plate 73 (FIGURE 15-122) Subvalvular and supravalvular aortic stenosis. *A*. Apical three-chamber view of discrete subaortic stenosis. A fibromuscular ridge (*arrow*) is present in the left ventricular outflow tract. LV = left ventricle; LA = left atrium; A = aortic root. *B*. Apical five-chamber view of discrete subaortic stenosis with color-flow Doppler, demonstrating aliasing and proximal flow convergence in the left ventricular outflow tract. LV = left ventricle; LA = left atrium. *C*. Transesophageal image of discrete subaortic stenosis. A fibrous ridge in the outflow tract of the left ventricle (LV) is present (arrow). LA = left atrium. *D*. Transesophageal image with color-flow Doppler, demonstrating mild aortic insufficiency associated with discrete subaortic stenosis. LV = left ventricle; LA = left atrium; Ao = aortic root. *E*. Transesophageal image of supravalvular aortic stenosis. A fibrous ridge extends into the aortic lumen just above the sinus of Valsalva.

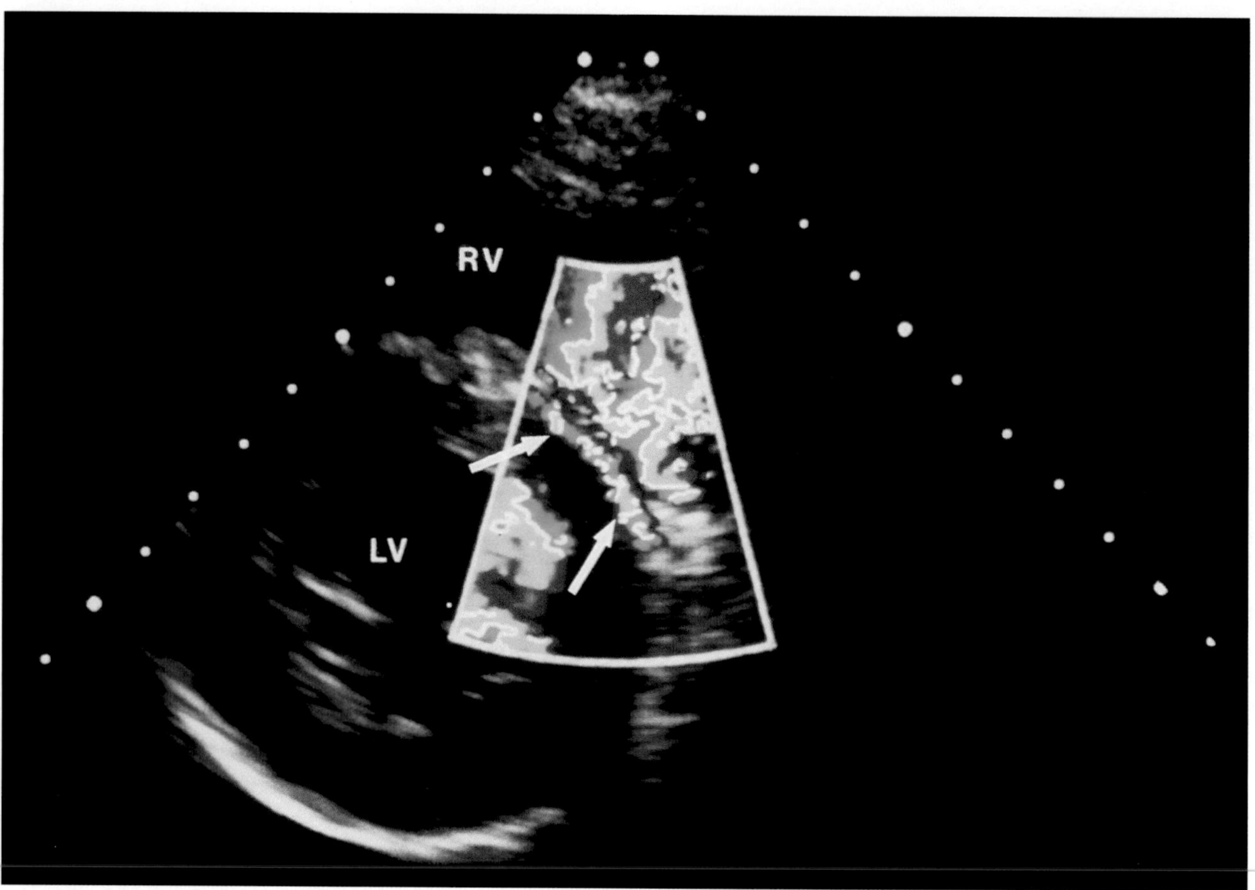


Plate 74 (FIGURE 15-141) *A*. Transthoracic short-axis image of a coronary artery within the interventricular septum (*arrows*). LV = left ventricle; RV = right ventricle. *B*. Pulsed-wave spectral Doppler tracing of flow within the distal left anterior descending artery. Diastolic flow is predominant. (Courtesy of Ajit Raisinghani, MD.)

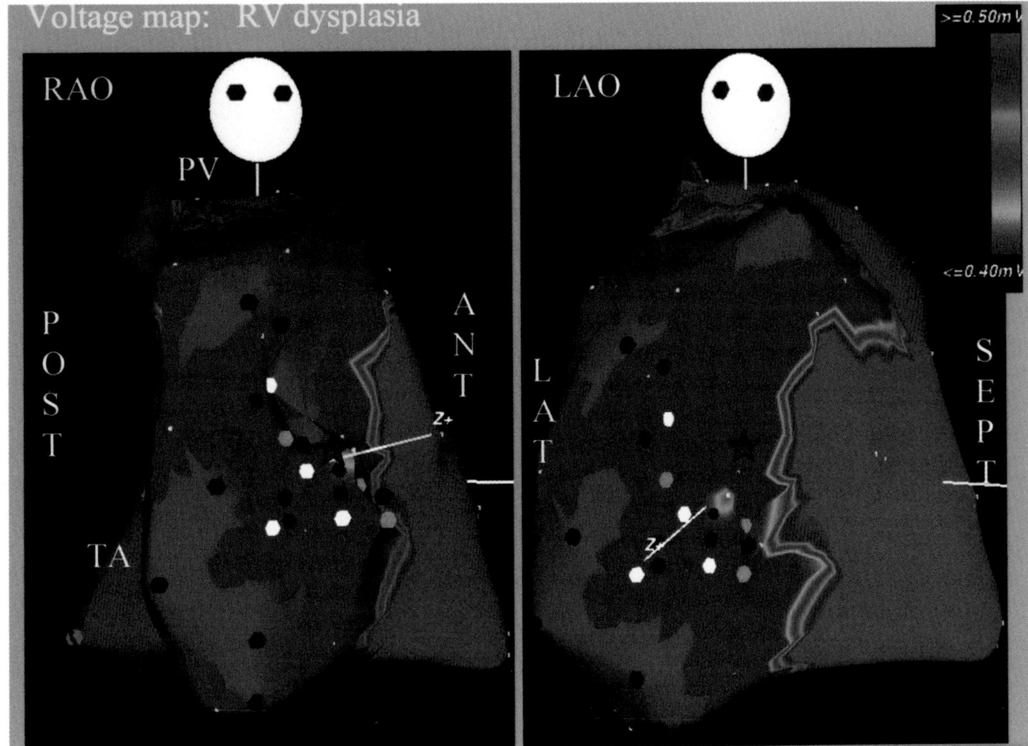


*A*

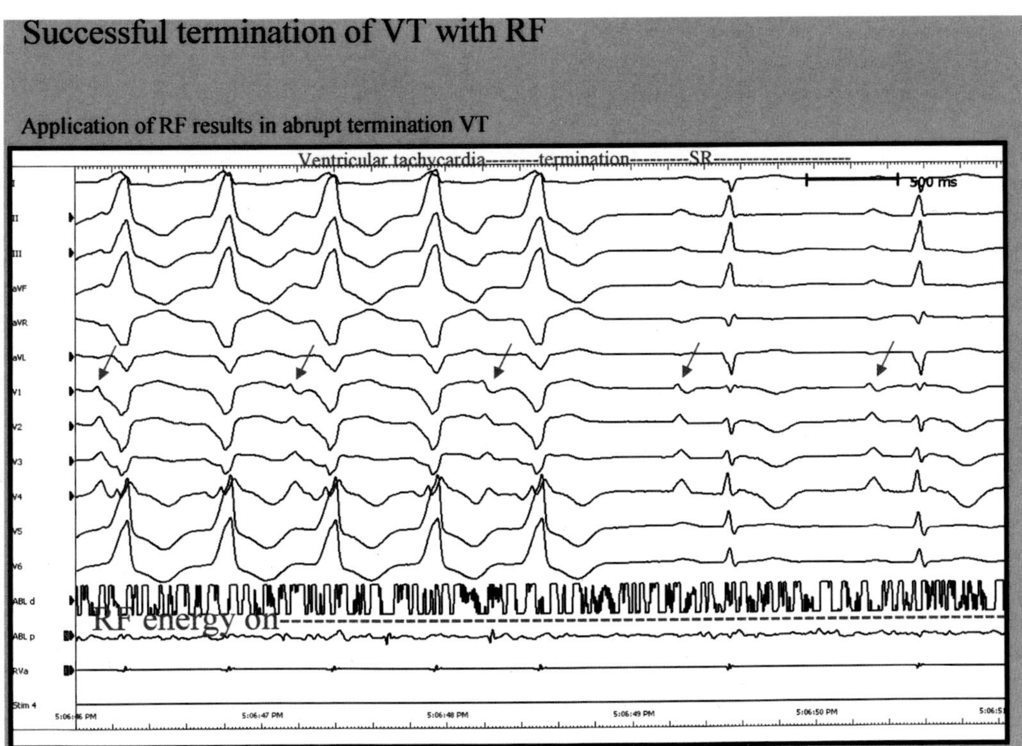


*B*

Plate 75 (FIGURE 31-5) *A*. Voltage map of the right ventricle, acquired using the Biosense Webster Carto, the three-dimensional electroanatomic mapping system. The red and gray areas indicate scar (low-voltage intracardiac electrograms) and the purple area represents healthy tissue (>0.5 mV intracardiac electrogram amplitude). The right anterior oblique (RAO) and left anterior oblique (LAO) projections are shown. A large basal free wall scar is present, extending from the base to beyond the midcavity of the right ventricle. TA = tricuspid annulus; Post = posterior; Ant = anterior; Lat = lateral; Sept = septal. The blue star represents the site where the vulnerable isthmus of the ventricular tachycardia (VT) circuit is mapped and where application of a radiofrequency lesion terminates VT (*B*).

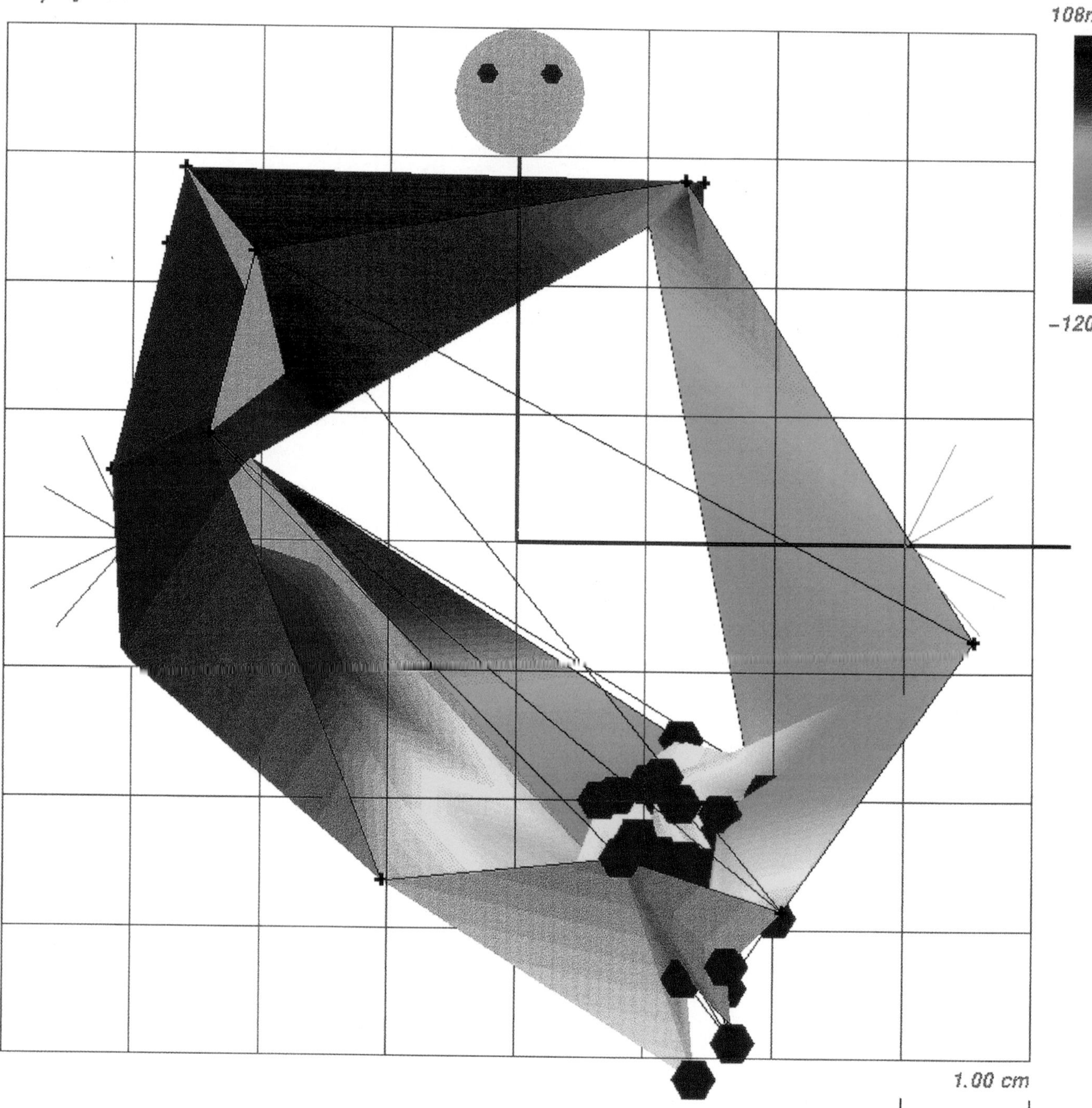


Plate 76 (FIGURE 34-3) Anterior-posterior view of the right atrium during typical, inferior vena cava (IVC)-tricuspid valve annulus isthmus-dependent atrial flutter using the Biosense CARTO system. The red shows the earliest activation with respect to the timing reference (typically the proximal coronary sinus recording), and the blue and the violet represent areas of late activation. The gray areas are where early activation meets late activation, a characteristic of reentrant tachycardias. The brown hexagons mark the location of radiofrequency lesions positioned on the isthmus to ablate the atrial flutter. RA = right atria.

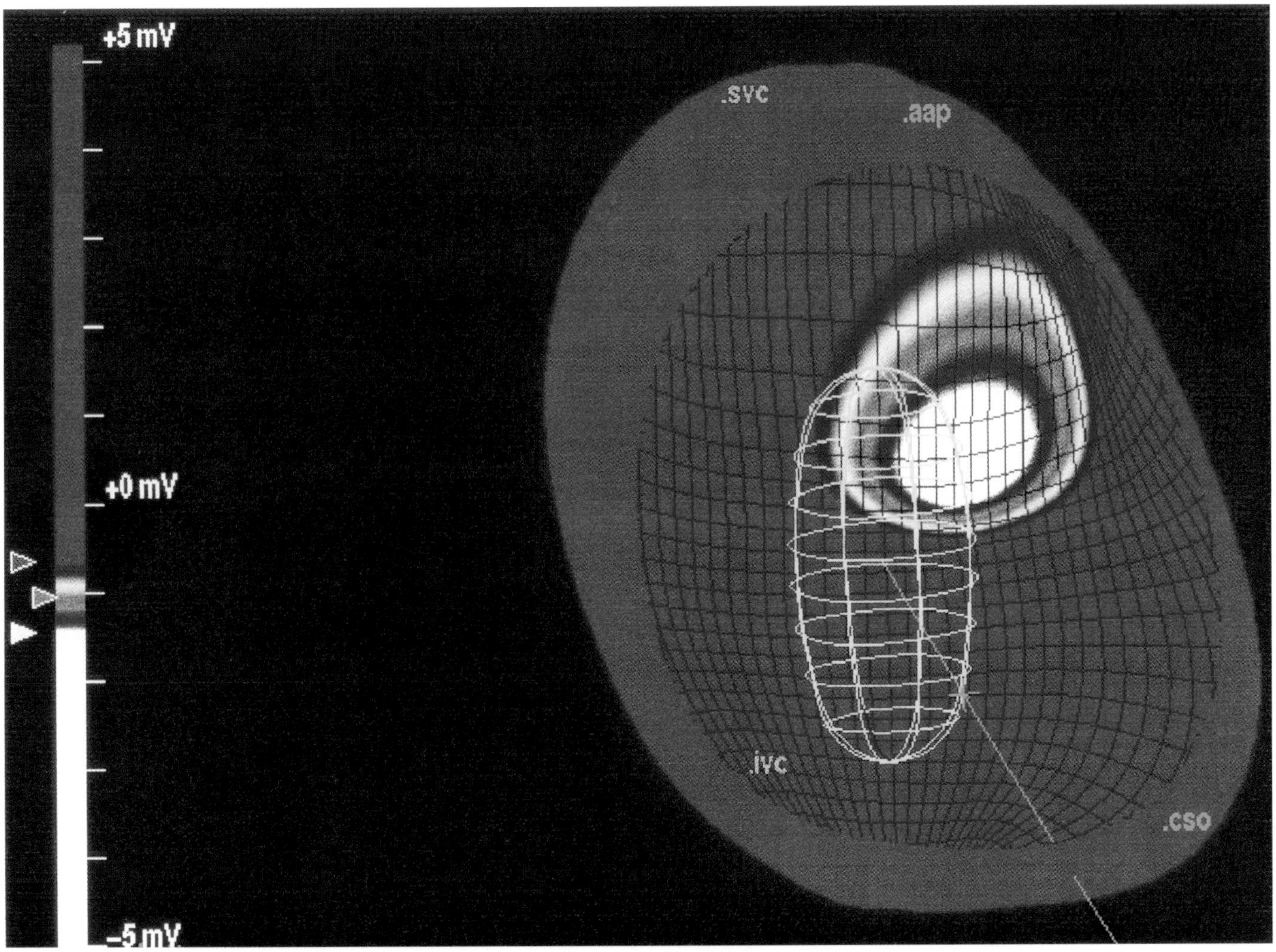

Plate 77 (FIGURE 34-4) Activation of the right atrium during focal atrial tachycardia, mapped with the Endocardial Solutions EnSite 3000 system. The white represents tissue that is fully activated, and purple is tissue that is not yet activated. SVC = superior vena cava; IVC = inferior vena cava.

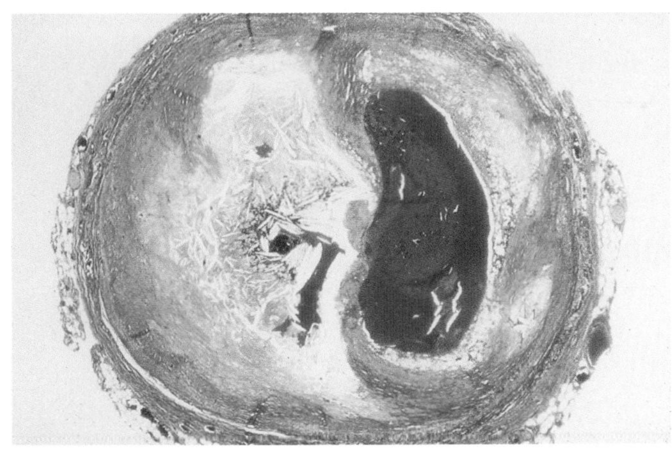

Plate 78 (FIGURE 44-1) Cross-sectioned coronary artery containing a ruptured plaque with a nonocclusive thrombosis superimposed. The actual defect in the fibrous cap is not seen in this section but is located nearby, documented by the presence of extravasated radiographic contrast medium (postmortem coronary angiography) in the soft, lipid-rich core just beneath the thin, inflamed fibrous cap. Trichrome stain, rendering thrombus red, collagen blue, and lipid colorless.

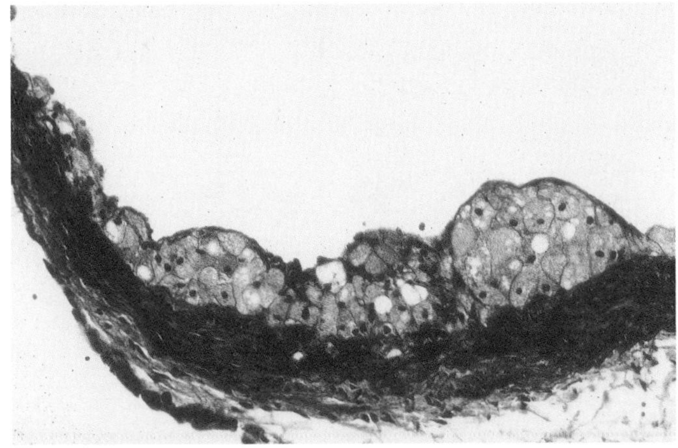

Plate 79 (FIGURE 44-3) An early atherosclerotic lesion (fatty streak) in the aortic root of a 3-month-old apolipoprotein E–deficient mouse fed a high-fat western-type diet for 6 weeks. The lesion consists of lipid-filled monocyte-derived macrophages (foam cells) and a few lymphocytes (T cells) beneath an intact endothelium. Elastin trichrome stain.

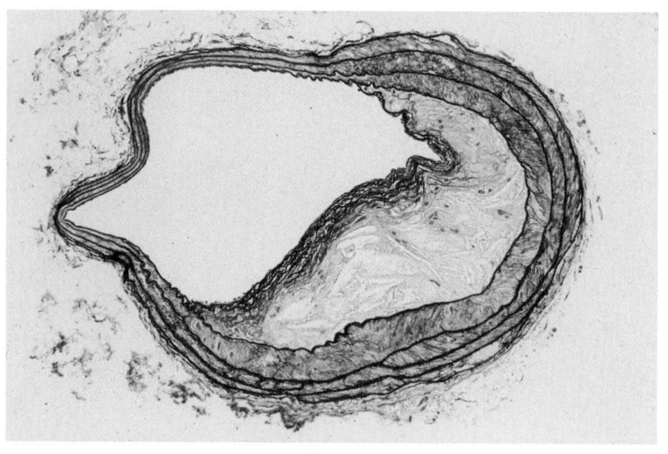

Plate 80 (FIGURE 44-4) An advanced atherosclerotic plaque in the brachiocephalic trunk of a 6-month-old apolipoprotein E–deficient mouse fed normal chow. The plaque appears vulnerable morphologically, consisting of a lipid-rich core with cholesterol crystals covered by a thin but intact fibrous cap. Orcein, staining elastic tissue black.

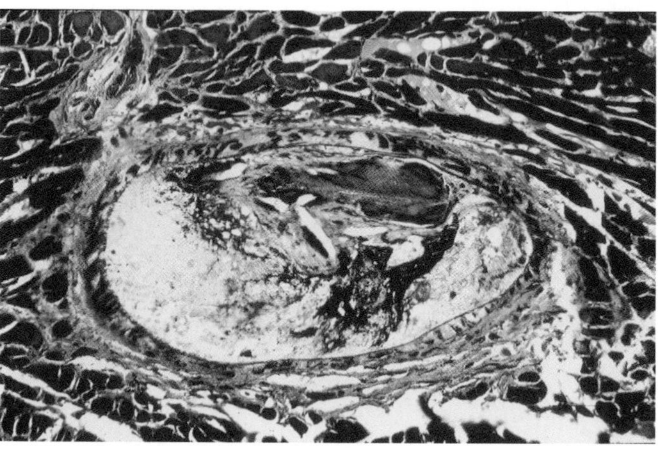

Plate 81 (FIGURE 44-5) Ruptured coronary plaque with occlusive thrombosis superimposed (natural death of a 21-month-old apolipoprotein E–deficient mouse). Spontaneous plaque rupture and/or luminal thrombosis are extremely rare in animal models of atherosclerosis. Elastin trichrome stain.

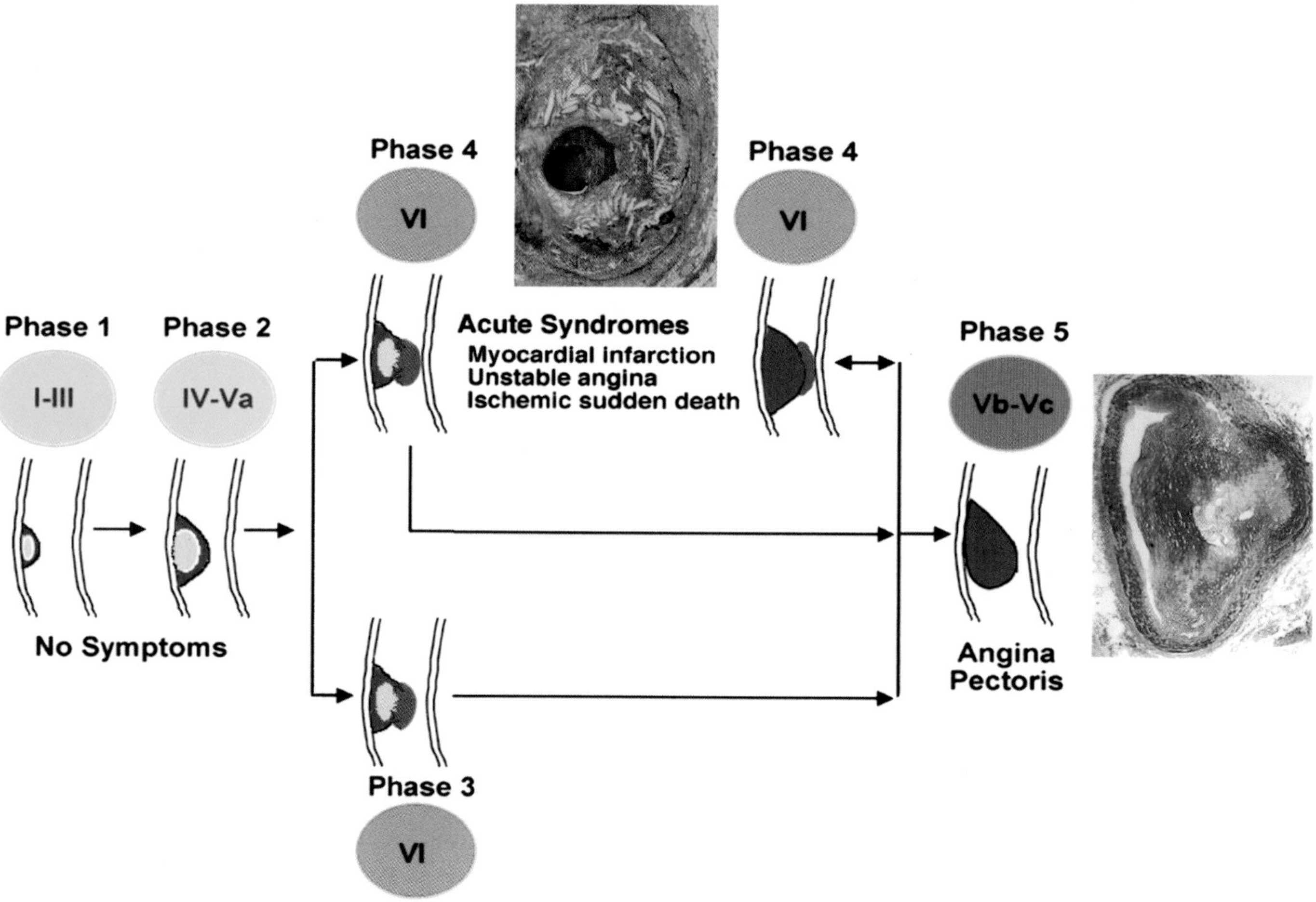

Phase 1
I-III
Phase 2
IV-Va
No Symptoms
Phase 4
VI
Acute Syndromes
Myocardial infarction
Unstable angina
Ischemic sudden death
Phase 4
VI
Phase 3
VI
Phase 5
Vb-Vc
Angina
Pectoris

Plate 82 (FIGURE 45-1) Simplified diagram of the evolution of coronary atherosclerosis. Phases and morphology of lesion progression.

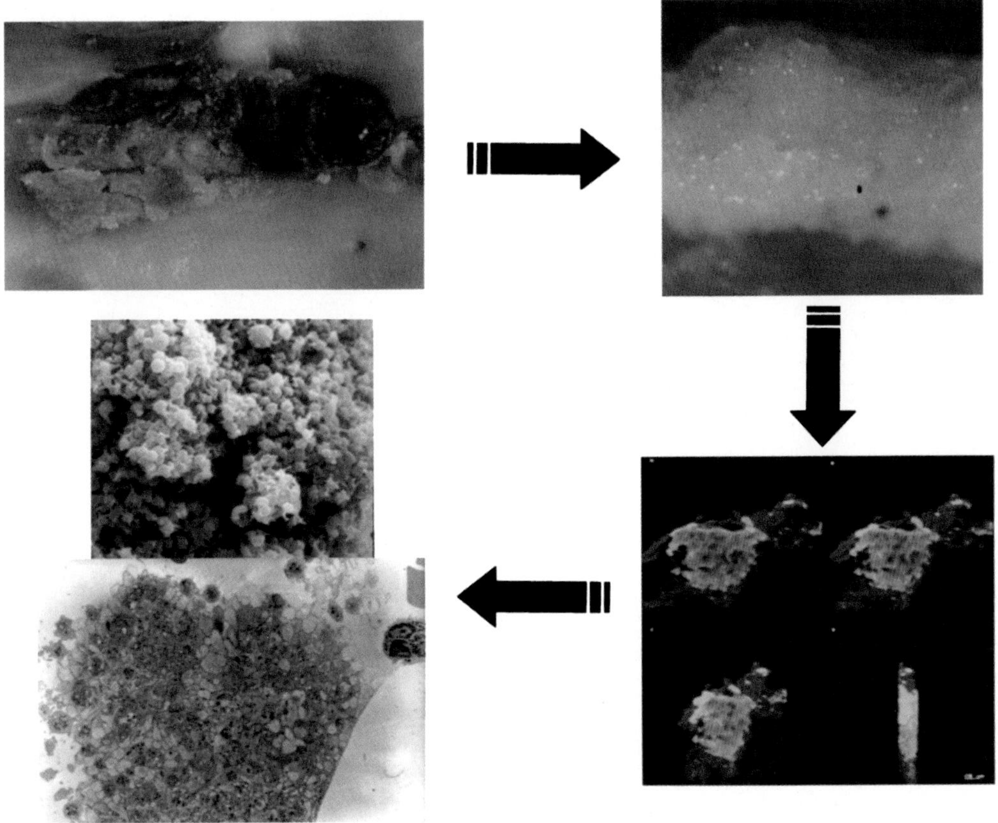

Plate 83 (FIGURE 45-3) Images of thrombosis. From naked eye observation to immunohistochemistry [green, platelets; red, fibrin(ogen)] and electronic microscopy (top, scanning; bottom, transmission).

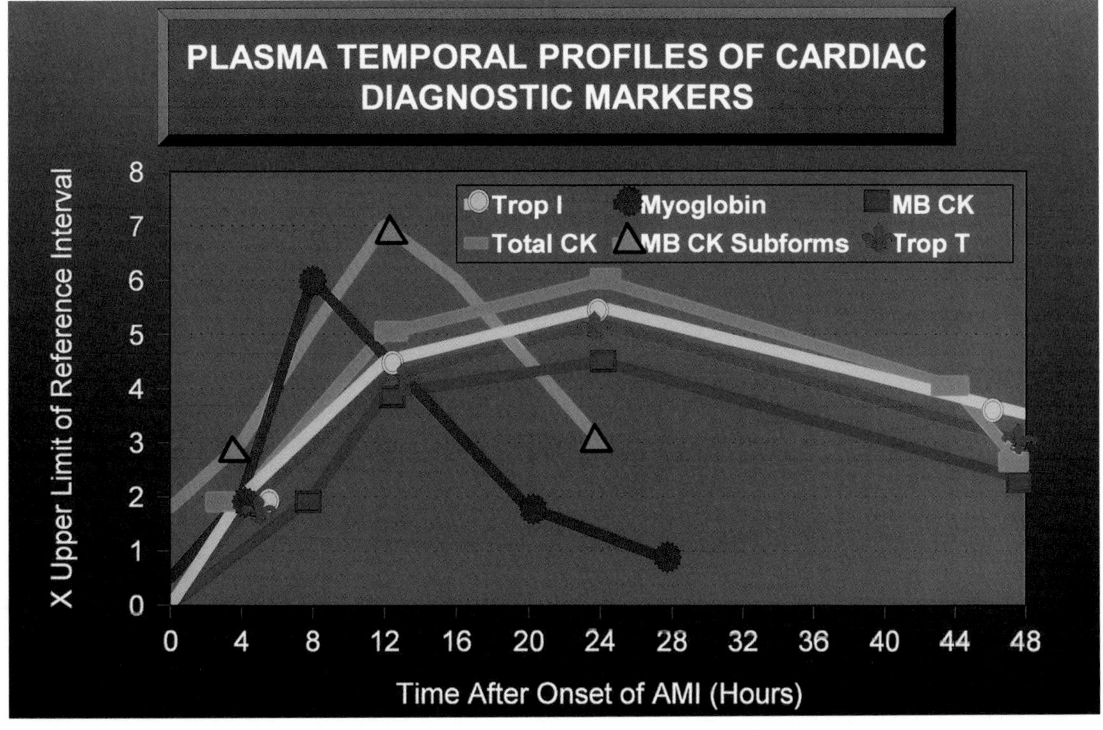


Plate 84 (FIGURE 52-1) Shown here is the temporal profile of the diagnostic biomarkers used for detecting myocardial infarction. The plasma temporal profile for early detection is illustrated for myoglobin and MB-CK subforms. The markers MB-CK, total CK, and cardiac troponins I and T are all released with a similar initial time profile. However, troponins I and T remain elevated for 10 to 14 days and thus are better markers for late diagnosis than that of MB-CK.

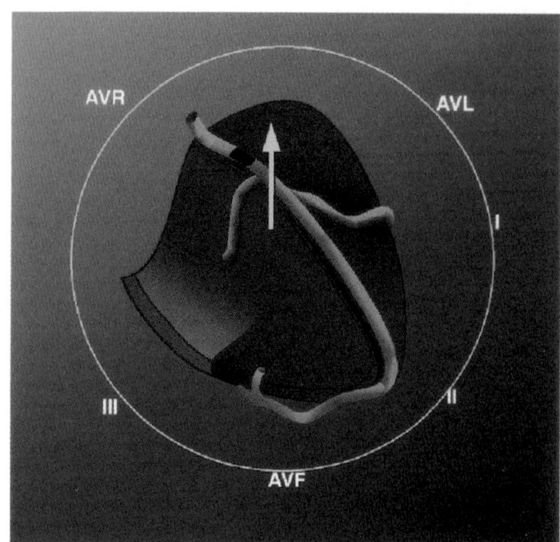


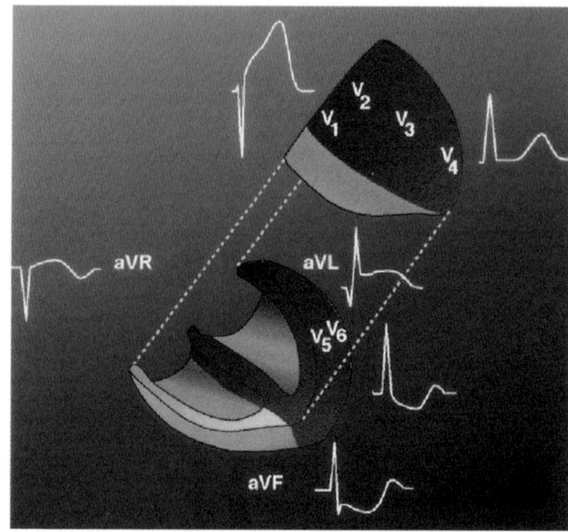


Plate 85 (FIGURE 53-2) Areas of left ventricular ischemia in LAD occlusion proximal to the first septal and first diagonal branch. *Left panel:* There is ischemia of the left ventricle. The ST-segment vector points in a superior direction because ischemia predominates in the basal areas. *Right panel:* The superiorly oriented ST vector leads to ST-segment elevation in lead aVR and lead $V_1$ and ST-segment depression in the inferior leads and in $V_5$ and $V_6$.

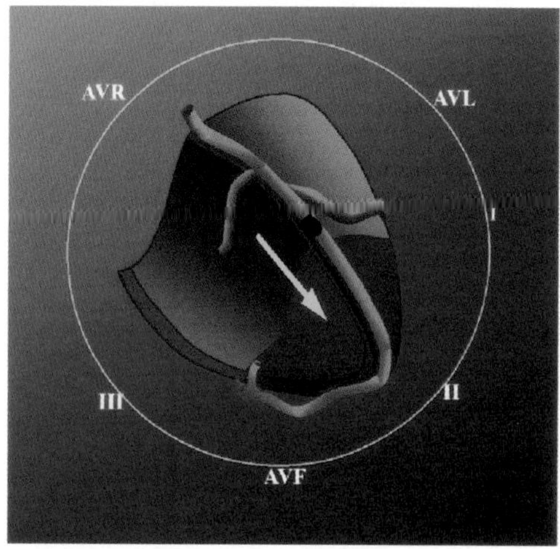


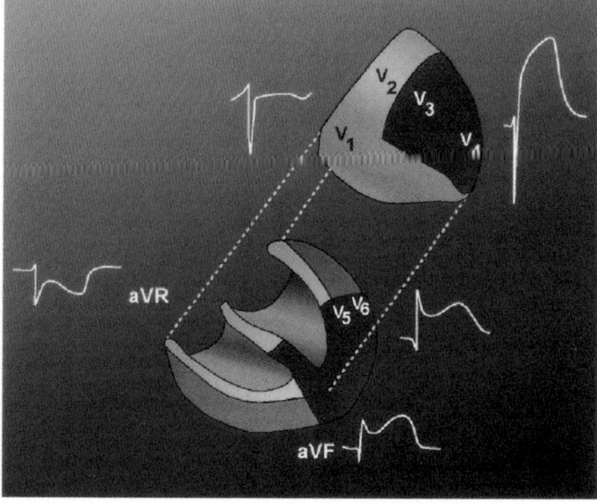


Plate 86 (FIGURE 53-4) Ischemic areas in distal LAD occlusion. *Left panel:* The ST vector points inferiorly due to ischemia of the inferoapical area. *Right panel:* The inferiorly directed ST vector leads to ST-segment depression in lead aVR and ST-segment elevation in the inferior leads.

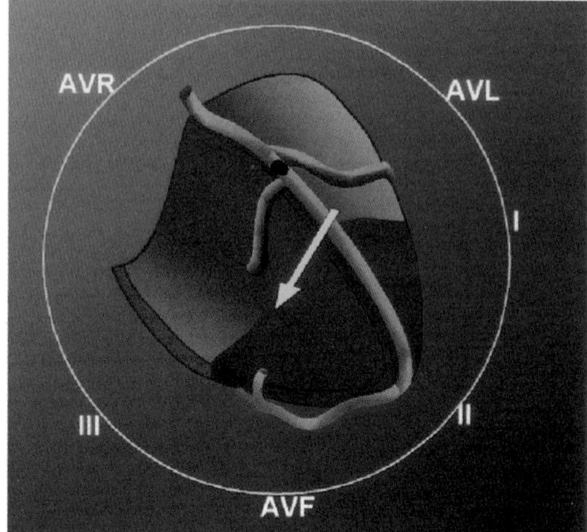


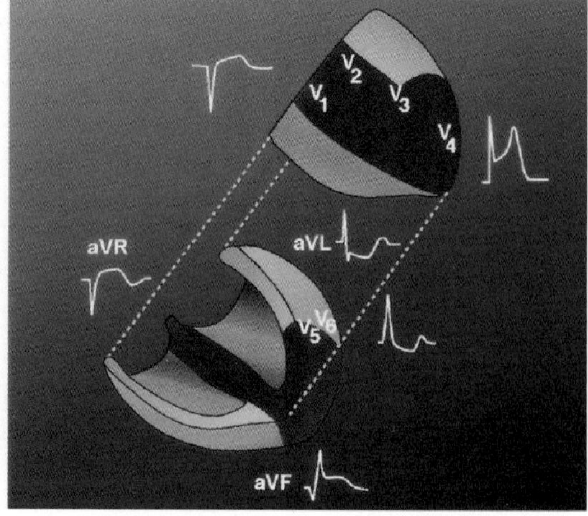


Plate 87 (FIGURE 53-6) Ischemic areas in LAD occlusion between the first diagonal (or intermediate) and first septal branch. *Left panel:* Predominance of ischemia in the septal-apical area leads to an ST-segment vector pointing in a rightward direction. *Right panel:* Apart from ST-segment elevation in the precordial leads, ST-segment elevation is also seen in leads III and aVR. Negativity of the ST segment is seen in lead aVL.

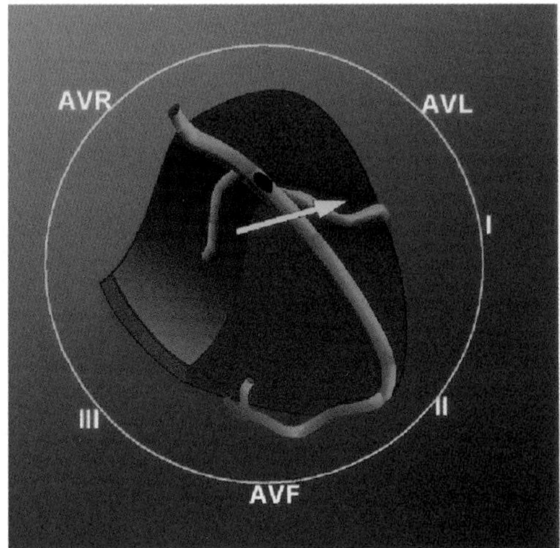

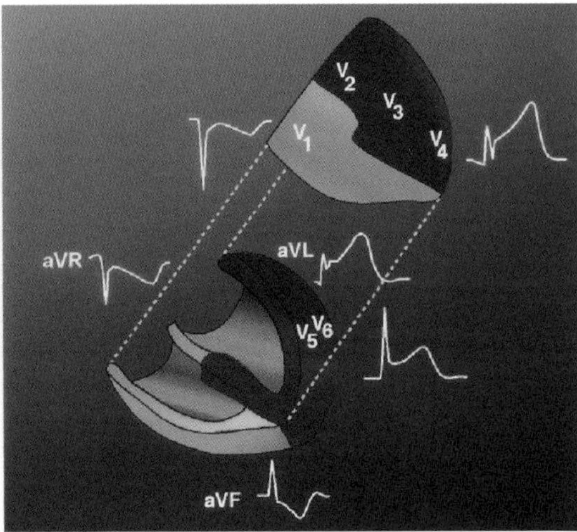


Plate 88 (FIGURE 53-8) Ischemic areas in LAD occlusion distal to the septal and proximal to the first diagonal branch. *Left panel:* Predominance of ischemia in the lateral area leading to an ST vector pointing in that direction. *Right panel:* The lateral orientation of the ST vector leads to ST-segment negativity of leads III and aVR. Lead II is isoelectric due to the perpendicular orientation of the ST vector in that lead. The lateral leads I and aVL show ST-segment elevation.

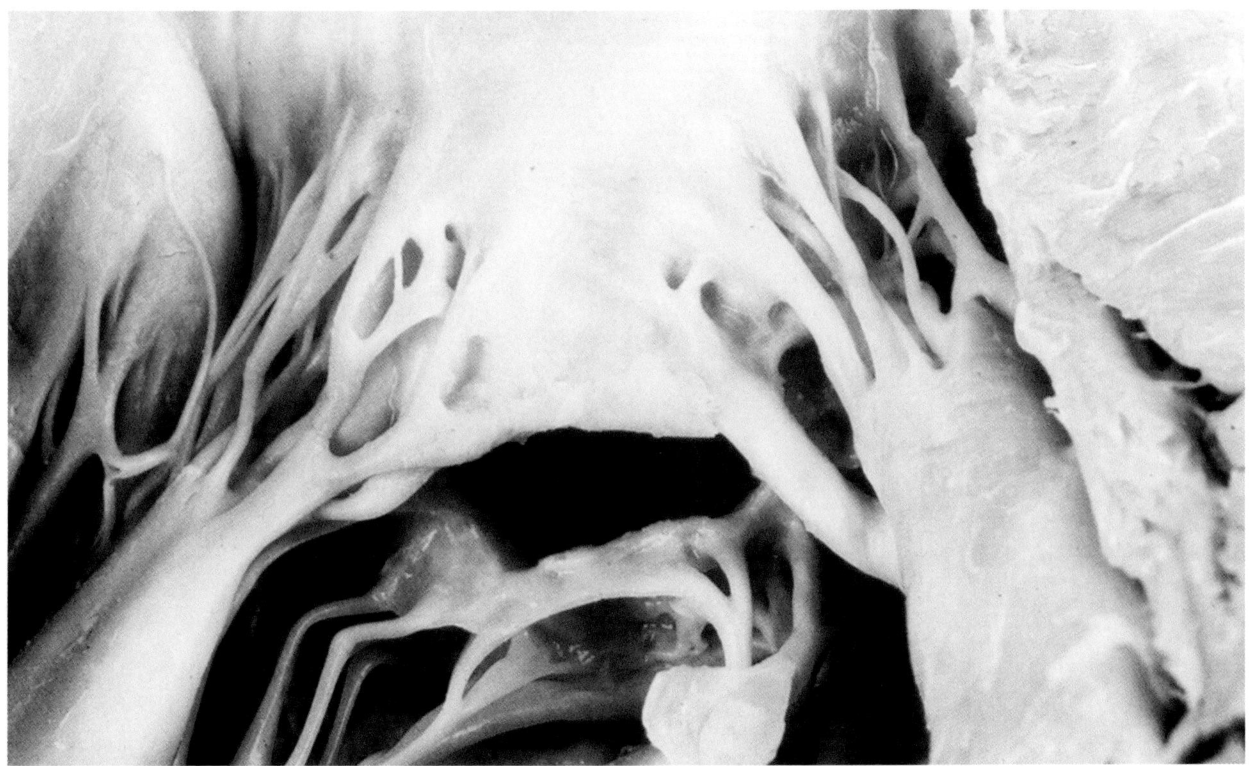

Plate 89 (FIGURE 67-7) Anatomic example of rheumatic mitral regurgitation. Note the thickening of the leaflet and chordae and the retraction of the mitral tissue. (Courtesy of WD Edwards.)

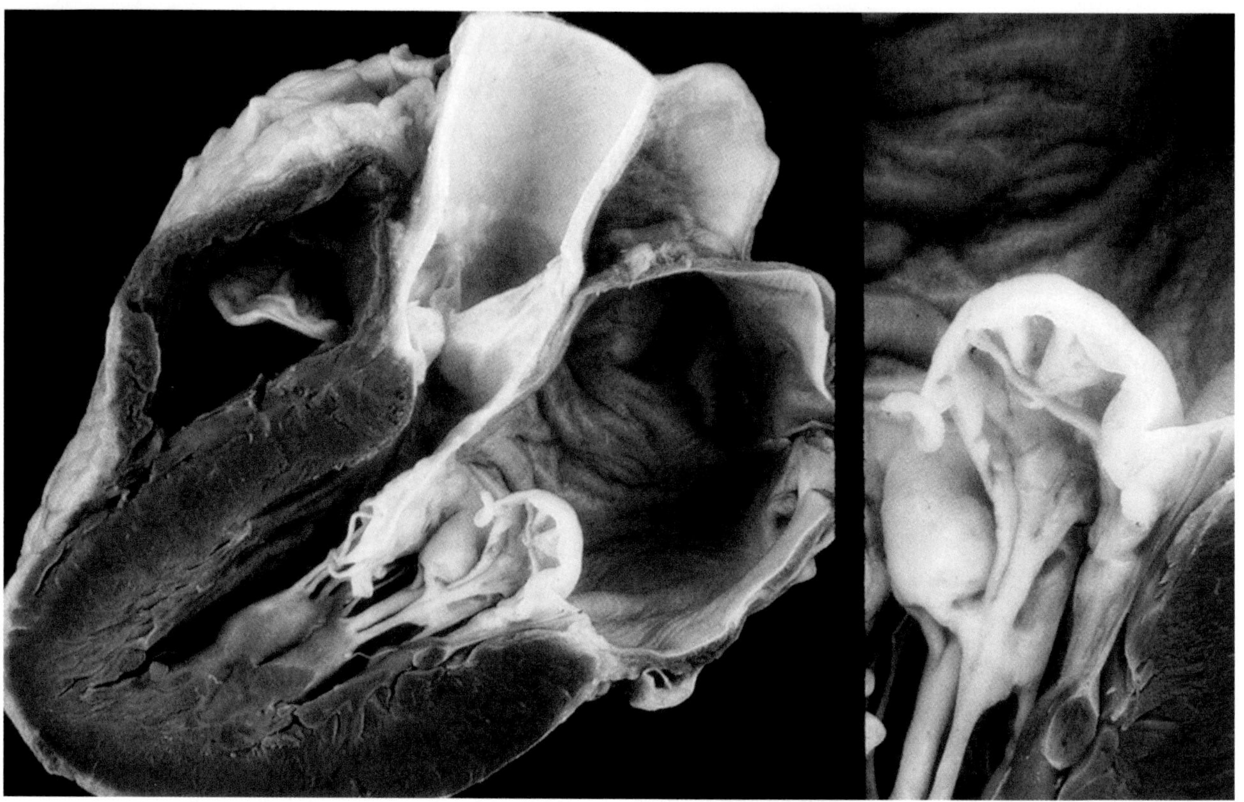

Plate 90 (FIGURE 67-8) Anatomic example of a flail posterior leaflet with ruptured chord. On the right of the picture, close-up view of the ruptured chord. Otherwise the left atrium is enlarged and the valvular tissue normal. (Courtesy of W. D. Edwards.)

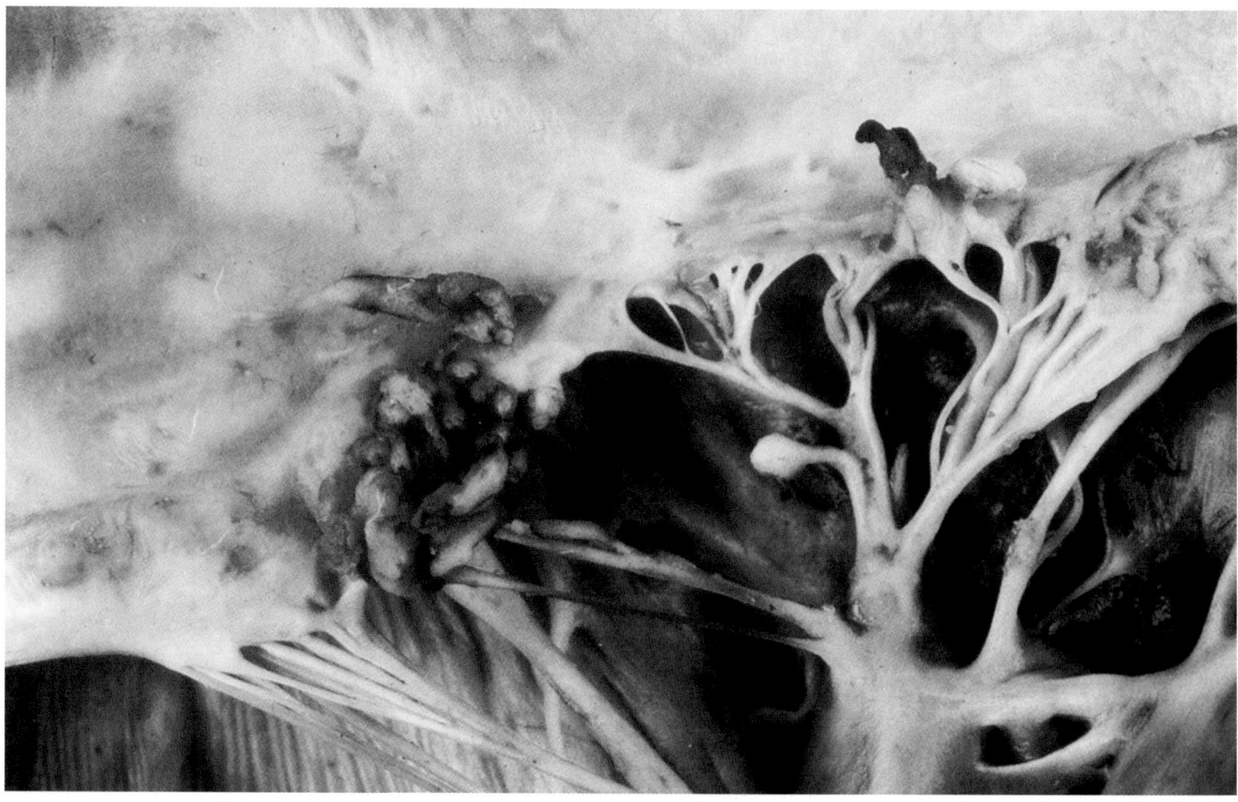

Plate 91 (FIGURE 67-9) Anatomic example of mitral regurgitation due to endocarditis. Note the vegetations of the anterior leaflet and the ruptured chords. (Courtesy of WD Edwards.)

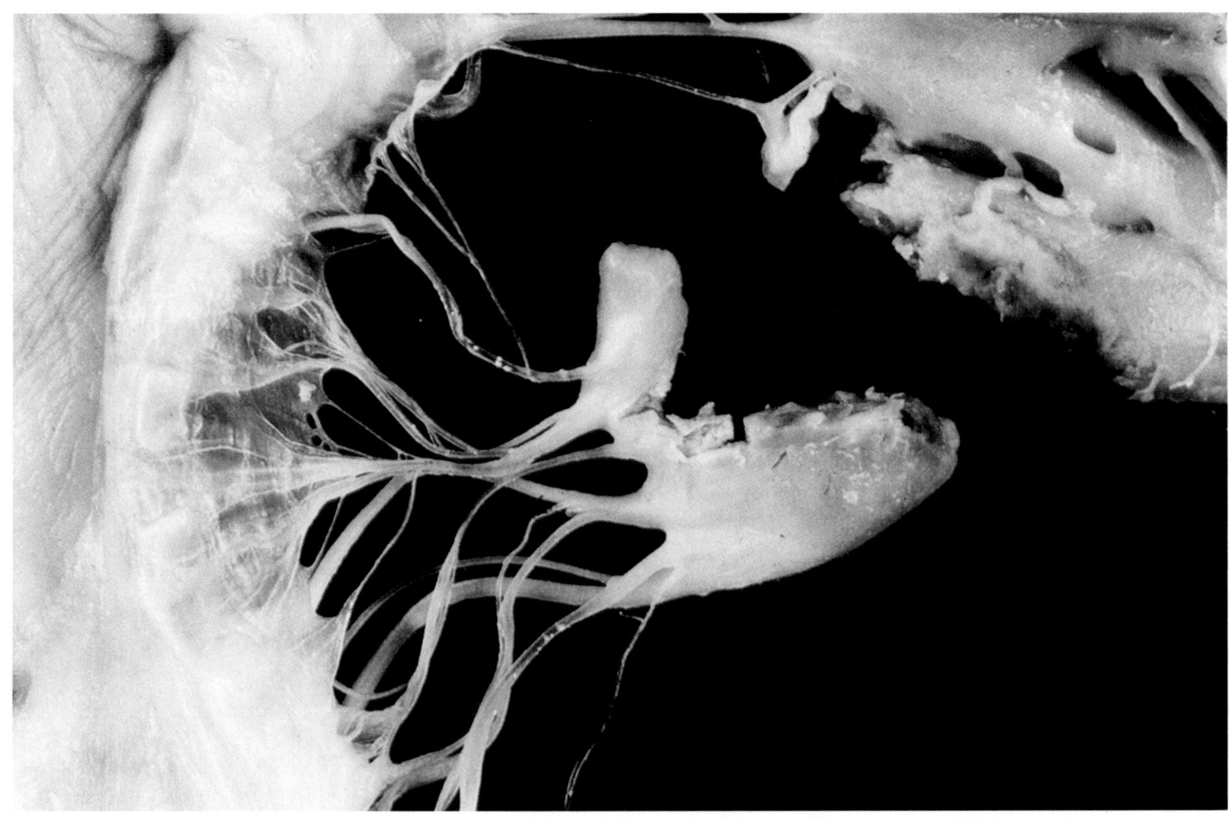

Plate 92 (FIGURE 67-10) Anatomic example of a ruptured posterior papillary muscle. Note the normal valvular tissue otherwise. (Courtesy of WD Edwards.)

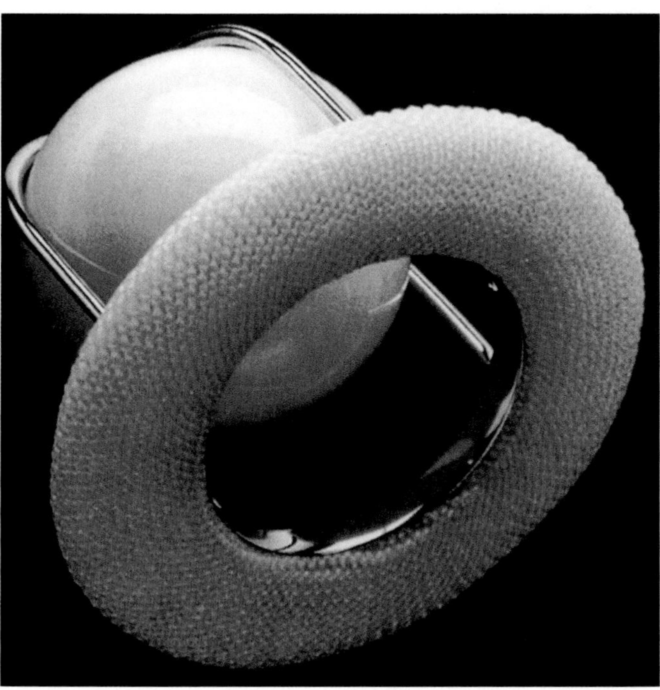

Plate 93 (FIGURE 70-1) Starr-Edwards caged ball valve. The ball is a silicone rubber polymer, impregnated with barium sulfate for radiopacity, which oscillates in a cage of cobalt-chromium alloy. When the valve opens, blood flows through the circular primary orifice and a secondary orifice between the ball and the housing. In the aortic position, there is a tertiary orifice between the ball and the aortic wall.

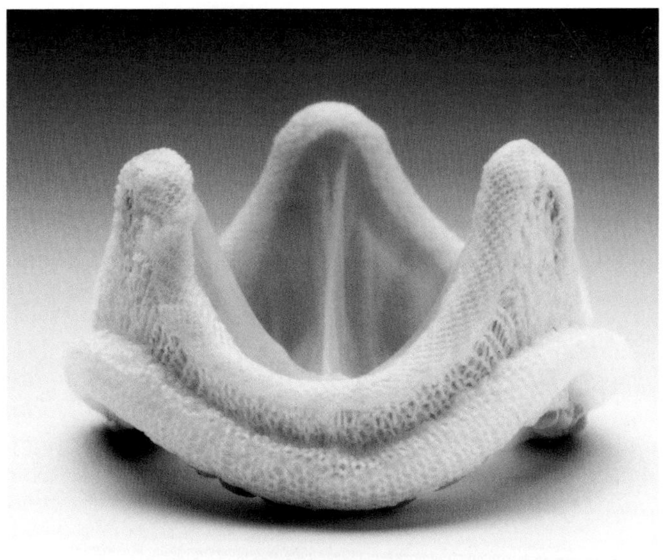

Plate 94 (FIGURE 70-3) Stented porcine valves. The Carpentier-Edwards Supra Annular Valve is designed to be implanted above rather than within the aortic annulus. It has low-pressure fixation and a cone-shaped stent, which flares out at the top to improve leaflet durability.

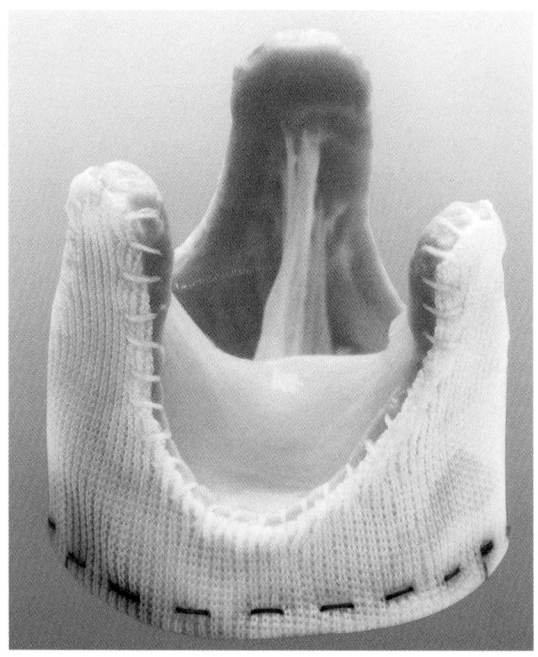

A

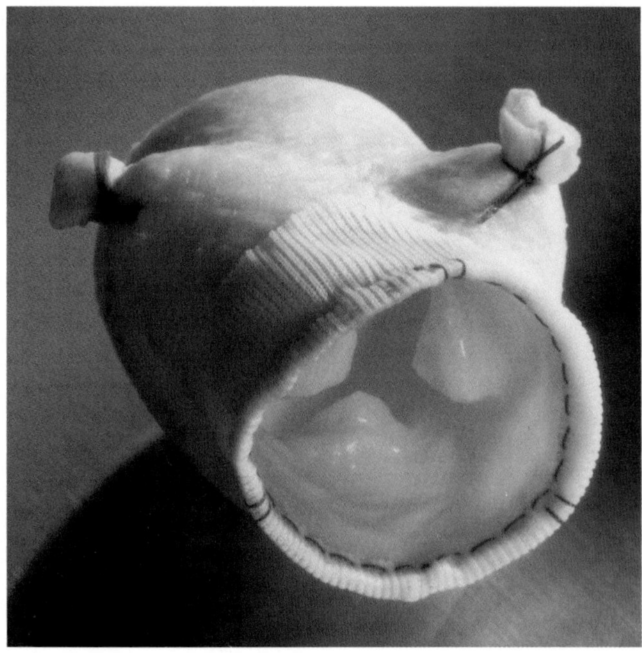

B

Plate 95 (FIGURE 70-4) St. Jude Toronto SPV (*A*) and Medtronic Freestyle (*B*) stentless porcine valves. The Toronto SPV is designed to be used as a subcoronary valve replacement. The Freestyle can be implanted using any of the methods of implantation used for homografts: subcoronary implantation of the valve alone, aortic root replacement, or cylinder (root) inclusion.

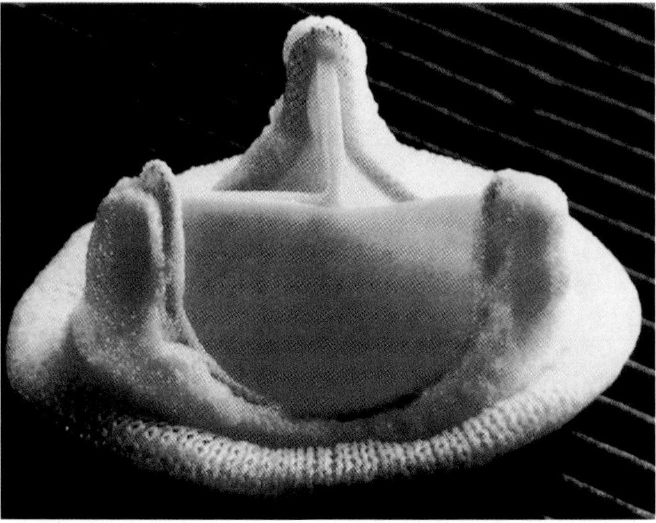

Plate 96 (FIGURE 70-5) The Carpentier-Edwards Perimount pericardial bioprosthesis uses a method of mounting the leaflets to the stent, which does not depend on retaining stitches passed through the pericardium—a design weakness of previous pericardial valves. Instead, the leaflets are anchored behind the stent pillars.

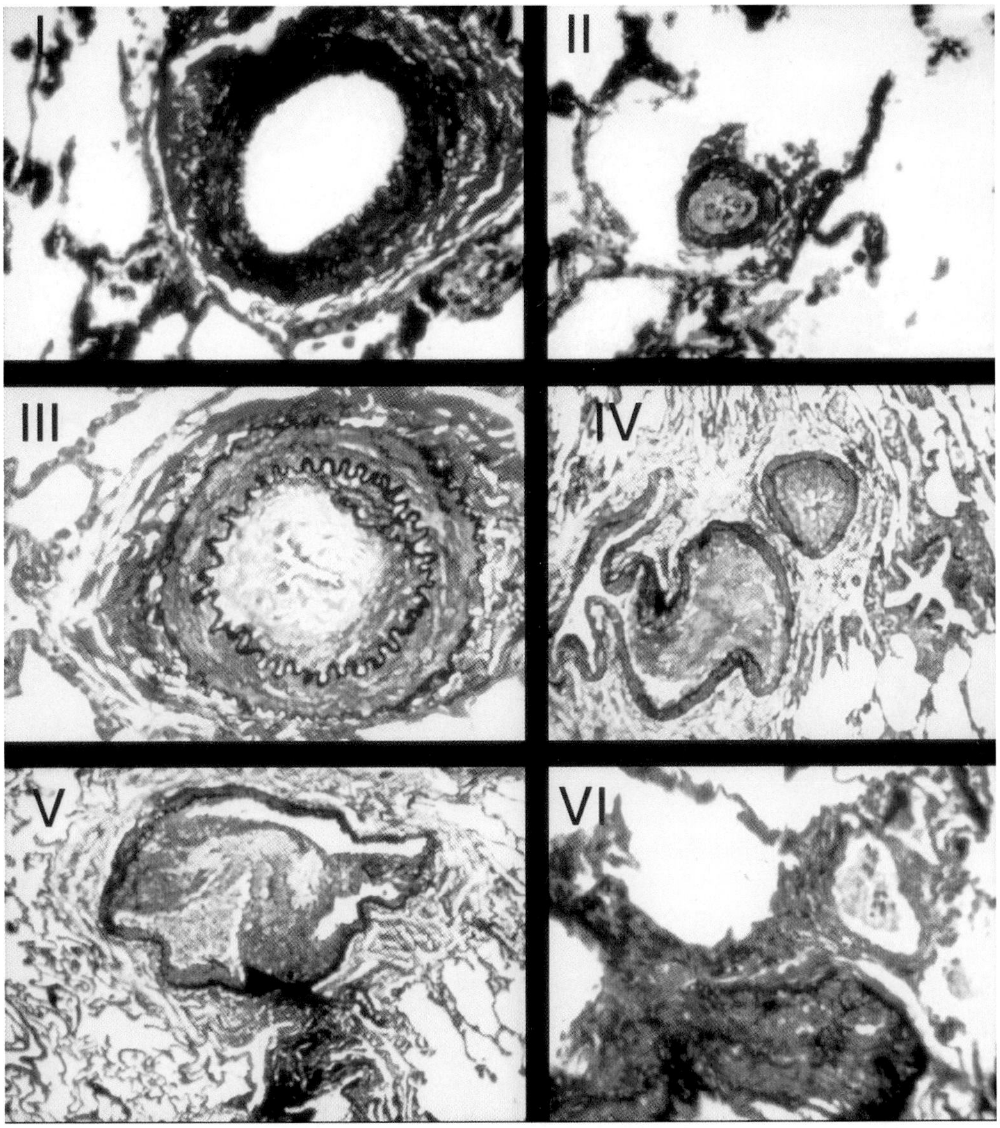

Plate 97 (FIGURE 73-4) Pulmonary vascular changes by the Heath and Edwards criteria (see text). Grades 1 to 6 are represented by panels I to VI, respectively.

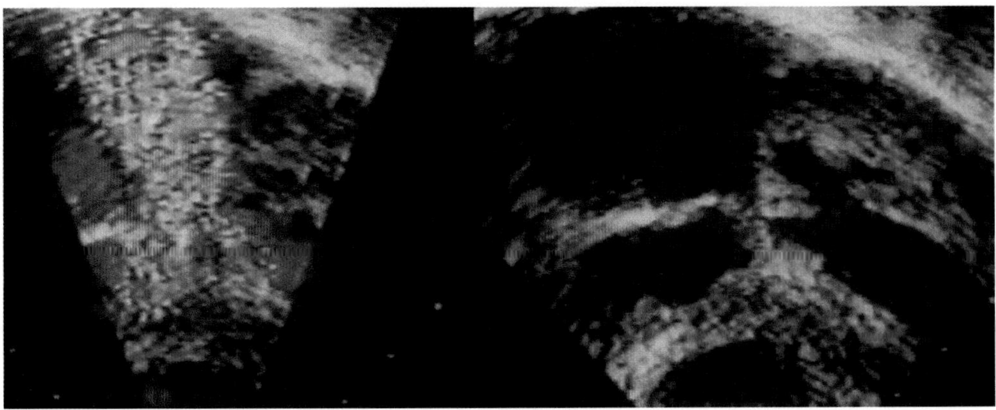

Plate 98 (FIGURE 77-14) Color flow Doppler imaging of a patient with hypertrophic cardiomyopathy, severe systolic anterior motion of the mitral valve, and secondary mitral regurgitation. Right: A still frame two-dimensional echocardiogram from the parasternal view showing systolic anterior motion of the mitral valve. Left: Color flow imaging demonstrating a large mosaic jet of mitral regurgitation directed posteriorly.

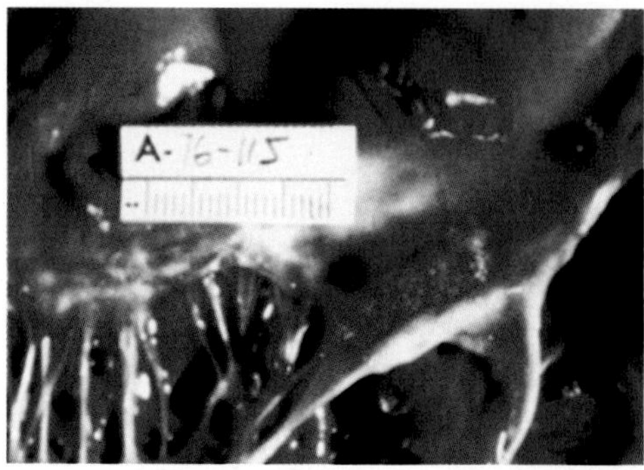


Plate 99 (FIGURE 81-3) Typical vegetation of nonbacterial thrombotic endocarditis found at necropsy in a cachectic patient who died with disseminated lung cancer.

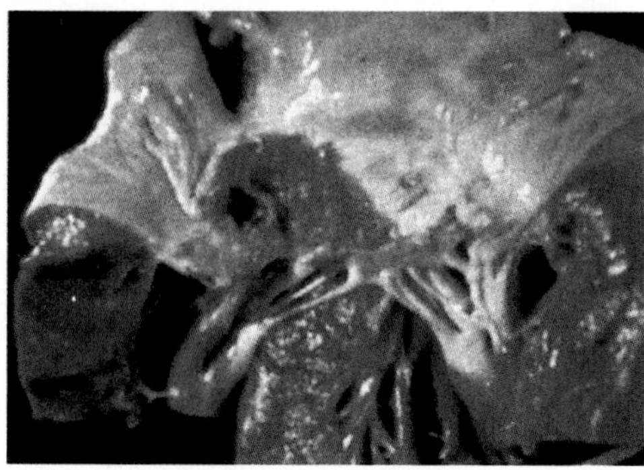

Plate 100 (FIGURE 81-5) Typical vegetation of bacterial endocarditis, complicated by perforation of the anterior mitral valve leaflet. Note that the valve shows preexisting chronic rheumatic disease, with thickening, deformity, and fusion of the chordae tendineae.

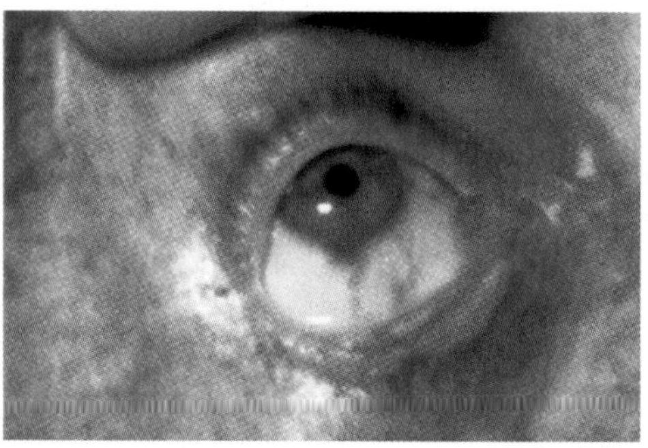

Plate 101 (FIGURE 81-7) Typical conjunctival petechiae in a patient with subacute bacterial endocarditis due to *Streptococcus sanguis*.

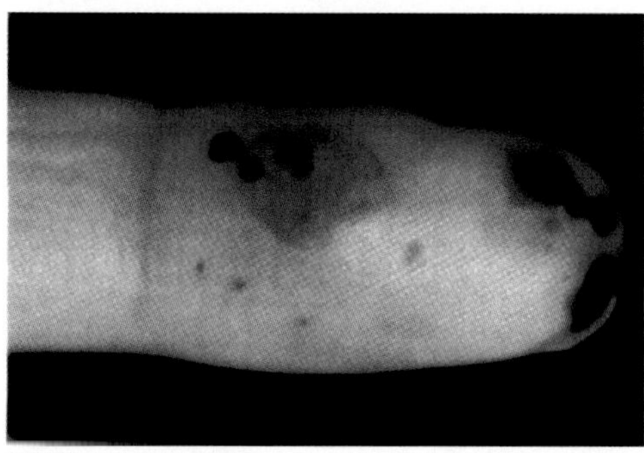

Plate 102 (FIGURE 81-8) Ischemic, hemorrhagic, and pustular lesions on the extremities in acute *Staphylococcus aureus* endocarditis.

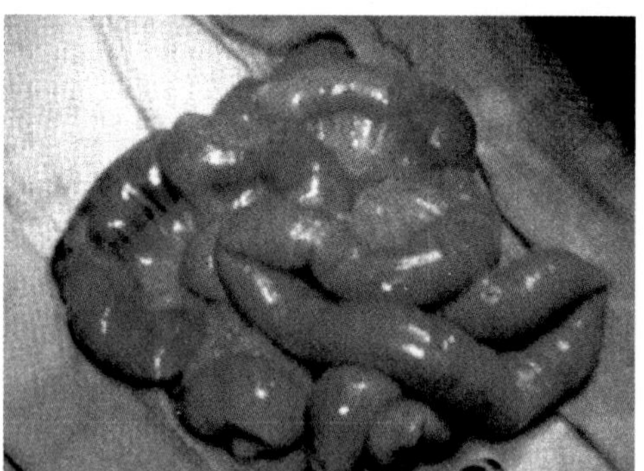

Plate 103 (FIGURE 81-9) Segmental ischemia and necrosis in the gut, presenting as acute abdomen.

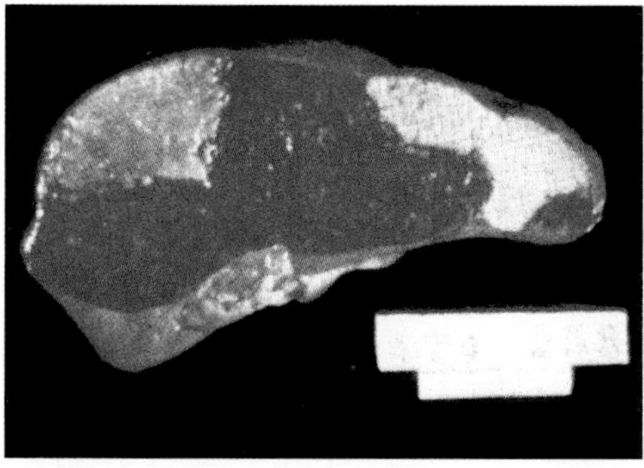

Plate 104 (FIGURE 81-10) Infarctions in the spleen.

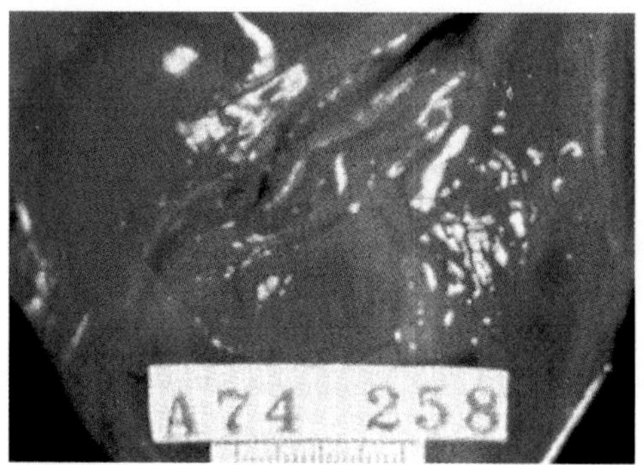


Plate 105 (FIGURE 81-11) An infected embolus in a coronary artery.

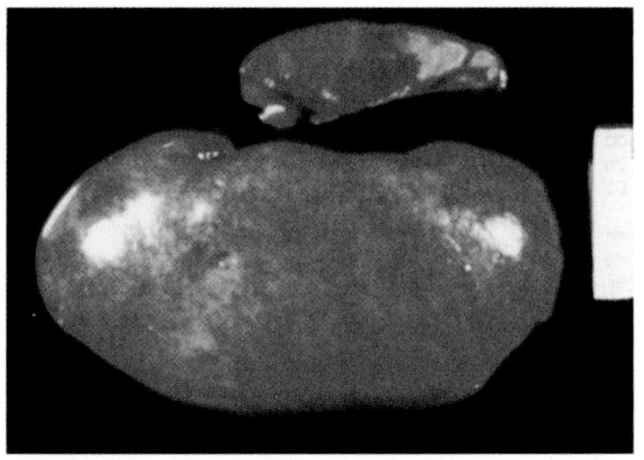

Plate 106 (FIGURE 81-12) Kidney from a patient with subacute bacterial endocarditis showing two abnormalities: (1) typical ischemic infarctions due to emboli and (2) swelling and petechiae (flea-bitten kidney) due to immune-complex glomerulonephritis.

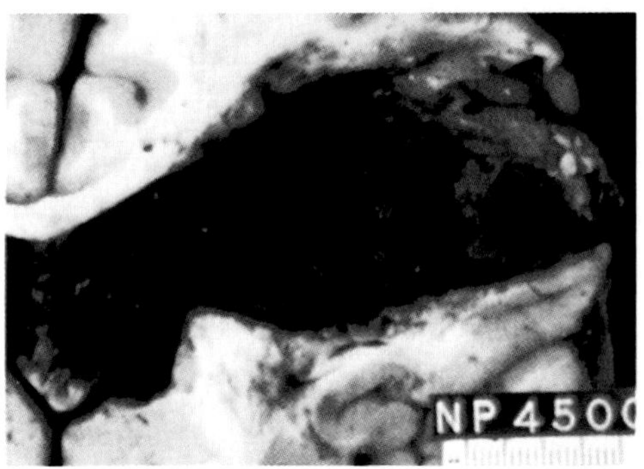

Plate 107 (FIGURE 81-13) Massive cerebral hemorrhage with intraventricular extension due to rupture of a small, peripheral mycotic aneurysm. The patient had been bacteriologically cured of *Staphylococcus epidermidis* endocarditis several weeks previously. Cultures of the blood, valve, and aneurysm taken at necropsy were negative.

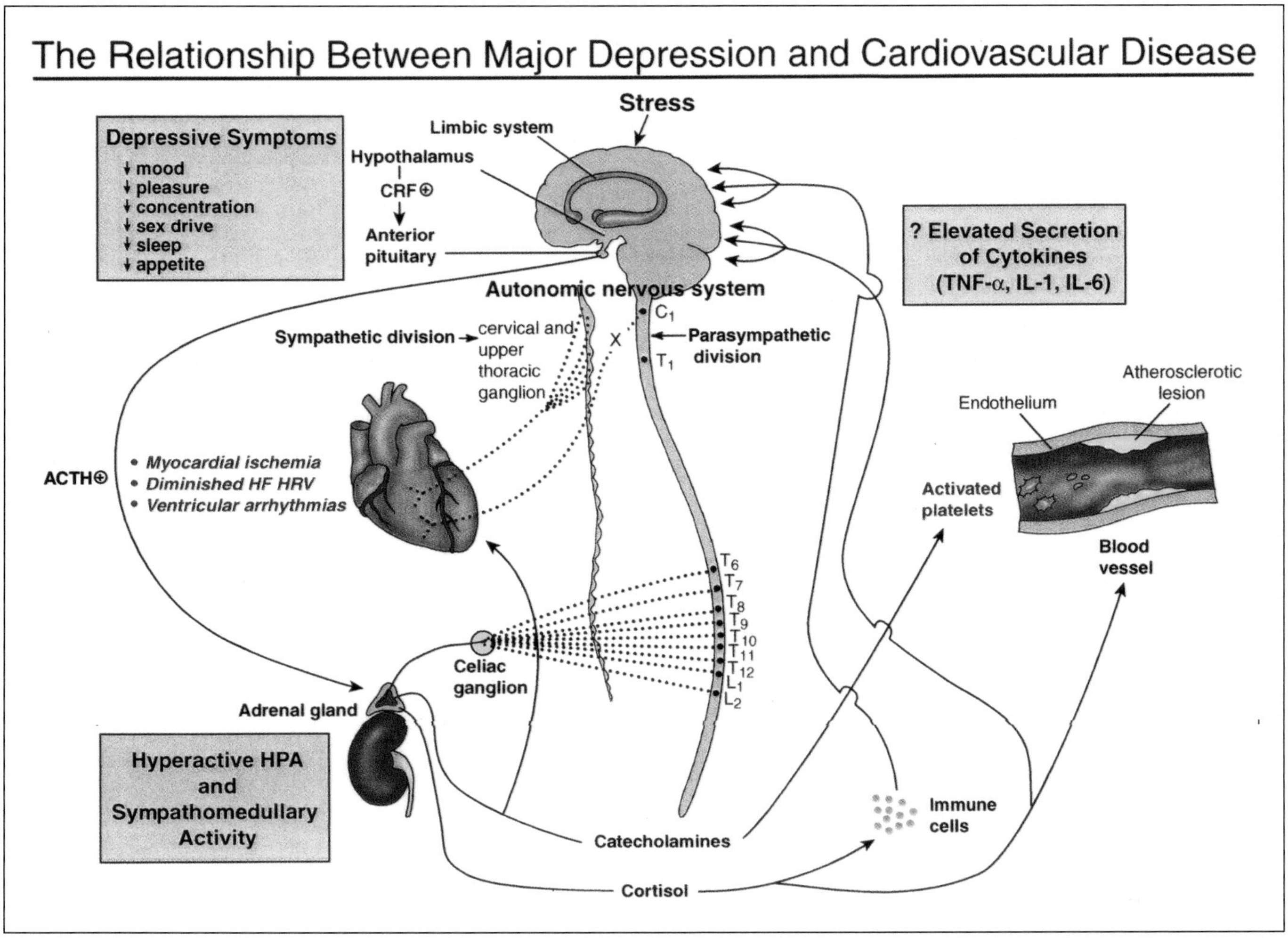

## The Relationship Between Major Depression and Cardiovascular Disease

Stress

**Depressive Symptoms**
- ↓ mood
- ↓ pleasure
- ↓ concentration
- ↓ sex drive
- ↓ sleep
- ↓ appetite

Limbic system
Hypothalamus
CRF ⊕
Anterior pituitary
Autonomic nervous system
$C_1$
$T_1$
Sympathetic division → cervical and upper thoracic ganglion
X
← Parasympathetic division

? Elevated Secretion of Cytokines (TNF-α, IL-1, IL-6)

Atherosclerotic lesion
Endothelium
Activated platelets
Blood vessel

ACTH ⊕
- *Myocardial ischemia*
- *Diminished HF HRV*
- *Ventricular arrhythmias*

$T_6$ $T_7$ $T_8$ $T_9$ $T_{10}$ $T_{11}$ $T_{12}$ $L_1$ $L_2$
Celiac ganglion
Adrenal gland

Hyperactive HPA and Sympathomedullary Activity

Immune cells
Catecholamines
Cortisol

Plate 108 (FIGURE 91-1) Hypothetical schema of pathophysiologic findings associated with depression that probably contributes to increased susceptibility to cardiovascular disease. Autonomic nervous system innervation of the heart via the parasympathetic vagus (X) nerve and sympathetic (postganglionic efferents from the cervical and upper thoracic paravertebral ganglia) nerves is shown. ACTH = corticotropin; CRF = corticotropin-releasing factor; HRV = heart rate variability; HPA = hypothalamic-pituitary-adrenocortical axis; IL-1 = interleukin-1; IL-6 = interleukin-6; TNF-$\alpha$ = tumor necrosis factor-$\alpha$. (From *Arch Gen Psychiatry*, July 1998;55: p 583. Copyright (1998), American Medical Association.)

# GENES ON CHIPS

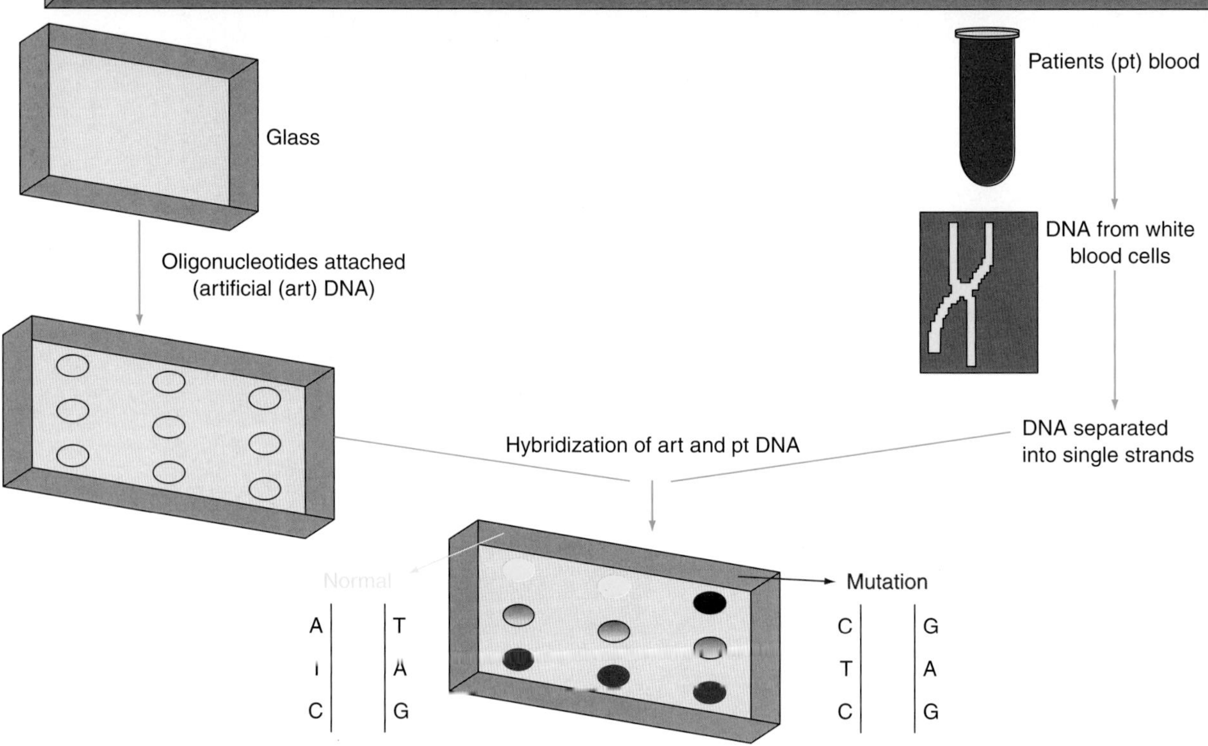


Plate 109 (FIGURE 9-1) Illustrated here is the means of detecting genes or their mutations. Oligonucleotides are single short strands of DNA of about 15 to 30 bases artificially synthesized to have the sequence of the desired gene. These oligonucleotides are bound to glass, with each of the four bases labeled with a distinct fluorescent color. The DNA extracted from the patient's white blood cells is denatured into separate strands and brought in contact with the artificial oligonucleotides' DNA. If the sequence in the patient's DNA is complementary to the oligonucleotide, hybridization will occur and the laser beam will detect the appropriate colors. If there is a mutation present, there will be a mismatch and a different color will be exhibited by the laser, indicating the site of the mutation.

Age-related annular dilatation of the aortic valve can result in aortic regurgitation.[20] Mitral annular calcification is rare before age 70 but is present in 40 percent of women over age 90.[20] Mitral annular calcification almost invariably involves only the posterior leaflet and forms a C-shaped ring of annular and subannular calcium.[17] *Mitral annular calcification may impede subannular ventricular contraction, thereby resulting in mitral regurgitation. Because of the proximity of the posteromedial commissure to the atrioventricular (His) bundle, mitral annular calcification may be associated with atrioventricular block.*[20] *With the increasing size of the aging population, degenerative calcific aortic disease is increasing in frequency.*[20]

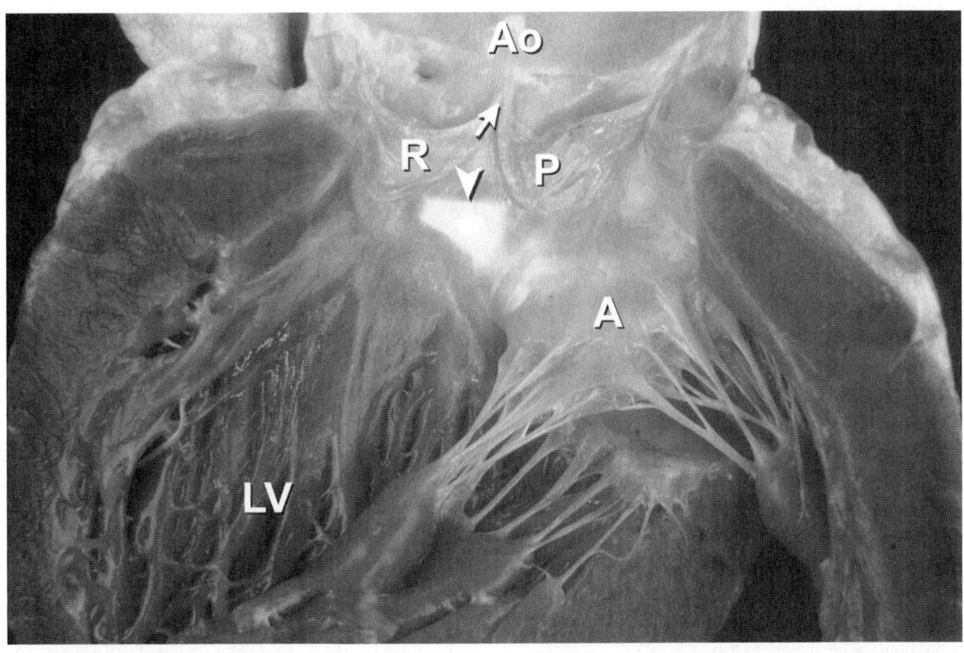


FIGURE 3-30 The commissure between the right and posterior aortic cusps (arrow) overlies the transilluminated membranous septum (arrowhead). A, anterior mitral leaflet; Ao, ascending aorta; LV, left ventricle; P, posterior aortic cusp; R, right aortic cusp.

## Cardiac Grooves, Crux, and Margins

The atrioventricular groove encircles the heart and defines its base. It separates the atria from the ventricles (Fig. 3-31). The two ventricles are separated by the anterior and posterior (inferior) interventricular grooves, which define the plane of the ventricular septum (see Figs. 3-5*A* and 3-31).

With age, fat tends to accumulate in increasing amounts in the epicardium, particularly in the atrioventricular grooves.[20,23] *Increased epicardial fat deposits may be associated with increased risk of cardiac rupture after acute transmural myocardial infarction.*[23] Excess fat in the atrial septum is called *lipomatous hypertrophy* (Fig. 3-45) and may result in a thickness that exceeds that of the ventricular septum. Fat in the right ventricular free wall is difficult to detect accurately clinically; its excess accumulation may be associated with increasing age, obesity, or arrhythmogenic right ventricular cardiomyopathy.[24]

Along the surface of the heart, the right and circumflex coronary arteries travel in the right and left atrioventricular grooves, respectively, and the left anterior and posterior descending coronary arteries course along the anterior and posterior (or inferior) interventricular grooves, respectively (see Figs. 3-5*A* and 3-31). The *external cardiac crux* is the cross-shaped intersection between the atrioventricular, posterior interventricular, and interatrial grooves (see Fig. 3-31). Its internal counterpart (*internal crux*) is the posterior intersection between the mitral and tricuspid annuli and the atrial and ventricular septa (see Figs. 3-16*B* and 3-34, Plate 12).

The junction between the anterior and inferior free walls of the right ventricle forms a sharp angle known as the *acute margin*. The rounded lateral wall of the left ventricle forms the *obtuse margin*.[15]

## Right Ventricle

The right ventricle is a right-anterior structure. It is comprised of an inlet and trabecular and outflow segments[15] (Fig. 3-32). The inlet

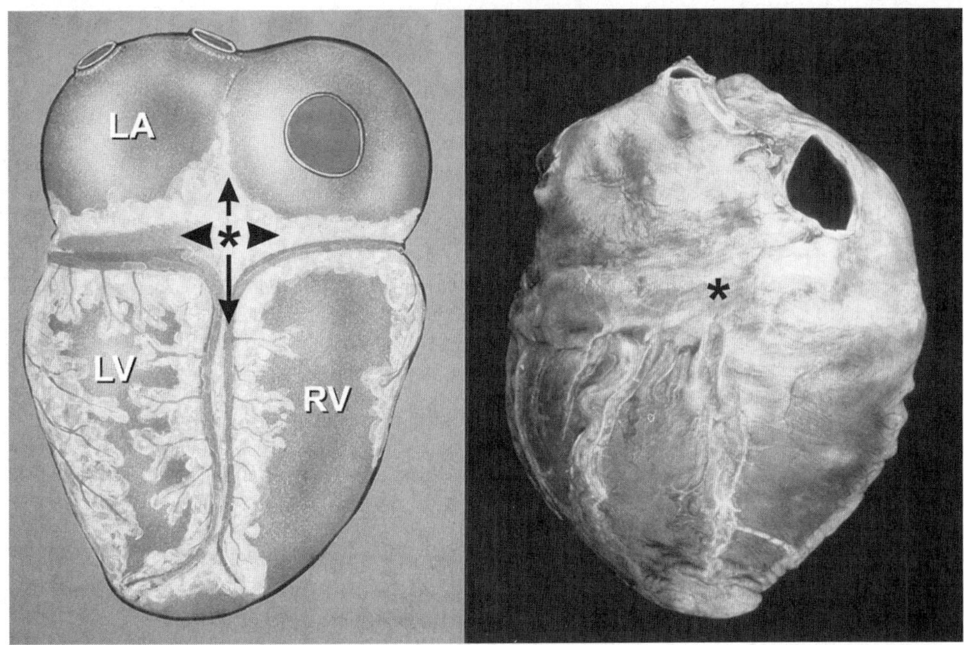


FIGURE 3-31 External cardiac crux. View of the diaphragmatic aspect of the heart shows the intersection of the atrioventricular (arrowheads), posterior interventricular (long arrow), and interatrial (small arrow) grooves at the external cardiac crux (*). (*Left*) Diagram. (*Right*) Cardiac specimen. LA, left atrium; LV, left ventricle; RV, right ventricle.

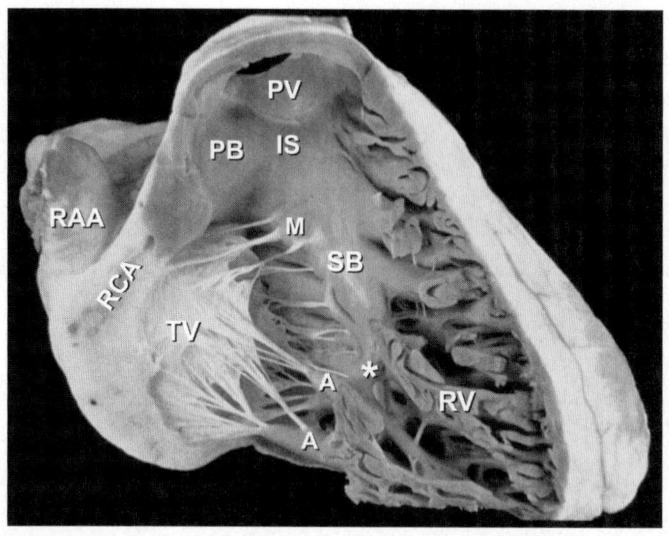


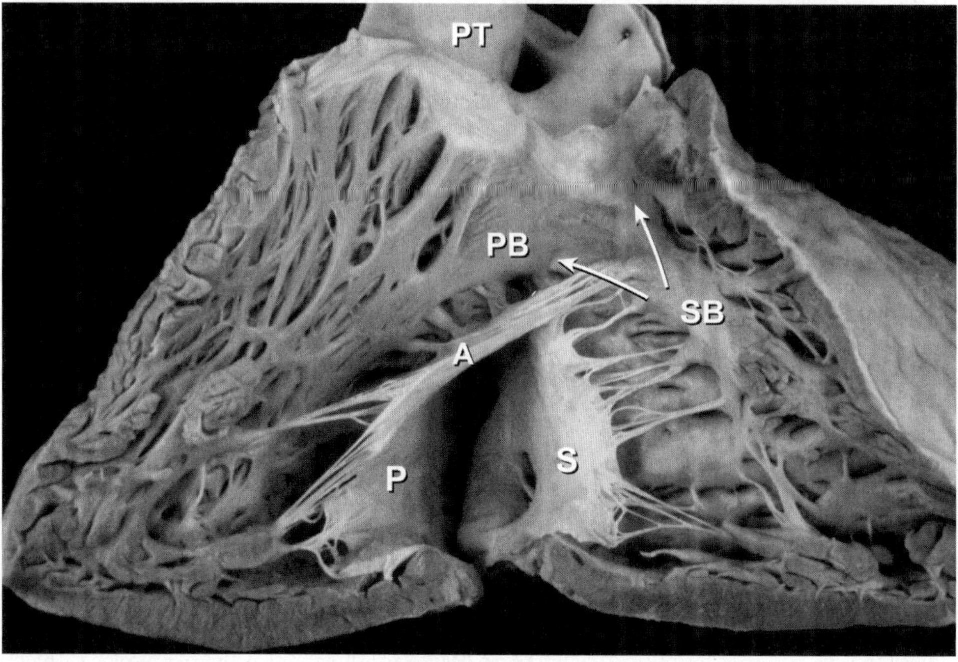


FIGURE 3-32 Right ventricle. *A*. The right ventricular free wall has been removed to show the arch-like crista supraventricularis (CSV), which consists of the parietal band (PB), infundibular septum (IS), and septal band (SB). The moderator band (*) joins the septal band to the anterior tricuspid papillary muscle (*A*). The anteroapical portion of the chamber is heavily trabeculated. M, medial tricuspid papillary muscle; PV, pulmonary valve; RAA, right atrial appendage; RCA, right coronary artery; TV, tricuspid valve. *B*. The right ventricle has been opened by the inflow-outflow method to show the parietal band (PB) separating the tricuspid and pulmonary valves, as well as the two upper limbs (arrows) of the septal band (SB). *A*, anterior leaflet of the tricuspid valve; P, posterior leaflet of the tricuspid valve; PT, pulmonary trunk; S, septal leaflet of the tricuspid valve; other abbreviations as in *A*.

component extends from the tricuspid annulus to the insertions of the papillary muscles. An apical trabecular zone extends inferiorly beyond the attachments of the papillary muscles toward the ventricular apex and about halfway along the anterior wall.[15] *This muscular meshwork is the site of insertion of transvenous ventricular pacemaker electrodes. During right ventricular endomyocardial biopsy, tissue generally is obtained from the trabeculated apex. Disruption of a portion of the tricuspid support apparatus is a potential complication of right-sided heart instrumentation (e.g., right ventricular endomyocardial biopsy).*[17] The outflow portion, also known as the conus (meaning "cone") or *infundibulum* (meaning "funnel"), is a smooth-walled muscular subpulmonary channel[15,17] (see Fig. 3-32).

A prominent arch-shaped muscular ridge known as the *crista supraventricularis* separates the tricuspid and pulmonary valves. It is made up of three components (i.e., parietal band, infundibular septum, and septal band) that may appear as distinct structures or may merge together[15,17] (see Fig. 3-32). The parietal band is a free-wall structure, whereas the adjacent infundibular septum is intracardiac and separates the two ventricular outflow tracts beneath the right and left cusps of both semilunar valves[15,17] (Figs. 3-12*D* and 3-33). The septal band forms a Y-shaped muscle, the two upper limbs of which cradle the infundibular septum. From this branching point of the septal band emanates the medial tricuspid papillary muscle[15,17] (see Fig. 3-32). The moderator band forms an intracavitary muscle that connects the septal band with the anterior tricuspid papillary muscle (see Fig. 3-32*A*).

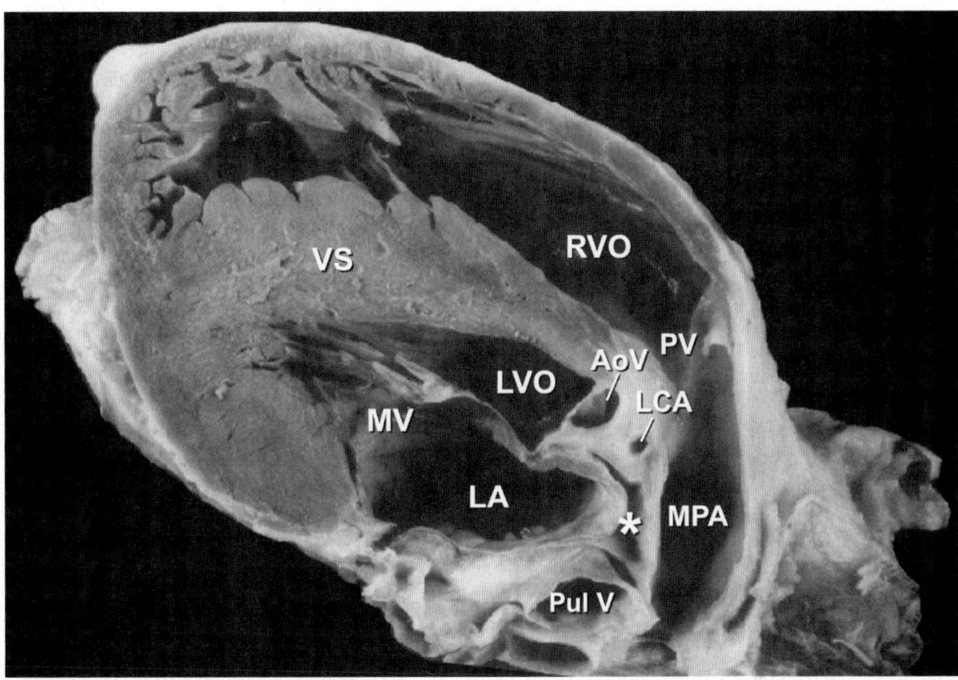


FIGURE 3-33 Long-axis view of the right ventricular outflow (RVO) tract showing the pulmonary valve (PV) and main pulmonary artery (MPA). AoV, aortic valve; LA, left atrium; LCA, left coronary artery; LVO, left ventricular outflow; MV, mitral valve; PulV, pulmonary vein; VS, ventricular septum; *, transverse pericardial sinus.

## Left Ventricle

The left ventricle, like the right ventricle, is made of an inlet portion comprised of the mitral valve apparatus, a subaortic outflow portion, and a finely trabeculated apical zone.[17] The left ventricular free wall is normally thickest toward the base and thinnest toward the apex, where it averages only 1 to 2 mm in thickness, even in hypertrophied hearts.[17] Structurally, the left and right ventricles differ considerably.[15,17] Normally, the left ventricular free-wall and septal thicknesses are three times the thickness of the right ventricular free wall. The mitral and aortic valves share fibrous continuity, whereas the parietal band separates the tricuspid and pulmonary valves. Whereas the mitral valve has an elliptical orifice and no septal attachments, the tricuspid valve has a triangular orifice and numerous direct septal attachments (see Fig. 3-23). The right ventricular apex is much more trabeculated than its counterpart on the left (see Figs. 3-9*B* and 3-18*C*). *The distinctive differences in apical trabeculations persist even in markedly hypertrophied or dilated hearts.*[17]

The annular attachment of the septal leaflet of the tricuspid valve inserts more apically than that of the anterior mitral leaflet, allowing distinction between the right and left ventricles by four-chamber imaging (Fig. 3-34, Plate 12). *Exceptions include partial atrioventricular septal defects and double-inlet ventricles in which the two valve annuli are at the same level. Ebstein's anomaly is characterized by exaggeration of apical displacement of the septal and posterior tricuspid leaflets*

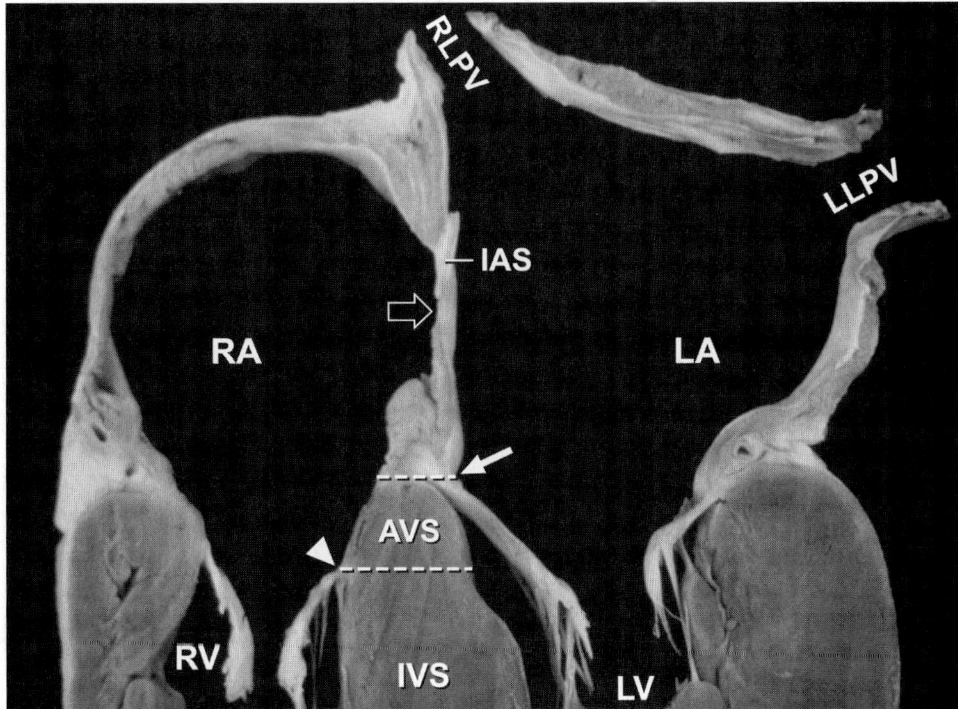


FIGURE 3-34 (Plate 12) Internal cardiac crux. Four-chamber slice of the heart shows the characteristic normal apical displacement of the tricuspid valve septal leaflet insertion (arrowhead) when compared with septal insertion of the mitral valve (solid arrow). This tomographic section also shows the interatrial septum (IAS), atrioventricular septum (AVS), and interventricular septum (IVS). Open arrow points to fossa ovalis. LA, left atrium; LLPV, left lower pulmonary vein; LV, left ventricle; RA, right atrium; RLPV, right lower pulmonary vein; RV, right ventricle.

*resulting in an atrialized portion of the right ventricular chamber.*[16,17] *Morphologic differentiation of the right and left ventricles is particularly important in congenital heart disease.* The morphologic tricuspid valve virtually always connects to a morphologic right ventricle, whereas the morphologic mitral valve connects to a morphologic left ventricle.[15,16] Because of the rightward bulging of the ventricular septum, the left ventricular chamber appears circular in cross section, whereas the right ventricular chamber has a crescentic appearance (see Fig. 3-23). Tomographic segmental left ventricular anatomy is reviewed in the section on the coronary arteries, below.

Left ventricular false tendons, also referred to as *pseudotendons* or *bands*,[25] are discrete, thin, cordlike fibromuscular structures that connect two walls, the two papillary muscles, or a papillary muscle to a wall, usually the ventricular septum (Fig. 3-35). However, false

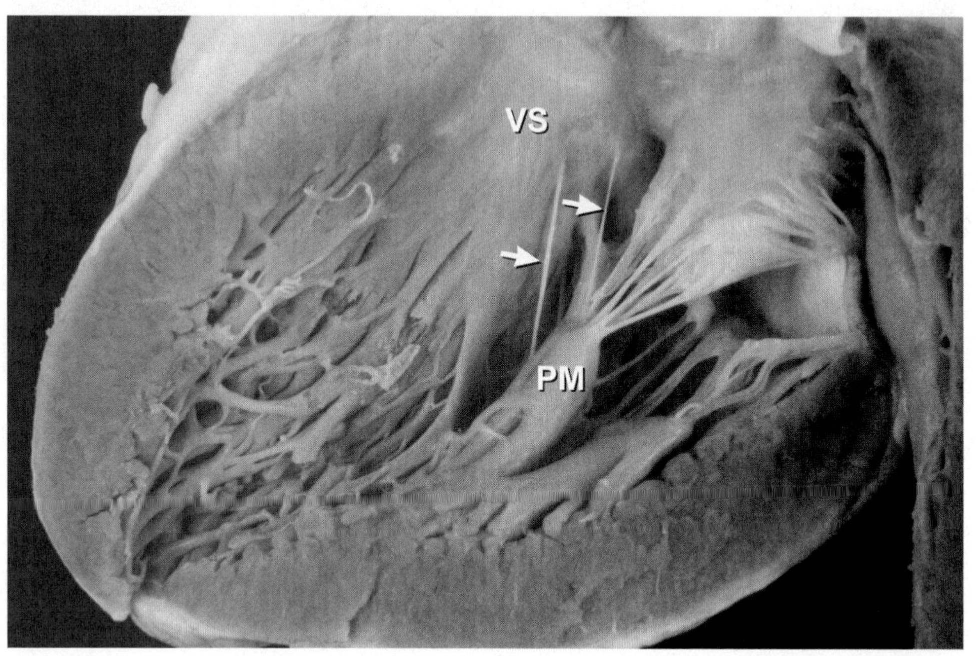


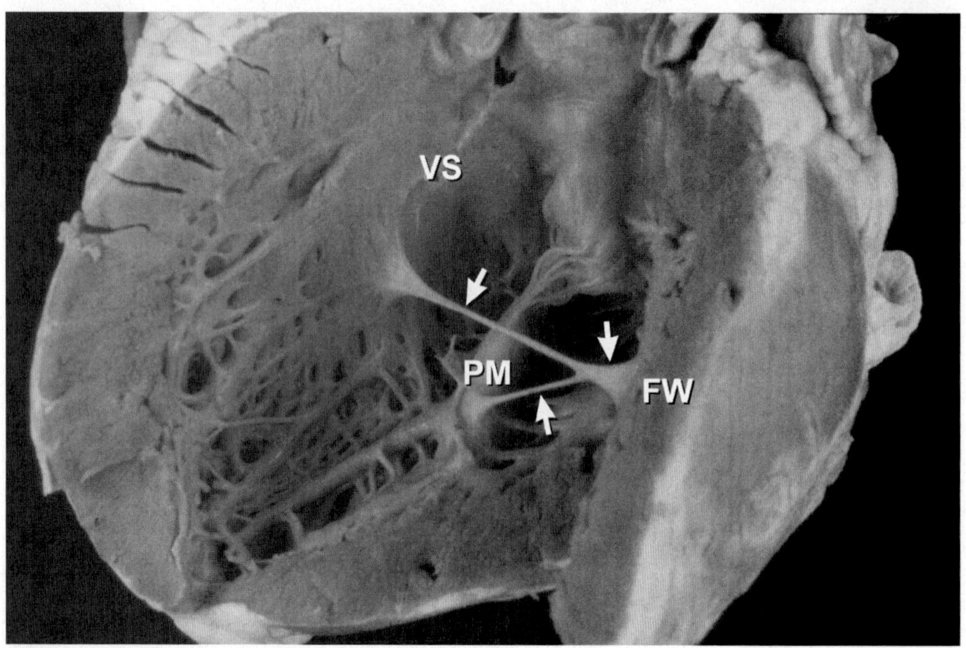


FIGURE 3-35 Various locations of left ventricular false tendons. *A.* Two false tendons (arrows) from posteromedial mitral papillary muscle (PM) to ventricular septum (VS), representing the most common location. *B.* Complex branching false tendon (arrows) with origin from the left ventricular free wall (FW) and insertions into the ventricular septum (VS) and base of posteromedial mitral papillary muscle (PM).

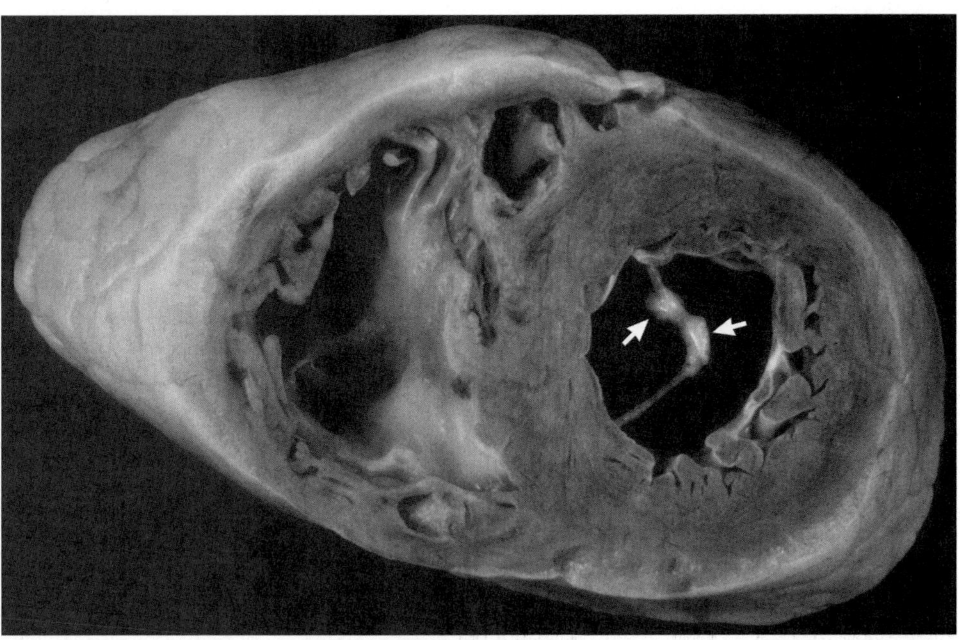

FIGURE 3-36 (Plate 13) Calcified left ventricular false tendon (arrows) seen in short-axis view.

tendons, as the name implies, are not attached to the mitral leaflets. *Chordal attachments between the mitral leaflets and the ventricular septum are abnormal and are usually associated with atrioventricular septal defects or straddling atrioventricular valves.*[16] False tendons are common anatomic variants of the normal left ventricle, occurring in 50 percent of hearts, and may become calcified with age (Fig. 3-36, Plate 13). They are more frequently observed in men, but their incidence does not appear to be age-related.[25] *It has been suggested that they may be the cause of innocent systolic musical murmurs.*[25] *Although they are readily detectable by echocardiography, they may be misinterpreted by the inexperienced sonographer as pathologic structures such as ruptured chords, mural thrombi, or vegetations.*[17,25]

Prominent left ventricular trabeculations[26] are another common anatomic normal variant that may be an even greater source of misinterpretation by two-dimensional echocardiography in patients with suspected mural thrombus. They are defined as discrete, thick muscle bundles that generally connect the free wall to the septum (Fig. 3-37).

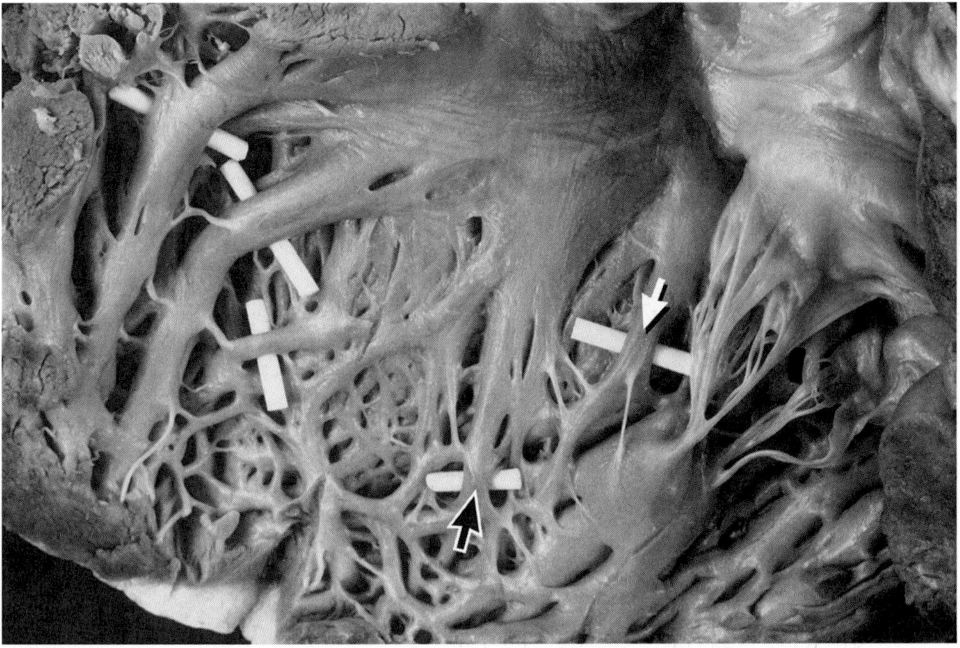

FIGURE 3-37 Prominent left ventricular trabeculations. Multiple large muscle bundles extend from the anterior free wall to the septum (probes). A single muscle bundle extends from the posteromedial mitral papillary muscle to the posterior septum (probe with white arrow), and one bundle extends from one portion of the posterior septum to another (probe with black arrow). Such trabeculations are more prominent in noncompaction cardiomyopathy.

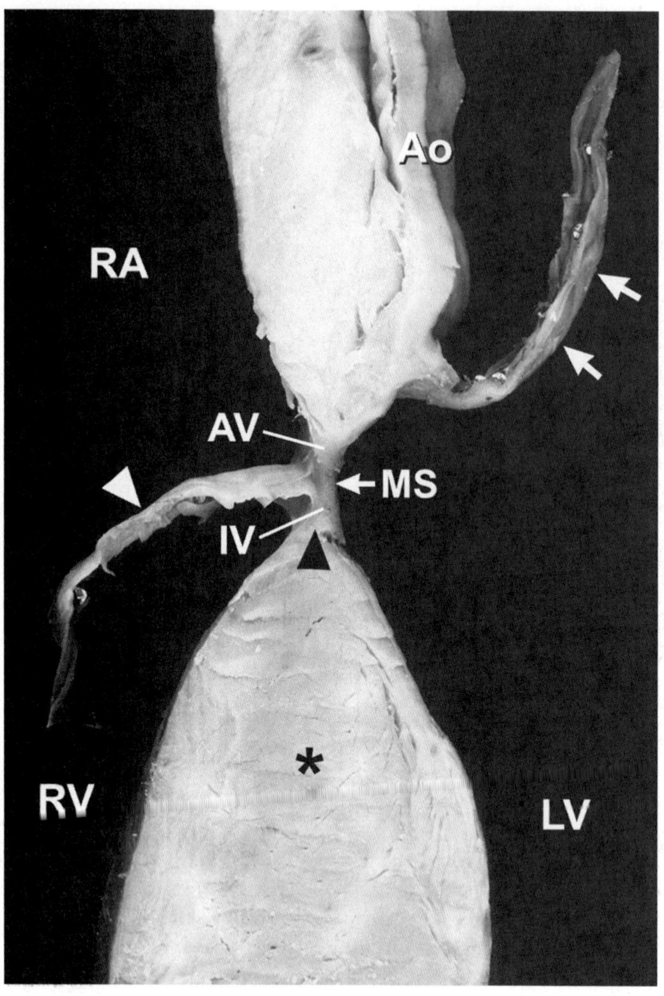


FIGURE 3-38 (Plate 14) Four-chamber tomographic slice through the aortic root (Ao) and aortic valve (arrows) showing the small membranous (MS) and large muscular (*) portion of the ventricular septum. The membranous septum is divided into atrioventricular (AV) and interventricular (IV) components by the septal tricuspid leaflet (white arrowhead). Black arrowhead points to the expected location of the AV (His) bundle. LV, left ventricle; RA, right atrium; RV, right ventricle.

Less common attachments include papillary muscle to the septum, septum to septum, or free wall to free wall. *In noncompaction of the left ventricular myocardium,*[27,28] *also known as* spongy myocardium, *there is persistence of multiple prominent ventricular trabeculations and deep intertrabecular recesses caused by arrest in the normal in utero process of myocardial compaction. The associated clinical manifestations and age at onset of symptoms (i.e., typically a dilated cardiomyopathy) are highly variable.*

## Ventricular Septum

The ventricular septum is a complex intracardiac partition that can be considered to comprise four parts: inlet, trabecular, membranous, and infundibular. The plane of the infundibular portion (see Figs. 3-12*D* and 3-33) is different from that of the three other portions. *This anatomic relationship is important in many forms of congenital heart disease in which the infundibular septum is dissociated from the remainder of the ventricular septum (e.g., malalignment forms of ventricular septal defects in tetralogy of Fallot and in double-outlet right ventricle).*[15–17]

The ventricular septum also may be divided into muscular and membranous portions[15–17] (Figs. 3-38, Plate 14, and 3-39). The membranous septum lies beneath the right and posterior (noncoronary) aortic cusps (see Fig. 3-30) and contacts the mitral and tricuspid annuli (Fig. 3-40, Plate 15). The membranous septum in conjunction with the right fibrous trigone with which it is continuous fuses the commissure between the right and posterior aortic cusps to the commissure between the anterior and septal tricuspid leaflets (see Fig. 3-21*B*). *The majority of clinically significant ventricular septal defects involve the membranous septum.*[17] Owing to normal angulation between the infundibular septum and remaining ventricular septum, the septal surface follows the course of an inverted S (moving from apex to aortic valve). The basal half of the ventricular septum is smooth-walled, while the apical half is characterized by numerous small and irregularly arranged trabeculations.[15–17]

Clinically relevant age-related anatomic changes include a disproportionate increase in ventricular septal thickness regardless of gender and in the absence of a history of hypertension.[20] This is associated with an appreciable increase in the ratio of ventricular septal to left ventricular free-wall thickness often exceeding 1.3 in patients above age 60[20] (Fig. 3-41, Plate 16). This may be due in part to accentuation of the sigmoid shape of the basal septum[15,20] (Fig. 3-42). *Age-related ventricular septal angulation may have clinical importance because it may mimic certain features of hypertrophic cardiomyopathy,*[15,20] *particularly if complicated by the indiscriminate use of volume depleting diuretics or afterload-reducing agents.*

## Atrial Septum

When viewed from its right aspect, the atrial septum is composed of interatrial and atrioventricular regions16,17 (see Fig. 3-34, Plate 12). The interatrial portion is characterized by the fossa ovalis, which is the anatomic hallmark of a morphologic right atrium (Fig. 3-43A). Its outer muscular rim is a horseshoe-shaped limbus, and its central depression is the valve of the fossa ovalis16,17 (see Fig. 3-43A). The potential interatrial passageway between the limbus and the valve (which is patent throughout fetal life) is the foramen ovale (Figs. 3-43B and 3-44). When viewed from the left atrium, the atrial septum is entirely interatrial, since the atrioventricular component lies below the mitral annulus, between the left ventricle and right atrium. Likewise, the limbus of the fossa ovalis is completely covered by its opaque valve and is not directly visible from the left atrium.[15]

*The foramen ovale is anatomically closed in about two-thirds of adults, but in the remaining one-third it remains patent and, therefore, a potential source for shunts and paradoxical embolism. Stretching of the atrial septum, when the atria are markedly dilated, can transform a patent foramen ovale into an acquired atrial septal defect. The posterior aortic sinus abuts against the interatrial septum* (see Fig. 3-12*D*). *During transseptal procedures, care must be taken to stay within the confines of the valve of the fossa ovalis in order to avoid perforation of an aortic sinus.*[16] *Echocardiography may help guide transseptal puncture during balloon mitral valvuloplasty or closure of an atrial septal defect with an occluder device.*[13] *Fenestrations of the valve of the fossa ovalis are the most common cause of congenital atrial septal defects. Redundant valve tissue may form an aneurysm of the valve of the fossa ovalis.*

The atrioventricular (AV) portion of the atrial septum is made of major muscular and minor membranous components and separates the right atrium from the left ventricle[16,17] (see Figs. 3-34, Plate 12, and 3-38, Plate 14). *This explains why there is a potential for left-ventricular-to-right-atrial shunts.*[16,17] *The AV septum corresponds*

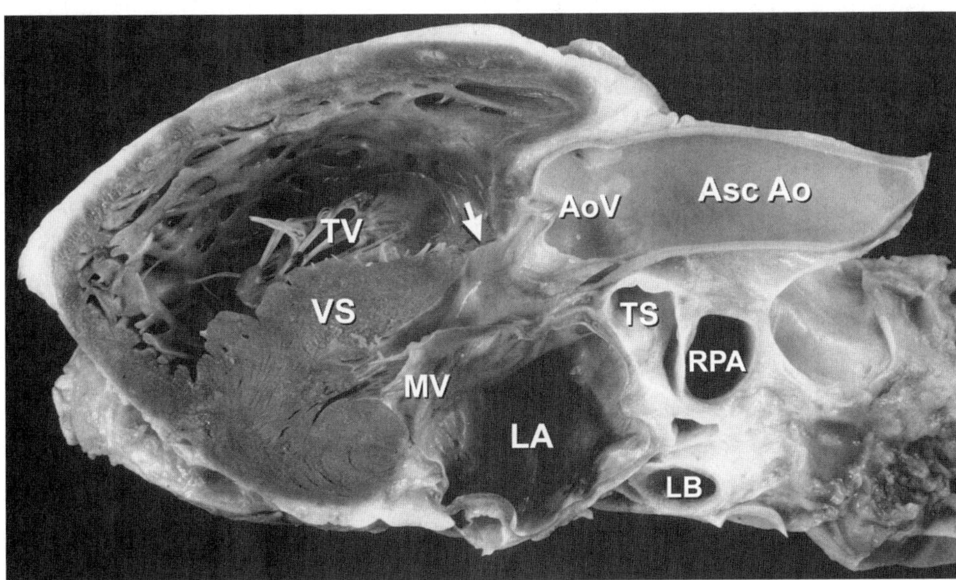


FIGURE 3-39 Tomographic section of the heart along a long-axis plane of the body. The aortic root lies in this plane. The left ventricle and aortic valve are cut obliquely. The membranous ventricular septum (arrow) lies beneath the right and posterior aortic cusps. AoV, aortic valve; Asc Ao, ascending aorta; LA, left atrium; LB, left bronchus; MV, mitral valve; RPA, right pulmonary artery; TS, transverse sinus; TV, tricuspid valve; VS, muscular ventricular septum.

*roughly to the triangle of Koch, an important anatomic surgical landmark because it contains the AV node and proximal portion of the AV (His) bundle. Thus, during tricuspid annuloplasty procedures and patch closures of membranous ventricular septal defects, care must be taken to avoid injury to the conduction system.*[16,17] The muscular component of the AV septum is interposed between the membranous septum anteriorly and the internal cardiac crux posteriorly.

*When defects occur in the muscular AV septum, the mitral annulus usually drops to the same level as the tricuspid annulus, so the defect becomes primarily interatrial (primum atrial septal defect), and the AV conduction tissues are displaced inferiorly.* Lipomatous hypertrophy of the atrial septum is characterized by excessive accumulation of adipose tissue within the limbus of the fossa ovalis but always sparing the valve of the fossa[7,15–17] (Fig. 3-45, Plate 17).

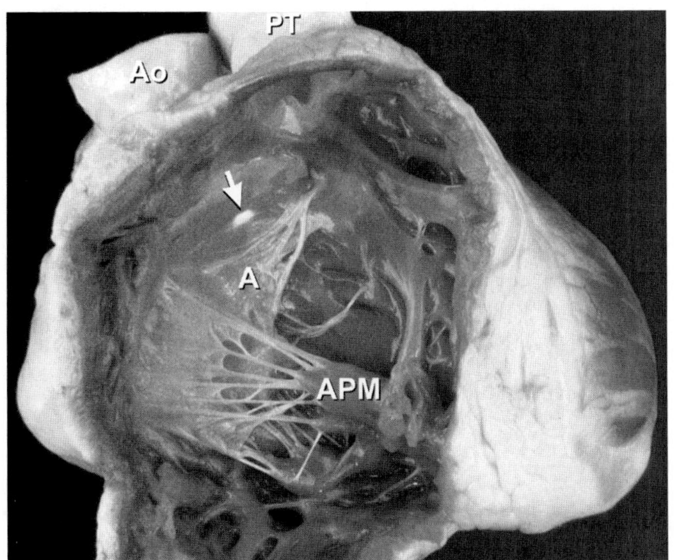


FIGURE 3-40 (Plate 15) A view of the right ventricle. Transilluminated membranous ventricular septum (arrow) in contact with the commissure between the anterior and septal leaflets of the tricuspid valve. A, anterior tricuspid leaflet; Ao, ascending aorta; APM, anterior tricuspid papillary muscle; PT, pulmonary trunk.

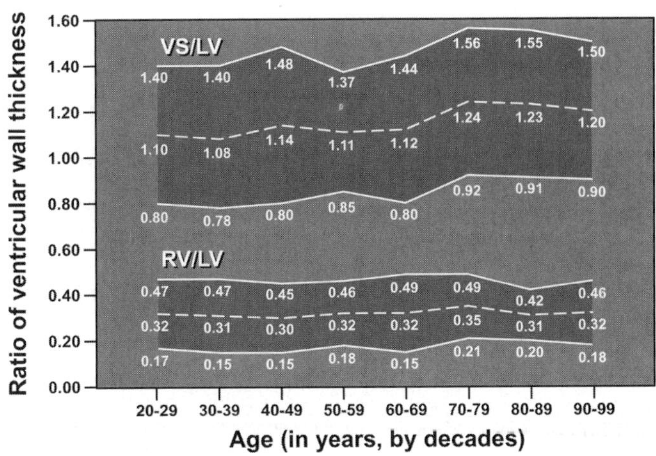


FIGURE 3-41 (Plate 16) Ratios of ventricular wall thicknesses (means ± 2 standard deviations) versus age. RV/LV, ratio of right to left ventricular wall thickness; VS/LV, ratio of ventricular septal to left ventricular free wall thickness. (From Kitzman DW, et al. *Mayo Clin Proc* 1988; 63:137–146. Reproduced with permission of Mayo Foundation.)

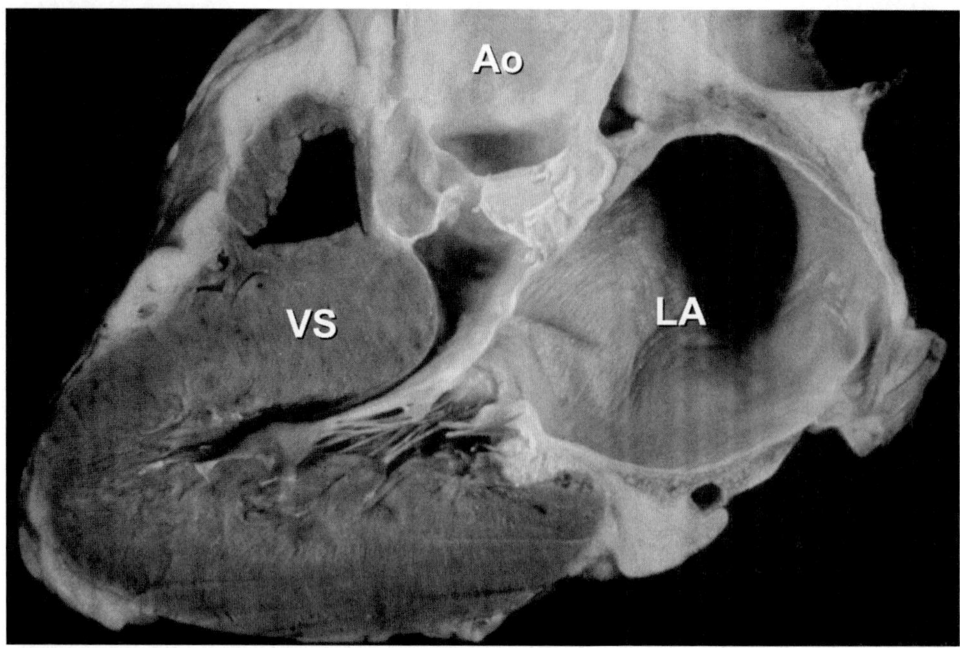


FIGURE 3-42 Age-related changes in the left-sided cardiac structures. Normal heart from an 84-year-old man demonstrates shortening of the base-to-apex (long-axis) dimension, decreased internal left ventricular dimension, aortic root dilatation, left atrial enlargement, and sigmoid-shaped septum. (Compare with Fig. 3-15 from an 18-year-old man.) Ao, ascending aorta; LA, left atrium; VS, ventricular septum.

Lipomatous hypertrophy of the atrial septum occurs commonly but not exclusively in older and obese persons.[15–17] *Although readily detected by echocardiography, it may be misinterpreted as a thrombus or tumor.*[7]

## Right Atrium

A prominent internal muscle ridge, the crista terminalis (Fig. 3-46), separates the right atrial free wall into a smooth-walled posterior region that receives the venae cavae and coronary sinus and a muscular anterior region that is lined by parallel pectinate muscles and from which the right atrial appendage emanates.[15–17] *Pectinatus* is Latin for "comb," and the pectinate muscles and crista terminalis resemble the teeth and backbone of a comb, respectively.[17] The right atrial appendage abuts the right aortic sinus and overlies the proximal right coronary artery (see Fig. 3-52). *The right atrial free wall is paper-thin between pectinate muscles and therefore can be perforated easily by stiff catheters.*[15–17]

Inferior vena caval blood flow is directed by the eustachian valve toward the foramen ovale, and superior vena caval blood is directed toward the tricuspid valve[15] (Fig. 3-47, Plate 18). *Thus transseptal cardiac catheterization is more easily accomplished via the inferior vena cava, whereas instrumentation of the right ventricular apex (e.g., endomyocardial biopsy, placement of ventricular pacemaker lead) is more easily accomplished via the superior vena cava.*[15]

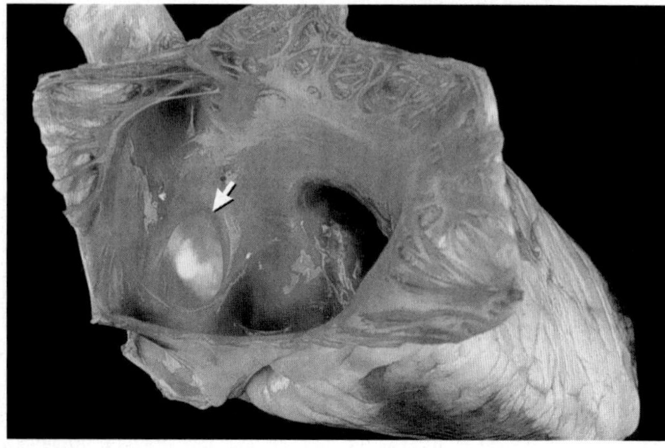


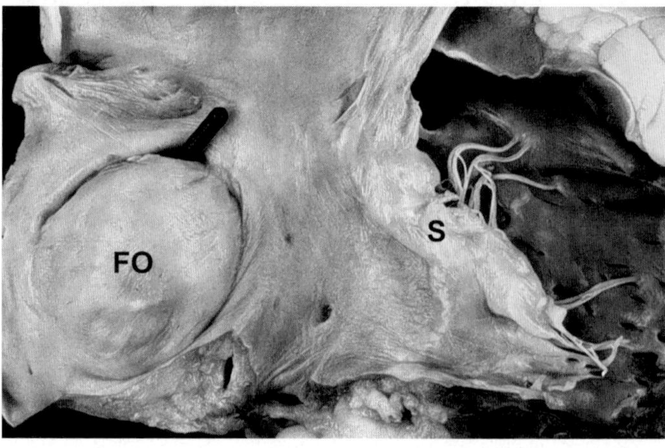


FIGURE 3-43 *A.* Fossa ovalis. Opened right atrium shows the thick muscular limbus of the atrial septum (arrow), in contrast to the thin valve of the fossa ovalis (transilluminated). *B.* Patent foramen ovale (black probe) as seen from the right atrium. There is also an aneurysm of the valve of the fossa ovalis (FO). S, septal leaflet of the tricuspid valve.

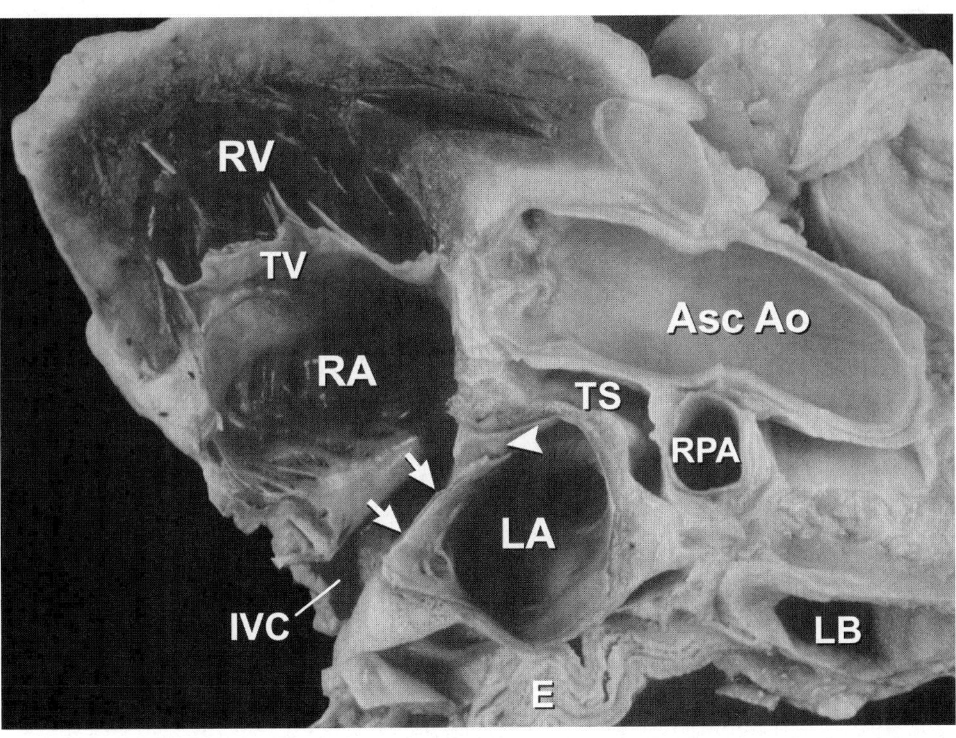


FIGURE 3-44 Tomographic section of the heart along a long-axis of the body. The valve of the fossa ovalis (arrows) and a patent foramen ovale (arrowhead) are seen in this view. Asc Ao, ascending aorta; E, esophagus; IVC, inferior vena cava; LA, left atrium; LB, left bronchus; RA, right atrium; RPA, right pulmonary artery; RV, right ventricle; TS, transverse sinus; TV, tricuspid valve.

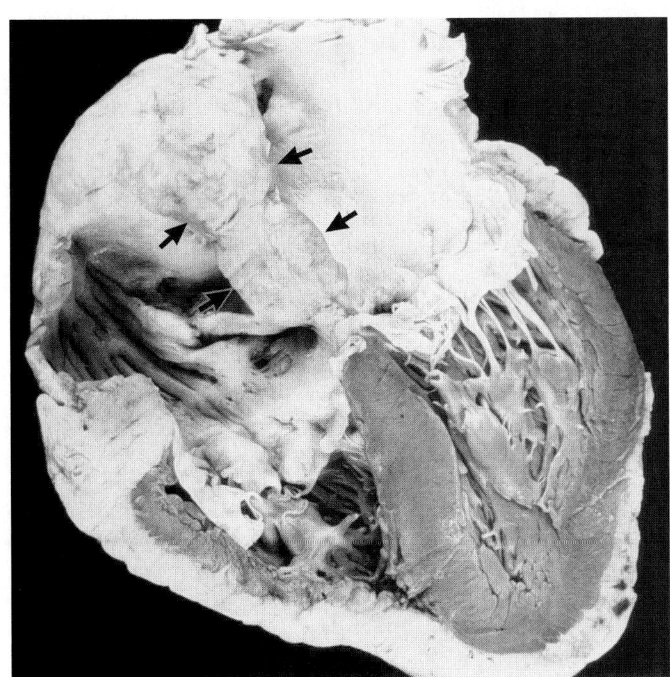

FIGURE 3-45 (Plate 17) Four-chamber slice through the heart showing lipomatous hypertrophy of the atrial septum (arrows).

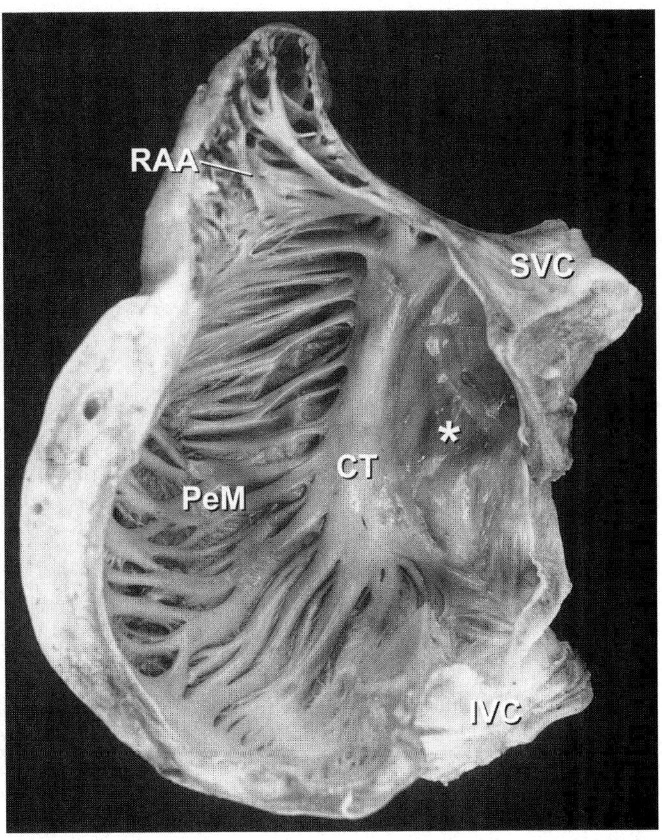


FIGURE 3-46 Right atrial free wall showing separation of the posterior smooth-walled (*) portion from the anterior muscular portion with its pectinate muscles (PeM) and right atrial appendage (RAA) by the crista terminalis (CT). IVC, inferior vena cava; SVC, superior vena cava.

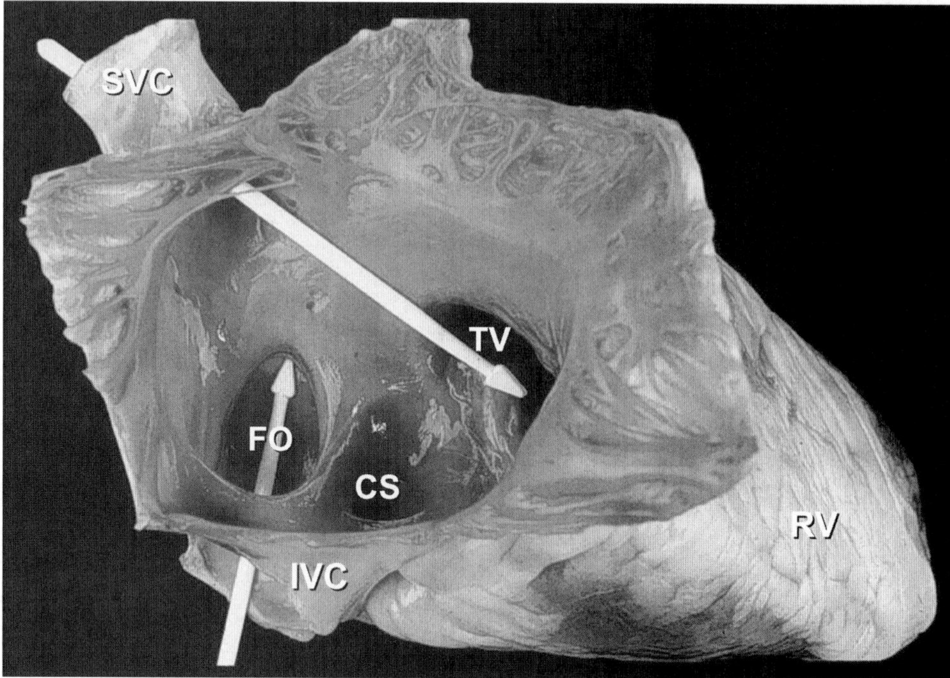


FIGURE 3-47 (Plate 18) Opened right atrium. Two arrow-shaped probes show that superior vena caval flow is directed toward the tricuspid orifice and inferior vena caval flow is directed toward the fossa ovalis (FO). CS, coronary sinus; IVC, inferior vena cava; RV, right ventricle; SVC, superior vena cava; TV, tricuspid valve.

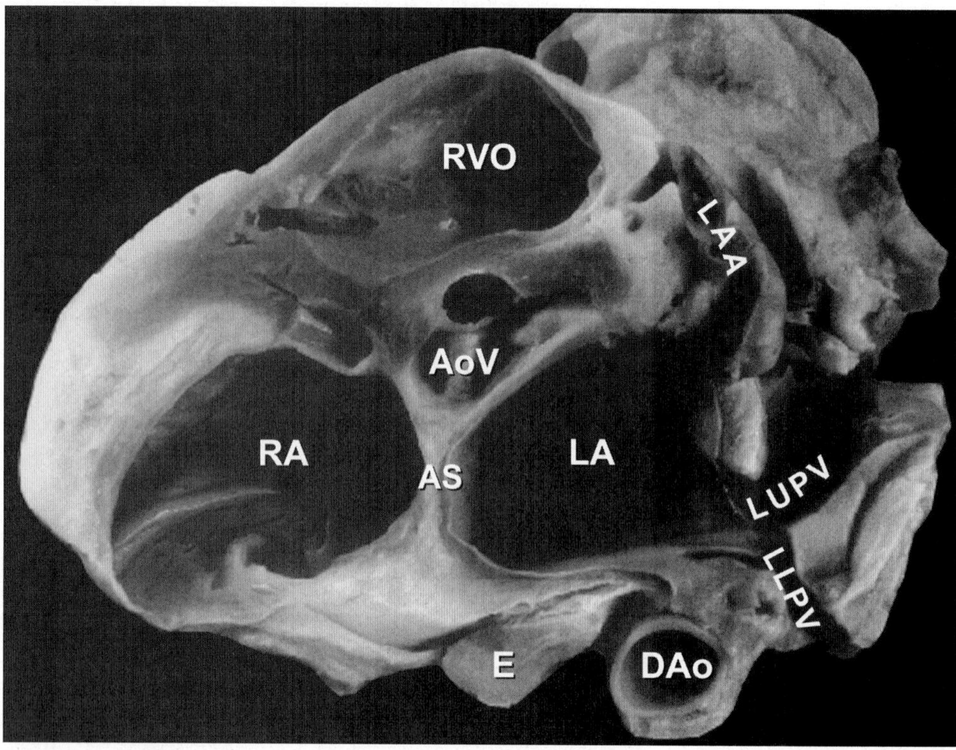


FIGURE 3-48 Oblique, short-axis cut at the base of the heart. The esophagus (E) is posterior and adjacent to the left atrium (LA) and adjacent to the descending thoracic aorta (DAo). The left upper pulmonary (LUPV) and left lower pulmonary vein (LLPV) are clearly seen. The right ventricular outflow tract (RVO) is anterior. AS, atrial septum; AoV, aortic valve; LA, left atrium; LAA, left atrial appendage; RA, right atrium.

## Left Atrium

The pulmonary vein orifices lie on the posterolateral (left pulmonary veins) and posteromedial (right pulmonary veins) aspects of the left atrial cavity. The left and right upper pulmonary veins are directed anterosuperiorly, whereas the lower veins enter the left atrium nearly perpendicular to the posterior atrial wall[15–17] (Figs. 3-15 and 3-48). *Left atrial muscle extends some distance within the pulmonary veins. The resultant cuff of muscle acts as a sphincter during atrial systole and may be the source of focal atrial fibrillation that is amenable to catheter ablation*[9–13] (see Fig. 3-2).

The atrial appendage arises anterolaterally and lies in the left atrioventricular groove atop the proximal portion of the left circumflex coronary artery and, in some individuals, the left main coronary artery[16] (see Figs. 3-21*A*, Plate 9, and 3-48). The left atrial appendage is smaller, more tortuous, and less pyramidal than its right atrial counterpart.[15–17] At least [illegible] per cent are multilobed (up to four lobes, but the most frequent finding is two lobes)[29] (Fig. 3-49, Plate 19). There are also age- and sex-related differences in the dimensions of the appendage.[20] *With increasing use of transesophageal echocardiography to search for a cardiac source of embolism and to guide cardioversion and percutanous balloon valvuloplasty procedures, a thorough appreciation of the variations in normal left atrial appendage morphology has become important because a thrombus may be missed if all lobes in the appendage are not visualized.* In contrast to the right atrial free wall, the left has no crista terminalis and no pectinate muscles outside its appendage.[15–17]

The coronary sinus travels along the posterior wall of the left atrium within the left atrioventricular groove (see Fig. 3-21*A*, Plate 9). *In patients with persistent left superior vena cava, which most commonly drains into a dilated coronary sinus, the left-sided cava courses between the left atrial appendage and the left upper pulmonary vein.*[17] *The venous structure can be misinterpreted as the descending thoracic aorta, a mass, or a pathologic cavity.*

The esophagus and descending thoracic aorta are in contact with the posterior left atrial wall (see Figs. 3-20

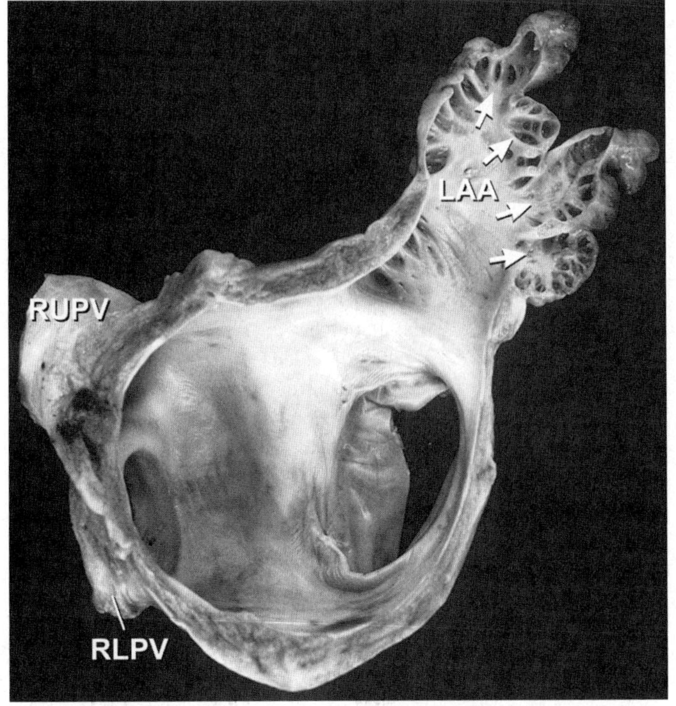


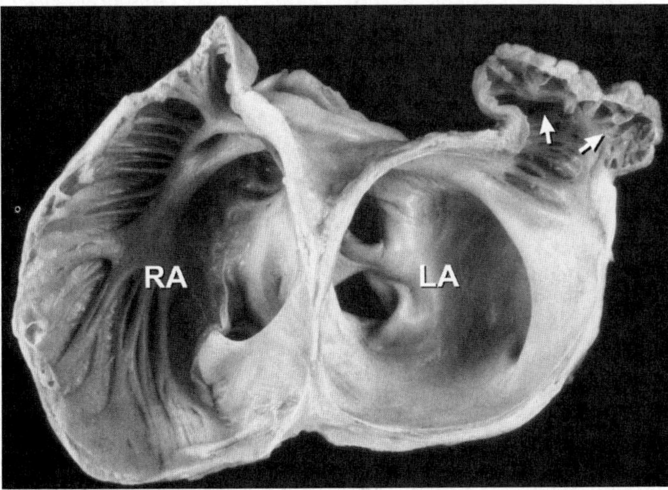


FIGURE 3-49 (Plate 19) Left atrial appendages (LAA). *A.* Left atrial free wall showing appendage with four lobes (arrows). *B.* Biatrial specimen demonstrating left atrial appendage with two lobes (arrows). LA, left atrium; RA, right atrium; RLPV, right lower pulmonary vein; RUPV, right upper pulmonary vein.

and 3-48). *Accordingly, esophageal carcinomas may compress, infiltrate, or perforate the left atrium, and descending thoracic aortic aneurysms may compress this chamber.*[15] *A large hiatal hernia also can abut against the left atrium and resemble a mass.*

*The marked increase in the incidence of atrial fibrillation from the fourth to the ninth decades of life may be due in part to the age-associated dilatation of the left atrium.*[20]

## Coronary Arteries and Veins

A detailed description of the spectrum of coronary artery anatomy including the many variations in the number and size of branches and course of the different arteries is beyond the scope of this chapter. The interested reader is referred to the elegant anatomic work by McAlpine published in 1975.[30] The focus of the following discussion, therefore, is to introduce the reader to the clinically relevant anatomy of the coronary circulation, with special emphasis on tomographic analysis of regional blood flow.

From the right and left aortic sinuses arise the right and left coronary arteries, respectively, and their ostia, normally originate about two-thirds the distance from the aortic annulus to the sinotubular junction and about midway between the aortic commissures[15–17] (Figs. 3-28 and 3-50, Plate 20). Whereas the right coronary artery arises nearly perpendicularly from the aorta, the left arises at an acute angle[15] (Fig. 3-51). Rarely, the anterior descending and circumflex arteries arise separately from a double-barrel left coronary ostium.[15–17] *Ostial stenosis most commonly results from atherosclerosis and degenerative calcification of the aortic sinotubular junction, which often overlies the right aortic sinus.*[17] *Less often it is due to aortic dissection or to aortitis associated with syphilis or ankylosing spondylitis. Stenosis of the right coronary ostium is much more frequent than that of the left. Iatrogenic ostial injury may complicate coronary angiography, intraoperative coronary perfusion, or aortic valve replacement.*[15–17] *Atherosclerosis or thrombosis of the most proximal portion of either coronary artery may mimic true ostial stenosis.*

The right coronary artery is embedded in adipose tissue throughout its course within the right atrioventricular groove. *Tricuspid annuloplasty or replacement may be complicated by injury to the right coronary artery.*[17] In 50 to 60 percent of persons, its first branch is the conus artery (Fig. 3-52), which supplies the right ventricular outflow tract and forms an important collateral anastomosis (circle of Vieussens), just below the pulmonary valve, with an analogous branch from the left anterior descending coronary artery (LAD).[15–17] In about a third of patients, the conus artery arises independently from the aorta[17] (see Fig. 3-28). The infundibular septum is supplied by the descending septal artery, which usually originates from the proximal right or conus coronary artery.[15–17] Among the numerous marginal branches of the right coronary artery that supply the remainder of the right ventricular free wall, the largest branch travels along the acute margin from base to apex[15–17] (see Fig. 3-50). In at

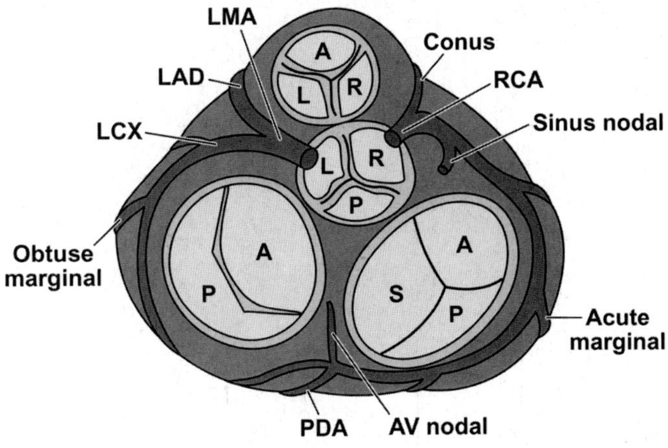


FIGURE 3-50 (Plate 20) Schematic diagram of coronary artery distribution viewed at the base of the heart. In this right-dominant system, the right coronary artery (RCA) gives rise to the posterior descending artery (PDA), and the left main coronary artery (LMA) gives rise to the left anterior descending (LAD) and left circumflex (LCX) branches. A, anterior; AV, atrioventricular; L, left; P, posterior; R, right; S, septal.

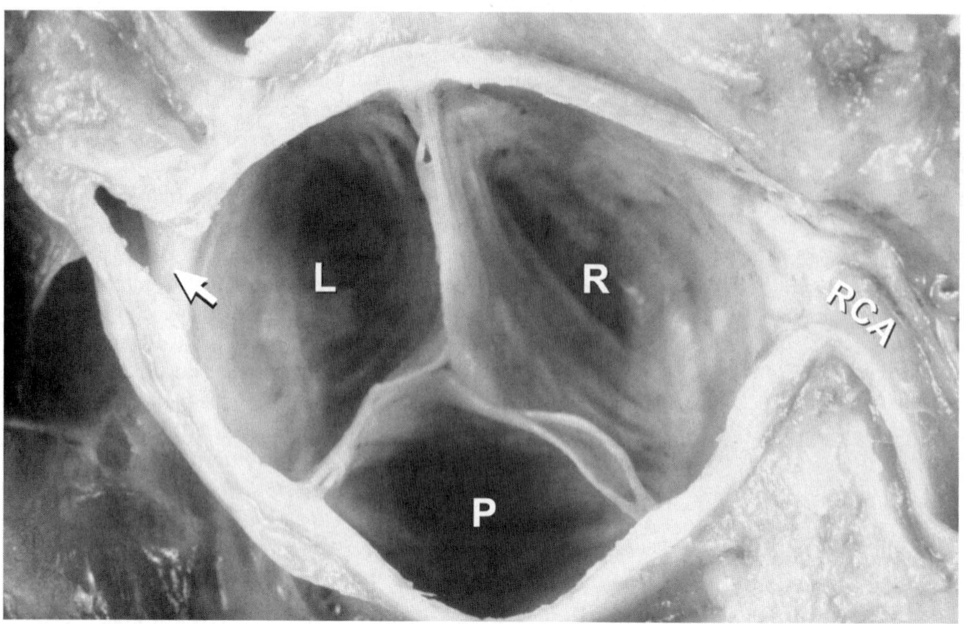


FIGURE 3-51 Differences in angulation at the origins of the right (RCA) and left main (arrow) coronary arteries. L, left aortic cusp; P, posterior aortic cusp; R, right aortic cusp.

least 70 percent of human hearts, the posterior descending artery arises from the distal right coronary artery (see Fig. 3-50, Plate 20). The posterior descending and distal posterolateral branches of a dominant right coronary artery supply the basal and middle inferior wall, basal (inlet) inferior septum, right bundle branch, AV node, AV (His) bundle, posterior portion of the left bundle branch, and posteromedial mitral papillary muscle.[17]

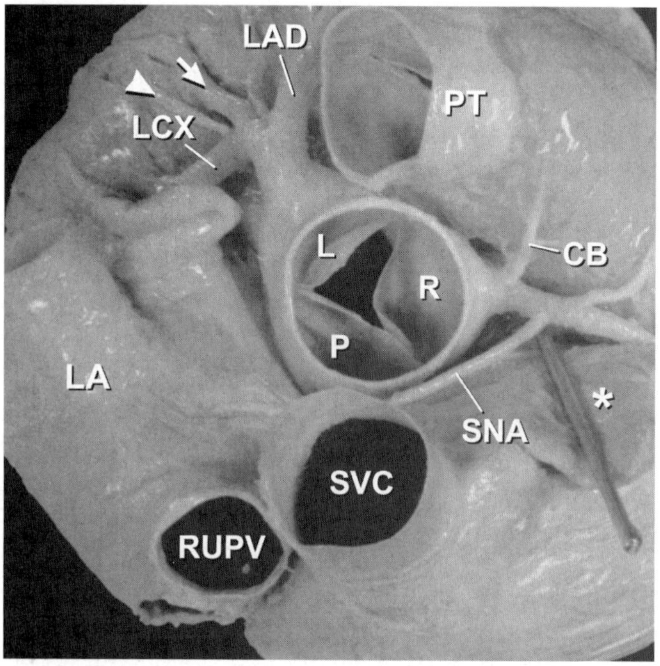

FIGURE 3-52 The right coronary artery gives rise to the conus branch (CB). A rod retracts the right atrial appendage (*) to disclose the sinus node artery (SNA). Arrow points to an intermediate left coronary artery; arrowhead points to a circumflex marginal branch. L, left aortic cusp; LA, left atrium; LAD, left anterior descending coronary artery; LCX, left circumflex coronary artery; P, posterior aortic cusp; PT, pulmonary trunk; R, right aortic cusp; RUPV, right upper pulmonary vein; SVC, superior vena cava. (From McAlpine,[30] with permission.)

The left main coronary artery travels for a very short distance along the epicardium between the pulmonary trunk and left atrium (see Figs. 3-50 and 3-52). It then divides into anterior descending and circumflex arteries (see Figs. 3-50 and 3-52). An intermediate artery also may arise at this division, thus forming a trifurcation rather than a bifurcation, and follows the course of a circumflex marginal branch[15–17] (see Fig. 3-52).

The LAD courses within the epicardial fat of the anterior interventricular groove, wraps around the cardiac apex, and travels a variable distance along the inferior interventricular groove toward the cardiac base. Its septal perforating branches supply the anterior septum and apical septum. The first septal perforating branch supplies the AV (His) bundle and proximal left bundle branch[17] (Fig. 3-53, Plate 21). *In patients with symptomatic hypertrophic obstructive cardiomyopathy, nonsurgical septal reduction by percutaneous transluminal occlusion of septal branches of the LAD is a new therapeutic approach aimed at reducing the outflow gradient.*[31] *The long-term effects of this procedure are currently unknown.* The epicardial diagonal branches of the LAD supply the anterior left ventricular free wall, part of the anterolateral mitral papillary muscle, and the medial one-third of the anterior right ventricular free wall.[15–17] Although short segments of the LAD may travel within the myocardium (covered by a so-called myocardial bridge) (Fig. 3-54), the resulting systolic luminal narrowing is probably benign in the vast majority of people.[17] *However, whereas*

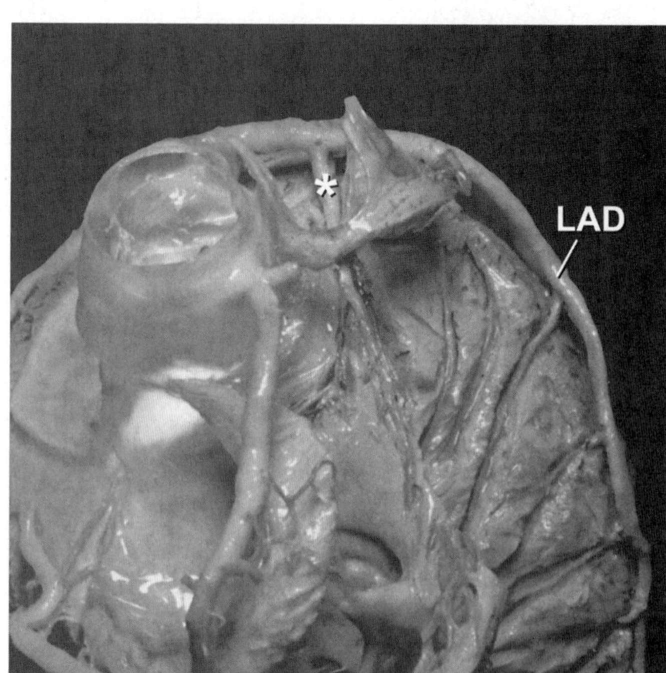


FIGURE 3-53 (Plate 21) Septal branches of the left anterior descending coronary artery (LAD);* points to the first septal perforator. (From McAlpine,[30] with permission.)

*the prevalence of myocardial bridging is only 0.5 to 1.6 percent in the general population, it is reported to be 28 percent in children and 30 to 50 percent in adults with hypertrophic cardiomyopathy.*[32] *More important, myocardial bridging appears to be associated with a poor prognosis (higher incidence of myocardial ischemia and sudden death) in patients with hypertrophic cardiomyopathy regardless of age.*[32]

The left circumflex coronary artery courses within the adipose tissue of the left atrioventricular groove (see Fig. 3-21*A*) and commonly terminates just beyond its large obtuse marginal branch (see Fig. 3-50). It supplies the lateral left ventricular free wall and a portion of the anterolateral mitral papillary muscle.[15–17]

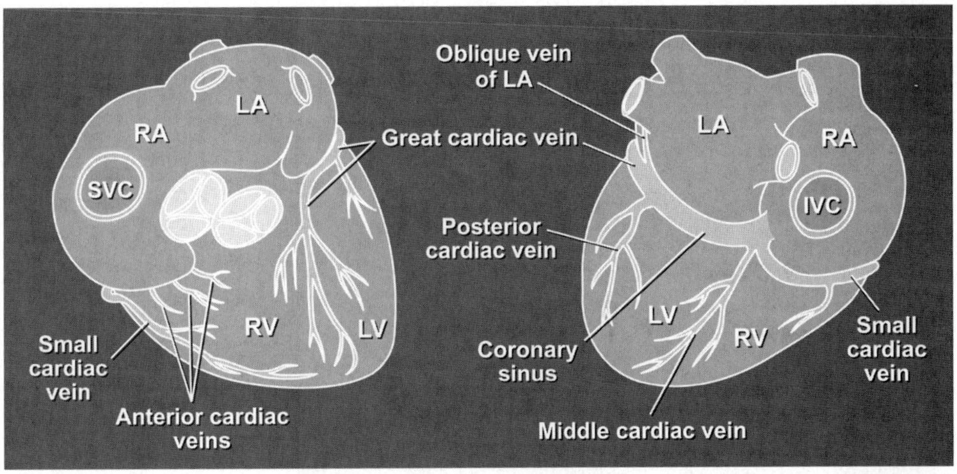

FIGURE 3-55 (Plate 22) Schematic diagram of the coronary venous circulation. IVC, inferior vena cava; LA, left atrium; LV, left ventricle; RA, right atrium; RV, right ventricle; SVC, superior vena cava.

Along the inferior surface of the heart, the length of the right coronary artery varies inversely with that of the circumflex artery. The artery that crosses the cardiac crux and gives rise to the posterior descending branch represents the dominant coronary artery. Dominance is right in 70 percent of human hearts, left in 10 percent, and shared in 20 percent.[15–17] *In patients with a congenitally bicuspid aortic valve, the incidence of left coronary dominance is 25 to 30 percent.*[17]

The coronary venous circulation is comprised of coronary sinus, cardiac veins, and thebesian venous systems[15–17] (Fig. 3-55, Plate 22). The great cardiac vein travels in the anterior interventricular groove beside the left anterior descending coronary artery and in the left atrioventricular groove beside the left circumflex artery.[15–17] The great cardiac vein and other cardiac veins, such as the left posterior and middle cardiac veins, drain into the coronary sinus, which courses along the posteroinferior aspect of the left atrioventricular groove and empties into the right atrium[15–17] (see Fig. 3-21*A*). The ostium of the coronary sinus is guarded by a crescent-shaped valvular remnant, the thebesian valve. Rarely, the coronary sinus drains directly into the left atrium.[17]

*During cardiac operations, cardioplegic solution may be administered retrogradely into the coronary sinus. In patients with the Wolff-Parkinson-White preexitation syndrome and left-sided bypass tracts, the ablation catheter during electrophysiologic studies can be positioned within the coronary sinus and great cardiac vein adjacent to the mitral valve ring in order to localize the aberrant conduction pathway.*[17] *The coronary veins, via the coronary sinus, provide access to percutaneous epicardial mapping and pacing of the ventricles and ablation of subepicardial arrhythmogenic foci*[33] (Fig. 3-56, Plate 23). *Some patients with ischemic cardiomyopathy may be poor candidates for conventional revascularization procedures (e.g., coronary*

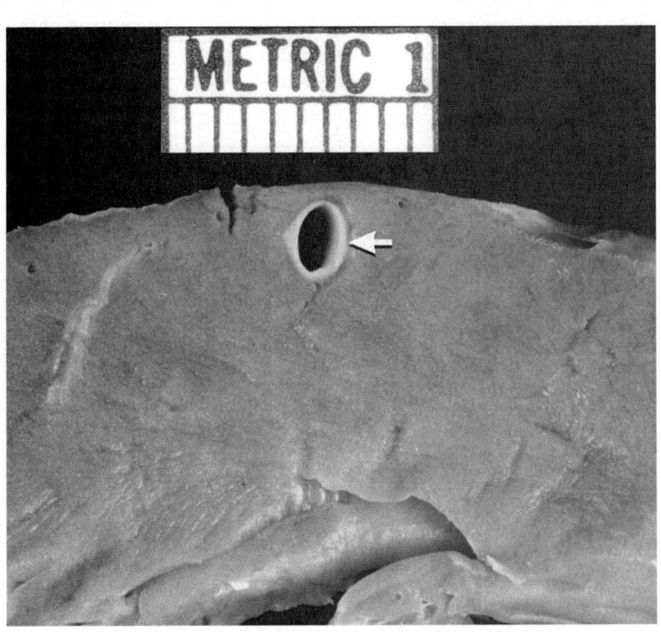


FIGURE 3-54 Intramyocardial course of the left anterior descending coronary artery (arrow).

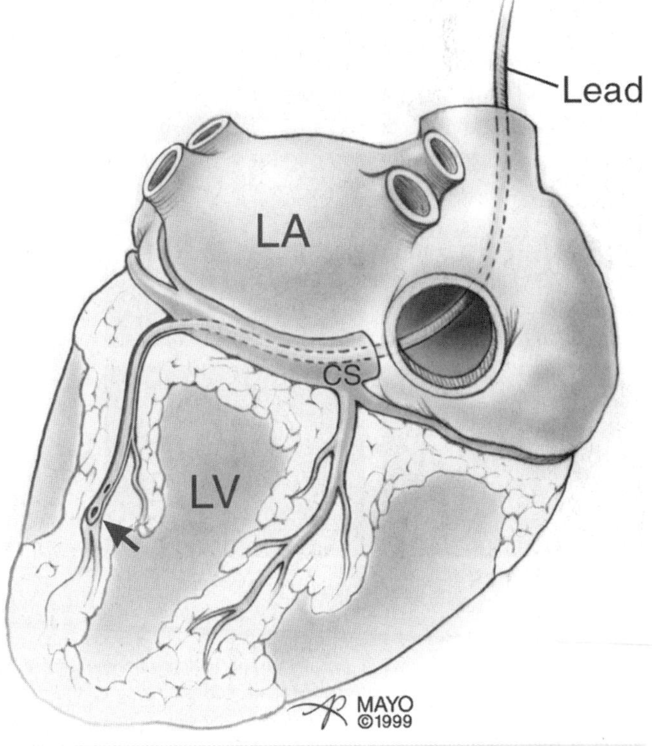


FIGURE 3-56 (Plate 23) Schematic diagram shows placement of the tip of a pacing/mapping catheter within a coronary vein (arrow) via the coronary sinus (CS). LA, left atrium; LV, left ventricle.

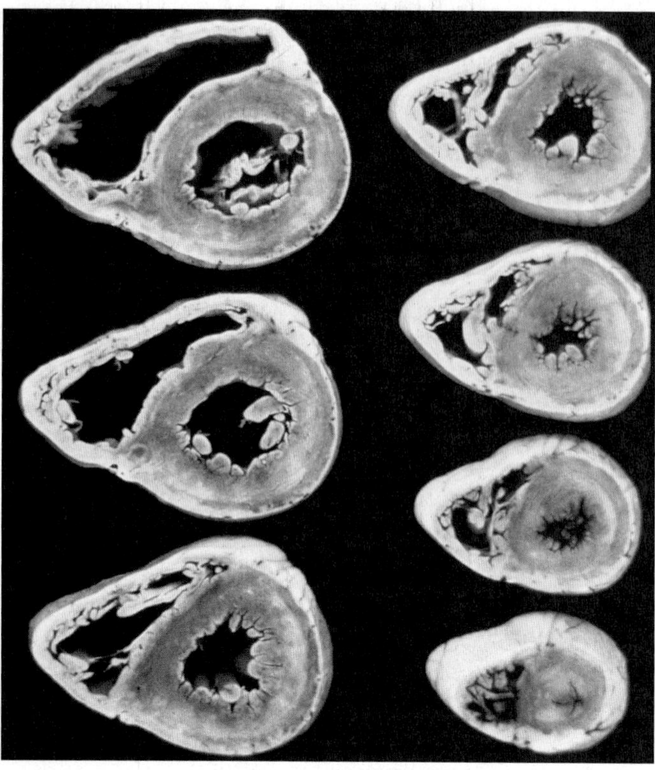

A

SA Apex

SA Mid

SA Base

Stress

Rest

B

FIGURE 3-57 Short-axis views. *A*. Collage of anatomic sections obtained by "bread slicing" the heart in its short-axis plane, corresponding to the tomographic sections obtained by echocardiography and SPECT imaging, viewed from the apex toward the base of the heart. *B*. Comparable sestamibi SPECT images of the left ventricle showing normal myocardial perfusion at rest and with exercise. SA, short axis

*artery bypass graft surgery or angioplasty) because their epicardial coronary arteries are diffusely diseased. Since in virtually all people the coronary veins run parallel to the entire course of coronary arteries, alternative percutaneous revascularization methods that use the coronary veins as a bypass conduit for coronary arterial flow are being explored.*[34–36] *Myocardial revascularization is achieved by either connecting the coronary artery proximal and distal to a stenosis to its companion coronary vein (similar to a conventional bypass graft) or by retroperfusion through the venous microvasculature if the artery and vein are only connected proximal to the stenosis. Coronary veins, unlike saphenous veins, are not removed, thus preserving their adventitia and blood supply.*[34–36]

Coronary artery disease is associated with regional abnormalities in ventricular structure and function. Because analysis of segmental myocardial perfusion or contractility is the cornerstone of tomographic imaging techniques [stress echocardiography, SPECT imaging, positron emission tomography (PET), and MRI], for clinicopathologic correlations (Fig. 3-57), a combination tomographic and segmental approach to coronary artery anatomy is recommended.[17,37,38] Ventricular mass is made of the left and right ventricular free walls and the partitioning ventricular septum. Three levels (i.e., basal, midventricular, and apical) are used to divide the base-apex length of the left ventricle into thirds (Fig. 3-58). The basal third includes that portion between the mitral annulus and the tips of the papillary muscles. The midventricular third is from the papillary muscle to the most apical insertion point of these muscles into the left ventricular free wall. The apical third includes the remainder of the ventricle, from the insertion of the papillary muscles to the left ventricular apex. A similar approach can be applied to the right ventricle.[15–17,37] The ventricular septum can be divided into anteroseptal, septal, and inferoseptal segments, and the left ventricular free wall is divided into anterior, lateral, and inferior segments at the basal and midventricular levels (see Fig. 3-58). The left ventricular apical level consists of four segments (i.e., septum, inferior, lateral, and anterior) (see Fig. 3-58).

This regional approach is not arbitrary and has been verified by studies of normal, dilated, and hypertrophied hearts. According to this system, there are 16 left ventricular segments that can be evaluated for regional abnormalities. This regional approach can also be used to assess transmural infarct size, because the percentage of left ventricular mass contributed by any particular region is not altered in any significant manner by symmetric hypertrophy or dilatation.[17]

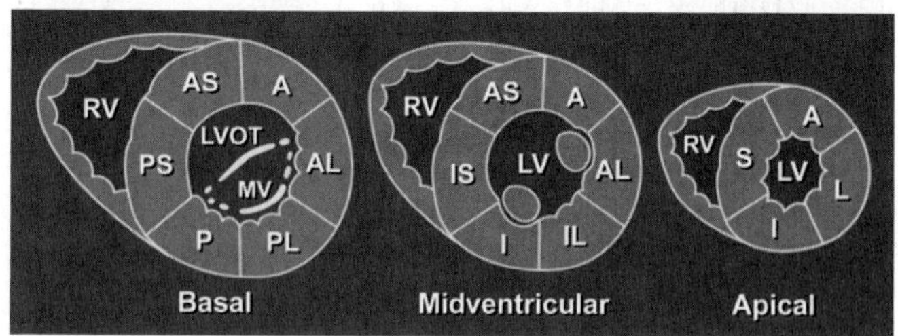


FIGURE 3-58 Schematic diagram of the three levels of short-axis tomographic views used in echocardiography for 16-segment wall motion analysis. A, anterior; AL, anterolateral; AS, anterior ventricular septum; I, inferior; IL, inferolateral; IS, inferior ventricular septum; L, lateral; LV, left ventricle; LVOT, left ventricular outflow tract; P, posterior; PL, posterolateral; PS, posterior ventricular septum; RV, right ventricle; S, septum. The most basal segment of the inferior wall is the anatomically true posterior segment. At this level, the adjacent ventricular septum is commonly referred to as either the *basal posterior septum* or the *basal inferior septum* and the adjacent lateral wall as either the *basal posterolateral wall* or the *basal inferolateral wall*.

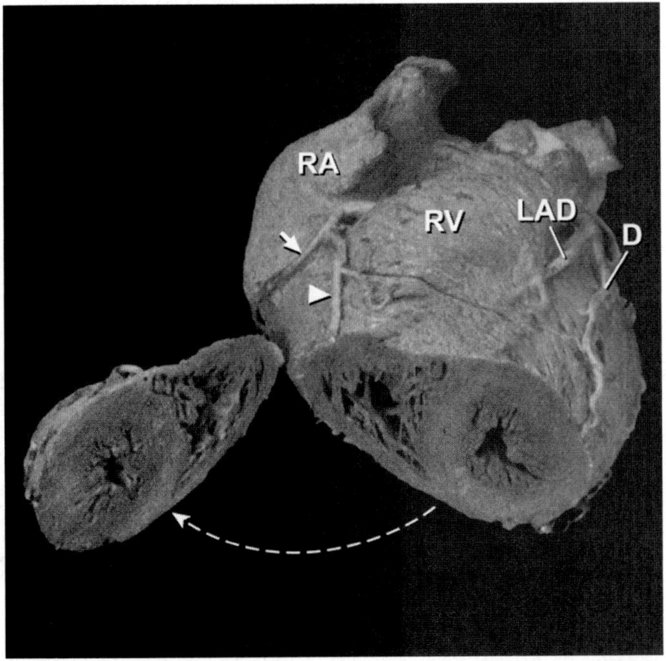


FIGURE 3-59 Regional coronary flow, with a short-axis slice of the heart. A large diagonal branch (D) of the left anterior descending coronary artery (LAD) supplies the lateral wall, and an acute marginal branch (arrowhead) of the right coronary artery (arrow) supplies the anterior right ventricular free wall. The distal segment of the LAD is intramural. RA, right atrium; RV, right ventricle. (From McAlpine,[30] with permission.)

## Regional Coronary Artery Supply

The ventricular regions described tend to correlate well with common patterns of coronary arterial distribution[15–17] (Figs. 3-59 and 3-60, Plate 24). Any specific epicardial coronary artery generally will supply a certain cluster of regions. For example, in a typical right-dominant system, the LAD would supply the midventricular and basal segments of the anterior and anterolateral walls and anterior septum and all apical segments. The left circumflex artery would supply the midventricular and basal inferolateral segments, and the right coronary artery would supply the midventricular and basal inferior wall and inferior septum (see Fig. 3-60, Plate 24). However, because the patterns of coronary distribution are so highly variable, these correlations between coronary blood flow and regional anatomy are not precise. For example, a hyperdominant right coronary artery may supply the apex, and a large, obtuse marginal branch of the circumflex artery may supply the anterolateral or inferior wall. Also, any given myocardial region may, in some people, receive its blood supply from the branches of two independent major epicardial arteries.[15–17] In old age, the coronary arteries become dilated and tortuous (Fig. 3-61).

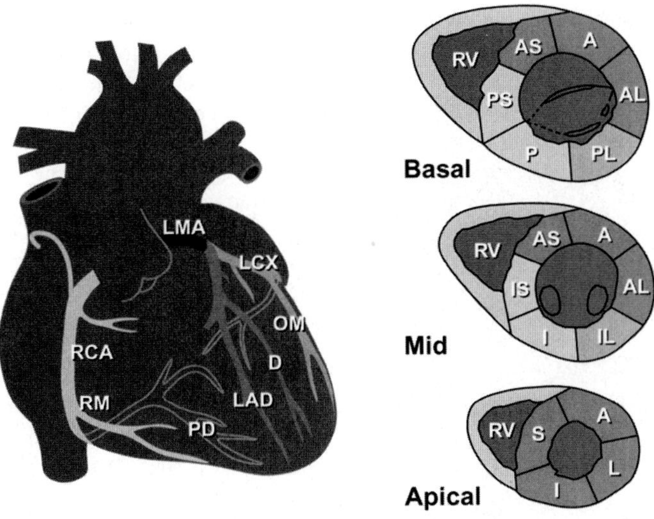


FIGURE 3-60 (Plate 24) Coronary distribution using a 16-segment model. D, diagonal branch of the left anterior descending coronary artery; LAD, left anterior descending coronary artery; LCX, left circumflex coronary artery; LMA, left main coronary artery; OM, obtuse marginal branch of the circumflex coronary artery; PD, posterior descending coronary artery; RCA, right coronary artery; RM, right marginal branch; other abbreviations as in Fig 3-58.

## Coronary Collaterals and Microcirculation

Collateral channels provide communication between the major coronary arteries and their branches.[17] If stenosis of an epicardial coronary artery produces a pressure gradient across such a vessel, the collateral channel may dilate with time and provide a bypass avenue for

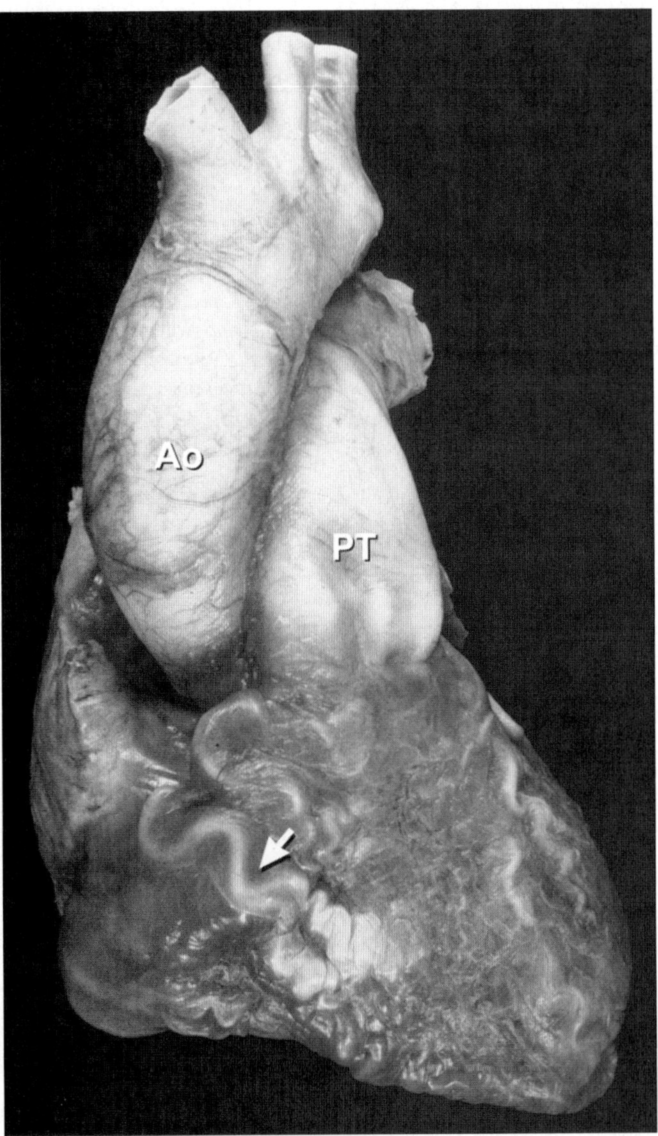


FIGURE 3-61 Tortuous coronary arteries (arrow) typically seen in the elderly with nondilated hearts. Ao, ascending aorta; PT, pulmonary trunk.

blood flow beyond the obstruction. Such functional collaterals may develop between the terminal extensions of two coronary arteries, between the side branches of two arteries, between branches of the same artery, or within the same branch (via the vasa vasorum). These are most common in the ventricular septum (between septal perforators of the anterior and posterior descending arteries), in the ventricular apex (between anterior descending septal perforators), in the anterior right ventricular free wall (between anterior descending and right or conus arteries), in the anterolateral left ventricular free wall (between anterior descending diagonals and circumflex marginals), at the cardiac crux, and along the atrial surfaces (between the right and left circumflex arteries).[17]

The intramural coronary vessels form the microcirculation. There are age-related variations in the pattern of distribution of the coronary microcirculation.[39] *Angina-like chest pain in some patients with angiographically normal epicardial coronary arteries (i.e., syndrome X, or microvascular angina) may be secondary to abnormal vasodilator reserve or vasoconstriction of the coronary microcirculation.*[40] *Abnormal flow reserve of the coronary microcirculation is seen in both dilated and hypertrophied hearts. In the latter, structural changes in the coronary arterioles can be found on histologic examination of the myocardium.*[41–43] *In patients with symptomatic hypertrophic cardiomyopathy without angiographic evidence of epicardial coronary artery disease, myocardial tissue obtained during surgical myectomy may show smaller than normal coronary arteriolar lumina.*[43] *Postmortem analysis of hearts with hypertrophic cardiomyopathy also has revealed coronary arterioles with abnormally thick walls.*[43] *With contrast echocardiography, it may be possible to noninvasively visualize intramyocardial arterioles and study coronary flow reserve.*[44] *Demonstration of an intact microvascular circulation in akinetic myocardium following acute myocardial infarction, using PET or SPECT imaging or contrast echocardiography, is evidence of viability of the affected segment.*[44] *The creation of intramyocardial channels with $CO_2$ laser transmyocardial revascularization has been associated with augmentation of collateral flow to ischemic myocardium through angiogenesis.*[45]

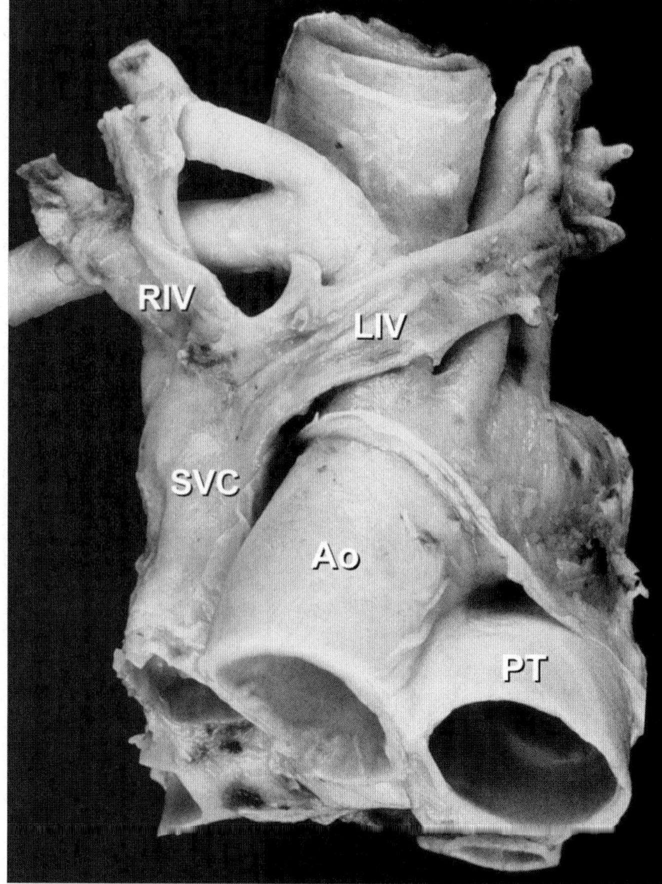


FIGURE 3-62 The longer left (LIV) and shorter right (RIV) innominate veins normally join to form the right superior vena cava (SVC). Ao, ascending aorta; PT, pulmonary trunk.

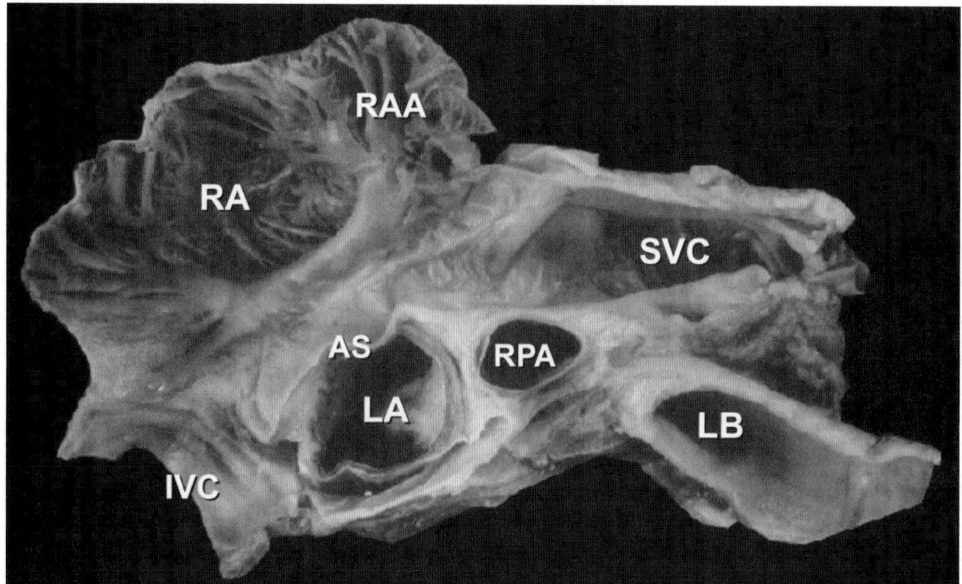


FIGURE 3-63 Long-axis view of the superior vena cava (SVC) and inferior vena cava (IVC). The specimen is viewed from the left looking toward the free wall of the right atrium. The right atrium (RA) and its appendage (RAA) are anterior. This is a commonly used tomographic plane in transesophageal echocardiography (TEE). AS, atrial septum; LA, left atrium; LB, left bronchus; RPA, right pulmonary artery.

## Cardiac Lymphatics

The myocardial lymphatics drain toward the epicardial surface, where they merge to form the right and left lymphatic channels, which travel in retrograde fashion with their respective coronary arteries. These two lymphatic channels travel along the ascending aorta and merge before draining into a pretracheal lymph node beneath the aortic arch. This single lymphatic channel then travels through a cardiac lymph node, between the superior vena cava and innominate artery, and finally empties into the right lymphatic duct. Metastatic tumor obstruction of epicardial lymphatics can produce a pericardial effusion.[15–17]

## Great Vessels

The subclavian and internal jugular veins merge bilaterally to form the right and left innominate veins (Fig. 3-62). Valves in the subclavian and internal jugular veins, near their junctions with

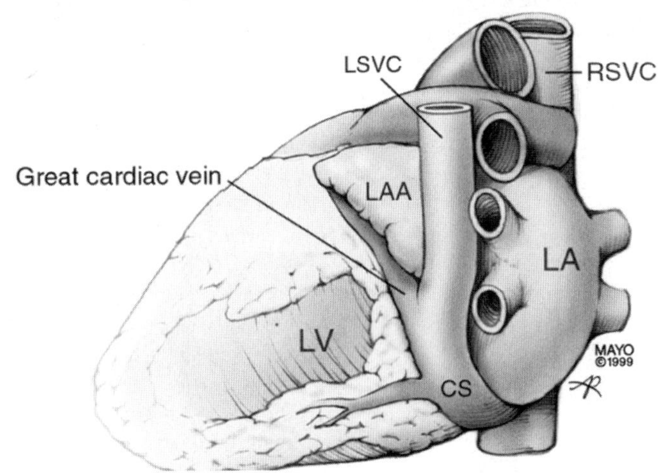


FIGURE 3-64 (Plate 25) Schematic diagrams showing the ligament/vein of Marshall in normal hearts (*left*) and persistent left superior vena cava (LSVC) (*right*). CS, coronary sinus; LA, left atrium; LAA, left atrial appendage; LV, left ventricle; RA, right atrium; RSVC, right superior vena cava.

the innominate veins, are important anatomic structures that help maintain unidirectional antegrade blood flow not only in the normal state but also in the setting of elevated right-sided heart filling pressures.[46] Subclavian and internal jugular venous valves are absent in 2 and 6 percent of people, respectively, and venous valves may be damaged by catheter-induced trauma or by age.[46] *Absent or malfunctioning valves may interfere with the success of closed-chest cardiopulmonary resuscitation and contribute to the development of brain edema during such a procedure.*[46]

The left innominate vein is two to three times the length of its right-sided counterpart. It travels anteriorly to the aortic arch along the right anterolateral border of the ascending aorta, where it joins the shorter right innominate vein to form the superior vena cava[15–17] *(see Fig. 3-62). Transesophageal echocardiographic imaging of the upper ascending aorta may show a double lumen (i.e., aorta and adjacent innominate vein) that can be misinterpreted as aortic dissection by an inexperienced echocardiographer.*[7]

The superior vena cava lies anterior to the right pulmonary artery (Fig. 3-63) and receives the azygos vein posteriorly before draining into the superior aspect of the right atrium, just posterior to the atrial appendage[15–17] (see Figs. 3-46, 3-47, Plate 18, and 3-63). *The vein of Marshall forms the terminal connection between a persistent left superior vena cava and the coronary sinus. Its vestigial remnant in normal adults is the ligament of Marshall (Fig. 3-64, Plate 25). Both vein and ligament are a potential source of arrhythmias.* The ostium of the inferior vena cava is guarded by a crescent-shaped, often fenestrated flap of tissue, the eustachian valve[15–17] (see Fig. 3-16*A*, Plate 8), which is readily seen by echocardiography. Although generally small, the eustachian valve may become so large that it can produce a double-chambered right atrium.[16] Also, when either the eustachian or thebesian valve is large and fenestrated, it is referred to as a *Chiari net.*[15–17] *By echocardiography, a Chiari net may be misinterpreted as a mass.* The thoracic aorta arises at the level of the aortic valve and is divided into three segments: ascending aorta, aortic arch, and descending thoracic aorta (Fig. 3-65). The ascending aorta consists of sinus and tubular portions, which are demarcated by

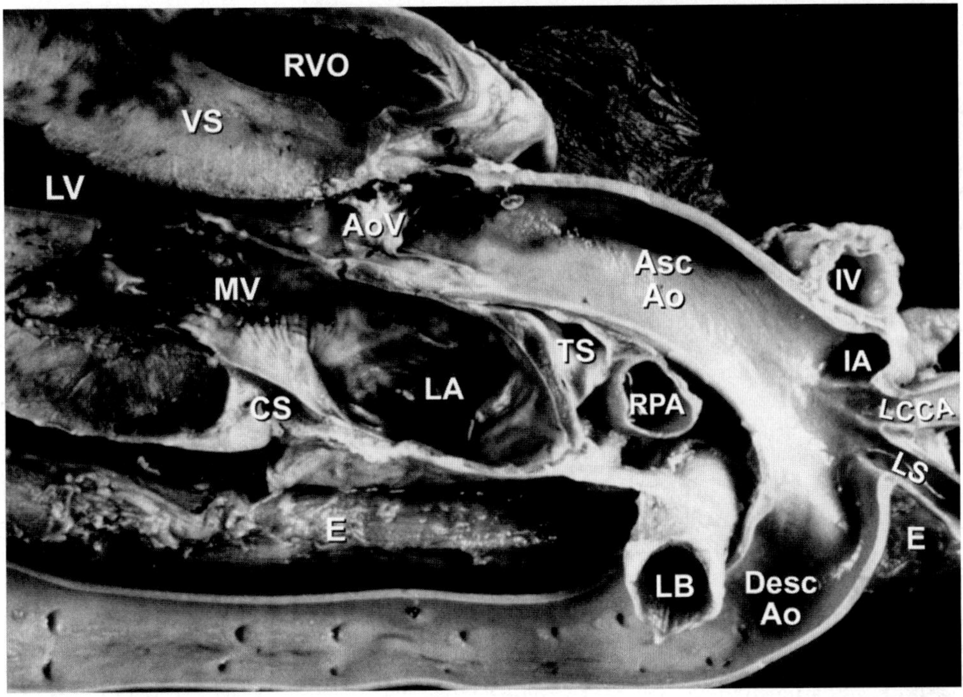


FIGURE 3-65 Thoracic aorta. The entire thoracic aorta has been cut in a tomographic manner. The aortic arch travels over the left bronchus and the right pulmonary artery. Asc Ao, ascending aorta; AoV, aortic valve; CS, coronary sinus; Desc Ao, descending thoracic aorta; E, esophagus; IA, innominate artery; IV, innominate vein; LA, left atrium; LB, left bronchus; LCCA, left common carotid artery; LS, left subclavian artery; LV, left ventricle; MV, mitral valve; RPA, right pulmonary artery; RVO, right ventricular outflow; TS, transverse sinus; VS, ventricular septum.

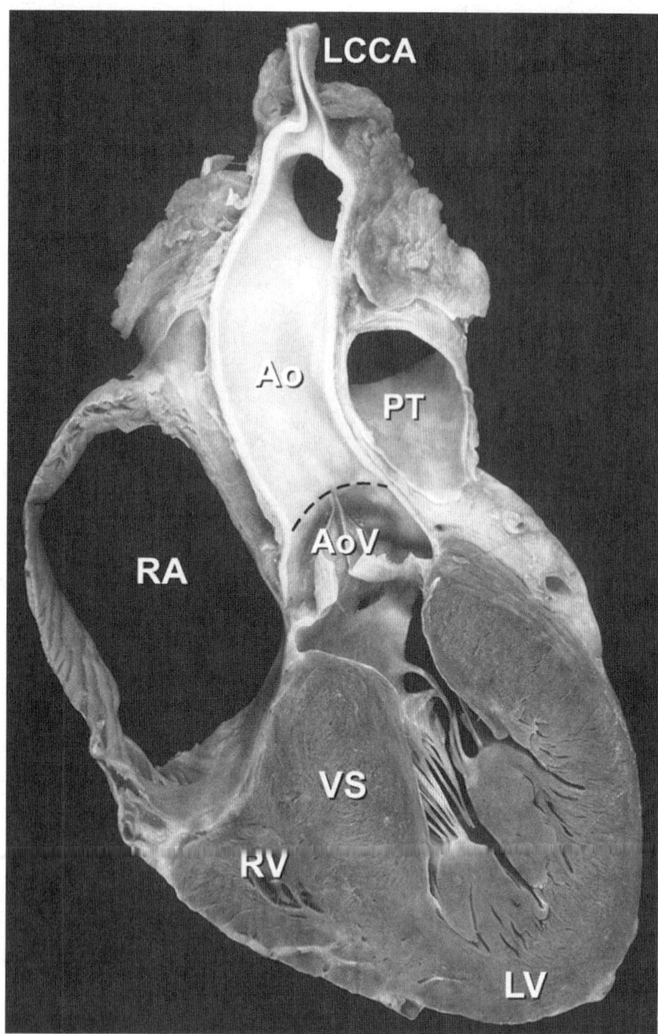


FIGURE 3-66 Tomographic section of the heart in the frontal plane of the body showing the aortic sinotubular junction (dashed line). Ao, ascending aorta; AoV, aortic valve; LCCA, left common carotid artery; LV, left ventricle; PT, pulmonary trunk; RA, right atrium; RV, right ventricle; LV, left ventricle; VS, ventricular septum.

the sinotubular junction (Figs. 3-28 and 3-66). *This is the site at which supravalvular aortic stenosis is often most severe.*[15–17]

Behind the aortic valve cusps are three outpouchings, or sinuses (of Valsalva). The right aortic sinus abuts against the ventricular septum and right ventricular parietal band and is covered in part by the right atrial appendage (see Figs. 3-30 and 3-52). In contrast, the left aortic sinus rests against the anterior left ventricular free wall and a portion of the anterior mitral leaflet, abuts the left atrial free wall, and is covered in part by the pulmonary trunk and left atrial appendage (see Figs. 3-20 and 3-21*A*, Plate 9). The posterior (noncoronary) aortic sinus overlies the ventricular septum and a part of the anterior mitral leaflet, forms part of the transverse sinus, abuts the atrial septum, and indents both atrial free walls[15–17] (see Figs. 3-12*D* and 3-22). *Rupture of the right and posterior aortic sinuses of Valsalva may result in a communication with the right ventricular outflow tract or right atrium, whereas rupture of the left aortic sinus of Valsalva leads to a communication with the left atrium or left ventricular outflow tract. Annuloaortic ectasia is associated with hypertension, aortic medial degeneration, and advanced age and may produce aortic regurgitation, ascending aortic aneurysm, or aortic dissection.*[15–17]

The aortic arch gives rise to the innominate, left common carotid, and left subclavian arteries in that order (see Fig. 3-65). In about 10 percent of people, the innominate and left common carotid arteries share a common ostium, and in 5 percent of people, the left vertebral artery arises directly from the aortic arch, between the left common carotid and left subclavian arteries.[17] The ligamentum arteriosum (ductal artery ligament) represents the vestigial remnant of the fetal ductal artery, which, when patent, connects the proximal left pulmonary artery to the undersurface of the aortic arch.[17] *Most coarctations occur just distal to the left subclavian artery (see Fig. 3-69). When thoracic aortic dissection does not involve the ascending aorta (DeBakey type III and Stanford type B), the intimal tear is commonly near the ligamentum arteriosum or the ostium of the left subclavian artery.*[17] *Nonpenetrating deceleration chest trauma, as may occur in motor vehicle accidents, commonly involves the aorta in the region between the aortic arch and descending thoracic aorta and may be associated with aortic transection or pseudoaneurysm formation.*[17]

The descending thoracic aorta lies adjacent to the left atrium, esophagus, and vertebral column. The pulmonary trunk (or main pulmonary artery) emanates from the right ventricle and travels to the left of the ascending aorta. As it bifurcates, the left pulmonary artery courses over the left bronchus, whereas the right pulmonary artery travels beneath the aortic arch and behind the superior vena cava (see Figs. 3-11*A* and 3-63). Thus the *left* bronchus and the *right* pulmonary artery normally travel beneath the aortic arch.

## Cardiac Conduction System

The cardiac conduction system consists of the sinus node, internodal tracts, AV node, AV (His) bundle, and right and left bundle branches[15–17] (Fig. 3-67, Plate 26). The sinus node is located subepicardially in the terminal groove, close to the junction between the superior vena cava and right atrium. The sinus node artery arises from the right coronary artery in 55 percent of people. Its course may place it in contact with the base of the right atrial appendage and the superior vena cava–right atrial junction (see Fig. 3-52). When the sinus node artery arises from the left circumflex artery (45 percent), it may course close to the left atrial appendage. *During such surgical operations as the Mustard and Fontan procedures, the sinus node and its artery are susceptible to injury.*[16,17] By light microscopy, there are no morphologically distinct conduction pathways between the sinus and AV nodes.[17] However, electrophysiologic studies support the concept of functional preferential pathways that travel along the crista terminalis and atrial septum including the limbus but not the valve of the fossa ovalis.[17] *Internodal conduction disturbances therefore are not expected as a result of transseptal procedures. With the Mustard operation for complete transposition of the great arteries, there may be severe disturbance of internodal conduction because the entire septum is resected, and the surgical atriotomy may disrupt the crista terminalis.*[17] *Lipomatous hypertrophy of the atrial septum may interfere with internodal conduction and induce a variety of atrial arrhythmias. Ventricular preexcitation is most commonly associated with aberrant bypass tracts that span the annulus of the tricuspid or mitral valve* (see Fig. 3-2).

The AV node, in contrast to the sinus node, is a sub*endo*cardial structure that is located within the triangle of Koch[15–17] (Fig. 3-68, Plate 27). The triangle of Koch is bordered by the coronary sinus ostium posteroinferiorly and the septal tricuspid annulus anteriorly. *Because of its right atrial location near the tricuspid annulus, the AV node is susceptible to injury during tricuspid annuloplasty and during plication procedures for Ebstein's anomaly.*[15–17]

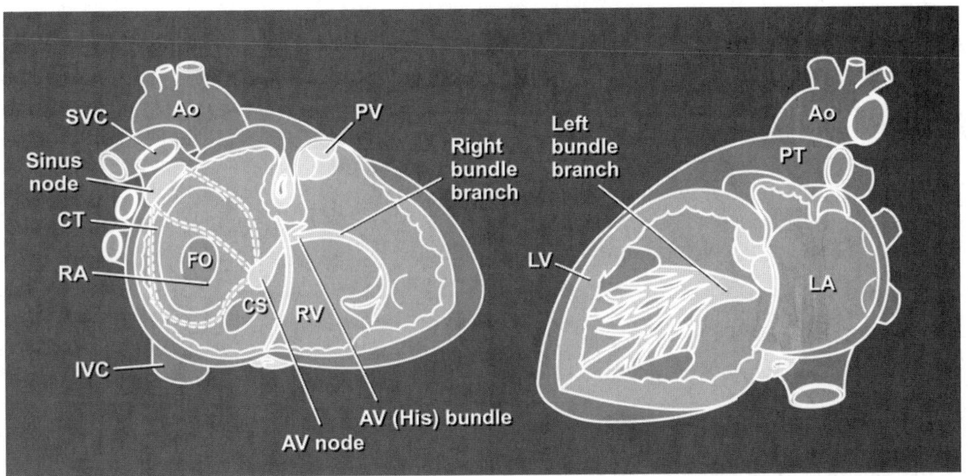


FIGURE 3-67 (Plate 26) Schematic diagram of the cardiac conduction system. The right side of the heart (*left*) showing the sinus node, atrioventricular (AV) node, AV (His) bundle, and right bundle branch. The left side of the heart (*right*) showing incomplete anatomic separation of the left bundle into antero and posterior fascicles. Ao, ascending aorta; AV, atrioventricular; CS, coronary sinus; CT, crista terminalis; FO, fossa ovalis; IVC, inferior vena cava; LA, left atrium; LV, left ventricle; PT, pulmonary trunk; PV, pulmonary valve; RA, right atrium; RV, right ventricle; SVC, superior vena cava.

The AV (His) bundle arises from the distal portion of the AV node and travels along the ventricular septum adjacent to the membranous septum[15–17] *(see Fig. 3-68, Plate 27). The AV conduction tissue is generally remote from the defect in the outlet, inlet, and muscular forms of ventricular septal defect but travels along the inferior margin of a membranous ventricular septal defect.* The AV bundle travels through the central fibrous body (right fibrous trigone) and therefore is closely related to the annuli of the aortic, mitral, and tricuspid valves. *Thus, during operative procedures involving these valves or a membranous ventricular septal defect, care must be taken to avoid injury to the His bundle. Whereas in normal hearts the AV bundle courses along the posteroinferior rim of the membranous septum, it courses along the anterosuperior rim of the membranous septum in hearts with AV discordance.* The AV bundle receives a dual blood supply from the AV nodal artery and the first septal perforator of the left anterior descending coronary artery.[17]

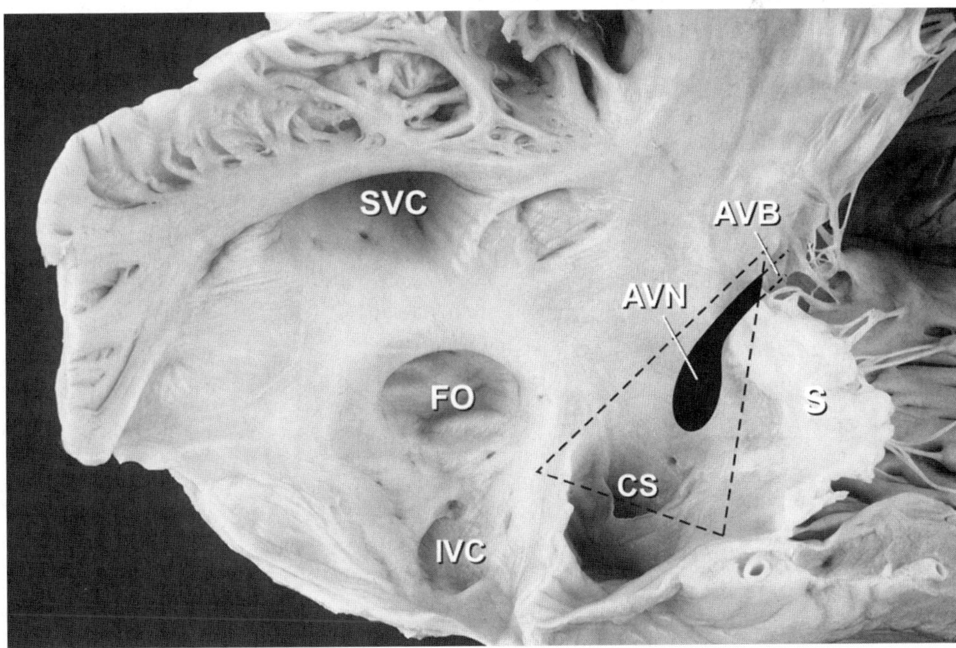


FIGURE 3-68 (Plate 27) The atrioventricular node (AVN) lies within the triangle of Koch (dashed triangle), and the AV (His) bundle (AVB) travels through the tricuspid annulus to rest along the summit of the ventricular septum. CS, coronary sinus; FO, fossa ovalis; IVC, inferior vena cava; S, septal leaflet of the tricuspid valve; SVC, superior vena cava.

The right bundle branch emanates from the distal portion of the AV bundle and forms a cord-like structure that travels along the septal and moderator bands toward the anterior tricuspid papillary muscle (see Fig. 3-67). In contrast, the left bundle branch represents a broad fenestrated sheet of subendocardial conduction fibers that spread along the septal surface of the left ventricle[15–17] (see Fig. 3-67). The right and left bundle branches receive dual blood supply from the septal perforators of the left anterior descending coronary artery and posterior descending coronary arteries.[17] Left ventricular pseudotendons may contain conduction tissue from the left bundle branch.[17] *Following right ventriculotomy for reconstruction of the right ventricular outflow tract, the electrocardiogram shows a pattern of right bundle-branch block even though the right bundle is not disrupted.*[16]

## NEW DEVELOPMENTS AND FUTURE CHALLENGES

The future holds promise for an integrated multidimensional approach to the study of cardiac anatomy that incorporates static three-dimensional data, the elements of time (the fourth dimension) and motion, and physiologic (pressure and perfusion) and metabolic parameters.[47–49] Until recently, the geometric fusion of anatomy and function was not possible without physically invading the body. With the currently available imaging techniques, multidimensional anatomy and physiology are mentally reassembled from the sequential tomographic images using echocardiography, MRI or CT, or multiple scintigraphy, as with SPECT imaging.[47] With the advances made in medical technology propelled by the rapid developments in computer technology, digital imaging, and data-storage techniques, it has become possible to electronically perform virtual dissection and reconstruction of the heart and cardiovascular system[47–49] (Fig. 3-69). Furthermore, multidimensional imaging allows continued study of any human organ of interest because of the ability to permanently store anatomic images and physiologic features for retrieval, comparison for change, and ultimately, physical replication.[47–49]

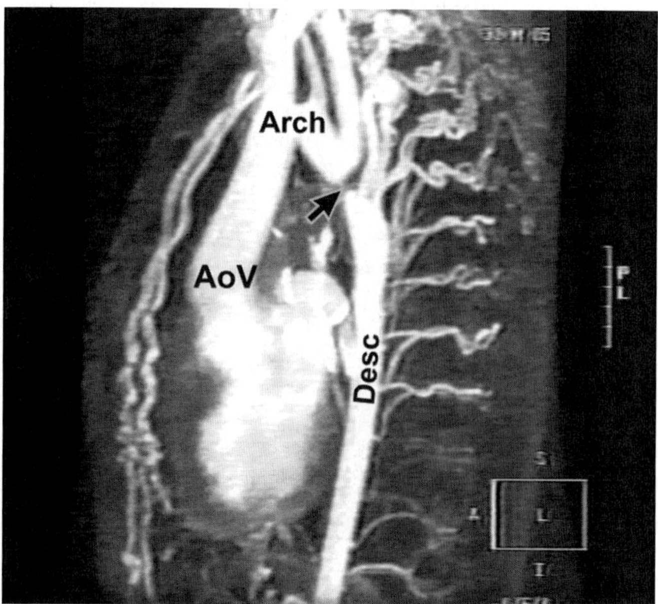


FIGURE 3-69 Real-time three-dimensional CT reconstruction of the thoracic aorta in a patient with coarctation (arrow) distal to the left subclavian artery. AoV, aortic valve. Desc, descending thoracic aorta. Note the tortuous intercostal and mammary arteries which collateralize the coarctation.

The potential realization of virtual anatomy notwithstanding, standardization of the various tomographic approaches to image acquisition in a manner that conforms with anatomic correctness remains a major challenge that has to be overcome if multidimensional cardiac imaging is to become a clinical reality. There is current progress in this direction. Real-time three-dimensional reconstruction of the heart using identical CT and two-dimensional tomographic sectioning of the heart is now possible. Virtual vivisection may soon become reality. It will allow virtual surgery (dry runs prior to the actual operation) and dissection of the heart into its various functional components, be it anatomic, physiologic, or metabolic, either separately or in various combinations. Because of these advances in multimedia technology, the centuries-old great divide between physiologists and anatomists has been relegated to the history books.

## ANATOMY NOT ADDRESSED AND QUANTUM COMPUTING

Fine-detailed anatomy such as that of the conduction system and microvasculature is not available to the usual anatomic dissection. Additionally, tissue histology or molecular biological assessment is not obtained routinely by the dissectionist. At the other end of the spectrum three-dimensional gross anatomic dissection of contiguous structures is also normally not available. How does metastatic cancer throughout the system relate to a primary tumor in the gut?

These and other desirable anatomic and histologic dissections await the future of increasingly sophisticated computer technology and information management. Both pathologic and living tissues someday will be dissected and analyzed not by destructive cutting but by higher-dimensional imagery. Today's computers have introduced the information era. Information has become a commodity expanding our ability to access useful data. Within the next two decades, however, we will have evolved to the "Quantum Era," where all that has been discussed in this chapter plus gross and microscopic anatomy will be possible within an electronic environment. Reality will be broken down into its base parts or characteristics (quanta, molecules, pixels, etc.) and then reformatted in three-dimensional geometry relative to the desired information. Gross anatomy, physiology, tissue characteristics, and even histopathology can be dissected and presented as a quantifiable geometric image. The concept of a "living autopsy" will be a reality.

## References

1. Callahan JA, Key JD. Foundations of cardiology. In: Giuliani ER, Fuster V, Gersh BJ, et al, eds. *Cardiology Fundamentals and Practice,* 2d ed: Vol 1. St Louis: Mosby–Year Book; 1991:3–25.
2. O'Malley CD, Saunders JB. *Leonardo da Vinci on the Human Body.* New York: Greenwich House; 1982:223.
3. Ackermann DM, Edwards WD. Anatomic basis for tomographic analysis of the pediatric heart at autopsy. *Perspect Pediatr Pathol* 1988; 12:44–68.
4. Landefeld CS, Goldman L. The autopsy in clinical medicine. *Mayo Clinic Proc* 1989; 64:1185–1189.
5. Hurst JW, King SB, Friesinger GC, et al. Atherosclerotic coronary heart disease: Angina pectoris, myocardial infarction, and other manifestations of myocardial ischemia. In: *Hurst's The Heart,* 6th, ed. New York: McGraw-Hill; 1986:882–1008.

6. Edwards WD. Anatomic basis for tomographic analysis of the heart at autopsy. *Cardiol Clin* 1984;2:485–506.
7. Seward J. Transesophageal echocardiographic anatomy. In: Freeman W, Seward J, Khandheria B, Tajik AJ, eds. *Transesophageal Echocardiography*. Boston: Little, Brown; 1994:55–101.
8. Stewart W. Intraoperative echocardiography. In: Topol EJ, ed. *Textbook of Cardiovascular Medicine*. Philadelphia: Lippincott-Raven; 1998: 1497–1525.
8a. Katsnelson Y, Raman J, Katsnelson F, et al. Current state of intraoperative echocardiography. *Echocardiography* 2003;20(8): 771–780.
8b. Szili-Torok T, Krenning BJ, Voormolen MM, Reclandt JR. Dynamic three-dimensional echocardiography combined with semiautomated border detection offers advantages for assessment of resynchronization therapy. *Cardiovasc Ultrasound* 2003;1(1):14.
9. Packer DL, Johnson SB. Intracardiac ultrasound guidance of linear lesion creation for ablation of atrial fibrillation. *J Am Coll Cardiol* 1998; 31:333A.
10. Chu E, Fitzpatrick AP, Chin MC, et al. Radio-frequency catheter ablation guided by intracardiac echocardiography. *Circulation* 1994; 89:1301–1305.
11. DeLurgio DB, Frohwein SC, Walter PF, et al. Anatomy of atrioventricular nodal reentry investigated by intracardiac echocardiography. *Am J Cardiol* 1997;80:231–234.
12. Bruce CJ, Packer DL, Seward J. Transvascular imaging: Feasibility study using a vector phased array ultrasound catheter. *Echocardiography* 1999;16:425–430.
13. Fu M, Hung JS, Lo PH, et al. Intracardiac echocardiography via the transvenous approach with use of 8F 10-MHz ultrasound catheters. *Mayo Clin Proc* 1999;74:775–783.
13a. Corsi C, Lamberti C, Sarti A, et al. Real-time 3D echocardiographic data analysis for left ventricular volume estimation. *Comput Cardiol* 2000;27:107–110.
13b. Abidov A, Bax JJ, Hayes SW, Hachamovitch R, et al. Transient ischemic dilation ratio of the left ventricle is a significant predictor of future cardiac events in patients with otherwise normal myocardial perfusion SPECT. *J Am Coll Cardiol* 2003;42(10):1818–1825.
14. Nazarian GK, Julsrud PR, Ehman RL, et al. Correlation between magnetic resonance imaging of the heart and cardiac anatomy. *Mayo Clinic Proc* 1987;62:573–583.
15. Edwards WD. *Anatomy of the Cardiovascular System: Clinical Medicine:* Vol 6. Philadelphia: Harper & Row; 1984:1–24.
16. Edwards WD. Cardiac anatomy and examination of cardiac specimens. In: Emmanouilides G, Reimenschneider T, Allen H, Gutgesell H, eds. *Moss & Adams' Heart Disease in Infants, Children, and Adolescents,* 5th ed. Baltimore: Williams & Wilkins; 1995:70–105.
17. Edwards WD. Applied anatomy of the heart. In: Giuliani ER, Fuster V, Gersh BJ, et al, eds. *Cardiology Fundamentals and Practice,* 2d ed: Vol 1. St Louis: Mosby-Year Book; 1991:47–112.
18. McAfee MK, Schaff HV. Valve repair for mitral insufficiency. *Cardiology* 1990; 20:35–43.
19. Arom KV, Edwards JD. Relationship between right ventricular muscle bundles and pulmonary valve: Significance in pulmonary atresia with intact ventricular septum. *Circulation* 1976; 54:79–83.
20. Kitzman D, Edwards WD. Minireview: Age-related changes in the anatomy of the normal human heart. *J Gerontol Med Sci* 1990; 45:M33–M39.
21. Freedberg RS, Goodkin GM, Perez JL. Valve strands are strongly associated with systemic embolization: A transesophageal echocardiographic study. *J Am Coll Cardiol* 1995;26:1709–1712.
22. Burke A, Virmani R. *Atlas of Tumor Pathology: Tumors of the Heart and Great Vessels in Papillary Fibroelastoma*. Washington DC: Armed Forces Institute of Pathology; 1996:47–54.
23. Roberts WC, Roberts JD. The floating heart too fat to sink: Analysis of 55 necropsy patients. *Am J Cardiol* 1983;52:1286–1289.
24. Cristina B, Gaetano T, Domenico C, et al. Arrhythmogenic right ventricular cardiomyopathy: Dysplasia, dystrophy, or myocarditis. *Circulation* 1996;94:983–991.
25. Luetmer PH, Edwards WD, Seward JB, et al. Incidence and distribution of left ventricular false tendons: An autopsy study of 483 normal human hearts. *J Am Coll Cardiol* 1986;8:179–183.
26. Boyd MT, Seward JB, Tajik AJ, et al. Frequency and location of prominent left ventricular trabeculations at autopsy in 474 normal human hearts: Implications for evaluation of mural thrombi by two-dimensional echocardiography. *J Am Coll Cardiol* 1987;9:323–326.
27. Ritter M, Oechslin E, Sutsch G. Isolated noncompaction of the myocardium in adults. *Mayo Clin Proc* 1997;72:26–31.
28. Agmon Y, Connolly H, Olson L, et al. Noncompaction of the ventricular myocardium. *J Am Soc Echocardiogr* 1999;20:859–863.
29. Veinot JP, Harrity PJ, Gentile F, et al. Anatomy of the normal left atrial appendage: A quantitative study of age-related changes in 500 autopsy hearts: Implications for echocardiographic examination. *Circulation* 1997;96:3112–3115.
30. McAlpine W. *Heart and Coronary Arteries: An Anatomic Atlas for Radiologic Diagnosis and Surgical Treatment*. New York: Springer-Verlag; 1975.
31. Naqueh SF, Lakkis NM, He ZX, et al. Role of myocardial contrast echocardiography during nonsurgical septal reduction therapy for hypertrophic obstructive cardiomyopathy. *J Am Coll Cardiol* 1988; 32:225–229.
32. Yetman AT, McCrindle BW, MacDonald C, et al. Myocardial bridging in children with hypertrophic cardiomyopathy: A risk factor for sudden death. *N Engl J Med* 1998;339:1201–1209.
33. Gras D, Mabo P, Tang T, et al. Multisite pacing as a supplemental treatment of congestive heart failure: Preliminary results of the Medtronic Inc in Sync Study. *PACE* 1998;21:2249–2255.
34. Kar S, Nordlander R. Coronary veins: An alternate route to ischemic myocardium. *Heart Lung* 1992;21:148–157.
35. Kar S, Drury JK, Hajduczki I, et al. Synchronized coronary venous retroperfusion for support and salvage of ischemic myocardium during elective and failed angioplasty. *J Am Coll Cardiol* 1991;18:271–282.
36. Lazar HL, Haan CK, Yang X, et al: Reduction of infarction size with coronary venous retroperfusion. *Circulation* 1992;86:11351–11352.
37. Schiller NB, Shah PM, Crawford M, et al. Recommendations for quantitation of the left ventricle by two-dimensional echocardiography: American Society of Echocardiography Committee on Standards, Subcommittee on Quantitation of Two-Dimensional Echocardiograms. *J Am Soc Echocardiogr* 1989;2:358–367.
38. Nagel E, Lehmkuhl H, Bocksch W, et al. Noninvasive diagnosis of ischemia-induced wall motion abnormalities with the use of high-dose dobutamine stress MRI comparison with dobutamine stress echocardiography. *Circulation* 1999;99:763–770.
39. Ichikawa H, Matsubara O. Studies on the microvasculature of human myocardium. *Bull Tokyo Med Dent Univ* 1977;24:53–65.
40. Cannon RO, Leon MB, Watson RM, et al. Chest pain and "normal" coronary arteries: The role of small coronary arteries. *Am J Cardiol* 1985;55:50B–60B.
41. Parodi O, Sambuceti G. The role of coronary microvascular dysfunction in the genesis of cardiovascular diseases. *Q J Nucl Med* 1996;40:9–16.
42. Schwartzkopff B, Motz W, Frenzel H, et al. Structural and functional alterations of the intramyocardial coronary arterioles in patients with arterial hypertension. *Circulation* 1993;88:993–1002.
43. Krams R, Kofflard MJM, Duncker DJ, et al. Decreased coronary flow reserve in hypertrophic cardiomyopathy is related to remodeling of the coronary microcirculation. *Circulation* 1998;97:23–233.
44. Oh JK, Seward JB, Tajik AJ. Contrast echocardiography. In: Weinberg RW, Simmons LA, Madrigal R, eds. *The Echo Manual,* 2d ed. Philadelphia: Lippincott-Raven; 1999:245–249.
45. Kantor B, McKenna CJ, Caccitolo JA, et al. Transmyocardial and percutaneous myocardial revascularization: Current and future roles in the treatment of coronary artery disease. *Mayo Clin Proc* 1999; 74:585–592.
46. Harmon J Jr, Edwards WD. Venous valves in subclavian and internal jugular veins. *Am J Cardiovasc Pathol* 1987;1:51–54.
47. Maclellan-Tobert SG, Buithieu J, Belohlavek M, et al: Three-dimensional imaging used for virtual dissection, image banking and

physical replications of anatomy and physiology. *Echocardiography* 1998;15:89–98.

48. Bruining N, Roelandt J, Grunst G, et al. Three-dimensional echocardiography: The gateway to virtual reality. *Echocardiography* 1999;16:417–423.

49. Seward JB, Belohlavek M, Kinter T, et al. Evolving era of multidimensional medical imaging. *Mayo Clin Proc* 1999; 74:399–414.

C H A P T E R 4

# NORMAL PHYSIOLOGY OF THE CARDIOVASCULAR SYSTEM

Martin M. LeWinter / George Osol



The cardiovascular system functions to deliver oxygen, nutrients, and other essential molecules to the tissues and carry waste products (e.g., $CO_2$, metabolic end products) to the organs responsible for their elimination (lungs, liver, kidney). Two separate circulations in series have evolved. The pulmonary circulation is a low-resistance, high-capacitance vascular bed specialized for bidirectional gas exchange with the environment. The systemic circulation consists of multiple, relatively high resistance vascular beds specialized for delivery of oxygen and nutrients to tissues and extraction of $CO_2$ and metabolic waste products. Blood flows sequentially through the two circulations by the action of two highly adapted pumps in series that together form the heart. Each side of the heart is composed of two chambers: (1) a thin-walled atrium that accepts venous blood from its respective circulation and also has a booster pump function and (2) a thicker-walled ventricle that pumps the blood to its respective circulation.

The cardiovascular system must function under a wide variety of demands. During exercise, the amount of blood pumped, the *cardiac output* (CO), increases fourfold or more.[1,2] Extremes of temperature require that the system function to maximize heat loss or conservation. Beat-to-beat variation in loading of the heart—related to functions such as respiration—require exquisitely fine tuning of the stroke volume (SV) produced by each side. There is no room for error; even a slight, sustained mismatch of left- and right-sided SV would be catastrophic. This chapter reviews the cellular and organ-level cardiac and vascular mechanisms nature has devised to accomplish these tasks.

## CARDIAC FUNCTION

### The Cardiac Cycle

First, consider the sequence of events that occur during a single heartbeat, or cardiac cycle (Fig. 4-1, Plate 28). Before mechanical activity begins, an electrical signal is delivered to the myocardium. Electrical signaling is accomplished by specialized conduction system (SCS) tissue that controls heart rate (HR) in response to various influences (especially sympathetic and parasympathetic stimulation); it provides a normal sequence of activation of the chambers that maximizes efficient contraction and filling. At the cellular level, the electrical signal initiates biochemical processes underlying contraction. With respect to HR, SCS cells have the property of spontaneous electrical depolarization; they function as pacemakers that control the rate of beating. The sinoatrial node (SAN), located in the right atrium (RA), is the component of the SCS that has the fastest spontaneous depolarization rate and therefore normally controls HR. It is directly influenced by the autonomic nervous and neuroendocrine systems, which modulate beat-to-beat and longer-term variation in HR.

At the body surface, activity of the SCS and spread of the electric impulse is represented by the electrocardiogram (ECG) (Chap. 13). At the cellular level, electrical excitation consists of transmission of a membrane-based depolarizing-repolarizing current called the *action potential* (AP), which is propagated through the heart by way of the SCS, ultimately reaching individual myocytes.

The AP begins in the SAN, traverses SCS tissue in both atria, and spreads to atrial myocytes, causing atrial contraction (ECG P wave). Atrial SCS tissue then converges at the atrioventricular node (AVN) region, consisting of the AVN itself and the more distal His bundle. These structures are located in the junctional region where interatrial and interventricular septa meet. The AVN is an area of relatively slow conduction that is responsible for most of the normal delay between atrial and ventricular contraction (PR interval). A properly timed delay maximizes the booster pump function of the atria and protects the ventricles from excessively rapid stimulation. From the His bundle, electrical excitation spreads through large intraventricular fascicles, the left and right bundles. The left bundle then branches into the left anterior and posterior fascicles. The bundle-branch systems ramify within the ventricular myocardium. Their smallest branches are Purkinje system fibers. The electrical signal is transmitted from Purkinje fibers to ventricular myocytes, which contract after a series of cellular events. Depolarization of ventricular myocardium

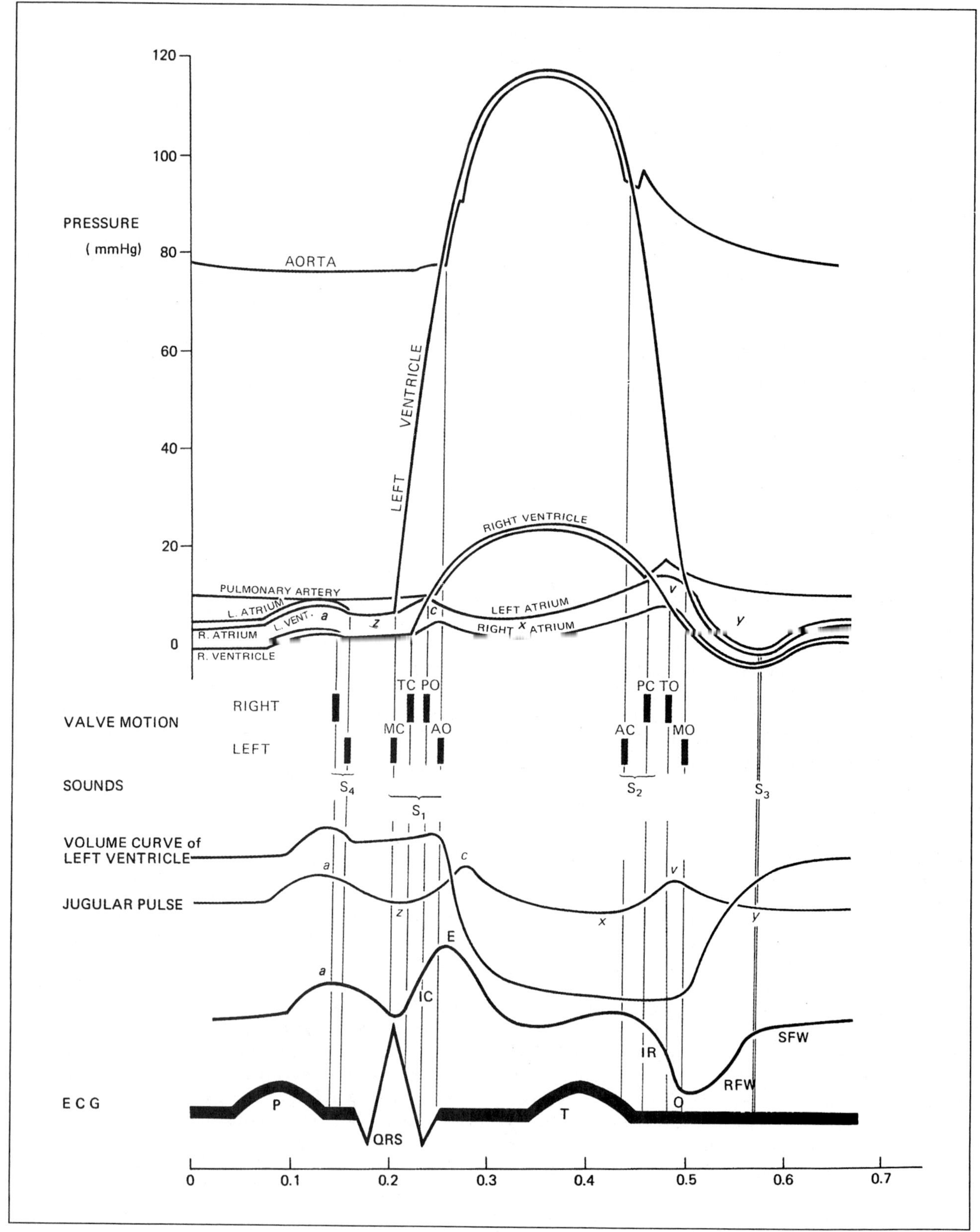


FIGURE 4-1 (Plate 28) Electrical and mechanical events during the cardiac cycle. Shown are pressure curves of great vessels and cardiac chambers, valvular events, timing of heart sounds, LV volume curve, jugular venous pulse wave, and electrocardiogram (ECG). MC and TC, mitral and tricuspid valve closure; PO and AO, pulmonic and aortic valve opening; AC and PC, aortic and pulmonic valve closure; TO and MO, tricuspid and mitral valve opening.

accounts for the ECG QRS complex. Within the myocardium, the AP spreads from myocyte to myocyte through specialized structures called *intercalated disks,* containing low-resistance gap junctions that allow preferential current flow. The left ventricle (LV), the most massive cardiac chamber, is the largest source of electrical potential differences. Electrical activation of the LV begins in the interventricular septum, spreads toward the anteroapical region, and reaches the posterior base last. Right ventricular (RV) activation begins slightly after the LV. Normal electrical activation causes a coordinated sequence of contraction and relaxation of the cardiac chambers, resulting in ejection of blood by the ventricles into the aorta and pulmonary artery (PA), followed by relaxation and filling.

By convention, the mechanical cycle (Fig. 4-1, Plate 28) begins at ventricular end diastole (ED), the instant just before active tension generation, or systole. Onset of systole is signaled by a sudden, rapid rise in intraventricular pressure. Soon thereafter, ventricular systolic pressure exceeds atrial pressure, at which time mitral and tricuspid valves close. Ventricular pressures then continue to rise rapidly until aortic (Ao) and PA pressures are exceeded, resulting in opening of Ao and pulmonic valves and onset of *ejection* of blood into the systemic and pulmonary circulations. Between mitral/tricuspid valve closure and Ao/pulmonic valve opening, ventricular volume is constant. This phase is termed *isovolumic contraction.* During ejection, ventricular and Ao/PA pressures rise and then fall together. Ao and pulmonic valves close and ejection ends when ventricular pressure falls below Ao and PA pressure, signaled by the *dicrotic notch* of the respective arterial pressures. In the LV, a period then ensues during which pressure continues to fall rapidly until it drops below left atrial (LA) pressure, when the mitral valve (MV) opens. Since Ao and MV are closed and volume is constant, this period is termed *isovolumic relaxation.* Although pulmonic valve closure and tricuspid valve opening are shown as separated in time in Fig. 4-1, the point at which RV pressure falls below PA pressure is so low that the RV isovolumic relaxation period is almost nonexistent.[3]

When ventricular pressure falls below atrial pressure, the atrioventricular (AV) valves open, signaling the onset of the *ventricular filling period.* Initially there is very rapid inflow of blood into the ventricles. The latter is caused by an AV pressure gradient (typically several millimeters of mercury) that develops immediately after the AV pressure crossover (Fig. 4-2). Ventricular pressure normally declines by at least several millimeters of mercury immediately after the onset of filling and then rises rapidly after reaching its minimum. Following this initial *rapid filling phase,* ventricular pressure plateaus, the AV gradient diminishes, and filling slows and may even stop (*diastasis*). Diastasis is immediately succeeded by atrial contraction, which results in a second increase in the AV gradient and injection of an additional bolus of blood into the ventricle. The increase in pressure caused by atrial contraction is the *a wave.* Because of its brief duration, it has relatively little effect on *mean* atrial pressure. Thus atrial pump function augments ventricular filling with little risk of an excessive increase in atrial pressure.

Ventricular volume changes are similar on both sides, except for the virtual absence of RV isovolumic relaxation (Fig. 4-1). The thick-walled LV generates a much higher pressure than the RV, reflecting the high-resistance systemic vascular bed. Pressure waveforms during filling are qualitatively similar in both ventricles but may be up to 7 to 8 mmHg higher in the thicker-walled LV. Table 4-1 lists hemodynamic values in normal adult humans.

LA and RA pressure waveforms are also qualitatively similar (Figs. 4-1 and 4-2). Mean LA pressure is normally higher than RA pressure. The waveforms of atrial contraction and relaxation are detailed in Chap. 12 and Fig. 4-2. Normally, the *a* wave is larger than the *v* wave in the RA, with the reverse in the LA. The *v* wave is followed by a second pressure decline, the *y* descent, that begins with AV valve opening and is more gradual than the simultaneous decline in ventricular pressure occurring at the onset of filling (Fig. 4-2).

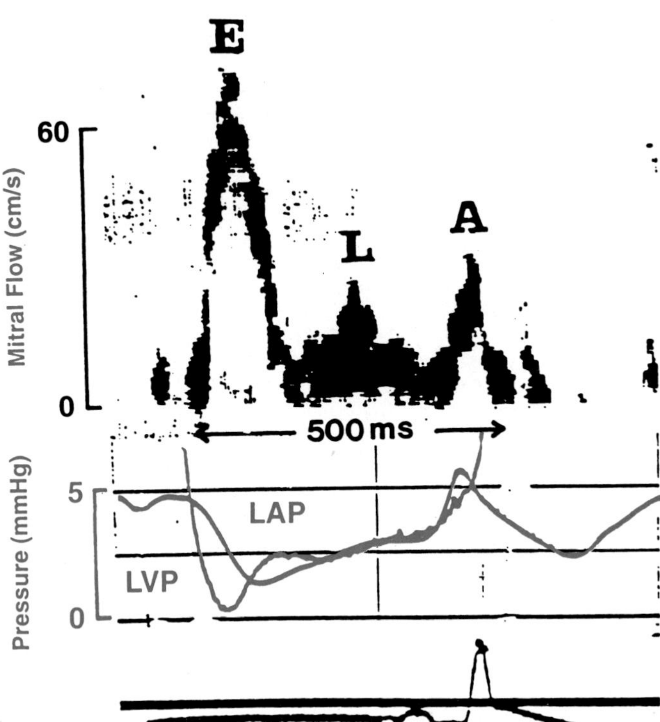


FIGURE 4-2 Mitral flow recorded with a Doppler probe in the mitral annulus and simultaneous LA (LAP) and LV (LVP) pressures in a dog. Note initial gradient immediately after LV pressure crosses LA pressure. As shown here, when recorded with high-fidelity manometers, this is typically followed by a brief reversal of the gradient and then, following the slow-filling phase, by atrial contraction and a second increase in the gradient. Note rapid, early transmitral mitral flow (E wave) and smaller contribution of atrial contraction (A wave). The record also reveals a middiastolic increase in flow (L wave) that is occasionally observed. (From Yellin EL, Nikolic SD. Diastolic suction and the dynamics of LV filling. In: Gaasch WH, LeWinter MM, eds. LV Diastolic Dysfunction and Heart Failure. *Philadelphia: Lea & Febiger, 1994:92. Reproduced with permission of the publisher.*)

The most important beat-to-beat variation in loading of the cardiac chambers is caused by normal respiration. The inspiratory decrease in intrathoracic pressure causes an *increase* in venous return to the right heart and pooling of blood in the pulmonary circulation in association with a small decrease in venous return to the left side of the heart. As a result of these changes in filling during inspiration, RV SV increases in relation to LV SV. This prolongs RV ejection time and delays pulmonic valve closure, accounting for the inspiratory increase in splitting of the second heart sound (Chap. 12).

## The Cellular Basis of Cardiac Contraction

Cardiomyocytes consist of three systems: (1) a sarcolemmal excitation system that participates in spread of the AP and functions as a switch initiating intracellular events giving rise to contraction, (2) an intracellular excitation-contraction coupling (ECC) system that converts the electric excitation signal to a chemical signal and activates the (3) contractile system, a molecular motor based on formation of chemical bridges between actin and myosin (Fig. 4-3, Plate 29).

TABLE 4-1 Hemodynamic Values in Normal Recumbent Adults

| Measurement | Range | Mean |
|---|---|---|
| Cardiac index, L/min/m$^2$ | 2.8–4.2 | 3.4 |
| SV, mL/beat | 30–65 | 47 |
| Arteriovenous oxygen difference, mL per liter of blood | 30–48 | 38 |
| Intravascular pressure,[a] mmHg | | |
| Brachial artery | | |
| Systolic | 90–140 | — |
| Diastolic | 60–90 | — |
| Mean | 70–105 | 85 |
| LV | | |
| Systolic | 90–140 | — |
| ED | 5–12 | — |
| LA or PA wedge | | |
| Mean | 5–12 | — |
| PA | | |
| Systolic | 15–28 | — |
| Diastolic | 5–16 | — |
| Mean | 10–22 | 16 |
| RV | | |
| Systolic | 15–28 | — |
| ED | 0–8 | — |
| RA | | |
| Mean | 0–8 | — |
| LV volume index (mL/m$^2$) | | |
| ED | 50–90 | — |
| ES | 15–25 | — |
| Resistance, dyn·s/cm$^5$ | | |
| Total systemic | 900–1400 | 1150 |
| Systemic arteriolar | 600–900 | 850 |
| Total pulmonary | 150–250 | 200 |
| Pulmonary arteriolar | 45–120 | 70 |

[a]Baseline for pressure measurements one-half of anteroposterior chest diameter. 1 mmHg = 133.332; Pa = 0.133 kPa.

## EXCITATION SYSTEM

This system is discussed in more detail in Chap. 27. The cellular AP consists of a transient, local transsarcolemmal depolarizing current that raises transmembrane potential from its resting value of negative 80 to 90 mV to slightly positive values, followed by a depolarizing current that returns the potential to the rest value[4–7] (Fig. 4-4). The AP is initiated within SCS tissue and propagates to individual myocytes. It results from a series of coordinated changes in conductance of specific ionic species through gated sarcolemmal channels. The earliest and largest component of depolarization is caused by a rapid, inward Na current. The resting potential is established and maintained by the transsarcolemmal Na-K-ATPase, which uses energy from ATP hydrolysis to pump Na ions out of the cytoplasm. The most important component of the AP-initiating contraction is a relatively *slow, inward Ca current* through voltage-sensitive, L-type Ca channels[5,7,8] ($Ca^{2+}$ influx in Fig. 4-4). These channels open and the current begins when transmembrane potential reaches −35 to −20 mV and continues well after the Na current has ceased. The Ca current is mainly responsible for the AP plateau and ceases when L-type channels become inactivated and regenerative currents begin repolarization. L-type channels, also termed *dihydropyridine* (*DHP*) *receptors,* are concentrated in invaginations of the sarcolemma (the *transverse-tubule system*) in close proximity to sarcoplasmic reticulum (SR) membrane-associated *ryanodine receptor* (RyR) Ca release channels.

The AP results in net movement of Ca ions into and net movement of Na ions out of the cytoplasm. Ionic balance is restored mainly by another sarcolemmal ion-transport mechanism, the *Na–Ca exchanger.*[7,9–11]

## EXCITATION-CONTRACTION COUPLING SYSTEM

ECC is accomplished by the *sarcotubular system,* an arrangement of specialized sarcolemmal and intracellular membranes that controls and amplifies the ability of the AP to switch the contractile system on and off by creating electrochemical signals between the sarcolemma and intracellular organelles.

The sarcotubular system consists of two main components, transverse or T tubules and the SR[7,12,13] (Fig. 4-3, Plate 29). T tubules are transverse invaginations of the sarcolemma concentrated at the Z line of the sarcomere. The SR is a longitudinally oriented system of intracellular sacs and tubules consisting of collar-like structures encircling the myofibrils at 1- to 2-$\mu$m spacings, forming repeating closed compartments that extend along the length of each myofibril. At the end of each collar is a bulge (*cistern*) that closely abuts a T tubule, creating a *dyad* or sometimes a *triad* structure. The gap between cistern and T tubule is bridged by structures called *feet.*

The SR contains a large store of Ca ions released into the cytoplasm as a result of a process termed *Ca-induced Ca release* (CICR)[7,8,14–21] that takes place within or near the dyad. The details of CICR have been revealed by Ca "spark" studies employing Ca concentration-sensitive bioluminescent dyes in conjunction with confocal microscopy[17–21] (Fig. 4-5). These studies have allowed delineation of fundamental events underlying the increase in Ca during systole. As noted earlier, DHP receptor channels are concentrated in the T-tubule region of the dyad. Adjacent SR membranes in the dyad contain the Ca release RyR channels [7,8,16,22–25] that bridge the cisternal membrane near the foot structures. RyR channels are organized into functional groupings containing more than 100 individual RyRs. When the AP depolarizes the membrane in the dyad region, the voltage-sensitive DHP receptor channel gate opens, allowing movement of Ca across the sarcolemma into the gap region of the dyad. The nearby RyR channels are activated (opened) by the local rise in Ca concentration,[7,22–25] resulting in rapid release of much larger amounts of Ca ions from the SR cisternae into the cytoplasm[26] (Fig. 4-6). In addition to being a Ca release channel, the RyR is also a scaffolding protein that localizes several regulatory proteins to the junctional area.[21,24] These include calmodulin, FK-506 binding protein, protein kinase A (PKA), and phosphatases 1 and 2A.

Amplification of Ca release is inherent in CICR because each DHP channel induces release of Ca from about 6 to 20 RyRs and because of the large Ca concentration gradient between SR and cytoplasm.[7,8,16,21–25] The CICR increase in intracellular Ca concentration is very transient, because Ca ions rapidly bind to contractile proteins and are removed from the cytoplasm by the Na-Ca exchanger and the SR Ca ATPase pump (SERCA2).

In order for contraction to be turned off (i.e., relaxation) Ca ions bound to contractile proteins must be returned to their SR storage sites and the relatively small number that enter during the AP must be transported back to the extracellular space. As noted earlier, the Na-Ca exchanger is primarily responsible for extrusion of Ca; the sarcolemmal Ca pump has a minimal role. The most important mechanism of reuptake of Ca ions by the SR is pumping by SERCA2, a SR membrane-spanning protein[7,13,21,27] (Fig. 4-3, Plate 29). SERCA2 uses energy from ATP hydrolysis to pump the bulk of

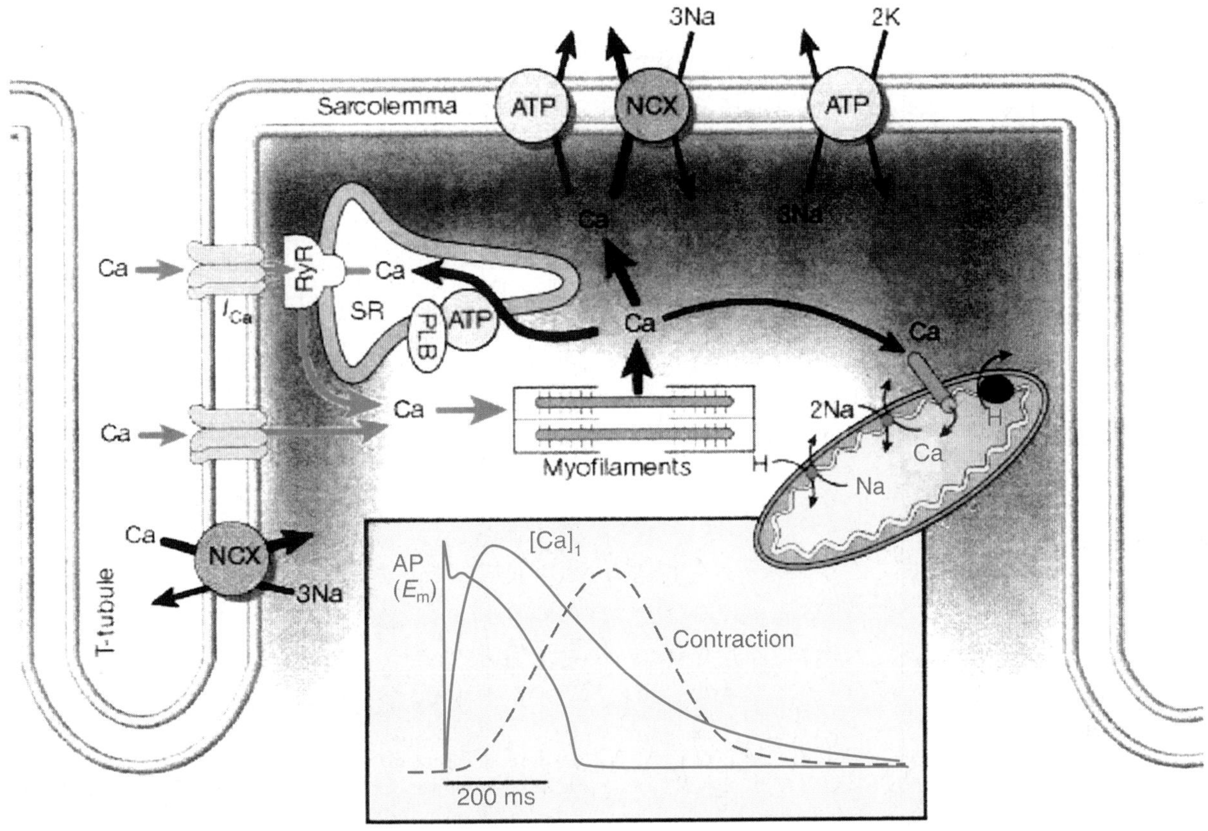


FIGURE 4-3 (Plate 29) Schematic diagram of the major cellular components involved in contraction of the myocyte, with emphasis on calcium transport mechanisms. SR, sarcoplasmic reticulum; RyR, ryanodine receptor; ATP, sarcolemmal and SR ATPase pumps, PLB, phospholamban; NCX, sodium-calcium exchanger. Mitochondrion shown lower right. Inset, time course of myocyte AP (action potential), intracellular calcium transient, force of contraction. (From Bers.[21] Reprinted with permission of the publisher.)

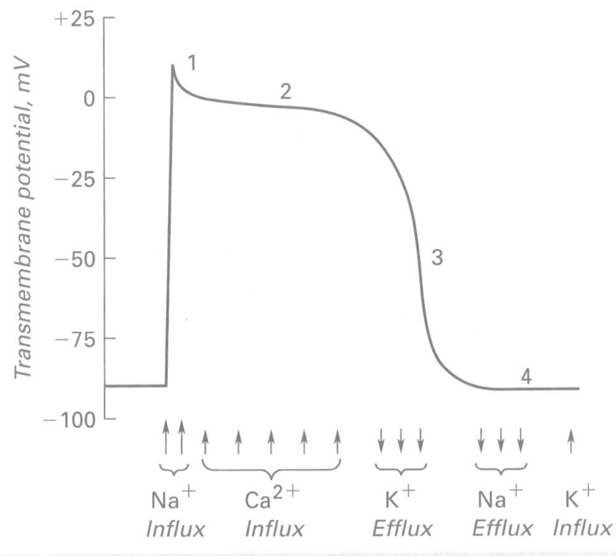


FIGURE 4-4 Phases of cellular AP and major associated currents in ventricular myocyte. Initial phase zero spike (not labeled) and overshoot (phase 1) is caused by rapid inward Na current, the plateau (phase 2) by slow inward Ca current through L-type Ca channels, and repolarization (phase 3) by outward K current. Phase 4 resting potential (Na efflux, K influx) is maintained by the Na-K-ATPase. Na-Ca exchanger is mainly responsible for Ca extrusion. In specialized conduction system tissue, there is spontaneous depolarization during phase 4 until the voltage resulting in opening of the Na channel is reached.

Ca ions released during CICR back into the SR. Ca ions pumped back into the SR enter a "reuptake pool" and move to a "release" pool.

SERCA2 pumping is partially self-regulating, since its speed increases in proportion to free Ca concentration. It is also regulated by a closely associated protein, phospholamban (PLB), a key modulator of responses to adrenergic signaling.[21,28–33] PLB inhibits SERCA2.[30,31] $\beta$-Adrenergic stimulation results in phosphorylation of PLB by activation of cyclic AMP–dependent PKA, which reduces PLB inhibition of SERCA2 and increases Ca cycled per beat and reuptake rate. Adrenergic stimulation also causes PKA-mediated phosphorylation of L-type Ca channels,[8,15,34] resulting in increased transsarcolemmal Ca current and the RyR channel itself,[21] the latter resulting in gating changes that further increase Ca release.

## CONTRACTILE SYSTEM

The building block of the contractile system is the sarcomere[12] (Fig. 4-7), a recurring arrangement of the proteins responsible for mechanical activity. Each sarcomere is composed of two bundles of longitudinally oriented filaments.[12] *Thick filaments,* ~1.6 $\mu$m long, are composed of cardiac myosin, a complex of proteins in a trigonal array at the center of the sarcomere's length. In addition to myosin, two other proteins are associated with the thick filament, titin and myosin-binding protein C (see below). At each end of this array, a set of ~1 $\mu$m–long *thin filaments* composed of actin and the proteins tropomyosin (Tm) and troponin (Tn) interdigitates with the thick filaments. The other ends of the thin filaments extend to the ends of the sarcomere, where they attach to a transverse structure, the *Z line*. The distance between sequential Z lines is sarcomere length (SL). At SL

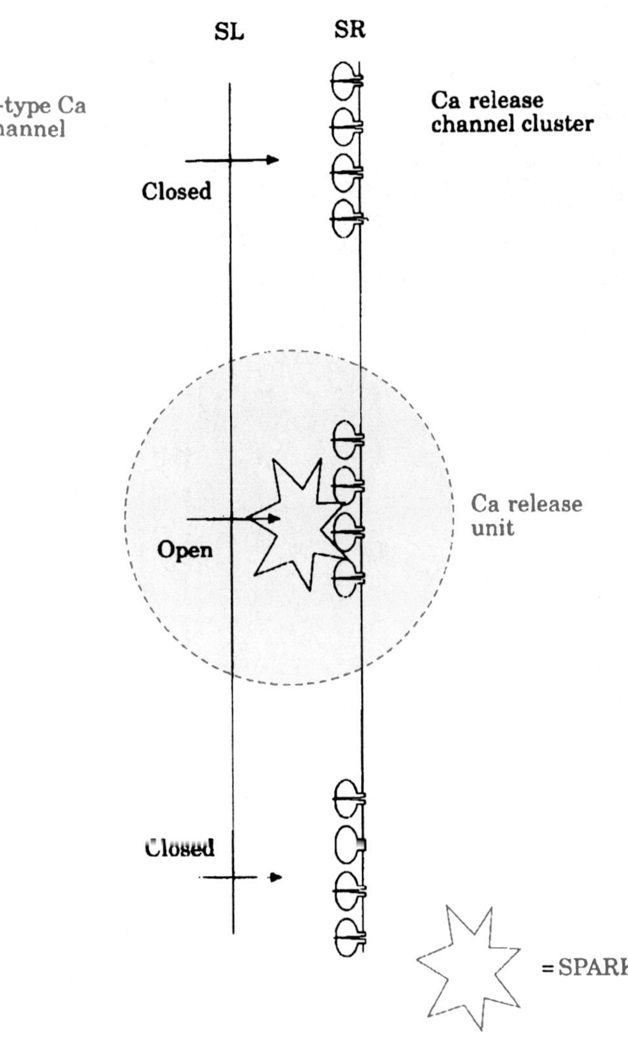


FIGURE 4-5 Schematic of Ca-induced Ca release from SR resulting in a Ca "spark." Opening of sarcolemmal (SL) L-type Ca channel results in movement of a relatively small amount of Ca ions into the cell. The latter causes opening of a number of nearby RyR channels (Ca release unit) with local release of a large amount of Ca ions from the SR and appearance of a "spark," as bioluminescent dye responds to change in local Ca concentration. (From Williams.[8] Reproduced with permission of the publisher.)

~2.2 μm, at which maximal force is produced, the central end of each thin filament overlaps 0.7 μm of the distal ends of the thick filaments (the *overlap zone*). The 0.3-μm length of nonoverlapped thin filaments extending to the Z line and the corresponding 0.3 μm of nonoverlapped thin filaments in the adjacent sarcomere constitute the *I band*. The centrally positioned thick filaments constitute the *A band*. Alternating A and I bands are responsible for the *striated* appearance of cardiac muscle.

In addition to the portion of each myosin molecule oriented longitudinally to form the thick filament, myosin *heads* protrude from the thick filament surface and can move freely in the space between thick and thin filaments (Fig. 4-8, Plate 30). This protruding portion includes the *heavy chain* that forms the crossbridge, the molecular structure that interacts with actin and is responsible for conversion of chemical energy to mechanical energy.[35,36] Myosin heavy chains contain a domain that binds with actin and a site of ATPase activity.[37,39] They also contain a "neck" region, consisting of essential and

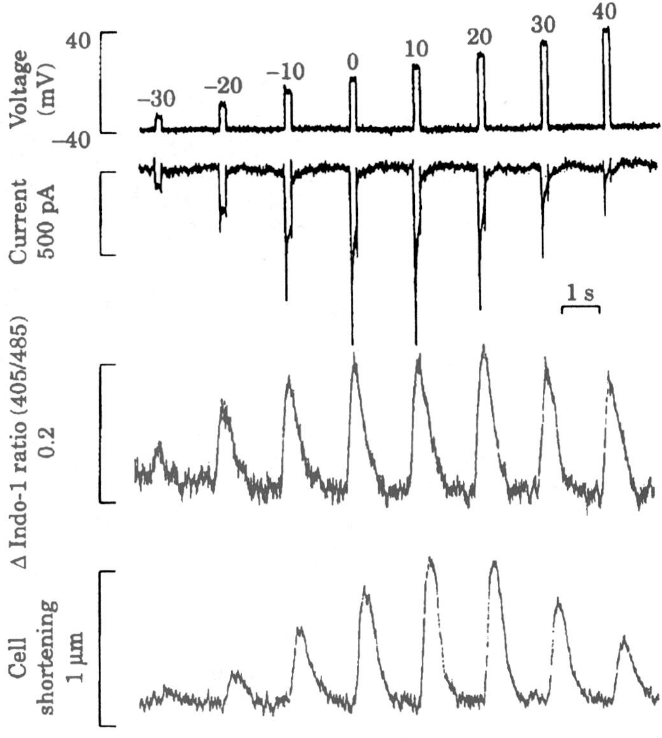


FIGURE 4-6 Intracellular Ca transient obtained with the bioluminescent dye Indo-1 is shown in the middle of this figure. It reflects the average instantaneous intracellular Ca ion concentration. The L-type Ca channel current modified by voltage clamping is shown in the top panel, and myocyte shortening is shown in the bottom panel. Note the voltage dependence of the Ca current and the parallel changes in both the Ca transient and shortening. (From Williams.[8] Reproduced with permission of the publisher.)

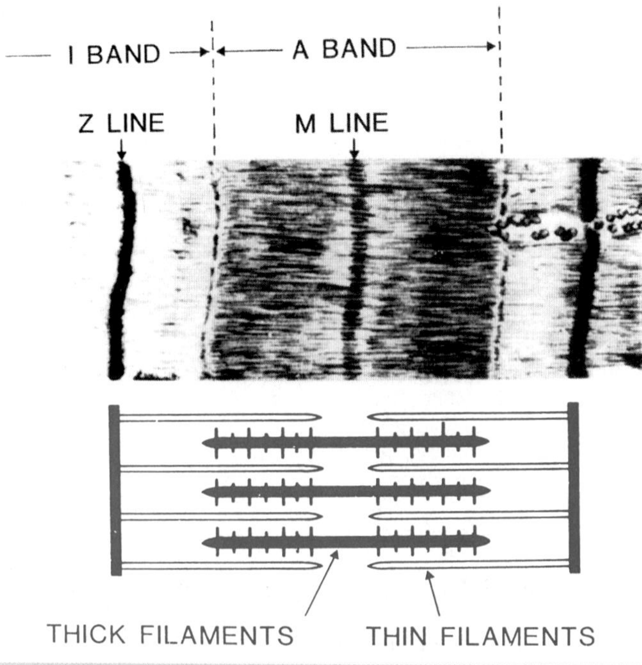


FIGURE 4-7 (*Top*) Electronmicrograph of sarcomere. (*Bottom*) Schematic (see text). (From Woledge RC, Curtin NA, Homsher E. *Energetic Aspects of Muscle Contraction*. London: Academic Press; 1985. Reproduced with permission of the publisher.)

regulatory light chains that connect the head to the thick filament. In mammalian cardiac muscle, myosin heavy chain exists primarily as two isoforms, alpha and beta.[37] The alpha isoform has higher ATPase activity and more rapid rates of crossbridge formation and velocity than beta and is dominant in adult small mammals but not in humans.[38–42]

Titin is a giant sarcomeric protein anchored in the Z line on one end and closely associated with both myosin and myosin-binding protein C on its other end.[43] Titin functions as a molecular spring and is a major determinant of the passive stiffness of the myocyte[43,44] and myocardium. Titin also likely has a role in diastolic suction. Myosin-binding protein C (MyBPC) is bound to both myosin and titin. MyBPC appears to have a role in sarcomere assembly, and its phosphorylation may modulate myosin ATPase activity.[45]

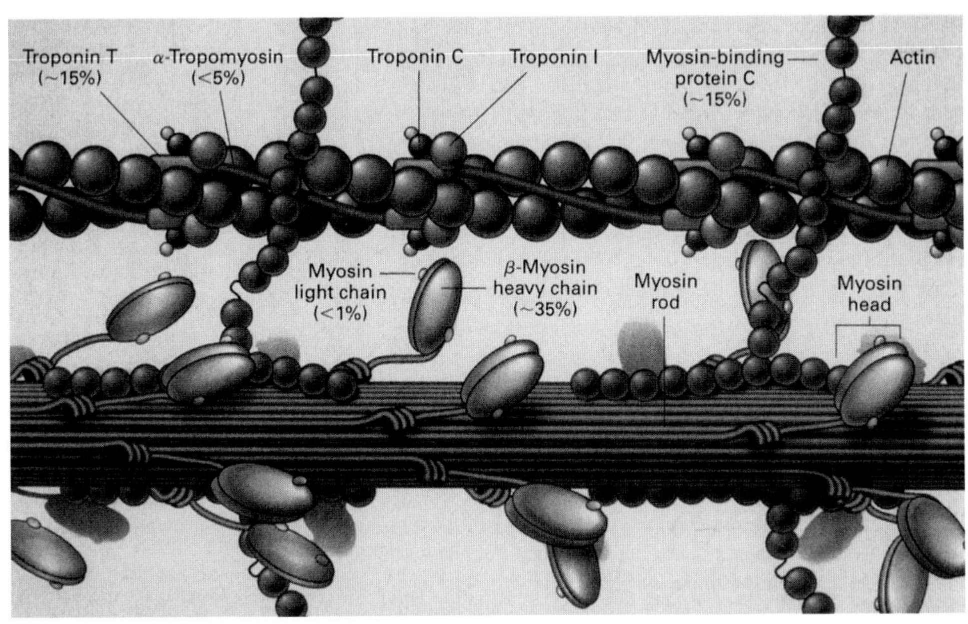


FIGURE 4-8 (Plate 30) Cartoon of sarcomeric proteins (titin not shown). (From Spirito P, Seidman CE, McKenna WJ, Maron BJ. The management of hypertrophic cardiomyopathy. *N Eng J Med* 1997; 336:775. Reprinted with permission of the publisher.)

Actin monomers are arranged in a double helix to form the core of the thin filament[46,47] (Figs. 4-8, Plate 30, and 4-9). Tm is adsorbed longitudinally along the thin filament. Each Tm spans seven actin monomers, with a short overlap segment at the ends of adjacent Tms. Tn, composed of three subunits, TnC, TnI, and TnT, is adsorbed on Tm, also in a ratio of one per seven actin monomers. TnC contains a Ca-binding site, TnI variably binds to Tm and TnC, and TnT links Tn to Tm at the overlap zone. The combined Tm-Tn complex is responsible for the ability of Ca ions, binding to TnC, to act as a switch initiating crossbridge formation. TnI and TnT, myosin regulatory light chain, and MyBPC all have phosphorylation sites.[49,50] Phosphorylation of these proteins, especially TnI and TnT, modulates the activity of myosin ATPase.

The sequence of events that ensues when the contractile system is activated by Ca ions entering the cytoplasm as a result of CICR may be summarized as follows[46,47] (Fig. 4-9): in diastole, with low [Ca], Tm occupies a position on actin that inhibits actin-myosin interaction. It has been proposed that at diastolic [Ca] crossbridges exist in both a truly detached or *blocked* state and a weakly attached, non–force producing state.[47,49,50] Weakly attached crossbridges may exist in two states, *closed* and *open,* depending on the position of Tm on actin. With activation, Ca ions bind to TnC and cause a complex rearrangement of the Tn complex and consequently a change in the position of Tm on actin that releases inhibition of actin-myosin. Also, the kinetics of crossbridge formation are affected by increasing the rate of transitions from non–force producing to force-producing states.

Two other factors are important in *thin filament activation.* One is *nearest-neighbor interaction*[47] along actin monomers. Thus, binding

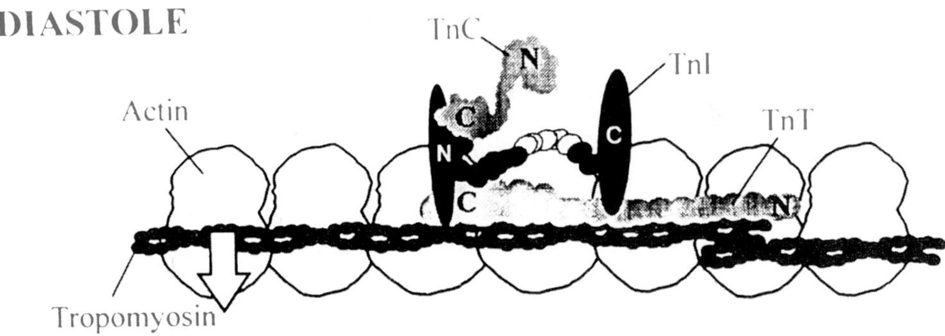


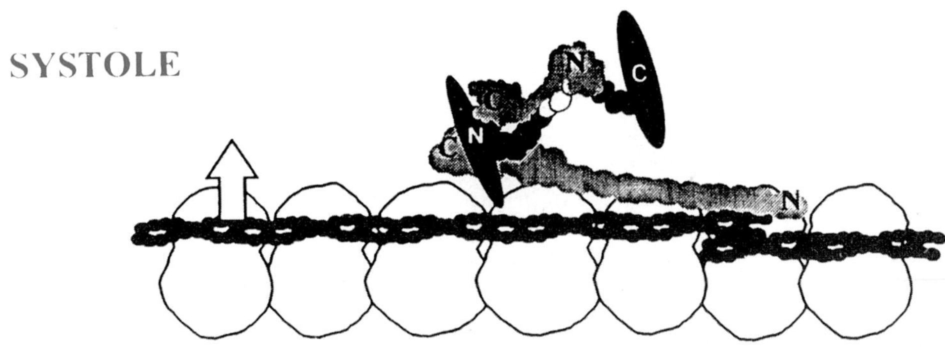


FIGURE 4-9 Cartoon of the thin filament with actin and regulatory proteins, Tm and Tn complex, showing conformational differences between inactive state (diastole) and activation (systole). C, COOH terminus; N, $NH_2$ terminus. (From Solaro RJ, Rarick. HM. *Circ Res* 1998;83:471. Reproduced with permission from the publisher.)

of Ca to Tn causes the process of crossbridge formation to spread down the thin filament. A second is strong binding of actin to myosin,[47,51,52] which begins once inhibition of actin-myosin interaction is relieved. Under most conditions, systolic [Ca] is not high enough to achieve maximum force and/or shortening; i.e., the muscle is *submaximally* activated. The relation between [Ca] and force/shortening between diastole and maximal activation is very steep (Fig. 4-10). This property is thought to be due to both nearest-neighbor interactions and strong actin-myosin binding. As a result, contractile reserve can be recruited with modest changes in Ca concentration.

When Ca binds to TnC, the crossbridge cycle is switched on, and actin and myosin undergo a chemical reaction powered by ATP hydrolysis, in which a series of transitions are made from detached/weakly bound states to force-producing states and back.[35,36,38,53] ATP hydrolysis occurs in conjunction with the transition from force-producing to detached/weakly bound states. While the myosin head is strongly bound to actin on the activated thin filament, conformational energy is released, causing it to rotate like the oar of a rower seated on the actin filament (Fig. 4-11). This motion generates a force propelling the thin filament along the thick filament toward the center of the sarcomere. This process occurs repeatedly and randomly at millions of actin-myosin crossbridges, causing large-scale force and/or motion.

The amount of force and/or shortening due to crossbridge formation is related to the restraints, or *load,* placed on the muscle.[53,54] If no external restraint is applied, crossbridges propel the filaments at the maximum speed their chemical reactions permit and a maximum amount of displacement occurs with no force generation. If shortening is opposed by an external load, as occurs during physiologic contraction, crossbridge motion is slowed, allowing time for force to develop and more crossbridges to find binding sites on the thin filaments. At the extreme of an *isometric* contraction, where the muscle is so restrained that there is no external shortening or work, crossbridge energy is used almost exclusively for force development. This trade-off between force and motion is reflected in the hyperbolic shape of the force-versus-velocity relation and the parabolic shape of the power or work-versus-load relation in isolated cardiac muscle

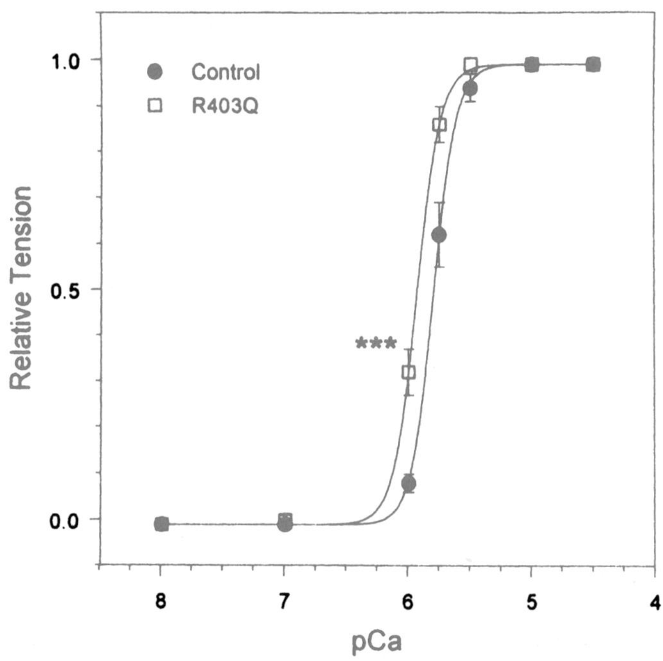


FIGURE 4-10 Relation between log Ca concentration (pCa) and isometric tension in detergent-treated ("skinned") strips of mouse cardiac muscle. R403Q indicates a transgenic animal with a mutation causing hypertrophic cardiomyopathy; control is wild type. Skinning results in loss of integrity of the sarcolemma and all intracellular membranes, leaving sarcomeric proteins intact. In skinned strip, the ionic milieu of the contractile proteins can be manipulated and their behavior studied in isolation from the excitation and ECC systems. Note very steep relation between isometric tension and pCa between relaxing (pCa > 7) and fully activating Ca concentrations (pCa 5) in both strips. The relation is shifted to the left in R403Q mice. (From Blanchard E, Seidman C, Seidman JG, et al. Altered crossbridge kinetics in the $\alpha$MHC$^{403/+}$ mouse model of familial hypertrophic cardiomyopathy. *Circ Res* 1999;84:475. Reprinted with permission of the publisher.)

(Fig. 4-12). There is also a reciprocal relation between load and the crossbridge cycling rate.[53,54]

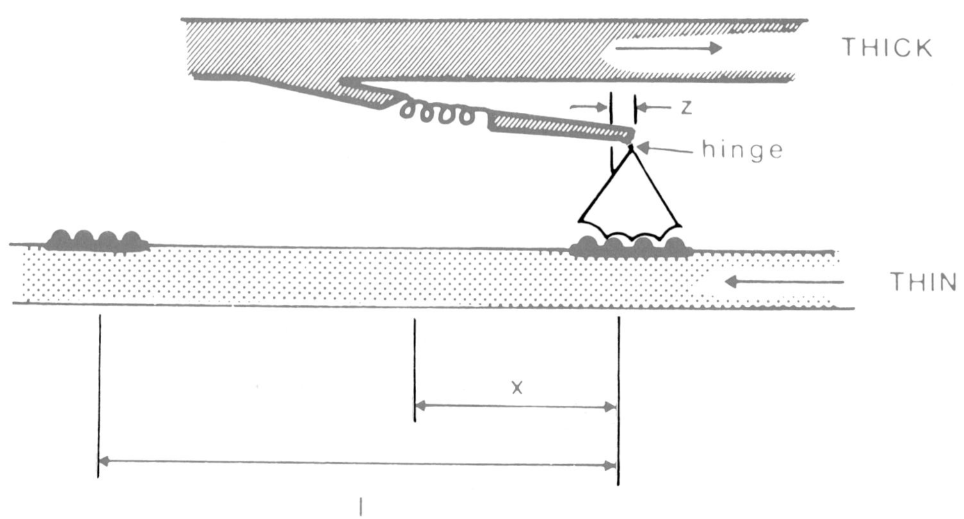


FIGURE 4-11 Schematic of the mechanical interaction between the myosin head (triangular structure) and actin located on the thin filament. Letter *z* denotes the distance moved by the thick filament as a result of rotation of the head region (see text). (From Woledge RC, Curtin NA, Homsher E. *Energetic Aspects of Muscle Contraction*. London: Academic Press; 1985. Reproduced with permission of the publisher.)

Another key determinant of mechanical performance of an activated sarcomere is its initial SL, as reflected by the muscle's initial length (its *preload*)[47,48,55,56] (Fig. 4-13). Force (or shortening) is maximal at initial SL ~2.2 $\mu$m and falls off very rapidly below approximately 2.0 $\mu$m. The ascending length–active tension/force relation is mainly caused by changes in Ca activation of crossbridges as a function of SL.[55,56] This may be related to the fact that thick and thin filaments move farther apart at shorter SLs.[57] The resulting change in geometry causes a decrease in effective activation at any [Ca]. However, alternative mechanisms have been proposed.[58] Regardless of the mechanism, *length-dependent activation* is the primary mechanism at the sarcomere level of the Frank-Starling law of the heart. Although a *descending limb* of the length-tension relation is evident in isolated muscle, it is not present in the intact ventricle.

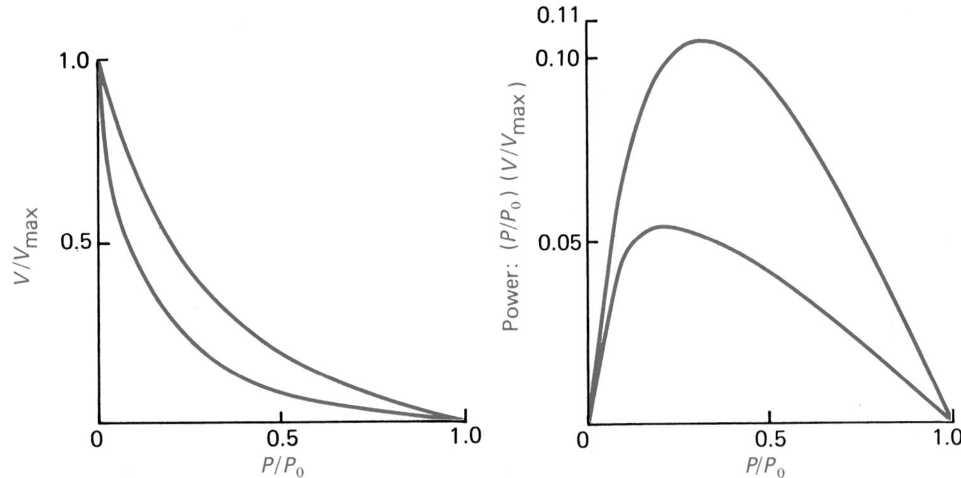


FIGURE 4-12 *(Left)* Force (*P*) versus velocity (*V*) relation for two muscles with differing contractile performance. Velocity normalized to maximum unloaded value ($V_{max}$) and force to maximum isometric value ($P_0$). *(Right)* Normalized force versus power (force × velocity) for same muscles. Power is maximal at midrange force values. (Modified from Woledge RC, Curtin NA, Homsher E. *Energetic Aspects of Muscle Contraction.* London: Academic Press; 1985. Reproduced with permission of the publisher.)

## MYOCYTE RELAXATION

Myocyte relaxation is a complex process whose rate is determined by three main factors: the kinetics of crossbridge cycling (the rate at which crossbridges transition from a force-producing to a non–force producing state), the sensitivity of the myofilament to calcium, and the activity of the main Ca reuptake and extrusion mechanisms.[57,60] Thus, slower kinetics of crossbridge cycling, increased Ca sensitivity of force production, and reduced activity of SERCA2 and/or the Na-Ca exchanger slow relaxation. Relaxation is also partly modulated by the load on the myocyte.

## ENERGY METABOLISM AND MECHANOENERGETICS

Cardiomyocytes are heavily dependent on oxidative metabolism and contain large numbers of mitochondria. Under basal conditions, fatty acids are preferentially taken up and oxidized to generate ATP.[61] During stress, glucose uptake, glycogenolysis, and glycolysis become more important. Certain ion pumps—e.g., SERCA2—may be especially dependent on glycolytic ATP.[62] Nitric oxide (NO) generated by vascular endothelium decreases myocardial oxygen consumption ($\dot{V}_{O_2}$) due to a direct effect on mitochondrial respiration and may have a role in normal control of energy production and utilization.[63]

The processes accounting for the majority of myocardial energy consumption are crossbridge cycling, Ca reuptake by the SR (SERCA2), and basal metabolism. Each crossbridge cycle consumes one high-energy phosphate bond, although at very rapid cycling rates one ATP may fuel more than one cycle. SERCA2 uses one high-energy phosphate bond for every two Ca ions pumped. The rate of energy consumption is dependent on loading conditions and resulting work and power generation.[64] The thermodynamic efficiency of heart muscle, (total mechanical energy output divided by total chemical energy input) is uncertain.

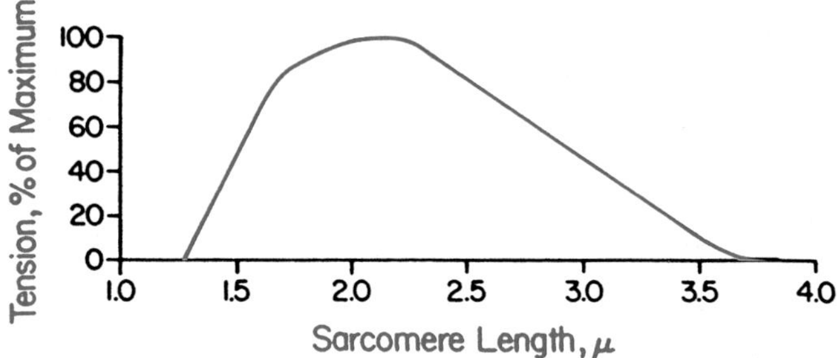


FIGURE 4-13 Schematic of relation between sarcomere length and developed tension (or force). Note fall in tension at lengths below approximately 2.2 μm.. At very long sarcomere lengths, thick-thin filament overlap is reduced, resulting in descending limb of relation (not observed in ventricle). (Modified from Braunwald E, Ross J Jr, Sonnenblick EH, eds. *Mechanisms of Contraction of the Normal and Failing Heart.* Boston: Little, Brown; 1976:77.)

## Cellular Control of Contractility

This section is divided into intrinsic and extrinsic control systems. *Intrinsic control* includes processes that are components of the normal mechanical behavior of cardiac muscle. *Extrinsic control* includes mechanisms that require elaboration/secretion of cardioactive substances by the myocyte or some other cell and classic neurohumoral modulation of function.

### INTRINSIC CONTROL SYSTEMS

The most obvious is *length-dependent activation* underlying the Frank-Starling relation. This allows heart muscle to adjust its performance on a beat-to-beat basis and is taken up further in the discussion of ventricular function, below.

An important intrinsic mechanism is the *force-frequency relation* (FFR) (Fig. 4-14).[65] At a basal rate of 60/min, the duration of myocardial contraction is such that relaxation would be incomplete at rates achieved during exercise and cause impaired diastolic filling. Therefore mechanisms that speed contraction and relaxation at rapid rates are required. With this abbreviation of contraction, the strength of contraction is markedly enhanced, allowing maintenance of SV even though less time is available for filling and emptying. The mechanism of the positive FFR involves increased and more rapid Ca cycling per beat as frequency increases.[8,21,64,67] Contributing factors include the direct effect of a greater number of APs per unit time, causing intracellular accumulation of Ca ions, and increased SR Ca pumping. Thus, Ca entry increases directly with more frequent opening of L-type Ca channels and indirectly when the Na-Ca exchanger extrudes excess Na ions arising from the increased frequency of sarcolemmal Na channel opening. Operating in isolation, these factors would risk elevation of diastolic [Ca]. However, SR pump speed increases concomitantly, increasing relaxation rate and abbreviating contraction. Besides PLB, SERCA2 activity is under the control of *Ca-activated calmodulin kinase,*[21] which increases SERCA2 activity in response to increased Ca concentration and has built-in frequency sensitivity. Small, transient increases in Ca ions are held in binding sites long enough that repeated increases are summated. This averaging process results in increased speed of the SERCA2 pump in response to increased average and instantaneous Ca concentration.

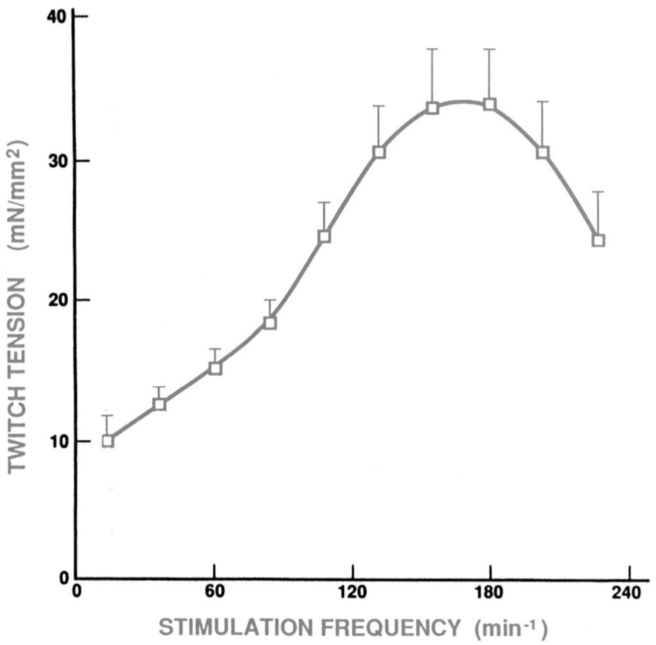


FIGURE 4-14 Example of average relation between developed force and stimulation frequency in strips of human myocardium obtained by epicardial biopsy from a group of patients undergoing coronary bypass surgery, all with normal LV contraction patterns. Note the marked increase in force as contraction frequency increases from typical basal level of 60/min to a value of 170–180/min, at which force is maximal (see text).

The normal FFR depends on the intactness of multiple elements of Ca handling and is depressed in a number of conditions in which the myocardium is diseased or subjected to chronic stress.[66,68] The ratio of SERCA2 pumps to PLB protein has been proposed as an important determinant of magnitude of the FFR. The FFR is markedly amplified by increased $\beta$-adrenergic stimulation.[65] Thus, during stress, increased adrenergic stimulation not only increases HR but also increases the magnitude of FFR occurring in response to increased HR.

### EXTRINSIC CONTROL SYSTEMS

The best-understood and most important extrinsic control is modulation of contractility by adrenergic and cholinergic neural discharge and circulating catecholamines.[65,69,70] Increased adrenergic stimulation markedly increases contractile strength, relaxation, and HR. These effects on the myocardium may be explained as follows: Normal myocytes contain predominantly $\beta_1$ receptors and a minority of $\beta_2$ receptors. Agonist binding to $\beta_1$- or $\beta_2$-adrenergic receptors on the sarcolemma results in an interaction between membrane-associated G protein and guanosine triphosphate (GTP), in which GTP combines with active subunit $G_s$, which activates enzymatic conversion of ATP to cyclic AMP by *adenylate cyclase* on the cytoplasmic side of the receptor complex. Cyclic AMP, in turn, activates PKA, which phosphorylates the L-type Ca channel, altering its gating to allow more Ca ion entry per AP, and PLB, which increases SERCA2 pumping. This results in more rapid removal of Ca from the contractile proteins (faster relaxation), a larger amount of Ca cycled per beat (increased activation), and potentiation of the FFR. Recently $\beta_3$ receptors were reported in myocardium.[70] Here, agonist binding actually decreases contractility.

Increased cholinergic stimulation decreases contractility, possibly by activating nitric oxide synthase-3 (NOS-3). Cholinergic discharge has a weak direct influence on contractile performance but is an important modulator of HR.

A number of other substances influence myocyte function, including circulating neurohormones and molecules produced by myocytes themselves and vascular endothelium. With the possible exception of NO, they are much less important in the normal cardiovascular system than in the intrinsic and extrinsic control systems already discussed. These substances and their signaling pathways are also discussed in Chaps. 6 and 7.

NO is produced in endothelial cells in proximity to cardiac myocytes and in myocytes themselves.[63,71,72] NOS-3 is the predominant form of nitric oxide synthase in the myocyte. NOS-3 is Ca-sensitive and activated by levels of intracellular Ca achieved during normal beating and by muscarinic cholinergic agonists. NO has a negative inotropic effect, which is mediated via cyclic GMP.[63,71,73] NOS-3 activation also blunts catecholamine responses. Inflammatory cytokines also activate NOS-3,[73] which may be important in disease. Endothelial-derived NO may have somewhat different effects than myocyte-derived NO. Thus endothelial-selective, NO-dependent vasodilators cause early and accelerated relaxation with only a modest negative inotropic effect. *Atrial natriuretic peptide* (ANP) and *brain natriuretic peptide* (BNP) produced in atria and ventricles, respectively, are naturally occurring vasodilators and diuretics. These substances have effects on myocyte function that are mediated by endothelial-derived NO. While increased secretion of these hormones has great significance in *heart failure,* their role in physiologic control of myocyte function is likely minor.

A number of substances—including *$\alpha_1$ adrenergic agonists*,[74] *endothelin-1* (ET-1),[75] and *angiotensin II* (ATII)[76,77]—influence myocyte function through activation of phospholipase, with resulting production of inositol triphosphate ($IP_3$) and diacylglycerol (DAG).[78] Although $IP_3$ increases the release of intracellular Ca during contraction, DAG appears to be more importantly involved in myocyte functional responses. Its effects are mediated through activation of protein kinase C (PKC).[78–80] The effects of DAG and PKC activation have been variable. PKC in general has functionally opposite effects on the activation and contractile systems, resulting in increased activator calcium combined with phosphorylation of TnT and TnI,[81] the latter resulting in decreases in crossbridge cycling rate.

## Structure and Function of the Ventricles

### ARCHITECTURE

The LV is a thick-walled chamber with a truncated ellipsoid shape composed of spiraling, sheetlike layers of myocyte bundles (Fig. 4-15). The orientation of the bundles progressively changes from subepicardium to subendocardium, from relatively longitudinal to roughly circumferential in the middle two-thirds of the wall, to longitudinal fibers once again in the subendocardium.[82] Regional wall thickness parallels the local radius of curvature. Thus, near the apex, radius and wall thickness are relatively small.

Contraction of the LV is associated with a wringing motion (torsion) characterized by counterclockwise rotation that is greatest near the apex.[83] Torsion is important for normal ejection and is an inherent feature of the normal spread of excitation and connections between the fiber bundles.[84] This complex architecture results in efficient conversion of shortening of individual myocytes and fibers to wall thickening, which is ultimately responsible for ejection of blood. Thus, even though individual fibers shorten only about 10 percent, the normal LV ejects about two-thirds of its ED volume. Inter-

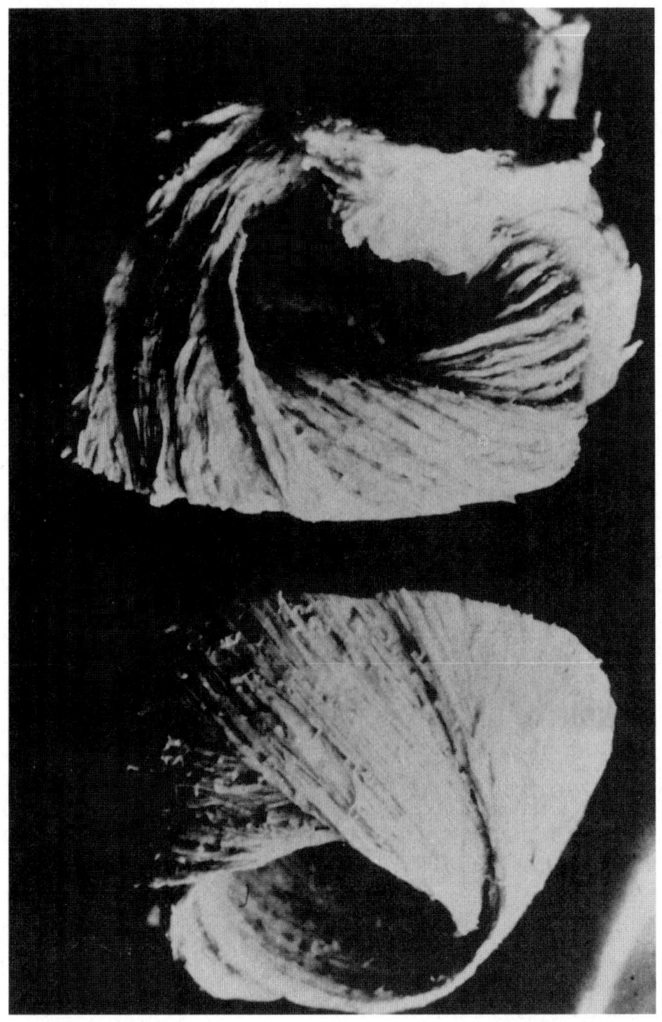

FIGURE 4-15 Three-dimensional architecture of LV, illustrating spiraling bundles of myofibers (see text). (From Streeter.[82] Reprinted with permission of the publisher.)

ventricular septal fibers have a similar orientation and are continuous with those of the LV free wall.

In line with the high-capacitance/low-resistance pulmonary vascular bed, the RV is thinner-walled than the LV and appears crescentic in cross section.[82] A fraction of the mechanical output of the RV results from energy transfer from the LV (systolic ventricular interaction).[83]

Ventricular myocardium also has a well-developed connective tissue matrix.[86] Cardiac collagen is organized into a weave of fibers forming a net-like structure around the myofibers (groups of six or more myocytes) as well as connections that link adjacent myofibers and strutlike projections connecting to adjacent blood vessels. The collagen network of the ventricles is an important determinant of their passive filling properties. The last major component of the ventricles is the vascular bed, described below.

## THE VENTRICLE AS A PUMP

Normal pump function requires that the ventricles deliver appropriate amounts of blood to the tissues at acceptably low filling pressures (FPs). Thus a useful means of characterizing the pump is to construct a *function curve* relating FP to a measure of mechanical output (SV,

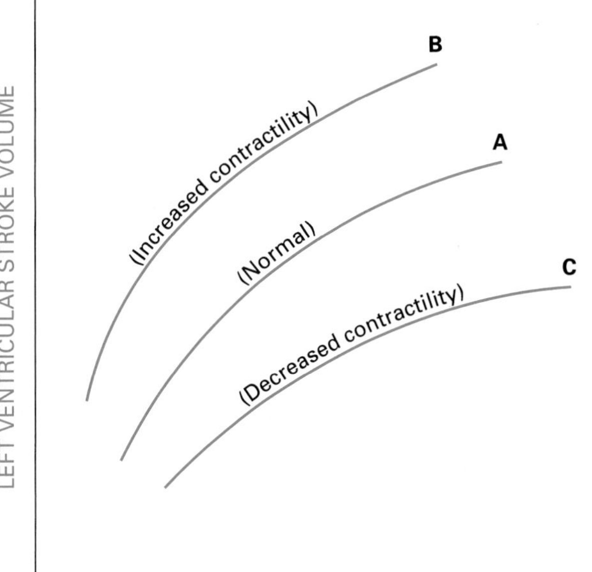


FIGURE 4-16 LV function curves relating SV to ED pressure (see text). *A*. Normal function. *B, C*. Augmented and depressed contractility, respectively, as occur with increases or decreases in adrenergic stimulation. Because ED pressure is plotted, identical shifts could be observed with altered diastolic compliance.

minute volume, EW, power). Ventricular function curves display a prominent *Frank-Starling effect,* i.e., a curvilinear relationship between FP and output with no descending limb in the ventricle (Fig. 4-16). A function curve relating ED *volume* (*preload*) to mechanical output more accurately represents the ventricular Frank-Starling effect. However, in the clinical setting FP (pulmonary capillary wedge, RA pressure) is more readily measurable than volume. Changes in intrinsic contractile performance result in upward or downward shifts of ventricular function curves. However, characterization of ventricular performance in terms of the relation between FP and output is a "black box" approach; effects caused by altered diastolic compliance (see below) are indistinguishable from those caused by altered contractile performance.

The normal heart can pump adequate amounts of blood to meet the needs of the body under extremely stressful conditions. Indeed, maximal CO normally is not limited by pumping capacity but by the ability of the systemic circulation, via venoconstriction and the systemic venous system of valves and muscular pumps, to return blood to the heart.[87]

## THE VENTRICLE AS A MUSCLE

For convenience, it is useful to consider myocardial contraction (systolic performance) as distinct from relaxation and filling (diastolic performance). This distinction is arbitrary, however. The two aspects of function overlap and interact.

***Systolic Function*** Systolic performance of the ventricle is traditionally characterized in terms of loading conditions (preload, afterload) and contractility.[88] We use the term *contractility* here as a *comparative concept* to connote differences in the intrinsic level of contractile performance either before or after some intervention *in the same heart* or *between different hearts* that cannot be accounted for by differences in loading conditions. Thus a change or difference in contractility is a change or difference in contractile performance when loading conditions are unchanged or can be accounted for—e.g., increased shortening despite increased afterload.

Loading Conditions and Contractile Performance In classic, isolated muscle experiments,[64] a force in the form of a weight is applied to one end of a quiescent, quasi-linear muscle (e.g., a cardiac papillary muscle) whose other end is tethered (Fig. 4-17). This force is the *preload,* which stretches the muscle to some initial length preceding contraction. The muscle is then stimulated electronically to contract and lift an additional weight, the *afterload.* Once stimulated, the muscle develops tension or force until it just meets and then exceeds the opposing force of the afterload. At this point, the muscle can begin to lift the afterload and shortening commences. In this system, once shortening begins, the developed force and afterload are constant (*isotonic* contraction). Force or afterload is reciprocally related to the magnitude and velocity of shortening; muscle performance is often characterized as the force-velocity or force-shortening relation (Fig. 4-12), with upward or downward shifts reflecting changes in contractility. If both ends of the muscle are tethered or if the afterload simply exceeds the force-generating capacity of the muscle, an *isometric* contraction ensues, in which tension is generated, but no shortening occurs. By varying preload, the Frank-Starling effect (Fig. 4-13) can be delineated by relating the initial length to shortening (isotonic contraction) or developed tension or force (isometric contraction).

In isolated muscle, load also can be expressed as *stress* (force normalized to cross-sectional area). Normalization allows comparison of muscles of different size and can be transferred to the ventricle. Thus, estimation of LV wall stress can be accomplished by using the LaPlace law.[89] For a relatively thick-walled sphere, the LaPlace law states that average wall stress = (pressure × internal radius)/ 2 × wall thickness. Variants of this equation can be employed to account

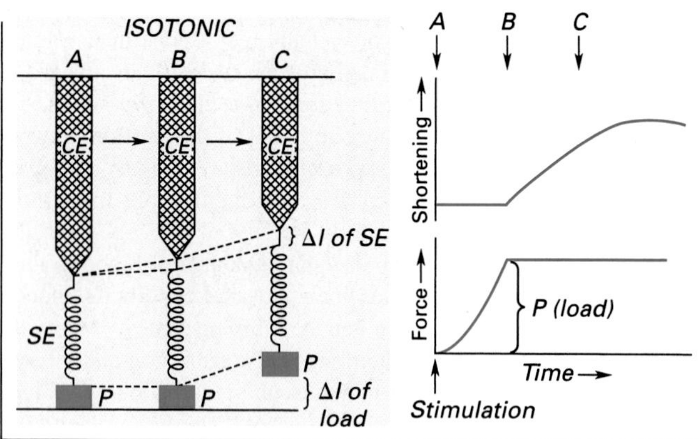


FIGURE 4-17 Schematic illustrating concept of preload and afterload during isotonic contraction. (*Left*) Linear muscle is depicted as consisting of contractile element (CE) (i.e., thick and thin filaments) and spring in series (SE). (*Right*) Shortening and force are depicted. *A*. Muscle is at rest, with one end tethered and the other connected to a weight (P). P is supported, however, so that muscle is only subjected to a fraction of weight (or load). This relatively small load is the preload, which stretches the muscle to the initial, resting length. *B*. Muscle begins to contract. In order to shorten, it must lift the entire weight P, which is the afterload. Initially, force increases but is insufficient to lift the weight. During this period, the CE shortens and reciprocally lengthens the SE, while total muscle length remains constant. Eventually, the developed force just exceeds the afterload, and the muscle begins to shorten (*C*). Once shortening begins, force is constant and essentially equal to the afterload. In an isometric contraction, the muscle cannot lift the load and therefore does not shorten (although the CE shortens and SE lengthens by the same amount).

for the actual shape of the LV, fiber orientation, and other geometric and structural features. Thus, for an ellipsoid, the long/short axis ratio (a measure of how ellipsoidal the shape is) modifies stress; as shape changes from less to more spherical, wall stress increases.

Use of the LaPlace law provides an estimate of the stress "seen" by the myofibers as the ventricle fills and then contracts against its afterload. Total systolic load presented to the LV by the vascular system has two components, a resistive load determined at the level of small systemic arteries and arterioles by microvascular tone and a smaller capacitive load determined by the properties of the large arteries, which absorb a certain amount of blood pumped via expansion of their walls.[90] A component of vascular load is caused by reflection of pressure waves back to the heart from the periphery.

Estimates of *systolic* stress using the LaPlace law are useful clinically in assessing and comparing contractile performance.[91] This can be accomplished by relating a measure of shortening [e.g., ejection fraction (EF) (SV/ED volume)] or shortening velocity [e.g., mean velocity of circumferential fiber shortening ($V_{cf}$); to estimated systolic stress. The ventricle behaves in a qualitatively similar fashion as isolated muscle; i.e., afterload (wall stress) is reciprocally related to shortening. As shown in Fig. 4-18, the stress-shortening relation can be characterized in a normal population with single data points obtained invasively or noninvasively (echocardiography combined with cuff sphygmomanometry). If the value in a patient falls above or below the normal range, this implies an alteration in intrinsic contractile performance.

Clinically, the most commonly employed index of ventricular contractile function is the EF, which can be estimated with several methods. Fractional shortening (minor axis diameter shortening/ED minor axis diameter) is calculated routinely from the echocardiogram and is interchangeable with EF, provided there are no regional wall motion abnormalities. Both shortening measurements are sensitive to alterations in preload and afterload.[88] Thus normal values indicate normal intrinsic contractile function only if loading conditions are also normal.

Elastance Concepts in the Assessment of Ventricular Contractile Function As an alternative to characterization of systolic function in terms of stress and shortening, Suga and Sagawa proposed an elastance approach [92–94] based on the empiric observation that during systole, the ventricle behaves like a spring with a time-varying elastance (or stiffness) that increases from a minimum at ED to a maximum at ES (Fig. 4-19). Elastance of a spring is the slope of its linear relation between the stress or force applied to stretch it and its length normalized to its unstressed or rest length. By analogy, ventricular elastance is the relation between pressure and volume at any time during systole normalized to a volume at which the pressure is zero (*dead volume,* $V_0$ or $V_d$).

At any specified time during contraction, elastance can be estimated by varying loading conditions and generating a series of pressure-volume loops with varying ES volumes. In their original studies, Suga and Sagawa used isolated, perfused canine ventricles.[92,93] Analysis of such a series of pressure-volume loops (Fig. 4-19) reveals that at any time $t$ during *each of the series of variably loaded contractions* (e.g., 100 ms after start of contraction), the relation between pressure and volume is linear, and its slope reaches a maximum (maximal elastance) at ES, or $t_{max}$. Elastance then decreases as the ventricle relaxes. The slope ($E_{max}$) of the end-systolic pressure-volume relationship (ESPVR) changes with acute inotropic interventions, increasing with positive and decreasing with negative inotropic interventions. Based on these observations and initial studies suggesting that ED volume did not influence the ESPVR, it was proposed that $E_{max}$ was a "load independent" index of contractility. Subsequent studies, especially those performed in the in situ heart and circulation, have modified these original conclusions.[94] Thus, the ESPVR is often significantly curvilinear, especially with augmented or depressed contractility. Also, it is influenced by preload (ED volume) and can be modified by the method by which afterload is varied (e.g., resistive versus capacitive load change). Systolic interaction also can modify the ESPVR.[95] Also, $E_{max}$ must be used with caution in comparing different hearts because of difficulties in normalizing for size and variable curvilinearity. To overcome these problems, the ESPVR has been modified by calculating ES stiffness based on wall stress estimates, and comparative analyses have been devised that take curvilinearity into account.[96,97]

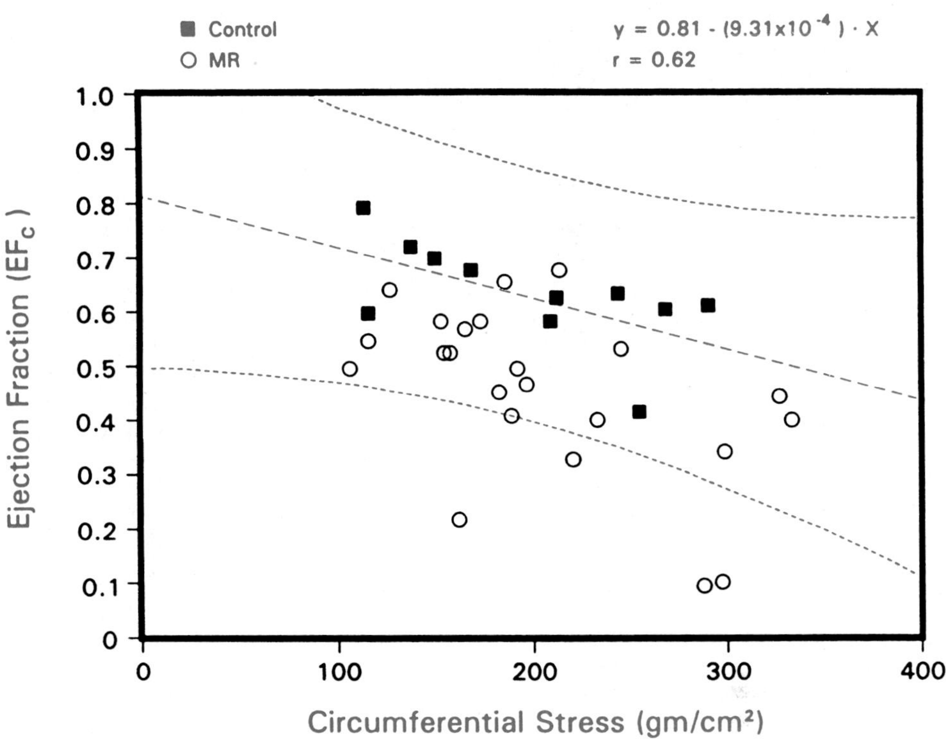


FIGURE 4-18 Relation between EF and circumferential stress (with 95 percent confidence intervals) in human subjects with normal ventricular function (control, filled squares) and mitral regurgitation (MR, open circles) (see text). Some MR patients fall below confidence intervals. (From Starling et al.[91] Reproduced with permission of the publisher.)

Despite the aforementioned cautions, the ESPVR remains a useful conceptual approach to assessment of contractile function in the experimental laboratory and the clinic. Although it corresponds to only a single point on the ESPVR, the ratio of systolic arterial pressure (a surrogate for ES pressure) to ES volume determined *noninvasively* using cuff sphygmomanometry and echocardiography also has been used as an index of ventricular function.

As proposed by Suga,[98] use of elastance theory to quantify mechanoenergetics is based on quantification of the *total mechanical energy* of contraction. Total mechanical energy consists of two components (Fig. 4-20, top), *external work* (EW), quantified as the area enclosed within the pressure-volume loop of a contraction, and *potential energy* (PE), which is dissipated as heat during relaxation. To understand PE in this context, consider an isovolumic contraction, which can be produced experimentally. Such a contraction obviously generates mechanical energy, but none of it is EW. As afterload is reduced and shortening and work increase, the ratio of EW to PE increases. The novelty of elastance theory in quantifying total mechanical energy is that it provides a basis for quantifying PE. In elastance theory, the PE stored in a spring is the area under its elastance relationship between its rest length and its actual length. Correspondingly, in the ventricle, PE for any beat can be considered the area under the ESPVR between its ES point and $V_0$ (Figs. 4-19 and 4-20). The sum of EW and PE is total mechanical energy and is termed *pressure-volume area* (PVA). The relation between PVA and $\dot{V}_{O_2}$ requires knowledge of the ESPVR and can be delineated by varying loading conditions while measuring LV $\dot{V}_{O_2}$. This is done most easily in isolated, perfused heart preparations.[98,99] PVA has a remarkably high linear correlation with $\dot{V}_{O_2}$ in several species, under a variety of loading conditions, and in both normal and abnormal hearts[98,99] (Fig. 4-20, bottom).

The linear $\dot{V}_{O_2}$-PVA relation has a positive $\dot{V}_{O_2}$ axis intercept (Fig. 4-20), where virtually no mechanical energy is produced. Unloaded $\dot{V}_{O_2}$ is largely accounted for by basal metabolism and Ca

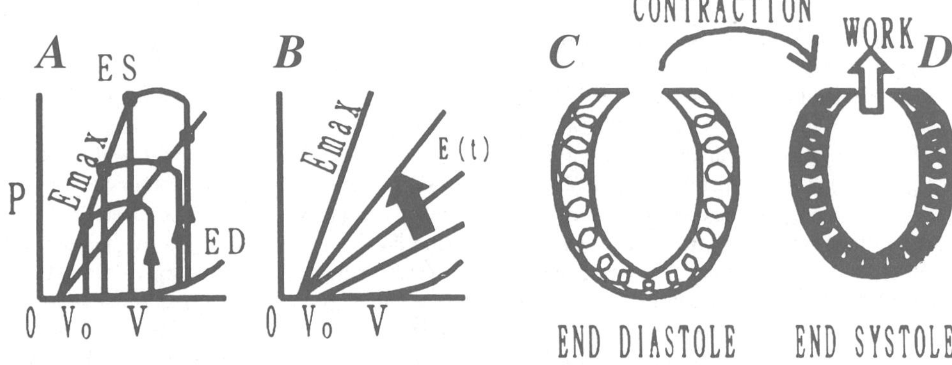


FIGURE 4-19 Schematic of elastance concept (see text). *A*. Series of variably loaded pressure-volume loops. Filled circles connected by straight lines occur at same time *t* during contraction. $E_{max}$ is line connecting points at ES. *B*. Elastance $E(t)$ increases at each time *t* during contraction until it reaches maximal value at ES. Increased contractility increases slope at any time *t*, including ES ($E_{max}$); vice versa for decreased contractility. *C*, *D*. The concept that the ventricle behaves like a spring of increasing stiffness (increased slope of elastance relations) during contraction. (From Suga H, Takaki M, Matsubara H, Goto Y. Energy costs of PVA and $E_{max}$: Constancy and variability. In: LeWinter MM, Suga H, Watkins MW, eds. *Cardiac Energetics: From $E_{max}$ to Pressure-Volume Area.* Boston: Kluwer; 1996:2. Reprinted with permission of the publisher.)

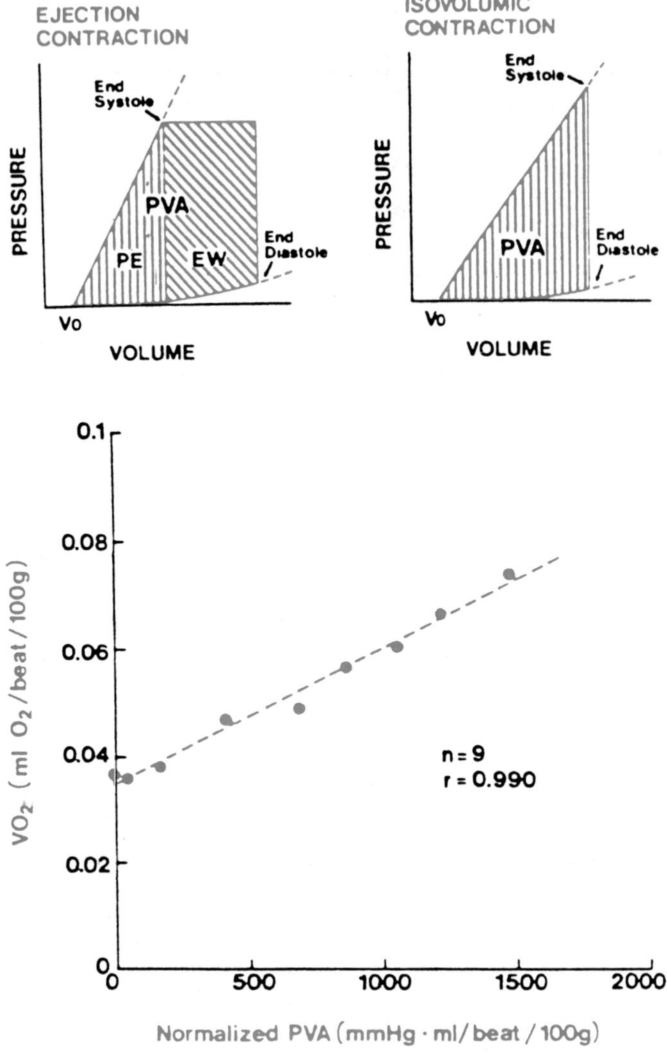


FIGURE 4-20 (*Top*) Schematic of $\dot{V}_{O_2}$-PVA concept (see text). In ejecting contraction, PVA = EW + PE; in isovolumic contraction, PVA = PE only. (*Bottom*) Correlation of PVA with $\dot{V}_{O_2}$. (From Goto et al.[99] Reproduced with permission of the publisher.)

pumping by SERCA2, which continue under unloaded conditions. Subtraction of unloaded $\dot{V}_{O_2}$ from total $\dot{V}_{O_2}$ is an estimate of $\dot{V}_{O_2}$ used by the contractile machinery, or PVA-dependent $\dot{V}_{O_2}$. Since $\dot{V}_{O_2}$ can be converted to units of energy, the ratio of PVA to PVA-dependent $\dot{V}_{O_2}$ (total mechanical energy output divided by total chemical energy input) is an estimate of the *efficiency* of conversion of $O_2$ to mechanical energy by the contractile machinery. Efficiency assessed in this fashion is inversely related to myosin ATPase activity.[100]

Based on the preceding analyses, it can be understood how changes in contractility and loading conditions alter myocardial energy demands and consumption (Fig. 4-20). Assuming no change in ED volume or afterload, increased contractility increases $E_{max}$, resulting in a smaller ES volume and increased EW at any preload. Even though ES volume is smaller, which in and of itself decreases PE, this is at least partially compensated by increased $E_{max}$, which serves to increase the area under the ESPVR. Many positive inotropic interventions increase the amount of Ca cycled per beat and, in turn, energy consumption by SERCA2, resulting in increased unloaded $\dot{V}_{O_2}$. Increased afterload increases the level of pressure at which the pressure-volume loop intersects the ESPVR, increasing PE with variable effects on EW but a net increase in PVA. In the LV, increases in preload have not been considered to markedly alter myocardial energy demands. Under basal conditions, the intact LV likely operates at an ED volume not too far from the point at which the diastolic pressure-volume relation becomes relatively steep. Thus there is not much room for the LV to acutely increase its preload, explaining the modest effect of preload on $\dot{V}_{O_2}$.

A second application of elastance theory is ventricular-vascular coupling.[101,102] Just as the ventricle can be considered in terms of an elastance relationship, systemic arteries are also characterized by an elastance relationship. Arterial elastance is largely a function of the properties of the large arteries. It influences the point at which the pressure-volume loop intersects the ESPVR and therefore the proportion of PVA converted to EW. The normal heart and vascular system operate at nearly optimal ventricular-vascular coupling. Coupling is adversely affected in heart failure, resulting in less efficient transfer of energy from the heart to the vascular system.[134]

OTHER APPROACHES TO ASSESSMENT OF SYSTOLIC VENTRICULAR PERFORMANCE Maximal rate of pressure rise (max $dP/dt$) is very sensitive to changes in intrinsic contractile performance but varies with preload[104] and to a modest extent with afterload. Max $dP/dt$ is especially useful in quantifying acute changes. Its use for comparisons between patients is limited by large interindividual variation. *Mean circumferential fiber shortening* velocity ($V_{cf}$)[105] [LV internal minor axis shortening/(ejection time × ED minor axis dimension)] is readily calculated from echocardiograms. Although quite sensitive to changes in afterload, it is a useful measure of intrinsic contractile performance if afterload is normal. *Maximum ventricular power index*[106] is attractive because of its physiologic significance. This index has been normalized to minimize effects of loading and has the potential for noninvasive determination. Two empiric indexes have been devised that are relatively afterload-insensitive, the relation between ED volume (or strain) and stroke work,[107] termed *preload recruitable stroke work,* and the relation between ED volume and max $dP/dt$.[108,109] Both are linear representations of the Frank-Starling relation; by incorporating ED volume, length-dependent activation is an intrinsic component of these indexes.

***Diastolic Function*** The heart must operate at FP levels that do not result in circulatory congestion. This requires normal relaxation and filling. Ventricular relaxation begins at about ES, continues through isovolumic relaxation, and does not reach completion until after AV valve opening. Before filling commences, several factors combine to determine relaxation rate or isovolumic pressure decline (Fig. 4-21). After filling begins, other factors related to the level of ventricular volume and/or the rate of ventricular volume change also influence ventricular diastolic pressure. Once relaxation is complete, "passive" properties of the ventricle dominate the relation between pressure and volume as filling continues through ED.

*During isovolumic relaxation,* pressure falls exponentially. The rate of isovolumic pressure fall (a measure of relaxation rate) has been quantified as a time constant ($\tau$)[110,111] or as time to reach one-half of some starting value ($T_{1/2}$). Peak $-dP/dt$ is a less accurate measure of relaxation rate than $\tau$ or $T_{1/2}$. The determinants of the rate of isovolumic pressure fall are as follows.[110,112] First, myocyte relaxation rate is determined by the balance between the sensitivity and/or avidity of the contractile proteins for Ca and the rate at which SERCA2 and other uptake and extrusion mechanisms remove Ca from them and restore cytoplasmic concentration to normal diastolic levels. In some pathologic conditions—e.g., ischemia—diastolic Ca may not be restored to normal.[113] Cross-bridge cycling continues during diastole resulting in increased diastolic tension. Isovolumic relaxation is also modulated by the load on the myocardium.[110,114,115] Increased afterload through all of systole or beginning early in systole (*a contraction load*) delays relaxation. Changes in load late during systole (*a relaxation load*) cause opposite effects. Changes in relaxation load may be physiologically significant. Normal arterial waves reflected from the periphery return to the ventricle at about ES and may function to accelerate relaxation. When arteries become noncompliant reflected waves return earlier and may be converted to a contraction load, with delay of relaxation. Last, a normal temporal and spatial activation sequence results in the most rapid relaxation rate.[116]

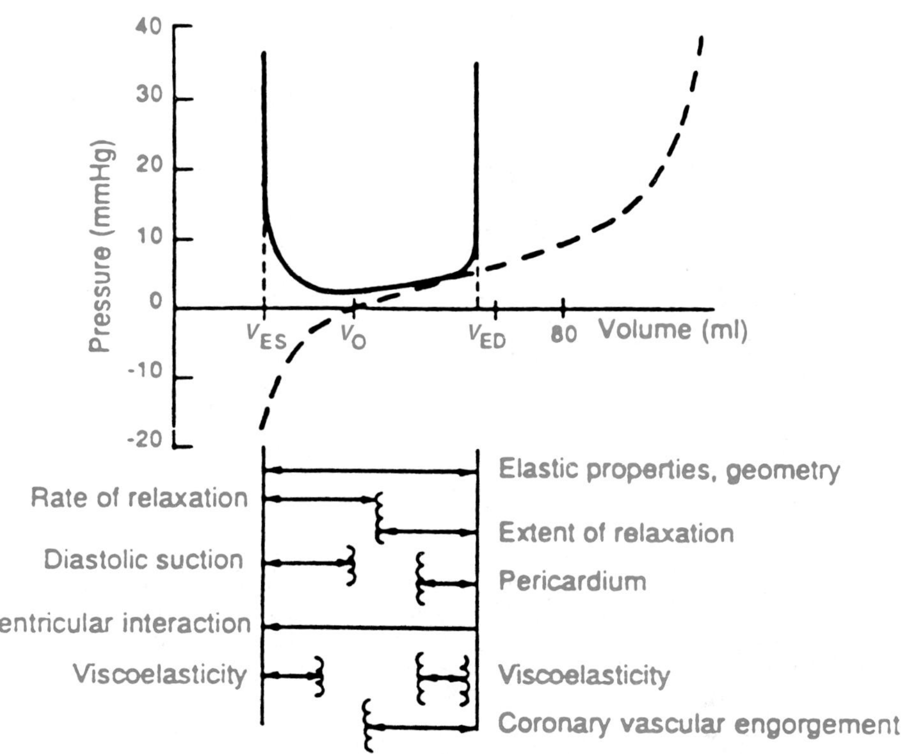


FIGURE 4-21 Determinants of relation between LV diastolic pressure and volume during filling. Solid line, LV pressure during isovolumic relaxation, filling, and isovolumic contraction; dashed line, positive and negative portions of passive pressure-volume relation. $V_{ES}$, ES volume; $V_O$, equilibrium volume or zero pressure intercept of passive pressure-volume relation (which is not same as dead volume of ESPVR); $V_{ED}$, ED volume. (From Gilbert JC, Glantz SA. Determinants of LV filling and of the diastolic pressure-volume relation. *Circ Res* 1989; 64:828. Reproduced with permission of the publisher.)

The magnitude and rate of ventricular filling are determined by the instantaneous AV pressure gradient (Fig. 4-2), which is determined by properties of both ventricle and atrium. Immediately after AV valve opening, rapid filling begins in association with a gradient of several millimeters of mercury (Fig. 4-2). This corresponds to the E wave of mitral inflow measured with Doppler ultrasound. During rapid filling, both ventricular and atrial pressures initially fall, but ventricular pressure falls faster. Ventricular pressure soon reaches a minimum and then increases throughout the rest of diastole. The peak AV gradient occurs at or near the time of minimum ventricular pressure. Rapid filling is succeeded by a variable slow filling phase, when the AV gradient is small to negligible. The length of slow filling is inversely related to HR and disappears at rapid rates. Atrial contraction increases the AV gradient once again and injects an additional volume of blood into the ventricle.

Ventricular properties that determine LV pressure and the AV gradient during filling are as follows: First, relaxation continues past the time of AV valve opening. Therefore the same factors (Ca reuptake, load) that modulate *isovolumic* pressure fall also influence pressure *after filling begins*.[112] In addition to ongoing relaxation, *restoring forces* generated during contraction also influence ventricular pressure during rapid filling.[117,118] By a *restoring force* we mean PE generated during contraction in the form of a deformation(s) of the myocyte and/or ventricle that is converted into kinetic energy during diastole, accelerating blood flow from atrium to ventricle. This energy-requiring driving force for filling results in lowering of ventricular pressure relative to atrial pressure and a larger AV gradient. Restoring forces are probably generated by two interrelated mechanisms. One is contraction of the ventricle to an ES volume below equilibrium volume ($V_{eq}$), the volume at which, in the *fully relaxed* state, transmural pressure = 0. With contraction below $V_{eq}$, the chamber may be considered to be "under compression". In this condition, PE stored in the walls can be converted to elastic recoil and assist filling. As noted earlier, titin appears to be responsible for a restoring force in the myocyte. The second mechanism involves complex, contraction-dependent three-dimensional deformations that return to the resting state during isovolumic relaxation and the early phase of ventricular filling. The magnitude of these deformations increases as ES volume decreases;[120] hence they parallel compressive forces related simply to contraction below $V_{eq}$. The sine qua non of suction is a negative transmural pressure early during diastole, but this is rarely observed because filling occurs rapidly and is driven simultaneously by the atrial pressure. However, suction appears to be important at diastolic volumes within the physiologic range and during exercise, when ES volume decreases.[83,84] A second myocardial property likely influencing ventricular pressure during rapid filling is *viscous resistance to stretch,*[120] but this does not appear to be important under physiologic conditions.

Relaxation and restoring forces are dynamic aspects of filling whose influence varies with time. Underlying these time varying properties is the passive ventricular pressure-volume relationship.[121] We refer to this as the *end-diastolic pressure-volume relationship* (EDPVR) (Fig. 4-22). The EDPVR has a negative-pressure portion where volume is less than $V_{eq}$. Passive *chamber compliance* is the ratio of change in volume to change in pressure at any point on the EDPVR. Because the EDPVR is exponential, passive compliance is inversely related to volume. The inverse of chamber compliance is *passive chamber stiffness*. The EDPVR is determined mainly by the geometry of the ventricular chamber, especially the volume to wall thickness ratio, and the passive stiffness of the myocardial tissue. All else being equal, increases in wall thickness or passive myocardial stiffness increase its slope. Passive stiffness is change in stress occurring in association with a given strain in the fully relaxed state. Passive myocardial stiffness is mainly accounted for by titin[43,44] at relatively low volumes and by a combination of connective tissue and titin at

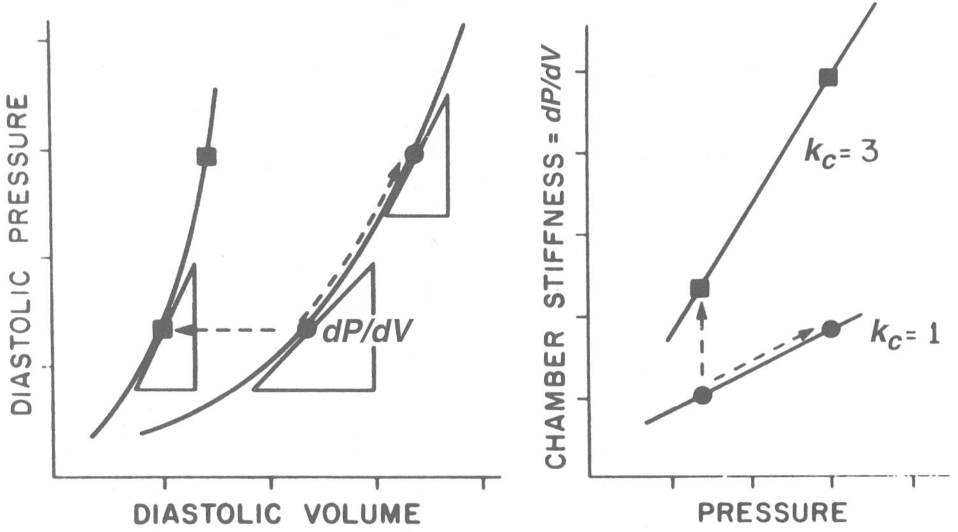


FIGURE 4-22 (*Left*) EDPVR in two ventricles with differing passive diastolic properties. Chamber stiffness is *dP/dV* at any point on the EDPVR. Chamber compliance is its inverse. Stiffer chamber (*left*) has steeper overall slope. (*Right*) Same data plotted as pressure versus chamber stiffness. Because of exponential nature of EDPVR, result is a straight line. Its slope ($k_c$) is a chamber-stiffness constant that characterizes the overall slope of the EDPVR. (From Gaasch.[114] Reprinted with the permission of the publisher.)

larger volumes. All through relaxation and filling, a portion of LV pressure is dictated by its position on its EDPVR. Early during filling, the actual relation between ventricular pressure and volume is determined by relaxation and elastic recoil, superimposed on the EDPVR; the EDPVR alone is the prime determinant of ventricular pressure once relaxation is complete.

The EDPVR is modified by external restraints, the most important being the parietal pericardium.[122] The pericardial sac has a relatively small reserve volume. At total heart volumes in the physiologic range, pericardial pressure is very low in relation to left-side FPs. However, with relatively modest increments in heart volume above the physiologic range, the *pericardial* pressure-volume relation becomes quite steep (noncompliant), and the pressure rises rapidly. This external pressure acting on the surface of the heart serves to restrain further filling; i.e., it decreases chamber compliance. Even under physiologic conditions, however, pericardial pressure is significant in relation to right-side FPs, which are normally lower than left-side FPs. Thus, pericardial pressure is normally responsible for a significant fraction of right-side FP. Restraint to filling by the pericardium becomes quite important when the heart dilates rapidly, as after RV myocardial infarction. The interventricular septum constitutes about one-third of the LV wall; diastolic pressure in the RV is therefore also an external restraint to filling of the LV. A component of LV diastolic pressure is transmitted from the RV, an effect termed *diastolic interaction.*[121]

An additional factor that influences the EDPVR is the volume of blood in the myocardial vascular bed, or *turgor.*[121] A significant component of pressure in the fully relaxed ventricle is accounted for by turgor. The significance of turgor is evident from the initial drop in diastolic pressure that occurs when coronary flow is terminated abruptly.[123]

Following rapid filling and the variable slow filling period, atrial contraction injects additional blood into the ventricle (typically one-quarter to one-third of the SV).

Atrial properties are also a key determinant of the AV gradient that drives filling.[124] Atrial pressure at the instant of AV valve opening is determined directly by atrial compliance; the lower the compliance, the higher the pressure and the larger the gradient. The relationship between ventricular pressure and volume as diastolic filling proceeds is also influenced by the properties of the atrium and even the pulmonary veins because LV, atrium, and pulmonary veins are an open system when the mitral valve is open. The ventricles, being much stiffer, are much more important determinants of the ED pressure-volume relation than the atria.

## SHORT-TERM MODULATION OF VENTRICULAR FUNCTION

***Heart Rate*** The ventricle has a positive FFR with an optimal frequency that parallels myocardial FFR.[65] This is an important means of modulating ventricular function that is intimately connected with changes in adrenergic stimulation. Changes in frequency also influence relaxation and filling. There is some shortening of relaxation in conjunction with the positive FFR even without concurrent increases in adrenergic stimulation. Moreover, with increased HR, diastole is shortened much more than systole, especially the slow-filling phase.

***Paracrine Modulation of Ventricular Function*** The significance of these factors with respect to *normal* ventricular function is not established. In the ventricle, they tend to have more prominent effects on relaxation than on contraction.[125] NO and endothelial-dependent vasodilators cause very modest depression of systolic function and an earlier onset of ventricular relaxation. Substances whose effects are mediated by the $IP_3$ second-messenger system (ET-1, $\alpha$-adrenergic agonists) have more or less opposite effects.

***Neurohumoral Responses*** The most important short-term neurohumoral modulation occurs as a result of variation in sympathetic and parasympathetic stimulation caused by both cardiac neural activity and circulating catecholamines. Stimulation of $\beta$-adrenergic receptors results in increased HR and contractility and more rapid relaxation. These effects are due to the influence of adrenergic stimulation on the sinus node and specialized conduction system and, within the myocyte, activation of adenyl cyclase with increased cyclic AMP. Increases in HR also allow utilitization of the FFR. Adrenergic stimulation interacts with the FFR not only by increasing HR but also by increasing FFR gain.[65] There are many other myocyte cell surface receptors, but none has a clearly delineated, significant role in normal, short-term modulation of ventricular function. Vagal stimulation, of course, has profound HR slowing effects as well as modest negative effects on contractility. Vagal withdrawal is an integral component of HR responses during exercise and other stresses.

A number of reflexes modulate HR and ventricular function in the short term.[126] These typically result in coordinated changes in parasympathetic and sympathetic stimulation. Thus the heart is a component of the efferent limb of arterial baro- and chemoreceptors. Acute increases in systemic arterial pressure result in slowing of HR due to increased vagal stimulation and decreased sympathetic neural stimulation with attendant effects on contractility; the reverse occurs with decreased arterial pressure. Vagal responses occur on a beat-to-beat time scale, whereas sympathetic responses are somewhat slower. Pulmonary stretch receptors are largely responsible for sinus arrhythmia. Atrial stretch receptors also may modulate HR via the Bainbridge reflex, tachycardia occurring with increased intravascular volume. Ventricular mechanoreceptors that discharge with deformation are activated when volume decreases. Their discharge causes vagally mediated bradycardia and hypotension and appears to be involved in vasovagal syncope. Chemoreceptors on the ventricular epicardium also connect to vagal efferents and may discharge in response to prostaglandins secreted into the pericardial sac.

***Ventricular Interaction*** Diastolic ventricular interaction has been discussed previously. The ventricles also interact during systole. Left-to-right systolic interaction was mentioned earlier. There is also a modest amount of right-to-left interaction.[95] Both diastolic and systolic ventricular interaction function as internal feedback mechanisms that modulate SV on a beat-to-beat basis to ensure that left- and right-side outputs remain equal over time.

***Coronary Perfusion and Ventricular Function*** Changes in coronary perfusion pressure and/or flow per se can influence ventricular function.[127] Increases augment systolic performance and may cause a decrease in passive compliance. Modest decreases insufficient to cause myocardial ischemia likely have opposite effects. A component of the influence of coronary perfusion on ventricular function is related to turgor. In addition to modulation of diastolic compliance, stretching of myocardial tissue due to increased turgor appears to augment the Frank-Starling effect. It is also possible that stretch-activated Ca channels[128] open as turgor increases, with resulting increased activation.

#### LONG-TERM MODULATION OF VENTRICULAR FUNCTION

Chronic nonphysiologic stresses modulate ventricular function by causing pathologic hypertrophy. Chronic alterations in the demands placed on the cardiovascular system within the physiologic range can cause modest changes in cardiac mass.[129,130] However, measurable changes require very substantially increased demand. Thus endurance athletes develop modest, physiologic hypertrophy characterized by increased chamber volume with little or no increase in wall thickness.

## THE PERIPHERAL CIRCULATION

Normal vascular function requires continual adjustment of both total and regional peripheral resistance to provide the proper distribution of blood flow in order to (1) ensure normal capillary pressures and fluid balance, (2) maintain systemic blood pressure and venous return to the heart, and (3) accommodate the metabolic demands of various organs.

### Physiology of the Peripheral Circulation

#### PRINCIPLES OF CAPILLARY EXCHANGE

Exchange of gases, nutrients, water, and waste material occurs at the capillary level and is governed by the interplay of two opposing but balanced forces. At the proximal end of a capillary, intravascular pressure slightly exceeds tissue pressure. The transmural gradient in hydrostatic pressure results in hydraulic *ultrafiltration,* a process characterized by the movement of fluid through the capillary wall and into the extracellular compartment. Composed of a single layer of endothelial cells, each capillary acts as a selective filter. The degree of selectivity varies within different tissues. Passage of large molecules such as proteins is largely impeded, although some leakage occurs with subsequent reabsorption into lymphatic vessels and return to the circulation.

As a result of ultrafiltration, the concentration of solute (plasma osmolarity) increases along the length of a capillary, and the associated force (termed *oncotic pressure*) acts to pull extracellular fluid back into the capillary lumen through the process of *reabsorption.*

This fundamental concept is known as the *Starling Hypothesis* and was first described by Ernest Starling in 1896. Mathematically, it is expressed as

$$Q_f = k[(P_c + \pi_i) - (P_i + \pi_p)]$$

where $Q_f$ = fluid movement across the capillary wall
$P_c$ = capillary hydrostatic pressure
$\pi_i$ = interstitial fluid oncotic pressure
$P_i$ = interstitial fluid hydrostatic pressure
$\pi_p$ = plasma oncotic pressure
$k$ = filtration constant for a capillary membrane

A positive $Q_f$ value indicates net filtration, while a negative value connotes net reabsorption. If filtration exceeds reabsorption an edematous state develops; conversely, if reabsorption is greater than filtration, plasma volume expands (primarily on the venous side) and thereby reduces cellular/extracellular volume. It should be noted, however, that not every capillary behaves in the idealized fashion predicted by the Starling hypothesis. Within the renal glomerulus, hydrostatic pressures are elevated along the entire length of the capillary, and filtration predominates; conversely, within the intestinal mucosa, the elevated oncotic forces result primarily in reabsorption, with little or no filtration.

*Transcapillary exchange* is modulated by a hierarchy of mechanisms including central neural control of cardiac output and total peripheral resistance, regional mechanisms within the microcirculation of each organ that modulate capillary hydrostatic pressure and blood flow, and localized events at the level of the capillary endothelium that govern its structural and metabolic properties.

Extravasation of fluid at the capillary level may occur through a combination of paracellular and transcellular routes. *Paracellular permeability* refers to a relatively nonselective component that may be caused by filtration through paracellular gaps between adjacent endothelial cells. Gap architecture is determined by the three-dimensional structure of the endothelial cell and by the types of junctions present between adjacent endothelial cells.[131] The presence of both actin and myosin in some endothelial cells, particularly those of postcapillary venules, supports the existence of a cytoskeletal mechanism for governing the geometry of interendothelial pores or clefts that facilitate paracellular exchange. The state of the cytoskeleton is, in turn, regulated by physical and chemical signals that impinge upon the capillary endothelium and govern the three-dimensional structure of cell-to-cell contact.

*Transcellular permeability* (also called *transcytosis*) involves the formation of plasmalemmal vesicles (caveolae) through endocytosis, vesicular transport from the luminal to the abluminal surface of the endothelial cell, and exocytosis from the basolateral (abluminal) membrane.[132]

It is clear that a variety of molecules—such as histamine, adenosine and nitric oxide—are able to alter the permeability characteristics of the endothelial layer, leading to rapid changes in permeability via different signal transduction mechanisms. For example, *vascular endothelial growth factor* (VEGF; formerly known as vascular permeability factor, or VPF) is a peptide that binds to receptors on the endothelial surface and initiates a series of intracellular signal transduction events that result in greatly augmented permeability. Recent observations suggest that this pathway involves the autophosphorylation of a receptor subtype (VEGF-R2) on endothelial cells, with subsequent activation of phospholipase C, whose activation leads to the generation of second messenger molecules that modulate both enzymatic and ionic events within the endothelial cell, including calcium release from the sarcoplasmic reticulum, activation of protein kinase C, and the generation of nitric oxide. The actions of VEGF appear to be quite complex, and may stimulate a variety of endothelial pathways, including formation of transcellular gaps, vesiculovacuolar organelle formation, and interendothelial fenestrations.[133] Finally, in some organs, such as the brain or kidney, capillary permeability may be subject to modulation by pericytes—highly specialized cells that encircle the capillary endothelium and secrete factors that modulate capillary endothelial function.[134]

From a more general standpoint, it is essential that the vascular resistance upstream of the capillary bed be regulated so as to maintain capillary hydrostatic pressure at levels where normal fluid exchange may occur. If this fails and the normal balance of ultrafiltration/reabsorption is altered, sufficient compensation by local capillary mechanisms is unlikely and dysregulation of fluid volume is likely to ensue. The remainder of this chapter is therefore devoted to reviewing the principal mechanisms by which the cells of the arterial and arteriolar wall regulate arterial tone and, hence, vascular resistance and capillary pressure.

## PERIPHERAL RESISTANCE AND ITS DETERMINANTS

Pressure, flow, and resistance are related through Poiseuille's equation, formulated in 1842 by the Parisian physician of the same name. Based on observations of water flowing through rigid tubes, Poiseuille demonstrated that the resistance ($R$) to flow through a cylinder is proportional to tube length ($L$) and fluid viscosity (**0**) and inversely proportional to the radius of the tube raised to the fourth power ($r^4$). These variables can be related to each other in the following way:

$$R = 8nL/\pi r^4$$

This equation is useful because it predicts that flow ($Q$) is proportional to the fourth power of the radius (and inversely proportional to resistance: $Q \propto 4r^4$, or $Q \propto 4x^1/R^4$ where $r$ = radius and $R$ = resistance)—i.e., given the same initial pressure, doubling the inner radius of a tube will result in a 16-fold ($2^4$) increase in flow. Estimates from intact vascular networks suggest this may be an overestimation, and that a third power equation may be more accurate.[135] Nevertheless, relatively minor changes in arterial caliber can produce large changes in resistance and flow.

The relationship between vascular resistance and blood flow may be defined through a simple equation that is analogous to Ohm's law for the flow of electrons, whereby flow = perfusion pressure/resistance. The complete formulation includes the main determinants of resistance (labeled as above in the Poiseuille formulation), and is called *Poiseuille's law:*

$$Q = (\text{PP})\ \pi r^4/8nL$$

where $Q$ = flow, PP = perfusion pressure, and the determinants of resistance (inverted during the simplification of the quotient) are signified as above in Poiseuille's formulation.

Although resistance can also be affected by the viscosity of the blood (**0**) and the vessel length ($L$), as predicted by the Poiseuille formula, these parameters are normally relatively invariant within the cardiovascular system. For this reason, lumen diameter is the single most powerful determinant of vascular resistance under physiologic conditions; its control is the primary endpoint for a variety of physiological mechanisms.

Most of the pressure drop between the large conduit arteries and capillaries occurs in vessels with lumen diameters of a few hundred microns or less. For this reason, small arteries and arterioles are considered to be of primary importance in regulating and determining peripheral resistance. These muscular vessels have a high ratio of wall thickness to lumen diameter and contain several layers of circumferentially oriented vascular smooth muscle cells. They also normally possess some degree of basal tone and are capable of changes in diameter that range from fully open to virtually closed. Hence, their potential to affect resistance is considerable. In contrast, large conduit arteries such as the aorta constrict by only 10 to 20 percent and are normally of minor importance to peripheral resistance and blood flow control. The relationship between blood pressure, blood flow velocity, and total cross-sectional area in various blood vessels of the systemic circulation is summarized in Fig. 4-23.

Larger vessels do contribute significantly to vascular resistance in some organs, such as the brain,[136] primarily due to the more linear geometry of the arterial vessels. In a *serial arrangement* of tubes, total resistance ($R_t$) is defined as the sum of individual resistance elements ($R_t = R_1 + R_2 + R_3$, etc.). Conversely, in regional circulations

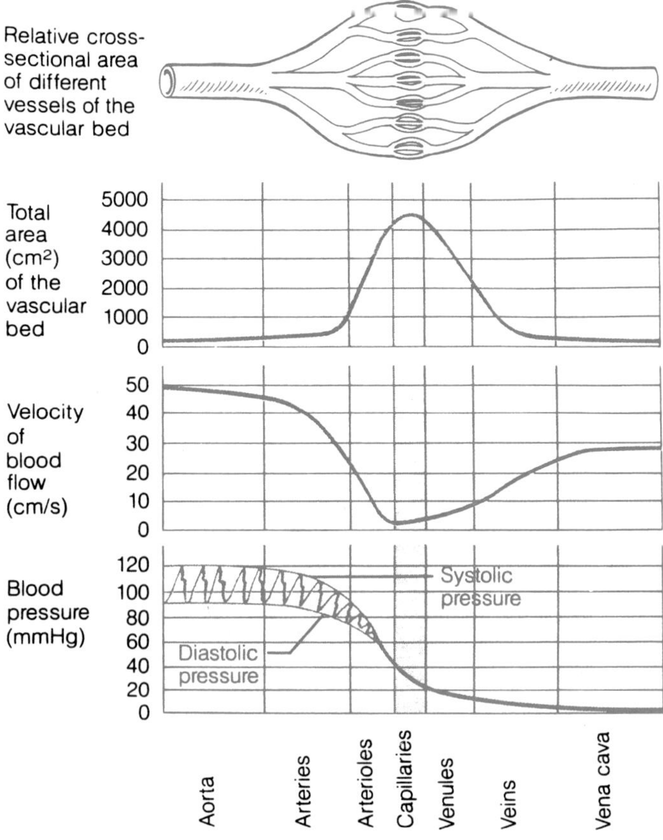


FIGURE 4-23 Relations between total cross-sectional area of the vascular bed (cm$^2$), velocity of blood flow (cm/s), and blood pressure (mmHg) in various vessels in systemic circulation. (From Marieb EN. *Human Anatomy and Physiology*. Redwood City, CA: Benjamin/Cummings; 1989:629. Reproduced with permission of the publisher.)

in which the vessels are highly and sequentially branched (e.g., the splanchnic arcade), resistance tends to be localized to smaller (<50-$\mu$m) arteries and arterioles. This occurs because a greater number of *parallel elements* lowers the overall resistance of the array. Given the same driving pressure, there are more tubes to conduct flow and, in this case, total resistance is defined by a reciprocal relationship ($1/R_t = 1/R_1 + 1/R_2 + 1/R_3$, etc). These concepts are shown in Fig. 4-24.

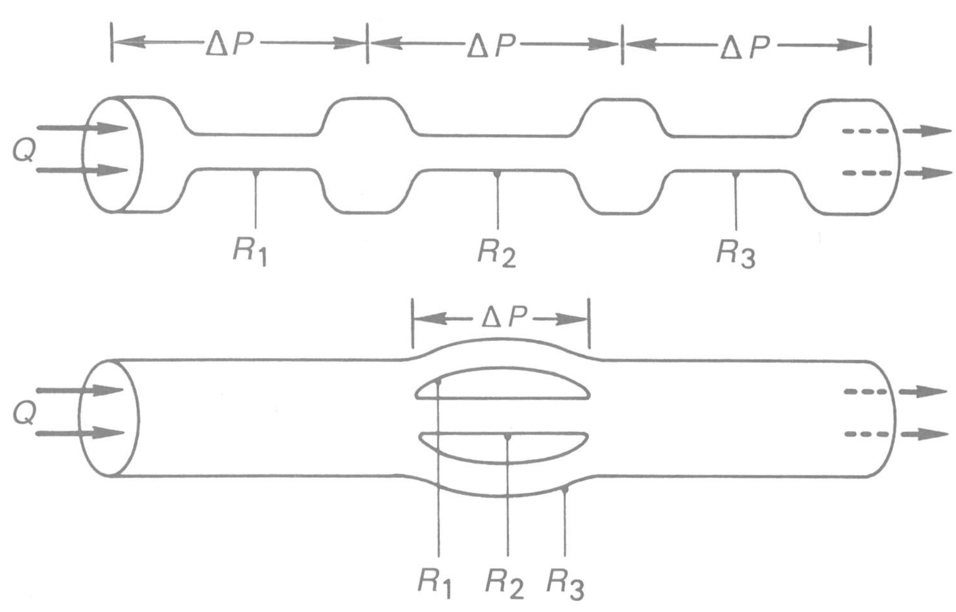


FIGURE 4-24 Illustration of principle of resistance elements arranged in series versus parallel. (*Top*) If the driving pressurer ($\Delta P$) across each series resistance is 3 mmHg, and flow ($Q$) is 1 mL/min, each resistance ($R$) would be $\Delta P/Q$, or 3 mmHg/mL per minute, and total resistance ($R_t$) would be 9 mmHg/mL per minute. (*Bottom*) In parallel resistances, if driving pressure ($\Delta P$) is 3 mmHg, and flow ($Q$) is 1 mL/min, total resistance is $1/R_1 + 1/R_2 + 1/R_3$, or 1 mmHg/mL per minute. When three resistances are in parallel, total resistance is only one-ninth that with resistances in series, so it would take a $\Delta P$ of only 1 mmHg to produce a 1 mL/min flow. (From Smith JJ, Kampine JP. *Circulatory Physiology: The Essentials*. Baltimore: Williams & Wilkins, 1990:20. Reprinted with permission of the publisher.)

## SYSTEMIC HEMODYNAMICS

In healthy adults, only one-sixth (15 percent) of the total blood volume is contained within the systemic arterial system. The remainder is distributed between capillaries (5 percent), veins (66 percent), the heart (6 percent in diastole), and the pulmonary circulation (8 percent). The peripheral circulation distributes cardiac output throughout the various tissues and organs of the body. The elasticity of large conduit arteries such as the aorta serves to absorb and dampen the highly pulsatile and discontinuous flow from the heart (a phenomenon termed the *Windkessel effect*). As a result, the amplitude of pressure pulsations is diminished in smaller vessels and capillaries and is virtually absent in the venous circulation. Intravascular pressure also decreases from a mean value of 90 to 95 mmHg in large arteries to about 30 mmHg in capillaries and <10 mmHg in veins.

It is essential that the peripheral circulation be able to adapt rapidly to changes in arterial pressure and end-organ metabolic demands. Even routine actions such as standing challenge the cardiovascular system: due to gravitational forces, cerebral perfusion pressure, and venous return are suddenly reduced, leading to transient feelings of dizziness in some individuals (orthostatic hypotension). At the same time, capillary pressures in the ankles may exceed 90 to 100 mmHg. The metabolic demands of exercise, another example, require a major redistribution of cardiac output to increase perfusion of coronary, pulmonary, and skeletal muscle circulations, diminish splanchnic flow, and still maintain cerebral blood flow (Table 4-2).

Regulatory mechanisms must therefore be bidirectional—i.e., allow blood flow to either increase or decrease upon demand. For this to occur, the venous circulation must be able to adjust its capacitance and modulate venous return and the arterial vasculature must operate at a point from which it can either dilate or constrict to increase or decrease flow, respectively. Because it is impossible to dilate a vessel that is already fully relaxed, some portion of the arterial circulation must operate in a state of partial constriction or tone.

### Integration of Circulatory Mechanisms: Blood Flow Autoregulation

Minute-to-minute control of the peripheral circulation involves a complex interplay between several physiologic mechanisms, mainly neural, myogenic, and humoral/endothelial. Metabolites released from adjacent tissues also impinge on the vascular wall (metabolic regulation). The importance of each varies with ambient conditions. Physical activity, such as jogging or swimming, results in many-fold increases in skeletal muscle blood flow due to a combination of increased cardiac output and arterial dilation, so that the proportion of cardiac output directed to skeletal muscles increases from 20 to >70 percent, and total blood flow is increased by a factor of 10 (Table 4-2).

During exercise, dilation of skeletal muscle arteries and arterioles occurs due to metabolic factors such as adenosine, potassium and hydrogen ions that diffuse from the adjacent myocytes into the vascular wall and induce hyperpolarization and relaxation of vascular smooth muscle either directly or indirectly, by stimulating the release of endothelial factors such as nitric oxide and prostacyclin.[137] Increased flow itself serves as a stimulus for further vasodilation, presumably through a shear stress–induced release of vasoactive substances from the endothelium as demonstrated in a number of studies.[138]

TABLE 4-2 Distribution of Tissue Blood Flow at Rest and during Exercise

| | Tissue Blood Flow (mL/min) | | |
|---|---|---|---|
| Organ | Rest | Light Exercise | Strenuous Exercise |
| Skeletal muscle | 1200 | 4500 | 12,500 |
| Heart | 250 | 350 | 750 |
| Brain | 750 | 750 | 750 |
| Skin | 500 | 1500 | 1,900 |
| Kidney | 1100 | 900 | 600 |
| Abdominal viscera | 1400 | 1100 | 600 |
| Miscellaneous | 600 | 400 | 400 |
| TOTAL CO | 5800 | 9500 | 17,500 |

SOURCE: Modified from Martini FH. *Fundamentals of Anatomy and Physiology*. Upper Saddle River, NJ: Prentice-Hall; 1998:735.

The degree of local circulatory control can be remarkable. For example, the act of speaking increases blood flow to the speech areas, solving mathematical equations augments flow to the frontal lobe, visual stimuli to the occipital cortex, and so on. At the same time, hemispheric and global cerebral blood flow is unaltered, and remains well preserved in the face of changing blood pressures, a phenomenon called *autoregulation*.

Autoregulation is the ability of an organ to maintain a relatively constant blood flow despite changes in systemic arterial pressure.[139] Although most organs possess this ability to some degree, it is particularly well developed in the cerebral, coronary, and renal circulations and is principally affected by adjustments in the caliber of smaller muscular arteries and arterioles. Autoregulatory effectiveness is determined by the ability of the arteries to constrict to increased pressure and dilate to decreased pressure so as to keep total flow relatively constant. This involves an interaction between several mechanisms, most notably myogenic, endothelial, neural, and metabolic; others—such as tissue pressure or tubuloglomerular feedback—may be invoked within the cranium and kidneys, respectively.

Autoregulation occurs over a range of perfusion pressures, with both upper and lower limits. If perfusion pressure falls below a certain point (lower limit of autoregulation), tissue hypoperfusion ensues. On the other hand, transmural pressures above the upper limit of autoregulation result in a "breakthrough" phenomenon in which *forced dilatation* of the arteries occurs, leading to loss of arterial and arteriolar tone. Large increases in organ blood flow, transmission of high intravascular pressures to capillaries and veins, and vessel leakage and rupture may potentially result. Experimental studies have shown that leakage occurs initially in postcapillary venules, although arteriolar damage and changes in permeability have been documented as well.[140]

The ability to autoregulate blood flow must be reserved for some (e.g., brain, heart, and kidney) but not all organs; if increased blood pressure stimulated arterial constriction throughout the body, total peripheral resistance would increase, raising pressure further via a positive feedback mechanism that could have dire consequences. An equally dangerous situation would occur in response to a fall in blood pressure, as unchecked reflex dilation could potentially lead to vascular collapse.

## Cellular Mechanisms Involved in the Regulation of Blood Flow

### VASCULAR TONE AND ITS DETERMINANTS

Vascular tone generally increases with decreasing arterial size and is greatest in the smaller "muscular" (as opposed to larger "conduit") arteries and arterioles that play the primary role in determining peripheral resistance and regulating regional blood flow. The level of tone at any time reflects an integration of multiple excitatory and inhibitory pathways that converge on the ultimate effector, vascular smooth muscle (VSM), to "set" the level of tone. Changes in the physical forces impinging on the vascular wall, neurotransmitter release from nerves, or the concentration of metabolites released from surrounding tissues all modulate the set point to either increase or decrease arterial tone and hence lumen diameter and resistance.

VSM itself is capable of constricting in response to pressure or stretch. Because this phenomenon occurs in isolated arterial segments that have been denuded of endothelium and in the absence of metabolic or neural factors, it is intrinsic to VSM and therefore termed *myogenic* tone (reviewed in Ref. 141).

The endothelium, situated at the interface between the flowing blood and VSM, is also an important modulator of tone through release of a number of vasoactive factors having both inhibitory (e.g., nitric oxide, prostacyclin) and excitatory (e.g., endothelin, thromboxane) effects on VSM.[142] Moreover, in many arteries, the endothelium is coupled to VSM through numerous myoendothelial junctions—areas in which the membranes of the endothelium and VSM are in close apposition.[143] Spontaneous vasomotion and, in some cases, upstream ("ascending") vasodilation have been observed in vivo in several circulatory beds and may involve cooperation between endothelial and VSM cells in determining network resistance.[144]

### MYOGENIC PROPERTIES OF VASCULAR SMOOTH MUSCLE

Arterial constriction to increased perfusion pressure was first described by Bayliss in 1902. Myogenic responses have been documented in arteries, arterioles, and veins, although the fundamental question of how a vessel is able to sense intravascular pressure has proven difficult to answer and the identity of the myogenic "sensor"—the structure(s) that convert physical force into VSM contraction—has thus far eluded investigators. Some putative candidates are integrins, stretch-activated cation channels, and cytoskeletal proteins.[145]

Recent studies have elucidated many of the intracellular signal transduction pathways involved in the generation and maintenance of myogenic tone. Myogenicity appears to involve cooperativity between ionic and enzymatic mechanisms, with calcium entry and activation of the phospholipase C (PLC)/PKC cascade central among them. Transmural pressure leads to depolarization of the VSM membrane through mechanisms as yet to be identified. Recent evidence points to a subset of nonselective cation channels [called *transient receptor potential* (TRP) channels] as being important in mediating depolarization.[146] Depolarization of VSM activates L-type calcium channels that are voltage-sensitive. Calcium entry into VSM promotes contraction through calmodulin-mediated myosin light-chain phosphorylation that initiates actomyosin ATPase activity and crossbridge (actin and myosin) cycling. At the same time, membrane enzymes such as PLC and PKC become activated. Many of these enzymes exist in multiple isoforms that may or may not be calcium-dependent. Enzyme activation leads to kinase-induced phosphorylation of a number of other enzymes and ion channels (e.g., potassium channels) as well as modulation of intracellular calcium stores through phosphoinositides such as $IP_3$.

Although calcium is required for constriction, enzymatic activity may "sensitize" the contractile proteins to calcium and lead to an increase in constriction without any change in cytosolic calcium. This may be accomplished at the crossbridge level by the inhibition of myosin light-chain phosphatase (MLCP), an enzyme that dephosphorylates myosin and leads to its inactivation. Consequently, the balance of inhibitory (MLCP) and stimulatory (MLCK, myosin light-chain kinase) activity shifts in favor of greater myosin phosphorylation and smooth muscle force production. The level of tone is therefore controlled by a combination of mechanisms that (1) regulate vascular smooth muscle calcium levels (calcium entry and extrusion) and (2) modulate the effect of calcium on the contractile proteins (calcium sensitivity). Feedback mechanisms for limiting pressure-induced myogenic constriction are poorly understood.

An intriguing concept, first reported in cardiac myocytes and discussed earlier in relation to them, invokes control of a subset of potassium channels that have been implicated in basal tone ($K_{ca}$, or calcium activated potassium channels) by highly localized intracellular "hot spots" of calcium, termed *calcium sparks*.[147–149] In this scenario, calcium is released from the VSM sarcoplasmic reticulum in a discrete fashion that leads to highly localized increases in the concentration of calcium within the cytoplasm (calcium sparks). The proximity of the sarcoplasmic calcium release site to the calcium-activated potassium channels, which are embedded in the plasma membrane, facilitates their activation. The resulting outward potassium current produces membrane hyperpolarization that in turn inhibits voltage-sensitive calcium channels, decreases calcium entry, and leads to vascular relaxation. Hence, calcium sparks produce vasodilation indirectly by activating $K_{Ca}$ channels.

### ENDOTHELIAL INFLUENCES ON VASCULAR SMOOTH MUSCLE CONTRACTILITY

Although the importance of the endothelium as a nonthrombogenic surface has been known for some time, its role in modulating arterial tone was not recognized until the early 1980s, when Furchgott and colleagues observed that this cell type was obligatory for the relaxation response to acetylcholine. In a landmark paper,[150] Furchgott reported that endothelial denudation abolished relaxation to acetylcholine and hypothesized that cholinergic stimulation led to the release of a substance as yet to be identified that relaxed VSM. This compound, initially called endothelium-derived relaxing factor (EDRF), was subsequently (1988) shown to be nitric oxide (NO). This simple gaseous molecule is produced during the conversion of the amino acid L-arginine into L-citrulline by the enzyme nitric oxide synthetase (NOS).[151] NO can be generated by several different isoforms of NOS that may vary in their dependence on calcium and type of regulation (constitutive versus inducible). For example, eNOS refers to endothelial NOS, while nNOS refers to the form of the enzyme that is contained within nerves.

The endothelium performs a variety of chemo- and mechanotransduction functions and releases a host of vasoactive molecules in response to both physical and chemical stimulation. Foremost in addition to NO are the peptide endothelin (a potent vasoconstrictor first isolated and sequenced in 1988)[152] and dilator and constrictor prostaglandins (e.g., prostacyclin and thromboxane, respectively). There is also experimental evidence for a non-NO factor that acts to hyperpolarize smooth muscle. In spite of a decade of effort, the chemical identity of this substance has not yet been determined and it is referred to as EDHF (endothelium-derived hyperpolarizing factor).[153]

Endothelial secretions diffuse to adjacent VSM to activate a variety of signal transduction mechanisms that alter intracellular concentrations of cAMP (e.g., via prostaglandins), cGMP (via nitric oxide), PLC (endothelin), and membrane potential (EDHF). The release of endothelium-derived vasoactive molecules is controlled by a variety of factors, both chemical and physical. By virtue of its location, the endothelium is exposed to much higher levels of shear stress than most other tissues. Shear is an important stimulus for a number of endothelial events, including hyperpolarization, calcium influx, up- and downregulation of mRNA for many different proteins, induction of G proteins and activation of a number of kinases, cytoskeletal rearrangement, and release of cytokines and growth factors.[154] There is also compelling evidence that shear stress can modulate arterial growth and expansive remodeling through an endothelium-dependent mechanism.[155] Described most simply, an increase in flow leads to elevated shear stress that can be normalized by increasing arterial diameter via vasodilation and/or expansive remodeling. Similarly, a decrease in blood flow (and shear stress) can be normalized by arterial narrowing via constriction (short term) or remodeling (long term). Thus, shear stress is an important signal for altering vascular structure based on tissue blood flow demand.

Aberrations in small artery endothelial function (most often characterized by diminished release of vasodilator substances) have been reported in several vascular diseases, such as hypertension and diabetes.[156] In larger arteries, abnormal flow patterns associated with lower than normal shear stress may also lead to metabolic derangements in endothelial function and accelerate the development of atherosclerosis.

## Autonomic Regulation of Peripheral Blood Flow

Most arteries and veins receive direct sympathetic innervation, which contributes to maintenance of arterial and venous pressure under normal and stressful conditions. Sympathetic efferent activity, which involves the release of norepinephrine, is determined by a complex interaction of neurons in the spinal cord, medulla, pons, hypothalamus, limbic system, and portions of the forebrain and by feedback signals arising from cardiovascular mechano- and chemoreceptors localized in discrete baroreceptor centers in the carotid sinuses, aortic arch and the heart.[157]

The two CNS areas that appear to be of principal importance in regulating sympathetic outflow are the nucleus tractus solitarius (NTS) and the rostral ventral lateral medulla (RVLM). The influence of the NTS on the RVLM is inhibitory.

Sympathetic denervation produces widely varying effects on organ blood flow. Cerebral and coronary circulations are virtually unaffected, most likely as a result of the aforementioned intrinsic autoregulatory mechanisms, whereas denervation of skin or skeletal muscle produces substantial increases in flow.

During intense sympathetic activation, the "fight or flight reaction," large amounts of epinephrine (and, to a lesser extent, norepinephrine) are released from the adrenal medulla in response to activation of sympathetic preganglionic afferents. Blood pressure increases markedly, and a significant redistribution of cardiac output occurs. Moreover, stimulation of the venous circulation increases venous return, thereby augmenting cardiac output considerably.

The efferent fibers of the cranial division of the parasympathetic system innervate the blood vessels of the head and viscera; those of the sacral division supply the vasculature of the large bowel, bladder, and genitalia. All release acetylcholine from postsynaptic nerve endings. The parasympathetic system generally produces effects opposite to those of the sympathetic division, i.e., decreased cardiac rate and output and vascular relaxation, but is thought to be of secondary importance in peripheral vascular regulation.

In summary, peripheral vascular control results from integration of a number of mechanisms both extrinsic and intrinsic to the vascular wall. VSM responds directly to pressure and stretch (myogenic constriction), the most fundamental source of basal vascular tone. The endothelium acts as an important transducer of physical stimuli such as shear stress and humoral signals that alter its release of vasoactive substances and modulate basal myogenic constriction. Extrinsic mechanisms include neural regulation via the sympathetic and, to a lesser extent, parasympathetic branches of the autonomic system, and metabolic regulation (through release of various vasodilator substances). Together, these mechanisms allow for the integrated regulation of total peripheral resistance and venous return. At the same time, by permitting bidirectional changes in regional resistance, they allow for a fine degree of local control of flow. This dynamic interaction between central and local mechanisms of vascular control is essential for normal hemodynamic function and fluid balance.

## THE CORONARY CIRCULATION

### Anatomic and Mechanical Considerations

The right and left main coronary arteries (CAs) arise at the root of the aorta. The right CA normally supplies the inferior surface of the LV, the RV, and RA, whereas the left CA divides into circumflex and anterior descending branches that perfuse the rest of LV and LA. In about 10 percent of cases, the left circumflex rather than the right CA supplies the inferior LV. Branches from the main CAs ramify and penetrate the myocardium, forming dense capillary beds. Most venous blood returns to the RA via the coronary sinus; there is also communication between the cardiac chambers and myocardium via arteriosinusoidal channels. Delivery of blood to the myocardium is complicated by compression of intramyocardial vessels during systole, which induces retrograde flow in epicardial CAs.[158–160] As a consequence, the bulk of coronary flow occurs during diastole, and the upstream perfusion pressure is the Ao *diastolic* pressure. The subendocardial layer of the myocardium is more susceptible to hypoperfusion because ventricular diastolic pressure opposes the driving pressure for flow. Moreover, compression of microvessels during systole is more prominent in the subendocardium. There has been some uncertainty about the actual driving pressure for nutrient flow, in particular whether the downstream pressure should be considered RA/coronary sinus pressure or a higher value related to tissue forces that cause collapse of the microcirculation (i.e., a critical closing pressure).

### Modulation of Coronary Vasomotor Tone and Flow

The distribution of coronary vascular resistance is complex and dependent on type of vessel, region, and specific vasomotor stimuli.[158] Arterioles are the main components of resistance, but small arteries and venules also contribute in a coordinated fashion to control regional flow. Some vasodilators and constrictors preferentially dilate small arteries rather than arterioles. Resistance in subendocardial microvessels appears to be significantly lower than in subepicardium. Modulation of coronary vascular resistance is complex; only a brief discussion can be undertaken here (see Ref. 158 and Chap. 46 for additional details). As the heart varies its mechanical performance over a range of demands, coronary flow must keep pace. Thus, nutritive coronary flow increases by as much as 400 percent during exercise. Since upstream Ao diastolic pressure does not change or decreases during exercise, this requires marked dilation of coronary resistance vessels. The most potent mechanism of modulation of coronary resistance and flow is endogenous autoregulation.[159] Autoregulation occurs at the level of small arteries, arterioles, and venules and appears to be both *myogenic* and *metabolically* mediated.[159,160] As discussed earlier, a myogenic response is an alteration in tone as a direct response to changes in pressure and/or flow. This is most prominent in arterioles, resulting in constriction when perfusion pressure is increased and dilatation when pressure is reduced. Although myogenic responses play a role in autoregulation, factors related to changes in metabolite washout are more important. The actual metabolites and effector mechanisms responsible for autoregulation are incompletely defined, but effects are most prominent in small arterioles. Locally released adenosine (a potent dilator) under conditions of increased metabolic demand appears to be a key mediator.[159,161] Other endogenous vasoactive mechanisms also contribute.[162] Local release of K and activation of ATP-sensitive K channels in small arteries and arterioles may have a role and adenosine itself may activate ATP-sensitive K channels.

Neurohumorally mediated responses also modulate coronary vascular resistance.[159] Their importance under *normal physiologic conditions* is uncertain. $\alpha$-Adrenergic responses are well documented in the coronary circulation. Agonists constrict large epicardial and small coronary arteries/arterioles (>100 $\mu$m in diameter) and dilate smaller arterioles. At physiologic perfusion pressure, the main effect is constriction of small arteries. While there is evidence of $\alpha$-adrenergic activity under physiologic conditions, endogenous mechanisms mask and/or counteract this vasoconstrictive influence. Thus, endothelial release of NO occurs concomitant with $\alpha$-adrenergic activity. $\beta$-Adrenergic receptors are present in coronary vessels and cause dilation of large arteries and resistance vessels, but this is likely of minor importance compared with autoregulation.

Vasoactive substances produced by endothelium play a key role in many of the changes in coronary tone occurring in response to a variety of stimuli, including autoregulation and responses to adenosine, serotonin, acetylcholine, and adrenergic stimulation.[159,163] These substances include prostaglandins, ET-1, endothelium-derived hyperpolarizing factor,[164] and NO.[159,162–164] At present, there is considerable information about NO, but little is known about the *physiologic* role of other substances. Although NO is a coronary vasodilator, it produces heterogeneous effects and may have quantitatively different influences on large arteries versus resistance vessels. NO is the key effector of autoregulatory responses to normal physiologic stimuli, including tachycardia and vasodilation during exercise,[165,166] and is intimately connected to responses to the endothelial-derived substances mentioned earlier as well as a variety of vasoactive drugs.

Coronary circulatory responses to changes in demand require coordination of the multiple modulatory mechanisms discussed earlier. The integrated response consists of heterogeneous effects that depend on the type of vessel and the region of the myocardium, which together increase nutritive flow. A scheme illustrating the complex interactions involved in the response to an increase in demand is shown in Fig. 4-25.

## INTEGRATION OF THE CARDIOVASCULAR SYSTEM: THE RESPONSE TO DYNAMIC EXERCISE

Integrated functioning of the heart and peripheral and coronary circulations is exemplified by responses to dynamic exercise—such as walking, running, and swimming—that entails repetitive shortening of skeletal muscle against relatively low loads. The coordinated response maximizes flow to working skeletal muscle and the heart; minimizes flow to nonworking muscle, visceral organs, and the kidneys; and ensures that flow to the brain is not compromised (Table 4-2). In the periphery, local vasodilatory influences reduce resistance in vascular beds of working muscle. Cutaneous beds dilate to facilitate heat transfer. In contrast, neurohumorally mediated responses cause vasoconstriction in nonworking skeletal muscle, abdominal viscera, and the kidneys. With isotonic exercise involving large muscle groups, total systemic vascular resistance usually decreases.

$O_2$ delivery to myocardium is augmented by increased coronary flow caused by autoregulatory vasodilatation in response to increased metabolic demands. $O_2$ consumption is augmented by increased extraction, with lowering of coronary sinus $O_2$ saturation. Myocardial glycolytic metabolism increases. NO produced in coronary endothelium may facilitate shifts in mitochondrial respiration that tend to minimize increases in energy demands.

In the normal circulation, the ability to return blood to the heart is the limiting factor for increased CO during exercise. In order to in-

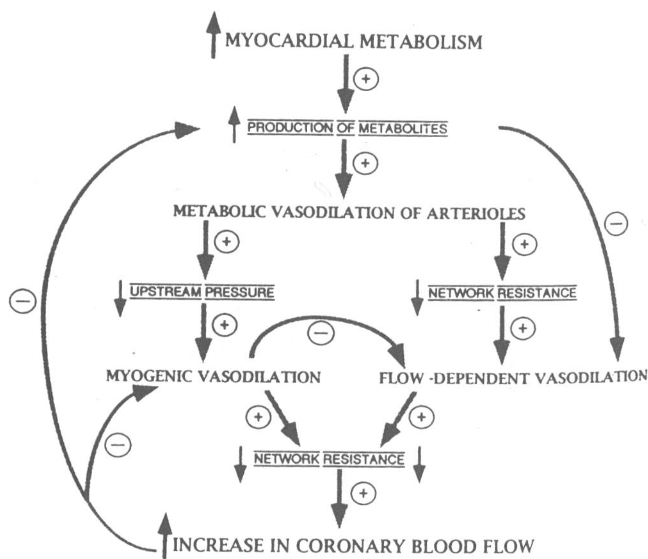


FIGURE 4-25 Schematic diagram of integrated response of metabolic, myogenic, and flow-mediated regulation of coronary vascular resistance and flow during increase in metabolic demand. Plus sign indicates vasodilatory feed-forward steps in response to initial increase in demand. Minus sign indicates negative-feedback processes that limit vasodilation. Events marked by lines ("Production of Metabolites") occur as a reaction to metabolic or vascular changes. Bolded items are metabolic or vasoactive adjustments. (From Muller et al.[158] Reprinted with permission of the publisher.)

crease venous return, systemic venoconstriction decreases the volume of blood in venous reservoirs, resulting in a shift of blood volume to the arterial circulation and the heart. Working skeletal muscles in conjunction with venous valves function as pumps to return blood to the heart. Increased respiratory rate causes intrathoracic pressure to be negative a larger proportion of the time, which directly assists venous return to the right side of the heart.

In the heart itself, increased adrenergic stimulation caused by the coordinated effects of increased central nervous outflow and circulating catecholamines, along with parasympathetic withdrawal, results in markedly increased HR, accelerated AV conduction, and enhanced contractility. Increased force and velocity of contraction and ultimately power are achieved through the effects of adrenergic stimulation (cyclic AMP) and the FFR. Associated effects on Ca reuptake and myofilament Ca sensitivity speed myocardial relaxation so that increased HR does not occur at the expense of incomplete relaxation. During upright exercise, ED volume remains relatively constant; during supine exercise, it increases somewhat.[167] Reflecting increased contractility, the ESPVR shifts leftward and ES volume decreases. The combination of relatively constant or modestly increased ED volume and reduced ES volume results in increased SV and EF. With respect to augmenting CO, however, the increase in HR is more important than increased SV.

The combination of increased HR and SV with resulting marked shortening of diastole means that ventricular filling must occur much more rapidly than at rest. This is partly accomplished by the increase in relaxation rate. However, an increase in the generation of restoring forces due to the smaller ES volume undoubtedly also increases suction. Thus, the same mechanisms causing increased force of contraction also result in more rapid diastolic filling at lower ventricular pressures.

Systolic systemic arterial pressure increases substantially during dynamic exercise as a result of increased contractility and SV, while diastolic arterial pressure decreases because systemic resistance decreases. Obviously, pulse pressure increases. Minimum ventricular diastolic pressure decreases with little or no change in ED pressure. Finally, coordinated changes in arterial elastance function to optimize ventricular-vascular coupling and efficiency of conversion of chemical energy to EW.

Predominantly isometric exercise involving relatively brief bursts of skeletal muscle shortening against a heavy load (e.g., weight lifting, handgrip) evoke different responses. This type of exercise does not require a marked and/or sustained increase in CO with selective distribution to working muscles and heart. However, isometric exercise does elicit reflex-mediated increases in sympathetic stimulation causing increased systemic vascular resistance and arterial pressure, HR, and cardiac contractility. The increases in systolic blood pressure are comparable to those during isotonic exercise, whereas the increases in HR are much smaller.

## References

1. Smith EE, Guyton AC, Manning RD, White RJ. Integrated mechanisms of cardiovascular response and control during exercise in the normal human. *Prog Cardiovasc Dis* 1976;18:421.
2. Brengelmann GL. Circulatory adjustments to exercise and heat stress. *Annu Rev Physiol* 1983;45:191.
3. Myhre ESP, Slinker BK, LeWinter MM. Absence of RV isovolumic relaxation in open-chest anesthetized dogs. *Am J Physiol* 1992;263: H1587.
4. Fozzard HA, Arnsdorf MF. Cardiac electrophysiology. In: Fozzard HA, Haber E, Jennings RB, et al, eds. *The Heart and Cardiovascular System,* 2d ed. New York: Raven Press; 1991:63.
5. Pelzer D, Pelzer S, McDonald TF. Ca channels in heart. In: Fozzard HA, Haber E, Jennings RB, et al, eds. *The Heart and Cardiovascular System,* 2d ed. New York: Raven Press; 1991:1049.
6. Fozzard HA, Hanck DA. Na channels. In: Fozzard HA, Haber E, Jennings RB, et al, eds. *The Heart and Cardiovascular System,* 2d ed. New York, Raven Press; 1991:1091.
7. Puglisi JL, Bers DM. LabHEART: An interactive computer model of rabbit ventricular myocyte ion channels and Ca transport. *Am J Physiol Cell Physiol.* 2001;281:C2049.
8. Williams AJ. The functions of two species of Ca channel in cardiac muscle ECC. *Eur Heart J* 1997;18 (suppl A):A27.
9. Yao A, Su Z, Nonaka A, et al. Effects of overexpression of the $Na^+$–$Ca^{2+}$ exchanger on $[Ca^{2+}]_i$ transients in murine ventricular myocytes. *Circ Res* 1998;82:657.
10. Sipido KR, Maes M, Van de Werf F. Low efficiency of $Ca^{2+}$ entry through the $Na^+$–$Ca^{2+}$ exchanger as trigger for $Ca^{2+}$ release from the SR. *Circ Res* 1997;81:1034.
11. Weber CR, Piacentino V III, Ginsburg KS, et al. Na(+)–Ca(2+) exchange current and submembrane [Ca(2+)] during the cardiac action potential. *Circ Res* 2002;90:182.
12. Sommer JR, Jennings RB. Ultrastructure of cardiac muscle. In: Fozzard HA, Haber E, Jennings RB, et al, eds. *The Heart and Cardiovascular System,* 2d ed. New York: Raven Press; 1991:3.
13. Lytton J, MacLennan DH Sr. In: Fozzard HA, Haber E, Jennings RB, et al, eds. *The Heart and Cardiovascular System,* 2d ed. New York: Raven Press; 1991:1203.
14. McDonald TF, Pelzer S, Trautwein W, Pelzaer DJ. Regulation and modulation of Ca channels in cardiac, skeletal, and smooth muscle cells. *Physiol Rev* 1994;74:365.
15. Carl SL, Felix K, Caswell AH, et al. Immunolocalization of sarcolemmal dihydropyridine receptor and SR triadin and RyR in rabbit ventricle and atrium. *J Cell Biol* 1995;129:673.
16. Cannell MB, Cheng H, Lederer WJ. The control of Ca release in heart muscle. *Science* 1995;268:1045.
17. Lopez-Lopez JR, Shacklock PS, Balke CW, Wier WG. Local Ca transients triggered by single L-type Ca channel currents in cardiac cells. *Science* 1995;268:1042.

18. Santana LF, Cheng H, Gomez MB, et al. Relation between the sarcolemmal $Ca^{2+}$ current and $Ca^{2+}$ sparks and local control theories for cardiac excitation-contraction coupling. *Circ Res* 1996;78:166.
19. Cheng H, Lederer MR, Xiao RP, et al. Excitation-contraction coupling in heart: New insights from $Ca^{2+}$ sparks. *Cell Calcium* 1996;20:129.
20. Wier WG, ter Keurs HEDJ, Marban E, et al. $Ca^{2+}$ "sparks" and waves in intact ventricular muscle resolved by confocal imaging. *Circ Res* 1997;81:462.
21. Bers DM. Cardiac excitation-contraction coupling. *Nature* 2002;415:198.
22. Sitsapesan R, Williams AJ. Gating of the native and purified cardiac SR $Ca^{2+}$-release channel with monovalent cations as permeant species. *Biophys J* 1994;67:1484.
23. Sitsapesan R, Williams AJ. Regulation of the gating of the sheep cardiac SR $Ca^{2+}$-release channel by luminal $Ca^{2+}$. *J Membr Biol* 1994;266:11144.
24. Marks AR, Marx SO, Reiken S. Regulation of ryanodine receptors via macromolecular complexes: A novel role for leucine/isoleucine zippers. *Trends Cardiovasc Med* 2002;12:166.
25. Ondrias K, Mojzisova A. Coupled gating between individual cardiac ryanodine calcium release channels. *Gen Physiol Biophys* 200;21:73.
26. Kao JPY, Harootunian AT, Tsien RY. Photochemically generated cytosolic Ca pulses and their detection by fluo-3. *J Biol Chem* 1989; 264:8171.
27. Schatzmann HJ. The Ca pump at the surface membrane and at the SR. *Annu Rev Physiol* 1989;51:473.
28. Luo W, Grupp IL, Harrer J, et al. Targeted ablation of the phospholamban gene is associated with markedly enhanced myocardial contractility and loss of $\beta$-agonist stimulation. *Circ Res* 1994;75:401.
29. Luo W, Wolska BM, Grupp IL, et al. Phospholamban gene dosage effects in the mammalian heart. *Circ Res* 1996;78:839.
30. Kadambi VJ, Ponniah S, Harrer J, et al. Cardiac-specific overexpression of phospholamban alters Ca kinetics and resultant cardiomyocyte mechanics in transgenic mice. *J Clin Invest* 1996;97:533.
31. Koss KL, Kranias EG. Phospholamban: A prominent regulator of myocardial contractility. *Circ Res* 1996;79:1059.
32. Frank KF, Bolck B, Brixius K, et al. Modulation of SERCA: Implications for the failing human heart. *Basic Res Cardiol* 2002; 97(Suppl 1):I72.
33. Hagemann D, Xiao RP. Dual site phospholamban phosphorylation and its physiological relevance in the heart. *Trends Cardiovasc Med* 2002;12:51.
34. Katz AM. Cardiac ion channels. *N Eng J Med* 1993;328:1244.
35. Huxley AF. Muscle structure and theories of contraction. *Prog Biophys Biophys Chem* 1957;7:255.
36. Spudich JA. How molecular motors work. *Nature* 1994;372:515.
37. McNally EM, Kraft R, Bravo-Zehnder M, et al. Full-length rat alpha and beta cardiac myosin HC sequences. *J Mol Biol* 1989;210:665.
38. Rayment L, Holden H, Whittaker M, et al. Structure of the actin-myosin complex and its implications for muscle contraction. *Science* 1993;261:58.
39. Pagani ED, Julian FJ. Rabbit papillary muscle myosin isozymes and the velocity of muscle shortening. *Circ Res* 1984;54:586.
40. VanBuren P, Harris DE, Alpert NR, Warshaw DM. Cardiac $V_1$ and $V_3$ myosins differ in their mechanical activities in vitro. *Circ Res* 1995;77:439.
41. Cuda G, Cooke R, Sellers JR. In vitro actin filament sliding velocities produced by mixtures of different types of myosin. *Biophys J* 1997; 72:1767.
42. Winegrad S. How actin-myosin interactions differ with different isoforms of myosin. *Circ Res* 1998;82:1109.
43. Wu Y, Labeit S, Lewinter MM, Granzier H. Titin: An endosarcomeric protein that modulates myocardial stiffness in DCM. *J Card Fail* 2002; 8(6 suppl):S276.
44. Helmes M, Trombitas K, Granzier H. Titin develops restoring force in rat cardiac myocytes. *Circ Res* 1996;79:619.
45. Winegrad S. Cardiac myosin binding protein C. *Circ Res* 1999;84:1117.
46. Tobacman LS. Thin filament-mediated regulation of cardiac contraction. *Annu Rev Physiol* 1996;58:447.
47. Craig R, Lehman W. Crossbridge and tropomyosin positions observed in native, interacting thick and thin filaments. *J Mol Biol* 2001; 311:1027.
48. Weisberg A, Winegrad S. Relation between crossbridge structure and actomyosin ATPase activity in rat heart. *Circ Res* 1998;83:60.
49. McKillop DFA, Geeves MA. Regulation of the interaction between actin and myosin subfragment 1: Evidence for three states of the thin filament. *Biophys J* 1993;65:693.
50. Geeves MA, Lehrer SS. Dynamics of the muscle thin filament regulatory switch: The size of the cooperative unit. *Biophys J* 1994; 67:273.
51. Swartz DR, Moss RL. Influence of a strong binding myosin analog on Ca sensitive mechanical properties of skinned skeletal muscle fibers. *J Biol Chem* 1992;267:20497.
52. Moss RL. $Ca^{2+}$ regulation of mechanical properties of striated muscle: Mechanistic studies using extraction and replacement of regulatory proteins. *Circ Res* 1992;70:865.
53. Baker JE, Thomas DD. A thermodynamic muscle model and a chemical basis for A.V. Hill's muscle equation. *J Muscle Res Cell Motil* 2000;21:335.
54. McMahon TA. *Muscles, Reflexes, and Locomotion*. Princeton, NJ: Princeton University Press; 1984.
55. Lakatta EG. Starling's law of the heart is explained by an intimate interaction of muscle length and myofilament Ca activation. *J Am Coll Cardiol* 1987;10:1157.
56. Lakatta EG. Length modulation of cardiac performance: Frank-Starling law of the heart. In: Fozzard HA, Haber E, Jennings RB, et al, eds. *The Heart and Cardiovascular System,* 2d ed. New York: Raven Press; 1991:1325.
57. McDonald KS, Moss RL. Osmotic compression of single cardiac myocytes eliminates the reduction in $Ca^{2+}$ sensitivity of tension at short sarcomere length. *Circ Res* 1995;77:199.
58. Konhilas JP, Irving TC, de Tombe PP. Myofilament calcium sensitivity in skinned rat cardiac trabeculae: Role of interfilament spacing. *Circ Res* 2002;90:11.
59. Apstein CS, Morgan JP. Cellular mechanisms underlying LV diastolic dysfunction. In: Gaasch WH, LeWinter MM, eds. *LV Diastolic Dysfunction and Heart Failure*. Philadelphia: Lea & Febiger; 1994:3.
60. Gillebert TC, Sys SU. Physiologic control of relaxation in isolated cardiac muscle and intact LV. In: Gaasch WH, LeWinter MM, eds. *LV Diastolic Dysfunction and Heart Failure*. Philadelphia: Lea & Febiger; 1994:25.
61. Stanley WC, Lopaschuk GD, Hall JL, McCormack JG. Regulation of myocardial carbohydrate metabolism under normal and ischaemic conditions: Potential for pharmacological interventions. *Cardiovasc Res* 1997;33:243.
62. Eberli FR, Weinberg EO, Grice WN, et al. Protective effect of increased glycolytic substrate against systolic and diastolic dysfunction and increased coronary resistance from prolonged global underperfusion and reperfusion in isolated rabbit hearts perfused with erythrocyte suspensions. *Circ Res* 1991;68:466.
63. Kelly RA, Balligand J-L, Smith TW. NO and cardiac function. *Circ Res* 1996;79:363.
64. Alpert NA, Mulieri LA, Hasenfuss G. Myocardial chemomechanical energy transduction. In: Fozzard HA, Haber E, Jennings RB, et al, eds. *The Heart and Cardiovascular System,* 2d ed. New York: Raven Press; 1991:111.
65. Ross J Jr, Miura T, Kambayashi M, et al. Adrenergic control of the force-frequency relation. *Circulation* 1995;92:2327.
66. Hasenfuss G, Schillinger W, Lehnart SE, et al. Relationship between $Na^+$–$Ca^{2+}$ exchanger protein levels and diastolic function of failing human myocardium. *Circulation* 1999;99:641.
67. Blanchard EL, Leavitt BJ, Mulieri LA, Alpert NR. Dynamic Ca requirements for activation of human ventricular muscle calculated from tension independent heat. *Basic Res Cardiol* 1992;87(suppl 1):245.
68. Mulieri LA, Leavitt BJ, Martin BJ, et al. Myocardial force-frequency defect in mitral regurgitation heart failure is reversed by forskolin. *Circulation* 1993;88:2700.

69. Xiao R-P, Avdonin P, Zhou Y-Y, et al. Coupling of $\beta_2$-adrenoceptor to $G_i$ proteins and its physiological relevance in murine cardiac myocytes. *Circ Res* 1999;84:43.
70. Gauthier C, Tavernier G, Charpentier F, et al. Functional $\beta_3$-adrenoceptor in the human heart. *J Clin Invest* 1998;98:556.
71. Kaye DM, Wiviott SD, Balligand J-L, et al. Frequency-dependent activation of a constitutive NO synthase and regulation of contractile function in adult rat ventricular myocytes. *Circ Res* 1996;78:217.
72. Ashley EA, Sears CE, Bryant SM, et al. Cardiac nitric oxide synthase 1 regulates basal and beta-adrenergic contractility in murine ventricular myocytes. *Circulation* 2002;105:3011.
73. Haque R, Kan H, Finkel MS. Effects of cytokines and NO on myocardial E-C coupling. *Basic Res Cardiol* 1998;93(suppl 1):86.
74. Graham RM, Perez DM, Hwa J, Piascik MY. $\alpha_1$-Adrenergic receptor subtypes: Molecular structure, function, and signaling. *Circ Res* 1996;78:737.
75. Endoh M, Fujita S, Yang H-T, et al. Endothelin: Receptor subtypes, signal transduction, regulation of $Ca^{2+}$ transients and contractility in rabbit ventricular myocardium. *Life Sci* 1998;62:1485.
76. Hoit BD, Shao Y, Kinoshita A, et al. Effects of angiotensin II generated by an angiotensin converting enzyme-independent pathway on LV performance in the conscious baboon. *J Clin Invest* 1985;95:1519.
77. Sadoshima J. Versatility of the angiotensin II type 1 receptor. *Circ Res* 1998;82:1352.
78. Pi Y, Sreekumar R, Xupei H, Walker JW. Positive inotropy mediated by diacylglycerol in rat ventricular myocytes. *Circ Res* 1997;81:92.
79. Rouet-Benzineb P, Mohammadi K, Perennec J, et al. Protein kinase C isoform expression in normal and failing hearts. *Circ Res* 1996;79:153.
80. Puceat M, Vassort G. Signalling by protein kinase C isoforms in the heart. *Mol Cell Biochem* 1996;157:65.
81. Solaro RJ, Van Eyk J. Altered interactions among thin filament proteins modulate cardiac function. *J Mol Cell Cardiol* 1996;28:217.
82. Streeter DD Jr. Gross morphology and fiber geometry of the heart. In: Berne RM, Sperelakis N, eds. *Handbook of Physiology,* Sec 2: *The Cardiovascular System,* Vol 1: *The Heart*. Bethesda, MD: American Physiological Society; 1979:61.
83. Buchalter MB, Weiss JL, Rogers WJ, et al. Noninvasive quantification of left ventricular rotational deformation in normal humans using magnetic resonance myocardial tagging. *Circulation* 1990;81:1236.
84. Arts T, Veenstra PC, Reneman RS. Epicardial deformation and LV wall mechanics during ejection in the dog. *Am J Physiol* 1982;243:H379.
85. Yaku H, Slinker BK, Bell SP, LeWinter MM. Effects of free wall ischemia and bundle branch on systolic ventricular interaction in dog hearts. *Am J Physiol* 1994;266:H1087–H1094.
86. Robinson TF, Cohen-Gould L, Factor SM. Skeletal framework of mammalian heart muscle: Arrangements of inter- and pericellular connective tissue structures. *Lab Invest* 1983;49:482.
87. Guyton AC. The circulation. In: Guyton AC, Nall JE, eds. *Textbook of Medical Physiology,* 9th ed. Philadelphia: Saunders; 1996:239.
88. Shroff SG, Janicki J, Weber KT. Mechanical and energetic behavior of the intact left ventricle. In: Fozzard HA, Haber E, Jennings RB, et al, eds. *The Heart and Cardiovascular System,* 2d ed. New York: Raven Press; 1991:129.
89. Mirsky I. Review of various theories for the evaluation of left ventricular wall stresses. In: Mirsky I, Ghista DN, Sandler H, eds. *Cardiac Mechanics*. New York: Wiley; 1974:381.
90. Cohn JN. Cardiac consequences of vasomotor changes in the periphery: Impedance and preload. In: Fozzard HA, Haber E, Jennings RB, et al, eds. *The Heart and Cardiovascular System*, 2d ed. New York: Raven Press; 1991:1369.
91. Starling MR, Kirsh MM, Montgomery DG, Gross MD. Impaired left ventricular contractile function in patients with long-term mitral regurgitation and normal EF. *J Am Coll Cardiol* 1993;22:239.
92. Suga H, Sagawa K, Shoukas AA. Load independence of the instantaneous pressure-volume ratio of the canine left ventricle and effects of epinephrine and HR on the ratio. *Circ Res* 1973;32:314.
93. Sagawa K. The ES pressure-volume relation of the ventricle: Definition, modifications and clinical use. *Circulation* 1981;63:1223.
94. Kass DA, Maughan WL. From "$E_{max}$" to pressure-volume relations: A broader view. *Circulation* 1991;77:1203.
95. Slinker BK, Goto Y, LeWinter MM. Systolic direct ventricular interaction affects left ventricular contraction and relaxation in the intact dog circulation. *Circ Res* 1989;65:307.
96. Mirsky I, Corin WJ, Murakami T, et al. Correction for preload in the assessment of myocardial contractility in aortic and mitral valve disease: Application of the concept of systolic myocardial stiffness. *Circulation* 1988;78:68.
97. Kameyama T, Chen Z, Bell SP, Maughan D, et al. Mechanoenergetic alterations during the transition from cardiac hypertrophy to failure in Dahl salt sensitive rats. *Circulation* 1998;98:2911.
98. Suga H. Ventricular energetics. *Physiol Rev* 1990;70:247.
99. Goto Y, Slinker BK, LeWinter MM. Similar normalized $E_{max}$ and $O_2$ consumption-pressure volume area relation in rabbit and dog. *Am J Physiol* 1988;255:H366.
100. Goto Y, Slinker BK, LeWinter MM. Decreased contractile efficiency and increased nonmechanical energy cost in hyperthyroid rabbit heart. *Circ Res* 1990;66:999.
101. Sunagawa K, Maughan WL, Sagawa K. Optimal arterial resistance for the maximal stroke work studied in isolated canine left ventricle. *Circ Res* 1985;56:586.
102. Hayashida K, Sunagawa K, Noma M, et al. Mechanical matching of the left ventricle with the arterial system in exercising dogs. *Circ Res* 1992;71:481.
103. Asanoi H, Sasayama S, Kameyama T. Ventriculoarterial coupling in normal and failing heart in humans. *Circ Res* 1989;65:483.
104. Peterson KL, Sklovan D, Ludbrook P, et al. Comparison of isovolumic and ejection phase indices of myocardial performance in man. *Circulation* 1974;49:1088.
105. Ross J Jr. Afterload mismatch and preload reserve: A conceptual framework for the analysis of ventricular function. *Prog Cardiovasc Dis* 1976;18:255.
106. Nakayama M, Chen CH, Nevo E, et al. Optimal preload adjustment of maximal ventricular power index varies with cardiac chamber size. *Am Heart J* 1998;136:281.
107. Glower DD, Spratt JA, Snow ND, et al. Linearity of the Frank-Starling relationship in the intact heart: The concept of preload recruitable stroke work. *Circulation* 1985;71:994.
108. Little WC. The left ventricular $dP/dt_{max}$-end-diastolic volume relation in closed chest dogs. *Circ Res* 1985;56:808.
109. Little WC, Park RC, Freeman GL. Effects of regional ischemia and ventricular pacing on left ventricular $dP/dt_{max}$-end-diastolic volume relation. *Am J Physiol* 1987;252:H993.
110. Weiss JL, Frederiksen JW, Weisfeldt ML. Hemodynamic determinants of the time-course of fall in canine left ventricular pressure. *J Clin Invest* 1976;58:751.
111. Karliner JS, LeWinter MM, Mahler F, et al. Pharmacologic and hemodynamic influences on the rate of isovolumic left ventricular relaxation in conscious dogs. *J Clin Invest* 1977;60:511.
112. Brutsaert DL, Sys SU. Relaxation and diastole of the heart. *Physiol Rev* 1989;69:1228.
113. Wexler LF, Weinberg EO, Ingwall JS, Apstein CS. Acute alterations in diastolic left ventricular chamber distensibility: Mechanistic differences between hypoxemia and ischemia in isolated perfused rabbit and rat hearts. *Circ Res* 1989;59:515.
114. Gaasch WH, Blaustein AS, Andrias CW, et al. Myocardial relaxation: II. Hemodynamic determinants of rate of left ventricular isovolumic pressure decline. *Am J Physiol* 1980;239:H1.
115. Zile MR, Gaasch WH. Load-dependent left ventricular relaxation in conscious dogs. *Am J Physiol* 1991;261:H691.
116. Gillebert TC, Lew WYW. Nonuniformity and volume loading independently influence isovolumic relaxation rates. *Am J Physiol* 1989;257:H1927.
117. Ingels NB Jr, Daughters GT II, Nikolic SD, et al. Left atrial pressure-clamp servomechanism demonstrates left ventricular suction in canine hearts with normal mitral valves. *Am J Physiol* 1994;267:H354.

118. Bell SP, Fabian J, Higashiyama A, et al. Restoring forces assessed with left atrial pressure clamps. *Am J Physiol* 1996;270:H1015.
119. Hansen DE, Daughters GT II, Alderman EL, et al. Torsional deformation of the left ventricular midwall in human hearts with intramyocardial markers: Regional heterogeneity and sensitivity to the inotropic effects of abrupt rate changes. *Circ Res* 1988;62:941.
120. Pouleur H, Karliner JS, LeWinter MM, Covell W. Diastolic viscous properties of the intact left ventricle. *Circ Res* 1979;45:410.
121. Gaasch WH. Passive elastic properties of the left ventricle. In: Gaasch WH, LeWinter MM, eds. *Left Ventricular Diastolic Dysfunction and Heart Failure*. Philadelphia: Lea & Febiger; 1994:143.
122. LeWinter MM, Myhre ESP, Slinker BK. Influence of the pericardium and ventricular interaction on diastolic function. In: Gaasch WH, LeWinter MM, eds. *Left Ventricular Diastolic Dysfunction and Heart Failure*. Philadelphia: Lea & Febiger; 1994:103.
123. Apstein CS, Grossman W. Opposite initial effects of supply and demand ischemia on left ventricular diastolic compliance: The ischemia-diastolic paradox. *J Mol Cell Cardiol* 1987;19:119.
124. Yellin EL, Nikolic S, Frater RWM. Left ventricular filling dynamics and diastolic function. *Prog Cardiovasc Dis* 1990;32:247.
125. Shah AM, Grocott-Mason RM, Pepper CB, et al. The cardiac endothelium: Cardioactive mediators. *Prog Cardiovasc Dis* 1996;39:239.
126. Waldrop TG, Eldridge FL, Iwamoto GA, et al. Central neural control of respiration and circulation during exercise. In: Rowell LB, Shepherd JT, eds. *Handbook of Physiology,* Sec 12: *Exercise Regulation and Integration of Multiple Systems*. Bethesda, MD: American Physiological Society; 1996:333.
127. Schulz R, Heusch G. The relationship between regional blood flow and contractile function in normal, ischemic, and reperfused myocardium. *Basic Res Cardiol* 1998;93:455.
128. Ruknudin A, Sachs F, Bustamente JO. Stretch-activated ion channels in tissue-cultured chick heart. *Am J Physiol* 1993;264:H960.
129. Maron BJ, Pelliccia A, Spataro A, Granata M. Reduction in LV wall thickness after deconditioning in highly trained Olympic athletes. *Br Heart J* 1993;69:125.
130. Maron BJ, Pelliccia A, Spirito P. Cardiac disease in young trained athletes: Insights into methods for distinguishing athlete's heart from structural heart disease, with particular emphasis on hypertrophic cardiomyopathy. *Circulation* 1995;91:1596.
131. Firth JA. Endothelial barriers: From hypothetical pores to membrane proteins. *J Anat* 2002;200:541.
132. Rippe B, Rosengren BI, Carlsson O, Venturoli D. Transendothelial transport: The vesicle controversy. *J Vasc Res* 2002;39:375.
133. Bates DO, Hillman NJ, Williams B, et al. Regulation of microvascular permeability by vascular endothelial growth factors. *J Anat* 2002; 200:581.
134. Brillault J, Berezowski V, Cecchelli R, Debouck MP. Intercommunications between brain capillary endothelial cells and glial cells increase the transcellular permeability of the blood-brain barrier during ischaemia. *J Neurochem* 2002;83:807.
135. Mayrovitz HN, Roy J. Microvascular blood flow: Evidence indicating a cubic dependence on arteriolar diameter. *Am J Physiol* 1983;245:H1031.
136. Heistad DD, Kontos HA. Cerebral Circulation:. In: Shephard JT, Abboud FM, eds. *Handbook of Physiology,* Sec 2: *The Cardiovascular System.* Bethesda, MD: American Physiological Society; 1983:137.
137. Koller A, Dornyei G, Kaley G. Flow-induced responses in skeletal muscle venules: Modulation by NO and prostaglandins *Am J Physiol* 1998;275:H831.
138. Burnstock G. Release of vasoactive substances from endothelial cells by shear: Stress and purinergic mechanosensory transduction. *J Anat* 1999;194:335.
139. Johnson PC. Autoregulation of blood flow. *Circ Res* 1986;59:483.
140. Mayhan WG. Disruption of blood brain barrier during acute hypertension in adult and aged rats. *Am J Physiol* 1990;258:H173.
141. Davis MJ, Hill MA. Signaling mechanisms underlying the vascular myogenic response. *Physiol Rev* 199;79:387.
142. Behrendt D, Ganz P. Endothelial function: From vascular biology to clinical applications. *Am J Cardiol* 2002;90:40L.
143. Little TL, Xia J, Duling BR. Dye tracers define differential endothelial and smooth muscle coupling patterns within the arteriolar wall. *Circ Res* 1995;75:519.
144. Segal SS, Welsh DG, Kurjiaka DT. Spread of vasodilation and vasoconstriction along feed arteries and arterioles of hamster skeletal muscle. *J Physiol* 1999;516:283.
145. Davis MJ, Wu X, Nurkiewicz TR, et al. Integrins and mechanotransduction of the vascular myogenic response. *Am J Physiol* 2001;280: H1427.
146. Welsh DG, Morielli AD, Nelson MT, et al. Transient receptor potential channels regulate myogenic tone of resistance arteries. *Circ Res* 2002;90:248–250.
147. Brayden JE, Nelson MT. Regulation of arterial tone by activation of calcium-dependent potassium channels. *Science* 1992;256:532.
148. Cheng HH, Lederer WJ, Cannell MB. Calcium sparks: Elementary events underlying excitation-contraction coupling in heart muscle. *Science* 1992;256:532.
149. Nelson MT, Cheng H, Rubart M, et al. Relaxation of arterial smooth muscle by calcium sparks. *Science* 1995;270:633.
150. Furchgott RF, Zawadski JV. The obligatory role of endothelial cells in the relaxation of arterial smooth muscle by acetylcholine. *Nature* 1980;288:373.
151. Ignarro LJ, Buga GM, Wood K, et al. Endothelium-derived relaxing factor produced and released from artery and vein is NO. *Proc Natl Acad Sci USA* 1987;84:2965.
152. Highsmith RF, Blackburn K, Schmidt DJ. Endothelin and calcium dynamics in vascular smooth muscle. *Annu Rev Physiol* 1992;54:257.
153. Feletou M, Vanhoutte PM. The alternative: EDHF. *J Mol Cell Cardiol* 1999;31:15.
154. Davies PF. Flow-mediated endothelial mechanotransdution. *Physiol Rev* 1995;75:519.
155. Driss AB, Benessiano JP, Levy BI, et al. Arterial expansive remodeling induced by high shear rates. *Am J Physiol* 1997;272:H851.
156. Arnal JF, Dinh-Xaun AT, Pueyo M, et al. Endothelium-derived NO and vascular physiology and pathology. *Cell Mol Life Sci* 1999;55:1078.
157. Yamauchi K, Tsutsui Y, Endo Y, et al. Sympathetic nervous and hemodynamic responses to lower body negative pressure in hyperbaria in men. *Am J Physiol* 2002;282:R38.
158. Austin RE Jr, Smedira NG, Squiers TM, Hoffman JI. Influence of cardiac contraction and coronary vasomotor tone on regional myocardial blood flow. *Am J Physiol* 1994;266:H2542.
159. Muller JM, Davis MJ, Chilian WM. Integrated regulation of pressure and flow in the coronary microcirculation. *Cardiovasc Res* 1996; 32:668.
160. Dube GP, Bemis KG, Greenfield JC Jr. Distinction between metabolic and myogenic mechanisms of coronary hyperemic response to brief diastolic occlusion. *Circ Res* 1991;68:1313.
161. Stepp DW, Van Bibber R, Kroll K, Feigl EO. Quantitative relation between interstitial adenosine concentration and coronary blood flow. *Circ Res* 1996;79:601.
162. Ishibashi Y, Duncker DJ, Zhang J, Bache RJ. ATP-sensitive $K^+$ channels, adenosine, and NO-mediated mechanisms account for coronary vasodilatation during exercise. *Circ Res* 1998;82:346.
163. DiCarlo PE, Gimbrone MA Jr. Vascular endothelium. In: Fuster V, Ross R, Topol EJ, eds. *Atherosclerosis and Coronary Artery Disease*. Philadelphia: Lippincott-Raven; 1996:387.
164. Popp R, Fleming I, Busse R. Pulsatile stretch in coronary arteries elicits release of endothelium-derived hyperpolarizing factor: A modulator of arterial compliance. *Circ Res* 1998;82:696.
165. Egashira K, Katsuda Y, Mohri M, et al. Role of endothelium-derived NO in coronary vasodilatation induced by pacing tachycardia in humans. *Circ Res* 1996;79:331.
166. Zhao G, Zhang X, Xu X, et al. Short-term exercise training enhances reflex cholinergic NO-dependent coronary vasodilatation in conscious dogs. *Circ Res* 1997;80:868.
167. Bar-Shlomo B–Z, Druck MN, Morch JE, et al. Left ventricular function in trained and untrained healthy subjects. *Circulation* 1982; 65:484.

C H A P T E R 5

# PRINCIPLES OF MOLECULAR CARDIOLOGY

Robert Roberts



## HISTORICAL PERSPECTIVE OF MOLECULAR BIOLOGY

In 1953, Watson and Crick[1] proposed the double-helix model for DNA structure based on the results of x-ray diffraction studies by Franklin and Wilkins. The implications of DNA being a double helix, in which each strand is a mirror image of the other, were evident—namely, that one strand could serve as a template for the synthesis of a daughter strand, thus providing the means whereby genetic information could be perpetuated from parent to offspring. In 1956, Schekman[2] described DNA polymerase, the enzyme necessary for the synthesis of DNA that was essential to recombinant DNA technology. Marmor and Lane showed that the double helix of DNA, when subjected to high temperatures,[3] could be separated into its separate strands (denatured), and decreasing the temperature resulted in the reannealing, or hybridizing, of the strands, thus returning them to their previous double-stranded nature. This specific hybridization, or "base pairing" of complementary nucleotide strands, provides both the rationale and the practical basis for much of recombinant DNA technology. Crick had suggested correctly that the genetic code would be written in codons of three nucleotides for each amino acid. The specific combination of three nucleotides that code for each amino acid was unraveled by Leder and Nirenberg[4] and Nishimura et al.[5] Several other necessary components were discovered subsequently, including the enzyme DNA ligase, which joins DNA fragments together.[6] All of this information was known in the 1960s, as was the complete DNA code, as well as the roles of messenger RNA and the cytoplasmic ribosomal RNA for protein synthesis. Recombinant technology was not yet born and, in fact, for the next few years did not appear promising.

Many important discoveries, including those from the 1950s, played a role in recombinant technology, but four that really brought it to fruition and made possible modern molecular biology occurred between the years of 1970 and 1977. A major obstacle to the manipulation of DNA was its large size with no means to cut it into smaller pieces of known specific size. This obstacle was overcome by the discovery of restriction endonucleases that made it possible to cut DNA into smaller pieces in a predictable fashion.[7] These endonucleases, more commonly referred to as *restriction enzymes,* recognize specific sequences of DNA consisting of anywhere from four to eight nucleotides and specifically cut the DNA molecules at their recognition sites, making it possible to use and manipulate DNA fragments in a variety of procedures and reactions. In 1970, the enzyme reverse transcriptase was discovered by Baltimore[8] and Temin and Mizutani[9] simultaneously, making it possible to translate messenger RNA (mRNA) into its complementary DNA (cDNA). Shortly after the first molecule was cloned,[10] recombinant DNA techniques were born, as was modern molecular biology. In 1975, Sanger and Coulson[11] and Maxam and Gilbert[12] developed techniques for the rapid sequencing of DNA. In addition to these four developments, polymerase chain reaction (PCR), a more recently developed technique to rapidly amplify small amounts of DNA or RNA several million-fold, is also having a revolutionary effect on medicine and other fields.

## TRANSCRIPTION AND TRANSLATION OF NUCLEIC ACIDS

### The Essentials of Nucleic Acids

DNA consists of four building blocks referred to as *nucleotides* or merely as *bases*. A nucleotide consists of a nitrogenous base, a 5-carbon sugar (deoxyribose), and a phosphate group.[13] There are two purine bases (adenine and guanine) and two pyrimidine bases (cytosine and thymine) (Fig. 5-1). The triphosphate molecule is bonded to the 5′ carbon of the sugar, and the base is bonded to the 1′ carbon of the sugar. Each DNA molecule consists of millions of nucleotides joined together in a linear fashion through the phosphate group, which forms a bond with the hydroxyl group of the 3′ carbon of the next sugar. The phosphate groups form the backbone of the molecule, but because they are water-soluble, they face outward. Attached to the inner side of the sugar is the hydrophobic base, which faces

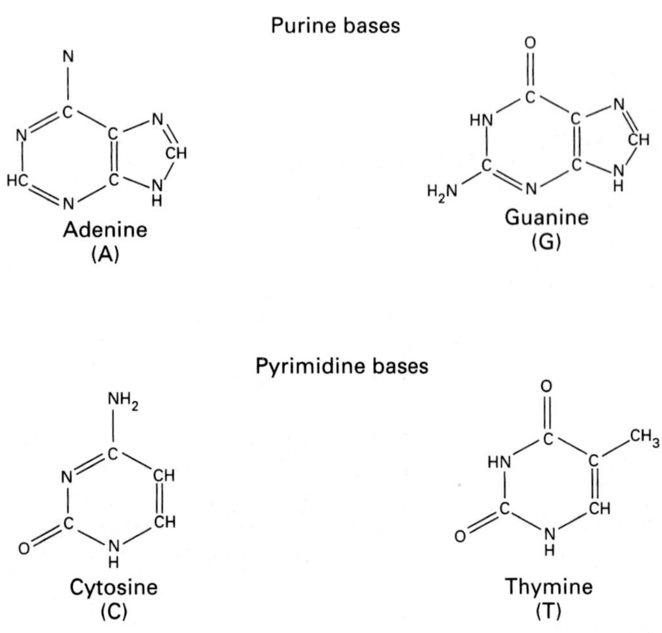


FIGURE 5-1 The common purine and pyrimidine bases found in DNA. Uracil is substituted for thymine in RNA. (From Mares A Jr, Towbin J, Bies RG, Roberts R. Molecular biology for the cardiologist. *Curr Probl Cardiol* 1992; 17:9–72. Reproduced with permission from the publisher and authors.)

inward to shield it from the aqueous environment. The molecule forms a right-sided spiral coil with a turn every 10 nucleotides (3.4 nm), referred to as a *right-sided α-helix,* and pairs with its complementary strand to form the so-called double helix (Fig. 5-2). The center of the molecule consists of the bases that face inward and are opposite to each other. This arrangement provides for the hydrogen bonding between the bases that keeps the two strands together. The hydrogen bonds are perpendicular to the helical axis. The directionality of the strands is referred to as *5′ to 3′* or *3′ to 5′*, which is based on the position of the carbons in the sugar. The end of the molecule with a phosphate or hydroxyl group on the 5′ carbon is termed the *5′ end,* whereas the end with a free terminal 3′ carbon is referred to as the *3′ end.* It is important to distinguish the two ends because the enzyme DNA polymerase always initiates replication of DNA from the 5′ end and proceeds to the 3′ end. There seems to be no constraints on which bases can be adjacent to each other; however, the hydrogen binding between the bases of the two chains is highly specific, since adenine (A) always pairs with thymine (T), and guanine (G) always pairs with cytosine (C). The sugars and the phosphate groups are always the same, whereas the sequence of the bases varies and determines the nature of the hereditary information to be passed onto the progeny. The specificity of this "base pairing" is the basis of the ability of DNA to replicate itself and pass on the genotype characteristics and also forms the basis for the specificity of essentially all the procedures used in recombinant DNA technology. During the process of DNA replication, the strands separate, and new strands form complementary to the original strands, resulting in two additional identical molecules.

## Transcription (from DNA to RNA)

The central dogma of molecular biology is that DNA produces RNA, which in turn produces a polypeptide, the latter being the molecules that make up proteins that provide the cell structure and perform the

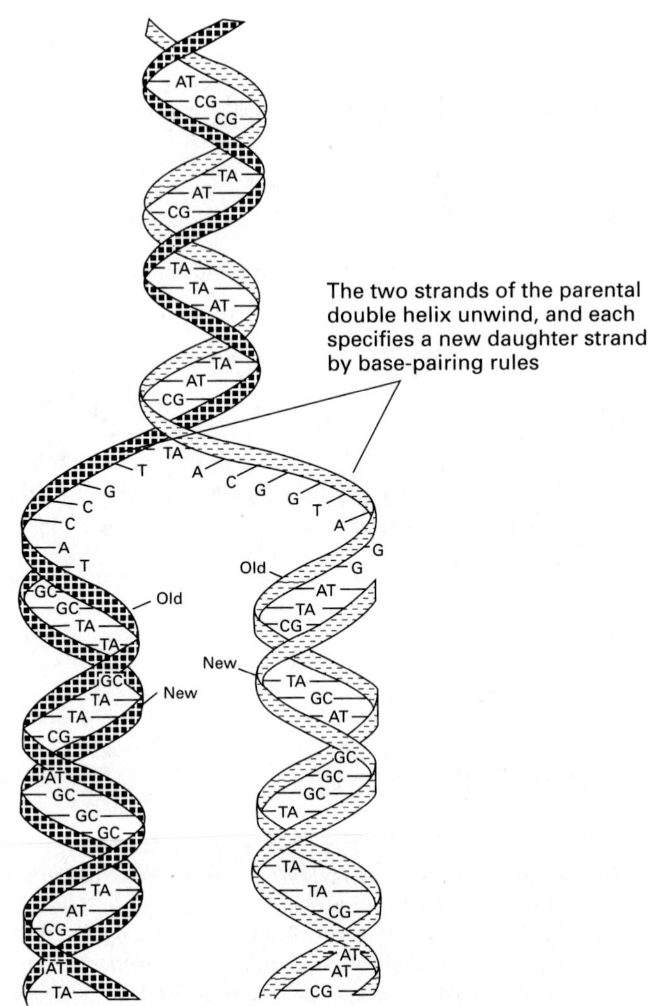


FIGURE 5-2 DNA replication conserves the nucleotide sequence. DNA is a double-stranded helical molecule bound together by the nucleotide bases contained on each individual strand. During cell division, two identical copies of the original parental strand are made by unwinding the DNA and then synthesis of a complementary second strand to make two identical new daughter strands.

functions of the cell (Fig. 5-3). The genetic information inherited by each individual is encoded by the sequence of the bases of the DNA (the genotype), which is translated into proteins and provides the observable characteristics of the individual (the phenotype). This overall process from DNA to protein, however, must first go through the intermediary step of RNA. The process whereby mRNA is synthesized using DNA as the template is referred to as *transcription*

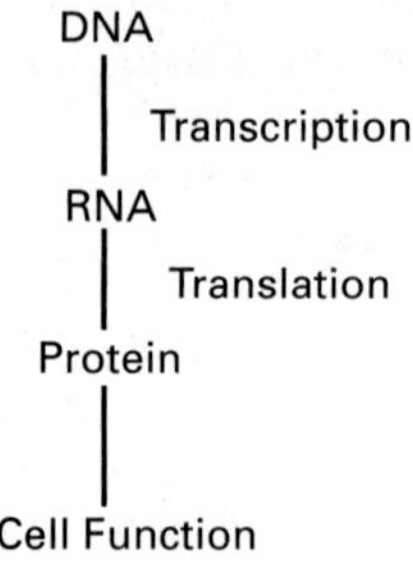


FIGURE 5-3 Central dogma of molecular biology.

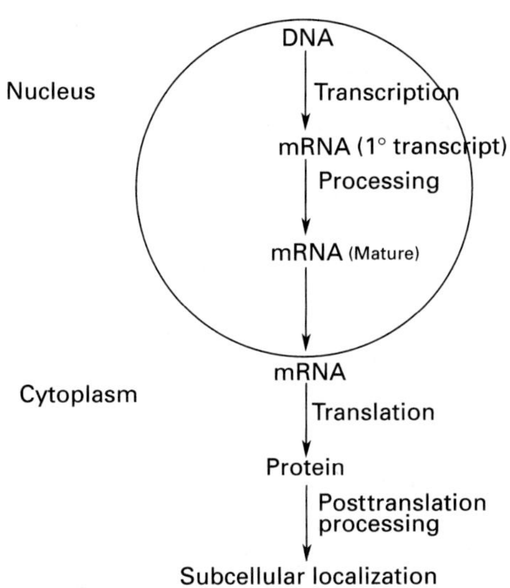


FIGURE 5-4 Schematic localization of the processes of transcription and translation.

(Fig. 5-4). Transcription and the processing of mRNA occur in the nucleus of the cell, separated by the nuclear membrane from the cytoplasm. The process of transcription is initiated by attachment of the enzyme RNA polymerase II to specific recognition sites where the DNA is double-stranded, but upon activation by the enzyme, the strands selectively unwind and separate. The binding site of RNA polymerase II is always located on the 5′ end of the gene, and the enzyme remains attached to a single strand of DNA as it travels in the 3′ direction. The DNA immediately in front of it separates into two strands with just one strand of DNA (antisense) acting as a template for the synthesis of mRNA. Thus, in contrast to DNA, mRNA is a single-stranded polynucleotide. Messenger RNA also differs from DNA in that deoxyribose, the sugar found in DNA, is replaced by ribose. Moreover, uracil (U) replaces thymine (T), and like thymine, uracil pairs exclusively with adenine (A).

The mRNA, as transcribed from the DNA, is referred to as the *primary transcript,* or sometimes as *immature mRNA,* and is a complementary copy of the DNA (Fig. 5-5). Since protein synthesis occurs in the cytoplasm, the mRNA must exit the nucleus, but prior to transport, it undergoes extensive posttranscriptional processing primarily through three main events: (1) addition of a methylated guanosine (4-methylguanosine residue) to the 5′ end, referred to as a *cap,* which is important for the initiation of translation; (2) addition of a long tail of repeated adenine nucleotides, called the *poly(A) tail,* to the 3′ region of the mRNA, which is essential for stability of the message in the cytoplasm; and (3) the primary transcript, which contains introns and exons, undergoes a specific splicing process whereby the introns are removed and the exons are properly respliced together prior to exit from the nucleus as mature mRNA. The process of splicing is, in part, performed by molecules referred to as *small nuclear ribonucleoproteins* (snRNPs), which consist of RNA molecules tightly associated with a group of about 10 different proteins. Exons survive the mRNA processing and exit the nucleus (hence the name) as part of the mature mRNA. The mature mRNA consists of three distinct regions. The exons of the 5′ end are not translated into protein but signal the beginning of mRNA translation and contain sequences that direct the mRNA to the ribosome in the cytoplasm for protein synthesis. The exons in the second region, referred to as the *coding region,* contain the information that determines the amino acid sequence of the protein. The exons of the 3′ end do not code for protein but for signals that terminate translation and direct the addition of the poly(A) tail. Introns are portions of the gene included in the primary mRNA transcript but which are spliced out of the mature mRNA. The process of splicing out introns and rejoining exons is an important means of introducing genetic diversity, since one mRNA may provide several different mRNAs that code for different polypeptides (this will be discussed further under gene regulation). The primary transcript undergoes extensive shortening such that the mature mRNA often represents only 10 percent of the primary transcript. The mature mRNA exits the nucleus through nuclear pores, enters the cytoplasm, and attaches to a ribosome to initiate protein synthesis.

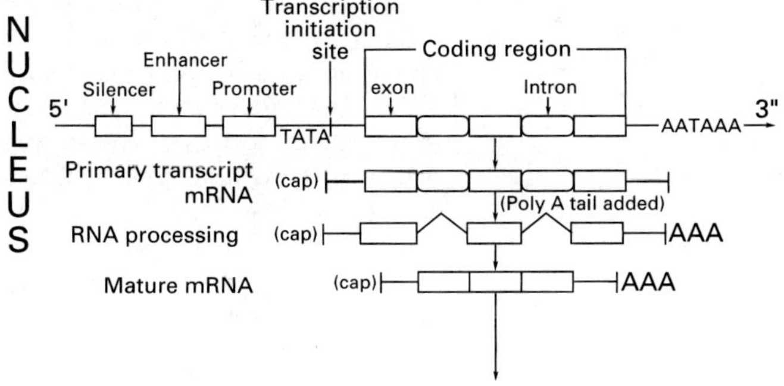


FIGURE 5-5 Transcription. Transcription occurs in the nucleus, producing mRNA that is processed into mature mRNA and transported to the cytoplasm. In the cytoplasm, translation occurs, with the mRNA coding for specific amino acids that are linked together to form a polypeptide and ultimately to form a mature protein. (From Mares A Jr, Towbin J, Bies RG, Roberts R. Molecular biology for the cardiologist. *Curr Probl Cardiol* 1992; 17:9–72. Reproduced with permission from the publisher and authors.)

## Translation

The final process, referred to as *translation,* is the most complex of the various processes that occur in the flow from genomic DNA (gene) to mature protein. The alphabet of the DNA or its single-stranded complementary mRNA is that of the four nucleotides (bases), whereas that of the protein is the 20 amino acids. To translate from the nucleic acids of DNA to the amino acids of protein, the genetic code is written in triplets of bases, with each amino acid being encoded by three base pairs referred to as a *codon.* The mRNA codons dictate which amino acids are to be selected, and the order of the codons dictates the sequence of the amino acids in the protein. There are four different nucleotides to form the triplets; thus the number of combinations ($4^3$) is 64, but there are only 20 amino acids. There is considerable redundancy, referred to as *degeneracy,* and this results in most of the amino acids having more than one codon. In addition to codons for each amino acid, there is also the codon AUG, which is the start codon that initiates protein synthesis and also codes for methionine. To stop translation, there are three codons, UAA, UAG, and UGA, that signal the end of a particular polypeptide. Translation into protein requires two other RNA species, ribosomal RNA (rRNA) and transfer RNA (tRNA). The mRNA, after exiting the nucleus, recognizes the ribosome, which is the site of protein synthesis. The ribosome moves along an mRNA molecule, translating each of its codons in a 5′ to 3′ direction to assemble the polypeptide from its amino (N-terminal) to its carboxy (C-terminal) ends. Their relative concentration of the types of RNAs in the cell, in large part, reflects their stability, with more than 80 percent being rRNAs, 15 percent being tRNAs, and less than 5 percent being mRNAs.

The mRNA does not interact directly with amino acids but rather through adaptor molecules referred to as *transfer RNA* (tRNA) to which amino acids are covalently joined by a highly specific enzyme (aminoacyl tRNA synthetase) using ATP. There is at least one tRNA species corresponding to each of the 20 naturally occurring amino acids. The aminoacyl tRNA synthetase performs a special function of activating the amino acids and ensuring that each amino acid is joined specifically to its tRNA. The structure of tRNA is now known in great detail, and its specificity is attributed to the sequence of three nucleotides complementary to the codon exposed at one end of the folded tRNA molecule, which, on the tRNA, is referred to as the *anticodon*. The amino acid receptor site is exposed at the other end. Amino acids thus are specified at two recognition steps: one in which a specific enzyme joins the amino acid to a specific tRNA and the other in which the tRNA serving as an adaptor molecule joins the amino acid to the ribosomal-mRNA complex through a codon-anticodon specific-base-pairing interaction between the mRNA and the tRNA. Once the process of protein synthesis is initiated, the ribosome moves along the mRNA joining the amino acids via peptide bonds in the sequence specified by the mRNA to form the mature polypeptide. The process of protein synthesis from this complex of mRNA and ribosome involves over 100 enzymes. The steps involved consist of initiation, elongation, and termination of the polypeptide, with each process having its own enzymes.[14]

Once a polypeptide is synthesized, many modifications occur referred to as *posttranslational modifications* (Fig. 5-6). It is estimated that over 200 modifications occur including: glycosylation; phosphorylation or dephosphorylation of serine, threonine or tyrosine; carboxylation; formation of thiol groups; prenylation; palmitoylation or oxidation. The polypeptide may also bind to other polypeptides and with the help of chaperone proteins undergo various conformational changes. Finally, the protein is destroyed usually through ubiquitization.[15] Leader sequences direct the protein to its destination of either the intracellular membranes, the plasma membrane, or organelle (e.g., mitochondria).

## Gene Structure, Expression, and Regulation

The concept that one gene leads to one protein remains basic to the central dogma of molecular biology but does, in some cases, need modification. In the classic sense, a gene consists of a discrete unit of DNA that encodes for a specific polypeptide. Two observations must be noted: First, transcription produces two end points—ribonucleic acid (RNA) and protein. The products, rRNA, tRNA, and small nuclear RNA (snRNA), do not get translated into protein but rather perform functions during posttranscription and translation that are pivotal to expression of the mRNA. The polymerases necessary for transcription of these genes are of three types—polymerase I for rRNA, polymerase II for mRNA, and polymerase III for tRNA and some other snRNAs. Second, in part because of snRNA and certain proteins, alternative splicing of the exons in the primary mRNA can lead to different mature mRNAs with each coding for a slightly different polypeptide which forms isoforms of the same protein.

The anatomy of a protein-coding gene is composed of introns and exons. The average exon is about 300 base pairs long, whereas introns are much larger and are spliced out of the mature mRNA and, thus, do not code for protein. A typical gene has three regions: the 5′ untranslated region that contains the *cis*-acting sequences that regulate transcription; the central portion, referred to as the *coding region*, that codes for protein; and the 3′ untranslated end, which also has regulatory sequences and coding signals for stability of the mature mRNA. The first nucleotide to be transcribed is given the +1 number, and everything 5′ to it is referred to as *upstream* or *proximal* and is numbered with the first base pair as −1, and so on. The initiation site for transcription is always upstream from the 5′ untranslated region. The 5′ regulatory untranslated region has variable sequences, but there are several consistent sequences present in the same position in most human genes. Polymerase II has no intrinsic affinity for DNA and can only bind after several transcription factors have bound. The site of transcription and its direction in most human genes are determined by a consensus sequence of TATAA(T)AA(T) referred to as the *TATA box* found at base pairs −25 to −30 upstream from the start site. A large complex of transcription factors (more than 25 proteins) binds to the TATA box in preparation for RNA polymerase II binding and transcription. Collectively, these transcription factors are referred to as *transcription factors for polymerase II*

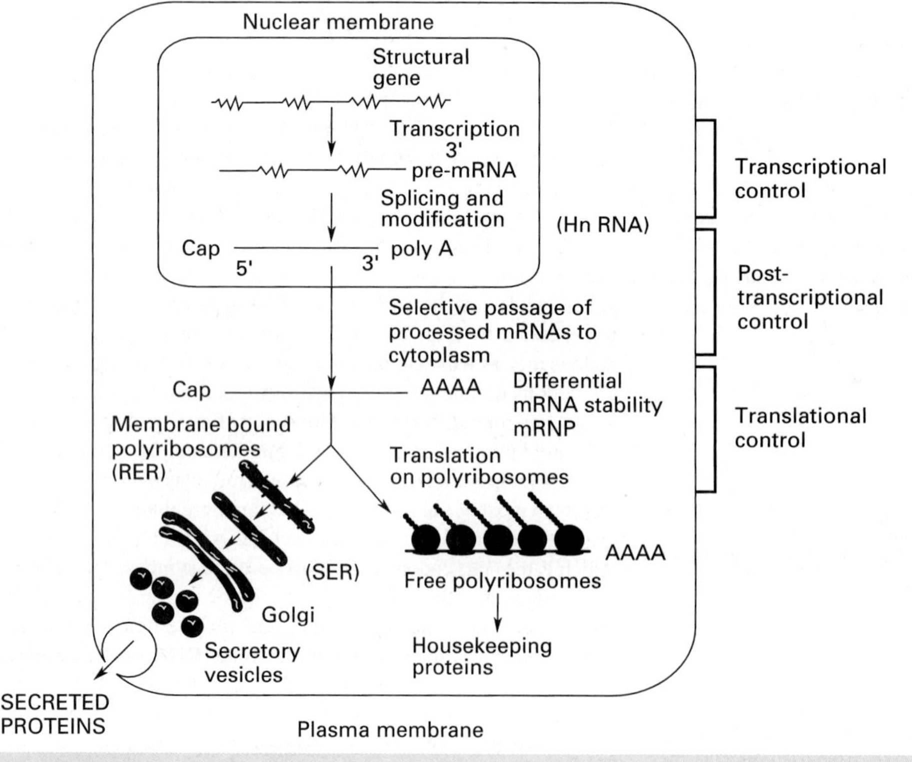


FIGURE 5-6 A summary of the multiple steps involved in gene expression from the genomic DNA to the protein showing how the protein destined for secretion follows a systematic path different from proteins destined to remain in the cytoplasm. RER = rough endoplasmic reticulum; SER = smooth endoplasmic reticulum. (From Mares A Jr, Towbin J, Bies RG, Roberts R. Molecular biology for the cardiologist. *Curr Probl Cardiol* 1992; 17:9–72. Reproduced with permission from the publisher and authors.)

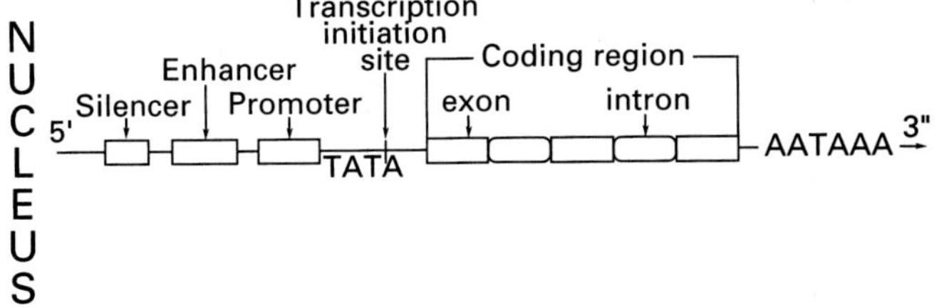


FIGURE 5-7 Structure of a gene. These small functional units within the nucleus contain the coding information for the synthesis of a polypeptide and on their 5′ ends have regulatory sequences that include silencers, enhancers, and promoters. The coding region consisting of exons (code for protein) as well as intervening noncoding sequences (introns) is followed by a 3′ noncoding region that is translated into the mRNA. The 3′ end appears important for exit of the mRNA from the nucleus and its stability in the cytoplasm but does not code for protein. The TATA is the initiation site for polymerase and is present in most eukaryotes at about 10 to 30 base pairs 5′ from the start codon (TAC) of the coding region. The AATAA will become the recognition site on the mRNA to which attaches an enzyme that cleaves the 3′ region and replaces the distal portion with a poly(A) tail. (From Mares A Jr, Towbin J, Bies RG, Roberts R. Molecular biology for the cardiologist. *Curr Probl Cardiol* 1992; 17:9–72. Reproduced with permission from the publisher and authors.)

(TFII), with letters designating the different factors. TFIID binds first, then TFIIB, followed by RNA polymerase II, followed by several TFII factors such as E, F, G, H, and J, etc. In addition, in many human genes, located at about base pair −200 upstream is the GGGCG box to which SP1 binds, and this is felt to be a regulator of housekeeping genes (Fig. 5-7).

*Gene expression* refers to all the processes required to go from DNA to protein, from the initial unfolding of the nuclear chromatin in preparation for transcription to the mature protein emerging following completion of posttranslational changes. Regulation of this process occurs at all levels in response to signals both from within the cell and from the environment. The cell maintains its integrity and responds to external stimuli through signals that activate receptors (generally in the cell membrane). These in turn use signaling proteins to transfer their message to the cytoplasm or nucleus, which in some way modifies gene expression. Delineation of the receptor, the signaling proteins, and where and how gene expression is altered are of prime importance.

The most fundamental level of gene regulation involves cell differentiation. The body contains at least 200 different types of cells that have been programmed by their genes to perform highly specialized functions. All cells have the same DNA and the same genes, but only those genes that are expressed determine the cell's phenotype. Cardiac myocytes, for example, are characterized by a set of proteins that specialize in contractile activity, whereas hepatocytes specialize in the synthesis and catabolism of proteins. Selective gene expression is the basis of cell differentiation. Cell growth and replication occur in what is termed the *undifferentiated cell* but, through complex mechanisms, give rise to cells that cease to replicate and are programmed to take on specialized functions (cell differentiation). In the process of cell differentiation, genes, particularly those concerned with cell proliferation and undifferentiated functions, are downregulated, whereas those genes coding for the proteins that perform the specialized functions are upregulated. Once cells are differentiated, protein synthesis, however, remains a dynamic process to maintain cell integrity. Most of gene regulation is concerned with the maintenance of cellular integrity, and the genes responsible for this basal function are referred to as *housekeeping genes.* Housekeeping genes are constitutively regulated, as opposed to genes responsible for cell differentiation and growth, which are developmentally regulated. It is estimated that organs use about 10,000 genes (constitutive) to maintain their integrity, with one exception, the brain, which is estimated to use around 20,000 genes. Gene regulation may be classified under the following headings: pretranscription, transcription, posttranscription, translation, and posttranslation.[16]

*Pretranscriptional regulation*[17] refers to the decompaction of the DNA and exposure of the region about to undergo transcription. The total DNA of a single cell would measure about 1m in length, yet in the nucleus it is markedly compacted and is folded around specific proteins, the dominant class being histones. The chromatin takes on a specific repeating structure called the *nucleosome*. The nucleosome is identical from gene to gene and highly conserved, being virtually identical from yeast to humans. This structure consists of core histones (two each of H2A, H2B, H3, and H4), around which are wrapped 146 bp in $1\frac{3}{4}$ superhelical turns.[18] Recently, it became evident that nucleosomes play a major role in the regulation of gene expression and can transmit epigenetic information from one cell generation to the next. The information storage function and gene regulation reside primarily in the amino terminal tails of the four core histones. The positive charge groups of the histone proteins related to, for example, lysine residues bind tightly to the negatively charged DNA to prevent exposure for transcription. Modification of histone binding to DNA is a major regulatory mechanism of gene expression.[19] A group of enzymes facilitates acetylation (HAC) of histone lysine tails exposed on the nucleosome surface, which decreases binding of the histone to the DNA (decompaction) and exposes the region for transcription. Similarly, another set of enzymes induces histone deacetylation (HDAC), removing the acetyl groups from the lysine to prevent transcription. Other modifications involved with binding between the histone proteins and DNA play a similar regulatory role in gene transcription including lysine and arginine methylation, serine phosphorylation, and attachment of the small peptide ubiquitin.[20,21] This pretranscriptional level of gene regulation is now an area of major research. Therapeutic targets are being sought to manipulate cell growth whether it be for cardiac disease or neoplastic disorders.

*Transcriptional control* is a major rate-limiting step to gene expression. The 5′ upstream region immediately adjacent to the transcription initiation site is referred to as the *promoter region*. This region contains sequences that are specific binding sites for proteins referred to as *transacting factors* or *transcriptional factors*. The protein-binding sites are often referred to as *cis-acting sequences* because they are on the same DNA molecule on which they act. The transcription factors (also referred to as *DNA-binding proteins*) are referred to as *transacting factors* (acting at a distance) because they are encoded by genes that may even be on another chromosome.

The promoter sequences and their corresponding DNA-binding proteins may act ubiquitously or may be tissue-specific. Promoters often increase transcription of a class of genes rather than a single gene. Another type of DNA sequence that increases transcription is referred to as an *enhancer* (see Fig. 5-7). Enhancers differ from promoter sequences in that they may be upstream or downstream from the coding region and be separated by as many as hundreds of thousand of base pairs and are effective in either the 5′ to 3′ or 3′ to 5′ direction. These enhancers, like promoters, consist of several small motifs of 4 to 10 base pairs and, when bound by their corresponding DNA-binding proteins (transcription factors), have a positive influence on gene transcription. Another regulatory DNA sequence that is similar to enhancers in size and location but exerts a negative influence on transcription is referred to as a *silencer* or *repressor*.

Several DNA-binding proteins are recognized (transcription factors) for their structure and include the zinc-finger, leucine-zipper, helix-loop-helix, and helix-turn-helix proteins. The zinc-finger type of protein is used by developmental genes called *GATA factors* and the receptors for circulating hormones, including the glucocorticoids, progesterones, androgens, mineralocorticoids, estrogen, thyroxine, vitamin $D_3$, and retinoic acid. These hormones, which are lipophilic, penetrate the cell membrane and activate an intracellular receptor or nuclear receptor, which, in turn, activates gene expression through the zinc-finger transcription proteins. Many of the growth-related signaling proteins, such as c-fos, jun-B, and c-jun, dimerize through leucine-zipper proteins prior to binding to DNA. For example, c-fos dimerizes with c-jun and subsequently binds to DNA. Transcription factors such as the *myo-D* family genes, which are the master genes for inducing differentiation of skeletal muscle, contain a helix-loop-helix motif. Several other transcription factors have a conserved sequence motif which is named MADS after the first four members identified MCMI, AGAMOUS, DEFICIENS, and SRF (serum response factor). This family also includes the myocyte enhancer factor 2 (MEF2). The helix-turn-helix proteins include homeodomain-containing proteins that are important in the development of prokaryotes and eukaryotes.

Another level at which gene expression is regulated is mRNA processing. The mature mRNA that exits the nucleus and migrates to the ribosome in the cytoplasm to serve as the template for protein synthesis is significantly altered from the original transcribed mRNA. The mature mRNA may be classified into three regions: the 5′ untranslated region (UTR) included in the first exon; the protein-coding region; and the 3′ untranslated region present in the last exon. The 5′ untranslated region (UTR) is capped by 7-methyl guanosine and occurs prior to completion of transcription. The CAP site is followed by a sequence (UTR sequence) that leads up to the initiation codon (ATG) to specify the start of translation. The protein-coding region undergoes significant modification with removal of the introns and subsequent splicing together of the exons to provide the mature mRNA. In the majority of instances, each exon present in the gene is incorporated into a mature mRNA via ligation of consecutive pairs of exons and removal of all introns. In other instances, however, nonconsecutive exons are joined in the processing of some gene transcripts, and this alternative pattern of primary mRNA splicing can exclude individual exons from mature mRNA in some transcripts and include them in others. The use of such differential splicing patterns creates mRNAs that generate a variety of proteins from a single gene. Differential splicing is particularly prevalent in genes of muscles and has been shown to occur in several sarcomeric proteins including myosin heavy chains, tropomyosin, and troponin T. The third region, the 3′ end, has a stop codon (TAA or TAG or TGA) to indicate the end of the translated region. This is followed by the UTR, which encodes for the poly(A) signal (AATAAA) that signals cleavage and the addition of adenosine residues [a poly(A) tail]. The number of adenosine residues added may vary from hundreds to thousands.

The 5′ *CAP,* subsequent to exit of the mRNA to the cytoplasm, plays a requisite role in being responsible for the initial binding of the mRNA to the ribosome to initiate translation. The 3′ non-protein-coding region of the mature mRNA contains the poly(A) tail, which is essential for message stability. It is believed that protein synthesis is, in part, regulated on the basis of alterations in message stability. The precise mechanism whereby an mRNA is induced to remain stable and encode several thousand polypeptides as opposed to being extremely unstable and encoding only a few molecules is not well understood. Nevertheless, it is likely to be an important step in regulating the response to cytoplasmic signals that require rapid synthesis of a particular polypeptide. Synthesis of a polypeptide initiated via transcription is estimated to take several minutes, whereas synthesis of a protein initiated through translation requires only seconds. Regulation of gene expression at the protein synthesis level is more fully discussed in Chap. 6.

## MOLECULAR AND RECOMBINANT DNA TECHNIQUES

### Overview

Modern molecular biology, initiated in the 1970s,[12,22] was in part due to four pivotal discoveries or inventions: restriction enzymes, reverse transcription, cloning, and DNA sequencing. The discovery of the restriction endonucleases provided the genetic scalpel to cut DNA into smaller pieces of predictable size that could be used in a variety of procedures. The unique feature of these enzymes is that each recognizes a specific sequence of DNA of 4 to 8 base pairs and cleaves the molecule at that particular site. Thus one knows precisely where the enzyme cuts, and using a number of different enzymes, one can identify the site and number of recognition sites for each enzyme in a fragment of DNA of interest and develop what is referred to as a *restriction map*. These enzymes also made it possible to cut DNA from different sources in a predictable manner in preparation for ligating them together into a recombinant molecule. Restriction endonucleases are obtained from bacteria, and enzymes have been purified that recognize more than 100 different cleavage sites.

The discovery that retroviruses contain an enzyme that catalyzes the formation of DNA from RNA, referred to as *reverse transcriptase,* revolutionized molecular biology (Fig. 5-8). Messenger RNA, as discussed previously, codes for a specific polypeptide and is derived from a discrete, specific unit of DNA referred to as a *gene*. Reverse transcriptase reverses this process so that a cDNA is generated from an mRNA (coding part of the gene) and can be used as a gene to express the protein. The cDNA is reinserted into the genome of a vector (virus or plasmid) and subsequently replicated in an appropriate host, such as a bacterium, which made possible the first cloning of a gene. Radioactive labeling of a cDNA provides an extraordinarily powerful tool to isolate and identify DNA fragments of interest including genes. The labeled cDNA, referred to as a *probe,* or *indicator molecule,* is a routine, essential tool used to identify and isolate DNA or RNA fragments of interest. Development of rapid-sequencing techniques made it possible to rapidly sequence fragments of DNA containing thousands of base pairs.

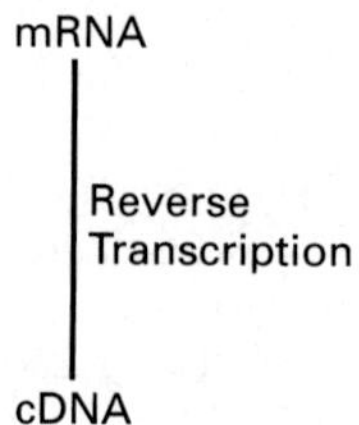


FIGURE 5-8 Generation of a complementary DNA (cDNA). Taking advantage of the enzyme reverse transcriptase, mRNA is converted to DNA, referred to as *complementary* DNA (cDNA). The DNA is single-stranded and complementary to the sequence of RNA, except thymine now replaces uracil. Using DNA polymerase, one can then make the single-stranded DNA into double-stranded cDNA. The cDNA can be used as a probe to identify specific sequences or genes of the genomic DNA, or it can be inserted into vectors to be cloned or expressed in a variety of hosts.

Three features essential to all techniques of recombinant DNA technology need to be highlighted: The first is the ability of DNA to denature and anneal, or hybridize. The double-stranded DNA, held together by hydrogen bonding of the corresponding complementary bases, will, on exposure to high temperatures (95°C), separate into two strands, but under appropriate conditions (55°C), the complementary strands will again anneal precisely as originally and return to their normal double-stranded state. The process of separating into separate strands is referred to as *denaturation,* and the recombining process is known as *annealment,* or *hybridization,* with the latter term preferred if the two DNA fragments are from different sources. Second, the strands come together identically to the parent molecule because of complementary base pairing, whereby A must bind to T and C to G. Third, the phosphorus present in DNA provides DNA with a net negative charge. This property is exploited in many techniques (e.g., electrophoresis) to separate and detect DNA molecules of different sizes. To understand the power of recombinant technology as it applies to cardiology, it is necessary to have knowledge of the terminology and methods. The starting material is usually DNA but could be RNA isolated from either a blood or tissue sample. DNA could be obtained from any source since DNA within the human body is the same regardless of the cell or organ from which it is obtained. Messenger RNA (mRNA) represents the expressed form of the DNA gene, and while it is identical throughout the body for a particular gene, certain mRNAs may or may not be expressed, depending on the organ source. Since DNA and RNA are negatively charged (phosphorus ion), this property is commonly used to separate DNA and RNA molecules of different size. Fragments of increasing size move slower through the pores of gels as they migrate toward the positive electrode during electrophoresis. One can alter the resolution of this technique by changing the size of the pores in the gel. For example, polyacrylamide gels with very small pores will separate fragments differing by only 100 base pairs (bp) whereas agarose gels of greater pores will separate only if the fragments differ by greater than 1000 base pairs. The gels can be stained by specific dyes, such as ethidium bromide, which would exhibit bands of DNA or RNA of different sizes. Thus, electrophoresis is the predominant method to separate RNA or DNA fragments. If one is interested, as is usually the case, in a specific DNA or RNA molecule, one can selectively detect that molecule of DNA or RNA based on specific complementary base pairing. One can use a short sequence complementary to the DNA of interest as a probe tagged with an identification marker such as radioactivity or fluorescence. The probe may be synthesized chemically, referred to as an *oligonucleotide,* or be a natural DNA or RNA fragment. The labeled sequence, referred to as a *probe,* will be used as bait to identify the RNA or DNA of interest. If the probe of interest is DNA, it is rendered single stranded. (RNA is single stranded.) Upon reannealling or hybridizing, the labeled probe will bind to complementary sequences of DNA or RNA of interest present in the sample. Upon electrophoresis, only the band with the attached marker (radioactivity or fluorescence) will be observed. The band will contain specifically only the DNA or RNA of interest because the probe will only bind to the specific and precise sequence that is complementary to the sequence of the probe.

Since gels used in electrophoresis are difficult to handle or store, Southern developed a method to transfer the DNA or RNA from the gel to a solid medium such as nylon by a wicking process. The RNA or DNA is transferred via a buffer from the gel to the nylon membrane through paper towels, which provide the absorbent or blotting effect. It was thus referred to as a blotting technique and hence the name, *Southern blot.* The pattern and location of the bands relative to each other on the gel are retained during the blotting transfer.

To obtain multiple copies of a gene, or any DNA sequence, one can insert the fragment of interest into various vectors which can be replicated in a host cell such as a bacteria to provide on average a million copies identical to the initial sequence. This process is referred to as cloning. Initially, it was thought one could only clone DNA based on the misconception that one could not go from RNA to DNA. The discovery of the enzyme reverse transcriptase (RT) made it possible to convert mRNA, which reflects a specific gene, into DNA referred to as *complementary DNA* (cDNA). This made it possible to isolate mRNA, which represents a specific gene; convert it to cDNA by RT; and clone it in cell culture or living organisms. This discovery has revolutionized biology and medicine and is routinely used to generate animal models of disease such as transgenic animals or to harvest specific drugs for the treatment of disease such as insulin, tissue plasminogen activator (t-PA), or vascular endothelial growth factor (VEGF). It is hoped that within the next 10 years cDNAs for all human genes will be available, which will further revolutionize the diagnosis, treatment, and prevention of human disease. Another technique routinely used to obtain multiple copies of a DNA or RNA sequence is referred to as the polymerase chain reaction (PCR). This is a technique whereby two primers of 15 to 20 bp are selected complementary to the sequence that is upstream and downstream to the sequence. The sequences between the two primers under appropriate conditions with a polymerase enzyme can be amplified to a million copies in 3 h and a billion copies in 24 h. If one needs to amplify copies of mRNA, the mRNA is converted to cDNA followed by amplification with PCR. This technique is much simpler, cheaper, and faster than cloning. Both techniques are necessary, since the size of the fragment amplified by PCR is limited (1000 to 20,000 bp). To provide multiple copies of larger fragments, cloning is necessary. Another useful and routinely used tool is a gene library. A library may consist of DNA sequences that would be the same for all organs or it may contain cDNAs specific for a particular organ. These libraries consist of genes stored in a host such as bacteria and are now commercially available. The library may consist of all the genes expressed in a particular organ or subspecialized region of the organ. An example is a cDNA library that contains supposedly all of the genes expressed in the heart and a library containing only those genes expressed in the cardiac Purkinje system.

## Unique Applications of Recombinant DNA Technology

The techniques of recombinant DNA are unique and are not limited by some of the restrictions imposed on other scientific techniques. Some of these are the abilities (1) to perform the structure-function analysis of a selected molecule or a portion thereof in the intact living cell or organism, (2) to isolate and identify genes responsible for hereditary diseases, (3) to unravel the molecular basis for the regulation of growth (including the heart), and (4) to generate large quantities of protein present only in trace amounts that otherwise would not be available, as well as the opportunity to genetically engineer proteins for maximum benefit with the least side effects. The techniques routinely used in molecular biology include electrophoresis, Southern and Northern blotting, DNA cloning, PCR, electrophoretic mobility shift assay, and the development of gene libraries.

## Isolation of DNA

Since the DNA of all human tissues is the same, practically any tissue can be used to obtain a DNA sample. It requires only a microgram for most procedures. In humans, lymphocytes are commonly used because they are very accessible and the DNA can be extracted easily. Lymphocytes are also used because they can be transformed by Epstein-Barr virus into an immortal cell line that can provide a continuous, renewable source of DNA. The cells can be grown in culture, frozen for years (from which samples can be obtained), thawed, and regrown, providing a renewable source of DNA for several decades. A sample of 10 to 15 mL of whole blood typically would yield about 50 to 100 $\mu$g of genomic DNA. If one's interest is restricted to the DNA sequences that are expressed, one would isolate mRNA and, using it as a template, employ reverse transcriptase to derive its cDNA. cDNA molecules represent the expressed form of a gene and thus can be used as probes to select the specific genomic DNA segments from which the mRNA was transcribed. Myocardial biopsies obtained under appropriate conditions provide adequate tissue for most DNA or RNA analyses.

## Detection of DNA

One of the important physical properties of the DNA molecule is that each individual nucleotide possesses a net negative charge resulting from the phosphate group. Thus, fragments of different sizes exposed to an electric field tend to migrate toward the positive electrode at differential rates depending on their size, with small fragments migrating faster than larger ones. This process of separation based on electric charge is called *electrophoresis*. The DNA sample, after being digested into fragments of different size by a restriction endonuclease, is added to a gel matrix such as agarose or acrylamide. After separation by electrophoresis, the pattern of the DNA can be visualized under an ultraviolet lamp with a fluorescent dye such as ethidium bromide (Fig. 5-9). Agarose gel electrophoresis will separate fragments from 1000 to 60,000 bp (60 kb) in size, and polyacrylamide gels effectively separate fragments smaller than 1000 bp (1 kb). The recent development of pulsed-field gel electrophoresis (PFGE) made possible the separation of DNA fragments even up to 2000 kb in size. In this technique, the electric field is alternated in different directions, forcing the molecules of DNA to reorient between each pulse of electric current. Thus this technique is particularly suitable for isolating and characterizing large segments of DNA, as to identify a known gene.

As noted previously, prior to electrophoresis, the DNA must be digested with one of the restriction endonucleases. The size of the fragments resulting from digestion will depend on the type of restriction endonuclease used—i.e., whether they recognize sequences of 4, 5, 6, or 8 bp. Enzymes recognizing a 4-bp sequence will cut the DNA into much smaller fragments than one that recognizes an 8-bp sequence.

## Development of a DNA Probe

A nucleic acid probe is a fragment of nucleic acid to which has been attached a label such as a radioisotope or a fluorescent compound, making it possible to easily detect and recognize the desired fragment among other native DNA molecules. The fragment labeled is usually cDNA or a synthetic oligonucleotide, although it could be RNA. It is now possible to synthesize DNA fragments of up to 30 to 40 bp, referred to as *oligonucleotides,* that, with an attached label, can be used as probes to identify cDNA in the human genome or mRNA. This takes advantage of the fact that at high temperatures, the double-stranded DNA probe and the native DNA will break into separate strands. On recombining at random, the labeled DNA probe can bind with either its original complementary strand or the native DNA that is complementary to the probe and thus provide a means of isolating a fragment of native genomic DNA. A probe is necessary in most recombinant DNA procedures to detect the molecule of interest following electrophoresis.

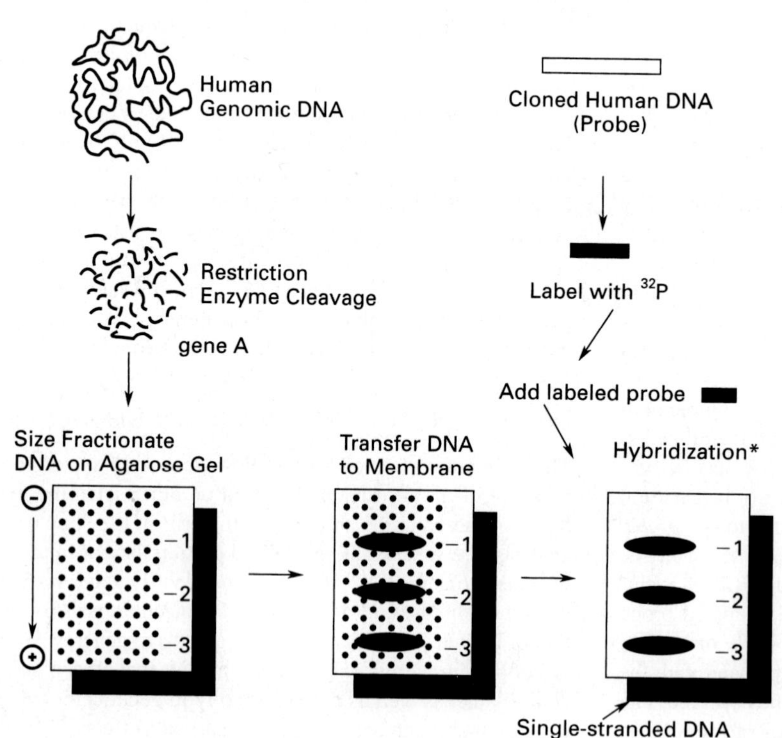


FIGURE 5-9 Southern blotting technique. The DNA is cleaved with an appropriately selected restriction endonuclease. The digested fragments are separated by electrophoresis on agarose gel, and the fragments of gene A are located at positions 1, 2, and 3 but cannot be seen against the background of many other randomly occurring DNA fragments. The DNA is denatured and transferred to a membrane in an identical pattern to what it was on the agarose gel. It is difficult to manipulate anything on a soft gel or to remove it. Once transferred to the membrane (filter), a solid support system, the DNA is much easier to handle. A DNA probe (cDNA) that has been labeled with $^{32}$P is hybridized to its cDNA and visualized after exposure of the nylon membrane to an autoradiograph. The transfer of the DNA from the gel to the membrane developed by Southern was a major innovation illustrated in the next figure. (From Mares A Jr, Towbin J, Bies RG, Roberts R. Molecular biology for the cardiologist. *Curr Probl Cardiol* 1992; 17:9–72. Reproduced with permission from the publisher and authors.)

## Southern, Northern, and Western Blotting

A procedure to separate and detect specific DNA fragments, referred to as *Southern blotting,* is named after E. M. Southern, who developed it in 1975.[23] Genomic DNA is isolated and digested into small fragments with restriction enzymes, and the fragments are separated by gel electrophoresis, as described previously. Following separation, DNA fragments are denatured chemically into single-strand fragments. It is very difficult to handle gels and even more difficult and also impractical to store them. Southern developed a technique whereby these separated single-stranded fragments in the gel could be transferred by capillary action to a solid support medium (nylon or nitrocellulose membrane) and fixed permanently by heating. The pattern on the membrane reflects identically the pattern induced by electrophoresis on the gel. The process used to produce a Southern blot is illustrated schematically in Fig. 5-9. The nylon membrane and its attached single-strand DNA fragments are then incubated with a radioactively labeled complementary probe. The hybridized, radioactive double-strand product, on exposure to x-ray film (autoradiography), will exhibit the pattern of the radiolabeled DNA fragments (Fig. 5-10). In summary, the electrophoretic separation of DNA followed by its transfer to a nylon membrane for subsequent identification by radioactive hybridization is referred to as *Southern blotting,* and the autoradiogram as a *Southern blot*. The same approach to detect mRNA is referred to as *Northern blotting*. This procedure also can be used for detection of proteins, in which case it is referred to as *Western blotting* (Table 5-1). The only significant difference in detecting protein versus nucleic acid by this procedure is the probe, which is an antibody rather than an oligonucleotide or cDNA. However, as in Southern and Northern blotting, the probe may be labeled with a radioactive isotope, a fluorescent tag, or some visual colorimetric substance.

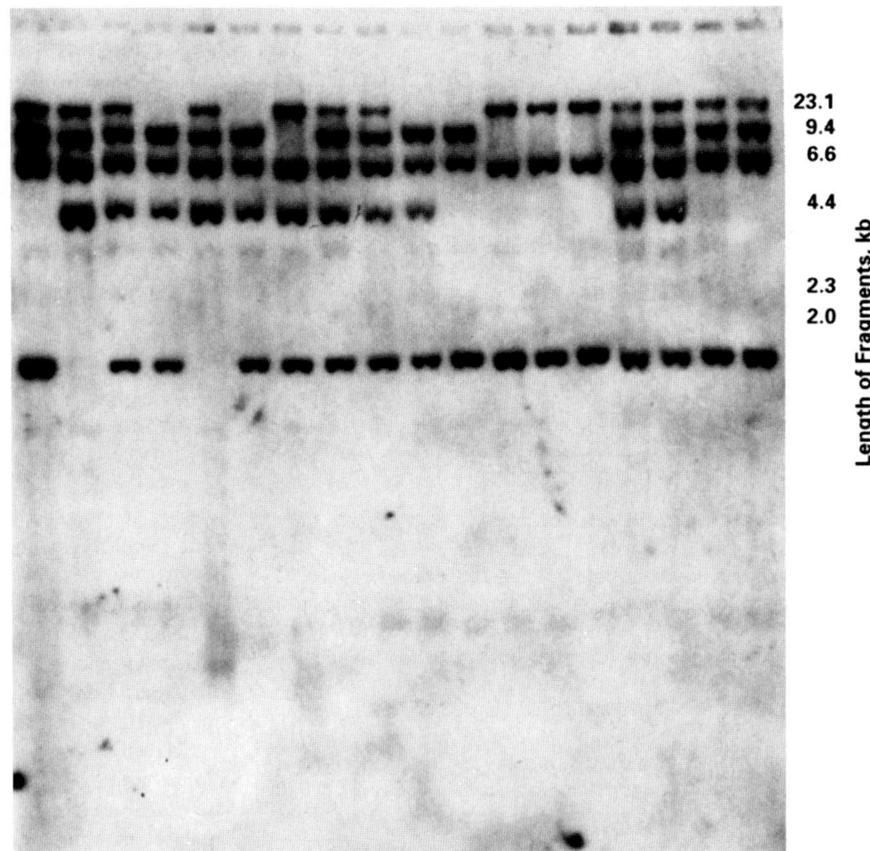


FIGURE 5-10 A typical Southern blot with distinct bands. Each vertical lane consists of DNA from a separate individual. All the individual DNAs were digested with the same restriction endonuclease. Following separation on electrophoresis and transfer to a nylon membrane, hybridization was performed with the selected radioactive probe, and thus only those fragments complementary to the probe are visualized. This is an analysis of a family with hypertrophic cardiomyopathy, and the different patterns reflect restriction fragment length polymorphisms (RFLPs) characteristic of the marker locus, which is linked to the disease locus. (From Mares A Jr, Towbin J, Bies RG, Roberts R. Molecular biology for the cardiologist. *Curr Probl Cardiology* 1992; 17:9–72. Reproduced with permission from the publisher and authors.)

## Cloning a Gene

DNA cloning is a technique used to produce large quantities of a specific DNA fragment of interest. It generally is quite feasible to produce a million copies of a DNA fragment by routine cloning techniques. The DNA fragment of interest to be cloned, referred to as the *insert,* is incorporated into the DNA of a vector and the vector is replicated in an appropriate host cell. The host provides replication of the DNA of both the vector and the insert. The prerequisites for cloning are (1) isolation of the DNA fragment (insert) of interest for cloning, (2) a vector for transferring the DNA fragment, (3) a restriction endonuclease to cut the DNA of the vector so the DNA ends will be compatible for ligating the insert (as illustrated in Fig. 5-11), (4) a DNA ligase to ligate the insert into the vector, (5) a means to introduce the vector into the host cell, and (6) a means to differentiate the host cells that have incorporated the vector from those which have not. Standard vectors used in cloning have circular DNA and fall into three classes: (1) plasmids harvested from bacterial cells (a *plasmid* is an extrachromosomal segment of DNA present in bacteria that is self-replicating and has been constructed to contain genes that express resistance to ampicillin or other antibiotics); (2) bacteriophages (commonly referred to merely as *phages,* which are viruses that invade and multiply in bacterial cells); and (3) an artificially developed vector (referred to as a *cosmid*). The usual host cell is bacteria, which has circular DNA as opposed to the linear DNA of the human genome. The circular DNA of the vector is cut by an appropriate restriction enzyme. The linear DNA is then incubated with the insert in the presence of a ligating enzyme, which induces the incorporation of the insert through attachment to each end of the vector's DNA to form a circle. The circularized recombinant product (hence

TABLE 5-1 Separation and Identification of Molecular Species

| Procedures | Molecule | Labeled Probe |
|---|---|---|
| Southern blotting | DNA | DNA or cDNA |
| Northern blotting | RNA | DNA or cDNA |
| Western blotting | Protein | Antibody |

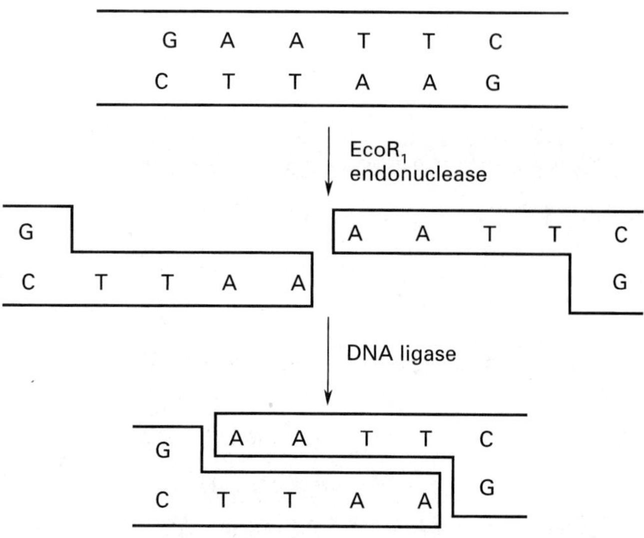


FIGURE 5-11 Restriction endonucleases recognize specific sequences and cut in a specific manner. The sequences recognized may be anywhere from 3 to 8 base pairs long and may cut to give a blunt end or a staggered end (EcoR1). Enzymes that provide staggered ends (cohesive or sticky ends) have unpaired bases that are easy to ligate together because they are complementary to each other, as shown in this illustration. This feature is exploited in cloning or in the formation of any recombinant DNA molecule. For cloning purposes, the fragment of DNA to be inserted is digested with the same restriction enzyme as is used to digest the DNA of the vector into which it will be inserted. Thus the sticky ends of the DNA insert and the vector will be complementary and easy to ligate together in the presence of the enzyme DNA ligase, as illustrated in Fig. 5-12.

the name *recombinant*) is inserted into a host such as a bacterium or a mammalian cell for amplification (Fig. 5-12). To increase uptake of the vector into the host, the pore sizes of the bacteria are increased, usually with heat shock treatment for about 45 s. In order to identify whether or not the particular DNA of interest has been replicated in the host, a so-called selection gene, such as one responsible for ampicillin resistance, is incorporated into the vector. The bacteria are grown in media containing ampicillin so only those bacteria with the resistance gene will survive. Since the resistance gene is attached to the DNA fragment being cloned, colonies (bacteria) or plaques (phage) that survive must contain the gene of interest. Some of the colonies or plaques may, however, contain the insert in the wrong direction or have circularized on itself without the insert, and thus, it is necessary to check and sometimes sequence the DNA to be certain the insert is in the appropriate direction. One can then transfer the colonies that contain the insert onto a petri dish and grow them for 24 h at 37°C. The colonies can be stored at 4°C. Replating for regrowth every few months will maintain a source of clones essentially indefinitely.

The size of the insert is a limitation in cloning. Plasmids as vectors can only accommodate inserts up to approximately 15,000 bp, phages up to 25,000 bp, and cosmids up to 45,000 bp. Recently, a new vector has been developed, namely, bacterial artificial chromosomes (BACs), that accommodates DNA fragments of up to 200,000 bp. The yeast artificial chromosome (YAC), developed several years ago, accommodates DNA inserts of up to 2 million bp but is extremely difficult to work with on a routine basis. In contrast, the BACs are as convenient as plasmids or phages. This has markedly accelerated the cloning of large fragments of DNA. Cloning, as discussed, is performed to obtain multiple copies of DNA, and unless specifically designed, the DNA is neither transcribed into mRNA nor translated into protein. If one desires to express a particular DNA fragment or gene, one must use what is referred to as an *expression vector*. It is imperative to provide a promoter element that is appropriate for the host, and the gene must contain the appropriate 5′ untranslated region for binding to the ribosome as well as the appropriate 3′ region for stability of the message. An example would be the expression of rt-PA in mammalian cells, whereby the protein is expressed and secreted to be harvested and processed commercially for use as a thrombolytic agent.

## Development of Gene Libraries

Gene libraries may be either genomic or cDNA libraries. A *genomic library* is one made from genomic DNA. A library is a collection of DNA fragments that have been cloned in an appropriate vector and grown in a particular host, usually bacteria. A major difference between a genomic and a cDNA library is that a genomic library contains DNA fragments composed of introns and exons, whereas a cDNA library is made from mRNA that represents genes expressed in a particular organ and does not have introns. The cDNA library contains genes specifically expressed in a particular tissue only. In contrast, a genomic library, whether derived from the heart or another tissue, will have the same genes. To make a human genomic library, one must first isolate the whole genome of a cell, cut it into fragments with a restriction enzyme, and insert the fragments into a vector to be replicated in an appropriate host, usually bacteria. To increase the odds that enough fragments are cloned to represent the whole genome, certain calculations are necessary. It is assumed that the recognition site for a particular restriction enzyme occurs at random. For the restriction enzyme EcoR1, with a 6-bp recognition site, the average size of each fragment will be $4^6 = 4096$ bp. In contrast, if the recognition site involves 4 bp, each fragment would be $4^4 = 256$ bp long. If the 6-bp cutter were used for the human genome, the result would be the 3 billion bp of the human genome divided by 4096 to produce roughly 750,000 fragments requiring 750,000 colonies or clones. However, the recognition sites are not evenly or randomly distributed. Thus some fragments are larger and others are smaller, so to be certain, at least 1 million colonies would be required. Other factors also must be considered, such as the choice of vector with respect to insert size. The library is a permanent, renewable source of DNA. cDNA libraries from all human tissues are now commercially available including the heart and specific structures of the heart such as the Purkinje system.

## Polymerase Chain Reaction

PCR has revolutionized application of the techniques of molecular biology. This technique was not developed until 1985,[24,25] but its impact has been felt throughout medicine and biotechnology. This procedure, conveniently and without the tedium of cloning, can provide 1 million copies of a DNA fragment in 3 to 4 h and 1 billion copies within 24 h. PCR simply and ingeniously takes advantage of the natural DNA replication process. One must know the sequence of the two ends of the DNA fragment that is to be amplified, but short sequences of 15 to 30 bp are adequate, and fragments in between these sequences as large as 20 kb can be amplified. The sequence is used to make two oligonucleotides, referred to as *primers,* with one for each end of the DNA fragment. The sequence of one primer is complementary to the sense direction, and the sequence of the other is made complementary to the antisense direction. The primers are used to prime the synthesis of cDNA strands and are designed such that the

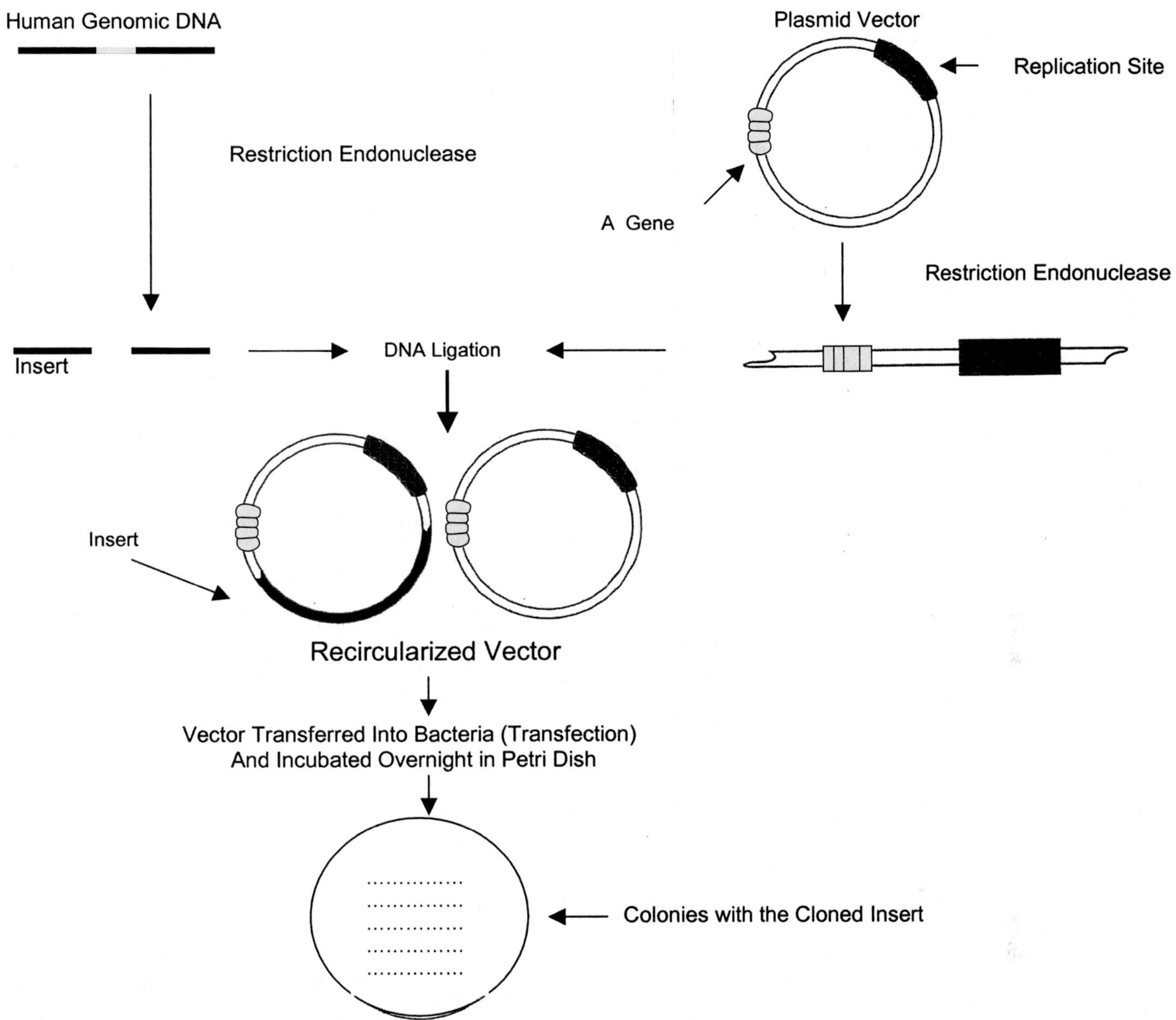


FIGURE 5-12 DNA cloning. The basic objective of cloning is to provide multiple copies of a DNA fragment of interest. The fundamental principles for cloning of a specific DNA fragment is as follows: (1) The human DNA fragment of interest is isolated from human DNA (shown on the left) by using a restriction endonuclease enzyme. The fragment obtained to be cloned is referred to as the *DNA insert* (*bottom*). (2) A DNA vector is selected (shown on the right), usually a plasmid, that has circular DNA and contains the necessary replication site (as indicated) and a drug resistance gene (A Gene, *top*). The vector's DNA is digested with a restriction endonuclease so that the circular DNA of the plasmid is linearized as shown on the right. (3) DNA ligase is selected to join both ends of the insert to both ends of the linearized vector DNA such that it is again recircularized. The vector DNA containing the insert along with the antibiotic resistance gene is transferred into a host cell which is usually bacteria. The bacteria are now plated on a petri dish and incubated (usually overnight) to grow colonies. The culture medium in the petri dish contains an antibiotic to which the bacteria containing the plasmid vector will be resistant. Thus, the only bacteria to form colonies will be those resistant to the antibiotic. Since the insert and the antibiotic resistance gene are together in the vector's DNA, the only bacteria to form colonies will be those that contain the insert. As the bacteria host proliferates, so will the insert of interest proliferate (cloned), usually to about 1 million copies after 24 h.

DNA between the primers is the fragment of interest to be amplified. If mRNA is to be amplified, it is first converted to a cDNA using the enzyme reverse transcriptase. The primers (oligonucleotides) and the necessary bases are added in excess, together with the enzyme Taq DNA polymerase (which catalyzes DNA synthesis) and a sample containing the DNA to be amplified. There are three steps to each cycle. Initially, one must denature the DNA (separate the primers and the native DNA) into separate strands, which is done by increasing the temperature to 95°C. The temperature is then decreased to 50°C so that the primers and native DNA will reanneal to their complementary base sequences. The native DNA strands will bind not only to each other but also to the primers. The temperature is now increased to 65°C for synthesis of the new DNA fragments. Synthesis in the presence of Taq1 polymerase is initiated at the 5′ end, and further nucleotides are added in the 5′ to 3′ direction to provide the desired double-stranded DNA fragment. Taq1 DNA polymerase, isolated from *Thermus aquaticus,* is thermostable, which is of tremendous advantage in performing the PCR reaction. Since the high temperatures of up to 95°C do not destroy this polymerase, it negates the need to add DNA polymerase between each cycle. Furthermore, since Taq polymerase has an optimal activity at around 70°C, one can significantly accelerate DNA synthesis. The cycle is then repeated, and after about 30 cycles over 3 h, one should have about 1 million copies. There are many clinical applications for PCR. To make a diagnosis of viral myocarditis, for example, one can use PCR to amplify from a myocardial biopsy any specific viral RNA or DNA for which primers can be made. The sensitivity of most conventional techniques is inadequate to detect molecules unless present in 50,000 to 100,000 copies per cell. In contrast, only one copy of RNA or DNA is needed for detection by PCR, and in 3 to 4 h, up to 1 million copies can be generated, which is adequate abundance for detection by most conventional techniques. PCR offers exquisite diagnostic sensitivity and specificity for determining the etiology of cardiac disorders such as myocarditis, and in patients undergoing cardiac transplantation, it is used for detecting infection or immunologic rejection. Another application of PCR is to detect and amplify mutations associated with hereditary disorders. One also can sequence DNA directly from PCR without the need for cloning.

### Electrophoretic Mobility Shift Assay (Band-Shift Assay)

This technique is used routinely to study transcriptional factors. On gel electrophoresis, DNA exhibits a certain migratory pattern owing to the large fragments moving more slowly. If a transcription factor is bound to its DNA-binding site, migration is further slowed compared to the control and the decreased mobility is detected as a shift in the migrating pattern through the gel (hence the name). Using an antibody to the protein, one also can study the protein specifically. It was this technique that identified a unique family of DNA- and RNA-binding proteins that are specific for the triplet repeat CTG (or CUG) known to cause myotonic dystrophy.[26]

## References


1. Watson JD, Crick FHC. Molecular structure of nucleic acids: A structure for deoxyribose nucleic acid. *Nature* 1953;171:737–738.
2. Schekman R, Weiner A, Kornberg A. Multienzyme systems of DNA replication. *Science* 1956;186:987–993.
3. Marmor J, Lane L. Strand separation and specific recombination of deoxyribonucleic acids: Biological studies. *Proc Natl Acad Sci USA* 1960;46:453–461.
4. Leder P, Nirenberg M. RNA codewords and protein synthesis: II. Nucleotide sequence of a valine RNA codeword. *Proc Natl Acad Sci USA* 1964;52:420–427.
5. Nishimura S, Jones DS, Khorana HG. The in vitro synthesis of a copolypeptide containing two amino acids in alternative sequence dependent upon a DNA-like polymer containing two nucleotides in alternating sequence. *J Mol Biol* 1981;146:1–21.
6. Olivera BM, Hall ZW, Lehman IR. Enzymatic joining of polynucleotides: V. A DNA adenylate intermediate in the polynucleotide joining reaction. *Proc Natl Acad Sci USA* 1968;61:237–244.
7. Smith HO, Wilcox KW. A restriction enzyme from *Hemophilus influenzae:* I. Purification and general properties. *J Mol Biol* 1970;51: 379–391.
8. Baltimore D. Viral RNA-dependent DNA polymerase. *Nature* 1970; 226:1209–1211.
9. Temin HM, Mizutani S. RNA-dependent DNA polymerase in virions of Rous sarcoma virus. *Nature* 1970;226:1211–1213.
10. Cohen S, Chang A, Boyer H, Helling R. Construction of biological functional bacterial plasmids in vitro. *Proc Natl Acad Sci USA* 1973;70: 3240–3244.
11. Sanger F, Coulson AR. A rapid method for determining sequences in DNA by primed synthesis and DNA polymerase. *J Mol Biol* 1975;94: 444–448.
12. Maxam AM, Gilbert W. A new method of sequencing DNA. *Proc Natl Acad Sci USA* 1977;74:560–564.
13. Metzler DE. The Nucleic Acids. In: Metzler DE, ed. *Biochemistry The Chemical Reaction of Living Cells,* 2nd ed. Burlington, MA: Harcourt/ Academic Press; 2001:198–279.
14. Lodish H, Berk A, Zipursky SL, et al. Nucleic acids, the genetic code, and the synthesis of macromolecules. In: *Molecular Cell Biology,* 4th ed. Houndsmills, Basingstoke, England: Freeman; 2000:100–137.
15. Lodish H, Berk A, Zipursky SL, et al. Regulation of the eukaryotic cell cycle. In: *Molecular Cell Biology,* 4th ed. Houndsmills, Basingstoke England: Freeman; 2000:500–505.
16. Roberts R. Modern molecular biology: Historical perspective and future potential. In: Roberts R, ed. *Molecular Basis of Cardiology.* Hamden, CT: Blackwell Scientific; 1992:1–15.
17. Ahmad K. Epigenetic consequences of nucleosome dynamics. *Cell* 2002;111:281–291.
18. Luger K, Mader AW, Richmond RK, et al. Crystal structure of the nucleosomes core particle at 2.8A resolution. *Nature* 1997;389: 251–260.
19. Zhang CL, McKinsey TA, Chang S, et al. Class II histone deacetylases act as signal-responsive repressors of cardiac hypertrophy. *Cell* 2002; 100(4):479–488.
20. Spotswood HT, Turner BM. An increasingly complex code. *J Clin Invest* 2002;110(5):577–582.
21. Sun ZW, Allis CD. Ubiquitination of histone H2B regulates H3 methylation and gene silencing in yeast. *Nature* 2002;418(6893): 104–108.
22. Brenner S. *Molecular Biology: A Selection of Papers*. San Diego, CA: Academic Press; 1989.
23. Southern EM. Detection of specific sequences among DNA fragments separated by gel electrophoresis. *J Mol Biol* 1975;98:503–517.
24. Saiki RK, Scharf S, Faloona F, et al. Enzymatic amplification of beta-globin genomic sequences and restriction site analysis for diagnosis of sickle cell anemia. *Science* 1985;230:1350–1354.
25. Saiki RK, Gelfand DH, Stoffel S, et al. Primer-directed enzymatic amplification of DNA with a thermostable DNA polymerase. *Science* 1988;239:487–491.
26. Timchenko LT, Timchenko NA, Caskey T, Roberts R. Novel proteins with binding specificity for DNA CTG repeats and RNA CUG repeats: Implications for myotonic dystrophy. *Hum Mol Genet* 1996;5:115–121.

CHAPTER 6

# MOLECULAR AND CELLULAR BIOLOGY OF THE NORMAL, HYPERTROPHIED, AND FAILING HEART

Richard A. Walsh



Growth of the heart is a dynamic process that occurs during embryogenesis, postnatal development, maturity, and senescence and in response to changing environmental and pathologic conditions. Cardiac growth occurs at the cellular level as a consequence of the interplay between *hyperplasia* (increase in cell number) and *hypertrophy* (increase in cell size) or a combination of both processes. The relative importance of each of these two mechanisms depends on the cell type, developmental stage, and nature of the growth stimulus. These two forms of cell growth are variably modulated by *apoptosis,* or programmed cell death.[1] This phenomenon is of importance in the determination of heart shape and chamber formation during cardiogenesis and may contribute to altered cardiac chamber geometry in response to pathologic stimuli. Physiologic and pathologic cardiovascular growth are generally mediated by developmental programs, mechanical deformation, and injury in various combinations. These processes stimulate a repertoire of biochemical signals that alter the cardiovascular phenotype. The application of molecular and cell biological approaches to this problem is rapidly defining the precise factors responsible for normal and pathologic growth of the heart and the mechanisms responsible for altered cardiac function.

## CARDIAC GROWTH AND HYPERTROPHY

Cardiac hypertrophy is a process wherein there is an increase in chamber mass produced largely by an increase in the size of terminally differentiated cardiomyocytes. Although cardiomyocytes make up only one-third of the total cell number, they are responsible in aggregate for over 70 percent of cardiac volume. Cardiac hypertrophy may be reasonably categorized as either physiologic or pathologic (Fig. 6-1).

### Physiologic Hypertrophy

Physiologic hypertrophy includes cardiogenesis during embryonic development, postnatal cardiac growth, a modest additional increase in heart size that evolves during senescence, and the increase in heart size that occurs in response to athletic conditioning. The earliest stage of cardiac growth in utero depends on a genetically determined developmental program, since it can occur in the absence of contractile activity. Subsequently, mechanical forces become increasingly important in the development of the normal cardiac phenotype. Throughout the embryonic period and for a few weeks after birth, cardiac growth occurs as a consequence of hyperplasia and hypertrophy of myocytes (see Chap. 8). Classically, adult myocytes have been described as terminally differentiated—that is, as incapable of reentering the cell cycle. This issue is currently undergoing reexamination. It is critical to make a distinction between DNA synthesis and cell division. In the adult cardiomyocyte, DNA synthesis may clearly result in either multinucleation or polyploidy (an increase in the DNA content of a single nucleus). By contrast, there is little evidence that cardiomyocytes are capable of division under normal conditions after the early postnatal period.[2] The capacity to reactivate hyperplasia in the terminally differentiated cardiomyocyte is an area of intense research interest, with potentially important therapeutic implications in the hypertrophied and failing heart.[3]

From birth to maturation, the mammalian heart undergoes a sixfold increase in mass. The normal heart/body weight ratio is species-specific. The largest hearts relative to body size occur in animals with survival requirements that depend on sustained exercise rather than on burst activity.[4] In humans, intense, prolonged exercise training can produce an increase in cardiac mass. Isotonic exercise, such as running, produces *eccentric hypertrophy,* characterized by a normal ratio of wall thickness to dimension; whereas isometric exercise,

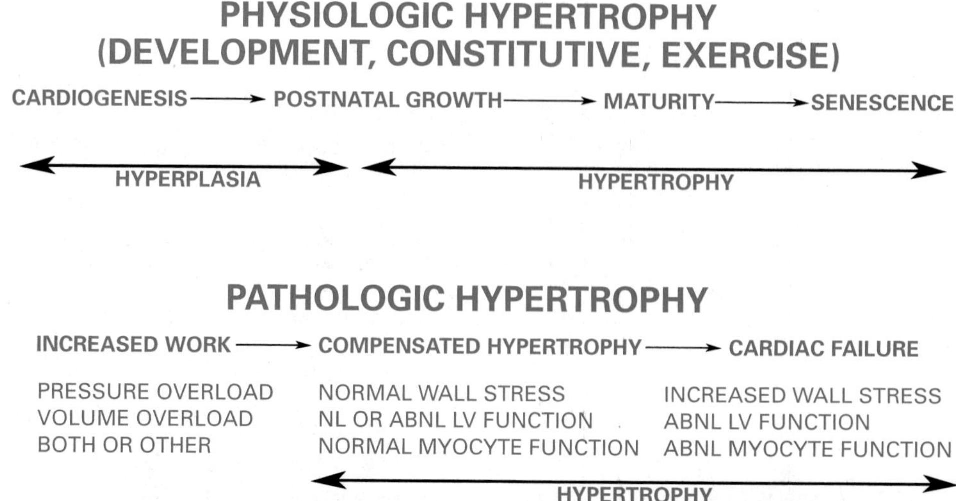


FIGURE 6-1 Relative roles of cardiomyocyte hypertrophy, hyperplasia, and apoptosis in physiologic and pathologic cardiac hypertrophy, along with the functional differences between compensated hypertrophy and heart failure.

such as weight lifting, stimulated *concentric hypertrophy,* associated with an increased ratio of wall thickness to dimension.[5] Senescent animals and humans free of organic heart disease develop mild concentric left ventricular hypertrophy as a consequence of age-related decreases in the distensibility of the peripheral vasculature. The molecular, biochemical, and physiologic changes associated with physiologic hypertrophy differ both qualitatively and quantitatively from those that occur during pathologic hypertrophy. Physiologic studies in animal models and humans have demonstrated no substantial alterations in isolated muscle or intact heart function. There is also little evidence of alterations in the molecular determinants of excitation-contraction coupling. Most importantly, epidemiologic data fail to demonstrate adverse risk associated with the modest hypertrophy that occurs as a consequence of athletic conditioning. It is, therefore, important clinically to distinguish physiologic hypertrophy from hypertrophic cardiomyopathy in athletes (see Chap. 77).

There are exceptions to the principle that pathologic hypertrophy occurs as a result of excessive increases in external work. For example, hypertrophic cardiomyopathy is produced by point mutations of the sarcomeric proteins, in particular the $\beta$-myosin heavy chain. These mutations result in massive asymmetric or concentric hypertrophy in the absence of augmented peripheral hemodynamic requirements (see Chap. 62). It is possible that the massive myofibrillar disarray that characterizes this genetic form of hypertrophy increases internal cardiac work, which, in turn, increases cardiac mass.[6] Genetically engineered mice with cardiac-specific postnatal overexpression of the $\beta_2$ adrenergic receptor[7] or targeted ablation of the phospholamban gene[8] have enhanced cardiac function throughout life but no significant increase in cardiac mass. By contrast, similar cardiac overexpression of the sarcoplasmic reticulum–binding protein calsequestrin in mice results in hypofunction of the heart, with decreased external work and substantial cardiac hypertrophy.[9] Finally, tachycardia-induced heart failure in animal models and humans is associated with increased external cardiac work, decreased cardiac function, and no alteration in cardiac mass. These recent observations suggest a critical reexamination of the primary role of mechanotransduction in the etiology of pathologic hypertrophy.

## Pathologic Hypertrophy

Pathologic hypertrophy is an important adaptive response to abnormal global or regional increase in cardiac work. Initially, the increase in cardiac mass serves to normalize wall stress and permit normal cardiovascular function at rest and during exercise in *compensated hypertrophy*. If the stimulus for pathologic hypertrophy is sufficiently intense or prolonged, *decompensated hypertrophy* and heart failure ensue. Pathologic hypertrophy may be caused by pressure overloading, as in systemic or pulmonary arterial hypertension, left ventricular outflow obstruction, or aortic coarctation. Pressure overloading produces an increase in systolic wall stress and results in concentric ventricular hypertrophy. Volume overloading, as occurs in mitral or aortic regurgitation or as a result of arteriovenous fistulas, also produces pathologic hypertrophy. These latter conditions induce an increase in either diastolic wall stress (mitral regurgitation) or both systolic and diastolic wall stress (aortic regurgitation and arteriovenous fistulas) and result in eccentric left ventricular hypertrophy. Regional hypertrophy that occurs in viable myocardium adjacent to and remote from an area of infarction has the characteristics of eccentric hypertrophy.

## Mechanisms for the Development of Cardiac Hypertrophy

### STIMULI AND SIGNAL TRANSDUCTION PATHWAYS

***Stretch-Induced Growth Factors*** Dynamic or static stretch of neonatal or adult cardiomyocytes, papillary muscle, isolated heart, or intact heart produces increased cardiac protein synthesis and resultant cellular hypertrophy. The process by which stimuli in the physical domain activate intracellular growth-signaling pathways is known as *mechanotransduction.*[10] There is evidence that this process may be accomplished in the cardiomyocyte by stretch-activated sarcolemmal ion channels, G protein–coupled receptors, $NA^+/H^+$ antiporters, tyrosine kinase–containing receptors, and/or an extracellular matrix–integrin linked pathway. These cell-surface mechanotransducers then activate cytosolic signal transduction pathways that initiate gene transcription and translation of increased quantities of protein (Fig. 6-2). Important signal transduction pathways that are clearly activated by mechanical deformation include protein kinase C (PKC), mitogen activated protein (MAP) kinases, stress-activated protein kinase, and possibly cyclic adenosine monophosphate (cAMP)–dependent protein kinase. In particular, stretch of neonatal cultured cardiomyocytes produces G protein–mediated activation of membrane-bound phospholipase C, which, in turn, hydrolyzes phosphatidylinositol bisphosphate ($PIP_2$) to inositol trisphosphate ($IP_3$) and diacylglycerol (DAG). Diacylglycerol then activates PKC. Phosphorylation of downstream cytosolic and nuclear proteins and transcription factors by PKC is known to be of critical importance for growth in a number of cell types, while inositol triphosphate is an important modulator of cytosolic calcium homeostasis by the interaction with its receptor on the sarcoplasmic reticulum. Angiotensin II receptor coupling appears to play a critical role in the activation of phospholipase C[11]; however, $\alpha_1$-adrenergic and endothelin receptor stimulation can also activate this pathway, with resultant hypertrophy in the neonatal cardiomyocytes and in transgenic mice.[12–13]

Current information suggests that mechanotransduction and a number of interrelated autocrine, paracrine, and endocrine effects of hormones and growth factors mediate cardiac hypertrophy (Fig. 6-2). The resultant activation of multiple signal transduction pathways, which have demonstrable cross talk and considerable redundancy, provides a powerful mechanism by which the heart can respond to changing chronic hemodynamic requirements. A point of downstream convergence of multiple signal transduction pathways in the heart and noncardiac systems appears to be the phosphorylation of mitogen-activated protein kinase [MAPK, also known as extracellular signal regulated kinase (ERK)].[14] Mammalian MAPKs are serine-threonine protein kinases that are activated by signal transduction pathways coupled to both phosphatidylinositol hydrolysis/PKC activation and receptor protein tyrosine kinases (Fig. 6-2). Of particular importance to cardiac hypertrophy is the observation that important transcription factors (c-*jun*, c-*myc*, p62[TCF]) are known substrates of MAPK phosphorylation. Recently, transfection of an antisense nucleotide to MAPK was shown to prevent hypertrophy in cardiomyocytes. Information from noncardiomyocyte cell systems, neonatal and adult myocytes, and genetically engineered mice has demonstrated considerable complexity, redundancy, and cross talk among these and other intracellular signaling pathways in the development of the cardiac hypertrophy phenotype in response to stretch and other stimuli.[15] In particular, ischemia, hypoxia, oxidative stress, neurohormones, and cytokines can activate downstream signaling and resultant nuclear transcriptional events, including cardiomyocyte hypertrophy and fibroblast hyperplasia.

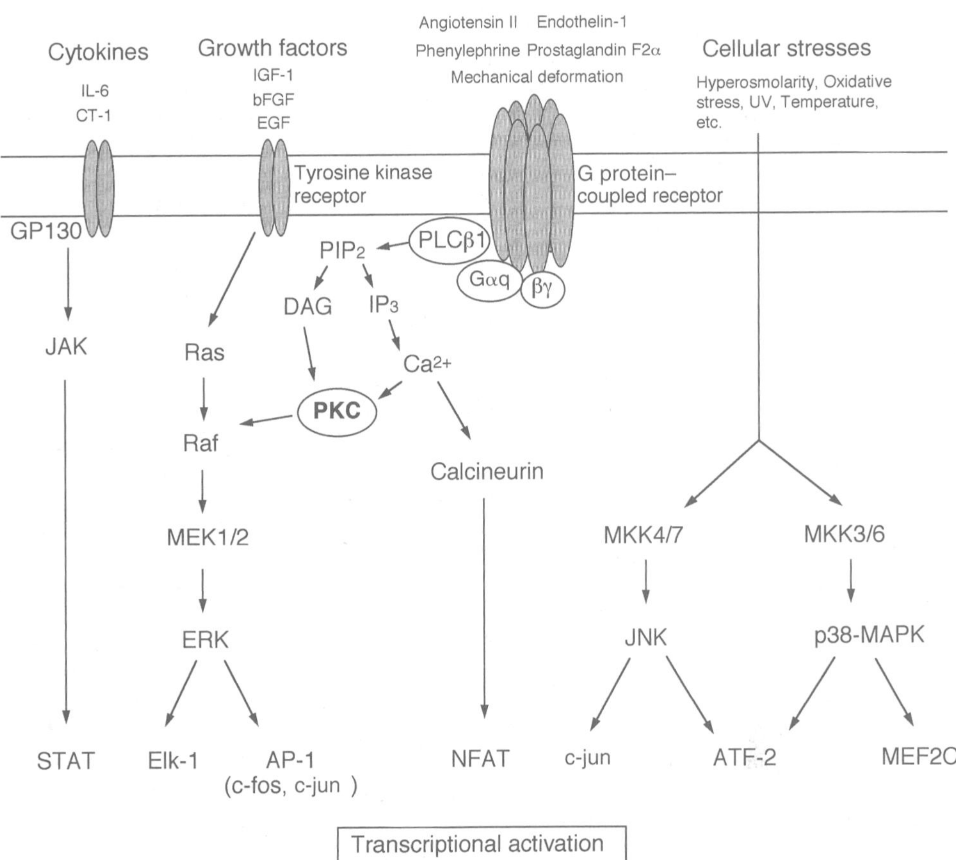


FIGURE 6-2 A schema for signal transduction pathways that activate transcriptional regulation and induce hypertrophic genes. G protein–coupled receptor agonists binding to their receptors activate phospholipase C (PLC) $\beta_1$ via the dissociated $\alpha$ subunit of a GTP-binding protein of the Gq class (G$\alpha$q). PLC$\beta_1$ catalyzes the hydrolysis of phosphatidylinositol bisphosphate ($PIP_2$) into diacylglycerol (DAG), which activates protein kinase C (PKC) and inositol trisphosphate ($IP_3$), which stimulates calcium release from intracellular stores. PKC activated by DAG and ± calcium initiates cascades of phosphorylation. One of the downstream targets of PKC is the ras-raf mitogen-activated protein kinase (MAPK) cascade. Insulin-like growth factor (IGF)-1, basic fibroblast growth factor (bFGF), or epidermal growth factor (EGF) interacts with cognate membrane tyrosine kinase receptors, which activate ras by the growth factor receptor–bound protein. Ras activates raf, MAPK/ERK-activating kinase (MEK), and extracellular signal regulated kinase (ERK). Cellular stresses activate other members of the MAPK family, c-jun N-terminal kinase (JNK) and p38-MAPK, but precise signaling elements are not as well defined as in the ERK cascade. The MAPK kinase (MKK) and small G proteins are likely to be involved. Ras, either directly or indirectly, may activate JNK and p38-MAPK. Signaling through interleukin-1 (IL-1) and cardiotrophin-1 (CT-1) receptors involves gp130, which acts as a signal transducing receptor component. The binding of ligands to their cognate receptors results in receptor dimerization, autophosphorylation, and activation of the associated Janus kinase (JAK). In turn, JAK activates members of the STAT (signal transducer and activator of transcription) family. PKC activation increases calcium concentration through phosphorylation of L-type calcium channel and $IP_3$ mediated calcium release from intracellular stores. This leads to stimulation of the calcium-dependent phosphatase calcineurin. Activated calcineurin dephosphorylates nuclear factor of activated T lymphocytes (NFAT), which translocates into the nucleus to interact with multiple transcription factors.

***Non-Stretch-Induced Growth Factors*** G$\alpha$q-coupled receptors—which include angiotensin II, phenylephrine, endothelin, prostaglandin F2$\alpha$, and thrombin—can induce hypertrophy of neonatal cardiomyocytes in culture in the absence of altered mechanical forces and in vivo in genetically engineered mice when the receptor is overexpressed.

## Cytokines

Cytokines were initially characterized by their pleiotropic effects on the cellular components of the immune system. They have recently been implicated in normal and pathologic cardiac growth by a variety of in vitro and in vivo animal studies and by clinical investigation. Cytokines of the interleukin-6 and cardiotrophin family activate the gp130 cardiomyocyte transmembrane receptor and rapidly stimulate cytoplasmic Janus kinases (JAK); these, in turn phosphorylate other cytoplasmic proteins called signal transducers and activators of transcription (STAT). Various components of gp130 and JAK-STAT pathways have induced hypertrophy in vitro and in vivo when overexpressed in transgenic mice. By contrast, interleukin-1 and tumor necrosis factor alpha (TNF-$\alpha$) use a distinct pathway that involves activation of a phosphatidylcholine-specific phospholipase C with generation of diacylglycerol. These cytokines are elevated in the plasma of patients with congestive heart failure, and inhibition of their effects is a current therapeutic target for clinical heart failure. There is increasing evidence that stimulation of cell-surface tyrosine-kinase receptors can elicit a hyperplastic or hypertrophic response in neonatal cardiomyocytes. Both acidic and basic fibroblast growth factors (FGFs), which act as ligands for tyrosine-kinase receptors, can induce myocyte growth. Acidic FGF produces a hyperplastic response, whereas basic FGF stimulates an increase in protein synthesis with resultant hypertrophy. In contrast to its role in vascular smooth muscle growth, transforming growth factor beta (TGF-$\beta$) does not induce a growth response under these conditions.[16]

In addition to FGF and TGF-$\beta$, insulin-like growth factor 1 (IGF-1) is expressed in the myocardium in response to pressure overload hypertrophy.[17] These and other peptide growth factors [neural growth factor (NGF), epidermal growth factor (EGF), platelet-derived growth factor (PDGF), and insulin] bind to receptor tyrosine kinases (RTK). These receptors undergo ligand-mediated homodimerization with resultant autophosphorylation of tyrosine residues on the cytoplasmic domain. These tyrosine complexes recruit signaling molecules such as the monomeric GTP-binding protein P21 ras to the membrane, where transient complexes stimulate downstream signaling to the nucleus. Increasing evidence using loss of function and gain of function in in vitro studies of neonatal myocytes implicates this signaling molecule and its downstream effector raf-1 as potential mediators of cardiac growth.

### Hormones

Thyroid hormone is generally considered the classic hormonal mediator of cardiac hypertrophy. Administration of excess thyroid hormone to experimental animals produces increased heart weight, which is associated with transcriptionally mediated alterations in the myosin heavy chains (MHCs), calcium-cycling proteins, and other functional constituents of the cardiomyocyte in small animals and primates.[18] Thyroid hormone–induced hypertrophy appears to be an indirect effect of the $T_3$-mediated increased oxygen consumption and resultant augmentation of cardiac work. For example, heterotopic transplantation of a nonworking rat heart into the abdominal aorta of the hyperthyroid animal is unassociated with hypertrophy, despite the presence of the transcriptionally mediated effects of the hormone in the transplanted organ and hypertrophy and typical transcriptional events in the native working heart.[19]

In addition to the indirect effects of thyroid hormone on cardiac growth, other endocrine mediators of hypertrophy have been examined. Growth hormone, which mediates its effects in large part though IGF-1, may be a mediator of physiologic hypertrophy. By contrast, there is preliminary evidence that retinoic acid and vitamin D may inhibit cardiac growth.[20]

### Calcium Signaling

Increases in intracellular calcium have been associated with hypertrophic cardiomyocyte growth in vitro (see Fig. 6-2).[21,22] For example, use of the calcium ionophore BAYK8644 enhances while application of a membrane-permeable calcium chelator inhibits the cellular hypertrophic response by affecting calcium-calmodulin–dependent protein kinase. In addition, calcineurin, a phosphatase activated by intracellular calcium, dephosphorylates nuclear factor for activation of transcription (NFAT), which translocates to the nucleus, where it activates numerous transcription factors such as GATA-4. In vitro and in vivo studies using genetically engineered mice have demonstrated that augmented levels of activity of calcineurin, NFAT, or both can initiate a hypertrophic response. However, the relative role of this pathway in normal and pathologic growth of the heart is unclear at this time.[23,24]

## PROTEIN CONTENT AND ISOFORM DIVERSITY

The hallmark of cardiac hypertrophy is a net increase in protein synthesis above protein degradation. Under normal circumstances, these two processes are matched and result in nitrogen balance. Since the average half-life of cardiac proteins is 5 days, the composition of the adult heart is regenerated approximately every 3 weeks. The more rapid rate of cardiac growth in response to increased hemodynamic load could result from an augmentation in either the efficiency or the capacity of protein synthesis or a combination of the two.[25,26] Efficiency of protein synthesis is usually measured as moles of amino acid incorporated per milligram of cellular RNA per hour; capacity is assessed by determining the number of milligrams of RNA per gram of tissue. Experiments in a variety of systems indicate that the critical determinant for cardiac hypertrophy is an increased capacity for protein synthesis, which is mediated by augmented ribosomal content. Protein degradation appears to be modestly increased in cardiac hypertrophy and may play a critical role in the distinctive geometry of the ventricles in response to pressure or volume overloading, regression of hypertrophy, and cardiac atrophy.[27] The mechanisms for protein degradation in the heart involve the activation of both lysosomal and cytosolic proteases. Posttranslational processes are increasingly being recognized as important factors in the production of the cardiac phenotype in cardiac hypertrophy and failure.[18,28]

In addition to increased total protein content, cardiac hypertrophy is characterized by alterations in the relative abundance and isoform composition of the cardiomyocyte contractile, regulatory, and calcium-cycling proteins and other subcellular constituents. These processes provide an additional degree of plasticity for the heart to adapt to changing functional requirements. It is clear that there is considerable species specificity in the capacity for isoform switching. In small mammals with rapid heart rates, such as mice and rats, imposition of a pressure overload produces a transcriptionally mediated shift from the $\alpha$- to the $\beta$-MHC and from cardiac to skeletal $\alpha$-actin.[29] $\alpha$-Myosin has a three- to sevenfold greater ATPase activity than $\beta$-myosin. The greater abundance of $\beta$-MHC in response to pressure overload in small animals increases the efficiency of force development by producing the same absolute muscle tension at a slower rate.[30] Despite identical cardiac muscle mechanics in response to hypertrophy, large animals with slower heart rates, including humans, possess $\beta$-MHC almost exclusively throughout embryogenesis and postnatal development. It is possible that, in higher mammalian species, altered myosin ATPase in response to pressure-overload hypertrophy may be mediated in part by a posttranslationally produced low-molecular-weight variant of the $\beta$-MHC or isoform shifts in other myofibrillar proteins. For example, cardiac isoforms exist for essential and regulatory light chains, troponin (I, C, and T), tropomyosin, and the sarcolemmal $Na^+$, $K^+$-ATPase. Isoform switching of each of the components of the cardiomyocyte has been reported in hypertrophy and failure, but the functional significance of this has been unclear. The ability to ablate or overexpress these isoforms in genetically engineered mice will more clearly elucidate their role in the normal and hypertrophied heart.

### Extracellular Matrix and the Cytoskeleton

Although cardiomyocytes make up the bulk of cardiac mass by volume, they are tethered in an extensive extracellular network of collagen and other structural proteins, including fibronectins and proteoglycans. The extracellular and intracellular myofibrillar scaffolding is a critical determinant of cardiac shape during normal and pathologic cardiac growth.[31,32] Collagen is synthesized principally by fibroblasts but also by vascular smooth muscle cells in response to a variety of pathologic stimuli, including increased oxidative and mechanical stress, ischemia, and inflammation. Most of the molecules and signal transduction pathways operant in cardiomyocyte growth play a role in hyperplasia of fibroblasts and in the elaboration of collagen. The resultant fibrosis produces altered myocardial stiffness and arrhythmogenesis in ischemic heart disease, cardiac hypertrophy, and congestive heart failure. Collagen synthesis is continuously and variably offset by extracellular matrix resorption mediated by matrix metalloproteinases (MMPs). The activity of these enzymes is increased in dilated cardiomyopathy. Conversely, the activity of a class of enzymes known as tissue inhibitors of matrix metalloproteinases (TIMPs) is reduced in this setting. The resultant excessive collagenolyses may induce myofibrillar slippage and contribute to the dilated thin-walled chamber geometry that characterizes acute and chronic heart failure. This process has been termed *chamber remodeling* by clinicians.[33]

Cardiomyocytes are tethered to the extracellular matrix by membrane-spanning proteins called *integrins*. The extracellular portion of these molecules binds to fibronectins in the extracellular matrix while the cytoplasmic domain is associated with a nonreceptor tyrosine kinase called focal adhesion kinase (FAK).[34] Downstream targets for FAK phosphorylation are the SRC kinases src and fyn. This pathway is differentially activated by mechanical stretch ischemia and oxidative stress in the myocardium and provides an additional mechanism for altered growth during pathologic conditions.[35] Perimyocyte extracellular proteins such as dystrophin and dystrophin-related proteins contribute to normal cardiogenesis; when altered in abundance, they can produce a cardiomyopathy in Duchenne's muscular dystrophy and some familial cardiomyopathies, respectively (see Chap. 62).

The cardiomyocyte cytoskeleton is the intracellular scaffolding that provides a framework for the orderly arrangement of sarcomeres in striated cardiac and skeletal muscle. Titin—the third most abundant protein in the heart, desmin, and vinculin have differing intracellular spatial distributions that contribute to resting tension of cardiac muscle. The amount and polymerization status of the proteins that make up the microtubular network of the cardiomyocyte cytoplasm (tubulin and $\beta$ actin) are important determinants of the viscous properties of heart muscle and contribute to altered cardiac function in pathologic states.[36,37]

Cardiac hypertrophy and failure are associated with changes in the relative abundance of the various intra- and extracellular structural proteins. All forms of cardiac hypertrophy are associated with increased collagen deposition in the extracellular matrix, which contributes to the observed alterations in passive chamber and muscle properties. Pressure overload (but not volume overload) hypertrophy has been associated with changes in the levels of the cytoskeletal proteins titin, desmin, and tubulin. Depolymerization of tubulin with colchicine reversed abnormalities in cardiac function in feline right ventricular hypertrophy but not in guinea pig left ventricular hypertrophy.[36,37]

### Excitation-Contraction Coupling and Calcium Homeostasis

Cardiomyocyte membrane depolarization is initiated by the intracellular movement of sodium through its ion channel, while repolarization is achieved by the extracellular movement of potassium via a family of sarcolemal $K^+$ channels. Membrane depolarization enhances the transmembrane conductance of calcium through a dihydropyridine-sensitive *l*-channel. The resultant increase in cytosolic calcium concentration permits binding of this cation to the ryanodine receptor on the surface of the sarcoplasmic reticulum. This process results in release of calcium from sarcoplasmic reticulum stores and further elevation of cytosolic calcium concentrations. The resultant hundredfold elevation of calcium permits binding to the myofilament regulatory protein troponin C. Calcium binding to troponin C promotes a steric movement of troponin I away from the actin binding site on the myosin molecule. This permits actin-myosin crossbridge formation and resultant tension development. The activity of troponin I can be modulated via phosphorylation by protein kinase A and C, while the affinity of troponin C for calcium is altered by intracellular pH. These processes may result in substantial alteration of myofilament calcium. Energy for crossbridge cycling is produced by hydrolysis of ATP via myosin ATPase. Calcium is released from troponin C and resequestered into the sarcoplasmic reticulum by a specific SR-ATPase. The activity of this enzyme is inhibited by the phosphoprotein phospholamban. Phosphorylation of phospholamban by cAMP (PKA)-dependent protein kinases, protein kinase C, or calcium-calmodulin–dependent protein kinase results in disinhibition and resultant enhancement of calcium uptake in the SR. Steady-state sarcoplasmic reticulum calcium content is determined by the abundance of the anionic storage proteins calsequestrin and calreticulum. Reequilibration of cytosolic sodium and potassium levels produced by the depolarization and repolarization cycle is facilitated by the activity of the sarcolemmal $Na^+$, $K^+$-ATPase. Extrusion of transarcolemmal mediated calcium influx is mediated by the coordinated interplay between the membrane situated $Na^+$-$H^+$ and $Na^+$-$Ca^{2+}$ exchangers. Isolated changes in the stoichiometry between the sarcoplasmic reticulum ATPase and its inhibitor, phospholamban, have been demonstrated to have functional significance in genetically engineered mice. Targeted ablation of phospholamban enhanced cardiac inotropic and lusitropic function, whereas cardiac-specific overexpression produced the opposite result.[38]

## CARDIAC FUNCTION OF THE HYPERTROPHIED HEART

The phenotypic consequences of the increased cardiac mass and altered protein abundance and composition of the hypertrophied heart are considerable and depend on the model utilized; the animal species; and the nature, intensity, and duration of the hypertrophic stimulus. Taken together, available clinical and animal studies suggest that functional alterations evolve along a continuum from normal chamber and myocyte function to abnormal chamber and normal myocyte function to abnormalities of both chamber and myocyte function (Fig. 6-1).

## Electrical Properties

The most typical electrical abnormality of the hypertrophied heart is prolongation of the duration of the action potential.[39] Recent studies using the single-cell voltage-clamp technique have begun to elucidate the ionic mechanisms responsible for this phenomenon. In mild hypertrophy, increases in calcium and calcium-activated currents (including the $NA^+/Ca^{2+}$ exchanger) appear to be important. In severe hypertrophy, prolongation of the action potential is also determined importantly by a reduction in the potassium currents Ik*l* and Ito. The relations between these changes in membrane current properties of hypertrophied hearts and altered mechanical behavior at the myocyte and whole-heart level are not clearly understood at present. Hypertrophied myocardium is more likely than normal tissue to precipitate arrhythmias. The mechanisms for arrhythmogenesis are multifactorial and are operant at the tissue and cardiomyocyte levels. Increased dispersion of refractoriness and slowed conduction results from myocyte loss and fibrosis. Prolongation of the duration of the action potential increases the likelihood of early afterdepolarizations, which may result in triggered arrhythmias. Reduced coronary artery flow reserve and accelerated atherosclerosis of epicardial coronary vessels predispose toward ischemia-induced arrhythmias. In concert, these mechanisms contribute to the finding of cardiac hypertrophy as the most powerful predictor of cardiovascular mortality in the Framingham Study (see Chap. 1).

The application of molecular biological and molecular genetic approaches is providing increasing insight into the cellular mechanisms of arrhythmogenesis. Normal cardiomyocyte excitation and arrhythmogenesis involve voltage-dependent ion channels, mechanosensitive channels, sarcolemmal electrogenic transporters, and gap junctions. The latter are two channels or connexins that enable ion current flow between and among cardiomyocytes. Connexins are composed of a class of molecules called *connexins*. Isoform diversity of the connexins are determinants of ion conductance and sensitivity.[40] The genes for each of the cardiomyocyte ion channels, transporters, and connexins have been cloned. Structure-function relations are being defined in vitro using site-directed mutagenesis and in vivo using loss of function or gain of function mutations in genetically engineered mice. In parallel, the abundance and/or function of the molecular determinants of excitability and arrhythmogenesis are beginning to be elucidated in animal models and human cardiovascular disease (see Chap. 23).

Genetic linkage analysis of familial arrhythmias and resultant identification of culprit gene defects of cardiomyocyte ion channels or channel modulators has provided complementary insight into the cellular mechanisms of arrhythmogenesis. The long-QT syndrome is now known to result from mutations in genes responsible for various outwardly rectifying potassium channels and the cardiomyocyte sodium channel.[41] Analyses of other inherited arrhythmias are under way.

## Mechanical Properties

Mechanical function of the hypertrophied heart has been studied at the isolated myocyte, muscle, and chamber levels and in the intact circulation.[42–44] The results of these studies have revealed variable alterations in the rate and extent of contraction and relaxation, in the amount of force development, and in resting muscle and chamber properties. In the intact circulation, altered systolic and diastolic function is a composite result of subcellular changes in the myocyte, changes in the extracellular matrix, altered chamber geometry and mass, altered ventricular-vascular coupling, and the modulatory effects of neural and hormonal influences.

The earliest changes in mechanical performance observed in isometrically contracting papillary muscles extracted from hypertrophied hearts consist of a prolongation of time to peak tension and relaxation, despite normal peak twitch tension normalized for cross-sectional area of the muscle. Afterloaded isotonically shortening papillary muscle preparations from hypertrophied hearts of a variety of animal species typically reveal a decrease in the force-velocity relationship and a depression of $\dot{V}_{max}$ (the extrapolated maximal unloaded shortening velocity). $\dot{V}_{max}$ has been directly related to the calcium-activated myosin ATPase activity. Both myosin and myofibrillar ATPase activity are typically depressed in hypertrophied myocardium. In small rodents, this is due to the transcriptionally mediated switch from $\alpha$- to $\beta$-MHC. In higher mammals including humans, the decreased myosin ATPase activity of the hypertrophied heart may be due to alterations in the troponin isoform composition or the posttranslational generation of a lower molecular variant of the $\beta$-MHC.[28]

The dissociation between depressed rate-dependent indices of contraction and relaxation and normal maximal force development and extent of shortening in early cardiac hypertrophy has also been demonstrated in isolated cardiomyocytes and in the intact circulation of the nonhuman primate.[42,43] *These results suggest that the rate of crossbridge cycling is reduced but that the effective number of active crossbridges per unit of myocardium is preserved in compensated cardiac hypertrophy.* In decompensated hypertrophy, reduced absolute levels of force development and diminished contractility ultimately ensue.

In addition to alteration in excitation-contraction coupling and relaxation, the increased cardiac mass and changes in geometry significantly affect passive muscle and chamber properties of the hypertrophied heart. Concentric hypertrophy is characterized by an increased resting muscle and chamber stiffness, which results in an increase in pulmonary venous pressure for any given left ventricular volume. The resultant pulmonary congestion at rest or with exercise is an important determinant of symptoms in patients with hypertensive left ventricular hypertrophy or hypertrophic cardiomyopathy and normal or elevated ejection fraction. Pure volume overload hypertrophy, as occurs with mitral regurgitation, is typically associated with no change or a decrease in passive muscle or chamber stiffness. As a result, patients with chronic volume overload may remain asymptomatic for long periods despite appreciable increase in regurgitant fraction (see also Chaps. 56 and 57).

## Coronary Circulation

Clinicians have long recognized that myocardial blood flow may be abnormal in the hypertrophied heart, since such patients may have exertional angina, resting or exercise-induced electrocardiographic or perfusion abnormalities, or pathologic evidence of subendocardial fibrosis, despite the presence of angiographically normal epicardial coronary arteries.

Morphologic studies of hypertrophied hearts from experimental animals and patients with pressure-overload hypertrophy demonstrate that the ratio of capillaries to myocytes remains unchanged.[45] Since myocyte cross-sectional area is increased, there is a resultant increase in nutrient diffusion distance in the hypertrophied heart. This anatomic change results in a reduced vasodilatory reserve in response to various stimuli in experimental and clinical studies. Myocardial blood flow and oxygen consumption per unit of myocardium are normal in compensated pressure overload–left ventricular hypertrophy, where wall stress has been normalized by an increase in wall thickness. The impairment in vasodilatory reserve produces evidence of ischemia during increased myocardial oxygen demand. In right ventricular pressure–overload hypertrophy, differences in perfusion between the ventricles result in increased right ventricular blood flow per unit of myocardial mass at rest and no increase in minimum coronary resistance of hypertrophied right ventricular myocardium.[46]

Few data are available regarding changes in the coronary circulation in experimental or clinical volume-overload hypertrophy. Most studies have reported normal resting flow values per unit of myocardial mass. In contrast to pressure overload, volume-overload hypertrophy has been associated with normal or mildly increased minimum coronary resistance and normal or mildly decreased coronary reserve. The coronary circulatory abnormalities associated with cardiac hypertrophy appear to be reversible with removal of the hypertrophic stimulus and resultant decreased chamber mass.[47]

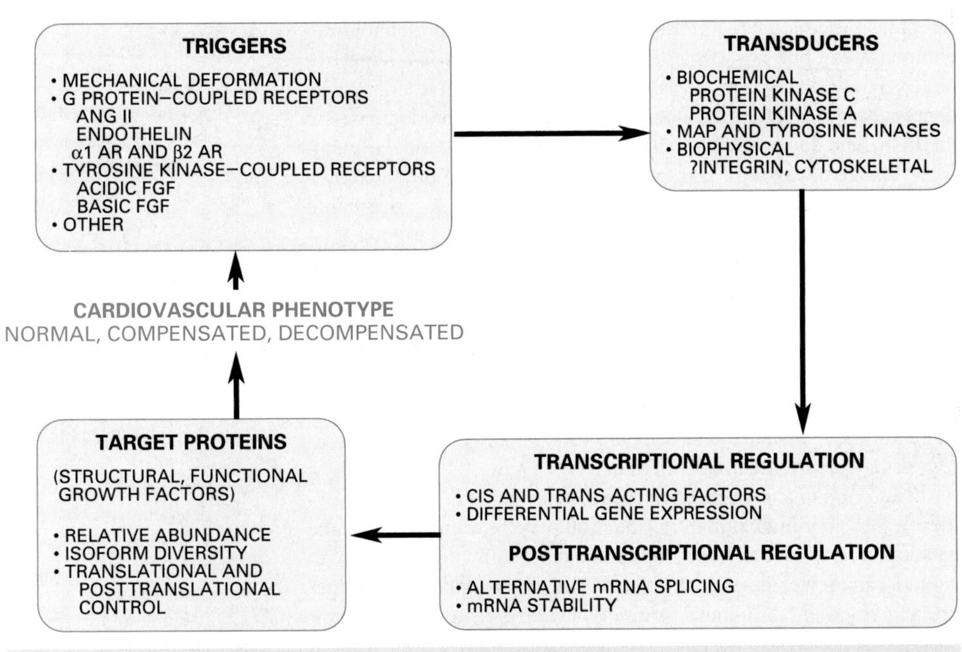


FIGURE 6-3 Schematic diagram of the mechanisms responsible for the development of the anatomic and functional cardiac phenotypes in physiologic and pathologic hypertrophy. Abnormalities at one or multiple levels in this putative closed-loop system may be responsible for the transition between compensated and decompensated hypertrophy.

Important recent studies have begun to elucidate the molecular and cellular mechanisms responsible for reversible functional consequences of ischemia and ischemia reperfusion. The syndrome of *myocardial stunning,* which refers to the variable period of regional or global myocardial hypofunction consequent to ischemia and reperfusion, is believed to involve two mechanisms. Either hydroxy-free radical generation, calcium overload, or both may be involved.[48] Downstream effects of these two pathologic processes include activation of protein kinase C, tyrosine kinases, and stress-activated kinases. In addition, proteolytic degradation of troponin I has been observed and is associated with uncoupling of excitation from contraction due to reduced myofilament calcium sensitivity. Transgenic overexpression either of a PKC isoform or the proteolytic degradation product of troponin I in mice produces both myocardial dysfunction and reduced myofilament calcium sensitivity responsiveness.[49]

Brief repetitive periods of ischemia and reperfusion also produce a powerful cardioprotective effect against myocardial necrosis. This process, called *ischemic preconditioning,* is also associated with activation of similar signal transduction pathways. The precise mechanism(s) for reduced myocyte cell death from necrosis, apoptosis, or both are presently unclear. *Hibernation* or myocardial hypofunction associated with reduced steady-state coronary blood flow may, in fact, result from repetitive periods of stunning.

## MECHANISMS FOR THE TRANSITION FROM COMPENSATED HYPERTROPHY TO HEART FAILURE

In contrast to hypertrophied skeletal muscle, chronically increased work eventually results in depressed contractility and relaxation of the hypertrophied heart. Compensated hypertrophy, which is characterized by abnormal chamber function but preserved muscle and myocyte function, evolves into a decompensated phase characterized by abnormal chamber, muscle, and myocyte function (Fig. 6-1). Attempts to elucidate the underlying mechanisms for this transition have involved multidisciplinary studies of clinical end-stage heart failure, longitudinal studies in experimental animals, and characterization of cardiovascular function in genetically engineered mice, where attempts are made to mimic human disease (Fig. 6-3).[50]

Current information suggests that decompensated hypertrophy may result from a number of mechanisms that are both intrinsic and extrinsic to the cardiomyocyte. These include necrosis; apoptosis[51]; altered growth secondary to altered signal transduction pathways; alterations in cardiomyocyte contractile, regulatory, calcium-cycling, and structural proteins; alterations in the extracellular matrix, and remodeling (Fig. 6-3). Because of the complex combinatorial alterations that occur in human heart failure and conventional animal models of hypertrophy, studies in genetically engineered mice in which a protein of interest is either overexpressed or ablated using homologous recombination hold particular promise in determining the relative importance of various candidate genes. For example, mice bearing the mutation in the $\beta$-MHC that occurs in familial cardiomyopathy have many features of the human disease.[52] Overexpression of the $\alpha$ subunit of the G protein that couples to the $\beta$-adrenergic receptor has produced dilated fibrotic hearts with altered cardiovascular function.[53] Overexpression or ablation of genes involved in cardiomyocyte calcium-cycling proteins has been associated with altered heart function and abnormal calcium kinetics. It is of interest that, with few exceptions, the resultant cardiac phenotype has failed to reproduce completely human decompensated hypertrophy and failure. This observation further supports the multifactorial nature of the condition and the importance of genetic background on the phenotype observed after loss-of-function or gain-of-function genetic engineering.

A common prominent feature of many experimental and clinical studies of decompensated hypertrophy and failure is a derangement of cardiomyocyte calcium homeostasis (Fig. 6-3). Studies of human cardiomyocytes extracted from the hearts of patients with end-stage heart failure have revealed elevated diastolic calcium levels with either no change or a reduction in the amplitude of the calcium transient.[54,55] Longitudinal studies of hypertrophy in experimental animals have revealed depression of steady-state mRNA levels and sarcoplasmic reticulum ATPase and phospholamban proteins in decompensated, but not compensated, pressure-overload hypertrophy.[43] These changes were associated with distinctive contractile depression of isovolumically contracting heart function, increases in the $EC_{50}$, and decreases in the $\dot{V}_{max}$ for sarcoplasmic reticular membrane uptake of calcium. Transgenic overexpression of the sarcoplasmic reticulum ATPase inhibitor phospholamban depressed cardiomyocyte function and calcium kinetics, whereas targeted ablation of the phosphoprotein produced the opposite result. Whether altered levels of the calcium-cycling proteins occur by transcriptional, translational, or posttranslational levels is currently unknown. In addition to altered levels of the various calcium-cycling proteins in hypertrophy and heart failure, there is evidence that abnormal spatial organization of the *l*-channel and SR may be contributory. Specifically, increased distance between the *l*-channel and the ryanodine receptor may contribute to abnormal calcium cycling.[56]

In addition to altered calcium homeostasis, there is increasing evidence that abnormal signal transduction plays a critical role in the development of cardiac hypertrophy and failure. In vitro studies with neonatal myocytes have demonstrated that phenylephrine, endothelin, and angiotensin II cause cardiomyocyte hypertrophy. These vasoactive peptides have cognate receptors that signal via the $\alpha$ subunit of the Gq protein (see Fig. 6-2). Cardiac-specific overexpression of G$\alpha$q produced cardiac hypertrophy, apoptosis, and contractile depression in transgenic mice.[57] By contrast, overexpression of a protein inhibitor of G$\alpha$q in a similar manner prevented cardiac hypertrophy due to pressure overload.[58] Transgenic overexpression of receptors that couple through G$\alpha$q, such as $\alpha_1$ and angiotensin II, produces a similar phenotype: cardiac-specific postnatal overexpression of the calcium-sensitive PKC isoform B produced cardiac hypertrophy and failure. Pretreatment of mice overexpressing PKC B with a highly specific inhibitor prevented or reversed this hypertrophy–heart failure phenotype.[59] Part of the contractile depression observed with excess PKC B activity was due to phosphorylation of troponin I and resultant reduced myofilament calcium sensitivity.[60] Augmented PKC activity and elevated levels of the calcium-sensitive PKC $\alpha$ and $\beta$ isoforms, but not G$\alpha$q, were found in human end-stage cardiomyopathic heart failure.[61,62] It is also known that PKC may be stimulated by pathophysiologic levels of stretch[63] and ischemia-reperfusion and directly by oxidative stress.[17] Taken together, these lines of evidence suggest that *PKC-mediated signal transduction plays a critical role in the development of cardiac hypertrophy and failure.*[64]

A variety of studies with end-stage human cardiomyopathic heart tissue, conventional animal models, and genetically engineered mice suggest that apoptosis may contribute to the heart failure phenotype.[65] The key issue that remains unclear is the quantitative importance of the phenomenon. This problem is further complicated by the fact that a number of signaling molecules (e.g., G$\alpha$q and TNF-$\alpha$) produce both hypertrophy and apoptosis. By contrast, gp130 heterodimerizes with LIF (leukemia inhibitory factor) receptor to permit binding of the interleukin-6 family of cytokines, such as cardiotrophin-1. Receptor binding stimulates the hypertrophic response while inhibiting apoptosis. Elimination of the gp130 by loss of function mutations of the gene results in mice that have structurally normal hearts. However, when a pressure overload is imposed, a rapidly progressive dilated cardiomyopathy ensues, which is associated with massive apoptosis. The application of molecular genetic and biologic approaches to elucidate mechanisms responsible for myocardial hypertrophy, cardiac failure, arrhythmogenesis, and ischemic dysfunction will permit improved diagnostic and therapeutic approaches to congenital and acquired heart diseases (Fig. 6-3).[66,66a–66c]

## References


1. Thompson CB. Apoptosis in the pathogenesis and treatment of disease. *Science* 1995;267:1456–1462.
2. Peter M, Herskowitz I. Joining the complex: Cyclin dependent kinase inhibitory proteins and the cell cycle. *Cell* 1994;79:181–184.
3. Field LJ. Atrial natriuretic factor-SV40 T antigen transgenes produce tumors and cardiac arrhythmias in mice. *Science* 1988;239:1029–1033.
4. Clark AJ. General physiology of hearts of cold-blooded vertebrates. In: Barcroft JSJ, ed. *Comparative Physiology of the Heart.* New York: Macmillan; 1927:151.
5. Ford LE. Heart size. *Circ Res* 1976;39:297–303.
6. Marian AJ, Roberts R. Recent advances in the molecular genetics of hypertrophic cardiomyopathy. *Circulation* 1995;92:1336–1347.
7. Milano CA, Allen LF, Rockman HA, et al. Enhanced myocardial function in transgenic mice overexpressing the $\beta_2$-adrenergic receptor. *Science* 1994;264:582–586.
8. Hoit BD, Khoury SF, Kranias EG, et al. In vivo echocardiograph detection of enhanced left ventricular function in gene-targeted mice with phospholamban deficiency. *Circ Res* 1995;77:632–637.
9. Sato Y, Ferguson DG, Sako H, et al. Cardiac-specific overexpression of mouse cardiac calsequestrin is associated with depressed cardiovascular function and hypertrophy in transgenic mice. *J Biol Chem* 1998;273: 28470–28477.
10. Watson PA. Mechanical activation of signaling pathways in the cardiovascular system. *Trends Cardiovasc Med* 1996;6:73–79.
11. Yamazaki T, Komuro I, Kudoh S, et al. Angiotensin II partly mediates mechanical stress-induced cardiac hypertrophy. *Circ Res* 1995;77: 258–265.
12. Knowlton KU, Michel MC, Itani M, et al. The $\alpha_{1A}$-adrenergic receptor subtype mediates biochemical, molecular, and morphologic features of cultured myocardial cell hypertrophy. *J Biol Chem* 1993;268: 15374–15380.
13. Bogoyevitch MA, Glennon PE, Andersson MB, et al. Endothelin 1 and fibroblast growth factors stimulate the mitogen-activated protein kinase signaling cascade in cardiac myocytes. *J Biol Chem* 1994;269:1110–1119.
14. Sugden PH, Clerk A. Regulation of mitogen-activated protein kinase cascades in the heart. *Adv Enzyme Regul* 1998;38:87–98.
15. Hunter JJ, Chien KR. Signaling pathways for cardiac hypertrophy and failure. *N Engl J Med* 1999;341:1276–1283.
16. Roberts AB, Roche NS, Winokur TS, et al. Role of transforming growth factor-$\beta$ in maintenance of function of cultured neonatal cardiac myocytes. *J Clin Invest* 1992;90:2056–2062.
17. Sacca L, Fazio S. Cardiac performance: Growth hormone enters the race. *Nat Med* 1996;1:29–31.
18. Khoury SF, Hoit BD, Dave V, et al. Effects of thyroid hormone on left ventricular performance and regulation of contractile and $Ca^{2+}$ cycling proteins in the baboon: Implications for the force-frequency and relaxation-frequency relationships. *Circ Res* 1996;79:727–735.
19. Klemperer JD, Ojamaa K, Klein I. Thyroid hormone therapy in cardiovascular disease. *Prog Cardiovasc Dis* 1996;38:329–336.
20. Wu J, Garami M, Cheng T, et al. 1,25$(OH)_2$ vitamin $D_3$ and retinoic acid antagonize endothelin-stimulated hypertrophy of neonatal rat cardiac myocytes. *J Clin Invest* 1996;97:1577–1588.
21. Sei CA, Irons CE, Sprenkle AB, et al. The alpha-adrenergic stimulation of atrial natriuretic factor expression in cardiac myocytes requires calcium influx, protein kinase C, and calmodulin-regulated pathways. *J Biol Chem* 1991;266:15910–15916.
22. Sadoshima J, Qiu Z, Morgan JP, et al. Angiotensin II and other hypertrophic stimuli mediated by G protein–coupled receptors activate tyrosine kinase, mitogen-activated protein kinase, and 90-kD S6 kinase in cardiac myocytes: The critical role of $Ca^{2+}$-dependent signaling. *Circ Res* 1995;76:1–15.
23. Sugden PH. Signaling in myocardial hypertrophy: Life after calcineurin? *Circ Res* 1999;84:633–646.
24. Walsh RA. Calcineurin inhibition as therapy for cardiac hypertrophy and heart failure: Requiescat in pace? *Circ Res* 1999;84:741–743.
25. Morgan HE, Gordon EE, Kira Y, et al. Biochemical mechanisms of cardiac hypertrophy. *Annu Rev Physiol* 1987;49:533–543.

26. Hannan R, Luyken J, Rothblum LI. Regulation of ribosomal DNA transcription during contraction-induced hypertrophy of neonatal cardiomyocytes. *J Biol Chem* 1996;271:3213–3220.
27. Samarel AM. Hemodynamic overload and the regulation of myofibrillar protein degradation. *Circulation* 1993;87:1418–1420.
28. Henkel RD, VandeBerg JL, Shade RE, et al. Cardiac beta myosin heavy chain diversity in normal and chronically hypertensive baboons. *J Clin Invest* 1989;83:1487–1493.
29. Walsh RA, Henkel R, Robbins J. Cardiac myosin heavy- and light-chain gene expression in hypertrophy and heart failure. *Heart Failure* 1990;6: 238–243.
30. Cooper G IV. Load and length regulation of cardiac energetics. *Annu Rev Physiol* 1990;52:505–522.
31. Borg T, Rubin K, Carver W, et al. The cell biology of the cardiac interstitium. *Trends Cardiovasc Med* 1991;6:65–70.
32. Prockop DJ, Kivirikko KI. Collagens: Molecular biology, diseases, and potentials for therapy. *Annu Rev Biochem* 1995;64:403–434.
33. Swynghedauw B. Molecular mechanisms of myocardial remodeling. *Physiol Rev* 1999;79:215–262.
34. Schlaepfer DD, Hanks SK, Hunter T, et al. Integrin-mediated signal transduction linked to Ras pathway by GRB2 binding to focal adhesion kinase. *Nature* 1994;372:786–791.
35. Takeishi Y, Abe J, Lee JD, et al. Differential regulation of p90 ribosomal S6 kinase and big mitogen-activated protein kinase 1 by ischemia/reperfusion and oxidative stress in perfused guinea pig hearts. *Circ Res* 1999;85:1164–1172.
36. Collins JF, Pawloski-Dahm C, Davis MG, et al. The role of the cytoskeleton in left ventricular pressure overload hypertrophy and failure. *J Mol Cell Cardiol* 1996;28:1435–1443.
37. Tsutsui H, Kshihara K, Cooper G. Cytoskeletal role in the contractile dysfunction of hypertrophied myocardium. *Science* 1993;260:682–687.
38. Kadambi VJ, Ponniah S, Harrer JM, et al. Cardiac-specific overexpression of phospholamban alters calcium kinetics and resultant cardiomyocyte mechanics in transgenic mice. *J Clin Invest* 1996;97:533–539.
39. Hart G. Cellular electrophysiology in cardiac hypertrophy and failure. *Cardiovasc Res* 1994;28:933–946.
40. Severs NJ. Pathophysiology of gap junctions in heart disease. *J Cardiovasc Electrophysiol* 1994;5:462–475.
41. Curran ME, Splawski I, Timothy KW, et al. A molecular basis for cardiac arrhythmia: *HERG* mutations cause long QT syndrome. *Cell* 1995;80:795–803.
42. Dorn GW II, Robbins J, Ball N, et al. Myosin heavy chain regulation and myocyte contractile depression after LV hypertrophy in aortic banded mice. *Am J Physiol* 1994;267:H400–H405.
43. Kiss E, Ball N, Kranias EG, et al. Differential changes in cardiac phospholamban and sarcoplasmic reticular $Ca^{2+}$-ATPase protein levels: Effects on $Ca^{2+}$ transport and mechanics in compensated pressure-overload hypertrophy and congestive heart failure. *Circ Res* 1995;77: 759–764.
44. Hoit BD, Shao Y, Gabel M, et al. Disparate effects of early pressure overload hypertrophy on velocity-dependent and force-dependent indices of ventricular performance in the conscious baboon. *Circulation* 1995;91:1213–1220.
45. Bache RJ. Effects of hypertrophy on the coronary circulation. *Prog Cardiovasc Dis* 1988;31:403–440.
46. Murray PA, Vatner SF. Reduction of maximal coronary vasodilator capacity in conscious dogs with severe right ventricular hypertrophy. *Circ Res* 1981;48:25–33.
47. Isoyama S, Ito N, Kuroha M, et al. Complete reversibility of physiological coronary vascular abnormalities in hypertrophied hearts produced by pressure overload in the rat. *J Clin Invest* 1989;84:288–294.
48. Bolli R, Marban E. Molecular and cellular mechanisms of myocardial stunning. *Physiol Rev* 1999;79:609–634.
49. Murphy AM, Kogler H, Georgakopoulos D, et al. Transgenic mouse model of stunned myocardium. *Science* 2000;287:488–491.
50. *Cardiovascular Physiology in the Genetically Engineered Mouse.* Norwell, MA: Kluwer, 1998.
51. Cheng W, Li B, Kajstura J, et al. Stretch-induced programmed myocyte cell death. *J Clin Invest* 1995;96:2247–2259.
52. Geisterfer-Lowrance AAT, Christe M, Conner DA, et al. A mouse model of familial hypertrophic cardiomyopathy. *Science* 1996;272:731–734.
53. Iwase M, Bishop SP, Uechi M, et al. Adverse effects of chronic endogenous sympathetic drive induced by cardiac Gs $\alpha$ overexpression. *Circ Res* 1996;78:517–524.
54. Schwinger RHG, Böhm M, Schmidt U, et al. Unchanged protein levels of SERCA II and phospholamban but reduced $Ca^{2+}$ uptake and $Ca^{2+}$-ATPase activity of cardiac sarcoplasmic reticulum from dilated cardiomyopathy patients compared with patients with nonfailing hearts. *Circulation* 1995;92:3220–3228.
55. Hasenfuss G, Reinecke H, Studer R, et al. Relation between myocardial function and expression of sarcoplasmic reticulum $Ca^{2+}$-ATPase in failing and nonfailing human myocardium. *Circ Res* 1994;75:434–442.
56. Gomez AM, Valdivia HH, Cheng H, et al. Defective excitation-contraction coupling in experimental cardiac hypertrophy and heart failure. *Science* 1997;276:800–806.
57. D'Angelo DD, Sakata Y, Lorenz NJ, et al. Transgenic G alpha q overexpression induces cardiac contractile failure in mice. *Proc Natl Acad Sci USA* 1997;94:8121–8126.
58. Akhter SA, Luttrell LM, Rockman HA, et al. Targeting the receptor-Gq interface to inhibit in vivo pressure overload myocardial hypertrophy. *Science* 1998;280:574–577.
59. Wakasaki H, Koya D, Schoen FJ, et al. Targeted overexpression of protein kinase C $beta_2$ isoform in myocardium causes cardiomyopathy. *Proc Natl Acad Sci USA* 1997;94:9320–9325.
60. Takeishi Y, Chu G, Kirkpatrick DM, et al. In vivo phosphorylation of cardiac troponin I by protein kinase C $beta_2$ decreased cardiomyocyte calcium responsiveness and contractility in transgenic mouse hearts. *J Clin Invest* 1998;102:72–78.
61. Bowling N, Walsh RA, Song G, et al. Increased protein kinase C activity and expression of $Ca^{2+}$-sensitive isoforms in the failing human heart. *Circulation* 1999;99:384–391.
62. Jalili T, Takeishi Y, Song G, et al. PKC translocation without changes in G alpha q and PLC-beta protein abundance in cardiac hypertrophy and failure. *Am J Physiol* 1999;277:H2298–H2304.
63. Paul K, Ball N, Dorn GW II, et al. Left ventricular stretch stimulates angiotensin II–mediated phosphatidylinositol hydrolysis and protein kinase C epsilon isoform translocation in adult guinea pig hearts. *Circ Res* 1997;81:643–650.
64. Jalili T, Takeishi Y, Walsh RA. Signal transduction during cardiac hypertrophy: The role of G alpha q, PLC beta I, and PKC. *Cardiovasc Res* 1999;44:5–9.
65. Guerra S, Leri A, Wang X, et al. Myocyte death in the failing human heart is gender dependent. *Circ Res* 1999;85:856–866.
66. Cohn JN, Bristow MR, Chien KR, et al. Report of the National Heart, Lung, and Blood Institute Special Emphasis Panel on Heart Failure Research. *Circulation* 1997;95:766–770.
66a. Kiatchoosakun S, Lawrence E, Nakada S, et al. Effect of angiotensin type I-receptor blockade on left ventricular remodeling in pressure overload hypertrophy. *J Card Fail* 2001;7:342–347.
66b. Hoit BD, Takeishi Y, Cox MJ, et al. Remodeling of the left atrium in pacing-induced atrial cardiomyopathy. *Mol Cell Biochem* 2002;238: 145–150.
66c. Takeishi Y, Walsh RA. Cardiac hypertrophy and failure: Lessons learned from genetically engineered mice. *Acta Physiol Scand* 2001;173: 103–111.

CHAPTER 7

# BIOLOGY OF THE VESSEL WALL

Kathy K. Griendling / David G. Harrison / R. Wayne Alexander



It has become apparent that a diverse number of pathologic processes contribute to common vascular diseases, such as atherosclerosis and hypertension. During the past several years, these pathologic events have been defined with increasing clarity at a cellular and molecular level, and strategies are emerging to treat these primary processes rather than simply treating the secondary manifestations of vascular disease. Because of this, an understanding of the normal functions of vascular cells and how they are altered by various vascular insults has become essential for both basic investigators and clinicians caring for patients with peripheral vascular disease coronary artery disease, and hypertension. This chapter introduces important concepts in vascular biology and emphasizes how fundamental aspects of vascular control are altered by common disease conditions.

## THE ENDOTHELIAL CELL

Normal endothelial cell function is crucial to homeostasis in the vascular system. During the past 15 years, it has become apparent that diseases such as atherosclerosis are ultimately manifestations of endothelial dysfunction. Normally, the endothelium has three major roles: (1) it is a metabolically active secretory tissue; (2) it serves as an anticoagulant, antithrombotic surface; and (3) it provides a barrier to the indiscriminate passage of blood constituents into the arterial wall. The implications of these physiologic properties for vascular biology are considered separately.

### Endothelial Cell Metabolism and Secretion of Vasoactive Factors

As discussed in more detail below, endothelial cells secrete vasoactive substances that play a major role in the control of vascular tone. These molecules include vasodilators such as prostacyclin, endothelial-derived relaxing factor (EDRF), and endothelial-derived hyperpolarizing factor (EDHF).[1–3] In addition, the endothelium produces vasoconstrictor substances, including endothelin[4] and vasoconstrictor prostanoids.[5]

Endothelial cells also manufacture and secrete substances such as factor VIII antigen, von Willebrand's factor, tissue factor, thrombomodulin, and tissue plasminogen activator, which are all involved in coagulation/fibrinolytic pathways. Structural components of the extracellular matrix synthesized by these cells include collagen, elastin, glycosaminoglycans, and fibronectin.[6,7] The composition of the extracellular matrix is dynamically modulated by matrix metalloproteinases, enzymes that degrade matrix protein and participate in its remodeling. These enzymes are secreted by both endothelial and smooth muscle cells.[8,9] In addition, endothelial cells synthesize and secrete heparans and growth factors that regulate smooth muscle cell proliferation.[10–13] Finally, endothelial cells are able to clear and metabolically alter bloodborne and locally produced substances, including plasma lipids and lipoproteins,[14] adenine nucleotides and nucleosides,[15] serotonin, catecholamines, bradykinin, and angiotensin I.[16]

Endothelial cells are involved in the metabolism of plasma lipids in several ways. Lipoprotein lipase, an enzyme that hydrolyzes triglycerides into constituent fatty acids, is bound to the endothelial cell surface by heparan sulfates.[17] The interaction of this enzyme with chylomicrons or very low density lipoprotein (VLDL) particles results in the release of free fatty acids, which can then cross the subendothelial space to the underlying smooth muscle or inflammatory cells in atherosclerosis. In addition, endothelial cells possess receptors for low-density lipoprotein (LDL),[18] which regulate the transport and modification of LDL. Normally, LDL receptors are downregulated because receptor processing is inhibited in the nonproliferating monolayer.[18] There are, however, two other pathways for uptake of LDL. First, LDL can be transported across the endothelium by an active process that is likely independent of plasmalemmal vesicles but may utilize paracellular gaps or fixed transendothelial channels.[19] Second, modified, or oxidized LDL can be taken up by "scavenger" LDL receptors,[20] which include SRA, SR-BI, CD36, and the lectin-like oxidized LDL receptor 1 (LOX-1).[21,22] Endothelial cells also have the capacity to modify LDL,[23] thus enhancing its uptake, ultimately leading to an increase in cholesterol esters in the vessel wall.

## The Endothelial Cell and Thrombosis

Quiescent endothelial cells normally present an antithrombotic surface that inhibits platelet adhesion and coagulation. (For a more detailed discussion of thrombosis, see Chap. 44.) Endothelial cells are, however, capable of synthesizing and secreting prothrombotic factors, especially when stimulated with cytokines or other inflammatory agents. The endothelium thus represents a functional antithrombotic-thrombolytic/thrombotic balance. Potent anticoagulants elaborated by the endothelium include prostacyclin and nitric oxide, which inhibit platelet aggregation[24]; antithrombin III[25]; heparin-like molecules[26]; thrombomodulin, which activates protein C and is also expressed by the endothelium[27]; and tissue plasminogen activator (t-PA). Procoagulant factors that can be produced by the endothelium include tissue factor,[28] factor VIII, factor Va, and PAI-1 (Fig. 7-1). Conditions of injury or inflammation enhance the prothrombotic state of the endothelium by stimulating production of tissue factor and PAI-1. There has been considerable interest in the role of PAI-1 in vascular disease. PAI-1 levels are substantially elevated in humans with atherosclerosis and even higher in the setting of acute coronary syndromes. Moreover, the metabolic syndrome—consisting of dyslipidemia, obesity, and insulin resistance—is associated with higher levels of PAI-1. Angiotensin II and thrombin likewise stimulate endothelial PAI-1 production, promoting thrombosis.[29] Thus, under inflammatory conditions, endothelial cells can amplify the prothrombotic response. Not all of the factors controlling the expression of pro- and antithrombotic/fibrinolytic molecules are known, but it is clear that the endothelium functions as a major regulator of hemostasis.

## Endothelial Cell Permeability

A very important role of the endothelium is regulation of permeability to macromolecules. The consequences of fluid and macromolecular transport vary depending on vessel size. In large vessels, these processes contribute to vessel nutrition and act as a selective barrier. In the microcirculation, endothelial permeability regulates delivery of nutrients to target organs and exchange of metabolic by-products.

The major two mechanisms regulating endothelial barrier function involve modulation of intercellular contacts and transendothelial vesicular transport in caveolae. Two types of junctions regulate endothelial cell contact: adherin junctions and tight junctions. Adherin junctions contain the protein VE-cadherin, which is essential for maintenance of inter-endothelial cell contacts. VE-cadherin associates with catenins, plakoglobulin, and the actin cytoskeleton to support cell adhesion. Tight junctions are composed of occludins, claudins, and junctional adhesion molecule-1 (JAM-1). Regulation of these inter-endothelial cell contacts is dynamic and important in modulation of new vessel growth, the extravasation of leukocytes, and macromolecule leakage. The nature of these intercellular contacts varies substantially depending on the vessel size and location. For example, tight junctions are well developed in the blood-brain barrier but are less structurally defined in postcapillary venules, where fluid and solute transport is active. Capillaries and postcapillary venules respond to vasoactive agents—including the vascular endothelial cell growth factor (VEGF), histamine, and prostaglandins—with increased flux through these sites.[30] The tight junctions found in arteries tend to be more occlusive but may also be influenced by various agonists. Dynamic regulation of these pathways enables the endothelium to serve as a selective barrier, modulating access of highly mitogenic, thrombotic, or vasoactive substances to the underlying vascular smooth muscle.

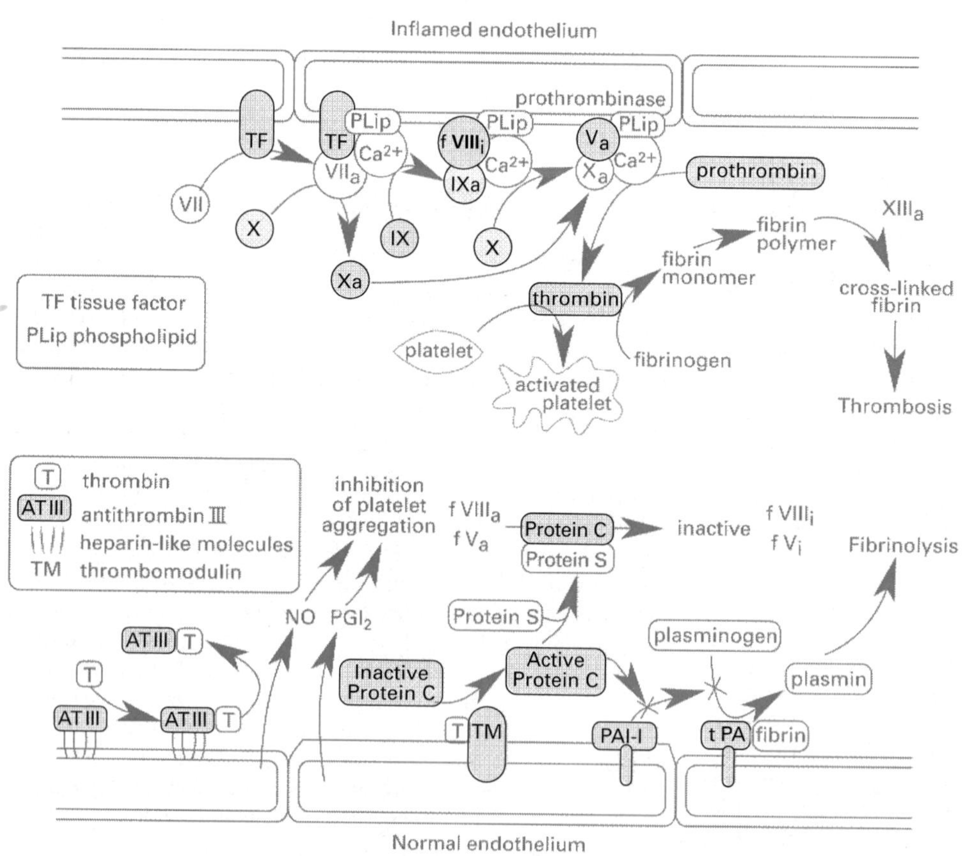


FIGURE 7-1 Pathways of thrombosis and thrombolysis. Under normal conditions, the endothelium is antithrombotic. Antithrombin III (ATIII) binds thrombin and serves to clear thrombin from the circulation. Prostacyclin (prostaglandin $I_2$, $PGI_2$) inhibits platelet aggregation, and thrombomodulin (TM) activates protein C, which inhibits plasminogen activator inhibitor I (PAI-I) and interacts with protein S to inactivate activated factors V and VIII, thus limiting thrombosis. Since PAI-I inhibits the tissue plasminogen activator (t-PA)–catalyzed conversion of plasminogen to plasmin, PAI-I inhibition leads to accumulation of plasmin and fibrinolysis. Upon stimulation with inflammatory cytokines, there is increased expression of tissue factor on the endothelial cell surface. Tissue factor participates in the activation of factor X, which, in turn, promotes assembly of the prothrombinase complex, producing thrombin. Under these conditions, endothelial cells thus amplify the thrombotic response. (Courtesy of Bernard Lassègue, Ph.D.)

Transendothelial vesicular transport is mainly utilized by the cell to transfer water-soluble macromolecules from the luminal surface to the abluminal surface. It has recently been shown that caveolae, vesicles containing the structural protein caveolin that are pinched off from the plasma membrane, are involved in transendothelial transport of macromolecules.[31,32] Caveolae are also sites where a variety of kinases, docking proteins, G proteins, and receptors reside[33] and therefore play an extremely important role in endothelial cell signal transduction.

Another major mechanism modulating endothelial barrier formation is endothelial cell contraction, analogous to smooth muscle contraction. This occurs in response to a variety of agonists, including thrombin, histamine, and ionomycin, and results in changes in cell shape that open gap junctions between cells. It is likely that this contractile response is a major mechanism for edema formation in response to histamine and bradykinin and is also involved in solute transport. This phenomenon is mediated by a series of intracellular signaling events, including activation of protein kinase C, myosin light-chain phosphorylation, activation of tyrosine kinases, and stimulation of the small G protein Rho.[34–36]

Thus, the endothelium has both passive and active roles in the control of vascular permeability by acting as a physical permeability barrier and by modulating the expression of cell surface and secreted agonists and molecules that are capable of altering permeability.

## Endothelial Control of Vascular Tone

The endothelium serves a dual function in the control of vascular tone (Fig. 7-2). It secretes relaxing factors such as nitric oxide, prostacyclin, and the endothelium-derived hyperpolarizing factor as well as constricting factors such as endothelin. Vessel tone thus depends on the balance between these factors as well as on the ability of the smooth muscle cell to respond to them. The most important regulatory molecules are discussed separately.

### NITRIC OXIDE

An endothelium-derived relaxing factor, (EDRF) was first described by Furchgott and Zawadzki,[2] who observed that aortic rings dilated in response to acetylcholine only when the rings maintained an intact endothelium. The EDRF was subsequently found to be nitric oxide (NO).[37]

NO is produced by the action of the enzyme NOS, which oxidizes the guanidino nitrogens of L-arginine to form citrulline and NO. This enzyme has been cloned from brain (nNOS, for neuronal NOS, type I),[38] macrophages (iNOS, for inducible NOS, type II),[39] and endothelial cells (eNOS, for endothelial NOS, type III).[40] The three isoforms of NOS share important consensus sequences for NADPH, flavin adenine dinucleotide, and flavin mononucleotide cofactor-binding sites, as well as a $Ca^{2+}$-calmodulin–binding site. An important cofactor for the NO synthases is tetrahydrobiopterin, which participates in electron transfer from the heme group of the enzyme to L-arginine. Interestingly, when tetrahydrobiopterin or L-arginine is absent, electron transfer is shunted to molecular oxygen, resulting in formation of the superoxide anion.[41] This phenomenon has been termed *uncoupling* of NOS, and there are substantial data that this may occur in a variety of disease states.[42]

Many factors have been shown to regulate the release of NO.[43] These include hormones such as acetylcholine, norepinephrine, bradykinin, thrombin, ATP, and vasopressin; the platelet-derived factors, serotonin and histamine; fatty acids; ionophores; and shear stress. NO easily crosses the smooth muscle cell membrane and binds to the heme moiety of the soluble guanylate cyclase, thereby enhancing the formation of cyclic GMP. Cyclic GMP, in turn, reduces intracellular $Ca^{2+}$ concentrations, leading to dephosphorylation of the myosin light chain and relaxation.[44] It should be noted that the drug nitroglycerin exerts its vasodilator effects by being converted to NO, thus substituting for a natural product.

Although increases in intracellular calcium in response to the above agents clearly activate eNOS via binding of calcium/calmodulin, phosphorylation of the enzyme is important in regulating its activity. For example, shear stress acutely stimulates the release of NO from the endothelium, and this depends only on calcium during the first few seconds of the response.[45] The continued activation of eNOS in response to several minutes or hours of shear is maintained by serine phosphorylation.[46]

While expression of the endothelial enzyme (eNOS) was originally thought to be constitutive, it is now clear that its expression is highly regulated. Increases in shear stress rather markedly enhance expression of eNOS.[47] Likewise, low shear is associated with a decrease in eNOS expression. Exercise training dramatically increases

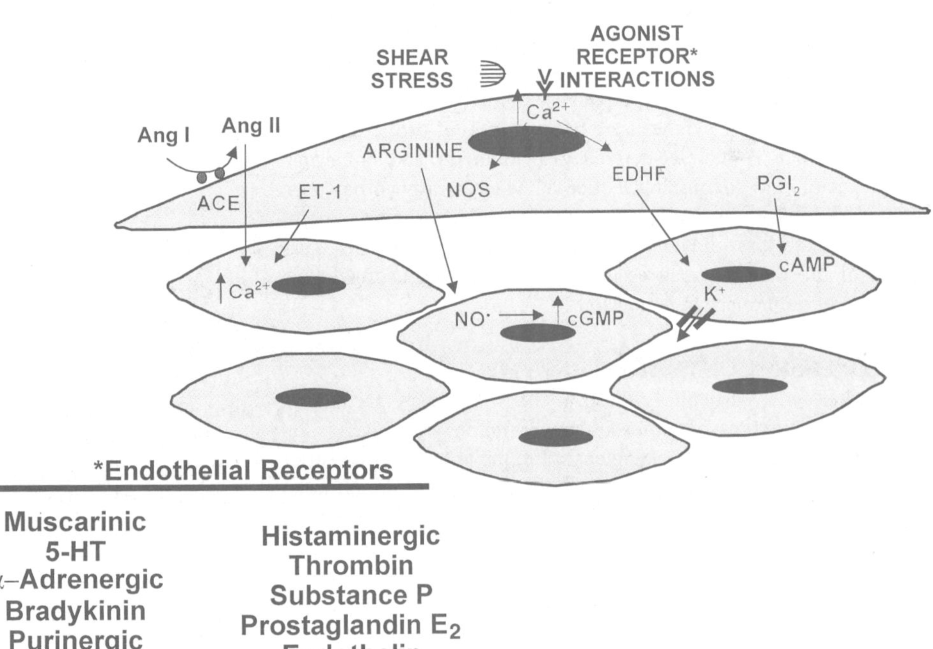


FIGURE 7-2 Endothelial control of vascular tone. Endothelial cells synthesize and secrete both vasodilator substances (NO, EDHF, and $PGI_2$) and vasoconstrictor compounds (Ang II and ET-1). Secretion of these factors occurs in response to receptor stimulation and hemodynamic forces such as shear stress. Vessel tone depends on the balance between these factors as well as on the ability of the smooth muscle cells to respond to them. NO = nitric oxide; NOS = nitric oxide synthase; EDHF = endothelial-derived hyperpolarizing factor; $PGI_2$ = prostaglandin $I_2$; ACE = angiotensin-converting enzyme; Ang = angiotensin; ET-1 = endothelin-1; cGMP = cyclic guanosine monophosphate; cAMP = cyclic adenosine monophosphate; 5-HT = 5-hydroxytriptamine.

eNOS expression in endothelial cells, likely because of the increased shear stress caused by the high cardiac output that accompanies sustained exercise.[48] In contrast, oxidized LDL, hypoxia and inflammatory cytokines such as TNF-$\alpha$ decrease eNOS expression.[40,49,50] The HMG-CoA reductase inhibitors increase eNOS levels by stabilizing the eNOS mRNA. This is thought to be an important component of the so-called pleiotropic effects of the statins, which may contribute to their therapeutic effects.

### ENDOTHELIUM-DERIVED HYPERPOLARIZING FACTOR

Shortly after the identification of NO, it was suspected that the endothelium could release more than one relaxing factor, depending on the vessel size, the stimulus, and the species studied. Initial studies showed that some vasodilators produce hyperpolarization of the vascular smooth muscle membrane in an endothelium-dependent manner. It is now clear that this is due to the release of a hyperpolarizing factor from the endothelium that is almost certainly different from NO.[51] Its production is stimulated by many of the same stimuli that evoke the release of NO and depends on intracellular calcium. While there is some debate regarding the nature of this factor, increasing evidence suggests that it is a cytochrome P450 metabolite of arachidonic acid and perhaps other fatty acids.[52] When released from the endothelium, this epoxide opens calcium-activated potassium channels in the adjacent vascular smooth muscle, resulting in vasodilation.[53] Hydrogen peroxide has also been suggested to be a hyperpolarizing factor and has recently been shown to be responsible for flow-induced dilatation of human coronary arterioles.[54]

### PROSTACYCLIN

Prostacyclin, or prostaglandin $I_2$ ($PGI_2$), a prostanoid derived from the action of cyclooxygenase on arachidonic acid, is released by the endothelium and relaxes vascular smooth muscle by increasing its intracellular content of cyclic AMP.[55] Prostacyclin is also platelet suppressant and antithrombotic and reduces the release of growth factors from endothelial cells and macrophages.[24] Among the agonists that stimulate prostacyclin synthesis are bradykinin (one of the most potent), substance P, platelet-derived growth factor and epidermal growth factor, and adenine nucleotides,[24] whereas aspirin has been shown to inhibit it transiently. Prostacyclin has been shown to compensate for the loss of NO in the eNOS knockout mouse.[56] Analogues of prostacyclin such as iloprost have proven useful in the treatment of pulmonary hypertension.[57]

### ANGIOTENSIN-CONVERTING ENZYME

Endothelial cells, particularly those in the pulmonary vasculature, synthesize and express angiotensin-converting enzyme (ACE)[58] on their surface. ACE converts angiotensin I to the potent vasoconstrictor angiotensin II and degrades and inactivates bradykinin. Of note, vascular and cardiac cells contain almost all components of the renin/angiotensin system[59]; thus local production of angiotensin II can contribute importantly to vascular function. This local production of angiotensin II can explain why ACE inhibitors and angiotensin receptor antagonists are often effective even when the circulating levels of renin or angiotensin II are not elevated.

### ENDOTHELINS

The endothelins are a family of closely related peptides made and secreted by many cells, including endothelial cells. There are three endothelins (ET-1, 2, and 3), all of which comprise 18 amino acid peptides. The endothelins are initially synthesized as preproendothelin, which undergoes preprocessing to big endothelin. Big endothelin is released and converted to active endothelin by the endothelin-converting enzyme. The vascular effects of endothelin are mediated by endothelin receptors, of which three subtypes have been identified (ET-A, B, and C). The receptors have differing specificity for the individual endothelin peptides, and activate different signaling pathways. In the vessel, the ET-A receptor is predominantly found on vascular smooth muscle, whereas the ET-B receptor resides on endothelial cells. Activation of the former stimulates potent vasoconstriction, whereas activation of the latter stimulates release of NO and thus favors vasodilation.[60]

The slow, intense, and sustained contraction caused by ET-1 appears to be the result of activation of the phosphoinositide/protein kinase C signaling pathway, as well as of opening voltage-dependent L-type calcium channels.[61] Importantly, even low, subthreshhold concentrations of ET-1 enhance vasoconstriction to a variety of other vasoconstrictor agents, including serotonin, angiotensin II, and $\alpha$-adrenergic agonists, seemingly via activation of protein kinase C. This has been suggested to contribute to the *rebound phenomenon* that occurs after nitroglycerin has been administered for several days and is suddenly discontinued.[62]

ET-1 is also a potent growth factor for VSMCs[63] and a chemoattractant for monocytes.[64] Importantly, angiotensin II has been shown to stimulate the production of ET-1 by VSMCs in culture[65]; in vivo, some of the hypertensive effect of angiotensin II is mediated by endothelin.[66] There is substantial interest in the notion that ET-1 and angiotensin II may act in concert in conditions such as hypertension and heart failure, or that many of the effects of angiotensin II are mediated by ET-1.[67]

## Endothelial Responses to Hemodynamic Influences

Many of the endothelial functions described above are modulated by the physical forces of stretch, strain, and shear stress imposed by the hemodynamics of the circulation. Flow-mediated, endothelium-dependent vasodilation has been described in many vascular beds,[68] and shear stress has been proposed to play a role in controlling endothelial cell proliferation.[69] Both stretch of the vessel wall (as observed in hypertension) and shear stress have been shown independently to affect endothelial cell morphology and/or function. Studies in cultured cells have shown that stretching endothelial cells leads to changes in cell shape,[70] intracellular signal generation with an increase in calcium and superoxide levels,[71] and proliferation.[69] Shear stress has numerous effects on endothelial cells. Initially, it was found that exposure of endothelial cell monolayers to elevated shear stresses in vitro caused them to align in the direction of flow. This reorientation was accompanied by changes in the cytoskeleton of the cells, including reorganization and alignment of the actin filaments and microtubules (Fig. 7-3). Similar mechanisms presumably also account for the orientation of endothelial cells parallel to the longitudinal axis in areas of laminar flow in the arterial system. The function of the endothelium is also altered by shear stress. Some of the cellular responses to shear stress include activation of $K^+$ currents; increased secretion of vasoactive and growth factors, including NO, endothelin, prostacyclin, and basic fibroblast growth factor (bFGF); enhanced tissue factor expression; elevation of LDL uptake; and increased tPA secretion.[72]

The importance of these observations lies in the variation in hemodynamic forces throughout the circulation. Areas of the vasculature exposed to low shear stress (branch points and curvatures) exhibit a predilection to the formation of atherosclerotic lesions.[73] True oscillations of flow have also been shown to occur in the carotid bulb, the proximal coronary arteries, and the distal aorta.[74] Studies in cul-

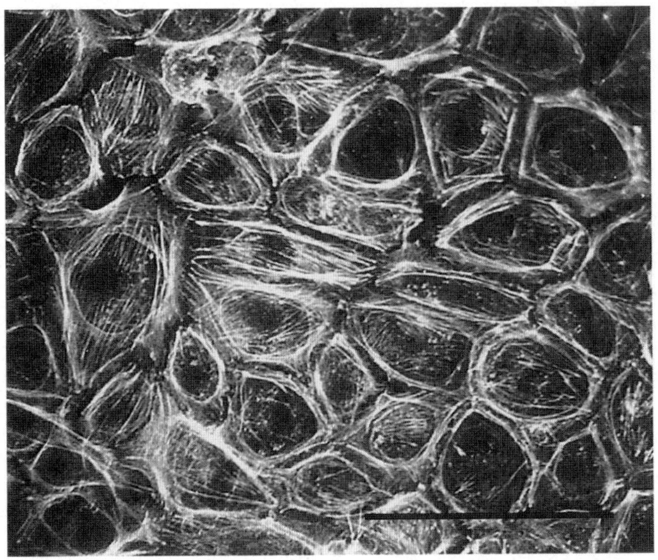

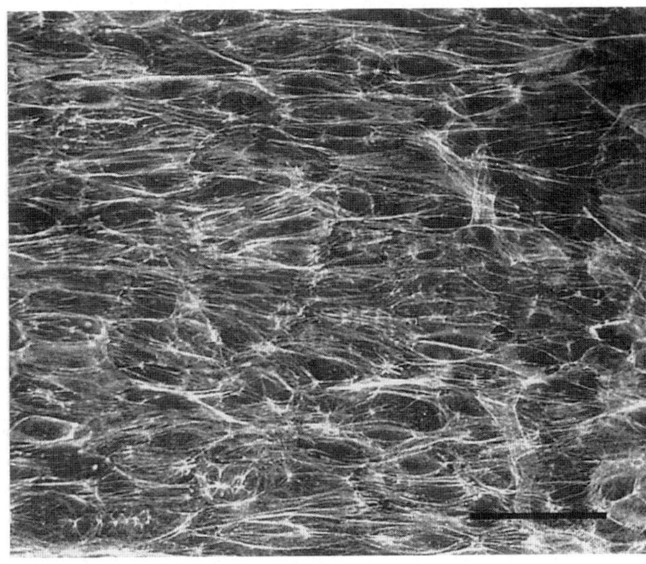

FIGURE 7-3 Effect of shear stress on endothelial cells. In bovine aortic endothelial cells grown in static conditions, F-actin filaments assume a random orientation as visualized by rhodamine-labeled phalloidin staining (left). Upon exposure to shear stress (30 dynes/cm$^2$, 24 h), these filaments align (right). Bars = 100 $\mu$m. (Courtesy of Lula Hilenski, Ph.D.)

tured endothelial cells have shown that oscillatory shear stress increases endothelial cell production of reactive oxygen species,[75] enhances adhesion molecule expression, and stimulates monocyte adhesion.[76]

The mechanisms by which the endothelial cell can sense and transduce mechanical signals have not been definitively determined. An attractive hypothesis deals with the concept that mechanical forces are transduced by integrin-mediated modifications of the endothelial cell cytoskeleton. Changes in the cytoskeleton, in turn, may have enormous effects on the biology of the endothelium. As an example, integrin activation leads to stimulation of kinases and phosphatases in focal adhesion complexes.[77] Changes in the actin cytoskeleton may affect RNA stability and translation.[78] In addition, flow-sensitive ion channels[79] and G proteins may be involved in mechanotransduction.[80] Furthermore, caveolae, which are flask-shaped membrane vesicular structures, are rich in signaling molecules such as G proteins and may be involved in signal generation in response to shear stress.[81]

## PHYSIOLOGY OF THE VASCULAR SMOOTH MUSCLE CELL

The smooth muscle cell normally responds to hormonal stimulation with contraction or relaxation. In certain disease states, however, growth and/or hypertrophy and migration to the intima are the predominant responses. Some of the biochemical signals generated by these vasoactive agonists are similar for both types of responses, with the final physiologic response dictated by the phenotype and environment of the cell and the exact biochemical pathways activated.

### Mechanisms of Vascular Smooth Muscle Cell Contraction

Some of the earliest signals generated within the cell following stimulation with calcium-mobilizing vasoactive agonists involve hydrolysis of a specific class of membrane lipids, the phosphoinositides, by phospholipase C.[82] This event leads to production of inositol trisphosphate ($IP_3$) and diacylglycerol (Fig. 7-4). $IP_3$ binds to a specific receptor on the sarcoplasmic reticulum, initiating release of $Ca^{2+}$ from intracellular stores.[83] $Ca^{2+}$, in turn, activates a cascade of enzymes leading to contraction or growth (see below). Diacylglycerol is a potent activator of protein kinase C, a $Ca^{2+}$- and phospholipid-dependent enzyme that phosphorylates numerous cellular proteins and thereby enhances contraction at any given level of intracellular calcium.[84] Diacylglycerol can be further metabolized to phosphatidic acid or to glycerol, fatty acids, and, ultimately, eicosanoids and leukotrienes that may themselves modulate tone. Additionally vasoconstrictor agents cause an influx of extracellular $Ca^{2+}$,[85] which serves to sustain and enhance vasoconstriction.

Contractions induced by various vasoactive hormones differ not only in magnitude and time course, but also differ between vessels. In general, there is an initial, rapid component of force generation and a more sustained phase of contraction. Some agonists, such as angiotensin II, induce only a transient constriction of many vessels, whereas others, including norepinephrine and vasopressin, nearly always cause a sustained contraction. The initial phase of force development has been shown to depend on the formation of actin-myosin crossbridges in response to acute elevations of intracellular calcium, whereas the sustained phase of contraction persists even after calcium levels return toward baseline.

A sliding-filament mechanism similar to that found in skeletal muscle is thought to regulate phasic contraction of smooth muscle. Tension development is regulated by the phosphorylation of the myosin light chain (Fig. 7-5) by an enzyme known as myosin light-chain kinase (MLCK). This protein associates with calmodulin, a calcium-binding protein required for activation of numerous cytoplasmic enzymes. Thus, when $Ca^{2+}$ increases within the cell in response to hormonal stimulation, it binds to calmodulin, which, in turn, associates with MLCK, converting it from an inactive to an active form. MLCK then phosphorylates the myosin light chain, enabling actin activation of the $Mg^{2+}$-ATPase and ultimately resulting in crossbridge formation. When the intracellular $Ca^{2+}$ concentration drops below about 100 n*M*, $Ca^{2+}$ dissociates from calmodulin,

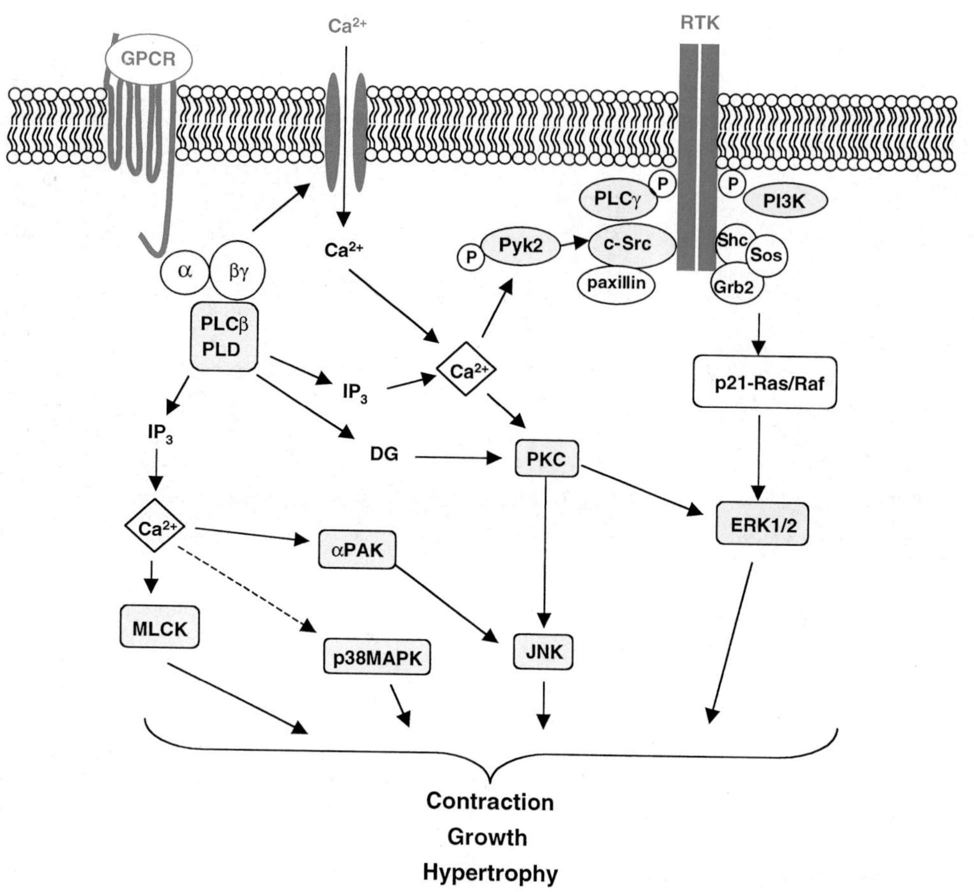


FIGURE 7-4 Signaling pathways in vascular smooth muscle. Vasoconstrictor agonists interact with specific G protein-coupled receptors (GPCRs) on vascular smooth muscle. These receptors are linked to a heterotrimeric G protein ($\alpha\beta\gamma$), which then couples to one or more phospholipase Cs (PLCs) or phospholipase D (PLD). PLC cleaves the inositol phospholipids to yield diacylglycerol (DG) and inositol phosphates, in particular, inositol trisphosphate ($IP_3$). $IP_3$ releases calcium from intracellular stores, and, along with DG, activates the $Ca^{2+}$- and phospholipid-dependent enzyme protein kinase C (PKC). $Ca^{2+}$ activates numerous other kinases, including p21-activated kinase ($\alpha$-PAK), Pyk2, and myosin light chain kinase (MLCK). PLD cleaves phosphatidylcholine to release phosphatidic acid, which is converted to DG. PKC is involved in activation of the mitogen-activated protein kinase (MAPK) cascade, including extracellular signal-regulated kinases (ERK1/2) and Jun kinase (JNK). Growth factors activate receptor tyrosine kinases (RTKs), Src, PLC-$\gamma$, and phosphatidylinositol 3-kinase (PI3K). RTKs also phosphorylate and form a signaling complex with paxillin and adapter proteins such as Shc, which binds Grb-2 and Sos and ultimately mediates the conversion of Ras to its active form. Ras phosphorylates Raf1, which in turn leads to activation of the MAP kinase cascade.

calmodulin detaches from MLCK, and MLCK becomes inactive. Myosin light chain phosphatase activity then predominates, myosin is dephosphorylated, and cross-bridge cycling ceases. During sustained contraction, however, the intracellular $Ca^{2+}$ concentration is low, and energy consumption is reduced, suggesting the development of a latch-bridge, or a low cycling state.[86] Alternatively, the sensitivity of the contractile apparatus to $Ca^{2+}$ may be increased, a response posited to be regulated by protein kinase C.[87] Recent evidence indicates that this latch state is also modulated by the actin-binding proteins caldesmon and calponin.[88] Caldesmon tonically inhibits contraction. Agonists such as phenylephrine stimulate extracellular regulated kinase (ERK1/2) mediated phosphorylation of caldesmon and enhance binding of calcium/calmodulin, removing its inhibitory effect and increasing tension.[89] Calponin has been suggested to directly inhibit the ATPase activity of myosin and to act as a signaling molecule that facilitates agonist-stimulated activation of protein kinase C.[90,91]

Recently it has become apparent that the small GTPase Rho, initially described as a modulator of the actin cytoskeleton, plays an important role in vascular smooth muscle contraction. In its active GTP-bound form, Rho activates Rho kinase, which inhibits myosin phosphatase type 1.[92] This inhibition in turn sustains MLC phosphorylation and sensitizes the contractile apparatus to calcium.[93] Rho kinase has become a target of therapeutic interventions. Its activity seems to be increased in hypertension,[94] and inhibitors of Rho kinase such as fasudil have been shown to lower vascular resistance in hypertension.[95]

## Factors Modulating Vascular Smooth Muscle Growth and Hypertrophy

Normally, vascular smooth muscle cells are relatively refractory to growth stimuli and exist in a quiescent, differentiated state. The healthy endothelium is critically important in maintaining this phenotype. Products of the endothelium such as nitric oxide,[96] prostacyclin,[96] heparan sulfates,[97] and transforming growth factor beta (TGF-$\beta$)[98] directly inhibit vascular smooth muscle growth. The endothelium is also an effective barrier limiting access of bloodborne growth factors to vascular smooth muscle. For example, the antithrombotic properties of the endothelium prevent access of promitogenic factors such as platelet-derived growth factor (PDGF) and thrombin to the underlying smooth muscle. Endothelial disruption allows initiation of a mitogenic smooth muscle response and regrowth of normal endothelium inhibits further proliferation.[99] In addition to these effects of the normal endothelium, the healthy vascular matrix minimizes vascular smooth muscle proliferation. It is impossible for cells to hypertrophy or proliferate without initial degradation of the matrix.

Under pathophysiologic conditions, the vascular milieu begins to favor vascular smooth muscle growth. Matrix metalloproteinases released by activated cells intrinsic to the vessel as well as invading inflammatory cells degrade the matrix to allow smooth muscle cell migration, proliferation, and hypertrophy. In addition, endothelial cells have the capacity to secrete several promitogenic agents. The best-studied of these factors is PDGF, so named because it was originally isolated from platelets. PDGF is a dimer, composed of two distinct peptide chains (designated A and B chains), and can be produced as an AB heterodimer or as an AA or BB homodimer. Endothelial cells contain the mRNA for both peptides.[100] Release of PDGF from the endothelium is regulated by growth factors, including TGF-$\beta$, fibroblast growth factor (FGF), and tumor necrosis factor

(TNF); circulating factors; and locally produced factors such as thrombin.[100] A second growth factor made and secreted by endothelial cells is insulin-like growth factor 1 (IGF-1),[13] which is a progression factor that facilitates movement of cells through the cell cycle and enhances the mitogenic effect of PDGF on smooth muscle.[101] IGF-1 production by endothelium is regulated by PDGF and plays a major role in vascular hypertrophy and hyperplasia.[102]

Other endothelial factors that affect smooth muscle proliferation include interleukin 1 (IL-1), FGF, and endothelin. IL-1 is an inflammatory cytokine that has numerous vascular effects in addition to mitogenesis, including the stimulation of procoagulant activity,[103] induction of leukocyte adhesiveness (see below), and inhibition of contraction.[104] Basic FGF has been detected in endothelial cells,[17] and acts as a potent smooth muscle mitogen, particularly after denuding injury.[105] It is stored in the subendothelial matrix and may be released by heparin and proteinases,[106] suggesting that the matrix may serve as a store for rapidly mobilizing this growth factor. FGF released from VSMCs may be particularly important in the growth response induced by injury to the arterial wall. Finally, endothelin-1, through its action on the ET-A receptor, induces smooth muscle cell growth by stimulating increases in intracellular calcium, activating protein kinase C and increasing intracellular production of reactive oxygen species. Diverse stimuli such as elevated insulin,[107] oscillatory shear stress and pressure,[108] and angiotensin II[109] potently induce endothelial production of ET-1.

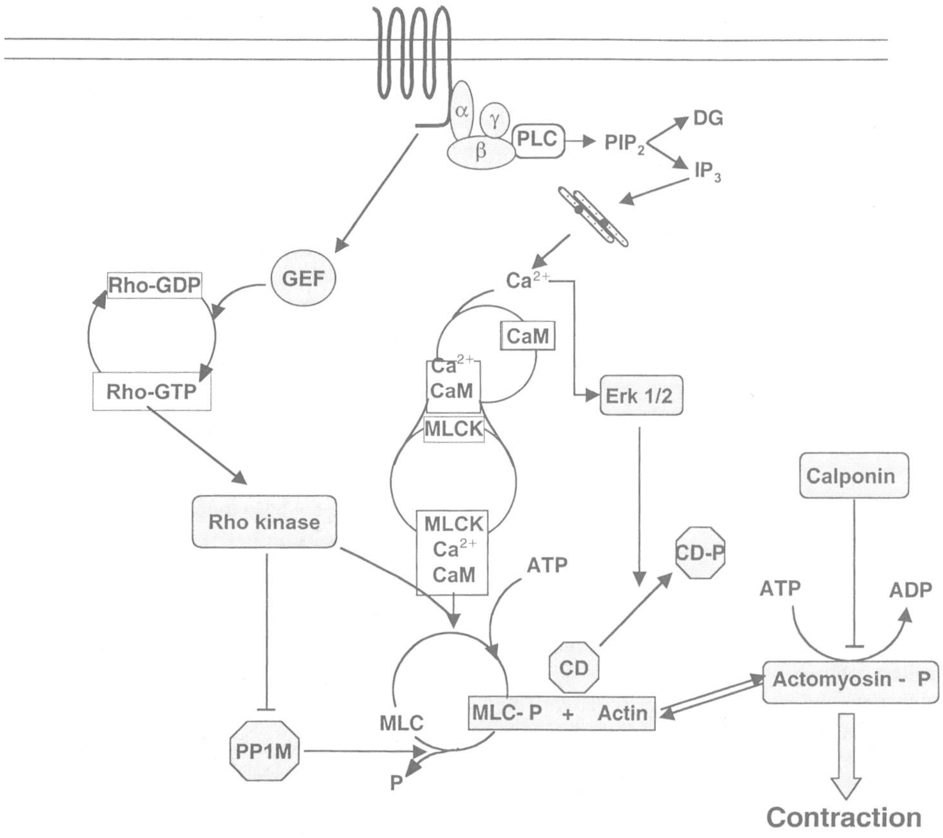

FIGURE 7-5 Contraction cascade. Activation of smooth muscle by a vasoconstrictor hormone leads to a cascade of biochemical signals, ultimately resulting in phosphorylation of actomyosin, crossbridge formation, and force generation. The release of $Ca^{2+}$ from intracellular stores is one of the major initiating events, since $Ca^{2+}$ combines with calmodulin (CaM) to activate myosin light chain kinase (MLCK). This enzyme phosphorylates the myosin light chain (MLC), which is then able to interact with actin. In addition, activation of a guanine nucleotide exchange factor (GEF) for the low-molecular-weight G protein Rho leads to stimulation of Rho and Rho kinase, which inhibits myosin phosphatase (PP1M), thus enhancing myosin light chain phosphorylation (MLC-P). Caldesmon (CD), which normally inhibits actin-myosin interaction, becomes phosphorylated by extracellular signal regulated kinase (Erk1/2) and is released from this complex. Calponin acts by inhibiting myosin ATPase activity. $\alpha\beta\gamma$ = heterotrimeric G protein; PLC = phospholipase C; DG = diacylglycerol; $PIP_2$ = phosphatidylinositol 4,5-bisphosphate; $IP_3$ = inositol trisphosphate; $Ca^{2+}$ = calcium; ATP = adenosine triphosphate; P = phosphate. (Courtesy of Bernard Lassègue, Ph.D.)

## Mechanisms of Vascular Smooth Muscle Growth

Vascular smooth muscle cell growth occurs via two processes: hypertrophy and hyperplasia. In general, hypertrophy occurs in response to long-term stimulation with vasoconstrictor-type agents, whereas hyperplasia occurs in response to the classic growth factors. Hypertrophy is characterized by an increase in smooth muscle cell mass due to increased protein synthesis and has been shown to occur in response to angiotensin II[110] and thrombin[111] and in large vessels during hypertension. Hyperplasia is characterized by cell replication and is stimulated by growth factors such as PDGF and FGF following vascular injury.[105,112,113] The biochemical processes leading to hypertrophy and hyperplasia have been extensively investigated.

Classic growth factors, such as PDGF, activate many of the same signaling pathways as do vasoconstrictors: phosphoinositide hydrolysis, $Ca^{2+}$ mobilization and influx, $Na^+/H^+$ exchange and intracellular alkalinization. Receptors for these growth factors are intrinsic tyrosine kinases, leading to the tyrosine phosphorylation of numerous proteins that are essential for growth. There is also increasing evidence that tyrosine phosphatases can counteract the mitogenic effects of growth factors by inhibiting tyrosine phosphorylation of specific substrates.[114]

A complex of substrates becomes associated with activated growth factor receptors and subsequently activates multiple signaling cascades leading to the final cellular response.[115] Upon stimulation, growth factor receptors dimerize and phosphorylate themselves on tyrosine residues. Some proteins, such as phospholipase C-$\gamma$, the tyrosine kinase c-Src, and phosphatidylinositol-3-kinase, bind directly to receptor tyrosine kinases, whereas others, including the tyrosine kinase Pyk-2 and the cytoskeletal protein paxillin, associate with the receptor via linker proteins such as Grb and Shc. Shc and Grb2 link these receptors to Ras, a ubiquitous GTPase that initiates a serine/threonine kinase cascade that includes mitogen-activated protein kinase (MAP kinase) and ultimately leads to growth. Recent evidence suggests that many of these proteins are also activated by seven-transmembrane-spanning G protein–coupled receptors,[116,117] an observation that may partially explain the growth-promoting properties of vasoconstrictor hormones like angiotensin II, thrombin and ET-1.

TABLE 7-1 Components of the Extracellular Matrix

| Matrix Component | Function |
|---|---|
| Proteoglycans | • Resistance to deformation<br>• Arterial permeability, filtration, ion exchange<br>• Transport and deposition of plasma elements<br>• Regulation of cellular metabolism |
| Collagens (types I and III) | • Mechanical strength |
| Collagens (types IV, V and VI) | • Attachment of vascular cells to the matrix<br>• Components of the basal lamina<br>• Linking collagens to noncollagenous structures |
| Elastin | • Regulation of vascular elasticity |
| Fibronectin | • Cell-cell adhesion<br>• Cell-substrate adhesion<br>• Cell motility<br>• Specific binding of collagen, heparin |
| Laminin | • Attachment of endothelial cells to type IV collagen |

In the past several years, it has become evident that reactive oxygen species play a crucial role in modulation of growth-related signaling pathways. Growth-promoting agonists stimulate the vascular NAD(P)H oxidases to produce superoxide and hydrogen peroxide, which may serve as progenitors to numerous other reactive oxygen species.[118,119] Of these, hydrogen peroxide seems to be particularly important in the growth process. Production of small concentrations of endogenous hydrogen peroxide activates specific mitogenic signaling pathways, such as p38 mitogen-activated protein kinase and Akt/protein kinase B, and promotes entry into the cell cycle.[120–122]

## THE EXTRACELLULAR MATRIX

The extracellular matrix is a major component of the vessel wall. It is the medium through which nutrients are transported, a repository for products secreted by the cells of the vascular wall, the site of accumulation of cell debris, and a substrate for migration and proliferation of endothelial cells, monocytes, and vascular smooth muscle cells. The matrix consists of several proteins that have distinct functions in maintaining the integrity of the wall (Table 7-1).

Extracellular matrix degradation and reformation is an extremely important biological process with profound clinical implications. It is impossible for vascular cells to hypertrophy, proliferate, or migrate without an initial degradation of the matrix. One of the earliest events in angiogenesis is the degradation of the extracellular matrix to enable tube (capillary) formation. Vascular cells—including endothelial cells, VSMCs, resident macrophages, and fibroblasts—may secrete matrix metalloproteinases (MMPs), enzymes that selectively digest the individual components of the matrix. In addition, these cells elaborate tissue inhibitors of metalloproteinases (TIMPs).[8]

MMPs belong to three main groups: the type IV collagenases (also called *gelatinases*), the stromelysins, and interstitial collagenase. The characteristics of these proteins are described in Table 7-2.

TABLE 7-2 Matrix Metalloproteinases and Inhibitors

| Class | Nomenclature | Molecular Weight (kDa)[a] | Vascular Cell Type | Expression |
|---|---|---|---|---|
| Interstitial collagenase | MMP-1 | ~45 | VSMC, EC, microvascular EC | Inducible by PDGF, PMA, IL-1, VEGF |
| Type IV collagenase | MMP-9<br>gelatinase B<br>type V gelatinase | 92 | VSMC<br>EC | Inducible by IL-1$\alpha$, PMA<br>Inhibited by retinoic acid |
| | MMP-2<br>gelatinase A<br>type IV gelatinase | 72 | VSMC<br>wounded EC<br>microvascular EC | Constitutive<br>↑ by TNF-$\alpha$, IL-1$\alpha$ (VSMC)<br>↑↓ by retinoic acid (EC) |
| Stromelysin | MMP-3 | 50 | VSMC<br>EC<br>microvascular EC | Inducible by IL-1 (VSMC); TNF-$\alpha$, PMA (EC) |
| Matrilysin | MMP-7 | — | VSMC, macrophage | Hypercholesterolemia |
| Membrane-type metalloproteinase | MT-MMP | — | VSMC, macrophage, EC | ? |
| TIMP-1 | Inhibits MMPs | 30 | VSMC<br>EC<br>microvascular EC | Constitutive |
| TIMP-2 | Inhibits MMP-2 | ~20 | VSMC<br>EC<br>microvascular EC | Constitutive<br>↑ by retinoic acid (EC) |

[a]The molecular weight of MMP-1 and MMP-3 depends on the species.

ABBREVIATIONS: EC = endothelial cell; IL = interleukin; MMP = matrix metalloproteinase; MT-MMP = membrane type MMP; PDGF = platelet-derived growth factor; PMA = phorbol 12,13-myrisate acetate; TIMP = tissue inhibitor of metalloproteinase; TNF = tumor necrosis factor; VEGF = vascular endothelial growth factor; VSMC = vascular smooth muscle cell.

MMPs are produced as inactive zymogens that can be activated by plasmin.[9] The activity of MMPs is also regulated by cytokines at transcriptional and posttranslational levels as well as by the relative levels of TIMPs. MMP-2 is usually found complexed with TIMP-2, its specific inhibitor.

In venous or microvascular endothelial cells, MMP-1 (interstitial collagenase), MMP-2 (72-kDa gelatinase), and TIMPs-1 and 2 are constitutively expressed. Although MMP-3 is only weakly expressed, it can be induced synergistically by incubation of the cells with the cytokine TNF-$\alpha$ and with phorbol ester tumor promoters.[8] This treatment also induces MMP-9 expression. Since MMP-2 and TIMP-2 are unaffected by TNF-$\alpha$, cytokine activation of endothelial cells can change the complement of metalloproteinases produced. In VSMCs, MMP-2 is constitutively expressed, whereas MMP-1, MMP-9 (92-kDa gelatinase), and MMP-3 (stromelysin) are induced by cytokines such as interleukin 1 and TNF-$\alpha$.[9] Cytokines can also activate MMP-2 zymogen.[123] Thus, cytokine stimulation increases the range of active metalloproteinases secreted by smooth muscle cells to encompass proteases capable of degrading all the major matrix components. In contrast, although TIMP-1 and TIMP-2 are constitutively expressed by vascular smooth muscle, their expression is unaffected by cytokines.[9] The net effect of cytokines on the vascular wall may be to tip the balance between the production of MMPs and TIMPs in favor of extracellular matrix degradation and remodeling.

Of particular importance, several reactive oxygen species have been shown to stimulate both activation and expression of MMPs, in particular MMP-9.[124,125] This is likely to be very important in diseases like atherosclerosis and hypertension, where vascular oxidant stress is increased. Activated macrophages accumulate at shoulder regions of the atherosclerotic plaque and secrete both MMPs and reactive oxygen species,[125,126] contributing to plaque rupture in this region.

There has been a great deal of interest recently in the pivotal role of MMPs and TIMPs in vascular remodeling and atherogenesis.[127] A considerable body of evidence now exists that suggests vascular remodeling, as reflected in outcomes as disparate as a stenotic atherosclerotic lesion or an atherosclerotic aneurysm, is caused by varying combinations of major drivers of MMP-mediated remodeling–oxidative stress, inflammation, injury, and hemodynamics. The relative strengths of these different modulators of MMPs and their inhibitors appear to be major determinants of clinical outcomes, including atherosclerotic plaque regression, progression, or rupture, aneurysm formation, and adaptive or maladaptive angiogenic responses.[127–130]

## ANGIOGENESIS

The development of the vascular support for organogenesis during embryogenesis (vasculogenesis) is coming to be well understood at the most basic levels (see also Chap. 8).[131] A great interest in this process has developed among cardiovascular scientists and clinical investigators recently as it has become apparent that the normal vasculature is not necessarily, as previously assumed, a totally stable, static system, with minimal turnover of the endothelial and vascular smooth muscle cells. Although vascular remodeling in, for example, atherosclerosis was widely appreciated, it was thought previously that any new arterial formation, such as collaterals in ischemic coronary disease, arose only from cells from the existing vascular structures (angiogenesis and arteriogenesis), and the processes involved were poorly understood. These general perceptions have changed radically and rapidly with dramatic increases in understanding of the cellular and molecular mechanisms involved in blood vessel formation (Fig. 7-6). Another major impetus for a paradigm shift has been the appreciation that endothelial and vascular smooth muscle progenitor cells, which are likely derived from the bone marrow, contribute to and perhaps guide not only new blood vessel development in adults but also probably contribute to continuous renewal of existing vasculature.[132]

### Vascular Development

The angioblast/hemangioblast is a very early endothelial cell progenitor and is also the progenitor cell for hematopoietic cells and skeletal muscle. Many of the genes and gene products (proteins) that are involved in vasculogenesis have been defined using mouse gene

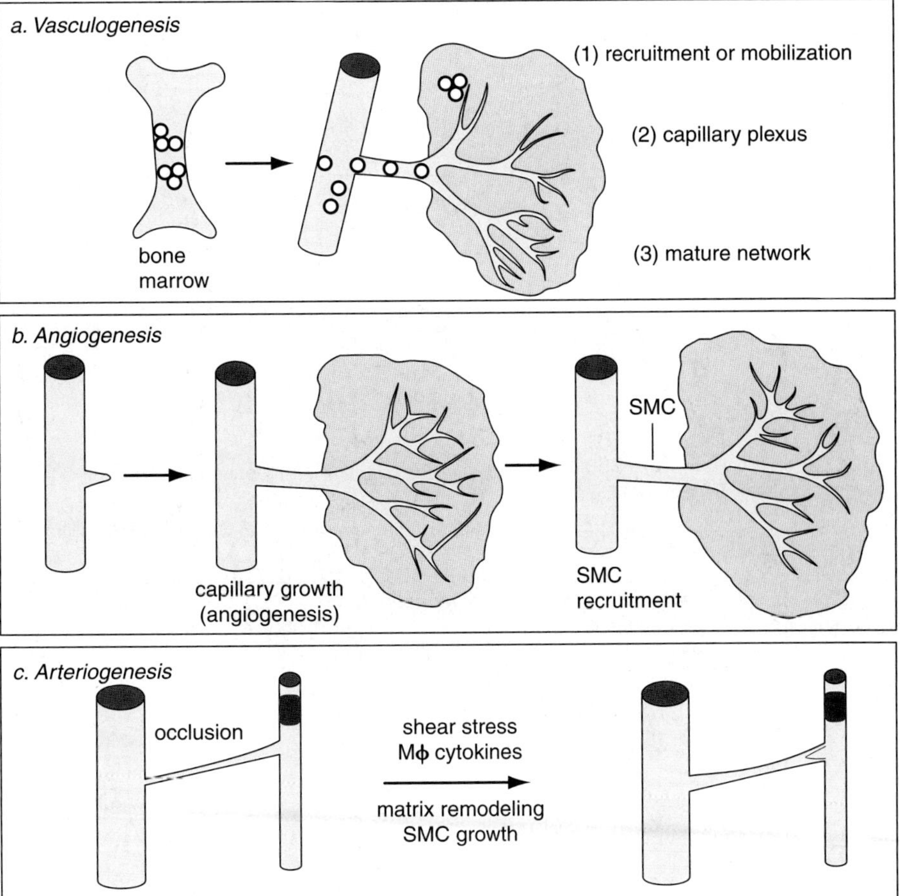


FIGURE 7-6 Pathologic vascular growth in the adult may occur via vasculogenesis [endothelial progenitor cell (EPC) moblization], angiogenesis (sprouting), or arteriogenesis (collateral growth). M$\phi$ = macrophages; SMC = smooth muscle cells. (From Luttun et al.[132] With permission.)

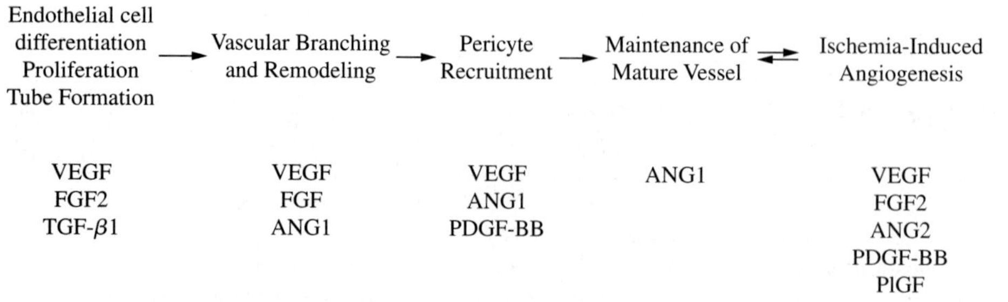

| Endothelial cell differentiation Proliferation Tube Formation → | Vascular Branching and Remodeling → | Pericyte Recruitment → | Maintenance of Mature Vessel ⇄ | Ischemia-Induced Angiogenesis |
|---|---|---|---|---|
| VEGF<br>FGF2<br>TGF-$\beta$1 | VEGF<br>FGF<br>ANG1 | VEGF<br>ANG1<br>PDGF-BB | ANG1 | VEGF<br>FGF2<br>ANG2<br>PDGF-BB<br>PlGF |

FIGURE 7-7 A simplified scheme of vasculogenesis and angiogenesis. Examples of angiogenic factors that are critical at each step are shown. VEGF, vascular endothelial growth factor; FGF, fibroblast growth factor; TGF-$\beta$1, transforming growth factor-$\beta$1; ANG1, angiopoietin-1; PDGF-BB, platelet-derived growth factor-BB (B = B chain); PlGF, placenta-derived growth factor. (From Semenza.[133] With permission.)

knockout models.[133] Of the large number of genes involved, a smaller number are particularly interesting because of the magnitude of the effects on vasculogenesis of knocking out the gene or of the potential of the encoded protein to promote angiogenesis in disease states. The vascular endothelial growth factor (VEGF) family is among the most important and VEGF is required for initial endothelial cell differentiation and proliferation.[134,135] VEGF binds to its cognate tyrosine kinase receptor VEGF receptor-2 (VEGFR-2), which is also known as flk1 or kdr.[136] Other homologues of VEGF include VEGF-B and placental growth factor (PlGF), and all three growth factors bind to VEGFR-1 or flt-1. The PlGF-flt-1 interaction is likely to be very important in pathological angiogenesis in the adult as discussed subsequently. Other growth factors, the angiopoietins (1 and 2), are important in the development and maintenance of mature blood vessels including the recruitment of pericytes, which are essential to the maturation process. An additional family of molecules that are important in blood vessel development into a network of arteries and veins are the ephrins, which are involved in cell-cell recognition.[134,135] Other growth factors that play a role in vascular development include platelet-derived growth factor BB (PDGF-BB), fibroblast growth factor (FGF), FGF2, and TGF-$\beta$1. The process of embryonic vasculogenesis, angiogenesis, and arteriogenesis is depicted sequentially with the involved growth factors in Fig. 7-7 and graphically in Fig. 7-8.

## Angiogenesis and Arteriogenesis in the Adult

### GROWTH FACTORS

In animal models of ischemic heart disease, VEGF expression is stimulated after coronary artery occlusion and is associated with the development of collateral formation.[137,138] VEGF expression is regulated, at least in part, by hypoxia-inducible factor 1 (HIF-1), which is a transcription factor that acts as a molecular switch for angiogenesis genes.[139] HIF-1 expression is upregulated by conditions of

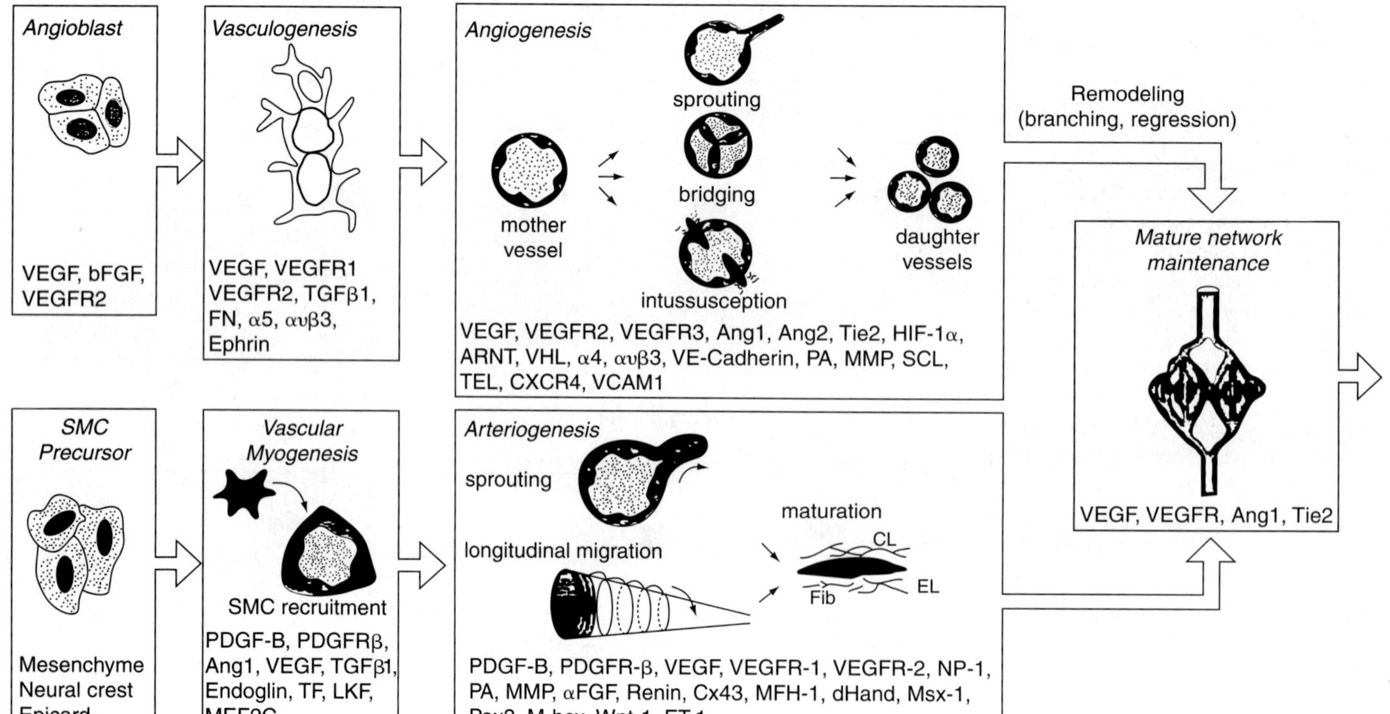


FIGURE 7-8 Endothelial precursors (angioblasts) in the embryo assemble in a primitive network (vasculogenesis) that expands and remodels (angiogenesis). Smooth muscle cells cover endothelial cells during vascular myogenesis and stabilize vessels during arteriogenesis. CL = collagen; EL = elastin, Fib = fibrillin. (From Carmeliet.[225] With permission.)

TABLE 7-3 Clinical Trials of Therapeutic Angiogenesis

| Angiogenic Factor | Mode of Administration |
|---|---|
| FGF-1 | Protein |
| FGF-2 | Protein |
| FGF-4 | Adenovirus |
| $VEGF_{121}$ | Adenovirus |
| $VEGF_{165}$ | Plasmid |
| $VEGF_{165}$ | Protein |
| VEGF-2 | Plasmid |
| **Transcription factor** | **Mode of administration** |
| HIF-lα/VP-16 fusion protein | Adenovirus |

ABBREVIATIONS: FGF = fibroblast growth factor; VEGF = vascular endothelial growth factor; HIF = hypoxia-inducible factor
SOURCE: From Semenza.[133] With permission.

hypoxia and ischemia. The response of this system, which is considerably more complicated than outlined here, is obviously very variable, as reflected in clinical experience in which different patients may have robust or no obvious collateralization with apparently similar degrees of coronary artery obstruction. This heterogeneity of individual responses appears to be dependent in part upon age as determined in animal experiments.[140–142] In addition to age-related factors, evidence suggests that individual genetic or environmental factors, predictably, may determine the responsiveness of the systems controlling collateralization in humans.[133,143]

The logic that inadequate collateralization clinically could be compensated for by the administration of either angiogenic growth factors or the genes encoding them has led to a number of clinical trials (Table 7-3).[144,145] Clinical efficacy has not been clearly demonstrated as yet. The approaches in these trials of using a single angiogenic factor such as VEGF or FGF may be conceptually flawed. As noted earlier, the generation of a mature blood vessel requires mutiple factors in addition to VEGF or FGF. The potential problem is perhaps illustrated by the fact that angiopoietin 1, which interacts with the receptor Tie-2, is essential to stabilize mature blood vessels, which are, among other things, very leaky in its absence.[146] In animal models, VEGF infusion not only stimulates formation of leaky blood vessels but can stimulate formation of hemangioma-like structures.[132] On the other hand, it has recently been shown in animal models that infusion of PlGF is more robust than VEGF in revascularization of ischemic tissues and in the induction of formation of stable, mature (imbued with vascular smooth cells and pericytes) blood vessels in this setting.[136] The effect of PlGF was attributed, in part, to its stimulation of flt-1 and to mobilization of bone marrow–derived inflammatory cells to ischemic regions. PlGF thus may be a more attractive candidate than VEGF (or FGF) for therapeutic angiogenesis using growth factor delivery to ischemic tissues as the principal strategy.

### BONE MARROW–DERIVED PROGENITOR CELLS

As noted, neovascularization in the adult previously was thought to result exclusively from angiogenesis.[132] Vascular progenitor cells (hemangioblasts) were identified earlier and were characterized as endothelial progenitor cells (EPCs) in studies of embryonic vasculogenesis.[147] Several recent studies, moreover, have described EPCs circulating in the peripheral blood postnatally that incorporated into the neovasculature and were associated with tumors, ischemic myocardium and hindlimbs, cutaneous wounds, and injured corneas.[148–151] Utilization of EPCs, whether derived from the bone marrow directly (or indirectly by stimulating the release out of the marrow with cytokines or growth factors) or by expanding the relatively small population of circulating EPCs in vitro, has enormous biological significance and therapeutic potential. The burgeoning literature on the subject has recently been reviewed in detail generally[132] and specifically with respect to clinical applications.[152,153]

## VASCULAR INFLAMMATION

Endothelial cells actively participate in the development of inflammatory reactions. The recruitment of leukocytes to sites of inflammation is initiated by endothelial secretion of chemotactic molecules and enhanced expression of adhesion molecules that interact with surface proteins on leukocytes.[154] Cytokines and arachidonic acid metabolites of the leukotriene pathway derived from cells of the vessel wall, the infiltrating macrophages and T-lymphocytes stimulate endothelial secretion of many of these molecules.[154] An important new class of molecules that mediate the vascular inflammatory response comprises the chemokines, of which more than 50 have been identified.[155] Two classes of the chemokines exist, known as the CXC and CC, based on differences in the position of the first two cysteines in their amino acid sequence. These interact with at least 20 G-protein receptors, classified as CXCR and CCR, according to their corresponding ligand.

It has been suggested that the sequential accumulation of different leukocyte classes at sites of inflammation can be explained by the differential induction of these endothelial cell adhesion molecules.[156] An early step in the inflammatory response is capture of leukocytes from the flowing blood, mediated by the L and P selectins.[157,158] A second step is leukocyte rolling, which is mediated by interaction with E and P selectins.[157,158] Ultimate adhesion of leukocytes is dependent on interactions with $\beta$2-integrins PECAM and ICAM-1.[157,158] At the site of atherosclerotic lesions, recruitment of leukocytes is markedly enhanced by the surface expression of VCAM-1 and interactions between the monocyte chemotactic protein MCP-1 with its monocyte receptor CCR2.[159,160] IL-8 and its receptor CXCR2, as well as fractalkine and its receptor $CX_3CL1$, also contribute to this response.[161,162] The list of proinflammatory molecules contributing to these endothelial/leukocyte interactions continues to grow, and it is likely that the complete inflammatory response depends on the concerted action of many such molecular mediators. This is supported by the observation that genetic knockout of either the IL-8 receptor, MCP-1, or CX3CR1 each leads to a >50 percent reduction in lesion formation in atherosclerotic mice.[161,162]

## ENDOTHELIAL DYSFUNCTION AND VASCULAR SMOOTH MUSCLE ABNORMALITIES

In general, the normal endothelium is in an inhibitory mode—inhibiting contraction, thrombosis, white cell adhesion, and vascular smooth muscle growth (Figs. 7-2 and 7-9). A common feature of many different vascular diseases is that these functions of the endothelium are either lost or disrupted, a phenomenon often referred to as *endothelial dysfunction*. Implicit in this term is the recognition that the fundamental or normal functions of the endothelium are not fixed but are mutable. Thus, the endothelium in a given area may lose its vasodilator predominance, become prothrombotic or less thrombolytic, begin to support leukocyte adherence (which may be a normal response in the inflammatory process), or stimulate rather than inhibit smooth muscle migration and proliferation.

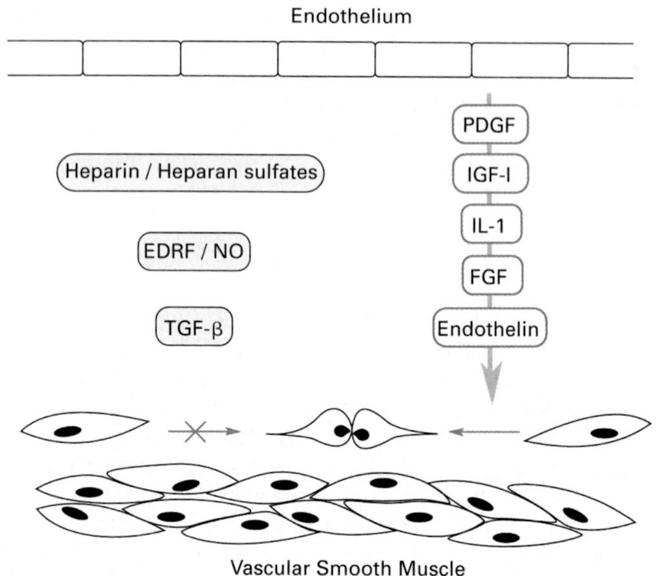


FIGURE 7-9 Endothelial control of vascular growth. As with vasoactive substances, endothelial cells make and secrete both growth-promoting (*white boxes*) and growth-inhibitory (*shaded boxes*) compounds. Under normal conditions, the net effect of the endothelium is growth-inhibitory. EDRF = endothelial-derived relaxing factor; NO = nitric oxide; TGF-$\beta$ = transforming growth factor beta; PDGF = platelet-derived growth factor; IGF-I = insulin-like growth factor-I; IL-1 = interleukin-1; FGF = fibroblast growth factor. (Courtesy of Bernard Lassègue, Ph.D.)

## Oxidative Stress and Vascular Disease

In the past several years, it has become clear that vascular cells—including endothelial, vascular smooth muscle, and adventitial cells—can produce reactive oxygen species (ROS).[163] These include the superoxide anion, hydrogen peroxide, NO, and peroxynitrite. In numerous pathophysiologic conditions, the production of ROS in the vascular wall is increased, resulting in a situation commonly referred to as *oxidant,* or *oxidative, stress.* Several enzyme systems have been implicated in production of ROS.

Recent studies suggest that NAD(P)H oxidases are major sources of ROS in endothelial and vascular smooth muscle cells.[163] These are multisubunit enzymes that have partial similarity to the neutrophil respiratory burst oxidase. In phagocytic cells, two membrane components, p22$^{phox}$ and gp91$^{phox}$, comprise the cytochrome b558, which is regulated by cytoplasmic subunits, including p47$^{phox}$, p67$^{phox}$, and the small G protein Rac.[164] On a molecular level, the vascular oxidases share limited homology with the neutrophil respiratory burst oxidase. Many of the neutrophil components including p22$^{phox}$, p47$^{phox}$, and the small GTPase Rac are present in vascular cells. During the past few years, a family of proteins termed the Nox proteins with homology to gp91$^{phox}$, the neutrophil oxidase catalytic subunit, has been shown to play a critical role in function of both the smooth muscle and endothelial cell NAD(P)H oxidases.[165–167] Endothelial cells contain Nox1, Nox2, and Nox4, while vascular smooth muscle cells express Nox1, Nox4, and Nox5.[167,168] The adventitia also contains fibroblasts and macrophages that express multiple oxidase subunits.[169]

Importantly, the NAD(P)H oxidases are activated by several pathophysiologic stimuli, including angiotensin II, mechanical stretch, cytokines, and thrombin.[71,119,170,171] Recent studies have shown that the low-molecular-weight G protein Rac1 is a central regulator of oxidase activity.[172] Rac1 geranylation can be inhibited by the HMG- CoA reductase inhibitors,[173] suggesting one mechanism whereby these agents can have vasculoprotective effects.

A second source of ROS is eNOS. As discussed previously, in the absence of tetrahydrobiopterin or L-arginine, this enzyme becomes "uncoupled," so that it produces hydrogen peroxide and superoxide rather than NO.[41,174] Importantly, this uncoupling process seems to occur in several common disease states, including hypercholesterolemia,[175] hypertension,[42] and diabetes,[176] although the mechanisms responsible for this process are poorly understood.

An important source of radicals in the vasculature is the lipoxygenases, in particular 12,15-lipoxygenase.[177] These do not form superoxide but react directly with unsaturated fatty acids (e.g., linoleic and arachidonic acids) to form a lipid radical (L·), which in turn can react with molecular oxygen to produce alkoxy-radicals (LO·), and lipid peroxy radicals (LOO·). These lipid radicals are biologically very active and can stimulate gene expression, consume NO, oxidize NADH, and serve as a source of other radicals.[178]

Other sources of ROS in vascular cells are xanthine oxidase, cytochrome P450, cyclooxygenase, and mitochondrial electron transport.[178] There is now substantial interest in the role of these various sources of ROS and how they contribute to vascular oxidant stress.

In the next several paragraphs, we consider how endothelial dysfunction and vascular smooth muscle abnormalities contribute to several vascular diseases. A recurring theme in these conditions is that ROS play a central role. For example, superoxide rapidly reacts with NO, forming the strong oxidant peroxynitrite. The latter can oxidize lipids, damage lipid membranes, deplete cellular thiols, and alter function of several enzymes.[179] This inactivation of NO alters vasomotion and can predispose one to or even cause hypertension.[180] Other ROS such as the hydroxyl radical and lipid radicals can react with NO. Recently it has been recognized that peroxidases, upon reaction with $H_2O_2$, can consume NO. A substantial component of VSMC hypertrophy caused by angiotensin II is mediated by hydrogen peroxide.[181] ROS also contribute to vascular inflammation by stimulating expression of adhesion molecules in endothelial cells.[182] These issues are discussed in the context of several vascular diseases.

## Atherosclerosis

Atherosclerosis is the prototypical disease characterized by endothelial dysfunction, which may explain many of its cardinal features. Thus, mononuclear and lymphocytic infiltration, vascular smooth muscle hypercontractility, modification of low-density liporotein (LDL), smooth muscle cell growth, and intimal migration are likely related to abnormalities of the endothelium induced by hyperlipidemia, hypertension, smoking, and unknown hereditary factors. The pathogenesis of atherosclerosis viewed as a disease of endothelial dysfunction is depicted in Fig. 7-10. (For a more detailed discussion, see Chap. 44.)

Clinically, endothelial dysfunction in atherosclerosis has primarily been defined by impairment of endothelium-dependent relaxation.[183,184] Coronary endothelium-dependent vasodilator function is impaired in patients with risk factors such as hypercholesterolemia and prior to angiographically demonstrable coronary disease.[185] As previously discussed, increased inactivation of NO by the superoxide anion is likely one cause of this abnormality.[186,187] Other causes may include "uncoupling" of the eNOS enzyme, altered calcium signaling of eNOS, and diminished expression of the eNOS enzyme, which clearly occurs late in the atherosclerotic process.[188] Of note, LDL and cytokines have been shown to downregulate eNOS by destabiliz-

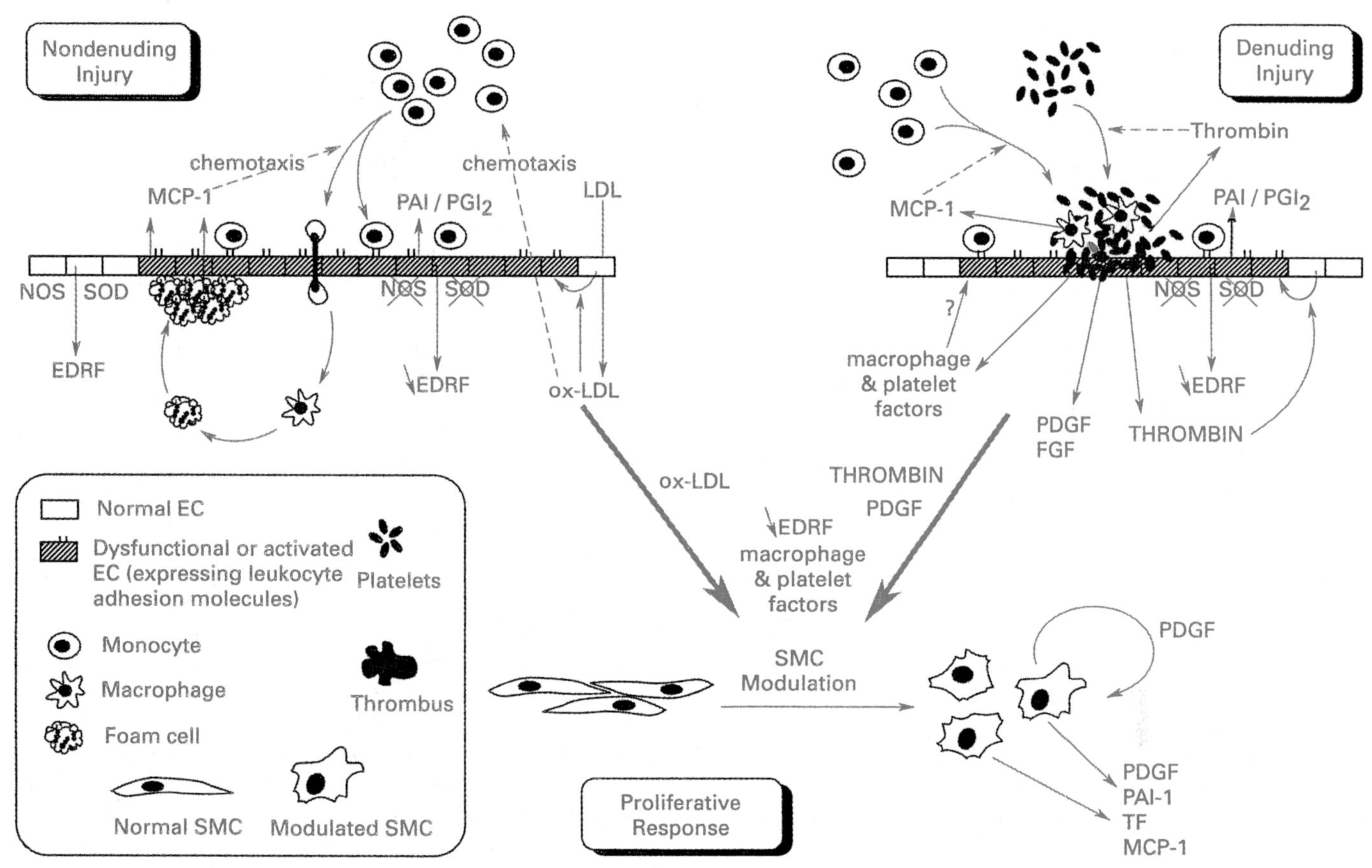


FIGURE 7-10 Theoretical initiating events in vascular lesion formation. Nondenuding injury: Low-density lipoprotein (LDL) enters the subendothelial space where it is converted to oxidized LDL (ox-LDL), which induces monocyte chemoattraction and endothelial dysfunction. Dysfunctional endothelial cells (ECs) express cell adhesion molecules (ICAM, ELAM, and VCAM), leading to increased monocyte adhesion and movement into the vessel wall. Monocytes in the vessel wall differentiate into macrophages, take up lipids, and remain locally as foam cells, subsequently evolving into fatty streaks. The foam cells in the fatty streak and the overlying endothelium express monocyte chemotactic protein 1 (MCP-1), resulting in further enhanced monocyte chemoattraction and adhesion. Dysfunctional ECs may synthesize less nitric oxide synthase (NOS) or superoxide dismutase (SOD, an enzyme that metabolizes oxygen radicals, which have been shown to inactivate NO). This decreases endothelium-derived relaxing factor (EDRF) release/activity. The loss of EDRF together with the direct effects of ox-LDL, or growth factors secreted by the foam cells or endothelium, act on the quiescent contractile smooth muscle cells in the vessel wall, giving rise to the proliferative phenotype, with division and migration into the intima. Denuding injury: Loss of endothelium leads to platelet deposition, tissue factor–mediated activation of extrinsic coagulation to generate thrombin, cleavage of fibrinogen to fibrin, and the formation of thrombus. Thrombin gives rise to endothelial expression of adhesion molecules and consequent monocyte attachment, together with secretion of platelet granular constituents. Monocytes enter the thrombus and differentiate into phagocytic macrophages expressing tissue factor and MCP-1. This leads to further monocyte chemoattraction into the vessel wall. Smooth muscle cell proliferation is produced by (1) thrombin generation at the site of denuding injury, (2) platelet-derived growth factor (PDGF) or other growth factors released from platelets in the thrombus, (3) factors secreted by the macrophages ingesting the thrombus, and (4) the loss of EDRF activity caused by endothelial dysfunction. *Proliferative response*: Modulated smooth muscle cells (SMCs) proliferate and synthesize factors that promote plaque development. SMCs synthesize (1) PDGF and other growth factors that cause self-perpetuating autocrine or paracrine stimulation of SMC proliferation, (2) tissue factor (TF) and plasminogen activator inhibitor 1 (PAI-1) that act locally to produce thrombin or inhibit fibrinolysis of the fibrin network used to facilitate cell migration, and (3) MCP-1, which increases monocyte chemoattraction into the lesion, thereby leading to lesion development. (We thank Drs. Laurence Harker, Josiah Wilcox, and Bernard Lassègue for their creative and intellectual contributions to the development of this figure.)

ing the eNOS mRNA. This is prevented by HMG-CoA reductase inhibitors even without lowering of cholesterol. New evidence suggests that this process involves the lipid modification of the small GTPase Rho by the attachment of a geranylgeranyl and lipid moiety which facilitates its localization to the cell membrane, suggesting a new target for the HMG-CoA reductase inhibitors.[189]

A second manifestation of a dysfunctional endothelium that is apparent very early after initiation of cholesterol feeding in animals is the recruitment of monocytes and macrophages into the vessel wall.[190] This recruitment is likely the result of induction of VCAM-1 expression[191] as well as secretion of MCP-1.[192] The molecular linkage between hyperlipidemia and MCP-1/adhesion molecule expression is unknown, but may reflect in part the oxidative stress imposed by this change in milieu. Inflammatory cytokines are also important mediators of adhesion molecule expression,[193] and their production by the endothelium and inflammatory cells in the vessel wall may also contribute to adhesion molecule expression in both the early and the late stages of the disease. Inhibition of MCP-1 or its receptor attenuates the development of early atherosclerotic lesions in experimental animals.[159,194] In addition, deletion of the fractalkine receptor (CX3CR1) reduces macrophage recruitment into the vessel wall and diminishes lesion formation in ApoE-deficient mice.[162] Moreover, a common polymorphism of the fractalkine receptor has been shown to have reduced adhesive and chemoattractant properties and is associated with a lower incidence of human atherosclerosis and acute coronary syndromes.[195]

The intimal proliferation observed in atherosclerotic lesion formation results from migration and hyperplasia of vascular smooth muscle cells and myofibroblasts[196] and accumulation of extracellular matrix.[197] Proliferation has been attributed to growth factors such as PDGF, FGF, and IGF-1. Since these growth factors can be produced by the endothelium in vitro, it is very likely that the dysfunctional endothelium in atherosclerosis also produces growth factors while shifting from a growth-inhibitory to a growth-promoting mode. Furthermore, there is evidence that products of oxidative metabolism may increase matrix metalloproteinase activation[124] and expression,[125] thus contributing to intimal lesion formation on multiple levels.

The recent advances in our understanding of vessel wall biology provide insight into the biological mechanisms responsible for the pathogenesis of atherosclerosis. A unifying concept of the disease has arisen that revolves around endothelial dysfunction mediated by changes in oxidative metabolism. Oxidative stress and oxidatively modified LDL thus assume central roles in atherogenesis (Fig. 7-10). As discussed previously, a major source of lipid oxidation is lipoxygenases. Knockout of 12,15 lipoxygenase or the NAD(P)H oxidase subunit p47*phox*[198,199] reduces atherosclerosis in ApoE-deficient mice. These data indicate that 12- and 15-lipoxygenases and the NAD(P)H oxidases are almost certainly involved in the atherosclerotic process. The role of oxidized LDL and the relationship of the cell biology of atherosclerosis to coronary ischemic syndromes are discussed in Chap. 44.

## Hypertension

Hypertension is characterized by dysfunction of both endothelium and vascular smooth muscle. In chronic hypertension, endothelium-dependent relaxations are impaired in both conduit and resistance arteries.[200–203] Relaxations to some platelet factors are also altered, but have been found to be augmented or diminished, depending on the hypertensive model studied.[204] Furthermore, the endothelium-dependent constrictor activity is increased in some models of hypertension.[204] These alterations in endothelial function would tend to increase the tone of hypertensive vessels. Recently, it has been shown that hypertension is associated with oxidation of tetrahydrobiopterin by NAD(P)H oxidases, a critical cofactor for NO synthase. This leads to eNOS uncoupling, reducing NO production and increasing endothelial superoxide production. Removing the oxidant stress by either knockout of p47*phox* or by replacement of tetrahydrobiopterin lowered blood pressure in experimental animals.[42,205]

Hypertension is also characterized by an increase in vessel wall mass. In the aortas of spontaneously hypertensive and Goldblatt hypertensive rats, this increase can be attributed to an increase in the size of the existing smooth muscle cells.[206,207] Hypertrophy is accompanied by an increase in ploidy; that is, an increased DNA content per cell.[206,207] In contrast, resistance vessels from these same animals appear to increase their mass by hyperplasia of the smooth muscle cells.[208] The stimuli responsible for these changes in the hypertensive vascular wall are unknown. Vascular remodeling appears to have two stages: (1) an initial, reversible, intense vasoconstriction mediated by neural or endogenous signals, followed by (2) a remodeling of the vessel wall characterized by increased smooth muscle mass and narrowing of the vessel lumen. There is some evidence that this response is dependent on the presence of the endothelium.[209]

## Vasospasm

When the endothelium becomes dysfunctional, as in atherosclerosis, the underlying smooth muscle cells often become hyperreactive to certain vasoconstrictor stimuli, including serotonin and ergonovine.[210] Coronary spasm leading to myocardial infarction is one of the most clinically relevant problems arising from this phenomenon. Proposed mechanisms underlying this vasoconstrictor abnormality that can result in total occlusion include supersensitivity of the smooth muscle cells to constrictor stimuli and loss of endothelium-dependent relaxing mechanisms. The increased tendency toward thrombus formation in dysfunctional endothelium, due to a loss of the normal anticoagulant properties, also promotes the release of thrombus-related factors (serotonin, thromboxane $A_2$, ADP, thrombin, and PDGF) in the vicinity of the smooth muscle cells, which can promote vasoconstriction.[211]

## Restenosis

Restenosis is the development of a neointima that occurs following angioplasty, often leading to reocclusion of the initial lesion. The response of the arterial wall to the injury induced by angioplasty (removal of the endothelium and stretching of the vessel wall) involves several distinct events. Removal of the endothelium not only alters the paracrine hormonal environment in which VSMCs exist, but it also exposes a thrombogenic surface to which platelets and other circulating factors can adhere, resulting in the formation of a thrombus. In addition, injury to the underlying smooth muscle may release factors such as FGF, which have mitogenic effects on the remaining smooth muscle cells. Finally, infiltration and subsequent activation of macrophages into the denuded vessel wall bring an additional set of hormonal influences to bear on the vascular smooth muscle. The pathophysiologic consequences of these complex events include migration and proliferation of smooth muscle cells into the intimal area, resulting in the formation of a neointima over a period of weeks to months.

Balloon injury has been extensively studied in several animal models, including pigs, rabbits, rats, and baboons. In the rat carotid artery, the events following injury can be divided into three stages: initial (injury to 48 h), migratory (3 to 7 days), and proliferative (7 days to 3 to 4 weeks). During the initial response to injury, growth-related genes in the smooth muscle cells are induced, including c-fos, PDGF-A, PDGF-$\beta$ receptor and MCP-1.[212,213] It also appears that deep injury to smooth muscle cells results in an outpouring of FGF, a potent smooth muscle mitogen.[214] This initial response does not appear to depend on platelet factors, but does appear to be directly related to the removal of the endothelium.[99] During the migratory phase, a large increase of thymidine incorporation in the vessel wall occurs, accompanied by further increases in the mRNA encoding IGF-1[215] and the PDGF-$\beta$ receptor.[212] This phase of the response can be modulated by platelet factors and inhibited by the endothelium.[99] Finally, the proliferative phase is characterized by marked intimal thickening, with a decreased percentage of thymidine-labeled cells. Some of the increased area is due to deposition of extracellular matrix, and the majority of the proliferative activity occurs at the luminal surface of the vessel. This proliferative phase seems ultimately to be inhibited by regrowth of normal-functioning endothelium.

Thus, during the process of restenosis after angioplasty, both the loss of endothelium and the transformation of smooth muscle cells appear to contribute to neointimal formation. At least two lines of evidence implicate the endothelium as having a crucial role in the response of the vessel wall to injury. First, removal of the endothelium allows initiation of the mitogenic response and, second, regrowth of normal endothelium inhibits further proliferation. Furthermore, gentle denudation with a nylon loop accompanied by rapid regeneration of endothelium results in significantly less neointimal proliferation.[216] In addition, proliferating smooth muscle cells have characteristics distinct from those of the differentiated smooth muscle cells in the medial layer. Their cytoskeleton is similar to that found in cultured cells. It seems likely, therefore, that two of the most important causes of restenosis are the loss of endothelium-derived growth-inhibitory factors and the transformation of smooth muscle cells into a phenotype able to respond to platelet- and endothelium-derived factors with proliferation.

ROS are thought not only to be centrally involved in the pathogenesis of atherosclerosis but very likely also to be major mediators of the proliferative, hypertrophic, and fibrotic responses that frequently occur in arteries after percutaneous transluminal coronary angioplasty (PTCA), resulting in renarrowing or restenosis of the lumen (see Chap. 55). Migration and growth of VSMCs into the intima contribute significantly to restenosis, and intracellular signaling pathways mediating growth, hypertrophy, and migration are stimulated by ROS.[217,218] As discussed previously, both proinflammatory pathways and matrix metalloproteinases, which facilitate vascular remodeling, involve redox-sensitive controlling mechanisms. The apparent broad role for oxidative signaling mechanisms in the vascular wall led to testing of the concept that antioxidants might inhibit restenosis. The production of superoxide is increased in vessels following balloon injury.[219,220] Several clinical studies have shown that the potent antioxidant probucol and a newer, soluble probucol derivative can prevent restenosis after either balloon angioplasty or coronary stent placement.[221–224]

## FUTURE DIRECTIONS

Defining the molecular and cellular basis for dysfunction of the arterial wall in vascular diseases provides information critical to developing clinical strategies for patient management, as well as to finding new therapeutic targets. It is now clear that both endothelial function and smooth muscle function are compromised by a variety of risk factors for vascular disease, due in part to oxidative stress. Further research is required to determine at a more basic level the molecular events that link these risk factors to these diseases. The human genome has been fully sequenced, and via the use of bioinformatics it will be possible to identify genetic profiles that predispose people to the development of vascular pathologies. Clinical trials in the future will be targeted to these populations in new and powerful ways, and basic research will address the roles of these newly identified genes in vascular physiology and pathophysiology. In addition, the advent of stem cell technology opens new avenues for therapeutic treatment. Once researchers understand the mechanisms controlling stem cell targeting and differentiation, genetic and pharmacologic manipulation of these cells may be the treatment of the future.

## References


1. Moncada S, Vane JR. Arachidonic acid metabolites and the interaction between platelets and blood vessel walls. *N Engl J Med* 1979;300: 1142–1147.
2. Furchgott RF, Zawadzki JV. The obligatory role of endothelial cells in the relaxation of arterial smooth muscle by acetylcholine. *Nature* 1980;228:373–376.
3. Taylor SG, Weston AH. Endothelium-derived hyperpolarizing factor: A new endogenous inhibitor from the vascular endothelium. *Trends Pharmacol Sci* 1988;9:272–274.
4. Yanagisawa Y, Kurihara H, Kimura S, et al. A novel potent vasoconstrictor peptide produced by vascular endothelial cells. *Nature* 1988; 332:411–415.
5. Lin L, Balazy M, Pagano PJ, et al. Expression of prostaglandin H2–mediated mechanism of vascular contraction in hypertensive rats. Relation to lipoxygenase and prostacyclin synthase activities. *Circ Res* 1994;74:197–205.
6. Stenmark KR, Orton EC, Reeves JT, et al. Vascular remodeling in neonatal pulmonary hypertension. *Chest* 1988;93:127S–133S.
7. Sato T, Arai K, Ishiharajima S, et al. Role of glycosaminoglycan and fibronectin in endothelial cell growth. *Exp Mol Pathol* 1987;47: 202–210.
8. Hanemaaijer R, Koolwijk P, le Clercq L, et al. Regulation of matrix metalloproteinase expression in human vein and microvascular endothelial cells. Effects of tumor necrosis factor alpha, interleukin 1 and phorbol ester. *Biochem J* 1993;296:803–809.
9. Galis ZS, Muszynski M, Sukhova GK, et al. Cytokine-stimulated human vascular smooth muscle cells synthesize a complement of enzymes required for extracellular matrix digestion. *Circ Res* 1994;75: 181–189.
10. Castellot JJ, Jr., Addonizio ML, Rosenberg R, et al. Cultured endothelial cells produce a heparin-like inhibitor of smooth muscle cell growth. *J Cell Biol* 1981;90:372–379.
11. Zerwes HG, Risau W. Polarized secretion of a platelet-derived growth factor–like chemotactic factor by endothelial cells in vitro. *J Cell Biol* 1987;105:2037–2041.
12. Hannan RL, Kourembanas S, Flanders KC, et al. Endothelial cells synthesize basic fibroblast growth factor and transforming growth factor beta. *Growth Factors* 1988;1:7–17.
13. Delafontaine P, Bernstein KE, Alexander RW. Insulin-like growth factor I gene expression in vascular cells. *Hypertension* 1991;17: 693–699.
14. Wang-Iverson P, DeRosa PM, Brown W V.Plasma lipoprotein interaction with endothelial cells. In: Ryan U, ed. *Endothelial Cells.* Boca Raton, FL: CRC Press; 1988:179–187.
15. Gordon EL, Pearson JD, Slakey LL. The hydrolysis of extracellular adenine nucleotides by cultured endothelial cells from pig aorta. *J Biol Chem* 1986;33:15496–15504.
16. Cary DA, Mendelsohn FA. Effect of forskolin, isoproterenol and IBMX on angiotensin converting enzyme and cyclic AMP production by cultured bovine endothelial cells. *Mol Cell Endocrin* 1987;53:103–109.
17. Shimada K, Gill PJ, Silbert JE, et al. Involvement of cell surface heparan sulfate in the binding of LPL to cultured bovine endothelial cells. *J Clin Invest* 1981;68:995–1002.
18. Vlodavsky I, Fielding PE, Johnson LK, et al. Inhibition of low density lipoprotein uptake in confluent endothelial cell monolayers correlates with a restricted surface receptor redistribution. *J Cell Physiol* 1979; 100:481–495.
19. Rippe B, Rosengren BI, Carlsson O, et al. Transendothelial transport: The vesicle controversy. *J Vasc Res* 2002;39:375–390.
20. Baker DP, van Lenten BJ, Fogelman AM, et al. LDL, scavenger and beta-VLDL receptors on aortic endothelial cells. *Arteriosclerosis* 1984;4:357–364.
21. Krieger M, Stern DM. Series introduction: Multiligand receptors and human disease. *J Clin Invest* 2001;108:645–647.
22 Hayashida K, Kume N, Minami M, et al. Lectin-like oxidized LDL receptor-1 (LOX-1) supports adhesion of mononuclear leukocytes and a monocyte-like cell line THP-1 cells under static and flow conditions. *FEBS Lett* 2002;511:133–138.
23. Morel DW, DiCorleto PE, Chisolm GM. Endothelial and smooth muscle cells alter low density lipoprotein in vitro by free radical oxidation. *Arteriosclerosis* 1984;4:357–364.
24. Gryglewski RJ, Botting RM, Vane JR. Mediators produced by the endothelial cell. *Hypertension* 1988;12:530–548.
25. van Iwaarden F, Acton DS, Sixma JJ, et al. Internalization of antithrombin III by cultured human endothelial cells and its subcellular localization. *J Lab Clin Med* 1989;113:717–726.

26. Rosenberg RD, Rosenberg JS. Natural anticoagulant mechanisms. *J Clin Invest* 1984;74:1–6.
27. Esmon CT, Owen WG. Identification of an endothelial cofactor for thrombin-catalyzed activation of protein C. *Proc Natl Acad Sci USA* 1981;78:2249–2252.
28. Schorer AE, Moldow CF. Production of tissue factor. In: Ryan US, ed. *Endothelial Cells*. Boca Raton, FL: CRC Press; 1988:85–105.
29. Vaughan DE. Fibrinolytic balance, the renin-angiotensin system and atherosclerotic disease. *Eur Heart J* 1998;19 Suppl G:G9–G12.
30. Svensjo E, Grega GJ. Evidence for endothelial cell–mediated regulation of macromolecular permeability by post-capillary venules. *Fed Proc* 1986;45:89–95.
31. Schnitzer JE. Caveolae: from basic trafficking mechanisms to targeting transcytosis for tissue-specific drug and gene delivery in vivo. *Adv Drug Deliv Rev* 2001;49:265–280.
32. Gumbleton M, Abulrob AG, Campbell L. Caveolae: An alternative membrane transport compartment. *Pharm Res* 2000;17:1035–1048.
33. Simons K, Toomre D. Lipid rafts and signal transduction. *Nat Rev Mol Cell Biol* 2000;1:31–39.
34. Garcia JG, Davis HW, Patterson CE. Regulation of endothelial cell gap formation and barrier dysfunction: role of myosin light chain phosphorylation. *J Cell Physiol* 1995;163:510–522.
35. Garcia JG, Schaphorst KL, Shi S, et al. Mechanisms of ionomycin-induced endothelial cell barrier dysfunction. *Am J Physiol* 1997;273: L172–184.
36. Garcia JG, Verin AD, Schaphorst K, et al. Regulation of endothelial cell myosin light chain kinase by rho, cortactin, and p60. *Am J Physiol* 1999;276:L989–998.
37. Palmer RMJ, Ferrige AG, Moncada S. Nitric oxide release accounts for the biological activity of endothelium-derived relaxing factor. *Nature* 1987;327:524–526.
38. Bredt DS, Hwang PM, Glatt CE, et al. Cloned and expressed nitric oxide synthase structurally resembles cytochrome P-450 reductase. *Nature* 1991;351:714–718.
39. Lyons CR, Orloff GJ, Cunningham JM. Molecular cloning and functional expression of an inducible nitric oxide synthase from a murine macrophage cell line. *J Biol Chem* 1992;267:6370–6374.
40. Nishida K, Harrison DG, Navas JP, et al. Molecular cloning and characterization of the constitutive bovine aortic endothelial nitric oxide synthase. *J Clin Invest* 1992;90:2092–2096.
41. Vasquez-Vivar J, Kalyanaraman B, Martasek P, et al. Superoxide generation by endothelial nitric oxide synthase: The influence of cofactors. *Proc Natl Acad Sci USA* 1998;95:9220–9225.
42. Landmesser U, Dikalov S, Price SR, et al. Oxidation of tetrahydrobiopterin leads to uncoupling of endothelial cell nitric oxide synthase in hypertension. *J Clin Invest* 2003;111:1201–1209.
43. Furchgott RF, Vanhoutte PM. Endothelium-derived relaxing and contracting factors. *FASEB J* 1989;3:2007–2018.
44. Rappoport RM, Draznin MB, Murad F. Endothelium-dependent relaxation in rat aorta may be mediated through cyclic GMP-dependent protein phosphorylation. *Nature* 1983;306:174–176.
45. Kuchan MJ, Frangos JA. Role of calcium and calmodulin in flow-induced nitric oxide production in endothelial cells. *Am J Physiol* 1994;266:C628–C636.
46. Gallis B, Corthals GL, Goodlett DR, et al. Identification of flow-dependent endothelial nitric-oxide synthase phosphorylation sites by mass spectrometry and regulation of phosphorylation and nitric oxide production by the phosphatidylinositol 3–kinase inhibitor LY294002. *J Biol Chem* 1999;274:30101–30108.
47. Uematsu M, Ohara Y, Navas JP, et al. Regulation of endothelial cell nitric oxide synthase mRNA expression by shear stress. *Am J Physiol* 1995;269:C1371–C1378.
48. Sessa WC, Pritchard K, Seyedi N, et al. Chronic exercise in dogs increases coronary vascular nitric oxide production and endothelial cell nitric oxide synthase gene expression. *Circ Res* 1994;74:349–353.
49. Liao JK, Shin WS, Lee WY, et al. Oxidized low-density lipoprotein decreases the expression of endothelial nitric oxide synthase. *J Biol Chem* 1995;270:319–324.
50. Liao JK, Zulueta JJ, Yu FS, et al. Regulation of bovine endothelial constitutive nitric oxide synthase by oxygen. *J Clin Invest* 1995;96: 2661–2666.
51. Feletou M, Vanhoutte PM. The alternative: EDHF. *J Mol Cell Cardiol* 1999;31:15–22.
52. Fisslthaler B, Popp R, Kiss L, et al. Cytochrome P450 2C is an EDHF synthase in coronary arteries. *Nature* 1999;401:493–497.
53. Hayabuchi Y, Nakaya Y, Matsuoka S, et al. Endothelium-derived hyperpolarizing factor activates $Ca^{2+}$-activated $K^+$ channels in porcine coronary artery smooth muscle cells. *J Cardiovasc Pharmacol* 1998;32:642–649.
54. Miura H, Bosnjak JJ, Ning G, et al. Role for hydrogen peroxide in flow-induced dilation of human coronary arterioles. *Circ Res* 2003;92: e31–e40.
55. Ito T, Ogawa K, Enomoto I, et al. Comparison of the effects of PGI2 and PGE1 on coronary and systemic hemodynamics and coronary arterial cyclic nucleotide level in dogs. *Adv Prostagl Thrombox Leukotr Res* 1980;7:641–646.
56. Sun D, Huang A, Smith CJ, et al. Enhanced release of prostaglandins contributes to flow-induced arteriolar dilation in eNOS knockout mice. *Circ Res* 1999;85:288–293.
57. Galie N, Manes A, Branzi A. Emerging medical therapies for pulmonary arterial hypertension. *Prog Cardiovasc Dis* 2002;45:213–224.
58. Gumkowski F, Kaminska F, Kaminiski M, et al. Heterogeneity of mouse vascular endothelium: In vitro studies of lymphatic, large blood vessel and microvascular endothelial cells. *Blood Vessels* 1987;24: 11–23.
59. Danser AH. Local renin-angiotensin systems: The unanswered questions. *Int J Biochem Cell Biol* 2003;35:759–768.
60. Luscher TF, Wenzel RR. Endothelin and endothelin antagonists: Pharmacology and clinical implications. *Agents Actions Suppl* 1995; 45:237–253.
61. Simonson MS, Dunn MJ. Cellular signaling by peptides of the endothelin gene family. *FASEB J* 1990;4:2989–3000.
62. Münzel T, Giaid A, Kurz S, et al. Evidence for a role of endothelin 1 and protein kinase C in nitroglycerin tolerance. *Proc Natl Acad Sci USA* 1995;92:5244–5248.
63. Hafizi S, Allen SP, Goodwin AT, et al. Endothelin-1 stimulates proliferation of human coronary smooth muscle cells via the ET(A) receptor and is co-mitogenic with growth factors. *Atherosclerosis* 1999;146:351–359.
64. Achmad TH, Rao GS. Chemotaxis of human blood monocytes toward endothelin-1 and the influence of calcium channel blockers. *Biochem Biophys Res Commun* 1992;189:994–1000.
65. Sung CP, Arleth AJ, Storer BL, et al. Angiotensin type 1 receptors mediate smooth muscle proliferation and endothelin biosynthesis in rat vascular smooth muscle. *J Pharmacol Exp Ther* 1994;271:429–437.
66. Rajagopalan S, Bech-Laursen J, Borthayre A, et al. A role for endothelin-1 in angiotensin II-mediated hypertension. *Hypertension* 1997;30:29–34.
67. Luft FC. Proinflammatory effects of angiotensin II and endothelin: Targets for progression of cardiovascular and renal diseases. *Curr Opin Nephrol Hypertens* 2002;11:59–66.
68. Marshall JJ, Kontos HA. Endothelium-derived relaxing factors: A perspective from in vivo data. *Hypertension* 1990;16:371–386.
69. Nerem RM, Girard PR. Hemodynamic influences on vascular endothelial biology. *Toxicol Pathol* 1990;18:572–582.
70. Dartsch PC, Betz E. Response of cultured endothelial cells to mechanical stimulation. *Basic Res Cardiol* 1989;84:268–281.
71. Howard AB, Alexander RW, Nerem RM, et al. Cyclic strain induces an oxidative stress in endothelial cells. *Am J Physiol* 1997;272: C421–C427.
72. Gimbrone MA Jr, Topper JN, Nagel T, et al. Endothelial dysfunction, hemodynamic forces, and atherogenesis. *Ann N Y Acad Sci* 2000;902: 230–239; discussion 239–240.
73. Asakura T, Karino T. Flow patterns and spatial distribution of atherosclerotic lesions in human coronary arteries. *Circ Res* 1990;66: 1045–1066.

74. Ku D, Giddens D, Zarins C, et al. Pulsatile flow and atherosclerosis in the human carotid bifurcation: Positive correlation between plaque location and low and oscillating shear stress. *Arteriosclerosis* 1985;5: 293–302.
75. De Keulenaer GW, Chappell DC, Ishizaka N, et al. Oscillatory and steady laminar shear stress differentially affect human endothelial redox state. *Circ Res* 1998;82:1094–1101.
76. Chappell DC, Varner SE, Nerem RM, et al. Oscillatory shear stimulates adhesion molecule expression in cultured human endothelium. *Circ Res* 1998;82:532–539.
77. Giancotti FG, Ruoslahti E. Integrin signaling. *Science* 1999;285: 1028–1032.
78. Takemoto M, Sun J, Hiroki J, et al. Rho-kinase mediates hypoxia-induced downregulation of endothelial nitric oxide synthase. *Circulation* 2002;106:57–62.
79. Clapham DE, Neer EJ. New roles for G-protein $\beta\gamma$-dimers in transmembrane signaling. *Nature* 1993;365:403–406.
80. Traub O, Berk BC. Laminar shear stress: Mechanisms by which endothelial cells transduce an atheroprotective force. *Arterioscler Thromb Vasc Biol* 1998;18:677–685.
81. Rizzo V, McIntosh DP, Oh P, et al. In situ flow activates endothelial nitric oxide synthase in luminal caveolae of endothelium with rapid caveolin dissociation and calmodulin association. *J Biol Chem* 1998; 273:34724–34729.
82. Berridge MJ, Irvine RF. Inositol trisphosphate, a novel second messenger in cellular signal transduction. *Nature* 1984;312:315–321.
83. Yamamoto H, van Breeman C. Inositol 1,4,5-trisphosphate releases calcium from skinned cultured smooth muscle cells. *Biochem Biophys Res Commun* 1985;130:270–274.
84. Nishizuka Y. The role of protein kinase C in cell surface signal transduction and tumour promotion. *Nature* 1984;308:693–698.
85. Brock TA, Alexander RW, Ekstein LS, et al. Angiotensin increases cytosolic free calcium in cultured vascular smooth muscle cells. *Hypertension* 1985;7:I-105–I-109.
86. Dillon PF, Aksoy MO, Driska SP, et al. Myosin phosphorylation and the cross-bridge cycle in arterial smooth muscle. *Science* 1981;211: 495–497.
87. Morgan KG. Role of calcium ion in maintenance of vascular smooth muscle tone. *Am J Cardiol* 1987;59:24A–28A.
88. Morgan KG, Gangopadhyay SS. Invited review: Cross-bridge regulation by thin filament-associated proteins. *J Appl Physiol* 2001;91: 953–962.
89. Dessy C, Kim I, Sougnez CL, et al. A role for MAP kinase in differentiated smooth muscle contraction evoked by alpha-adrenoceptor stimulation. *Am J Physiol* 1998;275:C1081–1086.
90. Je HD, Gangopadhyay SS, Ashworth TD, et al. Calponin is required for agonist-induced signal transduction—Evidence from an antisense approach in ferret smooth muscle. *J Physiol* 2001;537:567–577.
91. Winder SJ, Allen BG, Clement-Chomienne O, et al. Regulation of smooth muscle actin-myosin interaction and force by calponin. *Acta Physiol Scand* 1998;164:415–426.
92. Sward K, Mita M, Wilson DP, et al. The role of RhoA and Rho-associated kinase in vascular smooth muscle contraction. *Curr Hypertens Rep* 2003;5:66–72.
93. van Nieuw Amerongen GP, van Hinsbergh VW. Cytoskeletal effects of rho-like small guanine nucleotide-binding proteins in the vascular system. *Arterioscler Thromb Vasc Biol* 2001;21:300–311.
94. Kitazono T, Ago T, Kamouchi M, et al. Increased activity of calcium channels and Rho-associated kinase in the basilar artery during chronic hypertension in vivo. *J Hypertens* 2002;20:879–884.
95. Masumoto A, Hirooka Y, Shimokawa H, et al. Possible involvement of Rho-kinase in the pathogenesis of hypertension in humans. *Hypertension* 2001;38:1307–1310.
96. Newby AC, Southgate KM, Assender JW. Inhibition of vascular smooth muscle cell proliferation by endothelium-dependent vasodilators. *Herz* 1992;17:291–299.
97. Ettenson DS, Koo EW, Januzzi JL, et al. Endothelial heparan sulfate is necessary but not sufficient for control of vascular smooth muscle cell growth. *J Cell Physiol* 2000;184:93–100.
98. Ueba H, Kawakami M, Yaginuma T. Shear stress as an inhibitor of vascular smooth muscle cell proliferation. Role of transforming growth factor-beta 1 and tissue-type plasminogen activator. *Arterioscler Thromb Vasc Biol* 1997;17:1512–1516.
99. Clowes AW, Clowes MM, Fingerle J, et al. Regulation of smooth muscle cell growth in injured artery. *J Cardiovasc Pharmacol* 1989; 14: S12–S15.
100. Kavanaugh WM, Harsh GR, IV, Starksen NF, et al. Transcriptional regulation of the A and B chain genes of PDGF in microvascular endothelial cells. *J Biol Chem* 1988;263:8470–8472.
101. Clemmons DR. Exposure to platelet-derived growth factors modulate the porcine aortic smooth muscle cell response to somatomedin-C. *Endocrinology* 1985;117:77–83.
102. Delafontaine P. Insulin-like growth factor I and its binding proteins in the cardiovascular system. *Cardiovasc Res* 1995;30:825–834.
103. Bevilaqua MP, Gimbrone MA Jr. Modulation of endothelial cell procoagulant and fibrinolytic activities by inflammatory mediators. In: Ryan US, ed. *Endothelial Cells,* Boca Raton, FL: CRC Press; 1988:107–118.
104. Beasley D, Cohen RA, Levinsky NG. Interleukin 1 inhibits contraction of vascular smooth muscle. *J Clin Invest* 1989;83:331–335.
105. Lindner V, Lappi DA, Baird A, et al. Role of basic fibroblast growth factor in vascular lesion formation. *Circ Res* 1991;68:106–113.
106. Bashkin P, Doctrow S, Klagsbrun M, et al. Basic fibroblast growth factor binds to subendothelial extracellular matrix and is released by heparinase and heparin-like molecules. *Biochemistry* 1989;28: 1737–1743.
107. Nagai M, Kamide K, Rakugi H, et al. Role of endothelin-1 induced by insulin in the regulation of vascular cell growth. *Am J Hypertens* 2003;16:223–228.
108. Ziegler T, Bouzourene K, Harrison VJ, et al. Influence of oscillatory and unidirectional flow environments on the expression of endothelin and nitric oxide synthase in cultured endothelial cells. *Arterioscler Thromb Vasc Biol* 1998;18:686–692.
109. Seeger H, Lippert C, Wallwiener D, et al. Valsartan and candesartan can inhibit deteriorating effects of angiotensin II on coronary endothelial function. *J Renin Angiotensin Aldosterone Syst* 2001;2: 141–143.
110. Geisterfer A, Peach MJ, Owens GK. Angiotensin II induces hypertrophy, not hyperplasia of cultured rat aortic smooth muscle cells. *Circ Res* 1988;62:749–756.
111. Berk BC, Taubman MB, Griendling KK, et al. Thrombin-stimulated events in cultured vascular smooth muscle cells. *Biochem J* 1991;274: 799–805.
112. Golden MA, Au YPT, Kirkman TR, et al. Platelet-derived growth factor activity and mRNA expression in healing vascular grafts in baboons. *J Clin Invest* 1991;87:406–414.
113. Myers PR, Minor RL, Guerra R, Jr., et al. The vasorelaxant properties of the endothelium-derived relaxing factor more closely resemble S-nitrosocysteine than nitric oxide. *Nature* 1990;345: 161–163.
114. Liebow C, Reilly C, Serrano M, et al. Somatostatin analogues inhibit growth of pancreatic cancer by stimulating tyrosine phosphatase. *Proc Natl Acad Sci USA* 1989;86:2003–2007.
115. Ullrich A, Schlessinger J. Signal transduction by receptors with tyrosine kinase activity. *Cell* 1990;81:203–212.
116. Luttrell LM, Daaka Y, Lefkowitz RJ. Regulation of tyrosine kinase cascades by G-protein–coupled receptors. *Curr Opin Cell Biol* 1999;11: 177–183.
117. Kalmes A, Daum G, Clowes AW. EGFR transactivation in the regulation of SMC function. *Ann N Y Acad Sci* 2001;947:42–54; discussion 54–45.
118. Sundaresan M, Zu-Xi Y, Ferrans VJ, et al. Requirement for generation of $H_2O_2$ for platelet-derived growth factor signal transduction. *Science* 1995;270:296–299.
119. Griendling KK, Minieri CA, Ollerenshaw JD, et al. Angiotensin II stimulates NADH and NADPH oxidase activity in cultured vascular smooth muscle cells. *Circ Res* 1994;74:1141–1148.

120. Ushio-Fukai M, Alexander RW, Akers M, et al. p38MAP kinase is a critical component of the redox-sensitive signaling pathways by angiotensin II: Role in vascular smooth muscle cell hypertrophy. *J Biol Chem* 1998;273:15022–15029.
121. Ushio-Fukai M, Alexander RW, Akers M, et al. Reactive oxygen species mediate the activation of Akt/protein kinase B by angiotensin II in vascular smooth muscle cells. *J Biol Chem* 1999;274:22699–22704.
122. Deshpande NN, Sorescu D, Seshiah P, et al. Mechanism of hydrogen peroxide–induced cell cycle arrest in vascular smooth muscle. *Antioxid Redox Signal* 2002;4:845–854.
123. Sato H, Takino T, Okada Y, et al. A matrix metalloproteinase expressed on the surface of invasive tumor cells. *Nature* 1994;370:61–65.
124. Rajagopalan S, Meng XP, Ramasamy S, et al. Reactive oxygen species produced by macrophage-derived foam cells regulate the activity of vascular matrix metalloproteinases in vitro. *J Clin Invest* 1996;98: 2572–2579.
125. Galis ZS, Asanuma K, Godin D, et al. N-acetyl-cysteine decreases the matrix-degrading capacity of macrophage-derived foam cells: New target for antioxidant therapy? *Circulation* 1998;97:2445–2453.
126. Galis ZS, Sukhova GK, Lark MW, et al. Increased expression of matrix metalloproteinases and matrix degrading activity in vulnerable regions of human atherosclerotic plaques. *J Clin Invest* 1994;94:2493–2503.
127. Galis ZS, Khatri JJ. Matrix metalloproteinases in vascular remodeling and atherogenesis: The good, the bad, and the ugly. *Circ Res* 2002; 90:251–262.
128. Bendeck MP. Matrix metalloproteinases: Are they antiatherogenic but proaneurysmal? *Circ Res* 2002;90:836–837.
129. Silence J, Collen D, Lijnen H. Reduced atherosclerotic plaque but enhanced aneurysm formation in mice with inactivation of the tissue inhibitor of matrix metalloproteinase-1 (TIMP-1) gene. *Circ Res* 2002; 90:897–903.
130. Visse R, Nagase H. Matrix metalloproteinases and tissue inhibitors of metalloproteinases: Structure, function and biochemistry. *Circ Res* 2003;92:827–839.
131. Risau W, Flamme I. Vasculogenesis. *Annu Rev Cell Dev Biol* 1995;11: 73–91.
132. Luttun A, Carmeliet G, Carmeliet P. Vascular progenitors: From biology to treatment. *Trends Cardiovasc Med* 2002;12:88–96.
133. Semenza GL. Angiogenesis in ischemic and neoplastic disorders. *Annu Rev Med* 2003;54:17–28.
134. Gale N, Yancopoulos G. Growth factors acting via endothelial cell-specific receptor tyrosine kinases: VEGFs, angiopoietins, and ephrins in vascular development. *Genes Dev* 1999;13:1055–1066.
135. Yancopoulos G, Davis S, Gale N, et al. Vascular-specific growth factors and blood vessel formation. *Nature* 2000;407:242–248.
136. Luttun A, Tjwa M, Moons L, et al. Revascularization of ischemic tissues by PlGF treatment, and inhibition of tumor angiogenesis, arthritis and atherosclerosis by anti-Flt1. *Nature Medicine* 2002;8:831–840.
137. White F, Carroll S, Magnet A, et al. Coronary collateral development in swine after coronary artery occlusion. *Circ Res* 1992;71:1490–1500.
138. Banai S, Shweiki D, Pinson A, et al. Upregulation of vascular endothelial growth factor expression induced by myocardial ischemia: Implications for coronary angiogenesis. *Cardiovasc Res* 1994;28: 1176–1179.
139. Semenza GL. Surviving ischemia: Adaptive responses mediated by hypoxia-inducible factor 1. *J Clin Invest* 2000;106:809–812.
140. Frenkel-Denkberg G, Gershon D, Levy A. The function of hypoxia-inducible factor 1 (HIF-1) is impaired in senescent mice. *FEBS Lett* 1999;462:341–344.
141. Rivard A, Fabre J, Silver M, et al. Age-dependent impairment of angiogenesis. *Circulation* 1999;99:111–120.
142. Rivard A, Berthou-Soulie L, Principe N, et al. Age-dependent defect in vascular endothelial growth factor expression is associated with reduced hypoxia-inducible factor 1 activity. *J Biol Chem* 2000;275: 29643–29647.
143. Schultz A, Lavie L, Hochberg I, et al. Interindividual heterogeneity in the hypoxic regulation of VEGF: Significance for the development of the coronary artery collateral circulation. *Circulation* 1999;100:547–552.
144. Epstein S, Fuchs S, Zhou Y, et al. Therapeutic interventions for enhancing collateral development by administration of growth factors: Basic principles, early results, and potential hazards. *Cardiovasc Res* 2001;49:532–542.
145. Isner J. Myocardial gene therapy. *Nature* 2002;415:234–239.
146. Thurston G, Rudge JS, Ioffe E, et al. Angiopoietin-1 protects the adult vasculature against plasma leakage. *Nat Med* 2000;6:460–463.
147. Asahara T, Murohara T, Sullivan A, et al. Isolation of putative progenitor endothelial cells for angiogenesis. *Science* 1997;275: 964–967.
148. Asahara T, Masuda H, Takahashi T, et al. Bone marrow origin of endothelial progenitor cells responsible for postnatal vasculogenesis in physiological and pathological neovascularization. *Circ Res* 1999;85: 221–228.
149. Takahashi T, Kalka C, Masuda H, et al. Ischemia- and cytokine-induced mobilization of bone marrow-derived endothelial progenitor cells for neovascularization. *Nat Med* 1999;5:434–438.
150. Kalka C, Masuda H, Takahashi T, et al. Transplantation of ex vivo expanded endothelial progenitor cells for therapeutic neovascularization. *Proc Natl Acad Sci USA* 2000;97:3422–3427.
151. Schatteman G, Hanlon H, Jiao C, et al. Blood-derived angioblasts accelerate blood-flow restoration in diabetic mice. *J Clin Invest* 2000;106:571–578.
152. Perin EC, Dohmann HFR, Borojevic R, et al. Transendocardial, autologous bone marrow cell transplantation for severe, chronic ischemic heart failure. *Circulation* 2003;107:2294–2302.
153. Perin EC, Geng Y-J, Willerson JT. Adult stem cell therapy in perspective. *Circulation* 2003;107:935–938.
154. Rosenfeld ME. Leukocyte recruitment into developing atherosclerotic lesions: The complex interaction between multiple molecules keeps getting more complex. *Arterioscler Thromb Vasc Biol* 2002;22: 361–363.
155. Baggiolini M. Chemokines in pathology and medicine. *J Intern Med* 2001;250:91–104.
156. Pober JS, Cotran RS. The role of endothelial cells in inflammation. *Transplantation* 1990;50:537–544.
157. Tailor A, Granger DN. Role of adhesion molecules in vascular regulation and damage. *Curr Hypertens Rep* 2000;2:78–83.
158. Steeber DA, Tedder TF. Adhesion molecule cascades direct lymphocyte recirculation and leukocyte migration during inflammation. *Immunol Res* 2000;22:299–317.
159. Egashira K. Molecular mechanisms mediating inflammation in vascular disease: special reference to monocyte chemoattractant protein-1. *Hypertension* 2003;41:834–841.
160. Nakashima Y, Raines EW, Plump AS, et al. Upregulation of VCAM-1 and ICAM-1 at atherosclerosis-prone sites on the endothelium in the ApoE-deficient mouse. *Arterioscler Thromb Vasc Biol* 1998;18: 842–851.
161. Boisvert WA, Santiago R, Curtiss LK, et al. A leukocyte homologue of the IL-8 receptor CXCR-2 mediates the accumulation of macrophages in atherosclerotic lesions of LDL receptor-deficient mice. *J Clin Invest* 1998;101:353–363.
162. Lesnik P, Haskell CA, Charo IF. Decreased atherosclerosis in CX3CR1-/- mice reveals a role for fractalkine in atherogenesis. *J Clin Invest* 2003;111:333–340.
163. Griendling KK, Sorescu D, Ushio-Fukai M. NAD(P)H oxidase: role in cardiovascular biology and disease. *Circ Res* 2000;86:494–501.
164. Babior BM. NADPH oxidase: An update. *Blood* 1999;93:1464–1476.
165. Suh Y, Arnold RS, Lassègue B, et al. Cell transformation by the superoxide-generating oxidase mox1. *Nature* 1999;401:79–82.
166. Lassègue B, Sorescu D, Szöcs K, et al. Novel gp91phox homologues in vascular smooth muscle cells: Nox1 mediates angiotensin II-induced superoxide formation and redox-sensitive signaling pathways. *Circ Res* 2001;88:888–894.
167. Sorescu D, Weiss D, Lassegue B, et al. Superoxide production and expression of nox family proteins in human atherosclerosis. *Circulation* 2002;105:1429–1435.
168. Banfi B, Molnar G, Maturana A, et al. A Ca(2+)-activated NADPH oxidase in testis, spleen, and lymph nodes. *J Biol Chem* 2001;276: 37594–37601.

169. Pagano PJ, Clark JK, Cifuentes-Pagano ME, et al. Localization of a constitutively active, phagocyte-like NADPH oxidase in rabbit aortic adventitia: Enhancement by angiotensin II. *Proc Natl Acad Sci USA* 1997;94:14438–14488.
170. De Keulenaer GW, Alexander RW, Ushio-Fukai M, et al. Tumor necrosis factor A activates a p22phox-based NADH oxidase in vascular smooth muscle cells. *Biochem J* 1998;329:653–657.
171. Patterson C, Ruef J, Madamanchi NR, et al. Stimulation of a vascular smooth muscle cell NAD(P)H oxidase by thrombin. Evidence that p47(phox) may participate in forming this oxidase in vitro and in vivo. *J Biol Chem* 1999;274:19814–19822.
172. Seshiah PN, Weber DS, Rocic P, et al. Angiotensin II stimulation of NAD(P)H oxidase activity: upstream mediators. *Circ Res* 2002;91: 406–413.
173. Laufs U, Kilter H, Konkol C, et al. Impact of HMG CoA reductase inhibition on small GTPases in the heart. *Cardiovasc Res* 2002;53: 911–920.
174. Xia Y, Tsai AL, Berka V, et al. Superoxide generation from endothelial nitric-oxide synthase. A $Ca^{2+}$/calmodulin-dependent and tetrahydrobiopterin regulatory process. *J Biol Chem* 1998;273: 25804–25808.
175. Verhaar MC, Wever RM, Kastelein JJ, et al. 5-methyltetrahydrofolate, the active form of folic acid, restores endothelial function in familial hypercholesterolemia. *Circulation* 1998;97:237–241.
176. Hink U, Li H, Mollnau H, et al. Mechanisms underlying endothelial dysfunction in diabetes mellitus. *Circ Res* 2001;88:E14–E22.
177. Cyrus T, Pratico D, Zhao L, et al. Absence of 12/15-lipoxygenase expression decreases lipid peroxidation and atherogenesis in apolipoprotein e–deficient mice. *Circulation* 2001;103:2277–2282.
178. Harrison DG, Galis Z, Parthasarathy S, et al. Oxidative stress and hypertension. In: Izzo JL, Black HR, eds. *Hypertension Primer,* Baltimore: Lippincott, Williams & Wilkins; 1999:163–166.
179. Beckman JS, Koppenol WH. Nitric oxide, superoxide, and peroxynitrite: The good, the bad, and ugly. *Am J Physiol* 1996;271: C1424–1437.
180. Bech-Laursen J, Rajagopalan S, Galis Z, et al. Role of superoxide in angiotensin II-induced but not catecholamine-induced hypertension. *Circulation* 1997;95:588–593.
181. Zafari AM, Ushio-Fukai M, Akers M, et al. Novel role of NADH/NADPH oxidase-derived hydrogen peroxide in angiotensin II–induced hypertrophy of rat vascular smooth muscle cells. *Hypertension* 1998;32:488–495.
182. Marui N, Offerman M, Swerlick R, et al. Vascular cell-adhesion molecule-1 (VCAM-1) gene-transcription and expression are regulated through an antioxidant sensitive mechanism in human vascular endothelial cells. *J Clin Invest* 1993;92:1866–1874.
183. Ludmer PL, Selwyn AP, Shook TL, et al. Paradoxical vasoconstriction induced by acetylcholine in atherosclerotic coronary arteries. *N Engl J Med* 1986;315:1046–1051.
184. Freiman PC, Mitchell GG, Heistad DD, et al. Atherosclerosis impairs endothelium-dependent vascular relaxation to acetylcholine and thrombin in primates. *Circ Res* 1986;58:783–789.
185. McLenachan JM, Williams JK, Fish RD, et al. Loss of flow-mediated endothelium-dependent dilation occurs early in the development of atherosclerosis. *Circulation* 1991;84:1273–1278.
186. Minor RL, Myers PR, Guerra R, et al. Diet-induced atherosclerosis increases the release of nitrogen oxides from rabbit aorta. *J Clin Invest* 1990;86:2109–2116.
187. Mügge A, Elwell JH, Peterson TE, et al. Chronic treatment with polyethylene-glycolated superoxide dismutase partially restores endothelium-dependent vascular relaxations in cholesterol-fed rabbits. *Circ Res* 1991;69:1293–1300.
188. Harrison DG. Cellular and molecular mechanisms of endothelial cell dysfunction. *J Clin Invest* 1997;100:2153–2157.
189. Laufs U, Liao JK. Post-transcriptional regulation of endothelial nitric oxide synthase mRNA stability by Rho GTPase. *J Biol Chem* 1998;273: 24266–24271.
190. Hansson GK, Seifert PS, Olsson G, et al. Immunohistochemical detection of macrophages and T lymphocytes in atherosclerotic lesions of cholesterol-fed rabbits. *Arterioscler Thromb* 1991;1:745–750.
191. Cybulsky MI, Gimbrone MAJ. Endothelial expression of a mononuclear leukocyte adhesion molecule during atherogenesis. *Science* 1991;251:788–791.
192. Wang JM, Sica A, Peri G, et al. Expression of monocyte chemotactic protein and interleukin-8 by cytokine-activated human vascular smooth muscle cells. *Arterioscler Thromb* 1991;11:1166–1174.
193. Meager A. Cytokine regulation of cellular adhesion molecule expression in inflammation. *Cytokine Growth Factor Rev* 1999;10: 27–39.
194. Eto Y, Shimokawa H, Tanaka E, et al. Long-term treatment with propagermanium suppresses atherosclerosis in WHHL rabbits. *J Cardiovasc Pharmacol* 2003;41:171–177.
195. McDermott DH, Fong AM, Yang Q, et al. Chemokine receptor mutant CX3CR1-M280 has impaired adhesive function and correlates with protection from cardiovascular disease in humans. *J Clin Invest* 2003;111:1241–1250.
196. Ross R. The pathogenesis of atherosclerosis—An update. *N Engl J Med* 1986;314:488–500.
197. Stary HC. Changes in components and structure of atherosclerotic lesions developing from childhood to middle age in coronary arteries. *Basic Res Cardiol* 1994;89:17–32.
198. Cyrus T, Witztum JL, Rader DJ, et al. Disruption of the 12/15-lipoxygenase gene diminishes atherosclerosis in apoE-deficient mice. *J Clin Invest* 1999;103:1597–1604.
199. Barry-Lane PA, Patterson C, van der Merwe M, et al. p47phox is required for atherosclerotic lesion progression in ApoE(-/-) mice. *J Clin Invest* 2001;108:1513–1522.
200. Alexander RW. Hypertension and the pathogenesis of atherosclerosis. Oxidative stress and the mediation of arterial inflammatory response: A new perspective. *Hypertension* 1995;25:155–161.
201. Li J, Zhao SP, Li XP, et al. Non-invasive detection of endothelial dysfunction in patients with essential hypertension. *Int J Cardiol* 1997;61:165–169.
202. Panza JA, Quyyumi AA, Brush JE Jr, et al. Abnormal endothelium-dependent vascular relaxation in patients with essential hypertension. *N Engl J Med* 1990;323:22–27.
203. Panza JA, Quyyumi AA, Callahan TS, et al. Effect of antihypertensive treatment on endothelium-dependent vascular relaxation in patients with essential hypertension. *J Am Coll Cardiol* 1993;21:1145–1151.
204. Luscher TF, Vanhoutte PM. Endothelium-dependent contractions to acetylcholine in the aorta of the spontaneously hypertensive rat. *Hypertension* 1986;8:344–348.
205. Landmesser U, Cai H, Dikalov S, et al. Role of p47(phox) in vascular oxidative stress and hypertension caused by angiotensin II. *Hypertension* 2002;40:511–515.
206. Owens GK, Schwartz SM. Alterations in vascular smooth muscle mass in the spontaneously hypertensive rat. Role in cellular hypertrophy, hyperploidy and hyperplasia. *Circ Res* 1982;51:280–289.
207. Owens GK, Schwartz SM. Vascular smooth muscle cell hypertrophy and hyperploidy in the Goldblatt hypertensive rat. *Circ Res* 1983;53: 491–501.
208. Halpern W, Warshaw DM, Mulvany MJ. Mechanical and morphological properties of arterial resistance vessels in young and old spontaneously hypertensive rats. *Circ Res* 1979;45:250–259.
209. Schwartz SM, Majesky MW, Dilley RJ.Vascular remodeling in hypertension and atherosclerosis. In: Laragh JH, Brenner BM, eds. *Hypertension: Pathophysiology, Diagnosis and Management,* New York: Raven; 1990:521–539.
210. Vita JA, Treasure CB, Nabel EG, et al. Coronary vasomotor response to acetylcholine relates to risk factors for coronary artery disease. *Circulation* 1990;81:491–497.
211. Rubanyi GM. Endothelium-derived relaxing and contracting factors. *J Cell Biochem* 1991;46:27–36.
212. Majesky MW, Reidy MA, Bowen-Pope DF, et al. PDGF ligand and receptor gene expression during repair of arterial injury. *J Cell Biol* 1990;111:2149–2158.
213. Taubman MB, Rollins BJ, Poon M, et al. JE mRNA accumulates rapidly in aortic injury and in platelet-derived growth factor–stimulated vascular smooth muscle cells. *Circ Res* 1992;70:314–325.

214. Lindner V, Reidy MA. Proliferation of smooth muscle cells after vascular injury is inhibited by an antibody against basic fibroblast growth factor. *Proc Natl Acad Sci USA* 1991;88:3739–3743.
215. Cercek B, Fishbein MC, Forrester JS, et al. Induction of insulin-like growth factor I messenger RNA in rat aorta after balloon denudation. *Circ Res* 1990;66:1755–1760.
216. Fingerle J, Au YP, Clowes AW, et al. Intimal lesion formation in rat carotid arteries after endothelial denudation in absence of medial injury. *Atherosclerosis* 1990;10:1082–1087.
217. Berk BC. Redox signals that regulate the vascular response to injury. *Thromb Haemost* 1999;82:810–817.
218. Griendling KK, Ushio-Fukai M. Redox control of vascular smooth muscle proliferation. *J Lab Clin Med* 1998;132:9–15.
219. Souza HP, Souza LC, Anastacio VM, et al. Vascular oxidant stress early after balloon injury: evidence for increased NAD(P)H oxidoreductase activity. *Free Radic Biol Med* 2000;28:1232–1242.
220. Szöcs K, Lassegue B, Sorescu D, et al. Upregulation of Nox-based NAD(P)H oxidases in restenosis after carotid injury. *Arterioscler Thromb Vasc Biol* 2002;22:21–27.
221. Cote G, Tardif JC, Lesperance J, et al. Effects of probucol on vascular remodeling after coronary angioplasty. Multivitamins and Protocol Study Group. *Circulation* 1999;99:30–35.
222. Rodes J, Cote G, Lesperance J, et al. Prevention of restenosis after angioplasty in small coronary arteries with probucol. *Circulation* 1998;97:429–436.
223. Tardif JC, Gregoire J, Schwartz L, et al. Effects of AGI-1067 and probucol after percutaneous coronary interventions. *Circulation* 2003;107:552–558.
224. Tardif J-C, Cote G, Lesperance J, et al. Prevention of restenosis by pre and post-PTCA probucol therapy: A randomized clinical trial. *Circulation* 1996;94:I-91.
225. Carmeliet P. Mechanisms of angiogenesis and arteriogenesis. *Nat Med* 2002;6:389–395.

CHAPTER 8

# MOLECULAR DEVELOPMENT OF THE HEART AND VASCULATURE

Bradley B. Keller / Andy Wessels / Roger R. Markwald



The wide spectrum of congenital cardiovascular anomalies found from the prenatal period into adulthood has challenged clinicians and scientists for centuries.[1,2] Equally daunting historically have been the complex and varied descriptions of cardiac embryology and the pathogenesis of congenital cardiovascular malformations.[3–6] Fortunately, scientific advances—including the availability of cell-specific immunohistochemistry, rapid advances in molecular biologic techniques, expansion of investigations into integrated embryonic cardiovascular physiology, and, finally, dramatic improvements in the three-dimensional imaging of embryonic cardiovascular anatomy—make the specific determination of pathogenesis for most cardiovascular anomalies a realistic goal within the near future.[7–11]

The goal of this chapter is to present a condensed summary of our current understanding of the normal development of heart and vasculature and to illustrate how this knowledge allows us to define the pathogenesis of congenital cardiovascular malformations. As with all complex developmental events, cardiovascular morphogenesis must be defined in a stepwise fashion, and this chapter details many of the pivotal developmental events. Although many of the mechanisms that lead to the fully septated, four-chambered vertebrate heart are interdependent (e.g., the formation of the muscular ventricular septum and the membranous portion of the atrioventricular septum), many of these events are discussed in separate sections for clarity. It must be emphasized, however, that none of these remodeling events are isolated processes (e.g., formation of outflow tract and closure of interventricular foramen). This chapter focuses on human development; however, numerous vertebrate and invertebrate animal models are now available to accelerate the investigation of genetic and epigenetic normal and aberrant cardiovascular morphogenesis.

## MOLECULAR DEVELOPMENT OF THE HEART TUBE

### Molecular Embryo Patterning

Morphogenesis of the heart begins at the earliest stage of development with the initial patterning of the embryo to determine the three axes of the embryo: anteroposterior, dorsoventral, and left-right.

These axes are imprinted onto the cellular program as cell populations expand to form the embryo and extraembryonic tissues. Specific genes have been identified that alter axis determination in a range of species including the mouse.[12,13] Following determination of the embryo axes, subpopulations of cells are programmed in a segmental body plan. Much of our understanding of the body plan comes from developmental studies of *Drosophila,* an insect with head, thorax, and abdomen.[14] In mammals, maternal gene products control the cell through the first two cell cycles; then control switches to the embryonic genome. These patterning (homeobox) genes are arranged along the anteroposterior axis of the embryo.[15] Structural asymmetry is apparent at the blastodisk stage, when the primitive streak defines the anteroposterior axis and the dorsoventral axis is defined by the position of the yolk sac. Myocyte commitment in the chick embryo occurs in the early blastula stage, followed by clonal expansion in the bilateral heart, forming regions located in the lateral splanchnic folds following gastrulation. Recent molecular studies confirm the segmental patterning of the cardiac tube, linking gene products with morphologic boundaries between segments that eventually integrate to form the future atria, ventricles, and outflow tract in chick, mouse, and human hearts.[16]

The process of mesoderm formation is integral to the organization of the primary axis of the embryo and the differentiation of right and left sides. At the blastodisk stage of development, there are two primitive germ layers, endoderm and ectoderm; the endoderm layer then splits into splanchnic and visceral layers, with interposed mesodermal cells (Fig. 8-1). Mesoderm is formed as ectodermal cells migrate through the primitive streak coursing adjacent to Hensen's node. Hensen's node contains retinoic acid and serves as an embryonic organizer that confers information required to direct the ultimate fate of these mesodermal cells.[17] At this critical phase in cell determination, exogenous retinoic acid is extremely teratogenic. Interestingly, retinoic acid has a gradient-like effect on determination of the heart tube, with the greatest effect at the arterial pole and least effect at the venous pole.[18] Following migration, this crescent of mesodermal cells forms the precardiac region from which heart and great vessels precursor cells originate.

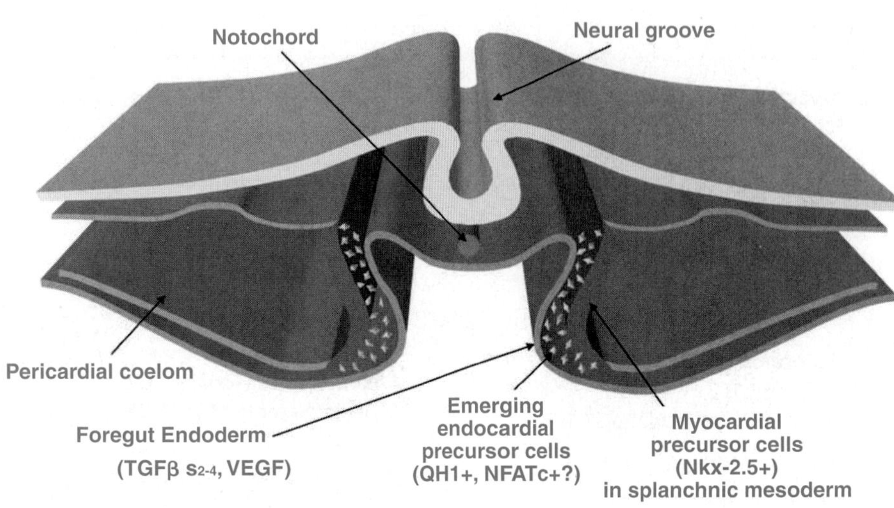


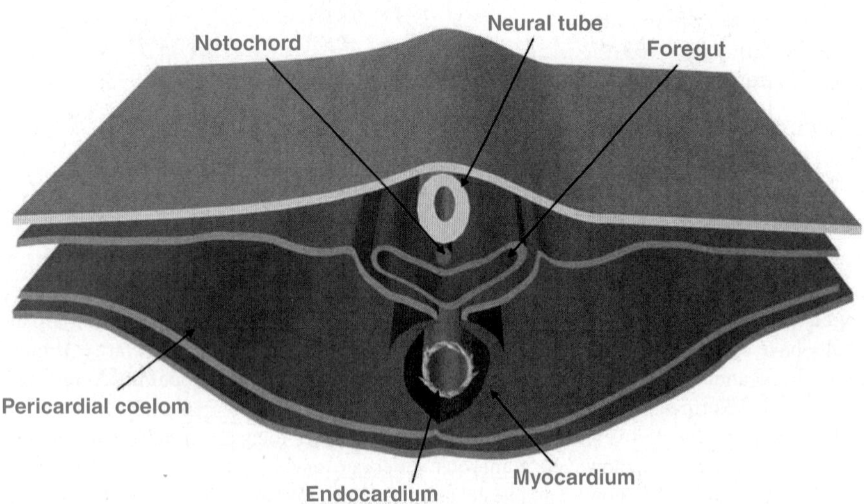


FIGURE 8-1 This figure illustrates the postgastrulation morphogenetic events involved in the formation of the tubular heart. The upper panel represents a quail embryo at stage 7/8 H/H, demonstrating the emergence of endocardial precursor mesenchymal cells, characterized by the expression of the antigen QH1 and the transcription factor NFATc, from the splanchnic mesoderm. This mesoderm is also the source for the future myocardium, which, for instance, expresses the trancription factor Nkx-2.5. It is proposed that the formation of both endocardium and myocardium are induced by growth factors, such as transforming growth factor (TGF) beta isoforms and vascular endothelial growth factor (VEGF) in the adjacent endoderm. The lower panel shows that, subsequent to the migration and assembly of endocardial precursor mesenchymal cells during stages 7 to 8 H/H, the cellular plexus coalesces to form the definitive endocardial tube enveloped by the myocardial tube. Note that the endocardium is still in close proximity to the ventral side of the foregut. (Courtesy of Yukiko Sugi, Cardiovascular Developmental Biology Center, Medical University of South Carolina.)

## Molecular Factors Involved in Cardiogenesis

Defining the molecular basis underlying the establishment and maintenance of cardiac muscle differentiation has presented a fundamental challenge in developmental biology and molecular genetics. Despite the shared expression of numerous contractile protein genes by both cardiac and skeletal striated muscles, the molecular mechanisms for cell determination, differentiation, and tissue patterning between these two "organs" are quite distinct. The following text summarizes some of the relevant information on molecular cardiogenesis and the molecular defects that are associated with structural and/or functional heart diseases in children and adults (Fig. 8-2).

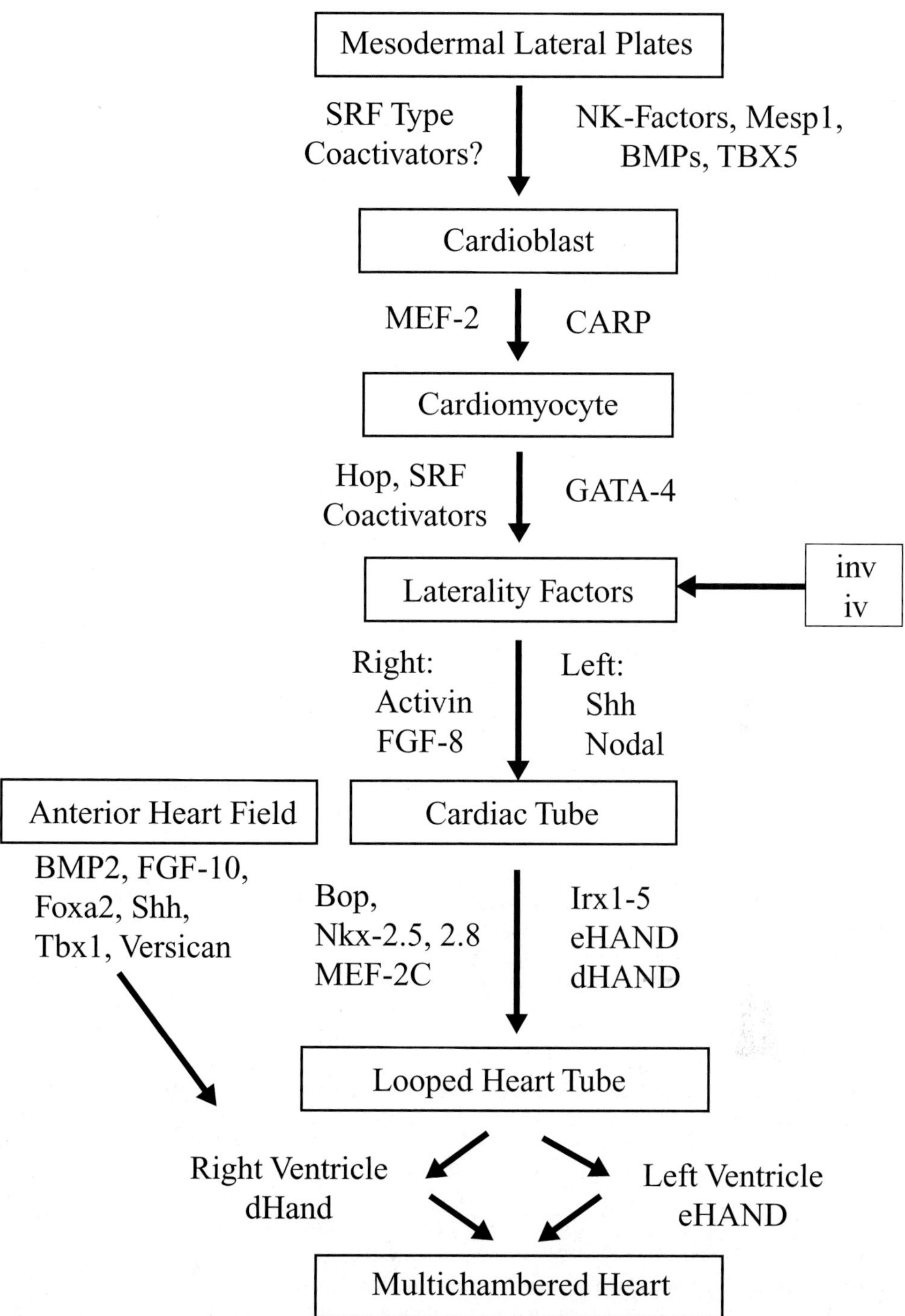


FIGURE 8-2 Schematic cascade of some of the major genes and transcription factors proven to regulate cardiomyocyte determination, differentiation, and final phenotype. This outline is intended to display the concept of temporal and spatial regulation of a complex developmental process rather than to be comprehensive, as there are now over 200 genes and proteins identified to affect cardiovascular morphogenesis.

## Basic Helix-Loop-Helix Factors and Muscle Development

One of the initial, critical discoveries related to muscle development was the observation that a specific transcription factor, Myo-D, expressed in myoblasts[19] is sufficient to convert a variety of mesodermal and nonmesodermal cell types to stable myoblasts with active muscle specific gene expression. Using Myo-D as a probe, several additional regulatory factors that specify skeletal muscle cell lineage in fibroblasts have been identified: myogenin,[20-21] Myf5,[22] MRF4-herculin, and Myf6.[23–25] These factors share extensive homology within a basic region and an HLH motif that mediate DNA-binding and dimerization, respectively.[26] HLH proteins share the ability to recognize the DNA consensus sequence CANNTG, known as an *E-box,* first identified with the immunoglobulin enhancer[26] and subsequently found in regulatory regions of most muscle-specific genes. Thus, the regulatory paradigm for skeletal muscle differentiation is centered upon the bHLH myogenic regulatory factors, but neither Myo-D, myogenin, Myf5, MRF4, or Myf6 are expressed in the heart.[27]

Additional bHLH factors are present in the developing mammalian heart. dHAND and eHAND are two bHLH transcription factors that share sequence homology in their bHLH regions and show segment-specific expression patterns.[28] In the mouse, HAND expression coincides with that of other cardiac transcription factors under the regulation of a cardiac specific SET domain protein, BOP, that interacts with histone deacetylases. dHAND expression in the myocardium is maintained throughout the straight heart tube but is restricted to the conotruncus and future RV as the heart tube forms a loop. eHAND expressed in the myocardium becomes rapidly restricted to the conotruncus and LV.[29] Expression of dHAND and eHAND precedes separation of the two ventricles, representing early chamber specification. In addition to cardiac expression, dHAND (HAND1) is expressed in early trophoblast tissue and is required for the nutritional support of the developing mouse embryo.[30] It is of interest that Nkx-2.8 has an expression pattern that overlaps eHAND, being restricted to the rostral and caudal regions of the heart tube following looping and expressed in the endoderm of the pharyngeal arches while Nkx-2.5 has a wider expression pattern within the heart. The recent deletion of dHAND by gene targeting showed that dHAND expression is necessary for RV formation.[29,31] Thus, it appears that dHAND may specify the RV and eHAND the LV. In addition, dHAND and eHAND specify RV and LV specific morphology independent of situs.[32] Expression of cardiac-specified genes, *αMHC, MLC2A, MLC2V, ANF,* and *Nkx-2.5,* were unaffected by elimination of the dHAND gene. GATA-4 in the myocardium was downregulated by dHAND-deficient hearts and appears to be a downstream target of dHAND. Elimination of dHAND or *Nkx-2.5* result in mouse embryos with single ventricles, while the double mutants lacks ventricular chamber development and fail to express the ventricular specific transcription factor Irx4.[33–35]

### *Drosophila Tinman* Is Required for Insect Heart Development

The identification of molecular mechanisms involved specifically in heart development has depended on the investigation of simpler biological models, including the fruit fly, *Drosophila melanogaster;* the zebrafish, *Danio rerio;* and the frog, *Xenopus laevis.* Homeotic genes are genes that determine a change in structure and have in common a 60–amino acid coding region. Genes with this sequence, referred to as homeobox (Hox) genes, are generally upregulated during early differentiation in a time-dependent sequence. Homeobox genes have been studied extensively in *Drosophila,* where they are involved in the commitment of cells to specific developmental pathways and play an important role in pattern formation.[36,37] Nkx-2 factors are DNA-binding proteins (transcription factors) capable of activating transcription; their 60–amino acid homeodomain comprises three helices, in which helixes II and III form a helix-turn-helix motif.[38] Helix III fits across the AT-rich major groove of the DNA binding site. Nkx-2.5 has been shown to bind to novel NKE sites,[39] certain serum response elements of the cardiac a-actin promoter,[40] and the NKE sites in the cardiac atrial natriuretic factor promoter.[41] Gajewski et al.[42] showed that two NKE promoter sites direct *Drosophila* MEF2 (dMEF2) expression in response to *tinman.* Mutations in the *tinman* gene result in loss of heart formation in the *Drosophila* embryo.[43] In addition, *tinman* is known to regulate NK-3/bagpipe expression in the visceral mesoderm[44] and the expression of dMEF2.[42] These observations suggest that *tinman* may be involved in cardiac mesoderm patterning and make it a candidate marker for cardiac mesoderm induction.

### *Tinman* and Other Related NK-2 Genes Are Required for Vertebrate Heart Morphogenesis

Murine NK homeobox genes (*NK-1/S59, NK-2/vnd, NK-3/bagpipe,* and *NK-4/msh-2/tinman* and *H6*) have been identified to have similar functions during early cardiac development in vertebrates.[37] The murine NK-2 homeobox gene *Nkx-2.5/Csx* is expressed in early cardiac progenitor cells prior to cardiogenic differentiation and continues through adulthood.[45,46] Superimposed upon the appearance of Nkx-2.5 in cardiac progenitor cells is the sequential expression of the cell type–restricted cardiac *α-actin* and *MHC* genes.[45] The Nkx-2.5 factors identified in other vertebrates such as zebrafish,[47] *Xenopus,*[48] and chickens[49] were highly related in sequence and expression pattern to the mouse gene and to cardiac development.

The similarity in expression patterns between *Nkx-2.5, XNkx-2.5, ceh-22, tinman,* and *bagpipe* suggested that the function of these genes might be conserved. Another member of the Nkx-2 family, Nkx-2.8, recently isolated from avian species, is closely related to *Xenopus,* chicken, and zebrafish *Nkx-2.5* homeoboxes and is expressed in the developing embryo in the lateral plate mesoderm and underlying pharyngeal endoderm.[50] An attractive hypothesis is that these homeodomain factors function in phylogenetically conserved myogenic pathways occurring in muscle types that do not utilize the Myo-D family. Whether the vertebrate Nkx-2.5 or other Nkx-2-related genes expressed in the early heart play a role in heart specification or whether they are downstream regulators of cardiac gene expression remains to be determined. In this respect it is interesting to note that, although it does not inhibit formation of the cardiac tube, homologous recombination knockouts of the endogenous murine *Nkx-2.5* gene do result in cardiac dysmorphogenesis at the looping stages of development and embryonic lethality.[51]

The partially overlapping expression pattern of Hox genes in embryos has led to the concept of a "Hox code."[52] The term *Hox code* means that a particular combination of Hox genes is functionally active in a region and thereby specifies the developmental fate of this region. The existence of eight Nkx-2 family members, their overlapping DNA binding specificities, and, most importantly, their partially overlapping patterns of expression raise the possibility of an "Nkx code."[50] Overexpression of Nkx-2.5 in zebrafish embryo results in an enlarged heart.[47] Thus, inactivation of the Nkx genes by homologous recombination and overexpression as transgenes offer promise to address the functional significance of the expression domains and thus also of the Nkx code. As mentioned below, patients with secundum atrial septal defect have now been identified to have specific mutations in the human homolog to the *Nkx2.5* gene.[52]

### Cardiac-Restricted Ankyrin Repeat Protein (CARP) Genes

The *CARP* gene encodes a nuclear coregulator for cardiac gene expression, which lies downstream of the cardiac homeobox gene, *Nkx-2.5,* and is an early marker of the cardiac muscle cell lineage.[53] The expression of the *CARP* gene is developmentally down regulated and dramatically induced as part of the embryonic gene program during cardiac hypertrophy. A distinct 5' cis regulatory element directs heart segment-specific expression, such as atrial versus ventricular and left versus right. In addition, a 213 base pair sequence element of the gene confers conotruncal segment-specific expression.[53] In addition, an essential GATA-4 binding site is present in the proximal upstream regulatory region of the gene and cooperative transcriptional regulation is mediated by Nkx-2.5 and GATA-4. This cooperative regulation is dependent on binding of GATA-4 to its cognate DNA sequence in the promoter, which suggests that Nkx-2.5 controls CARP expression, at least in part, through GATA-4.[53]

### SRF and MEF2, MADS Box Factors Involved with Cardiogenesis

Serum response factor (SRF) was generally assumed to be an ubiquitous and constitutive trophic factor[54] but is also highly expressed in the embryonic heart.[55] SRF represents an ancient DNA-binding protein, whose relatives shared a highly conserved DNA-binding/dimerization domain of 90 amino acids, termed the *MADS box.* SRF-related proteins capable of binding to sites found in the regulatory regions of both non-muscle- and muscle-specific genes also belong to the MADS box family of trophic factors.[56] SRF-related proteins are capable of binding MEF2 sites, CTA(A/T)4TAG, which can be found in the regulatory regions of both non-muscle- and muscle-specific genes.[57,58] Like SRF, MEF2 factors contain a MADS box and an adjacent MEF2 box. Expression and mutagenesis studies in *Drosophila* have shown that MEF2 proteins are necessary for myogenic differentiation during development[59,60] and are activated by *tinman.*[42]

In the mouse embryo, MEF2 genes are highly expressed in the early heart and skeletal muscle progenitor cells prior to the induction of cardiac and skeletal muscle structural genes, implicating MEF2 as key regulator of cardiac and skeletal muscle differentiation programs.[61–63] Four MEF2 genes have been isolated in vertebrate species and are referred to as *MEF2A-MEF2D*.[63,64] The four MEF2 gene products are highly homologous in the MADS box domain but divergent in the carboxy termini, arising from alternative splicing mechanisms. *MEF2C* shows a tissue-restricted expression pattern being expressed exclusively in skeletal muscle, brain, and spleen and is induced by myogenin in fibroblasts during myogenic differentiation in tissue cultures.[65]

## Transactivation of the Cardiac $\alpha$-Actin Gene by Nkx-2.5 and SRF

Grueneberg and coworkers[66,67] showed that human SRF interacts with a novel human homeodomain protein, Phox, which shows similarity to the homeodomains of two murine *Pax* genes. The highest similarity is to a partial murine cDNA termed S8[68] and to MHox, a novel homeodomain protein expressed in mesoderm.[69] Phox interacts with SRF to enhance the exchange of SRF with its binding site in the *c-fos* gene. Recently, it was shown that Nkx-2.5 transactivates the cardiac *α-actin* gene by binding to SRF, but only after SRF has bound to DNA.[70]

## The Role of the GATA Family and FOG Cofactors in Cardiogenesis

The GATA family of proteins has been subdivided, with GATA-1/2/3 being linked to hematopoiesis and GATA-4/5/6 thought to be involved with cardiac, gut, and blood vessel formation. Each of the six GATA proteins contains a highly specific DNA-binding domain, consisting of two C4 zinc fingers that bind to the DNA sequence element (A/T)GATA(A/G) and that may be able to interchange with each other. GATA-4 and 6 has been found to be expressed in a developmentally and lineage-specific pattern within cardiac mesoderm and gut epithelium.[71–73] GATA-5 expression is restricted to the epicardium. Experiments have shown that GATA-4 regulates expression of cardiac-specific genes, such as cardiac *troponin C*[74] and *α MHC*.[75] Mice without the *GATA-4* gene display a severe defect in formation of the cardiac tube. Several studies have demonstrated that the GATA-4 transcription factor plays an important role in regulating cardiac-specified genes and appears to be downstream to the *Nkx-2.5* gene. Transcriptional repressors have also been found to regulate cardiac development. FOG-2 a zinc-finger repressor protein, expressed in the developing heart tube, functions to suppress GATA-4–mediated activation of a cardiac-restricted gene.[76]

## Cardiogenesis, an Nkx-2-Dependent Paradigm

An attractive hypothesis from the analysis of these NK-2 homologues is that these homeodomain factors function in phylogenetically conserved pathways in muscle cell types that do not utilize the Myo-D family. Expression of Nkx-2.5 in fibroblasts demonstrated that downstream targets such as the cardiac *α-actin* gene were not directly activated by Nkx-2.5 alone but required the collaboration of additional factors, such as SRF.[40,70] Whether the vertebrate *Nkx-2.5* or other Nkx-2-related genes with SRF are sufficient to play the primary role in heart specification and serve as regulators of other downstream cardiac genes remains to be determined. It is reasonable to postulate that the vertebrate MEF2C genes and the GATA-4 factor are high in the hierarchical order of regulatory factors that in combination with Nkx-2.5 and SRF specify the cardiac cell lineage.

## Role for Bone Morphogenic Proteins in Initiating Early Myocardial Cell Differentiation

One type of signaling molecule responsible for cardiogenic commitment was recently identified to be composed of the bone morphogenic proteins (BMPs), which are members of the transforming growth factor $\beta$ family of signaling molecules. BMP-2 and -4 appear to be capable of inducing the cardiac regulatory factors Nkx-2.5 and GATA-4 when ectopically applied to regions of chick embryos that are not usually specified to become heart tissue.[49] In mice lacking the BMP-4 gene there was little or no mesoderm differentiation. Some of the mice deficient for BMP-2 gene that lacked Nkx-2.5 expression also failed to develop beyond the early stages of looping.[77] Thus, BMPs appear to have an early influence on cardiogenesis and Nkx-2.5 expression.

## Laterality of the Cardiac Tube

Correct laterality is a fundamental aspect of normal embryonic development and situs solitus has the lowest risk of congenital cardiovascular malformations.[78] The first grossly asymmetric feature to develop is the heart tube, which forms from the fusion of cardiac primordia at the midline, initiates rhythmic contractions at about day 28 in humans and then undergoes rightward looping (see Fig. 8-1). However the asymmetric expression of molecular markers occurs much earlier in development. This pattern of left-right asymmetry occurs in all vertebrate internal organs due to a signaling cascade present prior to gastrulation. The characterization of asymmetric transcription factor and gene expression prior to gastrulation is under intense investigation in zebrafish, frog, and mouse embryos. The earliest identified "morphogen" regulating L-R patterning in *Xenopus* is the asymmetric phosphorylation of syndecan-2 by protein kinase C gamma.[79,80] The critical timing of this patterning process has been shown to vary phenotype between L-R reversal and randomized L-R patterning within a one-hour window. The function of surface cilia on cells termed dorsal forerunner cells in the region of the neural tube prior to gastrulation drive unilateral extraembryonic "nodal flow" of fluid containing secreted morphogens. Mutant mouse embryos that lack the kinesin motor protein, KIF3, have immotile epithelial nodal cilia, randomized localization of the laterality gene *lefty2,* and randomized left-right determination.[81] These epithelial monocilia can be subdivided into a subclass that contain or lack the motor protein left-right dynein, lrd. The subclass of monocilia that contain lrd is targeted by the mutant *iv* gene in mice which display situs inversus.[82–84] A second mouse *inv* mutant shows consistent reversal of left-right patterning, which may be dependent in part on calcium-calmodulin signaling.[85–87]

On the right side of Hensen's node, the secreted morphogen activin represses Sonic hedgehog, *Shh,* expression and induces expression of the genes for the activin receptor and fibroblast growth factor 8. On the left side, *Shh* induces *Nodal* expression in lateral plate mesoderm and subsequent left-sided expression of the bicoid-type transcription factor Pitx2. Targeted disruption of *Pitx2c* in mice results in a complex phenotype including body plan laterality defects associated with complex cardiac anomalies associated with right atrial isomerism and complex intracardiac defects.[88] It is important to note that *Pitx2c* is also expressed later in development in the secondary heart forming field responsible for expanding and remodeling the outflow tract; therefore the "cardiac" phenotype in this mouse mutant is related to more than disrupted laterality.[89] Misexpression of the normally left-sided signals *Nodal, Lefty2* and *Shh* on the right side, or ectopic application of retinoic acid, results in upregulation of NKX-3.2 contralateral to its normal expression on the left.[90] FGF8 is an important negative determinant of asymmetric NKX-3.2 and ectopic application of FGF8 on the left side blocks NKX-3.2 expression, whereas an FGF receptor-1 antagonist implanted on the right side results in bilateral NKX-3.2 expression in the lateral plate mesoderm.[90]

## Myocardial Expansion and Differentiation

Retroviral labeling studies have demonstrated that the ventricular myocardium expands by a process of clonal expansion of myocytes within the cardiac tube as well as the recruitment of mesenchymal cells into a cardiomyocyte lineage from an anterior or secondary heart forming region.[91–94] The regulation of myocyte specification and differentiation in the anterior heart forming region likely involves cell adhesion molecules, including N-cadherin, extracellular proteases, and morphogenetic signals from the transforming growth factor beta (TGF-$\beta$) and fibroblast growth factor (FGF) families of growth and differentiation factors.[92,95–98] Recent data suggest major roles for the T-box transcription factor, Tbx-1, and both FGF 8 and FGF10 in regulating the fate of these cells in contributing to the aortic arches and expanding outflow tract.[89,99–101] The transcription factor Tbx-1 has been identified in the pharyngeal arch under the regulation of Shh and the forkhead transcription factor Foxa2. Tbx-1–expressing cells are recruited from the anterior heart-forming region to expand the developing outflow tract.[102] Cardiomyocyte maturation is associated with regionally specific gene and protein expression that correlates both with structure and function.[103] Cardiomyocyte clonal expansion and cell death are regionally regulated in response to mechanical loading conditions.[104–107]

Expansion of unique RV and LV myocardium is under the tight regulation of molecular pathways. For example, expression of the T-box gene, *Tbx5,* is responsible for the specific identity of LV myocardium via interactions with both eHAND and eHAND-sensitive elements and is negatively regulated by the related *Tbx20* gene that is normally expressed in the developing RV myocardium. When *Tbx5* expression is suppressed in the embryo, the ventricular septum does not form resulting in a single ventricle, and when expression is only partially reduced the ventricular septum is shifted rightward resulting in a small RV and enlarged LV. The differential effects of changes in Tbx expression in the embryo reflects differences between the concept of heterochrony (similar genes expressed under differential temporal schemes) versus heterotopy (similar genes with differential effects based on spatial context). Mice that lack a single copy of *Tbx-5* have the atrial septal defect and conduction abnormality found in patients with Holt-Oram syndrome and the zebrafish mutant, heartstrings, has a similar defect.[108] *Tbx-5* directly regulates forelimb development via direct activation of the Fgf-10 gene.[109–111]

## The Neural Crest and Cardiac Development

The neural crest functions as the origin for migrating pluripotent cell populations with broad developmental fates. The "cardiac" neural crest is an important migratory cell population contributing to CV morphogenesis. The cardiac neural crest arises from the dorsal margin of the neural tube prior to fusion and migrates ventrally to form the autonomic ganglia, melanocytes and Schwann cells. The crest cells move in waves through the branchial arches during the first 4 weeks of human development. The eventual fate of the neural crest cells is likely determined long before the initial phenotypic expression of a heart tube by activation of the cellular gradients of Hox genes and other morphoregulating factors.[112,113] The cranial neural crest region defines a developmental field that includes the heart, hind brain, face, and branchial arch derivatives.

Experimental disruption of cranial neural crest produces a spectrum of abnormalities. In a series of elegant ablation and chick/quail chimera studies, Kirby and colleagues defined the region of cardiac neural crest that is integral to the septation of the conotruncal region of the heart and branchial arch derivatives including facial abnormalities, thymus, parathyroid and autonomic derivatives.[112] These neural crest cells migrate to specific sites from the neural crest through the pharyngeal arches to the developing heart and carry information critical both to normal CV morphogenesis and function.

Several genes have been identified to be important in the proper migration and differentiation of the cardiac neural crest. Transgenic mouse mutants lacking the endothelin peptide, ET-1, or endothelin receptors ET-A and ET-B express abnormal cardiac neural crest phenotypes including abnormal pharyngeal arches and outflow tract septation similar to the avian neural crest ablation model.[113,114] The *splotch* mutant mouse contains a mutated *Pax-3* gene and homozygote splotch mutants have a complete neural crest ablation phenotype, including persistent truncus arteriosus and aortic arch anomalies[114,115] similar to the CV phenotype of neural crest ablation in the chick embryo. Hox gene abnormalities are also associated with defects in the derivatives of cranial neural crest.[116] A transgenic murine model of Hox 1.1 overexpression has neural crest ectomesenchymal tissue abnormalities including cleft palate, nonfused pinnae and open eyes. *Hox 1.5* deficient mice have features of DiGeorge syndrome.[113] In humans, DiGeorge syndrome, velo-cardio-facial syndrome, and conotruncal anomaly face syndrome are associated with chromosomal deletions in the 22q11 region on long arm of chromosome 22.[117–120] Recent studies have indicated a number of candidate factors being involved in the pathogenesis of these syndromes (referred to as Catch-22 syndrome), including *Tbx-1*. Interestingly, *Tbx-1* is expressed in the pharyngeal endoderm but not in migrating neural crest cells and so this gene regulates morphogenesis via second messengers, including FGF-8 and FGF-10, in determining neural crest cell fate.[121,122] Another secreted factor, semaphorin 3C, and the associated coreceptor, Plexin A2, are also required for normal migration of pharyngeal and cardiac neural crest cells.[123,124] In addition to genetic mechanisms, exogenous dosing of retinoic acid acts as a potent teratogen in humans and produces a syndrome involving all the derivatives of the cranial neural crest.[125]

## Myocyte Differentiation

In the human embryo, the heart begins to contract at day 17, as the electromechanical machinery of contraction and relaxation become functional. These functional units include the sarcomere, containing the contractile elements; the mitochondria, containing the enzymes for energy production and modulation; and the sarcolemma, including the cell envelope with specialized components of the t-tubular system linked to the sarcoplasmic reticulum. In the mature myocardium, sarcomeres are organized parallel to the lines of peak systolic stress. In the embryonic myocyte, myofibrils initially appear disarrayed and become aligned in response to mechanical load as development proceeds.[126] Confocal microscopic studies of the early looping heart reveal a circumferential pattern of premyofibril distribution with randomized surface focal adhesions.[127,128] Despite this disordered appearance, the contraction pattern of the early embryonic heart is isotropic for only a brief period and then the contraction and relaxation patterns of the embryonic heart become regionally anisotropic.[107,129] This contraction pattern also depends on the temporal and spatial expression of the rho family of small G proteins found to regulate actin cytoskeletal organization.[130]

The temporal and spatial expression of contractile proteins in the developing heart is similar across a range of species. At the precardiac tube stage, smooth muscle *α-actin* is the only isoform present. The onset of cardiac contractions is associated with a progressive increase in the expression of the cardiac form of sarcomeric actin. Smooth muscle *α-actin* may act as a scaffolding during assembly of the sarcomere.[131,132] Much additional work is required to define the regulation of myofibrillogenesis during cardiac morphogenesis.

Mitochondria multiply concurrently with the myofibrils in the differentiating myocyte. In the mature heart, mitochondrial enzymes are the major source of high-energy phosphate necessary for contraction and likely begin this function during embryonic development. In the chick, mitochondria account for about 10 percent of myocyte volume.[126] In the rat embryo, the total volume increases from 22 to 34 percent between days 6 and 10, and the mitochondria also change morphologically with development, becoming larger with more cristae and denser matrix.[133] The myocyte mitochondrial volume fraction correlates directly with heart rate and oxygen consumption among animals.[134]

Maturation of the sarcoplasmic reticulum and apparatus for excitation-contraction coupling occurs coincident with the structural morphogenesis of the embryonic heart. The sarcolemma contains ion pumps, channels, and exchangers that maintain chemical and charge differences between extracellular and intracellular spaces.[135] During maturation of the heart, the resting potential increases (becomes more negative) in both birds and mammals[136,137] and $Ca^{2+}$ influx through $Ca^{2+}$ channels may play a relatively important role in transsarcolemmal $Ca^{2+}$ influx in the immature heart.[114] However, peak $Ca^{2+}$ current density is actually decreased as compared to that measured in mature cells.[138,139] Although $Ca^{2+}$ influx by way of the $Na^+$-$Ca^{2+}$ exchanger is less important for excitation-contraction coupling in mature myocardium, $Na^+$-$Ca^{2+}$ exchange plays an important role in the developing myocyte. In contrast to the mature myocardium, T-type $Ca^{2+}$ channels also play an important role in regulating both heart rate and myocardial contractility in the embryonic myocardium.[140] The molecular regulation of ion channels has been identified in the pathogenesis of several adult dysrhythmias and this process is likely to be as critical in the regulation of ion channels and embryo fate during cardiac morphogenesis.

Relaxation, an active process by which the myocardium returns to a passive, steady state after contraction, depends on the rapid removal of $Ca^{2+}$ from troponin C, mediated primarily by active transport of $Ca^{2+}$ back into the SR. The SR $Ca^{2+}$ pump ATPase (SERCA2a) usually couples hydrolysis of ATP to active $Ca^{2+}$ transport. The rate of SR $Ca^{2+}$ uptake correlates well with the observed rate of myocardial relaxation. Regulation of SR $Ca^{2+}$ pump activity is mediated by the intrinsic SR protein, phospholamban. $Ca^{2+}$ is also removed from the myofilaments by extrusion across the cell membrane. In the steady state, the amount of $Ca^{2+}$ removed from the myocyte equals the amount entering through the $Ca^{2+}$ channels.[141]

## Segmental Basis of Heart Tube Formation

Formation of the cardiac tube is a complex morphogenetic sequence. Initially, primitive, bilateral heart tubes form from lateral plate mesoderm and each contains an inner layer of endocardium, a middle layer of cardiac jelly, and an outer layer of myocardium. At the cephalic end of the embryo (on each side of the midsagittal plane), myocytes within a section of each heart tube acquire contractile elements as the position of the heart tubes shifts to be parallel and then adjacent to each other within the cephalic part of the developing body cavity (intraembryonic coelom), ventral to the foregut. The primitive heart tubes then fuse in the ventral midline to form the linear or "straight" heart tube.[4,5,142–144]

It is important to note the primitive linear heart tube does not contain all of the cardiac segments present in the mature heart. During morphogenesis, the proximate portion of the aortic sac is incorporated into the outflow tract of the right ventricle (along with migrating neural crest cells) and the proximate sinus venosus is incorporated into developing atria. Thus, each "segment" of the mature heart arises at a unique time during embryogenesis.[145] One critical aspect of this segmental assembly and maturation of the heart is that there are temporal and spatial "windows" that are developmentally regulated, partially explaining why morphogens such as retinoic acid can also function as potent teratogens to produce a embryowide spectrum of defects depending upon the time in gestation of exposure. Another aspect of this segmental paradigm for molecular cardiogenesis is that normal cardiac morphogenesis depends on complex molecular, cellular, and mechanical interactions between the respective segments during cardiogenesis.[145]

## Cardiac Jelly and Extracellular Matrix

Prior to looping, the acellular space between the myocardium and endocardium in the heart is filled with a deformable extracellular matrix. This "cardiac jelly" forms prior to cardiac tube fusion and is closely associated with the primordial myocytes.[146] At the pretubular heart stages, the extracellular matrix contains collagen types I and IV, fibronectin, and laminin. The primordial endothelial cells destined to form the endocardium interact and migrate through this matrix during the establishment of the primitive, bilateral heart tubes. Radioactive labeling demonstrates that proteins produced in the myocardium flow toward the endocardium and are incorporated into the basal lamina.[147] The cardiac jelly has a variety of functions related to hemodynamic performance, cardiac looping, and cell migration in cardiac septation and formation of the endocardial cushion valves at the atrioventricular (AV) junction and outflow tract of the heart.

More than a hundred genes have been identified in the formation of endocardial cushions, and these genes function to either stimulate or repress competitive molecular pathways.[148] The protein composition of the cardiac jelly regulates endothelial differentiation via the TGF-$\beta$ family of peptide growth factors.[149] TGF-$\beta$2 proteins in the extracellular matrix are required to coordinate the morphogenetic changes that occur in the AV cushions by acting through second messengers, including protein kinase C and Smad6.[150] In addition, the unique radial distribution of fibronectin within the AV cushions likely serves to set up migratory pathways in the cardiac jelly. The fibronectin strands are oriented in response to mechanical stress and may serve as a template for the fibrous skeleton of the AV valve leaflets.[151–153] Some extracellular matrix proteins stimulate transdifferentiation of the endocardium in these regions by prompting endothelial cells to transform into mesenchymal cells and then migrate into the cushion matrix. Blockade of the TFG-$\beta$ type I (activin receptor–like kinase, or ALK2), type II, and type III receptors can block this cell transformation.[154,155] Smad6 negatively regulates AV cushion transformation and myocyte proliferation.[150,156] Conversely, laminin and type IV collagen are likely to be stabilizing signals or markers, since these compounds are absent in the cushion regions but their presence in adjacent regions stimulates endocardial cells to maintain epithelial integrity. Periostin, the osteoblast-specific factor 2, functions to promote the differentiation of cells along a fibroblastic cell lineage toward the formation of the primary fibrous rings in the developing heart under the negative regulation of BMP-2.[157]

The extracellular matrix also presents a complex three-dimensional, antigenic, structural environment that directly influences cell migration, differentiation, and response to cyclic mechanical loads. The temporal and spatial secretion and remodeling of the extracellular matrix influences the fate of numerous cell populations with dramatic effects on CV phenotype and function.[158–160] Errors in matrix composition and in the cellular responses to matrix molecules will be as relevant to cardiac morphogenesis as to acquired cardiac diseases in adults.

## Endocardial Maturation

The endothelial cells that make up the lining of the embryonic heart are initially arranged as a single sheet. This squamous-like sheet has the morphologic features of an active tissue, including microvilli, ruffles, and intercellular openings.[161] The endocardium participates in the formation of endocardial cushions at the AV junction and in the outflow tract.[162] Transdifferentiation of the endocardium occurs in the endocardial cushions, where cells round up, produce pseudopodia, and migrate into the cardiac jelly.[163] These cells eventually make up a portion of the fibrous skeleton of the cardiac valves. Inductive chemical signals from the myocardium contribute to the endocardial transdifferentiation and regulate the migration of the mesenchymal cells.[163] In addition, hemodynamic alterations can influence the orientation of endocardial cells on the endocardial cushions[164,165] and the loci of dead and dying cells in the chick and zebrafish embryos.[166] These interactions are similar to the relationship between the endothelium and smooth muscle of the mature vascular bed.[167] Endocardial cells are also involved in patterning and remodeling of the developing outflow tract under the regulation of nuclear transcription factor NFATc1.[168] Finally, expansion of the endocardium is critical to the process of ventricular trabeculation, as discussed below.

## Looping

Following the formation of the straight heart tube, the human embryo is about 2 mm long and 23 days old. At the cephalic (or cranial) end of the myocardial heart tube, the nonmyocardial aortic sac can be recognized. The aortic sac is connected to the first pair of aortic arches and, later, also to the second, third, fourth, and sixth arches (the fifth pair of aortic arches does not normally develop in mammals). The caudal end of the myocardial tube receives the paired confluence of veins that lie extrapericardially and embedded in mesenchyme. In the early tubular stage, the heart hangs suspended from the ventral foregut by a dorsal mesocardium. During heart tube looping, the midportion of the dorsal mesocardium disintegrates, leaving the heart connected at the anterior pole at the level of the aortic sac and at the posteriorly located venous pole (atria and sinus venosus). At least three distinct biomechanical mechanisms may act in combination to generate the characteristic rightward bend in the cardiac tube: locally constrained growth, active cell deformation and the release of the prestressed dorsal mesocardium.[169]

As the tubular heart continues to grow, it bends to the right and anteriorly (Fig. 8-3). This results in a compound sigmoid structure with a d-loop (dextro- or rightward) configuration. At this stage it is easy to distinguish the sinus venosus, the common atrium, the atrioventricular canal, the future LV and RV, and the outflow segment. Internally, the developing muscular interventricular septum is recognizable, its crest characteristically expressing the molecular marker GLN2/HNK-1.[170,171] It is important to note that, at this stage, all the future segments of the heart are still basically connected in series and that the common atrium connects via the atrioventricular canal exclusively to the LV, while the outflow tract is exclusively committed to the RV (Fig. 8-4.) If cardiac morphogen-

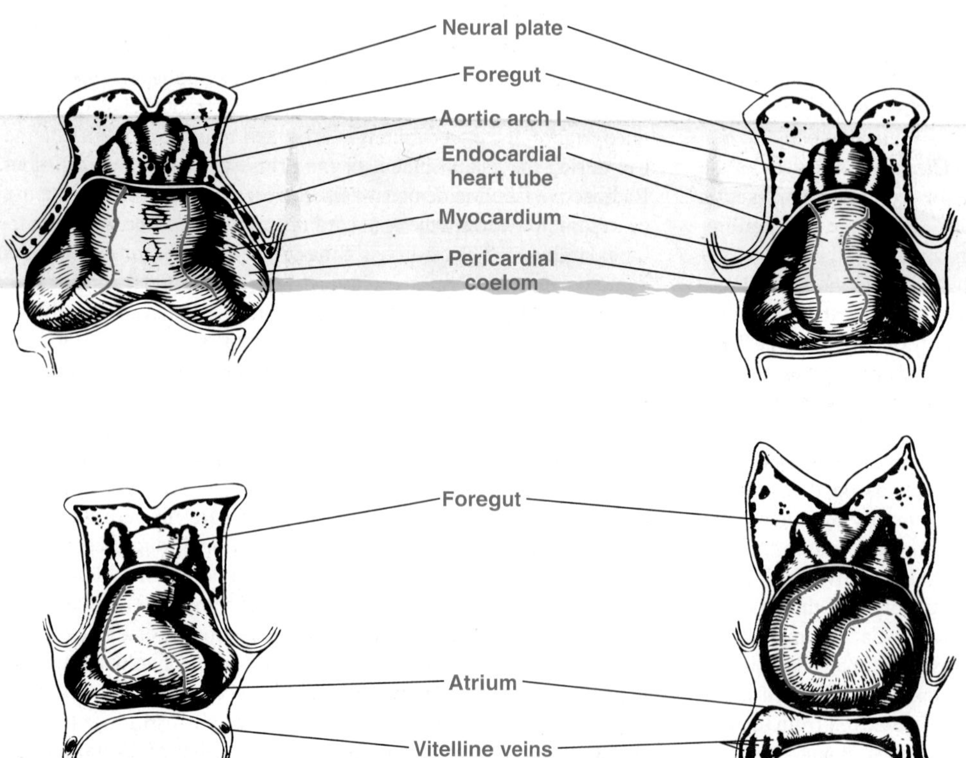


FIGURE 8-3 Schematic ventral dissections of human embryos of different ages, showing formation of the heart loop. (Adapted from CL Davis: Development of the human heart from its first appearance to the state found in embryos of 20 paired somites. *Contrib Embryol* 1927;19:245. Reproduced with permission from the Carnegie Institution of Washington, D.C.)

esis fails to progress beyond this state, then the cardiac anatomy will include a double-inlet left ventricle (DILV) and a double-outlet right ventricle (DORV), as discussed further on in this chapter.

The transition from a tubular heart, in which the future segments are arranged in series (atrium to LV to RV to outflow tract), into a four-chambered heart, in which the definitive chambers are arranged in parallel separated by septa and valves, raises two important questions. The first is how the right atrium becomes connected to the RV and the second is how the LV gains access to the aortic portion of the outflow tract. The remodeling of the so-called inner curvature of the looping heart tube plays an important role in this process and involves a rightward expansion of the AV canal and a concomitant leftward shift of the aorta. Immunohistochemical studies have demonstrated that this remodeling is intimately related to the development of the so-called primary ring (Fig. 8-5).[170,171] In the postnatal human heart, derivatives of the primary ring are found in the AV conduction system, in the right AV junction (the right AV ring), and behind the aorta (the retroaortic root branch) (Fig. 8-6).[171]

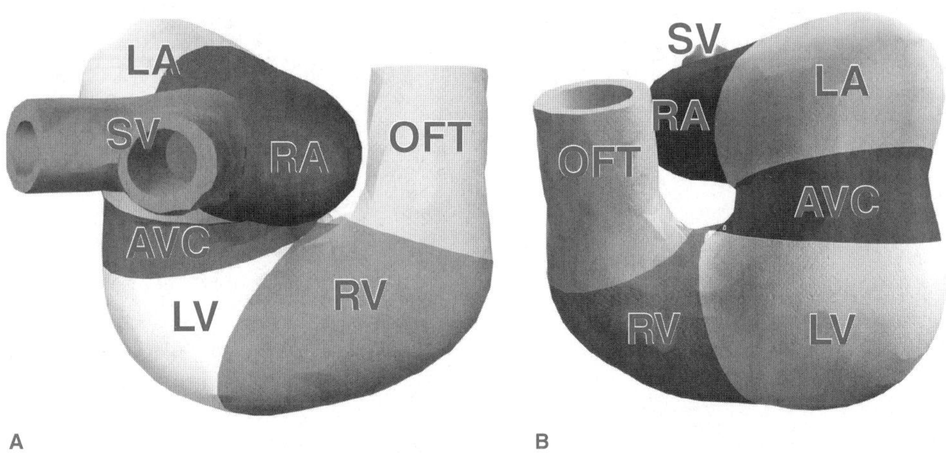


FIGURE 8-4 Schematic representation of the tubular heart during looping. *A* and *B.* Inferior and superior views of the heart. Note that at this stage (approximately 4 weeks of development in the human), all the segments are more or less arranged in series. From inflow to outflow: SV = sinus venosus, RA = right atrium, LA = left atrium, AVC = atrioventricular canal, LV = left ventricle, RV = right ventricle, OFT = outflow tract.

## STRUCTURAL ANOMALIES

***Ventricular Inversion with Transposition of the Great Arteries*** If the cardiac tube loops to the left and anterior (L loop) rather than to the right and anterior, most of the structures adjacent to and including ventricular segments of the heart tube (the AV valves, ventricles, and arterial roots) will develop in an inverted position. Subsequently the right atrium is connected via a morphologic mitral valve to a morphologic left ventricle and the left atrium is connected via a morphologic tricuspid valve to a morphologic right ventricle. Within the aortic sac, the aorticopulmonary septum develops in a normal fashion. However, as partitioning of the inverted conotruncus (outflow track) takes place in mirror image, the end result is L-transposition of the great arteries, with the aorta arising anteriorly from a left-sided, morphologically right (systemic) ventricle and the pulmonary trunk arising posteriorly from a right-sided, morphologically left (venous) ventricle. Because systemic and pulmonary venous return are still routed to the pulmonary and systemic arterial circulations, respectively, this anomaly is commonly referred to as "corrected" transposition.

***Double-Outlet Right Ventricle*** This anomaly is due to a failure in the leftward repositioning of the aortic portion of the outflow tract, resulting in persistence of the more "primitive" embryonic morphology in which the entire outflow tract originates from the right ventricle. One morphologic hallmark of the failure of completion of the leftward shift of the aorta is the presence of myocardial tissue between the left AV valve and the aorta (mitral-aortic separation). This anomaly is found following a wide range of hemodynamic, metabolic, and genetic insults to the embryo, suggesting that the phenotype of double-outlet right ventricle may be a final common expression of a range of primary abnormalities that result in persistence of the embryonic configuration.[172]

### Myocardial Trabeculation

The processes of primary myocardial trabeculation, expansion of secondary and tertiary myocardial trabeculae, and myocardial compaction are critical to the structural maturation of the ventricular chambers. This process results in the transformation of the smooth walled endocardial lining into complex three-dimensional structure of the right and left ventricular myocardium. Rapid cell division and interposition of endothelial cells along the right and left ventrolateral borders of the endocardial tube is associated with a rapid resorption of cardiac jelly resulting in myocardial ridges and trabeculae lined with single layers of endocardial cells.[173] The initial number and orientation of the myocardial ridges differs between species.[174] In general, myocardial trabeculation begins at the ventricular outer curvature (future apex) and then extends proximally and distally. The intersection between the outer, compact myocardium and the base of the trabeculae is likely a site of peak wall stress and myocyte division is most active at this site.[175,176] Retroviral marker studies have also shown that ventricular myocardial growth is associated with a transmural distribution of clonally related myocardial cells extending from the epi- to endocardium.[91,92] Of note, these cells reside in muscle bundles that are oriented at an angle to the longitudinal axis of the heart, consistent with the adult myocardial architecture, which results in efficient twist and contraction.[91,92] However, the mechanisms that regulate clonal myocardial expansion and compaction remain undefined.

With the onset of myocardial trabeculation, diverticula first appear as two sharply defined areas along the right and left ventrolateral borders of the endocardial tube (Fig. 8-7).[177] These diverticula develop initially at the expense of the cardiac jelly and later also penetrate the myocardium as the latter increases in thickness, producing a spongy mass of trabeculae.[173] The filling capacity of the heart is increased by the added intertrabecular spaces. The trabeculating embryonic heart can now be divided into primitive right and left

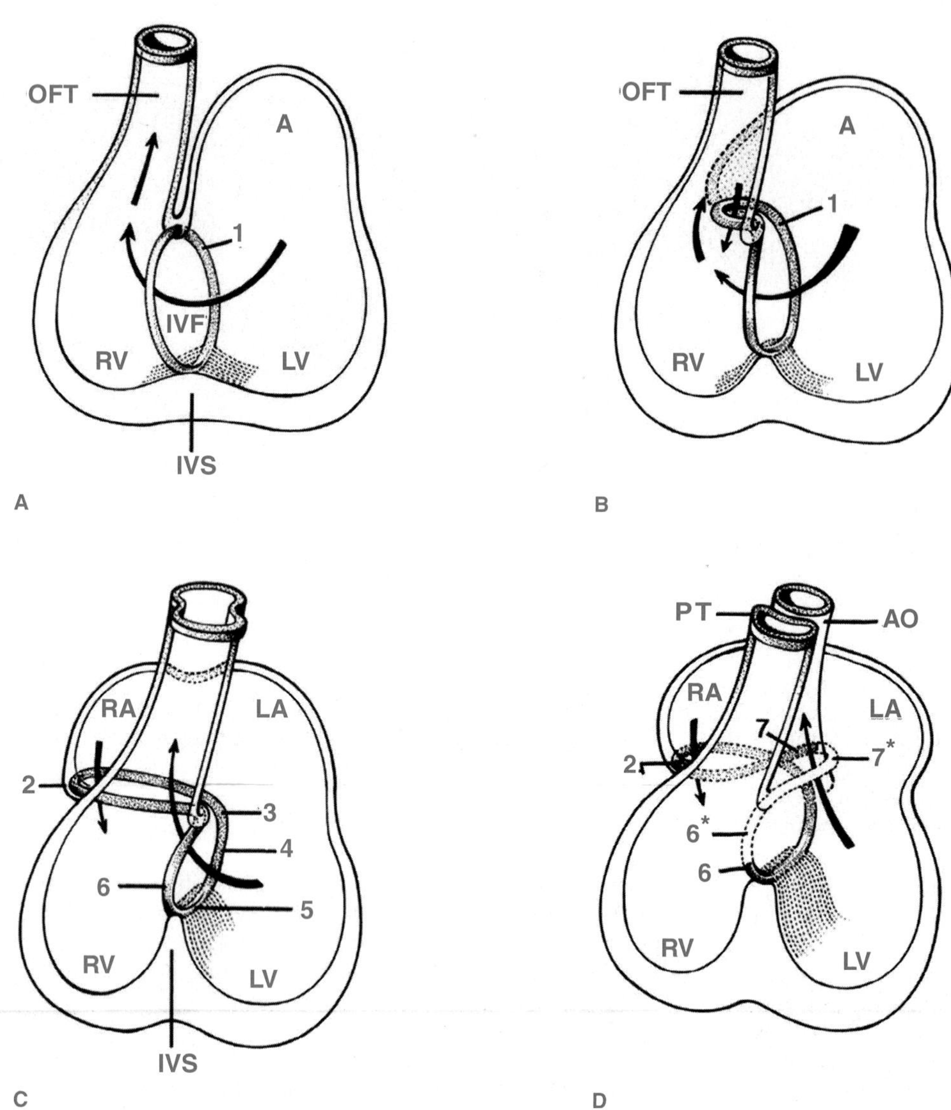


FIGURE 8-5 Schematic representation of the location of the "primary ring" (characterized by the expression of the antigen G1N2) in different stages of human development. The drawings illustrate the development of the conduction system as a derivative of the primary ring but also show that the changes in the topography of the ring-tissue is reflecting (1) the rightward expansion of the atrioventricular canal and (2) the leftward shift ("wedging") of the developing aorta. 1 = primary ring, 2 = right atrioventricular ring, 3 = atrioventricular nodal area, 4 = penetrating His bundle, 6 = septal branch, 7 = retroaortic branch. Those areas marked with an asterisk have lost their expression. The Carnegie stages of development presented in drawings A to D are as follows: A = stage 14, B = stage 15, C = stage 17, D = stage18–19. (Adapted from Wessels et al.[170])

ventricles, as there are distinct morphologic differences between the trabecular architecture of the developing ventricular chambers. The developing left ventricle is trabeculated along the majority of its greater curvature, while the developing right ventricle has a significant portion of the greater curvature that is smooth-walled.[178] At this stage of development, the embryo is approximately 3 mm long and has an ovulation age of about 25 days.[142] The common outflow tract of the developing heart can be classified as having a proximal (conus) segment and a distal (truncus) segment. The conus eventually septates into the outflow portions of each ventricle as the fused conal cushions become "myocardialized" to form the muscular portion of the outlet septum. The truncus contributes to the formation of the semilunar valves and to the development of the aortic and pulmonary roots. Migrating neural crest cells contribute to aortic sac and septation of the distal truncus.

## STRUCTURAL ANOMALIES

***Noncompaction of the Ventricular Myocardium*** Noncompaction of the ventricular myocardium is a rare familial congenital cardiomyopathy resulting from incomplete compaction of the trabecular embryonic myocardium.[179,180] The characteristic echocardiographic findings consist of multiple prominent myocardial trabeculations and deep intertrabecular recesses communicating with the left ventricular cavity. The disease uniformly affects the left ventricle, with or without concomitant right ventricular involvement, and results in systolic and diastolic ventricular dysfunction and clinical heart failure. Recent studies have characterized this disease in both children and adults. A higher incidence of Wolff-Parkinson-White syndrome was found in the children, whereas left bundle branch block was rarer in children than reported in adults. Familial recurrence is high.[181] Recently, a case of ventricular noncompaction was identified in a patient who also had a haplotype deletion on the long arm of chromosome 5.[182] The affected region included the locus for *Nkx-2.5,* the cardiac-specific homeobox gene, suggesting an association between ventricular myocardial noncompaction and haploinsufficiency of *Nkx-2.5.*

## MECHANISMS OF CARDIAC SEPTATION

### Cardiac and Extracardiac Orientation

Because of rapid growth and the progressive curvature of the longitudinal axis of the embryo during organogenesis, it is critical to define cardiac morphogenesis, including septation, with reference to extracardiac morphologic landmarks that relate to the longitudinal axis of the embryo.[183] In the following discussion on cardiac septation, therefore, the diaphragm (septum transversum) is assumed to maintain an approximately horizontal position, as in the mature heart. The terms *anterior, posterior, superior,* and *inferior* are employed accordingly. Although the formation of the various cardiac septa occurs almost simultaneously, for clarity it is necessary to consider their development separately.

## Cardiac Septation

Cardiac septation involves the formation of several septal (myocardial and mesenchymal/fibrous) and valvar structures. All the original tissues of the tubular heart (myocardium, endocardium, endocardial cushion tissues) as well as the "extracardiac" cell populations, which arrive in the heart at relatively late stages of development (neural crest, epicardium, ventral neural tube cells), appear to play a role during valvuloseptal morphogenesis. Multiple genetic factors—including *Tbx-5, Nkx-2.5, Evc,* and *Prk-AR1*—have been identified in patients with abnormal atrial morphogenesis.[184]

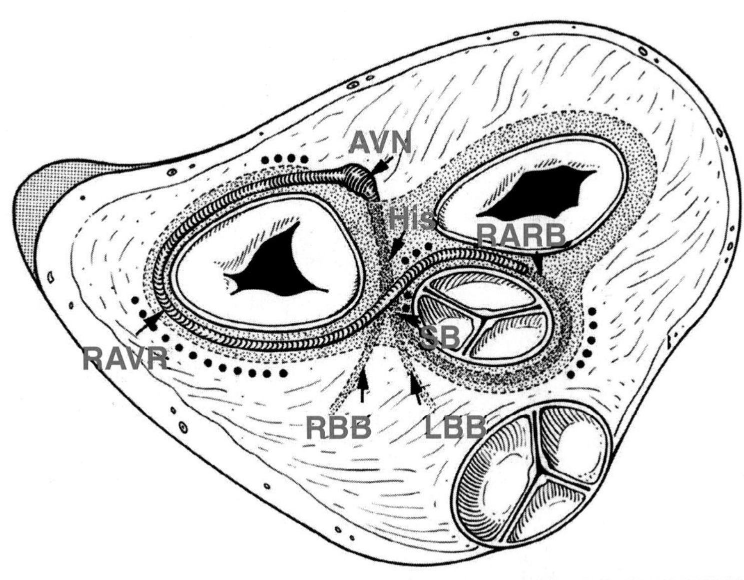


FIGURE 8-6 Schematic representation of the localization of remnants of the primary ring in the neonatal human heart. The ring is projected on a superior view of the aortic mitral fibrous unit of the heart. The black dots indicate the areas in which remnants of the ring are detected in a series of neonatal hearts as described in Wessels et al.[171] AVN = atrioventricular node, His = bundle of His, LBB = left bundle branch, RARB = retroaortic root branch, RAVR = right atrioventricular ring, RBB = right bundle branch, SB = septal branch.

## The Sinus Venosus

In the 3-mm human embryo, the sinus venosus consists of a central transverse portion and of the right and left sinus horns (Fig. 8-8). The sinus venosus receives three pairs of veins: the omphalomesenteric (vitelline) veins, the umbilical (allantoic) veins, and the common cardinal veins. The proximal portions of the umbilical veins soon disappear. As a result of the increased blood flow associated with the right and left systemic veins, the right sinus horn and proximal cardinal and vitelline veins attain a vertical position, increase in size, and form the smooth-walled, intercaval part of the atrium. The transverse

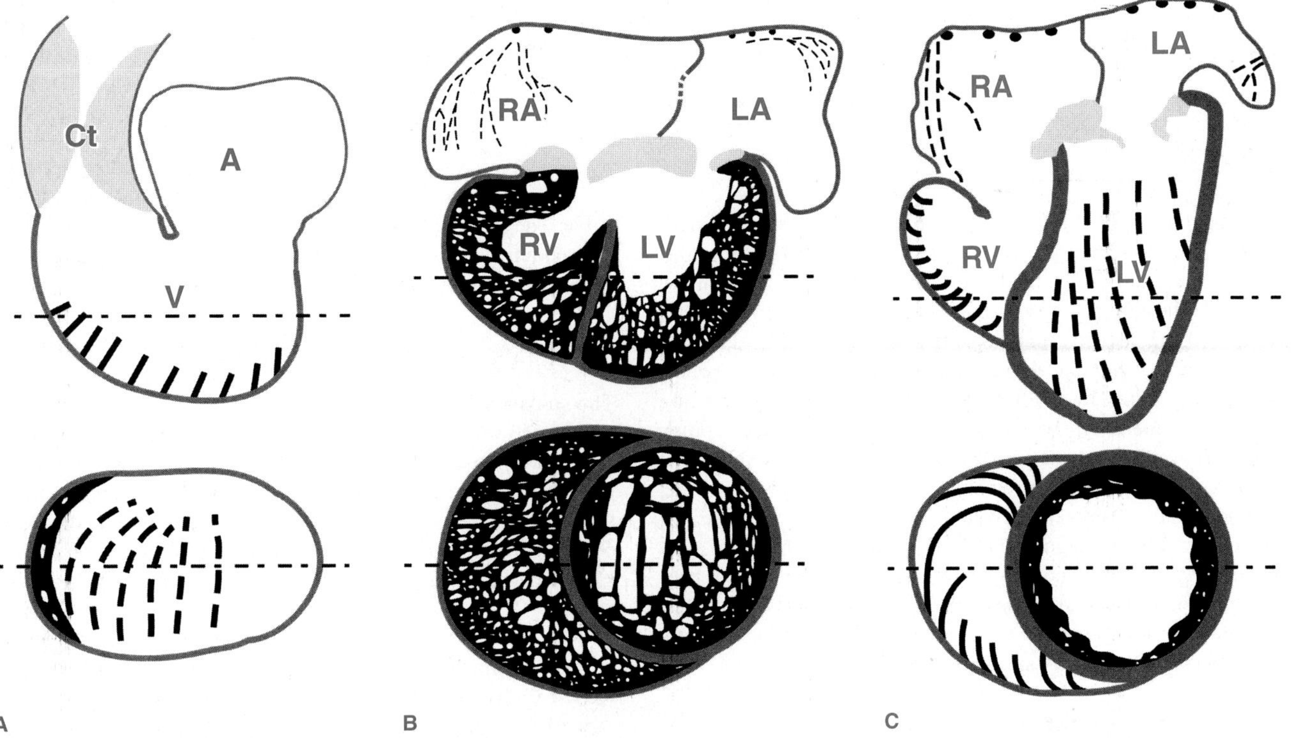


FIGURE 8-7 Schematic representation of myocardial trabecular development in the chick embryo. The top row of diagrams represents frontal (four-chamber) long-axis views; the bottom row of diagrams represents transverse (two-chamber) short-axis views. *A*. At the onset of ventricular trabeculation (around Hamburger-Hamilton stage 17), the trabeculation process is limited to the apex of the primitive ventricle (V), while the inner curvature of the cardiac loop, the primitive atrium (A), and the conotruncus (Ct) remain smooth. *B*. Pattern of secondary trabeculae (around Hamburger-Hamilton stage 29). A complex three-dimensional network of fine trabeculae fills most of the ventricular cavities. LA = left atrium; LV = left ventricle; RA = right atrium; RV = right ventricle. *C*. Mature tertiary trabecular pattern (Hamburger-Hamilton stage 45). In both ventricles, the trabeculae are arranged in a counterclockwise apicobasal spiral (viewed from base to apex). Differences between the right and left ventricle relate primarily to geometric differences (cone/crescent versus cylinder/prolate ellipsoid). The trabeculae and pectinate muscles in the atria are shown in black, the rest of the myocardium in dark gray, and mesenchymal structures in light gray. (Adapted from Sedmera et al.[192])

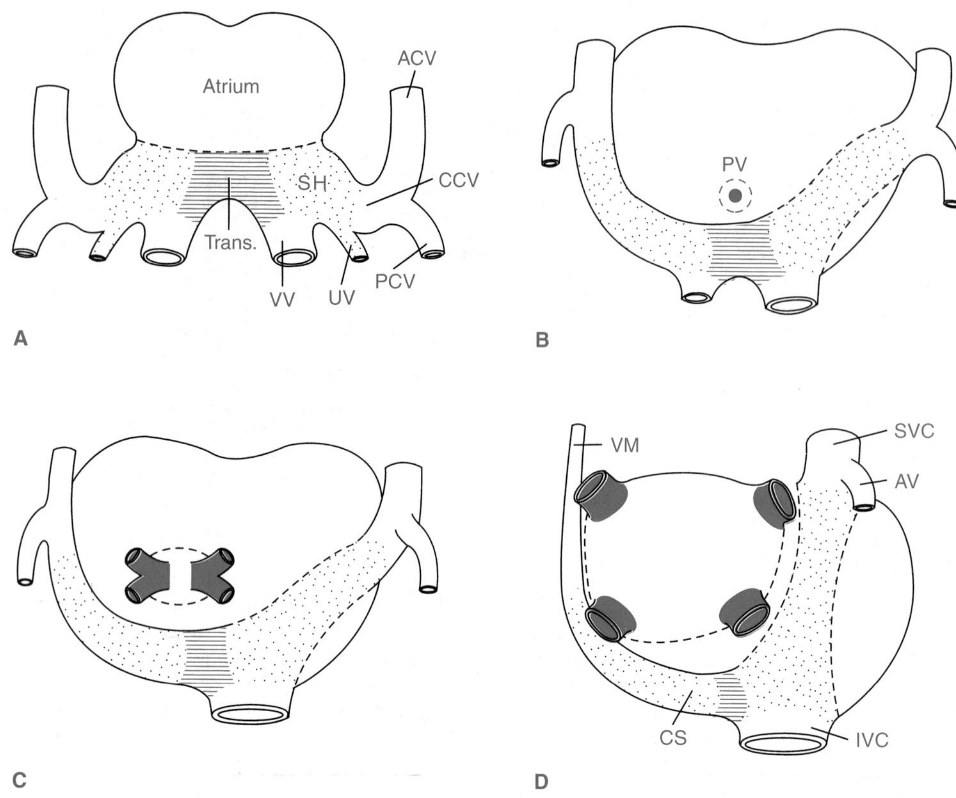


FIGURE 8-8 Posterior view of the atria and sinus venosus in embryos. *A*. 3 mm CR length; *B*. 5 mm CR length; *C*. 12 mm CR length; *D*. Newborn, diagrammatic view. A(C)CV = anterior (common) cardinal vein; AV = azygos vein, CS = coronary sinus, IVC = inferior vena cava, PCV = posterior cardinal vein, PV = pulmonary vein, SH = sinus horn, trans. = transverso portion, UV = umbilical vein, VM = vein of Marshall, VV = vitelline vein. (From Van Mierop LHS, Wiglesworth FW. Isomerism of the cardiac atria in the asplenia syndrome. *Lab Invest* 1962;11:1303. Copyright by the U.S. and Canadian Academy of Pathology.)

portion and the proximal left sinus horn become the coronary sinus. Infolding of the sinoatrial junctional tissue at the right border of the sinoatrial foramen results in the formation of the right venous valve.[185,186] The left valve develops as a result of active growth, similar to that of the primary atrial septum (i.e., the left valve does not develop as a fold) (see Fig. 8-9). Thus, the vertical sinoatrial orifice is flanked on each side by a valve-like structure in the 4- to 6-mm human embryo. Superiorly, the venous valves join to form the septum spurium. The venous valves, particularly the right venous valve, are relatively large in the 16-mm embryo. The superior aspect of the right venous valve eventually develops into the crista terminalis, or terminal crest. The left sinus valve fuses partly with the atrial septum. Inferiorly, the left venous valve intersects with the inferior part of the right venous valve. As a result, the right venous valve becomes divided into the relatively large inferior vena caval (or eustachian) valve and a smaller coronary sinus (or thebesian) valve.

## STRUCTURAL ANOMALIES

***Cor Triatriatum Dexter*** Complete persistence of the right venous valve of the embryonic heart produces a septum in the right atrium separating the intercaval part of the right atrium from the atrial body. The remaining opening may be quite small and restrictive.

***Persistent Left Superior Vena Cava*** Persistence of the left common cardinal vein and left sinus horn results in a left superior vena cava draining into the coronary sinus.

## Atrial Septation

Septation of the embryonic common atrium involves two distinct mechanisms.[185] The primary atrial septum (septum primum) forms by active growth of a myocardial septum. Initially the primordium of this septum can be seen as a ridge in the medial roof of the common atrium. The leading edge of the ridge is covered with a mesenchymal cap termed the *spina vestibuli*, which is contiguous superiorly with the superior AV cushion and inferiorly with the inferior AV cushion. As the primary septum descends from roof of the atrium toward the atrioventricular canal, thereby decreasing the size of the primary interatrial foramen, the mesenchymal leading edge continues to fuse with the AV cushions, which themselves are also in the process of fusing. These events result in closure of the primary interatrial foramen (or ostium primum) and the formation of the central fibrous body (Fig. 8-10). Concomitantly, perforations appear in the superior aspect of the primary. The perforations coalesce, resulting in the secondary atrial foramen (or ostium secundum). Next, the secondary atrial septum develops as an infolding of the atrial roof located between the primary septum and the left venous valve. The foramen ovale is the opening bordered by the free edge of the septum secundum. After fusion of the septum primum with the septum secundum, the foramen ovale becomes the fossa ovalis.

## Development of the Pulmonary Veins

The so-called pulmonary pit, the future portal of entry for the main pulmonary vein, is recognizable at around 28 days of human gestation and is situated in the midline of the inferior portion of the common atrium. The orifice of the nonlumenized common pulmonary vein is positioned within the sinus venosus segment and development of the muscular septum primum and ventral proliferation of the dorsal mesocardium positions the common pulmonary vein in the left atrium.[187,188]

Remodeling of the tissues surrounding the pulmonary pit results in incorporation of the ostium of the pulmonary vein in the wall of the left ventricle. The rightward wall of the common pulmonary vein contributes to the posterior part of the atrial septum and is continuous with the dorsal sinoatrial fold (future left venous valve).[187]

## STRUCTURAL ANOMALIES

***Atrial Septal Defect at the Fossa Ovalis*** This defect, often referred to as a secundum-type atrial septal defect, is due to malformation of the primary atrial septum, resulting in an oversized ostium secundum. Frequently, the atrial defect is further enlarged by a hypoplastic septum secundum. Total absence of both septum primum and septum secundum (common atrium) is rare and almost always associated with a form of persistent AV canal.

***Sinus Venosus Defect*** Deficiency of the wall of the common pulmonary vein results in communication between the pulmonary veins, left atrium, and right atrium. This defect can be located superior and posterior (superior sinus venosus defect) and is commonly associated with preferential drainage of the right upper lobe pulmonary vein into the right atrium. Less frequently, the defect is inferior and posterior (inferior sinus venosus defect) and is associated with drainage of the right lower lobe pulmonary vein to the right atrium.

***Anomalous Pulmonary Venous Connection*** The total form of anomalous pulmonary venous connection presumably is due either to lack of development or to a premature involution of the common pulmonary vein. A number of types of pulmonary venous to systemic venous connections occur, depending on which of the early embryonic channels connecting the pulmonary venous bed to the systemic venous circulation remains patent. In addition to the abnormal anatomic connection between the pulmonary veins and the heart, there is usually an intrinsic dysregulation of pulmonary venous growth and remodeling, which results in inadequate pulmonary venous growth despite "successful" surgical management. The mortality associated with anomalous pulmonary venous connections remains high due to recurrent pulmonary vein stenosis and secondary pulmonary hypertension.

***Cor Triatriatum Sinister*** If incorporation of the common pulmonary vein into the left atrium does not take place and the common pulmonary venous ostium remains narrow, the result is a septum-like structure that might derive from the left pulmonary ridge and divides the left atrium into two components: one receiving the pulmonary veins and the other giving access to the mitral valve and left atrial appendage.

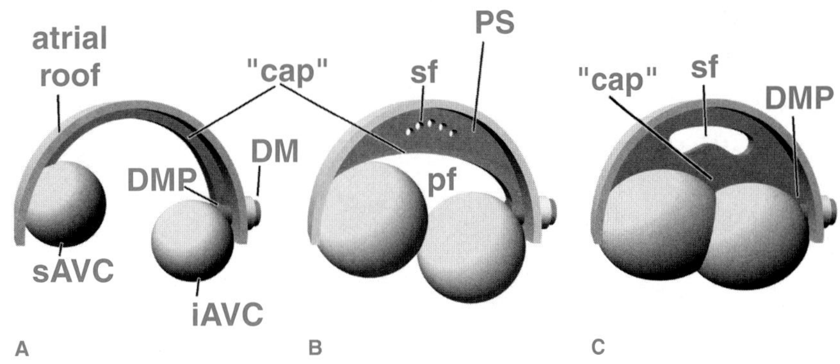


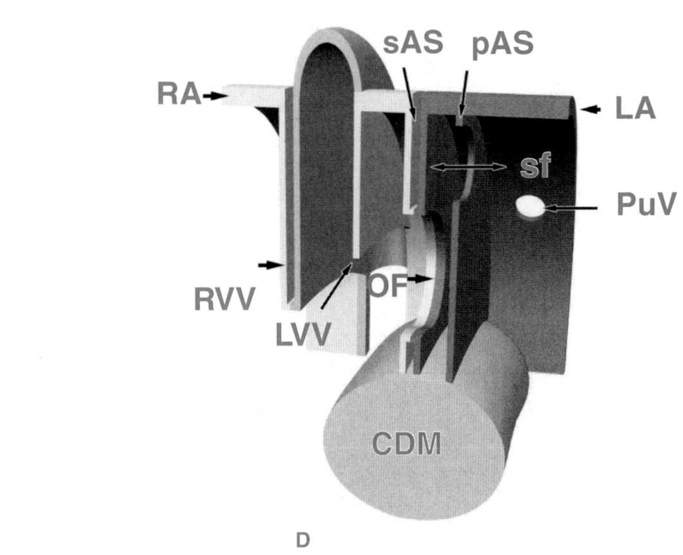


FIGURE 8-9 A model for the development of the atrial septal complex in the human heart. *A*. A heart at approximately 4 1/2 weeks of development. The atrioventricular cushions can be distinguished but have not yet fused. The leading edge of the primary septum is covered by a mesenchymal cap, which is in continuity with the dorsal mesenchymal protrusion of the dorsal mesocardium. *B*. A heart at approximately 6 weeks of development. The leading edge of the primary atrial septum, covered with a mesenchymal cap, is now approaching the atrioventricular cushions, which themselves are in the process of fusing. Within the myocardial portion of the primary septum, multiple fenestrations represent the developing secondary foramen. Completion of fusion of the mesenchymal tissues, at 6 to 7 weeks of development (as seen in *C*) results in the closure of the primary interatrial foramen. At this time a prominent secondary foramen can be found within the superior portion of the primary septum. *D*. Schematic diagram showing the formation of the atrial septum and venous valves. Formation of the secondary atrial septum results from infolding of the atrial roof. This occurs at the margin between myocardium with left and right atrial expression domain. The myocardium of the primary atrial septum is part of the left atrial expression domain; the orifice of the pulmonary vein is also surrounded by myocardium with a left atrial molecular phenotype. This panel also illustrates that, based on the gene expression patterns, the left venous valve develops as a myocardial structure with a right atrial molecular phenotype, whereas the right venous valve (like the secondary atrial septum) develops by infolding, in this case of the junctional tissue between the right atrium and the sinus venosus. (From Wessels et al.[185]) iAVC = inferior atrioventricular cushion, sAVC = superior atrioventricular cushion, DM = dorsal mesocardium, DMP = dorsal mesenchymal protrusion, pf = primary foramen, PS = primary atrial septum, sf = secondary foramen, LA = left atrium, RA = right atrium, OF = oval fossa, pAS = primary atrial septum, sAS = secondary atrial septum, PuV = pulmonary vein, LVV = left venous valve, RVV = right venous valve.

## The Atrioventricular Canal

Division of the AV canal into left- and right-sided orifices occurs as a result of fusion of the superior and inferior AV cushions, which are first evident in the 6-mm CR-length human embryo. At this stage, the common AV canal is located exclusively over the left ventricle. The superior aspect of the developing interventricular septum is continuous with the right aspect of the AV junctional myocardium. The communication between the developing right atrium and right ventricle is established by the rightward expansion of the AV canal. This expansion, combined with tissue remodeling, brings the right margin of the original AV junction, still being in continuity with the posterior part

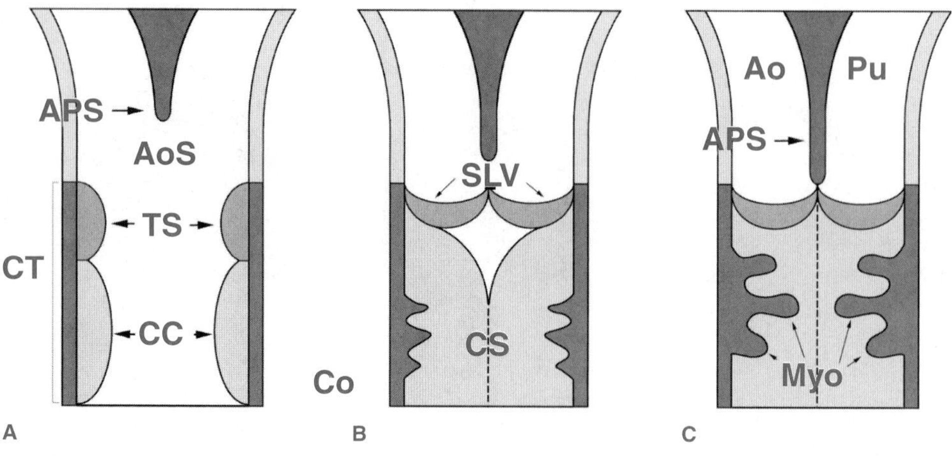


FIGURE 8-10 Schematic diagram of some of the developmental events involved in the septation of the outflow tract. *A.* The stage at which the endocardial cushion tissues in the outflow tract (conal cushions and truncal swellings) and the aortopulmonary septum have not yet fused. *B.* The truncal swellings contribute to the formation of the semilunar valves of aorta and pulmonary trunk, whereas the fusing conal cushions form the mesenchymal outlet septum. At this stage the conal myocardium starts to myocardialize the outlet septum. *C.* One of the final stages. The aortopulmonary septum has now completely separated the aorta and pulmonary trunk above the level of the semilunar valves while below the valves the outlet septum divides the outlet segment of the heart in a subaortic and sub-pulmonary outlet. Ao = aorta, AoS = aortic sac, APS = aorticopulmonary septum, CC = conal cushions, CS = conal septum, CT = conotruncal segment, Myo = myocardialization, Pu = pulmonary trunk, SLV = semilunar valves, TS = truncal swellings.

of the interventricular septum toward the posteromedial aspect of the AV junction, where it will form the AV node.[16,126]

## Myocardialization

The term *myocardialization* refers to the process of active ingrowth of existing myocardium into mesenchymalized tissues of the heart. In the human heart, it primarily takes place in the conal septum, where it transforms the mesenchymal outlet septum, formed as a result of fusion of the conal ridges of the outflow tract, into the muscular outlet septum (Fig. 8-11).[189] It is believed that myocardialization is the driving force for the incorporation of the aortic portion of the outflow tract into the left ventricle and for the rightward expansion of the AV junction. Absence or inhibition of myocardialization is associated with structural congenital heart disease in a number of experimental animal models.[190] Most of these malformations involve malalignment of the outlet septum with the muscular interventricular septum, resulting in ventricular septal defects with varying of great vessel size disparity.[145]

Meanwhile, the AV canal has enlarged to the right while the growing endocardial cushions project into the lumen. Smaller cushions appear on the lateral borders of the AV canal. In the 10-mm CR-length embryo, the major cushions reach each other and fuse, resulting in a complete division of the canal into right and left AV orifices. At the same time, the cushions also bend, and after fusion they form an arch that is concavely directed anteriorly and toward the left ventricle[190] and its convexity directed anteriorly and toward the atria. The mesenchymal cap on the free margin of the atrial septum primum fuses with the convex atrial side of the fused endocardial cushions. The left limb of the fused AV cushion eventually becomes incorporated into the anterior cusp (aortic leaflet) of the mitral valve. The right half of the fused endocardial cushions comes to lie within the ventricles in a sagittal orientation somewhat to the right of the muscular interventricular septum. Thus the communication remaining between right and left ventricles, the secondary interventricular foramen, is bordered by the muscular ventricular septum inferiorly and anteriorly, the right extremity of the fused endocardial cushions posteriorly, and the conal septum superiorly. The plane of the secondary interventricular foramen, therefore, inclines somewhat to the right; that of the primary interventricular foramen, as we have seen, has come to deviate to the left. Both interventricular foramens share the top of the muscular septum as part of their inferior borders.

## STRUCTURAL ANOMALIES

***Partial and Complete AV Canal Defect*** The several forms of persistent AV canal are due to various degrees of failure of fusion of the superior and inferior AV canal cushions. The muscular septum primum and venous valves develop normally and the size and histology of the nonfused endocardial cushions are normal.[191] However, the mass of extracardiac mesenchyme (vestibular spine) located in the dorsal mesocardium is reduced and, as a result, does not protrude ventrally toward the right wall of the common pulmonary vein. Total lack of fusion results in a single AV ostium—i.e., the complete form of the anomaly. Since the arch or bay, normally formed after the fusion of the endocardial cushions, fails to develop, the lower mesenchymal border of the atrial septum cannot fuse with the endocardial cushions. The result is a low-lying, large interatrial communication,

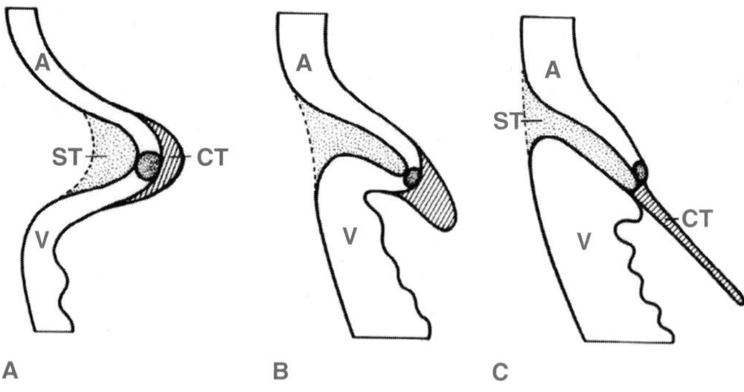


FIGURE 8-11 Schematic diagrams of formation of atrioventricular junction in the human heart. *A.* The atrioventricular junction at 4 to 5 weeks of development. Myocardial continuity between atrium and ventricle occurs through the myocardium of the atrioventricular canal. The atrioventricular junction is sandwiched between the tissues of the atrioventricular sulcus at the epicardial side and the atrioventricular cushion at the endocardial side. *B.* With progressive remodeling of the atrioventricular junction, the sulcus tissues expand toward the midline of the atrioventricular canal as the cushion tissue remodels. *C.* On completion of this process, continuity is lost between atrial and ventricular myocardium. A = atrium, V = ventricle, ST = sulcus tissue, CT = cushion tissue.

with the AV part of the cardiac septum absent. The upper part of the ventricular septum remains deficient to a greater or lesser degree, and there is an interventricular communication. In the partial forms, the endocardial cushions fuse only centrally. The result is an interatrial communication or so-called ostium primum–type atrial septal defect. The upper part of the muscular ventricular septum remains deficient, but this area of the ventricular septum is closed by fibrous tissue. Because the left side of the endocardial cushions does not fuse, the anterior or aortic cusp of the mitral valve is cleft. AV septal defects are frequently associated with trisomy 21 in humans and trisomy 16 in mice.[172] Genetic markers in patients without trisomy 21 are also under investigation.

***Ventricular Septal Defect*** Some forms of perimembranous ventricular septal defect may be due to failure of fusion of the right extremity of the fused endocardial cushions, the upper border of the muscular ventricular septum and the conal septum. Since the endocardial cushions fuse normally, there is no cleft in the anterior mitral valve cusp, nor is there an interatrial communication.

***Single Ventricle, Left Ventricular Type with Rudimentary Outflow Chamber, or Double-Inlet Left Ventricle*** If the AV canal becomes divided into two separate ostia (by the fusing AV cushions) but fails to expand to the right, thus retaining its far leftward position, then both ostia connect only to the primitive left ventricle. As a result, a communication between right atrium and right ventricle does not develop. The communication between the large ventricular chamber (i.e., left ventricle) and the rudimentary outflow chamber (i.e., right ventricle) represents the persistence of the primary interventricular foramen.

## The Ventricles

As mentioned above, the AV canal communicates exclusively with the primitive (or embryonic) left ventricle in the 5-mm CR-length human embryo and blood from the left ventricle reaches the primitive (or embryonic) right ventricle only by way of the primary interventricular foramen. In the developing human heart, the myocardium surrounding the interventricular foramen is characterized by expression of the GFlN2/HNK antigen and is called the *primary interventricular ring*.[170]

The ventricles enlarge by centrifugal growth or "ballooning" of the myocardium along the greater curvature of the heart. The trabecular myocardium progresses from primary to secondary to tertiary trabeculations, while the compact outer myocardial layer remains relatively thin.[192] Coalescence of the secondary trabeculations into larger tertiary trabeculations occurs following septation, coincident with formation of the AV valve leaflets.[193] The trabeculae positioned at the border between the developing left and right ventricle coalesce to form the major portion of the muscular ventricular septum.[193] On the right side, a large trabecula, the trabecula septomarginalis,[194] appears early (in embryos of about 9 mm in CR length) and runs from the anteroinferior border of the primary interventricular foramen toward the apex.

### STRUCTURAL ANOMALIES

***Muscular Ventricular Septal Defect*** Failure of compaction and fusion of the trabecular portion of the ventricular septum results in the most common congenital cardiovascular anomaly, the isolated muscular ventricular septal defect.

## The Truncus Arteriosus

The embryonic "outflow tract" consists of the conus, truncus, and aortic sac and functions as the conduit between the primitive right ventricle and the aortic arches. Septation of the conotruncal area of the outflow tract begins in embryos of about 6 mm in CR length with the appearance of two opposing truncal cushions. One of these is located along the dextrosuperior truncal endocardium (dextrosuperior truncal cushion) and the other on the sinistroinferior wall (sinistroinferior truncal cushion). Coincident with the expansion of the conotruncus, the cushions rapidly enlarge and fuse to form the truncal septum, thus dividing the truncus into aortic and pulmonary channels. The truncus is the first part of the heart to septate (at the 7-mm CR-length stage). Proximally, the truncal cushions merge with the superior aspects of the conal cushions, which are the comparable mesenchymal masses within the conus. Distally, the undivided portion of the truncus and the aortic sac enlarge to form the truncoaortic sac. Simultaneously, the origin and course of the sixth arches shift leftward, aligning with right ventricular outflow and the origin and course of the fourth aortic arches shift rightward, aligning with left ventricular outflow. At the same time, a population of cells located between the fourth and sixth aortic arches and derived from the cardiac neural crest contributes to the formation of a vertical septum, the aortopulmonary septum (APS), in the aortic sac.[115] The APS fuses with the truncal septum to complete septation of the posterior aorta and the anterior pulmonary trunk.[172,178,190,194,195] The role of altered cell number, migration, and differentiation of cells from the anterior heart-forming region on altered conotruncal septation remains unknown.

### STRUCTURAL ANOMALIES

***Persistent Truncus Arteriosus*** If the truncal cushions remain hypoplastic and fail to fuse, partitioning of the truncus arteriosus does not take place. If, in addition to the hypoplastic truncal cushions, both intercalated valve cushions persist, the result is a quadricuspid truncal valve. Usually, fusion occurs between adjacent valve anlagen, resulting in an apparently tricuspid truncal valve with one larger cusp containing a fused raphe. In the great majority of cases, a truncated aortopulmonary septum does develop, and a short common pulmonary trunk arises from the persistent trunk. The ductus arteriosus is almost always absent except when associated with interruption of the aortic arch. In experimental models, persistent truncus arteriosus can be produced following selected ablation of neural crest tissue, as mentioned above.[112]

***Aortopulmonary Septal Defect*** This anomaly may be due to malalignment and/or failure of fusion between the distal truncal septum and the aortopulmonary septum. Both arterial valves are present, but there is a communication of varying size (aortopulmonary window) between the ascending aorta and the pulmonary trunk.

## The Conus

The conal cushions make their appearance slightly before the truncal cushions. One cushion is located on the dextrodorsal wall and the other on the sinistroventral wall of the conus. On the right side, the dorsal conal cushion becomes continuous with the superior truncal cushion; on the left side, the ventral conal cushion becomes continuous with the inferior truncal cushion. Fusion of the conal cushion begins proximally and then progresses rapidly, completing the partition of the conal septum by the 14- to 15-mm CR-length stage in the human embryo. Conal septation reduces and then closes the small secondary interventricular foramen, which was bordered by the conal septum, the top of the muscular ventricular septum, and the right extremities of the fused endocardial cushions. The mesenchymal conal septum and infundibulum eventually become "myocardialized," resulting in the muscular outlet septum.[189]

**STRUCTURAL ANOMALIES**

***Ventricular Septal Defect, Eisenmenger Type*** A large basilar septal defect, dextroposition of the aortic valve, and a hypoplastic or absent infundibular septum is likely due to hypoplasia or absence of the conal cushions. If mitral-aortic separation occurs, then this ventricular septal defect can be included under the heading of double-outlet left ventricle.

***Ventricular Septal Defect, Supracristal Type*** The supracristal type of ventricular septal defect is likely due to either simple failure of conal septal fusion or to septal malalignment, which prevents fusion.

***Tetralogy of Fallot*** The primary anomaly in tetralogy of Fallot is likely an anterior displacement to a varying degree of the conal septum, which leads to unequal partitioning of the conus and reduction of the right ventricular infundibulum. A large basilar ventricular septal defect and dextroposition of the aortic valve result from failure of the displaced conal septum to participate in closure of the interventricular foramen. Pulmonary vascular hypoplasia is likely a secondary result of diminished forward blood flow. As mentioned above, tetralogy of Fallot is frequently associated with 22q11 deletion, particularly in the setting of severe pulmonary atresia or in the presence of extracardiac anomalies.

## DEVELOPMENT OF THE HEART VALVES

### The Atrioventricular Valves

Initially the tubular embryonic heart functions as a peristaltoid pump, relying on endocardial cushions to function as valves and regional variations in conduction velocity to facilitate forward flow. The endocardial cushions develop in the areas characterized by slow contraction and relaxation and, in combination with the specialized myocardium with which they are associated, serve to promote antegrade blood flow. Initially, we can distinguish only two AV cushions, the inferior (iAVC) and the superior (sAVC) cushions. Fusion of these two cushions result in the formation of the two AV orifices. At later stages the so-called lateral AV cushions appear. Over time, the cushion-derived tissues develop into the thin mature AV valve cusps.[196] The sAVC contributes to the aortic leaflet of the mitral valve, the iAVC to the septal and posteroinferior leaflet of the tricuspid valve. The right lateral AVC contributes to the formation of the anterosuperior leaflet of the tricuspid valves, and the left lateral AVC is involved in the formation of the parietal leaflet of the mitral valve. Although the cushion derived tissues form the main component of the leaflets (Fig. 8-10), it is important to note that an essential step in the morphogenesis of the valves is the delamination of the developing leaflets from the underlying ventricular myocardium.[197,198]

**STRUCTURAL ANOMALIES**

***Tricuspid Valve Atresia, Mitral Valve Atresia*** Tricuspid and mitral valve atresias are anomalies that may be caused by incomplete expansion of the common AV canal toward the right during remodeling of the inner curvature of the heart or caused by abnormal formation and/or premature fusion of endocardial cushion tissue that borders the AV canal.

***Ebstein's Anomaly of the Tricuspid Valve*** Ebstein's anomaly of the tricuspid valve is likely due to an abnormality in the process of myocardial delamination required for AV valve and chordal formation.

### The Arterial Valves

The primordia of the semilunar valves become visible as small tubercles on the distal extensions of each truncal cushion after truncal partitioning in the 9-mm embryo. One of each pair is assigned to pulmonary and aortic channels, respectively. On the walls of both aortic and pulmonary channels, opposite the fused truncus cushions, a third small cushion appears.[194] These two intercalated valve cushions form the third member of each arterial valve primordium. Both the aortic and pulmonary roots, consisting of the sinuses of Valsalva and the semilunar valves, are likely derived from the truncus arteriosus and the truncal and intercalated valve cushions.

**STRUCTURAL ANOMALIES**

***Bicuspid Arterial Valves*** A bicuspid aortic or pulmonary valve is due to a failure of development of an intercalated valve cushion, resulting in a valve with two equal sized cusps, neither containing a raphe, or to fusion of adjacent valve anlagen, in which case the cusps are generally unequal in size with the larger containing a raphe of varying length.

***Arterial Valve Stenosis or Atresia*** Fusion of two or all three of the arterial valve anlagen likely results in stenosis or atresia of the valve. Pulmonary valve stenosis is associated with several autosomal dominant genetic syndromes including Noonan's syndrome, due to an altered non-receptor-type tyrosine phosphatase, PTPN11, mapped to 12q24.1,[199] and Costello syndrome.

***Absent Arterial Valves*** Failure of the arterial valve anlagen to develop likely explains the rare occurrence of absence of the pulmonary or aortic valve.

## AORTIC ARCH DEVELOPMENT

Aortic arch development involves the sequential development and then involution of six arch pairs. The first pair of arches in the 3-mm CR-length embryo is large when the second pair is just forming (Fig. 8-12*A*). Caudally, the dorsal aortas fuse to form a single vessel, and then vessel fusion progresses cranially. In a 4-mm embryo, the first and second arches have largely disappeared (Fig. 8-12*B*). The third aortic arch is well developed, and the fourth and sixth arches are being formed as ventral and dorsal sprouts of the aortic sac and dorsal aorta, respectively. The ventral portion of the sixth arch already has as its major branch the primitive pulmonary artery, even though the arch itself has not yet been completed. Of note, in mammals, the fifth aortic arch is rudimentary. By the 10-mm embryonic stage, the first two aortic arches have regressed; and the third, fourth, and sixth are present; and the truncoaortic sac has been divided by the formation of the aortopulmonary septum, so that the sixth arches are now continuous with the pulmonary trunk (Fig. 8-12*C*). Of note, the seventh cervical intersegmental arteries arise from the dorsal aorta near

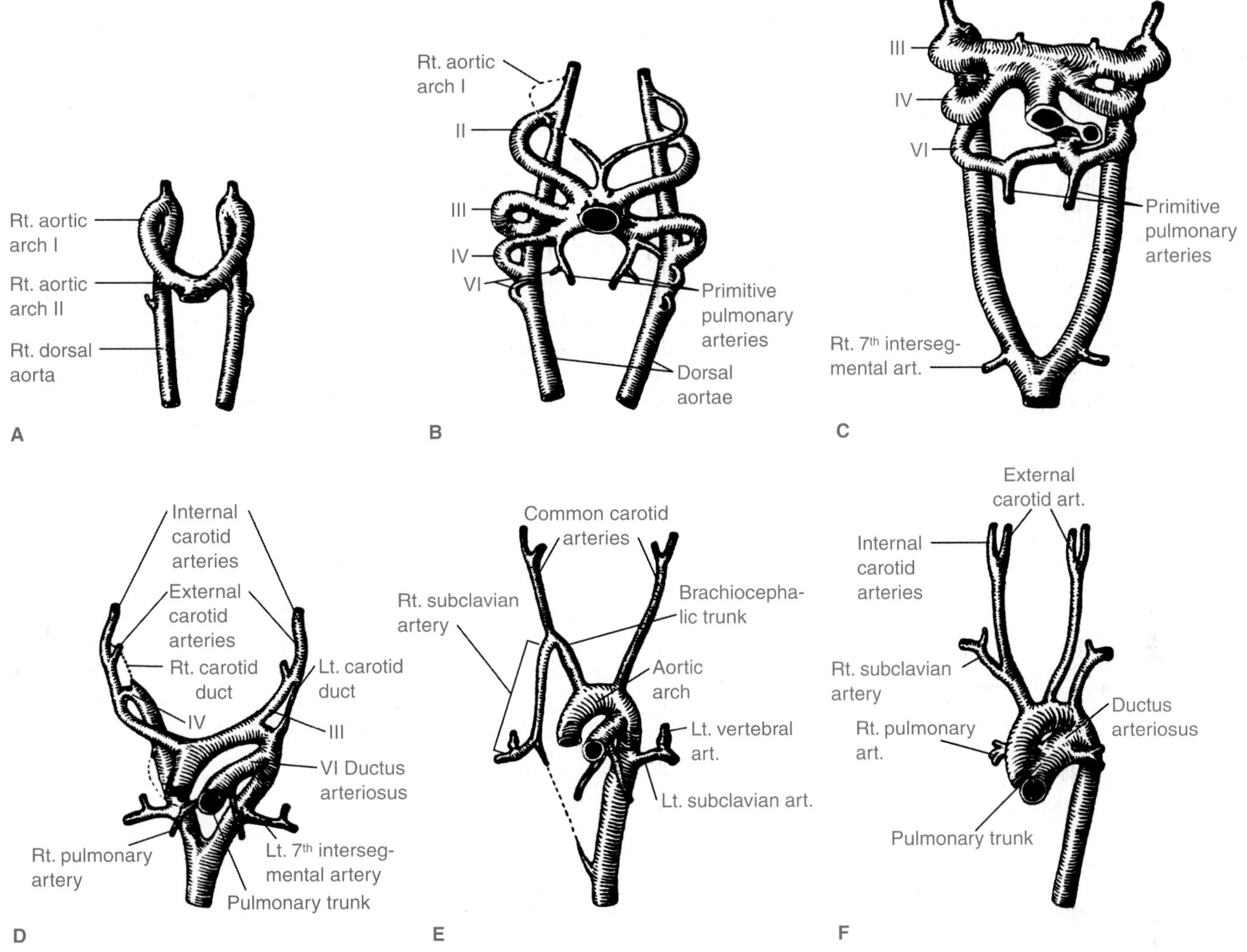


FIGURE 8-12 Development of the aortic arch system. Sizes of embryos: *A.* 3 mm, *B.* 4 mm, *C.* 10 mm, *D.* 14 mm, *E.* 17 mm, and *F.* neonate. (Adapted from Congdon ED. Transformation of the aortic arch system during development of the embryo. *Carnegie Contrib Embryol* 1922;14:47.)

the midline and form the subclavian arteries. In a 14-mm embryo, the dorsal aortas, between the third and fourth arches, have disappeared and the third arches begin to elongate (Fig. 8-12*D*). At this point, the dorsal portion of the right sixth arch has disappeared, though the left sixth arch persists as the ductus arteriosus. The aortic sac has been broadened to contribute to the brachiocephalic trunk on the right and part of the definitive aortic arch up to the origin of the left third arch (common carotid artery). Finally, by the 17-mm embryo stage, the right dorsal aorta has become atrophic between its junction with the left dorsal aorta; the origin of the right seventh intersegmental artery has now become attenuated and later disappears (Fig. 8-12*E*). The remaining components of the right dorsal aorta and right fourth aortic arch form the proximal subclavian artery. After birth, the distal part of the left sixth aortic arch, the ductus arteriosus, normally also involutes to form the ligamentum arteriosum. Thus, most aortic arch anomalies are secondary to abnormal retention or disappearance of various embryonic segments.

## STRUCTURAL ANOMALIES

***Patent Ductus Arteriosus*** Persistence of the ductus arteriosus postnatally frequently occurs in premature infants due to delayed ductal involution. Ductal closure involves the prostaglandin cascade[200] as well as mitochondrial oxygen sensing and altered voltage-gated $K^+$ channels.[201] However, persistence of a large ductus arteriosus also occurs in isolation and in association with a variety of congenital cardiovascular malformations. Patent ductus also occurs as a component of Char syndrome, an autosomal dominant syndrome that also includes facial dysmorphism and hand abnormalities. Mutations in the neuroectoderm transcription factor TFAP2B gene on chromosome 6p12-p21 have been identified in Char syndrome.[202] TFAP2B protein is expressed in the neural fold, lateral head mesenchyme, and developing third, fourth, and sixth aortic arches, but the direct pathogenesis of ductal patency has not yet been defined.[202]

***Coarctation of the Aorta*** Coarctation of the aorta is defined as a luminal narrowing of the aortic arch, usually posterior and adjacent to the insertion of the ductus arteriosus.[203] Coarctation of the aorta is often associated with abnormal aortic valve morphologies, abnormal dimensions of the transverse aortic arch (isthmus) and with abnormal antegrade left ventricular output in utero. The functional consequence of reduced antegrade left ventricular output in utero is a bifurcation of flow from the fetal ductus arteriosus, resulting in retrograde flow from the ductus toward the ascending aorta and abnormal shear stress to the juxtaductal aortic wall. The final phenotype of the coarctation can be "preductal," in the setting of associated transverse arch hypoplasia, or "juxtaductal."[203]

***Double Aortic Arch*** Double aortic arch is the result of persistence and continued patency of the segment of the right dorsal aorta between the origin of the right seventh intersegmental artery and its junction with the left dorsal aorta.

***Right Aortic Arch*** In the right aortic arch anomaly, the right rather than the left dorsal aorta is maintained in its entirety. The branching pattern of the aortic arch, therefore, will be the mirror image of normal with the brachiocephalic (innominate) artery arising as the first vessel on the left rather than the right side.

***Anomalous Subclavian Artery*** The origin of the right subclavian artery is the right fourth aortic arch. When this neural crest patterned segment is absent, the right subclavian artery can arise from the aortic arch distal to the left subclavian artery if the right dorsal aorta between the origin of the right seventh intersegmental artery and the junction with the left dorsal aorta is maintained to form the proximal portion of the right subclavian artery.[198]

***Interrupted Aortic Arch*** Interrupted aortic arch anomaly type B results from the disappearance of the left fourth aortic arch (type A is a form of coarctation of the aorta), which has been shown in the mouse embryo to represent a unique population of neural crest cells.[198] The ascending aorta terminates as the brachiocephalic and left common carotid arteries and is isolated from the descending aorta, which is perfused by the pulmonary trunk by way of a patent ductus arteriosus. In the setting of interrupted aortic arch, an anomalous right subclavian artery is frequently present due to comparable unique neural crest patterning of this vessel.[198]

***Absent Left Pulmonary Artery*** The left pulmonary artery can be absent when it arises from a left-sided ductus arteriosus (or ligamentum arteriosum). This anomaly is the result of disappearance of the proximal left sixth arch. If, in this anomaly, the aortic arch is on the left side, the ductus arteriosus that feeds the intrapulmonary part of the left pulmonary artery arises from the usual position on the underside of the arch. If the aortic arch is on the right, the ductus arteriosus usually arises from the brachiocephalic trunk, with the left common carotid and left subclavian arteries as a trifurcation or, rarely, from a diverticulum of the descending aorta. Usually the left subclavian artery in such cases also arises from the diverticulum.

## CORONARY ARTERY DEVELOPMENT

### Endothelial Cell Origin

Coronary vascular endothelial maturation closely parallels the development of the embryonic epicardium.[204] A series of cell-fate studies has revealed that the coronary endothelial cells as well as coronary smooth muscle cells derive from the so-called proepicardium organ, a cluster of cells attached to the ventral wall of the sinus venosus. As cells from the proepicardium spread out and cover the surface of the heart, a subpopulation of epicardially derived cells (EPDCs) transdifferentiate and migrate into the myocardial cell layers,[205–209] where they contribute to the formation of the coronary network. Recent studies have shown that these future coronary epithelial cells express *Tbx-5* and retroviral studies show that overexpression of *Tbx-5* in these cells suppresses cell migration and coronary formation. A part of this network reaches the mesenchymal border of the aortic annulus.[204] Initially, multiple connections between the coronary vascular plexus and the aortic root are present; however, only two connections persist. It is interesting to note that the heart begins to pump blood before perfusion by the coronary vasculature occurs, indicating that, in these early stages, local diffusion of nutrients is sufficient for the early trabecular myocardium.

### Vascular Smooth Muscle Cell Origin

Antibodies to smooth muscle $\alpha$-actin document that the maturation of coronary smooth muscle precedes the maturation of the outflow vessels.[210] Several studies have demonstrated that coronary smooth muscle is derived from the epicardially derived cells. Interestingly, the orderly development of the coronary arterial branching pattern and elastic lamina is dependent upon the presence of the neural crest (NC), demonstrating that the perturbation in the development of one subpopulation of "extracardiac" cells (NC-derived cells) can lead to the abnormal development of another (epicardially derived cells).[211] Following experimental NC ablation in the chick embryo, persistent truncus arteriosus associated with a single origin of the coronary arterial tree occurs.[210] The distribution and symmetry of the coronary vascular is distinctly abnormal following injury to the NC. In addition, the elastic lamina and collagen organization of the great vessels is markedly abnormal following NC ablation, as has been noted in some congenital cardiovascular anomalies.[212]

### Vasculogenesis and Adaptation

It is important to note that the maturation of the coronary vasculature, as with the systemic vasculature, represents both angiogenesis (sprouting of existing vessels) and vasculogenesis (fusion of precursor cells).[213] Following increased ventricular pressure loading in the chick embryo, myocardial vasculogenesis increases to match increased ventricular mass.[214] This finding is consistent with the investigation of children with pressure-overload left ventricular hypertrophy, where capillary density remains unchanged.[215]

#### STRUCTURAL ANOMALIES

***Anomalous Origin of the Left Coronary Artery*** Occasionally, the left coronary artery is found to arise from the pulmonary artery and rarely from other aortic arch vessels. The developing coronary vessels perforate the aortic annulus in association with specific immunohistochemical markers, so anomalies are likely to occur when this patterning event is altered.

***Abnormal Origin and Course of Coronary Arteries*** Numerous variations in the architecture and course of the coronary arteries occur in association with structural cardiovascular malformations. For example, an anomalous origin of the left anterior descending coronary artery from the right coronary artery occurs in association with tetralogy of Fallot. Unfortunately, the mechanisms for these associations have not yet been defined.

***Coronary Arterial Fistulas*** Coronary arterial fistulas occasionally occur in isolation and occur in association with pulmonary valve atresia with intact ventricular septum. The development of coronary artery fistula to the right ventricle may be due to reduced antegrade coronary artery flow during early cardiac development.[216]

## CONDUCTION SYSTEM DEVELOPMENT

The development of the conduction system has fascinated cardiovascular embryologists from the moment it became clear that a subpopulation of specialized myocytes is responsible for the regulation of the cardiac impulse in the heart.[217] The cardiac conduction system is composed of central and peripheral components and, during the last decade, several studies have revealed new aspects regarding the development of the conduction system. Immunohistochemical studies have shown that the developing conduction system in human and other vertebrates is characterized by the expression of a unique set of antigens and genes—some of which are also expressed in the nervous system—sometimes referred to as *neuromuscular markers* (Fig. 8-13).[170,218,219] Methods of retroviral cell targeting and tracing have defined subpopulations of cardiomyocytes that differentiate into Purkinje cells within the trabecular myocardium.[170,220,221] Mikawa and colleagues have shown that a subpopulation of myocytes within the trabecular myocardium differentiate into a Purkinje lineage under the regulation of endothelin secreted by adjacent coronary epithelial cells.[222,223] These developing Purkinje cells express unique molecular markers, and their fate is dynamically influenced by the local environment.[224]

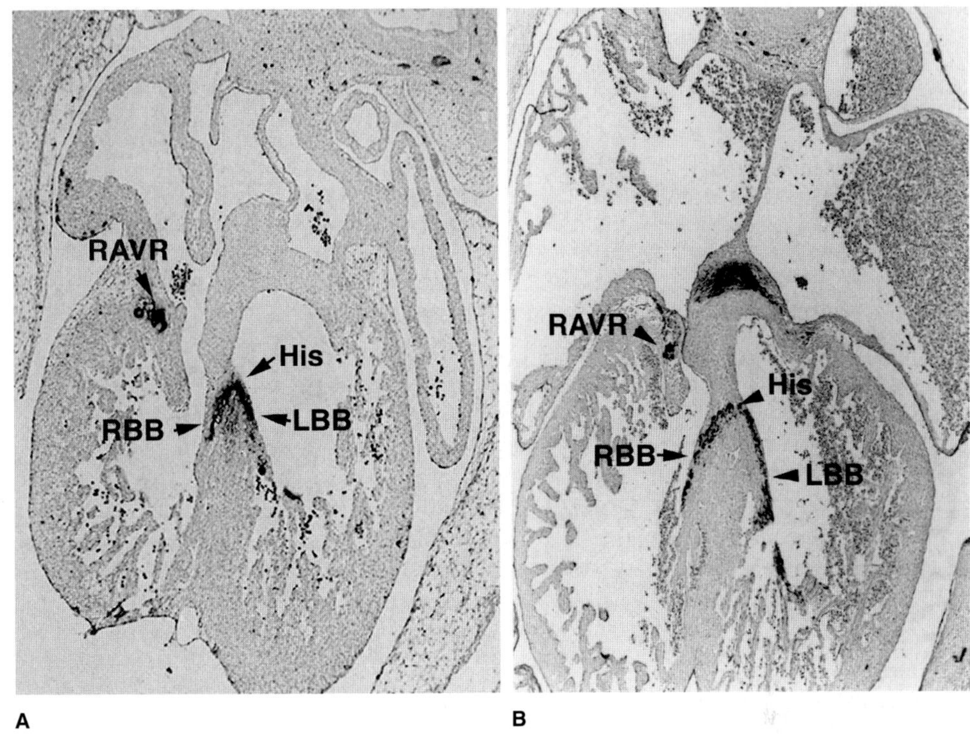


FIGURE 8-13 Expression of neuromuscular markers in the developing vertebrate heart. *A.* A transverse section of a human heart at 6 weeks of development immunohistochemically stained for the presence of a carbohydrate moiety recognized by the monoclonal antibody G1N2 (see also Ref. 170). *B.* Section of a rabbit embryo at 15 days of development that was immunohistochemically stained for the presence of neurofilaments. (Adapted from Wessels et al. *Anat Rec* 1992;223:97. With permission.) RAVR = right atrioventricular ring bundle, His = bundle of His, LBB = left bundle branch, RBB = right bundle branch.

Altered patterns of atrial and ventricular depolarization have been recognized in association with structural heart defects, such as the pattern of depolarization noted with endocardial cushion defects, and conduction abnormalities associated with atrial septum defects are observed in patients with mutations in the *Nkx-2.5*[225] and *TBX5* (Holt-Oram syndrome) genes.[226]

## CARDIOVASCULAR INNERVATION

Despite numerous descriptive studies regarding the location of cardiac ganglia, little was known regarding the immunohistochemical cues required for the patterning of myocardial innervation until relatively recently. NC cell migration is critical for this process, as NC cells serve as precursors for the cardiac nerves and ganglia.[112] Cardiac ganglia and nerves are present in the human embryo at 7 weeks of gestation.[227] The density of cardiac innervation exhibits a gradient of decreasing density from the atrium to the ventricle. It is interesting to note that functional adrenergic receptors are present on the embryonic heart prior to histologic evidence of autonomic nerves.[228] The differential appearance and distribution of peptide-containing nerves indicates that there is a maturational order to the autonomic and sensory components of the developing human heart.[222]

## FUNCTIONAL MATURATION OF THE EMBRYONIC HEART

Obviously, cardiovascular morphogenesis is directly influenced by the dynamic mechanical environment of the pulsatile embryonic heart. Unfortunately, an overview of functional maturation, while critical, is beyond the scope of this chapter. The reader is therefore referred to several recent reviews of embryonic functional maturation in vertebrate and invertebrate species.[229,230]

## MOLECULAR MECHANISMS OF CONGENITAL HEART DISEASE

The list of congenital and acquired cardiovascular diseases identified to have specific molecular mechanisms continues to expand rapidly (Table 8-1). The challenge now is to correlate specific changes in genotype with the dynamic process of CV morphogenesis and subsequent phenotype. Many of the molecular mechanisms involved in CV development are spatially and temporally restricted, so that a conserved set of transcription factors can have dramatically disparate effects during morphogenesis. The developing CV system also adapts to altered morphogenetic events via evolutionarily conserved mechanisms to preserve CV function, which result in structural and functional remodeling. Finally, epigenetic maternal factors likely play a critical role in influencing embryonic and fetal development.

TABLE 8-1 Molecular Mechanisms of Congenital Heart Disease[a]

| | |
|---|---|
| **Situs** | |
| Heterotaxy, Kartagener | DNAH11 (7p21), connexin 43, NKX-2.5 |
| **Atrioventricular canal** | |
| Atrioventricular canal defect: | Trisomy 21, 18, 13 (del8p) |
| Heterotaxy syndrome: | ZIC3, LEFTYA, ACVR2B, DFC1 |
| Ellis-van Creveld | EvC, EvC2 (4p16) |
| Holt-Oram | TBX5 (12q24.1) |
| Smith-Lemli-Opitz | DHCR7 (11q12-13) |
| **Pulmonary valve** | |
| Noonan's syndrome | PTPN11 (12q24.1) |
| Costello's syndrome | |
| **Pulmonary vasculature** | |
| Primary pulmonary hypertension | BMPR-II |
| **Hypoplastic left heart syndrome** | |
| Jacobsen's syndrome | 11q23 (terminal deletions), OBCAM |
| **Tetralogy of Fallot** | |
| Catch-22 syndrome | (22q11) |
| DiGeorge's syndrome | (22q11) |
| Velo-cardio-facial syndrome | (22q11) |
| Alagille syndrome | JAGGED1 (20p12) |
| 8p deletion syndrome | |
| **Aortic valve** | |
| Turner's syndrome | 45 (X,O) |
| **Aortic vasculature** | |
| Williams' syndrome | Elastin (7q11.23) |
| Marfan's syndrome | Fibrillin-1 (15q21) |
| **Cardiomyopathy/tumors** | |
| Hypertrophic/dilated | beta-myosin heavy-chain (14q11), dystrophin, G4.5, titin (2q31), actin, desmin, lamin A/C, Delta-sarcoglycan, troponin, tropomyosin |
| Arrhythmogenic | Plakoglobin, 14q23, 10p12, 1q42 |
| Mitochondrial | Numerous mtDNA deletions |
| Metabolic | VLCAD (17p11.2), LCHAD |
| Histiocytoid | (Xp22) |
| Barth's syndrome | G4.5 (Xq28) |
| Tuberous sclerosis | TSC1 (9q34), TSC2 (16p13) |
| Ventricular noncompaction | CSX (del5q35.1-3) |
| Carney complex (atrial myxoma) | (2p16) |
| **Conduction System** | |
| Wolf-Parkinson-White syndrome | PRKAG2 |
| Kearns-Sayre syndrome | mtDNA (deletions) |
| Friedreich's ataxia | Frataxin (9q13) |
| Long-QT syndrome | HERG, SCN5A, numerous others |

[a]Recognized genes and transcription factors identified in human patients with congenital heart disease. Some molecular markers are multipurpose transcription factors, e.g., NKX-2.5, associated with atrial septal defect, and the specific genotype-phenotype correlation is unproven. For other molecular markers, such as the structural protein elastin in Williams' syndrome or the fibrillin protein in Marfan's syndrome, the correlation is more straightforward. However, many of these genes have been identified to have a range of coding errors that can result in pleiotropic phenotypes, thus further complicating genomewide screening for molecular mechanisms of congenital heart disease.

Thus, the identification of molecular mechanisms of congenital heart disease constitutes an important advance in our understanding of this complex, dynamic, and critical developmental process.

## References


1. Von Haller A. *Sur la formation du coeur dans le poulet.* Lausanne, 1758.
2. Neill CA, Clark EB. Tetralogy of Fallot: The first 300 years. *Texas Heart Inst J* 1994;21:272–279.
3. Anderson RH. Simplifying the understanding of congenital malformations of the heart. *Int J Cardiol* 1991;32:131–142.
4. Van Mierop LHS. Morphological development of the heart. In: Berne RM, ed. *Handbook of Physiology:* Sec 2, Vol I. Bethesda, MD: American Physiological Society; 1979:1–28.
5. Clark EB, Van Mierop LHS. Cardiac development. In: Adams FH, Emmanoulides GC, Riemenschneider TA. eds. *Heart Disease in Infants, Children, and Adolescents*, 4th ed. Baltimore: Williams & Wilkins; 1989:1–22.
6. Wenick ACG. Embryology of the heart. In: Anderson RH, Macartney FJ, Shinebourne EA, Tynan M, eds. *Pediatric Cardiology:* Vol 1 New York: Churchill Livingstone; 1987:83–107.
7. Ferrens VJ, Rosenquist GC, Weinstein C. *Cardiac Morphogenesis.* New York: Elsevier; 1985.
8. Nora JJ, Takao A. *Congenital Heart Disease: Causes and Processes.* Mount Kisco, NY: Futura; 1984.
9. Clark EB, Takao A. *Developmental Cardiology: Morphogenesis and Function.* Mount Kisco, NY: Futura; 1990.
10. Bockman DE, Kirby ML. *Embryonic Origins of Defective Heart Development.* New York: NY Academy of Sciences; 1990.
11. Clark EB, Markwald RR, and Takao A. *Developmental Mechanisms of Heart Disease.* Mount Kisco, NY: Futura; 1995.
12. Brueckner M, D'Eustachio P, Horwich AL. Linkage mapping of a mouse gene, *iv,* that controls left-right asymmetry of the heart and viscera. *Proc Natl Acad Sci USA* 1989;86:5035–5038.
13. Yokoyama T, Copeland NG, Jenkins NA, et al. Reversal of left-right asymmetry: A situs inversus mutation. *Science* 1993;260:679–682.
14. Akam M, Dawson I, Tear G. Homeotic genes and the control of segment diversity. *Development* 1988;104:123–168.
15. Hunt P, Krumlauf R. HOX codes and positional specification invertebrate embryonic axes. *Annu Rev Cell Biol* 1992;8:227–256.
16. Lamers WH, Wessels A, Verbeek FJ, et al. New findings concerning ventricular septation in the human heart: Implications for maldevelopment. *Circulation* 1992;86:1194–1205.
17. Osmond MK, Butler AJ, Voon FCT, et al. The effects of retinoic acid on heart formation in the early chick embryo. *Development* 1991;113:1405–1417.
18. Chen Y, Solursh M. Comparison of Hensen's node and retinoic acid in secondary axis induction in the early chick embryo. *Dev Dyn* 1992;195:142–151.
19. Davis RL, Weintraub H, Lassar AB. Expression of a single transfected cDNA converts fibroblasts to myoblasts. *Cell* 1987;51:987–1000.
20. Edmondson DG, Olson EN. A gene with homology to the myc similarity region of MyoD1 is expressed during myogenesis and is sufficient to activate the muscle differentiation program. *Genes Dev* 1989;3:628–640.
21. Wright WE, Sassoon DA, Lin VK. Myogenin, a factor regulating myogenesis, has a domain homologous to Myo D. *Cell* 1989;56: 607–617.
22. Braun T, Buschhausen-Denker G, Bober E, et al. A novel human muscle factor related to but distinct from MyoD1 induces myogenic conversion in 10T1/2 fibroblasts. *EMBO J* 1989;8:701–709.
23. Rhodes SJ, Konieczny SF. Identification of *MRF4:* A new member of the muscle regulatory factor gene family. *Genes Dev* 1989;3: 2050–2061.
24. Miner JH, Wold B. *Herculin,* a fourth member of the MyoD family of myogenic regulatory genes. *Proc Natl Acad Sci USA* 1990;87:1089–1093.
25. Braun T, Bober E., Winter B, et al. *Myf-6,* a new member of the human gene family of myogenic determination factors: Evidence for a gene cluster on chromosome 12. *EMBO J* 1990;9:821–831.
26. Murre C, McCaw PS, Baltimore D. A new DNA binding and dimerization motif in immunoglobulin enhancer binding, daughterless, MyoD, and myc proteins. *Cell* 1989;56:777–783.
27. Sassoon D, Lyons G, Wright WE, et al. Expression of two myogenic regulatory factors myogenin and MyoD1 during mouse embryogenesis. *Nature* 1989;41:303–307.
28. Srivastava, D. Genetic assembly of the heart: Implications for congenital heart disease. *Annu Rev Physiol* 2001;63:451–469.
29. Srivastava D, Thomas T, Lin Q, et al. Regulation of cardiac mesodermal and neural crest development by the bHLH transcription factor, dHAND. *Nat Genet* 1997;16:154–160.
30. Riley P, Anson-Cartwright L, Cross JC. The Hand1 bHLH transcription factor is essential for placentation and cardiac morphogenesis. *Nat Genet* 1998;18:271–275.
31. Lin Q, Schwarz J, Bucana C, et al. Control of mouse cardiac morphogenesis and myogenesis by transcription factor MEF2C. *Science* 1997;276:1404–1407.
32. Thomas T, Yamagishi H, Overbeek PA, et al. The bHLH factors, dHAND and eHAND, specify pulmonary and systemic cardiac ventricles independent of left-right sidedness. *Dev Biol* 1998; 15;196:228–236.
33. Bao ZZ, Bruneau BG, Seidman JG, et al. Regulation of chamber-specific gene expression in the developing heart by *Irx4. Science* 1999;283:1161–1164.
34. Christoffels VM, Keijser AG, Houweling AC, et al. Patterning the embryonic heart: Identification of five mouse Iroquois homeobox genes in the developing heart. *Dev Biol* 2000;224:263–274.
35. Wang GF, Nikovits W Jr, Bao ZZ, et al. Irx4 forms an inhibitory complex with the vitamin D and retinoic X receptors to regulate cardiac chamber-specific slow MyHC3 expression. *J Biol Chem* 2001:276:28835–28841.
36. Harvey RP. *NK-2* homeobox genes and heart development. *Dev Biol* 1996;178:203–216.
37. Kim Y, Nirenberg M. Drosophila NK-homeobox genes. *Proc Natl Acad Sci USA* 1989;86:7716–7720.
38. Scott MP, Tamkun JW, Hertzell GW III. The structure and function of the homeodomain. *Biochem Biophys Acta* 1989; 989:25–48.
39. Chen CY, Schwartz RJ. Identification of novel DNA binding targets and regulatory domains of a murine tinman homeodomain factor, *Nkx-2.5. J Biol Chem* 1995;270:15628–15633.
40. Chen CY, Croissant J, Majesky M, et al. Activation of the cardiac α-actin promoter depends upon serum response factor, tinman homologue, *Nkx-2.5,* and intact serum response elements. *Dev Genet* 1996;19:119–130.
41. Durocher D, Chen CY, Ardati A, et al. The atrial natriuretic factor promoter is a downstream target for *Nkx-2.5* in the myocardium. *Mol Cell Biol* 1996;16:4648–4655.
42. Gajewski K, Kim Y, Lee YM, et al. *D-mef2* 8s a target for *tinman* activation during Drosophila heart development. *EMBO J* 1997;16: 515–522.
43. Bodmer R. The gene *tinman* is required for specification of the heart and visceral muscles in *Drosophila. Development* 1993;118:719–729.
44. Azpiazu N, Frasch H. *Tinman* and *bagpipe:* Two homeobox genes that determine cell fates in the dorsal mesoderm of *Drosophila. Genes Dev* 1993;7:1325–1340.
45. Lints TJ, Parsons LM, Hartley L, et al. Nkx-2.5: A novel murine homeobox gene expressed in early heart progenitor cells and their myogenic descendants. *Development* 1993;119:419–431.
46. Komuro I, Izumo S. *Csx:* A murine homeobox-containing gene specifically expressed in the developing heart. *Proc Natl Acad Sci USA* 1993;90:8145–8149.
47. Chen JN, Fishman MC. Zebrafish *tinman* homolog demarcates the heart field and initiates myocardial differentiation. *Development* 1996;122:3809–3816.

48. Tonissen KF, Drysdale TA, Lints TJ, et al. *XNkx-2.5,* a Xenopus gene related to *Nkx-2.5* and *tinman*: Evidence for a conserved role in cardiac development. *Dev Biol* 1994;162:325–328.
49. Schwartz RJ, Olson EN. Building the heart piece by piece: Modularity of cis-elements regulating *Nkx-2.5* transcription. *Development* 1999;126:4187–4192.
50. Reecy JM, Yamada M, Cummings K, et al. Chicken *Nkx-2.8:* A novel homeobox gene expressed in early heart progenitor cells and pharyngeal pouch-2 and -3 endoderm. *Dev Biol* 1997;188:295–311.
51. Lints TJ, Parsons LM, Hartley L, et al. *Nkx-2.5:* A novel murine homeobox gene expressed in early heart progenitor cells and their myogenic descendants. *Development* 1993;119:969.
52. Schott JJ, Benson DW, Basson CT, et al. Congenital heart disease caused by mutations in the transcription factor *NKX2-5*. *Science* 1998;281:108–111.
53. Kuo H, Chen J, Ruiz-Lozano P, et al. Control of segmental expression of the cardiac-restricted ankyrin repeat protein gene by distinct regulatory pathways in murine cardiogenesis. *Development* 1999; 126:4223–4234.
54. Teisman R. Identification of a protein-binding site that mediates transcription response of the c-*fos* gene to serum factors. *Cell* 1986; 46:567–574.
55. Croissant JD, Kim JH, Eichele G, et al. Avian serum response factor expression restricted primarily to muscle cell lineages is required for α-actin gene transcription. *Dev Biol* 1996;177:250–264.
56. Dalton S, Treisman R. Characterization of SAP-1, a protein recruited by serum response factor to the *c-fos* serum response element. *Cell* 1992;68:597–612.
57. Pollock R, Treisman R. Human SRF-related proteins: DNA-binding properties and potential regulatory targets. *Genes Dev* 1991;5: 2327–2341.
58. Gossett LA, Kelvin DJ, Sternberg EA, et al. A new myocyte-specific enhancer-binding factor that recognizes a conserved element associated with multiple muscle-specific genes. *Mol Cell Biol* 1989; 9:5022–5033.
59. Bour BA, O'Brien MA, Lockwood ML, et al. *Drosophila* MEF2, a transcription factor is essential for myogenesis. *Genes Dev* 1995; 9:730–741.
60. Lilly B, Zhao B, Ranganayakulu G, et al. Requirement of MADS domain transcription factor D-MEF2 for muscle formation in *Drosophila*. *Science* 1995;267:688–693.
61. Edmondson DG, Lyons GE, Martin JF, et al. *Mef-2* gene expression marks the cardiac and skeletal muscle lineages during mouse myogenesis. *Genes Dev* 1994;120:1251–1263.
62. Yu Y-T, Breitbart RE, Smoot LB, et al. Human myocyte-specific enhancer factor 2 comprises a group of tissue restricted MADS box transcription factors. *Genes Dev* 1992;6:1783–1798.
63. Chien KR, Zhu H, Knowlton KU, et al. Transcriptional regulation during cardiac growth and development. *Annu Rev Physiol* 1993;55:77–95.
64. Breitbart RE, Liang C, Smott LB, et al. A fourth human MEF-2 transcription factor, hMEF-2d, is an early marker of the myogenic lineage. *Development* 1993;118:1095–1106.
65. Martin JF, Miano JM, Hustad CM, et al. *Mef2* gene that generates a muscle-specific isoform via alternative mRNA splicing. *Mol Cell Biol* 1994;14:1647–1656.
66. Grueneberg DA, Natesan S, Alexandre C, et al. Human and *Drosophila* homeodomain proteins that enhance the DNA-binding activity of serum response factor. *Science* 1992;257:1089–1095.
67. Grueneberg DA, Simon KJ, Brennan K, et al. Sequence-specific targeting of nuclear signal transduction pathways by homeodomain proteins. *Mol Cell Biol* 1995;15:3318–3326.
68. Opstelten DJ, Vogels R, Robert B, et al. The mouse homeobox gene, *S8,* is expressed during embryogenesis predominantly in mesenchyme. *Mech Dev* 1991;34:29–42.
69. Cserjesi P, Lilly B, Bryson L, et al. MHox: A mesodermally-restricted homeodomain protein that binds an essential site in the muscle creatine kinase enhancer. *Development* 1992;115:1087–1101.
70. Chen CY, Schwartz RJ. Recruitment of the *tinman* homolog *Nkx*-2.5 by serum response factor activates cardiac α-actin gene transcription. *Mol Cell Biol* 1996;16:6372–6384.
71. Charron F, Nemer M. GATA transcription factors and cardiac development. *Semin Cell Dev Biol* 1999;10:85–91.
72. Laverriere AC, MacNeill C, Mueller C, et al. GATA4/5/6 a subfamily of three transcription factors transcribed in developing heart and gut. *J Biol Chem* 1994;269:23177–23184.
73. Morrisey EE, Ip HH, Lu MM, et al. GATA-6: A zinc finger transcription factor that is expressed in multiple cell lineages derived from lateral mesoderm. *Dev Biol* 1996;177:309–322.
74. Ip HS, Wilson DB, Heikinheimo M, et al. The GATA-4 transcription factor transactivates the cardiac muscle specific troponin C promoter-enhancer in nonmuscle cells. *Mol Cell Biol* 1994;14:7515–7526.
75. Mokentin JD, Lin Q, Duncan S, et al. Requirement of the transcription factor GATA4 for heart tube formation and ventral morphogenesis. *Genes Dev* 1997;11:1061–1072.
76. Crispino JD, Lodish MB, Thurberg BL, et al. Proper coronary vascular development and heart morphogenesis depend on interaction of GATA-4 with FOG cofactors. *Genes Dev* 2001;15(7):839–844.
77. Zhang HB, Bradley A. Mice deficient for BMP2 are nonviable and have defects in amnion/chorion and cardiac development. *Development* 1996;122:2977–2986.
78. Bisgrove BW, Yost HJ. Classification of left-right patterning defects in zebrafish, mice, and humans. *Am J Med Genet* 2001;101:315–323.
79. Schneider H, Brueckner M. Of mice and men: Dissecting the genetic pathway that controls left-right asymmetry in mice and humans. *Am J Med Genet* 2000;97:258–270.
80. Kramer KL, Yost HJ. Ectodermal Syndecan-2 regulates left-right axis formation in migrating mesoderm as a cell non-autonomous Vg1 co-receptor. *Dev Cell* 2002;2:115–124.
81. Miki H, Setou M, Kaneshiro K, et al. All kinesin superfamily protein, *KIF,* genes in mouse and human. *Proc Natl Acad Sci USA* 2001; 98:7004–7011.
82. Layton WM. Random determination of developmental process: Reversal of normal visceral asymmetry in the mouse. *J Hered* 1976;67:336–338.
83. Supp DM, Brueckner M, Kuehn MR, et al. Targeted deletion of the ATP binding domain of left-right dynein confirms its role in specifying development of left-right asymmetries. *Development* 1999;126: 5495–5504.
84. Essner JJ, Vogan KJ, Wagner MK, et al. Conserved function for embryonic nodal cilia. *Nature* 2002;418:37–38.
85. Yokoyama T, Copeland NG, Jenkins NA, et al. Reversal of left-right asymmetry: A situs inversus mutation. *Science* 1993;260:679–682.
86. Morgan D, Turnpenny L, Goodship J, et al. *Inversin,* a novel gene in the vertebrate left-right axis pathway, is partially deleted in the *inv* mouse. *Nat Genet* 1998;20:149–156.
87. Yasuhiko Y, Imai F, Ookubo K, et al. Calmodulin binds to inv protein: Implication for the regulation of *inv* function. *Dev Growth Differ* 2001;43:671–681.
88. Liu C, Liu W, Palie J, et al. *Pitx2c* patterns outflow myocardium and aortic arch vessels and is required for local cell movement into atrioventricular cushions. *Development* 2000;129:5081–5091.
89. Kelly RG, Brown NA, Buckingham NE. The arterial pole of the mouse heart forms from Fgf10-expressing cells in pharyngeal mesoderm. *Dev Cell* 2001;1:435–440.
90. Schneider A, Mijalski T, Schlange T, et al. The homeobox gene NKX-3.2 is a target of left-right signaling and is expressed on opposite sides in chick and mouse embryos. *Curr Biol* 1999;9:911–914.
91. Mikawa T, Borisov A, Brown AM, et al. Clonal analysis of cardiac morphogenesis in the chicken embryo using a replication-defective retrovirus: I. Formation of the ventricular myocardium. *Dev Dyn* 1992;193:11–23.
92. Mikawa T, Cohen-Gould L, Fischman DA. Clonal analysis of cardiac morphogenesis in the chicken embryo using a replication-defective retrovirus. III: Polyclonal origin of adjacent ventricular myocytes. *Dev Dyn* 1992;195:133–141.

93. Mjaatvedt CH, Nakaoka T, Moreno-Rodriquez R, et al. The outflow tract of the heart is recruited from a novel heart-forming field. *Dev Biol* 2001;238:97–109.
94. Kruithof BP, Van Den Hoff MJ, Tesink-Taekema S, et al. Recruitment of intra- and extracardiac cells into the myocardial lineage during mouse development. *Anat Rec* 2003;271:303–314.
95. Linask KK. N-Cadherin localization in early heart development and polar expression of Na+, K+-ATPase, and integrin during pericardial coelom formation and epithelialization of the differentiating myocardium. *Dev Biol* 1992;151:213–224.
96. Parlow MH, Bolender DL, Kokan-Moore NP, et al. Localization of bFGF-like proteins as punctate inclusions in the preseptation myocardium of the chicken embryo. *Dev Biol* 1991;146: 139–147.
97. Lyons KM, Jones CM, Hogan BL. The TGF-beta-related DVR gene family in mammalian development. *Ciba Found Symp* 1992;165: 219–230.
98. Sugi Y, Sasse J, Lough J. Inhibition of precardiac mesoderm cell proliferation by antisense oligodeoxynucleotide complementary to fibroblast growth factor-2 (FGF-2). *Dev Biol* 1993;157:28–37.
99. Lindsay EA, Vitelli F, Su H, et al. *Tbx1* haplo-insufficiency in the DiGeorge syndrome region causes aortic arch defects in mice. *Nature* 2001;410(6824):97–101.
100. Vitelli F, Morishima M, Taddei I, et al. *Tbx1* mutation causes multiple cardiovascular defects and disrupts neural crest and cranial nerve migratory pathways. *Hum Mol Genet* 2002;11(8):915–922.
101. Szeto DP, Griffin KJ, Kimelman D. *HrT* is required for cardiovascular development in zebrafish. *Development* 2002;129:5093–5101.
102. Yamagishi H, Maeda J, Hu T, et al. *Tbx1* is regulated by tissue-specific forkhead proteins through a common Sonic hedgehog-responsive enhancer. *Genes Dev* 2003;17:269–281.
103. Franco D, Lamers WH, Moorman AFM. Patterns of expression in the developing myocardium: Towards morphologically integrated transcriptional model. *Cardiovasc Res* 1998;38:25–53.
104. Clark EB, Hu N, Frommelt P, et al. Effect of increased pressure on ventricular growth in stage 21 chick embryos. *Am J Physiol* 1989;257: H55–H61.
105. Sedmera D, Pexieder T, Rychterova V, et al. Remodeling of chick embryonic ventricular myoarchitecture under experimentally changed loading conditions. *Anat Rec* 1999;254:238–252.
106. Miller CE, Donlon KJ, Toia L, et al. Cyclic strain induces proliferation of cultured embryonic heart cells. *In Vitro Cell Dev Biol Anim* 2000;36:622–639.
107. Tobita K, Keller BB. Right and left ventricular wall deformation patterns in normal and left heart hypoplasia chick embryos. *Am J Physiol* 2000:279:H959–969.
108. Garrity DM, Childs S, Fishman MC. The heartstrings mutation in zebrafish causes heart/fin *Tbx5* deficiency syndrome. *Development* 2002;129(19):4635–4645.
109. Li QY, Newbury-Ecob RA, Terrett JA, et al. Holt-Oram syndrome is caused by mutations in *TBX5*, a member of the Brachyury (T) gene family. *Nat Genet* 1997;15:21–29.
110. Basson CT, Bachinsky DR, Lin RC, et al. Mutations in human *TBX5* [corrected] cause limb and cardiac malformation in Holt-Oram syndrome. *Nat Genet* 1997;15:30–35.
111. Bruneau BG, Logan M, Davis N, et al. Chamber-specific cardiac expression of *Tbx5* and heart defects in Holt-Oram syndrome. *Dev Biol* 1999;211:100–108.
112. Kirby ML, Waldo KL. Role of neural crest in congenital heart disease. *Circulation* 1990;82:332–340.
113. Chisaka O, Capecchi MR. Regionally restricted developmental defects resulting from targeted disruption of the mouse homeobox gene Hox-1.5. *Nature* 1991;350:473–474.
114. Conway SJ, Godt RE, Hatcher CJ, et al. Neural crest is involved in development of abnormal myocardial function. *J Mol Cell Cardiol* 1997;29:2675–2685.
115. Epstein JA. *PAX3*, neural crest and cardiovascular development. *Trends Cardiovasc Med* 1996;6:255–261.
116. Kirby ML. Contribution of neural crest to heart and vessel morphology. In: Harvey RP, and Rosenthal N, eds. *Heart Development.* San Diego, CA: Academic Press; 1999:179–193.
117. Lammer EJ, Opitz JM. The DiGeorge anomaly as a developmental field defect. *Am J Med Genet Suppl* 1986;2:113–127.
118. Wilson DI, Cross IE, Goodship JA, et al. DiGeorge syndrome with isolated aortic coarctation and isolated ventricular septal defect in three sibs with a 22q11 deletion of maternal origin. *Br Heart J* 1991;66:308–312.
119. Scambler PJ, Kelly D, Lindsay E, et al. Velo-cardio-facial syndrome associated with chromosome 22 deletions encompassing the DiGeorge locus. *Lancet* 1992;339:1138–1139.
120. Driscoll DA, Budarf ML, Emanuel BS. A genetic etiology for DiGeorge syndrome: Consistent deletions and microdeletions of 22q11. *Am J Hum Genet* 1992;50:924–933.
121. Kochilas LK, Li J, Jin F, et al. *p57Kip2* expression is enhanced during mid-cardiac murine development and is restricted to trabecular myocardium. *Pediatr Res* 1999;45:635–642.
122. Kochilas L, Merscher-Gomez S, Lu MM, et al. The role of neural crest during cardiac development in a mouse model of DiGeorge syndrome. *Dev Biol* 2002;251:157–166.
123. Feiner L, Webber AL, Brown CB, et al. Targeted disruption of semaphorin 3C leads to persistent truncus arteriosus and aortic arch interruption. *Development* 2001;128:3061–3070.
124. Brown CB, Feiner L, Lu MM, et al. Plexin A2 and semaphorin signaling during cardiac neural crest development. *Development* 2001;128:3071–3080.
125. Lammer EJ, Chen DT, Hoar R, et al. Retinoic acid embryopathy. *N Engl J Med* 1985;313:837–841.
126. Clark EB, Hu N, Dummett JL, et al. Ventricular function and morphology in the chick embryo stage 18 to 29. *Am J Physiology* 1986;250:H407–H413.
127. Shiraishi I, Takamatsu T, Minamikawa T, et al. 3-D observation of actin filaments during cardiac myofibrinogenesis in chick embryo using a confocal laser scanning microscope. *Anat Embryol* 1992; 185:401–408
128. Price RL, Chintanawonges C, Shiraishi I, et al. Local and regional variations in myofibrillar patterns in looping rat hearts. *Anat Rec* 1996;245:83–93.
129. Taber LA, Keller BB, Clark EB: Cardiac mechanics in the stage 16 chick embryo. *J Biomech Eng* 1992;114:427–434.
130. Wei L, Roberts W, Wang L, et al. Rho kinases play an obligatory role in vertebrate embryonic organogenesis. *Development* 2001;128: 2953–2962.
131. Ruzicka DL, Schwartz RJ. Sequential activation of alpha actin genes during avian cardiogenesis: Vascular smooth muscle alpha actin gene transcripts mark the onset of cardiomyocyte differentiation. *J Cell Biol* 1988;107:2575–2586.
132. Sugi Y, Lough J. Onset of expression and regional deposition of alpha-smooth and sarcomeric actin during avian heart development. *Dev Dyn* 1992;193:116–124.
133. Sordahl LA, Crow CA, Draft GH, et al. Some ultrastructural and biochemical aspects of heart mitochondria associated with development. *J Mol Cell Cardiol* 1972;4:1–10.
134. Barth E, Stammler G, Speiser B, et al. Ultrastructural quantitation of mitochondria and myofilaments in cardiac muscle from 10 different animal species including man. *J Mol Cell Cardiol* 1992;24: 669–681.
135. Mahony L. Cardiac membrane structure and function. In: Burggren WW, Keller BB, eds. *Development of Cardiovascular Systems: Molecules to Organisms.* New York: Cambridge University Press. In press.
136. Bernard C: Establishment of ionic permeabilities of the myocardial membrane during embryonic development of the rat. In: Lieberman M, Sano T, eds. *Development and Physiological Correlates of Cardiac Muscle.* New York: Raven Press; 1975;169–184.
137. Artman M, Henry G, Coetzee WA. Cellular basis for age-related differences in cardiac excitation-contraction coupling. *Prog Pediatr Cardiol* 2000;11:185–194.

138. Osaka T, Joyner RW: Developmental changes in calcium currents of rabbit ventricular cells. *Circ Res* 1991;68:788–796.
139. Wetzel GT, Chen F, Klitzner TS. $Ca^{2+}$channel kinetics in acute isolated fetal, neonatal and adult rabbit cardiac myocytes. *Circ Res* 1993;72:1065–1074.
140. Takehima H. Intracellular $Ca^{2+}$ store in embryonic cardiac myocytes. *Front Biosci* 2002;7:1642–1652.
141. Bridge JHB, Smolley JR, Spitzer KW. The relationship between charge movements associated $I_{Ca}$ and $I_{Na\text{-}Ca}$ in cardiac myocytes. *Science* 1990;248:376–378.
142. Davis CL. Description of a human embryo having 20 paired somites. *Contrib Embryol* 1923;15:1–52.
143. Davis CL. The cardiac jelly of the chick embryo. *Anat Rec* 1924; 27:201–202.
144. Van Mierop LHS: Embryology of the heart. In: Netter FH, ed. *The CIBA Collection of Medical Illustrations*: Vol 5, Pt 1. Summit, NJ: CIBA Pharmaceutical Co; 1969:112–130.
145. Markwald RR, Trusk T, Gittenberger-de Groot AC, et al. Cardiac morphogenesis: Formation and septation of the primary heart tube. In: Kavlock R, Datson G, eds. *Handbook of Experimental Pharmacology.* Berlin: Springer-Verlag; 1998:11–40.
146. Drake CJ, Davis LA, Walters L, et al. Avian vasculogenesis and the distribution of collagens I, IV, laminin and fibronectin in the heart primordia. *J Exp Zool* 1990;255:309–322.
147. Markwald RR, Mjaatvedt CH, Krug EL. Induction of endocardial cushion tissue formation by adheron-like molecular complexes derived from the myocardial basement membrane. In: Clark EB, Takao A, eds. *Developmental Cardiology: Morphogenesis and Function.* Mt. Kisco, NY: Futura; 1990:191–204.
148. Eisenberg LM, Markwald RR. Molecular regulation of atrioventricular valvuloseptal morphogenesis. *Circ Res* 1995;77:1–6.
149. Lyons KM, Jones CM, Hogan BLM. The TGF-$\beta$-related DVR gene family in mammalian development. In: *Postimplantation Development in the Mouse.* Ciba Foundation Symposium 165. Chichester, UK: Wiley 1992;219–234.
150. Runyan RB, Potts JD, Sharma RV, et al. Signal transduction of a tissue interaction during embryonic heart development. *Cell Regul* 1990; 1:301–313.
151. Chin C, Gandour-Edwards R, Oltjen S, et al. Fate of the atrioventricular endocardial cushions in the developing chick heart. *Pediatr Res* 1992;32:390–393.
152. Garcia-Martinez V, Sanchez-Quintana D, Hurle JM. Histogenesis of the semilunar valves: An immunohistochemical analysis of tenascin and type-I collagen distribution in developing chick heart valves. *Cell Tissue Res* 1990;259:299–304.
153. Potts JD, Vincent EB, Runyan RB, et al. Sense and antisense TGF beta 3 mRNA levels correlate with cardiac valve induction. *Dev Dyn* 1992;193:340–345.
154. Brown CB, Boyer AS, Runyan RB, et al. Requirement of type III TGF-beta receptor for endocardial cell transformation in the heart. *Science* 1999;283:2080–2082.
155. Lai YT, Beason KB, Brames GP, et al. Activin receptor–like kinase 2 can mediate atrioventricular cushion transformation. *Dev Biol* 2000;222:1–11.
156. Izumi M, Fujio Y, Kunisada K, et al. Bone morphogenetic protein-2 inhibits serum deprivation-induced apoptosis of neonatal cardiac myocytes through activation of Smad1 pathway. *J Biol Chem* 2001;276:31133–31141.
157. Kruzynska-Frejtag A, Machnicki M, Rogers R, et al. Periostin (an osteoblast-specific factor) is expressed within the embryonic mouse heart during valve formation. *Mech Dev* 2001;103:183–188.
158. Simpson DG, Majeski M, Borg TK, et al. Regulation of cardiac myocyte protein turnover and myofibrillar structure in vitro by specific directions of stretch. *Circ Res* 1999;85:59–69.
159. Ross RS, Borg TK. Integrins and the myocardium. *Circ Res* 2001;88: 1112–1119.
160. Sussman MA, McCulloch A, Borg TK. Dance band on the Titanic: Biomechanical signaling in cardiac hypertrophy. *Circ Res* 2002;91: 888–898.
161. Pexieder T. Prenatal development of the endocardium: A review. *Scan Electron Microsc* 1981;2:223–253.
162. Noden DM. Origins and patterning of avian outflow tract endocardium. *Development* 1991;111:867–876.
163. Markwald RR, Mjaatvedt CH, Krug EL, et al. Inductive interaction in heart development: Role of cardiac adherons in cushion tissue formation. In: Bockman DE, Kirby ML, eds. *Embryonic Origins of Defective Heart Development. Ann NY Acad Sc* 1990;588:13–25.
164. Icardo JM, Hurle JM, Ojeda JL. Endocardial cell polarity during the looping of the heart in the chick embryo. *Dev Biol* 1982;90:203–209.
165. Hove JR, Koster RW, Forouhar AS, et al. Intracardiac fluid forces are an essential epigenetic factor for embryonic cardiogenesis. *Nature* 2003;421:172–177.
166. Pexieder T. Cell death in the morphogenesis and teratogenesis of the heart. *Adv Anat Embryol Cell Biol* 1975;51:1–100.
167. Dzau VJ, Krieger JE. Molecular biology of hypertension. In: Roberts R, ed. *Molecular Basis of Cardiology.* Boston: Blackwell; 1993: 325–354.
168. Zhou B, Cron RQ, Wu B, et al. Regulation of the murine *NFATc1* gene by NFATc2. *J Biol Chem* 2002;277:10704–10711.
169. Taber LA, Lin IE, Clark EB: Mechanics of cardiac looping. *Dev Dyn* 1995;203:42–50.
170. Wessels A, Vermeulen JLM, Verbeek FJ, et al. Spatial distribution of "tissue-specific" antigens in the developing human heart and skeletal muscle: III. An immunohistochemical analysis of the distribution of the neural tissue antigen GlN2 in the embryonic heart: Implications for the development of the atrioventricular conduction system. *Anat Rec* 1992;232:97–111.
171. Wessels A, Mijnders TA, de Gier-de Vries C, et al. Expression of myosin heavy chain in neonatal human hearts. *Cardiol Young* 1992; 2:318–334.
172. Gittenberger-de Groot A. Principles of abnormal cardiac development. In: Burggren WW, Keller BB, eds. *Development of Cardiovascular Systems: Molecules to Organisms.* New York: Cambridge University Press; 1996;259–267.
173. Icardo JM, Fernandez-Teran A. Morphologic study of ventricular trabeculation in the embryonic chick heart. *Acta Anat* 1987;130: 264–274.
174. Pexieder T, Christen Y, Vuillemin M, et al. Comparative morphometric analysis of cardiac organogenesis in chick, mouse, and dog embryos. In: Nora JJ, Takao A, eds. *Congenital Heart Disease: Causes and Processes.* Mount Kisco, NY: Futura; 1984;423–438.
175. Taber LA, Hu N, Pexieder T, et al. Residual strain in the ventricle of the stage 16-24 chick embryo. *Circ Res* 1993;72:455–462.
176. Thompson RP, Lindroth JR, Wong YMM. Regional differences in DNA-synthetic activity in the preseptation myocardium of the chick. In: Clark EB, Takao A, eds. *Developmental Cardiology: Morphogenesis and Function.* Mount Kisco, NY: Futura; 1990:219–234.
177. Streeter GL. Developmental horizons in human embryos: Description of age groups XI, 13-20 somites, and age group XII, 21-29 somites. *Contrib Embryol* 1942;30:211–246.
178. Van Mierop LHS, Alley RD, Kausel HW, et al. The anatomy and embryology of endocardial cushion defects. *J Thorac Cardiovasc Surg* 1962;43:71–83.
179. Chin TK, Perloff JK, Williams RG, et al. Isolated noncompaction of left ventricular myocardium. A study of eight cases. *Circulation* 1990;82:507–513.
180. Agmon Y, Connolly HM, Olson LJ, et al. Noncompaction of the ventricular myocardium. *J Am Soc Echo* 1999;12:859–863.
181. Ichida F, Hamamichi Y, Miyawaki T, et al. Clinical features of isolated noncompaction of the ventricular myocardium: Long-term clinical course, hemodynamic properties, and genetic background. *J Am Coll Cardiol* 1999;34:233–240.
182. Pauli RM, Scheib-Wixted S, Cripe L, et al. Ventricular noncompaction and distal chromosome 5q deletion. *Am J Med Genet* 1999;85:419–423.
183. Pexieder T, Christen Y. Quantitative analysis of the shape development in the chick embryo heart. In: Pexieder T, ed. *Mechanisms of Cardiac Morphogenesis and Teratogenesis.* New York: Raven Press; 1981: 49–67.

184. Hatcher CJ, Kim MS, Basson CT. Atrial form and function: Lessons from human molecular genetics. *Trends Cardiovasc Med* 2000;10: 93–101.
185. Wessels A, Anderson RH, Markwald RR, et al. Atrial development in the human heart: An immunohistochemical study with emphasis on the role of mesenchymal tissues. *Anat Rec* 2000;259:288–300.
186. Seo JW, Kim AEK, Brown NA, et al. Section directed cryosectioning of specimens for scanning electron microscopy: A new method to study cardiac development. *Microsc Res Tech* 1995;30:491–495.
187. Blom NA, Gittenberger-de Groot AC, Jongeneel TH, et al. Normal development of the pulmonary veins in human embryos and formation of a morphogenetic concept for sinus venosus defects. *Am J Cardiol* 2001;87:305–309.
188. Webb S, Kanani M, Anderson RH, et al. Development of the human pulmonary vein and its incorporation in the morphologically left atrium. *Cardiol Young* 2001;11:632–642.
189. Van den Hoff MJB, Bennington RW, Moorman AFM, et al. Myocardialization in the developing heart. *Dev Biol* 1999;212:477–490.
190. Van Mierop LHS, Alley RD, Kausel HW, et al. Pathogenesis of transposition complexes: I. Embryology of the ventricles and great arteries. *Am J Cardiol* 1963;12:216–225.
191. Blom NA, Ottenkamp J, Wenink AG, et al. Deficiency of the vestibular spine in atrioventricular septal defects in human fetuses with down syndrome. *Am J Cardiol* 2003;91:180–184.
192. Sedmera D, Pexieder T, Hu N, et al. Developmental changes in the myocardial architecture of the chick. *Anat Rec* 1997;248:421–432.
193. Streeter GL. Developmental horizons in human embryos: Description of age groups XV, XVI, XVII, XVIII, being the third issue of a survey of the Carnegie Collection. *Contrib Embryol* 1948;32:133–204.
194. Pexieder T. Conotruncus and its septation at the advent of the molecular biology era. In: Clark EB, Markwald RR, Takao A, eds. *Developmental Mechanisms of Heart Disease.* Mount Kisco, NY: Futura; 1995:227–247.
195. Dor X, Corone P. Embryologie cardiaque: Malformations (I). In: *Embryologie Cardiaque—Editions Techniques—Encyclopedie Medico-Chirurgicale.* Paris; 1992:1–20.
196. Wessels A, Markman MWM, Vermeulen JLM, et al. The development of the atrioventricular junction in the human heart; an immunohistochemical study. *Circ Res* 1996;78:110–117.
197. Oosthoek PW, Wenink ACG, Vrolijk BCM, et al. Development of the atrioventricular valve tension apparatus in the human heart. *Anat Embryol* 1998;198:317–329.
198. Bergwerff M, Verberne ME, DeRuiter MC, et al. Neural crest cell contribution to the developing circulatory system: Implications for vascular morphology? *Circ Res* 1998;82:221–231.
199. Tartaglia M, Mehler EL, Goldberg R, et al. Mutations in *PTPN11,* encoding the protein tyrosine phosphatase SHP-2, cause Noonan syndrome. *Nat Genet* 2001;29:465–468.
200. Leonhardt A, Glaser A, Wegmann M, et al. Expression of prostanoid receptors in human ductus arteriosus. *Br J Pharmacol* 2003;138: 655–659.
201. Michelakis ED, Rebeyka I, Wu X, et al. O2 sensing in the human ductus arteriosus: Regulation of voltage-gated K+ channels in smooth muscle cells by a mitochondrial redox sensor. *Circ Res* 2002;91: 478–486.
202. Zhao F, Weismann CG, Satoda M, et al. Novel *TFAP2B* mutations that cause Char syndrome provide a genotype-phenotype correlation. *Am J Hum Genet* 2001;69:695–703.
203. Elzenga NJ, Gittenberger-de Groot AC, Oppenheimer-Dekker A. Coarctation and other obstructive aortic arch anomalies: Their relationship to the ductus arteriosus. *Int J Cardiol* 1986;13:289–308.
204. Poelmann RE, Gittenberger-de Groot AC, Metlink MMT, et al. Development of the cardiac/coronary vascular endothelium, studied with antiendothelial antibodies, in chicken-quail chimeras. *Circ Res* 1993;73:559–568.
205. Perez-Pomares JM, Macias D, Garcia-Garrido L, et al. Contribution of the primitive epicardium to the subepicardial mesenchyme. *Dev Dyn* 1997;210:96–105.
206. Perez-Pomares JM, Macias D, Garcia-Garrido L, et al. The origin of the subepicardial mesenchyme in the avian embryo: An immunohistochemical and quail-chick chimera study. *Dev Biol* 1998: 200:57–68.
207. Dettman RW, Denetclaw W Jr, Ordahl CP, et al. Common epicardial origin of coronary vascular smooth muscle, perivascular. *Dev Biol* 1998;193:169–181.
208. Gittenberger-de Groot AC, Vrancken Peeters MP, Mentink MM, et al. Epicardium-derived cells contribute a novel population to the myocardial. *Circ Res* 1998;82:1043–1052.
209. Perez-Pomares JM, Phelps A, Sedmerova M, et al. Experimental studies on the spatiotemporal expression of WT1 and RALDH2 in the embryonic avian heart: A model for the regulation of myocardial and valvuloseptal development by epicardially derived cells (EPDCs). *Dev Biol* 2002;247:307–326.
210. Hood LC, Rosenquist TH. Coronary artery development in the chick: Origin and deployment of smooth muscle cells, and the effects of neural crest ablation. *Anat Rec* 1992;234:291–300.
211. Li We, Waldo K, Linask KL, et al. An essential role of connexin 43 gap junctions in mouse coronary artery development. *Development* 2002;129:2031–2042.
212. Rosenquist TH, Modis L. Spatial disorder of collagens in the great vessels, associated with congenital heart defects. *Anat Rec* 1991; 229:116–124.
213. Risau W. Vasculogenesis, angiogenesis and endothelial cell differentiation during embryonic development. In: Feinberg RN, Sherer GK, Auerbach R, eds. *The Development of the Vascular System.* Issues Biomed. Basel: Karger, 1991;14:58–68.
214. Rakusan K, Flanagan MF, Geva T, et al. Morphometry of human coronary capillaries during normal growth and the effect of age in left ventricular pressure-overload hypertrophy. *Circulation* 1992;86:38–46.
215. Tomanek RJ, Phan BP, Hu N, et al. Myocardial vascularization is accelerated in chick embryos with increased afterload and ventricular mass (abstr). *FASEB J* 1996;10:A579.
216. Lie-Venema H, Gittenberger-de Groot AC, Van Empel LJ, et al. Ets-1 and ETS-2 transcription factors are essential for normal coronary and myocardial development in chicken embryos. *Circ Res* 2003;92: 749–756.
217. Anderson RH, Becker AE, Wenink ACG. The development of the conducting tissues. In: Roberts EA, ed. *Cardiac Arrhythmias in the Neonate, Infant and Child.* New York: Appleton-Century-Crofts; 1978.
218. Gorza L, Vitadello M. Distribution of conduction system fibers in the developing and adult rabbit heart revealed by an anti-neurofilament antibody. *Circ Res* 1989;65:360–369.
219. Ikeda T, Iwasaki K, Shimokawa I, et al. Leu-7 immunoreactivity in human and rat embryonic hearts, with special reference to the development of the conduction tissue. *Anat Embryol* 1990;182: 553–562.
220. Wessels A, Vermeulen JLM, Verbeek FJ, et al. Spatial distribution of "tissue-specific" antigens in the developing human heart and skeletal muscle: III. An Immunohistochemical analysis of the distribution of the neural tissue antigen GlN2 in the embryonic heart: Implications for the development of the atrioventricular conduction system. *Anat Rec* 1992;231:97–111.
221. Gourdie RG, Mima T, Thompson RP, et al. Terminal diversification of the myocyte lineage generates Purkinje fibers of the cardiac conduction system. *Development* 1995;121:1423–1431.
222. Hyer J, Johansen M, Prasad A, et al. Induction of Purkinje fiber differentiation by coronary vascularization. *Proc Natl Acad Sci USA* 1999;96:13214–13218.
223. Reese DE, Mikawa T, Bader DM. Development of the coronary vessel system. *Circ Res* 2002;91:761–768.
224. Kanzawa N, Poma CP, Takebayashi-Suzuki K, et al. Competency of embryonic cardiomyocytes to undergo Purkinje fiber differentiation is regulated by endothelin receptor expression. *Development* 2002; 129:3185–3194.
225. Benson DW, Silberbach GM, Kavanaugh-McHugh A, et al. Mutations in the cardiac transcription factor NKX-2.5 affect diverse cardiac developmental pathways. *J Clin Invest* 1999;104:1483–1484.

226. Li QY, Newbury-Ecob RA, Terrett JA, et al. Holt-Oram syndrome is caused by mutations in *TBX5,* a member of the Brachyury (T) gene family. *Nat Genet* 1997;15:21–29.
227. Gordon L, Polak JM, Moscoso GJ, et al. Development of the peptidergic innervation of human heart. *J Anat* 1993;183:131–140.
228. St Petery LB, Van Mierop LHS. Evidence for the presence of adrenergic receptors in 3-day-old chick embryo. *Am J Physiol* 1977;232:H250–H254.
229. Keller BB: Functional maturation and coupling of the embryonic cardiovascular system. In: Clark EB, Markwald RR, Takao A, eds. *Developmental Mechanisms of Heart Disease.* Mount Kisco, NY: Futura; 1995:367–386.
230. Keller BB: Embryonic cardiovascular function, coupling, and maturation: A species view. In: Burggren W, Keller BB, eds. *Development of Cardiovascular Systems: Molecules to Organisms.* New York: Cambridge University Press; 1996:65–87.

CHAPTER 9

# THE HUMAN GENOME AND ITS FUTURE IMPLICATIONS FOR CARDIOVASCULAR DISEASE

Robert Roberts / Richard P. Lifton



## THE HUMAN GENOME

The term *genome* refers to all of the DNA including the genes responsible for an organism. The term *proteome* refers to all of the proteins responsible for an organism. The genes exert all of their influence through the proteins they produce. Each gene produces a unique protein, preferably referred to as a *polypeptide,* since some proteins are made of two or more polypeptides, and a significant proportion of genes, through alternative splicing, produce more than one polypeptide. The human genome contains 23 pairs of chromosomes, of which 22 pairs are homologous (one from the father and one from the mother), referred to as *autosomes,* and the remaining pair contain the sex chromosomes. In the male, these consist of X and Y; in the female, they consist of two X chromosomes. Each pair of autosomal homologous chromosomes carries the same set of genes, with one inherited from each parent. Despite their homology and potentially identical function, some of the genes have a slightly different DNA sequence from that of the corresponding gene on its homologous partner, which may slightly or markedly alter its function. An example of this would be the gene encoding for the angiotensin-converting enzyme (ACE), which, in the general population, exists in three forms or alleles: D, DI, and II. One may inherit the D form from the mother and the I form from the father. While both genes encode for ACE and convert angiotensinogen to angiotensin II, there is increased plasma enzyme activity associated with the D form, and studies suggest if you are homozygous for the D gene (DD), you are predisposed to develop cardiac hypertrophy.[1,2] These minor differences give rise to an individual's genetic distinguishing features and in some instances predispose him or her to the disease. The difference in the DNA sequence between all humans is about 0.1 percent, which means that 99.9 percent of the DNA sequence is identical. However, this means that there is a difference in over 3 million bases of the DNA sequence. Each chromosome is a long molecule made of DNA, which is comprised of only four bases: adenine (A), guanine (G), cytosine (C), and thymidine (T) (see Chap. 5). A chromosome consists of monotonous repeats of these four bases. Nevertheless, the sequence of these four bases determines all of a person's inherited characteristics. The average length of a chromosome is about 135 million base pairs (bp). The longest chromosome, chromosome 1, has over 250 million bp. The smallest, chromosome 21, has only 50 million bp. The 23 chromosomes together contain a total of 3 billion bp (Table 9-1). Genes themselves are discrete units with a start and stop point and vary in size from 10,000 to 2 million bp. The estimated average is about 20,000 bp. Thus, only about 2 percent of the DNA is used to make genes.[3] Genes themselves do not participate in specific functions but function through an intermediary, its single-stranded template being referred to as *messenger RNA* (mRNA). The mRNA leaves the nucleus and goes to the ribosome in the cytoplasm, where it provides the template for protein synthesis. It is estimated there are about 30,000 genes; however, alternative splicing provides for other forms of the same gene.

The intervening DNA between the genes, which does not exit the nucleus, is referred to as *introns,* whereas the DNA transcribed into mRNA that exits the nucleus to form the template for protein synthesis is referred to as *exons*. The function of the introns is largely unknown. A small proportion of the introns has the important regulatory function of determing when and how often the gene will make mRNA. Another function of the introns is presumably maintaining the structure and integrity of the DNA molecule. The introns, on a simple mathematical basis, also offer some protection from mutations to the genes. The natural mutation rate is one every 200,000 years per gene. The mutation rate is higher in the introns, but since it is not expressed in the protein, it tends to be benign and not disease-producing. Introns with repeating units of the same sequence occur throughout the genome. The most frequent example is the ALU repeat, a 300-bp repeat with over 500,000 copies scattered throughout the human genome. The role of these repeat sequences is also not known but may play a role as replication or initiation sites for duplication of DNA. While foreign DNA is usually destroyed, some, such as the genomes of retroviruses, do become incorporated into the human genome. It is estimated that 46 percent of the human genome is composed of DNA from mobile DNA elements with no known function transposed into the human genome over the past 150 to 200 million years.[4] Mutations that induce single-gene disease, inherited

TABLE 9-1 The Human Genome

| | |
|---|---|
| Base pairs | 3 billion |
| Genes estimated | 30,000 |
| Percent of DNA contained in genes | <2% |

as Mendelian disorders, occur at a frequency of less than 1 percent. In contrast, mutations that induce more subtle changes (genes that predispose to polygenic diseases; e.g., DD versus II) occur more frequently, in the range of 10 to 20 percent. One form of these polymorphisms, referred to as *single nucleotide polymorphisms,*[5,6] occurs every 1000 bp and is thought to account for most individual phenotypic differences. These polymorphisms also provide the most promising markers for identifying genes responsible for polygenic diseases.

## THE HUMAN GENOME PROJECT

The Human Genome Project, the first large international effort in the history of biological research, was initiated on October 1, 1990, to be completed in the year 2005.[7,8] However, with improvements in technology and increasing demands, the timetable was accelerated. A rough draft of 90 percent was completed in 2000,[7] and the complete sequence became available in 2001.[9] At the end of the millennium (2000), less than 1000 human genes responsible for human disease were available in GenBank. It is expected that 10,000 to 20,000 genes will be available by 2008. It is part of the policy of the Human Genome Project that all of these genes will be available to the public. Each gene, as it is sequenced, is entered into a publicly accessible database and available at no cost. In the United States, GenBank (at http://www.ncvi.nlm.nih.gov) is run by the National Center for Biotechnology Information and serves as the public repository of sequence information. The results of the efforts of the publicly funded Human Genome Project consist of not only DNA sequences of the various genes but also the intervening sequences. In addition but very important is that each sequence is anchored to one of the known genetic markers integrating the physical and genetic maps.

The Human Genome Project contains the blueprint for the development of a single fertilized egg into a complex organism of more than $10^{13}$ cells. This blueprint is written in a coded message given by the sequence of nucleotide bases—the A's, C's, G's, and T's—that are strung along the DNA molecules in the human genome. However, while the overall objective was to sequence the human genome, other goals were completed along the way that markedly accelerated the efforts of all investigators involved in biological or medical research. The first goal was to develop a genetic map. This meant developing markers (a unique DNA sequence) along each chromosome that would have a readily identifiable chromosomal position to provide highly informative signposts for the identification of nearby genes. This goal has been reached, with thousands of markers spaced less than 1 million bp apart, spanning the entire human genome.[10] Thus, the complete set of genetic markers available for each chromosome provides a complete genetic map of the human genome. The genetic map was the necessary tool for widespread application of genetic linkage analysis, a technique that has led to the mapping of numerous genes responsible for diseases of the cardiovascular system (Chap. 72) and other organs.

Another goal was to develop a physical map of that part of the DNA that is expressed as genes. These markers are referred to as *expressed sequence tags* (ESTs) and contain short sequences of 200 to 300 bp. These sequences are unique and represent a specific gene. One may wonder how it is possible to obtain such ESTs and be certain that they represent only sequences expressed in genes. As indicated previously, genes are transcribed as single-stranded mRNA, which leaves the nucleus to travel to the ribosome in the cytoplasm where it serves as a template for synthesis of its unique protein product. Thus, if one extracted all of the mRNAs, it would include all of the genes expressed in that cell. The mRNA can be converted to cDNA with the enzyme reverse transcriptase and the sequences amplified by the polymerase chain reaction, from which unique sequences are selected and entered into GenBank as ESTs. These ESTs, cloned and stored in vehicles such as bacteria, are referred to as *a library of human ESTs*. Many of the ESTs have been mapped to their chromosomal locations and can be used as markers to find genes responsible for disease. The development of the genetic map (chromosomal markers), followed by the physical map (ESTs), has tremendously accelerated the efforts of investigators to identify genes responsible for disease.

## FUNCTIONAL GENOMICS (PROTEOMICS)

One of the great accomplishments of the twenty-first century or even the new millennium will be the identification of all the genes responsible for humankind. This is often compared to another great landmark, which occurred in physics—namely, the identification of the table of periodic elements. The identified genes will provide the tools for determining gene function and how to manipulate them to benefit humankind. In understanding the gene and its function, one must consider genomic sequences. A gene nestled in its genomic origin contains the sequences to form the protein template and also the regulators which will determine if it is expressed as mRNA. The mRNA can be converted to a cDNA, which is used in expression studies to determine its function and to generate genetic animal models of disease. The cDNA is also used for gene therapy. However, the mRNA or cDNA is only a fraction of the genomic sequence. The additional genomic sequences represent intervening sequences of known and unknown function. Some of the sequences of known function are regulatory elements to which proteins bind (in the 5′ promoter region) to regulate gene expression and in the 3′ region to promote stability. While ultimate function requires knowledge of the protein, much of its function can be derived from its genomic sequence, a process referred to as *functional genomics*. In a workshop at Cold Spring Harbor,[11] it was estimated that determining the function of genes by conventional techniques—namely, eliminating the gene from the mouse by homologous recombination or overexpressing the gene (transgenic mouse)—would require most of this century. New approaches have emerged from the Genome Project to markedly accelerate this timetable.[12]

Paralleling the sequencing of the human genome was the effort to sequence simpler genomes of single and multicellular organisms, which interestingly has accelerated determining the function of human genes. The first organism for which the genome was sequenced and its genes identified was that of *Haemophilus influenzae* in 1995, consisting of 1.4 million bp and 1740 genes. Since then, the genomes of many single-celled and multicellular organisms have been determined—including *Saccharomyces cerevisiae,*[13] the cause of vaginitis, and the spirochete *Treponema pallidum,*[14] the cause of syphilis. Identification of the genes responsible for these various organisms has ushered in a new era for antibiotics based on a variety of different molecular mechanisms made possible through the identification of genes and the various pathways they regulate. A major step forward

TABLE 9-2 Comparison of Human and Mouse Genomes

| | Human | Mouse |
|---|---|---|
| Genome size | 3.0 billion bp | 2.5 billion bp |
| Number of genes | 30,000 | 30,000 |
| Nucleotide sequence homology | 40% | 40% |
| Genes with identifiable orthologues | 80% | 80% |
| Genes with some homologous sequence | 99% | 99% |

in our understanding of the function of human genes came with the sequencing of the first multicellular organism, namely *Caenorhabtidis elegans,*[15] which was recently followed by the sequencing of the fruit fly (*Drosophila*),[16] the mouse,[17] the rat,[18] and others. *C. elegans,* though a tiny a worm that is not visible to the naked eye, has 959 cells, all of which have been identified and characterized. Its genome consists of over 97 million bp with a total of over 19,000 genes, which is half the number of genes present in the human genome. Importantly, 36 percent of the genes in *C. elegans* are virtually identical to human genes. *C. elegans* is a transparent worm; thus it is possible to observe its development under the microscope from a single cell to a multicellular organism in the context of knowing all of the genes. It should therefore be possible, by determining the function of many genes in *C. elegans* homologous to humans, to learn of their approximate function in humans.

Genomes of organisms such as the mouse and rat provide an immense opportunity for determining the function of similar human genes.[19] All mammals have a similar size genome of 2.5 to 3.0 billion bp and approximately 30,000 genes. The mouse genome consists of 2.5 billion bp and has 30,000 genes.[20] The human and mouse diverged about 75 million years ago. Comparative genomics is a blossoming field, and with both the mouse and the human genomes sequenced, it will provide an avalanche of new information relative to gene function and epigenetic control. The following features have emerged to support this claim (Table 9-2): At the nucleotide sequence level, 40 percent of the human genome can be aligned to the mouse genome; over 80 percent of the mouse genes have an identifiable orthologue in the human genome; and 99 percent of all mouse genes have a homologous sequence in the human genome. The mouse routinely used for genetic manipulation is ideal for determining gene function.[19,21] Ultimately, in addition to determining the function of a single gene (a reductionist concept), we must also understand epigenetics—namely, what is responsible for determining the hierarchal function and regulation of genes for the overall organism. What determines how 30,000 genes, most of which are identical, in one instance generates a mouse and in another a human? Comparison of the differences between the mouse and human sequences may provide the first necessary clue.[22]

## COMPUTERIZED GENE BANK NETWORKS AND THEIR ROLE IN DETERMINING GENE FUNCTION (BIOINFORMATICS)

The information derived from unraveling genomes made it necessary to develop a computerized network of gene databases in which information would be rapidly entered worldwide and available at no cost.[23] Such a computerized network of gene banks (GenBank) was established in the United States, Britain, and Japan, and all investigators have agreed to input their data daily. Information on DNA and genes from all species are entered into this network and catalogued for readily accessibility. Billions of DNA bases collected from over 30,000 species are available and expanding on a daily basis. The function of certain genes is often first determined in simple organisms such as single-cell bacteria or viruses. It is also well recognized that certain genes, because of their function, have been conserved throughout evolution. Thus, a DNA sequence identified in the human genome with a consensus sequence to one of the genes of known function in simpler organisms can immediately provide an important clue to the function of that sequence in humans. A DNA sequence from the human genome with unknown function can be entered into a gene bank network such as GenBank (http://www.ncvi.nlm.nih.gov) and a consensus sequence sought. With GenBank, it is possible to travel back in time over 1 billion years to very simple organisms whose genes and their function are much better known. Although the human genome may contain 30,000 genes, it is highly likely that many of these genes can be grouped into families that have a common function.[24] An example would be the genes that encode for kinases. These proteins all have a common function—namely, the transfer of high-energy phosphate from one compound to another; thus, genes encoding for kinases share a common sequence that encodes for this motif. The functional unit referred to as a *motif* has an amino acid sequence with a distinct function conserved throughout evolution. The sequence of this common motif can be used to identify unknown genes with this sequence that belong to the family of kinases. It is estimated that over 3000 genes code for kinases. Another is the grouping of genes that have in common a functioning network,[24] whether it be that of metabolism or signaling. The cascade of signaling proteins responsible for the growth and development of the heart are likely to be very similar across the invertebrate, vertebrate, and mammalian cardiac genetic systems. It is well recognized that proteins have certain domains, essential to their function, that have been conserved throughout evolution. In structural biology, a domain is defined as a distinct, compact, and stable unit that folds independently of other units.[25] Over 1000 folds have already been identified, and this probably accounts for over half of all proteins.[26–28] It is anticipated that, in terms of human illnesses, all of this information on genes and their function will be transmitted to the nursing station and thus be readily available to physicians, nurses, and genetic counselors. How this will be achieved and individual privacy maintained remains to be determined.

## PREDICTION OF GENES FROM DNA SEQUENCES

Since only 2 percent of DNA codes for genes, it remains a challenge to identify genes responsible for specific functions or diseases. Various computerized programs have been developed to determine whether a particular DNA sequence encodes for a gene. In general, these programs are based on detecting components known to make up genes. All genes have a start codon ATG and one of the stop codons (AAU, AGU, AUG). A sequence that has an open reading frame, meaning no stop codon for thousands of sequences, is more likely to reflect a gene. The exon-intron junctions have a specific sequence, beginning with GT and ending with AG, that, when present, reflects sequences of a gene. Other features include identifying start codons (ATG), stop codons (AAU, AGU, AUG), and sequences encoding for polyadenylation. Certain sequences code for motifs of known function, such as kinases. Genes are not randomly distributed throughout the genome but occur in clusters. These clusters of genes tend to be preceded by sequences rich in CpG nucleotides, referred to as *CpG islands,* and thus can be used to identify regions rich in genes.

## THE DNA CHIP TECHNOLOGY

A major obstacle in applying the progress made in molecular genetics to the practice of medicine is our inability to detect mutations rapidly and accurately. There are over 1000 genes in GenBank known to cause disease. To perform genetic screening for known mutations and determine individuals at risk for disease is still a formidable task carrying an unacceptable cost. The various techniques for detecting mutations are time-consuming, expensive, and ideally require confirmation by DNA sequencing. Technologies to perform these tasks on a daily basis with results available within a reasonable time, from hours to days, are essential. Several technologies are evolving, the most promising being the DNA microarray chip.[29] Several thousand genes are attached to glass or plastic, and each base is color-coded to detect mismatches in hybridization (mismatch mutations) (Fig. 9-1, Plate 109). This technique has the potential for robust high-throughput detection of thousands of mutations within hours. Other techniques include high-pressure liquid chromatography and mass spectrometry, both of which also have the potential for high-throughput analysis. Genetic testing of individuals, for example, those with familial hypertrophic cardiomyopathy (FHCM) or arrhythmogenic right ventricular dysplasia (ARVD), could help to identify thousands of individuals who die each year in combative sports. Another use of the DNA chip technology is that of pharmacogenomics—namely, genotyping to individualize drug therapy. This technique is used also to screen for genes up- or downregulated during the response of a particular organ to various physiologic or pathologic stimuli.

## RESTORATIVE BIOLOGY

It is highly likely that, within the first decade of the new millennium, significant progress will be made in our ability to generate organs. While the average human has over 200 trillion cells, it is estimated there are only about 200 distinct cells as defined by a unique function. These cells are derived from stem cells that are totipotent, which means that with appropriate stimulation, they can develop into any kind of cell. There are two types of these: embryonic and adult stem cells.[30] Embryonic stem cells have not yet specialized into any type of cell and are obtained from two sources: (1) fetal tissues from mis-

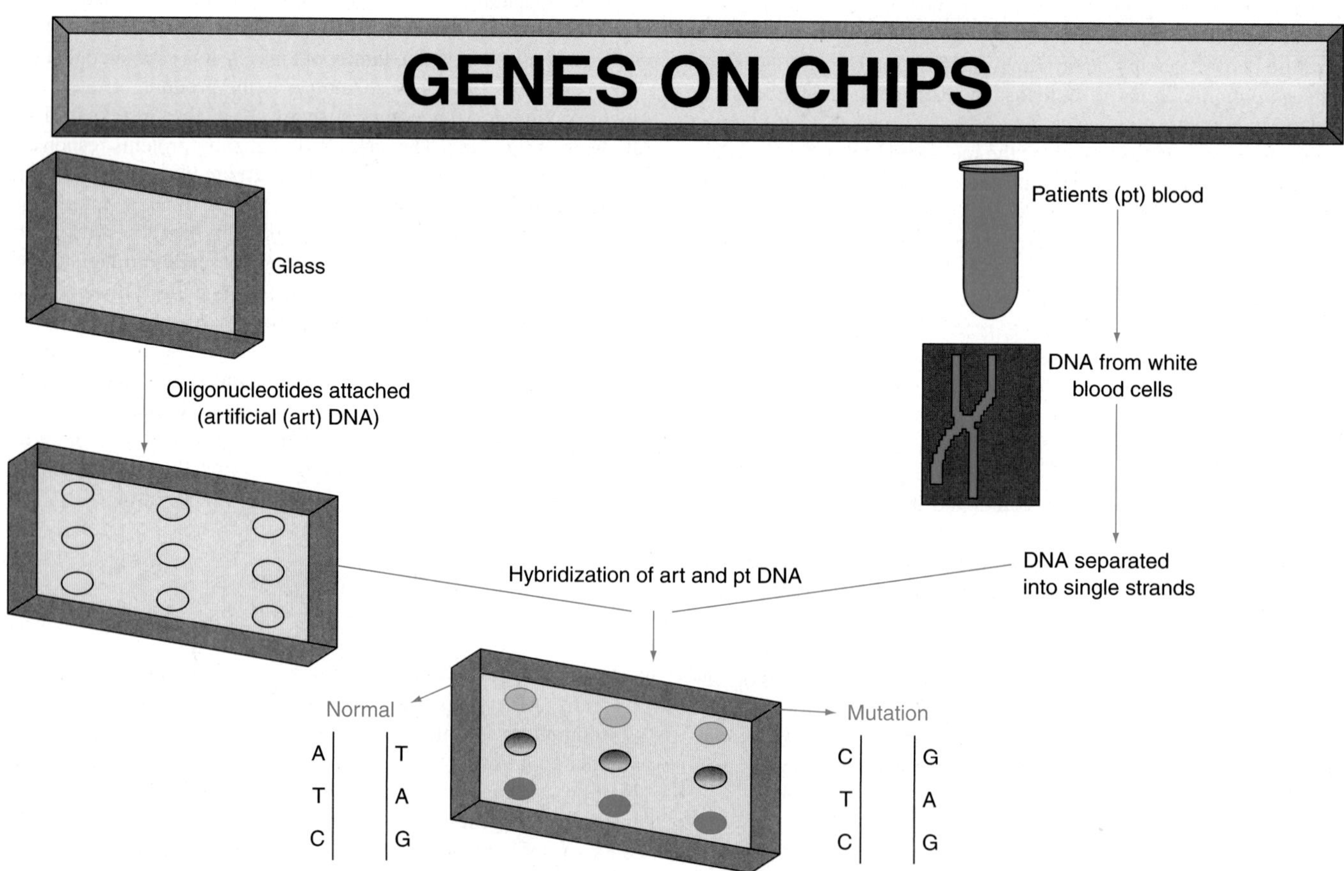


FIGURE 9-1 (Plate 109) Illustrated here is the means of detecting genes or their mutations. Oligonucleotides are single short strands of DNA of about 15 to 30 bases artificially synthesized to have the sequence of the desired gene. These oligonucleotides are bound to glass, with each of the four bases labeled with a distinct fluorescent color. The DNA extracted from the patient's white blood cells is denatured into separate strands and brought in contact with the artificial oligonucleotides' DNA. If the sequence in the patient's DNA is complementary to the oligonucleotide, hybridization will occur and the laser beam will detect the appropriate colors. If there is a mutation present, there will be a mismatch and a different color will be exhibited by the laser, indicating the site of the mutation.

carriages or abortions and (2) in vitro embryos that cannot be implanted and are discarded by fertility clinics. Adult stem cells have some limited capacity to be directed to develop into more than one cell type. At present, investigators have been relatively unsuccessful in obtaining stem cells from most organs in adults. Stem cells in limited numbers have been obtained from bone marrow, liver, brain, and skeletal muscle.[30] These stem cells, exposed to the appropriate cardiac growth factor, would be expected to develop into cardiac myocytes. Bone marrow stem cells have been used with considerable success in regenerating bone marrow in the treatment of leukemias. The National Institutes of Health has already developed goals to begin the pursuit of research to repair or regenerate human organs (www.bioethics.gov). Extensive research will be required to understand the molecular factors necessary to convert stem cells into a pretargeted specific cell (see Chap. 11). Another approach is to elucidate the molecular basis for organ regeneration and target the barriers to be surpassed to induce regeneration in the adult heart. Recently, it has been shown that the heart in the zebrafish routinely regenerates itself after injury.[31] Unraveling the molecular basis permitting regeneration in the heart of the adult zebrafish is likely to provide insights fundamental to human cardiac regeneration.

## A NEW ERA FOR UNRAVELING POLYGENIC DISORDERS

The extraordinary similarities in the height, weight, body habitus, and facial features of identical twins underscore the extremely limited variation in physical features of individuals who share complete genetic identity. The wide variation that is seen in these features among unrelated individuals in the general population strongly implies that much of this variation is attributable to variation in DNA sequence. Therefore, it comes as no surprise that this same principle applies to variation in disease susceptibility and that virtually all human diseases have an inherited component. In some cases, referred to as *Mendelian diseases,* mutation in a single gene is sufficient to produce disease in a high proportion of individuals inheriting that mutation. For other diseases, the inherited contribution is more subtle, requiring inheritance of variants in a number of genes, with disease development also being influenced by environmental factors. In this setting, inheritance of a particular genetic variant may be neither necessary nor sufficient for disease development. These genetically complex diseases are of multifactorial determination.

With the development of complete genetic maps of the human genome, a new approach to identifying genes contributing to Mendelian diseases, called *positional cloning,* became available.[32] Positional cloning proceeds in several stages: (1) the collection of families segregating traits of interest; (2) determination of the chromosomal location of disease genes by comparing the inheritance of chromosome segments to the inheritance of disease in families; (3) refinement of the interval containing the disease gene and identification of genes in the disease interval; and (4) screening genes in the interval for mutations that alter the structure or expression of the encoded protein. In the Mendelian paradigm, independent mutations that alter the encoded protein and segregate specifically with the disease in families constitute proof that the disease gene has been identified. This approach to date, and mostly within the last decade, has resulted in the identification of over 1000 human disease genes, of which over 100 are associated with cardiac diseases. While these Mendelian disorders are typically uncommon or rare, they have in many cases provided fundamental new insight into disease biology, which has proved relevant to the understanding of more common forms of disease.

Nonetheless, the truly common diseases—such as coronary artery disease, stroke, diabetes, and hypertension—are believed to be generally multifactorial in nature. For these diseases, the positional cloning paradigm that has been so successful for Mendelian diseases may have limited power, since within even single families affected individuals may have different combinations of inherited and acquired risk factors; moreover, the number of factors and the magnitude of the impact of any single risk locus is unknown. These barriers to identifying the genes underlying common diseases are formidable. Evidence that these diseases have an inherited component comes from a variety of studies, including studies of twins, demonstrating that monozygotic twins, who share 100 percent of their genes, are more concordant in disease status than dizygotic twins, who share only 50 percent of their genes, or studies of familial aggregation, showing that diseases occur within families more often than expected from their prevalence in the general population. A relatively simple means of assessing recurrence risk in families is determination of the so-called $\lambda$sib, defined as the risk of disease recurrence in a sibling of a disease case divided by the prevalence in the general population.[33] A $\lambda$sib of 1.0 would indicate no familial contribution to disease risk, while a $\lambda$sib of 10 would indicate that all familial factors together increase the risk of disease tenfold. Importantly, while these approaches can provide strong evidence for the impact of inheritance on disease risk, none indicates how many genes underlie the inherited disease risk, their mode of transmission, or the magnitude of the effect imparted by any single locus. For example, the same 10-fold familial increase in disease risk could be determined by the effects of two genes, each imparting a 5-fold increased risk, or alternatively 50 genes, each imparting a 1.2-fold increased risk. The best study design for identifying underlying disease genes is considerably confounded by this imprecise knowledge.

There are a number of potential approaches to unraveling the inherited contribution to these complex disorders. One is to simplify the analysis by identifying subordinate or intermediate phenotypes in which the genetic contribution is relatively more homogeneous or contributes to a larger fraction of disease risk. For example, the considerable etiologic heterogeneity of coronary artery disease can be reduced by focusing on cases sharing diabetes, hypertension, or hypercholesterolemia as contributing factors. Similarly, further refinement of these subgroups might define physiologic subsets with more homogeneous genetic contribution, potentially defining Mendelian subsets to which the power of Mendelian genetics can be applied.[34] Despite this potential, few useful intermediate phenotypes have been defined for common diseases. In this setting, linkage approaches like those used for Mendelian diseases might be successful if any single locus imparts a relatively large effect on disease risk, and collecting large extended kindreds may be worthwhile. In the absence of evidence of a substantial Mendelian component, a modification of the linkage approach analyzing large numbers of sibling or relative pairs concordant or discordant for disease has potential advantages. In this approach one scans the genome for chromosome segments that are shared among phenotypically concordant sibs more often than expected by chance. This approach has the advantage that it can detect linkage despite complications in which a disease locus does not contribute to disease in every affected individual and not all individuals inheriting a disease allele develop disease. Nonetheless, success with this approach requires that individual risk loci impart relatively large effects on disease risk.[35]

Another approach that will be increasingly used for complex trait analysis is identification of risk alleles by the study of cases and

TABLE 9-3 Single Nucleotide Polymorphisms (SNPs)

- 3 million SNPs per human genome
- 1 SNP per 1000 bp
- Approximately 40,000 SNPs present in coding regions

controls. There are estimated to be approximately 10 million common single nucleotide polymorphisms (SNPs) in the human population; however, there are only 3 million in any particular human genome (Table 9-3). A fraction of these will ultimately prove to underlie multifactorial traits by altering the expression or function of the gene in which they reside. The ability to identify and genotype these SNPs motivates their use for genetic studies. It is anticipated that the vast majority of common SNPs in human populations will be identified by 2008 and that many of the alleles contributing to common diseases will be found among these. If one tested an SNP whose variation contributes to, for example, coronary artery disease, comparison of SNP allele frequencies in disease cases and a matched cohort of controls free of disease would demonstrate a significantly different distribution of allele frequencies. This approach has substantially higher power than linkage to detect variants with small effects on disease risk.[35] This case-control approach also has a number of important caveats, however. One of these is that cases and controls must be well matched for genetic background. If they are not, many SNPs will show a false-positive association with disease. This is a current and serious problem with case-control studies. Unless disease associations are highly reproducible using the same SNP alleles and the same clinical phenotype, their significance should be regarded with caution. One means of eliminating this vexing problem is to collect the parents of affected individuals so as to permit use of transmission disequilibrium.[36] If an SNP allele contributes to disease risk, it ought to be transmitted from a heterozygous parent to an affected offspring more often than the expected Mendelian proportion of 0.5. This test thus eliminates the problem of poorly matched cases and controls and holds considerable promise for the investigation of complex genetic traits. Proof that a disease-associated SNP is itself a functional variant contributing to disease may be problematic, as some of these may well be common alleles in the population. Proof can be pursued by clinical studies of the physiology of individuals with and without the disease allele, biochemical studies of the wild-type and variant gene and gene product in vitro, as well as by the construction and investigation of animal models based on the variant gene.

A second caveat to this SNP approach is that at present we have limited capacity for SNP genotyping. As a result, we cannot readily perform comprehensive genomewide searches for disease variants by this approach but instead are limited to the investigation of candidate genes. While this approach may prove successful, we are presently largely limited to implicating genes in pathways that can already be associated with disease. There are two approaches to extending this case-control approach to a genomewide analysis. One is to investigate populations that have been established from a small number of founders in relatively recent time. In this case, one expects relatively long ancestral chromosome segments to be preserved in the present-day population, such that genetic markers at considerable distance from one another remain in *linkage disequilibrium*. In this case, one may be able to screen for the chromosomal location of disease susceptibility loci using a relatively modest number of SNPs distributed across the genome; proceeding from initial map location would be analogous to the positional cloning paradigm for Mendelian traits. Alternatively, with identification of complete SNP maps of the human genome, we will have many or all of the common SNPs in hand; one can contemplate performing extremely high density SNP genotyping in outbred populations to identify disease susceptibility alleles. In order to retain analytic power, this approach may require the performance of $10^9$ to $10^{10}$ genotypes; such a study is clearly beyond the capacity of present implemented technology but is not inconceivable in the future.[35]

Ultimately, one can envision that alleles contributing to susceptibility to common diseases will be identified and that these findings will have important consequences for clinical medicine. First, they will permit identification of individuals with specific inherited disease susceptibility before the disease has become manifest, affording new opportunity for targeted lifestyle or pharmacologic intervention in individual patients. Second, identification of these susceptibility alleles will define the physiologic pathways that contribute to disease, providing "validated targets" whose altered activity can be predicted with high likelihood to alter disease development; these will highlight opportunities for the development of new therapies. Third, we presently treat multifactorial diseases as though they were of homogeneous causation, with largely empiric therapies. The ability to identify specific risk alleles in individual patients may afford the opportunity to tailor treatment in individual patients to the specific inherited abnormalities underlying their disease susceptibility.

## References


1. Marian AJ. Genetic risk factors for myocardial infarction. *Curr Opin Cardiol* 1999;13:171–178.
2. Schunkert H, Dzau VJ, Tank SS, et al. Increased rat cardiac angiotensin converting enzyme activity and mRNA levels in pressure overload left ventricular hypertrophy: Effects on coronary resistance, contractility and relaxation. *J Clin Invest* 1990;86:1913–1920.
3. The Chromosome 21 Mapping and Sequencing Consortium. *Nature* 2000;405:311–319.
4. Bestor TH, Bycko B. Creation of genomic methylation patterns. *Nat Genet* 1996;12:363–367.
5. Halushka MK, Fan J-B, Bentley K, et al. Patterns of single-nucleotide polymorphisms in candidate genes for blood-pressure homeostasis. *Nat Genet* 1999;22:239–247.
6. Cargill M, Altshuler D, Ireland J, et al. Characterization of single-nucleotide polymorphisms in coding regions of human genes. *Nat Genet* 1999;22:231–238.
7. Collins FS. Shattuck lecture—Medical and societal consequences of the human genome project. *N Engl J Med* 1999;341(1):28–37.
8. Department of Health and Human Services, Department of Energy. *Understanding Our Genetic Inheritance: The U.S. Human Genome Project*. Washington, DC: USDHS; 1990.
9. Katsanis N, Worley KC, Lupski JR. An evaluation of the draft human genome sequence. *Nat Genet* 2001;29(1):88–91.
10. Murray JC, Buetow KH, Weber JL, et al. A comprehensive human linkage map with centimorgan density. Cooperative Human Linkage Center (CHLC). *Science* 1994;265(5181):2049–2054.
11. Abboud FM, Bassingthwaighte JB, Bond EC, et al. The Banbury Conference. Genomics to physiology and beyond: How do we get there? *Physiologist* 1997;40:205–211.
12. Collins FS, McKusick VA. Implications of the Human Genome Project for medical science. *JAMA* 2001;285(5):540–544.
13. Holstege FC, Jennings EG, Wyrick JJ, et al. Dissecting the regulatory circuitry of a eukaryotic genome. *Cell* 1998;95(5):717–728.
14. Fraser C, Norris S, Weinstock G, et al. Complete genome sequence of *Treponema pallidum*, the syphilis spirochete. *Science* 1999;281:375–388.
15. Hodgkin J, Horowitz RS, Jasny BR, Kimble J. *C. elegans*: Sequence to biology. *Science* 1998;282:2011.
16. Garza DAJ, Burke D, Hartl D. Mapping the *Drosophila* genome with yeast artificial chromosomes. *Science* 1989;246:641–646.

17. Waterston RH, Lindblad-Toh K, Birney E, et al. Initial sequencing and comparative analysis of the mouse genome. *Nature* 2002;420:520–562.
18. Dressel R, Walter L, Gunther E. Genomic and funtional aspects of the rat MHC, the RT1 complex. *Immunol Rev* 2001;184:82–95.
19. Bradley A. Commentary: Mining the mouse genome. *Nature* 2002;420: 512–514.
20. Okazaki Y, Furuno M, Kasukawa T, et al. Analysis of the mouse transcriptome based on functional annotation of 60,770 full-length cDNAs. *Nature* 2002;420:563–573.
21. Boguski MS. The mouse that roared. *Nature* 2002;420:515–516.
22. Fortna A, Gardiner K. Genomic sequence analysis tools: A user's guide. *Trends Genet* 2001;17(3):158–164.
23. Roberts RD. Bioinformatics analysis of gene banks provides a treasure trove for the functional genomist. *J Mol Cell Cardiol* 2000;32(11): 1917–1919.
24. Manning G, Whyte DB, Martinez R, et al. The protein kinase complement of the human genome. *Science* 2002;298(5600): 1912–1934.
25. Koonin EV, Wolf YI, Karev GP. The structure of the protein universe and genome evolution. *Nature* 2002;420(6912):218–223.
26. Orengo CA, Jones DT, Thornton JM. Protein superfamilies and domain superfolds. *Nature* 1994;372(6507):631–634.
27. Chothia C. Proteins. One thousand families for the molecular biologist. *Nature* 1992;357(6379):543–544.
28. Wolf YI, Grishin NV, Koonin EV. Estimating the number of protein folds and families from complete genome data. *J Mol Biol* 2000;299(4): 897–905.
29. Bumol TF, Watanabe AM. Genetic information, genomic technologies, and the future of drug discovery. *JAMA* 2001;285(5):551–555.
30. Kaji EH, Leiden JM. Gene and stem cell therapies. *JAMA* 2001;285(5): 545–550.
31. Poss KD, Wilson LG, Keating MT. Heart regeneration in zebrafish. *Science* 2002;298(5601):2188–2190.
32. Botstein D, White RL, Skolnick M, Davis RW. Construction of a genetic linkage map in man using restriction fragment length polymorphisms. *Am J Hum Genet* 1980;32:314–331.
33. Risch N. Linkage strategies for genetically complex traits: II. The power of affected relative pairs. *Am J Hum Genet* 1990;46:229–241.
34. Lipton RP. Molecular genetics of human blood pressure variation. *Science* 1996;272:676–680.
35. Risch N, Merikangas K. The future of genetic studies of complex human diseases. *Science* 1996;273:1516–1517.
36. Spielman RS, McGinnis RE, Ewens WJ. Transmission test for linkage disequilibrium: The insulin gene region and insulin-dependent diabetes mellitus (IDDM). *Am J Hum Genet* 1993;52:506–516.

CHAPTER 10

# GENETIC BASIS OF CARDIAC ARRHYTHMIAS

Fadi G. Akar / Gordon F. Tomaselli



Gene expression and genomics may be important in the genesis of cardiac arrhythmias in a number of ways. Most cardiac arrhythmias occur in the context of structural heart disease, such as myocardial ischemia, infarction, and cardiomyopathy. The overwhelming majority of these diseases are acquired and the result of the interaction of a genetic predisposition and environmental influences. Indeed, it is the maladaptive interaction between an individual's genetic constitution and the environment that produces disease. Most common structural heart disease is genetically complex; that is, a number of genes are involved in the phenotypic manifestations of disease.

Monogenic inherited diseases are characterized by a well-defined pattern of inheritance and in some cases may serve as a model for more complex acquired heart disease. Monogenic diseases may heighten the predisposition to cardiac arrhythmias by directly altering the electrophysiology of the heart, for example in the long-QT syndrome (LQTS) and idiopathic ventricular fibrillation (IVF). Alternatively, single gene defects may alter myocardial structure and function and, in doing so, enhance the risk of serious cardiac arrhythmias in a manner analogous to that of complex, polygenic heart disease.

The phenotypic expression of even monogenic diseases is quite variable. This may be the result of interactions of the expressed genes with the environment or the effect of other "modifier genes." Modifier genes alter the susceptibility of an individual to the expression of a specific phenotype. It is likely that the specific alleles of a number of genes will influence the probability of developing a specific arrhythmia without directly producing a disease phenotype. For example, known polymorphisms and phenotypically silent mutations of ion channel genes have been associated with acquired or drug-induced LQTS (see below). Similarly it has been suggested that a polymorphism in *KCNE1* (minK) predisposes to the development of atrial fibrillation (AF).[1] There are likely to be a number of genes and specific polymorphisms that contribute to the probability of expressing a specific trait; therefore a promise of the human genome is the ability to develop genetic/genomic profiles of risk.

Finally there is a reprogramming of the expression of a number of genes and an alteration in the function of a number of gene products that are central to normal cardiac electrophysiology in structural heart disease. This "electrical remodeling" figures prominently in the predisposition to both atrial[2] and ventricular[3] arrhythmias in the diseased heart and the high incidence of potentially lethal proarrhythmic complications of antiarrhythmic drugs. This electrical remodeling is likely to be a consequence rather than a cause of myocardial disease, implying that upstream signaling molecules and pathways are responsible for maladaptive electrophysiologic changes in the heart.

This chapter focuses on our current understanding of monogenic diseases that predispose to cardiac arrhythmias.

## Molecular and Cellular Basis of Cardiac Excitability

Many of the heritable diseases that produce arrhythmias are the result of mutations that alter the active membrane properties of the cardiac myocyte. Therefore it is useful to consider the molecular basis of excitability in the heart. An elementary and distinctive signature of any excitable tissue is its action potential (AP) profile. Myocardial cells have a characteristically long AP that is sculpted by the orchestrated activity of a number of ion channels and transporters (Fig. 10-1). Depolarizing currents, primarily Na and Ca, are responsible for the AP upstroke; repolarizing currents, primarily K, in combination with a reduction in depolarizing currents are responsible for restoration of the normal intracellular negativity of the heart cell at rest. The plateau of the AP is a time of very high membrane resistance or low current flow; thus any perturbation of the balance between depolarizing and repolarizing currents can dramatically influence the duration of the plateau and therefore the duration of the AP. In the past two decades, most of the relevant ion channel genes encoding the major ($\alpha$) subunits and many of the ancillary ($\beta$) subunits of the corresponding ionic currents in the heart have been cloned, sequenced, and functionally characterized. A number of inherited arrhythmias result from mutations in ion channel subunit genes. Other heritable cardiac diseases that alter the structure of the heart may change the level of expression or function of one or more of these ion channel genes, enhancing the risk of arrhythmias. Furthermore, many of these molecules serve as molecular targets for drugs used in the treatment of cardiovascular disease. Indeed, we are just beginning to discover that functionally inconsequential changes in the gene sequence that occur in a significant proportion of the population (i.e., polymorphisms) may dramatically and potentially lethally alter the response to drugs that act on ion channels.

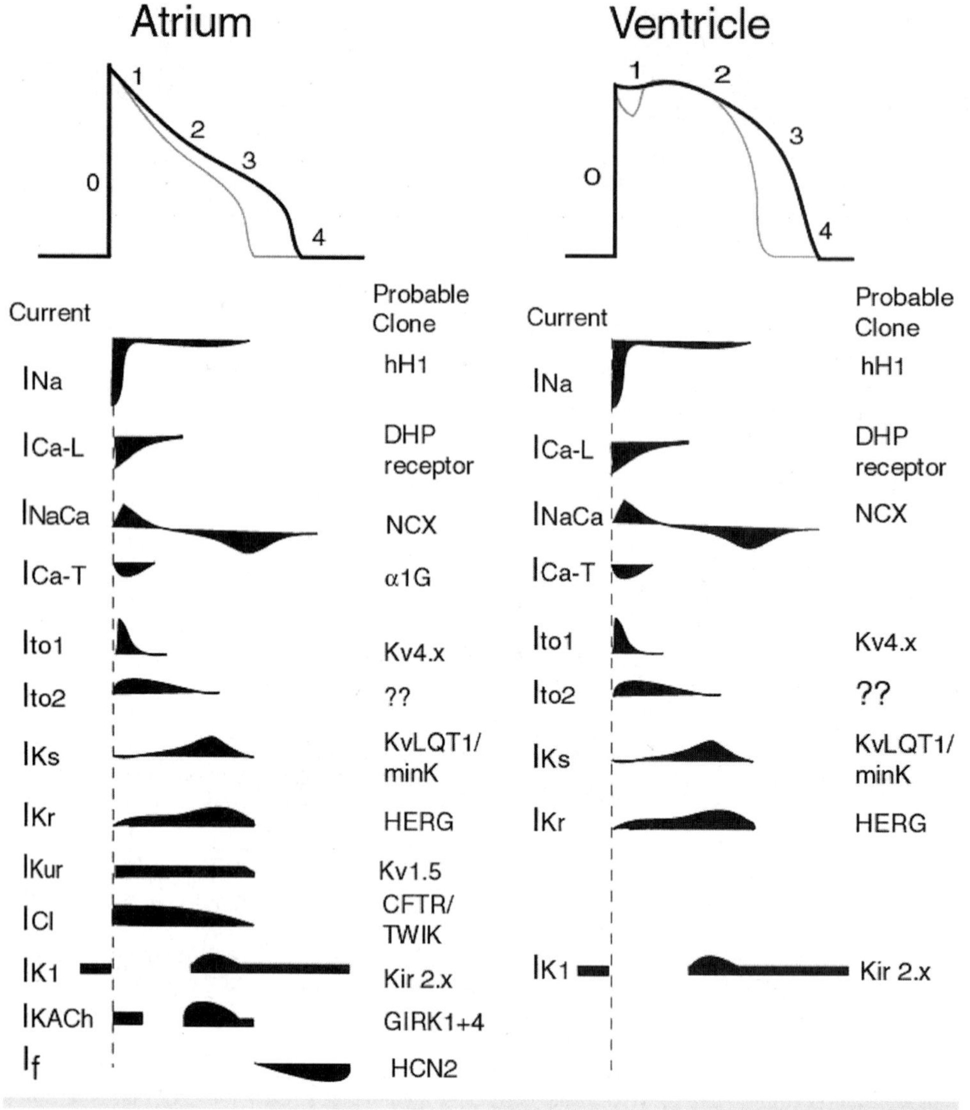


FIGURE 10-1 Schematic of inward and outward ionic currents, pumps, and exchangers that underlie atrial and ventricular action potentials in the mammalian heart. Control and failing (*bold line*) action potential profiles are shown on top. Each phase of the action potential is labeled. Under the action potentials, a schematic of the time course of each current is shown, and the gene product (probable clone) that underlies the current is indicated.

## GENETICALLY DETERMINED CARDIAC ARRHYTHMIAS

### Conduction System Disease

Familial clustering of atrioventricular (AV) block has been known for over a century, with the first descriptions by Osler[4] and Morquio.[5] Block at multiple levels of the cardiac conduction system is a common occurrence in a number of inherited diseases of the myocardium and heart rhythm (Table 10-1). There are a number of monogenic and polygenic structural heart diseases with conduction block as a prominent feature. For example, mutations in the homeobox transcription factor *CSX/NKX2.5* (OMIM #600584) produce significant abnormalities in folding of the heart tube during development, with consequent defects in septation such as atrial septal defects (ASD), ventricular septal defects (VSD), and tetralogy of Fallot.[6] Mutations in *CSX/NKX2.5* have also been associated with isolated AV conduction block.[7] As one might anticipate, AV conduction block also frequently accompanies other defects of cardiac septation, such as familial ASD (OMIM *108800)[8] and the heart-hand syndromes typified by the Holt-Oram syndrome (OMIM #142900).[9]

Progressive familial heart block [PFHB, also known as progressive cardiac conduction defect (PCCD) or Lenegre-Lev disease] of two types, distinguished primarily by the duration of the QRS complex of the escape rhythm, have been described.[10] PFHB type I (OMIM #113900), characterized by wide QRS escape complexes, has been linked to two genetic loci. In a large South African kindred, PFHB I maps to a 10-cM region of chromosome 19 (19q13.2-q13.3). A number of genes reside in this region and at least one, myotonin protein kinase, has been ruled out by a recombination event.[11] Another family has been described that exhibits a mutation in *SCN5A*, the gene that encodes the cardiac sodium channel.[12] The mechanism(s) by which mutations in this channel gene produce conduction disease is uncertain. PFHB I is distinct from PFHB II in that the former is characterized by disease in the bundle branches and a wide QRS escape rhythm. The escape rhythm in PFHB II has a narrow QRS complex and presumably originates above the bundle of His, but verification by intracardiac recording has not been reported.[10,11]

A number of AV conduction abnormalities have been reported in heritable diseases with prominent extracardiac manifestations, such as the muscular dystrophies (Table 10-2). Mutations in dystrophin, a protein that links the extracellular matrix with the cytoskeleton through the membrane-associated dystrophin-associated complex, produce muscular the X-linked Duchenne (OMIM #310200) and Becker forms of muscular dystrophy. Patients with these muscular dystrophies exhibit AV conduction block of varying severity both in and below the AV node. AV block is a prominent feature of other muscle diseases, such as myotonic dystrophy (Steinert disease, OMIM #160900) and limb-girdle dystrophy.[13] Patients with myotonic dystrophy most often exhibit first- or second-degree AV block, which is not correlated with age or size of the CTG expansion. In addition to AV conduction block, atrial standstill has been described in limb-girdle muscular dystrophy. Inherited neuromuscular diseases such as Kearn-Sayre (OMIM #530000),[14] McArdle (OMIM 153460), and Kugelberg-Welander (OMIM *158600)[15] syndromes have also been associated with AV block.

### Supraventricular Arrhythmias

There are a number of familial atrial tachy- and bradyarrhythmias with Mendelian inheritance (see Table 10-1). Atrial fibrillation (AF) is the most common sustained arrhythmia in humans. The vast majority of cases of AF are polygenic and occur in the context of structural heart disease. However, familial forms of AF were first recognized over six decades ago.[16,17] Since then, a number of families with heritable AF in the absence and presence of structural atrial abnormalities have been described.

There are a number of changes in the active membrane properties of the atrial myocyte as well as the interstitium that have been observed in human and animal models of AF.[18] However, it is unclear if such alterations in gene expression cause AF or are a consequence of the arrhythmia. It seems reasonable to assume that remodeling of atrial structure and electrophysiology supports the maintenance of or the predisposition to AF, thus identifying classes of possible candidate genes.

TABLE 10-1 Genetic Disorders Associated with Supraventricular Arrhythmias and Conduction Block

| Arrhythmia | Inh | Chromosome | Gene | OMIM | Reference |
|---|---|---|---|---|---|
| Atrial fibrillation | AD | 11p15.5 | *KCNQ1(KvLQT1)* | #607554 | 21 |
| | AD | 10q23 | ? | | 22 |
| | AD | ? | ? | | |
| WPW, AF | AD | 7q35-q36 | *PRKAG2* | #194200 | 27 |
| Atrial asystole, AF | AD | ? | ? | | 100 |
| Nodal rhythm | AD | ? | ? | #163800 | 101 |
| AV block (PFHB I) | AD | 19q13.3 | ? | #113900 | 11 |
| | AD | 3p21 | *SCN5A* | #113900 | 12 |
| PFHB II | AD | ? | ? | 140400 | 10 |
| AV block/±ASD | AD | 5q34 | *CSX/NKX2.5* | *600584 | 7 |
| AV block/ASD | AD | 6p21.3 | ? | *108800 | 8 |
| Familial BBB | ? | ? | ? | | 102 |
| | AD | ? | ? | *113950 | 103 |

ABBREVIATIONS: OMIM: Online Mendelian inheritance in man; Inh: inheritance pattern; WPW: Wolff-Parkinson-White syndrome; AF: atrial fibrillation; ASD: atrial septal defect; PFHB I: progressive familial heart block type I; PFHB II: type II; BBB: bundle branch block.

In human AF, atrial action potential duration (APD) is shortened due to reduced functional expression of L-type Ca channels[19] and an increase in inward rectifier ($I_{K1}$) and acetylcholine-gated ($I_{KACh}$) potassium currents.[20] Similar APD shortening is possible with increased activity of repolarizing K currents (see Fig. 10-1). Indeed, a family with autosomal dominant AF (OMIM #607554) has been described with a gain-of-function mutation in the slow component of the delayed rectifier current ($I_{Ks}$) encoded by *KCNQ1* (*KvLQT1*) on chromosome 11p15.5.[21] Interestingly patients with AF in this family did not exhibit QT shortening but instead had modest prolongation, which was felt to be secondary to the arrhythmia.[21] Familial AF is a genetically heterogeneous disease. Linkage analysis has identified 10q22 as a disease locus for AF that occurs early in life and segregates as an autosomal dominant trait.[22] This locus was subsequently excluded in a number of other families with early-onset AF in the absence of structural heart disease (e.g., Ref. 23). The identification of other AF disease genes has thus far proven to be elusive.

Ventricular preexcitation with supraventricular tachycardia, or Wolff-Parkinson-White syndrome (WPW), has rarely been described as an autosomal dominant, inherited arrhythmia.[24,25] Familial WPW with (OMIM #600858)[24–26] and without (OMIM #194200)[27] hypertrophic cardiomyopathy (HCM) has been linked to mutations in the regulatory gamma subunit (*PRKAG2*) of the heterotrimeric metabolic stress sensing protein kinase 5′-AMP-activated protein kinase (AMPK). However, 5 to 10 percent of patients with HCM not linked to *PRKAG2* have ventricular preexcitation, with a significant number of those patients exhibiting WPW syndrome.

Supraventricular tachycardia, particularly AF, complicates a number of other inherited cardiac diseases, such as the myopathies described in the subsequent section, heart-hand syndromes typified by the Holt-Oram syndrome,[9] familial amyloidosis, and inherited ASD. In many instances, AF may arise as a consequence of the structural heart disease produced by the gene defect rather than a direct consequence of the genetic abnormality. A number of muscular dystrophies—such as Duchenne, fascioscapulohumeral, and Emery-Dreifuss dystrophies and Barth syndrome—are complicated by atrial tachycardia and fibrillation.[28]

## Ventricular Arrhythmias

Heritable diseases of the myocardium may produce potentially lethal ventricular arrhythmias. In aggregate, such heritable disorders account for the majority of sudden deaths in the young. In about 80 to 85 percent of cases, unexplained sudden death in the young is the result of unsuspected heart disease. Most often, unrecognized structural heart diseases—such as HCM, dilated cardiomyopathy (DCM), arrhythmogenic right ventricular dysplasia (ARVD), myocarditis, congenital anomalies (of both the heart and coronary arteries) and premature coronary artery disease (CAD)—are the cause of sudden cardiac death (SCD) in the young. Primary electrical diseases—such as LQTS, IVF, ARVD, catecholaminergic polymorphic ventricular tachycardia (CPVT), WPW, and congenital conduction system disease—constitute a significant minority of cases of SCD in the young. Less frequently, noncardiac causes—such as aortic rupture, cerebral hemorrhage, pulmonary embolus, and respiratory arrest—may be the culprit.

## Structural Diseases of the Myocardium Associated with Arrhythmias

### FAMILIAL HYPERTROPHIC CARDIOMYOPATHY (HCM, ASH, HOCM, IHSS)—OMIM #192600

A number of excellent reviews, cited in Chap. 77, have been published on various aspects of HCM. The following section (see Table 10-2) focuses on the arrhythmic phenotype. Familial HCM is a relatively common disease of the myocardium transmitted as an autosomal dominant trait. The incidence in the general population is about 1 per 500,[29] which may be an underestimate due to the low penetrance of some disease-causing mutations. HCM is genetically and phenotypically heterogeneous. The hallmark features are myocardial hypertrophy without chamber dilation and myofiber disarray on histologic examination of the heart.[30] Diastolic dysfunction is the major mechanical defect in patients with HCM, with a minority exhibiting an obstruction to left ventricular outflow.[31,32] HCM is a substantial cause of morbidity in affected patients, but clearly the most devastating complication is sudden death. HCM is among the most common causes of unexplained death in the young (<35 years).

TABLE 10-2 Genetic Disorders Producing Structural Heart Disease with Arrhythmias as a Prominent Feature

HCM (AF AND SCD)

| Locus | Gene | Protein (# mutations) | Freq | Misc | Reference |
|---|---|---|---|---|---|
| 14q11-q12 | *MYH7* | β-Myosin HC (>70) | 35% | | 104 |
| 1q32 | *TNNT2* | cTroponin T (14) | 15% | | 105 |
| 11p11.2 | *MYBPC3* | Myosin BP-C (29) | 20% | | 106,107 |
| 15q22 | *TPM1* | α-Tropomyosin (4) | ~5% | | 105 |
| 3p21 | *MYL3* | MEsLC (2) | <1% | MVC | 108 |
| 12q23-q24.3 | *MYL2* | Myosin light chain 2 (8) | <5% | MVC | 108 |
| 14q12 | *MYH6* | α-MHC (2) | Rare | Elderly | 109 |
| 19q13.4 | *TNNI* | cTNI (8) | ~5% | Apical | 110 |
| 3p21-p14 | *TNNC1* | cTNC | Rare | | 111 |
| 2q24.3 | *TTN* | Titin (1) | Rare | DCM | 112 |
| 15q14 | ACTC | α-Actin (2) | <5% | DCM | 113 |
| 7q36 | *PRKAG2* | AMP-PK$_{\gamma 2}$ (1) | Rare | WPW | 25,26 |

DCM (AD)—NO EXTRACARDIAC MANIFESTATIONS (AF AND VENTRICULAR ARRHYTHMIAS)

| Locus | Gene | Protein | Reference |
|---|---|---|---|
| 1q32 | *TNNT2* | cTroponin T | 114 |
| 2q24.3 | *TTN* | Titin | 115 |
| 2q35 | *DES* | Desmin | 116 |
| 5q33 | *SGCD* | δ-Sarcoglycan | 117 |
| 10q22-q23 | *VCL* | Metavinculin | 118 |
| 11p11.2 | *MYBPC3* | MyPBC | 119 |
| 14q11-q12 | *MYH7* | β-MHC | 114 |
| 15q22 | *TPM1* | α-TM | 120 |
| 15q14 | *ACTC* | α-Actin | 121 |
| 6q12-q16 | ? | ? | 122 |
| 9q13-q22 | ? | ? | 123 |
| 9q22-q31 | ? | ? | |

DCM AND CONDUCTION SYSTEM DISEASE (AD)

| Locus | Gene | Protein | Reference |
|---|---|---|---|
| 1p1-q21 | *LMNA* | Lamins A & C | 124 |
| 2q14-q22 | ? | ? | 125 |
| 3p22-p25 | ? | ? | 126 |

DCM + SKM MYOPATHY + CSD (AD)

| Locus | Gene | Protein | Reference |
|---|---|---|---|
| 1p1-q21 | *LMNA* | Lamins A & C | 127 |
| 6q23 | ? | ? | 128 |

DCM + DEAFNESS

| Locus | Gene | Protein | Reference |
|---|---|---|---|
| 6q23 | ? | ? | 129 |

(Continued)

The genetic heterogeneity of HCM is underscored by the fact that over 150 different mutations in 12 genes have been described to date (see Table 10-2), although mutations in *PRKAG2*, which cause HCM and WPW, are more properly glycogen storage diseases.[33] In general, the mutated genes encode proteins that are part of the cardiac sarcomere or contractile apparatus. Causative mutations in sarcomeric proteins are intellectually appealing; however, the mechanism by which these mutations cause disease and in particular cardiac hypertrophy and myofibrillar disarray is uncertain.

Cardiac arrhythmias are a significant determinant of the clinical course of patients with HCM.[34] Some patients are at high risk for sudden death, while others may develop AF with morbid consequences, such as stroke. Several factors may enhance the propensity for developing AF in HCM, including an elevation in filling pressures, remodeling of active membrane properties of atrial myocytes and connectivity of these cells, and alterations in the interstitium.

A significant minority of patients (10 to 20 percent) with HCM are at high risk of sudden death.[35] The mechanisms of sudden cardiac death in HCM patients are likely to be heterogeneous and include malignant ventricular arrhythmias as well as bradycardia resulting from sinus node disease and AV conduction block. It is not surprising that no single factor is highly predictive of sudden death in HCM; however, a number of factors have been associated with increased risk of sudden death. Importantly, specific mutations have been reported to increase the propensity for sudden death, including mutations in the *βMHC* (R403Q, R453C, R719W) and *TnT* genes and to a lesser extent mutations in *MBPC* (InsG791) and *αTM* (D175N). Detection of *TnT* mutations may be particularly relevant in that these mutations are often associated with mild ventricular hypertrophy.[36,37] However because of the limited number of patients with HCM, such data may be biased toward high-risk families and should be interpreted with caution.

A number of clinical features are associated with an increased risk of sudden death in HCM, including a family history of premature sudden death; personal history of cardiac arrest, sustained VT, or syncope; a decrease in BP with exercise; extreme hypertrophy (LV thickness > 30 mm); and younger age at diagnosis. The presence of two or more risk factors is associated with an almost 30 percent 6-year mortality rate, which supports the use of prophylactic therapy with an implantable cardioverter defibrillator (ICD).[32] The role of inducibility at electrophysiologic (EP) study to risk-stratify patients for sudden death remains controversial; however, EP studies may be useful in patients with HCM with conduction system disease, ventricular preexcitation, and monomorphic VT. In light of the imperfect risk stratification for premature death from HCM, it is important to focus on phenotypic features associated with a low risk of dying suddenly. Indeed, adult patients (and gene carriers) who exhibit none of the clinical risk factors described above are at low risk (< 1 percent per year) of sudden death.[32]

TABLE 10-2 Genetic Disorders Producing Structural Heart Disease with Arrhythmias as a Prominent Feature (Continued)

X-LINKED INHERITANCE

| | Locus | Gene | Protein | Reference |
|---|---|---|---|---|
| Xp21 | *DMD* | Dystrophin | | 130 |
| Xp28 | *G4.5* | Tafazzin | Infantile DCM | 131 |

ARRHYTHMOGENIC RIGHT VENTRICULAR DYSPLASIA (ARVD, ARVC)

| | Locus | Gene | Protein | Reference |
|---|---|---|---|---|
| ARVD1 | 14q23-q24 | ? | | 132 |
| ARVD2* | 1q42-q43 | *RYR2* | Cardiac RyR | 53 |
| ARVD3 | 14q12-q22 | ? | | 133 |
| ARVD4 | 2q32 | ? | | 134 |
| ARVD5 | 3p23 | ? | | 135 |
| ARVD6 | 10p12-p14 | ? | | 136 |
| ARVD8 | 6p23 | *DSP* | Desmoplakin | 52 |
| Naxos (AR) | 17q21 | *PKGB* | Plakoglobin | 51 |

ABBREVIATIONS: MVC: midventricular chamber; DCM: both HCM and DCM are caused by mutations in these genes; WPW: Wolff-Parkinson-White syndrome and HCM; AF: atrial fibrillation or flutter; CSD: carotid sinus denervation; SCD: sudden cardiac death; DCM: dilated cardiomyopathy; HCM: hypertrophic cardiomyopathy.

## DILATED CARDIOMYOPATHY (DCM)

Other inherited structural heart diseases such as DCM are frequently associated with arrhythmias, including a high risk of sudden death. DCM is a disorder of contractile function of the left or right ventricle and may have a number of varied etiologies. The incidence of idiopathic DCM is estimated to be 5 to 8 per 100,000 per year.[38] In systematic studies of first-degree relatives of probands, it has been estimated that 35 percent of DCM is inherited (e.g., Ref. 39). The reasons for underestimates in other studies are age-related penetrance or nonpenetrance; that is, patients who have a mutation but develop disease late or not at all.

Familial forms of DCM can be inherited in an autosomal dominant (AD) fashion (most frequently), more rarely as autosomal recessive and X-linked traits, and maternally via mutations in the mitochondrial genome. The role that DCM-causing mutations play in other etiologies of systolic dysfunction and heart failure is unknown. In addition, the diagnosis of familial forms of DCM may be confounded by more common multigenic causes of cardiomyopathy, such as ischemic heart disease, infectious and infiltrative causes, and alcoholic cardiomyopathy.

Inherited DCM exhibits marked genotypic and phenotypic variability and is often associated with a number of other cardiac and extracardiac manifestations.[40] The mutations that cause only DCM, involving no extracardiac manifestations, are listed in Table 10-2. Note that some of the genes that cause HCM are mutated in different regions to cause DCM. There are a number of loci that have been linked to DCM for which the disease genes have not yet been identified.

Lamins (A type: A, C, A$\delta$10, C2; and B type: B1 and B2) are intermediate filament proteins located at the nuclear lamina. The precise function of lamins is unknown, but they are thought to be involved in nuclear membrane integrity and are important in nuclear reassembly in dividing cells. A total of 19 different mutations typically in the central rod domain common to lamins A and C have been found in patients with DCM+ conduction system disease with no evidence of skeletal myopathy. Mutations (>30) in lamins also cause two forms of AD skeletal myopathy (Emery-Dreifuss and limb-girdle muscular dystrophies). X-linked Emery-Dreifuss muscular dystrophy is caused by mutations in emerin, an inner nuclear membrane protein. Mutations in the intermediate filament protein desmin cause DCM, and different mutations are associated with desmin-related myopathy—a skeletal myopathy with cardiac conduction system disease and restrictive CM (OMIM #601419).

Dystrophin is a large cytoskeletal protein that interacts with cytoskeletal actin and the dystrophin-associated glycoprotein complex in the sarcolemma and is thought to contribute to intracellular organization, force transduction, and membrane stability. Mutations in dystrophin were first identified in Duchenne and Becker muscular dystrophies. Mutations in dystrophin have also been found in males without evidence of skeletal myopathy but rapidly progressive DCM.

The mitochondrial genome is minute compared to the nuclear genome (16 kb compared to $6 \times 10^6$ kb) and encodes 13 structural genes, 22 tRNAs, and 2 rRNAs. Point mutations in mitochondrial DNA have been found in a number of systemic disorders associated with cardiac abnormalities, including adult-onset HCM, childhood-onset DCM, and fatal infantile DCM. The role of mitochondrial DNA mutations in the pathogenesis of DCM is uncertain, but the maternal transmission in some families suggests that they are etiologic. However, it is important to note that there is a high mutation rate in mitochondrial DNA in normal aging and in DCM of other etiologies, such as that associated with alcohol and ischemia.

As with HCM, the arrhythmic natural history of inherited DCM is variable across and even within families, highlighting the importance of the individual's genetic makeup in the phenotypic expression of the disease. However, unlike HCM, there are no specific mutations that have been linked to a high rate of sudden death predating systolic dysfunction. In patients with familial DCM and conduction system disease (see Table 10-2), AV block often precedes symptomatic systolic dysfunction and can produce sudden death, which can be aborted by permanent pacemaker implantation.

In addition to structural remodeling, there are significant EP changes in the failing heart, regardless of etiology, that may predispose to life-threatening ventricular arrhythmias.[3] In patients with ischemic cardiomyopathy, several large clinical trials have demonstrated the utility of the ICD in the primary prevention of sudden death (e.g., Ref. 41; also see Chap. 38). There are presently insufficient data to guide the management of patients with nonischemic cardiomyopathy, including familial DCM, with respect to the primary prevention of sudden death. Two large ongoing clinical trials (SCD-HeFT and DEFINITE) address this question. In a small study of patients with recently diagnosed idiopathic DCM, the ICD produced a nonsignificant increase in survival when compared with the best pharmacologic management of heart failure.[42] The role of cardiac resynchronization therapy (CRT) in patients with DCM is evolving; clinical trial data suggest an improvement in symptoms in patients with advanced heart failure, but no mortality benefit. A recent met-analysis of the major CRT trials suggests an overall reduction in mortality.[43] Antiarrhythmic drug therapy has a limited role in the treatment of ventricular arrhythmias in patients with DCM because of the substantial proarrhythmic risk (see Chap. 41). Therefore treatment of ventricular arrhythmias and prevention of sudden death in patients with familial DCM must be individualized. Clinical features such as the patient's presentation and family history are helpful in guiding antiarrhythmic therapy, primarily the use of the ICD.

## ARRHYTHMOGENIC RIGHT VENTRICULAR DYSPLASIA (ARVD, ARVC) (OMIM *107970, #600996, #602086, #602087, *604400, *604401, #607450)

ARVD is an unusual cardiomyopathy that prominently but not exclusively affects the right ventricle, with histologic features of myocyte necrosis and apoptosis.[44–46] The pathologic hallmarks are right ventricular thinning and aneurysm formation (50 percent of cases), the extreme manifestation being so-called parchment RV (Uhl's anomaly). ARVD is somewhat (but not extremely) rare, with a prevalence of 1 per 5000, and up to 4.4 per 1000 in northern Italy.[47] It is thought to account for about 5 percent of unexplained sudden deaths in the young in the United States and up to 20 percent in Italy (< 35 years of age). It is a highly lethal disease with an annual mortality of up to 3 percent per year.[45,47]

The typical case of ARVD is that of a young man (2–3 : 1 male predominance), presenting with ventricular ectopy [premature ventricular contractions (PVCs), nonsustained ventricular tachycardia (VT)]. In rare cases, syncope and sudden death, typically occurring with exercise, are the initial manifestations of ARVD. Ventricular ectopy in ARVD typically exhibits a left bundle branch block (LBBB) morphology, reflecting its origin in the right ventricle. PVCs and VT are often of multiple morphologies, distinguishing ARVD from idiopathic VT originating from the right ventricular outflow tract (RVOT). ARVD rarely causes frank right heart failure and commonly affects the left ventricle but infrequently produces left heart failure. Patients with ARVD and left heart failure are typically older and have macroscopic fibrofatty replacement of left ventricular myocardium.[45]

Most presentations of ARVD are not typical and indeed can be quite challenging, with a number of crucial differential diagnoses. In 1994, the European Society of Cardiology Working Group[48] proposed a set of diagnostic criteria (both major and minor) that included mechanical, electrical, and historical features of ARVD. The major and minor mechanical/functional criteria included severe dilation and reduction of the right ventricular ejection fraction, localized right ventricular aneurysms, segmental dilation of the right ventricle, and fibrofatty replacement of the myocardium on biopsy as major criteria. Minor structural criteria included mild global right ventricular dilation or reduced ejection fraction, mild segmental dilation of the right ventricle, and regional right ventricular hypokinesia.

Historically, angiography has been used to define contractile abnormalities in the right heart.[49] However, magnetic resonance imaging (MRI), particularly cine gradient-echo MRI, provides a comparable assessment of right ventricular function as well as superior morphology, and it permits the noninvasive assessment of tissue composition.[50]

The functional electrical abnormalities that constitute the major diagnostic criteria for ARVD include epsilon waves or localized QRS prolongation (> 110 ms) in the right precordial leads ($V_1$ to $V_3$). The minor electrocardiographic criteria for ARVD include inverted T waves ($V_2$ and $V_3$) in absence of a RBBB, late potentials on the signal-averaged electrocardiogram (SAECG), LBBB-morphology VT, and frequent LBBB ventricular extrasystoles (> 1000 per 24 h).

The diagnostic scheme also includes historical features: the major criterion is a pathologically confirmed family history of ARVD; minor criteria are a family history of premature sudden death and ARVD without pathologic confirmation. The presence of two major or one major plus two minor criteria is consistent with a positive diagnosis of ARVD.

ARVD is genetically heterogeneous, and most forms are inherited in an autosomal dominant fashion. An unusual variant associated with woolly hair and palmoplantar keratoderma that is prevalent on the island of Naxos segregates in a recessive manner and has been associated with mutations in the intercalated disk protein plakoglobin (OMIM #601214)[51] (see Table 10-2). Another form of ARVD (ARVD8, OMIM #607450) that is inherited in a dominant fashion results from mutations in desmoplakin, another protein associated with the intercalated disk.[52] The mechanism by which mutations in these genes produce the structural features of ARVD is not known.

A mutation in the cardiac ryanodine receptor (*RYR2*) has been described in four independent families with ARVD2 (OMIM #600996).[53] A large number of distinct mutations in *RYR2* are responsible for catecholaminergic polymorphic ventricular tachycardia (CPVT, OMIM #604772), an inherited arrhythmia that is not associated with structural heart disease.[54,55] The ryanodine receptor (and calsequestrin, a $Ca^{2+}$-binding sarcoplasmic reticulum protein; see CPVT2) is critical for normal $Ca^{2+}$ homeostasis in the cardiac myocyte. Aberrant $Ca^{2+}$ handling is prominent in a number of acquired heart diseases and may be associated with abnormalities of cellular repolarization and malignant ventricular arrhythmias. Similarly, mutations in *RYR2* may predispose to ventricular tachyarrhythmias resulting from abnormal $Ca^{2+}$ handling in ARVD2 and CPVT2. The mechanism by which dysplastic changes in the right ventricle are produced is uncertain.

A prognostically important differential diagnosis of ARVD is idiopathic ventricular tachycardia that originates from the right ventricular outflow tract (RVOT). The importance of distinguishing these entities is that the latter has a benign prognosis, can be cured by radiofrequency catheter ablation, and is well controlled by beta-adrenergic receptor blockers. This may be a difficult distinction if the right ventricular anatomic abnormalities are subtle and monomorphic ventricular tachycardia is the major presenting feature of ARVD. The other distinguishing features of idiopathic VT are the absence of Mendelian inheritance, a single morphology of VT, and a normal resting ECG and SAECG; moreover, the presumed mechanism of RVOT is triggered automaticity and not reentry. A related question is whether ventricular ectopy emanating from the right ventricular outflow tract represents a forme fruste of ARVD. In the absence of an abnormal ECG, SAECG, and MRI, the majority of patients with idiopathic VT appear not to be a subset of ARVD patients with early, localized disease.[56]

There are few data to guide the management of patients with ARVD. Small studies have examined all of the conventional modalities used to suppress or treat VT. However, because of the risk of sudden death,[45,47] catheter ablation alone or antiarrhythmic drug therapy is seldom relied on in patients with severe presentations such as cardiac arrest or syncope that is presumed to be arrhythmic. Because of the progressive nature of this cardiomyopathy, radiofrequency catheter ablation is likely to be limited in its palliative effect. In light of the frequency of exercise-induced arrhythmias and sudden death, vigorous physical activity is generally proscribed. The clinical features that favor ICD implantation in ARVD include a malignant family history, syncope presumed due to VT, evidence of extensive right ventricular disease, left ventricular involvement, polymorphic VT, and right ventricular apical aneurysms.

TABLE 10-3 Primary Electrical Diseases Producing Ventricular Arrhythmias

| AUTOSOMAL DOMINANT VARIANTS OF LQTS | | | | | |
|---|---|---|---|---|---|
| Arrhythmia | Chromosome | Gene | Protein | Frequency | Reference |
| LQT1 | 11p15 | *KCNQ1* | KvLQT1($I_{Ks}$) | ~50% | 137 |
| LQT2 | 7q35 | *KCNH2* | HERG ($I_{Kr}$) | 30–40% | 84 |
| LQT3 | 3p21 | *SCN5A* | Na Channel | 5–10% | 85 |
| LQT4 | 4q25 | *ANK2* | Ankyrin B | Rare | 86 |
| LQT5 | 21q22 | *KCNE1* | MinK ($I_{Ks}$) | Rare | 138 |
| LQT6 | 21q22 | *KCNE2* | MiRP1($I_{Kr}$) | Rare | 93 |
| LQT7 | 17 | *KCNJ2* | $I_{K1}$ | Rare | 88 |
| **IDIOPATHIC VF WITH RIGHT CONDUCTION ABNORMALITY (BRUGADA SYNDROME)** | | | | | |
| Arrhythmia | Chromosome | Gene | Protein | Inh[a] | Reference |
| IVF | 3 | *SCN5A* (>30) | Na channel | AD | 73 |
| **CATECHOLAMINE-DEPENDENT POLYMORPHIC VENTRICULAR TACHYCARDIA (CPVT)** | | | | | |
| Arrhythmia | Chromosome | Gene | Protein | Inh[a] | Reference |
| CPVT1 | 1q42-43 | *RYR2* | Cardiac RyR | AD | 54,55 |
| CPVT2 | 1p11-p13.3 | *CASQ2* | Calsequestrin | AR | 59 |
| CPVT3-? | ? | ? | ? | AD | |

[a]Inheritance pattern.

## Primary Electrical Disease

CPVT is a heritable disorder that presents as exercise- or stress-induced ventricular arrhythmias, syncope, or sudden death. It was originally described in children,[57] but more recent studies suggest that ventricular arrhythmias may also begin in adulthood.[54,55,58] In patients with CPVT who have been monitored during exercise, several types of malignant ventricular arrhythmias have been described, including polymorphic VT, bidirectional VT (exhibiting a beat-to-beat alternation of the QRS axis), and ventricular fibrillation. This syndrome is genetically heterogeneous, with both autosomal dominant and autosomal recessive transmission. Disease-causing mutations in *RYR2*[54,55] and calsequestrin (*CSQ*)[59] have been identified, the former segregating as dominant and the latter as recessive traits. Over 20 different mutations in functionally important domains of *RYR2* have already been described in CPVT.[54,55,58] There are a number of families that do not map to either the *RYR2* or *CSQ* loci; thus there may be at least one and probably several other disease genes (Table 10-3). *RYR2* and *CSQ* are molecules that are central to normal $Ca^{2+}$ homeostasis of the cardiac myocyte. Mutations that produce functional abnormalities in either of these molecules can produce cellular $Ca^{2+}$ overload and lead to arrhythmias induced by abnormalities of repolarization known as afterdepolarizations. This type of afterdepolarization-induced ventricular arrhythmia is most akin to the mechanism of arrhythmias that occurs in patients or animal models that have been rendered digitalis-intoxicated.

## Channelopathies

Idiopathic ventricular fibrillation (IVF) in the setting of right ventricular ECG abnormalities and the absence of structural heart disease is a lethal arrhythmia often referred to as Brugada syndrome (OMIM #601144). The syndrome of sudden death with unexplained right precordial ECG abnormalities was described in the 1950s.[60] A number of reports emerged in the late 1980s describing patients with potentially lethal ventricular arrhythmias and similar ECG abnormalities.[61] This was a mixed group of patients, some of whom had ARVD but others who had minimal structural heart disease and likely had IVF. In the early 1990s, Brugada and Brugada described a cohort of patients who had no apparent structural heart disease, right venticular ECG abnormalities, and a propensity to die suddenly.[62] It is now recognized that IVF with right bundle branch block is worldwide in distribution, with a high prevalence in Southeast Asia,[63,64] where is it known as *lai tai* (death during sleep) in Thailand, *bangungut* (to rise and moan in sleep) in the Philippines, and *pokkuri* (sudden unexpected death at night) in Japan. There is a striking male predominance (8 : 1) of IVF in the Southeast Asian population[63]; this is less pronounced in western cohorts.[65,66]

Syncope or sudden death may be the only symptoms in IVF; less commonly, patients present with palpitations and nonsustained arrhythmias. Syncope, particularly in the presence of spontaneous ECG changes, identifies patients at high risk for sudden death,[65,66] which typically occurs when patients are at rest, often in the early morning hours.[67] The typical age of presentation is in the third and fourth decades of life,[65,66] but cases have been described presenting

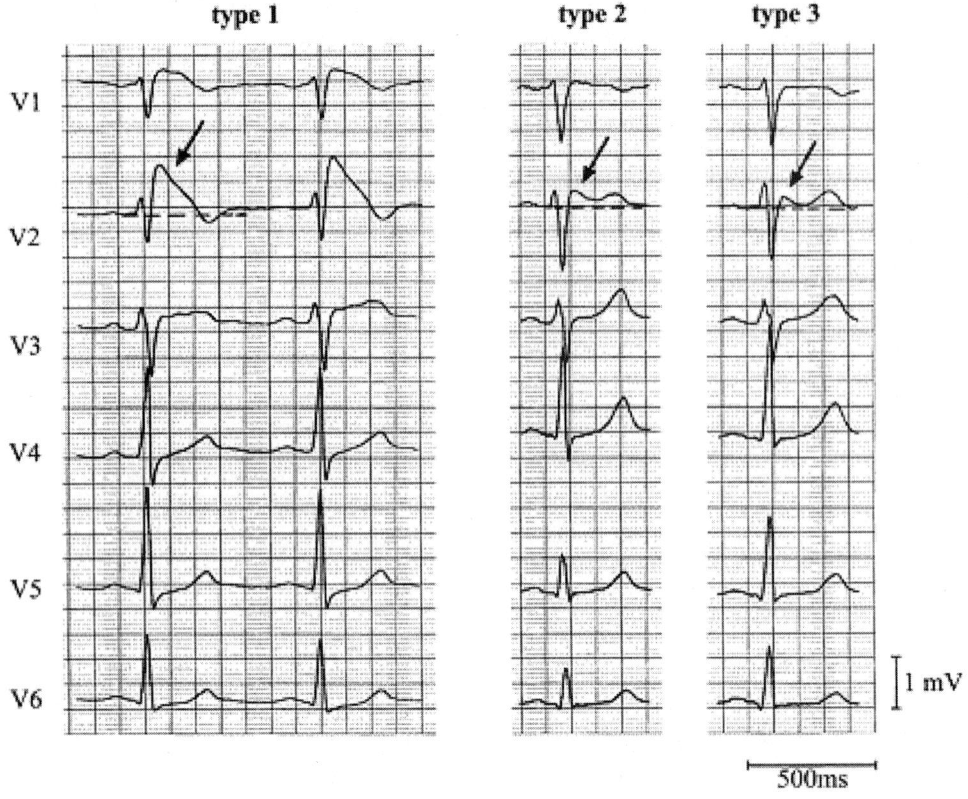


FIGURE 10-2 Variation in the precordial lead ST and T waves in a patient with IVF (Brugada syndrome). See text for details.

in infancy,[68] childhood,[69] and late life.[62] IVF is a highly lethal disease, with only a 40 percent survival at 5 years in high-risk patients.[65,66,70]

The hallmark ECG features of IVF are shown in Fig. 10-2.[70] Patients with IVF exhibit a spectrum of right precordial repolarization abnormalities in leads $V_1$ to $V_3$, from most severe (type I) to least severe (type III), both in appearance and prognosis. The type I ECG is characterized by an r′ wave with J-point elevation of greater than or equal to 2 mm (0.2 mV) and a coved ST segment with little separation from the subsequent negative T wave. The type II ECG exhibits a similar degree of J-point elevation but a downwardly sloping ST segment followed by a biphasic or upright T wave, producing a "saddleback" appearance. In the type III ECG, the J-point elevation is less than 1 mm (0.1 mV) and the ST segment may be saddleback, coved, or both. The J-point and ST-segment changes may be subtle and, in some cases, can be unmasked in patients with placement of the right precordial leads in a superior intercostal space.[71] These changes must be interpreted with caution in the presence of a true RBBB, and the type I pattern may itself mimic a RBBB, but other evidence of right ventricular conduction delay (S waves in the left precordial leads) is absent. An ST-segment pattern is referred to as spontaneous if it is present on the resting ECG; however, the ECG changes are dynamic and patterns may vary in the same patient; thus repeated recordings may be required. Antiarrhythmic drugs with class I action (flecainide, procainamide, ajmaline) have been used to unmask and exaggerate the ST-segment changes in IVF. Other ECG abnormalities that have been described include RBBB and other intraventricular conduction disturbances, QT-interval prolongation, and AV conduction delay in some cases associated with prolongation of the HV interval.[64,72] A variety of supraventricular tachycardias, including AV reentry in the Wolff-Parkinson-White syndrome, have been associated with IVF.[72]

A number of clinical features identify patients at greatest risk for sudden death, including a prior history of VF or aborted sudden death and syncope in the presence of spontaneous ECG changes.[65,66] The absence of effective pharmacotherapy mandates ICD implantation in these patients. A major dilemma is in risk stratification of asymptomatic individuals with a diagnostic or suspicious ECG. In small numbers of individuals, usually identified in the course of screening family members of probands, there was a 14 percent incidence of potentially lethal arrhythmic events in 27 months of follow-up. The utility of electrophysiologic study in this group of patients is controversial, although the absence of inducibility was reported to have a good negative predictive value in a small number of patients during a limited follow-up period.[66]

The major role of pharmacologic challenge in IVF appears to be in confirming the diagnosis in symptomatic patients (typically cardiac arrest or syncope, less commonly palpitations) with a nondiagnostic ECG.[66] Although pharmacologic challenge may aid in the diagnosis in asymptomatic patients with nondiagnostic ECGs, the unmasking of a diagnostic ECG by drug does not appear to be prognostically significant.[65,66]

IVF has been linked to mutations in the $\alpha$ subunit of the cardiac Na-channel gene, *SCN5A*,[73] but the syndrome is genetically heterogenous. In the largest genotyped cohort reported to date, only 84 of 200 (42 percent) subjects (probands and family members) and only 20 percent of probands harbored *SCN5A* mutations.[65] There have been over 30 different mutations in *SCN5A* associated with IVF. A consistent theme has been the functional reduction in peak Na current; however, mutations have been described that produce overlap syndromes of IVF and LQTS that are associated with multiple defects in channel function.[74] The proposed mechanisms of the ECG abnormalities and arrhythmia induction in the *SCN5A*-linked forms of IVF involve the imbalance of ionic currents during phase 1 repolarization, resulting in a steep voltage gradient across the ventricular wall (J-point elevation and ST-segment changes) and in the extreme, short-circuiting of the epicardial action potential and phase 2 reentry.[75] The deep phase 1 notch in the epicardial action potential, particularly in the right ventricle, renders it susceptible to the effects of a reduction in the Na current. Support for this hypothesis in humans comes from a small study of monophasic action potential recordings in patients with IVF during chest surgery.[76]

Right precordial ECG abnormalities may be observed in a number of congenital and acquired conditions that increase the risk of sudden death, such as myocardial ischemia, muscular dystrophies, cocaine intoxication, LQTS, and ARVD. The distinction between IVF and ARVD may be problematic, particularly when structural right ventricular disease is subtle. The clinical features that are helpful in distinguishing these entities are outlined in Table 10-4.

TABLE 10-4 ARVD versus IVF

| Feature | ARVD | IVF |
|---|---|---|
| Age at presentation (years) | 25–35 | 35–40 |
| Gender (M:F) | 2–3:1 | 5–8:1 |
| Distribution | Worldwide (NE Italy) | Worldwide (Southeast Asia) |
| Inheritance | AD, AR | AD |
| Symptoms | Palpitations, syncope, CA | Syncope, CA |
| Circumstances of CA | Exertion, emotion | Rest |
| Imaging | Functional RV > LV abnormal | Normal |
| Pathology | Fibrofatty replacement | Normal |
| ECG | e Waves | J-point elevation |
| | Right precordial TWI | RBBB/LAD |
| | Right ventricular IVCD | |
| ECG changes | Fixed | Variable |
| AV conduction | Normal | 50% prolonged |
| Atrial arrhythmias | Secondary, late | Primary, early |
| Ventricular arrhythmias | LBBB monomorphic VT[a] VF | PM-VT, VF |
| Arrhythmia mechanism | Scar-related reentry | Functional, phase 2 reentry |
| Effect on ST-segment elevation | | |
| Class I drug | Decrease | Increase |
| β-Adrenergic stimulation | Increase | Decrease |

[a]Multiple morphologies are possible.

ABBREVIATIONS: AD: autosomal dominant; AR: autosomal recessive; RV: right ventricle; LV: left ventricle; RBBB: right bundle branch block; LAD: left anterior descending coronary artery; CA: cardiac arrest; PM-VT: polymorphic VT; TWI: T-wave inversion; VF: ventricular fibrillation or flutter; IVCD: intraventricular conduction defect.

SOURCE: Modified from Wilde et al.,[70] with permission.

IVF and another inherited arrhythmia LQTS share the common feature that they are diseases of ion channels, which span the gamut from cystic fibrosis (CF) to familial migraine to some forms of hypertension and abnormalities of glucose regulation.

## LONG-QT SYNDROME (OMIM #192500, *152427, #603830, #600919, *176261, *603796)

The congenital long-QT syndrome (LQTS) is an inherited disease characterized by prolongation of ventricular repolarization and a high risk of sudden death from ventricular arrhythmias. Like IVF, LQTS is referred to as a primary electrical disease because it occurs in the absence of structural abnormalities in the heart. The LQTS was first formally described by Anton Jervell and Fred Lange-Nielsen in 1957, but several reports in the medical literature predate this description.[77] Most of the early reports described the variety of LQTS associated with deafness, referred to by Jervell as the surdocardiac syndrome and now known as the Jervell and Lange-Nielsen syndrome. The first description of the syndrome was probably that of Meissner in 1856, who related the case of a female pupil at the Leipzig school for the deaf who collapsed and died after being publicly admonished by the director.

In 1963–1964, two independent accounts by Romano and coworkers[78] and Ward[79] appeared, reporting a similar syndrome of syncopal attacks and ECG abnormalities but with no concomitant hearing loss. It soon became apparent that the Romano-Ward syndrome was more prevalent than that described by Jervell and Lange-Nielsen and that it was inherited through an autosomal dominant rather than recessive mechanism. In the next three decades, the clinical and ECG description of the syndrome was refined and an international registry of congenital LQTS patients was established.[80]

The detailed clinical characterization led to the positing of the sympathetic imbalance hypothesis as the mechanism for LQTS[81]; although this hypothesis was not supported by genetic analysis of the disease, sympathetic nervous system activity is a central determinant of the phenotypic manifestations of LQTS.[82] A major breakthrough came in 1991, when Keating and colleagues began to unravel the molecular basis of the LQTS, reporting genetic linkage of a disease gene to chromosome 11p15.5 (LQTS1).[83] In 1995, through a combination of positional cloning and candidate gene approaches, mutations in two ion channel genes were identified in the autosomal dominant form of the LQTS.[84,85] In the past decade, disease genes at five additional loci linked to the LQTS have been defined by similar approaches (see Table 10-3). Of the seven disease genes that have been identified, two encode K channel α subunits, the third encodes the voltage-gated Na channel, and two others encode K channel accessory (β) subunits. Most recently, a mutation in ankryin B (*ANK2*) a scaffolding protein, has been described in LQTS4, the only nonchannel disease gene thus far described.[86] Mutations in ankryin B disrupt the subcellular distribution of a number of ion transporters that are essential to normal $Ca^{2+}$ homeostasis in the heart cell, providing the link to abnormal repolarization and QT prolongation.

Andersen syndrome is a rare sporadic or autosomal dominant disorder characterized by periodic paralysis, cardiac arrhythmias, short stature, scoliosis, clinodactyly, and dysmorphic facies.[87] Patients with Andersen syndrome exhibit a number of ventricular arrhythmias, such as the distinctive ventricular arrhythmia called torsades de pointes (TdP) and bidirectional ventricular tachycardia. Mutations in *KCNJ2* the gene that encodes Kir2.1, the α subunit of the inward rectifier K channel ($I_{K1}$), have been identified in several families with this syndrome.[88] Thus an ion channel that is essential to normal cardiac excitability also appears to play a critical role in normal development.

Syncope and sudden death in LQTS patients result from TdP, which was originally described by Dessertenne.[90] This polymorphic VT has a characteristic undulating axis and may be nonsustained or may degenerate into VF, culminating in death. TdP is typically initiated with sudden increases in sympathetic tone, as might occur with fright, anger, or physical activity. However, some families have been reported in which cardiac arrests occur almost exclusively at rest or during sleep, and this has been associated with mutations in the Na channel in patients with LQTS3.[82] Data from the International Long QT Registry have also suggested that mortality may vary in a disease gene–specific fashion. For example, patients with LQTS3 have the lowest event rate but the highest frequency of lethal events.[91]

TABLE 10-5 Diagnostic Criteria for LQTS

| ECG Findings | Points | Clinical history | Points |
|---|---|---|---|
| QTc > 480 $ms^{1/2}$ | 3 | Syncope w/ stress | 2 |
| QTc 460–470 $ms^{1/2}$ | 2 | Syncope w/out stress | 1 |
| QTc: 450 $ms^{1/2}$ (m) | 1 | Congenital deafness | 0.5 |
| Torsades de pointes | 2 | FAMILY HISTORY | |
| T-wave alternans | 1 | | |
| Notched T in three leads | 1 | Positive family history LQTS | 1 |
| Heart rate <2% for age | 0.5 | Unexplained sudden death <30 y | 0.5 |

KEY: ≤1 Point: low probability; 2–3 points: intermediate probability; 4 points: high probability; (m): male.

Typical presentations of LQTS, with QT-interval prolongation and TdP, are unmistakable, but exceptions to the rule are commonplace and became more prevalent when large families with sudden death and linkage to LQT loci were studied. In order to enhance diagnostic accuracy, a set of clinical and electrocardiographic criteria were developed.[92] ECG criteria in addition to QT-interval prolongation include TdP, time-varying changes in the T wave and abnormal T-wave morphology, and bradycardia. Clinical criteria include syncope, deafness, and a compatible family history. Four or more points are associated with a high probability of the diagnosis (Table 10-5).

Not all patients with congenital QT prolongation are at equal risk for SCD or cardiac arrest. In addition to the specific genotype, several clinical factors are associated with a particularly high incidence of TdP, syncope, and SCD. They include congenital deafness, a prior history of syncope and/or tachyarrhythmia (with risk of SCD approaching 5 percent per year), female gender, and the degree of QT prolongation; the relative risk increases 1.1 to 1.2 times for each 10-ms prolongation of the QTc above the normal value for age and gender.

The genetic heterogeneity of the LQTS emphasizes the fact that there are a number of ways to prolong the ventricular AP (and therefore the QT interval) by single gene defects. In LQTS, both increases in depolarizing and decreases in repolarizing current may contribute to AP prolongation (see Fig. 10-1). The details of the changes depend on the specific genotype, but the final common pathway is AP prolongation and decreased repolarizing reserve, resulting in a diminished capacity of the ventricular heart cell to respond to additional stresses that alter repolarization, such as hypokalemia, hypomagnesemia, and drugs that prolong the AP.

The Na channel and K channels have opposite effects on the AP duration. The Na channel tends to depolarize the cell. Most of the Na channel activity occurs during the upstroke of the AP, but a small amount of current is active during the plateau (late current) that tends to depolarize the cell, thus lengthening the APD. K channels generate repolarizing currents; when they are active, they tend to restore the internal negativity of the cell. If K currents predominate during the plateau, repolarization will occur, shortening the APD; if Na currents predominate during the plateau, depolarization is favored and the AP is prolonged. The prediction is that LQTS-associated defects in the K-channel genes should reduce the function of the gene product and in the Na-channel gene should increase it, both of which would result in APD and QT prolongation, and this is indeed the case. In fact, as predicted by the autosomal dominant inheritance, only one copy of the mutated gene is necessary to produce the clinical syndrome.

The rapid and slow components of the delayed rectifier, $I_{Kr}$ and $I_{Ks}$ respectively, are abnormal in LQTS. LQTS2 is due to a defective potassium channel known as HERG (*KCNH2*) or the human ether a-go-go related gene. This gene product putatively combines with *KCNE2* (MiRP-1) to produce $I_{Kr}$.[93] $I_{Kr}$ is the target of a number of clinically used antiarrhythmic drugs with class III action—such as sotalol, amiodarone, and dofetilide—that are known to prolong the QT interval. The HERG channel also has a cyclic nucleotide-binding domain in its C-terminus, providing a link to the adrenergically mediated triggering of arrhythmic events.

The K-channel gene that is defective in chromosome 11–linked LQTS1 is a gene called *KvLQT1* (*KCNQ1*), which, when coexpressed with *KCNE1* (minK), forms $I_{Ks}$, a target of compounds such as chromanol, amiodarone, and diuretics such as indapamide. *KCNE1* on chromosome 21 encodes the accessory subunit known as minK and is one of two genes mutated in LQTS5. Mutations in *KCNQ1*, *KCNE1*, and *KCNE2* have been associated with both the Romano-Ward (autosomal dominant) and the Jervell and Lange-Nielsen (autosomal recessive) variants of LQTS. Additionally, a number of polymorphisms in *KCNQ1*, *KCNH2*, and *KCNE2* have been linked to acquired, drug-induced TdP. More recently, other single-nucleotide polymorphisms in other ion channel genes (e.g., *Y1102*) of the cardiac Na channel (*SCN5A*) in African Americans has been linked to an increased incidence of acquired LQTS.[94]

Over 200 different mutations in K-channel subunits have been described in patients with LQTS. The mutations are either point mutations in regions of the channel critical for its function or frameshift mutations; thus they are likely to represent loss-of-function mutations. Loss-of-function mutations may be sufficient to explain the phenotype if the amount of repolarizing current is significantly reduced by the loss of one functional allele. However, in some cases, the mutation's autosomal dominance is explained by the structure of the K channel. The HERG and *KvLQT1* gene products are $\alpha$ subunits that tetramerize with three other similar or identical subunits. Some of the HERG mutations, despite their inability to form functional channels, retain the ability to combine with normal subunits; in doing so, they render the holochannel nonfunctional and reduce the pool of functional subunits from which intact functional HERG channels can be synthesized.

The cardiac Na channel encoded by *SCN5A* is a large glycoprotein of about 250 kDa made up four internally homologous repeats analogous to each subunit of a K channel. A number of regions of the channel, particularly on its cytoplasmic face, are involved in proper closure of the pore and turning off ion flux. A common functional consequence of most mutations in *SCN5A* that produce LQTS is that closure of the channel is incomplete; residual $Na^+$ current is present long after ion flux should have ceased. This defect results in a persistent small pedestal of Na current causing depolarization, which is sufficient to produce AP prolongation; it is essentially a gain-of-function mutation, thus accounting for the autosomal dominant behavior. Drugs like ibutilide (and a number of naturally occurring toxins) have a similar effect on Na channels.

Distinct mutations in the same gene may produce distinct phenotypes. For example, the cardiac Na channel is the disease gene in two distinct inherited arrhythmias, IVF and LQTS3, with distinct mutations producing each syndrome. A single large family has been described that experienced nocturnal death and ECG features of both

IVF and LQT3. Genetic analysis revealed that a single mutation in affected individuals was associated with the overlap syndrome with features of both phenotypes.[74] Experimental and simulation studies of this *SCN5A* mutation suggest that it may indeed produce both electrical phenotypes.[74,95]

Understanding the molecular basis of LQTS affords the possibility of genotype-directed therapy. Patients in the registry with LQTS3 have been treated with lidocaine and its oral congeners mexiletine or tocainide, with success in normalizing the QT intervals and eliminating symptoms; however, the effect of these agents on mortality is unknown.[96] Furthermore, the existence of overlap syndromes with the same mutations producing features of both LQTS and IVF suggests that caution should be exercised when contemplating such a therapeutic strategy.[97] Restoring the activity of the K channels pharmacologically is more challenging, and one therapeutic approach is to attempt to increase the activity of other repolarizing K currents to compensate for the defective current.[98] Strategies that have been tested include increasing extracellular K, which increases the activity of several K channels found in the heart, and the use of a class of drugs with vasodilating properties that has been useful in hypertension; these open up the ATP-sensitive K channel, thereby hastening repolarization.

The management of patients with LQTS depends to a great extent on the presentation. Recent data suggest that for those with serious presenting arrhythmias, syncope, or aborted SCD, the ICD should be first-line therapy. In patients with milder presentations and for family members of probands, the therapeutic approach is to use anti-adrenergic interventions as a first-line therapy and are associated with a 70 to 95 percent reduction in the rate of adverse cardiac events. It is important to determine the genotype of these patients and family members because of the possibility of genotype-specific antiarrhythmic therapy at least for the chromosome 3–linked form. For patients who remain symptomatic and are bradycardic on beta-adrenergic receptor blockers, permanent pacemaking is indicated; alternatively, with the reduction in size and ease of implantation, ICDs should be considered early for the patient who remains symptomatic despite medical therapy.[99]

## References


1. Lai LP et al. Association of the human minK gene 38G allele with atrial fibrillation: Evidence of possible genetic control on the pathogenesis of atrial fibrillation. *Am Heart J* 2002;144(3):485.
2. Nattel S. Ionic determinants of atrial fibrillation and $Ca^{2+}$ channel abnormalities: Cause, consequence, or innocent bystander? *Circ Res* 1999;85(5):473.
3. Tomaselli GF, Marban E. Electrophysiological remodeling in hypertrophy and heart failure. *Cardiovasc Res* 1999;42(2):270.
4. Osler W. On the so-called Stokes-Adams disease. *Lancet* 1903;II:516.
5. Morquio L. Sur une maladie infantile et familiale caracterisee par des modifications permanetes du pouls, des attaques syncopales et epileptiformes et la mort subite. *Arch Med Enfants* 1901;4:467.
6. Schott JJ, Benson DW, Basson CT, et al. Congenital heart disease caused by mutations in the transcription factor NKX2-5. *Science* 1998;281(5373):108–111.
7. Benson DW, Silberbach GM, Kavanaugh-McHugh A, et al. Mutations in the cardiac transcription factor NKX2.5 affect diverse cardiac developmental pathways. *J Clin Invest* 1999;104(11):1567.
8. Mohl W, Mayr WR. Atrial septal defect of the secundum type and HLA. *Tissue Antigens* 1977;10(2):121.
9. Basson CT, Solomon SD, Weissman B, et al. Genetic heterogeneity of heart-hand syndromes. *Circulation* 1995;91(5):1326.
10. Brink AJ, Torrington M. Progressive familial heart block—two types. *S Afr Med J* 1977;52(2):53.
11. Brink PA, Ferreira A, Moolman JC, et al. Gene for progressive familial heart block type I maps to chromosome 19q13. *Circulation* 1995; 91(6):1633–1640.
12. Schott JJ, Alshinawi C, Kyndt F, et al. Cardiac conduction defects associate with mutations in SCN5A. *Nat Genet* 1999;23(1):20.
13. Champion P, Harrison RJ. Limb-girdle dystrophy and heart block. *Proc R Soc Med* 1969;62(7):733.
14. Ross A, Lipschutz D, Austin J, et al. External ophthalmoplegia and complete heart block. *N Engl J Med* 1969;280(6):313.
15. Tanaka H, Uemura N, Toyama Y, et al. Cardiac involvement in the Kugelberg-Welander syndrome. *Am J Cardiol* 1976;38(4):528.
16. Wolff L. Familial auricular fibrillation. *N Engl J Med* 1943;229:396.
17. Gould WL. Auricular fibrillation: Report on a study of a familial tendency 1920–1956. *Arch Intern Med* 1957;100:916.
18. Nattel S. New ideas about atrial fibrillation 50 years on. *Nature* 2002;415(6868):219.
19. Van Wagoner DR, Pond AL, Lamorgese M, et al. Atrial L-type $Ca^{2+}$ currents and human atrial fibrillation. *Circ Res* 1999;85(5):428.
20. Dobrev D, Graf E, Wettwer E, et al. Molecular basis of downregulation of G-protein-coupled inward rectifying K(+) current I(K,ACh) in chronic human atrial fibrillation: decrease in GIRK4 mRNA correlates with reduced I(K,ACh) and muscarinic receptor-mediated shortening of action potentials. *Circulation* 2001;104(21):2551.
21. Chen YH, Xu SJ, Bendahhou S, Wang XL, et al. KCNQ1 gain-of-function mutation in familial atrial fibrillation. *Science* 2003;299(5604):251.
22. Brugada R, Tapscott T, Czernuszewicz GZ, et al. Identification of a genetic locus for familial atrial fibrillation. *N Engl J Med* 1997;336(13):905.
23. Darbar D, Herron KJ, Ballew JD, et al. Familial atrial fibrillation is a genetically heterogeneous disease. *J Am Coll Cardiol* 2003;41(12): 2185.
24. MacRae CA, Ghaisas N, Kass S, et al. Familial hypertrophic cardiomyopathy with Wolff-Parkinson-White syndrome maps to a locus on chromosome 7q3. *J Clin Invest* 1995;96(3):1216.
25. Gollob MH, Green MS, Tang AS, et al. Identification of a gene responsible for familial Wolff-Parkinson-White syndrome. *N Engl J Med* 2001;344(24):1823.
26. Blair E, Redwood C, Ashrafian H, et al. Mutations in the gamma(2) subunit of AMP-activated protein kinase cause familial hypertrophic cardiomyopathy: evidence for the central role of energy compromise in disease pathogenesis. *Hum Mol Genet* 2001;10(11):1215.
27. Gollob MH, Seger JJ, Gollob TN, et al. Novel PRKAG2 mutation responsible for the genetic syndrome of ventricular preexcitation and conduction system disease with childhood onset and absence of cardiac hypertrophy. *Circulation* 2001;104(25):3030.
28. Roberts R, Brugada R. Genetic aspects of arrhythmias. *Am J Med Genet* 2000;97(4):310.
29. Maron BJ, Gardin JM, Flack JM, et al. Prevalence of hypertrophic cardiomyopathy in a general population of young adults. Echocardiographic analysis of 4111 subjects in the CARDIA Study. Coronary Artery Risk Development in (Young) Adults. *Circulation* 1995;92(4):785.
30. Teare RD. Asymmetrical hypertrophy of the heart in young adults. *Br Heart J* 1958;20:1.
31. Maron BJ, Bonow RO, Cannon RO, et al. Hypertrophic cardiomyopathy. Interrelations of clinical manifestations, pathophysiology, and therapy. *N Engl J Med* 1987;316(14):844.
32. Spirito P, Seidman CE, McKenna WJ, et al. The management of hypertrophic cardiomyopathy. *N Engl J Med* 1997;336(11):775.
33. Arad M, Benson DW, Perez-Atayde AR, et al. Constitutively active AMP kinase mutations cause glycogen storage disease mimicking hypertrophic cardiomyopathy. *J Clin Invest* 2002;109(3):357.
34. Maron BJ. Hypertrophic cardiomyopathy: a systematic review. *JAMA* 2002;287(10):1308.
35. Elliott PM, Poloniecki J, Dickie S, et al. Sudden death in hypertrophic cardiomyopathy: Identification of high risk patients. *J Am Coll Cardiol* 2000;36(7):2212.
36. Watkins H, McKenna WJ, Thierfelder L, et al. Mutations in the genes for cardiac troponin T and alpha-tropomyosin in hypertrophic cardiomyopathy. *N Engl J Med* 1995;332(16):1058.

37. Moolman JC, Corfield VA, Posen B, et al. Sudden death due to troponin T mutations. *J Am Coll Cardiol* 1997;29(3):549.
38. Dec GW, Fuster V. Idiopathic dilated cardiomyopathy. *N Engl J Med* 1994;331(23):1564.
39. Michels VV, Moll PP, Miller FA, et al. The frequency of familial dilated cardiomyopathy in a series of patients with idiopathic dilated cardiomyopathy. *N Engl J Med* 1992;326(2):77.
40. Fatkin D, Graham RM. Molecular mechanisms of inherited cardiomyopathies. *Physiol Rev* 2002;82(4):945.
41. Moss AJ, Zareba W, Hall WJ, et al. Prophylactic implantation of a defibrillator in patients with myocardial infarction and reduced ejection fraction. *N Engl J Med* 2002;346(12):877.
42. Bansch D, Antz M, Boczor S, et al. Primary prevention of sudden cardiac death in idiopathic dilated cardiomyopathy: The Cardiomyopathy Trial (CAT). *Circulation* 2002;105(12):1453.
43. Bradley DJ, Bradley EA, Baughman KL, et al. Cardiac resynchronization and death from progressive heart failure: A meta-analysis of randomized controlled trials. *JAMA* 2003;289(6):730.
44. Marcus FI, Fontaine GH, Guiraudon G, et al. Right ventricular dysplasia: A report of 24 adult cases. *Circulation* 1982;65(2):384.
45. Corrado D, Basso C, Thiene G, et al. Spectrum of clinicopathologic manifestations of arrhythmogenic right ventricular cardiomyopathy/dysplasia: A multicenter study. *J Am Coll Cardiol* 1997;30(6):1512.
46. Thiene G, Basso C. Arrhythmogenic right ventricular cardiomyopathy: An update. *Cardiovasc Pathol* 2001;10(3):109.
47. Thiene G et al. Arrhythmogenic right ventricular cardiomyopathy. *Trends Cardiovasc Med* 1997;7:84.
48. McKenna WJ, Thiene G, Nava A, et al. Diagnosis of arrhythmogenic right ventricular dysplasia/cardiomyopathy. Task Force of the Working Group Myocardial and Pericardial Disease of the European Society of Cardiology and of the Scientific Council on Cardiomyopathies of the International Society and Federation of Cardiology. *Br Heart J* 1994;71(3):215.
49. Fontaine G, Fontaliran F, Hebert JL, et al. Arrhythmogenic right ventricular dysplasia. *Annu Rev Med* 1999;50:17.
50. Auffermann W, Wichter T, Breithardt G, et al. Arrhythmogenic right ventricular disease: MR imaging vs angiography. *Am J Roentgenol* 1993;161(3):549.
51. McKoy G, Protonotarios N, Crosby A, et al. Identification of a deletion in plakoglobin in arrhythmogenic right ventricular cardiomyopathy with palmoplantar keratoderma and woolly hair (Naxos disease). *Lancet* 2000;355(9221):2119.
52. Rampazzo A, Nava A, Malacrida S, et al. Mutation in human desmoplakin domain binding to plakoglobin causes a dominant form of arrhythmogenic right ventricular cardiomyopathy. *Am J Hum Genet* 2002;71(5):1200.
53. Tiso N, Stephan DA, Nava A, et al. Identification of mutations in the cardiac ryanodine receptor gene in families affected with arrhythmogenic right ventricular cardiomyopathy type 2 (ARVD2). *Hum Mol Genet* 2001;10(3):189.
54. Priori SG, Napolitano C, Tiso N, et al. Mutations in the cardiac ryanodine receptor gene (hRyR2) underlie catecholaminergic polymorphic ventricular tachycardia. *Circulation* 2001;103(2):196.
55. Laitinen PJ, Brown KM, Piippo K, et al. Mutations of the cardiac ryanodine receptor (RyR2) gene in familial polymorphic ventricular tachycardia. *Circulation* 2001;103(4):485.
56. Grimm W, List-Hellwig E, Hoffmann J, et al. Magnetic resonance imaging and signal-averaged electrocardiography in patients with repetitive monomorphic ventricular tachycardia and otherwise normal electrocardiogram. *Pacing Clin Electrophysiol* 1997;20(7):1826.
57. Leenhardt A, Lucet V, Denjoy I, et al. Catecholaminergic polymorphic ventricular tachycardia in children. A 7-year follow-up of 21 patients. *Circulation* 1995;91(5):1512.
58. Priori SG, Napolitano C, Memmi M, et al. Clinical and molecular characterization of patients with catecholaminergic polymorphic ventricular tachycardia. *Circulation* 2002;106(1):69.
59. Lahat H, Pras E, Olender T, et al. A missense mutation in a highly conserved region of CASQ2 is associated with autosomal recessive catecholamine-induced polymorphic ventricular tachycardia in Bedouin families from Israel. *Am J Hum Genet* 2001;69(6):1378.
60. Osher HL, Wolff L. Electrocardiographic pattern simulating acute myocardial injury. *Am J Med Sci* 1953;226:541.
61. Martini B, Nava A, Thiene G, et al. Ventricular fibrillation without apparent heart disease: Description of six cases. *Am Heart J* 1989; 118(6):1203.
62. Brugada P, Brugada J. Right bundle branch block, persistent ST segment elevation and sudden cardiac death: A distinct clinical and electrocardiographic syndrome. A multicenter report. *J Am Coll Cardiol* 1992;20(6):1391.
63. Nademanee K, Veerakul G, Nimmannit S, et al. Arrhythmogenic marker for the sudden unexplained death syndrome in Thai men. *Circulation* 1997;96(8):2595.
64. Alings M, Wilde A. Brugada syndrome: Clinical data and suggested pathophysiological mechanism. *Circulation* 1999;99(5):666.
65. Priori SG, Napolitano C, Gasparini M, et al. Natural history of Brugada syndrome: Insights for risk stratification and management. *Circulation* 2002;105(11):1342.
66. Brugada J, Brugada R, Antzelevitch C, et al. Long-term follow-up of individuals with the electrocardiographic pattern of right bundle-branch block and ST-segment elevation in precordial leads $V_1$ to $V_3$. *Circulation* 2002;105(1):73.
67. Matsuo K, Kurita T, Inagaki M, et al. The circadian pattern of the development of ventricular fibrillation in patients with Brugada syndrome. *Eur Heart J* 1999;20(6):465.
68. Suzuki H, Torigoe K, Numata O, et al. Infant case with a malignant form of Brugada syndrome. *J Cardiovasc Electrophysiol* 2000; 11(11):1277.
69. Priori SG, Napolitano C, Giordano U, et al. Brugada syndrome and sudden cardiac death in children. *Lancet* 2000;355(9206):808.
70. Wilde AA, Antzelevitch C, Borggrefe M, et al. Proposed diagnostic criteria for the Brugada syndrome: Consensus report. *Circulation* 2002;106(19):2514.
71. Shimizu W, Matsuo K, Takagi M, et al. Body surface distribution and response to drugs of ST segment elevation in Brugada syndrome: Clinical implication of eighty-seven-lead body surface potential mapping and its application to twelve-lead electrocardiograms. *J Cardiovasc Electrophysiol* 2000;11(4):396.
72. Eckardt L, Kirchhof P, Loh P, et al. Brugada syndrome and supraventricular tachyarrhythmias: A novel association? *J Cardiovasc Electrophysiol* 2001;12(6):680.
73. Chen Q, Kirsch GE, Zhang D, et al. Genetic basis and molecular mechanism for idiopathic ventricular fibrillation. *Nature* 1998; 392(6673):293.
74. Bezzina C, Veldkamp MW, van Den Berg MP, et al. A single $Na^+$ channel mutation causing both long-QT and Brugada syndromes. *Circ Res* 1999;85(12):1206.
75. Antzelevitch C, Yan GX, Shimizu W. Transmural dispersion of repolarization and arrhythmogenicity: The Brugada syndrome versus the long QT syndrome. *J Electrocardiol* 1999;32(suppl):158.
76. Kurita T, Shimizu W, Inagaki M, et al. The electrophysiologic mechanism of ST-segment elevation in Brugada syndrome. *J Am Coll Cardiol* 2002;40(2):330.
77. Jervell A, Lange-Nielsen F. Congenital deaf-mutism, functional heart disease with prolongation of the Q-T interval and sudden death. *Am Heart J* 1957;54:59.
78. Romano C, Gemme G, Pongiglione R. Aritmie cardiache rare in eta pediatrica. *Clin Pediatr* 1963;45:656.
79. Ward OC. A new familial cardiac syndrome in children. *J Irish Med Assoc* 1964;54:103.
80. Moss AJ, Schwartz PJ, Crampton RS, et al. The long QT syndrome: A prospective international study. *Circulation* 1985;71(1):17.
81. Schwartz PJ, Periti M, Malliani A. The long QT syndrome. *Am Heart J* 1975;89:378.
82. Schwartz PJ, Priori SG, Spazzolini C, et al. Genotype-phenotype correlation in the long-QT syndrome: Gene-specific triggers for life-threatening arrhythmias. *Circulation* 2001;103(1):89.

83. Keating M, Atkinson D, Dunn C, et al. Linkage of a cardiac arrhythmia, the long QT syndrome, and the Harvey *ras*-1 gene. *Science* 1991;252(5006):704.
84. Curran ME, Splawski I, Timothy KW, et al. A molecular basis for cardiac arrhythmia: HERG mutations cause long QT syndrome. *Cell* 1995;80(5):795.
85. Wang Q, Shen J, Splawski I, et al. SCN5A mutations associated with an inherited cardiac arrhythmia, long QT syndrome. *Cell* 1995;80(5):805.
86. Mohler PJ, Schott JJ, Gramolini AO, et al. Ankyrin-B mutation causes type 4 long-QT cardiac arrhythmia and sudden cardiac death. *Nature* 2003;421(6923):634.
87. Andersen ED, Krasilnikoff PA, Overvad H. Intermittent muscular weakness, extrasystoles, and multiple developmental anomalies. A new syndrome? *Acta Paediatr Scand* 1971;60(5):559.
88. Plaster NM, Tawil R, Tristani-Firouzi M, et al. Mutations in Kir 2.1 cause the developmental and episodic electrical phenotypes of Andersen's syndrome. *Cell* 2001;105(4):511.
89. Roden DM, Lazzara R, Rosen M, et al. Multiple mechanisms in the long-QT syndrome. Current knowledge, gaps, and future directions. The SADS Foundation Task Force on LQTS. *Circulation* 1996;94(8): 1996.
90. Dessertenne F. La tachycardie ventriculaire a deux foyers opposes variables. *Arch Mal Coeur* 1966;59:263.
91. Zareba W, Moss AJ, Schwartz PJ, et al. Influence of genotype on the clinical course of the long-QT syndrome. International Long-QT Syndrome Registry Research Group. *N Engl J Med* 1998;339(14):960.
92. Schwartz PJ, Moss AJ, Vincent GM, et al. Diagnostic criteria for the long QT syndrome. An update. *Circulation* 1993;88(2):782.
93. Abbott GW, Sesti F, Splawski I, et al. MiRP1 forms IKr potassium channels with HERG and is associated with cardiac arrhythmia. *Cell* 1999;97(2):175.
94. Splawski I, Timothy KW, Tateyama M, et al. Variant of SCN5A sodium channel implicated in risk of cardiac arrhythmia. *Science* 2002;297(5585):1333.
95. Clancy CE, Rudy Y. $Na^+$ channel mutation that causes both Brugada and long-QT syndrome phenotypes: a simulation study of mechanism. *Circulation* 2002;105(10):1208.
96. Schwartz PJ, Priori SG, Locati EH, et al. Long QT syndrome patients with mutations of the SCN5A and HERG genes have differential responses to $Na^+$ channel blockade and to increases in heart rate. Implications for gene-specific therapy. *Circulation* 1995;92(12): 3381.
97. Priori SG, Napolitano C, Schwartz PJ, et al. The elusive link between LQT3 and Brugada syndrome: The role of flecainide challenge. *Circulation* 2000;102(9):945.
98. Compton SJ, Lux RL, Ramsey MR, et al. Genetically defined therapy of inherited long-QT syndrome. Correction of abnormal repolarization by potassium. *Circulation* 1996;94(5):1018.
99. Dorostkar PC, Eldar M, Belhassen B, et al. Long-term follow-up of patients with long-QT syndrome treated with beta-blockers and continuous pacing. *Circulation* 1999;100(24):2431.
100. Balaji S, Till J, Shinebourne EA. Familial atrial standstill with coexistent atrial flutter. *Pacing Clin Electrophysiol* 1998;21(9):1841.
101. Bacos JM, Eagan JT, Orgain ES. Congenital familial nodal rhythm. *Circulation* 1960;22:887.
102. Combrink JM, Davis WH, Snyman HW. Familial bundle branch block. *Am Heart J* 1962;64:397.
103. Esscher E, Hardell LI, Michaelsson M. Familial, isolated, complete right bundle-branch block. *Br Heart J* 1975;37(7):745.
104. Geisterfer-Lowrance AA, Kass S, Tanigawa G, et al. A molecular basis for familial hypertrophic cardiomyopathy: A beta cardiac myosin heavy chain gene missense mutation. *Cell* 1990;62(5):999.
105. Thierfelder L, Watkins H, MacRae C, et al. Alpha-tropomyosin and cardiac troponin T mutations cause familial hypertrophic cardiomyopathy: A disease of the sarcomere. *Cell* 1994;77(5):701.
106. Bonne G, Carrier L, Bercovici J, et al. Cardiac myosin binding protein-C gene splice acceptor site mutation is associated with familial hypertrophic cardiomyopathy. *Nat Genet* 1995;11(4):438.
107. Watkins H, Conner D, Thierfelder L, et al. Mutations in the cardiac myosin binding protein-C gene on chromosome 11 cause familial hypertrophic cardiomyopathy. *Nat Genet* 1995;11(4):434.
108. Poetter K, Jiang H, Hassanzadeh S, et al. Mutations in either the essential or regulatory light chains of myosin are associated with a rare myopathy in human heart and skeletal muscle. *Nat Genet* 1996;13(1):63.
109. Niimura H, Patton KK, McKenna WJ, et al. Sarcomere protein gene mutations in hypertrophic cardiomyopathy of the elderly. *Circulation* 2002;105(4):446.
110. Kimura A, Harada H, Park JE, et al. Mutations in the cardiac troponin I gene associated with hypertrophic cardiomyopathy. *Nat Genet* 1997;16(4):379.
111. Hoffmann B, Schmidt-Traub H, Perrot A, et al. First mutation in cardiac troponin C, L29Q, in a patient with hypertrophic cardiomyopathy. *Hum Mutat* 2001;17(6):524.
112. Satoh M, Takahashi M, Sakamoto T, et al. Structural analysis of the titin gene in hypertrophic cardiomyopathy: Identification of a novel disease gene. *Biochem Biophys Res Commun* 1999;262(2):411.
113. Mogensen J, Klausen IC, Pedersen AK, et al. Alpha-cardiac actin is a novel disease gene in familial hypertrophic cardiomyopathy. *J Clin Invest* 1999;103(10):R39.
114. Kamisago M, Sharma SD, DePalma SR, et al. Mutations in sarcomere protein genes as a cause of dilated cardiomyopathy. *N Engl J Med* 2000;343(23):1688.
115. Gerull B, Gramlich M, Atherton J, et al. Mutations of TTN, encoding the giant muscle filament titin, cause familial dilated cardiomyopathy. *Nat Genet* 2002;30(2):201.
116. Li D, Tapscoft T, Gonzalez O, et al. Desmin mutation responsible for idiopathic dilated cardiomyopathy. *Circulation* 1999;100(5):461.
117. Tsubata S, Bowles KR, Vatta M, et al. Mutations in the human delta-sarcoglycan gene in familial and sporadic dilated cardiomyopathy. *J Clin Invest* 2000;106(5):655.
118. Olson TM, Illenberger S, Kishimoto NY, et al. Metavinculin mutations alter actin interaction in dilated cardiomyopathy. *Circulation* 2002; 105(4):431.
119. Daehmlow S, Erdmann J, Knueppel T, et al. Novel mutations in sarcomeric protein genes in dilated cardiomyopathy. *Biochem Biophys Res Commun* 2002;298(1):116.
120. Olson TM, Kishimoto NY, Whitby FG, Michels VV. Mutations that alter the surface charge of alpha-tropomyosin are associated with dilated cardiomyopathy. *J Mol Cell Cardiol* 2001;33(4):723.
121. Olson TM, Michels VV, Thibodeau SN, et al. Actin mutations in dilated cardiomyopathy, a heritable form of heart failure. *Science* 1998;280(5364):750.
122. Sylvius N, Tesson F, Gayet C, et al. A new locus for autosomal dominant dilated cardiomyopathy identified on chromosome 6q12-q16. *Am J Hum Genet* 2001;68(1):241.
123. Krajinovic M, Pinamonti B, Sinagra G, et al. Linkage of familial dilated cardiomyopathy to chromosome 9. Heart Muscle Disease Study Group. *Am J Hum Genet* 1995;57(4):846.
124. Fatkin D, MacRae C, Sasaki T, et al. Missense mutations in the rod domain of the lamin A/C gene as causes of dilated cardiomyopathy and conduction-system disease. *N Engl J Med* 1999;341(23):1715.
125. Jung M, Poepping I, Perrot A, et al. Investigation of a family with autosomal dominant dilated cardiomyopathy defines a novel locus on chromosome 2q14-q22. *Am J Hum Genet* 1999;65(4):1068.
126. Olson TM, Keating MT. Mapping a cardiomyopathy locus to chromosome 3p22-p25. *J Clin Invest* 1996;97(2):528.
127. Muchir A, Bonne G, van der Kooi AJ, et al. Identification of mutations in the gene encoding lamins A/C in autosomal dominant limb-girdle muscular dystrophy with atrioventricular conduction disturbances (LGMD1B). *Hum Mol Genet* 2000;9(9):1453.
128. Messina DN, Speer MC, Pericak-Vance MA, et al. Linkage of familial dilated cardiomyopathy with conduction defect and muscular dystrophy to chromosome 6q23. *Am J Hum Genet* 1997;61(4):909.
129. Schonberger J, Levy H, Grunig E, et al. Dilated cardiomyopathy and sensorineural hearing loss: A heritable syndrome that maps to 6q23-24. *Circulation* 2000;101(15):1812.

130. Towbin JA, Hejtmancik JF, Brink P, et al. X-linked dilated cardiomyopathy. Molecular genetic evidence of linkage to the Duchenne muscular dystrophy (dystrophin) gene at the Xp21 locus. *Circulation* 1993;87(6):1854.
131. D'Adamo P, Fassone L, Gedeon A, et al. The X-linked gene G4.5 is responsible for different infantile dilated cardiomyopathies. *Am J Hum Genet* 1997;61(4):862.
132. Rampazzo A, Nava A, Danieli GA, et al. The gene for arrhythmogenic right ventricular cardiomyopathy maps to chromosome 14q23-q24. *Hum Mol Genet* 1994;3(6):959.
133. Severini GM, Krajinovic M, Pinamonti B, et al. A new locus for arrhythmogenic right ventricular dysplasia on the long arm of chromosome 14. *Genomics* 1996;31(2):193.
134. Rampazzo A, Nava A, Miorin M, et al. ARVD4, a new locus for arrhythmogenic right ventricular cardiomyopathy, maps to chromosome 2 long arm. *Genomics* 1997;45(2):259.
135. Ahmad F, Li D, Karibe A, et al. Localization of a gene responsible for arrhythmogenic right ventricular dysplasia to chromosome 3p23. *Circulation* 1998;98(25):2791.
136. Li D, Ahmad F, Gardner MJ, et al. The locus of a novel gene responsible for arrhythmogenic right-ventricular dysplasia characterized by early onset and high penetrance maps to chromosome 10p12-p14. *Am J Hum Genet* 2000;66(1):148.
137. Wang Q, Curran ME, Splawski I, et al. Positional cloning of a novel potassium channel gene: KVLQT1 mutations cause cardiac arrhythmias. *Nat Genet* 1996;12(1):17.
138. Duggal P, Vesely MR, Wattanasirichaigoon D, et al. Mutation of the gene for IsK associated with both Jervell and Lange-Nielsen and Romano-Ward forms of long-QT syndrome. *Circulation* 1998;97(2):142.

C H A P T E R 11

# CARDIOVASCULAR TISSUE MODIFICATION BY GENETIC APPROACHES

Elizabeth G. Nabel / Victor J. Dzau



The field of cardiovascular gene therapy had its origins in the mid-1980s because of rapid advances in the molecular genetics of the cardiovascular system. The cloning of genes important for the development and function of the cardiovascular system increased our understanding of the normal biology and pathology of cardiac diseases. In turn, this genetic information has provided new opportunities for novel therapeutics using gene-transfer approaches.

*Somatic gene transfer* is the introduction of recombinant genetic material (DNA or RNA) into host cells such that gene expression within the host cell is altered to achieve a therapeutic effect. The genetic material includes eukaryotic genes (often with transcriptional regulatory elements) and RNA that encodes intracellular or secreted gene products. *Vectors* are used commonly to introduce the genetic material into cells (Table 11-1). These vectors include replication-incompetent viruses and biochemical substances. The genetic material can be delivered directly into vascular or myocardial cells in vivo, referred to as *direct gene transfer,* or into tissues, such as a venous bypass graft ex vivo that in turn is returned to the host. This latter approach is termed *indirect gene transfer.* Local delivery catheters are required for the introduction of vectors and cells (Fig. 11-1).

This chapter reviews our current understanding of genetic therapies, including stem cell biology, for cardiovascular diseases. This discussion will examine vector systems for delivering genes, disease

TABLE 11-1 Gene Transfer Vectors

| Viral Vectors | Nonviral Vectors |
|---|---|
| Retrovirus | Cationic liposomes |
| Adenovirus | Fusigenic liposomes |
| Adeno-associated virus | DNA plasmid vectors |

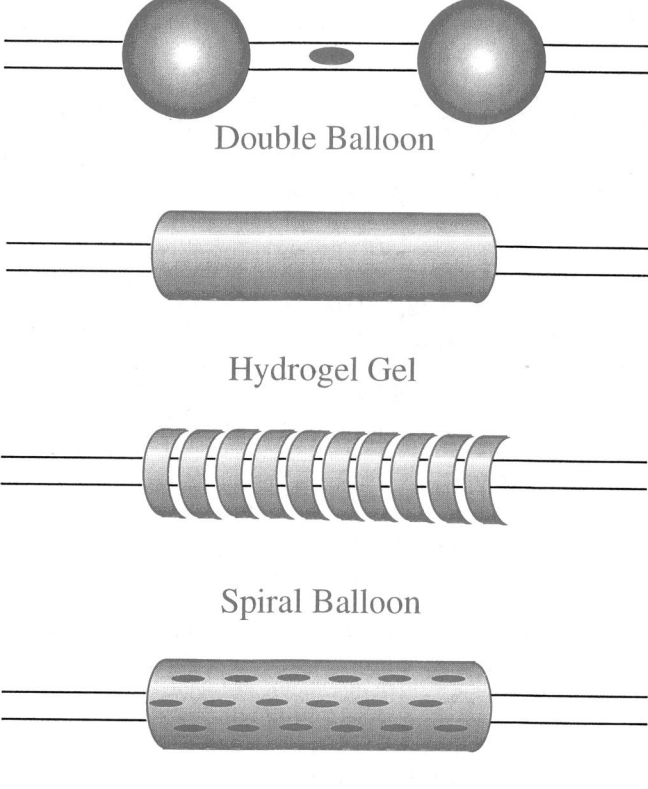

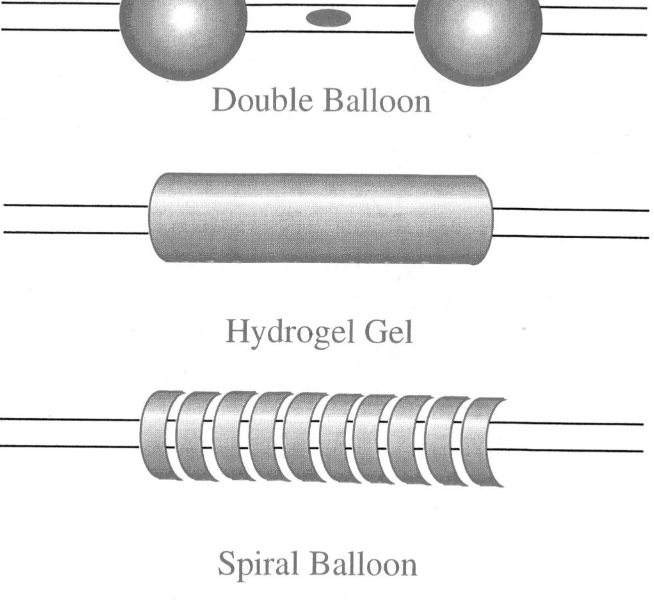


FIGURE 11-1 Catheters for cardiovascular gene therapy. (From Nabel,[111] with permission.)

targets and preclinical animal models, recent results of clinical trials, and new, emerging opportunities for cell transplantation with pluripotent stem cells.

## VECTORS FOR GENE TRANSFER

### Viral Vectors

#### RETROVIRAL VECTORS

Retroviruses were the first viruses adapted for use as vectors owing to the simplicity of their genomes and their capacity to integrate stably their genome into the host chromosome. A retroviral vector is constructed in several steps.[1,2] First, the structural genes required for viral replication are deleted to render the vector nonreplicating. After insertion of the exogenous gene of interest into the viral backbone, the recombinant retrovirus contains the exogenous gene, regulatory sequences, and packaging signals but lacks the actual structural genes required to produce a complete virion. It requires a helper cell to produce infectious viral particles. Nabel et al. demonstrated the feasibility of transfecting blood vessels with foreign DNA in vivo by transfecting pig iliofemoral arteries with a recombinant amphotropic retroviral vector containing a $\beta$-galactosidase gene.[3,4] Several cell types in the vessel wall were transduced, including endothelial and vascular smooth muscle cells. Using a $\beta$-galactosidase retroviral vector to modify endothelial cells, Wilson et al.[5] demonstrated $\beta$-galactosidase expression up to 5 weeks after transfection in prosthetic vascular grafts seeded with the genetically transformed cells. Retroviral vectors have not been effective vectors for cardiovascular applications because they require actively dividing cells for integration and expression of the viral genome. Since most myocardial and vascular cells are not dividing, transfection efficiency with retroviral vectors in these cells has been low.

#### ADENOVIRAL VECTORS

Adenoviral vectors are widely used for cardiovascular gene transfer because adenoviruses infect nondividing cells and do not integrate into the host genome. Adenoviruses are double-stranded linear DNA viruses that in their wild type cause a self-limited respiratory tract infection in humans.[6] The wild-type adenovirus genome is a 36-kDa DNA molecule that is divided into 100 map units. The majority of adenoviral vectors are derived from adenovirus serotypes 2 and 5. These vectors are constructed by deletion of the E1 region (map units 1 to 9) of the genome that normally encodes E1A and E1B motifs that are required for the expression of late viral genes and for the induction of the lytic phase of the virus. Without the E1 region, the virus cannot replicate. This region is replaced with the transgene of interest, up to 7.5 kb in size. Because the E1 deletion renders them replication-incompetent, adenoviral vectors are propagated in a helper cell line that expresses E1 protein in transfection. These vectors can be produced in high titers for in vivo delivery.[7] Adenoviral vectors enter mammalian cells by receptor-mediated endocytosis and $\alpha 2\beta 3$ integrins.[8] Aortic smooth muscle cells[9] and cardiac myocytes[10] were transfected successfully using replication-defective adenovirus carrying the $\beta$-galactosidase or chloramphenicol acetyltransferase reporter gene, respectively. In vivo transfection by adenoviral vectors was demonstrated in vascular tissue by direct infusion into vessels,[9,11,12] in myocardial tissue by direct injection into the myocardium,[10,13] and in the circulation after adenoviral infection of skeletal muscle.[14] Limitations of the first-generation adenoviral vectors include transient gene expression and host inflammatory and immune responses against the transgene[15] and viral antigens.[16,17] These limitations are being overcome by the development of "gutted" adenoviral vectors.[18] These vectors retain viral coat proteins for receptor attachment and internalization but lack other viral proteins that are immunogenic.

#### ADENO-ASSOCIATED VIRAL VECTORS

Adeno-associated virus (AAV) is a defective human parvovirus that is not able to replicate unless a helper virus, such as adenovirus, is also present.[19] There are several features that make AAV an attractive vector. The virus can be prepared at high titer, is not pathogenic in humans, and infects a broad range of cell lines.[20] Wild-type AAV integrates in a site-specific manner in a 7-kb region of human chromosomes.[20,21] The AAV genome is a single-stranded linear 5-kb DNA molecule. The genome is flanked by two 145-bp inverted terminal repeats (ITRs) that contain the sequences required for packing, integration, and DNA replication. The coding region contains two open reading frames (ORFs). Either of these ORFs is replaced with the transgene and regulatory elements to construct an AAV vector. The ORF can only accept a transgene of 4 to 5 kb, thus limiting the size of the transgene insert. Propagation of AAV vectors requires AAV Rep and Cap proteins and five adenoviral proteins: E1A, E1B, E2A, E4, and VA. These are complex packaging requirements, and thus it has been difficult to construct a packaging cell line. Instead, AAV vectors are propagated by cotransfection of the AAV vector with a plasmid wild-type or mutant helper adenovirus. AAV vectors have been used very successfully when injected into skeletal muscle to produce proteins secreted into the circulation, such as factor IX for hemophilia B.[22] Cardiovascular applications include cardiac myocytes, where Svensson et al. have demonstrated stable expression.[23] Whether AAV vectors can be adapted to efficiently transduce vascular endothelial cells and smooth muscle cells is not known.

### Nonviral Vectors

#### CATIONIC LIPOSOMES

The encapsulation of DNA in artificial lipid membranes (i.e., liposomes) can facilitate its uptake and cellular transport. Cationic liposomes have been used for cellular delivery of DNA[24] and antisense oligonucleotides.[25] The activity of cationic liposomes is postulated to be mediated by (1) spontaneous capture of the negatively charged polynucleotides with cationic lipids by a condensation reaction, (2) increased cellular uptake due to interaction of positively charged complexes with negatively charged biologic membranes, and (3) membrane fusion (or transient membrane destabilization) with the plasmalemma or the endosome to achieve delivery into the cytoplasm while avoiding degradation in the lysosomal compartment. Recent data indicate that movement of DNA from the cytoplasm to the nucleus and successful dissociation of DNA from the lipid complex appear to be important variables for lipid-mediated gene transfer.[26] Expression of recombinant genes after cationic lipid-mediated gene transfer has been demonstrated in vivo in several animal models.[27–29] Gene expression after liposome-mediated arterial gene transfer may be augmented in the presence of ongoing proliferation (e.g., intimal proliferation after balloon injury).[30]

#### FUSIGENIC LIPOSOMES

This method uses a combination of fusigenic proteins of the Sendai virus (hemagglutinating virus of Japan) and neutral liposomes. Hemagglutinating virus of Japan (HVJ) is an RNA virus that belongs to the paramyxovirus family, which has HN and F glycoproteins on its envelope. HN binds with glycol-type sialic acid and degrades the receptor by its own neuraminidase activity. F glycoprotein is cleaved to generate a hydrophobic fusion peptide by proteases, and the activated F protein can interact directly with the cellular lipid bilayer and induces fusion. A nuclear protein, namely, high-mobility group 1

(HMG-1), that binds DNA enhances the integration of transfected DNA into the nucleus.[31] HVJ liposomes consist of neutral liposomes complexed with ultraviolet (UV) light-inactivated HVJ virus. It is postulated that after fusion of the liposome complex with the cell membrane, the DNA is released directly into the cytosol without undergoing endocytosis, thereby reducing lysosomal destruction of the DNA construct and facilitating the nuclear uptake.[32] HVJ liposome methods have been employed successfully for gene transfer in vivo to liver,[31] kidney,[33] and vasculature.[34,35]

### PLASMID DNA

Direct injection of plasmid DNA in cardiac or skeletal muscle results in stable transfection of a small percentage of cells.[36] Following direct injection to the heart muscle, expression of a reporter gene was demonstrated for up to 4 weeks.[37] Expression of injected genes can be targeted to specific cell types in vivo (e.g., cardiac muscle cells) and can be modulated by the hormonal status of the animal.[38]

### SYNTHETIC OLIGONUCLEOTIDES

Antisense oligonucleotides (ASOs) are short 10- to 30-bp chemically synthesized DNA molecules designed to be complementary to the coding sequence of a target RNA. ASOs are introduced into cells simply by diffusion or complexed with liposomes, such as HVJ.[32] Inside the cell, ASOs form double-stranded complexes with their complementary RNA and decrease translation of RNA. Mechanisms of antisense inhibition include interference with ribosome binding and processing of mRNA, interference with mRNA conformation or mRNA splicing, and RNase-H activation of mRNA digestion.[39,40]

ASOs are attractive agents for in vivo gene therapy. They are chemically synthesized in large quantities and do not require a viral component for in vivo delivery. However, there are several limitations to their use in vivo. ASOs have a short half-life in vivo due to nuclease degradation. Chemical modifications, such as substitution of sulfur for one of the nonbridging oxygens of a phosphate group (phosphorothiorates), render ASOs more stable to degradation in serum.[41] Several nonspecific effects of ASOs have been noted that account in part for their biologic effect.[39,42] ASOs can have nonspecific cytotoxic effects due to binding to intracellular and cell surface proteins. Some ASOs affect the expression of multiple genes in addition to the gene of interest. This effect is sequence-specific and is not controlled with scrambled oligonucleotides. ASOs containing $C_pG$ dinucleotides have been shown to have nonantigen activation of the humoral immune system.[43] Despite these relative limitations, ASOs are well suited to the treatment of diseases where transient reductions in gene expression are required. ASOs theoretically are used to reduce specifically the expression of one or more genes. The uptake of ASOs can be enhanced by complexing the oligonucleotide with cationic liposomes[25] or HVJ liposomes.[34,35]

Synthetic double-stranded oligonucleotides containing binding sites for transcription factors serve as "decoys" to block the binding of nuclear factors to promoter regions of targeted genes, resulting in the inhibition of gene transactivation.[41,44] Morishita et al.[45] have shown that a single administration of an E2F decoy (containing the E2F cis element) that binds the transcription factor E2F inhibits smooth muscle cell hyperplasia in a rat carotid balloon injury model[45] (Fig. 11-2). The binding of E2F prevents it from transactivating the gene expression of cell cycle regulatory proteins such as PCNA, c-myc, and cdk2, thereby inhibiting vascular smooth muscle cell proliferation and subsequent neointimal formation in vivo.

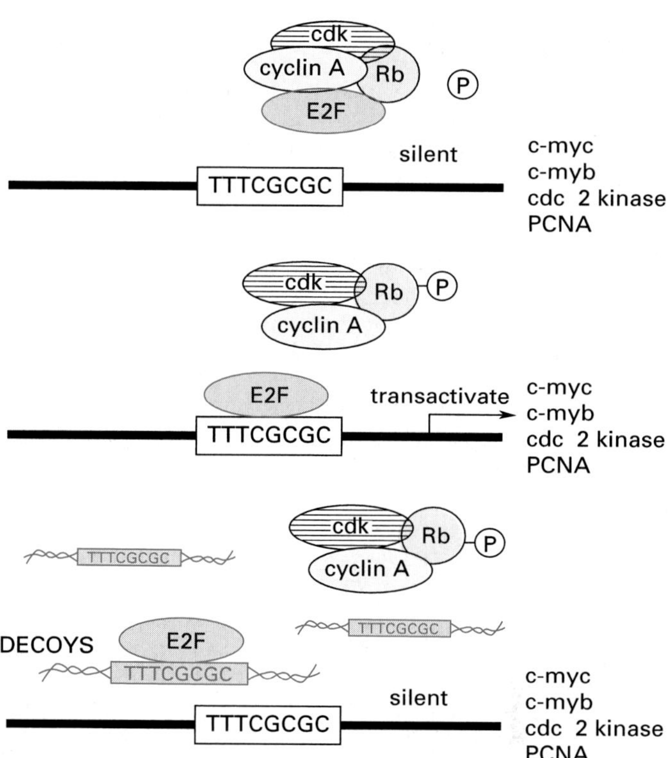


FIGURE 11-2 Principal of E2F "decoy" strategy. TTTCGCGC is the consensus sequence for the E2F binding site. In the quiescent cell state, the transcription factor E2F is complexed with Rb (retinoblastoma gene product), cyclin A, and the cyclin-dependent kinase cdk2 (*top*). Phosphorylation of Rb releases free E2F, which binds to cis elements of the cell cycle regulatory genes, resulting in the transactivation of these genes (*middle*). The E2F decoy cis-element double-stranded oligonucleotide binds to free E2F, preventing E2F-mediated transactivation of cell cycle regulatory genes (*bottom*). (From Morishita et al.[45] With permission.)

## CELLULAR TRANSPLANTATION

The implantation of cells expressing recombinant genes into the heart or vasculature is termed *ex vivo gene transfer*. Nabel et al.[3] demonstrated a cell-based vascular gene-transfer technique. By reimplanting endothelial cells transfected ex vivo with a retroviral $\beta$-galactosidase vector on the surface of balloon-injured porcine iliofemoral arteries, genetically modified cells are detected up to 2 to 4 weeks following reimplantation. Wilson et al.[5] demonstrated expression of a reporter gene from endothelial cells implanted on a Dacron graft and placed in the carotid arteries of dogs. In addition to endothelial cells, ex vivo–transfected smooth muscle cells have been introduced in the vasculature.[46] Lynch et al.[47] reported the seeding of smooth muscle cells transfected with the adenosine deaminase gene into endothelium-denuded blood vessels. Another application of ex vivo gene transfer is the engineering of vascular grafts seeded with endothelial cells previously transfected in a culture dish.[48] Seeding of vascular grafts with soluble vascular cell adhesion molecules (sVCAMs) (see Chap. 5) using adenoviral ex vivo gene transfer was reported by Chen et al.[49]

Implantation of genetically modified myoblasts or fibroblasts into skeletal muscle is an attractive gene-transfer method because the gene product is delivered systemically. Indeed, several investigators have reported successful gene delivery using these approaches.[50–52] In a mouse model, myoblasts were transplanted and supported sustained delivery of functionally active erythropoietin to correct anemia associated with renal failure.[53] The myoblast method potentially could provide an approach for the delivery of insulin (diabetes), atrial natriuretic peptide (hypertension or heart failure), or apolipoprotein AI (atherosclerosis).

## GENE TRANSFER AND VASCULAR DISEASE

Gene transfer into the vasculature is used to investigate the pathophysiology of vascular diseases and to develop novel therapies for these diseases. This field has expanded rapidly in the past decade. A number of models in the mouse, rat, rabbit, dog, and pig have been created to dissect vascular pathophysiology in peripheral, coronary, renal, pulmonary, and cerebral blood vessels. A full discussion of these animal models is beyond the scope of this chapter; the reader may consult pertinent reviews.[54–58]

### Experimental Applications of ASOs

#### INTIMAL HYPERPLASIA

Simons et al.[59] reported that the administration of ASOs against *c-myb* applied by pluronic gel to the adventitial layer of rat carotid arteries inhibited neointimal hyperplasia in response to balloon injury. Data from Morishita et al.[34] demonstrated that a single HVJ liposome–mediated administration of ASOs against proliferating cell nuclear antigen (PCNA) and cdc2 kinase inhibited neointimal lesion formation after balloon injury for at least 8 weeks after transfection. The combination of antisense cdc2 kinase and cdk2 kinase oligonucleotides also resulted in almost complete inhibition of neointima formation.[35] Bennett et al.[60] showed an inhibition of vascular smooth muscle cell proliferation by administration of *c-myc* ASOs to the adventitial surface of injured carotid arteries in a pluronic gel solution. Two other studies reported inhibition of neointima formation after application of ASOs. Delivery of antisense PCNA oligonucleotides by pluronic gel (in a rat carotid model) and of antisense c-myc oligonucleotides by direct application through a porous balloon (in a porcine coronary artery model) resulted in significant inhibition of neointimal hyperplasia.[61,62]

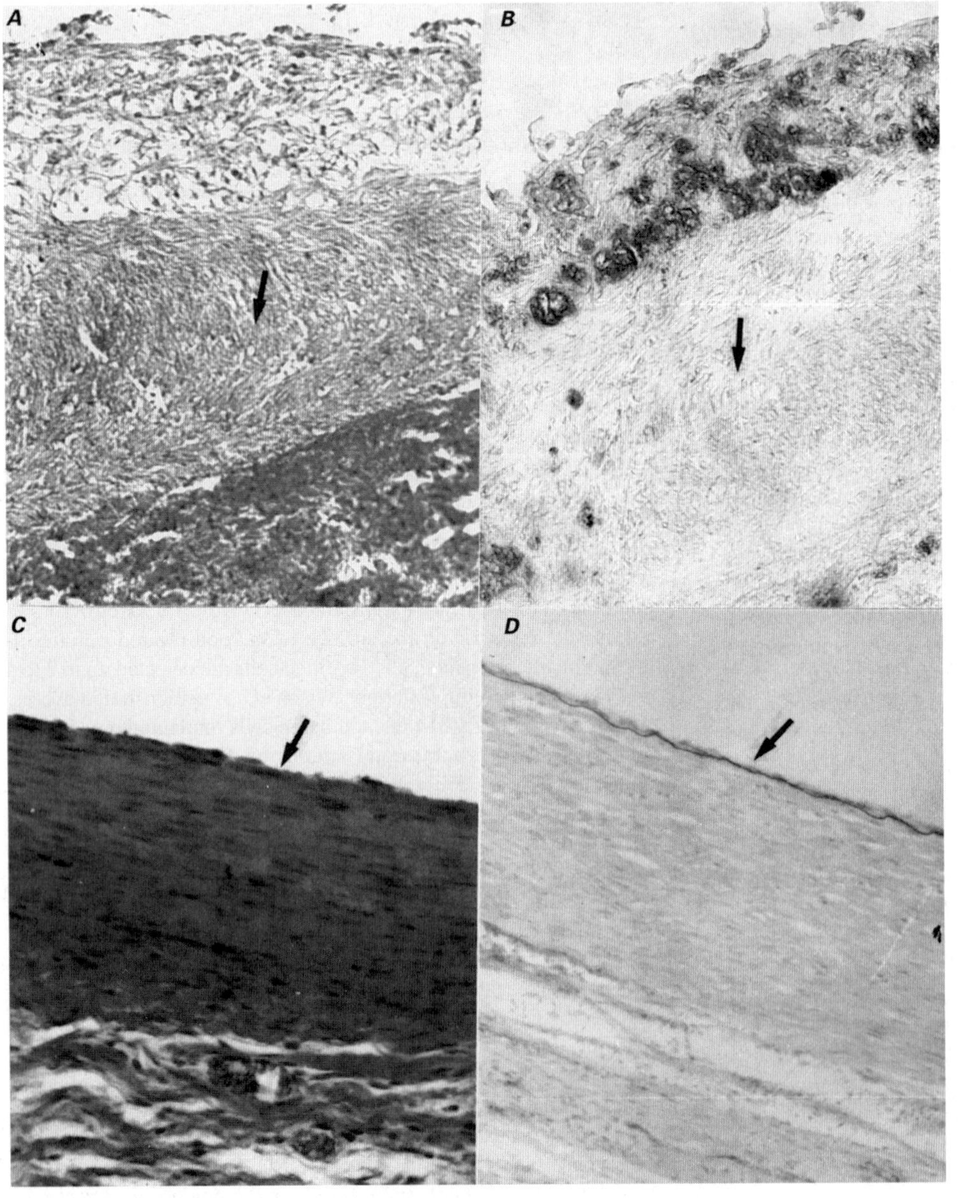


FIGURE 11-3 Control oligonucleotide-treated (*A* and *B*) and ASO (against cdc2 kinase/PCNA)-treated vein grafts (*C* and *D*) in hypercholesterolemic rabbits 6 weeks after surgery (×70). Sections of 5 mm were stained with hematoxylin/van Gieson (*A* and *C*) and a monoclonal antibody against rabbit macrophages (*B* and *D*). Arrows indicate the location of the internal elastic lamina. (From Mann et al.[63] With permission.)

#### VEIN GRAFT DISEASE

Autologous vein grafts remain the most commonly used conduits for surgical revascularization of the heart and lower extremities. Given the failure of traditional therapies at improving long-term vein graft function, gene therapy offers a new opportunity for reducing the morbidity and increased costs associated with the current limitations on functional graft survival. The vein graft offers an unusual opportunity for combining intact tissue in vivo gene-transfer techniques with the increased safety of an ex vivo application of the transfection medium. Manipulation of transfection conditions, including increased exposure time and controlling components of the transfection medium, can also be more easily achieved. Some researchers have begun to explore the possibility of ex vivo virus-mediated gene transfer in autologous vein grafts. Chen et al.[49] demonstrated the expression of the marker gene $\beta$-galactosidase along the luminal surface and in the adventitia of porcine vein grafts infected with a replication-deficient adenoviral vector at the time of surgery. In this same study, short-term expression of soluble VCAM-1 was documented after transfection of vein grafts.

The Dzau laboratory hypothesized that genetic engineering could alter the ability of the grafts to mount a hyperplastic response to acute injury while leaving intact their ability to respond to chronic hemodynamic stress via a hypertrophic response, such as that seen in arteries exposed to hypertension. This group used HVJ liposomes to deliver a combination of ASOs to cdc2/PCNA to rabbit veins at the time of grafting into the carotid artery and observed a greater than 90 percent inhibition of smooth muscle cell (SMC) proliferation during the first postoperative week[63] (Fig. 11-3).

This blockade of cell cycle progression resulted in the nearly complete inhibition of neointimal hyperplasia. Instead, the vein graft wall was shifted to an adaptive process of medial hypertrophy. Having redirected the genetically engineered grafts away from neointimal hyperplasia and toward medial hypertrophy as an adaptation to the arterial environment, the susceptibility of these ASO-treated grafts to accelerated atherogenesis was tested. Control ASO-treated and untreated grafts placed in cholesterol-fed rabbits developed significant foam cell lesions and plaque within 6 weeks after surgery. ASO-treated grafts that had remained free of neointima formation, however, resisted macrophage invasion and the development of macroscopic plaque. This inhibition of cell cycle progression is likely to have effects on the phenotypes of the vascular cells undergoing remodeling after vein grafting, and these changes are likely to affect the proatherogenic environment of the normal graft wall. For example, the endothelium of ASO-treated grafts retained more of its capacity to produce nitric oxide and resist monocyte adhesion in comparison with untreated or control ASO-treated grafts.[64]

## Gene Transfer and Vascular Remodeling

Molecular cardiovascular research has resulted in significant gains in the knowledge of disease processes at cellular and molecular levels and has led to the characterization of expressed genes in diseased blood vessels. These gene products play autocrine and/or paracrine roles in vascular pathophysiology.

Nabel et al.[65] overexpressed an expression vector encoding a secreted form of fibroblast growth factor 1 (FGF-1) in porcine arteries. FGF-1 expression was associated with intimal thickening of the transfected vessels together with neocapillary formation in the expanded intima. These findings suggest that FGF-1 induces intimal hyperplasia in the arterial wall in vivo and, through its ability to stimulate angiogenesis in the neointima, FGF-1 could stimulate neovascularization of atherosclerotic plaques. In the same porcine model, the overexpression of transforming growth factor $\beta$1 (TGF-$\beta$1) in normal arteries resulted in substantial production of extracellular matrix accompanied by intimal and medial hyperplasia.[65] These findings demonstrated that TGF-$\beta$1 differentially modulates extracellular matrix production and cellular proliferation in the arterial wall and plays a reparative role in response to arterial injury. The increased production of extracellular matrix that accompanied the intimal and medial hyperplasia was not observed following expression of other growth factor genes in the vessel wall, including genes for platelet-derived growth factor (PDGF-BB)[27,66] or the secreted form of FGF-1.[62] Porcine arteries transfected with human PDGF-BB demonstrated intimal hyperplasia with increased numbers of intimal smooth muscle cells. An increased deposition of procollagen, however, as seen in TGF-$\beta$1-transfected vessels, was not observed. By stimulating the formation of extracellular matrix, it is possible that TGF-$\beta$1 could promote healing following vascular injury, limiting the extensive cellular intimal hyperplasia observed with PDGF-BB.[66]

The pathogenesis of vascular diseases such as hypertension involves a process of vascular remodeling associated with increased vascular hypertrophy and activation of the local angiotensin system. Angiotensin II has been shown to stimulate the growth and proliferation of vascular smooth muscle as well as collagen biosynthesis in vitro. Its in vivo role has been inferred from experiments using angiotensin converting enzyme (ACE) inhibitors. Since these drugs produce hemodynamic effects, a direct role of local angiotensin in vascular remodeling was not clear. To study the local effects of angiotensin, Morishita et al.[67] overexpressed ACE within the vascular wall. Immunoreactive ACE activity was noted in medial vascular smooth muscle cells as well as in intimal endothelial cells. Vascular ACE activity was associated with increased DNA synthesis and vascular protein content via the local production and action of vascular angiotensin II without changes in systemic blood pressure. Parallel to these biochemical changes, medial thickening of ACE-transfected vessel segments was noted, without changes in luminal diameters, implying medial wall hypertrophy by local production of angiotensin II. In a subsequent study, Nakajima et al.[68] demonstrated that overexpression of the type 2 angiotensin II ($AT_2$) receptor in balloon-injured rat carotid arteries exerts an antiproliferative effect, counteracting the growth action of $AT_1$ receptors.

One approach to the treatment of vascular diseases that are characterized by excessive cell proliferation is to overexpress a gene that inhibits cellular proliferation. It is important that expression of the gene proceed during the time period when intimal cells undergo proliferation following vascular injury. This may vary between animal models, and it is likely that in humans, cell proliferation following angioplasty, stent placement, or bypass graft surgery may proceed over a longer period of time than in animal models. Nonetheless, several gene products have proven efficacious in appropriate animal models of vascular injury. Most of these approaches are based on arresting vascular cells in G1 or S phase of the cell cycle (Fig. 11-4). One approach is to express the herpes simplex virus thymidine kinase gene (*HSVtk*). *HSVtk* encodes for the enzyme thymidine kinase that phosphorylates the nucleoside analog ganciclovir or acyclovir into a metabolite that disrupts replication of DNA during S phase of the cell cycle. A by-product of this biochemical reaction is diffusible to adjacent cells, where it is incorporated in replicating cells, leading to inhibition of cell replication. This property is termed a *bystander effect* and allows for inhibition of replication in a greater number of cells than transfected. This model was established initially in a pig peripheral artery model of vascular injury, where intimal hyperplasia was decreased by 50 percent.[69] Subsequent investigations in the rat, rabbit, and a transplant model also demonstrated reductions in cell proliferation and lesion formation by about 50 percent.[70–73] This

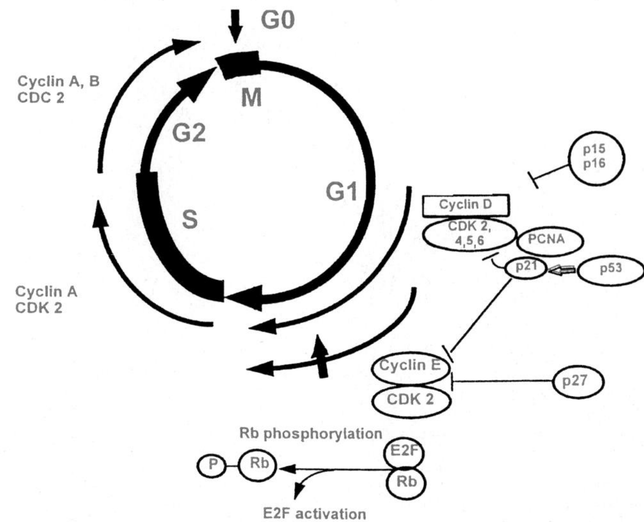


FIGURE 11-4 Regulation of the cell cycle. Progression through the G1 phase of the cell cycle is regulated by the assembly and phosphorylation of cyclins and cyclin-dependent kinases (CDKs). The cyclin-CDK complexes are inhibited by cyclin-dependent kinase inhibitors (CKIs), of which p21 and p27 are examples. These CKIs lead to G1 arrest. Inhibition of Rb phosphorylation, inactiviation of E2F, or inhibition of cyclin A and B also lead to disruption of DNA synthesis and inhibition of cell proliferation. (From Tanner et al.[112] With permission.)

approach is currently being investigated in a model of in-stent restenosis. Chang et al.[74] demonstrated that localized arterial infection with a replication-defective adenovirus encoding a nonphosphorylatable, constitutively active form of the retinoblastoma gene product at the time of angioplasty significantly reduced SMC proliferation and neointima formation in both the rat carotid and porcine femoral artery models of restenosis. The cyclin-dependent kinase inhibitors p21 and p27 that arrest smooth muscle cells in G1 phase of the cell cycle are also potent negative regulators of lesion formation after vascular injury.[75–78] Ras proteins are key transducers of mitogenic signals from the cell membrane to the nucleus. The local delivery of vectors expressing *ras* transdominant negative mutants, which interfere with the function of *ras,* reduced neointimal lesion formation in a rat carotid artery balloon-injury model.[79] To assess the effect of endothelial cell nitric oxide synthase (ecNOS) on vessel lesion formation, a DNA vector encoding ecNOS was expressed in a rat model of arterial injury[80] (Fig. 11-5). Four methods were used to verify ecNOS expression: transgene protein expression by Western blot, localization of enzyme expression by in situ histochemical staining, enzymatic activity of the transgene product, and vascular reactivity in response to the transgene. Overexpression of ecNOS led to vasorelaxation and 70 percent inhibition of neointima formation after balloon injury. This same approach has been investigated in a pig coronary model.[81] The loss of ecNOS may play a fundamental role in the pathogenesis of vascular diseases, including atherosclerosis. The overexpression of ecNOS may be useful for gene therapy of neointimal hyperplasia and associated local vasospasm after vascular injury.

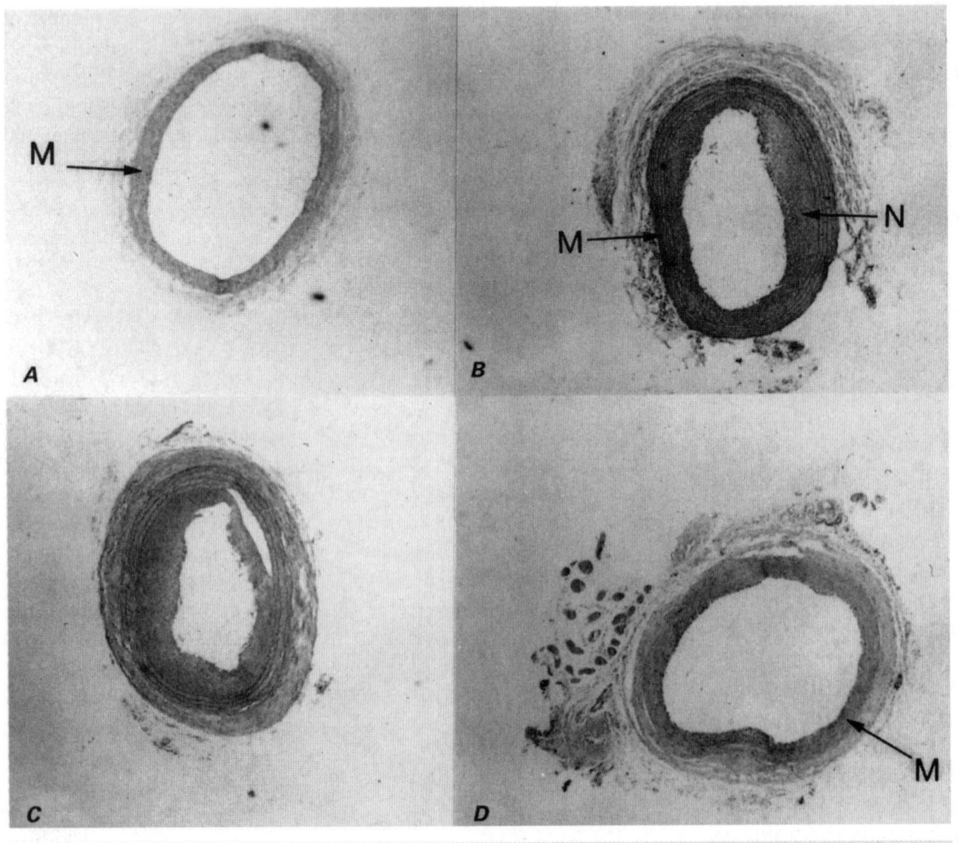


FIGURE 11-5 Inhibition of neointimal hyperplasia by in vivo gene transfer of endothelial cell nitric oxide synthase (ecNOS) in balloon-injured rat carotid arteries. *A.* Normal artery. *B.* Injured untransfected artery. *C.* Injured control vector-transfected artery. *D.* Injured ecNOS-transfected artery. M, media; N, neointima. (From von der Leyen et al.[80] With permission.)

## Angiogenesis

Angiogenic growth factors may be useful to augment collateral artery development in animal models of myocardial and hindlimb ischemia. Initial studies—using intramuscular injections of angiogenic proteins, including basic fibroblast growth factor (bFGF) and acidic fibroblast growth factor (aFGF) into the hindlimbs of rabbits with surgically induced ischemia—led to increased capillary densities and augmented blood flow.[82,83] These findings have been extended to gene-transfer approaches using vascular endothelial growth factor (VEGF). Following gene transfer of VEGF via a hydrogel balloon, increased numbers of capillary vessels were also observed in a rabbit model of hindlimb ischemia, and the improvement of resting and maximum flow achieved was comparable with that of a single administration of VEGF protein.[84] Intracoronary delivery of a recombinant adenovirus that encodes FGF-5 has been shown to induce collateral blood flow and restore myocardial function in a pig model of myocardial ischemia.[85] While these studies are encouraging, our understanding of the process by which VEGF, angiopoietin, and other angiogenic proteins lead to blood vessel formation and maturation is still incomplete.

# MYOCARDIAL GENE TRANSFER

Direct injection of DNA into myocardial tissue has been shown to be effective in local delivery of a transgene to the heart. Lin et al.[37] reported in vivo expression of β-galactosidase in cardiac myocytes for at least 4 weeks after direct injection into the left ventricle. Direct injections of a major histocompatibility complex gene (*MHC*) and the reporter gene *luciferase* under the control of an MHC promoter also resulted in the regulated expression of these genes.[38] Subsequent studies also showed increased gene expression after myocardial injection of adenoviral vectors.[10,13]

Healing and remodeling of the ventricle after myocardial infarction remain important clinical problems. Some candidate genes (e.g., those for TGF-β1 and myogenin) may enhance the healing and recovery of myocytes after injury associated with infarction. The induction of neovascularization or angiogenesis in ischemic myocardium after coronary artery occlusion using gene transfer may salvage myocardium at risk by enhancing blood supply to the ischemic areas. Indeed, intracardiac myoblast grafts stably transfected with an inducible TGF-β1 construct were associated with increased DNA synthesis in vascular endothelial cells, consistent with a sustained angiogenic response.[86] The success of intracardiac grafting with genetically modified cardiomyocytes depends on the ability of grafts to couple with host myocytes. Soonpaa et al.[87] demonstrated that fetal cardiomyocytes isolated from transgenic mice carrying a fusion protein of the cardiac $\alpha$-MHC promoter with a $\beta$-galactosidase reporter gene were connected to the host myocardium by nascent intercalated disks formed after grafting. Chronic heart failure is accompanied by a reduction in the number of myocardial $\beta$-adrenergic receptors and inotropic responsiveness. Cardiac-specific overexpression of a $\beta_2$-adrenergic receptor in a transgenic animal model with subsequent increased myocardial function suggests a potential gene-therapy approach to heart failure.[88]

## CLINICAL TRIALS

Cardiovascular diseases are excellent candidates for gene- and cell-based therapies. Arterial lesions are focal, facilitating delivery of vector and gene through a catheter and/or stent. Devices are being modified for delivery of recombinant genes directly into the myocardium, using an injection catheter inserted into the left ventricle. Short-term expression will likely be sufficient to treat the disease, avoiding systemic side effects. Clinical trials have gone forward in two areas: vascular proliferative diseases and angiogenesis. Investigators have identified a number of candidate therapeutic genes for vascular and myocardial gene therapy. In addition, since the 1995 review of gene therapy by the National Institutes of Health (NIH), there have been significant improvements in the basic science of gene vectors, enhancing their safety profile. Considerable efforts have now gone into the development of vascular and myocardial delivery catheters, including polymer-coated stents.

In a phase I/II randomized study, cell cycle blockade by ex vivo gene therapy of experimental vein grafts was accomplished with E2F, a dominant negative transcription decoy, which leads to G1 arrest and inhibition of cell proliferation.[89] The investigators hypothesized that this transcription decoy would inhibit the neointimal hyperplasia and subsequent accelerated atherosclerosis leading to the failure of human bypass grafts. This hypothesis was tested in a prospective randomized controlled trial to investigate the safety and biological efficacy of intraoperative gene therapy in patients receiving bypass vein grafts. Patients undergoing infrainguinal bypass grafting were randomized to decoy oligodeoxynucleotide (which binds to and inactivates E2F), scrambled oligodeoxynucleotides, or no treatment. Oligonucleotide was delivered to grafts intraoperatively by ex vivo pressure-mediated transfection. Since this was a phase I/II study, the primary endpoints were safety and inhibition of target cell cycle–regulatory genes and of DNA synthesis in the grafts. The investigators found that the E2F decoy treatment reduced proliferating–cell nuclear antigen and c-myc mRNA concentrations as well as cell proliferation indices. Twelve months later, there were fewer clinical complications in the E2F treatment group, defined as fewer graft occlusions, revisions, or severe lesions. The investigators concluded that the intraoperative transfection of human bypass vein grafts with E2F decoy oligodeoxynucleotide was not only safe and feasible but that it also achieved inhibition of cell cycle genes and cell replication.[89]

Angiogenic growth factors have been tested in phase I studies by gene transfer or with recombinant protein to promote development of supplemental collateral blood vessels around occluded or severely stenosed native arteries. The concept of therapeutic angiogenesis dates back almost 30 years to the pioneering work of Judah Folkman on neovascularization.[90] While many growth factors and cytokines have angiogenic activity, the two growth factors most widely studied in preclinical animal models and in human studies are vascular endothelial growth factor (VEGF) and fibroblast growth factor (FGF). Several phase I studies aimed at stimulating angiogenesis in the coronary and peripheral circulation have been conducted using VEGF or FGF gene transfer or recombinant protein. A trial of intra-arterial gene transfer of plasmid DNA encoding for human $VEGF_{165}$, coded onto an angioplasty balloon, reported the safe delivery of the vector/gene and indirect angiographic evidence of angiogenesis in the peripheral circulation.[91] Plasmid DNA coated onto an angioplasty balloon was mechanically delivered into an atherosclerotic lesion at the time of angioplasty in the peripheral superficial femoral artery with the goal of stimulating angiogenesis distal to the angioplasty site. This delivery method was not optimal, since the gene delivery was not at the site of ischemic tissue. An improved approach is the direct injection of vectors into peripheral skeletal muscle near the site of the arterial lesion. This approach has been tested with two trials of VEGF gene therapy. In a phase I study, 400 $\mu$g of plasmid DNA encoding $VEGF_{165}$ was injected intramuscularly in patients with severe peripheral vascular disease.[92] Adverse events related to the vector or gene were not observed. Some indices of clinical efficacy were measured, including increased pain-free walking time and increased ankle-brachial index in some patients—an indirect measure of improved circulation. Subsequent clinical trials of $VEGF_{165}$ to stimulate angiogenesis in peripheral vascular disease in patients with rest pain or ischemic foot ulcers have noted some lower extremity edema in one-third of patients and indirect evidence of clinical improvement in 60 to 70 percent of patients.[93] These phase I studies, again, are promising and provide the safety basis for proceeding with phase II/III dose escalation and efficacy trials. More recently, a phase I study of $VEGF_{121}$, delivered by adenoviral vectors into peripheral skeletal muscle, reported improvement of endothelial cell function in treated patients, suggesting a benefit to peripheral arterial circulation.[94] Phase I clinical trials of adenoviral delivery of FGF5 to the coronary circulation have also demonstrated safety and minimal toxicity.[95]

Several phase I studies have been conducted in patients with severe myocardial ischemia to stimulate coronary angiogenesis. Vectors encoding VEGF have been delivered by a transepicardial approach at the time of bypass surgery or directly into the left ventricle or transendocardially by a catheter.[96,97] Other phase I studies have been conducted in patients with inoperable coronary artery disease, not suitable for revascularization (PTCA or CABG); in these, plasmid $VEGF_{165}$ was administered by direct injection via a limited anterior thoracotomy.[98] This approach was shown to be safe, and some measures of improved symptoms—an increase in exercise time and reduced ischemia on myocardial perfusion scanning—were obtained. In another study, adenoviral vectors encoding $VEGF_{121}$ were directly injected into the myocardium of patients undergoing coronary artery bypass surgery.[96] The adenoviral vectors were well tolerated. Symptoms and exercise duration improved, while myocardial perfusion studies were not changed in this phase I study. In a small pilot phase I study of plasmid VEGF2 delivered percutaneously by a left ventricular injection catheter, the plasmid DNA was delivered safely[99]; on the basis of these findings, a phase II/III study has been initiated.

In summary, these phase I studies of angiogenesis in the peripheral and coronary circulation have demonstrated that delivery of plasmid or adenoviral vectors encoding VEGF by direct injection or through a catheter have been safe and well tolerated.[100] Indirect measures of improved perfusion and a reduction in symptoms in this small number of patients are encouraging and provide the impetus for phase II/III studies, which will be required to determine optimal dosing and clinical efficacy.[101]

## STEM CELL BIOLOGY

Advances in stem cell biology are progressing at a rapid pace and are providing a new platform of technologies for the introduction of recombinant genes into human tissues. Both embryonic and adult stem cells are under study and characterization (Table 11-2). This field is still in early stages, and considerable research is required to fully elucidate the potential risks and benefits of these therapies prior to wide-scale implementation of human trials (reviewed in Refs. 102 and 103).

Embryonic stem (ES) cells are pluripotent cells derived from the inner cell mass of the blastocyst that can be propagated indefinitely in an undifferentiated state. ES cells differentiate to all cell lineages in vivo and differentiate into many cell types in vitro. Although ES cells have been isolated from humans, their use in research as well as therapeutics is encumbered by ethical considerations. Current research focuses on characterization of the growth properties of murine and human ES cells; the factors that lead to differentiation of ES cells into different cell types, such as cardiac myocytes, neurons and hepatocytes; and avoidance of undesired outcomes of ES cell growth in culture, like teratomas.

Adult stem cells exist for most tissues, including hematopoietic, neural, gastrointestinal, epidermal, hepatic, and mesenchymal stem cells. Compared with ES cells, tissue-specific stem cells have less self-renewal ability, and although they differentiate into multiple lineages, they are not pluripotent. Until recently, it was thought that tissue-specific stem cells could differentiate only into cells of the tissue of origin; however, recent studies suggest that tissue-specific stem cells can differentiate into lineages other than the tissue of origin. After transplantation of bone marrow or enriched hematopoietic stem cells, skeletal myoblasts, cardiac myoblasts, endothelium, hepatic epithelium, lung, gut and skin epithelia, and neuroectodermal cells of donor origin have been detected. In addition, a multipotent adult progenitor cell (MAPC) has been identified within human bone marrow mesenchymal stem cell cultures that differentiates into mesenchymal, endothelial, and endodermal lineages.[104]

In the vasculature, endothelial progenitor cells (EPCs) functionally contribute to revascularization of ischemic tissues and may be a source for therapeutic angiogenic cell transplantation.[105,106] Circulating endothelial progenitor cells derived from bone marrow have a role on ongoing endothelial repair, and impaired mobilization or depletion of these cells, as occurs in patients with cardiovascular risk factors, contributes to endothelial cell dysfunction and cardiovascular disease progression.[107] Hematopoietic stem cells differentiate into mesenchymal cells that give rise to smooth muscle cells during arterial remodeling in postangioplasty restenosis, graft vasculopathy, and hyperlipidemia-induced atherosclerosis.[108,109] The extent to which mobilized bone marrow cells repair the infarcted heart and improve function and survival is being investigated.[110]

TABLE 11-2 Properties of Human Adult and Embryonic Stem Cells

| | Human Adult | Human Embryonic |
|---|---|---|
| Pluripotent | − | + |
| Self-renewal | +/− | + |
| Rejection | + | − |
| Teratomas | − | + |

## SUMMARY AND FUTURE DIRECTIONS

Since the 1980s, there has been remarkable progress in the design of vectors, the enhancement of gene expression by optimizing regulatory units, the development of animal models, and the translation of basic science studies into clinical applications. Despite this progress, there are still significant hurdles and challenges that must be met if the promise of gene therapy is to be fulfilled. There is a persistent need for improved vectors that increase transgene expression and program expression specifically to cardiovascular tissues. Cell-specific promoters are being studied. Improved catheters are needed to deliver vectors and transgenes in vascular and myocardial tissues.[94] A better understanding of the pathways leading to cardiovascular diseases will permit more careful delineation of candidate target genes. There is no doubt, however, that enthusiasm and optimism that this technology can lead to successful cardiovascular therapies remain high.

### References


1. Boris-Lawrie K, Temin HM. The retroviral vector: Replication cycle and safety considerations for retrovirus-mediated gene therapy. *Ann NY Acad Sci* 1994;716:59–70.
2. Danos O, Mulligan RC. Expression of retroviral trans-acting functions from complementary crippled genomes: A system for helper free packaging of retroviral vectors. *J Cell Biochem* 1988;12:172–178.
3. Nabel EG, Plautz G, Boyce FM, et al. Recombinant gene expression in vivo within endothelial cells of the arterial wall. *Science* 1989;244: 1342–1344.
4. Nabel EG, Plautz G, Nabel GJ. Site-specific gene expression in vivo by direct gene transfer into the arterial wall. *Science* 1990;249:1285–1288.
5. Wilson JM, Birinyi LK, Salomon RN, et al. Implantation of vascular grafts lined with genetically modified endothelial cells. *Science* 1989;244:1344–1346.
6. Horwitz M. The adenoviruses. In: Fields B, Knipe D, eds. *Virology*. New York: Raven Press; 1990:1723–1742.
7. Wilson JM. Adenoviruses as gene-delivery vehicles. *N Engl J Med* 1996;334:1185–1187.
8. Wickman TJ, Mathias P, Cheresh DA, et al. Integrins $\alpha v\beta 3$ and $\alpha v\beta 5$ promote adenovirus internalization but not virus attachment. *Cell* 1983;73:309–319.
9. Guzman RJ, Lemarchand P, Crystal RG, et al. Efficient and selective adenovirus-mediated gene transfer into vascular neointima. *Circulation* 1993;88:2838–2848.
10. Kass-Eisler A, Falck-Pedersen E, Alvira M, et al. Quantitative determination of adenovirus-mediated gene delivery to rat cardiac myocytes in vitro and in vivo. *Proc Natl Acad Sci USA* 1993;90: 11,498–11,502.
11. Barr J, Kalynych AM, Tripathy SK, et al. Efficient catheter-mediated gene transfer into the heart using replication-defective adenovirus. *Gene Ther* 1994;1:51–58.
12. Lemarchand P, Jones M, Yamada I, et al. In vivo gene transfer and expression in normal uninjured blood vessels using replication-deficient recombinant adenovirus vectors. *Circ Res* 1993;72:1132–1138.
13. Guzman RJ, Lemarchand P, Crystal RG, et al. Efficient gene transfer into myocardium by direct injection of adenovirus vectors. *Circ Res* 1993;73:1202–1207.
14. Tripathy SK, Goldwasser E, Lu MM, et al. Stable delivery of physiological levels of recombinant erythropoietin to the systemic circulation by intramuscular injection of replication-defective adenovirus. *Proc Natl Acad Sci USA* 1994;91:11,557–11,561.
15. Tripathy SK, Black HB, Goldwasser E, et al. Immune responses to transgene-encoded proteins limit the stability of gene expression after injection of replication-defective adenovirus vectors. *Nat Med* 1996;2: 545–550.

16. Yang Y, Ertl J, Wilson JM. MHC class 1-restricted cytotoxic T lymphocytes to viral antigens destroy hepatocytes in mice infected with E1-deleted recombinant adenoviruses. *Immunity* 1994;1:433–442.
17. Yang Y, Li Q, Ertl HC, et al. Cellular immunity to viral antigens limits E1-deleted adenoviruses for gene therapy. *Proc Natl Acad Sci USA* 1994;91:4407–4411.
18. Hartigan-O'Connor D, Amalfitano A, Chamberlain JS. Improved production of gutted adenovirus in cells expressing adenovirus preterminal protein and DNA polymerase. *J Virol* 1999;73:7835–7841.
19. Muzyczka N. Use of adeno-associated virus as a general transduction vector for mammalian cells. *Curr Top Microbiol Immunol* 1992;158: 97–129.
20. Rolling F, Samulski RJ. AAV as a viral vector for human gene therapy: Generation of recombinant virus. *Mol Biotechnol* 1995;3:9–15.
21. Kotin R, Linden R, Berns K. Characterization of a preferred site on human chromosome 19q for integration of adeno-associated virus DNA by nonhomologous recombination. *EMBO J* 1992;11:5071–5078.
22. Herzog RW, Yang EY, Couto LB, et al. Long-term correction of canine hemophilia B by gene transfer of blood coagulation factor IX mediated by adeno-associated viral vector. *Nat Med* 1999;5(1):56–63.
23. Svensson EC, Marshall DJ, Woodard K, et al. Efficient and stable transduction of cardiomyocytes after intramyocardial injection or intracoronary perfusion with recombinant adeno-associated virus vectors. *Circulation* 1999;99:201–205.
24. Felgner PL, Gader TR, Holm M, et al. Lipofectin: A highly efficient, lipid mediated DNA-transfection procedure. *Proc Natl Acad Sci USA* 1987;84:7413–7417.
25. Bennett CF, Chiang MY, Chan H, et al. Cationic lipids improve antisense oligonucleotide uptake and prevent degradation in cultured cells and in human serum. *Mol Pharmacol* 1992;41:1023–1033.
26. Zabner J, Fasbender AJ, Moninger T, et al. Cellular and molecular barriers to gene transfer by a cationic lipid. *J Biol Chem* 1995;270: 189–197.
27. Nabel EG, Yang Z, Liptay S, et al. Recombinant platelet-derived growth factor B gene expression in porcine arteries induces intimal hyperplasia in vivo. *J Clin Invest* 1993;91:1822–1829.
28. Nabel EG, Yang Z, Plautz G, et al. Recombinant fibroblast growth factor-1 promotes intimal hyperplasia and angiogenesis in arteries in vivo. *Nature* 1993;362:844–846.
29. Leclerc G, Gal D, Takeshita S, et al. Percutaneous arterial gene transfer in a rabbit model: Efficiency in normal and balloon-dilated atherosclerotic arteries. *J Clin Invest* 1992;90:936–944.
30. Takeshita S, Gal D, Leclerc G, et al. Increased gene expression after liposome-mediated arterial gene transfer associated with intimal smooth muscle cell proliferation. *J Clin Invest* 1994;93:652–661.
31. Kaneda Y, Iwai K, Uchida T. Increased expression of DNA cointroduced with nuclear protein in adult rat liver. *Science* 1989;243:375–378.
32. Okada Y, Koseki I, Kim J, et al. Modification of cell membranes with viral envelopes during fusion of cells with HVJ (Sendai virus). *Exp Cell Res* 1975;93:368–378.
33. Isaka Y, Fujiwara Y, Ueda N, et al. Glomerulosclerosis induced by in vivo transfection of transforming growth factor-$\beta$ or platelet-derived growth factor gene into the rat kidney. *J Clin Invest* 1993;92:2597–2601.
34. Morishita R, Gibbons GH, Ellison KE, et al. Single intraluminal delivery of antisense cdc2 kinase and proliferating-cell nuclear antigen oligonucleotides results in chronic inhibition of neointimal hyperplasia. *Proc Natl Acad Sci USA* 1993;90:8474–8478.
35. Morishita R, Gibbons GH, Ellison KE, et al. Intimal hyperplasia after vascular injury is inhibited by antisense cdk2 kinase oligonucleotides. *J Clin Invest* 1994;93:1458–1464.
36. Wolff J, Malone R, Williams P, et al. Direct gene transfer into mouse muscle in vivo. *Science* 1990;247:1465–1468.
37. Lin H, Parmacek MS, Morle G, et al. Expression of recombinant gene in myocardium in vivo after direct injection of DNA. *Circulation* 1990;82:2217–2221.
38. Kitsis RN, Buttrick PM, McNally EM, et al. Hormonal modulation of a gene injected into rat heart in vivo. *Proc Natl Acad Sci USA* 1991; 88:4138–4142.
39. Stein CA, Cheng YC. Antisense oligonucleotides as therapeutic agents: Is the bullet really magical? *Science* 1993;261:1004–1012.
40. Cohen JS. Oligonucleotide therapeutics. *Trends Biotechnol* 1992; 10:87–91.
41. Bielinska A, Schivdasani RA, Zhang L, et al. Regulation of gene expression with double-stranded phosphothiolate oligonucleotides. *Science* 1990;250:997–1000.
42. Epstein SE, Speir E, Finkel T. Do antisense approaches to the problem of restenosis make sense? *Circulation* 1993;88:1351–1353.
43. Krieg AM, Yi A, Matson S, et al. CpG motifs in bacterial DNA trigger direct B-cell activation. *Nature* 1995;374:546–549.
44. Sullenger BA, Gallardo HF, Ungers GE, et al. Overexpression of TAR sequences renders cells resistant to human immunodeficiency virus replication. *Cell* 1990;63:601–608.
45. Morishita R, Gibbons GH, Horiuchi M, et al. A novel molecular strategy using cis element "decoy" of E2F binding site inhibits smooth muscle proliferation in vivo. *Proc Natl Acad Sci USA* 1995;92: 5855–5859.
46. Plautz G, Nabel EG, Nabel GJ. Introduction of vascular smooth muscle cells expressing recombinant genes in vivo. *Circulation* 1991; 83:578–583.
47. Lynch CM, Clowes MM, Osborne RA, et al. Long-term expression of human adenosine deaminase in vascular smooth muscle cells of rats: A model for gene therapy. *Proc Natl Acad Sci USA* 1992;89:1138–1142.
48. Dichek DA, Neville RF, Zwiebel JA, et al. Seeding of intravascular stents with genetically engineered endothelial cells. *Circulation* 1989; 80:1347–1353.
49. Chen S, Wilson JM, Muller DWM. Adenovirus-mediated gene transfer of soluble vascular cell adhesion molecule to porcine interposition vein grafts. *Circulation* 1994;89:1922–1928.
50. Yao SN, Smith KJ, Kurachi K. Primary myoblast-mediated gene transfer: Persistent expression of human factor IX in mice. *Gene Ther* 1994;1:99–107.
51. Barr E, Leiden JM. Systemic delivery of recombinant proteins by genetically modified myoblasts. *Science* 1991;254:1507–1509.
52. Dhawan J, Pan LC, Pavlath GK, et al. Systemic delivery of human growth hormone by injection of genetically engineered myoblasts. *Science* 1991;254:1509–1512.
53. Hamamori Y, Samal B, Tian J, et al. Myoblast transfer of human erythropoietin gene in a mouse model of renal failure. *J Clin Invest* 1995;95:1808–1813.
54. Barr E, Leiden JM. Somatic gene therapy for cardiovascular diseases: Recent advances. *Trends Cardiovasc Med* 1994;4:57–63.
55. Nabel EG. Gene therapy for cardiovascular disease. *Circulation* 1995;91:541–548.
56. Ooboshi H, Welsh MJ, Rios CD, et al. Adenovirus-mediated gene transfer in vivo to cerebral blood vessels and perivascular tissue. *Circ Res* 1995;77:7–13.
57. Muller DW, Gordon D, San H, et al. Catheter-mediated pulmonary vascular gene transfer and expression. *Circ Res* 1994;75: 1039–1049.
58. Crystal RG. Transfer of genes to humans: Early lessons and obstacles to success. *Science* 1995;270:404–410.
59. Simons M, Edelman ER, DeKeyser JL, et al. Antisense c-*myb* oligonucleotides inhibit intimal arterial smooth muscle cell accumulation in vivo. *Nature* 1992;359:67–70.
60. Bennett MR, Anglin S, McEwan JR, et al. Inhibition of vascular smooth muscle cell proliferation in vitro and in vivo by c-*myc* antisense oligonucleotides. *J Clin Invest* 1994;93:820–828.
61. Shi Y, Fard A, Galeo A, et al. Transcatheter delivery of c-*myc* antisense oligomers reduces neointimal formation in a porcine model of coronary artery balloon injury. *Circulation* 1994;90:944–951.
62. Simons M, Edelman ER, Rosenberg RD. Antisense proliferating cell nuclear antigen oligonucleotides inhibit intimal hyperplasia in a rat carotid artery injury model. *J Clin Invest* 1994;93:2351–2356.
63. Mann MJ, Gibbons GH, Kernoff RS, et al. Genetic engineering of vein grafts resistant to atherosclerosis. *Proc Natl Acad Sci USA* 1995; 92:4502–4506.

64. Mann MJ, Gibbons GH, Tsao PS, et al. Cell cycle inhibition leads to preservation of endothelial function in genetically engineered vein grafts. *J Clin Invest* 1997;99:1295–1301.
65. Nabel EG, Shum L, Pompili VJ, et al. Direct transfer of transforming growth factor $\beta1$ gene into arteries stimulates fibrocellular hyperplasia. *Proc Natl Acad Sci USA* 1993;90:10,559–10,563.
66. Pompili VJ, Gordon D, San H, et al. Expression and function of a recombinant PDGF B gene in porcine arteries. *Arterioscler Thromb Vasc Biol* 1995;15:2254–2264.
67. Morishita R, Gibbons GH, Ellison KE, et al. Evidence for direct local effect of angiotensin in vascular hypertrophy: In vivo gene transfer of angiotensin converting enzyme. *J Clin Invest* 1994;94:978–984.
68. Nakajima M, Hutchinson HG, Fujinaga M, et al. The angiotensin II type 2 (AT2) receptor antagonizes the growth effects of the AT1 receptor: Gain-of-function study using gene transfer. *Proc Natl Acad Sci USA* 1995;92:10,663–10,667.
69. Ohno T, Gordon D, San H, et al. Gene therapy for vascular smooth muscle cell proliferation after arterial injury. *Science* 1994;265:781–784.
70. Chang MW, Ohno T, Gordon D, et al. Adenovirus-mediated transfer of the herpes simplex virus thymidine kinase gene inhibits vascular smooth muscle cell proliferation and neointima formation following balloon angioplasty. *Mol Med* 1995;1:172–181.
71. Guzman RJ, Hirschowitz EA, Brody SL, et al. In vivo suppression of injury-induced vascular smooth muscle cell accumulation using adenovirus-mediated transfer of the herpes simplex virus thymidine kinase gene. *Proc Natl Acad Sci USA* 1994;10:732–736.
72. Simari R, San H, Rekhter M, et al. Regulation of cellular proliferation and intimal formation following balloon injury in atherosclerotic rabbit arteries. *J Clin Invest* 1996;98:225–235.
73. Rekhter MD, Shah N, Simari RD, et al. Graft permeabilization facilitates gene therapy of transplant atherosclerosis in a rabbit model. *Circulation* 1998;98:1335–1341.
74. Chang MW, Barr E, Seltzer J, et al. Cytostatic gene therapy for vascular proliferative disorders with a constitutively active form of the retinoblastoma gene product. *Science* 1995;267:518–522.
75. Chang MW, Barr E, Lu MM, et al. Adenovirus-mediated overexpression of the cyclin/cyclin-dependent kinase inhibitor, p21 inhibits vascular smooth muscle cell proliferation and neointima formation in the rat carotid artery model of balloon angioplasty. *J Clin Invest* 1995;96:2260–2268.
76. Yang Z, Simari R, Perkins N, et al. Role of the p21 cyclin-dependent kinase inhibitor in limiting intimal cell proliferation in response to arterial injury. *Proc Natl Acad Sci USA* 1996;93:1905–1910.
77. Chen D, Krasinski K, Sylvester A, et al. Down regulation of cyclin-dependent kinase 2 activity and cyclin A promoter activity in vascular smooth muscle cells by p27(KIP1), an inhibitor of neointima formation in the rat carotid artery. *J Clin Invest* 1997;99:2334–2341.
78. Tanner FC, Boehm M, Akyurek LM, et al. Differential effects of the cyclin-dependent kinase inhibitors p27(Kip1), p21(Cip1), and p16(Ink4) on vascular smooth muscle cell proliferation. *Circulation* 2000;101: 2022–2025.
79. Indolfi C, Avvedimento EV, Rapacciuolo A, et al. Inhibition of cellular *ras* prevents smooth muscle cell proliferation after vascular injury in vivo. *Nat Med* 1995;1:541–545.
80. von der Leyen HE, Gibbons GH, Morishita R, et al. Gene therapy inhibiting neointimal vascular lesion: In vivo gene transfer of endothelial-cell nitric oxide synthase gene. *Proc Natl Acad Sci USA* 1995;92:1137–1141.
81. Varenne O, Pislaru S, Gillijns H, et al. Local adenovirus-mediated transfer of human endothelial nitric oxide synthase reduces luminal narrowing after coronary angioplasty in pigs. *Circulation* 1998;98: 919–926.
82. Pu LQ, Sniderman AD, Brassard R, et al. Enhanced revascularization of the ischemic limb by means of angiogenic therapy. *Circulation* 1993;88:208–215.
83. Unger EF, Banai S, Shou M, et al. Basic fibroblast growth factor enhances myocardial collateral flow in a canine model. *Am J Physiol* 1994;266:H1588–H1595.
84. Takeshita S, Weir L, Chen D, et al. Therapeutic antiogenesis following arterial gene transfer of vascular endothelial growth factor in a rabbit model of hindlimb ischemia. *Biochem Biophys Res Commun* 1996;227:628–635.
85. Giordano FJ, Ping P, McKirnan MD, et al. Intracoronary gene transfer of fibroblast growth factor-5 increases blood flow and contractile function in an ischemic region of the heart. *Nat Med* 1996;2:534–539.
86. Koh GY, Kim S, Klug MG, et al. Targeted expression of transforming growth factor-$\beta1$ in intracardiac grafts promotes vascular endothelial cell DNA synthesis. *J Clin Invest* 1995;95:114–121.
87. Soonpaa MH, Koh GY, Klug MG, et al. Formation of nascent intercalated disks between grafted fetal cardiomyocytes and host myocardium. *Science* 1994;264:98–101.
88. Milano CA, Allen LF, Rockman HA, et al. Enhanced myocardial function in transgenic mice overexpressing the $\beta_2$-adrenergic receptor. *Science* 1994;264:582–586.
89. Mann MJ, Whittemore AD, Donaldson MC, et al. Ex-vivo gene therapy of human vascular bypass grafts with E2F decoy: The PREVENT single-centre, randomised, controlled trial. *Lancet* 1999; 354:1493–1498.
90. Folkman J. Addressing tumor blood vessels. *Nat Biotechnol* 1997; 15:510–512.
91. Isner JM, Pieczek A, Schainfeld R, et al. Clinical evidence of angiogenesis following arterial gene transfer of phVEGF$_{165}$. *Lancet* 1996;348:370–374.
92. Baumgartner I, Pieczek A, Manor O, et al. Constitutive expression of phVEGF$_{165}$ following intramuscular gene transfer promotes collateral vessel development in patients with critical limb ischemia. *Circulation* 1998;97:1114–1123.
93. Baumgartner I, Rauh G, Pieczek A, et al. Lower-extremity edema associated with gene transfer of naked DNA vascular endothelial growth factor. *Ann Intern Med* 2000;132:880–884.
94. Rajagopalan S, Shah M, Luciano A, et al. Adenovirus-mediated gene transfer of VEGF(121) improves lower-extremity endothelial function and flow reserve. *Circulation* 2001;104:753–755.
95. Grines CL, Watkins MW, Helmer G, et al. Angiogenic gene therapy (AGENT) trial in patients with stable angina pectoris. *Circulation* 2002;105:1291–1297.
96. Rosengart TK, Lee LY, Patel SR, et al. Six-month assessment of a phase I trial of angiogenic gene therapy for the treatment of coronary artery disease using direct intramyocardial administration of an adenovirus vector expressing the VEGF$_{121}$ cDNA. *Ann Surg* 1999;230: 466–472.
97. Vale PR, Losordo DW, Milliken CE, et al. Randomized, single-blind, placebo-controlled pilot study of catheter-based myocardial gene transfer for therapeutic angiogenesis using left ventricular electromechanical mapping in patients with chronic myocardial ischemia. *Circulation* 2001;103:2138–2143.
98. Losordo DW, Vale PR, Symes J, et al. Gene therapy for myocardial angiogenesis: Initial clinical results with direct myocardial injection of phVEGF$_{165}$ as sole therapy for myocardial ischemia. *Circulation* 1998;98:2800–2804.
99. Vale PR, Losordo DW, Milliken CE, et al. Randomized, single-blind, placebo-controlled pilot study of catheter-based myocardial gene transfer for therapeutic angiogenesis using left ventricular electromechanical mapping in patients with chronic myocardial ischemia. *Circulation* 2001;103:2138–2143.
100. Baumgartner I, Isner JM. Somatic gene therapy in the cardiovascular system. *Annu Rev Physiol* 2001;63:427–450.
101. Laitinen M, Hartikainen J, Hiltunen MO, et al. Catheter-mediated vascular endothelial growth factor gene transfer to human coronary arteries after angioplasty. *Hum Gene Ther* 2000;11:263–270.
102. Weissman IL. Stem cells—Scientific, medical and political issues. *N Engl J Med* 2002;346:1576–1579.
103. Blau HM, Brazelton TR, Weimann JM. The evolving concept of a stem cell: Entity or function? *Cell* 2001;105:829–841.
104. Jiang Y, Jahagirdar BN, Reinhardt RL, et al. Pluripotency of mesenchymal stem cells derived from adult marrow. *Nature* 2002;418:41–49.

105. Nabel EG. Stem cells combined with gene transfer for therapeutic angiogenesis. *Circulation* 2002;105:672–674.
106. Luttun, A, Carmeliet G, Carmeliet P. Vascular progenitors: From biology to treatment. *Trends Cardiovasc Med* 2002;12:88–96.
107. Hill JM, Zalos G, Halcox JPJ, et al. Circulating endothelial progenitor cells, vascular function, and cardiovascular risk. *N Engl J Med* 2003; 348:593–600.
108. Sata M, Saiura A, Kunisato A, et al. Hematopoietic stem cells differentiate into vascular cells that participate in the pathogenesis of atherosclerosis. *Nat Med* 2002;4:403–409.
109. Boehm M, True AL, San H, et al. Deletion of the $p27^{Kip1}$ and $p21^{Cip1}$ loci accelerates cellular proliferation and impairs arterial wound repair. *Circulation* 2001;104:1553.
110. Orlic D, Kajstura J, Chimenti S, et al. Mobilized bone marrow cells repair the infarcted heart, improving function and survival. *Proc Natl Acad Sci USA* 2001;98:344–349.
111. Nabel EG. Gene therapy for cardiovascular diseases. *J Nucl Cardiol* 1999;6:69–75.
112. Tanner FC, Yang ZY, Simari RD, et al. Gene transfer and vascular remodeling. In: LaFont A, Topol E, eds. *Arterial Remodeling*. Boston: Kluwer; 1997:549–556.

PART TWO

# EVALUATION OF THE PATIENT

CHAPTER 12

# THE HISTORY, PHYSICAL EXAMINATION, AND CARDIAC AUSCULTATION

Robert A. O'Rourke / Mark E. Silverman / James A. Shaver



In the assessment of patients with definite or suspected heart disease, relevant information can be acquired from the history, physical examination, chest roentgenogram, electrocardiogram, and other routine laboratory tests. These data, when integrated properly, facilitate an accurate diagnosis and appropriate decisions regarding therapy in many patients. When more information is necessary, additional, more expensive noninvasive cardiac tests such as echocardiography or radionuclide studies are often indicated. In some patients, the general assessment indicates the need for cardiac catheterization and contrast angiography with or without additional noninvasive cardiac testing. For example, the proper approach to certain patients with symptomatic coronary artery disease may include both coronary arteriography and cardiac catheterization (anatomy and hemodynamics) as well as myocardial perfusion imaging with thallium or technetium sestamibi (extent of inducible ischemia).

*Not all patients need every test;* the skillful use of low-technology approaches, including the history and general examination, may preclude the need for additional testing or may indicate which of a variety of available sophisticated tests should be selected for a particular patient. This chapter is divided into three sections. The first concerns the proper application of the history and its use to delineate the differential diagnosis in patients who present with certain common cardiovascular symptoms. The second details the essential components of the *physical examination* and their usefulness in establishing a likely diagnosis when specific abnormal findings are detected. Finally, the third section focuses on cardiac auscultation.

## THE HISTORY

### Components of Accurate History Taking

A carefully obtained history is the cornerstone for evaluating a patient with known or suspected cardiac disease.[1,2] A deliberate, compassionate interview forms the basis for a patient-physician relationship that may continue indefinitely. Unfortunately, the interview may result in adversarial roles for physician and patient if the interviewer appears hurried, shows impatience, fails to establish eye contact, seems to treat dreaded diseases casually, or appears to be unsympathetic.[2] When the medical interview is unsatisfactory due to poor communication and lack of rapport, inaccurate information will often be obtained.[2] Also, important facts not revealed during a meticulous initial history are usually not detected later, since both the patient and physician become focused on high-technology studies and more aggressive therapeutic interventions.[1]

The patient's chief complaint, which requires further elaboration and investigation, may not identify his or her most serious problem. Therefore symptoms other than the patient's chief complaint must be defined.[2] The interviewer should note all existing symptoms and establish a present illness for each of these.[2]

A medical questionnaire given to the patient well in advance of the interview is useful and may record important data more accurately because of the time thus made available to reflect and check details.[2] Abnormalities indicated on the questionnaire should be defined more completely during the interview.[2]

A proper interpretation of the past history is important; the physician should not accept a past event as a fact when the evidence is not well established. Information obtained from family members about the patient's symptoms and his or her response to the illness is extremely important.[2]

Serious heart disease can occur in patients with mild or no symptoms. The physician must determine whether or not the history obtained is sufficient to support a decision-making process about the patient.[2] While many patients with severe heart disease have no symptoms, others have many symptoms associated with minor or no disease.

Some patients deny symptoms because they cannot accept the reality of the situation, whereas others may purposely withhold information so as not to jeopardize their jobs.[2] Some patients may overstate their symptoms for personal gain. Elderly patients, sedentary patients, and those with other illnesses may have no symptoms because they are not physically active enough to induce them.[2]

### Past and Family History

The past history may provide important clues to the presence of cardiovascular disease. A definite history of rheumatic fever may be useful in defining the cause of a heart murmur (Chap. 65), whereas a negative history does not exclude it.[2] A history of hypertension in a family member increases the likelihood that the patient has essential hypertension.[2] Previous trauma may be the cause of constrictive pericarditis, a thoracic aortic aneurysm, an arteriovenous fistula, and other types of cardiac lesions. A detailed history of the use of medications, addicting drugs, and alcohol, each of which may cause heart disease, is essential. A past history of pulmonary embolism, thrombophlebitis, or systemic embolism should be ascertained.

A history of dental work, some other diagnostic or therapeutic procedure, or recent infection suggests infective endocarditis in a patient with valvular heart disease. Patients often give a history of having had a "heart attack" that, in fact, may have been an episode of unstable angina, heart failure, or arrhythmia. The "heart attack" history often becomes "myocardial infarction" in the patient's medical record unless more information is obtained or documentation of the event is reviewed.[1]

*Many patients are referred who have had several catheterizations, percutaneous coronary interventions, and one or more coronary bypass operations in addition to multiple noninvasive tests.* A thorough and often time-consuming review of records from other institutions, operative notes, cineangiographic films, and noninvasive studies will often provide an accurate assessment of the patient's current status without the *unnecessary repetition* of expensive and potentially risky procedures.[1]

Past and present therapeutic regimens must be reviewed carefully. Various treatment programs have often been inappropriate or suboptimal. Drugs used for the treatment of cardiovascular diseases have potential side effects that can produce both cardiovascular and noncardiovascular symptoms (Chap. 90).

Multiple risk factors for developing coronary heart disease (CHD) have been identified, including age, male sex, hypertension, hypercholesterolemia, a low level of high-density lipoprotein (HDL) cholesterol, cigarette smoking, diabetes, and a family history of premature atherosclerosis (Chap. 43).

Information from previous health evaluations should be sought. Patients have often been examined for military service, athletics, or insurance, and they may have been told of a heart murmur or hypertension on those occasions[2] or are rejected for medical insurance or military service. Many patients have never had a careful examination of the cardiovascular system.

The increasing hemodynamic burden of pregnancy may cause an otherwise marginally compensated cardiac patient to become symptomatic (Chap. 92). Specific inquiry should be made about heart failure, edema, dyspnea, or prescribed prolonged periods of bed rest during pregnancy.[1] Many normal women have had a murmur detected during pregnancy. A history of illicit parenteral drug use should raise the suspicion of infective endocarditis, especially in a febrile patient (Chap. 81). Cocaine can cause coronary artery vasospasm and also raise myocardial oxygen demand by increasing heart rate and blood pressure (BP). Angina, myocardial infarction, and sudden cardiac death after cocaine use have been well documented (Chap. 90).

A history of moderate to excessive alcohol consumption, an enlarged heart on a prior chest roentgenogram, periods of rapid weight gain or loss, and other illnesses may provide important information.[1]

A family history of congenital heart disease indicates a higher risk of a congenital heart lesion (Chap. 73). The patient's mother may give a history of rubella during the first few months of pregnancy; this increases the likelihood that the patient has patent ductus arteriosus, pulmonic valve stenosis, coarctation of the pulmonary arteries, or atrial septal defect.

Although many of the common cardiovascular diseases are sporadic, there are a rapidly increasing number of disease entities in which genetic transmission has been documented. These are detailed elsewhere. (Chaps. 9, 10, 72, and 73).

## Symptoms Due to Cardiovascular Disease

### CHEST PAIN

Chest pain or chest discomfort is the foremost manifestation of myocardial ischemia and results from a disparity between myocardial oxygen demand and coronary blood flow in patients with coronary artery disease (CAD).[3] The most common causes of myocardial ischemia are coronary atherosclerosis, coronary vasoconstriction, and coronary artery thrombosis, the latter occurring particularly in patients with acute coronary syndromes such as acute myocardial infarction and unstable angina (Chaps. 51 and 52). An increase in myocardial oxygen demand ($M\dot{V}O_2$) or demand ischemia, a decrease in or inadequate blood flow (supply ischemia), or their combination may be responsible for anginal chest pain (Chap. 57).

The mechanism responsible for cardiac pain is not clearly understood. Nonmedullated small sympathetic nerve fibers that parallel the coronary arteries are thought to provide the afferent sensory pathway for angina; these enter the spinal cord in the C8–T4 segments.[4] Impulses are transmitted to corresponding spinal ganglia and then through the spinal cord to the thalamus and cerebral cortex. Angina pectoris, like other pain of visceral origin, is often poorly localized and is commonly referred to the corresponding segmental dermatomes.

The differential diagnosis of chest pain is extensive.[5] In addition to angina pectoris and myocardial infarction, other cardiovascular diseases, gastrointestinal diseases, psychogenic diseases, neuromuscular diseases, and diseases of the pulmonary system must be considered (Table 12-1). An accurate interpretation of the etiology and significance of chest discomfort is critically dependent on a carefully taken history. Important, clinically relevant information may be missed if the *overenthusiastic use of noninvasive or invasive diagnostic methods* replaces rather than augments direct physician-patient communication (Chap. 57).

The original subjective description of angina pectoris by William Heberden[6] in the late eighteenth century has not been surpassed. It is quoted in Chap. 57.

*Angina pectoris* is defined as chest pain or discomfort of cardiac origin that usually results from a temporary imbalance between myocardial oxygen supply and demand.[7] It may occur only with exertion or spontaneously at rest; various subtypes are defined in Chap. 57. The quality of the chest discomfort is usually described as "tightness," "pressure," "burning," "heaviness," "aching," "strangling," or "compression." Usually the patient is able to describe a deep rather than a superficial origin of the pain. Since the qualitative description of the pain is greatly influenced by the patient's intelligence, education, and social/cultural background, a delineation of the other characteristics of the chest discomfort is often extremely important in evaluating the symptoms appropriately. The most important of these characteristics are the *precipitating factors* for the onset of pain, its mode of onset and duration, *its pattern of disappearance,* and its *location.* Classically, the discomfort is induced by exercise, emotion, eating, or cold weather.

TABLE 12-1 Differential Diagnosis of Chest Pain

1. Angina pectoris/myocardial infarction
2. Other cardiovascular causes
    a. Likely ischemic in origin
        (1) Aortic stenosis
        (2) Hypertrophic cardiomyopathy
        (3) Severe systemic hypertension
        (4) Severe right ventricular hypertension
        (5) Aortic regurgitation
        (6) Severe anemia/hypoxia
    b. Nonischemic in origin
        (1) Aortic dissection
        (2) Pericarditis
        (3) Mitral valve prolapse
3. Gastrointestinal
    a. Esophageal spasm
    b. Esophageal reflux
    c. Esophageal rupture
    d. Peptic ulcer disease
4. Psychogenic
    a. Anxiety
    b. Depression
    c. Cardiac psychosis
    d. Self-gain
5. Neuromusculoskeletal
    a. Thoracic outlet syndrome
    b. Degenerative joint disease of cervical/thoracic spine
    c. Costochondritis (Tietze's syndrome)
    d. Herpes zoster
    e. Chest wall pain and tenderness
6. Pulmonary
    a. Pulmonary embolus with or without pulmonary infarction
    b. Pneumothorax
    c. Pneumonia with pleural involvement
7. Pleurisy

A recognizable pattern of reproducibility of chest pain by certain activities is an important characteristic of angina. Often, patients develop pain with exertion after meals, and there is a greater tendency for arm work (a greater degree of isometric exercise) to produce distress.[8–10] Occasionally, angina will dissipate despite continued exercise (the "walk-through" phenomenon) or will not occur when a second exercise effort is undertaken that previously produced chest discomfort (warmup phenomenon). Both circumstances may be attributed to the opening of functioning coronary arterial collaterals during the initial myocardial ischemia. This is consistent with ischemic preconditioning as described elsewhere (Chap. 57).[11]

Angina commonly occurs after the patient has eaten a heavy meal or when he or she is excited, angry, or tense. Cold showers increase BP and heart rate, whereas hot showers cause an augmented cardiac output in response to vasodilation. Either may precipitate angina after exercise. The chest pain during any activity is often made worse by the use of tobacco. All the hemodynamic changes due to the use of nicotine increase myocardial oxygen demand.

Angina pectoris characteristically has a crescendo pattern at onset and "builds up." Pains, often described as "shooting" or "stabbing," that reach their maximum intensity virtually instantaneously are often not angina but are of musculoskeletal or neural origin. Angina is usually relieved within 5 to 20 min by rest, with or without the use of vasodilator drugs such as nitroglycerin, although sublingual nitroglycerin or nitroglycerin spray characteristically hastens relief. Failure to obtain relief with rest or nitroglycerin suggests another cause of pain or actual impending myocardial infarction. The reproducible relief of chest pain in an appropriate time frame (usually within 10 min) is strong evidence favoring ischemia. A trial of nitroglycerin can be a useful diagnostic strategy. Patients with angina pectoris are usually classified functionally from class I to class IV (Table 12-2), depending on the amount of activity necessary to induce chest pain.[12]

Localizing the *site* of chest discomfort provides additional information as to its cause. Anginal pain is ordinarily retrosternal or felt slightly to the left of the midline, beside or partly under the sternum. It is rarely isolated to the cardiac apex in the inframammary region. The chest pain of myocardial ischemia tends to radiate bilaterally across the chest into the arms (left more than right) and into the neck and lower jaw. Occasionally, radiation to the back or occiput is noted. In the arms, the pain passes down the ulnar and volar surface to the wrist and then only into the ulnar fingers, rarely into the thumb or down the outer (extensor) surface of the arm, which has a different dermatome pattern. Pain may occasionally be felt only in the arm or may start in the arm and radiate to the chest. Noting the patient's gestures in characterizing and localizing the site of pain may be useful. One or two clenched fists held by the patient over the sternal area (Levine's sign) is much more indicative of ischemic pain than is a finger pointed to a small, circumscribed area in the left inframammary region. The latter is likely an indicator of psychogenic pain.

The *duration* of chest pain may also be a useful differentiating feature. Angina pectoris rarely lasts less than 1 min or more than 20 min in the absence of myocardial infarction or persistent arrhythmias. Most patients with angina report *prompt relief* in less than 5 min after cessation of activity or with the use of sublingual or spray nitroglycerin.[13] Carotid sinus massage should be performed only in the absence of extracranial occlusive cerebrovascular disease as indicated by carotid bruits or decreased carotid arterial pulsations and with careful auscultatory monitoring of the heart rate. The Valsalva maneuver may also relieve anginal pain by decreasing myocardial wall stress due to the reduced venous return and left ventricular (LV) volume accompanying the increase in intrathoracic pressure. *Associated symptoms*—such as nausea, vomiting, faintness, fatigue, or diaphoresis—often accompany severe episodes of myocardial ischemia.[12] Severe myocardial ischemia often produces marked dyspnea due to a large increase in LV diastolic filling pressure, sometimes producing an "angina equivalent" in the absence of chest discomfort.

TABLE 12-2 Canadian Cardiovascular Society Functional Classification of Angina Pectoris

I. Ordinary physical activity, such as walking and climbing stairs, does not cause angina. Angina results from strenuous or rapid or prolonged exertion at work or recreation.

II. Slight limitation of ordinary activity. Walking or climbing stairs rapidly, walking uphill, walking or stair climbing after meals, in cold, in wind, or when under emotional stress, or only during the few hours after awakening. Walking more than two blocks on the level and climbing more than one flight of ordinary stairs at a normal pace and under normal conditions.

III. Marked limitations of ordinary physical activity. Walking one to two blocks on the level and climbing more than one flight under normal conditions.

IV. Inability to carry on any physical activity without discomfort—anginal syndrome may be present at rest.

SOURCE: Modified from Campeau L. Letter to the editor. *Circulation* 1976; 54:522. Reproduced with permission from the American Heart Association, Inc., and the author.

*Linked angina* is a term applied to definite episodes of angina in patients with established CAD caused by gastrointestinal factors not related to an increase in cardiac work.[15] Episodes are typically induced by stooping or occur after eating; they can be mimicked by esophageal acid stimulation, which can reduce coronary blood flow.[15]

No consideration of myocardial ischemia as a likely cause of chest discomfort is complete without carefully considering the chest pain in the context of *known risk factors* for CAD (Chap. 43).

Angina pectoris should be considered a symptom and not a specific disease. Coronary arteriographic studies have demonstrated that more than 90 percent of patients with chest pain precipitated by exercise and relieved by rest have angiographic evidence of significant CAD. However, other diseases may be associated with classic angina pectoris.

Several reports have described certain patients with typical exertional chest discomfort and arteriographically normal coronary arteries.[16,17] These patients are more likely to be females, have fewer coronary risk factors, and have variable responses to various antianginal agents, including nitroglycerin. Although the underlying cause of this condition remains unsettled, the life expectancy of these patients appears no different from that of an age- and sex-matched population without chest discomfort[18] (Chap. 57).

There is some evidence that abnormal function of small coronary arteries may cause limited coronary blood flow (CBF) responses to stress or pharmacologic vasodilators in a subset of patients with anginal chest pain despite angiographically normal coronary arteries (*microvascular angina*).[19–25] In the past, investigators arguing for or against the existence of this syndrome have often used the term *syndrome X* to describe their patient cohort.[26] Syndrome X appears to include a heterogeneous group of patients with a wide spectrum of chest pain and a variety of hypersensitive vascular and smooth muscle constrictor responses. Multiple research studies continue in an effort to explain syndrome X.[27–33] The term *syndrome X* is a poor substitute for chest pain in patients with normal large vessel coronary arteriography. It is likely to represent a polyglot of disorders.[18] It must be distinguished from the *metabolic syndrome (X)* of insulin resistance (glucose intolerance), hypertension, hyperlipidemia, and upper body obesity[18] (Chaps. 86 and 87). The latter is often associated with severe vascular disease and frequently abnormal coronary arteriography.

Some patients with CAD experience angina at rest as a complication or an isolated clinical manifestation of ischemic heart disease.[14] Myocardial ischemic pain at rest more likely results from an acute reduction in CBF than from an increase in $M\dot{V}O_2$. Possible causative factors include isolated coronary artery spasm or embolism, coronary artery spasm superimposed on coronary atherosclerosis (a common occurrence),[4] and coronary thrombosis with spontaneous thrombolysis.[34–37] In patients with progressive coronary atherosclerosis, however, ischemic rest pain also may result from intermittent arrhythmias that increase $M\dot{V}O_2$ or decrease CBF or from labile hypertension, with its increased wall stress. Chest pain at rest may occur only as nocturnal angina. In addition, nocturnal angina (also known as *angina decubitus*) may be produced by the increase in wall stress and $M\dot{V}O_2$ due to the redistribution of the intravascular blood volume in the recumbent position.

The relative hypercapnia and acidosis that occur during sleep may also contribute to nocturnal angina. Nocturnal angina has been accompanied by concomitant rapid-eye-movement sleep patterns on the electroencephalogram, which may be associated with augmented sympathetic discharge increasing $M\dot{V}O_2$ and/or causing coronary constriction[11–14] (Chap. 57).

The quality of pain with rest angina is usually similar to that of exertional angina, but the discomfort may be more severe and its duration longer. In addition, angina at rest is commonly associated with nausea, vomiting, and diaphoresis. The onset of shortness of breath during or after the beginning of chest discomfort suggests that the pain is due to extensive myocardial ischemia and results from an acute elevation of LV filling pressure secondary to the development of a large, transiently ischemic myocardial segment. Such patients commonly have multivessel occlusive CAD on arteriography.

Chest pain or discomfort resulting from *myocardial infarction* (MI) is qualitatively similar to angina at rest. Differentiation between the pain resulting from ischemia and that due to MI is often impossible based on the history alone.[11–13] Pain associated with acute coronary syndromes (ACS) is usually more severe and longer-lasting than anginal pain and is often associated with nausea, vomiting, and diaphoresis. In addition, MI or other ACS is frequently accompanied by symptoms of sustained LV dysfunction (dyspnea, orthopnea) and evidence of autonomic nervous system hyperactivity (tachycardia, diaphoresis, bradycardia).[11–13] Painless or atypical presentations of MI, however, occur in up to 30 percent of patients, particularly in diabetic patients and the elderly. Thus, determination of serial serum enzymes, isoenzymes, and other serum markers (e.g., troponin I or T), providing evidence of myocardial necrosis, and serial electrocardiograms (ECGs), indicating myocardial injury, are necessary to establish the diagnosis (Chaps. 51 and 52).

There are two groups of *cardiovascular diseases causing chest pain that is not due to coronary atherosclerosis* (Table 12-1). The first group consists of cardiac diseases causing myocardial ischemia-related angina in the absence of CAD. Ischemia is due to hemodynamic changes associated with an inadequate CBF in relation to a normal or increased myocardial oxygen demand. Among these are *aortic valve stenosis* (Chap. 66), *hypertrophic cardiomyopathy* (Chap. 77), and *systemic arterial hypertension* (Chap. 61), in which LV systolic pressure and LV wall tension are greatly increased or LV hypertrophy is present.[11–13] Chest pain due to myocardial ischemia also can occur with severe aortic regurgitation (AR) (Chap. 66). The large LV volume load and increased LV dimensions augment $M\dot{V}O_2$, and the reduced diastolic perfusion pressure results in a relatively inadequate CBF. Occasionally, very severe anemia or hypoxia may also produce myocardial ischemia due to inadequate oxygen blood supply even in the absence of associated CAD. Both also may increase angina in the presence of obstructive CAD.[11–13] In addition, severe right ventricular (RV) systolic hypertension, as often occurs with pulmonic stenosis (PS) or pulmonary hypertension (PH), may cause exertional angina, presumably on the basis of RV subendocardial ischemia.[38]

A second group of cardiac diseases causing chest pain not usually due to myocardial ischemia includes *pericarditis* (Chap. 80), aortic dissection (Chap. 98), and mitral valve prolapse (MVP) (Chap. 68). Pericarditis is a relatively common cause of chest pain.[39] It is most often sharp and penetrating in quality; patients often obtain relief by sitting up and bending forward (Chap. 80). The cardinal diagnostic feature of pericardial pain is its frequent worsening by changes in body position, during deep inspiration, and occasionally on swallowing. The chest discomfort may radiate to the shoulders, upper back, and neck because of irritation of the diaphragmatic pleura, which is innervated through the phrenic nerve by fibers originating in sympathetic ganglia C3–C5. Therefore the chest discomfort associated with pericarditis is due predominantly to parietal pleural irritation. Occasionally, the pain of acute benign, presumptive viral pericarditis may mimic that observed in acute MI. Importantly, the most common cause of pericarditis in middle-aged or older people is acute MI. The pericarditis usually occurs several days after the myocardial necrosis and must be distinguished from recurrent infarction or ischemia. Pericarditis may also be a cause of chest pain after cardiac surgery and may be a complication of aortic dissection, with leakage into the pericardium.

Aortic dissection (Chap. 98) may be misdiagnosed on initial presentation as an acute MI; indeed, MI is a recognized complication of aortic dissection. The pain with dissection, however, is usually of sudden onset as compared with that of myocardial ischemia, which builds in intensity with time.[40] Patients frequently characterize the pain as excruciating, as having a tearing quality and commonly localized to the interscapular area. The discomfort may radiate widely into the neck, back, abdomen, flanks, and legs and may migrate, depending on the location and progression of the aortic dissection and the amount of arterial luminal compression. Neurologic symptoms and signs may occur when dissection involves the cerebral arteries. With the exception of patients with Marfan's syndrome (Chaps. 84 and 98) or idiopathic cystic medial necrosis, most patients with aortic dissection have a history of long-standing systemic arterial hypertension or evidence of it on physical examination, or by ECG (LV hypertrophy).

*Psychogenic chest discomfort* is a common type of recurrent chest pain that may be difficult to separate from angina pectoris, particularly when it occurs in patients with multiple risk factors for CAD or in otherwise asymptomatic patients with well-documented CAD. The most common psychogenic cause of chest discomfort is anxiety[41] (Chap. 91). Psychogenic chest pain is often described as sharp or stabbing, localized to the left inframammary area, and usually sharply circumscribed. Descriptors such as "stabbing" or "lightning-like" may be used to describe extremely short (<1 min) episodes of pain. At times, the pain may persist for many hours or several days. Patients often note psychogenic pain at rest. Also, nonvocal communication—such as a flat or worried facial expression, retarded motor activity, and hand wringing—may indicate underlying depression. Observation of the patient during pain that occurs spontaneously or during exercise testing often provides insight into a potential psychogenic etiology. Patients with anxiety often have multiple complaints. Associated symptoms—such as air hunger, circumoral paresthesias, globus hystericus, and multiple somatic complaints—may suggest a neurasthenic personality or hyperventilation syndrome.

*Pain originating in the gastrointestinal tract,* particularly that of esophageal origin, is commonly confused with ischemic chest pain.[42] *Diffuse esophageal spasm,* a neuromuscular motor disorder of the esophagus characterized by chest pain, is the extracardiac condition most frequently confused with angina pectoris. Esophageal spasm may occur at any age but is more common in individuals in the fifth decade. The pain is usually retrosternal; may be burning, squeezing, or aching in quality; and often radiates to the back, arms, and jaw. It usually begins during or after a meal and can last minutes or hours. The pain may be relieved by nitroglycerin, which also relaxes esophageal smooth muscle. A useful diagnostic feature in esophageal spasm is its frequent association with pain as a result of swallowing, dysphagia, and the regurgitation of gastric contents. The diagnosis of diffuse esophageal spasm is based on the history, the exclusion of cardiac and musculoskeletal causes of chest pain and the demonstration of abnormal esophageal motility on cineesophagograms or by esophageal manometry.

*Reflux esophagitis* results from mucosal irritation produced by failure of the lower esophageal sphincter to prevent regurgitation of highly acidic gastric contents into the distal esophagus.[43–45] The pain is usually epigastric or retrosternal, burning in quality, and frequently precipitated by the recumbent position or by bending over. "Heartburn" and regurgitation often occur after meals or ingestion of coffee or after postural changes. Patients are often awakened by chest discomfort due to acid reflux occurring in the recumbent position. Dysphagia may result from stricture formation secondary to longstanding esophageal reflux. An upper gastrointestinal x-ray series may demonstrate hiatal hernia, but this does not establish the diagnosis of esophagitis or esophageal reflux. Esophagoscopy and esophageal biopsy may demonstrate mucosal lesions and are useful for assessing the severity of inflammation and for excluding malignancy. Sphincter incompetence may be documented by the use of esophageal manometry. Esophageal acid perfusion testing (Bernstein test) often will provoke the patient's characteristic symptoms, and distal esophageal pH monitoring will detect gastroesophageal reflux.[44]

*Acute esophageal rupture,* a serious and often rapidly lethal event, causes severe retrosternal pain secondary to the chemical mediastinitis produced by acidic gastric contents.[8–11] Spontaneous rupture usually results from a prolonged bout of vomiting or retching after a heavy meal. The pain varies in location depending on the rupture's site and position. The diagnosis is based on symptoms and signs of mediastinal air following vomiting or esophageal instrumentation.

Although peptic ulcer disease and biliary colic are less commonly confused with chest pain of cardiac origin, myocardial ischemic pain may occasionally be described as burning in character and located near the epigastrium.

*Diseases involving the neuromuscular-skeletal systems* may cause pain affecting dermatomal patterns similar to those occurring with angina pectoris.[8–11] The thoracic outlet syndromes, in which various neural and vascular structures are compressed, may produce symptoms that are sometimes confused with cardiac chest pain. Although compression of the neurovascular bundle by a cervical rib or the scalenus anterior muscle may cause discomfort radiating to the head and neck, the shoulder region, or the axilla, most patients experience pain in the upper extremity ulnar distribution resulting from somatic nerve compression. The presence of associated paresthesias, of pain unrelated to physical exercise, and the worsening of discomfort with certain body positions are useful differentiating characteristics.

*Tietze's syndrome,* or idiopathic costochondritis, is an occasional cause of anterior chest wall pain that is aggravated by movement and deep breathing. Reproducing the chest pain syndrome by direct pressure over the involved costochondral junction or the relief of pain after local infiltration with lidocaine is a helpful diagnostic maneuver.[46] Degenerative arthritis of the cervical and thoracic vertebrae may cause band-like pain confined to the chest, neck, or back that often radiates to the arms.[8–10] Radiologic evidence of degenerative changes involving the cervical and thoracic vertebrae is often found in asymptomatic elderly patients. The production or exacerbation of pain by various postures, movement, sneezing, or coughing is more useful in the diagnosis of chest discomfort due to vertebral disease.[8–10]

The *preeruptive stage of herpes zoster* may be characterized by band-like chest pain over one or more dermatomes. The advanced age of the patient; additional symptoms of malaise, headache, and fever; the presence of hyperesthesia of the involved area on physical examination; and the eventual eruption of typical lesions 4 or 5 days after the onset of symptoms will result in the correct diagnosis. Chest wall pain and tenderness may occur for unknown reasons.[47] The discomfort may be reproduced by pressure over the painful area and by movements of the thorax such as bending, twisting, or turning.

The syndrome of acute massive *pulmonary embolism* with its associated acute PH and low cardiac output occasionally may simulate acute MI, since myocardial ischemia may be present in both conditions. The quality of chest pain may be identical to that observed in patients with nonradiating ischemic chest pain or may be pleuritic. The associated signs of severe dyspnea, tachypnea, and intense cyanosis, accompanied by profound anxiety and agitation, however, favor the diagnosis of pulmonary embolism[9–12] (Chap. 63). Measurements of arterial blood gases, abnormal pulmonary ventilation/perfusion scans, and, if needed, pulmonary arteriography will establish the correct diagnosis.[8–10]

*Other pulmonary conditions associated with chest discomfort,* such as pneumothorax, are rarely confused with ischemic chest pain because of additional characteristic clinical features. Spontaneous pneumothorax usually occurs in otherwise healthy males in the third and fourth decades. The clinical presentation is usually characterized by the abrupt onset of agonizing unilateral pleuritic chest pain associated with severe shortness of breath. The plain or expiratory chest film provides the definitive diagnosis. Chest pain associated with pneumonias of various etiologies, as well as pulmonary infarctions as a consequence of pulmonary embolus, may result from pleural irritation. The discomfort is sharp, varies acutely with breathing, and is frequently accompanied by a reduced inspiratory effort. Associated signs of pulmonary parenchymal infection or infarction usually indicate the underlying diagnosis.

## EXTRATHORACIC PAIN

Intermittent claudication of the lower extremities due to peripheral atherosclerosis (Chap. 101) may present as discomfort during exercise in the arch of the foot, calf of the leg, thighs, hips, or gluteal region.[8–11] Acute arterial occlusion in the lower extremities due to systemic embolism may cause the sensation of hypesthesia.[2] The pain of Raynaud's disease may be noted in the fingers after exposure to cold, with pallor of the fingers prior to the sensation of pain. Pain and swelling of lower extremities may be caused by thrombophlebitis (Chap. 101).

*Head pain* secondary to myocardial ischemia may be felt in the jaw, hard palate, cheek, and sometimes deep in the ear canals. The pain of temporal arteritis, commonly localized to the temporal area, often is associated with abnormal vision and polymyalgia rheumatica. A severe headache may be present in patients with uncontrolled hypertension (Chap. 61).

*Pain in the abdomen,* often localized to the midabdomen and lower portion of the back, may be produced by an expanding or rupturing atherosclerotic abdominal aneurysm. Abdominal angina due to vascular disease of the mesenteric arteries is discussed in Chap. 98. The liver is often painful and tender in severe right-sided heart failure, with worsening of the pain during activity.[2]

Various types of *joint pain* may be associated with heart disease. Rheumatic fever, rheumatoid arthritis, lupus erythematosus, psoriatic arthritis, ankylosing spondylitis, gonococcal arthritis, Reiter's syndrome, and Lyme disease may be associated with valvular, myocardial, or pericardial disease.[2]

## RESPIRATORY SYMPTOMS

*Dyspnea* is defined as difficult or labored respiration or the unpleasant awareness of one's breathing. A clue to the etiology is obtained from the factors that precipitate or relieve it.[1] Chronic dyspnea can be caused by heart failure, pulmonary disease, anxiety, obesity, poor physical fitness, pleural effusions, and asthma.[2] Acute dyspnea may occur with acute pulmonary edema, hyperventilation, pneumothorax, pulmonary embolism, pneumonia, and airway obstruction.[2]

*Dyspnea on effort,* a frequent symptom, is usually due to congestive heart failure, chronic pulmonary disease, or physical deconditioning (Chap. 25). A recent or dramatic increase in the dyspnea is more likely to be due to the development of heart failure than to lung disease. When heart and lung disease coexist, however, determination of the relative contribution of pulmonary and cardiac dysfunction to dyspnea can be very difficult.

*Cheyne-Stokes respiration* is a form of periodic breathing characterized by cycles beginning with shallow respirations that increase in rate and depth to significant hyperpnea, followed by decreasing rate and depth of respiration, and then a period of apnea that may last 15 s or longer. This form of respiration occurs in advanced congestive heart failure and in some forms of central nervous system disease. Cheyne-Stokes respiration often occurs during sleep without the patient's awareness and is often reported by others.

*Orthopnea results* from an increase in hydrostatic pressure in the lungs that occurs with assumption of the supine position. It consists of cough and dyspnea in some patients with LV failure or mitral valve (MV) disease and necessitates the use of two or more pillows on lying down. The patient with severe obstructive lung disease, especially acute asthma, also cannot lie flat comfortably.

*Paroxysmal nocturnal dyspnea* (PND) is the occurrence of dyspnea during sleep, commonly 2 to 3 h after going to bed, that is relieved by assuming the upright position. Dyspnea usually does not recur after the patient goes back to sleep. Episodes can be mild, or they can be severe with wheezing, coughing, gasping, and apprehension.[1] Some episodes will progress to pulmonary edema. The probable mechanism for this *relatively specific symptom* of left-sided heart failure is the increase in central blood volume in the supine position.

A dry, unproductive cough, occurring with effort or at rest, may be related to the pulmonary congestion associated with heart failure (Chap. 25). Although dyspnea is usually present, cough may dominate the clinical picture. The cough that accompanies acute pulmonary edema is often associated with frothy, pink-tinged sputum, whereas the sputum associated with chronic bronchitis is usually white and mucoid.[2] Sputum associated with pneumonia is often thick and yellow and due to pulmonary infarction may be bloody, as may the sputum associated with cancer of the lung or bronchiolectasis. Cough also may be caused by angiotensin-converting enzyme inhibitors.

Recurrent coughing due to heart failure is often thought to be due to bronchitis, and patients with chronic bronchitis may cough more when heart failure ensues.[2] Patients with a high pulmonary blood flow due to congenital left-to-right shunts are subject to pulmonary infection. Patients with a high pulmonary venous pressure (e.g., mitral stenosis) are more vulnerable to pulmonary edema when they have viral pneumonitis than are patients with normal pulmonary venous pressure.

*Hemoptysis* occurs in many cardiac disorders. Posterior epistaxis due to systemic hypertension may cause blood-streaked sputum; patients on anticoagulants may have epistaxis that mimics hemoptysis. Bright red pulmonary venous blood from rupture of submucosal pulmonary venules may be expectorated by patients with pulmonary venous hypertension due to mitral stenosis (MS) or severe LV failure.[2] Darker blood or clots often occur with pulmonary emboli.

Pink, frothy sputum may be produced during acute pulmonary edema. Blood-streaked sputum is a feature of the "winter bronchitis" of mitral stenosis.[2] Massive hemoptysis with exsanguination can follow rupture of an aortic aneurysm or one of the cardiac chambers into the bronchial tree.[2] Rupture of a pulmonary artery by the balloon of an indwelling pulmonary artery catheter can cause abrupt, severe hemoptysis in hospitalized patients.

*Wheezing* associated with dyspnea may be due to lung or heart disease. If the symptoms have developed recently in an adult over age 40, other clues indicating heart disease (cardiac asthma) should be sought.

## EDEMA AND ASCITES

*Edema* is a common symptom or finding in patients with right- or left-sided heart failure. Fluid retention in heart failure results from increased venous pressure and abnormal activity of salt-retaining hormones (Chap. 25). In an average-sized person, 5 to 10 lb of excess fluid is required for edema to become apparent; a history of recent weight gain will often correlate with deterioration in clinical status. The amount of weight loss in response to treatment for heart failure in the past will relate to the severity of the problem. Minor degrees of edema are evident only after a period of dependency of the legs and will decrease after rest. Presacral edema may be most obvious when the patient has been at bed rest. Although edema of cardiac origin may progress to anasarca, cardiac edema rarely involves the face or upper extremities. Persistent edema in the legs from which veins were harvested at the time of bypass surgery is common. Other causes of edema—such as varicosities, obesity, tight girdle, renal insufficiency, or cirrhosis with hypoproteinemia—must be considered.[1] A patient with chronic congestive heart failure may detect edema of the ankles and lower legs during the day and note that it diminishes during the night. It is important to ascertain whether edema of the extremities preceded or followed dyspnea on effort. The calcium antagonists may produce bilateral edema of the lower legs. Edema may occur in one or both legs following the harvesting of veins for conduits in patients undergoing coronary artery bypass graft (CABG) surgery.

Patients will be aware of ascites because of increased abdominal girth. Previously comfortable trousers or skirts may no longer fit. Bending at the waist is uncomfortable, with ill-defined abdominal fullness. Patients with severe edema due to congestive heart failure may develop ascites; however, ascites is particularly common in patients with constrictive pericardial disease, sometimes occurring before peripheral edema becomes obvious (Chap. 80). Ascitic fluid is formed when elevated venous pressure leads to transudation of fluids from the serosal surfaces.

## FATIGUE AND WEAKNESS

*Fatigue* and *weakness* may be due to many causes and therefore are not specific symptoms for heart disease. The most common cause of these symptoms is anxiety and depression. Anemia, thyrotoxicosis, and other chronic disease states may be associated with fatigue and weakness.

When a patient with heart disease is volume overloaded, or when there is pulmonary congestion due to heart disease, the patient is likely to complain of dyspnea. With vigorous diuretic therapy, this complaint may be replaced by symptoms of fatigue and weakness,[2] probably related to inadequate cardiac output (Chap. 25). As congestive heart failure worsens, fatigue may replace dyspnea as the major symptom. Beta blockers used to treat angina or hypertension often cause fatigue and lethargy. Hypotension or hypokalemia caused by diuretics can result in fatigue and weakness, as can relative hypovolemia due to the use of angiotensin-converting enzyme inhibitors.

Severe fatigue related to effort may result from transient global myocardial ischemia in patients with extensive CAD. Dyspnea and hypotension also may occur at the same time as the severe fatigue as *angina equivalents.*[2]

## PALPITATION

Most normal individuals are intermittently aware of their heart action, particularly at the time of physical and emotional stress. When the heart action is more vigorous than usual or its perception is unpleasant, the term *palpitation* is appropriate.[1] The patient may complain of a "pounding," "stopping," "jumping," or "racing" in the chest. Palpitation is frequently a benign symptom without any serious cardiac disease present; at other times it may indicate a potentially life-threatening condition. Simple premature beats may be perceived as a "floating" or "flopping" sensation in the chest due to the more forceful beat that occurs after the pause following the premature beat. Sometimes a transient feeling of fullness in the neck (due to cannon a waves) is perceived with premature beats. Certain patients perceive almost every premature beat, whereas others are totally unaware of frequent or advanced arrhythmias. A report of skips or irregularity during uninterrupted sinus rhythm is not uncommon. Generally, thin, tense individuals are likely to be more aware of their cardiac activity than others. Individuals with and without arrhythmias often are aware of their cardiac activity when they first lie down to sleep, especially if they lie on their left side.[1]

Rapid heart action of a paroxysmal tachycardia usually begins and terminates abruptly and causes a pounding sensation in the chest.[1] Patients often will indicate whether the tachycardia is regular or irregular and may be able to tap out the rate and rhythm of the episode (Chap. 28). Chest pressure suggesting angina may occur with an episode of tachycardia even in young, healthy patients without CAD. Patients with CAD, however, often develop severe angina with a sustained arrhythmia because of increased $M\dot{V}O_2$. Depending on the rate and mechanism of the arrhythmia, faintness and syncope may be described during questioning. Nevertheless, sustained ventricular tachycardia can occur in the setting of serious underlying cardiac disease without a significant compromise in hemodynamics (Chap. 28). Syncope due to tachyarrhythmias may occur without the patient being aware of palpitations.

## SYNCOPE

Cardiac *syncope* (fainting) is defined as the transient loss of consciousness due to inadequate cerebral blood flow secondary to an abrupt decrease in cardiac output (Chap. 40). *Near syncope* refers to the clinical situation in which the patient feels dizzy and weak and tends to lose postural tone but does not lose consciousness. In assessing the patient with syncope, one determines if there were precipitating factors, premonitory symptoms, injury with the episode, seizure activity or incontinence, or a postictal state.[1] Injury during an episode suggests a sudden profound loss of body tone and increases the likelihood of more serious causes. Brief, unsustained seizure activity can occur with syncope due to a cardiac arrhythmia.

The patient may be incontinent during cardiogenic syncope, but an aura, sustained tonic-chronic movements, tongue biting, and confusion or drowsiness after the event are more characteristic of syncope due to central nervous system disease. In contrast, return of consciousness to the alert state is prompt after reversal of the arrhythmia causing cardiac syncope.[1] The common faint (*vasovagal syncope*) results from bradycardia and hypotension caused by excessive vagal discharge. It is often associated with some precipitating event such as a "heavy" meal in a warm room and has brief premonitory signs and symptoms such as nausea, yawning, diaphoresis, and sometimes the feeling of decreased hearing or vision.[1] The results of head-up tilt-table testing indicate a vasovagal mechanism in some patients with syncope who do not have premonitory symptoms (Chap. 40). Following a fainting episode, the patient may be pale and diaphoretic and have a slow heart rate. A history of similar episodes during the preceding several years is common in patients with vagal syncope.

A hypersensitive carotid sinus can cause syncope. A history of episodes during an activity such as shaving, wearing of a tight collar, or extreme turning of the head may occur but is unusual even when a sensitive carotid sinus is shown to be the cause of syncope. Syncope following urination (micturition syncope) may occur at the time of rapid decompression of a distended bladder, which typically occurs after a period of sleep. Paroxysms of coughing, usually in patients with underlying pulmonary disease, can result in syncope. Very fast or slow arrhythmias may decrease the cardiac output enough to cause alterations in consciousness, ranging from abrupt profound syncope to mild light-headedness. Stokes-Adams syncope is caused by intermittent complete heart block, sinus arrest, or ventricular tachyarrhythmias (Chap. 40). It is characterized by abrupt loss of consciousness without warning, a variable period of unconsciousness (seconds to minutes), and then a rapid return of normal mental status without amnesia or a postictal state.

In the presence of severe LV outflow obstruction (aortic stenosis or hypertrophic cardiomyopathy), loss of consciousness with effort may occur. Syncope can be due either to the heart's inability to increase its output in response to the peripheral vasodilatation that occurs during exercise or to a tachyarrhythmia. Intermittent obstruction of a cardiac valve by an intracavitary tumor or thrombus is a rare cause of syncope that occasionally may be precipitated when the patient changes position (Chap. 85).

Many normal subjects experience transient light-headedness with rapid changes in position. This is more common in older patients, since the ability of the peripheral vasculature to respond is attenuated with aging (Chap. 96). Postural hypotension is a well-defined cause of fainting or dizziness that usually occurs when the individual is upright and often just after rising from a supine or sitting position. Possible causes include peripheral neuropathy, autonomic dysfunction, volume depletion, or drug side effects.

## OTHER CEREBRAL SYMPTOMS

Patients with decreased cardiac output secondary to heart failure may become mentally confused and disoriented. Such symptoms also may be due to hypoxia, to drugs that are invariably prescribed for such patients, and to renal or hepatic failure.[2] A completed stroke may be caused by a lacunar infarct, cerebral hemorrhage, cerebral arterial thrombosis, or a cerebral embolus (Chap. 99). A transient cerebral ischemic attack is commonly due to an embolus. The embolus may originate in an atheromatous ulcer in the carotid artery system or the aortic arch; be related to infective endocarditis, a recent MI, atrial fibrillation, or clots on a prosthetic valve; or originate in the leg veins and pass through a patent foramen ovale to the brain (Chap. 99).

The patient with cardiogenic shock or with a severe tachyarrhythmia who also has considerable intracranial or extracranial vascular disease may develop such severe cerebral hypoxia that coma occurs. Hypoxic encephalopathy may follow cardiac resuscitation and occasionally occurs after cardiopulmonary bypass for cardiac surgery. A cerebral abscess may occur in patients with congenital heart disease and a right-to-left shunt.[2]

## FEVER, CHILLS, AND SWEATS

Fever with chills is common in patients with bacterial endocarditis. Symptoms of fever, chills, or sweats in any patient with a heart murmur should lead one to suspect infective endocarditis (Chap. 81). A history of valvular heart disease is not a prerequisite since previously normal valves become infected. A history of recent dental work, genitourinary surgery, or illicit drug use increases the suspicion of infective endocarditis. Fever may accompany rheumatic fever or pericarditis. An intracardiac tumor (myxoma) may produce systemic symptoms in the absence of infection. Low-grade fever in a patient with heart failure may be a sign of pulmonary emboli.[2] Excessive sweating may occur in patients with severe aortic regurgitation (AR) or acute MI. Diaphoresis is often a sign of congestive heart failure in infants.

### HOARSENESS

*Hoarseness* can occur in patients with an aortic aneurysm that involves the left recurrent laryngeal nerve. MS occasionally may produce hoarseness due to the pressure of a large pulmonary artery on the recurrent laryngeal nerve. Pericardial effusion may be related to myxedema, which may be associated with a coarse, low-pitched voice. Hoarseness and loss of voice may occur following the use of an endotracheal tube during cardiac surgery.

### INDIGESTION, HICCUPS, AND DYSPHAGIA

Many patients with angina pectoris due to CAD erroneously attribute their symptoms to *indigestion* or heartburn. Also, patients with heartburn, esophageal reflux, and esophageal spasm may believe they have angina pectoris. *Hiccups* occasionally may occur in patients with MI and are common during the postoperative period after cardiac surgery. *Dysphagia* may occur in patients with progressive systemic sclerosis, an aortic arch anomaly, or an extremely large left atrium.

### GASTROINTESTINAL SYMPTOMS

Anorexia, nausea, and vomiting may occur as a result of digitalis excess. Hepatomegaly associated with tricuspid valve disease or severe right-sided heart failure may cause right-upper-quadrant epigastric pain and fullness as well as anorexia. Abdominal pain due to visceral ischemia or infarction may occur in a patient who has had a period of very low cardiac output.

### ABNORMAL SKIN COLOR

Although *cyanosis* is a sign rather than a symptom, patients or family members may describe cyanosis during the history. *Cyanosis* is a bluish color of the skin or mucous membranes caused by excess amounts of reduced hemoglobin. About 4 g of reduced hemoglobin is required for cyanosis to be apparent (Chap. 73). Severely anemic patients will not exhibit cyanosis. A distribution of cyanosis involving the mucous membranes as well as the periphery (central cyanosis) is caused by the admixture of venous blood at the level of the heart or great vessels. A patient or a family member may detect that the cyanosis is more intense in the feet than in the hands. This differential cyanosis suggests a right-to-left shunt through a patent ductus arteriosus in a patient with Eisenmenger physiology (Chap. 73). Peripheral cyanosis does not involve the mucous membranes but is the result of slow peripheral flow with accumulation of excess reduced hemoglobin in the setting of circulatory failure, shock, or peripheral vasospasm.

Jaundice may be detected by a patient or by a member of the family. As a rule, hepatic congestion due to heart failure will not produce jaundice. When jaundice does occur in a patient with heart failure, it is appropriate to consider pulmonary infarction in addition to hepatic congestion or cirrhosis of the liver. Hemolysis of red blood cells may occur in patients with prosthetic valves and can produce jaundice.[2]

A history of flush of face and trunk, sometimes accentuated by alcohol, should lead one to search for the other signs and symptoms of carcinoid heart disease[2] (Chap. 85). Cardiomyopathies due to hemochromatosis should be considered in the patient with diabetes whose skin color has changed from normal to bronze.[2] A slate-like color of the skin, hands, and nose may develop in patients who take amiodarone.

### EMBOLIZATION

The entry of a blood clot, vegetation, or tumor fragment from the heart into the systemic circulation results in arterial embolus. Clots may occur in the left atrium behind a stenotic mitral valve, within a ventricular aneurysm, or in the LV of a patient with cardiomyopathy. While many emboli originate in the heart, arteriosclerotic material in the ascending and descending aorta often embolizes to the periphery.[1] Many emboli are asymptomatic. Symptoms of a stroke occur with emboli to the cerebral vessels. MI can result from an embolus to a coronary artery. Hematuria, flank pain, and hypertension can result from embolization to a renal artery. The abrupt development of a cold, painful extremity follows embolic obstruction of an arm or leg artery.[1] Emboli from the vegetations of acute endocarditis may produce characteristic areas of vascular necrosis in the fingers or toes (Chap. 81). Severe atherosclerosis in the abdominal aorta and iliac vessels can be responsible for showers of peripheral emboli with multiple small, reddish blue lesions on the lower extremities sometimes causing small areas of gangrene. An embolic event may be the presenting manifestation of previously unrecognized cardiac disease.

### INSOMNIA

The most common causes of insomnia are mental conflict, emotional disturbances, and depression. Heart failure, however, may also cause insomnia. The patient with Cheyne-Stokes respirations (see above) may sleep during the apneic phase and wake during the hyperpneic phase of the condition. Occasionally, patients with pulmonary congestion due to heart failure have insomnia before they develop nocturnal dyspnea. Central and obstructive sleep apnea are discussed elsewhere (Chaps. 25, 76, and 87).

## Classification of Cardiac Disability

Several classifications have been proposed and used for the systematic and reproducible grading of disability due to cardiac disease. Although the complete New York Heart Association method of classifying cardiac diagnoses, originally proposed many years ago, is not widely used now, the portion of the classification that concerns functional capacities[48] in heart failure is still commonly used (Table 12-3). Although the Canadian Cardiovascular Society's grading system for angina (see Table 12-2) is more widely used for patients with chest pain, both classifications continue to be used in the medical literature and in clinical practice, particularly as criteria for the inclusion of heart patients in multicenter clinical trials.

TABLE 12-3 The Old New York Heart Association Functional Classification

| | |
|---|---|
| Class 1 | No symptoms with ordinary physical activity. |
| Class 2 | Symptoms with ordinary activity. Slight limitation of activity. |
| Class 3 | Symptoms with less than ordinary activity. Marked limitation of activity. |
| Class 4 | Symptoms with any physical activity or even at rest. |

SOURCE: The Criteria Committee of the New York Heart Association. *Diseases of the Heart and Blood Vessels: Nomenclature and Criteria for Diagnosis of the Heart and Great Vessels,* 6th ed. New York: New York Heart Association/Little, Brown; 1964. Reproduced with permission from the New York Heart Association, Inc., and the publisher.

## THE PHYSICAL EXAMINATION

Important information concerning the patient with heart disease is often obtained by a careful and deliberate physical examination, which includes a general inspection of the patient, an indirect measurement of the arterial blood pressure (BP) in both arms and one or both lower extremities, an examination of central and peripheral arterial pulses, an evaluation of the jugular venous pressure and pulsations, palpation of the precordium, and cardiac auscultation. Based on the results of this rather inexpensive evaluation, a definite diagnosis often is made; selected noninvasive and invasive testing is ordered only when appropriate.

### General Inspection of the Patient

Bedside examination begins with a careful general appraisal of the patient. This visual inspection may provide important information leading to the etiology of cardiovascular disease.

Clues to the diagnosis of underlying congenital heart disease may be obtained from careful observation of the thorax and extremities. Bilateral prominence of the anterior chest with bulging of the upper two-thirds of the sternum is commonly present in children with a large ventricular septal defect (VSD). A unilateral bulge at the fourth and fifth intercostal spaces at the lower left sternal border is found in adults with VSD. Scoliosis may be present in cyanotic congenital heart disease. Underdeveloped musculature of the lower extremities compared with the upper extremities occurs with coarctation of the aorta. Clubbing of the digits and cyanosis of the skin or nails suggest congenital heart disease with right-to-left shunting of blood (Fig. 12-1, Plate 31). Differential cyanosis provides information about anatomy.[49] Cyanosis and clubbing of the toes associated with pink fingernails of the right hand and cyanosis and clubbing of the left hand are due to a patent ductus arteriosus with normally related great vessels and a reversed shunt due to pulmonary hypertension, with the patent ductus arteriosus delivering cyanotic blood to the left arm and lower extremities (Figs. 12-2 and 12-3, Plates 32 and 33). The same color pattern results from interruption of the aortic arch and a patent ductus arteriosus delivering desaturated blood to the legs. However, if the right subclavian artery arises proximal to the aortic obstruction, the right hand may be pink and the left hand cyanotic. When an anomalous right subclavian artery originates from the descending aorta, both hands are cyanotic. Cyanosis of the fingers greater than in the toes indicates complete transposition of the great vessels with preductal coarctation or complete interruption of the aortic arch, pulmonary hypertension, and a reverse shunt through a patent ductus arteriosus, in this case delivering oxygenated blood to the lower extremities.

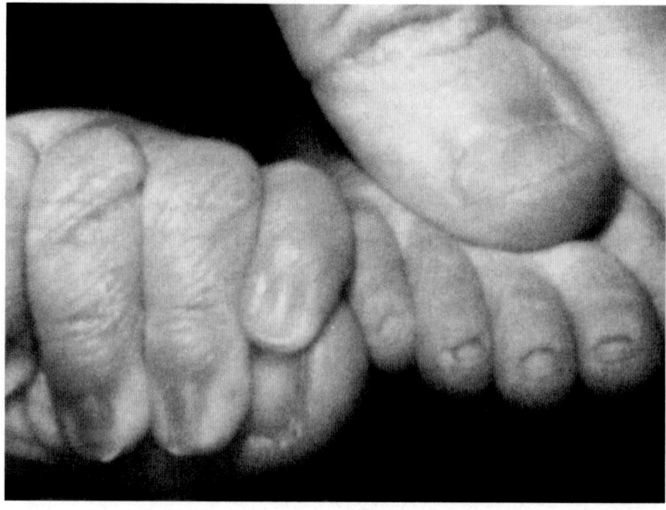

FIGURE 12-2 (Plate 32) *Differential cyanosis*. Clubbing of left hand (compare thumbs) and cyanosis of left hand and all toes due to patent ductus arteriosus with pulmonary hypertension and normally related great vessels. (Courtesy of Dr. Joseph K. Perloff, University of California, Los Angeles.)

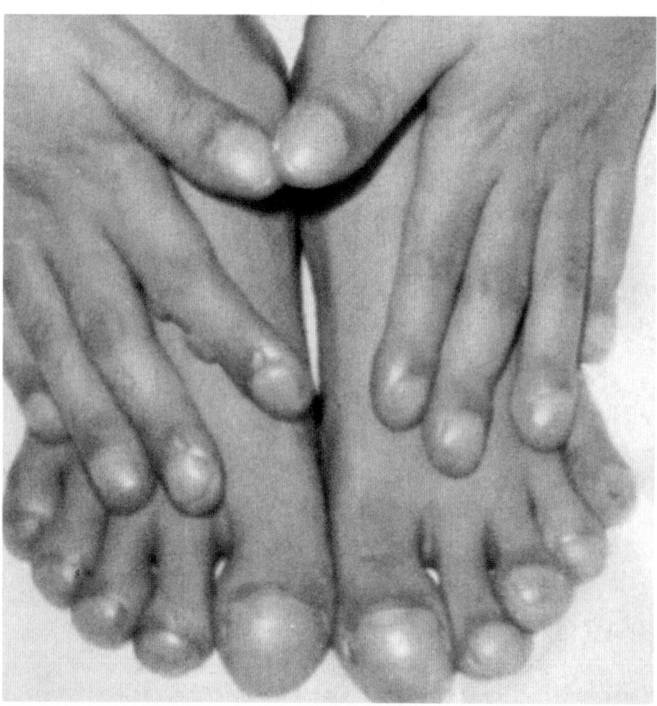

FIGURE 12-1 (Plate 31) *Symmetric cyanosis*. Equal cyanosis and clubbing of hands and feet due to transposition of the great vessels and a ventricular septal defect without patent ductus arteriosus.

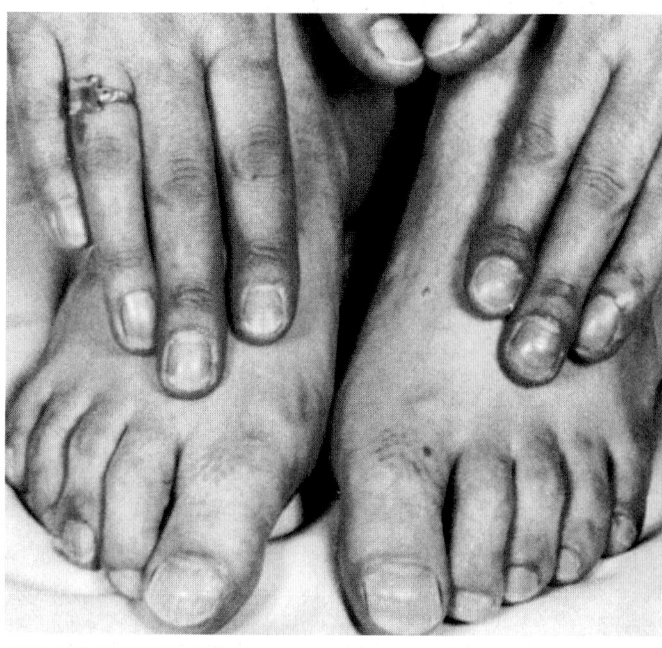

FIGURE 12-3 (Plate 33) *Differential cyanosis*. Cyanosis of fingers (*left*) greater than that of toes due to transposition of the great vessels with patent ductus arteriosus.

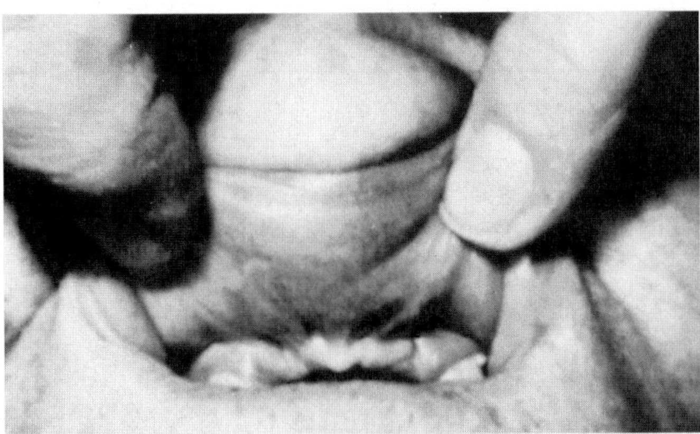

A

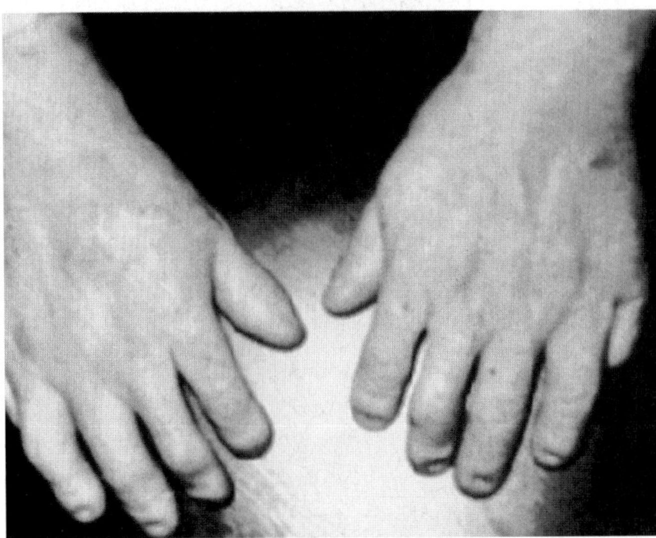

B

FIGURE 12-4 *Ellis-van Creveld syndrome. A.* Typical "lip tie" due to multiple frenulum. *B.* Polydactyly. This patient has a large septal defect.

The presence of any congenital somatic abnormality should prompt a search for congenital heart disease.

## Syndromes Associated with Congenital Heart Disease

The Ellis-van Creveld syndrome is a heritable form of dwarfism characterized by short extremities, polydactyly, dysplastic teeth and nails, and multiple frenula binding the upper lip to the alveolar ridge (Fig. 12-4*A* and *B*). Over half the patients have heart disease, usually a large atrial septal defect or a single atrium.

The thrombocytopenia–absent radius (TAR) syndrome includes bilateral radial aplasia with a persistent thumb and thrombocytopenia and may be associated with an ostium secundum atrial septal defect (ASD) and/or tetralogy of Fallot. The Holt-Oram syndrome, an autosomal dominant condition, combines an ASD or other congenital heart disease with an abnormal thumb[50] (Fig. 12-5). In the Laurence-Moon-Bardet-Biedl syndrome, mental retardation, polydactyly, obesity, retinitis pigmentosa, and hypogonadism occur with a variety of congenital heart diseases.

The Cornelia de Lange syndrome is characterized by bushy, confluent eyebrows, downward-slanting eyes, a small mandible, low-set ears, hirsutism, long eyelashes, a broad, flat, upturned nose, severe growth and mental retardation, and a peculiar "chicken wing" extremity with a single thumblike digit (Fig. 12-6). A VSD, patent ductus arteriosus, pulmonic stenosis, anomalous venous return, or ASD may be present.

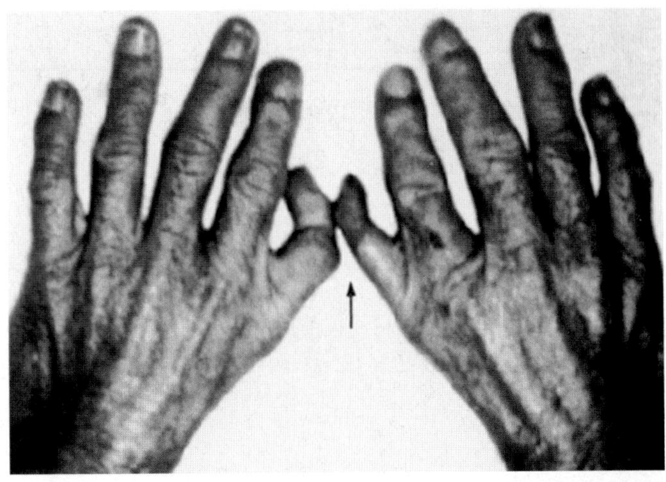

FIGURE 12-5 *Holt-Oram syndrome:* fingerized thumb (*arrow*) associated with an atrial septal defect.

There is an increased incidence of congenital heart disease in children with a cleft palate or lip. In the Pierre Robin syndrome (Fig. 12-7) the cleft palate is associated with a hypoplastic mandible causing a "shrewlike" face. Patients with the Ehlers-Danlos syndrome (Fig. 12-8*A* and *B*) have hyperextensible joints and hyperelastic and

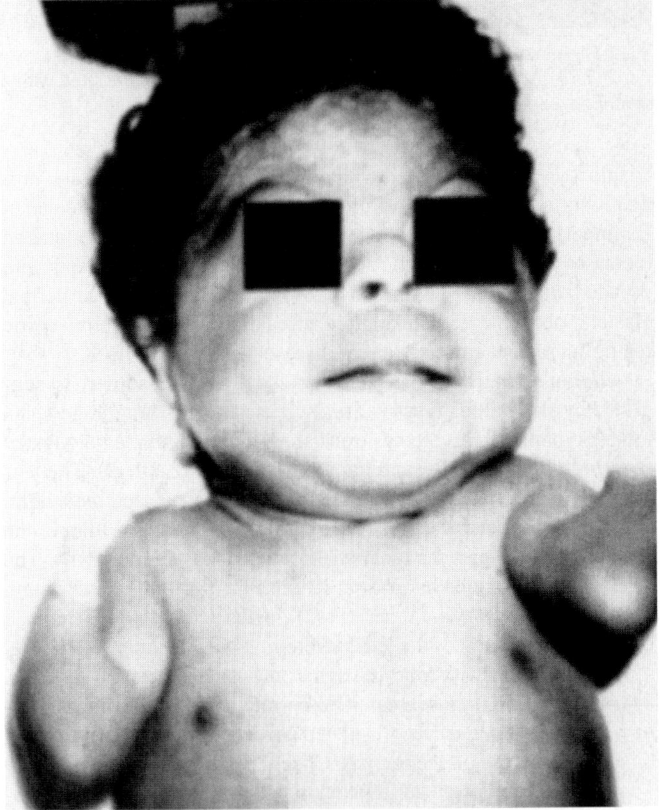

FIGURE 12-6 *Cornelia de Lange's syndrome:* low hairline, hirsutism, bushy brows, phocomelia, and a single thumb-like digit. May be associated with ventricular septal defect.

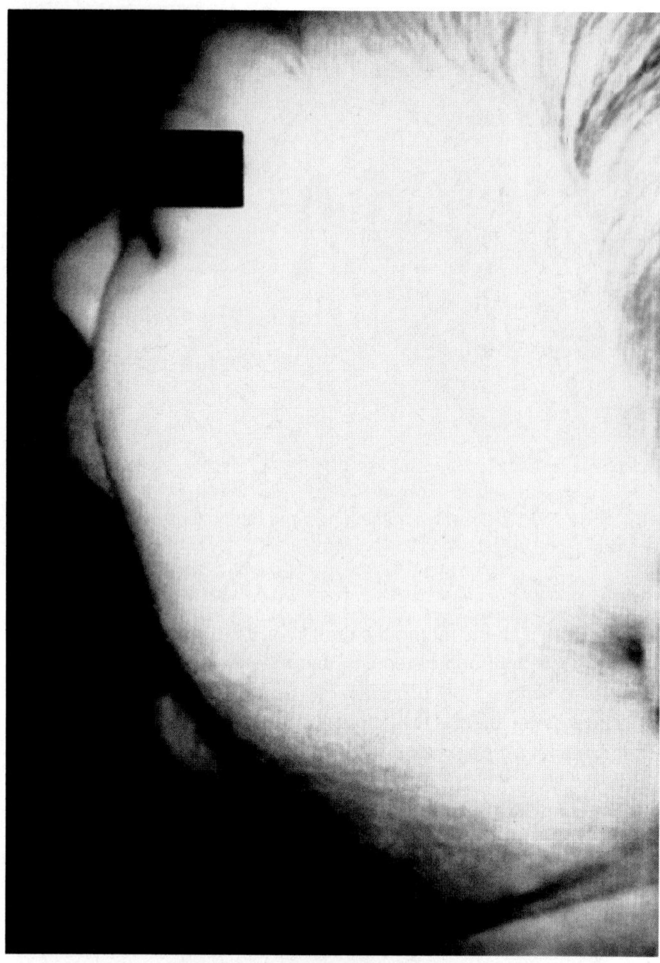

FIGURE 12-7 *Pierre Robin syndrome:* hypoplastic mandible associated with a ventricular septal defect.

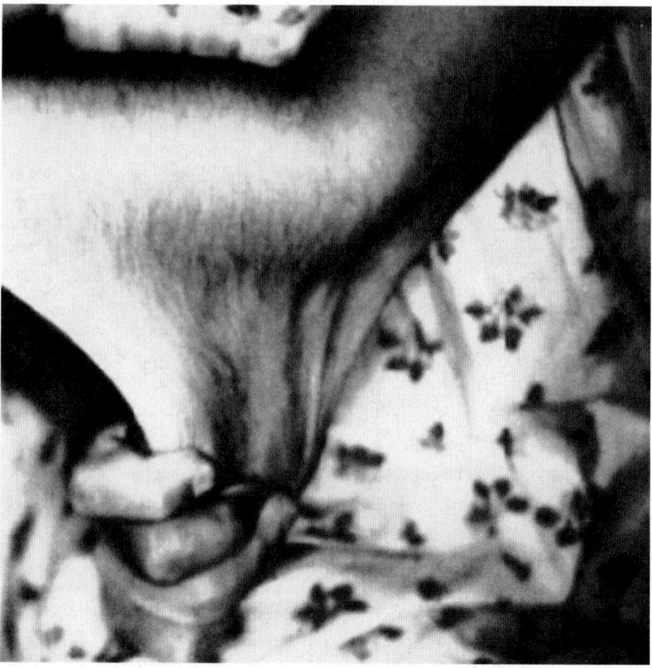

A

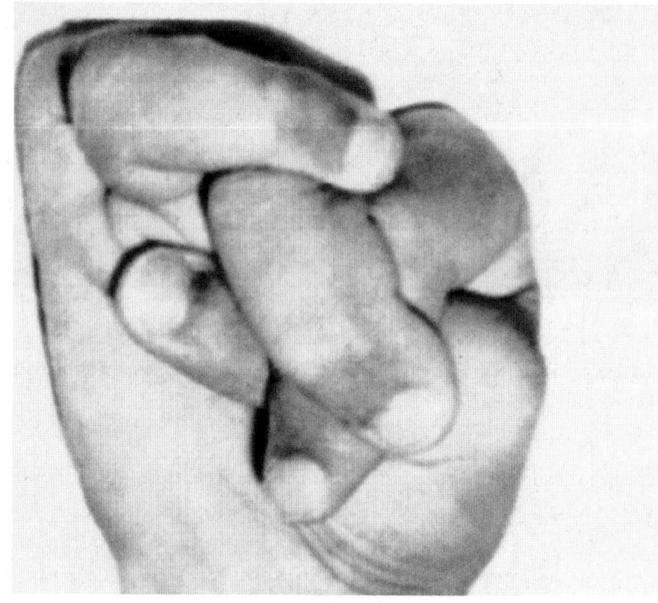

B

FIGURE 12-8 *Ehlers-Danlos syndrome. A.* Hyperextensible skin. *B.* Lax joints. Redundant chordae tendineae and arterial rupture may occur.

friable skin often associated with arterial dilatation and rupture, aortic regurgitation, or mitral valve prolapse.[51] Patients with osteogenesis imperfecta have brittle bones, blue sclera, and short legs and an increased incidence of aortic and mitral regurgitation.[52] Patients with pseudoxanthoma elasticum (Chap. 84) have degeneration of dermal elastic fibers and retinal angioid streaks and can develop aortic regurgitation and coronary artery disease (CAD) (Fig. 12-9).

Marfan's syndrome, an autosomal dominant disorder, is suggested by skeletal features such as increased height, long fingers, lax joints, kyphoscoliosis, pectus excavatum or carinatum, an elongated face, high-arched palate, and flat feet[53] (Fig. 12-10*A* to *D*). The legs are disproportionately long and the arm span may exceed the height. When a patient clenches the fingers around their flexed thumb, the thumb protrudes past the ulnar side of the hand ("thumb sign"). The wrist can be encircled by grasping it with the fifth finger and thumb of the other hand ("wrist sign") (Fig. 12-10*B*). Other findings include bilateral subluxation of the lens, severe myopia, and blue sclera (Fig. 12-10*D*). Patients with Marfan's syndrome usually have MVP (Chap. 84), mitral regurgitation, a calcified mitral annulus, and chordal rupture. AR is a consequence of a dilated aortic root, prolapse of the aortic cusps, or aortic dissection (see Chap. 84).

AR has been described in patients with inborn errors of metabolism, including Morquio's syndrome (mucopolysaccharidosis IV) and Scheie's syndrome (mucopolysaccharidosis V). Patients with Morquio's syndrome are identified by their short stature, short neck, barrel chest, broad mouth, short nose, widely spaced teeth, and cloudy cornea. In Scheie's syndrome, growth retardation, sternal protrusion, facial abnormalities, and cloudy cornea are present. In Fabry's disease, angiokeratomas—purplish pinpoint skin lesions—occur on the lips, underarm, buttocks, scrotum, and penis (Fig. 12-11). Cardiomyopathy, ischemic heart disease, and conduction defects are associated with this sex-linked recessive disorder in which there is a genetic deficiency of the enzyme alpha-galactosidase A.[54]

Many chromosomal abnormalities cause congenital heart disease. The well-recognized characteristics of Down's syndrome (trisomy 21) include a small head, shallow orbits, epicanthal folds, low-set ears, widely spaced eyes (hypertelorism), Brushfield's white spots of

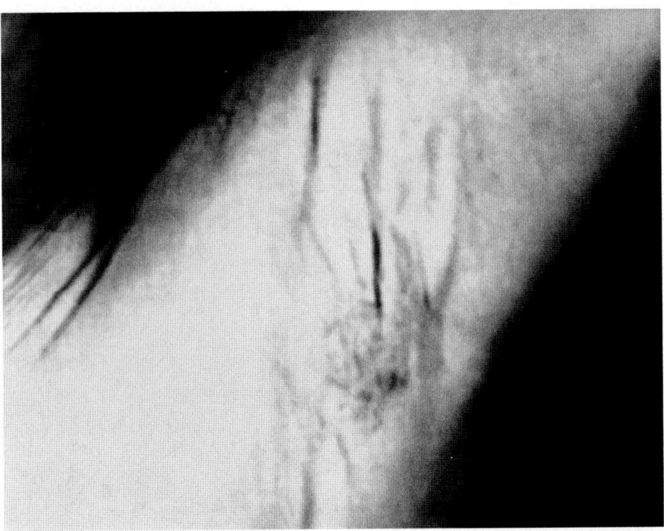

FIGURE 12-9 *Pseudoxanthoma elasticum:* grooved skin in a typical location. Arterial calcification may occur.

the iris, protruding tongue, transverse palmar creases, and mental retardation (Chaps. 72 and 73). Congenital heart disease occurs in 40 to 60 percent of patients; a VSD or endocardial cushion defect are the most frequent. Klinefelter's syndrome is characterized by gynecomastia, small testicles, a eunuchoid appearance, tall stature, and long extremities septum, proximum and secundum. ASDs have been described.

Congenital heart disease of varied types is common in trisomy 13 and trisomy 18 syndromes.[55] In trisomy 13 syndrome, the child has a cleft palate and lip; the ocular tissue and the nose may be missing. Polydactyly, retroflexible thumbs, transverse creases, hyperconvex narrow nails, and flexion of the fingers and hands are characteristic of this syndrome. The features of the trisomy 18 syndrome are a small, triangular mouth with receding chin, small mandible, webbed neck, and tightly clenched fists with the index finger overlapping the third finger and the fifth finger over the fourth (Fig. 12-12).

Low hairline, low-set ears, deafness, small jaw, and short, webbed neck are physical findings common to both Turner's syndrome and the Klippel-Feil syndrome. Turner's syndrome (Fig. 12-13) also includes short stature, broad chest with widely spaced nipples, epicanthal folds, widely spaced eyes, pigmented moles, ptosis, clinodactyly (curved fifth finger), and a shortened fifth finger.[56] Coarctation of the aorta, aortic stenosis, and hypertrophic cardiomyopathy are the cardiovascular considerations. The Klippel-Feil syndrome may cause facial asymmetry, cleft palate, torticollis, scoliosis, deafness, strabismus, and hydrocephaly. VSD is the most common cardiac disorder.

There are sporadic disorders associated with congenital heart disease. The VATER association includes vertebral defect, tracheoesophageal fistula, and radial and renal dysplasia. A ventricular defect occurs in 80 percent of these patients. The asplenia syndrome is associated with a high incidence of complex congenital heart disease. Cardiovascular malformations are found in 15 to 25 percent of newborns with omphalocele.

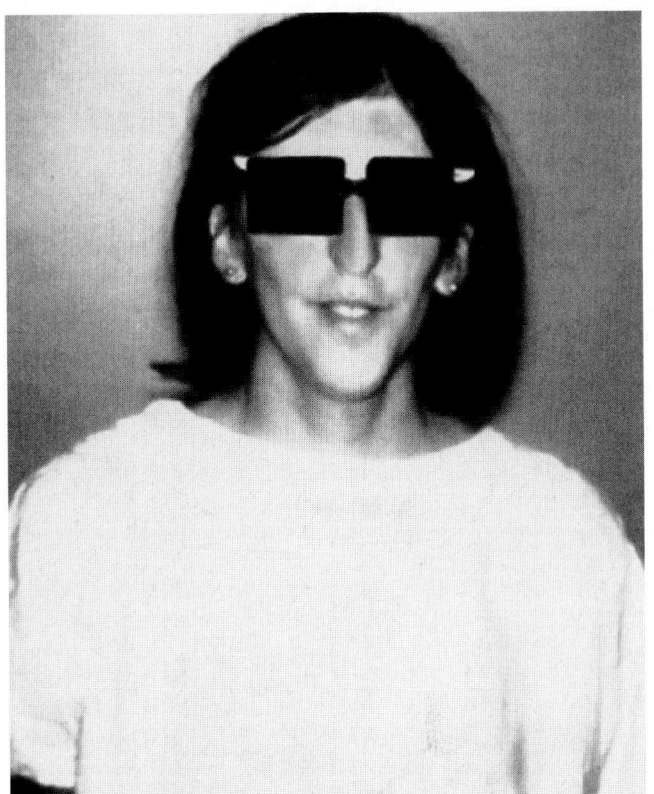

A

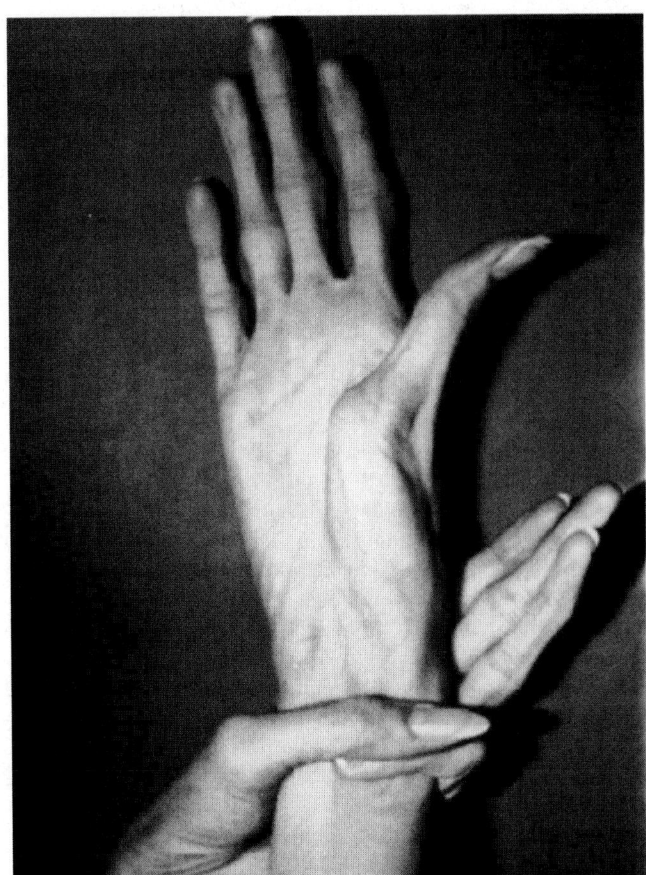

B

FIGURE 12-10 *Marfan's syndrome. A.* Long, narrow face. *B.* Arachnodactyly and positive wrist sign. *C.* High-arched palate. *D.* Ectopia lentis associated with aortic aneurysm and severe aortic regurgitation in a teenage girl.

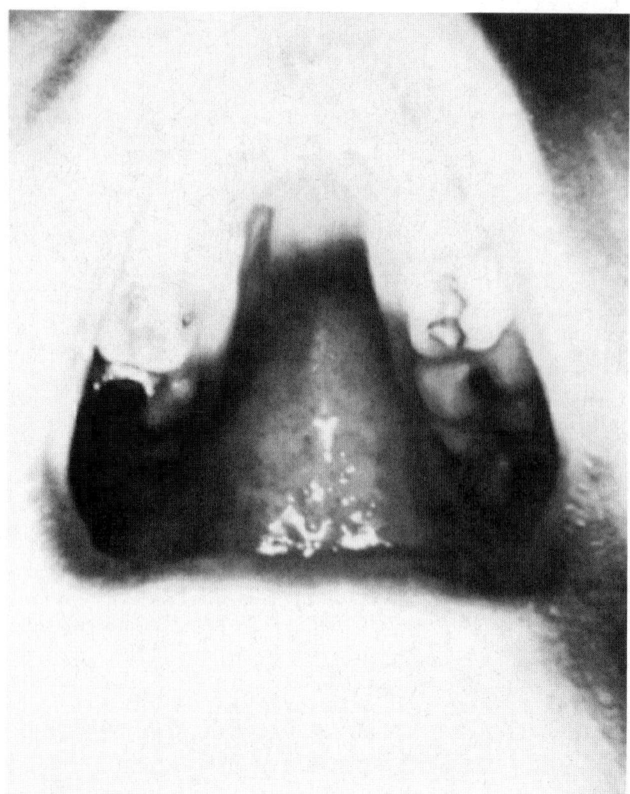

C

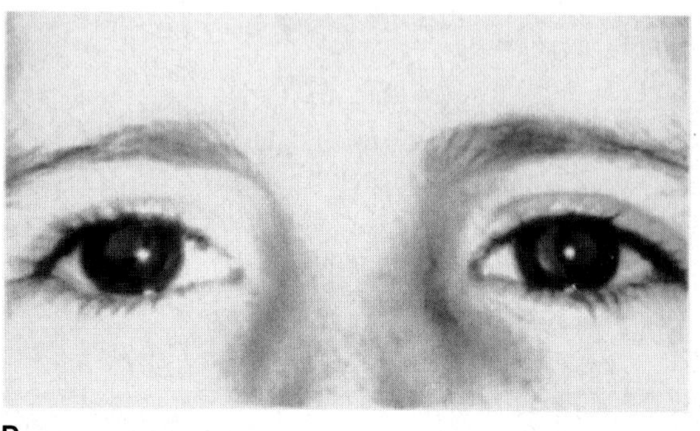

D

FIGURE 12-10 *(Continued)*

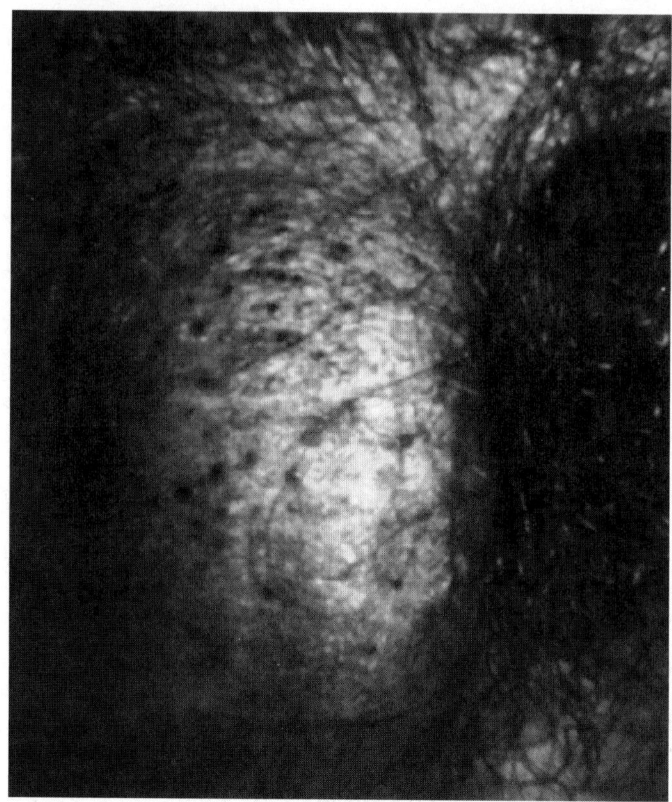

FIGURE 12-11 *Fabry's disease:* dark-red angiokeratomas on the penis may be linked with coronary artery disease.

Teratogenic effects resulting in congenital heart disease may be alcohol-related, the result of rubella during pregnancy, or induced by phenytoin, thalidomide, or lithium. From 30 to 40 percent of children born to alcoholic mothers are affected with the fetal alcohol syndrome. These children have an undeveloped-appearing central face because of maxillary hypoplasia, a small and upturned nose, an indistinct or smooth philtrum, micrognathia, and a thin upper lip and vermilion (Fig. 12-14). ASDs and VSDs are most common. The teratogenic effects of the rubella syndrome include cataracts, deafness, microcephaly, patent ductus arteriosus, pulmonic valvular and/or arterial stenosis, and ASD.

## Disorders Affecting the Valves

The cutaneous manifestations of infective endocarditis (Chap. 81) include Osler's nodes, Janeway lesions, clubbing of the fingers (Fig. 12-15*A* and *B*, Plate 34), splinter hemorrhages of the nails, and petechiae.[57] Osler's nodes are reddish purple, tender nodules typically found in the distal pad of the finger or toe (Fig. 12-15*A* and *B*, Plate 34). Janeway lesions are hemorrhagic, nontender, and involve the palms or soles. Splinter hemorrhages are linear, black, and appear in the distal third of the fingernail.

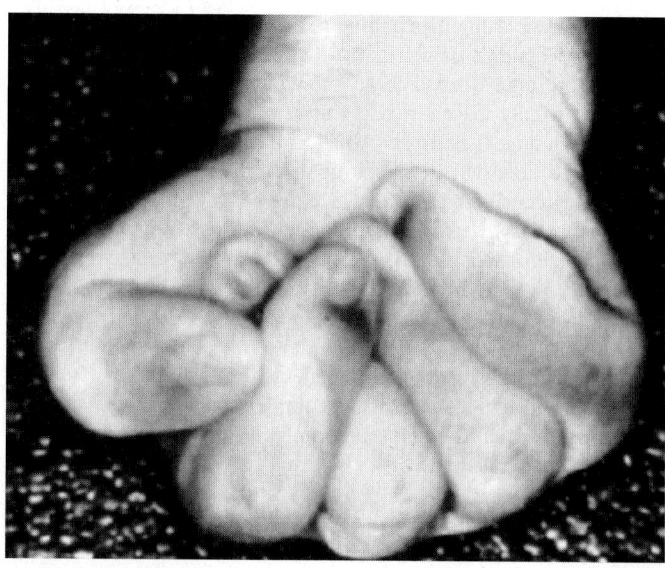

FIGURE 12-12 *Trisomy 18 syndrome:* tightly clenched fist with overlapping index and fifth fingers. A ventricular septal defect was present.

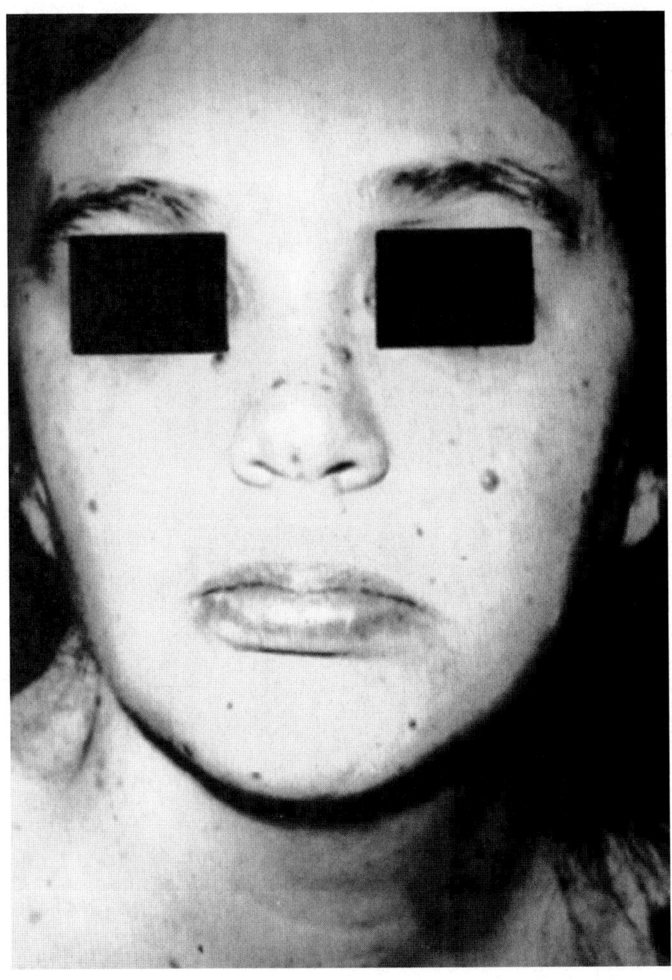

FIGURE 12-13 *Turner's syndrome:* epicanthal folds, pigmented moles, hypertelorism, and scars on the neck where webs have been removed. May be associated with coarctation of the aorta.

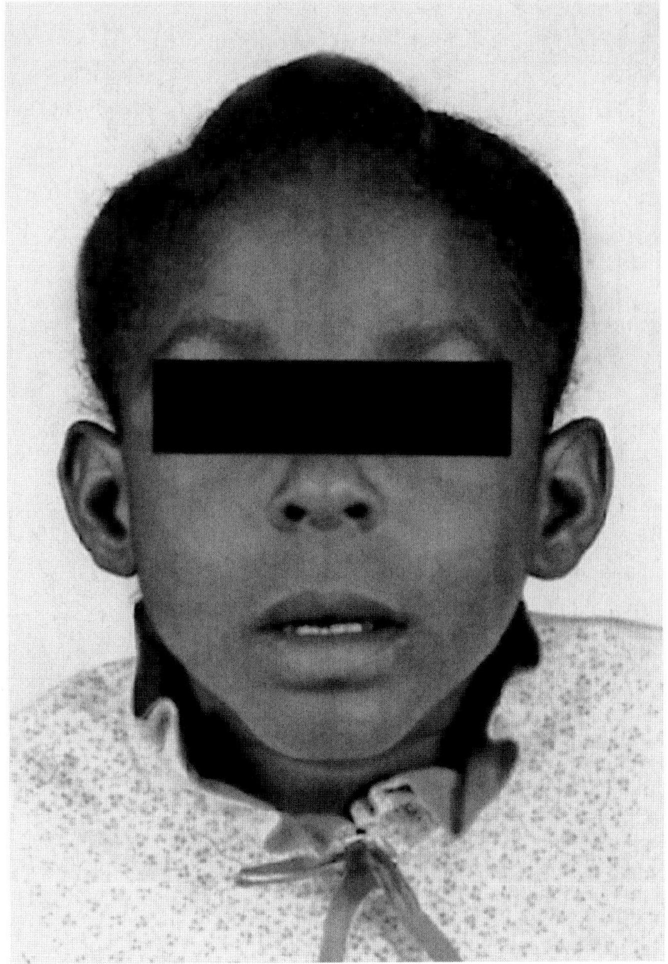

FIGURE 12-14 *Fetal alcohol syndrome:* midface hypoplasia, absent philtrum, and microcephaly associated with a ventricular septal defect.

Pulmonic stenosis may be part of Noonan's syndrome, Turner's syndrome, Rubinstein-Taybi syndrome, rubella syndrome, the multiple-lentigines syndrome, pulmonary valve dysplasia, or Watson's syndrome. In Noonan's syndrome,[58] the characteristic findings include ptosis, low-set ears, downward-slanting eyes, webbed neck, hypertelorism, low posterior hairline, short stature, mental retardation, normal chromosomes, and a dysplastic pulmonic valve (Fig. 12-16). Broad toes and thumbs, a slanting forehead, a thin, beaked nose, and large, low-set ears are seen in Rubinstein-Taybi syndrome (Fig. 12-17*A* and *B*).

The multiple lentigines syndrome is identified by the presence of multiple dark brown macules varying in size from pinpoint to 5 cm (Fig. 12-18). They cover the entire body but are most heavily concentrated on the neck and upper thorax.

The carcinoid syndrome (Chaps. 69 and 85) may present as intense flushing of the face and a chronic cyanotic hue. Telangiectasia may be present. Stenosis and/or regurgitation of the tricuspid and/or pulmonic valves can result when hepatic metastases are present.[59] When a patent ductus arteriosus, lung metastases, or a patent foramen ovale is present, the left-sided heart valves can also be affected.

In scleroderma, there is tightening of the skin of the fingers and then the hands, forearms, upper chest, and face. Subcutaneous tissue and skin creases disappear. Flexion contractures of the fingers may cause a clawlike hand deformity (Fig. 12-19). Raynaud's phenomenon is an early manifestation. The CREST syndrome (calcinosis, Raynaud's, esophageal involvement, sclerodactyly and telangiectasia) is a variant of scleroderma (Fig. 12-20). Valvular changes, including thickening of the edges of the mitral, aortic, and tricuspid valves, as well as thickening and shortening of the mitral chordae, are rarely significant.[60]

Joint disease is often associated with cardiac valvular disease and can occur with systemic lupus erythematosus (SLE), rheumatoid arthritis, rheumatic fever, polychondritis, ankylosing spondylitis, alkaptonuria, and Whipple's disease. In SLE, the joint inflammation is usually symmetric and nondeforming. Typical skin lesions include an erythematous, scaling eruption over the cheeks and bridge of the nose, circumscribed reddish purple plaques, telangiectasia, and patchy hair loss (Fig. 12-21). Verrucous endocarditis may involve any of the four cardiac valves; however, severe valvular dysfunction is unusual.[61]

In patients with rheumatoid arthritis, the wrists, shoulders, knees, ankles, and elbows may become inflamed. Advanced disease results in ulnar deviation of the fingers and flexion of the distal interphalangeal joints with hyperextension of the proximal interphalangeal joints, producing a "swan neck" deformity and a Z-shaped configuration of the thumb (Fig. 12-22, Plate 35). Granulomatous aortic or

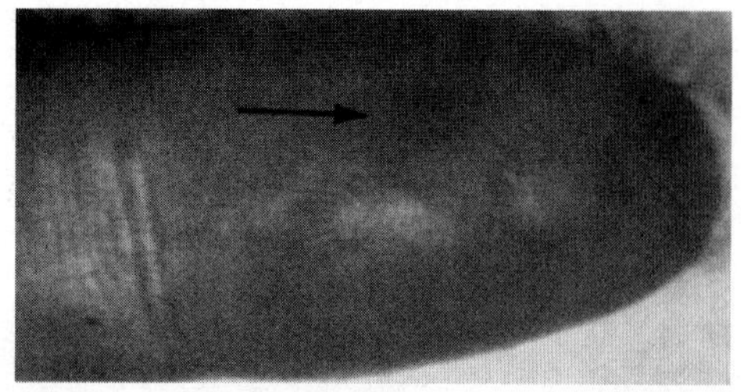


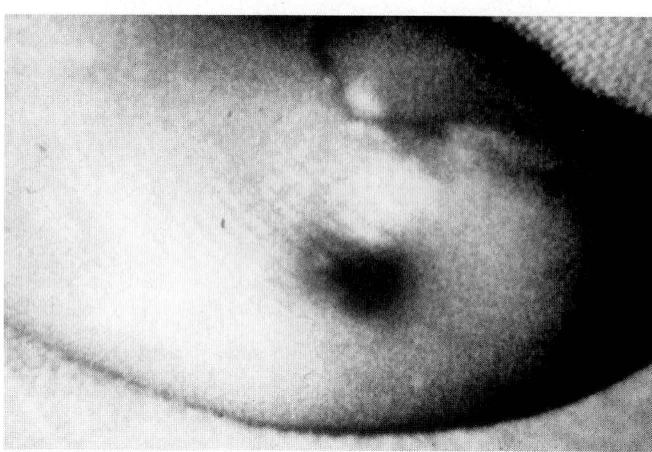


FIGURE 12-15 (PLATE 34) *Bacterial endocarditis: A.* Valvular infection associated with a tender, purplish nodule (Osler's node) in the finger pad (*arrow*). *B.* Osler's node from another patient.

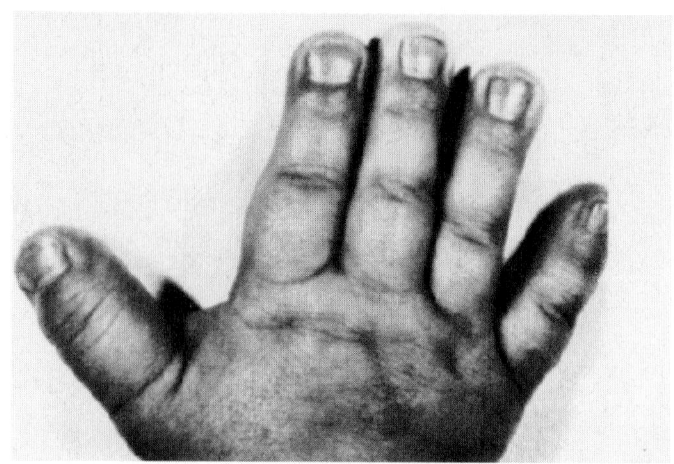

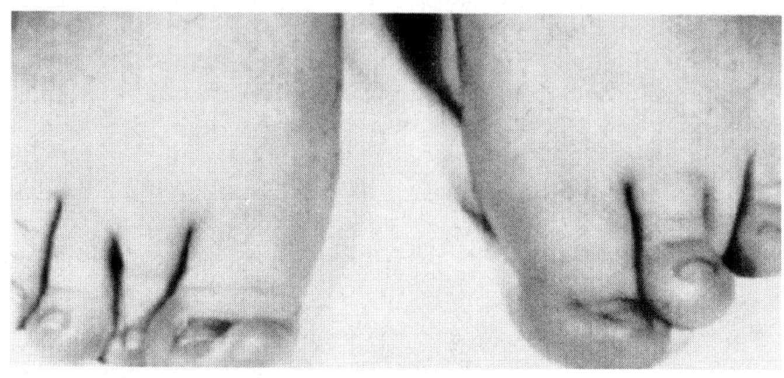

FIGURE 12-17 *Rubinstein-Taybi syndrome* may be associated with a variety of congenital heart defects. (From Silverman ME, Hurst JW. The hand and heart. *Am J Cardiol* 1968;22:718. Reproduced with permission from the publisher and authors.)

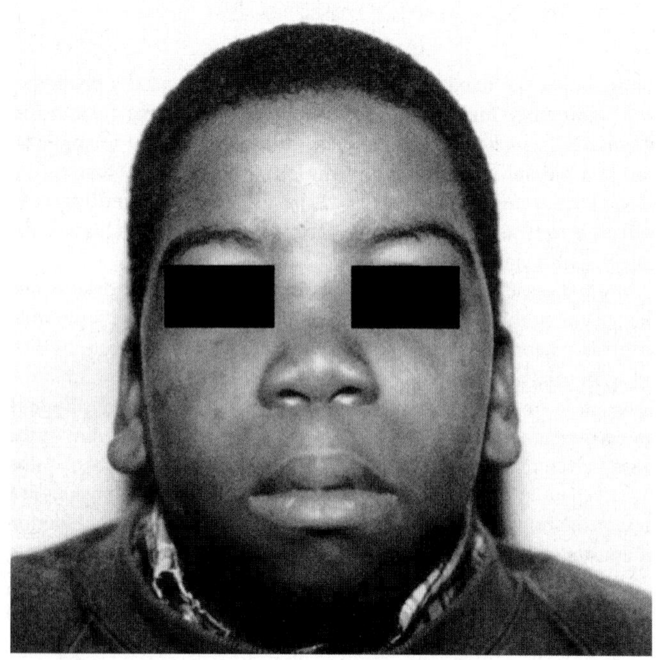

FIGURE 12-16 *Noonan's syndrome:* ptosis, hypertelorism, and low-set ears associated with valvular pulmonic stenosis.

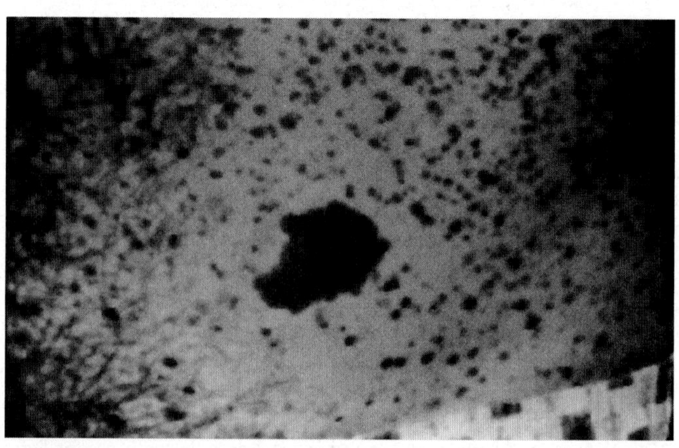

FIGURE 12-18 *Multiple lentigines syndrome:* dark-brown macular lesions of the abdomen associated with hypertrophic obstructive cardiomyopathy. (From Silverman ME. Visual clues to diagnosis. *Prim Cardiol* 1986;. Reproduced with permission from the publisher and author.)

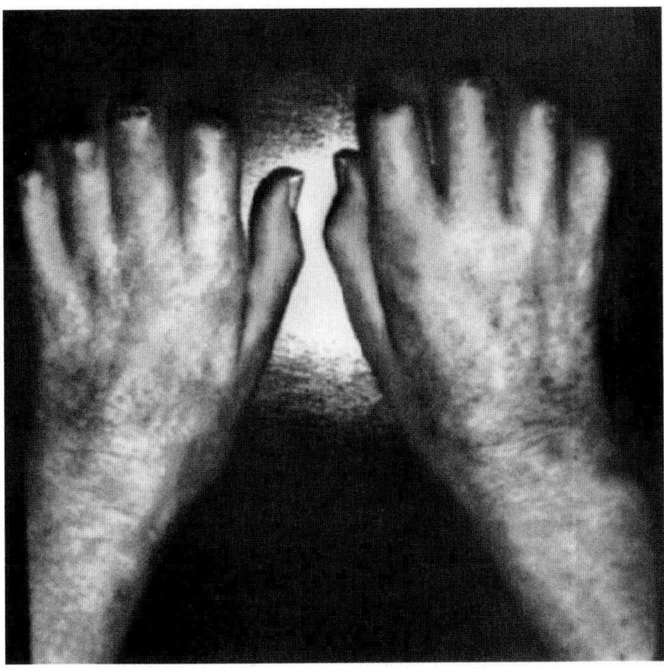

FIGURE 12-19 *Scleroderma:* clawlike hand deformity and shiny, tight skin. May be linked with myocardial fibrosis.

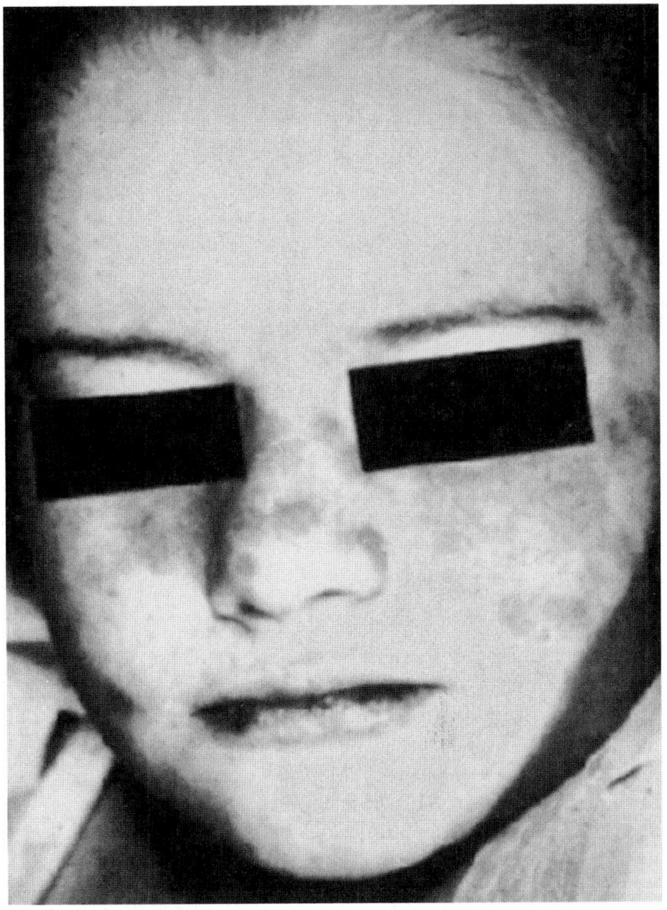

FIGURE 12-21 *Systemic lupus erythematosus:* butterfly rash associated with pericardial, myocardial, and endocardial disease.

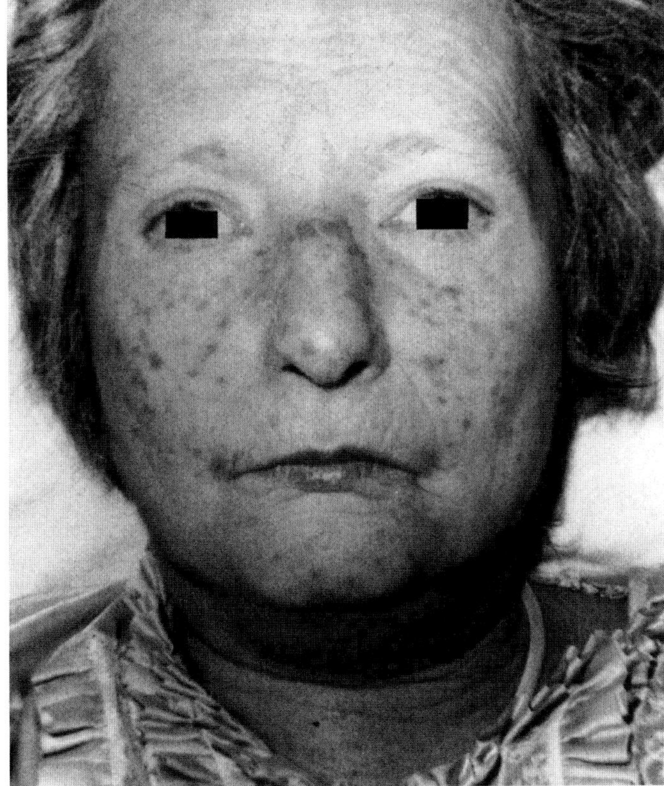

FIGURE 12-20 *CREST syndrome*. Telangiectasia of the face in a patient with Raynaud's phenomenon and sclerodactyly.

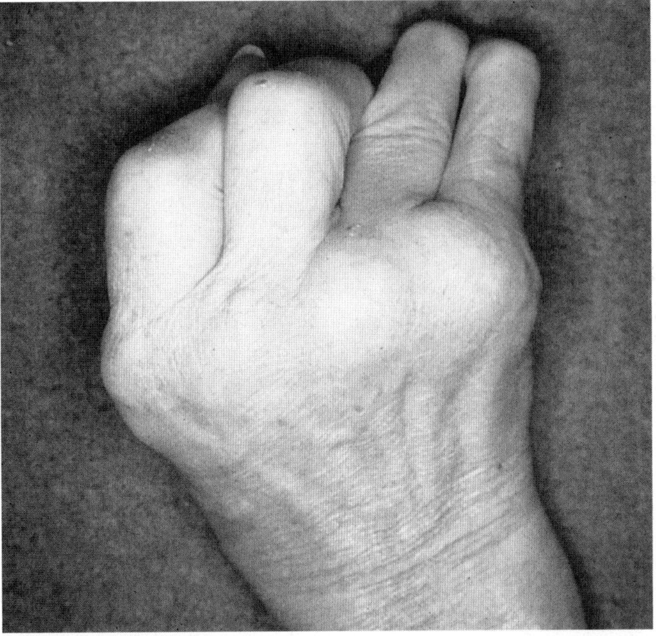

FIGURE 12-22 (Plate 35) *Rheumatoid arthritis:* with ulnar deviation of the fingers and flexion of the distal interphalangeal joints with hyperextension of the proximal interphalangeal joints.

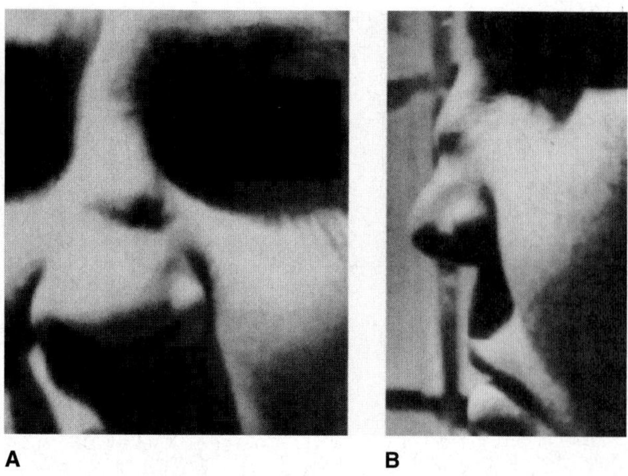

FIGURE 12-23 *Polychondritis. A* and *B*. Destruction of cartilage of the nose, producing a "saddle nose" deformity in association with aortic regurgitation. (Courtesy of Dr. Warren Sarrell, Anniston, AL.)

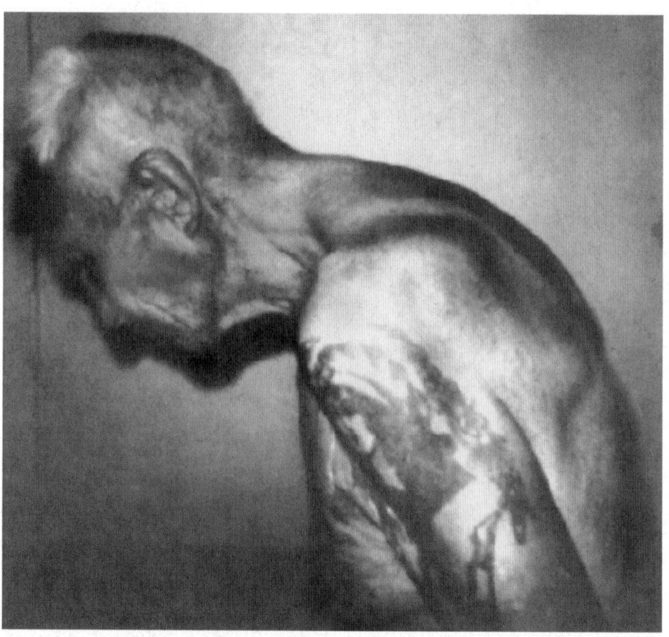

FIGURE 12-24 *Ankylosing spondylitis:* immobile, curved spine with forward jutting of head. May be seen with AV block or aortic regurgitation. (From Silverman ME. Visual clues to diagnosis. *Prim Cardiol* 1987;. Reproduced with permission from the publisher, author, and patient.)

mitral valve disease with regurgitation is most common in patients who are seropositive and have subcutaneous nodules or classic rheumatoid deformities. Rheumatic fever should be suspected in patients with erythema marginatum and migratory polyarthritis involving the large joints (Chap. 65). Marked ulnar deviation, suggesting rheumatoid arthritis, can be due to repeated attacks of rheumatic fever and is known as Jaccoud's arthritis. In contrast to rheumatoid arthritis, the fingers can be moved freely back into a correct alignment.

Polychondritis causes an inflammatory destruction of cartilage, resulting in a saddle-shaped collapse of the nose or a cauliflower ear. Aortic root dilatation and rarely dissection are associated[62] (Fig. 12-23*A* and *B*).

Chronic synovitis of the spine occurs in patients with ankylosing spondylitis. The patient with advanced disease is bent forward, unable to stand upright, and walks with a stiff and halting gait (Fig. 12-24). Aortic regurgitation, due to thickening and shortening of the aortic cusps from perivascular inflammation and fibrosis, mitral regurgitation, and complete heart block may occur.[63]

Whipple's disease is suggested by polyarthritis, abdominal pain, and diarrhea. Aortic and mitral regurgitation and endocarditis are known complications. Aortic or mitral valvular disease may be due to an accumulation of homogentisic acid in alkaptonuria. Blue-black, stiff ears and joints are important clues to this inherited disorder of tyrosine metabolism.

Patients with the MVP syndrome (Chap. 59) may have a straight thoracic spine, pectus excavatum, scoliosis, micromastia, and joint laxity (Fig. 12-25, Plate 36). Systolic and rarely diastolic murmurs have been described with chest wall deformities due to a straight-back syndrome and pectus excavatum that may impinge on or displace the heart.

## Disorders Associated with Cardiomyopathy

Hypertrophic cardiomyopathy (see Chap. 77) that may be concentric or asymmetric has been associated with Friedreich's ataxia, Turner's syndrome, Noonan's syndrome, Fabry's disease, neurofibromatosis, and the multiple-lentigines syndrome. Friedreich's ataxia is a spinocerebellar degenerative disorder that results in a broad-based, lurching gait, impaired vibration, position, and joint sense and incoordination.[64] Kyphoscoliosis and pes cavus (high instep, retraction of the toes at the metatarsophalangeal joints, and hammer toes) are two important physical signs (Fig. 12-26*A* and *B*).

Cor pulmonale may be secondary to pulmonary hypertension caused by kyphoscoliosis, restrictive lung disease, scleroderma, upper airway blockade by enlarged tonsils and adenoids, or the sleep apnea syndrome.[65]

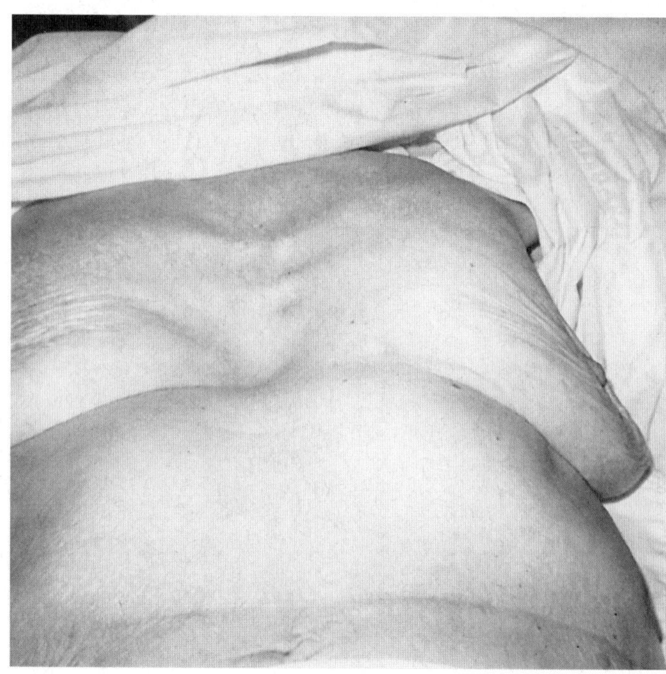

FIGURE 12-25 (Plate 36) Marked pectus excavatum.

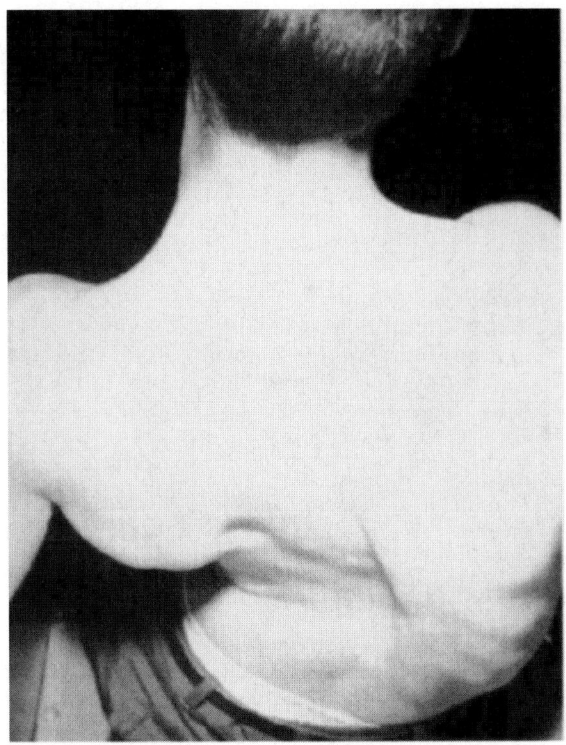

A

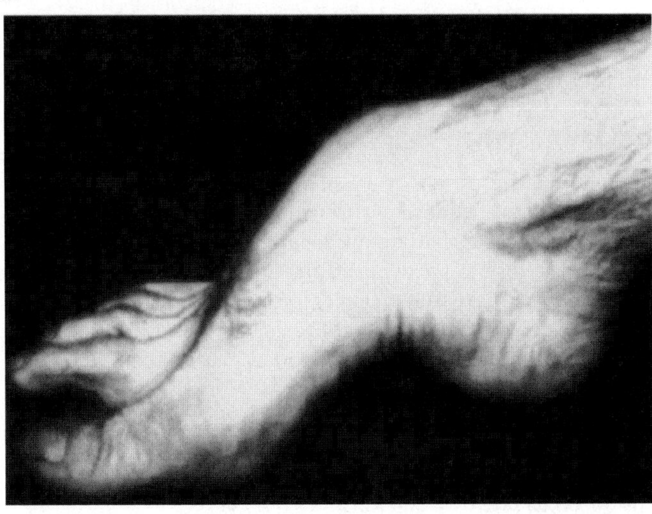

B

FIGURE 12-26 *Friedreich's ataxia* (photographs from different patients). *A.* Kyphoscoliosis. *B.* Pes cavus. Myocardial fibrosis and hypertrophy are often present. (From Silverman ME. Visual clues to diagnosis. *Prim Cardiol* 1987; . Reproduced with permission from the publisher and authors.)

Myocarditis (Chap. 79) occurs with SLE, rheumatic fever, Reiter's syndrome, Kawasaki's disease, Lyme arthritis,[66] and, occasionally, Whipple's disease. In Reiter's syndrome, conjunctivitis and hyperkeratotic coalescing lesions encrusted on the soles and palms, known as hyperkeratosis blenorrhagicum, are associated with arthritis and urethritis (Fig. 12-27, Plate 37). Kawasaki's disease begins with fever; nonexudative conjunctivitis; dry, fissured lips; cervical adenopathy; and a strawberry tongue. Later, the palms and soles become indurated, purplish red, and then peel. A widespread erythematous rash may appear and then desquamate. Lyme arthritis, caused by the spirochete *Borrelia burgdorferi,* begins with a red macule or papule and then develops into an expanding erythematous rash with a bright red border known as erythema migrans (Fig. 12-28). The center of the rash may clear, indurate, blister, or become necrotic. Multiple annular lesions may develop.[66]

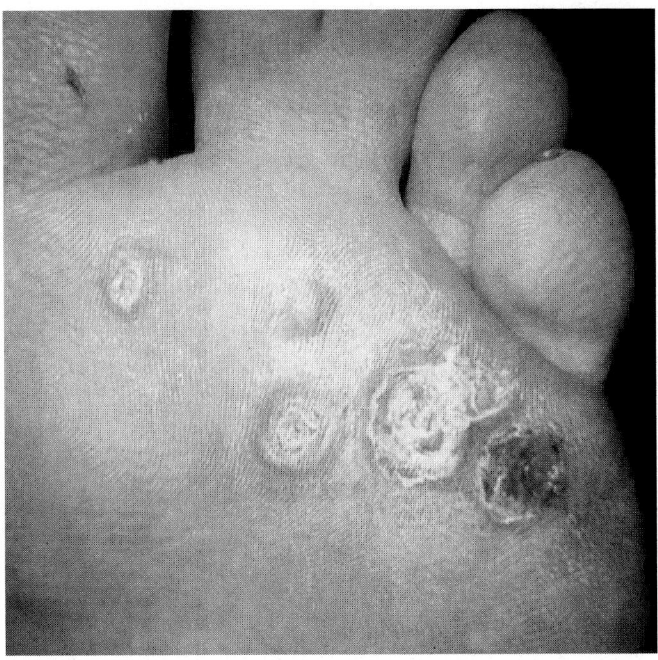

FIGURE 12-27 (Plate 37) *Hyperkeratotic lesions* encrusted on the soles of the feet in Reiter's syndrome.

Diseases that cause myocardial fibrosis include dermatomyositis, Duchenne's and Becker's muscular dystrophy, myotonic muscular dystrophy, Kearns-Sayre's syndrome, Friedreich's ataxia, sarcoidosis, and scleroderma (Chaps. 78 and 79). With dermatomyositis, a heliotropic discoloration is displayed on the upper eyelids (Fig. 12-29, Plate 38), and a scaly, erythematous papular rash—"Gottron's

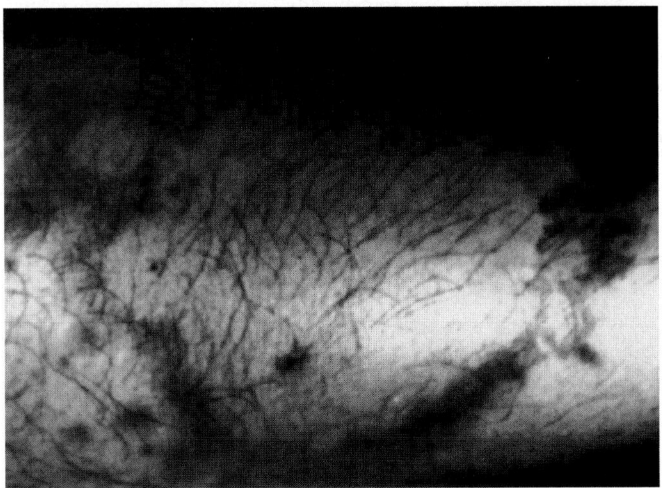

FIGURE 12-28 *Lyme arthritis:* annular expanding rash with a clear central area. May be associated with pericarditis and AV block. (From Silverman ME. Visual clues to diagnosis. *Prim Cardiol* 1986;. Reproduced with permission from the publisher and author.)

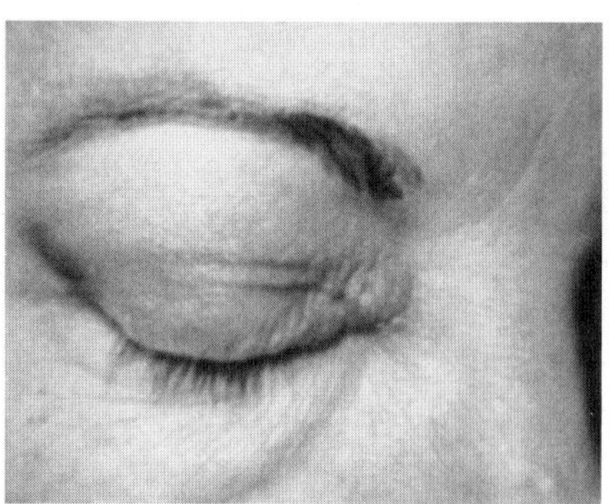

FIGURE 12-29 (Plate 38) *Dermatomyositis.* A violaceous hue and edema of upper eyelid may be associated with myocardial disease.

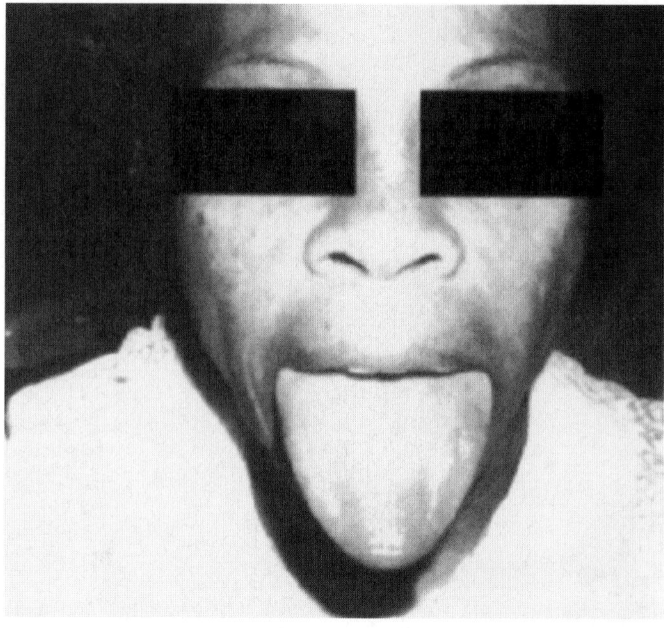

FIGURE 12-30 *Amyloidosis.* Enlarged tongue may be a sign of an infiltrative cardiomyopathy. (From Silverman ME. Visual clues to diagnosis. *Prim Cardiol* 1987;. Reproduced with permission from the publisher, author, and patient.)

papules"—may cover the knuckles, sparing the interphalangeal region. A waddling gait and pseudohypertrophic calves are characteristic of Duchenne's muscular dystrophy which may lead to fibrosis of the posterior left ventricle. In myotonic dystrophy, drooping eyelids, cataracts, a receding hairline, and a mask-like expression are present. The Kearns-Sayre syndrome is a form of ocular muscular dystrophy in which external ophthalmoplegia, ptosis, and retinitis pigmentosa occur.[67] Skin manifestations of sarcoidosis are common and include erythema nodosum, lupus pernio (a red or violet plaque formation with a predilection for the nasolabial folds, eyelids, and ears), and waxy translucent papules found on the cheeks, periorbital area, ears, and elsewhere.[68] Uveitis, bilateral parotid and lacrimal gland enlargement, and arthritis are other signs (Chap. 78).

Infiltrative diseases of the myocardium include Wilson's disease, Cori's disease, Fabry's disease, hemochromatosis, amyloidosis, glycogen storage disease, and sarcoidosis (Chap. 78). Wilson's disease is an autosomal recessive disorder in which copper accumulates in tissues, including the myocardium.[69] Arrhythmias, autonomic dysfunction, and cardiomyopathy have been reported. Kayser-Fleischer rings, usually golden-brown in color and circling the edge of the cornea, provide a major clue to the correct diagnosis.

In hemochromatosis, the skin has a bronze or slate-gray coloration; myocardial infiltration with iron deposits can cause a dilated or rarely a restrictive cardiomyopathy associated with arrhythmias and heart failure. Macroglossia with indentations, waxy nodules of the skin and eyelids due to fibrillar protein deposition, and "pinch purpura" are clues to the diagnosis of amyloidosis[70] (Fig. 12-30) (Chap. 78).

## Disorders Associated with Pericardial Disease

Pericarditis may be a result of Reiter's syndrome, Whipple's disease, Kawasaki's disease, SLE, rheumatoid arthritis,[71] rheumatic fever, sarcoidosis, scleroderma, dermatomyositis, hemochromatosis, Behçet's syndrome, Degos' disease, uremia, mulibrey nanism, polychondritis, hypothyroidism, or metastatic disease (Chap. 80). The components of Behçet's syndrome include erythema nodosum, superficial phlebitis, oral and genital ulcers, and iritis.[72] Patients with Degos' disease (malignant atrophic papulosis) present with painless, oval cutaneous lesions that have a white center and surrounding erythema. In this rapidly fatal disease, occlusive fibrosis of small and medium-sized arteries produces pleuritis and pericarditis. In far-advanced renal disease, urochrome pigmentation of the skin and uremic frost can be cutaneous manifestations. Hypothyroidism, a cause of massive pericardial effusion, thickens the face and causes dry hair, puffy eyelids, and an enlarged tongue. Pericarditis is common in SLE but only rarely the presenting manifestation.[61]

## Disorders Causing Conduction System Disease

Acquired causes of atrioventricular (AV) block or bundle branch block include sarcoidosis,[68] rheumatic fever, gout, Reiter's syndrome,[73] dermatomyositis, polychondritis, amyloidosis, Kawasaki's disease, ankylosing spondylitis, SLE, and Lyme arthritis.[66] In gout, uric acid crystals may form nodules affecting the conduction system. AV block may be an early cardiac manifestation of ankylosing spondylitis. Maternal lupus is an important cause of congenital complete AV block in the newborn.[61]

Inherited disorders associated with conduction defects include Fabry's disease, Friedreich's ataxia, Kearns-Sayre syndrome, the multiple-lentigines syndrome, muscular dystrophy, myotonic dystrophy, tuberous sclerosis, and Refsum's disease.

There is a high incidence of paroxysmal complete AV block with myotonic dystrophy, and pacing is often necessary.[74]

## Disorders Affecting the Vascular System

Aortic aneurysms and dissection (Chap. 98) are frequent cardiovascular complications of Marfan's and Ehlers-Danlos syndromes. Aneurysms of other vessels and arterial rupture may also occur. A progressive looseness of skin producing pendulous folds and droopy eyelids can be due to cutis laxa, a generalized destruction of elastic tissue that can cause dilatation of the aorta or rupture of the pulmonary artery and aorta. Coronary aneurysms and occlusion—leading to arrhythmia, infarction, and sudden death—are late sequelae of Kawasaki disease which may present in a young adult.[75]

Coronary atherosclerosis can be associated with hyperlipidemia, cerebrotendinous xanthomatoses, Werner's syndrome, uremia, progeria, acromegaly, and diabetes mellitus. Hyperlipidemia may be suspected when xanthomas or arcus senilis are present. Xanthelasma is a skin condition usually involving lipid-laden plaques on the upper eyelid. When it occurs before age 50, there is a strong association with familial hyperlipidemia and premature CAD. Eruptive xanthomata are recognized as 1- to 4-mm papules with yellow centers surrounded by an erythematous halo. They often appear with a sudden outbreak of discrete lesions on the buttocks, back, thighs, and exterior surfaces of the knees and elbows. They indicate a very high level of triglycerides and are associated with hyperlipidemia, diabetes mellitus, pancreatitis, myxedema, and the nephrotic syndrome. Tendon xanthomata are firm, painless nodules that thicken the exterior tendons of the hand, the Achilles tendons, and sometimes the tendons of the knees and elbows in patients with familial type II hyperlipidema (Fig. 12-31*A* and *B*).

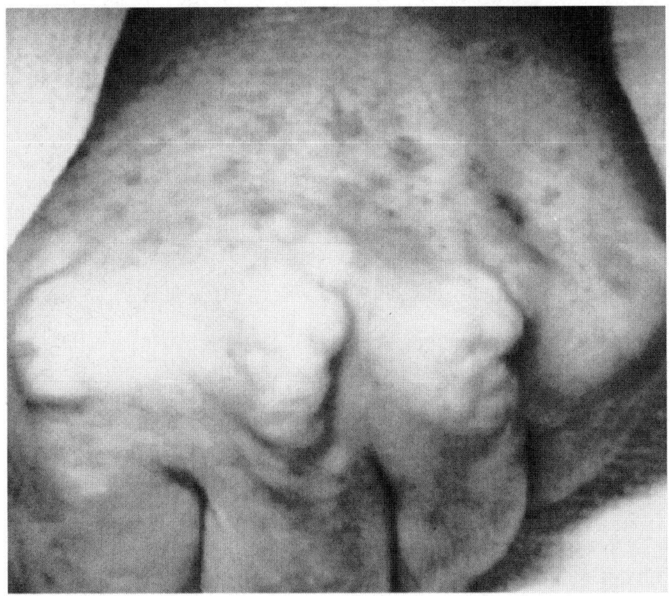

A

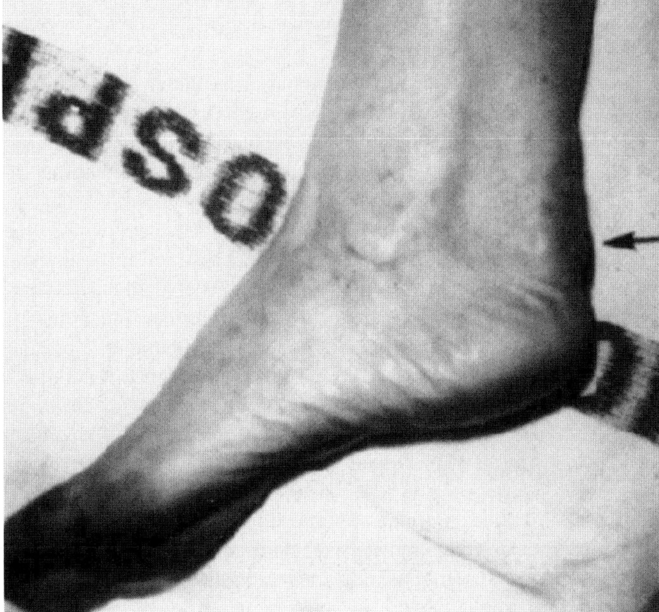

B

FIGURE 12-31 *Hyperlipidemia:* xanthomata associated with coronary artery disease. *A*. On the extensor tendons of the hand. *B*. On the Achilles tendon (*arrow*).

In Werner's syndrome, the skin is tightly stretched over the underlying bones. There is marked loss of subcutaneous tissue, and ulcerations occur over the legs. Severe coronary atherosclerosis often results in myocardial infarction at an early age. Physical findings in diabetes mellitus may include tight skin and necrobiosis diabeticorum, an atrophy of the skin of the lower extremities characterized by ovoid plaques with central telangectasia and a violet, indurated perimeter. Progeria is a rare disorder in which the face is small and prematurely aged, the eyes bulge, and the nose is beaked. Severe atherosclerosis is a common cause of death in early life. A diagonal earlobe crease is curiously associated with coronary artherosclerosis and stroke[76] and present in 60 percent of patients, including virtually all with onset before age 40 (Fig. 12-32, Plate 39). Patients with homocystinuria resemble those with Marfan's syndrome because they have long extremities, pectus carinatum, and kyphoscoliosis. Their cardiac disease differs from Marfan's, with homocystinuria causing premature coronary disease. Pseudoxanthoma elasticum has been associated with fibrosis of the coronary artery and calcification of peripheral arteries (Chap. 84). A glycosphingolipid is deposited in the arterial endothelium of patients with Fabry's disease and may result in angina pectoris or MI. Patients with Hurler's syndrome have mental retardation; a large, boat-shaped head; a broad nose; large lips; small, widely spaced teeth; and a large, protuberant tongue. Glycosaminoglycan deposition in the coronary arteries is present.[77] Myocardial fibrosis due to repeated spasm of the small coronary vessels has been postulated to be a result of scleroderma.[60]

Vasculitis may be due to SLE, rheumatoid arthritis, Behçet's syndrome, Kawasaki disease, and polyarteritis. Cutaneous infarction, nodules, petechiae, livedo reticularis, gangrenous digits, MI, heart failure, and hypertension may be due to polyarteritis (Chap. 84). Cholesterol emboli, due to extensive aortic atherosclerosis, causes livedo reticularis and embolic/gangrenous changes in the toes simulating polyarteritis.

Arteriovenous shunts may be found in extensive skin disease, hereditary hemorrhagic telangiectasia, and the Klippel-Trenaunay-Weber

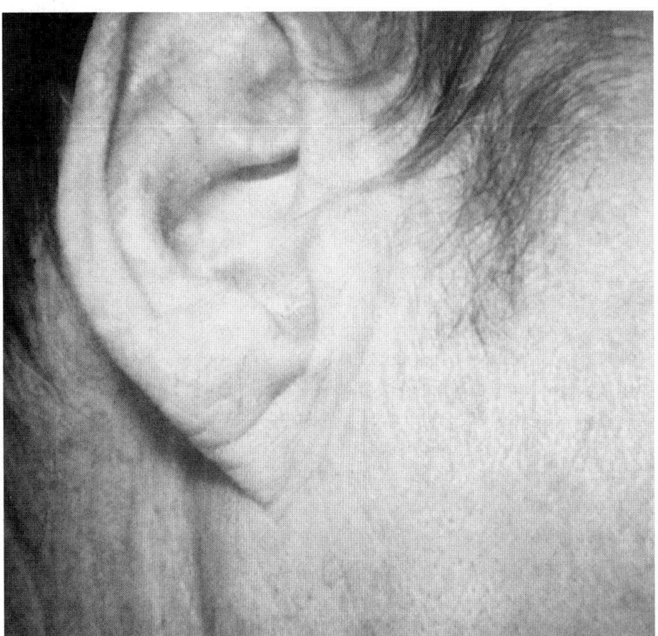

FIGURE 12-32 (Plate 39) Horizontal ear creases are often associated with the presence of extensive CAD.

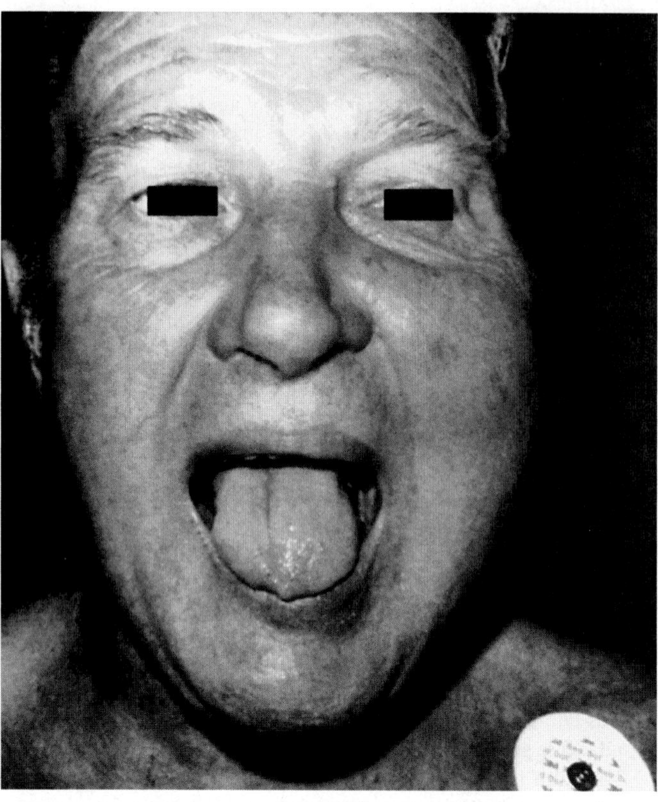

FIGURE 12-33 *Klippel-Trenaunay syndrome:* hypertrophy of left side of face and tongue in a patient with port-wine stains, gigantism of digits, and varicose veins.

syndrome. Kaposi's sarcoma or exfoliative dermatitis due to psoriasis may divert the blood supply through shunts in the skin to produce high-output cardiac failure. Telangiectasias of the fingertips, face, palate, lips, and tongue, as well as pulmonary and hepatic arteriovenous fistulas, are components of hereditary hemorrhagic telangiectasia (Osler-Weber-Rendu syndrome).[78] The triad of anomalies that Klippel-Trenaunay-Weber syndrome comprises are vascular nevus, large varices, and bony or soft tissue hypertrophy (Fig. 12-33). Marked enlargement of a limb(s) and facial hemihypertrophy are features of this disorder, in which part or all of the deep venous system is absent and arteriovenous malformation is often present. Hemangiomas of the skin also may indicate multinodular hemangiomatosis of the liver, a cause of high-output heart failure in infancy.

Stenosis of large arteries may occur with supravalvular aortic stenosis, rubella syndrome, Turner's syndrome, and neurofibromatosis. The face of a child with supravalvular aortic stenosis (Williams syndrome) is diagnostic (Fig. 12-34). The head is small, with an elflike appearance; the cheeks are full and baggy; and the mouth and forehead are large.[79] Curved lips and peg-shaped, widely spaced teeth are typical. Mental retardation is often present. Pulmonic artery branch stenosis is frequently present. Coarctation of the aorta is a common cardiac lesion in Turner's syndrome,[53] and neurofibromatosis has been associated with renal artery stenosis.

## Miscellaneous Disorders

Multiple lentigines, cutaneous myxomas, myxoid fibroadenomas of the breast, and various endocrine abnormalities are features of an inherited disorder in which single or multiple cardiac myxomas occur.

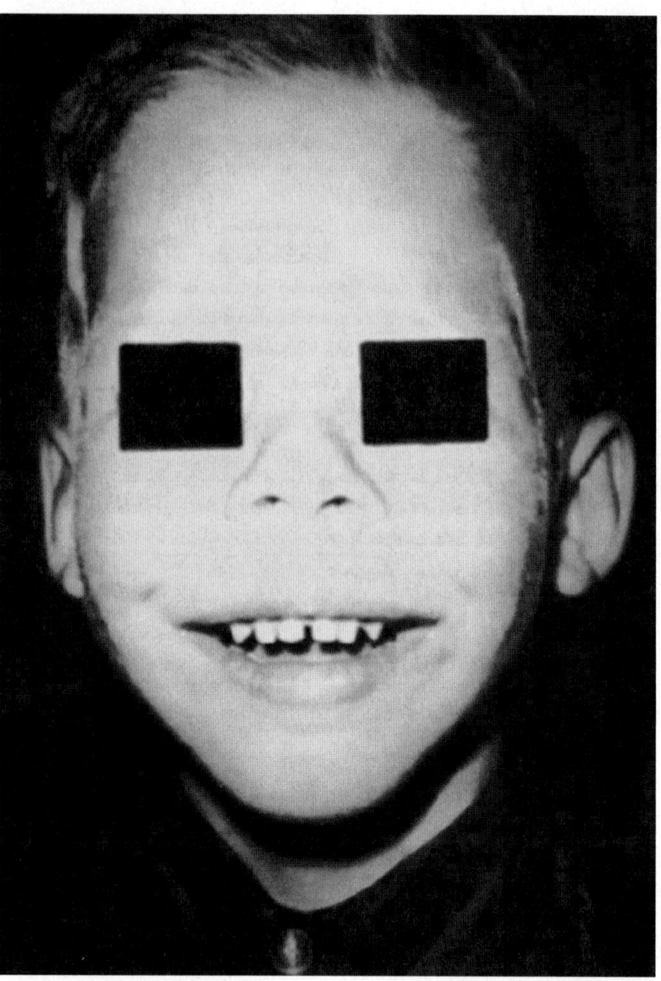

FIGURE 12-34 *Supravalvular aortic stenosis:* turned-up nose, broad cheeks, large mouth with peg-shaped teeth, and large ears.

A susceptibility to atrial fibrillation and atrial flutter has been documented in patients who have facioscapulohumeral muscular dystrophy.[80] Sinus node dysfunction with atrial paralysis, elbow contractures, and humeroperoneal weakness are manifestations of Emery-Dreifuss muscular dystrophy.[81]

Single or multiple rhabdomyomas may develop within the myocardium and cause heart failure, valvular obstruction, or arrhythmias in patients with tuberous sclerosis.[82] The diagnosis is suggested by the presence of yellow-brown angiofibromas (adenoma sebaceum) on the face (Fig. 12-35, Plate 40), subungual fibromas around the fingernail, café-au-lait spots, and subcutaneous nodules.

# MEASUREMENT OF ARTERIAL BLOOD PRESSURE

For the noninvasive assessment of arterial BP, a pneumatic cuff with a mercury or aneroid manometer is the most commonly used method for assessing the status of the circulation and the interaction between the heart and arterial system. BP measurements outside normal limits often provide important diagnostic information in patients with a variety of cardiac and noncardiac diseases. Accordingly, the BP is best recorded by the *physician* during his or her *initial physical examination*.

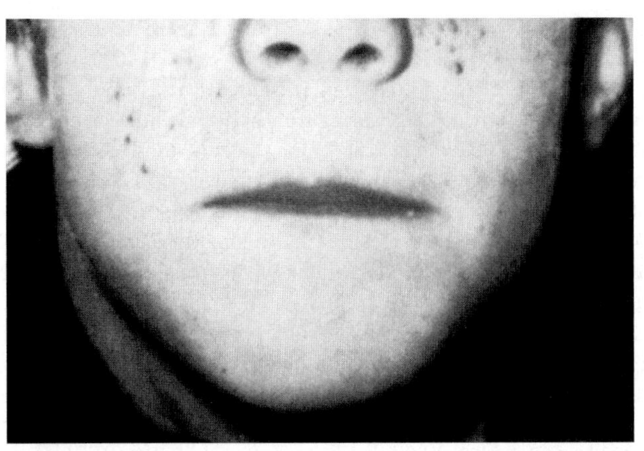

FIGURE 12-35 (Plate 40) Tuberous sclerosis. Adenoma sebaceum may be associated with rhabdomyomas of the myocardium.

## Physical Determinants of the Arterial Pressure

The arterial BP, a measure of lateral force per unit area of vascular wall, is quantitated as millimeters of mercury (mmHg) or dynes per square centimeter (d/cm$^2$). The factors responsible for the peak systolic BP include the volume and velocity of LV ejection, the peripheral arteriolar resistance, the distensibility of the arterial wall, the viscosity of the blood, and the end-diastolic volume in the arterial system.[83] The subsequent diminution in pressure during diastole is determined by blood viscosity, arterial distensibility, peripheral resistance to flow, and length of the cardiac cycle.[84] Important physical factors affecting arterial distensibility include (1) the elastic modulus of the arterial wall, the ratio of stress (force acting to deform the wall) to strain (the proportional deformation produced), and (2) the geometry of the arterial wall, i.e., the internal radius ($r$) and wall thickness ($h$), which govern wall tension ($T$) according to the modified Laplace equation $T = Pr/h$, where $P$ is intravascular pressure. A decrease in elasticity or an increase in radius results in diminished distensibility and a greater rise in pressure per unit volume of blood.[85]

The mean arterial pressure is the product of the cardiac output and the total peripheral resistance, the latter often being increased by several mechanisms, including $\alpha$-adrenergic stimulation, the renin-angiotensin system, or other circulating hormonal or humoral factors.[86]

## Methods for Measuring the Arterial Pressure

### DIRECT METHODS

In 1733, Stephen Hales recorded the arterial pressures in animals by cannulation and use of a blood-filled glass column.[86] Current methods for the direct and continuous measurement of arterial pressure use the electromanometer, a transducer that converts mechanical energy into an electric signal that is amplified, displayed, and recorded. The artery is cannulated with a saline-filled catheter or needle that mechanically couples the circulation to the arterial manometer. Pressures are recorded using atmospheric pressure as the "zero" reference level, and intravascular pressures are further referenced to the level of the heart by addition or subtraction of a gravitation factor. The gravitation factor is expressed as $pgh$, where $p$ is the density of blood (in grams per milliliter), $g$ is the acceleration due to gravity (980 cm/s), and $h$ is the transducer height (centimeters) above or below the horizontal plane of the heart.

The strain-gauge manometer is commonly used for the precise and accurate measurement of the arterial pressure. However, error may originate in the catheter or coupling system when the properties of inertia, friction, and elasticity interact to produce damping of the frequency response. Systems may be overdamped or underdamped; either can result in signal distortion. Nevertheless, the appropriate combination of an inelastic cardiac catheter and connecting tube filled with bubble-free fluid produces "critical" damping with the system response constant to some desirable frequency level and adequate for the clinical recording of intravascular pressures.[83]

Measurement errors also occur when an end-hole catheter is positioned axial to flow in a vessel and may become especially important during high arterial flow, when kinetic energy may exceed 10 percent of the total fluid energy. Also, pressure transients due to catheter whip can falsely elevate the measured arterial pressure.[83]

Miniature, self-flushing strain-gauge manometers attached directly to an intravascular catheter or needle eliminate many of the problems related to transducer mounting and flushing and overdamping by connective tubing. A more effective method for reducing measurement errors, however, is the use of intravascular electromanometers mounted on cardiac catheters or surgically implanted in the vascular wall.

### INDIRECT METHODS

The invention of the pneumatic cuff manometer (Riva-Rocci, 1896) and the subsequent discovery and use of the arterial sounds (Korotkoff, 1905) enabled indirect measurement of the arterial pressure. The mercury manometer is the "gold standard," and the more fragile aneroid manometer should be calibrated against the mercury manometer at least every 6 months. Semiautomatic electronic devices, if used, should be validated according to Association for the Advancement of Medical Instrumentation (AAMI) guidelines.[87] The most commonly used noninvasive method is based on the auscultatory detection of low-pitched Korotkoff sounds over a peripheral artery at a point distal to cuff compression of the artery. McCutcheon and Rushmer[88] defined two major components of these sounds: the initial transient ($k_{-i}$) and the compression murmur ($k_c$), which coincide with the opening tap and rumble sounds of Rodbard.[89] The initial sound, $k_{-i}$, occurs when cuff pressure reaches arterial pressure and likely results from abrupt arterial opening and vascular distention. The intensity of this initial sound depends on the slope of the pressure pulse and the level of the distal arterial pressure at the time of arterial opening, the sound being louder with vasodilatation and high-velocity flow and softer with arterial constriction or circulatory collapse. The initial transient is probably caused by oscillation of the arterial walls as the occluded segment is suddenly opened by systolic pressure, and the compression murmur is caused by a turbulent jet of flow distal to the partially compressed segment.

The Korotkoff sounds have been divided into five phases occurring in sequence as the occluding pressure declines (Table 12-4). To avoid error, the observer must be prepared to recognize two normal Korotkoff sound variations associated with BP reading: (1) The *auscultatory gap* is a period of silence occurring during Korotkoff phases I and II. This disappearance of sound is temporary and is usually short, but the gap can occur over a period of 40 mmHg. It seems to be more prominent with higher BP readings. (2) An absent Korotkoff phase V occurs when sounds are heard to "0." When this is the case, phase IV should be recorded along with phase V. In this case, phase IV is the best reference for diastolic pressure.

Proper technique is important for accurate measurement. The inflatable rubber bag within the compression cuff should have a width that is 20 percent greater than the limb diameter and a length

TABLE 12-4 Phases of the Korotkoff Sounds

Phase I
The pressure level at which the first faint, consistent tapping sounds are heard. The sounds gradually increase in intensity as the cuff is deflated. The first of at least two of these sounds is defined as the systolic pressure.
Phase II
The time during cuff deflation when a murmur of swishing sounds are heard.
Phase III
The period during which sounds are crisper and increase in intensity.
Phase IV
The time when a distinct, abrupt, muffling of sound (usually of a soft blowing quality) is heard. This is defined as the diastolic pressure in anyone in whom sounds continue to zero.
Phase V
The pressure level when the last regular blood pressure sound is heard and after which all sound disappears. This is defined as the diastolic pressure unless sounds are heard to zero.

adequate to encompass two-thirds the limb. The cuff should be applied snugly, with the inflatable bag positioned over the artery, at the level of the heart. Before auscultation, the cuff is quickly inflated to a pressure 20 mmHg above the systolic, as indicated by obliteration of the radial pulse. The stethoscope is then applied lightly but firmly over the artery, and auscultatory pressure is determined by noting the onset (peak systole) and behavior of the Korotkoff sounds as the cuff is deflated at a rate of about 3 mmHg/s. When the sounds disappear, the bag should be rapidly decompressed and 1 or 2 min allowed to pass before repeat determinations are made. When possible, the BP should be taken with the subject upright as well as supine. Measurement of the BP in both arms is recommended, especially in the elderly. An American Heart Association hypertension primer recommends that the systolic pressure be recorded as the point at which the first tapping sounds occur for two consecutive beats (phase I) and that the diastolic pressure *in adults* be recorded as the point at which sounds become inaudible. *In children* and in adults with a hyperkinetic circulation, the diastolic pressure should be recorded as the point at which muffling of the sounds occurs (onset of phase IV). The arterial pressures at both the onset of muffling (phase IV) and the disappearance of sound (phase V) should be recorded. The mean BP can be estimated by the addition of one-third the pulse pressure (systolic pressure minus diastolic pressure) to the diastolic pressure.

Patients with atrial fibrillation may have a significant beat-to-beat variation in their arterial pressure. Accordingly, the indirect BP should be measured several times and the average noted.

This indirect method provides several potential sources of error due to improper equipment, inaccurate detection of the Korotkoff sounds, and observer techniques.[83] The standard pneumatic cuff often may be unsatisfactory for pressure measurement in the arms or in the legs of very obese subjects.[90] The arterial pressure may be underestimated if the cuff is deflated too rapidly, or if inadequate inflation does not result in complete arterial occlusion. When the cuff is deflated too slowly or is immediately reinflated for multiple pressure determinations, the resulting venous congestion may elevate the diastolic pressure artificially and falsely decrease the systolic pressure by decreasing the intensity of phase I or phase II sounds to an inaudible level.

Studies correlating direct and indirect BP measurements have, in general, shown a good correlation between indirect and direct measurements of BP in the arm. The indirect method tends to underestimate systolic pressure by several millimeters of mercury, to overestimate diastolic pressure by several millimeters of mercury when phase IV is used as an endpoint, and to slightly underestimate diastolic pressure in normal individuals when phase V is taken as the endpoint.

Home BP recordings using manual or automatic inflation and deflation of the cuff and detection of Korotkoff sounds by a microphone, stethoscope, or ultrasonic transducer are being used with increasing frequency for the ambulatory assessment of patients with hypertension. Although clinically useful, ambulatory BP devices in general do not meet the standards for automated devices of the Association for the Advancement of Medical Instrumentation.[87,91–93]

More recently, arterial tonometry has been used as a completely noninvasive method for monitoring the arterial pressure. This probe, with a micromanometer in its tip, operates on the principle of a piezo-resistive transducer of cantilever construction.[94–99]

## Normal Arterial Pressure

Normal pressures have been defined on the basis of values included within two standard deviations of the mean of pressures obtained in a large population of apparently healthy individuals. The normal BP range varies with age, sex, and socioracial grouping.[100] In the United States, the pressure increases rapidly during the first few days of life and then increases gradually, with a slightly greater increment in systolic than in diastolic values, throughout life. The pressure tends to be higher in western industrialized societies than in Asian, African, and technically undeveloped societies.

With increasing age and into senescence, the aorta undergoes progressive dilatation and elongation, with increasing stiffness of its walls.[101] Resulting from this diminished vascular distensibility, there is an increase in systolic arterial pressure with less change in diastolic pressure.[102]

The normal BP limits for adults living in the United States are approximately 100 to 140 mmHg systolic and 60 to 90 mmHg diastolic. In an individual subject, however, baseline pressures above or below these levels do not define a pathologic state, since the physiologic range of normal for an individual may overlap with the statistical range of abnormality.[83] The systolic arterial pressure rises slowly and progressively in most Americans between the ages of 20 and 60 and more rapidly later, increasing by about 20 mmHg between the ages of 60 and 80.[103] Diastolic pressure usually rises very little after age 45. Data from the Framingham Study and more recent studies (e.g., MRFIT, SHEP, Syst-Eur) have shown a clear correlation between systolic BP and cardiovascular events, a reduction in events with reduction of systolic BP,[104–109] or even a negative association between diastolic BP and events.[110]

In mildly to moderately hypertensive persons, the BP "casually" recorded by a physician is significantly higher than the average value of a series of intermittent, indirect determinations or continuous direct recordings made during normal activity.[111] To estimate basal BP, measurements have been obtained during sleep, when the subject first awakens in the morning while still recumbent, or after several hours of reclining.

Factors contributing to variations in an individual's BP during daily activities include (1) body posture; (2) state of muscular, cerebral, or gastrointestinal activity; (3) emotional or painful stimuli;

(4) environmental factors such as temperature and noise level; and (5) the use of tobacco, coffee, alcohol, and other drugs with direct or neurally mediated vasomotor properties.[83,112] Twenty-four-hour pressures, obtained from normal and hypertensive subjects with an automatic recorder, have shown considerable variability with activity and emotional stimuli.[113,114] The average diurnal pattern of BP consists of an increase throughout the day and early evening and a significant, rapid decline to a low point during the early, deep stage of sleep. This is an important fact to remember in prescribing medications for systemic hypertension (Chap. 61).

With normal respiration, the peak systolic BP is greater during expiration than during inspiration by as much as 10 mmHg. An augmentation of this difference occurs in patients with pericardial tamponade (pulsus paradoxus; Chap. 80) and during hyperventilation.

Isotonic exercise in both the supine and upright positions produces a moderate increase in BP (systolic pressure greater than mean pressure, which is greater than diastolic pressure). Sustained isometric muscular contractions produce an abrupt increase in systolic, mean, and diastolic BP that depends on the strength of the contraction.[115]

## Abnormal Arterial Pressure

### INCREASED PULSE PRESSURE

An increase in arterial pulse pressure is commonly observed during routine BP recordings. This usually is due to an increase in stroke volume and ejection velocity, often with a decrease in peripheral resistance. Fever, anemia, hot weather, exercise, pregnancy, hyperthyroidism, or arteriovenous fistulas may produce this change. Several cardiac diseases, such as AR, patent ductus arteriosus, and truncus arteriosus, also can result in a widened pulse pressure. An increased pulse pressure due to a large stroke volume may occur with complete heart block or marked sinus bradycardia.[83]

Atherosclerosis of the large arteries often reduces arterial compliance and results in an elevated systolic pressure with a normal or even decreased stroke volume. The systolic hypertension of the elderly does not necessarily represent a change in arteriolar resistance. Efforts to lower this type of systolic pressure elevation are often appropriate but can result in diminished peripheral perfusion (Chap. 61). The increased pulse pressure associated with systemic arteriovenous fistulas is less common; a relative tachycardia may be the only clinical clue. Compression of a systemic arteriovenous fistula can produce a prompt slowing of the heart rate (Branham's sign).

### REDUCED PULSE PRESSURE

A narrow pulse pressure is uncommon in normal subjects but may result from an increased peripheral resistance (increased circulating catecholamines in heart failure), decreased stroke volume [severe (AS)], and/or markedly decreased intravascular volume (diabetic ketoacidosis).[83]

### UNEQUAL PULSE PRESSURES

The diagnostic importance of BP differences between the right and left arms may occur due to supravalvular AS as well as the "choanal effect" in children and the subclavian steal syndrome in adults.[116] Most patients with the former have greater than 20 mmHg higher BP in the right arm. The subclavian steal syndrome, often accompanied by symptoms of cerebrovascular insufficiency, usually results in a pronounced lowering or absence of brachial artery pressure in the ipsilateral extremity.[83] There is diminished vertebral blood flow to the brain, since flow is diverted to the involved subclavian artery distal to the stenosis.

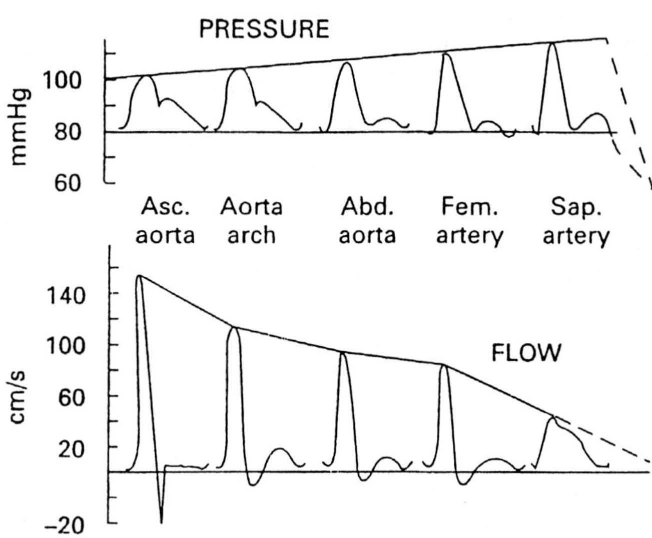


FIGURE 12-36 Micromanometer and catheter tip flow velocity as change in contour of pressure waves (above) and flow waves (below) between the ascending aorta and the saphenous artery. (From Vlachopoulos C, O'Rourke MF. The arterial pulse. *Curr Probl Cardiol* 2000; 25:296–346. Used with permission from the publisher.)

A progressive increase in systolic pressure normally occurs as the point of measurement is moved peripherally from the central aorta (Fig. 12-36); the increment is similar in the large arteries of the upper arm and the thigh. Direct recordings of femoral and brachial arterial pressures (systolic, diastolic, and mean) in adults[117] and children[118] and indirect measurement of popliteal and brachial artery pressures have demonstrated that mean pressures are equal at these sites.[119] A difference in arm and leg pressures may occur because of coarctation of the aorta or acquired disease, such as aortic dissection, aortic arch syndrome, or the subclavian steal syndrome.[83]

## Pulsus Alternans

Pulsus alternans may be detected by palpating a peripheral artery, preferably the femoral artery, when the heart rhythm is normal. The sphygmomanometer can be used to measure accurately the beat-to-beat variation in pressure that characterizes pulsus alternans.

Pulsus alternans occurs in patients with severe heart disease who exhibit impaired LV contraction. It can also occur for several beats following supraventricular tachycardia in normal persons or when the respiratory rate is half the pulse rate.

## Pulsus Paradoxus

A normal person may exhibit a 10 mmHg drop in systolic pressure during normal inspiration. A greater decline may be identified in patients with acute cardiac tamponade, constrictive pericarditis, severe obstructive lung disease, and restrictive cardiomyopathy.

Pulsus paradoxus is best detected by inflating the BP cuff above systolic pressure and then slowly releasing it. As the cuff pressure is gradually reduced, the BP sounds become audible during expiration. The difference in pressure between the first audible sound heard on expiration and the pressure level at which the sounds are heard during all phases of respiration gives a measurement of magnitude of pulsus paradoxus. The mechanism of pulsus paradoxus is discussed in Chap. 80.

## THE ARTERIAL PULSE

The arterial pulse, like any periodic fluctuation that is caused by the heart, occurs at the same frequency as the heartbeat. Ejection of blood with every cardiac contraction is converted to *flow, pressure,* and *dimension* pulsations in arteries throughout the body. While the term *pulse* refers to any such pulsation, the arterial pulse perceived by a clinician is the pressure pulse in a large, accessible artery. Palpation of the arterial pulse is a basic and important element of the physical examination.[120–124]

### Physical Determinants of the Arterial Pulse

#### GENESIS OF THE ARTERIAL PULSE

Pressure and blood flow in the ascending aorta result from the interaction between the heart and arterial system. When LV pressure exceeds the aortic pressure, it becomes the driving force for the movement of blood into the ascending aorta.[121] This driving force depends on the intrinsic contractility of ventricular muscle, the size and shape of the LV, and the heart rate. It is opposed by several forces that impede the development of flow and are interrelated in a complex manner. Three major determinants of arterial impedance include (1) resistance, (2) inertia, and (3) compliance.

Resistance is related to blood viscosity and the geometry of the vasculature; it opposes flow and is unaffected by changes in heart rate. Inertia, which is related to the mass of the column of blood, opposes the rate of change of arterial blood flow (i.e., acceleration) and depends on the heart rate. Compliance is related to the distensibility of the vascular walls, opposes changes in arterial blood volume, and also depends on the heart rate. The heart rate dependency of inertia and compliance introduces phase shifts between instantaneous pressure and flow in a pulsatile system.[125] Inertia and compliance are important determinants of the character of ventricular ejection, especially in early systole, when flows and pressures are changing rapidly.

The arterial pulse wave begins with aortic valve opening and the onset of LV ejection. Aortic pressure rises rapidly in early systole because the LV stroke volume enters the aorta faster than it flows to distal sites. The rapid-rising portion of the arterial pressure curve is often termed the *anacrotic limb* (from the Greek meaning "upbeat"). In experimental animals and in humans, peak proximal aortic flow velocity occurs slightly earlier than peak pressure.[126] After its peak, aortic pressure declines as LV ejection slows and peripheral blood flow continues. During isovolumic relaxation, a transient reversal of flow from the central arteries toward the ventricle just prior to aortic valve closure is associated with an incisura on the descending limb of the aortic pressure pulse. The subsequent smaller, secondary positive wave has been attributed to the elastic recoil of the aorta and aortic valve but is partially due to reflected waves from more distal arteries. Subsequently, aortic pressure decreases again as further "runoff" in the peripheral circulation occurs in diastole.

The proximal aortic pulse pressure is directly proportional to the ratio of stroke volume to arterial distensibility, but multiple factors influence this complex relationship.[127] Arterial distensibility diminishes as the distending arterial pressure increases. Accordingly, the pulse pressure for a constant stroke volume will be larger if the mean BP is elevated. Also, arterial distensibility varies inversely with the rate of rise of intraluminal pressure. When the systolic ejection rate increases, the stiffer arterial wall results in a greater pulse pressure. Finally, the arterial pulse pressure is modified by reflected pressure waves and by the rate of blood flow from arterioles to veins.

#### CONTOUR OF THE ARTERIAL PULSE

Pulsatile changes in arterial diameter are virtually identical to the pressure pulse, with minor differences explained in terms of nonlinear elasticity and viscosity of the arterial wall. In 1939, Hamilton and Dow defined the pressure wave contour in different arteries in terms of wave reflection between the aortic valve and peripheral sites.[128] The pulse waveform recorded at any site of the arterial tree is the sum of a forward waveform and a backward-traveling one that is the "echo" of the incident wave reflected at peripheral sites. *Wave reflection is an important determinant of LV load and CBF.* A reflected wave occurring at systole increases systolic pressure and thereby increases ventricular afterload. In contrast, occurrence of the reflected wave at diastole is highly desirable because augmentation of pressure during diastole aids coronary perfusion.

Conventionally, the pulse is described in the *time domain,* where it is considered as a change in arterial pressure with time. An alternative, quantitative approach is to analyze the pulse in the *frequency domain.* Pulse is conceived as a composite wave that can be resolved into component harmonics like a musical wave. Impedance is the measure of the opposition to flow presented by a system and can be measured when harmonic analysis is used to relate frequency components of pressure and flow pulses.[131–136]

Usually there is a linear relation between pressure and flow at the same point in an artery and between pressures at different points in the arterial system. From impedance curves, it is possible to identify the factors responsible for the relation between the pulsatile pressure and flow. The peripheral arterial pressure wave recorded is the summation of the incident (initial) and reflected waves. The systemic circulation has been represented by a simple asymmetric T-tube model that emphasizes the importance of wave reflection at two arteriolar reflecting sites in the upper and lower parts of the body.[127] An important patient study indicates major reflection sites at the aortic level of the renal arteries and at a point distal to the terminal abdominal aorta bifurcation.[128]

#### PERIPHERAL TRANSMISSION OF THE ARTERIAL PULSE

As the normal aortic pulse wave is transmitted peripherally, significant changes in its contour occur due to (1) distortion and damping of pulse wave components, (2) different rates of transmission of various components, (3) distortion or exaggeration by reflected, resonant, or standing waves, (4) conversion of kinetic energy into hydrostatic or potential energy, (5) differences in distensibility and caliber of the arteries, and (6) changes in the vessel wall due to age and/or disease.[134]

The arterial pressure pulse enters the proximal aorta and travels distally at a velocity many times faster than that of maximum blood flow. The pressure wave is accompanied by a traveling wave distending the arterial wall, the pulse wave velocity increasing as arterial wall distensibility diminishes.[129]

The pulse wave arrives progressively later at more peripheral sites when timed from the QRS complex on the ECG. Representative time delays from the central aorta are as follows: carotid, 30 ms; brachial, 60 ms; radial, 80 ms; and femoral, 75 ms.

The arterial pulse wave undergoes a progressive change in shape during its transmission distally (Fig. 12-36). The pulse pressure and systolic amplitude increase, and the ascending limb of the pulse wave becomes steeper. The incisura of the central aorta pulse is gradually replaced by a smoother, somewhat later dicrotic notch that occurs at lower pressure levels. The dicrotic notch and the following positive secondary or dicrotic wave probably result from the summation of the forward pulse wave and reflected waves from the peripheral vessels.[120]

## EXAMINATION OF THE ARTERIAL PULSE

All major arterial pulses should be examined bilaterally for both patency and waveform characteristics. The thickness and hardness of the arterial walls often can be assessed by "rolling" the vessel against underlying tissue. A pulse in the foot should not be considered absent unless examined with the foot in a dependent position. Otherwise, the arterial pulses usually are examined with the patient supine and with the trunk of the body slightly elevated.

The examiner uses tactile receptors in the tips of the fingers to sense movement of the arterial wall associated with the pressure pulse as it passes the site of palpation. Measurements in the proximal aorta show cyclic movement in both diameter and length proportional to the pulse pressure. In more peripheral arteries with connective tissue attachments, however, the detectable movement is small and variable, with radial expansion by only about 2 percent of the end-diastolic cross-sectional area.[120]

The usual technique for palpating the arterial pulse is to press with the examining fingers until the maximum pulse is sensed. The pulse is felt as changing displacement superimposed on the "baseline" displacement produced by compressing the artery. The examiner should apply varying degrees of pressure while concentrating on the separate phases of the pulse wave. This method, referred to as *trisection,* is useful for assessing the upstroke, systolic peak, and diastolic slope of the arterial pulse.[131]

Palpation of the carotid artery is preferred for assessing cardiac performance, since the carotid pulse corresponds more closely to the central aortic pressure. In certain cardiac diseases (e.g., AR), however, the abnormalities detected in the carotid pulse are accentuated in the more peripheral pulses. To evaluate the integrity of the peripheral arterial blood supply and to localize any lesions that exist, the arterial pulses in all four extremities should be examined and compared (Chap. 101).

Inspection of the carotid arterial and jugular venous pulsations should be performed at the same time. The carotid pulse is usually best examined with the sternocleidomastoid muscles relaxed and the head rotated slightly toward the examiner. The carotid pulse may be timed from the first heart sound, which is heard slightly before the pulsation. The carotid pulse should be palpated in the lower half of the patient's neck in order to avoid carotid sinus compression. Occasionally, it is useful to palpate two arteries simultaneously (e.g., radial and femoral) to detect an apparent pulse wave delay, such as occurs in patients with coarctation of the aorta.

The examination of arterial pulses in the abdomen and upper and lower extremities should be performed carefully in all patients and compared using a scale such as the following: 0 = complete absence of pulsation; 1+ = small or reduced pulsation; 2+ = normal or average pulsation; and 3+ = large or bounding pulsation. Furthermore, auscultation over the major arteries should be performed, since an audible bruit may be a clue to partial occlusion or may indicate transmission (e.g., carotid) of a cardiac murmur (Chap. 101).

## NORMAL ARTERIAL PULSE

The normal carotid pulse has a smooth, rapid upstroke or ascending limb to a smooth, dome-shaped summit (Fig. 12-37). Then a downstroke occurs that is somewhat less rapid than the upstroke. The dicrotic notch and secondary diastolic wave are usually not felt but may be palpable in some normal individuals, particularly during fever, exercise, or excitement. The dicrotic notch usually occurs about 300 ms after the onset of the pulse wave when corrected for heart rate.

In arteries distal to the carotid, the pulse wave arrives later and has a steep initial wave that rises to a high peak pressure, whereas the diastolic and mean pressures are slightly lower. The systolic upstroke time (onset of pulse wave to its peak) tends to be shorter, but the apparent LV ejection time (onset of pulse wave to incisura) is longer in more peripheral arterial pulses. In the brachial artery, the heart rate-corrected systolic upstroke time averages 120 ms (range, 90 to 160 ms), and the systolic ejection time averages about 320 ms (range, 280 to 360 ms).

Graphic recordings of the arterial pulses frequently show two positive deflections during systole, the first shoulder being referred to as the *percussion wave* and the second as the *tidal wave*. In the normal proximal aortic pulse, the percussion wave is due to arrival of the impulse generated by LV ejection, the tidal wave may represent its echo from the upper part of the body, and the dicrotic or diastolic wave is a reflection from the lower part of the body.[124]

With aging, there is a relative increase in the second (tidal) systolic wave and the height of the incisura relative to the first systolic wave.[120,135,140] The systolic upstroke time is longer, and the amplitude and duration of the diastolic wave tend to be less prominent.

## ABNORMAL ARTERIAL PULSES

In hypertension and arteriosclerosis, the pressure pulse amplitude is increased, the tidal wave is prominent, and the diastolic wave is absent. All features of the pulse can be explained by increased wave velocity.[120,135,139,140] Reflected waves return to the proximal aorta during late systole, augmenting the tidal wave and increasing systolic pressure. With systemic hypotension, the pulse-wave velocity is decreased, and the later tidal and diastolic waves are further displaced from the percussion wave.

Impairment of the pulse of one or both carotid arteries is usually produced by atherosclerosis, but multiple other causes include

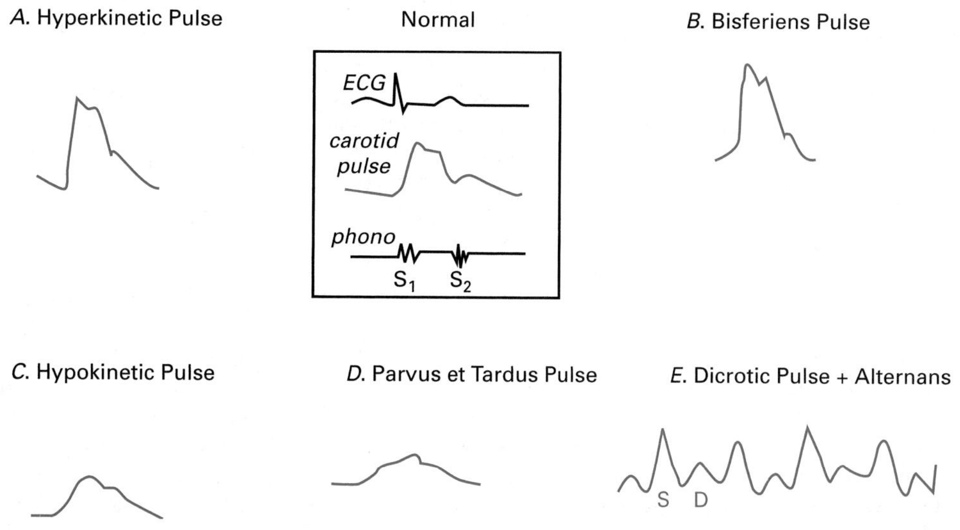

FIGURE 12-37 Schematic representation of the normal carotid arterial pulse, five types of abnormal pulses, and pulsus alternans. ECG = electrocardiogram; phono = phonocardiogram; $S_1$, $S_2$ = first and second heart sounds; S = systole; D = diastole.

thrombosis, embolus, arteritis, and diseases of the aortic arch. Kinking of the carotid or brachiocephalic artery is relatively frequent, particularly in hypertensive patients, and may simulate aneurysmal dilatation. Femoral pulses may be diminished in the child or young adult as a result of coarctation of the aorta. In most adults, however, the diminution of the femoral pulsation is caused by atherosclerosis of the abdominal aorta, aortic bifurcation, or ileofemoral arteries (Chap. 101).

### HYPERKINETIC ARTERIAL PULSE

Large, bounding arterial pulses usually indicate the rapid ejection of an increased volume of blood from the LV (Fig. 12-37*A*). Commonly, the arterial pulse pressure is increased, and the peripheral arterial resistance diminished. The hyperdynamic arterial pulse is sometimes referred to in terms that describe a particular component of the pulse wave. Thus the *water-hammer pulse,* named after a Victorian toy, refers to an extremely rapid, forceful ascending limb of the arterial pulse wave.[139] By contrast, *collapsing pulse* refers to a quick, marked decrease in the arterial pulse wave following its peak. The term *Quincke pulse* refers to visible small pulsations in the nail bed of patients with hyperdynamic arterial pulses from any cause, including AR.

Hyperkinetic arterial pulses occur in normal subjects with a hyperkinetic circulation (e.g., exercise, fever), patients with cardiovascular diseases associated with increased stroke volume, and subjects with marked bradycardia and an extremely large stroke volume (e.g., athletes). A hyperdynamic arterial pulse also occurs in patients with an abnormally rapid runoff of blood from the arterial system (e.g., patent ductus arteriosus, arteriovenous fistulas). Patients on chronic hemodialysis often have hyperdynamic pulses produced by the combination of a surgical arteriovenous fistula, anemia, and hypertension.

In AR, the rapid-rising, bounding arterial pulse results from increases in both stroke volume and the rate of LV ejection. The early systolic flow often produces palpable vibrations manifest as a thrill on the steep ascending limb. Later in systole, the rate of ventricular ejection and the arterial pulse wave decrease sharply, often resulting in systolic collapse.

### BISFERIENS ARTERIAL PULSE

The bisferiens (from the Latin "twice beating") pulse has a waveform characterized by two positive waves during systole (Fig. 12-37*B*).[141] The pulse wave upstroke rises rapidly and forcefully, producing the first systolic peak (percussion wave). A brief decline in pressure is followed by a smaller and somewhat slower-rising positive pulse wave (tidal wave). Abnormalities of LV ejection and reflected waves from peripheral arteries contribute to the prominence of the second systolic wave in the bisferiens pulse. The bisferiens pulse is sometimes more easily palpable in a brachial or radial artery. A bisferiens pulse often occurs in patients with pure AR and in patients with combined AS and severe AR.[142] It also occurs in association with the rapid ejection of an increased stroke volume from the LV (e.g., exercise, fever, patent ductus arteriosus).

The bisferiens pulse often is present in patients with hypertrophic cardiomyopathy, many of whom have a pressure gradient in the LV outflow tract.[142] In this syndrome, the midsystolic negative wave usually coincides with a marked decrease in the rate of LV ejection. The second systolic wave, or tidal wave, most likely is produced by reflected waves from the periphery. The bisferiens pulse may be elicited by maneuvers that decrease the LV size or increase its contractility. The most characteristic aspect of the arterial pulse in hypertrophic cardiomyopathy is its rapid rate of rise. A physical finding nearly specific for hypertrophic cardiomyopathy is a much smaller arterial pressure pulse in the cardiac cycle following a premature ventricular beat (Chap. 77).

### HYPOKINETIC ARTERIAL PULSE

A small, weak arterial pulse is frequently present in patients with a diminished stroke volume (Fig. 12-37*C*). Usually, the decreased stroke output is associated with decreased rate and duration of LV ejection, and there is a narrow arterial pulse pressure despite an increased arterial resistance. Common causes include hypovolemia, LV failure, and mitral or aortic valve stenosis.

### PARVUS ET TARDUS PULSE

Patients with moderate or severe valvular AS often have an arterial pulse that is small and has a delayed systolic peak.[143–145] Occasionally, there may be a detectable shoulder on the upstroke of the carotid pulse, referred to as *anacrotic*[146] (Fig. 12-37*D*). Palpable coarse vibrations often are present as a systolic thrill over the slowly rising carotid pulse. The parvus et tardus pulse is much easier to detect in the carotid arteries than in more distal arteries.

Most middle-aged patients with uncomplicated severe AS have a parvus et tardus pulse, but this pulse also may occur in relatively mild stenosis. Conversely, an apparently normal arterial pulse is not unusual in elderly patients with severe AS who have decreased distensibility of the large arteries.[120,122] Severe LV failure often results in a small, weak pulse that may be difficult to distinguish from that of AS.

### DICROTIC ARTERIAL PULSE

The dicrotic (from the Greek *dikrotos,* "double beating") pulse is a twice-peaked pulse with one peak in systole and the second in diastole, the latter due to an accentuated and palpable dicrotic wave that follows the second heart sound[147] (Fig. 12-37*E*). It is usually best felt in the carotids, although it also may be palpated over more peripheral arteries. Major abnormalities include a short systolic ejection phase, a low dicrotic notch, a large diastolic wave, a narrow pulse pressure, a diminished rate of rise of the pulse, and the lack of distinct percussion and tidal waves. The dicrotic pulse is most common in young or middle-aged patients with impaired LV performance. It is usually associated with a low cardiac output, markedly diminished stroke volume, elevated LV end-diastolic pressure, and high systemic arterial resistance. Rarely, the dicrotic wave can be palpated in young, febrile patients in whom none of the other abnormal features of the dicrotic pulse are present.

### PULSUS ALTERNANS

In pulsus alternans, beats occur at regular intervals with a regular alternation of the systolic height of the pressure pulses[148,149] (Fig. 12-37*E*). Rarely, pulsus alternans is so marked that the weaker pulses are not felt at all. When pulsus alternans is noticed first after a premature beat, the extent of the difference in systolic pressure in alternating beats may decline for several cycles until the pulse amplitude is again constant. The initiation of post-premature ventricular beat pulsus alternans is probably related to the increased duration of LV filling after the premature beat.

Sustained pulsus alternans is seen in severe depression of LV performance with an alteration in aortic flow, systolic LV pressure, aortic systolic pressure, LV *dP/dt,* and LV end-diastolic pressure. Sustained pulsus alternans likely is due to alteration of the contractile state of at least part of the myocardium, which may be caused by the failure of electromechanical coupling in some cells during the weaker contraction.[147] A subsequent stronger contraction would then represent contraction of all cells, some of which were potentiated.[150]

Pulsus alternans may be better appreciated when palpating a distal artery, which normally has a slightly wider pulse pressure than the carotid artery. The patient's respiration should be held, since the small changes in arterial pressure caused by normal respiration may obscure the recognition of pulsus alternans. Pulsus alternans can be confirmed by using a sphygmomanometer and is usually associated with a LV third heart sound.

## PULSUS PARADOXUS

A *paradoxical pulse* is defined as a marked decrease in the pulse amplitude during normal quiet inspiration or a decrease in the systolic arterial pressure by more than 10 mmHg.[151] The normal small decline in systolic BP probably is produced predominantly by relative pooling of blood in the pulmonary vessels during inspiration and also may reflect the delayed transmission through the lungs of the preceding expiratory fall in venous pressure and RV cardiac output.[133]

In patients with cardiac tamponade, fluid accumulation in the pericardium increases intrapericardial pressure, and the heart's filling capacity is reduced. During inspiration, the expected augmentation of venous return to the right side of the heart occurs despite the elevated intrapericardial pressure.[152] The diminished thoracic pressure also causes a pooling of blood in the pulmonary veins and capillaries and diminishes pulmonary venous return to the left atrium. Since the high intrapericardial pressure limits flow to the heart and the total cardiac filling capacity is limited, the increase in right-sided heart volume with inspiration causes an obligatory decrease in left-sided heart filling. This, along with the pooling of blood in the pulmonary bed, produces a decline in LV stroke volume and systolic BP during inspiration.[152]

Pulsus paradoxus is common with cardiac tamponade but infrequent with constrictive pericarditis (Chap. 80). Different hemodynamic mechanisms contribute to the production of a paradoxical pulse in certain patients with superior vena cava obstruction, asthma, or obstructive airways disease; in some patients with pulmonary embolism or shock; and in some patients after thoracotomy.[134]

The extent of pulsus paradoxus can be quantitated by cuff sphygmomanometry as the pressure difference between the first discernible Korotkoff sound on expiration and the pressure level at which Korotkoff sounds are audible during all phases of respiration.

## EFFECTS OF ARRHYTHMIAS ON THE ARTERIAL PULSE

***Premature Ventricular Depolarizations*** A premature ventricular depolarization may be associated with no pulse, a small-amplitude pulse, or a normal arterial pulse, depending on timing and whether or not the LV pressure generated is able to open the aortic valve.[153,154] The arterial pulse following a premature beat usually is greatly enhanced because of decreased aortic impedance, increased LV filling, and augmented LV contractility. At times, premature ventricular beats are so common as to produce an irregularly irregular pulse. Then the presence of cannon *a* waves in the jugular venous pulse (JVP) should alert one to the correct diagnosis.

***Tachyarrhythmias*** The ECG is usually needed for the definitive diagnosis of any abnormality of heart rate or rhythm. On the other hand, careful observation of the arterial and JVP frequently leads to the correct diagnosis. Simultaneous cardiac auscultation is also frequently helpful.

Most tachycardias associated with a regular pulse are of supraventricular origin. In sinus tachycardia, the arterial pulse will slow gradually with carotid sinus pressure and then again increase gradually. Paroxysmal atrial tachycardia has an "all or none" response. In patients with atrial flutter, carotid sinus pressure will increase the block at the AV junction, the pulse rate slowing and subsequently returning to its original rate in a "jerky" fashion.

In patients with ventricular tachycardia and AV dissociation, the variation in the atrial ventricular sequence of contraction and resulting variation in pulse amplitude often may be detected by palpation.[153–155]

An irregularly irregular pulse with a varying pulse pressure is usually the result of atrial fibrillation; however, multifocal atrial tachycardia is also a common cause of this finding in patients with severe chronic obstructive lung disease.

***Bradyarrhythmias*** An unusually slow heart rate frequently is associated with a decrease in the rate of rise and amplitude of the arterial pressure pulse. Complete heart block often is readily diagnosed by the variability in the arterial pulse amplitude, changing intensity of the first heart sound, and intermittent cannon *a* waves in the JVP. These are all due to the time-dependent variable contribution of atrial contraction to ventricular filling.

## EFFECTS OF DRUG THERAPY ON THE ARTERIAL PULSE

*Pulse wave analysis* provides important information about the actions of drugs that, most importantly, may not be apparent with conventional methods.[120] *Nitrates* decrease central systolic pressure substantially while they have no or minimal effect on peripheral systolic pressure (Fig. 12-38).[121] *Beta-blocking* agents have variable effect, depending on their intrinsic properties. Nonselective agents tend to increase late systolic pressure augmentation; in contrast, those agents with vasodilating properties have the opposite effect.

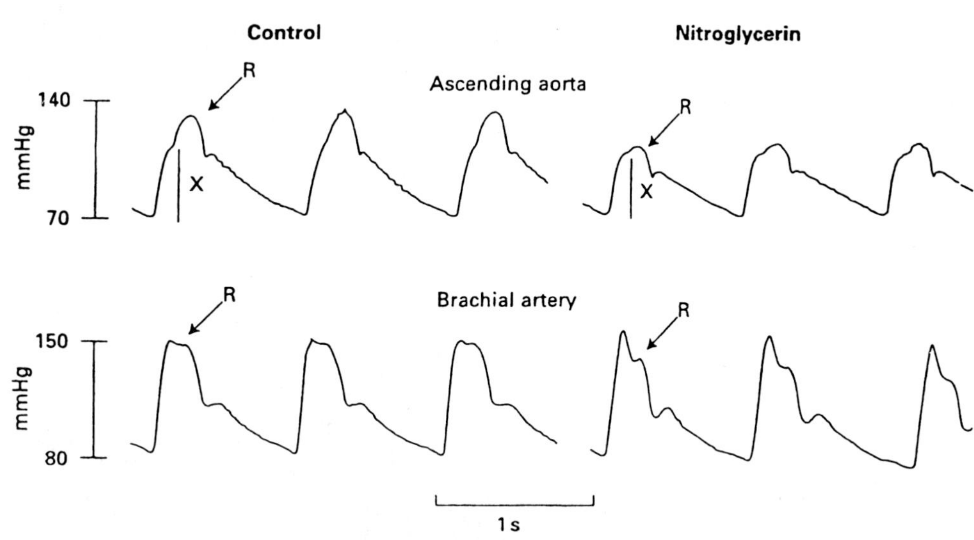


FIGURE 12-38 Pressure waves recorded directly in the ascending aorta (*top*) and brachial artery (*bottom*) under control conditions (*left*) and after 0.3 mg sublingual nitroglycerin (*right*) in a human adult. X, height the pressure would have without reflection (R). (From Kelly RP, Gibbs HH, O'Rourke MF, et al. Nitroglycerin has a favorable effect on left ventricular afterload than apparent from measurement of pressure in a peripheval artery. *Eur Heart J* 1990;11:138–144, with permission.)

Both angiotensin-converting enzyme (ACE) inhibitors and calcium channel blockers have significant effects on the arterial pulse by reducing late systolic pressure augmentation. These actions can be explained on the basis of wave reflection. Reduction of wave reflection is an important advantage in the logical treatment of hypertension and heart failure.

## THE VENOUS PULSE

An accurate assessment of the venous pulse is an integral part of the physical examination because it provides information concerning both the mean right atrial pressure and the hemodynamic events in the right atrium.[123] Factors influencing the right atrial and central venous pressure (CVP) include the total blood volume, the distribution of blood volume, and the strength of right atrial contraction.

Venous blood returning from the systemic capillaries is nonpulsatile. Changes in volume flow created by skeletal muscles and the respiratory pump are nonsynchronous with the pulsatile activity of the heart. Changes in flow and pressure caused by right atrial and ventricular filling, however, produce pulsations in the central veins that are transmitted toward the peripheral veins, opposite to the direction of blood flow. With the possible exception of the *c* wave, which is the combined result of carotid arterial impact and an upward movement of the tricuspid valve, the pulsations observed in the neck are produced by right atrial and ventricular activity.[154]

### Examination of the Jugular Venous Pulse

The two main objectives of the bedside examination of the neck veins are estimation of the CVP and inspection of the waveform.[154] Usually, the right internal jugular vein (IJV) is superior for both purposes. In most normal subjects, the maximum pulsation of the IJV is observed when the trunk is inclined by less than 30 degrees. In patients with an elevated CVP, it may be necessary to elevate the trunk further, sometimes to as much as 90 degrees. When the neck muscles are relaxed, shining a beam of light tangentially across the skin overlying the IJV often exposes its pulsations. Simultaneous palpation of the left carotid artery aids the examiner in deciding which pulsations are venous.

### Measurements of Venous Pressure

The difference between venous distention and venous pressure elevation must be considered. Veins may be markedly dilated with minimal increase in pressure or may not be visibly distended despite a very high venous pressure.[154,155] Venous pressure may be estimated by examining the veins on the dorsum of the hand. With the patient sitting or lying at 30 degrees of elevation or greater, the arm is slowly and passively raised from a dependent position. When the CVP is normal, the veins collapse when the dorsum of the hand reaches the level of the sternal angle of Louis. Unfortunately, local venous obstruction or augmented peripheral venous constriction may diminish the accuracy of estimating CVP by this method.

The external or internal jugular veins may also be used to estimate venous pressure.[154] Because of its more direct route to the right atrium, the IJV is superior for the estimation of venous pressure and assessment of the venous waveform. The patient is examined at the optimal degree of trunk elevation for visualization of venous pulsations. The vertical distance from the top of the oscillating venous column to the level of the sternal angle is generally less than 3 cm. Greatly elevated venous pressure may be missed by failing to elevate the patient's head adequately. It may be necessary to actually have the patient sit upright. If the "pulsating meniscus" is very high, pulsations may not be apparent in the lower neck. When venous engorgement is marked, the patient's earlobe may pulsate, and even the veins on the top of the head may be distended.

In patients suspected of RV failure but with a normal resting venous pressure, the abdominojugular test is useful.[156,157] With the patient breathing normally, firm pressure is applied with the palm of the hand to the upper right quadrant of the abdomen for 10 s or more. The patient should be instructed to continue to breathe normally during the test. In most subjects, the jugular venous pressure is not altered significantly. In some normal patients there is a transient increase in jugular venous pressure with a rapid return to or near baseline in less than 10 s. The dysfunctioning RV, however, is unable to accept the increment in blood volume due to enhanced venous return without a marked increase in its filling pressure, which is transmitted to the neck veins. In patients with RV failure, often due to left-sided heart failure, the venous pressure either rises rapidly and then partially declines slowly during continued abdominal compression or remains elevated by 4 cm of blood or more until the abdominal pressure is released (Fig. 12-39). Ducas et al.[158] also studied the abdominojugular test and confirmed its clinical value.

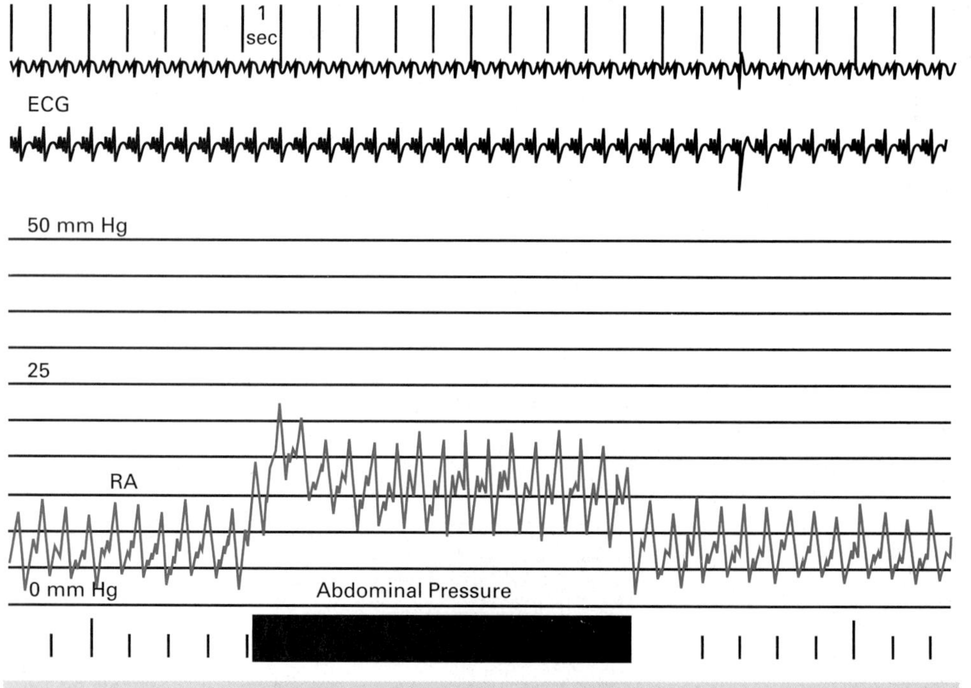


FIGURE 12-39 Elevation in RA pressure observed during abdominal pressure in patient with mild congestive heart failure. (From Ewy GA. The abdominojugular test: Technique and hemodynamic correlates. *Ann Intern Med* 1989; 109:456. Used with permission from the publisher and author.)

## Analysis of Venous Waveforms

Again, the patient's trunk should be inclined to whatever elevation is necessary to reveal the top of the oscillating venous column.[159] Slow, deep inspiration will increase the amplitude of the presystolic *a* wave while decreasing the mean right atrial pressure. This is a useful technique for identifying the site at which the pulsations will be best visualized. Simultaneous palpation of the left carotid artery and cardiac auscultation aid the examiner in relating the venous pulsations to the timing of the cardiac cycle.

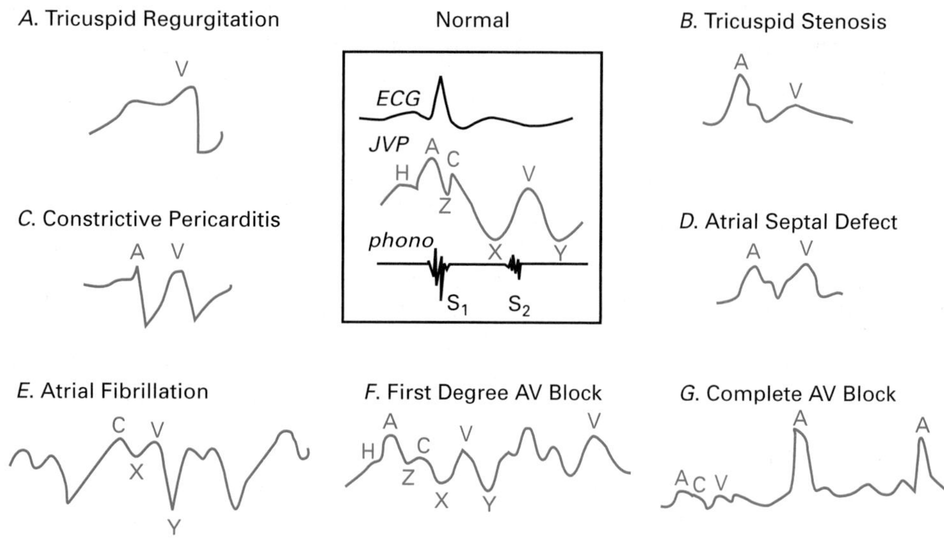


FIGURE 12-40 Schematic representation of the normal jugular venous pressure (JVP), four types of abnormal JVP, and the JVP in three arrhythmias. See text under "Normal Venous Pulse" for definition of H, A, Z, C, X, V, and Y.

## Normal Venous Pulse

The normal *jugular venous pulse* (JVP) reflects phasic pressure changes in the right atrium and consists of three positive waves and two negatives troughs (Fig. 12-40). It is useful to refer to the events of the cardiac cycle (see Fig. 3-5, Plate 3). The positive presystolic *a* wave is produced by right atrial (RA) contraction and is the dominant wave in the JVP, particularly during inspiration. During atrial relaxation, the venous pulse descends from the summit of the *a* wave. Depending on the PR interval, this descent may continue until a plateau (*z* point) is reached just prior to RV systole. More often, the descent is interrupted by a second positive venous wave, the *c* wave, that is produced by bulging of the tricuspid valve into the right atrium during RV isovolumic systole and by the impact of the carotid artery adjacent to the jugular vein.[158] Following the summit of the *c* wave, the JVP contour declines, forming the normal negative systolic wave, the *x* wave. The *x* descent is due to a combination of atrial relaxation, the downward displacement of the tricuspid valve during RV systole, and the ejection of blood from both ventricles (see Chap. 3).

The positive, later systolic *v* wave in the JVP results from the increase in blood volume in the venae cavae and right atrium during ventricular systole when the tricuspid valve is closed. After the peak of the *v* wave is reached, the RA pressure decreases because of the diminished bulging of the tricuspid valve into the right atrium and the decline in RV pressure that follows tricuspid valve opening. In the JVP, the latter occurs at the peak of the *v* wave. Following the summit of the *v* wave, there is a negative descending limb, referred to as the *y* descent or diastolic collapse, which is due to the tricuspid valve opening and the rapid inflow of blood into the RV. The initial *y* descent corresponds to the RV rapid-filling phase. The trough of the *y* wave occurs in early diastole and is followed by the ascending limb of the *y* wave, which is produced by the continued diastolic inflow of blood into the right side of the heart. The velocity of this ascending pressure curve depends on the rate of venous return and the distensibility of the chambers of the right side of the heart. When diastole is long, the ascending limb of the *y* wave is often followed by a small, brief, positive wave, the *h* wave, which occurs just prior to the next *a* wave. At times, there is a plateau phase rather than a distinct *h* wave. With increasing heart rate, the *y* trough and *y* ascent are followed immediately by the next *a* wave.

Usually, there are three visible major positive waves (*a*, *c*, and *v*) and two negative waves (*x* and *y*) when the pulse rate is below 90 beats per minute and the PR interval is normal. With faster heart rates, there is often fusion of some of the pulse waves, and an accurate analysis of the waveform is more difficult.

## Abnormal Venous Pulse

### ELEVATED VENOUS PRESSURE

The most common cause of an elevated jugular venous pressure is an increased RV pressure such as occurs in patients with PS, PH, or RV failure secondary to left-sided heart failure or RV infarction. The venous pressure also is elevated when obstruction to RV inflow occurs, as with tricuspid stenosis (TS) or RA myxoma, or when constrictive pericardial disease impedes RV inflow. It also may result from vena cava obstruction and, at times, an increased blood volume. Patients with obstructive pulmonary disease may have an elevated venous pressure only during expiration.

### KUSSMAUL'S SIGN

Normally, during inspiration, there is an increase in the *a* wave of the JVP but a decrease in the mean JVP as a result of the increased filling of the right-sided chambers associated with the decrease in intrathoracic pressure. *Kussmaul's sign* denotes an inspiratory increase in the venous pressure, which may occur in patients with severe constrictive pericarditis when the heart is unable to accept the increase in RV volume without a marked increase in the filling pressure. Although Kussmaul's sign was first described in patients with constrictive pericarditis, its most common cause is severe right-sided heart failure, regardless of etiology. The presence of Kussmaul's sign is also useful in the diagnosis of RV infarction[159] (Chap. 80).

### ABNORMALITIES OF THE *a* WAVE

The *a* wave in the JVP is absent when there is no effective atrial contraction, such as in atrial fibrillation (Fig. 12-40*E*). In certain other conditions, the *a* wave may not be apparent. In sinus tachycardia, the *a* wave may fuse with the preceding *v* wave, particularly if the PR interval is prolonged. In some patients with sinus tachycardia, the jugular *a* wave may occur during the *v* or *y* descent and may be small or absent. In the presence of first-degree AV block, a discrete *a* wave with ascending and descending limbs is often completed prior to the first heart sound, and the *ac* interval is prolonged (Fig. 12-40*F*).

Large *a* waves are of considerable diagnostic value (Fig. 12-40*B*). When giant *a* waves are present with each beat, the right atrium is contracting against an increased resistance. This may result from obstruction at the tricuspid valve (TS or atresia, right atrial myxoma) or conditions associated with increased resistance to RV filling.[160] A giant *a* wave is more likely to occur in patients with PS or PH in whom both the atrial and ventricular septa are intact.

Cannon *a* waves occur when the right atrium contracts while the tricuspid valve is closed during RV systole.[158] Cannon *a* waves may occur either regularly or irregularly and are most common in the presence of arrhythmias (Fig. 12-40*G*).

**ABNORMALITIES OF THE *x* WAVE**

The most important alteration of the normally negative systolic collapse (*x* wave) of the JVP is its obliteration or even replacement by a positive wave, usually due to TR. Although atrial relaxation may contribute to the normal *x* descent, the development of atrial fibrillation does not obliterate the *x* wave except in the presence of TR. Accordingly, the occurrence of a positive wave in the JVP during ventricular systole is strong evidence of TR (Fig. 12-40*A*). Mild TR lessens and shortens the downward *x* wave as the regurgitation of blood into the right atrium produces a positive wave that diminishes the usual systolic fall in venous pressure. In some patients with moderate TR, there is a fairly distinct positive wave during ventricular systole between the *c* and *v* waves. This abnormal systolic waveform is usually referred to as a *v* or *cv* wave, although it has also been referred to as an *r* (regurgitant) or an *s* (systolic) wave. In patients with constrictive pericarditis, the *x* descent wave during systole is often more prominent than the early diastolic *y* wave (Fig. 12-40*C* and Chap. 80).

**ABNORMALITIES OF THE *v* WAVE**

The positive, late systolic *v* wave results from the increasing RA blood volume during ventricular systole when the tricuspid valve normally is closed. With mild TR, the *v* wave and the obliteration of the *x* descent result in a single, large positive systolic wave (ventricularization) (Figs. 12-40*A* and 12-41).

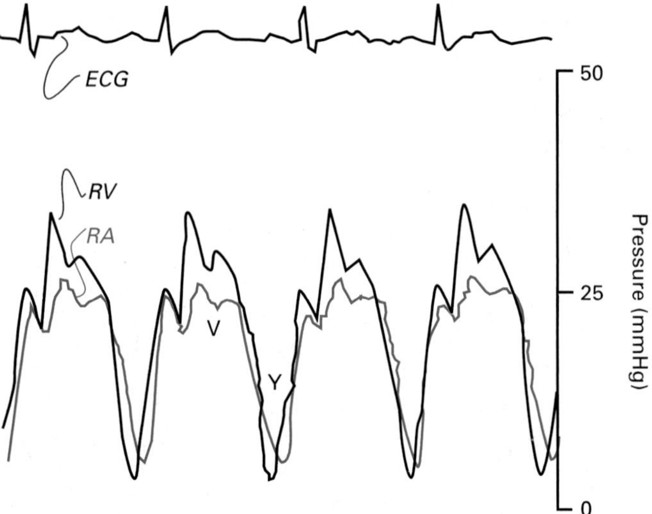


FIGURE 12-41 Right ventricular (RV) and right atrial (RA) pressure curves and simultaneous ECG from a patient with severe tricuspid regurgitation. Note ventricularization of the RA pressure curve.

Normally in the JVP the *v* wave is lower in amplitude than the *a* wave. In patients with an ASD, however, the *a* and *v* waves are often equal in the right atrium and the JVP (Fig. 12-40*D*). In patients with constrictive pericarditis and sinus rhythm, the RA *a* and *v* waves also may be equal, but the venous pressure is increased, which is unusual with isolated ASD. In patients with constrictive pericarditis who are in atrial fibrillation, the *cv* wave is prominent and the *y* descent rapid.

**ABNORMALITIES OF THE *y* TROUGH**

The *y* descent, or diastolic collapse, is produced mainly by tricuspid valve opening and the rapid inflow of blood into the RV. A rapid, deep *y* descent in early diastole occurs with severe TR (Fig. 12-40*A*). A venous pulse characterized by a sharp *y* descent, a deep *y* trough, and a rapid ascent to the baseline is seen in patients with constrictive pericarditis or with severe right-sided heart failure. A slow *y* descent in the JVP suggests an obstruction to RV filling and may be the *only* abnormal finding in patients with TS or right atrial myxoma (Fig. 12-40*B*). In both constrictive pericarditis and severe right-sided heart failure, the venous pressure is elevated with a sharp *y* dip in the JVP (Chap. 80). The presence of a large positive systolic venous wave favors the diagnosis of severe heart failure.

## Effects of Arrhythmias on the Venous Pulse

Large *a* waves in the JVP during arrhythmias are present when the *P* wave (atrial contraction) occurs between the onset of the QRS complex and the termination of the T wave (Fig. 12-40*G*). Such cannon *a* waves may occur regularly in junctional rhythm. More commonly, they occur irregularly when AV dissociation accompanies premature ventricular beats, ventricular tachycardia, or complete heart block. The *a* wave is absent in patients with atrial fibrillation, and flutter *a* waves at a regular rate of 250 to 300 per minute occasionally are observed in patients with atrial flutter and varying degrees of AV block. Patients with multifocal atrial tachycardia often have prominent and somewhat variable *a* waves in the JVP. In these patients, many of whom have PH secondary to lung disease, the *a* waves are often very large.

# EXAMINATION OF THE RETINA*

Inspection of the smaller vessels of the body is possible in only three areas: the retina, conjunctiva, and nail beds. The ophthalmoscope[161] has made the retina by far the easiest and most rewarding site.[161] Viewing this two-dimensional vascular display is generally much easier if the pupils are dilated. Pulse and BP determinations should be made prior to the instillation of rapidly acting mydriatics, since both may increase after absorption of the drops. Examination of the retina should proceed methodically. Best pupillary dilatation is maintained if the optic disk is observed first. Assess for evidence of edema and blurred margins and for cupping with sharp contours. Rule out neovascularization or the pallor of optic atrophy. Next, scan along the superior temporal arcade and inspect the arteries carefully for embolic plaques at each bifurcation. Observe the arteriovenous crossing for obscuration of the vein and for pronounced nicking and banking of the vessels. The lower arcade and the nasal vessels may be inspected next. Avoid the macular area until all else has been viewed because the pupil constricts most intensely when this area is illumi-

*This text is modified from Chap. 11 by N. Banks Anderson, Jr., in the ninth edition of *The Heart.*

TABLE 12-5 Retinal Topography

| Finding | Most Common Location |
|---|---|
| Arteriovenous crossings | Upper temporal quadrant |
| Cotton-wool spots | Around optic disk |
| Hard exudates | Between disk and fovea |
| Microaneurysms | Temporal to fovea |
| Emboli | Arterial bifurcations |
| Diabetic new vessels | Nerve head and arcades |

nated. To discover diabetic microaneurysms early, look just temporal to the fovea, along the horizontal raphe. To find cotton-wool infarcts, look circularly around the disk two disk diameters out. Using this method, the retina can be efficiently searched for evidence of cardiovascular disease[161](Table 12-5).

Variations in the caliber of a single vessel are more important than determinations of arteriovenous ratios. These changes may take the form of focal narrowing, sometimes called *beading* or *spasm*.

### Thickening of the Vascular Wall

Normally, only the blood column is visible when the retinal vessels are viewed. When changes in the walls do occur, they are most visible along the sides of the vessels, since the location of the tangential line of sight presents a greater thickness to the viewer. Fatty exudate (hard exudate) may collect along venous walls (never arteries), particularly in diabetic exudative retinopathy.

### Arteriosclerosis

In arteriosclerosis, medial smooth muscle (which may hypertrophy in chronic hypertension) becomes hyalinized with the deposition of collagen. As the wall thickens, the vessel takes on a burnished coppery luster; with further thickening, this may transmute to silver.

### Arteriovenous Compressions

Arteriovenous compressions or "nicking" results from the sharing by the artery and vein of a common adventitial sheath at their crossings. Arteriosclerotic thickening impedes venous outflow at these locations, with venous tortuosity, engorgement, and darkening of the flood column distal to the compression.[161]

### Atherosclerosis

Retinal atheromata have a predilection for the bifurcation and bends within the first two branches of the central retinal artery, appearing as segments of irregular yellowish sheathing and having the crystalline knobbiness of a salted pretzel stick.[161]

### Cotton-Wool Spots

Cotton-wool spots are generally a sign of serious systemic disease. They may be seen in patients with severe hypertension, blood dyscrasias, collagen diseases, or hemorrhagic shock. Cotton-wool spots also are seen frequently in patients with acquired immunodeficiency syndrome (AIDS) (Fig. 12-42, Plate 41). Cotton-wool "exudates" are not exudates but consist of a cluster of cell-like swollen ends of fragmented axons (cytoid bodies) in an area of edematous retina.[161]

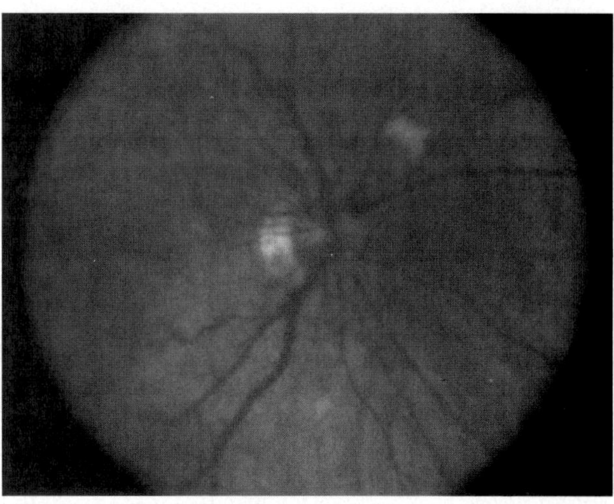

FIGURE 12-42 (Plate 41) Retinal cotton-wool spot. Cotton-wool spots are most frequently found close to the optic disk. Although they occur in acute uncontrolled systemic hypertension, the more common cause now, in younger patients, is infection with the human immunodeficiency virus (HIV). This normotensive 37-year-old man had no visual symptoms and no other retinopathy. There is a myopic crescent at the temporal disk edge, which is not abnormal. He died of complications related to the acquired immunodeficiency syndrome (AIDS) 2 years later.

### Hard Exudates

Hard exudates are most likely residues of edema. They occur in situations where the vessels become leaky, and as the more watery component of the extravasation is resorbed, the lipid residue forms a hard, yellow, waxy deposit. These deposits may surround the leaking vessel in a circinate ring or may accumulate in the macula, radiating from the fovea in the spokes of a macular "star" (Fig. 12-43, Plate 42).

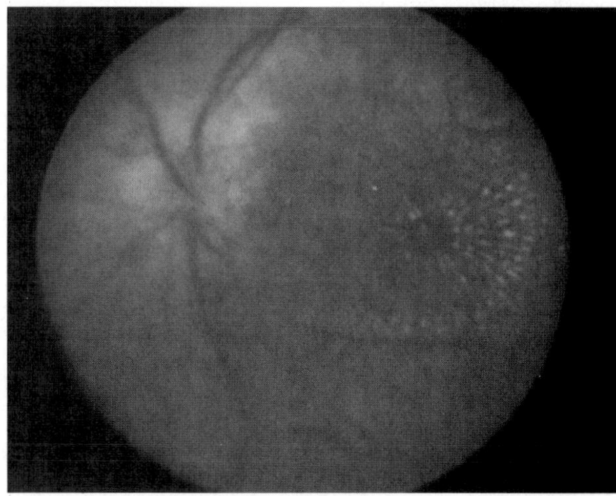

FIGURE 12-43 (Plate 42) Disk swelling and hard exudate in a macular "star" pattern. In this hypertensive patient with periarteritis nodosa, vascular leakage has led to the deposition of hard exudates around the fovea. The star pattern of the exudate is due to radial perifoveal connective tissue. Note also that the optic disk is edematous, with blurred margins, secondary to hypertension.

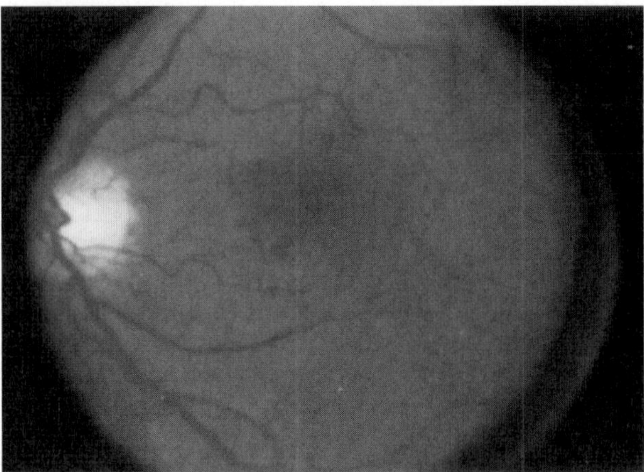

FIGURE 12-44 (Plate 43) Background diabetic retinopathy. Retinal microaneurysms, dot-and-blot hemorrhages, and a few fine upper temporal hard exudates are diagnostic of early diabetic retinopathy. The patient had no visual symptoms, but retinopathy of this magnitude can often be seen in patients with insulin-requiring diabetes of 15 or more years' duration.

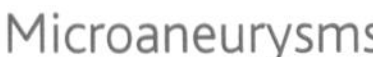

## Microaneurysms

Microaneurysms occur in many disease states, including retinal venous obstructive disease, sickle cell disease, the dysproteinemias, Behcet's disease, sarcoidosis, and other forms of uveitis. They may represent abortive attempts at revascularization of compromised capillary bed in diabetics (Fig. 12-44, Plate 43).

## Neovascularization

In neovascularization the new vessels generally originate from capillaries from the venous side of the circulation and are associated with greater or lesser degrees of fibrosis. In all cases, however, the new vessels are incorporated in an associated fibrous membrane (Figs. 12-45, Plate 44, and 12-46).

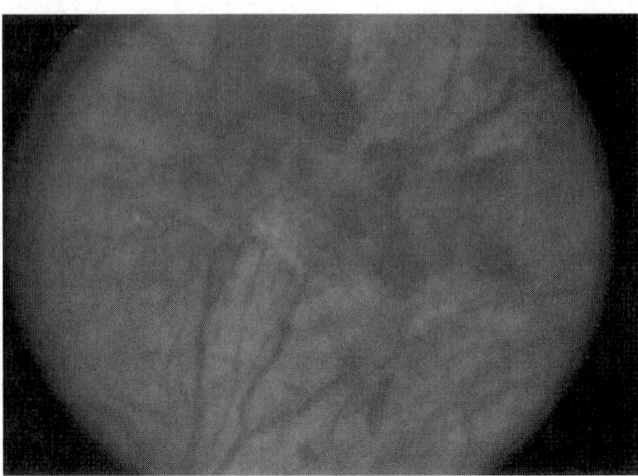

FIGURE 12-45 (Plate 44) Proliferative diabetic retinopathy with preretinal hemorrhage. When neovascularization develops, preretinal and vitreous hemorrhages are much more likely to occur. Easily visible neovascularization either in the periphery of the retina, as in this diabetic patient, or at the disk is an indication for immediate panretinal laser photocoagulation.

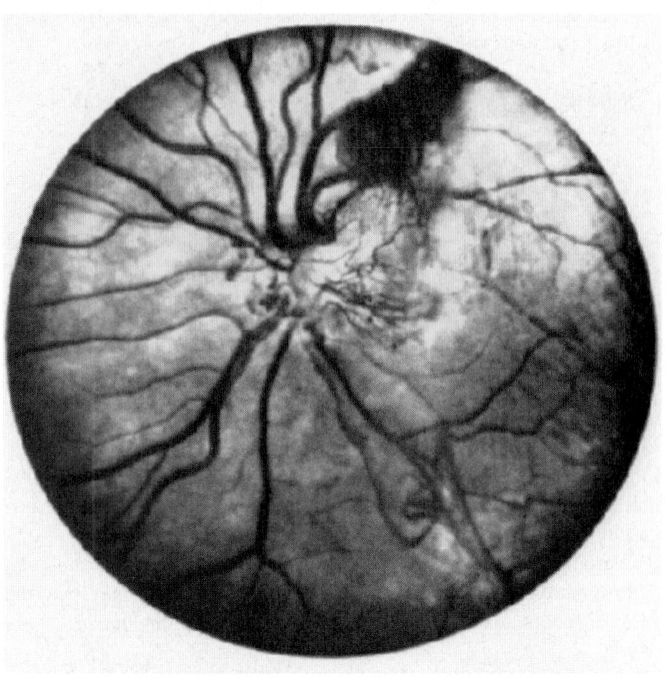

FIGURE 12-46 Proliferative diabetic retinopathy, left eye. There is extensive neovascularization of the disk with an associated small intravitreal hemorrhage that obscures the upper temporal vessels. Along the inferior temporal arcade is another area of neovascularization. These new vessels are incorporated into fibrous membranes, which may tent up the vessels and cause traction detachments of the retina, as at the lower right edge of the photograph.

## Retinal Hemorrhage

Hemorrhage into the retina indicates further breakdown in the integrity of the vascular wall. When the hemorrhage occurs in the inner retina, as in hypertension, it assumes a feathery flame shape as it is molded and dispersed by the nerve fibers coursing toward the disk. In obstruction of the central retinal vein, the fundus may be splattered with blood (Fig. 12-47, Plate 45).

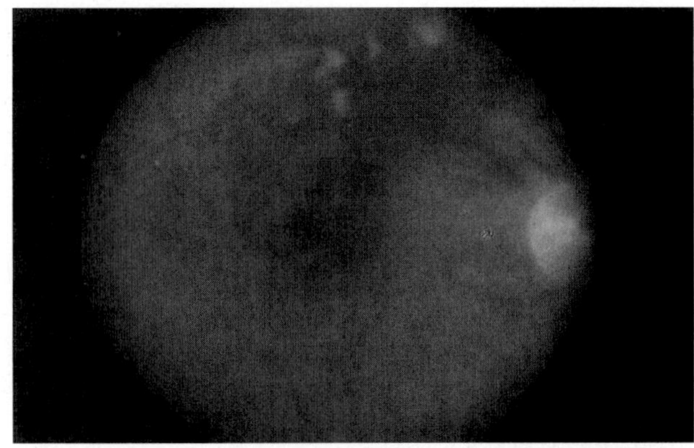

FIGURE 12-47 (Plate 45) Branch retinal vein obstruction. Thickening of the retinal arterial wall in diabetes and hypertension may compromise the lumen of the vein, where artery and vein share a common adventitial sheath at an arteriovenous crossing. The resulting obstruction produces hemorrhage retinopathy in the drainage area of the affected vein. Note how the flame-shaped pattern of blood outlines the arcuate pattern of the nerve fibers as they run toward the optic disk.

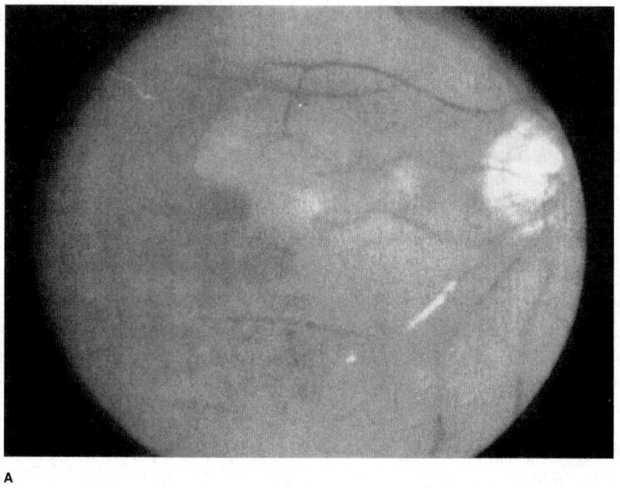

A

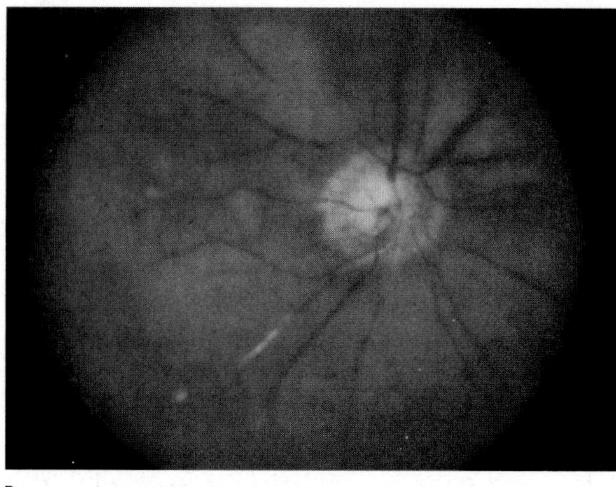

B

FIGURE 12-48 (Plate 46) Embolic retinal arterial obstruction (*A* and *B*). Cholesterol crystals may dislodge from the walls of the heart, aortic arch, or carotids. Carried into the retinal circulation as Hollenhorst plaques, they seldom obstruct the arterioles completely. Although amaurosis fugax is more common, the embolic burden may occasionally be so large as to produce retinal infarction. Note in the photograph of the macular area (*A*) that this patient's fovea remains red, while there is a pale, cloudy swelling nasal to it. This has produced a half "cherry-red" spot. With complete central retinal artery occlusion, the red foveal area is completely surrounded by pale swollen retina. Hollenhorst cholesterol plaques can be seen in both the upper and lower temporal retinal arteries. In *A*, the inferior temporal arteriole demonstrates "boxcar" segmentation of the blood column, indicative of very slow flow.

## Vascular Occlusion

When the central artery or one of its branches is occluded, the nonperfused retinal area becomes cloudy in a matter of minutes. At the fovea, where the retina is one cell layer thick and nourished by the choroid, the normal color and transparency persist. By contrast with the surrounding pallor, the fovea then has a cherry-red appearance (Fig. 12-48, Plate 46). Occlusions of branches of the central vein produce edema and hemorrhage in the drained area. As collateral drainage channels develop (Fig 12-47 and Plate 45), the edema and hemorrhagic retinopathy subside, leaving white-walled veins, neovascularization, and microaneurysms in the affected area (Fig. 12-49, Plate 47).

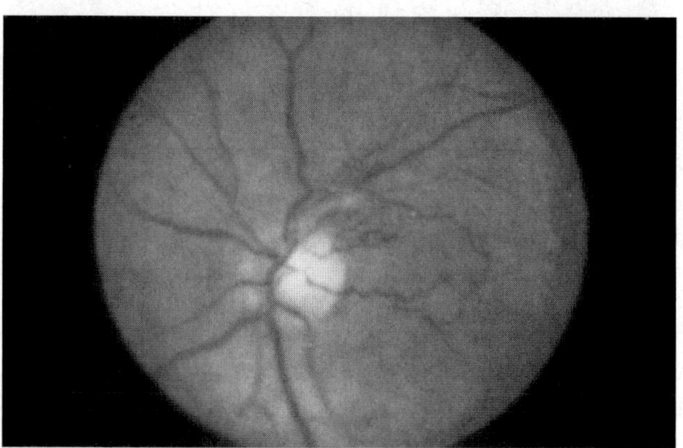

FIGURE 12-49 (Plate 47) Neovascularization after branch retinal vein obstruction. New vessels may develop late after obstruction of a branch of the central retinal vein. These most often serve to shunt flow around the obstructed vessel site and are thus not as exuberantly proliferative as those seen in diabetic retinopathy.

## Optic Disk Edema

The term *papilledema* is reserved for the form of disk edema that is the result of increased intracranial pressure. It therefore has an etiologic connotation. *Papillitis* is the term applied to inflammatory disk edema. Patients with anterior ischemic optic neuropathy commonly have a pale, edematous disk with an altitudinal field effect.

## Embolism

The characteristics of retinal emboli of cardiovascular significance are listed in Table 12-6. Of these, platelet emboli are at once the most common and the most evanescent. Hollenhorst cholesterol plaques may be identified at the same bifurcations for months to years after the embolic shower. Platelet emboli, Hollenhorst plaques (Fig. 12-48, Plate 46; Fig. 12-50), and calcium emboli (Fig. 12-51, Plate 48) are usually seen along the course of a retinal artery. Roth spots (Fig. 12-52, Plate 49) and fat emboli may not appear to be intravascular and may not be associated with a vessel that is ophthalmoscopically visible (Table 12-6).[159]

## Diabetes Mellitus

In diabetes mellitus, focal loss of a portion of the capillary bed is followed by microaneurysm formation and vascular dilatation around the borders of the area of capillary dropout (Fig. 12-44 and Plate 43). Vascular leakage occurs with dot-and-blot hemorrhages and deposits of hard exudate (Fig 12-53). New blood vessels develop along the vascular arcades and at the optic nerve head (Figs. 12-45, Plate 44, and 12-46).

Vasoconstriction of the arterial tree and thickening of the arterial vessel walls with consequent reduction in lumen diameter are homeostatic responses to hypertension. Arteriosclerotic narrowing of the vessels acts to insulate the capillary bed from the elevated pressure of the arterial supply. These arteriosclerotic changes are visible as

TABLE 12-6 Emboli of Cardiovascular Significance

| Type | Appearance | Significance |
|---|---|---|
| Platelet | Dull pink to gray often with associated fibrin | Downstream vegetations, mural thrombi |
| Hollenhorst plaque | Glistening yellow-orange plaques at bifurcations | Downstream atheroma (containing cholesterol) |
| Calcium plaque | Glistening white plaques | Calcific aortic stenosis |
| Roth spot | Hemorrhage with gray-white center | Blood dyscrasia or septic embolus as in subacute bacterial endocarditis |
| Fat embolus | Fuzzy-bordered gray-white spot without hemorrhage | Severe trauma with long-bone fractures |
| Myxoma | Disk edema, retinal edema in arterial supply zone | Life-threatening atrial myxoma |

narrowing, increases in central light reflexes, and copper and silver "wiring" of the arteries (Fig. 12-54, Plate 50). Radial arrangement of such exudate deposits in the macula produces a "star" (Fig 12-43 and Plate 42). Hemorrhage may occur in the retinal layers in a characteristic flame pattern, and focal ischemia in the nerve fiber may result in cotton-wool microinfarcts. In severe hypertensive decompensation, the optic nerve head becomes swollen and edematous (Fig. 12-43, Plate 42).

Hypertensive patients should be classified as to whether or not their retinal circulation is compensated or has decompensated with observable edema, cotton-wool spots, flame hemorrhages, or swelling of the optic disk.[161]

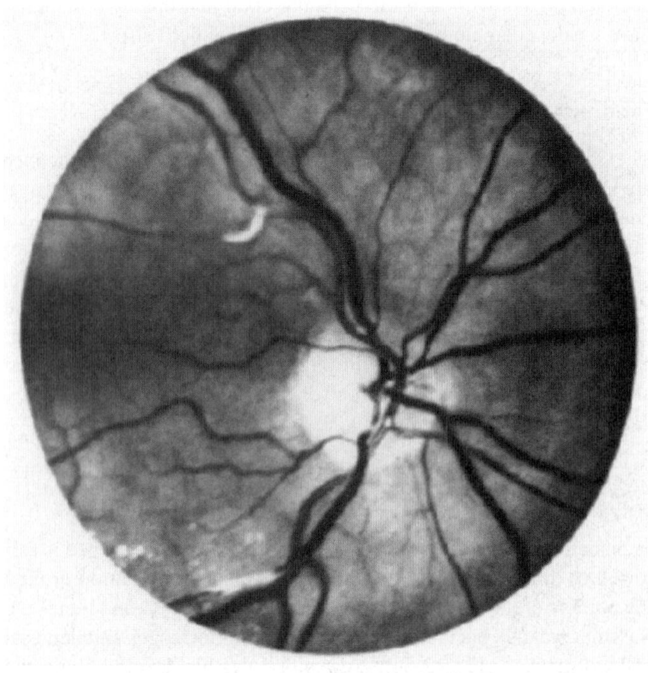

FIGURE 12-50 Retinal emboli often lodge at bifurcations, as in this patient with carotid atherosclerosis. Note that the embolic material often seems larger than the containing vessel, as in the embolus at the lower left edge of the photograph. Emboli may damage the vessel wall and cause leakage, as can be seen by the exudate deposited about the inferior embolus. Hollenhorst cholesterol plaques rarely obstruct arterial flow completely, and this patient maintained vision.

## PHYSICAL EXAMINATION OF THE CHEST, ABDOMEN, AND EXTREMITIES

Physical examination of the lungs is an important noninvasive technique requiring only a stethoscope.[162] Wheezing and a pleural friction rub are detected only by the clinical evaluation. The pleural friction rub may be a clue to the diagnosis of pulmonary infarction. Pleural fluid due to heart failure is usually located in the right pleural space. When pleural fluid is localized predominately to the left, a cause other than or in addition to heart failure, such as pulmonary infarction, should be considered.

A pneumothorax may develop as a consequence of spontaneous mediastinal emphysema or may be iatrogenic, due to procedures.[162] Hyperresonance and diminished breath sounds may be due to pulmonary emphysema. Signs of pulmonary consolidation may be due to pneumonia or pulmonary infarction. Wheezing and rales may be due to bronchial disease. Heart failure may be associated with rales in the lung bases, wheezing, and pleural fluid. Importantly, heart failure frequently is not associated with rales, since interstitial pulmonary edema usually does not produce rales.[162]

The diameter of the *abdominal* aorta should be determined in every patient[162] (Chap. 98). An abdominal aortic aneurysm may be missed if the examiner fails to assess the area above the umbilicus.

Specific abnormalities of the abdomen may be secondary to heart disease. A large, tender liver is common in patients with heart failure or constrictive pericarditis. Systolic hepatic pulsations are frequent in patients with tricuspid regurgitation (TR). A palpable spleen is a common but late sign in patients with severe heart failure and is also often present in patients with infective endocarditis.

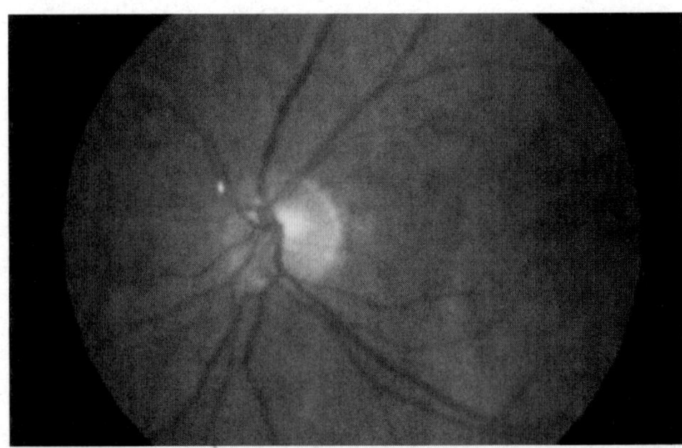

FIGURE 12-51 (Plate 48) Calcific retinal embolus associated with aortic valvular disease. Calcific aortic valvular disease and valve replacement surgery may give rise to retinal emboli. Like cholesterol emboli, these calcific flecks lodge at arterial bifurcations but seldom obstruct flow completely. They are white and glitter in the ophthalmoscope beam. Somewhat similar emboli may be seen after the intravenous injection of illicit drugs expanded with talc.

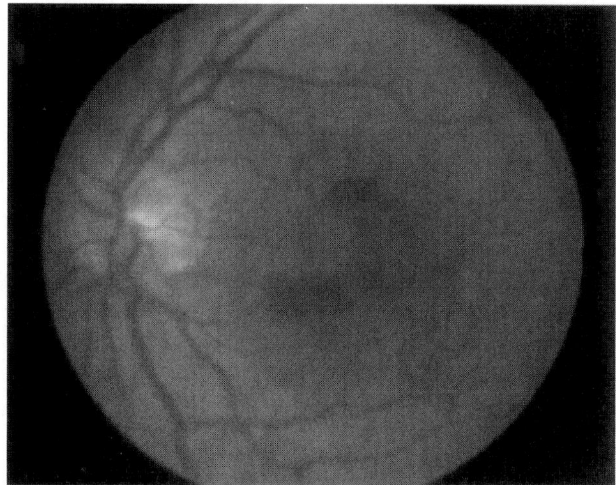

FIGURE 12-52 (Plate 49) Retinal hemorrhages, such as may occur after cardiac catheterization. They can be either symptomatic or asymptomatic, although the latter are more common. Presumably these are the result of embolic events. Note, in this recently catheterized patient, the two oval hemorrhages and a small area of cloudy swelling just inferior and temporal to the fovea.

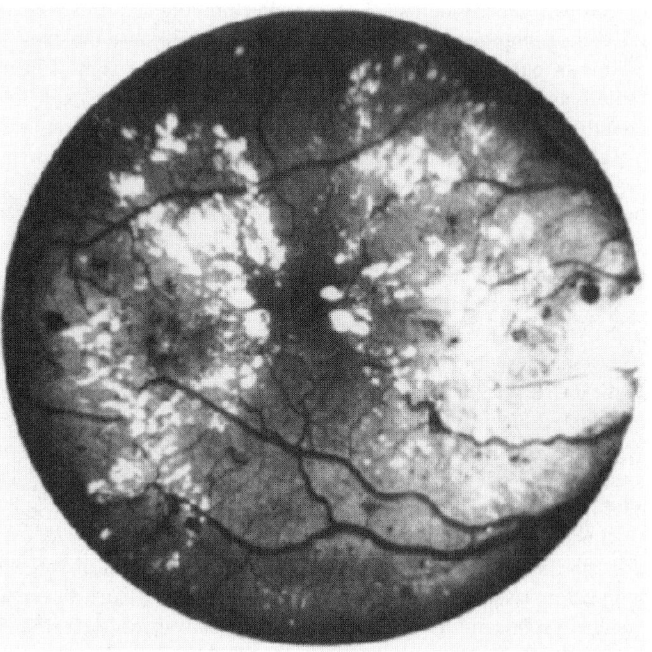

FIGURE 12-53 Exudative diabetic retinopathy, right eye, illustrating microaneurysms, dot-and-blot hemorrhages, and venous engorgement with extensive deposits of hard yellow exudate.

Although hepatic cirrhosis is the most common cause of ascites, the latter may occur with heart failure alone, although it is less common with the use of diuretic therapy. Severe TR, as caused by infective endocarditis in drug addicts, may produce prominent systolic pulsation of the internal jugular veins in the neck; a large, moving, and pulsating liver; and ascites. Constrictive pericarditis should be considered when the ascites is out of proportion to peripheral edema. In many such patients, the heart is normal in size or only slightly enlarged, a pericardial "knock" is heard, and there is a rapid $x$ and/or $y$ descent in the internal jugular vein pulsation.[162] Restrictive cardiomyopathy can mimic constrictive pericarditis, but the heart is usually moderately large in patients with restrictive cardiomyopathy. When there is an arteriovenous fistula in the abdomen, a continuous murmur may be heard over the abdomen. Fistulas due to trauma and surgery may occur.

A systolic bruit may be heard over the kidney areas and may signify renal artery stenosis, particularly in patients with systemic hypertension. A systolic bruit often is auscultated over the abdominal aorta, but its presence does not indicate the severity of disease of the aorta.[162]

Examination of the upper and lower extremities may provide important diagnostic information (Chap. 90). Atherosclerosis of the peripheral arteries may produce intermittent claudication of the buttock, calf, thigh, or foot, with severe disease resulting in tissue damage of the toes. Peripheral atherosclerosis is an important risk factor for ischemic heart disease, and its presence increases the likelihood

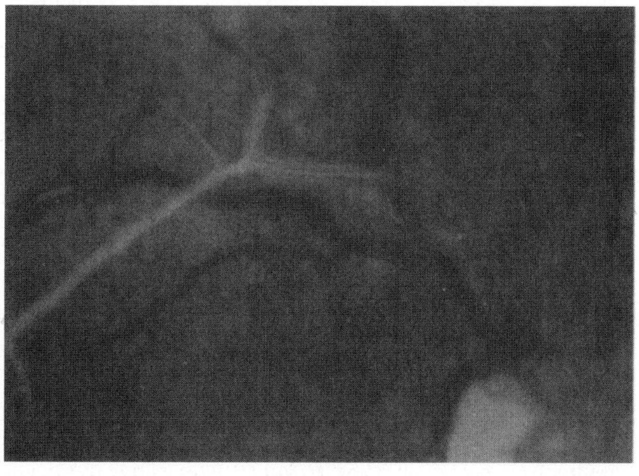

A

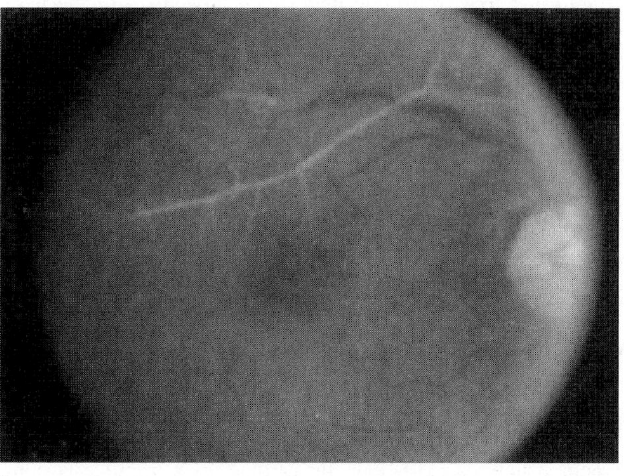

B

FIGURE 12-54 (Plate 50) *A.* Retinal arteriosclerosis. This 75-year-old hypertensive woman has marked arteriosclerosis of the upper temporal retinal arteriole and its branches. When the narrowed blood column can no longer be seen, the thickened wall produces the "silver wire" appearance seen here. Where the arteriole crosses its associated vein, the course of the vein is altered and its blood column cannot be seen. This venous "nicking" and "banking" is associated with impairment of outflow, and the affected veins become darker, larger, and more tortuous. *B.* Low-power view showing the silver-wire arteriole.

of coronary atherosclerosis. Thrombophlebitis often causes pain in the calf or thigh or edema, and its presence should raise the consideration of pulmonary emboli as well. Edema is a late sign of heart failure, and its predictive value as a diagnostic sign is poor. It frequently involves the right leg prior to the left. Considerable heart failure and a resulting weight gain may be present without edema being present. Edema of the lower extremities may be secondary to local factors such as varicose veins or thrombophlebitis or the removal of veins at CABG surgery. Under such circumstances, the edema often occurs in only one leg.

Edema may result from restrictive garments, and venous stasis often is secondary to a long trip in a car or airplane.[157] Edema may be due to salt and water retention in patients with primary renal disease. In the differential diagnosis of edema, local factors should be considered first. If local factors can be excluded, an assessment for evidence of primary renal disease is indicated. Rarely, peripheral edema can be an early sign of lymphatic obstruction produced by metastatic disease in the pelvis or abdomen.

Since the invention of the stethoscope by Laennec in 1826, cardiac auscultation has played a key role in the evaluation of patients with cardiovascular disease and is unlikely to be replaced by small handheld echocardiographic detectors. The analysis of heart sounds and murmurs by phonocardiography, together with information obtained by cardiac catheterization, angiography, echocardiography, and cardiac surgery, has made cardiac auscultation a *precise discipline* based on firm physiologic principles.[163]

## INSPECTION AND PALPATION OF THE PRECORDIUM

Inspection and palpation of the cardiac pulsations of the anterior chest have been practiced by physicians since ancient times and have a solid scientific basis. The results of precordial inspection and palpation have been correlated with noninvasive studies, hemodynamic data, and surgical and autopsy studies[164,165] and remain an important part of the cardiovascular examination.

### Precordial Pulsations Due to the Heartbeat

Precordial pulsations, reflecting underlying movement of the heart and great vessels, occur principally in seven areas of the anterior chest[164,165] (Fig. 12-55):

1. The sternoclavicular area
2. The aortic area
3. The pulmonic area
4. The RV (left parasternal) area
5. The LV (apical) area
6. The epigastric area
7. Ectopic (variable-location) areas

While the cardiac apex is usually produced by the LV, it is sometimes produced by an enlarged RV that displaces the LV laterally and posteriorly. Occasionally, the cardiac position is abnormal due to dextroposition, dextroversion, dextrocardia, or other changes in intrathoracic structures. Although the cardiac apex impulse is commonly referred to as the *point of maximal impulse* (PMI), the two terms are not necessarily synonymous, since the maximal precordial pulsation may be produced by an enlarged or hypertrophied RV, a dilated aorta or pulmonary artery, or an LV wall-motion abnormality.

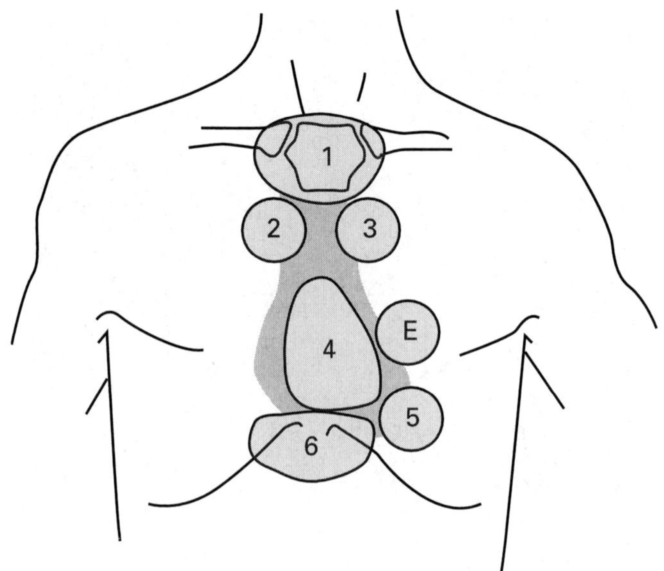


FIGURE 12-55 Seven areas to be examined for abnormal cardiovascular pulsations by inspection and palpation. (From Schlant RC, Hurst JW. *Examination of the Precordium: Inspection and Palpation*. New York: American Heart Association; 1990:1–28. Used with permission from the publisher and authors.)

Therefore, precordial pulsations should be described by their location, timing, contour, and duration.

### Inspection of the Precordium

The examiner should first inspect the thorax from the foot of the bed with the subject supine, the legs horizontal, and the head and trunk elevated to approximately 30 degrees.[162–167] The patient may have a barrel-shaped chest with an increased anteroposterior diameter, a straight-back syndrome, pectus excavatum, pectus carinatum, kyphoscoliosis, or ankylosing spondylitis. Each may produce or be associated with cardiac abnormalities. Asymmetry of the thorax due to convex bulging of the precordium suggests the presence of heart disease since childhood. Exaggerated movements of the cardiac apex often can be detected from this observation point.

Next, the examiner should move to the patient's right side and observe the patient's chest tangentially rather than from above. A light beam directed across the precordium may enhance subtle findings.[163,164] Precordial movements frequently can be recognized more easily if the tip of an applicator stick, tongue blade, or light pencil is held against the impulse as a fulcrum. Motion of the underlying chest wall is transmitted to the free end of the instrument and exaggerated, making the movements more obvious.

In patients with an abnormally prominent apical impulse and in some thin, normal individuals, the apex beat can be seen. The presystolic apical motion associated with the atrial contribution to ventricular filling (a fourth heart sound) sometimes may be visualized, as may the diastolic waveform due to rapid ventricular filling (a third heart sound). A late systolic bulge either at the apex or in an ectopic area, usually located either medial and superior or lateral to the apical impulse, may be observed in patients with a large dyskinetic ventricular aneurysm.[168] When precordial pulsations are exaggerated, they become visible as well as palpable. In general, outward movements are best discerned by palpation, whereas inward movements usually are seen more easily than felt.[164,165]

## Palpation of the Precordium

With Tietze's syndrome, pain, sometimes with swelling and tenderness, may affect the costochondral, chondrosternal, or xiphosternal joints and may be reproduced by touching. Palpation also may reveal tender superficial veins on the anterior chest (Mondor's disease), a rare etiology of chest discomfort.[166] Collateral vessels in the posterior intercostal spaces may be palpable in patients with aortic coarctation.

Palpation of the precordium is also best performed from the right side, with the patient supine and the upper trunk elevated 30 degrees. Palpation with the right hand usually provides more information. Patients with suspected cardiovascular disease also should be examined in the left lateral decubitus position, rotated 45 to 90 degrees.[162] In this position, the normal LV impulse may be displaced several centimeters leftward and may appear more prominent and sustained. The size of the apex impulse rather than its distance from the midsternal or midclavicular line determines its normality.[162] Often, the apex impulse and other palpable events such as an LV rapid filling wave ($S_3$) or presystolic *a* wave ($S_4$) may be felt only in this position.

The location and size of the cardiac apex impulse should be defined, its contour characterized, and any abnormal precordial pulsations identified. The palm of the hand, ventral surface of the proximal metacarpals, and fingers should all be used for optimal appreciation of specific movements. The fingers appear to be particularly insensitive to movements of relatively large amplitude and very low frequency. Thus, an examiner's hand occasionally can be seen to move up and down with precordial motion, although the same movements are imperceptible by palpation alone. By contrast, higher-frequency events, such as the vibrations associated with abnormally loud aortic or pulmonic components of the second heart sound, are easily palpable, but the amplitude of their movement is not readily visible.[162]

The pads of the fingers are most useful for detecting LV and normal RV motion, whereas the palm and proximal metacarpals are usually best used for palpating larger, low-frequency movements such as the parasternal systolic lift of RV hypertrophy.[162] High-frequency movements such as ejection sounds, valve closure sounds, and mitral opening snaps are detected more easily with the hand held firmly against the chest, whereas low-frequency movements such as ventricular diastolic filling events are best recognized with light pressure with the fingertips.

Thrills are palpable vibrations from murmurs or bruits ordinarily associated with grade 4/6 murmurs or louder. The location of a thrill often helps identify its origin. Thrills are palpated most easily using either the palm of the hand or the proximal metacarpals. Sometimes thrills are felt better during a held end-expiration with moderate pressure applied from the right hand on top of the left hand.[163]

To detect abnormal RV motion, the heel of the hand should be placed over the lower half of the sternum with the patient's breath held at end-expiration. The parasternal lift due to RV hypertrophy is often better visualized than actually felt. In patients with chronic obstructive pulmonary disease, subxiphoid and epigastric palpation with the patient's breath held at end-inspiration is useful for assessing RV motion.

Proper patient positioning is important. The location of the apex impulse is usually described in terms of its distance from the midsternal or midclavicular line and the intercostal space in which it is located. The apex impulse is often faint or not palpable with the patient supine because of the distance of the ventricular apex from the chest wall. Palpation of the cardiac apex with the patient in the left lateral position, however, permits optimal assessment of the size (diameter) and contour of the systolic outward movement at the apex; diastolic movements are also best appreciated with the patient in this position. Since the apex impulse may shift several centimeters laterally when the patient rotates to the left lateral position, however, the location of the apex impulse may be incorrect in this position. Palpation with simultaneous cardiac auscultation often is useful for identifying the systolic or diastolic timing of precordial pulsations. Simultaneous palpation of the apical impulse and carotid pulse may be helpful in assessing the severity of AS. An appreciable lag time between the onset of the apex impulse and carotid pulse usually indicates severe AS.

## Physiology of Precordial Motion

Although only the apical impulse is palpable normally, a brief RV systolic motion can be felt at the left sternal edge in asthenic individuals. With the onset of isovolumic LV contraction, there is anterior movement of the LV toward the chest walls (Fig. 12-56). Counterclockwise rotation of the LV along its longitudinal axis occurs as the cardiac apex moves anteriorly and makes contact with the chest wall in early systole.[166] The maximal outward movement occurs coincident with or just after aortic valve opening. After rapid early ejection, the LV moves away from the chest wall, and the apex retracts during later systole and returns to baseline well before the second heart sound.[162] The outward apex movement in early systole normally is palpable, but the later systolic inward movement is only visible (Fig. 12-56). Palpable movements of the apex in diastole result from LV filling. The early diastolic outward movement due to rapid ventricular filling (F wave), which corresponds to the normal $S_3$, is occasionally palpable in normal children and young adults (Fig. 12-56). Later diastolic filling due to left atrial contraction (*a* wave) is not normally palpable. Precordial motion is modified by age, chest wall thickness, lung disease, and pleural or pericardial effusion.

### AREA 1: STERNOCLAVICULAR AREA PULSATIONS

The sternoclavicular area (Fig. 12-55) includes the right and left sternoclavicular joints, the manubrium, and the upper sternum. Usually, no pulsation is noted in this area. A slight, brief systolic pulsation of a sternoclavicular joint or the manubrium may be due to AR. Abnormal pulsations and movements in the sternoclavicular area are commonly produced by enlargement, dilatation, or diseases of the aorta, particularly aortic dissection, atherosclerotic aneurysm, or syphilitic aneurysm. An abnormal pulsation of a sternoclavicular joint in patients with chest pain may be an early clue to diagnosis of aortic dissection. A slight pulsation in the right sternoclavicular area may suggest a right-sided aortic arch in patients with cyanotic heart disease, particularly tetralogy of Fallot.[162] A kinked, tortuous right carotid artery or dilatation and tortuosity of other brachiocephalic vessels may produce visible and palpable pulsations in the suprasternal notch or the supraclavicular areas.

### AREA 2: AORTIC AREA PULSATIONS

Vibrations of the aortic component ($A_2$) of the second heart sound may be palpated when they are accentuated, as in arterial hypertension. With valvular AS, a systolic thrill is present frequently in the second and less commonly in the first and third right intercostal spaces near the sternum (Fig. 12-55). It often radiates upward toward the right side of the neck and to the suprasternal notch and right supraclavicular area. Less frequently, the thrill is palpable at the second

| Type of movement and associated clinical condition | Graphic Representation (palpable features in heavy line) | Location and accompanying features |
|---|---|---|
| **NORMAL ADULT APEX IMPULSE** | 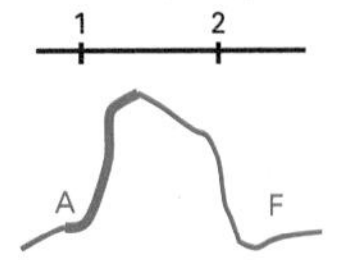 1 2 A F | Cardiac apex; moderate systolic thrust; A and F waves usually imperceptible |
| **HYPERKINETIC APEX IMPULSE**<br>°°Normal Child<br>°°Hyperdynamic states<br>°°Ventricular septal defect<br>°°Patent ductus arteriosus<br>°°Mitral regurgitation<br>°°Aortic regurgitation | 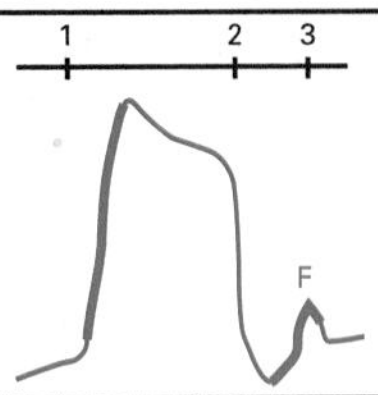 1 2 3 F | Exaggerated thrust at cardiac apex; F wave may be palpable, coincident with third heart sound |
| **HYPERKINETIC RIGHT VENTRICULAR IMPULSE**<br>°°Atrial septal defect<br>°°Pulmonary regurgitation | Same as above | Maximal at left sternal edge in third and fourth intercostal spaces |
| **SUSTAINED APEX IMPULSE**<br>°°Left ventricular hypertrophy,<br>°°°°as in:<br>°°Aortic stenosis<br>°°Hypertension<br>°°Insert: a variation that<br>°°°°may occur in hypertrophic<br>°°°°cardiomyopathy | 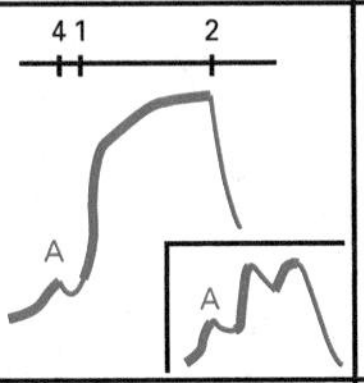 4 1 2 A A | Maximal at cardiac apex; A wave may be visible and palpable coincident with fourth heart sound |
| **SUSTAINED RIGHT VENTRICULAR IMPULSE**<br>°°Right ventricular<br>°°°°hypertrophy, as in:<br>°°Pulmonary hypertension<br>°°Pulmonary stenosis | Same impulse as in Sustained above | Maximal at left sternal edge in third and fourth intercostal spaces |
| **ECTOPIC LEFT VENTRICULAR IMPULSE**<br>°°Ventricular aneurysm | Same impulse as in Sustained above | Maximal over mid-precordium rather than at apex |
| **LEFT ATRIAL EXPANSION**<br>°°Severe mitral regurgitation | 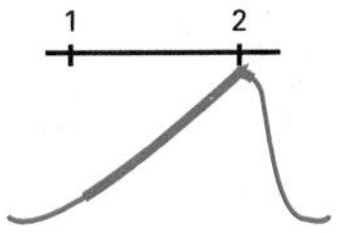 1 2 | Left sternal edge or entire precordium; hyperkinetic apex impulse due to left ventricular volume overload |
| **PULMONARY ARTERY PULSATION**<br>°°Pulmonary hypertension | 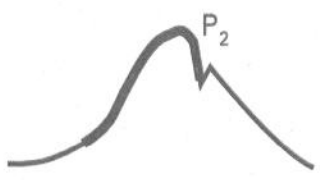 $P_2$ | Second left intercostal space; palpable $P_2$ |
| **INWARD MOVEMENT DURING SYSTOLE**<br>°°Constrictive pericarditis<br>°°Tricuspid regurgitation;<br>°°°°primary | 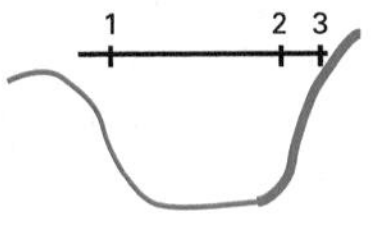 1 2 3 | Cardiac apex or entire precordium; reversal of direction during systole as compared with preceding examples |
| **DIASTOLIC MOVEMENTS**<br>°°Cardiomyopathy | 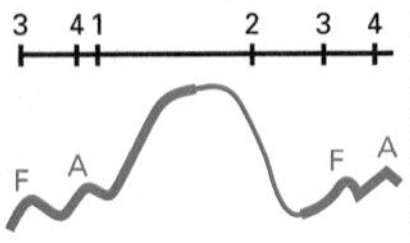 3 4 1 2 3 4 F A F A | Cardiac apex; systolic movement may be inconspicuous; diastolic movements F and A correspond to 3rd and 4th heart sounds which may merge in tachycardia to form a summation gallop |

FIGURE 12-56 Graphic representation of apical movements in health and disease. Heavy line indicates palpable features. $P_2$ = pulmonary component of second heart sound; A = atrial wave, corresponding to a fourth heart sound ($S_4$) or atrial gallop; F = filling wave, corresponding to third heart sound ($S_3$) or ventricular gallop. (From Willis P IV. Inspection and palpation of the precordium. In: Hurst JW, ed. *The Heart*, 7th ed. New York: McGraw-Hill; 1990:164. Reproduced with permission from the publisher and author.)

or third left interspaces next to the sternum or at the apex. A systolic thrill in the aortic area and in the right carotid artery also can occur in patients with severe AR without stenosis. Abnormal systolic pulsations in the aortic area may be due to dilatation of the ascending aorta due to aneurysm and/or chronic AR.

## AREA 3: PULMONIC AREA PULSATIONS

Vibrations associated with a loud pulmonic component of $S_2$ (Fig. 12-55) often are palpable in patients with PH from any cause. During simultaneous palpation of the carotid pulse, a palpable $P_2$ or $A_2$ coincides with the early downslope of the carotid pulse. A systolic thrill in the second and third left intercostal spaces near the sternum often occurs with pulmonic valve stenosis. The thrill often radiates toward the left side of the neck, in contrast to the thrill with AS, which radiates upward and to the right.

Pulsations of a dilated pulmonary artery may be seen or felt in the second or third left intercostal space near the sternum. In normal infants and children or anxious adults with thin chest walls, a slight, brief, early systolic pulsation may be present in this area. This pulsation is accentuated by conditions that cause an increased cardiac output (e.g., fever, pregnancy). Idiopathic dilatation of the pulmonary artery also may cause a palpable systolic impulse in the same area.[163]

The common causes of an accentuated and sustained systolic pulsation in the pulmonary artery area are PH, increased pulmonary blood flow, and their combination. In general, PH causes a relatively slow, sustained, and forceful pulmonary artery pulsation, whereas a large pulmonary blood flow (e.g., ASD) produces an extremely active, more vigorous, but less sustained pulsation. Valvular pulmonary stenosis with poststenotic dilatation of the pulmonary artery may be associated with a palpable, sustained pulsation in this area, often with a slow rise of the initial phase.

## AREA 4: LEFT PARASTERNAL–RIGHT VENTRICULAR OR TRICUSPID AREA PULSATIONS

A systolic thrill in the third, fourth, or fifth intercostal space in the parasternal area to the left of the sternum (Fig. 12-55) is characteristic of VSD, although TR also can produce a thrill here.

Normally, the lower left parasternal region retracts very slightly during systole, and RV activity is not palpable. Slight, gentle outward pulsations of the lower sternum and left parasternal area may be recorded in normal children and young adults, in thin adults with a small anteroposterior thoracic diameter, or in patients with pectus excavatum.

Abnormal pulsations of the sternal and left parasternal areas most commonly are due to RV hypertrophy or dilatation. The pulsation associated with RV hypertension is usually more sustained throughout systole and tends to rise more gradually than the pulsation produced by an RV volume load, which usually is more vigorous but often briefer.[161,166]

A predominant RV pressure load occurs with PS and PH due to LV failure, mitral valve disease, a left-to-right shunt, or pulmonary vascular disease. The sustained anterior precordial pulsation associated with isolated valvular PS may not occur with tetralogy of Fallot because the thick RV is not excessively dilated. ASD and VSD are two congenital lesions frequently associated with an RV volume load.

Moderate or severe MR may produce an abnormal late systolic anterior left parasternal pulsation even in the absence of PH.[164] This precordial lift is brisk, and its greatest force coincides with the accentuated *v* wave in the left atrial pressure wave. It likely is due to the large volume of blood regurgitated into the expanding left atrium, which is located centrally behind the RV and anterior to the spine. While expansion of the left atrium may contribute somewhat to the anterior motion of the heart, it is likely that most of the anterior motion and force is the result of a jet or squid effect.

Conditions associated with a decrease in RV compliance, such as RV hypertrophy due to PH, may be associated with a palpable "right-sided" $S_4$ in this area or, occasionally, in the epigastric area. Although a palpable $S_3$ in this area may reflect a large RV volume load, it usually indicates RV dysfunction or failure. RV $S_3$ and $S_4$ vibrations may be augmented during inspiration and may be attenuated or even disappear during expiration.

### AREA 5: APICAL AREA PULSATIONS

As mentioned earlier, the apex impulse (Fig. 12-55) is not necessarily synonymous with maximum impulse or point of maximum impulse (PMI). The location, size, and character of the apex impulse should be determined.[165] The examiner should focus on one phase of the cardiac cycle at a time and correlate the findings with other cardiovascular events.

The normal apex (apical) impulse usually is located within 10 cm of the sternal midline, at or within the left midclavicular line in the fifth intercostal space, when the patient is supine. It may be located lateral to the midclavicular line when associated with a high diaphragm, pregnancy, marked pectus excavatum, or other conditions that displace a normal heart to the left. The normal apex impulse is *less than 3 cm in diameter* and in most instances is considerably smaller. The early systolic outward movement of the apical area (Fig. 12-56) begins at about the same time as that of the $S_1$, just before the upstroke of the carotid pulse. Peak outward motion normally occurs with or just after blood is ejected into the aorta; then the apex normally moves inward. The outward movement of the apical impulse is normally not excessively forceful and is felt only during the first third of systole.

The apex impulse may be hyperkinetic or hyperdynamic with increased amplitude in normal individuals who have a thin chest wall, a flat chest, or a depressed sternum. Lying on the left side may cause a normal apical impulse to move laterally and to have increased amplitude and duration[165]; however, it still should not exceed a diameter of >3 cm. A hyperdynamic apex impulse also may be found in anxious children, in patients with high cardiac output states, and in patients with a mild to moderate LV volume load from mitral or AR. The apex impulse is more sustained when mitral or AR is severe or when LV systolic function is decreased.[162] In general, a greatly sustained apex impulse indicates either marked LV hypertrophy or depressed LV systolic function, whereas LV dilatation displaces the apex impulse laterally and inferiorly[165,168] (Fig. 12-56).

Concentric LV hypertrophy without an increase in LV cavity size may occur in systemic hypertension, valvular AS, and hypertrophic cardiomyopathy. Characteristically, the apex impulse is not displaced but is both abnormally forceful and sustained.[162,168] An $S_4$ vibration may be palpable or visible or both.

Severe LV dilatation—whether due to volume load or ventricular failure—may displace the apex impulse laterally and inferiorly and cause a marked increase in size and duration.

Important information about relative amounts of ventricular hypertrophy and dilatation often can be obtained from the apex impulse. Thus, in valvular AS, with marked concentric LV hypertrophy but little or no dilatation, the apex impulse characteristically is small, forceful, and sustained but not displaced. A presystolic $S_4$ often is palpable at the apex. By contrast, in severe AR with marked dilatation of the LV plus considerable eccentric hypertrophy, there is a diffuse apex impulse with increased force, duration, and amplitude, and it is displaced laterally and inferiorly.[163]

In some patients with acute MI, a sustained apex impulse may simulate that due to LV hypertrophy.[204] Those developing mitral regurgitation (MR) secondary to MI (papillary muscle dysfunction) may manifest LV dilatation and hypertrophy by a displaced and sustained, forceful, large apex impulse.[169] A late systolic bulge at the cardiac apex may be due to a functional LV aneurysm, occasionally resulting in a bifid apex impulse. In other patients, a late systolic bulge may be palpable in an ectopic area between the apex impulse and the left parasternal area.

A bifid apex impulse during systole also may be due to marked LV dilatation and hypertrophy in patients with both AS and regurgitation or in patients with hypertrophic cardiomyopathy.[170] Infrequently, a faint systolic notch is palpable in the apex impulse of patients with MVP at the moment of a midsystolic click. Systolic retraction of the apical impulse usually indicates either constrictive pericarditis or severe TR with marked RV dilatation (Fig. 12-56). An apical systolic thrill most commonly is produced by MR and often is diffuse, whereas a diastolic thrill is usually produced by MS and is localized to a small, discrete periapical area.

## Diastolic Events: Palpable Third and Fourth Heart Sounds

During early diastole, brief outward chest wall movement corresponding to an LV filling or a third heart sound ($S_3$) occasionally may be seen or felt, even if it is not audible with a stethoscope (Fig. 12-56). In children and young adults, the presence of an early diastolic ventricular filling sound ($S_3$) and movement is usually normal. On the other hand, the presence of such a movement or sound in a sedentary adult or a patient with heart disease usually indicates an elevated LV diastolic pressure and volume and likely ventricular decompensation, often with a decreased ejection fraction. Patients with acute MI or transient myocardial ischemia during angina pectoris frequently develop a transient palpable and audible ventricular filling $S_3$, which reflects the acutely decreased ventricular compliance. A palpable ventricular rapid filling wave ($S_3$) may be present in patients with LV failure from any cause; however, hemodynamic systolic ventricular failure is often not always present when a ventricular filling wave or sound occurs in the presence of volume loading and dilatation of the left ventricle, as with MR or AR.

The presystolic left atrial contribution to the apical impulse (referred to as the *atrial impulse* or *a* wave) may be detected during late diastole, just prior to $S_1$ (Fig. 12-56). Usually, a palpable atrial impulse coincides with an audible fourth heart ($S_4$) sound and is associated with an increased LV end-diastolic pressure and decreased compliance. In general, an LV $S_4$ presystolic impulse is not normally palpable but may be felt at the apex with its associated $S_4$ in some normal adults if the PR interval is long and circulation is hyperdynamic.[160] In some patients with ischemic heart disease, a palpable apical $S_4$ may develop or become more prominent during an episode of angina pectoris or even during exertion without chest pain. A palpable presystolic impulse, $S_4$, or both occur frequently in patients with acute MI, but these are also often present in other conditions producing a decrease in LV compliance and increased end-diastolic pressure.

A double, or bifid, apical impulse may be present in various circumstances, most commonly in the combination of an outward movement during ventricular systole and a second outward pulsation during diastole.[163] The diastolic impulse may occur either in early diastole ($S_3$) or in late diastole or presystole ($S_4$).

A bifid apical impulse with two systolic impulses may be present in patients with hypertrophic obstructive cardiomyopathy, complete left bundle branch block (LBBB), or MI. If these patients also develop a palpable impulse during either early ($S_3$) or late ($S_4$) diastole, a triple or trifid apical impulse may occur. When such patients develop both a palpable $S_3$ and a palpable $S_4$, it is occasionally possible to see and feel a quadruple apical impulse.

#### AREA 6: EPIGASTRIC AREA PULSATIONS

Some normal and many hyperkinetic individuals have visible or palpable pulsations of the aorta in the epigastric area (Fig. 12-56). Abnormally large pulsations of the aorta may be due to an aortic aneurysm or AR. Hepatic movements may be identified in the epigastric area, particularly in patients with TR, tricuspid stenosis, or marked RV dilatation, hypertrophy, and hyperactivity.

In some patients with PH due to chronic lung disease, the detection of RV hypertrophy by precordial palpation is difficult because the shape of the chest often conceals the enlarged RV. To detect abnormal RV pulsations in patients with emphysema, the palm of the right hand should be placed on the epigastric area and moved cephalad while gently sliding the fingers under the rib cage. Aortic pulsations can be detected by the palmar surface of the fingers, and pulsations due to RV hypertrophy can be felt in the fingertips.

#### AREA 7: ECTOPIC AREA PULSATIONS

Occasionally, cardiac pulsations are encountered in areas other than those described previously, i.e., between the pulmonary and apical areas (Fig. 12-56). Ischemic heart disease is the most common cause of an ectopic systolic pulsation, which may occur transiently during an episode of angina pectoris. A similar paradoxical systolic outward movement may be detected after acute MI and may persist; more commonly, it disappears within a few weeks. A persistent paradoxical ectopic pulsation also may be found in patients who develop a ventricular aneurysm after MI. Ectopic pulsations on the anterior chest wall also can be found in patients with cardiomyopathies of varying etiologies. In patients with severe MR and a giant left atrium that extends to the right, an ectopic systolic pulsation of the atrium occasionally may be felt in the right anterior or lateral chest or in the left axilla.[163]

### Percussion versus Inspection and Palpation of the Precordium

When performed by a skilled examiner, percussion of the heart can provide an estimate of cardiac size and shape. Percussion of the heart only gives information about the location of the borders of cardiac dullness, whereas precordial inspection and palpation provide both information about the location of the outer limits of cardiac pulsations and a determination of the size and character of the pulsations. Although percussion has been used in the diagnosis of pericardial effusion, it has limited value when the results are objectively correlated with the diagnosis as determined by more sensitive and specific noninvasive and invasive testing.

## CARDIAC AUSCULTATION

### The Stethoscope

The physician must choose a stethoscope that fits the ears comfortably with the right angulation, has only a short segment of flexible tubing, and is equipped with a diaphragm and a bell. Selection of the proper earpieces for comfort and the best transmission of sound is based on individual preference. A snug, comfortable fit depends on the size of the earpieces as well as the angle at which they enter the ear canal. The rubber tubing should be as short as possible; experience indicates that tubing about 12 in. (30 cm) long is the best compromise. Rapaport and Sprague[173] have shown that thick-walled tubing about 3 mm in diameter is best suited to transmit sounds and murmurs.

The human ear is most sensitive to auditory vibrations that occur in the frequency range between 1000 and 4000 to 5000 Hz; the sensitivity falls off sharply when the frequency of vibration is below 1000 Hz. This is particularly true of low-frequency sounds, which must be of considerably greater amplitude to reach the threshold of audibility than sounds of higher frequency. Most cardiovascular sounds and murmurs of diagnostic importance are between 30 and 1000 Hz, thereby placing the auscultator at considerable disadvantage.[174] Therefore, a stethoscope requires *both a diaphragm and a bell,* and each must be applied to the chest wall with optimal pressure. The diaphragm, which is fairly rigid, brings out the high frequencies and attenuates the lows. When the diaphragm is used to accentuate high-pitched sounds, it should be pressed very firmly against the skin. This technique will make a high-frequency murmur, such as the faint diastolic blowing murmur of AR, audible along the left sternal border when it would otherwise be missed. The bell tends to accentuate the low-frequency sounds and to filter out the high-pitched tones. Often, low-frequency sounds are more easily appreciated by palpation than by auscultation; in these situations, the stethoscope should be placed very lightly on the skin, with just enough pressure to seal the edge at the point of maximal impulse. With very light pressure of the bell, the low-pitched sounds are accentuated; however, with firm pressure of the bell against the skin, the skin itself becomes a relatively tight diaphragm, and the low-frequency sounds are suppressed.

### Examination of the Patient

The examination should take place in a quiet room that is well lighted and comfortably heated. The patient should be properly gowned, with adequate exposure to the waist. The examining table should be large enough that the patient can be instructed to lie flat, sit up, or roll to one side with complete ease. Usually, the physician will examine from the right side, and it is equally important that the physician be comfortable.

Prior to auscultation, the clinician should take advantage of the information obtained from the history as well as from the examination of the arterial, venous, and cardiac pulsations. When abnormalities are found, their auscultatory counterparts should be pursued diligently. For example, prominent *a* waves in the JVP should alert the clinician to search carefully for a low-pitched, right-sided $S_4$ or the subtle presystolic murmur of TS, whereas large *v* waves that augment with inspiration should suggest TR. The presence of pulsus alternans should always demand a careful search for third and fourth heart sounds ($S_3$, $S_4$) as well as for the presence of functional mitral or TR, often present in severe cardiac decompensation. A rapid, jerky rise of the carotid pulse may be the clue to the diagnosis of hypertrophic cardiomyopathy, which can be confirmed by manipulating the systolic murmur with maneuvers that change the pre- and afterloading conditions of the heart.

There are four primary areas of cardiac auscultation: (1) the primary and secondary aortic areas in the second right interspace and the third left interspace adjacent to the sternum, respectively, (2) the pulmonary area in the second left interspace, (3) the tricuspid area in the fourth and fifth interspaces adjacent to the left sternal border, and (4) the mitral area at the cardiac apex. This does not imply that auscultatory events arising from each valve are heard only in these respective areas. The murmur of AS in the elderly is often heard best (and at times only) at the apex, whereas the murmur of a flail posterior mitral leaflet may radiate to the base and simulate the murmur of AS. Ejection sounds arising from the stenotic aortic valve are usually most prominent at the apex, whereas the opening snap of MS is heard best midway between the tricuspid and mitral areas. The murmur of TR may be appreciated best at the classic mitral area if the RV occupies the apex. Furthermore, cardiac auscultation should not be restricted to just these four areas. For example, the murmur of AR secondary to abnormalities of the aortic root may be heard best to the right of the sternum, whereas the murmur of TR in the emphysematous patient with PH may be heard best in the epigastrium. The continuous murmur of a patent ductus arteriosus is heard just below the left clavicle, whereas the murmur of large bronchial collaterals may be most prominent in the posterior thorax.

During auscultation, one listens both specifically and selectively for heart sounds and then for murmurs, first during systole and then during diastole. As described by Levine and Harvey,[176] the physician should adopt a *systematic approach* to listening. The patient should be lying on his or her back, and each area should be surveyed with both chest pieces. In each area examined, the physician listens specifically for the first heart sound ($S_1$). This is followed by selective listening for the second heart sound ($S_2$), noting the presence of splitting and variation with respirations. Then extra sounds are searched for and carefully listened to, first in systole and then in diastole, with mental notations as to their time of appearance, pitch, and other characteristics that may identify them as gallop sounds, ejection sounds, or valve-opening sounds. Of greater importance is that the examination be performed in a methodical, systematic way, with the physician listening intently for one event at a time. Attention is then first turned to systole and then to diastole for the presence of murmurs. After this general survey, the physician listens selectively for certain sounds and murmurs. With the bell applied lightly to the skin at the apex, the patient is instructed to roll onto the left side, and the clinician selectively "tunes in" to diastole and the low-frequency range. This allows the physician to determine the presence or absence of diastolic filling sounds or diastolic rumbles arising from the AV valves. The examination is continued with the patient in the sitting position. While the patient leans slightly forward during quiet respiration, the clinician can optimally appreciate splitting of $S_2$. With the patient's breath held in deep expiration, the physician examines the aortic and pulmonic areas with the diaphragm firmly pressed against the chest wall, selectively tuning in to the high-frequency range in an effort to hear the faint blowing diastolic murmur of AR or, if the clinical situation warrants, the presence of a pericardial friction rub. Sounds and murmurs such as these are discovered only when they are searched out carefully with intent listening and concentration.

Auscultation of the heart should be considered a dynamic exercise. In addition to being auscultated in the left lateral decubitus position, the patient should, when possible, also be examined while standing, squatting, and during the Valsalva maneuver and following its release. This type of dynamic examination changes the pre- and afterloading conditions of the heart and may yield diagnostic information because of the typical responses of various heart sounds and murmurs using these maneuvers.

## HEART SOUNDS

Heart sounds are of two types: high-frequency transients associated with the abrupt terminal checking of valves that are closing or opening and low-frequency sounds related to early and late diastolic filling events of the ventricles. Sounds related to closing and opening of the AV valves include mitral and tricuspid closing sounds ($M_1$, $T_1$), nonejection sounds, and the opening snaps; sounds related to closing and opening of the semilunar valves include aortic and pulmonic closure sounds ($A_2$, $P_2$) and early valvular ejection sounds or clicks. Low-frequency sounds include the physiologic heart sound ($S_3$) and the pathologic $S_3$ gallop associated with early ventricular filling events and the presystolic atrial $S_4$ gallop associated with late diastolic events resulting from the atrial contribution to ventricular filling. With tachycardia, these sounds may fuse, producing a summation gallop.[174,175]

### The First Heart Sound

The first heart sound ($S_1$) as recorded by high-resolution phonocardiography consists of four sequential components. The two *major components normally audible* at the left lower sternal border are the louder $M_1$ followed by $T_1$. They are separated by only 20 to 30 ms, and at the apex in the normal subject only a single sound ($M_1$) is usually appreciated. Splitting of the first heart sound is less evident with the tachycardia following coughing or with sustained handgrip exercise.

#### ECHOCARDIOGRAPHIC CORRELATES AND SPLITTING OF $S_1$

The first high-frequency component of $S_1$ coincides with the complete coaptation of the anterior and posterior leaflets of the mitral valve. This sound is due to the sudden deceleration of blood setting the entire cardiohemic system into vibration when the elastic limits of the closed, tensed valves are met. It is unlikely that complete coaptation of the complex valve leaflets and final tensing are simultaneous; presumably it is the latter event that is associated with vibrations perceived as $M_1$. When $T_1$ is more widely separated from $M_1$, however, identical echocardiographic correlates have been demonstrated in patients with wide splitting of $S_1$ due to Ebstein's anomaly of the tricuspid valve.[177] This exaggerated $T_1$, or "sail sound," and its wide separation from $M_1$ have been a helpful sign in the diagnosis of this entity.[178] Wide splitting of $S_1$ with normal sequencing ($M_1$, $T_1$) is also present in right bundle branch block of the proximal type as well as in LV pacing, ectopic beats, and idioventricular rhythms originating from the LV due to a delayed contraction of the RV. Similarly, pacing from the RV and ectopic beats and idioventricular rhythms originating from the RV will produce reversed splitting of $S_1$ ($T_1$, $M_1$) due to delay in LV contraction. Reversed splitting of $S_1$ also may be present in patients with hemodynamically significant obstruction of the mitral valve, since mitral valve closure is delayed due to the increased left atrial pressure, which must be overcome by the rising LV pressure before closure can occur. Similar delay in $M_1$ also may be found in mitral obstruction secondary to left atrial myxoma.

## HEMODYNAMIC CORRELATES OF $S_1$

Figure 12-57 illustrates the sound and pressure correlates of $M_1$. The first high-frequency component of $M_1$ coincides with the downstroke of the left atrial *c* wave and is delayed from the LV–left atrial pressure crossover by 30 ms. However, the elegant studies of Laniado et al[179] have established that forward flow continued for a short period following LV–left atrial pressure crossover due to the inertia of mitral flow, with $M_1$ occurring 20 to 40 ms later, coincidentally with cessation of mitral flow and closure of the valve. An even greater delay between the occurrence of $T_1$ and RV–right atrial pressure crossover has been shown.[180] Also, $T_1$ coincides with the downstroke of the right atrial *c* wave.[181] These hemodynamic data, together with the echocardiographic correlates of $M_1$ and $T_1$, confirm the prime role played by the AV valves in the genesis of $S_1$.

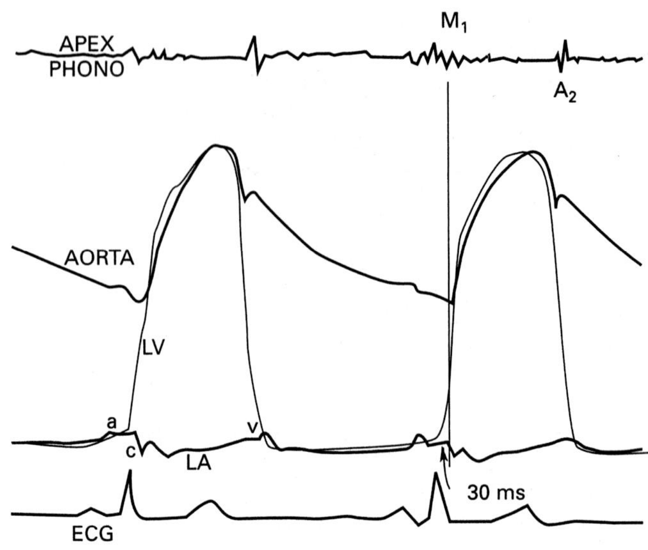


FIGURE 12-57 The apex phonocardiogram is displayed simultaneously with the cardiac cycle, as recorded by high-fidelity catheter-tipped micromanometers in the central aorta, left ventricle (LV), and left atrium (LA). The first high-frequency component of $M_1$ is coincident with the downstroke of the left atrial *c* wave and is separated from LV–left atrial pressure crossover by an interval of 30 ms. (From Shaver JA, Salerni R, Reddy PS. Normal and abnormal heart sounds in cardiac diagnosis: I. Systolic sounds. *Curr Probl Cardiol* 1985; 10:10–53. Reproduced with permission from the publisher and authors.)

## INTENSITY OF $S_1$

The primary factors determining intensity of $S_1$ are (1) integrity of valve closure, (2) mobility of the valve, (3) velocity of valve closure, (4) status of ventricular contraction, (5) transmission characteristics of the thoracic cavity and chest wall, and (6) physical characteristics of the vibrating structures.

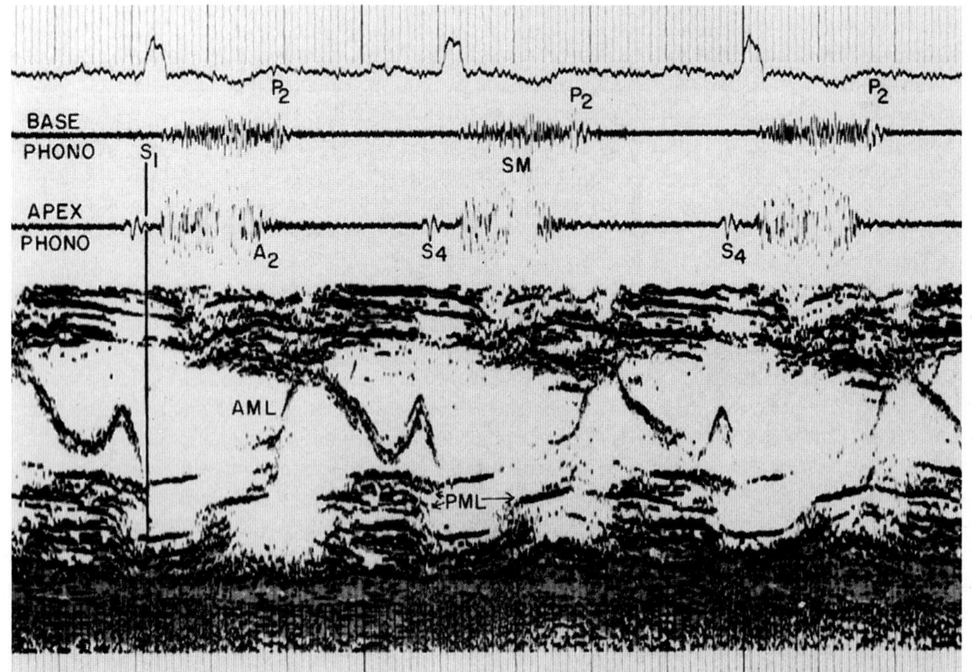


FIGURE 12-58 Base and apex phonocardiograms are recorded simultaneously with the mitral valve echocardiogram in a 62-year-old man who developed acute mitral regurgitation (MR) secondary to rupture of the chordae tendineae of a myxomatous valve. During diastole, multiple echoes arise from the flail posterior mitral leaflet (PML); during early ventricular systole, effective mitral valve closure does not occur, resulting in an inaudible low-frequency vibration on the apex phonocardiogram. During systole, there is separation of the anterior mitral leaflet (AML) and PMLs, resulting in severe MR. The murmur has a crescendo-decrescendo contour simulating the murmur of aortic stenosis (AS) ending prior to $A_1$. Wide physiologic splitting of $S_1$ is present. The prominent $S_4$ present on the apex phonocardiogram was associated with an apical presystolic impulse. (From Shaver JA. The physical examination in cardiac diagnosis. *Cardiol Consult* 1985;6:3. Reproduced with permission from the publisher and author.)

***Integrity of Valve Closure*** In rare situations, usually in the setting of severe MR, there is inadequate coaptation of the mitral leaflets to a degree that valve closure is not effective. As a result, abrupt halting of the retrograde blood column during early ventricular contraction does not occur, and $S_1$ may be markedly attenuated or absent. Such may be the case in severe MR due to a flail mitral leaflet, as shown in Fig. 12-58.

***Mobility of the Valve*** Severe calcific fixation of the mitral valve with complete immobilization will cause a markedly attenuated $M_1$. This is seen most commonly in the setting of longstanding severe MS.

***Velocity of Valve Closure*** The velocity of valve closure is the most important factor affecting the intensity of $S_1$ and is determined by the timing of mitral valve closure in relation to the LV pressure rise in early systole.[179] The relative timing of left atrial and LV systole may vary this relationship. As the PR interval progressively decreases from 130 to 30 ms, there is a progressive increase in the intensity of $M_1$ and progressive delay in $M_1$ relative to the onset of LV contraction. When left atrial and LV systole occur almost simultaneously, at a PR interval of 10 ms, however, $S_1$ again becomes soft. At short PR intervals (30 to 70 ms), the mitral valve leaflets are maximally separated by atrial contraction at the onset of LV systole. With LV contraction, the mitral valve closes at a high velocity with a large excursion. This results in a loud, late $M_1$ occurring on a steeper part of the LV pressure curve when the retrograde blood column is suddenly decelerated at the moment the elastic limits of the mitral valve are met. At longer PR intervals, there is less separation of the mitral valve leaflets, which have already begun to close with atrial relaxation. When LV systole begins, there is less excursion of the mitral valve until tensing occurs, and $S_1$ occurs earlier relative to the onset of LV contraction at a lower LV pressure. Thus less force is applied to the mitral valve, its closing velocity is decreased, and less energy is generated when a column of retrograde blood is abruptly halted, resulting in a softer $M_1$.

The clinical finding of marked variation in the intensity of $S_1$ in a patient with a slow heart rate often will alert the clinician at the bedside to the diagnosis of complete AV block with AV dissociation. Other conditions in which there are beat-to-beat variations in the intensity of $S_1$ include Mobitz type I AV block and ventricular tachycardia with AV dissociation. Variations in the intensity of $S_1$ also occur with atrial fibrillation with both normal and stenotic AV valves. The loud $S_1$ occurs at short RR intervals, whereas a softer $S_1$ occurs at longer RR intervals when the valve leaflets have closed partially.[180]

The position of the mitral valve at the onset of ventricular systole may be altered not only by the relative timing of atrial and ventricular systole but also by altering the rate of LV filling during atrial systole. The timing and intensity of both $S_1$ and $S_4$ in hypertensive patients can be influenced by variations in venous return.[179] It is suggested that the mitral leaflets have a greater separation when venous return is *decreased* to the noncompliant hypertensive LV because there is more effective atrial volume transport into a relatively underfilled ventricle. This results in a softer $S_4$ that migrates toward an increased $S_1$. When venous return is *increased,* the atrial contribution of ventricular filling is now operating on the steeper portion of the LV pressure-volume curve. The $S_4$ becomes louder and earlier, and $S_1$ is decreased in amplitude due to partial atriogenic closure of the mitral valve. This is the most likely explanation of a soft $S_1$ frequently noted in hypertensive patients with normal PR intervals.

***Status of Ventricular Contraction*** The status of ventricular contractility is also an independent factor determining the amplitude of $S_1$.[179,180] In normal subjects, both exercise and catecholamine infusion increase the amplitude of $S_1$, whereas administration of beta-blocking agents decreases it.[179] In both situations, the prime factor in altering the intensity of $S_1$ is the rate of pressure development in the ventricle. This increased rate of pressure development partially explains why $S_1$ is increased in patients with anemia, arteriovenous fistulas, pregnancy, anxiety, and fever. It is also likely that these high-output states, often associated with tachycardia, result in wider separation of the AV valves at the onset of ventricular systole due to high flow through a shortened diastolic period. Similarly, the loud $T_1$ in an ASD is due to high flow through the tricuspid valve, secondary to the left-to-right shunt at the atrial level. A decrease in the intensity of $S_1$ associated with a decrease in the rate of LV pressure development may be found in myxedema, cardiomyopathy, and acute MI.[178,179] Beat-to-beat variation in the intensity of $S_1$ (auscultatory alternans) also has been found in patients with pulsus alternans, when beat-to-beat alteration in the rate of LV pressure development occurs.

***Transmission Characteristics of the Thoracic Cavity and Chest Wall*** The degree of attenuation of heart sounds generated by the vibrating cardiohemic system is a function of both sound frequency and the distance of the heart from the chest wall. The higher-frequency heart sounds are attenuated to a greater extent than are lower-frequency sounds. Conditions such as obesity, emphysema, and large pleural or pericardial effusions will decrease the intensity of all auscultatory events, whereas a thin body habitus would tend to increase the intensity.

***Physical Characteristics of the Vibrating Structures*** Alterations in the physical characteristics of the vibrating structures also may vary the intensity of $S_1$. Both MI and ischemia induced by pacing have been shown to decrease the intensity of $S_1$ secondary to these alterations.[182]

## $S_1$ IN PATHOLOGIC CONDITIONS

Careful attention to the intensity of $S_1$ is an extremely important aspect of cardiac auscultation, often giving clues to the proper diagnosis and degree of abnormality of the involved structures.[184–186] In the following conditions, alterations in the intensity of $S_1$ may play a key role in the correct diagnosis.

***$S_1$ in Mitral Stenosis*** A loud, late $M_1$ is the hallmark of hemodynamically significant mitral stenosis.[183] When $M_1$ is loud, it is associated with a loud opening snap, and the intensity of both $M_1$ and the opening snap correlates with valve motility (Fig. 12-59, *left*). When calcific fixation of the stenotic mitral valve occurs, $M_1$ is soft, and the opening snap is absent. The relationship between sound and pressure and echocardiographic mitral valve motion is shown in Fig. 12-60. The increased left atrial pressure delays the time of pressure crossover between the left atrium and the LV. As a result, $M_1$ occurs later and at a much higher than normal LV pressure, at a time when there is a more rapid rate of development of LV pressure. The presystolic gradient between the left atrium and the LV prevents preclosure of the mitral valve leaflets. As a result, the closure of the leaflet begins from a domed position within the LV cavity and takes place over a much greater distance following the onset of LV contraction. Both these factors increase the velocity of mitral valve closure and the momentum of blood directed toward the mitral valve leaflets, resulting in a loud $M_1$. A similar mechanism is responsible for the booming $S_1$ with after vibrations in left atrial myxoma (Fig. 12-59, center).

***$S_1$ in Mitral Valve Prolapse*** Tei et al.[187] have reported a loud $M_1$ heard over the apex in patients with nonrheumatic MR; this is indicative of holosystolic MVP (Fig. 12-59, right). Patients with the more common middle to late systolic prolapse have a normal $S_1$, whereas a soft or absent $S_1$ may indicate a flail mitral leaflet (Fig. 12-60). The increased amplitude of leaflet excursion with prolapse beyond the line of closure explains the loud $M_1$ associated with holosystolic prolapse. An alternate explanation may be a summation of a normal $M_1$ and an early nonejection click of valvular prolapse.

***$S_1$ and LBBB*** In LBBB, $M_1$ is decreased in intensity and is frequently delayed, at times resulting in reversal of sequence of $S_1$.[188] The reason for the delay and the decreased intensity of $M_1$ in this condition is multifactional.[189] The primary factors involved are (1) delay in onset of LV contraction, (2) degree of LV dysfunction, (3) presence of concomitant first-degree heart block, and (4) presence of a noncompliant LV facilitating atriogenic preclosure of the mitral valve. It is likely that more than one factor is operative in most patients with LBBB, with one or two factors predominating.

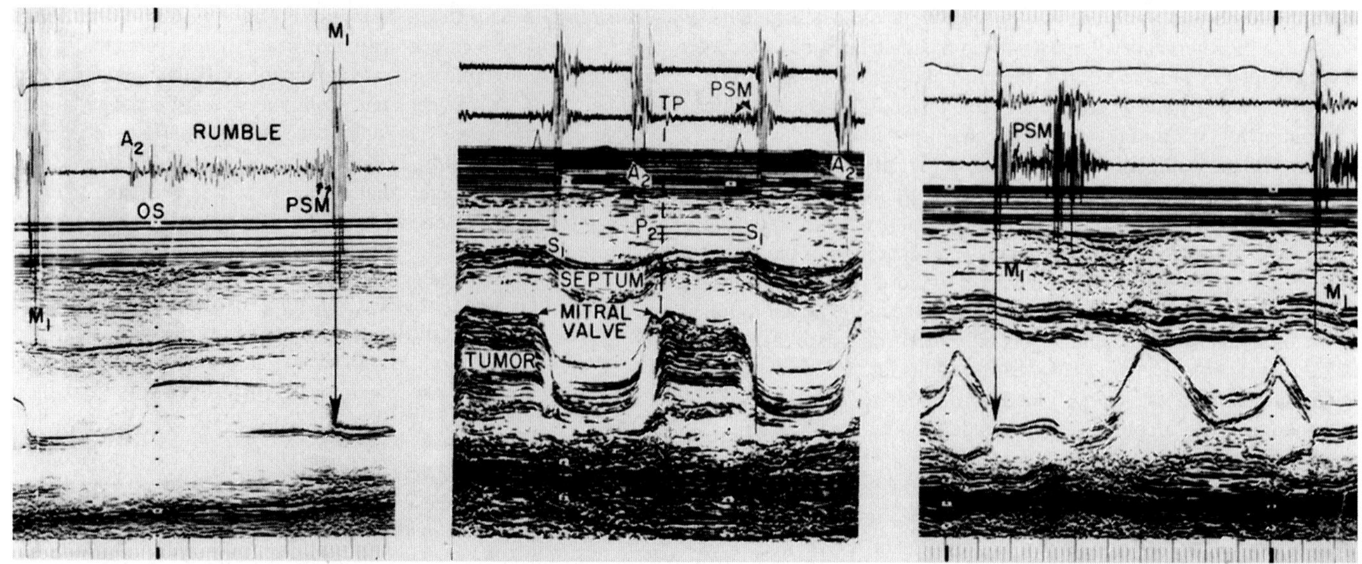


FIGURE 12-59 Simultaneous phonocardiograms are recorded with the mitral valve echocardiograms in three patients: mitral stenosis (MS) (*left*), left atrial myxoma (*center*), and prolapse of the mitral valve (*right*). In each condition, a loud $M_1$ is present and coincident with the closing point of the mitral valve echocardiogram. Common to each condition is wide separation of the mitral leaflets at the onset of LV systole, with high-velocity closure occurring over a large excursion. In the left panel, a mobile stenotic valve is demonstrated, and a loud opening snap (OS) is coincident with the E point. In the center panel, an early diastolic tumor plop (TP) is coincident with the maximal excursion of the tumor during its rapid descent into the ventricle. Note the presystolic crescendo murmur (PSM) occurring during the rapid closure of the mitral valve in both MS and left atrial myxoma. In the right panel, a pansystolic murmur (PSM) with late systolic accentuation is secondary to the prolapse of the mitral valve with late systolic hammocking. (From Shaver JA. Current uses of phonocardiography in clinical practice. In: Rapaport E, ed. *Cardiology Update: Reviews for Physicians*. New York: Elsevier; 1981:370. Reproduced in part (*center panel*) with permission from the publisher and author. Copyright 1981 by Elsevier Science Publishing Co, Inc.)

***$S_1$* in Acute Aortic Regurgitation** One of the important auscultatory findings in acute AR is attenuation or absence of $M_1$.[180] Severe regurgitation into an LV that has not had time to adapt to the acute volume overload causes an marked increase in the LV end-diastolic pressure, resulting in premature closure of the normal mitral valve in middiastole. With the onset of LV systole, minimal mitral valve excursion occurs, causing a marked reduction in the intensity of $M_1$.

## Systolic Ejection Sounds

Ejection sounds are early systolic ejection events that can originate from either the left or the right side of the heart. These sounds may be classified as *valvular*, arising from deformed aortic or pulmonic valves, or as *vascular* or *root* events caused by the rapid, forceful ejection of blood into the great vessels.[190–192] The presence or absence of valvular ejection sounds is of great benefit in defining the level of RV or LV outflow tract obstruction, whereas root ejection sounds indicate abnormalities of the great vessels with or without systemic or PH.

### AORTIC VALVULAR EJECTION SOUNDS

Aortic valvular ejection sounds are found in nonstenotic congenital bicuspid valves and in the entire spectrum of mild to severe stenosis of the aortic valve. This sound introduces the typical ejection murmur of AS, is widely transmitted, and is often heard best at the apex. The aortic valvular ejection sound is delayed 20 to 40 ms after the onset of pressure rise in the central aorta and is coincident with the sharp anacrotic notch on the upstroke of the aortic pressure curve. The sound is coincident with the maximal excursion of the domed valve when its elastic limits are met.[193] The abrupt deceleration of the oncoming column of blood sets the entire cardiohemic system into vibration, the lower-frequency components being recorded as the anacrotic notch and the high-frequency components representing the valvular ejection sound. Inherent in this mechanism of sound production is the ability of the deformed valve to move. With severe calcific fixation of the valve, no sudden tensing of the valve leaflets or abrupt deceleration of the column of blood occurs. Sound and motion correlates identical to those demonstrated by cineangiography have been found with phonoechocardiography, clearly showing the onset of the ejection sound to be coincident with the maximal opening of the valve[194] (Fig. 12-61). The intensity of the ejection sound correlates directly with the mobility of the valve, but there is no correlation between intensity and the severity of the obstruction. In mobile, nonstenotic bicuspid valves, the ejection sound is not only loud but also widely separated from $S_1$ due to the prolonged excursion of the mobile valve. The presence of an aortic valvular ejection sound is a valuable physical finding at the bedside; it not only defines the LV outflow obstruction at the valvular level but also gives insight into the mobility of the valve (Fig. 12-61).

### PULMONIC VALVULAR EJECTION SOUNDS

Pulmonic valvular ejection sounds have identical sound and pressure correlates as aortic valvular ejection sounds.[192] Echocardiographic correlations also show that the onset of the pulmonary ejection sound occurs at the maximal excursion of the stenotic pulmonic valve. In contrast to the aortic valvular ejection sounds and to most right-sided auscultatory events, the *pulmonic sound or ejection click decreases in intensity or disappears with inspiration* in mild to moderate PS. In very mild valvular PS, respiratory variation may be absent.[192] In very severe valvular obstruction, a vigorous atrial contraction can completely preopen the pulmonic valve in diastole, causing a crisp pre-ejection sound. In this situation, RV pressure at the time of the atrial kick actually can exceed pulmonary artery end-diastolic pressure.[192] As the severity of the PS increases, both the excursion of the de-

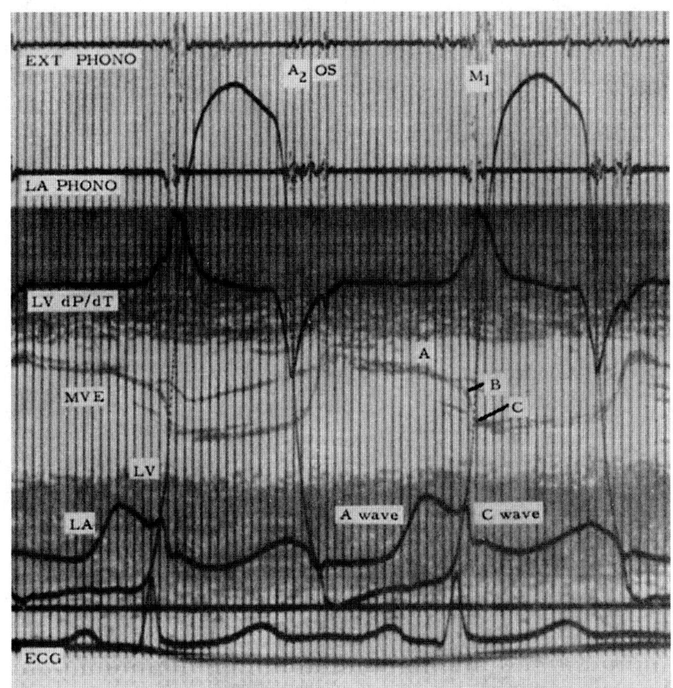


FIGURE 12-60 External sound, equisensitive left ventricular (LV) and left atrial pressures (catheter-tipped micromanometer), LV *dP/dt*, and left atrial sound are recorded simultaneously with the mitral valve echocardiogram in a patient with hemodynamically significant mitral stenosis. A significant presystolic gradient is present due to atrial contraction, and the onset of the rapid closure of the mitral valve (*B*) is delayed until the LV pressure exceeds left atrial pressure. This occurs 40 ms after the beginning of the LV pressure rise at a time when LV *dP/dt* is much higher than normal. Following left atrial–LV pressure crossover, there is rapid ventriculogenic closure of the mitral valve (*B* and *C*), resulting in a very loud $M_1$ coincident with the *C* point of the mitral valve echocardiogram. Its separation from $A_2$ is determined by both the level of the left atrial pressure and the rate of LV pressure decline. (From Shaver JA, et al. Normal and abnormal heart sounds in cardiac diagnosis: I. Systolic sounds. *Curr Probl Cardiol* 1985;10:10–53. Reproduced with permission from the publisher and the authors.)

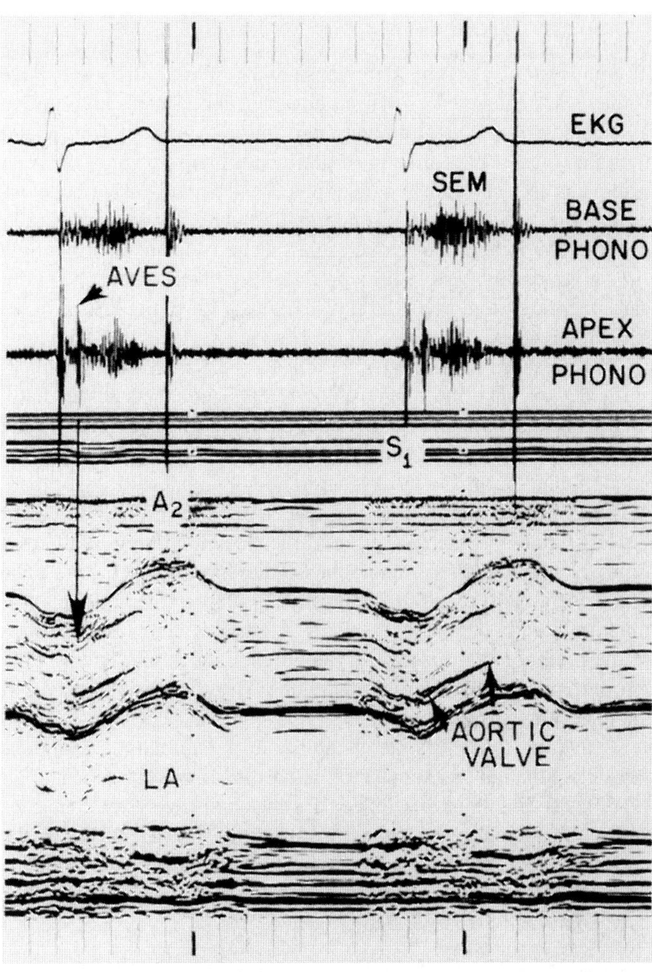


FIGURE 12-61 Base and apex phonocardiograms are recorded simultaneously with the aortic valve echocardiogram in a young man with valvular aortic stenosis. A prominent aortic valvular ejection sound (AVES) is recorded at the apex and is coincident with the maximal excursion of the aortic valve in early systole. It is followed by a crescendo-decrescendo systolic ejection murmur (SEM) that ends well before a loud $A_2$.

formed valve and the RV isovolumic contraction time decrease. The net effect of both these events is migration of the pulmonic ejection sound toward $S_1$.

## AORTIC VASCULAR EJECTION SOUNDS

Ejection sounds originating from the aortic root are common in systemic arterial hypertension in the setting of a tortuous sclerotic aortic root, a tight, noncompliant arterial tree, and forceful LV ejection. They are coincident with the upstroke of the high-fidelity central aortic pressure and have been interpreted as an exaggeration of the ejection component of the normal $S_1$. Echocardiographic correlations by Mills et al.,[191] show that this sound occurs at the moment of complete opening of the aortic valve and always on the pressure upstroke of the high-fidelity aortic pressure curve. Thus, this sound probably originates from the valve leaflets.

In contrast to the ejection sound of the stenotic aortic valve, these aortic root sounds tend to be poorly transmitted from the aortic area and are not heard well at the apex. It should be emphasized that the benign $S_1$ ejection sound or $M_1$-$T_1$ complex is frequently misinterpreted as a pathologic $S_4$-$S_1$ sequence. Factors that favor the presence of an $S_4$-$S_1$ complex are an associated palpable presystolic apical impulse, optimal audibility of the $S_4$ with the stethoscope bell applied lightly at the apex, and a change in the intensity of the $S_4$ with maneuvers that vary venous return.

## PULMONARY VASCULAR EJECTION SOUNDS

Vascular or root ejection sounds also may arise from the pulmonary artery, and the common denominator is dilatation of the pulmonary artery.[192] This dilatation can be idiopathic or secondary to severe PH. Although it has been stated that this sound is louder during expiration, *there is no consensus on this point*. Unlike splitting of $S_1$, which is heard best at the mitral or tricuspid area, this sound is louder in the second and third left intercostal spaces.

Echocardiographic correlates of the pulmonic root ejection sound show it to be coincident with complete opening of the pulmonary valve and occurring during the upstroke of the high-fidelity pulmonary artery pressure recording. This has led to the conclusion that these vascular ejection sounds may originate from semilunar valve cusps that have undergone changes in structure in response to increased pressure. In both idiopathic dilatation of the pulmonary artery and ASD, this sound occurs during the upstroke of the pulmonary pressure tracing.[192]

## Nonejection Sounds

The midsystolic click due to prolapse of the mitral or tricuspid valve is the most frequent cause of systolic nonejection sounds and is often associated with a systolic regurgitant murmur. Although originally thought to be extracardiac in origin, confirmation of their valvular origin has been shown by angiographic,[193,194] intracardiac phonocardiographic,[195,196] and echocardiographic studies.[197,198] As originally proposed by Reid,[199] the cause of this sound is due to tensing of the AV valves during systole. It is produced by vibrations of the entire cardiohemic system when the elastic limits of the prolapsed valve are suddenly reached.

The presence of a nonejection click on physical examination is sufficient to make the diagnosis of MVP. The sound has a sharp, high-frequency clicking quality and, although often confined to the apex, can be transmitted widely on the precordium. It may be an isolated finding, occurring most often in middle to late systole, or there may be multiple clicks, presumably as a result of different areas of the large, redundant, scalloped mitral leaflets prolapsing at different times. Numerous echocardiographic studies have shown the presence of the characteristic mid- to late-systolic prolapse as well as holosystolic prolapse in patients with clicks. All these patterns may be seen in the presence of an isolated systolic click, click and late systolic murmur, or a late systolic murmur alone. The click usually occurs at the time of maximal prolapse.

A feature of MVP is the variability of the auscultatory findings from examination to examination and even from beat to beat (Fig. 12-62). The timing of the click or the click and late systolic murmur varies considerably with changes in posture[200] (Fig. 12-63). In the upright posture, the heart becomes smaller due to decreased venous return, and the click moves earlier in systole. Angiographic studies have confirmed an earlier and greater degree of prolapse in the upright posture compared with the supine position. Squatting, which causes an immediate increase in venous return and afterload, increases LV volume, resulting in later prolapse and movement of the click toward $S_2$. At the bedside, these simple maneuvers are helpful in differentiating the nonejection click from early ejection sounds, a split $S_2$, or an $S_3$ (Chap. 68).

In general, maneuvers that decrease LV volume such as sitting, standing, or strain of the Valsalva maneuver cause the click to move closer to $S_1$. Maneuvers that increase LV volume move the click toward $S_2$ (Chap. 68).

Although the most common cause of nonejection clicks is prolapse of the AV valves, systolic sounds have been reported in patients with left-sided pneumothorax, adhesive pericarditis, atrial myxomas, LV aneurysm, aneurysm of the membranous ventricular septum associated with a VSD, and incompetent heterograft valves. The presence of these conditions usually can be recognized by the clinical setting and by the absence of the typical changes in the timing of the click associated with physiologic and pharmacologic maneuvers.

## The Second Heart Sound

Leatham[201] has emphasized the importance of the $S_2$ in the cardiac examination by labeling it as the "key to auscultation of the heart." To appreciate the significance of the normal and abnormal $S_2$, knowledge of its relationship to the hemodynamic events of the cardiac cycle is essential.[202,203] Figure 12-64 records the two components of $S_2$ simultaneously with the cardiac cycle by high-fidelity catheter-tipped micromanometers. The $A_2$ and $P_2$ are coincident with the incisura of the aorta and pulmonary artery pressure trace, respectively, and terminate the LV and RV ejection periods. RV ejection begins prior to LV ejection, has a longer duration, and terminates after LV ejection, resulting in $P_2$ normally occurring after $A_2$. RV and LV sys-

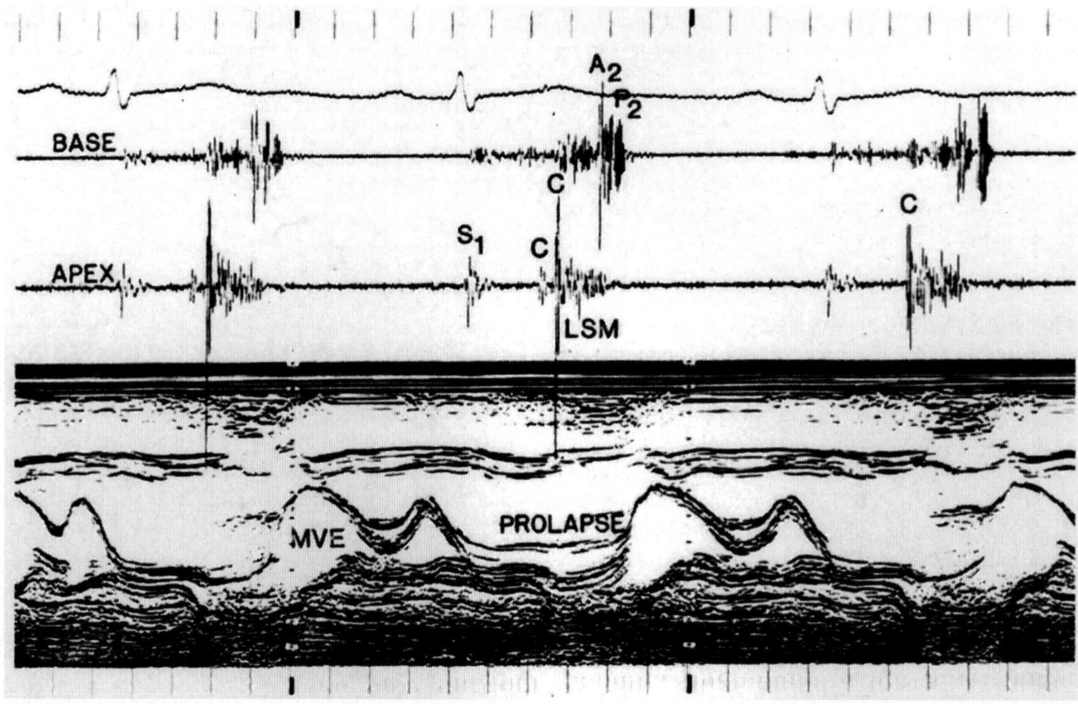


FIGURE 12-62 Simultaneously recorded base and apex phonocardiograms and mitral valve echocardiogram (MVE) demonstrating the frequent association of a late systolic murmur with a prominent late systolic click. Although the murmur is well transmitted to the base, the click transmits poorly. In the first two complexes, an additional softer click precedes the click murmur complex. The last complex shows only a single click, demonstrating the variability of the auscultatory findings even at rest. The large click occurs at maximal prolapse, and the smaller click occurs near the onset of echocardiographic prolapse.

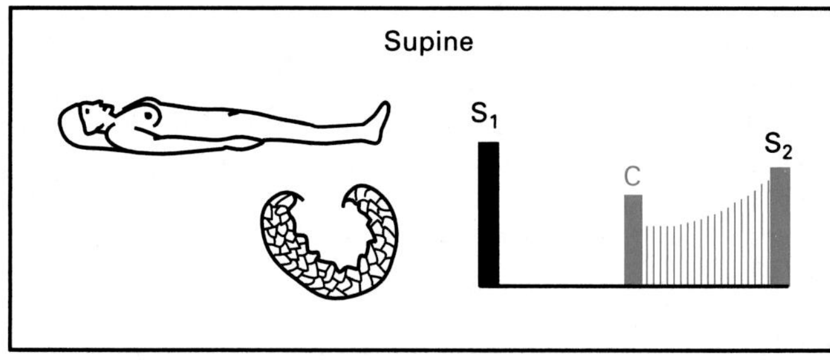


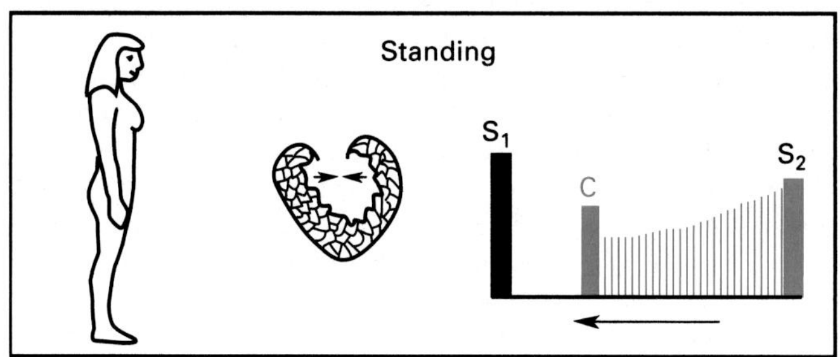


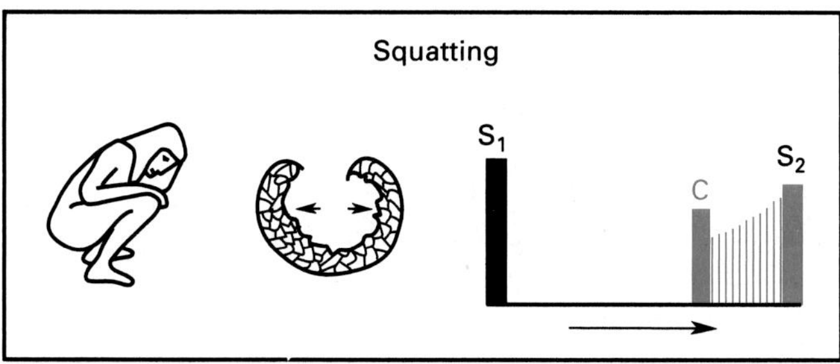


FIGURE 12-63 A midsystolic nonejection sound (*C*) occurs in mitral valve prolapse and is followed by a late systolic murmur that crescendos to $S_1$. With assumption of the upright posture, venous return decreases, the heart becomes smaller, the *C* moves closer to $S_1$, and the mitral regurgitant murmur has an earlier onset. With prompt squatting, both venous return and afterload increase, the heart becomes larger, the *C* moves toward $S_2$, and the duration of the murmur shortens. (From Shaver JA. *Examination of the Heart*, Part IV: Auscultation. Dallas: American Heart Association; 1990:13. Reproduced with permission from the publisher and the authors.)

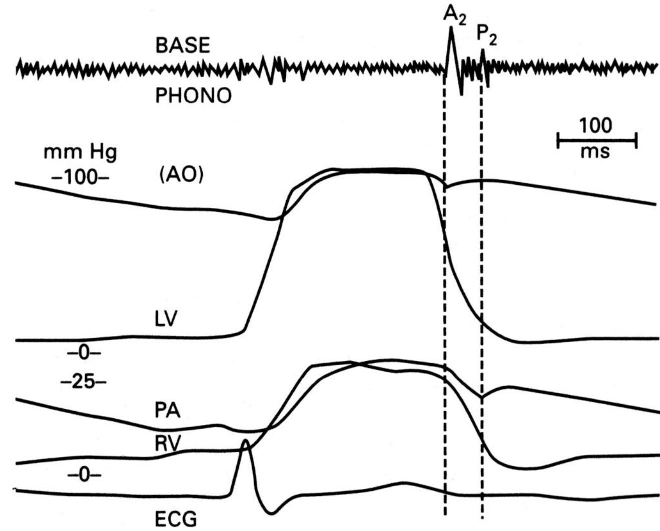


FIGURE 12-64 The cardiac cycle recorded by high-fidelity catheter-tipped micromanometers. The aortic ($A_2$) and pulmonic ($P_2$) closure sounds are coincident with the incisurae of their respective arterial traces. Although the left and right ventricular (LV and RV) mechanical systoles are nearly equal in duration, the RV systolic ejection period terminates after LV ejection because of an increased right-sided "hangout" interval. (From Shaver JA. The second heart sound: Newer concepts: I. Normal and wide physiological splitting. *Mod Concepts Cardiovasc Dis* 1997;46:7. Reproduced with permission from the American Heart Association and the authors.)

tole are nearly equal in duration, and the pulmonary artery incisura is delayed relative to the aortic incisura, primarily due to a larger interval separating the pulmonary artery incisura from the RV pressure compared with the same left-sided event. This interval has been called the "hangout" interval, a purely descriptive term coined in Shaver's laboratory over 15 years ago. Its duration is felt to be a reflection of the impedance of the vascular bed into which the blood is being received.[204] Normally, it is less than 15 ms in the systemic circulation and only slightly prolongs the LV ejection time. In the low-resistance, high-capacitance pulmonary bed, however, this interval is normally much greater than on the left, varying between 43 and 86 ms, and therefore contributes significantly to the duration of RV ejection.

## ECHOCARDIOGRAPHIC CORRELATIONS AND MECHANISMS OF SOUND PRODUCTION

Figure 12-65 illustrates the relationship between the aortic and pulmonary valve echocardiogram and $A_2$ and $P_2$. The first high-frequency component of both $A_2$ and $P_2$ is coincident with completion of closure of the aortic and pulmonic valve leaflets. $A_2$ and $P_2$ are produced by the sudden deceleration of retrograde flow of the blood

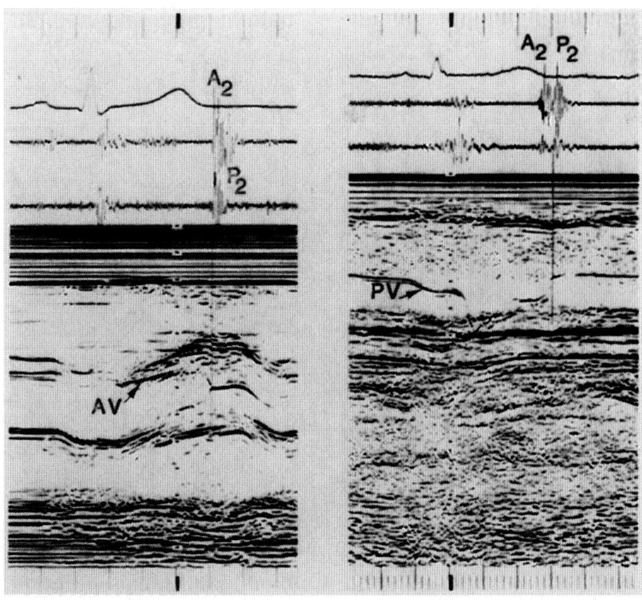


FIGURE 12-65 *Left.* The base and apex phonocardiograms are recorded simultaneously with the aortic valve echocardiogram. The first high-frequency component of $A_2$ is coincident with the completion of closure of the aortic valve. *Right.* Base and apex phonocardiograms are recorded with the pulmonary valve echocardiogram. The first high-frequency component of $P_1$ is coincident with the completion of closure of the pulmonic valve. (From Shaver JA, Salerni R, Reddy PS. Normal and abnormal heart sounds in cardiac diagnosis: I. Systolic sounds. *Curr Probl Cardiol* 1985:10:43. Reproduced with permission from the publisher and the authors.)

column in the aorta and pulmonary artery when the elastic limits of the tensed leaflets are met. This abrupt deceleration of flow sets the cardiohemic system into vibration and the higher-frequency components result in $A_2$ and $P_2$. This pressure gradient across the valves is the result of both the level of the diastolic pressure in the great vessel and the rate of pressure decline in the ventricle and is consistent with the well-known clinical observation of increased intensity of $A_2$ and $P_2$ in systemic and PH.

## NORMAL PHYSIOLOGIC SPLITTING

Normally during expiration, $A_2$ and $P_2$ are separated by an interval of less than 30 ms and are heard by the clinician as a single sound.[205] During inspiration, both components become distinctly audible as the splitting interval widens, primarily due to a delayed $P_2$, although an earlier $A_2$ contributes to a lesser degree[206] (Fig. 12-66). More recent studies have shown that the delayed $P_2$ and early $A_2$ associated with inspiration are due to a complex interplay between dynamic changes in pulmonary vascular impedance and changes in systemic and pulmonary venous return.[206]

On auscultation, splitting of $S_2$ is usually best heard at the second or third left intercostal space; the normal $P_2$ is softer than $A_2$ and is rarely audible at the apex. When $P_2$ is heard at the apex, either significant PH is present or the apex is occupied by the RV, a situation seen commonly in normotensive ASD. The absolute value of inspiratory splitting varies with age and depth of respiration. In younger subjects, maximal splitting during inspiration averages 40 to 50 ms; with age, this value decreases such that a single $S_2$ during both phases of respiration may be normal in subjects older than age 40.[207,208]

## ABNORMAL SPLITTING

All conditions in which abnormal splitting of $S_2$ exists can be identified at the bedside by the presence of audible expiratory splitting (>30 ms), i.e., the ability to hear two distinct sounds during expiration[208] (Fig. 12-66). This finding must be present when the patient is auscultated in both the supine and upright positions. There are three causes of audible expiratory splitting: (1) wide physiologic splitting primarily due to delayed $P_2$, (2) reversed splitting primarily due to delayed $A_2$, and (3) narrow physiologic splitting as seen in PH, where $A_2$ and $P_2$ are heard as two distinct sounds during expiration at a narrow splitting interval. Tables 12-7 and 12-8 classify the common causes of wide physiologic splitting and reversed splitting of $S_2$ ac-

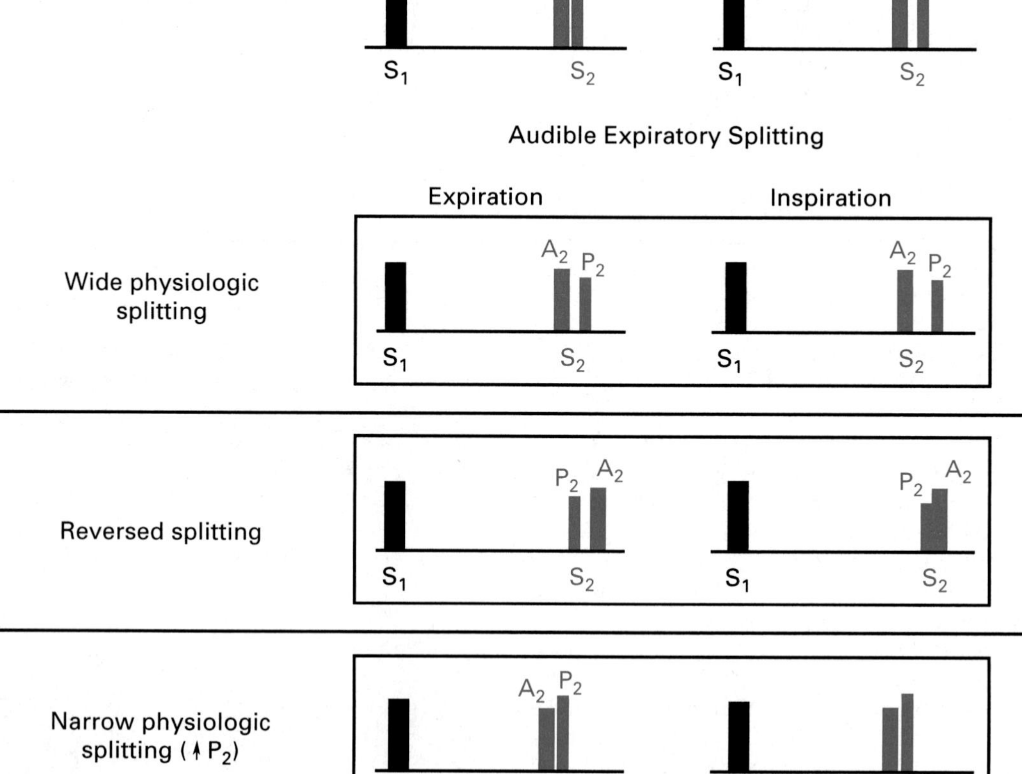


FIGURE 12-66 *Top.* Normal physiologic splitting. During expiration, $A_2$ and $P_2$ are separated by less than 30 ms and are appreciated as a single sound. During inspiration, the splitting interval widens, and $A_2$ and $P_2$ are clearly separated into two distinctly audible sounds. *Bottom.* Audible expiratory splitting. In contrast to normal physiologic splitting, two distinct sounds are easily heard during expiration. Wide physiologic splitting is due to delay in $P_2$. Reversed splitting is due to delay in $A_2$, resulting in paradoxical movement; i.e., with inspiration, $P_2$ moves toward $A_2$, and the splitting interval narrows. Narrow physiologic splitting is seen in pulmonary hypertension, and both $A_2$ and $P_2$ are heard during expiration at a narrow splitting interval due to an increased intensity and high-frequency composition of $P_2$. (From Shaver JA. *Examination of the Heart*, Part IV: Auscultation. Dallas: American Heart Association; 1990:17. Reproduced with permission from the publisher and the authors.)

TABLE 12-7 Wide Physiologic Splitting of the Second Heart Sound

- Delayed pulmonic closure
  - Delayed electrical activation of the right ventricle
    - Complete RBBB (proximal type)
    - Left ventricular paced beats
    - Left ventricular ectopic beats
  - Prolonged right ventricular mechanical systole
    - Acute massive pulmonary embolus
    - Pulmonary hypertension with right heart failure
    - Pulmonic stenosis with intact septum (moderate to severe)
  - Decreased impedance of the pulmonary vascular bed (increased "hangout")
    - Normotensive atrial septal defect
    - Idiopathic dilation of the pulmonary artery
    - Pulmonic stenosis (mild)
    - Atrial septal defect, postoperative (70%)
    - Unexplained AES in normal subjects
- Early aortic closure
  - Shortened left ventricular mechanical systole (LVET)
    - Mitral regurgitation
    - Ventricular septal defect

ABBREVIATIONS: RBBB = right bundle branch block; AES = audible expiratory splitting; LVET = left ventricular ejection time.

SOURCE: From Shaver JA et al. The second heart sound: Newer concepts: 1. Normal and wide physiological splitting. *Mod Concepts Cardiovasc Dis* 1977;46:9. Reproduced with permission from the American Heart Association, Inc., and the authors.

TABLE 12-8 Reversed Splitting of the Second Heart Sound

- Delayed aortic closure
  - Delayed electrical activation of the left ventricle
    - Complete LBBB[a] (proximal type)
    - Right ventricular paced beat
    - Right ventricular ectopic beats
  - Prolonged left ventricular mechanical systole
    - Complete LBBB (peripheral type)
    - Left ventricular outflow tract obstruction
    - Hypertensive cardiovascular disease
    - Arteriosclerotic heart disease
      - Chronic ischemic heart disease
      - Angina pectoris
  - Decreased impedance of the systemic vascular bed (increased "hangout")
    - Poststenotic dilation of the aorta secondary to aortic stenosis or regurgitation
    - Patent ductus arteriosus
- Early pulmonic closure
  - Early electrical activation of the right ventricle
    - Wolff-Parkinson-White syndrome, type B

[a]LBBB = left bundle branch block.

SOURCE: From Shaver JA et al. The second heart sound: Newer concepts: 2. Paradoxical splitting and narrow physiological splitting. *Mod Concepts Cardiovasc Dis* 1977;46:13. Reproduced with permission from the American Heart Association, Inc., and the authors.

cording to the abnormality of the cardiac cycle responsible for the altered timing of $A_2$ and $P_2$. In each table, the cardiac cycle has been divided into three phases (Fig. 12-64): (1) the electromechanical couple interval, the time from the onset of the Q wave to the rise of ventricular pressure; (2) ventricular mechanical systole, the sum of the isovolumic contraction time plus the ejection period minus the "hangout" interval (abnormalities of this interval exclude those conditions in which prolongation of the "hangout" interval is primarily responsible for the increased ejection time); and (3) "hangout" or impedance interval, the time between the incisura of the arterial trace and the ventricular pressure at the same level as the incisura (includes all conditions in which prolongation of this interval is primarily responsible for the increased ejection time).

***Wide Physiologic Splitting of $S_2$*** An example of wide physiologic splitting of $S_2$ due to delayed electrical activation of the RV secondary to right bundle branch block is shown in Fig. 12-67. Prolongation of RV mechanical systole secondary to severe PH and PS are also responsible for a delayed $P_2$. Classic wide, fixed splitting of $S_2$ is found in patients with ASD. A composite in Fig. 12-68 documents the role played by decreased impedance of the pulmonary vascular bed in the audible expiratory splitting found in ASD, idiopathic dilatation of the pulmonary artery, and mild PS with aneurysmal dilatation of the pulmonary artery. In each case, there is a marked increase in the "hangout" interval, as measured by high-fidelity pressure tracings. Wide physiologic splitting secondary to a decreased LV ejection time occurs in patients with acute MR.

***Reversed Splitting of $S_2$*** Almost all cases of reversed splitting of $S_2$ are due to a delay in $A_2$. As a result, the sequence of closure sounds is reversed, with $P_2$ preceding $A_2$. This abnormality is recognized by paradoxical movement of $A_2$ and $P_2$ with respiration.[208] During inspiration, $P_2$ moves toward $A_2$, and the splitting interval narrows, whereas during expiration, the two components separate, and audible expiratory splitting is present (Fig. 12-66). The presence of reversed splitting of $S_2$ almost always indicates significant underlying cardiovascular disease.

Both RV ectopic and paced beats produce a delay in the onset of LV contraction, resulting in reversed splitting of $S_2$. The mechanism responsible is a delayed activation of the LV, prolonging the Q to LV pressure rise interval. The most common cause of reversed splitting is complete LBBB, which can be due either to delayed activation of the LV, as seen in isolated proximal block, or to prolonged mechanical systole (primarily isovolumic contraction time), as seen in proximal or peripheral block invariably associated with significant LV dysfunction.

Reversed splitting of $S_2$ may occur in a patient with hypertrophic cardiomyopathy and is due to the large systolic pressure gradient and prolonged LV relaxation.[209] Although both these mechanisms may contribute to the reversed splitting observed in patients with valvular AS, an additional mechanism is an exaggerated "hangout" interval.[210]

In hypertensive cardiovascular disease, splitting is usually physiologic, with the intensity of $A_2$ being increased; however, rare instances of reversed splitting do occur. Reversed splitting of $S_2$ also has been reported in ischemic heart disease and during episodes of angina pectoris. The latter is extremely uncommon and rarely has been documented by phonocardiography. It is most likely due to a prolonged isovolumic contraction time of the ischemic LV, although during angina it also may be due to an increase in systemic arterial pressure or transient LBBB.[211]

Decreased impedance in the systemic vascular bed also can contribute to the delayed $A_2$ seen in poststenotic dilatation of the aorta. It

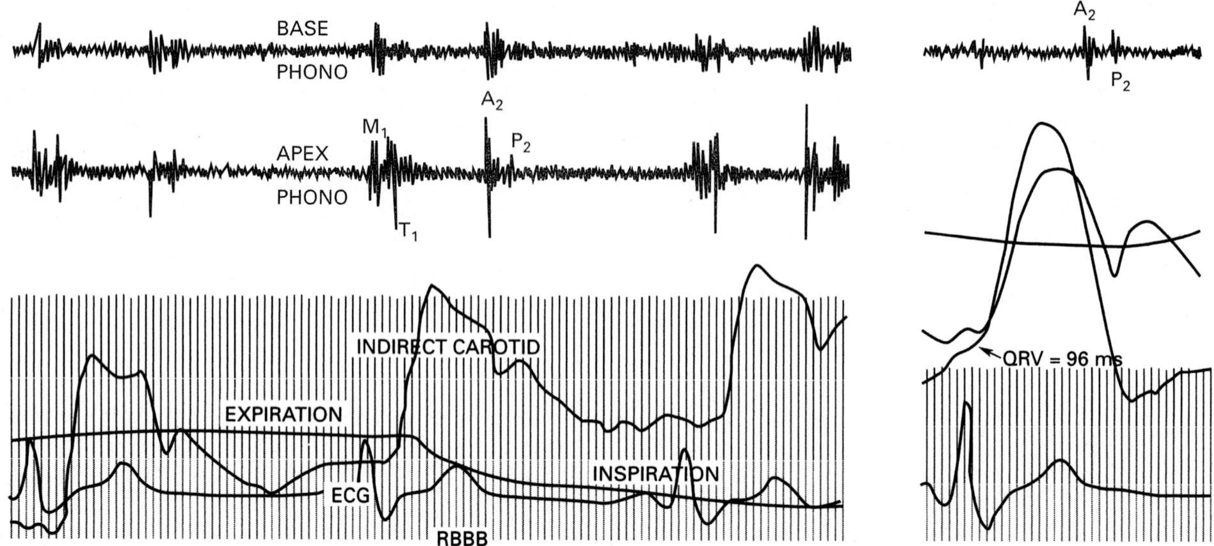


FIGURE 12-67 *Left.* Wide physiologic splitting of $S_2$ is seen in a patient with complete right bundle branch block. Audible expiratory splitting, which widens normally with inspiration, is present. Note also the wide splitting of the first heart sound into its mitral ($M_1$) and tricuspid ($T_1$) components, as recorded at the apex. *Right.* The base phonocardiogram is recorded simultaneously with high-fidelity catheters in the right ventricle (RV) and pulmonary artery during cardiac catheterization. There is marked prolongation of the Q to the onset of the RV pressure rise of 96 ms, resulting in wide physiologic splitting of $S_2$. The delayed $P_2$ is secondary to delayed activation of the RV. (From Shaver JA. Current uses of phonocardiography in clinical practice. In: Rapaport E, ed. *Cardiology Update: Reviews for Physicians*. New York: Elsevier; 1981:337. Reproduced originally in part (*left panel*) with permission from the publisher and author, and from Shaver JA, Salerni R, Reddy PS. Normal and abnormal heart sounds in cardiac diagnosis: I. Systolic sounds. *Curr Probl Cardiol* 1985;10:48. Reproduced in total with permission from the publisher and authors.)

also plays a role in the reversed splitting occasionally seen in both chronic AR and patent ductus arteriosus. Reversed splitting of $S_2$ also has been reported in some cases of type B Wolff-Parkinson-White syndrome, where early activation of the RV through an accessory pathway has caused $P_2$ to occur prematurely.

***Narrow Physiologic Splitting*** Narrow physiologic splitting of $S_2$ is a common finding in severe PH, as shown in Fig. 12-66.[211] In contrast to the normal situation, where only a single sound is heard during expiration, both $A_2$ and $P_2$ are easily heard, even though the splitting interval is less than 30 ms because of the increased intensity and high-frequency composition of $P_2$. Narrow splitting, although common in severe PH, is not always the case, and wide splitting with an increased amplitude of $P_2$ is often present. Wide, persistent splitting becomes a useful sign of abnormal RV performance in patients with primary PH. In order to reconcile these different responses in $S_2$ when PH develops, it is essential to appreciate that normally the duration of RV and LV systole is nearly equal and that a potential interval (the normally wide right-sided "hangout" interval) can be encroached on as the PH progressively decreases the capacitance and increases the resistance of the pulmonary vascular bed[212,213] (Fig. 12-64). Thus a spectrum of the width of splitting may be seen in PH, depending on the degree of selective prolongation of RV systole, always in the setting of a narrow "hangout" interval. Similar hemodynamic correlates have been found in patients having hyperkinetic PH secondary to large ASDs. Fixed splitting of $S_2$ occasionally has been documented in severe RV failure secondary to PH.

**SINGLE $S_2$**

All conditions listed in Table 12-8 that delay $A_2$ may produce a single $S_2$ when the splitting interval becomes less than 30 ms. Also, conditions in which one component of $S_2$ is either absent or inaudible will produce a single $S_2$ (e.g., truncus arteriosus, severe tetralogy of Fallot, severe semilunar valve stenosis, pulmonary atresia, and most cases of tricuspid atresia). In Eisenmenger's VSD, the duration of RV and LV systole is necessarily equal, and a loud, single $S_2$ is appreciated because $A_2$ and $P_2$ occur simultaneously. The most common cause of an apparently single $S_2$ is the inability to hear the fainter of the two components of the sound (usually $P_2$) because of emphysema, obesity, or respiratory noise. Single $S_2$ often is seen in individuals over age 50. Although this has been attributed to a delayed $A_2$, a decreased inspiratory delay in $P_2$ also has been reported.

## Opening Snaps

Opening of the normal AV valve is almost always a silent event. With thickening and deformity of the leaflets, usually rheumatic in origin, however, a sound is generated in early diastole in a manner analogous to ejection sounds arising from deformed semilunar valves. The term *opening snap* was first used by Thayer[214] in 1908 to describe the high-frequency early diastolic sound in MS. Thayer also recognized that the sound had been absent in those patients who, on autopsy, had markedly thickened and essentially immobile valves. This mechanism was confirmed by hemodynamic and angiographic studies that showed sudden checking of the early diastolic descent of the funnel-shaped stenotic valve when its elastic limits were met.[215] Phonoechocardiography has shown an even more precise correlation of the opening snap with the maximum opening motion of the anterior mitral leaflet (Fig. 12-59, *left*).

The opening snap is a crisp, sharp sound that can be heard in the midprecordial location, usually best in the area from the left sternal border to just inside the apex. Often it is heard well at the base of the heart and frequently is not well heard at the maximal intensity of the diastolic murmur. The diastolic rumble generally follows the opening snap by a short interval. There is no variation in the intensity or timing of the mitral opening snap with respiration.

As with ejection sounds of valvular origin, the intensity of the mitral opening snap correlates well with the mobility of the valve. A loud opening snap is found in mobile stenotic valves with good excursions (Fig. 12-59, *left*), whereas the opening snap is absent with severe calcific fixation of the valve. The intensity of $M_1$ parallels the intensity of the opening snap. Although the presence of valvular calcification decreases valve mobility and the audibility of the opening snap, the sound is actually found in 50 to 60 percent of patients with calcific valves.

The opening snap follows $A_2$ by an interval of 0.03 to 0.15 s. In patients with mild MS, the interval is usually long, whereas in patients with more severe stenosis, the $A_2$–opening snap interval is shorter. The $A_2$–opening snap interval in atrial fibrillation can vary with cycle length. With a short preceding RR interval, the left atrium has not had time to empty, the left atrial pressure remains high, and the $A_2$–opening snap interval is short. With a longer preceding RR interval, the left atrial pressure falls, and the $A_2$–opening snap interval widens.

The opening snap occurs at the maximal mitral valve opening shortly after LV–left atrial pressure crossovers. Factors that influence the timing of the opening snap relative to $A_2$ are (1) the rate of LV pressure decline, (2) the level of the LV pressure at the time of $A_2$, and (3) the level of the left atrial pressure.[216] Increasing severity of MS is usually accompanied by a shortening of the $A_2$–opening snap interval. Because this interval is multifactorially determined, there is an imperfect correlation between the $A_2$–opening snap interval and the mitral valve area.[217] Tricuspid valve stenosis also can produce an opening snap. This sound is frequently not detected because the findings of coexisting MS, which is almost invariably present, overshadow those of TS. When present, it generally follows the mitral opening snap.[218] An early diastolic sound can also be caused by a right or left atrial myxoma. Although the clinical findings of a left atrial myxoma may be similar to those of MS, the echocardiographic picture is classic (Fig. 12-59, *center*). The tumor "plop" occurs at the maximal diastolic descent of the myxoma.

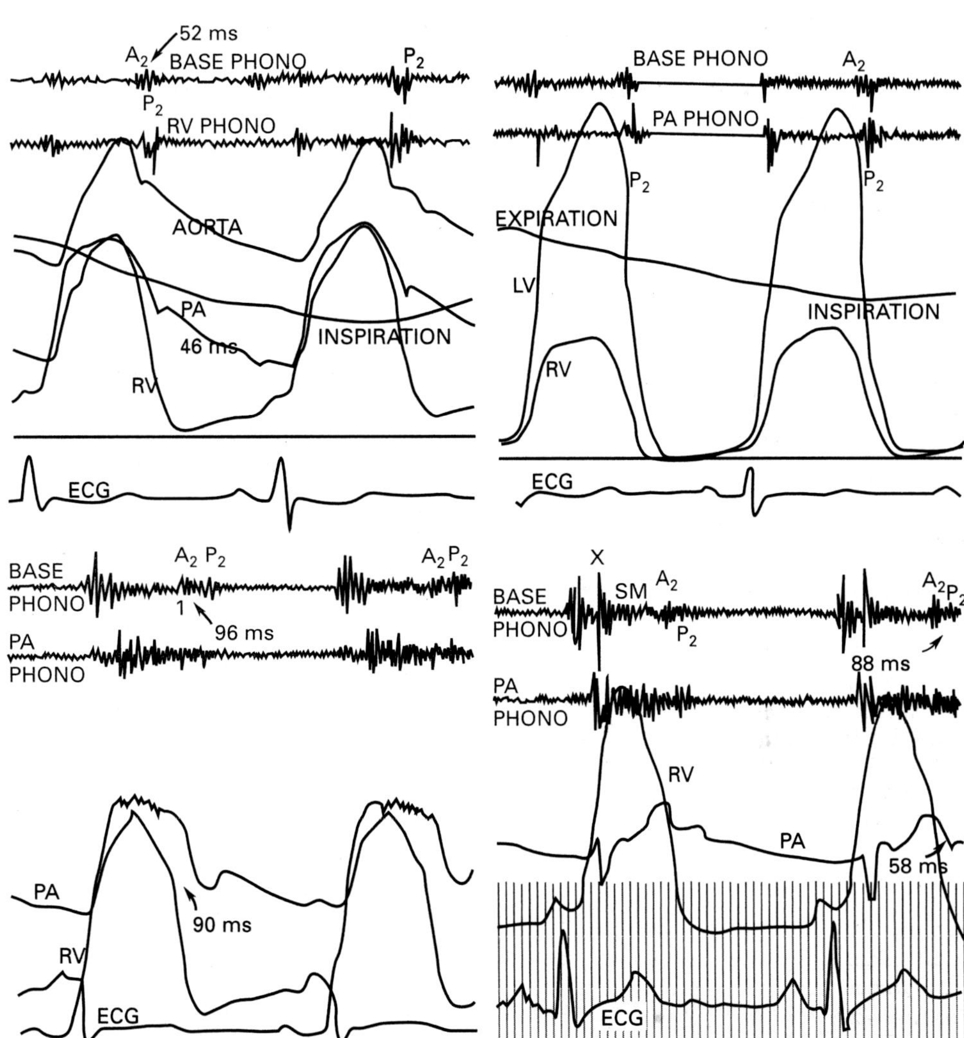


FIGURE 12-68 *Upper left.* Sound and pressure correlates of $S_2$ in a 45-year-old woman with a normotensive atrial septal defect (shunt 2:1). Wide, fixed splitting of $S_2$ is demonstrated; $P_2$ and $A_2$ are coincident with their respective incisurae, and the duration of the "hangout" interval is nearly equal to the $A_2$–$P_2$ interval. *Upper right.* Simultaneous RV and LV pressures clearly show that the duration of RV and LV systole is equal. *Lower left.* Sound and pressure correlates of a patient with idiopathic dilatation of the pulmonary artery. $P_2$ is coincident with the incisura of the pulmonary artery and separated from the RV pressure tracing by a "hangout" interval of 90 ms (almost identical to the splitting interval). *Lower right.* Similar sound and pressure correlates in a patient with mild valvular pulmonic stenosis and aneurysmal dilatation of the pulmonary artery. Most of the delay in $P_2$ is due to a wide "hangout" interval of 56 ms. In each patient all pressures are recorded by catheter-tipped micromanometers. (From Shaver JA, O'Toole JD. Second heart sound: The role of altered greater and lesser circulation. In: Leon DF, Shaver JA, eds. *Physiologic Principles of Heart Sounds and Murmurs*. Monograph 46. New York: American Heart Association; 1975:63. Reproduced originally in part (*top panel*) with permission from the publisher and the authors, and from Shaver JA. The second heart sound: Hemodynamic determinants. *Acta Cardiol* 1985;40:12. Reproduced in total with permission from the publisher and authors.)

Although an opening snap is rarely heard with normal valves, it may be heard in situations where high flow exists across the AV valves.[219] An early diastolic sound is frequently present in large ASDs coincident with maximal opening of the tricuspid valve. The opening snap must be differentiated from other early diastolic sounds such as the $S_3$, the pulmonary component of a widely split $S_2$, and a pericardial knock. At the bedside, differentiation of an opening snap from $P_2$ is made by noting that the maximal intensity is near the apex rather than at the pulmonary area and that there is lack of movement with respiration. During continuous respiration, it is often possible to appreciate three sounds on inspiration, occurring in rapid sequence in the pulmonary area, and only two components on expiration.

## The Third and Fourth Heart Sounds

The third and fourth heart sounds ($S_3$, $S_4$) are low-frequency events related to early and late diastolic filling of the ventricles (Fig. 12-69). When they are heard in disease states, they are called *gallop sounds,* and their presence gives valuable information to the clinician regarding the status of ventricular function and compliance.

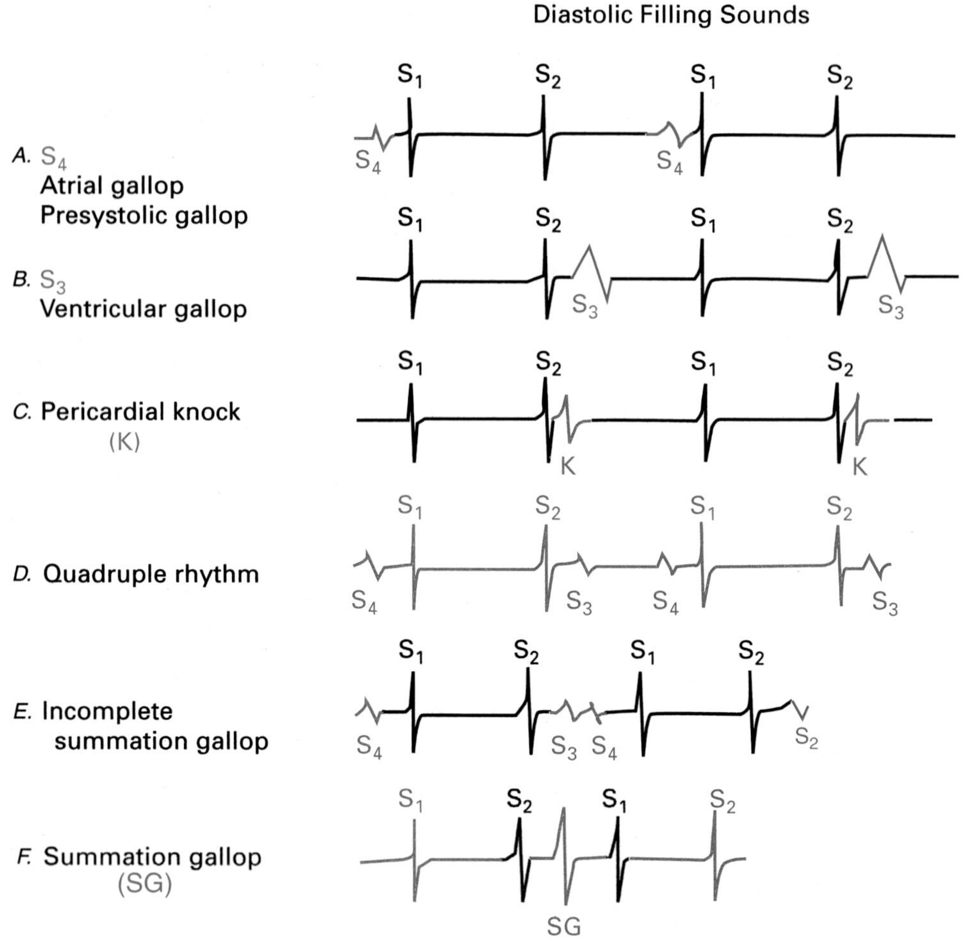


FIGURE 12-69 *A.* The $S_4$ occurs in presystole and is frequently called an atrial, or presystolic, gallop. *B.* The $S_3$ occurs during the rapid phase of ventricular filling. It is a normal finding and is commonly heard in children and young adults, disappearing with increasing age. When it is heard in a patient with cardiac disease, it is called a pathologic $S_3$, or ventricular gallop, and usually indicates ventricular dysfunction or AV valvular incompetence. *C.* In constrictive pericarditis, a sound in early diastole, the pericardial knock (K), is heard earlier and is louder and higher pitched than the usual pathologic $S_3$. *D.* A quadruple rhythm results if both $S_4$ and $S_3$ are present. *E.* At faster heart rates, the $S_3$ and $S_4$ occur in rapid succession and may give the illusion of a middiastolic rumble. *F.* When the heart rate is sufficiently fast, the two rapid phases of ventricular filling reinforce each other, and a loud summation gallop (SG) may appear; this sound may be louder than either the $S_3$ or $S_4$ alone. (From Shaver JA. *Examination of the Heart*, Part IV: Auscultation. Dallas: American Heart Association; 1990:27. Reproduced with permission from the publisher and the authors.)

## THE THIRD HEART SOUND

***Physiologic $S_3$*** The physiologic $S_3$ is a benign finding commonly heard in children, adolescents, and young adults, but it is rarely present in adults after age 40 and, when present, is often associated with a thin, asthenic body habitus. This is a low-frequency sound that follows $A_2$ by 120 to 200 ms and occurs during rapid filling of the ventricle.[220,221] It is best heard at the apex in the left lateral position with the stethoscope's bell pressed lightly against the skin and is differentiated from the pathologic $S_3$ primarily by the "company it keeps."[222]

***Pathologic $S_3$*** Most agree that the pathologic $S_3$ is an exaggeration of the physiologic $S_3$, with a common mechanism of production.[223] The exact genesis of the $S_3$ remains controversial. Three major mechanisms of production have been proposed: the valvular theory, the ventricular theory, and the impact theory. The most popular theory has indicated that these sounds have their origins within the left or RV or their walls.[224] The dynamic interplay between the force of delivery of blood into the ventricle and the ability of the ventricle to accept this flow is an important factor in the genesis of this sound. When there is appropriate interaction between these factors, the $S_3$ occurs when the ventricle suddenly reaches its elastic limits and abruptly decelerates the onrushing column of blood, thereby setting the entire cardiohemic system into vibration. Thus an $S_3$ may be produced by excessive rapid filling into a ventricle with normal or increased compliance, as with high-output states and MR, or by a normal or less than normal rate of filling into a ventricle with decreased compliance, as in patients with hypertrophic cardiomyopathy. Likewise, decreased rates of filling into overfilled ventricles with large end-systolic volumes, as seen in patients with LV systolic dysfunction, will produce this sound.[225]

Although this mechanism is likely responsible for the sound recorded within the ventricular cavity and on its epicardial surface, Reddy et al.[178,226] have reported convincing data that the sound heard with the stethoscope can be due to the dynamic impact of the heart with the chest wall. This theory explains the $S_3$ present in hyperdynamic states as well as those with an increased end-systolic volume secondary to LV dysfunction. In the latter, the space between the enlarged heart and the lateral chest wall is diminished, thereby facilitating a more forceful impact in early diastole. This results in an exaggerated rapid filling wave on the apexcardiogram and the prominent $S_3$ pathognomonic of congestive failure (Fig. 12-70, lower panel). Table 12-9 tabulates the major factors responsible for the production of the $S_3$ as recorded within the LV and on the chest wall.

A convenient classification of physiologic and pathologic states with an $S_3$ is presented in Table 12-10. Both the intensity and timing of the pathologic $S_3$ associated with LV dysfunction are related to the patient's volume status. With diuresis, the $S_3$ may decrease in intensity or disappear, and it tends to move away from $A_2$. A loud, persistent $S_3$ with cardiomyopathy or acute MI is an ominous sign associated with high mortality, whereas prompt subsidence with therapy suggests a more favorable outlook. LV third heart sounds are heard best at the apex, whereas RV third heart sounds are heard at the lower left sternal edge and may increase in intensity with inspiration.

In chronic AR, even though end-diastolic volume is increased, end-systolic volume may not be increased until LV dysfunction develops. As LV dysfunction develops, the ejection fraction decreases, resulting in an increased end-systolic volume, and a pathologic $S_3$ appears in these patients.[223] An $S_3$ is very common in acute AR and is usually followed by the middiastolic component of the Austin Flint rumble.

A pathologic $S_3$ resulting from excessive early diastolic filling is common in hyperkinetic states and AV valve regurgitation and often initiates a short flow rumble.[227] It is often present in large left-to-right shunts due to high flow across the mitral valve with VSD or patent ductus arteriosus and with high flow across the tricuspid valve with ASD. The presence of this sound in these conditions does not imply congestive heart failure, and such patients may maintain normal myocardial contractility for years after the $S_3$ is detected.[228] Pathologic third heart sounds are heard in both restrictive and hypertrophic cardiomyopathy. In constrictive pericarditis, an early prominent sound of a somewhat higher frequency is heard, the *pericardial knock*. The evidence to date points to the simultaneous occurrence of the pericardial knock and the termination of rapid filling of the ventricles. The apex cardiac pulsation may show systolic retraction followed by an exaggerated diastolic impulse. The pericardial knock usually increases in intensity with inspiration and occurs near the nadir of the *y* descent of the JVP. Atrial fibrillation is commonly present in severe constrictive pericarditis, and at times the loud early knock may be confused with the opening snap of MS.

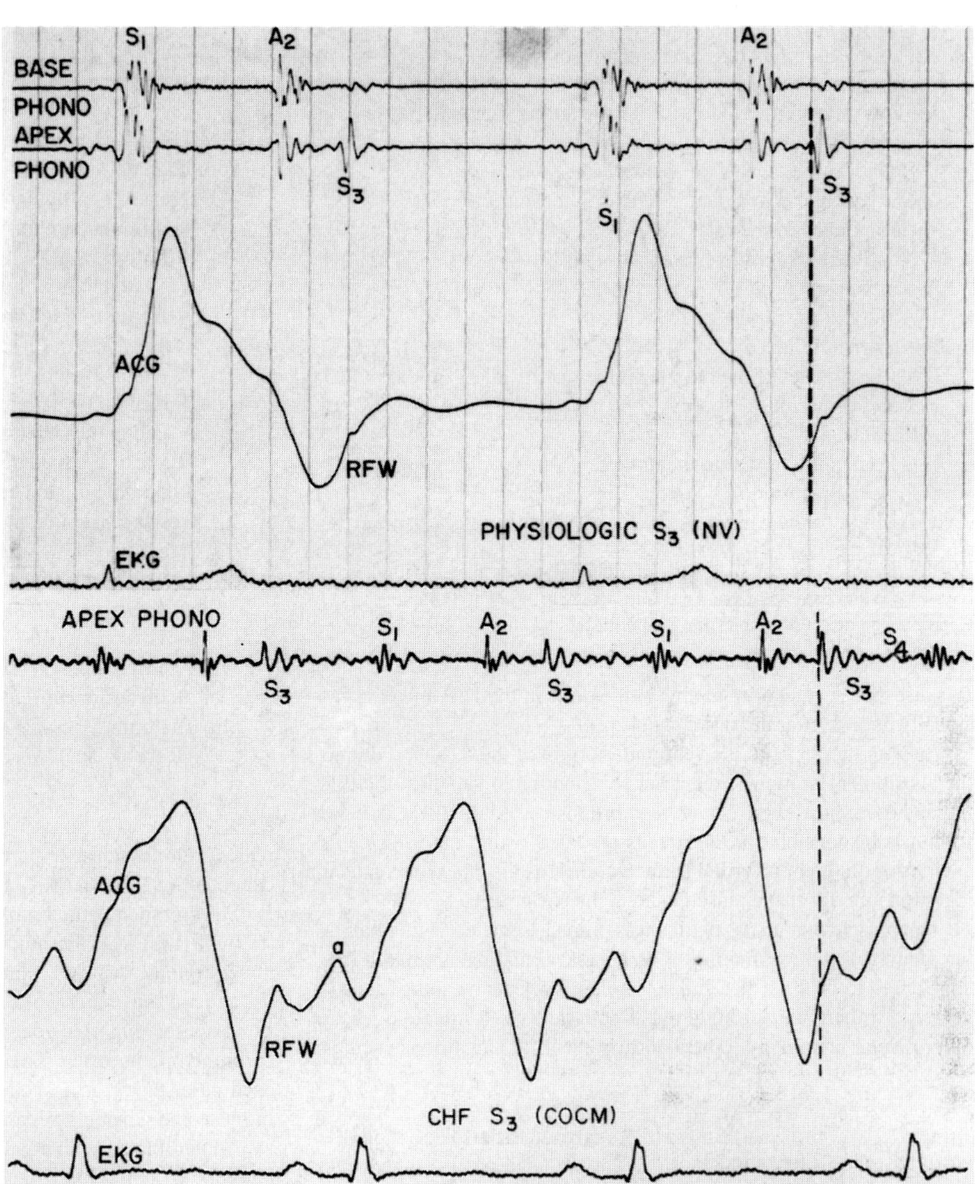


FIGURE 12-70 *Top.* A physiologic $S_3$ (normal variant) recorded in a 24-year-old woman without evidence of cardiovascular disease. The onset of the $S_3$ occurs during the rapid filling wave (RFW) of the ACG between the *O* and *F* points. The remainder of the cardiovascular examination was entirely within normal limits. *Bottom.* A very prominent $S_3$ gallop is recorded in a patient with severe congestive cardiomyopathy (COCM). On physical examination, there was a small-volume carotid pulse and marked engorgement of the neck veins with elevated venous pressure. The apexcardiogram (ACG) shows a very prominent presystolic pulsation (a), and an extremely rapid filling wave is present. The onset of the $S_3$ occurs during the RFW of the ACG. The first heart sound is soft. (From Shaver JA. Early diastolic events associated with the physiologic and pathologic $S_3$. *J Cardiogr* 1984;14(suppl 5):30. Reproduced with permission from the publisher and the authors.)

## THE FOURTH HEART SOUND

Precordial vibrations resulting from atrial contraction are normally neither palpable nor audible. Under pathologic conditions, forceful atrial contraction generates a low-frequency sound ($S_4$) just prior to $S_1$ (also termed the *atrial diastolic gallop* or the *presystolic gallop*). Atrial contraction must be present for production of an $S_4$. It is absent in atrial fibrillation and in other rhythms in which atrial contraction does not precede ventricular contraction. The $S_4$ follows the onset of the P wave of the ECG by approximately 70 ms. Audibility of the $S_4$ depends not only on its intensity and frequency but also on its separation from $S_1$. The degree of this separation is determined primarily by the PR interval, but it is also somewhat influenced by the P-$S_4$ and the Q-$S_1$ intervals. A loud $S_1$ also may mask the audibility of a preceding softer $S_4$. The $S_4$ is best heard at the apex impulse with the patient turned in the left lateral position. It varies considerably with respiration, usually being heard best during expiration. A left-sided $S_4$ may radiate to the brachiocephalic and carotid vessel and be best heard in the areas in patients with severe lung disease or who are very obese. A left-sided $S_3$ may do likewise. A left-sided $S_4$ and $S_3$ may also be augmented post-tussively and with sustained handgrip exercise. Both the intensity and timing of the $S_4$ are closely related to the end-diastolic volume of the ventricle. Maneuvers that increase venous return increase the audibility by increasing the intensity of the sound and by causing it to occur earlier, thereby separating it further from $S_1$. Decreased venous return does the opposite. Audible fourth heart sounds are usually accompanied by a palpable presystolic apical impulse in the absence of obesity, emphysema, etc., but occasionally, palpable presystolic impulses are not audible. The $S_4$ generated by a forceful right atrial contraction is usually heard best at the lower left sternal border. Unlike the left-sided $S_4$, it tends to be accentuated with inspiration.

TABLE 12-9 Hemodynamic Determinants of the $S_3$

Ability of the ventricle to accept flow during the rapid phase of diastolic filling
- Rate of relaxation of the ventricle
- End-systolic or residual volume of the ventricle
- Compliance of the relaxed ventricle
- Nonobstructed atrioventricular valve

Atrial pressure head
- Atrial blood volume
- Atrial compliance

Dynamic impact of the heart with the chest wall
- Architecture of the thorax
- Cardiac size
- Cardiac motion within the thorax
- Phase of respiration
- Position of the patient

SOURCE: From Shaver JA et al. Early diastolic events associated with the physiologic and pathologic $S_3$. *Am J Cardiol* 1984;14(suppl 5):45. Reproduced with permission from the publisher and authors.

It is also accompanied by prominent *a* waves in the JVP and is occasionally audible over the right jugular vein.[229]

As with the $S_3$, both the ventricular origin of the $S_4$ sound due to the abrupt deceleration of the atrial contribution to late diastolic filling and the impact theory have been proposed.[230] It is likely that the former is responsible for the sounds recorded within the ventricular cavities or on their epicardial surfaces, whereas the latter mechanism is responsible for the $S_4$ auscultated at the chest wall.

The presence of an $S_4$, particularly when associated with a palpable presystolic apical impulse, is an abnormal finding. Although it is considered to be a normal finding in older subjects by some investigators,[230] others feel strongly that a definite $S_4$ in a middle-aged or older person is unlikely to be a normal event.[229] Conditions such as obesity, emphysema, or barrel-chest deformity may hinder the clinical detection of both an $S_4$ and an apical presystolic impulse.

TABLE 12-10 Third Heart Sound ($S_3$), Ventricular Diastolic Gallop, Protodiastolic Gallop, and Pericardial Knock

- Physiologic $S_3$—children and young adults
  - Decreased prevalence with increasing age
- Pathologic $S_3$
  - Ventricular dysfunction—poor systolic function, increased end-diastolic and end-systolic volume, decreased ejection fraction, and high filling pressures
    - Idiopathic dilated cardiomyopathy
    - Ischemic heart disease
    - Valvular heart disease
    - Congenital heart disease
    - Systemic and pulmonary hypertension
  - Excessively rapid early diastolic ventricular filling
    - Hyperkinetic states
      - Anemia
      - Thyrotoxicosis
      - Arteriovenous fistula
    - Atrioventricular valve incompetence
    - Left-to-right shunts
  - Restrictive myocardial or pericardial disease
  - Constrictive pericarditis (pericardial knock)
  - Restrictive cardiomyopathy
  - Hypertrophic cardiomyopathy?

TABLE 12-11 Fourth Heart Sound ($S_4$), Atrial Diastolic Gallop, and Presystolic Gallop

- Physiologic—recordable, but rarely audible
- Pathologic
  - Decreased ventricular compliance
    - Ventricular hypertrophy
      - Left or right ventricular outflow obstruction
      - Systemic or pulmonary hypertension
      - Hypertrophic cardiomyopathy
    - Ischemic heart disease
      - Angina pectoris
      - Acute myocardial infarction
      - Old myocardial infarction
      - Ventricular aneurysm
    - Idiopathic dilated cardiomyopathy
  - Excessively rapid late diastolic filling secondary to
    - Vigorous atrial systole
    - Hyperkinetic states
      - Anemia
      - Thyrotoxicosis
    - Arteriovenous fistula
    - Acute atrioventricular valve incompetence
  - Arrhythmias
    - Heart block

The common pathologic conditions in which $S_4$ is heard are listed in Table 12-11. A forceful atrial contraction into a hypertrophied, noncompliant ventricle almost always produces an early and easily audible and recordable $S_4$. The severe LV hypertrophy present in systemic hypertension, severe valvular AS, and hypertrophic cardiomyopathy often is responsible for a loud $S_4$ (Fig. 12-71). In each case, the $S_4$ is associated with a prominent apical presystolic impulse and is widely separated from $S_1$.

An audible $S_4$ with a palpable presystolic impulse is common in patients with ischemic heart disease during an acute episode of angina and in the early phases of transmural MI. Its prevalence is also increased with prior MI; however, audible fourth heart sounds in patients with ischemic heart disease without prior infarction or hypertension are uncommon.[178] In patients with LV aneurysm or idiopathic or ischemic cardiomyopathy, abnormal fourth heart sounds are commonly present and often associated with an $S_3$, producing a quadruple rhythm. If tachycardia is present, or if the PR interval is prolonged, $S_3$ and $S_4$ may fuse, giving rise to a loud summation gallop (Fig. 12-69).

Quadruple rhythms are common in hyperkinetic states where the $S_3$ is due to excessively rapid early diastolic filling and the $S_4$ results from a forceful atrial contraction into a volume-loaded ventricle. With varying degrees of tachycardia, incomplete summation may occur, simulating a diastolic rumble, or complete fusion may occur, generating a loud summation gallop (Fig. 12-69). In acute AV valve regurgitation, vigorous atrial contraction into an acutely volume-loaded ventricle can produce an $S_4$ associated with a presystolic apical impulse. At times it may be difficult to appreciate because of the masking effect of the loud systolic murmur. This contrasts with most patients with chronic MR, who do not have an $S_4$ but frequently have an $S_3$.

Presystolic and isolated diastolic fourth heart sounds as well as summation gallops may be heard with varying degrees of heart

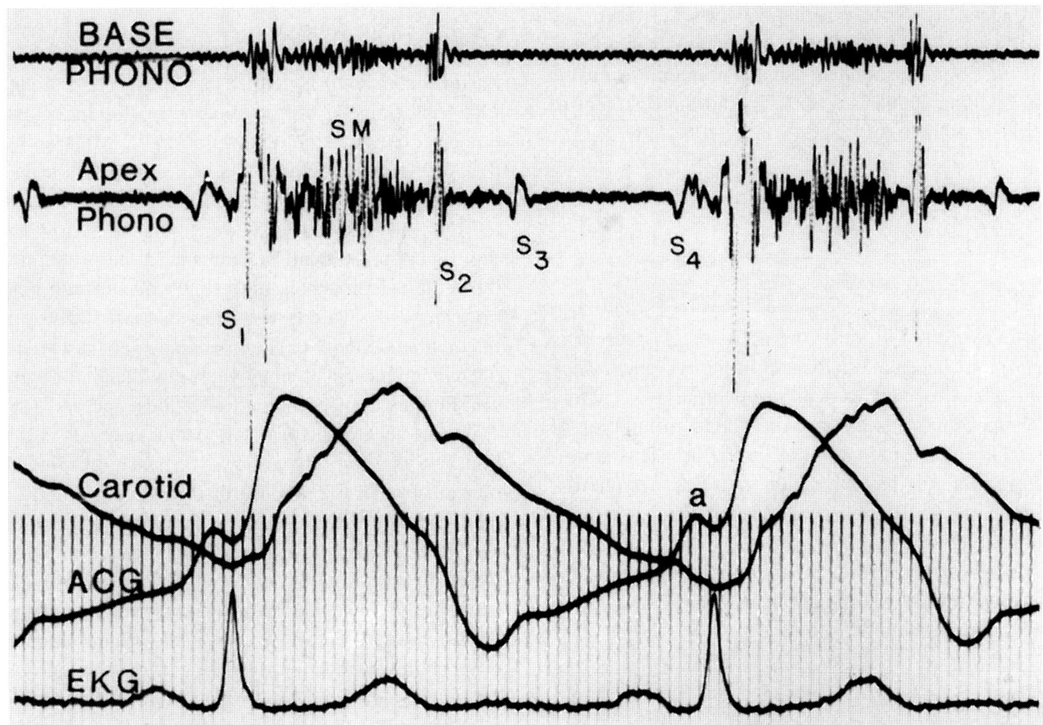


FIGURE 12-71 Atrial diastolic gallop (ADG) and ventricular diastolic gallop (VDG) recorded in an adult with severe calcific aortic stenosis. The ADG is associated with a prominent presystolic apical impulse (a); the VDG occurs during the rapid filling wave of the apexcardiogram (ACG). The carotid pulse has a very slow rate of rise and a markedly prolonged LV ejection time. The classic diamond-shaped systolic ejection murmur (SM) is present at the base and apex. Note the higher-frequency composition of the SM at the apex but preservation of the crescendo-decrescendo pattern. (From Shaver JA. Current uses of phonocardiography in clinical practice. In: Rapaport E, ed. *Cardiology Update: Reviews for Physicians*. New York: Elsevier; 1981:356. Reproduced with permission from the publisher and author. Copyright 1981 by Elsevier Publishing Co., Inc.)

block. First-degree heart block facilitates audibility of the $S_4$ because it further separates $S_4$ from $S_1$. In 2:1 heart block, an isolated $S_4$ may be heard in diastole, and a presystolic $S_4$ may be audible because of the increase in diastolic volume. In complete heart block, $S_4$ may be heard randomly throughout diastole, and when it occurs simultaneously with rapid early ventricular filling, a loud summation gallop may occur.

## Prosthetic Valve Sounds

The sounds produced by prosthetic valves are varied, depending on the type of valve, its position, and whether or not it is functioning normally (Chap. 70). Mechanical valves produce opening and closing clicks that are easily audible and in many patients can be heard even without a stethoscope. Ball-in-cage valves such as the Starr-Edwards produce the loudest and most distinctive opening and closing clicks in any position as long as there is normal valve and ventricular function. In the aortic position, a crisp opening click occurs 0.06 to 0.07 s after $S_1$ and is coincident with maximal ball excursion, as demonstrated by echocardiography. The metallic ball of the Starr-Edwards valve also produces multiple early systolic clicks when the freely moving ball bounces against the cage during early systolic ejection. These clicks occur *during* the harsh systolic ejection murmur. Absence or decrease in intensity of these clicks can occur with valve obstruction or LV dysfunction. A decrease in the intensity of the opening and closing clicks, which normally have an intensity ratio of more than 0.5, and the absence of the opening click are also indications of valve malfunction.

In the mitral position, a prominent opening click occurs 0.05 to 0.15 s after $A_2$. Narrowing of this interval indicates an elevation of left atrial pressure, which may be due to either relative MS or MR. Interference with ball motion also can produce prolongation or significant beat-to-beat variation of this interval. A closing click is also prominent. Just as is seen with the normal $S_1$, there is variability in the intensity of the closing click, with the changing RR intervals of atrial fibrillation being louder with short RR intervals and softer with long intervals. A decreased intensity with first-degree AV block also occurs due to partial atriogenic closure of the valve, thus reducing the ball excursion and therefore the click intensity. Although a decreased intensity of the valve clicks occurs with valve malfunction, the presence of normal ball motion on an echocardiogram suggests that a nonvalvular cause such as severe LV dysfunction is responsible for the decreased intensity.

The auscultatory findings of disk valve prostheses vary, depending on the type of disk valve. Central occluder valves such as the Beall valve, which was used predominantly in the mitral and tricuspid positions, produce distinct, audible opening and closing sounds. The more commonly used tilting-disk valves do not ordinarily produce audible opening sounds in either the aortic or mitral position.[165] The closing sounds of disk valves are distinct and easily heard in both aortic and mitral positions. LV dysfunction, first-degree AV block, or another arrhythmia that causes the disk to move to a partially closed position prior to the onset of ventricular contraction will result in a softer sound. This finding must be distinguished from malfunction caused by either fibrosis or thrombus disturbing the disk motion. Auscultation of the bileaflet St. Jude valve is similar to that of the tilting-disk valve.

The sounds produced by tissue prosthetic valves are more like normal heart sounds than the sounds from a mechanical valve.[165] In the aortic position, an opening sound is usually not audible. In the mitral position, an opening sound is audible in about 50 percent of patients at an interval of 0.07 to 0.11 s after $A_2$.

## EXTRACARDIAC SOUNDS

### Pacemaker Sounds

High-frequency sounds of brief duration are occasionally present in patients with transvenous pacemakers located in the RV apex. They are extracardiac in origin, occurring nearly synchronously (within 6 to 10 ms) with the pacemaker spike, and are due to stimulation of intercostal nerves adjacent to endocardial electrodes.[231] This stimulus results in contraction of the intercostal muscles; frequently, twitching of the muscle can be observed. The presence of these sounds should suggest myocardial perforation by the endocardial lead, although this is not always present. Stimulation of the pectoral muscles, as well as diaphragmatic stimulation, also has been reported to produce these extracardiac sounds.

### Pericardial Friction Rub

Inflammation of the pericardial sac with or without fluid may cause a pericardial friction rub. These friction sounds are very high pitched, leathery, and scratchy in nature. They seem close to the ear and are auscultated best with the patient leaning forward or in the knee-chest position, holding his or her breath after forced expiration. The pericardial rub may have three components during the intervals of the cardiac cycle when the heart has the greatest excursions within the pericardial sac—at the time of atrial systole, at the time of ventricular contraction, and during rapid early diastolic filling. The usual friction rub occurs during the first two intervals, although three-component rubs may be heard. Triple-component friction rubs are common in uremic pericarditis, particularly when the underlying cardiac disease is hypertension. In this situation, the heart is hyperkinetic due to both pressure and volume overload as well as to the anemia associated with renal failure. Pericardial friction rubs are very common in the acute phase of transmural MI, although they often last for only a few hours. There is a common misconception that friction rubs are not heard when there is a large amount of fluid in the pericardial sac; this is not the case, because usually some portions of the visceral and parietal pericardial surfaces are in contact despite the large amount of fluid (Chap. 80).

Occasionally, certain midsystolic (ejection) murmurs have a scratchy character and may be misinterpreted as friction rubs. This is particularly true of the short, scratchy pulmonic ejection murmur heard in hyperthyroidism (Means-Lerman sign).[235] Such scratchy sounds should not be interpreted as a friction rub unless both systolic and diastolic components are heard.

### Mediastinal Crunch: Hamman's Sign

When air is present in the mediastinum, a series of scratchy sounds (Hamman's sign[233]) may occur, related indirectly to both heartbeat and respiratory excursion. These sounds occur most frequently during ventricular systole and in a random fashion. The diagnosis of mediastinal emphysema may be confirmed by crepitation in the neck secondary to subcutaneous air. These crunching sounds due to air in the mediastinum are common following cardiac surgery.

## HEART MURMURS

A *cardiac murmur* is defined as a relatively prolonged series of auditory vibrations of varying intensity (loudness), frequency (pitch), quality, configuration, and duration.[234] Most authorities now agree that turbulence is the prime factor responsible for most murmurs. Turbulence occurs when blood velocity becomes critically high due to high flow, flow through an irregular or narrow area, or a combination of both. Leatham has attributed the production of murmurs to three main factors: (1) high flow rate through normal or abnormal orifices, (2) forward flow through a constricted or irregular orifice or into a dilated vessel or chamber, and (3) backward or regurgitant flow through an incompetent valve, septal defect, or patent ductus arteriosus. Frequently, a combination of these factors is operative.

While the intensity of a systolic murmur is not always proportional to the hemodynamic disturbance, grading the loudness of a murmur from 1 to 6 as described by Freeman and Levine[235] is generally used. A *grade 1 murmur* is so faint that it can be heard only with special effort. A *grade 2 murmur* is faint but can be heard easily. A *grade 3 murmur* is moderately loud, a *grade 4 murmur* is very loud, and a *grade 5 murmur* is extremely loud and can be heard if only the edge of the stethoscope is in contact with the skin but cannot be heard if the stethoscope is removed from the skin. A *grade 6 murmur* is exceptionally loud and can be heard with the stethoscope just removed from contact with the chest. Experience has shown that systolic murmurs of grade 3 or more in intensity are usually hemodynamically significant.[236] Systolic thrills usually are associated with murmurs of grade 4 or louder. The intensity of the murmur varies directly with the velocity of blood flow across the area of murmur production. The velocity, in turn, is directly related to the pressure head that drives the blood across the murmur-producing area. For example, high velocity of flow through a small VSD produces a loud murmur, whereas a large flow at low velocity through an ASD produces no murmur. The *intensity* of a murmur as auscultated at the chest wall is also determined by the transmission characteristics of the tissues intervening between the source of the murmur and the stethoscope. Obesity, emphysema, and the presence of significant pericardial or pleural effusion will decrease the intensity of a murmur, whereas a thin, asthenic body habitus often will accentuate it.

The frequency of a murmur bears a direct relationship to the velocity of blood flow, as does the intensity of the murmur. The low-velocity flow resulting from a small pressure head across a stenotic mitral valve produces a low-pitched rumbling murmur, whereas the large diastolic pressure gradient across a regurgitant aortic valve causes a high-pitched murmur. Occasionally, the frequency composition of the same systolic murmur may vary, depending on the area auscultated. For example, the systolic murmur of AS frequently sounds higher-pitched at the apex than at the base.[237] Some murmurs—such as the "cooing dove" regurgitant murmur of a ruptured or retroverted aortic cusp, the systolic "whoop" or "honk" of MVP, or the high-pitched systolic murmur of a degenerated bioprosthetic valve—have a very distinctive musical quality.

In addition to the intensity and frequency of murmurs, their *timing* should also be described. There is seldom any difficulty distinguishing between systole and diastole, since systole is considerably shorter at normal heart rates. At rapid heart rates, however, the durations of these two intervals approach each other. Under such circumstances, the examiner can usually time the murmur by simultaneous palpation of the lower right carotid artery or can rely on the fact that the second heart sound ($S_2$) is usually the louder sound at the base. Once $S_2$ is identified, murmurs can be located properly in the cardiac cycle as systolic or diastolic. If the murmur in question is at the apex, the proper timing can be ensured by the "inching" technique popularized by Harvey and Levine.[176] This consists of slowly moving the stethoscope down from the base to the apex while repeatedly fixing the cardiac cycle in mind, using $S_2$ as a reference point. With sinus tachycardia, carotid sinus pressure may temporarily slow the rate and make it possible to differentiate systole from diastole. Continuous murmurs are heard throughout the cardiac cycle in systole and diastole and usually have their peak intensity around $S_2$.

The *location* and *radiation* of a murmur are determined multifactorially by the site of origin, intensity, and direction of blood flow, as well as by the physical characteristics of the chest. The duration and time intensity contour (murmur *envelope*) of a specific murmur are intimately related to the instantaneous pattern of blood flow velocity causing the murmur.

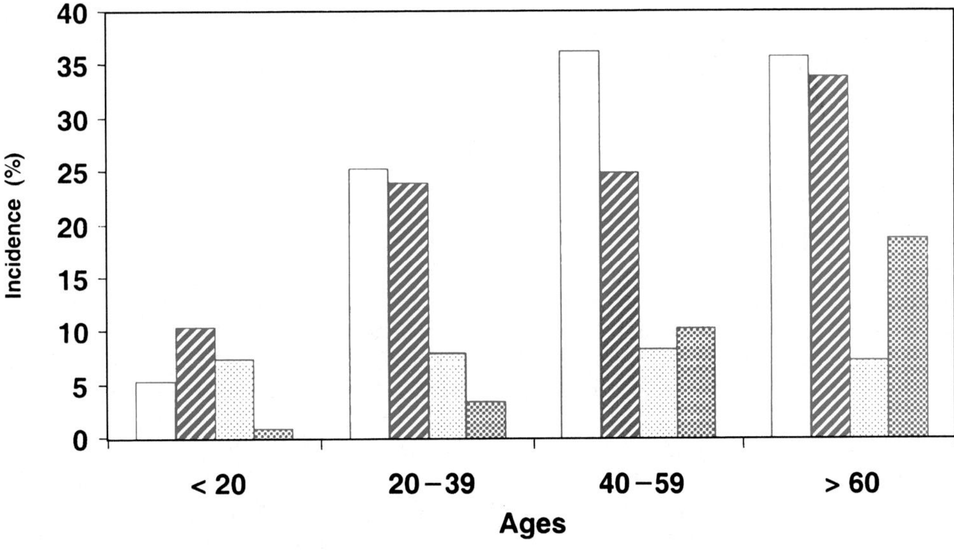


FIGURE 12-72 Percent incidence of mitral, tricuspid, pulmonic, and aortic regurgitation, respectively, by Doppler echocardiography in clinically normal subjects at various ages.

## Accurate Auscultation versus Echocardiography

The availability of echocardiography doe not eliminate the need for properly performed auscultation of the heart. While echocardiography provides additional information in many patients and may even provide the correct etiology of various systolic and diastolic murmurs, it is an unnecessary step in many patients with "innocent" murmurs. Echocardiography may even lead to a false diagnosis of "echocardiographic heart disease."

Often, a mild valvular regurgitant jet, detected by color-flow Doppler techniques, is not associated with an audible murmur despite optimal auscultation. Such regurgitant jets usually do not indicate clinical heart disease. Trivial mitral regurgitation can be detected by Doppler in up to 45 percent of normal individuals; tricuspid regurgitation in up to 70 percent; and pulmonic regurgitation in up to 88 percent. Normal aortic regurgitation is encountered much less frequently, and its incidence increases with advancing age (Fig. 12-72). Newly developed small handheld echocardiographic detectors are highly unlikely to replace the stethoscope.

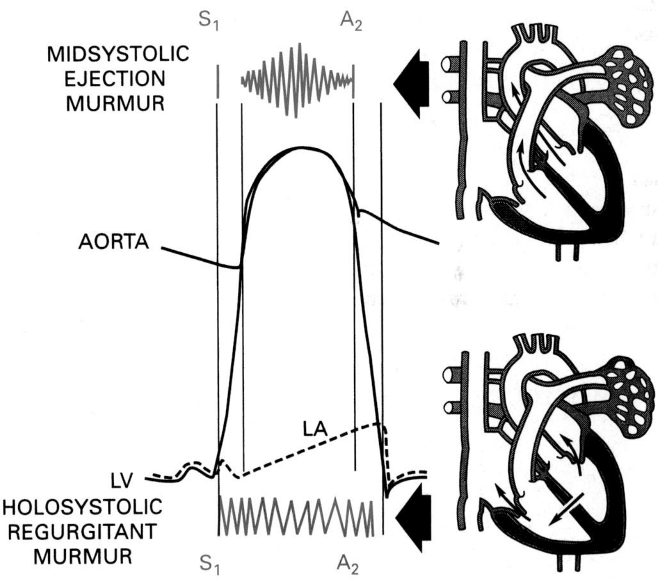


FIGURE 12-73 Midsystolic ejection murmurs are caused by forward flow across the left ventricular (LV) or right ventricular (RV) outflow tract, whereas pansystolic regurgitant murmurs are caused by retrograde flow from a high-pressure cardiac chamber to a low-pressure one. *Left.* Diagrammatic representation of the midsystolic ejection murmur and the pansystolic regurgitant murmur as related to LV, aortic, and left atrial (LA) pressures. The systolic ejection murmur occurs during the period of LV ejection; the onset of the murmur is separated from $S_1$ by the period of isovolumic contraction and the crescendo-decrescendo murmur terminates before $A_2$. The pansystolic regurgitant murmur begins with or may replace $S_1$, and the murmur continues up to and through $A_2$ as LV pressure exceeds left atrial pressure during the period of isovolumic relaxation. The murmur has a plateau configuration and varies little with respiration. *Right.* Flow diagram. (Left panel reproduced from Reddy PS, Shaver JA, Leonard JJ. Cardiac systolic murmurs: Pathophysiology and differential diagnosis. *Prog Cardiovasc Dis* 1971;14:19. Entire figure reproduced with permission from Shaver JA. Systolic murmurs. *Heart Dis Stroke* 1993; 2:10.)

## Systolic Murmurs

Systolic murmurs may be classified into two basic categories—ejection (midsystolic) murmurs and regurgitant murmurs. This simple classification is attractive because it has a physiologic as well as a descriptive basis. Systolic *ejection* murmurs are due to forward flow across the LV or RV outflow tract, whereas systolic *regurgitant* murmurs are due to retrograde flow from a high-pressure cardiac chamber to a low-pressure chamber.[238]

### SYSTOLIC EJECTION (MIDSYSTOLIC) MURMURS

The systolic *ejection* murmur begins shortly after the pressure in the left or RV exceeds the aortic or pulmonic diastolic pressure sufficiently to open the aortic or pulmonic valve. There is a delay between the $S_1$, which occurs shortly after AV pressure crossover, and the beginning of the murmur (Fig. 12-73). The murmur then waxes and wanes in a crescendo-decrescendo fashion often described as "diamond-shaped" or "spindle-shaped" in configuration. The murmur ends before the semilunar valve closure on the side from which it originates. The contour of the time-intensity pattern or *envelope* of the murmur corresponds to the contour of the flow velocity, and the murmur is heard when the sound produced during the peak turbulence exceeds the audible threshold. Thus, not only is the overall intensity of the murmur proportional to the rate of ventricular ejection, but also its shape depends on the instantaneous flow velocity during the period of ejection. As can be seen in Fig. 12-74, during normal LV ejection, a disproportionately large volume flow occurs in early systole. If velocity of flow exceeds the murmur threshold, a short midsystolic or ejection murmur results, and its envelope corresponds to the flow velocity pattern. If the stroke volume of the ventricle is increased, this pattern of ejection persists in an exaggerated fashion; the resulting murmur has a tendency to peak early in systole and fade out about halfway through the ejection phase. Such murmurs have been referred to as "kite-shaped" and are common in high-output states or conditions such as AR or heart block, where stroke volume is high.

The flow characteristics of normal RV ejection are somewhat different. Early ejection rates are not nearly as high, and the flow curve peaks somewhat later, having a more rounded contour. This flow pattern may well explain some of the long systolic ejection murmurs heard in ASDs and the straight-back syndrome, where only minimal gradients are found across the RV outflow tract.[239] With true valvular obstruction, rapid early ejection is no longer possible; the aortic flow velocity patterns become rounded, resulting in the more symmetric murmur of AS. In such cases, the instantaneous flow pattern is determined by the instantaneous pressure head with the resulting high correlation between the contour of the pressure gradient and the murmur envelope. If LV or RV obstruction is severe, systole is prolonged, and closure sound of the semilunar valve is delayed. The murmur, however, always stops before the closure sound on the side from which it originates, although it may envelop the closure sound of the *opposite side* of the circulation.

The intensity of ejection murmurs closely parallels changes in cardiac output. Any condition that increases forward flow—such as exercise, anxiety, fever, or increased stroke volume associated with the long diastolic filling period after a premature beat—increases the intensity of the murmur. Likewise, conditions that decrease cardiac output—congestive heart failure, beta blockade, or other negative inotropic agents—will decrease the intensity of the ejection murmur. Furthermore, definitive diagnosis of the systolic murmur often can be made during auscultation by careful attention to the response of the murmur to various bedside maneuvers that alter the flow and loading conditions of the heart.[240] These maneuvers include respiration, the strain and release phases of the Valsalva maneuver, standing, squatting, passive leg elevation, isometric hand-grip exercise, and transient arterial occlusion (Fig. 12-72).

## Innocent Murmurs

Innocent murmurs are always systolic ejection in nature and occur without evidence of physiologic or structural abnormalities in the cardiovascular system when peak flow velocity in early systole exceeds the murmur threshold.[236] These murmurs are almost always less than grade 3 in intensity and vary considerably from examination to examination and with body position and level of physical activity. They are not associated with a thrill or with radiation to the carotid arteries or axillae. They may arise from flow across either the normal LV or RV outflow tract and always end well before semilunar valve closure.

Innocent murmurs are found in approximately 30 to 50 percent of all children. In young children, especially children aged 3 to 8 years, the vibratory systolic (Still's) murmur is common. It has a very distinctive quality described as "groaning," "croaking," "buzzing," or "twanging." It is heard best along the left sternal border at the third or fourth interspace and disappears by puberty. Considerable controversy exists as to the origin of the vibratory systolic murmur. Regardless of the exact cause, most authorities agree that this murmur originates from flow in the LV outflow tract.

Innocent systolic ejection murmurs also have been attributed to flow in the normal RV outflow tract and have been termed *innocent pulmonic systolic murmurs* because the site of their maximal intensity is auscultated best in the pulmonic area at the second left interspace with radiation along the left sternal border. These are low to medium in pitch, with a blowing quality, and are common in children, adolescents, and

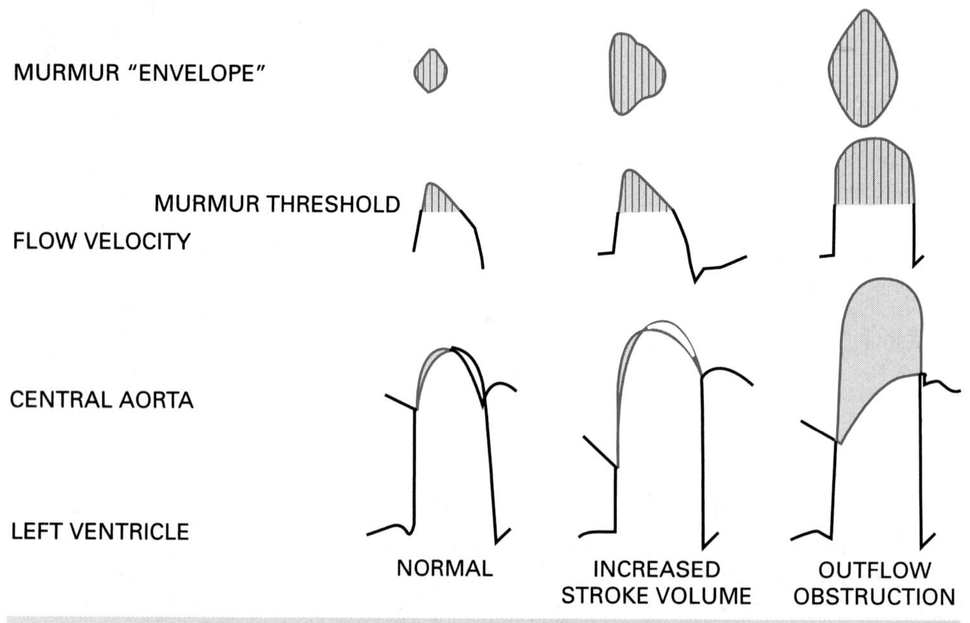


FIGURE 12-74 The simultaneous time-intensity course of the murmur "envelope," aortic flow velocity, and left ventricular (LV) and central aortic pressure. During normal LV ejection (*left*), peak flow velocity is early, with two-thirds of the ventricular volume ejected during the first half of systole. The murmur threshold may be exceeded during the early peak flow and the corresponding murmur envelope inscribed. *Center.* Exaggeration of the normal pattern of LV ejection with a high stroke volume, as in high-output states. With critical aortic stenosis (AS) (*right*), rapid early ejection is no longer possible; the flow velocity is increased, and the contour becomes rounded and prolonged, producing the typical diamond-shaped murmur of AS. (Modified from Reddy PS, Curtis EI, Salerni R, et al. Cardiac systolic murmurs: Pathophysiology and differential diagnosis. *Prog Cardiovasc Dis* 1971;14:4. Reproduced with permission from the publisher and the authors.)

young adults. Stein et al.,[244] who used high-fidelity catheter-tipped micromanometers to record intracardiac sound and pressure in the aorta and pulmonary artery in adults with normal valves, invariably recorded the ejection murmur in the region of the aortic valve. They concluded that these murmurs, despite their pulmonic precordial location, were aortic in origin.

In adults over age 50, innocent murmurs due to flow in the LV outflow tract are often heard and may be of a higher frequency, with a musical quality, and frequently loudest at the apex. They may be associated with a tortuous, dilated sclerotic aortic root, often in the setting of systolic hypertension. Mild sclerosis of the aortic valve also may be present.

The preceding descriptive breakdown of innocent murmurs is based primarily on age, precordial location, and distinctive acoustic qualities. Since both innocent and pathologic ejection murmurs have the same mechanism of production, it is "the company the murmur keeps" that affords the differential diagnosis of the pathologic systolic ejection murmur from the innocent murmur[242] (Fig. 12-75).

For a murmur to be considered innocent, the examination of the cardiovascular system must disclose no abnormalities. BP and contour of the carotid, femoral, and brachial arteries always should be evaluated carefully. There should be no elevation of the JVP, and the contour of the jugular pulse should be normal, without exaggeration of either the *a* or *v* wave. Evidence of cardiac enlargement on physical examination should be absent, and palpation of the apex in the left lateral position should show no evidence of a presystolic impulse, sustained systolic motion, or hyperdynamic circulation. On auscultation, normal physiologic splitting should be present. A physiologic $S_3$ is often present in association with an innocent murmur in children and young adults but should not be heard after age 30. An $S_4$ is rarely heard in normal children and adults (younger than 50 years) and always should be considered to be abnormal when associated with a palpable presystolic impulse. Systolic ejection sounds of valvular origin as well as midsystolic nonejection sounds should be absent because their presence points to minor abnormalities of the semilunar and AV valves, respectively (Fig. 12-75). The remainder of the physical examination should show no evidence of a cardiac cause of pulmonary or systemic congestion.

The supraclavicular arterial murmur or bruit is a common finding in normal individuals, particularly children and adolescents. These murmurs are maximal in intensity above the clavicles and tend to be louder on the right, although they are often heard bilaterally. The bruit begins shortly after $S_1$, is diamond-shaped, and is of brief duration, usually occupying less than half of systole. Although the exact mechanism is unknown, it is related to peak flow velocity near the origin of the normal subclavian, brachiocephalic, or carotid artery. Unlike the cardiac ejection murmur, the supraclavicular murmur is always louder above the clavicles than below them. Complete compression of the subclavian artery may cause the murmur to disappear completely, whereas partial compression occasionally may intensify it. Hyperextension of the shoulders is a simple bedside maneuver that may decrease the intensity of the murmur and cause it to disappear completely. In the adult, the supraclavicular murmur must be distinguished from the murmur of true organic carotid obstruction, this latter murmur being longer, often extending through $S_2$, and frequently associated with a history suggestive of transient ischemic attacks.

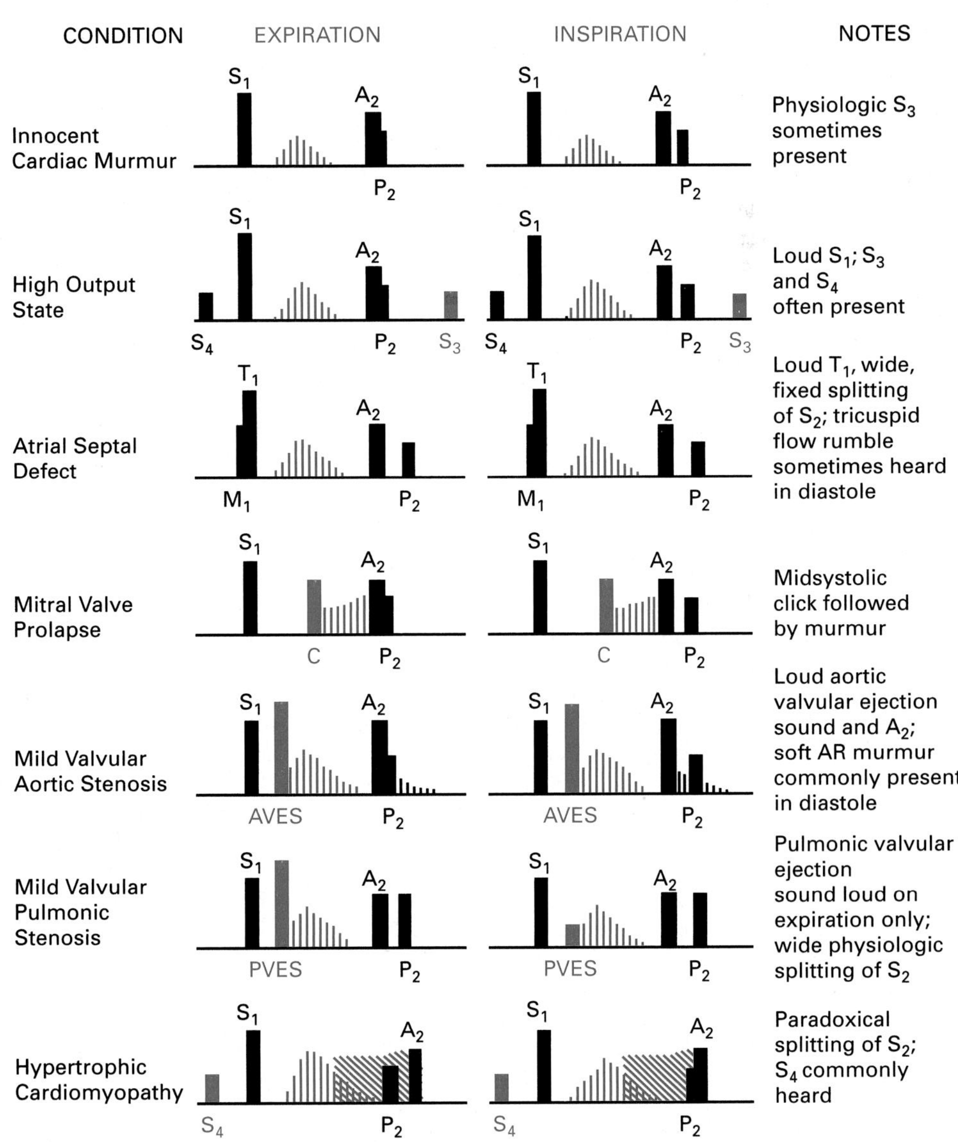


FIGURE 12-75 The differential diagnosis of the innocent murmur versus the pathologic systolic murmur is made by the "company the murmur keeps." The innocent murmur must be found in the setting of an otherwise normal cardiovascular examination. C = midsystolic nonejection sound; AVES = aortic valvular ejection sound; PVES = pulmonic valvular ejection sound; AR = aortic regurgitation. (From Shaver JA, et al. *Examination of the Heart*, Part IV. Auscultation. Dallas: American Heart Association; 1990:40. Reproduced with permission from the publisher and the authors.)

## Functional Systolic Ejection Murmurs

Systolic ejection murmurs produced by high-cardiac-output states are functional and flow-related but are excluded from the category of innocent murmurs because of their associated altered physiologic state. These include the cardiac murmurs of thyrotoxicosis, pregnancy, anemia, fever, exercise, and peripheral arteriovenous fistula, which are best interpreted in light of the total presentation of the patient (Fig. 12-73). Although these murmurs are often grade 3 and occasionally grade 4 in intensity, they always end well before $S_2$ and are only rarely confused with obstruction of the LV or RV outflow tract. The large stroke volume associated with high-degree heart block often produces a functional systolic murmur; when found in the setting of complete heart block, beat-to-beat variations in the intensity of the murmur are present due to the random contribution of atrial systole to LV filling.

The functional systolic murmur in patients with a hemodynamically significant ASD is due to the increased flow in the RV outflow tract secondary to the left-to-right shunt at the atrial level. It is easily diagnosed at the bedside "by the company it keeps." The hallmark of this condition is wide, fixed splitting of $S_2$. When the shunt is large (more than 2.5:1), a hyperdynamic parasternal impulse is usually present, and a diastolic flow rumble is often heard in the tricuspid area. In addition, the tricuspid closure is loud, and prominent *a* and *v* waves are seen in the JVP. An important condition to be differentiated from an ASD is narrowing of the anteroposterior diameter of the bony thorax. Prominent systolic murmurs—often grade 3 or 4—are heard in patients who have the straight-back syndrome and/or pectus excavatum.[243] Audible expiratory splitting is frequently present and, coupled with a prominent pulmonary artery on the chest x-ray [secondary to the narrow anteroposterior (AP) diameter], can lead to additional unnecessary procedures to rule out an ASD. Careful attention at the bedside to the physical examination of the spine, thoracic cage, and sternum should be part of the routine evaluation of any patient with a murmur. Often, confirmation of the thoracic abnormality with a lateral chest film is all that is necessary for definitive evaluation.

Prominent systolic ejection murmurs are the rule in patients with significant AR secondary to the large forward stroke volume. Although no significant LV outflow pressure gradient is found in these patients, the intensity of such murmurs may be grade 4 or 5, and occasionally they are associated with a thrill. They always end well before aortic closure and are clearly separated from the early regurgitant murmur. Such a murmur is rarely confused with significant valvular obstruction because of the peripheral findings of wide-open AR. When true valvular obstruction is present (mixed AS and AR), the longer systolic ejection murmur is often associated with a prominent thrill. Systolic ejection murmurs due to large RV stroke volume are also seen in severe organic pulmonic valvular regurgitation.

Ventricular ejection into a dilated great vessel is commonly associated with a systolic ejection murmur. In the elderly, such murmurs are due to ejection into a dilated, sclerotic aorta and often are best heard at the apex. Frequently, degenerative changes of the aortic valve are also present, and the clinician is faced with a difficult decision as to whether or not true obstruction exists. The presence of significant calcification on fluoroscopic examination favors true obstruction and can be confirmed when a significant gradient is demonstrated by Doppler studies. A systolic ejection murmur due to RV ejection into a massively dilated pulmonary artery is frequently present in idiopathic dilatation of the pulmonary artery (Fig. 12-68), which is often confused with an ASD due to the wide auditory expiratory splitting present in this condition. Short systolic ejection murmurs, frequently associated with a prominent late pulmonary ejection sound, are also seen in dilated pulmonic arteries secondary to severe pulmonary hypertension (PH) of any cause. Physical findings of severe PH are always present, including a prominent parasternal impulse and increased intensity of the pulmonic component of $S_2$, which is well heard at the apex. Prominent *a* waves in the neck and a right-sided $S_4$ that increases with inspiration are present if the ventricular septum is intact. If the PH is associated with intracardiac shunting, cyanosis frequently is present. A high-pitched, early diastolic murmur of pulmonic regurgitation secondary to severe PH often is present.

## Left Ventricular Outflow Tract Murmurs

Obstruction to LV outflow may be congenital or acquired and may be located at the valvular, supravalvular, or subvalvular level. Stenosis is occasionally present at more than one level. In the clinical evaluation, one should attempt to define the severity and the level of obstruction. A summary of this differential diagnosis can be found in Table 12-12 (Chap. 66).

The murmur of fixed stenosis of the LV outflow tract, regardless of the site, is crescendo-decrescendo, and its contour closely parallels the instantaneous pressure gradient. As long as cardiac output is maintained, there is an excellent correlation between the intensity and length of the murmur with severity of obstruction. Although there is a tendency toward late peaking of the murmur with increasing severity of the obstruction, this delayed peaking has not been found to correlate as well with the severity of valvular obstruction in AS as it has in PS.[244] The murmur of significant fixed LV outflow tract obstruction usually is best heard in the second right and second and third left interspaces near the sternum. It radiates widely into the neck and along the great vessels. With radiation to the apex, particularly in the elderly patient, the high-frequency components of the murmur predominate, and the apical murmur has a high pitch and often a musical quality. This characteristic change in the pitch between the proximal and distal radiation of the murmur is often a source of confusion on auscultation. There is an urge to call it a separate murmur of MR; however, observations repeatedly demonstrate that this murmur, regardless of its harmonics, retains a spindle-shaped configuration whenever it is heard or recorded. The murmur of AS varies directly with the length of the preceding diastole; the longer the preceding ventricular filling period, the louder is the systolic murmur (Fig. 12-76). In contrast, the apical murmur of MR is associated with little or no variation in intensity with varying cycle lengths. This observation is useful in patients with atrial fibrillation or frequent premature contractions for identifying whether an apical murmur is due to radiation of an AS murmur or is an additional murmur of MR. Beat-to-beat variations in the intensity of the murmur of AS have been noted in both pulsus alternans and AV dissociation.

A loud early systolic valvular ejection sound or click is the hallmark of congenital valvular AS, and its presence defines the obstruction at the valvular level (Fig. 12-61). Its intensity correlates well with the mobility of the valve, and there is little correlation with the severity of the obstruction. It disappears when the valve becomes immobile due to calcific fixation and is absent in fixed subaortic stenosis. With progressive increase in the severity of the outflow obstruction, the duration of LV ejection is prolonged, resulting in narrow, single, or reversed splitting of $S_2$. Reversed splitting of $S_2$ in AS in the absence of LBBB is always associated with severe obstruction (Chap. 66).

Regardless of the site of obstruction, significant AS always results in LV hypertrophy, with a decreased diastolic compliance. Clinically, this is manifest as a presystolic apical pulsation on palpation and as an $S_4$ on auscultation (Fig. 12-71). The relationship between the severity of obstruction and the presence of $S_4$ gallops is indirect, reflecting hypertrophy and decreased compliance of the LV rather than obstruction per se.

Because of the frequent coexistence of hypertensive or arteriosclerotic heart disease in elderly patients with calcific AS, the presence of an $S_4$ is nonspecific and correlates poorly with the severity of obstruction. $S_3$ gallops also may be heard in LV outflow tract obstruction, particularly when decompensation occurs (Fig. 12-71).

The diagnosis of hemodynamically significant AS in the elderly presents a particularly difficult problem.[247,248] The murmur is often of low intensity due to the decreased cardiac output and poor LV function. An ejection sound or click is rarely present, due to calcific fixation of the valve leaflets, and $S_2$ is of low amplitude. The murmur is often loudest at the apex, has a high-frequency content, and may be difficult to define as ejection in nature because $S_1$ and $A_2$ may be poorly heard.[244] In most patients with severe AS, no $A_2$ is heard, and the systolic murmur obliterates $P_2$. In the elderly, the rate of rise of the carotid pulse may be nearly normal due to the hard, sclerotic vessels even with severe obstruction. As shown in Fig. 12-76, the response of the murmur following a premature ventricular contraction (PVC) may be very helpful in confirming the ejection nature of the murmur. Differentiation from the benign murmur of mild aortic sclerosis may be difficult and often necessitates confirmation of obstruction and its quantitation by echo-Doppler examination[245] (Chaps. 15 and 66).

## Right Ventricular Outflow Tract Obstruction

Obstructions to RV outflow are congenital anomalies and may be at the level of the valve, infundibulum, and proximal or distal branches of the pulmonary artery. Isolated infundibular PS with an intact septum is rare and is usually associated with a large VSD (tetralogy of Fallot). When the ventricular septum is intact, there is an excellent correlation between both the intensity and duration of the murmur and the severity of obstruction.[246] Figure 12-77 contrasts the auscultatory findings of progressively more severe valvular PS with an intact ventricular septum with those in tetralogy of Fallot with progressively more severe RV outflow obstruction.[246] As with valvular AS, an early systolic ejection sound defines the level of obstruction at the valve. In mild to moderate valvular obstruction, the intensity of this sound is markedly attenuated or may disappear with inspiration. In more severe valvular obstruction, this sound may fuse with $S_1$ or actually may present as a presystolic click when the pressure generated by a forceful right atrial contraction exceeds RV end-diastolic pressure, causing doming of the stenotic valve in late diastole. Although obstruction to RV outflow in tetralogy of Fallot is usually at

TABLE 12-12 Differential Diagnosis of Left Ventricular Outflow Obstruction

| | Congenital Aortic Stenosis | | | | |
|---|---|---|---|---|---|
| Parameter | Valvular | Subvalvular | Supravalvular | Acquired Aortic Stenosis | Hypertrophic Obstructive Cardiomyopathy |
| Physical appearance | Normal | Normal | Characteristic facies | Normal | Normal |
| Arterial pulse | Slow rise, sustained peak | Slow rise, sustained peak | Right brachial and carotid > left | Slow rise, sustained peak | Brisk rise, unsustained double peak |
| $S_4$ presystolic impulse | Yes | Yes | Yes | Yes | Yes |
| Left ventricular systolic impulse | Sustained, single | Sustained, single | Sustained, single | Sustained, single | Sustained, may be double |
| Aortic ejection sound | Typical ↓ with calcif.[a] | Rare | Rare | Common ↓ with calcif.[a] | Rare exception |
| Midsystolic ejection murmur; maximal site | First or second right interspace | First or second right interspace | First right interspace and over right carotid | First or second right interspace; apex in elderly | Apex, lower left sternal edge |
| Second sound splitting | Usually normal or single | Usually normal or single | Usually normal or single | Usually single or reversed | Usually reversed or single |
| Intensity of aortic closure | Normal or increased or ↓ with calcif.[a] | Normal or decreased | Normal or decreased | Decreased or absent with calcif[a] | Normal |
| Murmur of aortic regurgitation | Common | Common | Uncommon | Common | Rare exception |

[a]Calcif. = calcification.

Source: Modified from Reddy PS et al. Cardiac systolic murmurs: Pathophysiology and differential diagnosis. *Prog Cardiovasc Dis* 1971;14:6 Reproduced with permission from the publisher and authors.

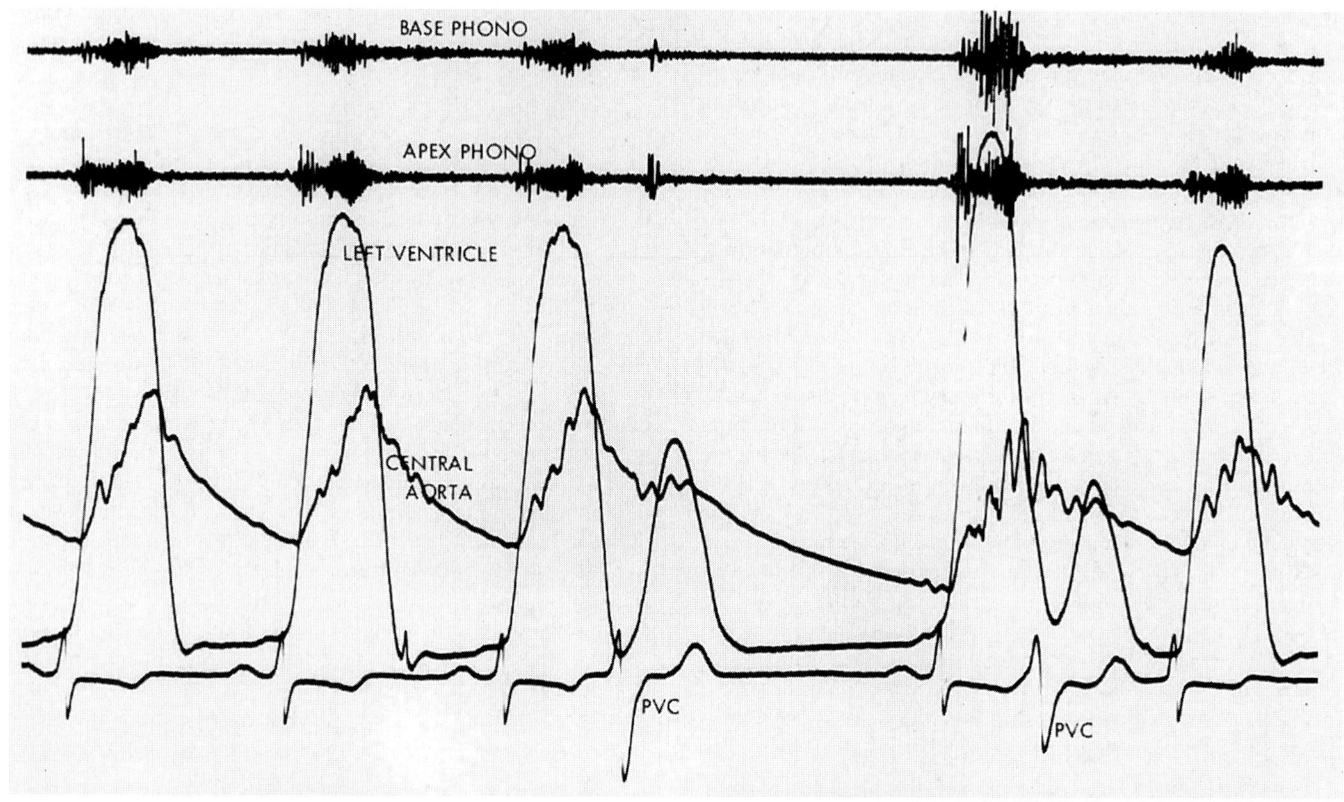


FIGURE 12-76 Effect of the long diastolic filling period following a premature ventricular contraction (PVC) on the intensity of a systolic ejection murmur. There is a marked increase in the intensity of the aortic stenosis: murmur recorded at the base and at the apex. Despite the higher-frequency content of the apical murmur, this response clearly identifies this murmur as ejection in nature. (From Paley H. Left ventricular outflow tract obstruction: Heart sounds and murmurs. In: Leon DF, Shaver JA, eds. *Physiologic Principles of Heart Sounds and Murmurs*. Monograph 46. Dallas: American Heart Association; 1975:112. Reproduced with permission from the publisher and the author.)

the infundibular level, valvular stenosis also may be present. In this setting, a pulmonary valvular ejection sound introduces a systolic murmur, and little variation in the intensity of the ejection sound is found with respiration.

The classic late peaking of the systolic ejection murmur of severe PS with an intact ventricular septum is demonstrated in Fig. 12-78. Note that the late vibrations of the murmur completely envelop $A_2$, whereas $P_2$ is markedly delayed and decreases in intensity secondary to the low pulmonary artery closing pressure. In moderate to severe valvular PS, an excellent correlation has been found between the $A_2$-$P_2$ interval and the RV peak pressure. When the ventricular septum is intact in severe RV outflow obstruction, prominent *a* waves are present in the JVP in association with a right-sided $S_4$ that may increase with inspiration. Neither of these is present in uncomplicated tetralogy of Fallot.

In isolated infundibular obstruction, a pulmonic ejection sound is usually not encountered, and the pulmonic closure ($P_2$) is usually not audible except in the mildest cases.

In branch stenosis of the pulmonary artery, there is a systolic murmur of varying intensity at the upper left sternal border that is widely transmitted to the right side of the chest, back, and both axillae. The murmur is usually less harsh and of higher pitch than the murmur of valvular PS. With more peripheral branch stenosis, systolic ejection murmurs or even continuous murmurs may be heard over the lung fields. The wide radiation of this murmur is particularly helpful in alerting the clinician to this type of right-sided obstruction.

## Systolic Regurgitant Murmurs

Systolic regurgitant murmurs are produced by retrograde flow from a chamber of high pressure to a chamber of lower pressure. The classic examples of such murmurs are the holosystolic (pansystolic) murmur of MR, TR, and VSD. Since there is usually a high-pressure differential between the two chambers throughout systole, the murmurs are holosystolic in duration, high-pitched and blowing in quality, and plateau-like in configuration.

### HOLOSYSTOLIC REGURGITANT MURMURS

The murmur of chronic MR is the prototype of the holosystolic regurgitant murmur, as shown in Fig. 12-73. It begins with or replaces $S_1$ and continues throughout systole in a plateau-like fashion beyond $A_2$, finally terminating when the LV pressure drops to the level of the left atrial pressure during isovolumic relaxation.[245] In contrast to the systolic ejection murmur, there is little variation in its intensity with varying cycle lengths.[249] It is heard best at the apex and radiates well into the axilla; only the loudest murmurs are associated with a thrill at the apex. There is little variation in its intensity with respiration, and it is frequently accompanied by a loud diastolic filling sound followed by a short rumble. In this situation, the loud $S_3$ is not a manifestation of congestive failure but a reflection of hemodynamically significant MR. Likewise, the short rumble does not mean concomitant obstruction at the mitral valve but rather is secondary to extremely rapid early diastolic filling. The intensity of the murmur is directly related to the pressure gradient between the LV and the left atrium.

The diagnosis of hemodynamically significant MR is established by the presence of the holosystolic regurgitant murmur and loud $S_3$ associated with a short flow rumble. The etiology, however, is determined by the clinical presentation and associated physical findings and is best confirmed by echocardiography (Chap. 15).

The classic holosystolic (pansystolic) murmur of TR in the setting of RV pressure overload is best heard at the lower left sternal border. At times it may be heard laterally to the midclavicular line, indicating that the RV occupies the region of the cardiac apex. Furthermore, it generally can be differentiated from MR because its intensity is usually strongly influenced by respiration.[250] During continuous and accentuated respiration, the murmur increases in intensity with inspiration due to the increased venous return and RV filling associated with inspiration. The inspiratory increase in loudness of right-sided auscultatory events is known as *Carvallo's sign*. Careful inspection of the JVP while auscultating the murmur will be of further help in defining its tricuspid origin, showing a prominent *v* wave with a rapid *y* descent that augments during inspiration. In severe RV failure, this respiratory variation may be absent, but it may reappear as the state of compensation improves. With severe TR, a short flow rumble introduced by an $S_3$ can be present, just as with MR, and both will increase with inspiration.[251]

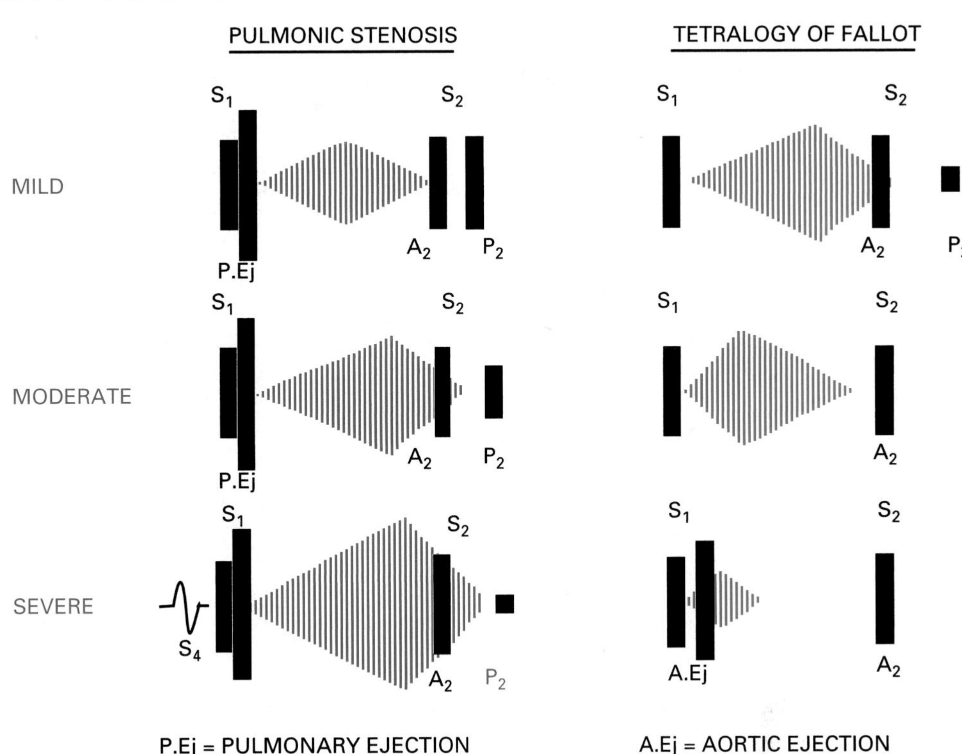


FIGURE 12-77 In valvular pulmonic stenosis (PS) with intact ventricular septum, right ventricular (RV) systolic ejection becomes progressively longer with increasing obstruction to flow. As a result, the murmur becomes louder and longer, enveloping the aortic closure sound. At the same time, pulmonic closure occurs later; splitting becomes wider but is more difficult to appreciate because the aortic closure sound is lost in the murmur; and the pulmonic closure sound becomes progressively softer due to the low pulmonary artery pressure. With increasing severity of PS, the pulmonary ejection sound may fuse with $S_1$. In severe obstruction with concentric hypertrophy and decreased RV compliance, an $S_4$ appears. In tetralogy of Fallot, with increasing obstruction at the infundibular area, more and more RV blood is shunted across a silent ventricular septal defect with less flow across the obstructed RV outflow tract. With increasing obstruction, the murmur becomes shorter, earlier, and fainter. The pulmonic closure sound is absent in severe tetralogy of Fallot. The dilated aorta receives almost all the cardiac output from both ventricular chambers, and there is an aortic ejection sound (Aej). (From Leonard J. *Examination of the Heart*, Part 4: Auscultation. Dallas: American Heart Association; 1974:45. Reproduced with permission from the publisher and authors.)

The holosystolic murmur of VSD is heard best just off the sternal border in the fourth, fifth, and sixth intercostal spaces and is usually accompanied by a forceful thrill.[252] The murmur does not radiate to the axilla as with MR and does not have the respiratory variation characteristic of TR. Wide physiologic splitting with an easily heard $P_2$ is usually present when the left-to-right shunt is hemodynamically significant. When the shunt is large, there is an LV $S_4$ followed by a short flow rumble. The regurgitant murmur is due to high-velocity flow from the high-pressure LV to the lower-pressure RV, and its intensity correlates poorly with the degree of left-to-right shunting. For example, a grade 5 murmur may be associated with a very high velocity flow through a small hemodynamically insignificant muscular VSD. On the other hand, an equally loud murmur associated with a thrill may be present with a larger defect having massive left-to-right shunting. When the defect is very large and the RV and LV pressures are equal, however, no murmur may be produced across the defect; instead, the short pulmonary ejection murmur of severe PH is present (Eisenmenger's VSD).

## EARLY SYSTOLIC REGURGITANT MURMURS

Rarely, a regurgitant murmur confined to early systole is seen in the presence of a small VSD. This murmur begins in the usual manner at the onset of ventricular systole and stops suddenly in early or middle systole.[253] The sudden cessation of the murmur is due to the fact that as ejection continues and ventricular size decreases, the small defect is sealed shut as the ventricular septum thickens during systole and the flow ceases. This murmur is important because it is characteristic of the type of VSD that may disappear with age.

In contrast to the holosystolic murmur of chronic MR, acute severe MR may present as an early systolic spindle-shaped murmur.[254] Common conditions producing acute MR include spontaneous rupture of the chordae tendineae of a myxomatous valve, acute or subacute bacterial endocarditis of the mitral valve, papillary muscle rupture or dysfunction secondary to acute MI, and disruption of the mitral apparatus due to chest trauma.[255] In each of these conditions, large-volume flow regurgitates into a relatively normal left atrium that has not had the time to make the adaptive changes in compliance seen in chronic long-standing MR. As a result, an extremely high *v* wave is generated in the left atrium.

This high *v* wave abolishes the LV–left atrial gradient during the latter part of systole, resulting in termination of retrograde flow and abbreviation of the systolic murmur. As shown in a patient with acute MR secondary to spontaneous rupture of the chordae tendineae of a myxomatous valve, the murmur ends before $A_2$. Audible expiratory splitting with an accentuated $P_2$ is present at the base, and a loud $S_4$

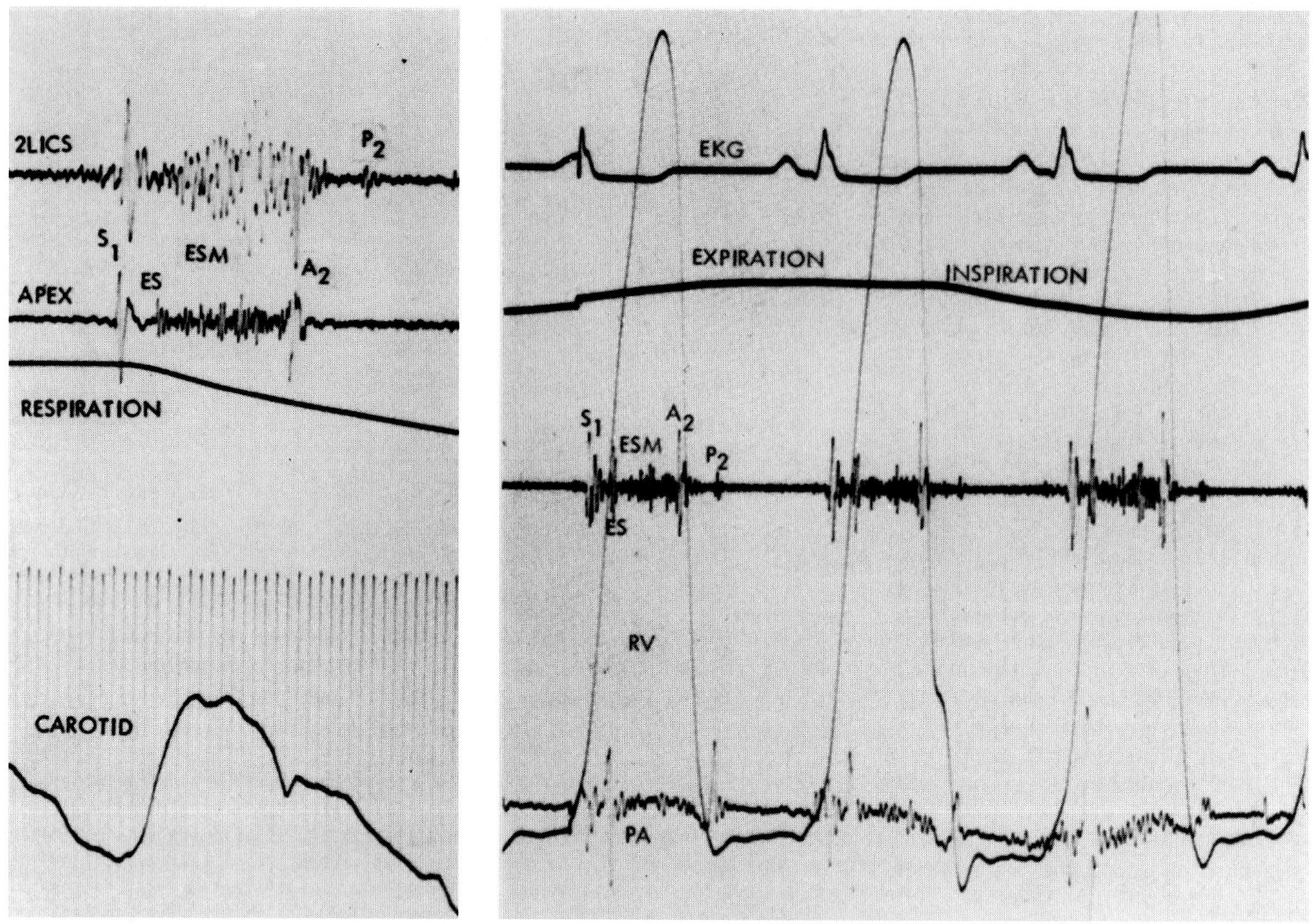


FIGURE 12-78 *Left.* The phonocardiogram of a patient with severe valvular pulmonic stenosis (PS) as recorded at the second left intercostal space (2LICS) and the apex. The long ejection murmur (ESM) has late systolic peaking and spills through $A_2$. There is a marked delay in $P_2$, which is very small in amplitude. *Right.* At cardiac catheterization, the markedly delayed $P_2$ is shown to be secondary to a very large systolic pressure gradient, and its decreased intensity is due to the low pulmonary artery pressure at the time of valve closure. The late peaking of the ejection murmur correlates with the maximal pressure gradient between the RV and the pulmonary artery. (From Curtiss EI. First and second heart sound. In: Horwitz LD, ed. *Signs and Symptoms in Cardiology.* Philadelphia: Lippincott; 1985:200. Reproduced with permission from the publisher and authors.)

is recorded at the apex. The presence of the $S_4$ associated with a prominent presystolic impulse on palpation is an important clue that indicates the acute nature of the MR and is rarely present in MR of a chronic nature. The systolic murmur of acute MR, which can mimic ejection murmurs, may have classic radiation to the axilla and back, especially if it is due to prolapse of the anterior leaflet of the mitral valve with flow directed over the posterior leaflet. When the murmur is loud, it may be conducted to the top of the head and to the sacrum along the spinal column. Occasionally, the murmur is conducted to the base of the heart and great vessels, simulating AS. The quick-rising carotid pulse with rapid falloff, as well as the wide physiologic splitting of the $S_2$, helps differentiation from AS.[256]

The systolic murmur of organic TR is often unimpressive and presents as an early systolic murmur ending well before $A_2$, even in the presence of severe regurgitation.[257] In this condition, the RV pressure is nearly normal, and massive regurgitation may be present with only a small pressure differential between the RV and the right atrium. The small pressure head results in a low-velocity flow, minimal turbulence, and a soft, abbreviated murmur. Occasionally, only minimal early systolic vibrations are heard. In most patients, large *v* waves are readily apparent in the JVP. The murmur retains the characteristic inspiratory augmentation seen in right-sided regurgitant murmurs and is frequently associated with an $S_4$ that increases in intensity with inspiration. A right-sided $S_4$ and a prominent diastolic tricuspid flow rumble are the rule when the TR is acute, as with endocarditis of the tricuspid valve. After total excision of the tricuspid valve for infective endocarditis related to intravenous drug abuse, the systolic murmur is often very unimpressive or may be completely absent. Giant *v* waves in the neck are easily visible, however, and palpable venous thrills and a murmur at the base of the neck may be present secondary to rapid retrograde flow in the jugular system.[258] Other causes of organic TR include carcinoid heart disease, RV infarction, chest trauma, and damage of the tricuspid valve during open heart surgery.

### MID- AND LATE-SYSTOLIC REGURGITANT MURMURS

Midsystolic murmurs can occur with MR due to papillary muscle dysfunction.[259] The timing of the murmur of papillary muscle dysfunction also may be late systolic, and the murmur may be either intermittent or constant. It occurs with ischemia or infarction of either the posteromedial or anterolateral papillary muscle. Often these murmurs are transient, being provoked by episodes of ischemia.

Varying degrees of MVP are the most frequent cause of a late-systolic murmur, and this entity is one of the most common causes of systolic murmurs seen in clinical practice[260] (Chap. 68). The murmur is best heard at the apex and often has a tendency to a late systolic crescendo. It is frequently introduced or accompanied by nonejection clicks. These clicks may be single or multiple, and they can occur independently without an accompanying systolic murmur. As shown in Fig. 12-62, the click occurs near the time of maximal prolapse in midsystole, and the late-systolic murmur continues up to and through $A_2$ due to prolapse of the posterior leaflet during the remainder of systole.

The timing and intensity of these murmurs vary with physiologic and pharmacologic maneuvers that alter the end-diastolic volume of the heart (Fig. 12-63). These murmurs are also sensitive to conditions that alter the peripheral vascular impedance as well as the inotropic state of the heart. These variations in the timing and duration of the murmur can be understood most easily by considering MVP as a condition in which the valve is too big for the ventricle (Chap. 68). This valvuloventricular disproportion manifests itself at a given geometric size and configuration during LV contraction. These dynamic changes can best be appreciated at the bedside by examining the patient in the supine, left lateral, sitting, and standing positions as well as during prompt squatting. Late-systolic murmurs also may originate from prolapse of the tricuspid valve (Chap. 69).

Levine and Harvey[176] described a musical, apical systolic murmur that they called a "whoop" because it simulated the "whoop" of whooping cough. These murmurs are loud, high-pitched, musical, sonorous, and vibratory; are best heard at the apex in late systole; and are frequently intermittent. They are often preceded by clicks and originate in the mitral valve. They are associated with ballooning of the mitral valve or MR (or both), and their unusual quality is secondary to the high-frequency vibrations of the mitral apparatus. The systolic "whoop" or "honk," together with late systolic murmurs, with or without associated clicks, is part of a continuum representing abnormalities of the mitral valve apparatus of varying etiologies. Similar honking noises, with or without clicks, may arise from the tricuspid valve and also have been produced by transvenous pacemaker catheters situated across the valve. These murmurs are best auscultated at the fourth left intercostal space and have the typical inspiratory augmentation of tricuspid murmurs (Chap. 69).

## MURMUR OF HYPERTROPHIC "OBSTRUCTIVE" CARDIOMYOPATHY

The classic cardiac findings of hypertrophic cardiomyopathy (HCM) with an LV outflow gradient are demonstrated in Fig. 12-79; the echocardiogram gives insight into the mechanism of production of the systolic murmur (Chap. 77). Systolic anterior motion (SAM) of the mitral apparatus impinges on the massively thickened septum, producing high-velocity flow in middle and late systole, resulting in a midsystolic ejection murmur usually with its maximal intensity at the left sternal edge.[261] Varying degrees of MR also may be present during systole due to the distorted mitral apparatus. Frequently, on auscultation, there is difficulty deciding whether the systolic murmur found in HCM is ejection or regurgitant in nature.[262] Usually, the murmur recorded by the precordial phonocardiogram is actually the summation of the murmurs of LV outflow obstruction and MR as transmitted to the chest wall.[263]

In patients with dynamic LV outflow gradients, the intensity of both the systolic ejection murmur and the MR murmur varies directly with the magnitude of the pressure gradient. Thus physiologic maneuvers and pharmacologic interventions that increase the pressure gradient will increase the intensity of the precordial murmur, and vice versa. Decreases in LV preload and afterload or increases in LV contractility are associated with increases in the pressure gradient and the intensity of the murmur, whereas increases in LV preload and afterload or decreases in LV contractility will decrease the pressure gradient and the intensity of the murmur.[264,265] For example, the upright posture and the strain phase of the Valsalva maneuver decrease venous return and LV preload, and the murmur increases in intensity. On reclining or with prompt squatting, augmented venous return increases LV preload, and the murmur decreases in intensity.

In the absence of an LV outflow gradient at rest or with provocation, the murmur of HCM is less impressive. Although a short ejection murmur is usually recorded due to rapid early LV ejection, it is often softer and extends through less of systole than when a gradient is present. There is also little variation in the intensity with changes in preload, afterload, or contractility.

In HCM with and without a gradient across the LV outflow tract, massive LV hypertrophy is present, and a prominent presystolic impulse associated with an LV $S_4$ is the rule when normal sinus rhythm is present. An $S_3$ is also a common finding in patients with HCM, and

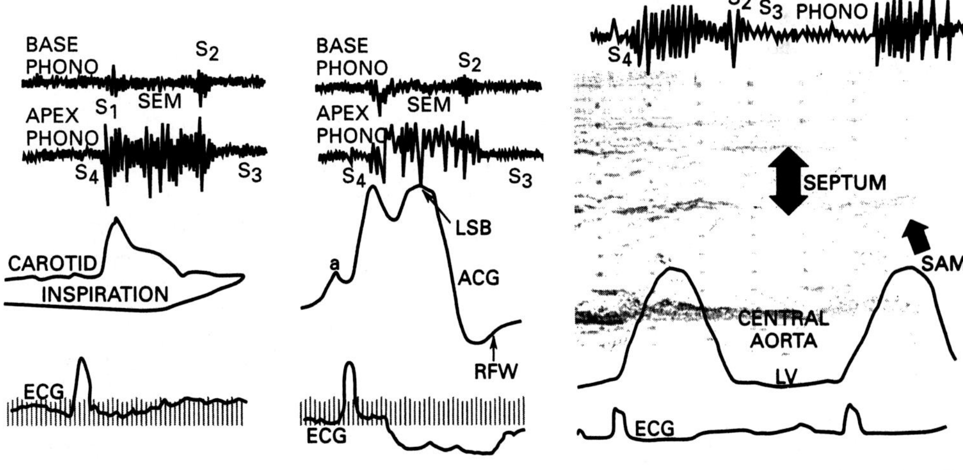


FIGURE 12-79 Simultaneous base and apex phonocardiograms are recorded with the carotid pulse and apexcardiogram in the left and center panels, respectively, in a 54-year-old man with hypertrophic cardiomyopathy. The carotid pulse rises rapidly and has a late systolic plateau and a prolonged ejection period. Prominent $S_4$ and $S_1$ are demonstrated and are associated with the *a* wave and the rapid filling wave (RFW), respectively, of the ACG. Note the late systolic bulge (LSB) on the ACG. $S_2$ is single. A loud grade 5 systolic ejection murmur is present and is of greatest intensity at the apex. In the right panel, the apical systolic murmur is recorded together with the M-mode echocardiogram. Simultaneous high-fidelity LV and central aortic pressures are recorded by catheter-tipped micromanometers. Marked thickening of the interventricular septum and systolic anterior motion of the mitral valve are present on the echocardiogram. A large systolic pressure gradient is demonstrated beginning shortly after the onset of the SAM. (From Shaver JA, et al. Phonoechocardiography and intracardiac phonocardiography in hypertrophic cardiomyopathy. *Postgrad Med J.* 1986;62:538. Reproduced with permission from the publisher and the authors.)

occasionally there is an early diastolic rumble that may mimic the diastolic murmur of MS. Such rumbles are felt to be due to the increased impedance to LV filling secondary to the decreased diastolic compliance of the LV.

## Diastolic Murmurs

Diastolic murmurs have two basic mechanisms of production. Diastolic filling murmurs or rumbles are due to forward flow across an AV valve, whereas diastolic regurgitant murmurs are due to retrograde flow across an incompetent semilunar valve[266] (Fig. 12-80).

### DIASTOLIC FILLING MURMURS (RUMBLES)

Diastolic rumbles are caused by forward flow across the AV valves and are delayed from their respective semilunar closure sound by the isovolumic relaxation period. Only following this period, when the atrial pressure exceeds the declining ventricular pressure, do the AV valves open and filling begins. Since there are two phases of rapid ventricular filling—early diastole and presystole—these murmurs have a tendency to be most prominent during these two filling periods. Because the velocity of flow is relatively low, these murmurs have a low-frequency content and are rumbling in character.

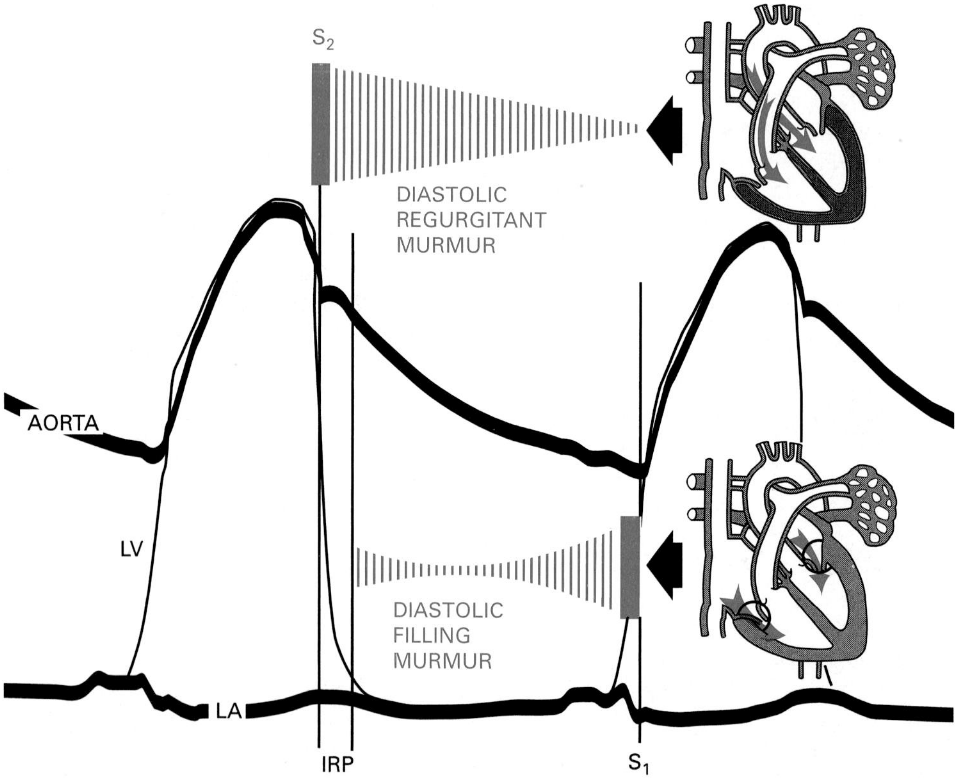

***Diastolic Rumbles Due to Obstruction of the AV*** The murmur of mitral stenosis (MS) is heard best at the apex in the left lateral position, and its duration correlates well with the duration of the mitral diastolic gradient. Its intensity is related to the severity of the obstruction and to the flow across the valve.[267] As a result, there is poor correlation between the intensity of the murmur and the severity of the obstruction; i.e. high flow across a mild obstruction may produce a loud rumble, whereas low flow across a severely stenotic valve may produce a very soft murmur or may be silent. When the stenotic mitral valve is mobile, the murmur is introduced by a prominent opening snap (Fig. 12-59, *left*). The duration of the interval between $A_2$ and the opening snap (OS) correlates well with the level of left atrial pressure; the shorter the $A_2$–OS interval, the higher is the left atrial pressure, and vice versa. The $S_1$ is also loud when the stenotic valve is mobile and is usually preceded by a crescendo murmur. Although originally attributed to increased flow secondary to left atrial systole, phonoechocardiographic studies have suggested that this short "presystolic" murmur is actually due to high-velocity antegrade flow through a progressively narrowing mitral orifice during very early (isovolumic) ventricular systole (Fig. 12-59, *left*). This mechanism also may be responsible for the brief crescendo presystolic murmur observed in patients with MS in atrial fibrillation following a short cycle length.

Although the intensity of the diastolic rumble in MS correlates poorly with the severity of obstruction, there is an excellent correlation of severity with the duration of the murmur. When sinus tachycardia or rapid atrial fibrillation is present, a rumble starting with an OS and continuing to $S_1$ may not be meaningful because of the short diastolic time. Carotid sinus pressure may be very helpful in temporarily slowing the heart rate, thereby allowing the clinician to uncover the potential length of the rumble.

Obstruction of the mitral orifice also can be produced by a left atrial tumor. The diastolic murmur may be very similar to that produced by MS (Fig. 12-59, *center*). A loud tumor "plop" is present instead of the OS, and the presystolic crescendo murmur occurs as the protruding tumor mass returns rapidly through the mitral orifice into the left atrium during early ventricular systole. A systolic murmur of MR also may be present, and both murmurs may vary from examination to examination and with changes in body position.

The murmur of tricuspid stenosis (TS) is usually heard in the xiphoid area just off the sternal border. Since right atrial systole occurs earlier than left, the diastolic murmur of TS may have a crescendo-decrescendo configuration. Even when the PR interval is normal, the presystolic accentuation of the diastolic rumble may terminate before $S_1$. Since TS almost al-

FIGURE 12-80 Diastolic filling murmurs or rumbles are caused by forward flow across the AV valves, whereas diastolic regurgitant murmurs are caused by retrograde flow across incompetent semilunar valves. *Left.* Diagrammatic representation of the diastolic filling murmur and the diastolic regurgitant murmur as related to left ventricular (LV), aortic, and left atrial (LA) pressures. The diastolic filling murmur occurs during the diastolic filling period and is separated from $S_2$ by the isovolumic relaxation period. The rumbling murmur is most prominent during rapid early ventricular filling and presystole, terminating with $S_1$. The diastolic regurgitant murmur begins immediately after $S_2$ and continues in a decrescendo fashion up to $S_1$, closely paralleling the aortic LV diastolic pressure gradient. *Right.* Flow diagram. (From Shaver JA. Diastolic murmurs. *Heart Dis Stroke* 1993;1:98–103. Reproduced with permission from the American Heart Association.)

ways occurs in the presence of MS, this diastolic diamond-shaped murmur, which augments during inspiration, and the presence of large *a* waves in the JVP are clues to this additional diagnosis. When atrial fibrillation is present, the murmur is in middiastole and has the typical inspiratory augmentation. A tricuspid OS, which usually follows the mitral OS, also may be present and may initiate the murmur.

***Diastolic Rumbles Due to High Flow Across the Atrioventricular Valves*** High-velocity flow across the normal or regurgitant AV valve may result in short middiastolic rumbles often accompanied by an $S_3$ and should not be confused with murmurs produced by true obstruction of the AV valves. Such rumbles are common in both VSD and patent ductus arteriosus due to the large flow across the MV secondary to the left-to-right shunt.[268] Likewise, the left-to-right shunt in a large ASD often produces a tricuspid rumble. Similar low-pitched rumbling murmurs also may be present in hyperkinetic states and occasionally are heard in patients with complete heart block and increased diastolic blood flow in each cardiac cycle. Common to all these conditions is high-volume flow during the latter phase of the rapid filling period. Phonoechocardiography indicates that these murmurs occur during the rapid closing motion of the mitral valve, suggesting a functional "obstruction" during the period of rapid early diastolic filling.[269] Identical phonoechocardiographic correlates also have been shown with MR and TR, where early diastolic filling is also extremely rapid. With TR, the early rumble will increase with inspiration, typical of right-sided murmurs. During rapid atrial fibrillation, ventriculogenic closure of the normal mitral valve during the rapid filling phase of a short cardiac cycle may cause a "presystolic" murmur by a similar mechanism.

Mitral valvulitis during an episode of acute rheumatic fever may cause a short diastolic rumble, the *Carey Coombs murmur*.[270] This rumble, especially in children or in the presence of fever and anemia, may be introduced by an $S_3$ rather than by an OS. This combination of an $S_3$ with a short rumble indicates that there is not enough obstruction to the valve to alter the characteristics of rapid early ventricular filling.

The Austin Flint murmur, as originally described in 1862,[271–275] consisted of an apical presystolic murmur observed in two patients with considerable AR and no evidence of MS at autopsy. Since its original description, the timing of this murmur has been extended to include a middiastolic component. It is heard best at the apex and has many of the qualities of the murmur of MS. It is introduced by an $S_3$ rather than by an OS, however, and $S_1$ is of normal or decreased amplitude. Maneuvers that increase the degree of AR, such as hand grip or transient arterial occlusions will increase the intensity of the rumble. In most cases of severe AR, particularly when acute, the presystolic component of the Austin Flint murmur is lost. In this situation, there is marked elevation of the LV end-diastolic pressure, and the reverse pressure gradient between the LV and the left atrium causes premature closure of the mitral valve.

Elegant phonoechocardiographic studies have shown that the murmur is associated with the rapid closing motion of the mitral valve leaflets during middiastole and presystole, presumably due to antegrade flow across a closing orifice in a manner similar to the flow rumble of AV valvular regurgitation and high-output states.[272] Austin Flint murmurs have been observed in the absence of rapid closing of the mitral valve, however, and Reddy et al.[276] have suggested that incomplete valve opening rather than excessively rapid closure rates may be the essential requirement for producing the increased mitral flow velocity. One echo-Doppler study has suggested that patients with an Austin Flint murmur usually have an aortic regurgitant jet aimed directly at the mitral valve, causing deformity and shuddering of the valve, in contrast to patients with equally severe regurgitation, in whom the murmur is absent.[274] Right-sided Austin Flint murmurs of similar quality have been reported in association with severe pulmonic regurgitation associated with PH.[275]

## DIASTOLIC REGURGITANT MURMURS

***Holodiastolic Aortic Regurgitant Murmurs*** The early diastolic murmur of AR is blowing and high-pitched and is often more difficult to record than to hear because of its high-frequency content. Since isovolumic relaxation of the LV is very rapid, a large gradient quickly develops between the aortic and LV diastolic pressures, and the murmur builds up to maximum intensity almost immediately after $A_2$. As diastole progresses, the gradient between the two chambers falls slowly, and the murmur envelope closely parallels the pressure drop in a decrescendo fashion up to $S_1$. When the AR is valvular in origin, the murmur is usually best heard at the third and fourth left parasternal areas. If the murmur is heard best to the right of the sternum, it should alert the clinician to an aortic root etiology of the regurgitation.[276] It should be pointed out that this finding is helpful only if present, since many patients with AR secondary to dilatation of the aortic root have the usual radiation with peak intensity to the left of the sternum. The murmur may be faint and overlooked if the examiner does not listen with the patient sitting up and leaning forward and does not listen with the diaphragm of the stethoscope pressed firmly against the chest wall. One should listen while the patient holds his or her breath after deep expiration.

The degree of AR is directly proportional to the pressure head driving the flow in a retrograde fashion. Maneuvers that increase or decrease the diastolic aortic LV pressure gradient will increase or decrease the intensity of the regurgitant murmur. Prompt squatting often will bring out a very faint AR blowing murmur at the bedside, and transient arterial occlusion with two BP cuffs will also markedly increase its intensity. It should be remembered that the murmur of mild AR often disappears during the latter stages of pregnancy due to the low peripheral vascular resistance. Pure AR without associated valvular stenosis may present with a prominent systolic ejection murmur as well as an Austin Flint rumble at the apex. The carotid pulse is rapid-rising and has a large volume. The $A_2$ is often diminished or even absent when the regurgitation is valvular in origin.

The etiology of the AR usually cannot be determined by the quality of the murmur. An exception to this rule is the presence of a "cooing dove" or musical diastolic murmur, which usually denotes a rupture or retroversion of an aortic cusp. Such ruptures occur secondary to trauma, infective endocarditis, and occasionally in the presence of arteriosclerosis of the aortic valve. Retroversion and subsequent rupture of the aortic valve with a musical murmur are also a complication of syphilitic AR (Chap. 66).

***Abbreviated Aortic Diastolic Regurgitant Murmur*** The murmur of very mild AR may be abbreviated and may end by middiastole. This is particularly true of the functional AR murmur of systemic arterial hypertension. As the volume of blood in the aorta decreases during diastole, the aortic annulus becomes smaller, and coupled with the decreasing aortic LV diastolic gradient, retrograde flow ceases, and the murmur disappears.

The murmur of AR also may be abbreviated if the AR is acute. Acute regurgitation of blood into an LV that has not had time to adapt to a large-volume load results in marked elevation of the LV end-diastolic pressure with equilibration of the aortic and LV diastolic pressures. As a result, retrograde flow ceases, and the murmur disap-

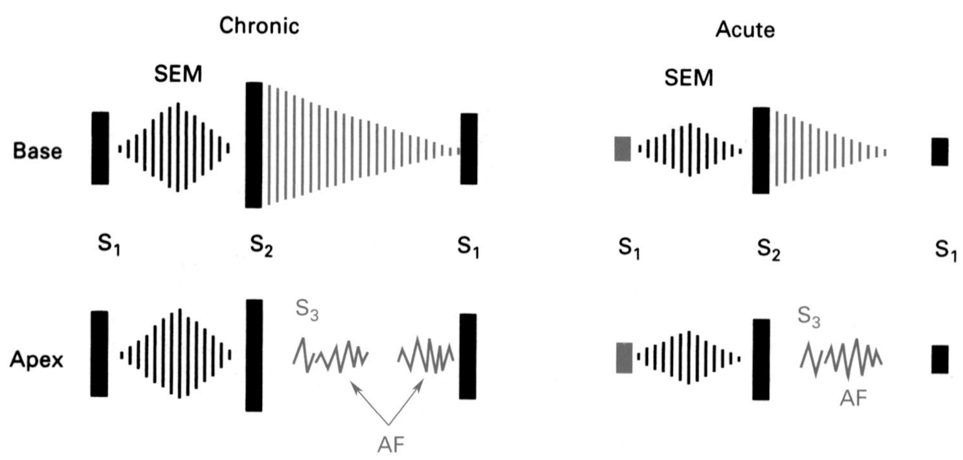


FIGURE 12-81 Diagram contrasting the auscultatory findings in chronic and acute aortic regurgitation (AR). In chronic AR, a prominent systolic ejection murmur (SEM), resulting from the large forward stroke volume, is heard at the base and apex and ends well before $S_2$. The aortic diastolic regurgitant murmur begins with $S_2$ and continues in a decrescendo fashion, terminating before $S_1$. At the apex, the early diastolic component of the Austin Flint (AF) murmur is introduced by a prominent $S_3$. A presystolic component of the AF is also heard. In acute AR, there is a significant decrease in the intensity of the SEM compared with chronic AR because of the decreased forward stroke volume. $S_1$ is markedly decreased in intensity because of preclosure of the mitral valve; at the apex, the presystolic component of the AF murmur is absent. The early diastolic murmur at the base ends well before $S_1$ because of the equilibration of the LV and aortic end-diastolic pressure. Significant tachycardia is usually present. (From Shaver JA. Diastolic murmurs. *Heart Dis Stroke* 1993;1:98–103. Reproduced with permission from the American Heart Association.)

pears in the latter part of diastole. When AR is acute, there may be preclosure of the mitral valve, resulting in a soft or absent $S_1$ as well as absence of the presystolic component of the Austin Flint murmur. The auscultatory findings of acute versus chronic AR are contrasted in Fig. 12-81. Common causes of acute AR include aortic valve endocarditis, trauma, acute aortic dissection, and dehiscence of an aortic valve prosthesis (Chap. 66).

***Holodiastolic Pulmonic Regurgitant Murmur*** Pulmonic regurgitation (PR) is found most commonly in the setting of severe PH and dilatation of the pulmonary artery with inadequate coaptation of the leaflets of the pulmonic valve. The functional murmur of PR (Graham Steell's murmur)[281] is similar in both frequency and contour to that of AR because the hemodynamics responsible for their production are identical. The differential diagnosis is made by the "company the murmur keeps," and when it is associated with the peripheral signs of hemodynamically significant AR or with the findings of severe PH, there is rarely a problem. However, when rheumatic MS is the primary lesion, the semilunar regurgitant murmur may be secondary either to associated rheumatic AR or to the Graham Steell murmur if the PH is severe. Careful investigation of the semilunar blowing murmur in the setting of MS has shown that it is usually due to AR, even when significant PH is present.[278] More common causes of the Graham Steell murmur of functional PR are primary PH and Eisenmenger's syndrome.

Early diastolic murmurs occasionally are heard in end-stage renal failure, particularly when there is concurrent anemia, hypertension, and fluid overload. Doppler echocardiography demonstrated that these murmurs are usually pulmonic in origin.[282] They are often transient in nature and are related to fluid overload. Such murmurs are diminished by extracellular fluid removal and reflect correctable PH.[282]

***Delayed Pulmonic Regurgitant Murmur*** The murmur of organic (nonpulmonary hypertensive) PR is quite different in quality and duration as compared with either AR or the Graham Steell murmur of PH.[281] The murmur is delayed from $P_2$ by a short interval and then builds up quickly to a crescendo followed by a decrescendo that ends well before $S_1$. In organic PR, the pulmonary artery pressure may be normal, and the diastolic gradient between the pulmonary artery and RV may be very small, resulting in low-velocity retrograde flow and a *lower-pitched murmur*. The murmur is heard only during the period of maximal gradient in early and middle diastole. This type of murmur may be congenital or acquired, as with pulmonic valve endocarditis, carcinoid syndrome, or surgical procedures on the pulmonic valve. It is often associated with a prominent systolic ejection murmur secondary to the large RV stroke volume.

## CONTINUOUS MURMURS

A *continuous murmur* is defined as one that begins in systole and extends through $S_2$ into part or all of diastole. It need not occupy the entire cardiac cycle; therefore, a systolic murmur that extends into diastole without stopping at $S_2$ is considered to be continuous even if it fades completely before the subsequent $S_1$. A physiologic classification of continuous murmurs as described by Myers[284] is detailed in Table 12-13.

***Continuous Murmurs Due to Rapid Blood Flow*** High-velocity blood flow through veins and arteries may cause a continuous murmur. The cervical venous hum is a continuous murmur with diastolic accentuation and is easily heard in most children. It is best heard with the patient sitting and the neck rotated laterally. This murmur also can be heard in healthy adults and is present in nearly all women in the later stages of pregnancy. High cardiac output states such as thyrotoxicosis and anemia are also associated with easily heard cervical venous hums. Peak intensity is in the supraclavicular fossa just lateral to the sternocleidomastoid muscle, and it is usually more prominent on the right side. When the murmur is loud, it may radiate below the clavicles and occasionally can be confused with the continuous murmur of patent ductus arteriosus. This error should never be made, however, because the cervical venous hum can be terminated easily by digital compression of the JVP.

The mammary souffle is a continuous murmur occurring in 10 to 15 percent of pregnant women during the second and third trimesters and in the early postpartum period, particularly in lactating women, and is heard between the second and sixth anterior intercostal spaces. This murmur may be obliterated by firm pressure on the stethoscope or by digital pressure applied just lateral to the site of auscultation and therefore should not be confused with the continuous murmur of patent ductus arteriosus or with an arteriovenous fistula. The mammary souffle disappears after termination of lactation. Other causes of continuous murmurs due to rapid blood flow through arterial or venous channels are outlined in Table 12-13.

***Continuous Murmurs Due to High- to Low-Pressure Shunts*** A group of congenital cardiovascular anomalies has shunting from the

TABLE 12-13 Physiologic Classification of Continuous Murmurs

Continuous murmurs due to rapid blood flow
- Venous hum
- Mammary souffle
- Hemangioma
- Hyperthyroidism
- Acute alcoholic hepatitis
- Hyperemia of neoplasm (hepatoma, renal cell carcinoma, Paget's disease)

Continuous murmurs due to high- to low-pressure shunts
- Systemic artery to pulmonary artery (patent ductus arteriosus, aortopulmonary window, truncus arteriosus, pulmonary atresia, anomalous left coronary, bronchiectasis, sequestration of the lung)
- Systemic artery to right heart (ruptured sinus of Valsalva, coronary artery fistula)
- Left-to-right atrial shunting (Lutembacher's syndrome, mitral atresia plus atrial septal defect)
- Venovenous shunts (anomalous pulmonary veins, portosystemic shunts)
- Arteriovenous fistula (systemic or pulmonic)

Continuous murmurs secondary to localized arterial obstruction
- Coarctation of the aorta
- Branch pulmonary stenosis
- Carotid occlusion
- Celiac mesenteric occlusion
- Renal occlusion
- Femoral occlusion
- Coronary occlusion

SOURCE: From Myers JD. The mechanisms and significances of continuous murmurs. In: Leon DF, Shaver JA, eds. *Physiologic Principles of Heart Sounds and Murmurs.* Monograph 46. New York: American Heart Association; 1975:202. Reproduced with permission from the American Heart Association, Inc., and author.

high-pressure systemic (aortic) circulation to the low-pressure pulmonary arterial circulation, resulting in a large gradient between the two systems throughout the cardiac cycle. The murmur of patent ductus arteriosus is the classic example of this type of anomaly. It is heard best in the left infraclavicular area and the second left intercostal space. The peak intensity of the murmur is at the time of $S_2$, after which it gradually wanes until it terminates before $S_1$.[227] The length of the murmur is determined by the difference in the vascular resistance between the greater and lesser circulation. As the pulmonary vascular resistance increases, the diastolic pressure in the pulmonary artery approaches and finally reaches systemic levels, diminishing and finally abolishing diastolic flow and the diastolic portion of the murmur. With equilibration of aortic and pulmonary artery pressure, systolic flow across the shunt diminishes and finally disappears, leaving the ductus silent (Eisenmenger's patent ductus arteriosus). Surgically produced aortopulmonary connections (Blalock, Waterston, and Potts shunts), as well as the murmur of aortic pulmonary window, have identical qualities, and the effect of PH on their length is analogous. These types of continuous murmurs must be distinguished from to-and-fro murmurs. The latter is a combination of the systolic ejection murmur and a semilunar diastolic murmur. The classic example of a to-and-fro murmur is the murmur of AS and AR. The continuous murmur builds to a crescendo around $S_2$, whereas the to-and-fro murmur has two components. The midsystolic ejection component decrescendos and may disappear as it approaches $S_2$, leaving a silent period before the onset of the regurgitant murmur. Truncus arteriosus is a rare congenital anomaly and probably produces a continuous murmur only if there is coexisting pulmonary artery stenosis (Chap. 73). In the presence of severe RV outflow obstruction, bronchial collateral arteries can enlarge their normal precapillary anastomoses with pulmonary arteries, and the resulting aortic pulmonary fistula can produce a continuous murmur. This murmur can be heard in the same location as the patent ductus but radiates widely, especially over the posterior thorax. Large bronchial collateral arteries producing such continuous murmurs are more common with pulmonary atresia but also occur with tetralogy of Fallot. Bronchial artery–pulmonary artery collaterals sufficient to produce continuous murmurs are also found in far-advanced bronchiectasis and sequestration of the lung (Chap. 73).

An anomalous left coronary artery arising from the pulmonary artery may cause a continuous murmur when the left-to-right shunt flow is large; it is usually best heard at the left sternal border. In this condition, the origin of the right coronary artery is from the aorta, and the left-to-right shunt is from the high-pressure right coronary arterial bed through large arterial collaterals to the left coronary system, which empties into the low-pressure pulmonary artery.

Sinus of Valsalva aneurysms may cause continuous murmurs when they rupture into the right side of the heart. In almost all cases, rupture occurs from the right and noncoronary sinuses into the right atrium or the RV.[282] The murmur is heard maximally at the lower sternal border or xiphoid over the area corresponding to the fistulous tract. Diastolic accentuation of this murmur is an important sign to differentiate ruptured sinus from patent ductus arteriosus or arteriovenous fistula. Systolic suppression of the murmur is due to both mechanical narrowing of the fistulous tract during systole as well as the probable Venturi effect created by the rapid ejection of blood past the aortic origin of the fistula.

Coronary artery fistulas usually empty into the right atrium or ventricle and may cause a continuous murmur that is best heard to either the left or the right of the lower sternal area. Since the majority of coronary flow occurs during diastole, the diastolic component of the murmur is louder. When the coronary artery fistula empties into a high-pressure RV, only a diastolic murmur may be heard because the pressure gradient across the shunt is reduced during systole. Left-to-right shunting through an uncomplicated ASD produces no murmur audible on the chest wall because of the minimal pressure gradient and absence of turbulence. When mitral valve obstruction is present, as with Lutembacher's syndrome or mitral atresia, however, there can be a high-pressure gradient between the left and right atria across a small defect, and a continuous murmur may be present.[283] This murmur increases in intensity with inspiration and decreases with the Valsalva maneuver. Occasionally, a small ASD is produced following transseptal catheterization or balloon valvuloplasty for MS, and a continuous murmur is produced due to high-velocity flow resulting from the large pressure gradient from the left to the right atrium.

Total anomalous pulmonary venous drainage into a systemic vein may produce a continuous venous hum usually heard in the pulmonary area or the left infraclavicular area. Frequently, a constriction at the junction of the anomalous venous conduit and the innominate vein or superior vena cava may cause augmentation of the murmur (Chap. 73).

Arteriovenous fistulas between peripheral vessels produce a classic continuous murmur with systolic accentuation caused by shunting of a large volume of blood at rapid flow rates from a high-pressure artery into a low-pressure vein. These murmurs are best

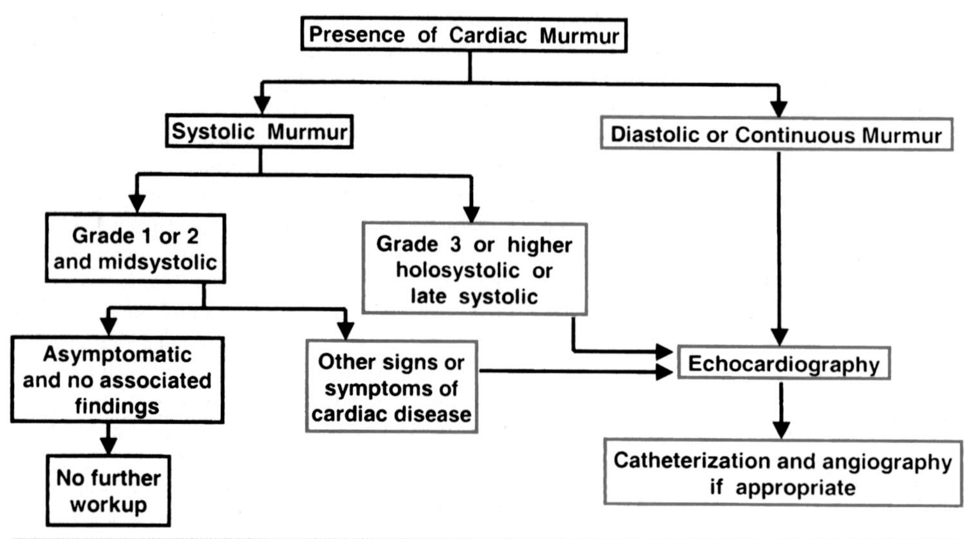


FIGURE 12–82 Algorithm for the evaluation of a cardiac murmur.

## Approach to Patient with a Heart Murmur

The majority of heart murmurs are midsystolic and soft (grades 1 to 3). When such a murmur occurs in an asymptomatic child or young adult *without* other evidence of heart disease on clinical examination, it is usually benign and echocardiography is not generally required. On the other hand, echocardiographic examination is indicated in patients with loud systolic murmurs (grade 3), especially when those are holosystolic or late systolic; in most patients with diastolic or continuous murmurs and in patients with additional unexplained physical findings on cardiac examination (Fig. 12-82).

heard at the site of the fistula. Local compression of the veins may decrease the intensity of the murmur by raising venous pressure and reducing the arteriovenous pressure gradient. Complete obliteration of the fistula will terminate the murmur, and if the shunt is of considerable magnitude, a baroreceptor-mediated reflex bradycardia may occur (Branham's sign). Likewise, a reflex tachycardia will occur on release of the obstruction. Pulmonary arteriovenous fistulas usually produce only a systolic murmur because the peripheral vascular resistance of the normal lung is very low, and the normally small diastolic pressure gradient from pulmonary artery to pulmonary vein is not significantly increased by the presence of the fistula.

***Continuous Murmur Secondary to Localized Arterial Obstruction***
Localized stenosis of systemic or pulmonary arteries may produce a continuous murmur if the obstruction is critical and adequate collateral flow is not available.[284] Most partially obstructed arteries have only systolic murmurs that are delayed relative to cardiac systole, depending on the transit time of pulsatile flow from the heart to the site of obstruction. This lack of diastolic gradient is due to the collateral arteries around the obstruction that deliver adequate flow such that the diastolic pressure on either side of the localized obstruction is essentially equal. Thus a localized, partial arterial obstruction characteristically produces only a systolic murmur. If adequate collateral flow is not present, there is a continuous murmur with systolic accentuation. In severe coarctation of the aorta, a continuous murmur may also be produced at the site of the coarctation (Chap. 73). This latter murmur is best heard over the back midline between the scapulae.

Continuous murmurs also may result from branch pulmonary stenosis or partial obstruction of a major pulmonary artery occluded by a massive pulmonary embolus. Other common locations of continuous murmurs secondary to localized arterial obstructions are listed in Table 12-13. Common to all these murmurs is critical narrowing of the vessel with inadequate collateral flow such that a continuous pressure gradient is produced throughout the cardiac cycle. Murmurs produced by obstruction of major coronary arteries are rarely loud enough to be transmitted to the chest wall. When audible, they produce only diastolic murmurs, even with inadequate collateral circulation.

## References

1. Vanden Belt RJ. The history. In: Chizner M, ed. *Classic Teachings in Clinical Cardiology: A Tribute to W. Proctor Harvey.* Cedar Grove, NJ: Laennec; 1996:41–54.
2. Hurst JW, Morris DC. The history: Symptoms and past events related to cardiovascular disease. In: Schlant RC, Alexander RW, O'Rourke RA, et al., eds. *The Heart,* 8th ed. New York: McGraw-Hill; 1994:205–216.
3. O'Rourke RA. Chest pain. In: Fuster V, Alexander RW, O'Rourke RA, et al., eds. *The Heart,* 10th ed. New York: McGraw-Hill; 2001: 195–199.
4. Sampson JJ, Cheitlin M. Pathophysiology and differential diagnosis of cardiac pain. *Prog Cardiovasc Dis* 1971;13:507–531.
5. O'Rourke RA. Diagnostic approach to the patient with chest pain compatible with definite or suspected angina pectoris. In: Sobel BE, ed. *Medical Management of Heart Disease.* New York: Marcel Dekker; 1996:4–22.
6. Heberden W. Some accounts of a disorder of the breast. *Med Trans* 1772; 2:59.
7. Goswami N, O'Rourke RA. The pathophysiology of chronic stable angina, In: Fuster V, Nabel E, Topol EJ, eds. *Atherothrombosis and Coronary Heart Disease,* 2d ed. Philadelphia: Lippincott. In press.
8. Murray DR, O'Rourke RA, Walling AD, Walsh RA: History and physical examination in myocardial ischemia and acute myocardial infarction. In: Francis G, Alpert J, eds. *Coronary Care,* 2d ed. Boston: Little, Brown; 1995:73–95.
9. Dell'Italia LJ. Chest pain. In: Stein JH, ed. *Internal Medicine,* 5th ed. Boston: Little, Brown; 1998:125–129.
10. Christie LG Jr, Conti CR. Systemic approach to evaluation of angina-like chest pain: Pathophysiology and clinical testing with emphasis on objective documentation of myocardial ischemia. *Am Heart J* 1981; 102:897–912.
11. Taggart P, Yellon D. Preconditioning and arrhythmias. *Circulation* 2002;106:2999–3001.
12. Campeau L. Letter to the editor. *Circulation* 1976;54:522.
13. Levine SA. Carotid sinus massage: A new diagnostic test for angina pectoris. *JAMA* 1962;182:1332–1356.
14. Douglas PS, Ginsberg GS. The evaluation of chest pain in women. *N Engl J Med* 1996;334:1311–1315.
15. Chauhan A, Mullins PA, Taylor G, et al. Cardioesophageal reflux: A mechanism for "linked angina" in patients with angiographically proven coronary artery disease. *J Am Coll Cardiol* 1996;27: 1621–1628.

16. Epstein SE, Talbot TL. Dynamic coronary tone in precipitation, exacerbation and relief of angina pectoris. *Am J Cardiol* 1981;48:797–803.
17. Proudfit WL, Shrey ED, Sones FM Jr. Selective cine coronary arteriography: Correlation with clinical findings in 1000 patients. *Circulation* 1996;33:901–910.
18. Gibbons R, Abrams J, Chatterjee K, et al. ACC/AHA 2002 guideline update for the management of patients with chronic stable angina. Available on line only: www.acc.org/clinical/guidelines/stable/stable.pdf
19. Cannon RO III: Microvascular angina: Cardiovascular investigations regarding pathophysiology and management. *Med Clin North Am* 1991;75:1097–1118.
20. Cannon RO III, Cattau EL Jr, Yakshe PN, et al. Coronary flow reserve, esophageal motility, and chest pain in patients with angiographically normal coronary arteries. *Am J Med* 1990;88:217–222.
21. Panza JA, Epstein S, Quyyumi AA. Circadian variation in vascular tone and its relation to $\alpha$-sympathetic vasoconstrictor activity. *N Engl J Med* 1991;325:986–990.
22. Crake T, Canepa-Anson R, Shapiro L, Poole-Wilson PA. Continuous recording of coronary sinus oxygen saturation during atrial pacing in patients with coronary artery disease or with syndrome X. *Br Heart J* 1988;59:31–38.
23. Cannon RO III, Schenk WH, Quyyumi A, et al. Comparison of exercise testing with studies of coronary flow reserve in patients with microvascular angina. *Circulation* 1991;83(suppl III):III-77–III-81.
24. Kaski JC, Tousoulis D, Galassi AR, et al. Epicardial coronary artery tone and reactivity in patients with normal coronary arteriograms and reduced coronary flow reserve (syndrome X). *J Am Coll Cardiol* 1991;18:50–54.
25. Cannon RO III, Peden DB, Berkebile C, et al. Airway hyper-responsiveness in patients with microvascular angina: Evidence for a diffuse disorder of smooth muscle responsiveness. *Circulation* 1990; 82:2011–2017.
26. Kemp HG. Left ventricular function in patients with the anginal syndrome and normal coronary arteries. *Am J Cardiol* 1973;32:375–376.
27. Attilio M. Syndrome X: Still an appropriate name. *J Am Coll Cardiol* 1991;17:1471–1472.
28. Levy RD, Cunningham D, Shapiro LM, et al. Diurnal variation in left ventricular function: A study of patients with myocardial ischemia, syndrome X, and of normal controls. *Br Heart J* 1987;57:148–153.
29. Spinelli L, Ferro G, Genovese A, et al. Exercise-induced impairment of diastolic time in patients with X syndrome. *Am Heart J* 1990;119: 829–833.
30. Kern MJ. Extracting the coronary artery from syndrome X: Is epicardial vasomotion physiologic in patients with normal coronary arteriograms and reduced coronary flow reserve? *J Am Coll Cardiol* 1991;18:55–56.
31. Galassi AR, Kaski JC, Pupita G, et al. Lack of evidence for alpha-adrenergic receptor-mediated mechanisms in the genesis of ischemia in syndrome X. *Am J Cardiol* 1989;64:264–269.
32. Epstein SE, Cannon RO III, Bonow RO. Exercise testing in patients with microvascular angina. *Circulation* 1991;83(suppl III):III-73–III-76.
33. Cannon RO III, Quyyumi AA, Schenke WH, et al. Abnormal cardiac sensitivity in patients with chest pain and normal coronary arteries. *J Am Coll Cardiol* 1990;16:1359–1366.
34. Maseri A, ed. *Ischemic Heart Disease.* New York: Churchill-Livingstone; 1995:1–713.
35. Hillis DL, Braunwald E. Medical progress: Coronary-artery spasm. *N Engl J Med* 1978;229:695–702.
36. Prinzmetal M, Kennamer R, Merliss R, et al. Angina pectoris: 1. A variant form of angina pectoris. *Am J Med* 1959;26:375–388.
37. Herrick JB. Clinical features of sudden obstruction of the coronary arteries. *JAMA* 1912;59:2015–2020.
38. Ross RS, Babe BM. Right ventricular hypertension as a cause of angina. *Circulation* 1960;22:801–802.
39. Spodick DH. Pitfalls in the recognition of pericarditis. In: Hurst JW, ed. *Clinical Essays on the Heart,* Vol V. New York: McGraw-Hill; 1985:95–111.
40. Eagle KA, DeSanctis RW. Dissecting aortic aneurysm. *Curr Probl Cardiol* 1989;14:227–228.
41. Katon W, Hall ML, Russo J, et al. Chest pain: Relationship of psychiatric illness to coronary arteriographic results. *Am J Med* 1988; 84:1–9.
42. Mellow MH. A gastroenterologist's view of chest pain. *Curr Probl Cardiol* 1983;9:1–36.
43. Rose S, Achkar E, Easley KA. Follow-up of patients with noncardiac chest pain: Value of esophageal testing. *Dig Dis Sci* 1994;39: 2063–2068.
44. Bernstein LM, Grain RC, Pacini R. Differentiation of esophageal pain from angina pectoris: Role of esophageal acid perfusion test. *Medicine* 1962;41:145–162.
45. Atkinson M. Monitoring esophageal pH. *Gut* 1987;28:509–514.
46. Wolf E, Stern S. Costosternal syndrome: Its frequency and importance in differential diagnosis of coronary heart disease. *Arch Intern Med* 1976;136:1289–1291.
47. Epstein SE, Gerber LN, Boren JS. Chest wall syndrome: A common cause of unexpected pain. *JAMA* 1979;241:2793–2797.
48. The Criteria Committee of the New York Heart Association. *Diseases of the Heart and Blood Vessels: Nomenclature and Criteria for Diagnosis of the Heart and Great Vessels,* 6th ed. New York: New York Heart Association/Little, Brown; 1964.
49. Aziz K, Sanyal SK, Goldblatt E. Reversed differential cyanosis. *Br Heart J* 1968;30:288–290.
50. Basson CT, Cowley GS, Solomon SD, et al. The clinical and genetic spectrum of the Holt-Oram syndrome (heart-hand syndrome). *N Engl J Med* 1994;330:885–891.
51. Takahashi T, Koide T, Yamaguchi H, et al. Ehlers-Danlos syndrome with aortic regurgitation, dilation of the sinuses of Valsalva, and abnormal dermal collagen fibrils. *Am Heart J* 1992;123:1709–1712.
52. Hortop J, Tsipouras P, Hanley JA, et al. Cardiovascular involvement in osteogenesis imperfecta. *Circulation* 1986;73:54–61.
53. Marsalese DL, Moodie DS, Vacante M, et al. Marfan's syndrome: Natural history and long-term follow-up of cardiovascular involvement. *J Am Coll Cardiol* 1989;14:422–428.
54. Fisher EA, Desnick RJ, Gordon RE, et al. Fabry disease: An unusual cause of severe coronary disease in a young man. *Ann Intern Med* 1992;117:221–223.
55. Musewe NN, Alexander DJ, Teshima I, et al. Echocardiographic evaluation of the spectrum of cardiac anomalies associated with trisomy 13 and trisomy 18. *J Am Coll Cardiol* 1990;15:673–677.
56. Subramaniam PN. Turner's syndrome and cardiovascular anomalies. *Am J Med Sci* 1989;297:260–262.
57. Proudfit WL. Skin signs of infective endocarditis. *Am Heart J* 1983; 106:1451–1453.
58. Burch M, Sharland M, Shinebourne E, et al. Cardiologic abnormalities in Noonan syndrome: Phenotypic diagnosis and echocardiographic assessment of 118 patients. *J Am Coll Cardiol* 1993;22:1189–1192.
59. Pellikka PA, Tajik AJ, Khandheria BK, et al. Carcinoid heart disease: Clinical and echocardiographic spectrum in 74 patients. *Circulation* 1993;87:1188–1196.
60. Goldman AP, Kotler MN. Heart disease in scleroderma. *Am Heart J* 1985;110:1043–1046.
61. Moder KG, Miller TD, Tazelaar HD. Cardiac involvement in systemic lupus erythematosus. *Mayo Clin Proc* 1999;74:275–284.
62. Trentham DE and Le CH. Relapsing polychondritis. *Ann Intern Med* 1998;129:114–122.
63. Roldan CA, Chavez J, Wiest PW, et al. Aortic root disease and valve disease associated with ankylosing spondylitis. *J Am Coll Cardiol* 1998; 32:1397–1404.
64. Casazza F, Morpurgo M. The varying evolution of Friedreich's ataxia cardiomyopathy. *Am J Cardiol* 1996;77:895–898.
65. Parish JM, Shepard JW. Cardiovascular effects of sleep disorders. *Chest* 1990;97:1220–1225.
66. Cox J, Krajden M. Cardiovascular manifestations of Lyme disease. *Am Heart J* 1991;122:1449–1455.
67. Kenny D, Wetherbee J. Kearns-Sayre syndrome in the elderly: Mitochondrial myopathy with advanced heart block. *Am Heart J* 1990; 120:440–443.

68. Shammas RL, Movahed A. Sarcoidosis of the heart. *Clin Cardiol* 1993;16:462–472.
69. Kuan P. Cardiac Wilson's disease. *Chest* 1987;91:579–583.
70. Kyle RA. Amyloidosis. *Circulation* 1995;91:1269–1271.
71. Hara KS, Ballard DJ, Ilstrup DM, et al. Rheumatoid pericarditis: Clinical features and survival. *Medicine* 1990;69:81–91.
72. Di Eusanio G, Mazzola A, Gregorini R, et al. Left ventricular aneurysm secondary to Behçet's disease. *Ann Thorac Surg* 1991;51: 131–135.
73. Deer T, Rosencrance JG, Chillag SA. Cardiac conduction manifestations of Reiter's syndrome. *South Med J* 1991;84:799–800.
74. Lazarus A, Varin J, Babuty D, et al. Long-term follow-up of arrhythmias in patients with myotonic dystrophy treated by pacing. A multicenter diagnostic pacemaker study. *J Am Coll Cardiol* 2002;40: 1645–1652.
75. Burns JC, Shike H, Gordon JB, et al. Sequelae of Kawasaki disease in adolescents and young adults. *J Am Coll Cardiol* 1996;28:253–257.
76. Elliott WJ, Powell LH. Diagonal earlobe creases and prognosis in patients with suspected coronary artery disease. *Am J Med* 1996;100: 205–211.
77. Braunlin EA, Hunter DW, Krivit W, et al. Evaluation of coronary artery disease in the Hurler syndrome by angiography. *Am J Cardiol* 1992;69:1487–1489.
78. Jacob AG, Driscoll DJ, Shaughnessy WJ, et al. Klippel-Trénaunay syndrome: Spectrum and management. *Mayo Clin Proc* 1998;73: 28–36.
79. Pagon RA, Bennett FC, LaVeek B, et al. Williams syndrome. *J Pediatr* 1987;80:85–91.
80. Stevenson WG, Perloff JK, Weiss JN, Anderson TL. Facioscapulohumeral muscular dystrophy: Evidence for selective, genetic electrophysiologic cardiac involvement. *J Am Coll Cardiol* 1990;15: 292–299.
81. Buckley AE, Dean J, Mahy IR. Cardiac involvement in Emery Dreifuss muscular dystrophy: A case series. *Heart* 1999;82:105–108.
82. Gibbs JL. The heart and tuberous sclerosis. *Br Heart J* 1985;54: 596–599.
83. Nutter DO. Measurements of the systolic blood pressure. In: Hurst JW, ed. *The Heart,* 5th ed. New York: McGraw-Hill; 1982.
84. Asmar R, Benetos A, London G, et al. Aortic distensibility in normotensive, untreated and treated hypertensive patients. *Blood Pressure* 1995;4:48–54.
85. Frohlich ED. Hypertension in the elderly. *Curr Probl Cardiol* 1988;13: 313–367.
86. Hales S. *Statistical Essays: Containing Haema-staticks; or, an Account of Some Hydraulick and Hydrostatical Experiments Made on the Blood and Blood-Vessels of Animals.* London: Innys W, Manby R;1733.
87. Grim NC, Grim CE. Blood pressure measurements. In: Izzo JL, Black HE, eds. *AHA Hypertension Primer,* 2d ed. New York: American Heart Association; 1998:295–298.
88. McCutcheon EP, Rushmer RF. Korotkov sounds: An experimental critique. *Circ Res* 1967;20:149–161.
89. Rodbard S. The components of the Korotkov sounds. *Am Heart J* 1967;74:278–282.
90. Neilsen PR, Janniche H. The accuracy of auscultatory measurement of arm blood pressure in very obese subjects. *Acta Med Scand* 1974;196: 403–409.
91. Littler WA, Komsuoglar B. Which is the most accurate method of measuring blood pressure? *Am Heart J* 1989;117:723–728.
92. Messerli FH, White WW, Staessen JA. If only cardiologists did properly measure blood pressure. *J Am Coll Cardiol* 2002;40: 2201–2203.
93. Evans CE, Haynes RB, Goldsmith CH, Hewson SA. Home blood pressure-measuring devices: A comparative study of accuracy. *J Hypertens* 1989;7:133–142.
94. White SB, Berson AS, Robbins C, et al. National standard for measurement of resting and ambulatory blood pressure with automated sphygmomanometers. *Hypertension* 1993;21:504–509.
95. Kelly RP, Haywood C, Ganis J, et al. Noninvasive registration of the arterial pressure waveform using high-fidelity applanation tonometry. *J Vasc Med Biol* 1989;1:142–149.
96. Nichols WW, O'Rourke MF, eds. *McDonald's Blood Flow in Arteries,* 4th ed. London: Edward Arnold; 1998.
97. Chen CH, Ting CT, Nussbacher A, et al. Validation of carotid artery tonometry as a means of estimating augmentation index of ascending aortic pressure. *Hypertension* 1996;27:168–175.
98. Liang YL, Teede H, Kotsopoulos D, et al. Noninvasive measurements of arterial structure and function: Repeatability, interrelationships and trial sample size. *Clin Sci* 1998;95:669–679.
99. Wilkinson IB, Fuchs SA, Jansen IM, et al. Reproducibility of pulse wave velocity and augmentation index measure by pulse wave analysis. *J Hypertens* 1998;16:2079–2084.
100. Siebenhofer A, Kemp C, Sutton A, Williams B. The reproducibility of central aortic blood pressure measurements in healthy subjects using applanation tonometry and sphygmocardiography. *J Hum Hypertens* 1999;13:625–629.
101. Frohlich ED, Gifford RW, Hall WD. Hypertensive cardiovascular disease. In: 18th Bethesda Conference Report: Cardiovascular Disease in the Elderly. *J Am Coll Cardiol* 1987;10(suppl A):57A–59A.
102. Cohn JN, Finkelstein SM. Abnormalities of vascular compliance in hypertension, aging and heart failure. *J Hypertens* 1992;10: S61–S64.
103. O'Rourke MF. *Arterial Function in Health and Disease.* New York: Churchill-Livingstone; 1982.
104. Wei Y, Gersh BJ. Heart disease in the elderly. *Curr Probl Cardiol* 1987;12:1–65.
105. Kannel WB. Historic perspectives on the relative contributions of diastolic and systolic blood pressure elevation to cardiovascular risk profile. *Am Heart J* 1999;138:205–210.
106. Kannel WB, Wolf PA, McGee DL. Systolic blood pressure, arterial rigidity, and risk of stroke: The Framingham Study. *JAMA* 1998;245: 1225–1229.
107. Rutan GH, Kuller LH, Neaton JD, et al. Mortality associated with diastolic hypertension among men screened for Multiple Risk Factors Intervention Trial (MRFIT). *Circulation* 1988;77:504–514.
108. SHEP Cooperative Research Group. Prevention of stroke by antihypertensive drug treatment in older persons with isolated hypertension: Final results of the Systolic Hypertension in the Elderly Program (SHEP). *JAMA* 1991;265:3255–3264.
109. Staessen JA, Fagard R, Thijs L, et al. Randomised double-blind comparison of placebo and active treatment for older patients with isolated systolic hypertension. The Systolic Hypertension in Europe (syst-Eur) trail investigators. *Lancet* 1997;350;757–764.
110. O'Rourke MF. Isolated systolic hypertension, pulse pressure, and arterial stiffness as risk factors for cardiovascular disease. *Curr Hypertens Reps* 1999;3:204–211.
111. Franklin SS, Khan SA, Wong ND, et al. The importance of pulse pressure and systolic blood pressure in predicting coronary heart disease in older adults: The Framingham Heart Study. *Circulation* 1999;100:354–360.
112. Kaplan NM. *Clinical Hypertension,* 5th ed. Baltimore: Williams & Wilkins; 1990.
113. Safar ME, Frohlich ED. The arterial system in hypertension: A prospective view. *Hypertension* 1995;26:10–14.
114. Littler WA, Honour AJ, Pugsley DJ, Sleight PL. Continuous recording of direct arterial pressure in unrestricted patients. *Circulation* 1975;51: 1101–1106.
115. Richardson DW, Honour AJ, Fenton DW, et al. Variation in arterial pressure throughout the day and night. *Clin Sci* 1964;26:445–460.
116. Donald KW, Lind AR, McNicol GW, et al. Cardiovascular response to sustained contractions. *Circ Res* 1967;20(suppl 1):15–30.
117. Wooley CF, Hosier DM, Booth RW, et al. Supravalvular aortic stenosis. *Am J Med* 1961;31:717–725.
118. Pascarelli EF, Bertrand CA. Comparison of blood pressure in the arms and legs. *N Engl J Med* 1964;270:693–698.

119. Park MK, Guntheroth WG. Direct blood pressure measurements in brachial and femoral arteries in children. *Circulation* 1979;42: 231–237.
120. Felix WR, Hochbert HM, George MED, et al. Ultrasound measurement of arm and leg blood pressure. *JAMA* 1973;226:1096–1099.
121. Vlachopoulos C, O'Rourke M. Genesis of the normal and abnormal arterial pulse. *Curr Probl Cardiol* 2000;25:306–367.
122. Kelly RP, Gibbs HH, O'Rourke MF, et al. Nitroglycerin has a favorable effect on left ventricular afterload than apparent from measurement of pressure in a peripheral artery. *Eur Heart J* 1990;11: 138–144.
123. Crawford MH. Inspection and palpation of venous and arterial pulses: In: *Examination of the Heart,* Part 2. New York: American Heart Association; 1990.
124. O'Rourke MF, Kelly R, Avolio A. *The Arterial Pulse*. Philadelphia: Lea & Febiger; 1992.
125. Ewy GA. Venous and arterial pulsations: Bedside insights into hemodynamics. In: Chizner M, ed. *Classic Teachings in Clinical Cardiology: A Tribute to W. Proctor Harvey.* Cedar Grove, NJ: Laennec; 1996:65–84.
126. O'Rourke MF. The arterial pulse in health and disease. *Am Heart J* 1971;82:687–702.
127. Murgo JP, Westerhof N, Giolma JP, Altobelli SA. Aortic input impedance in normal man: Relationship to pressure wave shapes. *Circulation* 1980;62:105–116.
128. Hamilton WF, Dow P. An experimental study of the standing waves in the pulse propagated through the aorta. *Am J Physiol* 1939;125:48.
129. O'Rourke MF. Pressure and flow waves in systemic arteries and the anatomic design of the arterial system. *J Appl Physiol* 1967;23: 139–149.
130. O'Rourke MF, Auido AP. Pulsatile flow and pressures in human systemic arteries: Studies in man and in a multibranched model of the human systemic arterial tree. *Circ Res* 1980;46:363–372.
131. Murgo JP, Westerhof N, Giolma JO, Altobelli SA. Effects of exercise on aortic impedance and pressure wave shapes in normal man. *Circ Res* 1981;48:334–343.
132. Marx HJ, Yu PN. Clinical examination of the arterial pulse. *Prog Cardiovasc Dis* 1967;10:207–235.
133. O'Rourke MF. Vascular impedance in studies of arterial and cardiac function. *Physiol Rev* 1982;62:570–623.
134. O'Rourke MF, Mancia G. Arterial stiffness. *J Hypertens* 1999;17:1–4.
135. O'Rourke MF, Taylor MG. Input impedance of the systemic circulation. *Circ Res* 1967;20:365–380.
136. Schlant RC, Felner MJ. The arterial pulse: Clinical manifestations. *Curr Prob Cardiol* 1977;2:1–50.
137. Franklin SS, Gustin W IV, Wong ND, et al. Hemodynamic patterns of age-related changes in blood pressure: The Framingham Heart Study. *Circulation* 1997;96:308–315.
138. Benetos A, Laurent S, Hoeks AP, et al. Arterial alterations with aging and high blood pressure: A noninvasive study of carotid and femoral arteries. *Arterioscler Thromb* 1993;13:90–97.
139. Armentano R, Megnien JL, Simon A, et al. Effects of hypertension on viscoelasticity of carotid and femoral arteries in humans. *Hypertension* 1995;26:48–54.
140. Safar ME, Frohlich ED. The arterial system in hypertension: A prospective view. *Hypertension* 1995;26:10–14.
141. Corrigan DJ. On permanent patency of the mouth of the aorta, or inadequacy of the aorta valves. *Edinburgh Med Surg* 1832;37: 225–245.
142. Ikram H, Nixon PGF, Fox JA. The hemodynamic implications of the bisferiens pulse. *Br Heart J* 1964;26:452–459.
143. Wigle ED. The arterial pressure pulse in muscular subaortic stenosis. *Br Heart J* 1963;25:97–105.
144. Deane CR, Needleman L. The cause of pulsus tardus in arterial stenosis. *Radiology* 1995;194:28–30.
145. Bude RO, Rubin JM, Platt JF, et al. Pulsus tardus: Its cause and potential limitations in detection of aortic stenosis. *Radiology* 1994;190: 779–784.
146. Dow P. The development of the anacrotic and tardus pulse of aortic stenosis. *Am J Physiol* 1940;131:432.
147. Ewy GA, Rios JC, Marcus FI. The dicrotic arterial pulse. *Circulation* 1969;39:655–661.
148. Mitchell JH, Sarnoff SJ, Sonnenblock EH. The dynamics of pulsus alternans: Alternating end-diastolic fiber length as a causative factor. *J Clin Invest* 1963;42:55–63.
149. Freeman GL, Widman LE, Campbell JM, Colston JT. An evaluation of the onset of pulsus alternans in closed-chest dogs. *Am J Physiol* 1992; 262:H278–H284.
150. White PD. Alternation of the pulse: A common clinical condition. *Am J Med Sci* 1915;150:82–96.
151. Shabetai R, Fowler NO, Fenton JC, Masangkay M. Pulsus paradoxus. *J Clin Invest* 1965;44:1882–1898.
152. Shabetai R, Fowler NO, Guntheroth WG. The hemodynamics of cardiac tamponade and constrictive pericarditis. *Am J Cardiol* 1970; 26: 480–498.
153. Otsuji Y, Toda H, Kisanuki A, et al. Influence of left ventricular filling profile during preceding control beats on pulse pressure during ventricular premature contractions. *Eur Heart J* 1994;15: 462–467.
154. Hurst JW, Schlant RC. Examination of the veins and their pulsation. In: Hurst JW, ed. *The Heart,* 4th ed. New York: McGraw-Hill; 1978: 193–201.
155. Garratt CJ, Griffith MJ, Young G, et al. Value of physical signs in the diagnosis of ventricular tachycardia. *Circulation* 1994;90:3103–3107.
156. Ewy GA, Marcus FI. Bedside estimation of the venous pressure. *Heart Bull* 1968;17:41.
157. Ewy GA. The abdominojugular test: Technique and hemodynamic correlates. *Ann Intern Med* 1989;108:456–460.
158. Ducas J, Magder S, McGregor M. Validity of the hepatojugular reflux as a clinical test for congestive heart failure. *Am J Cardiol* 1983;52: 1299–1303.
159. Dell'Italia L, Starling MR, O'Rourke RA. Physical examination for exclusion of hemodynamically important right ventricular infarction. *Ann Intern Med* 1983;99:608–612.
160. Stonjic BB, Brecker SJ, Xiao HB, Gibson DG. Jugular venous *a* wave in PH: New insights from a Doppler echocardiographic study. *Br Heart J* 1992;68:187–191.
161. Anderson WB. Examination of the retina: In: Alexander AW, Schlant RC, Fuster W, eds. *Hurst's The Heart,* 9th ed. New York: McGraw-Hill; 1998:343–349.
162. Hurst JW, Robinson PH. Physical examination of the chest, abdomen and extremities. In: Hurst JW, et al., eds. *The Heart,* 7th ed. New York: McGraw-Hill; 1990:242–243.
163. Shaver JA. Cardiac auscultation: A cost-effective diagnostic skill. *Curr Probl Cardiol* 1995;20:443–530.
164. Willis PW IV. Inspection and palpation of the precordium. In: Hurst JW, ed. *The Heart,* 7th ed. New York: McGraw-Hill; 1990:163–169.
165. Schlant RC, Hurst JW. *Examination of the Precordium: Inspection and Palpation.* New York: American Heart Association; 1990:1–28.
166. Abrams J. Precordial palpation: Let your fingers do the walking. In: Chizner M, ed. *Classic Teachings in Clinical Cardiology: A Tribute to W. Proctor Harvey.* Cedar Grove, NJ: Laennec; 1996:85–103.
167. Eilen SD, Crawford MH, O'Rourke RA. Accuracy of precordial palpation for detecting increased left ventricular volume. *Ann Intern Med* 1983;99:628–630.
168. Abrams J. *Essentials of Cardiac Physical Diagnosis.* Philadelphia: Lea & Febiger; 1987.
169. Ronon JA Jr, Steelman RB, DeLeon AC Jr, et al. The clinical diagnosis of acute severe mitral insufficiency. *Am J Cardiol* 1971;27:284–290.
170. Abrams J. Precordial palpation. In: Horwitz LD, Graves BM, eds. *Signs and Symptoms in Cardiology.* Philadelphia: Lippincott; 1985: 156–177.
171. Harvey WP. Some pertinent physical findings in the clinical evaluation of acute myocardial infarction. *Circulation* 1969;39/40(suppl IV):IV-175–IV-181.

172. Shah PM. Newer concepts in hypertrophic obstruction cardiomyopathy, part II. *JAMA* 1979;242:1771–1776.
173. Rapaport MB, Sprague HB. The effects of tubing bore on stethoscope efficiency. *Am Heart J* 1951;42:605–609.
174. Butterworth JS, Chassin MR, McGrath R, et al. *Cardiac Auscultation.* New York: Grune & Stratton; 1960.
175. Clement DL,Cohn JN: Salvaging the history, physical examination and doctor-patient relationship in a technological cardiology environment. *J Am Coll Cardiol* 1999;33:892.
176. Levine SA, Harvey SP. *Clinical Auscultation of the Heart,* 2d ed. Philadelphia: Saunders; 1959.
177. Shaver JA, Salerni R, Reddy PS. Normal and abnormal heart sounds in cardiac diagnosis: I. Systolic sounds. *Curr Probl Cardiol* 1985;10: 1–68.
178. Reddy PS, Salerni R, Shaver JA. Normal and abnormal heart sounds in cardiac diagnosis: II. Diastolic sounds. *Curr Probl Cardiol* 1985;10: 1–55.
179. Laniado S, Yellin EL, Miller H, Frater WM. Temporal relation of the first heart sound to closure of the mitral valve. *Circulation* 1973;47: 1006–1014.
180. Mills P, Craige E. Echophonocardiography. *Prog Cardiovasc Dis* 1978; 20:337.
181. O'Toole JD, Reddy PS, Curtiss EI, et al. The contribution of tricuspid valve closure to the first heart sound: An intracardiac micromanometer study. *Circulation* 1976;53:752–758.
182. Thompson ME, Shaver JA, Leon DF, et al. Pathodynamics of first heart sound. In: Leon DF, Shaver JA, eds. *Physiologic Principles of Heart Sounds and Murmurs* (Monograph 46). New York: American Heart Association; 1975:8–18.
183. Shah PM. Hemodynamic determinants of the first heart sound. In: Leon DF, Shaver JA, eds. *Physiologic Principles of Heart Sounds and Murmurs* (Monograph 46). New York: American Heart Association; 1975:2–7.
184. Delman AJ. Hemodynamic correlates of cardiovascular sounds. *Annu Rev Med* 1967;18:139–158.
185. Adolph RJ, Stephens JF, Tanaka K. The clinical value of frequency analysis of the first heart sound in myocardial infarction. *Circulation* 1970;41:1003–1014.
186. Thompson ME, Shaver JA, Heidenreich FP, et al. Sound, pressure and motion correlates in mitral stenosis. *Am J Med* 1970;49:436–450.
187. Tei C, Shah PM, Cherian G, et al. The correlates of an abnormal first heart sound in MVP syndromes. *N Engl J Med* 1982;307:334–339.
188. Burggraf GW. The first heart sound in left bundle branch block: An echophonocardiographic study. *Circulation* 1981;63:429–435.
189. Shaver JA, Rahko PS, Grines CL, et al. Effect of left bundle branch block on the events of the cardiac cycle. *Acta Cardiol* 1988;4: 459–467.
190. Shaver JA, Griff FW, Leonard JJ. Ejection sounds of left-sided origin. In: Leon DF, Shaver JA, eds. *Physiologic Principles of Heart Sounds and Murmurs* (Monograph 46). New York: American Heart Association; 1975:27–34.
191. Mills PG, Brodie B, McLaurin L, et al. Echocardiographic and hemodynamic relationships of ejection sounds. *Circulation* 1977;56: 430–436.
192. Martin CE, Shaver JA, O'Toole JD, et al. Ejection sounds of right-sided origin. In: Leon DF, Shaver JA, eds. *Physiologic Principles of Heart Sounds and Murmurs* (Monograph 46). New York: American Heart Association; 1975:35–44.
193. Barlow JB, Pocock WA, Marchand P, Denny M. The significance of late systolic murmurs. *Am Heart J* 1963;66:443–452.
194. Criley JM, Lewis KB, Humphries JO, Ross RS. Prolapse of the mitral valve: Clinical and cine-angiocardiographic findings. *Br Heart J* 1966; 28:488–496.
195. Ronan JA, Perloff JK, Harvey WP. Systolic clicks and the late systolic murmur. *Am Heart J* 1965;70:319–325.
196. Leon DF, Leonard JJ, Kroetz FW, et al. Late systolic murmurs, clicks, and whoops arising from the mitral valve. *Am Heart J* 1966;72: 325–336.
197. Kerber RE, Isaeff DM, Hancock EW. Echocardiographic patterns in patients with the syndrome of systolic click and late systolic murmur. *N Engl J Med* 1971;284:691–693.
198. Popp RL, Brown OR, Silverman JF, Harrison D. Echocardiographic abnormalities in the MVP syndrome. *Circulation* 1974;49:428–433.
199. Reid JVO. Mid-systolic clicks. *S Afr Med J* 1961;35:353–355.
200. Fontana ME, Pence HL, Leighton RF, Wooley CF. The varying clinical spectrum of the systolic click–late systolic murmur syndrome: A postural auscultatory phenomenon. *Circulation* 1970;41:807–816.
201. Leatham A. The second heart sound, key to auscultation of the heart. *Acta Cardiol* 1964;19:395–416.
202. Shaver JA, O'Toole JD. The second heart sound: Newer concepts: I. Normal and wide physiologic splitting. *Mod Concepts Cardiovasc Dis* 1977;46:7–12.
203. Shaver JA. Clinical implications of the hangout interval. *Int J Cardiol* 1984;5:391–398.
204. Shaver JA, Nadolny RA, O'Toole JD, et al. Sound pressure correlates of the second heart sound: An intracardiac sound study. *Circulation* 1974; 49:316–325.
205. Adolph RJ. Second heart sound: Role of altered electromechanical events. In: Leon DF, Shaver JA, eds. *Physiologic Principles of Heart Sounds and Murmurs* (Monograph 46). New York: American Heart Association; 1975:45–57.
206. Leatham A, Towers M. Splitting of the second heart sound in health. In: Proceedings of the Thirtieth Annual General Meeting of the British Cardiac Society, Glasgow, May 10, 1951. *Br Heart J* 1951;13:575.
207. Adolph RJ, Fowler NO. The second heart sound: A screening test for heart disease. *Mod Concepts Cardiovasc Dis* 1970;39:91–96.
208. Shaver JA, O'Toole JD. The second heart sound: Newer concepts: 2. Paradoxical splitting and narrow physiological splitting. *Mod Concepts Cardiovasc Dis* 1977;46:13–16.
209. Alvares RF, Shaver JA, Gamble WH, Goodwin JF. The isovolumic relaxation period in hypertrophic cardiomyopathy. *J Am Coll Cardiol* 1984;3:71–81.
210. Gamble WH, Shaver JA, Alvares RF, et al. A critical appraisal of diastolic time intervals as a measure of relaxation in left ventricular hypertrophy. *Circulation* 1983;68:76–87.
211. Martin CE, Shaver JA, Leonard JJ. Physical signs, apex cardiography, phonocardiography, and systolic time intervals in angina pectoris. *Circulation* 1972;46:1098–1114.
212. Wood P. Pulmonary hypertension. *Br Med Bull* 1952;8:348–353.
213. Dell'Italia LJ, Walsh RA. Acute determinants of the hangout interval in the pulmonary circulation. *Am Heart J* 1988;16:1289–1297.
214. Thayer WS. The early diastolic heart sound. *Trans Assoc Am Phys* 1908;13:326–357.
215. Ross RS, Criley JM, Morgan RH. Cineangiography in mitral valve disease. *Trans Assoc Am Phys* 1961;74:271–279.
216. Oriol A, Palmer WH, Nakhjavan F, McGregor M. Prediction of left atrial pressure from the second sound-OS interval. *Am J Cardiol* 1965; 16:184–188.
217. Rahko PS, Shaver JA, Salerni R, et al. Echophonocardiographic estimates of pulmonary artery wedge pressure in mitral stenosis. *Am J Cardiol* 1985;55:462–469.
218. Tavel ME. Opening snaps: Mitral and tricuspid. In: Leon DF, Shaver JA, eds. *Physiologic Principles of Heart Sounds and Murmurs* (Monograph 46). New York: American Heart Association; 1975: 85–91.
219. Millward DK, McLaurin LP, Craige E. Echocardiographic studies to explain opening snaps in the presence of nonstenotic mitral valves. *Am J Cardiol* 1973;31:64–70.
220. Sloan AW, Campbell FW, Henderson AS. Incidence of the physiological third heart sound. *Br Med J* 1952;2:853–855.
221. Harvey WP, Stapleton J. Clinical aspects of gallop rhythm with particular reference to diastolic gallops. *Circulation* 1958;18:1017–1024.
222. Craige E. Gallop rhythm. *Prog Cardiovasc Dis* 1967;10:246–260.
223. Shaver JA, Reddy PS, Alvares FR. Early diastolic events associated with the physiologic and pathologic $S_3$. *J Cardiol* 1984;14(suppl V):30–46.

224. Shah PM, Jackson D. Third heart sound and summation gallop. In: Leon DF, Shaver JA, eds. *Physiologic Principles of Heart Sounds and Murmurs* (Monograph 46). New York: American Heart Association; 1975:79–84.
225. Reddy PS, Meno F, Curtiss EI, O'Toole JD. The genesis of gallop sounds: Investigation by quantitative phono- and apex cardiography. *Circulation* 1981;63:922–933.
226. Shaver JA, Reddy PS, Alvares RF, Salerni R. Genesis of the physiologic third heart sound. *Am J Noninvas Cardiol* 1987;1:39–55.
227. Abdulla AM, Frank MJ, Erdin RA Jr, Canedo M. Clinical significance and hemodynamic correlates of the third heart sound gallop in AR. *Circulation* 1981;64:464–471.
228. Stapleton JF. Third and fourth heart sounds. In: Horwitz LD, Groves BM, eds. *Signs and Symptoms in Cardiology*. Philadelphia: Lippincott; 1985:214–226.
229. Fowler NO, Adolph RJ. Fourth sound gallop or split first sound? *Am J Cardiol* 1972;30:441–444.
230. Spodick DH, Quary-Pigotti VM. Fourth heart sound as a normal finding in older persons. *N Engl J Med* 1973;288:140–141.
231. Harris A. Pacemaker "heart sound." *Br Heart J* 1967;29:608–615.
232. Lerman J, Means JH. Cardiovascular symptomatology in exophthalmic goiter. *Am Heart J* 1932;8:55–65.
233. Hamman L. Spontaneous mediastinal emphysema. *Bull Johns Hopkins Hosp* 1939;64:1–21.
234. Soffer A, Feinstein A, Luisada AA, et al. Glossary of cardiologic terms related to physical diagnosis and history. *Am J Cardiol* 1967;20:285–286.
235. Freeman AR, Levine SA. Clinical significance of systolic murmurs: Study of 1000 consecutive "noncardiac" cases. *Ann Intern Med* 1933; 6:1371–1385.
236. Norton P, O'Rourke RA. Cardiac murmurs. In: Goldman L, Braunwald E, eds. *Cardiology for the Primary Physician,* Second Edition. Philadelphia: Saunders; 2003:151–168.
237. Etchells E et al: Does this patient have an abnormal systolic heart murmur? *JAMA* 1997;277(7):564.
238. Mangione S, Nieman LZ: Cardiac auscultatory skills of internal medicine and family practice trainees. A comparison of diagnostic proficiency. *JAMA* 1997;278(9):717.
239. Murgo JP: Systolic ejection murmurs in the era of modern cardiology. What do we really know? *J Am Coll Cardiol* 1998;32:1596.
240. Gallavardin L, Ravault P. Le souffle du retrecissement aortique puet changer de timbre et devenir musical dans sa propagation apexienne. *Lyon Med* 1925;135:523–529.
241. Shaver JA. Systolic murmurs. *Heart Dis Stroke* 1993;2:9–17.
242. Murgo JP, Altobelli SA, Dorethy JF, et al. Normal ventricular ejection dynamics in man during rest and exercise. In: Leon DF, Shaver JA, eds. *Physiologic Principles of Heart Sounds and Murmurs* (Monograph 46). New York: American Heart Association; 1975:92–101.
243. Lembo NJ, Dell'Italia LJ, Crawford MH, O'Rourke RA. Bedside diagnosis of systolic murmurs. *N Engl J Med* 1988;318:1572–1578.
244. Stein PD, Sabbah HN. Aortic origin of innocent murmurs. *Am J Cardiol* 1977;39:665–671.
245. Shaver JA. Innocent murmurs. *Hosp Med* 1978;8–35.
246. deLeon AC Jr. "Straight back" syndrome. In: Leon DF, Shaver JA, eds. *Physiologic Principles of Heart Sounds and Murmurs* (Monograph 46). New York: American Heart Association; 1975:197–208.
247. Gamboa R, Hugenholtz PG, Nadas AS. Accuracy of the phonocardiogram in assessing severity of aortic and PS. *Circulation* 1964; 30:35–46.
248. Aronow WS, Kronzon I. Correlation of prevalence and severity of valvular aortic stenosis determined by continuous-wave Doppler echocardiography with physical signs of aortic stenosis in patients aged 62 to 100 years with aortic systolic ejection murmurs. *Am J Cardiol* 1987;60:399–401.
249. Vogelpoel L, Schrire V. Auscultatory and phonocardiographic assessment of pulmonary stenosis with intact ventricular septum. *Circulation* 1960;22:55–72.
250. Zuberbuhler JR, Lenox CC, Neches WH, et al. Auscultatory spectrum of the tetralogy of Fallot. In: Leon DF, Shaver JA, eds. *Physiologic Principles of Heart Sounds and Murmurs* (Monograph 46). New York: American Heart Association; 1975:187–192.
251. O'Rourke RA, Crawford MH. Mitral valve regurgitation. *Curr Probl Cardiol* 1984;9:1–52.
252. Karliner JS, O'Rourke RA, Kearney DJ, Shabetai R. Hemodynamic explanation of why the murmur of MR is independent of cycle length. *Br Heart J* 1973;35:397–401.
253. Rivero Carvallo JM. Signo para el diagnostico de las insufficiencias tricuspideas. *Arch Inst Cardiol Mex* 1946;16:531–540.
254. Wooley CF. The spectrum of TR. In: Leon DF, Shaver JA, eds. *Physiologic Principles of Heart Sounds and Murmurs* (Monograph 46). New York: American Heart Association; 1975:139–148.
255. Leatham A, Segal BL. Auscultatory and phonocardiographic findings in ventricular septal defect with left-to-right shunt. *Circulation* 1962; 25:318–327.
256. Leatham A. The spectrum of ventricular septal defect. In: Leon DF, Shaver JA, eds. *Physiologic Principles of Heart Sounds and Murmurs* (Monograph 46). New York: American Heart Association; 1975: 135–138.
257. Ronan JA Jr, Steelman RB, DeLeon AC, et al. The clinical diagnosis of acute severe mitral insufficiency. *Am J Cardiol* 1971;27:284–290.
258. Perloff JW, Roberts WC. The mitral apparatus: Functional anatomy of MR. *Circulation* 1972;46:227–239.
259. Braunwald E. MR. *N Engl J Med* 1969;281:425–433.
260. Rios JC, Massumi RA, Breesmen WT, Sarin RK. Auscultatory features of acute TR. *Am J Cardiol* 1969;23:4–11.
261. Amidi M, Irwin JM, Salerni R, et al. Venous systolic thrill and murmur in the neck: A consequence of severe tricuspid insufficiency. *J Am Coll Cardiol* 1986;7:942–945.
262. Burch GE, DePasquale NP, Phillips HJ. Clinical manifestations of papillary muscle dysfunction. *Arch Intern Med* 1963;112: 158–163.
263. Barlow JB, Bosman CK, Pocock WA, Marchand P. Late systolic murmurs and nonejection ("mid-late") systolic clicks. *Br Heart J* 1968;30:203–217.
264. Wigle ED, Sasson Z, Henderson MA, et al. Hypertrophic cardiomyopathy: The importance of the site and the extent of hypertrophy. A review. *Prog Cardiovasc Dis* 1985;28:1–83.
265. Shaver JA, Alvares RF, Reddy PS, Salerni R. Phonoechocardiography and intracardiac phonocardiography in hypertrophic cardiomyopathy. *Postgrad Med J* 1986;62:537–543.
266. Murgo JP, Miller JW. Hemodynamic, angiographic and echocardiographic evidence against impeded ejection in hypertrophic cardiomyopathy. In: Goodwin JF, ed. *Heart Muscle Disease*. Lancaster, England: MTP Press; 1985:187–211.
267. Shah PM. Controversies in hypertrophic cardiomyopathy. *Curr Probl Cardiol* 1986;11:563–613.
268. Shaver JA, Salerni R, Curtiss EI, Follansbee WP. A clinical presentation and noninvasive evaluation of the patient with hypertrophic cardiomyopathy. In: Shaver JA, Brest AN, eds. *Cardiomyopathies: Clinical Presentation, Differential Diagnosis, and Management* (Cardiovascular Clinics). Philadelphia: Davis, 1988:149–192.
269. Shaver JA. Diastolic murmurs. *Heart Dis Stroke* 1993;2:98–103.
270. Wood P. An appreciation of mitral stenosis. *Br Med J* 1954;1: 1051–1063.
271. Craige E. Phonocardiography in interventricular septal defects. *Am Heart J* 1960;60:51–60.
272. Fortuin NJ, Craige E. Echocardiographic studies of genesis of mitral diastolic murmurs. *Br Heart J* 1973;35:75–81.
273. Coombs CF. *Rheumatic Heart Disease.* New York: William Wood; 1924:190.
274. Flint A. On cardiac murmurs. *Am J Med Sci* 1862;44:29–54.
275. Craige E. The Austin Flint murmur. In: Leon DF, Shaver JA, eds. *Physiologic Principles of Heart Sounds and Murmurs* (Monograph 46). NewYork: American Heart Association; 1970:160–165.
276. Reddy PS, Curtiss EI, Salerni R, et al. Sound pressure correlates of the Austin Flint murmur: An intracardiac sound study. *Circulation* 1976; 53:210–217.

277. Rahko PS. Doppler and echocardiographic characteristics of patients having an Austin Flint murmur. *Circulation* 1991;83:1940–1950.
278. Green EW, Agruss NS, Adolph RJ. Right-sided Austin Flint murmur. *Am J Cardiol* 1973;32:370–374.
279. Harvey WP, Corrado MA, Perloff JK. "Right-sided" murmurs of aortic insufficiency. *Am J Med Sci* 1963;245:533–543.
280. Steell G. The murmur of high pressure in the pulmonary artery. *Med Chron* 1888;9:182–188.
281. Runco V, Molnar W, Meckstroth CV, Ryan JM. The Graham Steell murmur versus AR in rheumatic heart disease. *Am J Med* 1961;31: 71–80.
282. Perez JE, Smith CA, Meltzer VN. Pulmonic valve insufficiency: A common cause of transient diastolic murmurs in renal failure. *Ann Intern Med* 1985;103:497–502.
283. Runco V, Levin HS. The spectrum of pulmonic regurgitation. In: Leon DF, Shaver JA, eds. *Physiologic Principles of Heart Sounds and Murmurs* (Monograph 46). New York: American Heart Association; 1975:175–182.
284. Myers JD. The mechanisms and significances of continuous murmurs. In: Leon DF, Shaver JA, eds. *Physiologic Principles of Heart Sounds and Murmurs* (Monograph 46). New York: American Heart Association; 1975:201–208.

CHAPTER 13

# THE RESTING ELECTROCARDIOGRAM

Agustin Castellanos / Alberto Interian, Jr. / Robert J. Myerburg



What is commonly called an *electrocardiogram* (ECG) is the graph obtained when the electrical potentials of an electrical field originating in the heart are recorded at the body surface.[1–7] Although the ECG gives very useful clinical information, it provides only an approximation of the voltage produced by the source. The ECG has not been able to achieve many interesting new insights into its own *basic* theoretic limitations, which some have considered as the solutions of the "forward" problem and the "inverse" problem of electrocardiography.[2,3] Whereas the former seeks the description of a specific ECG pattern in response to a specific local or regional intracardiac change in electrical activity, the latter seeks to predict the behavior of the cardiac generator from potentials recorded at the body surface.[2,3] Nevertheless, recent experimental studies have provided new information capable of expanding the clinical usefulness of the ECG. The ECG has many uses: it may serve as an independent marker of myocardial disease; it may reflect anatomic, hemodynamic, molecular, ionic, and drug-induced abnormalities of the heart; and it may provide information that is essential for the proper diagnosis and therapy of many cardiac problems[4] (Chap. 28). *It is not only the most commonly used laboratory procedure for the diagnosis of heart disease but also one of the most commonly employed tests in medicine.*[4,6] *Furthermore, it is a required portion of the subspecialty boards in cardiovascular diseases that must be passed by those taking the certifying examination.* Underreading or misreading due to insufficient knowledge of pathologic conditions, overreading due to an inability to recognize technical errors, and—most important—failure to correlate ECG findings with clinical findings may result in iatrogenic heart disease.[4,6]

## VENTRICULAR DEPOLARIZATION AND REPOLARIZATION

To understand the electrical forces produced by the heart as a whole at the body surface, it has been conventional to first discuss the electrical properties of a hypothetical muscle strip from the free wall of the left ventricle (LV) extending from endocardium to epicardium.[1,2] In the resting or polarized state, the charges are at rest. A unipolar electrode facing the epicardial side of the strip, such as $V_6$, registers an isoelectric line.[1,2,7–12] If activation of this relatively large muscle strip starts in the endocardial side, it initiates the process called *depolarization*.[1,2,7–12] The *sequence* of this process is from endocardium to epicardium. Depolarization has been described as a moving wave *with the positive charges in front of the negative charges*. The previously mentioned lead $V_6$ overlying the epicardium of the LV will record a positivity because it consistently faces positive charges throughout the entire depolarization sequence. On the other hand, the *sequence* of ventricular repolarization is from epicardium to endocardium. The *negative charges,* however, travel *in front* because repolarization tends to reestablish the resting, polarized state of the previously depolarized cells. Accordingly, $V_6$ will record a positive deflection (T wave) because it constantly faces positive charges throughout the entire repolarization sequence. The earlier epicardial end of repolarization has been attributed to the shorter duration of repolarization that epicardial cells have in comparison with endocardial cells. Thus repolarization finishes at the epicardium while still incomplete at the endocardium. Hence the *sequence* of repolarization is, as noted previously, from epicardium to endocardium. This simplistic view is of didactic value only because it fails to take into consideration the role played by the M cells, described by Antzelevitch et al.[13] The M cells play a determining role in the inscription of the T wave because currents flowing down voltage gradients on either side of the usual (but not necessarily) midmyocardial cells determine both the height and width of the T wave as well as the degree to which the ascending or descending limbs of the T wave are interrupted.

## ELECTROCARDIOGRAPHIC LEADS

To record an ECG, an electrical circuit between the heart and the electrocardiograph must be completed.[11] For this purpose, electrodes are placed on different parts of the body surface and are connected to the instrument by means of cables.[1,12,14] Thus the whole system consists of an instrument, electrodes, cables, and leads.[1,12,13]

### Bipolar Limb Leads

An ECG lead can be defined as a pair of terminals with designated polarity, each of which is connected either directly or through a passive-active network to recording electrodes. In 1913, Einthoven et al. developed a method of studying the electrical activity of the heart by representing it graphically in a two-dimensional (2D) geometric figure—namely, an equilateral triangle.[1,2,12] Einthoven's hypothesis is based on several oversimplifying assumptions[12,14]: (1) The body is a homogeneous volume conductor. (2) The sum of all the electrical forces, or the mean of all the forces generated during the cardiac cycle, can be considered as originating in a dipole located in the electrical center of the heart. (3) Electrodes placed on the right arm (RA), left arm (LA), and left leg (LL) are used to pick up the potential variations on these extremities to form an equilateral triangle. Attachment between these limb electrodes, on the forearms and limbs, corresponds to a position in the root of the corresponding limb. The latter do not form a true geometric equilateral triangle, but they do so because the distances from the dipole to the extremities are great enough to approach "infinity." Consequently, when the electrodes are placed proximally to the roots of the extremities, they lose their relatively "far" distance from the heart and Einthoven's equilateral theory does not hold. This explains why leads used for exercise testing and intensive care monitoring, by being only "equivalent" to the corresponding bipolar leads, are in some cases markedly different from the "true" standard bipolar leads.

### Wilson Central Terminal

The sum of the potentials from the right arm (RA), left arm (LA), and left leg (LL) is equal to zero throughout the cardiac cycle with respect to any point at the body surface.[1,8–12] Lead wires attached to electrodes on each limb are connected together, through 5000-Ω resistors, at a point. When this common point (*Wilson's central terminal*) is attached to the negative pole of the ECG machine and an "exploring" electrode is connected to the positive pole, the potential variations recorded will be those of the latter only.[12] A lead taken by this method is called a *unipolar lead.* Actually, the central terminal is not zero, because the RA, LA, and LL are not equidistant from each other and from the heart, the body tissues vary in resistance, and the heart and extremities do not lie in exactly the same plane in the body. The potential of the central terminal has been said to average around 0.3 mV.[14] That the potential between right leg (RL) and LL is not zero becomes evident when the RA or LA electrodes are erroneously misplaced (interchanged with) the RL electrode (see section on "Artifacts").

### Unipolar Extremity Leads

At present, unipolar extremity leads are obtained by disconnecting the input to the central terminal of Wilson from the extremity being explored. This results in a 1½ increase in their voltage. These *augmented* (a) extremity leads are the ones usually used for clinical electrocardiography and are labeled aVR, aVL, and aVF.[1,2,11,12,14]

### Unipolar Precordial Leads

The unipolar precordial ECG is obtained by placing the exploring electrode (connected to the positive pole of the ECG machine) on the classic six locations of the anterior and left portions of the chest.[1,2,8–12] The central terminal is used as the indifferent electrode. Precordial (V) leads yield a positive deflection when facing positive charges and negative deflections when facing negative charges.[1,2,5,10–12] They do this according to what Wilson called the *solid-angle concept*.[1,8,11,12,15] A solid angle is merely an imaginary cone extending from a site in the chest throughout the heart. The precordial electrode is at its apex, and its base is at the opposite epicardial surface.[12] This concept is most important in understanding precordial lead morphologies. According to Wilson's scalar concept of ECG, this occurs because the solid angle subtended by the corresponding lead records the electrical activity from the regions of the heart over which the lead is placed as well as from distant regions.[5,8,12,15] Thus, if $V_2$ is placed over (thereby facing) the right ventricle (RV), part of the initial positive ventricular deflection reflects RV activation, with the corresponding electrical forces moving toward the electrode.[5,12,15]

Most portions of the terminal S wave represent activation of muscle other than the RV (septum and free left ventricular wall), reflecting electrical forces moving away from the electrode.[12,15] Acceptance that the amount of muscle activity recorded by various unipolar leads is not the same implies different "real" duration of depolarization and repolarization, irrespective of that supposedly resulting from the projections of a vector on an idealized horizontal lead axis (see sections on "QT Dispersion" and "Vectorcardiography"). For practical purposes, the peak of the r (or R) wave in precordial leads gives a rough estimate of the moment of arrival of excitation (*intrinsicoid* deflection) at the muscle underneath the electrode.[12] This encompasses a considerable number of muscle fibers (given by the solid-angle concept) greater than if the electrode is placed directly on the epicardial surface.[12] In the latter case, the moment of arrival of excitation at the electrode affects a lesser number of fibers and is thus given by the *intrinsic* deflection.[12,14]

## NORMAL ACTIVATION OF THE HEART: VENTRICULAR DEPOLARIZATION

In normal individuals, intervals between sinus beats show different degrees of variations because of respiration, blood pressure regulation, thermoregulation, actions of the renin-angiotensin system, circadian rhythms, premature beats, etc. (Fig. 13-1).[16–20] This has led to the analysis of so-called heart rate variability and heart rate turbulence (Chap. 27).[16–20] After emerging from the sinus node, the cardiac impulse propagates throughout the atria in its journey toward the atrioventricular (AV) node. The sequence of atrial depolarization occurs in an inferior, leftward, and somewhat posterior direction. The normal P waves are always positive in leads I, II, aVF, and $V_3$ to $V_6$ and negative in lead aVR.[1,11,12,14] According to the anatomic position of the heart, the P wave may be diphasic in $V_1$ and aVL or negative in the latter lead. Atrial repolarization, also called $T_a$, is directly opposite in polarity to the P wave.[8,11,12] It is usually not seen because it coincides with the PR segment and QRS complex. The PR interval (used to estimate AV conduction time) includes conduction through the "true" AV structures (AV node, His bundle, bundle branches, and main divisions of the left bundle branch) as well as through those

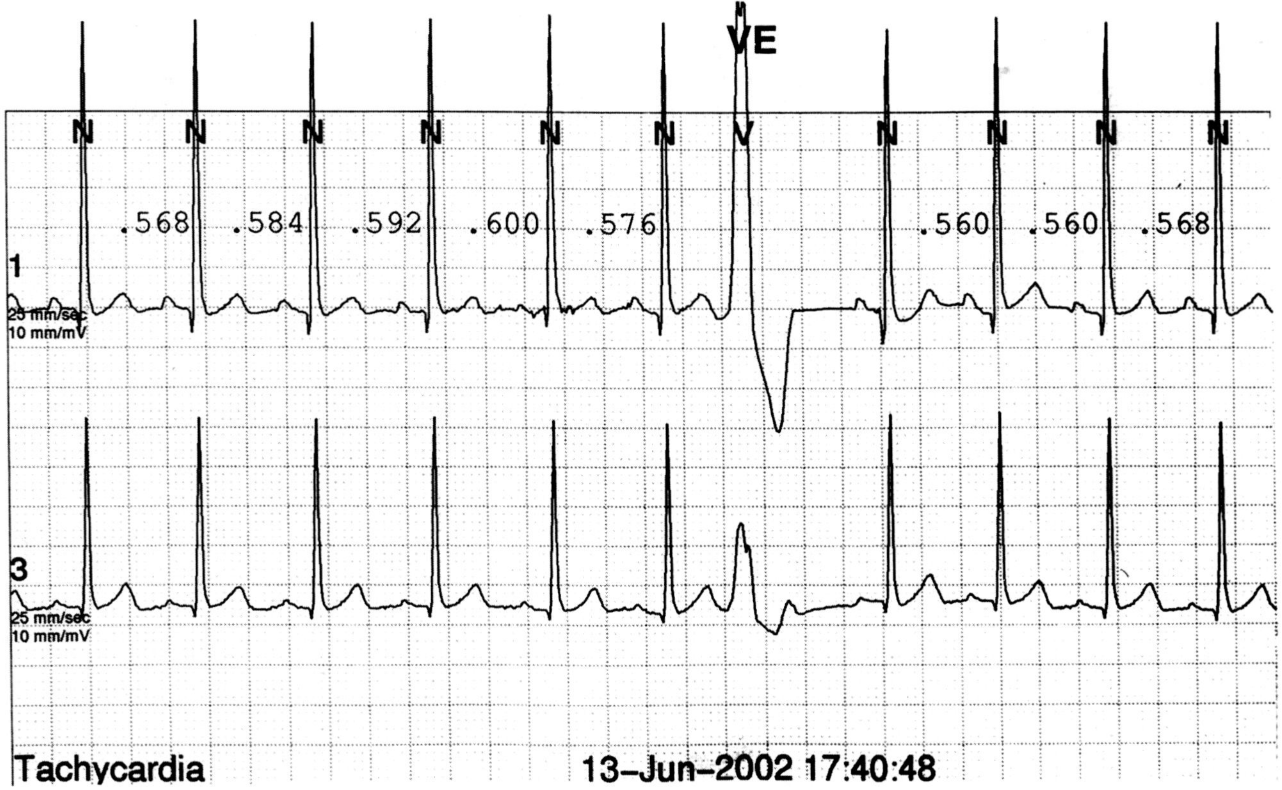


FIGURE 13-1 Rhythm strips showing that the RR intervals are slightly irregular even during sinus tachycardia (when sinus arrhythmia should not be marked). In addition, ventricular ectopic beats (VE) tend to affect (usually accelerate) the first two postextrasystolic intervals, a phenomenon known as *heart rate turbulence onset*.

parts of the atria located between sinus and AV nodes.[9] The onset of ventricular depolarization (given by the beginning of the normal q wave) reflects activation of the left side of the interventricular septum. This has been attributed to the fact that the left bundle system is shorter than the right bundle branch.[9,21] In addition, the large fanlike distribution of the ramifications of the fascicles of the left bundle branch on the left septal surface produces activation of a greater number of ordinary muscle cells per unit of time.[9,21] For this reason, the normal initial depolarization is oriented from left to right, therefore explaining the small q wave in lead $V_6$ and the small r wave in lead $V_1$. After the cardiac impulse descending through the right bundle branch reaches the right septal surface, the interventricular septum is activated in both directions. Septal activation is thereafter encompassed within or neutralized by free-wall activation.[8,9,11,12,14] The most distal ramifications of both bundle branches (Purkinje fibers) form networks within the subendocardial regions of both ventricular walls. The latter are activated as soon as the multiple ramifications emerge from the Purkinje fibers. The greater mass of the LV free wall explains why LV free-wall events overpower those of the interventricular septum and right ventricular free wall.

## ELECTRICAL AXIS

The *electrical axis* (EA) may be defined as a vector originating in the center of Einthoven's equilateral triangle.[8,11,12,14] When applied to the QRS complexes, the vector that represents it also gives the direction of the activation process as projected only in the (frontal) plane of the limb leads. Its length represents the manifest potential of the dipole in the center of the triangle. These general considerations apply either to the instantaneous EA (the vector indicating the direction of the impulse at the instant at which it is determined) or to the mean EA (which is the resultant of all instantaneous electrical axes). Although the term *EA* can be used in reference to any of the major components of the ECG (P, T, or QRS), it is generally applied to the QRS. There are many methods for determining the mean EA. The one recommended by electrocardiographers of the classic school consists of calculating the net areas enclosed by the QRS complex in leads I, II, and III.[1,2,7–12,14,22] One of the drawbacks of this method is that the absolute values of the net area cannot be determined *accurately* by inspection. A simpler though less precise method of calculating the quadrant (or parts of a quadrant) in which the EA is located consists of using the maximal QRS deflection in leads I and aVF and, when necessary, lead II. This method is inexact from the mathematical viewpoint but has the value of simplicity.[21–23]

## VENTRICULAR GRADIENT

The relationship between the EA of the QRS complex and the T wave was referred to by Wilson as the *ventricular gradient*.[22] In the isolated muscle strip, the *sequence* of ventricular depolarization occurs in the same direction as that of repolarization.[10,12] Although the QRS and T deflections have opposite polarity, the algebraic sum of QRS and T *areas* is zero. In the human heart, however, not only is the sequence different, but the pathways of ventricular depolarization and repolarization are not exactly the same. Thus the algebraic sum of QRS and T *areas* is no longer zero. Therefore, a *gradient* is said to exist.[10,12,23] The ventricular gradient *must* be calculated by determining the electrical axis of the QRS and T (using *areas*) and then obtaining the resultant by the parallelogram method (Figure 13-2, left). Its magnitude ranges between 8 and 88 $\mu$V/s with its direction being between −16 and +86 degrees in the frontal plane.[23] Although valid for the latter plane only, there are methods to calculate it in a spatial (tridimensional) space. Its main usefulness is the differentiation between primary and secondary changes in repolarization. Unfortunately, in practice, calculation of the ventricular gradient is difficult and time-consuming because it has to be determined by areas and not maximal amplitude.

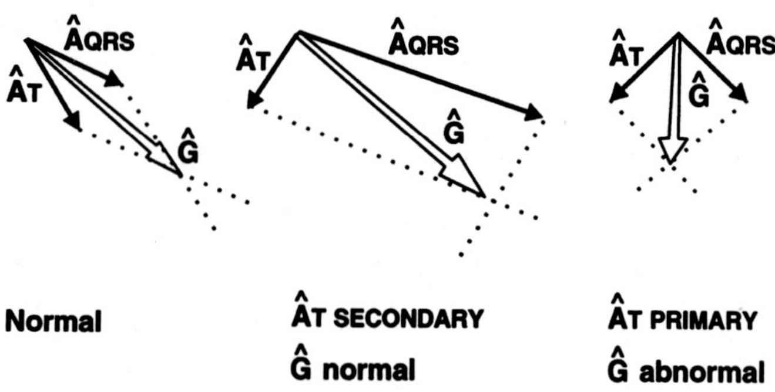


FIGURE 13-2 Ventricular gradient (Ĝ) calculated by areas of QRS complex and T waves in the frontal plane. Although the T vectors are abnormally located in the middle and right diagrams, secondary T-wave abnormalities do not produce an abnormally directed gradient, while primary abnormalities do.

## VENTRICULAR REPOLARIZATION

### Primary T-Wave Abnormalities

Primary T-wave abnormalities can be produced by a uniform change in the shape and/or the duration of all ventricular action potentials without a change in the sequence of repolarization or to nonuniform alterations in the shape and/or duration of the action potentials leading to an altered sequence of repolarization.[1,12,14] Figure 13-2, right, shows an abnormally located T vector with an abnormal gradient. This results from molecular, metabolic, or structural changes that induce alterations in repolarization having no dependence whatsoever on the sequence (and duration) of activation.

### Secondary T-Wave Abnormalities

Secondary T-wave abnormalities are generated mainly by changes in conduction and occur (for example) in left bundle branch block (LBBB) and RV pacing in leads with a predominant positive deflection (such as $V_6$), because repolarization (in contrast with what occurs normally) proceeds from endocardium to epicardium with negative changes in front.[1,10–12,14] Figure 13-2, middle, shows an abnormally oriented T vector with a normally located gradient.

### Pseudoprimary (?) T-Wave Changes, Cardiac Memory, Accumulation, and Dissipation

Rosenbaum et al.[24] studied the prolonged depolarization occurring during long periods of ventricular stimulation and found two types of altered ventricular repolarization. One, corresponding to Wilson's

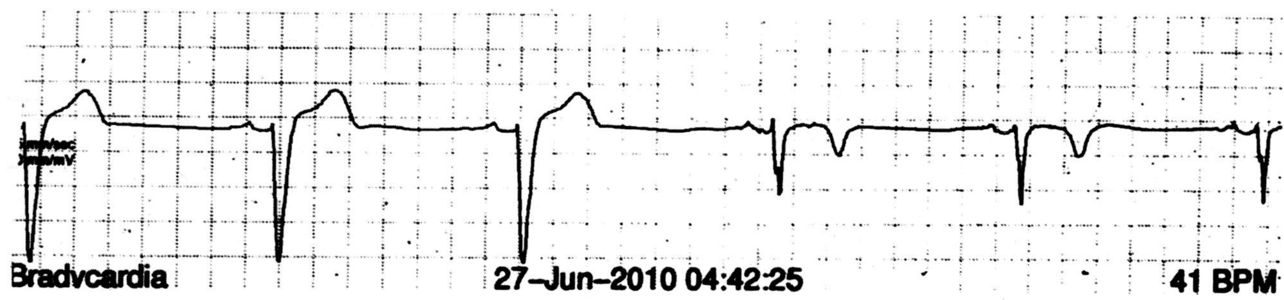


FIGURE 13-3 Rate-dependent complete LBBB (lead $V_1$). Negative T waves become manifest when the LBBB disappears in leads showing a predominant negative (S-wave) deflection. The patient had sclerodegenerative conduction system disease with no other evidence of organic heart disease.

classic theory, was transient and proportional in magnitude to the QRS complex but of opposite polarity.[24,25] The other, concealed by (but occurring during) the former, required a longer time to reach maximal effect—as well as to disappear—becoming apparent only when the ventricular complexes became narrow (Fig. 13-3).[24] They appeared to be modulated by electrotonic interactions occurring during cardiac activation in such a way that repolarization is accelerated at sites where depolarization starts and delayed in sites where depolarization ends.[24] Since in a single, static ECG the T waves seem to be primary (but occur only because the QRS complexes were previously wide, thus depending on this widening), Rosenbaum et al. categorized them as "pseudoprimary" (Fig. 13-3).[24,25] Moreover, considering that the ventricles were still "remembering" what had happened before, the concept of cardiac memory was used to categorize this form of electrophysiologic remodeling, characterized by (1) a T-wave vector having the same direction as that of the abnormally activated QRS complexes; (2) increased magnitude of this vector with repeated episodes of abnormal activation (accumulation); and (3) persistence of the abnormal T wave for variable periods (time to dissipation).[24–26]

Rosen defined the underlying mechanisms to be a likely variant on the same processes that determine memory in the central nervous system. Thus, cardiac memory can be classified as being of short, intermediate, or long-term duration.[26] These T-wave changes can be seen after disappearance of a variety of inciting events, such as complete LBBB, RV pacing, wide QRS tachycardias, and after spontaneous or radiofrequency-induced disappearance of preexcitation syndromes.[1,24–28] Interestingly, they have not been searched for or reported after disappearance of "complete" RBBB.[1]

## THE NORMAL QT INTERVAL

Although this interval has been considered as a surrogate of action potential duration, it yields a limited view of the complicated electrogenesis of ventricular repolarization.[29–32] The manual method of Lepeschkin and Surawicz consists of measuring from the beginning of the q wave to the end of the T wave, defined as the return to the isoelectric, or TP, baseline.[1,29] However, there are difficulties in determining the exact moment where the T wave ends in some leads, as when they are of low amplitude or merged with U (or even P) waves. Certain T-wave morphologies can also cause great difficulties.[1] Unfortunately, automatic measurements have not proven to be more reliable than human interpreters.[30] The most popular algorithm is the so-called tangent method, which defines the end of the T wave as the point in which one tangent drawn to the steepest portion of its terminal part crosses the isoelectric line.[30,31] For simplicity, when measured manually, a lead with a large T wave ($V_3$ has been said to be the best) and a distinct termination can be used, but obviously multichannel recordings are more helpful.[1,30,31] Some authors believe that QT intervals still can give useful information even if *during sinus rhythm* the QRS complexes are wide and accompanied by the obligatory, secondary T-wave changes.[7,32] For such cases Lepeschkin suggested that the "normal QRS duration for the heart rate must be subtracted from the actual QRS duration and the difference subtracted from the actual, total QT interval." This procedure yielded the "adjusted QT duration." On the other hand, studies performed when the QRS complexes were wide due to ventricular pacing from various sites at a different or the same time revealed that a pacing site-dependent change in ventricular activation in diffusely fibrotic hearts was able to produce varying degrees of differential prolongation of the QT intervals.[33] The latter were shorter during RV endocardial than during LV epicardial pacing, presumably in absence of abnormal action potential prolongation in these sites and without proportional changes in QRS duration. Different effects may occur in absence of severe myocardial disease[33] (see section on "Biventricular Pacing"). The QT interval is slightly longer in women than in men, is affected by autonomic tone as well as catecholamines, and it shows circadian variations.[1,30,32] Nevertheless, the most important aspect of this interval is its relation with heart rate.[32–48] Theoretically the task of describing the QT/RR relationship does not appear to be too complicated. Unfortunately the problem is far from simple.[31,35] This explains the large number of formulas that have been proposed to establish a rule allowing conversion of a pair of QT and RR durations into a standardized QTc value corresponding to a "basal" RR interval of 1 s. Bazett's is the most commonly used (in spite of its imperfection) formula, in which:

$$\text{QTc} = k\sqrt{\text{RR}} \text{ (in seconds)}$$

The $k$ value as modified is 0.397 for men and 0.415 for women. Values of 0.46 s for men and 0.47 s for women apply only when rates are within the normal range, since this formula tends to overcorrect at rapid rates and undercorrect at slower rates. Tables have been proposed by several authors with mean values ranging from 0.40 to 0.44 s at rates of 60/min and 0.31 to 0.34 s at rates of 100/min.[1,49] Whereas the uncorrected QT interval decreases with increasing rates including during exercise, the QTc first increases until reaching approximately a rate of 120/min, thereafter again decreasing.

Adjustment of the QT interval to changes in rate does not occur immediately but rather gradually. A steady state is not reached until

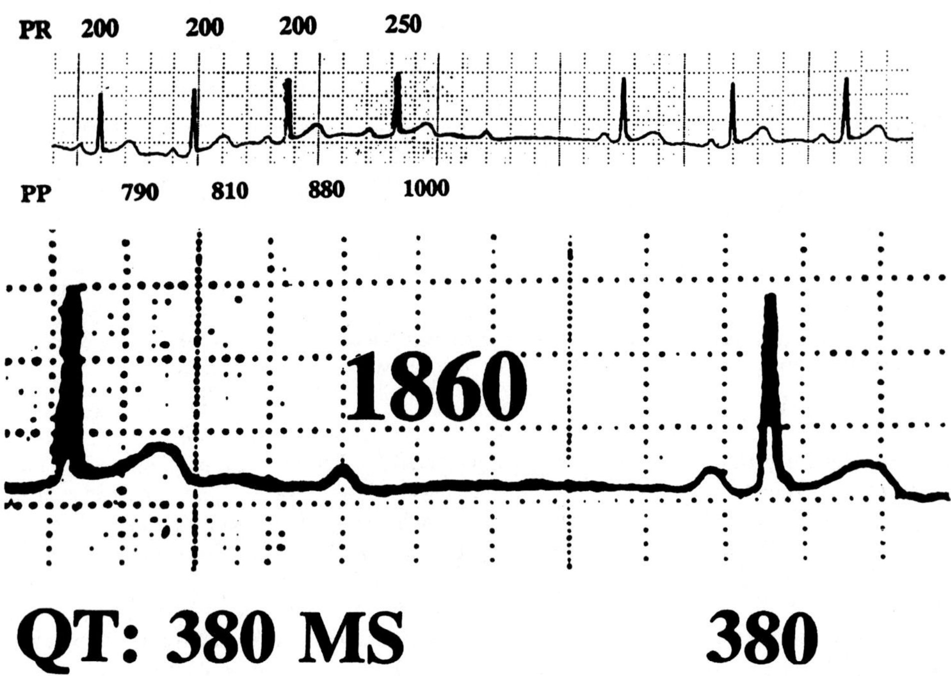


FIGURE 13-4 Vagally induced AV nodal block in a young person without structural heart disease. All values are expressed in milliseconds. The uncorrected QT interval does not increase at the end of an 1860-ms (RR) pause. This can be due to another form of cardiac memory, whereby the QT interval "remembers" its prepause values because of the slow adjustment to abrupt changes in cycle length due to cumulative effects of previous cycle lengths.

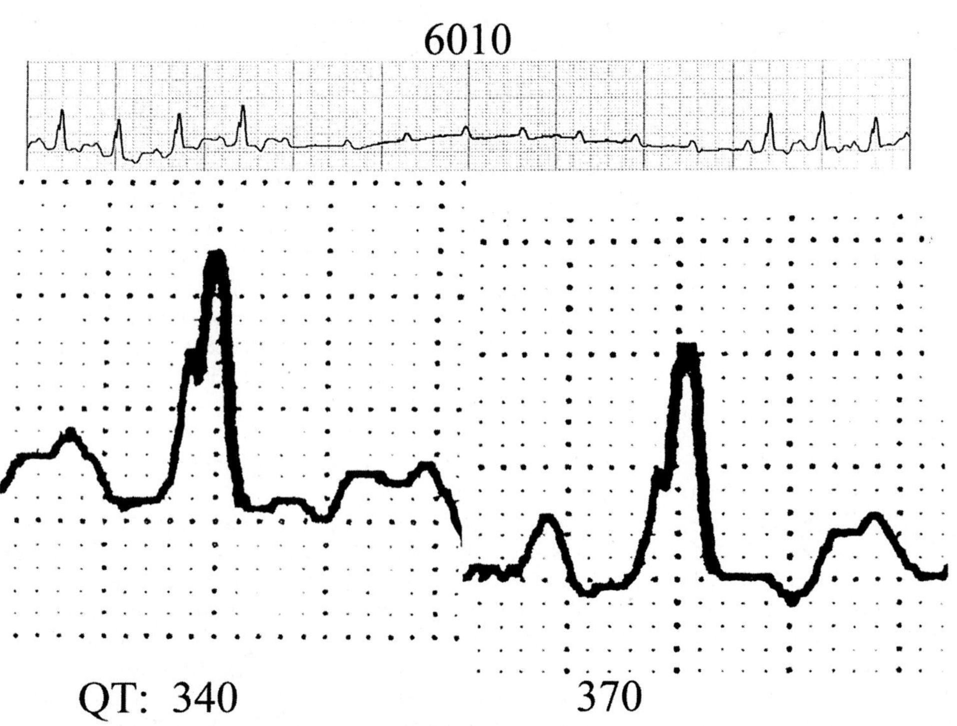


FIGURE 13-5 Lead I from a patient with complete LBBB due to sclerodegenerative conduction system disease without myocardial involvement. Note that a pause of 6010 ms due to paroxysmal AV block produces only a relatively small increment in the QT interval (30 ms) with restitution of the preblock duration in the second postpause beat. Magnified complexes on the bottom, left, and on bottom, right, correspond to the last preblock and the first postblock beats, respectively.

several cycles have elapsed. In normal subjects and even in persons with minimal myocardial abnormalities (with, mainly, conducting system disease) abrupt RR changes do not prolong the QT interval if the pauses are short (Fig. 13-4).[27,28,32,37,46,50,51] Longer pauses produce some prolongation but restitution tends to occur in the first postpause beat (Fig. 13-5).[32,37] Broadly interpreted, this behavior can be considered as that of another type of cardiac memory since the plateau currents seem to "remember" their previous status, due to the cumulative effects of previous cycle lengths or the influence of past history.[32,37,46,50,51] QT dispersion is discussed at the end of this chapter.

## THE ABNORMAL QT INTERVAL

Whereas shortening of the QT interval is discussed in the section on electrolytes, congenital and acquired causes of QT prolongation are dealt with in the corresponding chapters on arrhythmias.

## ST-SEGMENT CHANGES DUE TO ELECTROCARDIOGRAPHIC INJURY: MECHANISMS

The most common cause of acute abnormal ST-segment elevation in two consecutive leads is *physiologic* acute myocardial ischemia. The latter should not be necessarily equated with *electrocardiographic* ischemia, which is simply a pattern consisting of negative T waves symmetric in shape (Fig. 13-6). Severe physiologic ischemia shortens the action potential, reduces the resting membrane potential, and decreases the rate of rise of phase 0. The shortening and decreased amplitude of the action potential creates potential differences in voltage gradient between normal and ischemic regions, resulting in the systolic current injury. Conventionally, ST-segment changes have been explained by the existence of diastolic and systolic currents of injury. During the control (diastolic) period, both membrane resting potential and surface ECG baseline are at their normal level. At the onset of injury, the resting intracellular potential de-

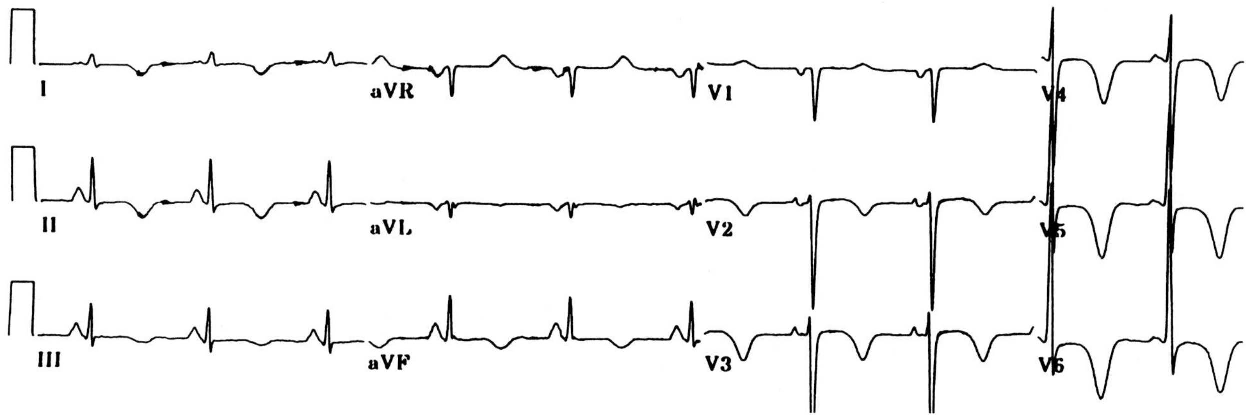


FIGURE 13-6 Pattern of electrocardiographic ischemia consisting of diffuse T-wave inversion and QT prolongation in all leads (except aVR) in a patient with acute intracerebral bleeding.

creases (e.g., from 90 to 70 mV), and the ECG baseline shifts below its preinjury level.[1,8,10–12,14,23,52–57] Because the injured cells leak negative ions, their exterior becomes relatively negative (or less positive) than that of the normal cells. Thus a "current of injury" flows between the negative ("injured") zone and the positive ("normal") region. This produces a negative displacement of the surface ECG baseline in the leads facing the injured region. In the surface ECG, depolarization (by virtue of the electrical negativization of the nonaffected area) practically reduces the potential difference between noninjured and injured regions. Therefore, the ST segment remains at the preinjury level, which is relatively elevated in reference to the injury baseline.[52–57] Consequently, the ST segment appears to be abnormally displaced above the latter so that the apparent presence of a systolic current of injury actually reflects disappearance of the diastolic current of injury. Finally, after the end of repolarization, the current of injury between injured and noninjured regions is reestablished, and the ECG baseline is again depressed (as it was immediately before depolarization). The abnormal ST-segment elevation in leads facing the affected zone does not merely represent the (passive) return of the baseline to its preinjury level but reflects a true, active, positive displacement.[1,14,52] Thus, when depolarization of both normal and injured regions has occurred, the surface of the normal cells will (on account of their greater initial polarization) be able to accumulate more negative ions so that the normal regions become more negative than the injured regions, which are relatively more positive. In consequence, the ST segment becomes actively elevated above and beyond the preinjury baseline because of the relative potential difference existing at the end of depolarization. Most likely, injury reflects both disappearance of diastolic baseline shifts and active ST-segment elevation.[1,2,7,8,10–12,14] One of the most important postulates in clinical ECG is that the *injury vector points toward the injured zone:* the epicardium in epicardial and transmural injury and the endocardium in subendocardial injury. Reciprocal changes occur in the (spatial) contralateral parts of the heart.

## LOCALIZATION OF THE AFFECTED SITES BY ANALYSIS OF LEADS SHOWING ABNORMAL ST-SEGMENT ELEVATION

In ECG interpretation and for the purpose of categorization, ST-segment elevation in leads I and aVL indicate anterolateral injury; in $V_1$, $V_2$, and $V_3$ anteroseptal injury; $V_4$, $V_5$, and $V_6$ apical or lateral injury; II, III, and aVF inferior injury, right-sided precordial leads (and occasionally in $V_1$, $V_2$, and $V_3$) RV injury.[1,2,10,12,53,54] Likewise, ST-segment depression in anterior leads may be reciprocal to ST-segment elevation (injury) in the posterior or posterolateral wall.[53,54] Importantly, the first ECG recorded from a patient with a new ST-segment elevation MI can also give information regarding the degree, size, and site of the injury (that is, of physiologic ischemia) as well as not only of the involved coronary artery but of the more proximal or distal affected site as discussed extensively in Chap. 53 and in a limited fashion in Figs. 13-7 to 13-9.[10,11,53–55]

## ABNORMAL Q WAVES

For abnormal Q waves to appear, the number of affected cells has to be large enough to produce changes reflected at the body surface. In general, the depth of the Q wave is proportional to wall-thickness involvement.[8,10–12,14] Thus, a QS complex is said to reflect transmural necrosis. On the other hand, clinical myocardial infarction (MI)

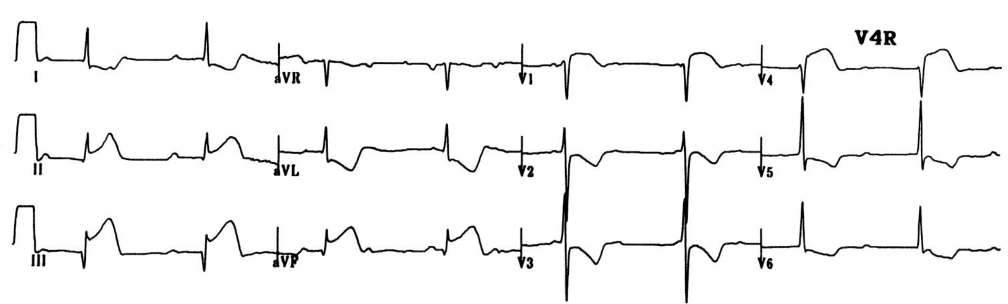


FIGURE 13-7 Acute inferior (diaphragmatic) injury showing ST-segment elevation in the inferior leads as well as in $V_1$ and $V_{4R}$ (due to right ventricular infarction). There are reciprocal changes from $V_2$ to $V_6$ as well as an AV junctional rhythm due to complete AV block. These changes were caused by proximal right coronary artery occlusion.

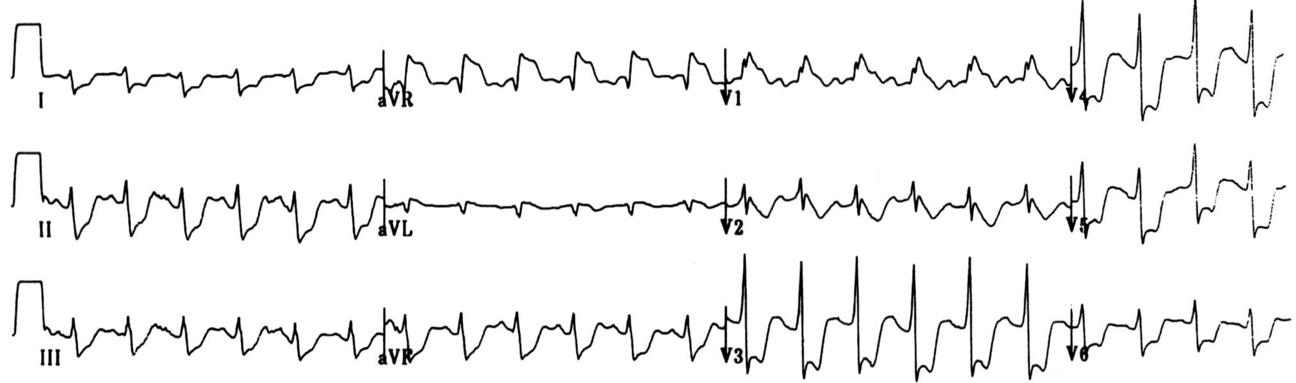


FIGURE 13-8 **Changes produced by occlusion of the left main coronary artery. Note RBBB with ST-segment elevation in aVR greater than in $V_1$ (features of an occlusion proximal to the first septal branch). There is extensive ST-segment depression in all other leads, with an injury vector pointing superiorly and to the right, indicating predominant severe posterobasal physiologic ischemia.**

without abnormal Q waves was categorized as subendocardial infarction. Presently, MIs are no longer classified as transmural or subendocardial (but as Q or non-Q MIs).[56] The duration of the Q wave is proportioned to the extent of the area of necrosis parallel to the epicardial surface. If the latter is large enough, starts in the subendocardium, and extends toward (but not quite reaching) the epicardium, the corresponding unipolar leads will record QR or Qr complexes, depending on the amount of living tissue located between dead tissue and the recording electrode. Therefore abnormal Q waves may occur in MIs that are not completely transmural.[8,14,56] The following changes have been said to be equivalent to Q waves in non-Q-wave MI: R/S ratio changes, acute frontal plane right axis deviation, new left axis deviation or LBBB, initial and terminal QRS notching, and some types of "poor r-wave progression."[56] Abnormal Q waves also can occur transiently in unstable angina, Prinzmetal's angina, coronary artery spasm (without chest pain), and exercise-induced ischemia. This has been attributed to an intensity of cellular affectation ("injury") severe enough to produce a significant degree of hypopolarization capable of rendering them electrically unexcitable (even though they are not anatomically, irreversibly necrotic).[8,9,21,57,58] Spontaneous recanalization of an occluded vessel, spontaneous reversion of the ischemia, or spasm and interventions (pharmacologic or mechanical) that improve cellular metabolism and oxygenation can restore the normal polarization. If these cells become again excitable, the abnormal Q waves may disappear or vanish.[57,58] Ischemic necrosis usually takes longer to appear than the accelerated abnormal Q waves seen in most patients with Q-wave MI after successful thrombolysis or effective coronary artery angioplasty performed early in its course.[59] The genesis of these Q waves is not well understood.[59,60] Some authors consider them an expression of the acceleration of necrosis secondary to explosive cell swelling in already irreversibly injured tissue.[58] Because some of these Q waves also tend to disappear quickly, other authors consider that they reflect factors other than myocardial necrosis, such as reversal of regional dysmetabolism or the occurrence of transient interstitial ischemia or hemorrhage.[59] Profound and prolonged ischemia can cause myocardial stunning with reversible functional, metabolic, ultrastructural, and electrophysiologic abnormalities.[61] Thus transient Q waves may be the ECG counterpart (electrical stunning) of the corresponding mechanical stunning.[58–61] Myocardial stunning often lags behind electrical recovery.[58] Myocardial *stunning* should be differentiated from myocardial *hibernation*. The latter is a term used in reference to

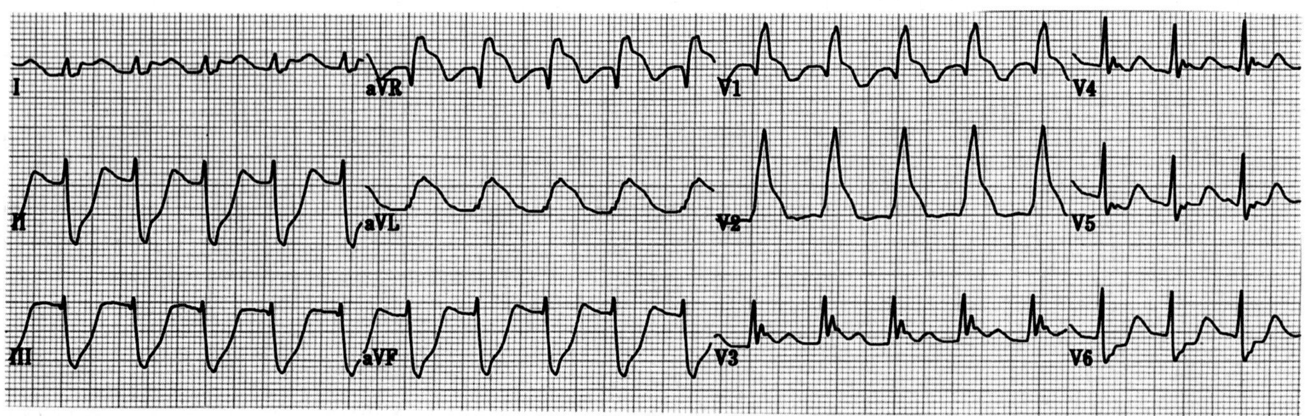


FIGURE 13-9 **Changes produced by occlusion of the proximal left anterior descending coronary artery. Note RBBB with ST-segment elevation in aVR greater than in $V_1$. The ST segment is also elevated in leads I and aVL, depressed in II, III, aVF, $V_5$, and $V_6$, with an injury vector pointing superiorly and to the left.**

mechanical dysfunction of an ischemic area that is not transient but chronic.[62,63] The ECG counterpart of this type of mechanical dysfunction requires further study.

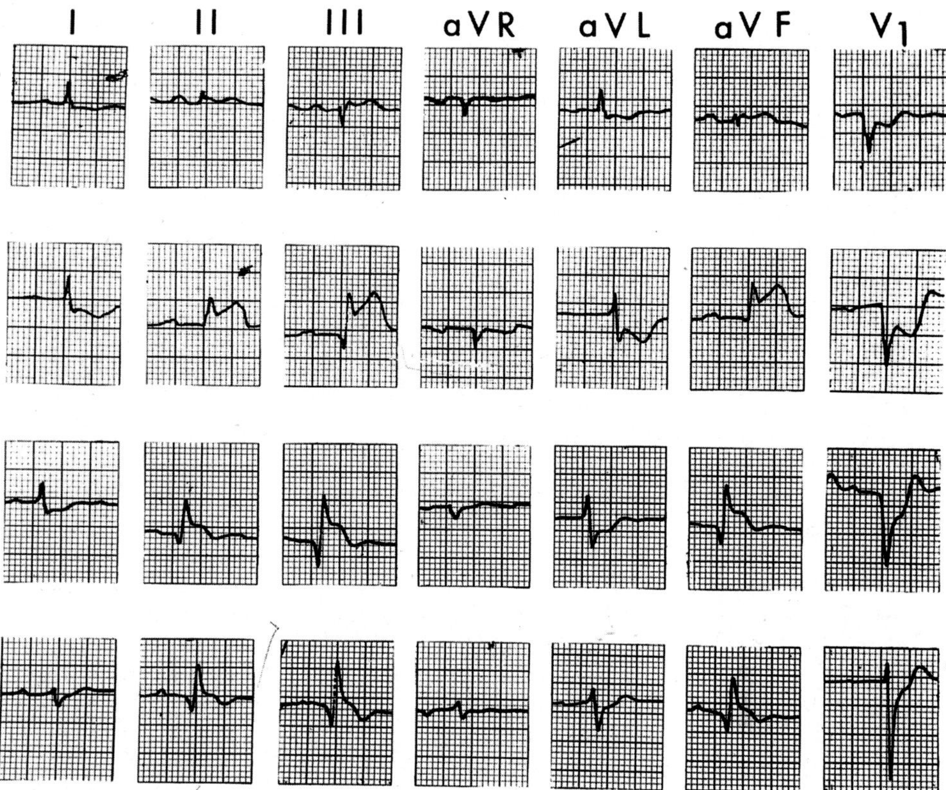


FIGURE 13-10 Spontaneous evolution of an acute inferior wall myocardial infarction in the preinterventional era, varying from isolated ST-segment changes on admission (*top strip*) to the development of abnormal Q waves, slight ST elevation, and negative T waves in the bottom strip. The latter also shows slight right axis deviation, which could be due to left posterior fascicular block.

## ACUTE MI

The "classic" ECG evolution of acute MI has been drastically transformed by relatively recently introduced laboratory studies, pharmacologic therapies, and interventional techniques. The succession of events in a course in what ends up as a Q-wave MI is from hyperacute T waves (on occasion) to ST-segment elevation to abnormal Q waves to T-wave inversion (Figure 13-10).[1–12,67,68] Commonly two or more of these findings appear together, depending on the timing of the first recorded static ECG. Acceleration of these phases is now common with intentional effective reperfusion.[60–67] The time course of regression of ST-segment elevation is a good predictor of reperfusion.[59] Because older 12-lead ECG studies on ST-segment evolution were based almost exclusively on static recordings obtained at fixed intervals, it became clear that continuous ECG monitoring (Chap. 33) was useful in evaluating the occurrence of reperfusion (Fig. 13-11).[68,69] In general, de Lemos and Braunwald support the hypothesis that ST-segment resolution is an acceptable surrogate for tissue-level reperfusion.[59] They accept that when "complete" ST resolution is seen 90 min after fibrinolysis, successful reperfusion has occurred at both epicardial and microvascular levels and prognosis is "excellent."[59] Persistent ST-segment elevation suggests either an occluded infarct-related artery or a patent artery with failure of myocardial and microvascular reperfusion.

### Location of Q-Wave MI

The Committee on Nomenclature of Myocardial Wall Segments of the International Society of Computerized Electrocardiography recommended adopting a 12-segment LV subdivision based on the works of Selvester et al.[1,11,70] The six most common locations of MI given are (1) large anterior, (2) anteroseptal, (3) anteroapical, (4) anterolateral, (5) inferior, and (6) posterior.[1,11]

### Right Ventricular MI

According to Braat et al.,[71] an ST-segment elevation of at least 1 mm in lead $V_{4R}$ in patients with *acute inferior MI* had a sensitivity of 100 percent, a specificity of 87 percent, and a predictive accuracy of 92 percent for the diagnosis of right ventricular infarction in patients with ST-segment elevation in leads II, III, and aVF (Fig. 13-7). In addition to $V_{4R}$, ST-segment elevation can be seen in leads $V_{5R}$ and $V_{6R}$ and in some cases (with decreasing amplitude) in $V_1$, $V_2$, and even $V_3$ (Chap. 53).

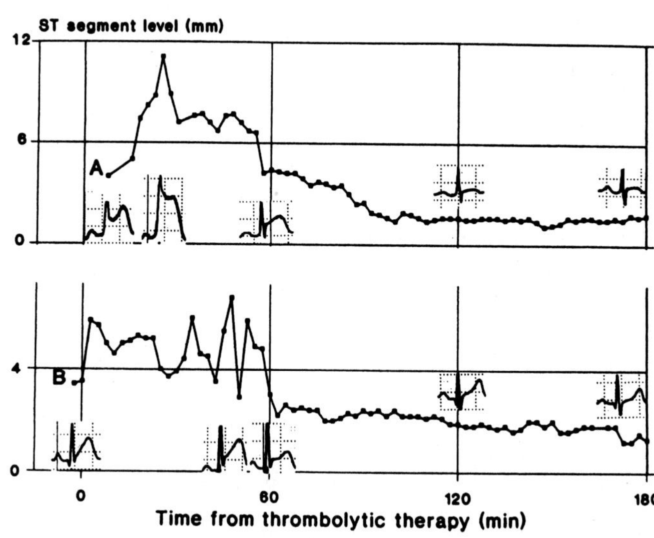


FIGURE 13-11 Plots of ST-segment levels versus time from therapy in two selected patients with patency of the infarct-related vessel at 60 min. Note that a 50 percent decrease in ST-segment levels within 60 min occurred only when measurements were made from the peak ST-segment level (highest ST-segment level measurement within the first 60 min).

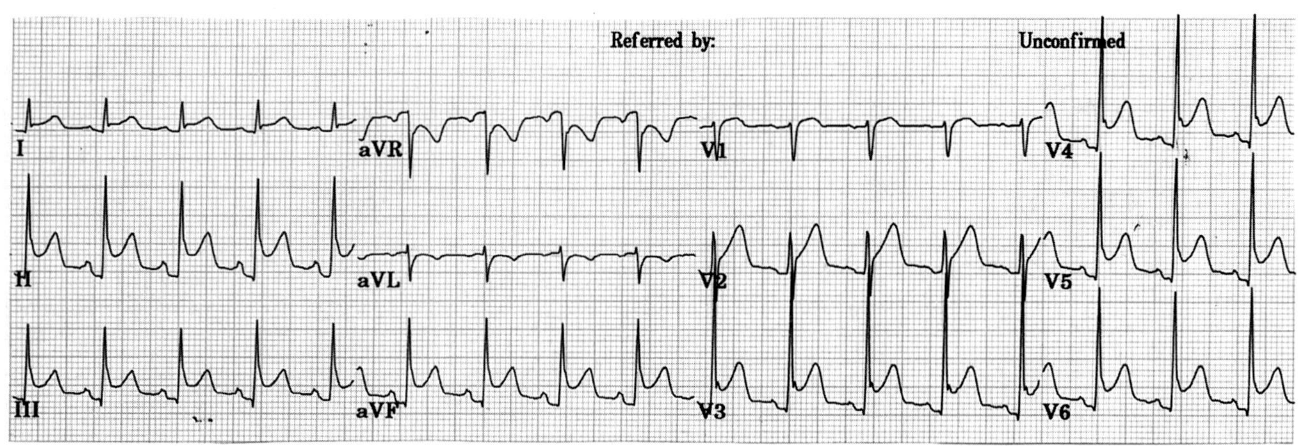


FIGURE 13-12 Acute nonspecific pericarditis showing ST-segment elevation in all leads except aVR and $V_1$.

## PERICARDITIS

In pericarditis, ST segments can be elevated in all leads except $aV_R$ and, rarely, in $V_1$ (Fig. 13-12). Symmetric T-wave inversion (due to epicardial "ischemia") usually develops after the ST segments have returned to the baseline (but can appear during the injury stage).[1] Neither reciprocal ST-segment changes nor abnormal Q waves are seen. In most cases of acute pericarditis, the PR segment is depressed (Fig. 13-12). Average ECG resolution occurs in close to 2 weeks.[72] In some young individuals the pattern of acute pericarditis can be difficult to differentiate from that of the normal variant referred to as *early repolarization* (Chap. 80).

## EARLY REPOLARIZATION

ST-segment elevation also results from the benign "early repolarization" pattern, a normal variant[73,74] (Fig. 13-13). In its classic form, there is J-point elevation (of no more than 3 mm) with an upwardly concave ST segment. R waves may be tall and at times have a distinct notch and slur on the downstroke (Fig. 13-13). ST-segment elevation is more frequent in chest leads but can occur in leads I and II. These dynamic ECG changes may be affected by exercise and hyperventilation. Isoproterenol reduces and propranolol increases ST-segment elevation.[74,75]

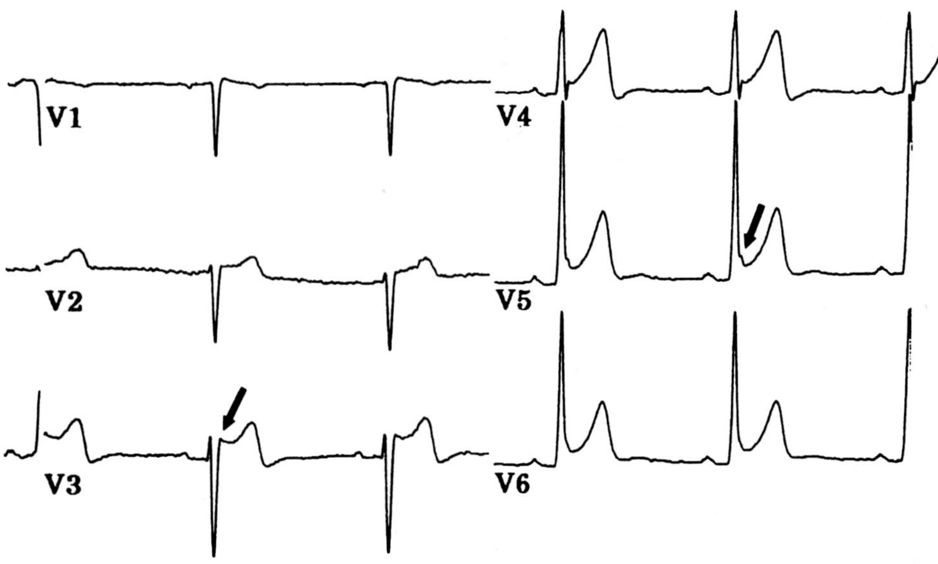


FIGURE 13-13 Early repolarization. This normal variant is characterized by narrow QRS complexes with J-point and ST-segment elevation in the chest leads. Left chest leads often show tall R waves with a distinct notch or slur in their downstroke (arrow in $V_5$), while the right chest leads may display ST segments having a "saddleback" or "humpback" shape (arrow in $V_3$).

## SELECTIVE NONISCHEMIC ST-SEGMENT ELEVATION IN THE RIGHT PRECORDIAL LEADS

The foremost cause is the Brugada syndrome, which is a familial disease causing ventricular fibrillation.[76,77] ECG abnormalities constituting the hallmark of this entity have recently been proposed by a consensus report.[78] They occur in absence of identifiable structural heart disease or electrolyte abnormalities. The three types of dynamic repolarization abnormalities are shown in Figs. 13-14 and 13-15.[78] The QT interval is usually normal but can be prolonged.[78,79] Strong Na channel blocking drugs can produce ST-segment elevations even in patients without any evidence of syncope or ventricular fibrillation.[80] The changes produced by potassium (dyalizable current of injury) are discussed in the section of hyperkalemia. Very slight ST-segment elevation with an incomplete RBBB pattern showing an epsilon wave has been described in arrhythmogenic right ventricular dysplasia[81] (Fig. 13-15). Negative T waves (not due to a "juvenile" pattern) are seen in leads $V_1$, $V_2$, and $V_3$.

## NONSPECIFIC ST-SEGMENT–T-WAVE CHANGES

It seems more appropriate to discuss ST-segment and T-wave changes separately, although they occur together most frequently (Fig. 13-16). While nonspecific (or rather, nondiagnostic) ST-segment–T-wave changes are the most commonly diagnosed ECG abnormalities, they have not been categorized adequately and represent different findings for various interpreters.[82,83] In the classic paper, Friedberg and Zager[82] considered depth of ST-segment depression and T-wave inversion as well as their contour (Fig. 13-16). When analyzed without clinical information, this diagnosis was made in 40 percent of 410 abnormal ECGs. The number was reduced to 10 percent, however, when clinical data became available. In the absence of structural heart disease, these changes can be due to a variety of physiologic (i.e., hyperventilation, anxiety, body position, food, neurogenic influences, and temperature), pharmacologic (i.e., antiarrhythmic and psychotropic drugs, digoxin), and extracardiac (i.e., electrolyte abnormalities, upper gastrointestinal processes, allergic reactions, etc.) factors.

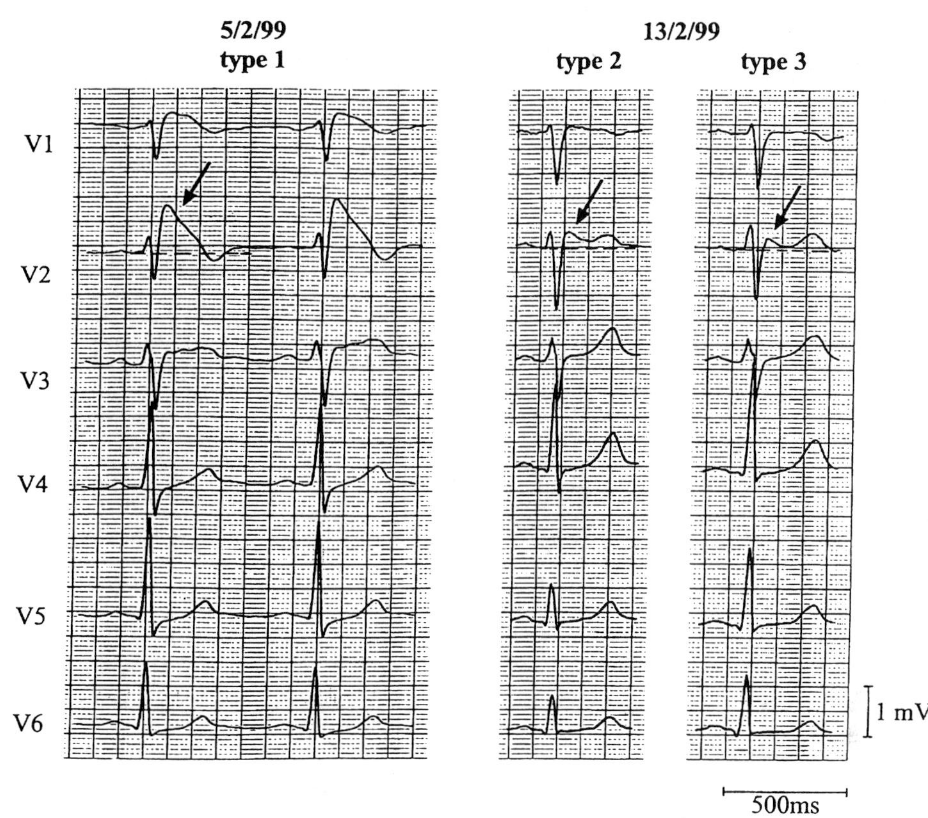


FIGURE 13-14 The three types of repolarization patterns proposed in the Consensus Report.[78] Type 1 is characterized by a prominent coved ST-segment elevation displaying a J wave or ST segment ≥2 mm at its peak followed by a negative T wave with little or no isoelectric separation. Type 2 also has a high takeoff ST elevation with J-wave amplitude ≥2 mm, giving rise to descending ST-segment elevation followed by a T wave with a saddleback configuration. Type 3 shows ST-segment elevation of <1 mm of saddleback type, coved type, or both. (From Wilde et al.[78] Reproduced with permission.)

## ST-SEGMENT DEPRESSION DURING SUPRAVENTRICULAR TACHYCARDIAS

Marked ST-segment depression can occur during paroxysmal supraventricular tachycardias in young individuals and even children.[84] Their mechanism probably differs from that producing posttachycardia T-wave changes, which are seen when sinus rhythm is reestablished. Figure 13-17 is an example occurring when the rate was 214/min. Note that the ST vector is pointing superiorly, posteriorly, and to the right, indicating severe injury. Lactate studies in cases similar to this showed no evidence of physiologic metabolic MI in spite of the resemblance to the changes observed in main left coronary artery disease occlusion (Fig. 13-8). These changes probably reflect rapid-rate, incomplete filling–related, purely electrical injury due to differences in action potential duration between subendocardium and epicardium.

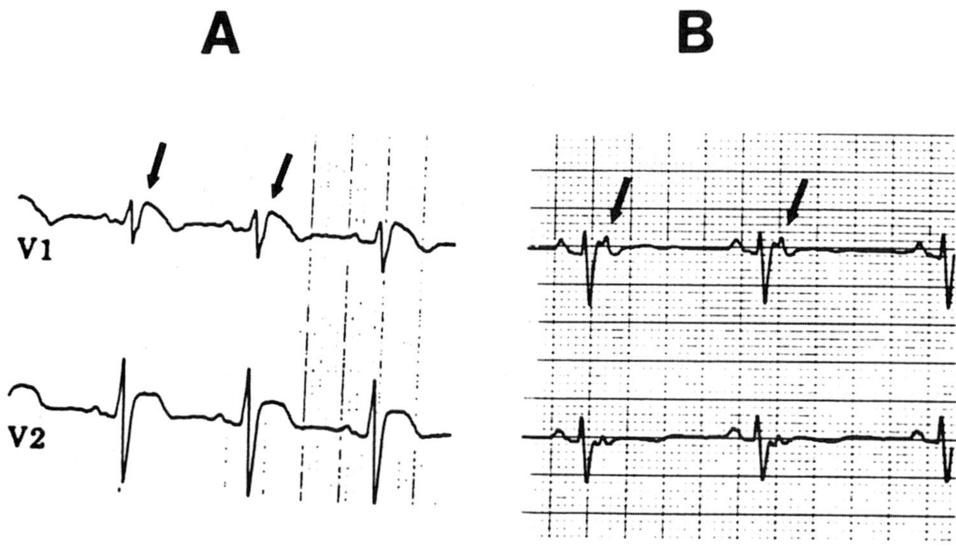


FIGURE 13-15 *A.* Nonischemic ST-segment elevation in the right precordial leads in a young patient with the Brugrada syndrome. *B.* Epsilon wave of a patient with arrhythmogenic right ventricular dysplasia.

## FASCICULAR BLOCKS

### Left Anterior Fascicular Block

Criteria for the diagnosis of uncomplicated left anterior fascicular block

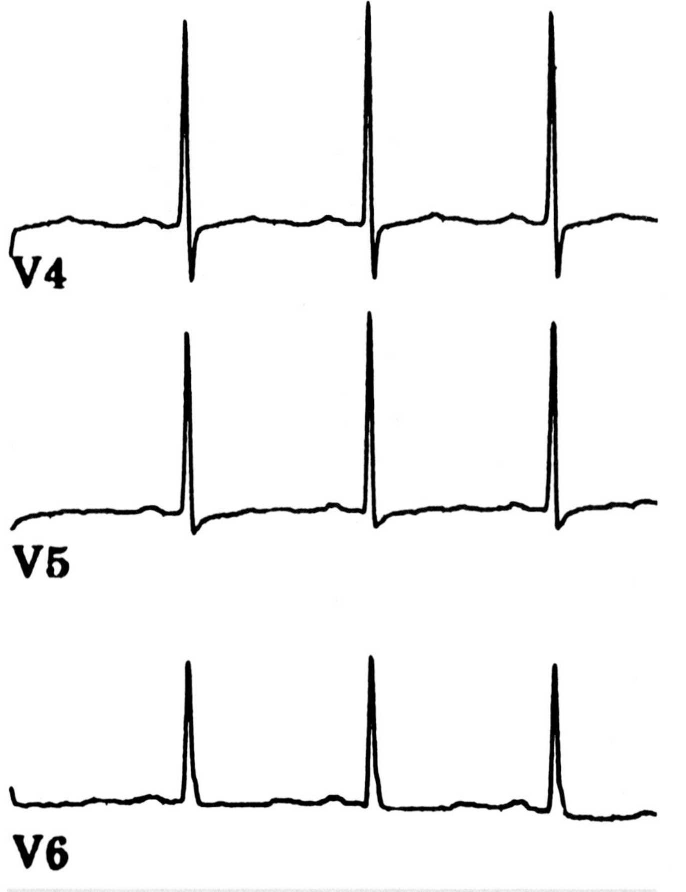


FIGURE 13-16 Nonspecific (nondiagnostic) ST-segment–T-wave changes, the most common abnormalities in ECG interpretation.

TABLE 13-1 Criteria for Diagnosis of Pure Left Anterior Fascicular Block

1. Abnormal left-axis deviation (usually between −45 and −60°), but right superior axis deviation can occur with atypical right bundle-branch blocks or extensive anterolateral myocardial infarction (Fig. 13-19*C*)
2. rS complexes in leads II, III, and aVF and qR complexes in leads I and aVL
3. Delayed intrinsicoid deflection in leads I and aVL
4. Peak of r wave in lead III occurring earlier than peak of r wave in lead II
5. Peak of R wave in lead aVL occurring earlier than peak of R wave in aVR
6. Exclusion of other causes of abnormal left axis deviation (Fig. 13-18)

SOURCE: From Castellanos and Myerburg[21] and Milliken,[88] with permission.

(LAFB) are given in Table 13-1 and Fig. 13-18, top. The constant feature of the axis deviation produced by LAFB is its *superior* orientation, not its superior and leftward orientation (abnormal left axis deviation).[9,21,85–89] Because of the multiple interconnections between the fascicles of the LBB system, the appearance of LAFB does not increase QRS duration by more than 0.025 s.[8] Therefore an LAFB pattern with a wider QRS complex generally indicates the presence of additional conduction disturbances such as RBBB, MI, or nonspecific intraventricular conduction delays due to free wall fibrosis.[9,21,85–89]

## Left Anterior Fascicular Block Coexisting with MI

The ECG changes imposed by MIs of different locations on LAFB are shown in Fig. 13-19.[9,21]

## Left Posterior Fascicular Block

In pure left posterior fascicular block (LPFB), the impulse emerges from the unblocked anterosuperior division, thus producing small q waves in leads II, III, and aVF[9,21](Fig. 13-20, top). Thereafter, the impulse moves through the electrically predominant LV in an inferior and rightward direction, thus explaining the S waves in leads I and aVL as well as the R waves in leads II, III, and aVF.[9,21,85] The degree of right axis deviation produced by pure LPFB is of lesser magnitude than that of left axis deviation produced by LAFB.[9,21,85] The hall-

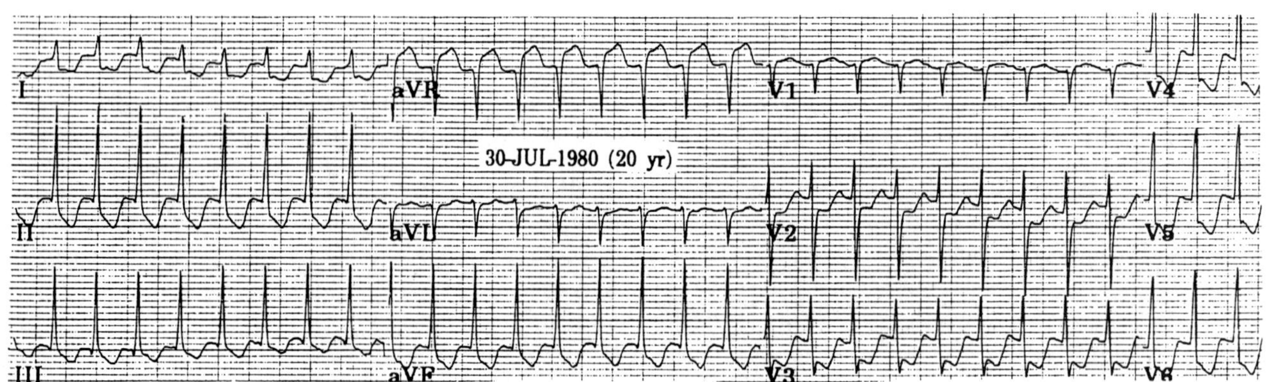


FIGURE 13-17 Paroxysmal supraventricular tachycardia. Marked ST-segment depression in an otherwise normal 20-year-old female presumably not due to physiologic (metabolic) ischemia but to predominantly a rate-related ECG injury, which could have been produced by differential duration and morphologies of endocardial and epicardial action potentials.[84]

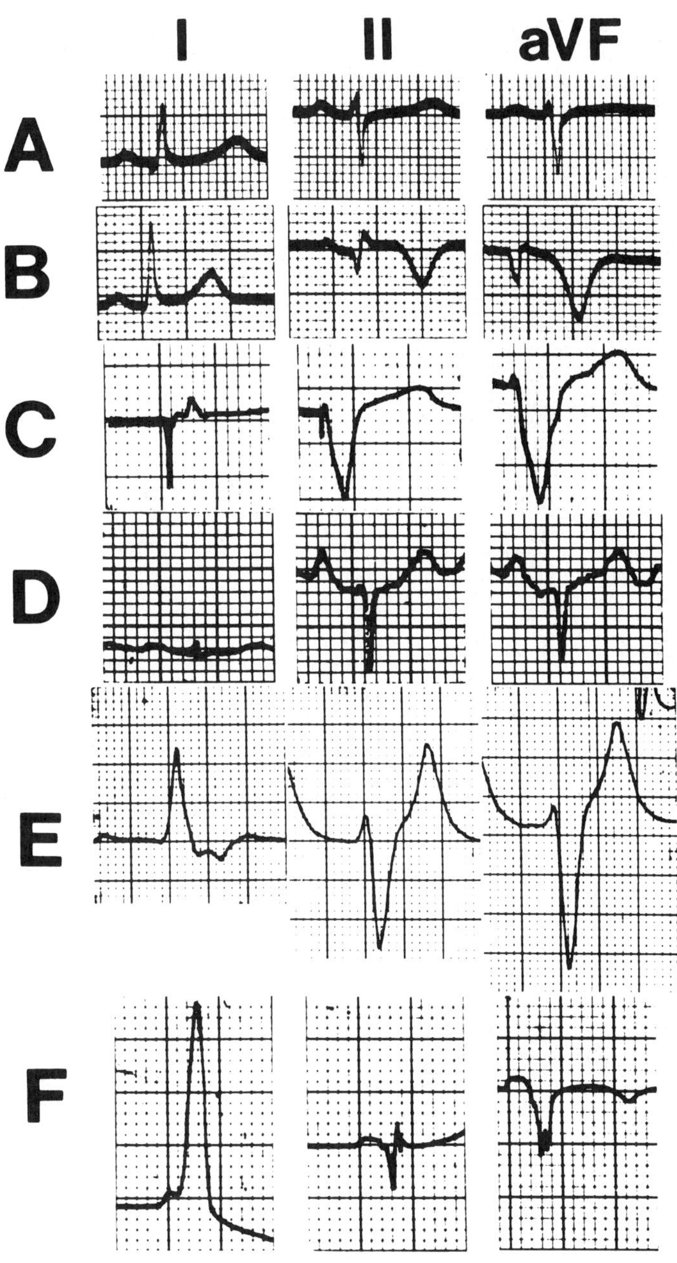


FIGURE 13-18 Causes of abnormal left axis deviation. *A*. Left anterior fascicular block. Note rS complexes in II and aVF. *B*. Extensive inferior wall MI showing Qr complexes in II. *C*. pacing from the spatial inferior regions of the heart, as from the right ventricular apex and middle cardiac or inferior or posterolateral veins. *D*. Rare cases of pulmonary emphysema with very low voltage in lead I and "P pulmonale." *E*. Hyperkalemia. *F*. Ventricular preexcitation due to posteroseptal accessory pathways.

mark of LPFB, therefore, is an "inferior" axis shift as much as a "right" axis deviation. Because a similar sequence of ventricular activation can also occur in RV hypertrophy, pleuropulmonary disease (acute or chronic), and extremely vertical anatomic heart positions due to a slender body build or chest wall deformities, it is evident that the diagnosis of "pure" LPFB cannot be made from the ECG alone. Additional clinical, ECG, or pathologic information is required for this purpose.[9,21,85] The changes imposed in LPFB by MIs of different locations are depicted in Fig. 13-20.[9,21,85]

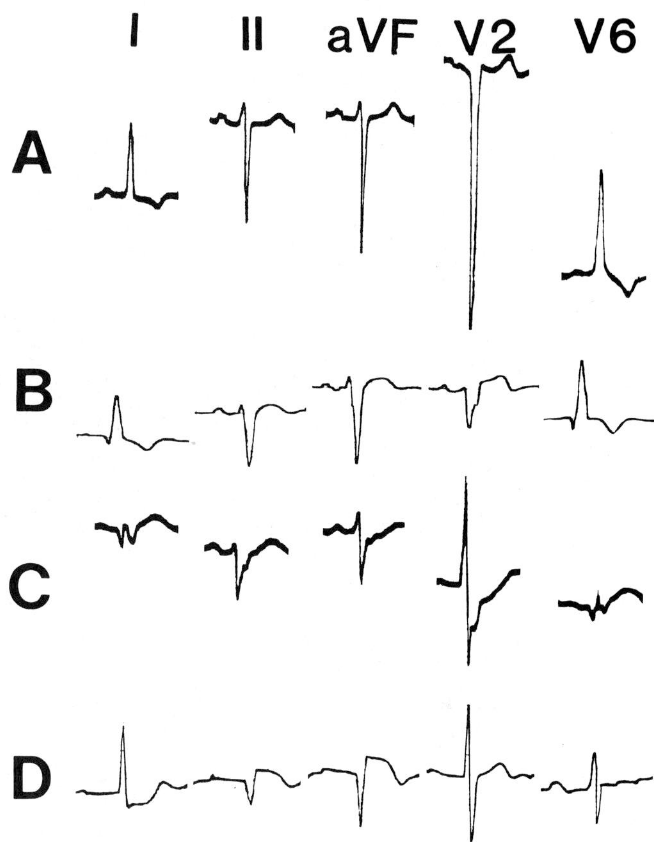


FIGURE 13-19 Diagnosis of LAFB associated with MI. Diagnostic feature given in parentheses. *A*. LAFB and anteroseptal MI (QR or QS complex in right chest leads). *B*. LAFB and anterolateral MI (abnormal q wave in leads I and $V_6$). *C*. LAFB and anterolateral MI with electrical axis in the right superior quadrant (Q wave in leads I and $V_6$). *D*. LAFB and inferior wall MI (QR or QS complexes and elevation of J point and ST segments in leads II and III).

### Left-Middle (Septal) Fascicular Blocks

While some authors consider that the right precordial leads show prominent R waves (similar to those found in true posterior, basal MI), others have described Q waves in leads $V_1$, $V_2$, and $V_3$.[90,91] It also has been considered that left-middle (septal) fascicular blocks are manifest by the absence of the expected q waves in leads $V_5$ and $V_6$ in ECG-intermediate or horizontal hearts. Such a diversity of diagnostic criteria shows that there are marked discrepancies regarding the ECG characteristics of this conduction disturbance. The unmasking of the trifascicular conduction system by catheter ablation of the right bundle branch with a diseased left intraventricular conduction system reported by Dhala et al. may reflect an ablation-induced damage of "predestined" fibers in a diseased His bundle.[92]

## NONSPECIFIC INTRAVENTRICULAR CONDUCTION DELAYS

Several names have been applied to the conduction disturbances occurring in the left-sided Purkinje-myocardial junctions, left septal surface, or free wall of the left ventricle: *arborization block, diffuse (nonspecific) intraventricular block, peri-infarction block, parietal block,* and *focal block.*[9,21,95–98] The morphologies are not those of

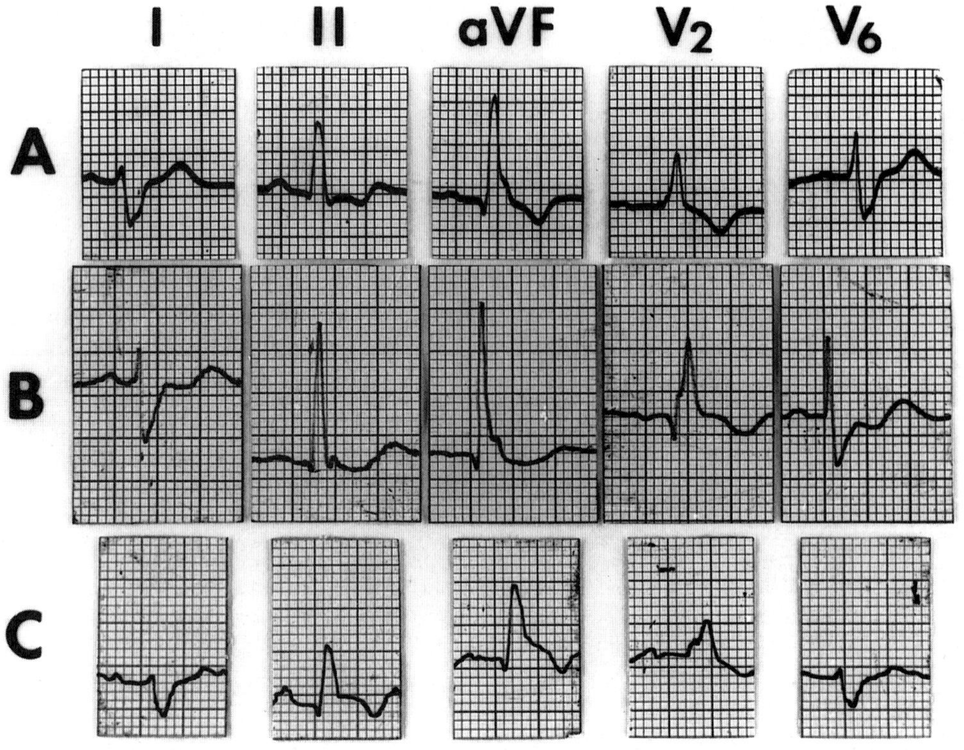


FIGURE 13-20 LPFB with RBBB. *A.* No MI. *B.* Anteroseptal MI (note q wave in $V_2$). *C.* Inferior MI (note ST-segment elevation and T-wave inversion in leads II and aVF with slight ST-segment depression in lead I). The differences in QRS complexes between *A* and *C* are not very marked because pure LPFB may produce an almost abnormal Q wave in the inferior leads.

fascicular or bundle branch blocks. These conduction disturbances have different electrogenetic mechanisms. Thus the cellular "affectation" due to acute injury resulting from coronary artery disease, hyperkalemia, drugs, and intracoronary injections of contrast material occurs within (inside) the affected regions.[5,9,21,97] Blocks occurring in subacute or chronic MI after the appearance of abnormal Q waves (peri-infarction block) (Fig. 13-21) as well as those occurring in the presence of diffuse myocardial fibrosis are due to the circuitous and irregular activation of living cells surrounding areas of fibrotic tissue.[21,95–98]

## BUNDLE BRANCH BLOCKS

### Complete RBBB

A "complete" RBBB pattern (with QRS duration of ≥0.12 s) does not necessarily reflect the existence of a total conduction block in the right branch. This pattern indicates only that the entire or major parts of both ventricles are activated by the impulse emerging from the left branch.[5,9,21] Thus a significant degree of conduction delay ("high-grade" or "incomplete" RBBB) can produce a similar pattern. In pure complete RBBB, the EA should not be deviated abnormally either to the left or to the right. These axis deviations reflect coexisting fascicular blocks (Fig. 13-20) or right ventricular hypertrophy.[21]

### Incomplete RBBB Patterns

For many years what has been proven with endocardial (catheter) and epicardial mapping is that incomplete RBBB "patterns" can be produced by various mechanisms[99–103]: (1) different degrees of conduction delays through the main trunk of the RBB, (2) an increased con-

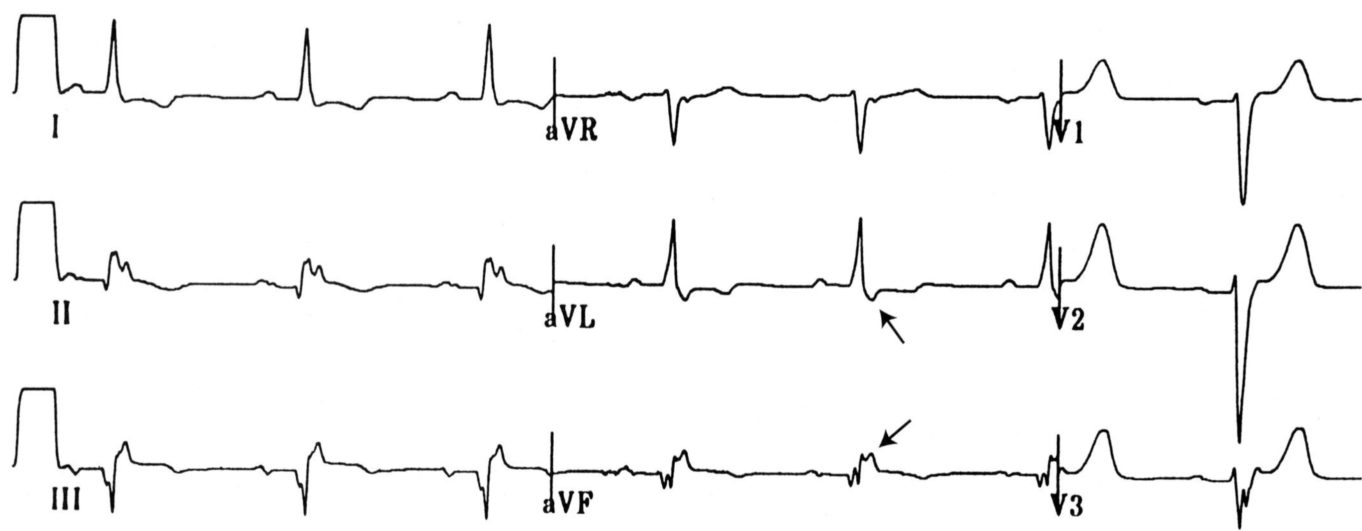


FIGURE 13-21 Type of nonspecific intraventricular conduction delay known as *peri-infarction block*. The patient had an evolving inferior wall MI. The wide (0.14s) ventricular complexes show a predominantly terminal delay (*arrows*) and notching (more evident in the inferior leads) without a typical LBBB or RBBB morphology.

duction time through an elongated RBB that is stretched because of a concomitant enlargement of the right septal surface, (3) a diffuse Purkinje-myocardial delay due to right ventricular stretch or dilatation, (4) surgical trauma or disease-related interruption of the major ramifications of the right branch ("distal" RBBB), or (5) congenital variations of the distribution of the major distal ramifications resulting in a slight delay in activation of the crista supraventricularis.[102]

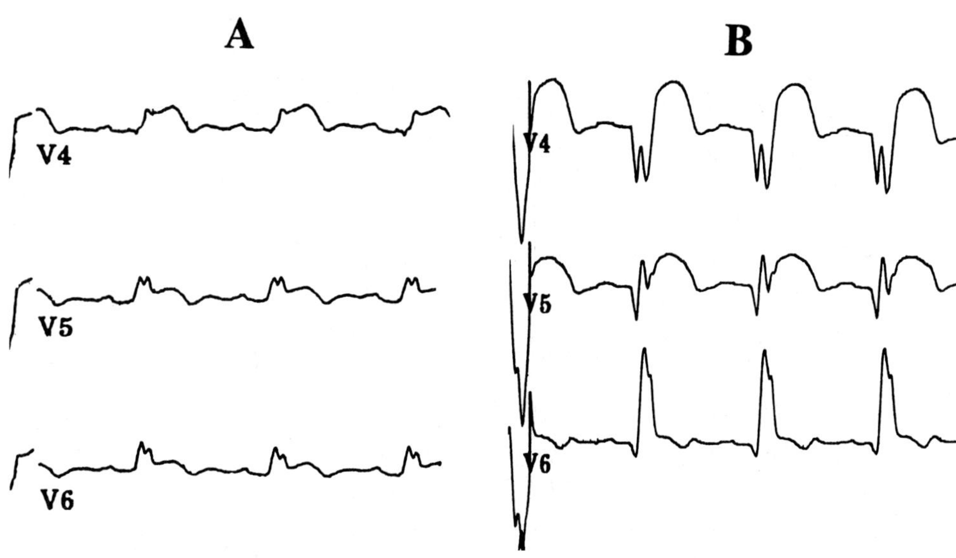


FIGURE 13-22 Morphologic characteristics of complete LBBB complicated by acute anterior MI. *A*. Abnormal ST-segment elevation without Q waves (QRS duration: 0.14 s). *B*. Abnormal ST-segment elevation, obtained from another patient, persisted after the appearance of abnormal Q waves (QRS duration: 0.13 s).

## Complete LBBB

The diagnostic criteria consist of prolongation of the QRS complexes (>0.11 s) with neither a q nor an S wave in leads I, $aV_L$, and a properly placed $V_6$. A wide R wave with a notch on its top ("plateau") is seen in these leads. Apparently, the EAs of most uncomplicated complete LBBBs usually are not located beyond −30°.[9,21,89] Complete LBBB with abnormal left axis deviation indicates a great degree of left Purkinje and myocardial disease.[9,21,89]

## Complete LBBB with Acute MI

The classic pattern of LBBB may not be modified by a small area of myocardial necrosis. It is known that occlusions of a coronary artery by either an angioplasty balloon or (a presumably large) MI can produce ST-segment changes as in the absence of a conduction disturbance. Sgarbossa[104] has suggested that ST-segment elevation of 1 mm or more concordant with QRS polarity has a high specificity and sensitivity. ST-segment elevation of 5 mm or more discordant with QRS polarity, ST-segment depression of 1 mm or more in $V_1$, $V_2$, and $V_3$, and (sudden) positive (primary) T waves in $V_4$ and $V_5$ have a high specificity but a low sensitivity.[104–106] Examples of LBBB complicated by acute anterior and inferior MI are shown in Figs. 13-22 and 13-23. The above-mentioned criteria also can be applied to diagnose acute MI in patients with pacemakers.[104,105]

## Complete LBBB with Old MI

Normally, in complete LBBB, the impulse emerges from the RBB and propagates inferiorly, to the left, and slightly anteriorly. This orientation of the initial forces tends to abolish previously present inferiorly and laterally located abnormal Q waves characteristic of inferior and lateral wall MIs.[1,2,21] If the infarction is anteroseptal, however, the impulse cannot propagate toward the left. Instead, the initial vectors point toward the free wall of the RV because now the RV free-wall forces are not neutralized by the normally preponderant septal and/or initial LV free-wall forces.[1,2,8,11,12,14] Thus a small q wave will be recorded in leads I, $V_5$, and $V_6$, where it is not normally present in complete LBBB. Similar findings can be seen in paced beats when in lead I the spike is followed by a well-defined q wave. Several studies reported that Q waves in lead I or in two or more lateral leads (I, aVL, or $V_5$ and $V_6$) have high specificity but moderate sensitivity.[104–106] The sign of Cabrera and Friedland (late notching of S waves in $V_3$ through $V_5$) has been found to have higher to moderate specificity and moderate to low sensitivity.[106] Notching of the upstroke of the R wave in leads I, $aV_L$, $V_5$, and $V_6$ has a sensitivity of 21 percent and a specificity of 82 percent.[106]

## Complete LBBB with Left Ventricular Hypertrophy

This is discussed under "Left Ventricular Hypertrophy."

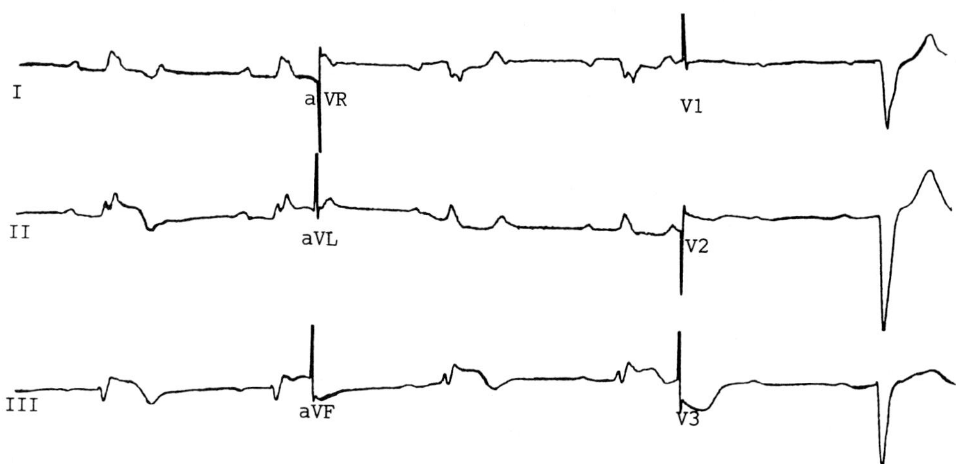


FIGURE 13-23 Morphologic features of complete LBBB complicated by acute inferior MI. There is abnormal ST-segment elevation in leads II, III, and aVF (QRS duration: 0.14 s). AV block is also present.

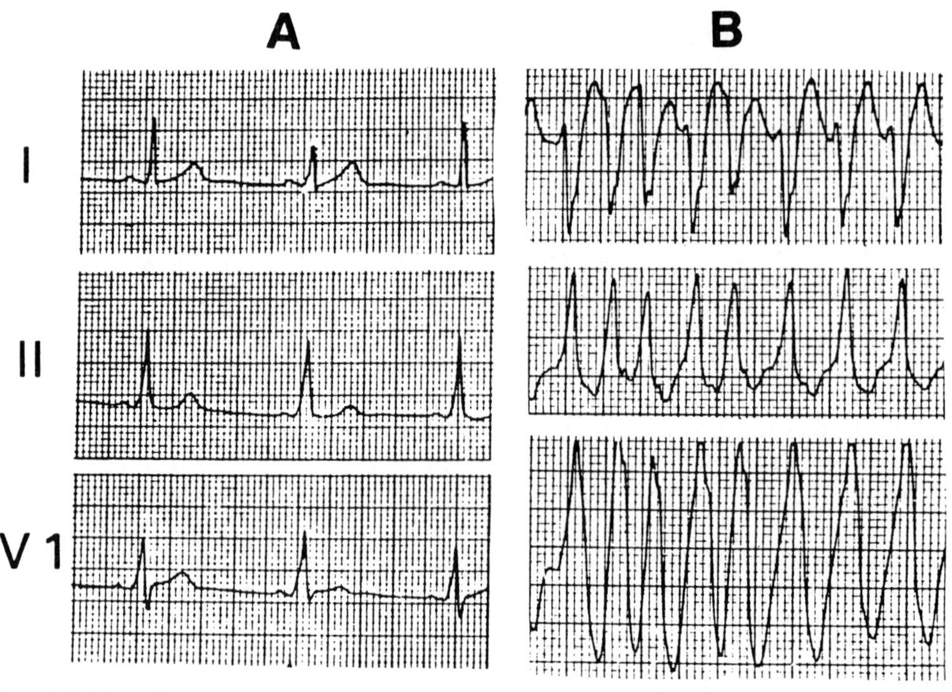


FIGURE 13-24 Wolff-Parkinson-White syndrome in a patient with a left free-wall accessory pathway. *A*. Sinus rhythm with fusion beats showing different degrees of preexcitation. *B*. Maximal preexcitation during atrial fibrillation. Note marked change in QRS duration and electrical axis now pointing inferiorly and to the right.

## Incomplete LBBB Pattern

An incomplete LBBB pattern can be diagnosed if leads I and an appropriately placed $V_6$ show an R wave not preceded by a q wave but followed by a negative T wave.[8,21] There are rS or QS complexes in lead $V_1$ and even $V_2$. Although QRS duration usually ranges between 0.10 and 0.11 s, this pattern can be observed with QRS durations of 0.12 and 0.13 s.

## WIDE QRS COMPLEXES DUE TO MANIFEST PREEXCITATION SYNDROMES

As a rule the ventricular complex is a fusion beat resulting from ventricular activation by two wavefronts.[107–113] The degree of preexcitation (amount of muscle activated through the accessory pathway) can be extremely variable and depends on many factors: distance between the sinus node and atrial insertion of the accessory pathway, differences in refractory period duration, and differences in conduction time through the normal pathway and the accessory pathway. If there is total block at the AV node or His-Purkinje system, the impulse will be conducted exclusively via the accessory pathway bundle.[111,112] Consequently the QRS complexes are different from fusion beats, although the direction of the delta wave remains the same. Moreover, the QRS complexes are as wide as (and really simulating) those produced by artificial or spontaneous beats arising in the vicinity of the ventricular end of the accessory pathway.

Not surprisingly, toward the end of the millennium, Basiouny et al.[114] reported that there were 41 publications dealing with methods for localizing the accessory pathways of patients with preexcitation syndrome. Of these, they analyzed what they considered the most important algorithms available for this purpose. For the purposes of this chapter, we cite the pioneer study of Milstein et al.,[113] who analyzed the direction of the delta wave and divided the mitral and tricuspid ring areas where the pathways are located into various segments. These investigators considered that only four segments were necessary. When this method was proposed, most ablations were performed surgically.[112,113] Left free-wall accessory pathways are characterized by positive or isoelectric delta waves in leads I, aVL, $V_5$, or $V_6$. Lead $V_1$ shows R or Rs complexes (Fig. 13-24). Posteroseptal accessory pathways show negative delta waves in leads III and aVF and R waves in $V_2$. A QS complex in $V_1$ suggests a right posteroseptal pathway (Fig. 13-25), whereas R, RS, or Rs complexes in the same lead may correspond to a left posteroseptal pathway. Right free wall accessory pathways display an LBBB pattern, defined—for purposes of accessory pathway localization—by an R wave greater than 0.09 s in lead I and rS complexes in leads $V_1$ and $V_2$, with an electrical axis ranging between +30 and −60°.[112]

Right anteroseptal accessory pathways show an LBBB pattern (as defined) with an electrical axis ranging between +30 and +120° (usually around +60°). A q wave may be present in lead aVL but not in leads I and $V_6$. Mixed patterns resulted from the existence of two separate accessory pathways.[112]

Since accessory pathways can traverse almost any part of the atrioventricular regions, this classification is obviously insufficient when catheter ablation is contemplated. Since the most useful algorithms are complex, electrocardiographers find them difficult to memorize. They are also not completely satisfactory, since smaller degrees of preexcitation seem to limit diagnostic accuracy, and the polarity of delta waves [positive, biphasic (+ or −), negative, and isoelectric] has to be properly categorized. Figure 13-26 illustrates a useful algorithm to predict accessory pathway location from the 12-lead ECG.[115]

The currently used nomenclature for accessory pathway location was discussed extensively (and has been challenged) by experts in the field of preexcitation.[116]

## WIDE QRS COMPLEXES PRODUCED BY VENTRICULAR PACING FROM DIFFERENT SITES

### Monoventricular Pacing

In determining the location of the stimulating electrodes, one should take special care not to consider that the distortion produced by large unipolar spikes constitutes parts of the pacing-induced QRS complexes. It is best not to describe the electrically produced ventricular beats as having an RBBB or LBBB morphology, since what is relevant is the polarity of the properly positioned $V_1$ and $V_2$ electrodes and the direction of the EA[117,118] (Fig. 13-27). For example, endocardial or epicardial stimulation of the anteriorly located RV at any site [apical (inferior), or mid/outflow tract (superior)] yields predom-

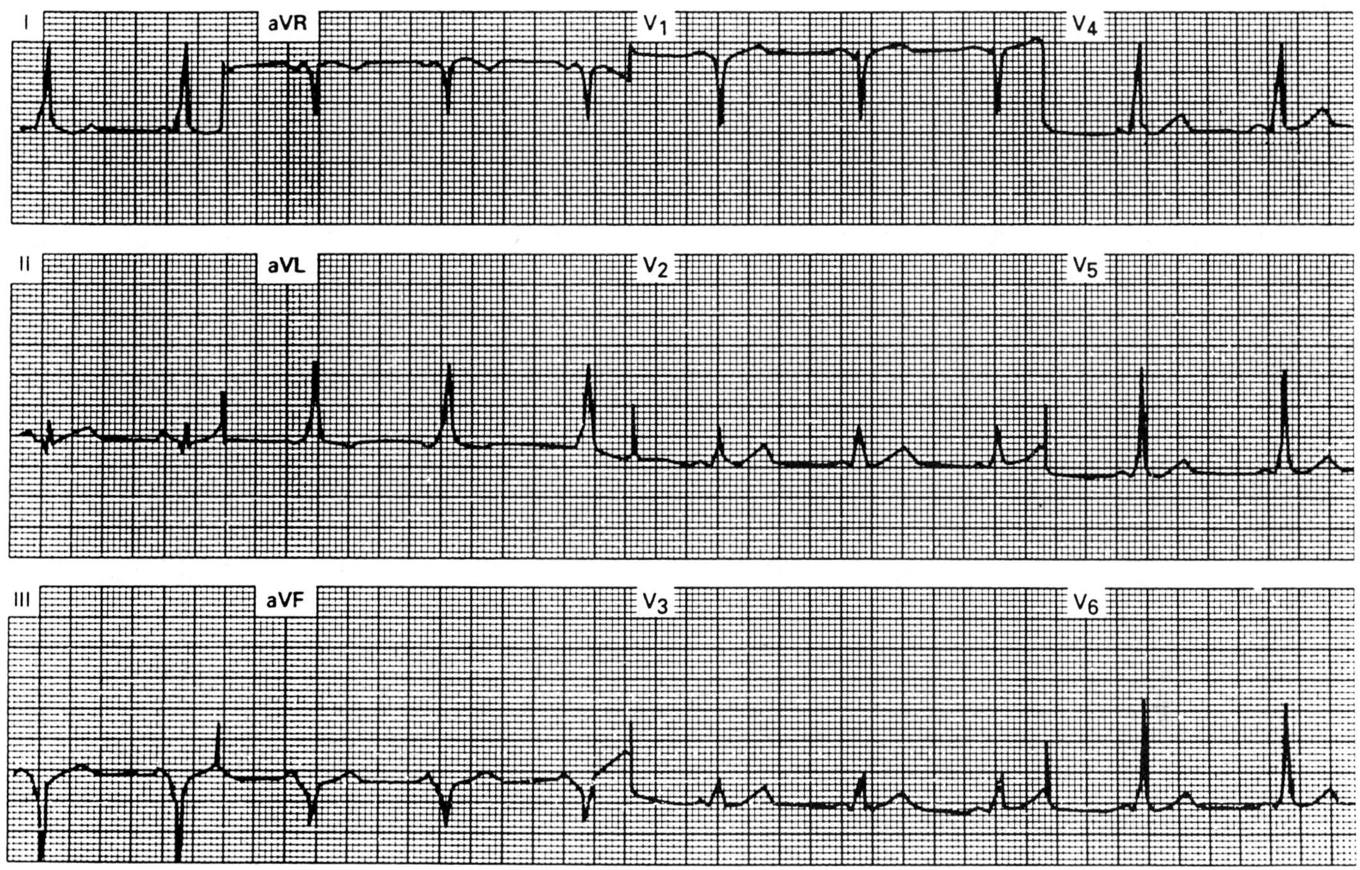


FIGURE 13-25 Wolff-Parkinson-White syndrome in a patient having a right posteroseptal accessory pathway. Note short PR intervals with negative delta waves in leads III and aVF (false pattern of inferior MI). Lead $V_1$ shows all-negative QRS complexes.

inantly negative deflections in the right chest leads due to the posterior spread of activation (first and second vertical rows in Fig. 13-27). The reverse (positive deflections in $V_1$ and $V_2$) occurs when the epicardial stimulation of the superior and lateral portions of the posterior LV by catheter electrodes in the distal coronary sinus or great and middle cardiac veins (or by implanted electrodes in the nearby muscle) results in anteriorly oriented forces (third and fourth vertical rows in Fig. 13-27). RV apical pacing may produce positive deflections in $V_1$ in rare cases if this lead is (mis)placed above its usual level. On the other hand, superior deviation of the electrical axis only indicates that a spatial inferior ventricular site has been stimulated, regardless of whether this site is the apical portion of the RV or the inferior part of the LV, the latter being paced through the middle cardiac vein (first and fourth vertical rows in Fig. 13-27). Conversely, an inferior vertical axis is simply a consequence of pacing from a superior site, which can be the endocardium of the RV outflow tract or the epicardium of the posterosuperior and lateral portions of the left ventricle (second and third vertical rows in Fig. 13-27).

### Biventricular Pacing

Although with this technique the right-sided electrode is usually in a single site—namely, the endocardium of the RV apex pacing—the location of the epicardial left-sided electrode varies with the vein (or segment of the latter) in which it is placed (posterior or anterior great cardiac vein, lateral or posterolateral veins, or even middle cardiac vein), depending on the preference and nomenclature of the implanting physician.[119–122] Because of this and due to the several and unevenly distributed, severe myocardial fibroses that these patients have, various different and difficult-to-interpret wide QRS patterns occur (right axis deviation with usually an RS, but also QS and, rarely, R waves in $V_1$; right superior axis with similar waves in the latter lead and, infrequently, left axis deviation with a QS in $V_1$). Persons with less severe myocardial disease have narrower ventricular complexes with possibly a shorter depolarization conduction time. Consequently the QT intervals are shorter.[119]

## LEFT VENTRICULAR HYPERTROPHY

As emphasized by Surawicz,[123] the advent of other noninvasive techniques has changed the role of the ECG in the diagnosis of ventricular hypertrophy. Necropsy studies have exposed the superiority of echocardiography (Chap. 15) with respect to the ECG for detecting LVH.[123] Echocardiography is also a better method for serial follow-up of changes during progression or regression of LVH. Multiple criteria have been proposed to diagnose LVH using necropsy or ECG information[1,123–135] (Tables 13-2 and 13-3). Of these, the Sokolow-Lyon criterion ($SV_1 + RV_{5-6} \geq 35$ mm) is very specific (>95 percent) but not very sensitive (see Table 13-2). The Romhilt-Estes score has a specificity of 97 percent and a sensitivity of 60 percent in studies correlated with echocardiography.[64,127] The following are some of the other criteria[64]: The Casale (modified Cornell) criterion

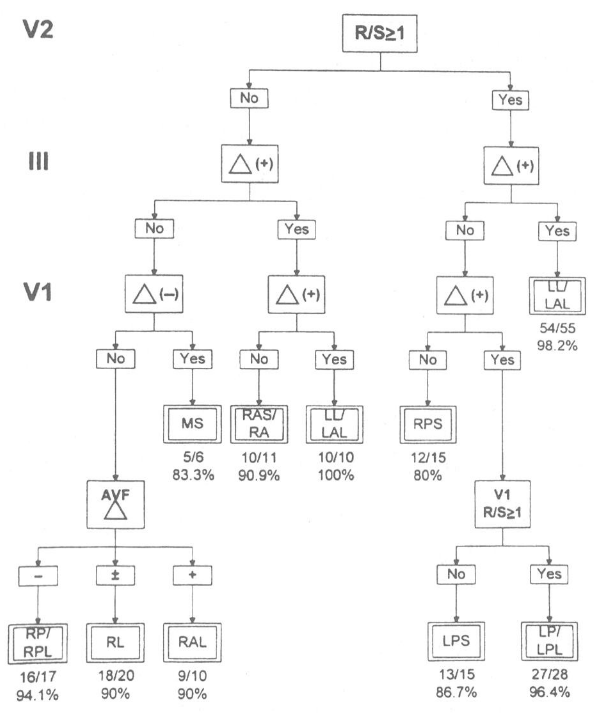


FIGURE 13-26 Useful algorithm to predict accessory pathway location from the 12-lead ECG. Step 1: Analysis of R/S ratio in $V_2$. Step 2: Existence of positive (+) delta wave in lead III (initial 40 ms). Step 3: Existence of positive or negative (−) delta wave in $V_1$ (initial 60 ms). Step 4: Delta-wave polarity in $aV_F$ (initial 40 ms) or analysis of R/S ratio in $V_1$ (+ = biphasic or isoelectric). The accuracy of the algorithm for each location in 187 prospective patients is also shown at the bottom. LAL, left anterolateral; LL, left lateral; LP, left posterior; LPL, left posterolateral; LPS, left posteroseptal; MS, midseptal; RA, right anterior; RAL, right anterolateral; RAS, right anteroseptal; RL, right lateral; RP, right posterior; RPL, right posterolateral; RPS, right posteroseptal. (From Chiang et al.[115] Reproduced with permission from the publisher and authors.)

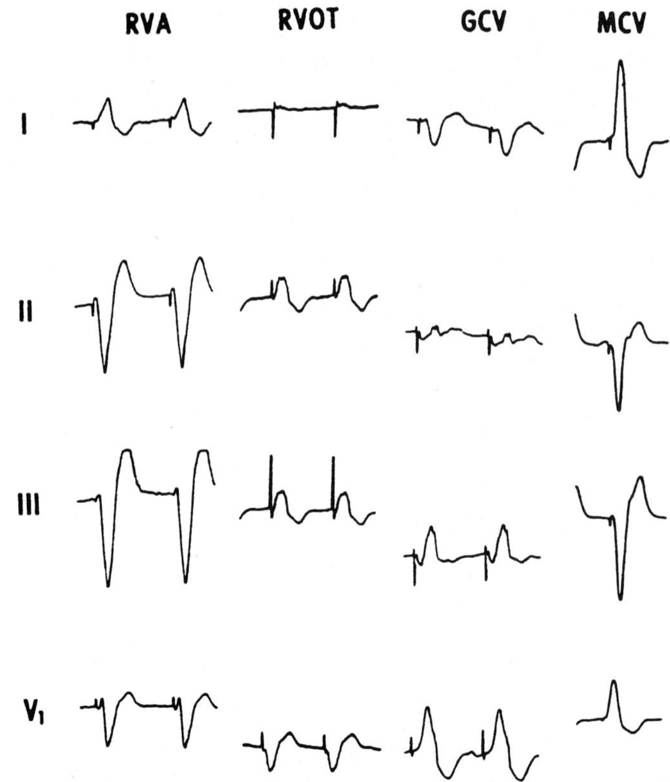


FIGURE 13-27 QRS changes (location of the electrical axis and polarity of lead $V_1$) produced by monoventricular pacing from right ventricular apex (RVA), right ventricular outflow tract (RVOT), great cardiac vein (GCV), and middle cardiac vein (MCV).

($RaVL + SV_3 > 28$ mm in men and >20 mm in women) is somewhat more sensitive but less specific than the Sokolow-Lyon criterion.[128] The Talbot criterion[129] (R ≥ 16 mm in aVL) is very specific (>90 percent), even in the presence of MI and ventricular block, but not very sensitive.[129] The Koito and Spodick criterion[130] ($RV_6 > RV_5$) claims a specificity of 100 percent and a sensitivity of more than 50 percent. According to Hernandez Padial,[131] a total 12-lead QRS voltage of greater than 120 mm is a good ECG criterion of LV hypertrophy in systemic hypertension and is better than the criteria most frequently used. Finally, the Cornell voltage criterion is $SV_3 + RaVL \geq 28$ and 20 mm for men and women, respectively.[132,133]

With echocardiography as the gold standard, several authors have postulated ECG criteria for diagnosis of LV hypertrophy in the presence of complete LBBB and LAFB[134,135] (Tables 13-4 and 13-5). The high sensitivity and specificity reported by Gertsch et al.[135] for diagnosis of LV hypertrophy with LAFB have not been corroborated in preliminary studies performed in our department.

TABLE 13-2 Electrocardiographic Criteria for Left Ventricular Enlargement

| Voltage Criteria | Sensitivity (%) | Specificity (%) | Accuracy (%) |
|---|---|---|---|
| $RI + S_{III} > 25$ mm | 10.6 | 100 | 55 |
| RVL > 7.5 mm | 22.5 | 96.5 | 59.5 |
| RVL > 11 mm | 10.6 | 100 | 55 |
| RVF > 20 mm | 1.3 | 99.5 | 50 |
| $SV_1 + RV_{5–6} \geq 35$ mm (Sokolow-Lyon) | 42.5 | 95 | 74 |
| $SV_1 + RV_{5–6} > 30$ mm | 55.6 | 89.5 | 73 |
| In $V_1–V_6$, the tallest S + tallest R > 45 mm | 45 | 93 | 69 |
| $RV_{5–6} > 26$ mm | 25 | 98 | 62 |
| Romhilt-Estes score | 60 | 97 | 78 |

SOURCE: From Bayes de Luna,[64] with permission.

## PROCESSES PRODUCING OR LEADING TO RV HYPERTROPHY AND ENLARGEMENT

RV hypertrophy is manifest in the ECG only when the RV forces predominate over those of the LV. Since the latter has roughly three times more mass than the former, the RV may

TABLE 13-3 Romhilt-Estes Score.[64] There Is Left Ventricular Enlargement if 5 or More Points Are Obtained. Left Ventricular Enlargement Is Probable if the Sum Is 4 Points

| | | |
|---|---|---|
| A. | *Criteria based on QRS modifications* | |
| 1. | Voltage criteria<br>One of the following should be present:<br>• R or S in the FP $\geq$ 20 mm<br>• S in $V_1$–$V_2 \geq$ 30 mm<br>• R in $V_5$–$V_6 \geq$ 30 mm | 3 points |
| 2. | ÂQRS at $-30°$ or more to the left | 2 points |
| 3. | Intrinsicoid deflection in $V_5$–$V_6 \geq$ 0.05 s | 1 point |
| 4. | QRS duration $\geq$ 0.09 s | 1 point |
| B. | *Criteria based on ST-T changes* | |
| 1. | ST-T vector opposite to QRS without digitalis | 3 points |
| 2. | ST-T vector opposite to QRS with digitalis | 1 point |
| C. | *Criteria based on P-wave abnormalities* | |
| 1. | Negative terminal P mode in $V_1 \geq$ 1 mm in depth and 0.04 s in duration | 3 points |

SOURCE: From Bayes de Luna,[64] with permission.

TABLE 13-4 Criteria for Diagnosis of Left Ventricular Hypertrophy in Presence of Complete Left Bundle Branch Block

| | | Sensitivity (%) | Specificity (%) |
|---|---|---|---|
| 1. | R in aVL $\geq$ 11 mm | 24 | 100 |
| 2. | Electrical axis $\geq$ 40° (or $S_2 \geq R_1$) | 39 | 100 |
| 3. | $SV_1$ + $RV_5$ or $RV_6 \geq$ 40 mm | 58 | 97 |
| 4. | $SV_2 \geq$ 30 mm and $SV_3 \geq$ 25 mm | 75 | 90 |

SOURCE: From Kafka et al.,[134] with permission.

double in size (when the LV is normal) or triple its weight (when there is significant RV hypertrophy) and still not result in the necessary requirements to pull the electrical forces anteriorly and to the right. For these reasons, RV hypertrophy cannot be recognized easily in adult patients. Despite these limitations, the ECG manifestations of RV hypertrophy or enlargement can be subdivided into the following main types: (1) the posterior and rightward displacement of the QRS forces associated with low voltage, as seen in patients with pulmonary emphysema (Fig. 13-28); (2) the incomplete RBBB pattern with right axis deviation occurring in patients with some congenital cardiac malformations, resulting in volume overloading of the RV (Fig. 13-29); (3) the true posterior wall MI pattern with normal to low voltage of the R wave in $V_1$ and P mitrale of mitral stenosis (Fig. 13-30); and (4) the classic RV hypertrophy and strain pattern seen in young patients with congenital heart disease (producing pressure overload) or in adult patients with high-pressure ("primary" pulmonary) hypertension (Fig. 13-31). False patterns of RV hypertrophy may occur in patients with true posterior (basal) MI, complete RBBB with LPFB, and Wolff-Parkinson-White syndrome resulting from AV conduction through left free wall or left posteroseptal accessory pathways.[1,2,21]

## ELECTROLYTE IMBALANCES

In practice, the major problem with the ECG diagnosis of electrolyte imbalance is not the negative ECG with abnormal serum values but the production of similar changes by other conditions in patients with normal serum values.[136]

### Hyperkalemia

The initial effect of acute hyperkalemia is the appearance of peaked T waves with a narrow base (Fig. 13-32, left). The diagnosis of hyperkalemia is almost certain when the duration of the base is 0.20 s or less (with rates between 60 and 110 beats per minute).[1,136,137] As the degree of hyperkalemia increases, the QRS complex widens (Fig. 13-33), with the electrical axis usually being deviated abnormally to the left and only rarely to the right. In addition, the PR interval prolongs and the P wave flattens until it disappears.[1,2,136] If this condition is not treated, death ensues either due to ventricular standstill or coarse, slow ventricular fibrillation. Death also can result if wide QRS complexes occurring at fast rates are diagnosed as ventricular tachycardia and the patient is treated with antiarrhythmic drugs. On the other hand, class IA, IC, and III drugs as well as large doses of tricyclic antidepressants (especially when ingested for suicidal purposes) can also produce marked QRS widening.[137] These processes, however, do not coexist with narrow-based, peaked T waves. Rarely, hyperkalemia produces (in the absence of coronary artery disease) a degree of ST-segment elevation in the right chest leads capable of suggesting anteroseptal myocardial injury (Fig. 13-33). These constitute the "dialyzable currents of injury in potassium intoxication" reported by Levine et al.[138]

TABLE 13-5 Criteria for Diagnosis of Left Ventricular Hypertrophy in Presence of Left Anterior Fascicular Block[a]

| Study | ECG Criteria | Sensitivity (%) | Specificity (%) | Positive Predictive Value (%) | Negative Predictive Value (%) |
|---|---|---|---|---|---|
| Bozzi and Figini | $SV_1$ + ($RV_5$ + $SV_5$) $\geq$25 mm | 69 | 92 | 80 | 73 |
| Milliken | RaVL $\geq$13 mm | 35 | 92 | 82 | 56 |
| Milliken | SIII $\geq$15 mm | 38 | 87 | 77 | 57 |
| Gertsch et al. | SIII + maximal sum of R + S in any single precordial lead | 96 | 87 | 89 | 95 |
| Reevaluated[b] Gertsch criteria | | 80 | 55 | 78 | 58 |

[a]Left ventricular hypertrophy diagnosed by echocardiography when left ventricular mass is $\geq$ 124 g/m$^2$.
[b]Unpublished observations performed in our department.
SOURCE: From Gertsch et al.,[135] with permission.

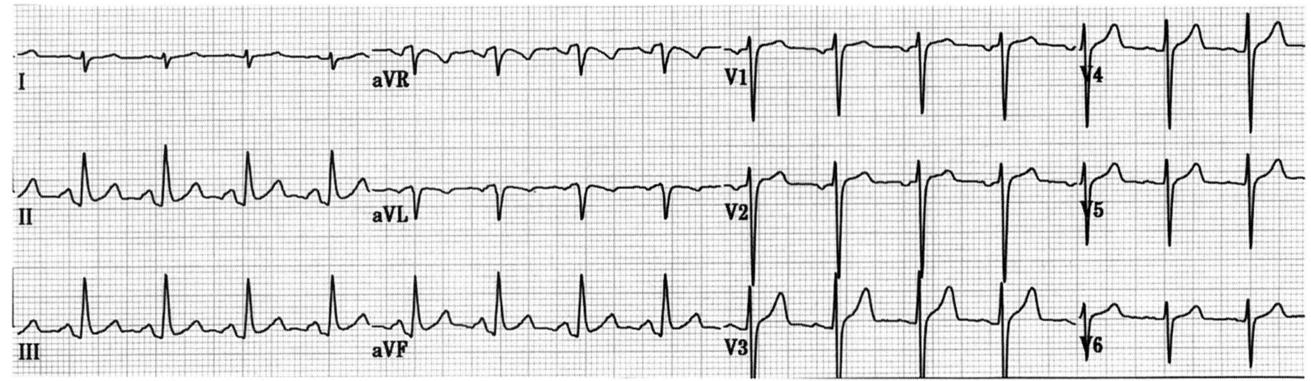


FIGURE 13-28 ECG taken on a patient with pulmonary emphysema showing slight right axis deviation with small rS complexes in lead I, an electrically vertical heart position (with aVL similar to aVR), overall tendency to low voltage, and rS complexes in all chest leads.

## Hypokalemia

The abnormal and delayed repolarization that occurs in hypokalemia is best expressed as QU rather than QT prolongation, since at times it can be difficult to differentiate between notching of the T wave and T- and U-wave fusion.[1,136] On the basis of the previously mentioned M cells, some of these U waves are part of notched T waves, suggesting that that term be used in place of U. As the serum potassium level falls, the ST segment becomes progressively more depressed and there is a gradual blending of the T wave into what appears to be a tall U wave (Fig. 13-34, top). An ECG pattern similar to that of hypokalemia can be produced by some antiarrhythmic drugs, especially quinidine and, experimentally, DL-sotalol.[1,13,137] In any case, when repolarization is greatly prolonged, ventricular arrhythmias, including torsades de pointes, can occur.

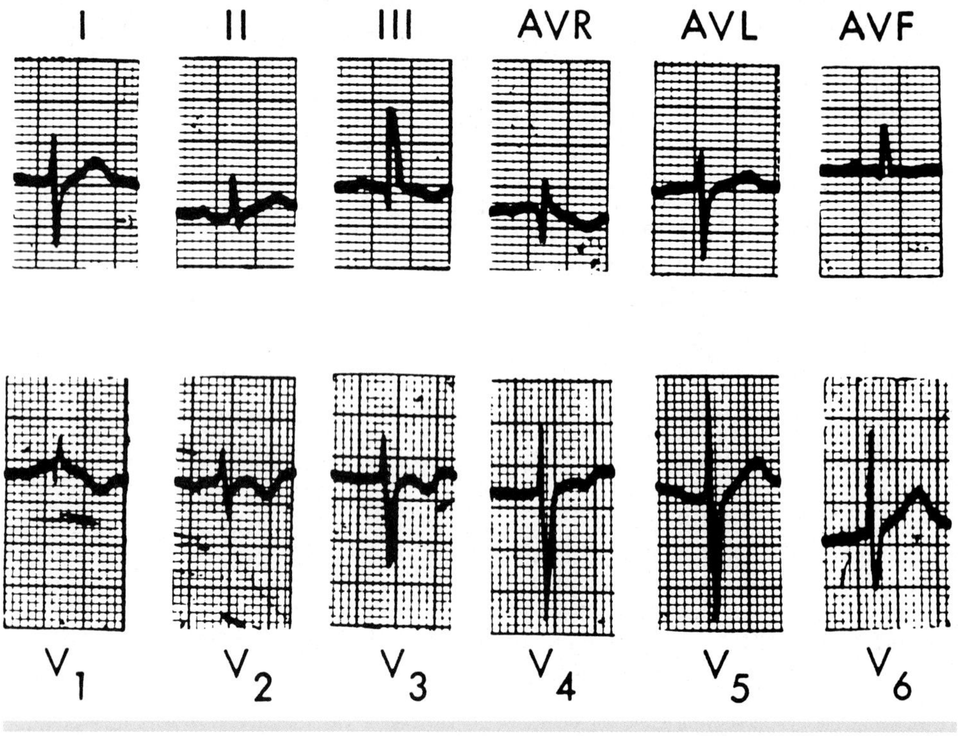

FIGURE 13-29 ECG from a patient with RV enlargement (volume overload in type) due to a small atrial septal defect (ostium secundum). Right axis deviation was associated with an incomplete RBBB pattern (rsR′ complexes in lead $V_1$). (From Lemberg and Castellanos.[155] Reproduced with permission from the publisher and authors.)

## Hypomagnesemia

Hypomagnesemia does not produce QU prolongation unless the coexisting hypokalemia (with which it is almost invariably associated) is severe.[136] Long-standing and very marked magnesium deficiency lowers the amplitude of the T wave and depresses the ST segment.[136] It may be difficult to differentiate the changes produced by magnesium from those produced by potassium. For this reason, it has been stated that hypomagnesemia does not cause any changes in the ECG.[137]

## Hypermagnesemia

Similarly, in clinical tracings, the effects of hypermagnesemia on the ECG are difficult to identify because the changes are dominated by calcium.[139] According to some authors, administration of intravenous magnesium to patients with normal ECGs may shorten the QT interval.[137] Other authors found no effects on ventricular refractoriness that could be reflected by changes in the QT interval.[140] Intravenous magnesium given to patients with torsades de pointes controls the arrhythmia in a high percentage without changing the prolonged QT interval significantly.[141] The calcium-blocking activity of magnesium was suggested to be one of the mechanisms responsible for this antiarrhythmic activity.[141]

## Hypercalcemia

During sinus rhythm with normal rates, the QT interval is short (see Fig. 13-34, bottom). In some cases, the Q-to-apex of T intervals is also short. If factors known to modify the QT interval are not present, it has been said that a reasonably accepted correlation exists between the duration of the interval and serum calcium levels.[137] Occasionally, the ST segment disappears and the T

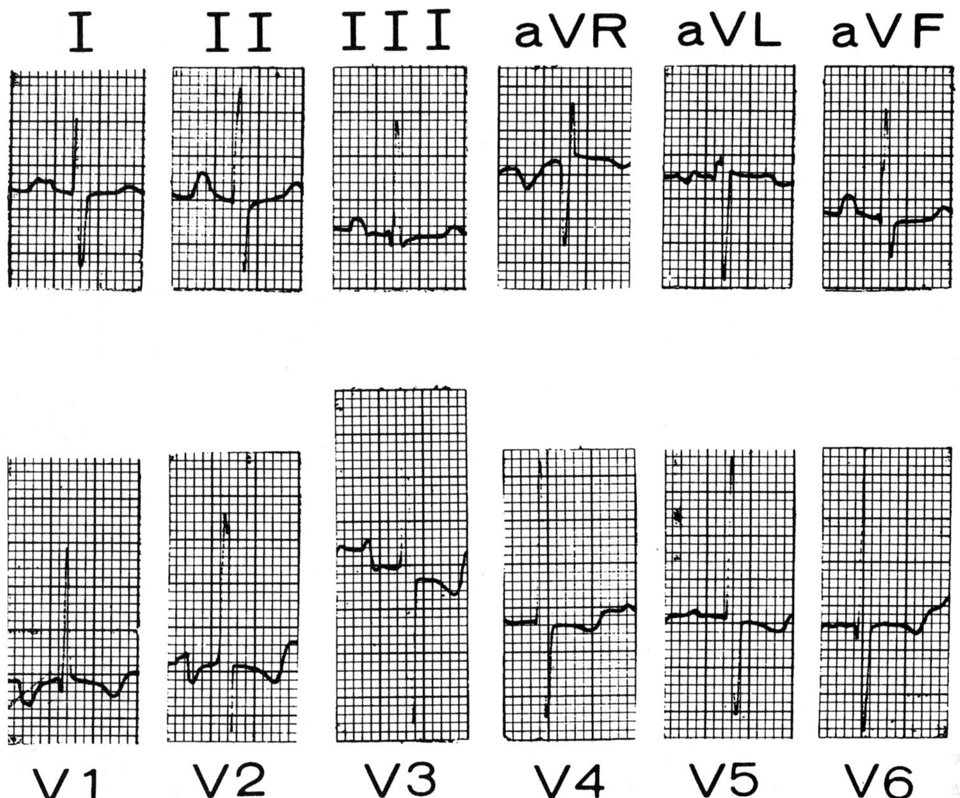


FIGURE 13-30 ECG from a patient with RV hypertrophy due to mitral stenosis showing P "mitrale," right axis deviation and R waves in $V_1$ and $V_2$. Negative T waves in $V_5$ and $V_6$ are due to coexistent left ventricular hypertrophy due to associated mitral regurgitation.

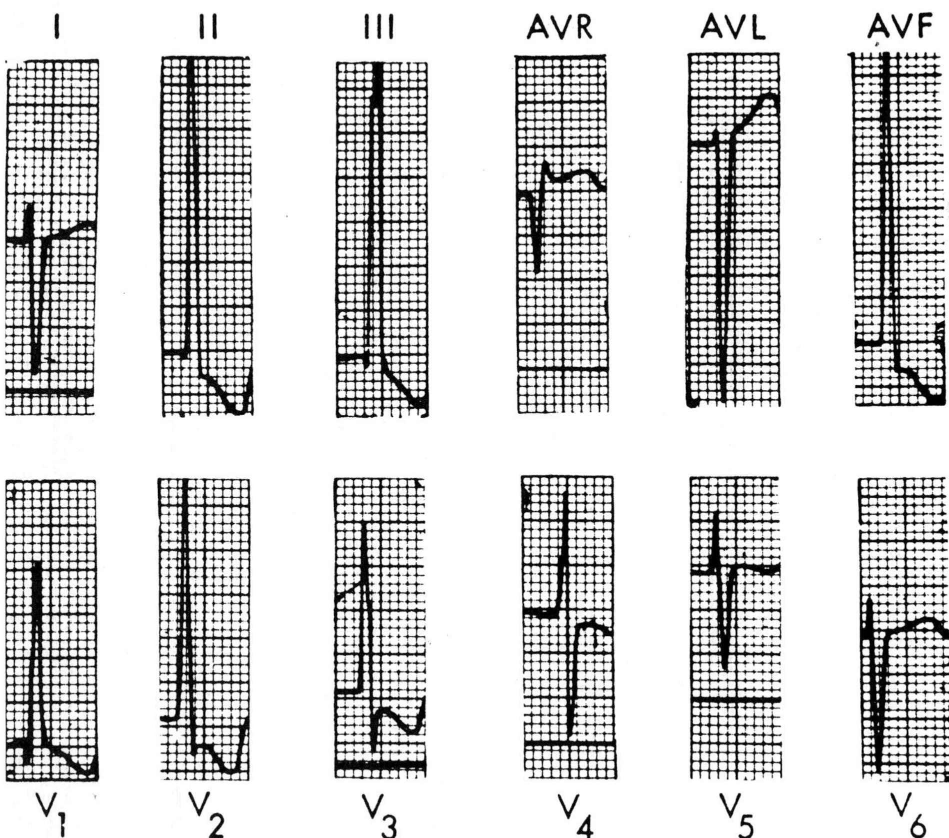


FIGURE 13-31 ECG from a 17-year-old patient who had RV enlargement (pressure overloading in type) due to severe pulmonic stenosis. Note extreme right axis deviation, overall high voltage, and qR complexes in lead $V_1$ without an incomplete RBBB pattern. (From Lemberg and Castellanos.[155] Reproduced with permission from the publisher and authors.)

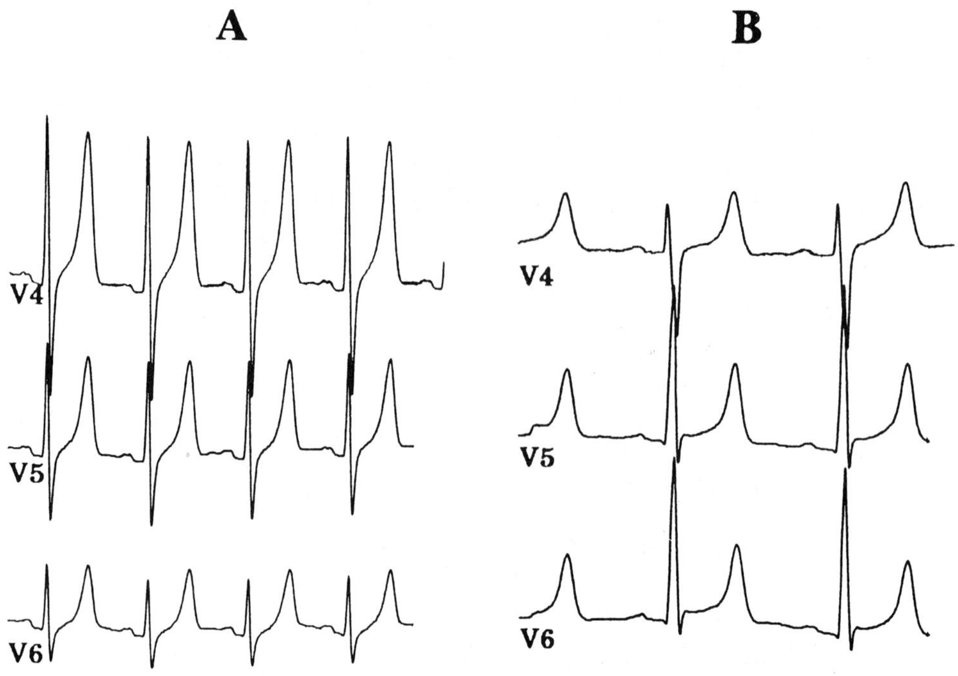


FIGURE 13-32 Electrocardiographic manifestations of early hyperkalemia. The slightly prolonged QRS complex is followed by a peaked T wave having a very narrow base. Uncorrected and corrected QT intervals of 0.32 and 0.44 s, respectively (*A*). Hyperkalemia with hypocalcemia characterized by prolongation of the QT interval at the expense of the ST segment preceding the narrow-based T wave. Uncorrected and corrected QT intervals of 0.52 and 0.53 s, respectively (*B*).

waves may become inverted in left and right chest leads. Digitalis also shortens the QT interval but produces its characteristic "effects" in leads where the R waves predominate.[137] The classic upward concavity of the ST segment is seen in the left chest leads in patients with LV hypertrophy and in leads $V_1$ and $V_2$ when there is RV hypertrophy (with predominantly positive deflections in these leads).

## Hypocalcemia

The typical ECG pattern of hypocalcemia consists of QT prolongation at the expense of the ST segment.[136,137] The T wave is usually of normal width but can be narrow if there is coexisting (moderate) hyperkalemia (see Fig. 13-32*B*). A very marked injury (with the so-called hyperacute ST-T changes) can produce a similar pattern, but in such cases the T wave, though peaked, is not as narrow-based. It has been said that hypocalcemia per se does not produce T-wave inversion. When present, the latter is usually a reflection of coexisting processes, such as LV hypertrophy and incomplete LBBB. An ECG pattern similar to that of hypocalcemia can be produced by some organic abnormalities of the central nervous system and by congenitally prolonged QT intervals.

## HYPOTHERMIA

Characteristic ECG changes develop when the body temperature drops to approximately 30°C.[11] The QT interval becomes prolonged. In addition, a deflection, called an *Osborn wave,* appears in a place said to be located between the end of the QRS complex and the beginning of the ST segment[142] (Fig. 13-35). This deflection has been attributed to delayed depolarization, to a current of injury, or to "early" repolarization. In leads facing the left ventricle, the deflection is positive, and its size is inversely related to body temperature. The role played by the intramyocardial M cells in its genesis has been discussed previously.[13]

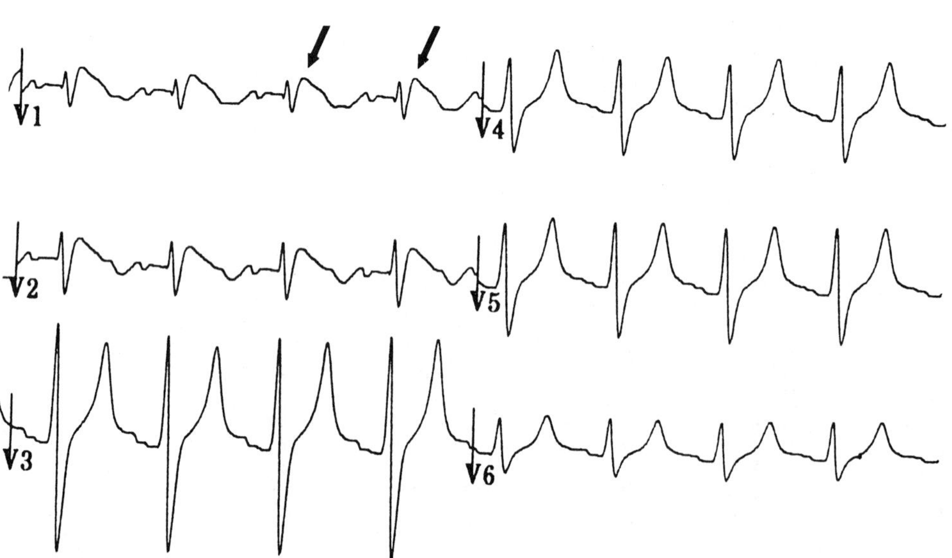


FIGURE 13-33 Advanced hyperkalemia. The wide (0.14-s) QRS complexes are followed by peaked T waves (best seen in lead $V_3$). The hyperkalemia-induced ST-segment elevation in lead $V_1$ (*arrows*), known as the *dialyzable current of injury*, disappeared after appropriate treatment. Note resemblance with the ST changes of the Brugada syndrome (Fig. 13-15*A*).

## ARTIFACTS

Muscle tremor and alternating-current interference are thought to be the most common artifacts.[137,143–148] But in clinical practice, worldwide experience in ECG has shown that recordings of precordial electrodes are made with astonishingly marked neglect as to the employment of the proper chest landmarks.[148] Simonson found that in a controlled study, placement of the $V_2$ electrode varied 10 cm vertically and 8 cm horizontally in 103 healthy subjects.[143] Moreover, Kerwin et al. found a rather large error in placement of chest electrodes (2 to 3 cm in both the horizontal and vertical directions) in repeated trials in the same patients by the same technicians.[144] A more recent study found that there was a superior displacement of more than 0.625 in. in $V_1$ and $V_2$ and inferior and upward displacement of more than 0.625 in. in $V_4$, $V_5$, and $V_6$.[146] Such a variability creates severe problems for computer interpretation of serial ECGs and considerable difficulties for the diagnosis of MI in the presence of LBBB.[146–148] In our institution, the most frequent cause of "poor r wave progression in the anteroseptal leads" is misplacement of the corresponding electrodes. Improper limb lead placement has gone beyond switching of right arm and left arm cables.[145] The method depicted in Fig. 13-36, based on the analysis of extremity leads only, is simpler than those incorporating the analysis of bipolar standard leads.[145] Not frequently recognized in ECG textbooks is the incontrovertible fact that, in some centers, even the "sanctity" of the attachment of the right leg (ground) cable to the right leg has been violated.[146]

Finally, overshooting, overdamping, the indiscriminate use of filters, the running down of standardization battery, the range and changing size as well as polarity of large unipolar pacemaker spikes, and the almost microscopic size of some bipolar spikes should be taken into consideration.

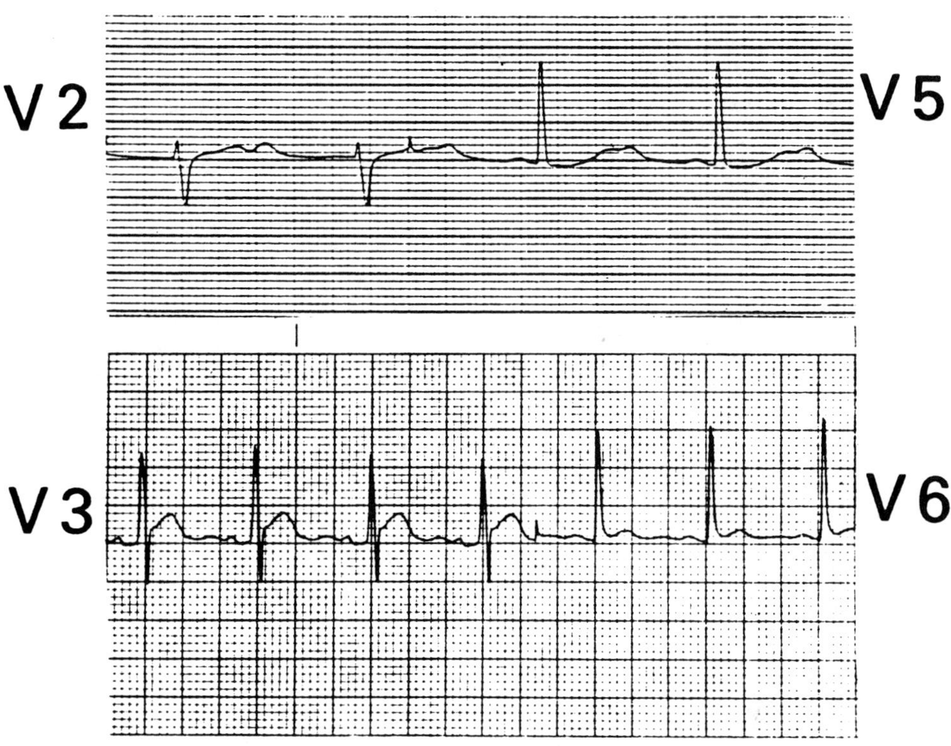


FIGURE 13-34 Electrocardiographic manifestations of hypokalemia (*upper strip*) and hypercalcemia (*lower strip*).

## Pseudoartifacts

The ECG changes produced by heart transplantation can be interpreted as artifacts. Orthotopic transplantation shows the small, barely visible P waves of the recipient's heart dissociated from the QRST complexes produced by the donor's heart. Heterotopic heart transplantation produces a unique interheart dissociation, resembling what in older Holter systems occurred when recordings were made on previously used unerased tapes (Fig. 13-37).

## COMPUTER APPLICATIONS

At the onset of the millennium, the use of computer technology in ECG interpretation has become universal.[150] Unfortunately (except in the case of arrhythmias) the frequent lack of value of these interpretations has received undue attention. Furthermore, the findings of the ACC/AHA Task Force on Guidelines for Electrocardiography have led to the statement that "no computer program can replace the skilled physician"; studies examining the accuracy of computer interpretations echo the thinking of most cardiologists.[6] The latest (2001) Clinical Competence statement restates the above.[151]

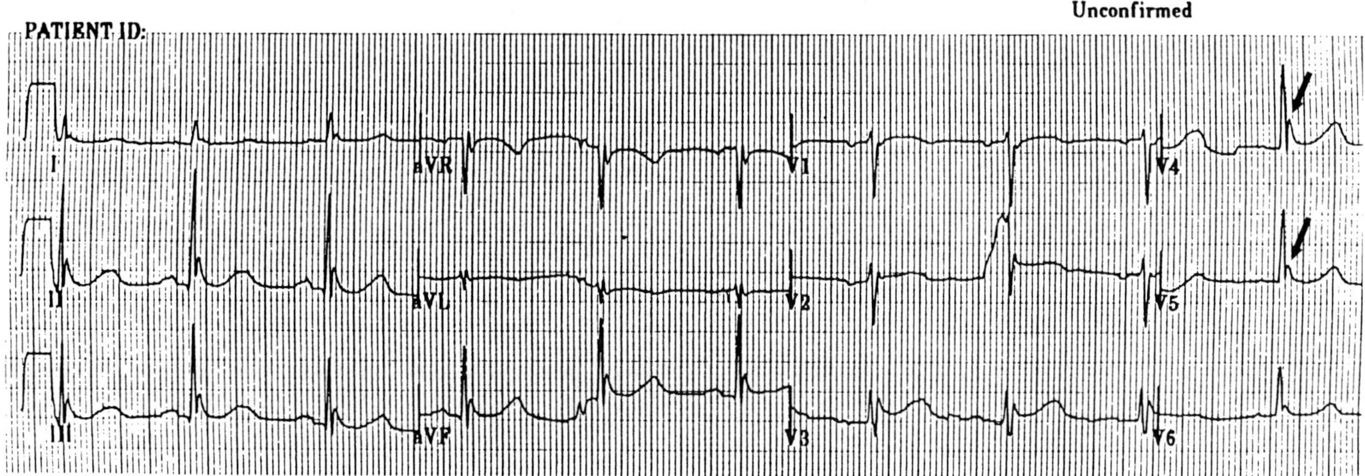


FIGURE 13-35 ECG obtained from a patient with hypothermia. The characteristic Osborn wave (*arrows*) is the terminal deflection inscribed between the slender part of the QRS complexes and the beginning of the ST segment. Note that it is not easy to determine where the ST segment starts. In addition, there is marked prolongation of the QT interval.

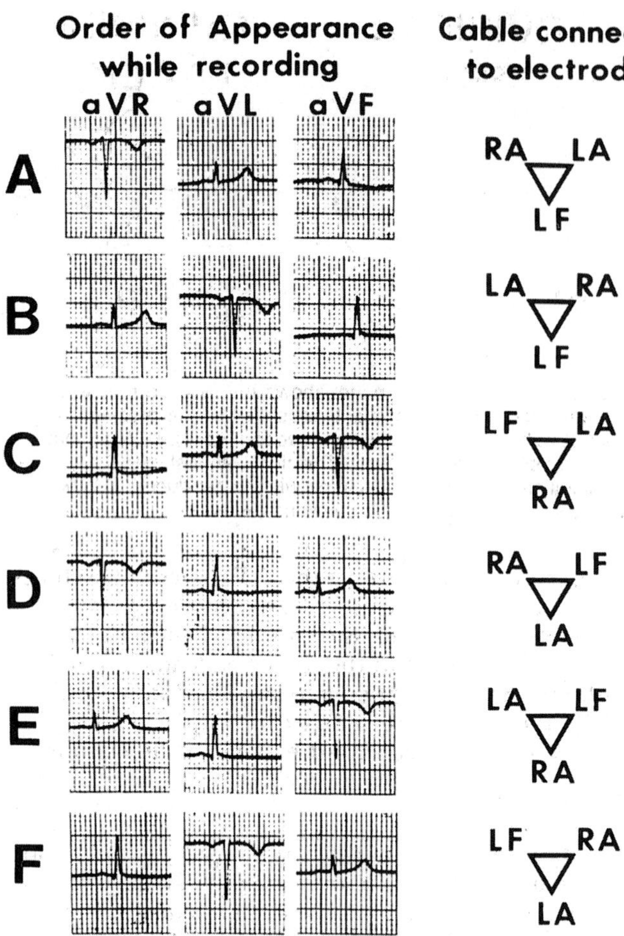


FIGURE 13-36 Identification of improper connections of the cables from the electrocardiographic machine to the corresponding electrodes placed on the patient's limbs. Note that aVR, aVL, and aVF invariably refer to whatever morphology is recorded while the ECG is being obtained. On the other hand, RA (*right arm*), LA (*left arm*), and LL (*left leg*) or LF (*left foot*) correspond to the normal morphology recorded by the cables so labeled, regardless of the limb to which they were connected. *A*. Normal. *B*. Since LA appears in aVR and RA appears in aVL (with LF being in its normal position), the right arm and left arm cables must have been switched. *C*. Since LF appears in aVR and RA appears in aVF (with LA in its normal position), the right arm and left leg cables must have been switched. *D*. Since LA appears in aVF and LF appears in aVL (with RA in its normal position), the left arm and left leg cables must have been switched. *E*. Counterclockwise switching of all three cables. *F*. Clockwise switching of all three cables.

However, in truth, this is not a failure of technology but of the programmers and tautologic attitude of electrocardiographers themselves who have not used the technology to its maximum. Better results can be assured with greater interest, improved programs, and better use of technology.

## SPATIAL VECTORCARDIOGRAPHY

### Generalities

Since the ECG deals with electrical forces, all ECGs can be considered vectorial. However, there are multiple methods to express the vectorial concept.[8,152–158] In analyzing the vectorcardiogram (VCG), one should consider the activation of each muscle cell as producing an electrical force that can be represented by a vector depicting the spatial orientation and magnitude of this force.[155–158]

During the spread of the activation process, innumerable electrical forces are generated. These multiple forces vary in magnitude and differ in direction. At any given moment, the resultant of these electrical forces can be represented by a spatial vector possessing magnitude, direction, and sense. This vector is referred to as an *instantaneous vector* and represents the resultant of all the forces of the heart acting at that particular moment.[155–158] Immediately afterward, the wave of accession spreads to different areas of the myocardium and the new instantaneous vector representing all the forces of the heart now occupies a different spatial position and has a different magnitude. This continues throughout the cardiac cycle, with the succeeding instantaneous vector occupying different spatial positions. If all manifest spatial vectors are diagrammatically represented as having a common point of origin and if the distal points of the vectors are joined, a single spatial loop is formed for ventricular depolarization (QRS), ventricular repolarization (ST-T), and the atrial complex (P). The VCG consists of four different loops. The electrical activity of the atria is recorded as a small loop designated the *P loop,* the depolarization of the ventricles is recorded as a large loop designated the *QRS loop,* while the repolarization of the ventricles is recorded as a smaller loop designated the *ST-T loop.* Finally, at high magnifications, even a small *U loop* also can be recorded.[155–158] A fundamental concept is that the term *loop* has a VCG, not an ECG, connotation.[155–158]

### Space: The Final Frontier and Multiple Dimensions

The theory of the truly spatial VCG is theoretically attractive.[155–158] Because the heart is a tridimensional structure (located in space), its electrical activity should best be recorded by a spatial method. Indeed, space, as conceived by human senses through objects and their motion, has three dimensions, and positions are characterized by three numbers. The instant of an event is the fourth number. Four definite numbers correspond to every event; a definite event corresponds to any four numbers. Therefore the world of events really forms a four-dimensional continuum.[159–161] Obviously what is perceived by the senses does not correlate with physical theories such as the almost Star Trekkian "string theory"; Hawking's M theories (p-branes), which involve 10 or 26 dimensions; or algebraic concepts dealing with more than three dimensions.[159–161]

To obtain the spatial VCG, electrodes are placed on the body surface so as to record three leads whose planes are at right angles to each other. The true spatial VCG requires three corrected orthogonal leads with the following features[155–158]: (1) Mutual perpendicularity, with each lead being parallel to one of the rectilinear coordinate axes of the human body. Such axes are the horizontal, *X* (left-to-right and right-to-left) axis; the vertical, *Y* (inferosuperior or superoinferior) axis; and sagittal, *Z* (anteroposterior or posteroanterior) axis. (2) Equal amplitude from the vectorial viewpoint. (3) Retention of the same magnitude and direction for all points where cardiac electromotive forces are generated. For example, even if the leads forming Einthoven's frontal plane were to be spatially correct, Einthoven's theory itself would make any electrodes placed for the purpose of obtaining the horizontal and sagittal planes (such as the tetrahedral system) spatially incorrect. The most widely used, corrected, truly spatial VCG method probably is the one introduced by Frank.[158] Because the spatial loop cannot be analyzed tridimensionally, it is customary to study its planar projections (Figs. 13-38 and 13-39).

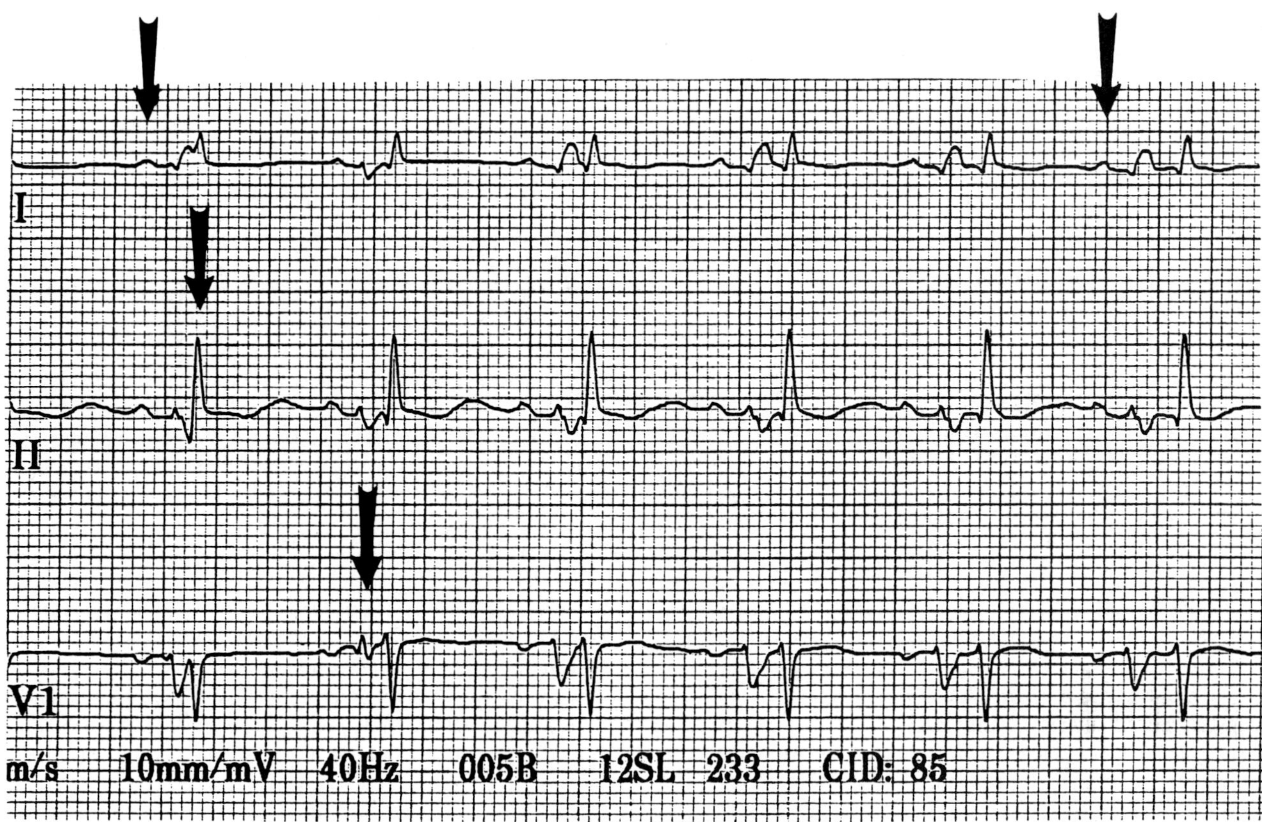


FIGURE 13-37 Pseudoartifact. Typical ECG pattern obtained after heterotopic heart transplantation. There is an "interheart" dissociation during which the ventricular activity of the recipient's heart (arrows in lead I) is totally independent from that of the donor's heart (arrow in lead II). To compound the problem, occasional ventricular ectopic beats (arrow in lead $V_1$) occasionally appear after the donor's P wave but with a shorter than normal PR interval.

Since the previous edition of this book, there has been a revival of the VCG using methods derived or reconstructed from the ECG. Some methods tended to duplicate the Frank system, such as the inverse Dower matrix and the Bjerle and Marquette (Marquette Electronics, Milwaukee system) methods.[162–164] It is commonly accepted that the Frank system does not record local or nondipolar components, since proximity effects do not apply.[155,158] Nondipolar components can be quantified from the 12-lead ECG, but whether they can be obtained from a reconstructed VCG is a subject of debate and speculation.[30,162–169] According to Malik this can be done in a way that requires the use of nonclinical, nonphysical, but valid mathematical terms, such as, for example, *dimension energy*.[31] Here, energy represents the variance of the projection of a vector into a dimension, whereas the latter, as previously stated, is used in reference to three spatial or eight algebraic dimensions.[31]

## Differences between Electrovectorcardiography and Spatial Vectorcardiography

Emphasis should be placed on the fact that previously mentioned VCG methods are distinctly different from the various nonspatial vectorial methods of ECG interpretation, such as those proposed by Sodi-Pallares et al.[8] and Grant.[152,153] Although the spatial VCG and the ECG should each be studied as distinct methods, most electrocardiographers either memorize loop patterns or attempt to derive the leads with which they are familiar from the corresponding QRS loops. Thus bipolar standard and unipolar extremity leads are derived from the frontal plane more or less as when, in clinical ECG, they are derived from the electrical axis. To do this in spatial vector loops, the electrical axis is equated with the maximal QRS vector that extends from the point of origin of the loop to its farthest point. The unipolar precordial leads are derived from the horizontal plane loops. Leads thus derived are different from the usual precordial ECG leads. The latter record electrical forces moving toward or away from them, including local potentials that can be of different duration in different precordial leads.[1,12,13,30] In the 12-lead ECG, however, these forces can move spatially not only in a left-to-right and anteroposterior direction but also in an inferosuperior direction, as in leads $V_5$ and $V_6$ in patients with a very superior and leftward deviation of the EA. On the other hand, the theory of truly spatial vectorcardiography states that the horizontal plane and unipolar leads derived from them just record left-to-right and anteroposterior forces and that they do not record local potentials, so that any differences in the duration of such derived measurements are an illusion due to the isoelectricity in a lead resulting from total perpendicularity of vectors.[155,164] In spatial VCG, electric forces moving superiorly or inferiorly cannot be reflected in the horizontal plane but only in the frontal or sagittal planes.

# QT DISPERSION AND NOVEL MODES OF REPOLARIZATION ANALYSIS

This problem is discussed after dealing with VCG because investigators have proposed the use of the previously mentioned reconstructed VCGs as improvements over this measurement. In fact, the concept

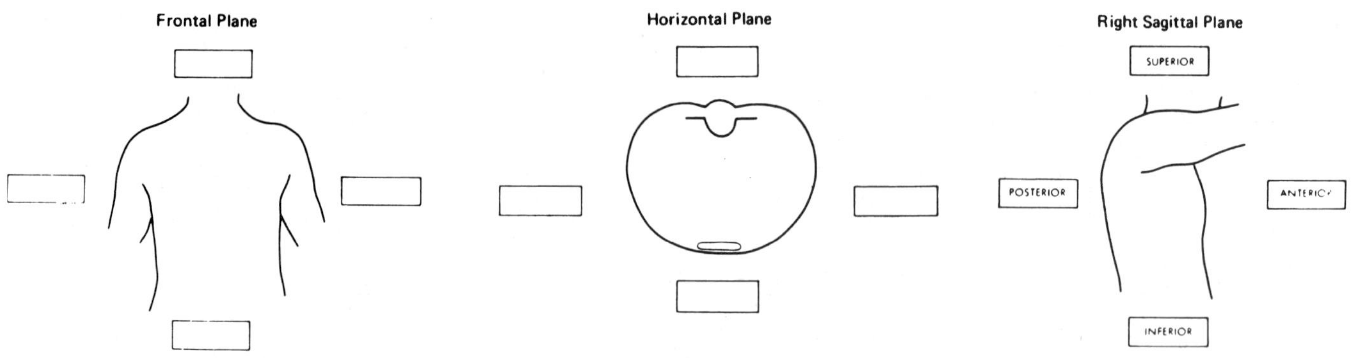


FIGURE 13-38 The spatial vectorcardiographic loops cannot be analyzed routinely in space with presently available techniques. Therefore it is customary to study their projections in three planes, seen as depicted in this figure. Note that (1) the frontal plane conforms to Einthoven's view of his equilateral triangle, (2) the horizontal plane is seen in such a way that the anterior surfaces of the heart and sternum are displayed in the inferior portions of the paper (in contrast to other noninvasive, nonelectrical methods), and (3) the sagittal plane is viewed from the right side of the patient. (From Lemberg and Castellanos.[155] Reproduced with permission from the publisher and authors.)

of QT dispersion (differences between the longest and the shortest QT intervals of the 12-lead ECG) has received considerable attention.[31] Increased dispersion has been reported to be associated with QT prolongation due to proarrhythmic drugs, with increased mortality in epidemiologic studies and after acute myocardial infarction, as well as as a marker of therapeutic efficiency in the congenital or acquired long QT syndromes.[31] Interestingly, more recent studies have challenged the usefulness of this measurement, which has even been considered an illusion.[30,31] Strictly speaking, if it is considered that vector loops lack nondipolar information, then the differences in QT interval in the various ECG leads simply reflect perpendicularity of vectors in some of them.[155,158,164] This is certainly true in regard to the bipolar and unipolar extremity leads but need not apply to the precordial leads, which can record local potentials.[30] More important, Malik and Batchvarov found that values are largely overlapping both between healthy and cardiac subjects as well as between patients with and without adverse outcome.[168] For these authors, QT dispersion is only a crude approximate method of determining the course of repolarization, and "probably grossly abnormal values (100 ms!) which are outside measurement error have practical value."[160]

QT dispersion was originally proposed as a measurement of spatial dispersion of ventricular recovery times. Lately this has been challenged by various investigators who consider that the so-called dispersion results from variations in T-loop morphology and from difficulties or errors in QT measurements as discussed in a previous section.[31]

They have hypothesized that certain novel spatial modes of repolarization analysis should be more accurate and clinically useful surface ECG markers of heterogeneity of repolarization than simple scalar intervals obtained from the ECG, such as QT dispersion. These articles,[31] though extremely original and intellectually stimulating, are complex, since they deal with semiconventional mathematical and physical concepts. More important, they interchange ECG and VCG terms and concepts. Novel descriptors include[164–169] (1) principal component analysis (essentially the ratio of the long and short axis of the three-dimensional (3D) T loop, which is equivalent to the length-to-width bidimensionally projected classical VCG concept); (2) T-loop dispersion (variation of interlead relationships); (3) normalized T-loop area [spatial area of the 3D loop projected in two dimensions (?)]; and (4) the so-called TCRT or vectorial deviation of R and T loops (equivalent to Wilson's ventricular gradient).

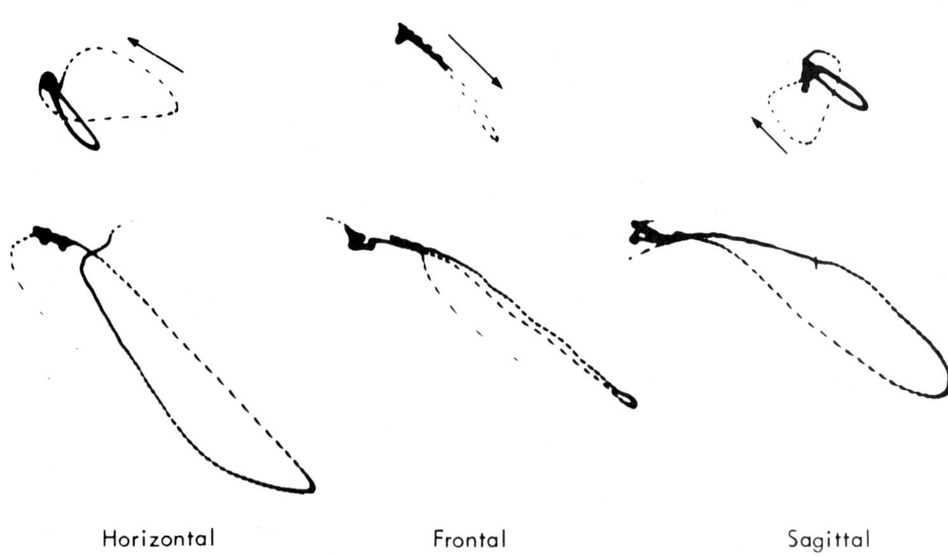


FIGURE 13-39 Planar projections of normal spatial VCG obtained with the Frank method. The ST-T loops are enlarged in the bottom view. In the horizontal plane, the QRS loop shows the expected normal, counterclockwise (CCW) rotation (*arrows*). Although the narrow frontal plane QRS loop has clockwise (CW) rotation, in this plane either CCW, CW, or figure-eight rotations can be normal. In the right sagittal plane, the QRS loop displays its normal (CW) rotation. Enlargement of the ST-T loop clearly shows that its first half is inscribed more slowly. Therefore, the dashes (each representing 0.0025 s, or 2.5 ms) are closer together. The rotation of the ST-T loop is similar to the rotation of the QRS loop in all planes. (From Lemberg and Castellanos.[155] Reproduced with permission from the publisher and authors.)

Regardless of whether QT dispersion is an illusion or not, if it can be superseded by these other measurements, all of them give "global" values different from the more "regional" transmural dispersion of repolarization in single precordial leads.[13] This is a reality given by the time elapsing between the peak of the T wave (reflecting the end of epicardial action potentials) and its termination (reflecting the end action potentials of M cells).[13]

## References


1. Surawicz B, Knilans TK. *Chou's Electrocardiography in Clinical Practice,* 5th ed. Philadelphia: Saunders; 2002:22,76,93,451–453.
2. MacFarlane PW, Lawrie TDV, eds. *Comprehensive Electrocardiology: Theory and Practice in Health and Disease.* New York: Pergamon Press; 1989.
3. Myerburg RJ, Castellanos A. Resolution of nonspecific repolarization patterns from body surface signals: A new horizon of clinical electrocardiography. *J Am Coll Cardiol* 1989;14:703–704.
4. Task Force Report of the American College of Cardiology and the American Heart Association. ACC/AHA Guidelines for Electrocardiography. *Circulation* 1992;19:473–481.
5. Castellanos A, Myerburg RJ. Electrocardiography. In: Schlant RC, Alexander RW, Lipton MJ, eds. *Diagnostic Atlas of the Heart.* New York: McGraw-Hill, 1996.
6. ACC/AHA guidelines for implantation of cardiac pacemakers and antiarrhythmia devices. A report of the American College of Cardiology/American Heart Association Task Force on practice guidelines (Committee on Pacemaker Implantation). *J Am Coll Cardiol* 1998; 31:1175–1209.
7. Lepeschkin E. *Modern Electrocardiography,* Vol 1. Baltimore, MD: Williams & Wilkins; 1951:180–186.
8. Sodi-Pallares D, Medrano GA, Bisteni A, et al. *Deductive and Polyparametric Electrocardiography.* Mexico City: Instituto Nacional Cardiologia Mexico; 1970:36,136.
9. Rosenbaum MB, Elizari MV, Lazzari JO. *The Hemiblocks.* Oldsmar, FL: Tampa Tracings, 1970.
10. Schamroth L. *The Electrocardiology of Coronary Artery Disease,* 2d ed. Oxford, England: Blackwell Scientific; 1984.
11. Wagner GS. Marriott's *Practical Electrocardiography,* 10th ed. Baltimore: Lippincott, Williams & Wilkins; 2001.
12. Barker JM. *The Unipolar Electrocardiogram: A Clinical Interpretation.* New York: Appleton-Century-Crofts; 1952.
13. Antzelevitch C, Shimizu W, Yan GX, et al. The M cell: Its contribution to the ECG and to normal and abnormal electrical function of the heart. *J Cardiovasc Electrophysiol* 1999;10:1124–1152.
14. Lipman BS, Massie E, Kleiger RE. *Clinical Scalar Electrocardiography,* 6th ed. Chicago: Year Book; 1972:210–215.
15. Holland RP, Arnsdorf MF. Solid angle theory and the electrocardiogram: Physiologic and quantitative interpretations. *Prog Cardiovasc Dis* 1997;19:6:431–456.
16. Task Force of the European Society of Cardiology and the North American Society of Pacing and Electrophysiology. Heart rate variability: Standards of measurement, physiological interpretation, and clinical use. *Circulation* 1996;93:1043–1065.
17. Schmidt G, Malik M, Barthel P, et al. Heart rate turbulence after ventricular premature beats as a predictor of mortality after acute myocardial infarction. *Lancet* 1999;353:130–196.
18. Malik M, Wichtele D, Schmidt G. Heart rate turbulence. *G Ital Cardiol* 1999;29:65–69.
19. Barthel P, Schneider R, Bauer A, Ulm K. Correlation coefficient of the heart rate turbulence slope: An independent risk stratifier in post-infarction patients. *Circulation* 2001(suppl II);285:511–603.
20. Ceri Davies L, France DP, Ponikowski P, et al. Relation of heart rate and blood pressure turbulence following premature ventricular complexes to baroreflex sensitivity in chronic congestive heart failure. *Am J Cardiol* 2001;87:737–742.
21. Castellanos A, Myerburg RJ. *The Hemiblocks in Myocardial Infarction.* New York: Appleton-Century-Crofts; 1976.
22. Wilson FN, MacLeod AG, Barker PS, et al. The determination and significance of the areas of the ventricular deflections of the electrocardiogram. *Am Heart J* 1934;10:46–61.
23. Cabrera E, Gaxiola A. *Teoria y Practica de la Electrocardiografia,* 2d ed. Mexico City: La Prensa Medica Mexicana; 1966.
24. Rosenbaum MB, Blanco HH, Elizari MV, et al. Electrotonic modulation of ventricular repolarization and cardiac memory. In: Rosenbaum MB, Elizari MV, eds. *Frontiers of Cardiac Electrophysiology.* Boston: Martinus Nijhoff; 1983:67–99.
25. Rosenbaum MB, Blanco HH, Elizari MV, et al. Electrotonic modulation of the T wave and cardiac memory. *Am J Cardiol* 1982;50:213–222.
26. Rosen MR. What is cardiac memory? *J Cardiovasc Electrophysiol* 2000;11:1289–1293.
27. Surawicz B. Transient T wave abnormalities after cessation of ventricular preexcitation: Memory of what? *J Cardiovasc Electrophysiol* 1996;7:51–59.
28. Surawicz B. Letters to the editor. *J Cardiovasc Electrophysiol* 2001; 12:390–391.
29. Lepeschkin E, Surawicz B. The measurement of the QT interval on the electrocardiogram. *Circulation* 1951;6:378–384.
30. Coumel P, Maison-Blanche P, Badilini F. Dispersion of ventricular repolarization: Reality? Illusion? Significance? *Circulation* 1998;97: 2491–2493.
31. Malik M, Acar B, Gang Y, et al. QT dispersion does not represent electrocardiographic interlead heterogeneity of ventricular repolarization. *J Cardiovas Electrophysiol* 2000;11:835–843.
32. Moleiro F, Castellanos A, Diaz JO, Myerburg RJ. Dynamics of the QT intervals encompassing secondary repolarization abnormalities during sudden but transient lengthening of the RR intervals. *Am J Cardiol* 2003;91:7:883–885.
33. Medina-Ravell VA, Lankipalli RS, Yan GX, et al. Effect of epicardial or biventricular pacing to prolong QT interval and increase transmural dispersion of repolarization. *Circulation* 2003;107:740–746.
34. Rautaharju PM, Zhang ZM. Linearly scaled, rate-invariant normal limits for QT interval: Eight decades of incorrect application of power functions. *J Cardiovasc Electrophysiol* 2002;13:1211–1218.
35. Malik M. Is there a physiologic QT/RR relationship? *J Cardiovasc Electrophysiol* 2002;13:1219–1221.
36. Moleiro F, Misticchio F, Torres JM, et al. Paradoxical behavior of the QT interval during exercise and recovery and its relationship with cardiac memory. *Clin Cardiol* 1999;22:413–416.
37. Castellanos A, Moleiro F, Lopera G, et al. Dynamics of the uncorrected QT interval during vagal-induced lengthening of RR intervals. *Am J Cardiol* 2000;86:1390–1392.
38. Boyett MR, Fedida D. Changes in the electrical activity of dog cardiac Purkinje fibers at high heart rates. *J Physiol* 1984;350:361–391.
39. Elharrar V, Surawicz B. Cycle length effect on restitution of action potential duration in dog cardiac fibers. *Am J Physiol* 1983;244: H782–792.
40. Coghlan JG, Madden B, Norell MN, et al. Paradoxical early lengthening and subsequent linear shortening of the QT interval in response to exercise. *Eur Heart J* 1992;13:1325–1328.
41. Kligfield P, Kevin GL, Okin PM. QTc behavior during treadmill exercise as a function of the underlying QT heart-rate relationship. *J Electrocardiol* 1996;28:206–210.
42. Mirvis DM. Spatial variation of QT intervals in normal persons and patients with acute myocardial infarction. *J Am Coll Cardiol* 1985; 5(3):625–631.
43. Ahvine S, Vallin H. Influence of heart rate and inhibition of autonomic tone on the QT interval. *Circulation* 1982;65:433–435.
44. ZaZa A, Malfatto G, Schwartz PJ. Sympathetic modulation of the relation between ventricular repolarization and cycle length. *Circ Res* 1991;68:1191–1203.
45. Cappato R, Alboni P, Pedroni P, et al. Sympathetic and vagal influences on rate-dependent changes of QT interval in healthy subjects. *Am J Cardiol* 1991;68:1188–1193.

46. Litovsky SH, Antzelevitch C. Rate dependence of action potential duration and refractoriness in canine ventricular endocardium differs from that of epicardium: Role of the transient outward current. *J Am Coll Cardiol* 1989:14:1053–1066.
47. Coumel P, Fayn J, Maison-Blanche P, et al. Clinical relevance of assessing QT dynamicity in Holter recordings. *J Electrocardiol* 1997; 27(suppl):62–66.
48. Shvilkin A, Danilo P Jr, Wang J, et al. Evolution and resolution of long-term cardiac memory. *Circulation* 1998;97:1810–1817.
49. The Criteria Committee of the New York Heart Association. *Nomenclature and Criteria for Diagnosis of Diseases of the Heart and Great Vessels,* 8th ed. New York: New York Heart Association; 1979:304.
50. Franz MR, Swerdlow CD, Liem LB, Schaefer J. Cycle length dependence of human action potential duration in vivo. Effects of single extrastimuli, sudden sustained rate acceleration and deceleration, and different steady-state frequencies. *J Clin Invest* 1988;82:972–979.
51. Jaeger JF Jr, Pinski SL, Trohman RG, Fouad-Tarazi FM. Paradoxical failure of QT prolongation during cardioinhibitory neurocardiogenic syncope. *Am J Cardiol* 1997;79:100–102.
52. Holland RP, Brooks H. QT-ST segment mapping: Critical review and analysis of current concepts. *Am J Cardiol* 1977;40:110–129.
53. Birbaum Y, Sclarovsky S. The grades of ischemia on the presenting electrocardiogram of patients with ST-segment elevation acute myocardial infarction. *J Electrocardiogr* 2001;34(suppl):17–26.
54. Sclarovsky S. *Electrocardiography of Acute Myocardial Ischaemic Syndromes.* London: Martin Dunitz; 1999.
55. Kim TY, Alturk N, Shaikh N, et al. An electrocardiographic algorithm for the prediction of the culprit lesion site in acute anterior myocardial infarction. *Clin Cardiol* 1999;22:77–83.
56. Phibbs B, Marcua F, Marriott HJC, et al. Q-wave versus non-Q-wave myocardial infarction: A meaningless distinction. *J Am Coll Cardiol* 1999;33:576–582.
57. Castellanos A, Lemberg L. *A Programmed Introduction to the Electrical Axis and the Action Potential.* Oldsmar, FL: Tampa Tracings; 1974:34: 114.
58. Barold SS, Falkoff MD, Ong LS, et al. Significance of transient electrocardiographic Q waves in coronary artery disease. *Cardiol Clin* 1987;5:367–380.
59. de Lemos JA, Braunwald E. ST segment resolution as a tool for assessing the efficacy of reperfusion therapy. *J Am Coll Cardiol* 2001; 38:1283–1294.
60. Timmis GC. Electrocardiographic effects of reperfusion. *Cardiol Clin* 1987;5:427–446.
61. Braunwald E, Kloner RA. The stunned myocardium: Prolonged postischemic ventricular dysfunction. *Circulation* 1982;66:1146–1149.
62. Rahimtoola SH. A perspective on the three large multicenter randomized clinical trials of coronary bypass surgery for chronic stable angina. *Circulation* 1985;72(suppl 5):123–135.
63. Braunwald E, Rutherford JD. Reversible ischemic left ventricular dysfunction: Evidence for the "hibernating myocardium." *J Am Coll Cardiol* 1986;8:1467–1470.
64. Bayes de Luna A. *Clinical Electrocardiography: A Textbook.* Mt. Kisco, NY: Futura;1993:450.
65. Califf RM, Mark DB, Wagner GS. *Acute Coronary Care in the Thrombolytic Era.* Chicago: Year Book, 1988.
66. Shah PK, Zahger D, Ganz W. Streptokinase in acute myocardial infarction. In: Francis GS, Alpert JS, eds. *Coronary Care,* 2nd ed. Boston: Little, Brown; 1995:409–450.
67. Goodman S. Q wave and non-Q wave myocardial infarction after thrombolysis (letter). *J Am Coll Cardiol* 1996;27(7):1817–1819.
68. Fernandez AR, Sequeira RF, Chakko S, et al. ST segment tracking for rapid determination of patency of the infarct-related artery in acute myocardial infarction. *J Am Coll Cardiol* 1995;26:675–683.
69. Veldkamp RF, Simoons ML, Pope JE, et al. Continuous multilead ST segment monitoring in acute myocardial infarction. In: Clements IP, ed. *The Electrocardiogram in Acute Myocardial Infarction.* Mt. Kisco, NY: Futura; 1998.
70. Selvester RH, Wagner GE, Iderker RE. Myocardial infarction. In: MacFarlane PW, Lawrie TD, eds. *Comprehensive Electrocardiology.* New York: Pergamon; 1989.
71. Braat SH, Brugada P, den Dulk K, et al. Value of lead $V_{4R}$ for recognition of the infarct coronary artery in acute inferior myocardial infarction. *Am J Cardiol* 1984;53:1538–1541.
72. Marriott HJL, ed. *Practical Electrocardiography,* 8th ed. Baltimore: Williams & Wilkins, 1998.
73. Wasserburger RH, Alt WJ. The normal RS-T segment elevation variant. *Am J Cardiol* 1961;8:184–192.
74. Goldberger AL. ST segment elevation: normal variants: Benign (functional) ST segment elevation, "early repolarization variant." In: Goldberger AL, ed. *Myocardial Infarction: ECG Differential Diagnosis,* 3d ed. St. Louis: Mosby; 1984:1970–1978.
75. Morace G, Padeletti L, Porciani MC, et al. Effect of isoproterenol on the early repolarization syndrome. *Am Heart J* 1979;97:343–347.
76. Miyazaki T, Mitamura H, Miyoshi S, et al. Autonomic and antiarrhythmic drug modulation of ST segment elevation in patients with Brugada syndrome. *J Am Coll Cardiol* 1996;27:1061–1070.
77. Brugada P, Brugada J. Right bundle branch block, persistent ST segment elevation and sudden cardiac death: A distinct clinical and electrocardiographic syndrome. *J Am Coll Cardiol* 1992;20:1391–1396.
78. Wilde AAM, Antzelevitch C, Borggrefe M, et al. Proposed diagnostic criteria for the Brugada syndrome. Consensus Report. *Circulation* 2002;106:2514–2519.
79. Corrado D, Nava A, Buja G, et al. Familial cardiomyopathy underlies syndrome of right bundle branch block, ST segment elevation and sudden death. *J Am Coll Cardiol* 1996;27:443–448.
80. Fujiki A, Usui M, Nagasawa H, et al. ST segment elevation in the right precordial leads induced with class IC antiarrhythmic drugs: Insight into the mechanism of Brugada syndrome. *J Cardiovasc Electrophysiol* 1999;10:214–218.
81. Fontaine G, Fontaliran F, Lascault P, et al. In: Zipes DP, Jalife J, eds. *Cardiac Electrophysiology: From Cell to Bedside,* 2d ed. Philadelphia: Saunders; 1995:754–768.
82. Friedberg CK, Zager A. Nonspecific ST- and T-wave changes. *Circulation* 1961;23:655–661.
83. Sequeira RF, Lemberg L. The electrocardiogram read as nonspecific ST-T waves. *ACC Curr J Rev* 1995; July/August: 36–40.
84. Nelson SD, Kou WH, Annesley T, et al. Significance of ST segment depression during paroxysmal supraventricular tachycardia. *J Am Coll Cardiol* 1988;12:383–387.
85. Castellanos A, Pina IL, Zaman L, et al. Recent advances in the diagnosis of fascicular blocks. *Cardiol Clin* 1987;5:469–488.
86. Rosenbaum MB, Corrado G, Oliveri R, et al. Right bundle branch block with left anterior hemiblock surgically induced in tetralogy of Fallot. *Am J Cardiol* 1970;26:12–19.
87. Cohen SI, Lau SH, Stein E, et al. Variations of aberrant ventricular conduction in man: Evidence of isolated and combined block within the specialized conduction system. *Circulation* 1968;38:899–916.
88. Milliken JA. Isolated and complicated left anterior fascicular block: A review of suggested electrocardiographic criteria. *J Electrocardiol* 1983;16:199–211.
89. Rosenbaum MB, Elizari MV, Lazzari JO. The differential electrocardiographic manifestations of hemiblocks, bilateral bundle branch blocks and trifasicular blocks. In: Schlant RC, Hurst JW, eds. *Advances in Electrocardiography.* New York: Grune & Stratton; 1972: 145–161.
90. Nakaya Y, Hiasa Y, Murayama Y, et al. Prominent anterior QRS forces as a manifestation of left septal fascicular block. *J Electrocardiol* 1978; 11:39–46.
91. Gambetta M, Childers RW. Rate-dependent right precordial Q waves: "Septal focal block." *Am J Cardiol* 1973;32:196–201.
92. Dhala A, Gonzalez-Zuelgaray J, Deshpande S, et al. Unmasking the trifascicular left intraventricular conduction system by ablation of the right bundle branch. *Am J Cardiol* 1996;77:706–712.
93. Grant RP. Peri-infarction block. *Progr Cardiovasc Dis* 1959;27: 237–247.

94. Oppenheimer BS, Rothschild MA. Electrocardiographic changes associated with myocardial involvement: With special reference to prognosis. *JAMA* 1997;69:429–431.
95. Castle CH, Keane WM. Electrocardiographic "peri-infarction block": A clinical and pathologic correlation. *Circulation* 1965;31:403–408.
96. Cotne RA, Parkin TW, Brandenburg RO, et al. Peri-infarction block: Postmyocardial infarction intraventricular conduction disturbance. *Am Heart J* 1965;69:150–153.
97. First SR, Bayley RH, Bedford DR. Peri-infarction block. *Circulation* 1950;2:31–36.
98. Wilson FN, Hill IGW, Johnston FD. The form of electrocardiogram in experimental myocardial infarction: III. The later effects produced by ligation of the anterior descending branch of the left coronary artery. *Am Heart J* 1935;10:903–915.
99. Barker JM, Valencia F. The precordial electrocardiogram in incomplete right bundle branch block. In: Johnson FD, Lepeschkin E, eds. *Selected Papers of Dr. Frank N. Wilson.* Ann Arbor, MI: Edwards Brothers; 1954; 884–914.
100. Blount SG, Munyan EA Jr, Hoffman MS. Hypertrophy of the right ventricular outflow tract: A contract of the electrocardiographic findings in atrial septal defect. *Am J Med* 1957;22:784–790.
101. Moore EN, Hoffman BF, Patterson DF, et al. Electrocardiographic changes due to delayed activation of the wall of the right ventricle. *Am Heart J* 1964;68:347–361.
102. Sung RJ, Tamer DM, Agha AS, et al. Etiology of the electrocardiographic pattern of "incomplete right bundle branch block" in atrial septal defect: An electrophysiologic study. *J Pediatr* 1975;87:1182–1186.
103. Castellanos A, Ramirez AV, Mayorga-Cortes A, et al. Left fascicular blocks during right-heart catheterization using the Swan-Ganz catheter. *Circulation* 1981;64:1271–1276.
104. Sgarbossa EB. Recent advances in the electrocardiographic diagnosis of myocardial infarction: Left bundle branch block and pacing. *PACE* 1998;21:120–131.
105. Kindwall KE, Brown JP, Josephson ME. Predictive accuracy of criteria for chronic myocardial infarction in pacing-induced left bundle branch block. *Am J Cardiol* 1986;57:1255–1260.
106. Wackers FJT. The diagnosis of myocardial infarction in the presence of left bundle branch block. *Cardiol Clin* 1987;5:393–401.
107. Wolff L, Parkinson J, White PD. Bundle-branch block with short P-R interval in healthy young people prone to paroxysmal tachycardia. *Am Heart J* 1930;5:685–704.
108. Castillo CA, Castellanos A Jr. His bundle recordings in patients with reciprocating tachycardias and Wolff-Parkinson-White syndrome. *Circulation* 1970;42:271–285.
109. Rosenbaum FF, Hecht HH, Wilson FN, et al. The potential variations of the thorax and esophagus in anomalous atrioventricular excitation (Wolff-Parkinson-White syndrome). *Am Heart J* 1945;29: 281–326.
110. Wallace AG, Sealy WC, Gallagher JJ, et al. Ventricular excitation in Wolff-Parkinson-White syndrome. In: Wellens HJJ, Lie KI, Janse MJ, eds. *The Conduction System of the Heart: Structure, Function and Clinical Implications.* Leiden: HE Stenfert Kroese; 1976:613–630.
111. Castellanos A, Agha AS, Portillo B, et al. Usefulness of vectorcardiography combined with His bundle recordings and cardiac pacing in evaluation of the preexcitation (Wolff-Parkinson-White) syndrome. *Am J Cardiol* 1972;30:623–628.
112. Wellens HJJ. Contribution of cardiac pacing to our understanding of the Wolff-Parkinson-White syndrome. *Br Heart J* 1975;37:231–241.
113. Milstein S, Sharma AD, Guiraudon GM, et al. An algorithm for the electrocardiographic localization of accessory pathways in the Wolff-Parkinson-White syndrome. *PACE* 1987;10:555–563.
114. Basiouny T, De Chillou D, Fareh S, et al. Accuracy and limitations of published algorithms using the twelve-lead electrocardiogram to localize over atrioventricular accessory pathways. *J Cardiovasc Electrophysiol* 1999;10:1340–1349.
115. Chiang CE, Chen SA, Teo WS, et al. An accurate stepwise electrocardiographic algorithm for localization of accessory pathways in patients with Wolff-Parkinson-White syndrome from a comprehensive analysis of delta waves and r/s ratio during sinus rhythm. *Am J Cardiol* 1995;76:40–46.
116. Cosio FG, Anderson RH, Kuck KH, et al. ESCWGA/NASPE/P experts consensus statement: living anatomy of the atrioventricular junctions. A guide to electrophysiologic mapping. *J Cardiovasc Electrophysiol* 1999;10:1162–1170.
117. Castellanos A Jr, Ortiz JM, Pastis N, et al. The electrocardiogram in patients with pacemakers. *Prog Cardiovasc Dis* 1970:13:190–209.
118. Castellanos A Jr, Lemberg L, Salhanick L, et al. Pacemaker vectorcardiography. *Am Heart J* 1968;75:6–18.
119. Befeler B, Berkovits BV, Aranda JM, et al. Programmed simultaneous biventricular stimulation in man, with special reference to its use in the evaluation of intraventricular reentry. *Eur J Cardiol* 1979;9:369–378.
120. Popovic ZB, Grimm RA, Perlic G, et al. Noninvasive assessment of cardiac resynchronization therapy for congestive heart failure using myocardial strain and left ventricular peak power as parameters of myocardial synchrony and function. *J Cardiovasc Electrophysiol* 2002; 13:1203–1208.
121. Akiyam M, Kaneko Y, Taniguchi Y, Kurabayashi M. Pacemaker syndrome associated with a biventricular pacing system. *J Cardiovasc Electrophysiol* 2002;13:1061–1062.
122. Varma C, Sharma S, Firoozi S, et al. Atriobiventricular pacing improves exercise capacity in patients with heart failure and intraventricular conduction delay. *J Am Coll Cardiol* 2003;41:582–588.
123. Surawicz B. Electrocardiographic diagnosis of chamber enlargement. *J Am Coll Cardiol* 1986;8:711–724.
124. Reichet N, Devereux RB. Left ventricular hypertrophy: Relationship of anatomic echocardiographic and electrocardiographic findings. *Circulation* 1981;63:1391–1399.
125. Bommer K, Weinert L, Neumann A, et al. Determinations of right atrial and right ventricular size by two-dimensional echocardiography. *Circulation* 1980;60:91–98.
126. Doxandabaratz J, Fort de Ribot R, Trilla E, et al. Miocardiopatia hipertrofica apical. *Rev Latina Cardiol* 1982;3:35–41.
127. Romhilt D, Estes E. A point score system for the ECG diagnosis of left ventricular hypertrophy. *Am Heart J* 1968;75:752.
128. Casale PN, Devereux R, Alonso D, et al. Autopsy validation of improved ECG criteria of left ventricular hypertrophy. *J Am Coll Cardiol* 1985;5:511–517.
129. Talbot S, Kilpatrick D. Diagnostic criteria for left ventricular hypertrophy. In: MacFarlane PW, ed. *Progress in Electrocardiology.* London: Pittman Medical; 1979:534–541.
130. Koito H, Spodick D. Electrocardiographic $RV_6/RV_1$ voltage ratio for diagnosis of left ventricular hypertrophy. *Am J Cardiol* 1989;63: 352–359.
131. Hernandez Padial L. Usefulness of total 12-lead QRS voltage for determining the presence of left ventricular hypertrophy in systemic hypertension. *Am J Cardiol* 1991;68:261–262.
132. Casale PN, Devereux RB, Kligfield P, et al. Electrocardiographic detection of left ventricular hypertrophy: Development and prospective validation of improved criteria. *J Am Coll Cardiol* 1985;6: 572–578.
133. Molloy TJ, Okin PM, Devereux RB, et al. Electrocardiographic detection of left ventricular hypertrophy by the simple QRS voltage-duration product. *J Am Coll Cardiol* 1992;20:1180–1186.
134. Kafka H, Burggraf GW, Milliken JA. Electrocardiographic diagnosis of left ventricular hypertrophy in the presence of left bundle branch block: An echocardiographic study. *Am J Cardiol* 1985;55:103–106.
135. Gertsch M, Theler A, Foglia E. Electrocardiographic detection of left ventricular hypertrophy in the presence of left anterior fascicular block. *Am J Cardiol* 1988;61:1089–1101.
136. Vander Ark CR, Ballantyne F III, Reynolds EW Jr. Electrolytes and the electrocardiogram. *Cardiovasc Clin* 1973;5:269–294.
137. Fisch C. Electrocardiography and vectorcardiography. In: Braunwald E, ed. *Heart Disease,* 4th ed. Philadelphia: Saunders; 1992:116–160.
138. Levine HD, Wanzer SH, Merrill JP. Dialyzable currents of injury in potassium intoxication resembling acute myocardial infarction or pericarditis. *Circulation* 1956;13:29–36.

139. Mosseri M, Porath A, Ovsyshcher I, et al. Electrocardiographic manifestations of combined hypercalcemia and hypermagnesemia. *J Electrocardiol* 1990;23:235–241.
140. Kulick DL, Hong R, Ryzen E, et al. Electrophysiologic effects of intravenous magnesium in patients with normal conduction systems and no clinical evidence of significant cardiac disease. *Am Heart J* 1988;148:367–373.
141. Tzivoni D, Keren A, Cohen AM, et al. Magnesium therapy for torsades de pointes. *Am J Cardiol* 1984;53:528–530.
142. Osborn JJ. Experimental hypothermia: respiratory and blood pH changes in relation to cardiac function. *Am J Physiol* 1953;175: 389–398.
143. Simonson E. *Differentiation between Normal and Abnormal in Electrocardiography*. St. Louis: Mosby; 1961:262.
144. Kerwin AJ, McLean R, Tegelaar H. A method for the accurate placement of chest electrodes in the taking of serial electrocardiographic tracings. *Can Med Assoc J* 1960;82:258–261.
145. Castellanos A, Saoudi NC, Schwartz A, et al. Electrocardiographic patterns resulting from improper connections of the right leg (ground) cable. *PACE* 1985;8:364–368.
146. Wenger W, Kligfield P. Variability of precordial electrode placement during routine electrocardiography. *J Electrocardiol* 1996;29(3): 179–184.
147. Schijvenaars BJ, Kors JA, van Herpen G, et al. Effect of electrode positioning on ECG interpretation by computer. *J Electrocardiol* 1997;30(3):247–256.
148. Madias JE. Serial ECG recordings via marked chest wall landmarks: An essential requirement for the diagnosis of myocardial infarction in the presence of left bundle branch block. *J Electrocardiol* 2002;35(4): 299–302.
149. Kadner A, Chen RH, Adams DH. Heterotopic heart transplantation: Experimental development and clinical experience. *Eur J Cardiothorac Surg* 2000;17:474–481.
150. Proceedings of the Engineering Foundation Conference "Computerized Interpretation of the Electrocardiogram XII." *J Electrocardiol* 1987;20 (suppl):preface.
151. ACC/AHA Clinical Competence Statement on Electrocardiography and Ambulatory Electrocardiography. A Report of the ACC/AHA/ ACP-ASIM Task Force on Clinical Competence (ACC/AHA Committee to Develop a Clinical Competence Statement on Electrocardiography and Ambulatory Electrocardiography). *J Am Coll Cardiol* 2001;38(7): 2091–2100.
152. Grant RP, Estes EH Jr. *Spatial Vector Electrocardiography*. New York: Blakistonl; 1951.
153. Hurst JM. Methods used to interpret the 12-lead electrocardiogram: Pattern memorization versus the use of vector concepts. *Clin Cardiol* 2000;24:4–13.
154. Wilson FN, Johnston FD. The vectorcardiogram. *Am Heart J* 1938;16: 14–28.
155. Lemberg L, Castellanos A Jr. *Vectorcardiography*, 2nd ed. New York: Appleton-Century-Crofts, 1975.
156. Massie E, Walsh TJ. *Clinical Vectrocardiography and Electrocardiography*. Chicago: Year Book; 1960.
157. Chou TC, Helm RA, Kaplan S. *Clinical Vectorcardiography*, 2nd ed. New York: Grune & Stratton; 1974.
158. Frank E. An accurate, clinically practical system for spatial vectorcardiography. *Circulation* 1956;13:737–749.
159. Kaku M, Trainer J. *Beyond Einstein. The Cosmic Quest for the Theory of the Universe.* New York: Bantam Books; 1987;13, 26.
160. Hawking S. *The Universe in a Nutshell.* New York: Bantam Books; 2001:88.
161. Castellanos A, Myerburg RJ. The dimensions of dimensions. *J Cardiovasc Electrophysiol* 2001;12(2):277–278.
162. Edenbrandt L, Pahlm O. Vectorcardiogram synthesized from a 12-lead ECG: Superiority of the inverse Dower matrix. *J Electrocardiol* 1988;21(4):361–367.
163. Kors JA, van Herpen G, Sittig AC, van Bemmel JH. Reconstruction of the Frank vectorcardiogram from standard electrocardiographic leads: Diagnostic comparison of different methods. *Eur Heart J* 1990;11: 1083–1092.
164. Kors JA, van Herpen G, van Bemmel JH. QT dispersion as an attribute of T-loop morphology. *Circulation* 1999;99:1458–1463.
165. Zabel M, Acar B, Klingenheben T, et al. Analysis of 12-lead T-wave morphology for risk stratification after myocardial infarction. *Circulation* 2000;102:1252–1257.
166. Malik M, Batchvarov V. The heart vector, the regional information in the electrocardiogram and QT dispersion. *Am J Cardiol* 2002;90: 1276–1277.
167. Somberg JC, Molnar J. Usefulness of QT dispersion as an electrocardiographically derived index. *Am J Cardiol* 2002;89:291–294.
168. Malik M, Batchvarov VN. Measurement, interpretation and clinical potential of QT dispersion. *J Am Coll Cardiol* 2000;36:1749–1766.
169. Takenaka K, Ai T, Shimizu W, et al. Exercise stress test amplifies genotype-phenotype correlation in the LQT1 and LQT2 forms of the long-QT syndrome. *Circulation* 2003;107:838–844.

CHAPTER 14

# THE CHEST ROENTGENOGRAM AND CARDIAC FLUOROSCOPY*

James T. T. Chen / Robert A. O'Rourke



Familiarity with the altered anatomy and understanding of the underlying pathophysiology of a diseased heart are the cornerstones to appropriate interpretation of its roentgen manifestations. The conventional four-view cardiac series is tabulated in Table 14-1 and the views are illustrated in Fig. 14-1*C, D, E, and F*.

The approach to the chest roentgenogram should be thorough and objective so that no clue is overlooked and no bias is incorporated in the process of radiographic analysis.[1–4] Rib notching (Fig. 14-1*A, B*) provides important clues to the diagnosis of coarctation of the aorta.[3,5] To prevent erroneous clinical information from misleading the radiographic interpretation, films should initially be interpreted without any knowledge about the patient.

A secundum atrial septal defect may be incorrectly diagnosed as mitral stenosis (MS) because of similar physical signs. The split-second sound may be misinterpreted as the opening snap (Chap. 12). The diastolic rumble due to increased flow through a normal tricuspid valve may mimic the murmur of MS. The x-ray signs of the two entities, however, are quite different (Fig. 14-2*B* versus 14-3*A*). The *final* radiologic diagnosis, however, should be made only after correlating the x-ray findings with clinical information and other laboratory data.[5a]

The radiologic examination for heart disease consists of six major steps. They are (1) roentgenographic examination for anatomy, (2) fluoroscopic examination for dynamics, (3) comparison, (4) statistical guidance, (5) clinical correlation, and (6) conclusion (Table 14-2).

*Acknowledgment: This chapter was adapted and modified from Chap. 12 of *Hurst's The Heart,* 10th edition, as originally authored by Dr. James T. T. Chen as the sole author. He has graciously given his coauthor (ROR) permission to revise this chapter.

## ROENTGENOGRAPHIC EXAMINATION FOR ANATOMY

### An Overview

The first step is to survey the roentgenogram and assess all the structures, searching particularly for noncardiac conditions that may reflect heart disease. For instance, a right-sided stomach with an absent image of the inferior vena cava may suggest the possibility of congenital interruption of the inferior vena cava with azygos continuation[6,7] (Fig. 14-4). A narrowed anteroposterior (AP) diameter of the thorax may be the cause of an innocent murmur[8] (Fig. 14-5).

### Pulmonary Vasculature

The lung may often reflect the underlying pathophysiology of the heart. For example, if uniform dilatation of all pulmonary vessels is present, the diagnosis of a left-to-right shunt (Fig. 14-2*B*) is more likely than a left-sided obstructive lesion. The latter typically shows a cephalic pulmonary blood flow pattern (Fig. 14-3*A*).

### Lung Parenchyma

With right heart failure, the lungs become unusually radiolucent because of decreased pulmonary blood flow (PBF). On the other hand, significant left heart failure is characterized by the presence of pulmonary edema and/or a cephalic blood flow pattern (Fig. 14-6). Long-standing, severe pulmonary venous hypertension may lead to hemosiderosis and/or ossification of the lung.[9,10] When right heart failure results from severe left heart failure, the preexisting pulmonary congestion may improve because of the decreased pulmonary blood flow (Fig. 14-6*B*).

TABLE 14-1 Conventional Four-View Cardiac Series

| | |
|---|---|
| Posteroanterior (PA) view | With barium |
| Left lateral (lateral) view | With barium |
| 45° Right anterior oblique (RAO) view | With barium |
| 60° Left anterior oblique (LAO) view | Without barium |

## Cardiac Size

An enlarged heart is always abnormal; however, mild cardiomegaly may reflect a higher-than-average cardiac output from a normal heart, as seen in athletes. The cardiothoracic ratio remains the simplest yardstick for assessment of cardiac size[1]; the mean ratio in upright posteroanterior (PA) view is 44 percent.

The nature of cardiomegaly can usually be determined by the specific roentgen appearance. As a rule, when the PBF pattern remains normal, volume overload tends to present a greater degree of cardiomegaly than lesions with pressure overload alone. For example, patients with aortic stenosis (AS) typically show features of left ventricular hypertrophy (LVH) without dilatation. On the other hand, the LV both dilates and hypertrophies in the case of aortic regurgitation (AR), producing a much larger heart even before the development of heart failure.

A smaller-than-average heart is encountered in patients with chronic obstructive pulmonary disease (Fig. 14-7*A*), Addison's disease, anorexia nervosa, and starvation. An abnormally small heart, however, is difficult to define except retrospectively, after successful therapy.

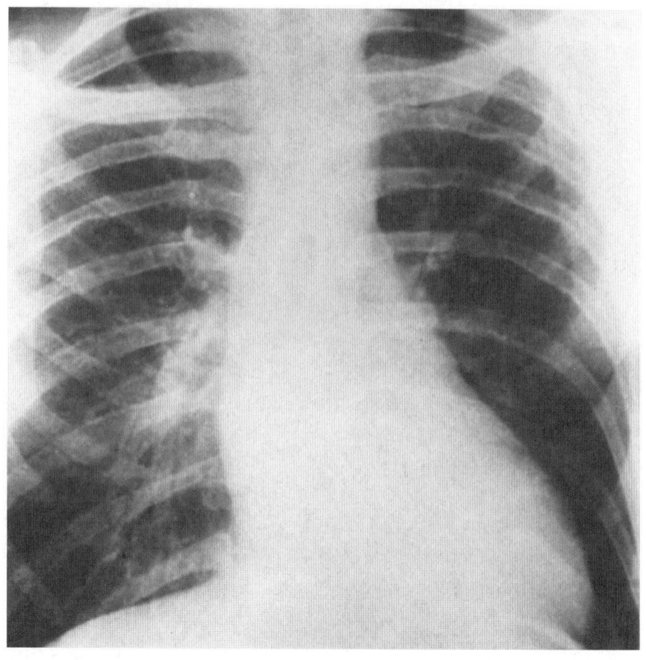


FIGURE 14-1 Practical application of four-view cardiac series. *A*. PA view in a patient with coarctation of the aorta showing areas of rib notching bilaterally and LV enlargement in the inferior and leftward direction. *B*. Magnified view of the left upper thorax of the same patient showing multiple areas of rib notching (*arrows*). *C*. PA view of another patient with aortic coarctation showing the "3 sign" of the deformed descending aorta and "E sign" on the barium-filled esophagus. The upper arrow points to the level of coarctation. The lower arrow marks the apex of the enlarged LV. The arrow on the patient's right indicates the dilated ascending aorta. *D*. Lateral view of a third patient with the same disease showing a barium-filled esophagus to be pushed forward (*upper arrow*) by the poststenotic dilatation of the descending aorta and pushed backward (*middle arrow*) by the enlarged LA. The very large LV (*lower arrow*) simply casts a shadow behind the esophagus without displacing it. The oblique arrow points to the calcified stenotic bicuspid aortic valve. *E*. RAO view of same patient whose PA view is shown in Fig. 14-7*D*. Note the huge RA casting a triangular density (*lower horizontal arrow*) behind the esophagus without displacing it. The esophagus is deviated posteriorly by the enlarged LA (*upper horizontal arrow*). The upper oblique arrows indicate the direction of the enlarging pulmonary trunk and RV. The lower oblique arrow points to the normal LV with the undisturbed left costophrenic sulcus. *F*. LAO view of a patient with valvular AS. The dilated ascending aorta (*upper white arrow*) is immediately above the flat anterior border of normal RV. The black arrow points to the calcified aortic valve. The lower white arrow marks the enlarged LV.

## Cardiac Contour

Any significant deviation from the normal cardiovascular contour may be a clue to the correct diagnosis. For instance, *coeur en sabot,* a "boot-shaped heart" (Fig. 14-2*C*), is characteristic of tetralogy of Fallot. A bulge along the left cardiac border with a retrosternal double density is virtually diagnostic of LV aneurysm (Fig. 14-8). A markedly widened right cardiac contour with a straightened left cardiac border is seen frequently in patients with severe MS leading to tricuspid regurgitation (TR) (Fig. 14-7*D*).

## Abnormal Densities

Besides the familiar double density cast by an enlarged left atrium (LA), other increased densities may be found within the confines of the heart, indicating a variety of dilated vascular structures [e.g., tortuous descending aorta, aortic aneurysm, coronary artery (CA) aneurysm, pulmonary varix].[2] Furthermore, large cardiac calcifications are readily seen, in lateral and oblique views. If smaller calcific deposits are suspected, they should be verified promptly, ruled out by cardiac fluoroscopy or computed tomography (CT) (Chap. 20). Any radiologically detectable calcification in the heart is clinically important. The heavier the calcification, the more significant it becomes (Fig. 14-1*F*). The extent of valvular calcification tends to be proportionate to the severity of the valve stenosis regardless of the other roentgen signs of the disease.[1,2,13,14] Calcification of the CA is almost always atherosclerotic in nature. A fluoroscopically detectable coronary calcification correlates with major vessel occlusion in 94 percent of patients *with chest pain*[15]; however, the sensitivity of the test is only 40 percent.

Recently, electron-beam CT (EBCT) scanning has proven to be a sensitive method for detection and quantifying coronary calcifications (Chaps. 20 and 57). While a negative result may indicate no need for further testing in asymptomatic individuals, a positive result does not necessarily denote obstructive CAD. The sensitivity for detecting any coronary calcifications is greater than 95 percent with a *specificity of less than 65 percent* for significant CA luminal stenosis. A calcified ascending aortic aneurysm with AR is highly suggestive of syphilitic aortitis[11] (Fig. 14-9).

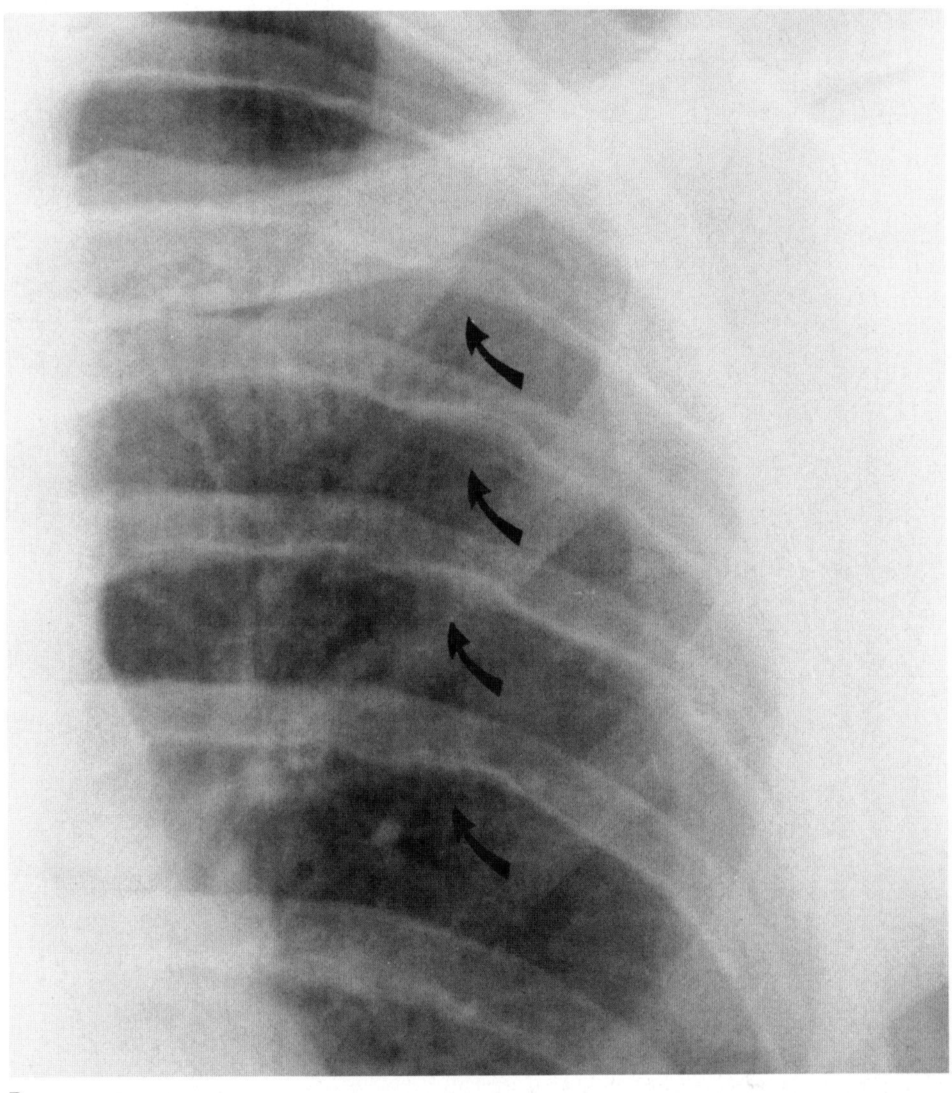


FIGURE 14-1 (*Continued*)

## Abnormal Lucency

The abnormal lucent areas in and about the heart include (1) displaced subepicardial fat stripes caused by effusion or thickening of the pericardium (Fig. 14-10), (2) pneumopericardium (Fig. 14-11), and (3) pneumomediastinum. Pneumomediastinum is differentiated from pneumopericardium by the fact that the former shows a superior extension of the air strip beyond the confines of the pericardium.

## Cardiac Malpositions

"Cardiac malpositions" are diagnosed only when either the heart or the stomach is out of the normal left-sided position. This definition is crucial in distinguishing an isolated right-sided aortic arch from a cardiac malposition.[6,7]

### DEXTROCARDIA WITH SITUS INVERSUS

Recently the term *dextrocardia* has been used to indicate any congenital right-sided heart regardless of the position of abdominal viscera. *Dextrocardia with situs inversus* means the mirror image of normal. In this situation, the incidence of congenital heart disease is only 5 percent, a ninefold increase over the general population. The combination of dextrocardia, sinusitis, and bronchiectasis is known as *Kartagener's triad.*

### DEXTROCARDIA WITH SITUS SOLITUS

This represents an anomaly with normal situs but a right-sided heart. Radiographically, normal situs (situs solitus) is a certainty when both the aortic knob and the gastric air bubble are on the left side. *Situs solitus* also means that both the abdominal viscera and the atria are in the normal position. Under these circumstances, if the ventricles fail to swing from the primitive right-sided position to the normal left-sided position, abnormal relationships between the ventricles and the rest of the cardiovascular structures are bound to develop. This entity was formerly termed *dextroversion.*

In patients with dextroversion, the incidence of congenital heart disease has been estimated at 98 percent. More than 80 percent have congenitally corrected (or L loop) transposition of great arteries. The

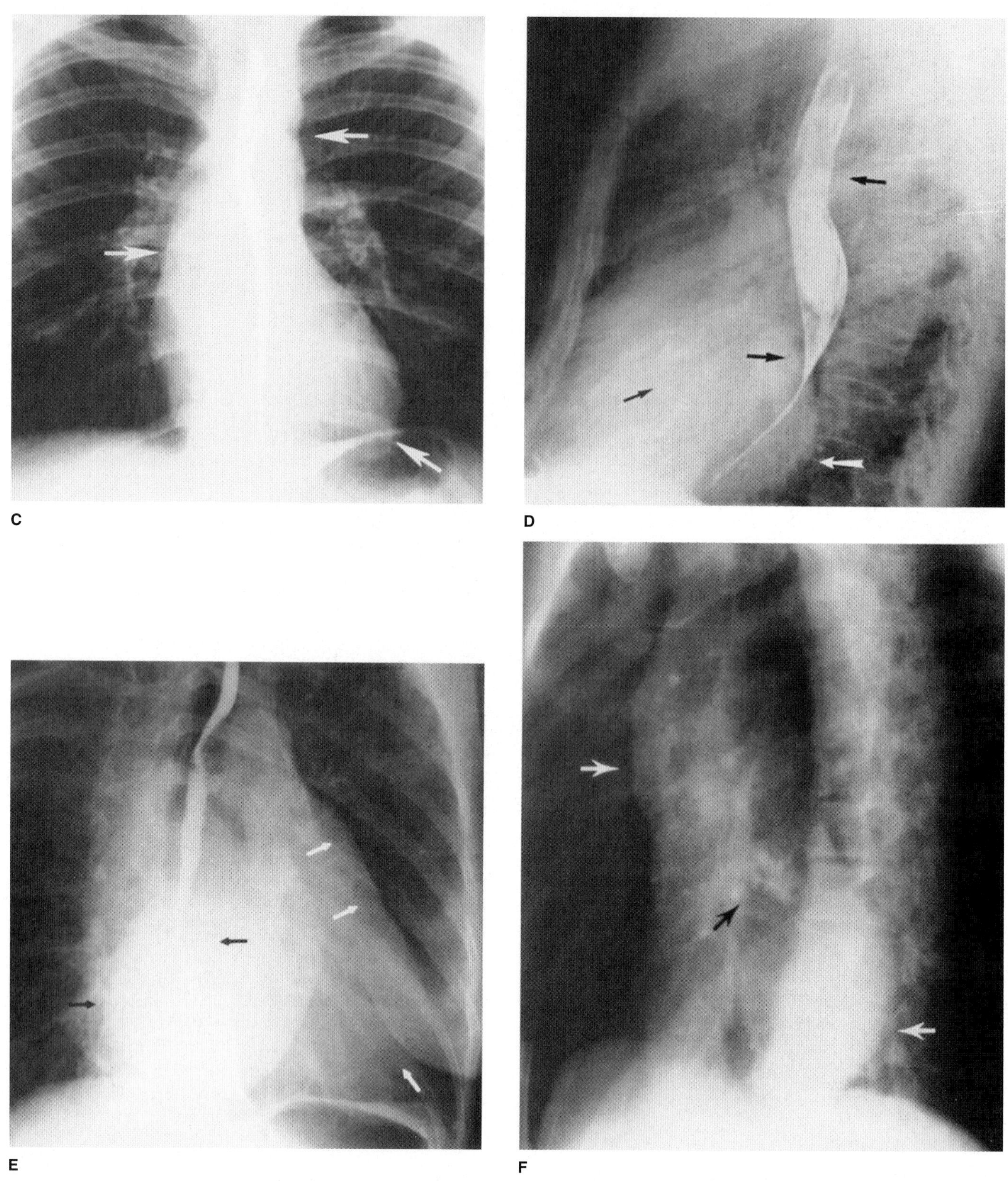


FIGURE 14-1 (*Continued*)

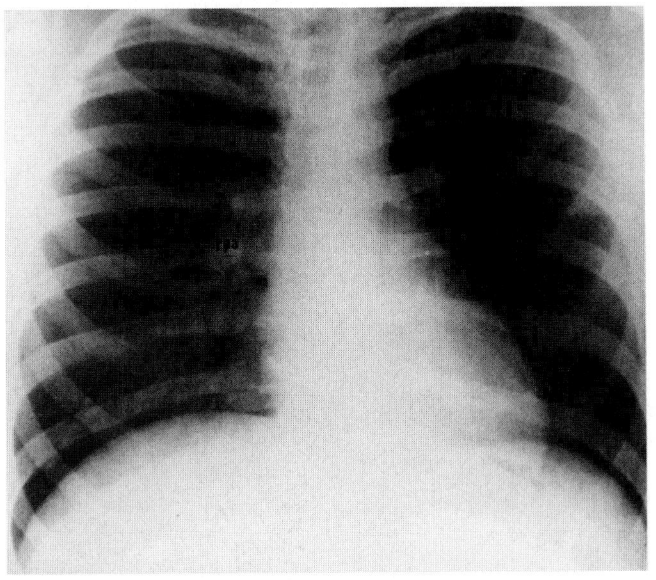

A

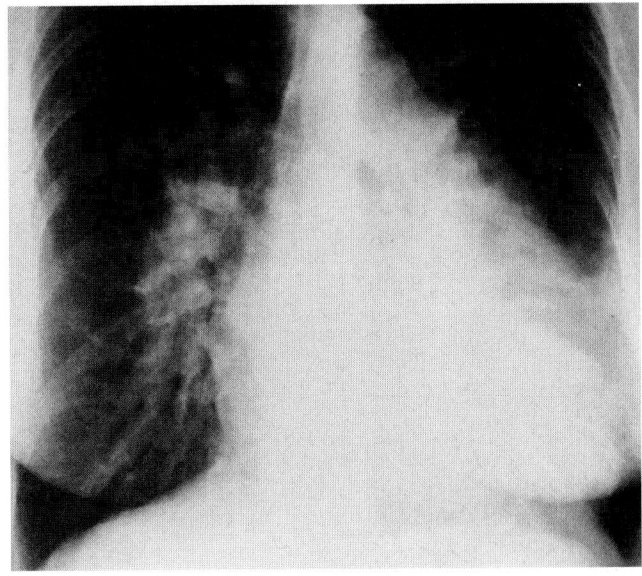

B

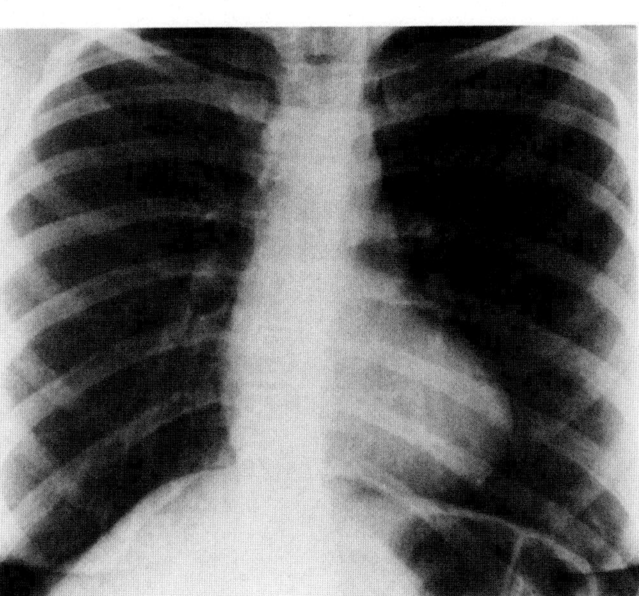

C

FIGURE 14-2 Roentgenographic assessment of the volume of pulmonary blood flow. *A. Normal*. There is caudalization of the pulmonary vascularity due to gravity. The right descending pulmonary artery (rpa) measures 13 mm in diameter in this young man. *B. Increased*. Patient with a secundum atrial septal defect showing uniform increase in pulmonary vascularity bilaterally. The right descending pulmonary artery is markedly enlarged, measuring 27 mm. *C. Decreased*. Patient with tetralogy of Fallot showing a boot-shaped heart and uniform decrease in pulmonary vascularity. The right descending pulmonary artery is much smaller than normal, measuring 6 mm in diameter.

next most commonly associated lesions are a combination of ventricular septal defect and pulmonary stenosis, a tetralogy-like pathophysiology (Fig. 14-12).

#### LEVOCARDIA WITH SITUS INVERSUS

This is a mirror image of dextroversion, and it is associated with nearly a 100 percent incidence of cyanotic congenital cardiac lesions similar to those seen in dextroversion. This entity was formerly termed *levoversion*.

#### LEVOCARDIA WITH SITUS SOLITUS

This is entirely normal.

#### CARDIAC MALPOSITIONS WITH SITUS AMBIGUUS

In this group, the patient's heart may be either left- or right-sided. The site is ambiguous because the aortic arch and the stomach are not on the same side. Under these circumstances, we are dealing with either asplenia or polysplenia syndrome. Patients with polysplenia syndrome tend to be acyanotic and frequently survive into adulthood. The associated lesions are bilateral left-sidedness, interruption of the inferior vena cava with azygos continuation (Fig.14-4), polysplenia, and a left-to-right shunt, most frequently an atrioventricular septal defect. Patients with asplenia tend to be cyanotic and critically ill; they die in infancy.

### Other Abnormalities

#### GREAT VESSELS

The roentgen appearance of the great vessels often provides valuable information for the diagnosis of heart disease.[2,3,16,17] For example, selective dilatation of the ascending aorta is the hallmark of valvular

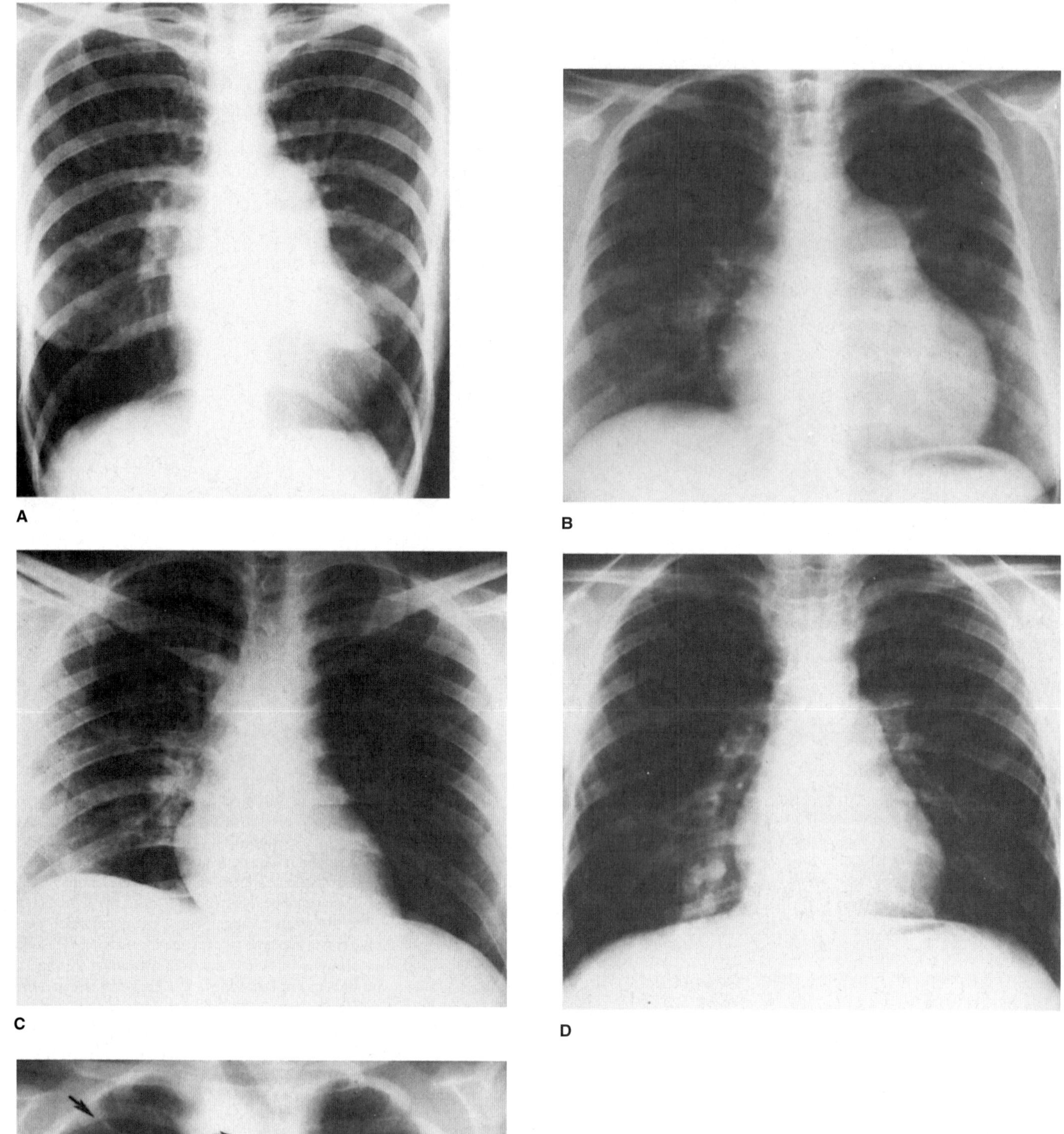


FIGURE 14-3 Abnormal pulmonary blood flow patterns. *A. Cephalization*. Patient with severe MS showing dilatation of the upper vessels with constriction of the lower vessels. *B. Centralization*. Patient with primary PH showing marked dilatation of the pulmonary trunk and the central segments of both pulmonary arteries with pruning of the peripheral branches. *C. Lateralization*. Patient with massive pulmonary embolism obstructing the left main pulmonary artery. Note the uneven distribution of pulmonary blood flow between the two lungs in favor of the right. *D. Localization*. A cyanotic child showing localized vascular changes representing a large pulmonary arteriovenous fistula in the right lower lobe. *E. Collateralization*. A child with pseudotruncus arteriosus with cardiomegaly and a right aortic arch (*small arrow*). Note severe pulmonary oligemia with numerous small tortuous vessels (*large arrow*) in upper medial lung zones, representing bronchial arterial collaterals.

TABLE 14-2 Major Steps of Roentgenologic Examination

Roentgenographic examination for anatomy
- Overview, e.g., rib notching
- Pulmonary vascularity, e.g., shunt vascularity in ASD
- Lung parenchyma, e.g., ossification in critical MS
- Cardiac size, e.g., huge right heart in Ebstein's anomaly
- Cardiac contour, e.g., boot-shaped heart in TOF
- Abnormal densities, e.g., calcification of LV aneurysm
- Abnormal lucency, e.g., conspicuous fat stripes in PE
- Cardiac malpositions, e.g., dextrocardia with SS
- Other abnormalities, e.g., Holt-Oram syndrome

Fluroscopic observation for dynamics

Comparison

Statistical guidance

Clincal correlation

Conclusion

ABBREVIATIONS: ASD = atrial septal defect; MS = mitral stenosis; TOF = tetralogy of Fallot; LV = left ventricle; PE = pericardial effusion; SS = situs solitus.

AS (Fig. 14-13); while generalized dilatation of the entire thoracic aorta (Fig. 14-14) suggests AR, systemic hypertension, or both, depending on the size of the LV. In atrial septal defect and MS, the pulmonary trunk is quite large and the aortic knob is usually small (Fig. 14-2*B*). A leftward cardiac rotation occurs when an enlarged RV coexists with a normal-sized LV. When the heart rotates to the left, the aorta folds on itself in the midline and becomes inconspicuous. Meanwhile, the pulmonary trunk is brought laterally and looks larger than it actually is. Aortic aneurysm (Fig. 14-15) and dissection are frequently associated with hypertensive and atherosclerotic disease.

Prominence of the pulmonary trunk is a reliable secondary sign of right ventricular (RV) enlargement (Fig. 14-16; also Fig. 14-2*B*), with the following exceptions: (1) tetralogy of Fallot with RV hypertrophy but pulmonary trunk hypoplasia, (2) idiopathic dilatation of the pulmonary artery, (3) patent ductus arteriosus with dilated pulmonary trunk but normal RV, and (4) straight-back syndrome, pectus excavatum, and scoliosis with narrowed AP diameter of the chest. Under the latter conditions, the heart is compressed, displaced, and rotated to the left, giving rise to a falsely enlarged pulmonary artery.

In coarctation of the aorta, the engorged aortic knob and the poststenotic dilatation of the descending aorta may cause a "3 sign" on the aorta and an "E sign" on the barium-filled esophagus, both depicting the site of coarctation[6] (Fig. 14-1*C*).

The abnormal size and distribution of both the pulmonary and systemic veins are important clues to the presence of certain conditions—e.g., anomalous pulmonary venous connections, pulmonary arteriovenous fistulas, pulmonary varix, persistent left superior vena cava, and interruption of inferior vena cava with azygos continuation (Fig. 14-4).

## MEDIASTINAL STRUCTURES

The mediastinal organs are frequently affected by the cardiovascular structures because of their close spatial interrelationships. An enlarged LA not only displaces the esophagus (Fig. 14-1*C, D, E*) and the descending aorta but also elevates and compresses the left mainstem bronchus. A double aortic arch may compress both the trachea and the esophagus. On the other hand, malignant processes may invade the heart and great vessels, causing cardiac tamponade or the

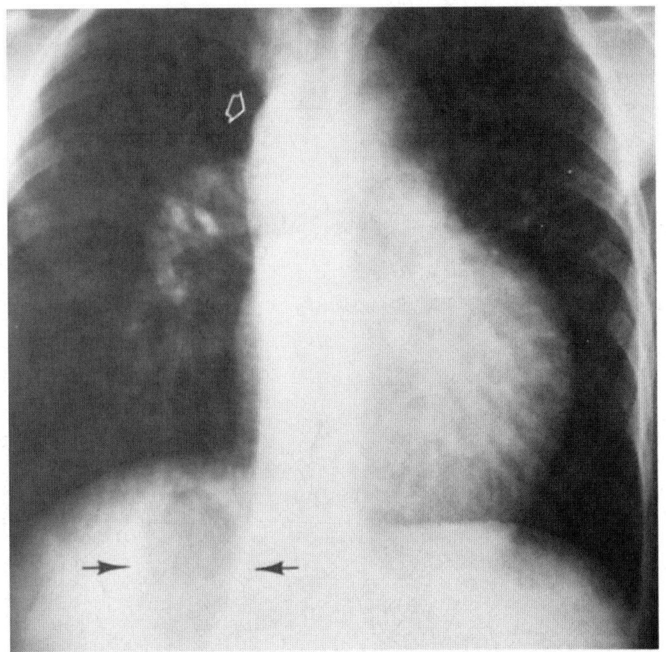

A

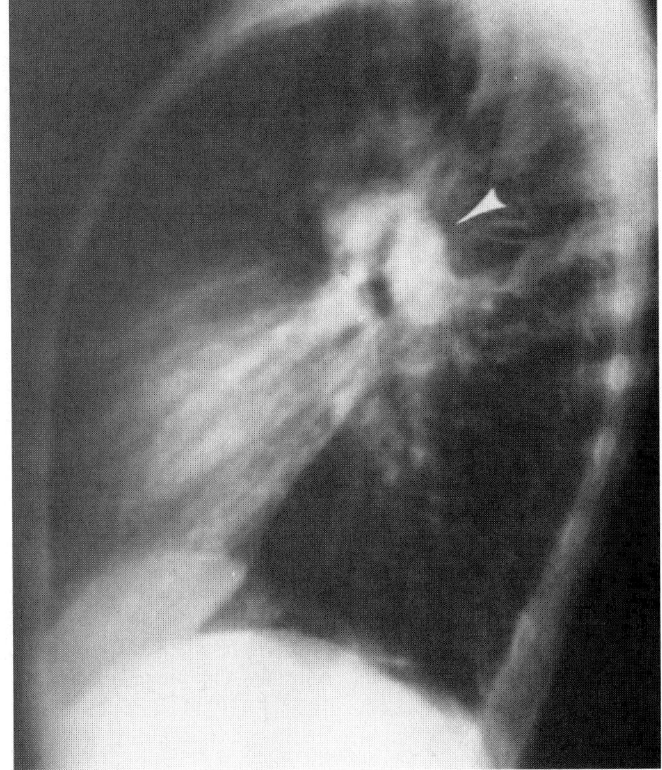

B

FIGURE 14-4 Patient with situs ambiguus, interruption of the inferior vena cava, ventricular septal defect, and polysplenia. *A*. PA view shows that the aortic arch and the heart are left-sided and the stomach (*lower arrows*) is right-sided. The azygos vein (*upper arrow*) is markedly enlarged. The heart is mildly enlarged, and there is a moderate increase in pulmonary vascularity. *B*. Lateral view shows an absent image of the inferior vena cava. The azygos arch (*arrow*) is markedly dilated.

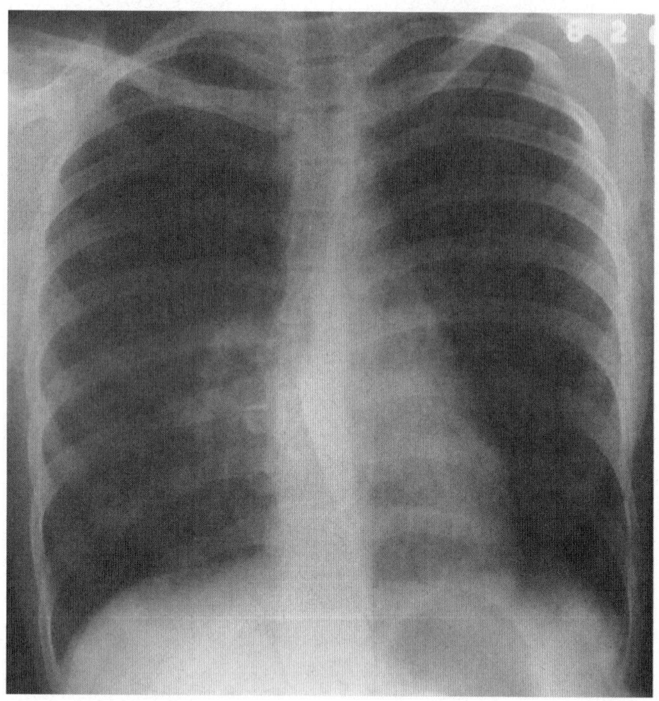

A

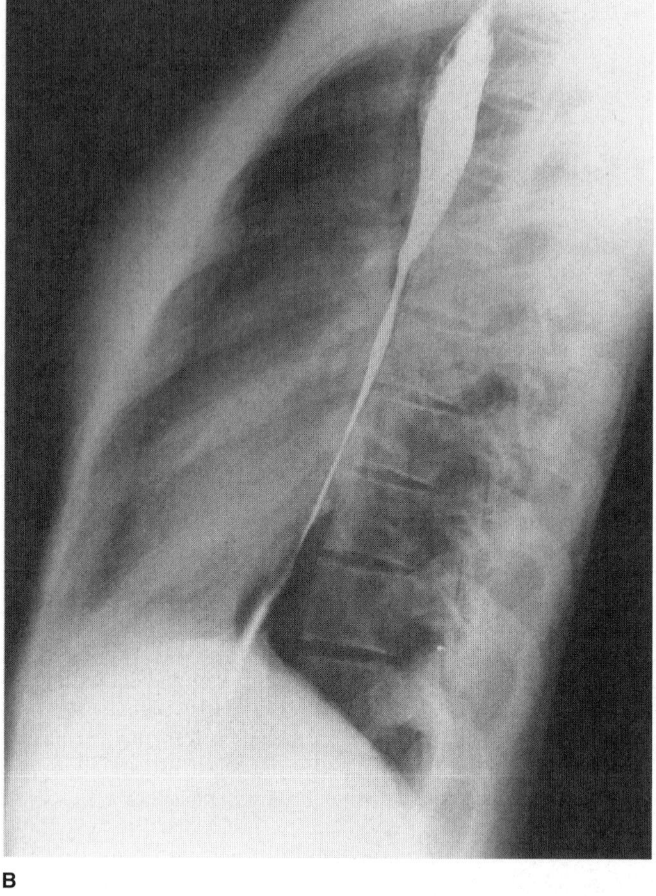

B

FIGURE 14-5 A 16-year-old girl with straight-back syndrome. *A*. PA radiograph shows normal pulmonary vascularity and normal heart size. Note leftward displacement and rotation of the heart, making its left border unusually prominent. *B*. Lateral view shows that the AP diameter of the chest is extremely narrow. The heart is squeezed, creating an innocent murmur.

superior vena cava syndrome. Usually, these mediastinal changes are evident on the chest roentgenogram and should be recognized promptly.[16–20]

### PLEURA

A right-sided pleural effusion is often present with left heart failure. A bilateral hydrothorax, on the other hand, suggests bilateral heart failure or a noncardiac etiology of the effusion. Congestive heart failure is also known to be associated with a pseudotumor or "vanishing" tumor, representing an interlobar collection of pleural fluid (Fig. 14-17). As congestive heart failure improves, the "tumor" disappears.

### BONES AND JOINTS

Notching of the ribs has many origins. Basically, any of the three major intercostal structures can enlarge, compress, and erode the lower borders of the ribs, producing areas of notching. They are intercostal arteries, veins, and nerves. Coarctation of the aorta[6] (Fig. 14-1*A*) represents the most common cause of rib notching due to dynamic dilatation and tortuosity of the arteries. Superior vena cava syndrome may cause a similar phenomenon of venous origin. Neurofibromatosis also can produce rib notching by numerous intercostal neurofibromas.

### SOFT TISSUES OVER THE CHEST

Patients with renal failure may show severe edema in the soft tissues over the chest as part of the picture of general anasarca (Fig. 14-18).

### EXTRATHORACIC STRUCTURES

In Holt-Oram syndrome (Fig. 14-19 and Chap. 12), the upper extremity abnormalities may be evident in a chest roentgenogram or on other films in the patient's x-ray folder (Chap. 63). A large arteriovenous malformation with curvilinear calcifications may be seen in the neck, thereby providing a clue as to the etiology of the patient's heart failure.[7,8]

## COMPARISON

To appreciate the acuteness or chronicity of the disease or its response to therapy, one must carefully compare serial roentgenograms. As demonstrated in Fig. 14-7*B,* the heart may be considered neither enlarged nor failing if the baseline study made 3 years earlier in Fig. 14-7*A* were not available for comparison. Similarly, an enlarging heart with normal pulmonary vascularity is highly suggestive of pericardial effusion. Conversely, a shrinking heart in the presence of normal vascularity is compatible with resolution of a pericardial effusion (Figs. 14-20*A, B*).

## STATISTICAL GUIDANCE

Certain roentgenologic findings are diagnostic of a disease; other signs are suggestive of a diagnosis on the basis of statistics only. Nevertheless, the latter can be quite useful by virtue of their high

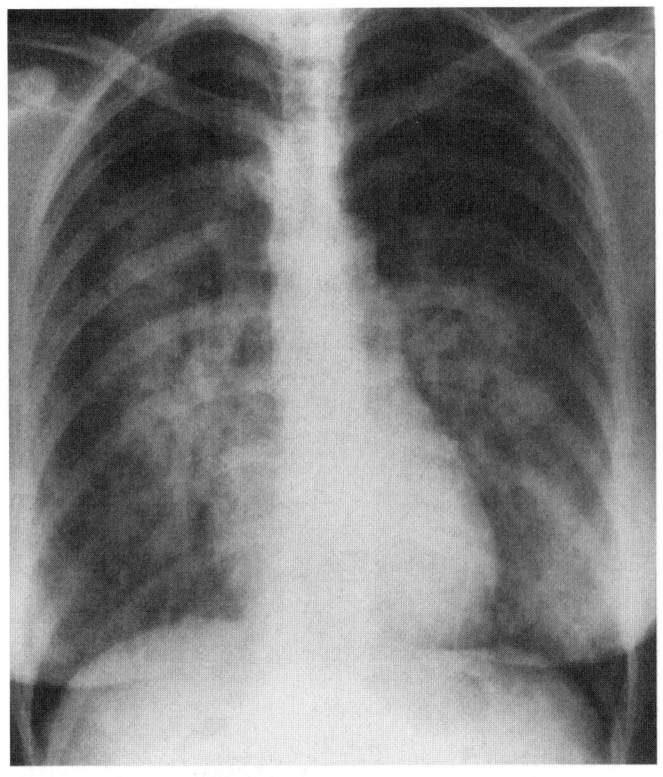

A

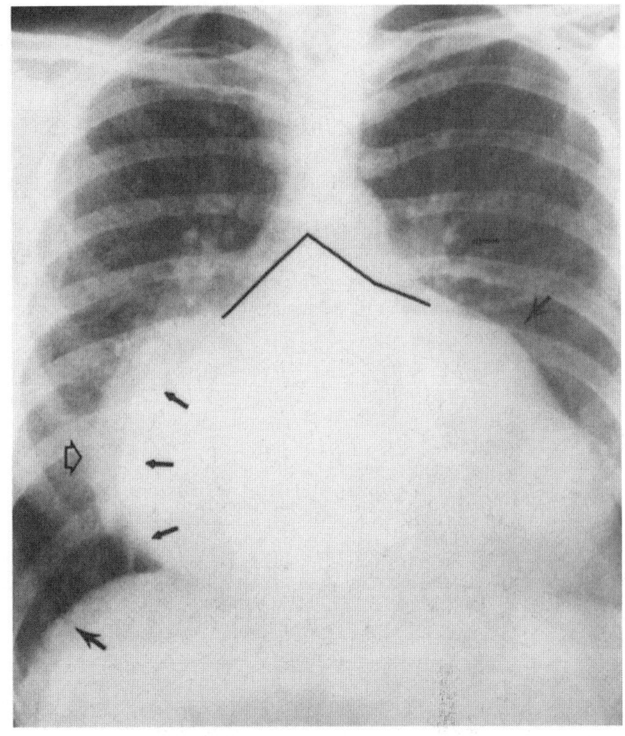

B

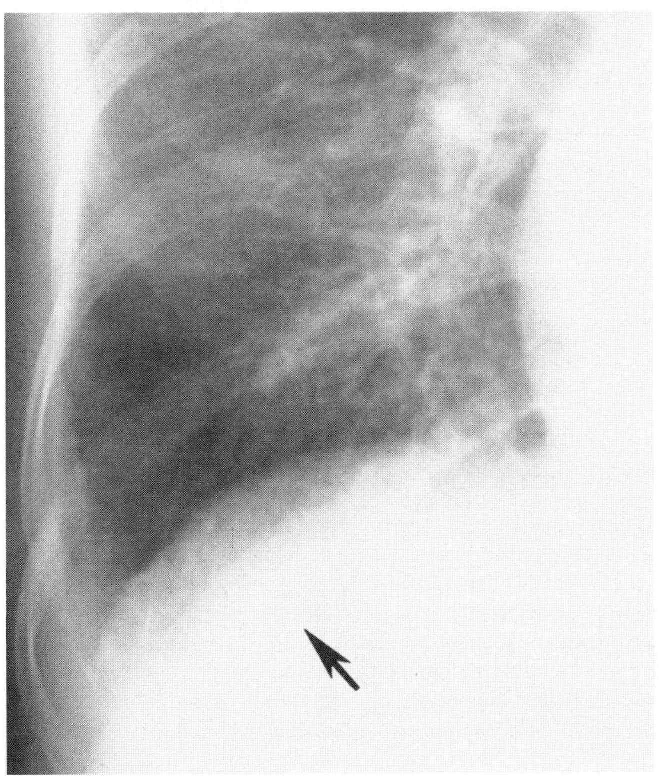

C

FIGURE 14-6 Roentgen appearance of left heart failure. *A. Acute*. Patient with acute mitral regurgitation due to rupture of chordae tendineae showing the "bat wings" appearance of a severe alveolar type of pulmonary edema and a normal-sized heart. *B. Chronic*. Patient with severe mitral and TR and mild AR. This is a predominantly left-sided failure pattern. Note gross cardiomegaly with striking cephalization and interstitial pulmonary edema. The giant LA forms the right cardiac border (*open arrow*), makes its appendage bulge outward on the left side (*upper large arrow*), and splays the mainstem bronchi wide apart (*solid lines*). The huge RA forms a double density within the right cardiac border (*three small arrows*). The upper small arrow marks the peribronchial cuffing of edema fluid. The lower large arrow points to multiple Kerley B lines. *C*. Magnified view of right costophrenic sulcus showing multiple Kerley B lines (*arrow*). *D*. A 44-year-old woman with severe MS. Her radiograph shows a diffuse stippling with fine nodules representing hemosiderosis. Hemosiderin-laden macrophages were found in her sputa. *E*. PA radiograph of a 63-year-old man with severe MS, status post mitral valve replacement, shows multiple scattered bony nodules (*arrows*) 2 to 10 mm in diameter throughout the lower two-thirds of both lungs, compatible with pulmonary ossification.

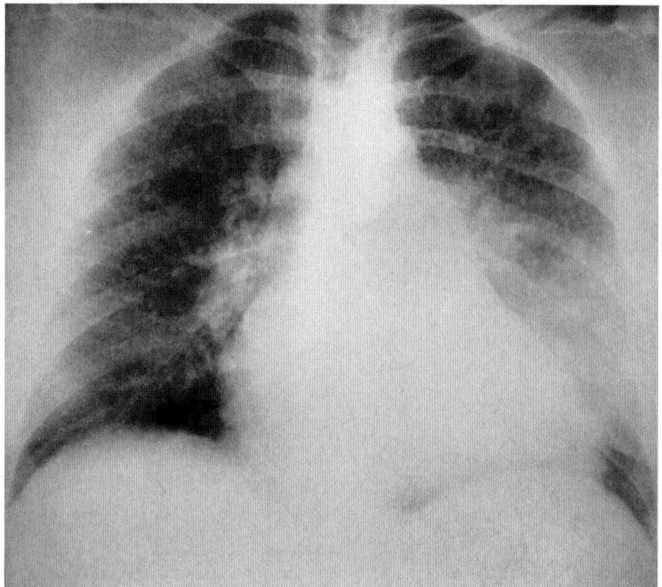

D

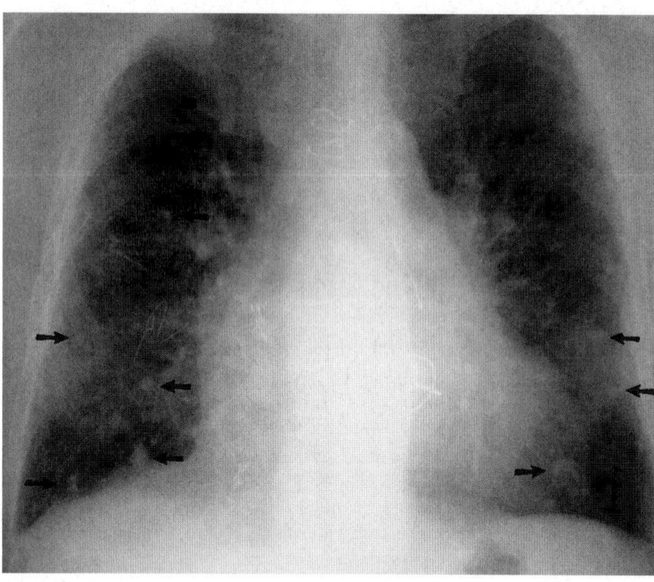

E

FIGURE 14-6 *(Continued)*

predictive value of a particular disease or a group of similar diseases. The incidence of congenital heart disease in patients with a right-sided aortic arch increases 10- to 100-fold depending on the anatomic details of the anomaly.[18,19] There are only two types of right-sided aortic arch. The first has been called the *avian type,* implying a normal status for birds but a detrimental one for humans. The overwhelming majority of patients with this type are born with cyanotic congenital heart disease. The second may be called the *common type* because of its higher incidence in the general population. Most patients with the common type are physiologically normal and have their anomaly incidentally diagnosed on chest radiographs or a barium meal study. The x-ray findings of the two types are similar in the PA view but quite different in the lateral view (Fig. 14-21). The incidence and list of congenital heart diseases with each type[19] are shown in Table 14-3. Only 2 percent of patients with the avian type are physiologically normal. Tetralogy of Fallot should be the diagnosis in these patients until proved otherwise.[18,19]

Patients with a double aortic arch rarely have congenital heart disease, although they tend to be symptomatic in infancy because of a compressing vascular ring.[19]

## CLINICAL CORRELATION

The roentgenologic findings must be correlated with the clinical information and other laboratory parameters for a final conclusion. It may become necessary at this point to reexamine the radiograph or review the fluoroscopic observation or both. After detailed analysis of some finer points, a wrong impression may be corrected or a correct diagnosis reinforced[1] (Table 14-2).

## PULMONARY VASCULARITY

### Normal

The normal roentgen appearance of the pulmonary vasculature of an upright human being is typified by a caudal flow pattern because of gravity. The pressure differential between the apex and the base of the lung is approximately 22 mmHg in adults in the upright position.[2,21] Therefore, more flow under higher distending pressure is expected in the lower-lobe vessels than in the upper. Normally, one sees very little vascularity above the hilum, whereas more and larger vessels are found below the hilum. Since the pulmonary resistance is normal, all vessels taper gradually in a tree-like manner from the hilum toward the periphery of the lung. The right descending pulmonary artery measures 10 to 15 mm in diameter in males and 9 to 14 mm in females[1,22] (Fig. 14-2).

### Abnormal

Abnormal pulmonary vascularity can be classified into two categories, either in terms of volume or in terms of distribution[2,10,23] (Table 14-4).

### Abnormalities in Volume

In the evaluation of pulmonary vasculature, the caliber of the vessels is more important than the length or the number. As long as the PBF pattern remains normal, with a greater amount of flow to the bases than to the apices, the volume of the flow is proportional to the caliber of the pulmonary arteries (Fig. 14-2). Besides measuring the right descending pulmonary artery, one may also assess the pulmonary blood volume by comparing the size of the pulmonary artery with that of the accompanying bronchus where they are viewed on end. Normally, the two structures have approximately equal diameters.[2,26] When the artery-bronchus ratio is greater than unity, increased blood flow is suggested. Conversely, when the ratio is smaller than unity (Fig. 14-2), decreased flow is likely.

**INCREASED PBF**

In the case of mild to moderate left-to-right shunts, for example, the vessels dilate in proportion to the increased flow with no significant change in pressure, resistance, or flow pattern. This phenomenon is

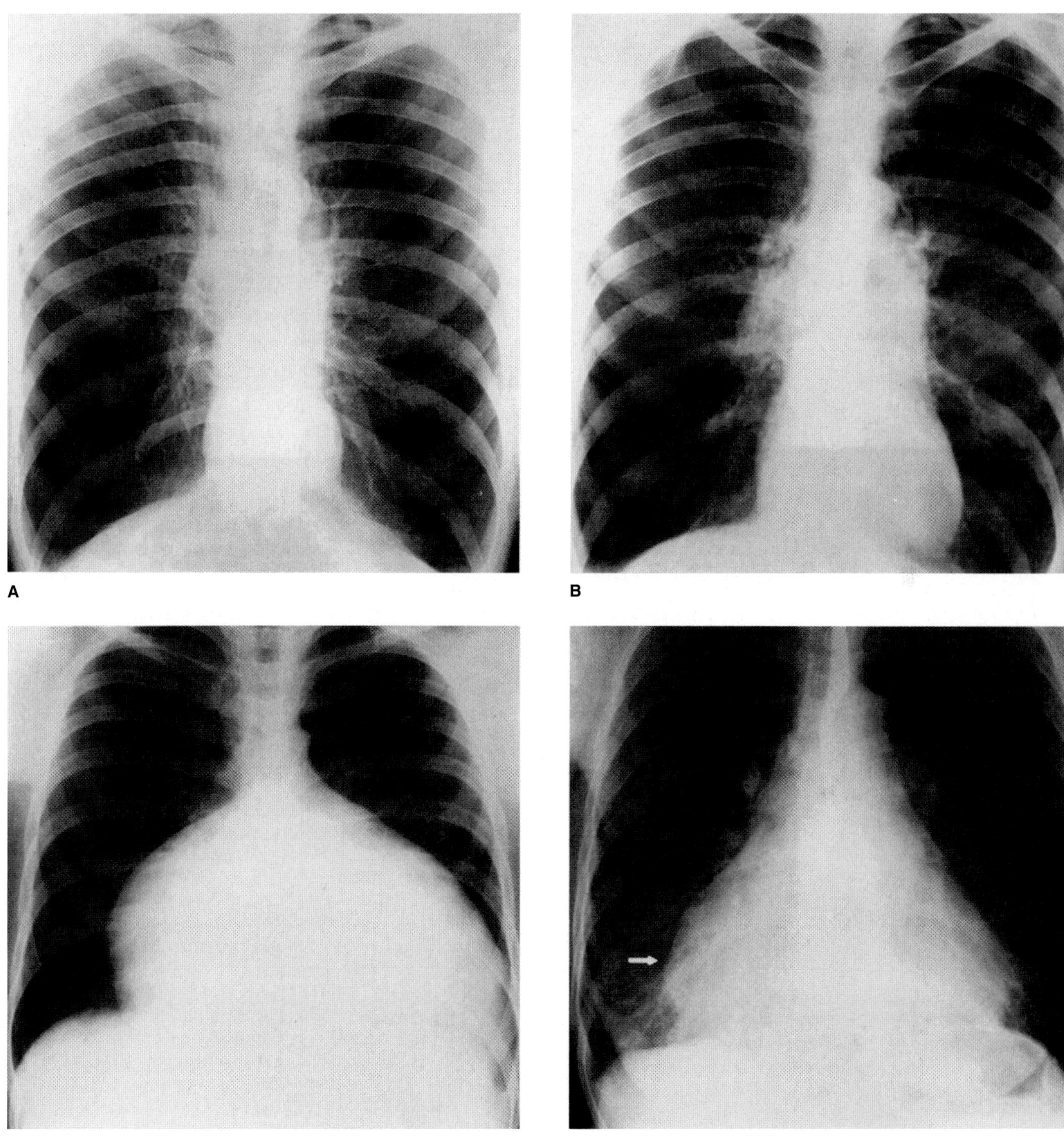


FIGURE 14-7 Roentgen appearance of right heart failure. *A*. Patient with severe obstructive emphysema showing overaeration of the lungs, centralized flow pattern, and a small heart size. *B*. Three years later, the patient was in frank right heart failure. Note that the heart got bigger as his emphysema got worse. The centralized flow pattern became more severe. *C*. Patient with Ebstein's anomaly showing gross cardiomegaly with severe decrease in pulmonary vascularity. The right cardiac border represents the huge RA, and the left cardiac border represents the giant RV. *D*. Patient with MS showing a giant RA (*arrow*) representing severe functional TR due to unrelenting left-sided failure. The pulmonary venous congestion had improved following the onset of right-sided heart failure.

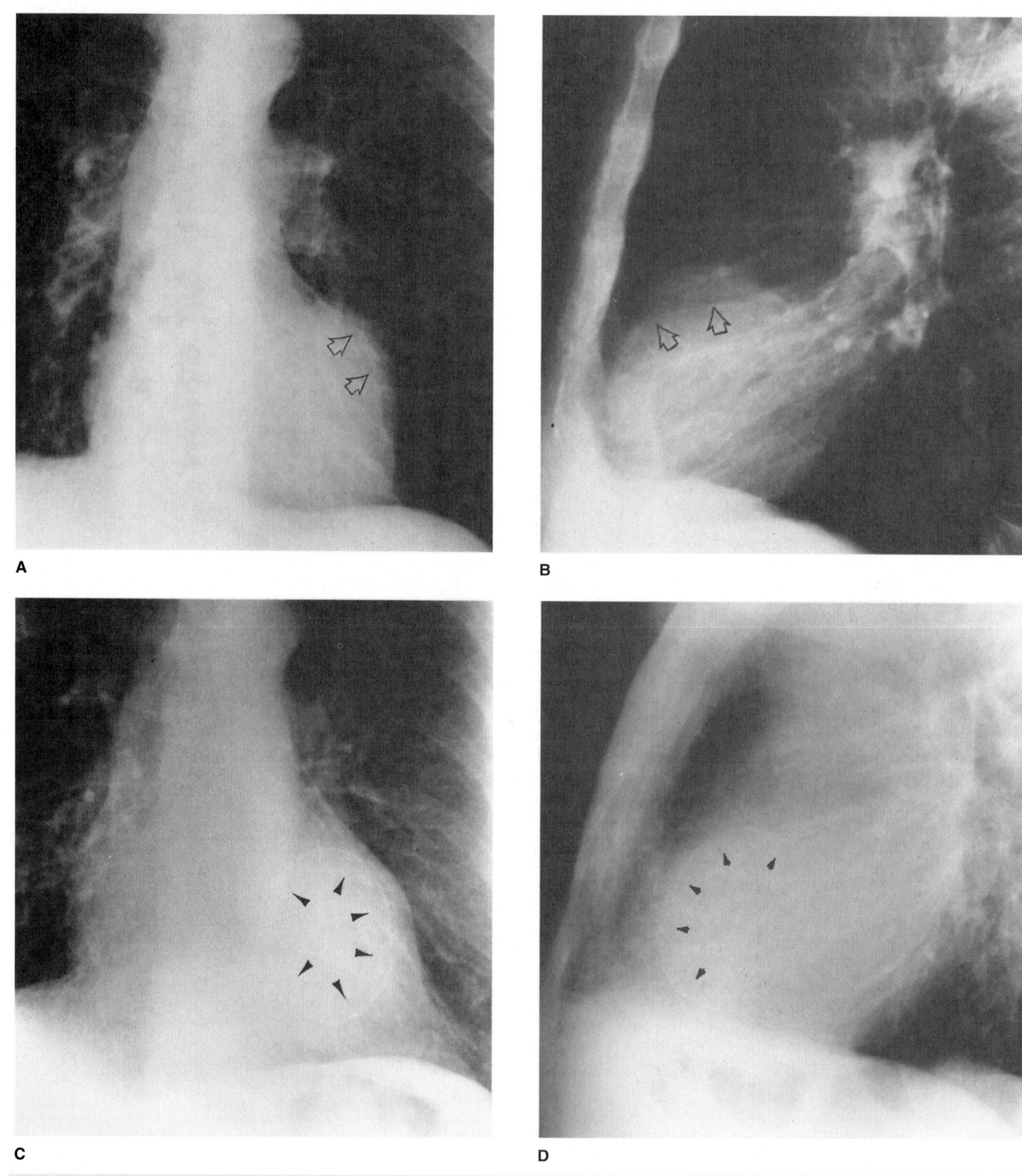


FIGURE 14-8 Left ventricular aneurysms. *A.* PA view of patient 1 shows a localized bulge (*arrows*) along the left cardiac border representing a left ventricular aneurysm from the anterolateral wall. *B.* Lateral view shows a double density with sharp borders anteriorly and superiorly (*arrows*). This is the left ventricular aneurysm that casts a shadow on the normal RV. Fluoroscopically, it is easy to confirm its origin and to separate it from the RV by rotating the patient under direct vision. *C.* PA view of patient 2, a 69-year-old man, shows total calcification of an anterolateral apical left ventricular aneurysm (*arrows*). *D.* Lateral view shows the same (*arrows*).

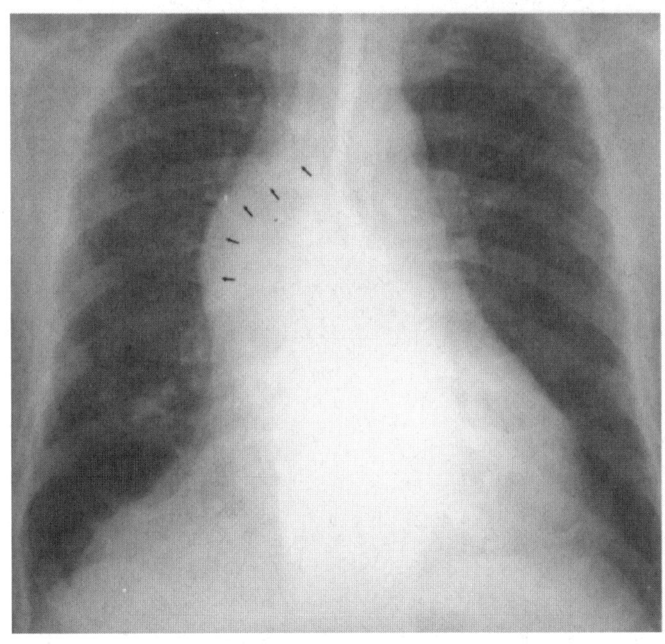


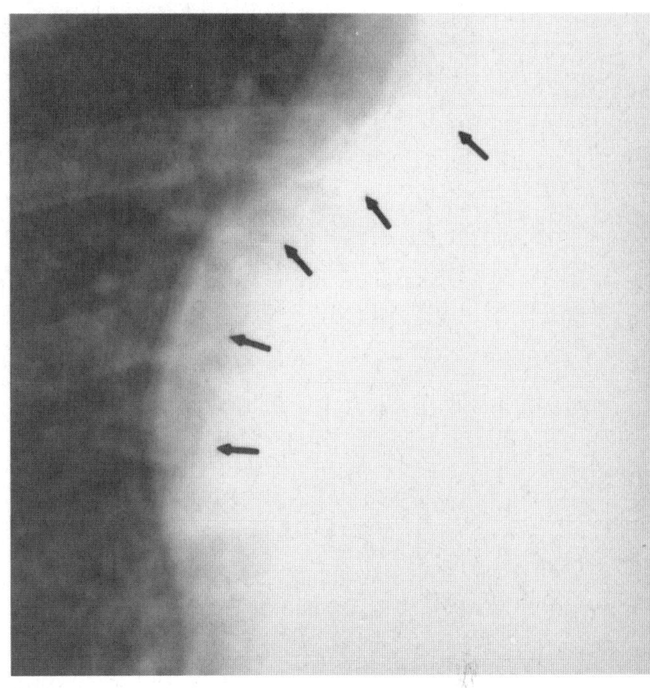


FIGURE 14-9 A 71-year-old woman with syphilitic aortitis. Her PA radiograph (*A*) shows a huge, calcified ascending aortic aneurysm (*arrows*). In addition, the entire aorta and the left ventricle are markedly dilated, compatible with severe AR (from Chen,[14] with permission.) A magnified view of the ascending aorta (*B*) shows the calcified aneurysm to better advantage.

also called *shunt vascularity* or *equalization*. Equalization of PBF between the upper and lower lung zones is only apparent rather than real, however; the lower lobes still receive a great deal more blood than the upper lobes, although the ratio of PBF between the two zones has changed—e.g., from 5:1 to 4:1 or 3:1. A mild increase in pulmonary vascularity with slight cardiomegaly is commonly found in pregnant women and trained athletes with increased cardiac output (Chap. 85).

### DECREASED PBF

Patients with tetralogy of Fallot frequently show decreased pulmonary vascularity with smaller and shorter pulmonary arteries and veins and more radiolucent lungs (Fig. 14-2*C*). Marked reduction in PBF is also encountered in patients with isolated right-sided heart failure without a right-to-left shunt (Fig. 14-7). This is attributed to the significant decrease in cardiac output from both ventricles.

## Abnormalities in Distribution

An abnormal distribution of PBF (or an abnormal PBF pattern) always reflects a changed pulmonary vascular resistance, either locally or diffusely.

### CEPHALIZATION

In the presence of postcapillary pulmonary hypertension (PH), physiologic disturbances begin when the total intravascular pressure exceeds the oncotic pressure of the blood. As a result, fluid leaks out of the vessels and collects in the interstitium before pouring into the alveoli.

Pulmonary edema interferes with gas exchange, resulting in a state of hypoxemia. Alveolar hypoxia has a profound influence on the pulmonary vessels, causing them to constrict. Since there is greater alveolar hypoxia in the lung bases than in the apices, the basilar vessels constrict significantly, forcing the blood to flow upward. This phenomenon actually represents a reversal of the normal PBF pattern: redistribution or cephalization of the pulmonary vascularity.

Cephalization occurs in any of three conditions: (1) left-sided obstructive lesions—e.g., MS[22] or AS; (2) LV failure—e.g., coronary heart disease or cardiomyopathies, and (3) severe mitral regurgitation (MR) even before pump failure of the LV occurs. It should be emphasized that unless there is obvious *constriction* of the lower-lobe vessels, the diagnosis of cephalization should not be made. Dilatation of the upper-lobe vessels is of secondary importance and can be found without narrowing of the basilar vessels in a number of entities, most noticeably left-to-right shunts.

### CENTRALIZATION

In the presence of precapillary PH, the pulmonary trunk and central pulmonary arteries dilate, whereas the distal pulmonary arteries constrict in a concentric fashion from the periphery of the lung toward the hilum. This phenomenon is called *centralization of the pulmonary vascularity*. It occurs in patients with primary PH, Eisenmenger's syndrome, recurrent pulmonary thromboembolic disease, or severe obstructive emphysema (Fig. 14-7*A*, *B*).

### LATERALIZATION

Massive unilateral pulmonary embolism may cause a lateralized PBF pattern. Since one major pulmonary artery is obstructed, the blood is

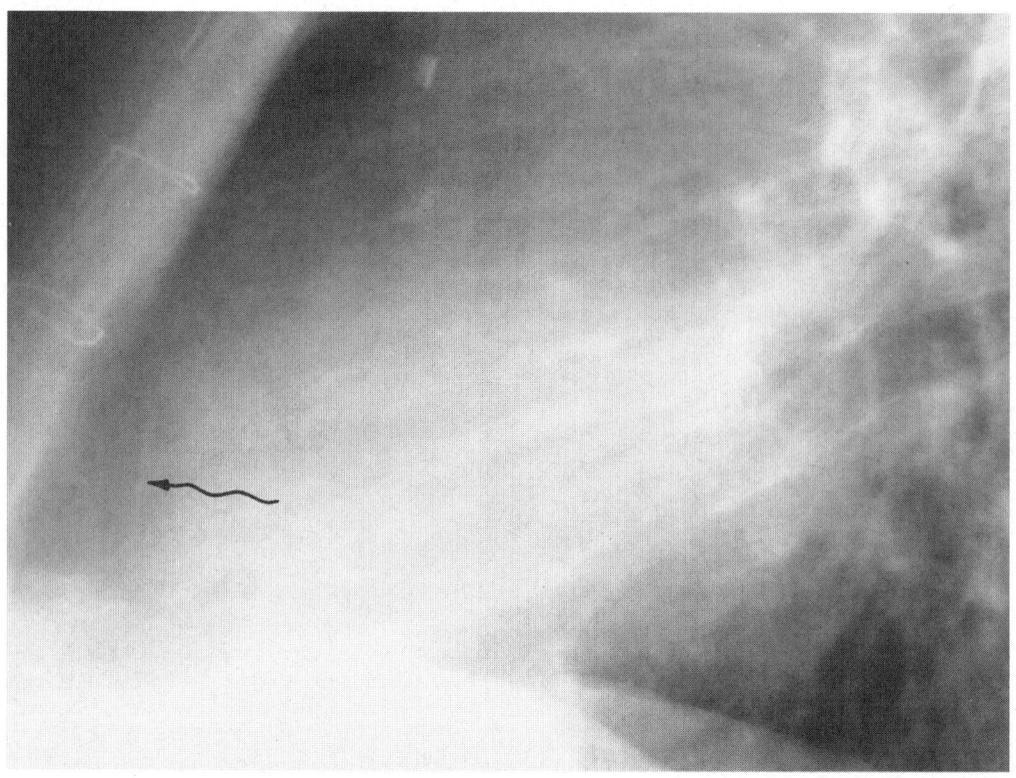

A

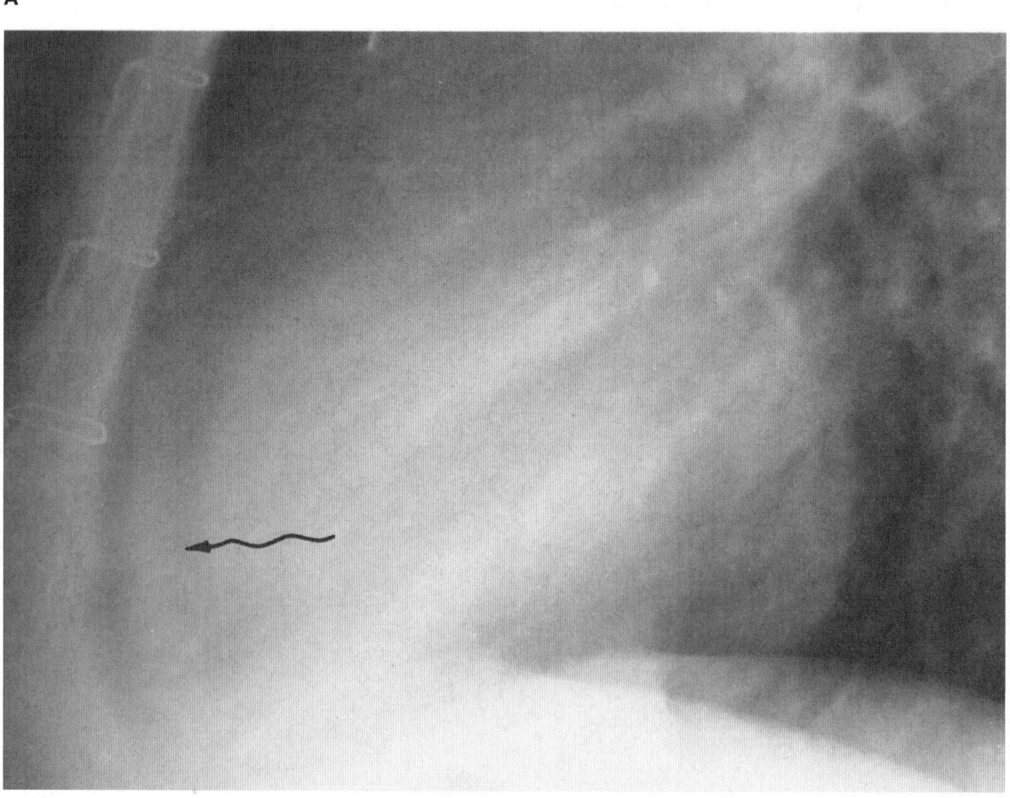

B

FIGURE 14-10 Developing pericardial effusion in 2 weeks. *A*. A magnified view of the retrosternal area showing the hairlike normal pericardium (*arrow*) sandwiched between the subepicardial fat stripe interiorly and the mediastinal fat stripe exteriorly. The maximal width of normal pericardium is 2 mm. *B*. The same patient 2 weeks later, with moderate pericardial effusion. The pericardial cavity now measured more than 1 cm in width (*arrow*).

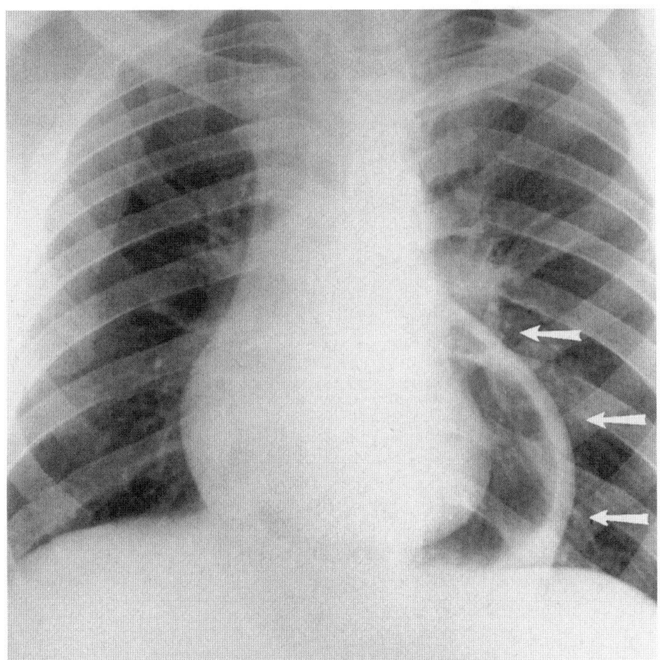

FIGURE 14-11 Traumatic constrictive-effusive pericarditis in a young man. Following emergent pericardiocentesis and injection of air, a radiograph was taken in the supine position. Air is confined to the left side of the pericardium. Note markedly thickened parietal layer (*arrows*).

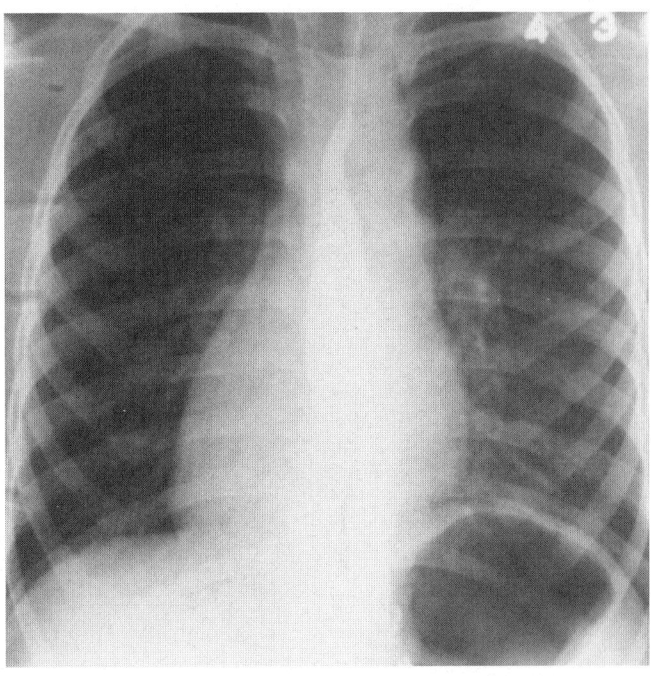

FIGURE 14-12 PA view of a patient with dextrocardia and situs solitus. Note that the aortic arch and the stomach air bubble are both on the left (*situs solitus*) and the apex of the ventricles is pointing to the right inferiorly. According to statistics and proved by cardiac catheterization, this patient had the typical combination of congenitally corrected transposition of the great arteries, ventricular septal defect, and pulmonary stenosis. He was cyanotic. The pulmonary vascularity appears decreased.

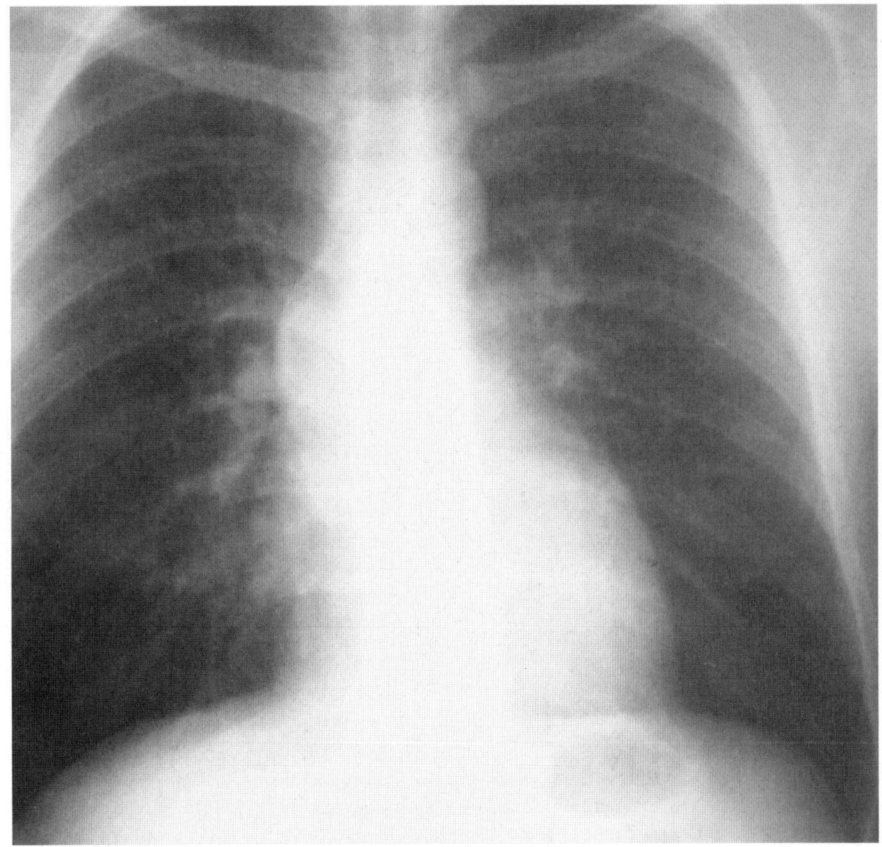

FIGURE 14-13 A 17-year-old boy with congenital aortic valve stenosis. Note dilatation of the ascending aorta, increased convexity of the left ventricle, and normal pulmonary vascularity. The systolic aortic pressure gradient was 100 mmHg.

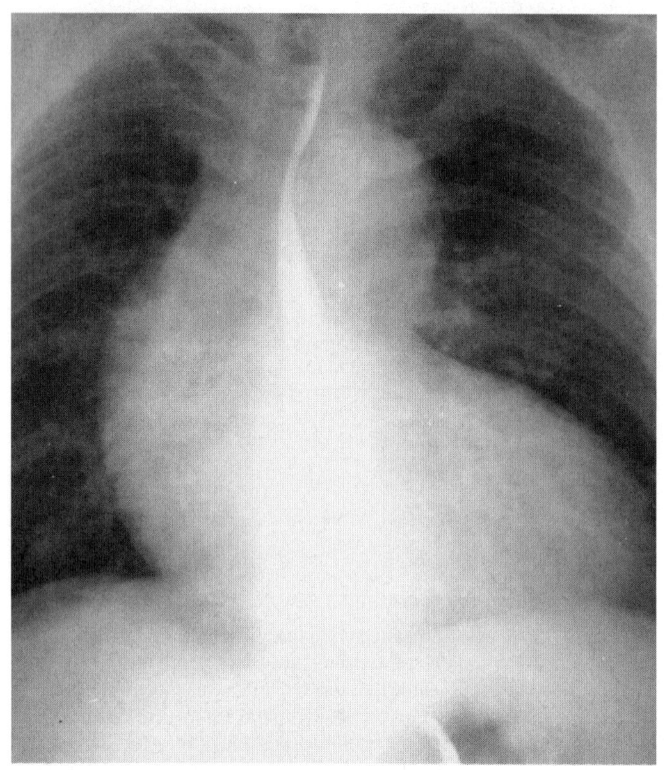

A

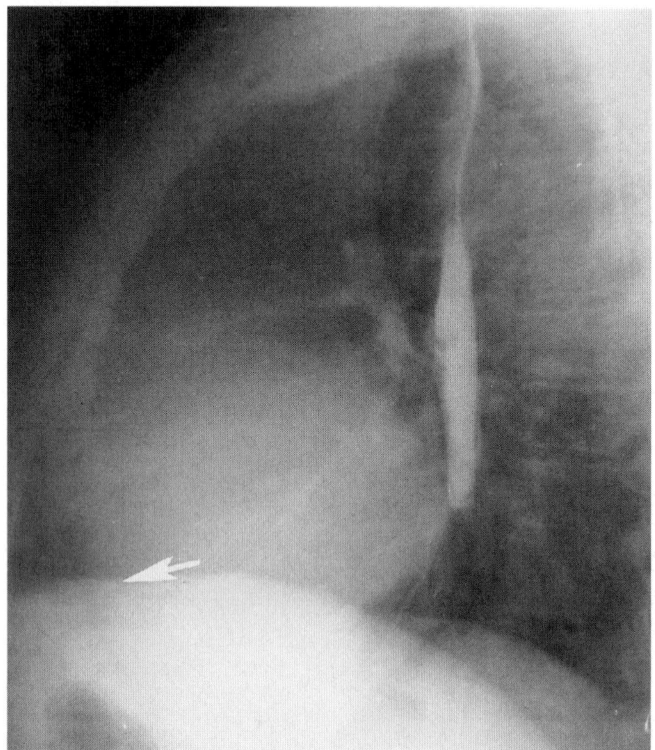

B

FIGURE 14-14 A 45-year-old man with Marfan's syndrome, severe AR, and proximal aortic dissection into the pericardial cavity. *A*. PA view shows a huge left ventricle and aneurysmal dilatation of the ascending aorta. There is no sign of heart failure. *B*. Lateral view shows a small pericardial effusion (*arrow*).

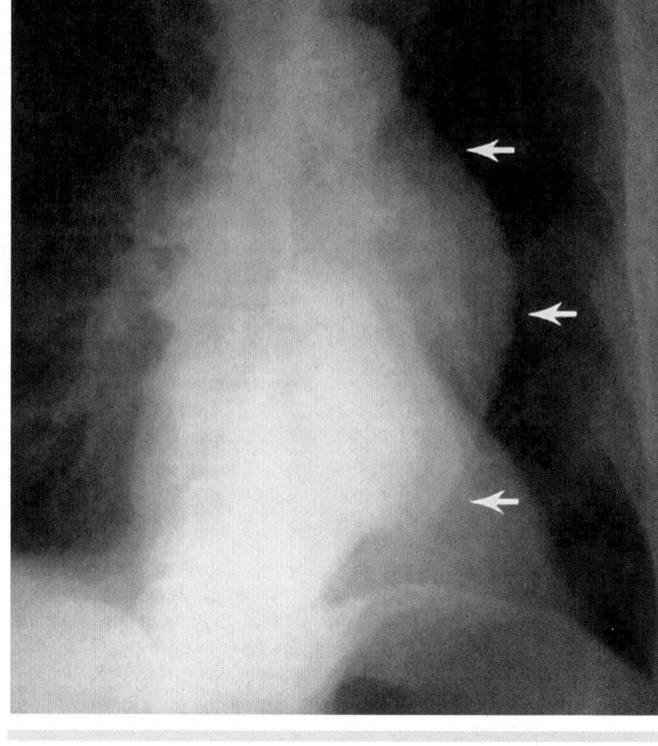

FIGURE 14-15 PA view of a 77-year-old man shows a huge descending aortic aneurysm (*arrows*).

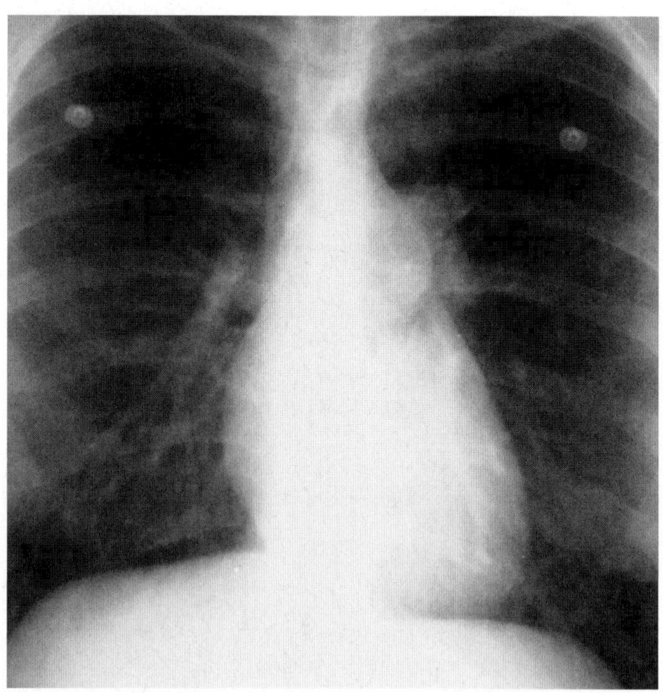

FIGURE 14-16 A 37-year-old woman with congenital valvular pulmonary stenosis. Note enlarged pulmonary trunk and left pulmonary artery versus diminished right pulmonary artery. Also note increased pulmonary blood flow on the left side and decreased pulmonary blood flow on the right side.

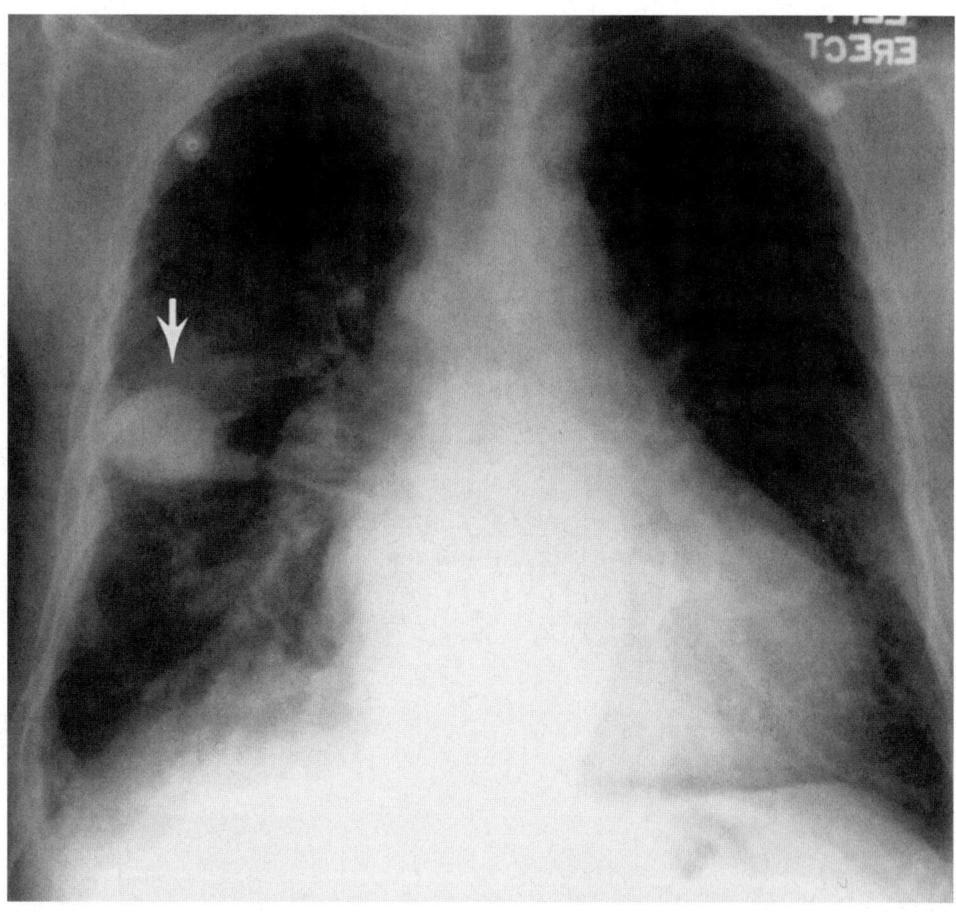

FIGURE 14-17 Patient with congestive heart failure. Note gross cardiomegaly, cephalization, interstitial pulmonary edema, and right-sided pleural effusion. Some of the fluid was loculated in the minor interlobar fissure (*arrow*), which disappeared with improved cardiac function.

forced to flow through the healthy lung only. The paucity of pulmonary vascularity in the diseased lung with the obstructed pulmonary artery is termed the *Westermark sign* (Fig. 14-3*C*). In the case of congenital valvular pulmonary stenosis, a jet effect from the stenotic valve can cause a lateralized PBF pattern in favor of the left side (Fig. 14-16).

**LOCALIZATION**
A localized abnormal flow pattern is exemplified by a congenital pulmonary arteriovenous fistula in a cyanotic child.

**COLLATERALIZATION**
Patients with markedly decreased PBF (e.g., severe tetralogy) tend to show numerous small, tortuous bronchial arterial collaterals in the upper medial lung zones near their origin from the descending aorta. The native pulmonary arteries are extremely small, although smooth and gracefully branching.

### Combined Abnormalities

In reality, an abnormal pulmonary vascularity is often a mixed type. There is a great variety of possible combinations—e.g., cephalization plus decreased flow in severe MS or centralization with increased PBF in Eisenmenger's atrial septal defect (Fig. 14-22).

## HEART FAILURE

In addition to specific chamber enlargement, the pulmonary vasculature uniquely portrays the underlying pathophysiology of heart failure. In the chronic setting, decreased flow with increased pulmonary lucency is the hallmark of right heart failure (Fig. 14-7); striking cephalization of the pulmonary vasculature is typical for left-sided decompensation (Fig. 14-3*A* and 14-6*B*).

### Left-Sided

**ACUTE LEFT-SIDED HEART FAILURE**
The pulmonary vascular changes associated with acute LV failure are usually not discernible for two reasons: (1) the resulting severe pulmonary edema obscures the pulmonary vasculature and (2) the redistribution of PBF secondary to acute left-sided heart failure is usually relatively mild. The combination of alveolar pulmonary edema and a normal-sized heart is the hallmark of acute left-sided heart failure[9] (Fig. 14-6*A*). The edema fluid tends to distribute in a butterfly pattern.[26]

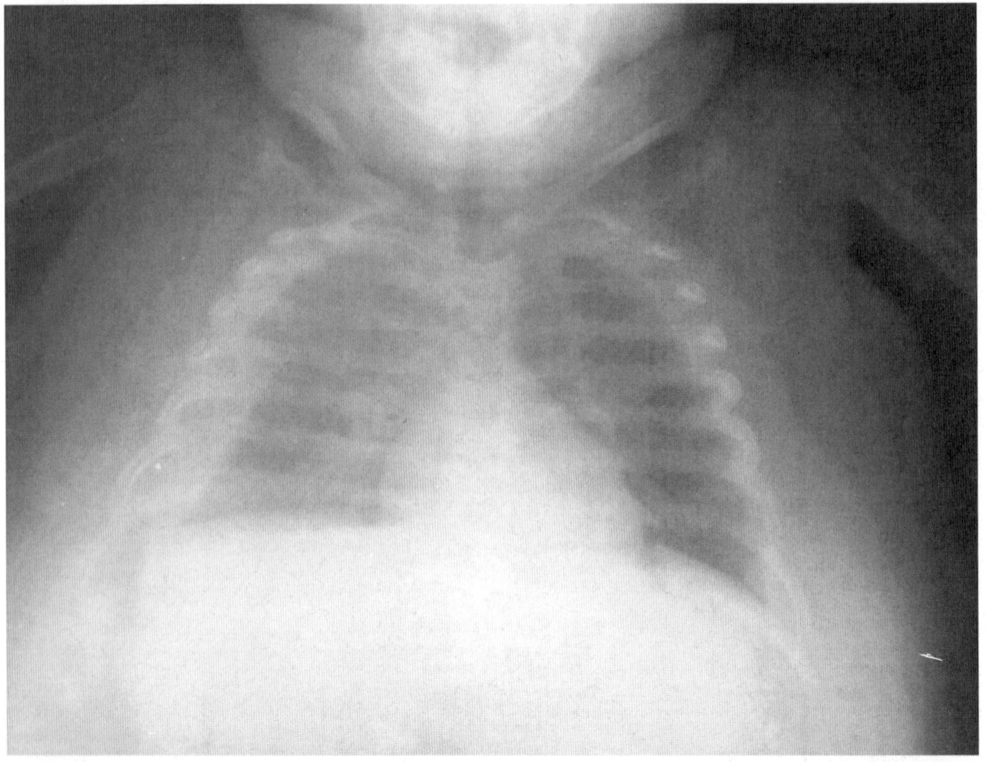

A

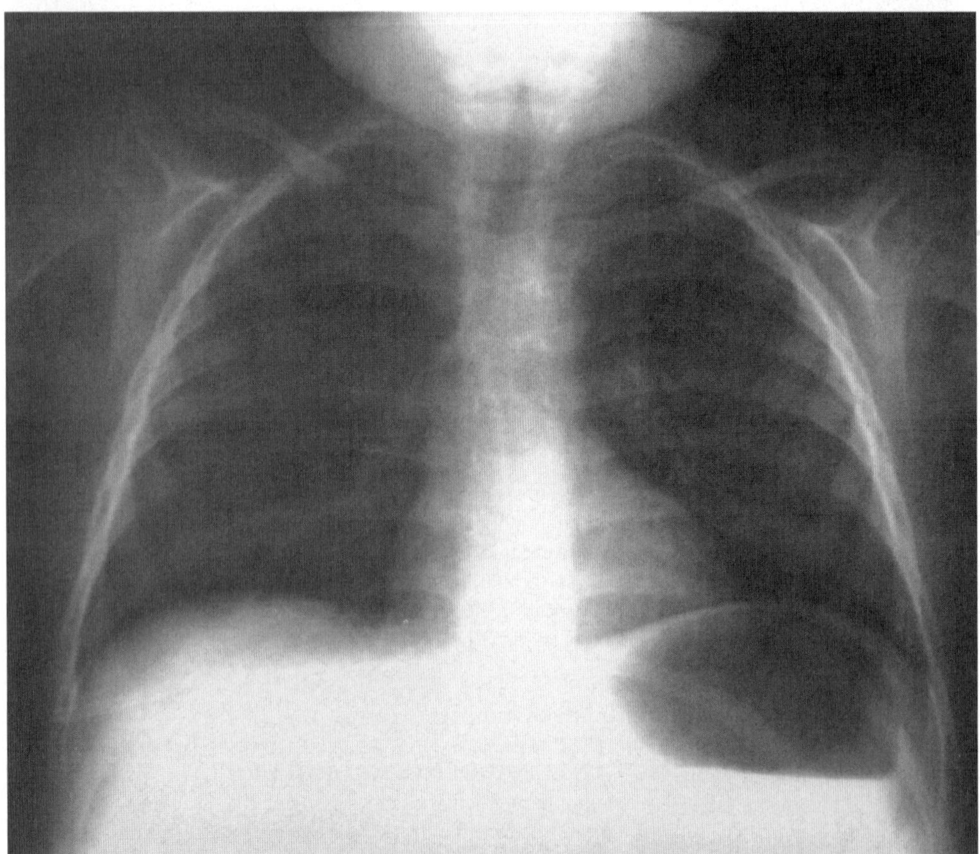

B

FIGURE 14-18 A child suffering from nephrotic syndrome, which was treated successfully. *A*. PA view during the worst period of his disease shows general anasarca, pulmonary edema, and pleural effusion. Note considerable soft tissue edema in the chest wall. *B*. With proper treatment, everything returned to normal in 2 weeks.

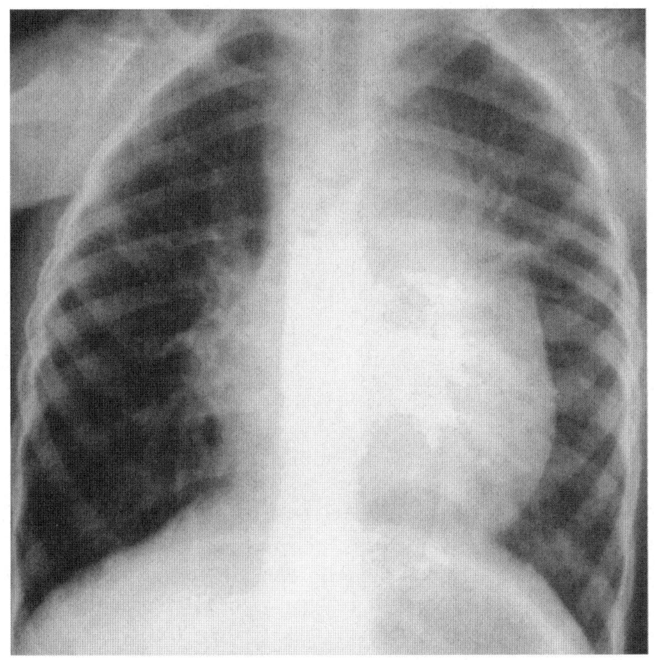
A

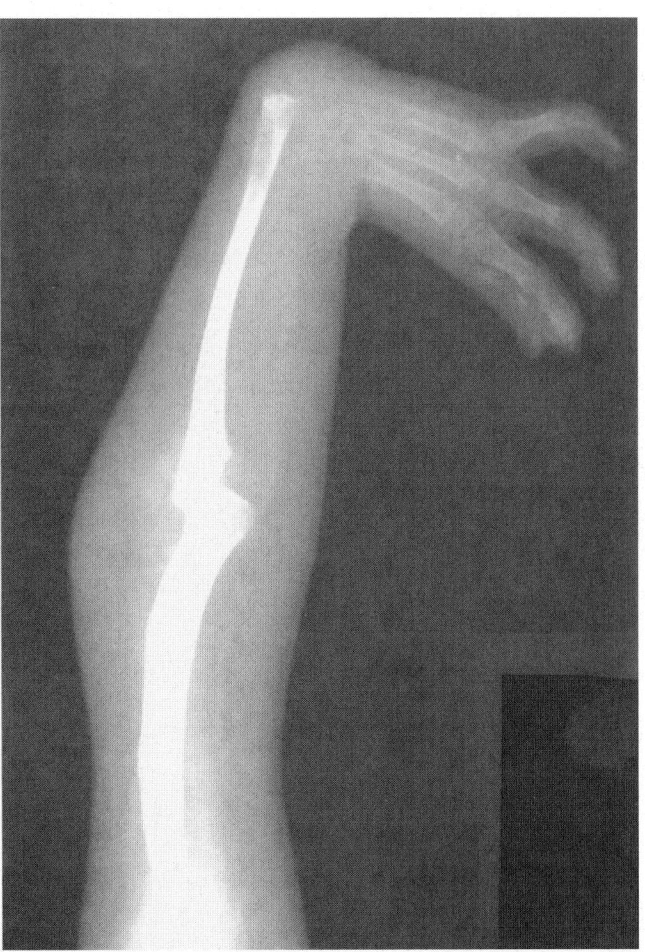
B

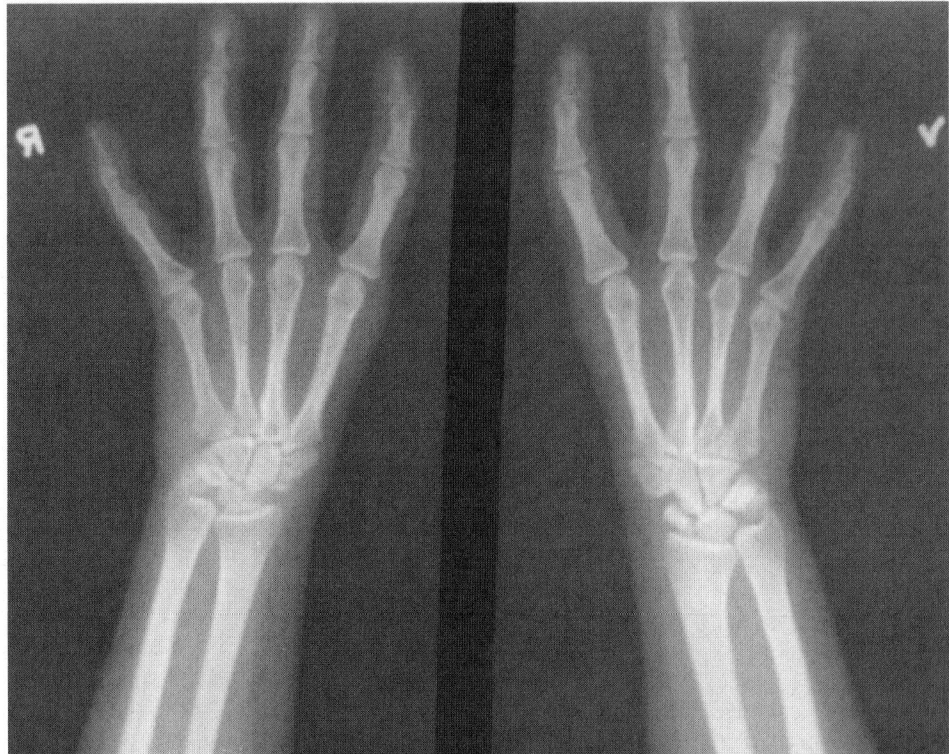

C

FIGURE 14-19 Patients with Holt-Oram syndrome. *A*. PA view of patient 1, a 7-year-old girl, shows a globular cardiac contour with increased pulmonary blood flow. The aortic arch is on the right side. Catheterization diagnosis: secundum atrial septal defect. *B*. Her left arm shows absent radius and thumb with radial clubhand. Her right arm is a mirror image of the left (not shown). *C*. Forearms of patient 2, a 33-year-old woman with secundum atrial septal defect, show bilateral absence of thumb.

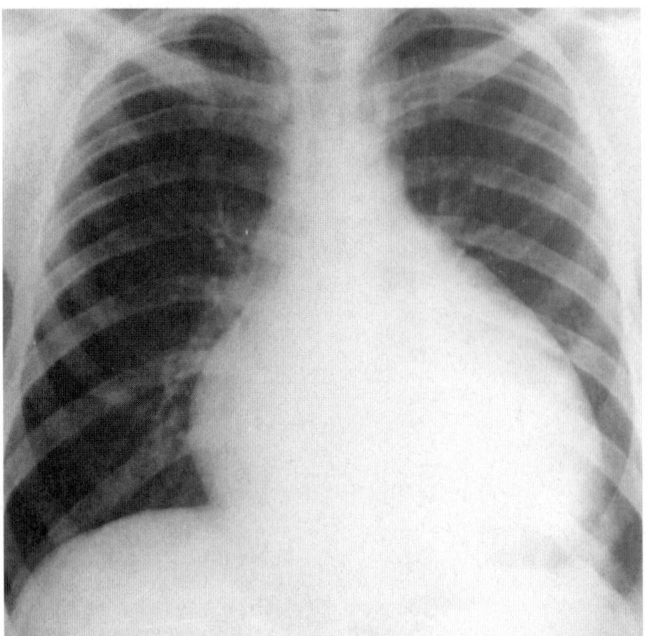

A

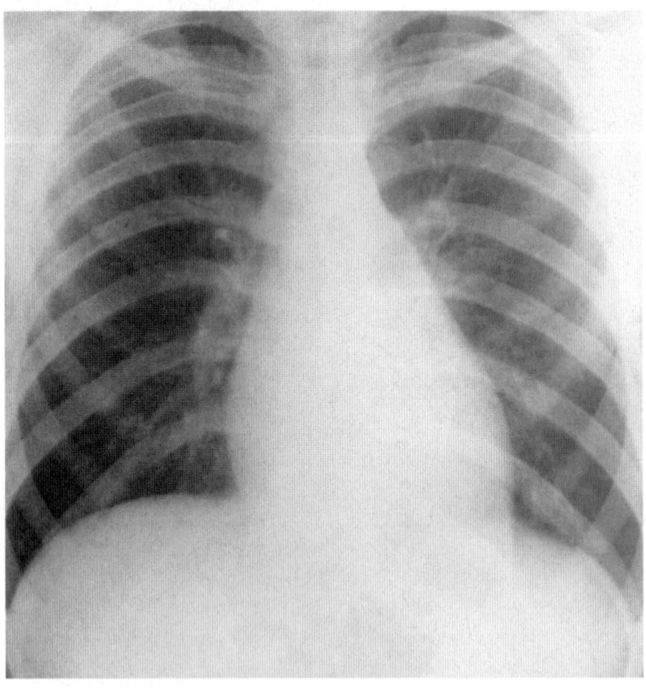

B

FIGURE 14-20 A young man with acute pericarditis with effusion. *A*. PA view shows a water bottle–shaped cardiomegaly, clear lungs, and normal pulmonary vascularity. *B*. Repeat film taken 5 days later shows excellent response to therapy.

#### CHRONIC LEFT-SIDED HEART FAILURE

Chronic left-sided heart failure is characterized by gross cardiomegaly, striking cephalization of the pulmonary vasculature, and interstitial pulmonary edema or fibrosis with multiple distinct Kerley B lines. Pulmonary hemosiderosis, ossification, or both may result from long-standing severe postcapillary PH (Figs. 14-6*B*–*E*).

### Right-Sided

#### ACUTE RIGHT-SIDED HEART FAILURE

Acute right-sided heart failure most commonly results from massive pulmonary embolism. The typical radiographic signs are rapidly developing centralization of the pulmonary vasculature and dilatation of the right-sided cardiac chambers and venae cavae. In addition, the lungs may show localized or lateralized oligemia (Fig. 14-3*C*). Eventually, opacities in either or both lungs may develop as a result of pulmonary infarction.

#### CHRONIC RIGHT-SIDED HEART FAILURE

Chronic right heart failure has many causes. The common ones include congenital pulmonary stenosis, Ebstein's anomaly, severe chronic obstructive pulmonary disease, and recurrent pulmonary thromboembolic disease. Diffusely decreased pulmonary vascularity with unusually lucent lungs is seen in patients with right heart failure without PH (Fig. 14-7*C*). Centralized PBF pattern is encountered when the right-sided heart failure is secondary to precapillary PH (Fig. 14-7*A*, *B*). A cephalized flow pattern with unusually lucent lungs is found in patients with right-sided heart failure secondary to long-standing severe left heart failure (Fig. 14-7*D*). The degree of right-sided chamber enlargement is proportional to the severity of TR.

### Combined

Right heart failure is caused most often by severe left heart failure. This is exemplified by patients with severe MS leading to severe TR (Fig. 14-7*D*). Other examples of bilateral heart failure are cardiac tamponade and constrictive pericarditis (Fig. 14-20).

## CARDIAC FLUOROSCOPY

Cardiac fluoroscopy explores the dynamic features of the organ that are discernible only in motion.[25] The two techniques are mutually complementary.

### Description

A good-quality image intensifier is a prerequisite for the proper performance of cardiac fluoroscopy.[1,16] The modern intensifier with cesium iodide phosphorus has increased the brightness of the fluoroscopic image at least 10,000 times. Television viewing permits cone vision under dim light with better perception of detail. The attached videotape or videodisk recorder provides a means for instant playback as well as future analysis of the fluoroscopic observations.

The milliamperage ranges from 1.5 to 3.5 mA, and the kilovoltage varies between 90 and 120 kV. Too high a kilovoltage tends to reduce the contrast, and excessive milliamperage blurs the margin of the image. The shortest fluoroscopic time and the smallest shutter opening are employed to keep the dose of radiation to the patient to the minimum.

The patient is routinely examined in the erect position with four views. The patient should be asked to stop breathing during the brief moment of fluoroscopy. A barium meal is given only after a thorough search for cardiac calcifications is completed. Occasionally, a recumbent position is used for better visualization of small calcifications as well as for a critical evaluation of cardiac asynergy.

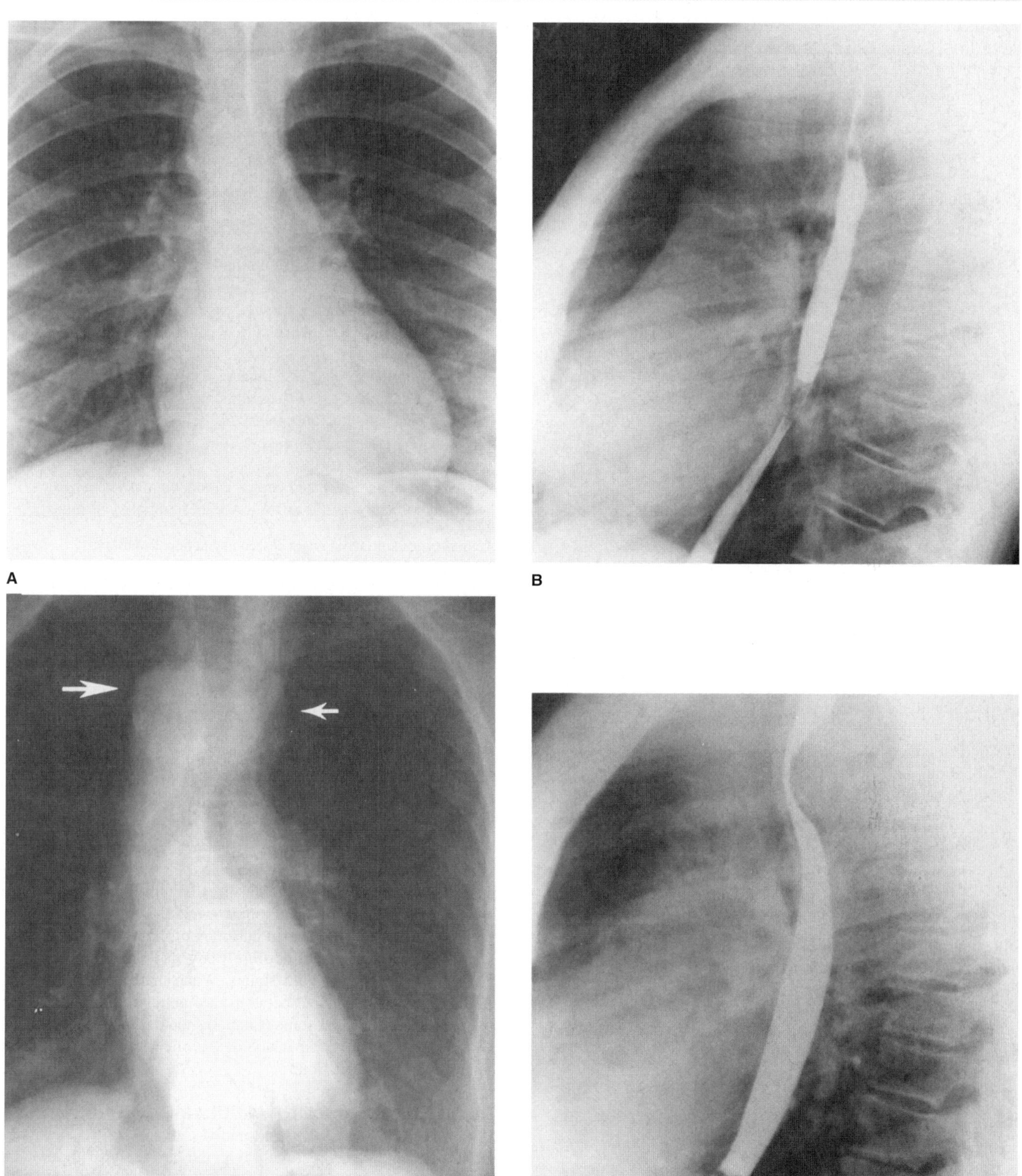


FIGURE 14-21 Statistical guidance focusing on the best diagnostic possibilities. *A*. PA view of a patient with tetralogy of Fallot showing a right aortic arch, avian type. Note that the esophagus and trachea are deviated to the left. The cardiovascular structures are otherwise within normal limits. *B*. Lateral view of the same patient showing the aortic arch normally situated, in front of the trachea and esophagus. *C*. PA radiograph of a healthy woman shows a right aortic arch (*large arrow*) with a large aortic diverticulum (*small arrow*) that protrudes to the left of the midline. The distal segment of the trachea is deviated to the left side by the right arch. Unlike double aortic arch, the left lateral margin of the trachea is not indented because the diverticulum is posterior and not lateral in position. *D*. Lateral view of a similar patient, a healthy man. Note that both the esophagus and the trachea are markedly displaced anteriorly by a huge diverticulum, which invariably gives rise to the aberrant left subclavian artery.

TABLE 14-3 Cardiac Defects Associated with Each Type of Right-sided Aortic Arch

| | Type of Anomaly | |
|---|---|---|
| | Avian | Common |
| Anatomic details | With mirror-image branching; the arch is anterior to the trachea | With aberrant left subclavian artery arising from a large aortic diverticulum that is posterior to the esophagus |
| Patients with cardiac defects, % | 98 | 12 |
| Type of defects, % | | |
| Tetralogy of Fallot | 90 | 71 |
| Truncus arteriosus | 2.5 | |
| Transposition of great arteries | 1.5 | |
| Atrial septal defect and/or ventricular septal defect | 0.5 | 21 |
| Coarctation of aorta | | 7 |
| Others | 5.5 | 1 |

## Results

When performed properly, cardiac fluoroscopy is useful in the following areas of investigation: (1) assessment of cardiovascular dynamics; (2) detection of small cardiovascular calcifications; (3) visualization of important anatomic landmarks—e.g., subepicardial fat stripes; (4) differentiation of cardiac from noncardiac disease; and (5) evaluation of cardiac valve prostheses, pacemakers, and radiopaque foreign bodies.

## Precautions

Both the patient and the examiner should be protected from excessive radiation. Even with an image intensifier, a routine cardiac fluoroscopy still involves more radiation than two-view chest roentgenography.

## Applications

### ASSESSMENT OF CARDIOVASCULAR DYNAMICS

The chest roentgenogram that is taken at random largely records the diastolic image of the heart. Fluoroscopy, on the other hand, provides a continuous vision of the pulsating organ throughout the entire cardiac cycle. Once familiar with the normal cardiovascular movements, the fluoroscopist will find any deviation from the norm to be obvious.[4,26–29]

TABLE 14-4 Pulmonary Vascularity

| Pulmonary Vascularity |
|---|
| Normal |
| Caudal PBF pattern in upright position (PBF controlled by gravity) |
| Gradual branching, treelike |
| RDPA = 10–15 mm in males |
| RDPA = 9–14 mm in females |
| A/B ratio = 1 |
| Abnormal |
| Volume with normal PBF pattern (distribution) |
| Increased, larger vessels, e.g., ASD |
| Decreased, smaller vessels, e.g., TOF |
| Distribution with anbormal PBF pattern |
| Cephalic, e.g., MS |
| Centralized, e.g., Eisenmenger syndrome |
| Lateralized, e.g., Westermark sign |
| Localized, e.g., pulmonary AV fistulas |
| Collateralized, e.g., severe TOF |
| Combined |
| Decreased volume and cephalization, e.g., cricitcal MS |
| Lateralization and localization, e.g., scimitar syndrome |

ABBREVIATIONS: RDPA = right descending pulmonary artery; A/B = artery/bronchus; PBF = pulmonary blood flow; ASD = atrial septal defect; TOF = tetralogy of Fallot; AV = arteriovenous; MS = mitral stenosis.

The telltale x-ray signs of many cardiac lesions manifest themselves only in ventricular systole. Therefore what may be missed on the film is often readily seen and diagnosed under the fluoroscope. For instance, LV enlargement may be the only radiographic abnormality of severe aortic regurgitation (AR) in children or young adults. On fluoroscopy, however, the aorta is vigorously expanding in systole and rapidly collapsing in diastole. This dynamic alternation is characteristic of AR (Fig. 14-21). In valvular pulmonary stenosis, vigorous pulsation of the pulmonary trunk and its left branch is in bold contrast to the diminished pulsation of the right pulmonary artery.[29] Increased pulsation of diffusely enlarged pulmonary arteries is characteristic of left-to-right shunts. When marked discrepancy in size and pulsation is noted between the central and peripheral vessels, Eisenmenger's syndrome (Chap.3) should be considered. Exaggerated left atrial (LA) expansion in ventricular systole is a reliable sign of mitral regurgitation.[29]

### DETECTION OF CARDIOVASCULAR CALCIFICATIONS

Heavy calcifications of the heart and vessels are easily detected by chest roentgenography, particularly in the lateral and oblique views (Fig. 14-23). Small calcifications can be registered only by fluoroscopy by virtue of their rhythmic movements from the pulsating heart.[3,8] The combination of chest pain and coronary calcification results from major vascular obstruction 94 percent of the time.[14] Since the major coronary arteries are embedded in the subepicardial fat stripes in the grooves between cardiac chambers, such fat stripes can be used effectively to locate the calcified arteries. Under the fluoroscope, the fat stripes present as pulsating radiolucent (bright) lines, in contrast to the accompanying pulsating radiopaque (dark) lines of calcified coronary arteries.

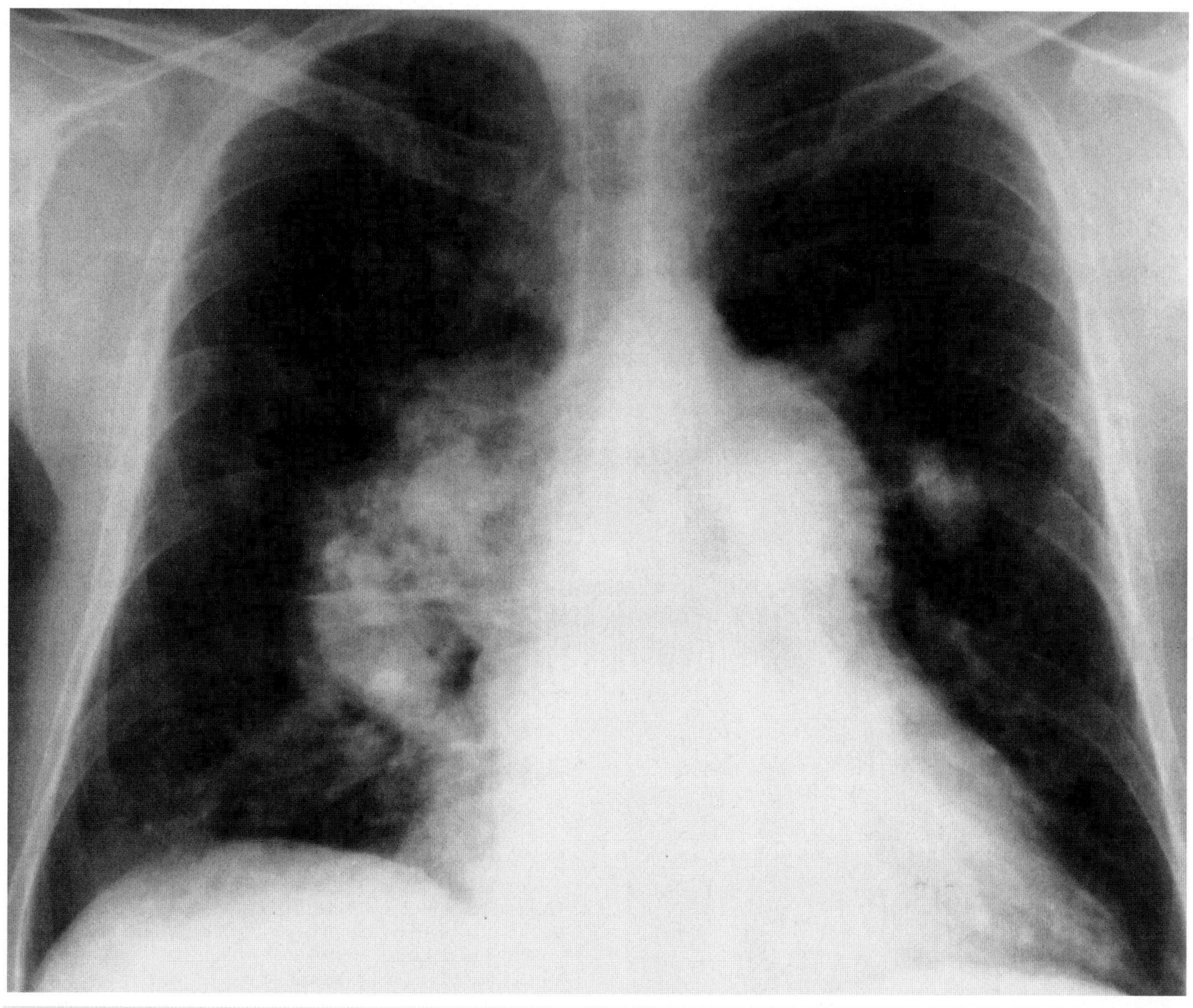

FIGURE 14-22 A 42-year-old man with Eisenmenger's atrial septal defect. Note increased pulmonary blood flow with a centralized pattern.

The lateral view is the best or only view for the detection of a calcified right CA. The left anterior oblique view at 20 to 30 degrees is the one most suitable for localizing the bifurcation of the left CA. In this view, the left CA is brought into relief between the hilar shadow anteriorly and the spinal column posteriorly. A ring-like density is seen frequently in this view, representing the end-on image of the calcified anterior descending CA. The right anterior oblique angle is used to view a calcified left main CA. If both the anterior descending and the circumflex branches are also calcified, a Y-shaped density may be seen. The calcified cardiac valves, myocardium, and pericardium are easily confirmed by fluoroscopy.[1,26]

### VISUALIZATION OF SUBEPICARDIAL FAT STRIPES

The subepicardial fat lines are important landmarks in the diagnosis of heart disease. The fat stripe is a cushion-like structure separating the myocardium from the pericardium. Normally, it is difficult to see the fat line because of the adjacent similar radiolucency of the air-filled lung. The in-between hairline density of the normal pericardium is delicate and also difficult to see except in the left lateral view. In the presence of pericardial effusion or thickening, the subepicardial fat line is displaced interiorly and becomes more visible because of the added background of water density (Fig. 14-10*B*). The subepicardial fat pulsates with the contracting myocardium within the immobile band of pericardial fluid. This is diagnostic of pericardial effusion.[32] In contrast, when pericardial thickening alone is present, the exterior border of the heart pulsates with the fat line. This, in turn, suggests the diagnosis of pericardial constriction.

### DIFFERENTIATION OF CARDIAC FROM NONCARDIAC DISEASE

When respiration is suspended, any structures that are moving are likely to be cardiovascular in nature. Conversely, noncardiac structures are immobile. This is exemplified by a bullet in the heart versus another in the chest wall. A pulmonary varix or an azygos vein

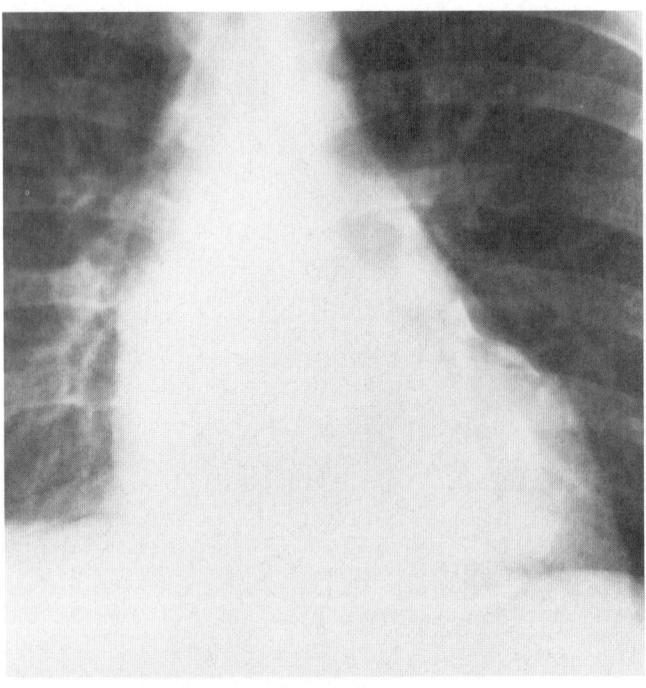

A

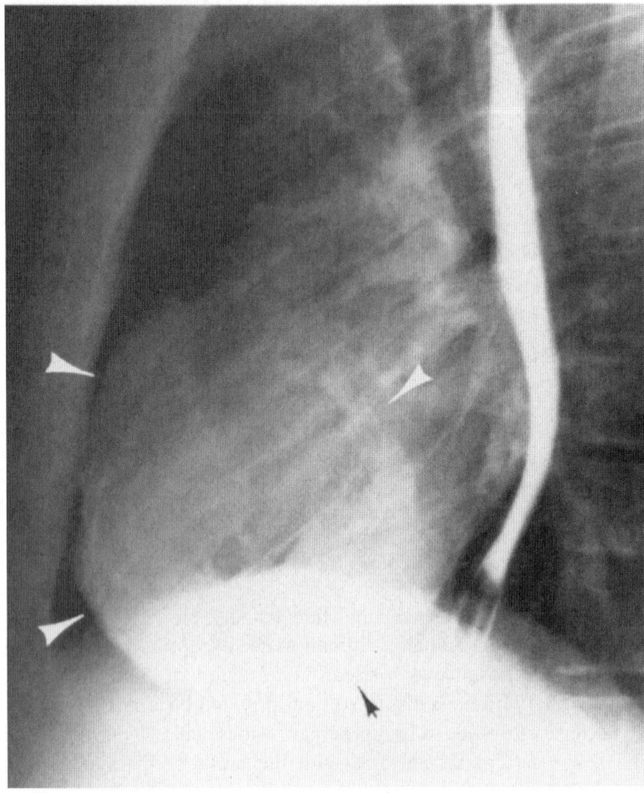

B

FIGURE 14-23 Patient with calcific constrictive pericarditis. Typically there is only mild postcapillary PH due to left-sided constriction. Severe pulmonary venous congestion is prevented by the concurrent right-sided constriction. *A*. PA view shows moderate cardiomegaly and mildly cephalic pulmonary blood flow pattern. *B*. Lateral view shows heavy calcification of the pericardium (*arrows*) and LA enlargement deviating the barium-filled esophagus posteriorly.

collapses on Valsalva maneuver, with exaggerated pulsation following release of the breath. Enlarged lymph nodes in these areas, on the other hand, will not change with such a maneuver.

## EVALUATION OF VALVE PROSTHESES AND PACEMAKERS

The normal movements of cardiac valve prostheses are parallel between the two phases of the cardiac cycle. If a significant angle of tilt (more than 12 degrees) is formed between the two phases, instability of the valve with associated regurgitation is nearly always present.[1,26,29,31]

The bileaflet St. Jude valve is used in both mitral and aortic positions. The valve is difficult to see radiographically but is readily detected under the fluoroscope.[1] When the leaflets move sluggishly, thrombotic stenosis of the valve should be suspected. Rarely, one leaflet may dislodge and embolize distally, causing acute valvular regurgitation.[33]

The position of the pacemaker can be determined promptly under the fluoroscope and recorded on film.[1,33] The subepicardial fat line overlies the myocardium and underlies the pericardium. If the pacing catheter is found within the fat stripe, it may have passed through the coronary sinus and entered one of the major cardiac veins. If the tip of the catheter is seen outside the fat stripe, however, it may have perforated the myocardium and thus be lying in the pericardium or beyond.[2] Although the wires and electrodes of a transmediastinal pacemaker may look normal on the films, minor breakage can be appreciated only in ventricular systole with the aid of fluoroscopy.[34]

## References


1. Chen JTT. *Essentials of Cardiac Imaging,* 2d ed. Philadelphia: Lippincott-Raven Press; 1997.
2. Chen JTT. The plain radiograph in the diagnosis of cardiovascular disease. In: Putman C, ed. Symposium on cardiopulmonary imaging. *Radiol Clin North Am* 1983;21:609–621.
3. Juhl JH, Grummy AB. *Essentials of Radiologic Imaging,* 6th ed. Philadelphia: Lippincott; 1993:1065–1138.
4. Meschan I, Formanek A. Roentgenology of the heart inclusive of major vessels. In: Meschan I, ed. *Roentgen Signs in Diagnostic Imaging,* 2d ed. Philadelphia: Saunders; 1987:784–925.
5. Figley M. Accessory roentgen signs of coarctation of the aorta. *Radiology* 1954;62:671–686.

5a. Durkman W, Vander Belt RJ. The chest x-ray in heart disease. In: Chissner M, ed. *Classic Teachings in Clinical Cardiology*. Washington, D.C: Laennec Publishing; 1996:241–258.

6. Elliott LP, Jue KL, Amplatz K. A roentgen classification of cardiac malpositions. *Invest Radiol* 1966;1:17–28.
7. Elliott LP, Schiebler GL. *X-ray Diagnosis of Congenital Cardiac Disease,* 2d ed. Springfield, IL: Charles C Thomas; 1979.
8. deLeon AC, Perloff JK, Twigg HL. The straight back syndrome: Clinical and cardiovascular manifestations. *Circulation* 1965;32: 193–203.
9. Chen JTT, Capp MP, Johnsrude IS, Goodrich JK, Lester RG. Roentgen appearance of pulmonary vascularity in the diagnosis of heart disease. *AJR* 1971;112:559–570.
10. Woodley K, Stark P. Pulmonary parenchymal manifestations of mitral valve disease. *Radiographics* 1999;19:965–972.
11. Chen JTT. The significance of cardiac calcifications. *Appl Radiol* 1992;21:11–19.
12. Stanford W, Rumberger JA. *Ultrafast Computed Tomography in Cardiac Imaging: Principles and Practice*. Mt. Kisco, NY: Futura; 1992.
13. Margolis JR, Chen JTT, Kong Y, et al. The diagnostic and prognostic significance of coronary artery calcification: A report of 800 cases. *Radiology* 1980;137:609–616.

14. Applegate KE, Goske MJ, Pierce G, Murphy D. Situs revisited: Imaging of the heterotaxy syndrome. *Radiographics* 1999;19:837–852.
15. Meszaros WT. *Cardiac Roentgenology*. Springfield, IL: Charles C Thomas; 1969.
16. Cooley RN. *Radiology of the Heart and Great Vessels,* 3d ed. Baltimore: Williams & Wilkins; 1978.
17. Swischuck LE. *Plain Film Interpretation in Congenital Heart Disease,* 2d ed. Baltimore: Williams & Wilkins; 1979.
18. Shuford WH, Sybers RG. *The Aortic Arch and Its Malformations*. Springfield, IL: Charles C Thomas; 1974:18.
19. Stewart JR, Kincaid OW, Titus JL. Right aortic arch: Plain film diagnosis and significance. *AJR* 1966;97:377–389.
20. Fraser RG, Pare JAP, Pare PD, et al. Factors influencing pulmonary circulation. In: Fraser RG, Pare JAP, Pare PD, et al, eds. *Diagnosis of Diseases of the Chest,* 3d ed: Vol I. Philadelphia: Saunders; 1988: 128–129.
21. Chen JTT, Behar VS, Morris JJ, et al., Correlation of roentgen findings with hemodynamic data in pure mitral stenosis. *AJR* 1968;102: 280–292.
22. Milne ENC, Pistolesi M. *Reading the Chest Radiograph: A Physiologic Approach*. St Louis: Mosby; 1993:164–241,343–369.
23. Wojtowicz J. Some tomographic criteria for an evaluation of the pulmonary circulation. *Acta Radiol [Diagn] (Stockh)* 1964;2:215–224.
24. Fleischner FG. The butterfly pattern of acute pulmonary edema. *Am J Cardiol* 1967;20:39–46.
25. Jeffers K, Rees S, eds. *Clinical Cardiac Radiology,* 2d ed. London: Butterworth; 1980.
26. Chen JTT. Cardiac fluoroscopy. In: Kelley MJ, ed. Symposium on chest radiography for the cardiologist. *Cardiol Clin* 1983;1:565–573.
27. Chen JTT, McIntosh HD, Capp MP, et al. Intercalative angiocardiography: A method for recording cardiovascular dynamics on a single film. *Radiology* 1969;93:499–506.
28. Chen JTT, Robinson AE, Goodrich JK, Lester RG. Uneven distribution of pulmonary blood flow between left and right lungs in isolated valvular pulmonary stenosis. *AJR* 1969;107:343–350.
29. Chen JTT, Lester RG, Peter RH. Posterior wedging sign of mitral insufficiency. *Radiology* 1974;113:451–453.
30. Jorgens J, Kundel R, Lieber A. The cinefluorographic approach to the diagnosis of pericardial effusion. *AJR* 1962;87:911–916.
31. Gimenez JL, Soulen RL, Davila JC. Prosthetic valve detachment: Its roentgenographic recognition: Report of cases. *AJR* 1968;103:595–600.
32. Kotler MN, Panidis J, Mintz GS, et al. The role of noninvasive technique in the evaluation of the St. Jude cardiac prosthesis. In: DeBakey ME, ed. *Advances in Cardiac Valves: Clinical Perspectives*. New York: Butterworth-Heinemann; 1983:213–226.
33. Sorkin RP, Schuurmann BJ, Simon AB. Radiographic aspects of permanent cardiac pacemakers. *Radiology* 1976;119:281–286.

C H A P T E R 15

# THE ECHOCARDIOGRAM

Anthony N. DeMaria / Daniel G. Blanchard



The term *echocardiography* refers to the evaluation of cardiac structure and function with images and recordings produced by ultrasound. In the past three decades it has rapidly become a fundamental component of the cardiac evaluation. Currently, echocardiography ("echo") provides essential (and sometimes unexpected) clinical information and has become the second most frequently performed diagnostic procedure after electrocardiography.[1] What began as a one-dimensional (1D) method performed from the precordial area to assess cardiac anatomy has evolved into a two-dimensional (2D) modality performed from either the thorax or from within the esophagus, capable of also delineating flow and deriving hemodynamic data.[2] Newly evolving technical developments likely will extend the capacity of ultrasound to routine 3D visualization[3] as well as to the assessment, in conjunction with contrast agents,[4] of myocardial perfusion.

The development of echocardiography is usually credited to Elder and Hertz in 1954.[5] Primitive cross-sectional images of the excised human heart were produced in 1957[6]; however, for nearly two additional decades, clinical echocardiography consisted primarily of 1D time-motion (M-mode) recordings, as popularized by Feigenbaum.[7] In the mid-1970s, Bom and associates developed a multielement linear-array scanner that could produce spatially correct images of the beating heart.[8] 2D images of superior quality were soon achieved by mechanical sector scanners[9,10] and ultimately by phased-array instruments as developed by Thurston and Von Ramm, which are the present-day standard.[11] In the past several years, 3D instruments capable of real-time volumetric imaging have been developed.[12] Miniaturization of ultrasound transducers has also led to their incorporation into gastroscopes and cardiac catheters to achieve transesophageal and intravascular images.[13,14]

Although efforts to use the Doppler principle to measure flow velocity by ultrasound were begun in the early 1970s by Baker et al.,[15] clinical application of this technique did not thrive until the work of Hatle in the early 1980s.[16,17] Pulsed and continuous-wave Doppler recordings soon were expanded to full 2D color-flow imaging. Most recently, Doppler velocity recordings have been obtained from myocardium itself, enabling measurement of tissue velocities and regional strain.

## PRINCIPLES OF ECHOCARDIOGRAPHY

### Physics and Instrumentation

Sound is an energy form that travels through a medium as a series of alternating compressions and rarefactions of the molecules (Fig. 15-1). Sound is typically characterized by its wavelength, which is the distance between any two consecutive phases of the cycle (e.g., peak compression to peak compression), and by its frequency, which is the number of wavelengths per unit time [customarily expressed as cycles per second, or hertz (Hz)]. The velocity of sound is the product of wavelength and frequency; thus there is an inverse relationship between these two characteristics: the greater the frequency, the shorter the wavelength. Ultrasound is sonic energy with a frequency above the audible range of the human ear (greater than 20,000 Hz) and is useful for diagnostic imaging, since, like light, it can be directed as a beam that will obey the laws of reflection and refraction.[12–14,17,18] Thus, an ultrasound beam will travel in a straight line through a homogeneous medium. If the beam meets an interface of different acoustic impedance, however, part of the energy will be reflected and the remaining attenuated signal will be transmitted. The reflected energy, or echo, is used to construct an image—in the case of echocardiography, an image of the heart (Fig. 15-2).

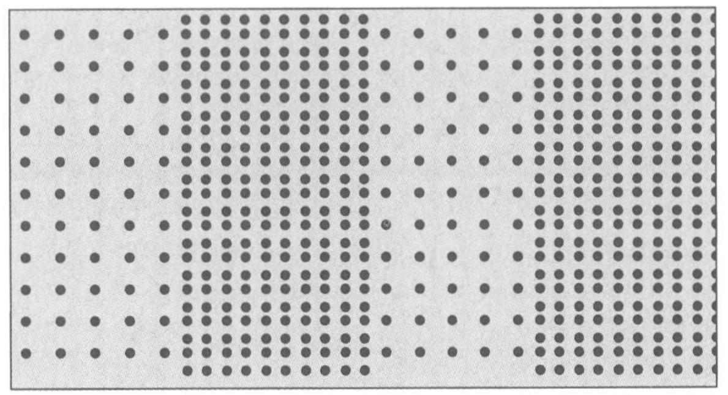

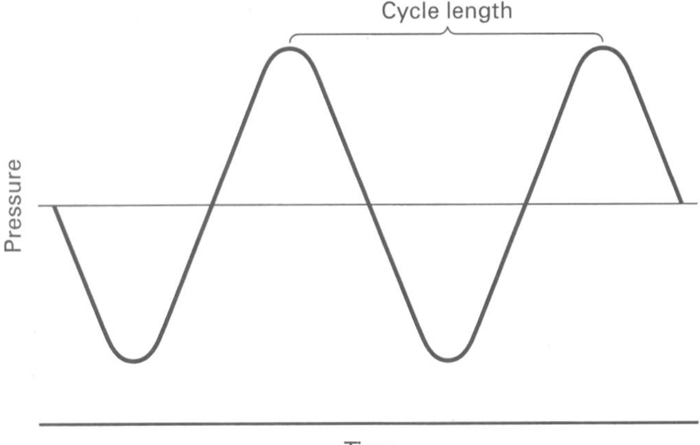


FIGURE 15-1 Sound energy results in alternating compression and rarefaction of particles in a conducting medium. This alternation, which can be plotted against time (or distance), conforms to a sine-wave pattern (*bottom panel*). (Modified from Hagan AD, DeMaria AN. *Clinical Applications of Two-Dimensional Echocardiography and Cardiac Doppler.* Boston: Little, Brown; 1989. With permission.)

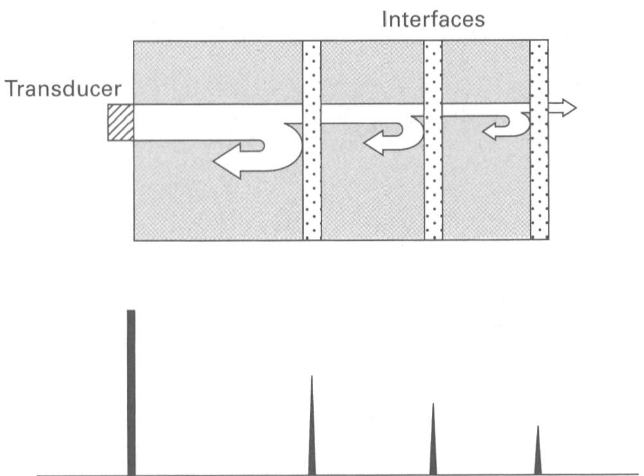


FIGURE 15-2 *Upper panel:* Attenuation of an ultrasound beam emitted from a transducer. There is reflection and progressive loss of energy at each interface encountered. *Lower panel:* the reflected wavefronts are recorded as signals of varying amplitudes (A mode) via the piezoelectric crystal. (Upper panel modified from Hagan AD, DeMaria AN. *Clinical Applications of Two-Dimensional Echocardiography and Cardiac Doppler.* Boston: Little, Brown; 1989. With permission.)

The most fundamental component of any echocardiographic instrument is the transducer, which is responsible for both transmitting and receiving the ultrasound signal. The transducer consists of electrodes and a piezoelectric crystal, whose ionic structure results in deformation of shape when exposed to an electric current.[18] Thus, piezoelectric crystals are composed of synthetic materials, such as barium titanate, that, when exposed to electric current from the electrodes, alternately expand and contract to create sound waves. When subjected to the mechanical energy of sound returning from a reflecting surface, the same piezoelectric element changes shape, thereby generating an electrical signal detected by the electrodes (Fig. 15-3). Thus the transducer both produces and receives ultrasonic signals.

In the past, echographs have both transmitted and received signals of the same frequency. Recently, *harmonic imaging* has been implemented, in which ultrasound energy is transmitted at a baseline (fundamental) frequency but then received at a higher harmonic of that frequency (usually the first harmonic). Harmonic imaging is based upon the change in the ultrasound frequency of a transmitted wave induced by the interaction with a reflecting target. The sinusoidal waveform becomes peaked as it travels through tissue, thereby undergoing a change in frequency. Similarly if a sound signal strikes a contrast microbubble, the periodic expansion and contraction (resonation) of the bubble will change the frequency of the wave. This change in frequency generates harmonic signals with frequencies which are multiples of the transmitted signal.

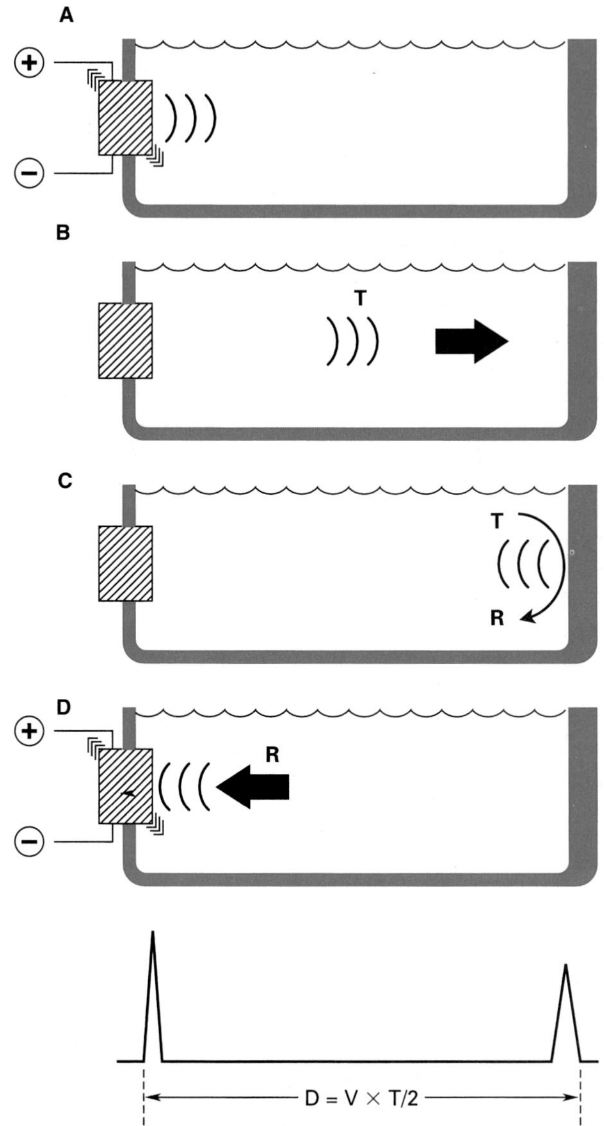


FIGURE 15-3 *A* through *D:* the basic principle of ultrasonic imaging. The piezoelectric crystal is activated, producing a transmitted pulse (T), which reflects off the interface. The reflected pulse (R) excites the crystal, producing an electric current. As the velocity of the pulse is constant, distance can be calculated based on the transit time. (Because the pulse must travel back and forth from the interface, the time is divided by 2.) (Modified from Weyman AE. *Principles and Practice of Echocardiography,* 2d ed. Philadelphia: Lea & Febiger; 1994. With permission.)

A simplistic analogy of this phenomenon would be the morphologic changes seen in ocean waves as they approach the shore and are affected by the rising ocean floor. The cresting of the waves and the changes in their height are analogous to the harmonic signals generated by the interaction of ultrasound and tissue.[19] Of note, these signals take some time (and distance) to develop. Therefore (and in sharp distinction to reflected *fundamental* ultrasound energy), structures very close to the transducer do not generate much harmonic signal at all. Thus, near-field artifacts and reverberation artifacts are minimized with tissue harmonic imaging.

Harmonic imaging has also been very useful in conjunction with intravascular echo contrast agents. The microbubbles in these agents resonate during ultrasound imaging, and demonstrate cyclic expansion and constriction: this resonance produces a large amount of harmonic energy.[20] In contrast, myocardial tissue does not resonate to any appreciable degree. The net effect of harmonic imaging with echocardiographic contrast is a marked enhancement of the signal from the left ventricular (LV) cavity compared to that of the myocardium, and thereby an improvement in endocardial definition.

As an imaging modality, ultrasound presents several unique technical difficulties. Sound energy is poorly transmitted through air and bone, and the ability to record adequate images is dependent upon a thoracic window that gives the interrogating beam adequate access to cardiac structures. The degree to which ultrasonic energy will be reflected when it strikes an interface of differential impedance depends on how perpendicular the interrogating beam is to the interface. When the ultrasound beam is directed to the interface, little or no sound energy will be reflected to the transducer. Therefore poor signal transmission, a nonorthogonal orientation of the ultrasound beam to the surface, and energy attenuation can cause failure to record signals from cardiac structures—a phenomenon referred to as *echo dropout*.[21] Conversely, some structures may be such strong ultrasonic reflectors—being perpendicular to the beam or extremely dense—that sufficient energy returns to the transducer to be reflected and again transmitted into the field. This phenomenon can lead to reverberations, or the reproduction of the echoes of anatomic structures at multiple locations within the image.[22] Also, background noise artifacts, or signals generated from the system rather than tissue, can also be encountered. Finally, targets lying on the periphery of the ultrasound beam may be recorded and displayed as if they were located along the central scan line (Fig. 15-4). This problem may be accentuated in the setting of very strong reflectors that result in the formation of *side lobes*.[23] Thus beam-width problems associated with ultrasound may result in the depiction of targets in erroneous locations and create problems in interpreting the images.[24]

The construction of a cardiac image from ultrasound signals is based on computation of the distance between an anatomic structure and the transducer (Fig. 15-3). Thus, an ultrasound beam is produced by a handheld transducer positioned on the thorax and directed into the heart. This beam will travel in a straight line until it reaches an interface between structures of different acoustic impedance, such as blood and myocardium. At this point, some ultrasonic energy will be

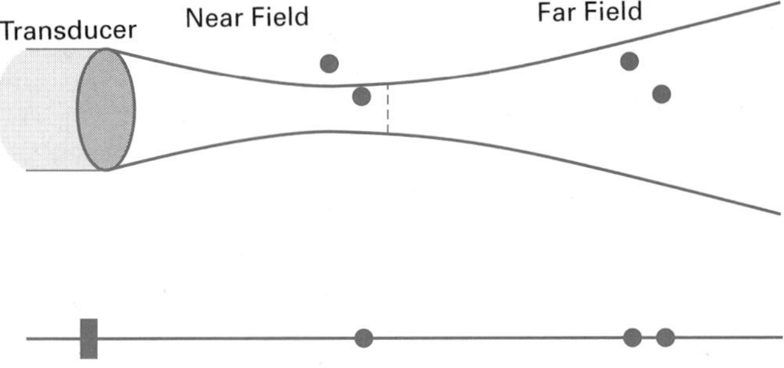


FIGURE 15-4 *Upper panel:* The transducer emits an ultrasonic beam that has a near field (where the beam is relatively focused) and a far field (where the beam width increases). *Lower panel:* B-mode diagram showing the effect of beam width. In the near field, the beam reflects off only one of two objects in close proximity to each other. In the far field, however, two similarly positioned objects are both within the beam width. Therefore, lateral resolution is compromised and the objects' positions are misrepresented.

reflected (depending on the density of interface); some will be scattered and some will continue forward. The amplitude of the propagating signal will be attenuated because of the reduction in energy at the interface (Fig. 15-2). The reflected sound waves return to the transducer and form the basis of the echogram. Electronic circuitry within the echograph measures the time interval required for the transit of the ultrasound beam from the transducer to the interface and back again. Since the velocity of sound in soft tissue is constant (approximately 1540 m/s), the instrument can calculate the total distance traveled to and from the reflecting surface as the product of transit time and velocity of sound. Interface location is derived as one-half of the total transit distance, and a signal is depicted on an oscilloscope or video monitor at that point (Fig. 15-3). The amplitude of ultrasonic energy reflected from each target interface is represented by the brightness of the signal that is displayed.

The 1D ultrasonic B- (or brightness) mode scan line resulting from a single transmitted beam is the cornerstone of echocardiographic imaging. In the most basic form of echocardiography, a single scan line produced by a piezoelectric crystal is passed through the heart (Fig. 15-5). At each structural interface, ultrasonic energy is reflected back and displayed at the appropriate distance as a signal, whose amplitude represents the acoustic impedance or density of the material encountered. These signals are subsequently displayed as dots, whose brightness is proportional to the amplitude of reflected ultrasonic energy. The distance from the transducer of these B-mode dots changes as the cardiac structures move during the cardiac cycle. Accordingly, if repetitive B-mode scan lines are produced and swept across the screen over time, the movement of the heart can be obtained as a time-motion (or M-mode) recording,[25] providing dynamic rather than merely static cardiac images (Fig. 15-5). In clinical use, the piezoelectric crystal within the transducer is activated by alternating electric current to transmit at a rate of approximately 1000 pulses per second. This same crystal also receives the returning echo reflections and actually spends most of the time (>90 percent) in the "receive" rather than the "transmit" mode. Because the beam is confined to a single location and transmits ultrasound signals at the pulse rate of the transducer, M-mode echocardiography provides *very high temporal resolution*. Importantly, M mode is an excellent modality for timing cardiac events or recording high-velocity motion.

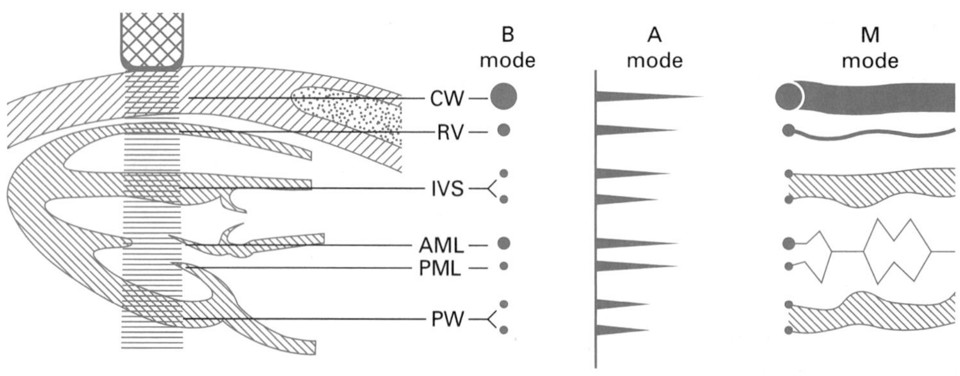


FIGURE 15-5 Formation of A-mode, B-mode, and M-mode echocardiograms. The transducer emits an ultrasound beam, which reflects at each anatomic interface. The reflected wavefronts can be represented as dots (B mode) or spikes (A mode). The dot brightness and spike magnitude vary with the amplitude of the reflected wave. If the B-mode scan is swept from left to right with time, an M-mode image is produced. CW = chest wall; RV = right ventricle; IVS = interventricular septum; AML = anterior mitral leaflet; PML = posterior mitral leaflet; and PW = posterior wall. (Modified from Hagan AD, DeMaria AN. *Clinical Applications of Two-Dimensional Echocardiography and Cardiac Doppler.* Boston: Little, Brown; 1989. With permission.)

As ultrasound technology advanced, multiple B-mode scan lines from different imaging angles were collected and displayed in proper alignment to create a 2D image. As opposed to B- or M-mode recordings, which are unidimensional (on an anteroposterior axis), 2D echocardiography provides additional information in either superoinferior or mediolateral directions. At present, M-mode recordings are derived from the 2D images rather than as a stand-alone signal.

Several characteristics of sound energy are of fundamental importance in determining the quality of the images obtained. High-quality images require optimal resolution—that is, the ability to distinguish two individual objects separated in space. Short wavelengths yield excellent resolution in echo imaging, since the shorter the cycle length, the smaller the object that will reflect the signal and be detected by the echo scanner. Since wavelength is inversely related to frequency, transducers that emit a high-frequency signal (3.5 to 7.0 MHz or greater) yield high-resolution images. High-frequency signals also overcome a limitation of ultrasonic imaging associated with lateral resolution. Since ultrasonic beams diverge as they propagate away from the transducer, the width of the beam can become sufficiently great to encompass multiple targets and decrease resolution (Fig. 15-4). The degree of beam divergence is less with high-frequency sonic energy than with low-frequency signals. The smaller wavelengths associated with high-frequency signals, however, are subject to greater reflection and scattering, with substantially higher attenuation as the beam propagates through tissue. The resultant attenuation is greater and leads to decreased sensitivity. Therefore, in clinical practice, echocardiographic examinations are performed utilizing the highest-frequency transducer capable of obtaining signals from all potential targets within the ultrasound field.[25]

## M-Mode Echocardiography

### THE STANDARD M-MODE EXAMINATION

Although largely supplanted by 2D imaging, M-mode echocardiography remains a useful part of a complete ultrasound examination. Figure 15-6*A* through *D* shows the typical views obtained when the transducer is placed at the left parasternal area and rocked through the heart from apex to base. Tissue typically reflects ultrasound at its surface (specular reflectors) and from internal inhomogenicity (backscatter), while blood is homogenous and does not produce reflections. Thus, blood is free of ultrasonic signals on the echocardiogram. At the mitral valve (MV) level (Fig. 15-6*C*), the cardiac structure seen closest to the transducer is the right ventricular (RV) free wall; it is followed by the RV cavity, the interventricular septum, the MV apparatus, and the LV posterior wall as the beam travels backward. At this level, MV excursion is well seen and is more easily recorded for the longer anterior leaflet. For the anterior leaflet, diastolic mitral opening is bipeaked (M-shaped), with maximal opening during early diastolic filling at the E point, a subsequent reclosure downslope to the F point, and a reopening with atrial contraction at the

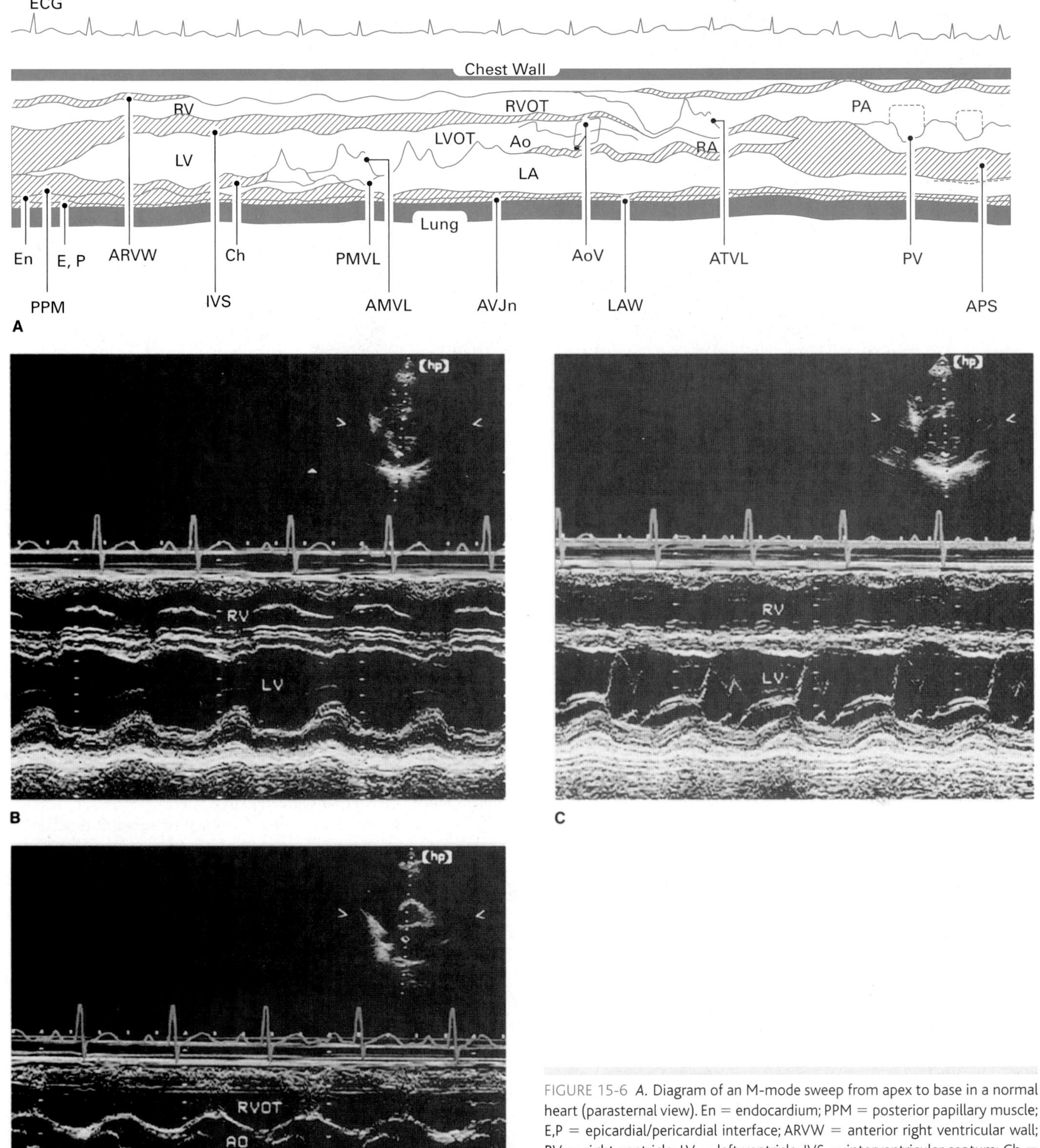


FIGURE 15-6 *A*. Diagram of an M-mode sweep from apex to base in a normal heart (parasternal view). En = endocardium; PPM = posterior papillary muscle; E,P = epicardial/pericardial interface; ARVW = anterior right ventricular wall; RV = right ventricle; LV = left ventricle; IVS = interventricular septum; Ch = chordae tendineae; PMVL = posterior mitral valve leaflet; AMVL = anterior mitral valve leaflet; LVOT = left ventricular outflow tract; AVJn = atrioventricular junction; RVOT = right ventricular outflow tract; Ao = aorta; LA = left atrium; AoV = aortic valve; LAW = left atrial wall; RA = right atrium; ATVL = anterior tricuspid valve leaflet; PA = pulmonary artery; PV = pulmonic valve; APS = atriopulmonic sulcus. (From Felner JM, Schlant RC. *Echocardiography: A Teaching Atlas*. New York: Grune & Stratton; 1976. With permission.) *B* to *D*. M-mode sweep from apex to base in a normal individual.

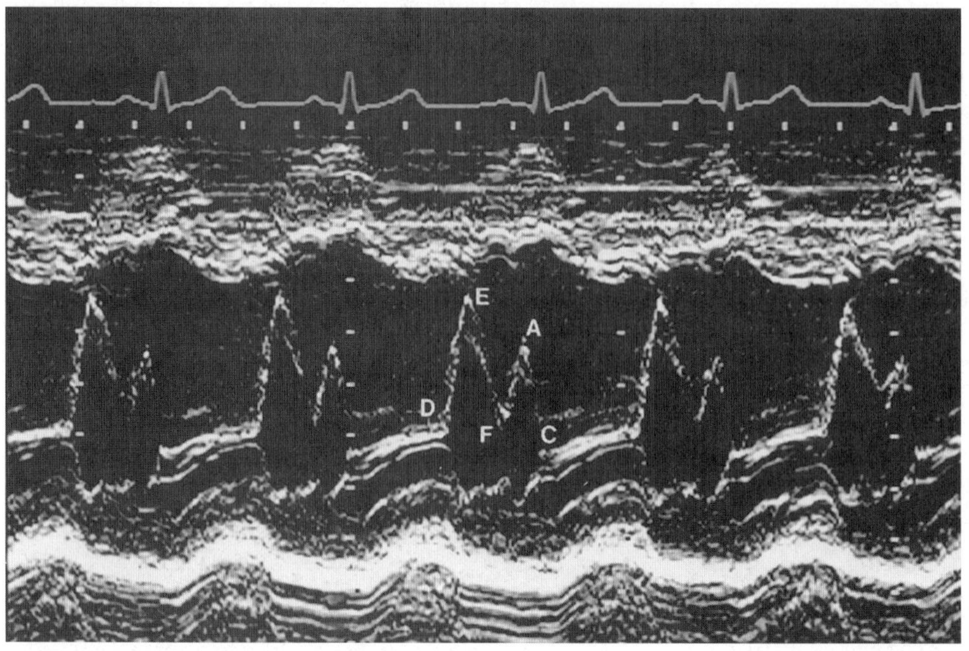


FIGURE 15-7 Standard M-mode image through the left ventricle at the level of the mitral valve. See text for discussion of nomenclature.

A point prior to valve closure at the C point[26] (Fig. 15-7). The posterior leaflet manifests a mirror-image W-shaped pattern. When LV end-diastolic pressure is elevated, a shoulder ("B" bump) is often present between the A and C points[27] (Fig. 15-8). If the transducer beam is directed inferolaterally from the MV level, the papillary muscles and LV apex will be imaged (Fig. 15-6*A*). With superior and medial angulation, the left atrium (LA), aortic valve (AoV), and aortic root are seen. The tricuspid valve (TV) can be imaged by angulating the transducer inferomedially and the pulmonic valve (PV) by angulating slightly superiorly and laterally.

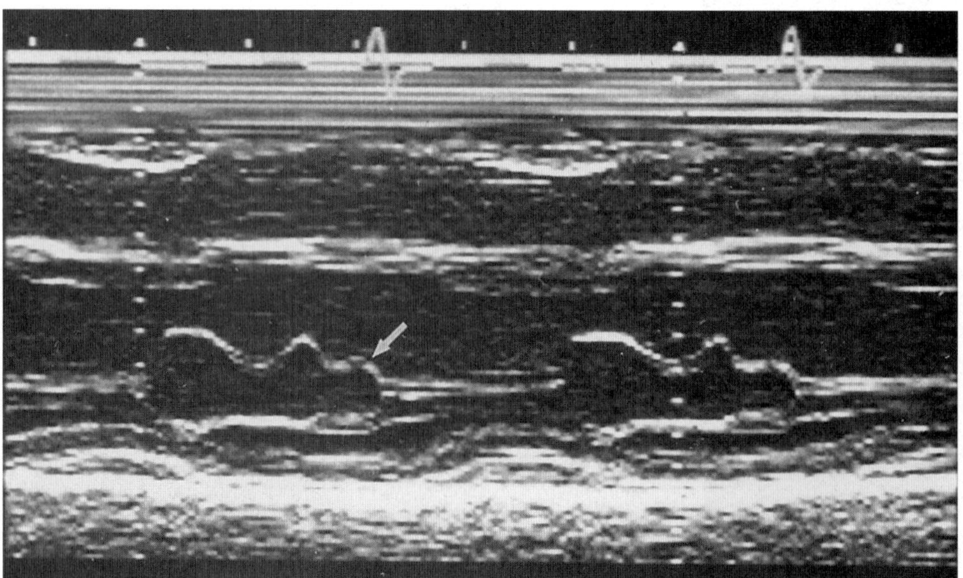

FIGURE 15-8 M-mode image through the mitral valve showing a "B bump", suggesting high left ventricular diastolic pressure (*arrow*). The E-point septal separation is also increased. (Transducer is in the left parasternal position.)

### ASSESSMENT OF SYSTOLIC FUNCTION BY M-MODE ECHOCARDIOGRAPHY

Measurements of the LV cavity dimension and wall thickness can be readily derived from M-mode recordings (Fig. 15-9) and are usually made according to the recommendations of the American Society of Echocardiography (ASE) at end diastole (the onset of the QRS complex) and end systole (the point of maximum upward motion of the LV posterior wall endocardium).[28] These measurements should be made from leading edge to leading edge to avoid incorporating artifacts and reverberations; they are accurate if the beam is orthogonal to the long axis of the ventricle. By convention, left atrial (LA) dimension is measured at end systole and aortic root diameter is recorded at end diastole at the level of the base of the heart (Fig. 15-9). During systole, opening of the aortic leaflets appears as a parallelogram produced by motion of the right coronary and (usually) the noncoronary AoV cusps.[29]

The M-mode LV cavity dimensions can be used to estimate ventricular volumes and ejection fraction (EF) if desired, most simply by merely cubing the value ($D^3$); but these calculations involve several assumptions regarding LV geometry that are not uniformly valid.[30,31] In addition, the M-mode dimension may not be representative of the entire ventricle. The fractional shortening can also be determined.[32] This value is often helpful in assessing systolic function, but it reflects the function of the LV in one chord and in one plane and can be misleading with asynchronous contraction [for example, left bundle branch block (LBBB)] or segmental dyssynergy.[33] An additional M-mode marker of systolic function is *E point–septal separation* (EPSS), or the distance between the anterior MV leaflet at its most anterior opening excursion (the E point) and the interventricular septum. A value of 8 mm or greater is abnormal.[34] The normal M-mode measurements are seen in Table 15-1.

## Two-Dimensional Echocardiography

A number of technical approaches exist by which multiple individual B-mode scan lines can be rapidly transmitted, received, and displayed in appropriate spatial orientation to construct a 2D image of the heart. The initial approach simply utilized a linear array of 20 piezoelectric crystals placed side by side, each of which transmitted and received signals independently[8] (Fig. 15-10*A*). The resulting scan lines were displayed

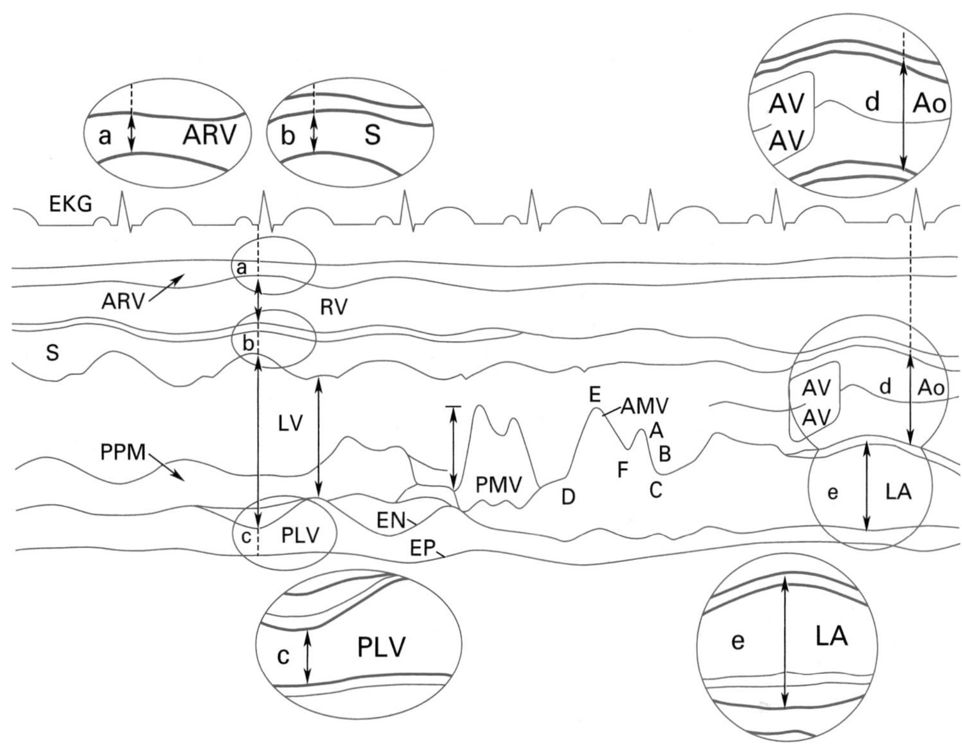


FIGURE 15-9 Recommended criteria for M-mode measurement of cardiac dimensions (see text for details). The figure and the elliptical inserts (*a, b, c, d,* and *e*) illustrate the leading-edge method. ARV = anterior right ventricular wall; RV = right ventricle; LV = left ventricle; PLV = posterior left ventricular wall; S = septum; PPM = papillary muscle; AMV and PMV = anterior and posterior mitral valve leaflets, EN: endocardium, EP: epicardium; AV = aortic valve; Ao = aorta; LA = left atrium. (Reproduced with permission from Sahn DJ, DeMaria AN, Kisslo J, Weyman AE. Recommendations regarding quantitation in M-mode echocardiography: Results of a survey of echocardiographic measurements. *Circulation* 1978;58;1072. With permission.)

TABLE 15-1 Normal Values

| | Mean ± Standard Deviation | Range | Mean ± Standard Deviation | Range |
|---|---|---|---|---|
| No. of patients | 25 | — | 50 | — |
| Age, years | 10 ± 3 | 4–18 | 24 ±. 6 | 1.10–2.53 |
| BSA, $m^2$ | 1.33 ± 0.38 | 0.72–2.04 | 1.81 ±. 34 | 1.10–2.53 |
| $LVID_d$, mm | 44 ± 6 | 32–50 | 50 ± 3 | 42–60 |
| $LVID_s$, mm | 28 ± 7 | 32–50 | 50 ± 3 | 22–43 |
| FSLV | 34 ± 4 | 25–42 | 33 ± 3 | 28–37 |
| IVS thickness, mm | 8 ± 2 | 5–10 | 9 ± 1 | 7–12 |
| IVS excursion, mm | 7 ± 1 | 5–9 | 9 ± 1 | 7–12 |
| $PW_d$ thickness, mm | 7 ± 2 | 4–9 | 9 ± 1 | 7–12 |
| $PW_s$ thickness, mm | 12 ± 3 | 8–17 | 16 ± 2 | 13–20 |
| Δ thickening PW | 0.70 ± 0.25 | 0.41–0.95 | 0.50 ± 0.19 | 0.32–0.69 |
| PW excursion, mm | 9 ± 2 | 7–14 | 11 ± 2 | 9–17 |
| $RVD_d$ supine, mm | — | — | 15 ± 6 | 7–22 |
| $RVD_d$ left lateral, mm | — | — | 20 ± 8 | 10–37 |
| $Aorta_d$ mm | 23 ± 4 | 15–27 | 28 ± 5 | 26–36 |
| $LAD_s$ mm | 25 ± 5 | 20–31 | 27 ± 6 | 12–35 |

ABBREVIATIONS: BSA = Body surface area; $LVID_d$ = left ventricular internal diameter, end diastole; $LVID_s$ = left ventricular internal diameter, end systole; FSLV = fractional shortening of left ventricle; PWV = posterior wall velocity; IVS = interventricular septum; PW = posterior wall; RVD = right ventricular dimension; LAD = left atrial dimension.

SOURCE: Felner JM, Schlant RC. *Echocardiography: A Teaching Atlas*. New York: Grune & Stratton; 1976. Reproduced with permission from the publisher and authors.

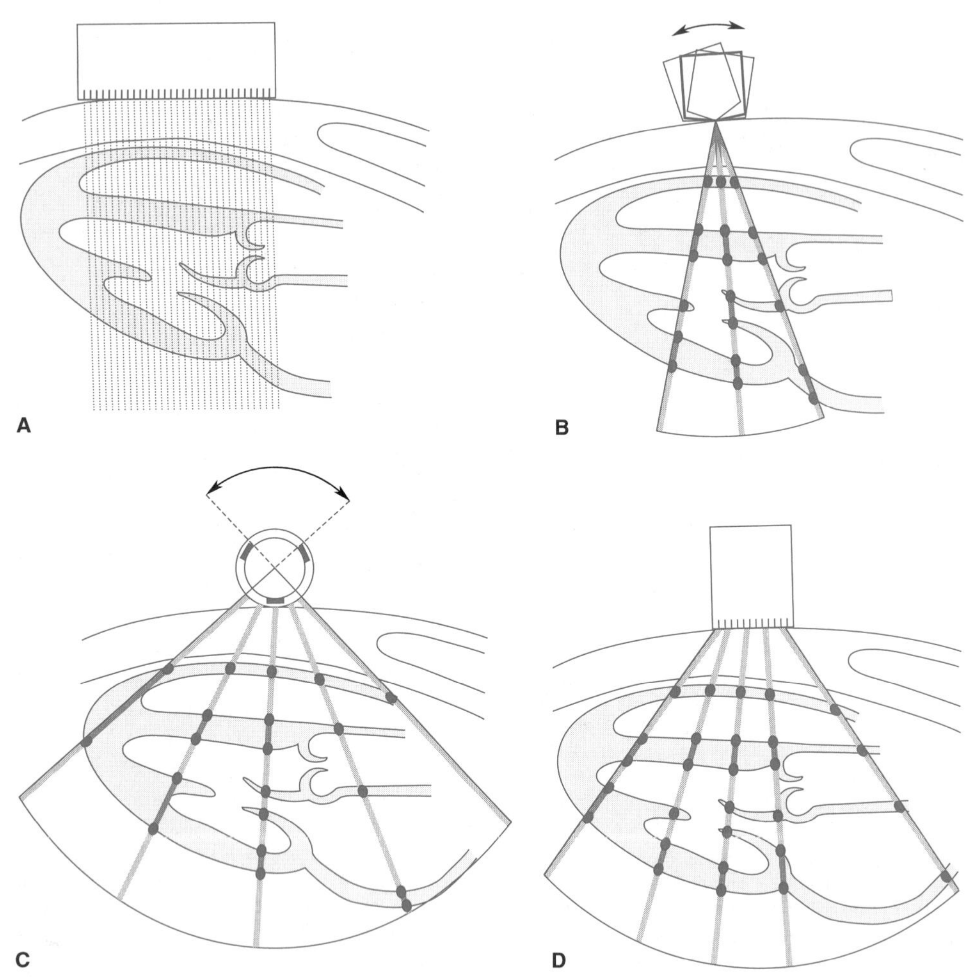


FIGURE 15-10 The four major types of ultrasonic scanners used to acquire 2D echocardiographic images. *A.* Linear-array scanner. *B.* Oscillating scanner. *C.* Rotating mechanical scanner. *D.* Phased-array scanner. (From Hagan AD, DeMaria AN. *Clinical Applications of Two-Dimensional Echocardiography and Cardiac Doppler.* Boston: Little, Brown; 1989. With permission.)

simultaneously to yield rectangular images. Unfortunately, transducer size and interaction between the elements resulted in images of unsatisfactory quality.

Current 2D scanners utilize B-mode scan lines that are independently transmitted and received and are directed through a wedge-shaped sector of cardiac anatomy by means of mechanical or electrical beam steering (Fig. 15-10*B* to *D*). A variety of motorized devices are available that, by rapidly oscillating or rotating one or more ultrasonic crystals through space, can mechanically direct multiple scan lines through a sector arc of the cardiovascular system.[9,10] The position of the beam in space is derived by determining the orientation of the piezoelectric crystal. Most current 2D scanners utilize a phased-array approach, where multiple ultrasonic crystals are employed in concert to create individual B-mode scan lines.[11] The piezoelectric crystals are activated in a closely coordinated temporal sequence, so that the individual wavelets produced by each element merge to form a single beam whose direction is determined by the sequence of crystal firing (Fig. 15-11). Since the direction of the resultant beam is determined by the sequence of activation of the individual elements, the beam can be electrically swept throughout a 90-degree sector arc. Also, a firing sequence can be employed that results in dynamic focusing of the beam along its length to achieve minimal beam width and increased resolution. Phased-array 2D scanners employ small transducers without moving parts that could require repair; however, these systems are more costly.

Originally, echocardiographic data were displayed in analogue form on a standard oscilloscope, transferred to a video monitor by a television camera, and hard-copied onto videotape or paper. Currently, computerized analogue-to-digital scan conversion is standard, so that the polar signals of individual scan lines are converted to a series of numerical gray-level values for individual box-like picture elements (pixels) aligned along *X*-*Y* coordinates.[35] The ability of a digital step-gradation technique to reproduce the continuous gradation of analog methods is a function of the density of pixels in the matrix and the shades of gray levels available. No loss of data is detected in current digitally converted images, and the digital format provides the opportunity for image processing, enhancement, and quantitation. More importantly, storage in digital format can avoid the image degradation inherent in videotape, provide random access and easy comparison of studies, enable rapid image transmission, and prevent deterioration with image copying and prolonged storage. Technology for fully digital echocardiography is now available, and fully digital acquisition and storage of echocardiograms will be commonplace in the near future, replacing analog videotape recordings.

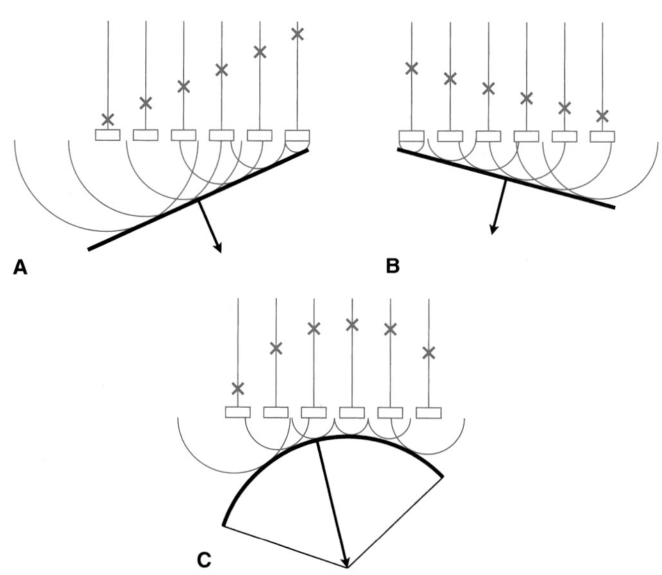


FIGURE 15-11 Electronic "steering" of a phased-array ultrasound beam. *A.* Elements are fired in sequence from left to right, resulting in a beam directed to the left. *B.* Elements are fired in sequence opposite to those in (*A*), producing a beam directed to the right. *C.* Elements are fired from the periphery toward the center, producing a beam that converges on a given focal point. (From Hagan AD, DeMaria AN. *Clinical Applications of Two-Dimensional Echocardiography and Cardiac Doppler.* Boston: Little Brown; 1989. With permission.)

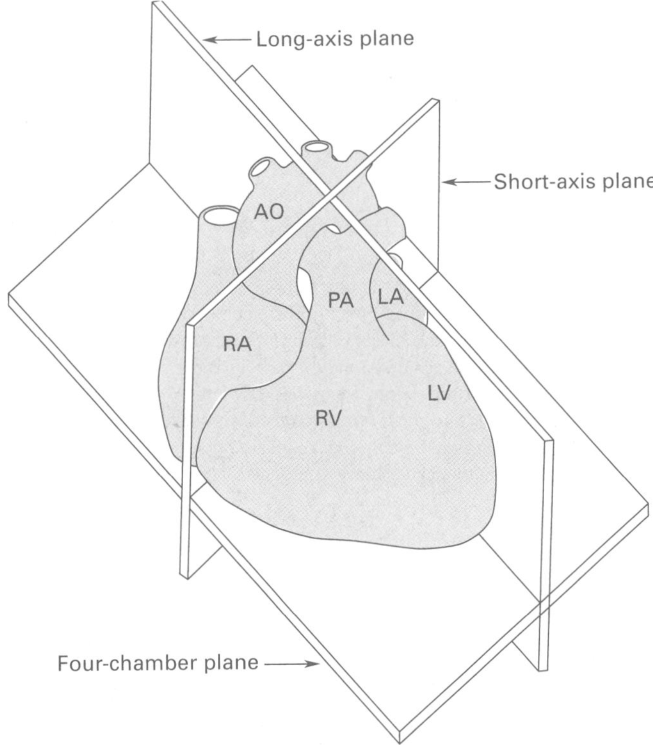


FIGURE 15-12 The three basic tomographic imaging planes used in echocardiography: long-axis, short-axis, and four-chamber. LV = left ventricle; LA = left atrium; RV = right ventricle; RA = right atrium; PA = pulmonary artery; AO = aorta. (From Hagan AD, DeMaria AN. *Clinical Applications of Two-Dimensional Echocardiography and Cardiac Doppler.* Boston: Little, Brown; 1989. With permission.)

## THE STANDARD TWO-DIMENSIONAL EXAMINATION

To help standardize the 2D examination, the ASE has recommended that cardiac imaging be performed in three orthogonal planes: long-axis (from aortic root to the apex), short-axis (perpendicular to long axis), and four-chamber (traversing both ventricles and atria through the mitral and TVs)[36] (Fig. 15-12). It is important to recognize that the long and short axes are those of the heart, not the body. These three planes can be visualized using four basic transducer positions: parasternal, apical, subcostal, and suprasternal[37,38] (Fig. 15-13*A*, *B*, and *C*). In general, the long-axis plane is best imaged from parasternal, apical, and occasionally the suprasternal positions, while the short-axis plane is best imaged in the parasternal and subcostal positions. The four-chamber views are obtained from the apical and subcostal positions. The ASE recognizes that these basic positions and planes may be modified somewhat and recommends that an image obtained within 45 degrees of a basic orthogonal plane be identified with that orthogonal plane. Table 15-2 lists the standard transducer positions and transthoracic echocardiographic (TEE) views. Anatomic drawings of the various imaging planes are seen in Figs. 15-13 through 15-20.

As opposed to other types of cardiac imaging, which are well standardized, the echocardiographic examination is iterative and largely determined by the anatomic characteristics of the patient and manual manipulation of the transducer by the operator. Of paramount importance is the identification of a thoracic site (window) that enables transmission of the ultrasound signal to the heart. In actual practice, the echocardiographic examination is performed with the operator either to the patient's left or right. The patient is in the left lateral decubitus position for most of the examination, with the head of the bed elevated 20 to 30 degrees. Alternate positioning may be employed for individual patients and views. Use of a thick foam rubber mattress (made expressly for echocardiography) that has a removable section under the area of the cardiac apex may facilitate the examination.

The examination customarily begins with the transducer in the left parasternal position in the long-axis view (Fig. 15-14). This provides excellent images of the LV, aorta, LA, and the mitral and aortic valves. By angling the beam slightly rightward and inferiorly (RV inflow view), the right atrium, RV, and TV are visualized (Fig. 15-15). If the beam is turned slightly leftward and rotated clockwise from the standard parasternal long-axis view, the RV outflow tract, PV, and main pulmonary artery (PA) appear (RV outflow view).

A 90-degree clockwise turn of the transducer produces the parasternal short-axis view. Slight axial angulation of the transducer enables visualization of the LV at various levels of the short axis, including the papillary muscle, mitral leaflets, and AoV (Fig. 15-16). With angulation toward the base, the LA, right heart structures, main PA, and occasionally the LA appendage are also recorded. The apical views are best acquired with the patient in a steep left lateral decubitus position and the transducer at the point of the apical impulse. The four-chamber view is obtained by turning the transducer so that both ventricles, atrioventricular valves, and atria are visualized (Fig. 15-17). In this view, the septal, apical, and lateral walls of the LV are visualized. Slight superior angulation of the transducer will add the AoV and proximal ascending aorta to the echocardiographic image (apical five-chamber view). From the four-chamber view, 90 degrees of counterclockwise transducer rotation will produce the apical two-chamber view (Fig. 15-18*A* and *B*). This imaging plane demonstrates the LA and the inferior, apical, and anterior wall segments of the LV (the right heart structures are absent). If the transducer is rotated slightly back toward the four-chamber plane, a three-chamber view similar to the parasternal long-axis view is produced (Fig. 15-18*C*)

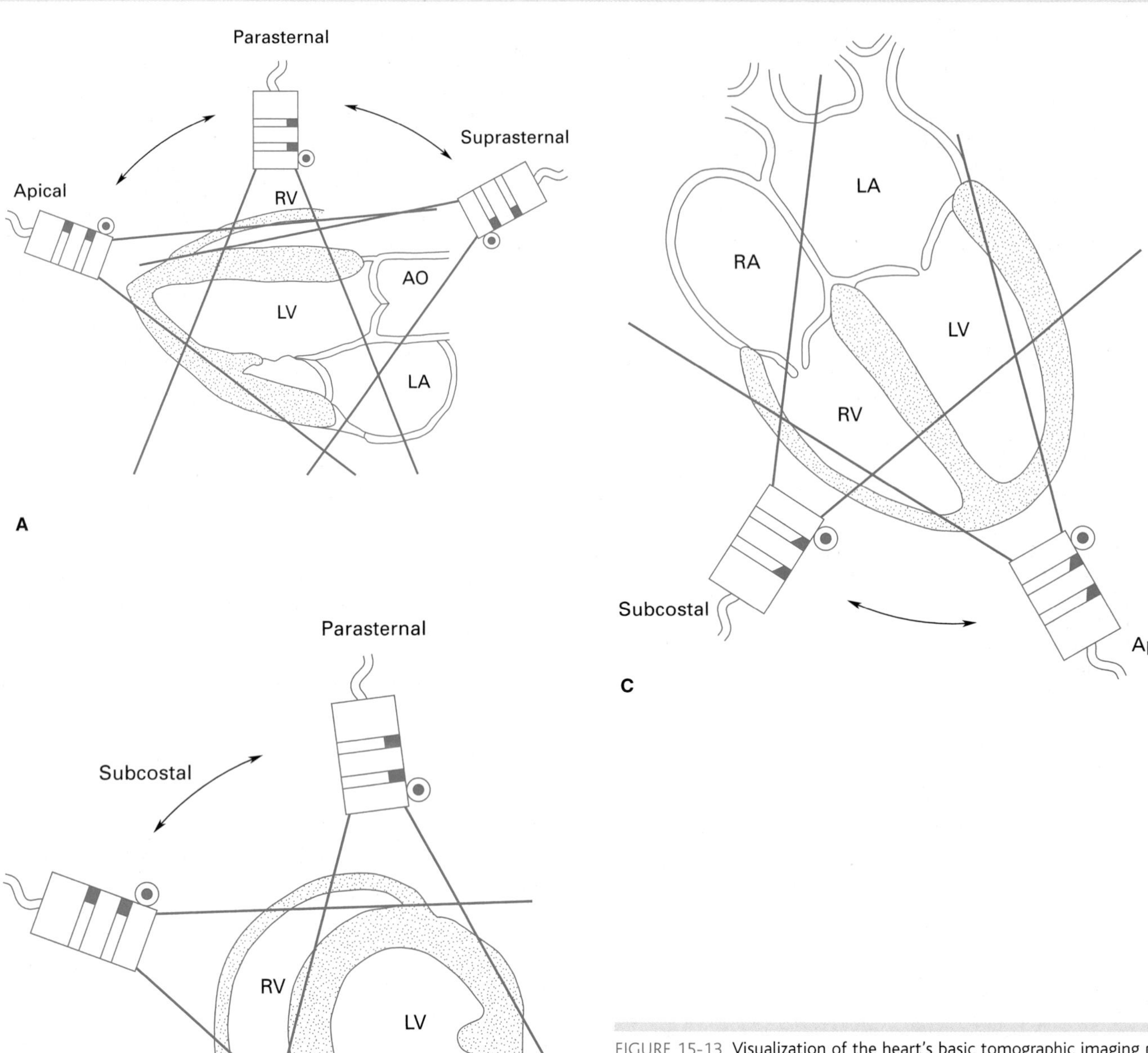

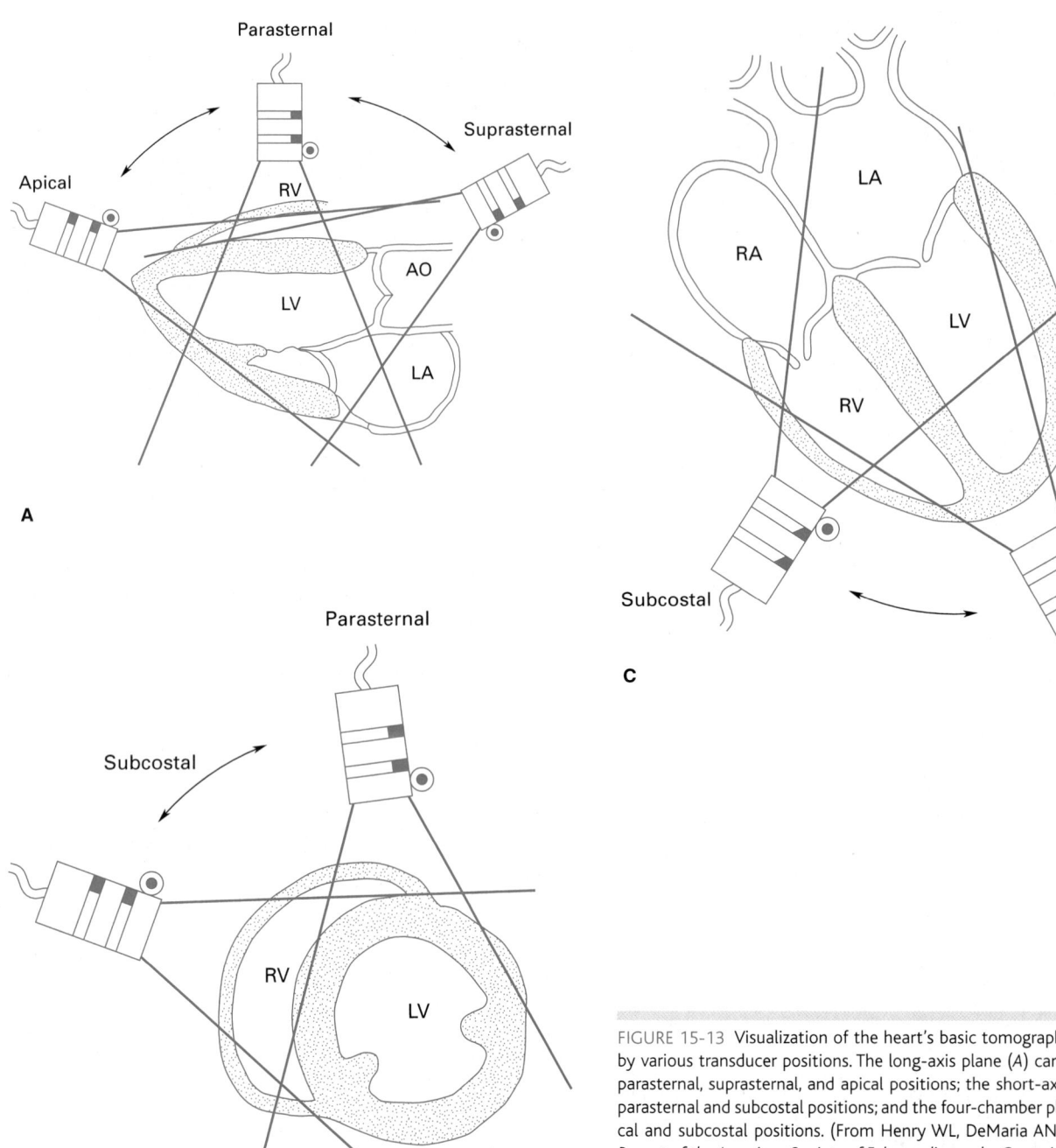

FIGURE 15-13 Visualization of the heart's basic tomographic imaging planes by various transducer positions. The long-axis plane (*A*) can be imaged in the parasternal, suprasternal, and apical positions; the short-axis plane (*B*) in the parasternal and subcostal positions; and the four-chamber plane (*C*) in the apical and subcostal positions. (From Henry WL, DeMaria AN, Gramiak R, et al. *Report of the American Society of Echocardiography Committee on Nomenclature and Standards in Two-Dimensional Echocardiography.* Reproduced with permission from the American Society of Echocardiography.)

and provides images of the posterior, apical, and anteroseptal LV wall segments as well as the LA, aorta, and mitral and aortic valves.

To facilitate subcostal imaging, the patient is moved into a supine position. The subcostal four-chamber view is much like the apical four-chamber view (Fig. 15-19), but because the ultrasound beam is now more perpendicular to the interventricular and interatrial septa, subcostal imaging is often helpful in the examination of these structures. A 90-degree rotation of the transducer will record a subcostal short-axis view. The transducer can also be angled to image the RV outflow and PA as well as the inferior vena cava (Fig. 15-19).

The long-axis suprasternal imaging plane is shown in Fig. 15-20. In adult echocardiography, the LV is usually not visualized satisfactorily from the suprasternal position, but these imaging planes are well suited for examination of the thoracic aorta, PA, and great vessels. Normal values for 2D echocardiographic measurements are shown in Table 15-3.

## Three-Dimensional Echocardiography

Several approaches exist to obtaining 3D echocardiographic images. The simplest approach is to merely move the transducer through a

TABLE 15-2 Standard Two-Dimensional Echocardiographic Transducer Positions

| Parasternal Position |
|---|
| Long axis |
| Left ventricular long axis |
| Right ventricular long |
| Right ventricular outflow |
| Short axis |
| Short axis through the plane of |
| The cardiac base |
| The mitral valve |
| The chordae tendineae |
| The papillary muscles |
| The apex |
| **Apical Position** |
| Four-chamber plane |
| Five-chamber plane |
| (Four-chamber plane angled superiorly to include the aorta) |
| Two-chamber plane |
| Three-chamber plane |
| **Subcostal Position** |
| Four-chamber plane |
| Short-axis through the plane of |
| The mitral valve |
| The papillary muscles |
| The cardiac base |
| Posteriorly directed planes through the venae cavae and atria |
| **Suprasternal Position** |
| Long axis (through the ascending and descending aorta) |
| Short axis |

defined space and align the tomographic slices appropriately. A variety of spatial locator devices can be attached to the transducer to provide spatial orientation. This enables the acquisition of data from many transducer positions. Images obtained in this way can be strikingly accurate, but they require computer reconstruction and therefore cannot be displayed in "real time." Several years ago, a probe with two orthogonally positioned crystal arrays was applied in conjunction with rapid parallel signal processing to achieve real-time 3D volumetric imaging. A pyramid-shaped ultrasound beam is produced that can often encompass the entire heart from one transducer location and acquire an entire data set in a single cardiac cycle (Fig. 15-20*C*). The resultant 3D data sets from any approach can be displayed as 2D tomographic cuts with 3D spatial orientation, as wire runs, or with surface rendering. This type of real-time 3D imaging has evolved considerably, and new software advances have improved tissue rendering and endocardial border definition (Fig. 15-20*D*). 3D images have been particularly of value in providing accurate quantitation, in assessing congenital heart disease and in evaluating structures of complex geometry such as the RV.[39,40]

## ASSESSMENT OF SYSTOLIC FUNCTION BY TWO-DIMENSIONAL ECHOCARDIOGRAPHY

Because 2D echocardiography enables visualization of the entire LV perimeter in multiple planes, it is significantly superior to M-mode approaches for the measurement of cardiac chamber volumes and EF.[41–44] Numerous algorithms have been applied to calculate LV volumes by echocardiography (Fig. 15-21). Most such algorithms have assumed that the LV conforms to the shape of a prolate ellipsoid and calculated volume by diameter-length or area-length formulas.[42,45] Multiple studies comparing LV volume calculated by area-length methods to those obtained by other techniques have yielded good correlations, with the best results obtained utilizing biplane apical views.[45,46] Other algorithms have assumed an LV cavity configuration that is a combination of geometric shapes, such as a cylinder-cone or a cylinder-hemiellipse.[45,47] Currently, the most

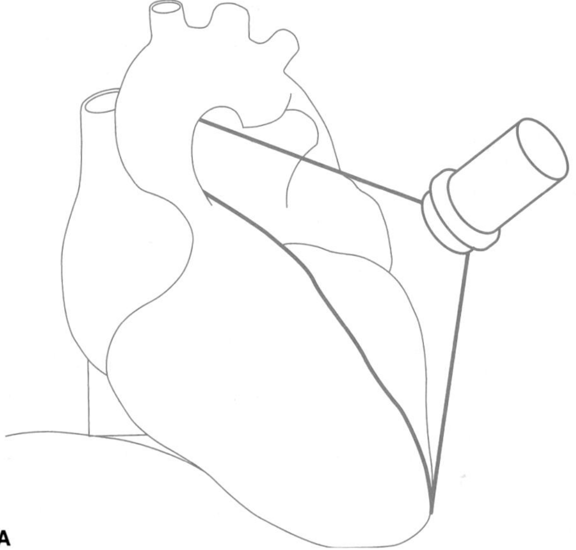


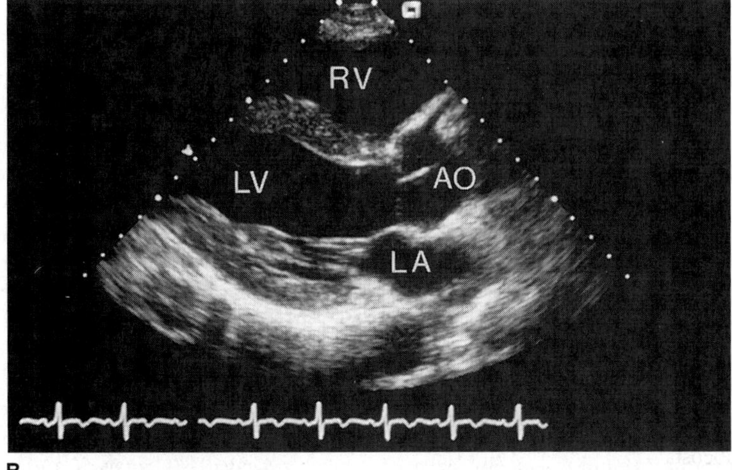


FIGURE 15-14 *A.* Orientation of the sector beam and transducer position for the parasternal long-axis view of the left ventricle. *B.* 2D image of the heart, parasternal long-axis view. LV = left ventricle; LA = left atrium; AO = aorta; RV = right ventricle.

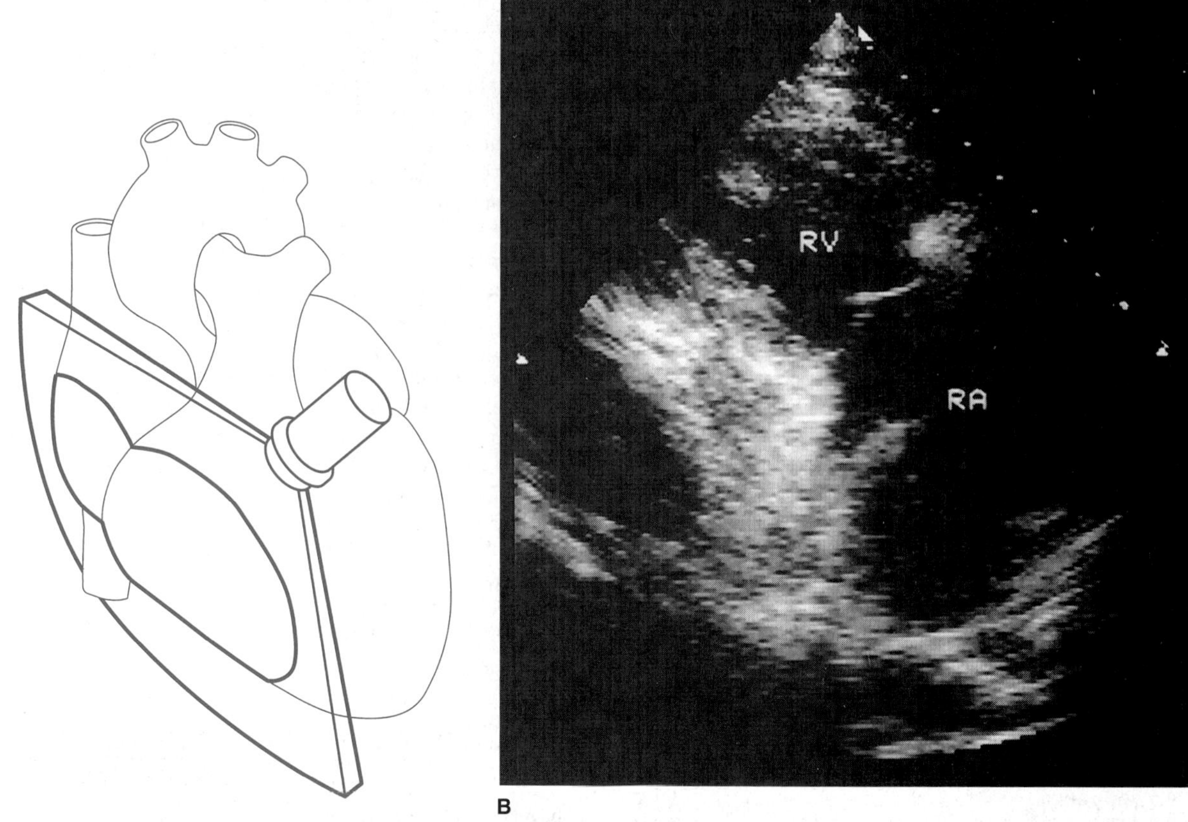


FIGURE 15-15 *A.* Orientation of the sector beam and transducer position for the parasternal RV inflow plane. (From Hagan AD, DeMaria AN. *Clinical Applications of Two-Dimensional Echocardiography and Cardiac Doppler.* Boston: Little, Brown; 1989. With permission.) *B.* Two-dimensional image of right ventricular inflow plane. RA = right atrium, RV = right ventricle.

commonly used algorithm to calculate LV volumes is based upon the Simpson rule, which derives measurements by dividing the LV by parallel planes into a number of small segments and then summating the area of the individual disks. This approach makes fewer assumptions about the geometry of the ventricle. Several modifications of the basic Simpson rule method have been applied to calculate LV volumes. Although all have yielded good results, the optimal correlations have been achieved with a modification that separately quantifies the volume of the apex as an ellipsoid.[44–46]

Regardless of the approach used, accurate calculations of LV volumes by echocardiography require attention to detail and are critically dependent upon high-quality images to delineate the endocardium and image the entire LV perimeter. Echocardiographic estimates of LV volumes underestimate those calculated by other techniques and are most accurate in the absence of significant alterations of LV size and contraction. End-systolic measurements are more accurate than those made at end diastole, probably owing to superior endocardial definition. Nevertheless, echocardiographic calculations of LV volumes have generally yielded correlation coefficients in excess of 0.75 as compared with radionuclide angiography, cineangiography, and autopsy studies regardless of the algorithm employed.[41–46] Calculation of LV volumes generally yields values with a standard error of estimate that renders these measurements suitable for clinical decision making in the care of most patients.

To refine and facilitate the derivation of LV volume measurements from echocardiography several technical developments have been evaluated. Images of the power spectrum of the Doppler signal produced by contraction/relaxation and colorization of the B-mode tissue image have been utilized to visualize the endocardial surface.[47] These techniques have been useful in identifying endocardial signals, particularly in patients with suboptimal tissue images. Greater enhancement of endocardial border delineation and improvement of the reliability of measures of LV size and contraction have been achieved through utilization of tissue harmonic imaging and by the injection of ultrasonic contrast agents to opacify the LV cavity.[19,48] A software package that provides instantaneous and automated endocardial border delineation throughout the cardiac cycle has been developed based upon the display of tissue signals as backscatter rather than specular reflection.[49] This technique of automated quantitation can yield continuous measurements of LV volume throughout the cardiac cycle and can derive values for ejection fraction, ejection rate, and rate of filling during diastole (Fig. 15-22). This same technology has been utilized to display endocardial excursion throughout systolic contraction or diastolic expansion in a color format superimposed upon the tissue image (Fig. 15-23, Plate 51). This technique has proved to be of value in the recognition of abnormalities of LV contraction and regional disturbances of LV diastolic function.[50–52] Finally, studies employing 3D echocardiography have reported improved reproducibility of measurements over 2D methods. These technical developments will likely facilitate the quantitative assessment of LV size and function from routine echocardiograms.

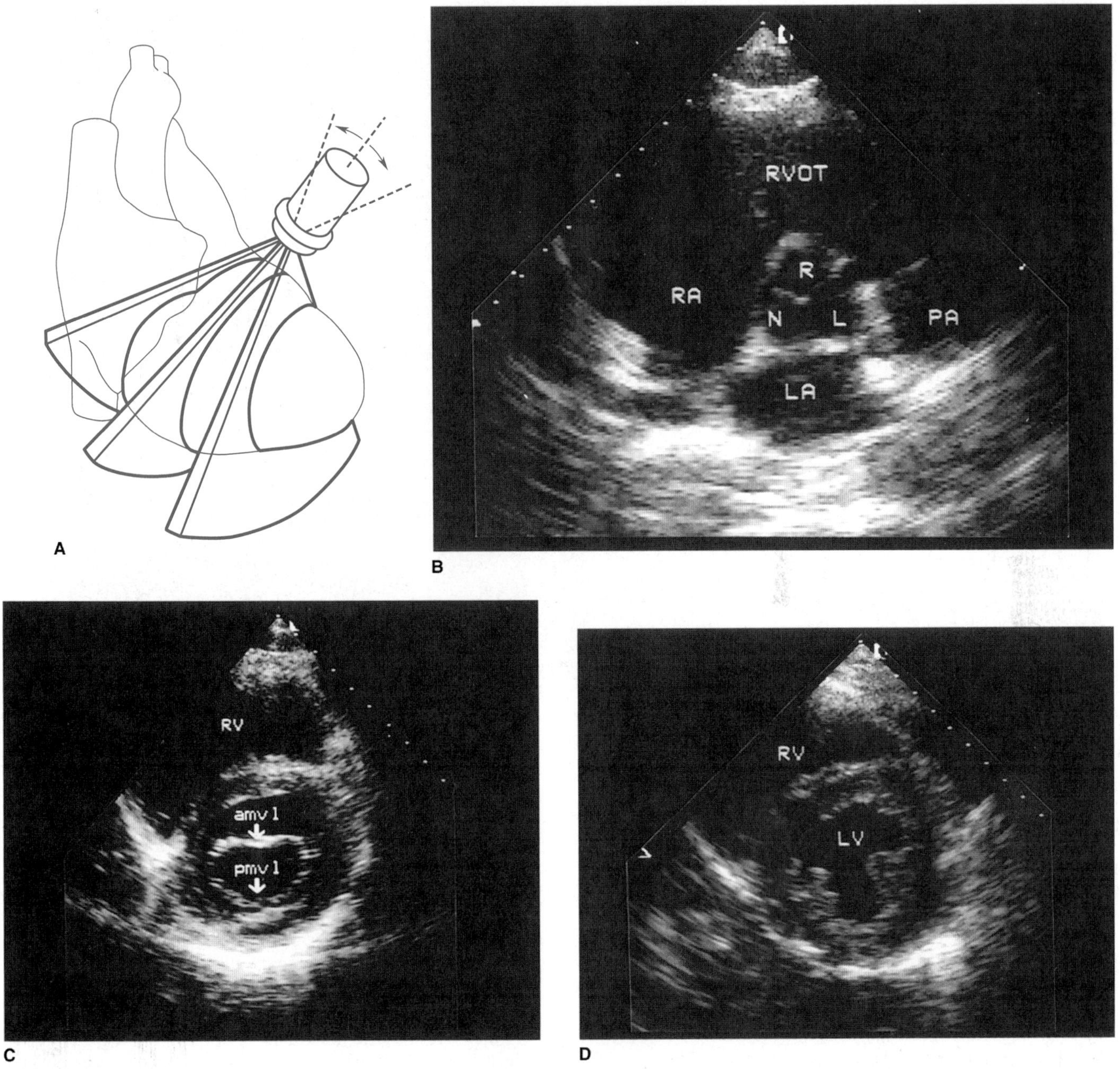


FIGURE 15-16 *A.* Orientation of various short-axis sector beams through the left ventricle obtained by angling the transducer in the parasternal position. (From Hagan AD, DeMaria AN. *Clinical Applications of Two-Dimensional Echocardiography and Cardiac Doppler.* Boston: Little, Brown; 1989. With permission.) *B.* Short-axis plane through the base of the heart. *C.* At the level of the mitral valve leaflets. *D.* At the papillary muscle level. LV = left ventricle; RV = right ventricle; LA = left atrium; RA = right atrium; RVOT = right ventricular outflow tract; PA = pulmonary artery; R, L, N = right, left, and noncoronary cusps of the aortic valve. RV = right ventricle; LV = left ventricle; amvl = anterior mitral valve leaflet; pmvl = posterior mitral valve leaflet.

## DOPPLER ECHOCARDIOGRAPHY: PRINCIPLES AND APPLICATIONS

### The Doppler Principle

Using the principle first delineated by the physicist Johann Christian Doppler,[53] one can use ultrasound to determine the velocity and direction of blood flow by measuring the change in frequency produced when sound waves are reflected from red blood cells.[54,55] In this way, information regarding the presence, direction, velocity, and turbulence of blood flow can be acquired by cardiac ultrasound.

The Doppler principle states that when a sound (or light) signal strikes a moving object, the frequency of that signal will be altered, and the increase or decrease in frequency will be proportional to the velocity and direction at which the object is moving. This is illustrated in Fig. 15-24. If a stationary transducer at the apex emits a sound wave with a transmitted frequency of $f_o$ and the wave is reflected by nonmoving red blood cells (RBCs) in an isovolumic phase of the cardiac cycle, then the received frequency $f_r$ will be identical to

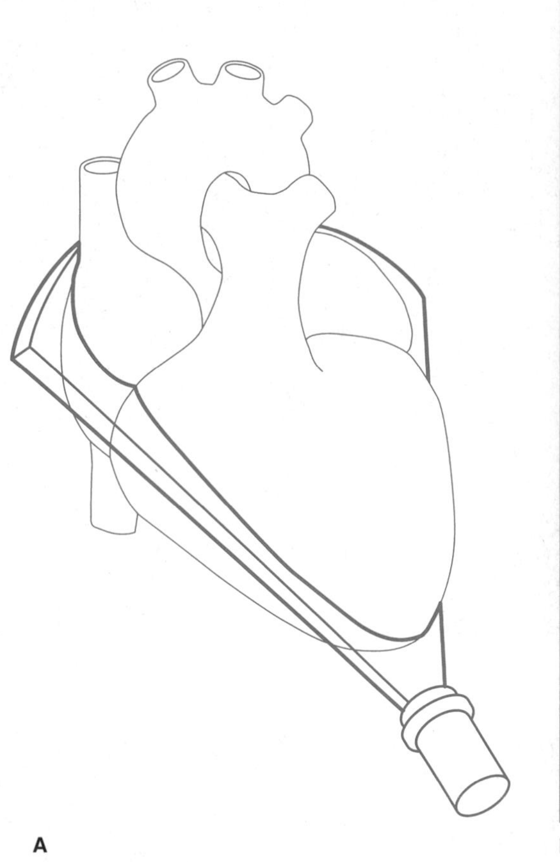


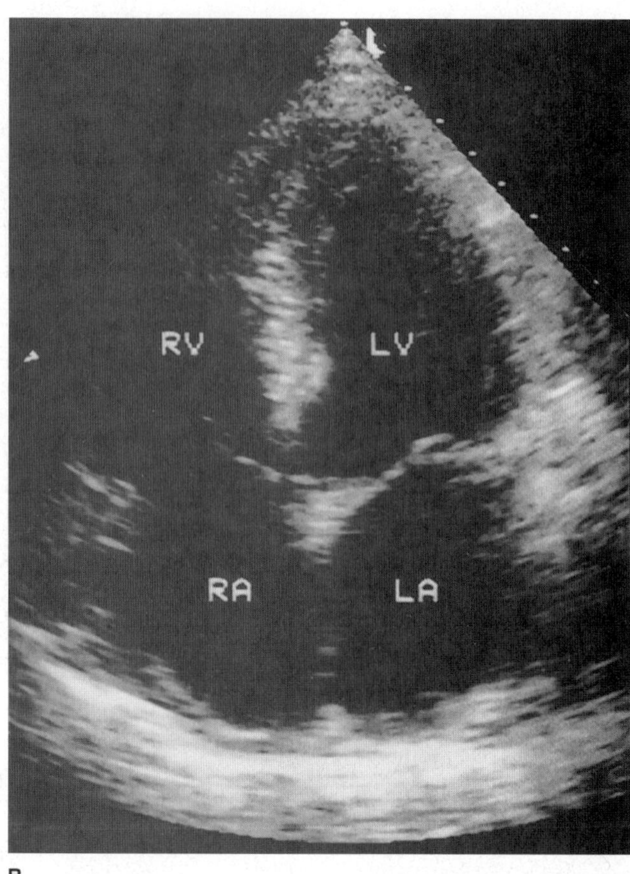


FIGURE 15-17 *A.* Orientation of the sector beam and transducer position for the apical four-chamber plane. (From Hagan AD, DeMaria AN. *Clinical Applications of Two-Dimensional Echocardiography and Cardiac Doppler.* Boston: Little, Brown; 1989. With permission.) *B.* 2D image of the apical four-chamber plane. RA = right atrium; RV = right ventricle; LV = left ventricle; LA = left atrium.

$f_o$. If the signal is reflected by RBCs that are moving toward the transducer, as through the MV in diastole, the returning waves will be compressed so that $f_r$ will be greater than $f_o$. Conversely, if the target RBCs are moving away from the transducer, as in the outflow tract in systole, the returning sound waves will be elongated and the received frequency will be decreased. Of importance, the magnitude of change in the received frequency is directly related to the velocity at which blood is flowing toward or away from the transducer.[55] If the velocity of sound and the angle $\theta$ between the direction of RBC flow and the beam path are known, then the velocity of the RBCs is described by the Doppler equation:

$$V = f_d(c)/2f_o(\cos\theta)$$

where $f_d$ is the frequency shift recorded, $f_o$ the transmitted frequency, and $c$ the velocity of sound. Note that the denominator is doubled because the sound wave does not originate with the RBC but must travel back and forth from the transducer. By measuring Doppler shift frequencies, the velocity and direction of blood flow can be calculated, displayed, and recorded.

The angle between the direction of blood flow and the course of the sound beam is a most important factor in Doppler ultrasound (Fig. 15-25). Velocity is a vectorial entity, having magnitude and direction, and Doppler will detect only those velocities parallel or near parallel to the interrogating signal. Since the relationship between velocity and the angle is a cosine function and the cosine of angles up to 20 degrees is 0.9, little error is introduced within this range.[55] Because the processor that calculates blood velocity assumes that the angle is 0 degrees, however, considerable errors occur when it is greater than 20 degrees. Moreover, the angle of incidence in 3D space usually cannot be determined with certainty from 2D echocardiographic images. Therefore, in order to obtain accurate velocity determination by Doppler, it is crucial to position and direct the transducer so that the beam is as parallel to flow as possible. In clinical use, the frequency of transmitted ultrasound is in the range of 2 to 7 MHz, the velocity of sound in tissue is approximately 1540 m/s, and the Doppler shift frequency is relatively small (approximately 1 to 4 kHz) as compared with the transmitted frequency. Because the Doppler shift frequencies are in the audible range, a speaker integrated into the Doppler echocardiography system can present them as an audible signal. Normal signals are tonal or musical. The Doppler shift can also be presented graphically to provide a hard copy printout and enable measurement.

Figure 15-26 shows the typical graphic pulsed Doppler pattern of normal systolic blood flow through the RV outflow tract into the PA, with flow velocity on the *y* axis and time on the *x* axis. The location and size of the area from which Doppler recordings are derived is determined by the operator by positioning a sample volume on the echo image. The absence of flow is represented by the zero or no-flow line, termed the *baseline.* By convention, flow toward the transducer is displayed above the baseline and flow away from the transducer is displayed below the baseline. The velocities above and below base-

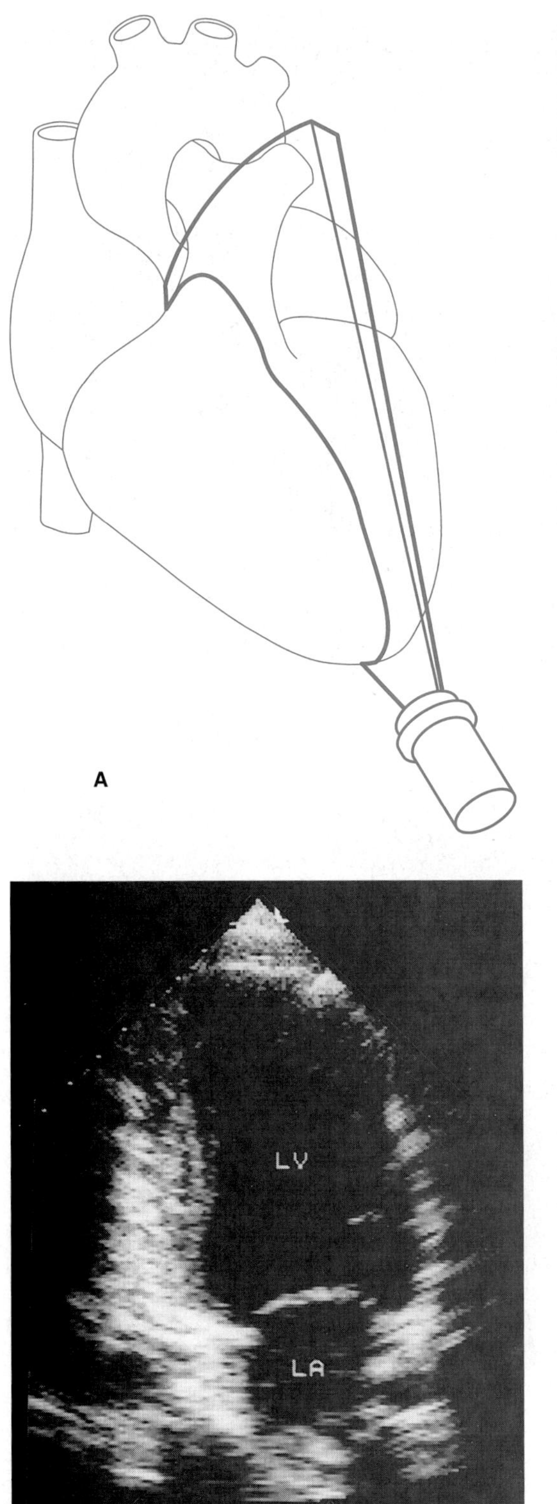


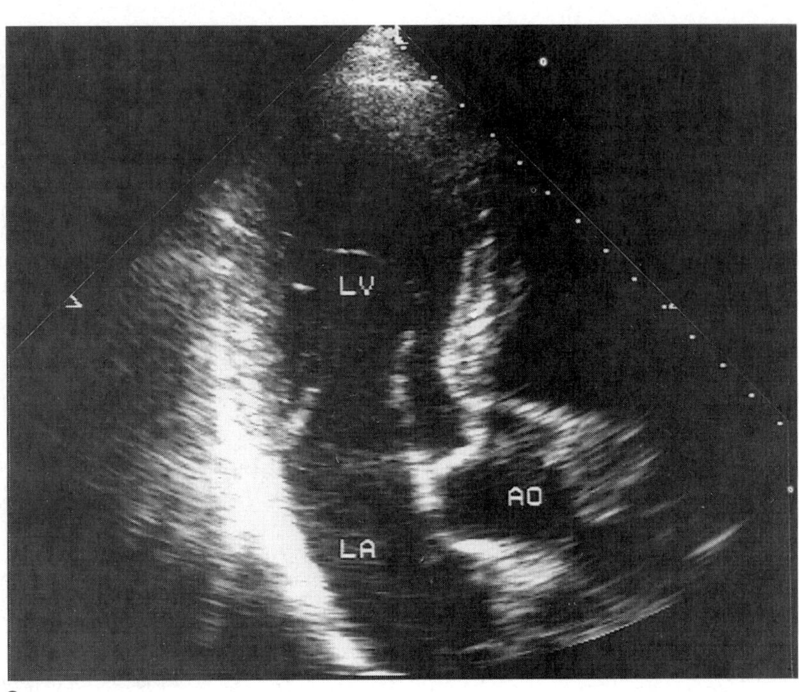


FIGURE 15-18 *A*. Orientation of the sector beam and transducer position for the apical two-chamber plane. (From Hagan AD, DeMaria AN. *Clinical Applications of Two-Dimensional Echocardiography and Cardiac Doppler*. Boston: Little, Brown; 1989. With permission.) *B*. 2D image of the apical two-chamber plane. LV = left ventricle; LA = left atrium. *C*. 2D image of the apical three-chamber view. LV = left ventricle; LA = atrium; AO = aorta.

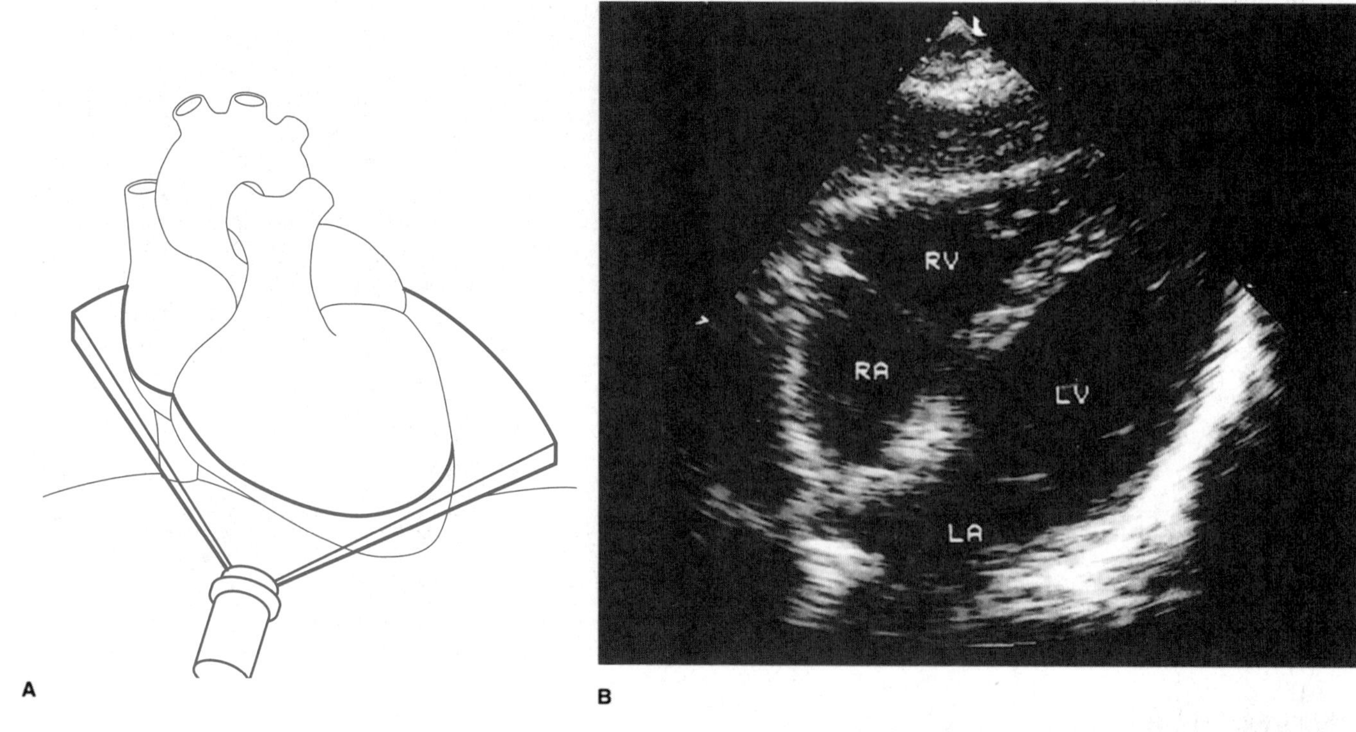


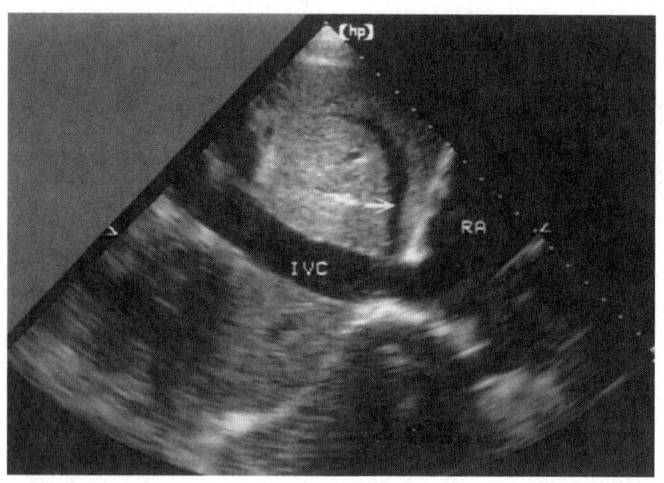


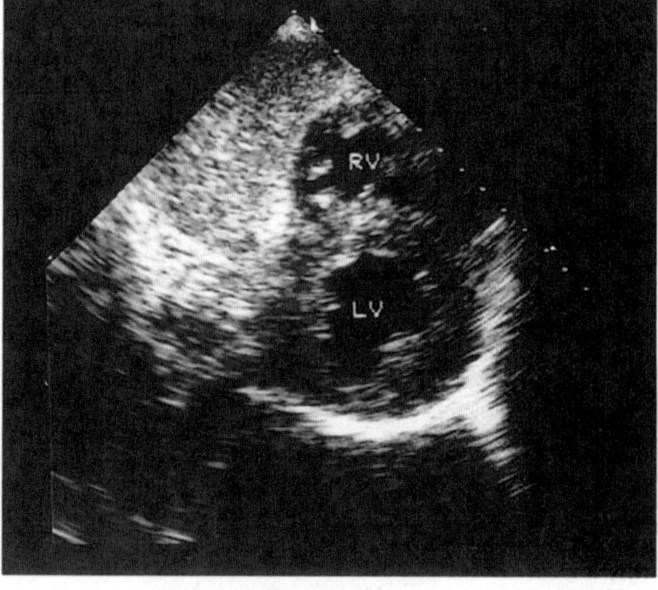


FIGURE 15-19 *A.* Orientation of the sector beam and transducer position for the subcostal four-chamber plane. (From Hagen AD, DeMaria AN. *Clinical Applications of Two Dimensional Echocardiography and Cardiac Doppler.* Boston: Little, Brown; 1989. With permission.) *B.* Two-dimensional image of the subcostal four-chamber plane. LV = left ventricle; LA = left atrium; RA = right atrium; RV = right ventricle. *C.* Subcostal 2D image demonstrating the right atrium (RA), inferior vena cava (IVC) and hepatic vein (arrow). *D.* 2D image of the subcostal short-axis plane. LV = left ventricle; RV = right ventricle.

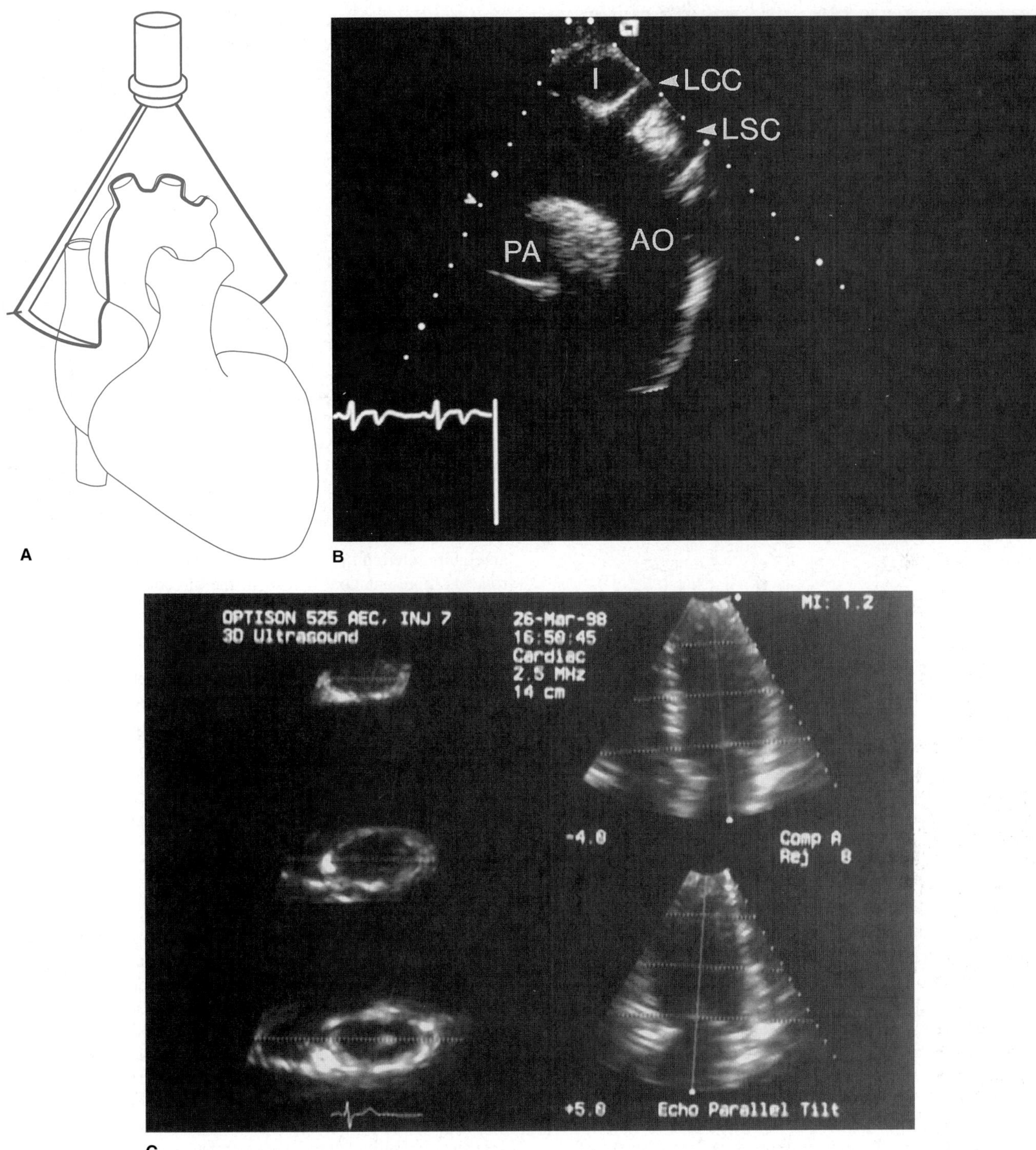


FIGURE 15-20 *A.* Orientation of the sector beam and transducer position for long-axis plane through the aorta from the suprasternal position. *B.* 2D image of the suprasternal long-axis view of the thoracic aorta. AO = aorta; PA = right pulmonary artery; I = innominate artery; LCC = left common carotid artery; LSC = left subclavian artery. *C.* Short-axis, apical four-chamber, and apical two-chamber images acquired simultaneously with a pyramidal 3D transducer system. *D.* Real-time 3D image, apical four-chamber plane. RV = right ventricle, RA = right atrium, LV = left ventricle.

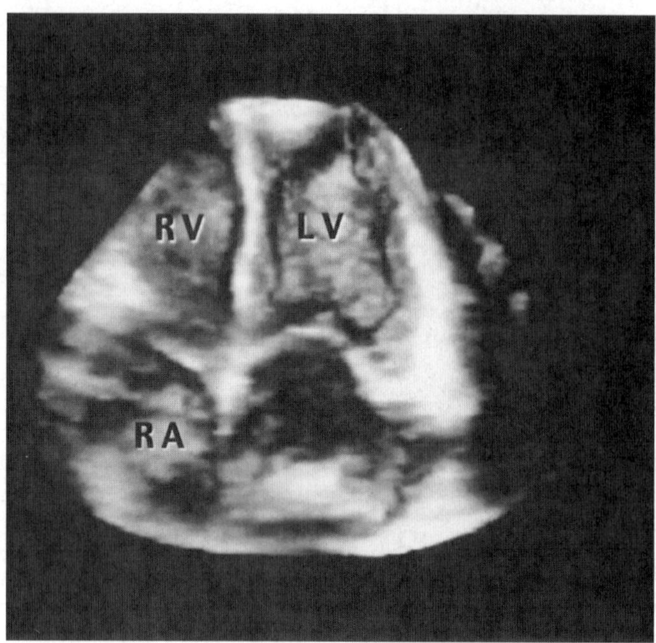


D

FIGURE 15-20 (*Continued*)

line represent flow toward or away from the transducer, not forward or backward in the circulation. Because of the effects of viscous friction, the sample volume almost invariably includes RBCs flowing at slightly different velocities. Even normal laminar blood flow in the great vessels varies in velocity across the lumen, as RBCs in the center of the vessel move at higher velocity than those exposed to viscous friction at the wall; this creates a parabolic rather than a flat flow profile. Therefore, any returning Doppler shifted signal contains a spectrum of velocities, each of which can be displayed by means of fast Fourier transform analysis. The graphic output of the Doppler signal displays the range of velocities within the sample volume site at any time in gray scale and the number of RBCs moving at any velocity as relative intensity. Normal laminar flow is characterized by a uniformity of velocity and direction of individual RBCs, and therefore a narrowly dispersed signal, while disturbed or turbulent flow is manifest by marked variability in velocity and direction and therefore a broad signal, which is multitoned, dissonant, and harsh.

Echographs have now been modified to enable recording of the low-velocity, high-amplitude Doppler signals produced by moving tissue as well as those of RBCs. The ability to assess tissue velocity provides an evaluation of transmural rate of contraction and relaxation.[56] Also, Doppler tissue recordings permit assessment of regional function and appear to be quite useful in the assessment of diastolic function (see below).[57,58] Finally, Doppler tissue recordings provide the basis for the derivation of regional strain measurements by echocardiography. Such measurements are independent of overall cardiac motion and passive motion due to tethering to adjacent myocardium and therefore enable the most accurate assessment of myocardial contractile performance.

## Continuous- and Pulsed-Wave Doppler

Time-velocity spectral recordings of blood flow are generally obtained with two types of Doppler interrogation: continuous- and pulsed-wave (Fig. 15-27).[59,60] In the *continuous-wave* (CW) mode, sound waves are both transmitted and received continuously. This requires two piezoelectric crystals in each transducer, one for transmitting and one for receiving. Because all flow velocities along the beam are recorded, CW Doppler cannot define individual signals at specific distances from the transducer—a problem referred to as *range ambiguity.* CW Doppler, however, has no upper limit of velocity that can be accurately recorded. Thus, a CW Doppler beam can accurately measure the direction and velocity of overall flow but cannot discern the precise site of origin of individual components within the signal (Fig. 15-28*B*).

The problem of range ambiguity can be overcome by *pulsed-wave* Doppler. In this mode, short bursts of signal are transmitted from the transducer at a given *pulse-repetition frequency* (PRF). The instrument then receives the signal for only a brief period—an interval that corresponds to the time required for sound energy to travel and return from a specific site along the beam path. In practice, the operator selects the location at which flow is to be examined by positioning a sample volume, and the instrument determines the period during which to receive the incoming reflected frequencies. With pulsed-wave Doppler, only a single piezoelectric crystal is needed and flow can be recorded in one small area within the heart or vasculature.[59,60] Unfortunately, pulsed Doppler techniques employ intermittent sampling and are therefore susceptible to a problem of range ambiguity referred to as *aliasing.*[61] By definition, aliasing is the erroneous representation of flow in the direction opposite to that in which it is actually occurring. To correctly record the velocity of blood flow by pulsed Doppler, the PRF must be at least double the Doppler shift frequency, a value known as the *Nyquist limit.* If the blood flow examined is of very high velocity or far from the transducer (requiring a long transit time), it may necessitate an unobtainably high PRF. In such cases, aliasing will occur as Doppler signals that depict flow at high velocity in ambiguous or opposite directions compared to actual flow (Fig. 15-28*A*). An intermediate mode between pulsed and CW methods, high-PRF Doppler, is also available. This mode enables higher-velocity recordings to be obtained at a compromise of depicting two to four sample sites simultaneously.

## Color-Flow Doppler

The major limitation of pulsed and CW Doppler (sometimes referred to as *spectral Doppler*) is that no spatial information regarding the size, shape, and 2D direction of flow is provided. An extension of pulsed-wave Doppler techniques, *color-flow Doppler* (CFD), provides real-time M-mode or 2D imaging of blood flow by presenting the velocity and direction of RBC movement as shades of color superimposed upon gray-level 2D tissue structure. Standard pulsed Doppler yields flow signals from a single site along a single scan line. In CFD, rapid pulsed-wave interrogations are performed at multiple sites for multiple scan lines to create a spatially correct and dynamic display of moving blood within the heart and vasculature (Fig. 15-29). Doppler signals are presented as colors assigned to individual sites (Fig. 15-30, Plate 52). Blood flow moving toward the transducer is displayed in red, flow away from the transducer is displayed in blue, and increasing velocity is depicted in brighter shades of each color. The variance within each signal is calculated as a statistical marker of turbulence and is presented by adding green to the image (Fig. 15-31, Plate 53). Therefore, turbulent flow jets appear as a mosaic mix of colors. CFD also can be superimposed onto M-mode tracings (Fig. 15-32, Plate 54), often termed *M/Q imaging,* and is helpful in clarifying the timing of flow phenomena. Given the time constraints imposed by collecting the large volume of data required by CFD, velocity estimates are performed by autocorrelation techniques

TABLE 15-3 Cardiac Dimensions by Two-Dimensional Echocardiography

| Cardiac Feature | Range | Mean | Index, cm/m$^2$ |
|---|---|---|---|
| | **Apical Four-Chamber View** | | |
| $LV_d$ major | 6.9–10.3 cm | 8.6 cm | 4.1–5.7 |
| $LV_d$ minor | 3.3–6.1 cm | 4.7 cm | 2.2–3.1 |
| $LV_s$ minor | 1.9–3.7 cm | 2.8 cm | 1.3–2.0 |
| $LV_d$ area | 21.2–40.2 cm$^2$ | 31.2 cm$^2$ | |
| $LV_s$ area | 8.0–21.1 cm$^2$ | 14.2 cm$^2$ | |
| RV major | 6.5–9.5 cm$^2$ | 8.0 cm | 3.8–5.3 |
| RV minor | 2.2–4.4 cm$^2$ | 3.3–3.5 cm | 1.0–2.8 |
| $RV_d$ area | 12.0–22.2 cm$^2$ | 18.6–2.1 cm$^2$ | |
| $RV_s$ area | 5.4–14.6 cm$^2$ | 9.9 cm$^2$ | |
| LA major | 4.1–6.1 cm | 5.1 cm | 2.3–3.5 |
| LA minor | 2.8–4.3 cm | 3.5 cm | 1.6–2.4 |
| LA area | 10.2–17.8 cm$^2$ | 14.7 cm$^2$ | |
| RA major (inf-sup) | 3.5–5.5 cm | 4.3–4.5 cm | 2.0–3.1 |
| RA minor | 2.5–4.9 cm | 3.7 cm | 1.7–2.5 |
| RA area | 11.3–16.7 cm$^2$ | 13.8–14 cm$^2$ | |
| | **Apical Two-Chamber View** | | |
| $LV_d$ major | 6.8–9.4 cm | 8.0 cm | |
| $LV_d$ minor | 3.8–5.7 cm | 4.6 cm | |
| $LV_d$ area | 19.4–48.0 cm$^2$ | 35.6 cm$^2$ | |
| $LV_s$ | 8.9–27.0 cm | 14.3 cm | |
| | **Parasternal Long-Axis View** | | |
| $LV_d$ | 3.5–6.0 cm | 4.8 cm | 2.3–3.1 |
| $LV_s$ | 2.1–4.0 cm | 3.1 cm | 1.4–2.1 |
| RV | 1.9–3.8 cm | 2.8 cm | 1.2–2.0 |
| LA (A-P) | 2.7–4.5 cm | 3.6 cm | 1.6–2.4 |
| LA (S-I) | 3.1–5.5 cm | 4.4 cm | |
| LA area | 9.0–19.3 cm$^2$ | 13.8 cm$^2$ | |
| Ao | 2.2–3.6 cm | 2.9 cm | 1.4–2.0 |
| | **Parasternal Short-Axis View** | | |
| Ao | 2.3–3.7 cm | 3.0–2.3 cm | 1.6–2.4 |
| RVOT | 1.9–2.2 cm | 2.7 cm | |
| RA | 1.5–2.5 cm | 1.9–2.2 cm | |
| LA | 2.6–4.5 cm | 3.6 cm | 1.6–2.4 |
| LA area | 7.2–13.0 cm$^2$ | 10.8 cm$^2$ | |
| $LV_d$ (PM level) | 3.5–5.8 cm | 4.7 cm | 2.2–3.1 |
| $LV_s$ (PM level) | 2.2–4.0 cm | 3.1 cm | 1.4–2.2 |
| $LV_d$ area (PM level) | 16.0–31.2 cm$^2$ | 22.2 cm$^2$ | |
| $LV_s$ area (PM level) | 5.2–13.4 cm$^2$ | 8.5 cm$^2$ | |
| $LV_d$ (Ch. level) | 3.5–6.2 | 4.8 cm | 2.3–3.2 |
| $LV_s$ (Ch. level) | 2.3–4.0 | 3.2 cm | 1.5–2.2 |
| $LV_d$ area (Ch. level) | 16.4–32.3 cm$^2$ | 22.5 cm$^2$ | |
| $LV_s$ area (Ch. level) | 6.1–16.8 cm$^2$ | 10.7 cm$^2$ | |
| | **Subcostal View** | | |
| IVC diameter | | 1.8 cm | |

ABBREVIATIONS: LV = left ventricle; $LV_d$ = left ventricle, end diastole; $LV_s$ = left ventricle, end systole; RV = right ventricle; $RV_d$ = right ventricle, end diastole; $RV_s$ = right ventricle, end systole; LA = left atrium; RA = right atrium; Ao = aorta; RVOT = right ventricular outflow tract; PA = pulmonary artery; IVC = inferior vena cava; PM = papillary muscle; Ch = chordal.

SOURCE: The values shown in this table represent a compilation of data from three sources: Schnittinger I, Gordon EP, Fitzgerald PJ, et al. Standardized intracardiac measurements of two-dimensional echocardiography. *J Am Coll Cardiol* 1983; 5:934. Triulzi M, Weyman A. Normal cross-sectional measurements in adults. In: Weyman A, ed. *Echocardiography*. Philadelphia: Lea & Febiger; 1982;497. Hagan AD, DiSessa TG, Bloor CM, et al. *Two-Dimensional Echocardiography: Clinical-Pathological Corrections in adult and Congenital Heart Disease*. Boston: Little, Brown; 1983;553.

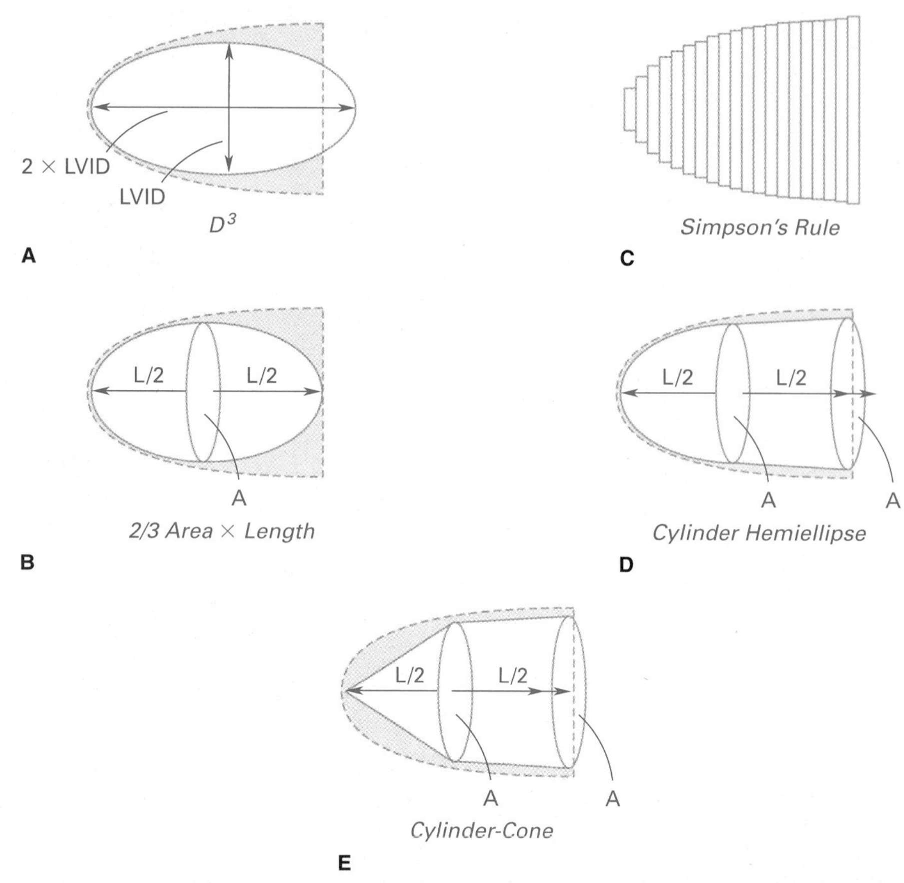


FIGURE 15-21 Various models used to estimate left ventricular volume. *A.* "D-cubed." *B.* Two-thirds area × length. *C.* Simpson's rule. *D.* Cylinder-hemiellipse. *E.* Cylinder-cone. A = cross-sectional area; LVID = left ventricular internal dimension (minor axis); L = length of LV major axis.

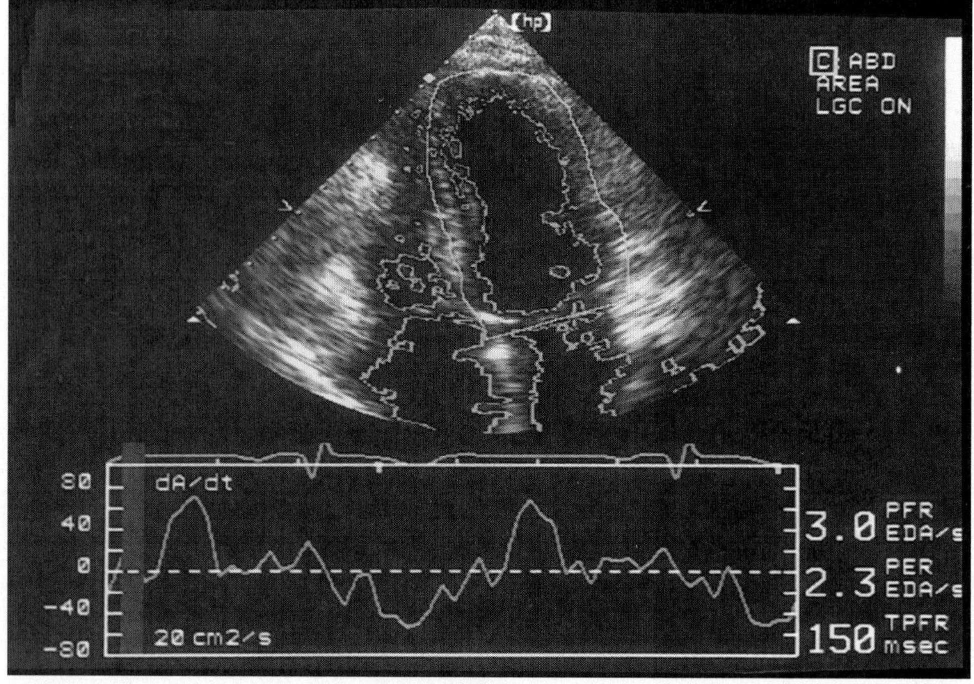


FIGURE 15-22 Example of endocardial border detection and on-line calculation of change in area over time (*dA/dt*).

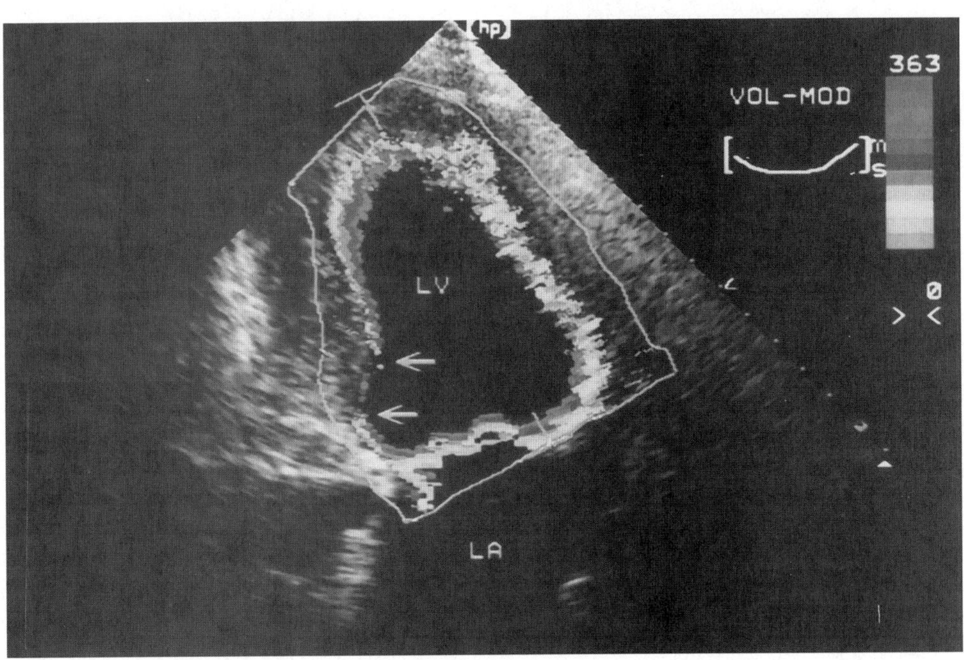


FIGURE 15-23 (Plate 51) Color kinesis image (apical two-chamber view) from a patient with an inferobasal infarction. Systolic motion in this area (*arrows*) is markedly diminished.

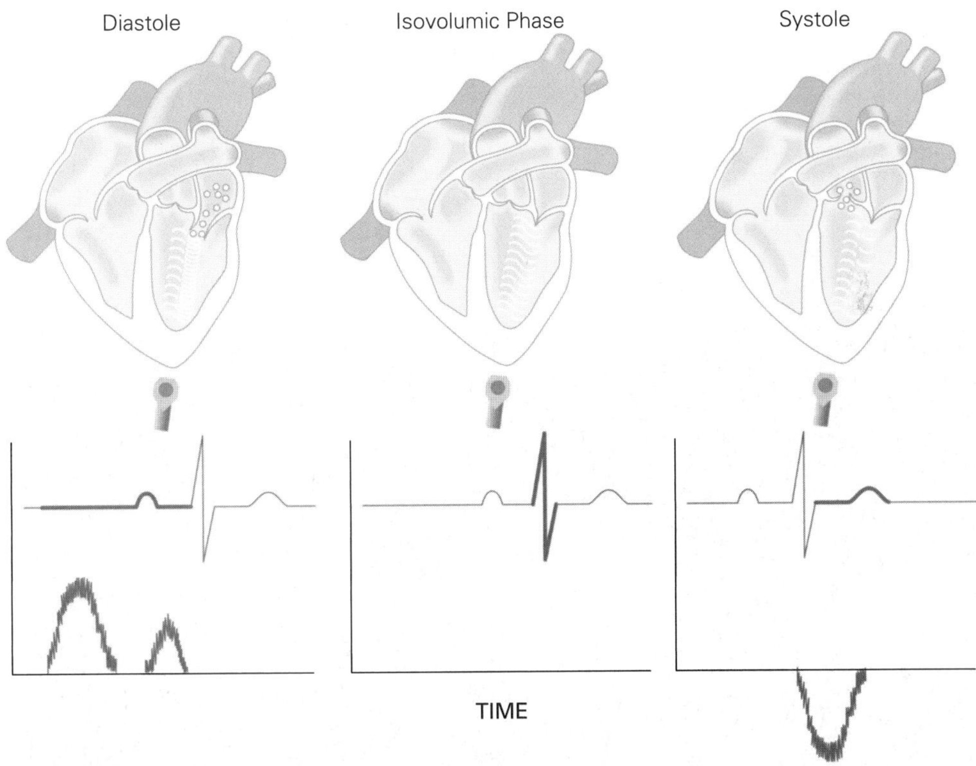


FIGURE 15-24 Basic principle of the Doppler shift. During diastole (*left panel*), an ultrasound beam directed toward the junction of the mitral and aortic annuli is reflected by red blood cells moving toward the transducer. The frequency of the received ultrasound is greater than that of the transmitted beam, and the spectral tracing is recorded above the baseline (i.e., flow is toward the transducer). During the isovolumic phase (*middle panel*), both the mitral and aortic valves are closed and little flow occurs within the left ventricle. Therefore, there are no significant changes in the transmitted and received frequencies of the Doppler beam and no spectral tracing is recorded. During systole (*right panel*), the transmitted beam is reflected by red blood cells moving away from the transducer. Therefore, the frequency of the received ultrasound is lower than that of the transmitted beam, and the spectral tracing is recorded below the baseline.

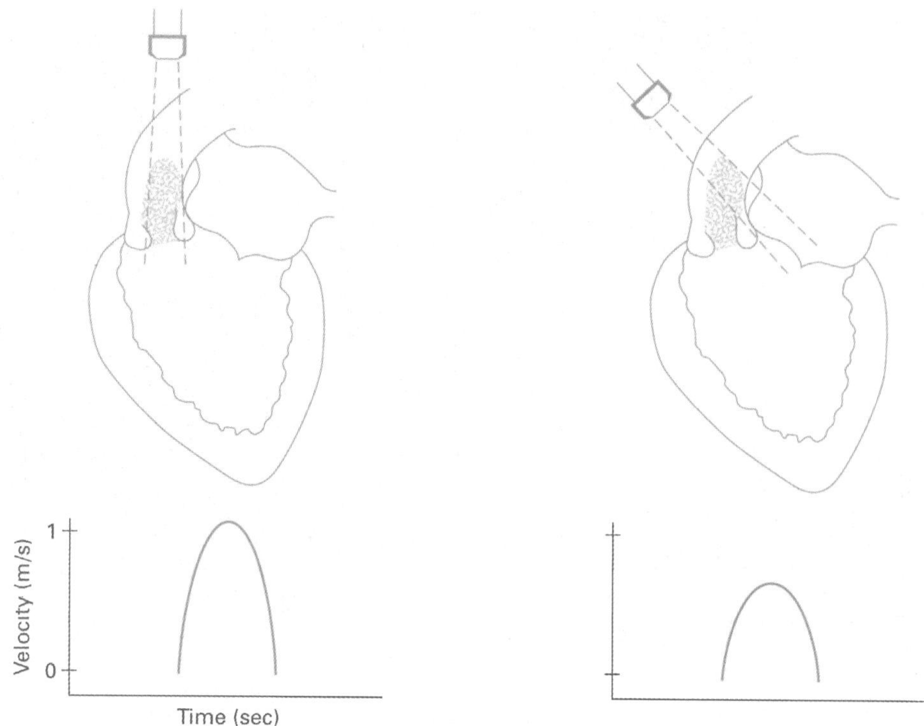


FIGURE 15-25 **Effect of the angle of incidence on the velocity recorded with Doppler analysis. The true velocity is underestimated when the ultrasound beam is not parallel to the direction of blood flow. (From Hagan AD, DeMaria AN. *Clinical Applications of Two-Dimensional Echocardiography and Cardiac Doppler.* Boston: Little, Brown; 1989. With permission.)**

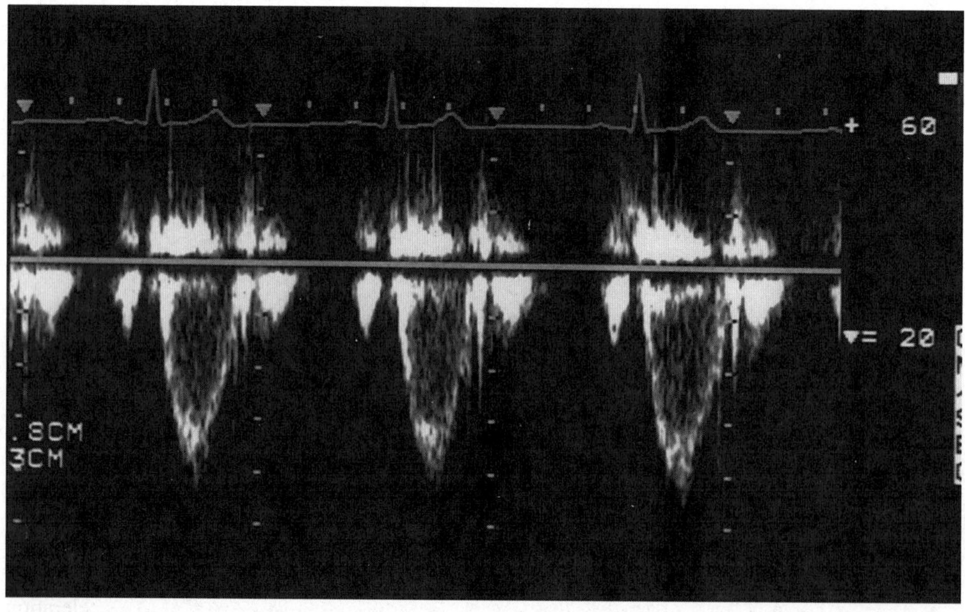


FIGURE 15-26 **Doppler spectral envelope of normal blood flow through the RVOT during systole. The transducer is in the parasternal position and the sample volume is placed just proximal to the pulmonic valve.**

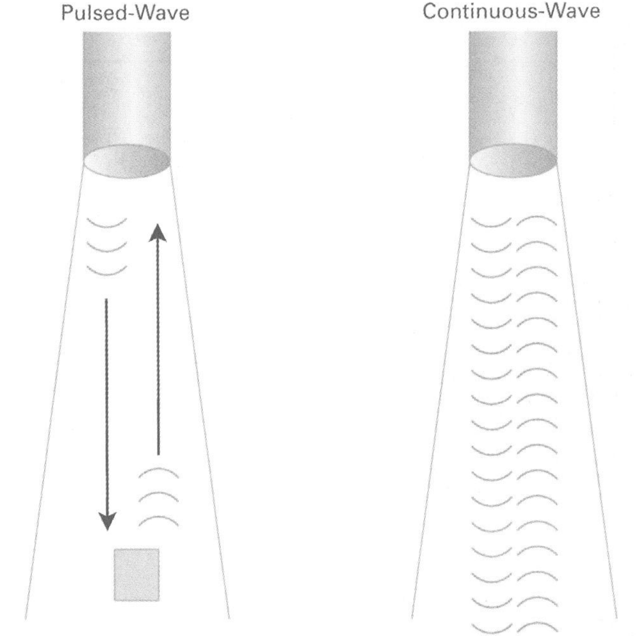


FIGURE 15-27 Pulsed-wave (PW) and continuous-wave (CW) Doppler. With PW, a single pulse of ultrasound energy is emitted and its reflection from a sample volume is received before the following pulse is transmitted. With CW, there is continuous transmission and reception of ultrasound energy.

that are less accurate than fast Fourier transform analysis. Nevertheless, CFD technology is a major advance that has improved the rapid detection of cardiac pathology, especially valvular regurgitation and intracardiac shunts.

## Normal and Abnormal Flow Dynamics

The clinical application of Doppler recordings is based on the fundamental differences between normal and disturbed blood flow. Normal flow is laminar, with all RBCs exhibiting the same velocity and direction of flow. Although some abnormalities, such as atrial septal defects, involve laminar flow, most pathologic conditions involve disturbed or turbulent flow and share a common hydrodynamic basis for the resultant flow dynamics. Specifically, nearly all circulatory disturbances (stenosis, regurgitation, shunt) involve blood flow from a high-pressure chamber to a lower-pressure chamber through a restricted orifice.[55] Aortic valve disease is a perfect example. Aortic stenosis is a forward flow disturbance in which turbulent blood travels from a high-pressure LV to a lower-pressure aorta through a restricted aortic orifice in systole. Aortic regurgitation (AR) is a retrograde flow disturbance in which turbulent blood regurgitates from a high-pressure aorta to a lower-pressure left ventricle through a small regurgitant orifice in diastole. In each case, the pressure gradient results in a high-velocity jet coursing through a restricted orifice, reaching its maximal velocity at a site just distal to the orifice, designated the *vena contracta,* at which time shear forces produce vortices resulting in flow of varying direction and velocity (Fig. 15-33). In each case, the velocity of the jet is related to the pressure gradient across the orifice. Thus, the hallmark of disturbed flow is a very high velocity jet with adjacent vortices of varying direction and velocity of flow. On pulsed Doppler recordings, these hemodynamic abnormalities cause broadening of the spectral signal and aliasing. On CW recordings, high velocity represents the primary abnormality. By color-flow imaging, the disturbance is manifest by the increased variance and higher velocities in the signal. With any of these techniques, of course, inappropriate timing of flow serves to highlight the abnormality (e.g., high-velocity LA flow during systole in mitral regurgitation).

## The Standard Doppler Examination

A clinical Doppler examination must be performed with full consideration of the three different Doppler modalities available, the types of information each can provide, the multiple sites for flow interrogation, and the spectrum of pathologic lesions that produces flow disturbances. In light of these considerations, it is understandable that the Doppler examination may not be as standardized as the format for 2D cardiac imaging. However, the vast majority of echocardiographic examinations include screening for flow disturbances by CFD. Since Doppler signals are best recorded with the ultrasound beam parallel to flow, screening is typically performed in long-axis or apical views. Any flow disturbances visualized are subsequently examined by CW spectral recordings and, in most laboratories, by pulsed-wave Doppler. Although CW examination is typically reserved for flow disturbances, pulsed-wave Doppler may also be of value in quantifying flow dynamics in the setting of laminar flow. In this regard, pulsed Doppler recordings obtained at the mitral, tricuspid, and aortic valvular orifices, PA, and pulmonary veins constitute part of a standard echocardiogram in many laboratories (Figs. 15-26 and 15-34 to 15-37).

The normal Doppler examination is characterized by uniformity of flow velocity and the absence of high-velocity turbulent flow. CFD recordings demonstrate laminar flow through the atrioventricular valves in diastole and the semilunar valves in systole. Since the Doppler examination is usually performed with a long-axis or apical transducer orientation, diastolic filling is characteristically encoded in red and ejection in blue (Fig. 15-30, Plate 52). Color aliasing is often observed at the levels of the mitral annulus and LV outflow tract as an abrupt change from bright red to bright blue or vice versa, usually in the center of the flow stream. Pulsed Doppler recordings of transmitral flow velocities are often recorded at the level of both the leaflet tips and annulus. Velocities are higher at the tips, while recordings at the annulus offer the ability to calculate flow through a cross-sectional area that is relatively uniform throughout the cardiac cycle. A sample volume positioned in the right upper pulmonary vein reveals systolic (S) and diastolic (D) flow velocities of nearly equal magnitude followed by a short, low-velocity reversal of flow into the pulmonary veins following atrial contraction (A) (Fig. 15-36). Flow in the LV outflow tract and aortic annulus area is characterized by a progressive increase of velocity peaking in early systole, followed by a more gradual deceleration of flow (Fig. 15-35). Minimal if any flow velocities are detected in the MV orifice and LV outflow tract in systole and diastole, respectively, in normal examinations. Examinations of the tricuspid and pulmonary valves give qualitatively similar results to those of the mitral and aortic valves (Figs. 15-26 and 15-37). Normal values for forward flow velocity are given in Table 15-4. As can be seen, velocity in normal individuals is highest in the aorta and is less than 2 m/s.[62] Other commonly made measurements include the acceleration time (from the beginning of flow to peak velocity of flow in the ascending aorta or PA); and the deceleration time, from LV inflow peak E-wave velocity extrapolated to baseline zero velocity.

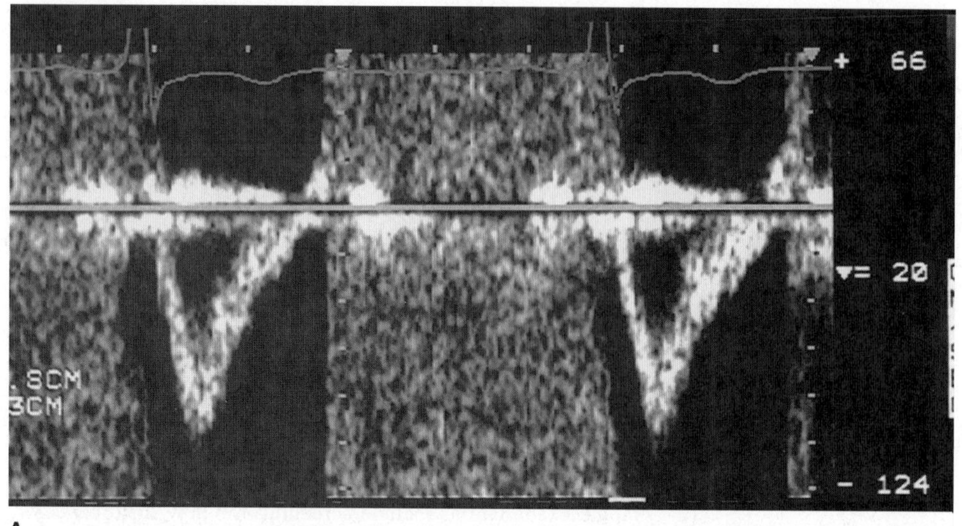


A

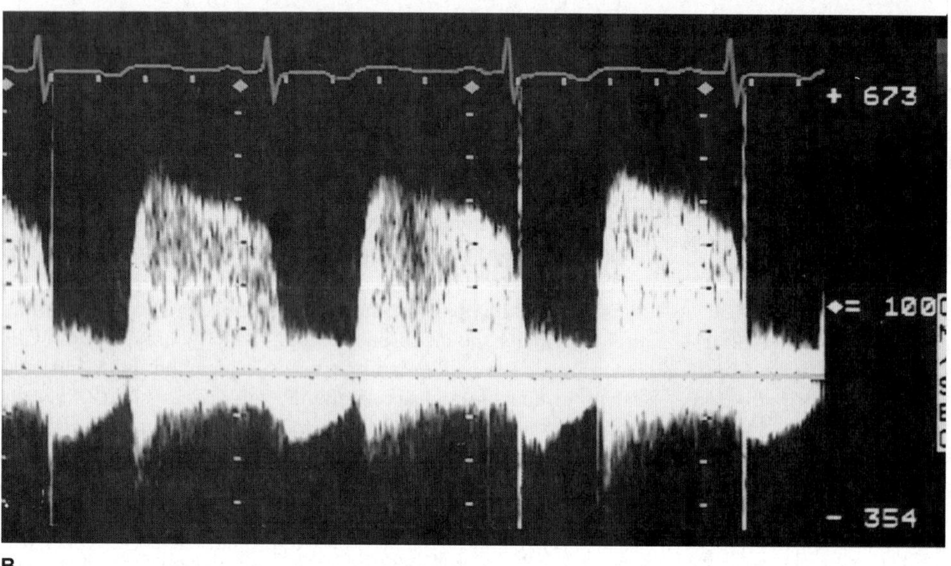


B

FIGURE 15-28 *A.* Pulsed-wave Doppler tracing from a patient with aortic regurgitation. The transducer is in the apical position and the sample volume is in the left ventricular outflow tract. A laminar envelope is seen during systole, while aliased flow is present during diastole because of high-velocity flow. *B.* Continuous-wave Doppler tracing through the left ventricular outflow tract (with transducer in the apical position). The maximal velocity of the aortic regurgitation is now measurable, but all other velocities along the Doppler beam are recorded as well.

## Doppler Assessment of Diastolic Function

In the last decade, there has been a great deal of interest in using mitral inflow velocity patterns to evaluate LV diastolic properties.[63–69] Transmitral filling velocities reflect the pressure gradient between the LA and LV during diastole[64] (Fig. 15-34). In early diastole, pressure in the LV normally falls below that in the LA, producing an increase in velocity due to rapid transmitral inflow (E wave). Flow decelerates as the pressures equilibrate in middiastole. In late diastole, LA contraction restores a small gradient, causing transmitral flow to accelerate to a second peak (A wave) that is of less magnitude than the E wave. In individuals in whom early LV relaxation is impaired, the transmitral pressure gradient is blunted, resulting in a decrease in both the velocity of early filling and rate of E-wave deceleration[65,67] (Fig. 15-38*A*). Conversely, in patients with marked increases of LA pressure and LV stiffness, early diastolic filling velocities are high, deceleration is rapid, and late filling following atrial contraction is markedly reduced. This is the so-called restrictive pattern of LV filling (Fig. 15-38*B*). Accordingly, an E-wave velocity that is substantially less than the A-wave velocity and is accompanied by a prolonged deceleration time represents evidence of impaired early diastolic relaxation by Doppler, while an increased E-wave velocity and decreased A-wave velocity (E/A ratio greater than 2.5 or 3 to 1) accompanied by a diminished deceleration time (less than 160 ms) is indicative of a noncompliant LV with markedly elevated lef atrial pressures.[66,67] Although a restrictive pattern can be seen with restrictive cardiomyopathy or advanced LV dysfunction of any cause, it also occurs in pericardial disease.[70] Of significance, a restrictive pattern of LV filling has been associated with an increased mortality rate in patients with advanced congestive heart failure,[71] and persistence

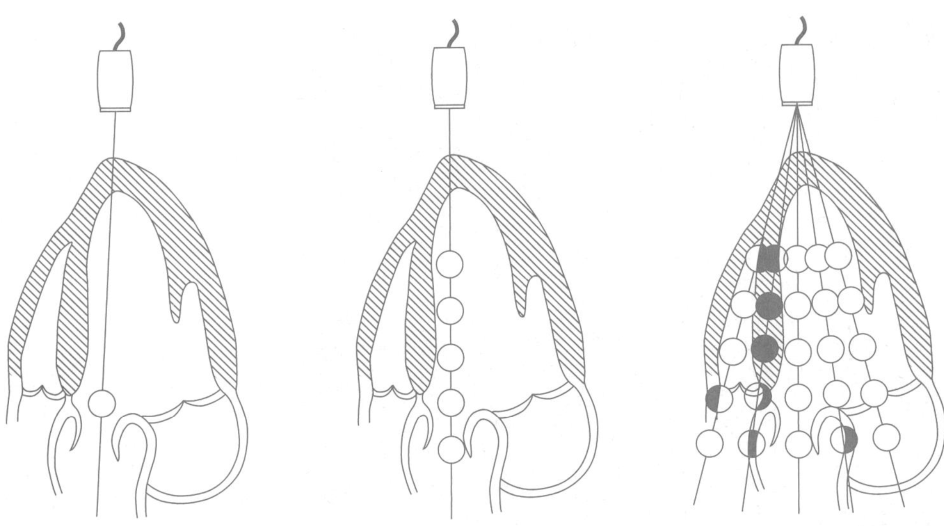

FIGURE 15-29 Simplified mechanism of color-flow Doppler imaging. Single-gate (*left*) or multiple-gate pulsed Doppler (*center*) can evaluate flow at points along a single ultrasound beam path. Color-flow imaging (*right*) assesses the velocity and direction of flow for multiple sample volumes along multiple beam paths and assigns a color indicative of velocity and direction at each sample volume site. (From Hagan AD, DeMaria AN. *Clinical Applications of Two-Dimensional Echocardiography and Cardiac Doppler.* Boston: Little, Brown; 1989. With permission.)

of this pattern despite changes in loading condition is an additional poor prognostic sign.[72]

These abnormal mitral inflow patterns can be clinically useful and, when they are markedly distorted, are generally reliable in identifying and characterizing diastolic dysfunction. Several variables other than diastolic function, however, are capable of influencing transmitral filling velocities. It has been shown that transmitral Doppler filling dynamics are affected by the age of the patient,[73] changes in heart rate,[74] respiration,[75] and even the position of the Doppler sample volume within the MV orifice.[76] Of greatest significance, transmitral inflow is very sensitive to loading conditions, and reductions in LV preload induced by nitroglycerin and/or lower-body negative pressure can induce a striking decrease in early transmitral filling velocities independent of changes in diastolic properties.[77] The influence of LV loading upon transmitral filling is most striking when an increase in LA pressure due to cardiac dysfunction restores early diastolic filling velocities and obscures impaired relaxation, thus inducing "pseudonormalization." Therefore, because Doppler transmitral filling dynamics have many limitations in assessing diastolic function, particular filling patterns should not be interpreted as "pathognomonic" findings of diastolic dysfunction but rather as components of a complete clinical and echocardiographic evaluation.

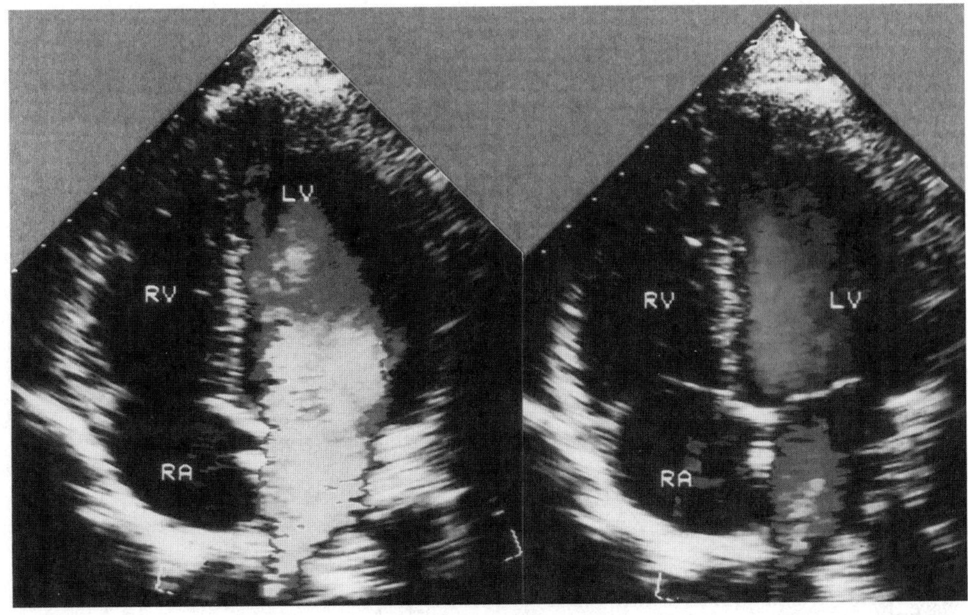


FIGURE 15-30 (Plate 52) Apical four-chamber images with color-flow Doppler during diastole and systole. Red flow indicates movement toward the transducer (diastolic filling); blue flow indicates movement away from the transducer (systolic ejection). LV = left ventricle; RA = right atrium; RV = right ventricle.

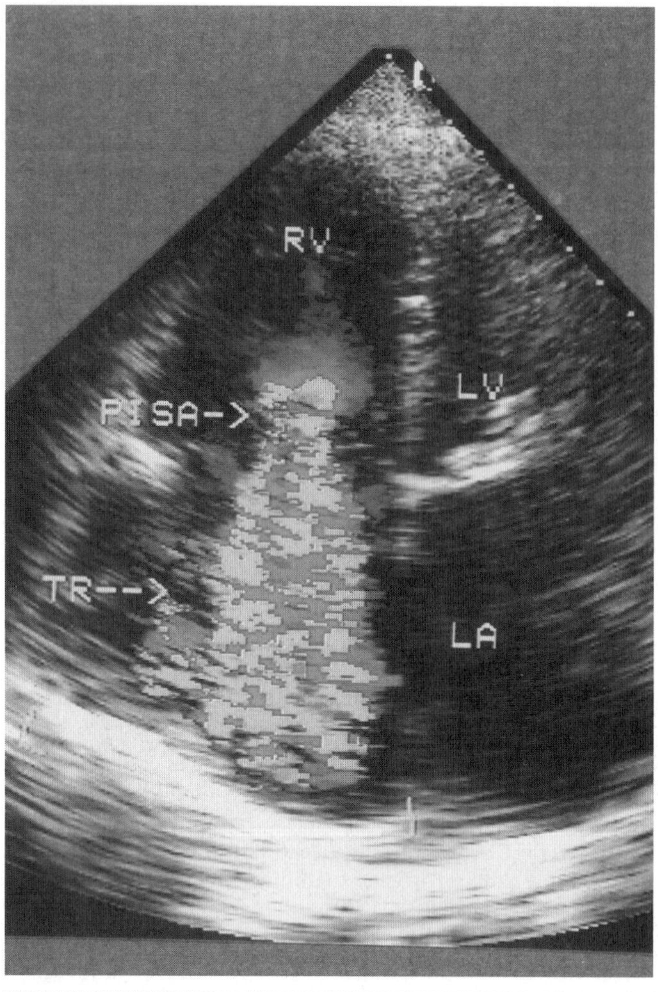


FIGURE 15-31 (Plate 53) Apical four-chamber view of severe tricuspid regurgitation. The Doppler color jet fills the right atrium (RA). PISA = proximal isovelocity surface area; LV = left ventricle; LA = left atrium; RV = right ventricle.

The recent addition of pulsed-wave tissue Doppler imaging (TDI) into the clinical arena has significantly enhanced the noninvasive assessment of diastolic function, especially when used together with transmitral and pulmonary venous PW Doppler. TDI measurements are obtained from the apical transducer position (four-chamber plane), with the sample volume placed on either the lateral or septal portion of the mitral annulus. Although TDI can assess systolic performance (i.e., by measuring systolic velocity of the mitral annulus toward the apex during systole), it is most often used to measure the motion of the annulus away from the transducer during diastole. The diastolic pattern is similar to the PW transmitral flow pattern, but the velocities are considerably less and in the opposite direction. The normal velocity of the early TDI motion ($E_m$) is 12 cm/s or greater at the lateral annulus and 8 cm/s or more at the septal annulus. In addition, the ratio of transmitral E velocity to $E_m$ is normally in the range of 8 to 15. TDI can be combined with other Doppler modalities to assess diastolic function and estimate LV filling pressure.

In a young, healthy individual, the E/A ratio is generally 1.5 to 2:1 (Fig. 15-34). Because of high LV compliance, the D velocity is greater than the S velocity in the pulmonary venous Doppler tracing (Fig. 15-36). With age, the LV compliance drops somewhat, so that by age 40 to 50, the S and D velocities are similar. As mentioned, TDI velocity is 12 cm/s or greater (Fig. 15-38*C*). In the setting of mild diastolic dysfunction, the E/A ratio is $<1$, the E deceleration time is prolonged ("relaxation abnormality," Fig. 15-38*A*), and the pulmonary venous S wave is considerably larger than the D wave (S/D ratio $>1$) (Fig. 15-38*D*). Tissue Doppler imaging shows blunting of the $E_m$ wave with relative preservation of the later atrial component ($A_m$) (Fig. 15-38*E*). As diastolic function worsens and LV filling pressures increase, a pseudonormal pattern occurs in the transmitral flow tracing (Fig. 15-39). Pulmonary venous and tissue Doppler imaging are especially helpful in this case: if the S/D ratio is $<1$ (except in the setting of a young individual), high LV filling pressure is likely present. Similarly, the presence of a low, blunted $E_m$ velocity in the setting of a "normal" transmitral E/A ratio strongly suggests diastolic dysfunction and elevated LV filling pressure. Of note, the Valsalva maneuver can be helpful in cases of pseudonormal

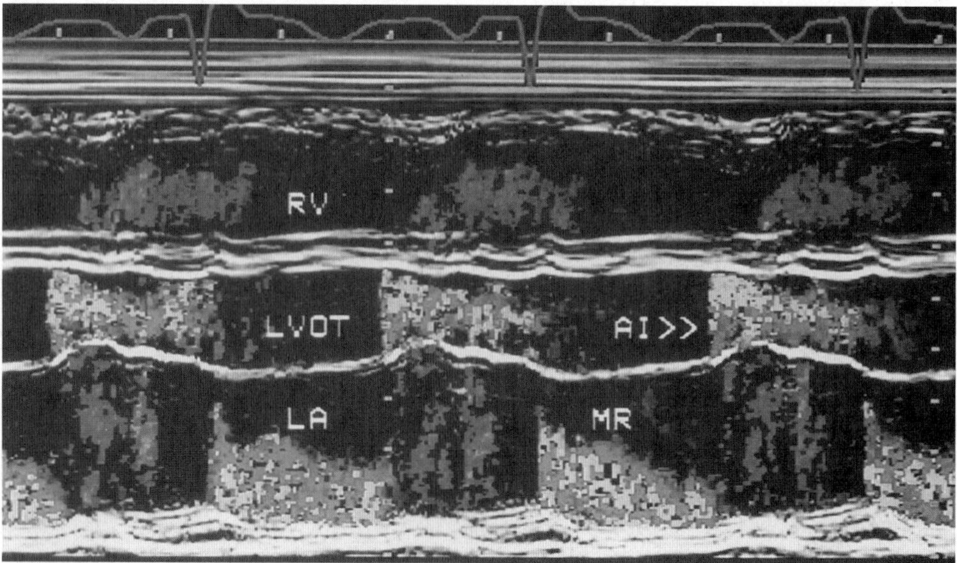


FIGURE 15-32 (Plate 54) Color-flow Doppler superimposed on an M-mode image. The transducer is in parasternal position, and the cursor is directed through the left ventricular outflow tract (LVOT) and left atrium (LA). The patient under study has both aortic insufficiency (AI) and mitral regurgitation (MR). RV = right ventricle.

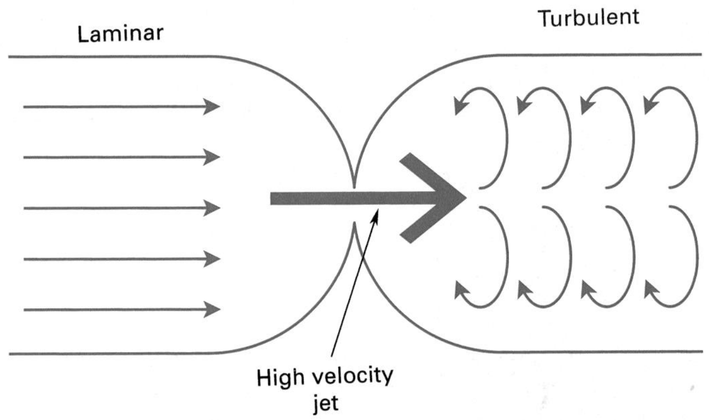


FIGURE 15-33 Flow characteristics through a stenotic orifice. Proximal to the stenosis, the flow is laminar. Near the point of maximal stenosis, the flow velocity is markedly increased. Turbulent flow is present distal to the stenosis.

transmitral flow patterns. In normal individuals, both E and A velocities drop to a similar degree with Valsalva. In pseudonormal cases, however, the drop in preload caused by the Valsalva maneuver changes the transmitral pattern to that of mild diastolic dysfunction (and the pseudonormal tracing changes to that of a "relaxation" abnormality).

In severe diastolic dysfunction, transmitral flow demonstrates a "restrictive" pattern, with an abnormally high E/A ratio and a markedly shortened E wave deceleration time (Fig. 15-38*B*). Concomitant pulmonary venous tracings show a very low S velocity and elevated D velocity (S ≪ D) (Fig. 15-38*F*). In some cases, the pulmonary venous atrial reversal wave can be very prominent and prolonged (this is not a universal finding, as atrial systolic dysfunction can sometimes occur along with severe LV diastolic failure). In this regard, an abnormally prolonged duration of reversed pulmonary venous flow during atrial contraction (i.e., a longer duration than that of the forward transmitral flow during the A wave) accurately predicts elevated LV filling pressures.[64] TDI in severe LV diastolic dysfunction shows marked blunting of both $E_m$ and $A_m$ velocities (Fig. 15-38*G*). An exception to this occurs in constrictive pericarditis, where early diastolic mitral annular motion is often preserved (as the myocardium is not inherently abnormal). Thus, when transmitral and pulmonary venous Doppler suggest severe diastolic dysfunction, a normal TDI pattern suggests constrictive rather than restrictive physiology.

Finally, color M-mode imaging has been used to assess the velocity of propagation of the transmitral filling stream into the left ventricle. This technique appears helpful in distinguishing constrictive pericarditis from restrictive cardiomyopathy. Some reports have suggested that the velocity of propagation is preload-independent,[58] but this has been questioned.

## Doppler Assessment of Systolic Function and Cardiac Output

Although measurements of LV volume and ejection fraction can be obtained by 2D echocardiography, Doppler interrogation provides a unique and complementary noninvasive assessment of systolic

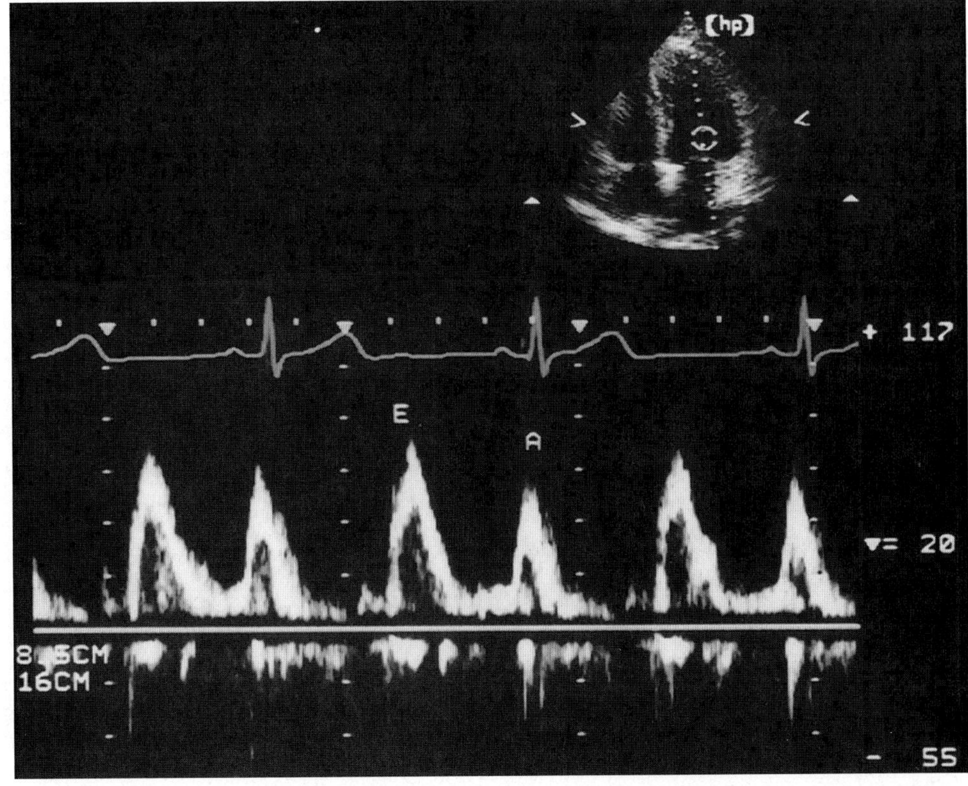


FIGURE 15-34 Normal pulsed-wave Doppler tracing from the left ventricular inflow tract, displaying the early rapid filling (E) and atrial contraction (A) phases of diastolic flow. The transducer is in the apical position and the sample volume is at the mitral leaflet tips.

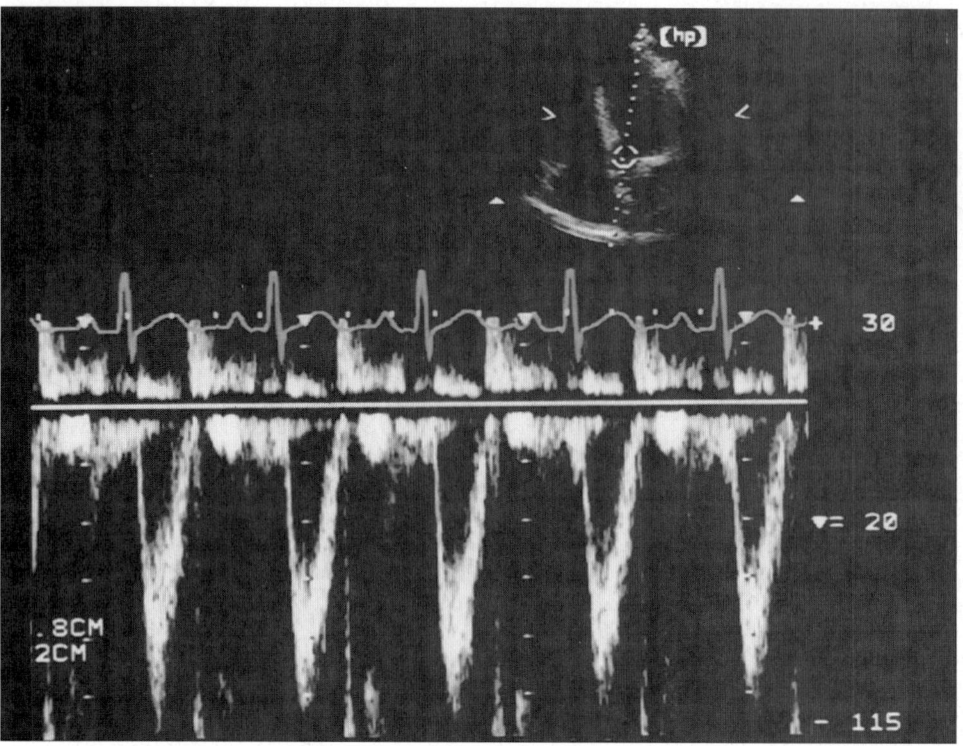


FIGURE 15-35 Normal pulsed-wave Doppler tracing with the sample volume in the left ventricular outflow tract (apical transducer position).

function. Thus, LV systolic dysfunction often results in decreased aortic velocity and acceleration time. As discussed below, in the presence of *mitral regurgitation* (MR), the acceleration of the MR jet can provide information regarding contractile function.[78]

One of the most important applications of Doppler is in the calculation of the stroke volume.[79] The theory involved is relatively simple. The volume of flow through any orifice or tube can be calculated as the product of the cross-sectional area through which flow occurs and the velocity of that flow (Fig. 15-40). Measurements of anatomic cross-sectional area can be derived from echocardiographic images, while velocity can be determined by Doppler. As the annulus of the aortic valve is nearly circular, its cross-sectional area can be estimated from a measurement of diameter as $\pi$ (diameter/2)$^2$. The pulsed-wave Doppler envelope also can be recorded at the same level. The *mean* flow velocity through the orifice is calculated by integrating velocity over time (that is, by measuring the area under the Doppler curve). This velocity-time integral, often called the *stroke distance,* is then multiplied by the cross-sectional area at the level of the Doppler interrogation to obtain the stroke volume.[79,80] The product of the stroke volume and heart rate then yields cardiac output.

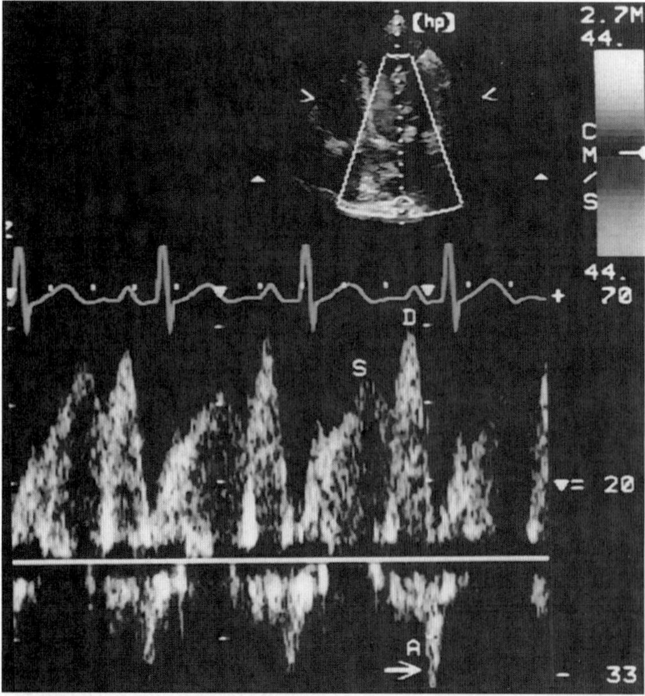


FIGURE 15-36 Pulsed-wave Doppler tracing from the right upper pulmonary vein (recorded from the apical transducer position). Flow toward the heart is biphasic, with peaks in systole (S) and diastole (D). A small amount of reversed flow is seen during atrial contraction (A).

Calculation of stroke volume by the Doppler method involves a number of assumptions. The orifice must be circular and constant in size, and the flow velocity must be uniform throughout the cross-sectional area. In addition, the angle between flow and the interrogating beam must be less than 20 degrees. Despite the uncertainty of these assumptions, Doppler-derived measurements of cardiac output and stroke volume have been shown to correspond well with thermodilution, Fick, and the angiographic calculations, though the correlation is not perfect.[79–81]

Theoretically, stroke volume can be calculated at any valve annulus.[80,82] In clinical practice, however, this is not always possible (e.g., it is difficult to obtain an accurate diameter of the PA in every patient). Because the measurement of annular radius is squared in the computation of area, it is the most important source of error of Doppler stroke-volume analyses. Stroke-volume analysis through the mitral annulus is cumbersome; it is uncertain whether the mitral annulus is best described as a circle or an ellipse, and the cross-sectional area of the annulus probably changes slightly during diastole. Calculations using the tricuspid annulus are hampered by similar problems. Despite these limitations, measurements of stroke volume through the various cardiac valves are clinically useful and can be used to calculate pulmonary-to-systemic shunt ratios, regurgitant volumes,[83,84] and orifice areas of stenotic valves by the continuity equation[85,86] (see below).

## The Bernoulli Equation

An important application of Doppler echocardiography is the calculation of pressure gradients within the cardiovascular system using a

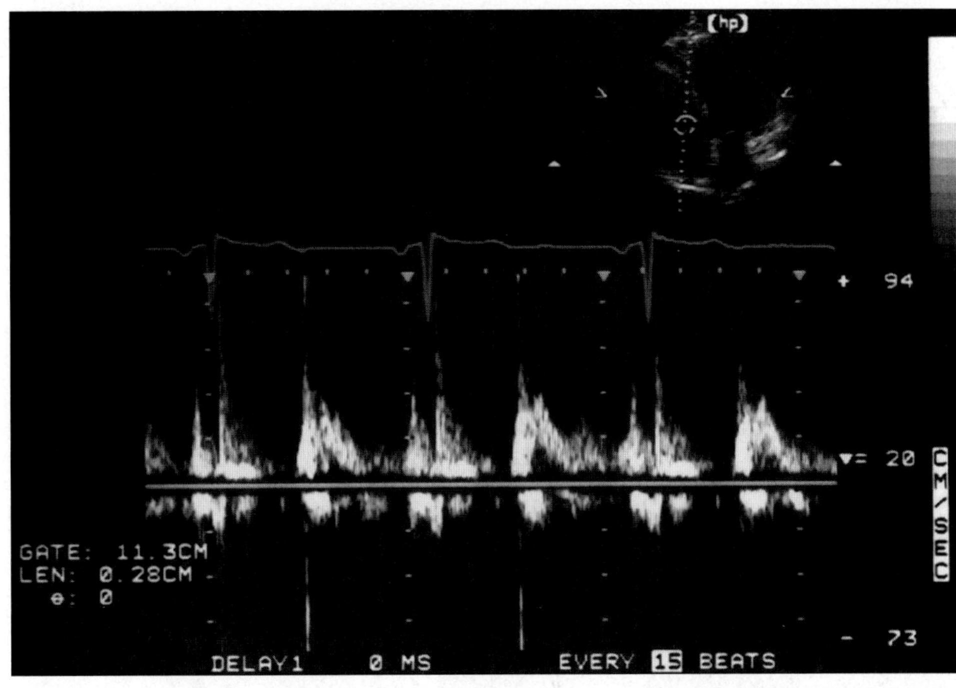


FIGURE 15-37 Pulsed-wave Doppler tracing from the right ventricular inflow tract (apical transducer position).

modification of the Bernoulli equation.[87] This theorem states that the pressure drop across a discrete stenosis in the heart or vasculature occurs because of energy loss due to three processes: (1) acceleration of blood through the orifice (*convective acceleration*), (2) inertial forces (*flow acceleration*), and (3) resistance to flow at the interfaces between blood and the orifice (*viscous friction*).[88] Therefore the pressure drop across any orifice can be calculated as the sum of these three variables (Fig. 15-41). In most clinical situations, the contribution of inertial forces and viscous friction are minimal and can be discounted. Since convective acceleration is determined by velocity, the pressure gradient can be calculated from the velocities of blood proximal to and at the level of an orifice as gradient = 4[(orifice velocity)$^2$ − (proximal velocity)$^2$]. If the blood velocity proximal to the stenosis is low (<1.0 m/s), this term can be ignored as well. The resulting modified equation states that the pressure gradient across a discrete orifice is equal to four times the square of the peak velocity ($V$) through the stenosis (PG = $4V^2$).[87,88]

TABLE 15-4 Normal Intracardiac Doppler Velocities

| | Velocity, m/s |
|---|---|
| Right ventricle | |
| Tricuspid flow | 0.3–0.7 |
| Pulmonary artery | 0.6–0.9 |
| Left ventricle | |
| Mitral flow | 0.6–1.3 |
| Aorta | 1.0–1.7 |

SOURCE: Hatle L, Angelsen B. *Doppler Ultrasound in Cardiology*, 2d ed. Philadelphia: Lea & Febiger; 1985.

The modified Bernoulli equation can be used to calculate pressure gradients across any flow-limiting orifice and has been validated against invasive measurements.[88,89] The method was originally applied to aortic, mitral, and pulmonic stenosis, but further uses have been identified. If at least trivial valvular regurgitation is present, systolic gradients across the tricuspid and end-diastolic gradients across the PV can be calculated.[90] If the RV diastolic pressure is known (or estimated as the right atrial or central venous pressure), peak RV and PA pressure (assuming pulmonic stenosis is absent) can be computed as follows[91]:

$$\text{Peak PA pressure} = 4(\text{TR velocity})^2 + \text{RA pressure}$$

End-diastolic PA pressure (PAD) also can be calculated:

$$\text{PAD} = 4(\text{end-diastolic pulmonary regurgitation velocity})^2 + \text{RA pressure}$$

In the presence of MR, a variety of calculations can be made. With measurement of peak systolic arterial pressure, systolic left atrial pressure can be estimated:

$$\text{Left atrial systolic pressure} = \text{systolic blood pressure} - 4(\text{MR velocity})^2$$

Further, the acceleration of the MR jet can be used to estimate LV systolic $dP/dt$.[92] Thus, from the Bernoulli equation, the LA-to-LV pressure gradients at regurgitant velocities of 1 and 3 m/s are 4 and 36 mmHg, respectively. Therefore $dP/dt$ can be calculated as 32 mmHg divided by the time (in seconds) required for the mitral regurgitant jet to accelerate from 1 to 3 m/s. In the case of ventricular septal defects or aortopulmonary shunts, measurements of the peak

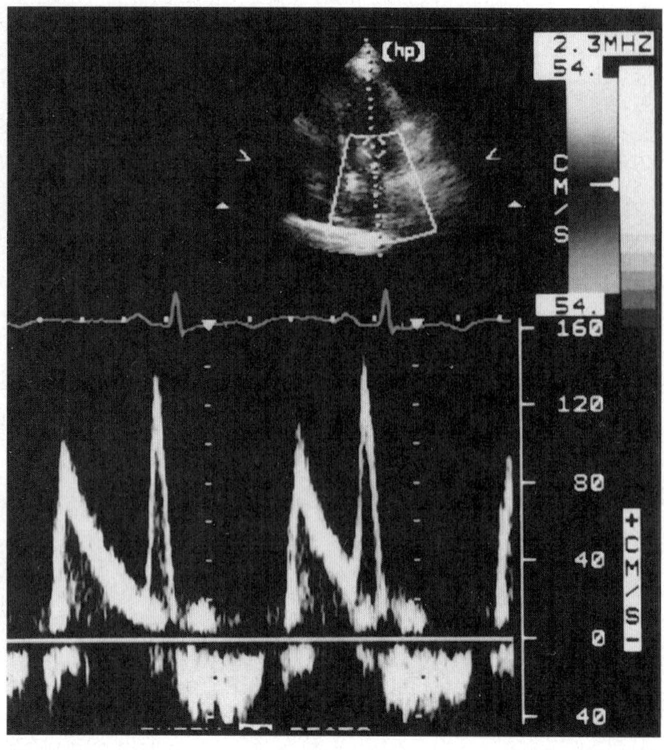


A

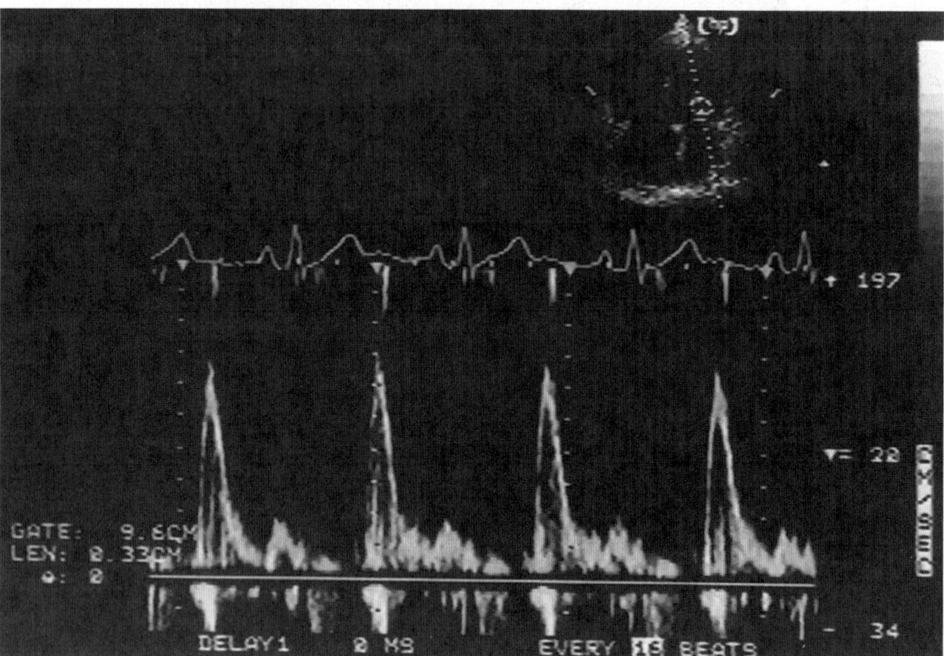


B

FIGURE 15-38 *A.* Pulsed-wave Doppler tracing of diastolic relaxation abnormality (see text for details). *B.* Pulsed-wave Doppler tracing of diastolic restrictive abnormality (see text for details). *C.* Tissue Doppler recording of normal lateral mitral annular motion (apical transducer position). Peak early diastolic annular velocity is 15 cm/s. *D.* PW Doppler recording of pulmonary venous flow in mild diastolic dysfunction (abnormal relaxation). The S wave is prominent while the D wave is small. *E.* Tissue Doppler image (lateral mitral annulus) in mild diastolic dysfunction. Early diastolic velocity is blunted (8 cm/s). *F.* PW Doppler recording of pulmonary venous flow in severe diastolic dysfunction. The S wave is small while the D wave is prominent. *G.* Tissue Doppler image in severe diastolic dysfunction. Both $E_m$ and $A_m$ velocities are abnormally low.

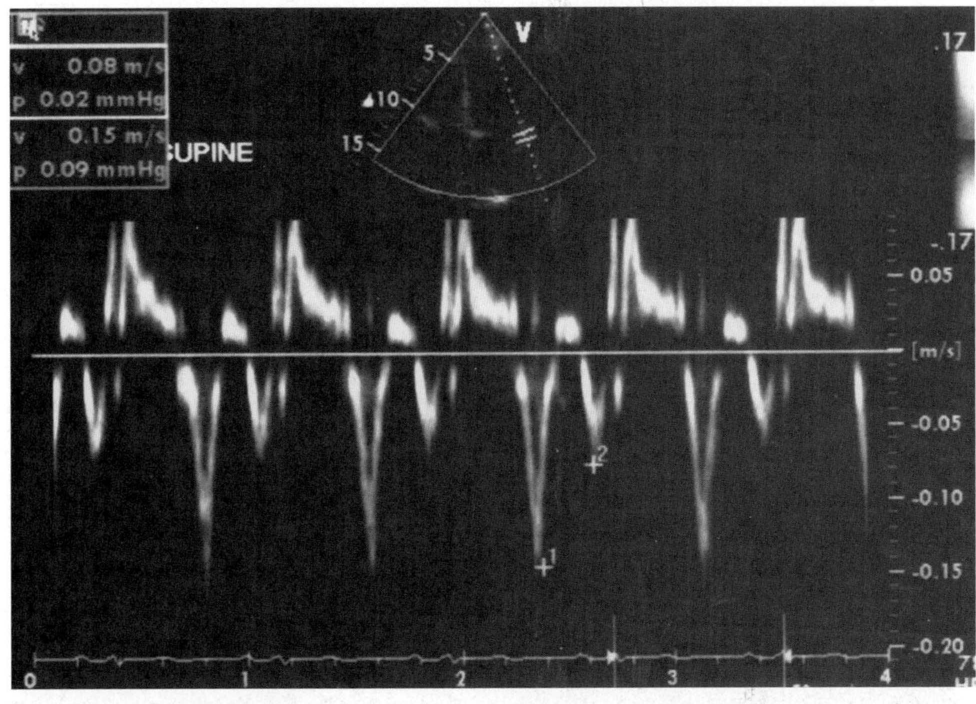


C

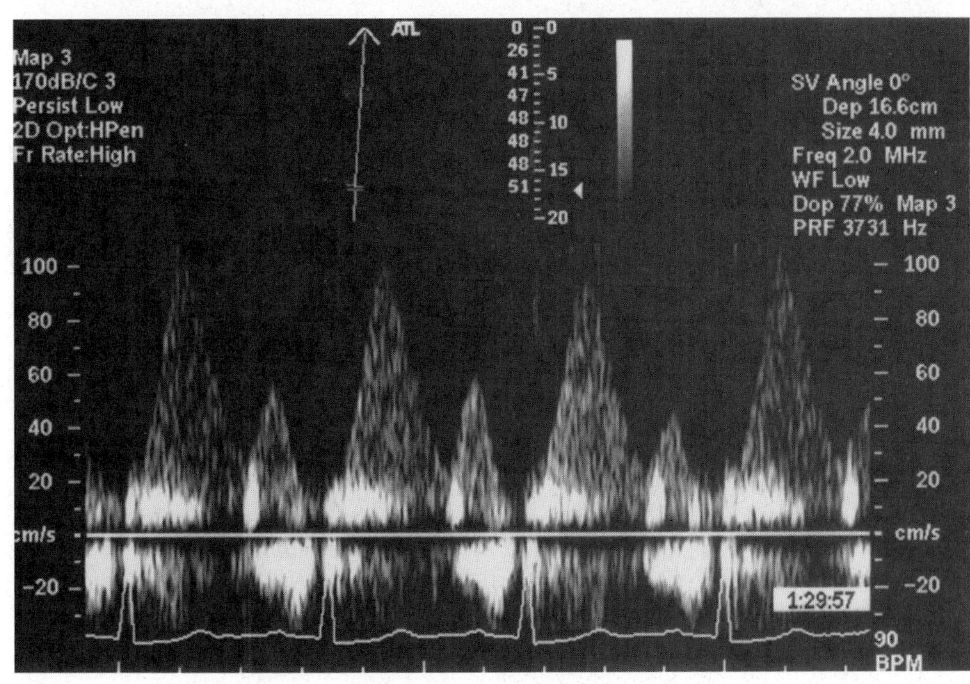


D

FIGURE 15-38 (*Continued*)

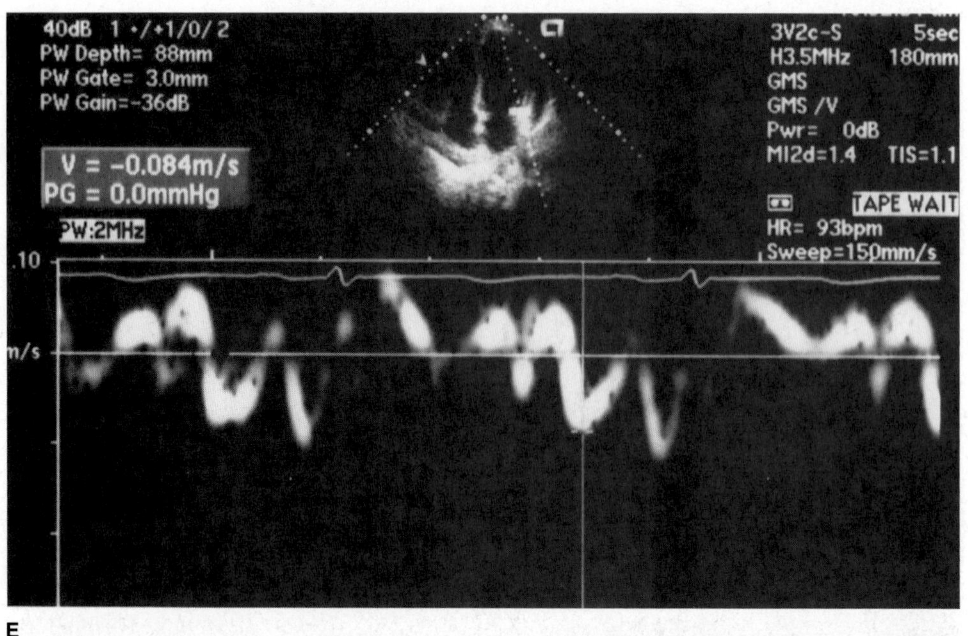


E

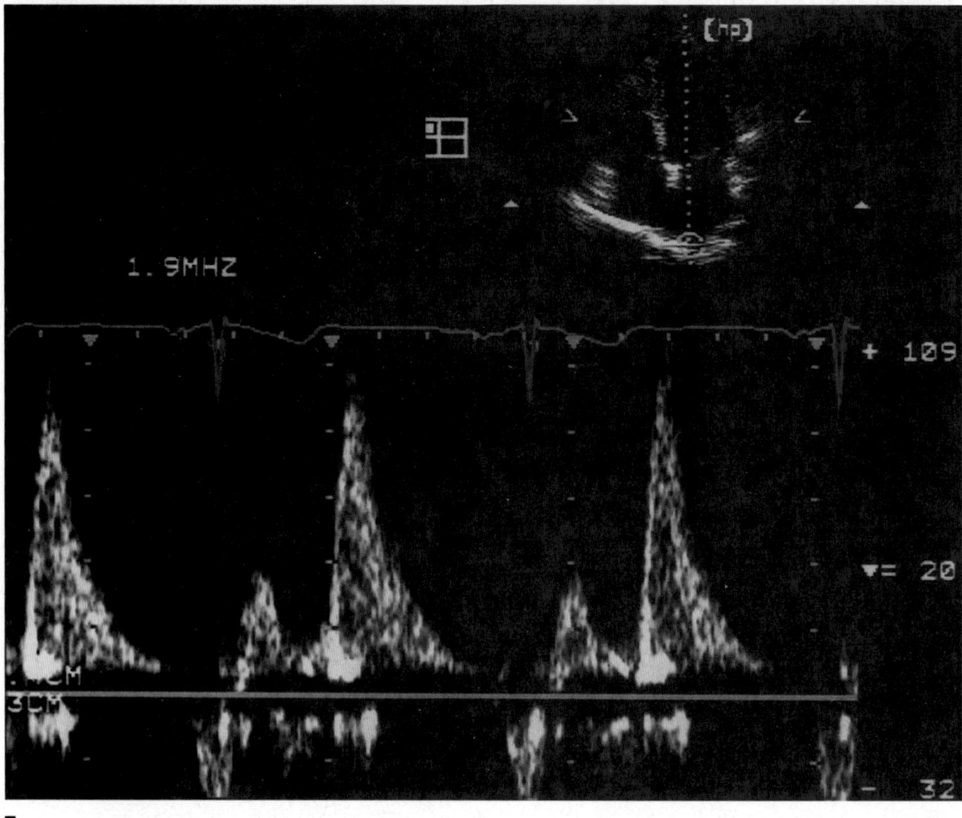


F

FIGURE 15-38 (*Continued*)

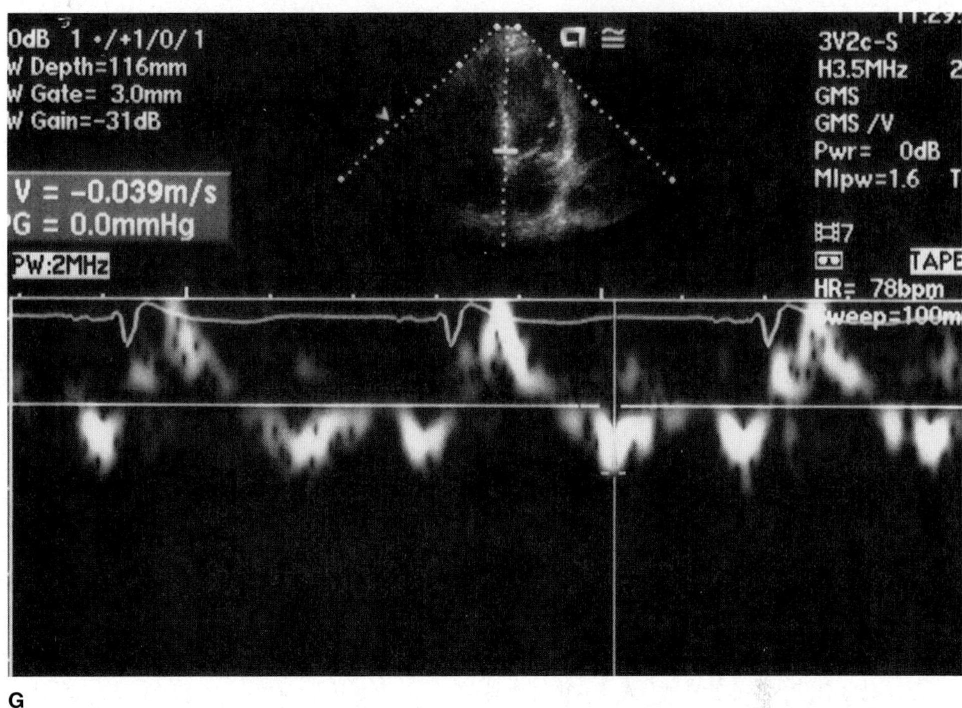


FIGURE 15-38 (*Continued*)

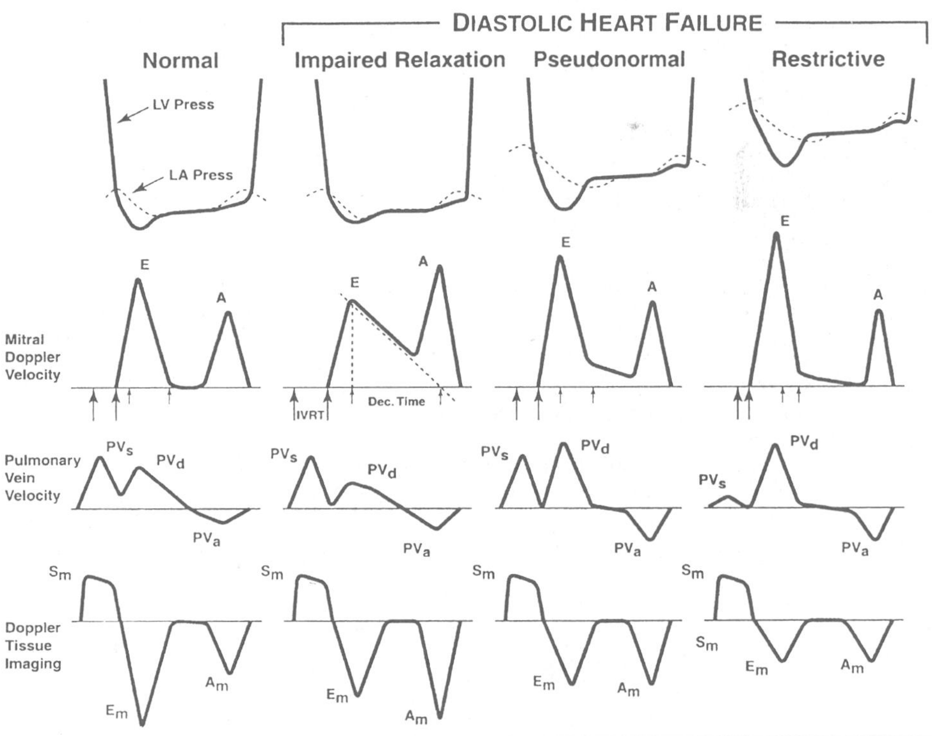


FIGURE 15-39 Doppler assessment of progressive diastolic dysfunction utilizing transmitral pulsed-wave Doppler, pulmonary venous Doppler, and mitral annular tissue Doppler imaging. IVRT = isovolumic relaxation time, Dec. Time = E wave deceleration time, E = early LV filling velocity, A = atrial component of LV filling, $PV_s$ = systolic pulmonary vein velocity, $PV_d$ = diastolic pulmonary vein velocity, $PV_a$ = pulmonary vein velocity resulting from atrial contraction, $S_m$ = systolic myocardial velocity, $E_m$ = early diastolic myocardial velocity, $A_m$ = myocardial velocity during LV filling produced by atrial contraction. (From Zile MR, Brutsaert DL. New concepts in diastolic dysfunction and diastolic heart failure: Part I. *Circulation* 2002;105:1387–1393. With permission).

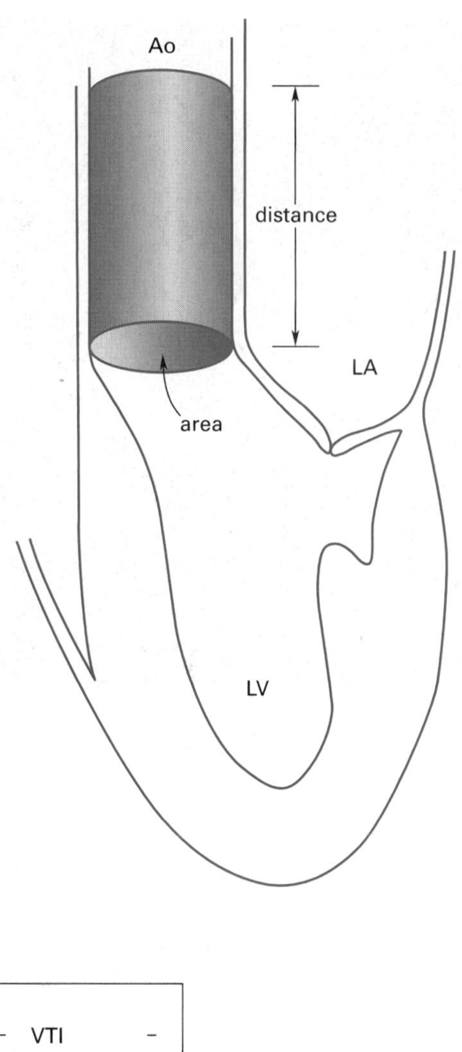


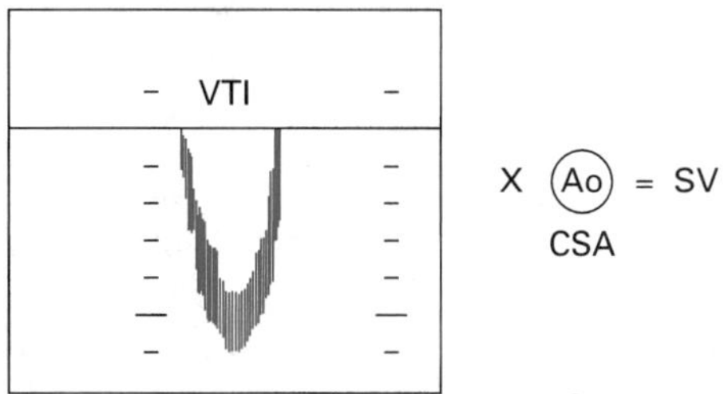


FIGURE 15-40 Calculation of stroke volume. Multiplying the cross-sectional area (CSA) of the blood column in the ascending aorta by the distance the column moves during a single cardiac contraction yields the stroke volume (SV). The velocity-time integral (VTI), expressed in units of length, represents the "stroke distance." (Modified from Pearlman AS. Technique of Doppler and color flow Doppler in the evaluation of cardiac disorders and function. In: Schlant RC, Alexander RW, eds. *The Heart, Arteries, and Veins*, 8th ed. New York: McGraw-Hill; 1994:2229. With permission.)

systolic arterial pressure and the peak Doppler velocity across the defect allows calculation of the RV (or pulmonary arterial) systolic pressure.

## The Continuity Equation

Although transvalvular pressure gradients can be calculated from CW Doppler recordings using the modified Bernoulli equation, gradients sometimes can be misleading in the evaluation of valvular stenosis. The transvalvular gradient is determined by both the size of

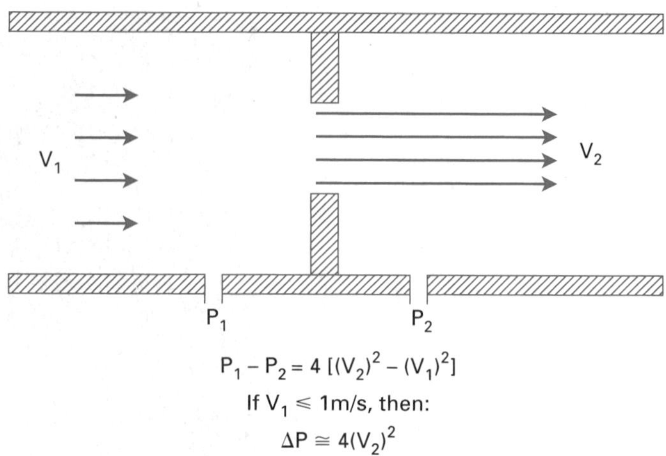


FIGURE 15-41 The modified Bernoulli equation. Pressure drop across a small orifice can be estimated as four times the square of the peak velocity (if the proximal velocity is less than 1 m/s). $V_1$ and $P_1$ = proximal velocity and pressure; $V_2$ and $P_2$ = distal velocity and pressure. (Modified from Pearlman AS. Technique of Doppler and color flow Doppler in the evaluation of cardiac disorders and function. In: Schlant RC, Alexander RW, eds. *The Heart, Arteries, and Veins*, 8th ed. New York: McGraw-Hill; 1994:2229. With permission.)

the stenotic orifice and the stroke volume traversing it. Severe aortic stenosis and accompanying LV systolic dysfunction may produce a low transvalvular gradient despite a small valve area, while coexistent AR may result in a large gradient with only mild aortic stenosis. The calculation of orifice area by Doppler echocardiography employs the *continuity equation*, which is derived from the law of the conservation of mass and states that the product of cross-sectional area and velocity is constant in a closed system of flow (Fig. 15-42). Thus, in the case of aortic stenosis, the product of the area and velocity of the left LV outflow tract equals the product of the area and velocity of the AoV orifice. Measurements of annular diameter and integrated velocity are derived by the standard volumetric approach, while the velocity across the stenotic orifice is derived by CW Doppler. The equation is then solved for the valve area.[85,86]

The continuity equation is simple and the constituent factors are readily measured, but a number of potential errors can occur. The most common pitfall is an inaccurate estimation of the cross-sectional area proximal to the stenosis. In addition, it is essential that blood velocity proximal to a stenosis be measured outside the area of flow acceleration. Finally, the continuity equation actually solves for the area of the vena contracta, which is usually just distal to the stenotic orifice. Although this area is very similar to the area of the stenotic orifice, occasional discrepancies occur.

## Determinants of the Size of Flow Disturbances

Although CFD yields primarily qualitative information, it is unique in its ability to provide measurements of the size of flow disturbances. The size of a turbulent jet should correlate with the volume of blood contained within the flow disturbance. Regardless of the lesion, however, the area of turbulence recorded by CFD has multiple determinants.[93,94] The volume of flow present in the disturbance is, of course, a major factor in its size. The pressure gradient operative in any flow disturbance is also an important determinant of the spatial distribution or "spray area" of turbulence.[94] Also, the size of a flow disturbance is influenced by the orifice through which flow oc-

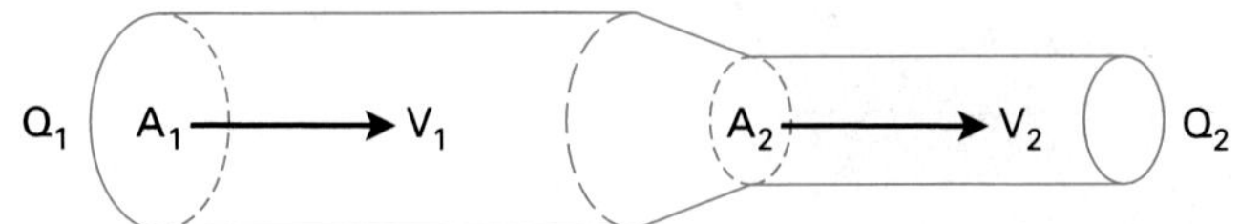


$$(A_1) = \pi r^2 = \pi\left(\frac{D}{2}\right)^2 = 0.785\ (D^2)$$

$$(A_2)(V_2) = (A_1)(V_1) \text{ or } (A_2) = \frac{(A_1)(V_1)}{(V_2)}$$

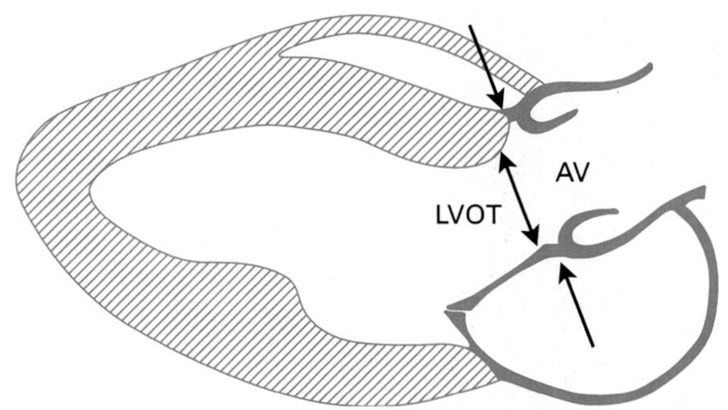


FIGURE 15-42 The continuity equation. In a closed system (*top*) with constant flow, $Q_1 = Q_2$. Therefore, $A_1 \times V_1$ must equal $A_2 \times V_2$. Determination of any three of the variables allows calculation of the fourth. Clinically (*bottom*), the area of the left ventricular outflow tract (LVOT) can be estimated and used to determine aortic valve area. (From Hagan AD, DeMaria AN. *Clinical Applications of Two-Dimensional Echocardiography and Cardiac Doppler.* Boston: Little, Brown; 1989. With permission.)

curs as well as the size and compliance of the receiving chamber.[93–96] Finally, a number of technical factors can influence jet size as imaged by CFD, including instrument gain, the angle of incidence of the interrogating beam, the frequency and pulse repetition rate of the transducer, and the temporal sampling rate.[97] Therefore measurements derived from the size of the turbulent jet recorded by color Doppler, are at best semiquantitative and should not be expected to correlate with the volume of blood contained in the flow disturbance.

## TRANSESOPHAGEAL ECHOCARDIOGRAPHY

*Transthoracic echocardiography* (TTE) usually defines cardiac anatomy and function satisfactorily, often obviating the need for further cardiac imaging. Occasionally, however, TTE does not provide complete or adequately detailed information. This is especially true in the evaluation of posterior cardiac structures (e.g., the LA, the left atrial appendage, the interatrial septum, the aorta distal to the root), in the assessment of prosthetic cardiac valves, and in the delineation of cardiac structures less than 3 mm in size (e.g., small vegetations or thrombi). Ultrasonic imaging from the esophagus is uniquely suited to these situations, as the esophagus is adjacent to the LA and the thoracic aorta for much of its course[98,99] and affords excellent access of the interrogating beam to these structures.

Over the past 15 years, a number of technologic advances have occurred in the field of *transesophageal echocardiography* (TEE), and flexible transesophageal ultrasound probes capable of multiplanar imaging of the heart are now widely available.[100] The current generation of probes also provide full pulsed-wave, CW, and CFD capabilities.

Although images can be recorded from a variety of probe positions most authorities recommend three basic positions: (1) posterior to the base of the heart, (2) posterior to the LA, and (3) inferior to the heart (transgastric position) (Fig. 15-43). Figures 15-44 through 15-47

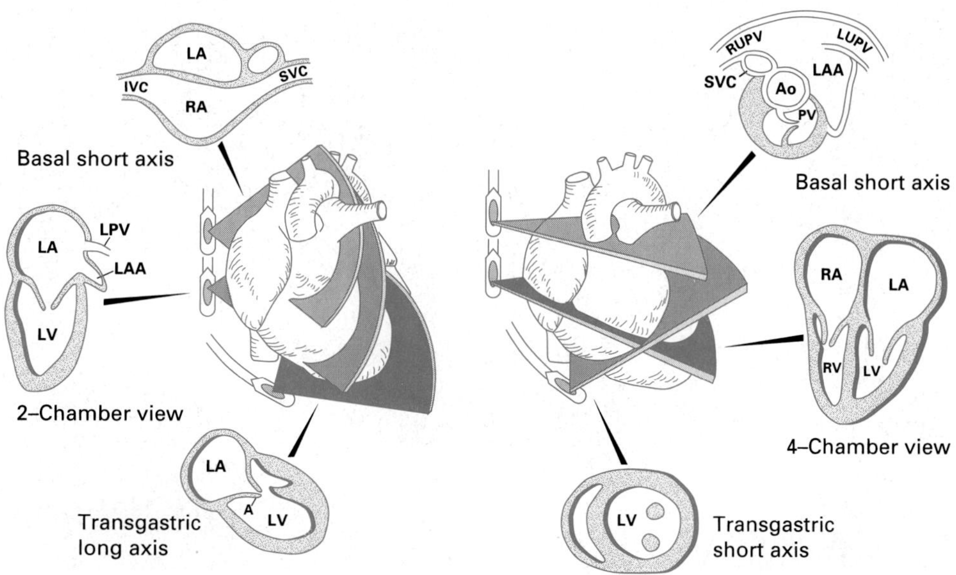


FIGURE 15-43 Standard TEE imaging planes in transverse and longitudinal axes. (From Fisher EA, Stahl JA, Budd JH, Goldman ME. Transesophageal echocardiography: Procedures and clinical applications. *J Am Coll Cardiol* 1991; 18:1333–1348. With permission.)

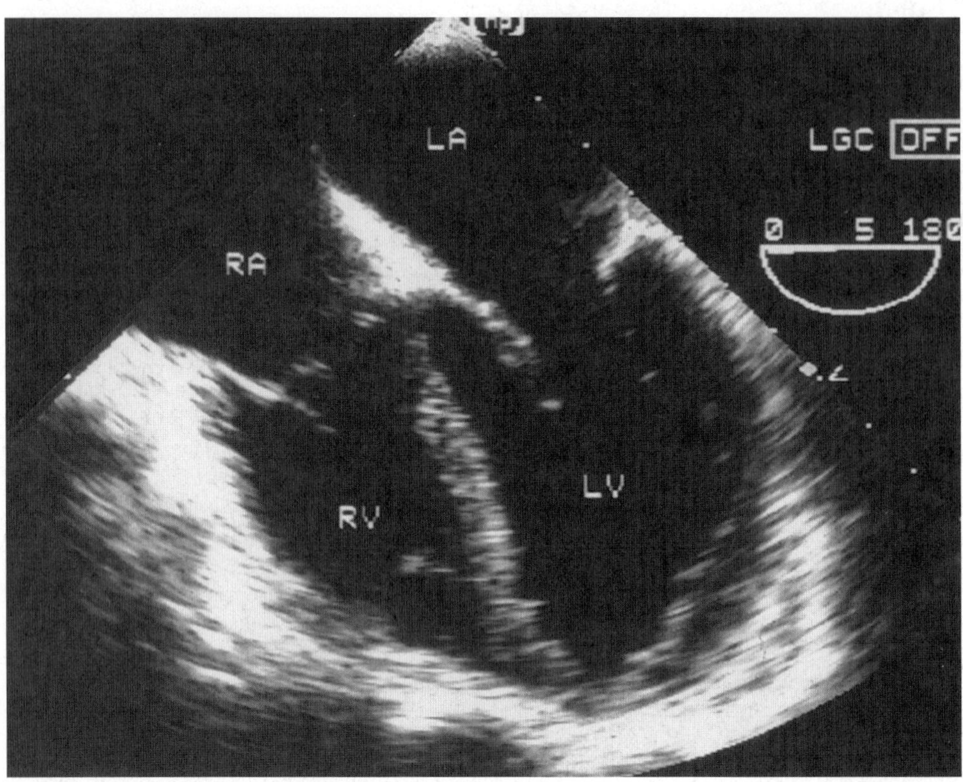


FIGURE 15-44 Transverse four-chamber TEE plane. LA = left atrium; LV = left ventricle; RA = right atrium; RV = right ventricle.

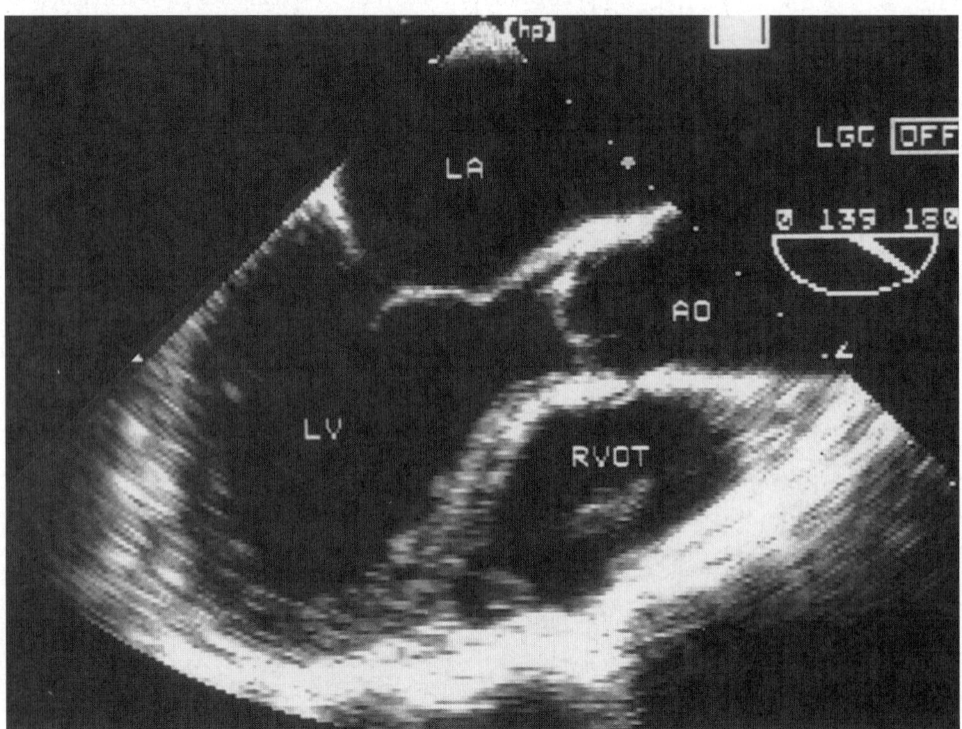


FIGURE 15-45 Modified longitudinal TEE plane (with transducer rotated to approximately 140 degrees), demonstrating a TEE apical "three-chamber" view. AO = ascending aorta; RVOT = right ventricular outflow tract; LA = left atrium; LV = left ventricle.

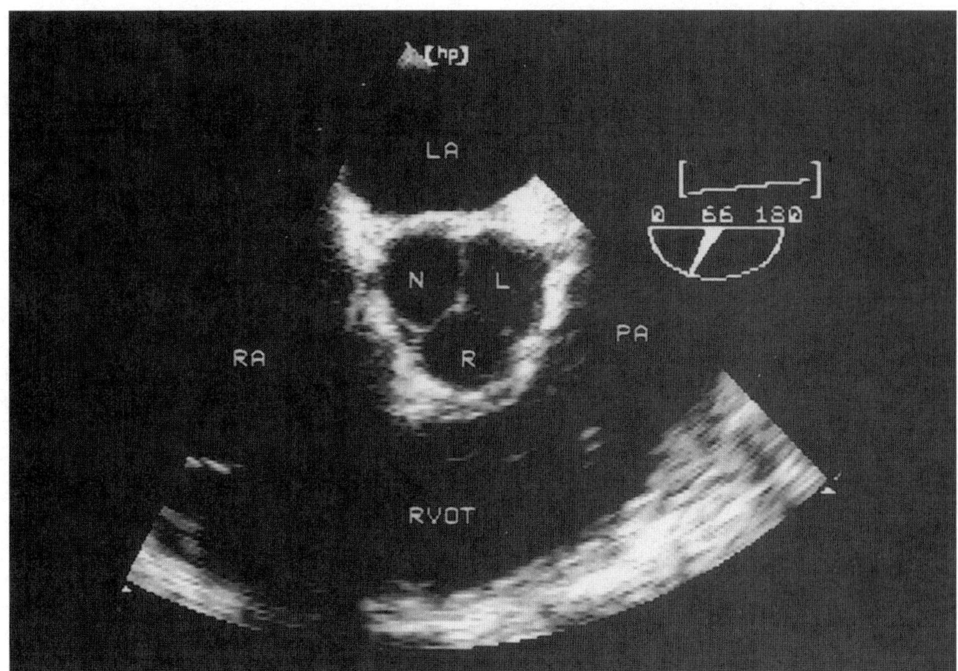


A

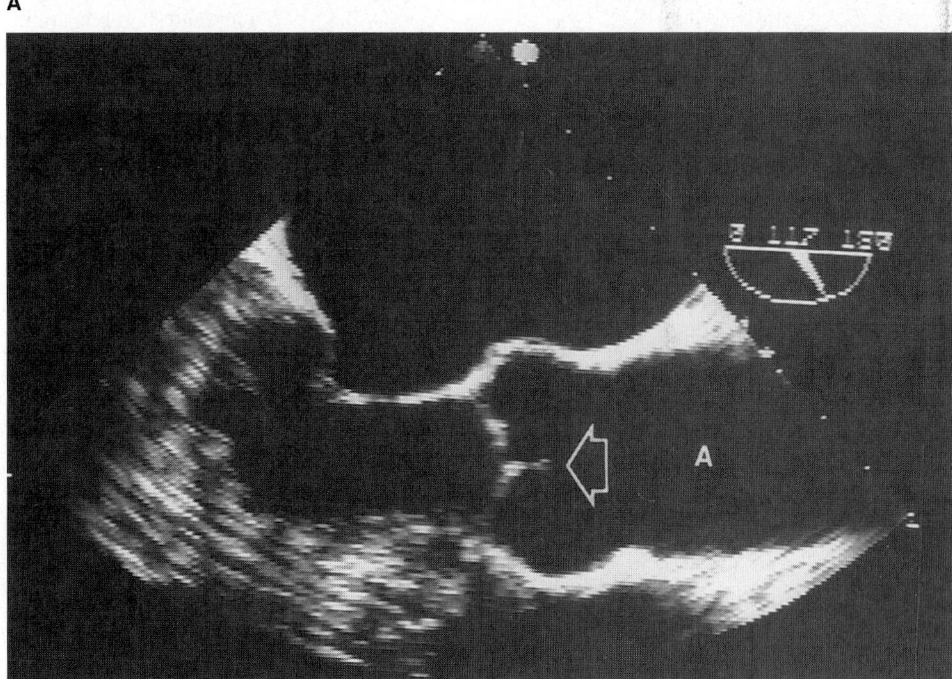


B

FIGURE 15-46 *A.* Modified short-axis view through the level of the aortic valve, demonstrating the left (L), right (R), and noncoronary (N) valvular cusps. LA = left atrium; RA = right atrium; RVOT = right ventricular outflow tract; PA = pulmonary artery. *B.* Magnified longitudinal view of the aortic valve (*arrow*) showing the coaptation of the cusps and the sinuses of Valsalva. A = aorta. (From Blanchard DG, Kimura BJ, Dittrich HC, DeMaria AN. Transesophageal echocardiography of the aorta. *JAMA* 1994;272:546–551. With permission.) *C.* Longitudinal image at level of the aortic arch, demonstrating the transverse aorta (A), the brachiocephalic vein (V), and the main pulmonary artery (PA). The pulmonic valve is visible as well (*arrow*).

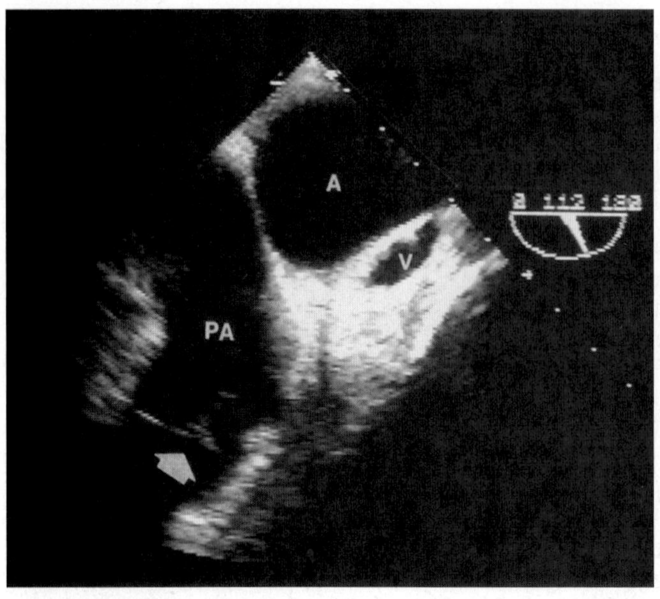


FIGURE 15-46 (*Continued*)

show TEE images obtained in various planes through the heart. It must be emphasized that, with the transducer in the esophagus, posterior structures appear at the top of the image. With the transducer in the stomach, a short-axis view is standardly obtained, with long-axis and apical views available to a variable degree. Upon withdrawing the transducer to the esophagus, one usually obtains apical-equivalent four-chamber and long-axis views, with multiple intermediate projections. Further withdrawal of the probe to the base yields excellent views of the atria, great vessels and semilunar valves, and pulmonary veins. Of particular value are views that delineate the LA appendage, all three leaflets of the aortic valve in short axis, and the transverse and descending aorta.[101]

TEE has become an important imaging modality for the diagnosis and management of infective endocarditis and its complications, including valvular vegetations, chordal rupture, fistulas, perivalvular abscesses, and mycotic aneurysms.[101,102] TEE is more accurate in detecting vegetations and abscesses than TTE[101,103,104] and provides prognostic information as well[104] (Fig. 15-48). In addition, TEE imaging may aid in accurate quantification of valvular disease (particularly MR) if TTE is inconclusive[105] (Fig. 15-49, Plate 55). TEE is especially useful for Doppler interrogation of the pulmonary veins (Fig. 15-50, Plate 56). Flow patterns in these vessels reflect LA pressure, and systolic reversal of pulmonary venous flow has been identified as an accurate marker of MR.[106,107] Although mitral regurgitant color jets are easier to see with TEE than TTE, they are usually larger, and care must be exercised not to overestimate the severity of the regurgitation.[108] Multiplane TEE can be used to planimeter the orifice area in AS.[109] The technique is also quite helpful in detection of aortic disease, including dissection, aneurysm, congenital malformations, and atherosclerosis.[99,110] Because of its portability, accuracy, and short preparation and procedural times, TEE is now recommended as the preferred diagnostic study in many cases of suspected aortic dissection (Fig. 15-51, Plate 57).[99,111]

Thromboemboli may originate from posterior cardiac structures such as the LA (LA) and appendage, interatrial septum, and aorta[112,113]; therefore TEE has received wide application in the evaluation of possible cardiogenic embolization. Since the most common

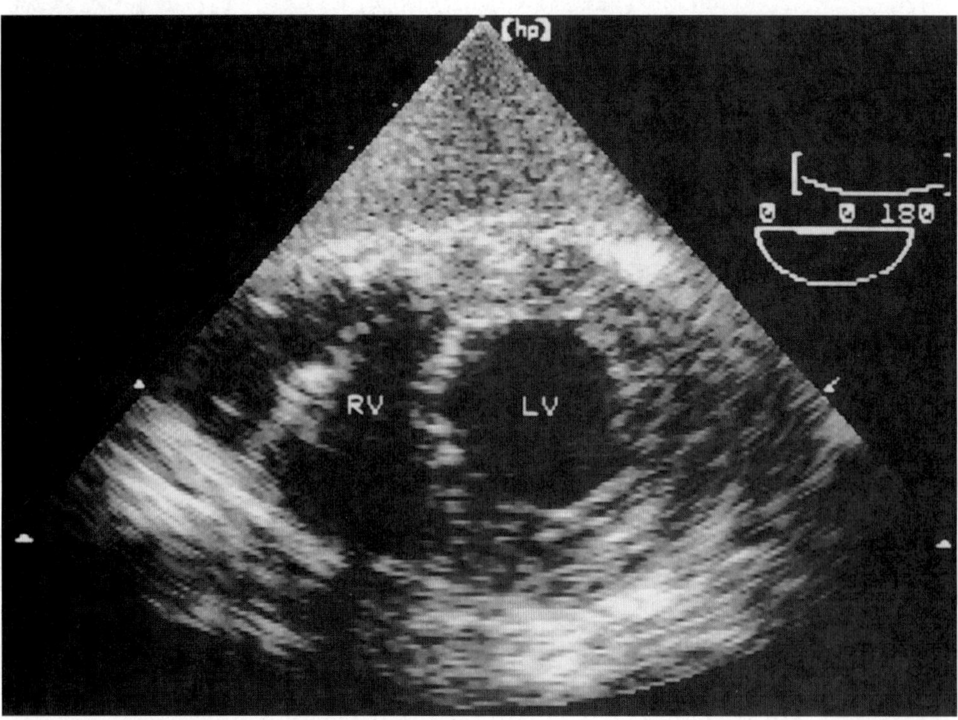


FIGURE 15-47 Short-axis TEE plane through the left ventricle from transgastric position. The inferior wall is closest to the transducer, the anterior wall farthest. The interventricular septum is to the reader's left, the lateral wall to the right. LV = left ventricle; RV = right ventricle.

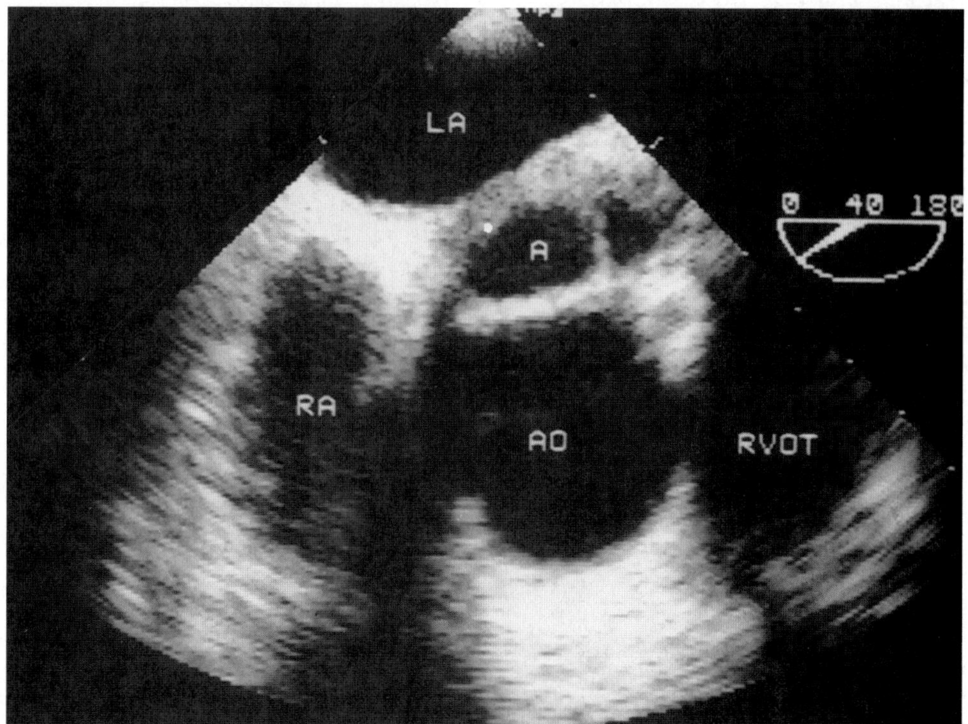


A

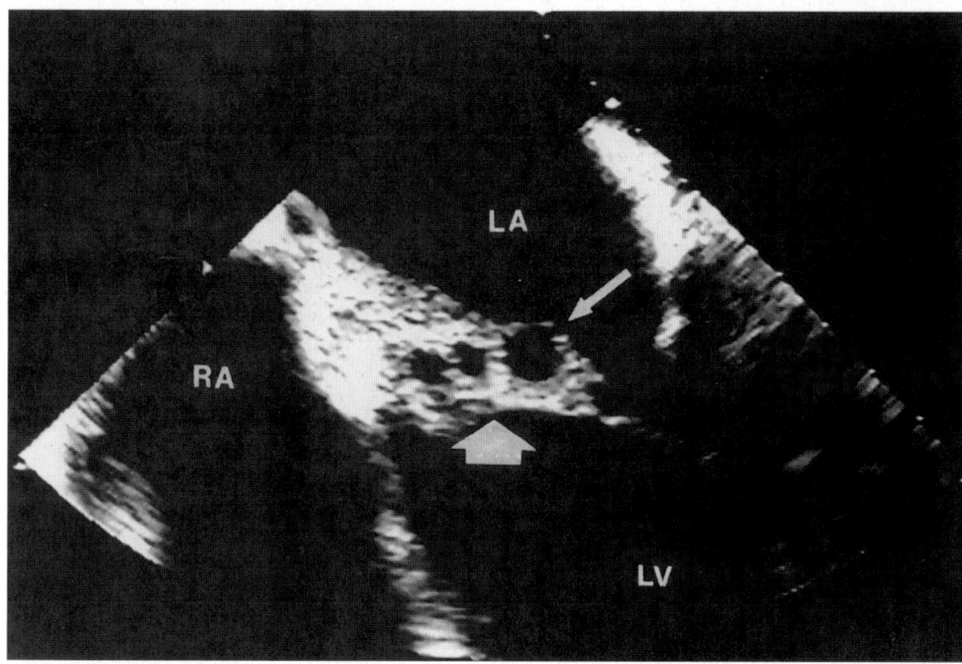


B

FIGURE 15-48 *A*. Short-axis TEE plane through the cardiac base. A large septated abscess cavity (A) is present between the aortic root (AO) and the left atrium (LA). RA = right atrium; RVOT = right ventricular outflow tract. *B*. Modified transverse four-chamber TEE plane showing a large abscess with several cavitations (*arrows*) involving the anterior mitral valve leaflet and the intervalvular fibrosa. RA = right atrium; LA = left atrium; LV = left ventricle. (From Sobel J, Maisel AS, Tarazi R, Blanchard DG. Gonococcal endocarditis: Assessment by transesophageal echocardiography. *J Am Soc Echocardiogr* 1997; 10:367–370. With permission.)

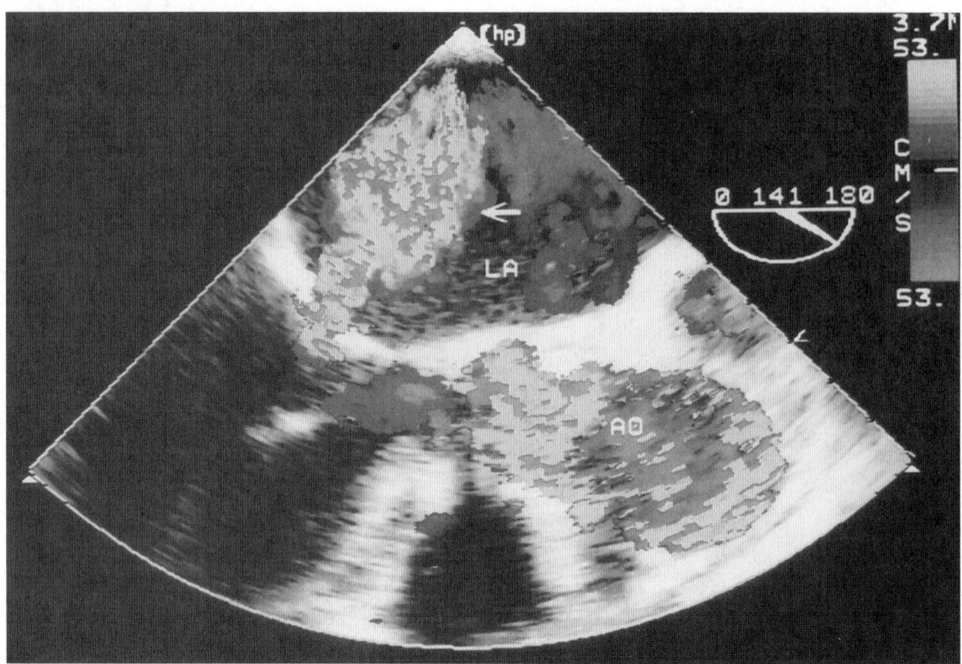


FIGURE 15-49 (Plate 55) Transesophageal echocardiography image (three-chamber plane) demonstrating a jet of mitral regurgitation (*arrow*) in the left atrium (LA). AO = aorta; LV = left ventricle.

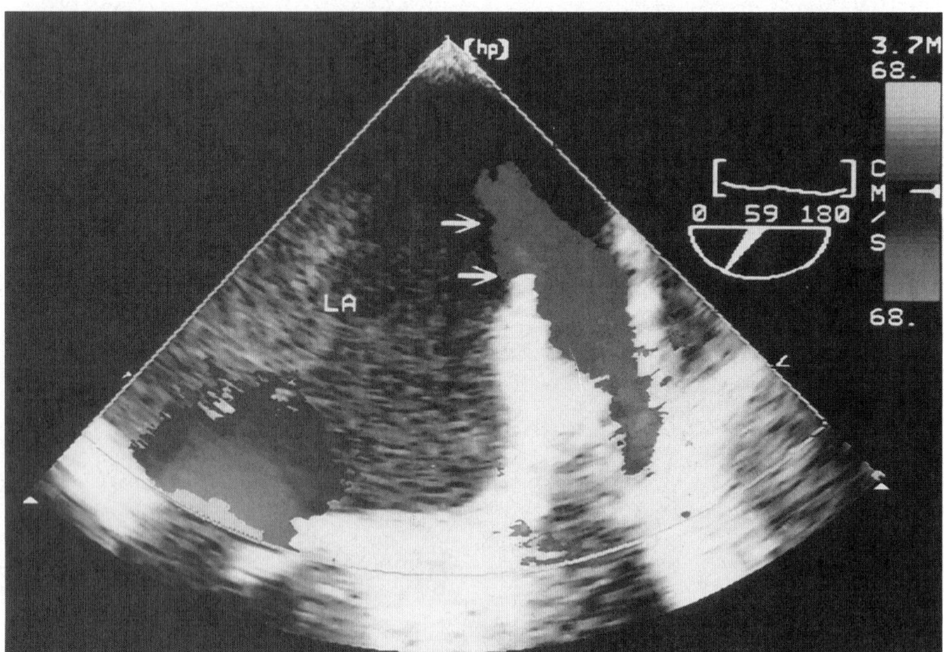


FIGURE 15-50 (Plate 56) Transesophageal echocardiography image of pulmonary venous flow (*arrows*) entering the left atrium (LA) during diastole.

site of LA thrombi is the appendage, the ability of TEE to visualize this structure is of particular value (Fig. 15-52). TEE can also detect spontaneous contrast signals (that appear to represent transient rouleaux formation and predispose to thromboemboli). In addition, TEE has provided unique real-time images of mobile, pedunculated, atherosclerotic "debris" in the thoracic aorta (Fig. 15-53*A* and *B*). Although the optimal therapy for this disorder is currently unknown, warfarin may be helpful and mobile or protruding aortic atheromas appear to be significant risk factors for embolic events.[113–115] The optimal role for TEE in the detection of intracardiac sources of emboli is controversial, and clinical trials are ongoing to evaluate the effect of treatment after discovery of potential embolic sources.

One of the proven applications of TEE is the evaluation of prosthetic valve dysfunction, particularly mechanical valves in the mitral

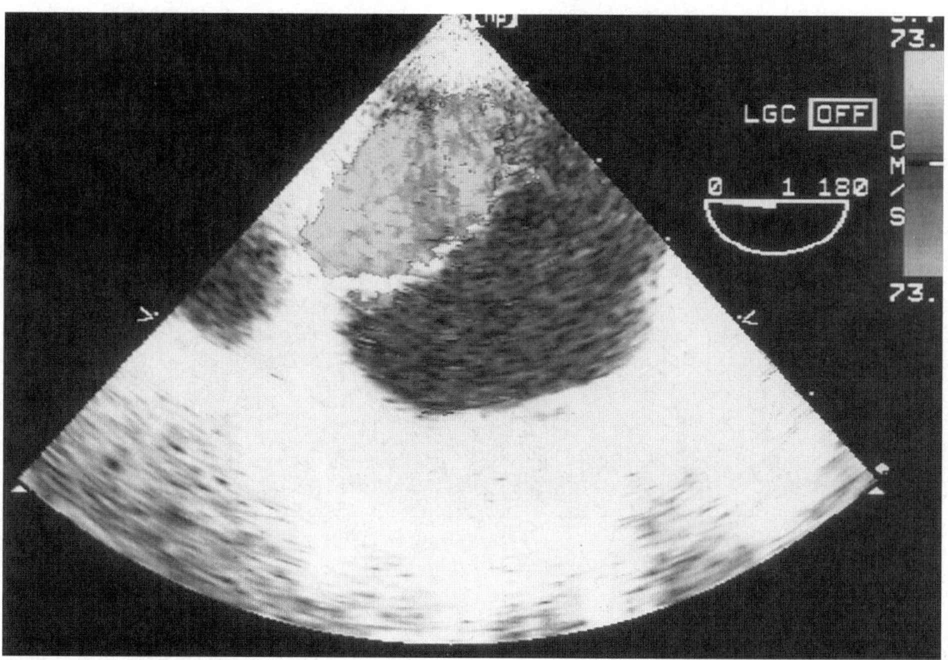


FIGURE 15-51 (Plate 57) Transverse TEE image of a descending aortic dissection. The true lumen is color-coded orange. The false lumen is mostly devoid of flow, but a small blue jet of communication between the two channels is present.

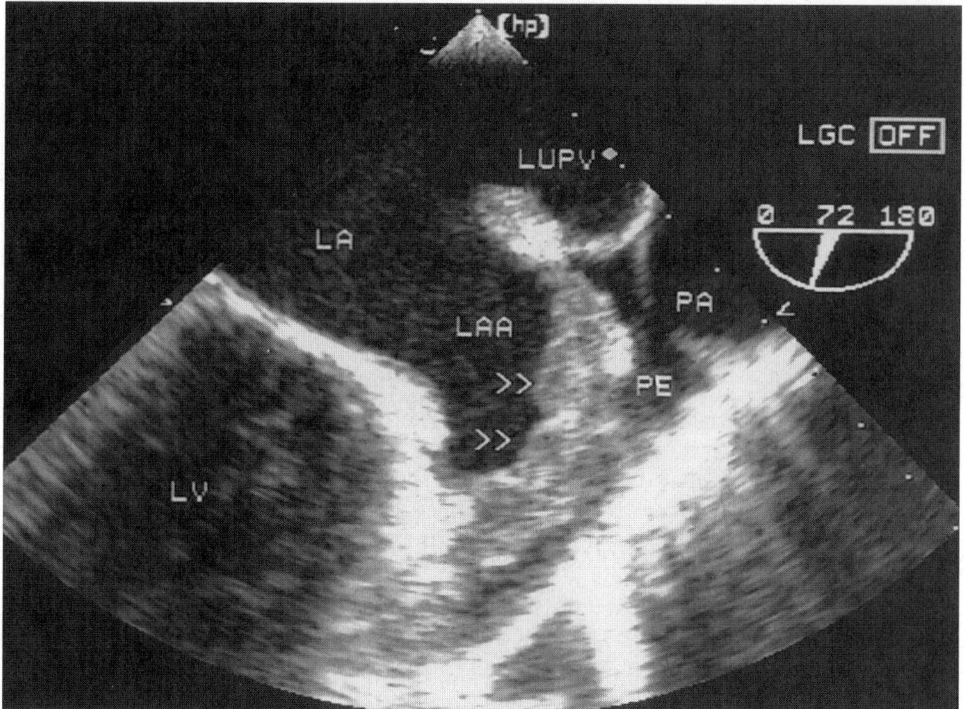


FIGURE 15-52 Transesophageal echocardiography image of a laminar thrombus (*arrows*) within the left atrial appendage (LAA). This thrombus was not visible with transthoracic echocardiography. LA = left atrium; LV = left ventricle; LUPV = left upper pulmonary vein; PA = pulmonary artery; PE = small pericardial effusion.

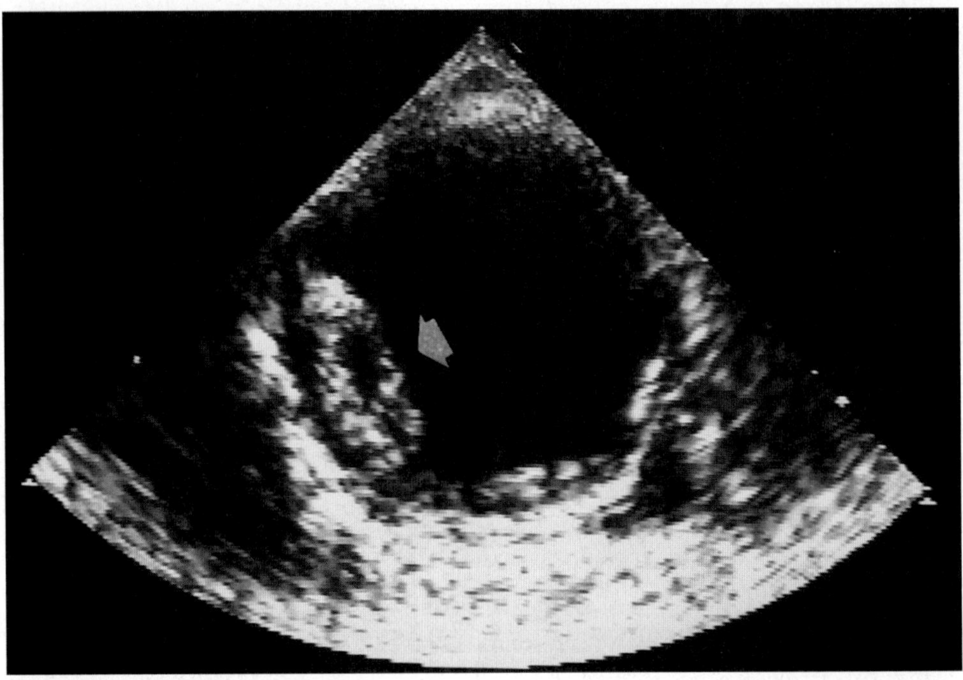

A

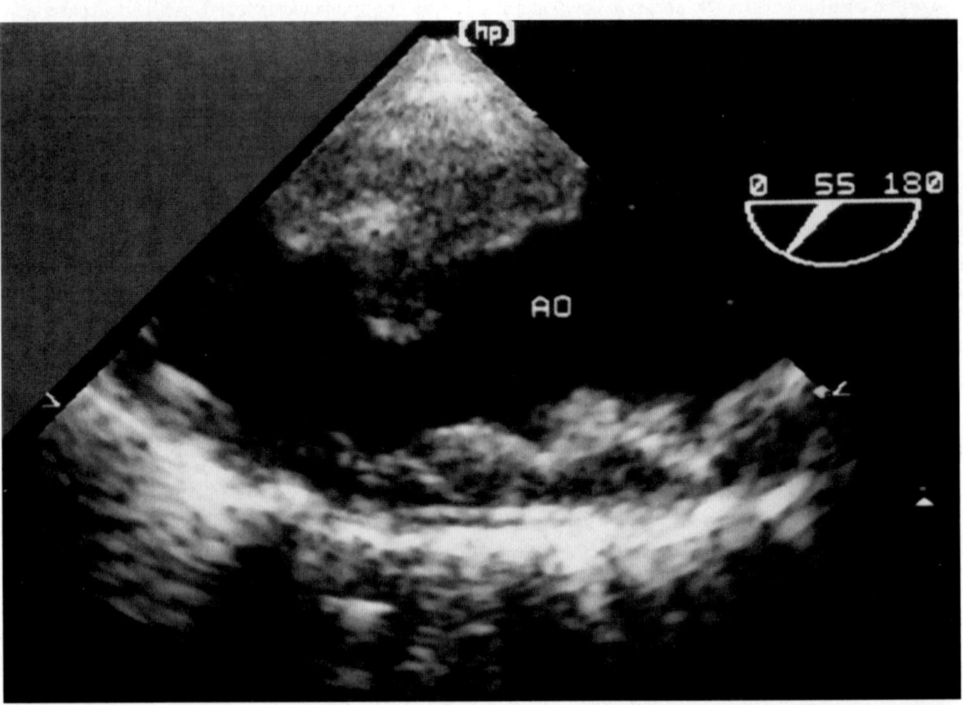


B

FIGURE 15-53 *A.* Transverse TEE image of the descending aorta, demonstrating atherosclerosis and a large atheroma (*arrow*). *B.* Longitudinal TEE image of the descending aorta, demonstrating severe, extensive atherosclerosis.

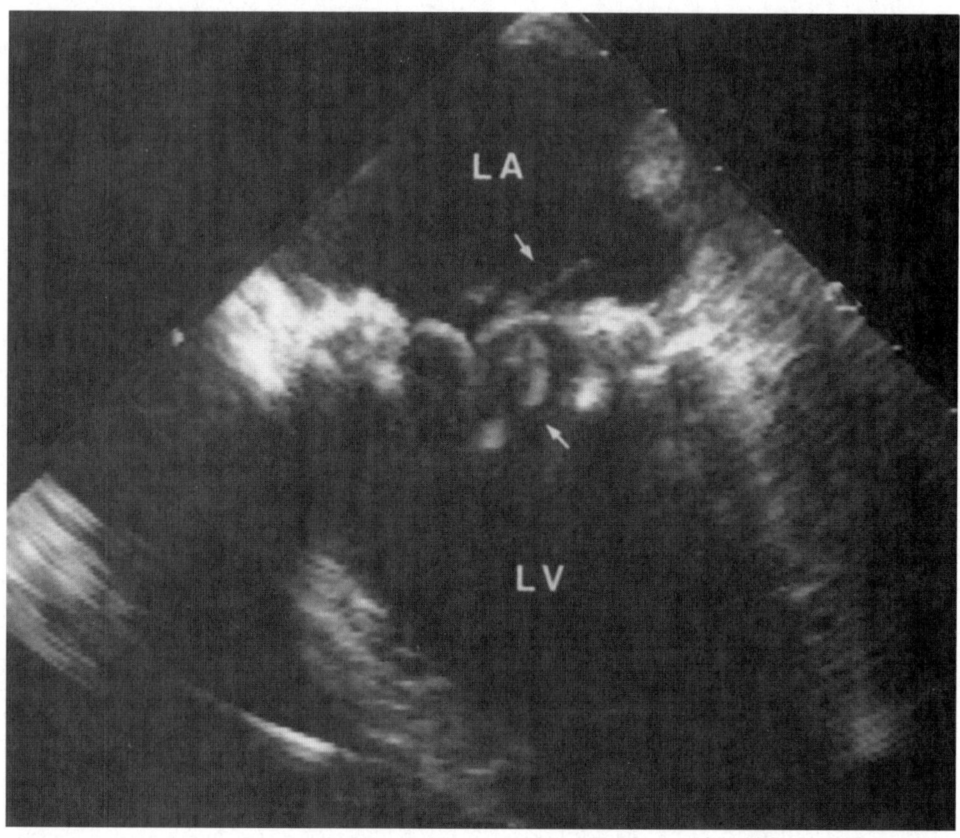


FIGURE 15-54 Transverse four-chamber TEE image of infective vegetations (*arrows*) on a porcine prosthesis in the mitral position. LA = left atrium; LV = left ventricle.

position.[116] Since the materials used in artificial valves are strong reflectors and often cause ultrasonic shadowing, the areas behind prosthetic valves are usually hidden from view when transthoracic imaging is used. Because of its unique window on the heart, TEE is clearly superior to TTE imaging for detection of prosthetic regurgitation, infection, tissue ingrowth, and thrombosis (Fig. 15-54).

TEE has also become an important intraoperative tool for the detection of cardiac ischemia, the evaluation of valve function after repair or replacement, and the delineation of congenital heart disease.[117,118] Cardiac surgeons often request intraoperative TEE for evaluation of cardiac anatomy and confirmation of a success of surgical repair before closing the chest. In this regard, TEE has almost completely replaced epicardial echocardiography. When TEE images are inadequate, TEE is helpful in managing critically ill patients and also can be used to monitor or guide interventional procedures, such as transseptal catheterization, mitral valvuloplasty, pericardiocentesis, and endomyocardial biopsy.

## Handheld Echocardiography

Recently, advances in electronic technology have led to production of small, relatively lightweight (5 to 6 lb) echocardiography units. These handheld devices can be carried to the clinic exam room or hospital bed, thereby facilitating point-of-care echo evaluation by the physician. Although the quality of images from these scanners has improved steadily, it still does not equal that of state-of-the-art standard ultrasound instruments. In addition, handheld scanners have marginal or nonexistent spectral and color Doppler capabilities (this will likely change in the future). The appropriate use of these scanners is *currently controversial,* and recommendations will certainly evolve over time. Experts in the field have raised numerous questions about the merits of handheld echocardiography: there are concerns about the sonographic skills required for accurate diagnosis (as physicians—rather than sonographers—will likely perform most studies with these devices), legal ramifications of potential misdiagnosis, added time commitments during clinic visits, and overall quality control (Chap. 12).[119]

Several studies have shown benefits from handheld scanning in the detection of cardiac and aortic pathology,[120] while others have shown a relative lack of utility, especially in critically ill patients. As the technical sophistication of these devices increases, they will likely become more useful in clinical practice. It is clear, however, that the sonographic skills of the person performing the study are critically important. To ensure adequate imaging competency, the ASE currently recommends that individuals performing handheld scanning have level 2 or 3 training in echocardiography.[121]

Many exams with handheld echo equipment are goal-directed and focused (rather than full, complete cardiac ultrasound studies), and this has spawned research into the arena of "targeted" or "limited" echocardiography.[121] A wide spectrum of opinion exists in this area. On one extreme, proponents argue that all echocardiographic studies should be complete and follow a standard and inclusive protocol to avoid missing incidental findings. Conversely, other experts recommend an increased use of limited echo exams, as a proportion of complete echocardiographic studies currently performed may be clinically unnecessary and therefore cost-ineffective.

This area is definitely in flux, but at present it may be best to view examinations with handheld echo devices as *limited extensions of the stethoscope.* Performed by a competent individual, the diagnostic capability of such an examination is at least equal to that of auscultation and *may be* significantly better (Chap. 12). In the future, examinations with this modality could be performed by various individuals, including physicians and even nursing staff, although medicolegal issues of clinical responsibility will likely play an important role in this evolution.[122]

## CONTRAST ECHOCARDIOGRAPHY

Opacification of the right heart cavities with dense ultrasonic reflectances during intravenous contrast injection was first applied clinically in 1968.[123] Subsequently, it became clear that the origin of the dense intracavitary echoes were microbubbles within the injectate, and that any agitated liquid injected intravenously caused the effect.[124] Since room-air microbubbles with the diameter of pulmonary capillaries persist intact in blood for less than 1 s before dissolving, agitated agents injected intravenously cannot cross the lungs and enter the left-sided cardiac chambers. Thus, the presence of echocardiographic contrast entering left heart chambers after intravenous injection of an agitated liquid indicates the presence of a right-to-left shunt.[125]

Identification of intracardiac shunts, particularly patent foramen ovale in patients with unexplained cerebral ischemia (Fig. 15-55), remains a frequent indication for contrast echocardiography. Simple agitated normal saline solution remains the most commonly used contrast agent for such studies.

Echocardiographic opacification of the LV cavity and myocardium by intracardiac or intravenous injection is now easily performed.[126–128] The presence of echocardiographic contrast within the myocardium after such injections reflects the spatial distribution of coronary blood flow (CBF) and is valuable in identifying collateral CBF and the absence of reflow following reperfusion therapy of acute myocardial infarction (AMI).[129,130] Of significance, the presence of microcirculatory flow and integrity in these studies was a reliable predictor of viable myocardium.[129]

Since direct injection of coronary contrast into the left heart or aorta (Fig. 15-56) is limited by its invasive nature, stabilized solutions of microbubbles have been developed which can traverse the pulmonary capillary bed in high concentration after intravenous injection. These new ultrasonic contrast agents have been designed to achieve prolonged bubble persistence or survival after injection into blood. The persistence time of a bubble prior to dissolving in blood can be increased by utilizing a shell or surface modifying agent which inhibits the leakage of gas across the bubble surface. Alternatively, prolonged bubble survival can be achieved by utilizing a dense, high-molecular-weight gas with a reduced capacity to diffuse across the bubble shell and a low saturation constant in blood, which favors return of gas back into the bubble. Therefore, the new ultrasonic contrast agents utilize shells made of human serum albumin, liposomes, or even biodegradable poliment materials, and the fluorocarbon gases, which are dense and poorly soluble. These new microbubble agents are all capable of producing dense, high-intensity signals not only within the LV but also within the myocardium following intravenous injection.[131,132]

Intravenous injection of stabilized solutions of microbubbles opacifies the LV in nearly all patients, thereby facilitating identification of the endomyocardial border. This capacity has found its greatest application in stress echocardiography, where detection of the endocardium is of fundamental importance in recognizing abnormal contraction produced by ischemia. By intensifying backscatter within the intracardiac cavities, new ultrasonic agents also enhance Doppler recording of flow abnormalities.[133] Marginal Doppler spectral tracings in cases of MR, tricuspid regurgitation, and aortic stenosis often improved dramatically after contrast injection, facilitating the quantitation of valvular lesions and pulmonary hypertension.[134]

In addition to new contrast agents, novel imaging technology directed to the amplification of contrast signals are also available. Harmonic imaging amplifies the ultrasonic backscatter from contrast microbubbles (which resonate in an ultrasonic field) relative to the returning signal from myocardium (which does not resonate). (Fig. 15-57). As discussed above, tissue harmonic imaging can also be used to visualize cardiac structures in the absence of contrast injection: this technique decreases clutter and other artifacts, often improving endocardial definition (Fig. 15-58).

Power Doppler imaging is a method that correlates signals between

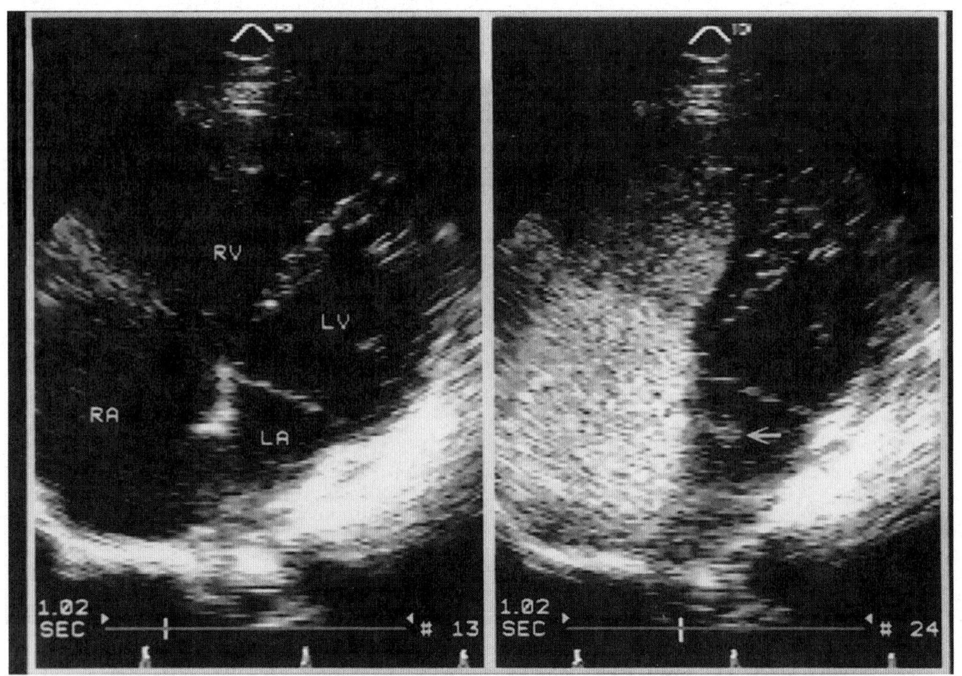


FIGURE 15-55 Contrast microbubble injection demonstrating a shunt (*arrow*) from the right atrium (RA) to left atrium (LA). RV = right ventricle; LV = left ventricle.

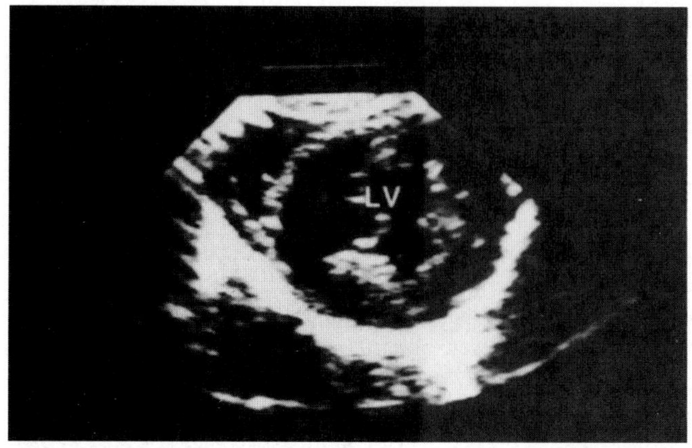


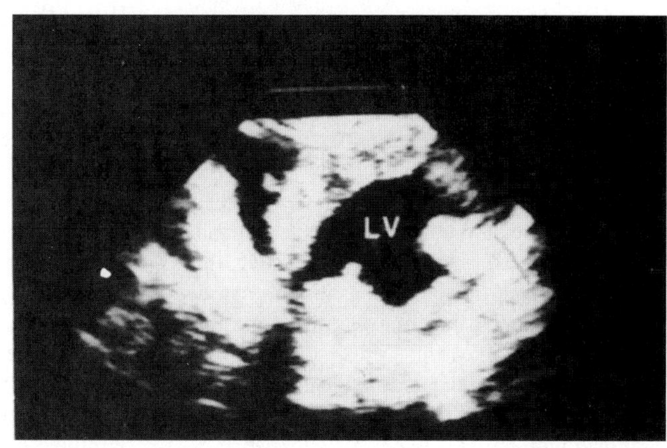


FIGURE 15-56 Short-axis plane through the left ventricle (LV) before (*left*) and after (*right*) injection of microbubbles into the aortic root. The myocardium is densely opacified on the right. (From Hagan AD, DeMaria AN. *Clinical Applications of Two-Dimensional Echocardiography and Cardiac Doppler.* Boston: Little, Brown; 1989. With permission.)

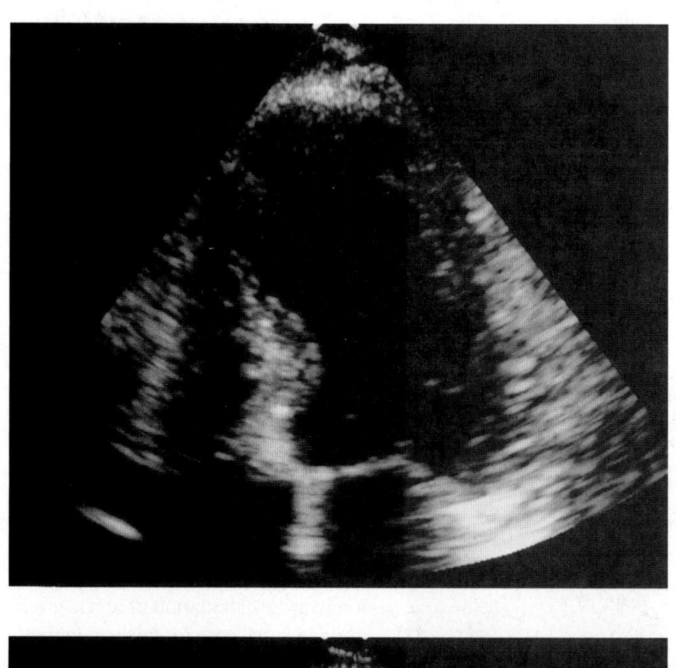

FIGURE 15-57 Harmonic imaging after intravenous injection of echocardiographic contrast. Endocardial border definition before injection is fair (*upper panel*) but is markedly improved with harmonic imaging following contrast injection (*lower panel*).

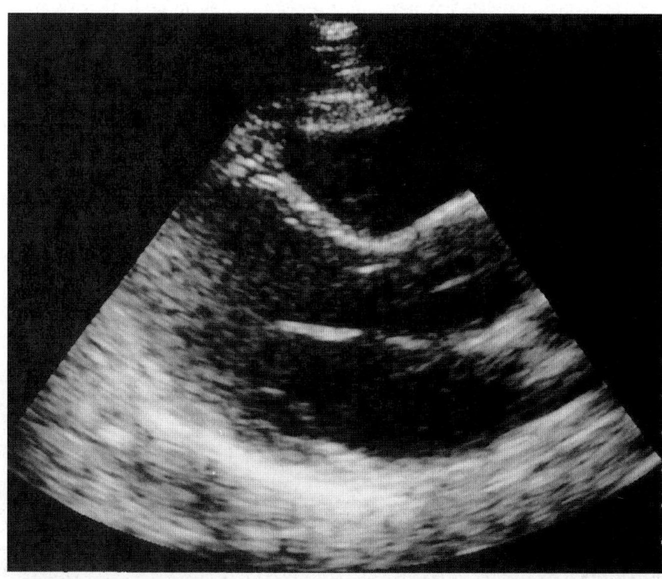

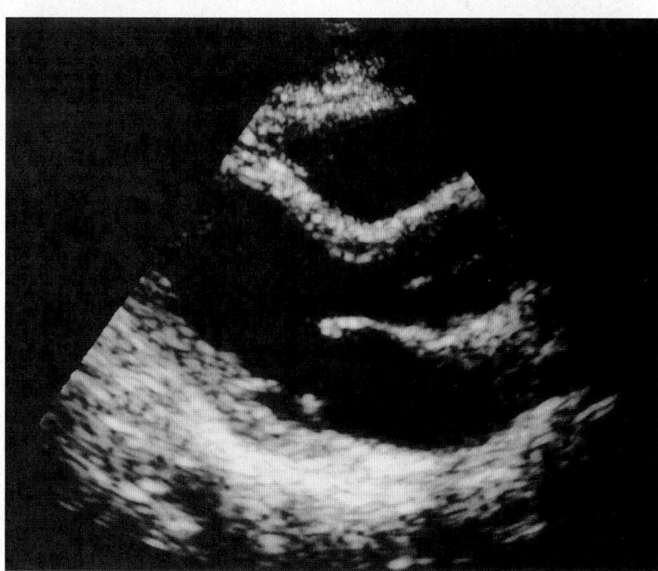

FIGURE 15-58 Tissue harmonic imaging. The upper panel shows a parasternal long-exis new figure view obtained with standard (fundamental) imaging. Endocardial definition is poor, but is markedly enhanced with tissue harmonic imaging (*lower panel*).

successfully transmitted pulses to derive images of moving blood or cardiac structures. Power Doppler techniques are especially well suited to detect the changing signals produced by movement and/or dissolution of contrast microbubbles.[47] Exposure to ultrasound energy can produce not only microbubble resonation but also destruction. Intermittent electrocardiographic (ECG-gated) imaging rather than continuous ultrasound transmission can also thereby prolong microbubble persistence and amplify contrast signals by limiting bubble destruction. Most recently, low power, real-time techniques have been developed that enable imaging of myocardial opacification without the need for ECG gating and intermittent imaging. When combined with the new ultrasonic contrast agents, these refined imaging modalities can achieve visualization of myocardial opacification following intravenous drug administration, thereby delineating myocardial perfusion.

Initial studies indicate that myocardial contrast echocardiography can yield information regarding myocardial perfusion comparable to that obtainable by radionuclide techniques and can be of value in delineating coronary artery stenoses.[135,136] Myocardial contrast echocardiography can identify infarct areas in AMI, document the absence of microcirculatory flow after epicardial coronary reperfusion ("no-reflow" phenomenon), and predict postinfarction viability.[129] Intravenous injection of contrast agents also permits visualization of intramyocardial vessels.[134,137] The ability to delineate regional myocardial perfusion is a major step forward in noninvasive imaging and can be expected to provide important information regarding coronary artery disease (CAD) in the near future.

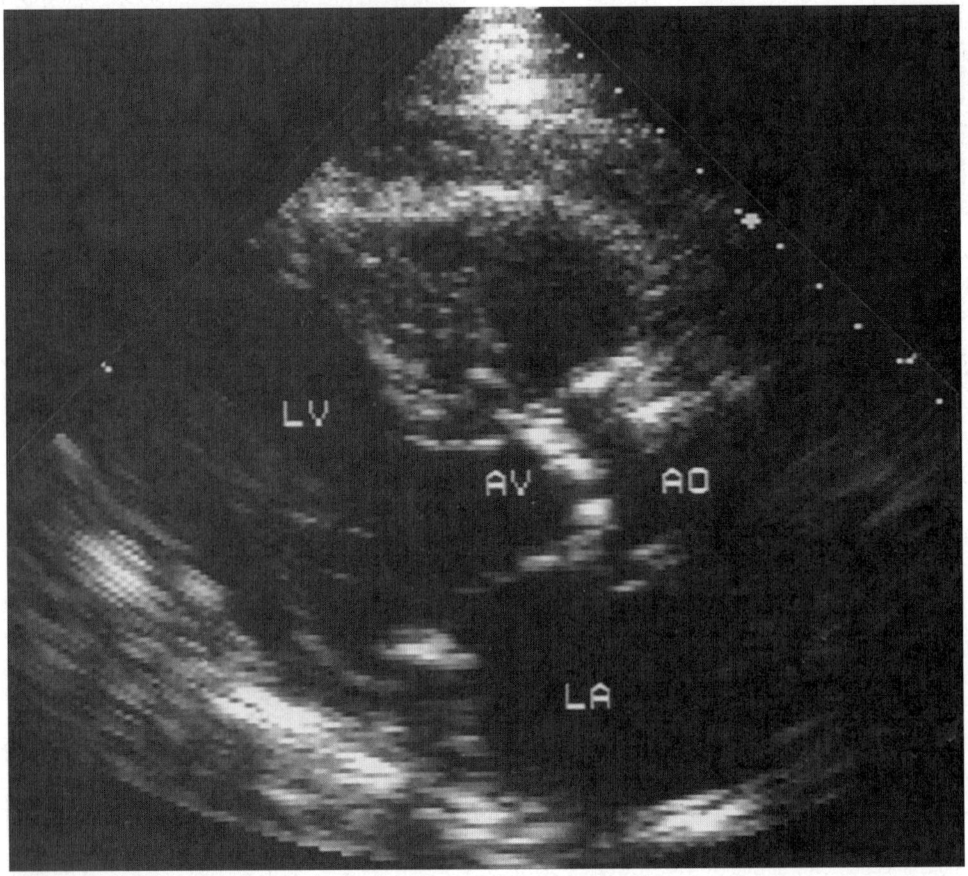

## DISEASES OF THE AORTIC VALVE AND AORTA

### Aortic Stenosis

The aortic valve is best imaged in the parasternal views.[138] The leaflets are thin, linear structures. All three can be visualized in the short-axis view and produce a triangular orifice during systolic opening. The long-axis view exhibits the right and usually the noncoronary leaflets, which normally open to the walls of the aorta. Mild thickening and reduction of mobility is often observed in the elderly (aortic sclerosis) and is associated with an increased risk of CAD. In older adults, acquired aortic stenosis (AS) is manifested by markedly thickened, often calcified, immobile aortic valve leaflets,[139] while doming of the leaflets suggests congenital aortic stenosis and is usually encountered in younger patients (Fig. 15-59). Echocardiography can distinguish valvular from sub- and supravalvular AS, can accurately identify bicuspid valves, and can delineate the presence of LVH.[140] Subaortic stenosis may be caused by asymmetrical septal hypertrophy with systolic anterior mitral motion, a subaortic membrane, or (less commonly) a subaortic tunnel. Bicuspid valves exhibit an oval rather than triangular orifice (Fig. 15-60). Although the severity of stenosis can be assessed semiquantitatively by 2D and M-mode image echocardiography, valvular calcification may shadow the leaflets or produce reverberations and obscure their motion.[139] Therefore, attempts to measure valve area by transthoracic planimetry have been unsuccessful, although multiplane TEE has been of greater value[109] (Fig. 15-61). Thus, 2D-echocardiographic imaging accurately detects the presence and etiology of AS but not the severity. Likewise, CFD demonstrates turbulent flow through the aortic valve and may guide continuous wave interrogation but provides little quantitative data. The use of Doppler echocardiography and the modified Bernoulli and continuity equations have now made noninvasive calculation of aortic gradients and valve area routine and have affected utilization of cardiac catheterization in AS patients (Chap. 66).

The cornerstone of the ultrasound evaluation of AS is CW Doppler interrogation through the aortic valve. The calculated gradient using the peak Doppler velocity [4(AS velocity)$^2$] correlates closely with the peak instantaneous gradient measured at catheterization[87,88] (Fig. 15-62). In interpreting echocardiographic studies, it is important to distinguish between the peak instantaneous pressure gradient, the mean gradient, and the peak-to-peak gradient. The first two physiologic parameters represent simultaneous pressure differences between LV and aorta and can be measured accurately by Doppler echocardiography. The *peak-to-peak gradient,* commonly used in the catheterization laboratory, compares the highest pressures reached in the LV and aorta (even though not

FIGURE 15-59 Parasternal long-axis plane demonstrating a thickened, stenotic aortic valve (AV). AO = aorta; LV = left ventricle; LA = left atrium.

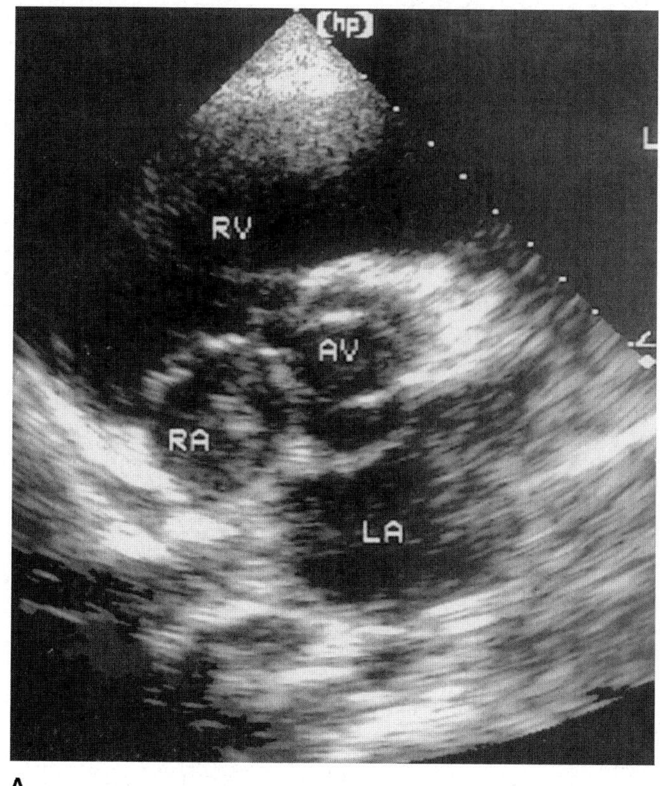


A

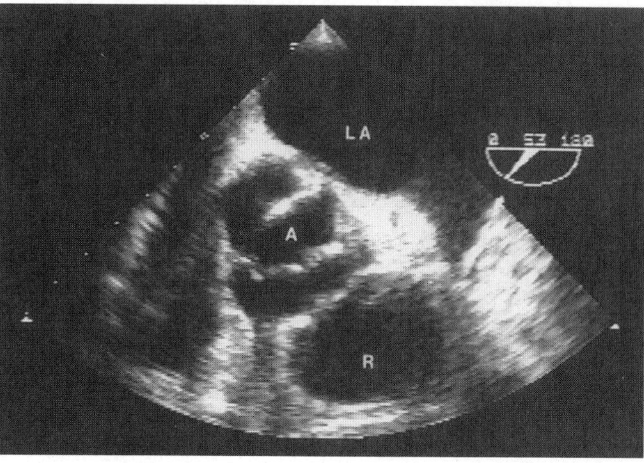


B

FIGURE 15-60 *A*. Parasternal short-axis image of a bicuspid aortic valve (AV) during systole. RV = right ventricle; RA = right atrium; LA = left atrium. *B*. Transesophageal image of a bicuspid aortic valve (A). LA = left atrium, R = right ventricular outflow tract. (From Blanchard DG, Kimura BJ, Dittrich HC, DeMaria AN. Transesophageal echocardiography of the aorta. *JAMA* 1994; 272:546–551. With permission.)

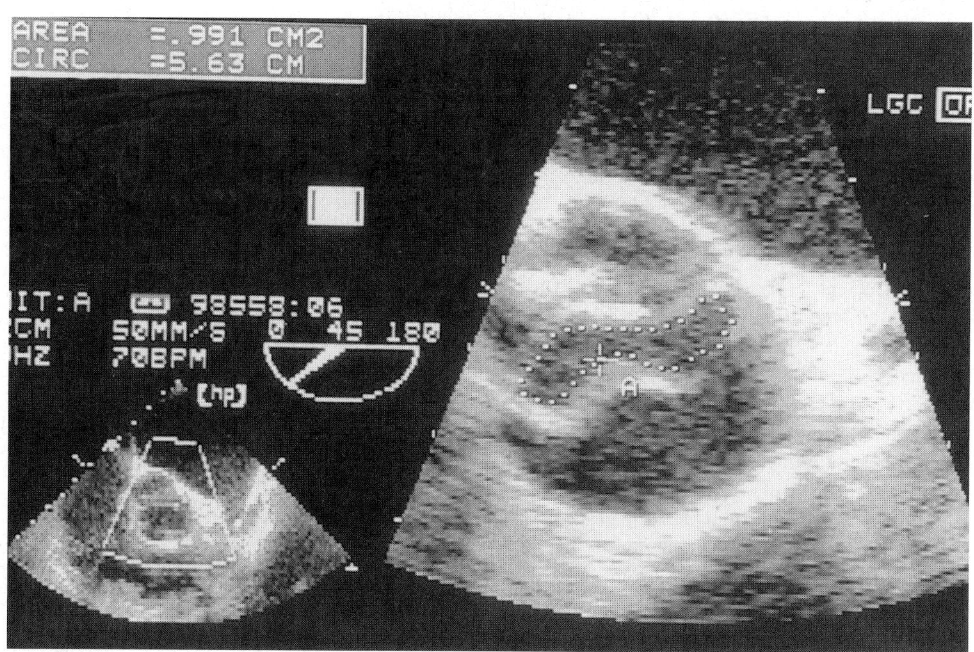


FIGURE 15-61 Transesophageal image of a stenotic bicuspid aortic valve (*A*) with superimposed planimetry of the valve area (approximately 1 $cm^2$).

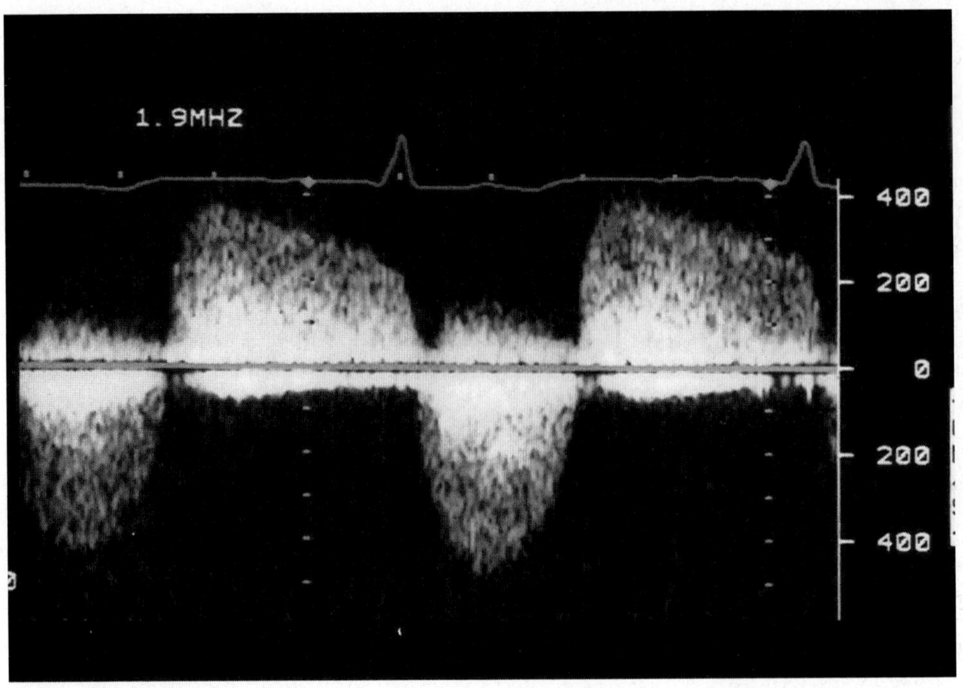


FIGURE 15-62 Continuous-wave Doppler tracing (from the apical transducer position) through the aortic valve in a case of combined aortic stenosis and insufficiency. The peak systolic velocity approaches 5 m/s.

simultaneous) and is uniformly lower than the peak instantaneous gradient recorded by Doppler. Therefore, the maximal Doppler gradient does not correlate with the peak-to-peak catheterization gradient, and comparisons between the two should be avoided (Chap. 66).

A number of potential sources of error exist in the estimation of the transvalvular aortic gradient by CW Doppler recordings. It is imperative that Doppler signals from the stenotic jet be obtained with an angle of incidence of less than 20 degrees. Since the direction of the jet rarely can be known with precision from 2D techniques, each examination must employ all possible windows and angulations, including apical, parasternal, and suprasternal transducer positions. Also, one must be careful to account for the proximal flow velocity in the Bernoulli equation if it is 1.5 m/s or greater. Finally, since some degree of pressure recovery occurs distal to the aortic valve leaflets, it is important to record continuous wave signals as close to these structures as possible. Values for the aortic valve area can be calculated using the continuity equation by measuring the velocity of the jet across the aortic valve with CW Doppler, the velocity in the LV outflow tract just proximal to the valve with PW Doppler, and by deriving the area of the outflow tract from the diameter of the aortic annulus. Results from the continuity equation have been found to correlate well with the area calculations based on catheterization data and the Gorlin formula.[85,86] CW Doppler can occasionally overestimate peak systolic pressure gradients, especially in patients with narrow aortic roots. As both AS jet velocity and aortic annular radius are squared in the continuity equation, accurate determination of these parameters is essential for reliable measurements. When atrial fibrillation is present, the peak Doppler velocity still correlates with peak instantaneous gradient through the aortic valve, but *calculations of valve area may be problematic,* as the outflow tract and peak aortic velocities are not measured simultaneously.

In summary, a comprehensive echocardiographic examination in a patient with AS should establish both the presence and severity of disease. Echocardiographic imaging should identify the structural abnormality involving either the subvalvular, valvular, or supravalvular area; distinguish congenital from acquired etiologies; and evaluate the state of LVH and function. CW Doppler recordings should provide accurate measurements of instantaneous and mean transaortic valvular gradients, and the continuity equation should provide reliable estimates of AoV area. In cases where the relative roles of orifice stenosis and LV dysfunction are uncertain, TEE imaging or Doppler recordings during inotropic stimulation with dobutamine may be of value.[109,141] In addition, dobutamine echocardiography is helpful in distinguishing high-risk patients with aortic stenosis and severe LV dysfunction. Cardiac catheterization is still necessary for the delineation of coronary anatomy.

## Aortic Regurgitation

In contrast to AS, the aortic valve leaflets are often anatomically normal by echocardiography in patients with aortic AR.[142] 2D and M-mode echocardiography often provide indirect evidence of the presence of AR, including signs of LV volume overload, diastolic fluttering of the anterior MV leaflet, aortic root enlargement, and incomplete coaptation of the aortic valve leaflets.[143] The important M-mode finding of premature diastolic closure of the MV prior to the onset of systole due to LV filling by the regurgitant jet signifies acute, severe AR (Fig. 15-63) and the need for surgery (Chap. 66).

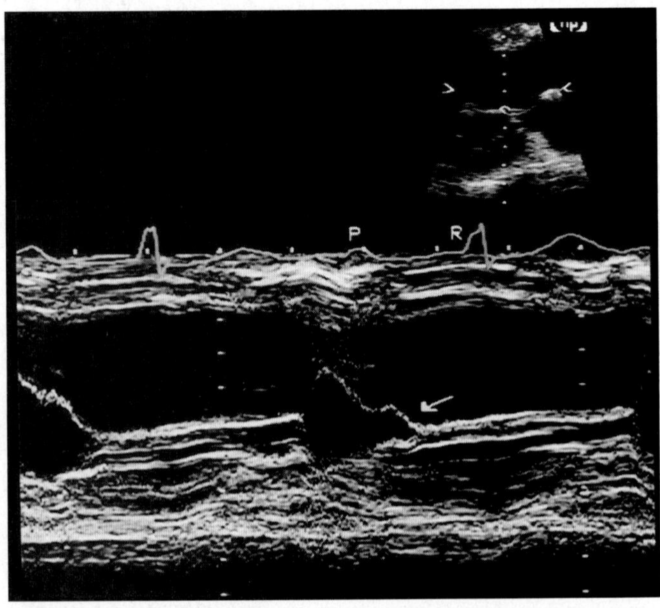


FIGURE 15-63 M-mode tracing (from the parasternal position) in a patient with acute severe aortic regurgitation. The mitral valve leaflets close (*arrow*) before ventricular contraction begins. P = p wave, R = QRS complex.

Perhaps the most important contribution of echocardiographic tissue imaging to the assessment of AR is in identifying the etiology. Thus, thickened leaflets that are restricted in movement are observed in patients with acquired AS, while oval doming of two functional leaflets will be observed in the presence of a bicuspid AoV (Fig. 15-60). AR due to infectious endocarditis can be identified by the presence of valvular vegetations, while regurgitation due to diseases of the aorta are manifest by anatomic changes of the vessel. Less common etiologies of AR, such as those associated with subvalvular pathology or ventricular septal defect, may also be recognized by echocardiographic imaging.

Although the findings yielded by echocardiographic imaging are useful, Doppler interrogation is necessary to obtain direct evidence of the presence and severity of AR. Screening with CFD demonstrates turbulent flow in the LV outflow tract during diastole in virtually all views[144] (Fig. 15-64*A*, *B*, and *C*, Plate 60). The jet is typically elliptical and may be located anywhere in the LV outflow tract. CW Doppler spectral recordings from this jet yield a high-velocity diastolic signal directed toward the apex (Fig. 15-62). Since AR jet velocity accurately reflects the diastolic pressure gradient between aorta and LV, it is maximum at the point of valve closure and decreases throughout diastole.[145] The flow pattern of AR may be readily distinguished from mitral inflow in that it is higher in velocity, begins immediately after aortic valve closure, generally has a much slower deceleration, and does not have an increased velocity following atrial contraction.

Several approaches exist for the quantitation of AR by echocardiography. Conventional echocardiographic imaging can provide evidence of the presence and extent of LV volume overload. More direct evidence of the severity of AR can be derived from the deceleration rate of the jet recorded by CW Doppler (Fig. 15-65).[145] In the presence of mild degrees of AR, the transvalvular pressure gradient will be maintained throughout diastole, creating a high-velocity jet with a minimal deceleration rate. Conversely, severe AR reduces aortic pressures and increases LV pressures in diastole, eliminating the pressure gradient and creating a rapid jet deceleration to a low velocity (Fig. 15-65). Severe, acute AR can also cause diastolic MR (Fig. 15-64*C*, Plate 58). The most common approach to assessing the deceleration rate of the AR jet is by calculating the time required for the velocity to fall to one-half of the maximal pressure equivalent, a technique similar to the pressure half-time measurements performed in the quantitation of mitral stenosis (MS). Previous studies have

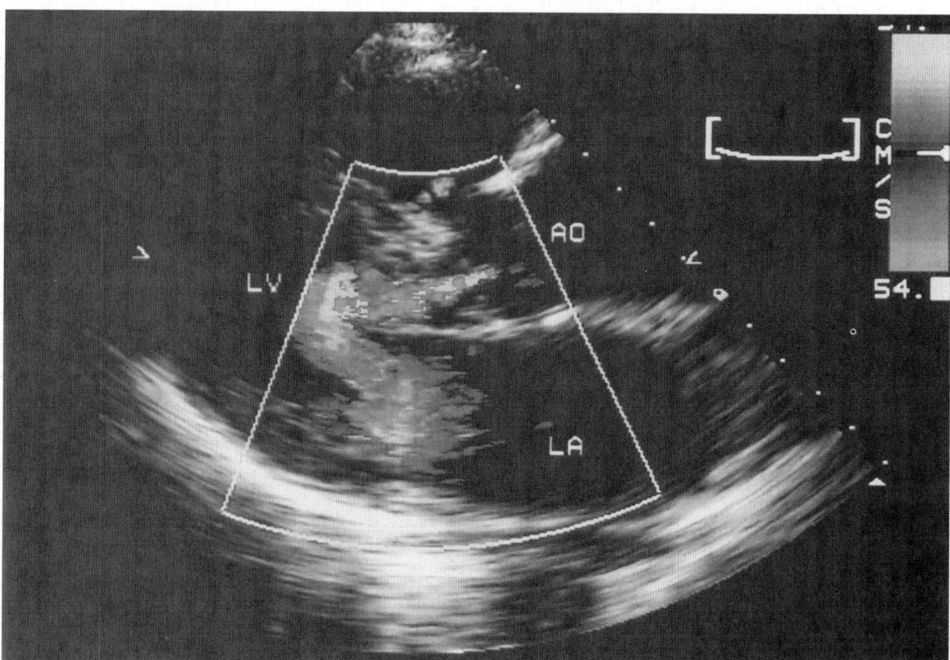


A

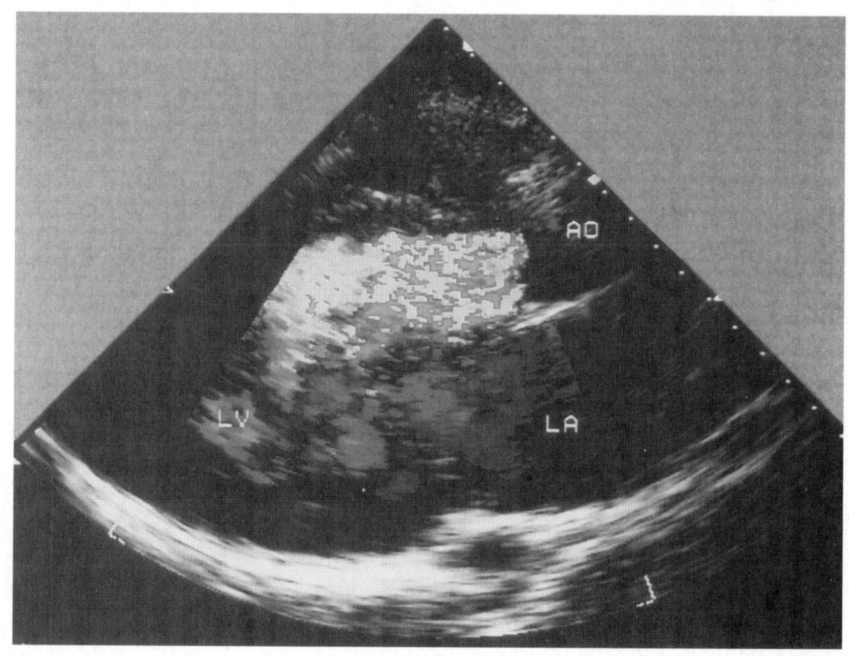


B

FIGURE 15-64 (Plate 58) *A*. Parasternal long-axis plane showing a multicolor jet (indicating turbulent flow) of aortic regurgitation in the left ventricular outflow tract. The jet is narrow in width, suggesting mild regurgitation. AO = aorta; LA = left atrium; LV = left ventricle. *B*. Parasternal long-axis plane with color-flow Doppler imaging. The aortic regurgitant (AR) color jet is as wide as the left ventricular outflow tract, suggesting severe AR. AO = aorta; LA = left atrium; LV = left ventricle. *C*. Parasternal long-axis image of acute severe aortic regurgitation (AI). The accompanying marked elevation of left ventricular (LV) diastolic pressure causes diastolic mitral regurgitation (MR). AO = aorta; LA = left atrium.

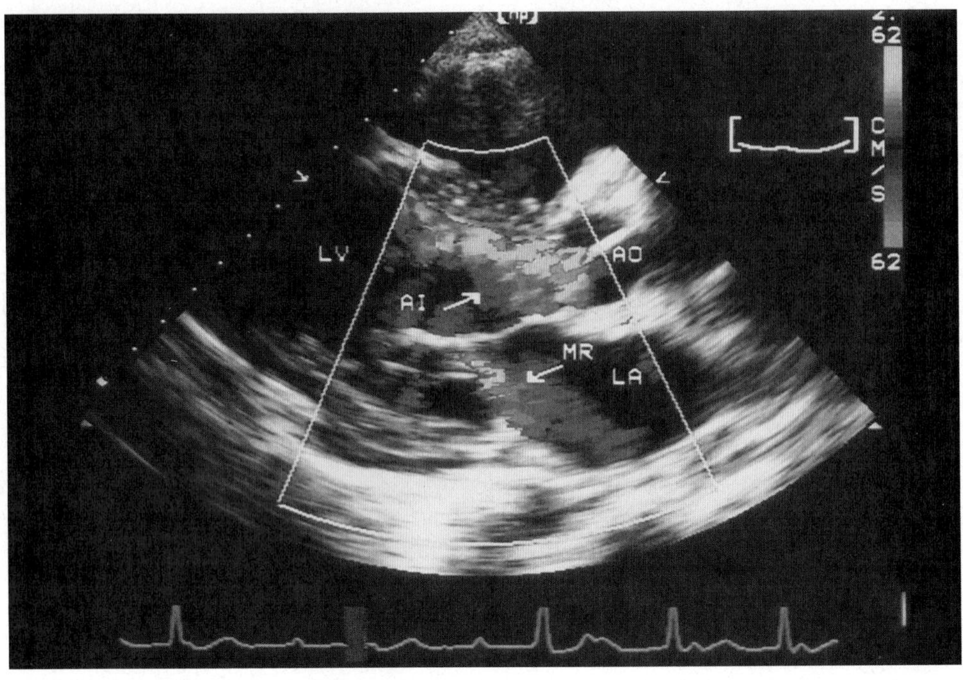


C

FIGURE 15-64 (*Continued*)

demonstrated that a pressure half-time of less than 250 ms reliably identifies patients with severe degrees of AR as assessed by invasive methods. Application of the pressure half-time approach to quantifying AR must take into account that, since the deceleration rate is a reflection of pressure gradient, it is determined by both the volume of AR and the LV compliance. Accordingly, ventricles that vary greatly in stiffness or distensibility will yield different AR deceleration rates for the same regurgitant volume.

The estimate of severity most commonly derived from echocardiography is the size of the AR jet by CFD.[144] Conceptually, jets that are distributed over a small area of the LV outflow tract represent lesser degrees of AR than jets that penetrate widely and to the level

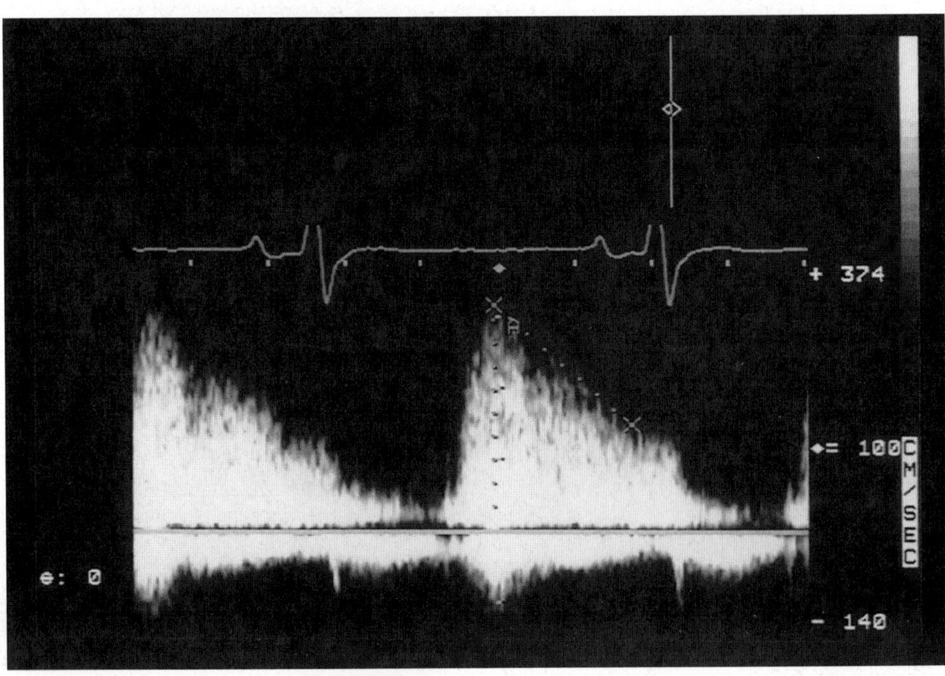


FIGURE 15-65 Continuous-wave Doppler tracing (from the apical transducer position) of severe AR. The pressure half-time of the AR envelope is approximately 200 ms.

of the papillary muscles. Some studies have demonstrated a general correlation between jet length and severity of AR.[146] The optimal results have been obtained when the width of the AR jet just proximal to the valve was expressed as a percentage of the width of the LV outflow tract; a jet occupying 50 percent or more of the outflow tract correlates with severe regurgitation by angiography.[144] Quantitation of AR based upon the size of the flow disturbance is subject to errors induced by the other factors that influence jet area: transvalvular pressure gradient, volume and compliance of the receiving chamber, regurgitant orifice, the Coanda effect (wall effect), and technical factors relating to the operator and instrument settings. In addition, entrainment and displacement of RBCs in the LV outflow tract also influence the size of the regurgitant jet. Finally, convergence of AR with normal transmitral filling may obscure the flow disturbance. Therefore, assessment of the severity of AR by analysis of the size and shape of the flow disturbance *is at best semiquantitative.*

The AR volume can be estimated by comparing volumetric measurements of LV inflow and LV outflow calculated from annular velocity and cross-sectional area (derived from pulsed Doppler and 2D images respectively).[84] This method is contingent upon the absence of valvular stenosis and of other regurgitant lesions. In the setting of AR, the volume ejected through the aortic annulus represents both systemic flow and regurgitant volume, while the volume coursing through the mitral annulus represents only systemic flow. Thereby, LV outflow will exceed LV inflow by the amount of the regurgitant volume.[84,147] This technique can provide useful estimates of regurgitant volume, but with any flow volume calculation by echocardiography, errors in technique and the assumptions involved in volume calculation can result in significant errors. An alternate *quantitative approach* derives estimates of regurgitant fraction from reverse diastolic flow in the aorta.[148] Assuming a constant cross-sectional aortic area, comparison of integrated flow velocities during forward systolic flow and retrograde diastolic flow should yield an estimate of regurgitant fraction. Although this is somewhat imprecise, the presence of a significant flow reversal in the aorta visualized by color or spectral Doppler is a reliable marker of severe AR (Fig. 15-66).

Determination of the optimal timing of surgical intervention in patients with AR remains a difficult problem in clinical medicine (Chap. 66). Several criteria derived from echocardiographic recordings have been proposed to guide this decision. Most prominently, an LV end-systolic dimension of 55 mm or greater with a shortening fraction of 25 percent or less have been advocated as sufficient criteria for surgical intervention in the absence of symptoms. However, no universally accepted echocardiographic criteria exist by which to determine the optimal role for surgical treatment.

## Diseases of the Aorta

The thoracic aorta is best visualized from the left and right parasternal positions and from the suprasternal notch. The descending aorta may also be imaged from subcostal and modified apical views. Normally, short-axis images of the aortic root yield a circular structure, while long-axis images exhibit two parallel linear walls with a maximal diameter of 35 mm.[149] Although 2D imaging is used most commonly, M-mode recordings of the aortic root facilitate precise measurement of its dimensions.

### AORTIC DISSECTION

Echocardiography has dramatically changed the diagnostic approach to aortic dissection. TTE is a convenient screening test (Fig. 15-67) and often enables accurate detection of ascending aortic dissection. The diagnostic findings include a dilated aorta with a mobile intimal flap that presents as a thin, linear signal within the lumen. Transthoracic imaging is unreliable for detection of descending aortic dissection, although it occasionally visualizes the complete length of the thoracic aorta (Chap. 98).

Although several noninvasive methods exist to diagnose aortic dissection, TEE has become the procedure of choice in many

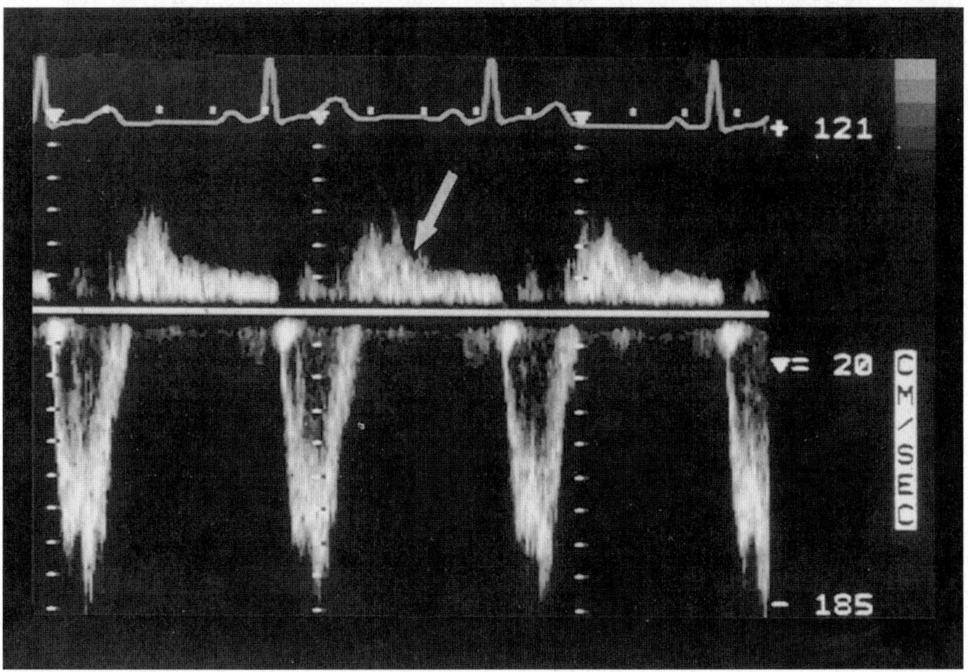


FIGURE 15-66 Pulsed-wave Doppler tracing (from the suprasternal transducer position) in a case of severe aortic regurgitation. The sample volume is in the descending thoracic aorta, and holodiastolic flow reversal (*arrow*) is present.

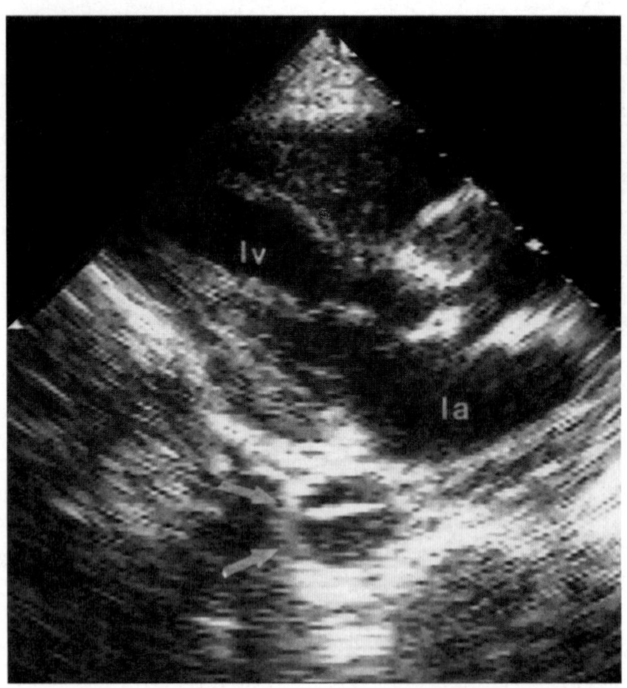


FIGURE 15-67 Transthoracic parasternal long-axis plane demonstrating a dissection of the descending thoracic aorta. The aortic root is dilated, the aortic valve is thickened, and an intimal flap is present in the descending aorta (*arrows*). LV = left ventricle; LA = left atrium.

hospitals because of its accuracy, portability, rapid procedural time, and ability to provide data regarding valvular regurgitation and LV function.[99,111,150,151] Except for *a short portion of the proximal aortic arch,* which is obscured by the bronchus, multiplane TEE provides excellent visualization of the entire thoracic aorta and high accuracy in detecting aortic enlargement, intimal tears, and false lumen thrombus (Fig. 15-68). CFD may reveal communications between true and false channels (Fig. 15-51, Plate 57; Fig. 15-69, Plate 59). TEE also appears useful for the diagnosis of aortic intramural hematoma, an increasingly recognized disorder which has a clinical prognosis similar to that of classic dissection. In this disorder, hemorrhage occurs within the aortic media, but an intimal tear (and a dissection flap) is absent. The finding of a curvilinear, asymmetric density within the aortic wall in a patient with typical symptoms of dissection strongly suggests a diagnosis of aortic intramural hematoma.[152]

## AORTIC ANEURYSM

Aneurysms of the aorta may be saccular or fusiform and are recognized as localized or circumferential areas of aortic enlargement, often with thin walls. TTE is especially useful in detecting ascending aortic dilatation but can also visualize descending thoracic and abdominal aortic aneurysms.[149,153] Echocardiography has been used extensively to assess aortic pathology in patients with Marfan's syndrome.[154] The nature of the lesion is relatively specific in that there is symmetrical dilatation of the annulus, sinuses of Valsalva, and aortic root (Fig. 15-70*A*). Aortic leaflet coaptation may be compromised leading to AR. Echocardiography is helpful in determining prognosis and optimal timing of aortic root replacement.

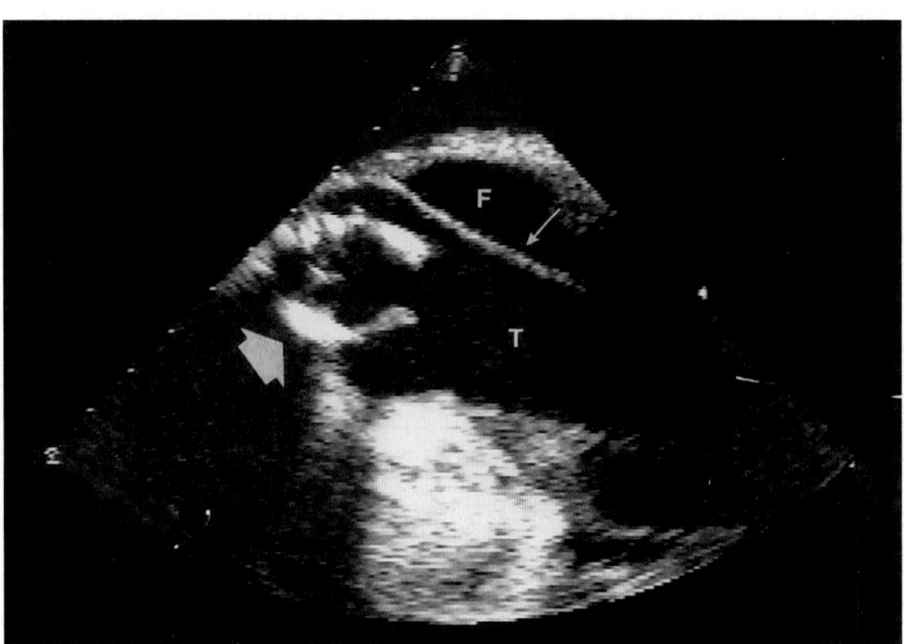


FIGURE 15-68 Longitudinal TEE view of an ascending aortic dissection in a patient with a porcine prosthetic valve in the aortic position (*large arrow*). The false (F) and true (T) lumens are separated by an intimal flap (*small arrow*). (From Blanchard DG, Kimura BJ, Dittrich HC, DeMaria AN. Transesophageal echocardiography of the aorta. *JAMA* 1994;272:546–551. With permission.)

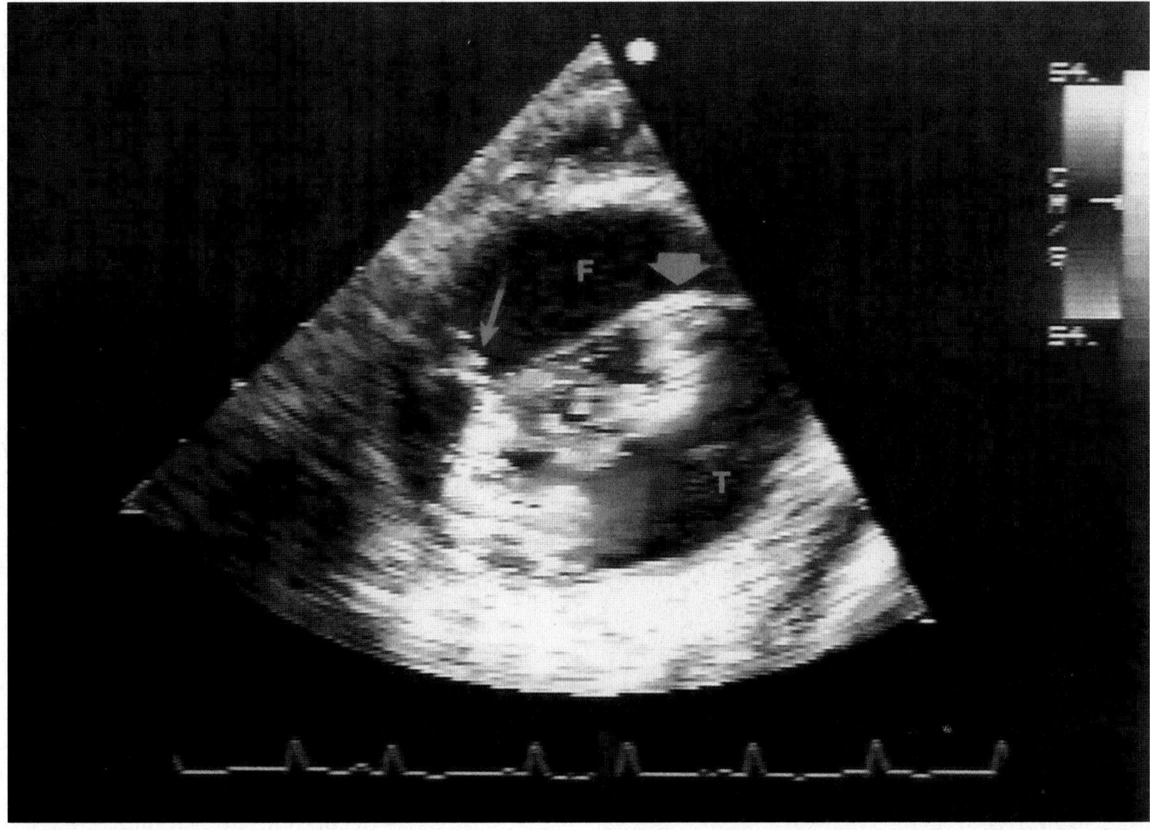


FIGURE 15-69 (Plate 59) Transverse TEE view of an aortic dissection. The false (F) and true (T) lumens are separated by an intimal flap (*large arrow*). The communication between the two channels is visible (*small arrow*).

Sinus of Valsalva aneurysms are also well visualized by both TTE and TEE.[155] These lesions cause asymmetric dilatation of the aortic root and seem to affect the right coronary sinus most frequently. They are prone to rupture, often into the right heart (Fig. 15-70*B*, Plate 60). Doppler echocardiography in such settings demonstrates fluttering of the TV, a color jet crossing from the aortic root into the right heart, and occasionally diastolic opening of the PV.

Congenital aortic disease, such as supravalvular aortic stenosis (SAS), aortic coarctation, patent ductus arteriosus, and truncus arteriosus also can be detected with echocardiography (see "Congenital Heart Disease," below, as well as Chaps. 63 and 64).[140] In these conditions, suprasternal and transesophageal imaging are often helpful. SAS is recognized as an "hourglass" narrowing or a discrete fibrous ridge just distal to the leaflets, while coarctation presents a more localized, abrupt luminal reduction in the descending aorta or distal portion of the aortic arch. Patent ductus arteriosus and truncus arteriosus are often best identified by virtue of the accompanying flow disturbance on CFD.[156]

A

FIGURE 15-70A Parasternal long-axis plane demonstrating severe aortic root (AO) enlargement. LV = left ventricle; LA = left atrium. (Courtesy of Kirk L. Peterson, MD.)

## AORTIC ATHEROSCLEROSIS

As mentioned in the section on TEE, recent studies suggest that aortic atherosclerosis is an important cause of stroke and embolic events.[113] Mobile and protruding intimal plaques have been detected by TEE (Fig. 15-53) in patients with stroke with a prevalence greater than in controls, a finding not previously appreciated by other imaging techniques. Optimal treatment for extensive aortic atherosclerosis is currently unknown, although warfarin appears useful.[115,157] It appears that the presence of aortic arch plaques and atherosclerosis increase the risk of perioperative stroke.[158] Given this, discovery of such plaques prior to cardiopulmonary bypass should prompt adjustment of cannula placement to avoid dislodging the aortic debris.

Penetrating aortic ulceration, which affects the descending aorta and mimics the clinical syndrome of acute aortic dissection, may also

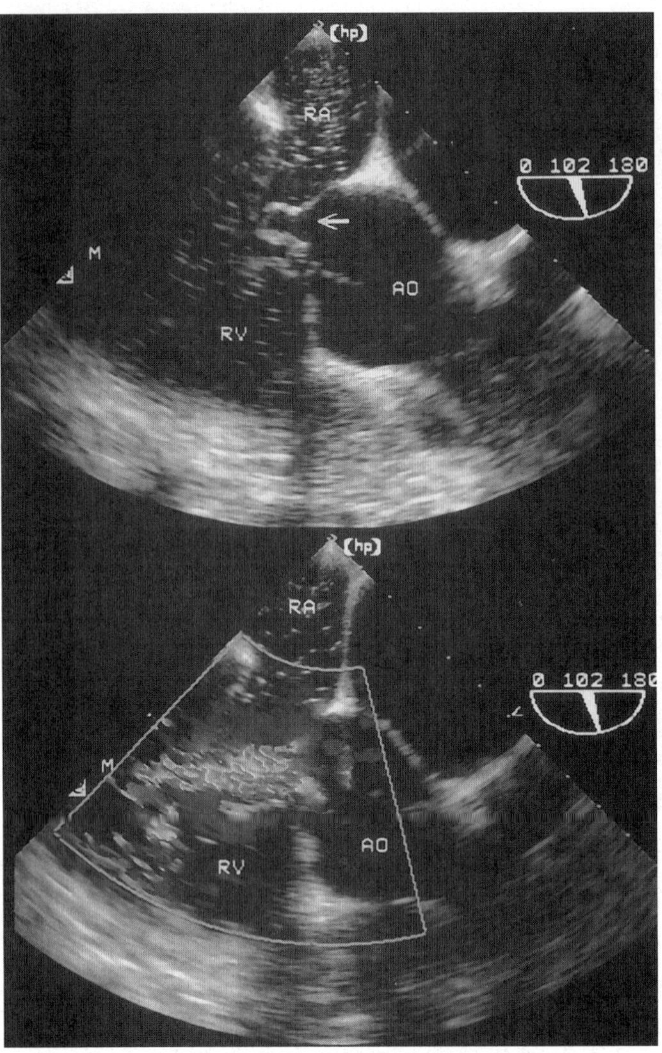


B

FIGURE 15-70B (Plate 60) TEE image of a ruptured sinus of Valsalva aneurysm. The upper image shows focal aneurysmal dilatation of the right coronary sinus with the appearance of a "windsock." Color Doppler (*lower image*) reveals a high-velocity flow jet from the aorta into the right ventricle. Agitated saline was injected intravenously to highlight right heart structures.

be diagnosed by TEE (Fig. 15-71, Plate 61). The diagnosis is based on visualization of a localized defect with protrusion of the ulcer into the vessel wall (in the absence of dissection). This disease entity, which occurs in the setting of atherosclerosis, warrants urgent surgery to avoid aortic rupture. Aortic tears induced by trauma are also accurately detected by TEE (Fig. 15-72).

## DISEASES OF THE MITRAL VALVE

### Mitral Stenosis

Detection of *mitral stenosis* (MS) was one of the earliest clinical applications of echocardiography[159] (see Chap. 67). In most individuals, the MV leaflets are easily visualized and yield thin linear echoes that exhibit wide bipeaked excursions as they open in early and late diastole.[26] The characteristic 2D ultrasound findings of MS are seen clearly in nearly all patients with this disorder.[160] The MV leaflets are thickened and often present bright, high-intensity reflections indicating calcification. The process may involve thickening and shortening of the chordal apparatus as well. There are varying degrees of commissural fusion restricting mitral leaflet separation, especially at the distal tips. This leads to diastolic "doming" or a right-angle bend of the anterior MV leaflet as high LA pressure creates a bulge in the leaflet's midportion (which is generally more pliable than the distal portion) (Fig. 15-73). The posterior leaflet actually may be pulled anteriorly during diastole because of commissural fusion with the longer anterior leaflet. Mitral doming may also occur in congenital valvular disease, but it is not seen when mitral leaflet opening is reduced due to low-flow states[34] or AR jets. The LA is nearly always enlarged with MS.

The effects of stenosis upon MV motion are often best demonstrated by M-mode recordings (Fig. 15-74). In addition to leaflet thickening and reduced excursion, M-mode tracings also depict a characteristic decrease in the reclosure rate of the anterior mitral leaflet in early diastole (reduced E-F slope) due to a persistent LA-LV pressure gradient and a slow rate of LV filling. The decrease of the E-F slope has been found to correlate grossly with the severity of MS. This finding is not specific for MS, however, and may occur whenever early diastolic filling is reduced.[26] Attempts to calculate the area of the MV orifice using the E-F slope have proved unsatisfactory.

The entire perimeter of the MV orifice can be visualized in the 2D parasternal short-axis view, and mitral leaflet excursion normally approaches the endocardial borders of the LV at the mitral tip level. In the setting of MS, the thickened leaflets form a fish-mouth orifice, which occupies only a small portion of the cross-sectional area of the left ventricle (Chap. 67).[160] Measurements of the area of the MV orifice may be obtained by planimetry of the orifice visualized in the parasternal short-axis view and correlate well with those obtained by cardiac catheterization (Fig. 15-73). Since the shape of the MV resembles that of a funnel, it is crucial to identify the smallest cross-sectional area and obtain recordings with orthogonal beam orientation at that point in order to avoid overestimation. Optimal gain settings must be employed to avoid encroachment of tissue signals upon the orifice.[161]

Doppler examination provides additional quantitation of MS.[162] Interrogation of mitral inflow with either PW or CW modes (depending on velocity and Nyquist limit) reveals elevated diastolic velocities, with a reduction in the rate of deceleration in early diastole yielding a pattern similar to the decreased E-F slope seen with M-mode in MS (Fig. 15-75). In a fashion similar to that of AS, the maximal gradient across the MV can be calculated from the peak diastolic velocity utilizing the Bernoulli equation. But since the maximal transmitral gradient is very sensitive to changes in heart rate and loading, the mean transmitral gradient obtained as the average of a number of individual gradients derived throughout diastole is customarily utilized to assess the severity of MS. In addition, Doppler technique may provide estimates of MV area (MVA) by means of the calculation of the pressure half-time.[162] The pressure half-time represents the interval required for transmitral velocity to decelerate from its highest point (E) to a velocity that yields one-half of the pressure equivalent (Fig. 15-75). As the severity of MS increases, the rate of deceleration decreases, prolonging the pressure half-time. Further, dividing an empiric constant of 220[163] by the pressure half-time yields an estimate of MVA, which correlates with values obtained during cardiac catheterization. Since Doppler estimates of MVA are indirect and involve the use of empiric constants, they are considered less accurate than direct measurements of MVA derived

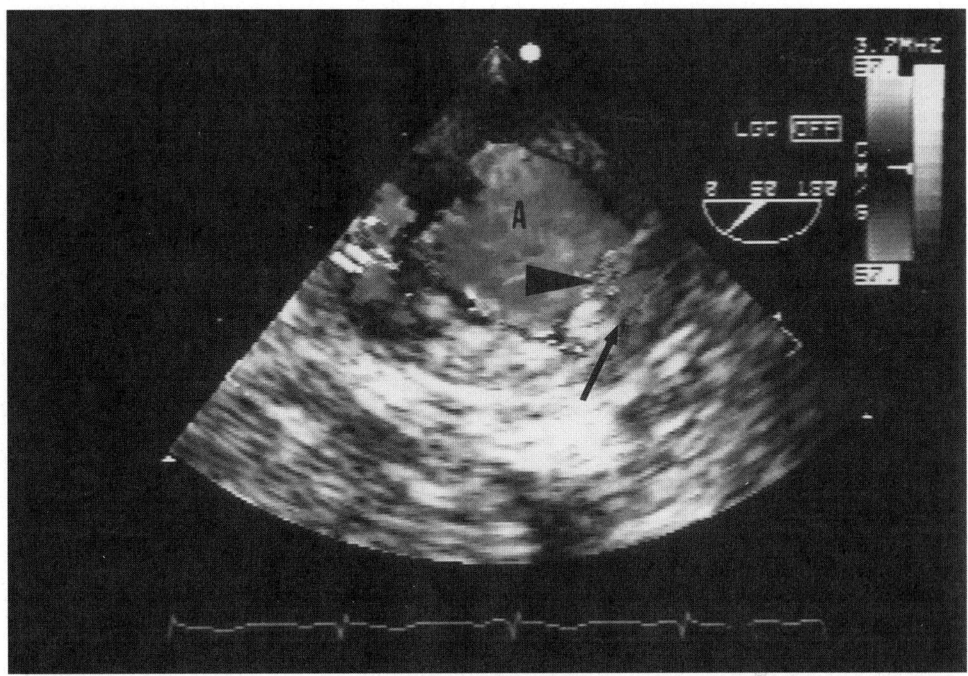


FIGURE 15-71 (Plate 61) Transverse TEE view of penetrating ulceration in the proximal portion of the descending aorta (A). The mouth of the ulcer crater is visible (*large arrowhead*), as is blood flow within the atheroma (*arrow*).

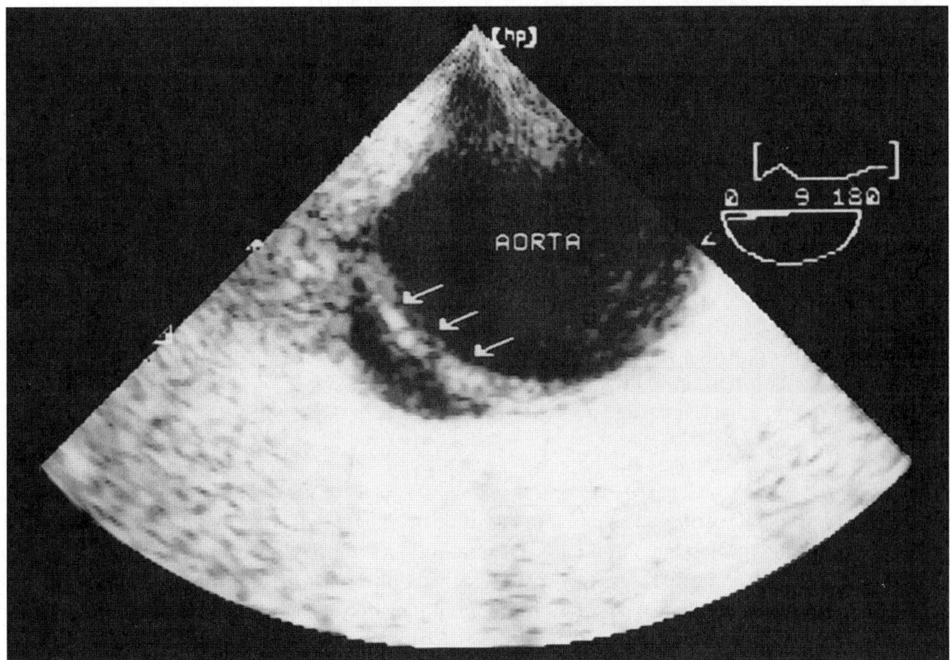


FIGURE 15-72 Transverse TEE image of traumatic aortic disruption and partial transection (*arrows*) involving the distal portion of the aortic arch.

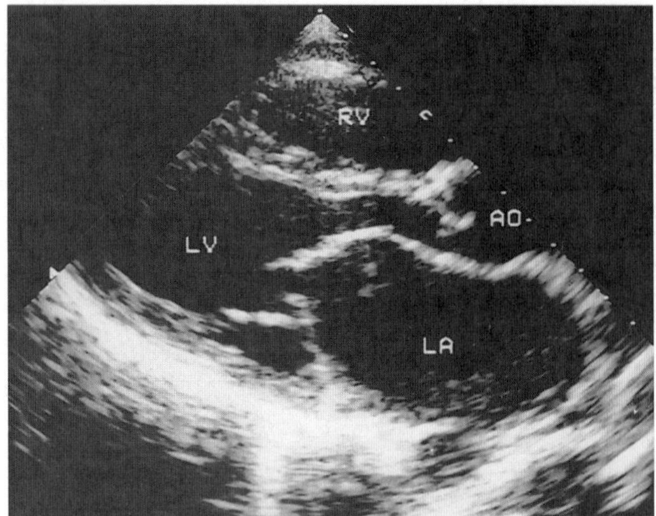


A

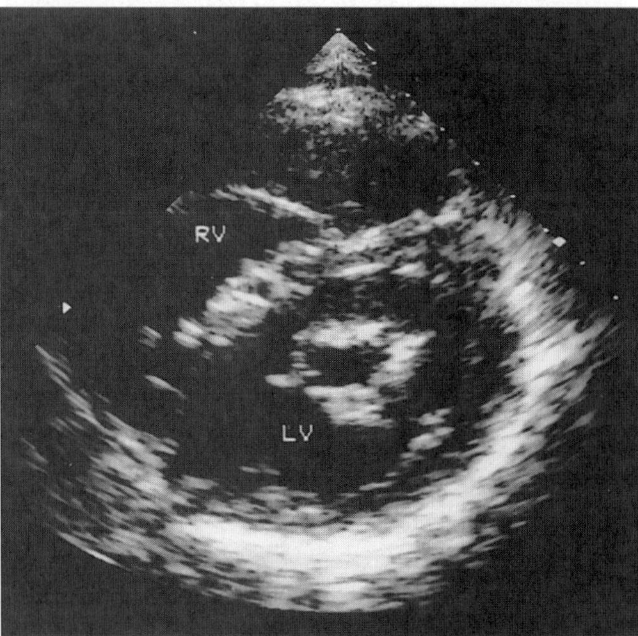


C

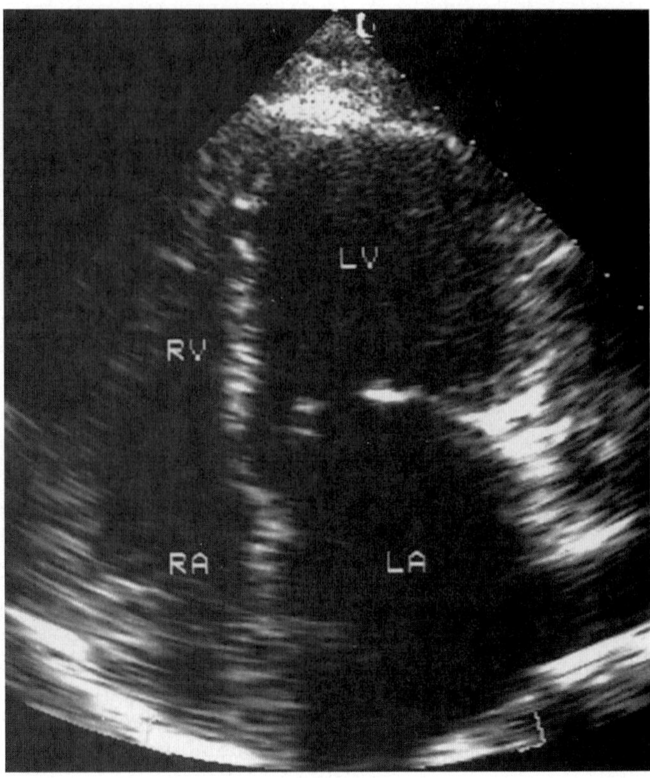


B

FIGURE 15-73 *A*. Parasternal long-axis view of MS. The left atrium (LA) is enlarged, mitral opening is limited, and "doming" of the anterior mitral leaflet is present. LV = left ventricle; RV = right ventricle; AO = aorta. *B*. Apical four-chamber view in mitral stenosis. The left artium is markedly dilated. RA = right atrium. *C*. Parasternal short-axis plane in mitral stenosis. *D*. Transesophageal image showing doming of the anterior mitral valve leaflet.

by planimetry of the MV orifice. The pressure half-time method is inaccurate immediately following mitral commissurotomy.

Echocardiography can help assess the feasibility and appropriateness of percutaneous catheter balloon mitral commissurotomy (CBMC) to treat individual patients with MS[164] (Chap. 46). An echocardiographic scoring system based on evaluation of mitral valvular thickening, calcification, mobility, and subvalvular involvement has been devised. Each variable is assigned a grade of 1 (minimal involvement) to 4 (severe), with a maximal score of 16. Although the prognostic capability of this method is limited, the outcome of balloon valvuloplasty in patients with higher scores, particularly greater than 12, is less satisfactory and involves a higher risk of complications than in patients with lower scores.[164] Therefore echocardiographic analysis is an important part of the decision-making process prior to CBMC. Preprocedural TEE is also often performed to detect left atrial thrombi, which can embolize during transseptal catheterization.[165] Following CBMC, echocardiography can identify complications including MR and atrial septal defect.

## Mitral Regurgitation

Although echocardiography is extremely accurate in the detection of mitral (and aortic) regurgitation, *quantitation* is more difficult. 2D imaging alone does not provide direct evidence of MR but usually reveals the etiology of the lesion.[166] Thus, 2D echocardiography reveals thickened, restricted leaflets in rheumatic disease, vegetations in infective endocarditis, flail mitral leaflets with torn chordae, and redundant leaflets with abnormal coaptation in MV prolapse. 2D echocardiography can also detect LA and LV abnormalities associated with MR, such as myxoma, papillary muscle dysfunction, and dilated cardiomyopathy. In addition, enlargement of these chambers offers indirect evidence of the severity of MR. In cases of chronic, severe MR, 2D echocardiography can also discern the presence of depressed LV function and decreased ejection fraction (Chap. 67).

Doppler echocardiography is the primary method for the detection and evaluation of MR[167–169] and reveals a disturbed flow jet in the LA during systole. Spectral Doppler recordings provide several indexes of severity, which are of semiquantitative value. Since the intensity of the Doppler signal is a function of the number of red blood cells (RBCs) in the sample volume, the videodensity of the jet correlates in a general way with regurgitant volume. Similarly, an increase

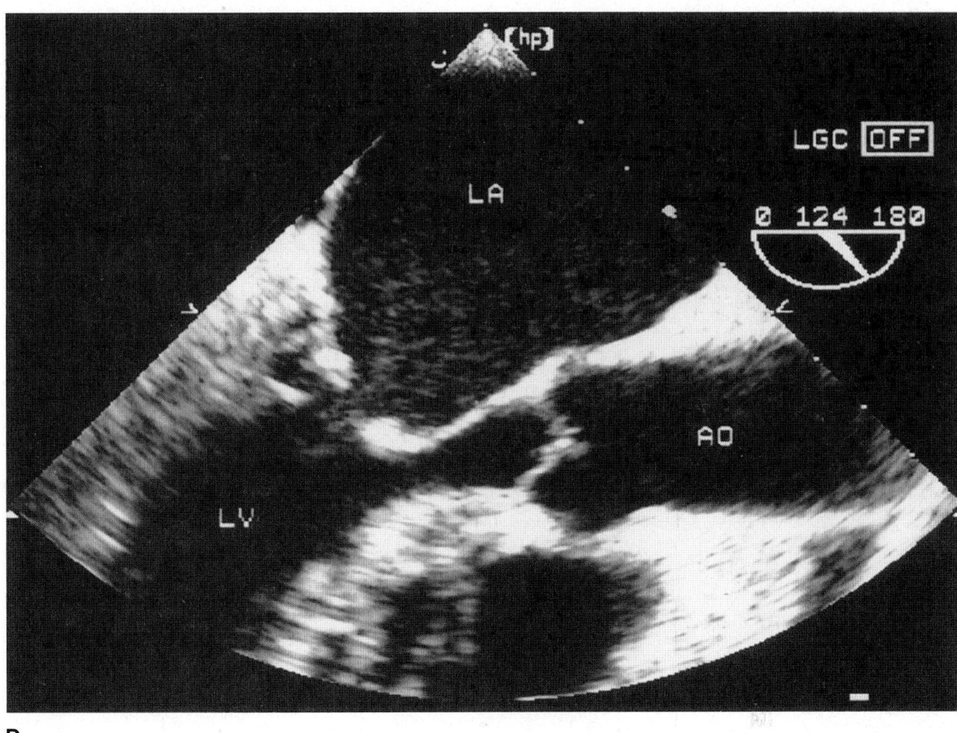


**D**

FIGURE 15-73 (*Continued*)

in transmitral filling velocities reflects increased forward flow and suggests a large regurgitant volume.[167] Measurements obtainable from the envelope of the CW Doppler recording of the MR jet include a slow rate of acceleration, indicative of a diminished LV $dP/dt$ (Fig. 15-76). Early peaking followed by rapid deceleration of the MR jet suggests a large V wave, increased left atrial pressure, and usually acute severe MR.

As in the case of AR, volumetric calculations of LV inflow and outflow by combined pulsed Doppler and 2D echocardiographic imaging techniques can be used to derive measurements of regurgitant volume.[168] In the case of MR, transmitral filling represents both systemic and regurgitant volume, while aortic outflow represents only systemic flow. Therefore mitral filling should exceed left ventricular ejection, and the difference will be regurgitant volume.

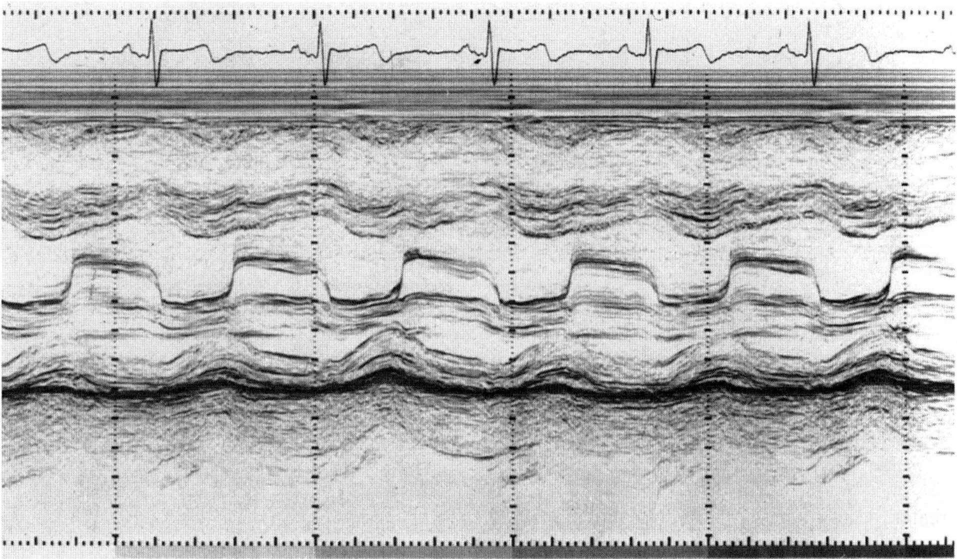

FIGURE 15-74 Parasternal M-mode image through the mitral valve in a patient with mitral stenosis. The normal rapid downslope of the anterior mitral leaflet after early rapid diastolic filling is absent.

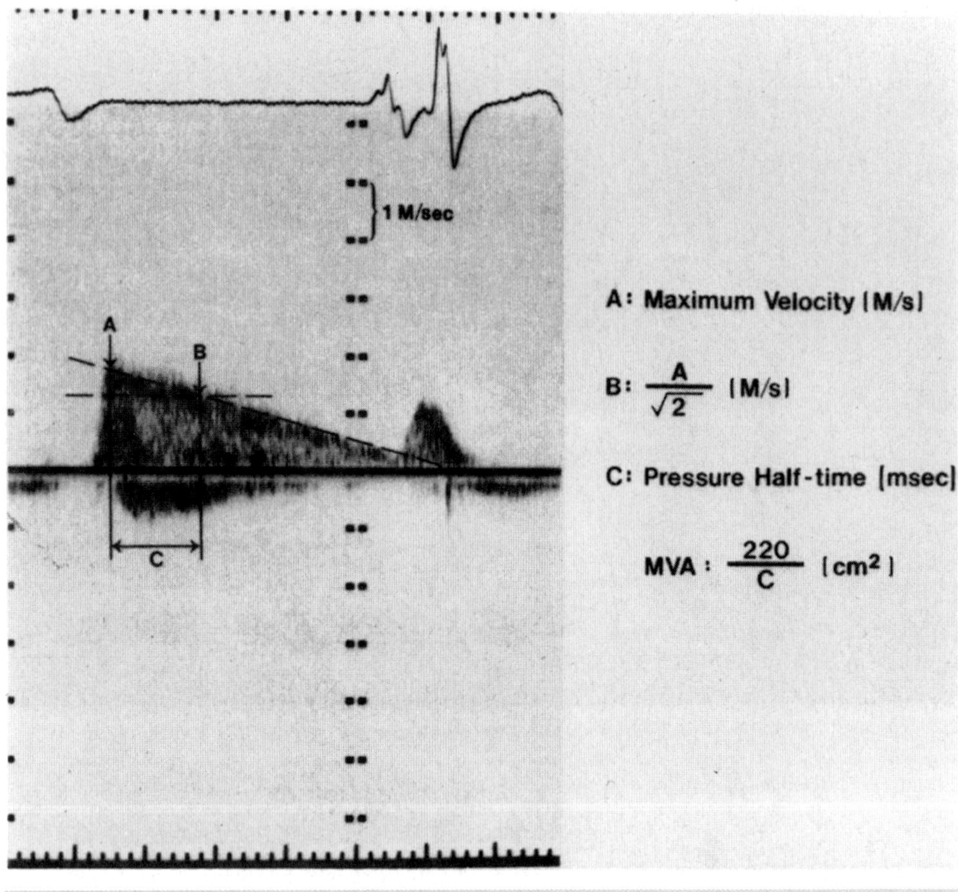


FIGURE 15-75 Pressure half-time method for calculation of mitral valve area (MVA). (From Hagan AD, DeMaria AN. *Clinical Applications of Two-Dimensional Echocardiography and Cardiac Doppler.* Boston: Little, Brown; 1989. With permission.)

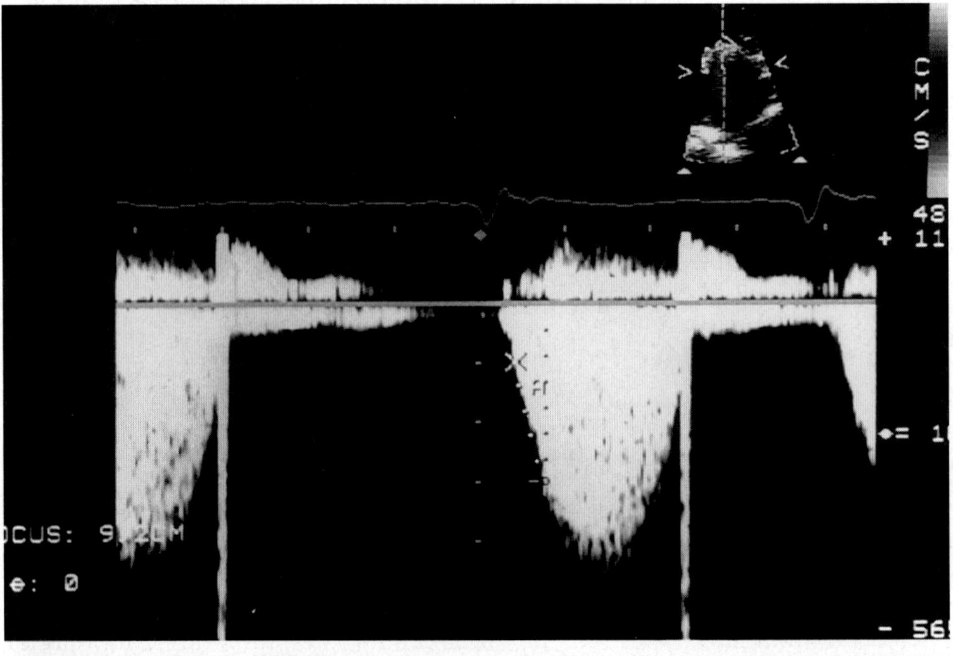


FIGURE 15-76 Continuous-wave tracing of mitral regurgitation with calculation of d*p*/d*t* (apical transducer position). The time period between velocities of 1 and 3 m/s is 0.07 s; the calculated d*p*/d*t* is approximately 460 mmHg/s. See text for details.

The most commonly applied method for the evaluation of MR is assessment of jet size by CFD.[169] Imaging of the LA in systole reveals a turbulent, mosaic jet of varying direction, size, and configuration (Fig. 15-77*A* and *B,* Plate 62). Previous studies have demonstrated that a mitral regurgitant jet whose absolute area exceeds 8 $cm^2$ or that fills at least 40 percent of the area of the LA is predictive of finding 3+ to 4+ MR by LV angiography. Unfortunately, neither jet size nor angiographic grade correlates closely with measurements of actual regurgitant volume.[169] The lack of correlation between CFD jet area and regurgitant volume is attributable to the additional variables that influence the distribution of the flow disturbance, such as the pressure gradient and the volume and compliance of the LA, as well as technical limitations. The Coanda effect is of particular significance in regard to MR, since jets into the LA are often eccentric (for example, in cases of MV prolapse and torn chordae tendineae). Due to differential frictional forces and resistance to flow, eccentric MR jets are drawn along the walls of the LA, resulting in cross-sectional jet areas that are smaller than centrally directed flow disturbances of comparable regurgitant volume (Figs. 15-77, Plate 62 and 15-78, Plate 63). This effect can lead to underestimation of the severity of regurgitation.

TEE is also useful for the assessment of MR, as the close proximity of the probe and its higher-frequency interrogating beam permit imaging of regurgitant jets in greater detail than with TTE.[170] Eccentric jets and mitral valvular anatomy are well visualized (Fig. 15-78*A* and *B,* Plate 63), and rightward bulging of the interatrial septum with severe MR is also sometimes apparent. As the regurgitant jets often appear larger with TEE than with TTE, one must avoid overestimation of MR severity.[108] TEE often yields Doppler interrogation of the pulmonary veins that is superior to that of TTE, and several recent studies have shown that systolic reversal of flow into the pulmonary veins is a reliable sign of severe MR[106] (Fig. 15-79).

Another color Doppler method of flow quantitation involves measurement of the zone of flow convergence proximal to the regurgitant orifice [or the *proximal isovelocity surface area* (PISA)]. The mechanism for this

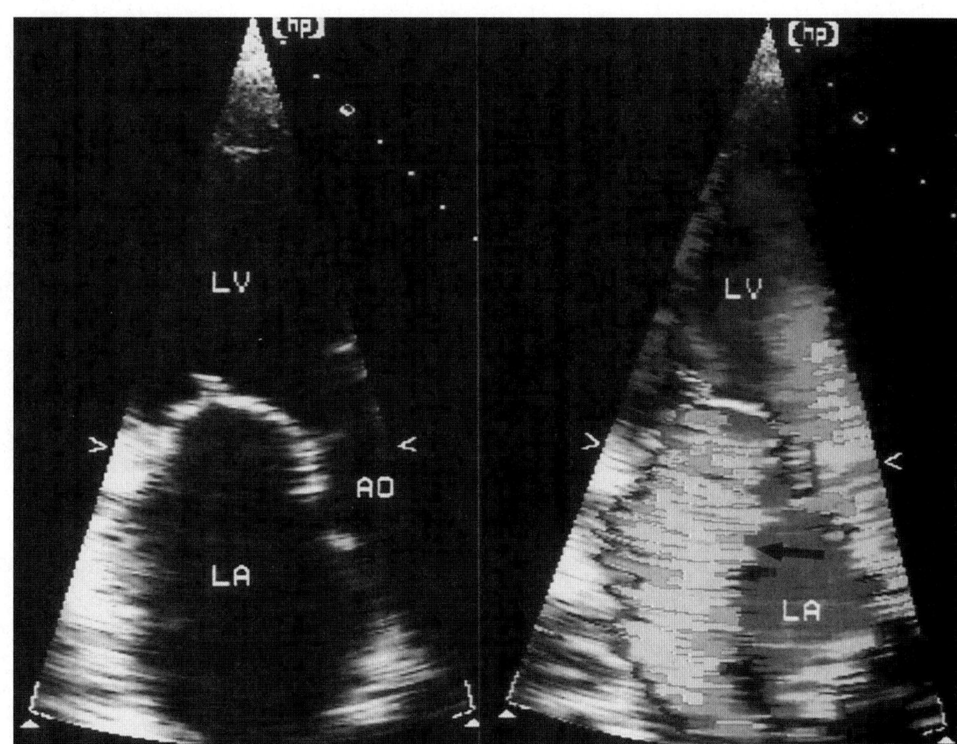


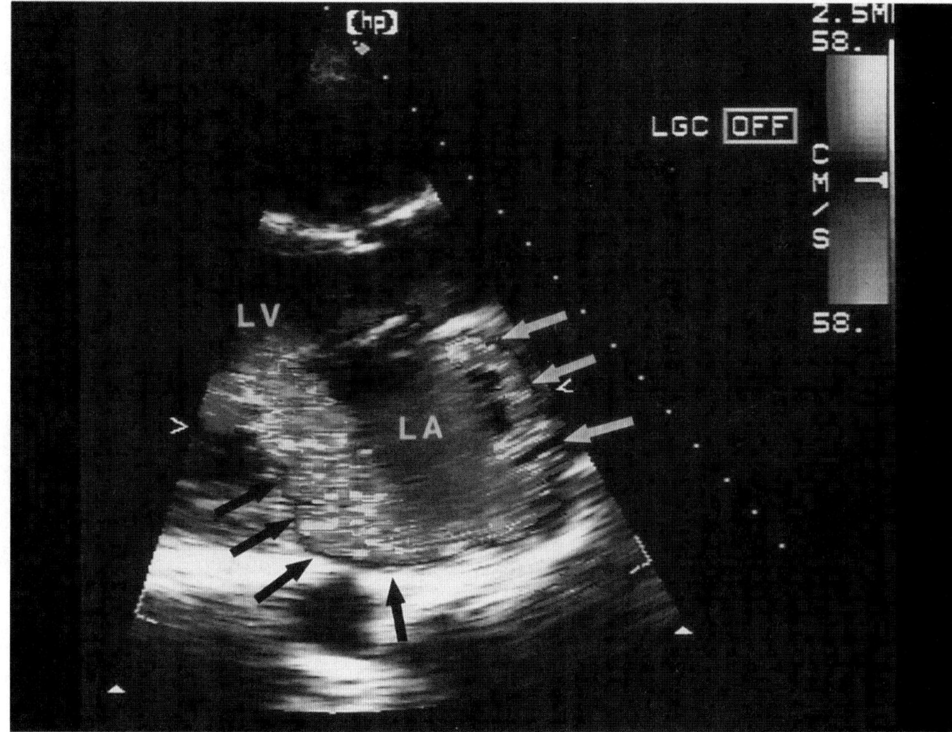


FIGURE 15-77 (Plate 62) *A.* Mitral regurgitation. *Left:* apical three-chamber plane. Right: same plane with color Doppler imaging. A large jet of mitral regurgitation (*arrow*) is present. AO = aorta; LA = left atrium; LV = left ventricle. *B.* Parasternal long-axis view from a patient with angiographically proved severe mitral regurgitation. The color Doppler jet in this case is directed posteriorly and eccentric (*black arrows*). The jet hugs the wall of the left atrium (LA) and wraps around all the way to the aortic root (*white arrows*). LV = left ventricle.

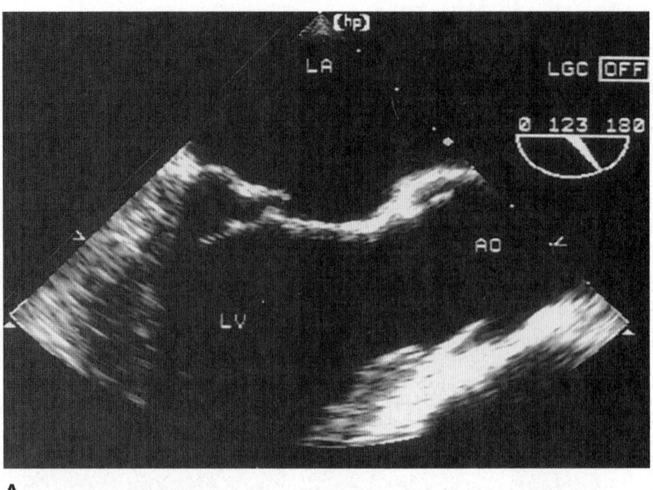


A

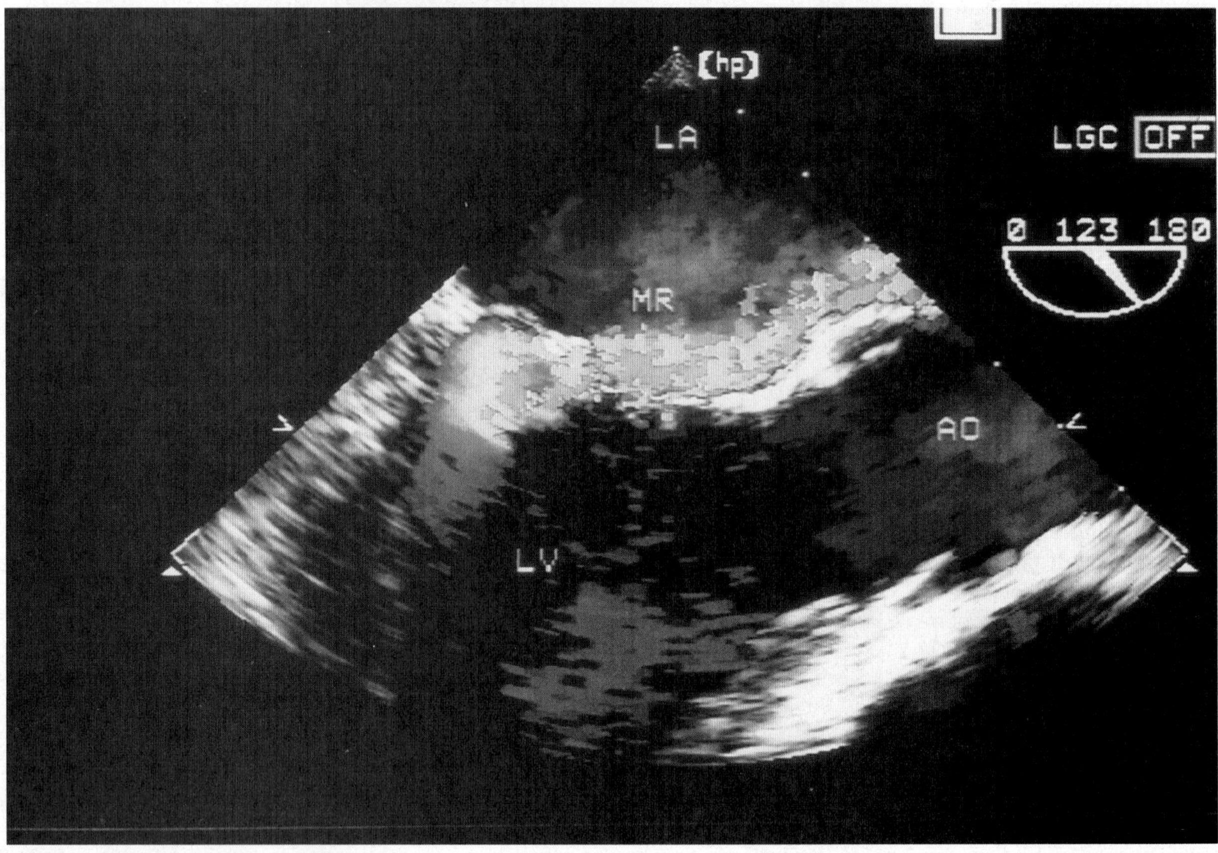


B

FIGURE 15-78 (Plate 63) TEE images from a case of severe mitral regurgitation secondary to a flail posterior mitral valve leaflet. *A.* abnormal coaptation and prolapse of the posterior leaflet is apparent. *B.* Color Doppler imaging demonstrates an eccentric jet of MR directed anteriorly toward the aortic root (AO). LA = left atrium; LV = left ventricle.

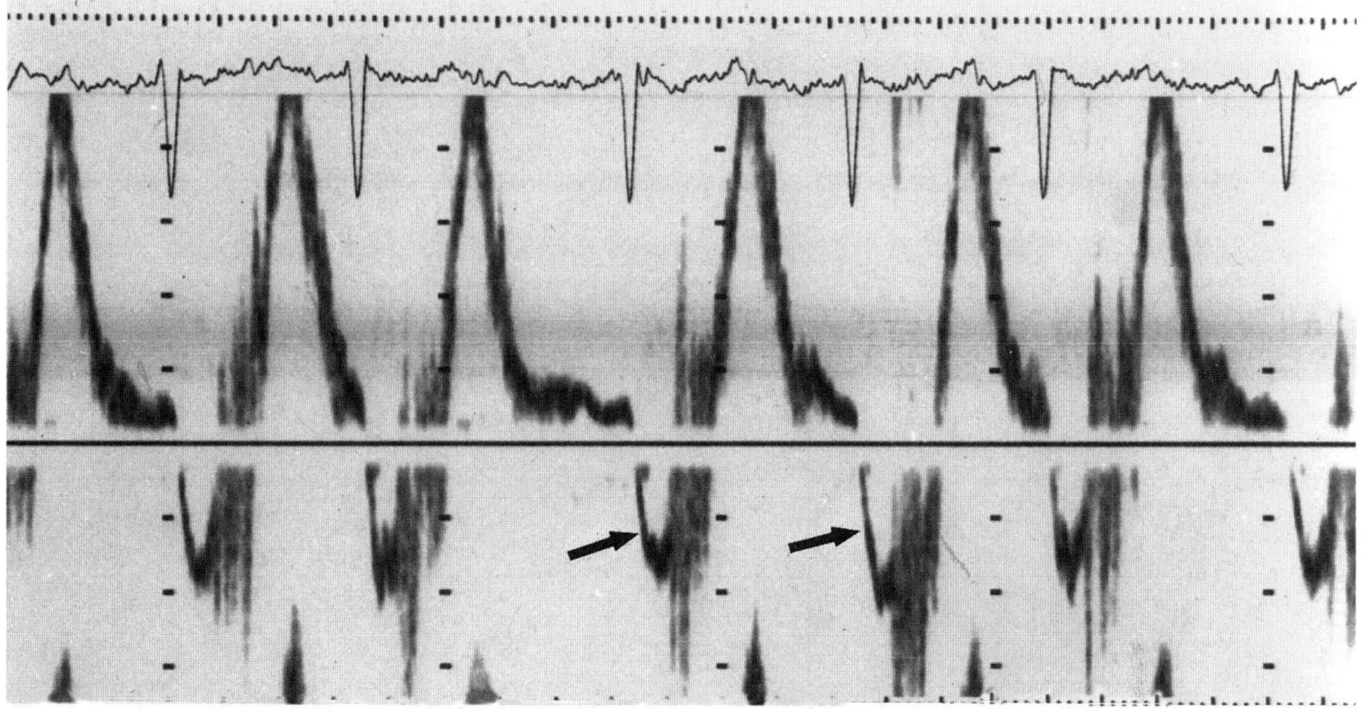

FIGURE 15-79 Pulmonary venous pulsed-wave Doppler in severe mitral regurgitation. Systolic flow reversal (i.e., systolic flow into the pulmonary vein) is present (*arrows*).

phenomenon is derived from the hydrodynamic principle that blood flow accelerates before passing through a small orifice under high pressure. If this increase in flow velocity exceeds the Nyquist limit, color aliasing occurs and the velocity aliasing border is equal to the Nyquist limit (Fig. 15-31 and Fig. 15-80*A* and *B;* Plate 64). If one assumes that the aliasing border conforms to the geometry of a hemisphere around the mitral orifice, then the instantaneous flow rate of blood through the orifice can be calculated as:

$$\text{Flow} = 2\pi r^2(V_r)$$

where $r$ is the radius of the hemisphere shell (distance from alias border to orifice) and $V_r$ is the velocity of blood at distance $r$ (the Nyquist limit velocity). If the maximal calculated flow rate is divided by the peak regurgitant flow velocity (measured with CW Doppler), the regurgitant orifice area is then obtained.[171] The product of regurgitant orifice area and integrated velocity of the MR jet by CW yields regurgitant volume. The PISA method avoids the variables associated with jet size and the assumptions and technical limitations of volumetric calculations. Numerous studies have shown a correlation between both flow rate and regurgitant orifice area calculated by PISA and the severity of MR assessed by standard methods.[171] In addition, flow convergence calculations have been applied to other valvular lesions, including AR and MS (Fig. 15-81, Plate 65), ventricular septal defect, and prosthetic heart valves.[172] The proximal flow convergence assumes a hemispheric geometry for the PISA signal and that the plane of the mitral leaflets is flat, two sources of potential error.[173] The method also assumes that regurgitant blood is flowing through only one orifice, an assumption often untrue in MR. Despite these limitations, the method can be useful in selected cases of valvular regurgitation.

## Mitral Valve Prolapse

As is true of so many aspects of MV prolapse (MVP), the echocardiographic findings in this disorder have been controversial for many years.[174] Recent insights into the anatomy of the mitral annulus and the significance of abnormal leaflet structure have established a central role for echocardiography in the diagnosis and prognosis of MVP.[175] The classic echocardiographic findings in overt MVP syndrome consists of mid- to late-systolic bulging of one or both mitral leaflets across the plane of the MV annulus into the LA (Fig. 15-82*A* to *C*). The leaflets are often observed to be structurally abnormal, with thickening, elongation, and hooding. Mid- to late-systolic MR is sometimes present, often eccentric, and generally directed away from the prolapsing leaflet. The chordae tendineae may be thickened and elongated, the aortic root may be dilated, and the TV leaflets may prolapse as well. LV function is usually normal, although the LA and LV may be enlarged if MR is significant. The greater temporal resolution of M-mode over 2D echocardiography often yields striking evidence of abrupt midsystolic posterosuperior motion of the MV leaflets in prolapse patients (Fig. 15-82*C*). Although such M-mode findings, which resemble a question mark on its side, are specific for MV prolapse, patients with classic MVP occasionally may demonstrate diagnostic findings only with 2D imaging (Chap. 68).

Although the diagnosis of classic, fully expressed MVP is straightforward by echocardiography, identification of mild prolapse is more difficult, and no absolute diagnostic criteria currently exist. This is largely related to the absence of any "gold standard" with which to validate findings, including auscultation, angiography, and even pathology. For prolapse to be present, the MV leaflets must cross the plane of the MV annulus after initial systolic coaptation. Recent studies have established that the MV annulus is not flat but

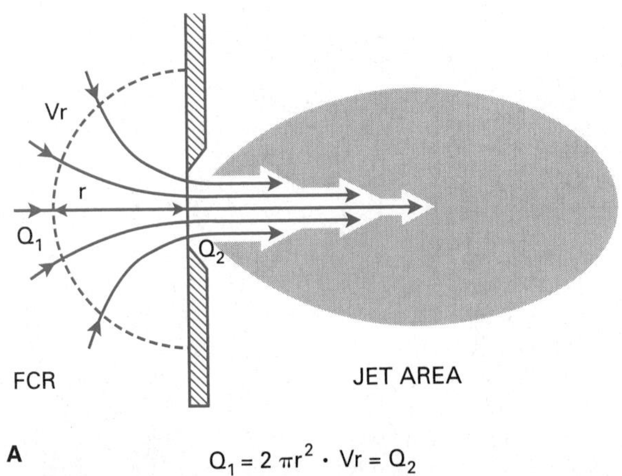


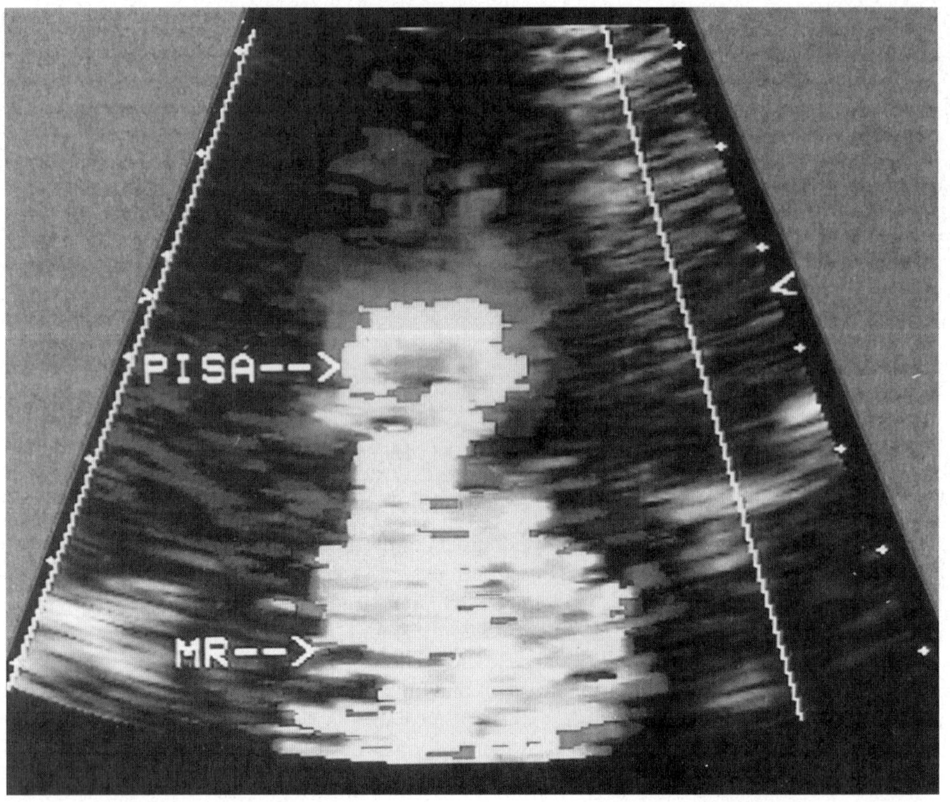


FIGURE 15-80 (Plate 64) *A.* Proximal isovelocity surface area (PISA). See text for details. Q = flow; FCR = flow convergence region; r = radius of isovelocity hemisphere; Vr = velocity of flow at distance r from the orifice. (From Bargiggia GS, Tronconi L, Sahn DJ, et al. A new method for quantitation of mitral regurgitation based on color flow Doppler imaging of flow convergence proximal to regurgitant orifice. *Circulation* 1991;84:1481–1489, with permission.) *B.* Magnified view (from the apical four-chamber plane) of mitral regurgitation (MR) demonstrating color Doppler flow convergence proximal to the mitral valve (PISA).

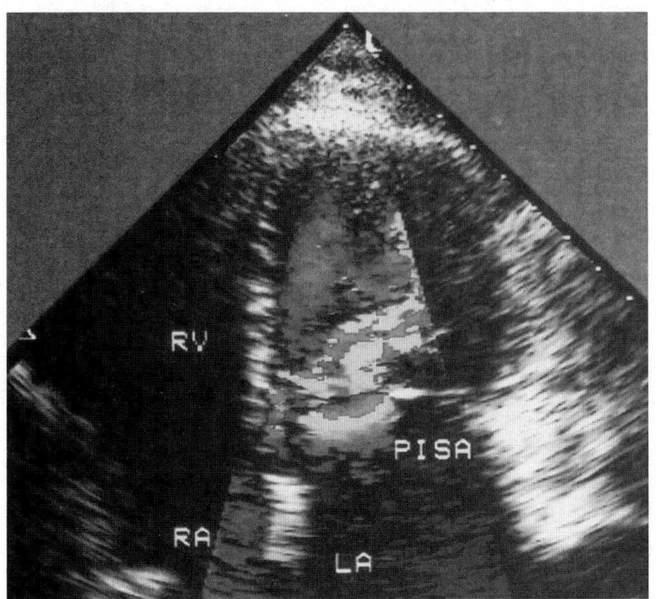


FIGURE 15-81 (Plate 65) Apical four-chamber plane in mitral stenosis. Color flow imaging in the mitral valve region shows flow convergence (PISA) proximal to the valve during diastole. LA = left atrium; RA = right atrium; RV = right ventricle.

rather saddle-shaped. The annulus reaches its nadir in the apical four-chamber view, and even normally coapting MV leaflets may appear to prolapse in this projection. Therefore, current criteria require that MVP be diagnosed only when one or both of the mitral leaflets clearly bulge past the plane of the MV annulus in the parasternal long-axis view.[175] Unfortunately, the degree to which the mitral leaflets must break the plane of the annulus is unclear. The greater the portion of the MV leaflets entering the LA, the more likely the existence of signs and symptoms related to this disorder; a peak distance behind the annulus of 2 mm almost invariably establishes the presence of MVP. The diagnosis of mild MVP may be assisted by examination of the structure of the leaflets and chordae tendineae, since it has been demonstrated that patients with redundant or thickening valve leaflets (greater than 5 mm in midleaflet) are at increased risk of complications, including severe MR and infective endocarditis (Chap. 78).

## Torn Chordae Tendineae

Rupture of chordae tendineae may occur spontaneously or in conjunction with MVP or endocarditis. This can result in a flail mitral leaflet and severe MR. Although TTE often detects these lesions, TEE is especially sensitive and accurate and often demonstrates free motion of the leaflet and ruptured chord into the LA even when the TTE is equivocal (Fig. 15-83*A* and *B*). As with MVP, the MR jet in this condition is usually eccentric and directed away from the affected leaflet, often "hugging" the adjacent left atrial wall (Coanda effect). Therefore, the jet's cross-sectional area may be misleadingly small. The findings of mitral valvular anatomy on TEE may also be helpful in predicting the feasibility and success of valve repair surgery.[176]

In the setting of ischemic heart disease, both LV enlargement and papillary muscle dysfunction (from infarction or transient ischemia) may cause MR. Both the MR and the contractile abnormality responsible for it are usually well visualized by 2D echocardiography. In rare cases, papillary muscle rupture (partial or complete) occurs in the postinfarction period. Rapid echocardiographic diagnosis often requires TEE and may be lifesaving in these cases.

## Mitral Annular Calcification

The finding of mitral annular calcification (MAC) is fairly common in adults and occurs more frequently with advancing age. Although ultrasound cannot discern histology, calcification typically appears as thickened, extremely high-intensity ("bright") signals (Fig. 15-84). The posterior portion of the mitral annulus is affected much more commonly than the anterior segment, and calcification often extends into the posterior mitral leaflet, sometimes restricting its motion. The abnormality, best visualized in the parasternal long- and short-axis views, is seen as a bright calcific density at the junction of the posterior mitral leaflet and the annulus. In the short-axis view, the posterior band of calcification often appears crescentic. Rarely, the calcification is extensive enough to cause marked valvular thickening and clinically significant MS. MAC has been associated with cardiogenic embolization, stroke, and cardiovascular events, although causality has not been established.[177,178]

# RIGHT-SIDED VALVULAR DISEASE AND PULMONARY HYPERTENSION

## Pulmonic Valve

Major structural abnormalities of the PV are relatively rare. *Pulmonic stenosis* (PS) is usually congenital in origin and resembles congenital AS in many respects. The stenotic valve does not open fully and exhibits characteristic thickening and systolic doming on 2D imaging (Fig. 15-85, Plate 66). M-mode recordings of the PV often show a large a wave, since RV diastolic pressure is often so high and PA pressure so low that the atrial "kick" is sufficient to open the PV. Doppler interrogation reveals turbulent flow distal to the valve, and CW measurements can be used to calculate gradients and valve areas with the Bernoulli and continuity equations much as in aortic stenosis.[179]

Although severe *pulmonic regurgitation* (PR) is rare, mild PR is common and appears as a flame shaped flow disturbance in the *RV outflow tract* (RVOT) in diastole. Many individuals have trivial PR on color Doppler examination; this is a physiologic, normal variant (Fig. 15-86). Hemodynamically significant PR is uncommon; when present, it is usually due to congenital heart disease, valvular tumors, endocarditis, or carcinoid heart disease (Chap. 59). The echocardiographic grading of PR is semiquantitative, based on the density of the CW envelope, area of the color Doppler jet, and width of the jet at the valve.[180] The PR pressure half-time by CW Doppler may be shorter with more severe PR, but this is not as well investigated as in the case of AR. Measurements derived from the CW Doppler recording also provide estimates of end-diastolic PA pressure using the Bernoulli equation, as follows:

$$[4(\text{PR end-diastolic velocity})^2] + \text{central venous pressure (CVP)}$$ [181]

## Tricuspid Valve

Tricuspid stenosis (TS) is usually rheumatic in origin, and coexistent mitral and aortic valvular disease is the rule. Congenital or acquired

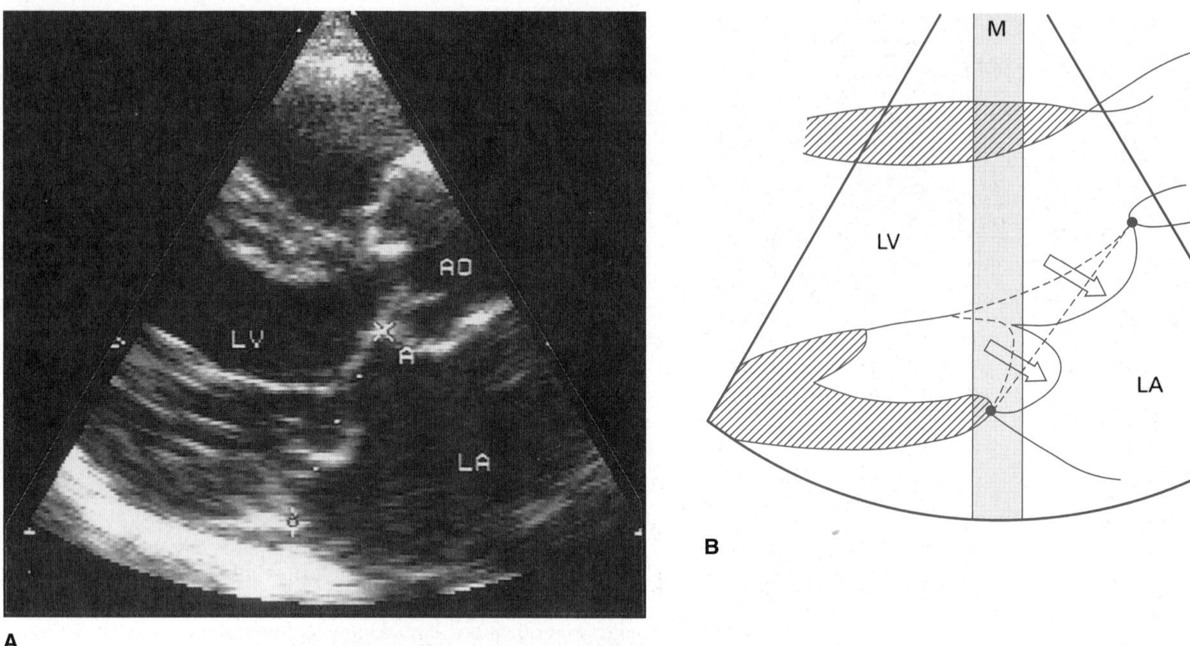


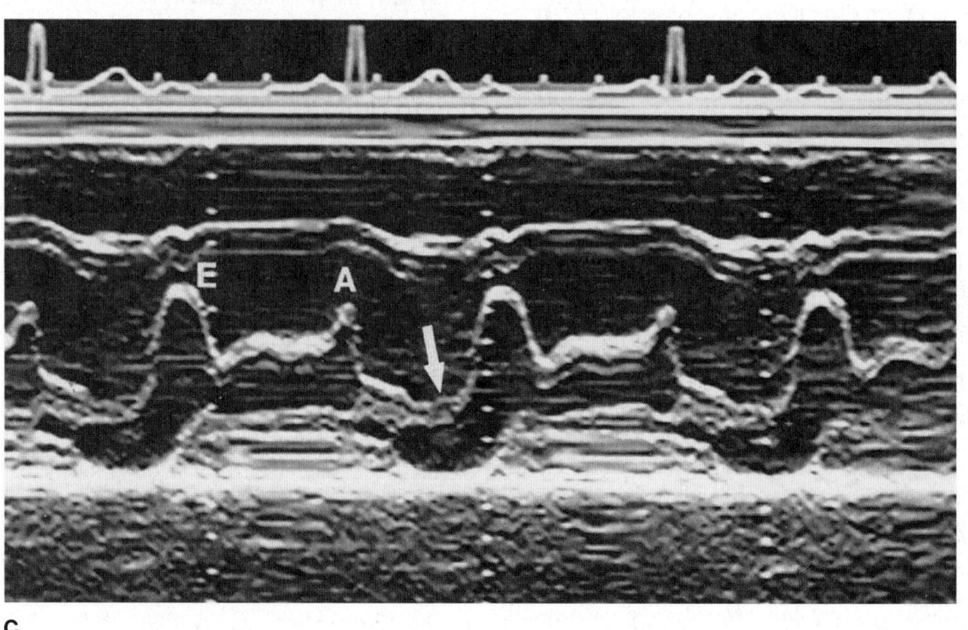


FIGURE 15-82 *A.* Parasternal long-axis plane through the mitral valve in late systole. The plane of the mitral annulus (A) is drawn in a dotted line. The posterior mitral leaflet prolapses past the level of the annulus into the left atrium (LA). AO = aorta; LV = left ventricle. *B.* Diagram of true mitral valve prolapse. The mitral leaflets clearly prolapse (*arrows*) posterior to the plane of the mitral annulus (*straight dotted line*). Ao = aorta; LV = left ventricle; LA = left atrium; M = m-mode imaging beam. (From Devereux RB, Kramer-Fox R, Kligfield P. Mitral valve prolapse: Causes, clinical manifestations, and management. *Ann Intern Med* 1989;111:305–317. With permission.) *C.* M-mode image through the plane of the mitral valve demonstrating posterior prolapse of the leaflets during systole (*arrow*). E = early diastolic filling; A = atrial component.

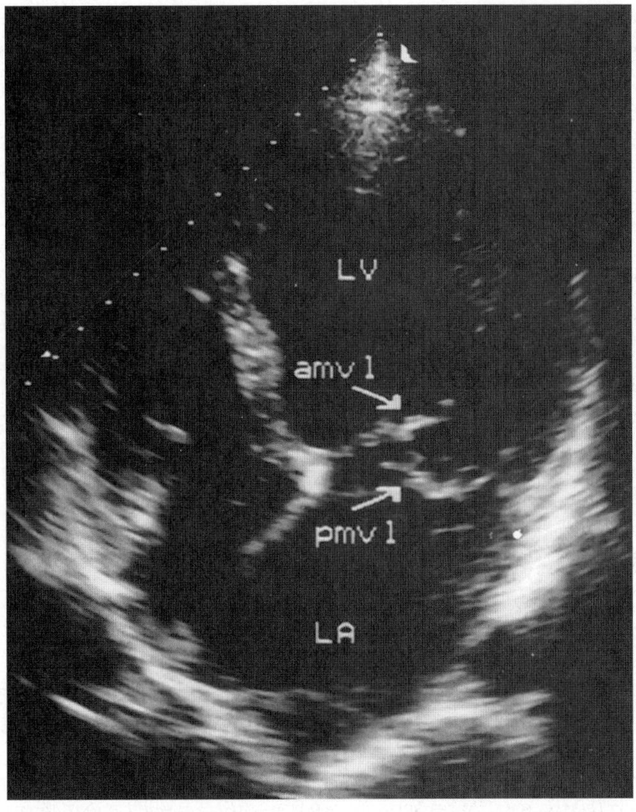


A

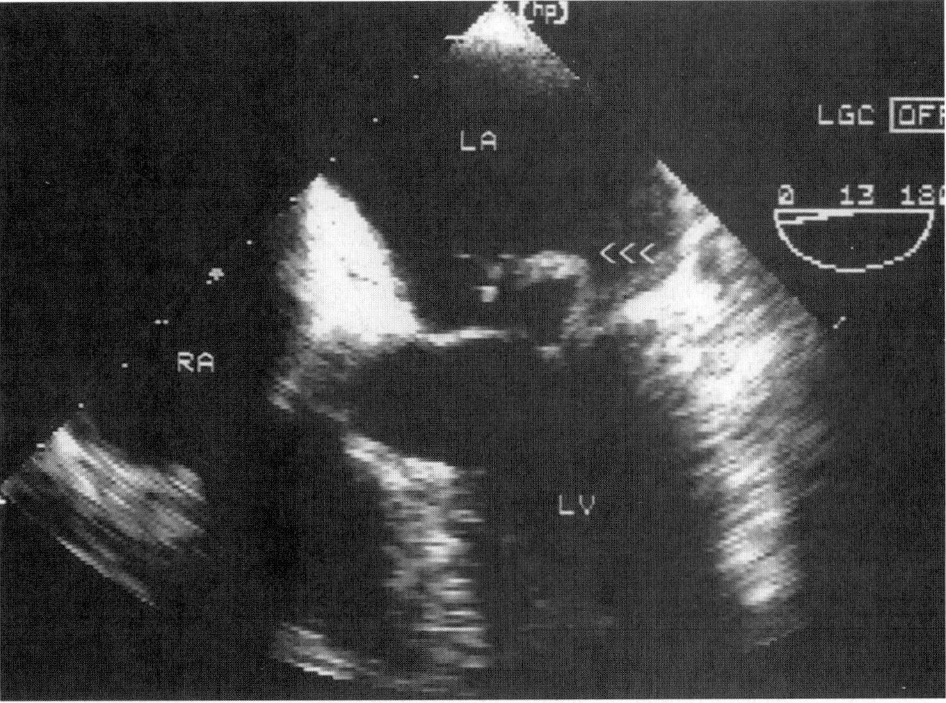


B

FIGURE 15-83 *A*. Apical four-chamber image of a flail posterior mitral valve leaflet (pmvl). The mitral valve is thickened and myxomatous. amvl = anterior mitral valve leaflet. *B*. Transesophageal echocardiography image (transverse four-chamber plane) of a flail posterior mitral valve leaflet (*arrows*) secondary to ruptured chordae. LA = left atrium; RA = right atrium; LV = left ventricle.

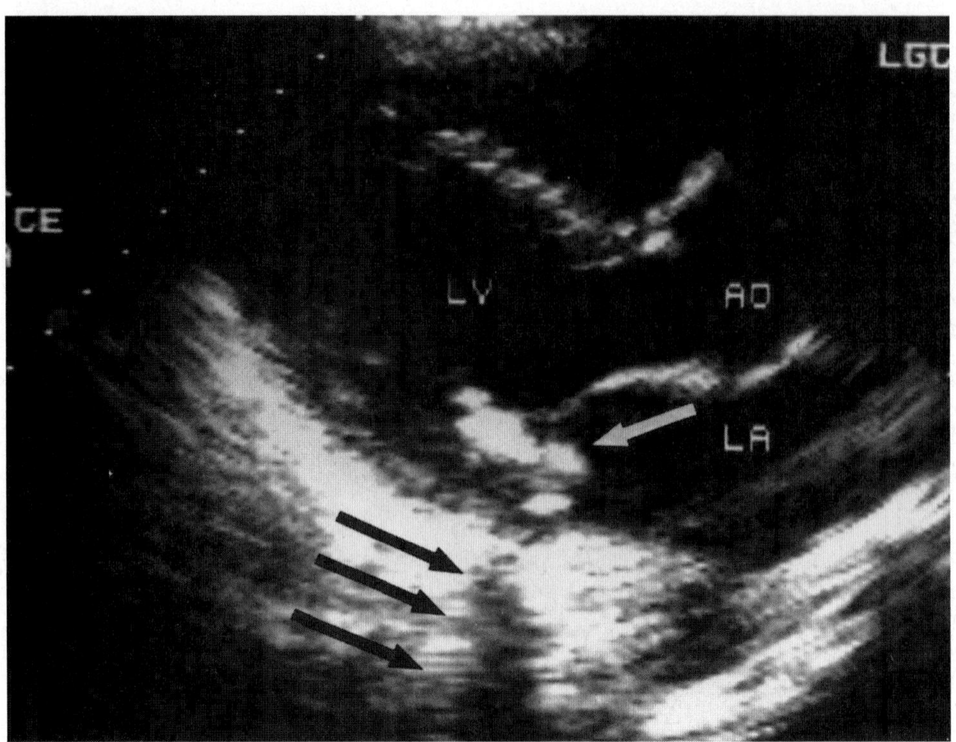


FIGURE 15-84 Parasternal long-axis plane demonstrating mitral annular calcification (*white arrow*) with ultrasonic shadowing posteriorly (*black arrows*). AO = aorta; LV = left ventricle; LA = left atrium. (From Blanchard DG, DeMaria AN. Cardiac and extracardiac masses: Echocardiographic evaluation. In: Skorton DJ, Schelber HR, Wolf GL, Brundage BH, eds. *Marcus' Cardiac Imaging*, 2d ed. Philadelphia: Saunders; 1996:452–480. With permission.)

(nonrheumatic) causes of TS are quite uncommon. On rare occasions, TS may be caused by carcinoid heart disease or by leaflet adhesions to permanent pacemaker leads. Because of the large size of the tricuspid annulus, obstruction by masses, even multiple vegetations, is unlikely to cause stenosis (Chap. 69).

Regardless of the etiology, diastolic doming of the valve leaflets suggests stenosis.[182] CW Doppler interrogation is also helpful and mimics the findings of MS (high diastolic velocity with prolonged pressure half-time).[182] The pressure half-time equation used to calculate the area of the MV orifice cannot be applied directly to the TV, and large studies comparing Doppler echocardiography with right heart catheterization in TS are not available.

*Tricuspid regurgitation* (TR) is much more common than TS, and, like PR, is present to a mild degree in many normal individuals (Chap. 59). Hemodynamically significant TR may be caused by endocarditis, rheumatic valvular disease, pulmonary hypertension (PH), congenital heart disease (for example, Ebstein's anomaly), carcinoid heart disease, flail TR leaflet (which can occur as a complication of cardiac trauma or endomyocardial biopsy), and TV prolapse. Echocardiographic findings in TR generally mirror those found in MR. Although 2D imaging can detect abnormalities associated with TR—such as incomplete leaflet coaptation, flail leaflet, and right-sided chamber enlargement—the technique cannot accurately quantify TR grade. Doppler echocardiography, especially color-flow mapping, has become the procedure of choice to detect TR and has reasonable accuracy for semiquantitation of severity.[183] As with MR, the severity of TR can be estimated by regurgitant jet area, ratio of jet area to right atrial area, and size of proximal flow convergence zones (Fig. 15-31). Doppler interrogation of the hepatic vein is also useful, as systolic flow reversal within the vein suggests severe TR[184] (Fig. 15-87). Peak RV (and PA) pressure can be estimated using measurements of peak TR velocity by CW Doppler (see "The Bernoulli Equation," above). If necessary, intravenous echocardiographic contrast agents can be injected to accentuate the TR Doppler jet and facilitate more accurate measurements of PA pressure.

## Right Ventricular Function and Pulmonary Hypertension

RV enlargement and PH can be diagnosed and assessed by echocardiography[185] (Fig. 15-88*A* and *B*). Because of the asymmetric and crescentic shape of the RV, accurate volume calculations are difficult. Nonetheless, 2D imaging provides useful general information regarding RV size and function. In the apical four-chamber view, the RV should appear somewhat smaller than the LV; therefore RV enlargement can be diagnosed qualitatively when the RV's cross-sectional area exceeds that of the LV. RV chamber area measurements in the apical four-chamber imaging plane can also be compared to standardized normal values. Although not well standardized, measurements of RV wall thickness can be performed from the parasternal view; a value of 5 mm is generally accepted as the upper limit of normal.[185] Systolic motion of the RV free wall and LV lateral wall toward the interventricular septum should be similar and roughly symmetric in normal situations. Asymmetric hypokinesis of the RV free wall indicates RV dysfunction. RV volume overload can lead to RVH, chamber enlargement, and, in advanced stages, depressed RV systolic function. TR can result from or cause RV overload, and the TR Doppler velocity allows estimation of the peak RV systolic pressure. The interventricular septum also becomes abnor-

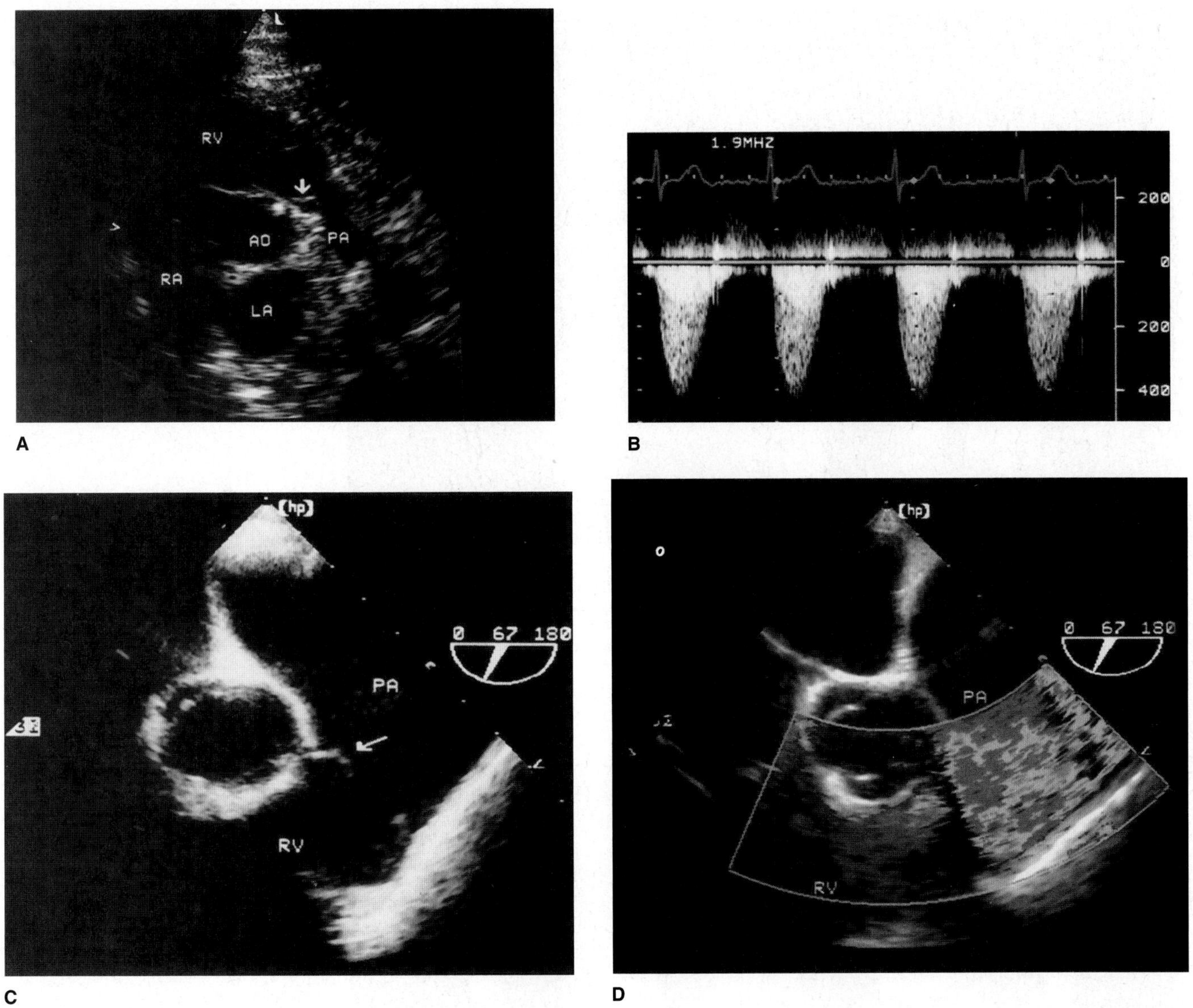


FIGURE 15-85 (Plate 66) *A.* Pulmonic stenosis. The pulmonic valve leaflet is thickened and echo-reflective, and does not open completely during systole (*arrow*). RA = right atrium; LA = left atrium; AO = aorta; PA = pulmonary artery; RV = right ventricle. *B.* Doppler interrogation reveals increased flow velocity (4 m/s) through the valve orifice. *C.* Transesophageal image of pulmonic stenosis. The valve leaflets exhibit doming during systole (arrow). *D.* TEE image with color Doppler, showing high-velocity, turbulent flow in the main pulmonary artery.

mal in RV overload and tends to flatten or even bulge toward the LV (Fig. 15-89). The pattern of septal movement can help distinguish between volume and pressure overload: in pure volume overload, the RV diastolic pressure may equal or exceed that of the LV, while the systolic pressure of the LV greatly exceeds that of the RV. Therefore the interventricular septum flattens during diastole and returns to its normal curvature during systole.[186] With RV pressure overload, however, the abnormally high RV pressures persist through the entire cardiac cycle and the interventricular septum remains deformed during both systole and diastole.[186]

The hallmark of PH by Doppler echocardiography is a high-velocity TR jet in the absence of PS. Peak TR jet velocity can be converted to peak systolic PA pressure as follows:

$$4(\text{TR velocity})^2 + \text{CVP}$$

where CVP = central venous pressure. In the setting of severe PH, the main PA and the inferior vena cava are often dilated. If RA pressure is elevated, the inferior vena cava (IVC) does not decrease in diameter with inspiration as normally expected. M-mode examination of the PV in PH may show a characteristic W-shaped motion of the valve leaflet during systole[187] (Fig. 15-90) and loss of the normal a dip caused by partial opening of the valve during atrial contraction. The loss of the a wave is probably due to the large pressure difference between the RV and PA during late diastole and the resulting inability of the atrial contraction to partially open the PV. The midsystolic closure of the valve and partial reopening in late systole (sometimes called the *flying W*) may be caused by elevated pulmonary vascular resistance and oscillation of a pressure wavefront within the PA.[188] Characteristic pulsed-wave Doppler abnormalities in PH include a decrease in the velocity-time integral of flow through the PV

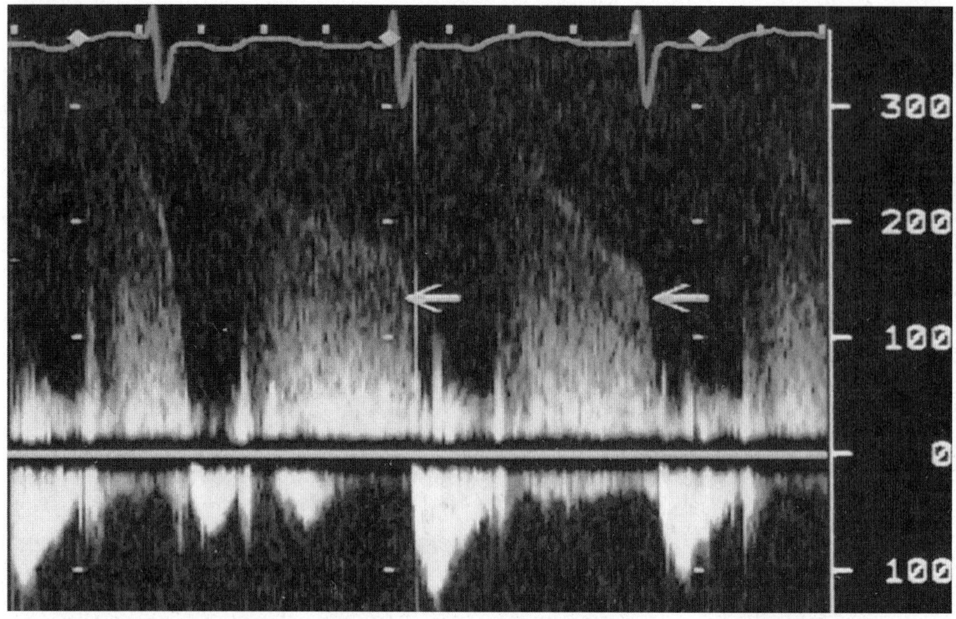


FIGURE 15-86 Continuous-wave Doppler tracing through the right ventricular outflow tract and pulmonary artery (left parasternal transducer position). Mild pulmonic regurgitation is present (*arrows*).

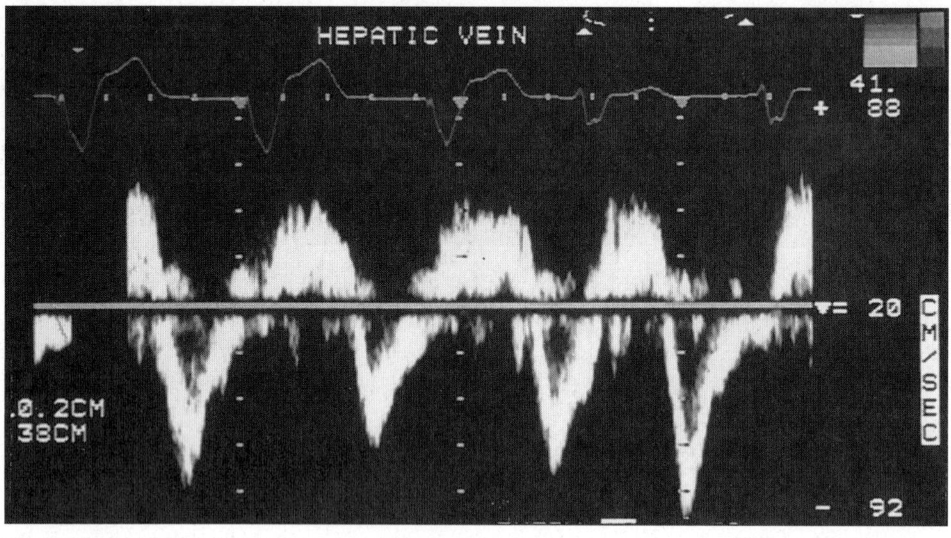


FIGURE 15-87 Pulsed-wave Doppler tracing of the hepatic vein in severe tricuspid regurgitation (TR) (subcostal transducer position). Systolic flow reversal into the hepatic vein is present.

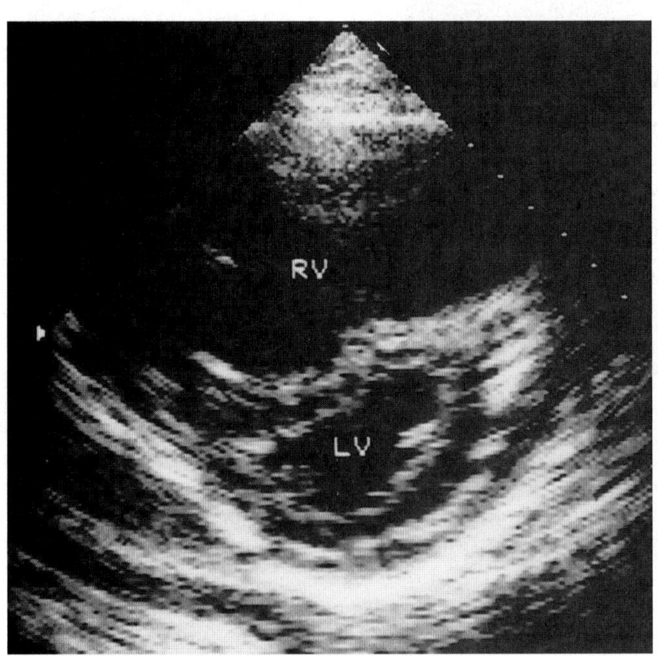


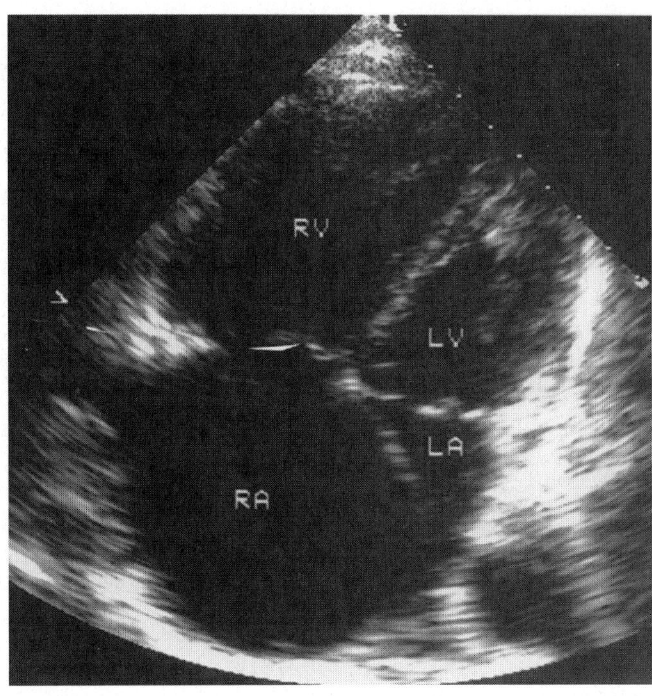


FIGURE 15-88 *A.* Parasternal short-axis view in severe pulmonary hypertension with marked enlargement of the right ventricle (RV). The left ventricle (LV) is small, and the interventricular septum is flattened. *B.* Apical four-chamber view in pulmonary hypertension. The right atrium (RA) and right ventricle (RV) are much larger than the left-sided chambers. LA = left atrium; LV = left ventricle.

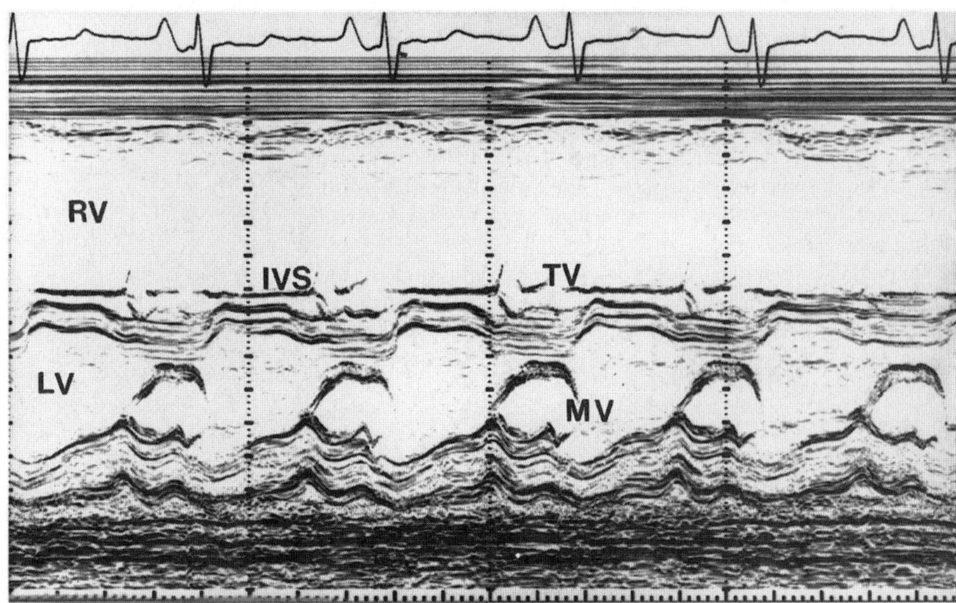


FIGURE 15-89 M-mode in severe pulmonary hypertension. The dimension of the right ventricle (RV) is larger than that of the left ventricle (LV). The interventricular septum (IVS) moves paradoxically—i.e., *toward* the mitral valve (MV) during diastole rather than away. TV = tricuspid valve.

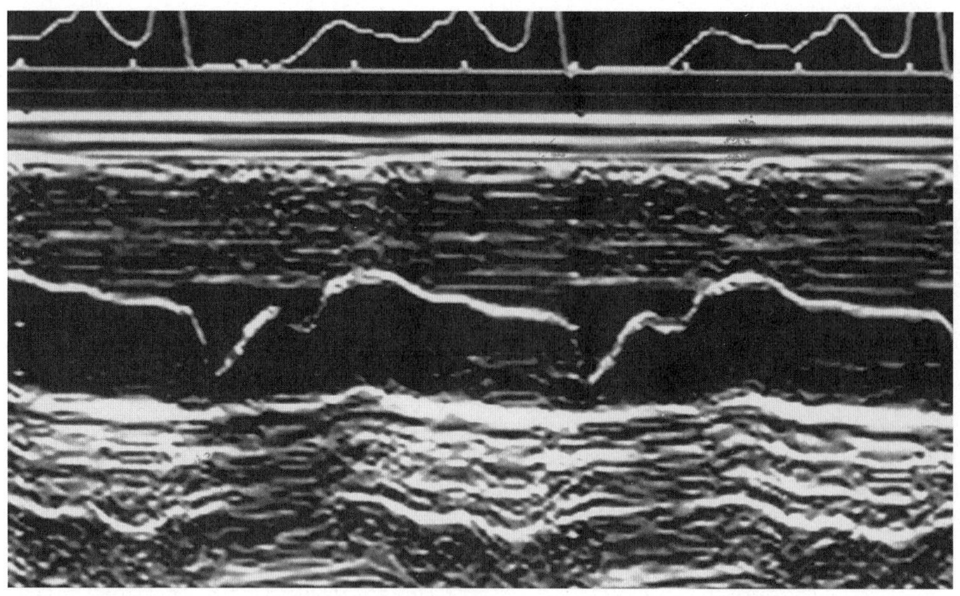

FIGURE 15-90 M-mode image of the pulmonic valve in severe pulmonary hypertension (parasternal transducer position). The a dip is absent, and a characteristic W-shaped motion of the leaflet is present during systole, indicating partial closure of the valve during midsystole followed by reopening prior to diastole.

(secondary to depressed RV stroke volume) and a shortening of the acceleration time (measured from beginning of flow through the PV to peak velocity). The acceleration time (in milliseconds) can be used to estimate the mean PA pressure as:

$$\text{Mean PA pressure} = 80 - (\text{acceleration time}/2)$$

Interestingly, RVH and severe PH affect LV diastolic filling characteristics, possibly through septal effects (or by relative underfilling of the left ventricle). Diastolic "abnormal relaxation" patterns of LV filling ($E < A$) are common in severe PH, and LV diastolic function often returns to normal if PH is reversed.[189] Several groups have attempted to differentiate various etiologies of PH with echocardiography. Although some reports have suggested some utility of echo in this regard, the diagnostic accuracy is insufficient to recommend its routine use.

Pulmonic regurgitation is also common in the setting of PH and is usually well recorded by pulsed Doppler. As discussed above, the end-diastolic PR velocity can be used to estimate PA end-diastolic pressure by the Bernoulli equation.

## PROSTHETIC CARDIAC VALVES

Echocardiography is a critically important tool in the evaluation and serial follow-up of mechanical and bioprosthetic valves. Unfortunately, the increased echo reflectivity of prosthetic valves (especially the mechanical models) causes extensive distal shadowing and reverberations that markedly limit the utility of transthoracic 2D echocardiography (Figs. 15-91 and 15-92). TTE imaging may detect partial ring dehiscence manifest as abnormal "rocking" motion of a prosthetic valve. TTE may also identify reduced movement of the valve disks or leaflets and may occasionally visualize adherent thrombi, tissue ingrowth, and vegetations.[190] Leaflet thickening, detachment, and flail motion also may be visualized for bioprosthetic valves.

Doppler interrogation is the cornerstone of the echocardiographic assessment of prosthetic valvular stenosis and regurgitation.[191] Color-flow imaging can document the presence, direction, and size of the forward flow stream. CFD can also detect regurgitant flow jets, but—like 2D imaging—it is limited by acoustic shadowing distal to the prosthesis. Doppler color jets due to prosthetic AR can be readily visualized from the transthoracic apical view, but jets produced by prosthetic mitral and tricuspid regurgitation are often obscured. Therefore, although detection of prosthetic regurgitation by transthoracic Doppler is usually feasible, quantitation is often difficult. A small flow signal shortly after valve closure may be observed frequently with prosthetic valves and is likely related to the blood caught behind the occluder as it closes.[192]

Doppler flow velocities and gradients (calculated by the Bernoulli equation) through normal prosthetic valves vary depending upon the type, position, and diameter of the prosthesis.[191] The velocities and gradients across prosthetic valves are flow-dependent as well and therefore related to LV function. Given these variables, it is not surprising that a wide range of transvalvular gradients exists for normally functioning prosthetic valves. Nevertheless, "normal"

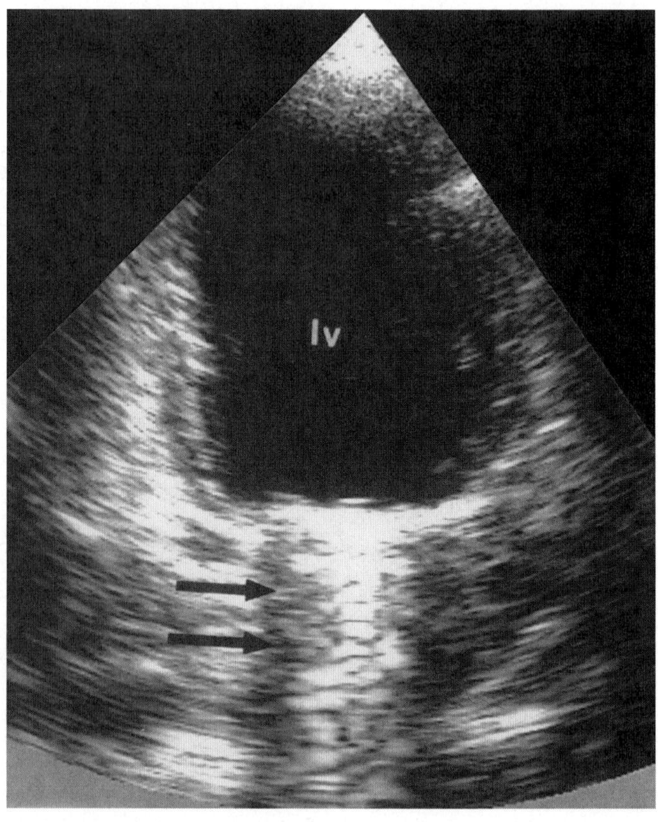


FIGURE 15-91 Apical two-chamber view of a mechanical prosthetic valve (mitral position) during systole. The left atrium is completely obscured by ultrasonic shadowing (*arrows*). LV = left ventricle.

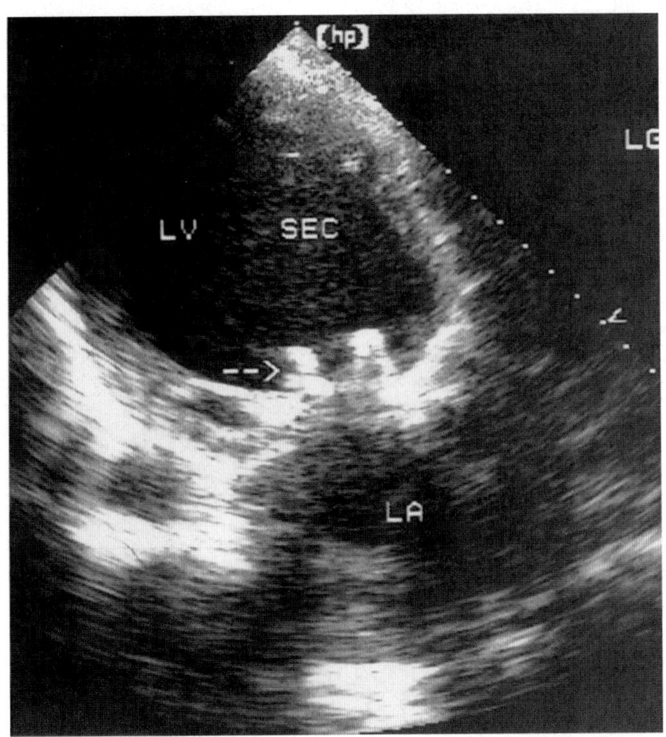


FIGURE 15-92 Apical view of a bioprosthetic valve (*arrow*) in the mitral position (two of the three prosthetic valve struts are apparent). Spontaneous echo contrast (SEC) is also present, secondary to systolic dysfunction and enlargement of the left ventricle (LV); LA = left atrium.

ranges have been reported for various valve types and can be used as a guide to recognize malfunction.[192] High prosthetic valvular gradients due to increased flow volume rather than stenosis can be recognized by high flow velocity across the remaining native valves, a short pressure half-time for mitral prostheses, and a short ejection time for aortic prostheses. With aortic valve prostheses, peak systolic Doppler velocities may indicate higher systolic pressure gradients than those actually found during cardiac catheterization.[193] This problem may be more prevalent with Starr-Edwards (ball-in-cage) and St. Jude (bileaflet tilting disk) valves than with Medtronic-Hall (single tilting disk) and bioprosthetic valves. The inaccuracies with Starr-Edwards and St. Jude valves are probably due to the presence of multiple flow channels (with various orifice areas) and the phenomenon of pressure recovery.[194] Because of these variabilities, an echocardiographic examination is warranted following prosthetic valve implantation to establish its baseline Doppler characteristics. As opposed to peak gradients, mean transvalvular gradients calculated by Doppler correlate reasonably well with direct catheter measurements.

TEE has dramatically changed the diagnostic approach to prosthetic valve dysfunction and is especially useful for assessing mitral prostheses, as it overcomes the problem of left atrial shadowing and reverberation (Fig. 15-93). TEE is extremely accurate in the detection of prosthetic regurgitation and impaired movement of the valve occluder, and it is the diagnostic procedure of choice in most cases of suspected prosthetic valve endocarditis.[195] Small thrombi, tissue ingrowth, infected or sterile vegetations, and even sutures in the sewing ring can usually be readily visualized. The enhanced sensitivity of TEE requires operator experience and judgment, as nearly all mechanical prostheses normally exhibit a small amount of regurgitation, which should not be misinterpreted as pathologic.[192] TEE may also visualize thin, fibrinous strands sometimes attached to prosthetic valves; these structures appear to be a potential source of cardiogenic embolization.[196] The technique is quite accurate in the diagnosis of prosthetic valve thrombosis, a potentially fatal medical emergency, and can assist clinical decision making in this disorder.[197]

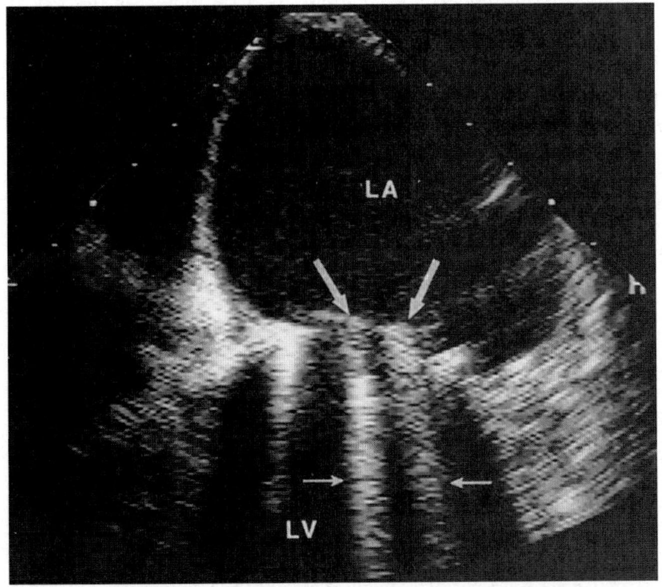


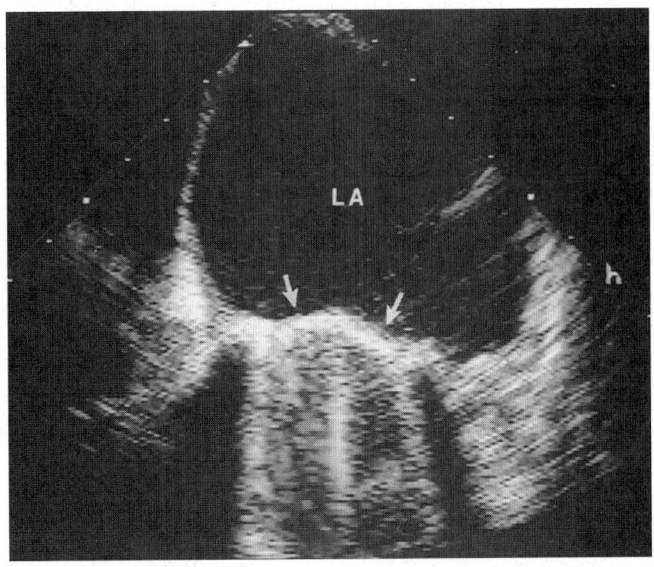


FIGURE 15-93 TEE images from a patient with a St. Jude prosthetic valve in the mitral position. *A*. Diastolic image. The two struts of the open valve are seen (*large arrows*) as well as their ultrasonic shadows (*small arrows*). LA = left atrium; LV = left ventricle. *B*. Systolic image. The two prosthetic leaflets are closed (*arrows*) and cast a dense ultrasonic shadow, obscuring the left ventricle.

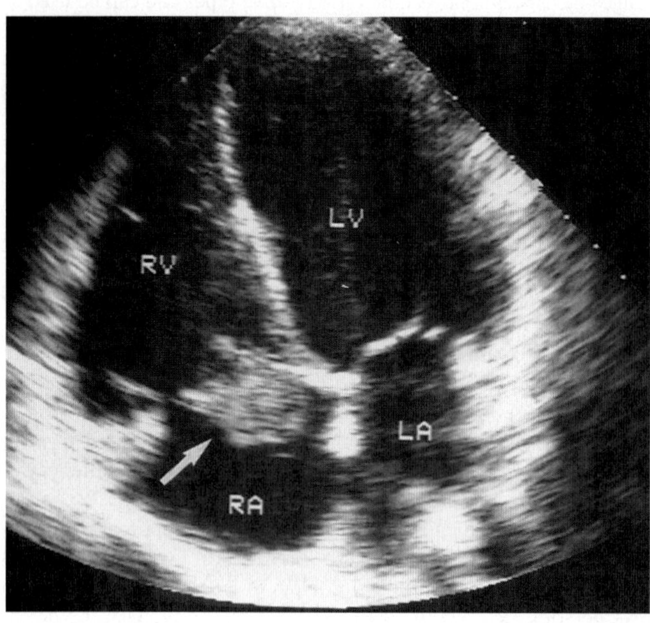


A

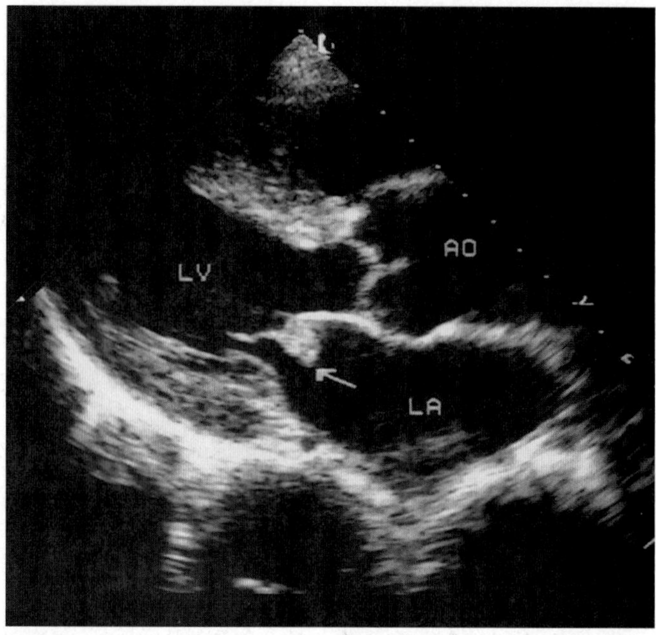


B

FIGURE 15-94 *A.* Apical four-chamber view demonstrating a large tricuspid valve vegetation (*arrow*). RA = right atrium; LA = left atrium; LV = left ventricle; RV = right ventricle. *B.* Parasternal long axis view demonstrating a vegetation (*arrow*) on the anterior valve leaflet; AO = aorta.

## INFECTIVE ENDOCARDITIS

Infective endocarditis remains an all too common illness, with a significant risk of morbidity and mortality (Chap. 86). Traditionally, the diagnosis has been based on either the cumulative results of blood cultures, physical examination, and laboratory findings or on pathologic proof of infected valvular vegetations at surgery or autopsy. Echocardiography may play an important role in infective endocarditis in regard to diagnosis, detection of associated cardiac abnormalities and hemodynamic dysfunction, prognosis, and the need for surgery. Vegetations can now be visualized noninvasively in many (but not all) cases of endocarditis and have become the echocardiographic hallmark of this disorder.[198,199] Thus even though TTE cannot exclude endocarditis, abnormal findings may strongly suggest the disorder, even in the presence of negative blood cultures. Since no single abnormality has 100 percent diagnostic accuracy for infective endocarditis, strategies for diagnosis have been devised based upon a number of criteria,[200] and definite echocardiographic vegetations are designated as a major criterion. Both TTE and TEE are valuable in the detection of perivalvular abscesses and prosthetic-valve endocarditis.[102] Although there is considerable debate concerning the most accurate diagnostic criteria for endocarditis, echocardiography has become one of the most commonly used techniques for the evaluation of potentially affected patients.[201] Echocardiography (both TTE and TEE) is also useful for evaluation of patients with systemic lupus erythematosus complicated by Libman-Sacks endocarditis.[202]

Even though M-mode recordings produced the first echocardiographic description of vegetations, this modality has been largely replaced by 2D imaging. With 2D echocardiography, valvular vegetations typically appear as irregular, usually localized masses of varying echocardiographic density attached to valvular or perivalvular structures (Figs. 15-94 and 15-95) without significantly altering their mobility. The vegetations may be small or quite large and may attach directly to the valve leaflets or the supporting chordal apparatus.[198,199,203] Occasionally, vegetations may be attached to unusual structures, such as the atrial wall or the eustachian valve.[204,205] Both small, nonmobile vegetations on a normal valve and large vegetations on a markedly abnormal valve may be difficult or impossible to identify with certainty. Aggressive infections often cause perforation or distortion of the affected leaflet, leading to varying degrees of valvular regurgitation. This is distinctly different from most cases of nonbacterial thrombotic (marantic) endocarditis, where the valvular vegetations are usually nondestructive. In cases of infective endocarditis, the presence of vegetations by TTE increases the risk of heart failure, embolic events, and the ultimate necessity of valve replacement.[206] Unfortunately, TTE is not 100 percent sensitive in

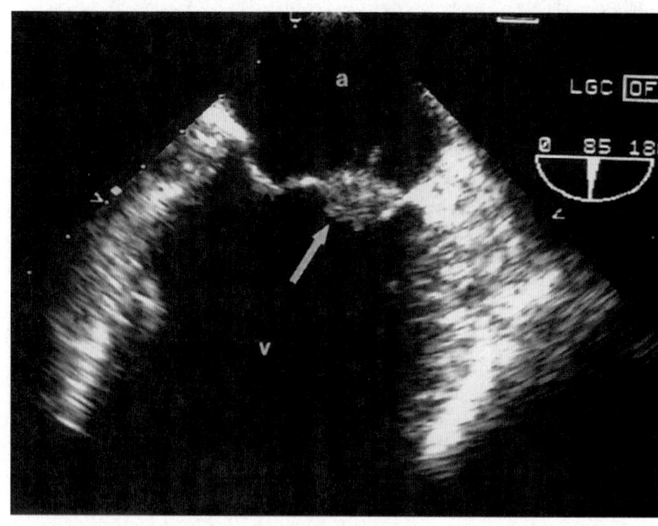


FIGURE 15-95 Longitudinal TEE view of a large mitral valve vegetation (*arrow*). a = left atrium; v = left ventricle. (Courtesy of William D. Keen, Jr., MD.)

detecting vegetations, and up to 20 percent of patients with proved native-valve endocarditis may have unremarkable examinations. The sensitivity of TTE in prosthetic valve endocarditis has been found to be even lower (approximately 60 percent) due to technical limitations in imaging.

TEE has proved significantly more sensitive than TTE for detection of infective vegetations and is extremely helpful for the diagnosis of perivalvular abscesses, mycotic diverticula, and prosthetic valve involvement.[102,207] The technique is also useful for assessing valvular regurgitation, fistulas (Fig. 15-96), other hemodynamic complications of endocarditis, and risk of embolization.[208] Although a negative TEE examination cannot completely exclude infective endocarditis, it confers a relatively good prognosis in those cases where the diagnosis is eventually confirmed. The optimal use of TEE in suspected endocarditis remains controversial: some authorities recommend routine TEE in all cases, but many do not. A reasonable approach may be to perform TTE as the first screening test in patients with suspected endocarditis. If the study is technically difficult or equivocal or detects vegetations in patients at high risk for perivalvular complications or hemodynamic compromise, TEE should be performed. If TTE is unremarkable or detects vegetations in patients at low risk for complications, TEE may not be necessary.[103] Exceptions to this last recommendation might include patients with prior antibiotic treatment or those with persistent bacteremia or fever of unknown etiology. In high-risk patients (i.e., with possible prosthetic valve involvement, congenital heart disease, or infection with especially virulent organisms), TEE is recommended even if TTE is normal.[103]

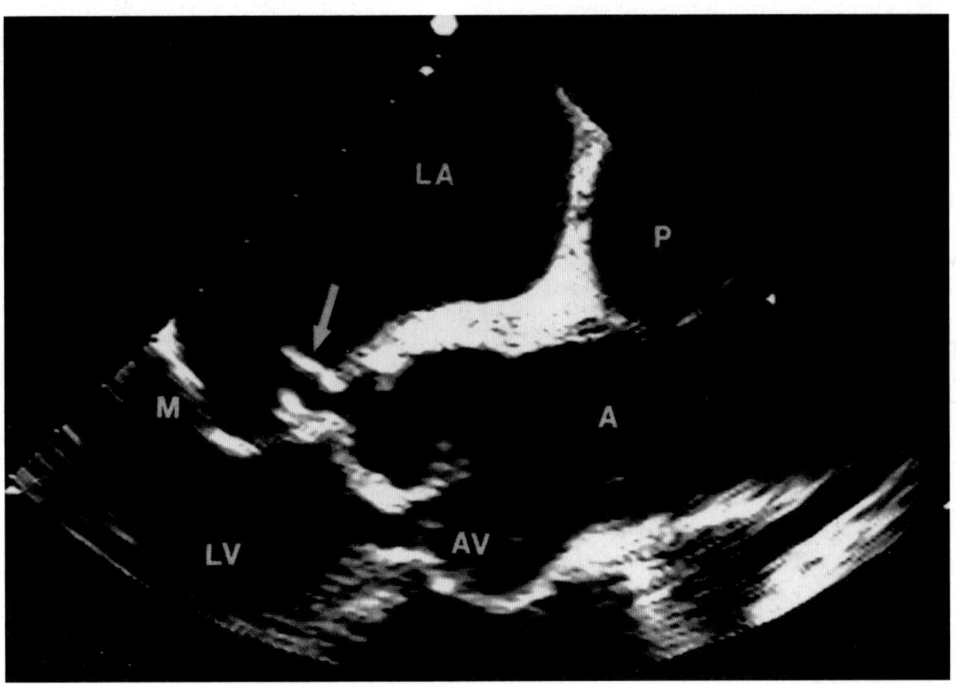


FIGURE 15-96 Longitudinal TEE image demonstrating a fistula between the aorta (A) and left atrium (LA) in a patient with endocarditis. AV = aortic valve; P = pulmonary artery; LV = left ventricle; M = mitral valve. (From Sobel J, Maisel AS, Tarazi R, Blanchard DG. Gonococcal endocarditis: Assessment by transesophageal echocardiography. *J Am Soc Echocardiogr* 1997;10:367–370. With permission.)

Echocardiographic evaluation of suspected endocarditis is not without pitfalls. It may be quite difficult to detect active vegetations in patients with preexisting valvular abnormalities such as calcification, myxomatous change, rheumatic involvement, and healed vegetations. Despite recent technologic advances, the diagnosis of infective endocarditis remains a clinical one, and overreliance on echocardiography may cause mistakes. Therefore, *echocardiographic results should be integrated with other clinical information* to diagnose this disorder accurately.[209]

## ISCHEMIC HEART DISEASE

### Echocardiography in Coronary Heart Disease

Although originally of greatest value in valvular heart disease and cardiomyopathy, echocardiography has now become one of the most important techniques for the detection and quantitative assessment of myocardial ischemia and infarction. Cardiac ultrasound—because it is rapid, portable, noninvasive, and inexpensive—is especially well suited to the evaluation of ischemic heart disease. Although visualization of coronary artery structure and flow has been achieved by echocardiography,[210] the application of this technique in ischemic heart disease continues to revolve primarily about the assessment of LV function. In addition, however, ongoing research with contrast agents has shown that echocardiography can be used to assess regional myocardial perfusion.

Currently, the primary application of echocardiography in patients with coronary heart disease is based upon the detection of the effects of myocardial ischemia and/or infarction upon LV structure and function. Interruption of coronary flow or imposition of an oxygen demand that exceeds oxygen supply quickly leads to impaired systolic thickening and excursion of the affected myocardium. If flow is not restored and transmural infarction occurs, the affected myocardium may become akinetic or dyskinetic and eventually thinned and fibrotic. In addition, myocardial ischemia produces diastolic dysfunction, which may be detected by analysis of transmitral Doppler flow recordings or tissue Doppler tracings.

The echocardiographic detection of myocardial ischemia was initially described using M-mode echocardiography, and this modality remains useful because of its excellent sensitivity and temporal resolution.[211] 2D imaging, however, is the primary technique for the examination of LV size, wall thickness, myocardial thickening, and regional wall motion, since it enables visualization of all LV wall segments. Therefore, in patients with CAD, standard echocardiographic approaches can be utilized to calculate LV diastolic and systolic volumes as well as ejection fraction. Digital echo analysis and 3D echocardiographic techniques can be used to enhance the accuracy of volume calculations and regional strain patterns.[212]

The echocardiographic manifestations of CAD consist of one or more of the following: reduction in systolic thickening, abnormal segmental wall motion during systole or diastole, alterations in the acoustic properties of the myocardium (usually termed *tissue characterization*), and diminished regional bloodflow (as measured during the LV myocardial phase after intravenous echo contrast injection).[213] These abnormalities may be expressed as a disturbance in global LV size and function, an increase in LV volume, and a decrease in LVEF calculated by standard approaches. In addition, using the standard tomographic planes, the LV can be divided into 16 wall segments according to the format recommended by the ASE (Fig. 15-97).[213] By grading the contraction of each of the 16 segments as hyperkinetic, normal, hypokinetic, akinetic, or dyskinetic (and assigning a numerical value to each grade), a semiquantitative wall motion score can be calculated as the mean numerical value for all segments. Wall motion scores of this kind have been used to assess prognosis in both AMI[214] and chronic coronary artery disease. When LV dysfunction is detected echocardiographically, the specific coronary artery responsible can often be inferred based upon the dyssynergy region(s).[215] The echocardiographic findings of akinesis with segmental myocardial thinning can also be used to distinguish CAD from dilated cardiomyopathy, which typically manifests global hypokinesis and decreased wall thickness. There is overlap in the echocardiographic findings between these two groups, however, as severe ischemic disease may cause global hypokinesis and nonischemic cardiomyopathy may sometimes cause heterogeneous dysfunction.[216]

## Myocardial Infarction and Postinfarction Complications

Cardiac ultrasound has achieved an important role in the evaluation of patients with AMI and is frequently used for diagnosis, quantitative functional assessment, risk stratification, and detection of complications[214] (Chap. 52). Echocardiography is especially valuable in *excluding* transmural infarctions, as these are almost always associated with regional akinesis or dyskinesis (Figs. 15-98 to 15-100).[217,218] Non-Q-wave infarctions are more difficult to diagnose with certainty, however, as the echocardiogram may show subtle regional hypokinesis or even normal wall motion in some cases. Thus echocardiography has been used to evaluate chest pain in the emergency department and appears to have a reasonable sensitivity and specificity in the diagnosis of MI.[218] It may also help to select patients for thrombolytic therapy. In addition, patients without contractile abnormalities who ultimately exhibit signs of MI have a low incidence of complications.[218]

Echocardiography is now the most commonly utilized approach to assess the effects of MI upon LV function. Ultrasound imaging studies of LV remodeling have demonstrated that infarct expansion occurs commonly with anterior infarctions, often beginning within the first 10 days, and conveys an adverse prognosis.[219] Similarly, calculation of the wall motion score has identified a cohort of post-MI patients at markedly increased risk for in-hospital complications.[218] This prognostic marker appears superior to conventional clinical criteria in predicting events.[218]

Echocardiography is probably of greatest value in the assessment of complications associated with AMI. Most such complications are quickly detected by echocardiography, and the fact that it is portable, rapid, and noninvasive render the technique extremely valuable in these circumstances. As indicated above, severe LV dysfunction resulting in advanced heart failure or shock can be readily identified by echocardiography. In addition, aneurysm formation is usually quite apparent in ultrasonic images.[220] By definition, postinfarction LV aneurysms are recognized as wide-mouthed, thin-walled myocardial segments that display dyskinetic expansion during systole. Aneurysms are a favored site for development of LV thrombi, which are covered in detail in the dis-

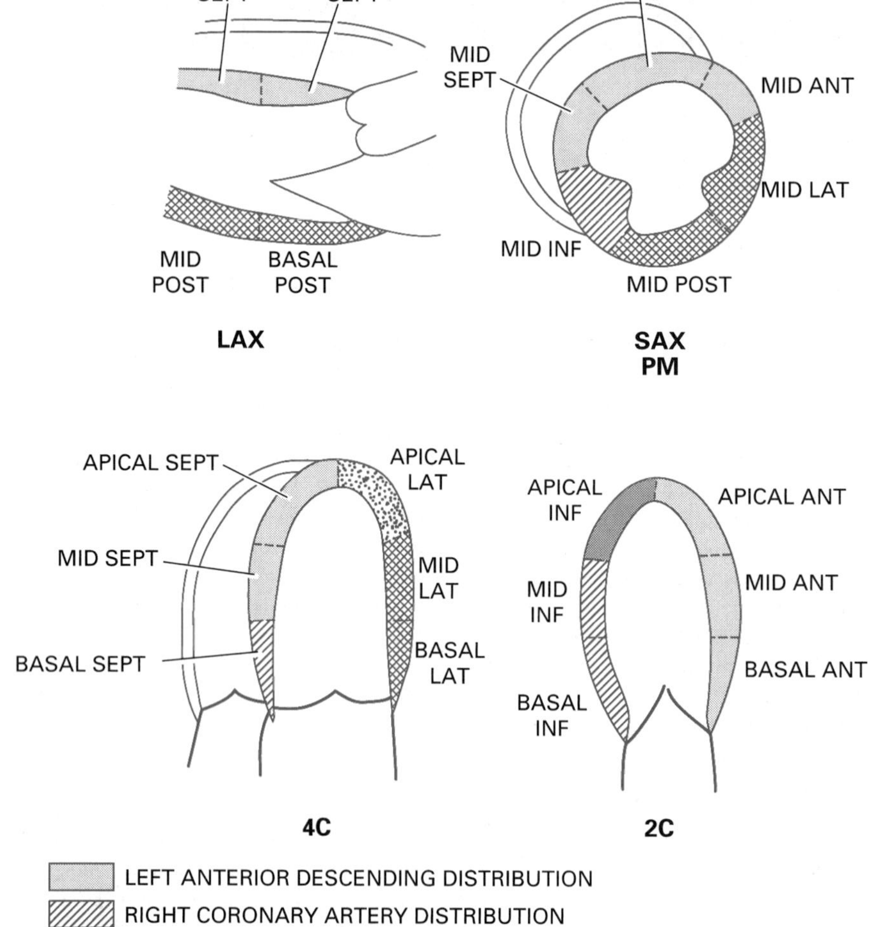


FIGURE 15-97 Sixteen-segment format for identification of left ventricular wall segments. Coronary arterial territories are also included. LAX = parasternal long axis; SAX PM = short axis at papillary muscle level; 4C = apical four-chamber; 2C = apical two-chamber; ANT = anterior; SEPT = septal; POST= posterior; LAT = lateral; INF = inferior. (From Segar D, Brown S, Sawada S, et al. Dobutamine stress echocardiography: Correlation with coronary lesion severity as determined by quantitative angiography. *J Am Coll Cardiol* 1992;19:1197. With permission.)

cussion of cardiac masses below. A less frequent complication is rupture of the LV free wall, which is usually rapidly fatal and therefore rarely imaged by echocardiography. However, the presence of significant pericardial effusion on echocardiography in patients with hemodynamic compromise in the postinfarction period should suggest this condition. If a free wall rupture is sealed off by clot and pericardial inflammation, a pseudoaneurysm is formed[221,222] (Fig. 15-101). This lesion is distinguished from a true aneurysm by its highly localized nature and the presence of a narrow neck connecting it with the ventricle. Pseudoaneurysms frequently have multilayered thrombi within them and exhibit characteristic Doppler flow signals at the junction with the ventricle.[222] Since the risk of rupture is high, accurate diagnosis and prompt surgical repair of pseudoaneurysms is important.

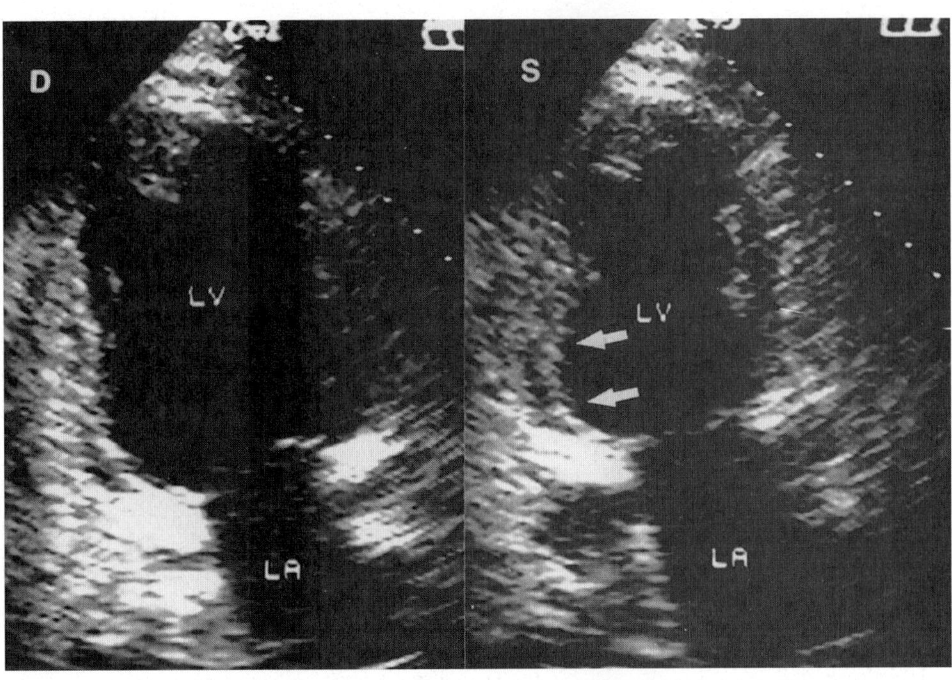


FIGURE 15-98 Diastolic (*left*) and systolic (*right*) images (apical two-chamber plane) from a patient with an inferior wall myocardial infarction. The inferobasal segment is dyskinetic (*arrows*). LV = left ventricle; LA = left atrium.

Although postinfarction free wall rupture does not lend itself well to echocardiographic detection, acquired defects of the interventricular septum are more commonly delineated by cardiac ultrasound.[223] Acquired ventricular septal defects often consist of a latticework of tissue rather than a discrete orifice, but nevertheless echocardiographic images can depict absence of myocardium and distinct flow jets communicating between the left and right ventricles (Fig. 15-102, Plate 67). These color jets are typically high-velocity and aliased, coursing from the septum into the RV. The echocardiographic location of the defect and jet correlate well with the location by cineangiography, surgery, or autopsy, and an apical location is most amenable to surgical correction.

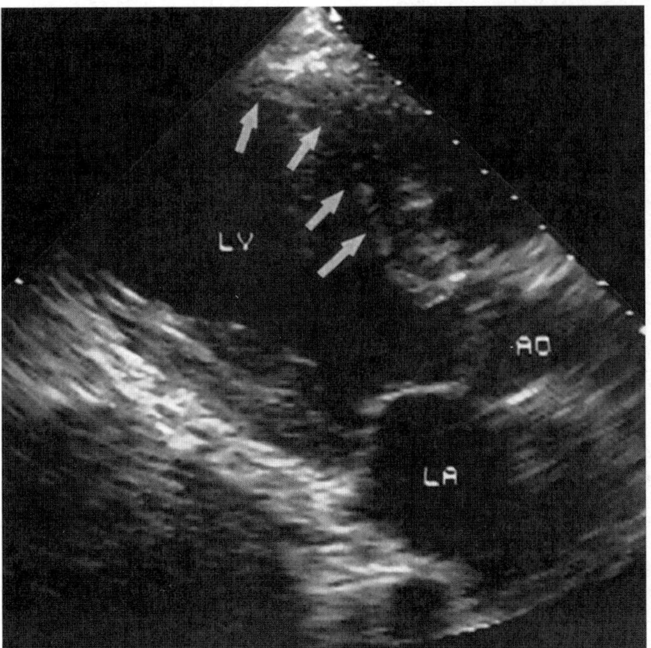


FIGURE 15-99 Parasternal long-axis view of a large anteroseptal myocardial infarction, with thinning and dyskinesis of the anteroseptal wall (*arrows*). LV = left ventricle; LA = left atrium; AO = aorta.

MR is a common sequela of AMI; if severe, it may result in profound congestive heart failure and shock. Several mechanisms may be responsible for the occurrence of postinfarction MR including dilation of the LV cavity and mitral annulus, papillary muscle dysfunction, and partial or complete rupture of a papillary muscle (Fig. 15-103).[224,225] MR from papillary dysfunction may lead to eccentric color jets within the LA. In general, the recognition and quantitation of MR occurring in the postinfarction period is no different from that of any other type of MR. Acute ischemic MR, however may cause a smaller flow disturbance by color Doppler than comparable grades of chronic MR, particularly with transthoracic imaging. Therefore, TEE may play an important role in the identification and quantitative assessment of this complication, as well as in ensuring adequate operative repair.[225]

In the setting of inferior wall infarction due to occlusion of the proximal right coronary artery, RV MI may occur. The most specific echocardiographic sign of RV infarction is a regional wall motion abnormality, which is usually best visualized in the RV free wall (Fig. 15-104). RV infarction is typically accompanied by RV enlargement and tricuspid regurgitation; associated inferior or posterior LV wall motion abnormalities are virtually always present.

Pericarditis is a common complication of AMI, typically occurring during the acute phase of the illness and much less often in the late phases as part of the Dressler syndrome. Postinfarction pericarditis, however, is not typically associated with marked echocardiographic abnormalities. If a pericardial effusion is present at all, the amount of fluid is usually quite small. Therefore, the absence of pericardial fluid on ECG cannot rule out pericarditis, and the presence of a large effusion with tamponade should raise the suspicion of a LV free wall rupture.

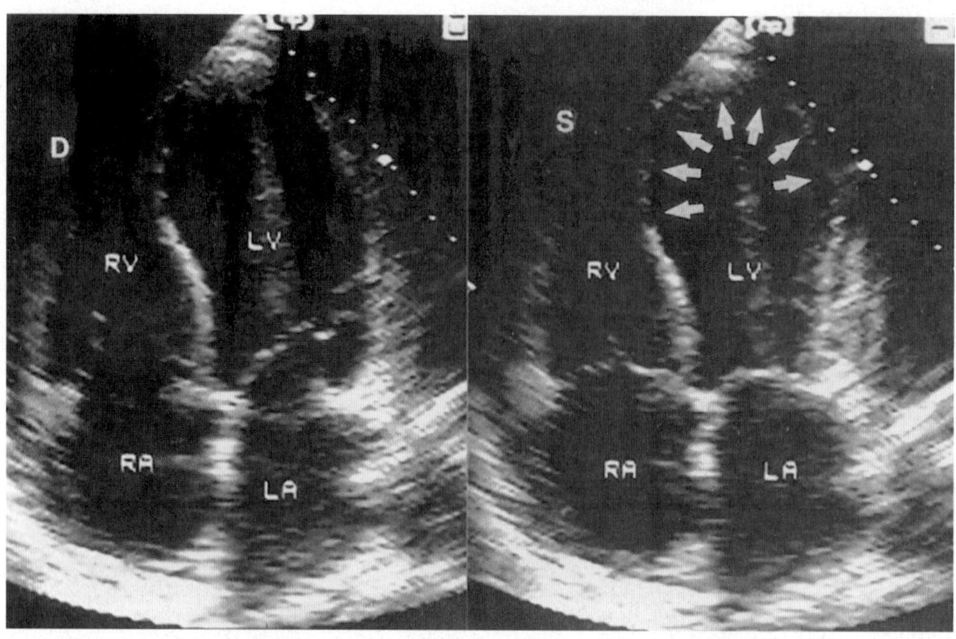


FIGURE 15-100 Apical four-chamber images of a large apical infarction. Diastole (D) is displayed on the left, systole (S) on the right. During systole, the base of the ventricle contracts, but the apex is dyskinetic (*arrows*).

TEE has assumed a central role in the evaluation of patients with significant hemodynamic abnormalities in the postinfarction period. When TTE is technically suboptimal, transesophageal images can rapidly identify LV dyssynergy, valvular dysfunction, and other abnormalities associated with infarction. TEE may enable direct visualization of acquired ventricular septal defects when the lesion is not obvious or seen only as a disturbed flow stream in the RV with transthoracic imaging. Perhaps of greatest significance, TEE can provide definitive identification of a ruptured papillary muscle and a quantitative assessment of postinfarction mitral regurgitation.

Echocardiography has been used to evaluate the extent of reperfusion after thrombolytic or interventional therapy for AMI. Several

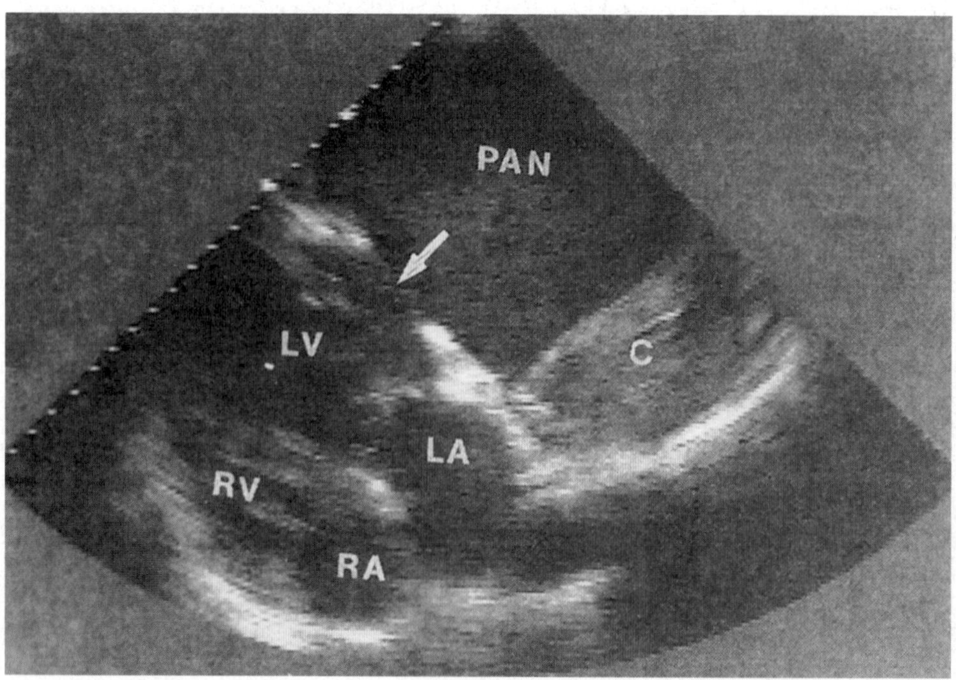


FIGURE 15-101 Modified apical four-chamber view of a large pseudoaneurysm (PAN) communicating with the left ventricle (LV). The rupture site is apparent (*arrow*); clot (C) is present within the aneurysm. (From Yucel G, Steinberg E, O'Reilly M, Kronzon I. Giant left ventricular pseudoaneurysm. *Circulation* 1996;94:848. With permission.)

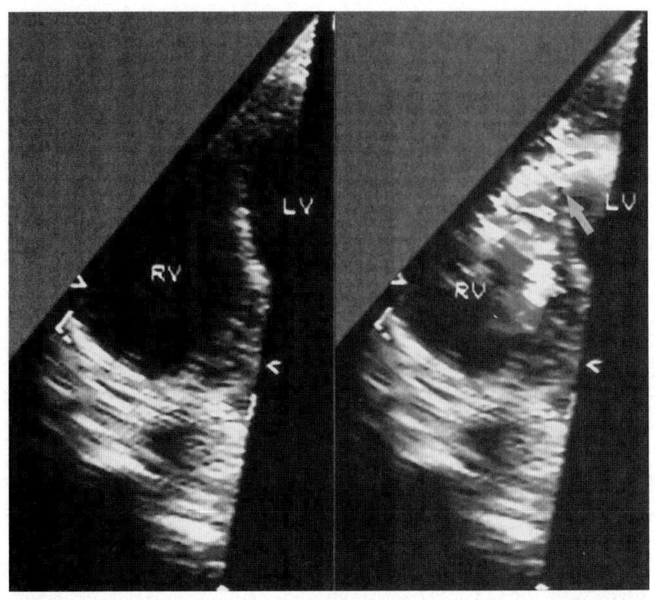


FIGURE 15-102 (Plate 67) Modified apical four-chamber image of a distal septal ventricular septal rupture. With 2D imaging (*left*), the distal septum is incompletely visualized. With color Doppler imaging, however, a high-velocity aliased color jet is seen in the right ventricle (RV). In addition, an area of flow convergence is seen on the left ventricular (LV) side of the rupture (*arrow*).

reports have demonstrated that LV systolic function assessed by 2D imaging improved within 24 h to 10 days of successful thrombolysis.[226] More recently, contrast echocardiograms obtained after intravenous or direct intracoronary injection have shown that reperfusion of the infarct-related epicardial coronary artery by angiography is not necessarily accompanied by evidence of normal flow in the downstream microcirculation. In addition, this "no-reflow" phenomenon on echocardiography heralds a poor prognosis, including failure of improvement of LV performance as well as increased late complications.[129,130,227]

## Stress Echocardiography

The combination of stress testing and echocardiography (stress echocardiography) has assumed an important role in the diagnosis of CAD[228] (Chap. 42). The utility of this technique improved dramatically when technologic advances permitted side-by-side viewing of rest and stress images together in a cine-loop format.[229,230] The application of stress echocardiography is based upon the concept that a stress-induced imbalance in the myocardial supply/demand ratio will produce regional ischemia and resultant abnormalities of regional contraction, which can be readily identified by echocardiography (Fig. 15-105). The location of wall motion abnormalities may be used to predict the stenosed coronary vessel(s), while the ratio of dyssynergic to normal myocardium can provide a quantitative assessment of LV ischemia.[215]

The types of stress employed fall into two basic groups, exercise and pharmacologic.[215] Other forms, such as mental stress and atrial pacing, are not widely used. Exercise testing can be performed either on a treadmill or a stationary bicycle (either upright or supine).[231] Treadmill testing involves a familiar activity, uses equipment that is widely available, and achieves greater oxygen consumption than bicycle ergometry. Echo imaging usually can be accomplished only before and after treadmill exercise, however, whereas bicycle exertion facilitates the acquisition of images during the exercise protocol. Thus far, treadmill has been the preferred exercise modality. Of importance, all postexertional images should be obtained within a 1- to 2-min window following exercise to avoid recording normal contractile function after recovery from ischemia.

Pharmacologic stress has the advantages of reducing the motion artifact of exercise, enabling continuous imaging throughout the protocol, and assessing myocardial viability.[232] Pharmacologic stress echocardiography can employ vasodilator agents such as dipyridamole or adenosine, which induce a heterogeneity of myocardial perfusion in ischemic heart disease, or inotropic agents such as dobutamine, which increase myocardial oxygen demand and directly produce ischemia.[232] As with exercise stress, diagnostic criteria include induction of regional wall motion abnormalities and LV dilatation. It is important to recognize that the normal response to exercise is hyperkinesis, and wall motion abnormalities may take the form of a lesser degree of hyperkinesis of a given segment in comparison with the rest of the LV myocardium. Dobutamine stress echocardiography appears to be of particular value in detecting myocardial viability,[229–234] and appears superior to PET and thallium scanning for the

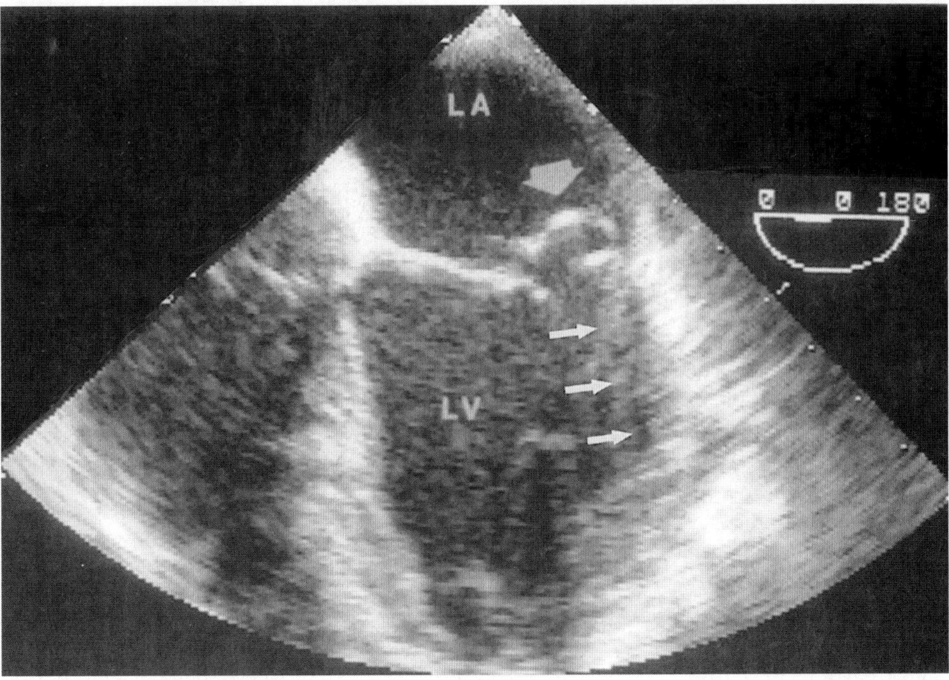


FIGURE 15-103 Transverse four-chamber TEE image of a posterolateral infarction causing posterior papillary muscle ischemia and partial rupture. The posterior mitral leaflet (*large arrow*) is poorly supported (but not actually flail) and prolapses into the left atrium (LA). The basal lateral wall segment (*small arrows*) of the left ventricle (LV) is dyskinetic.

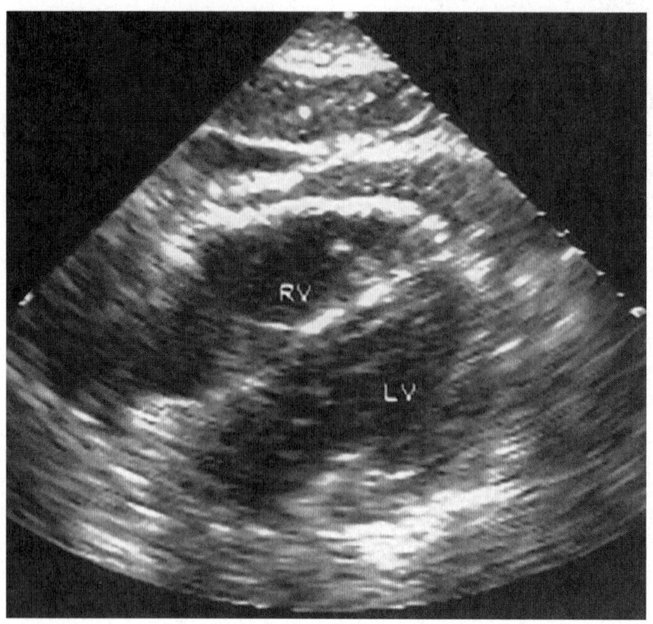


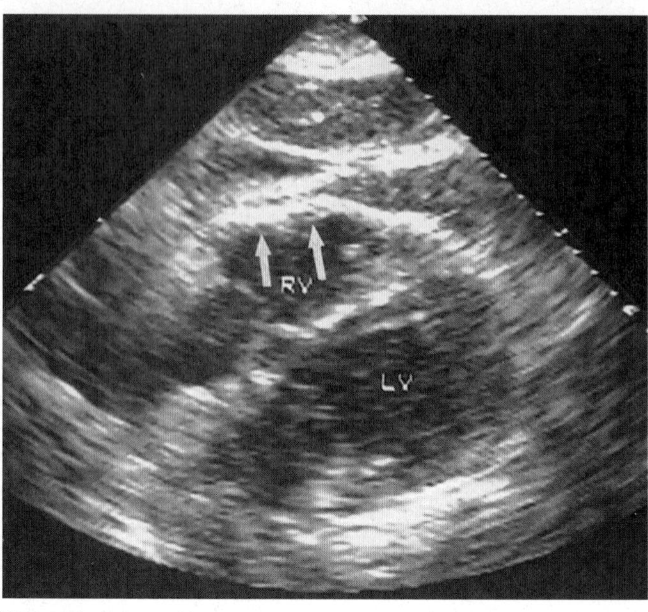


FIGURE 15-104 Diastolic (*A*) and systolic (*B*) subcostal four-chamber images of right ventricular (RV) myocardial infarction. The RV free wall is dyskinetic (*arrows*) during systole (*B*).

prediction of improvement in systolic function after coronary bypass surgery.[235]

The safety and accuracy of stress echocardiography for the diagnosis of myocardial ischemia has been examined in a number of studies.[228,233–236] Both exercise and pharmacologic stress carry an extremely low risk of arrhythmia or infarction, although dobutamine can result in hypotension or *systolic anterior motion of the MV* (SAM) with resultant LV outflow obstruction.[228,237,238] In general, stress echocardiography and nuclear scintigraphy yield similar results, although stress echocardiography may be slightly less sensitive

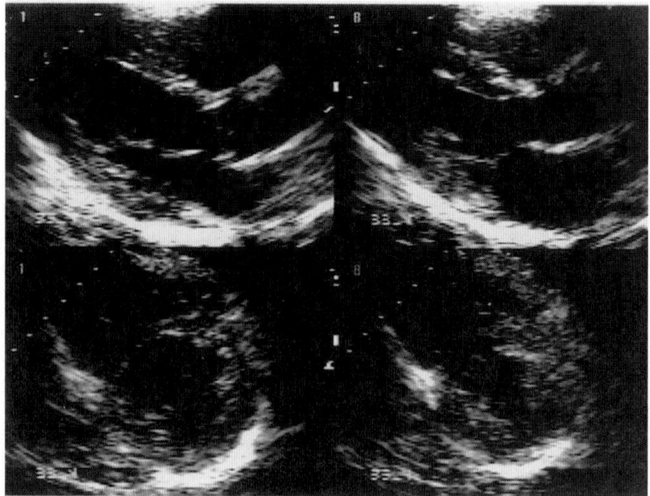


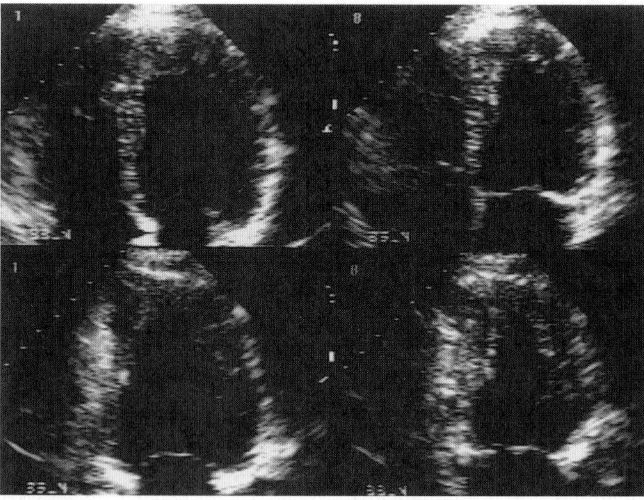


FIGURE 15-105 *A.* Digitized parasternal views during diastole (*left*) and systole (*right*) from a normal individual. *Upper panels:* long-axis plane; *lower panels:* short-axis plane. *B.* Digitized apical views during diastole (*left*) and systole (*right*) from a normal individual. *Upper panels:* four-chamber plane; *lower panels:* two-chamber plane. *C.* Digitized parasternal long-axis views at peak systole before (*left*) and immediately after exercise (*right*). The anteroseptal wall moves normally at rest (*arrows*) but becomes dyskinetic with exercise. LV = left ventricle; LA = left atrium; AO = aorta. *D.* Digitized apical four-chamber views at peak systole before (*left*) and immediately after exercise (*right*). The apical septal, apical, and apical lateral walls become dyskinetic with exercise, suggesting inducible ischemia in the left anterior descending artery territory. LA = left atrium; LV = left ventricle. *E.* Digitized parasternal short-axis views (all recorded at peak systole) during dobutamine echocardiography in a patient with three-vessel coronary artery disease. At baseline (*upper left panel*), the left ventricular systolic function is normal. With low-dose dobutamine (5 $\mu$g/kg/min, *upper right panel*), function improves. With 10 $\mu$g/kg/min, however (*lower left panel*), function is similar to that at baseline. At 20 $\mu$g/kg/min (*lower right panel*), systolic function deteriorates and the left ventricle dilates. This response suggests global ischemia induced by dobutamine infusion.

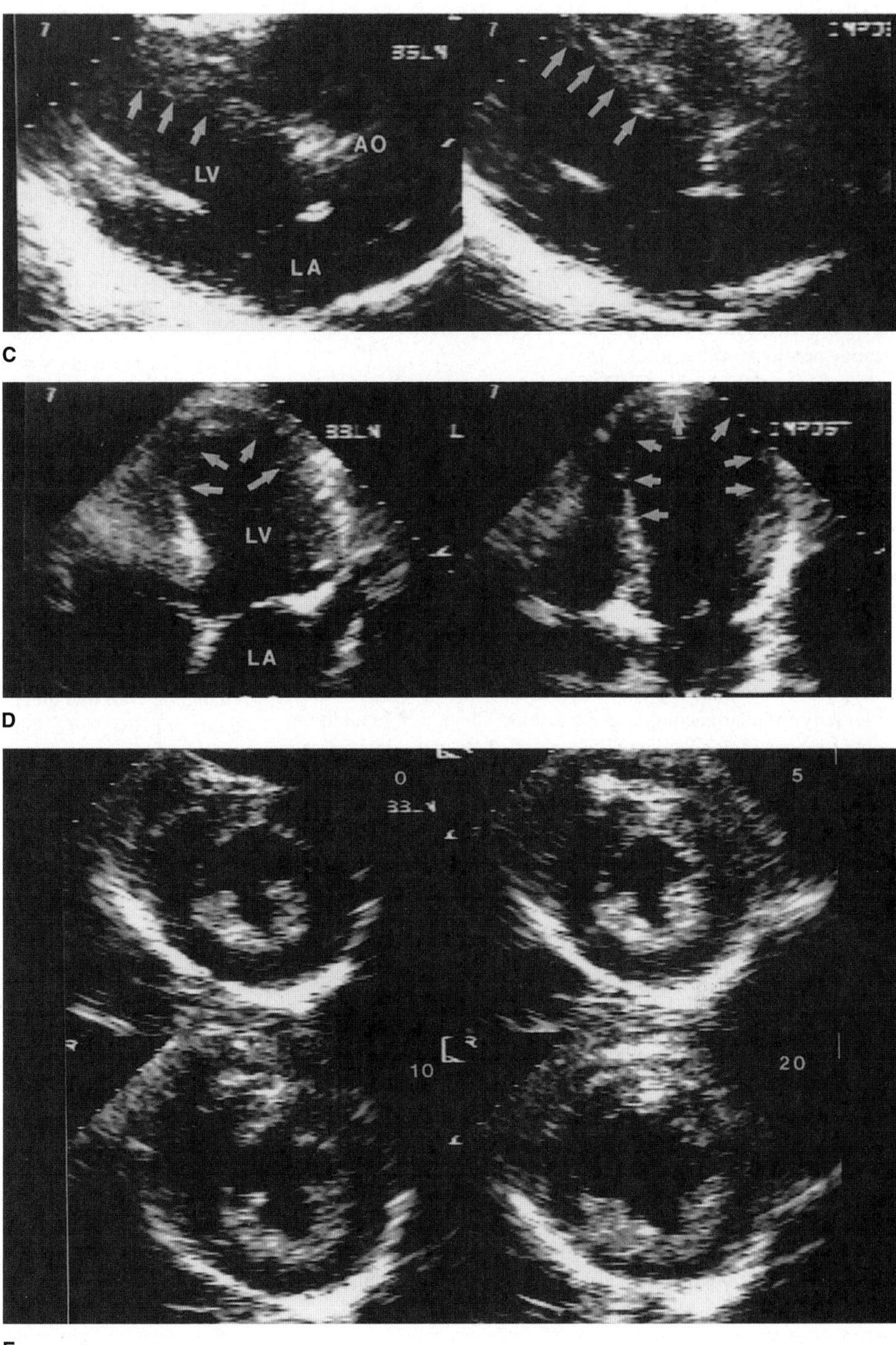


FIGURE 15-105 (*Continued*)

and slightly more specific than scintigraphy.[229] In a study performed in an institution with high volumes and expertise in both ultrasound and radionuclide stress imaging, the two techniques were found to be comparable in their accuracy of detecting coronary artery disease.[229] The most common clinical application of stress echocardiography is in the diagnosis of CAD, and it appears especially useful in cases where exercise *electrocardiography* (ECG) may be inaccurate or falsely positive (e.g., abnormal baseline ECG, LVH, or chronic digitalis administration).[228,136,239] In this regard, stress echocardiography appears especially useful for detection of ischemia in women,[240,241] in whom stress ECG yields a high incidence of false-positive results. Stress echocardiography also adds independent prognostic information to exercise ECG, even in multivessel CAD. Dobutamine echocardiography may aid in the detection of ischemia in patients with cardiac transplantation and allograft vasculopathy (chronic rejection).[242] In patients with known CAD, exercise echocardiography may facilitate localization and quantitation of ischemia, guide revascularization procedures, and assess the functional severity of coronary artery stenoses. Stress echocardiography can also demonstrate resolution of regional ischemia after successful coronary artery bypass surgery or angioplasty.[243]

Stress echocardiography can play an important role in determining the prognosis of patients with CAD.[244,245] Both exercise and pharmacologic stress echocardiography appear superior to exercise ECG for identification of patients at high risk of recurrent ischemic events after MI. In addition, dobutamine stress echocardiography is useful in predicting perioperative ischemic complications in patients undergoing noncardiac surgery[244] and appears to have a very strong negative predictive value.

In patients with chronic CHD, dobutamine stress echocardiography can identify hypokinetic yet viable myocardium and predicts improvement in function after successful revascularization.[233,234] Functional improvement in a hypokinetic segment with low-dose dobutamine infusion which then progresses to hypokinesis or akinesis with higher dobutamine dose (the so-called biphasic response) correlates well with the presence of ischemic yet viable ("hibernating") myocardium. Studies have suggested that dobutamine stress echocardiography compares well with positron emission tomography and thallium single-photon emission computed tomography (SPECT) imaging in this regard.[235,246,247] It is likely that this application of echocardiography will continue to evolve over time, particularly for pharmacologic stress testing (Chap. 58). In addition, quantitation of regional myocardial blood flow using intravenous echo contrast agents may enhance the usefulness of stress echocardiography in the detection of both ischemia and viability.

There is evidence that exercise echocardiography can provide useful information regarding the hemodynamic status and functional severity of valvular heart disease.[248] Specifically, stress echocardiography has been used to assess the degree of obstruction in patients with MS and to quantitate the severity of AS in patients with advanced LV dysfunction.[248] These data may help guide the timing of surgical valve repair or replacement.

As is true of all diagnostic modalities, stress echocardiography has certain limitations. High-quality ultrasound images may be difficult to acquire in some patients—a situation that may be exacerbated by exertion and the time constraints inherent to exercise stress testing. In addition, considerable expertise is required to interpret stress echocardiographic images accurately, and this learning curve precludes the use of stress echocardiography by all but experienced echocardiographers. Nevertheless, stress echocardiography has many advantages over alternate diagnostic approaches such as radionuclide scintigraphy and coronary angiography, including its noninvasive and relatively inexpensive nature, rapid acquisition and interpretation times, and freedom from ionizing radiation. Harmonic imaging (both with and without intravenous echocardiographic contrast) has also enhanced endocardial border definition, facilitating stress echo studies in many patients with suboptimal fundamental (nonharmonic) echo images. Therefore it is anticipated that the use of stress echocardiography will continue to increase in the foreseeable future.

## THE CARDIOMYOPATHIES

The evaluation of cardiomyopathy is complicated by the fact that few specific diagnostic criteria exist, and identification is often a process of exclusion. Further, many potential etiologies may be responsible for the myopathic process, and it may be possible to identify a specific etiology in only the minority of patients. Accordingly, a diagnostic strategy has evolved that initially seeks to place patients into one of three pathophysiologic categories: dilated, hypertrophic, or restrictive; then, the specific etiologies recognized as producing the individual pathophysiologic state are pursued. Thus, dilated cardiomyopathies are associated with myocyte loss and necrosis, a marked increase in LV volume, thinning of the myocardium, and profound systolic dysfunction.[249] *Hypertrophic cardiomyopathy* (HCM) (Chap. 77) is recognized by increased myocardial thickness, particularly involving the interventricular septum, with preserved systolic function. Restrictive cardiomyopathies may be due to infiltration of the myocardium by abnormal substances or fibrotic tissue; these cause symmetrical degrees of wall thickening with modest or no diminution of systolic function and little change in cavity size.[250] Echocardiography customarily serves as the cornerstone of such evaluations and provides data on cavity size, wall thickness, and systolic function. Thus, on echocardiogram, patients with dilated cardiomyopathy exhibit a marked increase in left LV and volume, little change in wall thickness, and severe contractile dysfunction.[249] Patients with HCM exhibit a dramatic increase in LV wall thickness, with the septum characteristically disproportionate to the posterior wall, and often subaortic stenosis induced by systolic anterior motion of the anterior MV leaflet. Patients with restrictive cardiomyopathy are identified by a symmetric increase in wall thickness accompanied by modest changes in contractile function and LV cavity size.[250]

### Hypertrophic Cardiomyopathy

HCM is a primary abnormality of the myocardium that exhibits myocyte disarray and unprovoked hypertrophy, often affecting the septum disproportionately (Chap. 77). The disorder, which is often transmitted in an autosomal dominant pattern, has been linked to a number of abnormalities in genes that code for myocardial proteins.[251] A number of classic echocardiographic findings occur in HCM (Fig. 15-106). The fundamental abnormality on echocardiogram in HCM is LVH, which is often severe. Although the hypertrophy may be confined to the septum, it may be concentric or involve any other portion of the LV.[252] The customary classic finding is *asymmetric septal hypertrophy* (ASH), defined as a disproportionate thickness of the interventricular septum compared to the posterobasal wall with a ratio of greater than 1.3 to 1.[253] In some cases the entire septum is hypertrophied, while in others the thickening may be localized to the proximal, mid-, or distal (apical) septum. Asymmetric hypertrophy of the proximal interventricular septum may lead to dynamic LV outflow tract obstruction—*hypertrophic obstructive cardiomyopathy* (HOCM) or *idiopathic hypertrophic subaortic stenosis* (IHSS). Although ASH is almost always present in cases of dynamic LV outflow tract obstruction, it is not a specific marker for

FIGURE 15-106 *A.* Parasternal long-axis view (during systole) of hypertrophic cardiomyopathy (HCM). Asymmetrical septal hypertrophy is present, as is systolic anterior motion of the anterior mitral valve leaflet (*arrow*). LV = left ventricle; LA = left atrium; RV = right ventricle; AO = aorta. *B.* Parasternal short-axis view of HCM. Asymmetrical septal hypertrophy is present (*arrows*). RV = right ventricle; LV = left ventricle. *C.* Parasternal M-mode image from a patient with HCM, demonstrating systolic anterior motion of the anterior mitral valve leaflet (*arrows*). RV = right ventricle; IVS = interventricular septum; LV = left ventricle. *D.* Transesophageal image of HCM. The anterior mitral valve leaflet appears normal during diastole (upper panel), but systolic anterior motion occurs during systole (lower panel). *E.* Transesophageal M-mode tracing through the aortic valve. Midsystolic notching and partial closure of the valve leaflets is present.

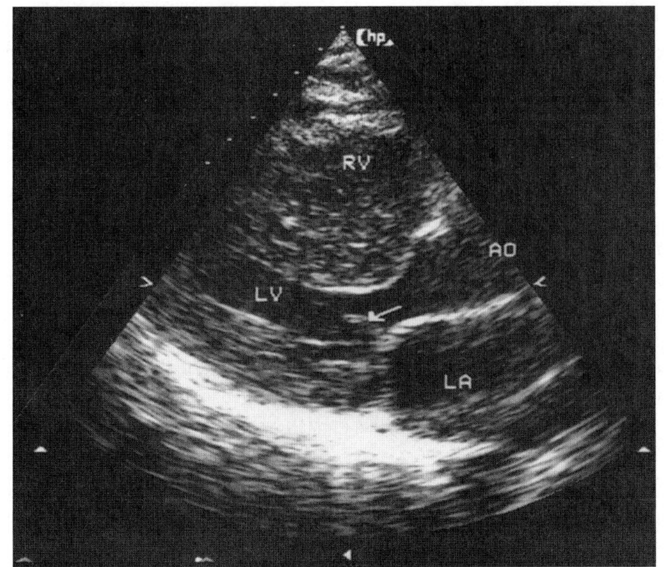
RV
AO
LV
LA

A

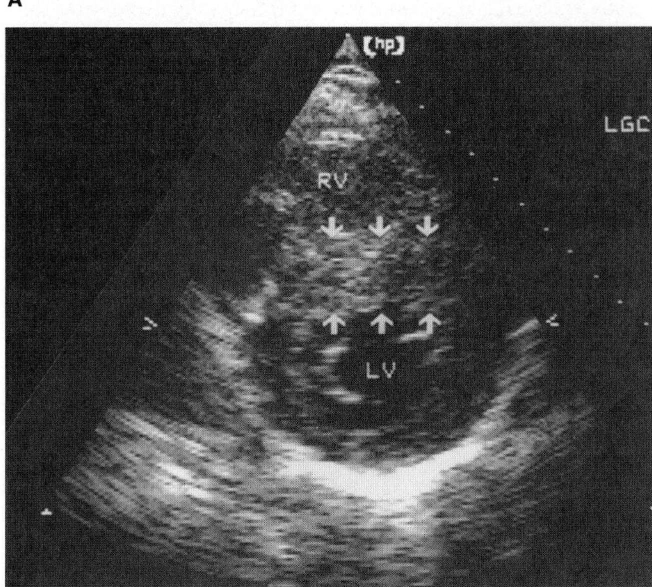
LGC
RV
LV

B

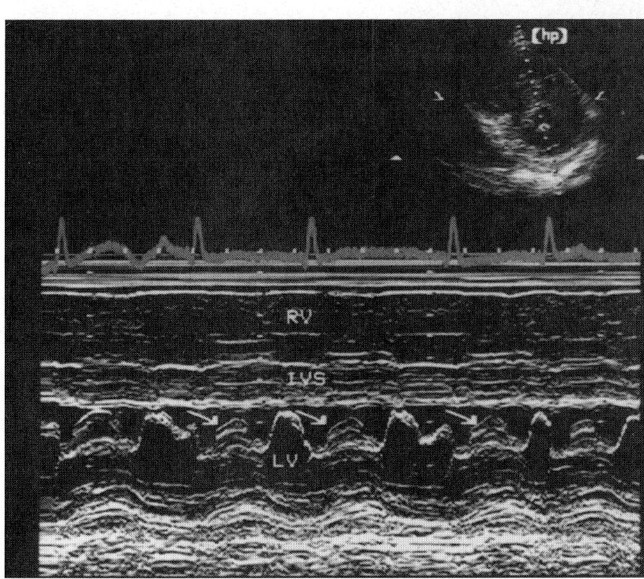
RV
IVS
LV

C

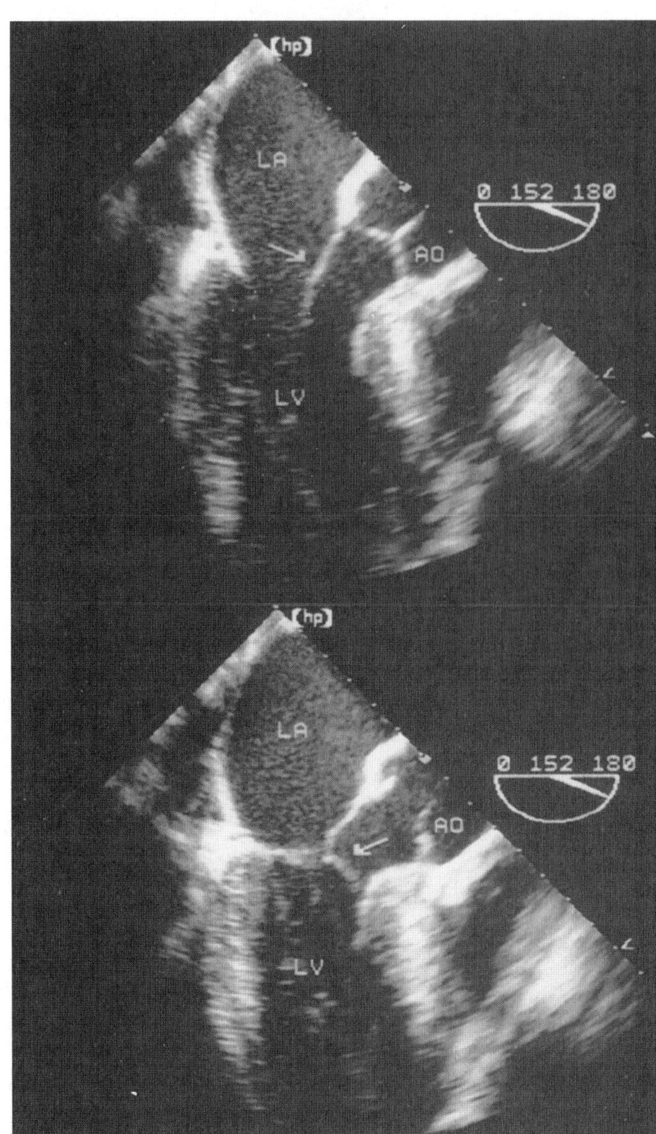
LA
0 152 180
AO
LV
LA
0 152 180
AO
LV

D

GAIN 60 COMP 58
CTR 49HZ 15CM
PROC 2/0/B/F3
84BPM
0:46:41.08
05 FEB 99
13:48:35
0 41 180

E

HCM and may occur in some patients with RV hypertrophy (RVH), inferior MI, and a minority with hypertensive LVH.[254] In general, the more extensive the hypertrophic process, the more severe the symptoms. Extent of hypertrophy, however, does not appear to correlate well with risk of sudden death, as patients with minimal hypertrophy may still be at significant risk.[255]

The second characteristic finding of HCM is systolic anterior motion of the MV, or SAM, which usually involves the anterior MV leaflet. Posterior-leaflet SAM also has been reported in HCM, as have a variety of MV deformities. Encroachment of the pathologically thickened septum upon the LV outflow tract creates a pressure drop by a Venturi effect, which draws the mitral leaflets toward the septum, creating dynamic (subaortic) LV outflow obstruction (Fig. 15-106). Recent work has also demonstrated the important effects of papillary muscle position and chordal tension on systolic mitral morphology and SAM.[256] Because of distorted mitral coaptation during systole, SAM generally causes MR of variable severity. The severity and duration of SAM directly influence the degree of both outflow tract obstruction and MR. Like asymmetrical septal hypertrophy, SAM (especially systolic motion of the chordae) is not pathognomonic for HCM, having been reported in other conditions such as hypovolemia, anemia, and states where LV outflow tract narrowing and hyperdynamic contraction are present.

The third manifestation of classic HCM is midsystolic closure of the aortic valve (Fig. 15-106*E*).[257] This finding is best seen on M-mode recordings, occurs only in the presence of outflow tract obstruction, and is probably a manifestation of the sudden pressure drop during mid- and late systole caused by SAM. As with ASH and SAM, midsystolic aortic closure is not specific for HCM and can occur in MR, aortic root dilatation, ventricular septal defect, and discrete subaortic stenosis. When HCM is present, however, midsystolic aortic valve closure suggests significant outflow tract obstruction.

The fourth important abnormality of HCM is observed on Doppler examination of the LV outflow tract (LVOT). Normally, Doppler interrogation of this area produces a spectral tracing that peaks early in systole and has a maximum velocity of less than 1.7 m/s. In many patients, HCM creates a high-pressure gradient coincident with SAM, which is detected by Doppler as a high-velocity systolic jet in the LVOT. As opposed to valvular aortic stenosis, however, the maximal velocity in obstructive HCM peaks late in systole, creating a characteristic "saber-tooth" pattern (Fig. 15-107). Although the subaortic gradient can be estimated using the modified Bernoulli equation, the assumptions used in this equation may not apply to HCM, as intraventricular gradient calculations can be spuriously high because of the phenomenon of pressure recovery.[258] Similar Doppler patterns also may be seen occasionally within the LV in patients with HCM if systolic obliteration of the hypertrophied LV causes localized areas of high flow velocity in the more distal portions of the ventricular cavity.

Diastolic dysfunction has been long recognized in HCM. Doppler interrogation of LV inflow often reveals a relaxation abnormality, with a reduced early diastolic (E) velocity, a prolonged deceleration slope of the E wave, and an increased velocity of the atrial systolic (A) component.[259] Color Doppler imaging can be used to demonstrate intraventricular flow characteristics.

## Dilated Cardiomyopathy

In cases of *dilated cardiomyopathy* (DCM), the heart is typically greatly enlarged and systolic function is markedly depressed (Chap. 66).[260] Four-chamber dilatation is a common but not uniform finding, as some patients may have relatively preserved RV size (this may confer an improved prognosis).[261] Marked LV enlargement and generalized dysfunction can also be caused by severe ischemic heart disease, chronic alcohol abuse, various infectious myocarditides, anthracyclines and other cardiotoxic agents, nutritional deficiencies, and hereditary myopathies.[262] Severe ischemic disease is often segmental and has been reported to spare the posterior wall frequently, while the LV dysfunction of DCM is usually global. The typical constellation of echocardiographic findings in DCM include an increased LV end-diastolic diameter and volume with decreased fractional shortening, thinning of the LV walls (Fig. 15-108), increased E point-septal separation, LA enlargement, and limited mitral and aortic valve opening (due to low stroke volume). Intracardiac thrombi are frequently observed and are most often found in the LV apex. M-mode imaging of the mitral leaflets may demonstrate a "B bump," or notch just before systolic valve closure, indicating elevated LV diastolic pressure (Fig. 15-8). The cardiac valves are usually normal, but mitral annular dilatation and secondary MR are common.

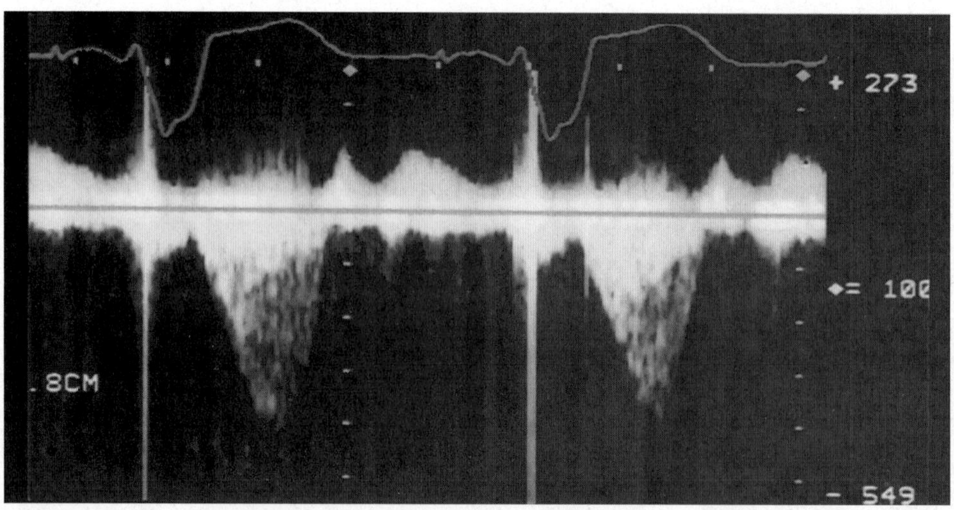


FIGURE 15-107 Continuous-wave Doppler tracing through the left ventricular outflow tract (from the apical transducer position) in hypertrophic obstructive cardiomyopathy (HOCM). In comparison to valvular aortic stenosis, the rise in velocity is delayed (reflecting dynamic rather than fixed outflow obstruction).

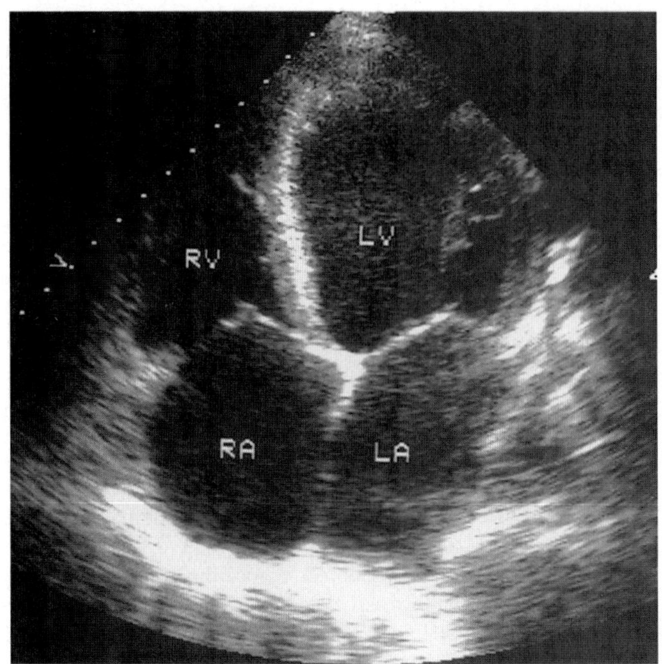


FIGURE 15-108 Apical four-chamber image of dilated cardiomyopathy. There is four-chamber enlargement as well as left ventricular (LV) spontaneous echo contrast. RV = right ventricle; RA = right atrium; LA = left atrium.

Doppler echocardiography often reveals an abnormally low-velocity time integral in the LV outflow or inflow tracts. Diastolic MR due to elevated LV diastolic pressure also may be present. Diastolic dysfunction is common, and pulsed-wave Doppler interrogation of mitral inflow may show an abnormal relaxation, restrictive, or pseudonormal pattern depending on LV diastolic pressures and loading conditions.[263] A restrictive pattern of mitral inflow Doppler confers a poor prognosis in patients with DCM.

## Restrictive Cardiomyopathy

Restrictive cardiomyopathy may be idiopathic or secondary to infiltrative diseases such as amyloidosis, hemochromatosis, hypereosinophilic syndrome and Loeffler endocarditis, sarcoidosis, radiation toxicity, glycogen storage diseases, and Gaucher disease (Chap. 83). Typical 2D echocardiographic features of these diseases include (1) a diffuse increase of ventricular thickness in the absence of marked ventricular chamber dilation and (2) marked biatrial enlargement[250] (Fig. 15-109). Systolic function is often modestly decreased. As with the other cardiomyopathies, these echocardiographic findings are nonspecific. Doppler examination may show a mitral inflow relaxation abnormality early in the course of restrictive cardiomyopathy, but restrictive pattern (E much greater than A, with shortened E deceleration time) is a more classic finding, which often evolves with time and indicates both a high LA pressure and poor prognosis.[265,266]

Amyloidosis is generally the most commonly encountered restrictive cardiac disease. In addition to biventricular hypertrophy, amyloidosis is also associated with diffuse thickening of the interatrial septum and cardiac valves. In advanced disease, depressed systolic function is also common. An abnormal "speckled" pattern or "ground glass" appearance of the myocardium has been described on 2D echocardiography, but this sign is absent in many cases and therefore has minimal clinical usefulness. The finding of a restrictive mitral inflow pattern (and an abnormally high diastolic component of pulmonary vein inflow) on Doppler echocardiography has been identified as a marker of advanced disease and poor prognosis.[266,267] In addition to increased myocardial thickness, endocardial thickening and fibrosis and restricted atrioventricular leaflet motion are common features of Loeffler endocarditis and endomyocardial fibroelastosis.[264] Intraventricular thrombi are also common in these processes.

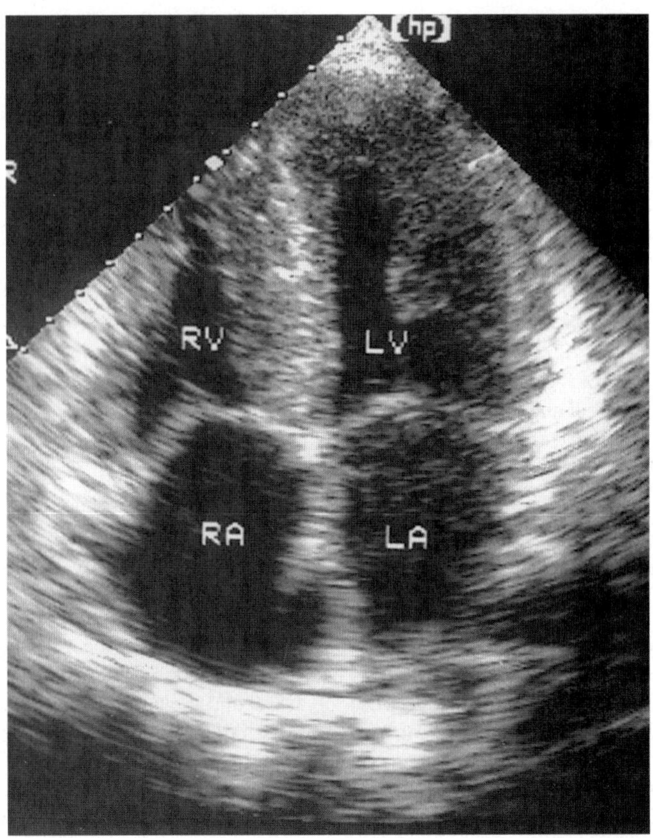


FIGURE 15-109 Apical four-chamber image of cardiac amyloid. RV = right ventricle; RA = right atrium; LA = left atrium; LV = left ventricle.

# CONGENITAL HEART DISEASE

## Echocardiographic Identification of Congenital Cardiac Anomalies

2D and Doppler echocardiography has had a major impact on the diagnosis and management of patients with congenital heart disease (Chaps. 63 and 64). From isolated congenital lesions to complex, extensive cardiac malformations, echocardiographic imaging (often with intravenous contrast injection) is usually sufficient to delineate cardiac anatomy. TEE is an important adjunctive technique as well; in many cases, a thorough echocardiographic evaluation may obviate the need for cardiac catheterization and angiography.[268]

The ultrasound diagnosis of a simple intracardiac shunt is usually straightforward, but the task of defining complex congenital cardiac abnormalities can be daunting. In these cases, it is useful to remember a few basic anatomic rules. The venae cavae and pulmonary veins generally empty into the morphologic right atrium and LA, respectively. The atrioventricular valves uniformly follow their ventricles through embryologic development: a TV accompanies the morphologic RV and a MV accompanies the left. Similarly, the semilunar valves follow the great vessels. The aorta and PA can be distinguished, regardless of their position, by the bifurcation of the PA.

Several features aid identification of the morphologic right and left ventricles. The RV has a tricuspid atrioventricular valve; in comparison with the mitral annulus, the tricuspid annulus is positioned slightly closer to the cardiac apex. The RV also has a moderator band, coarser trabeculations than those in the left ventricle, and an infundibulum that separates the inlet area from the RVOT.

## Cardiovascular Shunts

### ATRIAL SEPTAL DEFECT

Most secundum and primum *atrial septal defects* (ASDs) are easily visualized by echocardiography, although sinus venous defects are often difficult to detect without TEE. Apical echocardiographic views often show artifactual "dropout" in the region of the fossa ovalis, since the interatrial septum is thin in this area and runs parallel to the ultrasound beam. Therefore the subcostal view provides the optimal imaging plane to detect lesions of the atrial septum.[269] Ostium secundum defects are the most common form of ASD, and 2D imaging shows a localized absence of septal tissue in the midportion of the interatrial septum (Fig. 15-110*A*, Plate 68). Lack of any interatrial septal tissue between the defect and the base of the interventricular septum characterizes an ostium primum defect (Fig. 15-110*B*). Although ostium secundum defects are usually isolated, ostium primum (or partial AV canal) defects are often accompanied by other lesions, such as cleft anterior MV leaflet, MR, and atrioventricular canal ventricular septal defect.[270] Sinus venosus defects are strongly associated with partial anomalous pulmonary venous return (for example, drainage of the right upper pulmonary vein into the right atrium or superior vena cava) (Fig. 15-111*A*). Rarely, the atrial septum may be completely absent (Fig. 15-112). With all but small ASDs, the right atrium is enlarged and RV volume overload is present, with a dilated RV and paradoxical septal motion.

Intravenous contrast injection generally demonstrates shunting across the ASD, frequently with bidirectional flow.[271] Therefore "negative jets" of unopacified flow from the LA into the contrast-filled right atrium may alternate with the appearance of contrast bubbles flowing through the defect into the LA. When an ASD is present, contrast should appear quickly (within three to five heartbeats) in the LA after entering the right atrium. Delayed appearance of contrast in the LA may indicate an intrapulmonary shunt rather than an ASD.

Color Doppler imaging is also useful for detecting flow through ASDs (Fig. 15-110*A*, Plate 68), although the pressure drop between atria often does not produce turbulence. Inflow from the inferior vena cava and right-sided pulmonary veins may be prominent in normals and can be misinterpreted as a shunt.[272] Pulsed-wave Doppler recordings usually reveal continuous flow, which peaks in late systole. Pulmonary-to-systemic flow ratios can be estimated in ASD (and ventricular septal defects) by comparing volumetric flow measurements through the LVOT and RVOT. Such calculations are only moderately accurate in adults.[273] With the advent of umbrella or "clamshell" devices that permit percutaneous closure of ASDs, TEE has assumed an important role in defining the cross-sectional dimensions and exact position of the ASD (Fig. 15-111B, Plate 69). TEE is also useful in confirming accurate placement of closure devices and subsequent correction of the interatrial shunt.

### VENTRICULAR SEPTAL DEFECT

*Ventricular septal defects* (VSDs) may be classified as perimembranous, inlet, outlet, or trabecular. Echocardiography is quite useful for the detection and classification of VSDs.[274] The defect itself is sometimes visible with 2D imaging alone (Fig. 15-113*A*), but smaller VSDs are easily missed. Complete absence of the interventricular septum (single ventricle) is quite rare (Fig. 15-113*B*). Pulsed- or continuous-wave Doppler interrogation often reveals discrete areas of high-velocity flow across the interventricular septum. Measurement of the peak CW velocity through the shunt allows calculation of the interventricular pressure gradient (via the modified Bernoulli equation); subtraction of this gradient from the systolic blood pressure (in the absence of AoV disease) approximates the RV systolic pressure.

Overall, color-flow imaging is the most useful Doppler technique for the diagnosis of VSDs.[274] Typically, a high-velocity systolic color jet is seen traversing the interventricular septum, although the velocity is lower with large defects and in the presence of PH (Fig. 15-114, Plate 70). The appearance of the color jet in the standard imaging planes can be used to determine the type of VSD. Intravenous contrast injection may reveal a negative contrast jet in the RV, and contrast may cross the defect and partially opacify the left ventricle. In the absence of MR, contrast will not enter the LA, distinguishing an isolated VSD from an ASD. Doppler echocardiography can also be used to detect abnormalities associated with VSDs, such as ventricular septal aneurysm, MR and TR, ASD (especially with inlet VSDs), aortic insufficiency—with outlet (supracristal) VSDs—and "straddling" of the defect by the mitral or TV.[275] Accurate detection of such lesions is especially critical before surgical intervention.

### PATENT DUCTUS ARTERIOSUS

The ductus arteriosus originates just to the left of the PA bifurcation and inserts into the aorta slightly distal to and opposite from the ostium of the left subclavian artery. Given this posterior location, it is difficult to image a *patent ductus arteriosus* (PDA) itself with 2D TTE alone, and TEE is usually superior for direct visualization of the lesion[574] (Fig. 15-115*A* and *B*, Plate 71). In most cases, 2D imaging of the communication is not essential, as CFD reliably detects high-velocity diastolic flow within the PA in nearly all non-Eisenmenger patients.[276] The flow jet characteristically enters the distal left region of the main PA and streams anterior along the medial wall of the vessel (Fig. 15-115*B*, Plate 71). With large shunts, volume overload and subsequent dilation of the left ventricle occurs. Aortopulmonary window is a much rarer shunt involving the great vessels which presents as a communication anteriorly between the ascending aorta and proximal PA.[277] It is embryologically distinct from a PDA and more closely related to a truncus arteriosus defect.

## Venous Inflow Abnormalities

*Anomalous pulmonary venous return* (APVR) may be partial or total. Partial APVR is present in 80 percent of sinus venosus ASD cases and is a feature of the scimitar syndrome.[278] The usual finding on TTE is RV volume overload. TEE is quite useful in detecting these abnormal venous connections. In total APVR, the pulmonary veins may empty directly into the right atrium or into a common posterior chamber or vein. This structure and its connection with the right atrium may be visualized echocardiographically, along with the obligatory ASD.[279] In some cases, the collecting chamber posterior to the LA may mimic the appearance of *cor triatriatum,* an entity characterized by a membrane in the posterior LA which may obstruct pulmonary venous inflow, causing symptoms similar to those of MS[280] (Fig. 15-116).

*Persistent left superior vena cava* occurs in 0.5 percent of the normal population. In most cases, the anomalous vein empties into

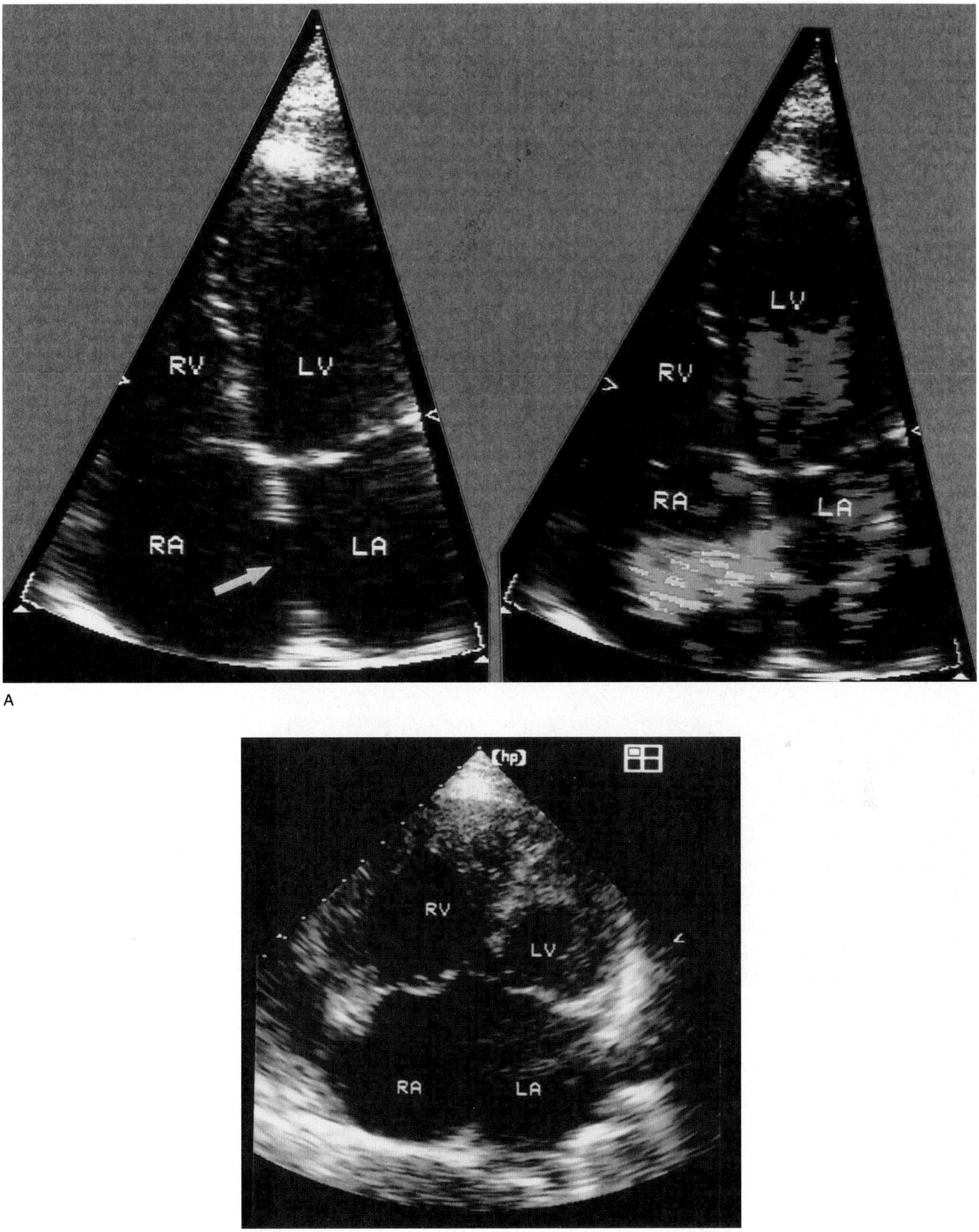

A

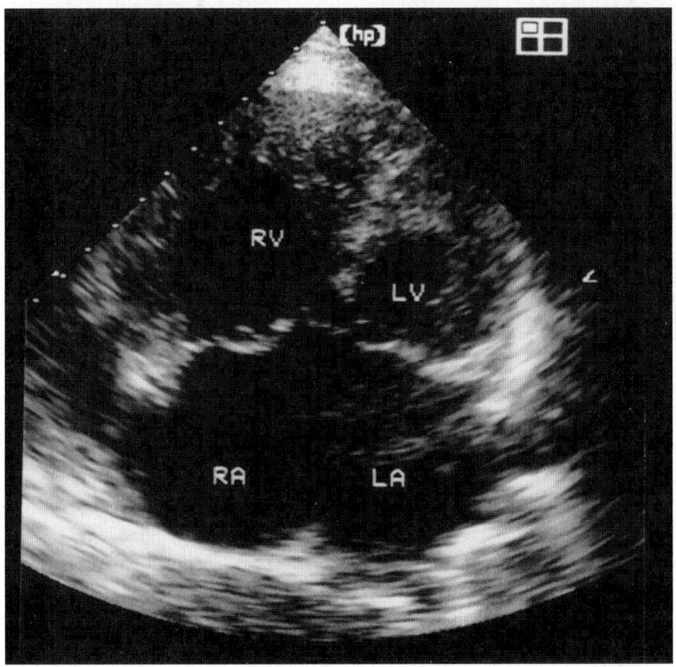


B

FIGURE 15-110 (Plate 68) *A*. Apical four-chamber view of an ostium secundum atrial septal defect (ASD). On the left, a defect in the mid atrial septum is apparent (*arrow*). On the right, there is color flow through the shunt. RV = right ventricle; RA = right atrium; LA = left atrium; LV = left ventricle. *B*. Apical four-chamber view of a large ostium primum atrial septal defect (as well as an inlet VSD) in a patient with Down's syndrome. RA = right atrium; LA = left atrium; LV = left ventricle; RV = right ventricle.

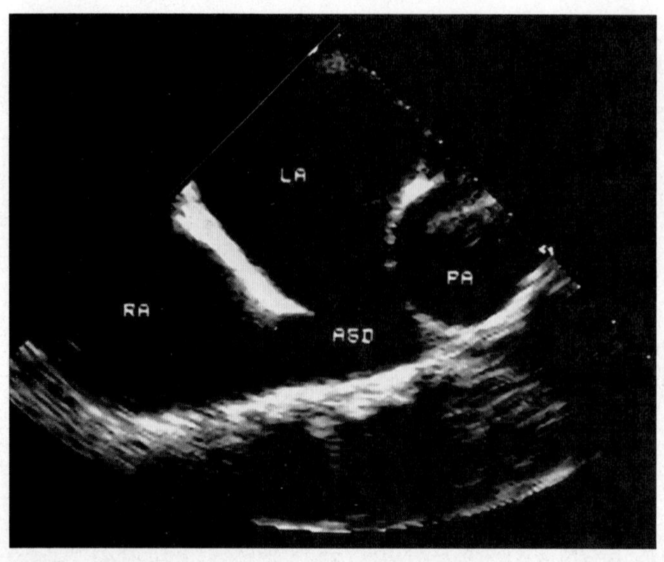


A

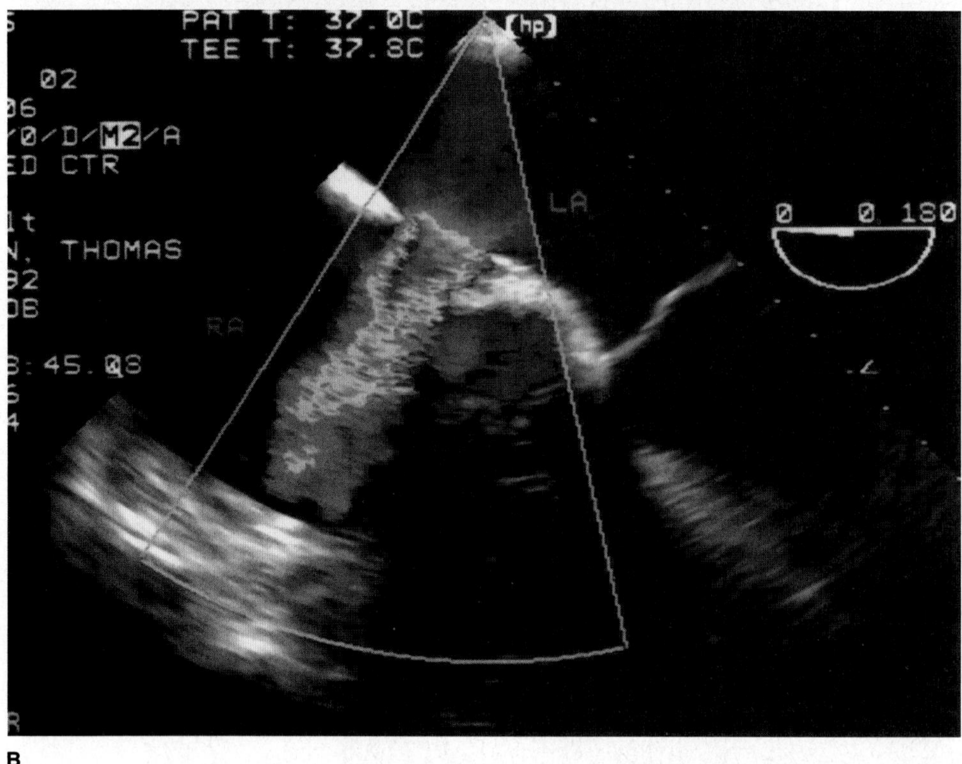


B

FIGURE 15-111 (Plate 69) *A*. Transesophageal image of a sinus venosus atrial septal defect (ASD) (longitudinal plane). The defect is present in the superior portion of the interatrial septum. RA = right atrium; LA = left atrium; ASD = atrial septal defect; PA = pulmonary artery. *B*. Transesophageal image of an ostium secundum ASD. Color-flow Doppler confirms a left to right shunt, and the size of the defect can be measured accurately.

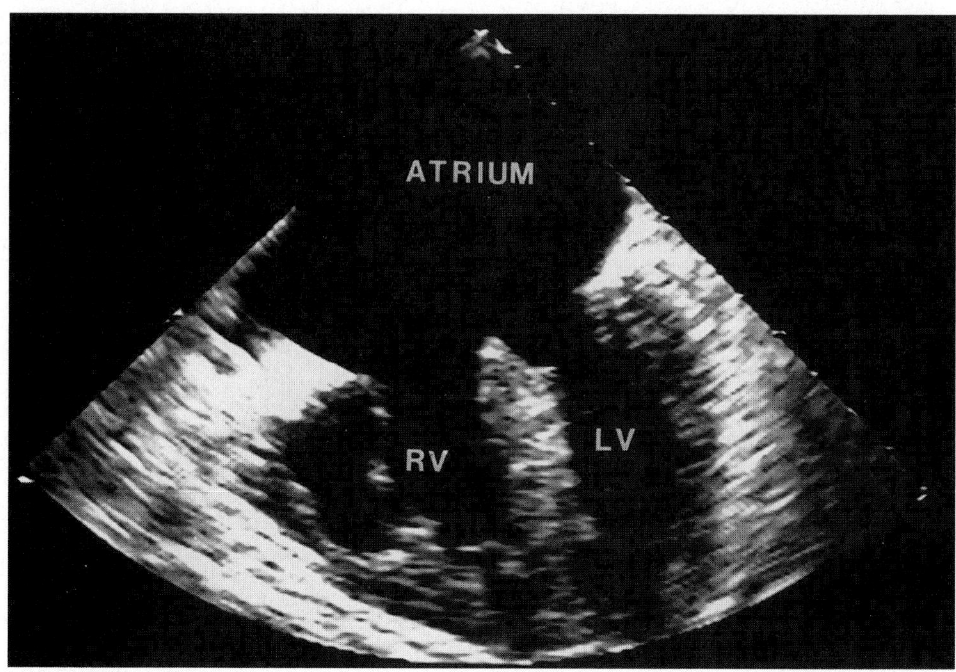


FIGURE 15-112 Transverse transesophageal image of single atrium. RV = right ventricle; LV = left ventricle. (From Blanchard DG, Scott ED. Single atrium. *Circulation* 1997;95:273. With permission.)

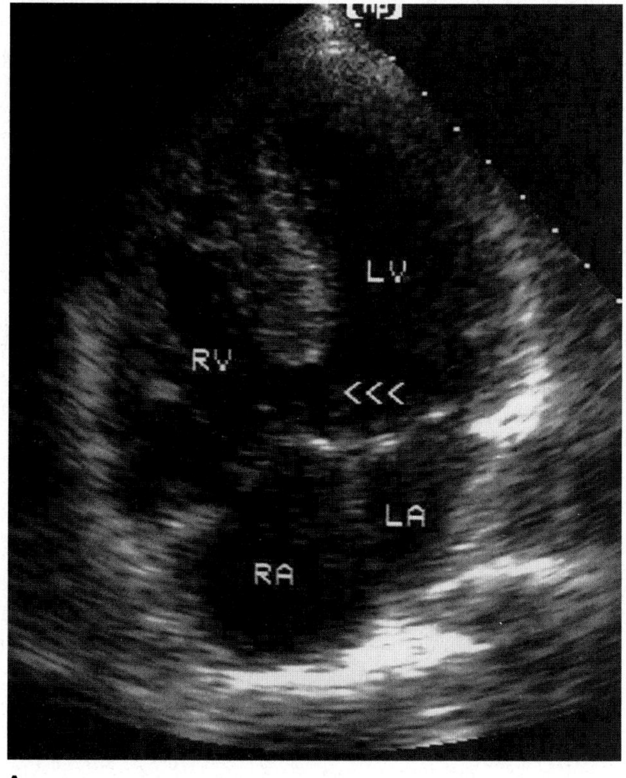


A

B

FIGURE 15-113 *A*. Apical four-chamber image of an inlet ventricular septal defect (VSD). The defect (*arrows*) is situated more inferiorly than the typical position of a perimembranous VSD. RV = right ventricle; RA = right atrium; LA = left atrium; LV = left ventricle. *B*. Apical image of single ventricle. RA = right atrium; LA = left atrium.

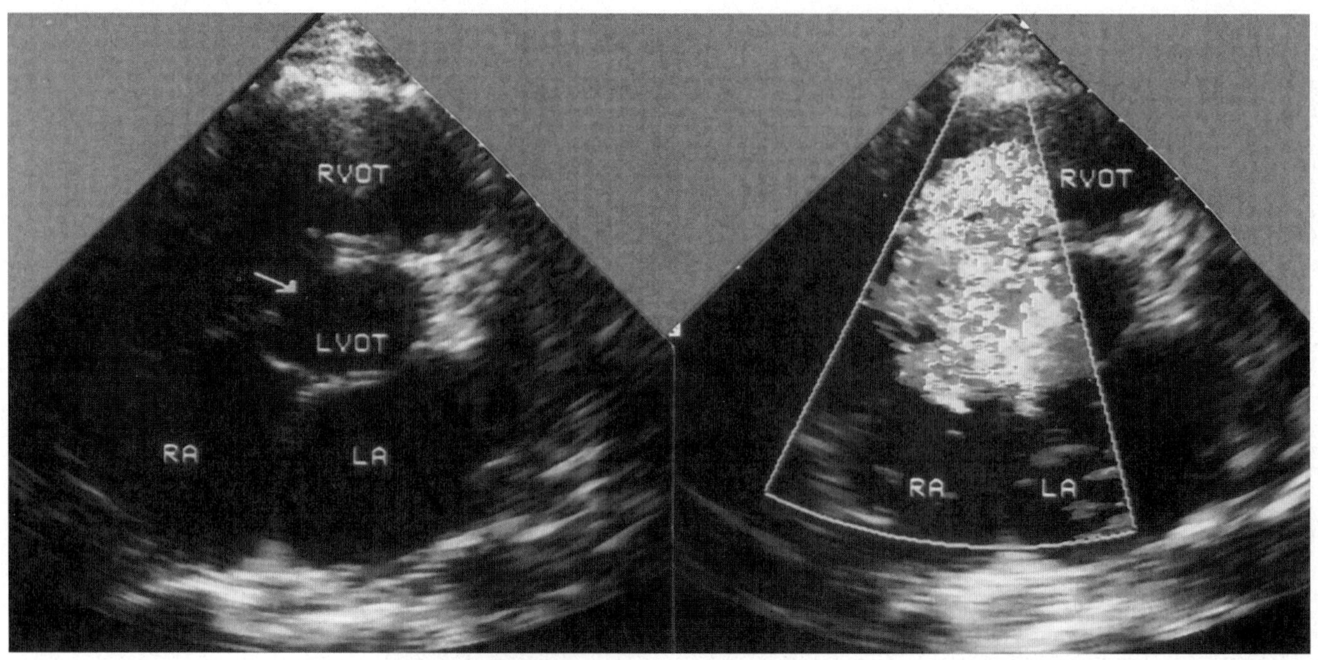


FIGURE 15-114 (Plate 70) Parasternal short-axis images of a large perimembranous ventricular septal defect (VSD) (*arrow*) without (*left*) and with (*right*) superimposed color flow Doppler. A large, turbulent color jet crosses the VSD during systole (*right*). RVOT = right ventricular outflow tract; RA = right atrium; LA = left atrium; LVOT = left ventricular outflow tract.

the coronary sinus, which then drains into the right atrium (Fig. 15-117). Unless the coronary sinus is unroofed and drains into the LA, no shunting occurs. The typical echocardiographic finding is a large coronary sinus, which is especially well seen on transesophageal or parasternal trans-thoracic views. The diagnosis may be confirmed by intravenous contrast injection from the left arm, as this will opacify the coronary sinus shortly before filling the right atrium.

## Conotruncal and Aortic Abnormalities

*Tetralogy of Fallot* is one of the more common conotruncal abnormalities, and affected individuals may sometimes survive to adulthood without surgical intervention. The classic echocardiographic features include a large perimembranous VSD, an anteriorly displaced aorta which overrides the VSD, RV enlargement and dysfunction, and pulmonic stenosis (either infundibular, valvular, or supravalvular) (Fig. 15-118).[281] The VSD and aorta are well visualized in the parasternal long-axis view, while the RVOT and proximal PA are best seen in the parasternal short-axis view at the base of the heart. Doppler interrogation can provide evaluation of the severity of pulmonic stenosis, both before and after surgery. Echocardiography may aid detection of infants with tetralogy who will require early surgical intervention as well as patients who are at high risk for sudden death after surgical repair.[282,283] Although *double-outlet RV* (DORV) shares several clinical characteristics with tetralogy of Fallot (VSD and anterior aortic displacement are invariably present, and pulmonic valvular stenosis and ASD are common in both), it is morphologically distinct (Fig. 15-119). Normal continuity of the posterior aortic wall with the anterior MV leaflet (always present in tetralogy of Fallot) is absent in DORV, and an interposed mass of fibrous tissue between the LA and the nearest great vessel is seen on 2D imaging. In addition, the great vessels may be transposed in DORV, resulting in a characteristic side-by-side appearance of the aorta and PA on parasternal short-axis images.[284]

Echocardiography has become a valuable tool for the detection, management, and postoperative follow-up of patients with *transposition of the great arteries.* Attention to the anatomic rules mentioned earlier is essential for accurate diagnosis of both D (classic) and L ("congenitally corrected") transposition. In D-transposition, the aorta arises from the RV, the PA arises from the LV, and one or more obligatory shunts are present. With L-transposition, the morphologic right and left ventricles are switched, and associated anomalies such as VSD and pulmonic stenosis are common. In both types of transposition, the normal echocardiographic orientation of the great vessels on parasternal short-axis images (a sausage-shaped RVOT and PA draped over a circular aorta) is no longer present, and the two great vessels are typically side by side and parallel (Fig. 15-120).[285] In general, the aorta is anterior and to the right of the PA in D-transposition and anterior and to the left in L-transposition. Both TTE and TEE are an important part of continuing care after surgical repair or palliation of transposition; they can detect valvular regurgitation, outflow tract narrowing, and stenosis of the atrial baffle systems used to palliate D-transposition surgically.[286]

FIGURE 15-115 (Plate 71) *A.* Transesophageal image of a patent ductus arteriosus (PDA). The upper panel shows a small communication (arrow) between the aorta (AO) and pulmonary artery (PA), which is confirmed with color-flow Doppler imaging (lower panel). *B.* Parasternal short-axis images at the aortic valve level. On the left, the pulmonary artery (PA) is somewhat enlarged. On the right, color imaging reveals diastolic flow within the PA, consistent with a patent ductus arteriosus. RV = right ventricle; RA = right atrium; LA = left atrium; AO = aorta.

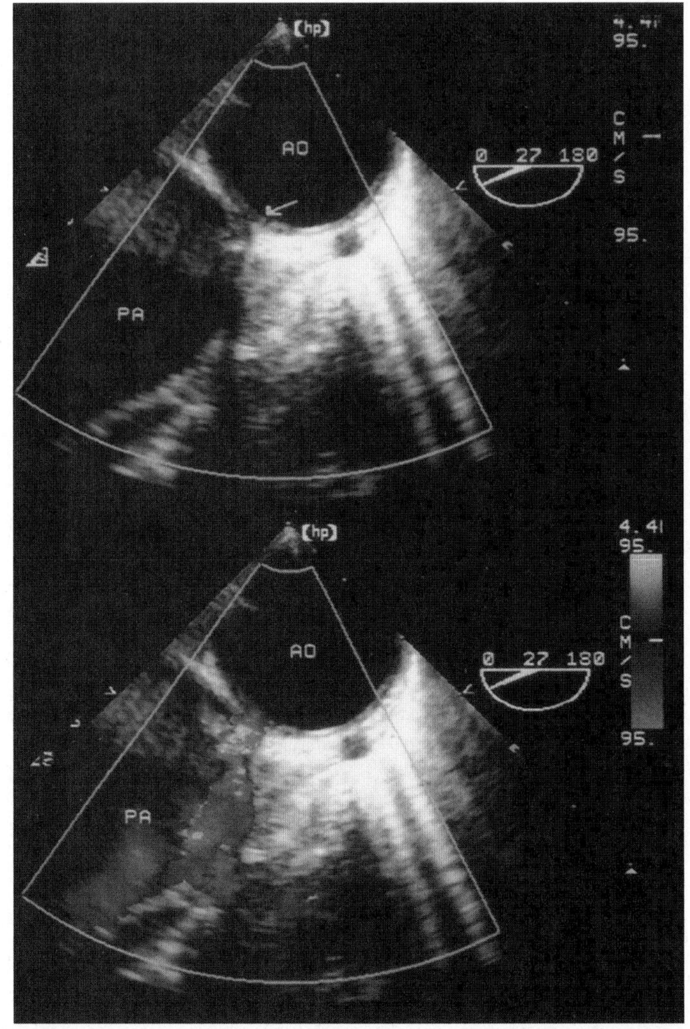


A

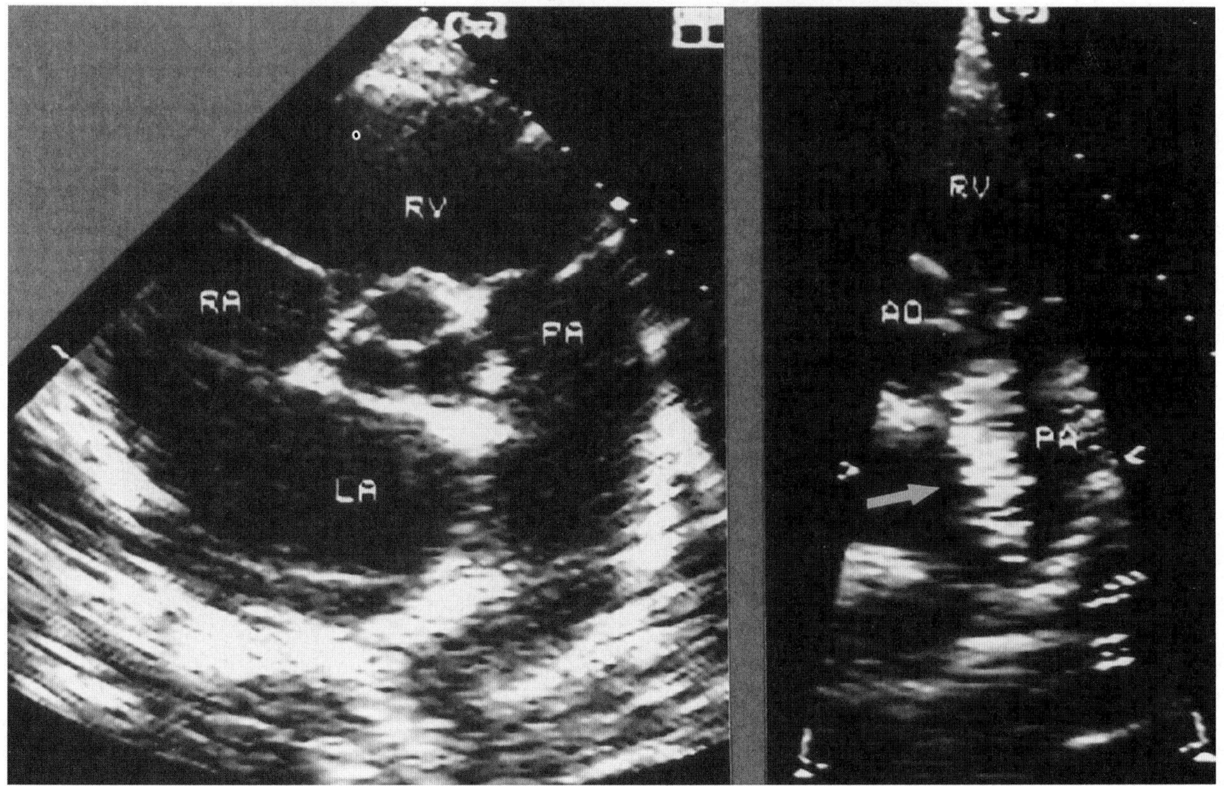


B

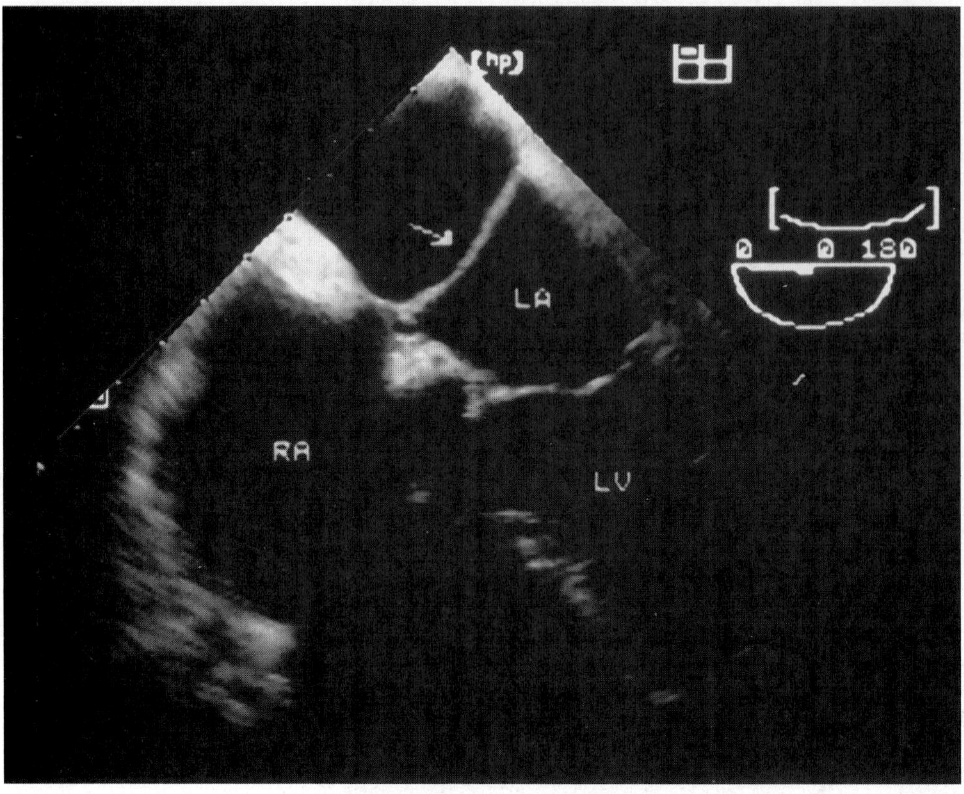


FIGURE 15-116 Transverse transesophageal image of cor triatriatum. A membrane (*arrow*) is present in the left atrium. RA = right atrium; LA = left atrium; LV = left ventricle.

*Truncus arteriosus* is a rare anomaly characterized by a large VSD, a single semilunar valve, and a single great vessel that divides into the ascending aorta and PA.[287] Ultrasound imaging can determine the anatomy of the great vessels and assist in defining the various subsets of truncus arteriosus.

*Coarctation of the aorta* is associated with a bicuspid aortic valve and is best visualized from the suprasternal position. 2D imaging may identify the site of coarctation, but the natural mild curving of the descending aorta can occasionally lead to a false-positive diagnosis. Clear visualization of narrowing in the proximal descending aorta with poststenotic dilatation, however, is pathognomonic of coarctation.[288] Doppler interrogation from the suprasternal notch demonstrates increased systolic velocity in the descending aorta and may also reveal a persistent flow gradient throughout diastole in cases of severe coarctation (Fig. 15-121*A*).[289] Color imaging may display flow acceleration proximal to the site of coarctation and aliasing distal to it (Fig. 15-121*B*, Plate 72). The maximum velocity through the coarctation can be used to estimate the pressure gradient, and this measurement can be particularly valuable for the detection of restenosis after surgical repair or percutaneous balloon aortic dilatation.[290] *Supravalvular aortic stenosis,* either isolated or associated with Williams syndrome (Chap. 12), is generally imaged best from the suprasternal and superior parasternal positions. Transesophageal imaging is also very helpful (Fig. 15-122*E*). Echocardiography reveals either an hourglass-shaped stenosis of the aorta above the sinuses of Valsalva, diffuse hypoplasia of the ascending aorta, or a focal fibrous ridge at the sinotubular junction (Fig. 15-122*E*). Doppler imaging can help estimate the gradient across the stenosis, and marked aliasing of color-flow imaging in the ascending aorta should raise suspicion of the diagnosis. Thickening of the aortic valve leaflets and stenoses of the coronary ostia are important associated findings that may be detectable by echocardiography.

## Abnormalities of the Ventricular Outflow Tract and Semilunar Valve

### RIGHT VENTRICLE

*Infundibular stenosis* is rare outside the setting of tetralogy of Fallot and is much less common than valvular PS. On 2D imaging, muscular hypertrophy is often visualized proximal to the PA, while Doppler interrogation reveals increased flow velocities through the infundibulum.[291] PS is reasonably common and may be either isolated or associated with other congenital lesions (such as VSD, transposition, and tetralogy of Fallot). Typical echocardiographic features include thickening of the leaflets, restricted leaflet motion, systolic doming of the valve, and elevated systolic flow velocity on Doppler (Fig. 15-85, Plate 66). As with other stenotic lesions, the gradient can be estimated using the modified Bernoulli equation. The PV is best visualized in the parasternal short-axis view through the base (or a modified parasternal view of the RVOT). In children, the subcostal position frequently provides excellent visualization of the RVOT and PV. When TTE is suboptimal, TEE can provide detailed images of the PV. In pulmonic stenosis, the valve leaflets may calcify over time, and poststenotic dilatation of the PA is often present.

### LEFT VENTRICLE

Subvalvular obstruction may be dynamic or fixed. *Hypertrophic cardiomyopathy,* which may present at any age, is discussed above. Discrete *subaortic stenosis* may be caused by a thin membrane in the

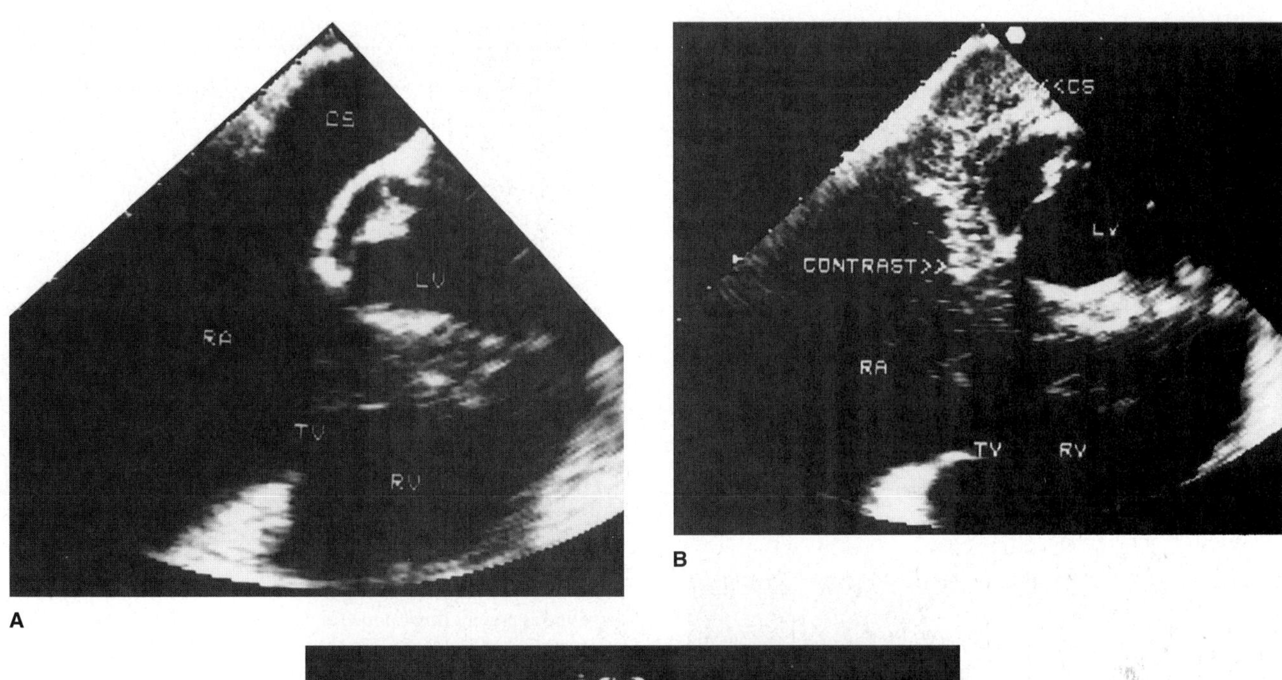


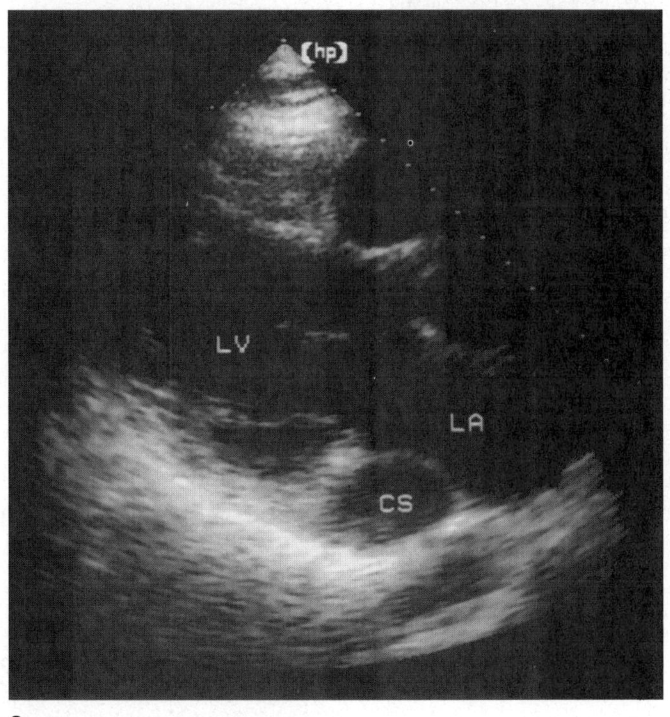


FIGURE 15-117 *A.* Transesophageal image (transverse plane) from a patient with persistent left superior vena cava. The coronary sinus (CS) is dilated. *B.* After injection of agitated saline into the left antecubital vein, contrast is seen entering the right atrium (RA) via the CS. TV = tricuspid valve; RV = right ventricle; LV = left ventricle. (From Blanchard DG, DeMaria AN. Cardiac and extracardiac masses: Echocardiographic evaluation. In: Skorton DJ, Schelbert HR, Wolf GL, Brundage BH, eds. *Marcus' Cardiac Imaging,* 2d ed. Philadelphia: Saunders; 1996:452–480. With permission.) *C.* Transthoracic parasternal long-axis image of persistent left superior vena cava. The coronary sinus is dilated.

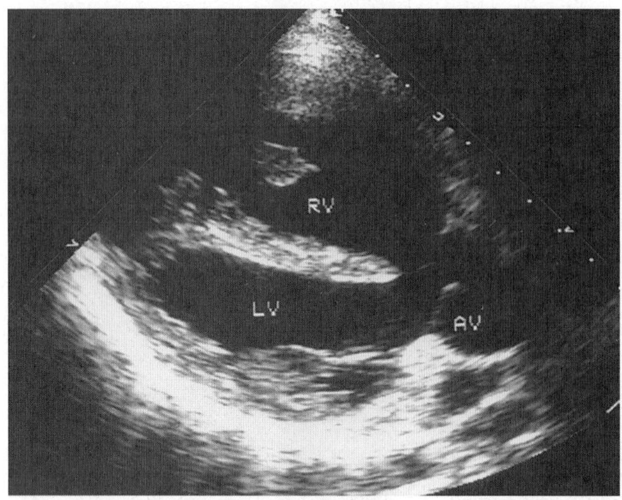


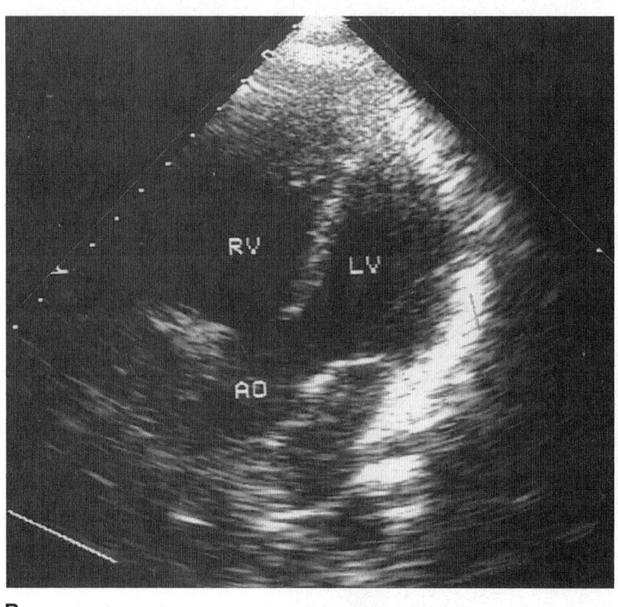


FIGURE 15-118 Parasternal long-axis (*A*) and apical four-chamber (*B*) images of tetralogy of Fallot. The right ventricle (RV) is enlarged, and a large VSD is present. The aorta (AO) overrides the interventricular septum. LV = left ventricle. (Courtesy of Reinaldo W. Beyer, MD.)

LVOT, a fibromuscular ridge, or diffuse muscular narrowing of the outflow tract (Fig. 15-122*A–D,* Plate 73). 2D echocardiographic imaging can distinguish these various forms of discrete subvalvular stenosis, and Doppler analysis permits estimation of the systolic gradient.[292] Color-flow imaging demonstrates increased turbulence in the LVOT as well as aortic valvular regurgitation in about 50 percent of cases (Fig. 15-122*D*). Apical views are sometimes more useful for detecting thin subaortic membranes, as these structures are parallel to the ultrasound beam on parasternal images. Subaortic fibromuscular ridges are sometimes associated with anomalous MV chordae connecting the papillary muscles or the anterior MV leaflet to the septum.[293] M-mode imaging may reveal midsystolic partial closure of the AoV, differentiating subvalvular from valvular AS.

*Bicuspid aortic valve* is the most common congenital cardiac lesion in adults and is present in 1 to 2 percent of all individuals (men are affected more often than women). Initially, eccentric diastolic coaptation of the aortic cusps was reported on M-mode in patients with bicuspid valves. However, M-mode findings are less accurate than 2D imaging, and the parasternal short-axis view is generally best for defining the fish-mouthed systolic aortic valvular anatomy (Figs. 15-60 and 15-61). Bicuspid valves are sometimes easy to detect in diastole as well, but raphes and remnants of commissures may obscure the diagnosis and mimic a trileaflet valve. In general, asymmetry of the aortic leaflets suggests congenital deformation. In equivocal cases, TEE is usually diagnostic (Fig. 15-61).

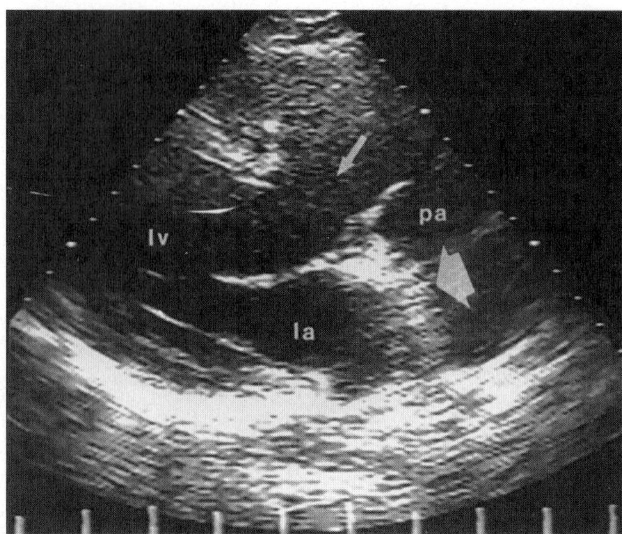


FIGURE 15-119 Parasternal long-axis image of double-outlet right ventricle. A large VSD is present (*small arrow*) and the normal continuity between the posterior aortic wall and the anterior mitral leaflet is absent. Fibrous tissue is seen (*large arrow*) between the left atrium (LA) and the nearest great vessel (in this case, the pulmonary artery (PA). LV = left ventricle.

## Abnormalities of the Ventricular Inflow Tract

*Ebstein's anomaly* is a congenital deformity of the TV in which the leaflets are displaced into the RV. Associated findings include TR,

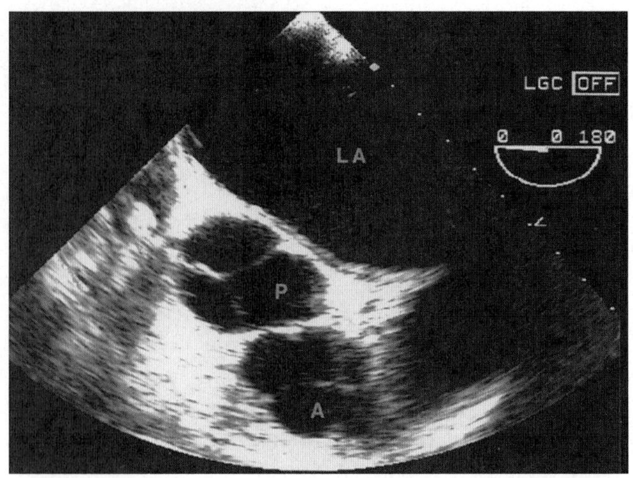


FIGURE 15-120 Transverse transesophageal image through the semilunar valves in L-transposition. The aortic valve (A) is anterior and to the left of the pulmonic valve (P). LA = left atrium.

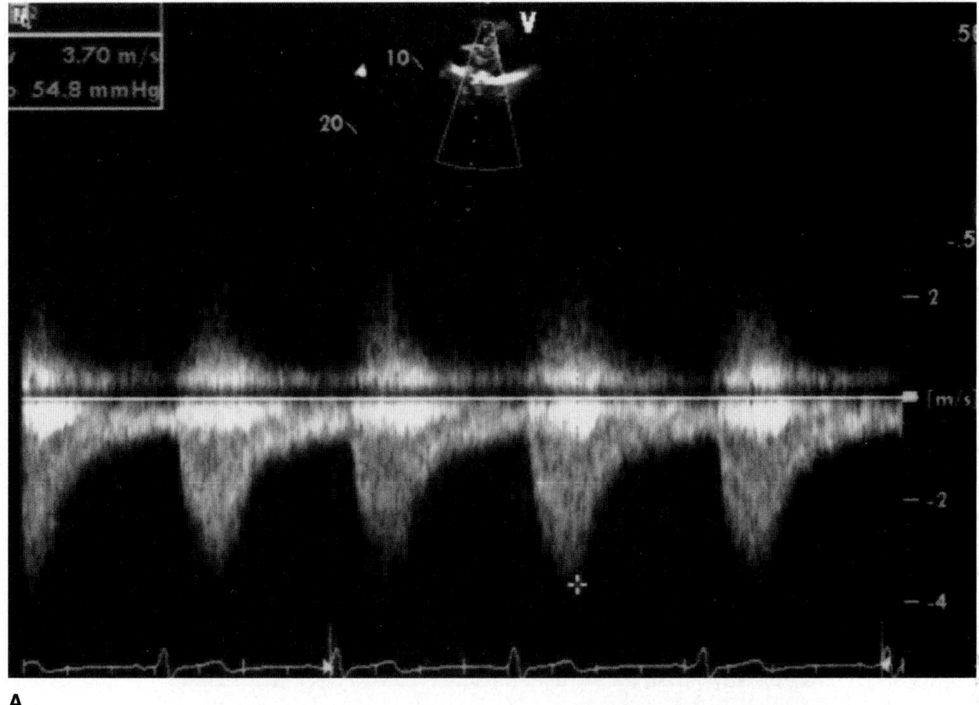


A

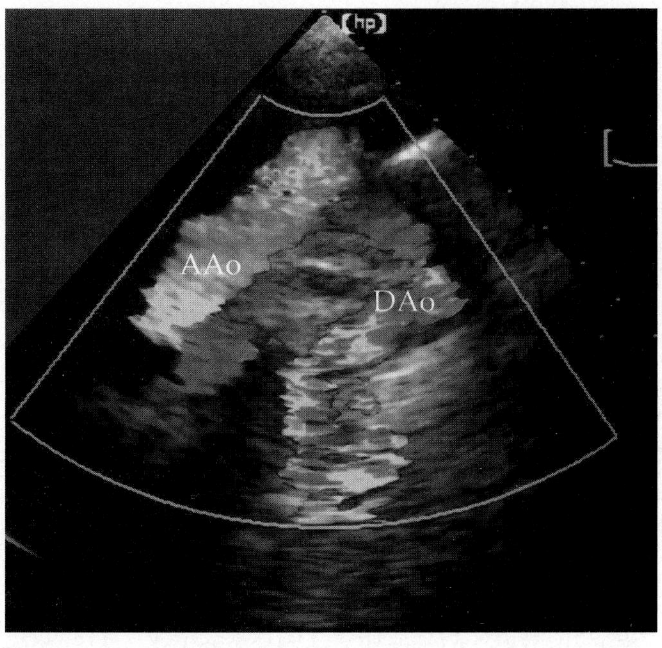


B

FIGURE 15-121 (Plate 72) *A.* Continuous-wave Doppler tracing of the descending aorta (from the suprasternal position) in aortic coarctation. Peak systolic velocity is 3.7 m/s, and there is persistent flow during diastole, suggesting severe coarctation. *B.* Suprasternal image of aortic coarctation. The descending aorta (DAo) is focally narrowed and tortuous, and turbulent (aliased) flow is present distal to the site of coarctation.

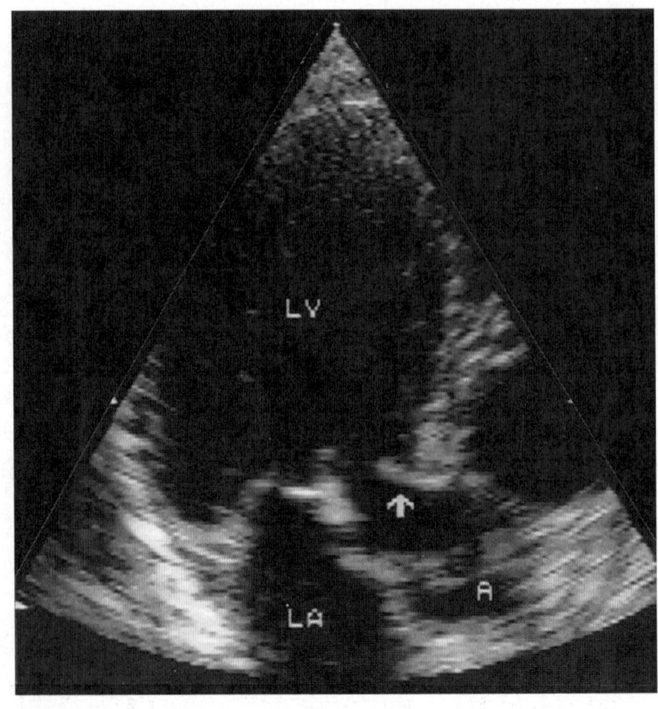


A

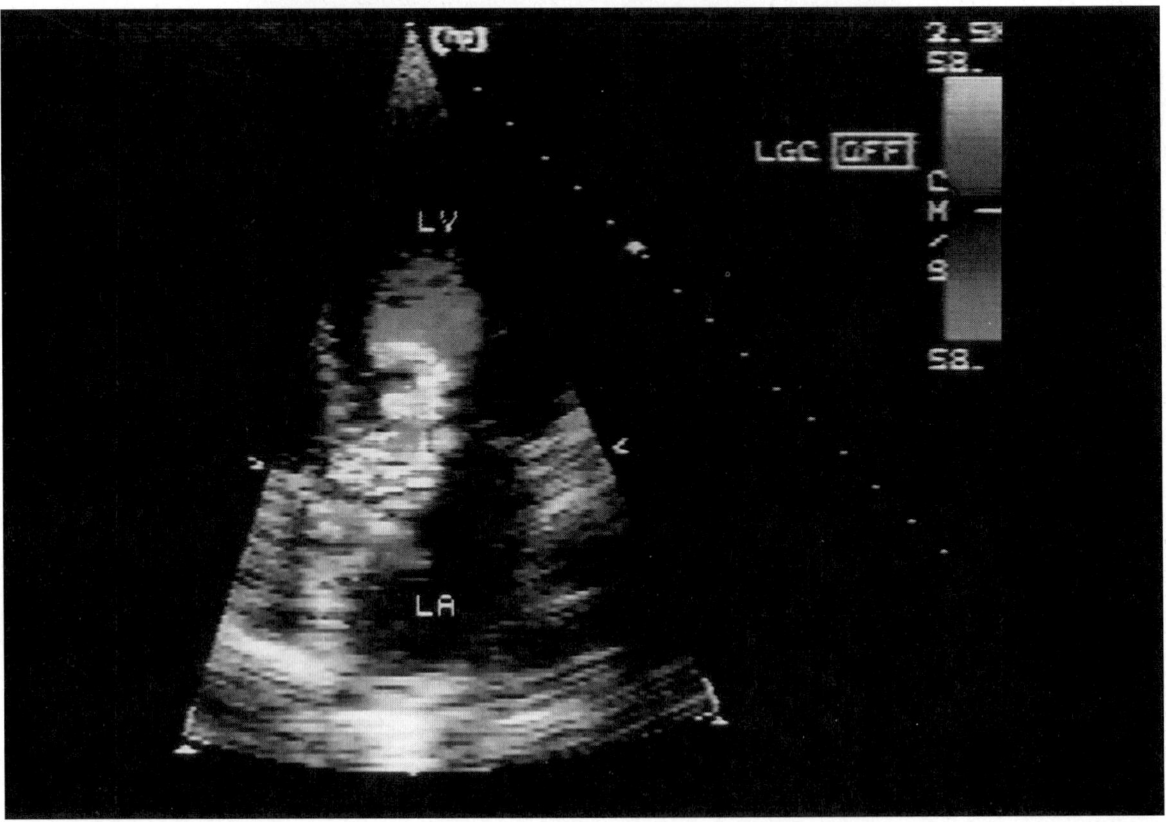


B

FIGURE 15-122 (Plate 73) Subvalvular and supravalvular aortic stenosis. *A*. Apical three-chamber view of discrete subaortic stenosis. A fibromuscular ridge (*arrow*) is present in the left ventricular out-flow tract. LV = left ventricle; LA = left atrium; A = aortic root. *B*. Apical five-chamber view of discrete subaortic stenosis with color-flow Doppler, demonstrating aliasing and proximal flow convergence in the left ventricular outflow tract. LV = left ventricle; LA = left atrium. *C*. Transesophageal image of discrete subaortic stenosis. A fibrous ridge in the outflow tract of the left ventricle (LV) is present (arrow). LA = left atrium. *D*. Transesophageal image with color-flow Doppler, demonstrating mild aortic insufficiency associated with discrete subaortic stenosis. LV = left ventricle; LA = left atrium; Ao = aortic root. *E*. Transesophageal image of supravalvular aortic stenosis. A fibrous ridge extends into the aortic lumen just above the sinus of Valsalva.

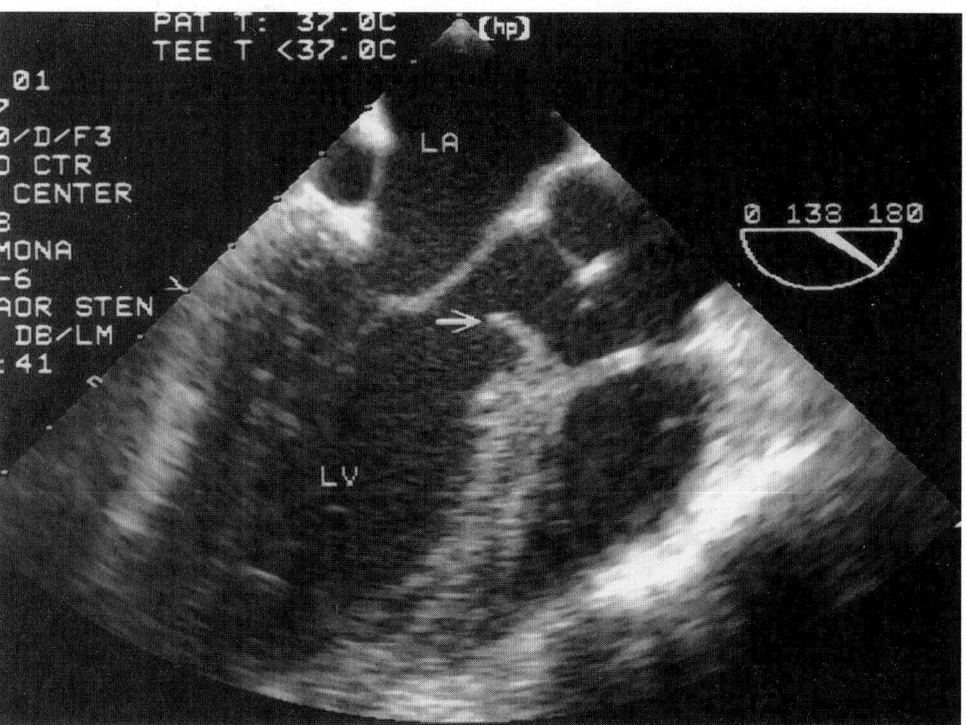


C

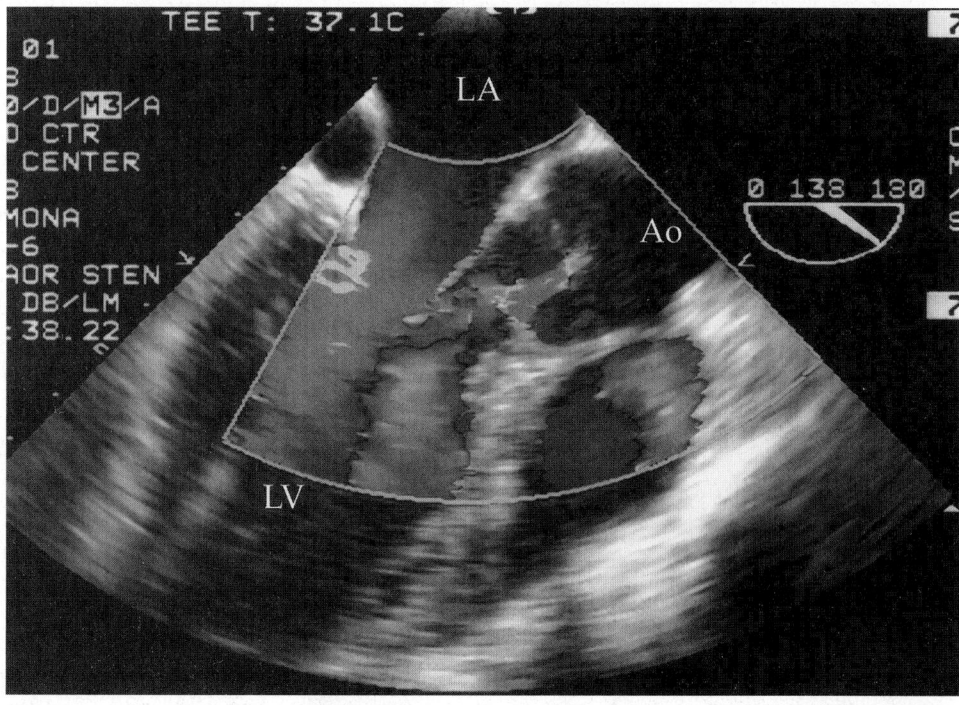

D

FIGURE 15-122 (*Continued*)

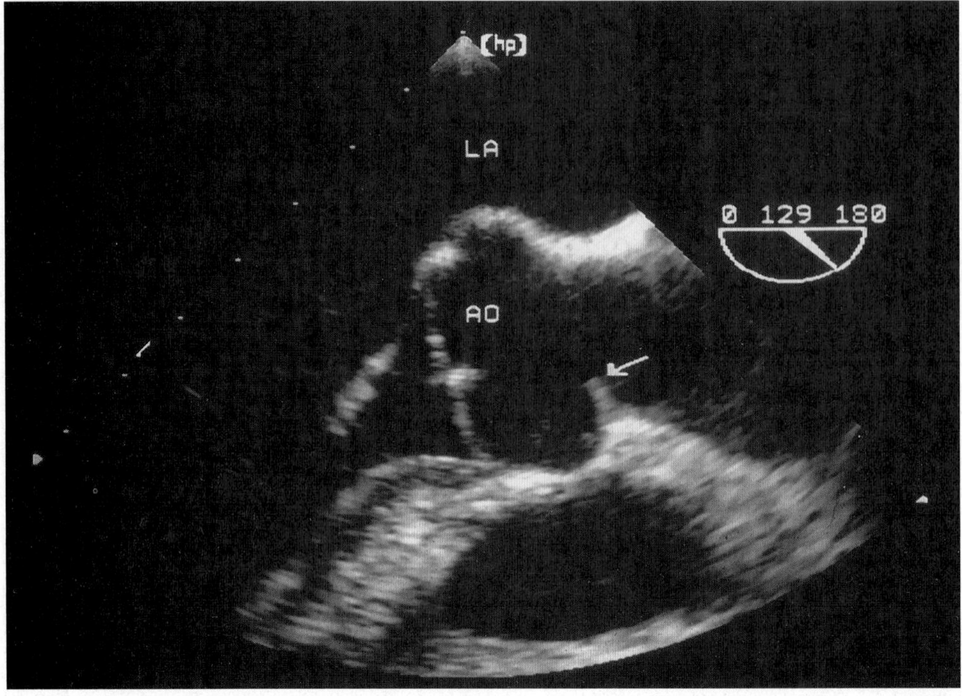


E

FIGURE 15-122 *(Continued)*

right atrial enlargement, and ASD.[294] 2D imaging typically shows abnormal apical displacement of the septal leaflet insertion, with variable deformity of the leaflet (Fig. 15-123). The anterior leaflet originates from the tricuspid annulus but is elongated and often tethered to the RV free wall by abnormal chordal attachments. The tricuspid deformity and regurgitation are best visualized in the apical four-chamber view, although the subcostal and modified parasternal views also may be helpful.

*Atrioventricular valvular atresia* is usually accompanied by hypoplasia of the corresponding ventricle. Echocardiographic images of tricuspid atresia characteristically show a small, nonfunctional RV, an interatrial communication of variable size, and a normally developed left ventricle. Associated lesions include VSD, transposition, and RV outflow obstruction. Echocardiography is an important tool in the management of patients with tricuspid atresia after palliation with the Fontan procedure. Mitral atresia is associated with a hypoplastic LV. Additional rare congenital mitral anomalies imaged by echocardiography include parachute MV and congenital MS.

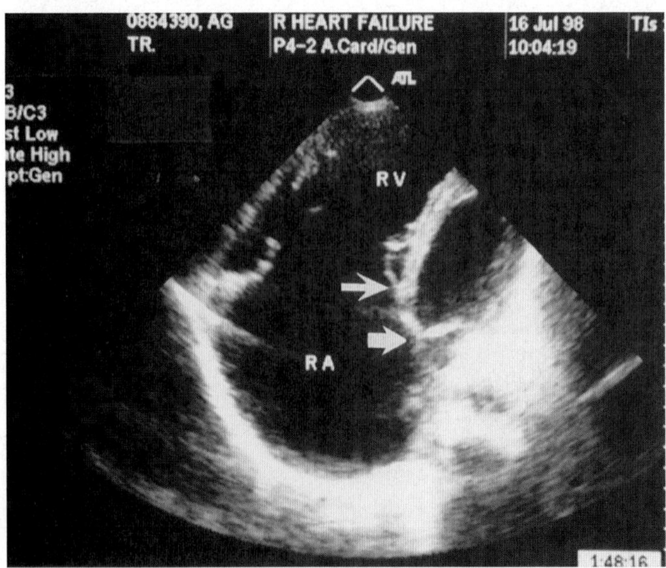


FIGURE 15-123 Ebstein's anomaly, apical four-chamber view. The tricuspid valve annulus (*thin arrow*) is apically displaced in comparison to the mitral annulus (*thick arrow*). The right ventricle (RV) and right atrium (RA) are enlarged.

## Fetal Echocardiography

The average risk for significant heart disease in the fetus is approximately 0.4 to 0.8 percent. Fetal echocardiography has evolved over the past 20 years into a sophisticated method for intrauterine detection of cardiac abnormalities[295] (Fig. 15-124). The technique has been advocated for the preterm diagnosis of congenital heart disease, especially in higher-risk cases [for example, maternal congenital heart disease or diabetes mellitus, maternal teratogen exposure, or TORCH (toxoplasmosis, other intrauterine infections, rubella, cytomegalovirus, and herpesvirus) infection, and familial syndromes that may affect the heart]. Fetal echocardiography has successfully identified a variety of congenital lesions including atrial and ventricular septal defect, pulmonic stenosis, transposition, tetralogy of Fallot, hypoplastic left heart, Ebstein's anomaly, and tricuspid atresia.[296] Prenatal detection of these lesions may improve prognosis and guide therapy. Although some have recommended routine limited fetal echocardiography during the second or third trimester, recent reports have suggested a low yield and limited diagnostic accuracy.[297,298] Like many imaging techniques, fetal echocardiography is evolving, and further study is required to define its optimal clinical use.

# CARDIAC MASSES, THROMBI, AND TUMORS

## Normal Variants and Masses of Uncertain Significance

When an abnormally localized accumulation of dense reflectances appears on the echocardiogram, it is said to represent a mass. Echocardiographic masses may be caused by technical artifacts or anomalous structures, but they are of greatest significance in representing true lesions of the heart such as tumors, thrombi, and vegetations. Echocardiography is the procedure of choice for the detection and evaluation of cardiac mass lesions; often, it is the only modality capable of delineating small lesions such as papillary fibroelastomas.[299] Accordingly, echocardiographic examinations are commonly performed to search for embolic sources, particularly in patients with cerebral ischemic events.

A number of technical artifacts are capable of appearing as masses on echocardiogram. For example, side lobe signals, reverberations, and noise artifact may lead to accumulations of ultrasonic reflectance within the cavities or adjacent to the myocardium of the heart.[22,23] Such structures usually lack distinct borders, do not move appropriately through the cardiac cycle, lack identifiable attachments to endocardial surfaces, and cannot be visualized in all views and at all depth settings. In seeking a way to distinguish artifacts from LV thrombi (a common clinical dilemma) the absence of wall motion abnormalities is of particular value.[300]

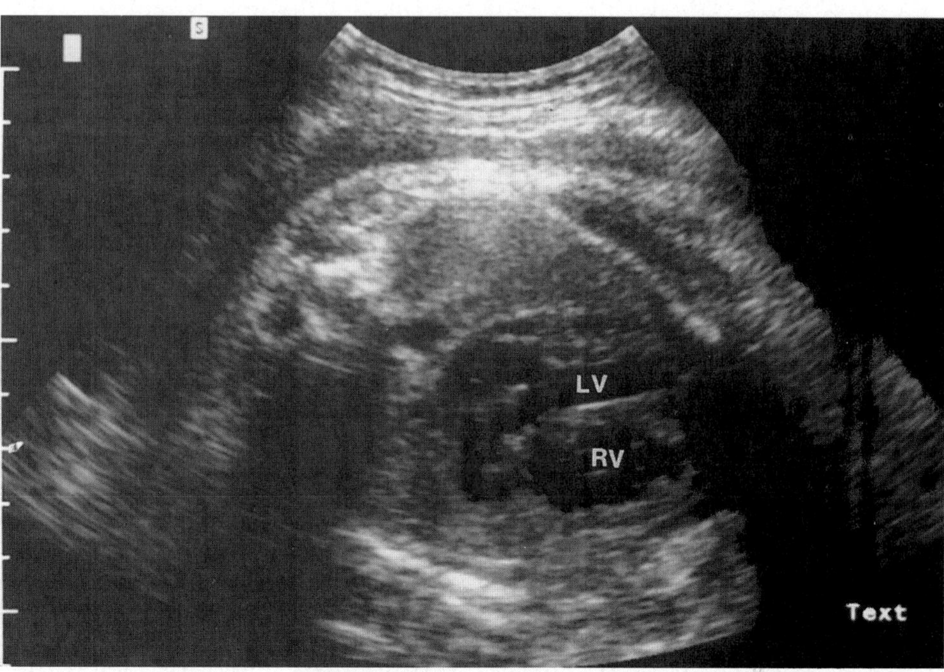


FIGURE 15-124 Fetal echocardiogram (four-chamber view). LV = left ventricle; RV = right ventricle.

Several benign normal variant findings can be observed during echocardiographic examination and must be distinguished from pathologic lesions. Thus, many adults manifest persistence of the eustachian valve (Fig. 15-125), a thin ridge of tissue at the junction of the inferior vena cava and right atrium.[301] The eustachian valve appears as a long, linear, freely mobile structure in the right atrium at the mouth of the inferior vena cava and is nearly always benign (although infective involvement has been reported).[302] An additional embryonic remnant that may be seen in the posterior right atrium is the Chiari network, which typically appears as a weblike mobile structure.[303] In some individuals, RVH may produce significant enlargement of the RV moderator band coursing along the interventricular septum to the apex of the RV.[304] Similarly, false chordae tendineae ("heartstrings") can occasionally be visualized as linear structures spanning the LV cavity attached to endomyocardium at both ends (Fig. 15-126).[305] Neither of the foregoing lesions has been conclusively associated with morbidity or mortality. On occasion, LVH or hypertrophied papillary muscles may simulate cardiac mass lesions.[304] Although TEE provides enhanced sensitivity and resolution in the delineation of cardiac mass lesions, this technique may be associated with variants and artifacts of its own.

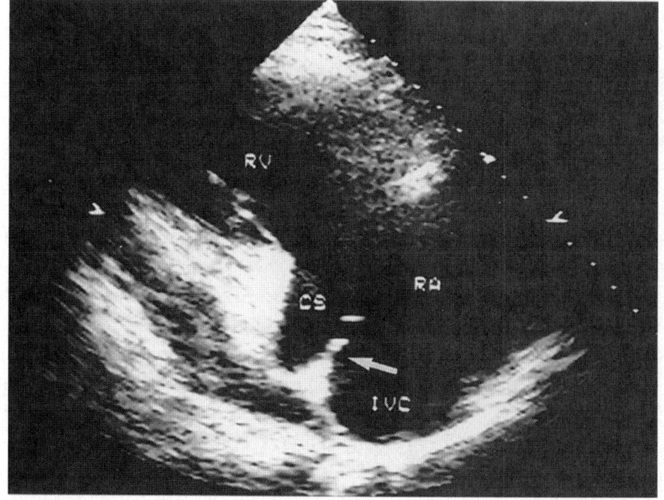


FIGURE 15-125 Right ventricular inflow view showing a prominent eustachian valve (*arrow*) at the junction of the inferior vena cava (IVC) and the right atrium (RA). RV = right ventricle; CS = coronary sinus. (From Blanchard DG, DeMaria AN. Cardiac and extracardiac masses: Echocardiographic evaluation. In: Skorton DJ, Schelbert HR, Wolf GL, Brundage BH, eds. *Marcus' Cardiac Imaging,* 2d ed. Philadelphia; Saunders; 1996:452–480. With permission.)

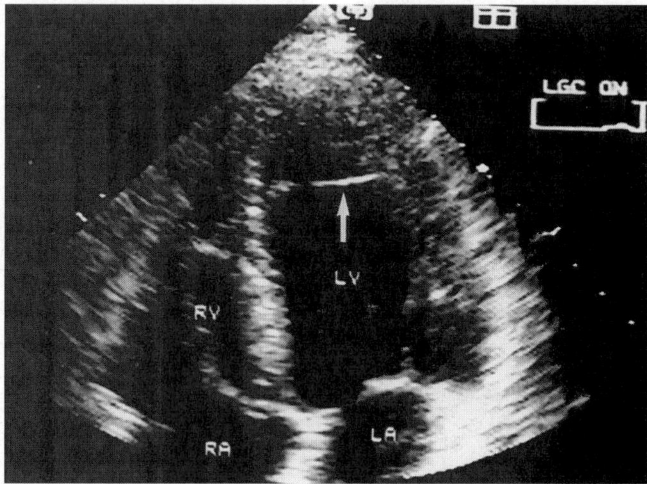


FIGURE 15-126 Apical four-chamber view demonstrating a false chord (*arrow*) within the left ventricle (LV). LA = left atrium; RA = right atrium; RV = right ventricle. (From Blanchard DG, DeMaria AN. Cardiac and extracardiac masses: Echocardiographic evaluation. In: Skorton DJ, Schelbert HR, Wolf GL, Brundage BH, eds. *Marcus' Cardiac Imaging,* 2d ed. Philadelphia: Saunders; 1996:452–480. With permission.)

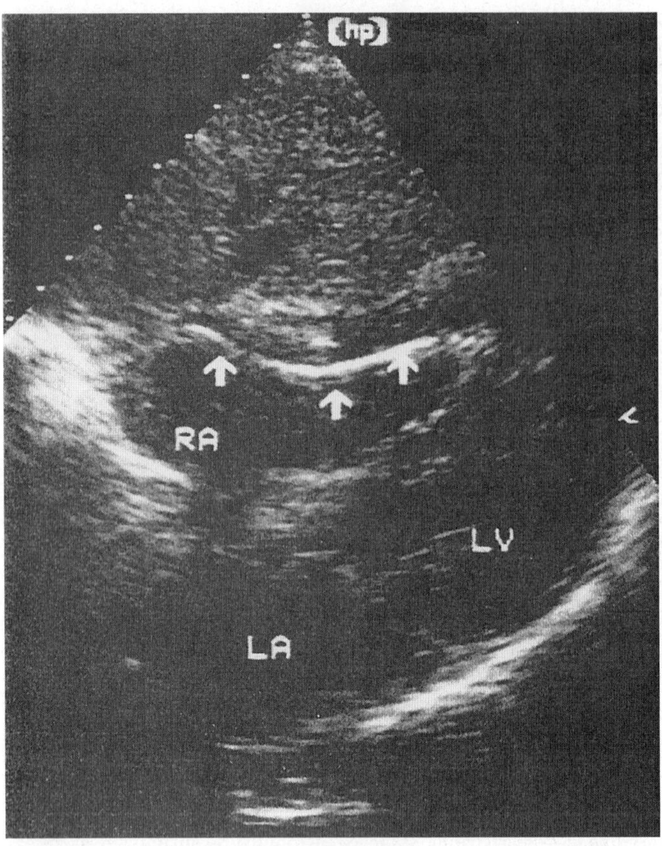


FIGURE 15-127 Subcostal four-chamber image demonstrating a pacemaker wire (*arrows*) in the right heart. RA = right atrium; LA = left atrium; LV = left ventricle.

A variety of foreign bodies and iatrogenically induced anatomic alterations may be visualized on echocardiogram and must be distinguished from pathologic lesions. Intracardiac catheters, pacemaker leads (Fig. 15-127), prosthetic valves or patches, and atrial suture lines after cardiac transplantation can be visualized during echocardiographic examination. These structures are usually easily recognized due to the highly reflective properties of the foreign material, which result in bright echoes, reverberations, and shadowing behind the structures. In this regard, endomyocardial biotomes and pericardiocentesis catheters can be readily visualized by cardiac ultrasound, and echocardiography can be employed to guide procedures utilizing these instruments in lieu of fluoroscopy.[306] Last, a variety of manufactured objects that have penetrated the heart have been described on echocardiography, including bullets, pellets, and nails.

Several morphologic changes involving the interatrial septum are often considered under the classification of cardiac mass lesions of uncertain significance. Aneurysms of the interatrial septum have been reported in about 1 percent of the population and are recognized on echocardiogram as a protrusion of the interatrial septum of at least 1.5 cm from its longitudinal plane dividing the left and right atrium (Fig. 15-128).[307] Although usually benign, interatrial septal aneurysms are often associated with a patent foramen ovale and have been implicated as a source of cardiogenic emboli. Interatrial septal aneurysms may be detected by TTE, but they are more readily imaged by the transesophageal approach.[307] Lipomatous hypertrophy of the interatrial septum, or accumulation of adipose tissue within this structure, is not an uncommon finding in elderly individuals. Lipomatous hypertrophy appears as a highly reflective thickening of the interatrial septum that typically spares the foramen ovale, thereby creating a characteristic dumbbell-shaped echocardiographic appearance.[308] No significant consequences or sequelae have been attributed to lipomatous infiltration of the interatrial septum.

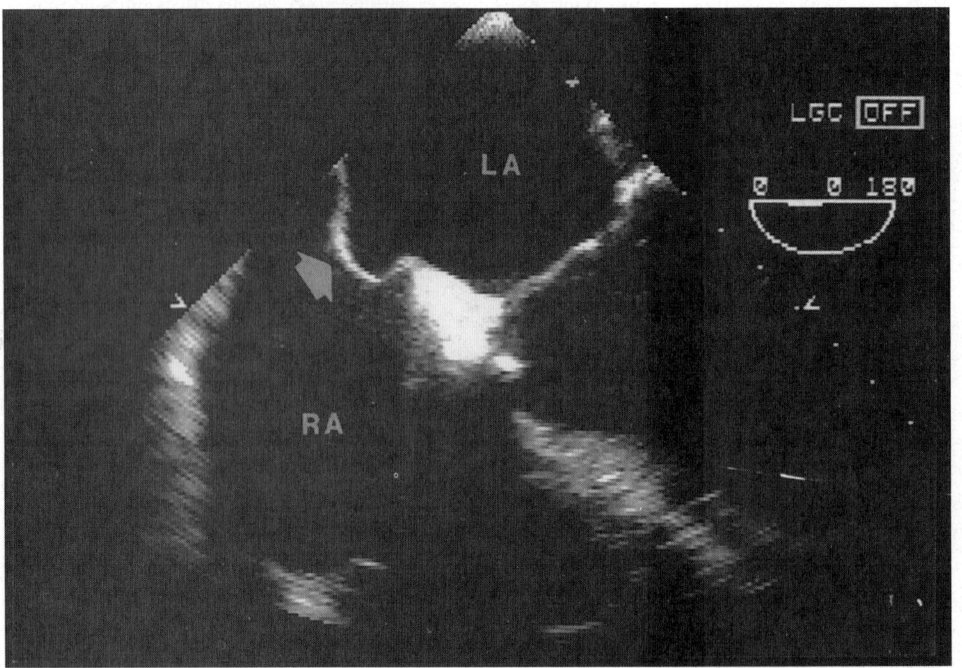


FIGURE 15-128 Transverse transesophageal image of an interatrial septal aneurysm (*arrow*). RA = right atrium; LA = left atrium. (From Blanchard DG, DeMaria AN. Cardiac and extracardiac masses: Echocardiographic evaluation. In: Skorton DJ, Schelbert HR, Wolf GL, Brundage BH, eds. *Marcus' Cardiac Imaging,* 2d ed. Philadelphia: Saunders; 1996:452–480. With permission.)

## Intracardiac Thrombi

Intracardiac thrombi occur commonly in a variety of cardiovascular disorders, may be visualized in any chamber of the heart, and frequently result in embolic events.[309] The major factors that predispose to the formation of intracardiac thrombi include localized stasis of flow, low cardiac output, and cardiac injury. In addition, migration of venous thrombi may also result in intracardiac clots. The appearance of intracardiac thrombi may vary considerably, and although they are typically attached to the endocardium, unrestricted and freely mobile thrombi occasionally may be encountered (particularly in the setting of valvular stenosis which prevents exit of the thrombus from the heart). Thrombi typically have identifiable borders and may be layered and homogeneous or heterogeneous, with areas of central liquefaction (Figs. 15-129 and 15-130).[310]

### RIGHT HEART

Thrombi within the right heart chambers may form locally or migrate from the venous circulation; they are found most commonly in the RA. As opposed to the laminar, relatively immobile nature of RA thrombi that form in situ, venous thromboemboli trapped in the RA tend to be serpentine and mobile. The potential for pulmonary embolism is high. Thrombi also can be seen within the main pulmonary arteries, although they are less well visualized by TTE than TEE.[311] RV thrombi are rare but may occur with RV infarction and endomyocardial fibrosis. Their appearance is similar to that of LV thrombi.

## LEFT ATRIUM

Left atrial thrombi occur in the setting of low cardiac output, mitral valvular disease (particularly MS), atrial fibrillation, and LA enlargement. Both TTE and TEE can detect thrombi within the main cavity of the LA (Fig. 15-131), but TEE is clearly superior for visualizing thrombi within the left atrial appendage. Since approximately 50 percent of LA thrombi are limited to the appendage, TEE is the diagnostic procedure of choice to detect this lesion.[312] LA thrombi appear as discrete masses, either fixed or mobile, and are usually of homogeneous echo density (Fig. 15-52). On TEE, normal pectinate muscular ridges in the appendage must be distinguished from small thrombi. In addition, the left atrial appendage may occasionally be multilobed. Although this anatomic variant may be a risk factor for appendage thrombi, the atrial tissue separating the lobes should not be mistaken for clot.[313] Left atrial thrombi are often accompanied by spontaneous echo contrast (or "smoke") within the LA. This finding, probably produced by transient aggregation of erythrocytes and plasma proteins, indicates stagnant blood flow and can occur in any cardiac chamber or the aorta. Left atrial spontaneous echo contrast, like LA thrombus, has been associated with embolic events[314]and may be a marker of regional prothrombotic activity.[315] On 2D imaging, the contrast signals are in constant motion and can be missed if gain settings are inappropriately low.

## LEFT VENTRICLE

Most LV thrombi occur in settings of abnormal systolic contraction (dilated cardiomyopathy, AMI, and chronic LV aneurysm).[316] LV thrombi have been reported in up to one-half of patients with large

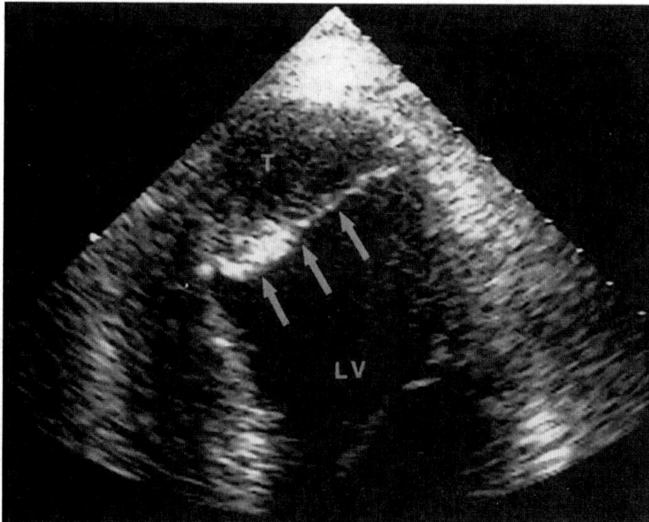


FIGURE 15-129 Magnified apical view of a large thrombus (T) in the apex of the left ventricle (LV). Although the thrombus is fairly homogeneous, its border is more echo-dense (*arrows*).

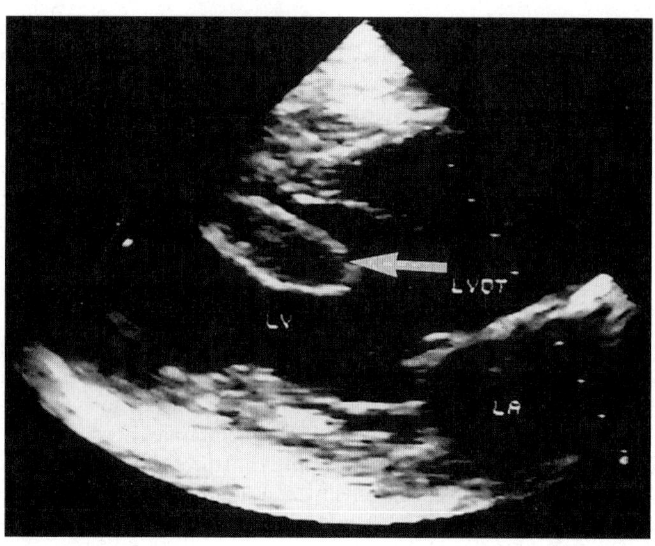


FIGURE 15-130 Parasternal long-axis view of a large mobile thrombus (*arrow*) attached to the anteroseptal segment of the left ventricle (LV). LVOT = left ventricular outflow tract; LA = left atrium. (From Blanchard DG, DeMaria AN. Cardiac and extracardiac masses: Echocardiographic evaluation. In: Skorton DJ, Schelbert HR, Wolf GL, Brundage BH, eds. *Marcus' Cardiac Imaging,* 2d ed. Philadelphia: Saunders; 1996:452–480. With permission.)

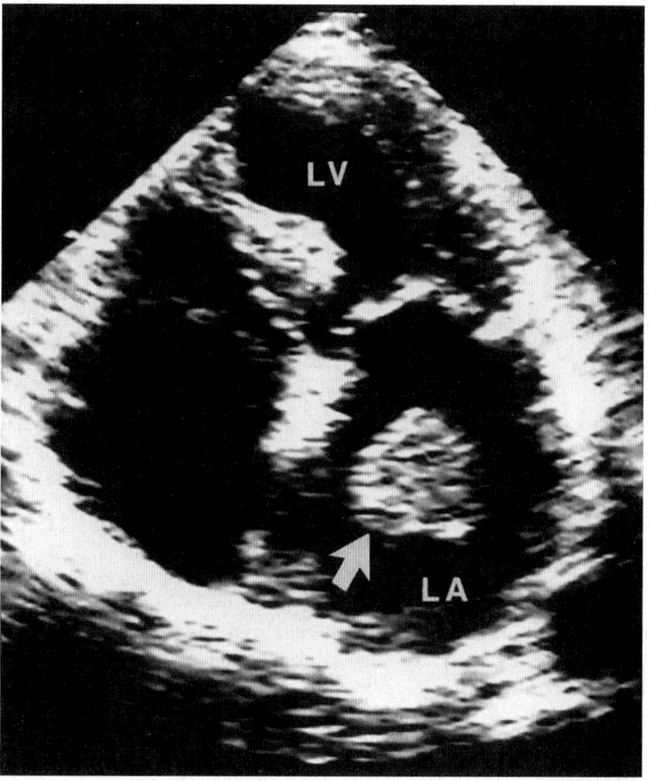


FIGURE 15-131 Apical four-chamber image of a large mobile "ball" thrombus (*arrow*) in the left atrium (LA). LV = left ventricle. (From Blanchard DG, DeMaria AN. Cardiac and extracardiac masses: Echocardiographic evaluation. In: Skorton DJ, Schelbert HR, Wolf GL, Brundage BH, eds. *Marcus' Cardiac Imaging,* 2d ed. Philadelphia: Saunders; 1996:452–480. With permission.)

myocardial infarctions and occur more frequently in anterior infarctions (up to 30 to 40 percent of such patients).[316] Most thrombi are located in the apex[300] and thus are best visualized in the apical views (Fig. 15-129). Although echocardiography is the procedure of choice for detecting LV thrombi, the technique's true sensitivity and specificity remains uncertain, since most patients included in validating studies had LV aneurysms and the echocardiographic criteria applied were subjective.[316]

LV thrombi may be laminar and fixed or protruding and mobile, and they may have a heterogeneous echo density (Figs. 15-129 and 15-130). Studies suggest that "immature" thrombi are often filamentous, with irregular borders, while older thrombi tend to be echodense and fixed.[300,309] The echocardiographic characteristics of thrombi may influence the risk of cardiogenic embolization, as irregularly shaped, mobile, and protruding thrombi are more likely to embolize than laminar, immobile clots.[309] True LV thrombi have a density distinct from the underlying myocardium, appear in multiple imaging planes, and move concordantly with the underlying myocardium. Suspected masses in areas of normally functioning myocardium are rarely thrombi.

## CARDIAC TUMORS

Although diagnosed infrequently, cardiac tumors often are included in the differential diagnosis of cardiac problems because of their protean clinical manifestations. Cardiac tumors may be intracavitary or intramural, and the location determines their echocardiographic appearance. Intracavitary tumors appear as sessile or mobile echo densities attached to the mural endocardium while intramural tumors appear as localized thickening of the LV wall. The pericardium also may be involved with cardiac tumors, with or without the presence of concomitant effusion (Chap. 85).

### Myxomas

Myxomas are the most common primary cardiac tumors, accounting for about 25 percent of all such lesions (Chap. 95).[317] Myxomas can occur in any cardiac chamber, but 75 percent are found in the LA.[317] On 2D imaging, myxomas usually appear as gelatinous, speckled, sometimes globular masses with frond-like projections (Figs. 15-132*A* and *B*). Tissue heterogeneity is common, but calcification is rare. Although they may be sessile, myxomas are usually attached to the endocardial surface by a pedicle. Typically, they are attached to the interatrial septum, but they can originate from the posterior or anterior atrial wall, the appendage, or even the cardiac valves. Large tumors are almost always mobile to some degree, and a sizable left atrial mass that appears fixed in position is therefore less likely to be a myxoma. Large left atrial myxomas may move back and forth into the MV annulus during the cardiac cycle, entering the orifice in diastole and the LA in systole. Accordingly, Doppler interrogation may demonstrate either obstruction of flow, valvular regurgitation, or both.[318] Most myxomas are visible on TTE, but TEE is superior for the delineation of tumor attachments and detection of small myxomas. Since approximately 5 percent of myxomas are biatrial, careful evaluation of the RA is mandatory.[317]

### Additional Primary Tumors

**BENIGN**

Rhabdomyomas are rare cardiac tumors associated with tuberous sclerosis (Chap. 80). There is a strong tendency for multiple tumors to occur within an affected heart (90 percent of cases). Fibromas are found most often in children and affect the left ventricle most frequently. The tumor may grow within the myocardium rather than expanding into a cardiac chamber. Papillary fibroelastomas are usually quite small in size (less than 1 cm in diameter) and often grow on cardiac valves or chordae (Fig. 15-133*A*). These rare tumors typically have multiple small fronds that tend to embolize.[299,319] Echocardiographic differentiation from vegetations can be difficult (Chap. 85).

**MALIGNANT**

Primary malignant cardiac tumors are quite rare and confer a very poor prognosis. Angiosarcoma is the most common and occurs most often in the right atrium (Fig. 15-133*B*). Rhabdomyosarcoma is an additional primary cardiac malignancy.[320] Echocardiography can be useful in monitoring response to therapy, but its diagnostic utility is limited as most findings are nonspecific.

### Metastatic and Secondary Tumors of the Heart and Pericardium

Metastatic tumors to the pericardium and heart occur 20 to 40 times more often than primary cardiac tumors (Fig. 15-134*A*).[321] Tumors that commonly involve the heart and pericardium include breast and lung carcinoma, melanoma, and lymphoma (Fig. 15-134*B*). Involvement may be secondary to hematogenous, lymphatic, or contiguous spread. Tumors such as hepatoma and renal carcinoma can also extend to the heart via the venae cavae. In these cases, tumor is often visible in the inferior vena cava and RA. Metastatic disease affects the pericardium more frequently than the heart itself, and pericardial effusion is the most common echocardiographic manifestation in patients with cardiac metastases.[321] Intracavitary and pericardial masses are easily visualized with 2D imaging, although intramural tumors are sometimes difficult to image. Echocardiographic findings are nonspecific, and metastatic tumors may be mistaken for primary cardiac neoplasms, vegetations, thrombi, or even prominent muscular trabeculations (Chap. 85).

### Additional Cardiac Masses

The heart is rarely involved in echinococcal disease (<2 percent of cases), but intracardiac or intrapericardial rupture of a cyst can lead to anaphylaxis and cardiac tamponade, respectively.[322] Echocardiographic detection of a multiseptated cyst in the left ventricle or interventricular septum suggests cardiac echinococcal disease. Simple pericardial cysts usually occur in the right costophrenic angle (posterior to the right atrium) and have a benign prognosis. The structures are nonseptated and fluid-filled; they do not compress the cardiac chambers.[323]

## PERICARDIAL DISEASE

In normal subjects, the pericardium is difficult to visualize since the pericardial cavity is only a potential space and visceral and parietal pericardial layers appear as a single echo. In the setting of pericardial effusion, the fluid appears as a sonolucent area (or clear space) separating epicardium from pericardium.[324] Pericarditis may be unaccompanied by pericardial effusion and in such cases may be undetectable by echocardiography. In addition, although thickening and/or calcification of the pericardium may be detectable by echocardiography in patients with constrictive pericarditis, cardiac ultrasound is limited in this capability. Therefore, the evaluation of constrictive pericarditis by echocardiography primarily involves Doppler flow recordings.[325]

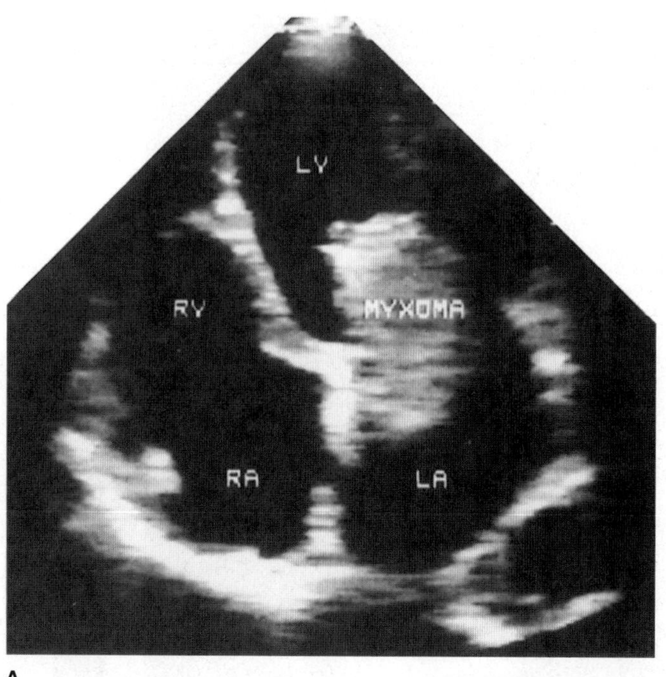


A

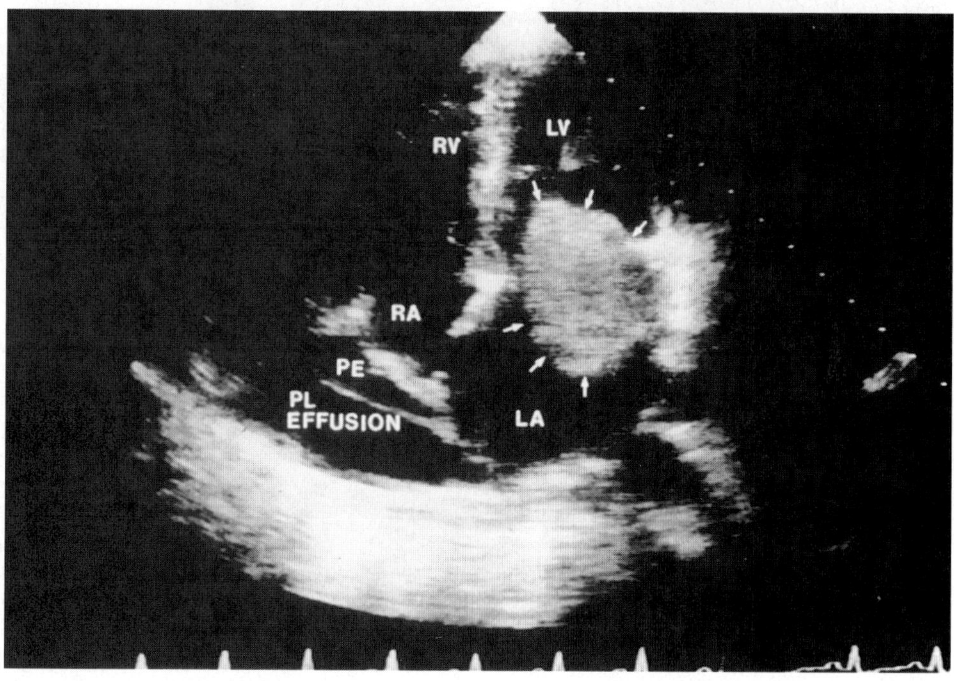


B

FIGURE 15-132 *A.* Apical four-chamber image of a left atrial myxoma which is attached to the interatrial septum and prolapses through the mitral valve. LA = left atrium; RA = right atrium; RV = right ventricle; LV = left ventricle. (From Blanchard DG, DeMaria AN. Cardiac and extracardiac masses: Echocardiographic evaluation. In: Skorton DJ, Schelbert HR, Wolf GL, Brundage BH, eds. *Marcus' Cardiac Imaging,* 2d ed. Philadelphia: Saunders, 1996:452–480. With permission.) *B.* Apical four-chamber image of a large left atrial myxoma (*arrows*), which is attached to the lateral wall of the atrium. LA = left atrium; RA = right atrium; RV = right ventricle; LV = left ventricle; PE = pericardial effusion; PL = pleural.

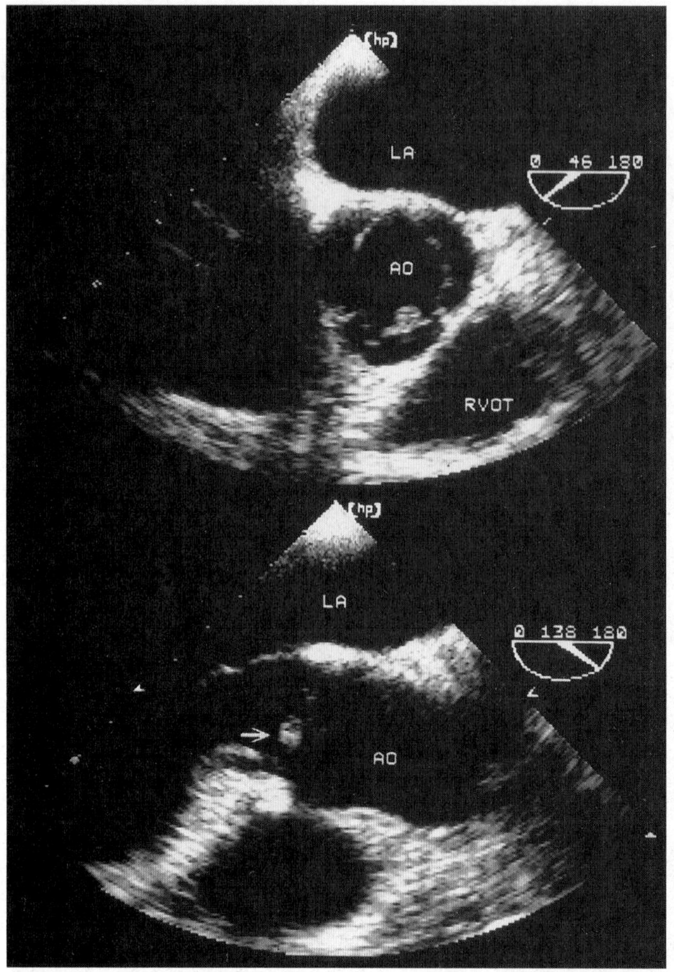


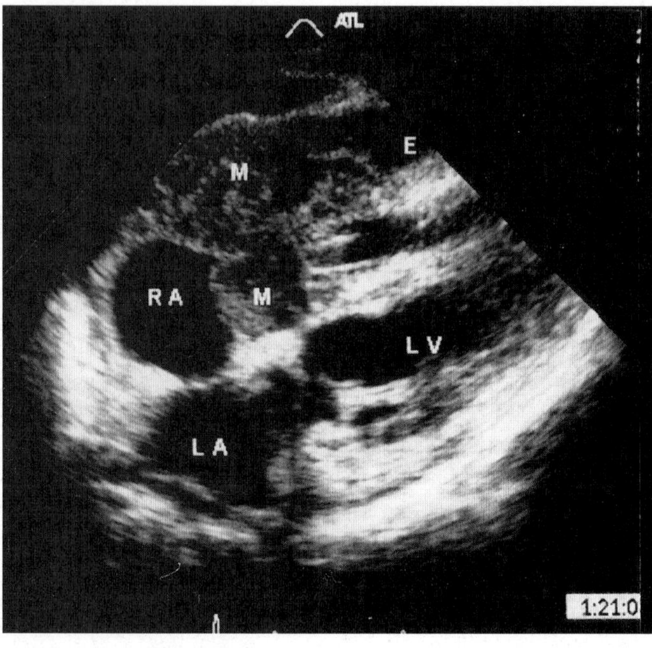


FIGURE 15-133 *A.* Transesophageal images of a surgically proven papillary fibroelastoma on the right coronary cusp of the aortic valve (*arrow*). The upper and lower panels show transverse and longitudinal planes through the aortic valve, respectively. *B.* Primary cardiac angiosarcoma (subcostal imaging plane). The tumor mass (M) is present in the right atrium (RA), and has extended through the atrial wall into the pericardial space. LA = left atrium; LV = left ventricle; E = pericardial effusion.

## Pericardial Effusion

Echocardiography is the diagnostic procedure of choice for detection of pericardial fluid (Fig. 15-135), and early M-mode studies demonstrated that volumes as small as 20 to 30 mL could be detected reliably.[325] As both myocardium and pericardium are echo-reflective and pericardial fluid is not, a sonolucent area between the epicardium and pericardium is diagnostic of a pericardial effusion. Although epicardial-pericardial separation may be seen during systole in normal cases, separation throughout the cardiac cycle is abnormal.[326] Descending aorta, coronary sinus, pleural effusion, pericardial cyst, and LV pseudoaneurysm occasionally may be mistaken for pericardial effusion.

Echocardiography can be used to identify pericardial loculations, fibrous strands, and pericardial tumors as well as to assess the size of effusions[324] (Fig. 15-136). Pericardial effusions may be concentric or loculated (the latter type is especially common with postoperative, infective, and malignant effusions). As pericardial tissue reflects upon itself behind the LA between the pulmonary veins (the oblique sinus), fluid is rarely seen in this area. Small, nonloculated effusions may move depending on patient position and thus are often drawn posteriorly and inferiorly by gravity during routine imaging. A rim of pericardial fluid surrounding the heart is evidence of a moderate or large effusion, and the heart can sometimes be seen "swinging" back and forth within the pericardial space, creating the mechanism of *electrical alternans.* In general, small effusions are seen posteriorly rather than anteriorly on supine imaging. Moderate-sized (100 to 500 mL) nonloculated effusions are present both anterior and posterior to the heart. Large nonloculated effusions (>500 mL) are circumferential and frequently allow free motion of the heart within the fluid-filled space.

Distinguishing between pericardial and pleural effusions is occasionally difficult with echocardiography.[327] If these conditions coexist, the pericardium usually can be identified as a linear density separating fluid in the two spaces. The parasternal long-axis view is often helpful in differentiating the disorders. The descending aorta is a mediastinal structure; therefore pericardial effusions will often separate the heart and descending aorta, while pleural effusions are seen inferior and posterior to the aorta[327] (Fig. 15-137). In cases of large pleural effusions, atelectatic lung tissue also may be present (Fig. 15-137). Subcostal views are often valuable and may yield the only satisfactory transthoracic images in postoperative or posttraumatic

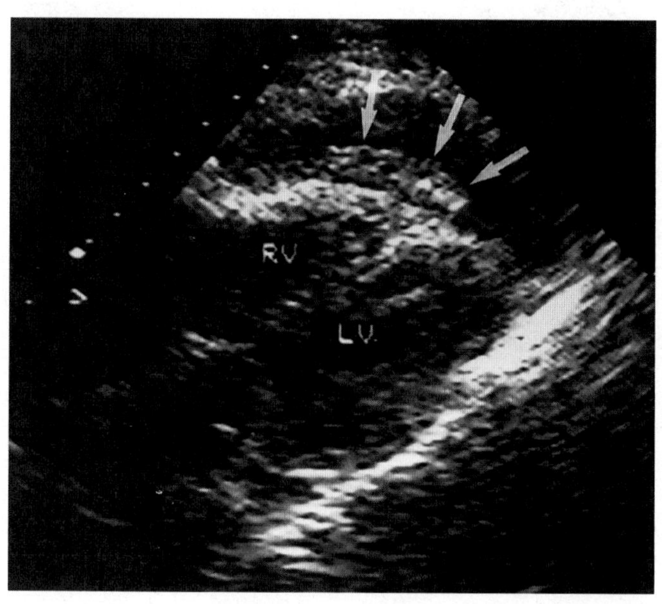


A

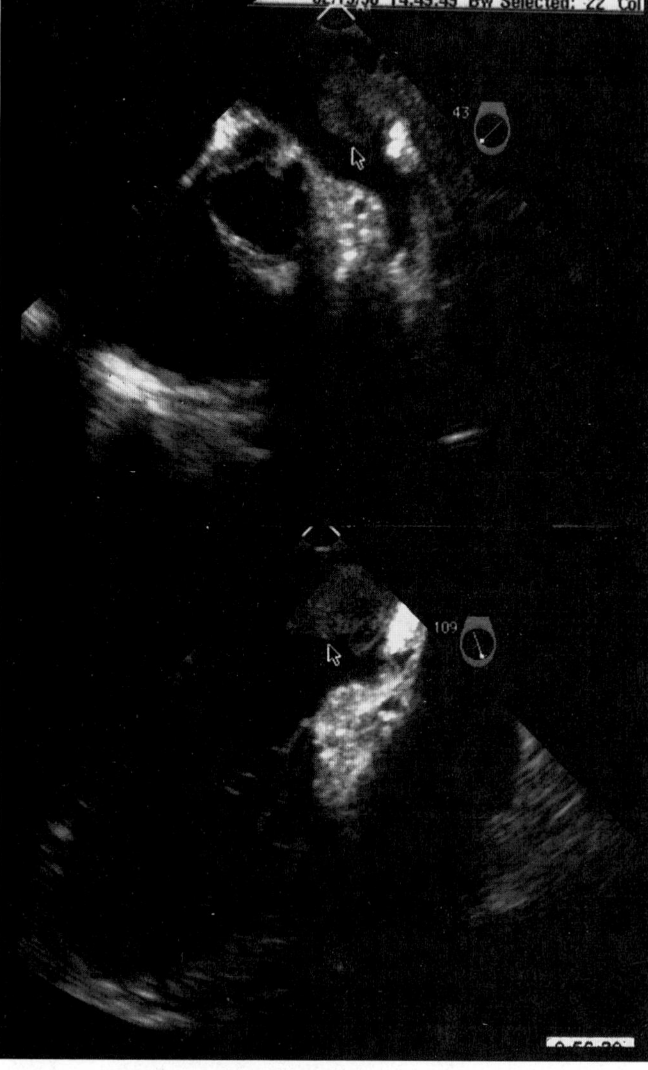


B

FIGURE 15-134 *A*. Modified subcostal image showing a metastatic tumor on the epicardium (*arrows*) and a malignant pericardial effusion. RV = right ventricle; LV = left ventricle. (From Blanchard DG, DeMaria AN. Cardiac and extracardiac masses: Echocardiographic evaluation. In: Skorton DJ, Schelbert HR, Wolf GL, Brundage BH, eds. *Marcus' Cardiac Imaging,* 2d ed. Philadelphia: Saunders; 1996:452–480. With permission.) *B*. Transesophageal images from a case of metastatic lung carcinoma. The tumor (*arrows*) has entered the left atrium via contiguous spread through the left upper pulmonary vein.

cases. The inferior vena cava also can be imaged in this view; if the vessel does not display inspiratory collapse greater than 50 percent of its maximum diameter, elevated RA pressure is present.

On parasternal images, an echolucent space is sometimes visualized anterior to the RV.[328] Although this finding may represent pericardial fluid, it usually is caused by epicardial fat (without effusion) and has no pathologic significance. Therefore the diagnosis of pericardial effusion based solely on the presence of this anterior clear space should be avoided.

## Cardiac Tamponade

As the pericardium is a relatively noncompliant membrane that adapts slowly to volume changes, pericardial effusions (especially those that accumulate rapidly) may limit cardiac filling and cause cardiac tamponade. Echocardiography can help diagnose this condition by detecting (1) morphologic signs of increased intrapericardial pressure and (2) abnormal intracardiac flow patterns caused by tamponade and enhanced ventricular interdependence.[329]

Because diastolic pressures are slightly lower in the right heart than the left, the RA and RV are usually the first chambers to exhibit evidence of increased intrapericardial pressure. High intrapericardial pressure can cause compression or collapse of right heart chambers.[329,330] Invagination of the right atrial wall during atrial systole is a sensitive (but not specific) sign of tamponade (Fig. 15-138).[330] Diastolic collapse or "buckling" of the RV free wall is a more specific sign of tamponade, and can be visualized both on 2D and M-mode imaging[329] (Fig. 15-135*B* and *C*). In cases of localized tamponade or severe RVH, left atrial or ventricular diastolic collapse may be the first sign of tamponade.[331]

Doppler echocardiographic recordings in patients with tamponade have demonstrated an enhancement or exaggeration of the normal

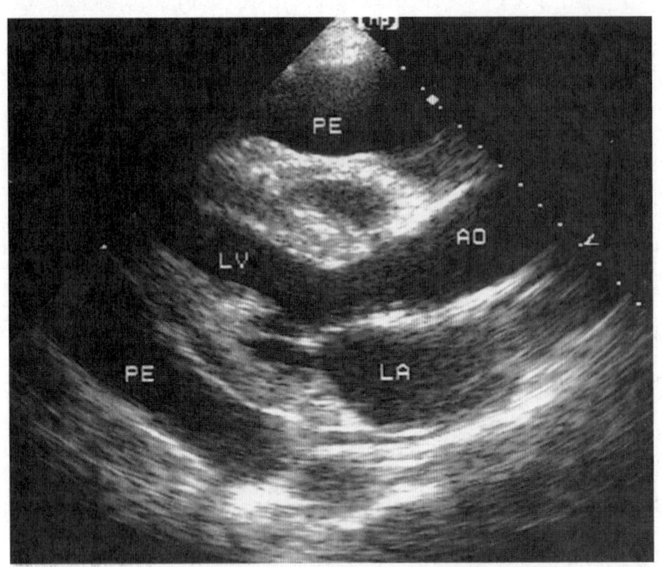


A

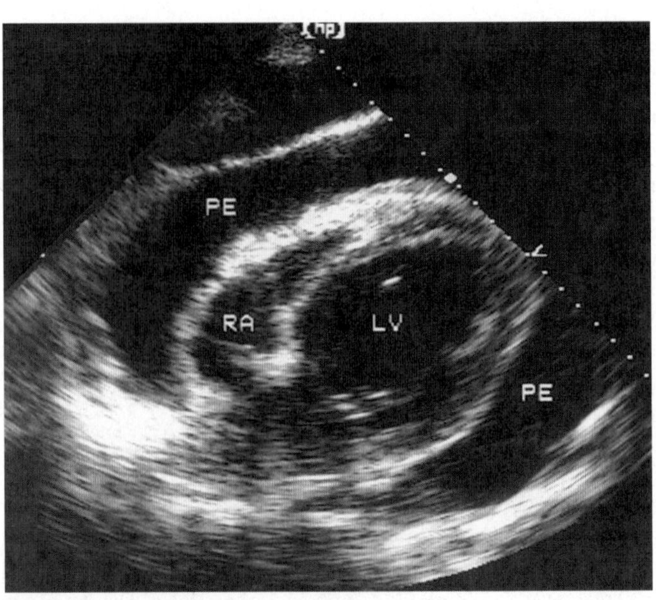


B

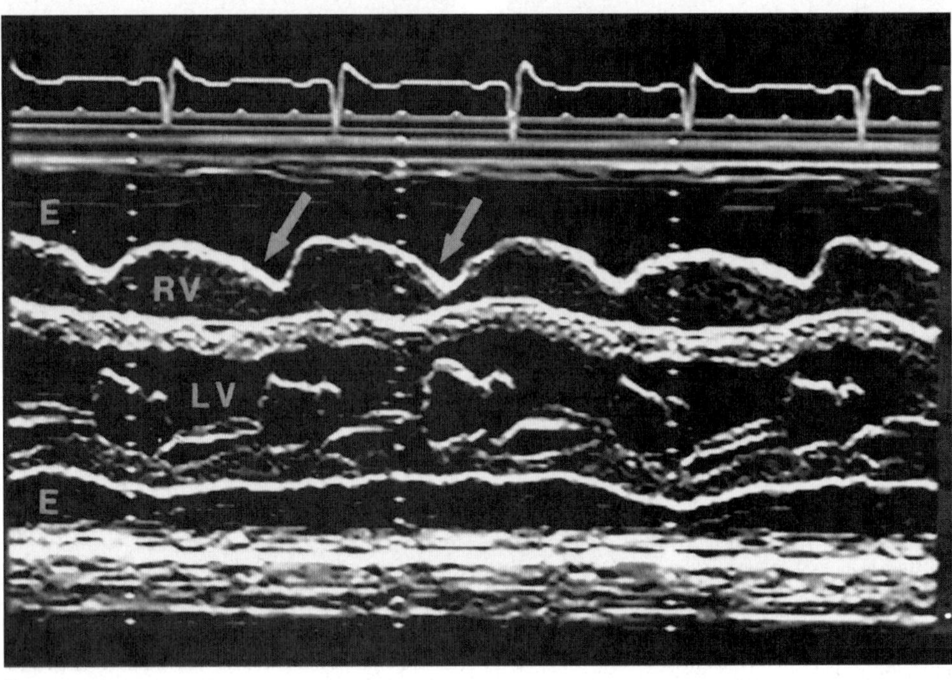


C

FIGURE 15-135 *A.* Moderate pericardial effusion (PE) on parasternal long-axis imaging. AO = aorta; LV = left ventricle; LA = left atrium. *B.* Right ventricular compression in cardiac tamponade (subcostal plane). RA = right atrium; LV = left ventricle; PE = pericardial effusion. *C.* M-mode image of cardiac tamponade and right ventricular diastolic collapse. The right ventricular (RV) free wall (*arrows*) moves posteriorly toward the interventricular septum during diastole. E = effusion; LV = left ventricle.

respiratory variation in ventricular inflow and outflow. Thus, transmitral and LVOT velocities decrease significantly with inspiration, most likely because of enhanced ventricular interdependence and a marked decrease in the transmitral diastolic gradient during inspiration (Fig. 15-139). The latter is caused both by high intrapericardial pressure as well as leftward motion of the interventricular septum from increased RV filling. Although cardiac tamponade remains a clinical diagnosis, echocardiography has significantly improved the detection of hemodynamic effects from pericardial fluid, especially in early and equivocal cases. Studies have also indicated that when echocardiography is used to direct pericardiocentesis to the site of greatest fluid accumulation, the risks associated with blind pericardial puncture are decreased.

## Constrictive Pericarditis

The diagnosis of constrictive pericarditis is sometimes difficult to establish, even by cardiac catheterization. 2D and M-mode echocardiography may provide evidence of thickened pericardial tissue by demonstrating increased reflectivity and multiple parallel moving echoes in the area of the pericardium. The criteria for pericardial thickening on echocardiogram are imperfect, however, as the normal

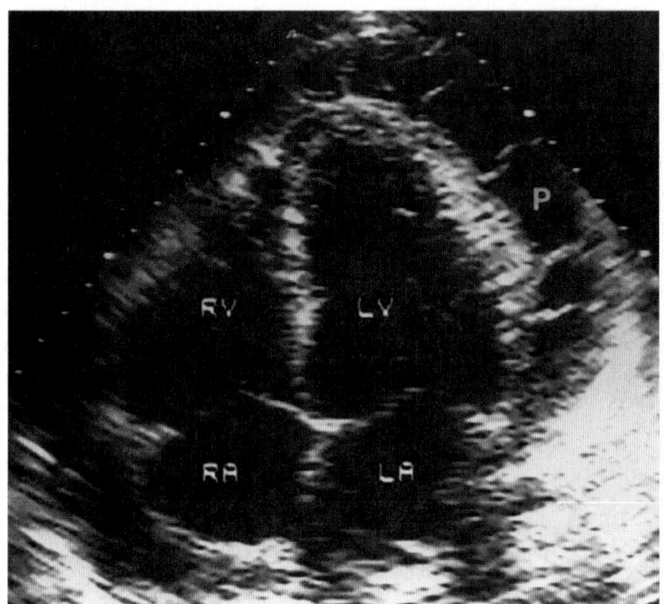


FIGURE 15-136 Apical four-chamber image in a case of malignant pericardial effusion (P). Numerous fibrinous strands are seen within the effusion. LA = left atrium; RA = right atrium; RV = right ventricle; LV = left ventricle. (From Blanchard DG, DeMaria AN. Cardiac and extracardiac masses: Echocardiographic evaluation. In: Skorton DJ, Schelbert HR, Wolf GL, Brundage BH, eds. *Marcus' Cardiac Imaging,* 2d ed. Philadelphia: Saunders,1996:452–480. With permission.)

pericardium is an echodense, highly reflective structure with a gain-dependent signal.[332] Paradoxical septal motion may be seen on M-mode with constriction, as can an abnormal inspiratory interventricular septal "bounce"[333] and limited diastolic motion of the posterior LV wall. A dilated inferior vena cava that does not collapse on deep inspiration is indicative of high RA pressure and may be observed on 2D imaging in constrictive pericarditis.[333]

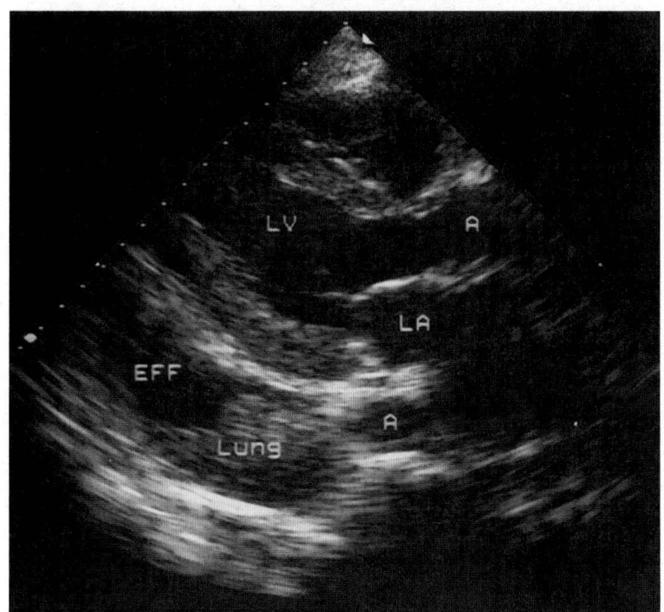


FIGURE 15-137 Parasternal long-axis view in a patient with a pleural effusion (EFF) posterior to the heart. Atelectatic lung tissue is present within the effusion. LA = left atrium; LV = left ventricle; A = aorta.

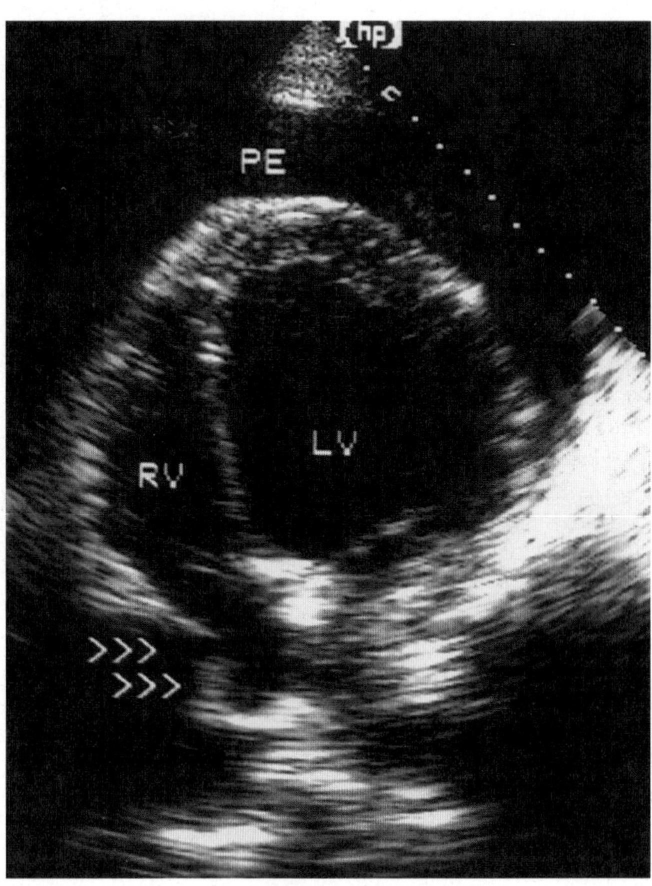


FIGURE 15-138 Right atrial collapse (*arrows*) in cardiac tamponade. PE = pericardial effusion; LV = left ventricle; RV = right ventricle.

The utility of Doppler recordings in evaluating constrictive pericarditis has been shown in several studies.[265,325,334] As with cardiac tamponade, pericardial constriction produces exaggerated respiratory variation in the isovolumic relaxation time and in flow velocities within right and left ventricles, pulmonary veins, and hepatic vein.[325] A respiratory variation of >20 percent in peak mitral E velocity favors the diagnosis of constriction over restrictive cardiomyopathy, while little respiratory variation favors restrictive physiology.[325] Doppler echocardiographic criteria for constriction have been validated prospectively and may help predict clinical response to pericardiectomy. Unfortunately, exaggerated respiratory flow variation is not specific for pericardial constriction and also can be seen in chronic obstructive pulmonary disease and asthma. In these cases, Doppler examination of superior vena cava flow is useful: patients with asthma will have increased flow toward the heart during inspiration, while limited forward flow will be seen in constriction (the echocardiographic equivalent of Kussmaul's sign).[335] In addition, tissue Doppler imaging of the mitral annulus is useful in differentiating constrictive vs restrictive physiology. As discussed in the above section on Doppler assessment of diastolic function, both of these forms of diastolic dysfunction typically exhibit restrictive patterns on transmitral ($E > A$) and pulmonary venous ($S < D$) spectral flow recordings. In cases of pericardial constriction, however, the early diastolic velocity of the mitral annulus ($E_m$) remains normal. In restrictive cardiomyopathy, this velocity is abnormally low. Finally, respiratory variation in the peak velocity and duration of continuous-wave Doppler TR spectral envelopes appear to reflect accurately the enhanced ventricular interdependence seen in constrictive pericarditis.[336]

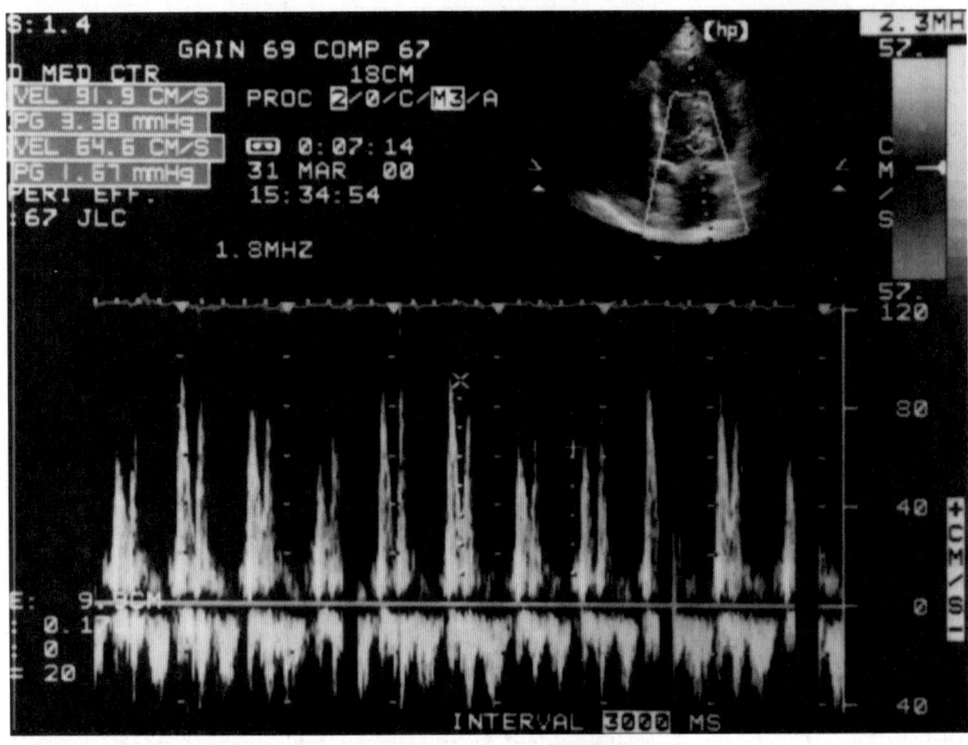


FIGURE 15-139 Pulsed-wave Doppler tracing of left ventricular inflow in cardiac tamponade (apical transducer position). There is abnormal respiratory variation in the peak E wave velocity (which varies from 92 to 65 cm/s).

## IMAGING OF THE CORONARY ARTERIES

The ability to visualize the proximal segments of the left and right coronary arteries was initially demonstrated by Weyman et al. Subsequent studies established the ability of color and spectral Doppler examination to image and record the velocity of flow from TTE and TEE approaches, particularly with regard to the left anterior descending coronary artery.[210] However, visualization of the coronary arteries by echocardiography has not achieved a significant role in clinical practice because the resolution of the technique is at the limit of vessel size and the vessels are circuitous and move vigorously, often coursing in and out of the beam path. Despite these limitations, transthoracic imaging has proven useful for the diagnosis and follow-up of patients with Kawasaki disease and coronary involvement[337] (Fig. 15-140) and may also help distinguish normal from atherosclerotic coronary arteries.

The coronary arteries are routinely imaged with TEE, which can detect proximal stenoses, atherosclerosis, and congenital abnormalities of the coronaries more accurately than surface imaging. Doppler TEE analysis also has been used to determine coronary flow reserve.[338]

Visualization of mid- and distal coronary arteries is problematic with both TTE and TEE. Recent advances in technology and contrast agents, however, have significantly improved capabilities in this area. Figure 15-141*A* (Plate 74) shows color flow within a septal coronary artery. Figure 15-141*B* shows a spectral Doppler recording of flow within the distal left

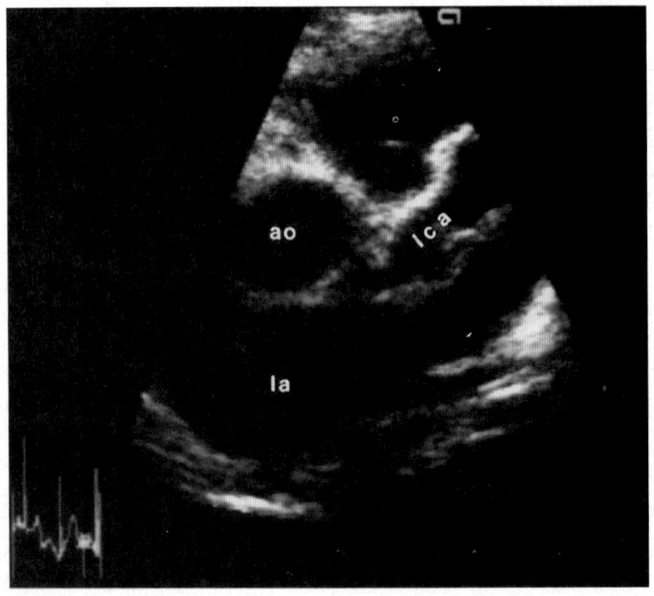


A

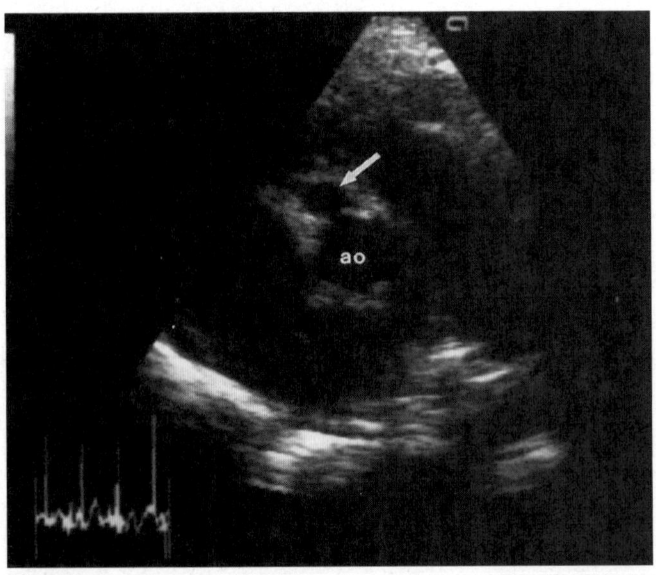


B

FIGURE 15-140 Parasternal short-axis images of coronary artery aneurysms associated with Kawasaki's disease. *A*. The proximal left coronary artery (LCA) is seen to be diffusely dilated and aneurysmal. *B*. A proximal right coronary artery aneurysm (*arrow*) is shown. AO = aorta, LA = left atrium. (Courtesy of Victor Lucas, MD and Paul Grossfeld, MD.)

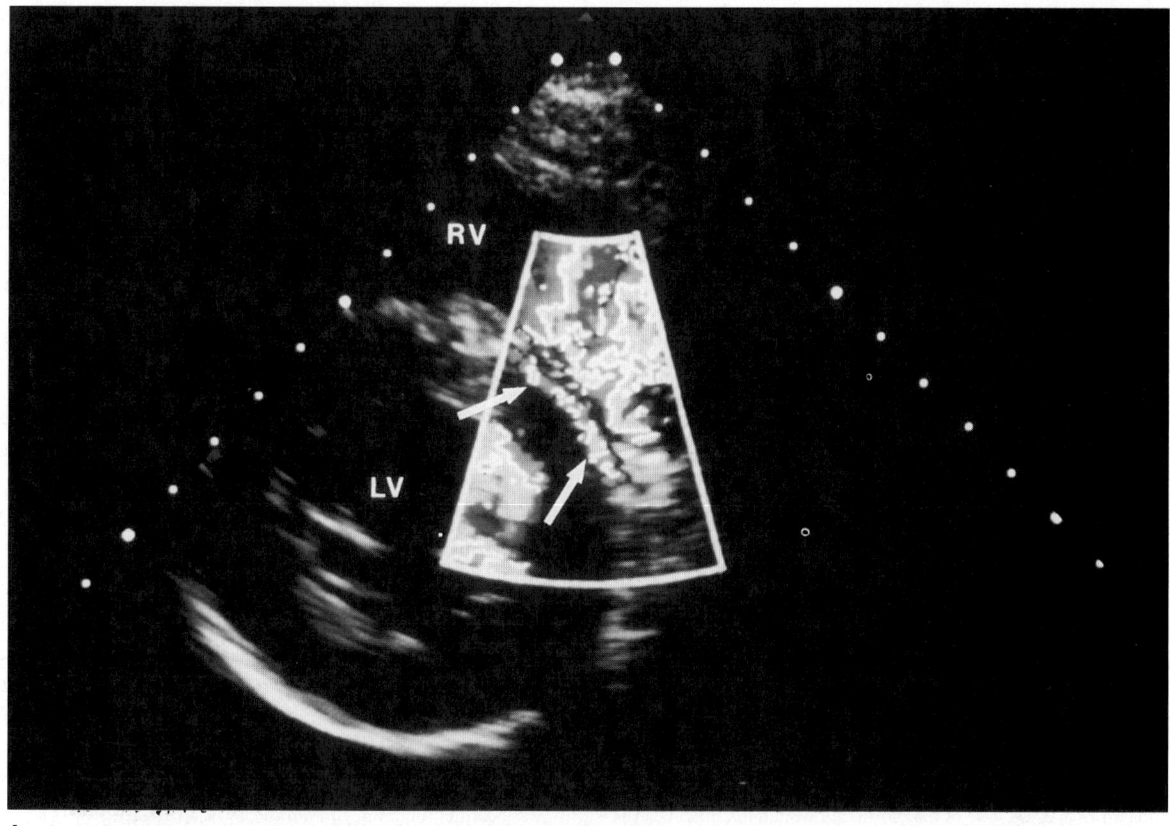


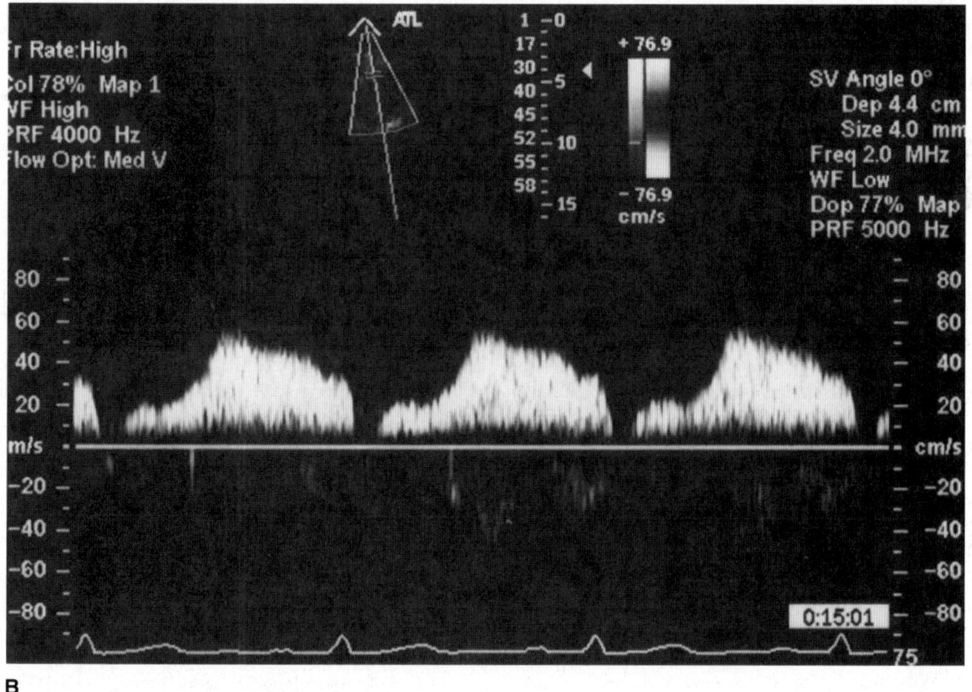


FIGURE 15-141 *A* (Plate 74). Transthoracic short-axis image of a coronary artery within the interventricular septum (*arrows*). LV = left ventricle; RV = right ventricle. *B*. Pulsed-wave spectral Doppler tracing of flow within the distal left anterior descending artery. Diastolic flow is predominant. (Courtesy of Ajit Raisinghani, MD.)

anterior descending coronary artery (note the predominance of diastolic flow). These images were produced by an instrument utilizing a fundamental frequency range of 5 to 7 MHz, rather than the more commonly used range of 2.5 to 5.0 MHz. This area of echocardiography is expanding rapidly and clinical applications will grow in the future.

## References


1. ACC/AHA Guidelines for the Clinical Application of Echocardiography: Executive Summary. A Report of the American College of Cardiology/American Heart Association Task Force on Practice Guidelines (Committee on Clinical Application of Echocardiography). *J Am Coll Cardiol* 1997;29:862–879.
2. Daniel WG, Mügge A. Transesophageal echocardiography. *N Engl J Med* 1995;332:1268–1279.
3. Handschumacher MD, Lethor JP, Siu SC, et al. A new integrated system for three-dimensional echocardiographic reconstruction: Development and validation for ventricular volume with application in human subjects. *J Am Coll Cardiol* 1993;21:743–753.
4. Rovai D, DeMaria AN, L'Abbate A. Myocardial contrast echo effect: The dilemma of coronary blood flow and volume. *J Am Coll Cardiol* 1995;26:12–17.
5. Elder I, Hertz CH. The use of ultrasonic reflectoscope for the continuous recording of movement of heart walls. *Kungl Fysiorgr Sallski Fund Forhandl* 1954;24:40–45.
6. Wild JJ, Crawford HD, Reid JM. Visualization of the excised human heart by means of reflected ultrasound or echocardiography. *Am Heart J* 1958;54:903–906.
7. Feigenbaum H, Zaky A. Use of diagnostic ultrasound in clinical cardiology. *J Indiana State Med Assoc* 1966;49:140–152.
8. Bom N, Lancee CT Jr, Van Zwieten G, et al. Multiscan echocardiography: I. Technical description. *Circulation* 1973;48;1066–1073.
9. Griffith JM, Henry WL. A sector scanner for real time two-dimensional echocardiography. *Circulation* 1974;49:1147–1152.
10. Eggelton RC, Johnston KW. Real time mechanical scanning system compared with array techniques. *IEEE Proc Sonics Ultrasounds* 1974;Cat. No. 74-CH0896-1:16.
11. VonRamm OT, Thurstone FL. Cardiac imaging using a phased array ultrasound system: I. System design. *Circulation* 1976;53:258–262.
12. Omoto R. *Color Atlas of Real-Time Two-Dimensional Doppler Echocardiography,* 2d ed. Tokyo: Sindan-to-Chiryo; 1987.
13. Hanrath P, Kremer P, Langenstein BA, et al. Transoesophageale Eckokardiographie: Ein neues Verfahren zur dynamischenVentrikelfunktionsanalyse. *Dtsch Med Wochenschr* 1981;106:523–525.
14. Seward JB, Khanderia BK, Oh JK, et al. Transesophageal echocardiography: Technique, anatomic correlations, implementation and clinical applications. *Mayo Clin Proc* 1988;63:649–680.
15. Baker DW. Pulsed ultrasonic Doppler blood-flow sensing. *IEEE Trans Sonics Ultrasonics* 1970;SU-17(3).
16. Hatle L, Angelsen B, Tromsdal A. Noninvasive assessment of atrioventricular pressure half-time by Doppler ultrasound. *Circulation* 1979; 60:1096–1104.
17. Hatle L, Angelsen BA, Tromsdal A. Noninvasive assessment of aortic stenosis by Doppler ultrasound. *Br Heart J* 1980;3:284–292.
18. Wells PNT. *Ultrasonics in Clinical Diagnosis,* 2d ed. New York: Churchill Livingstone; 1977.
19. Thomas JD, Rubin DN. Tissue harmonic imaging: Why does it work? *J Am Soc Echocardiogr* 1998;11:803–808.
20. Main ML, Asher CR, Rubin DN, et al. Comparison of tissue harmonic imaging with contrast (sonicated albumin) echocardiography and Doppler myocardial imaging for enhancing endocardial border resolution. *Am J Cardiol* 1999;83:218–222
21. Kremkau FW, Taylor KJW. Artifacts in ultrasound imaging. *J Ultrasound Med* 1986;15:227–237.
22. Yeh E. Reverberations in echocardiograms. *J Clin Ultrasound* 1977; 5:84–86.
23. Weyman AE. Physical principles of ultrasound. In: Weyman AE, ed. *Principles and Practice of Echocardiography,* 2d ed. Philadelphia: Lea & Febiger;1994:3–28.
24. Mann DL, Gillam LD, Weyman AE. Cross-sectional echocardiographic assessment of regional left ventricular performance and myocardial perfusion. *Prog Cardiovac Dis* 1986;29:1–52.
25. Rose JL, Goldberg BB. *Basic Physics in Diagnostic Ultrasound.* New York: Wiley; 1979.
26. DeMaria AN, Miller RR, Amsterdam EA, et al. Mitral valve early diastolic closing velocity in the echocardiogram: Relation to sequential diastolic flow and ventricular compliance. *Am J Cardiol* 1976;37: 693–700.
27. Konecke L, Feigenbaum H, Chang S. Abnormal mitral valve motion in patients with elevated left ventricular end diastolic pressure. *Circulation* 1973;47:989–996.
28. Sahn DJ, DeMaria A, Kisslo J, Weyman AE. Recommendations regarding quantitation in M-mode echocardiography: Results of a survey of echocardiographic measurements. *Circulation* 1978;58:1072–1083.
29. Nanda NC, Gramiak R, Manning EB. Echocardiographic recognition of the congenital bicuspid aortic valve. *Circulation* 1974;49:870–875.
30. Rasmussen S, Corya BC, Phillips JF, Black MJ. Unreliability of M-mode left ventricular dimensions for calculating stroke volume and cardiac output in patients without heart disease. *Chest* 1982;81: 614–619.
31. Teichholz LE, Kreulen T, Herman MV, Gorlin R. Problems in echocardiographic volume determinations: Echocardiographic-angiographic correlations in the presence or absence of synergy. *Am J Cardiol* 1976; 37:7–11.
32. McDonald IG, Feigenbaum H, Chang S. Analysis of left ventricular wall motion by reflected ultrasound: Application to assessment of myocardial function. *Circulation* 1972;46:14–25.
33. Feigenbaum H: Echocardiographic examination of the left ventricle. *Circulation* 1975;51:1–7.
34. Massie BM, Schiller NB, Ratshin RA, Parmley WW. Mitral-septal separation: New echocardiographic index of left ventricular function. *Am J Cardiol* 1977;39:1008–1016.
35. Ophir J, Maklad NF. Digital scan converters in diagnostic ultrasound imaging. *Proc IEEE* 1979;67–75.
36. Henry WL, DeMaria A, Gramiak R, et al. Report of the American Society of Echocardiography: Nomenclature and standards in two-dimensional echocardiography. *Circulation* 1980;62:212–217.
37. Feigenbaum H. The echocardiographic examination. In: Feigenbaum H. *Echocardiography,* 5th ed. Philadelphia: Lea & Febiger; 1994: 68–133.
38. Weyman AE. *Principles and Practice of Echocardiography,* 2d ed. Philadelphia: Lea & Febiger; 1994.
39. Sapin PM, Clarke GB, Gopal AS, et al. Validation of three-dimensional echocardiography for quantifying the extent of dyssynergy in canine acute myocardial infarction: Comparison with two-dimensional echocardiography. *J Am Coll Cardiol* 1996;27:1761–1770.
40. Shiota T, Jones M, Chikada M, et al. Real-time three-dimensional echocardiography for determining right ventricular stroke volume in an animal model of chronic right ventricular volume overload. *Circulation* 1998;97:1896–1900.
41. Teichholtz LE, Kreulen T, Herman MV, Gorlin R. Problems in echocardiographic volume determinations: Echocardiographic-angiographic correlations in the presence or absence of asynergy. *Am J Cardiol* 1976;37:7–11.
42. Wyatt HL, Heng MK, Meerbaum S, et al. Cross-sectional echocardiography: II. Analysis of mathematic models for quantifying volume of formalin fixed left ventricle. *Circulation* 1980;61:1119–1125.
43. Wyatt HL, Meerbaum S, Heng MK, et al. Cross-sectional echocardiography: III. Analysis of mathematic models for quantifying volume of symmetric and asymmetric left ventricles. *Am Heart J* 1980;100: 821–828.
44. Schiller NB, Acquatella H, Ports TA, et al. Left ventricular volume from paired biplane two-dimensional echocardiography. *Circulation* 1979;60:547–555.

45. Folland ED, Parisi AF, Moynihan PF, et al. Assessment of left ventricular ejection fraction and volumes by real-time, two-dimensional echocardiography and radionuclide techniques. *Circulation* 1979;60:760–766.
46. Stamm RB, Carabello BA, Mayers DL, Martin RP. Two-dimensional echocardiographic measurement of left ventricular ejection fraction: Prospective analysis of what constitutes an adequate determination. *Am Heart J* 1982;104:136–144.
47. Becher H, Tiemann K, Schlief R, et al. Harmonic power Doppler contrast echocardiography: Preliminary clinical results. *Echocardiography* 1997;14:637–642.
48. Spencer KT, Bednarz J, Rafter PG, et al. Use of harmonic imaging without echocardiographic contrast to improve two-dimensional image quality. *Am J Cardiol* 1998;82:794–799.
49. Perez JE, Waggoner AD, Barzilai B, et al. On-line assessment of ventricular function by automatic boundary detection and ultrasonic backscatter imaging. *J Am Coll Cardiol* 1992;19:313.
50. Lang RM, Vignon P, Weinert L, et al. Echocardiographic quantification of regional left ventricular wall motion with color kinesis. *Circulation* 1996;93:1877–1885.
51. Duong AM, Blanchard DG, Cotter B, et al. Endomyocardial movement in patients with disturbed diastolic filling dynamics: Assessment by acoustic quantitation color kinesis (abstr). *J Am Soc Echocardiogr* 1996;9:365.
52. Godoy IE, Mor-Avi V, Weinert L, et al. Use of color kinesis for evaluation of left ventricular filling in patients with dilated cardiomyopathy and mitral regurgitation. *J Am Coll Cardiol* 1998;31:1598–606.
53. Doppler JC. Ueber das farbige Licht der Dopplesterne und einiger anderer Gestirne des Himmels. *Abhandlungen der Konigl, Bohmischen Gesellschaft der Wissenschaften,* 5th ser. 1842;2:465.
54. Franklin DL, Schlegal W, Rushmer RF. Blood flow measured by Doppler frequency shift of backscattered ultrasound. *Science* 1961; 134:564.
55. Hatle L, Angelsen B. *Doppler Ultrasound in Cardiology: Physical Principles and Clinical Applications,* 2d ed. Philadelphia: Lea & Febiger; 1984.
56. Garcia MJ, Thomas JD, Klein AL. New Doppler echocardiographic applications for the study of diastolic function. *J Am Coll Cardiol* 1998;32:865–875.
57. Nagueh SF, Middleton KJ, Kopelen HA, et al. Doppler tissue imaging: A noninvasive technique for evaluation of left vertricular relaxation and estimation of filling pressures. *J Am Coll Cardiol* 1997;30:1527–1533.
58. Garcia MJ, Smedira NG, Greenberg NL, et al. Color M-mode Doppler flow propagation velocity is a preload insensitive index of left ventricular relaxation: Animal and human validation. *J Am Coll Cardiol* 2000;35:201–208.
59. Baker DW, Rubenstein SA, Lorch GS. Pulsed Doppler echocardiography: Principles and applications. *Am J Med* 1977;63:69–80.
60. Burns PM. The physical principles of Doppler and spectral analysis. *J Clin Ultrasound* 1987;15:567–590.
61. Bom K, deBoo J, Rijsterborgh H. On the aliasing problem in pulsed Doppler cardiac studies. *J Clin Ultrasound* 1984;12:559–567.
62. Feigenbaum H. Appendix: Echocardiographic measurements and normal values. In: Feigenbaum H, ed. *Echocardiography,* 5th ed. Philadelphia: Lea & Febiger; 1994:658–683.
63. Rakowski H, Appleton C, Chan K-L, et al. Canadian consensus recommendations for the measurement and reporting of diastolic dysfunction by echocardiography. *J Am Soc Echocardiogr* 1996;9:736–760.
64. Nishimura RA, Housmans PR, Hatle LK, Tajik AJ. Assessment of diastolic function of the heart: Background and current applications of Doppler echocardiography: Part I. Physiologic and pathophysiologic features. *Mayo Clin Proc* 1989;64:71–81.
65. Nishimura RA, Hatle LK, Abel MD, Tajik AJ. Assessment of diastolic function of the heart: Background and current applications of Doppler echocardiography: Part II. Clinical studies. *Mayo Clin Proc* 1989;4: 181–204.
66. Cohen GI, Pietrolungo JF, Thomas JD, Klein AL. A practical guide to assessment of ventricular diastolic function using Doppler echocardiography. *J Am Coll Cardiol* 1996;27;1753–1760.
67. Thomas JD, Weyman AE. Echocardiographic Doppler evaluation of left ventricular diastolic function: Physics and physiology. *Circulation* 1991;84:977–990.
68. Yamamoto K, Masuyama T, Doi Y, et al. Noninvasive assessment of left ventricular relaxation using continuous-wave Doppler aortic regurgitant velocity curve: Its comparative value to the mitral regurgitation method. *Circulation* 1995;91:192–200.
69. DeMaria AN, Blanchard D. The hemodynamic basis of diastology. *J Am Coll Cardiol* 1999;34:1659–1662.
70. Appleton CP, Hatle LK, Popp RL. Cardiac tamponade and pericardial effusion: Respiratory variation in transvalvular flow velocities studied by Doppler echocardiography. *J Am Coll Cardiol* 1988;11:1020–1030.
71. Xie G-Y, Berk MR, Smith MD, et al. Prognostic value of Doppler transmitral flow patterns in patients with congestive heart disease. *J Am Coll Cardiol* 1994;24:132–139.
72. Temporelli PL, Corra U, Imparato A, et al. Reversible restrictive left ventricular diastolic filling with optimized oral therapy predicts a more favorable prognosis in patients with chronic heart failure. *J Am Coll Cardiol* 1998;31:1591–1597.
73. Miyatake K, O'Kamoto M, Knoshita N, et al. Augmentation of atrial contribution to left ventricular inflow with aging as assessed by intracardiac Doppler flowmetry. *Am J Cardiol* 1984;53:586–589.
74. Harrison M, Clifton G, Pennell A, DeMaria A. Effect of heart rate on left ventricular diastolic transmitral flow velocity patterns assessed by Doppler echocardiography in normal subjects. *Am J Cardiol* 1991;67: 622–627.
75. Dabestani A, Takenaka K, Allen B, et al. Effects of spontaneous respiration on left ventricular filling assessed by pulsed Doppler echocardiography. *Am J Cardiol* 1988;61:1356–1358.
76. Dittrich HC, Blanchard DG, Wheeler K, et al. Influence of Doppler sample location on the assessment of changes in mitral inflow velocity profiles. *J Am Soc Echocardiogr* 1990;3:303–309.
77. Berk MR, Xie G, Kwan OL, et al. Reduction of left ventricular preload by lower body negative pressure alters Doppler transmitral filling patterns. *J Am Coll Cardiol* 1990;16:1387–1392.
78. Chen C, Rodriguez L, Guerrero JL, et al. Noninvasive estimation of the instantaneous first derivative of left ventricular pressure using continuous-wave Doppler echocardiography. *Circulation* 1991;83: 2101–2110.
79. William GA, Labovitz AJ. Doppler estimation of cardiac output: Principles and pitfalls. *Echocardiography* 1987;4:355–374.
80. Sahn DJ. Determination of cardiac output by echocardiographic Doppler methods: Relative accuracy of various sites for measurement. *J Am Coll Cardiol* 1985;6:663–664.
81. Looyenga DS, Liebson PR, Bone RC, et al. Determination of cardiac output in critically ill patients by dual beam Doppler echocardiography. *J Am Coll Cardiol* 1989;13:340–347.
82. Valdes-Cruz LM, Horowitz S, Goldberg SJ, Allen HD. The mitral valve orifice method for noninvasive two-dimensional echo Doppler determinations of cardiac output. *Circulation* 1983;67:872–877.
83. Barron JV, Sahn DJ, Valdes-Cruz LM, et al. Clinical utility of two-dimensional Doppler echocardiographic techniques for estimating pulmonary to systemic flow ratios in children with left to right shunting, atrial septal defect, ventricular septal defect and patent ductus arteriosus. *J Am Coll Cardiol* 1984;3:169–178.
84. Xie G-Y, Berk MR, Smith ND, DeMaria AN. A simplified method for determining regurgitant fraction by Doppler echocardiography in patients with aortic regurgitation. *J Am Coll Cardiol* 1994;24:1041–1045.
85. Richards KL, Cannon SR, Miller JF, Crawford MH. Calculation of aortic valve area by Doppler echocardiography: A direct application of the continuity equation. *Circulation* 1986;73:964–969.
86. Zoghbi WA, Farmer KL, Soto JG, et al. Accurate noninvasive quantitation of stenotic aortic valve area by Doppler echocardiography. *Circulation* 1986;73:452–459.
87. Currie PJ, Seward JB, Reeder GS, et al. Continuous wave Doppler echocardiographic assessment of severity of calcific aortic stenosis: A simultaneous Doppler-catheter correlative study in 100 adult patients. *Circulation* 1985;71:1162–1169.

88. Holen J, Waag RC, Gramiak R, et al. Doppler ultrasound in orifice flow: In vitro studies of the relationship between pressure difference and fluid velocity. *Ultrasound Med Biol* 1985;11:261–266.
89. Currie PJ, Hagler DJ, Seward JB, et al. Instantaneous pressure gradient: A simultaneous Doppler and dual catheter correlative study. *J Am Coll Cardiol* 1986;7:800–806.
90. Lee RT, Lord CP, Plappert T, Sutton MS. Prospective Doppler echocardiographic evaluation of pulmonary artery diastolic pressure in the medical intensive care unit. *Am J Cardiol* 1989;64:1366–1370.
91. Yock PG, Popp RL. Noninvasive estimation of right ventricular systolic pressure by Doppler ultrasound in patients with tricuspid regurgitation. *Circulation* 1984;70:657–662.
92. Pai RG, Bansal RC, Shah PM. Doppler-derived rate of left ventricular pressure rise: Its correlation with the postoperative left ventricular function in mitral regurgitation. *Circulation* 1990;84:514–520.
93. Krabill KA, Tamura T, Phil C, et al. The shape of regurgitant jets: In vitro flow visualization and color flow Doppler studies (abstr). *J Am Coll Cardiol* 1987;9:110A.
94. Simpson IA, Valdes-Cruz LM, Sahn DJ. Color Doppler flow mapping of simulated in vitro regurgitant jets: Evaluation of the effects of orifice size and hemodynamic variables. *J Am Coll Cardiol* 1989;13:1195.
95. Chao K, Moises VA, Shandas R, et al. Influence of the Coanda effect on color Doppler jet area and color encoding; In vitro studies using color Doppler flow mapping. *Circulation* 1992;85:333–341.
96. Chen C, Thomas JD, Anconina J, et al. Impact of impinging wall jet on color Doppler quantification on mitral regurgitation. *Circulation* 1991; 84:712–720.
97. Matsumura M, Wong M, Omoto R. Assessment of Doppler color flow mapping in quantification of aortic regurgitation—Correlations and influencing factors. *Jpn Circ J* 1989;53:735–746.
98. Dittrich HC, ed. *Clinical Transesophageal Echocardiography*. St. Louis: Mosby–Year Book; 1992.
99. Blanchard DG, Kimura BJ, Dittrich HC, DeMaria AN. Transesophageal echocardiography of the aorta. *JAMA* 1994;272:546–551.
100. Freeman WK, Seward JB, Khanderia BK, Tajik AJ, eds. *Transesophageal Echocardiography*. Boston: Little, Brown; 1994.
101. Daniel WG, Mügge A. Transesophageal echocardiography. *N Engl J Med* 1995;332:1268–1279.
102. Daniel WG, Mügge A, Martin RP, et al. Improvement in the diagnosis of abscesses associated with endocarditis by transesophageal echocardiography. *N Engl J Med* 1991;324:795–800.
103. Yvorchuk KJ, Chan K-L. Application of transthoracic and transesophageal echocardiography in the diagnosis and management of infective endocarditis. *J Am Soc Echocardiogr* 1994;14:294–308.
104. Mügge A, Daniel WG, Frank G, Lichtlen PR. Echocardiography in infective endocarditis: Reassessment of prognostic implications of vegetation size determined by the transthoracic and the transesophageal approach. *J Am Coll Cardiol* 1989;14:631–638.
105. Yoshida K, Yoshikawa J, Yamaura Y, et al. Assessment of mitral regurgitation by biplane transesophageal color Doppler flow mapping. *Circulation* 1990;82:1121–1126.
106. Klein AL, Obarski TP, Stewart WJ, et al. Transesophageal Doppler echocardiography of pulmonary venous flow: A new marker of mitral regurgitation severity. *J Am Coll Cardiol* 1991;18:518–526.
107. Castello R, Pearson AC, Lenzen P, Labovitz AJ. Effect of mitral regurgitation on pulmonary venous velocities derived from transesophageal echocardiography and color-guided pulsed Doppler imaging. *J Am Coll Cardiol* 1991;17:1499–1605.
108. Smith MD, Harrison MR, Pinton R, et al. Regurgitant jet size by transesophageal compared with transthoracic Doppler color flow imaging. *Circulation* 1991 83:79–86.
109. Hoffmann R, Flachskampf FA, Hanrath P. Planimetry of orifice area in aortic stenosis using multiplane transesophageal echocardiography. *J Am Coll Cardiol* 1993;22:529–534.
110. Keren A, Kim CB, Hu BS, et al. Accuracy of biplane and multiplane transesophageal echocardiography in diagnosis of typical acute aortic dissection and intramural hematoma. *J Am Coll Cardiol* 1996;28: 627–636.
111. Cigarroa JE, Isselbacher EM, DeSanctis RW, Eagle KA. Diagnostic imaging in the evaluation of suspected aortic dissection. *N Engl J Med* 1993;328:35–43.
112. Manning WJ, Weintraub RM, Waksmonski CA, et al. Accuracy of transesophageal echocardiography for identifying left atrial thrombi: A prospective, intraoperative study. *Ann Intern Med* 1995;123: 817–822.
113. Amarenco P, Duyckaerts C, Tzourio C, et al. The prevalence of ulcerated plaques in the aortic arch in patients with stroke. *N Engl J Med* 1992;326:221–225.
114. The French Study of Aortic Plaques in Stroke Group. Atherosclerotic disease of the aortic arch as a risk factor for recurrent ischemic stroke. *N Engl J Med* 1996;334:1216–1221.
115. Dressler FA, Craig WR, Castello R, Labovitz AJ. Mobile aortic atheroma and systemic emboli: Efficacy of anticoagulation and influence of plague morphology on recurrent stroke. *J Am Coll Cardiol* 1998;31:134–138.
116. Van den Brink RBA, Visser CA, Basart DCG, et al. Comparison of transthoracic and transesophageal color Doppler flow imaging in patients with mechanical prostheses in the mitral valve position. *Am J Cardiol* 1989;63:1471–1474.
117. Fyfe DA. Transesophageal echocardiography for congenital heart disease. *J Invas Cardiol* 1992;4;459–467.
118. Fyfe DA, Kline CH. Transesophageal echocardiography for congenital heart disease. *Echocardiography* 1991;8:573–586.
119. Schiller NB. Hand-held echocardiography: Revolution or hassle? *J Am Coll Cardiol* 2001;37:2023–2024.
120. Bruce CJ, Spittell PC, Montgomery SC, et al. Personal ultrasound imager: Abdominal aortic aneurysm screening. *J Am Soc Echocardiogr* 2000;13:674–679.
121. Seward JB, Douglas PS, Erbel R, et al. Hand-carried cardiac ultrasound (HCU) device: Recommendations regarding new technology. A report from the echocardiography task force on new technology of the nomenclature and standards committee of the American Society of Echocardiography. *J Am Soc Echocardiogr* 2002;15:369–373.
122. Kimura BJ, Blanchard DG, Willis CL, DeMaria AN. Limited cardiac ultrasound examination for cost-effective echo referral. *J Am Soc Echocardiogr* 2002;15:640–646.
123. Gramiak R, Shah PM: Echocardiography of the aortic root. *Invest Radiol* 1968;3:356–366.
124. Meltzer RS, Tichner EG, Shaines TP, Popp RL. The source of ultrasonic contrast effect. *J Clin Ultrasound* 1980;8:121–127.
125. Valdes-Cruz LM, Sahn DJ. Seminar on contrast two-dimensional echocardiography: Applications and new developments: Part II. *J Am Coll Cardiol* 1984;3:978–985.
126. DeMaria AN. Echocardiographic visualization of myocardial perfusion by left heart and intracoronary injection of echo contrast agents (abstr). *Circulation* 1980;60(suppl 3):II–143.
127. Kaul S, Jayaween AR, Glasheen WP, et al. Myocardial contrast echocardiography and the transmural distribution of flow: A critical appraisal during myocardial ischemia not associated with infarction. *J Am Coll Cardiol* 1992;20:1005–1016.
128. Crouse LJ, Cheirif J, Hanly DE, et al. Opacification and border delineation improvement in patients with suboptimal endocardial border definition in routine echocardiography: Results of the phase III Albunex multicenter trial. *J Am Coll Cardiol* 1993;22:1494–1500.
129. Ito H, Maruyama A, Iwakura K, et al. Clinical implications of "no reflow" phenomenon: A predictor of complications and left ventricular remodeling in reperfused anterior wall myocardial infarction. *Circulation* 1996;93:223–228.
130. Villanueva FS, Camarano G, Ismail S, et al. Coronary reserve abnormalities in the infarcted myocardium: Assessment of myocardial viability immediately versus late after reflow by contrast echocardiography. *Circulation* 1996;94:748–754.
131. Price RJ, Skyba DM, Kaul S, Skalak TC. Delivery of colloidal particles and red blood cells to tissue through microvessel ruptures created by targeted microbubble destruction with ultrasound. *Circulation* 1998;98:1264–1267.

132. Porter TR, Li S, Kricsfeld D, Armbruster RW. Detection of myocardial perfusion in multiple echocardiographic windows with one intravenous injection of microbubbles using transient response second harmonic imaging. *J Am Coll Cardiol* 1997;29:791–799.
133. vonBibra H, Becher H, Firschke C, et al. Enhancement of mitral regurgitation and normal left atrial color Doppler flow signals with peripheral venous injections of a saccharide-based contrast agent. *J Am Coll Cardiol* 1993;22:521–528.
134. Porter TR, Xie F, Kresfeld A, Kilzer K. Noninvasive identification of acute myocardial ischemia and reperfusion with contrast ultrasound using intravenous perfluoropropane-exposed sonicated dextrose albumin. *J Am Coll Cardiol* 1995;26:33–40.
135. Kaul S, Senior R, Dittrich H, et al. Detection of coronary artery disease with myocardial contrast echocardiography: Comparison with $^{99m}$Tc-sestamibi single-photon emission computed tomography. *Circulation* 1997;96:785–792.
136. Galiuto L, DeMaria AN, May-Newman K, et al. Evaluation of dynamic changes in microvascular flow during ischemia-reperfusion by myocardial contrast echocardiography. *J Am Coll Cardiol* 1998;32: 1096–1101.
137. Mulvagh SL, Foley DA, Aeschbacher BC, et al. Second harmonic imaging of an intravenously administered echocardiographic contrast agent. *J Am Coll Cardiol* 1996;27:1519–1525.
138. Tajik AJ, Seward JB, Hagler DJ, et al. Two-dimensional real-time ultrasonic imaging of the heart and great vessels: Technique, image orientation, structures, identification, and validation. *Mayo Clin Proc* 1978;53:271–303.
139. DeMaria AN, Bommer W, Joye JA, et al. Value and limitations of cross-sectional echocardiography of the aortic valve in the diagnosis and quantification of valvular aortic stenosis. *Circulation* 1980;62: 304–312.
140. Weyman AE, Feigenbaum H, Hurwitz RA. Localization of left ventricular outflow obstruction by cross-sectional echocardiography. *Am J Med* 1976;60:33–38.
141. DeFilippi CR, Willett DL, Brickner ME, et al. Usefulness of dobutamine echocardiography in distinguishing severe from nonsevere valvular aortic stenosis in patients with depressed left ventricular function and low transvalvular gradients. *Am J Cardiol* 1995;75: 191–194.
142. Ciobanu M, Abbasi AS, Allen M, et al. Pulsed Doppler echocardiography in the diagnosis and estimation of severity of aortic insufficiency. *Am J Cardiol* 1982;49:339–343.
143. Grayburn PA, Smith MD, Handshoe R, et al. Detection of aortic insufficiency by standard echocardiography, pulsed Doppler echocardiography and auscultation. *Ann Intern Med* 1986;104:599–605.
144. Perry GJ, Nelmcke F, Nanda NC, et al. Evaluation of aortic insufficiency by Doppler color flow mapping. *J Am Coll Cardiol* 1987;9:952–959.
145. Grayburn PA, Handshoe R, Smith MD, et al. Quantitative assessment of the hemodynamic consequences of aortic regurgitation. *J Am Coll Cardiol* 1987;10:135–141.
146. Omoto R, Yokote Y, Takamoto S, et al. The development of real-time two-dimensional Doppler echocardiography and its clinical significance in acquired valvular disease. *Jpn Heart J* 1984;25:325–340.
147. Touch T, Prasquier R, Nitenberg A, et al. Assessment and follow-up of patients with aortic regurgitation by an updated Doppler echocardiographic measurement of the regurgitant fraction in the aortic arch. *Circulation* 1985;72:819–824.
148. Perlman AS, Otto CM. Quantification of valvular regurgitation. *Echocardiography* 1987;4:271–287.
149. DeMaria AN, Bommer W, Newmann A, et al. Identification and localization of aneurysms of the ascending aorta by cross-sectional echocardiography. *Circulation* 1979;59:755–761.
150. Ballal RS, Nanda NC, Gatewood R, et al. Usefulness of transesophageal echocardiography in assessment of aortic dissection. *Circulation* 1991;84:1903–1914.
151. Nienaber CA, Spielman RP, von Kodolitsch Y, et al. Diagnosis of thoracic aortic dissection: Magnetic resonance imaging versus transesophageal echocardiography. *Circulation* 1992;85:434–447.
152. Sawhney NS, DeMaria AN, Blanchard DG. Aortic intramural hematoma: An increasingly recognized and potentially fatal entity. *Chest* 2001;120:1340–1346.
153. Eisenberg MJ, Geraci SJ, Schiller NB. Screening for abdominal aortic aneurysms during transthoracic echocardiography. *Am Heart J* 1995; 130:109–115.
154. Come PC, Fortuin NJ, White RI Jr, McKusick VA. Echocardiographic assessment of cardiovascular abnormalities in the Marfan syndrome. *Am J Med* 1983;74:465–474.
155. Kiefaber RW, Tabakin BS, Coffin LH, Gibson TC. Unruptured sinus of Valsalva aneurysm with right ventricular outflow obstruction diagnosed by two-dimensional and Doppler echocardiography. *J Am Coll Cardiol* 1986;7:438–442.
156. Rice MJ, Seward JB, Hagler DJ, et al. Definitive diagnosis of truncus arteriosus by two-dimensional echocardiography. *Mayo Clin Proc* 1982;57:476–481.
157. Tunick PA, Kronzon I. Atheromas of the thoracic aorta: Clinical and therapeutic update. *J Am Coll Cardiol* 2000;35:545–554.
158. van der Linden J, Hadjinikolaou L, Bergman P, Lindblom D. Postoperative stroke in cardiac surgery is related to the location and extent of atherosclerotic disease in the ascending aorta. *J Am Coll Cardiol* 2001;38:131–135.
159. Edler I. The diagnostic use of ultrasound in heart disease. *Acta Med Scand* 1955;308:32.
160. Nichol PM, Gilbert BW, Kisslo JA. Two-dimensional echocardiographic assessment of mitral stenosis. *Circulation* 1977;55:120–128.
161. Martin RP, Rakowski H, Kleinman JH, et al. Reliability and reproducibility of two-dimensional echocardiography measurement of the stenotic mitral valve orifice area. *Am J Cardiol* 1979;43:560–568.
162. Hatle L, Angelsen B, Tromsdal A. Noninvasive assessment of atrioventricular pressure half-time by Doppler ultrasound. *Circulation* 1979;60:1096–1104.
163. Libanoff AJ, Rodbard S. Atrioventricular pressure half-time: Measure of mitral valve area. *Circulation* 1968;38:144.
164. Cannon CR, Nishimura RA, Reeder GS, et al. Echocardiographic assessment of commissural calcium: A simple predictor of outcome after percutaneous mitral balloon valvotomy. *J Am Coll Cardiol* 1997;29: 175–180.
165. Manning WJ, Reis GJ, Douglas PS. Use of transesophageal echocardiography to detect left atrial thrombi before percutaneous balloon dilation of the mitral valve: A prospective study. *Br Heart J* 1992;67: 170–173.
166. Roberts WC, Perloff JK. Mitral valvular disease: A clinicopathologic survey of the conditions causing the mitral valve to function abnormally. *Ann Intern Med* 1972;77:939–975.
167. Thomas L, Foster E, Schiller NB. Peak mitral inflow velocity predicts mitral regurgitation severity. *J Am Coll Cardiol* 1998;31:174–179.
168. Rokey R, Sterling LL, Zoghbi WA, et al. Determination of regurgitant fraction in isolated mitral or aortic regurgitation by pulsed Doppler two-dimensional echocardiography. *J Am Coll Cardiol* 1986;7:1273.
169. Spain MG, Smith MD, Grayburn PA, et al. Quantitative assessment of mitral regurgitation by Doppler color flow imaging: Angiographic and hemodynamic correlations. *J Am Coll Cardiol* 1989;13:585.
170. Klein AL, Stewart WJ, Bartlett J, et al. Effects of mitral regurgitation on pulmonary venous flow and left atrial pressure: An intraoperative transesophageal echocardiographic study. *J Am Coll Cardiol* 1992;20: 1345–1352.
171. Vandervoort PM, Rivera JM, Mele D, et al. Application of color Doppler flow mapping to calculate effective regurgitant orifice area: An in vitro study and initial clinical observations. *Circulation* 1993;88: 1150–1156.
172. Yoshida K, Yoshikawa J, Akasaka T, et al. Value of acceleration flow signals proximal to the leaking orifice in assessing the severity of prosthetic mitral valve regurgitation. *J Am Coll Cardiol* 1992;19:333–338.
173. Simpson IA, Shiota T, Gharib M, Sahn DJ. Current status of flow convergence for clinical applications: Is it a leaning tower of "PISA"? *J Am Coll Cardiol* 1996;27:504–509.

174. DeMaria AN, King JF, Bogren HG, et al. The variable spectrum of echocardiographic manifestations of the mitral valve prolapse syndrome. *Circulation* 1974;50:33–41.
175. Levine RA, Triulzi MO, Harrigan P, Weyman AE. The relationship of mitral annular shape to the diagnosis of mitral valve prolapse. *Circulation* 1987;75:756–767.
176. Marwick TH, Stewart WJ, Currie PJ, et al. Mechanisms of failure of mitral valve repair: An echocardiographic study. *Am Heart J* 1991;122: 149–156.
177. Benjamin EJ, Plehn JF, D'Agostino RB, et al. Mitral annular calcification and the risk of stroke in an elderly cohort. *N Engl J Med* 1992; 327:374–379.
178. Fox CS, Vasan RS, Parise H, et al. Mitral annular calcification predicts cardiovascular morbidity and mortality. *Circulation* 2003;107: 1492–1496.
179. Johnson GL, Kwan OL, Handshoe S, et al. Accuracy of combined two-dimensional echocardiography and continuous wave Doppler recordings in the estimation of pressure gradient in right ventricular outlet obstruction. *J Am Coll Cardiol* 1984;3:1013–1018.
180. Waggoner AD, Quinones MA, Young JB, et al. Pulsed Doppler echocardiographic detection of right-side valve regurgitation. *Am J Cardiol* 1981;47:279–286.
181. Lee RT, Lord CP, Plappert T, Sutton MS. Prospective Doppler echocardiographic evaluation of pulmonary artery diastolic pressure in the medical intensive care unit. *Am J Cardiol* 1989;64:1366–1370.
182. Parris TM, Panidis IP, Ross J, Mintz GS. Doppler echocardiographic findings in rheumatic tricuspid stenosis. *Am J Cardiol* 1987;60: 1414–1416.
183. Curtius MM, Thyssen M, Breuer HWM, Loogen F. Doppler versus contrast echocardiography for diagnosis of tricuspid regurgitation. *Am J Cardiol* 1985;56:333–336.
184. Pennestri F, Loperfido F, Salvatori MP, et al. Assessment of tricuspid regurgitation by pulsed Doppler ultrasonography of the hepatic veins. *Am J Cardiol* 1984;54:363–368.
185. Baker BJ, Scovil JA, Kane JJ, Murphy MG. Echocardiographic detection of right ventricular hypertrophy. *Am Heart J* 1983;105:611–614.
186. Ryan T, Petrovic O, Dillon J, et al. An echocardiographic index for separation of right ventricular volume and pressure overload. *J Am Coll Cardiol* 1985;5:918–924.
187. Weyman AE, Dillon JC, Feigenbaum H, Chang S. Echocardiographic patterns of pulmonary valve motion with pulmonary hypertension. *Circulation* 1974;50:905–910.
188. Tahara M, Tanaka H, Nakao S, et al. Hemodynamic determinants of pulmonary valve motion during systole in experimental pulmonary hypertension. *Circulation* 1981;64:1249–1256.
189. Mahmud E, Raisinghani A, Hassankhani A, et al. Correlation of left ventricular diastolic filling characteristics with right ventricular overload and pulmonary artery pressure in chronic thromboembolic pulmonary hypertension. *J Am Coll Cardiol* 2002;40:318–324.
190. Come PC, Riley MF. Echocardiographic recognition of perivalvular infection complicating aortic bacterial endocarditis. *Am Heart J* 1984; 108:166–168.
191. Williams GA, Labovitz AJ. Doppler hemodynamic evaluation of prosthetic (Starr-Edwards and Bjork-Shiley) and bioprosthetic (Hancock and Carpentier-Edwards) cardiac valves. *Am J Cardiol* 1985;56:325–332.
192. Flachskampf FA, O'Shea JP, Griffin BP, et al. Patterns of normal transvalvular regurgitation in mechanical valve prostheses. *J Am Coll Cardiol* 1991;18:1493–1498.
193. Burstow DJ, Nishimura RA, Bailey KR, et al. Continuous wave Doppler echocardiographic measurement of prosthetic valve gradients: A simultaneous Doppler-catheter correlative study. *Circulation* 1980;8:504–514.
194. Voelker W, Reul J, Stelzer T, et al. Pressure recovery in aortic stenosis: An in vitro study in a pulsatile flow model. *J Am Coll Cardiol* 1992; 20:1585–1593.
195. Dittrich HC, McCann HA, Walsh T, et al. Transesophageal echocardiography in the evaluation of prosthetic and native aortic valves. *Am J Cardiol* 1990;66:758–761.
196. Freedberg RS, Goodkin GM, Perez JL, et al. Valve strands are strongly associated with systemic embolization: A transesophageal echocardiographic study. *J Am Coll Cardiol* 1995;26:1709–1712.
197. Hurrell DG, Schaff HV, Tajik AJ. Thrombolytic therapy for obstruction of mechanical prosthetic valves. *Mayo Clin Proc* 1996;71:605–613.
198. Wann LS, Dillon JC, Weyman AE, Feigenbaum H. Echocardiography in bacterial endocarditis. *N Engl J Med* 1976;295:135–139.
199. Gilbert BW, Haney RS, Crawford F, et al. Two-dimensional echocardiographic assessment of vegetative endocarditis. *Circulation* 1977; 55:346–353.
200. Habib G, Derumeaux G, Avierinos JF, et al. Value and limitations of the Duke criteria for the diagnosis of infective endocarditis. *J Am Coll Cardiol* 1999;33:2023–2029.
201. von Reyn CF, Arbeit RD. Case definitions for infective endocarditis. *Am J Med* 1994;96:220–222.
202. Roldan CA, Shively BK, Crawford MH. An echocardiographic study of valvular heart disease associated with systemic lupus erythematosus. *N Engl J Med* 1996;335:1424–1430.
203. Stewart JS, Silimpert D, Harris P, et al. Echocardiographic documentation of vegetative lesions in infective endocarditis: Clinical implications. *Circulation* 1980;61:374–380.
204. San Roman JA, Vilacosta I, Sarria C, et al. Eustachian valve endocarditis: Is it worth searching for? *Am Heart J* 2001;142:1037–1040.
205. Sawhney N, Palakodeti V, Raisinghani A, et al. Eustachian valve endocarditis: A case series and analysis of the literature. *J Am Soc Echocardiogr* 2001;14:1139–1142.
206. Steckelberg JM, Murphy JG, Ballard D, et al. Emboli in infective endocarditis: The prognostic value of echocardiography. *Ann Intern Med* 1991;114:635–640.
207. Birmingham GD, Rahko PS, Ballantyne F. Improved detection of infective endocarditis with transesophageal echocardiography. *Am Heart J* 1992;123:774–781.
208. Di Salvo G, Habib G, Pergola V, et al. Echocardiography predicts embolic events in infective endocarditis. *J Am Coll Cardiol* 2001;37:1069–1076.
209. Lindner JR, Case RA, Dent JM, et al. Diagnostic value of echocardiography in suspected endocarditis: An evaluation based on pretest probability of disease. *Circulation* 1996;93:730–736.
210. Raisinghani A, Ohmori K, Cotter B, et al. Does flow reversal within intramyocardial coronary vessels occur systole? Detection of biphasic flow in intramyocardial vessels by transthoracic echo (abstr). *J Am Coll Cardiol* 1997;29:365A.
211. Kerber R, Abboud F. Echocardiographic detection of regional myocardial infarction. *Circulation* 1973;47:997.
212. Franklin TD Jr, Cuddeback JK, Sanghn NT, et al. Differentiation of A-mode ultrasound signals from normal and ischemic myocardium by multivariate discriminant analysis of waveform parameters. (abstr). *Am J Cardiol* 1980;45:403.
213. Bourdillon PDV, Broderick TM, Sawada SG, et al. Regional wall motion index for infarct and noninfarct regions after reperfusion in acute myocardial infarction: Comparison with global wall motion index. *J Am Soc Echocardiogr* 1989;2:398–407.
214. Nishimura RA, Tajik AJ, Shub C, et al. Role of two-dimensional echocardiography in the prediction of in-hospital complications after acute myocardial infarction. *J Am Coll Cardiol* 1984;4:1080–1087.
215. Segar DS, Brown SC, Sawada SG, et al. Dobutamine stress echocardiography: Correlation with coronary lesions severity as determined by quantitative angiography. *J Am Coll Cardiol* 1992;19:1197–1202.
216. Corya BC, Feigenbaum H, Rasmussen S, Black MJ. Echocardiographic features of congestive cardiomyopathy compared with normal subjects and patients with coronary artery disease. *Circulation* 1974; 49:1153–1159.
217. Weiss JL, Buckley BH, Hutchins GM, Mason SJ. Two-dimensional echocardiographic recognition of myocardial injury in man: Comparison with postmortem studies. *Circulation* 1981;63:401–408.
218. Sabia P, Abbott RD, Afrookteh A, et al. Importance of two-dimensional echocardiographic assessment of left ventricular systolic function in patients presenting to the emergency room with cardiac-related symptoms. *Circulation* 1991;84:1615–1624.

219. Eaton L, Weiss JL, Bulkley BH, et al. Regional cardiac dilatation after acute myocardial infarction. *N Engl J Med* 1979;300:57–62.
220. Matsumoto M, Watanabe F, Gotto A, et al. Left ventricular aneurysm and the prediction of left ventricular enlargement studied by two-dimensional echocardiography: Quantitative assessment of aneurysm size in relation to clinical course. *Circulation* 1985;72:280–286.
221. Catherwood E, Mintz GS, Kotler MN, Two-dimensional echocardiographic recognition of left ventricular pseudoaneurysm. *Circulation* 1980;62:294–303.
222. Roelandt J, Sutherland GR, Yoshida K, Yoshikawa J. Improved diagnosis and characterization of left ventricular pseudoaneurysm by Doppler color imaging. *J Am Coll Cardiol* 1988;12:807–811.
223. Helmcke F, Mahan EF, Nanda NC, et al. Two-dimensional echocardiography and Doppler color flow mapping in the diagnosis and prognosis of ventricular septal rupture. *Circulation* 1990;81:1775–1783.
224. Kono T, Sabbah HN, Rosman H, et al. Mechanism of functional mitral regurgitation during acute myocardial infarction. *J Am Coll Cardiol* 1992;9:1101–1105.
225. Stoddard MF, Keedy DL, Kupersmith J. Transesophageal echocardiographic diagnosis of papillary muscle rupture complicating acute myocardial infarction. *Am Heart J* 1990;120:690–692.
226. Otto CM, Stratton JR, Maynard C, et al. Echocardiographic evaluation of segmental wall motion early and late after thrombolytic therapy in acute myocardial infarction: The Western Washington tissue plasminogen activator emergency room trial. *Am J Cardiol* 1990;65:132–138.
227. Porter TR, Li S, Oster R, Deligonul U. The clinical implications of no reflow demonstrated with intravenous perfluorocarbon containing microbubbles following restoration of Thrombolysis in Myocardial Infarction (TIMI) 3 flow in patients with acute myocardial infarction. *Am J Cardiol* 1998;82:1173–1177.
228. Marwick T, Nemec J, Pashkow F, et al. Accuracy and limitations of exercise echocardiography in a routine clinical setting. *J Am Coll Cardiol* 1992;19:74–81.
229. Quinones MA, Verani MS, Haichin RM, et al. Exercise echocardiography versus T1–201 single photon emission computerized tomography in evaluation of coronary artery disease: Analysis of 292 patients. *Circulation* 1992;85:1026–1031.
230. Roger VL, Pellikka PA, Oh JK, et al. Identification of multivessel coronary artery disease by exercise echocardiography. *J Am Coll Cardiol* 1994;24:109–114.
231. Ryan T, Segar DS, Sawada SG, et al. Detection of coronary artery disease with upright bicycle exercise echocardiography. *J Am Soc Echocardiogr* 1993;6:186–197.
232. Geleijnse ML, Floretti PM, Roelandt J. Methodology, feasibility, safety and diagnostic accuracy of dobutamine stress echocardiography. *J Am Coll Cardiol* 1997;30:595–606.
233. Cornel JH, Bax JJ, Elhendy A, et al. Diphasic response to dobutamine predicts improvement of global left ventricular function after surgical revascularization in patients with stable coronary artery disease. *J Am Coll Cardiol* 1998;31:1002–1010.
234. Afridi I, Grayburn PA, Panza JA, et al. Myocardial viability during dobutamine echocardiography predicts survival in patients with coronary artery disease and severe left ventricular systolic dysfunction. *J Am Coll Cardiol* 1998;32:921–926.
235. Bax JJ, Wijns W, Cornel JH, et al. Accuracy of currently available techniques for prediction of functional recovery after revascularization in patients with left ventricular dysfunction due to chronic coronary artery disease: Comparison of pooled data. *J Am Coll Cardiol* 1997;30:1451–1460.
236. Bach DS, Muller D, Gros BJ, Armstrong WF. False positive dobutamine stress echocardiograms: Characterization of clinical, echocardiographic, and angiographic findings. *J Am Coll Cardiol* 1994;24:928–933.
237. Anthopoulos LP, Bonou MS, Kardaras FG, et al. Stress echocardiography in elderly patients with coronary artery disease. *J Am Coll Cardiol* 1996;28:52–59.
238. Pellikka PA, Oh JK, Bailey KR, et al. Dynamic intraventricular obstruction during dobutamine stress echocardiography: A new observation. *Circulation* 1992;86:1429–1432.
239. Marwick T, Wilemart B, D'Hondt AM, et al. Selection of the optimal non-exercise stress for the evaluation of ischemic regional myocardial dysfunction and malperfusion: Comparison of dobutamine and adenosine using echocardiography and Tc-99m MIBI single photon emission computerized tomography. *Circulation* 1993;87:345–354.
240. Sawada SG, Ryan T, Feinberg NS, et al. Exercise echocardiographic identification of coronary artery disease in women. *J Am Coll Cardiol* 1989;14:1440–1447.
241. Heupler S, Mehta R, Lobo A, et al. Prognostic implications of exercise echocardiography in women with known or suspected coronary artery disease. *J Am Coll Cardiol* 1997;30:414–420.
242. Spes CH, Mudra H, Schnaak SD, et al. Dobutamine stress echocardiography for noninvasive diagnosis of cardiac allograft vasculopathy: A comparison with angiography and intravascular ultrasound. *Am J Cardiol* 1996;78:168–174.
243. Kafka H, Leach AJ, Fitzgibbon GM. Exercise echocardiography after coronary artery bypass surgery: Correlation with coronary angiography. *J Am Coll Cardiol* 1995;25:1019–1023.
244. Das MK, Pellikka PA, Mahoney DW, et al. Assessment of cardiac risk before nonvascular surgery: Dobutamine stress echocardiography in 530 patients. *J Am Coll Cardiol* 2000;35:1647–1653.
245. Pingitore A, Picano E, Varga A, et al. Prognostic value of pharmacological stress echocardiography in patients with known or suspected coronary artery disease. *J Am Coll Cardiol* 1999;34:1769–1777.
246. Bax JJ, Poldermans D, Elhendy A, et al. Improvement of left ventricular ejection fraction, heart failure symptoms and prognosis after revascularization in patients with chronic coronary artery disease and viable myocardium detected by dobutamine stress echocardiography. *J Am Coll Cardiol* 1999;34163–34169.
247. Senior R, Kaul S, Lahiri A. Myocardial viability on echocardiography predicts long-term survival after revascularization in patients with ischemic congestive heart failure. *J Am Coll Cardiol* 1999;33:1848–1854.
248. deFilippi CR, Willett DL, Brickner ME, et al. Usefulness of dobutamine echocardiography in distinguishing severe from nonsevere valvular aortic stenosis in patients with depressed left ventricular function and low transvalvular gradients. *Am J Cardiol* 1995;75:191–194.
249. Rihal CS, Nishimura RA, Hatle LK, et al. Systolic and diastolic dysfunction in patients with clinical diagnosis of dilated cardiomyopathy: Relation to symptoms and prognosis. *Circulation* 1994;90:2772–2779.
250. Siegel RJ, Shah PK, Fishbein MC. Idiopathic restrictive cardiomyopathy. *Circulation* 1984;70:165–169.
251. Watkins H, McKenna WJ, Thierfelder L, et al. Mutations in the genes for cardiac troponin T and atropomyosin in hypertrophic cardiomyopathy. *N Engl J Med* 1995;332:1058–1064.
252. Louie EK, Maron BJ. Apical hypertrophic cardiomyopathy: Clinical and two-dimensional echocardiographic assessment. *Ann Intern Med* 1987;106:663–670.
253. Henry WL, Clark CE, Epstein SE. Asymmetric septal hypertrophy (ASH): Echocardiographic identification of the pathognomonic anatomic abnormality of IHSS. *Circulation* 1973;47:225–233.
254. Maron BJ, Epstein SE. Hypertrophic cardiomyopathy: Recent observations regarding the specificity of three hallmarks of the disease: Asymmetric septal hypertrophy, septal disorganization and systolic anterior motion of the anterior mitral leaflet. *Am J Cardiol* 1980;45:141.
255. Blanchard DG, Ross J Jr. Hypertrophic cardiomyopathy: Prognosis with medical or surgical therapy. *Clin Cardiol* 1991;14:11–19.
256. Jiang L, Levine RA, King ME, Weyman AE. An integrated mechanism for systolic anterior motion of the mitral valve in hypertrophic cardiomyopathy based on echocardiographic observations. *Am Heart J* 1987;113:633–644.
257. Gilbert BW, Pollick C, Adelman AG, Wigle ED. Hypertrophic cardiomyopathy: Subclassification by M mode echocardiography. *Am J Cardiol* 1980;45:861–872.
258. Baumgartner H, Schima H, Tulzer G, Kühn P. Effect of stenosis geometry on the Doppler-catheter gradient relation in vitro: A manifestation of pressure recovery. *J Am Coll Cardiol* 1993;21:1018–1025.

259. Spirito P, Maron BJ. Relation between extent of left ventricular hypertrophy and diastolic filling abnormalities in hypertrophic cardiomyopathy. *J Am Coll Cardiol* 1990;15:808–813.
260. Keren A, Popp RL. Assignment of patients into the classification of cardiomyopathies. *Circulation* 1992;86:1622–1633.
261. Lewis JF, Webber JD, Sutton LL, et al. Discordance in degree of right and left ventricular dilation in patients with dilated cardiomyopathy: Recognition and clinical implications. *J Am Coll Cardiol* 1993;21: 640–654.
262. Frishman WH, Sung HM, Yee HCM, et al. Cardiovascular toxicity with cancer chemotherapy. *Curr Probl Cardiol* 1996;21:225–288.
263. Nishimura RA, Appleton CP, Redfield MM, et al. Noninvasive Doppler echocardiographic evaluation of left ventricular filling pressures in patients with cardiomyopathies: A simultaneous Doppler echocardiographic and cardiac catheterization study. *J Am Coll Cardiol* 1996;28:1226–1233.
264. Acquatella H, Schiller NB, Puigbo JJ, et al. Value of two dimensional echocardiography in endomyocardial disease with and without eosinophilia. *Circulation* 1983;67:1219–1226.
265. Klein AL, Cohen GI. Doppler echocardiographic assessment of constrictive pericarditis, cardiac amyloidosis, and cardiac tamponade. *Cleve Clin J Med* 1992;59:278–290.
266. Klein AL, Hatle LK, Taliercio CP, et al. Serial Doppler echocardiographic follow-up of left ventricular diastolic function in cardiac amyloidosis. *J Am Coll Cardiol* 1990;16:1135–1141.
267. Klein AL, Hatle LK, Taliercio CP, et al. Prognostic significance of Doppler measures of diastolic function in cardiac amyloidosis. *Circulation* 1991;83:808–816.
268. Lipschulz SE, Sanders SP, Mayer JE, et al. Are routine preoperative cardiac catheterization and angiography necessary before repair of ostium primum atrial septal defect? *J Am Coll Cardiol* 1988;11: 373–378.
269. Shub C, Dimopoulos IN, Seward JB, et al. Sensitivity of two-dimensional echocardiography in the direct visualization of atrial septal defect utilizing the subcostal approach: Experience with 154 patients. *J Am Coll Cardiol* 1983;2:127–135.
270. Hagler DJ, Tajik AJ, Seward JB, et al. Real-time wide-angle sector echocardiography: Atrioventricular canal defects. *Circulation* 1979; 59:140–150.
271. Franker TD, Harris PJ, Behar VS, Kisslo JA. Detection and exclusion of interatrial shunts by two-dimensional echocardiography and peripheral venous injections. *Circulation* 1979;59:379–384.
272. Pollick C, Sullivan H, Cujec B, Wilansky S. Doppler color-flow imaging assessment of shunt size in atrial septal defect. *Circulation* 1988; 78:522–528.
273. Dittman H, Jacksch R, Voelker W, et al. Accuracy of Doppler echocardiography in quantification of left to right shunts in adult patients with atrial septal defect. *J Am Coll Cardiol* 1988;11:338–342.
274. Linker DT, Rossvoll O, Chapman JV, Angelsen B. Sensitivity and speed of color Doppler flow mapping compared with continuous wave Doppler for the detection of ventricular septal defects. *Br Heart J* 1991;65:201–203.
275. Schmidt KG, Cassidy SC, Silverman NH, Stanger P. Doubly committed subarterial ventricular septal defects: Echocardiographic features and surgical implications. *J Am Coll Cardiol* 1988;12:1538–1546.
276. Liao P-K, Su W-J, Hung J-S. Doppler echocardiographic flow characteristics of isolated patent ductus arteriosus: Better delineation by Doppler color flow mapping. *J Am Coll Cardiol* 1988;12:1285–1291.
277. Balaji S, Burch M, Sullivan ED. Accuracy of cross-sectional echocardiography in diagnosis of aortopulmonary window. *Am J Cardiol* 1991;67:650–653.
278. Gao Y-A, Burrows PE, Benson LN, et al. Scimitar syndrome in infancy. *J Am Coll Cardiol* 1993;22:873–882.
279. Smallhorn JF, Burrows P, Wilson G, et al. Two-dimensional and pulsed Doppler echocardiography in the postoperative evaluation of total anomalous pulmonary venous connection. *Circulation* 1987;76:289–305.
280. Lengyel M, Arvay A, Biro V. Two-dimensional echocardiographic diagnosis of cor triatriatum. *Am J Cardiol* 1987;59:484–485.
281. Flanagan MF, Foran RB, VanPraagh R, et al. Tetralogy of Fallot with obstruction of the ventricular septal defect: Spectrum of echocardiographic findings. *J Am Coll Cardiol* 1988;11:386–395.
282. Geva T, Ayres NA, Pac FA, Pignatelli R. Quantitative morphometric analysis of progressive infundibular obstruction in tetralogy of Fallot: A prospective longitudinal echocardiographic study. *Circulation* 1995; 9:886–892.
283. Bricker JT. Sudden death and tetralogy of Fallot: Risks, markers, and causes. *Circulation* 1995;92:158–159.
284. Roberson DA, Silverman NH. Malaligned outlet septum with subpulmonary ventricular septal defect and abnormal ventriculoarterial connection: A morphologic spectrum defined echocardiographically. *J Am Coll Cardiol* 1990;16:459–468.
285. Daskalopoulos DA, Edwards WD, Driscoll DJ, et al. Correlation of two-dimensional echocardiographic and autopsy findings in complete transposition of the great arteries. *J Am Coll Cardiol* 1983;3:1151–1157.
286. Smallhorn J, Grow R, Freedom R, et al. Pulsed Doppler echocardiographic assessment of the pulmonary venous pathway after the Mustard or Senning procedure for transposition of the great arteries. *Circulation* 1986;73:765–774.
287. Marin-Garcia J, Tonkin ILD. Two-dimensional echocardiographic evaluation of persistent truncus arteriosus. *Am J Cardiol* 1982;50: 1376–1379.
288. Simpson IA, Sahn DJ, Valdes-Cruz LM, et al. Color Doppler flow mapping in patients with coarctation of the aorta: New observations and improved evaluation with color flow diameter and proximal acceleration as predictors of severity. *Circulation* 1988;77:736–744.
289. Shaddy RE, Snider AR, Silverman NH, Lutin W. Pulsed Doppler findings in patients with coarctation of the aorta. *Circulation* 1986;73:82–88.
290. Nihoyannopoulos P, Karas S, Sapsford RN, et al. Accuracy of two-dimensional echocardiography in the diagnosis of aortic arch obstruction. *J Am Coll Cardiol* 1987;10:1072–1077.
291. Johnson GL, Kwan OL, Handshoe S, et al. Accuracy of combined two-dimensional echocardiography and continuous wave Doppler recordings in the estimation of pressure gradient in right ventricular outlet obstruction. *J Am Coll Cardiol* 1984;3:1013–1018.
292. Valdes-Cruz LM, Jones M, Scagnelli S, et al. Prediction of gradients in fibrous subaortic stenosis by continuous wave two-dimensional Doppler echocardiography: Animal studies. *J Am Coll Cardiol* 1985;5: 1363–1367.
293. Zielinsky P, Rossi M, Haertel JC, et al. Subaortic fibrous ridge and ventricular septal defect: Role of septal malalignment. *Circulation* 1987;75:1124–1129.
294. Shiina A, Seward JB, Edwards WD, et al. Two-dimensional echocardiographic spectrum of Ebstein's anomaly: Detailed anatomic assessment. *J Am Coll Cardiol* 1984;3:356–370.
295. Copel JA, Pilu G, Green J, et al. Fetal echocardiographic screening for congenital heart disease: The importance of the four-chamber view. *Am J Obstet Gynecol* 1987;157:648–655.
296. Sharland GK, Chita SK, Allan LD. The use of color Doppler in fetal echocardiography. *Int J Cardiol* 1990;28:229–236.
297. Buskens E, Grobbee DE, Frohn-Mulder IME, et al. Efficacy of routine fetal ultrasound screening for congenital heart disease in normal pregnancy. *Circulation* 1996;94:67–72.
298. Chang AC, Huhta JC, Yoon GY, et al. Diagnosis, transport, and outcome in fetuses with left ventricular outflow tract obstruction. *J Thorac Cardiovasc Surg* 1991;102:841–848.
299. Hicks KA, Kovack JA, Frishberg DP, et al. Echocardiographic evaluation of papillary fibroelastoma: A case report and review of the literature. *J Am Soc Echocardiogr* 1996;9:353–360.
300. DeMaria AN, Bommer W, Neumann A, et al. Left ventricular thrombi identified by cross-sectional echocardiography. *Ann Intern Med* 1979; 90:14–18.
301. Limacher M, Gutgesell HP, Vick GW, et al. Echocardiographic anatomy of the eustachian valve. *Am J Cardiol* 1986;57:363–365.
302. Georgeson R, Liu M, Bansal RC. Transesophageal echocardiographic diagnosis of eustachian valve endocarditis. *J Am Soc Echocardiogr* 1996;9:206–208.

303. Werner JA, Cheitlin MD, Gross BW, et al. Echocardiographic appearance of the Chiari network: Differentiation from right-heart pathology. *Circulation* 1981;63:1104–1109.
304. Keren A, Billingham ME, Popp RL. Echocardiographic recognition and implications of ventricular hypertrophic trabeculations and aberrant bands. *Circulation* 1984;70:836–842.
305. Vered Z, Melzer RS, Benjamin P, et al. Prevalence and significance of false tendons in the left ventricle as determined by echocardiography. *Am J Cardiol* 1984;53:330–332.
306. French JW, Popp RL, Pitlick PT. Cardiac localization of transvascular biotome using two-dimensional echocardiography. *Am J Cardiol* 1983;51:219–223.
307. Pearson AC, Nagelhout D, Castello R, et al. Atrial septal aneurysm and stroke: A transesophageal echocardiographic study. *J Am Coll Cardiol* 1991;18:1223–1229.
308. Fyke III FE, Tajik AJ, Edwards WD, Seward JB. Diagnosis of lipomatous hypertrophy of the interatrial septum by two-dimensional echocardiography. *J Am Coll Cardiol* 1983;1:1352–1357.
309. Haugland JM, Asinger RW, Mikell FL, et al. Embolic potential of left ventricular thrombi detection by two-dimensional echocardiography. *Circulation* 1984;70:588–598.
310. Aschenberg W, Schluter M, Kremer P, et al. Transesophageal two-dimensional echocardiography for the detection of left atrial appendage thrombus. *J Am Coll Cardiol* 1986;7:163–166.
311. Klein AL, Stewart WC, Cosgrove DM III, et al. Visualization of acute pulmonary emboli by transesophageal echocardiography. *J Am Soc Echocardiogr* 1990;3:412–415.
312. Feltes TF, Friedman RA. Transesophageal echocardiographic detection of atrial thombi in patients with nonfibrillation atrial tachyarrhythmias and congenital heart disease. *J Am Coll Cardiol* 1994;24:1365–1370.
313. Galzerano D, Tucillo B, Lama D, et al. Does multilobularity of left atrial appendage represent an additional risk for thrombus formation in atrial fibrillation? (abstr). *J Am Coll Cardiol* 1997;29:212A.
314. Daniel WG, Nellessen U, Schroder E, et al. Left atrial spontaneous echo contrast in mitral valve disease: An indicator for an increased thromboembolic risk. *J Am Coll Cardiol* 1988;11:1204–1211.
315. Peverill RE, Harper RW, Gelman J, et al. Determinants of increased regional left atrial coagulation activity in patients with mitral stenosis. *Circulation* 1996;94:331–339.
316. Asinger RW, Mikell FL, Elsperger J, Hodges M. Incidence of left ventricular thrombosis after acute transmural myocardial infarction: Serial evaluation by two-dimensional echocardiography. *N Engl J Med* 1981;305:297–302.
317. Reynen K. Cardiac myxomas. *N Engl J Med* 1995;1610–1617.
318. Goli VD, Thadani U, Thomas SR, et al. Doppler echocardiographic profiles in obstructive right and left atrial myxomas. *J Am Coll Cardiol* 1987;9:701–703.
319. Topol EJ, Biern RO, Reitz BA. Cardiac papillary fibroelastoma and stroke. *Am J Med* 1986;80:129–132.
320. Hui KS, Green LK, Schmidt WA. Primary cardiac rhabdomyosarcoma: Definition of a rare entity. *Am J Cardiovasc Pathol* 1988;2:19–29.
321. Hanfling SM. Metastatic cancer to the heart. *Circulation* 1960;22:474.
322. Limacher MC, McEntee CW, Attart M, et al. Cardiac echinococcal cyst: Diagnosis by two dimensional echocardiography. *J Am Coll Cardiol* 1983;2:574–577.
323. McAllister HA Jr. Primary tumors and cysts of the heart and pericardium. *Curr Probl Cardiol* 1979;4:1–51.
324. Ling LH, OH JK, Tei C, et al. Pericardial thickness measured with transesophageal echocardiography: Feasibility and potential clinical usefulness. *J Am Coll Cardiol* 1997;29:1317–1323.
325. Hatle LK, Appleton CP, Popp RL. Differentiation of constrictive pericarditis and restrictive cardiomyopathy by Doppler echocardiography. *Circulation* 1989;79:357–370.
326. Horowitz MS, Schultz CS, Stinson EB. Sensitivity and specificity of echocardiographic diagnosis of pericardial effusion. *Circulation* 1974; 50:239–247.
327. Haaz WS, Mintz GS, Kotler MN, et al. Two dimensional echocardiographic recognition of the descending thoracic aorta: Value in differentiating pericardial from pleural effusion. *Am J Cardiol* 1980;46:739–743.
328. Isner JM, Carter BL, Roberts WC, Bankoff MS. Subepicardial adipose tissue producing echocardiographic appearance of pericardial effusion. *Am J Cardiol* 1983;51:565–569.
329. Schiller NB, Botvinick EH. Right ventricular compression as a sign of cardiac tamponade: An analysis of echocardiographic ventricular dimensions and their clinical implications. *Circulation* 1977;56:774–779.
330. Gillam LD, Guyer DE, Gibson TC, et al. Hydrodynamic compression of the right atrium: A new echocardiographic sign of cardiac tamponade. *Circulation* 1983;68:294–301.
331. Brodyn NE, Rose MR, Prior FP, Haft JI. Left atrial diastolic compression in a patient with a large pericardial effusion and pulmonary hypertension. *Am J Med* 1990;88:1–8.
332. Pandian NG, Skorton DJ, Kieso RA, Kerber RE. Diagnosis of constrictive pericarditis by two-dimensional echocardiography: Studies in a new experimental model and in patients. *J Am Coll Cardiol* 1984;4: 1164–1173.
333. Himelman RB, Lee S, Schiller NB. Septal bounce, vena cava plethora, and pericardial adhesion: Informative two-dimensional echocardiographic signs in the diagnosis of pericardial constriction. *J Am Soc Echocardiogr* 1988;1:333–340.
334. Oh JK, Tajik AJ, Appleton CP, et al. Preload reduction to unmask the characteristic Doppler features of constrictive pericarditis: A new observation. *Circulation* 1997;95:796–799.
335. Boonyaratavej S, Oh JK, Tajik AJ, et al. Comparison of mitral inflow and superior vena cava Doppler velocities in chronic obstructive pulmonary disease and constrictive pericarditis. *J Am Coll Cardiol* 1998; 32:2043–2048.
336. Klodas E, Nishimura RA, Appleton CP, et al. Doppler evaluation of patients with constrictive pericarditis: Use of tricuspid regurgitation velocity curves to determine enhanced ventricular interaction. *J Am Coll Cardiol* 1996;28:652–657.
337. Capannari TE, Daniels SR, Meyer RA, et al. Sensitivity, specificity, and predictive value of two-dimensional echocardiography in detecting coronary artery aneurysms in patients with Kawasaki disease. *J Am Coll Cardiol* 1986;7:355–360.
338. Redberg RF, Sobol Y, Chou TM, et al. Adenosine-induced coronary vasodilatation during transesophageal Doppler echocardiography: Rapid and safe measurement of coronary flow reserve ratio can predict significant left anterior descending coronary stenosis. *Circulation* 1995; 92:190–196.

CHAPTER 16

# ECG EXERCISE TESTING

Gregory Engel / Victor F. Froelicher



The number of exercise tests performed is increasing and the exercise test, alone and in combination with other modalities, remains an important testing method because of its high yield of diagnostic, prognostic, and functional information. The electrocardiographic (ECG) component remains critical not only for diagnosis and prognosis but also for arrhythmia assessment, safety, heart rate measurement, and as a reference point for processing ancillary technologies. Exercise test scores combining clinical and exercise data have been developed using multivariable statistical techniques and have significantly improved the diagnostic and prognostic power of the test. These enhancements have extended the utility of the exercise ECG to women, the elderly, and those on beta blockers or not reaching target heart rate.

This chapter reviews the general protocol for performing and evaluating an exercise test with an emphasis on the use of scores and heart rate to enhance the standard exercise ECG test. Indications for exercise testing are also discussed.

## METHODS OF EXERCISE TESTING

Updated guidelines are available from the American Heart Association and the American College of Cardiology (AHA/ACC) that are based on a multitude of research studies over the last 20 years and have led to greater uniformity in methods.[1,2,2a] These guidelines now form the basis for competency evaluation, appropriate clinical use of exercise testing, reimbursement, and malpractice concerns.

### Safety Precautions and Equipment

The safety precautions outlined in the guidelines are very explicit with regard to the requirements for exercise testing. Perhaps due to an expanded knowledge concerning indications, contraindications, and endpoints, maximal exercise testing appears safer today[3] (0.8 untoward events per 10,000 tests) than it did 20 years ago.[4] It has been shown that even in patients who develop ischemia during exercise testing, serum elevations in cardiac-specific troponins do not occur, demonstrating that myocardial damage does not occur.[5,6]

Besides emergency equipment, the safety and accuracy of the testing equipment should be considered. The treadmill should have front and side rails to help subjects steady themselves. It should be calibrated monthly. Some models can be greatly affected by the weight of the subject and will not deliver the appropriate workload to heavy individuals.

Although numerous clever devices have been developed to automate blood pressure measurement during exercise, none can be recommended except those that allow audible monitoring of the Korotkoff sounds and operator validation. The time-proven method of holding the subject's arm with a stethoscope placed over the brachial artery remains most reliable. The subject's arm should be free of the handrails so that noise is not transmitted up the arm.

### Pretest Preparations

When the test is scheduled, the patient should be instructed not to eat, drink, or smoke at least 2 h prior to the test and to come dressed for exercise, including proper footwear.

During the pretest evaluation, the patient's usual level of exercise activity should be established.[7] The response to signs or symptoms should be moderated by the information the patient gives regarding his or her usual activity. If abnormal findings occur at levels of exercise that the patient usually performs, it may not be necessary to stop the test because of them. Also, the patient's activity history should help determine the appropriate target workload for testing.

The physician should also review the patient's medical history, making note of any conditions that may increase the risk of testing. Table 16-1 lists the absolute and relative contraindications to exercise

TABLE 16-1 Contraindications to Exercise Testing

| Absolute |
|---|
| Acute myocardial infarction (within 2 days) |
| High-risk unstable angina |
| Uncontrolled cardiac arrhythmias causing symptoms or hemodynamic compromise |
| Symptomatic severe aortic stenosis |
| Uncontrolled symptomatic heart failure |
| Acute pulmonary embolus or pulmonary infarction |
| Acute myocarditis or pericarditis |
| Acute aortic dissection |
| **Relative[a]** |
| Left main coronary stenosis |
| Moderate stenotic valvular heart disease |
| Electrolyte abnormalities |
| Severe arterial hypertension[b] |
| Tachyarrhythmias or bradyarrhythmias |
| Hypertrophic cardiomyopathy and other forms of outflow tract obstruction |
| Mental or physical impairment leading to inability to exercise adequately |
| High-degree atrioventricular block |

[a]Relative contraindications can be superseded if the benefits of exercise outweigh the risks.
[b]In the absence of definitive evidence, the committee suggests systolic blood pressure of >200 mmHg and/or diastolic blood pressure of >110 mmHg.
SOURCE: Modified from Gibbons RJ, Balady GJ, Bricker JT, et al. ACC/AHA 2002 guideline update for exercise testing. *Circulation* 2002;106:1883–1892.

testing. The patient should be specifically questioned in appropriate areas. Testing patients with aortic stenosis should be done with great care because they may develop severe cardiovascular complications (see Chap. 66). *Thus, a physical examination—including assessment of systolic murmurs—should be performed before all exercise tests.* If a loud systolic murmur is heard, an echocardiogram should be considered prior to testing.

Specific questioning should determine which drugs are being taken, and potential electrolyte abnormalities should be considered. The patient should bring along his or her medication bottles so that medications can be identified and recorded. Because of a greater potential for cardiac events with the sudden cessation of beta blockers, they should not be automatically stopped prior to testing but tapered off gradually under physician guidance. Although the accuracy of standard ST criteria are significantly decreased in patients on beta blockers who do reach adequate heart rates, exercise scores or less strict ST-depression criteria can be used to maintain the sensitivity of the test.[8]

Pretest standard 12-lead ECGs are necessary in both the supine and standing positions. Good skin preparation usually causes some discomfort but is necessary for good conductance and to avoid artifacts. The changes caused by exercise electrode placement can be kept to a minimum by keeping the arm electrodes off the chest, placing them on the shoulders, and recording the baseline ECG supine.[9] The ground (green) electrode can be placed over the spine, low on the back, and the right leg electrode should be placed below the umbilicus. In this situation, the modified exercise limb lead placement can serve as the reference resting ECG prior to an exercise test.

## During the Test

Most complications can be avoided by measuring blood pressure, monitoring the ECG, questioning the patient about symptoms and levels of fatigue and assessing appearance during the test. Subjects should be reminded not to grasp the front or side rails because this decreases the work performed and creates noise in the ECG. The subject may rest his or her hands on the rails for balance but should not hang on. Hanging on the rails results in an overestimation of exercise capacity.

Target heart rates based on age should not be used because the relationship between maximal heart rate and age is poor and a wide scatter exists around the many different recommended regression lines. Such heart rate targets result in a submaximal test for some individuals, a maximal test for some, and an unrealistic goal for others. The absolute and relative indications for test termination are listed in Table 16-2. If none of these endpoints are met, the test should be symptom-limited. The Borg scales are an excellent means of quanti-

TABLE 16-2 Indications for Terminating Exercise Testing

| Absolute Indications |
|---|
| Drop in systolic blood pressure of >10 mmHg from baseline blood pressure despite an increase in workload when accompanied by other evidence of ischemia |
| Moderate to severe angina |
| Increasing nervous system symptoms (e.g., ataxia, dizziness, or near-syncope) |
| Signs of poor perfusion (cyanosis or pallor) |
| Technical difficulties in monitoring ECG or systolic blood pressure |
| Subject's desire to stop |
| Sustained ventricular tachycardia |
| ST-segment elevation (≥1.0 mm) in leads without diagnostic Q waves (other than $V_1$ or aVR) |
| **Relative Indications** |
| Drop in systolic blood pressure of (≥10 mmHg from baseline blood pressure despite an increase in workload in the absence of other evidence of ischemia |
| ST or QRS changes such as excessive ST-segment depression (>2 mm of horizontal or downsloping ST-segment depression) or marked axis shift |
| Arrhythmias other than sustained ventricular tachycardia, including multifocal PVCs, triplets of PVCs, supraventricular tachycardia, heart block, or bradyarrhythmias |
| Fatigue, shortness of breath, wheezing, leg cramps, or claudication |
| Development of bundle branch block or intraventricular conduction delay that cannot be distinguished from ventricular tachycardia |
| Increasing chest pain |
| Hypertensive response[a] |

[a]In the absence of definitive evidence, the committee suggests systolic blood pressure of >250 mmHg and/or a diastolic blood pressure of >115 mmHg.
SOURCE: Modified from Gibbons RJ, Balady GJ, Bricker JT, et al. ACC/AHA 2002 guideline update for exercise testing. *Circulation* 2002;106:1883–1892.

fying an individual's effort. Subjects should be monitored for perceived effort level by using the 6-to-20 Borg scale at 2-min intervals.[10]

To ensure the safety of exercise testing, the following list of the most dangerous circumstances in the exercise testing laboratory should be recognized:

- When patients exhibit ST-segment elevation (without baseline diagnostic Q waves), this can be associated with dangerous arrhythmias and infarction. The incidence is about 1 in 1000 clinical tests and usually occurs in $V_2$ or aVF rather than $V_5$.
- When a patient with an ischemic cardiomyopathy exhibits severe chest pain due to ischemia (angina pectoris), a cool-down walk is advisable.
- When a patient develops exertional hypotension accompanied by ischemia (angina or ST-segment depression) or when it occurs in a patient with a history of congestive heart failure, cardiomyopathy, or recent myocardial infarction, safety is a serious issue.
- When a patient with a history of sudden death or collapse during exercise develops premature ventricular depolarizations that become frequent, a cool-down walk is advisable.

### Recovery after Exercise

If maximal sensitivity is to be achieved with an exercise test, patients should be supine as soon as possible during the postexercise period (maximal wall stress). It is advisable to record about 10 s of ECG data while the patient is standing motionless but still at near-maximal heart rate and then have the patient lie down. Having the patient perform a cool-down walk after the test can delay or eliminate the appearance of ST-segment depression,[11] while having patients lie down enhances ST-segment abnormalities in recovery.

Monitoring should continue for at least 5 min after exercise or until changes stabilize. An abnormal response occurring only in the recovery period is neither unusual nor necessarily suggestive of a false-positive result.[12]

A cool-down walk can be helpful in performing tests on patients with an established diagnosis undergoing testing for other than diagnostic reasons, as in testing athletes or patients with CHF, valvular heart disease, or a recent MI.

### Exercise Test Modalities

Three types of exercise can be used to stress the cardiovascular system: isometric, dynamic, and a combination of the two. *Isometric exercise,* defined as constant muscular contraction without movement (such as handgrip), imposes a disproportionate pressure load on the left ventricle relative to the body's ability to supply oxygen. *Dynamic exercise* is defined as rhythmic muscular activity resulting in movement, and it initiates a more appropriate increase in cardiac output and oxygen exchange. This chapter considers only dynamic exercise testing, since a delivered workload can be calibrated accurately and the physiologic response measured easily. Isometric exercise is not recommended for routine exercise testing.

### Bicycle Ergometer versus Treadmill

The bicycle ergometer usually costs less, takes up less space, and makes less noise than a treadmill. Although bicycling is a dynamic exercise, most individuals perform more work on a treadmill because a greater muscle mass is involved, and most subjects are more familiar with walking than cycling. In most studies comparing exercise on an upright cycle ergometer versus a treadmill exercise, maximal heart rate values have been demonstrated to be roughly similar, whereas maximal oxygen uptake has been shown to be 6 to 25 percent greater during treadmill exercise.[13,14]

### Exercise Protocols

The many different exercise protocols in use have led to some confusion regarding how physicians compare tests between patients and serial tests in the same patient. The most common protocols, their stages, and the predicted oxygen cost of each stage are illustrated in Fig. 16-1. When treadmill and cycle ergometer testing were first introduced into clinical practice, practitioners adopted protocols used by major researchers.[15,16] The large and uneven work increments in some of these protocols have been shown to result in a tendency to overestimate exercise capacity.[17,18] Investigators have since recommended protocols with smaller and more equal increments.[19] Recent guidelines suggest that protocols should be individualized for each subject such that test duration is approximately 8 to 12 min. An approach to exercise testing that has gained interest is the ramp protocol, in which work increases constantly and continuously.[14]

## HEART RATE

### Methods of Recording Maximal Heart Rate

The different ways of recording rate and differences in the type of exercise used may affect measurements of maximal heart rate ($HR_{max}$). Premature beats can affect measurement, and most computerized systems attempt to eliminate them automatically. Cardiotachometers are incorporated into most exercise test devices but may fail to trigger or may trigger on T waves, artifacts, or aberrant beats, thus yielding inaccurate results.

### Factors Limiting Maximal Heart Rate

Several factors may affect the $HR_{max}$ during dynamic exercise. $HR_{max}$ declines with advancing years and is affected by gender. Height, weight, and even lean body weight apparently do not affect $HR_{max}$ very much.[20] Systole has a relatively fixed time interval; in contrast, relatively less time of the cardiac cycle is spent in diastole as heart rate increases. Many studies have reported $HR_{max}$ during treadmill testing in a variety of patients. Regressions with age have varied depending on the population studied and other factors. Figure 16-2 summarizes these studies of $HR_{max}$.[21] In an effort to clarify the relationship between $HR_{max}$ and age, a comprehensive review of the literature compiling over 23,000 subjects aged 5 to 81 years was performed.[20] A stepwise multiple regression revealed that age alone accounted for 75 percent of the variability; other factors added only about 5 percent and included the method of exercise and fitness. The 95 percent confidence interval for the regression of maximal heart rate on age is nearly 50 beats per minute wide for any age. Heart rates at maximal exercise were lower on bicycle ergometry than on the treadmill and lower still with swimming. Other factors that affect $HR_{max}$ include deconditioning and altitude.[22,23] Older patients may be restrained by poor muscle tone, pulmonary disease, claudication, orthopedic problems, and other noncardiac causes of limitation. The usual decline in $HR_{max}$ with age is not as steep in those who are free of myocardial disease and stay active.

Since prediction of maximal heart rate is inaccurate, exercise should be symptom-limited and not targeted on achieving a certain heart rate. A relatively low heart rate can be maximal for a patient of

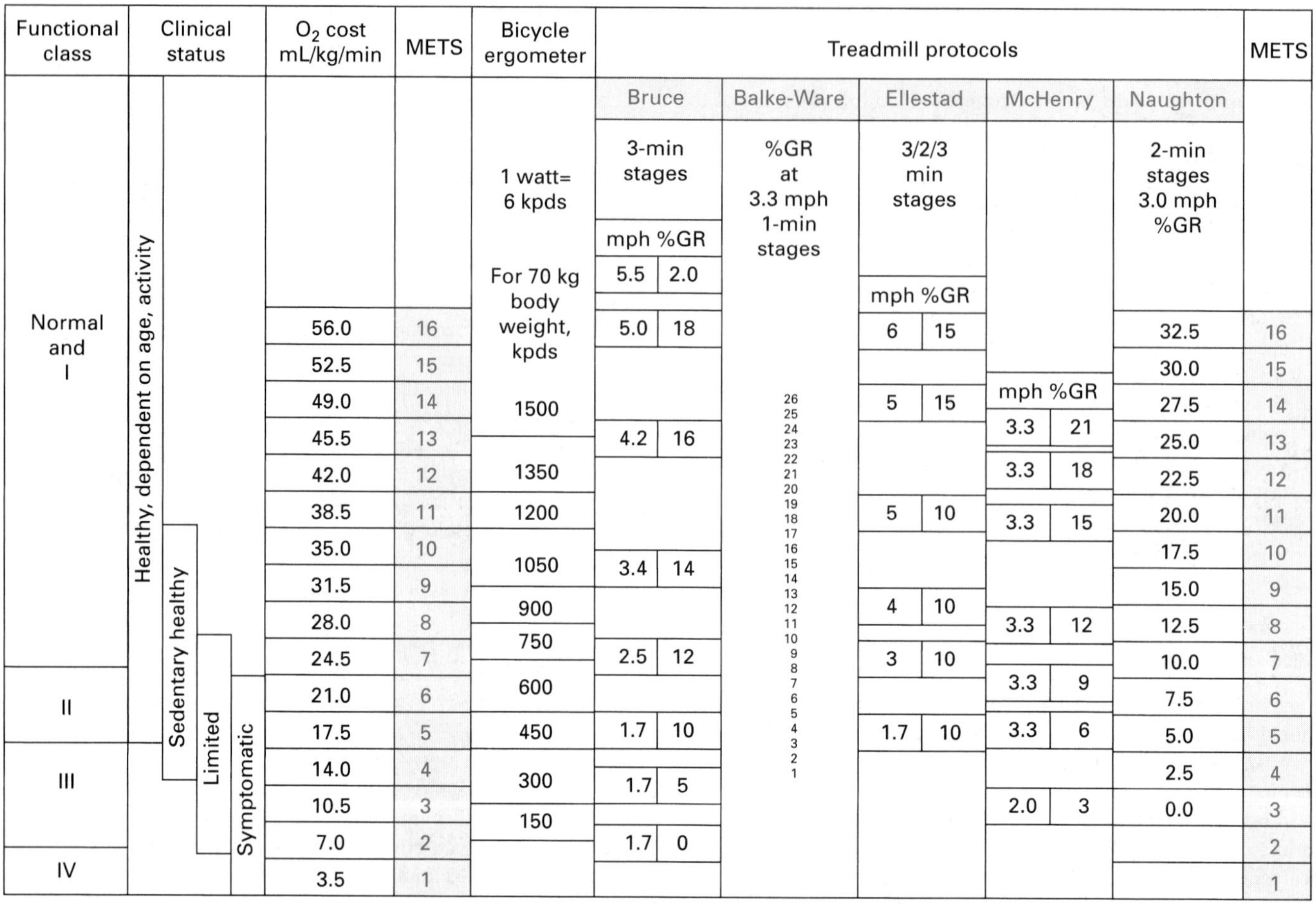

| Functional class | Clinical status | $O_2$ cost mL/kg/min | METS | Bicycle ergometer | Treadmill protocols: Bruce | Balke-Ware | Ellestad | McHenry | Naughton | METS |
|---|---|---|---|---|---|---|---|---|---|---|
| | | | | 1 watt= 6 kpds | 3-min stages | %GR at 3.3 mph 1-min stages | 3/2/3 min stages | | 2-min stages 3.0 mph %GR | |
| | | | | For 70 kg body weight, kpds | mph %GR | | mph %GR | mph %GR | | |
| | | | | | 5.5 2.0 | | | | | |
| Normal and I | Healthy, dependent on age, activity | 56.0 | 16 | | 5.0 18 | | 6 15 | | 32.5 | 16 |
| | | 52.5 | 15 | | | | | | 30.0 | 15 |
| | | 49.0 | 14 | 1500 | | 26 25 | 5 15 | | 27.5 | 14 |
| | | 45.5 | 13 | | 4.2 16 | 24 23 | | 3.3 21 | 25.0 | 13 |
| | | 42.0 | 12 | 1350 | | 22 21 | | 3.3 18 | 22.5 | 12 |
| | | 38.5 | 11 | 1200 | | 20 19 18 | 5 10 | 3.3 15 | 20.0 | 11 |
| | Sedentary healthy | 35.0 | 10 | | | 17 16 | | | 17.5 | 10 |
| | | 31.5 | 9 | 1050 | 3.4 14 | 15 14 | | | 15.0 | 9 |
| | Limited | 28.0 | 8 | 900 | | 13 12 11 | 4 10 | 3.3 12 | 12.5 | 8 |
| | | 24.5 | 7 | 750 | 2.5 12 | 10 9 8 | 3 10 | | 10.0 | 7 |
| II | Symptomatic | 21.0 | 6 | 600 | | 7 6 | | 3.3 9 | 7.5 | 6 |
| | | 17.5 | 5 | 450 | 1.7 10 | 5 4 | 1.7 10 | 3.3 6 | 5.0 | 5 |
| III | | 14.0 | 4 | 300 | 1.7 5 | 3 2 1 | | | 2.5 | 4 |
| | | 10.5 | 3 | 150 | | | | 2.0 3 | 0.0 | 3 |
| | | 7.0 | 2 | | 1.7 0 | | | | | 2 |
| IV | | 3.5 | 1 | | | | | | | 1 |

FIGURE 16-1 The most common protocols, their stages, and the predicted oxygen cost of each stage.

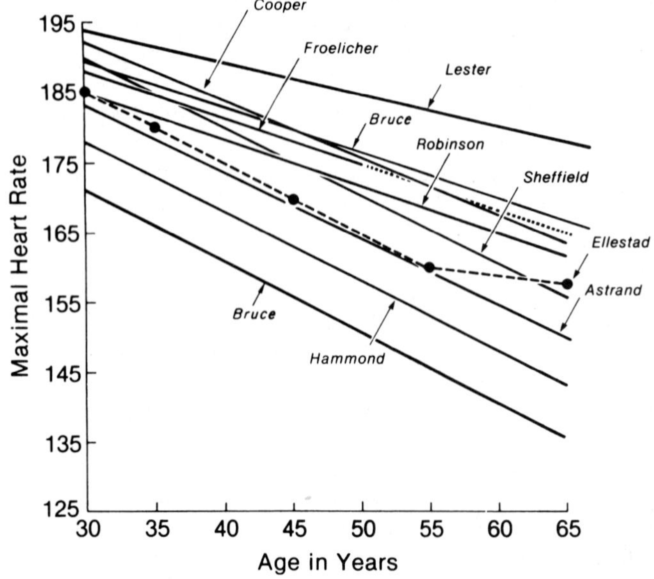


FIGURE 16-2 Many studies, as shown in this illustration, have reported $HR_{max}$ during treadmill testing in a variety of patients. Regressions with age have varied depending on the population studied and other factors.

a given age and submaximal for another. *Thus, a test should not be considered nondiagnostic if a percentage of age-predicted maximal heart rate (i.e., 85 percent) is not reached.*

## Recovery Heart Rate

Heart rate usually falls rapidly at the end of a bout of progressive exercise. While the rate of the drop in heart rate is related to fitness, it has more recently been shown to be inversely related to survival.[24] In general, a decline in heart rate of less than 20 beats per minute by the first or second minute of recovery is associated with an increased risk of death.[25]

## BLOOD PRESSURE RESPONSE

Systolic blood pressure should rise with increasing treadmill workload, whereas diastolic blood pressure usually remains about the same or drops (Fig. 16-3). A drop in systolic blood pressure (SBP) below preexercise values is the most ominous criterion; whereas a drop of 20 mmHg or more without a fall below preexercise values appears to have less predictive value.[26] Exercise-induced hypotension raises concern for left ventricular dysfunction, ischemia, or outflow obstruction. When exercise-induced hypotension occurs without association with these factors or in a patient with good exercise capacity, it can be benign.

The highest systolic blood pressure should be achieved at maximal workload. To avoid fainting, patients should not be left standing on the treadmill for more than the few seconds required to obtain a final ECG. A rise in SBP immediately after exercise has been suggested as a marker of ischemia.[27]

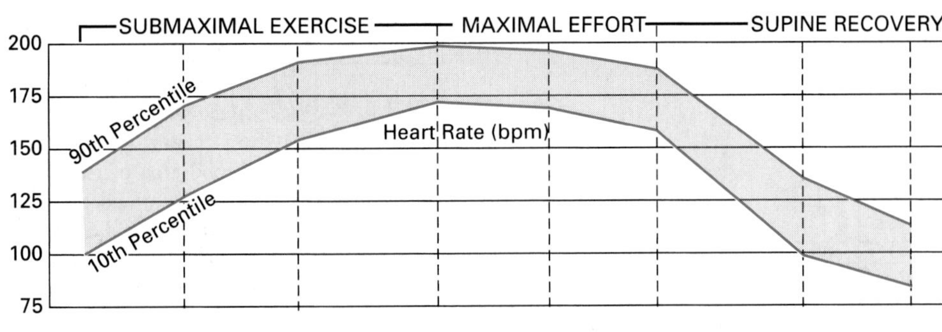


THE RESPONSE OF HEALTHY MEN TO TREADMILL EXERCISE

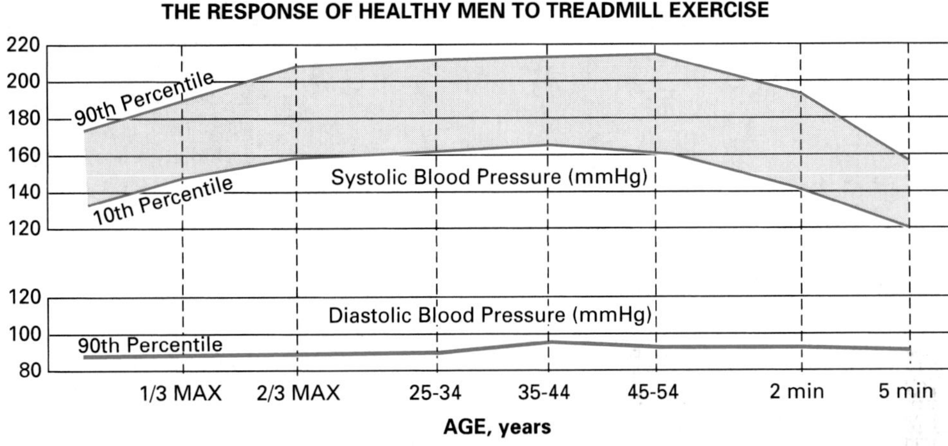


FIGURE 16-3 The results of a large number of normal individuals who underwent a progressive treadmill test show the response of heart rate and blood pressure according to age.

## EXERCISE CAPACITY

Maximal ventilatory oxygen uptake is the greatest amount of oxygen that a person can extract from inspired air while performing dynamic exercise involving a large part of the total-body muscle mass. Since maximal ventilatory oxygen uptake is equal to the product of cardiac output and arteriovenous oxygen difference, it is a measure of the functional limits of the cardiovascular system. Maximal arteriovenous difference is physiologically limited to roughly 15 to 17 mL/dL. Thus maximal arteriovenous difference behaves more or less as a constant, making maximal oxygen uptake an indirect estimate of maximal cardiac output.

Maximal oxygen uptake depends on many factors, including natural endowment, activity status, age, and gender, but it is the best index of exercise capacity and maximal cardiovascular function. The maximal oxygen uptake of the normal sedentary adult is often considered approximately 30 mL $O_2$/kg/min, and the minimal level for a physically fit adult is often considered roughly 40 mL $O_2$/kg/min. In general, aerobic training can increase maximal oxygen uptake by up to 25 percent. Individuals performing aerobic training such as distance running can have maximal oxygen uptakes as high as 60 to 90 mL $O_2$/kg/min. For convenience, oxygen consumption is often expressed in multiples of basal resting requirements. The metabolic equivalent (MET) is a unit of basal oxygen consumption equal to 3.5 mL $O_2$/kg/min. This is the approximate amount of oxygen required to sustain life in the resting state. Table 16-3 lists clinically meaningful METs for exercise, prognosis, and maximal performance.

An individual's maximal oxygen uptake is usually estimated from the workload reached while performing an exercise test using a formula based on speed and grade. Maximal oxygen uptake is most precisely determined by direct measurement using ventilatory gas-exchange techniques.

*Clinical exercise test results always should be reported in METs and not minutes of exercise.* In this way, the results from different protocols and exercise modalities can be compared directly. Achieved workload in METs has been shown to be a major prognostic variable and can be used to predict mortality with equal effectiveness in young and elderly patients.[28]

### Normal Values for Exercise Capacity

In measuring or estimating maximal oxygen uptake, it is useful to have reference values for comparison. Maximal oxygen uptake declines with increasing age, and higher values are observed among men than among women. "Normal" values are usually based on age and gender, but many other difficult-to-measure factors affect one's exercise capacity, such as genetics and the type and extent of comorbid disease.[29] Nomograms can be used to estimate expected exercise capacity (Fig. 16-4).[30] In using regression equations or nomograms for reference purposes, it is important to consider several points. First, the relationship between exercise capacity and age is rather poor ($r$ = 0.30 to 0.60). Second, nearly all equations are derived from different populations. Moreover, since treadmill time or workload tends to overpredict maximal METs, it is important to consider whether gas-exchange techniques were used in developing the

TABLE 16-3 Clinically Significant Metabolic Equivalents for Maximum Exercise

| | |
|---|---|
| 1 MET[a] | Resting |
| 2 METs | Level walking at 2 mi/h |
| 4 METs | Level walking at 4 mi/h |
| <5 METs | Poor prognosis; peak cost of basic activities of daily living |
| 10 METs | Prognosis with medical therapy as good as coronary artery bypass surgery |
| 13 METs | Excellent prognosis regardless of other exercise responses |
| 18 METs | Elite endurance athletes |
| 20 METs | World-class athletes |

[a]MET = metabolic equivalent, or a unit of sitting resting oxygen uptake. 1 MET = 3.5 mL/kg/min oxygen uptake.

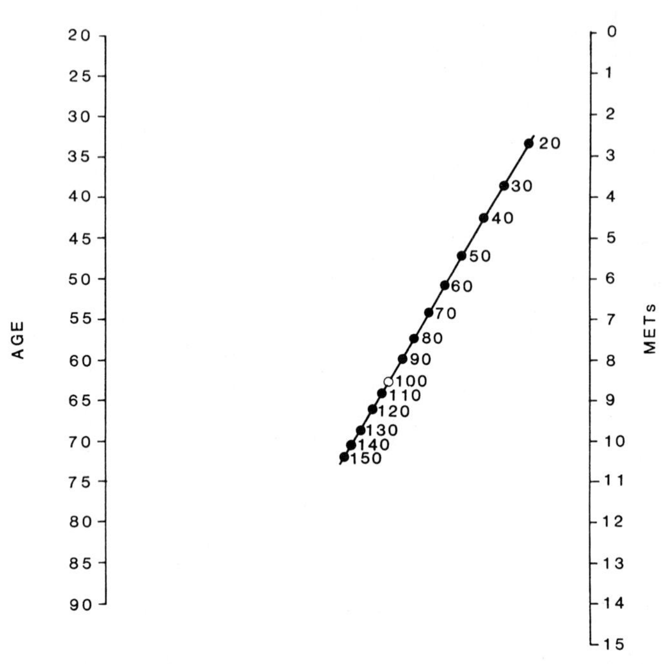


FIGURE 16-4 The exercise capacity nomogram, providing a relative estimate of normal for age, with 100 percent being as expected for age in a clinical population.

equations. When one is directly measuring oxygen uptake, the MET values are shifted downward roughly a MET for any given age, reflecting the lower but more precise measurement of exercise capacity. Within the above limitations, the nomograms can provide reasonable references.

## ECG INTERPRETATION

The ECG is the only component of the exercise test that has had its diagnostic characteristics demonstrated using a protocol to limit workup bias,[31] fulfilling one of the most important criteria for proper test evaluation.[32] Neither echocardiography nor nuclear scanning have been so evaluated.

### ST Analysis

ST-segment depression is a representation of global subendocardial ischemia. ST-segment depression does not localize coronary artery lesions. $V_5$ is the lead that most often exhibits significant ST-segment depression. The standard criterion for abnormal is 1 mm or more of horizontal or downsloping ST-segment depression below the PR isoelectric line or 1 mm of further depression if there is baseline depression. ST-segment depression in the inferior leads (II, aVF) is most often due to the atrial repolarization wave that begins in the PR segment and can extend to the beginning of the ST segment.[33] When ST-segment depression is isolated to these leads, it is usually a false-positive response.[34]

ST-segment depression limited to the recovery period does not generally represent a false-positive response. Inclusion of analysis during this time period increases the diagnostic yield of the exercise test. Maximal exercise and 3 min of recovery are critical and equally important times to look for ST-segment depression. ECG recordings should continue for 5 min in recovery or until any new changes from baseline stabilize. When the resting ECG shows Q waves of an old myocardial infarction, ST-segment elevation during exercise is most often associated with wall motion abnormalities. Less often, it is due to ischemia. Accompanying ST-segment depression can be due to a second area of ischemia or reciprocal changes. When the resting ECG is normal, exercise-induced ST-segment elevation is due to severe ischemia (spasm or a critical lesion), and accompanying ST-segment depression is usually reciprocal. Such ST-segment elevation is uncommon and very arrhythmogenic, and it localizes the involved coronary artery.

Exercise-induced ST-segment elevation and ST-segment depression can both represent ischemia, but they are quite distinctive. Elevation is due to transmural ischemia, is arrhythmogenic, occurs only about once in a thousand patients tested, and localizes to the artery where there is spasm or a tight lesion.[35] Depression is due to subendocardial ischemia, is not arrhythmogenic, has a 5 to 50 percent prevalence (depending upon age and chest pain symptoms), is rarely due to spasm, and does not localize. Figure 16-5 illustrates the various patterns.

While computer analysis can help interpretation, the raw data should always be considered first, because processing can cause artifacts.[36] Although numerous computerized ST-segment criteria have been studied, most appear to be equivalent to visual interpretation using standard criteria. Dividing ST-segment depression by heart rate has been studied the most and may be helpful.[37,38]

### Exercise-Induced Ventricular Arrythmias

Exercise-induced ventricular arrythmias (EIVA), mostly consisting of premature ventricular contractions (PVCs), are not uncommon during exercise testing. The prevalence of EIVA is greater in older patients and in those with cardiopulmonary disease, resting PVCs, or ischemia during exercise.[39] EIVA and resting PVCs are both independent predictors of mortality. Nonsustained ventricular tachycardia is uncommon during routine clinical treadmill testing (prevalence <2 percent).[40]

## EXERCISE TEST SCORES

A variety of statistical tools are available to create diagnostic and prognostic scores, and the use of exercise testing scores has been well studied.[41] The guidelines of the American College of Cardiology/American Heart Association (ACC/AHA) suggest the use of scores to enhance the predictive ability of exercise tests.

### Statistical Techniques to Develop Scores

In developing a score or prediction rule, investigators consider variables that they believe may predict the occurrence of an outcome and then make use of those variables found to have discriminating power.[42] The standard approach for creating an exercise test score is to use a combination of clinical information and exercise test results to form an algorithm for estimating the probability of disease. Although many mathematical techniques are available for demonstrating what variables are predictive as well as their relative predictive power, logistic regression is preferred, since it models the relationship to a sigmoid curve (the most common mathematical relationship between a probability variable and an outcome) and its output is between zero and one (i.e., from 0 to 100 percent probability of the predicted outcome).

## Application of Scores

The ability of any score or measurement to diagnosis a disease depends on how much the score differs among those with and without the disease.[43] Figure 16-6 shows the application of a simple treadmill score to an actual population of over 1000 male veterans who underwent both exercise testing and coronary angiography. Unfortunately, there is a great deal of overlap in scores between patients with and without coronary artery disease. Using a cut point of 50 may be a practical choice to separate patients but will not absolutely classify those with and without disease. The better the test or measurement, the further apart the curves of the measurement and the less they overlap.

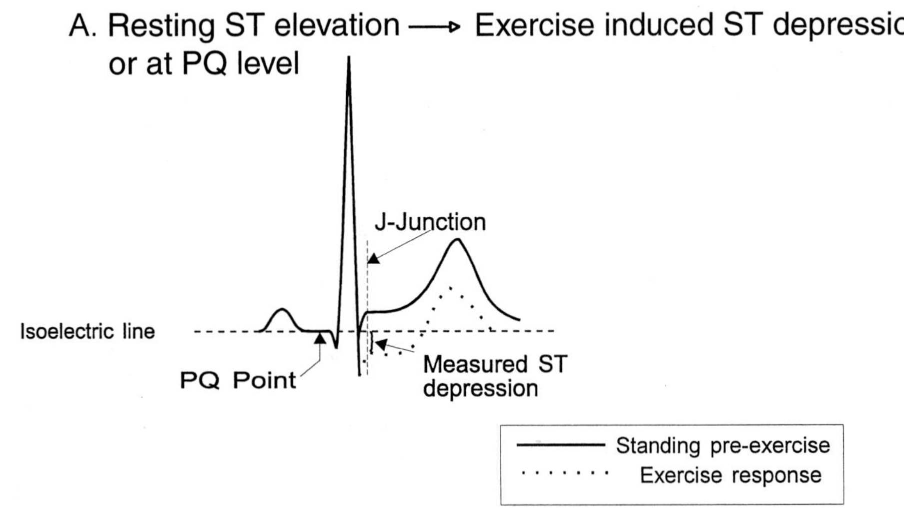


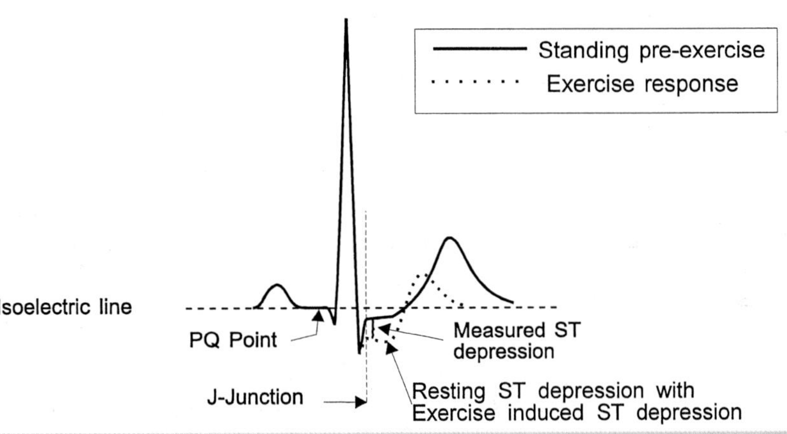


FIGURE 16-5 The various patterns of ST-segment shift. The standard criterion for abnormal is 1 mm of horizontal or downsloping ST-segment depression below the PR isoelectric line or 1 mm further depression if there is baseline depression.

## Score Evaluation

The accuracy of a model to separate patients with and without a certain disease or outcome is assessed by evaluating the receiver operating characteristic (ROC) curve. An ROC curve is a plot of the sensitivity and specificity for the full range of cut points (criteria for abnormal) for a test measurement or the value of a score. The shape of the curve shows the tradeoffs between sensitivity and specificity produced at different cutoff criteria with specificity and sensitivity being inversely related. The area under the ROC curve ranges from 0 to 1, with 0.5 corresponding to no discrimination (i.e., random performance), 1.0 to perfect discrimination, and values less than 0.5 to worse than random performance. Figure 16-7 is an ROC plot of the simple treadmill score ranging from 0 to 100 with two other cut points, 40 and 60, illustrated. These cut points could be appropriate for particular purposes of the test; i.e., the higher cut point of 60 would be useful for screening well people where a high specificity is needed while the lower cut point of 40 would be well suited for ruling out ischemia after presentation to an emergency department for chest pain where high sensitivity is required. Plotting ROC curves for different diagnostic techniques or scores allows their discriminatory or diagnostic value to be compared.[44]

## Pretest Scores

The exercise ECG test is the recommended test for diagnosing coronary artery disease in patients at intermediate probability for coronary artery disease. In the ACC/AHA exercise test guidelines, the Diamond-Forrester tabular method is used to determine pretest probability with consideration of age, gender, and chest pain characteristics (Table 16-4). The intermediate pretest probability category was assigned a class I indication, whereas the low and high pretest probabilities were assigned class IIb indications for exercise testing. The Morise score for categorizing patients as to pretest probability of angiographic disease (Fig. 16-8) appears superior to the tabular method.[45]

## Exercise Test Diagnostic Scores

### ANALYSIS OF VARIABLES FOR USE IN SCORES

Many investigators have proposed multivariable scores combining clinical and exercise parameters in addition to the ST responses to enhance the accuracy of the standard exercise test. Age, gender, chest pain symptoms, elevated cholesterol, ST-segment slope and depression, and maximum heart rate were the variables chosen as significant predictors in more than half of the studies.[46]

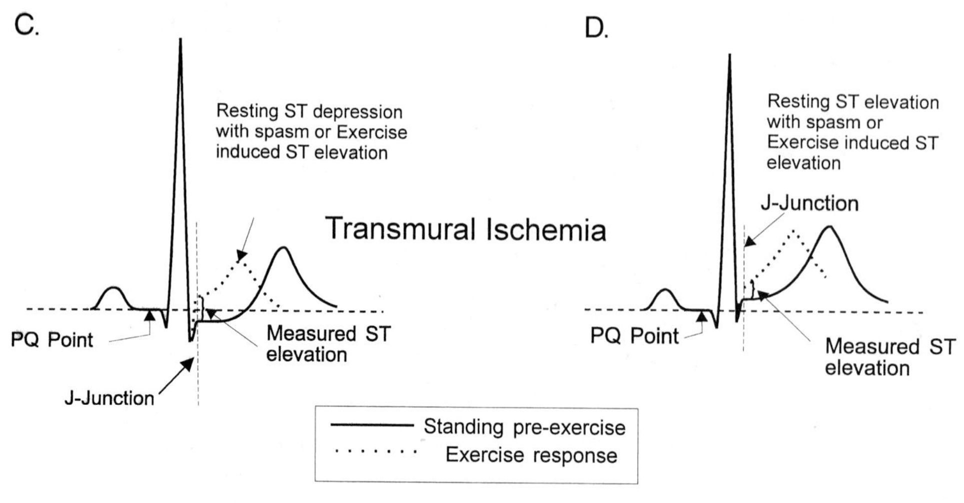


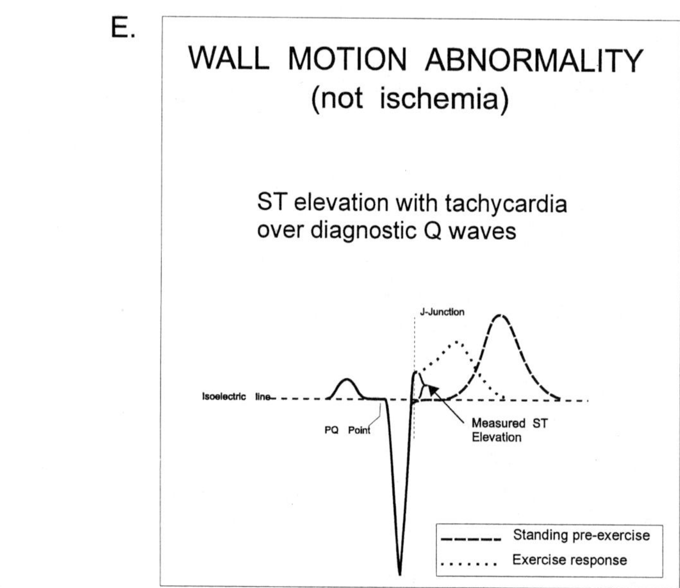


FIGURE 16-5 *(Continued)*

## MANAGEMENT STRATEGY USING SCORES

Exercise test scores can also assist in managing patients with possible coronary artery disease by placing them into three categories of risk rather than just dichotomizing them as positive or negative. Low-risk patients can be treated safely with medical management of coronary risk factors and watchful waiting prior to further testing. High-risk patients should be considered candidates for more aggressive management, which may include cardiac catheterization. In patients with an intermediate-probability treadmill score, myocardial perfusion imaging and other tests are of value for further risk stratification.

## CONSENSUS OF SCORES

A consensus approach was developed for the purpose of increasing accuracy and making the scores broadly applicable to different populations.[47] Three validated scores with established thresholds were used. If a patient was found to have a high probability in at least two of the three scores, he or she was considered "high probability"; similarly, if a low score was found in at least two of the three equations, he or she was considered "low risk." All others were considered "intermediate." Since the patients in the intermediate group would be sent for further testing and would eventually be correctly classified, both the sensitivity and specificity were greater than 90%.

## "SIMPLIFIED" SCORE DERIVATION

Simplified scores derived from multivariable equations have been developed to determine the probability of disease and prognosis. All variables are coded with the same number of intervals, so that the coefficients will be proportional. For instance, if 5 is the chosen interval, dichotomous variables are 0 if not present and 5 if present. Continuous variables like age and maximum heart rate are coded in five groups associated with increasing prevalence of disease. The relative importance of the selected variables is obvious and the health care provider merely compiles the variables in the score, multiples by the appropriate number, and then adds up the products. Calculation of the "simple" exercise test score can be done using Fig. 16-9[48] for men and Fig. 16-10[49] for women.

## PREDICTIVE ACCURACY

Some test results are dichotomous (normal vs. abnormal, positive vs. negative) rather than continuous, like a score. Predictive accuracy (true positive plus true negatives divided by the total population studied) can be used to compare dichotomous test results. Any score can also be dealt with as a dichotomous variable by choosing a cut point. An advantage of predictive accuracy is that it provides an estimate of the number of patients correctly classified by the test out of 100 tested. However, when predictive accuracy is used to compare tests, populations with roughly the same prevalence of disease should be considered. Table 16-5, based on published meta-nalyses, summarizes the predictive accuracy of the major diagnostic tests for coronary artery disease currently available.[50]

# Exercise Test Prognostic Scores

Different statistical techniques should be used to develop prognostic scores and predict mortality or cardiac events as opposed to the presence or absence of disease. The key features of survival analysis are consideration of time to event and censoring (ending the time of observation when an intervention occurs). A Cox proportional hazards model should be used to select significant variables and to determine the effect of a given independent variable on time to death or event.

## ENDPOINTS AND CENSORING

The relative importance of ischemic variables can be minimized if censoring for interventions does not occur. Patients who have an intervention to treat ischemia are not as likely to experience an outcome and should be removed from the analysis (i.e., censored). The use of all-cause mortality instead of cardiovascular mortality also decreases the significance of ischemic variables. While all-cause mortality has advantages over cardiovascular mortality as an endpoint,[51] exercise scores are more appropriately generated using endpoints such as infarction and cardiovascular death. Furthermore, interventions should not be used as endpoints, since the association of ischemic variables with endpoints is falsely strengthened because the ischemic symptoms clinically lead to the performance of the intervention.

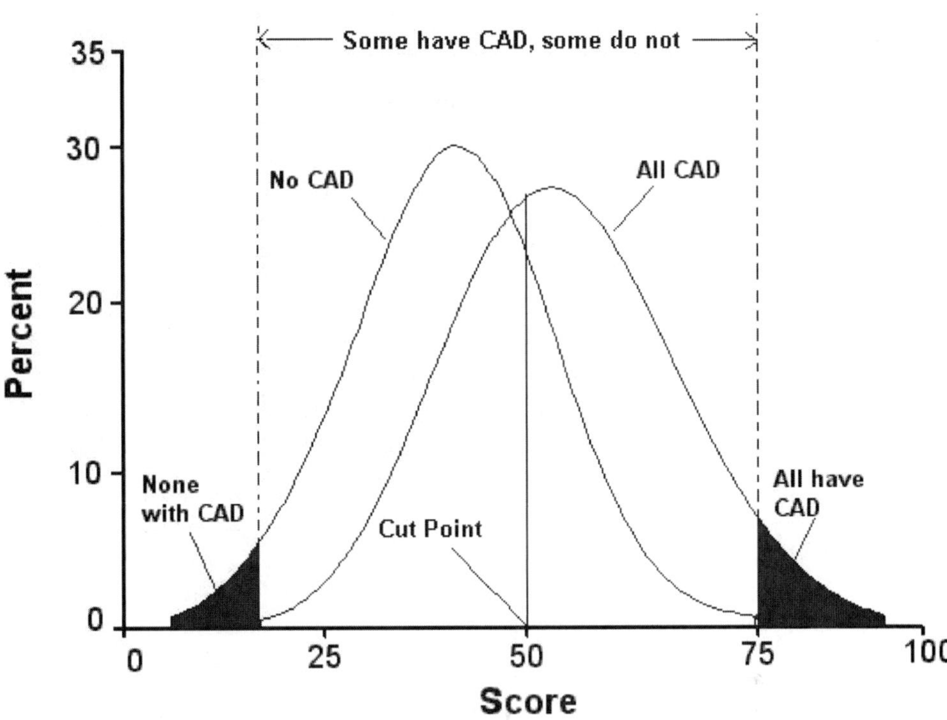


FIGURE 16-6 Distribution of those with and without angiographic coronary artery disease according to values for a simple exercise test diagnostic score.

## EVALUATION OF PROGNOSTIC SCORES

The most widely used exercise test score is the Duke treadmill score calculated as [exercise time, or METs − 5 × (amount ST depression) − 4 × (treadmill angina index (1 = occurred, 2 = reason for stopping))] possibly because it can be used both for prognosis and diagnosis.[52] It has been validated as a powerful prognostic tool for both men and women, and when the resting ECG exhibits ST-segment depression, however, it appears less effective in the elderly.[53] Many exercise scores have been developed and there is substantial overlap in most of the variables chosen; but maximum heart rate tends to have more diagnostic power, while METs achieved tends to have more prognostic power. In a study of a broad spectrum of over 6000 patients referred for testing, the following variables were shown to be associated with time to death: METs less than 5, age greater than 65, history of congestive heart failure, and history of myocardial infarction.[54] A score based on simply adding these variables classified patients into low-, medium-, and high-risk groups. Figure 16-11 shows improved survival curves with progressively higher scores.

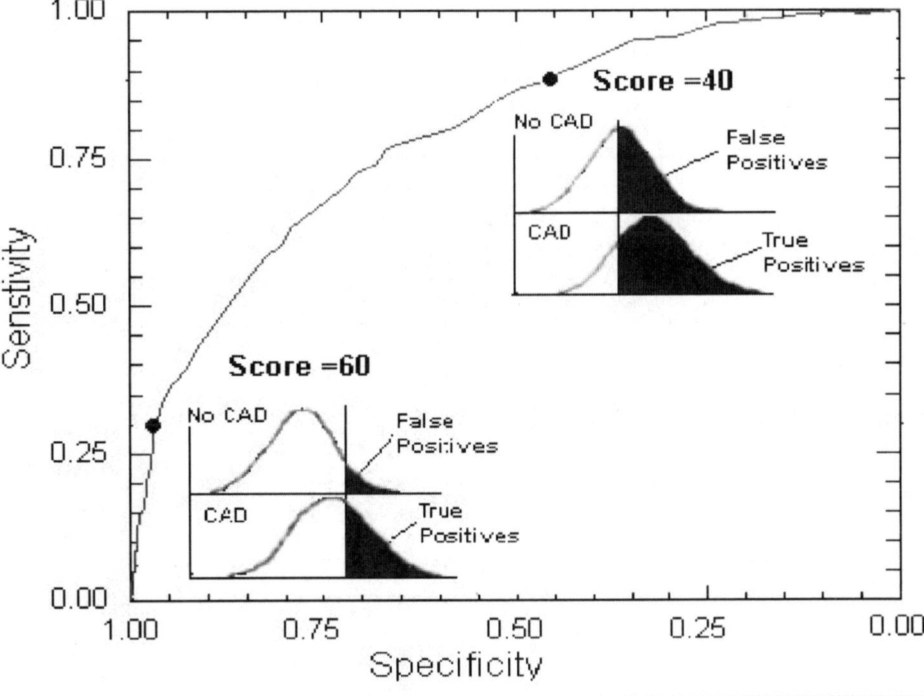


FIGURE 16-7 Illustration of an ROC curve and how it can help to choose cut points for different applications of a test or score.

### Comparing Scores and Physicians

Several studies have shown that scores perform at least as well as physicians in predicting angiographic coronary disease and estimating prognosis. In the largest study, clinical information and treadmill test results were sent to expert cardiologists and to two other groups, including randomly selected cardiologists and internists, who classified them in terms of high, low, or intermediate probability of disease in addition to estimating a numerical probability from 0 to 100%.[55] When probability estimates were compared,

TABLE 16-4 Pretest Probability of Coronary Artery Disease by Symptoms, Gender, and Age

| Age[a] | Gender | Typical/ Definite Angina[b] | Atypical/Probable Angina | Nonanginal Chest Pain | Asymptomatic |
|---|---|---|---|---|---|
| 30–39 | Men | Intermediate | Intermediate | Low | Very low |
| | Women | Intermediate | Very Low | Very low | Very low |
| 40–49 | Men | High | Intermediate | Intermediate | Low |
| | Women | Intermediate | Low | Very low | Very low |
| 50–59 | Men | High | Intermediate | Intermediate | Low |
| | Women | Intermediate | Intermediate | Low | Very low |
| 60–69 | Men | High | Intermediate | Intermediate | Low |
| | Women | High | Intermediate | Intermediate | Low |

[a]There are no data for patients younger than 30 or older than 69, but it can be assumed that the prevalence of coronary artery disease increases with age.
[b]High = >90%, intermediate = 10–90%, low = <10%, very low = <5%.

the scores were superior to all the physician groups both for diagnosing coronary disease and determining prognosis.

## THE ACC/AHA GUIDELINES FOR THE USE OF THE STANDARD EXERCISE TEST

The task force established guidelines for the use of exercise testing in 1986 and 1997 and most recently in 2002.[1] The full guidelines can be found on the American College of Cardiology website (www.acc.org). (See Chap. 106 for classification.)

### Exercise Testing to Diagnose Coronary Artery Disease

Class I indications for exercise testing include patients with an intermediate pretest probability of disease (see Table 16-4), including those with less than 1 mm of resting ST-segment depression and complete right bundle branch block. Patients with a complete left bundle branch block, greater than 1 mm of resting ST-segment depression, preexcitation, or paced rhythms should not undergo ECG exercise testing (class III).

Testing of patients with vasospastic angina is class IIa. Testing of patients with low or high pretest probability of disease is class IIb. Patients with less than 1 mm of resting ST-segment depression and evidence of left ventricular hypertrophy or on digoxin are class IIb as well.

### Exercise Testing for Risk Assessment and Prognosis

Class I indications for exercise testing in patients with known or suspected coronary artery disease include those patients undergoing initial evaluation or presenting with a significant change in clinical status. Patients with low-risk unstable angina 8 to 12 h after presentation and intermediate-risk unstable angina 2 to 3 days after presentation who do not have active ischemia or heart failure symptoms are also class I. Testing intermediate-risk unstable angina patients with negative cardiac markers 6 to 12 h after presentation and no evidence of active ischemia is class IIa.

Patients with a complete left bundle branch block, any interventricular conduction defect with QRS duration >120 ms, greater than 1 mm of resting ST-segment depression, preexcitation, or paced rhythms are class IIb for risk assessment and prognosis. High-risk unstable angina patients or those with severe comorbidities are class III.

### Exercise Testing after Myocardial Infarction

One of the major applications of the exercise ECG is for patients within 2 months of a myocardial infarction.[56] Appropriate evidence-based uses (class I) of the test are (1) before discharge for prognostic assessment, activity prescription, or evaluation of medical therapy (submaximal at about 4 to 7 days); (2) early after discharge if the predischarge exercise test was not done (symptom limited, about 14 to 21 days); and (3) late after discharge if the early exercise test was submaximal (symptom limited, about 3 to 6 weeks). Another use of the test is after discharge for activity counseling and/or exercise training as part of cardiac rehabilitation in patients who have undergone coronary revascularization (class IIa). Exercise testing can also be used in those with the ECG abnormalities, mentioned above, that interfere with the recognition of ischemia or for periodic monitoring in patients who continue to participate in exercise training or cardiac rehabilitation (class IIb).

| Variable | Circle response | Sum |
|---|---|---|
| Age | Men <40, Women <50 = 3 | |
| | Men 40-55, Women 50-65 = 6 | |
| | Men >55, Women >65 = 9 | |
| Estrogen Status | Positive = -3 | |
| | Negative = 3 | |
| Diabetes | Yes = 2 | |
| Obesity | Yes = 1 | |
| Family History | Yes = 1 | |
| Hypercholesterolemia | Yes = 1 | |
| Hypertension | Yes = 1 | |
| Smoking | Yes = 1 | |
| | Total Score: | |

**Pretest**

<9 = Low Probability

9-15 = Intermediate Probability

>15 = High Probability

FIGURE 16-8 Calculation of the simple pretest clinical score for angiographic coronary disease. Choose only one per group.

A metanalysis of 28 studies performed in the prethrombolytic era involving 15,613 patients found that exercise capacity and blood pressure response were more accurate predictors of adverse cardiac events after myocardial infarction than measures of exercise-induced ischemia.[57] A more recent study has validated these conclusions.[58]

## Exercise Testing Using Ventilatory Gas Analysis

The use of ventilatory gas analysis to directly measure maximal oxygen uptake is usually reserved for research-based exercise protocols, but there are a limited number of clinical scenarios where it may be appropriate.

Evidence supports the addition of ventilatory gas analysis to the exercise test for the evaluation of exercise capacity and response to therapy in patients with heart failure who are being considered for heart transplantation and when assistance is needed in differentiating cardiac versus pulmonary limitations as a cause of exercise-induced dyspnea or impaired exercise capacity (class I).

Another reason to add gas analysis to the exercise test (class IIa) is for the evaluation of exercise capacity when indicated for medical reasons in patients in whom subjective assessment of maximal exercise is unreliable.

Last, gas analysis can be used for evaluation of the patient's response to specific therapeutic interventions in which improvement of exercise tolerance is an important goal or endpoint or for determination of the intensity for exercise training as part of comprehensive cardiac rehabilitation (class IIb).

## Exercise Testing in Asymptomatic Individuals without Known Coronary Artery Disease

There are no class I indications for using the ECG exercise test to screen asymptomatic individuals. Testing diabetic patients who plan to start vigorous exercise is class IIa. Exercise testing can be used to evaluate men over age 45 and women over age 55 who plan to start exercise, are in occupations that affect public safety, or are at high risk for coronary disease due to other diseases such as

| Variable | Circle response | Sum | |
|---|---|---|---|
| Maximal Heart Rate | Less than 100 bpm = 30 | | Men |
| | 100 to 129 bpm = 24 | | |
| | 130 to 159 bpm = 18 | | |
| | 160 to 189 bpm = 12 | | |
| | 190 to 220 bpm = 6 | | |
| Exercise ST Depression | 1-2mm = 15 | | <40 = |
| | > 2mm = 25 | | Low |
| Age | >55 yrs = 20 | | Probability |
| | 40 to 55 yrs = 12 | | |
| Angina History | Definite/Typical = 5 | | 40-60 = |
| | Probable/atypical = 3 | | Intermediate |
| | Non-cardiac pain = 1 | | Probability |
| Hypercholesterolemia? | Yes = 5 | | |
| Diabetes? | Yes = 5 | | >60 = |
| Exercise Test Induced Angina? | Occurred = 3 | | High |
| | Reason for stopping = 5 | | Probability |
| | Total Score: | | |

FIGURE 16-9 Calculation of the simple score for angiographic coronary disease in men. Choose only one per group.

| Variable | Circle response | Sum | |
|---|---|---|---|
| Maximal Heart Rate | Less than 100 bpm = 20 | | Women |
| | 100 to 129 bpm = 16 | | |
| | 130 to 159 bpm = 12 | | |
| | 160 to 189 bpm = 8 | | |
| | 190 to 220 bpm = 4 | | |
| Exercise ST Depression | 1-2mm = 6 | | <37 = |
| | > 2mm =10 | | Low |
| Age | >65 yrs = 25 | | Probability |
| | 50 to 65 yrs = 15 | | |
| Angina History | Definite/Typical = 10 | | 37-57 = |
| | Probable/atypical = 6 | | Intermediate |
| | Non-cardiac pain = 2 | | Probability |
| Hypercholesterolemia? | Yes = 10 | | |
| Diabetes? | Yes = 10 | | >57 = |
| Exercise Test Induced Angina? | Occurred = 9 | | High |
| | Reason for stopping =15 | | Probability |
| Estrogen Status | Positive=-5, Negative=5 | | |
| | Total Score: | | |

FIGURE 16-10 Calculation of the simple score for angiographic coronary disease in women. Choose only one per group.

TABLE 16-5 Comparison of Diagnostic Tests for Coronary Artery Disease

| Diagnostic Technology Evaluated | Number of Studies | Total Number of Patients | Predictive Accuracy |
|---|---|---|---|
| ECG exercise test | 147 | 24,047 | 73% |
| Exercise test scores | 24 | 11,788 | 80% |
| Score strategy | 2 | >1000 | 88% |
| Thallium scintigraphy | 59 | 6,038 | 85% |
| Single photon emission computed tomography (SPECT) | 30 | 5,272 | 80% |
| Adenosine SPECT | 14 | 2,137 | 85% |
| Exercise echocardiography (ECHO) | 58 | 5,000 | 80% |
| Dobutamine ECHO | 5 | <1000 | 86% |
| Dobutamine scintigraphy | 20 | 1014 | 81% |
| Electron beam computed tomography (EBCT) | 16 | 3,683 | 65% |

peripheral vascular disease or chronic renal failure (class IIb). Evaluation of patients with multiple risk factors to guide therapy is also class IIb.

Routine screening of asymptomatic men or women is not recommended (class III).

## SUMMARY

The exercise test complements the medical history and the physical examination, and it remains the second most commonly performed cardiologic procedure next to the routine ECG. The addition of echocardiography or myocardial perfusion imaging does not negate the importance of the ECG or clinical and hemodynamic responses to exercise. The renewed efforts to control costs undoubtedly will support the role of the exercise test. Convincing evidence that treadmill scores enhance the diagnostic and prognostic power of the exercise test certainly has cost-efficacy implications.

Use of proper methodology is critical for safety and obtaining accurate and comparable results. The use of specific criteria for exclusion and termination, interaction with the subject, and appropriate emergency equipment is essential.

The following rules are important to follow for getting the most information from the standard exercise test:

- The exercise protocol should be progressive, with even increments in speed and grade whenever possible.
- The treadmill protocol should be adjusted to the patient, and one protocol is not appropriate for all patients; consider using a manual or automated ramp protocol.
- Report exercise capacity in METs, not minutes of exercise.
- Hyperventilation prior to testing is not indicated.
- ST-segment measurements should be made at ST0 (J-junction), and ST-segment depression should be considered abnormal only if horizontal or downsloping.
- Raw ECG waveforms should be considered first and then supplemented by computer-enhanced (filtered and averaged) waveforms when the raw data are acceptable.
- In testing for diagnostic purposes, patients should be placed supine as soon as possible after exercise, with a cool-down walk avoided.
- The 3-min recovery period is critical to include in analysis of the ST-segment response.
- Measurement of systolic blood pressure during exercise is extremely important and exertional hypotension is ominous; manual blood pressure measurement techniques are preferred.
- Age-predicted heart rate targets are largely useless because of the wide scatter for any age; exercise tests should be symptom limited.
- A treadmill score should be calculated for every patient; use of multiple scores or a computerized consensus score should be considered as part of the treadmill report.

The ACC/AHA guidelines for exercise testing clearly indicate the correct uses of exercise testing. Since the last guidelines, exercise testing has been extended as the first diagnostic test in women and in individuals with right bundle branch block and resting ST-segment depression. The use of diagnostic scores and prognostic scores such as the Duke treadmill score increases the value of the exercise test. In fact, the use of scores results in test characteristics that approach the nuclear and echocardiographic add-ons to the exercise test.

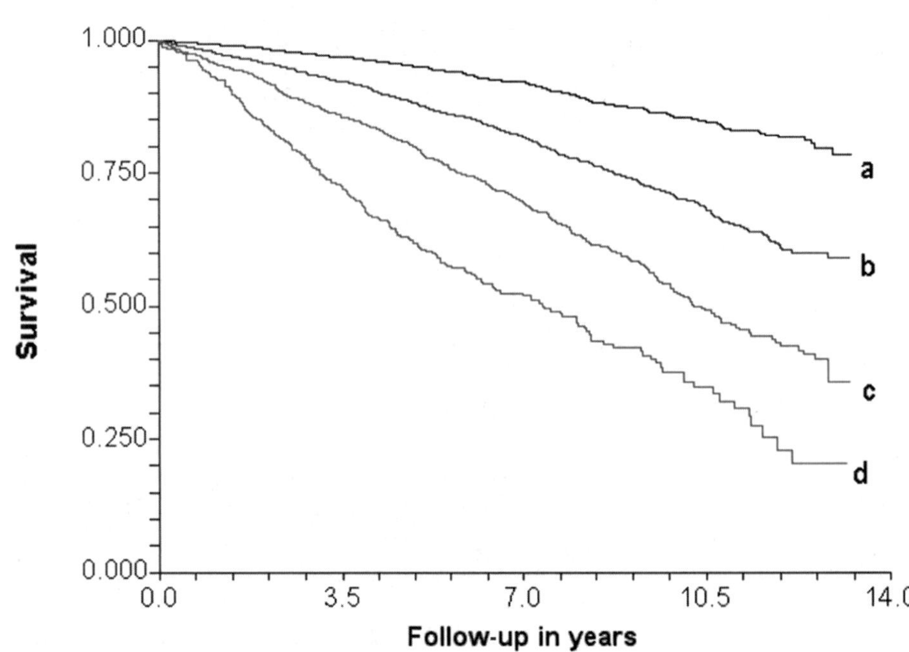


FIGURE 16-11 Kaplan-Meier survival curves for the "all comers" prognostic score. Score yes = 1 and no = 0 for METs < 5 + age > 65 + history of CHF + history of MI or Q waves. Curve a = 0, b = 1, c = 2, and d = more than 2.

## References


1. Gibbons RJ, Balady GJ, Bricker JT, et al. ACC/AHA 2002 guideline update for exercise testing: A report of the American College of Cardiology/American Heart Association Task Force on Practice Guidelines (Committee on Exercise Testing). *Circulation* 2002;106: 1883–1892.
2. Fletcher GF, Balady GJ, Amsterdam EA, et al. Exercise standards for testing and training: A statement for healthcare professionals from the American Heart Association. *Circulation* 2001;104:1694–1740.

2a. Froelicher V, Shetler K, Ashley E. Better decisions through science: Exercise Testing Scores. *Curr Probl Cardiol* 2003;28:621–656.

3. Gibbons L, Blair SN, Kohl HW, Cooper K. The safety of maximal exercise testing. *Circulation* 1989;80:846–852.
4. Rochmis P, Blackburn H. Exercise tests: A survey of procedures, safety, and litigation experience in approximately 170,000 tests. *JAMA* 1971; 217:1061–1066.
5. Akdemir I, Aksoy N, Aksoy M, et al. Does exercise-induced severe ischaemia result in elevation of plasma troponin-T level in patients with chronic coronary artery disease? *Acta Cardiol* 2002;57:13–18.
6. Ashmaig ME, Starkey BJ, Ziada AM, et al. Changes in serum concentrations of markers of myocardial injury following treadmill exercise testing in patients with suspected ischaemic heart disease. *Med Sci Monit* 2001;7:54–57.
7. Myers J, Bader D, Madhavan R, Froelicher V. Validation of a specific activity questionnaire to estimate exercise tolerance in patients referred for exercise testing. *Am Heart J* 2001;142:1041–1046.
8. Gauri AJ, Raxwal VK, Roux L, et al. Effects of chronotropic incompetence and beta-blocker use on the exercise treadmill test in men. *Am Heart J* 2001;142:136–141.
9. Gamble P, McManus H, Jensen D, Froelicher VF. A comparison of the standard 12-lead electrocardiogram to exercise electrode placement. *Chest* 1984;85:616–622.
10. Borg G. *Borg's Perceived Exertion Scales.* Champaign, IL: Human Kinetics; 1998.
11. Gutman RA, Alexander ER, Li YB, et al. Delay of ST depression after maximal exercise by walking for two minutes. *Circulation* 1970;42: 229–233.
12. Lachterman B, Lehmann KG, Abrahamson D, Froelicher VF. "Recovery only" ST-segment depression and the predictive accuracy of the exercise test. *Ann Intern Med* 1990;112:11–16.
13. Hambrecht RP, Schuler GC, Muth T, et al. Greater diagnostic sensitivity of treadmill versus cycle exercise testing of asymptomatic men with coronary artery disease. *Am J Cardiol* 1992;70:141–146.
14. Myers J, Buchanan N, Walsh D, et al. A comparison of the ramp versus standard exercise protocols. *J Am Coll Cardiol* 1991;17:1334–1342.
15. Bruce RA. Exercise testing of patients with coronary heart disease. *Ann Clin Res* 1971;3:323–330.
16. Ellestad MH, Allen W, Wan MCK, Kemp G. Maximal treadmill stress testing for cardiovascular evaluation. *Circulation* 1969;39:517–522.
17. Panza JA, Quyyumi AA, Diodati JG, et al. Prediction of the frequency and duration of ambulatory myocardial ischemia in patients with stable coronary artery disease by determination of the ischemic threshold from exercise testing: Importance of the exercise protocol. *J Am Coll Cardiol* 1991;17:657–663.
18. Webster MWI, Sharpe DN. Exercise testing in angina pectoris: The importance of protocol design in clinical trials. *Am Heart J* 1989;117: 505–508.
19. Sullivan M, McKirnan MD. Errors in predicting functional capacity for postmyocardial infarction patients using a modified Bruce protocol. *Am Heart J* 1984;107:486–491.
20. Londeree BR, Moeschberger ML. Influence of age and other factors on maximal heart rate. *J Cardiac Rehabil* 1984;4:44–49.
21. Hammond HK, Froelicher VF. Normal and abnormal heart rate responses to exercise. *Prog Cardiovasc Dis* 1985;27:271–296.
22. Hartley LH, Vogel JA, Cruz JC. Reduction of maximal exercise heart rate at altitude and its reversal with atropine. *J Appl Physiol* 1974;36: 362–365.
23. Convertino V, Hung J, Goldwater D, et al. Cardiovascular responses to exercise in middle-aged man after 10 days of bed rest. *Circulation* 1982;65:134–140.
24. Cole CR, Blackstone EH, Pashkow FJ, et al. Heart-rate recovery immediately after exercise as a predictor of mortality. *N Engl J Med* 1999; 341:1351–1357.
25. Shetler K, Marcus R, Froelicher VF, et al. Heart rate recovery: Validation and methodologic issues. *J Am Coll Cardiol* 2001;38: 1980–1987.
26. Dubach P, Froelicher VF, Klein J, et al. Exercise-induced hypotension in a male population: Criteria, causes, and prognosis. *Circulation* 1988;78:1380–1387.
27. Taylor AJ, Beller GA. Postexercise systolic blood pressure response: Clinical application to the assessment of ischemic heart disease. *Am Fam Phys* 1998;58:1126–1130.
28. Spin JM, Prakash M, Froelicher VF, et al. The prognostic value of exercise testing in elderly men. *Am J Med* 2002;112:453–459.
29. Wasserman K, Hansen JE, Sue DY, Whipp BJ. *Principles of Exercise Testing and Interpretation.* Philadelphia: Lea & Febiger; 1999:72–86.
30. Morris CK, Myers J, Kawaguchi T, et al. A nomogram based on metabolic equivalents and age for aerobic exercise capacity in men. *J Am Coll Cardiol* 1993;22:175–182.
31. Froelicher VF, Lehmann KG, Thomas R, et al. The electrocardiographic exercise test in a population with reduced workup bias: Diagnostic performance, computerized interpretation, and multivariable prediction. *Ann Intern Med* 1998;128:965–974.
32. Froelicher VF, Fearon W, Ferguson C, et al. Lessons learned from studies of the standard exercise test? *Chest* 1999;116:1442–1451.
33. Sapin PM, Blauwet MB, Koch GG, Gettes LS. Exaggerated atrial repolarization waves as a predictor of false positive exercise tests in an unselected population. *J Electrocardiol* 1995;28:313–321.
34. Miranda CP, Liu J, Kadar A, et al. Usefulness of exercise-induced ST-segment depression in the inferior lead. *Am J Cardiol* 1992;69:303–307.
35. Nosratian F, Froelicher VF. ST elevation during exercise testing: A review. *Am J Cardiol* 1989;63:986–988.
36. Milliken JA, Abdollah H, Burggraf GW. False-positive treadmill exercise tests due to computer signal averaging. *Am J Cardiol* 1990;65:946–948.
37. Lachterman B, Lehmann KG, Neutel J, Froelicher VF. Comparison of the ST/heart rate index to standard ST criteria for analysis of the exercise electrocardiogram. *Circulation* 1990;82:44–50.
38. Fletcher GF, Flipse TR, Klingfield P, Malouf JR. Current status of ECG stress testing. *Curr Probl Cardiol* 1998;23:353–423.
39. Parthington S, Cho S, Myers J, et al. Prevalence and prognostic value of exercise-induced ventricular, arrhythmias. *Am Heart J* 2003;145: 139–146.
40. Yang JC, Wesley RC, Froelicher VF. Ventricular tachycardia during routine treadmill testing: Risk and prognosis. *Arch Intern Med* 1991;151: 349–353.
41. Froelicher V, Shetler K, Ashley E. Better decisions through science: Exercise testing scores. *Prog Cardiovasc Dis* 2002;44:395–414.
42. Swets JA, Dawes RM, Monahan J. Better decisions through science. *Sci Am* 2000;283:82–87.
43. Ashley E, Myers J, Froelicher V. Exercise testing scores as an example of better decisions through science. *Med Sci Sports Exerc* 2002;34: 1391–1398.
44. Atwood JE, Do D, Froelicher V, et al. Can computerization of the exercise test replace the cardiologist? *Am Heart J* 1998;136:543–552.
45. Morise A. Comparison of the Diamond-Forrester method and a new score to estimate the pretest probability of coronary disease before exercise testing. *Am Heart J* 1999;138:740–745.
46. Yamada H, Do D, Morise A, Froelicher V. Review of studies utilizing multi-variable analysis of clinical and exercise test data to predict angiographic coronary artery disease. *Prog Cardiovasc Dis* 1997;39:457–481.
47. Do D, West JA, Morise A, Froelicher V. A consensus approach to diagnosing coronary artery disease based on clinical and exercise test data. *Chest* 1997;111:1742–1749.
48. Raxwal V, Shetler K, Do D, Froelicher V. A simple treadmill score. *Chest* 2000;113:1933–1940.

49. Morise AP, Lauer MS, Froelicher VF. Development and validation of a simple exercise test score for use in women with symptoms of suspected coronary artery disease. *Am Heart J* 2002;144:818–825.
50. O'Rourke RA, Brundage BH, Froelicher VF, et al. American College of Cardiology/American Heart Association Expert Consensus Document on electron-beam computed tomography for the diagnosis and prognosis of coronary artery disease. *J Am Coll Cardiol* 2000;36:326–340.
51. Lauer MS, Blackstone EH, Young JB, Topol EJ. Cause of death in clinical research: Time for a reassessment? *J Am Coll Cardiol* 1999;34: 618–620.
52. Shaw LJ, Peterson ED, Shaw LK, et al. Use of a prognostic treadmill score in identifying diagnostic coronary disease subgroups. *Circulation* 1998;98:1622–1630.
53. Kwok JM, Miller TD, Hodge DO, et al. Prognostic value of the Duke treadmill score in the elderly. *J Am Coll Cardiol* 2002;39:1475–1481.
54. Prakash M, Myers J, Froelicher VF, et al. Clinical and exercise test predictors of all-cause mortality: Results from >6,000 consecutive referred male patients. *Chest* 2001;120:1003–1013.
55. Lipinski M, Do D, Froelicher V, et al. Comparison of exercise test scores and physician estimation in determining disease probability. *Arch Intern Med* 2001;161:2239–2244.
56. Ashley EA, Froelicher V. The post myocardial infarction exercise test: Still worthy after all of these years. *Eur Heart J* 2001;22:273–276.
57. Froelicher VF, Perdue S, Pewen W, Risch M. Application of meta-analysis using an electronic spread sheet to exercise testing in patients after myocardial infarction. *Am J Med* 1987;83:1045–1054.
58. Shaw LJ, Peterson ED, Kesler K, et al. A meta-analysis of predischarge risk stratification after acute myocardial infarction with stress electrocardiographic, myocardial perfusion, and ventricular function imaging. *Am J Cardiol* 1996;78:1327–1337.

CHAPTER 17

# CARDIAC CATHETERIZATION, CARDIAC ANGIOGRAPHY, AND CORONARY BLOOD FLOW AND PRESSURE MEASUREMENTS

Morton J. Kern / Spencer B. King III / John S. Douglas, Jr. / Robert H. Franch



## CARDIAC CATHETERIZATION

In 1929, Werner Forssman, a resident surgeon at Eberswalde, Germany, inserted a urologic catheter into his right atrium from a left antecubital vein cutdown he performed on himself using a mirror. After walking downstairs to the radiology suite, the position of the catheter tip was verified by a roentgenogram.[1] From this beginning of cardiac catheterization, dramatic and innovative advances in methods and materials have occurred. Catheterization has long since moved from a specialized laboratory to the bedside enabling the clinician to employ physiologic data to guide treatment.[2–4]

Cardiac catheterization—the insertion and passage of small plastic catheters into arteries, veins, the heart, and other vascular structures—is performed to acquire radiographic images of coronary arteries and cardiac chambers and to measure cardiovascular hemodynamics (pressures, cardiac output, oximetry data). The catheterization laboratory not only performs diagnostic cardiac imaging but can also examine the aorta, pulmonary veins, and peripheral vessels for diseases, anomalies, or obstructions. Furthermore, in the last two decades, cardiac catheterization has evolved from a strictly diagnostic modality to one of therapeutics through numerous catheter-based interventions (like angioplasty, stenting, and closure of atrial septal defects). Now, a wide variety of palliative and corrective interventions may accompany a diagnostic catheterization study (Table 17-1).

### Indications and Contraindications

Cardiac catheterization is used to diagnose atherosclerotic artery disease, cardiomyopathy, infarction, and valvular or congenital heart abnormalities. The principal indications for cardiac catheterization are summarized in Table 17-2.

In general, cardiac catheterization is an elective diagnostic procedure and should be deferred if the patient is not prepared either psychologically or physically. For urgent procedures, especially if the patient is unstable from a suspected cardiac cause such as acute myocardial infarction, catheterization must proceed. In the event of

TABLE 17-1 Diagnostic and Therapeutic Interventional Procedures That May Accompany Coronary Angiography

| Diagnostic Procedures | Comment |
|---|---|
| Central venous access (femoral, internal jugular, subclavian) | Access for emergency medications or fluids, temporary pacemaker |
| Hemodynamic assessment | |
| Left heart pressures (aorta, left ventricle) | Routine for all studies |
| Right and left heart combined pressures | Not routine for coronary artery disease; mandatory for valvular heart disease; congestive heart failure (CHF), right ventricular dysfunction, pericardial diseases, cardiomyopathy, intracardiac shunts, congenital abnormalities |
| Transseptal or LV puncture | Valvular heart disease |
| Intracoronary pressure/flow | Coronary lesion assessment |
| Left ventricular angiography | Routine for all studies; may be excluded with high-risk patients, left main coronary or aortic stenosis, severe CHF, renal failure |
| Internal mammary artery and saphenous vein bypass graft selective angiography | Routine for coronary bypass conduit |
| Pharmacologic studies | |
| Ergonovine | Routine for suspected coronary vasospasm |
| IC/IV/sublingual nitroglycerin | Routine for all coronary angiography |
| Aortography | Routine for aortic insufficiency, aortic dissection, aortic aneurysm, with or without aortic stenosis, routine to locate bypass grafts not visualized by selective angiography |
| Renal and peripheral vascular angiography | For renovascular hypertension and peripheral vascular disease |
| Cardiac pacing and electrophysiologic studies | Arrhythmia evaluation |
| Therapeutic interventional procedures | |
| Coronary disease | Percutaneous coronary interventions (e.g., PTCA, stenting) |
| Valvular stenosis | Balloon catheter valvuloplasty |
| Atrial septal defect | Atrial septal defect closure |
| Hypertrophic obstructive cardiomyopathy (HOCM) | Transseptal alcohol septal ablation for HOCM |
| Arrhythmia | Electrophysiologic conduction tract catheter ablation |
| Arterial access site closure devices | Available for patients prone to access site bleeding |

SOURCE: From Kern MJ. *The Cardiac Catheterization Handbook*. St. Louis: Mosby; 2003. With permission.

decompensated congestive heart failure requiring cardiac catheterization for diagnosis and potential treatment, rapid medical management in the catheterization laboratory may be an expeditious option whereby endotracheal intubation, intraaortic balloon pumping, and vasopressors can be instituted rapidly before angiography and revascularization.

Relative contraindications to cardiac catheterization include fever, anemia, electrolyte imbalance (especially hypokalemia predisposing to arrhythmias), or other systemic illnesses needing stabilization (Table 17-3).

## Preparations for Cardiac Catheterization

The procedure should be explained in simple terms as to what will take place and for what reason each step of the procedure will occur. The operator or his or her assistant, usually a physician, obtains consent. The operator should explain the risks for routine cardiac catheterization to the patient and family. The incidence of major risks of stroke, death, and myocardial infarction is approximately 0.1 percent. The minor risks of vascular injury, allergic reaction, bleeding, hematoma, and infection range from 0.04 to 5 percent and should be discussed. Certain patient groups are at higher risk for complications (Table 17-4). There is no alternative to coronary angiography. Often the patient and family's concern of "not knowing" about coronary disease outweighs the risk of performing the test.

Patient preparations should be tailored to the specific individual and the associated clinical problems. Patients with diabetes mellitus, renal insufficiency, or previous reported hypersensitivity to iodinated contrast media constitute groups who need special considerations.

For diabetic patients, the dose of neutral protamine Hagedorn (NPH) insulin should be cut by 50 percent, because an overnight fast with their normal morning dose of insulin will cause hypoglycemia. Patients receiving NPH insulin are also at higher risk for protamine reactions. Some diabetic patients will be receiving an antihyperglycemic agent, metformin (Glucophage), an analogue of phenformin that was associated with a risk of lactic acidosis. Rare cases of metformin-associated lactic acidosis have been reported in diabetics with chronic renal insufficiency. Metformin is contraindicated in patients with renal dysfunction, as determined by elevated serum creatinine levels. However, there is no evidence that withholding metformin for 48 h before a contrast procedure in patients with normal renal function provides any clinical benefit. Table 17-5 lists conditions that require special patient preparations.

Some patients may be suitable for outpatient or same-day-discharge cardiac catheterization. Patients suitable for these studies require careful selection.[3] Patients with a high likelihood of needing a coronary intervention after the diagnostic study will require either transportation to a full-service laboratory or have to undergo a second procedure at a later time elsewhere. Although some physicians have performed cardiac catheterization on stable, low-risk patients in freestanding facilities, the lack of support in this environment is a potential liability.

## Techniques of Vascular Access

Vascular access is determined by the anticipated pathoanatomic and clinical conditions of the patient. Whenever possible, previous procedure notes of any difficulties, especially of vascular access, should be reviewed. Preprocedural assessment of all peripheral pulses is mandatory.

### PERCUTANEOUS FEMORAL ARTERY PUNCTURE

Percutaneous femoral arterial catheterization is the most widely used vascular access technique. In patients with claudication, chronic arterial insufficiency, diminished or absent pulses, or bruits over the iliofemoral area, alternate entry sites should be considered (Table 17-6).

A detailed explanation of percutaneous femoral puncture technique can be found elsewhere.[5–7] In brief, the proposed entry site into the femoral artery can be verified by fluoroscopy using the tip of a metal clamp and placing it near the medial edge of the middle of the head of the femur (Fig. 17-1). The index finger palpates the artery and a Seldinger needle punctures its front wall. A J -tipped guidewire is introduced into the needle and advanced gently into the artery. After the guidewire is advanced in the aorta, the arterial needle is removed and a valved catheter sheath is inserted over the guidewire. The sheath hub is held firmly in place and the dilator and guidewire are removed together. The sheath is flushed with heparinized saline solution.

TABLE 17-2 Indications for Cardiac Catheterization

| Indications | Procedures |
|---|---|
| Suspected or known coronary artery disease | |
| New onset angina | LV, COR |
| Unstable angina | LV, COR |
| Evaluation before a major surgical procedure | LV, COR |
| Silent ischemia | LV, COR, ERGO |
| Positive ETT | LV, COR, ERGO |
| Atypical chest pain or coronary spasm | LV, COR, ERGO |
| Myocardial infarction | |
| Unstable angina post infarction | LV, COR |
| Failed thrombolysis | LV, COR, RH |
| Shock | LV, COR, RH |
| Mechanical complications | |
| (Ventricular septal defect, rupture of wall or papillary muscle) | LV, COR, RH |
| Sudden cardiovascular death | LV, COR, R + L |
| Valvular heart disease | LV, COR, R + L, AO |
| Congenital heart disease (before anticipated corrective surgery) | LV, COR, R + L, AO |
| Aortic dissection | AO, COR |
| Pericardial constriction or tamponade | LV, COR, R + L |
| Cardiomyopathy | LV, COR, R + L, BX |
| Initial and follow-up assessment for heart transplant | LV, COR, R + L, BX |

ABBREVIATIONS: AO = aortography; BX = endomyocardial biopsy; COR = coronary angiography; ERGO = ergonovine provocation of coronary spasm; ETT = exercise tolerance test; LV = left ventriculography; RH = right heart oxygen saturations and hemodynamics (e.g., placement of Swan-Ganz catheter); R + L = right and left heart hemodynamics.
SOURCE: From Kern MJ. *The Cardiac Catheterization Handbook*. St. Louis: Mosby; 2003. With permission.

### PERCUTANEOUS FEMORAL VEIN PUNCTURE

The femoral vein is located approximately 1 cm medial to the femoral artery. The procedure for femoral vein percutaneous entry is similar to that for the femoral artery with only several minor differences.

Because venous pressure is low, it may be difficult to see unassisted backbleeding from the needle on entry. A syringe may be

TABLE 17-3 Contraindications to Cardiac Catheterization

- Absolute contraindications
  - Inadequate equipment or catheterization facility
- Relative contraindications
  - Acute gastrointestinal bleeding or anemia
  - Anticoagulation (or known uncontrolled bleeding diathesis)
  - Electrolyte imbalance
  - Infection/fever
  - Medication intoxication (e.g., digitalis, phenothiazine)
  - Pregnancy
  - Recent carebral vascular accident (<1 month)
  - Renal failure
  - Uncontrolled congestive heart failure, high blood pressure, arrhythmias
  - Uncooperative patient

SOURCE: From Kern MJ. *The Cardiac Catheterization Handbook,* St. Louis: Mosby; 2003. With permission.

TABLE 17-4 Conditions of Patients at Higher Risk for Complications of Catheterization

- Acute myocardial infarction
- Advanced age (>75 years)
- Aortic aneurysm
- Aortic stenosis
- Congestive heart failure
- Diabetes
- Extensive three-vessel coronary artery disease
- Left ventricular dysfunction (left ventricular ejection fraction <35%)
- Obesity
- Prior carebral vascular accident
- Renal insufficiency
- Suspected or known left main coronary stenosis
- Uncontrolled hypertension
- Unstable angina

SOURCE: From Kern MJ. *The Cardiac Catheterization Handbook*. St. Louis: Mosby; 2003. With permission.

TABLE 17-5 Conditions Requiring Special Preparations for Cardiac Catheterization

| Condition | Management |
|---|---|
| Allergy | Treat potential hypersensitivity |
| Prior contrast studies | Contrast premedication |
| Iodine, fish | Contrast reaction algorithm |
| Premedication allergy | Hold premedication |
| Lidocaine | Use Marcaine (1 mg/ML) |
| Patients receiving anticoagulation (INR > 1.5) | Defer procedure |
| | Vitamin K |
| | Fresh frozen plasma |
| | Hold heparin |
| | Protamine for heparin |
| Diabetes | Hydration, urine output >50 mL/hr |
| NPH insulin (protamine reaction) | Glucophage held 48 h |
| Renal function | If renal insufficiency postpone catheterization |
| (Prone to contrast-induced renal failure) | Consider urgency and risks of lactic acidosis |
| Glucophage usage | |
| Electrolyte imbalance ($K^+$, $Mg^{2+}$, or $Mg^{++}$) | Defer procedure, replenish/correct electrolytes |
| Arrthythmias | Defer procedure, administer antiarrhythmics |
| Anemia | Defer procedure |
| | Control bleeding |
| | Transfuse |
| Dehydration | Hydration |
| Renal failure | Limit contrast |
| | Maintain high urine output |
| | Hydrate |

SOURCE: From Kern MJ. *The Cardiac Catheterization Handbook,* St. Louis: Mosby; 2003. With permission.

attached to the Seldinger needle and gently aspirated during needle advancement. Once in the vein, the remainder of the venous sheath placement is completed in the same fashion as described for the femoral arterial sheath insertion.

**RADIAL ARTERY CATHETERIZATION**

Campeau first described the radial approach for coronary angiography in 1989.[8] The technique has gained widespread acceptance around the world. Kiemeneij, of the Netherlands, also pioneered the radial approach for coronary interventions.[9] The radial approach has several distinct advantages: (1) the radial artery is easily accessible in most patients and is not located near significant veins or nerves; (2) the superficial location of the radial artery makes for easy control of bleeding; (3) no significant clinical sequelae after radial artery occlusion occur in patients with a normal Allen test because of the collateral flow to the hand through the ulnar artery; (4) patient comfort is enhanced by the ability to sit up and walk immediately after the procedure; and (5) the radial artery access provides the most secure hemostasis in the fully anticoagulated patient.

Patients with a normal Allen test (Table 17-7) are candidates for the radial approach with 5F and 6F sheaths and catheters. Small or female patients are more likely to have spasm of the radial artery, but this can be treated effectively with the use of intraarterial nitroglycerin or verapamil. Specially coated hydrophilic sheaths reduce spasm on sheath insertion and removal.

Arterial puncture using a short 20-gauge needle, a 0.025-in. guidewire, and a radial artery sheath system (24 cm) is performed in a manner similar to femoral artery puncture. The point of puncture is over the radial artery pulsation on the wrist. After puncture, the small guidewire is inserted followed by a long arterial sheath. During arterial sheath insertion, 5000 U of heparin, 2 mL of 1% lidocaine, and 200 $\mu$g of nitroglycerin are often given through the partially positioned sheath. An additional intraarteriolar vasodilator—such as diltiazem, verapamil, papaverine, or adenosine—may be necessary to minimize spasm of the radial artery. After vascular access has been secured, angiographic and hemodynamic data are obtained, as discussed below.

TABLE 17-6 Possible Vascular Access Routes

- Arterial
  - Axillary
  - Brachial
  - Femoral
  - Radial
  - Subclavian—*not* used for cardiac catheterization
  - Translumbar—*not* used for cardiac catheterization
- Venous
  - Brachial
  - Femoral
  - Internal jugular
  - Subclavian

## Access Site Hemostasis

After the catheterization procedure has been completed and the catheters removed, the sheath is flushed. If heparin has been given, an activated clotting time (ACT) is obtained; if this is >200 s, protamine sulfate may be given before sheath removal (25 to 50 mg protamine IV reverses 10,000 U heparin). Caution should be used in giving protamine to patients receiving NPH insulin, who may have higher likelihood of a protamine reaction (Table 17-8).

To remove the femoral artery sheath, gentle pressure is applied over the puncture site while the sheath is removed, taking care not to crush the sheath and "strip" clot into the distal artery. Firm downward pressure is applied for 15 to 30 min, periodically evaluating distal pulses. After manual hemostasis is achieved, an adhesive bandage is used to cover the wound. Large pressure dressings are generally ineffective to prevent bleeding and obscure the puncture site. Additional methods to secure postprocedure arterial hemostasis include mechanical pressure clamps and vascular closure devices.

Four vascular closure devices are currently available.[10–12] These devices reduce the time to obtain hemostasis and early ambulation.

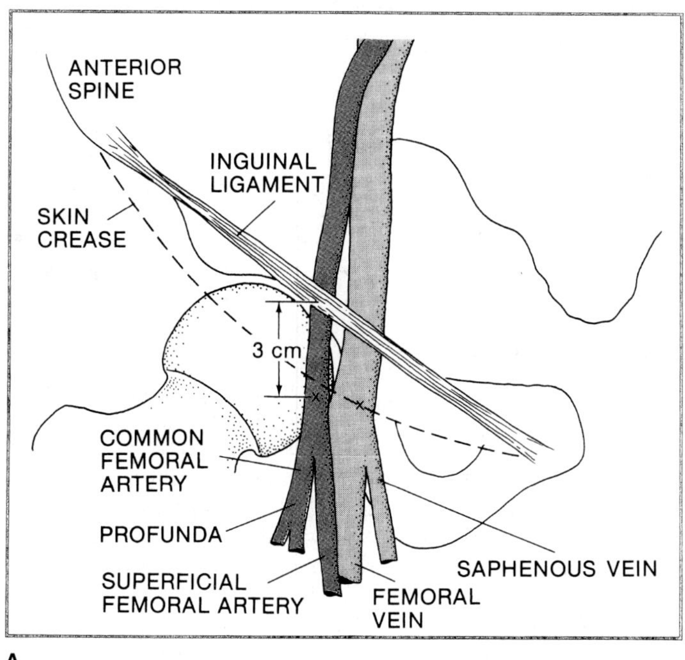


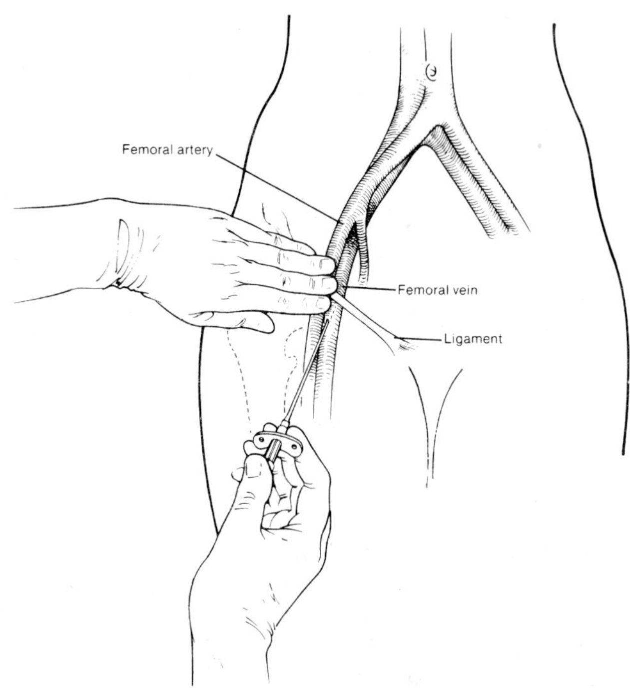


FIGURE 17-1 *A.* Anatomy relevant to percutaneous catheterization of the femoral artery and vein. The right femoral artery vein pass underneath the inguinal ligament, which connects the anterior-superior iliac spine and public tubercle. The arterial skin nick (indicated by X) should be placed approximately 1 ½ to two fingerbreadths (3 cm) below the inguinal ligament and directly over the femoral artery pulsation. The venous skin nick should be placed at the same level, but approximately one fingerbreadth medial. (From Baim DS, Grossman W. Percutaneous approach including transseptal and apical puncture. In: Baim DS, Grossman W, eds. *Grossman's Cardiac Catheterization, Angiography, and Intervention*, 6th ed. Baltimore: Lippincott, Williams & Wilkins; 2000. With permission.) *B.* Femoral vein puncture with the needle at a 30- to 45-degree angle aiming medially toward the umbilicus. (From Tilkian AG, Daily EK, *Cardiovascular Procedures: Diagnostic Techniques and Therapeutic Procedures*. St Louis: Mosby; 1986. With permission.)

Collagen, either plugs (Vasoseal and Angioseal) or liquid (Duett) can be delivered directly to the arterial puncture site through a special sheath system (Vasoseal or Duett) or anchored inside of the vessel (Angioseal). A percutaneous vascular suture delivery system (Perclose) also provides hemostasis and permits early ambulation. These devices may especially be helpful in anticoagulated patients and patients with back pain or an inability to lie flat. The advantages and disadvantages are summarized in Table 17-9. All vascular closure devices should be used with caution in patients with peripheral vascular disease or low arterial puncture (at or below the femoral bifurcation). Femoral angiography with an oblique angle will demonstrate the puncture site and any artery disease. Patients at high risk for groin hematoma and arterial complications who may need longer pressure application or may benefit with a vascular closure device are listed in Table 17-10.

For radial artery hemostasis, sheath removal utilizes a plastic bracelet with a pressure pad placed around the wrist.[9] While pressing the pad over the puncture site, the sheath is then gently withdrawn and the bracelet tightened. The bracelet should be tight enough to ensure hemostasis but not occlude the flow to the hand. An hour or two later, the patient is checked and the bracelet is loosened. The patient can be discharged 2 h later and the bracelet removed at home.

TABLE 17-7 The Allen Test

The Allen test assesses the circulation of an intact palmar arterial arch.

Method:

1. The radial and ulnar arteries are simultaneously occluded while the patient makes a fist.
2. The hand is opened appearing blanched.
3. The ulnar artery is released, and the hand observed for change in color.

Satisfactory ulnar flow is present if color returns to palm in 8 to 10 s or if pulse oximetry normalizes on release of the artery.

TABLE 17-8 Characteristics and Treatment of a Protamine Reaction[a]

Characteristics
- Shaking
- Flushing
- Chills
- Back, chest, or flank pain
- Vasomotor collapse

Treatment
1. Morphine (2 mg IV) or meperidine (25 mg IV),
2. Diphenhydramine (25 to 50 mg IV)
3. Saline administration
4. Support of low blood pressure

[a]Protamine reactions are usually self-limited (<1 h).

TABLE 17-9 Advantages/Disadvantages of Vascular Closure Devices

| Device | Mechanism | Vascular Closure Devices Advantages and Limitations |
|---|---|---|
| AngioSeal | Collagen seal | Secure hemostasis<br>Anchor may catch on side branch |
| Duett | Collagen-thrombin | Stronger collagen-thrombin seal<br>Intraarterial injection of collagen-thrombin |
| Perclose | Sutures | Secure hemostasis of suture<br>Device failure may require surgical repair |
| VasoSeal | Collagen plug | No intraarterial components<br>Positioning wire may catch on side branch |

## Equipment in the Catheterization Laboratory

### CATHETERS FOR ANGIOGRAPHY AND HEMODYNAMICS

Numerous shapes and sizes of catheters are available to the angiographer. Basic, routine catheters that are preshaped for normal anatomy are available for both the radial and femoral approaches. There is an array of shapes and sizes to aid the angiographer when abnormal anatomy is present (Fig. 17-2).

***Judkins-Type Coronary Catheters*** The Judkins catheters have unique preshaped curves and tapered end-hole tips. The Judkins left coronary catheter has a double curve. The length of the segment between the primary and secondary curve determines the size of the catheter (i.e., 3.5, 4.0, 5.0, or 6.0 cm). The proper size of the left judkins catheter is selected depending on the length and width of the ascending aorta. The ingenious design of the left Judkins catheter permits cannulation of the left coronary artery without any major catheter manipulation except the slow advance of the catheter under fluoroscopic control. The catheter tip follows the ascending aortic border and falls into the left main coronary ostium, often with an abrupt jump. In the words of its inventor, "The [Judkins] catheter knows where to go if not thwarted by the operator." A left 4-cm Judkins catheter fits in most adult patients. When catheter size is adequate, the catheter tip is aligned with the long axis of the left main coronary trunk. A smaller (3.5-cm) catheter in the same patient will tip upward toward the anterior descending artery and a larger (5.0-cm) catheter will tip downward into the circumflex ostium.

The Judkins right coronary catheter is sized by the length of the secondary curve and comes in 3.5-, 4.0-, and 5.0-cm sizes. The 4.0-cm catheter is adequate in the majority of cases. The right Judkins catheter is advanced into the ascending aorta (usually with LAO projection) with the tip directed caudally.

TABLE 17-10 Patients Who May Benefit from a Vascular Closure Device

| |
|---|
| Obese patients |
| Patients with hypertension |
| Elderly |
| Women |
| Patients with aortic insufficiency |
| Patients who have undergone prior arterial puncture |
| Patients with advanced peripheral atherosclerosis |
| Patients who suffer from coagulopathy or those receiving anticoagulant or antiplatelet agents |

SOURCE: From Kern MJ. *The Cardiac Catheterization Handbook*. St. Louis: Mosby; 2003. With permission.

***Amplatz-type catheters*** The left Amplatz-type catheter (Fig. 17-2) is a preshaped half circle with the tapered tip extending perpendicular to the curve. Amplatz catheter sizes (left 1, 2, and 3 and right 1 and 2) indicate the diameter of the tip's curve. In the LAO projection, the tip is advanced into the left aortic cusp. Further advancement of the catheter causes the tip to move upward into the left main trunk. It is necessary to push the Amplatz catheters slightly to disengage by backing the catheter tip upward and out of the left main ostium. If the catheter is pulled instead of first being advanced, the tip moves downward and into the left main or circumflex artery. Unwanted deep cannulation might tear this branch or the left main trunk. *Amplatz catheters have a higher incidence of coronary dissection than Judkins-style catheters.*

The right Amplatz (modified) catheter has a smaller but similar hook-shaped curve. The catheter is advanced into the right coronary cusp. As with Judkins right catheters, the catheter is rotated clockwise for 45 to 90 degrees. The same maneuver is repeated at different levels until the right coronary artery is entered. After coronary injections, the catheter may be pulled, advanced, or rotated out of the coronary artery.

***Multipurpose Catheters*** These catheters are mostly straight catheters with an end hole and two side holes placed close to the tapered tip. Preshaped, mildly angled configurations are also available. The multipurpose catheter can be used for both left and right coronary injections and left ventriculography.

***Special-Purpose Femoral Catheters for Bypass Grafts*** The right coronary vein graft catheter is similar to a right Judkins catheter with a wider, more open primary curve allowing cannulation of vertically oriented coronary artery vein graft. The left vein graft catheter is similar to the right Judkins catheter with a smaller and sharper secondary curve, allowing easy cannulation of left anterior descending [coronary artery] (LAD) and left circumflex vein grafts, which usually are placed higher and more anterior than the right coronary grafts with a relatively horizontal and upward takeoff from the aorta. The internal mammary artery graft catheter has a peculiar hook-shaped tip configuration that facilitates the engagement of internal mammary artery grafts, especially in patients with a very vertical origin of the internal mammary artery.

***Ventriculography Catheters*** The pigtail catheter has a tapered tip, preshaped to make a full circle 1 cm in diameter. Five to twelve side holes are located on the straight portion of the catheter above the curve. A pigtail catheter with an angled (145-degree) shaft is also available for horizontally oriented hearts. Another variation on the pigtail catheter is one with a helical tip with inward-directed side holes (Halo catheter, Angiodynamics, Inc.). Unlike a pigtail catheter, it has all side holes located at the coiled end and the end of the catheter points inward, reducing ectopy during ventriculography. The multipurpose catheter is also used for femoral ventriculography, but the high-pressure contrast jet from the end hole often produces sig-

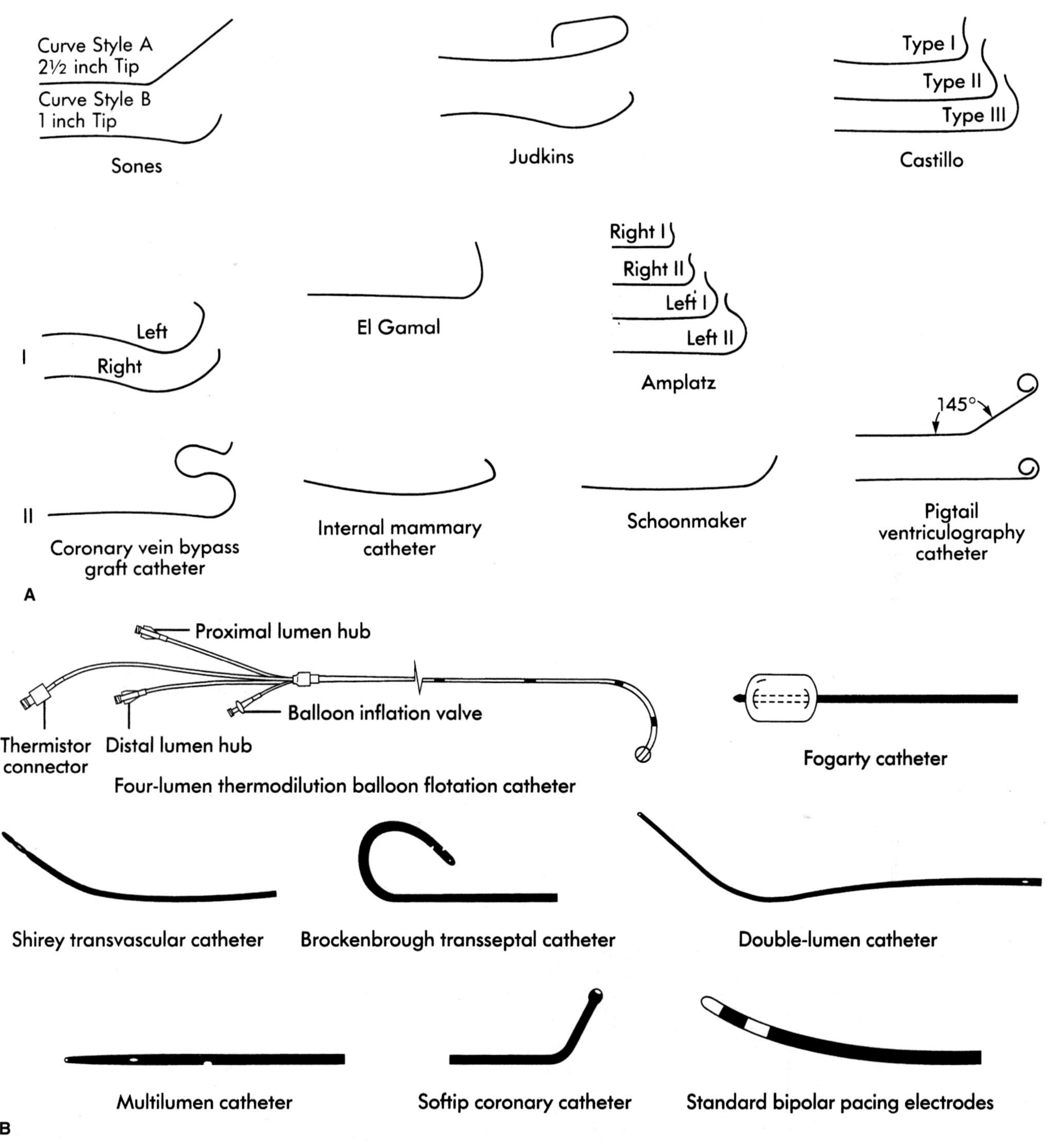


FIGURE 17-2 *A.* Left heart catheters in common use for selective coronary arteriography and ventriculography. (From Kern MJ. *Cardiac Catheterization Handbook.* St Louis: Mosby; 2003. With permission.) *B.* Various special-purpose catheters for right and left heart catheterization. (Modified from Tilkian AG, Daily EK. *Cardiovascular Procedures: Diagnostic Techniques and Therapeutic Procedures.* St. Louis: Mosby; 1986. With permission.)

nificant ventricular tachycardia; rarely, myocardial tissue contrast staining or perforation occurs.

A comprehensive discussion of left heart catheter types and techniques can be found elsewhere.[5–7] The new operator should concentrate on mastering a few types of catheters and gain extensive experience in using them effectively.

***Right Heart Catheters*** For right heart catheterization, a balloon-tipped flotation catheter (Fig. 17-2), originally designed by Drs. H.J.C. Swan and W. Ganz, is the most widely used. The balloon tip allows the catheter to float through the right side of the heart safely and easily in a majority of cases. The balloon "wedges" in the distal pulmonary artery to measure pressure and accurately reflects left atrial and ventricular filling pressures. Thermodilution cardiac output measurements are exclusive to this type of catheter. The balloon-tipped catheter can be introduced through any venous access route. The balloon is inflated with room air. The balloon-tipped catheters do not provide good torque control, making catheterization of the pulmonary artery in patients with right atrial or ventricular enlargement, pulmonary hypertension, or tricuspid regurgitation difficult from the femoral approach.

For right heart angiography, the Berman catheter, a large-lumen, balloon-tipped angiographic catheter with side holes placed proximally to the balloon, is introduced easily into the right heart. Keeping the balloon inflated increases the catheter stability during angiography. A regular pigtail catheter, or one with a special obtuse angle (Grollman), can also be used for right ventriculography.

### THE FLUOROSCOPIC IMAGING SYSTEM

Passage of catheters and acquisition of angiographic data requires a high-resolution image-intensifier television system with digital cineangiographic capabilities. The components are mounted on a C arm, which is a semicircular support with the x-ray tube beneath the patient and the image intensifier above. Rotation of the C arm allows viewing over a wide range of different angles. The patient is placed in the center of the semicircle, which can be moved 180 degrees around the patient. Some laboratories have two C arms perpendicular to one another (called "biplane" arms) and use a double monitoring system, providing simultaneous visualization of the heart from two different angles (Fig. 17-3).

### THE PHYSIOLOGIC MONITOR AND RECORDING SYSTEM

During catheterization, it is necessary to monitor and record electrocardiographic and hemodynamic signals. Digital recording systems incorporate physiologic data with digital angiographic data.

### CONTRAST POWER INJECTOR

A high-pressure contrast media injector is needed to administer a large bolus (20 to 50 mL) of contrast media into the left ventricle (10 to 20 mL/s), pulmonary arteries (10 to 25 mL/s), or aortic arch (40 to 60 mL/s). When properly set and flushed, the power injector can be used to inject contrast into the coronary arteries (3 to 8 mL/s). Some injector systems also incorporate a pressure transducer and have replaced traditional manifolds with stopcocks.

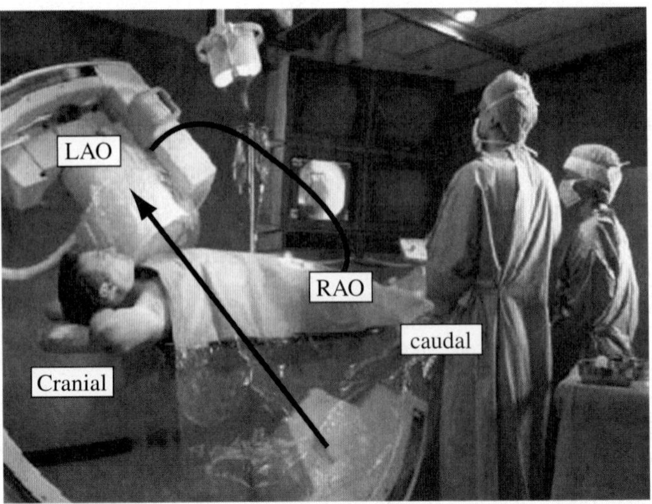


FIGURE 17-3 The cardiac catheterization laboratory. The operators stand on the patient's right side facing the fluoroscopic and hemodynamic monitors. The fluoroscope is positioned over the patient's left shoulder to produce a left anterior oblique (LAO) cranially angulated view of the heart. The image intensifier can be rotated to other positions (e.g., caudal or right anterior oblique (RAO) as well to visualize the cardiac structures from any angle.

### "CRASH CART" AND DEFIBRILLATOR

Every cardiovascular laboratory is equipped with an emergency crash cart containing emergency drugs, oxygen, airways, suction apparatus, and other emergency equipment. A defibrillator should be charged and ready for use during a procedure.

### STERILE EQUIPMENT AND SUPPLIES

The angiographer works from a sterile pack or tray that contains the various supplies needed to perform the procedure. The pack will contain syringes and needles, local anesthetic, basins for flushing solutions, small drapes and towels, clamps, scalpels, pressure manifolds and connecting tubings, and the like.

## Radiographic Contrast Media

### CHARACTERISTICS OF CONTRAST MEDIA

All contrast media contain three iodine molecules attached to a fully substituted benzene ring. The fourth position in the standard ionic agent is taken up by sodium or methylglucamine as a cation; the remaining two positions of the benzene ring have side chains of diatrizoate, metatrizoate, or iothalamate. All media are excreted predominantly by glomerular filtration. The normal half-time of excretion is 20 min; biliary excretion is 1 percent. A dose of 0.5 to 1.0 mL/kg of medium is selected based on total body weight, size of the heart chambers, systemic blood flow, degree of left-to-right shunting, severity of pulmonary vascular disease, and clinical status of the patient. The vasodilator effect and the transient decrease in systemic vascular resistance are directly related to the degree of osmolality of the contrast medium used. Transient hypervolemia and depressed contractility are related to both osmolality and ionic charge and in part responsible for the elevation of left atrial and left ventricular (LV) end-diastolic pressure after contrast injection.

To reduce the osmotic effects of contrast medium, the number of dissolved particles must be decreased or the molal concentration of iodine per particle must be increased. New-generation, nonionic, monomeric, and ionic dimeric contrast agents have approximately the same viscosity and iodine concentration but have only one-half or less of the osmolality of the ionic agents.[13–15] Ionic contrast media produce hypotension by peripheral arterial vasodilation, transient myocardial dysfunction, and decreasing circulating volume and blood pressure after osmotic diuresis. Initially contrast media increase circulating fluid volume by osmotically shifting fluid into vascular space. The advantages of the nonionic, low-osmolar agents include less hemodynamic loading, patient discomfort, binding of ionic calcium, depression of myocardial function and blood pressure, and possibly fewer anaphylactoid reactions.[13–15] Currently, nonionic, low-osmolar agents are preferred in all patients, but especially in adults with extremely poor LV function; in patients with renal disease, especially those with diabetes; and in patients with a history of serious reaction to contrast media or with multiple allergies.

Table 17-11 provides a summary of commonly used contrast agents for coronary and left ventricular angiographic studies. Although thousands of studies have been performed safely with conventional high-osmolar/ionic agents, considerable data exist indicating that low-osmolar/nonionic agents may be safer and provide satisfactory diagnostic quality, especially for high-risk patients[16] (Table 17-12).

### CONTRAST MEDIA REACTIONS

The Committee on Safety of Contrast Media of the International Society of Radiology report that in more than 300,000 patients the overall incidence of adverse reaction was <5 percent. Adverse reactions

TABLE 17-11 Commonly Used Iodinated Contrast Agents in Cardiac Angiography

| Product Category | Proprietary Name | Generic Constituent | Ratio to Iodine to Osmotically Active Particles | Calcium Chelation | Anticoagulation Effect |
|---|---|---|---|---|---|
| High-osmolar, ionic | Renografin-76 | Diatrizoate and citrate | 1.5 | (+) | (+++) |
| High-osmolar, ionic | Hypaque-76 | Diatrizoate only | 1.5 | (−) | (+++) |
| Low-osmolar, ionic | Hexabrix | Ioxaglate | 3.0 | (−) | (+++) |
| Low-osmolar, nonionic | Isovue | Iopamidol | 3.0 | (−) | (+) |
| Low-osmolar, nonionic | Omnipaque | Iohexol | 3.0 | (−) | (+) |
| Low-osmolar, nonionic | Optiray | Ioversol | 3.0 | (−) | (+) |

KEY: (+) = present; (+++) = strongly present; (−) = absent.
SOURCE: From Peterson KL, Nicod P. *Cardiac Catheterization: methods, diagnosis, and therapy*. Philadelphia: Saunders; 1997. With permission.

were found in 10 to 12 percent of patients with a history of allergy and in 15 percent of patients with reported reaction on previous examination. From these reports major life-threatening reactions do not tend to recur on reexamination, whereas minor reactions are more likely to be repeated.

There are three types of contrast allergies (Table 17-13): (1) minor cutaneous and mucosal manifestations, (2) smooth muscle and minor anaphylactoid responses, and (3) major cardiovascular and anaphylactoid responses. Major reactions involving laryngeal or pulmonary edema often are accompanied by minor or less severe reactions. Although some reactions to a pretest contrast dose may be violent (but rarely life-threatening), pretesting has been found to be of no value in determining who will have an adverse reaction. Nonionic contrast media has replaced ionic contrast media for most patients to minimize chance of allergic and other adverse contrast reactions.

Patients reporting allergic reactions to contrast media should be premedicated with prednisone and diphenhydramine. The routine for the laboratory may vary, but common dosages include 60 mg prednisone the night before, and 60 mg of prednisone the morning of, along with 50 mg oral diphenhydramine given at the time of call to the catheterization laboratory. Pretreatment with corticosteroids has been found to be helpful in reducing all types of reactions except those characterized predominantly by hives. Premedication may not prevent the occurrence of adverse reactions completely. Additional routine treatment of patients with prior allergic reactions with an $H_2$ blocker (e.g., cimetidine) does not appear to have any benefit. Patients with known prior anaphylacoid reactions to contrast dye should be pretreated with steroids and an $H_1$ blocker.

TABLE 17-12 Indications for Low-Osmolar/Nonionic Contrast Agents

Unstable ischemic syndromes
Congestive heart failure
Diabetes
Renal insufficiency
Hypotension
Severe bradycardia
History of contrast allergy
Severe valvular heart disease
Use for internal mammary artery and peripheral vascular injections

**CONTRAST-INDUCED RENAL FAILURE**

Patients with diabetes or renal insufficiency or those who are dehydrated from any cause are at risk for contrast-induced nephropathy (CIN). Advanced preparations to limit CIN include hydration and maintenance of large-volume urine flow (>200 mL/h). These patients should be hydrated intravenously the night before the procedure. Following the contrast study, intravenous fluids should be liberally continued unless intravascular volume overload is a problem. Furosemide (Lasix), mannitol and calcium channel blockers are not helpful in reducing CIN (see Table 17-14). Fenoldopam and *N*-acetylcysteine given intravenously before the procedure are associated with reduced CIN in some studies,[16a,b,c] but not in others.[16d] A decreased urine output after the procedure which is not responsive to increased intravenous fluids indicates that renal insufficiency is probable. A consultation with a nephrologist is often helpful. All types of contrast agents (ionic, nonionic, or low-osmolar) are associated with a similiar incidence of contrast-induced nephropathy.

## Complications of Cardiac Catheterization

Table 17-15 lists the major and minor complications of cardiac catheterization. For diagnostic catheterization, analysis of the complications in more than 200,000 patients indicates the incidence of risks as follows: death, <0.2 percent; myocardial infarction, <0.05 percent; stroke, <0.07 percent; serious ventricular arrhythmia, <0.5

TABLE 17-13 Anaphylactoid Reactions to Contrast Medium

- Cutaneous and mucosal
  - Angioedema
  - Flushing
  - Laryngeal edema
  - Pruritus
  - Urticaria
- Smooth muscle
  - Bronchospasm
  - Gastrointestinal spasm
  - Uterine contraction
- Cardiovascular
  - Arrhythmia
  - Hypotension (shock)
  - Vasodilatation

TABLE 17-14 Summary of Contrast Induced Renal Failure Prophylaxis Trials

| Beneficial | Deleterious | Conflicting Data | No Effect |
|---|---|---|---|
| IV hydration | Furosemide (without volume replacement) | Calcium channel blockers | Hemodialysis |
| Forced duresis | Ionic contrast | Dopamine | Atrial natriuretic peptide |
| Nonionic contrast | Endothelin receptor blocker | Theophylline | Allopurinol |
| Acetylcysteine | Mannitol (without volume replacement) | Captopril | |
| PGE-1 | | | |
| Fenoldopam | | | |

SOURCE: From McCullough, PA, Mauley HS. Prediction and prevention of contrast nephropathy. *J Intervent Cardiol* 2001;14:547–558. With permission.

percent; and major vascular complications (thrombosis, bleeding requiring transfusion, or pseudoaneurysm), <1 percent[17–20] (Table 17-16). Vascular complications are more frequent when the brachial approach is used. Risks are higher in well-described subgroups.

## COMPLICATIONS OF ARTERIAL ACCESS

The most common complication from femoral catheterization is hemorrhage and local hematoma formation, increasing in frequency with the increasing size of the sheath, the amount of anticoagulation, and obesity. Other common complications (in order of decreasing frequency) include retroperitoneal hematoma, pseudoaneurysm, arteriovenous (AV) fistula, arterial thrombosis, stroke,[19] sepsis with or without abscess formation, and cholesterol or air embolization.[20] The frequency of these complications is increased in obese patients; high-risk procedures; critically ill elderly patients with extensive atheromatous disease; patients receiving anticoagulation, antiplatelet, and fibrinolytic therapies; and concomitant interventional procedures. Compared to the femoral approach, the radial approach causes significantly fewer vascular complications.

A retroperitoneal hematoma should be suspected in patients with hypotension, tachycardia, pallor, a rapidly falling hematocrit postcatheterization, lower abdominal or back pain, or neurologic changes in the leg with the puncture. This complication is associated with *high femoral arterial puncture* and *full anticoagulation.*[18] Pseudoaneurysm is a complication associated with *low femoral arterial puncture* (usually below the head of the femur). With ultrasound imaging techniques the pseudoaneurysm can easily be identified and nonsurgical closure performed. Manual compression of the expansile growing mass guided by Doppler ultrasound with or without thrombin or collagen injection is an acceptable therapy for femoral pseudoaneurysm.[21]

## PROTAMINE REACTIONS

Protamine is commonly used in reversing the systemic effects of heparin. Minor protamine reactions may appear as back and flank pain or flushing with peripheral vasodilation and low blood pressure. Major protamine reactions simulate anaphylaxis. Although rare, major reactions involve marked facial flushing and vasomotor collapse, which may be fatal. The incidence of major protamine reactions in NPH insulin-dependent diabetics is 27 percent, compared to 0.5 percent in patients with no history of insulin use. It is recommended that diabetics on NPH insulin and patients with allergies to fish undergoing cardiac catheterization do so without use of protamine or, when necessary, that protamine be administered cautiously in anticipation of a major reaction.

## COMPLICATIONS OF RIGHT HEART CATHETERIZATION

Right heart catheterization may be complicated by arrhythmia due to stimulation of the right ventricular (RV) outflow tract, which may re-

TABLE 17-15 Complications of Cardiac Catheterization

- Major
  - Cerebrovascular accident
  - Death
  - Myocardial infarction
  - Ventricular tachycardia, fibrillation, or serious arrhythmia
- Other
  - Aortic dissection
  - Cardiac perforation, tamponade
  - Congestive heart failure
  - Contrast reaction/anaphylaxis/nephrotoxicity
  - Heart block, asystole
  - Hemorrhage (local, retroperitoneal, pelvic)
  - Infection
  - Protamine reaction
  - Supraventricular tachyarrhythmia, atrial fibrillation
  - Thrombosis/embolus/air embolus
  - Vascular injury, pseudoaneurysm
  - Vasovagal reaction

TABLE 17-16 Incidence of Major Complications of Diagnostic Catheterizations

| | Percent |
|---|---|
| Death | 0.11 |
| Myocardial infarction | 0.05 |
| Neurologic | 0.07 |
| Arrhythmia | 0.38 |
| Vascular | 0.43 |
| Contrast | 0.37 |
| Hemodynamic | 0.26 |
| Perforation | 0.03 |
| Other | 0.28 |
| Total (patients) | 1.98 |

SOURCE: Modified from Noto TJ, Johnson LW, Krone R, et al. Cardiac catheterization 1990: A report of the Registry of the Society for Cardiac Angiography and Interventions (SCA&I), *Cathet Cardiovasc Diagn* 1991;24:75–83 and Uretzky BF, Weinert HH. *Cardiac Catheterization: Concepts, Techniques, and Applications*. Walden, MA: Blackwell; 1997. With permission.

TABLE 17-17 Complications of Right Heart (Pulmonary Artery) Catheterization

| | Major | Minor |
|---|---|---|
| Access | Pneumothorax | Hematoma |
| | Hemothorax | Thrombosis |
| | Tracheal perforation (subclavian route) | |
| | Sepsis | Cellulitis |
| Intracardiac | Right ventricular perforation | Ventricular arrhythmia |
| | Heart block (right bundle branch block) pulmonary rupture | |
| | Pulmonary infarction | |

sult in atrioventricular block, or, rarely, right bundle branch block (Table 17-17). Significant but transient ventricular arrhythmias occur in 30 to 60 percent of patients undergoing right heart catheterization and are terminated when the catheter is readjusted. Sustained ventricular arrhythmias have been reported, especially in unstable patients or those with electrolyte imbalance, acidosis, or concurrent myocardial ischemia. In patients with left bundle branch block, a temporary pacemaker may be needed if right bundle branch block occurs during right heart catheterization.

## CARDIAC ANGIOGRAPHY

In 1923, Osborn noted that the urinary bladder of luetic patients treated with oral and intravenous sodium iodide became opaque to x-rays because of the absorption of photons by iodine. Contrast medium was first injected through a rubber catheter placed in the right ventricle by Chavez in 1947. *Cineangiography* is the term used to describe the x-ray photographing of cardiac and vascular structures. This term persists even though radiographic images are now stored electronically on digital computer imaging media (e.g., CD-ROM) rather than on cine film.[22] Angiographic images are the visual representation of the vascular conduits and networks connected to internal structures (organs) and, at times, predict cardiovascular function. Catheterization and angiography are performed as combined techniques to provide hemodynamic and anatomic data. Optimal angiographic data collection is a series of linked steps. Failure of any link may cause loss of all or part of the data. Angiography begins with the positioning of the patient on the table, performing the angiographic image recording, storing the digital image data, and finally displaying the images for review and analysis.

Angiography is the primary method of defining coronary anatomy in living patients, providing an anatomic map of the site, severity, shape and distribution of stenotic lesions. In addition, the characteristics of distal vessel size, intracoronary thrombus, diffuse atherosclerotic disease, mass of myocardium served, an approximate index of coronary flow, and identification of collateral vessels can be obtained. The presence of coronary spasm can be ascertained by using provocative maneuvers.[23] The functional significance of a coronary stenosis can be assessed by measuring coronary flow or pressure directly, using information obtained both at rest and during maximal coronary vasodilatation.[24] A full discussion of assessing the functional significance of coronary angiographic lesions is provided later in this chapter.

Included in nearly every coronary angiographic study is left ventriculography. Contrast opacification of the contracting ventricle enables one to make a visual analysis of wall motion. Ventricular systolic and diastolic volume and ejection fraction can be calculated. Examination of the left ventriculogram helps identify viable myocardium. LV wall motion can be further evaluated by the addition of stress such as atrial pacing, pharmacologic agents, or exercise. Assessing viability through augmenting LV contraction by the use of nitrates, catecholamines, or postextrasystolic beats facilitate decisions for revascularization.[25–27] LV angiography also documents mitral regurgitation.

### Coronary Arteriography

Sones ushered in the modern era of coronary arteriography in 1958 when he developed a safe and reliable method of selective coronary arteriography.[28] The Sones technique used an antecubital brachial artery incision and a woven Dacron catheter. The catheter was maneuvered into the ascending aorta and then the soft, tapered catheter tip was deflected off the aortic valve cusps up to the coronary orifices. Although the Sones technique has been surpassed by percutaneous femoral, brachial, and radial artery techniques with preformed angiographic catheters, manipulative skills and precise knowledge of the aortic root anatomy are still required for all coronary angiographic techniques.

Percutaneous arterial catheterization, described in 1953 by Seldinger,[29] was first used to study the coronary arteries, as reported by Ricketts and Abrams in 1962.[30] Modification of catheters was made by Amplatz et al.[31] and by Judkins[32] in 1967. The Judkins technique, the most popular coronary angiographic technique in the world, uses three preformed catheters: one for each coronary artery and a pigtail catheter for the LV injection. The Judkins technique is much easier to learn than the Sones technique (Fig. 17-4). The Judkins technique is highly successful because of the simplicity of using preshaped catheters from the femoral approach as compared to the Sones technique, where the operator must use more manipulation to position the catheter in the coronary ostia from the arm. A multipurpose (Sones-style) catheter is still used but its devotees are few. Coronary angiography can be completed using Judkins catheters from the femoral approach in more than 95 percent of patients.

In an attempt to combine the advantages of the Sones and Judkins techniques, the single-catheter percutaneous femoral approach was first applied by Schoonmaker in 1968, and use of this technique was reported by Schoonmaker and King.[33] This technique has also become obsolete and replaced nearly completely by the Judkins technique. A detailed description of the Judkins technique also has been published.[34]

The description of the performance of coronary arteriography provided herein is necessarily brief; more detailed descriptions are available.[5–7,35] Expertise in performing coronary arteriography is achieved by training in an active laboratory and performing hundreds of coronary arteriograms under close supervision. In this way the physician can gain needed skills and an appreciation of the potential hazards of coronary arteriography; The American College of Cardiology/American Heart Association (ACC/AHA) recommendations for the performance of coronary angiography[3] are provided in Appendix 17-1.

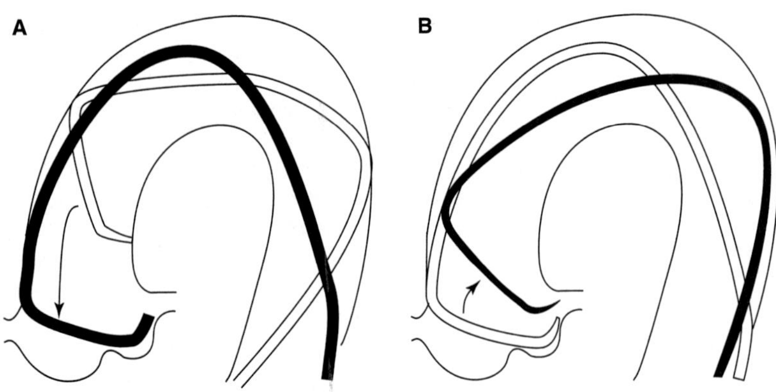


FIGURE 17-4 Push-pull technique for catheterizing the left coronary artery with the Judkins left catheter. *A.* In the left anterior oblique view, the coronary catheter is positioned in the ascending aorta over a guidewire and the guidewire is removed. The catheter is advanced so that the tip enters the left sinus of Valsalva. If the catheter does not selectively engage the ostium of the left coronary artery, further slow advancement into the left sinus of Valsalva imparts a temporary acute angle at the catheter. *B.* Prompt withdrawal of the catheter allows easy entry into the left coronary artery. (From Braunwald E, Zipes DP, Libby P, eds. *Heart Disease: A Textbook of Cardiovascular Medicine*, 6th ed. Philadelphia: Saunders; 2001. With permission.)

## Techniques of Cannulating Coronary Arteries and Grafts

### LEFT CORONARY ARTERY

A short left main and separate ostia for left anterior descending and circumflex arteries can present problems for cannulation. In these cases it may be necessary to cannulate the left anterior descending (LAD) and circumflex (CX) arteries separately. Slightly advancing the left Judkins catheter or using a left Judkins catheter that is one size smaller (i.e., 3.5 cm from 4.0 cm) permits cannulation of the LAD artery. Slight withdrawal and clockwise rotation of the catheter or use of a left Judkins catheter that is one size larger permit cannulation of the CX artery. An Amplatz-type catheter is especially useful to cannulate the CX artery separately but must be used with care to avoid arterial dissection. An unusually high origin of the left main coronary artery from the aorta usually can be cannulated using a multipurpose catheter or an Amplatz-type catheter (e.g., AL 2). To cannulate the high-origin left main trunk through the brachial approach, a long tapered-tip multipurpose catheter may be used. In patients with a relatively horizontal and wide aortic root with upward takeoff of the left main coronary artery, a large-curve left Judkins catheter (5 or 6 cm), an Amplatz-type left coronary catheter, or a multipurpose catheter may be required.

### RIGHT CORONARY ARTERY

The origin of the right coronary artery shows more variation than that of the left coronary artery. A contrast injection low into the right coronary cusp will show the origin of the right coronary artery and help the angiogapher direct the catheter. If the right coronary artery is not seen with this injection, it may be totally occluded or may have an anomalous origin, anteriorly on the aorta or from the left sinus of Valsalva. In this case the orifice usually is located above the sinotubular ridge. A left Amplatz catheter or a left bypass graft catheter can be used successfully to engage the right coronary artery orifice located anteriorly or in the left cusp. Minimal anterior displacement of the right coronary artery from the right coronary sinus is more common. In this case, the right Judkins catheter tip may not be directed toward the right, but appear foreshortened (seen on end) in the left anterior oblique (LAO) view. Directing the catheter tip to the right in the usual fashion using the lateral view permits easy cannulation of the anteriorly directed right coronary Rarely an aortogram will be needed to confirm the presence of the RCA. In a patient with a horizontal and wide aortic root or high ostial origin, cannulation of the right coronary orifice and right coronary cusp may require an Amplatz or multipurpose catheter.

### SAPHENOUS VEIN BYPASS GRAFTS

In general, saphenous vein bypass grafts are anastomosed to the anterior wall of the ascending aorta (Fig. 17-5). The right coronary artery graft usually is anastomosed a few centimeters above and anterior to the right coronary orifice. Left anterior descending and diagonal grafts usually are anastomosed somewhat higher and slightly to the left. Obtuse marginal grafts are usually the highest and furthest left.

### INTERNAL MAMMARY ARTERY GRAFT CANNULATION

The left internal mammary artery (IMA) originates anteriorly from the caudal wall of the subclavian artery distal to the vertebral artery

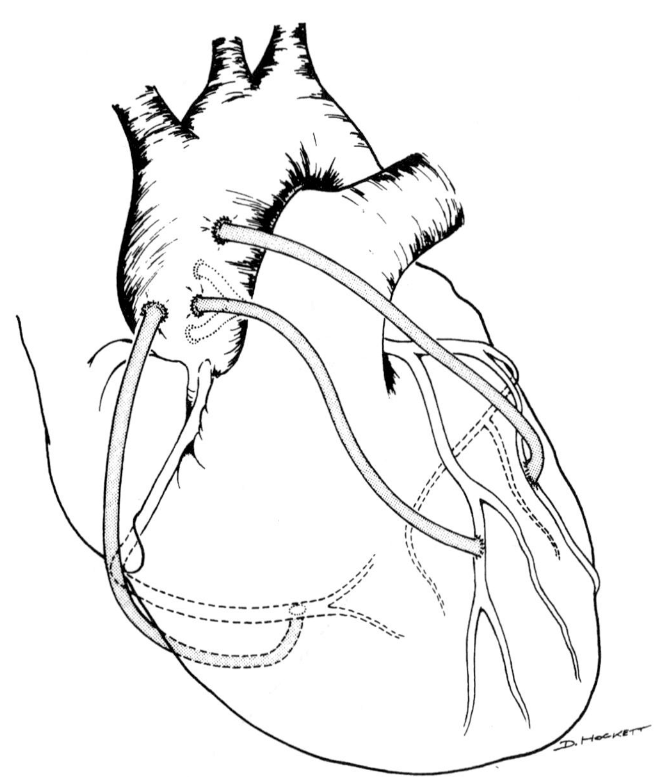


FIGURE 17-5 Usual insertion sites of vein grafts to coronary arteries. The proximal (aortic) anastomosis site of the graft to the right coronary artery is most anterior and usually the lowest. Grafts to the branches of the left coronary artery usually are inserted in a progressively higher and more posterolateral position. Variations frequently occur. (From Tilkian AG, Daily EK. *Cardiovascular Procedures: Diagnostic Techniques and Therapeutic Procedures*, St. Louis: Mosby; 1986. With permission.)

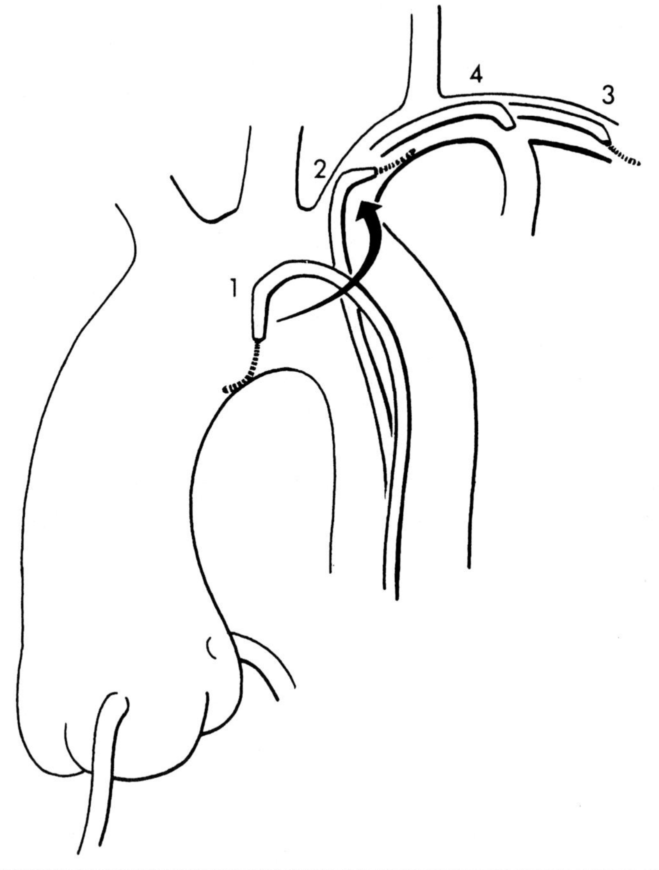


FIGURE 17-6 A guidewire is inserted in the internal mammary graft catheter until it is passed into the left subclavian. It is removed and withdrawn into the internal mammary artery. (From King SB, Douglas JS Jr. *Coronary Arteriography and Angioplasty.* New York: McGraw-Hill; 1985. With permission.)

origin (Fig. 17-6). The left subclavian artery can be entered using a right Judkins catheter but a more sharply angled catheter tip on the mammary artery catheter is preferred. The right Judkins or IMA catheter is advanced into the aortic arch up to the level of the right brachiocephalic truncus with the tip directed caudally. Subsequently, the catheter is withdrawn slowly and rotated counterclockwise. The catheter tip is deflected cranially, usually engaging the left subclavian artery at the top of the aortic knob in the anteroposterior projection. Once the subclavian artery is engaged, the catheter is advanced over a J-tipped or flexible straight tip guidewire beyond the internal mammary orifice. After the catheter has been advanced beyond the internal mammary artery takeoff, it is withdrawn slowly and small contrast injections are given to visualize the internal mammary artery orifice. The catheter tip should be directed caudally. At the level of the internal mammary orifice a slight counterclockwise rotation and advancement may be necessary to cannulate the artery. In cases with a vertically directed internal mammary artery, an internal mammary artery catheter and a more acute tip angle can be used. Sometimes this catheter cannot be introduced into the subclavian artery because of the tip angle. In this case the subclavian artery can be entered using a right Judkins catheter and then exchanged for an internal mammary artery catheter over an exchange guidewire. Because of the peculiar tip configuration, the internal mammary curve catheter and especially the C-type IMA catheter usually engages into the IMA ostium without much difficulty.

### RIGHT INTERNAL MAMMARY ARTERY GRAFT CANNULATION

Right internal mammary artery cannulation is less common and more difficult than left internal mammary artery cannulation. The right brachiocephalic truncus is entered using a right Judkins catheter by deflecting the tip with a counterclockwise rotation at the level of the brachiocephalic truncus. The catheter is advanced into the subclavian artery. The rest of the manipulation is similar to that described for left internal mammary artery graft cannulation. In patients for whom cannulation of the internal mammary artery is not possible because of excessive tortuosity or obstructive lesions, an internal mammary artery catheter can be introduced through the ipsilateral radial artery. The catheter is advanced beyond the mammary artery orifice over a guidewire. Withdrawing it slowly and making frequent, small contrast injections engage the catheter. A technique for cannulation of the contralateral internal mammary artery from the arm approach using a Simmons catheter also has been described.

## Angiographic Views (Fig. 17-7 and Table 17-18).

For all catheterization laboratories, the x-ray source is *under* the table and the image intensifier is directly *on top* of the patient. The x-ray source and image intensifier are moved in opposite directions in an imaginary circle around the patient, who is positioned in the center of this circle. The body surface of the patient that faces the observer determines the specific view. This relationship holds true whether the patient is supine, standing, or rotated.

*AP (anteroposterior) position.* The image intensifier is directly over the patient with the beam traveling perpendicular back to front, (i.e., from posterior to anterior) to the patient lying flat on the x-ray table. An oblique view is achieved by turning the left/right shoulder forward (anterior) to the camera (image intensifier) or in the cath lab, rotating the *image intensifier toward* the shoulder.

*RAO (right anterior oblique) position.* The image intensifier is to the right side of the patient.

*LAO (left anterior oblique) position.* The image intensifier is to the left side of the patient.

*Cranial/caudal position.* This nomenclature refers to image intensifier angles in relation to the patient's long axis.

*Cranial.* The image intensifier is tilted toward the *head* of the patient.

*Caudal.* The image intensifier is tilted toward the *feet* of the patient.

*Cranial* views are best for the *left anterior descending artery; caudal* views are best for the *circumflex artery.* Cranial and caudal views are used to "open" overlapped coronary segments that are *foreshortened* or obscured in regular views.

### THE LEFT CORONARY ARTERY

The ostium of the left coronary artery originates from the left sinus of Valsalva near the sinotubular ridge. The anterior descending artery is usually best visualized in a cranially angulated RAO view. If the orientation of the anterior descending artery is unusually superior, a caudally angulated LAO view or a straight lateral view may be helpful.

The circumflex coronary artery travels in the AV groove, after its right-angle origin from the left anterior descending artery. Its course is quite variable. The artery may terminate in one or more large, obtuse marginal branches coursing over the lateral to posterolateral LV free wall. The circumflex may continue as a large artery in the interventricular groove. In 10 to 15 percent of cases, the circumflex gives rise to a posterior descending artery[36] (Fig. 17-8). The artery that supplies the major posterior descending artery is commonly referred to as the *dominant* artery. The circumflex artery in the AV

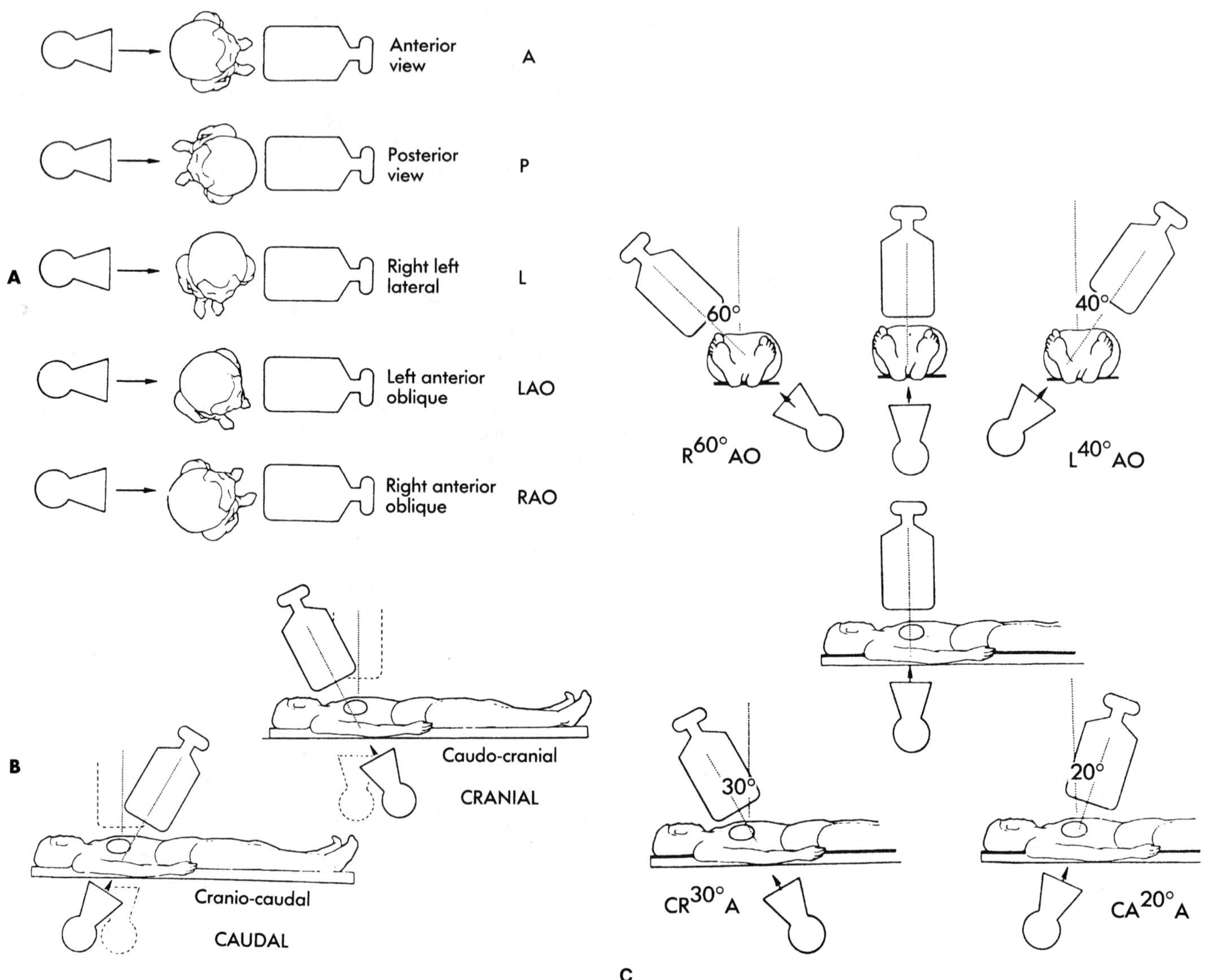


FIGURE 17-7 Nomenclature for radiographic projections. The small black arrowheads show the direction of the x-ray beam. *A*. Anterior, posterior, lateral, and oblique. *B*. If the intensifier is tilted toward the feet of the patient, a caudal view is produced. If the intensifier is tilted toward the head of the patient, a cranial view is produced. *C*. Cranial (CR) and caudal (CA) oblique views. (Redrawn from Paulin S. Terminology for radiographic projects in cardiac angiography. *Catheter Cardiovasc Diagn* 1981;7:341. With permission.)

groove is best seen in either caudally angulated LAO or RAO views (Fig. 17-9).

## THE RIGHT CORONARY ARTERY

The right coronary artery ostium normally is located in the right sinus of Valsalva. It may be high near the sinotubular ridge or above it, in the midsinus, or occasionally low near the aortic valve. The artery commonly courses upward from the plane of the aortic valve and then travels in the right AV groove to reach the posterior LV wall (Fig. 17-10). Along the way, several vessels arise. The conus branch and sinus node arteries branch first, followed by small RV branches, then a large branch that courses over the right ventricle. The right coronary continues to become the posterior descending artery before reaching the crux of the heart (junction of the interventricular and interatrial septa). The posterior descending artery sends branches at right angles into the posterior interventricular groove, providing the perforating branches to the basal and posterior one-third of the septum. A right coronary artery that supplies the major posterior descending branch has been referred to as a *dominant* right coronary artery. The posterior descending artery usually stops before reaching the apex, but it may curl around the apex in association with a short anterior descending artery. After giving rise to the posterior descending artery, the right coronary artery becomes intramyocardial at the crux, gives rise to the AV node artery. The LV branches of the right coronary artery are variable and cover the same area as the posterolateral branches of a large circumflex system. The proximal portion of the right coronary artery is well seen in standard RAO and LAO views. However, because of its horizontal orientation, the origin and length of the posterior descending artery, well seen in the RAO view, is foreshortened in the LAO view. Thus, cranial angulation provides a better view of the PDA.

## Interpretation of the Coronary Arteriogram

The coronary arteriogram should be viewed in a systematic fashion. Because coronary anatomy can be quite variable, the entire LV sur-

TABLE 17-18 Angiographic Views for Specific Coronary Artery Segments

| Coronary Segment | Origin/ Bifurcation | Course/ Body |
|---|---|---|
| Left main | AP | AP |
| | LAO cranial | LAO cranial |
| | LAO caudal[a] | |
| Proximal LAD | LAO cranial | LAO cranial |
| | RAO caudal | RAO caudal |
| Mid-LAD | LAO cranial | |
| | RAO cranial | |
| | Lateral | |
| Distal LAD | AP | |
| | RAO cranial | |
| | Lateral | |
| Diagonal | LAO cranial | RAO cranial, Caudal or straight |
| | RAO cranial | |
| Proximal circumflex | RAO caudal | LAO caudal |
| | LAO caudal | |
| Intermediate | RAO caudal | RAO caudal |
| | LAO caudal | Lateral |
| Obtuse marginal | RAO caudal | RAO caudal |
| | LAO caudal | |
| | RAO cranial (distal marginals) | |
| Proximal RCA | LAO | |
| | Lateral | |
| Mid-RCA | LAO | LAO |
| | Lateral | Lateral |
| | RAO | RAO |
| Distal RCA | LAO cranial | LAO cranial |
| | Lateral | Lateral |
| PDA | LAO cranial | RAO |
| Posterolateral | LAD cranial | RAO |
| | RAO cranial | RAO cranial |

[a]Horizontal hearts.

ABBREVIATIONS: AP = anteroposterior; LAD = left anterior descending artery; LAO = left anterior oblique; PDA = posterior descending artery (from RCA); RAO = right anterior oblique; RCA = right coronary artery.

face and septum should be adequately supplied with vessels. No gaps should exist. If significant vessels are missing, an occluded or anomalous artery is likely. Areas of foreshortening and overlap should be examined in other orthogonal or oblique views to demonstrate the region in question. Several observers should review an arteriogram. As each segment is viewed, a systematic scoring and reporting system is helpful to maintain a consistent and dependable report.

## ANGIOGRAPHIC ASSESSMENT OF CORONARY ARTERY NARROWINGS

An angiographic lumen narrowing is commonly referred to as a stenosis which may be due to atherosclerosis, vasospasm, or angiographic artifact (Fig. 17-11). The evaluation of a stenosis relates the percentage reduction in the diameter of the narrowed vessel site to the adjacent unobstructed vessel. The diameter stenosis is calculated in the projection where the greatest narrowing is seen. An exact evaluation of dimensions is impossible and, in fact, the severity of stenotic lesions are roughly classified. It should be noted that the stenotic lumen is compared to a nearby unobstructed lumen, which indeed may have diffuse atherosclerotic disease and thus is "angiographically" normal but may still be diseased (Fig. 17-12). This fact explains why postmortem examinations report much more plaque than is seen on angiography.[37–39] The angiographic "normal" adjacent proximal segments may be larger than distal segments, explaining the large disparity between several observer estimates of stenosis severity.[39] Also note that *area stenosis* is always greater than *diameter stenosis* and assumes the lumen is circular when in reality most of the time the lumen is eccentric.[40] In 1975, the American Heart Association recommended that the diameter method be adopted for grading coronary artery stenosis.[40a] A 50 percent reduction in diameter is equivalent to a 75 percent reduction in cross-sectional area, and a 75 percent reduction in diameter is equal to a 90 percent reduction in cross-sectional area.

Six categories of coronary narrowing have been commonly used:

1. Normal coronary artery
2. Irregularities of the vessel
3. Narrowing of less than 50 percent
4. Stenosis between 50 and 75 percent
5. Stenosis between 75 and 95 percent
6. Total occlusion

For nonquantitative reports, the length of a stenosis may be simply mentioned (e.g., LAD proximal segment stenosis diameter 25 percent, long or short). Other features of the coronary lesion (e.g., distribution eccentricity, calcification, true length) may not be appreciated by angiography and require intravascular ultrasound imaging (Fig. 17-13).

Because of the subjective nature of visual lesion assessment, there is a ±20 percent variation between readings of two or more experienced angiographers, especially for lesions 40 to 70 percent narrowed. Different angiographers may interpret the same angiographic image differently, and the same angiographer may render a different interpretation at a time remote from the first reading.[41,42] In addition, there may be disagreement about the number of major vessels with 70 percent stenosis about 30 percent of the time.[43] Angiographic narrowings of 40 to 75 percent narrowing do not always correspond to abnormal physiology and myocardial ischemia. For such lesions, noninvasive or direct physiologic measurements of impaired flow validate decisions for revascularization.

## QUANTITATIVE ANGIOGRAPHIC ASSESSMENT

The degree of coronary stenosis is usually a visual estimation of the percentage of diameter narrowing using the proximal assumed normal arterial segment as a reference. The ratio of normal to stenosis artery diameter is widely used in clinical practice, is inadequate for a true quantitative methodology. The intraobserver variability may range between 40 and 80 percent, and there is frequently a range as wide as 20 percent on interobserver differences. Quantitative methodologies include digital calipers, automated or manual edge detection systems, or densitometric analysis with digital angiography.[44]

## INTRAVASCULAR ULTRASOUND ASSESSMENT OF CORONARY ARTERY NARROWINGS

Intravascular ultrasound (IVUS) generates a tomographic, cross-sectional image of the vessel and lumen. IVUS enables the operator to make measurements of luminal dimensions, such as minimum and maximum diameter, cross-sectional area, vessel wall and plaque

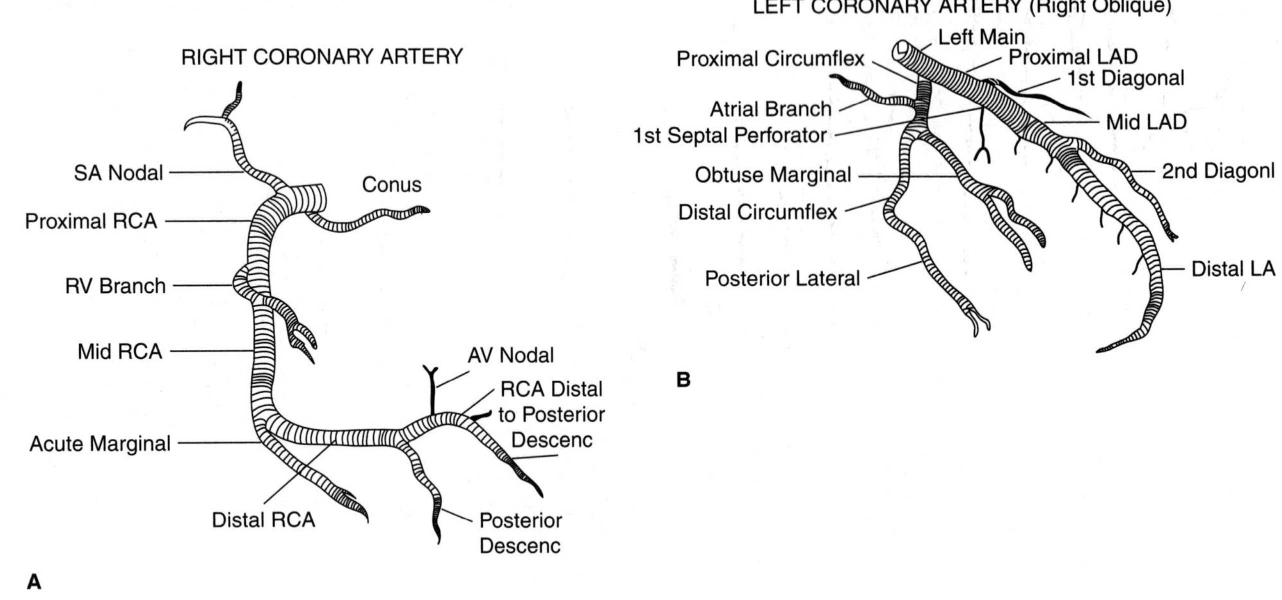


FIGURE 17-8 Diagrams of the anatomy of the right (*A*) and left (*B*) coronary circulation.

thickness. Intravascular coronary ultrasound images the soft tissues within the arterial wall enabling characterization of atheroma size, plaque distribution, and lesion composition during diagnostic or therapeutic catheterization.[45,46] The ACC/AHA recommendations for intravascular ultrasound imaging are provided in Appendix 17-2.[3]

## ASSESSMENT OF CORONARY SPASM

Coronary spasm can be demonstrated by angiographic narrowing, provoked by mechanical stimulation (Fig. 17-14), methylergonovine maleate, acetylcholine, cold pressor testing, or hyperventilation. The methylergonovine provocative test is the most reliable test for coronary spasm in patients with Prinzmetal variant angina. Optimally, nitrates and calcium antagonists should be withheld for 48 h before testing. Methylergonovine should be administered by an experienced operator in a laboratory with full resuscitative capabilities. Intracoronary acetylcholine has also been used as a provocative test for coronary spasm. Its effectiveness is comparable to methylergonovine. In patients with one episode of variant angina per day, the hyperventilation provocative test is nearly as effective as methylergonovine in causing vasospasm. The end point of a pharmacologic provocative test is focal coronary narrowing, which can be reversed with intracoronary nitroglycerin. In patients with ST-segment elevation with chest pain and a normal coronary angiogram, the diagnosis of coronary spasm is established and provocative tests are not necessary.[47]

FIGURE 17-9 *A.* Diagrammatic representation of the standard RAO view of the left coronary angiogram, the direction of the x-ray beam, and the position of the overhead image intensifier. Most of the left coronary artery is well visualized in this projection, although there is considerable overlap of the middle left anterior descending artery and the diagonal branches. When the left main, circumflex, and diagonal branches have a leftward initial course, the long axis of these arterial segments is projected away from the image intensifier, preventing optimal visualization from the RAO view. The image intensifier is placed anteriorly in an RAO position relative to the patient. (From King et al.[36] Reproduced with permission from the publisher, editor, and authors.) *B.* Diagrammatic representation of the LAO left coronary angiogram and the direction of the x-ray beam in this view. The value of this view depends in large part on the orientation of the long axis of the heart. When the heart is relatively horizontal, the left anterior descending (LAD) coronary artery and diagonal branches are seen end-on throughout much of the course. In this illustration, the longitudinal axis is an intermediate position and there is moderate foreshortening of the anterior descending and diagonal branches in their proximal portions (compare with Fig. 17-9*E*). The LAO projection is frequently inadequate to visualize the proximal LAD and its branches; the left main segment, which is directed toward the image tube and therefore foreshortened, and the proximal circumflex coronary artery, which may be obscured by overlapping vessels, as in this illustration. The LAO projection is frequently used to visualize the distal LAD and its branches, the midcircumflex coronary artery in the AV groove, and the distal right coronary artery that is filling via collaterals from the left coronary artery. The image intensifier is above the patient in an LAO position. (From King et al.[36] Reproduced with permission from the publisher, editor, and authors.) *C.* Diagrammatic illustration of the left coronary angiogram in the 45-degree LAO with 30 degrees of cranial angulation and the direction of the x-ray beam used to produce this view. This is the most valuable view of the left coronary artery in most patients. Foreshortening of the left main and proximal left anterior descending and diagonal branches present in the LAO view is usually overcome by cranial angulation of the image intensifier. The proximal left coronary arterial segments are frequently visualized at an angle almost perpendicular from their long axis. The ostium of the left main coronary artery, the most proximal portion of the LAD, and the origin of the diagonal branches are usually well visualized without overlap (compare with Fig. 17-9*B*). Some overlap may occur with branches of the proximal circumflex coronary artery, and this is frequently overcome by using a 60-degree LAO with 30 degrees of cranial angulation. The value of the LAO with cranial angulation is considerably less when the proximal left coronary artery is superiorly directed, in which case caudal angulation of the image intensifier is frequently helpful. The direction of the x-ray beam in the 45-degree LAO with 30 degrees of angulation is demonstrated. (From King et al.[36] Reproduced with permission from the publisher, editor, and authors.) *D.* Diagrammatic illustration of the direction of the x-ray beam and the left coronary angiogram in the 15-degree RAO with 30 degrees of cranial angulation. This view is particularly helpful in analyzing the mid–left anterior descending artery and the diagonal branch points. Overlap with diagonal branches is usually avoided. The origin of the circumflex artery may be well seen, as in this illustration. (From King et al.[36] Reproduced with permission from the publisher, editor, and authors.)

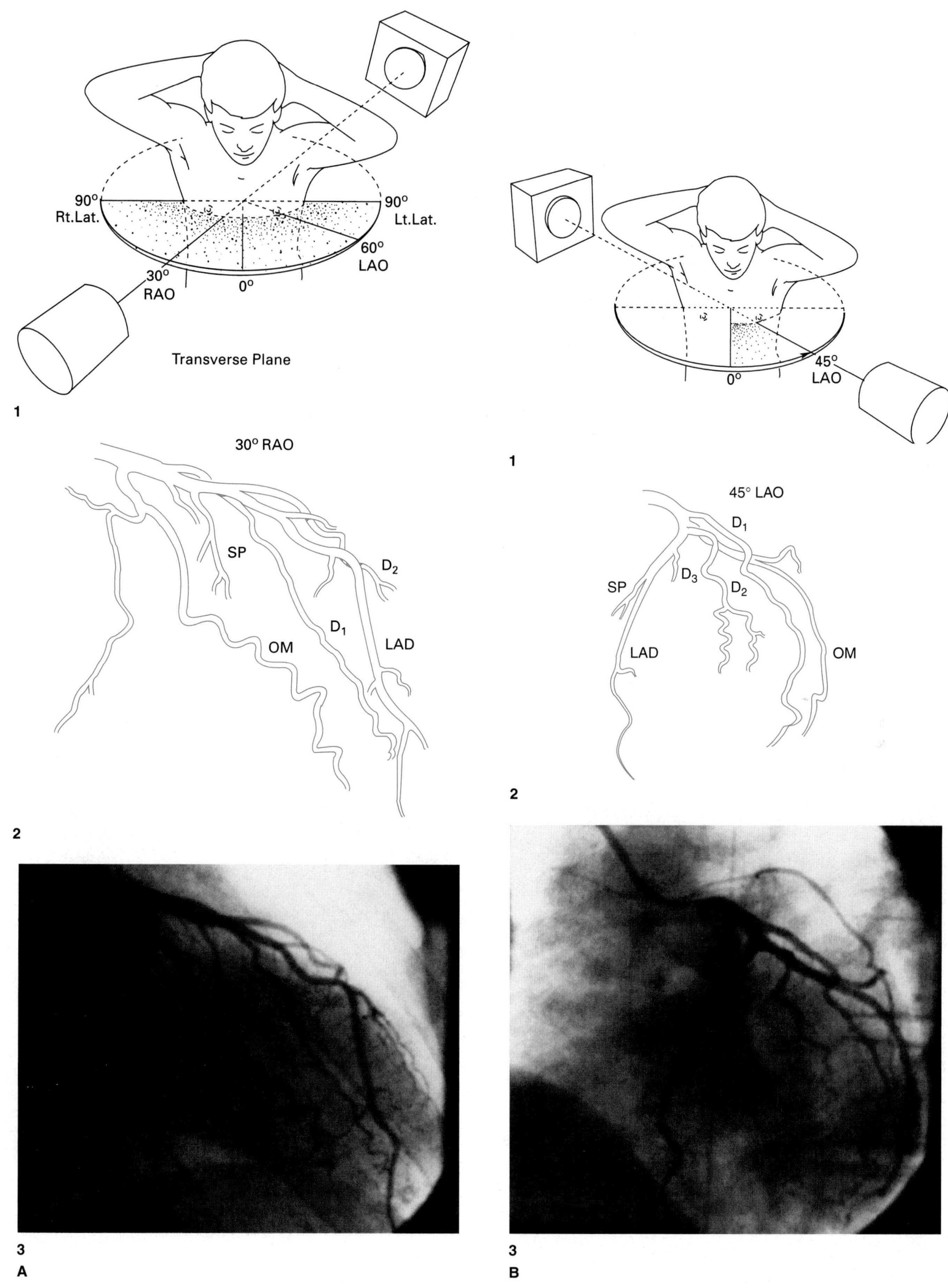
90°
Rt.Lat.
90°
Lt.Lat.
60°
LAO
30°
RAO
0°
Transverse Plane
1
30° RAO
SP
$D_2$
$D_1$
OM
LAD
2
45°
LAO
0°
1
45° LAO
$D_1$
SP
$D_3$
$D_2$
LAD
OM
2
3
A
3
B

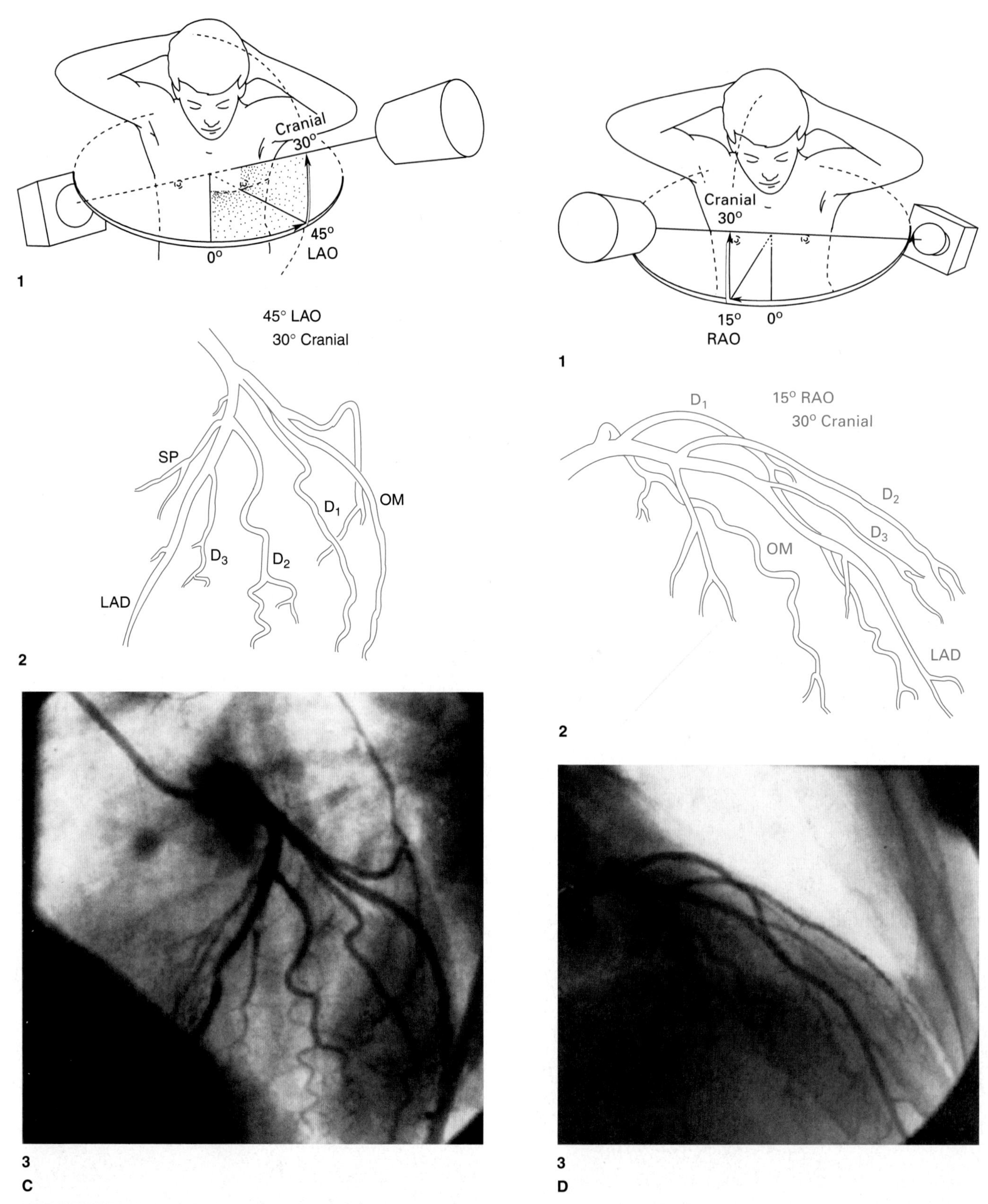


FIGURE 17-9 (*Continued*)

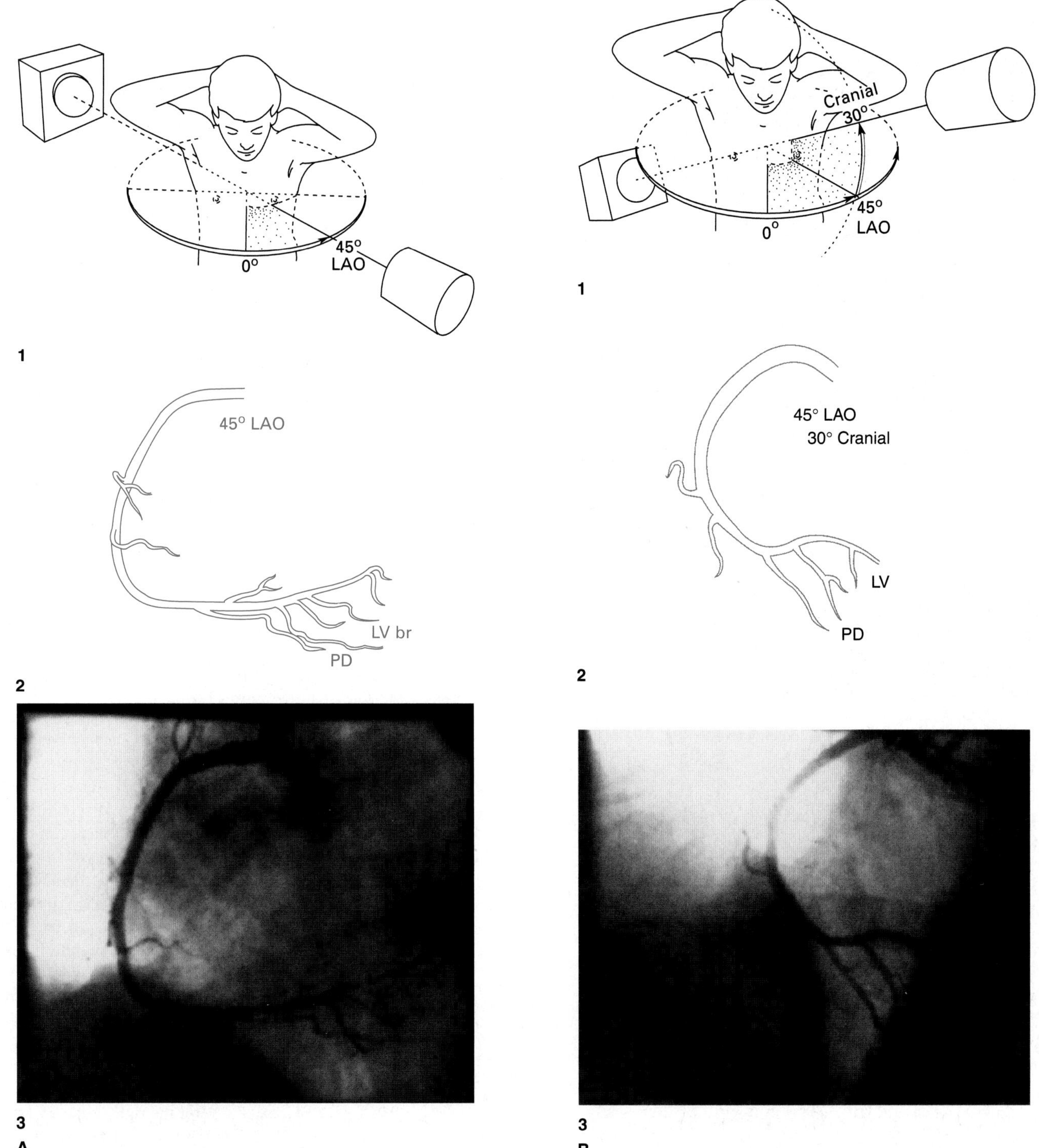


FIGURE 17-10 *A.* Diagrammatic illustration of the direction of the x-ray beam and the right coronary artery in the 45-degree LAO projection. This view is excellent for visualizing the proximal mid- and distal right coronary artery in the AV groove, since the direction of the x-ray beam is perpendicular to these arterial segments. Ostial lesions of the right coronary artery are now well visualized if the proximal right coronary artery takes an anterior direction from the aorta and therefore originates in a direction parallel to the x-ray beam. This usually can be overcome by turning to a more severe left oblique projection. The posterior descending and LV branches of the right coronary artery, which pass down the posterior aspect of the heart toward the apex, are severely foreshortened because the long axis of these vessels is in the same direction as the x-ray beam. The proximal posterior descending branches can be visualized by cranial angulation of the overhead intensifier or from a right oblique view. The image intensifier is in the standard LAO position. (From King et al.[36] Reproduced with permission from the publisher, editor, and authors.) *B.* Diagrammatic illustration of the direction of the x-ray beam and the right coronary artery in 30-degree LAO with 30 degrees cranial angulation. Cranial angulation of the image intensifier overcomes the problem of foreshortening of the posterior decending and left ventricular branches observed in Fig. 17-27. Lesions in the posterior decending or LV brances can be well visualized. When the right coronary artery originates anteriorly from the aorta, the proximal portion of the vessel is frequently well seen in this projection. With anomalous origin of the left anterior decending artery from the right coronary artery, this view is helpful because the standard LAO view produces considerable foreshortening of the anomalous artery. The direction of x-ray beam is the same as in Fig. 17-25. (From King et al.[136] Reproduced with permission from the publisher, editor, and authors.)

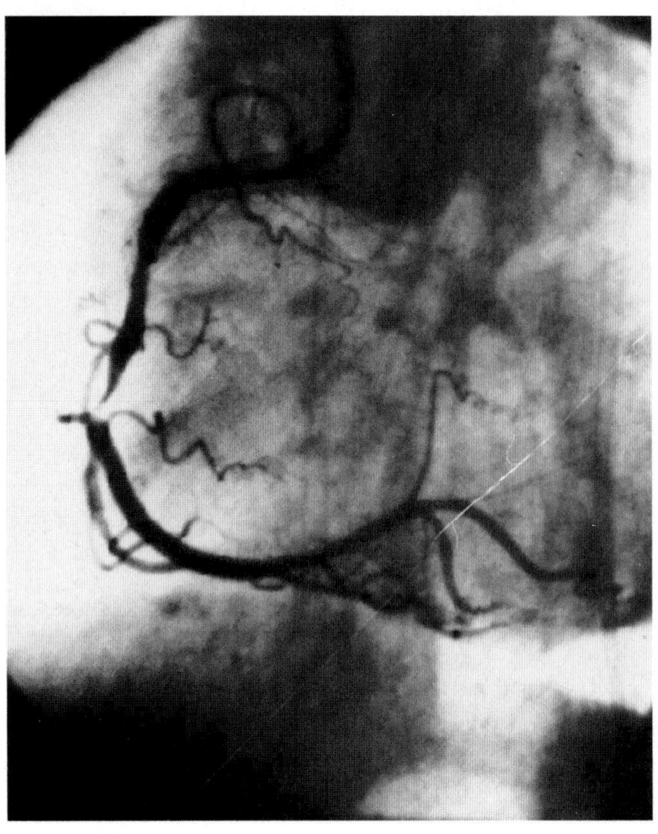

FIGURE 17-11 LAO view of the right coronary artery (RCA) with high-grade lesion in its midportion.

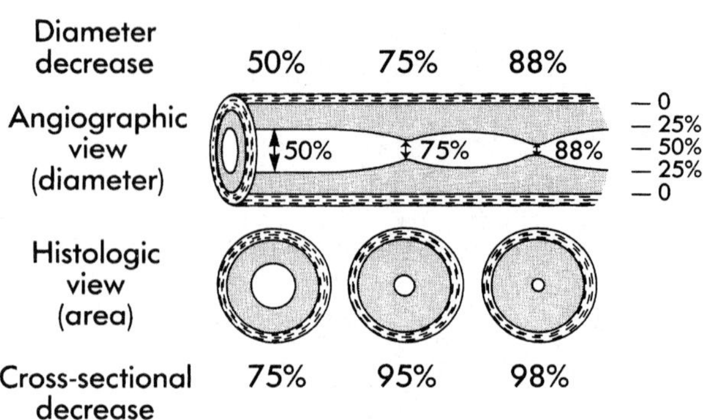


FIGURE 17-12 Diagrammatic representation of angiographic versus postmortem analysis of coronary artery stenosis. (From Robert WC. Coronary heart disease: A review of abnormalities observed in the coronary arteries. *Cardiovasc Med* 1977;2:29–38. With permission.)

## ANGIOGRAPHICALLY ESTIMATED CORONARY BLOOD FLOW (TIMI FLOW)

Myocardial blood flow has been assessed angiographically using the Thrombolysis in Myocardial Infarction (TIMI) score for qualitative grading of coronary flow. TIMI flow grades 0 to 3 have become a standard description of angiographic coronary blood flow in clinical trials. In acute myocardial infarction trials, TIMI grade 3 flows have been associated with improved clinical outcomes. The four grades of flow are described as follows:

1. Normal distal runoff (TIMI-3)
2. Good distal runoff (TIMI-2)
3. Poor distal runoff (TIMI-1)
4. Absence of distal runoff (TIMI-0)

The quantitative method of TIMI flow uses cineangiography with 6F catheters and filming at 30 frames per second. The number of cine frames from the introduction of dye in the coronary artery to a predetermined distal landmark is counted. The TIMI frame count for each major vessel is thus standardized according to specific distal landmarks. The first frame used for TIMI frame counting is that in which the dye fully opacifies the artery origin and in which the dye extends across the width of the artery touching both borders with antegrade motion of the dye. The last frame counted is when dye enters the first distal landmark branch. Full opacification of the distal branch segment is not required. Distal landmarks used commonly in analysis are (1) for the LAD, the distal bifurcation of the left anterior descending artery; (2) for the circumflex system, the distal bifurcation of the branch segments with the longest total distance; (3) for the right coronary artery, the first branch of the posterolateral artery.

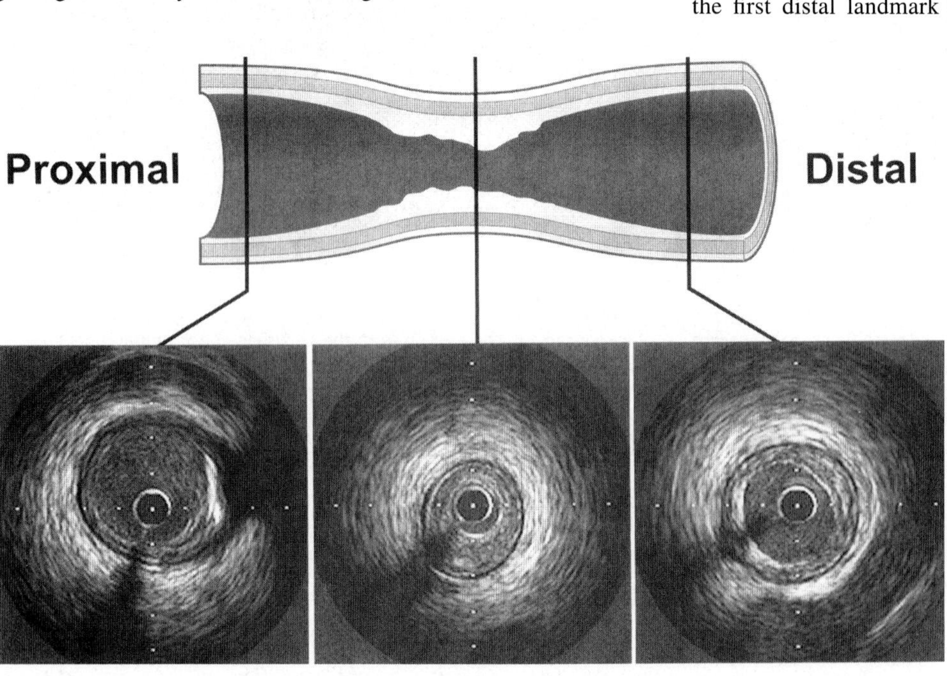


FIGURE 17-13 Intravascular ultrasound (IVUS) imaging of the coronary artery.

The TIMI frame count can further be quantitated for the length of the left anterior descending coronary artery for comparison to the two other major arteries; this is called the corrected TIMI frame count (CTFC).[48] The average left anterior descending coronary artery is 14.7 cm long, the right 9.8 cm, and the circumflex 9.3 cm, according to Gibson et al.[48] CTFC accounts for the distance the dye has to travel in the LAD relative to the other arteries. CTFC divides the absolute frame count in the LAD by 1.7 to

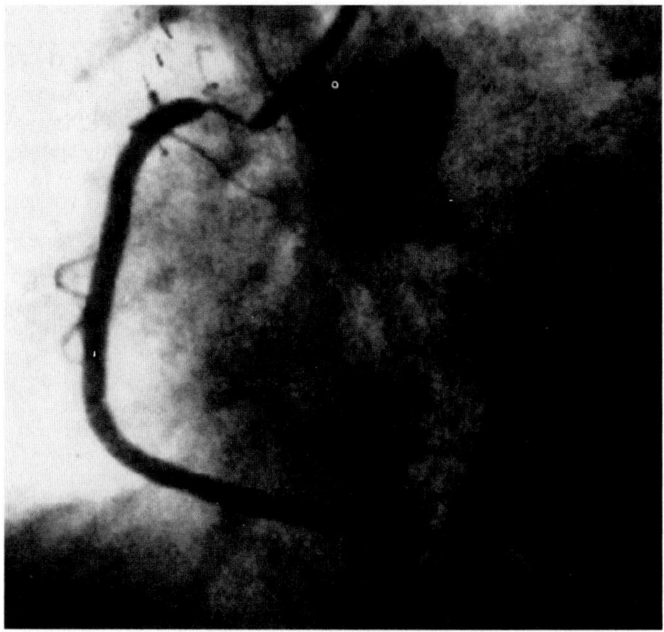

A

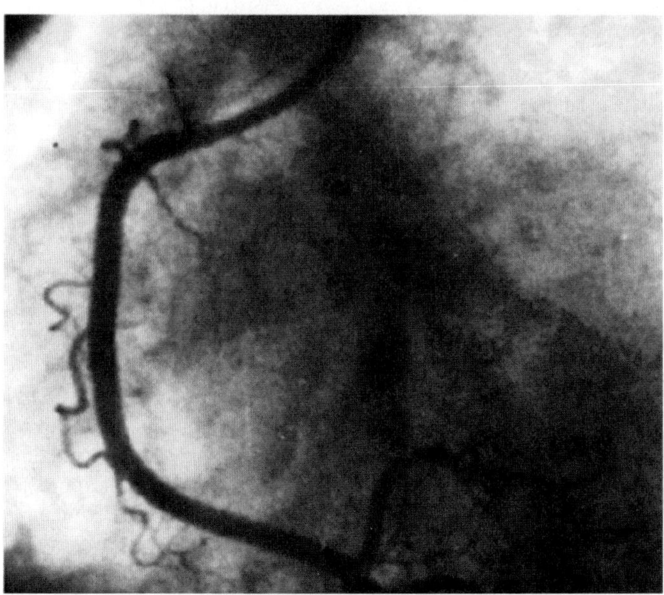

B

FIGURE 17-14 *A.* LAO view of right coronary injection showing pericatheter spasm. *B.* Same view following nitroglycerin, showing relief of spasm.

standardize the distance of dye travel in all three arteries. Normal TFC and CTFC for LAD is 36 ± 3 and CTFC 21 ± 2; for the CFX, TFC = 22 ± 4; for the RCA, TFC = 20 ± 3. TIMI flow grades do not correspond to measured Doppler flow velocity or the CTFC. High TFC may be associated with microvascular dysfunction despite an open artery. CTFC of $< 20$ frames were associated with low risk for adverse events in patients following myocardial infarction. A contrast injection rate increase of $\geq 1$ mL/s by hand injection can decrease the TIMI frame count by two frames. The TIMI frame count method provides valuable information relative to clinical responses after coronary interventions.

## COLLATERAL CIRCULATION

The reopacification of a totally or subtotally (99%) occluded vessel from antegrade or retrograde filling is defined as collateral filling. The collateral circulation is graded angiographically as follows:

| Grade | Collateral Appearance |
|---|---|
| 0 | No collateral circulation |
| 1 | Very weak (ghostlike) reopacification |
| 2 | Reopacified segment, less dense than the feeding vessel and filling slowly |
| 3 | Reopacified segment as dense as the feeding vessel and filling rapidly |

It is useful but difficult to establish the size of the recipient vessel exactly, whether the collateral circulation is ipsilateral (e.g., same side filling, proximal RCA to distal RCA collateral supply) or contralateral (e.g., opposite side filling, LAD to distal RCA collateral supply). Identification of exactly which region is affected by collateral supply will influence decisions regarding management of stenoses in the artery feeding the collateral supply. Collateral vessel evaluation is important for making decisions regarding which vessels might be protected or lost during coronary angioplasty.[49]

## PITFALLS IN CORONARY ARTERIOGRAPHY

There are a number of pitfalls in coronary arteriography that should be avoided.

***Short Left Main or Double Left Coronary Orifices*** When the left main orifice is very short or absent, selective injection of the anterior descending or circumflex arteries may be done. The absence of circumflex or anterior descending artery filling, either primarily or through collaterals from the right coronary artery, may indicate that the artery was missed by subselective injection, or an anomalous location.

***Ostial Lesions*** The left and right coronary artery orifices need to be seen on a tangent with the aortic sinuses. Some contrast reflux from the orifices is needed to fully opacific the ostium to see whether an ostial narrowing is present. Catheter pressure damping is an additional indication of an ostial stenosis.

***Myocardial Bridges*** The anterior descending, diagonal, and marginal branches occasionally run intramyocardially. The overlying myocardium may compress the artery during systole. If the coronary artery is not viewed carefully in diastole, this bridging may give the appearance of an area of stenosis.[50]

***Foreshortening*** Foreshortening is the viewing of a vessel in plane with its long axis. Vessels seen on end cannot display a lesion along its length. When possible, review arteries that are seen coming toward or away from the image intensifier in angulated (cranial/caudal) views. Dense opacification of segments seen end-on may produce the appearance of a lesion in an intervening segment.

***Coronary Spasm*** Catheter-induced spasm may appear as a lesion (Fig. 17-14). When spasm is suspected (usually at the catheter tip in the right coronary artery), intracoronary nitroglycerin (100 to 200 $\mu$g) should be given, and the angiogram should be repeated in 1 to 2 min. Spontaneous coronary artery spasm may also present as an atherosclerotic narrowing. When this is suspected, obtain an angiogram before and again after nitrates. If clinically indicated, provocation with ergot derivatives will identify most patients with spontaneous coronary artery spasm.

***Totally Occluded Arteries or Vein Grafts*** Absence of vascularity in a portion of the heart may indicate total occlusion of its arterial supply. Collateral channels often permit visualization of the distal occluded artery. Vessels filled solely by collaterals are under low pressure and may appear smaller than their actual lumen size. This finding should not exclude the possibilities for surgical anastomosis.

***Anomalous Coronary Arteries*** Coronary arteries may arise from anomalous locations, or a single coronary artery may be present.[51] Only by ensuring that the entire epicardial surface has an adequate arterial supply can one be confident that all branches have been visualized. Misdiagnosis of unsuspected anomalous origin of the coronary arteries is a potential problem for any angiographer. As the natural history of a patient with an anomalous origin of a coronary artery may be dependent on the initial course of the anomalous vessel, it is the angiographer's responsibility to define accurately the origin and course of the vessel. It is an error to assume a vessel is occluded when in fact it has not been visualized because of an anomalous origin. It is often difficult even for experienced angiographers to delineate the true course of an anomalous vessel.

For the most critical anomaly, the anomalous left main artery originating from the right cusp, a simple "dot and eye" method for determining the proximal course of anomalous artery from an RAO ventriculogram, an RAO aortogram, or selective RAO injection is proposed[52] (Table 17-19). The RAO view best separates the normally positioned aorta and pulmonary artery. Placement of right-sided catheters or injection of contrast in the pulmonary artery is unnecessary and often misleading. Figure 17-15 diagrams the four common pathways of anomalous left coronary arteries.

***Complications of Coronary Arteriography*** Minor complications of coronary angiography include local arterial complications, arterial occlusion or stenosis, hematoma formation, false aneurysm, and infection. Major complications are potentially lethal and include thromboembolic events or depression of myocardial function due to infarction or acute ischemia.

## Left Ventriculography

Left ventriculography is the standard method for evaluating LV performance in the cardiac catheterization laboratory. The normal pattern of LV contraction is a uniform and almost concentric inward movement of all points along the endocardial surface during systole. Harrison introduced the term *asynergy,* which has been used to indicate a disturbance of the normal contraction pattern. The Ad Hoc Committee for Grading of Coronary Artery Disease of the American Heart Association[52a] has recommended that five RAO segments and two LAO left ventricular segments be defined and characterized as to wall motion (Fig. 17-16). Herman et al.[52b] classified LV asynergy according to the severity of the contractile abnormality.

### VENTRICULAR WALL MOTION ANALYSIS

There are three distinct types of asynergy (Fig. 17-17):

1. *Hypokinesia*—a diminished but not absent motion of one part of the LV wall (also called weak or poor contraction).
2. *Akinesia*—total lack of motion of a portion of the LV wall (i.e., no contraction).
3. *Dyskinesia*—paradoxical systolic motion or expansion of one part of the LV wall (i.e., an abnormal bulging outward during systole).

There are several methods for analyzing LV wall motion. A point system based on the regional severity of abnormal wall motion from the Coronary Artery Surgery Study (CASS)[52a] is used to produce a wall motion score reflecting overall LV function. The RAO and LAO left ventriculrogams are divided into five segments. Points are assigned as follows: normal contraction = 1 point; moderate hypokinesis = 2; severe hypokinesis = 3; akinesis = 4; aneurysm-dyskinesis = 5. A normal score is 5. Higher scores indicate more severe wall motion abnormalities.

For determination of quantitative regional wall motion abnormalities, three methods have been commonly employed: (1) *Long axis method.* Determination of the major long axis and division of the long axis into equal segments with perpendicular lines; (2) *Center point method.* Midpoint of the major axis and division of the lines radiating out from the center point; (3) *Center line method.* A center line is established between the end-diastolic and end-systolic borders, 100 perpendicular chords are drawn, and shortening of these chords determines wall motion abnormalities. Results are corrected using a normal motion value for each chord length. Some of these methods of determining regional wall motion abnormality use computer planimetry available currently on most advanced x-ray systems.

TABLE 17-19 Radiographic Appearance of Anomalous Origin of the Left Main Coronary Artery from the Right Sinus of Valsalva

| Course of Anomalous Left Main Coronary | RAO Aortography or Ventriculography: Dot | RAO Aortography or Ventriculography: Eye | LAD Length | Septals Arising from LMCA |
|---|---|---|---|---|
| Septal | – | +(upper CFX) (lower LMCA) | Short | Yes |
| Anterior | – | +(upper LMCA) (lower CFX) | Short | No |
| Retroaortic | +(posterior) | – | Normal | No |
| Interarterial | +(anterior) | – | Normal | No |

ABBREVIATIONS: + = present; – = absent. Posterior and anterior are in reference to the aorta root. LAD = left anterior descending coronary artery; LMCA = left main coronary artery; CFX = circumflex coronary artery.

### INDICATIONS FOR LEFT VENTRICULOGRAPHY

1. Identify LV function for patients with coronary artery disease, myopathy, or valvular heart disease.
2. Identify ventricular septal defect.
3. Quantitate degree of mitral regurgitation.
4. Quantitate mass of myocardium for regression of hypertrophy or other similar research studies.

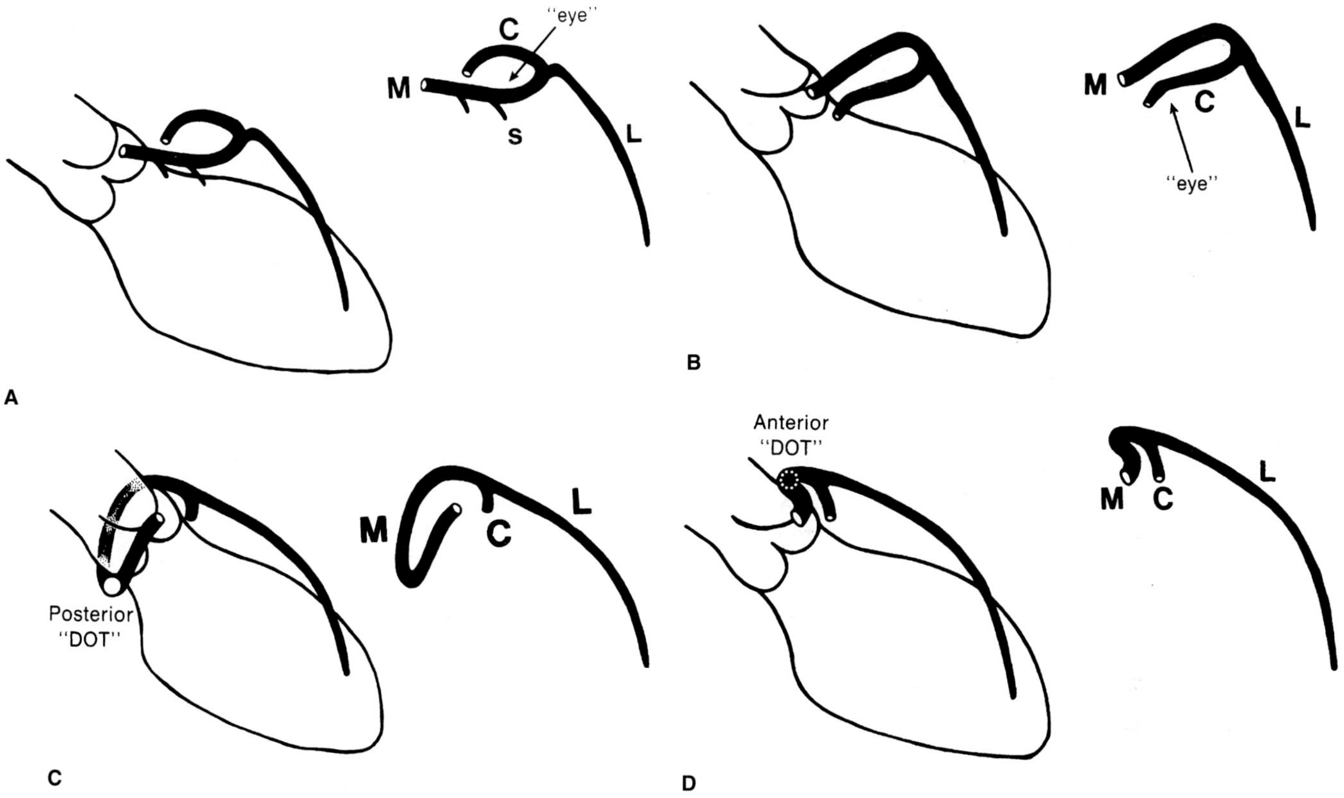

FIGURE 17-15 *A.* Diagram of septal course of anomalous left coronary artery. *M* = Left main; *S* = septals; *C* = circumflex; *L* = left anterior descending artery. *B.* Diagram of anterior course of anomalous left coronary artery. *C.* Diagram of retroaortic course of anomalous left coronary artery. *D.* Diagram of interarterial course of left main coronary artery. (From Kern MJ. *Cardiac Catheterization Handbook*. St. Louis: Mosby; 2003. With permission.)

## VENTRICULOGRAPHY TECHNIQUES

***Catheters*** The two most common ventriculography catheters are the pigtail and multipurpose sidehole catheters. *The pigtail catheter* has a tapered tip, shaped to make a full circle, 1 cm in diameter. Five to twelve side holes are located on the straight portion of the catheter above the curve. The catheter is placed in front of the mitral valve with the loop directed away from the valve (in the RAO position). A slight rotation, advancement, or withdrawal may be necessary to find a position that does not cause frequent premature ventricular contractions (Fig. 17-18).

*The multipurpose catheter* with sideholes is also used for ventriculography. This catheter should be positioned freely in the left ventricular chamber so that the high-pressure contrast jet does not produce ventricular tachycardia, contrast injection in the myocardial tissue (contrast staining), or perforation (Fig. 17-19). The pigtail catheter (and halo-modified pigtail) is safer and produces less ectopy contrast staining and perforation than a multipurpose catheter.

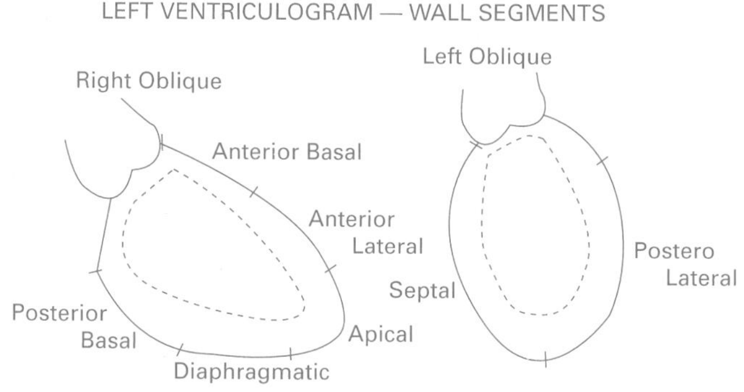


FIGURE 17-16 LV wall silhouette in RAO and LAO views.

***Left Ventriculography Views*** Standard left ventriculographic views are (1) a 30-degree RAO that visualizes the high lateral, anterior, apical, and inferior LV walls and (2) a 45- to 60-degree LAO, 20 degrees of cranial angulation that best identifies the lateral and septal LV walls. The degrees of axial obliquity and cranial angulation are used as follows: (1) The 40-degree left anterior oblique (LAO) and 30-degree cranial position (four-chamber view) outlines the posterior third of the ventricular septum, the valve plane in AV canal defects, and the four heart chambers without superimposition. (2) The 60-degree LAO and 30-degree cranial position (long-axial view) outlines the anterior two-thirds of the ventricular septum, the membranous ventricular septum, and the LV outflow tract. The LAO with cranial angulation provides a view of the interventricular septum, projected on edge and tilted downward to give the best view of ventricular septal defects and septal wall motion. An elongated RAO view, which is useful for seeing the RV infundibulum and supracristal ventricular septal defect, is obtained by a 30-degree axial RAO and 40 degrees of cranial angulation. The main pulmonary artery and its bifurcation are seen in the frontal position with 30 degrees of cranial angulation; a steep LAO position with marked cranial angulation is also used.

Biplane ventriculography may be available in some catheterization laboratories. It involves increased radiation and more time spent positioning equipment. These considerations are offset by providing

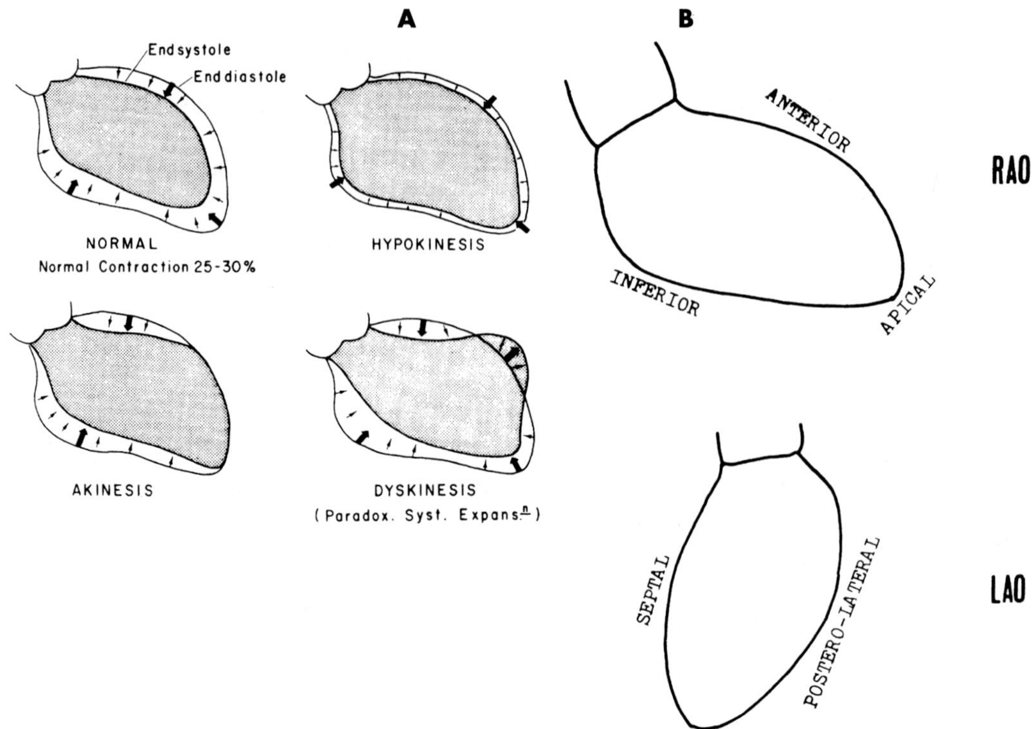


FIGURE 17-17 *A*. Types of ventricular asynergy. *B*. Diagrammatic representation of the zones of the left ventricular inner wall in the right anterior oblique (RAO) above and left anterior oblique (LAO) below left ventriculograms. (*A* from Herman MV et al. Localized disorders in myocardial contraction. Asynergy and its role in congestive heart failure. *N Engl J Med* 1967;227:225. With permission. *B* from Yang SS: *From Cardiac Catheterization Data to Hemodynamic Parameters*, 3d ed. Philadelphia: FA Davis; 1987. With permission.

more information with less contrast media, an important consideration in children and patients with renal failure. If a biplane system is unavailable, patients with coronary disease affecting the lateral wall should have a second left ventriculogram in the 45- to 60-degree LAO, 20-degree cranial view. Almost every such patient can tolerate an additional 30 to 40 mL of contrast.

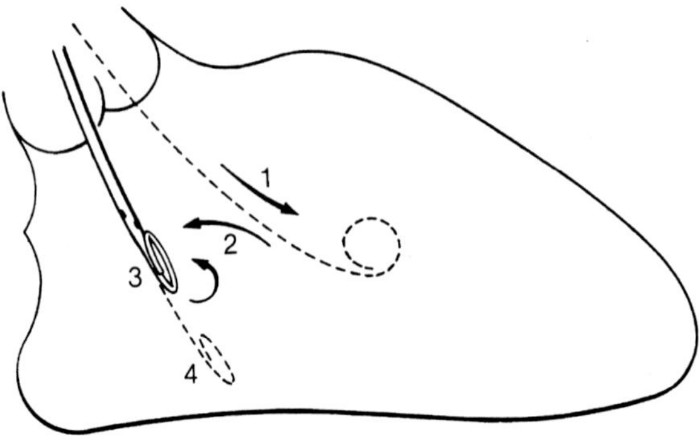


FIGURE 17-18 Judkins method of left ventricular catheterization: (1) Having crossed the aortic valve, the pigtail catheter will be in position. (2) The catheter is withdrawn 2 to 3 cm and rotated 70 to 90 degrees counterclockwise. (3) The coiled loop will be in the inflow tract of the mitral valve. (4) If the catheter moves excessively in this position, it should be advanced until it is stable. (From Judkins MP, Judkins E. Coronary arteriography and left ventriculographic Judkins technique. In: King SB III, Douglas JS Jr, eds. *Coronary Arteriography and Angioplasty*. New York: McGraw-Hill; 1985:201. With permission.)

## VENTRICULAR VOLUME MEASUREMENT

LV volume is estimated from the opacified image of the LV cavity. Although a single-plane mode using the frontal or RAO projection often is adequate,[53,54] biplane view image pairs including frontal and lateral, right and left anterior oblique, or half-axial left anterior oblique and conventional RAO may be more precise.[55,56] In the classic biplane technique, each image of the LV cavity is treated as an ellipse. The long axis of the ventricle ($L_m$) and the two mutually perpendicular short axes at its midpoint ($D_a$ and $D_i$) are measured, and

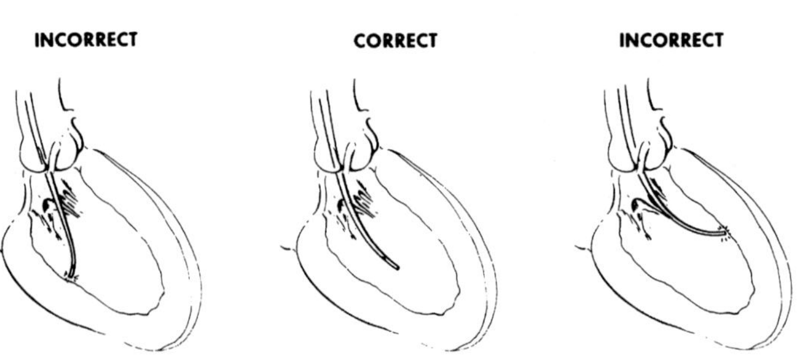


FIGURE 17-19 Multipurpose catheterization of the left ventricle in the 35-degree right anterior oblique projection. When positioned correctly (*center*), the catheter tip should be near the tip of the papillary muscles; aiming toward the apex. If it is touching the inferior or inferolateral wall (*left*) it should be rotated clockwise. If it is touching the anteroseptal wall (*right*), it should be rotated counterclockwise. (From King SB, Douglas JS Jr. *Coronary Arteriography and Angioplasty*, New York: McGraw-Hill; 1985. With permission.)

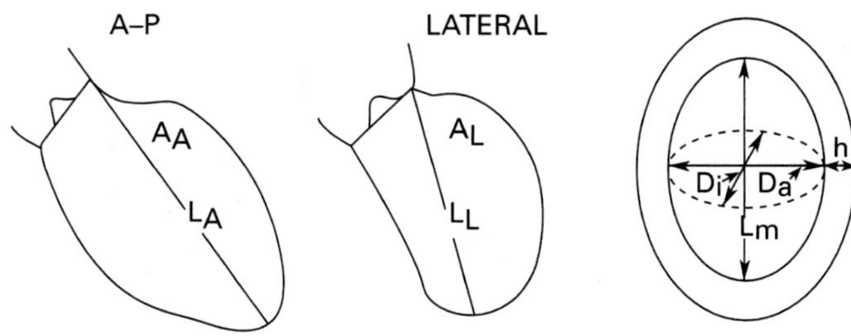


FIGURE 17-20 Dimensions of the left ventricular (LV) cavity in end-diastole used for the calculation of the ventricular volume by the area-length method, biplane technique. A-P = anteroposterior plane; $A_A$, $A_L$ = area, A-P and area lateral plane (planimetry); $L_A$, $L_L$ = length or long axis of the left ventricle (measured); $D_a$, $D_i$ = diameter of short axis, A-P lateral plane (derived); $L_m$ = maximum length or long axis whether from the lateral A-P or lateral plane; h = wall thickness, LV. See text for formulas. (Left and middle portion of figures from Sandler and Dodge. Right portion of figure from Dodge HT. Hemodynamic aspects of cardiac failure. *Hosp Pract* 1971; January:91. Illustration by B. Tagawa and A. Miller. Reproduced with permission from the publishers and authors.)

the volume ($V$) is calculated from the formula for volume of an ellipsoid (Fig. 17-20):

$$V = \frac{4}{3}\pi \times \frac{D_a}{2} \times \frac{D_i}{2} \times \frac{L_m}{2},$$

Also

$$V = \frac{\pi}{6} \times D_a \times D_i \times L_m$$

In the single-plane method, the long axis and one short axis are measured; the second nonvisible short axis is assumed to equal the first; thus

$$V = \frac{\pi}{6} \times L_m \times D^2$$

More often, in either the biplane or single-plane method, the short-axis dimension is derived from the measured long axis and the area ($A$) of the LV shadow, treated as an ellipse (area-length method of Dodge). Since

$$A = \pi L_m \frac{D}{4},$$

then,

$$D = \frac{4A}{\pi L_m}$$

and volume can be calculated from only the measured area and long axis by substituting for D, obtaining:

$$V = \frac{8\,A^2}{3\pi L_m}$$

Corrections must be made for magnification due to the divergence of the x-ray beam[55] using a calibrated grid or circular reference marker. Digital ventriculography provides rapid, computer-dervied ventricular volumes. Techniques for calculation of ventricular volumes have been validated using geometric and nongeometric count-based radionuclide methods as well as with magnetic resonance imaging.[56]

The methods for determination of ventricular volume by biplane ventriculography are described elsewhere.[57,58] Important parameters of LV volume measurements include: LV end-diastolic volume (normally 70 ± 20 mL/m$^2$), the end-systolic volume (24 ± 10 mL/m$^2$), and the ejection fraction (0.67 ± 0.08). LVEF values below 0.55 are considered abnormal. Diastolic LV wall thickness measured by angiography is 9 mm for women and 12 mm for men, and LV wall mass is 76 g/m$^2$ for women and 99 g/m$^2$ for men.[58]

The major measurements of left ventricular contractility are the ejection fraction (EF) and stroke volume (SV). Ejection fraction (EF, %) is calculated as

$$EF = \left(\frac{EDV - ESV}{EDV}\right) \times 100$$

The stroke volume is calculated as

$$SV = EDV - ESV$$

where EDV is end-diastolic volume, ESV is end-systolic volume, and SV is stroke volume. The velocity of circumferential fiber shortening (VCF, cm/s) is calculated as

$$VCF = \frac{\left(\frac{D_{ed} - D_{es}}{D_{ed}}\right)}{LVET}$$

where $D_{ed}$ is diameter end diastole, $D_{es}$ is diameter end systole, and LVET is LV ejection time (ms).

## ANGIOGRAPHIC ASSESSMENT OF VALVE REGURGITATION

1. Left ventricular opacification visualizes mitral but not aortic valvular regurgitation. For the aortic valve, contrast injections made low in the aortic root serve to quantify aortic regurgitation. In mild degrees of aortic regurgitation, a fine regurgitant jet or puff is noted; opacification is limited to the LV outflow tract, clearing with each systole (grade 1), or faint, persistent, incomplete opacification of the LV cavity (grade 2) occurs. In grades 3 and 4, no distinct jet is seen, and dense complete opacification of the left ventricle occurs either progressively or in one or two diastolic cycles, and LV density exceeds aortic density in the severe case (Fig. 17-21).
2. For the mitral valve, LV injection in the RAO view detects and quantifies mitral regurgitation. The angiographic criteria for grading mitral regurgitation are highly subjective. Mild grades 1 and 2 mitral regurgitation have a narrow-to-moderate width regurgitant jet of slight to moderate density with minimum-to-moderate opacification of the left atrium clearing quickly. Grades 3 and 4 have no well-defined jet with intense and persistant left atrial opacification (Fig. 17-22). The left atrium appears denser than the left ventricle or aorta in grade 4 mitral regurgitation. If there is associated mitral valve prolapse, shown best in a lateral projection, all or a portion of one or both leaflets

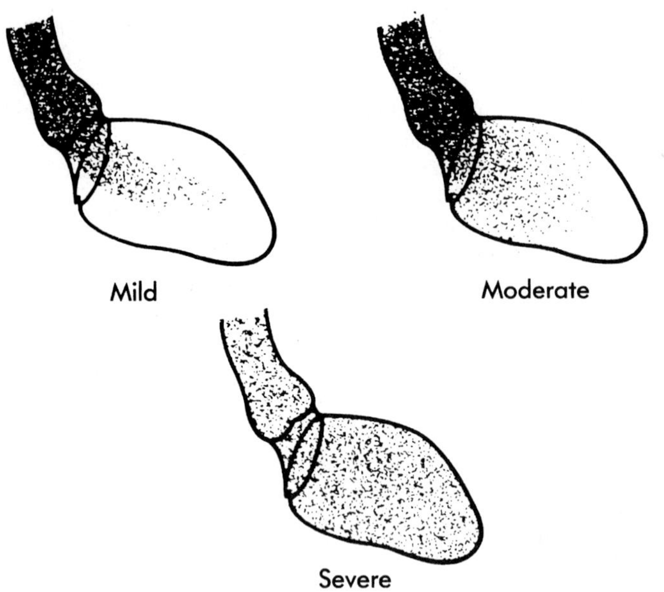


FIGURE 17-21 Angiographic evaluation of aortic regurgitation, right anterior oblique view. When the left anterior oblique view is used, overestimation of the aortic regurgitation occurs. (From Pujadas G. *Coronary angiography in the Medical and Surgical Treatment of Ischemic Heart Disease*. New York: McGraw-Hill; 1980. With permission.)

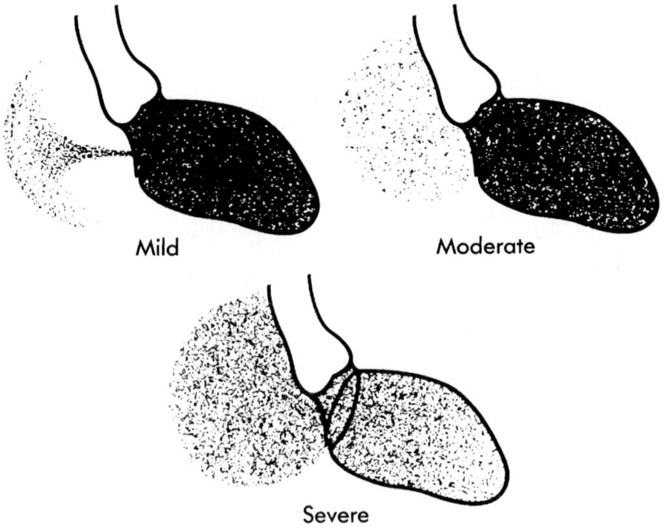

FIGURE 17-22 Angiographic evaluation of mitral regurgitation. (From Pujadas G. *Coronary Angiography in the Medical and Surgical Treatment of Ischemic Heart Disease*. New York: McGraw-Hill; 1980. With permission.)

balloons may appear above the mitral annulus in systole. A normal mitral valve may be transiently regurgitant if ectopic beating occurs.

Mitral regurgitation can also be quantitated by calculating a regurgitant fraction as follows:

The total stroke volume obtained by left ventriculography is used to assess the severity of mitral and aortic valve regurgitation. Total stroke volume minus forward stroke volume equals regurgitant stroke volume. The regurgitant fraction equals regurgitant stroke volume divided by total stroke volume. Severe valvular regurgitation has a regurgitant fraction of 0.50 or greater.

The angiographic quantitation of valvular regurgitation is shown in Table 17-20.

## RIGHT VENTRICULOGRAPHY

RV volume is estimated by applying Simpson's rule or the area-length method to the cavity silhouettes after biplane angiography.[59] The end-diastolic volume of the right ventricle in normal persons is $81 \pm 12$ mL/m$^2$. The opacified left atrial shadow is represented as an ellipsoid, so the left atrial volume also can be calculated in the biplane mode; the normal left atrial maximal volume is $63 \pm 16$ mL with a mean volume of $35 \pm 8.7$ mL. Indications for right ventriculography include (1) documentation of tricuspid regurgitation; (2) RV dysplasia for arrhythmias; (3) pulmonary stenosis; (4) abnormalities of pulmonary outflow tract; and (5) right-to-left ventricular shunts.

## COMPLICATIONS OF VENTRICULOGRAPHY

Cardiac arrhythmias, especially ventricular tachycardia and ventricular fibrillation, require immediate cardioversion. Intramyocardial "staining," injection of contrast into the myocardium, is generally transient and of no clinical importance unless it is deep or perforating (emergency pericardiocentesis may be required). Arrhythmias and staining are more common with end hole catheters than any pigtail catheters. Embolism from thrombi or air may occur. These events are minimized with careful catheter and injection syringe preparation, flushing,

TABLE 17-20 Angiographic Quantitation of Valvular Regurgitation

| | Mitral Regurgitation | | Aortic Regurgitation |
|---|---|---|---|
| | Mild LA opacification; clears rapidly, often jet-like | + | Small regurgitant jet only; LV ejects contrast each systole |
| ++ | Moderal LA opacification, < LV | ++ | Regurgitant jet faintly opacifies LV cavity; not cleared each systole |
| +++ | Diffuse contrast Regurgitant; LA Opacification = LV; LA Significantly enlarged[a] | +++ | Persistent LV Opacification = aortic root density; LV enlargement[a] |
| ++++ | LA opacification > LV, persistent; systolic pulmonary vein opacification may occur; often marked LV enlargement[a] | ++++ | Persistent LV Opacification > aortic root concentraton; often marked LV enlargement[a] |

[a]Chronic regurgitation.
KEY: ++ = mild; +++ = moderate; ++++ = severe.
ABBREVIATIONS: LA = left atrium; LV = left ventricle.

TABLE 17-21 Indications and Contraindications for Ascending Aortography

*Indications*
Aortic aneurysm/aortic dissection
- Aortic insufficiency
- Nonselective coronary or bypass graft arteriography
- Supravalvular aortic stenosis
- Brachiocephalic or arch vessel disease
- Coarctation of the aorta
- Aortic to pulmonary artery or right heart (e.g., sinus of Valsalva fistula) communication
- Aortic or periaortic neoplastic disease
- Arterial thromboembolic disease
- Arterial inflammatory disease

*Contraindications*
- Contrast media reaction
- Injection into false lumen of aortic dissection
- End-hole catheter malposition
- Inability to tolerate additional radiographic contrast media

and debubbling. Contrast-related complications including allergic-type vasomotor collapse may occur during this procedure. Transient hypotension (<15 to 30 s) was common with ionic contrast media.

## Other Cardiovascular Angiographic Studies

### RIGHT ATRIAL ANGIOGRAPHY INDICATIONS

1. Defining the tricuspid valve in Ebstein's anomaly and tricuspid atresia or stenosis.
2. Myxoma or thrombus.
3. Juxtaposition of right atrial appendage in cyanotic congenital heart disease.
4. The right atrial border in pericardial effusion or tumor.
5. Atrial septal defect with right-to-left shunting.

### ASCENDING AORTOGRAPHY

Although cut film is an established radiologic method, for cardiac catheterization laboratories cineangiography is acceptable in patients with suspected dissection of the aorta. Indications and contraindications are shown in Table 17-21.

#### *Radiographic Projections for Aortography*

LAO OR LATERAL PROJECTION This view is excellent for identifying dissection of the ascending aorta extending up to the neck vessels, optimally delineating the aortic arch, opening the aortic curvature, and providing clear views of the innominate, common carotid artery, and left subclavian arteries. The coronary arteries at the root of the aorta are displayed in a semilateral projection.

TABLE 17-22 Indications for Abdominal Aortography

- Nonselective evaluation of renal arteries and mesenteric vessels
- Abdominal aneurysm or dissection
- Abdominal aortic atherosclerotic disease
- Vascular assessment prior to IAB[a] counterpulsation
- Initial evaluation of claudication
- Evaluation of cause of difficult catheter movement for coronary angiography

[a]Intraaortic balloon.

RAO PROJECTION The descending thoracic aorta, and the ascending aorta may be superimposed across the arch in the AP or LAO projection. The RAO view is more helpful in delineating the effect of dissection on the lower thoracic arota and intercostal arteries as well as the origin of bypass grafts to the left coronary system. There are no advantages to cranial or caudal tilts for viewing the aorta. In nonselective coronary arteriography in which aortic root angiography may help to identify a vein graft takeoff, the cranial and caudal angulation may provide some increased detail.

### ABDOMINAL AORTOGRAPHY

Indications for abdominal aortography are shown in Table 17-22. A lateral projection is commonly needed for anteriorly angulated aneurysm, especially if stent graft repair of abdominal aortic aneurysm is being considered. Evaluation of peripheral lower extremity disease requires identification of iliac bifurcation and common femoral artery patency before subselective injections. The contraindications of abdominal aortography are the same as thoracic aortography Figure 17-23 shows typical findings in abdominal aortography in a patient with peripheral vascular disease.

### PULMONARY ANGIOGRAPHY

Pulmonary angiography, the visualization of vascular abnormalities of the lung vessels (e.g., intraluminal defects representing pulmonary

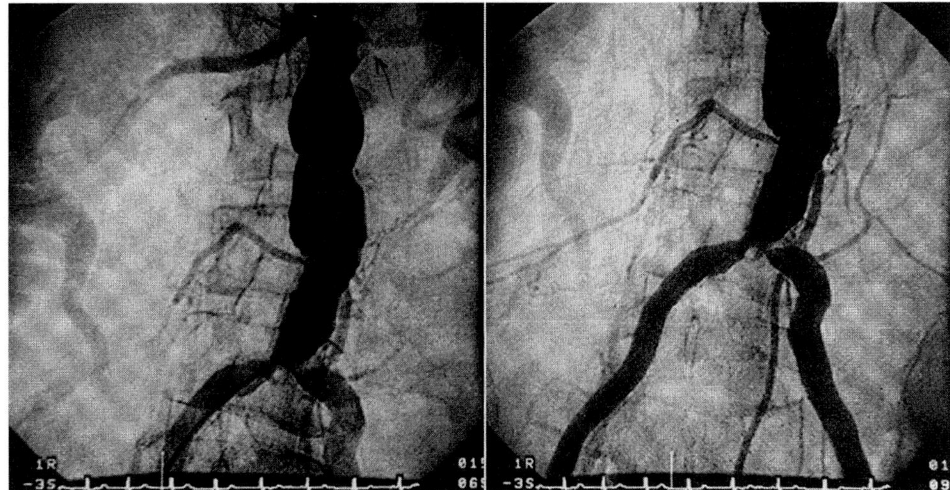

FIGURE 17-23 Aortography of the lower abdominal aorta demonstrating bilateral iliac stenosis at its origin from the most distal part of the abdominal aorta. (From Kern MJ. *Cardiac Catheterization Handbook,* St. Louis: Mosby; 2003. With permission.)

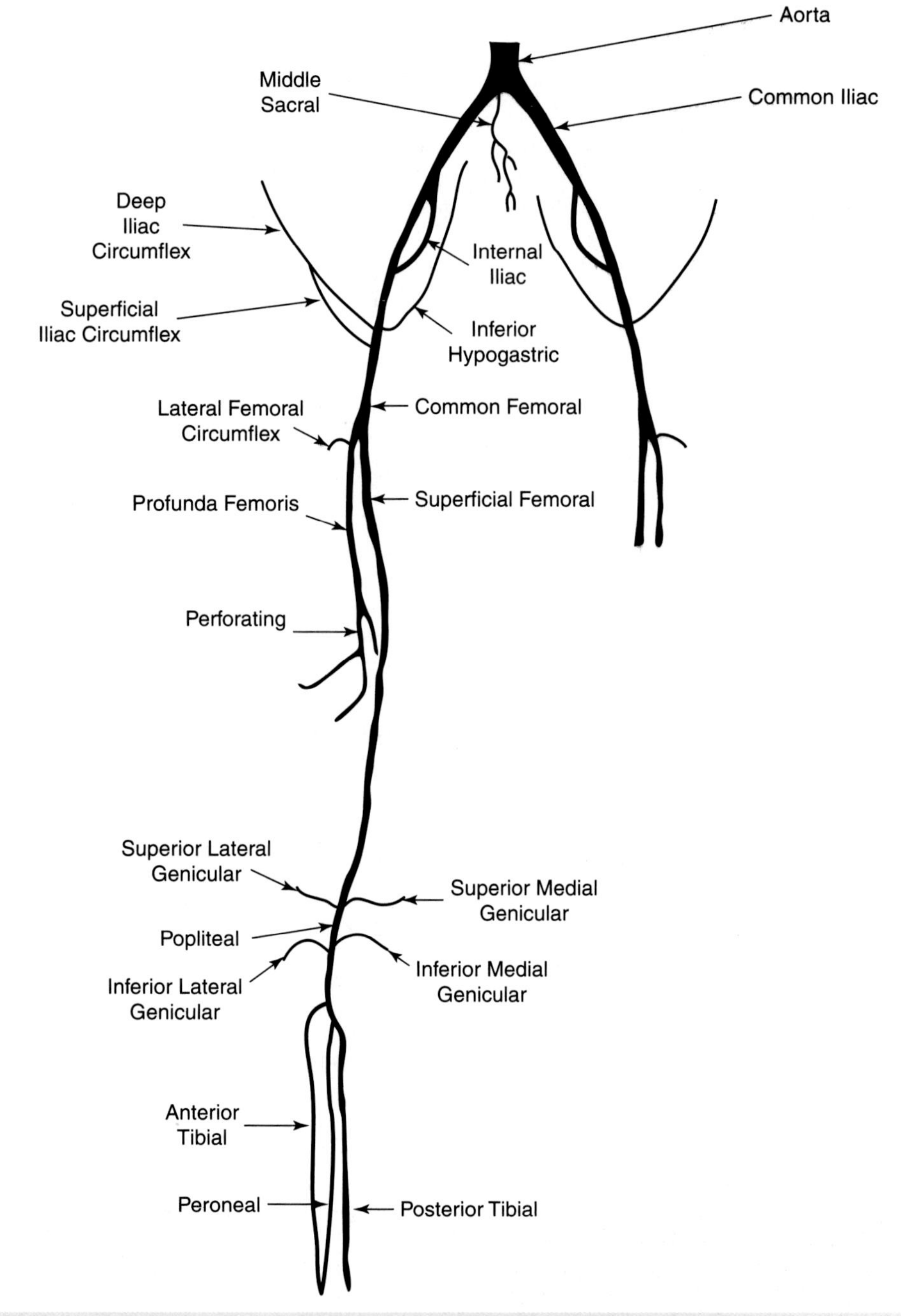


FIGURE 17-24 Peripheral vascular anatomy.

emboli, shunts, stenosis, AV malformation, and anomalous connections), should be preceded by the measurements of right heart pressures.

## PERIPHERAL VASCULAR ANGIOGRAPHY

Once the techniques of coronary angiography have been mastered, peripheral vascular angiography is not difficult. Digital subtraction angiography is the method of choice for identifying peripheral vascular disease. However, cineangiography can provide satisfactory information if the filming time, frame rates, and contrast dosages are properly established. Cine angiography is also helpful to detect the speed of vessel opacification and collateral filling.

Based on clinical signs and symptoms of arterial insufficiency to the legs, suspected obstructions of vessel are often screened with noninvasive studies (i.e., ankle brachial index) before angiography is performed. Small-diameter (5F) catheters are satisfactory. Reduced volume of contrast (10 to 20 mL over 1 to 2 s) are injected during filming with panning down the artery, following the course to the most distal locations. Angulated views may be necessary to open bifurcations and overlying vessels that obscure the vessel origin. When possible, angiographic filming should extend at least to the ankle. Nonionic contrast agents are less painful than ionic media for peripheral angiography.

The area most frequently involved in peripheral atherosclerotic disease involves the distal superficial femoral artery at the abductor canal (Fig. 17-24). The calf (tibial), and knee (popliteal) arteries are the next most commonly involved vessels after the superficial femoral artery. Disease in the deep femoral artery (femoral profunda) is rare. Pathways of collateralization are often rich and varied in patients with chronic distal femoral artery disease, especially in total occlusions of the superficial femoral artery that reconstitutes at or below the knee, close to the branching trifurcation of the tibial and deep peroneal arteries. Determining the level of reconstitution of collateralized vessels and distal runoff is crucial in determining the feasibility of revascularization.

## RENAL ARTERIOGRAPHY

Selective renal arteriography evaluates the renal artery origins and vasculature. Selective arterial injections provide the most detail and are easily obtained with a JR4 catheter. For screening aortography, the renal artery origins usually arise at L1 vertebra (just below the T12 ribs). The 30-degree ipsilateral oblique projection often provides the best view of the renal artery ostia in a majority of patients. Acutely angled takeoffs of the renal artery may require specially shaped catheters or an arm approach. Atherosclerotic disease of the renal artery usually involves the proximal one-third of the renal artery and is seldom present without abdominal atherosclerotic plaques. Delayed imaging to see the nephrogram is essential to exclude accessory renal arteries and to screen for presence of severe parenchymal disease. Measurement of a pressure gradient across ostial proximal lesion is recommended to determine the need for intervention.

## THE X-RAY IMAGE

### Generation of the X-ray Image

Cardiac angiography uses a complex interaction of radiographic x-ray elements, transforming energy into a visual image. The x-ray image generation chain can be simplified into three major components: (1) the x-ray generator; (2) the x-ray tube; and (3) the image intensifier. The details of x-ray equipment should be familiar to all personnel working in a catheterization laboratory.

#### X-RAY GENERATOR

The generator provides the power source necessary to accelerate the electrons through the x-ray tube. The duration of x-ray exposure is similar to the shutter speed on a regular camera. During the cardiac "photographic" examination, the exposure usually is set fast enough to stop blurring as a result of heart movement. During selective coronary arteriography, the shorter the exposure time, the better the image. Exposure times of 3 to 6 ms reduce movement blur. Most modern generators are capable of delivering adequate power while providing precise and automatically adjusted exposure timing. Current generators are equipped with either multiple phase (alternating on/off) or short/long pulse widths that are automatically adjusted for correct exposure. Manual settings, which are operator selected, are limited to film frame rates (e.g., 15, 30, or 60 frames per second).

#### X-RAY TUBES

The function of the x-ray tube is to convert electrical energy, provided from the generator, to an x-ray beam. Electrons emitted from a heated filament (cathode) are accelerated toward a rapidly rotating disc (anode) and at contact undergo conversion to x-radiation. This process generates extreme heat. The heat capacity of an x-ray tube is a major limiting factor in the design of x-ray tubes. Only 0.2 to 0.6 percent of the electrical energy provided to the tube eventually is converted to x-rays.

In addition to the exposure times (controlled by the generator system) and the size of the imaging field (controlled by the x-ray tube), two other factors of the x-ray determine the quality of x-ray for proper image exposures.

***Electrical Current (mA)*** The number of photons (electrical particles) generated per unit of time. The greater the electrical current the greater the number of photons, resulting in improved image resolution. If the photon volume if marginal, the resulting image may be "mottled" or have a spotty appearance. Increasing the milliamperage will improve this result, but the level of milliamperage is limited by the heat capacity of the x-ray tubes. Also, increasing the number of milliamperes markedly increases radiation exposure and scatter to patient and catheterization personnel.

***The Level of Kilovoltage (kV)*** The energy spectrum (wavelengths) of the x-ray beam. The higher the level of kilovoltage, the shorter the wavelength of radiation and the greater the ability of x-rays to penetrate target tissue. Increased kilovoltage is especially important in *obese* patients. To obtain better images through more tissue, a higher kilovolt level is required. Unfortunately, a high kilovolt level also will produce lower resolution because of wide scatter. There is also greater radiation exposure to patients and laboratory personnel. Modern radiographic equipment currently allows for variability of the amperage and voltage to attain optimal quality radiographic images. An automatic exposure control system sets exposure times to incorporate changes in voltage (kV) and, amperage (mA), providing the desired images at the best exposures possible (Fig. 17-25).

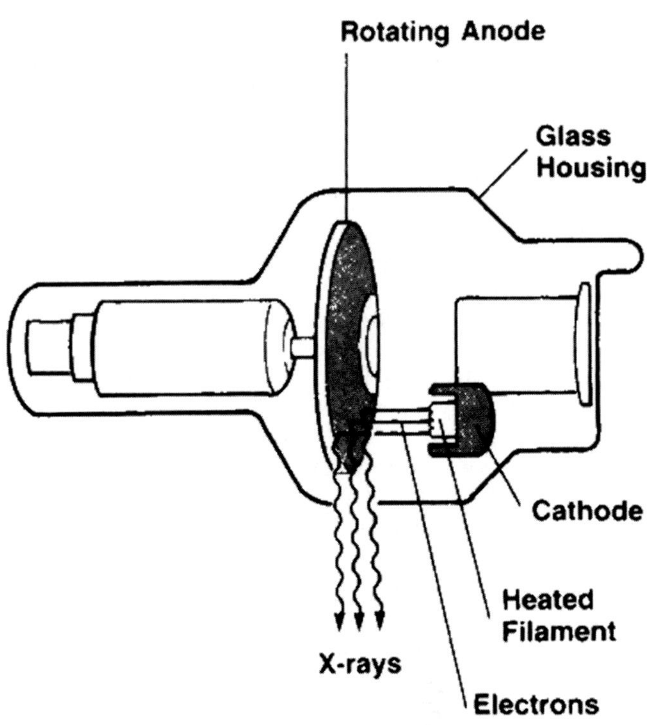


FIGURE 17-25 X-ray generation. (From Baim D, Grossman W, eds. *Grossman's Cardiac Catheterization, Angiography and Intervention,* 6th ed. Philadelphia: Lippincott Williams & Wilkins; 2000:19. With permission.)

#### IMAGE INTENSIFIER AND IMAGE DISTORTION

After the x-rays have penetrated the body, the partially absorbed beams are cast in a shadow fashion on the input screen of the image intensifier. The image intensifier converts the invisible x-ray image into a visual image. Each x-ray photon hits the phosphorous covered plate of the intensifier resulting in a light particle which is detected and its position and intensity noted. The sum of all events produces an image for video and digital recording. Image intensifiers are equipped with different-sized image fields that alter the image resolution. In general, the smaller the input screen diameter, the smaller the image field size and the sharper the resolution. Smaller input screen diameters (5- to 7-in. screens) are better suited for selective coronary cineangiography because of their enhanced resolution. For more detailed work, such as percutaneous transluminal coronary angioplasty, even smaller input diameter (4-in.) screens have been particularly useful. In contrast, large-screen (or field) examinations (i.e., left ventriculography, aortography, or peripheral angiography) use input screen diameters of 9 to 11 in. The trade-off, of course, is that detailed resolution is reduced.

Image distortion may be caused by magnification or foreshortening. The x-ray image casts an x-ray shadow onto the input screen of the image intensifier. The distance of the object from the screen produces an image that may be either sharp or indistinct, depending on the distance. Increasing the distance of the heart to the image intensifier also requires more kilovoltage, thereby further reducing image quality. Distortion of the object's perspective is called *foreshortening*. When the longitudinal axis is seen at an oblique angle, there is foreshortening of the length shadow, and when it is perpendicular to the x-ray beam (parallel to the film plane), there is a full and true image of the length and contour details. Because of foreshortening, arterial lesions that may appear severe in one projection may not appear at all or seem significantly less severe in other projections. For this reason multiple angulated projections are used to identify the severity of lesions within the coronary tree.

### DIGITAL ANGIOGRAPHY IMAGING

Digital angiography converts the x-ray image into a quantitative information format for storage and display on a computer. Digital angiography stores x-ray images on magnetic tapes, disks, or other electronic media rather than on x-ray film. Digital angiography permits compact storage and quantitative image analysis. Digital imaging also permits various manipulations to be performed to enhance the stored images. The contrast image can be amplified or enlarged or contrast adjusted. One image can be subtracted from another and then that image can be subtracted from a third image. Similar contrast adjustments and enlargements are not possible with film radiographs. The durability of some digital achival media has been questioned.

## Radiation Safety

The catheterization laboratory environment should be made as safe as possible for the staff and patient. Standards for radiation protection (from the Society for Cardiac Angiography and Intervention)[59a] include four basic principles:

1. The less exposure, the less chance of absorbed energy biologic interaction.
2. No known level of ionizing radiation is a permissible dose or absolutely safe.
3. Radiation exposure is cumulative. There is no washout phenomenon.
4. All participants in the cardiac catheterization laboratory have voluntarily accepted some degree of radiation exposure, but they are obliged to minimize and reduce risks to other personnel and themselves.

The primary x-ray beam, emanating from the under table x-ray tube upward through the patient and onto the image intensifier exposes all subjects to radiation in a dose geometrically inverse to the distance from the source. Radiation scatter is increased when the angle of the x-ray tube is set obliquely. A high degree of angulation increases the amount of radiation scatter (Fig. 17-26). Acrylic shields and table-mounted lead aprons reduce exposure from x-ray scatter. Fluoroscopy generates approximately *one-fifth* the x-ray exposure of cineangiography. The increased use of cineangiography for complex catheterization procedures has increased the total exposure and should be a consideration in procedures requiring extensive intracardiac manipulation, such as angioplasty, valvuloplasty, or electrophysiology studies.[60–62]

Practices to ensure radiation dose limitation should be routinely employed. Although no known threshold for radiation exposure exists to define specific risks, the National Council on Radiation Protection and Measurements (NCRP) indicates that no dose >3 rem should be allowed over a 3-month period. The eyes, gonads, and red bone marrow have a whole-body limit of 5 rem (roentgen equivalent man) per year; any specific organ, such as the thyroid or skin, has a yearly limit of 15 rem. The maximal permissible dose, or "safe" exposure, for catheterization laboratory personnel is 100 mrem per week monitored by an unshielded left collar badge. Definitions of radiation units are provided in Table 17-23.

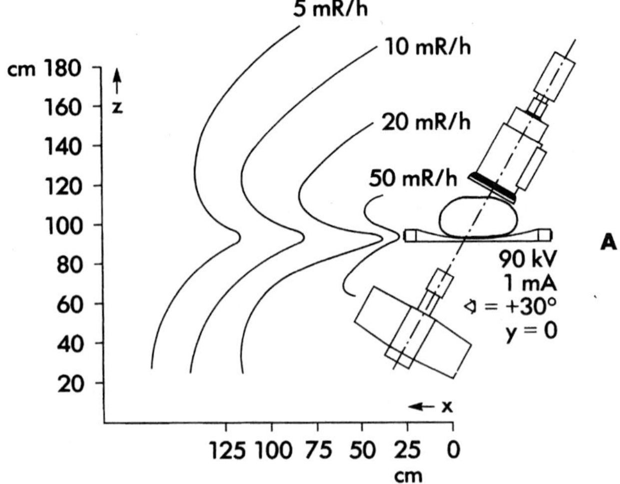


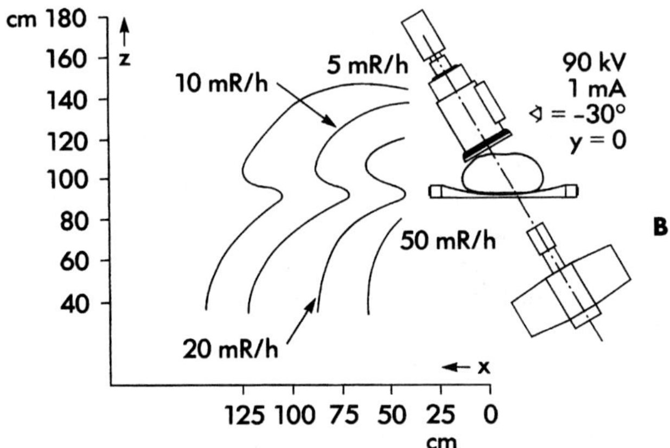


FIGURE 17-26 Isoexposure curves representing ranges of relative exposure in the position usually occupied by the operator performing an angiographic procedure from the right arm. *A*. 30-degree left anterior oblique. *B*. 30-degree right anterior oblique. (From Balter S, Sones FM, Brancato R. Radiation exposure to the operator performing cardiac angiography with U-arm systems. *Circulation* 1978;58:925. With permission.)

Radiation exposure is greater during angioplasty than during diagnostic catheterization. If the protective shields are employed

TABLE 17-23 Definitions or Radiation Units

*Roentgen (R)* is the measure of ionization delivered to a specific point (exposure). One chest x-ray equals 3 to 5 mR.

*Radiation absorbed dose (rad)* is the amount of radiation energy deposited per unit mass of tissue. The amount of absorbed dose per given exposure is dependent upon tissue type. For example, for soft tissue, 1 R = 1 rad; for bone, 1 R = 4 rad (i.e., greater absorption).

*Radiation equivalent dose in man (rem)* is used to express the biological impact of a given exposure. For x-radiation, 1 rad = 1 rem.

carefully, the radiation exposure for single- and double-vessel angioplasty as compared to diagnostic catheterization may be comparable. However, it should be understood that radiation exposures are generally higher for these procedures, especially when biplane angiography is performed.

## HEMODYNAMIC DATA FROM THE CARDIAC CATHETERIZATION LABORATORY

In conjunction with angiographic data gathered during the cardiac catheterization, hemodynamic information is recorded from catheters inside vascular structures. Hemodynamic data includes pressure measurements, blood flow, and blood oxygen saturation measurements.

Protocols for systematic hemodynamic data collection are available elsewhere.[5–7] Clinical indications for hemodynamic studies are summarized in Table 17-1.

### Pressure Measurements

#### PRESSURE-RECORDING SYSTEMS

Blood within the heart or vessels exerts pressure. A pressure wave is created by cardiac muscular contraction and is transmitted from the vessel or chamber along a closed, fluid-filled column (catheter) to a pressure transducer, converting the mechanical pressure to an electrical signal that is displayed on a video monitor. Cardiac pressure waveforms are cyclical, repeating the pressure change from the onset of one cardiac contraction (systole) to the onset of the next contraction. The complete description of the physiology of heart function is discussed in Chap. 4. An examination of the cardiac cycle and corresponding pressures will provide an understanding of basic hemodynamics in the cardiac catheterization laboratory.

The collection of hemodynamic data for cardiac catheterization is an integral part of every procedure. Even complex hemodynamic data recording can be accomplished accurately and rapidly if an efficient and consistently used methodology is established in the laboratory. A predetermined plan for data collection facilitates simultaneous pressure measurements across the heart, concentrating on the aortic and mitral valves, those that are affected most commonly by disease. Different hemodynamic measurements for specific clinical situations are necessary.

In conjunction with pressure measurements, cardiac output by thermodilution technique or the Fick (oxygen consumption) method is also obtained, especially for valvular heart disease or cardiomyopathy. To measure suspected cardiac shunts, arterial, vena caval, right atrial (RA), and pulmonary artery (PA) oxygen saturations are collected routinely. Multiple oxygen saturation samples are obtained throughout the right and left heart for intracardiac shunt identification.

Pressure wave fidelity depends on quality components that can transmit the pressure wave to a transducer without signal distortion. If the heart rate is 60 to 120 beats per minute, the fundamental frequency of the basic wave is 1 to 2 per s. The higher frequency sine-wave components of the pressure wave then occur at frequencies of up to 10 to 20 Hz; For best results, the transducer must detect these components without phase lag or amplitude distortion because their sum represents the rising and falling contours of the native pressure curve. A properly responding pressure-recording system should have a high natural frequency and optimal damping to minimize over- or undershoot of the waveform. A high natural frequency is obtained by using a bubble-free, saline solution–filled system of minimum length

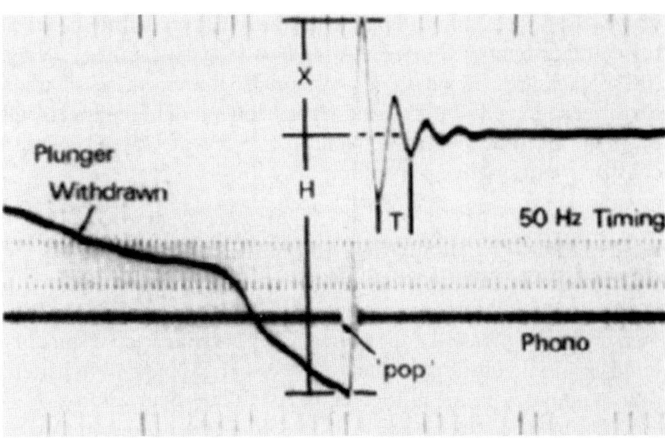


FIGURE 17-27 In order to measure the dynamic frequency response of a catheter transducer system, an abrupt transient input dynamic pressure is applied to the catheter tip (a plunger is pulled free of an air-filled syringe); the pressure oscillations are recorded at a fast paper speed and measured. X = height of the initial overshoot; H = end height of the recorded deflection; T = period of a free oscillation, 0.08 s. The natural frequency is 13 Hz; the useful range is 4 Hz. The amplitude ratio of two successive peak amplitudes is 0.59, and the damping coefficient is 0.17. This underdamped system is optimally damped to a coefficient around 0.64 by the addition of a narrow-bore tube between catheter and transducer. (Reproduced with the permission of Irex Corporation.)

whose catheter and connector tubings have stiff walls and wide bores. A frequency response and damping coefficient can be obtained by introducing a square-wave pressure input to the pressure system and measuring the amplitude ratio of any two successive peak pressure amplitudes and the time interval between peaks (Fig. 17-27). For clinical cardiac catheterization, a manometer system with a uniform dynamic response of greater than 20 Hz is desirable.

Clinically, the zero (atmospheric) position for an external pressure transducer is set at the lateral midchest level. Specifically, hydrostatic zero is considered to be at the level of most anterior surfaces of the LV blood pool.[63] An additional limiting factor in pressure recording is the superimposition of artifacts on the pressure pulse by the accelerating and decelerating movements imparted to the fluid-filled cardiac catheter by the beating heart. Distortion of the catheter-obtained phasic pressure waveform by motion or damping artifact can be avoided with the use of a catheter-tip, side-mounted, miniature semiconductor gauge. This manometer system is required for first- or second-derivative measurements of the pressure curve and is principally a research tool.

#### THE FEMORAL ARTERY AND LEFT VENTRICULAR PRESSURE

The most common pressure measurements include systemic pressure and LV pressure. The femoral artery sheath is often used to compare aortic pressure to LV pressure to assess the aortic valve. A delay in pressure transmission and overshoot of the systolic pressure compared to centrally measured aortic pressure are characteristic of femoral artery pressure measurements.

The LV pressure should be examined for waveform characteristics to insure all side holes are beneath the aortic valve and that the catheter system is flushed to permit accurate interpretation of the diastolic LV waveform.[64]

Right heart hemodynamics are easily obtained with balloon-tipped flotation catheter. Blood oxygen saturations in the inferior vena cava, right atrium and pulmonary artery are collected to screen for cardiac shunts. RA, RV, PA, and pulmonary capillary wedge (PCW) pressures are measured and cardiac output by thermodilution performed. If necessary during right heart pressure catheter pull back, the LV pressure can be compared to RV pressure to identify constrictive/ restrictive physiology.

### RIGHT HEART PRESSURES AND THE PULMONARY CAPILLARY WEDGE PRESSURE

PCW pressure closely approximates left atrial (LA) pressure. PCW pressure overestimates LA pressure in patients with acute respiratory failure, chronic obstructive lung disease with pulmonary hypertension, pulmonary venoconstriction, or LV failure with volume overload. Discrepancies between LA and PCW may be caused, in part, by different types of catheters: balloon-tipped flotation catheters are soft with small lumens; LA pressure catheters (e.g., Brockenbrough or Mullins-type sheath) are stiff with large lumens. In most patients, the PCW is sufficient to assess LV filling pressure. However, in patients with mitral valvular disease or mitral valve prostheses, the most accurate method is direct LA pressure measurement by transeptal puncture.

PCW pressure can be identified from adequate pressure waveforms. Correct catheter position can be confirmed with oximetry, since blood drawn from the wedge position should have an oxygen saturation of >90 percent. The best location of the PCW pressure has been questioned, but for practical purposes any of the four locations (left or right upper lobes or left or right lower lobes) within the pulmonary tree are generally acceptable. The right lower lobe is the most common location for positioning of the pulmonary artery balloon-tipped catheter. In patients with high pulmonary artery pressures (>50 mmHg), an inflated balloon should not be left in place for more than 10 min because prolonged balloon inflation may cause pulmonary infarction or damage to the pulmonary artery. Care should be taken not to inflate a balloon vigorously in distal portions of the lung, where the balloon may tear a small pulmonary vessel. PCW pressure can also be obtained with end-hole multipurpose catheters. A deep inspiration and gentle simultaneous catheter advancement with a cough facilitate a wedge placement with these catheters. Complications of pulmonary artery catheterization are described in Table 17-24.

## Computations for Hemodynamic Measurements

Once the hemodynamic data have been obtained, computations are made to clarify and enhance quantitation of cardiac function. The most often used computations involve quantitation of cardiac work, flow resistance, valve areas, and amount of shunting. Specific derivations and applications of these formulas can be found elsewhere.[5–7]

TABLE 17-24 Complications of Pulmonary Artery Catheterization

| |
|---|
| Complications of vascular access |
| Pulmonary infarction |
| Pulmonary artery rupture |
| Injury to chordae in right ventricle |
| Tricuspid regurgitation |
| Right bundle branch block |
| Dislodgment of pacemaker leads |

1. Cardiac output (CO) by the Fick ($O_2$ consumption) method is calculated as follows:

$$\text{CO} = \frac{O_2 \text{ consumption (mL/min)}}{\text{AV}O_2 \text{ difference (mL } O_2\text{/100 mL blood)} \times 10}$$

In 1870, Adolph Fick expounded a theory for the measurement of blood flow that he never used in the laboratory: "The total uptake or release of a substance by an organ is the product of the blood flow to the organ and of the arteriovenous concentration of the substance." Using total oxygen consumption of 300 mL/min, arterial blood oxygen content of 19 mL/100 mL of blood, and mixed venous blood oxygen content of 14 mL/100 mL of blood, the cardiac output, in liters per minute, is equal to the oxygen consumption divided by the arteriovenous oxygen difference multiplied by 10 (to convert the latter to liters). With these data, in this case, the cardiac output equals 6.0 L/min.

Oxygen consumption is measured from a metabolic "hood"; it also can be estimated as 3 $mLO_2$/min/kg or 125 mL/min/$m^2$. $AVO_2$ (arteriovenous oxygen) difference is calculated from arterial–mixed venous (pulmonary artery) $O_2$ content, where $O_2$ content = saturation × 1.36 × hemoglobin concentration. For example, if the arterial saturation is 95%, the pulmonary artery saturation is 65%, the hemoglobin concentration is 13.0 g/dL, and the $O_2$ consumption is 210 $mLO_2$/min (70 kg × 3 $mLO_2$/min/kg), then the cardiac output is:

$$\frac{210}{(0.95 - 0.65) \times 1.36 \times 13.0 \times 10} = \frac{210}{53} = 3.96 \text{ L/min}$$

2. Cardiac index (CI, L/min/$m^2$)

$$\text{CI} = \frac{\text{CO (L/min)}}{\text{BSA } (m^2)}$$

where CO is cardiac output and BSA is body surface area.

3. Stroke volume (SV, ml/beat)

$$\text{SV} = \frac{\text{CO (mL/min)}}{\text{HR (bpm)}}$$

where HR is heart rate.

4. Stroke index (SI, mL/beat/$m^2$)

$$\text{SI} = \frac{\text{SV (mL/beat)}}{\text{BSA } (m^2)}$$

5. Stroke work (SW, g · m)

$$\text{SW} = (\text{mean LV systolic pressure} - \text{mean LV diastolic pressure}) \times \text{stroke volume} \times 0.0144$$

6. Pulmonary arteriolar resistance (PAR, Wood units)

$$\text{PAR} = \frac{\text{mean pulmonary arterial pressure} - \text{mean LA pressure (or mean PCW)}}{\text{CO}}$$

7. Total pulmonary resistance (TPR, Wood units)

$$\text{TPR} = \frac{\text{mean pulmonary arterial pressure}}{\text{CO}}$$

8. Systemic vascular resistance (SVR, Wood units)

$$\text{SVR} = \frac{\text{mean systemic arterial pressure} - \text{mean right atrial pressure}}{\text{CO}}$$

Resistance calculations follow the form of Ohm's law, where

$$R = \Delta p/\dot{Q}$$

R = Resistance, Δp = mean pressure differential across the vascular bed, $\dot{Q}$ = blood flow. Resistance units (mmHg/L/min) are also called Hybrid resitance units (HRU) or Wood units. To convert Wood units to metric resistance (dynes-s-cm$^{-5}$), multiply by 80.

## Calculation of Valve Areas

Valvular or vascular obstruction produces a pressure gradient across a stenosis or vascular conduit/chamber narrowing. A pressure gradient is defined as the pressure difference across an area of valvular or vascular obstruction (such as a stenosis or an occlusion). The pressure gradient is influenced by physiologic variables such as rate of blood flow (cardiac output, coronary blood flow, etc.), resistance to flow, proximal chamber pressure and compliance, and anatomic variables, such as shape and length of valve ofice, tortuosities of the vessels (for arterial stenosis), or multiple or serial lesions (for both cardiac valves and arterial stenosis). In addition, pressure measurements may be influenced by artifactual variables which include miscalibrated pressure transducers, pressure leaks on catheter manifold or connecting tubing, pressure tubing type, length, and connectors, air in system, catheter sizes (especially small diameters), and fluid viscosity.

### VALVE AREA FORMULAS

A valve area can be calculated from standard hemodynamic data with the following formula:

$$\text{Area (cm}^2) = \frac{\text{valve flow (mL/s)}}{\text{K} \times \text{C} \times \sqrt{\text{MVG}}}$$

where MVG is mean valvular gradient (mmHg), K (44.3) is a derived constant by Gorlin and Gorlin,[65,66] C is an empiric constant that is 1 for semilunar valves and tricuspid valve and 0.85 for mitral valve, and valve flow is measured in milliliters per second during the diastolic or systolic flow period.

**For mitral valve flow :**

$$\frac{\text{CO (mL/min)}}{\text{(diastolic filling period) (HR)}}$$

**For aortic valve flow:**

$$\frac{\text{CO (mL/min)}}{\text{(systolic ejection period) (HR)}}$$

### CALCULATING AORTIC VALVE AREA

The method of calculating aortic valve area (AVA) from data obtained at catheterization for a patient with aortic stenosis (Fig. 17-28) is as follows. Assuming CO = 4000 mL/min, HR = 60 bpm.

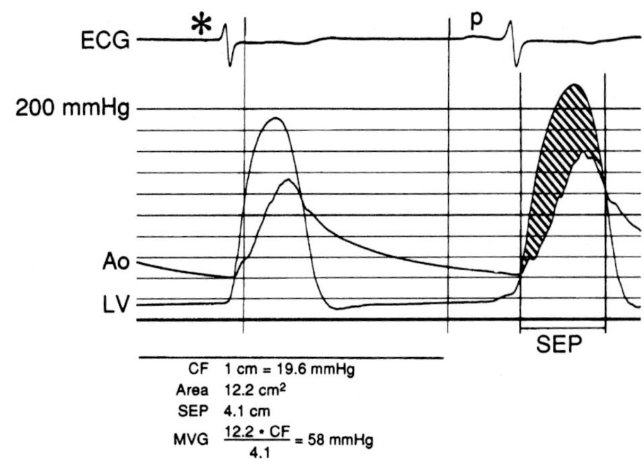


FIGURE 17-28 Aortic valve area is determined from the planimetered area of the aortic valve gradient. The aortic valve gradient area (*shaded area*) is bounded by the systolic ejection period (SEP). Ao = aortic pressure; LV = left ventricular pressure (scale 0 to 200 mmHg); CF = correction factor or scale factor; MVG = mean value gradient. See text for details. (From Kern MJ. *Cardiac Catheterization Handbook.* St. Louis: Mosby; 2003. With permission.)

1. Planimeter aortic-LV pressure gradients (area = 12.2 cm$^2$) and measure systolic ejection periods (SEP = 4.1 cm). Next convert cm to time and convert planimetered area to mean systolic pressure gradient.

   Systolic ejection period of 4.1 cm/beat at paper speed of 100 mm/s = 0.41 s/beat

   Mean valve gradient (MVG) = (area × scale factor)/SEP (Scale Factor: 1 cm = 19.6 mmHg [directly measured paper calibration lines of 200 mmHg])

$$\text{MVG} = 12.2\ \text{cm}^2 \times \frac{19.6\ \text{mmHg/1 cm}}{4.1\ \text{cm}} = \frac{239}{4.1} = 58\ \text{mmHg}$$

2. Compute aortic valve flow.

$$\text{Flow} = \frac{\text{CO}}{\text{SEP} \times \text{HR}} = \frac{4000\ \text{mL/min}}{0.41\ \text{s/beat} \times 60\ \text{bpm}} = \frac{4000}{24.6} = 162.6\ \text{mL/min}$$

3. Compute aortic valve area.

$$\text{AVA} = \frac{\text{Aortic valve flow}}{1.0 \times 44.3\sqrt{\text{MVG}}} = \frac{162.6}{44.3 \times \sqrt{58}} = \frac{162.6}{44.3 \times 7.6} = \frac{162.6}{336.6} = 0.48\ \text{cm}^2$$

Although mean pressure is used in the Gorlin formula, peak-to-peak pressure gradients are easily measured and also used to estimate valve area. The peak-to-peak gradient is *not* equivalent to mean gradient for mild and moderate stenosis but often approximates mean gradient for severe stenosis. The *delay* in pressure transmission and augmented pressure wave reflection from the proximal aorta to the femoral artery artificially *increases* the mean gradient. Femoral pressure overshoot (amplification) reduces the true gradient. If the femoral arterial pressure is used, phase shifting of the femoral arterial pressure to the left ventricle upstroke may be important. In patients with low gradients (i.e., <35 mmHg), more accurate valve areas were obtained with *unadjusted* LV-Ao pressure tracings.[67] Optimally, a second catheter can be positioned directly above the aortic valve to eliminate transmission delay and pressure amplification. Transseptal cardiac catheterization also can be performed to obtain LV pressure (via crossing mitral valve).

Aortic valve area can also be estimated closely by a simplified formula as cardiac output divided by the square root of the LV-Ao peak-to-peak pressure difference. For example, if peak-to-peak gradient = 65 mmHg and CO = 5 L/min, then Hakke valve area[68] =

$$\frac{5\text{ L/min}}{\sqrt{65}} = \frac{5\text{ L/min}}{8} = 0.63\text{ cm}^2$$

The simplified formula for valve area differs from the Gorlin formula by 18 ± 13 percent in patients with bradycardia (<65 bpm) or tachycardia (>100 bpm).[69,70] The Gorlin equation at *low* flow states *overestimates* the severity of valve stenosis. In low flow states (CO < 2.5 L/min), the Gorlin formula should be modified to employ the mean transvalvular gradient with new empirically derived constants.

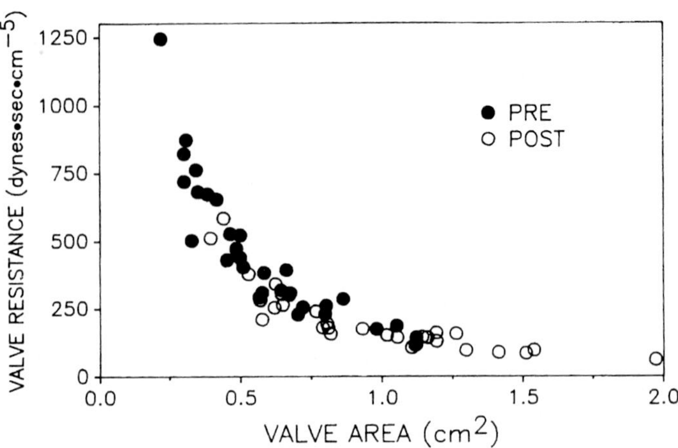


FIGURE 17-29 Comparison of valve area by Gorlin formula versus valve resistance before (*pre*) and after (*post*) aortic valvuloplasty. Valve resistance <200 dynes · s · cm$^{-5}$ is associated with minimal obstruction, >250 dynes · s cm$^{-5}$ with significant obstruction. This measure complements and refines valve area decision making. (From Feldman T, Ford L, Chiu YC, Carroll J. Changes in valvular resistance power dissipation and myocardial reserve with aortic valvuloplasty. *J Heart Valve Dis* 1992;1:55–64. With permission.)

## USE OF VALVE RESISTANCE FOR AORTIC STENOSIS

Valve resistance, a measure of valve obstruction, has recently been shown to have clinical use. Although proposed around the same time that the Gorlin valve area formula was initially reported, valve resistance has not been used because the units of dynes-s-cm-5 were not well related to clinical outcome.

Despite obvious strengths, valve area measurements have both practical and theoretical limitations. Area is a planar measurement without consideration of the funnel-like nature of the mitral inflow or the more tubelike configuration of the aortic outlet. Valve area is based on laminar flow of a noncompressible fluid. Turbulence is not considered. The constant in the denominator of the Gorlin formula is the square root of gravity, 2gH (acceleration of water due to gravity), and assumes that blood flow is gravity driven and nonpulsatile.[71]

Valve areas under 0.7 cm$^2$ are almost always associated with an important clinical syndrome, and areas greater than 1.1 cm$^2$ are usually not associated with significant symptoms, but the areas in between remain in a gray zone. One of the most common clinical situations is found in the patient with a valve area of 0.9 to 1.0 cm$^2$, a low transvalve pressure gradient, low cardiac output, and poor LV function. There is uncertainty regarding the outcome following valve replacement with a high mortality if ventricular function does not improve following surgery.

Valve resistance ($R$), as an alternative method to assess valve obstruction, is calculated using the same variables used for valve area measurement as:

$$R = \frac{\text{Mean gradient}}{(\text{CO/SEP}) \times \text{HR}} \times 80$$

where CO = cardiac output, SEP = systolic ejection period, HR = heart rate.

In contrast to valve area, the mean pressure gradient is considered to be a linear variable rather than taken as a square root term. Thus, the contribution of pressure gradient to the magnitude of valve resistance is greater. Resistance also has been shown to be more constant under conditions of changing cardiac output than valve area. Resistance thus necessarily has a close relationship to valve area. Fig. 17-29 shows resistance and area calculated in a group of patients before and after balloon aortic valve dilatation. Resistance rises sharply below a valve area of 0.7 cm$^2$. The shoulder of this curve is between 0.7 and 1.1 cm$^2$, which is the common area of indeterminate significance of Gorlin aortic valve area. Some patients in this gray zone tend to have higher valve resistance than others. It has been shown in this setting that the patients with resistance >250 dynes × s × cm$^{-5}$ are more likely to have significant obstruction while those with resistance below 200 dynes × sec × cm$^{-5}$ are less likely. There remains a gray zone using this index as well. In addition, some patients may have a resistance below 250 despite a planar valve area of 0.7 to 0.8 cm$^2$.

Resistance is a complementary index, not a replacement for valve area. Valve resistance is not expected to remain consistent. Some of the changes in valve area observed in a single patient under different conditions or at different times might be more acceptable when considered as changes in valve resistance than planar area. As with peripheral resistance, valve resistance is interpreted in the context of the clinical conditions under which it is measured. A peripheral resistance of 1000 dynes × s × cm$^{-5}$ has a greatly different significance in a patient with presumed sepsis than it does in a patient with LV failure. Similarly, we can expect valve resistance to vary as cardiac output changes.

## CALCULATIONS FOR MITRAL VALVE AREA

To calculate the most accurate valve area, use the direct LA pressure from transseptal measurement. Transseptal catheterization should be performed to confirm large pressure gradients, especially for suspected prosthetic mitral stenosis. The PCW pressure overestimates LA pressure (transseptal catheterization) in patients with prosthetic mitral valves (Fig. 17-30). Overestimation is caused, in part, by large v waves increasing the phase delay, making correction and alignment of pressure tracings difficult.[72] However, if the PCW pressure-LV pressure tracings show no significant gradients, transseptal catheterization is unnecessary. Mitral valve area from the following data is calculated below. Assuming CO = 3500 mL/min, HR = 80 bpm.

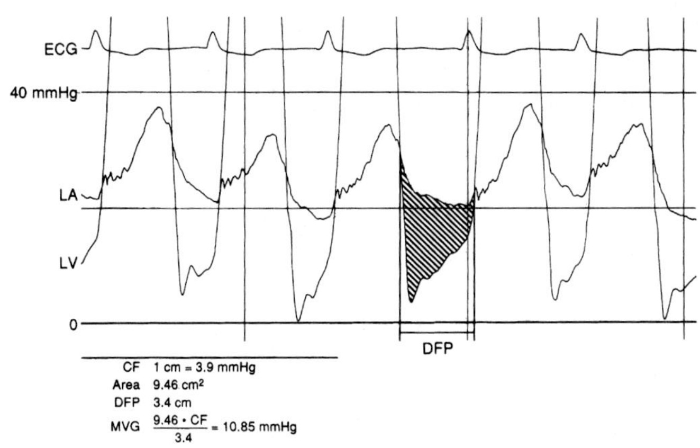


FIGURE 17-30 Hemodynamic tracing used to calculate mitral valve area. The shaded area is the diastolic mitral valve gradient surrounded by the diastolic filling period (DFP). CF = correction factor or scale factor; LA = left atrial pressure; LV = left ventricular pressure (scale 0 to 40 mmHg), MVG = mean value gradient. See text for details.

1. Planimeter LV-PCW areas (area = 9.46 cm$^2$) and measure diastolic filling period (DFP = 3.4 cm). Next convert cm to time and planimetered area to mean diastolic pressure gradient.

   Diastolic filling period of 3.4 cm/beat at paper speed of 100 mm/s = 0.34 s/beat

   Mean valve gradient (MVG) = (area × scale factor)/DFP (Scale Factor: 1 cm = 3.9 mmHg [directly measured paper calibration lines of 40 mmHg])

$$\text{MVG} = 9.46\ \text{cm}^2 \times \frac{3.9\ \text{mmHg}/1\ \text{cm}}{3.4\ \text{cm}} = 10.85\ \text{mmHg}$$

2. Compute mitral valve flow.

$$\text{Flow} = \frac{\text{CO}}{\text{DFP} \times \text{HR}} = \frac{3500\ \text{mL/min}}{0.34\ \text{s/beat} \times 80\ \text{bpm}}$$
$$= \frac{3500}{0.34 \times 80} = \frac{3500}{27.2} = 128.7\ \text{mL/min}$$

3. Compute mitral valve area.

$$\text{MVA} = \frac{\text{Mitral valve flow}}{0.85 \times 44.3\sqrt{10.85}} = \frac{128.7}{0.85 \times 44.3 \times 3.3}$$
$$= \frac{128.7}{124.3} = 1.0\ \text{cm}^2$$

## Cardiac Output Techniques

### THERMODILUTION TECHNIQUE

The thermodilution technique was introduced by Fegler in 1953 to measure volume flow rate. A multiple-lumen, balloon-tipped flow-directed thermistor catheter is placed in the pulmonary artery. Ten milliliters of room-temperature (22°C) 5% dextrose or normal saline solution is injected rapidly (<4 s) through a second lumen into the right atrium. As the injectate blood mixture initially passes from the right ventricle, the pulmonary artery blood temperature drops maximally and then progressively rises in a beat-to-beat disappearance slope as the residual injectate blood mixture is washed out of the right ventricle. The recirculation phase is negligible. The area under the time-temperature curve is electronically integrated, and the cardiac output is computed by the Stewart-Hamilton formula. Since there is no "gold standard" for cardiac output, the results have been compared with the dye-dilution and Fick techniques and have correlated well, except in low cardiac output states, where the Fick method is preferable. If severe tricuspid or pulmonary regurgitation or significant left-to-right shunting is present, the indicator (temperature loss) is attenuated and the downslope of the temperature curve is prolonged, so the thermal dilution cardiac output will be unreliable.[73–75] In general, when one uses thermal dilution, a true directional change in cardiac output is reflected by an observed change of ±10 percent.

Thermodilution is inaccurate in patients with low cardiac output. In low-flow states or in valvular regurgitation, recirculation of the indicator, (i.e., cold saline or green dye) may appear as a distortion on the curve downslope before reaching baseline. Failure to reach accurate baseline will result in inaccurate cardiac output determinations. Hillis and others found the Fick/thermodilution percentage difference averaged 10 ± 10 percent. In patients with aortic or mitral regurgitation, the Fick/thermodilution percentage difference was 7 ± 7 percent. Thermodilution is preferable to green dye indicator dilution technique because right-sided injection and right-sided sampling (of the cold indicator) yield a curve that is less subject to recirculation-induced distortion than right-sided injection and left-sided sampling of green dye. Fick, thermodilution, angiographic, and indocyanine green dye determinations all measure cardiac output. Significant variations among cardiac output techniques occur in patients with low cardiac output or in those with aortic or mitral regurgitation. In patients with mitral and aortic valve regurgitation, and low cardiac output, the dye dilution method varied by more than 20 percent from the Fick method.

### THE FICK METHOD OF CARDIAC OUTPUT

The Fick method most often utilizes an assumed oxygen consumption value or less frequently a metabolic wood to measure oxygen consumption. The Fick calculation is described above.

### ANGIOGRAPHIC CARDIAC OUTPUT

Cardiac output determined angiographically is computed as the stroke volume (end-diastolic volume minus the end-systolic volume) times the heart rate. Angiographic cardiac output provides the best estimate of cardiac output through a stenotic valve when any degree of regurgitation is present. Errors in stroke volume computation are increased with enlarged ventricles, especially when single-plane cineangiography is employed. Angiographic cardiac output is not determined simultaneously with a transvalvular gradient, therefore additional error may be introduced by delay in simultaneous measurements. A calibrated ventriculogram is also necessary.

## Intracardiac Shunts

A shunt is an abnormal communication between the left and right heart chambers. The direction of blood flowing through the shunt may be left to right, right to left, or sometimes bidirectional. In the absence of shunting, the pulmonary blood flow (right heart output) is equal to the systemic blood flow. Table 17-25 lists intracardiac shunt locations. A left-to-right shunt increases the amount of blood to the

TABLE 17-25 Shunt Locations and Oximetry Sampling Sites

| Locations | Earliest Step-Up Location (for left-to-right shunts) |
|---|---|
| **Atrial septal defects** | |
| Primum (low) | RA, RV |
| Secundum (mid) | RA |
| Sinus venosus (high) | RA |
| Partial anomalous pulmonary venous return (pulmonary veins entering right atrium) | RA |
| **Ventricular septal defects** | |
| Membranous (high) | RV |
| Muscular (mid) | RV |
| Apical (low) | RV |
| **Aorticopulmonary window (connection of aorta to pulmonary artery)** | PA |
| **Patent ductus arteriosus (normally closed Ao-PA connection at birth)** | PA |

ABBREVIATIONS: Ao = aortic; PA = pulmonary artery; RA = right atrium; RV = right ventricle.

right heart and increases pulmonary blood flow, now equal to the sum of the systemic blood flow plus shunt flow. With a right-to-left shunt, the amount of blood shunted from the right side to the left is added to that normally ejected into the systemic circulation. Systemic blood flow is then greater than pulmonary blood flow by the amount of the shunt (Fig. 17-31.).

Intracardiac shunts have been evaluated by four methods:

1. Oximetry
2. Indocyanine green dye dilution curves
3. Angiography
4. Radioactive tracers

## OXIMETRY FOR CARDIAC SHUNTS

An increase in the oxygen content of blood from the chambers of the right side of the heart in excess of the normal variation in oxygen content on serial sampling is used as evidence of a left-to-right shunt.[76] Oxygen content can be expressed as volumes percent (vol% = mL $O_2$/100 mL blood) or can be expressed from percent oxygen saturation where content is calculated from the hemoglobin concentration assuming a constant relationship for oxygen carrying capacity (1.36 mL $O_2$/g hemoglobin). Thus an oxygen step-up from the SVC to the right atrium of more than 1.9 vol% indicates shunting into the right atrium; a step-up from the right atrium to the right ventricle of 0.9 vol% or more and a step-up from the right ventricle to the pulmonary artery of 0.5 vol% or more indicates a left-to-right shunt at the RV and pulmonary artery levels, respectively. By these criteria, false-positive results are rare, but false-negative results can occur in patients with small shunts. In an anemic or polycythemic patient, the detection of shunting is best reflected by the step-up in percentage oxygen saturation rather than the step-up in volume percent, since the latter depends on the hemoglobin concentration.[77]

Studies show that sensitivity in detecting left-to-right shunts is improved if numerous serial paired blood samples are withdrawn in rapid succession for oximetry. Assuming an aterial saturation of 95%, a *9% saturation* increase between the SVC and the right atrium indicates a large atrial shunt, a *5% saturation* increase between the right atrium and the right ventricle indicates a ventricular shunt, and a *3% saturation* increase between the right ventricle and the pulmonary artery indicates a pulmonary artery shunt. The rise in oxygen saturation step-up for a given left-to-right shunt is related to the saturation of mixed venous blood (MVB). For example, if the MVB is

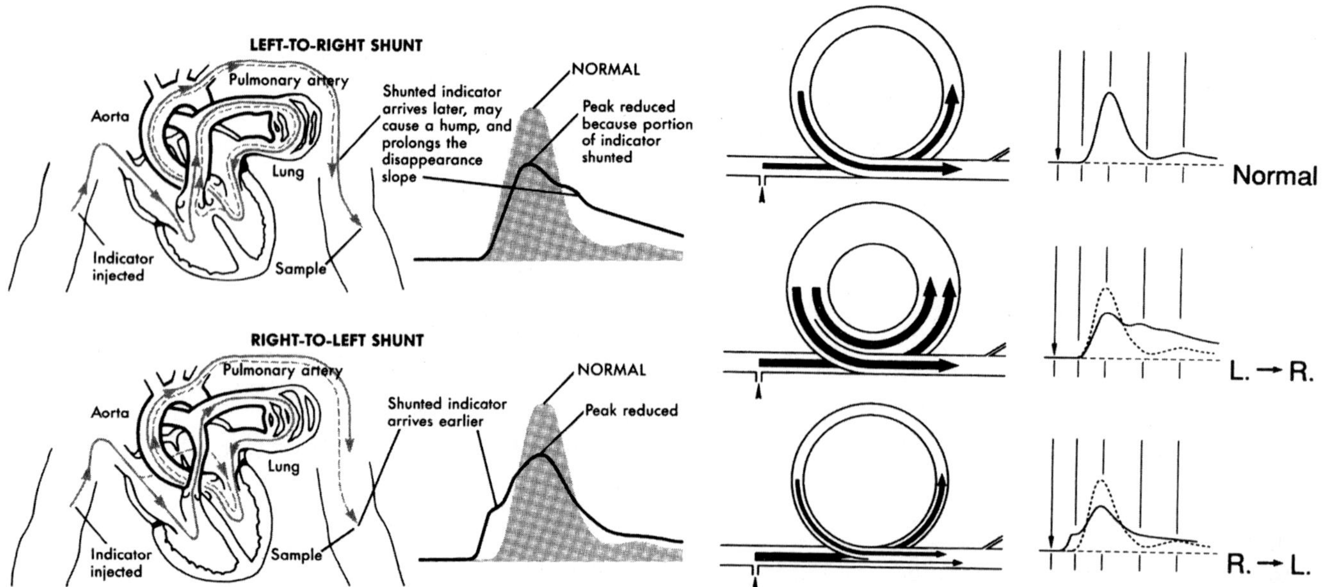


FIGURE 17-31 Indicator dilution curves for shunts. *Left-to-right shunt (increased pulmonic flow)*. Indicator is not cleared rapidly but recirculates through central circulation via defect. Based on magnitude of shunt, a constant fraction leaves the central pool with each circulation. Maximal deflection is reduced and the disappearance is prolonged as a result of slow clearance. *Right-to-left shunt (decreased pulmonic flow)*. A portion of the indicator passes directly to the arterial circulation via the defect without passing through the lungs and arrives at the arterial sampling site before the portion that did traverse the pulmonary circulation. (From Kern MJ. *Cardiac Catheterization Handbook*, St. Louis: Mosby; 2003. With permission.)

TABLE 17-26 Oxygen Saturation Values for Shunt Detection

| Level of Shunt | Significant Step-Up Different[a] $O_2$% Saturation |
|---|---|
| Atrial (SVC/IVC to right aorta) | 7 |
| Ventricular | 5 |
| Great vessel | 5 |

ABBREVIATIONS: SVC = superior vena cava; IVC = inferior vena cava; PA = pulmonary artery pressure.

[a]Difference distal-proximal chamber. For example, for atrial septal defect:

$$PA - \frac{3\ SVC + 1\ IVC}{4} \quad \text{(should be } <7\% \text{ normally)}$$

85%, a 5% step-up represents a 2:1 shunt; if MVB is 75%, a 10% step-up is needed; if the MVB is 65%, a 15% step-up indicates a 2:1 shunt. Left-to-right shunts of <20 percent of pulmonary flow are not detectable by oximetry.

Desaturation of arterialized blood samples from the left heart chambers and aorta suggests a right-to-left shunt. In determining the site of the right-to-left shunt, sequential sampling can be made from the left atrium, left ventricle, and aorta (Table 17-26). Mixed venous blood is assumed to be fully mixed PA blood. If there is a left-to-right shunt, mixed venous blood is measured one chamber proximal to the step-up. In the case of an atrial septal defect, the mixed venous oxygen content is computed from the weighted average of vena caval blood, (i.e., as the sum of three times the superior vena cava plus one inferior vena cava oxygen content and divided by 4). When pulmonary venous blood is not collected, $PVo_2$ (pulmonary vein) percentage saturation is assumed to be 95 percent. The oximetric technique has some well known limitations which include inability to detect small shunts, poor blood oxygen mixing, and inaccuracies with high flow states.[78]

## ANGIOGRAPHY AND RADIONUCLIDE SHUNT DETECTION

Angiography is nonquantitative method used to localize either left-to-right or right-to-left shunts. The angiographic method may be useful when origin of the shunt cannot be entered. To detect the shunt, contrast media can be injected into the closest proximal chamber. The LAO view with cranial angulation puts the interatrial and interventricular septae on edge, providing an ideal view for detection of contrast passage across the atrial and ventricular septal defects.

Radioactive tracers for shunts are administered by vein in the nuclear medicine department and provide a useful estimate of shunt flow. Radioactivity seen in the brain or kidneys after right-sided injection means the tracer has passed through an intracardiac shunt (right-to-left), escaping entrapment by the lungs. Intracardiac shunts have also been detected and quantified by indicator-dilution curves.

## SHUNT CALCULATIONS

The Fick or left-sided indicator dilution methods of cardiac output determination are employed to measure systemic flow. Using the Fick method, the following formulas apply:

1. Systemic flow,

$$Q_S\ (\text{L/min}) = \frac{O_2 \text{ consumption (mL/min)}}{(\text{arterial} - \text{mixed venous})\ O_2 \text{ content}}$$

2. Pulmonary flow, $Q_P$ (L/min)

$$= \frac{O_2 \text{ consumption (mL/min)}}{(\text{pulmonary venous} - \text{pulmonary arterial})\ O_2 \text{ content}}$$

Thus the effective pulmonary blood flow (EPB)

$$Q_{EPB} = \frac{O_2 \text{ consumption (mL/m)}}{(\text{pulmonary venous} - \text{mixed venous})\ O_2 \text{ content}}$$

The effective pulmonary blood flow is that volume of blood which, after returning to the right atrium, actually reaches the pulmonary capillaries.

It follows that

$$L \rightarrow R \text{ shunt} = Q_P - Q_{EPB}$$

and

$$R \rightarrow L \text{ shunt} = Q_S - Q_{EPB}$$

If arterial blood is fully saturated, then there is no R → L shunt, since arterial $O_2$ content is equal to pulmonary venous $O_2$ content and $Q_S = Q_{EPB}$.

The shunt ratio is defined as $Q_P/Q_S$. Shunt ratios of >1.5 are associated with anatomic defects that often require closure.

3. Example calculations for a simple left-to-right shunt in a patient with an atrial septal defect (ASD) using data obtained at catheterization are as follows:

Assume Hgb = 14.1 g/dL, $O_2$ consumption = 225 mL $O_2$/min and oxygen saturation data as follows:

| Location | Oxygen Saturation (%) |
|---|---|
| Arterial | 98 |
| SVC | 71 |
| Mid-RA | 71 |
| PA | 81 |
| Pulmonary vein | 98 |
| IVC | 70 |

a. Compute $O_2$ content.

$$\text{Arterial } O_2 \text{ content} = 0.98 \times 1.36 \text{ mL } O_2/\text{g} \times 14.1 \text{ g/dL} \times 10 = 188 \text{ mL } O_2/\text{liter}$$

Mixed venous $O_2$ content (Use estimate of $\frac{3\ SVC + 1\ IVC}{4}$ for mixed venous oxygen saturation.):

$$\frac{(.71 + .71 + .71 + .70)}{4} = 0.71$$

$$0.71 \times 1.36 \text{ mL } O_2/\text{g} \times 14.1 \text{ g/dL} \times 10 = 136 \text{ mL } O_2/\text{liter}$$

$$\text{Pulmonary artery } O_2 \text{ content} = (0.81 \times 1.36 \text{ mL } O_2/\text{gm} \times 14.1 \text{ g/dL} \times 10) = 155 \text{ mL } O_2/\text{liter}$$

$$\text{Pulmonary vein } O_2 \text{ content} = (0.98 \times 1.36 \text{ mL } O_2/\text{g} \times 14.1 \text{ g/dL} \times 10) = 188 \text{ mL } O_2/\text{liter}$$

b. Compute systemic flow [Equation (1)].

$$\frac{225 \text{ mL } O_2/\text{min}}{(188 - 136)\text{mL } O_2/\text{liter}} = \frac{225}{52} = Q_S = 4.3 \text{ L/min}$$

c. Compute pulmonary flow [Equation (2)].

$$\frac{225 \text{ mL } O_2/\text{min}}{(188 - 155)\text{mL } O_2/\text{liter}} = \frac{225}{33} = Q_P = 6.8$$

d. Compute $\frac{Q_P}{Q_S} = \frac{6.8}{4.3} = 1.6$, and the L → R shunt is 6.8 L/min − 4.3 L/min or 2.5 L/min

If absolute flows are not required, the $Q_P/Q_S$ ratio can be determined using saturations only as follows:

$$\frac{Q_P}{Q_S} = \frac{SAO_2 - MVO_2}{PVO_2 - PAO_2}$$

where, $SAO_2$; systemic arterial $O_2$ saturation; $PVO_2$; pulmonary venous $O_2$ saturation; $MVO_2$; mixed venous $O_2$ saturation; $PAO_2$; pulmonary artery $O_2$ saturation.

Using saturation data from the example of left-to-right shunt:

$$\frac{Q_P}{Q_S} = \frac{98 - 71}{98 - 81} = \frac{27}{17} = 1.6$$

Example calculations for a more complex, bidirectional shunt from data obtained at catheterization are as follows:

Assume Hgb = 15 g/dL, $O_2$ consumption = 195 ml $O_2$/min, and oxygen saturation data:

| Location | Oxygen Saturation (%) |
|---|---|
| Arterial | 89 |
| SVC | 81 |
| RA, mid | 83 |
| RA, low | 82 |
| LA | 88 |
| PA | 82 |
| Pulmonary vein | 96 |
| IVC | 70 |

a. Compute $O_2$ content.

Arterial = (0.89 × 15 g/100 mL × 1.36 mL $O_2$/g × 10)
= 182 mL $O_2$/L

Mixed venous estimated mixed venous saturation =
(.81 + .81 + .81 + .70) 4 = 0.78

Mixed venous = (0.78 × 15 g/dL × 1.36 m $O_2$/g × 10)
= 159 mL $O_2$/L

Pulmonary arterial = (0.82 × 15 g/dL × 1.36 mL $O_2$/g × 10)
= 167 mL $O_2$/L

Pulmonary venous = (0.96 × 15 g/dL × 1.36 mL $O_2$/gm × 10)
= 196 mL $O_2$/L

b. Compute systemic flow.

$$\frac{O_2 \text{ consumption}}{(\text{arterial} - \text{mixed venous})\, O_2 \text{ content}} = \frac{195 \text{ mL } O_2/\text{min}}{(182 - 159)\text{mL } O_2/\text{L}} = 8.5 \text{ L/min}$$

c. Compute pulmonary blood flow.

$$\frac{O_2 \text{ consumption}}{(\text{pulmonary venous} - \text{pulmonary arterial})\, O_2 \text{ content}} = \frac{195 \text{ mL } O_2/\text{min}}{(196 - 167) \text{ mL } O_2/\text{L}} = 6.7 \text{ L/min}$$

d. Compute effective pulmonary blood flow.

Effective pulmonary blood flow

$$= \frac{O_2 \text{ consumption}}{(\text{pulmonary venous} - \text{mixed venous})\, O_2 \text{ content}} = \frac{195 \text{ mL } O_2/\text{min}}{(196 - 159) \text{ mL } O_2/\text{L}} = 5.3 \text{ L/min}$$

Left-to-right shunt = $Q_P - Q_{EPB}$
= 6.7 − 5.3
= 1.4 L/min

Right-to-left shunt = $Q_S - Q_{EPB}$
= 8.5 − 5.3
= 3. 2 L/min

## Normal Hemodynamic Waveforms

### NORMAL RIGHT HEART PRESSURE WAVES

Simultaneous RV and RA pressures (Fig. 17-32) demonstrate the correspondence of the atrial contraction "a" wave and the "v" wave (caused by venous return to the RA while the tricuspid valve is closed) to the right ventricular pressure tracing. Following the a wave is the X descent and following the v wave is the normal Y descent. These features may be altered in the presence of disease or obscured in patients who have atrial arrhythmias. The notch (closed arrow) on the top of the RV tracing is the "ringing" (underdamping) of a fluid-filled catheter. This rebound or ringing also is evident on the early diastolic part of the pressure wave (open arrow, bottom of same beat).

During the continuous pressure on pullback (* on Fig. 17-33 denotes point of crossing from LA to RA) across the interatrial septum from the left atrium to the right atrium of a patient with aortic steno-

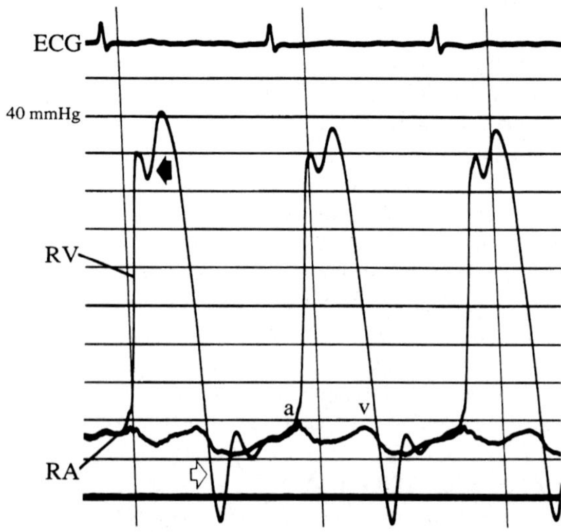


FIGURE 17-32 Right atrial (RA) and right ventricular (RV) tracings in a normal patient. Notch of ringing or overshoot on right ventricular pressure rise (*closed arrow*). Ringing and overshoot of decline in right ventricular pressure at early diastole (*open arrow*). a = atrial wave; v = ventricular filling wave. (From Kern MJ. *Cardiac Catheterization Handbook*. St. Louis: Mosby; 2003. With permission.)

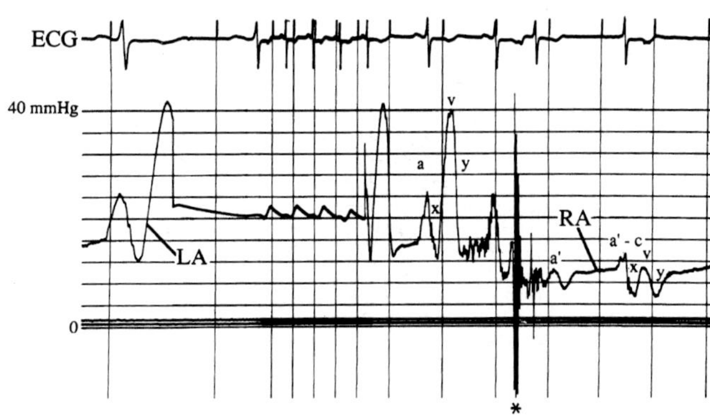


FIGURE 17-33 Hemodynamic tracing of left atrium (LA) with catheter pullback to right atrium (RA) across the intraatrial septum (* indicates site of pullback from LA to RA). See text for details of waveform analysis. (From Kern MJ. *Cardiac Catheterization Handbook*. St. Louis: Mosby; 2003. With permission.)

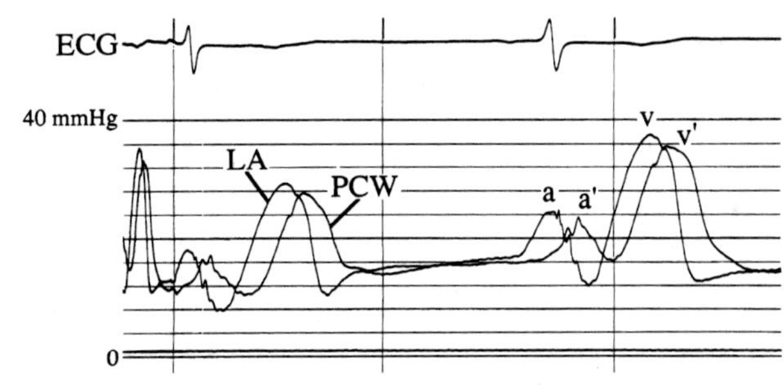


FIGURE 17-35 Simultaneous left atrial (LA) and pulmonary capillary wedge (PCW) tracings. (The patient has aortic stenosis with high ventricular filling pressure.) (From Kern MJ. *Cardiac Catheterization Handbook*. St. Louis: Mosby; 2003. With permission.)

sis (Fig. 17-33), the differences between LA and RA a and v waves are seen. The v waves on the left atrium are very prominent with their corresponding X and Y descents. In the right atrium, the a and v waves are present but less striking. In general, RA a waves are bigger than v waves. In the left atrium, v waves are more prominent than a waves. RA pressure can be markedly altered by respiration.

Normal right heart pressures during continuous pressure recording (using balloon-tipped pulmonary artery catheter) on catheter pullback from pulmonary artery to right ventricle and right atrium (0 to 40 mmHg scale) (Fig. 17-34) show the simultaneous LV and RV pressures for evaluation of constricture or restrictive myocardial physiology. The premature ventricular contractions in RV pressure are common when catheters contact the RV outflow tract.

### PCW PRESSURE AND LA PRESSURE WITH SIMULTANEOUS TRANSSEPTAL AND RIGHT HEART CATHETERIZATION

The PCW pressure measured through a 7F fluid-filled balloon-tipped catheter and the LA pressure measured through a Brockenbrough catheter (Fig. 17-35) demonstrate that the LA pressure rise precedes that of the PCW pressure for every waveform by approximately 100 to 150 ms. The good correspondence (generally) of these two pressures permits clinical use of PCW pressure for the majority of standard hemodynamic cases (a, a′- and v, v′ are the LA and PCW pressures, respectively).

### NORMAL FEMORAL ARTERIAL AND CENTRAL AORTIC PRESSURES

The femoral arterial pressure measured through the side arm of the femoral arterial sheath (8F) is matched against pressure in the pigtail catheter (7F) positioned above the aortic valve (Fig. 17-36). These pressures normally correspond closely with only a slight overshoot of the more peripheral FA pressure (open arrow). The timing of upstroke of the pressures distinguishes the central aortic (first tracing rising) from FA pressure. The mean of the two pressures is identical (closed arrow).

Simultaneous arterial pressure with LV pressures recorded before and after crossing the aortic valve permits satisfactory assessment of most aortic valvular lesions. Note the phase lag and normal overshoot of the arterial pressure compared to the LV pressure.

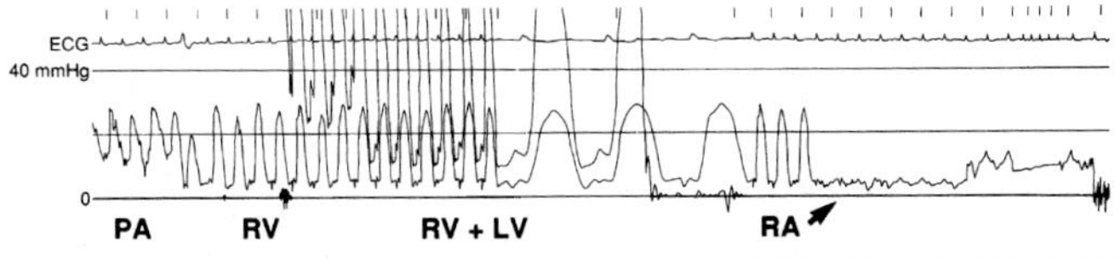


FIGURE 17-34 Continuous hemodynamic tracing during catheter pullback from the pulmonary artery (PA) to right atrium (RA). Differences in left ventricular (LV) and right ventricular (RV) pressures are shown (0 to 40 mmHg full scale). (From Kern MJ. *Cardiac Catheterization Handbook*. St. Louis: Mosby; 2003. With permission.)

## Pathologic Hemodynamic Waveforms

### RA PRESSURE WITH TRICUSPID REGURGITATION

Unlike the normal pattern, the right atrial pressure rises throughout right ventricular systole as a result of tricuspid valvular regurgitation pushing blood back into the right atrium (Fig.17-37). In this patient the RA pressure during diastole matches the RV pressure, indicating no tricuspid stenosis.

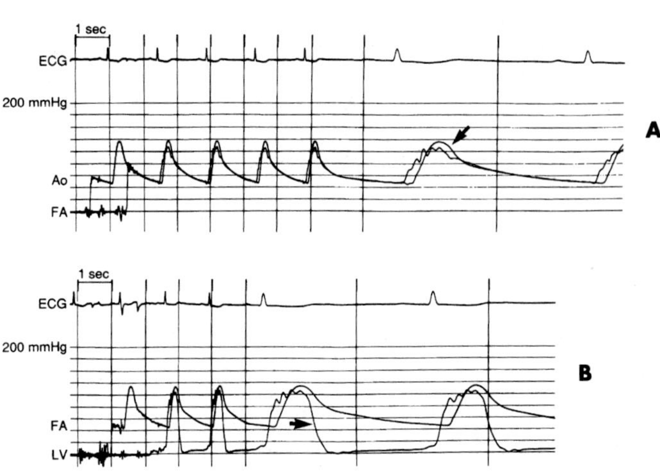


FIGURE 17-36 *A.* Simultaneous hemodynamic tracings of femoral artery (FA) pressure taken through the side arm of the 8F sheath and central aortic pressures. Central aortic (Ao) pressure is obtained through the 7F pigtail catheter. The overshoot of the femoral artery pressure (*arrow*) and lag in the pressure upstroke are the normal characteristics for the femoral tracings. *B.* Femoral artery and left ventricular (LV) pressure (*arrow*). (From Kern MJ. *Cardiac Catheterization Handbook*. St. Louis: Mosby; 2003. With permission.)

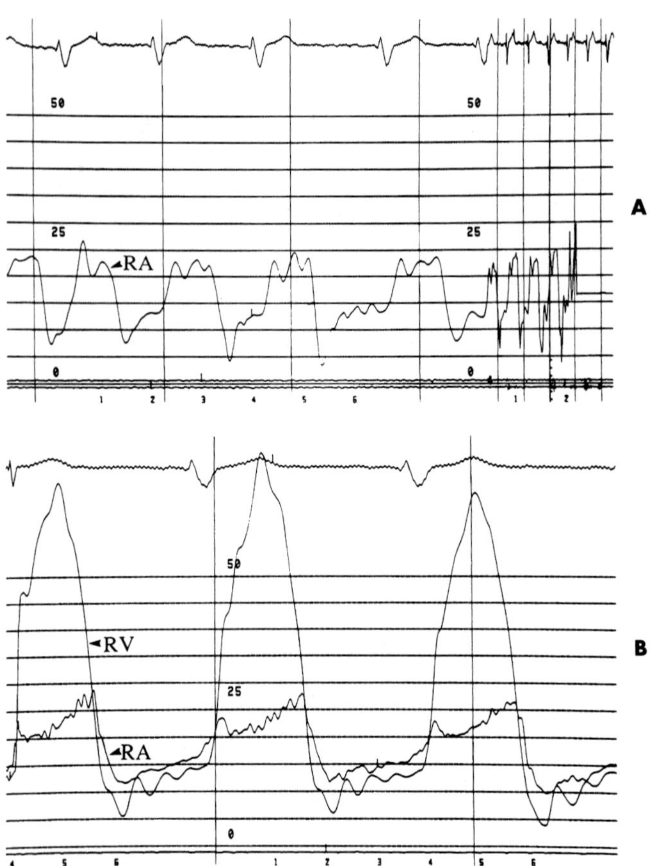


FIGURE 17-37 *A.* Right atrial (RA) pressure in a patient with severe tricuspid regurgitation. *B.* When paired with simultaneous right ventricular (RV) pressure, tricuspid regurgitation can now be seen associated with tricuspid stenosis as the separation (gradient) between the right atrial-right ventricular pressures during diastole. (From Kern MJ. *Cardiac Catheterization Handbook.* St. Louis: Mosby; 2003. With permission.)

## RA PRESSURE IN A PATIENT WITH ATRIOVENTRICULAR DISSOCIATION

Normal a waves represent atrial contraction into the ventricle with no obstruction to in-flow. In an atrioventricular block, the atria are not contracting at the proper time in relation to the ventricles (Fig. 17-38). Immediately after the QRS the ventricles contract and the tricuspid and mitral valves close. If the p wave (and atrial contraction) comes after the tricuspid valve is closed, a giant C or cannon wave can be seen. When atrioventricular synchrony (normal sequence) occurs on beats 6 and 7 the a waves return, proportional in size to the timing of the atrial contraction, emptying blood before ventricular systole (QRS). Similar findings may be seen when the dissociation is caused by a pacemaker. Giant C waves can occur during pacing.

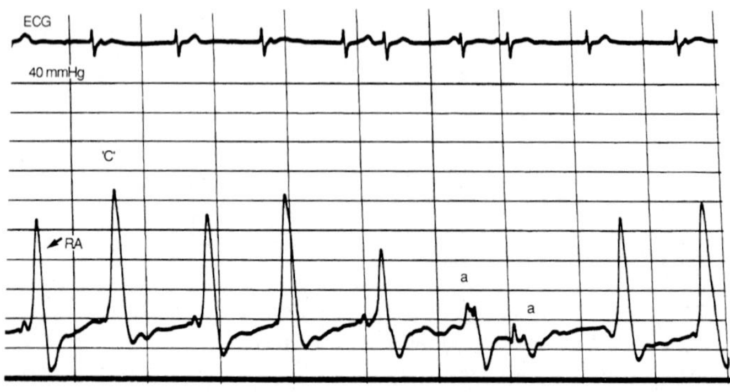


FIGURE 17-38 Right atrial (RA) pressure during atrial-ventricular dissociation. C = cannon wave; a = small a wave during synchrony of the atrial and ventricular activity. (From Kern MJ. *Cardiac Catheterization Handbook.* St. Louis: Mosby; 2003. With permission.)

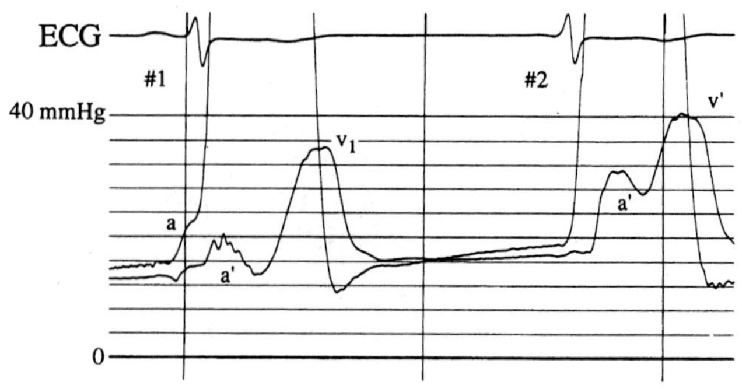


FIGURE 17-39 Simultaneous pulmonary capillary wedge and left ventricular pressures in a patient who has loss of atrial activity (beat 2). On beat 1 the a wave is evident on both left ventricle (a) and pulmonary capillary wedge pressure (a′). The a′ wave is considerably higher because of its contraction against the closed mitral valve. (From Kern MJ. *Cardiac Catheterization Handbook.* St. Louis: Mosby; 2003. With permission.)

## LARGE WAVES ON THE PCW TRACING

The PCW has moderate and large v waves (Fig. 17-39). On beat 2, the atrium contracts after the ventricle, resulting in a different initial upstroke of the LV pressure and a cannon wave. The v wave on a PCW pressure tracing usually is associated with significant mitral regurgitation. However, large v waves are not highly sensitive nor are they specific for mitral regurgitation. Large v waves also may be present with mitral stenosis or ventricular septal defect or any condition in which the left atrial volume [e.g., ventricular septal defect (VSD)] or left atrial pressure relationship (the stiffness or compliance) is increased (such as rheumatic heart disease, postcardiac surgery, and infiltrative heart diseases).

## AORTIC–LEFT VENTRICULAR GRADIENTS

The atrial contraction is important in patients with aortic stenosis (Fig. 17-40). Simultaneous aortic and LV pressure (transseptal

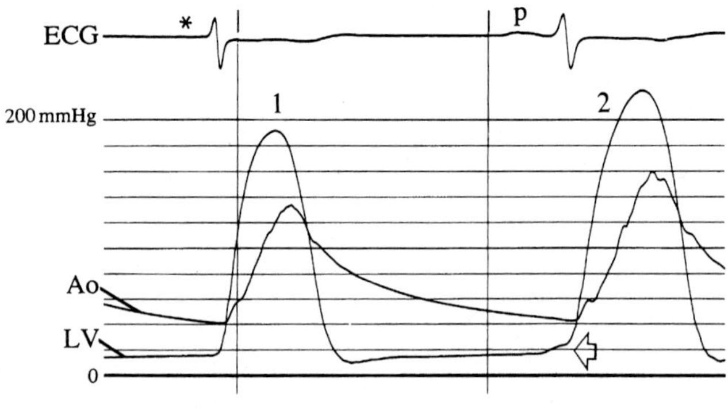


FIGURE 17-40 Simultaneous left ventricular (LV; obtained with transseptal technique) and aortic (Ao) pressures from fluid-filled catheter systems. Note the contribution of atrial contraction (*arrow*) to the change in left ventricular and systemic pressures on beat 2. p = p wave; * = absence of p wave on this tracing. The wide pulse pressure also is indicative of aortic insufficiency. (From Kern MJ. *Cardiac Catheterization Handbook*, St. Louis: Mosby; 2003. With permission.)

approach) shows that atrial activity is absent in the first beat, a junctional beat (* denotes specific beat on Fig. 17-40). With atrial contraction (second beat) LV pressure increases to 225 mmHg, an approximate 25 percent increase over the first beat.

Hypertrophic cardiomyopathy is a condition in which very thick heart muscle, especially inside the LV chamber, contracts so hard that it obstructs flow out of the ventricle, and thus by its own contraction produces a pressure gradient with a normal aortic valve. Figure 17-41 depicts simultaneous LV and aortic pressure showing a large aortic–LV gradient (LV= 220 mmHg; Ao = 120 mmHg). On pullback of the LV catheter (multipurpose) from the distal LV to a position just beneath the aortic valve the Ao–LV gradient disappears (see the LV pressure matching with aortic pressure) (arrow).

### LEFT ATRIAL–LEFT VENTRICULAR GRADIENTS

Simultaneous LV and PCW pressures (Fig. 17-42) demonstrate a mitral valve gradient throughout diastole. The a wave is absent in this patient in atrial fibrillation. As can be seen, mitral valve gradients are strongly influenced by heart rate. In Fig. 17-43 large v waves in the PCW tracing represent LV pressure transmitted backward through an incompetent mitral valve. The v wave (up to 60 mmHg) occurs on the downstroke of the LV pressure in a patient with mitral regurgitation. Matching of elevated diastolic pressures with an early dip followed by a plateau during diastole (first beat) is the characteristic pattern. Often, only during slow heart rates does the classic dip-and-plateau configuration appear. Tachycardia and respiratory effort obscure the pattern, but matching of both RV–LV pressures during diastole is consistent. Dynamic respiratory variation differentate constrictive from restrictive pathology (Fig. 17-44).

## Physiologic Maneuvers in the Catheterization Laboratory

### EXERCISE

Exercise evaluation of cardiac function is helpful to relate symptoms to hemodynamic changes, especially for patients with valvular heart disease (e.g., mitral stenosis). Hemodynamics are measured at rest and during peak exercise using bicycle ergometry, repeated leg or arm lifts, and, occasionally, arm bicycle ergometry. Commonly measured responses to exercise include minute ventilatory capacity, oxygen extraction, heart rate, cardiac output, ventricular volume and filling pressures, and metabolic substrate utilization (e.g., glucose concentration without lactate production).

Exercise may be *dynamic* or *isometric*. Measurement of each type demonstrates different features of left ventricular function. Dynamic exercise measures the ability of the cardiovascular system to supply oxygen in keeping with increased metabolic demands. Oxygen consumption and work load increases should be parallel until the maximal oxygen consumption for the patient is reached. Dynamic exercise in the cardiac catheterization laboratory requires simultaneous right and left heart pressure measurements during exercise (e.g., treadmill device mounted on the catheterization table). The patient's

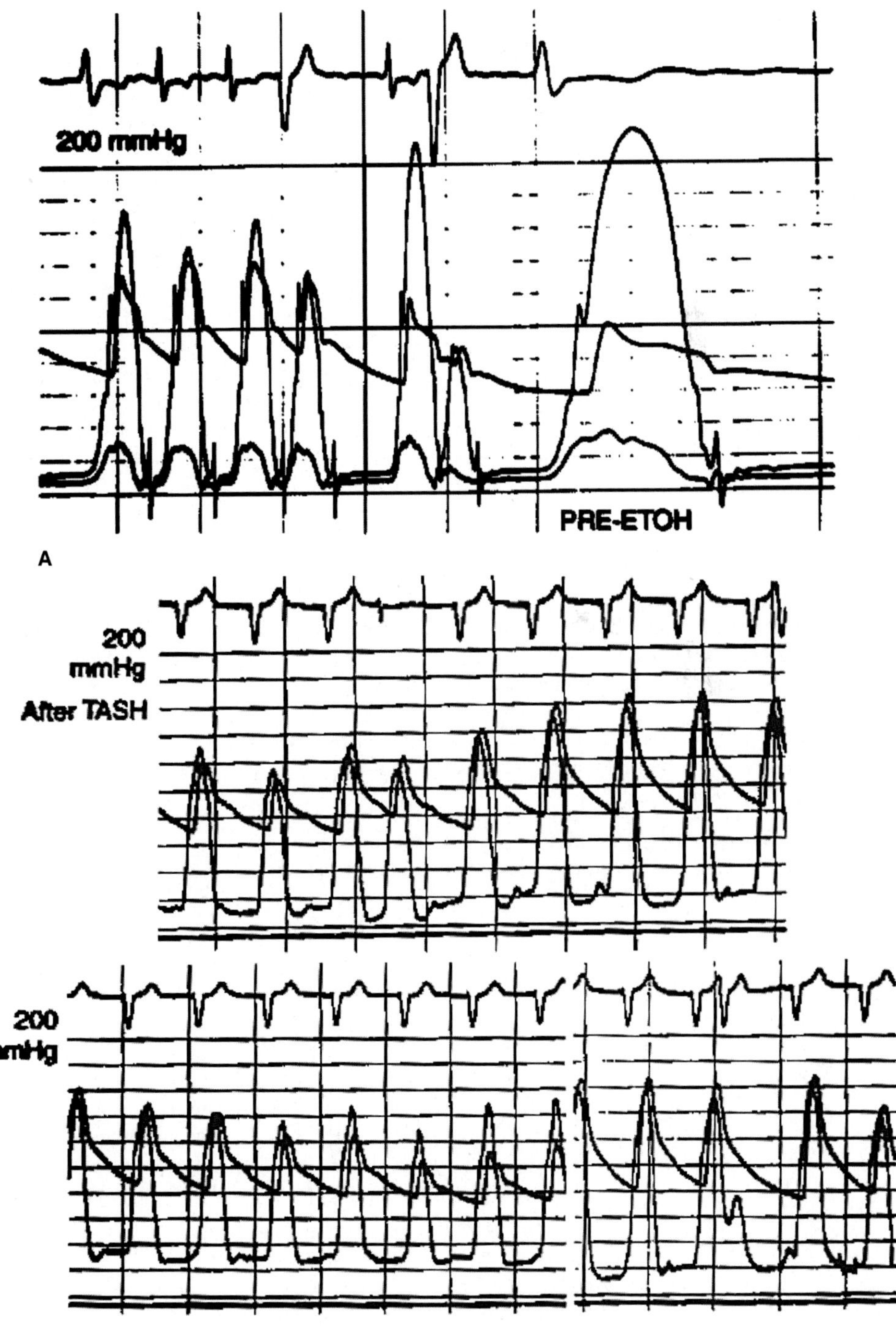


FIGURE 17-41 Hemodynamic tracings of patient with hypertrophic obstructive cardiomyopathy. *A*. Before alcohol septal ablation. *B*. After transluminal alcohol septal ablation (TASH).

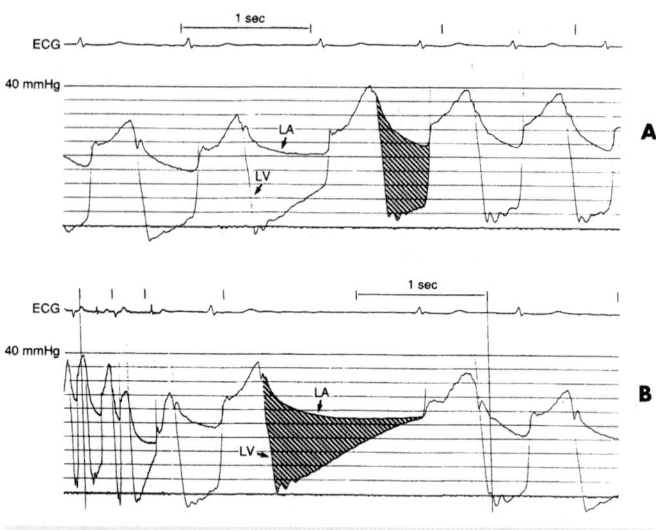


FIGURE 17-42 Changing mitral stenosis gradient with heart rate (RR interval). *A.* Short RR interval is associated with gradient (shaded area) of 22 mmHg. *B.* Long RR interval has a mean gradient of 29 mmHg. When computing mean valve area in atrial fibrillation, average 10 beats. LA = Left atrial pressure; LV = left ventricular pressure. (From Kern MJ, Aguirre F. Hemodynamic rounds: interpretation and cardiac pathophysiology from pressure waveform analysis: Mitral valve gradients. Part I. *Cathet Cardiovasc Diagn* 1992;26:308–315.

oxygen consumption also is measured by artery and vein oxygen saturations and is compared to the normal hemodynamic responses. Supine exercise in the catheterization laboratory differs from normal upright exercise in several ways:

1. Ventricular volumes are larger when the patient is supine rather than upright.
2. Heart rate and diastolic arterial pressure are higher when the patient is upright rather than supine.
3. Pulmonary and intracardiac filling pressures are lower when the patient is upright.
4. Stroke volume increases 100 percent with maximal exercise when the patient is upright and only 20 percent to 50 percent when the patient is supine.

It can be noted that both upright and supine exercise are normally associated with increases in LV end-diastolic volume and decreases in end-systolic volume with concomitant increase in ejection fraction. In patients with coronary artery disease, these finding may not occur.

Exercise data are analyzed with respect to change in hemodynamics (valve gradients), cardiac output, and oxygen consumption. Patients may be unable to exercise because of leg weakness, depressed cardiac function, peripheral vascular disease, or severe deconditioning. These factors may preclude determination of accurate exercise results in the catheterization laboratory and should be considered before undertaking the study.

Isometric exercise consists of skeletal muscle contraction without shortening. Isometric exercise commonly is performed using a hand grip with a graded hand dynamometer. Measurements of hemodynamics and ventricular function are obtained during sustained hand grip at a predetermined range (15 to 50 percent of the maximal handgrip contraction) for a period of 3 to 4 min. In patients with coronary artery disease, isometric exercise rarely precipitates ischemia but may induce new LV wall motion abnormalities, a decrease in LV ejection fraction, and an increase in end-systolic volume with no change in diastolic volume. Stroke volume (SV) and CO may decline during isometric exercise. In patients with congestive heart failure, heart rate and systemic pressure may rise appropriately with a fall in SV and CO resulting in increase in LV end-diastolic volume and pulmonary artery (PA) pressure.

Several measurements of the response to exercise are important. Cardiac output (CO) is useful measurement for studying practically all types of heart disease. Measurement of CO for the corresponding oxygen uptake allows categorization of a patient's physiologic cardiovascular response to activity. A predicted cardiac index (CI) with exercise can be determined as 2.99 + 0.0059 × (measured $O_2$ consumption index). The measured CI with exercise divided by the predicted CI is called the exercise (Dexter) index and expresses exercise capacity as a percentage of the normal response. An index of ≥ 0.8 indicates a normal CO response to exercise. An "exercise factor" can also be computed. For every 100 mL/min increase in $O_2$ consumption with exercise, the CO should increase by at least 600mL/min. The exercise factor is calculated directly from observed changes in CO and $O_2$ consumption and is normalized to BSA, thus normal exercise factor is calculated as follows:

$$\text{Exercise Factor} = \frac{\text{CO (mL/min)}}{O_2 \text{ consumption (mL/min)}} \geq 6$$

Appropriate increases in arterial blood pressure and heart rate should also be noted.

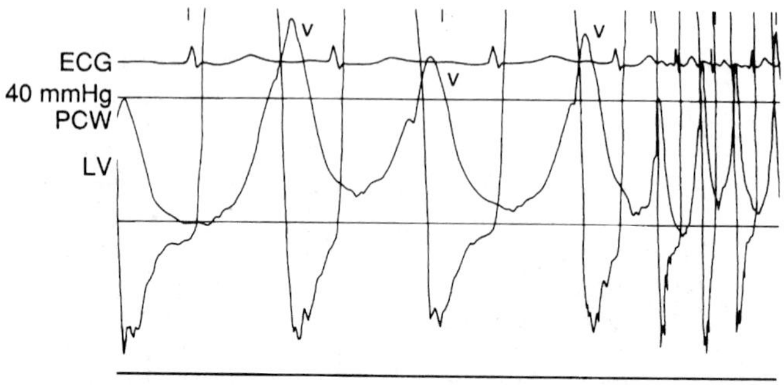


FIGURE 17-43 Simultaneous left ventricular (LV) and pulmonary capillary wedge (PCW) pressures in a patient with severe mixed mitral regurgitation and mitral stenosis. The large v wave and the persistent diastolic gradient are characteristic of mixed mitral valvular disease. (From Kern MJ. *Cardiac Catheterization Handbook.* St. Louis: Mosby; 2003. With permission.)

## VALSALVA, MUELLER, AND OTHER PHYSIOLOGIC MANEUVERS

The Valsalva maneuver is performed by having the patient forcibly expire against a closed glottis and straining as if having a bowel movement. The magnitude of the Valsalva can be quantitated by measuring the pressure against which the patient must expire. The Valsalva maneuver can be performed safely and without complications by almost every type of patient. The four phases of the normal Valsalva maneuver (strain, hypotension, release, and pressure overshoot) may be absent in patients with specific cardiac diseases (congestive heart failure, coronary artery disease, and obstructive cardiomyopathy). In addition, the hemodynamics demonstrated for different types of valvular lesions may be more pronounced during the Valsalva maneuver because of changes in ventricular filling.

The Mueller maneuver is performed by inspiring against a closed glottis, and it is considered the inverse or opposite of the Valsalva maneuver. The subject inhales and the force of inhalation is measured with a manometer, usually −30 to −60 mmHg for 30 s. Hemodynamic alterations of the Mueller maneuver include increased RV filling, increased period of diminished filling as result of the collapse of the venae cavae at thoracic inlets, increasing LV afterload with increase in LV end-diastolic and end-systolic volumes, diminished SV, reduced CO, and reduced ejection fraction. This maneuver is used to augment right-sided heart murmurs and to decrease the physical findings of obstructive cardiomyopathy by a reduction in LV outflow gradient. A reduction in the intensity of the systolic murmur in patients with echocardiographic evidence of anterior mitral valve leaflet motion also can be demonstrated with this maneuver.

Pharmacologic and physiologic stress on LV performance can be obtained in the cath lab by cold pressor testing, hyperventilation, or pharmacologic stimuli such as dobutamine, nitroglycerin, or any nitrates.

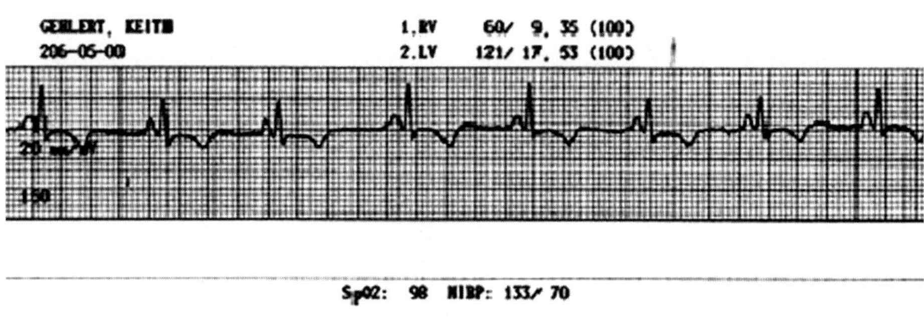


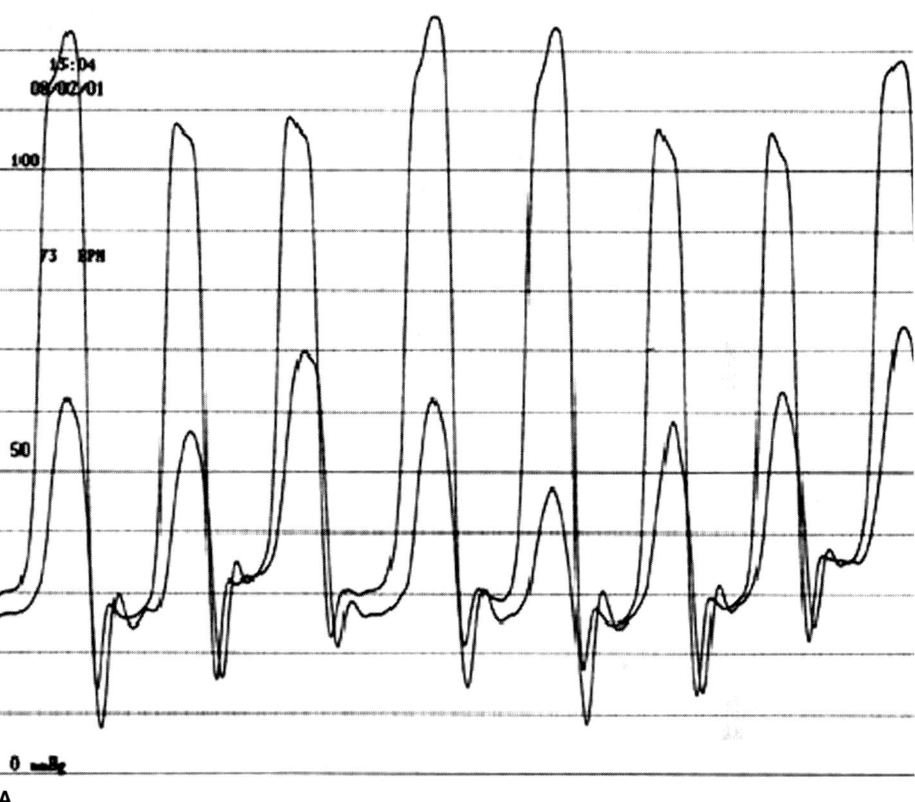


FIGURE 17-44 *A.* Hemodynamic tracings showing physiology of constrictive pericardial constraint. Simultaneous right and left ventricular pressures during respiration increase discordantly with LV increase and RV decreasing during expiration and vice versa. *B.* Hemodynamics of restrictive pathophysiology shows concordance of systolic pressure changes in both right and left ventricles during respiration.

## SPECIAL CATHETERIZATION TECHNIQUES

### Transseptal Heart Catheterization

Retrograde left heart catheterization for aortic or mitral stenosis or prosthetic valve dysfunction may not be suitable or possible in all patients. Transseptal access across the thin atrial septal membrane at the fossa ovalis into the left atrium and left ventricle is an established and safe technique in experienced hands (Fig. 17-45).[79–82]

#### INDICATIONS

1. Conditions that require direct left atrial (LA) or left ventricular (LV) measurement of pressure (such as mitral stenosis, pulmonary venous disease, left intraventricular gradient, aortic stenosis, or hypertrophic cardiomyopathy).
2. Access for mitral balloon-catheter valvuloplasty.
3. Access for deployment of atrial septal defect closure devices.
4. Prosthetic aortic or mitral heart valve dysfunction. Retrograde crossing of a tilting disk-type prosthetic valve has been associated with death from entrapped catheters and should not be attempted.

#### CONTRAINDICATIONS

1. Patients who cannot lie flat or fully cooperate
2. Anticoagulant therapy, low platelet count, or other hemostatic abnormalities
3. Left or right atrial thrombus
4. Atrial myxoma
5. Inferior vena cava mass or obstruction

Transseptal left heart catheterization should be considered carefully in patients with distorted cardiac anatomy secondary to congenital heart disease, dilated aortic root, marked atrial enlargement, or thoracic skeletal deformity.

#### RISKS

Punctures of the aortic root, coronary sinus (CS), or the posterior free wall of the atrium are potentially lethal problems. In patients who have not been given anticoagulants, the 21-gauge tip of the transseptal needle rarely causes a problem. However, if the large transeptal catheter is advanced into these spaces, cardiac tamponade may occur. A detailed description of the transseptal technique can be found elsewhere.[79–82]

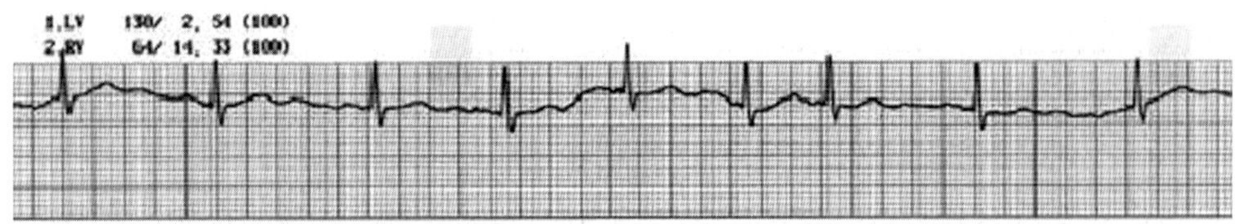


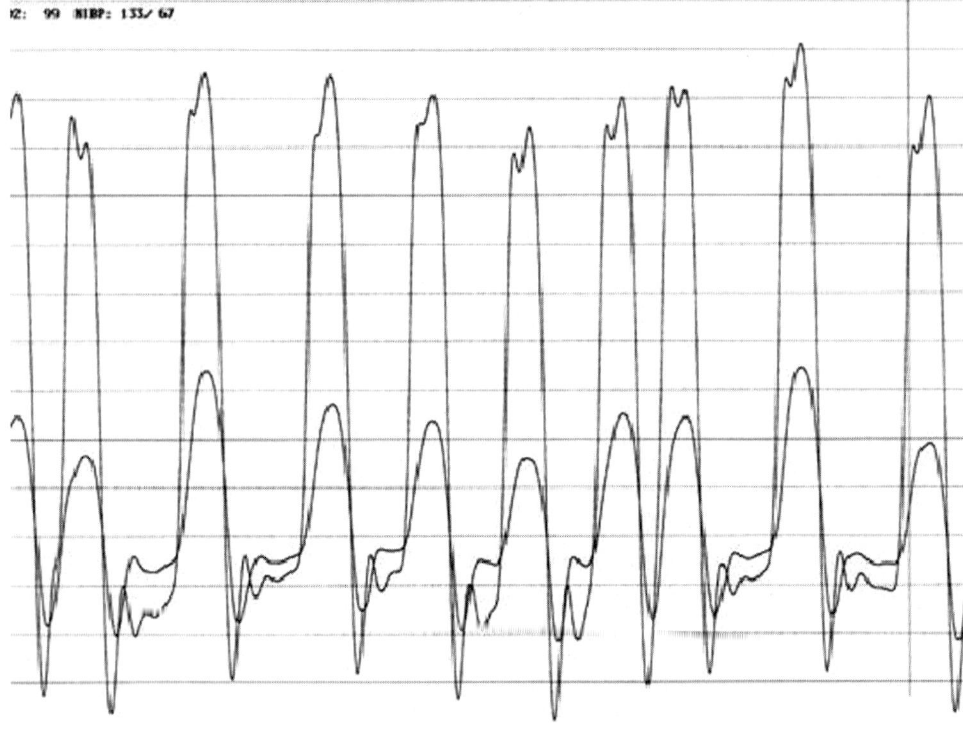


B

FIGURE 17-44 (*Continued*)

## Endomyocardial Biopsy

Endomyocardial biopsy is a common procedure in the catheterization laboratory. Monitoring of cardiac transplant rejection and anthracycline cardiotoxicity are the two major indications for endomyocardial biopsy. Other indications include diagnosis for secondary causes of cardiomyopathy, myocarditis (when there is a history of congestive heart failure in the preceding 6 months), and differentiation between restrictive and constrictive cardiomyopathies. The two major contraindications to endomyocardial biopsy are anticoagulation, anatomic abnormality precluding bioptome placement. Complications of endomyocardial biopsy include access-site related events (3 percent), biopsy related (3 percent), arrhythmia (1 percent), conduction abnormalities (1 percent), perforation (0.7 percent), and death (0.4 percent). All complication rates are higher for patients with cardiomyopathy compared to heart transplant recipients.

## Pericardiocentesis

Pericardiocentesis may be required for diagnosis and management of acute and chronic pericardial effusions. In cardiac tamponade this is a lifesaving technique. A sufficient degree of operator skill must be employed to prevent damage to the heart and pericardium.

Pericardiocentesis usually is preceded by echocardiographic confirmation of pericardial fluid. However, in cases in which a large pericardial effusion is known or suspected with hemodynamic compromise in which tamponade is acute, echocardiographical assessment is not required, and may be detrimental by delaying needed intervention. A Seldinger puncture technique is used from a subxyphoid approach to access the pericardial space, verify the position by echo-contrast or hemodynamics, and introduce a catheter to drain the pericardial effusion. Although monitoring of pericardial pressure is not essential for elective procedures, it is important to document evidence of cardiac tamponade and resolution of pericardial pressure restricting cardiac output.

## Intraaortic Balloon Counterpulsation

### MECHANISMS

Intraaortic balloon (IAB) counterpulsation was first introduced in 1967 by Kantrowitz and Moulopoulos,[83] positioning a balloon in the descending aorta to improve hemodynamics. It is the most commonly used system for temporary mechanical support of patients in a wide variety of clinical settings, such as the cardiac catheterization laboratory, operating room, and the intensive care unit.

IAB counterpulsation increases coronary blood flow and decreases myocardial oxygen demand. Balloon inflation in diastole, at the dicrotic notch on the central arterial pressure tracing, augments aortic diastolic pressure, increasing both coronary artery pressure and flow. Balloon deflation at end-diastole, the upstroke of arterial pressure tracing, decreases aortic volume and ventricular afterload, decreasing myocardial oxygen consumption and increasing cardiac output (CO) (Fig. 17-46). Augmented diastolic blood pressure typically produces a substantial increase in mean arterial blood pressure. Left ventricular end-diastolic pressures decrease during IAB counterpulsation with a preservation or increase in left ventricular stroke volume and ejection fraction. Left ventricular work is reduced by the reduction in afterload. Coronary perfusion occurs predominantly during diastole when the balloon is inflated causing a rise in the aortic pressure, causing the coronary perfusion pressure gradient (Aortic-LVEDP) to increase. However, coronary perfusion is determined not only by the perfusion gradient, but also by the degree of stenosis in the coronary vessels, the collateral circulation, and the duration of diastole. Kern et al.[84] showed that IAB counterpulsation augmented coronary flow velocity proximal but not distal to a high-grade stenosis. After a successful angioplasty of a stenotic lesion in the same vessel, the IAB augmented coronary flow velocity throughout the entire vessel. IAB increases diastolic flow velocity more in patients with a basal systolic blood pressure less than 90 mmHg.[85]

### INDICATIONS AND CONTRAINDICATIONS

The indications and contraindications for IAB counterpulsation are listed in Table 17-27. In high-risk or unstable patients, an IAB pump (IABP) may be inserted before catheterization. During catheterization or interventional procedures, IAB counterpulsation is indicated for hypotension (not responding to volume loading or intravenous vasopressors) or refractory angina.

### TECHNIQUE OF IABP INSERTION

Before IABP catheter insertion, the patient must be assessed for iliofemoral and aortic vascular disease. Significant peripheral vascular disease is a relative contradiction. An abdominal aortogram will identify the course and disease of iliac and femoral vessels before the IABP insertion. The 8F intraaortic balloon sheath is inserted into either femoral groin artery using standard Seldinger technique. Aortic dissection may occur if the balloon has not been advanced and positioned carefully over a guidewire. *Blind insertion of a counterpulsation balloon catheter without a leading guidewire is not recommended.* The tip of the IABP catheter should be positioned left 1 to 2 cm below the top of the aortic arch and then secured. After the patient has returned to the intensive care unit, IAB position is checked by chest x-ray.

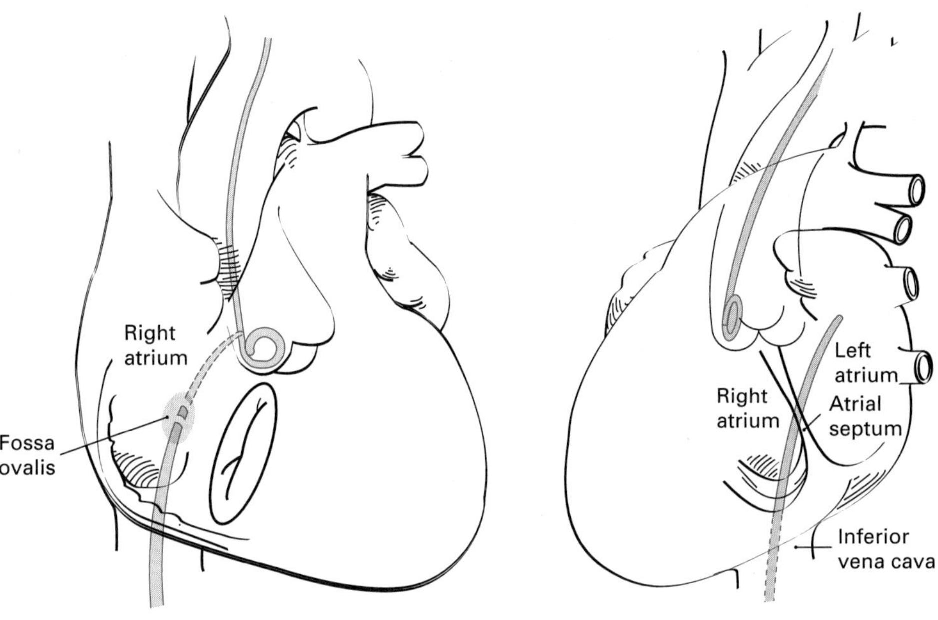


FIGURE 17-45 Anteroposterior (*left*) and lateral (*right*) views of a sheath and dilator positioned in the left atrium following needle puncture of the interatrial septum. The aortic root is defined by a pigtail catheter. Note that the septum is safely crossed posterior and inferior to the aortic valve. (From Roelke M, Conrad-Smith AJ, Palacios IF. The technique and safety of transseptal left heart catheterization. *Catheter Cardiovasc Diagn* 1994;32:332–339. Reproduced with permission from the publisher and authors.)

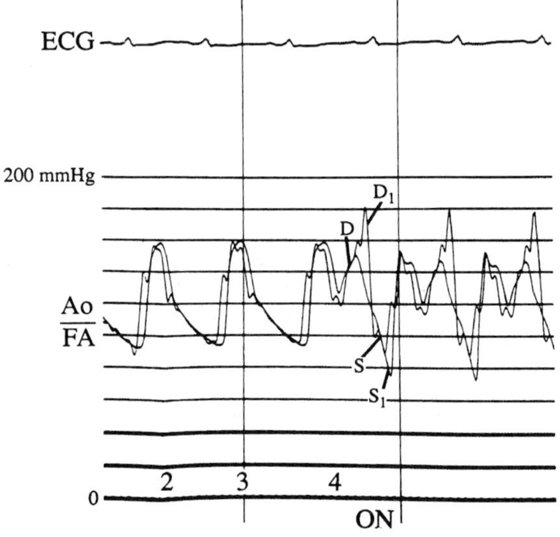


FIGURE 17-46 Hemodynamic tracings of femoral artery (FA) and central aortic (Ao) pressure during intraaortic balloon pumping, demonstrating the augmentation in diastole in the central position (D) and femoral artery position ($D_1$) and reduction in systolic load in the central position (S) and the femoral artery position ($S_1$). Moving the timing of inflation toward the dicrotic notch and the timing of deflation away from systolic upstroke will augment the diastolic pressure and optimally reduce systolic load. ON = the point at which the balloon pump is turned on. (From Kern MJ. *Cardiac Catheterization Handbook*. St. Louis: Mosby; 2003. With permission.)

### COMPLICATIONS OF IAB COUNTERPULSATION

Complications of IAB placement most commonly result from low site of puncture, perforation of the superficial femoral artery, or forceful arterial dissection due to advancement of the guidewire. The puncture site should be located similar to or slightly more proximal to a standard femoral puncture for diagnostic catheterization. A puncture lower than the prescribed site may involve a small superficial femoral artery and cause leg ischemia. Assessment of the patient during IAB counterpulsation includes evaluation for infection, thrombocytopenia, hemorrhage, hemolysis, and vascular obstruction with limb ischemia. Thrombus or dissection may be present at the puncture site or proximally. Heparin administration (5000-unit bolus with 1000 units/h) is standard practice in most institutions.

## Cardiac Catheterization in Heart Transplant Patients and Adults with Congenital Heart Disease

### TRANSPLANTATION

Cardiac transplantation is a common procedure in most tertiary care centers. Routine yearly follow-up of the posttransplant patient includes cardiac catheterization, coronary angiography, and assessment of LV function, PA pressures, and endomyocardial biopsy. Cardiac transplant patients have unique problems that may include altered anatomic relationships, absence of anginal pain, contrast allergic reactions, and high sensitivity to infection, all of which must be considered in the approach to this unusual patient population. Routine left and right heart catheterization is usually performed from the femoral approach. If femoral scar tissue is excessive on one side, approach from the opposite groin or arm may be necessary. If endomyocardial biopsy is considered, the internal jugular or femoral venous approach may be suitable using either fluoroscopy or echocardiographically guided biopsy.

Angiography of the heart transplant patient must account for the transplanted heart that is rotated clockwise. Thus, the right coronary

TABLE 17-27 Indications and Contraindications to Intraaortic Balloon Counterpulsation

| Indications | Contraindications |
|---|---|
| Acute myocardial infarction +/− cardiogenic shock | Severe peripheral vascular disease |
| Refractory unstable angina | Severe aortic incompetence |
| Stabilization of left main disease | Active bleeding |
| Complications of AMI—acute MR or VSD | Patients with contraindication to anticoagulation |
| Weaning from cardiopulmonary bypass | Thrombocytopenia (<50,000) |
| High-risk cardiac percutaneous revascularization | Acute stroke |
| Bridge to cardiac transplantation | |
| High-risk noncardiac surgery in coronary patients | |
| Refractory arrhythmias | |
| Myocardial contusion | |
| Right ventricular failure | |
| Septic shock | |

ABBREVIATIONS: AMI = acute myocardial infarction; VSD = ventricular septal defect.

ostium is anterior and the left coronary ostium is located in a more posterior plane than the normal heart. In addition, a suture ridge in the lower ascending aorta at the site of the aortic anastomosis may be encountered, causing the Judkins catheter to snag or bend as it is advanced. The anterior position of the right coronary ostia may be better engaged using an AP or slightly rightward oblique view. The multipurpose angiographic catheter may be required for unusual positions of the coronary ostia. These patients are generally preload-dependent and thus the recommended administration of intracoronary nitroglycerine before angiographic studies may result in a significant drop in blood pressure.

**CONGENITAL HEART DISEASE**

Adults with corrected congenital heart disease are encountered with increasing frequency by the adult cardiac catheterization physician. Detailed knowledge of previous cardiac surgery, catheterization and echocardiographic findings is necessary for the performance of a complete and accurate catheterization. Residual hemodynamic and electrophysiologic abnormalities must be identified in these patients to maintain long-term survival.

Among the most commonly encountered problems are those of ventricular septal defects and conditions resulting in cyanosis. Ventricular septal defects may occur at the muscular septum or the site of an old patch in corrected hearts. Great vessel shunts may occur from collateral supply, especially in those patients with repaired cyanotic heart disease or incompletely occluded shunts. Cyanosis in these individuals may from the following:

1. Persistent left SVC to left atrium shunting with or without coronary sinus or septal defect
2. Right pulmonary AV fistula (Glenn anastomosis)
3. Acquired lung disease
4. A combination of the above

Careful hemodynamic and oximetric measurements are important to examine cardiac or extracardiac shunting. Both right and left pulmonary arteries must be sampled for oxygen saturations during the oximetry run. Patients with cyanosis are placed on 100 percent oxygen to identify cardiac causes of cyanosis from noncardiac causes.

Large-format image intensifiers (9-in. screen) or biplane angiography may be needed to display both ventricles simultaneously. Coronary artery abnormalities may occur and contribute to ventricular dysfunction in the adult with congenital heart disease. The late natural history of coronary atherosclerosis in corrected forms of congenital heart disease is unknown. It is recommended that any patient over the age of 35 with evidence of ventricular dysfunction undergo coronary arteriography.

Patients with complex congenital heart disease—such as tetralogy of Fallot with an overriding aorta, ventricular septal defect, and pulmonary stenosis or truncus arteriosus (common arterial trunk with ventricular septal defect)—may have abnormally large aortic roots requiring modified coronary catheters. Single coronary arteries or anomalous origins of the left coronary from the right coronary artery may be part of the truncus arteriosus (a common pulmonary and aortic outflow tube) and transposition of the great vessels (switching of pulmonary artery and aorta).

## CORONARY BLOOD FLOW AND PRESSURE MEASUREMENTS

The inability to determine the functional significance of a coronary stenosis remains a well-recognized limitation of angiography,[86,87] repeatedly demonstrated anatomically by intravascular ultrasound (IVUS) imaging and physiologically by ischemia stress testing.[88–90] Measurements of coronary blood flow and pressure provide unique information that complements the anatomic (angiographic) evaluation and facilitates decision making regarding therapy in the catheterization laboratory.

### Coronary Blood Flow and Resistance

Coronary blood flow can increase from a resting level to a maximum depending on increases in myocardial oxygen demand or in response to neurogenic or pharmacologic hyperemic stimuli. The ratio of maximal to basal flow is coronary flow reserve (CFR), or coronary vasodilatory reserve (CVR). Resistance to flow increase occurs at three levels: epicardial conduits (R1), precapillary arterioles (R2), and intramyocardial resistance (R3). Normally, large epicardial vessel resistance (R1) is trivial. Most coronary flow is regulated by the myocardial precapillary arteriolar resistance vessels (R2). In a normal artery supplying normal myocardium, coronary blood flow reserve can exceed 3. However, several conditions, including left ventricular hypertrophy, myocardial ischemia, or diabetes can affect the microcirculatory resistance R3, blunting the maximal absolute increase in coronary flow. Increased R3 resistance may also be associated with increased resting flow above the expected level for myocardial oxygen demand at rest also resulting in reduced coronary flow reserve (Fig. 17-47).

Significant atherosclerotic stenosis produces epicardial conduit resistance. In response to the loss of perfusion pressure and flow to

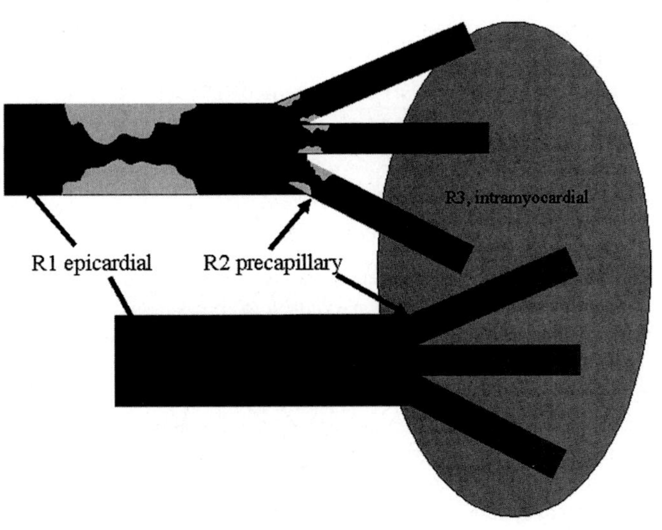


FIGURE 17-47 Coronary circulation. $R_1$, $R_2$, $R_3$ = epicardial, anteriolar, and microvascular resistance, respectively.

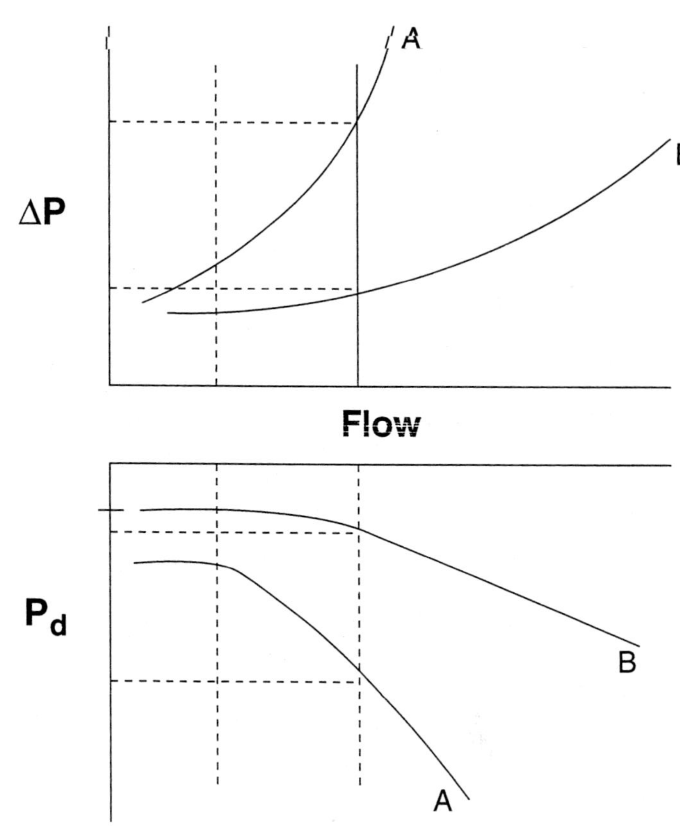


FIGURE 17-48 Coronary pressure-flow relationships for two stenoses of the same angiographic severity. *Top:* ΔP = pressure gradient (aortic-distal coronary pressure) versus coronary flow. *Bottom:* Absolute distal coronary pressure $P_d$ versus flow. Increasing flow produces marked loss of $P_d$ as well as an increase in ΔP. The loss of $P_d$ in absolute terms determines myocardial perfusion pressure ($P_d$ − venous pressure) and the potential for inducible ischemia.

the distal microcirculation bed, precapillary resistance vessels (R2) dilate to maintain satisfactory basal flow appropriate for myocardial oxygen demand. In parallel with resistance to flow, viscous friction, flow separation forces, and flow turbulence at the site of the stenosis produce energy loss at the stenosis. Energy (heat) is extracted reducing pressure distal to the stenosis, producing a pressure gradient between proximal and distal artery regions. The pressure loss increases with increasing coronary flow along an exponential pressure-flow relationship of the specific coronary stenosis resistance[91,92] (Fig. 17-48). There exists an absolute poststenotic myocardial perfusion pressure threshold below which myocardial ischemia may be easily induced. The hemodynamic significance of a given stenosis can be measured by the pressure-flow relationship using sensor angioplasty guidewires.[87]

## Coronary Flow Velocity and Reserve

The coronary flow velocity of red blood cells moving past the ultrasound emitter/receiver on the end of a 0.014-in. Doppler-tipped angioplasty guidewire can be determined from the frequency shift, defined by the Doppler equation as the difference between the transmitted and returning frequency:

$$V = (F_1 - F_0) \times (C)/(2F_0) \times (\mathrm{Cos}\, \varnothing),$$

where $V$ = velocity of blood flow, $F_0$ = transmitting (transducer) frequency, $F_1$ = returning frequency, C = constant for the speed of sound in blood, ∅ = angle of incidence. Flow velocity measurements have been validated by Doucette et al.[93] and Labovitz et al.[94] Volumetric flow is the product of vessel area ($cm^2$) and flow velocity (cm/s) yielding a value in $cm^3$/s. Absolute Doppler flow velocities represent changes in volumetric coronary flow when the vessel cross-sectional area remains constant over the measurement period. Compared to volumetric measurements, velocity may underestimate the volumetric flow reserve in some vessels, which demonstrated intact endothelial mediated vasodilation.

CVR is the ratio of maximal hyperemic to basal mean flow velocity in the target vessel obtained *distal* to the stenosis. As stenosis severity increases, hyperemic flow becomes attenuated, and CVR decreases. Absolute CVR measures the capacity of the two-component system of the R1 coronary artery resistance and the R2 vascular resistance to achieve maximal blood flow in response to a given hyperemic stimulation. Normal CVR in young patients with IVUS demonstrated normal arteries commonly exceeds 3.0.[95] In patients with chest pain undergoing cardiac catheterization with angiographically normal vessels, the normal absolute CVR is 2.7 ± 0.6,[96] suggesting a degree of patient to patient variability and distal microvascular disease that is beyond the threshold of angiographic detection. The values for CVR associated with nonobstructed coronary arteries in patients with chest pain syndromes, transplanted hearts, and in normal arteries in patients with obstructive coronary artery disease elsewhere are 2.8 ± 0.6, 3.1 ± 0.9, and 2.5 ± 0.95, respectively.[96] The incidence of impaired coronary vasodilatory reserve < 2.0 in 450 angiographically normal coronary arteries from 220 patients undergoing evaluation for chest pain or cardiac transplantation follow-up angiography is approximately 12 percent.[96]

### FACTORS INFLUENCING CORONARY FLOW RESERVE

Coronary flow reserve (CFR or CVR) is subject to variations in hemodynamics that may alter resting flow and land limit maximal hyperemic flow. Tachycardia increases basal flow; thus CFR is reduced by 10 percent for every 15 heartbeats.[97] Increasing mean arterial pressure reduces maximal vasodilatation, thus reducing hyperemia with less alteration in basal flow. CFR may be reduced in patients with essential hypertension and normal coronary arteries[97–99] and in patients with aortic stenosis and normal coronary arteries.[100] In some patients with moderate coronary artery disease, the stenotic configuration and surrounding vessel segments are subject to vasomotor stimuli. Thus vasoconstrictor, neurologic, or humoral influences, endothelial dysfunction, and extracardiac vasoconstrictor stimuli may produce dynamic or episodic ischemia-related symptoms with activities of daily life such as exercise, emotional stress, or adrenergic stimulation.[101,102]

The variability in CVR in unobstructed arteries may also be due to age.[103,104] To improve the assessment of CVR, Wieneke et al.[104] measured CVR in 141 patients in 242 unobstructed coronary arteries. Based on a regression model, individual CVR values obtained at different basal average peak velocities could be transformed and corrected for patient age relating them to a mean basal average peak velocity (BAPV) of 15 cm/s and age of 55 years ($CVR_{corr} = 2.85 \times CVR_{measured} \times 10^{x}$, where $X = 0.48 \log(\text{BAPV}) + 0.0025 \times \text{age} - 1.16$). The transformation by the correction formula showed that only patients with diabetes had a significant decrease of the traditional CVR and corrected CVR, whereas hypertension and current smoking had no influence on corrected CVR. Use of the corrected CVR standardizes for variations in basal average peak velocity and patient age and may discriminate between intrinsic and extra cardiac factors impairing CVR.

Coronary flow reserve is diminished in patients with diabetes, but especially so in those with diabetic retinopathy. Akasaka et al.[105] evaluated 29 patients with diabetes mellitus, 18 with and 11 without diabetic retinopathy and 15 control patients with chest pain and normal coronary arteries. The diabetic retinopathy was nonproliferative in all 18 patients studied. Coronary flow velocity was measured in the angiographically normal segment of the left anterior descending coronary artery in patients at rest and during maximal hyperemia induced with 0.014 mg/kg of intravenous adenosine. Volumetric coronary blood flow (velocity × vessel cross-sectional area) was significantly reduced during hyperemia (107 ± 23 and 116 ± 18 vs. 136 ± 17mL/min, respectively) and was higher at baseline (58 ± 16 and 45 ± 12 vs. 37 ± 10 mL/min, respectively) in diabetic patients with and without retinopathy compared to control groups ($p < 0.05$ for both diabetic groups). Coronary flow reserve was also significantly lower in those diabetic patients with and without retinopathy compared to the control patients (1.9 ± 0.4 and 2.8 ± 0.3 vs. 3.3 ± 0.4; $p < 0.01$, respectively).

**RELATIVE CORONARY FLOW VELOCITY**

CVR is the summed response of the major two coronary flow resistances and therefore an abnormal value (e.g.,< 2.0) cannot distinguish between increased resistance at R1 epicardial level or R2 microvascular level. A relative CVR (rCVR) can be determined in a fashion similar to that defined by Gould et al.[91,92] rCVR is defined as the ratio of maximal flow in the coronary with stenosis ($\dot{Q}^S$) to flow in a normal coronary without stenosis ($\dot{Q}^N$). It was shown that rCVR is independent of the aortic pressure and rate pressure product, and was well suited to assess the physiologic significance of coronary stenoses when an adjacent nondiseased coronary artery is available. For flow velocity studies, rCVR in the catheterization laboratory is defined as the ratio of $CVR_{target}$ to CVR in an angiographically normal reference vessel ($rCVR = (\dot{Q}^S/\dot{Q}_{base})/(\dot{Q}^N/\dot{Q}_{base}) = (CVR_{target}/CVR_{reference})$, and assumes basal flow in the two vessels is similar and thus, mathematically resembles Gould's derivation. The normal range for rCVR is 0.8 to 1.0.[106,107]

rCVR cannot be used in patients with three-vessel coronary disease who have no suitable reference vessel. rCVR relies on the assumption that the microvascular circulatory response is uniformly distributed among the myocardial beds, thus rCVR is of no value in patients with myocardial infarction, left ventricular regional dysfunction, or patients in whom the microcirculatory responses are heterogeneous.

## Pressure-Derived Fractional Flow Reserve of the Myocardium

Myocardial perfusion is closely linked to myocardial ischemia and is directly dependent on the coronary"driving" pressure associated with three major coronary vascular resistances. The myocardial perfusion pressure (aortic pressure minus left ventricular pressure or right atrial pressure) is reduced when an epicardial stenosis causes pressure loss distal to the stenosis. If the myocardial bed resistances are stimulated to maximal hyperemia and remain constant, then the poststenotic hyperemic coronary artery pressure represents the maximal achievable perfusion available in that vessel and can be used to produce an estimate of normal coronary blood flow and an ischemic threshold.

Using coronary pressure measured at constant and minimal myocardial resistances (i.e., maximal hyperemia), Pijls et al.[108–110] derived an estimate of the percentage of normal coronary blood flow expected to go through a stenotic artery. This pressure-derived ratio is called the fractional flow reserve (FFR). FFRcor is defined as the maximum coronary flow in the presence of a stenosis divided by the normal maximum flow of the artery (i.e., the maximum flow in that artery if no stenosis were present).[108] Similarly, FFRmyo is defined as maximum myocardial blood flow distal to an epicardial stenosis divided by its value if no epicardial stenosis were present. Stated another way, FFR represents that fraction of normal maximum flow that remains despite the presence of an epicardial lesion. The FFR of a coronary artery and its dependent myocardium can be calculated by:

$$FFR_{cor} = (P_d - P_w)/(P_a - P_w) \tag{1}$$

and

$$FFR_{myo} = (P_d - P_v)/(P_a - P_v) \tag{2}$$

where $P_a$, $P_d$, and $P_v$ are aortic, distal coronary, and venous pressures taken at maximum vasodilation. $P_w$ is coronary occlusion wedge pressure taken at coronary occlusion. Because of the necessity to know $P_w$, $FFR_{cor}$ can be calculated only during percutaneous transluminal coronary angioplasty (PTCA). $FFR_{myo}$, however, can also be calculated during diagnostic procedures. The difference between $FFR_{myo}$ and $FFR_{cor}$ represents the contribution of collateral flow to total myocardial perfusion and is called fractional collateral flow. Because $FFR_{myo}$ reflects both antegrade and collateral contribution to maximum myocardial perfusion, it is the most important flow index from a clinical point of view. It describes to what extent maximum myocardial perfusion is affected by the epicardial coronary stenosis.

The FFR is calculated as the ratio of the poststenotic coronary pressure to aorta pressure obtained at sustained minimal resistance (i.e., maximal hyperemia) (Fig. 17-49). FFR reflects both antegrade and collateral myocardial perfusion rather than merely transstenotic pressure loss (i.e., a stenosis pressure gradient). Because it is calculated only at peak hyperemia, FFR is also differentiated from CVR by being largely independent of basal flow, driving pressure, heart rate, systemic blood pressure, or status of the microcirculation[110] (Fig. 17-50). The FFR, but not the resting pressure or hyperemic pressure gradient, is strongly related to provocable myocardial ischemia demonstrated by comparisons to different clinical stress testing modalities in patients with stable angina.[109]

FFR and rCVR are more specific for flow limitations due to a stenosis than is CVR. FFR, rCVR, and CVR were determined in 21 patients in 24 target vessels for stenosis severity ranging from 40 to 95 percent, with an average of 74 ± 15 percent.[106] Absolute CVR did not correlate with percent area stenosis or FFR. FFR, as well as rCVR, showed a curvilinear relationship to percent area stenosis ($r = 0.89$ and $r = 0.79$; $p < 0.0001$) with a close linear relationship between FFR and rCVR ($r = 0.91$; $p < 0.0001$). rCVR closely correlated with FFR and percent area stenosis. Absolute CVR, as expected, varied due to the influence of microvascular flow status. An additional concern in interpreting FFR as well as absolute CVR, is the effect of an abnormal microcirculation. In patients with a nonuniform microcirculation, such as those with myocardial infarction, neither absolute CVR nor rCVR can be used for assessment of lesion severity. Likewise, in patients with severe hypertrophy, diabetes, or hypertension, the discriminatory capacity using rCVR with a markedly reduced CVR may be too low to allow for accurate assessment of a stenosis. In patients with potential microcirculatory impairment, a lesion is best assessed by FFR. In patients with an abnormal microcirculation, it can be argued that a normal FFR indicates the conduit resistance is not a major contributing factor to perfusion impairment, and that focal conduit enlargement (e.g., stenting) would not restore normal perfusion. The current physiologic criteria have not been completely examined in patients with profound microvascular disease.

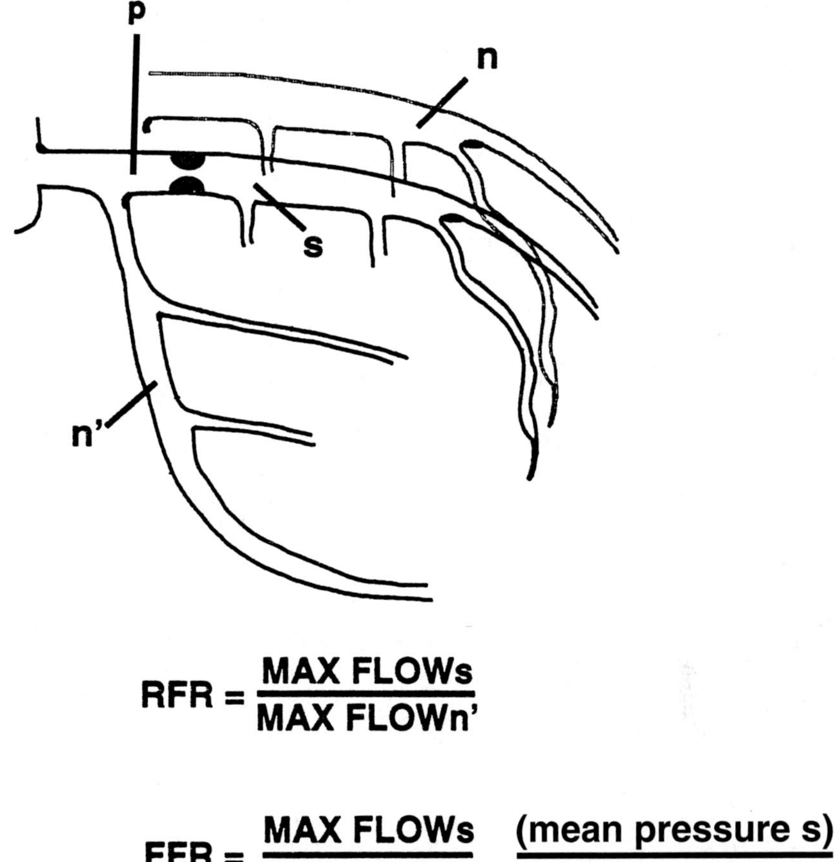


FIGURE 17-49 Schematic drawing illustrating the rationale of comparing relative and fractional myocardial flow reserve. The relative flow reserve (RFR) is the ratio of hyperemic flow in the anterior region (depending on the stenotic left anterior descending coronary artery) to the hyperemic flow in the normal region (depending on the left circumflex coronary artery). The myocardial fractional flow reserve (FFR) is the ratio of hyperemic flow in the anterior region (depending on the stenotic left anterior descending coronary artery) to hyperemic flow in that same region in the hypothetical case of a normal left anterior descending coronary artery (*faint lines*). These measurements are derived from the mean pressure distal to the stenosis divided by the mean pressure proximal to the stenosis at maximal hyperemia. In the case of a similar decrease of myocardial resistance during hyperemia in the left anterior descending area and the left circumflex area, the value of both the relative and the fractional myocardial flow reserves should be identical. n = the hypothetical normal left anterior descending coronary artery; n' = normal left circumflex coronary artery; s = stenotic left anterior descending coronary artery. (From de Bruyne B, Banohuin T, Melin J, et al. Coronary flow reserve calculated from pressure measurements in humans. Validation with positron emission tomography. *Criculation* 1994;89:1013–1022. With permission.)

## Method of Sensor Guidewire Use

After diagnostic angiography or during angioplasty, the sensor guidewire is passed through an angioplasty Y connector attached to a guiding catheter. Intravenous (IV) heparin 40 to 60 units/kg is given. IC nitroglycerin (100 to 200 $\mu$g) is also given several minutes before the guidewire is advanced into the artery.

For flow velocity, the sensor tip is advanced at least 5 to 10 artery-diameter lengths (>2 cm) beyond the stenosis to measure reestablished laminar flow. Resting flow velocity data are recorded. Induction of coronary hyperemia by intracoronary or intravenous adenosine is performed with continuous recording peak hyperemic flow velocity. CVR is computed as maximal hyperemic to basal average peak velocity (APV) (Fig. 17-51). Poor Doppler signal acquisition may occur in 10 to15 percent of patients even within normal arteries. As in transthoracic echo Doppler studies, the operator must adjust the guidewire's position (sample volume) to optimize the velocity signal. Several different tip orientations interrogating the maximal velocity spectra are necessary.[111]

For FFR, the guidewire is advanced in the guide catheter to the coronary ostium and the sensor pressure is matched to the guide catheter pressure. The wire is then advanced into the artery beyond the stenosis. Baseline pressure is recorded. Coronary hyperemia with

**Reproducibility of FFR vs CFR**

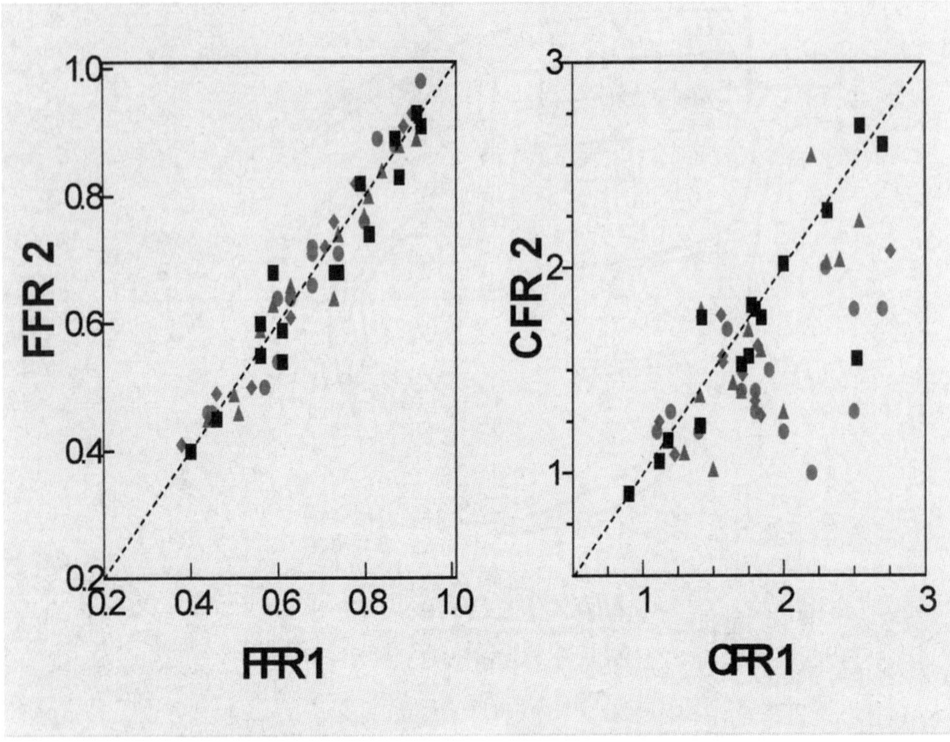


FIGURE 17-50 Reproducibility of FFR versus CVR for changing heart rate, blood pressure, and contractility. Circles = contractility; triangle = heart rate; diamond = MAP; square = duplicate measurement. (From de Bruyne Bartunek J, Sys SU, et al. *Circulation* 1996;94:1842–1849. With permission.)

intracoronary or intravenous adenosine is induced, while both guide catheter and sensor-wire pressures are continuously recorded. FFR is computed as the ratio $pressure_{distal}/pressure_{aorta}$ at maximal hyperemia (Fig. 17-52). Pressure signal artifacts may be reduced by careful attention to technique.[112] The safety of intracoronary sensor-wire measurements has been excellent, as reported by Qian et al.[113] in 906 patients. Complications included severe transient bradycardia after intracoronary adenosine (1.7 percent), coronary spasm during passage of the Doppler guidewire (1 percent), and ventricular fibrillation during the procedure (0.2 percent). All complications could easily be managed medically.

## Assessing Stenosis Severity with Pharmacologic Hyperemic Stimuli

Stenosis severity should always be assessed using measurements obtained during maximal hyperemia. The most widely used maximal vasodilator agents are dipyridamole, papaverine, and adenosine. The hyperosmolar ionic and low-osmolar nonionic con-

**N.L., CFX**

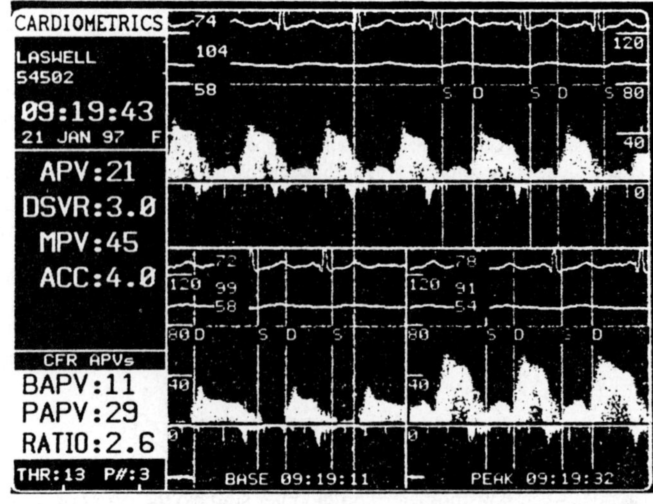


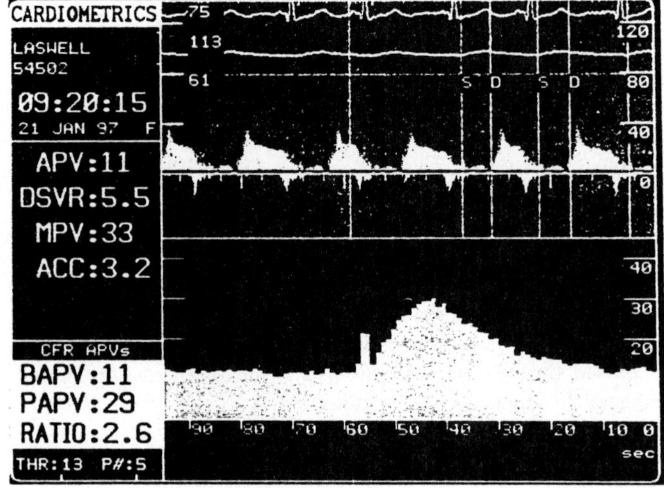


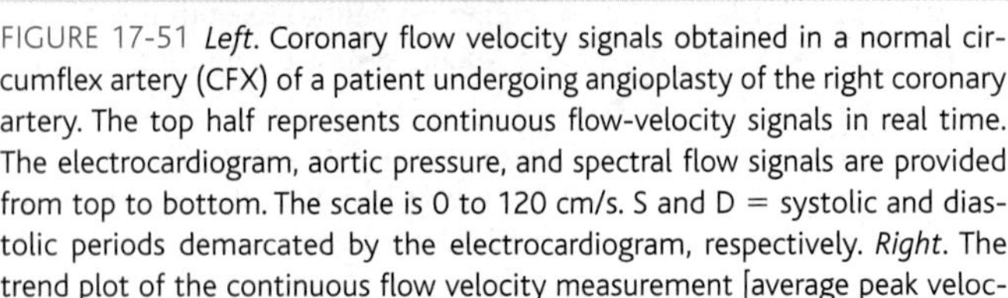

FIGURE 17-51 *Left.* Coronary flow velocity signals obtained in a normal circumflex artery (CFX) of a patient undergoing angioplasty of the right coronary artery. The top half represents continuous flow-velocity signals in real time. The electrocardiogram, aortic pressure, and spectral flow signals are provided from top to bottom. The scale is 0 to 120 cm/s. S and D = systolic and diastolic periods demarcated by the electrocardiogram, respectively. *Right.* The trend plot of the continuous flow velocity measurement [average peak velocity (APV)] is shown in the right-hand panel on the lower tracing. After intracoronary adenosine administration, APV increased from 11 to 29 cm/s, producing a coronary flow ratio (CFR) of 2.6. The duration of hyperemia is 45 s. The trend velocity scale is 0 to 40 cm/s. The time base is 90 s. (From Kern MJ, de Bruyne B, Pijls NHJ, et al. From Research to clinical practice: Current role of physiologically based decision making in the catheterization laboratory. *J Am Coll Cardiol* 1997;30:613–620. With permission.)

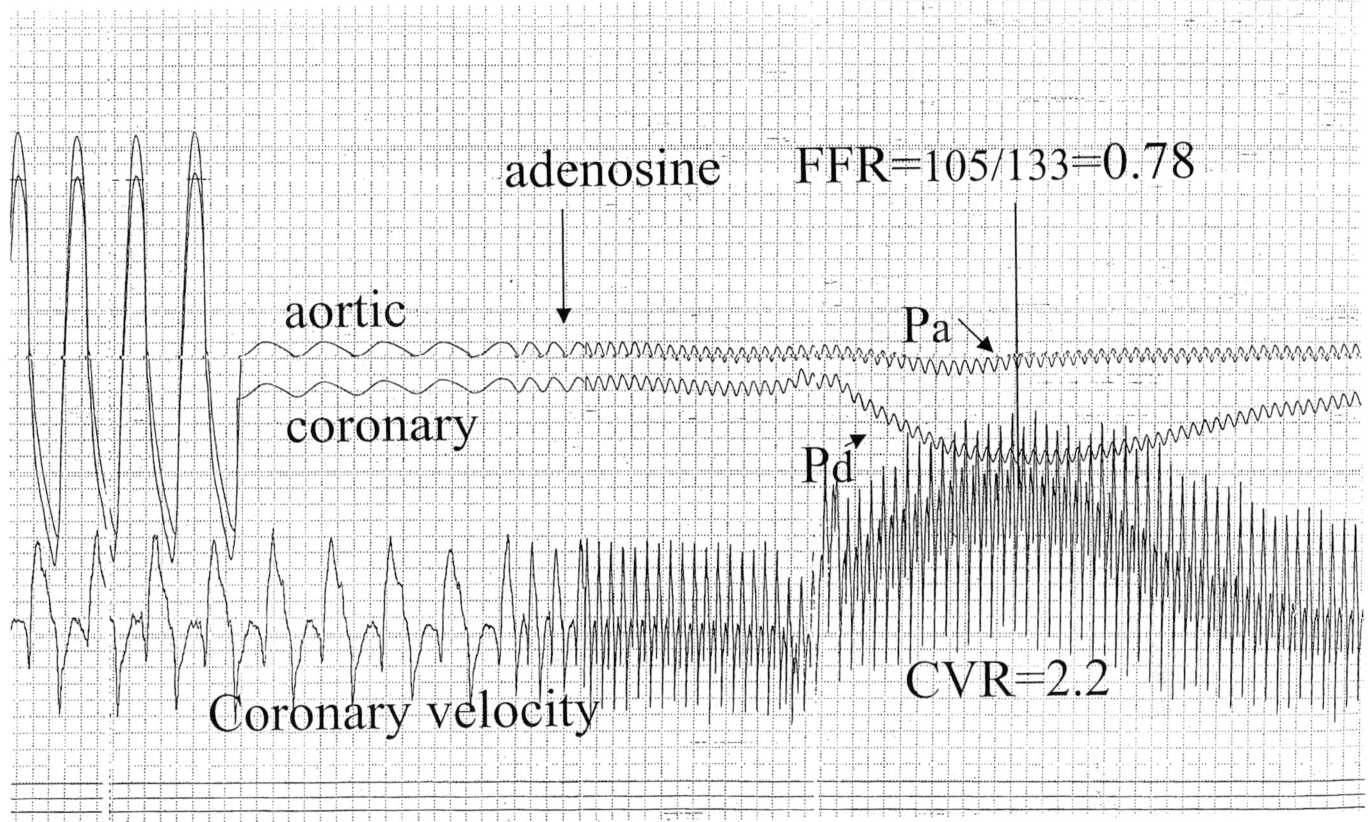


FIGURE 17-52 Hemodynamic and coronary flow velocity tracings demonstrating coronary flow reserve (CVR) and fractional flow reserve (FFR) data collection. Aortic ($P_a$) and distal coronary pressure ($P_d$) at baseline and during adenosine hyperemia (*at vertical line*). Coronary velocity shows a 2.2-fold increase with adenosine. FFR = 0.78.

trast media do not produce maximal vasodilatation. Nitrates increase volumetric flow, but since these agents also dilate epicardial conductance vessels, the increase in coronary flow velocity is less than with adenosine or papaverine. Intracoronary nitroglycerin (100 to 200 $\mu$g) should be given before flow velocity measurements to paralyze vasomotion and minimize any flow-mediated vasodilation. Intracoronary papaverine increases coronary blood flow velocity four to six times over resting values in patients with normal coronary arteries.[114] Papaverine (8 to 12 mg) produces a response equal to that of an intravenous infusion of dipyridamole in a dose of 0.56 to 0.84 mg/kg of body weight but can cause QT prolongation occasionally and ventricular tachycardia or fibrillation.[115]

Adenosine, both intracoronary and intravenous, has a short half-life. The total duration of the hyperemic response of intracoronary adenosine is only 25 percent that of papaverine or dipyridamole.[116,117] Adenosine is benign in the appropriate dosages (20 to 30 $\mu$g in the right coronary artery or 30 to 40 $\mu$g in the left coronary artery or infused intravenously at 140 $\mu$g/kg/min). Since bolus intracoronary adenosine does not increase vessel cross-sectional area,[118] coronary flow velocity reserve can be used as a surrogate for coronary volumetric flow reserve. In measuring FFR using intracoronary (15 to 20 $\mu$g in the right, and 18 to 24 $\mu$g in the left coronary artery) versus intravenous adenosine (140 $\mu$g/kg/min) in 52 patients with 60 lesions (mean percent stenosis of 56 $\pm$ 24 percent; range 0 to 95 percent), Jeremias et al.[119] found a linear relationship between the two methods ($r = 0.978$, $p < 0.001$). The mean measurement difference for FFR was $-0.004 \pm 0.03$. In 8 percent of the cases, intracoronary adenosine FFR was $\geq$ 0.05 units different from intravenous FFR. Thus, in a small percentage of cases, maximal coronary hyperemia may require increased intracoronary doses of adenosine.

Although it is unavailable in the United States, adenosine triphosphate (ATP) may also be used to stimulate maximal hyperemia.[120] There was significant correlation between coronary flow reserve with ATP and papaverine, indicating that maximal coronary vasodilation is safely obtained with intracoronary ATP doses $\geq$15$\mu$g. Intravenous dobutamine (10 to 40 $\mu$g/kg/min) has also been used to assess lesion severity with FFR.[121] Peak dobutamine infusion produced similar distal coronary pressure and pressure ratios ($P_d/P_a$ 60 $\pm$ 18 vs. 59 $\pm$ 18 mmHg; FFR 0.68 $\pm$ 0.18 and 0.68 $\pm$ 0.17, respectively; all $p$ = NS). High-dose intravenous dobutamine did not modify the angiographic area of the epicardial stenosis, and—much like adenosine—fully exhausted myocardial resistance regardless of inducible left ventricular dysfunction.

## Clinical Applications of Coronary Blood Flow and Pressure Measurements

### PHYSIOLOGIC CRITERIA

A hemodynamically significant coronary lesion is associated with one or more of the following: (1) poststenotic absolute coronary flow reserve (CVR) $< 2.0$; (2) relative coronary flow reserve (rCVR) $<$ 0.8; (3) proximal to distal flow velocity ratio ($P/D$) $< 1.7$; (4) diastolic-to-systolic velocity ration (DSVR) $< 1.8$; and (5) Using pressure sensor guidewires, the hyperemic translesional absolute pressure ratio, also known as the FFR $< 0.75$.[87,122] Coronary physiologic

TABLE 17-28 Catheter-Based Anatomic and Physiologic Criteria Associated with Clinical Outcomes

| Application | IVUS | CVR | rCVR | FFR |
|---|---|---|---|---|
| Ischemia detection | <3–4 $mm^2$ | < 2.0 | <0.8 | <0.75 |
| Deferred angioplasty | — | >2.0 | — | >0.75 |
| Endpoint of angioplasty | — | >2.0–2.5 With <35% DS | — | >0.90 |
| Endpoint of stenting | >9 $mm^2$ >80% ref. area, full apposition | — | — | >0.94 |

SOURCE: From Kern MJ. Coronary physiology revisited: Practical insights from the cardiac catheterization laboratory. *Circulation* 2000;101:1344–1351. With permission.

ABBREVIATIONS: CVR = coronary vasodilator reserve; DS = diameter stenosis; FFR = fractional flow reserve; IVUS = intravascular ultrasound; rCVR = relative coronary vasodilator reserve.

measurements associated with four major clinical outcomes supported by numerous studies[122] are summarized in Table 17-28. The recommendation for use of physiologic measurements during invasive procedures is provided in Appendix 17-3.

## ISCHEMIC STRESS TESTING

Strong correlations exist between myocardial stress testing and FFR or CVR.[123–137] An FFR of < 0.75 identified physiologically significant stenoses associated with inducible myocardial ischemia, with high sensitivity (88 percent), specificity (100 percent), positive predicted value (100 percent), and overall accuracy (93 percent). An abnormal CVR (< 2.0) corresponded to reversible myocardial perfusion imaging defects with high sensitivity (86 to 92 percent), specificity (89 to 100 percent), predictive accuracy (89 to 96 percent), and positive and negative predictive values (84 to 100 percent and 77 to 95 percent, respectively). A summary of ischemic stress testing and coronary physiologic measurements is provided in Table 17-29.

## DIFFUSE ATHEROSCLEROSIS

Coronary arteries without focal stenosis are generally considered non-flow-limiting. A diffusely diseased atherosclerotic coronary artery can be viewed as a series of branching units diverting and gradually distributing flow and reducing pressure longitudinally along the conduit. In such a vessel, a reduced CVR is not associated with any single location of stenotic pressure loss, Thus, mechanical therapy to treat presumed "culprit" plaque would be futile. De Bruyne et al.[138] examined patients with coronary artery disease in nonstenotic arteries with diffuse coronary atherosclerosis. Coronary pressure and fractional flow reserve were obtained in 37 arteries in 10 individuals without atherosclerosis, and from 106 nonstenotic arteries in 62 patients. Fractional flow reserve was normal, 0.97 ± 0.02, in group 1, with no resistance to flow in truly normal arteries but was significantly lower, 0.80 ± 0.08, in group 2, indicating

TABLE 17-29 Stress Testing and Directly Measured Coronary Blood Physiology

| Author | Ref no. | *n* | Ischemic Test | Physiologic Threshold | Sensitivity | Specificity | PV+ | PV− | Accuracy |
|---|---|---|---|---|---|---|---|---|---|
| *Poststenotic CVR/rCVR* | | | | | | | | | |
| Miller | 123 | 33 | Adeno/Dipy MIBI | <2.0 | 82 | 100 | 100 | 77 | 89 |
| Joye | 124 | 30 | Exercise thallium | <2.0 | 94 | 95 | 94 | 95 | 94 |
| Deychak | 125 | 17 | Exercise thallium | <1.8 | 94 | 94 | 100 | 91 | 96 |
| Heller | 126 | 100 | Exercise thallium | <1.8 | 89 | 92 | 96 | 89 | 92 |
| Danzi | 129 | 30 | Dipy echo | <2.0 | 91 | 84 | — | — | 87 |
| Schulman | 131 | 35 | Exercise ECG | <2.0 | 95 | 71 | — | — | 86 |
| Donahue | 146 | 50 | Exercise/pharm thallium | <2.0 | 98 | 76 | 88 | 88 | — |
| Duffy | 133 | 43 | Stress echo | <2.0 | 80 | 93 | — | — | 88 |
| | | | | rCVR <0.75 | 100 | 76 | — | — | 81 |
| Chamuleau | 134 | 127 | Dipy MIBI | CVR <2.0, | — | — | — | — | 69 |
| | | | | rCVR <0.75 | — | — | — | — | 75 |
| EL Shafei | 137 | 53 | Exercise /pharm thallium | CVR <0.20, | 71 | 83 | 81 | 74 | — |
| | | | | rCVR <0.75 | 63 | 88 | 83 | 70 | — |
| *FFR* | | | | | | | | | |
| Pijls | 112 | 45 | Four-test standard | <0.75 | 88 | 100 | 100 | 88 | 93 |
| de Bruyne | 127 | 60 | Exercise ECG | <0.72 | 100 | 87 | — | — | — |
| Bartunek | 130 | 37 | Dobu/exercise echo | <0.68 | 95 | 90 | — | — | — |
| Chamuleau | 134 | 127 | Dipy MIBI | <0.75 | — | — | — | — | 75 |
| Caymaz | 135 | 30 | Exercise thallium | <0.75 | — | — | 91 | 100 | — |
| Fearon | 136 | 10 | Exercise thallium | <0.75 | 90 | 100 | — | — | 95 |

ABBREVIATIONS: Adeno/Dipy MIBI = adenosine or dipyridamole sestamibi scan; CVR = coronary vasodilatory reserve; Dobu = dobutamine; FFR = fractional flow reserve; PV+/PV− = predictive value positive/negative.

significant resistance. In 57 percent of arteries in group 2, FFR was lower than the lowest value in group 1. In 8 percent of arteries in group 2, FFR was less than 0.75, well below the ischemic threshold (Fig. 17-53). Diffuse atherosclerosis on angiography was associated with a continuous pressure loss along the arterial length contributing to myocardial ischemia and a potential for ischemia, despite the absence of an epicardial focal stenosis.[138] Measuring continuous coronary pressure during wire pullback from a distal to proximal location

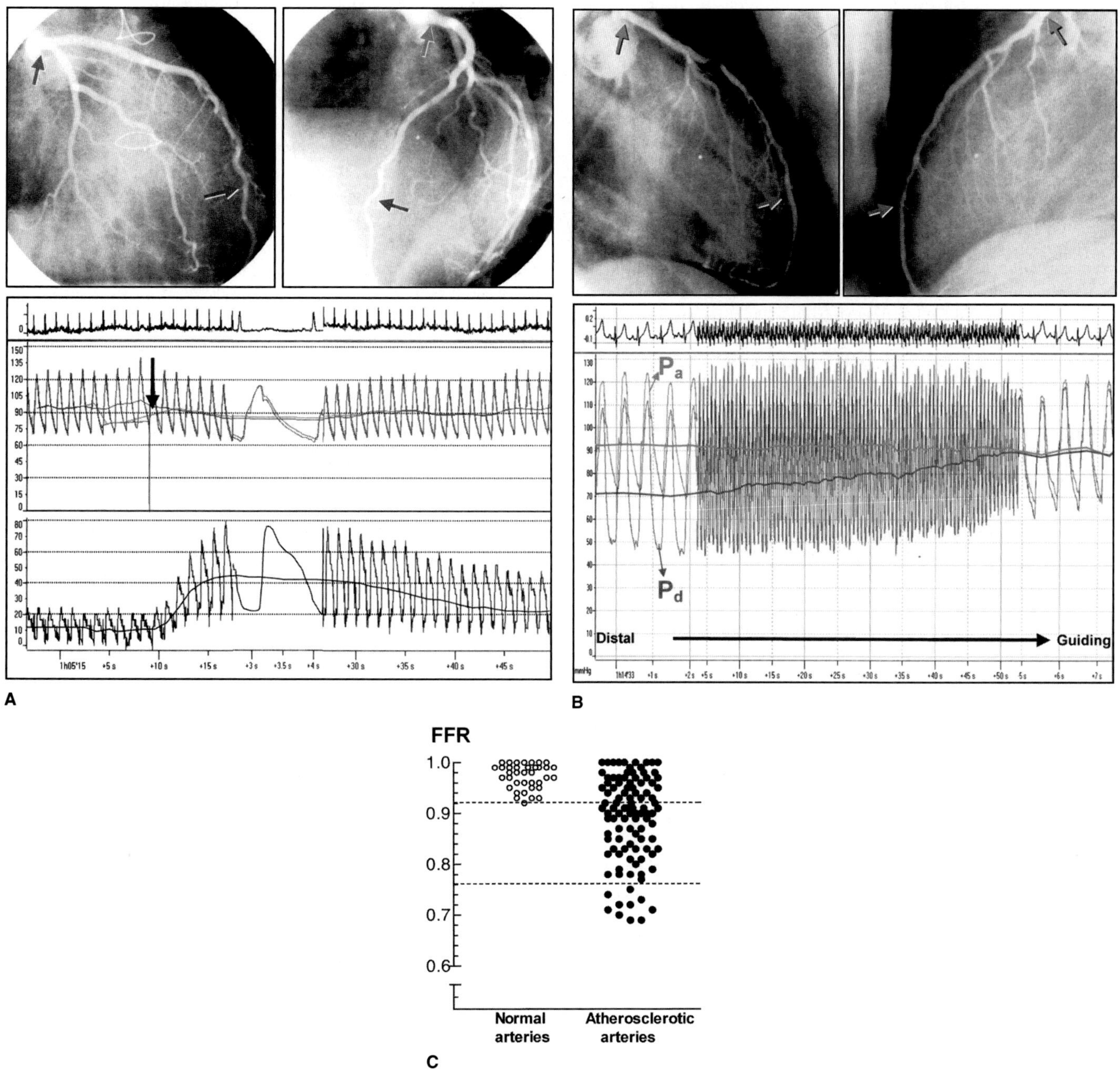


FIGURE 17-53 *A*. Normal coronary angiogram (*upper panels*) and simultaneous aortic and distal coronary pressures and coronary flow velocity recordings (*lower panel*) in a 55-year-old patient 3 weeks after orthotopic cardiac transplantation. Even during an adenosine-induced fourfold increase in coronary blood flow velocity, no pressure gradient was measured between the proximal and distal LAD, illustrating that normal coronary arteries do not cause appreciable resistance to blood flow. The exact locations of aortic and distal coronary pressure measurements are indicated by the arrows, respectively. (From De Bruyne.[138] With permission.) *B*. Example of a 44-year-old man with stable angina pectoris. A tight stenosis in the mid-RCA was treated by angioplasty. The coronary angiogram of the LAD (*upper panels*) did not show any focal stenosis, but luminal irregularities suggested diffuse atherosclerosis. Aortic and distal coronary pressures recordings (*lower panel*) during adenosine-induced maximal hyperemia show a pressure gradient of 23 mmHg (corresponding to a FFR of 0.76) when the pressure sensor is located in the distal LAD. This pressure gradient indicates that the diffusely atherosclerotic artery is responsible for approximately one-fourth of the total resistance to blood flow. When the sensor is slowly pulled back, a graded, continuous increase in distal coronary pressure is observed, which indicates diffuse atherosclerosis, not focal stenosis. The exact locations of aortic and distal coronary pressure measurements are indicated by the arrows, respectively. (From De Bruyne.[138] With permission.) *C*. Graphs of individual values of FFR in normal arteries and in atherosclerotic coronary arteries without focal stenosis on arteriogram. The uppper dotted line indicates the lowest value of FFR in normal coronary arteries. The lower dotted line indicates the 0.75 threshold level. (From De Bruyne.[138] With permission.)

permits assessment of both focal and diffusely diseased regions responsible for pressure loss and potential ischemia. Diffuse atherosclerosis, rather than a focal narrowing, is characterized by a continuous and gradual pressure recovery without localized abrupt increase in pressure related to an isolated stenosis. Diffuse atherosclerosis also explains a persistently abnormal distal FFR despite unobstructed proximal segments.

## DEFERRAL OF CORONARY INTERVENTION

The clinical outcomes of deferring coronary intervention for intermediate stenoses with normal physiology are remarkably consistent, with clinical event rates of <10 percent over a 2-year follow-up period.[139–145] No study reports results of deferred treatment in symptomatic patients with abnormal traslesional physiology. Despite excellent safety, some patients with deferred procedures may still have recurrent angina, requiring continued medical therapy. Nonetheless, when physiologically normal, the functional and clinical impact of angiographically intermediate stenoses is associated with as excellent clinical outcome. Like other tests at a single point in time, in-laboratory translesional hemodynamics may not reflect the episodic ischemia-producing conditions of daily life; particularly those related to vasomotor changes during exercise or emotional stress, Fortunately, most dynamic conditions are often highly responsive to medical therapy. Physiologic thresholds validated by ischemic stress testing and clinical outcomes support decisions to defer intervention while continuing medical therapy for endothelial dysfunction, hypertension, hyperlipidemia, and episodic coronary vasoconstriction.

Fractional flow reserve can be used to determine the appropriateness of angioplasty and moderate coronary stenosis. Bech et al.[144] studied 325 patients with intermediate coronary stenosis without documented myocardial ischemia. FFR was measured. When FFR was greater than 0.75, patients were randomly assigned to a deferral group of 91 patients or a performance group of 90 patients. If FFR was less than 0.75, PTCA was performed as planned. These patients were followed as a reference group of 144 patients. At clinical follow-up of 1, 3, 6, 12, and 24 months, the event-free survival was similar between the deferral and performance groups, 92 versus 89 percent at 12 months; 89 versus 83 percent at 24 months. However, these data were significantly lower in the reference group, 80 percent at 12 months and 78 percent at 24 months. The percentage of patients free from angina was similar between the deferral and the performance group at 12 and 24 months, but there was a significantly higher incidence of angina in the reference (PTCA) group; 67 versus 50 percent at 12 and 80 versus 50 percent at 24 months. These data indicated that in patients with coronary stenosis without evidence of ischemia, coronary pressure–derived FFR identifies those patients who will benefit from PTCA and also indicates that performance of PTCA in such individuals provides no additional benefit to their outcome.

## SIGNIFICANCE OF ABNORMAL PHYSIOLOGY AFTER PERCUTANEOUS CORONARY INTERVENTION (PCI)

Because balloon angioplasty usually converts a severe stenosis into an angiographically acceptable but physiologically intermediate stenosis, intracoronary physiologic measurements can help determine the adequacy of restoration and stabilization of flow following PTCA. Impaired postangioplasty CVR is often associated with residual lumen impairment undetected by angiography. Sequential flow velocity data have confirmed that the normalization of CVR occurs in only 50 percent of patients after PTCA alone and may be increased to 80 percent of patients after stenting.[146,147] Improving lumen area improves coronary blood flow. Serial measurements of CVR, rCVR, QCA, and IVUS in 55 patients were made after PTCA alone and again after stent placement.[148] The percent diameter stenosis decreased from 75 ± 13 percent to 40 ± 18 percent after PTCA and to 10 ± 9 percent after stent placement. CVR increased from 1.6 ± 0.7 to 1.9 ± 0.6 after PTCA, and to 2.5 ± 0.8 after stenting, with normalization of rCVR (0.64 ± 0.26 to 1.00 ± 0.34). In a 15-patient subset, IVUS cross-sectional area was significantly larger after stenting compared with PTCA alone ($7.6mm^2$ vs. $4.5mm^2$; $p < 0.01$), again demonstrating the relationship between lumen size and coronary flow. However, in 20 percent of patients, CVR remained < 2.0 despite widely patent target sites consistent with coexistent microvascular disease.

Coronary flow velocity reserve after PCI predicts periprocedural outcome. Albertal et al.[149] examined data from the Doppler endpoint balloon angioplasty trial Europe, DEBATE II study, in which 379 patients had Doppler flow–guided angioplasty. The patients were stratified by coronary flow reserve greater or less than 2.5 at the end of the procedure. Those with CVR less than 2.5 had an elevated baseline flow in both the target and reference vessel. A low CVR at the end of the procedure was an independent predictor of major adverse cardiac events at 30 days (odds ratio 4.7, $p = 0.034$) and at 1 year (odds ratio 2.06, $p = 0.014$). Excluding the major adverse cardiac events at 30 days, there was no difference in major adverse cardiac events in 1 year between patients with and without CVR of less than 2.5 at the end of the procedure, indicating that a low postprocedural CVR was associated with a worse periprocedural outcome related to microcirculatory disturbances without significant differences in late long-term follow-up.

A normal FFR after PTCA is associated with stent-like late clinical outcomes.[142] In 43 percent of patients with optimal quantitative coronary angiography, a residual diameter stenosis < 35 percent and good functional (FFR > 0.90) results (26 of 60 single vessel angioplasty), had event-free survival rates which were significantly better at 6 months (92 vs. 72 percent, $p = 0.047$), 12 months (92 vs. 69 percent, $p = 0.028$), and 24 months (88 vs. 59 percent, $p = 0.014$) compared to those patients with an FFR < 0.90. No improvement in clinical outcome was gained by additional stenting.

Coronary pressure measurements after stenting predict adverse cardiac events at follow-up. Pijls et al.[143] examined 750 patients with postprocedural FFR and related these findings to major adverse cardiac events at 6 months. In 76 patients (10.2 percent), one adverse event occurred. Five patients died, 19 experienced myocardial infarction, and 52 underwent at least one repeat target vessel revascularization. Fractional flow reserve immediately after stenting was an independent variable related to all types of events. In 36 percent of patients, FFR normalized (>0.95), with an event rate of 5 percent. In 32 percent of patients with post-FFR between 0.90 and 0.95, event rate was 6 percent. In the remaining 32 percent with FFR less than 0.90, event rates were 20 percent. In 6 percent of patients with FFR less than 0.80, the event rate was 30 percent (Fig. 17-54). The authors concluded that FFR after stenting is a strong predictor of outcome at 6 months. These data suggests that both edge stent subnormalization and diffuse disease are associated with worse long-term outcome.

## CORONARY PHYSIOLOGIC MEASUREMENTS FOR PROVISIONAL STENTING AND RESTENOSIS

The concept of provisional stenting was to use only balloon angioplasty guided by angiographic or IVUS anatomy and a physiologic end point to produce a result with an outcome equivalent or superior to stenting. A multicenter prospective trial, the Doppler End Point Balloon Angioplasty Trial Europe (DEBATE), demonstrated that the combination of optimal angiographic and coronary flow velocity measurements could identify a subset (22 percent) of patients in

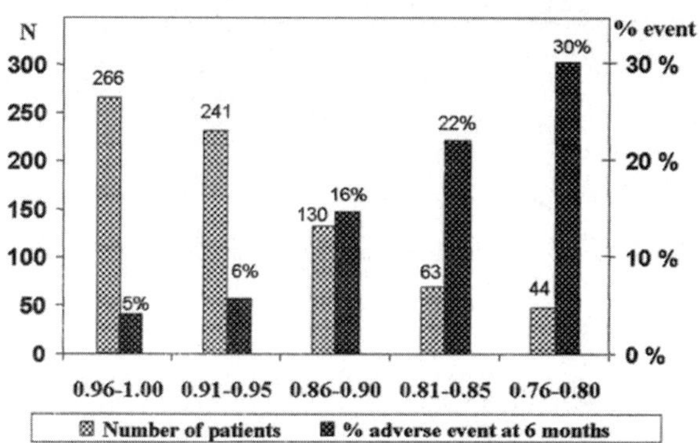


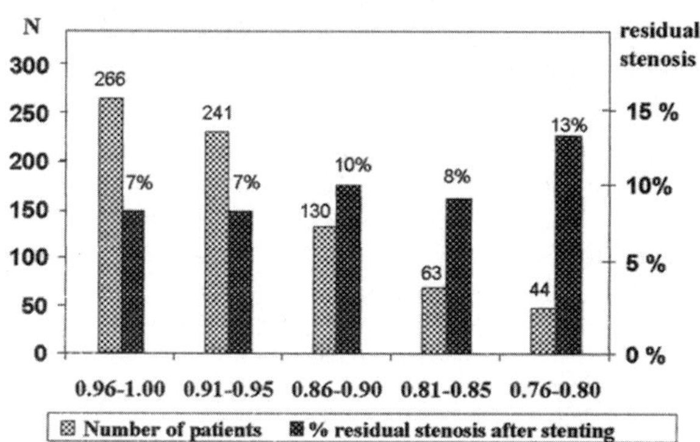


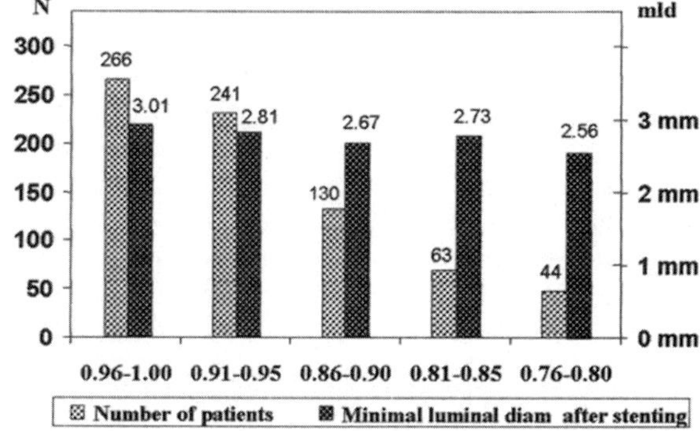


FIGURE 17-54 *Top.* Distribution of the study population over the 5 FFR categories. A strong inverse correlation was present between FFR after stenting and event rate at 6-month follow-up. *Middle.* Distribution of percentage residual stenosis in the five FFR categories. *Bottom.* Minimal luminal diameter (*mid*) in the five FFR categories. (From Pijls.[143] With permission.)

whom a clinical event rate after balloon angioplasty alone was low (<16 percent) at 6 months and comparable to results after coronary stenting.[150] A combined endpoint of quantitative coronary angiography (QCA) residual stenosis <35 percent and CVR > 2.5 immediately after balloon angioplasty was associated with reduced incidence of recurrent angina, need for repeat target lesion revascularization, and angiographic restenosis rates of <16 percent.[150] Similar results have been seen in multicenter trials.[151–155] Provisional stenting has not become common practice because (1) routine stenting results are excellent, (2) a large percentage of procedures require stenting due to suboptimal anatomic results, (3) provisional stenting uses more time than routine stenting, and (4) although QCA, intravascular ultrasound, Doppler, and FFR are valuable on an individual basis, routine stenting appears less costly than provisional stenting.[155] Since significant reductions in major adverse clinical events are expected after drug-eluting stents, the provisional stenting concept has become obsolete.

Major predictors of adverse cardiac events after stent implantation can be determined by intracoronary Doppler and quantitative coronary angiography. Haude et al.[156] examined both absolute and relative coronary reserve and angiographic results in 150 patients 6 months after stenting. After stenting, CVR, rCVR, and minimal luminal diameter were significantly higher than values after coronary angioplasty (3.0 ± .9 vs. 2.4 ± .7, 1.02 ± 0.24 vs. 0.81 ± 0.24, and 2.98 ± 0.56 vs. 2.11 ± 0.47 mm; all $p < 0.001$, respectively). Of the 150 patients, 33 developed adverse cardiac events with relative CVR < 0.88, defining an incidence of 6.8 percent. A combination of relative CVR > 0.88 and diameter stenosis <11 percent predicted adverse cardiac event rate of 1.5 percent. The measurement of relative CVR and percent diameter stenosis after stenting were highly significant for identifying those at risk for major adverse cardiac events 6 months after stenting.

## CORONARY PHYSIOLOGY IN PATIENTS WITH ACUTE MYOCARDIAL INFARCTION

A normal fractional flow reserve is indicative of reversal of myocardial perfusion defects in patients with prior myocardial infarction. De Bruyne et al.[157] examined FFR in 57 patients who had sustained a myocardial infarction more than 6 days prior to investigation. Sensitivity and specificity of an FFR of 0.75 to detect abnormal scintigraphic imaging were 82 and 87 percent, respectively; the concordance between FFR and scintigraphy was 85 percent ($p < 0.001$). Excluding false-positive and negative studies, the corresponding values increased to 87, 100, and 94 percent respectively, ($p < 0.001$). Patients with positive scintigraphic imaging before percutaneous coronary intervention (PCI) had lower FFRs than patients with negative imaging (0.52 ± 0.18 vs. 0.67 ± 0.16, $p < 0.008$) and had significantly higher ejection fraction (63 ± 10 percent vs. 52 ± 10 percent, $p < 0.0009$). An FFR > 0.75 distinguished patients after myocardial infarction with negative scintigraphic imaging (Fig. 17-55).

Phasic coronary blood flow characteristics correlate with TIMI perfusion grade and myocardial recovery after rescue PCI for acute myocardial infarction. Akasaka al.[158] examined 35 patients after successful recanulization for an acute anterior myocardial infarction. After PCI, average peak velocity (APV) was lower in patients with TIMI-2 flow ($n = 22$), and in those with TIMI-3 flow ($n = 13$) with APV values of 8 ± 4 cm/s versus 21 ± 5 cm/s ($p < 0.001$). Phasic patterns of coronary flow differentiated the patients with TIMI-2 versus TIMI-3. In TIMI 2, there were two subtypes of flow, 15 patients with reduced APV (8 ± 5 cm/s vs. 24 ± 7 cm/s) and prolonged diastolic deceleration time and small diastolic-to-systolic velocity ratio. Seven patients had TIMI II, which was subtype 2 systolic flow reversal, a rapid deceleration time, and negative diastolic-to-systolic flow velocity ratio. A significantly lower left ventricular wall motion chord index and greater number of effected chords was present in type 2 versus type 1 TIMI flow. Stenting increased TIMI-2 flow to TIMI-3 flow in more patients who had type 1 than type 2 abnormalities

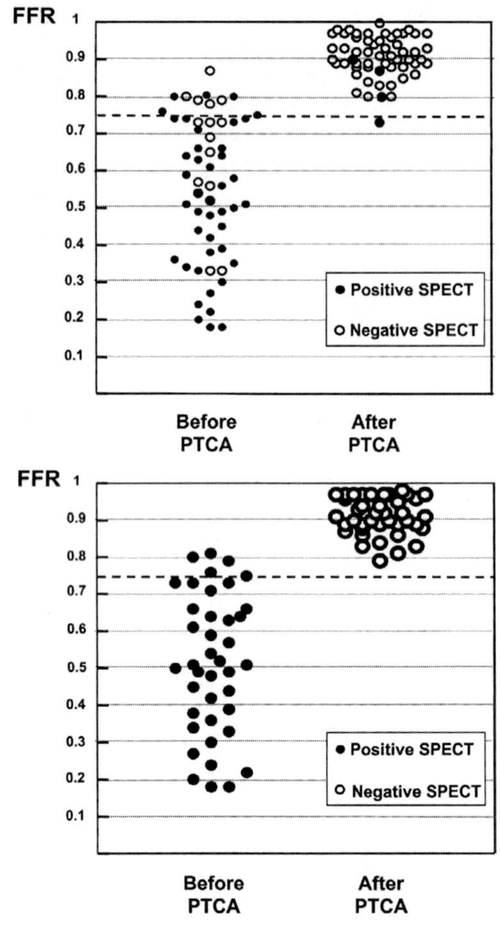


FIGURE 17-55 Values of FFR before and after angioplasty for myocardial infarction according to results of sestamibi SPECT myocardial perfusion imaging in patient population as a whole (*top*) and in patients with truly positive and truly negative SPECT imaging (*bottom*). (From De Bruyne.[157] With permission.)

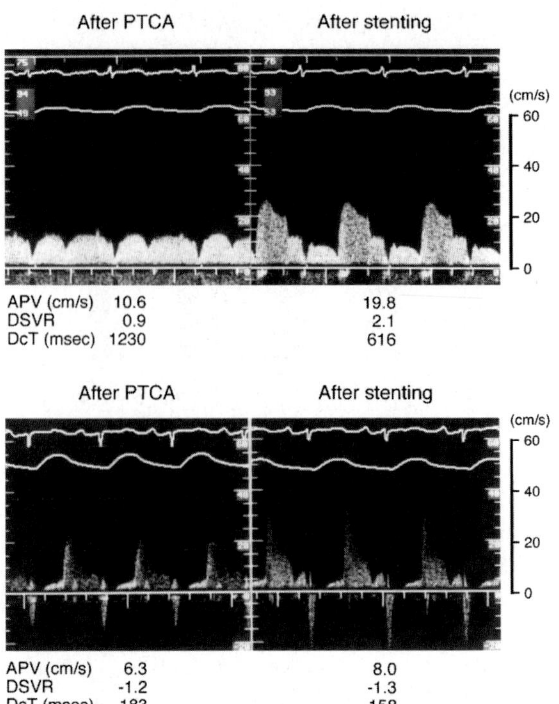


FIGURE 17-56 Examples of coronary flow velocity recordings in patient with TIMI-2 flow after angioplasty (PTCA) and TIMI-3 flow after stenting (*top*) and patients with TIMI-2 flow after both PTCA and rescue stenting *(bottom)*. Compared with values after PTCA (*top left*), greater APV, diastolic APV, and DSVR and improvement of diastolic deceleration time (DcT) were observed after stenting (*top right*) in cases with TIMI-2 flow after PTCA and TIMI-3 flow after rescue stenting. However, suppressed APV with early diastolic reversal flow and rapid diastolic deceleration time was demonstrated after PTCA and rescue stenting (*bottom*) in a case with TIMI-2 flow after both PTCA and rescue stenting. (From Akasaka.[158] With permission.)

of phasic flow (67 vs. 0 percent, $p = 0.003$). Patients with TIMI-2 flow after stenting continued to demonstrate the type 2 pattern and they had poor LV wall motion recovery. The differentiation between two types of TIMI flow velocity can predict left ventricular wall motion recovery after additional stenting.[158]

Postinfarction viability is associated with preservation of the microcirculation.[159–161] The capacitance of viable microcirculation would be reflected in phasic CVR flow characteristics (Fig. 17-56). To examine this hypothesis, Kawamoto et al.[160] measured systolic APV and diastolic flow velocity deceleration time (DDT) in 23 patients with acute anterior MI and demonstrated that if the systolic APV was >6.5 cm/s or the DDT >600 ms, there was greater recovery within the infarcted region and improved regional wall motion as assessed by echocardiography. Similarly, Tsunoda et al.[161] evaluated continuous flow velocity measurements for 18 ± 4 h after successful angioplasty in 19 patients with acute anterior myocardial infarction. Two divergent flow response groups were identified. In those patients in whom APV increased after only a transient decline, regional wall motion and overall left ventricular systolic function improved (ejection fraction increased 17 ± 9 percent), whereas if the APV progressively decreased throughout the next day, left ventricular systolic function did not improve (ejection fraction increased only 4 ± 9 percent; $p = 0.007$). These findings suggest that maneuvers, that might maintain or produce flow augmentation (e.g., intraaortic balloon counterpulsation or adenosine) might result in improved myocardial salvage.

Claeys et al.[162] found no relationship between CVR and residual viability by scintigraphy. However, improved microcirculation responses correlated with recovery of left ventricular function. Neumann et al.[163] examined CVR and regional left ventricular function immediately after stenting and again 14 days later in a group treated with standard therapy (heparin), and another group treated with standard therapy and glycoprotein IIb/IIIa inhibition with abciximab. Improved coronary hyperemia was coupled with improved regional systolic wall motion in the ReoPro group compared with the standard therapy group suggesting that agents such as glycoprotein IIb/IIIa antithrombotic therapy limit the degree of microvascular damage and may lead to improved left ventricular function and long-term outcomes.

Coronary blood flow reserve and left ventricular function and infarct size are related to the success of reperfusion. Feldman et al.[164] examined 21 patients with anterior myocardial infarction less than 12 h at the onset of coronary recannulization by PCI. CVR, left ventricular ejection fraction, infarct size, and LV end-diastolic volume were measured. Baseline ST-segment elevation and chest pain time were similar in patients with and without a reperfusion syndrome. In 10 patients with reperfusion syndrome, lower post-PCI coronary flow reserve was seen compared to 19 patients without reperfusion syndrome, even though previous CVR was similar in the two groups. Infarct size at 6 weeks was increased and predischarge LV end-systolic volume index was larger with lower ejection fraction in the reperfusion syndrome compared to those patients without reperfusion syndrome. Patients with reperfusion syndrome had significantly abnormal and lower CVR and left ventricular function as well as a larger infarct. Reperfusion syndrome was related with significant microvascular injury.

### MICROVASCULAR DISEASE

As part of the Women's Ischemic Syndrome Evaluation (WISE) study, Reis et al.[165] examined 48 women with chest pain, normal coronary arteries, or minimal luminal irregularities with CVR. Sixty percent of women with CVR $<2$ had a hyperemic velocity of 89 percent of baseline, but no change in cross-sectional vessel area. Forty percent of women with normal microcirculation with CVR on average of 3.24 were associated with increases in coronary flow velocity and a cross-sectional area by 179 and 17 percent, respectively. A CVR of 2.2 provided a high sensitivity and specificity (90 and 89 percent, respectively) for the diagnosis of microvascular dysfunction. Failure of epicardial coronary artery to dilate at least 9 percent was also a sensitive (79 percent) and specific (79 percent) surrogate marker of microvascular dysfunction. The attenuated epicardial coronary dilatory response likely represents significant microvascular dysfunction in women with chest pain and no obstructive coronary artery disease.

Similar data were reported by Hasdai et al.[166] in 203 patients with angiographically normal coronary arteries. CVR and endothelial vasodilatory response to intracoronary acetylcholine and adenosine were measured. Ninety-two percent of patients had at least one risk factor for atherosclerosis. Abnormal CVR was found in 59 percent of patients, 11 percent had impaired response to adenosine with CVR $\leq 2.5$, and 29 percent had impaired response to acetylcholine with CVR of $\leq 1.5$; 18 percent had a combined abnormality. There was no correlation between endothelium-dependent and endothelium-independent flow response. The authors concluded that most patients with chest pain syndromes and nonobstructive coronary artery disease had risk factors for coronary artery disease with diverse abnormalities and endothelium-dependent and independent function. A comprehensive evaluation of the endothelium and microvascular system can be obtained for a complete understanding of the chest pain syndrome.

### COLLATERAL CIRCULATION

The collateral circulation can be described by intracoronary pressure and flow relationships. Ipsilateral collateral flow and contralateral arterial responses have been described in numerous studies using both pressure and flow to provide new information regarding mechanisms, function, and clinical significance of collateral flow in patients[167–170] and provide new insights into coronary artery disease.[171] The reader is referred to excellent works elsewhere for details.[167–170]

In summary, coronary blood flow and pressure can be determined during cardiac catheterization to provide insight into pathophysiologic mechanisms as well as unique data, which may facilitate clinical decisions regarding coronary revascularization. In the laboratory, coronary physiologic measurements have a strong association with noninvasive ischemia testing. Clinical validation supports operator confidence that coronary physiology can be used to facilitate clinical decisions, especially for coronary arteries narrowed between 40 percent and 70 to 80 percent in diameter. Measurements of coronary physiology strongly complement coronary lumenography and permit exploration of the coronary microcirculation, collateral flow, myocardial infarction physiology, and mechanisms of interventions for coronary artery disease.

## NOTE

Portions of this chapter come from R.H. Franch, J.S. Douglas, S.B. King, and M.J. Kern, authors of chap. 15 in the 10th edition of *Hurst's The Heart.* Other portions come from M.J. Kern, ed. *The Cardiac Catheterization Handbook*, 3d ed. St. Louis: Mosby; 2001: 479–524. With permission.

## References


1. Forssman W. Die Sondierung des rechten Herzens. *Berl Klin Wochenschr* 1929;8:2058–2087.
2. Mueller HS, Chatteryee K, Davis KB, et al. Present use of bedside right heart catheterization in patients with cardiac disease. *J Am Coll Cardiol* 1998;32:840–864.
3. Scanlon PJ, Faxon DP, Auden AM, et al. A Report of the American College of Cardiology/American Heart Association Task Force on Practice Guidelines (Committee on Coronary Angiography) Developed in collaboration with the Society for Cardiac Angiography and Interventions Committee Members. ACC/AHA Guidelines for Coronary Angiography: Executive Summary and Recommendations. *Circulation* 1999;99:2345–2357.
4. Connors AF, Speroff T, Dawson NV, et al. The effectiveness of right heart catheterization in the initial care of critically ill patients. *JAMA* 1996;276:889–897.
5. Kern MJ. *The Cardiac Catheterization Handbook,* 4th ed. St. Louis; Mosby; 2003.
6. Baim DS, Grossman W, eds. *Grossman's Cardiac Catheterization, Angiograpy and Intervention,* 6th ed. Baltimore: Lippincott, Williams & Wilkins; 2000.
7. Pepine CJ, Hill JA, Lambert CR. *Diagnostic and Therapeutic Cardiac Catheterization,* 3d ed. Baltimore: Williams & Wilkins; 1998.
8. Campeau L. Percutaneous radial artery approach for coronary angiography. *Catheter Cardiovasc Diagn* 1989;16:3–7.
9. Kiemeneij F, Laarman GJ, Odekerken D, et al. A randomized comparison of percutaneous transluminal coronary angioplasty by the radial, brachial and femoral approaches: The Access Study. *J Am Coll Cardiol* 1997;29:1269–1275.
10. Silber S. Rapid hemostasis of arterial puncture sites with collagen in patients undergoing diagnostic and interventional cardiac catheterization. *Clin Cardiol* 1997;20:981–982.
11. Chamberlin JA, Lardi AB, McKeever LS, et al. Use of vascular sealing devices (Vasoseal and Perclose) versus assisted manual compression (Femostop) in transcatheter coronary interventions requiring abciximab (ReoPro). *Catheter Cardiovasc Interv* 1999;47:143–147.
12. Sanborn TA, Gibbs HH, Brinker JA, et al. A multicenter randomized trial comparing a percutaneous collagen hemostasis device with conventional manual compression after diagnostic angiography and angioplasty. *J Am Coll Cardiol* 1993;22:1273.
13. Kern MJ. Selection of radiocontrast media in cardiac catheterization: Comparative physiology and clinical effects of nonionic and ionic dimeric formulations. *Am Heart J* 1991;122:195–201.
14. Werner GS, Schmidt T, Scholz KH, et al. Comparison of hemodynamic and Doppler echocardiographic effects of new low osmolar nonionic and a standard ionic contrast agent after left ventriculography. *Catheter Cardiovasc Diagn* 1994;33:11–19.
15. Hirshfield JW Jr. Cardiovascular effects of contrast agents. *Am J Cardiol* 1990;66(suppl):9F–17P.
16. McClennan BL. Ionic and nonionic iodinated contrast media: Evolution and strategies for use. *AJR* 1990;155:225–233.

16a. Tepel M, va der Geit M, Schwarzfeld C, et al. Prevention of radiographic-contrast-agent-induced reductions in renal function by acetylcysteine. *N Engl J Med* 2000;343:180–184.

16b. Chu VL, Cheng JW. Fenoldopam in the prevention of contrast media-induced acute renal failure. *Ann Pharmacother* 2001;35:1278–1282.

16c. Madyoon H, CrushoreL, Weaver D, et al. Use of fenoldopam to prevent radiocontrast nephropathy in high-risk patients. *Catheter Cardiovasc Interv* 2002;53:341–345.

16d. Stone GW, McCullough PA, Tumlin JA, et al. Fenoldopam mesylate for the prevention of contrast-induced nephropathy: A randomized controlled trial: *JAMA* 2003;290(17):2284–2291.

17. Krone RJ, Johnson L, Noto T. Five year trends in cardiac catheterization: A report from the Registry of the Society for Cardiac Angiography and Interventions. *Catheter Cardiovasc Diagn* 1996;39:31–35.

18. Trerotola SO, Kuhlman JE, Fishman EK. Bleeding complications of femoral catheterization: CT evaluation. *Radiology* 1990;174:37–40.

19. Lazar JM, Uretsky BF, Denys BG, et al. Predisposing risk factors and natural history of acute neurologic complications of left-sided cardiac catheterization. *Am J Cardiol* 1995;75:1056–1060.

20. Douglas JS Jr, King SB III. Complications of coronary arteriography: Management during and following the procedure. In: King SB III, Douglas JS Jr, eds. *Coronary Arteriography*. New York: McGraw-Hill; 1984:302–313.

21. Chatterjee T, Do D, Kaufmann U, et al. Ultrasound-guided repair for treatment of femoral artery pseudoaneurysm. *Catheter Cardiovasc Diagn* 1996;38:335–340.

22. Holmes DR, Wondrow MA, Bell MR, et al. Cine angiographic image replacement digital archival requirements and remaining obstacles. *Catheter Cardiovasc Diagn* 1998;44:346–356.

23. Waters DD, Szlachcic J, Bonan R. Comparative sensitivity of exercise, coldpressor and ergonovine testing in provoking attacks of variant angina in patients with active disease. *Circulation* 1983;67:310–315.

24. Donohue TJ, Kern MJ, Aguirre FV, et al. Assessing the hemodynamic significance of coronary artery stenoses: Analysis of translesional pressure-flow velocity relations in patients. *J Am Coll Cardiol* 1993;22:449–458.

25. Helfant RH, Pine R, Meister SG, et al. Nitroglycerin to unmask reversible asynergy: Correlation with post coronary bypass ventriculography. *Circulation* 1974;50:108–113.

26. Horn HR, Teichholz LE, Cohn PF, et al. Augmentation of left ventricular contraction pattern in coronary artery disease by inotropic catecholamine: The epinephrine ventriculogram. *Circulation* 1974;49:1063–1071.

27. Dyke SH, Cohn PF, Gorlin R, Sonnenblick EH. Detection of residual myocardial function in coronary artery disease using post extrasystolic potentiation. *Circulation* 1974;50:694–699.

28. Sones FM Jr, Shriey Ek. Cine coronary arteriography. *Mod Concepts Cardiovasc Dis* 1962;31:735–738.

29. Seldinger SI. Catheter replacement of the needle in percutaneous arteriography: A new technique. *Acta Radiol* 1953;39:368–376.

30. Ricketts HJ, Abrams HL. Percutaneous selective coronary cine arteriography. *JAMA* 1962;181:620–626.

31. Amplatz K, Formanek G, Stranger P, Wilson W. Mechanics of selective coronary artery catheterization via femoral approach. *Radiology* 1967;89:1040–1047.

32. Judkins MP. Selective coronary arteriography: I. A percutaneous transfemoral technique. *Radiology* 1967;89:815–824.

33. Schoonmaker FW, King SB III. Coronary arteriography by the single catheter percutaneous femoral techniques: Experience with 6800 cases. *Circulation* 1974;50:735–740.

34. Judkins MP, Judkins EJ. The Judkins technique. In: King SB III, Douglas JS, Jr, eds. *Coronary Arteriography*. New York: McGraw-Hill; 1984:182–217.

35. King SB III, Douglas JS Jr. Catheterization techniques in coronary arteriography and left ventriculography: Multipurpose techniques: In: King SB III, Douglas JS Jr, eds. *Coronary Arteriography*. New York: McGraw-Hill; 1984:239–274.

36. King SB, Douglas JS, Morris DC. New angiographic views for coronary arteriography. In: Hurst JW, ed. *The Heart, Update IV*. New York: McGraw-Hill; 1980:275–287.

37. Arnett EN, Isner JM, Redwood DR, et al. Coronary artery narrowing in coronary heart disease: Comparison of cine angiographic and necropsy findings. *Ann Intern Med* 1979;91:350–356.

38. Grandin CM, Dyrda I, Pastemac A, et al. Discrepancies between cineangiographic and postmortem findings in patients with coronary artery disease and recent myocardial revascularization. *Circulation* 1974;49:703–708.

39. Roberts CS, Roberts WC. Cross-sectional area of the proximal portions of the three major epicardial coronary arteries in 98 patients with different coronary events: Relationship to heart, weight, age, and sex. *Circulation* 1980;62:953–959.

40. Isner JM, Kishel J, Kent KM, et al. Inaccuracy of angiographic determination of left main coronary arterial narrowing: Angiographic-histologic correlative analysis of 29 patients. *Circulation* 1979;59,60 (suppl 2):ii–161.

40a. Austin WG, Edwards JE, Frye RL, et al. A reporting system on patients evaluated for coronary artery disease: Report of the as hoc committee for grading coronary artery disease, Council on Cardiovascular Surgery, American Heart Association. *Circulation* 1975;51(suppl 4):5–40.

41. Zir LM, Miller SW, Dinsmore RE, et al. Interobserver variability in coronary arteriography. *Circulation* 1976;53:627–630.

42. DeRouen TA, Murray JA, Owen W. Variability in the analysis of coronary arteriograms. *Circulation* 1977;55:324–328.

43. Schwartz JN, King Y, Hackel DB, Bartel AG. Comparison of angiographic and postmortem findings in patients with coronary artery disease. *Am J Cardiol* 1975;36:174–178.

44. Hermiller JB, Cusma JT, Spero LA, et al. Quantitative and qualitative coronary angiographic analysis: Review of methods, utility and limitations. *Cathet Cardiovasc Diagn* 1992;25:110–131.

45. Nissen SE, Yock P. Intravascular ultrasound. Novel pathophysiological insights and current clinical applications. *Circulation* 2001;103:604–616.

46. Takahashi T, Honda Y, Russo RJ, Fitzgerald PJ. Intravascular ultrasound and quantitative coronary angiography. *Catheter Cardiovasc Intervent* 2002;55:118–128.

47. Heupler FA Jr. Syndrome of symptomatic coronary arterial spasm with nearly normal coronary arteriograms. *Am J Cardiol* 1980;45:873–881.

48. Gibson CM, Cannon CP, Daley WL, et al. TIMI frame count: A quantitative method of assessing coronary artery flow. *Circulation* 1996;93:879–888.

49. Levin DC. Pathways and functional significance of the coronary collateral circulation. *Circulation* 1974;50:831–837.

50. Kramer JR, Kitazume H, Proudfitt WL, Sones FM Jr. Clinical significance of isolated coronary bridges: Benign and frequent conditions involving the left anterior descending artery. *Am Heart J* 1982;103:283–288.

51. Douglas JS Jr, Franch RH, King SB III. Coronary artery anomalies. In: King SB III, Douglas JS Jr, eds. *Coronary Arteriography and Angioplasty*. New York: McGraw-Hill; 1985:33–85.

52. Serota H, Barth CW III, Seuc CA, et al. Rapid identification of the course of anomalous coronary arteries in adults: The "dot and eye" method. *Am J Cardiol* 1990;65:891–898.

52a. The Principal Investigators of CASS and their Associates. The National Heart, Lung, and Blood Institute Coronary Artery Surgery Study: Historical background, design, methods, the registry, the randomized trial, clinical database. *Circulation* 1981;63(suppl I):1–181.

52b. Herman MV Heinle RA, Klein MD, et al. Localized disorders in myocardial contraction. Asynergy and its role in congestive heart failure. *N Engl J Med* 1967:227:225.

53. Sandler H, Dodge HT. The use of single plane angiocardiograms for the calculation of left ventricular volume in man. *Am Heart J* 1968;75:325–334.

54. Kennedy JW, Trenholme SE, Kasser IS. Left ventricular volume and mass from single plane cineangiocardiograms. *Am Heart J* 1970;80:343–352.

55. Sheehan FH, Mitten-Lewis S. Factors influencing accuracy in left ventricular volume determination. *Am J Cardiol* 1989;64:661–664.

56. Lawson MA, Blackwell GG, Doves ND, et al. Accuracy of biplane long-axis left ventricular volume determined by cine magnetic resonance imaging in patients with regional and global dysfunction. *Am J Cardiol* 1996;77:1098–1104.
57. Kennedy JW, Baxley WA, Figley MM, et al. Quantitative angiocardiography: I. The normal left ventricle in man. *Circulation* 1966;34:272–278.
58. Kennedy JW, Trenholme SE, Kasser IS. Left ventricualr volume and mass from single plane cineangiocardiograms. *Am Heart J* 1970;80: 343–352.
59. Shimazaki Y, Kawashima Y, Mori T, et al. Angiographic volume estimation of right ventricle. *Chest* 1980;77:390–395.
59a. Johnson LW, Moore RJ, and Balter S. Review of radiation safety in the cardiac catheterization laboratory. *Catheter Cardiovasc Diagn* 1992; 25:186–194.
60. Limacher ML, Douglas PS, Germano G, et al. Radiation safety in the practice of cardiology. *J Am Coll Cardiol* 1998;31:892–893.
61. Cusma JT, Bell MR, Wondrow MA, et al. Real time measurement of radiation exposure during diagnostic coronary angiography and percutaneous interventional procedures. *J Am Coll Cardiol* 1999;33: 427–435.
62. Balter S. Radiation safety in the cardiac catheterization laboratory. *Catheter Cardiovasc Interv* 1999;47:347–353.
63. Courtois M, Faltal PG, Kovacs SJ, et al. Anatomically and physiologically based reference levels for measurement of intracardiac pressures. *Circulation* 1995;92:1994–2000.
64. Assey ME, Zile MR, Usher BW, et al. Effect of catheter positioning on the variability of measured gradient in aortic stenosis. *Catheter Cardiovasc Diagn* 1993;30:287–292.
65. Gorlin R, Gorlin G. Hydraulic formula for calculation of area of stenotic mitral valve, other cardiac valves and central circulatory shunts. *Am Heart J* 1951;41:1–29.
66. Cohen MV, Gorlin R. Modified orifice equation for the calculation of mitral valve area. *Am Heart J* 1972;84:839–840.
67. Folland ED, Parisi AF, Carbone C. Is peripheral arterial pressure a satisfactory substitute for ascending aortic pressure when measuring aortic valve gradients? *J Am Coll Cardiol* 1984;4:1207–1212.
68. Hakki AH. A simplified valve formula for the calculation of stenotic cardiac valve areas. *Circulation* 1981;63:1050–1055.
69. Bache RJ, Jorgensen CR, Wany Y. Simplified estimation of aortic valve area. *Br Heart J* 1972;34:408–411.
70. Angel J, Soler-Soler J, Anivarro I, Domingo E. I. Hemodynamic evaluation of stenotic cardiac valves. II. Modification of the simplified formula for mitral and aortic valve area calculation. *Catheter Cardiovasc Diagn* 1985;11:127–138.
71. Voelker W, Reul H, Niehaus G, et al. Comparison of valvular resistance, stroke work loss and Gorlin valve area for quantification of aortic stenosis. *Circulation* 1995;91:1196–1204.
72. Hosenpud JD, McAnulty JH, Morton MJ. Overestimation of mitral valve gradients obtained by phasic pulmonary artery wedge pressure. *Catheter Cardiovasc Diagn* 1983;9:283–290.
73. Hamilton MA, Stevenson LW, Woo RN, et al. Effect of tricuspid regurgitation on the reliability of the thermodilution cardiac output technique in congestive heart failure. *Am J Cardiol* 1989;64:945–948.
74. Lehmann KG, Platt MS. Improved accuracy and precision of thermodilation cardiac output measurement using a dual thermistor catheter system. *J Am Coll Cardiol* 1999;33:883–891.
75. Levett JM, Replogle RL. Thermodilution cardiac output: A critical analysis and review of the literature. *J Surg Res* 1979;27:392–404.
76. Hillis DL, Firth BG, Winniford MD. Variability of right-sided cardiac oxygen saturations in adults with and without intracardiac left-to-right shunting. *Am J Cardiol* 1986;58:129–132.
77. Freed MD, Miettinen OS, Nadas AS. Oximetric detection of intracardiac left-to-right shunts. *Br Heart J* 1979;42:690–694.
78. Shepherd AP, McMahan CA. Role of oximeter error in the diagnosis of shunts. *Catheter Cardiovasc Diagn* 1996;37:435–446.
79. O'Keefe JH, Vlietstra RE, Hanley PC, Seward JB. Revival of the transseptal approach for catheterization of the left atrium and ventricle. *Mayo Clin Proc* 1985;60:790–795.
80. Mullins CE. Transseptal left heart catheterization: Experience with a new technique in 520 pediatric and adults patients. *Pediatr Cardiol* 1983;4:239–246.
81. Laskey WK, Kusiak V, Untereker WJ, Hirshfeld JW. Transseptal left heart catheterization: Utility of a sheath technique. *Catheter Cardiovasc Diagn* 1982;8:535–542.
82. Croft CH, Lipscomb K. Modified technique of transseptal left heart catheterization. *J Am Coll Cardiol* 1985;5:904–910.
83. Nanas JN, Moulopoulos SD. Counterpulsation: Historical background, technical improvements, hemodynamic and metabolic effects. *Cardiology* 1994:84:156–167.
84. Kern MJ, Aguirre F, Bach R, et al. Augmentation of coronary blood flow by intra-aortic balloon pumping in patients after coronary angioplasty. *Circulation* 1993;87:500–511.
85. Kern MJ, Aguirre FV, Tatineni S, et al. Enhanced coronary blood flow velocity during intraaortic balloon counterpulsation in critically ill patients. *J Am Coll Cardiol* 1993;21:359–368.
86. Topol EJ, Nissen SE. Our preoccupation with coronary luminology. The dissociation between clinical and angiographic findings in ischemic heart disease. *Circulation* 1995;92:2333–2342.
87. Kern M. Curriculum in interventional cardiology: coronary pressure and flow measurements in the cardiac catheterization laboratory. *Catheter Cardiovasc Interv* 2002;54:378–400.
88. Toshihiko N, Amanullah AM, Luo H, et al. Clinical validation of intravascular ultrasound for assessment of coronary stenosis severity. *J Am Coll Cardiol* 1999;33:1870–1878.
89. White CW, Wright CB, Doty DB, et al. Does visual interpretation of the coronary arteriogram predict the physiologic importance of a coronary stenosis? *N Engl J Med* 1984;310:819–824.
90. Harrison DG, White CW, Hiratzka LF, et al. The value of lesion cross-sectional area determined by quantitative coronary angiography in assessing the physiologic significance of proximal left anterior descending coronary arterial stenoses. *Circulation* 1984;69:1111–1119.
91. Gould KL, Kirkeeide RL, Buchi M. Coronary flow reserve as a physiologic measure of stenosis severity. *J Am Coll Cardiol* 1990;15: 459–474.
92. Gould KL, Lipscomb K, Hamilton GW. Physiologic basis for assessing critical coronary stenosis: Instantaneous flow response and regional distribution during coronary hyperemia as measures of coronary flow reserve. *Am J Cardiol* 1974;33:87–94.
93. Doucette JW, Corl PD, Payne HM, et al. Validation of a Doppler guide wire for intravascular measurement of coronary artery flow velocity. *Circulation* 1992;85:1899–1911.
94. Labovitz AJ, Anthonis DM, Cravens TL, Kern MJ. Validation of volumetric flow measurements by means of a Doppler-tipped coronary angioplasty guide wire. *Am Heart J* 1993;126:1456–1461.
95. Baumgart D, Haude M, Liu F, et al. Current concepts of coronary flow reserve for clinical decision making during cardiac catheterization. *Am Heart J* 1998;136:136–149.
96. Kern MJ, Bach RG, Mechem C, et al. Variations in normal coronary vasodilatory reserve stratified by artery, gender, heart transplantation and coronary artery disease. *J Am Coll Cardiol* 1996;28:1154–1160.
97. McGinn AL, White CW, Wilson RF. Interstudy variability of coronary flow reserve: Influence of heart rate, arterial pressure, and ventricular preload. *Circulation* 1990;81:1319–1330.
98. Marcus ML, Mueller TM, Gascho JA, Kerber RE. Effects of cardiac hypertrophy secondary to hypertension on the coronary circulation. *Am J Cardiol* 1979;44:1023–1031.
99. Chauhan A, Millins PA, Petch MC, Schonfield PM. Is coronary flow velocity response really normal in syndrome X? *Circulation* 1994;89:1998–2004.
100. Marcus ML, Doty DB, Hiratzka LF, et al. Decreased coronary flow reserve: a mechanism for angina pectoris in patients with aortic stenosis and normal coronary arteries. *N Engl J Med* 1982;307:1362–1367.
101. Cobb F, McHale P, Remert J. Effects of acute cellular injury on coronary vascular reactivity in awake dogs. *Circulation* 1978;57:962–968.
102. Gould KL. Dynamic coronary stenosis. *Am J Cardiol* 1980;45: 286–292.

103. Czernin J, Muller P, Chan S, et al. Influence of age and hemodynamics on myocardial blood flow and reserve. *Circulation* 1993;88:62–69.
104. Wieneke H, Haude M, Ge J, et al. Corrected coronary flow velocity reserve: A new concept for assessing coronary perfusion. *J Am Coll Cardiol* 2000;35:1713–1720.
105. Akasaka T, Yoshida K, Hozumi T, et al. Retinopathy identifies marked restriction of coronary flow reserve in patients with diabetes mellitus. *J Am Coll Cardiol* 1997;30:935–941.
106. Baumgart D, Haude M, Goerge G, et al. Improved assessment of coronary stenosis severity using the relative flow velocity reserve. *Circulation* 1998;98:40–46.
107. Kern MJ, Puri S, Bach RG, et al. Abnormal coronary flow velocity reserve after coronary artery stenting in patients: Role of relative coronary reserve to assess potential mechanisms. *Circulation* 1999; 100:2491–2498.
108. Pijls NH, Van Gelder B, Van der Voort P, et al. Fractional flow reserve: A useful index to evaluate the influence of an epicardial coronary stenosis on myocardial blood flow. *Circulation* 1995;92:3183–3193.
109. Pijls NH, De Bruyne B, Peels K, et al. Measurement of fractional flow reserve to assess the functional severity of coronary-artery stenoses. *N Engl J Med* 1996;334:1703–1708.
110. De Bruyne B, Bartunek J, Sys SU, et al. Simultaneous coronary pressure and flow velocity measurements in humans: Feasibility, reproducibility, and hemodynamic dependence of coronary flow velocity reserve, hyperemic flow versus pressure slope index, and fractional flow reserve. *Circulation* 1996;94:1842–1849.
111. Kern MJ, Aguirre FV, Bach RG, et al. Interventional physiology rounds: Fundamentals of translesional pressure-flow velocity measurements. *Catheter Cardiovasc Diagn* 1994;31:137–143.
112. Pijls NHJ, Kern MJ, Yock PG, De Bruyne B. Practice and potential pitfalls of coronary pressure measurement. *Cathet Cardiovasc Intervent* 2000;49:1–16.
113. Qian J, Ge J, Baumgart D, et al. Safety of intracoronary Doppler flow measurement. *Am Heart J* 2000;140;502–510.
114. Wilson RF, Laughlin DE, Ackell PH, et al. Transluminal subselective measurement of coronary artery blood flow velocity and vasodilator reserve in man. *Circulation* 1985;72:82–92.
115. Wilson RF, White C. Serious Ventricular dysrhythmias after intracoronary papaverine. *Am J Cardiol* 1988;62:1301–1302.
116. Wilson RF, Wyche K, Christensen BV, et al. Effects of adenosine on human arterial circulation. *Circulation* 1990;82:1595–1606.
117. Kern MJ, Deligonul U, Tatineni S, et al. Intravenous adenosine: continuous infusion and low dose bolus administration for determination of coronary vasodilatory reserve in patients with and without coronary artery disease. *J Am Coll Cardiol* 1991;18:718–729.
118. Caracciolo EA, Wolford TL, Underwood RD, et al. Influence of intimal thickness on coronary blood flow responses in orthotopic heart transplant recipients: A combined intravascular Doppler and ultrasound imaging study. *Circulation* 1995;92:II-182–II-190.
119. Jeremias A, Whitbourn RJ, Filardo SD, et al. Adequacy of intracoronary versus intravenous adenosine-induced maximal coronary hyperemia for fractional flow reserve measurements. *Am Heart J* 2000;140:651–657.
120. Sonoda S, Takeuchi M, Nakashima Y, Kuroiwa A. Safety and optimal dose of intracoronary adenosine 5′-triphosphate for the measurement of coronary flow reserve. *Am Heart J* 1998;135:621–627.
121. Bartunek J, Winjs W, Heyndrickx GR, de Bruyne B. Effects of dobutamine on coronary stenosis. Physiology and morphology comparison with intracoronary adenosine. *Circulation* 1999;100:243–249.
122. Kern MJ. Coronary physiology revisited: Practical insights from the cardiac catheterization laboratory. *Circulation* 2000;101:1344–1351.
123. Miller DD, Donohue TJ, Younis LT, et al. Correlation of pharmacologic 99mtc-sestamibi myocardial perfusion imaging with poststenotic coronary flow reserve in patients with angiographically intermediate coronary artery stenoses. *Circulation* 1994;89:2150–2160.
124. Joye JD, Schulman DS, Lasorda D, et al. Intracoronary Doppler guide wire versus stress single-photon emission computed tomographic thallium-201 imaging in assessment of intermediate coronary stenoses. *J Am Coll Cardiol* 1994;24:940–947.
125. Deychak YA, Segal J, Reiner JS, et al. Doppler guide wire flow-velocity indexes measured distal to coronary stenoses associated with reversible thallium perfusion defects. *Am Heart J* 1995;129:219–227.
126. Heller LI, Popma J, Cates C, et al. Functional assessment of stenosis severity in the cath lab: A comparison of Doppler and tl-201 imaging. *J Interven Cardiol* 1995:7;23A.
127. de Bruyne B, Bartunek J, Sys SU, Hendrickx GR. Relation between myocardial fractional flow reserve calculated from coronary pressure measurements and exercise-induced myocardial ischemia. *Circulation* 1995;92:39–46.
128. Zilstra F, Fioretti P, Reiber J, Serruys PW. Which cineangiographically assessed anatomic variable correlates best with functional measurements of stenosis severity? A comparison of quantitative analysis of the coronary cineangiogram with measure coronary flow reserve and exercise/redistribution thallium-201 scintigraphy. *J Am Coll Cardiol* 1988;12:686–691.
129. Danzi GB, Pirelli S, Mauri L, et al. Which variable of stenosis severity best describes the significance of an isolated left anterior descending coronary artery lesion? Correlation between quantitative coronary angiography, intracoronary Doppler measurements and high dose dipyridamole echocardiography. *J Am Coll Cardiol* 1998;31:526–533.
130. Bartunek J, Van Schuerbeeck E, De Bruyne B. Comparison of exercise electrocardiography and dobutamine echocardiography with invasively assessed myocardial fractional flow reserve in evaluation of severity of coronary arterial narrowing. *Am J Cardiol* 1997;79: 478–481.
131. Schulman DS, Lasorda D, Farah T, et al. Correlations between coronary flow reserve measured with a Doppler guide wire and treadmill exercise testing. *Am Heart J* 1997;134:99–104.
132. Donohue TJ, Miller DD, Bach RG, et al. Correlation of poststenotic hyperemic coronary flow velocity and pressure with abnormal stress myocardial perfusion imaging in coronary artery disease. *Am J Cardiol* 1996;77:948–954.
133. Duffy SJ, Gelman JS, Peverill RE, et al. Agreement between coronary flow velocity reserve and stress echocardiography in intermediate-severity coronary stenoses. *Catheter Cardiovasc Interv* 2001;53: 29–38.
134. Chamuleau SAJ, Meuwissen M, van Eck-Smit BLF, et al. Fractional flow reserve, absolute and relative coronary blood flow velocity reserve in relation to the results of technetium-99m sestamibi single-photon emission computed tomography in patients with two-vessel coronary artery disease. *J Am Coll Cardiol* 2001;37:1316–1322.
135. Caymaz O, Fak AS, Tezcan H, et al. Correlation of myocardial fraction flow reserve with thallium-201 SPECT imaging in intermediate-severity coronary artery lesions. *J Invasive Cardiol* 2000;12:345–350.
136. Fearon WF, Takagi A, Jeremias A, et al. Use of fractional myocardial flow reserve to assess the functional significance of intermediate coronary stenosis. *Am J Cardiol* 2000;86:1013–1014.
137. El-Shafei A, Chiravuri R, Stikovac MM, et al. Comparison of relative coronary Doppler flow velocity reserve to stress myocardial perfusion imaging in patients with coronary artery disease. *Catheter Cardiovasc Interv* 2001;53:193–201.
138. De Bruyne B, Hersbach F, Pijls NHJ, et al. Abnormal epicardial coronary resistance in patients with diffuse atherosclerosis but "normal" coronary angiography. *Circulation* 2001;104:2401–2406.
139. Kern MJ, Donohue TJ, Aguirre FV, et al. Clinical outcome of deferring angioplasty in patients with normal translesional pressure-flow velocity measurements. *J Am Coll Cardiol* 1995;25:178–187.
140. Ferrari M, Schnell B, Werner GS, Figulla HR. Safety of deferring angioplasty in patients with normal coronary flow velocity reserve. *J Am Coll Cardiol* 1999;33:83–87.
141. Bech GJ, De Bruyne B, Bonnier HJRM, et al. Long-term follow-up after deferral of percutaneous transluminal coronary angioplasty of intermediate stenosis on the basis of coronary pressure measurement. *J Am Coll Cardiol* 1998;31:841–847.
142. Bech GJW, Pijls NHJ, De Bruyne B, et al. Usefulness of fractional flow reserve to predict clinical outcome after balloon angioplasty. *Circulation* 1999;99:883–888.

143. Pijls NHJ, Klauss V, Siebert U, et al. Coronary pressure measurement after stenting predicts adverse events at follow-up. A multicenter registry. *Circulation* 2002;105:2950–2954.
144. Bech GJW, De Bruyne B, Pijls NHJ, et al. Fractional flow reserve to determine the appropriateness of angioplasty in moderate coronary stenosis. A randomized trial. *Circulation* 2001;103:2928–2934.
145. Gruberg L, Kapeliovich M, Roguin A, et al. Deferring angioplasty in intermediate coronary lesions based on coronary flow criteria is safe: Comparison of a deferred group to an intervention group. *Int J Cardiovasc Interv* 1999;2:35–40.
146. Wilson RF, Johnson MR, Marcus ML, et al. The effect of coronary angioplasty on coronary flow reserve. *Circulation* 1998;77:873–885.
147. Kern MJ, Deligonul U, Vandormael M, et al. Impaired coronary vasodilatory reserve in the immediate post-coronary angioplasty period: analysis of coronary arterial velocity flow indices and regional cardiac venous efflux. *J Am Coll Cardiol* 1989;860–872.
148. Kern MJ, Dupouy P, Drury JH, et al. Role of coronary artery lumen enlargement in improving coronary blood flow after balloon angioplasty and stenting: A combined instravascular ultrasound Doppler flow and imaging study. *J Am Coll Cardiol* 1997;29:1520–1527.
149. Albertal M, Voskuil M, Piek JJ, et al. Coronary flow velocity reserve after percutaneous interventions is predictive of periprocedural outcome. *Circulation* 2002;105:1573–1578.
150. Serruys PW, Di Mario C, Piek J, et al for the DEBATE study Group. Prognostic value of intracoronary flow velocity and diameter stenosis in assessing the short- and long-term outcomes of coronary balloon angioplasty: the DEBATE study (Doppler Endpoints Balloon Angioplasty Trial Europe). *Circulation* 1997;96:3369–3377.
151. Lafont A, Dubois-Rande JL, Steg PG, et al for the FROST Study Group. The French Randomized Optimal Stenting Trial: A prospective evaluation of provisional stenting guided by coronary velocity reserve and quantitative coronary angiography. *J Am Coll Cardiol* 2000;36: 404–409.
152. DiMario C, Moses JW, Anderson TJ, et al on behalf of the DESTINI Study Group (Doppler Endpoint STenting INternational Investigation). Randomized comparison of elective stent implantation and coronary balloon angioplasty guided by online quantitative angiography and intracoronary Doppler. *Circulation* 2000;102:2938–2944.
153. Serruys PW, de Bruyne B, Carlier S, et al on behalf of the Doppler Endpoints Balloon Angioplasty Trial Europe (DEBATE) II Study Group. Randomized comparison of primary stenting and provisional balloon angioplasty guided by flow velocity measurement. *Circulation* 2000;102:2930–2937.
154. Dupouy P, Pelle G, Garot P, et al. Physiologically guided angioplasty in support to a provisional stenting strategy: Immediate and six-month outcome. *Catheter Cardiovasc Interv* 2000;49:369–375.
155. Anderson HV, Carabello BA. Provisional versus routine stenting—Routine stenting is here to stay. *Circulation* 2000;102:2910–2914.
156. Haude M, Baumgart D, Verna E, et al. Intracoronary Doppler and quantitative coronary angiography–derived predictors of major adverse cardiac events after stent implantation. *Circulation* 201;103: 1212–1217.
157. De Bruyne B, Pijls NHJ, Bartunek J, et al. Fractional flow reserve in patients with prior myocardial infarction. *Circulation* 2001;104: 157–162.
158. Akasaka T, Yoshida K, Kawamoto T, et al. Relation of phasic coronary flow velocity characteristics with TIMI perfusion grade and myocardial recovery after primary percutaneous transluminal coronary angioplasty and rescue stenting. *Circulation* 2000;101:2361–2367.
159. Mazur W, Bitar JN, Lechin M, et al. Coronary flow reserve may predict myocardial recovery after myocardial infarction in patients with TIMI grade 3 flow. *Am Heart J* 1998;136:335–344.
160. Kawamoto T, Yoshida K, Akasaka T, et al. Can coronary blood flow velocity pattern after primary percutaneous transluminal coronary angiography predict recovery of regional left ventricular function in patients with acute myocardial infarction? *Circulation* 1999;100: 339–345.
161. Tsunoda T, Nakamura M, Wakatsuki T, et al. The pattern of alteration in flow velocity in the recanalized artery is related to left ventricular recovery in patients with acute infarction and successful direct balloon angioplasty. *J Am Coll Cardiol* 1998;32:338–344.
162. Claeys MJ, Vrints CJ, Bosmans J, et al. Coronary flow reserve during coronary angioplasty in patients with recent myocardial infarction: Relation to stenosis and myocardial viability. *J Am Coll Cardiol* 1996;28:1712–1719.
163. Neumann FJ, Blasini R, Schmitt C, et al. Effect of glycoprotein IIb/IIIa receptor blockade on recovery of coronary flow and left ventricular function after the placement of coronary-artery stents in acute myocardial infarction. *Circulation* 1998;98:2695–2701.
164. Feldman LJ, Himbert D, Juliard JM, et al. Reperfusion syndrome: Relationship of coronary blood flow reserve to left ventricular function and infarct size. *J Am Coll Cardiol* 2000;35:1162–1169.
165. Reis SE, Holubkov R, Lee JS, et al for the WISE Investigators. Coronary flow velocity response to adenosine characterizes coronary microvascular function in women with chest pain and obstructive coronary disease. *J Am Coll Cardiol* 1999;33:1469–1475.
166. Hasdai D, Holmes DR, Higano ST, et al. Prevalence of coronary blood flow reserve abnormalities among patients with nonobstructive coronary artery disease and chest pain. *Mayo Clin Proc* 1998;73: 1133–1140.
167. Seiler C, Fleisch M, Billinger M, Meier B. Simultaneous intracoronary velocity- and pressure-derived assessment of adenosine-induced collateral hemodynamics in patients with one- to two-vessel coronary artery disease. *J Am Coll Cardiol* 1999;34:1985–1994.
168. Pijls NHJ, Bech GJW, el Gamal MIH, et al. Quantification of recruitable coronary collateral blood flow in conscious humans and its potential to predict future ischemic events. *J Am Coll Cardiol* 1995; 25:1522–1528.
169. Piek JJ, van Liebergen RAM, Koch KT, et al. Clinical, angiographic and hemodynamic predictors of recruitable collateral flow assessed during balloon angioplasty coronary occlusion. *J Am Coll Cardiol* 1997;29:275–282.
170. Billinger M, Kloos P, Eberli FR, et al. Physiologically assessed coronary collateral flow and adverse cardiac ischemic events: A follow-up study in 403 patients with coronary artery disease. *J Am Coll Cardiol* 2002;40:1545–1550.
171. Gruberg L, Mintz GS, Fuchs S, et al. Simultaneous assessment of coronary flow reserve and fractional flow reserve with a novel pressure-based method. *J Interv Cardiol* 2000;13:323–330.

APPENDIX 17-1 Class I Recommendations for Coronary Angiography

### In Stable Angina or Asymptomatic Individuals

| | Level of Evidence |
|---|---|
| 1. CCS class III and IV angina on medical treatment | B |
| 2. High-risk criteria on noninvasive testing regardless of anginal severity (Table 17-1) | A |
| 3. Patients who have been successfully resuscitated from sudden cardiac death or have sustained (>30 s) monomorphic ventricular tachycardia or nonsustained (<30 s) polymorphic ventricular tachycardia | B |

### In Unstable Coronary Syndromes

| | Level of Evidence |
|---|---|
| 1. High or intermediate risk for adverse outcome in patients with unstable angina (Table 17-2) refractory to initial adequate medical therapy or with recurrent symptoms after initial stabilization. Emergent catheterization is recommended. | B |
| 2. High risk for adverse outcome in patients with unstable angina (Table 17-2). Urgent catheterization is recommended. | B |
| 3. High- or intermediate-risk unstable angina that stabilizes after initial treatment. | A |
| 4. Initially low short-term–risk unstable angina (Table 17-2) that is subsequently high risk on noninvasive testing (Table 17-1). | B |
| 5. Suspected Prinzmetal variant angina. | C |

### During the Initial Management of Acute MI (MI Suspected and ST Elevation or BBB Present): Coronary Angiography Coupled with the Intent to Perform Primary PTCA

| | Level of Evidence |
|---|---|
| 1. As an alternative to thrombolytic therapy in patients who can undergo angioplasty of the infarct artery within 12 h of the onset of symptoms or beyond 12 h if ischemic symptoms persist, if performed in a timely fashion[a] by individuals skilled in the procedure and supported by experienced personnel in an appropriate laboratory environment. | A |
| 2. In patients who are within 36 h of an acute ST elevation/Q-wave or new LBBB MI who develop cardiogenic shock, are <75 years of age, and in whom revascularization can be performed within 18 h of the onset of shock. | |

### During the Risk-Stratification Phase of MI (Patients with All Types of MI)

| | Level of Evidence |
|---|---|
| Ischemia at low levels of exercise with ECG changes (1-mm ST-segment depression or other predictors of adverse outcome) (Table 17-3) and/or imaging abnormalities | B |

### In Perioperative Evaluation Before (or After) Noncardiac Surgery: Patients with Suspected or Known CAD

| | Level of Evidence |
|---|---|
| 1. Evidence for high risk of adverse outcome based on noninvasive test results (Table 17-1) | C |
| 2. Angina unresponsive to adequate medical therapy | C |
| 3. Unstable angina, particularly when facing intermediate or high-risk noncardiac surgery | C |
| 4. Equivocal noninvasive test result in a high-clinical-risk patient undergoing high-risk surgery | C |

APPENDIX 17-1 Class I Recommendations for Coronary Angiography (*Continued*)

| In Patients with Valvular Heart Disease | Level of Evidence |
|---|---|
| 1. Before valve surgery or balloon valvotomy in an adult with chest discomfort, ischemia by noninvasive imaging, or both | B |
| 2. Before valve surgery in an adult free of chest pain but of substantial age and/or with multiple risk factors for coronary disease | C |
| 3. Infective endocarditis with evidence of coronary embolization | C |

| In Patients with CHF | Level of Evidence |
|---|---|
| 1. CHF due to systolic dysfunction with angina or with regional wall motion abnormalities and/or scintigraphic evidence of reversible myocardial ischemia when revascularization is being considered | B |
| 2. Before cardiac transplantation | C |
| 3. CHF secondary to postinfarction ventricular aneurysm or other mechanical complications of MI | C |

[a]Performance standard: within 90 min. Individuals who perform >75 PTCA procedures per year. Centers that perform >200 PTCA procedures per year and have cardiac surgical capability.

ABBREVIVATIONS: BBB = bundle branch block; CCS = Canadian Cardiovascular Society; CHF = congestive heart failure; LBBB = left bundle branch block; MI = myocardial infarction; PTCA = percutaneous transluminal coronary angioplasty.

SOURCE: Modified and reproduced with permission from the American Heart Association. Scanlon PJ, Faxon DP, Auden AM, et al. A Report of the American College of Cardiology/ American Heart Association Task Force on Practice Guidelines (Committee on Coronary Angiography). Developed in collaboration with the Society for Cardiac Angiography and Interventions Committee Members. ACC/AHA Guidelines for Coronary Angiography: Executive Summary and Recommendations. *Circulation* 1999;99:2345–2357.

APPENDIX 17-2 ACC/AHA Recommendations for Coronary Intravascular Ultrasound

Class I None

| Class II A | Level of Evidence |
|---|---|
| 1. Evaluation of lesion severity at a location difficult to image by angiography in a patients with a positive functional study and a suspected flow-limiting stenosis | C |
| 2. Assessment of a suboptimal angiographic result after coronary intervention | C |
| 3. Diagnostic and management of coronary disease after cardiac transplantation | C |
| 4. Assessment of the adequacy of deployment of the Palmaz-Schatz coronary stent, including the extent of stent apposition and determination of the minimal luminal diameter within the stent | B |
| **Class II B** | |
| 1. Determination of plaque location and circumferential distribution for guidance of directional coronary atherectomy | C |
| 2. Further evaluation of patients with characteristic anginal symptoms and a positive functional study with no focal stenoses or mild CAD on angiography | C |
| 3. Determination of the mechanism of stent restenosis (inadequate expansion versus neointimal proliferation) and to enable selection of appropriate therapy (plaque ablation versus repeat balloon expansion) | C |
| 4. Preinterventional assessment of lesional characteristics as a means to select an optimal revascularization device | C |

SOURCE: Reproduced with permission from the American Heart Association. Scanlon PJ, Faxon DP, Auden AM, et al. A Report of the American College of Cardiology/American Heart Association Task Force on Practice Guidelines (Committee on Coronary Angiography). Developed in collaboration with the Society for Cardiac Angiography and Interventions Committee Members. ACC/AHA Guidelines for Coronary Angiography: Executive Summary and Recommendations. *Circulation* 1999;99:2345–2357.

APPENDIX 17-3 Recommendations for Intracoronary Physiologic Measurements (Doppler Ultrasound, FFR)

| Class I None<br>Class II a | Level of Evidence |
|---|---|
| 1. Assessment of the physiologic effects of intermediate coronary stenosis (30 to 70 percent luminal narrowing) in patients with anginal symptoms. Coronary pressure or Doppler velocimetry may also be useful as an alternative to performing noninvasive functional testing (e.g., when the functional study is absent or ambiguous) to determine whether an intervention is warranted. | B |
| Class II b | |
| 1. Evaluation of the success of percutaneous coronary revascularization in restoring flow reserve and to predict the risk of restenosis | C |
| 2. Evaluation of patients with anginal symptoms without an apparent angiographic culprit lesion | C |

SOURCE: From Smith SC, Jr, Dove JT, Jacobs AK, et al. ACC/AHA guidelines for percutaneous coronary intervention: a report of the American College of Cardiology/American Heart Association Task Force on Practice Guidelines (Committee to Revise the 1993 Guidelines for Percutaneous Transluminal Coronary Angioplasty). *J Am Coll Cardiol* 2001;37:2239i–lxvi. With permission.

CHAPTER 18

# CORONARY INTRAVASCULAR ULTRASOUND IMAGING

Steven E. Nissen



After more than a decade of continuous development, coronary intravascular ultrasound has achieved general acceptance as an essential element in all contemporary catheterization laboratories. Although angiography continues to serve as the primary imaging modality used to assess the anatomy of coronary artery disease, intravascular ultrasound represents an important alternative method for examination of the coronaries during diagnostic or interventional catheterization.[1–8] Studies comparing angiography and intravascular ultrasound have demonstrated important differences in quantitative and qualitative findings.[7–11] Unlike angiography, which portrays the vessel as a silhouette of the lumen, intravascular ultrasound provides tomographic images that depict not only the lumen but also the deeper intramural structures within the vessel wall.

The ability of ultrasound to penetrate and image soft tissue enables direct visualization of the atheroma, providing insights into the pathophysiology of coronary disease not obtainable by any other technique. Accordingly, intraluminal ultrasound imaging is now commonly utilized to confirm, refute, or supplement angiographic data in patients with coronary disease.[8] Recently, because of its ability to measure atherosclerosis progression and regression, intravascular ultrasound has been increasingly employed in clinical trials. Ongoing studies using this methodology offer the opportunity to develop new antiatherosclerotic therapies, supplementing traditional long-term morbidity and mortality trials.

## RATIONALE FOR INTRAVASCULAR ULTRASOUND

### Limitations of Angiography

Visual interpretation of angiograms is associated with significant observer variability, and necropsy examination is often discordant with the apparent angiographic severity of lesions.[12–18] In comparison to postmortem evaluation, angiography often significantly underestimates the extent of atherosclerosis.[13,18] Angiographic assessment of lesion severity is strikingly discordant with measurements of the physiologic effects of stenoses.[19] Angiography depicts coronary anatomy from a planar two-dimensional silhouette of the contrast-filled lumen. However, coronary lesions are often complex, with markedly distorted or eccentric luminal shapes, and mechanical interventions (other than stenting) exaggerate luminal eccentricity by fracturing or dissecting the atheroma.[9,20,21] The angiographic appearance of the postintervention vessel often reveals an enlarged but "hazy" lumen. This indistinct, broadened angiographic silhouette may overestimate actual vessel diameter and misrepresent the gain in luminal size.[21]

The traditional method for characterizing angiographic lesion severity depends on visual or computer measurements of the percentage stenosis. This process requires comparison of luminal dimensions within both the lesion and an adjacent, uninvolved "normal" reference segment. However, necropsy studies demonstrate that coronary disease is frequently diffuse and contains no truly normal reference segment.[18] In the presence of diffuse disease, calculation of percent stenosis will predictably underestimate disease severity. Diffuse, concentric, and symmetrical disease affecting the entire vessel may result in the angiographic appearance of a small but normal artery.[21] Angiography is also confounded by the phenomenon of coronary "remodeling," observed histologically as the outward displacement of the external vessel wall in segments with atherosclerosis.[22] This adventitial enlargement attenuates lumen encroachment, thereby concealing the presence of the atheroma on angiography. Although such lesions do not restrict blood flow, clinical studies have demonstrated that these minimal, nonobstructive lesions represent an important cause of acute coronary syndromes.[23] Angiographically unrecognized disease virtually always underlies an ergonovine-positive response in symptomatic patients with a "normal" coronary angiogram.[24]

### Theoretical Advantages of Ultrasound

Intravascular ultrasound has several unique properties of theoretical value in the detection and quantitation of coronary disease.[25,26] The cross-sectional perspective of ultrasound permits visualization of the full 360-degree circumference of the vessel wall. Accordingly, measurement of luminal area can be determined by planimetry, independent of the radiographic projection or magnification.[7,21,25,26] The tomographic perspective of ultrasound enables evaluation of vessels difficult to assess by angiographic techniques, including diffusely diseased segments and bifurcation or ostial lesions. The ability to directly image the atheroma within the vessel wall represents a truly unique capability not possible using any other commonly available imaging modality.

## IMAGING TECHNOLOGY

### Catheter Design

Intracoronary ultrasound equipment consists of two major components: a catheter incorporating a miniaturized transducer and a console containing the electronics necessary to reconstruct the image. High frequencies (20 to 50 MHz) are employed, resulting in excellent theoretical resolution (axially $<100$ $\mu$m and laterally $<250$ $\mu$m). Two dissimilar technical approaches to transducer design exist: mechanically rotated devices and multielement electronic arrays.[1–5] Each design has yielded small intravascular devices suitable for coronary imaging, typically ranging in size from approximately 2.6 to 3.5F (diameter of 0.86 to 1.17 mm). To facilitate subselective coronary cannulation and catheter exchanges, ultrasound catheters provide a lumen for a movable guidewire. Most systems generate images at a temporal frequency of 30 frames per second for recording on videotape.

### Limitations and Artifacts

Intravascular ultrasound devices generate artifacts that may adversely affect image quality, alter interpretation, or reduce quantitative accuracy (Fig. 18-1).[27] Ring-down artifact arises from acoustic oscillations in the piezoelectric transducer, resulting in high-amplitude signals that preclude imaging close to the transducer surface. Accordingly, the "acoustic" size of catheters is slightly larger than their physical size. Since the minimum size of current devices is approximately 0.9 mm, some severe stenoses cannot be imaged prior to intervention. Geometric distortion can result from imaging in an oblique plane (not perpendicular to the long axis of the vessel), resulting in an elliptical rather than circular imaging plane.[28]

Mechanical, but not electronic, transducers may exhibit cyclical oscillations in rotational speed, resulting in an artifact known as

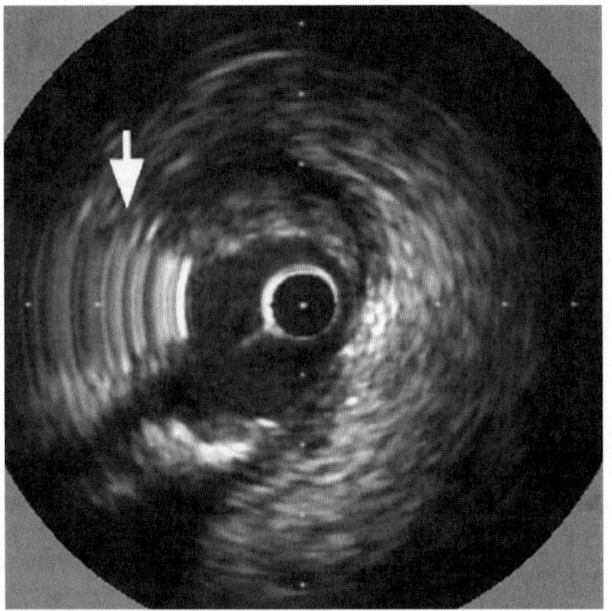

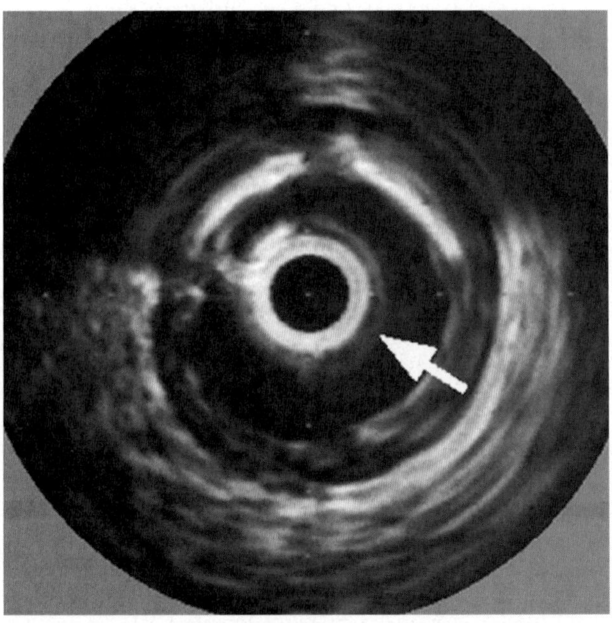

FIGURE 18-1 Intravascular ultrasound artifacts. In the left panel, there is an example of nonuniform rotational distortion (NURD) with circumferential "stretching" of the image from 8 to 10 o'clock (*arrow*). The right panel shows an example of ring-down artifact.

nonuniform rotational distortion (NURD).[27] This artifact arises from mechanical friction within the catheter drive shaft during the portions of its rotational cycle. This speed variation produces readily visible distortion, often observed as circumferential stretching of a portion of the image with compression of the contralateral vessel wall (Fig. 18-1). NURD is most evident when the drive shaft is bent into a small radius of curvature by a tortuous vessel. Improvements in the mechanical precision of ultrasound devices have reduced the impact of the artifact, but it still remains troublesome during some examinations.

## CORONARY IMAGING

### Examination Technique

Standard interventional techniques for intracoronary catheter delivery are used for intraluminal ultrasound examination. Intravenous heparin [to maintain activated clotting time (ACT) >200 to 250 s] and intracoronary nitroglycerin (100 to 300 $\mu$g) are routinely administered, although there are no controlled studies documenting the necessity for anticoagulation. Using a 6- or 7F guiding catheter, the operator advances a steerable guidewire to subselectively cannulate the vessel. A stable guiding catheter position with good support is desirable, since current ultrasound catheters have less trackability and a larger profile than modern angioplasty equipment. The operator carefully advances or retracts the imaging catheter over the wire to examine the vessel in real time, recording images on videotape for subsequent quantitative or qualitative analysis. Side branches, visualized with both angiography and ultrasound, are often used as landmarks to facilitate interpretation. Some practitioners advocate use of a uniform format, electronically rotating the ultrasound image so that branches appear in a standardized orientation. For example, imaging of the left anterior descending is often performed with the septal branches at 6 o'clock and the left circumflex appearing at about 9 o'clock. Some centers use a motorized pullback device to withdraw the catheter at a constant speed (between 0.25 and 1 mm/s, but most often 0.5 mm/s). In clinical practice, motorized pullback is often used to survey the coronary prior to more prolonged and thorough examination of sites of interest. However, in studies of atherosclerosis progression versus regression, the motorized pullback is an integral feature of the investigative procedure. In this application, during analysis of the motorized pulback, "slices" are selected at regular intervals (typically every 1 mm) and subsequently analyzed in a core laboratory. By comparing atheroma burden at a baseline examination with a similar study at follow-up, the extent of disease progression or regression can be precisely characterized.

### Safety of Coronary Ultrasound

Although intravascular ultrasound requires intracoronary instrumentation, studies have demonstrated few serious untoward effects.[29–31] The most frequently encountered complication is focal coronary spasm, which usually responds rapidly to intracoronary nitroglycerin. Data from European centers report a 1.1 percent complication rate in 718 ultrasound examinations.[30] Another report from 28 centers (2207 studies) documents spasm in 2.9 percent and major complications, such as occlusion or dissection, judged to have a "certain relation" to instrumentation in 0.4 percent.[29] In both studies, complications (spasm, vessel dissection, or guidewire entrapment) occurred in patients undergoing angioplasty rather than diagnostic imaging. In 170 cardiac transplant recipients (240 studies), there was no morbidity, but spasm occurred in 20 patients (8.3 percent) despite pretreatment with nitroglycerin.[31] Any intracoronary instrumentation carries the potential risk of intimal injury or vessel dissection. Accordingly, most laboratories limit credentialing for this procedure to personnel with interventional training.

### Normal Coronary Anatomy

Studies performed either in vivo or using excised, pressure-distended vessels have characterized the appearance of normal coronaries by intravascular ultrasound.[32–36] Important determinants of vessel wall appearance include both the normal arterial structure and the inherent properties of ultrasound. An ultrasound reflection occurs at a tissue boundary whenever there is an abrupt change in acoustic impedance. Normally, two strong acoustic interfaces are visualized by ultrasound, the leading edge of the intima (at the interface between the blood-filled lumen and the endothelium) and the outer border of the media (at the junction of media and external elastic membrane). Underlying the trailing edge of the intima, a middle sonolucent layer is usually evident, which is composed principally of the tunica media. The echodense intima and adventitia with a sonolucent medial layer often give the wall a trilaminar appearance. However, this pattern is not a universal finding; in 30 to 50 percent of normal segments, a thin intimal layer reflects ultrasound poorly, which results in a monolayer appearance (Fig. 18-2).[35] In a necropsy study, the ultrasound-derived intimal thickness in segments with three layers was significantly greater than for monolayered sites (0.24 ± 0.1 vs. 0.11 ± 0.06 mm, $p < 0.001$). The mean age in the three-layered group was greater, 42.8 ± 9.8 versus 27.1 ± 8.5 years ($p < 0.001$).[37] Other studies demonstrate that a trilaminar appearance is dependent not only on the age but also on the histologic characteristics of the vessel. A three-layered appearance is consistently observed if an internal elastic membrane is present.[38] However, if an internal elastic membrane is absent, a trilaminar appearance is observed only when the collagen content of the media is low. In older "normal" subjects, intimal thickening usually results in a pattern of two distinct echogenic layers "sandwiching" a sonolucent intermediate layer. In nearly all cases, the deepest arterial layers exhibit a characteristic onionskin pattern, representing the adventitia and periadventitial tissues with an indistinct outer vessel border (Fig. 18-2). In both normal and abnormal arteries, the lumen exhibits faint, finely textured, swirling echoes that arise from acoustic reflections from circulating blood elements. This blood "speckle" may assist image interpretation by providing a means to confirm the communication between dissection planes and the lumen. The pattern of blood speckle is dependent on the velocity of flow, showing increased intensity and a more coarse appearance when flow is reduced. In some cases, the coarse blood speckle can mimic the appearance of tissue, complicating image interpretation. The physical presence of the ultrasound catheter may exacerbate this problem, particularly if there exists a stenosis with relatively severe narrowing proximal to the imaged site. In such cases, the reduction of blood flow produced by partial obstruction of the proximal narrowing, may result in reduced blood flow at the imaged site, and the resulting coarse blood speckle may be misinterpreted at tissue protruding into the lumen.

## CHARACTERIZATION OF ATHEROSCLEROSIS

### Atheroma Composition

The subtle changes that occur early in the development of atherosclerosis, such as fatty streaks, are not visible using current ultrasound devices. Atherosclerotic arteries exhibit a variety of features

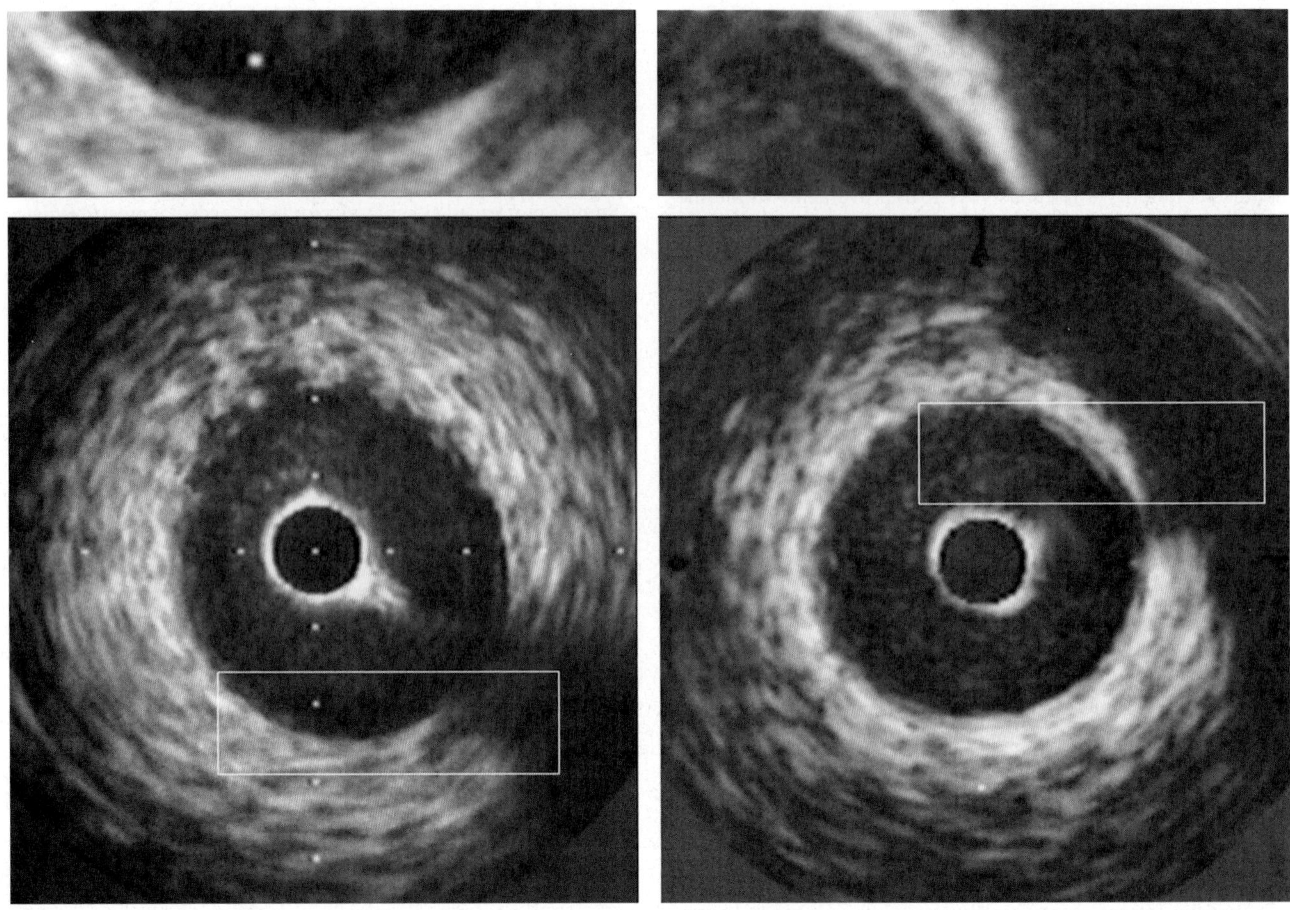

FIGURE 18-2 Two variants of normal coronary anatomy by intravascular ultrasound. In both images, a magnified view of the area contained within the rectangle is shown at the top. In the left panel, there is a monolayered artery; in the right panel, the artery has a trilaminar structure.

that reflect the distribution, severity, and composition of the atheroma.[32–34] Sites with limited disease exhibit generalized or focal thickening of the intimal leading edge, while advanced lesions appear as large echogenic masses encroaching on the lumen. A comparative study of ultrasound and histology in 1100 fresh necropsy sections demonstrated that lipid-laden lesions are usually hypoechoic.[32] Soft, low-intensity echoes most often represent fibromuscular lesions and very bright echoes are characteristic of dense fibrous or calcified tissues (Fig. 18-3). In highly echogenic plaques, areas of calcification are recognized by obstruction or severe attenuation of ultrasound penetration, which obscures deeper layers, a phenomenon known as *acoustic shadowing*. In lipid-laden or fibromuscular lesions, a prominent echogenic overlying "fibrous cap" may be observed.

The echogenicity of the plaque components is dependent not only on the acoustic properties of tissue, but also on the acquisition settings (gain, compression, etc.). Accordingly, most morphologic classification schemes compare the echogenicity of the plaque to the surrounding adventitia to adjust for differences in ultrasound technique. However, in plaques containing a zone of reduced echogenicity, it is not possible to determine whether these represent areas of lipid deposition, thrombus, or necrotic degeneration, all of which can appear as zones of low density. Plaque composition was accurately predicted by ultrasound imaging in 96 percent of 112 quadrants from 21 freshly explanted human coronary arteries.[38] Fibrous and calcified plaque quadrants were correctly identified in almost all cases (100 of 103, or 97 percent), but only 7 of 9 quadrants (78 percent) with predominantly lipid deposits were correctly identified. Accordingly, some caution is warranted in the intravascular ultrasound classification of atheroma composition. Although currently available devices produce detailed views of the vessel wall, interpretation employs visual inspection of acoustic reflections to impute morphology. Different histologic features may exhibit comparable acoustic properties, and well-validated methods for objective or automated classification of atheromatous lesions do not yet exist. Thus, intravascular ultrasound can delineate the thickness and echogenicity of vessel wall structures, but this technique does not provide actual histology.

More recently, sophisticated image processing techniques have been employed to classify the composition of atherosclerotic plaques. The most promising methods employ analysis of raw radiofrequency data from ultrasound studies to assess the morphology of the atheroma.[39] Using necropsy specimens, some recent investigations have demonstrated that automated methods for characterization of atheroma morphology are more accurate and reproducible than methods based on simple visual inspection.[40] By plotting morphologic characteristics as a color overlay superimposed on the ultrasound image, such methods facilitate relatively facile image interpretation. Accordingly, such methods are likely to achieve broader acceptance within the next few years.

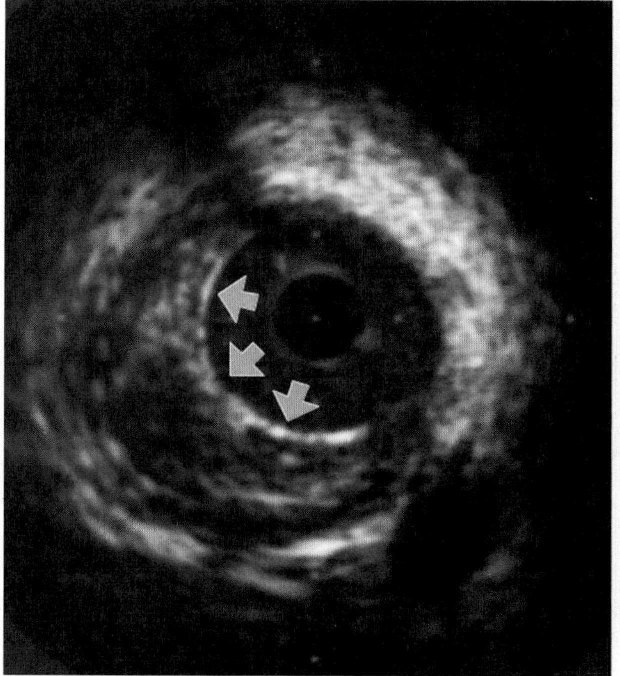

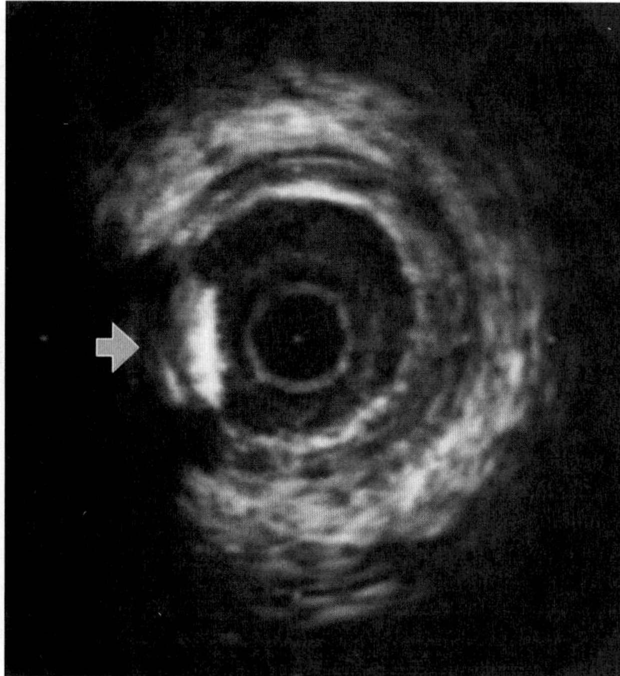

FIGURE 18-3 Atheroma morphology by intravascular ultrasound. In the left panel, a large, "soft," lipid-laden atheroma with a thin fibrous cap is seen (*arrows*). It is eccentric, involving only about 50 percent of the vessel wall. The right panel shows a circumferential atheroma with an area of focal calcification is evident (*arrow*).

## Detection of Calcification

Ultrasound imaging is more sensitive than fluoroscopy or angiography for the detection of coronary calcification. In a series of 110 patients undergoing intervention, target lesion calcification was detected by ultrasound and fluoroscopy in 84 and 50 patients, respectively (76 vs. 14 percent, $p < 0.001$).[41] Another retrospective study analyzed calcification by angiography and ultrasound in 183 interventional patients.[42] Assessment by the two techniques was concordant in 92 and discordant in 91 cases. Calcification was detected in 138 patients by ultrasound and 63 by fluoroscopy, showing a sensitivity and specificity for angiography of 46 and 82 percent, respectively. When calcium was detected angiographically, calcification by ultrasound often subtended >90 degrees and was superficial to the lumen in location. If no calcification could be visualized on the angiogram, the chance of detecting a large superficial arc of calcium by ultrasound was low (12 percent).

Ultrasound calcification is an important determinant of the arterial response to intervention, portending a greater risk of dissection following balloon angioplasty, less tissue retrieval with directional atherectomy, and potentially greater benefit with the use of rotational atherectomy.[43,44] Most classification schemes quantify the extent of calcification, usually by measuring the circumferential angle subtended by calcified plaque.[41] Commonly, the axial length of the calcified portion of the lesion is also reported. The depth of calcification is also assessed, described as superficial when the calcium remains in contact with the luminal surface and deep if no portion of the calcium deposit is superficial. During initial development of intravascular ultrasound, the extent of calcification was often utilized in the selection of interventional devices, particularly as a means to select vessels suitable for directional coronary atherectomy. However, in recent years, the reduced importance of directional atherectomy and the nearly universal application of coronary stenting has lessened the importance of calcification as a determinant of the interventional approach. Accordingly, in current practice, intravascular ultrasound is uncommonly performed solely as a means to detect coronary calcification.

## Arterial Remodeling

The term *arterial remodeling* refers to a change in arterial dimensions associated with the development of atherosclerosis. In a necropsy study of 136 human left main coronary arteries, Glagov et al. originally described focal arterial enlargement at atherosclerotic sites, reporting a positive correlation between external elastic membrane (EEM) area and the area occupied by atheroma ($r = 0.44$, $p < 0.001$).[22] At sites with area stenosis less than 40 percent, the increase in arterial size "overcompensated" for the plaque deposition, leading to an increase in absolute lumen area. With more advanced lesions (area stenosis >40 percent), the degree of arterial enlargement or remodeling was blunted, resulting in a smaller lumen area. The authors hypothesized that this phenomenon represented a compensatory mechanism to preserve lumen size.

The findings of Glagov et al. were later confirmed in vivo by intravascular ultrasound imaging (Fig. 18-4).[45,46] In 80 ultrasound cross sections obtained from 44 patients undergoing coronary interventions, EEM area correlated closely with plaque area ($r = 0.79$, $p = 0.0001$). In this study, lumen area increased with early atherosclerosis, confirming the phenomenon of overcompensation in early stages of the disease. With more advanced atherosclerosis, there was a correlation between increasing area stenosis and decreasing lumen area ($r = 0.58$, $p = 0.0001$).[45] Compensatory enlargement has also been demonstrated by ultrasound in superficial femoral arteries;

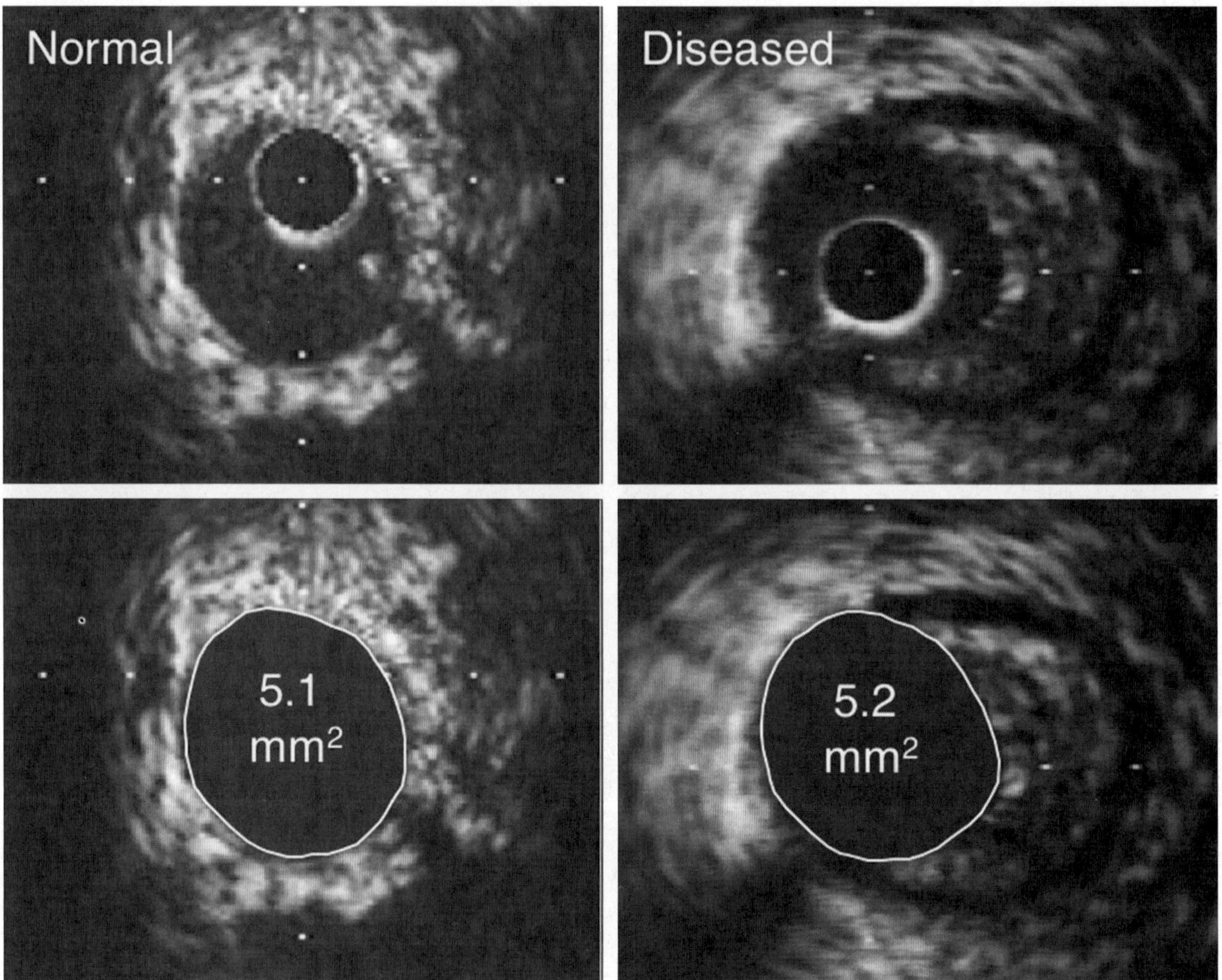


FIGURE 18-4 Example of coronary remodeling. The left upper panel shows a normal segment of the circumflex coronary. In the right upper panel, an atherosclerotic segment of the coronary a few millimeters proximal to the normal segment is shown. In the bottom two panels, measurements taken at each of the sites show very similar cross-sectional areas. The preservation of luminal area results in a coronary angiogram that is normal despite the presence of a large atherosclerotic plaque in the involved segment.

however, there was no difference between lesions less than, and greater than 40 percent stenosis.[47]

In recent years, ultrasound studies have demonstrated a new dimension to arterial remodeling, the phenomenon of "negative" remodeling.[48,49] At diseased sites, the EEM area may actually be reduced in size, contributing to luminal narrowing, rather than compensating for it. In 51 femoral arteries, EEM area was smaller at lesions than adjacent reference sites, with a negative correlation between stenosis severity and EEM area reduction ($r = 0.62$ by histology and 0.66 by ultrasound, $p < 0.001$ for both).[48] "Inadequate" remodeling, defined as an EEM area within the lesion less than 78 percent of a proximal reference site, has also been described in the coronaries of patients with stable angina.[49] Although 91 of 603 lesions (15 percent) fit this definition, there was a highly variable response among lesions within the same patient. However, when remodeling is defined in this fashion, there is an assumption that the reference EEM area represents the original vessel size, which may not be correct, since angiographic reference sites are frequently diseased by ultrasound.

Although the exact mechanisms of compensatory or negative remodeling remain unclear, these phenomena have important clinical implications. Compensatory remodeling represents an important factor in the underestimation of the severity of atherosclerosis by angiography. Thus, a vessel site may contain a very large atheroma but minimal stenosis if outward remodeling of the EEM has "compensated" for the plaque accumulation. Recent evidence suggest such sites may be particularly prone to plaque rupture. Because remodeling can affect both the lesion and adjacent reference segments, remodeling may also influence the estimation of the vessel size during coronary interventions. Recently, negative remodeling has been implicated in restenosis following atherectomy and balloon angioplasty.[50]

## Unstable Plaque and Thrombi

An emerging application of intracoronary ultrasound is the characterization of the atheroma associated with acute coronary syndromes (Fig. 18-5).[51–56] The typical angiographic appearance of a ruptured plaque is a stenosis with an eccentric or ulcerated lumen, often with overhanging edges (Ambrose type II lesion). However, retrospective reviews of angiograms of patients performed before an episode of unstable angina often reveal minimal stenosis severity within the cul-

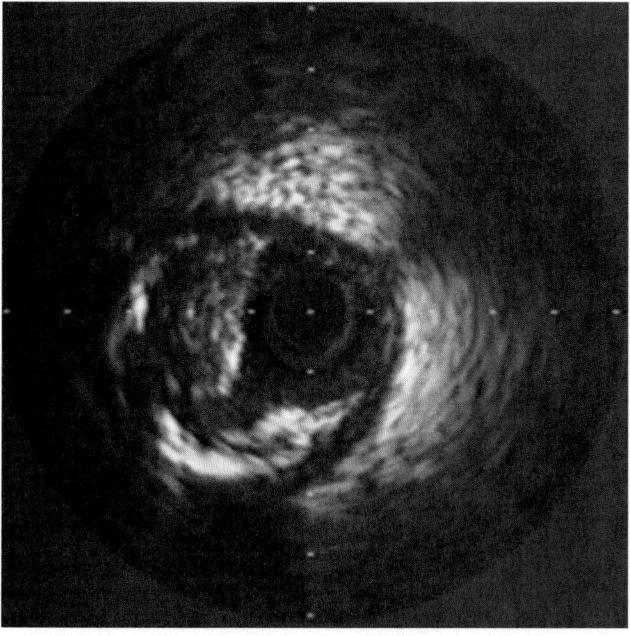

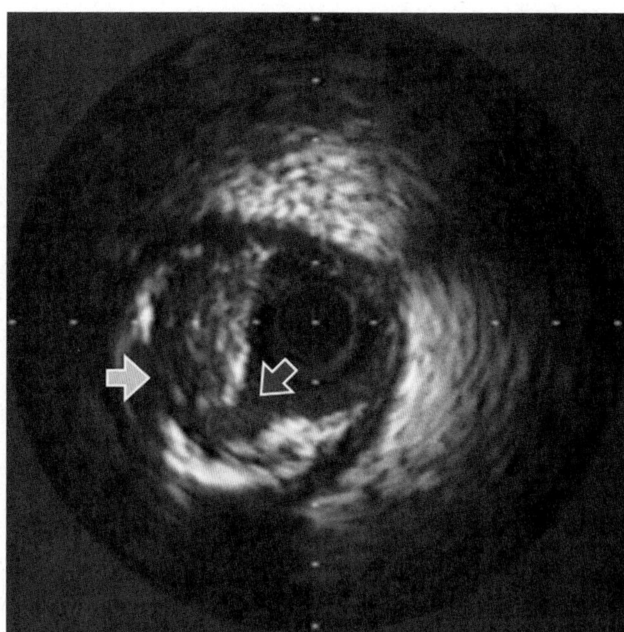

FIGURE 18-5 Ruptured coronary plaque. In these two identical images, the anatomy of a ruptured coronary plaque is seen. There is a large lipid core with a fracture of the fibrous cap (*right panel, arrow*). This image was obtained a few days after hospitalization of this patient for a unstable coronary syndrome.

prit lesion segment.[53] Such studies highlight the inability of angiography to identify "rupture prone" atherosclerotic lesions. Histologic examination of unstable plaques after rupture usually reveals a lipid-laden plaque with a thin fibrous cap.[51] Based on these observations, it has been postulated that the size of the lipid pool and the thickness of the fibrous cap are more important than severity of stenosis in predicting plaque rupture.[54] Some intravascular ultrasound studies have suggested the presence of an echolucent atheroma within culprit lesions in patients with acute coronary syndromes. In a very limited study of 22 stable and 43 unstable angina patients, type II eccentric lesions were detected on the angiograms in 18 percent of stable and 40 percent of unstable angina patients. Echolucent plaques were more frequently observed in patients with unstable than in those with stable angina syndromes (74 vs. 41 percent, $p < 0.01$).[11] However, this finding has not been confirmed by other investigators.

Recent intravascular ultrasound studies have examined the relationship between remodeling and the type of clinical presentation, suggesting difference in the remodeling pattern for unstable versus stable patients.[57] The culprit lesions in 76 patients with acute coronary syndromes were compared with lesions in 40 patients with stable angina. In the unstable patients, both EEM and plaque areas were significantly larger than the corresponding measurements in the stable patients ($p = 0.02$ for both). Positive remodeling was more prevalent in the unstable group (51 vs. 18 percent, $p = 0.002$) and negative remodeling more prevalent in the stable group (58 vs. 33 percent, $p = 0.002$). This finding provides further insight into the relationship between lesion severity and the likelihood of plaque rupture. Because angiographic studies suggested that minimal stenoses were associated with atheroma rupture, most investigators assumed that the culprit lesion represented a small plaque. However, the finding that rupture sites frequently exhibit positive remodeling suggests that such lesions are not particularly small plaques. Rather, the presence of remodeling enables the atheroma to reach a large size without compromising the lumen.

The formation of intraluminal thrombi at a ruptured or fissured plaque is considered to be the hallmark of acute coronary syndromes.[58] Angiographic criteria for diagnosis of a coronary thrombus, the presence of haziness, an intraluminal filling defect, and/or irregular lumen contour are not sensitive.[56] Small observational studies have attempted to differentiate the ultrasound appearance of thrombus, defined as hypoechoic material projecting into the lumen with a slight synchronous pulsation and a distinct acoustic interface, from more echogenic plaque (Fig. 18-6).[59] However, in vitro studies have revealed limitations in the reliability of intravascular ultrasound diagnosis of thrombi (sensitivity of 57 percent and specificity of 91

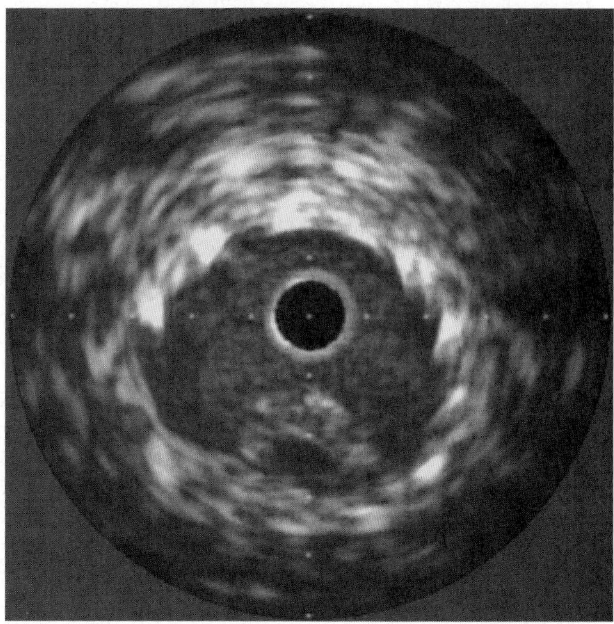

FIGURE 18-6 Thrombus within a coronary stent. In this intravascular ultrasound image, a stent is well visualized. There is a globular mass projecting into the lumen at 6 o'clock; it probably represents a large thrombus.

percent), considerably inferior to angioscopy (sensitivity and specificity of 100 percent).[58]

## DIAGNOSTIC CLINICAL APPLICATIONS

### Quantitative Luminal Measurements

A broad spectrum of therapeutic decisions hinge on assessment of coronary luminal dimensions. Accordingly, in diagnostic and interventional practice, quantitation of vascular dimensions represents a common clinical application of intravascular ultrasound. Recently, a committee of the American College of Cardiology and the European Society of Cardiology defined standards for the acquisition, measurement, and reporting of intravascular ultrasound studies.[60] This standards document precisely defines the terrminology and methodology for performing intravascular ultrasound measurements and constitutes the recognized standard for both clinical and research studies. The presence of standardized nomenclature and measurement methods represents a critical advance in the wider acceptance of intravascular ultrasound.

Several studies have compared luminal measurements by intravascular ultrasound and quantitative angiography.[6,7] For vessels without atherosclerosis, most studies document a relatively close correlation between angiographic and ultrasonic coronary dimensions, although a few studies suggest slightly larger measurements by ultrasound.[7] However, in patients with atherosclerotic arteries, most investigators report only a moderate correlation between ultrasonic and angiographic dimensions, with the greatest disparities in vessel segments with a noncircular lumen shape.[5,7,10] This reduced correlation is probably explained by the irregular, noncircular cross-sectional profile of diseased vessels, which cannot be adequately measured using angiography.[10]

### Quantitation of Atherosclerosis

Analysis of intravascular ultrasound images permits quantitative measurements of the extent and severity of coronary atherosclerosis (Fig. 18-7).[26] However, the inherent properties of ultrasound require utilization of different anatomic landmarks than those employed in classical histology. In all ultrasound imaging, reflections at the leading edge of any interface are located precisely at the boundary where acoustic impedance abruptly changes. However, the position of the trailing edge of any anatomic structure is determined by multiple nonanatomic factors, including ultrasound beam properties, particularly the wavelength (frequency). Thus, leading-edge measurements accurately describe the location of a boundary, whereas trailing-edge measurements are unreliable. As previously noted, strong reflections are generally produced at two locations, the leading edge of the intima and the border between the media and the external elastic membrane. The position of the trailing edge of the intima is not accurately localized in intravascular ultrasound images. Accordingly, quantitative measurements must calculate the atheroma's cross-sectional area by subtracting the area bounded by the intimal leading edge from the area enclosed by the external elastic membrane. This approach results in a slight overestimation of atheroma area (in comparison to histology) by including the area of the media within the calculation.

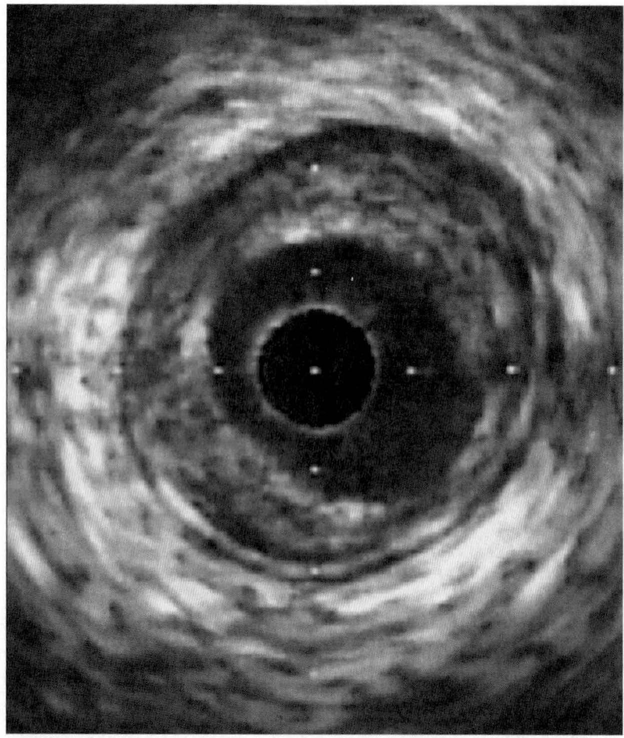

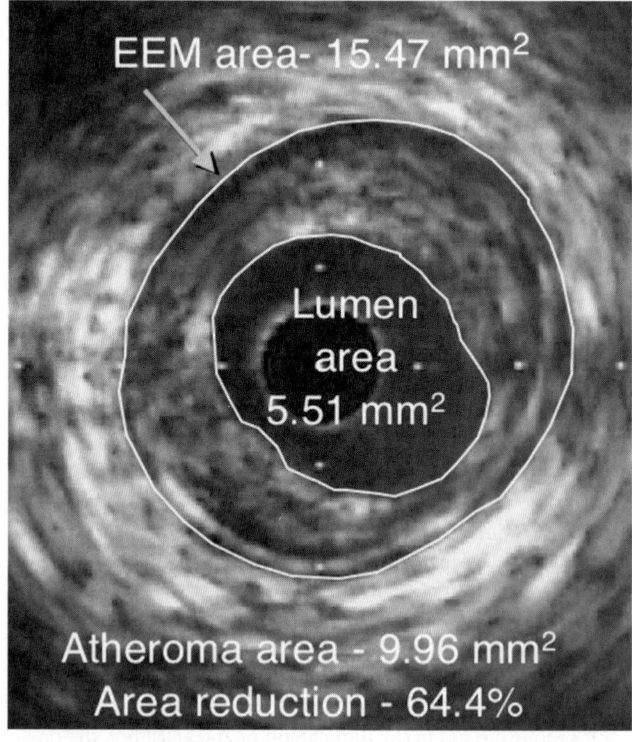


FIGURE 18-7 Boundaries for intravascular ultrasound measurements. In these two identical images, an atherosclerotic plaque is well visualized. The right panel illustrates the planimetry typically employed to measure the extent of atherosclerotic disease. Both the lumen and external elastic membrane (EEM) are measured. The atheroma area represents the difference between the EEM and the lumen areas. The area reduction is calculated as the atheroma area divided by the EEM area multiplied by 100.

## Normal Intimal Thickness

The threshold for abnormal intimal thickness by intravascular ultrasound is controversial, particularly since the categorical classification of a continuous variable intimal thickness as normal and abnormal is inherently arbitrary. In various histologic and ultrasound studies, normal intimal thickness ranges between 0.10 and 0.35 mm, and the normal medial thickness ranges from 0.15 to 0.25 mm. In a necropsy study, normal intimal thickness not including media was age-dependent, averaging 0.21 mm in 21- to 25-year-olds, 0.22 mm in 26- to 30-year-olds, and 0.25 mm in 36- to 40-year-olds.[37] In a comparative study, intravascular ultrasound measurements of the intima plus media averaged 20 percent greater than histologic measurements.[61,62] Considering the histologic and ultrasound data, most clinical studies have defined threshold for coronary disease by ultrasound as a measured intimal thickness ≥0.5 mm.[63–67] Currently, there is no well-defined threshold for normal values for other measures of atherosclerosis, such as intimal cross-sectional area.

## Assessment of Atheroma Burden

The tomographic orientation of intravascular ultrasound represents a problem in quantifying atherosclerosis. Since each image contains information from only a thin "slice" of the vessel, global measures of atheroma burden require the integration of multiple cross sections. One successful approach to this conundrum employs a motorized device to steadily and progressively withdraw the ultrasound catheter through the interrogated vessel, typically at 0.5 mm/s. Since motor speed is kept constant, the operator can obtain a series of cross sections separated by a constant, recurring time interval (fixed distance from each other). These slices are individually measured and then summated to calculate an approximate total atheroma burden using Simpson's rule. This method is increasingly employed in clinical trials designed to assess the effect of pharmacologic agents on atherosclerosis progression or regression. The first large scale trial, the REVERSAL study (Regression of Atherosclerosis with Aggressive Lipid Lowering), will compare the effects of atorvastatin 80 mg and pravastatin 40 mg on total atheroma burden in a single coronary artery.[68] This study, which randomized 655 patients to the two treatment cohorts, showed enhanced plaque stabilization in the high-dose statin group as reported by Nissen (AHA scientific session 2003). Many additional clinical trials of antiatherosclerotic therapies are ongoing. If such studies demonstrate the ability of intravascular ultrasound to determine the relative effectiveness of antiatherosclerotic therapies, the application is likely to grow rapidly in use during the coming years.

## Atheroma Distribution

The circumferential distribution of the atheroma varies from nearly symmetrical plaques to very eccentric lesions in which the entire atheroma is located on one side of the artery. Assessed by ultrasound, the majority of plaques are eccentric, with a maximum atheroma thickness more than twice the minimum plaque thickness.[69] Studies have demonstrated a poor correlation between the apparent circumferential pattern by angiography and the actual plaque distribution revealed by ultrasound examination.[69] Such studies demonstrate the inaccuracy inherent in determining plaque distribution from the projected two-dimensional silhouette of the lumen (angiography). Although previously advocated as means to guide directional atherectomy, the decreased popularity of this interventional method has reduced the value of eccentricity measurement as a clinical application for intravascular ultrasound.

## Angiographically Unrecognized Disease

In patients undergoing angiography for clinically suspected coronary artery disease, no angiographic evidence of narrowing is present in 10 to 15 percent of cases. In these patients, intravascular ultrasound commonly detects atherosclerosis at angiographically normal sites.[21,25,26,70,71] Using intravascular ultrasound, atherosclerotic abnormalities were documented in 21 of 44 patients (48 percent) with suspected coronary artery disease and normal coronary angiograms.[70] Combining ultrasound and functional assessment (coronary flow reserve and endothelium-mediated vasodilator response), only 36 percent of patients in this cohort were completely normal. Other studies demonstrate that, if any luminal irregularity is present by angiography, ultrasound will usually demonstrate atherosclerosis at nearly all other examined sites.[21] The prevalence of atherosclerosis at angiographically normal sites confirms the finding, previously reported from necropsy studies, that coronary involvement is frequently underestimated using angiographic evaluation methods (Fig. 18-8)[12,13].

There are several mechanisms by which angiography may underestimate the presence, extent, or severity of atherosclerosis.[21] First, to detect focal narrowing, angiography relies on comparison of the interrogated site to an adjacent uninvolved segment. However, the involved vessel is often reduced in caliber along its entire length, containing no truly normal segment for comparison. The angiographer may erroneously conclude that the vessel is simply "small in caliber." Overlapping structures and mechanical limits in x-ray positioning may prevent the angiographer from obtaining optimal radiographic projections (orthogonal to the lesion). Accordingly, eccentric plaques that occupy only a portion of the vessel circumference represent an important source of false-negative angiography. At atherosclerotic sites, compensatory enlargement of the vessel wall overlying the plaque often preserves lumen diameter, resulting in false-negative angiography, because the lumen size in the involved segment is identical to that of adjacent, uninvolved segments. Finally, radiographic foreshortening can conceal short "napkin ring" lesions.

For each of these mechanisms of false-negative angiography, intravascular ultrasound has been employed to confirm the presence and estimate the extent of atherosclerosis.[21] However, the long-term clinical implications of angiographically unrecognized atherosclerosis remain uncertain, since no outcomes-based research has demonstrated a worse prognosis for patients with atherosclerosis detected only by ultrasound. However, several investigators have demonstrated that plaques with minimal to moderate angiographic narrowing are the most likely lead to acute coronary syndromes. Accordingly, the presence of angiographically occult coronary disease may have prognostic significance. Studies are currently under way to determine the value of ultrasound in predicting the clinical outcome in patients with angiographically unrecognized coronary disease.

## Prevalence of Coronary Atherosclerosis

Recent intravascular ultrasound studies have demonstrated an extraordinary prevalence of coronary atherosclerosis in the general population, beginning at a relatively young age.[71] In the most thorough study, intravascular ultrasound was performed in 262 transplant recipients within 31 days of transplantation to determine the prevalence of atherosclerotic disease in the donor hearts. These heart transplant donors (116 women and 146 men) had a mean age of 33 years and no known coronary artery disease. Imaging of multiple coronary segments was performed to determine the greatest and least intimal thickness in each segment for an average of 2.3 coronary arteries per

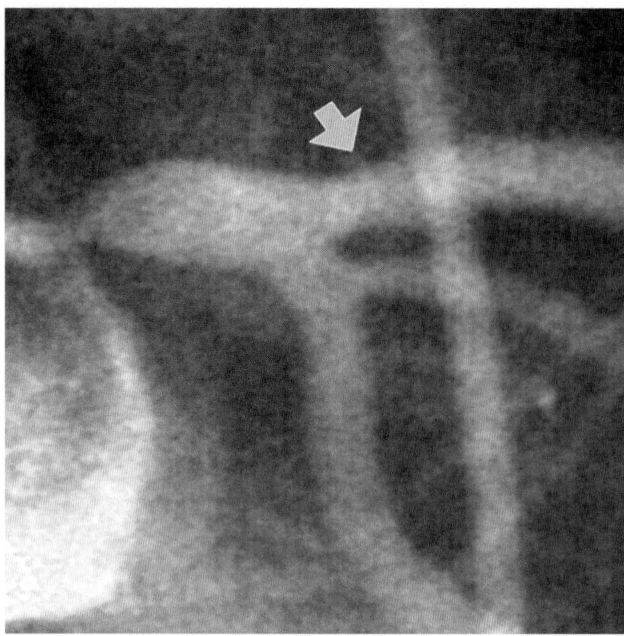

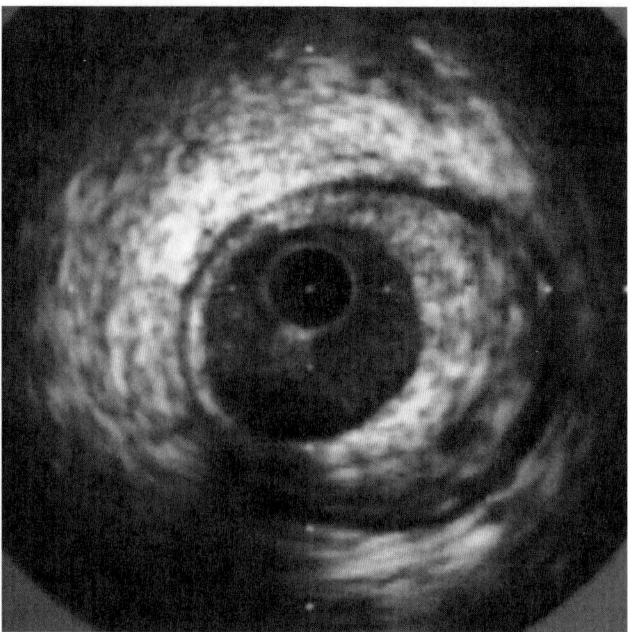

FIGURE 18-8 Underestimation of coronary atherosclerosis by angiography. In the angiogram in the left panel, a relatively minor lesion of the left anterior descending coronary is seen (*arrow*). In the right panel, this lesion is depicted by intravascular ultrasound and consists of a large eccentric atherosclerotic plaque that appears much more extensive than would be suspected from the angiogram.

patient. Assessment of 2014 sites in 1477 segments of 574 coronary arteries showed that atherosclerotic lesions, defined as an intimal thickness ≥0.5 mm, were present in 51.9 percent of donor hearts. Intimal thickness correlated with donor age with the prevalence of disease ranging from 17 percent for donors aged <20 years to 85 percent in those aged ≥50 years (Fig. 18-9). For all age groups, average intimal thickness was greater in male than female donors, although similar proportions (52 and 51.7 percent) had atherosclerosis. Coronary angiography was completely normal in 92 percent of these subjects and none of the donors aged <30 years had angiographic evidence of atherosclerosis. This study confirms previously reported necropsy findings showing a high prevalence of atherosclerosis in

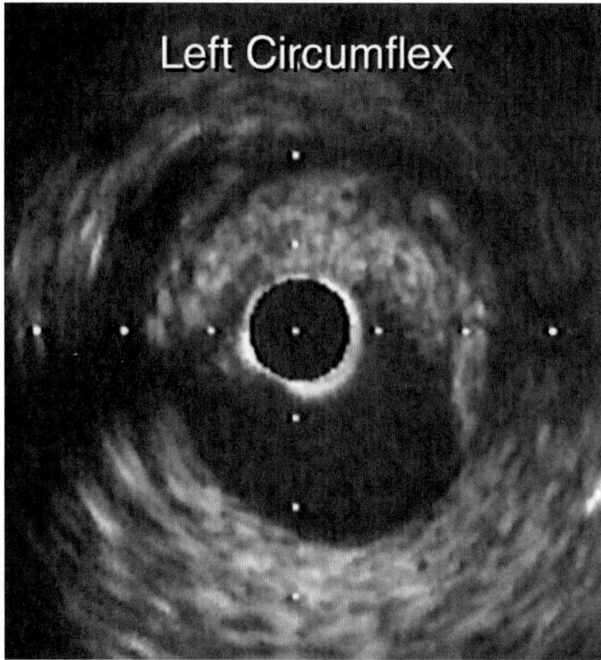


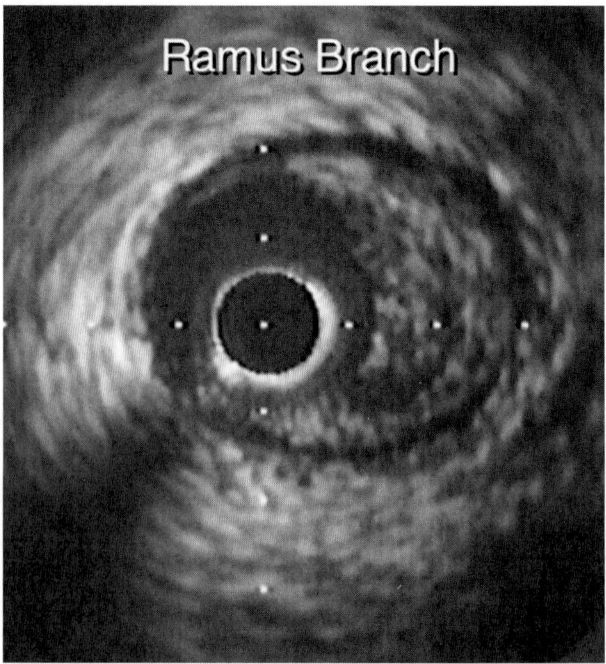


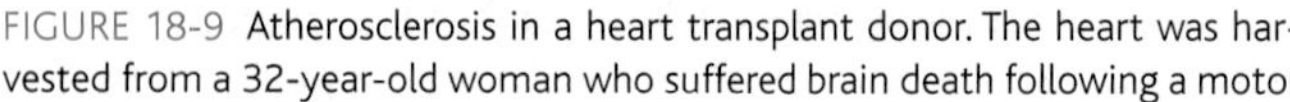

FIGURE 18-9 Atherosclerosis in a heart transplant donor. The heart was harvested from a 32-year-old woman who suffered brain death following a motor vehicle accident. In both the left circumflex coronary (*left panel*) and the ramus branch (*right panel*), there is extensive atherosclerosis.

young adults. However, unlike earlier postmortem studies, this intravascular ultrasound report demonstrates the extent of angiographic underestimation of the phenomenon.

## Lesions of Uncertain Severity

Angiographers commonly encounter lesions that elude accurate characterization despite thorough examination using multiple radiographic projections. Difficult-to-assess sites include ostial or bifurcation lesions and moderate stenoses (angiographic severity ranging from 40 to 75 percent) in patients whose symptomatic status is difficult to evaluate. For ambiguous lesions, ultrasound provides a tomographic perspective, independent of the radiographic projection, that may permit quantification of the lesion. In two prospective series, intracoronary ultrasound changed the management strategy in approximately 20 percent of the examinations performed immediately prior to coronary intervention.[73,74] In both studies, however, operator selection of patients for ultrasound examination may have resulted in an overestimation of the true impact of ultrasound imaging on clinical decision making.

Angiographic assessment of left main coronary artery (LMCA) obstruction represents a particularly vexing clinical problem.[14] Radiographic contrast in the aortic cusp can obscure the ostium, and "streaming" of contrast from the injection vortex can result in a false impression of luminal narrowing. The LMCA is often short in length, leaving no normal reference segment. The bifurcation or trifurcation of the LMCA into daughter branches may produce vessel overlap, thereby concealing a stenosis. Intravascular ultrasound is commonly used to quantify LMCA lesions when angiographic interpretation is uncertain.[75] The technique for examination consists of subselective placement of the ultrasound transducer in the circumflex or anterior descending, followed by slow pullback to the aorta with the guiding catheter disengaged. There is no consensus regarding the threshold for critical LMCA obstruction. However, an area stenosis >50 percent or an absolute area <9 mm$^2$ has been proposed as a threshold.[75]

## Cardiac Allograft Disease

Transplant coronary artery disease is the leading cause of death beyond the first year after cardiac transplantation, with a reported incidence of 15 to 20 percent per year.[76] Although most transplant centers perform arteriograms annually for screening, these surveillance studies often fail to detect atherosclerosis prior to a clinical event.[77,78] Necropsy studies have demonstrated that angiography systematically underestimates coronary atherosclerosis in transplant recipients.[78] Patients may have diffuse vessel involvement that, for reasons already enumerated, conceals the atherosclerosis from the angiographer. Many active transplant centers now routinely perform intravascular ultrasound at the time of annual catheterization in all recipients. Investigations using ultrasound to detect transplant vasculopathy report a very high incidence of abnormal intimal thickening, involving 80 percent of patients at 1 year and more than 92 percent studied 4 or more years after transplantation.[65–67,79–83]

Recent studies have revealed two pathways to transplant-associated atherosclerosis. Some patients receive atherosclerotic plaques transmitted via the donor heart, while others develop an immune-mediated vasculopathy.[67,72,81] The natural history of donor lesions after transplantation is largely unknown. Since angiography is relatively insensitive, ultrasound remains the most important method used to study the early atherosclerotic lesion. In the first year after transplantation, progression occurred in 42 percent of patients.[82]

# INTERVENTIONAL CLINICAL APPLICATIONS

## Preinterventional Imaging

Several studies have demonstrated that ultrasound imaging of interventional target lesions may influence the approach to therapy. In one study (313 lesions), the intended revascularization strategy before ultrasound imaging was compared with the treatment actually performed.[42] In 40 percent of cases, the intended strategy was altered based on the ultrasound findings, most often ultrasound assessment of lesion composition or eccentricity (26 percent). Although there was a relatively close correlation between angiographic and ultrasonic lumen diameter ($r = 0.83$), a disagreement between the two methods was cited as the reason for altering the procedure in 13 percent of lesions. In another small, non-randomized study ($n = 56$) of ultrasound guidance of balloon angioplasty or directional atherectomy, operators reclassified lesion characteristics after ultrasound in 68 percent of patients and the therapeutic approach was modified in 48 percent. Ultrasound measurements revealed a smaller lumen diameter than expected from angiography, leading to balloon "upsizing" in 34 percent of angioplasty cases.[84] Several studies have purported to show benefits of ultrasound imaging prior to implantation of coronary stents.[85,86] The preliminary results of one prospective study identified vessel calcification as one of the predictors of "inadequate" stent expansion.[85] For ostial lesions, ultrasound imaging is sometimes used to determine whether the lesion involves the "true" ostium or spares the most proximal few millimeters, which may assist optimal stent positioning. When stents are used to treat dissections, ultrasound may reveal involvement of a longer segment than can be appreciated by angiography. This may be particularly relevant in bailout stenting for threatened abrupt closure, where it may be preferred to cover the full length of the dissection.[86]

Despite promising data, reports on preinterventional imaging must be interpreted with caution. There are no prospective controlled trials demonstrating a superior outcome using an preinterventional ultrasound guidance. In most studies, patients were not randomized, allowing for bias in selection of more complex cases for ultrasound guidance, which would likely emphasize the contributions of imaging. Furthermore, cases in which the operators were unable to advance the ultrasound catheter through the lesion were systematically excluded. Finally, previous studies suggesting a benefit for preinterventional imaging were performed in an era when techniques such as directional atherectomy or rotational ablation were commonly performed. The preeminence of coronary stenting has reduced the likelihood that one of these alternative revascularization approached will be performed. Accordingly, device selection using intravascular ultrasound has diminished in importance in recent years.

## Imaging during Specific Interventions

### BALLOON ANGIOPLASTY

Ultrasound guidance of balloon sizing has been proposed as a means to improve procedural result and late clinical outcome for percutaneous transluminal coronary angioplasty (PTCA).[87] In a study of 104 lesions, ultrasound was performed after obtaining a "satisfactory" angiographic result and revealed remodeling at the lesion or extensive plaque within the reference segment in 73 percent of the cases. In this subset, the balloon-to-artery ratio was increased from 1.12 ± 0.15 to 1.30 ± 0.17 ($p < 0.0001$) and the resulting angiographic minimal lumen diameter increased from 1.95 ± 0.5 to 2.21 ± 0.5 mm.

Ultrasound lumen area improved from 3.16 ± 1.0 to 4.52 ± 1.1 $mm^2$ ($p > 0.0001$). Following ultrasound-guided balloon upsizing, the incidence of angiographic dissection was not increased (37 vs. 40 percent, $p = 0.67$). However, the study was too small to demonstrate any effect upon intermediate or long-term clinical restenosis rates.

Intravascular ultrasound studies have evaluated the mechanisms of luminal enlargement following balloon angioplasty. Prior necropsy studies in patients who expired shortly after balloon angioplasty have described plaque fracture or disruption as the most common mechanism of dilatation.[20] Most ultrasound studies have confirmed that dissection is an important mechanism of luminal enlargement, occurring in 40 to 80 percent of patients.[9,41,88–92] Identification of dissection or fracture is based on the visualization of blood flow in the newly created lumen, sometimes aided by injection of saline or iodinated contrast to opacify the lumen via microbubbles. Wall disruptions can be further defined by measuring the circumferential extent, length, and/or maximal depth of the dissection. One small study reported that calcified lesions had a higher incidence of dissection (67 vs. 25 percent, $p = 0.03$) with a trend toward restenosis in lesions with no dissection.[41] Following iliac artery angioplasty, ultrasound evidence of dissection was noted in all 40 cases, accounting for 72 percent of the total lumen gain.[89]

Several alternative mechanisms for luminal enlargement not discernible by angiography have been identified using ultrasound, including arterial wall stretching and plaque compression, or "axial redistribution."[93–95] The contribution of vessel stretch to lumen gain following balloon angioplasty has been validated in experimental and clinical investigations. A peripheral angioplasty study reported that plaque area was reduced by 33 percent, accounting for only 20 percent of luminal gain.[89] However, studies using automatic pullback devices have shown that "compression" actually represents redistribution of plaque along the long axis of the vessel.[95] The prognostic significance of different mechanisms of luminal enlargement remains uncertain.

### DIRECTIONAL ATHERECTOMY

Directional coronary atherectomy (DCA) is currently performed relatively uncommonly. DCA devices incorporate a rotating circular blade to remove atherosclerotic plaque from the luminal surface.[96] Because angiographic and/or ultrasound calcification is a well-documented predictor of failure of directional atherectomy, ultrasound imaging was advocated for guidance of atherectomy, particularly for preintervention lesion selection.[97,98] Some investigators have proposed that achieving a larger lumen after atherectomy using ultrasound guidance would result in a lower restenosis rate. This hypothesis was tested in a multicenter registry (the Optimal Atherectomy Restenosis Study, or OARS), in which residual stenosis was reduced from 64 to 7 percent with ultrasound guidance.[98] The angiographic restenosis rate at 6 months was 28.9 percent and the 1-year target lesion revascularization rate was 17.8 percent. However, in the larger CAVEAT trial, DCA failed to reduce late events as compared with PTCA, with or without ultrasound guidance.[99] The success of coronary stenting in reducing restenosis has largely rendered directional atherectomy obsolete.

### ROTATIONAL ABLATION

Rotational ablation employs a high-speed (up to 200,000 rpm) diamond-coated burr to debulk atheroma. Theoretically, this device minimizes injury to the normal arterial wall by "differential cutting," in which normal elastic tissue is deflected away from the burr while relatively inelastic atheroma is not displaced and is therefore abraded by rotation of the burr. Clinical indications for rotational ablation include calcified segments or lesions that resist balloon dilatation. Rotational ablation is also sometimes used in long lesions, ostial lesions, and in-stent restenosis.[100–104] Demonstration of a heavily calcified vessel by angiography or intravascular ultrasound is often cited by operators as an indication for rotational ablation. As previously noted, there is a poor correlation between ultrasound and fluoroscopy in assessing the presence and extent of calcification. Accordingly, ultrasound is sometimes employed prior to rotational ablation to confirm or refute the presence of calcification. Vessels revascularized using rotational ablation are often diffusely diseased, and the "normal" dimension can be difficult to determine by angiography. Therefore, ultrasound is sometimes used to size the vessel and determine the largest burr that can be safely employed.

Intravascular ultrasound studies have confirmed the principle of selective plaque removal or differential cutting. In 48 lesions treated with rotational ablation, atheroma area decreased from 15.7 ± 4 to 13.0 ± 5 $mm^2$ and the arc of calcium decreased slightly from 227 ± 107 to 209 ± 107 degrees, $p < 0.05$.[104] Vessel expansion or dissection was noted in a minority of cases and did not contribute significantly to lumen gain. The residual narrowing of the cross-sectional area measured by ultrasound averaged 74 percent. Following rotational ablation, the residual lumen is usually round or ellipsoid and may have a 15 to 20 percent greater area than the largest burr used, presumably due to lateral movement of the burr during the procedure.

## Luminal Measurements Postintervention

A poor correlation has been reported for comparisons of ultrasound and angiography in assessment of residual stenosis following balloon angioplasty, with measurements that are usually smaller by ultrasound than by angiography.[9,41,88–92] Two factors probably influence the overly optimistic tendency of angiographic imaging.[21] At the reference site, angiography tends to underestimate the diameter of the normal reference vessel because of the frequent presence of unrecognized atherosclerosis. At the target site, angiography tends to overestimate the actual gain in luminal diameter because contrast material penetrates into complex cracks and fissures produced by the intervention, giving the appearance of an enlarged lumen. To calculate a postprocedure percent diameter stenosis, the diameter at the target site (an overestimate) is divided by the reference diameter (an underestimate), resulting in a more favorable impression of the actual gain in luminal dimensions. Quantitative angiography showing a residual stenosis of 10 to 15 percent is commonly associated with a 60 to 80 percent atheroma burden by intravascular ultrasound.

## Coronary Stent Deployment

### INITIAL STUDIES OF ULTRASOUND GUIDANCE

The use of stents in percutaneous revascularization has increased exponentially over the last few years. Intravascular ultrasound imaging has played a pivotal role in understanding and optimizing the benefits of stent therapy.[105–107] In initial trials leading to approval by the U.S. Food and Drug Administration (FDA), articulated slotted-tube stents were deployed using moderate balloon pressures (6 to 10 atm).[108,109] To reduce subacute thrombosis, patients received aggressive anticoagulation with both antiplatelet and antithrombotic agents, including warfarin, for 3 to 6 months. Initial studies demonstrated a reduction in the restenosis rate compared with balloon angioplasty but reported a high incidence of hemorrhagic complications and longer hospital stays. A pioneering report detailing the intravascular ultrasound experience of Colombo et al. in Milan, Italy, significantly altered the understanding of optimal stent deployment and preven-

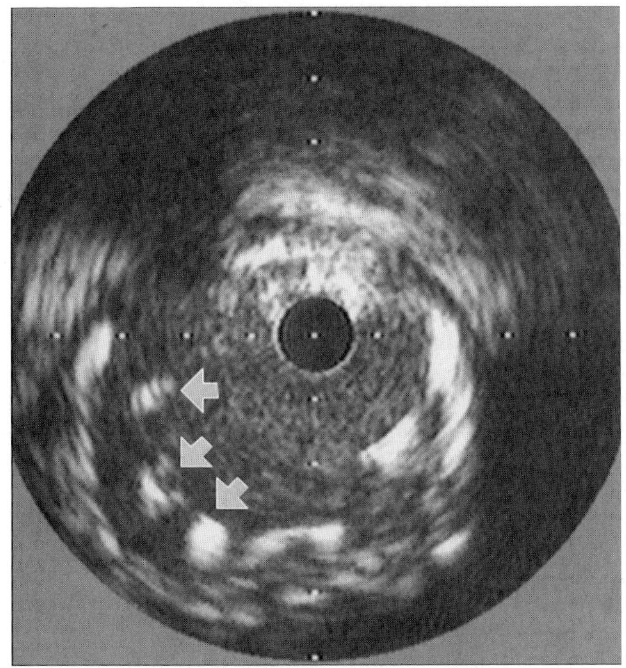

FIGURE 18-10 Underdeployed coronary stent. In this example, intravascular ultrasound images show several stent struts (*arrows*) that are not in full contact with the underlying vessel wall. This process is referred to as incomplete stent apposition.

tion of subacute thrombosis.[107] Ultrasound examination revealed a mean residual stenosis of 51 percent following angiographically guided stent deployment and a high prevalance of incomplete stent apposition (Fig. 18-10).

Because stents are porous structures, angiographic contrast can flow outside of a partially deployed stent, resulting in the angiographic appearance of full deployment despite the presence of incomplete apposition. In the Milan study, the operators performed additional balloon inflations at higher pressures (typically 18 to 20 atm) or used a larger balloon (or both), reducing final ultrasound residual stenosis to 34 percent and with a subacute thrombosis rate of only 0.3 percent using no systemic antithrombotic agents (antiplatelet therapy only). It is now widely accepted that high-pressure deployment of the stents dramatically reduces the incidence of subacute thrombosis and obviates the need for acute and chronic administration of antithrombotic agents.[110,111] Subsequently, routine high-pressure deployment without ultrasound imaging became the standard of therapy.

## ROUTINE VERSUS NONROUTINE ULTRASOUND

Following the widespread acceptance of high-pressure postdilatation with antiplatelet rather than anticoagulation regimens, the further benefit of ultrasound imaging has been debated.[86,110–114] Some investigators have suggested that despite routine use of high-pressure postdilatation, ultrasound-guided therapy could improve procedural results.[86,114] In a retrospective analysis of 315 lesions treated by high-pressure stenting, ultrasound was defined as "beneficial" if imaging resulted in further interventions that increased stent area by >25 percent or identified other lesions that required treatment.[115] Prior to ultrasound examination, the mean inflation pressure was 14.7 ± 3.2 atm, and only 47 percent of stents were considered "optimally" deployed. Additional ultrasound-triggered inflations improved in-stent lumen area by more than 25 percent in 83 lesions (26 percent of patients). Additional procedures were performed in other lesions identified by ultrasound in 51 (16 percent). Final in-stent area improved from 6.9 ± 2.2 to 8.0 ± 1.93 mm$^2$ ($p < 0.001$). Procedural results were "improved" in 39 percent of the cases following ultrasound imaging.[115] It is now generally accepted that after high-pressure coronary stenting, ultrasound imaging results in additional procedures in approximately 20 to 40 percent of cases.

Since in-stent restenosis is predominantly determined by the degree of intimal hyperplasia, a larger lumen could theoretically accommodate more tissue growth without flow-limiting obstruction.[116] However, it remains uncertain whether ultrasound-guided "optimal" expansion translates into better clinical outcome. A randomized trial in 164 patients of ultrasound-guided stenting demonstrated a 6.3 percent absolute reduction in restenosis rate, which was not statistically significant, because the study was powered to detect a 50 percent reduction of the restenosis rate.[117] A nonrandomized substudy of 538 patients from the Stent Anticoagulation Regimen Study (STARS) compared the outcome of ultrasound and angiographically guided stenting. The ultrasound arm achieved a significantly larger lumen area and a 39 percent relative reduction in clinical restenosis.[118] However, the impact of the more aggressive dilatation on restenosis rates has not been adequately examined by properly designed, prospective randomized clinical trials.

## ULTRASOUND IMAGING OF PERI-STENT SEGMENTS

Ultrasound imaging of reference segments following stenting may be useful in identifying reference segment disease or dissections that require additional interventions. The presence of significant peri-stent flow-limiting lesions or dissections has been linked to higher likelihood of stent thrombosis.[119] These findings are often angiographically occult or appear as areas of indistinct haziness at the vessel border. In 201 stent patients, 31 segments with peri-stent angiographic haziness were detected. Ultrasound imaging revealed an angiographically inapparent obstructive lesion in 15, a peri-stent wall injury in 14, and mild intimal thickening in the remaining 2 segments.[120] The extent of neointimal hyperplasia at the stent margins has been linked to preexisting disease in the reference segment.[121] In stenting as a bailout for dissection, intravascular ultrasound is more sensitive in detecting the extent of dissection, often revealing a greater true length than is evident from angiography, which may be helpful in guiding vessel salvage.

## OPTIMAL PROCEDURAL GOALS OF ULTRASOUND GUIDED STENTING

Although ultrasound guidance of stenting has been practiced for several years, there is no consensus regarding optimal procedural endpoints. Colombo initially recommended achieving ≥60 percent of the average proximal and distal reference areas but later altered the definition to ≥100 percent of the distal reference lumen area.[105–107] Other definitions of optimal expansion include ≥90 percent of the distal reference area, ≥80 percent or ≥90 percent of the average reference area, a "lumen symmetry index" >0.7, and/or full coverage of reference-segment disease or dissections.[122,123] In most clinical trials, procedural endpoints are not achieved in the majority of cases. In the Optimal Stent Implantation Trial, the target of >90 percent of the average reference or >100 percent of the smaller reference area were not achieved in half the patients at an inflation pressure of 15 atm and only 60 percent of patients at 18 atm.[122] In the Angiography Versus Intravascular Ultrasound Directed Stent Placement (AVID) trial, the target endpoint of ≥90 percent of the distal reference area was not achieved in >70 percent of 225 patients.[124]

Other reports have questioned the clinical relevance of using the stent-to-reference ratios as target for ultrasound-guided stenting. In

165 patients, target vessel revascularization was predicted by final in-stent lumen area (OR 1.4, 95 percent CI 1.1 to 1.9) and not the ratio of stent-to-reference area (OR 1.1, 95 percent CI 0.85 to 1.6).[112] Repeat revascularization was required in 30 percent of patients with a minimum in-stent lumen area $<5$ mm$^2$ but only 3 percent of cases with an area exceeding 9 mm$^2$. In another large cohort undergoing ultrasound-guided stenting, restenosis was inversely related to the minimum in-stent area.[125] An area of 9 mm$^2$ was achieved in 23 percent, but the incidence of restenosis in this subgroup was only 8 percent, compared with 29 percent in the remaining patients, $p < 0.0001$. Thus, commonly employed ultrasound endpoints based upon a predefined stent-to-reference ratio are both difficult to achieve and correlate weakly with clinical outcome.[125–127] Ultrasound studies have demonstrated that the degree of in-stent neointimal hyperplasia is independent of final lumen size, which may explain the higher restenosis rates in smaller vessels and poorly expanded stents.[116] If acute lumen gain is not adequate to accommodate subsequent tissue proliferation, there is significant late loss and restenosis.

## Intravascular Ultrasound and Restenosis

A more complete understanding of restenosis has evolved from serial ultrasound measurements of plaque and lumen areas following balloon angioplasty and directional atherectomy.[128,129] In some studies, serial ultrasound examinations have shown that a late reduction in total vessel area (chronic negative remodeling) is an important mechanism of restenosis after interventional procedures.[129] These observations suggest that mechanical interventions to prevent chronic recoil (such as stenting) may be more important in preventing restenosis than interventions designed to prevent intimal hyperplasia. This concept likely explains the lower restenosis rate observed in randomized multicenter studies comparing balloon angioplasty and stent implantation.[108,109]

In 212 native coronary lesions in 209 patients following intervention, the ultrasound cross-sectional area with the smallest lumen area at late follow-up was compared with the matching site obtained immediately following the intervention.[129] At follow-up examination, there was a significant decrease in EEM area and an increase in plaque area ($p < 0.0001$ for both) that combined to reduce lumen area. More than 70 percent of lumen loss was attributable to the decrease in EEM area, whereas the neointimal area accounted for only 23 percent of the decrease in lumen area. The change in lumen area correlated more strongly with the change in EEM area ($r = 0.75, p < 0.0001$) than with the change in plaque area ($r = 0.28, p < 0.0001$). At lesions that demonstrated an increase in EEM area at follow-up (47 percent), there was no change or an actual gain in lumen area and a reduction in angiographic restenosis (26 versus 62 percent for lesions with a decrease in EEM area at follow-up, $p < 0.0001$).

Other investigators have suggested a bidirectional remodeling response following percutaneous coronary interventions: early adaptive enlargement and late shrinkage of the vessel. In a unique study, 61 lesions in 57 patients who underwent balloon angioplasty or atherectomy were examined by intravascular ultrasound in a serial manner before and immediately after the intervention and after 24 h, 1 month, and 6 months.[48] The lumen area significantly improved during the first month following the intervention, but significantly decreased at 6 months. Simultaneously, the EEM area increased in the first month, but later decreased at 6 months. However, plaque area steadily increased from immediately postintervention to the 6-month follow-up. Thus the changes in lumen size closely tracked the changes in EEM area ($r = 0.72, p = 0.0001$). Although the increase in plaque area correlated with lumen loss, the correlation was not as strong ($r = 0.34, p = 0.0008$). The lumen gain observed during the first month was solely due to the compensatory vessel enlargement, whereas the late lumen loss was mostly caused by vessel shrinkage but also by progressive neointimal hyperplasia.

Investigations employing quantitative angiography have demonstrated that late lumen loss is significantly greater with stents than with balloon angioplasty. This, however, is offset by the much larger acute lumen gain, such that the net gain at follow-up is significantly greater with stenting.[108,109] Intravascular ultrasound has been employed to examine the mechanism of stent restenosis. Unlike the restenotic response to other percutaneous devices, which is a mixture of arterial remodeling and neointimal growth, stent restenosis is almost exclusively due to the neointimal proliferation.[129] In a serial study using intravascular ultrasound of stented coronary segments, there was no significant change in the area bound by stent struts, indicating that stents can withstand and resist the arterial remodeling process.[130] In some cases, restenosis develops at the margins of the stent. Predictors of stent restenosis have been identified by multivariate analysis, including the smaller reference vessel and lumen size, the larger plaque burden at the reference segments, and the smaller achieved in-stent lumen area at the stent margins.[121]

## Intravascular Ultrasound and Brachytherapy

Ultrasound has proven useful in clarifying the mechanisms of benefit and refining the techniques used for brachytherapy.[130,131] Intravascular ultrasound studies demonstrate that radiation inhibits neointimal proliferation within a stent. In a randomized study of 70 lesions with in-stent restenosis, at follow-up, 79 percent of stents in patients who received radiation had no measureable intimal proliferation, compared to 27 percent of those randomized to the "no radiation" cohort.[130] In the nonstented segments, some studies suggest that radiation initiates a process of vessel expansion (a type of positive remodeling).[131] These effects are strongly influenced by the dose delivered to the media or adventitia, which is dependent on the thickness and composition of the atheroma and the position of the catheter in the lumen. Current research is examining whether an ultrasound image-based dosing algorithm will be required to optimize therapeutic benefit. Ultrasound has already demonstrated the potential for radiation to accelerate restenosis at the edges of the treatment region where the dosing falls off ("candy-wrapper" effect).[131]

## Intravascular Ultrasound and Drug-Eluting Stents

Intravascular ultrasound has proven useful in assessing the mechanism of benefit of drug-eluting stents.[132,133] Studies consistently demonstrate that drug-eluting stents have the potential to markedly reduce neointimal proliferation within the stent at 6 to 9 months follow-up. In the RAVEL trial, a subset of 95 patients underwent intravascular ultrasound examination 6 months following stent implantation. The patients who received a sirolimus-eluting stent exhibited an average of only 2 mm$^3$ of intimal hyperplasia compared to 37 mm$^3$ for the control group ($p < 0001$).[132] More recently, similar although less pronounced results were reported for a paclitaxel-eluting stent.[133] Using paclitaxel, investigators reported a dose-dependent reduction in intimal hyperplasia at 4 to 6 months from 31 mm$^3$ in the control arm to 18 mm$^3$ in a low-dose cohort to 13 mm$^3$ in the highest dose paclitaxel group.

# FUTURE DIRECTIONS

Intravascular ultrasound is commonly but not routinely performed in the United States during coronary interventions. Approximately 5 to 8 percent of interventional procedures are currently performed with ultrasound guidance. Usage in Europe is considerably less than in the United States; in Japan it is considerably higher, reflecting differing reimbursement rates and practice patterns. Technical developments in both catheters and systems are continuing, but at a relatively slow pace.[134] Additional technologic advances in intravascular imaging are anticipated, including further reductions in the size of imaging catheters and higher-frequency ultrasound catheters, yielding significantly better spatial resolution.[135] Although high-frequency probes enable better axial and lateral resolution, there are significant tradeoffs in moving beyond the current 40-MHz frequency. For example, penetration is likely to be impaired in comparison with more conventional devices, and greater backscatter from blood cells at high frequencies may interfere with discrimination of the interface between lumen and vessel wall.

As previously discussed, analysis of backscattered ultrasound signals has been employed by several investigators to perform "tissue characterization."[39,40] Intrinsic properties of the backscattered ultrasound signals—including the amplitude distribution, frequency response, and power spectrum of the signal—may convey specific information about tissue types.[39] However, the ability of computer-based analysis of the unprocessed radiofrequency backscatter to differentiate the histologic layers of the normal vessel wall remains investigational. The promise of this research is the potential to identify "vulnerable" atherosclerotic plaques, defined as lesions at high risk for plaque rupture leading to thrombosis and acute coronary syndromes.

Three-dimensional reconstruction of intravascular ultrasound has been proposed as a means to facilitate understanding of the spatial relationship between the structures within different tomographic cross sections.[136,137] Despite the promise of these methods, many unresolved problems remain. The algorithms applied for three-dimensional reconstruction do not consider the presence of curvatures of the vessel and assume that the catheter passes in a straight line through the center of consecutive cross sections. The systolic expansion of the coronary vessel and the movements of the catheter within the vessel during the cardiac cycle also generate artifacts. Accordingly, the reconstructed images should not be considered faithful representations of the vessel and should not be used for volumetric plaque determination.

## SUMMARY

The equipment, technique, and applications for intravascular ultrasound imaging continue to evolve. The insights provided by the unique ability of intravascular ultrasound to directly image coronary plaques have contributed greatly to our understanding of the nature of atherosclerosis and the effects of interventional devices. Current studies using intravascular ultrasound to measure atherosclerosis progression and regression have the potential to further expand the utility of this important diagnostic method.

## References


1. Bom N, Lancee CT, Van Egmond FC. An ultrasonic intracardiac scanner. *Ultrasonics* 1972;10:72–76.
2. Yock PG, Johnson EL, Linker DT. Intravascular ultrasound: Development and clinical potential. *Am J Cardiac Imaging* 1988;2: 185–193.
3. Roelandt JR, Bom NY, Serruys PW. Intravascular high-resolution real-time, two-dimensional echocardiography. *Int J Cardiac Imaging* 1989;4:63–67.
4. Hodgson JM, Graham SP, Savakus AD, et al. Clinical percutaneous imaging of coronary anatomy using an over-the-wire ultrasound catheter system. *Int J Cardiac Imaging* 1989;4:187–193.
5. Nissen SE, Grines CL, Gurley JC, et al. Application of a new phased-array ultrasound imaging catheter in the assessment of vascular dimensions: In vivo comparison to cineangiography. *Circulation* 1990;81:660–666.
6. Tobis JM, Mallery J, Mahon D, et al. Intravascular ultrasound imaging of human coronary arteries in vivo. *Circulation* 1991;83:913–926.
7. Nissen SE, Gurley JC, Grines CL, et al. Intravascular ultrasound assessment of lumen size and wall morphology in normal subjects and patients with coronary artery disease. *Circulation* 1991;84:1087–1099.
8. Nissen SE, Di Mario C, Tuzcu EM. Intravascular ultrasound, angioscopy, Doppler, and pressure measurement. In: Topol EJ, ed. *Topol Cardiovascular Medicine*. Philadelphia: Lippincott-Raven; 1997.
9. Tobis JM, Mallery JA, Gessert J, et al. Intravascular ultrasound cross-sectional arterial imaging before and after balloon angioplasty in vitro. *Circulation* 1989;80:873–882.
10. Topol EJ, Nissen SE. Our preoccupation with coronary luminology: The dissociation between clinical and angiographic findings in ischemic heart disease. *Circulation* 1995;92:2333–2342.
11. Hodgson JM, Reddy KG, Suneja R, et al. Intracoronary ultrasound imaging: Correlation of plaque morphology with angiography, clinical syndrome and procedural results in patients undergoing coronary angioplasty. *J Am Coll Cardiol* 1993;21:35–44.
12. Arnett EN, Isner JM, Redwood CR, et al. Coronary artery narrowing in coronary heart disease: Comparison of cineangiographic and necropsy findings. *Ann Intern Med* 1979;91:350–356.
13. Grodin CM, Dydra I, Pastgernac A, et al. Discrepancies between cineangiographic and post-mortem findings in patients with coronary artery disease and recent myocardial revascularization. *Circulation* 1974;49:703–709.
14. Isner JM, Kishel J, Kent KM. Accuracy of angiographic determination of left main coronary arterial narrowing. *Circulation* 1981;63:1056–1061.
15. Vlodaver Z, Frech R, van Tassel RA, Edwards JE. Correlation of the antemortem coronary angiogram and the postmortem specimen. *Circulation* 1973;47:162–168.
16. Zir LM, Miller SW, Dinsmore RE, et al. Interobserver variability in coronary angiography. *Circulation* 1976;53:627–632.
17. Galbraith JE, Murphy ML, Desoyza N. Coronary angiogram interpretation: Interobserver variability. *JAMA* 1981;240:2053–2059.
18. Roberts WC, Jones AA. Quantitation of coronary arterial narrowing at necropsy in sudden coronary death. *Am J Cardiol* 1979;44:39–44.
19. White CW, Wright CB, Doty DB, et al. Does visual interpretation of the coronary arteriogram predict the physiologic importance of a coronary stenosis? *N Engl J Med* 1984;310:819–824.
20. Waller BF. "Crackers, breakers, stretchers, drillers, scrapers, shavers, burners, welders, and melters": The future treatment of atherosclerotic coronary artery disease? A clinical-morphologic assessment. *J Am Coll Cardiol* 1989;13:969–987.
21. Topol EJ, Nissen SE. Our preoccupation with coronary luminology: The dissociation between clinical and angiographic findings in ischemic heart disease. *Circulation* 1995;92:2333–2342.
22. Glagov S, Weisenberg E, Zarins CK, et al. Compensatory enlargement of human coronary arteries. *N Engl J Med* 1987;316:1371–1375.
23. Little WC, Constantinescu M, Applegate RJ, et al. Can arteriography predict the site of a subsequent myocardial infarction in patients with mild-to-moderate coronary artery disease? *Circulation* 1988;78: 1157–1166.
24. Yamagishi M, Miyatake K, Tamai J, et al. Detection of atherosclerosis at the site of focal vasospasm in angiographically normal or minimally narrowed coronary segments by intravascular ultrasound. *J Am Coll Cardiol* 1994;23:352–357.
25. Nissen SE, Gurley JC. Application of intravascular ultrasound to detection and quantitation of coronary atherosclerosis. *Int J Cardiac Imaging* 1991;6:165–177.
26. Nissen SE, DeFranco A, Tuzcu EM. Detection and quantification of atherosclerosis: The emerging role for intravascular ultrasound. In: Fuster V, ed. *Syndromes of Atherosclerosis: Correlations of Clinical Imaging and Pathology*. Armonk, NY: Futura; 1996:291.

27. TenHoff H, Korbijn A, Smit ThH, et al. Image artifacts in mechanically driven ultrasound catheters. *Int J Cardiac Imaging* 1989;4:195–199.
28. Di Mario C, Madretsma S, Linker D, et al. The angle of incidence of the ultrasonic beam: A critical factor for the image quality in intravascular ultrasonography. *Am Heart J* 1993;125:442–448.
29. Hausmann D, Erbel R, Alibelli-Chemarin MJ, et al. The safety of intracoronary ultrasound: A multicenter survey of 2207 examinations. *Circulation* 1995;91:623–630.
30. Batkoff BW, Linker DT. Safety of intracoronary ultrasound: Data from a multicenter European registry. *Cathet Cardiovasc Diagn* 1996; 38:238–241.
31. Pinto FJ, St Goar FG, Gao SZ, et al. Immediate and one-year safety of intracoronary ultrasonic imaging: Evaluation with serial quantitative angiography. *Circulation* 1993;88:1709–1714.
32. Gussenhoven EJ, Essed CE, Lancee CT, et al. Arterial wall characteristics determined by intravascular ultrasound imaging: An in vitro study. *J Am Coll Cardiol* 1989;4:947–952.
33. Potkin BN, Bartorelli AL, Gessert JM, et al. Coronary artery imaging with intravascular high-frequency ultrasound. *Circulation* 1990;81: 1575–1585.
34. Nishimura RA, Edwards WD, Warnes CA, et al. Intravascular ultrasound imaging: In vitro validation and pathologic correlation. *J Am Coll Cardiol* 1990;16:145–154.
35. Fitzgerald PJ, St Goar FG, Connolly AJ, et al. Intravascular ultrasound imaging of coronary arteries: Are three layers the norm? *Circulation* 1992;86:154–158.
36. St Goar FG, Pinto FJ, Alderman EL, et al. Intravascular ultrasound imaging of angiographically normal coronary arteries: An in vivo comparison with quantitative angiography. *J Am Coll Cardiol* 1991;18:952–958.
37. Velican D, Velican C. Comparative study on age-related changes and atherosclerotic involvement of the coronary arteries of male and female subjects up to 40 years of age. *Atherosclerosis* 1981;38: 39–50.
38. Maheswaran B, Leung CY, Gutfinger DE, et al. Intravascular ultrasound appearance of normal and mildly diseased coronary arteries: Correlation with histologic specimens. *Am Heart J* 1995; 130:976–986.
39. Bridal SL, Fornes P, Bruneval P, Berger G. Parametric (integrated backscatter and attenuation) images constructed using backscattered radio frequency signals (25–56 MHz) from human aortae in vitro. *Ultrasound Med Biol* 1997;23:215–229.
40. Nair A, Kuban BD, Tuzcu EM, et al. Coronary plaque classification with intravascular ultrasound radiofrequency data analysis. *Circulation* 2002;106(17):2200–2206.
41. Mintz GS, Popma JJ, Pichard AD, et al. Patterns of calcification in coronary artery disease: A statistical analysis of intravascular ultrasound and coronary angiography in 1,155 lesions. *Circulation* 1995;91:1959–1965.
42. Tuzcu EM, Berkalp B, DeFranco AC, et al. The dilemma of diagnosing coronary calcification: Angiography versus intravascular ultrasound. *J Am Coll Cardiol* 1996;27:832–838.
43. Honye J, Mahon DJ, Jain A, et al. Morphological effects of coronary balloon angioplasty in vivo assessed by intravascular ultrasound imaging. *Circulation* 1992;85:1012–1025.
44. Mintz GS, Pichard AD, Kovach JA, et al. Impact of preintervention intravascular ultrasound imaging on transcatheter treatment strategies in coronary artery disease. *Am J Cardiol* 1994;73:423–430.
45. Hermiller JB, Tenaglia AN, Kisslo KB, et al. In vivo validation of compensatory enlargement of atherosclerotic coronary arteries. *Am J Cardiol* 1993;71:665–668.
46. Ge J, Erbel R, Zamorano J, et al. Coronary artery remodeling in atherosclerotic disease: An intravascular ultrasonic study in vivo. *Coron Artery Dis* 1993;4:981–986.
47. Losordo DW, Rosenfield K, Kaufman J, et al. Focal compensatory enlargement of human arteries in response to progressive atherosclerosis: In vivo documentation using intravascular ultrasound. *Circulation* 1994;89:2570–2577.
48. Pasterkamp G, Wensing PJ, Post MJ, et al. Paradoxical arterial wall shrinkage may contribute to luminal narrowing of human atherosclerotic femoral arteries. *Circulation* 1995;91:1444–1449.
49. Mintz GS, Kent KM, Pichard AD, et al. Contribution of inadequate arterial remodeling to the development of focal coronary artery stenoses: An intravascular ultrasound study. *Circulation* 1997;95: 1791–1798.
50. Kimura T, Kaburagi S, Tamura T, et al. Remodeling of human coronary arteries undergoing coronary angioplasty or atherectomy. *Circulation* 1997;96:475–483.
51. Richardson PD, Davies MJ, Born GV. Influence of plaque configuration and stress distribution on fissuring of coronary atherosclerotic plaques. *Lancet* 1989;2:941–944.
52. Kalbfleisch SJ, McGillem MJ, Simon SB, et al. Automated quantitation of indexes of coronary lesion complexity: Comparison between patients with stable and unstable angina. *Circulation* 1990;82:439–447.
53. Ambrose JA, Winters SL, Arora RR, et al. Angiographic evolution of coronary artery morphology in unstable angina. *J Am Coll Cardiol* 1986;7:472–478.
54. Loree HM, Kamm RD, Stringfellow RG, Lee RT. Effects of fibrous cap thickness on peak circumferential stress in model atherosclerotic vessels. *Circ Res* 1992;71:850–858.
55. Levin DC, Fallon JT. Significance of the angiographic morphology of localized coronary stenoses: Histopathologic correlations. *Circulation* 1982;66:316–320.
56. Ambrose JA, Winters SL, Stern A, et al. Angiographic morphology and the pathogenesis of unstable angina pectoris. *J Am Coll Cardiol* 1985;5:609–616.
57. Shoenhagen P, Ziada KM, Kapadia SR, et al. Extent and direction of arterial remodeling in stable versus unstable coronary syndromes: An intravascular ultrasound study. *Circulation* 2000;101:598–603.
58. Siegel RJ, Ariani M, Fishbein MC, et al. Histopathologic validation of angioscopy and intravascular ultrasound. *Circulation* 1991;84: 109–117.
59. Bocksch W, Schartl M, Beckmann S, et al. Intravascular ultrasound imaging in patients with acute myocardial infarction. *Eur Heart J* 1995;16(suppl J):46–52.
60. Mintz G. Nissen SE, Anderson WD, et al. Standards for the acquisition measurement and reporting of intravascular ultrasound studies. *J Am Coll Cardiol* 2001;37(5):1478–1479.
61. Wong M, Edelstein J, Wollman J, Bond MG. Ultrasonic-pathological comparison of the human arterial wall: Verification of intima-media thickness. *Arterioscler Thromb* 1993;13:482–486.
62. Potkin BN, Bartorelli AL, Gessert JM, et al. Coronary artery imaging with intravascular high-frequency ultrasound. *Circulation* 1990; 81:1575–1585.
63. Tuzcu EM, Hobbs H, Rincon G, et al. Occult and frequent transmission of atherosclerosis coronary disease with cardiac transplantation. *Circulation* 1995;91:1706–1713.
64. Mehra MR, Ventura HO, Stapleton DD, Smart FW. The prognostic significance of intimal proliferation in cardiac allograft vasculopathy: A paradigm shift (review). *J Heart Lung Transplant* 1995;14(6 Pt 2): S207–S211.
65. Escobar A, Ventura HO, Stapleton DD, et al. Cardiac allograft vasculopathy assessed by intravascular ultrasonography and nonimmunologic risk factors. *Am J Cardiol* 1994;74:1042–1046.
66. Rickenbacher PR, Pinto FJ, Chenzbraun A, et al. Incidence and severity of transplant coronary artery disease early and up to 15 years after transplantation as detected by intravascular ultrasound. *J Am Coll Cardiol* 1995;25:171–177.
67. Tuzcu EM. DeFranco AC, Goormastic M, et al. Dichotomous pattern of coronary atherosclerosis 1 to 9 years after transplantation: Insights from systematic intravascular ultrasound imaging. *J Am Coll Cardiol* 1996;27:839–846.
68. Nissen SE: Application of intravascular ultrasound to characterize coronary artery disease and assess the progression or regression of atherosclerosis. *Am J Cardiol* 2001;87(4A):15A–20A.

69. Mintz GS, Popma JJ, Pichard AD, et al. Limitations of angiography in the assessment of plaque distribution in coronary artery disease: A systematic study of target lesion eccentricity in 1446 lesions. *Circulation* 1996;93:924–931.
70. Erbel R, Ge J, Bockisch A, et al. Value of intracoronary ultrasound and Doppler in the differentiation of angiographically normal coronary arteries: A prospective study in patients with angina pectoris. *Eur Heart J* 1996;17:880–889.
71. Mintz GS, Painter JA, Pichard AD, et al. Atherosclerosis in angiographically "normal" coronary artery reference segments: An intravascular ultrasound study with clinical correlations. *J Am Coll Cardiol* 1995;25:1479–1485.
72. Tuzcu EM, Kapadia SR, Tutar E, et al. High Prevalence of coronary atherosclerosis in asymptomatic teenagers and young adults: Evidence from intravascular ultrasound. *Circulation* 2001;103:2705–2710.
73. Lee DY, Eigler N, Luo H, et al. Effect of intracoronary ultrasound imaging on clinical decision making. *Am Heart J* 1995;129: 1084–1093.
74. Mintz GS, Pichard AD, Kovach JA, et al. Impact of preintervention intravascular ultrasound imaging on transcatheter treatment strategies in coronary artery disease. *Am J Cardiol* 1994;73:423–430.
75. Hermiller JB, Buller CE, Tenaglia AN, et al. Unrecognized left main coronary artery disease in patients undergoing interventional procedures. *Am J Cardiol* 1993;71:173–176.
76. Uretsky BF, Kormos RL, Zerbe TR, et al. Cardiac events after heart transplantation: Incidence and predictive value of coronary arteriography. *J Heart Transplant* 1992;11:S45–S50.
77. O'Neill BJ, Pflugfelder PW, Single NR, et al. Frequency of angiographic detection and quantitative assessment of coronary arterial disease one and three years after cardiac transplantation. *Am J Cardiol* 1989;63:1221–1226.
78. Johnson DE, Alderman EL, Schroeder JS, et al. Transplant coronary artery disease: Histopathological correlations with angiographic morphology. *J Am Coll Cardiol* 1991;17:449–457.
79. Yeung AC, Davis SF, Hauptman PJ, et al. Incidence and progression of transplant coronary artery disease over 1 year: Results of a multicenter trial with use of intravascular ultrasound. Multicenter Intravascular Ultrasound Transplant Study Group. *J Heart Lung Transplant* 1995;14(suppl 6):S215–S220.
80. Kerber S, Rahmel A, Heinemann-Vechtel O, et al. Angiographic, intravascular ultrasound and functional findings early after orthotopic heart transplantation. *Int J Cardiol* 1995;49:119–129.
81. St Goar FG, Pinto FJ, Alderman EL, et al. Detection of coronary atherosclerosis in young adult hearts using intravascular ultrasound. *Circulation* 1992;86:756–763.
82. Kapadia SR, Nissen SE, Ziada KM, et al. Development of transplant vasculopathy and progression of donor-transmitted atherosclerosis: A comparison by serial intravascular ultrasound imaging. *Circulation* 1998;8:2672–2678.
83. Kapadia SR, Crowe TD, Ziada KM, et al. Natural history of donor transmitted atherosclerosis in transplant patients: Serial intravascular ultrasound study. *J Am Coll Cardiol* 1998;31:856–862.
84. Impact of intravascular ultrasound on device selection and endpoint assessment of interventions: Phase I of the GUIDE trial (abstr). *J Am Coll Cardiol* 1993;21:134A.
85. Hoffmann R, Mintz GS, Popma JJ, et al. Treatment of calcified coronary lesions with Palmaz-Schatz stents: An intravascular ultrasound study. *Eur Heart J* 1998;19:1224–1231.
86. Russo RJ. Ultrasound-guided stent placement. *Cardiol Clin* 1997;15:49–61.
87. Stone GW, Hodgson JM, St Goar FG, et al. Improved procedural results of coronary angioplasty with intravascular ultrasound-guided balloon sizing: The CLOUT pilot trial: Clinical Outcomes with Ultrasound Trial (CLOUT) investigators. *Circulation* 1997;95:2044–2052.
88. Gil R, Di Mario C, Prati F, et al. Influence of plaque composition on mechanisms of percutaneous transluminal coronary balloon angioplasty assessed by ultrasound imaging. *Am Heart J* 1996;131: 591–597.
89. Losordo DW, Rosenfield K, Pieczek A, et al. How does angioplasty work? Serial analysis of human iliac arteries using intravascular ultrasound. *Circulation* 1992;86:1845–1858.
90. Potkin BN, Keren G, Mintz GS, et al. Arterial responses to balloon coronary angioplasty: An intravascular ultrasound study. *J Am Coll Cardiol* 1992;20:942–951.
91. Braden GA, Herrington DM, Downes TR, et al. Qualitative and quantitative contrasts in the mechanisms of lumen enlargement by coronary balloon angioplasty and directional coronary atherectomy. *J Am Coll Cardiol* 1994;23:40–48.
92. van der Lugt A, Gussenhoven EJ, Stijnen T, et al. Comparison of intravascular ultrasonic findings after coronary balloon angioplasty evaluated in vitro with histology. *Am J Cardiol* 1995;76:661–666.
93. Mintz GS, Pichard AD, Kent KM, et al. Axial plaque redistribution as a mechanism of percutaneous transluminal coronary angioplasty. *Am J Cardiol* 1996;77:427–430.
94. Botas J, Clark DA, Pinto F, et al. Balloon angioplasty results in increased segmental coronary distensibility: A likely mechanism of percutaneous transluminal coronary angioplasty. *J Am Coll Cardiol* 1994;23:1043–1052.
95. Mintz GS, Pichard AD, Kent KM, et al. Axial plaque redistribution as a mechanism of percutaneous transluminal coronary angioplasty. *Am J Cardiol* 1996;77:427–430.
96. Simpson JB, Selmon MR, Robertson GC, et al. Transluminal atherectomy for occlusive peripheral vascular disease. *Am J Cardiol* 1988;61:96G–101G.
97. Matar FA, Mintz GS, Pinnow E, et al. Multivariate predictors of intravascular ultrasound end points after directional coronary atherectomy. *J Am Coll Cardiol* 1995;25:318–324.
98. Simonton CA, Leon MB. Baim DS, et al. "Optimal" directional coronary atherectomy: Final results of the Optimal Atherectomy Restenosis Study (OARS). *Circulation* 1998;97:332–339.
99. Topol EJ, Leya F, Pinkerton CA, et al., on behalf of the CAVEAT Study Group. A comparison of coronary angioplasty with directional atherectomy in patients with coronary artery disease. *N Engl J Med* 1993;329:221–227.
100. MacIsaac AI, Bass TA, Buchbinder M, et al. High speed rotational atherectomy: Outcome in calcified and noncalcified coronary artery lesions. *J Am Coll Cardiol* 1995;26:731–736.
101. De Franco AC, Nissen SE, Tuzcu EM, Whitlow PL. Incremental value of intravascular ultrasound during rotational coronary atherectomy. *Catheter Cardiovasc Diagn* 1996;(suppl 3):23–33.
102. Sharma SK, Duvvuri S, Dangas G, et al. Rotational atherectomy for in-stent restenosis: Acute and long-term results of the first 100 cases. *J Am Coll Cardiol* 1998;32:1358–1365.
103. Schiele F, Meneveau N, Vuillemenot A, et al. Treatment of in-stent restenosis with high speed rotational atherectomy and IVUS guidance in small 3.0 mm vessels. *Catheter Cardiovasc Diagn* 1998;44:77–82.
104. Kovach JA, Mintz GS, Pichard AD, et al. Sequential intravascular ultrasound characterization of the mechanisms of rotational atherectomy and adjunct balloon angioplasty. *J Am Coll Cardiol* 1993;22:1024–1032.
105. Nakamura S, Colombo A, Galglione S, et al. Intracoronary ultrasound observations during stent implantation. *Circulation* 1994;89: 2026–2034.
106. Goldberg SL, Colombo A, Nakamura S, et al. Benefit of intracoronary ultrasound in the deployment of Palmaz-Schatz stents. *J Am Coll Cardiol* 1994;24:996–1003.
107. Colombo A, Hall P, Nakamura S, et al. Intracoronary stenting without anticoagulation accomplished with intravascular ultrasound guidance. *Circulation* 1995;91:1676–1688.
108. Serruys PW, de Jaegere P, Kiemeneij F, et al, on behalf of the Benestent Study Group. A comparison of balloon-expandable-stent implantation with balloon angioplasty in patients with coronary artery disease. *N Engl J Med* 1994;331:489–495.
109. Fischman DL, Leon MB, Baim DS, et al. A randomized comparison of coronary-stent placement and balloon angioplasty in the treatment of coronary artery disease. *N Engl J Med* 1994;331:496–501.

110. Morice MC, Breton C, Bunouf P, et al. Coronary stenting without anticoagulation, without intravascular ultrasound: Results of the French registry. *Circulation* 1995;92(suppl I):I-796.
111. Sandardas MA, McEniery PT, Aroney CN, Bett JHN. Elective implantation of intracoronary stents without intravascular ultrasound guidance or subsequent warfarin. *Catheter Cardiovasc Diagn* 1996; 37:355–359.
112. Goods CM, Al-Shaibi KF, Yadav SS, et al. Utilization of the coronary balloon-expandable coil stent without anticoagulation or intravascular ultrasound. *Circulation* 1996;93:1803–1808.
113. Karrillon GJ, Morice MC, Benveniste E, et al. Intracoronary stent implantation without ultrasound guidance and with replacement of conventional anticoagulation by antiplatelet therapy. 30-day clinical outcome of the French Multicenter Registry. *Circulation* 1996; 94:1519–1527.
114. Prati F, Gil R, Di Mario C, et al. Is quantitative angiography sufficient to guide stent implantation? A comparison with three-dimensional reconstruction of intracoronary ultrasound images. *G Ital Cardiol* 1997;27:328–336.
115. Allen KM, Undemir C, Shaknovich A, et al. Is there need for intravascular ultrasound after high pressure dilatation of Palmaz-Schatz stents (abstr). *J Am Coll Cardiol* 1996;27:138A.
116. Hoffmann R, Mintz GS, Pichard AD, et al. Intimal hyperplasia thickness at follow-up is independent of stent size: A serial intravascular ultrasound study. *Am J Cardiol* 1998;82:1168–1172.
117. Schiele F, Meneveau N, Vuillemenot A, et al. Impact of intravascular ultrasound guidance in stent deployment on 6-month restenosis rate: A multicenter, randomized study comparing two strategies—With and without intravascular ultrasound guidance. RESIST Study Group (REStenosis after IVUS guided STenting). *J Am Coll Cardiol* 1998;32:320–328.
118. Fitzgerald PJ, Oshima A, Hayase M, et al, for the CRUISE investigators. Final results of the Can Routine Ultrasound Influence Stent Expansion (CRUISE) study. *Circulation* 2000;102:523–530.
119. Schuhlen H, Hadamitzky M, Walter H, et al. Major benefit from antiplatelet therapy for patients at high risk for adverse cardiac events after coronary Palmaz-Schatz stent placement: Analysis of a prospective risk stratification protocol in the Intracoronary Stenting and Antithrombotic Regimen (ISAR) trial. *Circulation* 1997;95:2015–2021.
120. Ziada KM, Tuzcu EM, De Franco AC, et al. Intravascular ultrasound assessment of the prevalence and causes of angiographic "haziness" following high-pressure coronary stenting. *Am J Cardiol* 1997; 80:116–121.
121. Hoffmann R, Mintz GS, Kent KM, et al. Serial intravascular ultrasound predictors of restenosis at the margins of Palmaz-Schatz stents. *Am J Cardiol* 1997;79:951–953.
122. de Jaegere P, Mudra H, Figulla H, et al. Intravascular ultrasound-guided optimized stent deployment: Immediate and 6 months clinical and angiographic results from the Multicenter Ultrasound Stenting in Coronaries Study (MUSIC Study). *Eur Heart J* 1998;19:1214–1223.
123. Stone GW, St Goar F, Fitzgerald P, et al. The Optimal Stent Implantation Trial: Final core lab angiographic and ultrasound analysis (abstr). *J Am Coll Cardiol* 1997;29:369A.
124. Russo RJ, Nicosia A, Teirstein PS, Investigators AVID. Angiography versus intravascular ultrasound-directed stent placement. *J Am Coll Cardiol* 1997;29:369A.
125. Kasaoka S, Tobis JM, Akiyama T, et al. Angiographic and intravascular ultrasound predictors of in-stent restenosis. *J Am Coll Cardiol* 1998;32:1630–1635.
126. Ziada KM, Tuzcu EM, De Franco AC, et al. Absolute, not relative, post-stent lumen area is a better predictor of clinical events (abstr). *Circulation* 1996;94:I-453.
127. Moussa I, Di Mario C, Moses J, et al. The predictive value of different intravascular ultrasound criteria for restenosis after coronary stenting (abstr). *J Am Coll Cardiol* 1997;29:60A.
128. Mintz GS, Popma JJ, Pichard AD, et al. Intravascular ultrasound predictors of restenosis after percutaneous transcatheter coronary revascularization. *J Am Coll Cardiol* 1996;27:1678–1687.
129. Mintz GS, Popma JJ, Pichard AD, et al. Arterial remodeling after coronary angioplasty: A serial intravascular ultrasound study. *Circulation* 1996;94:35–43.
130. Morino Y, Limpijankit T, Honda Y, et al. Late vascular response to repeat stenting for in-stent restenosis with and without radiation: An intravascular ultrasound volumetric analysis. *Circulation* 2002; 105(21):2465–2468.
131. Mintz GS, Weissman NJ, Fitgerald PJ. Intravascular ultrasound assessment of the mechanisms and results of brachytherapy. *Circulation* 2001;104(11):1320–1325.
132. Serruys PW, Degertekin M, Tanabe K, et al Intravascular ultrasound findings in the multicenter, randomized, double blind RAVEL trial. *Circulation* 2002;106(7):798–803.
133. Park SJ, Shim WH, Ho DS, et al. A paclitaxel eluting stent for the prevention of coronary restenosis. *N Engl J Med* 2003;348(16): 1537–1545.
134. Nissen SE, Yock P. Intravascular ultrasound: Novel diagnostic insights and current clinical applications. *Circulation* 2001;103:604–616.
135. Lockwood GR, Ryan LK, Foster FS. A 45 to 55 MHz needle-based ultrasound system for invasive imaging. *Ultrasound Imaging* 1993;5:1–13.
136. von Birgelen C, de Vrey EA, Mintz GS, et al. ECG-gated three-dimensional intravascular ultrasound: Feasibility and reproducibility of the automated analysis of coronary lumen and atherosclerotic plaque dimensions in humans. *Circulation* 1997;96:2944–2952.
137. Evans JL, Ng KH, Wiet SG, et al. Accurate three-dimensional reconstruction of intravascular ultrasound data: Spatially correct three-dimensional reconstructions. *Circulation* 1996;93:567–576.

CHAPTER 19

# NUCLEAR CARDIOLOGY

Daniel S. Berman / Rory Hachamovitch / Leslee J. Shaw / Sean Hayes / Guido Germano



## OVERVIEW

Nuclear cardiology is an integral part of cardiovascular practice, with stress nuclear cardiology procedures accounting for over one-third of all stress tests performed by cardiologists and sustaining growth rates approaching 20 percent per year. This chapter provides a synopsis of nuclear cardiology procedures and the published evidence of their role in the diagnosis and risk assessment of patients with suspected or known coronary artery disease (CAD).

### Historical Perspectives in Nuclear Cardiology

The Anger scintillation camera, the imaging device used today for virtually all nuclear cardiology procedures except positron emission tomography (PET), became clinically available in the late 1960s. By providing dynamic images of the cardiac distribution of radioactivity, this camera marked the beginning of clinical nuclear cardiology. The commercial availability in 1976 of thallium 201 ($^{201}$Tl) initiated the broad application of clinical myocardial perfusion scintigraphy, which, with planar imaging was quickly shown to be useful for detection of CAD and, in the early 1980s, was demonstrated to be highly valuable in risk stratification of the CAD patient. Also in the early 1980s, single photon emission computed tomography (SPECT), using a rotating Anger camera, became widely available, increasing the ability to localize and quantify regional myocardial perfusion defects. In 1990, technetium 99m ($^{99m}$Tc)-sestamibi was approved for use in the United States. Its higher myocardial count rates improved image quality, so that adequate images could be obtained with SPECT from the different parts of the cardiac cycle (gated SPECT.) When coupled with the widespread use of multidetector cameras and dramatic increases in speed of computer systems, the availability of $^{99m}$Tc-sestamibi and tetrofosmin, another $^{99m}$Tc-based agent, in 1997, gated SPECT became clinically feasible.[1] By 2001, nearly 90 percent of myocardial perfusion SPECT (MPS) used a $^{99m}$Tc myocardial perfusion imaging agent and approximately 80 percent employed gated SPECT, providing routine objective clinical assessments of rest and stress myocardial perfusion and function. MPS makes up >95 percent of all nuclear cardiology procedures and thus is the focus of this chapter.

Although radionuclide angiography played a prominent role in noninvasive testing in decades past, in the 1990s the use of this modality was largely replaced by echocardiography and gated MPS. Some important clinical applications of this modality remain, however, and are discussed in the latter portion of this chapter. The recent American College of Cardiology/American Heart Association/American Society of Nuclear Cardiology (ACC/AHA/ASNC) Guidelines for the Clinical Use of Cardiac Radionuclide Imaging provide a useful, comprehensive review of the state of the art and current recommendations for the field of nuclear cardiology.[2]

## MYOCARDIAL PERFUSION SPECT

In general, MPS protocols consist of a combination of a stress modality (exercise or pharmacologic) with rest and stress administration and imaging of radiopharmaceuticals.

***Basics of Imaging*** The nuclear cameras consist of one or more scintillation detectors, typically made of high-density materials such as sodium iodide. Imaging can be performed with either planar or SPECT approaches. The planar technique generally consists of three two-dimensional (2D) image acquisitions, usually 10 to 15 min each. For SPECT, the camera detectors rotate around the patient in a circular or elliptical fashion, collecting a series of planar "projection images" at regular angular intervals. The 3D distribution of radioactivity in the myocardium is then mathematically "reconstructed" from the 2D projections, usually by a process called *filtered backprojection.*

***Gated SPECT*** What distinguishes the gated technique (Fig. 19-1) is that the projection images are acquired in 8 to 16 phases of the cardiac cycle based on electrocardiographic (ECG) triggering ("gating"). Hence, a gated MPS acquisition results in a standard SPECT data set (a summation of all of the gated SPECT data), from which perfusion is assessed, and a larger gated SPECT data set, from which function is evaluated. Gated SPECT's popularity is a direct result of the ease and modest expense with which perfusion assessment is "upgraded" to perfusion/function assessment and of the incremental information provided by the combined measurements.

## Radiopharmaceuticals

### THALLIUM 201

A cyclotron-generated radionuclide with a half-life of 73 h, $^{201}$Tl emits gamma rays from 68 to 80 keV (90 percent abundance) and at 167 keV (10 percent abundance). Owing to its relatively long half-life, the absorbed radiation dose is such that recommended injected doses are limited to about one-tenth of those used with $^{99m}$Tc agents. $^{201}$Tl has excellent physiologic properties for myocardial perfusion imaging. Being highly extracted during the first pass through the coronary circulation, a linear relationship between blood flow to viable myocardium and $^{201}$Tl uptake has been shown during exercise; however, at very high levels of flow, a "roll-off" in uptake occurs. As an unbound potassium analogue, $^{201}$Tl redistributes over time (see Ref. 32); its initial distribution is proportional to regional myocardial perfusion and, at equilibrium, the distribution of $^{201}$Tl is proportional to the regional potassium pool, reflecting viable myocardium. The mechanisms of $^{201}$Tl redistribution are differential washout rates between hypoperfused but viable myocardium and normal zones and wash-in to initially hypoperfused zones.

The washout rate of $^{201}$Tl is the concentration gradient between the myocardial cell and the blood. There is slower blood clearance of $^{201}$Tl following resting or low-level exercise injection. Diffuse slow washout rates, mimicking diffuse ischemia, may be observed in normal patients who do not achieve adequate levels of stress. Hyperinsulinemic states slow redistribution, leading to an underestimation of viable myocardium; thus fasting is recommended prior to and for 4 h following $^{201}$Tl injection.[3]

An inverse relationship between the degree of coronary stenosis and subsequent redistribution of $^{201}$Tl (i.e., late redistribution) has been reported.[4,5]

### $^{99m}$Tc-SESTAMIBI AND TETROFOSMIN

$^{99m}$Tc is produced from a molybdenum-99m generator, has a half-life of 6 h, and emits monoenergetic gamma rays at 140 keV. The whole-body radiation dose is estimated to be 16 mrad/mCi, in contrast to 240 mrad/mCi associated with $^{201}$Tl, allowing greater amounts of $^{99m}$Tc to be injected clinically. Following extraction from the blood, $^{99m}$Tc-sestamibi and tetrofosmin are quickly bound by mitochondria, and only a limited amount of myocardial washout (or wash-in) occurs over time.[6] As with $^{201}$Tl, the initial uptake of $^{99m}$Tc-sestamibi and tetrofosmin is a function of myocardial perfusion to viable tissue. The initial myocardial uptake among these agents (percent injected dose per gram of myocardium) differs, mainly due to differences in myocardial extraction fraction, which is highest with $^{201}$Tl and lowest with tetrofosmin.[7,8] The tracers also differ as to extracardiac (e.g., hepatic) uptake, which, early after injection, is highest with sestamibi and lowest with $^{201}$Tl.[9,10]

### OTHER $^{99m}$Tc MYOCARDIAL PERFUSION AGENTS

$^{99m}$Tc-teboroxime has a higher extraction fraction than $^{201}$Tl and a plateau at a higher flow rate than other agents.[11,12] However, very rapid myocardial washout[13] requires that initial imaging be completed within the first few minutes after injection. The technically demanding nature of $^{99m}$Tc-teboroxime MPS protocols limits their broad use.

$^{99m}$Tc NOET is a not-yet-available neutral lipophilic myocardial perfusion imaging agent based on a Tc-nitrido core.[14] Extraction fraction may be as high as 76 percent with this tracer,[15] which redistributes over time, related to the absence of intracellular binding.[15] $^{99m}$Tc NOET overall has kinetic properties very similar to those of $^{201}$Tl, with the advantage of the higher photon flux associated with the use of a $^{99m}$Tc agent[16]; however, variable lung uptake may be a limiting factor with this tracer.

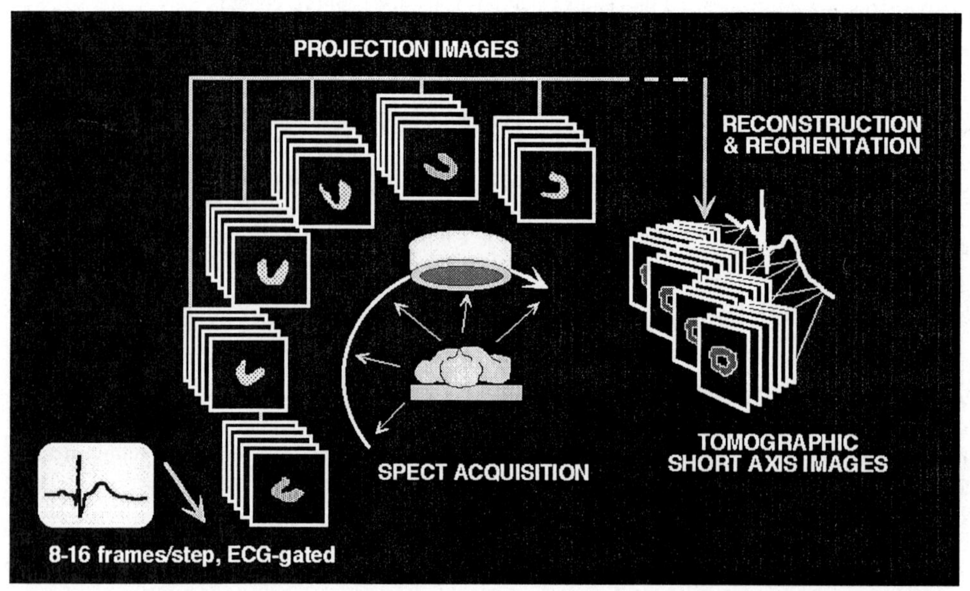


FIGURE 19-1 Schematic representation of ECG-gated perfusion SPECT acquisition and processing.

## Exercise Protocols

Exercise stress is preferred over pharmacologic stress for use with MPS in patients who can exercise adequately, since it allows assessment of exercise capacity and symptoms as well as ST-segment response. For exercise MPS, an indwelling intravenous line is inserted preexercise, the tracer is injected at maximal stress, and exercise is continued for an additional 1 min at peak workload and often 2 min more at a lower workload.[17]

## Pharmacologic Stress Protocols

### VASODILATOR STRESS

For patients who cannot achieve an adequate level of exercise (≥85 percent of maximal predicted heart rate),[2] pharmacologic stress testing is preferred.[18] The preferred pharmacologic stress agents for MPS are coronary vasodilators: adenosine or dipyridamole. These agents provide a three- to fivefold increase in coronary flow. Dipyridamole blocks the cellular reuptake of adenosine, increasing the extracellular adenosine concentration. Increased extracellular adenosine results in coronary vasodilation. Adenosine is growing in use more than dipyridamole, due predominantly to its rapid onset and offset of peak effect. Methylxanthines, such as theophylline or caffeine, block adenosine binding and can eliminate the coronary vasodilation effects of adenosine or dipyridamole, leading to false-negative stress perfusion studies. In general, being off caffeine-containing medicines, foods, or beverages for 24 h is recommended, since the half-life of caffeine is variable.[2,19]

One of the limitations of current vasodilator agents is the high frequency of uncomfortable systemic side effects and the risk of bronchoconstriction in asthmatics. Currently, several $A_2$ agonists—which are more cardioselective, resulting in a reduced systemic effect on heart rate and blood pressure, fewer side effects, and a reduced risk of bronchospasm—are in phase II and III clinical trials.[20,20a] The diagnostic accuracies of MPS using exercise or pharmacologic stress are equivalent, despite the higher coronary flow rates associated with the vasodilators.[21]

Regarding the clinical and hemodynamic responses to vasodilator stress, normally there is a mild rise in heart rate (HR) and fall in blood pressure (BP) with adenosine or dipyridamole infusion. However, clinical assessment and hemodynamic responses to vasodilators are not useful in identifying patients in whom the pharmacologic effects of adenosine or dipyridamole have been blocked by caffeine; failure of HR or BP to change with adenosine stress does not imply lack of myocardial perfusion response.[22] Recent data suggest that resting tachycardia and failure to mount a tachycardia in response to vasodilator stress is associated with a considerable increase in mortality risk.[23]

***Dipyridamole Infusion*** Dipyridamole is usually infused at 0.142 mg/kg/min for 4 min, although some investigators have recommended increasing the dose by 50 percent.[21] The maximal effect occurs approximately 3 to 4 min after end of the infusion. Mild transient side effects are common, including chest pain, shortness of breath, dizziness, and flushing. Severe side effects are rare, being noted in only 1 of 10,000 patients.[24] Side effects can usually be reversed by intravenous aminophylline, usually 75 to 125 mg. Due to the potential side effect of severe bronchospasm, dipyridamole is contraindicated for asthmatics.

***Adenosine Infusion*** Adenosine is infused intravenously (140 μg/kg/min), usually over 4 to 6 min, with radiopharmaceutical administration at 2 to 3 min of infusion.[17,25] Transient side effects occur more frequently than with dipyridamole,[25] but due to the duration of action of about 13 s, reversal with aminophylline is not needed. With adenosine, there is an increased incidence of advanced atrioventricular (AV) block. Adenosine is considered contraindicated for patients with greater than first-degree AV block, sick sinus syndrome, or bronchospasm.

### COMBINED PHARMACOLOGIC AND EXERCISE TESTING

It has become preferred to combine vasodilator stress with low-level exercise in patients able to walk, except in patients with left bundle branch block (LBBB) or paced rhythm. With dipyridamole, stress exercise begins at the end of the infusion. With adenosine stress, exercise is performed during the adenosine infusion.[26]

### DOBUTAMINE STRESS

An alternative to vasodilator stress is inotropic stress with dobutamine.[27] At the present time, dobutamine stress is usually reserved for patients with asthma, chronic obstructive pulmonary disease with bronchospasm, or those who have ingested caffeine. Dobutamine stress results in a lower rate pressure product than exercise and a lower peak coronary blood flow with vasodilator stress. Side effects, including ventricular irritability, are more common than with the vasodilator stress.

### ANTI-ISCHEMIC DRUG USE DURING STRESS TESTING

In general, for purposes of diagnosis or initial risk stratification, exercise nuclear testing is performed with the patient off of anti-ischemic medications.[2] Medications that decrease myocardial oxygen demand, such as beta-adrenergic or calcium channel blocking agents, may limit the development of ischemia during the exercise test. Consequently, the sensitivity of the exercise perfusion study for the diagnosis of CAD is lower in patients taking such agents. Nitrates may also decrease the extent of perfusion defects. When feasible use of beta blockers or long-acting calcium channel blockers should be discontinued at least 48 h before exercise and long-acting nitrates should be discontinued at least 12 h before testing.[2]

Whether antianginal drugs should be suspended before pharmacologic stress has not been widely studied, but an increasing body of evidence suggests that stopping these medications may be preferred. Sharir et al.[28] reported that compared to dipyridamole stress MPS performed off medications, MPS performed *on medications* was associated with smaller and less reversible perfusion defects and approximately a one-third lowering of overall and individual vessel sensitivities. A recent study has demonstrated that acute beta blockade reduces the size of adenosine stress myocardial perfusion defects.[28a]

### PATIENT PREPARATION FOR STRESS TESTING

Recommendations are that (in addition to not being under the influence of anti-ischemic medications) patients be off of caffeine prior to exercise MPS.[2] By preparing patients in this manner, if a patient fails to achieve 85 percent of maximal predicted heart rate (MPHR) during exercise, pharmacologic testing with adenosine or dipyridamole can be immediately substituted prior to stress tracer injection. This avoids nondiagnostic normal MPS studies associated with limited exercise (<85 percent MPHR). Recent findings have prognostically confirmed this threshold in that patients with normal scans who achieve less than 80 to 85 percent MPHR are at significantly greater risk than those who achieve maximal workload.[29] For patients unable to exercise adequately who have had caffeine, dobutamine is a reasonable form of stress for MPS.

### STRESS TESTING ON MEDICATIONS

While it is recommended that the *initial risk stratification* study be performed with the patients off of cardiac active medications, it is recognized that potentially useful clinical information can be derived from exercise or pharmacologic MPS study performed on cardiac medications.[2]

## Imaging Protocols

### $^{201}$Tl PROTOCOLS

With $^{201}$Tl, a variety of SPECT protocols are available (Fig. 19-2). When $^{201}$Tl is the only radiopharmaceutical, the usual protocol uses some combination of stress with redistribution and/or reinjection MPS (Fig. 19-2*A*). The latter improves detection of viable myocardium over standard-stress 4-h redistribution imaging[30] but requires three image acquisitions and a decision to reinject. A two-acquisition sequence with stress and redistribution/reinjection imaging is commonly performed but may still need 24-h imaging if fixed defects are found at 4 h[30] (Fig. 19-2*B*). A variation of this protocol is to give sublingual nitroglycerin prior to the reinjection of $^{201}$Tl. With this approach, the frequency of further improvement at 24-h imaging may be reduced.[31] Rest/redistribution $^{201}$Tl MPS is commonly used for resting ischemia/viability testing[32,33] (Fig. 19-2*C*). Even with rest thallium MPS, 24-h imaging can result in additional redistribution compared to 4-h imaging.[34]

With $^{201}$Tl SPECT, the timing of initial poststress acquisition is particularly important, since delay could result in early redistribution of the radiopharmaceutical, thus decreasing sensitivity for detection of CAD. With either $^{201}$Tl or $^{99m}$Tc agents, MPS should not begin <10 min after exercise because of the frequent observation of an artifactual perfusion defect due to "upward creep of the heart."[35] This phenomenon is related to the increased depth of respiration very early postexercise, which is associated with an average lower position of the diaphragm, causing the heart to gradually move cephalad during the early portion of SPECT acquisition. Gated SPECT can be performed with $^{201}$Tl, particularly with multidetector systems. LVEF by gated $^{201}$Tl MPS correlates highly with that of $^{99m}$Tc-sestamibi MPS.[36]

### $^{99m}$Tc-SESTAMIBI OR TETROFOSMIN PROTOCOLS

Due to the absence of clinically significant redistribution, separate rest and stress injections are standard with $^{99m}$Tc-sestamibi or tetrofosmin SPECT (Fig. 19-3).[37,38] An important benefit of the absence of redistribution is that there is an uncoupling of injection and imaging times. Hence, imaging can be delayed or repeated. In this regard, if imaging artifact is suspected, prone imaging as an adjunct to supine imaging increases the specificity of MPS with $^{99m}$Tc-sestamibi or tetrofosmin (Fig. 19-4).[38] A variety of protocols can be used with these agents, including 2-day stress/rest, same-day rest/stress, same-day stress/rest, and dual-isotope.

From the standpoint of defect contrast and image quality, the 2-day stress/rest protocol is ideal (Fig. 19-3*A*). Both stress and rest studies are obtained after injection of high doses of $^{99m}$Tc-sestamibi or tetrofosmin, allowing acquisition of consistent high-count images. The drawback is its requirement for 2 imaging days. The most common $^{99m}$Tc agent protocol is same-day low-dose rest/high-dose stress[39] (Fig. 19-3*B*). While convenient, it has the disadvantage of reduction in stress-defect contrast due to preexisting resting myocardial radioactivity. The same-day low-dose stress/high-dose rest sequence (Fig. 19-3*C*) has the advantage of image acquisition times the same as those used for stress $^{201}$Tl imaging, facilitating mixing of these two protocols. The principal drawback of this approach is that the count rates associated with the stress image set are low. With either the 1- or 2-day stress/rest sequences, an advantage is the ability to perform the stress image only.[40]

A common alternative to the standard $^{99m}$Tc-sestamibi or tetrofosmin protocols is a rest $^{201}$Tl/stress $^{99m}$Tc-sestamibi dual-isotope SPECT (Fig. 19-5).[17] Dual isotope MPS takes advantage of the Anger camera's ability to collect data in different energy windows. It is usually performed with separate rest/stress acquisitions, including redistribution thallium images either before the stress study (Fig. 19-5*B*) or at 24 h (after stress) (Fig. 19-5*C*). Advantages of this approach over other $^{99m}$Tc protocols are increased efficiency and the ability to assess resting perfusion defect reversibility (detecting resting ischemia by thallium redistribution images).[41] The separate

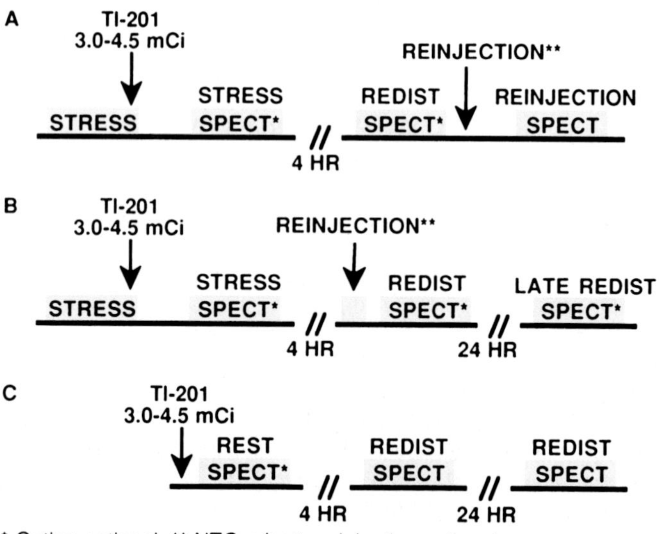


FIGURE 19-2 $^{201}$Tl, protocols. *A*. Stress/redistribution (redist), reinjection. *B*. Stress/reinjection/late redistribution. *C*. Rest/redistribution.

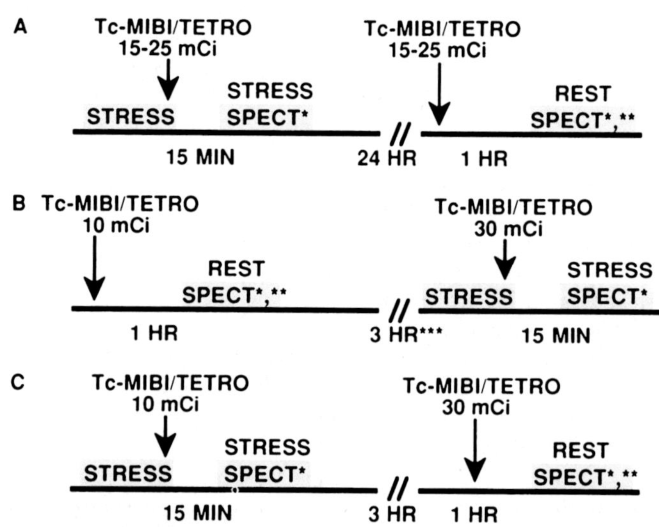


FIGURE 19-3 Two-day (*A*), same-day rest-stress (sequence interchangeable) (*B*), and same-day stress-rest (*C*), $^{99m}$Tc-sestamibi or tetrofosmin protocols. Tc = $^{99m}$Tc; MIBI = sestamibi; Tetro = tetrofosmin.

acquisition approach does not require correction for cross-contamination between the two radioisotopes,[17] which would be important for simultaneous dual-isotope approach,[42] a potentially efficient approach not yet in general clinical use.

In any protocol using the rest/stress sequence, inspection of the resting images prior to stress can identify patients with unexpected resting perfusion abnormality, obviating the need for a stress study[43] (Fig. 19-6).

### ATTENUATION CORRECTION

Several camera manufacturers have recently provided hardware and software implementation of attenuation-correction protocols. In general, these attenuation corrections are imperfect, reducing but not eliminating apparent perfusion defects due to soft tissue attenuation in normal patients.

Several reports have compared the diagnostic accuracy of attenuation-corrected and non-attenuation-corrected SPECT using a variety of commercially available approaches.[44–50] In general, these have demonstrated improved specificity with no change in overall sensitivity. Recently reported results from a multicenter blinded read of stress-only attenuation-corrected versus non-attenuation-corrected images suggest that this method increases reader confidence and obviates the need for rest images in many patients.[51] A similar conclusion has been reached in a recent study of 729 patients with a low to medium pretest probability of CAD being evaluated for chest pain.[40] Despite these considerations, attenuation correction is not yet widely used.

## BASICS OF INTERPRETATION

The interpretation of MPS is performed by visual or computer-based methods. Perfusion defects are characterized by their type as well as their extent and severity. The various defect types are illustrated in Fig. 19-7 for stress and

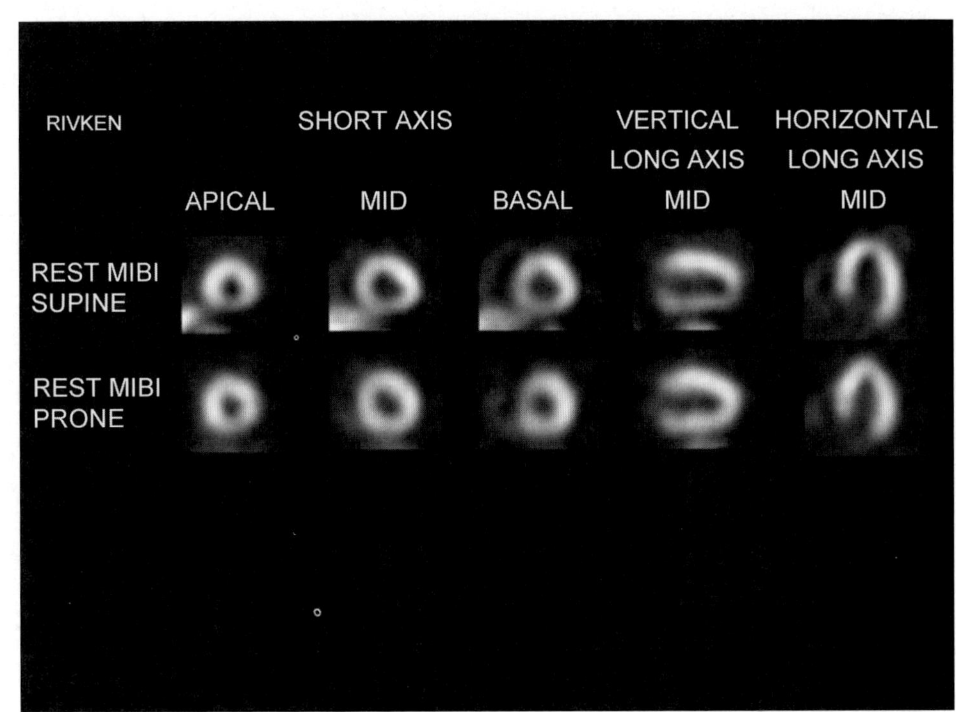


FIGURE 19-4 Rest sestamibi (MIBI) SPECT images in the supine position (*top*) and prone position (*bottom*) in a 55-year-old patient with a low likelihood of CAD. Prone images are normal, demonstrating that the apparent inferior wall perfusion defect on the supine images is secondary to soft tissue attenuation. Normal wall motion was noted on gated SPECT. (Reproduced with permission from Germano and Berman.[1])

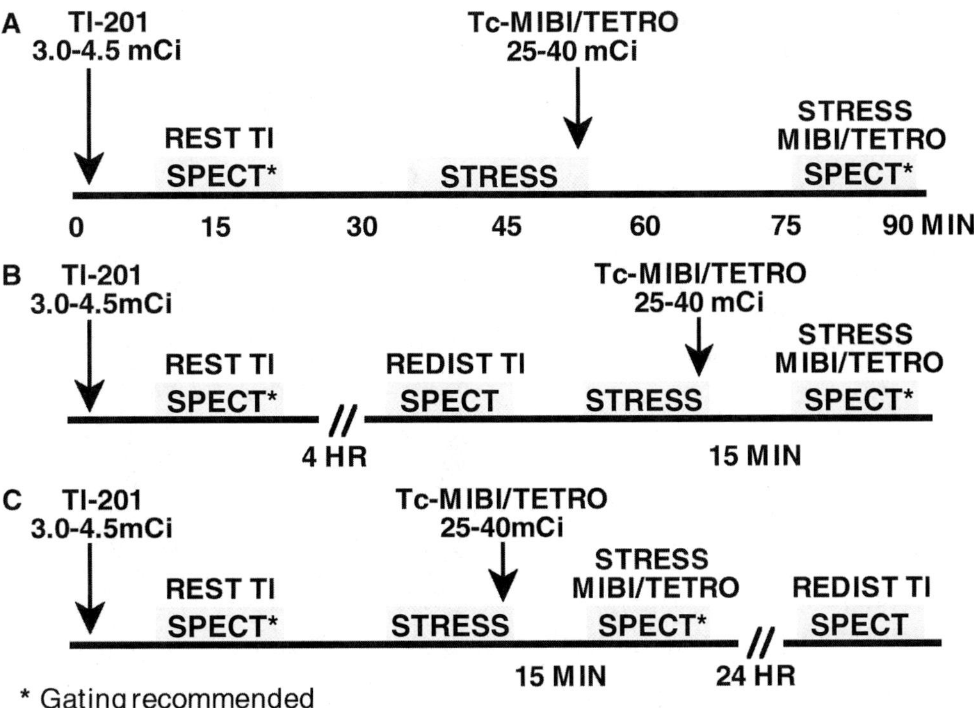


FIGURE 19-5 Variations of the resting $^{201}Tl/^{99m}Tc$-sestamibi or tetrofosmin dual-isotope MPS protocol. Most commonly, only rest and stress imaging is performed (*A*). When resting defects are present, redistribution imaging is recommended and may be performed before (*B*) or 24 h after (*C*) injection of the technetium perfusion agent.

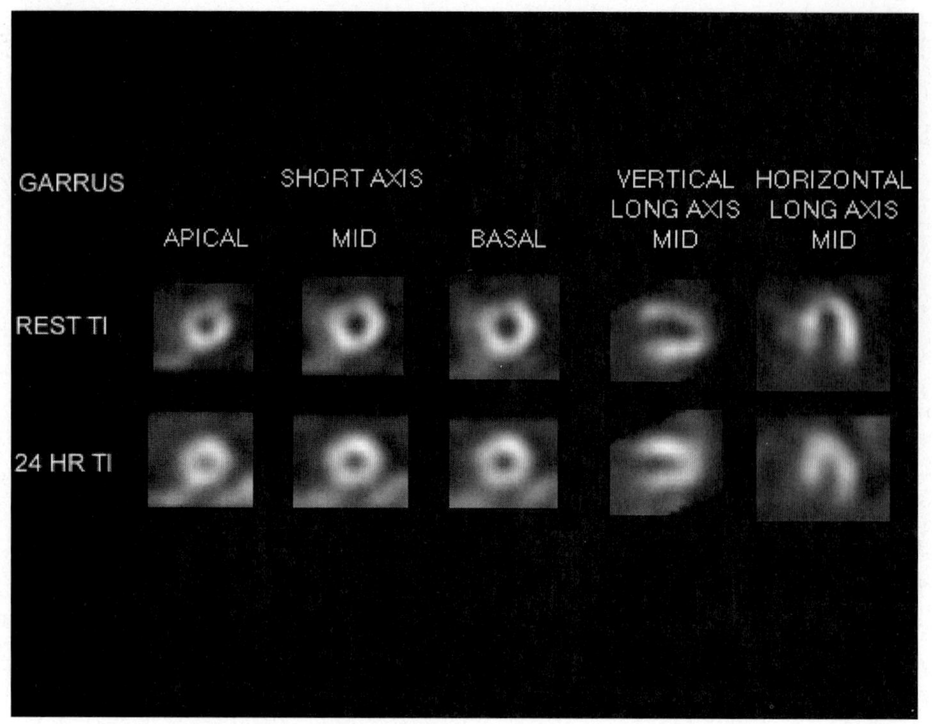


FIGURE 19-6 Rest and 24-h redistribution $^{201}Tl$ MPS of a 75-year-old male with atypical angina showing a large amount of resting ischemia in the left anterior descending territory, which subsequently revealed a 95 percent proximal stenosis by coronary angiography. Of note, the left ventricle was larger at rest than at the time of redistribution imaging. The stress MPS study was cancelled in this patient due to the unexpected perfusion defect (Adapted with permission from Aboul-Enein et al.[43])

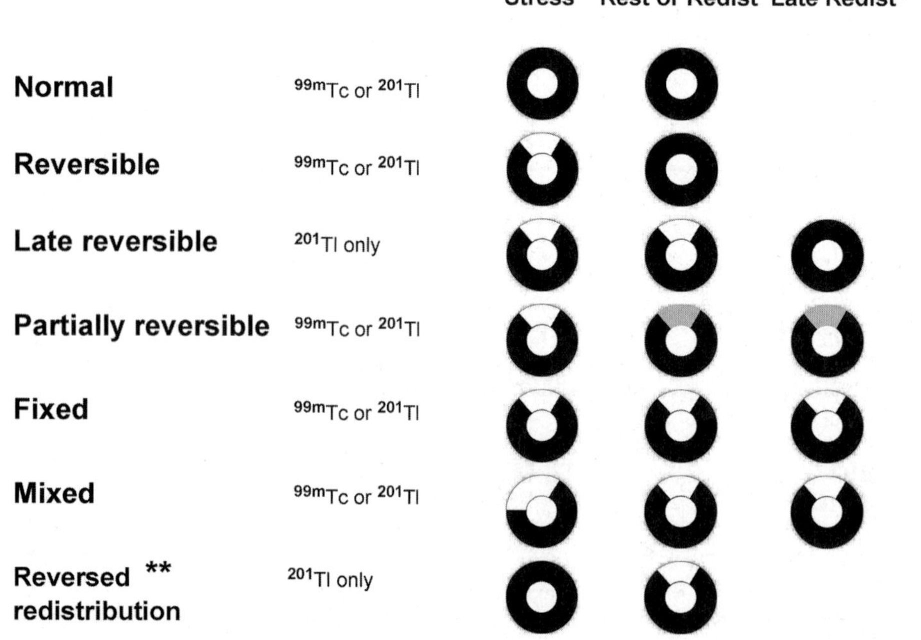


FIGURE 19-7 Patterns of stress/rest or redistribution MPS defects. Black represents normal tracer update; white represents a definite perfusion defect; gray represents less severe but still definite perfusion defect (seen in the partially reversible defect example).

rest MPS. For assessment of myocardial viability, rest/redistribution $^{201}Tl$ protocols are most common, with rest and NTG-enhanced $^{99m}Tc$ agent studies also valid alternatives. The patterns of myocardial viability associated with regional wall motion abnormality in these studies are shown in Fig. 19-8. The distribution of SPECT abnormalities provides information regarding the location of coronary artery stenoses. Representative examples of SPECT defect locations associated with individual coronary artery stenoses are illustrated in Figs. 19-9 and 19-10.

## SEMIQUANTITATIVE SEGMENTAL SCORING SYSTEMS

Semiquantitative perfusion scoring systems standardize the visual interpretation of scans, reduce the likelihood of overlooking significant defects, and provide global indices for overall assessment of extent and severity of perfusion abnormality. Further, they are more systematic and reproducible than simple qualitative evaluation.

***20-Segment Model*** A 20-segment scoring method for MPS is based on three short-axis slices [distal (apical), mid, and basal] representing the entire left ventricle (LV), with the two apical segments visualized in a midvertical long-axis image. Each of the 20 segments has a distinct name and is scored using a 5-point system [0 = normal, 1,2,3 = mild (equivocal), moderate, and severe reductions of a radioisotope, and 4 = absence of detectable tracer uptake].[52] Severe reversible perfusion defects with scores of 3 or 4 (Figs. 19-9*B* and *E*, 19-10*B* and *C*) can be reported as consistent with a critical (≥90 percent) coronary stenosis.[53]

***17-Segment Model*** A 17-segment scoring system for MPS that more accurately represents the size of each segment is now recommended (Fig. 19-11).[54,55] The only differences from the 20-segment model are that the smaller size of the distal short-axis slice is accounted for by 4 versus 6 segments and the apex is one rather than two segments.

***Summed Scores*** Segmental scoring systems lend themselves to the derivation of summed scores from the 17 to 20 segments (i.e., global indices of perfusion).[56] The overall extent and severity of perfusion defects are reflected by the summed stress score (SSS), the summed rest score (SRS), and the summed differences score (SDS), the latter defined by SSS-SRS and measuring the degree of reversibility. Risk groups may be defined using SSS categories[57,58] (Table 19-1).

More recently, we have shifted to percent myocardium involved, expressing overall perfusion defects as percent stress, percent reversible, and percent fixed.[59] The conversion of summed scores to percent myocardium is accomplished by dividing the summed scores by the worst segmental score possible (80 for 20 segments; 68 for 17 segments) and multiplying by 100 (5-point scoring). The benefits of this approach are that it provides a measure with intuitive implications (percent myocardium hypoperfused) not possible with the unitless summed scores, that it can easily be applied with scoring systems using varying numbers of segments (e.g., 20, 17, 14, 12) and that it is applicable to quantitative methods that directly measure these abnormalities as percent myocardium. Risk groups by the percent stress abnormal, which correlate with SSS risk groups, are <5 percent (normal or minimally abnormal), 5 to 9 percent mildly abnormal, 10 to 14 percent moderately abnormal, and ≥15 percent severely abnormal[41,59,60] (Table 19-1).

## QUANTITATIVE ANALYSIS

A variety of commercially available software packages are available to assist in image interpretation. These computer approaches generally operate by automatic determination of the amount of radioactivity at rest and stress within each pixel or small zone of the myocardium, scaling this amount by the maximal amount of radioactivity in the myocardium (normalization), and then comparing this scaled amount to the lower limit of normal. The change between rest and stress is usually also assessed and compared to normal, providing information about perfusion defect reversibility. The results are most commonly displayed using polar maps. Figure 19-12 displays polar maps associated with the various scan abnormalities shown in Figs. 19-9 and 19-10.

Because these computer-based quantitative programs do not take into

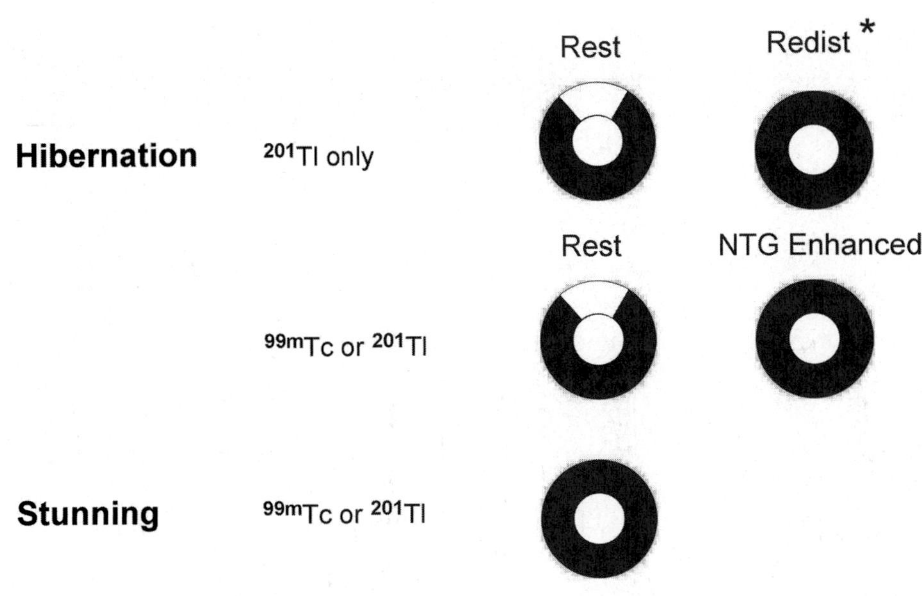


FIGURE 19-8 Patterns of myocardial viability associated with regional contractile abnormality. White represents perfusion defect.

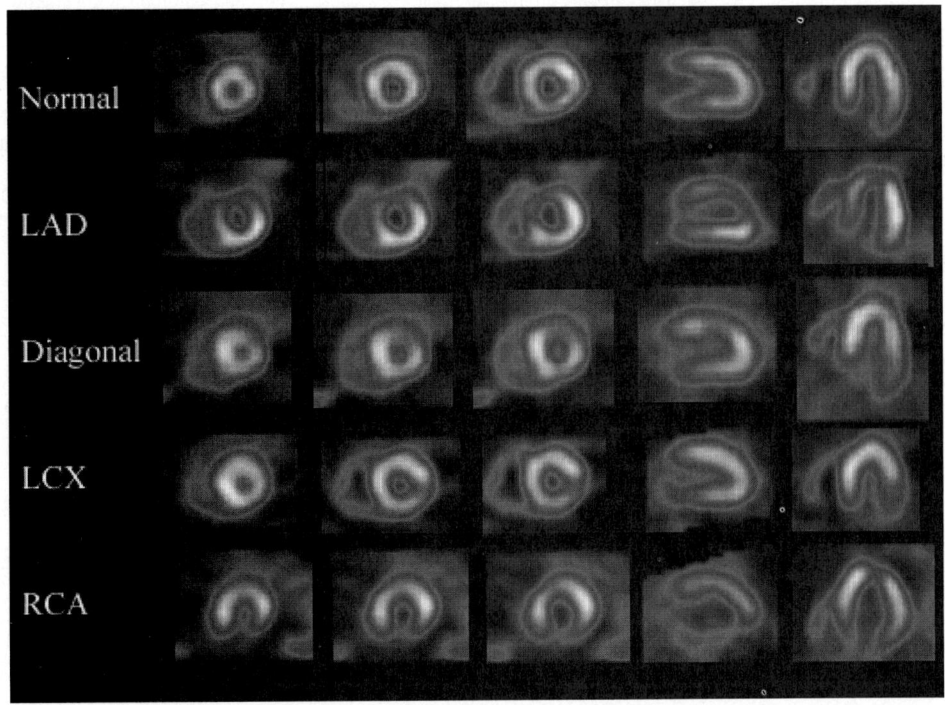


FIGURE 19-9 Examples of typical stress perfusion patterns corresponding to normal (*top*) and various single-territory abnormalities. Coronary angiographic findings in these patients were as follows: LAD (left anterior descending coronary artery) proximal 95 percent stenosis; diagonal (occluded proximal first diagonal artery); left circumflex coronary artery (LCX): occluded first marginal artery branch; right coronary artery (RCA): mid-95 percent stenosis. All patients had no evidence of myocardial infarction and normal MPS at rest. From left to right, the images represent distal short axis, mid-short axis, basal short axis, midvertical long axis, and midhorizontal long axis. These patients show the typical distributions of perfusion defects associated with the specific coronary arteries involved, as shown in Fig. 19-11.

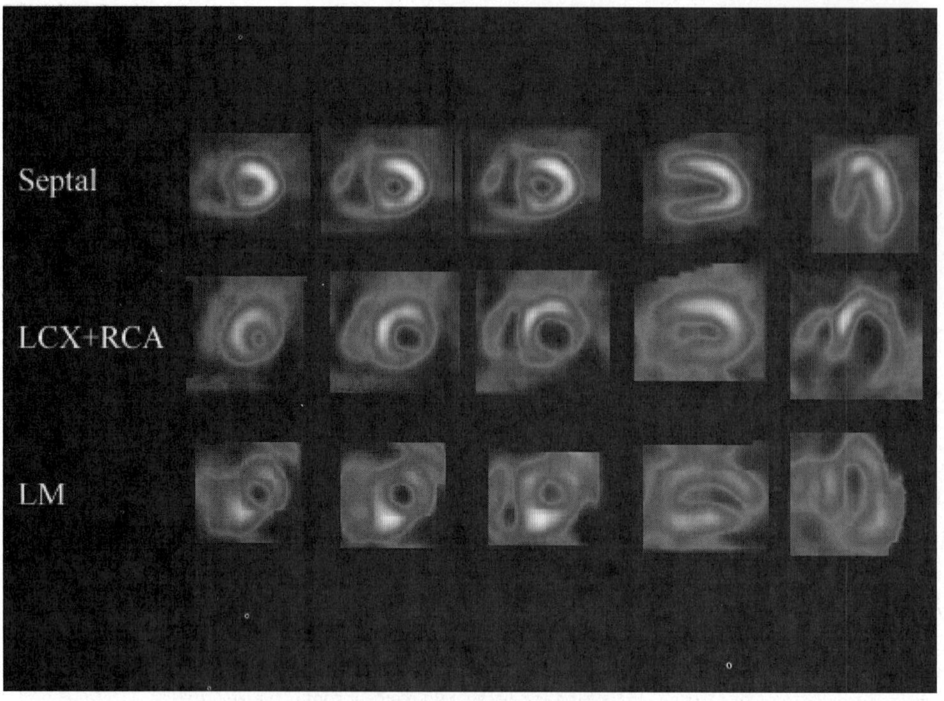


FIGURE 19-10 Stress MPS images demonstrating more complex patterns associated with known coronary lesions in patients with normal resting perfusion images and no history of prior myocardial infarction. Septal: trapped septal perforator coronary artery (occlusion of first septal coronary artery) in a patient with critical LAD stenoses proximal and distal to the septal perforator takeoff and patent right posterior descending coronary artery, vein grafts to the left circumflex marginal coronary artery, and patent LAD internal mammary graft. LCX plus RCA: occlusion of proximal left circumflex and proximal right coronary arteries; left main (LM): subtotal left main coronary artery stenosis.

account artifacts that may be easily detected visually (such as marked breast attenuation), it is generally recommended that they be used as a "second expert opinion," with the principal and final interpretation based on the visual assessment.

## CONSIDERATIONS FOR INTERPRETATION OF MYOCARDIAL VIABILITY

The assessment of myocardial viability with the myocardial perfusion tracers applies to segments with contractile dysfunction, and viability is considered present if the degree of uptake at rest, redistribution, or following nitrate-augmented rest injection[61–65] is normal. If a dysfunctional segment or region has severely reduced or absent uptake of radioactivity, it is considered to be nonviable. Areas with moderate reduction of counts in these conditions (score 2/4 at redistribution or nitrate-augmented rest) are usually partially viable, and patients in this group have a variable response in terms of postoperative improvement. Some investigators have utilized a cutoff percentage of maximal counts in the myocardium for predicting viability in a region in question[66,67]; given the regional count variability, due to varying soft tissue attenuation, use of the number of standard deviations below normal tracer activity may be preferable. When perfusion defects are seen at rest and not after redistribution or after separate injection following administration of nitroglycerin (NTG), MPS is commonly interpreted as showing "resting ischemia" and considered to represent regions of critically reduced blood flow to viable myocardium.[43]

## GATED SPECT FOR VENTRICULAR FUNCTION MEASURES

Gated MPS is used to quantify global function parameters, including left ventricular ejection fraction (LVEF), end-diastolic volumes, and end-systolic volumes. Regional LV myocardial wall motion and thickening can be quantitated from gated MPS images and is useful in the identification of hibernation, stunning, and infarction as well as distinguishing true perfusion defects from attenuation artifacts. Quantitation of gated MPS can be performed by a variety of algorithms. The most common approaches are fully 3D and are based on the automatic detection of endocardial and epicardial surface points.[68–70]

In validation studies of gated-perfusion SPECT LVEF published to date,[71] the agreement between gated SPECT and other standard measurements of LVEF has been shown to be generally very good to excellent. While LVEF measured by the various quantitative algorithms correlate highly,

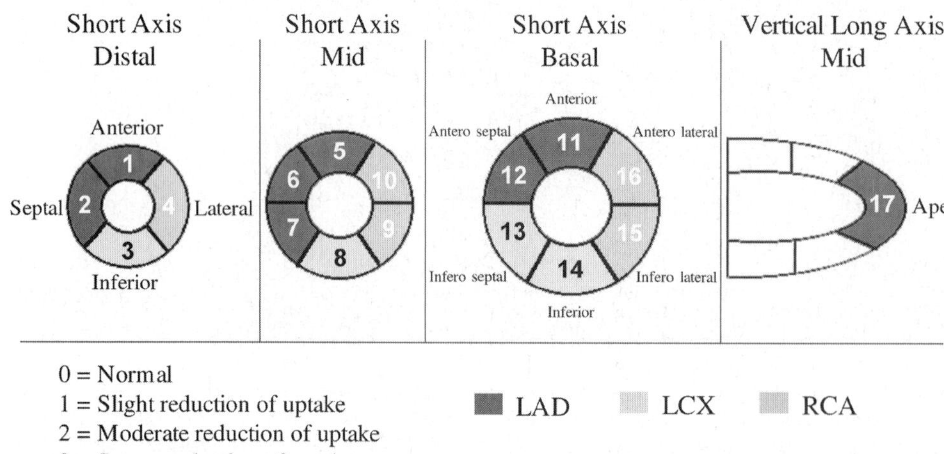


FIGURE 19-11 Diagrammatic representation of segmental division of the SPECT slices and assignment of the individual segments of the individual coronary arteries using the 17-segment model. LAD, left anterior descending coronary artery; LCX, left circumflex coronary artery; RCA, right coronary artery.

the thresholds for abnormality are different depending on the method used.[72] With some methods, the normal threshold for the global LVEF measured by gated MPS images is slightly lower than that measured using other imaging modalities (approximately 45 percent) due principally to the use of only eight gating intervals.[71] Recently, 16-frame gating has become more common, reducing the underestimation of LVEF. Normal limits for LVEF and LV volumes have been reported.[73–75]

TABLE 19-1 Definitions of Summed Perfusion Scores and Percent Myocardium Hypoperfused

| | | |
|---|---|---|
| Summed stress score (SSS)[a] | Sum of the segmental scores at stress | Amount of infarcted, ischemic, or jeopardized myocardium |
| Summed rest score (SRS)[a] | Sum of the segmental scores at rest | Amount of infarcted or hibernating myocardium |
| Summed difference score (SDS)[a] | SSS − SRS | Amount of ischemic or jeopardized myocardium |
| | 20-Segment | 17-Segment |
| Percent total | = SSS × 100/80 | = SSS × 100/68 |
| Percent ischemic | = SDS × 100/80 | = SDS × 100/68 |
| Percent fixed | = SRS × 100/80 | = SRS × 100/68 |

[a]Reflect the extent and severity of perfusion abnormality.
SOURCES: [59]Hachamovitch et al.

***Sources of Artifacts with Gated SPECT Measurements*** Several technical artifacts can affect the accuracy of LVEF measurement from gated MPS. LVEFs can be overestimated in analyzing gated SPECT images of small hearts,[76] due to the limitations of spatial resolution with SPECT. In patients with severe LVH, LVEF may also be underestimated due to failure to accurately determine the endocardial border in the presence of the large muscle mass.

## OTHER ABNORMALITIES: CAVITY SIZE, DILATION, AND LUNG UPTAKE

In addition to perfusion defects, several nonperfusion abnormalities can be observed with MPS, including size of the LV, transient ischemic dilation (TID) of the LV,[77,78] right ventricular (RV) myocardial uptake pattern, RV size, and abnormalities of lung uptake or other abnormal extracardiac activity.

***Transient Ischemic Dilation of the Left Ventricle*** TID is considered present when the LV cavity appears to be significantly larger in the poststress images than at rest[77,78] and may actually be an apparent cavity dilation secondary to diffuse subendocardial ischemia (obscuring the endocardial border). This explains why TID may be seen for several hours following stress, when true cavity dilation is probably no longer present. The correlation between LV TID and lung uptake is weak, suggesting that there may be different pathophysiologic mechanisms for each, and their measurements may be complementary in assessing the extent and severity of CAD for risk stratification.[79] TID is considered to represent severe and extensive ischemia and has been shown to be highly specific for critical stenosis (greater than 90 percent narrowing) in vessels supplying a large portion of the myocardium (i.e., proximal left anterior descending or multivessel 90 percent lesions).[77,78] Dipyridamole or adenosine-induced TID has similar implications as those associated with exercise.[80] Figure 19-13 illustrates an example of TID on MPS from a patient with severe disease of the left anterior descending artery. TID can easily be measured by the quantitative gated SPECT algorithms. The upper limit of normal for the TID ratio in dual-isotope imaging has been reported to be 1.22 for exercise MPS. Patients who have TID of the LV (TID > 1.22) are likely to have severe and extensive CAD (>90 percent stenosis of the proximal left anterior descending coronary artery or of multiple vessels).[78] For reasons that are not known, with vasodilator stress, the upper limit of normal in order to consider TID to be present is higher, approximately 1.30 with dual-isotope SPECT.

***Increased Lung Uptake of Perfusion Tracers*** It is generally accepted that increased pulmonary uptake of thallium reflects increased pulmonary capillary wedge pressure. Nonischemic causes of increased pulmonary capillary wedge pressure—such as mitral

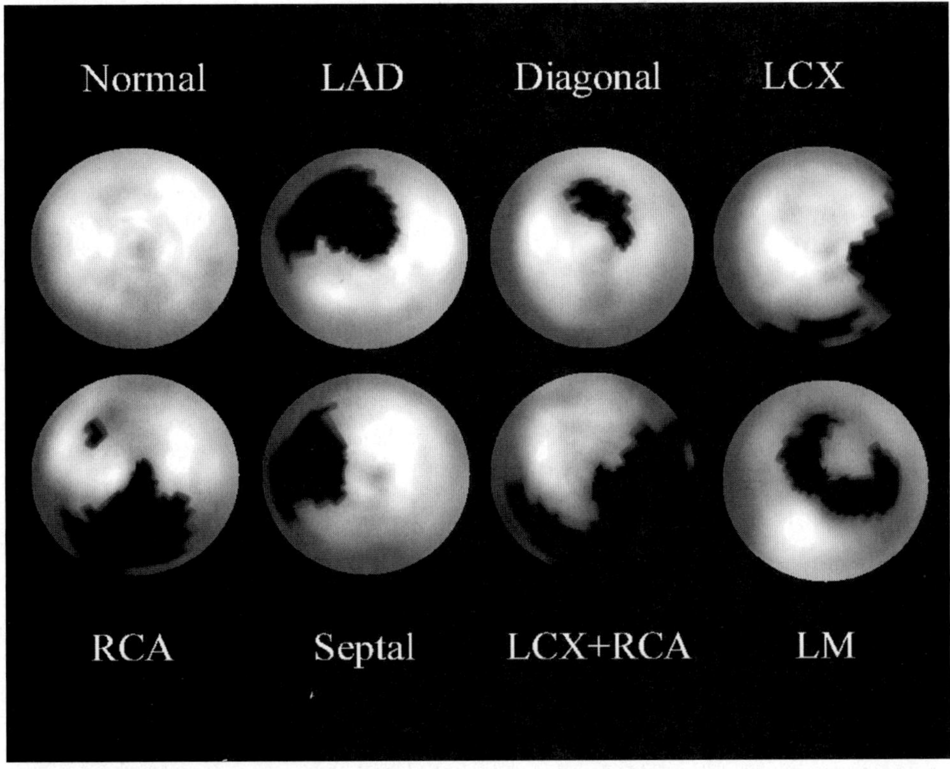


FIGURE 19-12 Quantitative stress polar maps of patients shown in Fig 19-10 and 19-11; black represents regions of quantitative perfusion defect when compared to normal limit files.

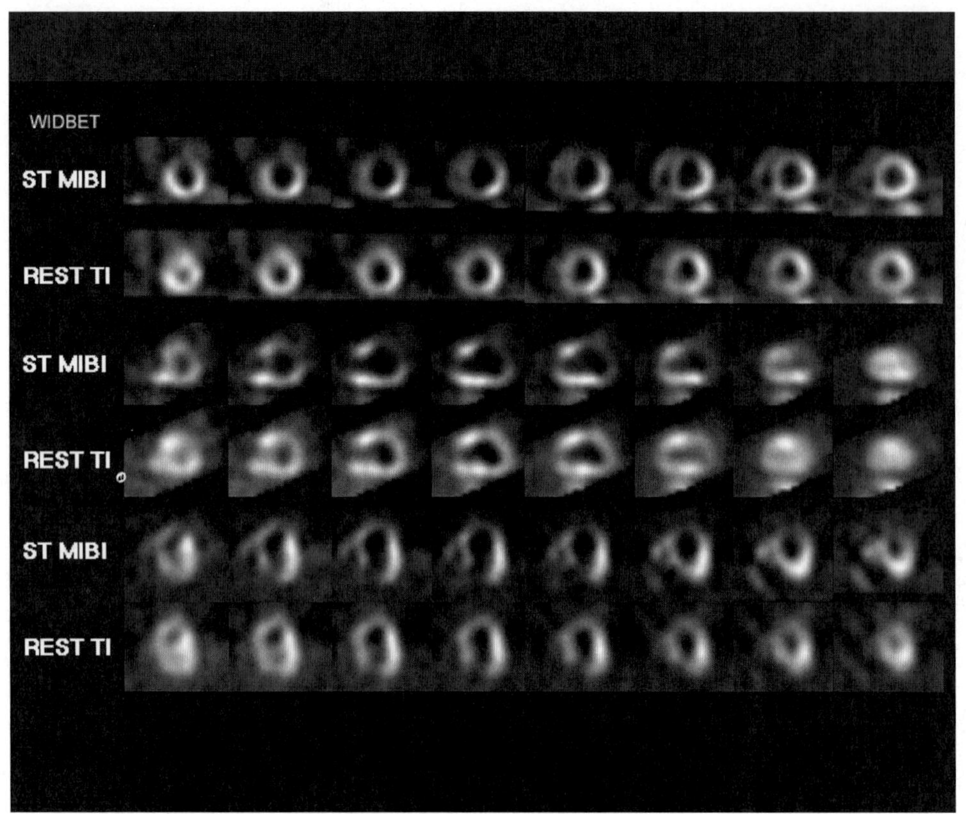


FIGURE 19-13 Adenosine stress $^{99m}$Tc-sestamibi/rest $^{201}$Tl-myocardial perfusion SPECT images in an 83-year-old female with typical angina. There is evidence of a severe and extensive reversible defect throughout the LAD coronary artery and transient ischemia dilation of the left ventricle. Angiography revealed proximal 95 percent stenosis of LAD.

regurgitation, mitral stenosis, etc.—are also associated with increased pulmonary thallium uptake. Increased thallium lung uptake after exercise has been shown to have incremental prognostic information over myocardial perfusion defect assessment.[81] Only a few studies have examined the implications of increased pulmonary uptake of $^{99m}$Tc-sestamibi, with differing results,[82–85] possibly explained by differences in imaging times after stress in various studies. If imaged very early after stress, sestamibi lung uptake may have similar implications to those of $^{201}$Tl.[82]

## CLINICAL APPLICATION OF MPS

The principles underlying the efficient use of stress nuclear techniques and the optimal use of the test results are discussed below. First, diagnostic testing is addressed, followed by the principles and applications of prognostic testing. Also, the evidence for the use of MPS and application of its results in specific patient populations commonly encountered in clinical cardiology settings are reviewed.

### Selecting the Appropriate Test Candidates for MPS

#### BAYESIAN THEORY: INTEGRATION OF PRETEST LIKELIHOOD OF CAD INTO SELECTION OF PATIENTS FOR TESTING AND TEST INTERPRETATION

Central to appropriate patient selection for nuclear imaging and the interpretation of test results is the ability to determine an individual patient's pretest likelihood of CAD based on demographic, clinical, and historical information. The accurate evaluation of pretest likelihood of CAD allows for the appropriate selection of patients who would most likely benefit from referral to nuclear imaging. The pretest likelihood or risk assessment may be estimated from published nomograms or by using available computerized programs (see Chaps. 14, 38, and 40). Several models have been developed to predict significant and extensive CAD as well as cardiac survival.[86–88]

The rationale for applying MPS to noninvasive diagnostic testing is based upon Bayesian theory (Chaps. 14 and 40), by which the posttest likelihood is a function of the patient's pretest likelihood of disease and the test's sensitivity and specificity. The ability of the test result to change posttest likelihood is strongly affected by the pretest likelihood of disease. The greatest shift in posttest likelihood of disease occurs in those patients with an intermediate pretest likelihood of CAD; hence, it is in these patients that nuclear myocardial perfusion imaging is most effective for diagnostic purposes.[88a]

#### MPS FOR THE DIAGNOSIS OF CAD

Detection of CAD is one of the most common indications for performing stress MPS. This referral is most appropriate in patients who have an intermediate likelihood of CAD. Exercise is the preferred form of stress due to the additional information derived from clinical, hemodynamic, and ECG responses to exercise. The principal exceptions to this are patients with LBBB or paced LV rhythms and patients with moderate aortic stenosis for whom vasodilator stress is preferred. Patients with LBBB may frequently demonstrate reversible septal defects in the absence of CAD.[89] The mechanism has been postulated to be true septal ischemia in LBBB in the presence of marked tachycardia. Hence, stress techniques that avoid tachycardia are preferred in LBBB—i.e., adenosine or dipyridamole testing without walking is generally considered preferable.[90–92]

***Diagnostic Accuracy*** Diagnostic testing for CAD is usually defined on the basis of sensitivity and specificity for identification of angiographically significant stenoses. Recent ACC/AHA/ASNC guidelines on cardiac radionuclide imaging show a pooled sensitivity and specificity of 87 and 73 percent for exercise stress (based on 33 published studies) and 89 and 75 percent for vasodilator stress (based on 17 published studies) for detection of angiographically significant CAD (≥50 to 70 percent stenosis). An improved predictive accuracy by nuclear testing over pretest information and ECG stress testing has been consistently documented.[93] By reducing attenuation artifacts, test specificity is increased with $^{99m}$Tc-based agents compared to $^{201}$Tl imaging in women.[94] The ability to immediately reacquire SPECT images with $^{99m}$Tc-based agents when either attenuation or motion artifact is suspected further increases specificity with these agents. Improvement in reader confidence and accuracy of scan final interpretation have been shown to be increased by the use of gated compared to ungated MPS (Fig. 19-14).

*Referral or Verification Bias* A major limitation to the measurement of diagnostic accuracy of CAD is the use of cardiac catheterization results as a "gold standard." In estimating the true sensitivity and specificity of noninvasive testing, referral or workup bias must be taken into account.[95] As routine patient workup results in preferential catheterization of patients with abnormal (ischemic) test results, this referral bias leads to an overestimation of test sensitivity and a reduction in test specificity,[96] with the latter showing the most dramatic change.

*Normalcy Rate* The normalcy rate has been advocated as an improved measure for this purpose,[38] defined as the percentage of patients with normal test results in a population with a low likelihood of disease. The recent ACC/AHA/ASNC guidelines show a normalcy rate for MPS of 91 percent.

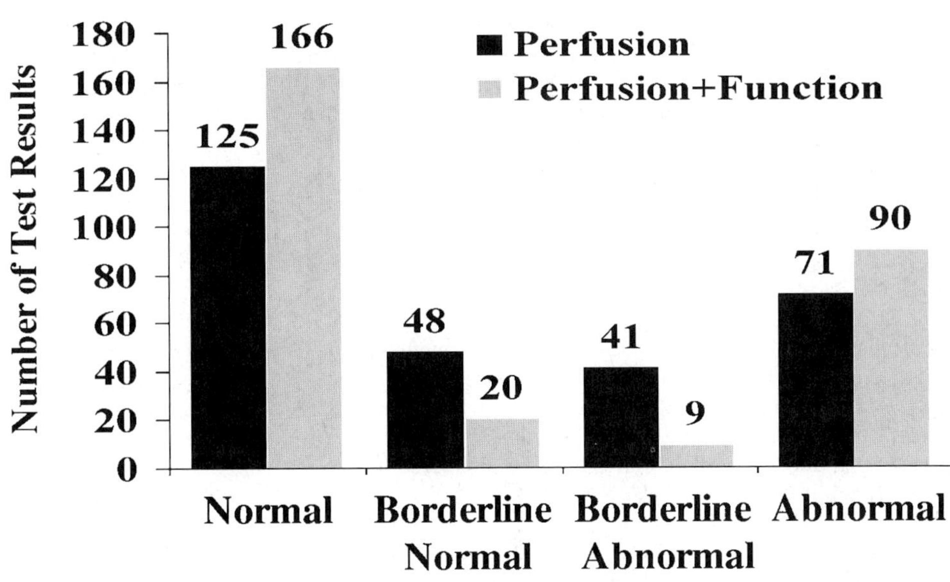


FIGURE 19-14 Distribution of categories of final interpretation of MPS based on perfusion images alone (black) or assessment of perfusion images in conjunction with gated SPECT images (gray). The use of gated SPECT reduced the frequency of borderline interpretations. (Reproduced with permission from Smanio et al.[269])

*Diagnostic Testing Algorithm* A clinical algorithm for the purpose of simple detection of CAD based on these concepts is as follows[97]: Patients with a low pre–exercise tolerance test (ETT) likelihood of CAD (<0.15) do not require further diagnostic testing, and primary CAD prevention is recommended. Patients with a low-intermediate pre-ETT likelihood of CAD (0.15 to 0.50) would undergo standard ETT, with those patients having low post-ETT likelihood having a primary prevention approach and those having intermediate to high likelihood going on to MPS. Although patients with pre-ETT likelihood of CAD in the 0.50 to 0.85 range are often considered ETT candidates in guidelines,[2,93] since even a negative ETT would not result in a low likelihood, many experts consider MPS to be the appropriate first test. Patients with a high pre-ETT likelihood of CAD (>0.85) would not need nuclear stress testing for *diagnostic* purposes, although they often do for risk stratification, as described below. Finally, patients with an indeterminate ETT result (e.g., intermediate-risk Duke treadmill score,[2,98]) as well as with ECG uninterpretable for ETT [e.g., left ventricular hypertrophy (LVH), digoxin, Wolff-Parkinson-White (WPW), >1-mm resting ST depression, LBBB, permanent pacemaker, etc.] are candidates for MPS rather than ETT.

*Guidelines for Testing of Patients with Suspected CAD* A variation of this approach was included in recent guidelines.[93] In patients who cannot exercise or have an uninterpretable ECG with respect to exercise and have an intermediate likelihood of CAD, nuclear testing for diagnosis of CAD has been given a class I indication (condition for which there is general agreement that a given procedure is useful and effective).[2,93,98]

## MPS for Risk Assessment

### PRINCIPLES OF RISK STRATIFICATION

A new paradigm in patient management is that of a *risk-based approach* to patients with suspected CAD in whom symptoms are nonlimiting. In patients referred directly to catheterization for any reason, precatheterization MPS may serve to identify the culprit lesion. However, in less symptomatic patients, precatheterization risk assessment is more important. With a risk-based approach, the focus is not on predicting who has CAD but on identifying patients at risk for specific adverse events. Subsequent management focuses on reducing the risk of these outcomes, whether cardiac death or nonfatal myocardial infarction (MI) or CAD progression. Invasive diagnostic and therapeutic procedures are limited to those patients who are most likely to benefit from them. The basic concept underlying the use of nuclear testing for risk stratification is that patients known to be at high or low risk for events would not be appropriate patients for cost-effective risk stratification with nuclear imaging since they are already stratified.

*Risk Thresholds* It has been suggested that a >3 percent annual mortality rate is a threshold to identify patients with symptoms whose mortality rate can be improved by coronary artery bypass surgery (CABS).[99] For the purposes of risk assessment, it has been proposed that low risk be defined as a <1 percent annual cardiac mortality rate and intermediate risk could be defined by the range of 1 to 3 percent per year.[93] Since the mortality risk for patients undergoing revascularization is greater than 1 percent per year,[100] symptomatic patients with a less than 1 percent mortality rate would not be candidates for revascularization to improve survival. MPS is most appropriate in patients with >1 percent annual mortality and intermediate or high likelihood of CAD. The exact level of these risk thresholds would vary according to the population being tested.

*Physiologic Basis of Risk Assessment in MPS* Many of the major determinants of prognosis in CAD are assessed by measurements of stress-induced perfusion and function, including infarcted and jeopardized myocardium (supplied by vessels with hemodynamically significant stenosis) and the degree of jeopardy (tightness of the individual coronary stenosis). Of additional importance is the stability (or instability) of the CAD process, a factor that may explain an apparent paradox. While nuclear tests in general are expected to identify only hemodynamically significant stenoses, it has been observed that most MIs occur in regions with less than 50 percent diameter narrowing.[101,102] Normal MPS, expected in patients with no or insignificant CAD, is associated with a low risk of either cardiac death or nonfatal MI. Several explanations may account for this apparent paradox. Patients with severe CAD may have more numerous mild plaques subject to potential instability and rupture than patients with no severe stenoses. Furthermore, a paradoxical vasoconstrictive response to stress due to endothelial dysfunction with unstable mild stenoses may also contribute.[103,104]

## RISK STRATIFICATION IN PATIENTS WITH SUSPECTED OR KNOWN CAD

Stress MPS is an integral part of the evaluation of symptomatic patients for CAD and is commonly used in patients at intermediate post-ETT risk or with resting ECG abnormalities. As with diagnostic testing, if the patient's rest ECG is uninterpretable for purposes of stress testing, direct referral to MPS is effective in prognostic stratification (Chap. 14).

***Incremental Prognostic Value*** The clinical value of MPS for prognostic assessment of CAD results from the incremental or added prognostic information yielded by this modality over all data available prior to the test (clinical, historical, and stress data), as first demonstrated by Ladenheim et al.[105]

***Event Risk after a Normal Scan*** A synthesis of available data reveals that a normal scan is generally associated with a $<1$ percent annual risk of cardiac death or MI.[29,58,106–108] A recent metanalysis of the prognostic value of a normal stress perfusion scan ($N = 29{,}788$) reveals that the annual risk of MI or cardiac death after a normal perfusion scan is 0.5 percent (95 percent CI 0.3 to 0.7 percent).[107,109] This uniformly low event rate is critical in applying nuclear test information to risk stratification, since in the absence of symptoms, patients with normal perfusion scans can be managed conservatively. This approach includes follow-up for signs of clinical worsening and treatment of cardiac risk factors and related symptoms (see Chap. 40). The recent study has suggested that when inferior wall defects seen on supine imaging are not seen on prone imaging and are thus considered to be attenuation artifacts, the event rate is as low as in patients with normal supine studies.[109a]

Despite the low risk associated with normal SPECT studies, a limited number of studies have reported somewhat higher levels of risk. Recently, a study examining predictors of risk and its temporal characteristics in a series of 7376 patients with normal stress MPS identified the use of pharmacologic stress and the presence of known CAD (Fig. 19-15), diabetes mellitus (in particular, female diabetics), and advanced age as markers of increased risk and shortened time to a hard event (e.g., risk in the first year of follow-up was less than in the second year).[29] Hence, a dynamic temporal component of risk was present and the existence of a "warranty" period for specific patient groups was defined (Fig. 19-16). This increased risk after normal SPECT in a small subset of patients is due to the presence of comorbidities that increase baseline risk of all patients (diabetes mellitus, age, inability to exercise, prior CAD) and, in some patients, the possibility that extensive CAD was "missed" due to balanced reduction of flow. The latter would lead to a severe underestimation of the extent of ischemia by MPS. While many of these patients can be detected by ancillary markers—such as LV transient ischemic dilation,[109b] a rest to poststress fall in LVEF, or increased lung tracer uptake—in some patients with high-risk anatomic lesions, MPS will appear completely normal.

## Event Risk with Abnormal Scans

Increasing scan abnormality is associated with an increasing risk of cardiac events.[58,93]

### MILDLY ABNORMAL PERFUSION SCANS

As shown in Fig. 19-17, a large study evaluating risk after MPS showed patients with moderately and severely abnormal scans to be at intermediate risk for both cardiac death and MI.[58] Importantly, patients with mildly abnormal scans were at intermediate risk for MI but at low risk for subsequent mortality (2.7 vs. 0.8 percent risk per year), hence could be considered as having "flow-limiting" CAD but unlikely to die of their disease. Due to this low mortality rate, and the observation that medical therapy, but not revascularization, lowers the risk of MI, acute ischemic syndromes, or cardiac hospitalizations,[110,111] we hypothesized that if not limited by symptoms, these patients would be candidates for aggressive medical therapy/risk-factor modification.

More recently we have further modified this approach. The presence of high-risk clinical or historical markers identifies a subset of patients at greater risk *for any level of SSS,* that is, prescan data yield incremental prognostic information over MPS results.[29,58–60,112–114] Hence, while patients with mildly abnormal MPS results generally are at low risk of cardiac death, this is not true in the

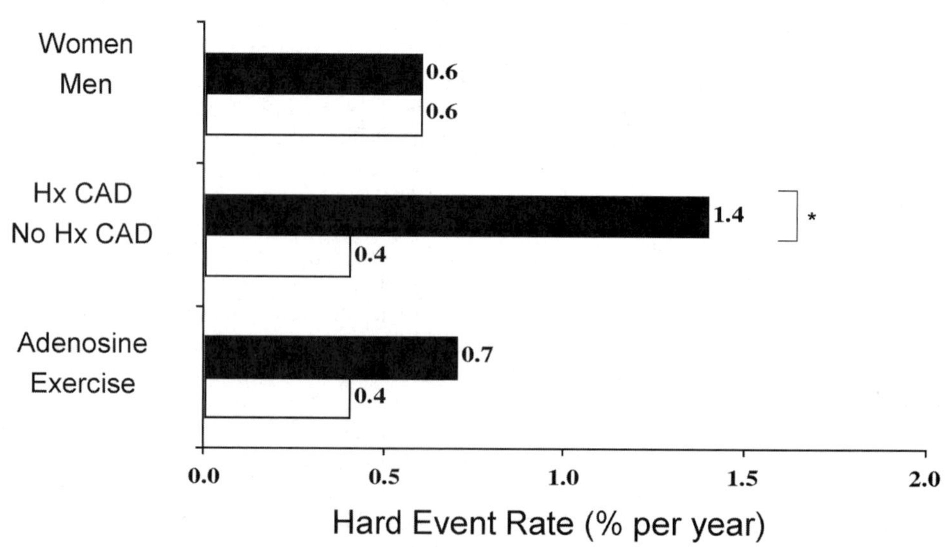


FIGURE 19-15 Annual rates of hard events in patients after normal MPS. The following subgroups are shown: women versus men, patients with and/without history (Hx) of CAD, and patients undergoing adenosine versus exercise stress. A significant risk is noted in the patients with Hx CAD. *$p < 0.001$. (Reproduced with permission from Hachamovitch et al.[29])

case of significant comorbidities (e.g., advanced age, diabetes mellitus, atrial fibrillation, pharmacologic stress).

### MODERATELY TO SEVERELY ABNORMAL PERFUSION SCANS

The relationship of varying extent and severity of perfusion abnormalities with cardiac outcomes has been reported in a variety of patient subsets.[57,58] Although both reversible and fixed stress perfusion defects are predictors of prognosis, those at highest risk of cardiac events are patients with extensive stress abnormalities. Prognosis is also dependent on both the severity and extent of perfusion defects, correlates of the stenosis magnitude, and the amount of myocardium subtended by the stenosed vessels.[115] As these parameters worsen, risk of major cardiac outcomes increase (Fig. 19-17). Annual cardiac event rates have been reported to range from 0.3 to 4.2 percent for patients with normal, mild, moderate, and severely abnormal perfusion scans.[58] Similar findings have been described with $^{201}$Tl (Fig. 19-18) and more recently with $^{99m}$Tc tetrofosmin.[116,117]

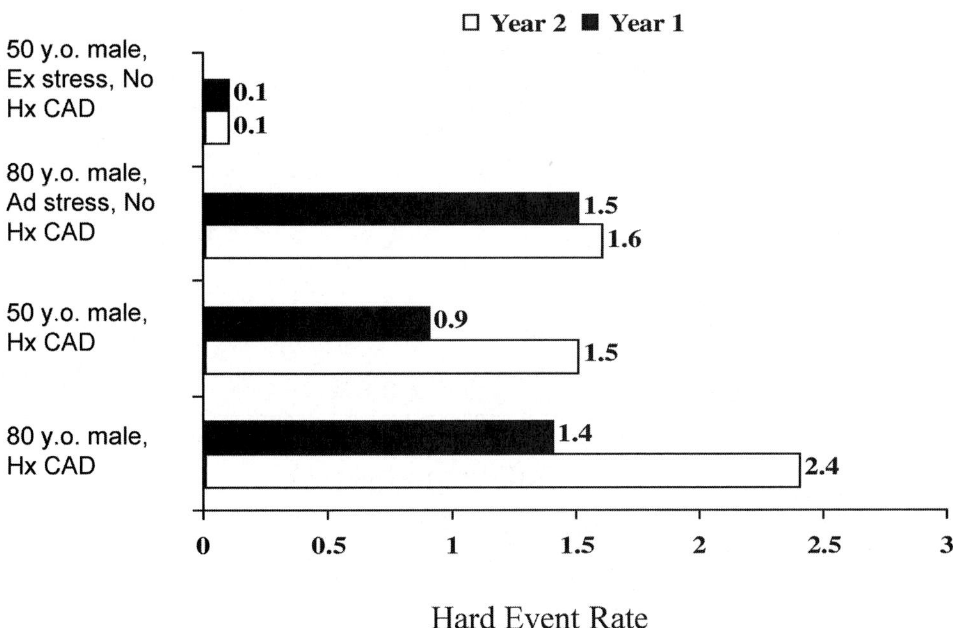


FIGURE 19-16 Rates of hard events in first and second years of follow-up after normal MPS. Four examples are given: a 50-year-old male undergoing exercise stress with no history of CAD, an 80-year-old male undergoing adenosine stress with no history of CAD, a 50-year-old male with a history of CAD, and an 80-year-old male with a history of CAD. In patients with no history of CAD, the event rates in the first and second years after MPS are not different; however, the event rate for normal MPS goes up significantly with increased patient risk. In patients with previous CAD, the event rates in the second year after MPS were greater than in the first year, and there is additional increase in the event rate with clinical risk. (Reproduced with permission from Hachamovitch et al.[29])

### USING MPS FOR MEDICAL DECISION MAKING: SURVIVAL BENEFIT

A major step forward is the recently evolved paradigm indicating that rather than identify patient risk, the goal of MPS in a testing strategy is the identification of patients who may have a *survival benefit* from revascularization as opposed to those who lack a survival benefit from this procedure. In 10,627 patients without prior MI or revascularization who underwent stress MPS, MPS identified a survival benefit for patients undergoing medical therapy versus revascularization in the setting of no or mild ischemia, whereas patients undergoing revascularization had an increasing survival benefit over patients undergoing medical therapy when moderate to severe ischemia was present (>10 percent of the total myocardium ischemic).[59] This survival benefit was particularly striking in higher-risk patients (elderly, requiring adenosine stress, and women, especially diabetics). These results have been extended to include information regarding gated MPS EF,[113] showing that EF and both the percent myocardium ischemic and the percent myocardium fixed are predictors of cardiac death. However, only inducible ischemia identified patients who would benefit from revascularization. With increasing amounts of ischemia, increasing survival benefit for revascularization over medical therapy was found. The absolute benefit associated with revascularization was also driven by EF and fixed defects, but the presence of this benefit was not impacted by results of these two markers.

## Integrating Clinical Data with MPS Results

A challenge facing clinicians attempting to apply MPS results to patient care is to distill all information reported after MPS—clinical, historical, stress test, perfusion, and function data—into an estimate of likelihood of CAD or risk of adverse events for an individual patient. Since MPS and pre-MPS data add incremental to each other, accurate final estimates of risk must also adjust for clinical data. Ideally, the development of validated scores will incorporate all available sources of information, including expressing MPS results in a

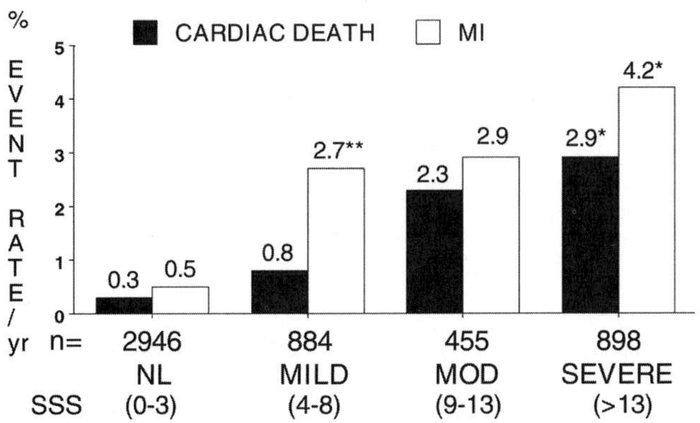


FIGURE 19-17 Rates of cardiac death (*solid bars*) and myocardial infarction (*open bars*) per year as a function of scan result. The numbers of patients within each scan category are shown underneath each pair of columns. *Statistically significant increase as a function of scan result. **Statistically significant increase in rate of MI versus cardiac death with scan category. NL = normal, MILD = mildly abnormal, MOD = moderately abnormal, SEVERE = severely abnormal. (Reproduced with permission from Hachamovitch et al.[58])

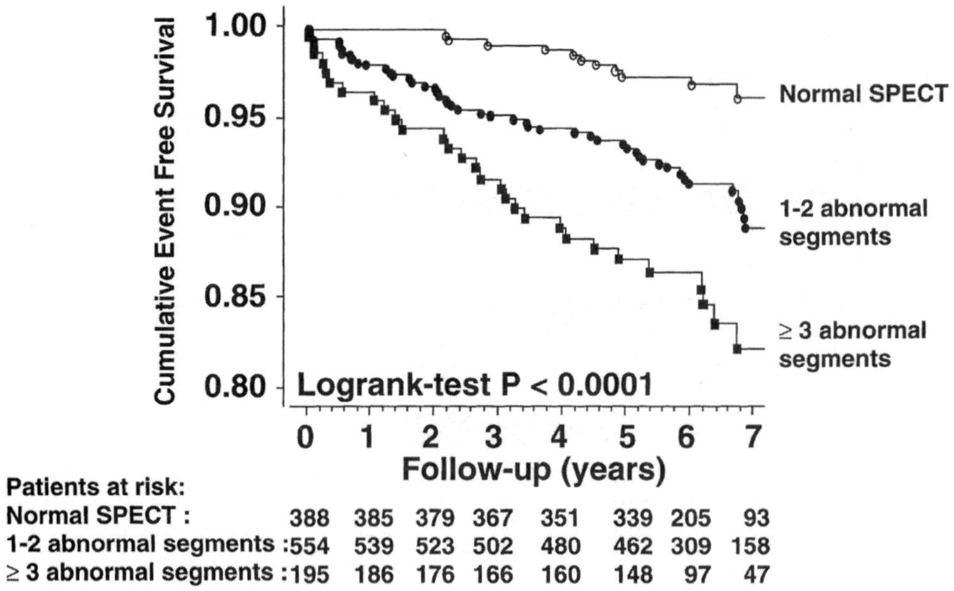


FIGURE 19-18 Kaplan-Meier survival curves for normal SPECT, abnormal SPECT in 1 to 2 segments, and abnormal SPECT in >2 segments from a large series of patients undergoing thallium MPS. The findings are similar to those observed with sestamibi.[270] (Reproduced with permission from the AHA.)

manner independent of the scoring system used (e.g., percent myocardium abnormal at stress, etc). Hence, by deriving the equivalent of the Duke treadmill score for stress MPS testing, accurate and reliable estimates of CAD likelihood or risk could be incorporated into MPS reporting. Table 19-2 summarizes the various clinical, stress test, and scintigraphic signs of elevated risk. It must always be recognized that clinical judgment is paramount in the application of these approaches due to imperfections in the data derived from populations in defining all variables that might be operative in determining the risk of an individual patient as well as limitations of the tests themselves.

## Use of MPS in Guiding Decisions for Catheterization

Several investigators have shown that MPS results appear to heavily influence post-MPS clinical decision making. Among patients with normal scans, only a small proportion undergo early post-MPS cardiac catheterization, usually as a result of clinical symptomatology.[56] As first shown by Hachamovitch and colleagues, the extent and severity of reversible defects shown by the MPS result is the dominant factor driving subsequent resource utilization[57] (Fig. 19-19). Similar results have been shown by other authors.[118,119] Furthermore, if catheterization were limited to patients with moderate to severe perfusion abnormalities, a 17 percent reduction in cardiac catheterization rate was shown in a study of 5183 patients.[58] It has become increasingly important to determine whether noninvasive testing can result in substantial cost savings in the diagnosis of CAD. Shaw et al.,[120] in a multicenter study of 11,249 patients, showed that strategies of direct referral to catheterization and referral to MPS with selective subsequent catheterization produced a substantial reduction (31 to 50 percent) in costs for all levels of pretest clinical risk in favor of the noninvasive approach (Fig. 19-20), with essentially identical outcomes (Fig. 19-21). Rates of revascularization were reduced by nearly 50 percent in the MPS strategy, as were rates of cardiac catheterization after normal MPS and the frequency of normal coronary angiographic findings.

## Estimating the True Prognostic Value of MPS and Posttest Referral Bias

Although there is compelling evidence that MPS is effective in the prognostic stratification of patients, the current data on risk stratification by MPS may actually underestimate the strength of this modality due to a prognostic counterpart to the diagnostic verification bias described above. Prognostic analyses performed to date are entirely comprised of patients undergoing medical therapy after testing, since prognostic assessment of noninvasive testing using observational data series dictate that patients undergoing early revascularization after testing be removed or censored from prognostic analyses due to the relationship between the referral to revascularization and the test results.[121–123] It has been hypothesized that with increasing physician acceptance and use of MPS, the strong dependence of post-MPS referral to revascularization on the MPS results, a posttest referral bias may develop that results in an underestimation of the prognostic value of this test due to the revascularization (and censoring) of the highest-risk patients.[57,118,124,124a]

## Added Value of Gated SPECT

Since gated SPECT has become routine only recently, there are few reports of its incremental value over perfusion in assessing prognosis. LV ejection fraction (at rest or rest/stress), measured by other modalities, has been shown to

TABLE 19-2 Markers of High Risk

| Clinical | Stress Test | SPECT |
|---|---|---|
| Diabetes mellitus | Severe ST-segment depression | TID |
| (esp. women) | Pharmacologic stress | Lung uptake |
| insulin dependence | Exercise hypotension | Stress-induced stunning or ↓EF |
| Atrial fibrillation | Blunted HR response to adenosine | Reduced EF |
| Elderly | Marked hypotension with adenosine stress | Severe and/or extensive defects |
| Marked resting ECG abnormalities | | |
| Dyspnea as presenting symptom | | |
| Typical angina | | |
| Unstable angina | | |

KEY: ECG, electrocardiogram; HR, heart rate; EF, ejection fraction; TID, transient ischemic dilation.

risk-stratify suspected disease patients for risk for cardiac death.[122,125,126]

Sharir et al.[127] demonstrated that poststress LVEF, as measured by gated SPECT, provided significant information over the extent and severity of perfusion defect in the prediction of cardiac death. Furthermore, LV end-systolic volume provided added information over poststress LVEF for prediction of cardiac death (Fig. 19-22). The relatively low cardiac death rate in patients with abnormal perfusion and normal LV function in this study is probably explained by a referral bias in which patients with greatest ischemia by SSS were preferentially sent for early revascularization and thus censored from assessment of the prognostic value of the test.[127a] In a subsequent report, in more than 2600 patients, Sharir et al. noted that perfusion variables are stronger predictors of nonfatal MI, while after risk adjustment, poststress EF was not predictive of nonfatal MI.[128] A preliminary report has shown that although EF best predicts cardiac mortality, only inducible ischemia identifies patients who are likely to benefit from revascularization at all levels of EF.[128a]

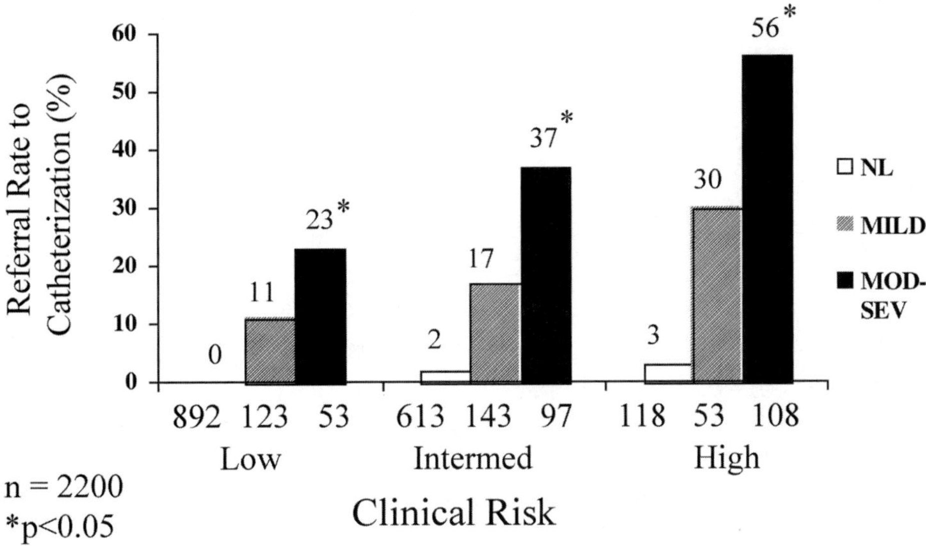


FIGURE 19-19 Referral rates to catheterization as a function of clinical risk in 2200 patients with no known CAD undergoing dual-isotope MPS. Low, intermediate (intermed), and high refer to the prescan likelihood of CAD. MPS findings are illustrated for each clinical risk category. NL: normal; mild: mild SSS (4 to 8); mod-sev (moderate to severely abnormal : SSS >8). A significant increase in referral rates to catheterization was observed in each category of clinical risk as a function of scan abnormality ($p < 0.05$). In patients with a normal scan, the referral rates were very low, even in the presence of a high prescan likelihood of CAD.[57]

## INTEGRATED CLINICAL ALGORITHMS FOR PERFUSION AND FUNCTION

In the future, complex algorithms will need to be developed that incorporate all of the information from gated SPECT for purposes of guiding patient management. With this regard, it is likely that poststress EF (related predominately to the size of MI) and summed difference score (an expression of the amount of stress-induced ischemia) will provide the greatest complementary information. Sharir et al. have reported the combination of the ejection fraction and reversible ischemia can be used in the prediction of cardiac events.[129]

Other important information that can be derived from MPS and may be related to risk has not been widely included in the prognostic assessment (Table 19-2). The assessment of poststress wall motion abnormalities on gated SPECT are a sign of exercise-induced stunning and a marker of severe CAD.[130,131] Transient ischemic dilation of the LV[77,78,109b] and pulmonary uptake of radioactivity as determined by the measurement of lung/heart ratios of radioactivity[82,132] have been shown to be of prognostic importance.[81,130,132] Extensive reversibility of resting defects (as determined by 24-h $^{201}$Tl imaging after rest $^{201}$Tl/stress $^{99m}$Tc-sestamibi MPS) has been shown to be predictive of a higher mortality rate than would be predicted by rest or stress perfusion defect abnormalities alone.[133] Finally, as noted above, inducible ischemia or viable myocardium—not EF— appears to identify patients who may benefit from revascularization.[113,134]

## USE OF MPS IN SPECIFIC PATIENT POPULATIONS

A principal strength of nuclear cardiology is that large databases have been accumulated resulting in evidence documenting the effectiveness of MPS for risk stratification of appropriately selected patients, comprising the full spectrum of patients with suspected or chronic CAD. This evidence has resulted in many class I indications for the use of stress MPS.[2] Several specific lines of evidence are described below.

**1. Evidence Supporting Nuclear Imaging for Patients with an Intermediate Risk or Indeterminate Treadmill Test.** Several recent reports support nuclear testing in patients with uninterpretable

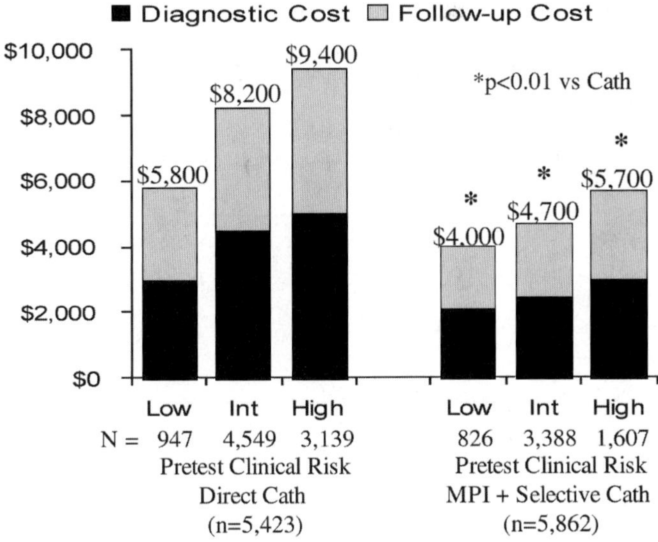


FIGURE 19-20 Comparative cost between screening strategies employing direct catheterization (Cath) and myocardial perfusion imaging (MPI) with selective Cath. Low, Int, and High represent low-, intermediate-, and high-risk subsets of the patients with stable angina. Shown are the initial diagnostic costs (*solid bars*) and follow-up costs including costs of revascularization (*gray bars*). A 30 to 41 percent reduction in costs was noted in each category. (Adapted with permission from Shaw.[271])

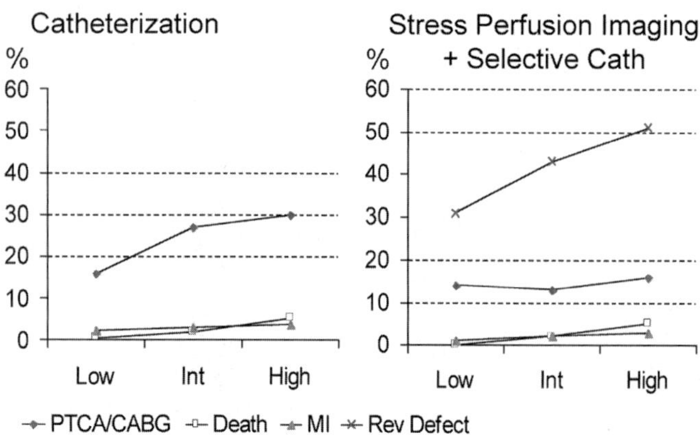


FIGURE 19-21 Subsequent event rates in the patient populations illustrated in Fig. 19-20. The rates of myocardial infarction and cardiac death were identical between the populations. The difference between the populations was an approximate 50 percent reduction in revascularization in the group approached with myocardial perfusion imaging and selective catheterization. Abbreviations as in Fig. 19-20. PTCA = percutaneous transluminal coronary angioplasty; CABS = coronary artery bypass surgery; Death = cardiac death; MI = myocardial infarction; Rev defect = reversible defect. (Adapted with permission from Shaw.[271])

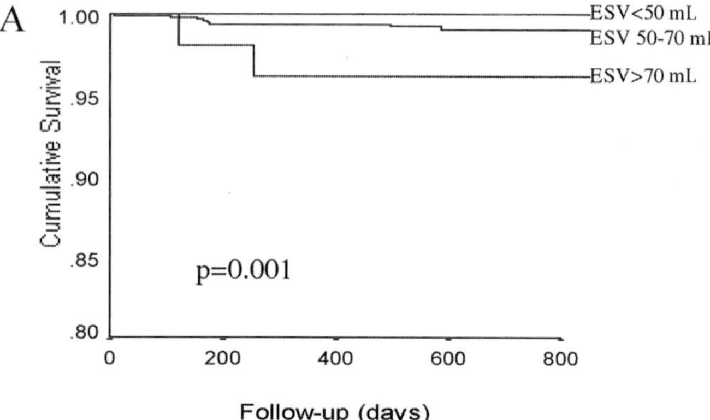


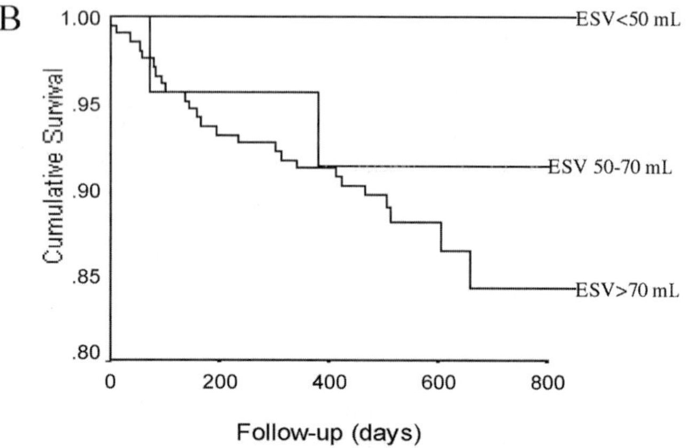


FIGURE 19-22 Cumulative survival of patients with poststress ejection fraction (EF) by quantitative gated SPECT greater than or equal to 45 percent (*left*) and less than 45 percent (*right*) stratified by end-systolic volume (ESV), also measured by gated SPECT. (Adapted with permission from Sharir et al.[127])

or intermediate exercise ECG response.[57,135,136] An initial report from Cedars-Sinai demonstrated that MPS was most effective in risk stratification and governing management of patients with intermediate Duke treadmill score.[57] Patients with a low (hard-event rate of less than 1 percent) or high (hard-event rate of 7.7 percent) Duke treadmill score did not benefit from MPS. Patients with an intermediate Duke treadmill score, the majority of patients studied, had an intermediate risk of hard events (also reported to have an intermediate risk of cardiac death) of 1.25 percent per year.[136] Patients with a normal scan had very low event rates and were infrequently catheterized, those with moderately abnormal scans had intermediate rates of events and catheterization, and those with moderately to severely abnormal scans had higher rates of events and catheterization. Thus, the nuclear tests were able to stratify patients who could not be differentiated according to risk by Duke treadmill score alone. Similar results were shown in two large multicenter studies reporting event rates and catheterization rates[98,135] (Fig. 19-23).

**2. Evidence Supporting Nuclear Imaging for Patients with Normal Resting ECG Able to Exercise.** Patients with normal resting ECGs represent a large and important subgroup who are commonly encountered in clinical practice in whom the use of MPS is controversial.[105,113,137–139] Generally speaking, patients with a normal resting ECG have an excellent prognosis[137] and are likely (92 to 96 percent) to have normal LV function.[140,141]

Several studies have examined the added value of exercise MPS over clinical and ETT data in this patient group.[105,113,138,139] The Mayo clinic demonstrated that although MPS yielded incremental value over clinical and ETT data for the prediction of left main or three-vessel disease, the yield was modest and not cost-effective.[138,142] A subsequent study reported incremental value for MPS in patients with an abnormal exercise ECG response, but only for the prediction of a combination of hard and soft events (including unstable angina).[139] More recently, a study of 3058 patients with normal resting ECGs showed that selective use of MPS in patients with intermediate to high post-ETT CAD likelihood yielded significant risk stratification, statistical incremental value, and cost-effectiveness in predicting hard events.[113] A subsequent study from the Mayo Clinic has shown that patients with a high clinical score (based on age, sex, prior MI, and diabetic state) are at too high pretest risk to be classified as low risk by exercise testing. The author suggests that initial stress MPS testing might be appropriate in this group.[142a] Complementary findings were also recently shown in the ability of stress MPS to define a low post-SPECT risk in the majority of patients with a high pretest likelihood of CAD.[124a]

**3. Evidence Supporting Nuclear Imaging for Patients with Normal Resting ECG Unable to Exercise.** In patients who have a normal resting ECG and an intermediate to high likelihood of CAD but are unable to exercise, adenosine or dipyridamole stress MPS has been shown to be effective for both CAD diagnosis and risk stratification. The risk of adverse events in these patients, however, is greater for any given MPS result when compared to patients undergoing exercise stress—i.e., the requirement of pharmacologic stress is an incremental predictor of adverse outcomes,[58] most likely related to an increased underlying risk of this population compared to patients who are able to exercise.

**4. Evidence Supporting Nuclear Imaging for Asymptomatic Patients.** Several studies have examined the diagnostic and prognostic value of stress MPS in asymptomatic populations. In a study examining asymptomatic siblings of patients with manifest CAD, a cohort acknowledged to be at increased risk of developing CAD, a relative risk of 4.7 for experiencing an adverse cardiac event was reported for individuals with an abnormal scan[143] and the presence of

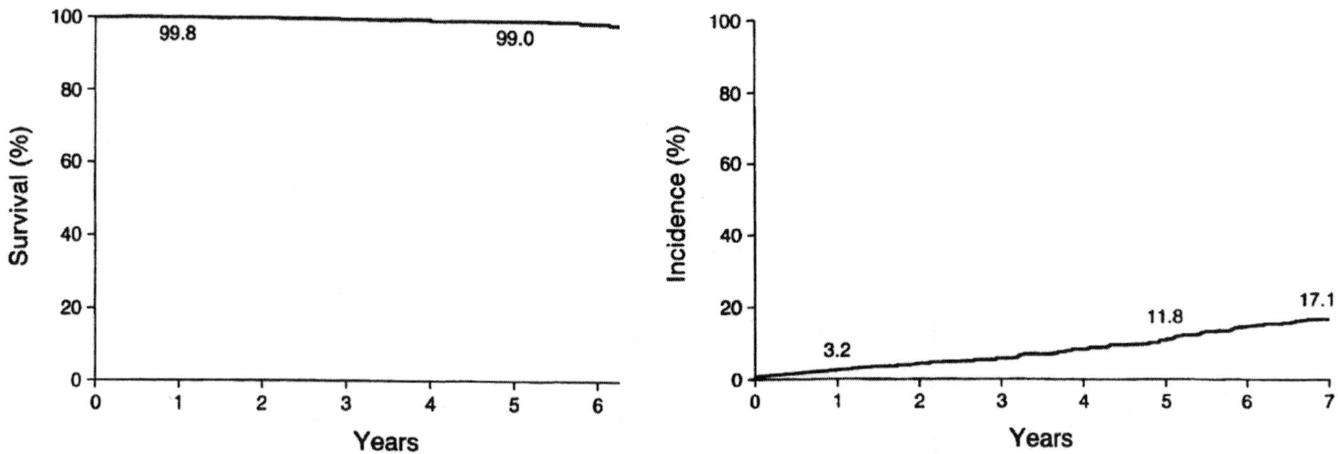


FIGURE 19-23 Kaplan-Meier and cumulative catheterization rate from 4649 patients with intermediate-risk Duke treadmill score and normal stress MPS showing a very low mortality rate (*left*) and a very low frequency of catheterization (*right*).[98] (With permission from the AHA.)

both an abnormal exercise ECG and abnormal perfusion scan yielded a relative risk of 14.5.

As predicted by Bayesian principles, however, the routine use of any test for detection of CAD in a low-risk/low prevalence of CAD asymptomatic population will be associated with high cost-effectiveness ratios and low positive predictive values. This was the case in studies attempting to detect CAD[144] and to predict future events[145] in this patient subgroup. Nonetheless, these evaluations are often performed for statutory reasons (e.g., pilots, truckers, etc.).[136] On the other hand, the use of MPS in asymptomatic individuals with high-risk clinical profiles, particularly in patients in whom classic anginal symptoms are infrequent or not predictive (e.g., diabetes mellitus, female sex, African Americans, the elderly), may be appropriate. Preliminary data have shown that MPS yields incremental value in asymptomatic patients referred to MPS and achieves significant risk stratification.[146] A recent large study has shown that 59 percent of asymptomatic diabetics have abnormal stress MPS studies, including 20 percent with a "high-risk" scan.[146a]

**5. Evidence Supporting Nuclear Imaging for Patients with Documented CAD (Prior Catheterization).** The functional implications of borderline stenoses, difficult to interpret from angiographic findings, can be determined by intravascular ultrasound or fractional flow reserve measurements during cardiac catheterization. When these measurements are not obtained, post-catheterization MPS can identify functionally significant lesions.[147]

**6. Evidence Supporting Nuclear Imaging for Patients with Diabetes Mellitus.** MPS has now been reported to be effective in risk stratification of patients with diabetes.[148–150] In a study comparing 1271 patients with diabetes to 5862 without, MPS risk stratified patients in both groups, but risk-adjusted event-free survival was worse in patients with diabetes than in those without.[148] These findings were confirmed in a multicenter series.[149] In this study, diabetic women had the worst outcome for any given extent of MI. In patients with normal MPS results, survival worsened sooner in diabetic compared to nondiabetic patients, suggesting that retesting of diabetics with normal studies might be needed earlier than in nondiabetics.

We have recently examined a cohort of 2656 women and 2677 men who underwent adenosine stress MPS and were followed up for 27.0 ± 8.8 months.[150] Multivariable models revealed that MPS results provided incremental prognostic value over prescan data for the prediction of cardiac death in both genders. Diabetic women had a greater risk of cardiac death than other patients, and risk of cardiac death for any MPS result was greater in patients with insulin-dependent diabetes mellitus than patients with non-insulin-dependent diabetes mellitus, who in turn had greater risk than non-diabetic patients (Fig. 19-24). Hayes et al. demonstrated that assessment of left

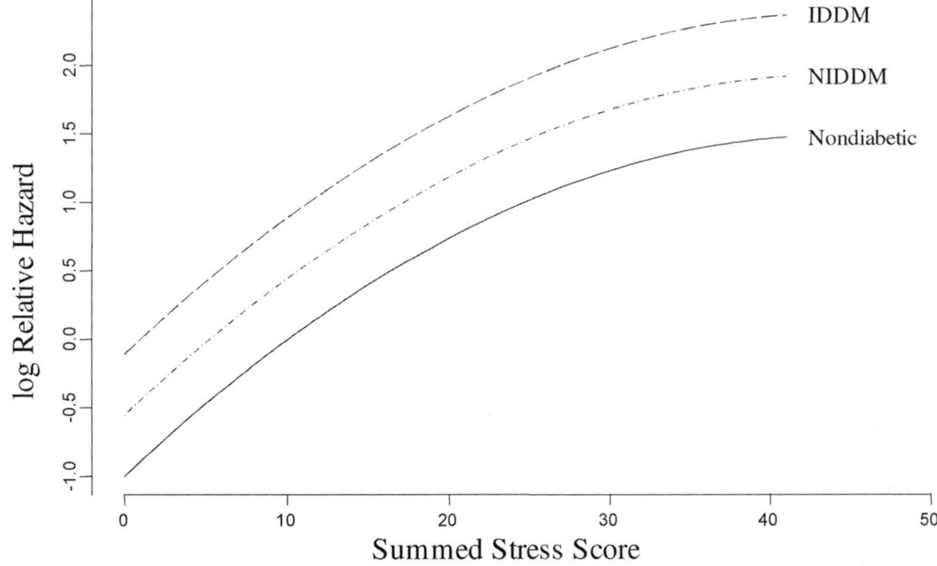


FIGURE 19-24 Risk of cardiac death (Y axis) versus summed stressed score (X axis) in patients with insulin-dependent diabetes mellitus (IDDM), non-insulin-dependent diabetes mellitus (NIDDM), and nondiabetics. An increase in cardiac risk was seen in all groups as a function of the summed stress score. For any given summed stress score, the risk of NIDDM was higher than in nondiabetics, and the risk in IDDM was higher than in NIDDM.[60] (Reproduced with permission from the ACC.)

ventricular EF from gated SPECT provides incremental value over perfusion SPECT parameters in predicting death in diabetic patients.[151]

**7. Evidence Supporting Nuclear Imaging for Patients with Left Bundle Branch Block.** A number of studies have found that vasodilator stress MPS was an excellent predictor of cardiac events in LBBB patients and achieves risk stratification.[152–155] A single study reported that dobutamine stress is accurate in CAD detection in combination with MPS in left branch block patients with LBBB.[156]

**8. Evidence Supporting Nuclear Imaging for Patients with LVH or Atrial Fibrillation.** In patients with LVH with or without resting ST-segment abnormality, ST-segment depression during exercise is frequently present in the absence of significant CAD, thus obfuscating the use of ETT. In these patients, MPS has been shown to have similar sensitivity and specificity to those observed in patients without LVH.[157] Others, however, have reported an increased frequency of "false-positive" studies in healthy athletes with LVH.[158] The prognostic value of MPS has been reported in patients with LVH.[159] A preliminary report has indicated increased risk in patients with atrial fibrillation for any degree of MPS abnormality and that MPS is able to effectively risk stratify AF patients.[159a]

**9. Gender-Based Differences in the Prognostic Value of MPS.** MPS in women has been found to have comparable diagnostic and accuracy as that in men, particularly with the use of $^{99m}$Tc for the stress images.[160–162] In a small randomized trial comparing the diagnostic accuracy of $^{201}$Tl with that of $^{99m}$Tc-sestamibi, test specificity was 67 versus 92 percent, respectively,[94] suggesting that gated SPECT with a $^{99m}$Tc perfusion agent may be the preferred form of SPECT in women. Amanullah and colleagues reported on 130 women undergoing adenosine $^{99m}$Tc-sestamibi SPECT, revealing that a moderately to severely abnormal perfusion scan was associated with a sensitivity and specificity of 91 and 70 percent for the detection of multivessel CAD.[162] Reports including large female populations reveal that there is an added prognostic value for MPS compared to clinical and exercise variables in women.[160,161,163] The added value of MPS in women may be greater than that in men with more efficient risk stratification.[160] Recently, guidelines for the use of MPS in women have been published, including an algorithm for test candidates.[164] Most likely due to a misperception on the part of clinicians regarding CAD in women, initial reports described a sex-related bias in referral to revascularization after nuclear testing,[165] which has been reduced with improved nuclear techniques and physician education.[124] ASNC guidelines currently recommend MPS in intermediate-high likelihood women with atypical or typical chest pain symptoms, dyspnea, or reduced activities of daily living. This would specifically include initial testing with MPS for diabetic women. MPS is also indicated for women who have an indeterminate ETT or who have an abnormal rest ECG. Of those women who are functionally impaired [i.e., cannot achieve 5 metabolic equivalents (METs)], the use of pharmacologic stress SPECT is indicated.

**10. Evidence Supporting Nuclear Imaging for Elderly Patients.** The prognostic value of perfusion scintigraphy in the elderly has been reported in several recent series.[166,167] These have shown that abnormal MPS identifies a high-risk population, enhances risk stratification, and yields incremental prognostic value.[166–169] Furthermore, the addition of myocardial perfusion imaging to test strategies reduced the overall cost of testing per patient. In general, for the elderly as well as for those patients with functional limitations, similar risk assessment is possible with exercise and pharmacologic stress SPECT.[58] Owing to the higher mortality rate of the general population in this age group, upward adjustment of the "intermediate-risk" group to levels higher than the 1 to 3 percent used for general populations may be appropriate. In this regard, Hayes et al. evaluated 1848 consecutive patients ≥80 years of age undergoing rest $^{201}$Tl/stress $^{99m}$Tc-sestamibi dual-isotope MPS. Annualized cardiac death rates ranged from 1.9 percent in normal scans to 9.3 percent in severely abnormal scans.[169]

**11. Evidence Supporting Nuclear Imaging for African-American Patients.** The role value of MPS in African Americans has been addressed in only two studies to date. Both studies found that although MPS yields added value and risk stratifies these patients, a normal MPS was associated with a rate of MI or cardiac death in African Americans of 2 percent per year.[170,171] This may be due to several factors, including inclusion of higher-risk patients (angina symptoms, prior MI) and an unusually high loss to follow-up. Given the considerably greater prevalence of hypertension and LVH and its contribution to mortality in African Americans,[172] a role for early, undetected cardiomyopathy is possible. Whether this higher risk is related to ethnicity or other factors (health care access, socioeconomic status) is unknown.

**12. Evidence Supporting Nuclear Imaging for Obese Patients.** The use of MPS in obese patients is associated with several problems. Most SPECT imaging tables have weight limits (often 300 lb). The use of planar scintigraphy as an alternative is less accurate than SPECT and many interpreting physicians are less familiar with its interpretation. While the problem of attenuation in these patients is lessened by use of $^{99m}$Tc agents, PET imaging may be superior to conventional MPS in these subjects. However, with a protocol using combined supine and prone imaging, sensitivity, specificity, and normalcy rates similar to those in nonobese patients have been described in the obese population in a preliminary report.[172a]

**13. Evidence Supporting Nuclear Imaging after Coronary Calcium Screening.** Increasing evidence is accumulating to support the use of CT derived coronary calcium scores (CCS) as a means to evaluate asymptomatic patients with multiple risk factors for detection of early, subclinical coronary atherosclerosis.

While most patients do not need further testing, some patients benefit from referral to MPS as a second test. He et al. evaluated 292 men and 78 women who had undergone electron beam tomography (EBT) calcium scoring and MPS.[173] Of patients with extensive CCS (>400), 47 percent had abnormal MPS, while abnormal MPS was rare with scores <400. Similar findings have been reported by others.[174] Nonetheless, the ACC/AHA/ASNC guidelines employ a more liberal threshold for MPS testing of these patients, giving a class IIB indication to the use of MPS in further assessment of patients in whom the CCS is >75th percentile for age and gender. A more conservative approach, which we currently follow, is to recommend MPS in those patients who are found to have CCS >75th percentile and >100 or CCS >400, concordant with the initial recommendations of Rumberger et al.[174a]

**14. Evidence Supporting Nuclear Testing for Patients after Percutaneous Coronary Intervention (PCI).** Post-PCI MPS can potentially play a number of roles, since MPS abnormalities post-PCI may reflect restenosis, periprocedural myocardial injury, side-branch compromise, de novo disease, or functionally significant angiographic disease in nonrevascularized vessels. As part of a staged procedure, MPS can assess the remaining ischemic burden after the initial PCI. Also, post-PCI MPS yields important prognostic information. In the Angioplasty Compared to Medicine (ACME) study,[175] the absence of reversible defects on 6-month follow-up planar $^{201}$Tl scintigraphy after randomization to medical therapy or PCI was associated with a reduction in risk compared to patients with defects (6 vs. 18 percent, $p = 0.02$).

Post-PCI MPS has been extensively used for the detection of silent or minimally symptomatic restenosis. Based on reviews of the literature and a metanalysis,[176–178] several statements can be made regarding the value of MPS. It is far superior to ETT for this application. It can detect silent restenosis; based on early studies, the presence of "false-positive" post-PTCA MPS is often predictive of future restenosis due to the abnormal endothelial properties of regions predisposed to restenosis. The role of MPS in detection of restenosis has been altered by the use of stenting. Stenting is associated with a rapid normalization of flow reserve in the intervened arteries,[179] but it also reduces absolute restenosis rate and prevalence of restenosis. As predicted by Bayesian theory, an increased false-positive rate has been found with MPS use in restenosis,[178] from 37 to 77 percent. Hence, the value of MPS for detecting silent restenosis is unclear.

The major indication for perfusion imaging in patients late after successful PCI is to evaluate symptoms suggesting new disease. While many experts recommend routine testing of asymptomatic patients 4 to 6 months after PCI, especially those with worrisome arteriographic patterns, its role requires further study. In a study of 211 low-risk patients tested 1 to 3 years after PTCA and followed for 7.3 years,[180] a low overall annual event rate of 1 percent per year was found, suggesting no need for testing, despite the predictive value of MPS for adverse events.

In general, when symptoms develop after PCI, MPS can be helpful in defining the culprit vessel and assessing the extent of ischemic abnormality. Routine nuclear testing after PCI is not currently recommended for asymptomatic patients.[2] The ACC/AHA 2002 Guideline Update for Exercise Testing favors only selective stress imaging in patients considered to be at particularly high risk (e.g., patients with decreased LV function, multivessel CAD, proximal LAD disease, previous sudden death, diabetes mellitus, hazardous occupations, and suboptimal PCI results). Whenever moderate to severe ischemia is found by nuclear testing, consideration should be given to repeat catheterization, even in the absence of symptoms.

**15. Evidence Supporting Nuclear Testing for Patients after CABS.** Nuclear testing has become central in the assessment of the post-CABS patient. It is known that >50 percent of vein grafts can be expected to be occluded by 10 years after surgery, hence an intermediate likelihood of vein graft disease.[181,182] Thus, a 5-year cutoff point to evaluate the postbypass patient may be considered appropriate.[177,179,183,184]

In patients studied with $^{201}$Tl MPS >5 years after CABS, inducible ischemia and abnormal lung uptake of $^{201}$Tl added incremental information to clinical variables in predicting outcome in 294 patients.[183] This was confirmed by Nallamothu et al. in 250 patients.[185] Even in asymptomatic patients, $^{201}$Tl-perfusion defects were independent predictors of subsequent death or MI.[179] Zellweger et al.[186] compared the prognostic value of MPS in patients early versus late after CABS, finding that symptomatic but not asymptomatic patients ≤5 years post-CABS benefit from routine MPS. Patients >5 years post-CABS appeared to benefit from MPS irrespective of symptoms, since if moderate to severe ischemia was present, at least a moderate mortality risk was present. In post-CABS patients with new symptoms, MPS can identify the presence and extent of ischemia. In asymptomatic patients, MPS should be considered 5 or more years after CABS. Whenever moderate to severe ischemia is present, catheterization should be considered.[177,184]

**16. Evidence Supporting Nuclear Imaging for Preoperative Risk Assessment in Noncardiac Surgery Patients.** Preoperative risk assessment is a common reason for cardiology consultation. Although clinical history, physical examination, and the resting ECG are highly useful, in many clinical settings these tools are insufficient. Assessment of LV function and/or jeopardized myocardium provides an accurate method to complement clinical assessment. It has been shown that peripheral vascular surgery, with its associated marked hemodynamic stresses, carries at least a moderate risk of perioperative events for patients with known CAD. A large body of literature exists documenting the effectiveness of nuclear stress testing in this context. Recent guidelines suggest that nuclear testing is best reserved for patients with an intermediate risk of a cardiac event undergoing an intermediate- to high-risk procedure. Data supporting this approach were first presented by Eagle et al.[187] and then expanded in 1996 to include 3368 operations.[188] Together with other data sets, these data led to the guidelines for perioperative cardiovascular evaluation, published by the ACC/AHA task force (see Chap. 74). Based on these guidelines, candidates for MPS include patients with two of three of the following: (1) intermediate clinical predictors (Canadian class I or II angina, prior MI, CHF, or diabetes mellitus), (2) poor functional capacity (<4 METs), or (3) high-risk surgical procedure (emergency major operation, aortic repair, peripheral vascular surgery, prolonged surgical procedure with large fluid shifts or blood loss).

## Assessment of Therapy

With the use of aggressive medical therapy (as an alternative to revascularization) in various subgroups of CAD patients, methods for evaluation of the efficacy of medical therapy become of increasing importance. In this regard, it is likely that nuclear cardiology techniques will find an additional area of growth in serial patient assessment. After a patient is defined as being an appropriate candidate for medical therapy, nuclear techniques can be effectively employed to determine whether therapy has been successful or whether the patient's risk status has worsened, thereby requiring a change in therapeutic regimen.

A requirement for serial applications is that the nuclear techniques being utilized be highly reproducible and that the degree of change in the assessed variables associated with measurement error be known. Multiple studies have found that repeat studies are associated with a variation of ≤10 percent in MPS results.[189–191] These data provide the initial validation for the clinical application of nuclear methods for sequential assessment of therapy. In this regard, reduction of defect size using nitrate preparations has been shown,[190,192] as has reduction of defect size in patients undergoing intensive medical therapy versus coronary angioplasty following acute MI.[193] Sequential assessment of perfusion and function with gated SPECT is also being applied in large, randomized trials comparing medical therapy with angioplasty [Clinical Outcomes Utilizing Revascularization and Aggressive Drug Evaluation (COURAGE), see Chap. 10] and in evaluating the response of stress myocardial perfusion to therapy with vascular endothelial growth factor.[194] Preliminary results from this trial indicated that dramatic improvement of MPS abnormalities can occur with maximal medical therapy alone (Fig. 19-25). Similar findings have recently been reported in two small randomized clinical trials of the effects of simvastatin and pravastatin on stress MPS.[195,196] An intriguing possibility, long held by "master clinicians," is that risk reduction with medical therapy parallels reduction of inducible ischemia. If this is supported by clinical trials, the use of MPS to define patients who are appropriate candidates for aggressive medical management despite the presence of stress-induced ischemia may increase, as may the use of MPS in monitoring therapy of these patients.

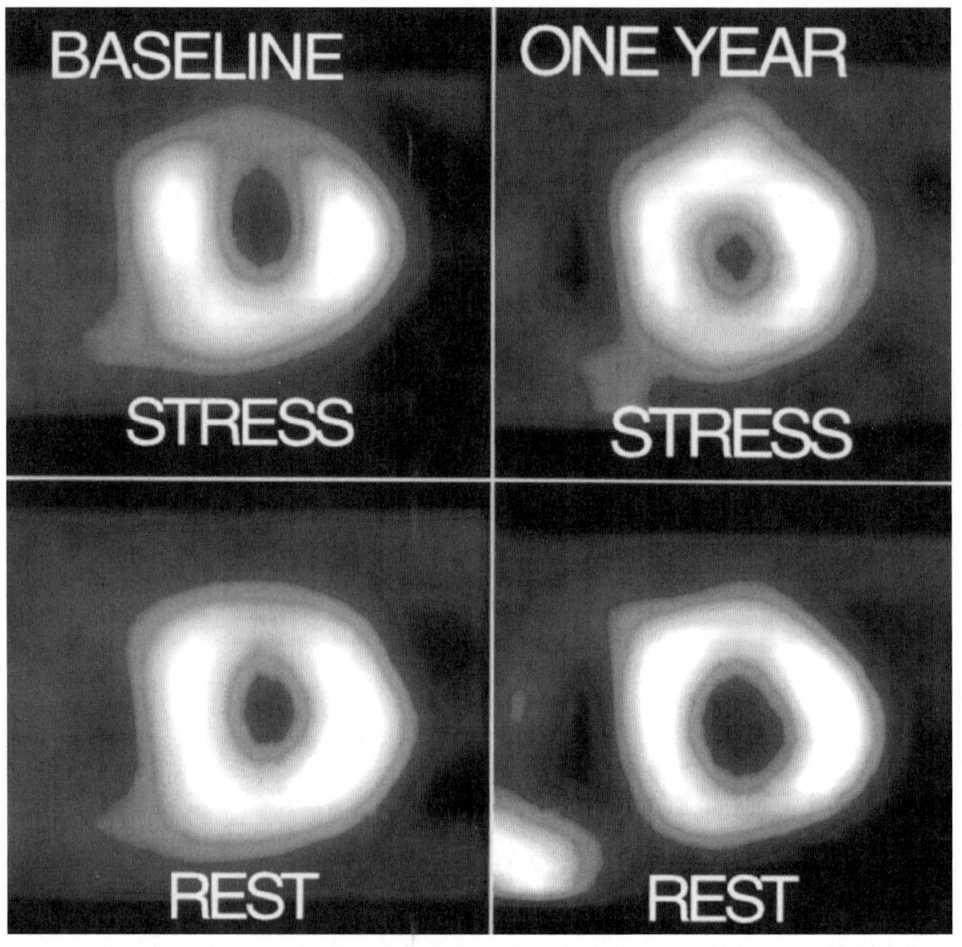


FIGURE 19-25 Case example of reversal of the stress myocardial perfusion defect with medical therapy. Baseline vasodilator stress and rest sestamibi mid-short-axis SPECT images (*left*) and repeat images 1 year after intensive medical therapy in a 50-year-old patient with baseline reversible defect in the LAD territory. One year into therapy, the stress perfusion defect is markedly improved. Baseline coronary angiography revealed an 80 percent mid-LAD stenosis, which improved angiographically on repeat coronary angiography at 1 year.[272] Two years later there are no reversible imaging defects and the patient is asymptomatic. (Reproduced with permission from the AHA.)

## ROLE OF NUCLEAR CARDIOLOGY IN PATIENTS WITH LV DYSFUNCTION: DETECTION OF CAD, ASSESSMENT OF MYOCARDIAL VIABILITY, AND PREDICTION OF LV RECOVERY AND SURVIVAL

Due to the high mortality rate and increasing prevalence of heart failure and the need to tailor therapy to the etiology and the stage of the condition, testing of patients with heart failure will become increasingly common. Radionuclide methods are useful in initial staging CHF (measurement of EF and ventricular volumes), in ruling out CAD as an etiology, and in determining the likelihood of response to interventional therapies. The recent recommendations of the ACC/AHA/ASNC task force regarding the general applications of radionuclide imaging[2] in patients with heart failure are summarized in Table 19-3.

***Detection of CAD as the Etiology of CHF*** Since CAD represents the largest etiology of CHF and since the therapy of CAD is so distinct from that of the general management of patients with CHF from other etiologies, ruling out CAD as the cause of CHF is of great importance. MPS is highly useful in this regard. Abnormalities of MPS are observed more frequently in CHF patients without CAD than in the general population—i.e., the specificity of MPS in CHF patients is low.

Patients with nonischemic cardiomyopathy may have patchy fibrosis or asymmetric hypertrophy, and the perfusion defects due to these causes are mild and small. Recent data suggest that the finding of only mild *regional* dysfunction defined by regional wall motion variability by gated SPECT coupled with mild perfusion defects is useful in identifying patients with CHF secondary to non-CAD etiologies.[197] On the other hand, patients with ischemic LV dysfunction or cardiomyopathies usually have large, severe perfusion defects (fixed, reversible, or a combination) associated with prominent regional myocardial dysfunction. If the perfusion defects are fixed, CHF and the reduced EF are considered to represent ventricular remodeling.

It has been stated recently that the sensitivity has been 100 percent in all studies for detecting CAD as the cause of CHF.[197–199]

TABLE 19-3 Use of RNI in Patients With Heart Failure: Fundamental Assessment

| Indication | Test | Class | Level of Evidence |
|---|---|---|---|
| 1. Initial assessment of LVF and RVF at rest[a] | Rest RNA | I | A |
| 2. Assessment of myocardial viability for consideration of revascularization in patients with CAD and LV systolic dysfunction who do not have angina | Myocardial perfusion imaging | I | B |
| 3. Assessment of the copresence of CAD in patients without angina | Myocardial perfusion imaging | IIa | B |
| 4. Routine serial assessment of LVF and RVF at rest | Rest RNA | IIb | B |
| 5. Initial or serial assessment of ventricular function with exercise | Exercise RNA | IIb | B |

KEY: CAD, coronary artery disease; LV, left ventricular; LVF, left ventricular function; PET, positron emission tomography; RNA, radionuclide angiography; RNI, radionuclide imaging; RVF, right ventricular function.
SOURCE: Klocke et al.[2]

However, the number of patients in whom this has been tested is small. Nonetheless, in the appropriate setting, a normal MPS study might obviate the need for coronary angiography.

***Noninvasive Identification of Hibernating Myocardium*** In patients with CAD and heart failure, the role of MPS is expanded because of the need to identify viable but nonfunctioning myocardium. Although chronic rest LV dysfunction in patients with CAD was previously thought to represent scarred myocardium, extensive evidence now supports the concept that myocardium subjected to acute or chronic ischemia may remain viable and demonstrate prolonged alterations in regional and global LV function that can be improved with revascularization.[200–203] Consequently, the distinction of ventricular dysfunction caused by fibrosis from that arising from viable myocardium has important implications for patients with low LVEF. Failure to identify patients with these potentially reversible causes of heart failure may lead to progressive cellular damage, heart failure, and death.

A number of reliable noninvasive imaging markers can be employed for determining the presence and extent of viable myocardium in patients with CAD and LV dysfunction. Radionuclide techniques have focused on indices of regional myocardial perfusion and cell membrane integrity (resting $^{99m}$Tc agent studies) and indices of regional cellularity as defined by the potassium space (redistribution $^{201}$Tl imaging). The latter approach has advantages over assessment of regional wall motion and regional systolic wall thickening, since in patients with underperfused but viable myocardium, blood flow, wall motion, and wall thickening may be severely reduced or absent at rest and with inotropic stimulation.[200–203]

***The Likelihood of Improvement with Revascularization: Assessment of Myocardial Viability and Stress-Induced Ischemia*** Mortality associated with LV dysfunction in the setting of severe CAD is quite high.[204–207] In general, patients with LV dysfunction who undergo CABS receive a greater proportional risk reduction compared to patients with preserved function.[93] The clinical setting in which viability assessment is most commonly used is the evaluation of CAD patients with poor LV function in whom revascularization is being considered. Excellent reviews of radionuclide techniques for assessment of myocardial viability have recently been provided by Bonow[204,205] and Arrighi and Dilsizian.[206]

As early as 1989, positron emission tomographic (PET) imaging was studied to examine the differential benefit of identifying viable from nonviable myocardium (see Chap. 19). Improved regional function postsurgery occurs more often in the setting of myocardial viability. Various protocols utilizing combinations of rest, redistribution, and reinjection $^{201}$Tl imaging have been validated to assess the presence of hibernating myocardium optimally. When reversibility of defects is noted on stress/rest or stress/redistribution studies, the likelihood of postrevascularization improvement of regions with abnormal ventricular function is high. Improvement would also be expected in patients with significant angiographic CAD if normal or mildly reduced tracer uptake is noted on rest scintigraphy. When severe reduction in uptake of radioactivity is noted on redistribution $^{201}$Tl imaging, the likelihood of improvement in regional ventricular function is low; a moderate defect on rest (or redistribution) has an intermediate likelihood of improvement.

Many studies have demonstrated rest-redistribution or stress-redistribution-reinjection $^{201}$Tl protocols to be nearly as accurate as PET in assessing myocardial viability.[206] Summary data of the positive and negative predictive value of $^{201}$Tl and $^{99m}$Tc-sestamibi in estimating functional recovery following CABS have shown that the positive predictive value ranged from 69 to 79 percent and the negative predictive value ranged from 72 to 85 percent, with neither having radioisotope differences. These results are dependent on underlying risk (with higher predictive values noted for higher-risk populations).[204–207]

PREDICTING RECOVERY OF RESTING LV FUNCTION The overall accuracies of PET, SPECT, and dobutamine echocardiography for predicting recovery of regional LV function after myocardial revascularization are similar based on the results of multiple studies published to date, although dobutamine echocardiography and PET appear to have greater specificity and positive predictive value compared to SPECT imaging, while SPECT has greater sensitivity and negative predictive value.[9,208]

PREDICTING IMPROVED PATIENT SURVIVAL The demonstration of viable myocardium in patients with CAD and LV dysfunction appears to identify patients with enhanced survival with revascularization but with particularly poor prognosis with medical therapy. A metanalysis of observational studies based on either radionuclide or echocardiographic assessments that dichotomize patients into groups with or without myocardial viability suggest that only those patients with extensive myocardial viability have survival improvement with CABS compared to medical therapy[134] (Fig. 19-26).

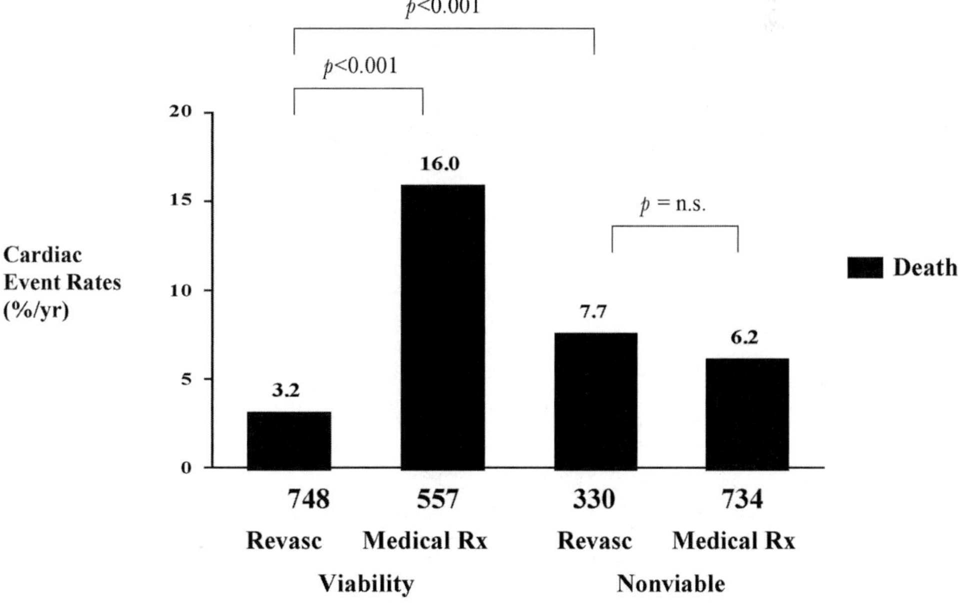


FIGURE 19-26 Metanalysis of studies examining rates of cardiac death in patients undergoing revascularization (revasc) vs medical therapy (Rx). When viability was present by noninvasive testing, a significant reduction in cardiac death rates was present in patients undergoing revascularization compared to those undergoing medical therapy. No such difference was present in patients without viability. Further, patients with viability undergoing revascularization had a significantly lower cardiac death rate compared to patients without viability. (With permission from the AHA.)

Several technical changes could improve the use of MPS in the assessment of myocardial viability. As mentioned above for $^{99m}$Tc agents, the possibility of further enhancing the viability information of reinjection $^{201}$Tl through the administration of nitroglycerin has been described.[31,209] Furthermore, in many of the studies assessing viability, a single cutoff point for myocardial counts in the region in question compared to the maximal observed value is employed: e.g., 50 or 60 percent of the maximal counts.[66,67] Finally, the use of combined rest-redistribution $^{201}$Tl/stress $^{99m}$Tc-sestamibi or tetrofosmin SPECT may be particularly effective in assessing myocardial viability, since the protocol can combine what may be the optimal rest MPS protocol (rest/redistribution $^{201}$Tl) with a stress imaging assessment.[17]

Table 19-4 illustrates conceptually the relationship between several different myocardial states associated with chronic CAD and the patterns that might be observed on MPS. In the presence of myocardial hibernation, resting blood flow would be expected to be mildly to even severely reduced, with corresponding reductions in resting $^{201}$Tl or $^{99m}$Tc perfusion agent uptake.[201–203,210,211] With $^{201}$Tl, the equilibrium uptake of radioactivity would also be expected to be normal or potentially slightly reduced if true equilibrium was not achieved or if prolonged hibernation had resulted in cellular degeneration.[201–203,211] Thus these patients often demonstrate resting reversibility of perfusion defects. For the $^{99m}$Tc agents, resting perfusion (and thus viability assessment) can be enhanced by nitroglycerin administration prior to the resting injection of the tracer.[64,65] If patients with hibernation are subjected to stress, an even greater degree of reduction in flow would be expected, causing a greater degree of defect reversibility in most cases. The likelihood of improvement with revascularization is great in these patients.

The extensive literature describing the relationship between viability testing, patient treatment assignment, and subsequent survival was recently assessed by a metanalysis of 24 published studies examining late survival with revascularization versus medical therapy after myocardial viability testing in patients with severe CAD and LV dysfunction.[134] In patients in whom viability was detected, revascularization was associated with an 80 percent reduction in annual mortality (16 vs. 3.2 percent, $p < 0.0001$) compared with medical treatment. In patients in whom no viability was detected by noninvasive testing, no difference in survival between therapies was noted (7.7 vs. 6.2 percent, $p =$ NS). Patients with viability showed a direct relationship between severity of LV dysfunction and magnitude of revascularization benefit ($p < 0.001$). Although no adjustment was made for the lack of randomization to treatment assignment, this metanalysis suggests that a strong association between myocardial viability on noninvasive testing and improved survival after revascularization in patients with chronic CAD and LV dysfunction. The degree of benefit appears to be related to the extent of LV dysfunction, with greater relative risk reductions noted with patients with EF <35 percent. These findings are similar to those based on randomized trial data showing a greater improvement in life expectancy for patients with abnormal systolic function.[99]

The ACC/AHA/ASNC recommendations[2] for radionuclide techniques in assessing myocardial viability are shown in Table 19-5.

## ACUTE CORONARY ISCHEMIC SYNDROMES

### Evaluation of Acute Chest Pain

Because of the relationship to closure of a coronary artery, MPS is an effective means of detecting patients with acute ischemic syndromes. Although the diagnosis of acute MI is frequently straightforward, in many patients it is not. For patients with normal or nondiagnostic initial ECGs on presentation to the emergency department (ED), an important clinical problem is to distinguish those with acute coronary syndromes requiring hospital admission from those who may be safely discharged.

Because most patients presenting with acute chest pain subsequently "rule out" for acute ischemic syndromes, chest pain units have been instituted for the acute evaluation of chest pain patients presenting to the ED. $^{99m}$Tc-sestamibi or tetrofosmin SPECT, with injection during chest pain, provides an excellent opportunity to reduce clinical indecision in the acute evaluation of chest pain (Fig. 19-27). A number of studies have demonstrated a role for MPS in the initial evaluation of these patients.[212,213] With a predictive model of index MI or revascularization based on multivariable risk-adjusted logistic regression in 532 patients with acute chest pain, an abnormal $^{99m}$Tc-sestamibi MPS was the strongest predictor of MI or revascularization (odds ratio = 14), with a negative predictive value of 99 percent.[212]

A recent prospective, randomized, controlled multicenter trial examined whether incorporating acute rest MPS into an ER evaluation

TABLE 19-4 Scintigraphic and Clinical Characteristics of Hypocontractile Regions According to Their Viability Status

| Viability Status | Rest | Redistribution ($^{201}$Tl) | Rest Reversibility | Stress/Rest/RI Reversibility | Likelihood of Improvement with Revasc |
|---|---|---|---|---|---|
| Q MI | ↓↓↓ | ↓↓↓ | — | — | — |
| Non-Q MI | ↓–↓↓ | ↓–↓↓ | — | ±[a] | ±[a] |
| Hibernation | ↓ to ↓↓↓ | → to ↓ | + | +++ | +++ |
| Stunning (with ACS) | → | → | → | ±[a] | ++ |
| Stunning (with exercise) | → | → | → | +++ | +++ |
| Remodeled | → | → | → | → | → |
| Nonischemic CM with incidental CAD | → | → | → | → | → |

KEY: Q = Q wave; MI = myocardial infarction; CM = cardiomyopathy; RI = reinjection; Revasc = revascularization; ACS = acute coronary syndrome.
[a]Depends on stenosis of IRA and the degree of transmurality of the infarct.

TABLE 19-5 Radionuclide Techniques for Assessing Myocardial Viability

| Indication | Test | Class | Level of Evidence |
|---|---|---|---|
| 1. Predicting improvement in regional and global LV function after revascularization | Stress/redistribution/reinjection $^{201}$Tl | I | B |
| | Rest-redistribution imaging | I | B |
| | Perfusion plus PET FDG imaging | I | B |
| | Resting sestamibi imaging | I | B |
| | Gated SPECT sestamibi imaging | IIa | B |
| | Late $^{201}$Tl redistribution imaging (after stress) | IIb | B |
| | Dobutamine RNA | IIb | C |
| | Postexercise RNA | IIb | C |
| | Postnitroglycerin RNA | IIb | C |
| 2. Predicting improvement in heart failure symptoms after revascularization | Perfusion plus PET FDG imaging | IIa | B |
| 3. Predicting improvement in natural history after revascularization | $^{201}$Tl imaging (rest-redistribution and stress/redistribution/reinjection) | I | B |
| | Perfusion plus PET FDG imaging | I | B |

KEY: FDG, flurodeoxygulcose; PET, positron emission tomography; RNA, radionuclide angiography; SPECT, single photon emission computed tomography; $^{201}$Tl, thallium 201.
SOURCE: Klocke et al.[2]

strategy of patients presenting with suspected acute ischemia but no initial ischemic ECG changes improved clinical decision making for initial ER triage.[214] A total of 2475 patients were randomly assigned to either usual ER evaluation strategy ($n$ = 1260) or to this same strategy supplemented with the results from acute resting $^{99m}$Tc-sestamibi SPECT ($n$ = 1215). There were no differences in hospitalization rates between these two groups in patients with acute MI ($n$ = 56) or unstable angina ($n$ = 273). However, among patients without acute cardiac ischemia ($n$ = 2146), hospitalization rates were reduced from 52 percent with usual care to 42 percent with SPECT imaging (odds ratio = 0.68, 95 percent CI = 0.57 – 0.82). See Table 19-6.

## Guidelines for SPECT Imaging in the ED

Several considerations are important for effective application of acute MPS. In patients with prior MI, the studies are generally not useful, unless patients had previously undergone MPS and the results of which are immediately available for comparison. Also, combined assessment of perfusion and function should be routinely performed in order to minimize the false negative rate. Additionally, with these agents, combined supine and prone imaging or attenuation correction is very useful in reducing the false-positive rate. If no abnormality is seen, patients are usually discharged with recommendations for follow-up stress MPS. Many centers are now routinely performing a stress MPS study immediately following the negative rest MPS if discharge is being contemplated. Of note, $^{99m}$Tc-based MPS agents ($^{99m}$Tc-sestamibi or tetrofosmin) are preferable in this application, since they may be injected during chest pain and imaged up to several hours later.

The accuracy of this approach for detecting an acute ischemic syndrome is probably affected by the timing of injection with respect

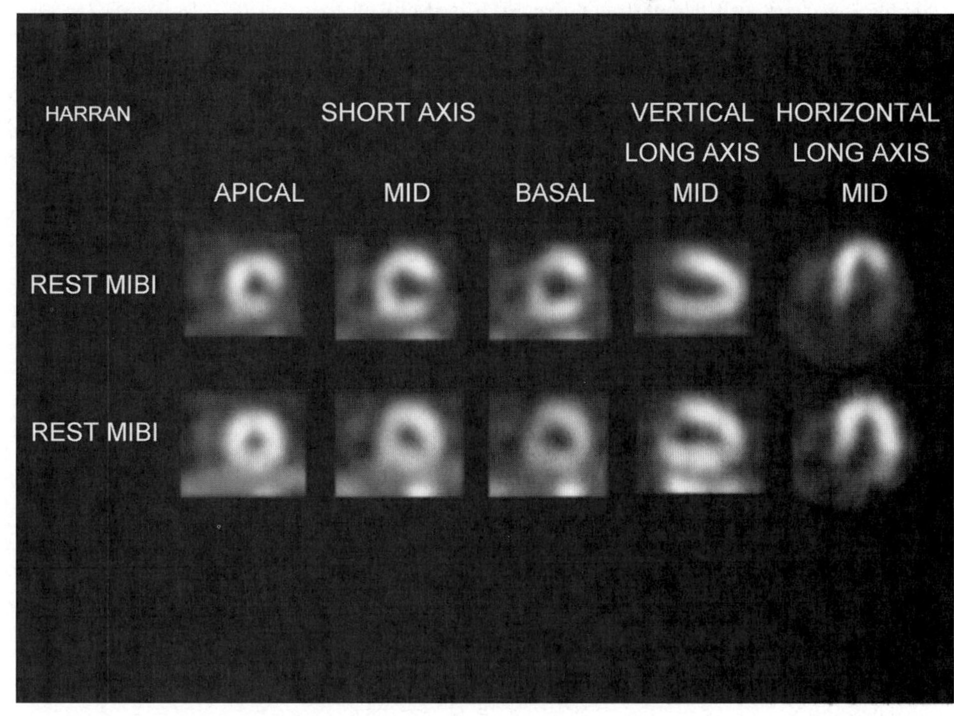


FIGURE 19-27 Resting sestamibi (MB) injected during chest pain in emergency department (*top*) and 3 days post-PCI of the left circumflex coronary artery (LCX) (*bottom*) in a patient with no EGG or enzyme abnormalities. Clear evidence of extensive myocardial salvage in LCX territory is shown.

TABLE 19-6 Effect of Sestamibi Imaging on ED Triage Decisions in Patients without ACI

| | Number (%) | | | |
|---|---|---|---|---|
| | Scan Strategy ($n$ = 1050)[a] | Usual Care ($n$ = 1096)[b] | RR (95% CI) | $p$ Value |
| Hospital admission rate | 438 (42) | 567 (52) | 0.84 (0.77–0.92) | <0.001 |
| Triage disposition | | | | |
| CCU | 43 (4) | 27 (3) | | 0.002 |
| Telemetry ward | 282 (27) | 379 (35) | | |
| Chest pain unit | 112 (11) | 160 (15) | | |
| Home from ED | 610 (58) | 529 (48) | | |

KEY: ED, emergency department; ACI, acute cardiac ischemia; RR, relative risk; CI, confidence interval; CCU, coronary care unit.
[a]Two patients missing data for admission status; three patients missing data for triage disposition.
[b]One patient missing data for triage disposition.

to the patient's chest pain, ideally with injection during chest pain. Patients with unstable angina would be expected to have perfusion defects during pain, but might have normalization of myocardial perfusion in pain-free periods, especially if intermittent occlusion is occurring. An alternate protocol may be preferable for patients whose chest pain has been relieved prior to injection[215] in whom rest $^{201}$Tl injection and MPS would be performed instead of using a $^{99m}$Tc agent. An abnormal resting $^{201}$Tl study would trigger admission and therapy for an acute ischemic syndrome. Patients with normal rest studies would not be discharged but, after negative enzymes are obtained, would undergo stress $^{99m}$Tc-sestamibi MPS to evaluate underlying CAD (Figs. 19-28 and 19-29).

### EVALUATION OF THERAPY

It has by now been well demonstrated that MPS is useful in the assessment of therapeutic efficacy for patients undergoing thrombolytic therapy or PCI. Several investigators demonstrated this application using $^{201}$Tl planar scintigraphy in the early 1980s.[216,217] Subsequently, Gibbons et al.[218] reported similar findings using $^{99m}$Tc-sestamibi. On the basis of extensive work, MPS can be used in patients with acute MI before and after therapy (or even simply after therapy) and represents an efficient, less expensive endpoint for examining the efficacy of a variety of therapies compared to conventional mortality endpoints.

***Assessment of Myocardial Viability*** In the setting of acute MI, at times it becomes clinically relevant to assess the viability of abnormally contracting segments as well as the presence of ongoing ischemia. In this regard, the finding of normal or nearly normal perfusion after initial therapy (thrombolytic therapy or PCI) can be used to accurately predict the return of ventricular function in a patient with an acute ischemic syndrome, whereas ongoing resting ischemia might indicate the need for urgent revascularization.[219]

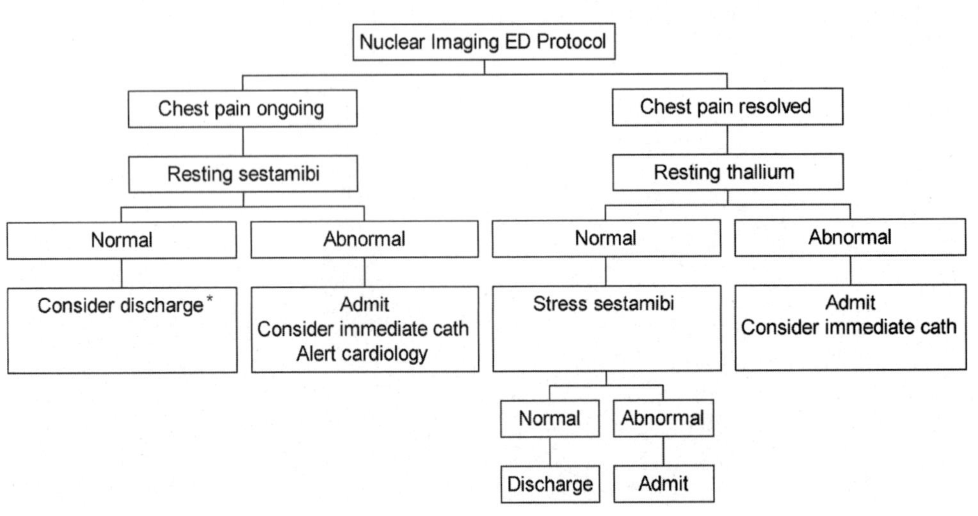


FIGURE 19-28 Nuclear imaging protocol for ED patients with low to intermediate risk of acute coronary syndrome. In patients with normal resting study being considered for discharge, immediate high-dose stress MPS is often useful to rule out significant ischemia. (Reproduced with permission from Ziffer et al.[215])

## Discharge Planning Post–Unstable Angina

Although most patients admitted with unstable angina are referred to catheterization, in medically stabilized patients, stress MPS can be effective in risk stratification.[220] This strategy is of particular importance in the presence of comorbidities that increase the risk of angiography or decrease the likelihood of using an invasive strategy (e.g., very advanced age or debilitation).

## Discharge Planning after Uncomplicated Acute MI

### CANDIDATES FOR INVASIVE VERSUS CONSERVATIVE MANAGEMENT

Recent AHA/ACC guidelines for exercise testing post-MI indicate that clinically low-risk MI patients remain candidates for predischarge stress testing,[136] despite the usual use of early coronary angiography in the United States. Both exercise[221] and pharmacologic stress testing post-MI have been shown to effectively identify patients at low and high risk of subsequent events.[222,223] This early post-MI application is one in which pharmacologic stress for MPS is particularly advantageous. Although either type of stress would be recommended by guidelines, evidence that favors the use of vasodilator stress includes the following: (1) vasodilator stress does not require that the patient be able to exercise; (2) it can be easily and safely employed as early as 2 days following MI[224]; (3) it lowers rather than raises blood pressure, avoiding possible myocardial rupture; and (4) it produces a maximal hyperemic stimulus, thereby obviating the need for maximal stress testing after recovery.

Overall, high-risk MPS results (indicating the need for angiography) in the predischarge patient include reversible defects in the MI zone, a multivessel defect pattern, large nonreversible defects, transient LV dilation, increased lung uptake, and reduced LV ejection fraction.[225] Two recent multicenter, randomized trials evaluated the prognostic value of MPS in the post-MI setting. Brown et al. initially compared submaximal $^{99m}$Tc-sestamibi SPECT at discharge to early dipyridamole $^{99m}$Tc-sestamibi SPECT performed 2 to 4 days after acute MI[226] in 451 patients presenting with first acute MI. The very early use of dipyridamole testing was associated with no adverse events, indicating the safety of this approach in appropriately selected post-MI patients. Multivariable predictors of postdischarge cardiac events included the SSS, the summed difference score, the summed rest score, and anterior MI. Dipyridamole sestamibi imaging showed better risk stratification than submaximal exercise myocardial perfusion imaging. Importantly, the submaximal exercise ECG had no significant predictive value for cardiac events. Additionally, the amount of ischemia (SDS) provided incremental prognostic information over the total defect size (SSS), particularly in patients with an intermediate SSS (Fig. 19-30). The prognostic value of perfusion versus function data in the post-MI patient was compared in 753 patients who underwent both rest radionuclide angiography (RNA) [for end-systolic volume index (ESVI) and EF] and rest $^{99m}$Tc-sestamibi MPS (for infarct size measurement) as part of the Collaborative Organization for RheothRx Evaluation (CORE) trial.[227] This study reported that EF was a superior predictor of outcome compared to ESVI or $^{99m}$Tc-sestamibi MPS infarct size. This study, however, was limited in that only 13 deaths occurred in the cohort undergoing both examinations and stress MPS was not performed.

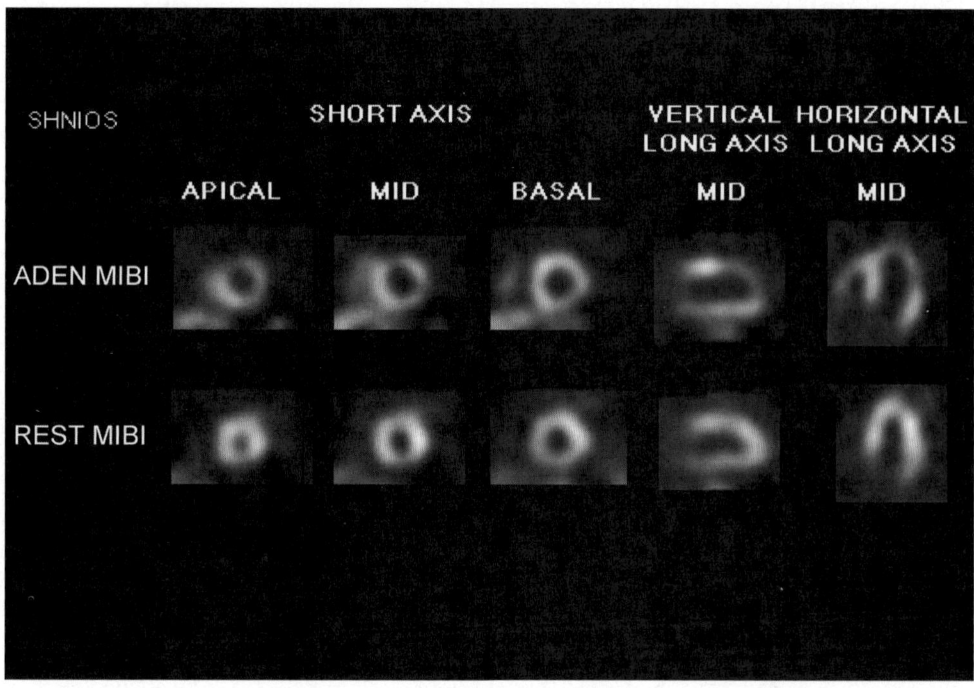


FIGURE 19-29 Normal rest $^{201}$Tl SPECT (*bottom*) followed by adenosine $^{99m}$Tc-sestamibi (ADEN MIBI) (*top*) in a patient with intermittent chest pain which had resolved prior to rest $^{201}$Tl injection. Reversible defects are seen in the left anterior descending and left circumflex territories. Angiography revealed 50 percent left main, 100 percent left anterior descending, 90 percent left circumflex, and 50 percent right coronary artery stenoses.

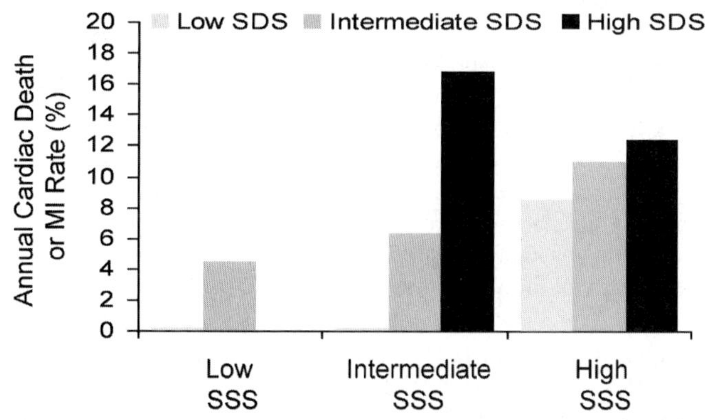


FIGURE 19-30 Annual cardiac death or MI rate as a function of SDS for a given SSS. For each SSS subgroup, cardiac event risk increased as SDS increased. The effect of SDS was greatest in the intermediate (intermed) SSS group. (Reproduced with permission from Brown et al.[226])

Recently, the Adenosine Sestamibi SPECT Post-Infarction Evaluation (INSPIRE) trial, a prospective randomized multicenter trial evaluating MPS in assessing risk and therapeutic outcomes in post-MI survivors,[228] was completed. Patients were randomized to medical therapy or revascularization if their baseline MPS study day 2 to 5 post-MI revealed preserved EF (>35 percent and total perfusion defect size >20 percent with >10 percent ischemia). Preliminary results reveal a 67 percent reduction in quantitative SPECT total amount of ischemia following aggressive management using either optimal anti-ischemic therapy alone or coronary revascularization.[229] Whether the reduction in perfusion defect size observed with medical therapy in these patients with postinfarction jeopardized myocardium is associated with a reduction in risk comparable to that achieved by revascularization has yet to be defined.

## RADIONUCLIDE ANGIOGRAPHY

Among the first applications of nuclear cardiology techniques was the assessment of cardiac function using radionuclide angiography (RNA) or radionuclide ventriculography (RNV). RNA is considered one of the "gold standards" for assessing LVEF on the basis of its accuracy and reproducibility.[230,231] The techniques of RNA can be performed by either equilibrium or first-pass methods, with assessments of LVEF, RVEF, LV regional wall motion, and LV volumes.

Equilibrium RNA uses ECG-gated acquisition, in which each frame corresponds to a specific portion (interval or gate) of the cardiac cycle, identified relative to the R wave on the patient's ECG. Because of the use of a multiple-gated acquisition, the term *MUGA scan* has also been applied to this technique. The cardiac cycle is divided in as many as 32 to 64 intervals and data from multiple cardiac cycles are averaged to ensure adequate count statistics. With the equilibrium approach, a blood-pool tracer (usually $^{99m}$Tc-labeled red blood cells) is used and must stay within the vascular compartment during the imaging period. Red blood cells can be labeled either through in vivo or in vitro methods. The latter provides the highest target-to-background ratio. Acquisition typically takes 5 to 10 min per view and multiple planar views are obtained. For exercise RNA, image acquisition can be as brief as 2 min.

For the equilibrium RNA, EFs of the LV[230,232] or RV[233] can be measured. The preferred method for measurement of EF from equilibrium RNA is referred to as the "area counts" technique. This method takes advantage of the proportionality between the volume of a cardiac chamber and the number of counts emitted from that chamber following injection of a blood-pool radiopharmaceutical. Thus, a background-corrected curve of ventricular activity versus time is a curve of relative volume versus time of the corresponding ventricle. From this curve, EF can be measured as a function of the peak (relative end-diastolic) and the nadir (relative end-systolic) volumes by the formula $(EDC - ESC)/EDC$, where EDC and ESC represent background-corrected counts in the end-diastolic and end-systolic frames, respectively. It is generally accepted that for most accurate measurement of LVEF, $\geq$16 frames per cardiac cycle are required. For measurement of RVEF, it has been demonstrated that carefully placed regions of interest over the RV at end-diastole and end-systole, using a left periventricular background region of interest, provide an effective method for assessment of RVEF. Very high degrees of correlation have been reported between LVEF using equilibrium RNA and contrast ventriculography. Good correlation has been demonstrated between RVEF measurements using equilibrium RNA and RV first-pass measurements.[233]

With the first-pass approach, imaging is performed only during the initial transit of radioactivity through the central circulation. This technique is a type of dynamic acquisition that uses rapid temporal sampling (20 to 100 frames per second) to look at the initial transit of a radionuclide bolus through the central circulation. The perfusion agents $^{99m}$Tc-sestamibi and $^{99m}$Tc-tetrofosmin can be used with success in first-pass studies as adjuncts to conventional perfusion studies. These are most commonly performed in either the anterior or right anterior oblique view and most commonly employ a multicrystal camera,[234] with either bicycle[234] or treadmill[235,236] exercise. The advantage of first-pass over equilibrium RNA is that LV function assessment is at the true peak of exercise.

Because of the ability to image the blood-pool radiopharmaceuticals for a substantial time period, SPECT acquisition is also practical with equilibrium radionuclide angiography. It has recently been shown that equilibrium blood-pool SPECT acquisition and processing are essentially the same as for MPS, and thus can be easily adopted in the laboratory where MPS is being performed. Methods for automatically assessing LVEF from gated blood-pool SPECT have been developed and validated.[237] Since the SPECT approach avoids the overlap of cardiac chambers inherent in planar imaging, it enhances assessment of regional function and may well become the method of choice for radionuclide angiography.

## The Role of RNA in Chronic CAD

In chronic CAD, the principal application of RNA at the present time is measurement of rest function. Resting RNA using either equilibrium or first-pass techniques can be effective in defining the presence of a reduced LVEF, and thereby a patient population for whom ACE inhibitors can be effective. Following initial observations in patients with MI,[238] subsequent randomized trials in patients with chronic CAD demonstrated that patients who have reduced LVEF obtain a distinct beneficial effect from the long-term administration of angiotensin-converting enzyme (ACE) inhibitors. Thus, the available evidence would suggest that patients with suspected acute or chronic CAD are candidates for ACE inhibitor therapy if LVEF is low. The other manner in which patients with CAD can benefit from RNA is with serial assessment of ventricular function. This is important in assessing the efficacy of treatments such as ACE inhibitor therapy and has been used in many trials of a variety of approaches to patients with severe reductions of LVEF. Commonly, a measurement of LVEF by equilibrium RNA is required as a method of documenting severe reduction of LVEF prior to admission into heart failure trials.

For the detection of CAD and management of patients with this condition, exercise RNA continues to play a role in some centers. The most commonly utilized measurement derived from RNA for these decisions is the peak exercise LVEF, whether from first-pass or equilibrium techniques. Many studies have reported the predictive power of this measure for cardiovascular death or nonfatal MI.[122,125,126,239–241] In a recent report by Shaw et al., the prognostic value of LV function during exercise was examined in 863 consecutive patients undergoing exercise gated equilibrium RNA within 90 days of catheterization who were followed up for subsequent events, with 99 percent of survivors completing 5 years of follow-up.[240] In a multivariable analysis, the resting or exercise EF contained significant predictive information ($p < 0.0001$). The rest or exercise EF contained similarly predictive information (exercise EF provided 63 percent of the information of the exercise model and resting EF provided 60 percent). In considering the addition of the presence and extent of CAD observed at catheterization, rest and exercise RNA data still provided significant improvement in the prediction of cardiac death. An inverse relationship between peak exercise LVEF and survival has been demonstrated.[240,242]

## Nuclear Cardiology Applications Unique to RNA

### ASSESSMENT OF ANTHRACYCLINE CARDIOTOXICITY

RNA is commonly used for evaluating the effects of doxorubicin and other anthracyclines on LV function in patients with suspected cardiotoxicity. In an early report, Alexander and colleagues demonstrated that patients with normal LVEF that had not fallen by more than 15 points did not develop cardiotoxicity with continued doxorubicin therapy; however, once EF fell below 45 percent or by more than 15 percent, continued doxorubicin therapy was commonly associated with irreversible cardiac failure.[243] In a subsequent report of a large high-risk population from the same group, guidelines were established for the use of continued doxorubicin therapy.[244] In a group of 70 high-risk patients in whom these guidelines were strictly followed, 2.9 percent developed subsequent congestive heart failure (CHF) that responded to therapy. Of 212 high-risk patients in whom the recommendations were not closely followed, 21 percent developed CHF ($p < 0.001$ versus the strict-guideline group). The CHF in the majority of these patients was considered moderate to severe.

### DETERMINING THE TIME FOR VALVE REPLACEMENT IN AORTIC REGURGITATION

It has been demonstrated that resting LVEF, as measured by equilibrium RNA, provides an excellent method for the sequential follow-up of asymptomatic patients with aortic regurgitation. For patients with chronic aortic regurgitation, a fall in LVEF has been shown to be strongly predictive of the development of subsequent progressive severe deterioration in LV function.[245] These investigators have suggested that asymptomatic patients with severe aortic regurgitation whose EFs at rest fall below normal should be considered for elective valve replacement.

## New Developments in MPS Tracers

### NONPERFUSION MYOCARDIAL SPECT

Radionuclide imaging has an inherent advantage over other cardiac imaging techniques for assessment of myocardial metabolic and biochemical processes. Two nonperfusion myocardial scintigraphic applications in common use in countries outside of the United States are fatty-acid imaging and imaging of myocardial innervation. The most commonly used radionuclide for these purposes is iodine 123 ($^{123}$I). From a biochemical standpoint, $^{123}$I is an excellent metabolic imaging tracer, since it is easily incorporated into a wide variety of compounds by a halogen exchange reaction in which the iodine replaces a methyl group. From a physical standpoint it has half-life, photon energy, and radiation exposure characteristics almost as favorable as those of $^{99m}$Tc for gamma camera imaging. While none of the $^{123}$I-labeled compounds is currently commercially available for routine use in the United States, clinical trials involving their use are beginning.

***Fatty-Acid Imaging*** A comprehensive review of this subject has been provided by Tamaki.[246] The principal fatty acid currently in clinical use with SPECT in Japan and Europe is betamethyl iodophenylpentadecanoic acid (BMIPP), a modified branched-chain fatty acid first introduced by Knapp et al.[247] This tracer appears to have "ischemic memory" properties offering unique capability for the assessment of previously severely ischemic myocardium. Discordant myocardial fatty acid uptake/perfusion findings, with less BMIPP uptake than $^{201}$Tl, has been described in patients with unstable angina and those with acute MI who were acutely revascularized.[248] This finding likely represents a persistent metabolic abnormality out of proportion to the perfusion abnormality at the time of injection. Furutani et al.[249] have suggested that this finding allows assessment of the amount of myocardium at risk in the subacute phase of the MI. A possible clinical application of BMIPP would be assessment of patients presenting several hours to days after a possible severe ischemic episode, potentially providing direct evidence of the recent severe ischemia at a time when perfusion had returned to normal. Despite the number of published papers dealing with BMIPP and this potential application, its added clinical value over conventional imaging remains unclear.

***Imaging of Myocardial Innervation*** Imaging of myocardial innervation is another application of the tracer technique to cardiac imaging recently reviewed by Dae.[250] The sympathetic nerves of the myocardium take up exogenously administered catecholamines with high affinity.[251] Metaiodobenzylguanidine (MIBG) is an analog of a false nerve transmitter, which when labeled with $^{123}$I, is also in common use in Japan. MIBG is taken up in myocardial sympathetic nerve endings in a manner similar to norepinephrine, but it is not metabolized. In regionally denervated myocardium, MIBG uptake is decreased while perfusion is unchanged.[252] In "syndrome X," abnormal cardiac MIBG uptake has been reported in 75 percent of patients, with the abnormality out of proportion to perfusion defects supporting the cardiac origin of chest pain in this syndrome.[252a] Furthermore, in diabetic patients, assessment of myocardial MIBG uptake may be useful in defining autonomic dysfunction.[253] Asymmetric uptake of MIBG has been shown in patients with ventricular tachycardia and no CAD[254,255] and potentially may be of value in determining patient subsets who may benefit from the use of ICD implantation. Abnormal MIBG uptake has been reported in idiopathic ventricular tachycardia and ventricular fibrillation.[256]

In nonischemic cardiomyopathy, abnormalities of MIBG distribution and washout has been reported. Recent studies have suggested that impaired cardiac sympathetic innervation in heart failure patients can be assessed by MIBG.[257] The late myocardial-to-mediastinal MIBG uptake 4 h after injection was shown to be the most powerful predictor of cardiac death, providing incremental information over clinical variables in clinical studies.[257,258] Furthermore, MIBG imaging may be useful in predicting the effectiveness of beta-blocker therapy for patients with dilated cardiomyopathies.[259,260] It appears that excessive norepinephrine levels result in rapid washout of the MIBG and a pattern of a low heart-to-mediastinal ratio on 4-h delayed MIBG images, which appears to be predictive of a poor response to beta-blocker therapy.[250] There is widespread interest in investigating the potential clinical role of MIBG in assessing patients with heart failure and patients at risk for sudden cardiac death.

***Direct Imaging of Myocardial Necrosis*** Hot-spot (infarct-avid) imaging methods for detecting acute MI are among the oldest techniques in nuclear cardiology. These techniques have included $^{99m}$Tc-pyrophosphate myocardial scintigraphy,[261,262] indium-111 ($^{111}$In) antimyosin antibody scintigraphy,[263] and $^{99m}$Tc-glucarate imaging.[264] Although these methods have been documented to be sensitive and specific for the detection of myocardial necrosis, they are not widely utilized. Antimyosin antibody, not available in the United States, is highly specific for myocardial necrosis and has been shown to be useful in the assessment of myocarditis[265] and the necrosis associated with cardiac transplant rejection.[266] A new agent, $^{99m}$Tc-glucarate, a small molecule similar to glucose with rapid blood-pool clearance, is taken up acutely in the necrotic myocardium[264,267] and unlike previous tracers becomes positive in the very early hours after onset of necrosis.

### MOLECULAR IMAGING

The current explosion of information in cell biology has led to initial formulations of imaging agents with specific molecular targets. While most work has occurred with PET in this regard, some SPECT tracers have recently become of interest. Most prominent in this regard is $^{99m}$Tc-annexin, an agent which allows imaging of apoptosis by specific binding to the exteriorized phosphatidylserine molecules, normally only found in the inner leaflet of the cell membrane and which become exteriorized during apoptosis.[268] Initial clinical trials with this agent have suggested high sensitivity for MI. In addition to acute MI, clinical settings in which the usefulness of this tracer might occur in cardiology include myocarditis, transplant rejection, and possibly congestive heart failure. Specific agents targeting components of the atherosclerotic process are also currently being developed. Many consider it likely that over the next decade nuclear cardiology will migrate toward molecular imaging, taking advantage of this modality's picomolar sensitivity, which allows external monitoring of tracer concentrations several orders of magnitude less than those associated with MRI methods.

### THE FUTURE OF GATED MPS IN NONINVASIVE CARDIAC IMAGING

The last decade has seen new developments in noninvasive imaging technology and improvements in existing modalities. The options for imaging in known or suspected CAD include echocardiography, cardiac magnetic resonance imaging, multidetector and electron beam computed tomography, and positron emission tomography as alternative or complementary modalities to MPS. In the future, it is likely that each of these modalities will play an important role, and in many cases their use will be complementary rather than competitive.

The ability of nuclear cardiology to provide standardized procedures that are not highly dependent on the hand-eye coordination of a technologist and which provide objective assessments of myocardial perfusion and function with equipment of only moderate expense offers strengths that are likely to ensure the continued growth of this field for many years. Recently this growth has been sustained predominantly by a rapid upsurge in the United States of nuclear cardiology practice in cardiology offices. Small dual-detector SPECT cameras, which can fit in standard office examination rooms and be dedicated to cardiac imaging without sacrifice of major quality, are becoming increasingly popular. In addition to the observed rise in office-based nuclear cardiology practice, it is expected that inpatient utilization of MPS will also increase, particularly in the setting of triage of emergency department chest pain presentations and in planning cost- and time-effective management of the hospitalized cardiac patient.

## ACKNOWLEDGEMENTS

The authors gratefully acknowledge the invaluable assistance in the preparation of this chapter of Helen Dailey; Xingping Kang, MD; Ling de Yang, MD; Aiden Abidov, MD; and Louise Thomson, MBChB.

## References


1. Germano G, Berman DS. Clinical applications of nuclear cardiology. In: Germano G, Berman DS, eds. *Clinical Gated Cardiac SPECT.* Armonk, NY: Futura; 1999:1–71.
2. Klocke FJ, Baird MG, Lorell BH, et al. ACC/AHA/ASNC Guidelines for the Clinical Use of Cardiac Radionuclide Imaging-Executive Summary. A Report of the American College of Cardiology/American Heart Association Task Force on Practice Guidelines (ACC/AHA/ASNC Committee to Revise the 1995 Guidelines for the Clinical Use of Cardiac Radionuclide Imaging). *Circulation* 2003;108:1404–1418.
3. Angello DA, Wilson RA, Palac RT. Effect of eating on thallium-201 myocardial redistribution after myocardial ischemia. *Am J Cardiol* 1987;60:528–533.
4. Berman D, Maddahi J, Charuzi Y, et al. Rate of redistribution in Th-201 exercise myocardial scintigraphy: Inverse relationship to degree of coronary stenosis (abstr). *Circulation* 1978;58(suppl 2):63.
5. Gutman J, Berman DS, Freeman M, et al. Time to completed redistribution of thallium-201 in exercise myocardial scintigraphy: relationship to the degree of coronary artery stenosis. *Am Heart J* 1983;106: 989–995.
6. Sinusas AJ, Bergin JD, Edwards NC, et al. Redistribution of $^{99m}$Tc-sestamibi and $^{201}$Th in the presence of a severe coronary artery stenosis. *Circulation* 1994;89:2332–2341.
7. Leppo JA, Meerdink DJ. Comparison of the myocardial uptake of a technetium-labeled isonitrile analogue and thallium. *Circ Res* 1989;65:632–639.
8. Hurwitz GA, Blais M, Powe JE, et al. Stress/injection protocols for myocardial scintigraphy with $^{99m}$Tc-sestamibi compared with $^{201}$Tl: Implications of early post-stress kinetics. *Nucl Med Commun* 1996;17:400–409.
9. Jain D, Wackers FJ, Mattera J, et al. Biokinetics of technetium-99m-tetrofosmin: Myocardial perfusion imaging agent: Implications for a one-day imaging protocol. *J Nucl Med* 1993;34:1254–1259.
10. Wackers FJ, Berman DS, Maddahi J, et al. Technetium-99m hexakis 2-methoxyisobutyl isonitrile: Human biodistribution, dosimetry, safety, and preliminary comparison to thallium-201 for myocardial perfusion imaging. *J Nucl Med* 1989;30:301–311.
11. Meerdink DJ, Leppo JA. Experimental studies of the physiologic properties of technetium-99m agents: Myocardial transport of perfusion imaging agents. *Am J Cardiol* 1990;66:9E–15E.
12. Leppo JA, Meerdink DJ. Comparative myocardial extraction of two technetium-labeled BATO derivatives (SQ30217, SQ32014) and thallium. *J Nucl Med* 1990;31:67–74.
13. Chua T, Kiat H, Germano G, et al. Technetium-99m teboroxime regional myocardial washout in subjects with and without coronary artery disease. *Am J Cardiol* 1993;72:728–734.
14. Pasqualini R, Duatti A, Bellande E, et al. Bis(dithiocarbamato) nitrido technetium-99m radiopharmaceuticals: A class of neutral myocardial imaging agents. *J Nucl Med* 1994;35:334–341.
15. Ghezzi C, Fagret D, Arvieux CC, et al. Myocardial kinetics of TcN-NOET: A neutral lipophilic complex tracer of regional myocardial blood flow. *J Nucl Med* 1995;36:1069–1077.
16. Vanzetto G, Calnon DA, Ruiz M, et al. Myocardial uptake and redistribution of 99mTc-N-NOET in dogs with either sustained coronary low flow or transient coronary occlusion: comparison with $^{201}$Tl and myocardial blood flow. *Circulation* 1997;96:2325–2331.
17. Berman DS, Kiat H, Friedman JD, et al. Separate acquisition rest thallium-201/stress technetium-99m sestamibi dual-isotope myocardial perfusion single-photon emission computed tomography: A clinical validation study. *J Am Coll Cardiol* 1993;22:1455–1464.
18. Verani MS, Mahmarian JJ, Hixson JB, et al. Diagnosis of coronary artery disease by controlled coronary vasodilation with adenosine and thallium-201 scintigraphy in patients unable to exercise. *Circulation* 1990;82:80–87.
19. Smits P, Thien T, van't Laar A. Circulatory effects of coffee in relation to the pharmacokinetics of caffeine. *Am J Cardiol* 1985;56: 958–963.
20. Glover DK RM, Sansoy V, Barrett RJ, Beller GA. Effect of N-0861, a selective adenosine Al receptor antagonist, on pharmacologic stress imaging with adenosine. *J Nucl Med* 1995;36(2):270–5.

20a. Udelson JE, Heller GV, Wackers FJT, et al: A randomized, controlled dose-ranging study of the selective adenosine $A_{2A}$ receptor agonist binodenoson for pharmacologic stress as an adjunct to myocardial perfusion imaging. *Circulation* 2003. In press.

21. Iskandrian AE. State of the art for pharmacologic stress imaging. In: Zaret BL, Beller G, eds. *Nuclear Cardiology: State of the Art and Future Directions,* 2d ed. St. Louis: Mosby; 1998:312–330.
22. Amanullah AM, Berman DS, Kiat H, et al. Usefulness of hemodynamic changes during adenosine infusion in predicting the diagnostic accuracy of adenosine technetium-99m sestamibi single-photon emission computed tomography (SPECT). *Am J Cardiol* 1997;79: 1319–1322.
23. Abidov A, Hachamovitch R, Hayes SW, et al. Prognostic impact of hemodynamic response to adenosine in patients older than age 55 years undergoing vasodilator stress myocardial perfusion study. *Circulation* 2003;107:2894–2899.
24. Lette J, Tatum JL, Fraser S, et al. Safety of dipyridamole testing in 73,806 patients: the Multicenter Dipyridamole Safety Study. *J Nucl Cardiol* 1995;2:3–17.
25. Cerqueira MD, Verani MS, Schwaiger M, et al. Safety profile of adenosine stress perfusion imaging: Results from the Adenoscan Multicenter Trial Registry. *J Am Coll Cardiol* 1994;23:384–389.
26. Pennell DJ, Mavrogeni SI, Forbat SM, et al. Adenosine combined with dynamic exercise for myocardial perfusion imaging. *J Am Coll Cardiol* 1995;25:1300–1309.
27. Pennell DJ, Underwood SR, Swanton RH, et al. Dobutamine thallium myocardial perfusion tomography. *J Am Coll Cardiol* 1991;18: 1471–1479.
28. Sharir T, Rabinowitz B, Livschitz S, et al. Underestimation of extent and severity of coronary artery disease by dipyridamole stress thallium-201 single-photon emission computed tomographic myocardial

perfusion imaging in patients taking antianginal drugs. *J Am Coll Cardiol* 1998;31:1540–1546.

28a. Taillefer R, Ahlberg AW, Masood Y, et al. Acute beta blockade reduces the extent and severity of myocardial perfusion defects with dipyridamole Tc-99m sestamibi imaging. *J Am Coll Cardiol* 2003;42(8):1475–1483.

29. Hachamovitch R, Hayes SW, Friedman J, et al. Determinants of risk and its temporal variation in patients with normal stress myocardial perfusion scans: What is the warranty period of a normal scan? *J Am Coll Cardiol* 2003;41:1329–1340.

30. Dilsizian V, Smeltzer WR, Freedman NM, et al. Thallium reinjection after stress-redistribution imaging. Does 24-hour delayed imaging after reinjection enhance detection of viable myocardium? *Circulation* 1991;83:1247–1255.

31. Basu S, Senior R, Raval U, et al. Superiority of nitrate-enhanced $^{201}$Tl over conventional redistribution $^{201}$Tl imaging for prognostic evaluation after myocardial infarction and thrombolysis. *Circulation* 1997; 96:2932–2937.

32. Pohost GM, Zir LM, Moore RH, et al. Differentiation of transiently ischemic from infarcted myocardium by serial imaging after a single dose of thallium-201. *Circulation* 1977;55:294–302.

33. Pagley PR, Beller GA, Watson DD, et al. Improved outcome after coronary bypass surgery in patients with ischemic cardiomyopathy and residual myocardial viability. *Circulation* 1997;96:793–800.

34. Wagdy HM, Christian TF, Miller TD, et al. The value of 24-hour images after rest thallium injection. *Nucl Med* Commun 2002;23:629–637.

35. Friedman J, Van Train K, Maddahi J, et al. "Upward creep" of the heart: A frequent source of false-positive reversible defects during thallium-201 stress-redistribution SPECT. *J Nucl Med* 1989;30: 1718–1722.

36. Germano G, Erel J, Kiat H, et al. Quantitative LVEF and qualitative regional function from gated thallium-201 perfusion SPECT. *J Nucl Med* 1997;38:749–754.

37. Berman DS, Kiat H, Maddahi J. The new 99mTc myocardial perfusion imaging agents: 99mTc-sestamibi and 99mTc-teboroxime. *Circulation* 1991;84:I7–21.

38. Berman D, Kiat H, Germano G, et al. 99m Tc-sestamibi SPECT. In: DePuey EG, Berman DS, Garcia EV, eds. *Cardiac SPECT Imaging.* New York: Raven Press; 1995:121–146.

39. Van Train KF, Areeda J, Garcia EV, et al. Quantitative same-day rest-stress technetium-99m-sestamibi SPECT: definition and validation of stress normal limits and criteria for abnormality. *J Nucl Med* 1993;34: 1494–1502.

40. Gibson PB, Demus D, Noto R, et al. Low event rate for stress-only perfusion imaging in patients evaluated for chest pain. *J Am Coll Cardiol* 2002;39:999–1004.

41. Berman DS, Germano G. Myocardial perfusion single photon approaches. In: Pohost GM, O'Rourke RA, Berman DS, Shah PM, eds. *Imaging in Cardiovascular Disease.* Philadelphia: Lippencott Williams & Wilkins; 2000:159–194.

42. Nakamura M, Takeda K, Ichihara T, et al. Feasibility of simultaneous stress 99mTc-sestamibi/rest 201Tl dual-isotope myocardial perfusion SPECT in the detection of coronary artery disease. *J Nucl Med* 1999;40:895–903.

43. Aboul-Enein FA, Hayes SW, Matsumoto N, et al. Rest perfusion defects in patients with no history of myocardial infarction predict the presence of a critical coronary artery stenosis. *J Nucl Cardiol* 2004. In press.

44. Ficaro EP, Fessler JA, Shreve PD, et al. Simultaneous transmission/emission myocardial perfusion tomography. Diagnostic accuracy of attenuation-corrected 99mTc-sestamibi single-photon emission computed tomography. *Circulation* 1996;93:463–473.

45. Kluge R, Sattler B, Seese A, et al. Attenuation correction by simultaneous emission-transmission myocardial single-photon emission tomography using a technetium-99m-labelled radiotracer: Impact on diagnostic accuracy. *Eur J Nucl Med* 1997;24:1107–1114.

46. Gallowitsch HJ, Sykora J, Mikosch P, et al. Attenuation-corrected thallium-201 single-photon emission tomography using a gadolinium-153 moving line source: clinical value and the impact of attenuation correction on the extent and severity of perfusion abnormalities. *Eur J Nucl Med* 1998;25:220–228.

47. Hendel RC, Berman DS, Cullom SJ, et al. Multicenter clinical trial to evaluate the efficacy of correction for photon attenuation and scatter in SPECT myocardial perfusion imaging. *Circulation* 1999;99: 2742–2749.

48. Links JM, Becker LC, Rigo P, et al. Combined corrections for attenuation, depth-dependent blur, and motion in cardiac SPECT: A multicenter trial. *J Nucl Cardiol* 2000;7:414–425.

49. Duvernoy CS, Ficaro EP, Karabajakian MZ, et al. Improved detection of left main coronary artery disease with attenuation-corrected SPECT. *J Nucl Cardiol* 2000;7:639–648.

50. Gerson MC, Singh BKM, Lukes J, et al. Comparison of attenuation and Compton scatter corrected to uncorrected thallium-201 tomograms for diagnosis of coronary artery disease (CAD) (abstr). *J Nucl Med* 1999;40:89P.

51. Heller GV, Bateman TM, Botvinick EH, et al. Value of attenuation correction in interpretation of stress only exercise Tc-99m sestamibi SPECT imaging: results of a multicenter trial (abstr). *J AM Coll Cardiol* 2002;39:343A.

52. Berman DS, Kiat H, Van Train K, et al. Technetium 99m sestamibi in the assessment of chronic coronary artery disease. *Semin Nucl Med* 1991;21:190–212.

53. Matzer L, Kiat H, Van Train K, et al. Quantitative severity of stress thallium-201 myocardial perfusion single-photon emission computed tomography defects in one-vessel coronary artery disease. *Am J Cardiol* 1993;72:273–279.

54. Port S. Imaging guidelines for nuclear cardiology procedures: Part 2. *J Nucl Cardiol* 1999;6:G49–G84.

55. Cerqueira MD, Weissman NJ, Dilsizian V, et al. Standardized myocardial segmentation and nomenclature for tomographic imaging of the heart. A statement for healthcare professionals from the Cardiac Imaging Committee of the Council on Clinical Cardiology of the American Heart Association. *Int J Cardiovasc Imaging* 2002;18:539–542.

56. Berman DS, Hachamovitch R, Kiat H, et al. Incremental value of prognostic testing in patients with known or suspected ischemic heart disease: A basis for optimal utilization of exercise technetium-99m sestamibi myocardial perfusion single-photon emission computed tomography. *J Am Coll Cardiol* 1995;26:639–647.

57. Hachamovitch R, Berman DS, Kiat H, et al. Exercise myocardial perfusion SPECT in patients without known coronary artery disease: Incremental prognostic value and use in risk stratification. *Circulation* 1996;93:905–914.

58. Hachamovitch R, Berman DS, Shaw LJ, et al. Incremental prognostic value of myocardial perfusion single photon emission computed tomography for the prediction of cardiac death: Differential stratification for risk of cardiac death and myocardial infarction. *Circulation* 1998;97:535–543.

59. Hachamovitch R, Hayes SW, Friedman JD, et al. Comparison of the short-term survival benefit associated with revascularization compared with medical therapy in patients with no prior coronary artery disease undergoing stress myocardial perfusion single photon emission computed tomography. *Circulation* 2003:107:2900–2906.

60. Berman DS, Kang X, Abidov A, et al. Prognostic value of myocardial perfusion SPECT comparing 17-segment and 20-segment scoring systems (abstr). *J Am Coll Cardiol* 2003;41:445A.

61. Bisi G, Sciagra R, Bull U, et al. Assessment of ventricular function with first-pass radionuclide angiography using technetium 99m hexakis-2-methoxyisobutylisonitrile: A European multicentre study. *Eur J Nucl Med* 1991;18:178–183.

62. He ZX, Darcourt J, Guignier A, et al. Nitrates improve detection of ischemic but viable myocardium by thallium-201 reinjection SPECT. *J Nucl Med* 1993;34:1472–1477.

63. Sciagra R, Bisi G, Santoro GM, et al. Comparison of baseline-nitrate technetium-99m sestamibi with rest-redistribution thallium-201 tomography in detecting viable hibernating myocardium and predicting postrevascularization recovery. *J Am Coll Cardiol* 1997;30:384–391.

64. Galli M, Marcassa C, Imparato A, et al. Effects of nitroglycerin by technetium-99m sestamibi tomoscintigraphy on resting regional myocardial hypoperfusion in stable patients with healed myocardial infarction. *Am J Cardiol* 1994;74:843–848.
65. Maurea S, Cuocolo A, Soricelli A, et al. Enhanced detection of viable myocardium by technetium-99m-MIBI imaging after nitrate administration in chronic coronary artery disease. *J Nucl Med* 1995;36:1945–1952.
66. Bonow RO. Assessment of myocardial viability with thallium-201. In: Zaret BL, Beller G, eds. *Nuclear Cardiology: State of the Art and Future Directions,* 2d ed. St. Louis: Mosby; 1998;503–512.
67. Udelson JE, Coleman PS, Metherall J, et al. Predicting recovery of severe regional ventricular dysfunction. Comparison of resting scintigraphy with $^{201}$Tl and $^{99m}$Tc-sestamibi. *Circulation.* 1994;89:2552–2561.
68. Germano G, Kiat H, Kavanagh PB, et al. Automatic quantification of ejection fraction from gated myocardial perfusion SPECT. *J Nucl Med* 1995;36:2138–2147.
69. Faber TL, Cooke CD, Folks RD, et al. Left ventricular function and perfusion from gated SPECT perfusion images: An integrated method. *J Nucl Med* 1999;40:650–659.
70. Goris ML, Thompson C, Malone LJ, et al. Modelling the integration of myocardial regional perfusion and function. *Nucl Med Commun* 1994;15:9–20.
71. Germano G, Berman D. Quantitative gated perfusion SPECT. In: Germano G, Berman DS, ed. *Clinical Gated Cardiac SPECT.* Armonk, NY: Futura; 1999;115–146.
72. Nichols K, Lefkovitz D, Faber T, et al. Ventricular volumes compared among three gated SPECT methods and echocardiography (abstr). *J Am Coll Cardiol* 1999;33:409A.
73. Kang X, Berman D, Germano G, et al. Normal parameters of left ventricle volume and ejection fraction measured by gated myocardial perfusion SPECT (abstr). *J Am Coll Cardiol* 1999;33:409A.
74. Case J, Bateman TM, Moutray K, et al. Establishing normal limits for LVEF from ECG-gated resting Tl-201 myocardial perfusion SPECT imaging (abstr). *J Am Coll Cardiol* 1999;6:S116.
75. Fujino S, Masuyama K, Kanayama S, et al. Early and delayed technetium-99m-labeled sestamibi myocardial ECG-gated SPECT by QGS program in normal volunteers (abstr). *J Nucl Med* 1999;40:180P.
76. Case J, Cullom S, Bateman TM, et al. Overestimation of LVEF by gated MIBI myocardial perfusion SPECT in patients with small hearts (abstr). *J Am Coll Cardiol* 1998;31:43A.
77. Weiss AT, Berman DS, Lew AS, et al. Transient ischemic dilation of the left ventricle on stress thallium-201 scintigraphy: A marker of severe and extensive coronary artery disease. *J Am Coll Cardiol* 1987;9:752–759.
78. Mazzanti M, Germano G, Kiat H, et al. Identification of severe and extensive coronary artery disease by automatic measurement of transient ischemic dilation of the left ventricle in dual-isotope myocardial perfusion SPECT. *J Am Coll Cardiol* 1996;27:1612–1620.
79. Hansen CL, Sangrigoli R, Nkadi E, et al. Comparison of pulmonary uptake with transient cavity dilation after exercise thallium-201 perfusion imaging. *J Am Coll Cardiol* 1999;33:1323–1327.
80. Chouraqui P, Rodrigues EA, Berman DS, et al. Significance of dipyridamole-induced transient dilation of the left ventricle during thallium-201 scintigraphy in suspected coronary artery disease. *Am J Cardiol* 1990;66:689–694.
81. Gill JB, Ruddy TD, Newell JB, et al. Prognostic importance of thallium uptake by the lungs during exercise in coronary artery disease. *N Engl J Med* 1987;317:1486–1489.
82. Bacher-Stier C, Sharir T, Kavanagh PB, et al. Postexercise lung uptake of 99mTc-sestamibi determined by a new automatic technique: validation and application in detection of severe and extensive coronary artery disease and reduced left ventricular function. *J Nucl Med* 2000;41:1190–1197.
83. Hurwitz GA, Fox SP, Driedger AA, et al. Pulmonary uptake of sestamibi on early post-stress images: Angiographic relationships, incidence and kinetics. *Nucl Med Commun* 1993;14:15–22.
84. Hurwitz GA, Ghali SK, Husni M, et al. Pulmonary uptake of technetium-99m-sestamibi induced by dipyridamole-based stress or exercise. *J Nucl Med* 1998;39:339–345.
85. Giubbini R, Campini R, Milan E, et al. Evaluation of technetium-99m-sestamibi lung uptake: correlation with left ventricular function. *J Nucl Med* 1995;36:58–63.
86. Diamond GA, Forrester JS. Analysis of probability as an aid in the clinical diagnosis of coronary-artery disease. *N Engl J Med* 1979;300:1350–1358.
87. Grundy SM, Pasternak R, Greenland P, et al. Assessment of cardiovascular risk by use of multiple-risk-factor assessment equations: A statement for healthcare professionals from the American Heart Association and the American College of Cardiology. *Circulation.* 1999;100:1481–1492.
88. Pryor DB, Harrell FE Jr, Lee KL, et al. Estimating the likelihood of significant coronary artery disease. *Am J Med* 1983;75:771–780.
88a. Berman DS, Garcia EV, Maddahi J. Thallium-201 myocardial scintigraphy in the detection and evaluation of coronary artery disease. In: Berman DS, Mason DT, eds. *Clinical Nuclear Cardiology.* New York: Grune & Stratton; 1981:49–106.
89. Hirzel HO, Senn M, Nuesch K, et al. Thallium-201 scintigraphy in complete left bundle branch block. *Am J Cardiol* 1984;53:764–769.
90. Rockett JF, Magill HL, Loveless VS, et al. Intravenous dipyridamole thallium-201 SPECT imaging methodology, applications, and interpretations, *Clin Nucl Med* 1990;15:712–725.
91. O'Keefe JH Jr, Bateman TM, Barnhart CS. Adenosine thallium-201 is superior to exercise thallium-201 for detecting coronary artery disease in patients with left bundle branch block. *J Am Coll Cardiol* 1993;21:1332–1338.
92. Burns RJ, Galligan L, Wright LM, et al. Improved specificity of myocardial thallium-201 single-photon emission computed tomography in patients with left bundle branch block by dipyridamole. *Am J Cardiol* 1991;68:504–508.
93. Gibbons RJ, Chatterjee K, Daley J, et al. ACC/AHA/ACP-ASIM guidelines for the management of patients with chronic stable angina: A report of the American College of Cardiology/American Heart Association Task Force on Practice Guidelines (Committee on Management of Patients With Chronic Stable Angina). *J Am Coll Cardiol* 1999;33:2092–2197.
94. Taillefer R, DePuey EG, Udelson JE, et al. Comparative diagnostic accuracy of Tl-201 and Tc-99m sestamibi SPECT imaging (perfusion and ECG-gated SPECT) in detecting coronary artery disease in women. *J Am Coll Cardiol* 1997;29:69–77.
95. Rozanski A, Diamond GA, Berman D, et al. The declining specificity of exercise radionuclide ventriculography. *N Engl J Med* 1983;309:518–522.
96. Roger VL, Pellikka PA, Bell MR, et al. Sex and test verification bias. Impact on the diagnostic value of exercise echocardiography. *Circulation* 1997;95:405–410.
97. Berman D, Hachamovitch R, Lewin H, et al. Risk stratification in coronary artery disease: implications for stabilization and prevention. *Am J Cardiol* 1997;79:10–16.
98. Gibbons RJ, Hodge DO, Berman DS, et al. Long-term outcome of patients with intermediate-risk exercise electrocardiograms who do not have myocardial perfusion defects on radionuclide imaging. *Circulation* 1999;100:2140–2145.
99. Yusuf S, Zucker D, Peduzzi P, et al. Effect of coronary artery bypass graft surgery on survival: Overview of 10-year results from randomised trials by the Coronary Artery Bypass Graft Surgery Trialists Collaboration. *Lancet* 1994;344:563–570.
100. Hlatky MA, Rogers WJ, Johnstone I, et. al. Medical care costs and quality of life after randomization to coronary angioplasty or coronary bypass surgery. Bypass Angioplasty Revascularization Investigation (BARI) Investigators. *N Engl J Med* 1997;336(2)92–99.
101. Little WC, Constantinescu M, Applegate RJ, et al. Can coronary angiography predict the site of a subsequent myocardial infarction in patients with mild-to-moderate coronary artery disease? *Circulation* 1988;78:1157–1166.

102. Ambrose JA, Tannenbaum MA, Alexopoulos D, et al. Angiographic progression of coronary artery disease and the development of myocardial infarction. *J Am Coll Cardiol* 1988;12:56–62.
103. Zeiher AM, Krause T, Schachinger V, et al. Impaired endothelium-dependent vasodilation of coronary resistance vessels is associated with exercise-induced myocardial ischemia. *Circulation* 1995;91: 2345–2352.
104. Kinsella JP, Torielli F, Ziegler JW, ct al. Dipyridamole augmentation of response to nitric oxide. *Lancet* 1995;346:647–648.
105. Ladenheim ML, Kotler TS, Pollock BH, et al. Incremental prognostic power of clinical history, exercise electrocardiography and myocardial perfusion scintigraphy in suspected coronary artery disease. *Am J Cardiol* 1987;59:270–277.
106. Shaw L, Hachamovitch R, Papatheofanis FJ. *Outcomes and Technology Assessment in Nuclear Medicine.* Reston, VA: Society of Nuclear Medicine Press; 1999.
107. Hachamovitch R, Schnipper J, Young-Xu Y. Are patients with known or suspected coronary artery disease and normal stress imaging studies at low risk for adverse outcomes? Meta-analysis of stress echocardiography and SPECT. *J Am Coll Cardiol* 2000.
108. Iskander S, Iskandrian AE. Risk assessment using single-photon emission computed tomographic technetium-99m sestamibi imaging. *J Am Coll Cardiol* 1998;32:57–62.
109. Shaw LJ, Hendel R, Borges-Neto S, et al, for the Myoview Multicenter Registry. Prognostic value of normal exercise and adenosine Tc-99m tetrofosmin SPECT imaging: results from the multicenter registry of 4,728 patients. *J Nucl Med* 2003;44(2):134–139.
109a. Hayes SW, De Lorenzo A, Hachamovitch R, et al. Prognostic implications of combined prone and supine acquisitions in patients with equivocal or abnormal supine myocardial perfusion SPECT. *J Nucl Med* 2003;44:1633–1640.
109b. Abidov A, Bax JJ, Hayes SW, et al. Transient ischemic dilation ratio of the left ventricle is a significant predictor of future cardiac events in patients with otherwise normal myocardial perfusion SPECT. *J Am Coll Cardiol.* In press.
110. Pasternak RC, Brown LE, Stone PH, et al. Effect of combination therapy with lipid-reducing drugs in patients with coronary heart disease and "normal" cholesterol levels. A randomized, placebo-controlled trial. Harvard Atherosclerosis Reversibility Project (HARP) Study Group. *Ann Intern Med* 1996;125:529–540.
111. Shepherd J, Cobbe SM, Ford I, et al. Prevention of coronary heart disease with pravastatin in men with hypercholesterolemia. West of Scotland Coronary Prevention Study Group. *N Engl J Med* 1995;333: 1301–1307.
112. Hachamovitch R, Berman DS, Lewin HC, et al. Stress SPECT in asymptomatic patients: Incremental prognostic value and risk stratification. *J Nucl Med* 1997;38:40P.
113. Hachamovitch R, Berman DS, Kiat H, et al. Value of stress myocardial perfusion single photon emission computed tomography in patients with normal resting electrocardiograms: An evaluation of incremental prognostic value and cost-effectiveness. *Circulation* 2002;105:823–829.
114. Santos MM, Abidov A, Hayes, SW, et al. Prognostic implications of myocardial perfusion SPECT in patients with atrial fibrillation (abstr). *J Nucl Med* 2002;43:98P.
115. Ladenheim ML, Pollock BH, Rozanski A, et al. Extent and severity of myocardial hypoperfusion as predictors of prognosis in patients with suspected coronary artery disease. *J Am Coll Cardiol* 1986;7:464–471.
116. Galassi AR, Azzarelli S, Tomaselli A, et al. Incremental prognostic value of technetium-99m-tetrofosmin exercise myocardial perfusion imaging for predicting outcomes in patients with suspected or known coronary artery disease. *Am J Cardiol* 2001;88:101–106.
117. Schinkel A, Elhendy A, van Domburg JJ, et al. Incremental value of exercise technetium-99m tetrofosmin myocardial perfusion single-photon emission computed tomography for the prediction of cardiac events. *Am J Cardiol* 2003;91:408–411.
118. Bateman TM, O'Keefe JH Jr, Dong VM, et al. Coronary angiographic rates after stress single-photon emission computed tomographic scintigraphy. *J Nucl Cardiol* 1995;2:217–223.
119. Nallamothu N, Pancholy SB, Lee KR, et al. Impact on exercise single-photon emission computed tomographic thallium imaging on patient management and outcome. *J Nucl Cardiol* 1995;2:334–338.
120. Shaw LJ, Hachamovitch R, Berman DS, et al. The economic consequences of available diagnostic and prognostic strategies for the evaluation of stable angina patients: an observational assessment of the value of precatheterization ischemia. Economics of Noninvasive Diagnosis (END) Multicenter Study Group. *J Am Coll Cardiol* 1999;33: 661–669.
121. Staniloff HM, Forrester JS, Berman DS, et al. Prediction of death, myocardial infarction, and worsening chest pain using thallium scintigraphy and exercise electrocardiograph. *J Nucl Med* 1986;27: 1842–1848.
122. Pryor DB, Harrell FE Jr, Lee KL, et al. Prognostic indicators from radionuclide angiography in medically treated patients with coronary artery disease. *Am J Cardiol* 1984;53:18–22.
123. Hachamovitch R, Shaw L, Berman DS. Methodological considerations in the assessment of noninvasive testing using outcomes research: Pitfalls and limitations. *Prog Cardiovasc Dis* 2000;43: 215–230.
124. Hachamovitch R, Berman DS, Kiat H, et al. Gender-related differences in clinical management after exercise nuclear testing. *J Am Coll Cardiol* 1995;26:1457–1464.
124a. Hachamovitch R, Hayes SW, Friedman JD, et al. Stress myocardial perfusion SPECT is clinically effective and cost-effective in risk stratification of patients with a high likelihood of CAD but no known CAD. *J Am Coll Cardiol.* In press.
125. Lee KL, Pryor DB, Pieper KS, et al. Prognostic value of radionuclide angiography in medically treated patients with coronary artery disease. A comparison with clinical and catheterization variables. *Circulation* 1990;82:1705–1717.
126. Jones RH, Johnson SH, Bigelow C, et al. Exercise radionuclide angiocardiography predicts cardiac death in patients with coronary artery disease. *Circulation* 1991;84:I52–I58.
127. Sharir T, Germano G, Kavanagh PB, et al. Incremental prognostic value of post-stress left ventricular ejection fraction and volume by gated myocardial perfusion single photon emission computed tomography. *Circulation* 1999;100:1035–1042.
127a. Hachamovitch R, Hayes SW, Friedman JD, et al. Is there a referral bias against revascularization of patients with reduced LV ejection fraction? Influence of ejection fraction and inducible ischemia on post-SPECT management of patients without history of CAD. *J Am Coll Cardiol* 2003;42:1286–1294.
128. Sharir T, Germano G, Lewin H, et al. Prognostic value of myocardial perfusion and function by gated SPECT in the prediction of non-fatal myocardial infarction and cardiac death (abstr). *Circulation* 1999; 100:I383.
128a. Hachamovitch R, Hayes SW, Cohen I, et al. Inducible ischemia is superior to EF for identification of short-term survival benefit with revascularization vs. medical therapy. *Circulation* 2002;106:II523.
129. Sharir T, Germano G, Kang X, et al. Prediction of myocardial infarction versus cardiac death by gated myocardial perfusion SPECT: Risk stratification by the amount of stress-induced ischemia and the post-stress ejection fraction. *J Nucl Med* 2001;42:831–837.
130. Sharir T, Bacher-Stier C, Dhar S, et al. Identification of severe and extensive coronary artery disease by postexercise regional wall motion abnormalities in Tc-99m sestamibi gated single-photon emission computed tomography. *Am J Cardiol* 2000;86:1171–1175.
131. Ambrosio G, Betocchi S, Pace L, et al. Prolonged impairment of regional contractile function after resolution of exercise-induced angina. Evidence of myocardial stunning in patients with coronary artery disease. *Circulation* 1996;94:2455–2464.
132. Bacher-Stier C, Kavanagh PB, Sharir T, et al. Post-exercise Tc-99m sestamibi lung uptake determined by a new automatic technique (abstr). *J Nucl Med* 1998;39:104P.
133. Sharir T, Berman DS, Lewin HC, et al. Incremental prognostic value of rest-redistribution (201)Tl single-photon emission computed tomography. *Circulation* 1999;100:1964–1970.

134. Allman KC, Shaw LJ, Hachamovitch R, et al. Myocardial viability testing and impact of revascularization on prognosis in patients with coronary artery disease and left ventricular dysfunction: A meta-analysis. *J Am Coll Cardiol* 2002;39:1151–1158.
135. Shaw LJ, Hachamovitch R, Peterson ED, et al. Using an outcomes-based approach to identify candidates for risk stratification after exercise treadmill testing. *J Gen Intern Med* 1999;14:1–9.
136. Gibbons RJ, Balady GJ, Bricker JT, et al. ACC/AHA 2002 guideline update for exercise testing: summary article: A report of the American College of Cardiology/American Heart Association Task Force on Practice Guidelines (Committee to Update the 1997 Exercise Testing Guidelines). *Circulation* 2002;106:1883–1892.
137. Elveback LR, Connolly DC, Melton LJ III. Coronary heart disease in residents of Rochester, Minnesota: VII. Incidence, 1950 through 1982. *Mayo Clin Proc* 1986;61:896–900.
138. Christian TF, Miller TD, Bailey KR, et al. Exercise tomographic thallium-201 imaging in patients with severe coronary artery disease and normal electrocardiograms. *Ann Intern Med* 1994;121:825–832.
139. Mattera JA, Arain SA, Sinusas AJ, et al. Exercise testing with myocardial perfusion imaging in patients with normal baseline electrocardiograms: Cost savings with a stepwise diagnostic strategy. *J Nucl Cardiol* 1998;5:498–506.
140. O'Keefe JH Jr, Zinsmeister AR, Gibbons RJ. Value of normal electrocardiographic findings in predicting resting left ventricular function in patients with chest pain and suspected coronary artery disease. *Am J Med* 1989;86:658–662.
141. Christian TF, Miller TD, Chareonthaitawee P, et al. Prevalence of normal resting left ventricular function with normal rest electrocardiograms. *Am J Cardiol* 1997;79:1295–1298.
142. Gibbons RJ, Zinsmeister AR, Miller TD, et al. Supine exercise electrocardiography compared with exercise radionuclide angiography in noninvasive identification of severe coronary artery disease. *Ann Intern Med* 1990;112:743–749.
142a. Poornima I, Miller T, Christian T, et al. Utility of myocardial perfusion imaging in patients with low-risk treadmill scores. *J Am Coll Cardiol* 2004. In press.
143. Blumenthal RS, Becker DM, Moy TF, et al. Exercise thallium tomography predicts future clinically manifest coronary heart disease in a high-risk asymptomatic population. *Circulation* 1996;93: 915–923.
144. Schwartz RS, Jackson WG, Celio PV, et al. Accuracy of exercise $^{201}$Tl myocardial scintigraphy in asymptomatic young men. *Circulation* 1993;87:165–172.
145. Fleg JL, Gerstenblith G, Zonderman AB, et al. Prevalence and prognostic significance of exercise-induced silent myocardial ischemia detected by thallium scintigraphy and electrocardiography in asymptomatic volunteers. *Circulation* 1990;81:428–436.
146. Wackers FJ, Zaret BL. Detection of myocardial ischemia in patients with diabetes mellitus. *Circulation* 2002;105:5–7.
146a. Miller TD, Rajagopalan N, Hodge DO, et al. The yield of stress single photon emission computed tomography in asymptomatic diabetic patients. *Am Heart J* 2003. In press.
147. Miller DD, Donohue TJ, Younis LT, et al. Correlation of pharmacological 99mTc-sestamibi myocardial perfusion imaging with post-stenotic coronary flow reserve in patients with angiographically intermediate coronary artery stenoses. *Circulation* 1994;89:2150–2160.
148. Kang X, Berman DS, Lewin HC, et al. Incremental prognostic value of myocardial perfusion single photon emission computed tomography in patients with diabetes mellitus. *Am Heart J* 1999;138: 1025–1032.
149. Giri S, Shaw LJ, Murthy DR, et al. Impact of diabetes on the risk stratification using stress single-photon emission computed tomography myocardial perfusion imaging in patients with symptoms suggestive of coronary artery disease. *Circulation* 2002;105:32–40.
150. Berman DS, Kang X, Hayes SW, et al. Adenosine myocardial perfusion SPECT in women compared to men: Incremental prognostic value, effect on patient management and impact of diabetes mellitus. *J Am Coll Cardiol* 2003; 41:1125–1133.
151. Hayes SW SE, Lewin HC, Kang X, et al. Gated myocardial perfusion SPECT has incremental value for predicting cardiac death in diabetic patients (abstr). *J Am Coll Cardiol* 2001;37:381A.
152. Wagdy HM, Hodge D, Christian TF, et al. Prognostic value of vasodilator myocardial perfusion imaging in patients with left bundle-branch block. *Circulation* 1998;97:1563–1570.
153. Nallamothu N, Bagheri B, Acio ER, et al. Prognostic value of stress myocardial perfusion single photon emission computed tomography imaging in patients with left ventricular bundle branch block. *J Nucl Cardiol* 1997;4:487–493.
154. Nigam A, Humen DP. Prognostic value of myocardial perfusion imaging with exercise and/or dipyridamole hyperemia in patients with preexisting left bundle branch block. *J Nucl Med* 1998;39:579–581.
155. Gil VM, Almeida M, Ventosa A, et al. Prognosis in patients with left bundle branch block and normal dipyridamole thallium-201 scintigraphy. *J Nucl Cardiol* 1998;5:414–417.
156. Vaduganathan P, He ZX, Raghavan C, et al. Detection of left anterior descending coronary artery stenosis in patients with left bundle branch block: Exercise, adenosine or dobutamine imaging? *J Am Coll Cardiol* 1996;28:543–550.
157. Elhendy A, van Domburg RT, Sozzi FB, et al. Impact of hypertension on the accuracy of exercise stress myocardial perfusion imaging for the diagnosis of coronary artery disease. *Heart* 2001;85:655–661.
158. Bartram P, Toft J, Hanel B, et al. False-positive defects in technetium-99m sestamibi myocardial single-photon emission tomography in healthy athletes with left ventricular hypertrophy. *Eur J Nucl Med* 1998;25:1308–1312.
159. Amanullah AM, Berman DS, Kang X, et al. Enhanced prognostic stratification of patients with left ventricular hypertrophy with the use of single-photon emission computed tomography. *Am Heart J* 2000;140:456–462.
159a. Santos MM, Abidov A, Hayes SW, et al. Prognostic implications of myocardial perfusion SPECT in patients with atrial fibrillation (abstr). *J Nucl Med* 2002;43:98P.
160. Hachamovitch R, Berman DS, Kiat H, et al. Effective risk stratification using exercise myocardial perfusion SPECT in women: Gender-related differences in prognostic nuclear testing. *J Am Coll Cardiol* 1996;28:34–44.
161. Marwick TH, Shaw LJ, Lauer MS, et al. The noninvasive prediction of cardiac mortality in men and women with known or suspected coronary artery disease. Economics of Noninvasive Diagnosis (END) Study Group. *Am J Med* 1999;106:172–178.
162. Amanullah AM, Berman DS, Hachamovitch R, et al. Identification of severe or extensive coronary artery disease in women by adenosine technetium-99m sestamibi SPECT. *Am J Cardiol* 1997;80:132–137.
163. Giri S, Shaw L, Miller DD, et al. Stress SPECT myocardial perfusion imaging for predicting cardiac events in diabetic women (abstr). *J Am Coll Cardiol* 1999;35:338A.
164. Mieres JH, Shaw LJ, Hendel RC, et al. A report of the American Society of Nuclear Cardiology Task Force on Women and Heart Disease (writing group on perfusion imaging in women). *J Nucl Cardiol* 2003;10:95–101.
165. Tobin JN, Wassertheil-Smoller S, Wexler JP, et al. Sex bias in considering coronary bypass surgery. *Ann Intern Med* 1987;107:19–25.
166. Hilton TC, Shaw LJ, Chaitman BR, et al. Prognostic significance of exercise thallium-201 testing in patients aged greater than or equal to 70 years with known or suspected coronary artery disease. *Am J Cardiol* 1992;69:45–50.
167. Amanullah A, Hachamovitch R, Erel J, et al. Prognostic value of exercise and adenosine myocardial perfusion SPECT in the very elderly (abstr). *J Am Coll Cardiol* 1997;29:362A.
168. Hachamovitch R, Diamond G, Kiat H, et al. Noninvasive risk stratification of the elderly patient: Use of nuclear testing to identify high risk patient populations (abstr). *Circulation* 1994;90:I-102.
169. Hayes SW, Lewin H, Friedman J, et al. Prognostic significance of rest Tl-201/stress Tc-technetium-99m sestamibi dual-isotope myocardial perfusion SPECT in very elderly patients (abstr). *J Am Coll Cardiol* 2000;35:455A.

170. Alkeylani A, Miller DD, Shaw LJ, et al. Influence of race on the prediction of cardiac events with stress technetium-99m sestamibi tomographic imaging in patients with stable angina pectoris. *Am J Cardiol* 1998;81:293–297.
171. Akinboboye OO, Idris O, Onwuanyi A, et al. Incidence of major cardiovascular events in black patients with normal myocardial stress perfusion study results. *J Nucl Cardiol* 2001;8:541–547.
172. Liao Y, Cooper RS, McGee DL, et al. The relative effects of left ventricular hypertrophy, coronary artery disease, and ventricular dysfunction on survival among black adults. *JAMA* 1995;273: 1592–1597.
172a. Kang X, Berman DS, Nishina H, et al. Comparison of normal weight and obese patients of myocardial perfusion SPECT without attenuation correction to detect coronary artery disease. *J Nucl Cardiol* 2003;10:S5.
173. He ZX, Hedrick TD, Pratt CM, et al. Severity of coronary artery calcification by electron beam computed tomography predicts silent myocardial ischemia. *Circulation* 2000;101:244–251.
174. Miranda RS SE, Gallagher AM, Lewin HC, et al. The extent of coronary calcium by electron beam computed tomography discriminates the likelihood of abnormal myocardial perfusion SPECT. *Circulation* 2000;102:II-543.
174a. Rumberger JA, Brundage BH, Rader DJ, Kondos G. Electron beam computed coronary calcium scanning: A review and guidelines for use in asymptomatic persons. *Mayo Clin Proc* 1999;74:243–252.
175. Parisi AF, Hartigan PM, Folland ED. Evaluation of exercise thallium scintigraphy versus exercise electrocardiography in predicting survival outcomes and morbid cardiac events in patients with single- and double-vessel disease. Findings from the Angioplasty Compared to Medicine (ACME) study. *J Am Coll Cardiol* 1997;30:1256–1263.
176. Miller DD, Verani MS. Current status of myocardial perfusion imaging after percutaneous transluminal coronary angioplasty. *J Am Coll Cardiol* 1994;24:260–266.
177. Berman D, Zellweger MJ, Shaw L, et al. Evaluation of patients after intervention. In: Pohost G, et al, eds. *Imaging in Cardiovascular Medicine.* Philadelphia: Lippincott Williams & Wilkins; 2000.
178. Garzon PP, Eisenberg MJ. Functional testing for the detection of restenosis after percutaneous transluminal coronary angioplasty: A meta-analysis. *Can J Cardiol* 2001;17:41–48.
179. Lauer MS, Lytle B, Pashkow F, et al. Prediction of death and myocardial infarction by screening with exercise-thallium testing after coronary-artery-bypass grafting. *Lancet* 1998;351:615–622.
180. Ho KT, Miller TD, Holmes DR, et al. Long-term prognostic value of Duke treadmill score and exercise thallium-201 imaging performed one to three years after percutaneous transluminal coronary angioplasty. *Am J Cardiol* 1999;84:1323–1327.
181. Grondin CM, Campeau L, Lesperance J, et al. Comparison of late changes in internal mammary artery and saphenous vein grafts in two consecutive series of patients 10 years after operation. *Circulation* 1984;70:I208–I212.
182. FitzGibbon GM, Leach AJ, Kafka HP, et al. Coronary bypass graft fate: long-term angiographic study. *J Am Coll Cardiol* 1191;17: 1075–1080.
183. Palmas W, Bingham S, Diamond GA, et al. Incremental prognostic value of exercise thallium-201 myocardial single-photon emission computed tomography late after coronary artery bypass surgery. *J Am Coll Cardiol* 1995;25:403–409.
184. Zellweger MJ, Lewin H, Lai S, et al. Risk stratification in patients early and late post-CABG using stress myocardial perfusion SPECT: Implications of appropriate clinical strategies. *J Am Coll Cardiol* 2001;37:144–152.
185. Nallamothu N, Johnson JH, Bagheri B, et al. Utility of stress single-photon emission computed tomography (SPECT) perfusion imaging in predicting outcome after coronary artery bypass grafting. *Am J Cardiol* 1997;80:1517–1521.
186. Zellweger MJ, Lewin HC, Lai S, et al. When to stress patients after coronary artery bypass surgery? Risk stratification in patients early and late post-CABG using stress myocardial perfusion SPECT: Implications of appropriate clinical strategies. *J Am Coll Cardiol* 2001;37:144–152.
187. Eagle KA, Coley CM, Newell JB, et al. Combining clinical and thallium data optimizes preoperative assessment of cardiac risk before major vascular surgery. *Ann Intern Med* 1989;110:859–866.
188. Eagle KA, Rihal CS, Mickel MC, et al. Cardiac risk of noncardiac surgery: influence of coronary disease and type of surgery in 3368 operations. CASS Investigators and University of Michigan Heart Care Program. Coronary Artery Surgery Study. *Circulation* 1997;96: 1882–1887.
189. Prigent FM, Berman DS, Elashoff J, et al. Reproducibility of stress redistribution thallium-201 SPECT quantitative indexes of hypoperfused myocardium secondary to coronary artery disease. *Am J Cardiol* 1992;70:1255–1263.
190. Mahmarian JJ, Fenimore NL, Marks GF, et al. Transdermal nitroglycerin patch therapy reduces the extent of exercise-induced myocardial ischemia: Results of a double-blind, placebo-controlled trial using quantitative thallium-201 tomography. *J Am Coll Cardiol* 1994;24:25–32.
191. Lewin H, Hachamovitch R, Harris AG, et al. Reproducibility of isotope myocardial perfusion SPECT using a new quantitive perfusion SPECT (QPS) approach (abstr). *J Am Coll Cardiol* 1999;33: 483A.
192. Lewin HC, Hachamovitch R, Harris AG, et al. Sustained reduction of exercise perfusion defect extent and severity with isosorbide mononitrate (Imdur) as demonstrated by means of technetium 99m sestamibi. *J Nucl Cardiol* 2000;7:342–53.
193. Dakik HA, Kleiman NS, Farmer JA, et al. Intensive medical therapy versus coronary angioplasty for suppression of myocardial ischemia in survivors of acute myocardial infarction: A prospective, randomized pilot study. *Circulation* 1998;98:2017–2023.
194. Henry T, Annex B, Azrin M. Double blind, placebo controlled trial of recombinant human vascular endothelial growth factor—The VIVA trial (abstr). *J Am Coll Cardiol* 1999;33:384A.
195. Schwartz RG, Pearson TA, Kalaria VG, et al. Prospective serial evaluation of myocardial perfusion and lipids during the first six months of pravastatin therapy: coronary artery disease regression single photon emission computed tomography monitoring trial. *J Am Coll Cardiol* 2003;42(4):600–610.
196. Mostaza JM, Gomez MV, Gallardo F, et al. Cholesterol reduction improves myocardial perfusion abnormalities in patients with coronary artery disease and average cholesterol levels. *J Am Coll Cardiol* 2000; 35:76–82.
197. Danias PG, Ahlberg AW, Clark BA III, et al. Combined assessment of myocardial perfusion and left ventricular function with exercise technetium-99m sestamibi gated single-photon emission computed tomography can differentiate between ischemic and nonischemic dilated cardiomyopathy. *Am J Cardiol* 1998;82:1253–1258.
198. Tauberg SG, Orie JE, Bartlett BE, et al. Usefulness of thallium-201 for distinction of ischemic from idiopathic dilated cardiomyopathy. *Am J Cardiol* 1993;71:674–680.
199. Saltissi S, Hockings B, Croft DN, et al. Thallium-201 myocardial imaging in patients with dilated and ischaemic cardiomyopathy. *Br Heart J* 1981;46:290–295.
200. Braunwald E, Kloner RA. The stunned myocardium: prolonged, postischemic ventricular dysfunction. *Circulation* 1982;66:1146–1149.
201. Bonow RO. The hibernating myocardium: Implications for management of congestive heart failure. *Am J Cardiol* 1995;75: 17A–25A.
202. Camici PG, Wijns W, Borgers M, et al. Pathophysiological mechanisms of chronic reversible left ventricular dysfunction due to coronary artery disease (hibernating myocardium). *Circulation* 1997;96: 3205–3214.
203. Vanoverschelde JL, Wijns W, Borgers M, et al. Chronic myocardial hibernation in humans. From bedside to bench. *Circulation* 1997;95: 1961–1971.
204. Bonow RO. Identification of viable myocardium. *Circulation* 1996; 94:2674–2680.

205. Bonow RO. Clinical value of combined assessment of perfusion and function for the evaluation of myocardial viability. In: Germano G, Berman DS, eds. *Clinical Gated Cardiac SPECT.* 1999:307–324.

206. Arrighi JA, Dilsizian V. Myocardial viability: radionuclide-based methods. In: Pohost GM, O'Rourke RA, Berman DS, Shah PM, eds. In:Imaging in Cardiovascular Disease. Philadelphia: Lippencott Williams & Wilkins; 2000:213–232.

207. Bax JJ, Wijns W, Cornel JH, et al. Accuracy of currently available techniques for prediction of functional recovery after revascularization in patients with left ventricular dysfunction due to chronic coronary artery disease: Comparison of pooled data. *J Am Coll Cardiol* 1997;30:1451–1460.

208. Udelson JE. Choosing a thallium-201 or technetium 99m sestamibi imaging protocol. *J Nucl Cardiol* 1994;1:S99–S108.

209. He ZX, Medrano R, Hays JT, et al. Nitroglycerin-augmented $^{201}$Tl reinjection enhances detection of reversible myocardial hypoperfusion. A randomized, double-blind, parallel, placebo-controlled trial. *Circulation* 1997;95:1799–1805.

210. Tubau JF, Rahimtoola SH. Hibernating myocardium: A historical perspective. *Cardiovasc Drugs Ther* 1992;6:267–271.

211. Elsasser A, Schlepper M, Klovekorn WP, et al. Hibernating myocardium: An incomplete adaptation to ischemia. *Circulation* 1997;96: 2920–2931.

212. Kontos MC, Jesse RL, Schmidt KL, et al. Value of acute rest sestamibi perfusion imaging for evaluation of patients admitted to the emergency department with chest pain. *J Am Coll Cardiol* 1997;30: 976–982.

213. Heller GV, Stowers SA, Hendel RC, et al. Clinical value of acute rest technetium-99m tetrofosmin tomographic myocardial perfusion imaging in patients with acute chest pain and nondiagnostic electrocardiograms. *J Am Coll Cardiol* 1998;31:1011–1017.

214. Udelson JE, Beshansky JR, Ballin DS, et al. Myocardial perfusion imaging for evaluation and triage of patients with suspected acute cardiac ischemia: A randomized controlled trial. *JAMA* 2002;288: 2693–2700.

215. Ziffer J, Nateman D, Janowitz W, et al. Myocardial perfusion imaging is a routinely effective triage tool to evaluate ongoing and recently resolved chest pain in a dedicated center (abstr). *J Nucl Med* 1997;38: 131P.

216. Christian TF, Schwartz RS, Gibbons RJ. Determinants of infarct size in reperfusion therapy for acute myocardial infarction. *Circulation* 1992;86:81–90.

217. O'Keefe JH Jr, Grines CL, DeWood MA, et al. Factors influencing myocardial salvage with primary angioplasty. *J Nucl Cardiol* 1995;2: 35–41.

218. Gibbons RJ, Verani MS, Behrenbeck T, et al. Feasibility of tomographic $^{99m}$Tc-hexakis-2-methoxy-2-methylpropyl-isonitrile imaging for the assessment of myocardial area at risk and the effect of treatment in acute myocardial infarction. *Circulation* 1989;80: 1277–1286.

219. Lew AS, Maddahi J, Shah PK, et al. Critically ischemic myocardium in clinically stable patients following thrombolytic therapy for acute myocardial infarction: Potential implications for early coronary angioplasty in selected patients. *Am Heart J* 1990;120:1015–1025.

220. Braunwald E, Antman EM, Beasley JW, et al. ACC/AHA 2002 guideline update for the management of patients with unstable angina and non-ST-segment elevation myocardial infarction—Summary article: A report of the American College of Cardiology/American Heart Association task force on practice guidelines (Committee on the Management of Patients With Unstable Angina). *J Am Coll Cardiol* 2002;40:1366–1374.

221. Gibson RS, Watson DD, Craddock GB, et al. Prediction of cardiac events after uncomplicated myocardial infarction: a prospective study comparing predischarge exercise thallium-201 scintigraphy and coronary angiography. *Circulation* 1983;68:321–336.

222. Dakik HA, Mahmarian JJ, Kimball KT, et al. Prognostic value of exercise $^{201}$Tl tomography in patients treated with thrombolytic therapy during acute myocardial infarction. *Circulation* 1996;94:2735–2742.

223. Shaw LJ, Peterson ED, Kesler K, et al. A metaanalysis of predischarge risk stratification after acute myocardial infarction with stress electrocardiographic, myocardial perfusion, and ventricular function imaging. *Am J Cardiol* 1996;78:1327–1337.

224. Heller GV, Brown KA, Landin RJ, et al. Safety of early intravenous dipyridamole technetium 99m sestamibi SPECT myocardial perfusion imaging after uncomplicated first myocardial infarction. Early Post MI IV Dipyridamole Study (EPIDS). *Am Heart J* 1997;134: 105–115.

225. Beller GA, Zaret BL. Contributions of nuclear cardiology to diagnosis and prognosis of patients with coronary artery disease. *Circulation* 2000;101:1465–1478.

226. Brown KA, Heller GV, Landin RS, et al. Early dipyridamole (99m)Tc-sestamibi single photon emission computed tomographic imaging 2 to 4 days after acute myocardial infarction predicts in-hospital and postdischarge cardiac events: comparison with submaximal exercise imaging. *Circulation* 1999;100:2060–2066.

227. Burns RJ, Gibbons RJ, Yi Q, et al. The relationships of left ventricular ejection fraction, end-systolic volume index and infarct size to six-month mortality after hospital discharge following myocardial infarction treated by thrombolysis. *J Am Coll Cardiol* 2002;39:30–36.

228. Dakik HA, Filipchuk NG, Pratt CM, et al. Suppression of post-infarction myocardial ischemia with medical and revascularization therapies: results form the adenosine sestamibi post-infarction evaluation (INSPIRE) trial (abstr). *Circulation* 2003;108:IV-635.

229. Iskander S, Pratt, CM, Filipchuk, NG, et al. Medical and revascularization therapies for suppression of post-infarction myocardial ischemia. Preliminary results from the Adenosine Sestamibi Post-Infarction Evaluation (INSPIRE) trial (abstr). *Circulation* 2001;104: II-455.

230. Hains AD, Al-Khawaja I, Hinge DA. Radionuclide left ventricular function ejection fraction. A comparison of three methods. *Br Heart J* 1987;57(3):242–246.

231. Maddahi J, Berman D, Silverberg R, et al. Validation of a two-minute technique for multiple gated scintigraphic assessment of left ventricular ejection fraction and regional wall motion. *J Nucl Med* 1978;19:669.

232. Borer JS, Bacharach SL, Green MV, et al. Real-time radionuclide cineangiography in the noninvasive evaluation of global and regional left ventricular function at rest and during exercise in patients with coronary-artery disease. *N Engl J Med* 1977;296:839–844.

233. Maddahi J, Berman DS, Matsuoka DT, et al. A new technique for assessing right ventricular ejection fraction using rapid multiple-gated equilibrium cardiac blood pool scintigraphy. Description, validation and findings in chronic coronary artery disease. *Circulation* 1979;60: 581–589.

234. Jones RH. Use of radionuclide measurements of left ventricular function for prognosis in patients with coronary artery disease. *Semin Nucl Med* 1987;17:95–103.

235. Borges-Neto S, Coleman RE, Jones RH. Perfusion and function at rest and treadmill exercise using technetium-99m-sestamibi: Comparison of one- and two-day protocols in normal volunteers. *J Nucl Med* 1990;31:1128–1132.

236. Friedman JD, Berman DS, Kiat H, et al. Rest and treadmill exercise first-pass radionuclide ventriculography: Validation of left ventricular ejection fraction measurements. *J Nucl Cardiol* 1994;1:382–388.

237. Van Kriekinge SD, Berman DS, Germano G. Automatic quantification of left ventricular ejection fraction from gated blood pool SPECT. *J Nucl Cardiol* 1999;6:498–506.

238. Sharp N, Murphy J, Smith H. Treatment of patients with symptomless left ventricular dysfunction after myocardial infarction. *Lancet* 1988;255–259.

239. Moriel M, Rozanski A, Klein J, et al. The differing prognostic utility of exercise radionuclide ventriculography in coronary artery disease patients with and without prior myocardial infarction. *Int J Card Imaging* 1997;13:403–413.

240. Shaw LJ, Heinle SK, Borges-Neto S, et al. Prognosis by measurements of left ventricular function during exercise. Duke Noninvasive Research Working Group. *J Nucl Med* 1998;39:140–146.

241. Bonow RO, Bacharach SL, Green MV, et al. Prognostic implications of symptomatic versus asymptomatic (silent) myocardial ischemia induced by exercise in mildly symptomatic and in asymptomatic patients with angiographically documented coronary artery disease. *Am J Cardiol* 1987;60:778–783.
242. Peterson ED, Shaw LJ, Califf RM. Risk stratification after myocardial infarction. *Ann Intern Med* 1997;126:561–582.
243. Alexander J, Dainiak N, Berger HJ, et al. Serial assessment of doxorubicin cardiotoxicity with quantitative radionuclide angiocardiography. *N Engl J Med* 1979;300:278–283.
244. Schwartz RG, McKenzie WB, Alexander J, et al. Congestive heart failure and left ventricular dysfunction complicating doxorubicin therapy. Seven-year experience using serial radionuclide angiocardiography. *Am J Med* 1987;82:1109–1118.
245. Bonow RO, Rosing DR, Maron BJ, et al. Reversal of left ventricular dysfunction after aortic valve replacement for chronic aortic regurgitation: Influence of duration of preoperative left ventricular dysfunction. *Circulation* 1984;70:570–579.
246. Tamaki N, Tadamura E. Fatty acid imaging. In: Pohost GM, O'Rourke RA, Berman DS, Shah PM. eds. In: *Imaging in Cardiovascular Disease*. Philadelphia: Lippencott Williams & Wilkins; 2000: 295–306.
247. Knapp FF Jr, Goodman MM, Callahan AP, et al. Radioiodinated 15-(*p*-iodophenyl)-3,3-dimethylpentadecanoic acid: A useful new agent to evaluate myocardial fatty acid uptake. *J Nucl Med* 1986;27: 521–531.
248. Saito T, Yasuda T, Gold HK, et al. Differentiation of regional perfusion and fatty acid uptake in zones of myocardial injury. *Nucl Med Commun* 1991;12:663–675.
249. Furutani Y, Shiigi T, Nakamura Y, et al. Quantification of area at risk in acute myocardial infarction by tomographic imaging. *J Nucl Med* 1997;38:1875–1882.
250. Dae MW. Imaging of myocardial innervation. In: Pohost GM, O'Rourke, RO, Berman D, Shah P, eds. *Imaging in Cardiovascular Disease*. Philadelphia: Lippincott Williams & Wilkins; 2000:307–314.
251. Whitby LG, Axelrod J, Weil-Malherbe H. The fate of 3H-norepinephrine in animals. *J Pharmacol Exp Ther* 1961;132:193–201.
252. Dae MW, O'Connell JW, Botvinick EH, et al. Scintigraphic assessment of regional cardiac adrenergic innervation. *Circulation.* 1989;79:634–644.
252a. Lanza GA, Giordano A, Pristipino C, et al. Abnormal cardiac adrenergic nerve function in patients with syndrome X detected by [123] metaiodobenzylquanidine myocardial scintigraphy. *Circulation* 1977; 96:821–826.
253. Schnell O, Muhr D, Dresel S, et al. Partial restoration of scintigraphically assessed cardiac sympathetic denervation in newly diagnosed patients with insulin-dependent (type 1) diabetes mellitus at one-year follow-up. *Diabet Med* 1997;14:57–62.
254. Mitrani RD, Klein LS, Miles WM, et al. Regional cardiac sympathetic denervation in patients with ventricular tachycardia in the absence of coronary artery disease. *J Am Coll Cardiol* 1993;22: 1344–1353.
255. Gill JS, Hunter GJ, Gane J, et al. Asymmetry of cardiac [123I] metaiodobenzyl-guanidine scans in patients with ventricular tachycardia and a "clinically normal" heart. *Br Heart J* 1993;69:6–13.
256. Schafers M, Wichter T, Lerch H, et al. Cardiac 123I-MIBG uptake in idiopathic ventricular tachycardia and fibrillation. *J Nucl Med.* 1999: 40:1–5.
257. Nakata T, Miyamoto K, Doi A, et al. Cardiac death prediction and impaired cardiac sympathetic innervation assessed by MIBG in patients with failing and nonfailing hearts. *J Nucl Cardiol* 1998;5:579–90.
258. Merlet P, Benvenuti C, Moyse D, et al. Prognostic value of MIBG imaging in idiopathic dilated cardiomyopathy. *J Nucl Med* 1999;40: 917–923.
259. Suwa M, Otake Y, Moriguchi A, et al. Iodine-123 metaiodobenzylguanidine myocardial scintigraphy for prediction of response to beta-blocker therapy in patients with dilated cardiomyopathy. *Am Heart J* 1997;133:353–358.
260. Yamazaki J, Muto H, Kabano T, et al. Evaluation of beta-blocker therapy in patients with dilated cardiomyopathy—Clinical meaning of iodine 123-metaiodobenzylguanidine myocardial single-photon emission computed tomography. *Am Heart J* 2001;141:645–652.
261. Krause T, Kasper W, Zeiher A, et al. Relation of technetium-99m pyrophosphate accumulation to time interval after onset of acute myocardial infarction as assessed by a tomographic acquisition technique. *Am J Cardiol* 1991;68:1575–1579.
262. Bonte FJ, Parkey RW, Graham KD, et al. A new method for radionuclide imaging of myocardial infarcts. *Radiology* 1974;110:473–474.
263. Tamaki N, Yamada T, Matsumori A, et al. Indium-111-antimyosin antibody imaging for detecting different stages of myocardial infarction: Comparison with technetium-99m-pyrophosphate imaging. *J Nucl Med* 1990;31:136–142.
264. Gerson MC, McGoron AJ. Technetium 99m glucarate: What will be its clinical role? *J Nucl Cardiol* 1997;4:336–340.
265. Narula J, Khaw BA, Dec GW, et al. Diagnostic accuracy of antimyosin scintigraphy in suspected myocarditis. *J Nucl Cardiol* 1996;3: 371–381.
266. Ballester M, Bordes R, Tazelaar HD, et al. Evaluation of biopsy classification for rejection: Relation to detection of myocardial damage by monoclonal antimyosin antibody imaging. *J Am Coll Cardiol* 1998;31:1357–1361.
267. Narula J, Petrov A, Pak KY, et al. Very early noninvasive detection of acute experimental nonreperfused myocardial infarction with 99mTc-labeled glucarate. *Circulation* 1997;95:1577–1584.
268. Narula J, Acio ER, Narula N, et al. Annexin-V imaging for noninvasive detection of cardiac allograft rejection. *Nat Med* 2001;7: 1347–1352.
269. Smanio PE, Watson DD, Segalla DL, et al. Value of gating of technetium-99m sestamibi single-photon emission computed tomographic imaging. *J Am Coll Cardiol* 1997;30:1687–1692.
270. Vanzetto G, Ormezzano O, Fagret D, et al. Long-term additive prognostic value of thallium-201 myocardial perfusion imaging over clinical and exercise stress test in low to intermediate risk patients: Study in 1137 patients with 6-year follow-up. *Circulation* 1999;100: 1521–1527.
271. Shaw L. Cost effectiveness of gated and nongated cardiac SPECT imaging. In: Germano G, Berman D, eds. *Clinical Gated Cardiac SPECT.* Armonk, NY: Futura; 1999:325–338.
272. O'Rourke RA, Chaudhuri T, Shaw L, et al. Resolution of stress-induced myocardial ischemia during aggressive medical therapy as demonstrated by single photon emission computed tomography imaging. *Circulation* 2001;103:2315.

C H A P T E R 20

# COMPUTED TOMOGRAPHY OF THE HEART

John J. Mahmarian



Computed tomography (CT) has emerged as a technique that can fully evaluate both cardiac structure and function. Recent advances in imaging speed have allowed for more complete evaluation of relatively stationary structures, such as the thoracic aorta, and rapidly moving structures, such as the myocardium. When combined with electrocardiographic (ECG) gating, "freeze-frame" images of the heart can be obtained, obviating most of the blur caused by motion artifact during systole and diastole. This is particularly important in obtaining contrast-enhanced images of the coronary arteries or quantifying coronary artery calcium.

Two general types of CT scanners are currently available for performing cardiac evaluations. Mechanical CT scanners can acquire images within 300 ms, whereas exposure times have been markedly reduced to 50 ms with the advent of electron beam computed tomography (EBCT).

## TECHNICAL CONSIDERATIONS

### Mechanical Computed Tomography

Advancements in CT technology have improved image acquisition speed and patient throughput. Traditional mechanical CT scanners produce images by rotating an x-ray tube around a circular gantry through which the patient advances on a moving couch. In the step-and-shoot CT mode, an obligatory 15-s delay occurs between each slice acquisition. In order to complete a standard 40-slice cardiac study, two scan acquisitions of 20 slices each must be obtained from two separate breathholds. This may lead to spatial misalignment of CT data from motion artifacts and differences in the depth of inspiration. With spiral CT scanners, the x-ray tube rotates continuously around the patient as the couch moves through the gantry, thus eliminating incremental stops and allowing completion of a cardiac scan within one breathhold. The introduction of multirow spiral CT detector systems (i.e., multislice CT) currently allow acquisition of typically 4 but up to 16 simultaneous images 2.5 mm thick.

Improvements in gantry rotation speeds and the development of partial reconstruction algorithms have reduced effective single-image acquisition time to <300 ms. However, image acquisition within 50 msec is required to completely avoid cardiac motion artifacts.[1–2] The coronary arteries also move independently throughout the cardiac cycle and even at slow heart rates (i.e., <70 beats per minute) exhibit significant translational motion of up to 60 mm/s for the right coronary artery and 20 to 40 mm/s for the left anterior descending and circumflex coronary arteries[2–3] (Fig. 20-1).

In order to potentially compensate for image blur, retrospective and prospective gating can be performed with either spiral or nonspiral CT using single or multirow detector arrays. Retrospective gating with spiral CT employs acquisition of multiple images throughout each cardiac cycle. With multidetector spiral systems, temporal resolution may be further improved by selecting specific partial image sector data from different heart beats and detector rings so as to reconstruct a complete 240-degree image data set. With retrospective gating, several hundred images can be acquired during a single cardiac study, allowing one to "pick and choose" images with the least amount of motion-related distortion prior to final image reconstruction. However, this oversampling leads to significant and unnecessary excess radiation exposure to the patient. The typical radiation exposure from an EBCT study is <1.0 rad,[4] whereas multidetector CT scanners using retrospective gating can increase exposure about 13-fold.[5] Prospective gating during either spiral or nonspiral acquisitions employs image triggering only at a specific

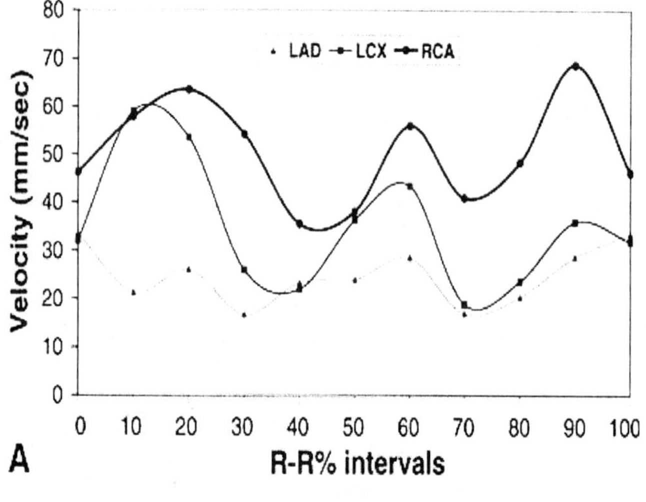


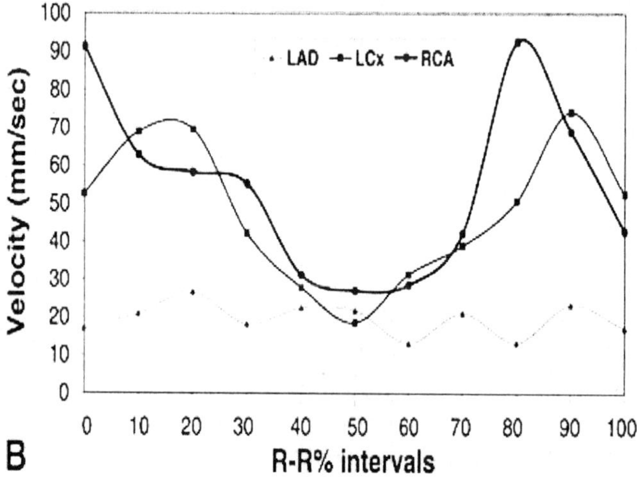


FIGURE 20-1 Coronary artery velocity varies substantially throughout the cardiac cycle, depending on whether the heart rate is relatively slow (*A*, 72 bpm) or fast (*B*, 89 bpm). The greatest motion occurs in the right coronary artery (RCA), followed by the left circumflex (LCx) and left anterior descending (LAD) coronary arteries. In (*A*), a biphasic pattern of rest is found during end-systole (at 40 to 50 percent of the RR interval) and middiastole (at 70 to 80 percent of the RR interval). In (*B*), a monophasic rest period pattern was found near end systole (at 40 to 60 percent of the RR interval). (From Lu, et al.[2] Reproduced with permission from the publisher and the authors.)

temporal location of the cardiac cycle, thereby significantly reducing radiation exposure. Gating works relatively well at slow heart rates (i.e., <60 beats per minute), where the R to R interval is >1000 ms and the fastest imaging protocols are utilized. However, at faster heart rates, a 300- to 500-ms acquisition effectively covers most of the cardiac cycle, thus obviating any potential benefit from gating the image acquisition.

## EBCT

EBCT utilizes an electron beam (current 630 mA, voltage 130 kV), which is deflected via a magnetic coil and focused to strike a series of four tungsten targets located beneath the patient (Fig. 20-2). The electron beam is magnetically swept along the tungsten targets at a 210-degree arc, and each target ring is separated by a 4-mm distance. The resultant x-rays generated beneath the patient are then attenuated as they pass through the thorax and recorded by a series of two twin fixed detector arrays arranged in a semicircle above the patient. Since EBCT has no moving parts, as found in conventional and spiral CT scanners, imaging time is complete within 50 ms, which is the time required for the electron beam to sweep along the tungsten targets. With a 100-ms acquisition time, a freeze-frame image of the myocardium and coronary arteries in end-diastole can be achieved with little if any motion blur.

EBCT is commonly operated using three different acquisition modes. The cine mode creates real-time cross-sectional views of the beating heart and is commonly used to assess both global and regional right and left ventricular function (Fig. 20-3). The volume mode allows acquisition of a single image with each preselected movement of the patient couch. Up to 40 continuous slices can be obtained scanning 12 to 32 cm of anatomy, depending on the couch speed selected (Fig. 20-4). This imaging mode is commonly gated to the ECG to obtain high-resolution static images for detailed evaluation of cardiovascular anatomy, such as coronary artery calcification. The triggered (flow) mode is used to assess blood flow through specific cardiac chambers and the myocardium itself. This mode allows acquisition of some 20 to 40 consecutive scans where imaging occurs at a designated time during each cardiac cycle. From these consecutive scans, time-density curves can be constructed, which can estimate blood flow through specific cardiac chambers and within the myocardium.

## EVALUATION OF MYOCARDIAL STRUCTURE AND FUNCTION

Both the left and right ventricles are well visualized by mechanical CT and EBCT, allowing excellent spatial separation between the two structures. Delineation of the epicardial and endocardial surfaces allows accurate and reproducible measurement of left and right ventricular wall thickness and myocardial mass.[6–8] Left ventricular hypertrophy can be quantified and serially assessed. Right ventricular dysplasia is accurately diagnosed based on the characteristic EBCT findings of an enlarged right ventricle, with a scalloped appearance, trabeculations with low attenuation characteristics, and abundant epicardial adipose tissue.[9]

EBCT can assess left and right ventricular hemodynamics[10] as well as regional myocardial wall motion and thickening.[11–13] The cine mode is used to acquire multiple gated images of the right and left ventricles during maximal contrast enhancement of the cavities.[12–13] This affords accurate and reproducible quantification of left and right ventricular end-diastolic and end-systolic volumes and ejection fraction.[10,12] EBCT is comparable to first-pass radionuclide angiography for the calculation of left ventricular ejection fraction (LVEF) in patients with myocardial infarction[14] (Fig. 20-5). Serial changes in right and left ventricular volumes and diastolic parameters are well defined in patients following acute myocardial infarction.[15–17] Ventricular remodeling can be assessed by using EBCT in a similar fashion to gated blood-pool radionuclide angiography[18,19] and echocardiography.[20] Cine EBCT can identify wall thinning and impaired LV thickening in an area of previous myocardial infarction[21] and delineate the presence of anterior and posterior LV aneurysms and associated mural thrombus[22–23] (Fig. 20-6).

Stress-rest EBCT imaging can detect underlying ischemic heart disease based on changes in global LVEF and regional wall motion. One small study compared semisupine bicycle exercise contrast-enhanced EBCT to technetium-99m ($^{99m}$Tc) single photon emission computed tomography (SPECT) of the myocardium in patients with suspected coronary artery disease (CAD), all of whom underwent angiography.[12] An abnormal EBCT study was defined as a <5 percent increase in LVEF during exercise. Regional LVEF was assessed by computer analysis of end-diastolic and end-systolic images. The sensitivity and specificity of exercise EBCT for detecting CAD were 81 and 76 percent, respectively, when the global LVEF criteria for abnormalcy were used, but these percentages improved to 88 and 100 percent when regional wall motion abnormalities were considered. EBCT was as accurate as $^{99m}$Tc SPECT in the diagnosis of CAD.

Although echocardiography is generally used to assess valvular heart disease, EBCT is an alternative modality in patients with poor acoustic windows. In patients with mitral or aortic regurgitation, EBCT can accurately determine left and right ventricular stroke volumes and thereby calculate valvular regurgitant fractions.[10,24] When possible need for valvular surgery is being considered, EBCT can delineate the important parameters of LV chamber size, wall thickness, and LVEF. As with gated blood-pool radionuclide angiography, EBCT cannot distinguish mitral from aortic regurgitation and cannot calculate the regurgitant fraction if significant right-sided valvular insufficiency is present. A complication of mitral valve disease is the development of left atrial thrombi. One study showed greater accuracy of EBCT as compared to transthoracic echocardiography in demonstrating such thrombi[25] (Fig. 20-7). Whether EBCT can detect thrombi as well as transesophageal echocardiography remains to be determined.

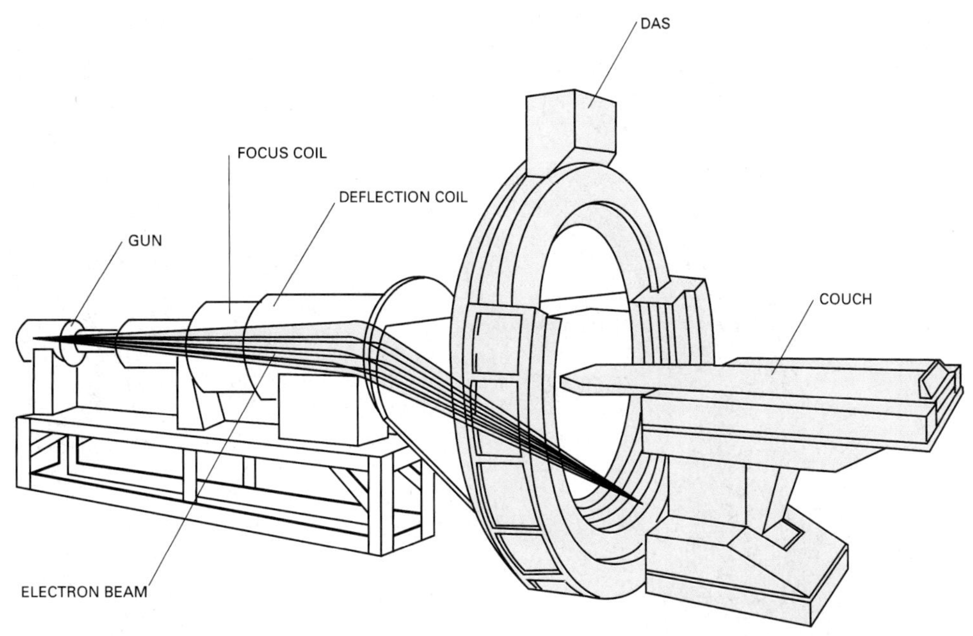


FIGURE 20-2 Diagram of the EBCT scanner. The electron beam is emitted from the electron gun and focused onto the tungsten targets by the magnetic deflection coil. DAS = immediate memory.

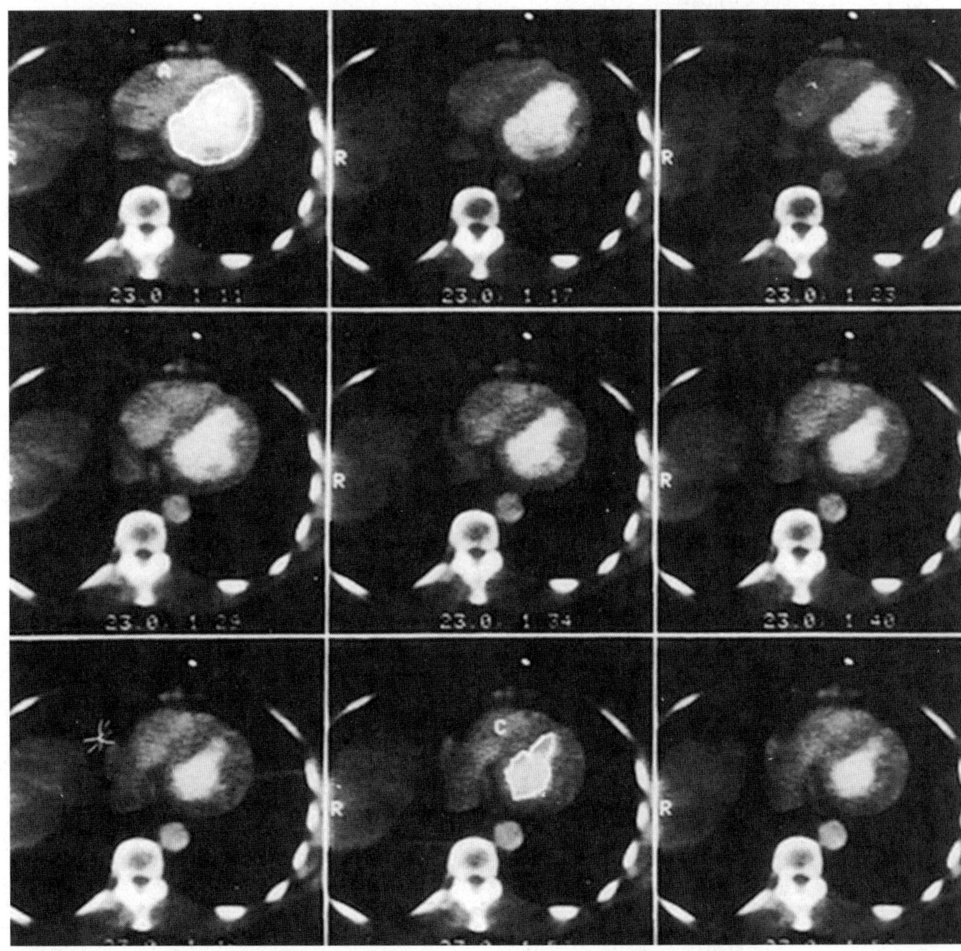

FIGURE 20-3 An 8-mm-thick CT slice of the mid–left ventricle imaged for one complete cardiac cycle at 58-ms intervals. A = end-diastole; C = end-systole.

## EVALUATION OF CORONARY ARTERY DISEASE

### Detection of Coronary Artery Calcification

The standard EBCT imaging protocol is to acquire 40 consecutive 3-mm-thick images at a rate of 100 ms per image from the base of the heart to just below the carina. Images are obtained at end-inspiration, with ECG triggering typically at 80 percent of the RR interval (end-diastole). Image pixel size using a 512 × 512 reconstruction matrix is 0.26 or 0.34 mm$^2$ based on a 26- or 30-cm field of vision, respectively.

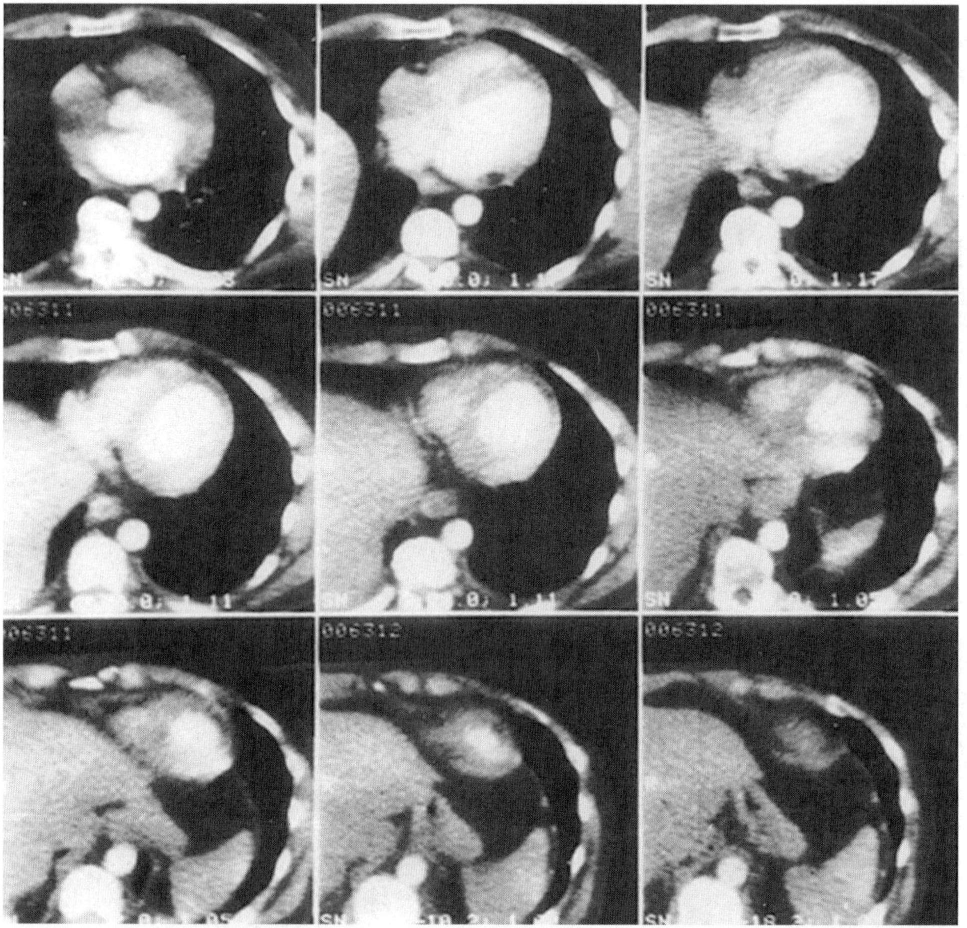

FIGURE 20-4 Fifty-millisecond contrast-enhanced EBCT images gated to end-diastole include the left ventricle from base (*top left*) to apex (*bottom right*). (From Brundage BH, Chomka E. Evaluation of acute myocardial infarction by computed tomography. In: Brundage BH, ed. *Comparative Cardiac Imaging*. Rockville, MD: Aspen; 1990:223–229. Reproduced with permission from the publisher and the authors.)

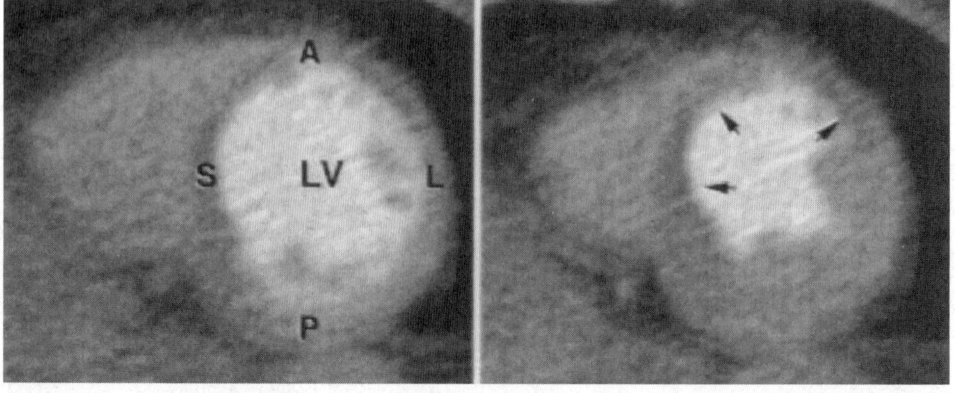


FIGURE 20-5 EBCT image of a mid–left ventricular (LV) slice in diastole (left) and systole (right), with an area of anteroseptal dyskinesis (*arrows*). The LVEF by EBCT was 37 versus 39 percent by first-pass radionuclide angiography. A = anterior; L = lateral; P = posterior; S = septal LV wall. (From Gerber TC, Behrenbeck T, Allison T, Mullan BP, Rumberger JA, Gibbons RJ. Comparison of measurement of left ventricular ejection fraction by Tc-99m sestamibi first-pass angiography with electron beam computed tomography in patients with anterior wall acute myocardial infarction. *Am J Cardiol* 1999;83:1022–1026. Reproduced with permission from the publisher and authors.)

A calcified lesion is generally defined as either two or three adjacent pixels (0.68 to 1.02 $mm^2$ for a $512^2$ reconstruction matrix and camera field size of 30 cm) of >130 Hounsfield units (HU). Using the traditional Agatston method, each calcified lesion is multiplied by a density factor as follows: 1 for lesions with a maximal density between 130 and 199 HU; 2 for lesions between 200 and 299 HU; 3 for lesions between 300 and 399 HU; and 4 for lesions >400 HU. The total coronary artery calcium score (CACS) is calculated as the sum of each calcified lesion in the four main coronary arteries over all the consecutive tomographic slices (Fig. 20-8). The EBCT-derived CACS correlates well with calcified areas found in individual coronary arteries as determined by histomorphometric measurements ($r = 0.96$, $p < 0.0001$)[26] (Fig. 20-9). No such comparative data are available using conventional or spiral mechanical CT.

Mechanical CT imaging protocols vary widely among different camera systems and manufacturers. Generally 40 consecutive 2.5- to 3-mm-thick images are acquired per cardiac study. Calcified lesions are defined as two or three adjacent pixels with a tomographic density of either >90 or >130 HU. Effective pixel size for a reconstruction matrix of 512 × 512 pixels with a common field of view of 26 cm is 0.26 $mm^2$. Calcium scoring is based on either the traditional Agatston method (i.e., initial density of >130 HU) or a modified system beginning at the 90-HU threshold. As with EBCT scoring, the total CACS is calculated as the sum of each calcified plaque over all the tomographic slices.

## Mechanical versus Electron Beam CT

The comparability of mechanical CT- and EBCT-derived coronary artery calcium scores has been explored in seven separate studies involving approximately 400 patients.[27–33] The mechanical CT protocols vary considerably in these studies, ranging from conventional CT to single-slice spiral CT (with either retrospective or prospective gating) to multislice CT (Table 20-1). EBCT imaging was performed using the standard protocol conventionally used in routine clinical

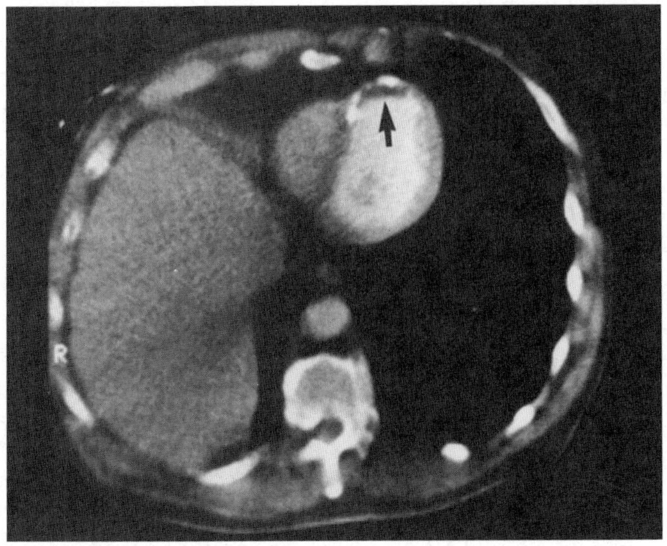

FIGURE 20-6 A single frame from a contrast-enhanced cine CT demonstrates thrombus in a left ventricular aneurysm. Also note that the wall of the aneurysm is calcified.

practice. Coronary calcification was defined as >130 HU for EBCT but varied from 90 to 130 HU for mechanical CT. Although high correlation coefficients were reported between EBCT and mechanical CT CACS, there was significant variability in individual CACS results (range 17 to 84 percent) (Table 20-1).

In the study by Goldin et al., EBCT showed significantly less interobserver variability for measuring calcium (4.5 percent) than spiral CT at either the 90 (46.8 percent) or 130 (41.5 percent) HU cutoff ($p < 0.001$). A 28 percent difference was noted in EBCT versus spi-

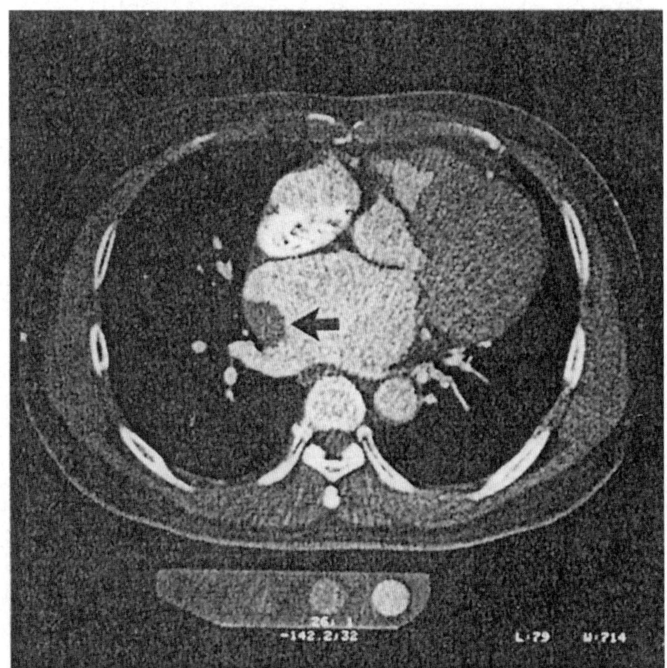

FIGURE 20-7 A left atrial thrombus (*arrow*) anterior to the right superior pulmonary vein is well described in this contrast-enhanced EBCT scan. The transthoracic echocardiogram did not detect any left atrial thrombus.

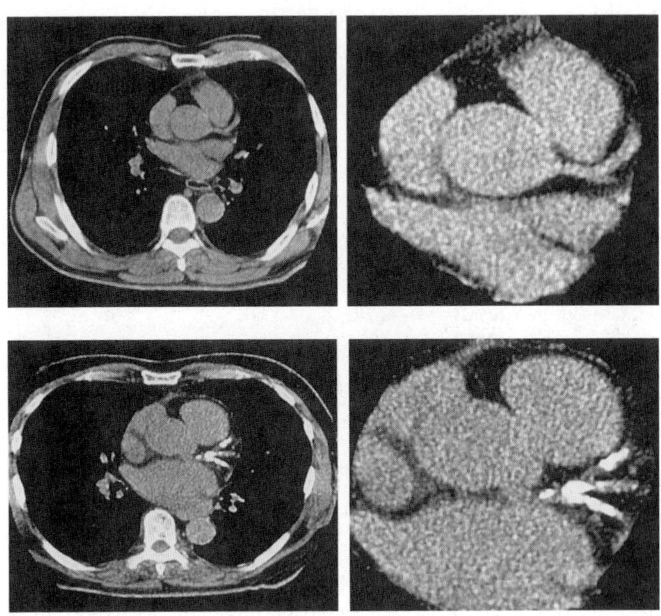

FIGURE 20-8 Single-level noncontrast EBCT scan of a normal subject (*left*) and an individual with severe coronary artery calcification (*right*). Calcium is shown as intensely white areas within the coronary arteries.

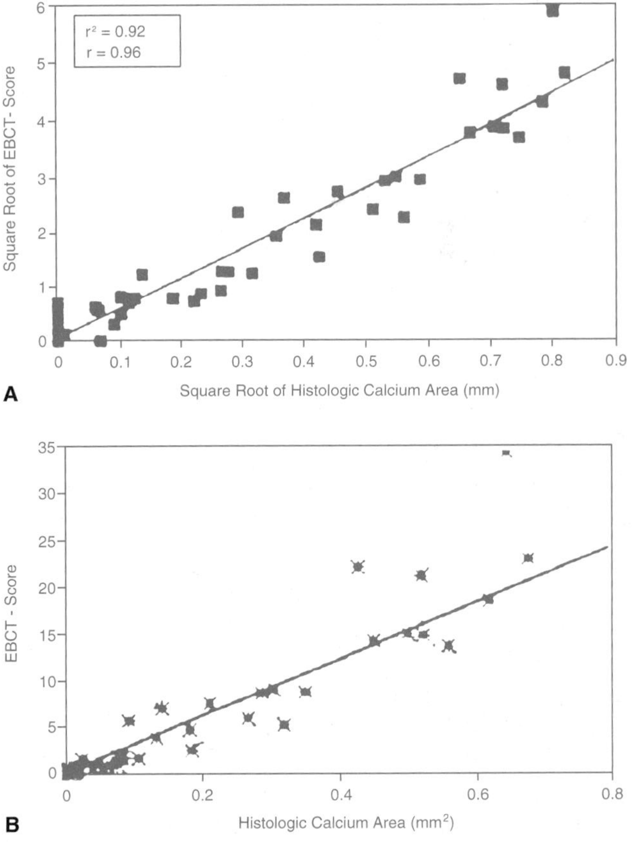


FIGURE 20-9 Linear regression comparing the EBCT CACS [square root transformation (A) and actual data (B)] versus the calcium area measured at histomorphometric examination. There is an apparent high-positive correlation between the EBCT calcium score and histomorphometric calcium area ($r^2 = .92$, $r = .96$; $p < 0.0001$). (From Mautner et al.[26] Reproduced with permission from the publisher and authors.)

TABLE 20-1 EBCT vs. Mechanical CT[a]

| Author | Year | Number of Patients | Age | Average $Ca^{2+}$ Score | Mechanical CT Technique | Gating | Number of Detectors | Correlation Coefficient | Mean % Difference |
|---|---|---|---|---|---|---|---|---|---|
| Becker,[27] | 1999 | 50 | 61 | 983 | Nonspiral | No | Single | 0.98 | 42% |
| Budoff,[28] | 2001 | 33 | 54 | 52 | Nonspiral | No | Single | 0.68 | 84% |
| Becker,[29] | 2000 | 50 | 62 | — | Nonspiral | Prosp | Single | 0.98 | 25% |
| Carr,[30] | 2000 | 36 | 68 | 432 | Spiral | Retrosp | Single | 0.96 | 17% |
| Goldin,[31] | 2001 | 70 | 48 | 70 | Spiral | Retrosp | Single | NA | 28% |
| Becker,[32] | 2001 | 88 | 63 | 793 | Spiral | Prosp | 4 | 0.99 | 32% |
| Knez,[33b] | 2002 | 99 | 60 | 722 | Spiral | Prosp | 4 | 0.99 | 17% |

[a]Agatston score except as indicated.
[b]Volumetric score.
ABBREVIATIONS: $Ca^{2+}$ = calcium; CT = computed tomography; prosp = prospective; retrosp = retrospective.

ral CT CACS results.[31] These authors further compared concordance between EBCT and spiral CT based on clinically accepted CACS risk categories: very low (CACS 0); low (CACS 1 to 10); moderate (CACS 11 to 100); moderately high (CACS 101 to 400); and high (CACS >400). Concordance in risk category between these two imaging modalities using either the 90- or 130-HU cutoff was only 73 and 76 percent, respectively. The 90-HU cutoff overestimated risk, whereas the 130-HU cutoff underestimated risk by mechanical CT as compared to EBCT. A more recent study by Knez et al. compared multislice spiral CT to EBCT using prospective ECG gating for both techniques.[33] The CACS was calculated using the volumetric (rather than the Agatston) calcium scoring method. Variability in CACS between the two techniques ranged from 20 percent (CACS <100) to 15 percent (CACS >100), with a mean variability of 17 percent. These results are encouraging and indicate that multislice mechanical CT may be more comparable to EBCT than either conventional or single-slice spiral CT. Further research is still needed to determine which mechanical CT technique, imaging protocol, calcium criterion, and scoring system best approximates the values determined by EBCT. A standardized and validated mechanical CT imaging protocol is required before this technique can be accepted for routine clinical use.

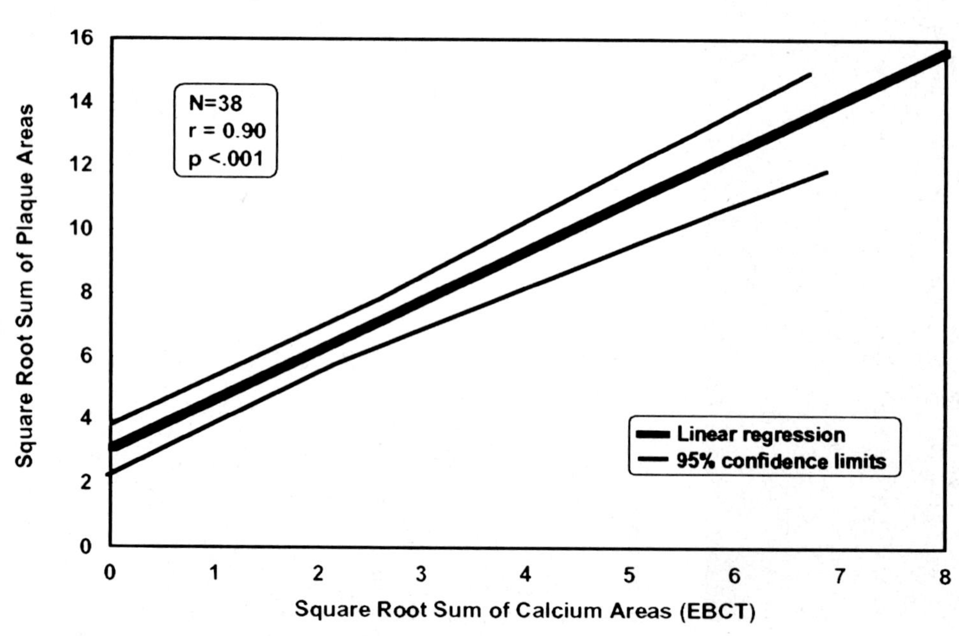


FIGURE 20-10 Comparison of the square root sum of total coronary calcium area (mm) by EBCT to actual atherosclerotic plaque area (mm) for 38 individual coronary arteries. The linear regression line and 95 percent confidence intervals are shown. (From Rumberger et al.[34] Reproduced with permission from the publisher and authors.)

## Coronary Artery Calcification and Atherosclerotic Plaque Burden

The presence of coronary artery calcification is clearly indicative of coronary atherosclerosis.[34–35] Furthermore, the CACS severity, as assessed by EBCT, is directly related to the total atherosclerotic plaque burden present in the epicardial coronary arteries.[34–35] Coronary calcification is thought to begin early in life, but it progresses more rapidly in older individuals who have further advanced atherosclerotic lesions.[36] Calcification is an active, organized, and regulated process occurring during atherosclerotic plaque development where calcium phosphate in the form of hydroxyapatite precipitates in atherosclerotic coronary arteries in a similar fashion as observed in bone mineralization.[37–39] Although lack of calcification does not categorically exclude the presence of atherosclerotic plaque, calcification occurs exclusively in atherosclerotic arteries and is not found in normal coronary arteries.

The presence and extent of histologically determined plaque area has been compared to the total calcium area as assessed by EBCT in individual coronary arteries derived from autopsied hearts.[34] A strong linear correlation exists between total coronary artery plaque area and the extent of coronary artery calcification as found in individual hearts ($r$ = 0.93, $p < 0.001$) and in individual coronary arteries ($r$ = 0.90, $p < 0.001$) (Fig. 20-10). However, the total calcium area underestimates total plaque area, with approximately five times as many noncalcified as calcified plaques.[34]

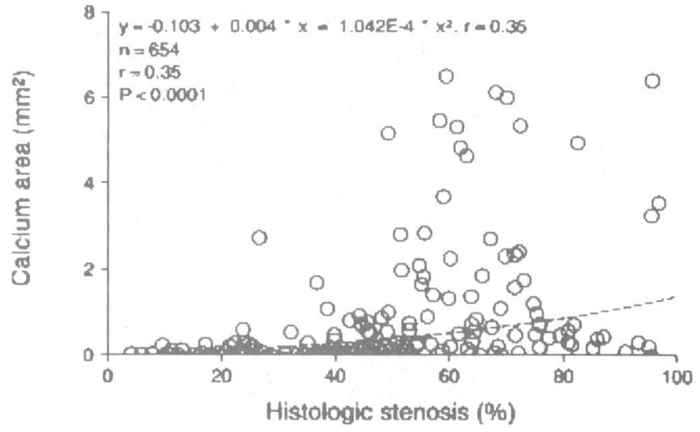


FIGURE 20-11 Graph showing the polynomial regression analysis of coronary calcium area (mm$^2$) versus percent histologic stenosis for 654 coronary artery segments with calcium >0 mm$^2$. (From Sangiorgi et al.[35] Reproduced with permission from the publisher and authors.)

## Coronary Artery Calcification and Stenosis Severity

Significant (>50 percent) coronary artery stenosis by angiography is almost universally associated with the presence of coronary artery calcium as assessed by EBCT. However, the severity of angiographic coronary artery stenosis is not directly related to the total CACS. A recent study compared calcium extent to coronary artery luminal diameter stenosis determined by morphologic examination of 723 coronary artery segments.[35] Although coronary stenosis severity increased with increasing coronary artery calcification, this relationship was poor and could not be used to estimate angiographic stenosis severity on a segment-by-segment basis (Fig. 20-11). One explanation is that coronary artery remodeling occurs with increasing plaque burden so as to increase luminal diameter and maintain arterial patency.[40,41] Although the extent of coronary calcification does not precisely predict stenosis severity, noncalcified plaques are almost universally associated with <50 percent diameter stenosis and typically <20 percent stenosis.[35] These data indicate that lack of coronary calcification predicts a very low likelihood of obstructive CAD.

Clinical angiographic trials confirm the relationship between CACS severity and the presence of significant (≥50 percent) CAD.[42–56] Although the diagnostic accuracy of EBCT improves with age, most younger patients (<50 years) with obstructive CAD also have coronary calcification (85 percent).[48,50] To date there are 15 studies evaluating EBCT with coronary angiography where obstructive CAD was defined as >50 percent luminal diameter stenosis[42–56] (Table 20-2). In these studies, the overall sensitivity and specificity for detecting obstructive CAD were 97 and 39 percent, respectively. In the largest series, Haberl et al. performed EBCT within 30 days of coronary angiography in 1764 patients who had suspected CAD.[56] Only 5 of 940 patients (0.5 percent) with significant (≥50 percent) coronary artery stenosis had a normal EBCT. Although differences in CACS were noted among men and women, EBCT predicted CAD equally well in both genders, based on age-specific CACS thresholds[56] (Fig. 20-12). EBCT may also be useful for detecting CAD in heart transplant recipients.[57]

The poor specificity of EBCT can be reconciled by the fact that the presence of coronary calcification confirms the presence of atherosclerotic plaque which may not necessarily be obstructive in nature (Fig. 20-13). The CACS severity may be a better barometer of obstructive CAD than the mere presence of calcium. Budoff et al. observed that specificity increased with the number of calcified coronary arteries (i.e., high calcium scores).[48] Two separate reports in patients referred for coronary angiography found that a CACS > 100 best predicted obstructive CAD with an equally high sensitivity and specificity of 80 percent.[58–59] There appears to be a threshold CACS above which most patients will have significant coronary artery stenosis. The accuracy for identifying significant CAD based on CACS may be further improved by incorporating age, gender,[54,56,60] and traditional risk-factor information[59,61] (Fig. 20-14). However, despite the relationship between obstructive CAD and CACS severity, the latter is still too imprecise in itself to be used as a definitive criterion for proceeding directly to coronary angiography. The current American College of Cardiology/American Heart Association (ACC/AHA) guidelines on coronary angiography do not recommend coronary angiography on the basis of a positive EBCT.

## Coronary Artery Calcification and Myocardial Ischemia

A recent trial explored the complementary role of EBCT and myocardial perfusion SPECT for identifying both subclinical CAD and silent myocardial ischemia in a generally asymptomatic population who had risk factors for CAD development.[62] The purpose of this study was to identify (1) patients with subclinical CAD who might benefit from aggressive risk factor modification and (2) those who are at relatively higher short-term risk for cardiac events based

TABLE 20-2 Accuracy of EBCT Coronary Artery Calcification in Detecting Significant (>50%) Coronary Artery Stenosis as Defined by Angiography

| Investigator | Year | Number of Subjects | Sensitivity (%) | Specificity (%) | Positive Predictive Accuracy | Negative Predictive Accuracy |
|---|---|---|---|---|---|---|
| Agatston,[42] | 1990 | 584 | 96 | 51 | 31 | 98 |
| Breen,[43] | 1992 | 100 | 100 | 47 | 63 | 100 |
| Bielak,[44] | 1994 | 160 | 96 | 45 | 57 | 93 |
| Kaufman,[45] | 1995 | 160 | 93 | 67 | 81 | 86 |
| Rumberger,[46] | 1995 | 139 | 98 | 39 | 59 | 97 |
| Braun,[47] | 1996 | 102 | 93 | 73 | 93 | 73 |
| Budoff,[48] | 1996 | 710 | 95 | 44 | 72 | 84 |
| Detrano,[49] | 1996 | 491 | 95 | 31 | 51 | 89 |
| Fallavollita,[50] | 1996 | 106 | 85 | 45 | 66 | 70 |
| Baumgart,[51] | 1997 | 57 | 97 | 21 | 56 | 86 |
| Schmermund,[52] | 1997 | 118 | 95 | 88 | 99 | 58 |
| Kennedy,[53] | 1998 | 368 | 96 | 31 | 51 | 90 |
| Bielak,[54] | 2000 | 213 | 99 | 39 | 64 | 98 |
| Shavelle,[55] | 2000 | 97 | 96 | 47 | 80 | 82 |
| Haberl,[56] | 2001 | 1764 | 99 | 30 | 62 | 98 |
| Total | | 5169 | 97 | 39 | 61 | 92 |

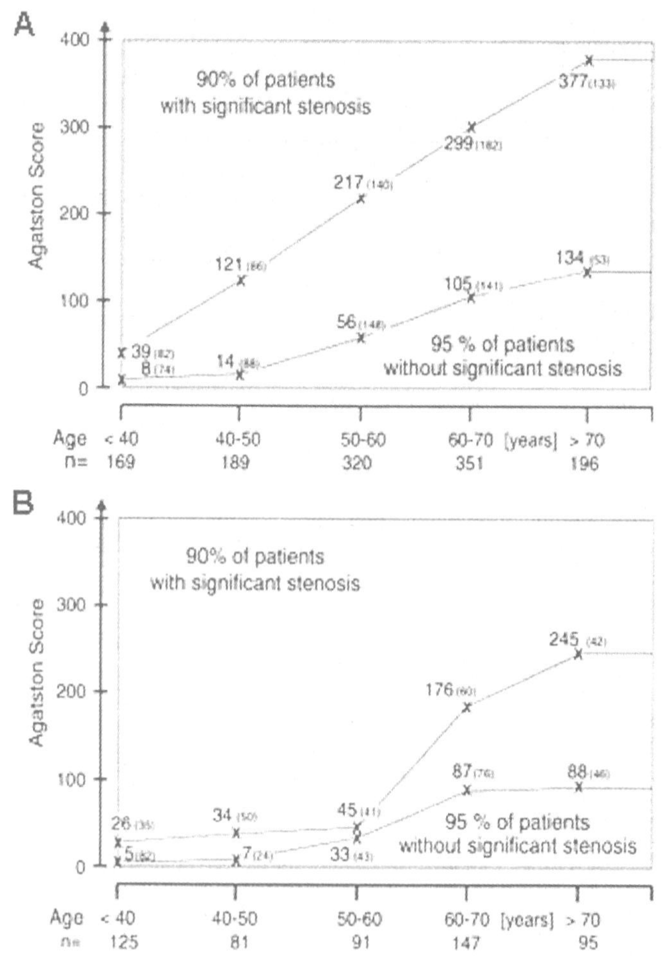


FIGURE 20-12 Diagnostic yield of calcium screening in symptomatic men (*A*) and women (*B*). The lower scores define the calcium score thresholds for the 95 percent of patients without significant stenoses. The higher scores give the calcium score thresholds for the 90 percent of patients with significant stenoses. Within the central area the diagnosis is uncertain. The numbers in parentheses give the number of patients within the area. For example, a man at the age of 50 years is probably free of coronary stenosis if his score is <56. At score values ≥217, he bears a high risk of stenosis. (From Haberl et al.[56] Reproduced with permission from the publisher and the authors.)

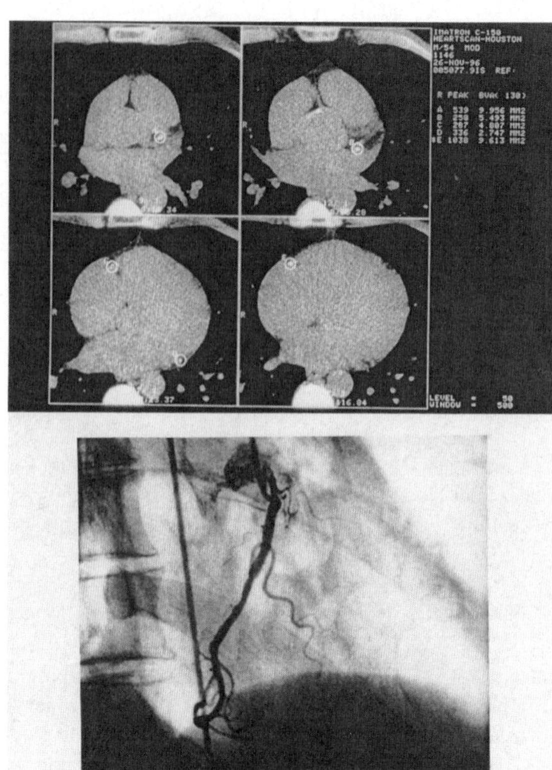

FIGURE 20-13 Four noncontrast EBCT images of a patient demonstrating calcification in all 3 major coronary arteries (*left*). Circles define regions of coronary calcification. The total CACS is moderate at 271 and highest in the right coronary artery. (176). Coronary arteriogram demonstrates a nonobstructive plaque in the mid–right coronary artery (*right*). The left anterior descending and circumflex coronary arteries were normal. The patient also had a normal exercise myocardial perfusion scan.

on the presence of silent myocardial ischemia. Among the 3895 subjects who had EBCT, 411 also underwent stress SPECT within a close temporal period (median 17 days). The mean CACS was significantly higher in the 81 subjects (20 percent) who had an abnormal (1065 ± 983) as compared to a normal (286 ± 394, $p < 0.00001$) SPECT. The likelihood of an abnormal SPECT increased dramatically with the total CACS (Fig. 20-15). Whereas only 1 percent of subjects with a total CACS <100 had an abnormal SPECT, this was observed in 46 percent of those with scores ≥400. Only 10 percent of all 3895 subjects scanned with EBCT had a CACS ≥400. Large ischemic perfusion defects were virtually confined to subjects who had a CACS score of 400 or higher. Patients with large ischemic perfusion defects by SPECT are known to be at high risk for subsequent cardiac events; whereas patients with small perfusion defects or those with normal scans, have an exceedingly low cardiac event rate.[63–68] Although a similar percentage of subjects had an abnormal SPECT (16.1 percent) or stress ECG (17.5 percent, $p =$ NS) only the former was related to the total CACS (Fig. 20-16), further illustrating the poor predictive accuracy of treadmill testing for detecting CAD in asymptomatic subjects.

Miranda et al. recently confirmed these findings in 233 consecutive asymptomatic patients who had EBCT and SPECT. No patients with a CACS <100 had an abnormal SPECT, whereas 4.1 percent with a moderate (101 to 400) CACS and 15 percent with a CACS ≥400 had an abnormal SPECT. The best CACS cutoff for predicting an abnormal SPECT in this study was also 400.[69]

## Coronary Artery Calcification: Prognostic Implications

The likelihood of plaque rupture and the development of acute cardiovascular events is related to the total atherosclerotic plaque burden.[70–72] Although controversy exists as to whether calcified or noncalcified plaques are more prone to rupture,[73–74] extensive calcification indicates the presence of both plaque morphologies.[34–35] Since there is a direct relationship between the CACS severity, the extent of atherosclerotic plaque, and the presence of silent myocardial ischemia, the calcium score should predict risk for subsequent cardiovascular events among otherwise heterogeneous patient populations with cardiac risk factors. Many studies have now demonstrated an increased risk for cardiac events in asymptomatic patients who have extensive silent myocardial ischemia.[63,64,75–77] In this regard, the CACS could be useful for risk assessment of asymptomatic individuals and potentially guide therapeutics.

Several recent trials in both symptomatic[78,79] and asymptomatic [80–87] patients have studied whether the extent of coronary artery calcification as assessed by EBCT can predict subsequent patient outcome. Detrano et al. followed 422 symptomatic patients for 30 ± 12 months following EBCT and coronary angiography.[78] Cardiac events were 10-fold higher in patients with a CACS above the 75th percentile for age (9.5 percent) versus those below the 25th percentile (0.9 percent). Patients with a CACS >100 had a significantly lower infarct-free survival than those with lower scores ($p$ = 0.009). Keelan et al. studied 288 symptomatic patients referred for coronary angiography.[79] Patients with a CACS >100 had a 3.2-fold higher relative risk of death or myocardial infarction than those with a lower CACS (95 percent confidence limit: 1.17 to 8.71). Patient age and the CACS were the only independent predictors of these hard cardiac events.

In an early series by Secci et al., 324 initially asymptomatic subjects were followed for 32 ± 4 months.[80] Eleven patients died or had a nonfatal myocardial infarction (3.3 percent) and an additional 12 patients (3.7 percent) underwent coronary revascularization. A threefold higher event rate was observed in patients in the highest quartile of CACS (>506). In another report from the same group, 1196 asymptomatic patients were followed for 41 ± 5 months after undergoing EBCT.[81] Subjects with a CACS >44 (median value in this trial) were 2.3 times more likely to suffer myocardial infarction or cardiovascular death than subjects with lower scores. Patients were enrolled only if they had >10 percent risk for developing cardiovascular events over an 8-year period as determined by the Framingham risk model. In this group at relatively high pretest clinical risk for cardiovascular events, the CACS results did not add to the Framingham risk model for predicting patient outcome.

Arad et al. followed 1173 asymptomatic patients for 19 months after an initial screening EBCT.[82] During follow-up, 18 patients (1.53 percent) had 26 cardiac events, including one death, 7 nonfatal myocardial infarctions, and 17 coronary revascularization procedures. No events occurred in patients with a normal study and the negative

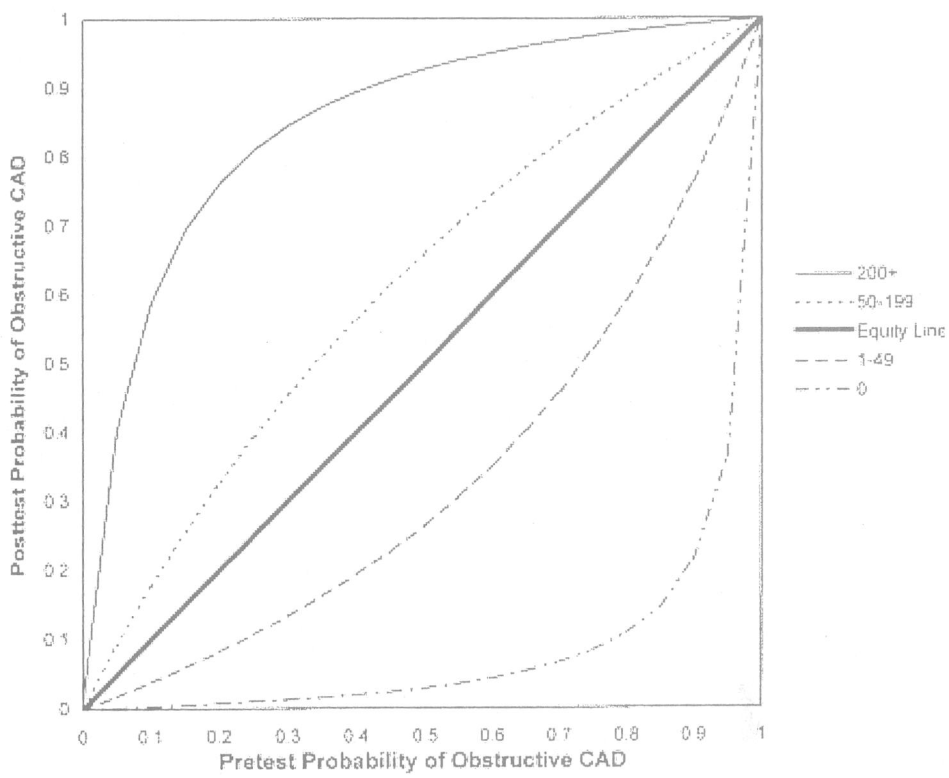


FIGURE 20-14 Influence of calcium score on probability of obstructive CAD as a function of pretest probability and stratum-specific likelihood ratio among men ≥50 years old. (From Bielak et al.[54] Reproduced with permission from the publisher and the authors.)

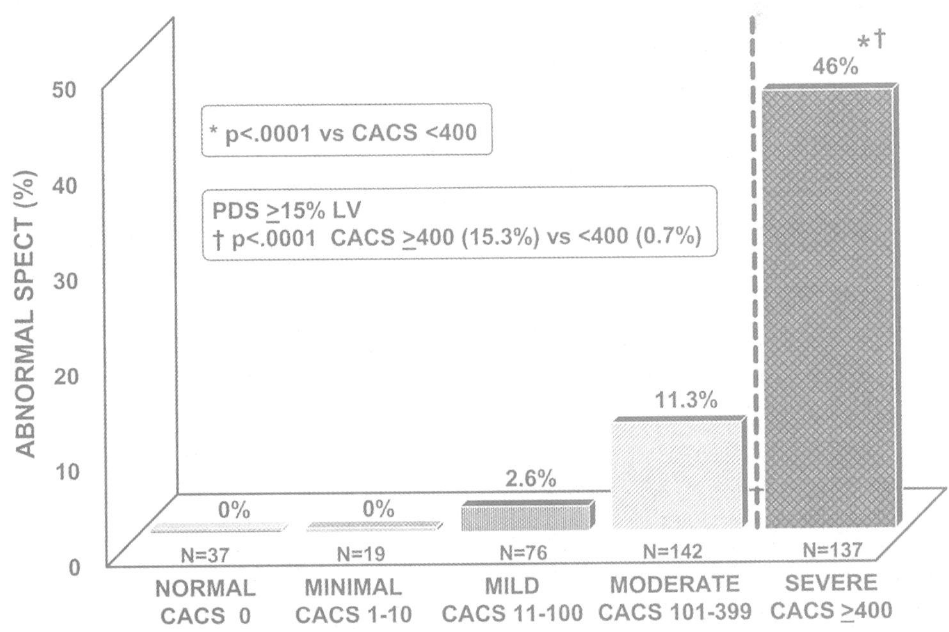


FIGURE 20-15 Single photon emission computed tomography (SPECT) results based on total coronary artery calcium score (CACS). Few subjects with CACS <400 had abnormal SPECT (6.6 percent), and most (99.3 percent) had only a small (<15 percent) perfusion defect size (PDS). LV indicates left ventricle. (From He et al.[62] Reproduced with permission from the publisher and authors.)

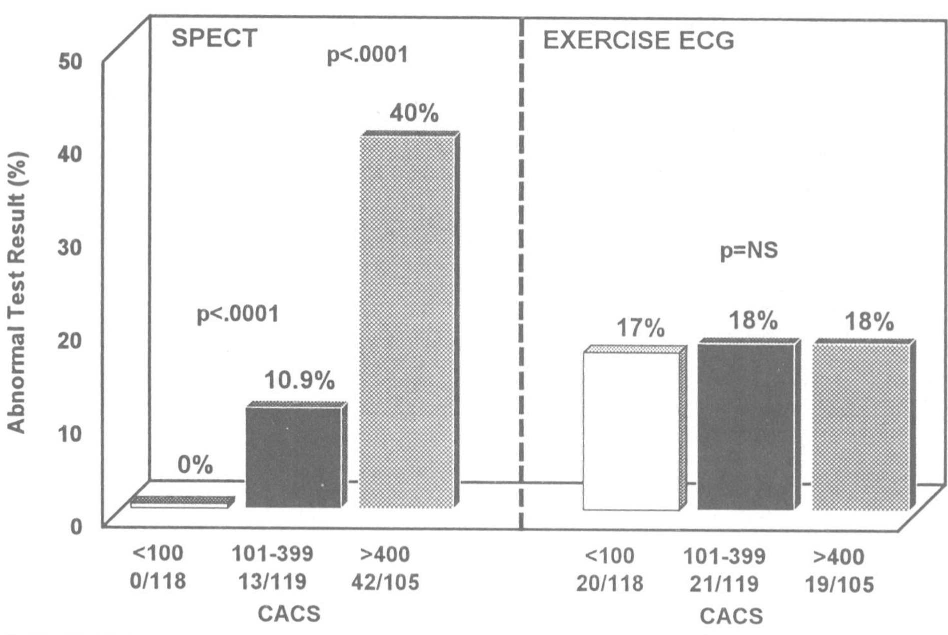


FIGURE 20-16 Exercise SPECT and ECG results based on total CACS. Same abbreviations as in Fig. 20-15. (From He et al.[62] Reproduced with permission from the publisher and authors.)

predictive value was 99.8 percent in patients with a CACS <100. However, the cardiac event rate progressively increased as the CACS increased from >100 (5.5 percent) to 160 (7.1 percent), to >680 (14 percent). These results have now been extended to 3.6 years with a 5, 7, and 13 percent hard cardiac event rate in individuals with a CACS ≥80, ≥160 and ≥600, respectively.[83] Subjects with a CACS ≥80 had a 22-fold higher risk of death or myocardial infarction than those with lower scores (95 percent CI 5.1 to 77.4). The total event rate was 10.9 percent among individuals in the highest (>75th) percentile of CACS (i.e., >97) versus 0.8 percent for those below this threshold. Multivariate analysis identified patient age, hypertension, diabetes, and hyperlipidemia as significant clinical risk predictors. The CACS remained the best single predictor of risk after adjustment for these variables (Table 20-3). Wong et al. also showed that the CACS severity predicted subsequent events independent of age, gender, and patient risk-factor profile[84] (Fig. 20-17).

Raggi et al. reported on 172 patients who had EBCT within 60 days of an unheralded myocardial infarction and on 632 asymptomatic patients who were referred for a screening EBCT and then followed for 32 ± 7 months.[85] Ninety-six percent of all patients with infarction were abnormal by EBCT, and the CACS was ≥100 in 62 percent and ≥400 in 47 percent of patients. In the cohort of 632 asymptomatic patients, both the absolute CACS and the relative CACS percentiles adjusted for age and gender predicted subsequent death and nonfatal myocardial infarction. The relative CACS percentiles for age and gender are now well defined from EBCT results in over 58,000 patients.[86] Hard cardiac events occurred in only 0.3 percent of subjects with a normal EBCT, but this increased to 13 percent in those with a CACS >400. Likewise, in patients in the lower 50th percentile for CACS severity based on age and gender, the total cardiac event rate was only 1.1 percent, as compared to 8.2 percent in those with a CACS greater than the 50th percentile (Table 20-4). A very high CACS ≥1000 may portend a particularly high risk of death or myocardial infarction (i.e., 25 percent per year).[87]

In the largest observational trial to date, Callister et al. reported all-cause mortality among 10,377 asymptomatic patients (4191 women and 6186 men) who had a baseline EBCT and were then followed for 5.0 ± 3.5 years.[88] Most subjects had cardiac risk factors including a family history of CAD (69 percent), hyperlipidemia (62 percent), hypertension (44 percent), and current cigarette smoking (40 percent). Risk-adjusted survival models were developed incorporating all traditional risk factors for CAD development and the CACS. The CACS was a strong independent predictor of mortality ($\chi^2 = 36.6$, $p < 0.00001$) with 43 percent additional predictive value contained within the CACS be-

TABLE 20-3 Multivariate Analyses of the Association of Coronary Artery Calcium Scores and Self-Reported Traditional Coronary Disease Risk Factors with All Events[a]

| | Variable | Odds Ratio (95% CI) |
|---|---|---|
| Independent of EBCT | Elevated cholesterol | 3.9 (1.3–11.7) |
| | Hypertension | 2.8 (1.2–6.5) |
| | Diabetes | 5.4 (2.0–14.9) |
| With EBCT CACS ≥80 | CACS >80 | 14.3 (4.9–42.3) |
| | Age >55 years | 3.3 (1.3–8.4) |
| | Elevated cholesterol | 4.0 (1.3–12.2) |
| | Hypertension | 2.6 (1.1–6.1) |
| | Diabetes | 4.8 (1.6–13.9) |
| With EBCT CACS ≥160 | CACS >160 | 19.7 (6.9–56.4) |
| | Age >55 years | 4.5 (1.6–12.2) |
| | Elevated cholesterol | 3.7 (1.2–11.5) |
| | Hypertension | 3.0 (1.2–7.4) |
| | Diabetes | 5.8 (2.1–19.7) |
| With EBCT CACS ≥600 | CACS >600 | 20.2 (7.3–55.8) |
| | Age >55 years | 2.9 (1.1–7.9) |
| | Elevated cholesterol | 3.5 (1.1–10.8) |
| | Hypertension | 2.9 (1.2–7.3) |
| | Diabetes | 4.4 (1.4–13.7) |

[a]Analyses were performed with and without the coronary artery calcium scores (CACS). CI = confidence interval; EBCT = electron beam computed tomography.
SOURCE: Reprinted from Arad Y et al.,[83] with permission.

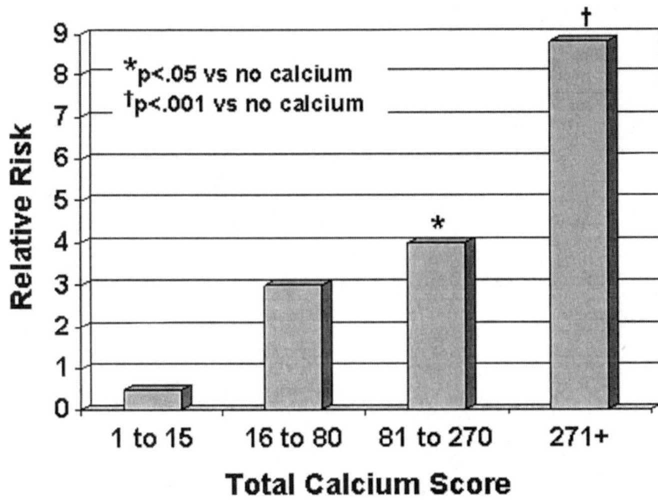


FIGURE 20-17 Relative risks for total cardiovascular events in patients at various total calcium score quartiles versus those without calcium, adjusting for age, gender, hypertension, hyperlipidemia, smoking history and diabetes. (Redrawn from Wong et al.[84])

yond risk factors alone. Mortality significantly increased with increasing CACS (Fig. 20-18).

The exceedingly low cardiac event rate in subjects with a CACS <100 is consistent with angiographic studies indicating a comparably low likelihood of significant CAD and an extremely low incidence of stress-induced myocardial ischemia (<1 percent) in such individuals.[62,69] The increasing number of cardiac events with an ever-increasing CACS is also consistent with the dramatic increase in the incidence of stress-induced myocardial ischemia when scores are >100, and particularly >400.[62,69] The CACS may provide complementary prognostic information to that obtained by the Framingham risk model.[89] Combining EBCT results with biochemical markers, such as C-reactive protein, may more precisely define risk than either test alone.[90] Since cardiac event rates are known to be very low in asymptomatic individuals with cardiac risk factors[76,82,91–94] (Table 20-5), the prognostic value of EBCT needs to be clarified in larger prospective trials enrolling men and women of greater ethnic diversity who are followed for a longer period of time.[95,96] There are currently no published data using mechanical CT–derived CACS for assessing prognosis.

A

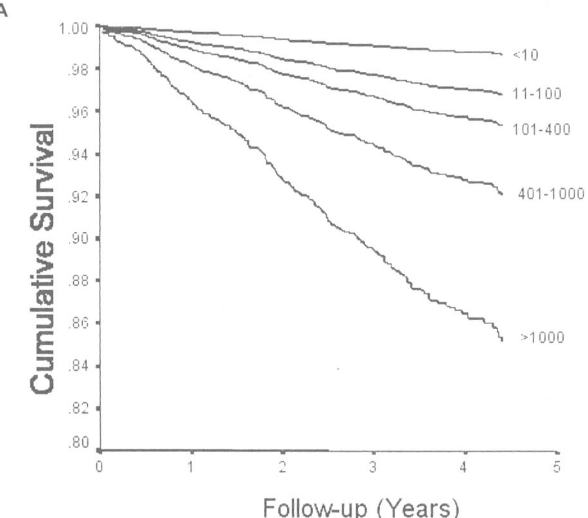


B

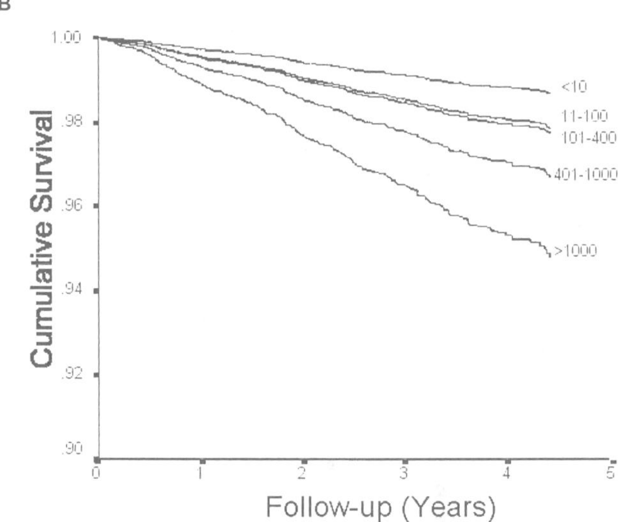


FIGURE 20-18 Risk factor unadjusted (*A*) and risk factor-adjusted (*B*) cumulative survival curves in 10,377 asymptomatic individuals based on EBCT-derived coronary artery calcium score results. (From Callister et al.[88] Reproduced with permission from the publisher and the authors.)

TABLE 20-4 Cardiac Event Rates in Asymptomatic Subjects Based on Absolute and Relative Coronary Artery Calcium Scores

| Absolute Calcium Score | Event Rate Death/NFMI[a] |
|---|---|
| 0 | 0.3% (1/292) |
| 1–99 | 5.5% (12/219) |
| 100–400 | 10.8% (8/74) |
| >400 | 12.8% (6/47) |
| Calcium Score Percentile | |
| <50th | 1.1% (4/351) |
| >50th | 8.2% (23/281) |
| >75th | 10.5% (19/181) |
| >90th | 11.8% (11/93) |

[a]NFMI = nonfatal myocardial infarction.

SOURCE: From Raggi et al.[85] Adapted with permission of the publisher and authors.

## Screening for Subclinical Coronary Artery Disease

The early detection of coronary atherosclerosis with risk-factor analysis and/or cardiac imaging modalities would seem desirable, particularly in light of recent primary prevention trials that have demonstrated reduced cardiac event rates following aggressive risk-factor modification and treatment of hyperlipidemia.[91,92,97]

### RISK-FACTOR ANALYSIS

Traditional risk-factor analysis is commonly used to identify individuals who are at increased risk for developing cardiovascular disease based on standard clinical criteria.[98,99] Implicit in this risk model is the assumption that a certain combination of risk factors will promote atherosclerosis, which, in turn, will result in cardiovascular

TABLE 20-5 Cardiac Event Rates in Asymptomatic Patients

| | N | Percent Men | Age (years) | F/U | Total Deaths per Year | CV Deaths per Year | Nonfatal MIs per Year | Angina Pectoris per Year |
|---|---|---|---|---|---|---|---|---|
| Arad et al.[82] | 1,173 | 71% | 53 ± 11 | 1.6 years | — | 0.05% | 0.37% | 2.3% |
| Shepherd et al.[91] | 6,595 | 100% | 55 ± 5 (45–64) | 5 years | 0.73% | 0.27% | 1.0% | — |
| Detrano et al.[93] | 1,462 | 88% | 63 ± 8 (≥45) | 1 year | — | 0.40% | 0.7% | 2.5% |
| Ekelund et al.[76] | 3,806 | 100% | 48 (35–59) | 7.4 years | 0.49% | 0.24% | 1.0% | — |
| MRFIT[94] | 12,866 | 100% | 46 (35–57) | 7.0 years | 0.58% | 0.31% | 0.7% | 1.6% |
| Gordon et al.[92] | 3,640 | 100% | 46 (30–70) | 8.5 years | 0.58% | 0.27% | — | — |
| Total | 29,541 | 98% | | | 0.60% | 0.28% | 0.8% | 1.74% |

ABBREVIATIONS: CV = cardiovascular; MI = myocardial infarction.

events. However, among individuals with a similar risk-factor profile, the presence and severity of atherosclerosis will vary enormously, thereby overestimating risk in certain subjects and underestimating it in others. This discrepancy will be most apparent among individuals with several risk factors who are members of a more heterogeneous population at risk than in those without risk factors (a more uniformly low-risk group) or those with multiple risk factors (a more uniformly high-risk group). The imprecision of risk-factor analysis for identifying patients with significant atherosclerosis is probably related to the fact that traditional risk factor analysis fails to incorporate presently unknown biochemical, environmental, and genetic factors that promote the development of CAD.

Since the development of symptomatic cardiovascular disease occurs almost exclusively in patients with atherosclerosis, it would seem advantageous in risk assessment to use a technique that directly measures the presence and severity of atherosclerotic burden rather than estimating its presence through indirect measures. For example, although there is a clear relationship between the number of cardiac risk factors and the presence and extent of coronary artery calcification, 40 percent of men and 30 percent of women without risk factors in one recent series had coronary artery calcification, whereas 26 percent of men and 36 percent of women with more than three traditional risk factors did not.[100] Likewise, Newman et al. showed great heterogeneity in the EBCT-derived CACS even among elderly men and women, which was only weakly associated with the presence of cardiac risk factors.[101] In this series, 9 percent of patients had a normal EBCT and 31 percent had a CACS <100 (Fig. 20-19). Increasing age and tobacco use were significantly associated with increasing CACS in both men and women, whereas hypertension, diabetes, and hyperlipidemia were not.

Hecht et al. demonstrated that 76 percent of asymptomatic subjects with an abnormal EBCT had a low-density lipoprotein (LDL) cholesterol <160 mg/dL and therefore would not meet National Cholesterol Education Program (NCEP) II guidelines for lipid-lowering therapy.[102] Conversely, 52 percent of patients with an LDL cholesterol <130 mg/dL and 46 percent with an LDL <100 mg/dL had an abnormal EBCT. Similarly, in the Healthy Women Study, risk-factor analysis was imprecise at predicting coronary calcification in postmenopausal women.[103] Although the combination of a high LDL cholesterol, a low high-density lipoprotein (HDL) cholesterol, and a history of cigarette smoking was a strong predictor of coronary artery calcification, this risk-factor profile was observed in only 6 percent of all women studied. Furthermore, only 6 of 21 women with the highest calcium scores (>101) had this risk-factor profile. Conversely, 20 percent of women in the lowest risk profile (i.e., nonsmokers, LDL cholesterol <130 mg/dL, and HDL cholesterol >60 mg/dL) had calcium by EBCT. Hecht et al. likewise showed that 42 percent of women aged ≤55 and 48 percent aged >55 years who were at low risk based on NCEP II guidelines (i.e., LDL cholesterol <130 and HDL ≥35 mg/dL) had evidence of

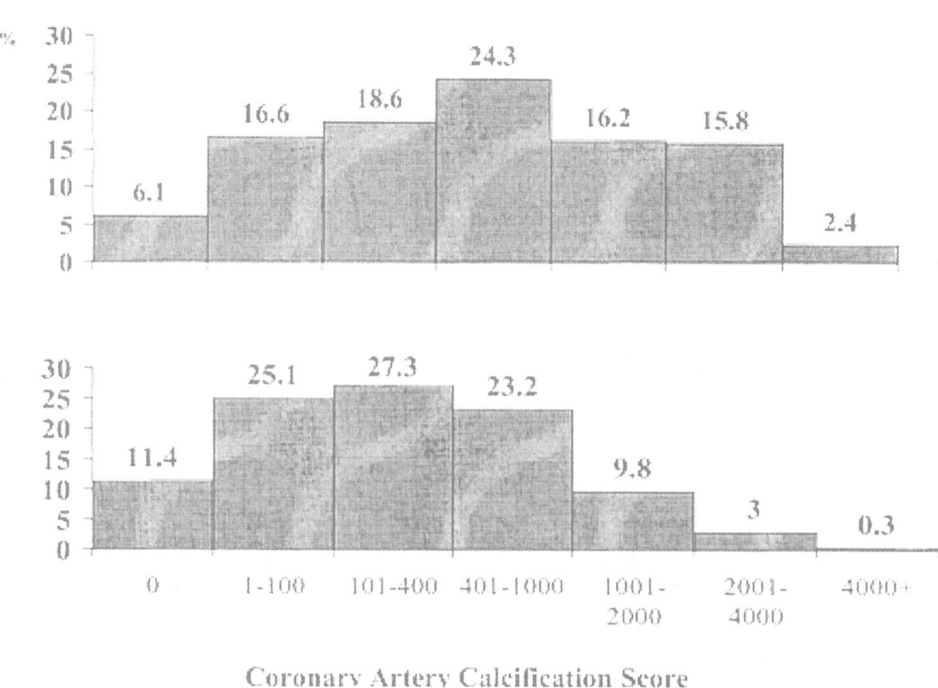


FIGURE 20-19 Distribution of the coronary artery calcification score in elderly men (*top*) and women (*bottom*). (From Newman et al.[101] Reproduced with permission from the publisher and the authors.)

coronary atherosclerosis based on an abnormal EBCT study.[104]

## DETECTION OF SUBCLINICAL CAD AND STRESS TESTING

Noninvasive techniques, such as exercise treadmill testing and myocardial perfusion imaging, can identify patients with coronary atherosclerosis. However, unlike EBCT, which can detect coronary atherosclerosis at its earliest stages, these techniques can identify only patients with advanced CAD who manifest myocardial ischemia. Although the presence and extent of ischemia can accurately identify asymptomatic individuals at high risk for cardiac events[63,64,76] (Fig. 20-20), the very low prevalence of a positive test result (<5 percent) precludes the use of these methodologies as primary screening tests for the early detection and treatment of CAD. In fact, both exercise treadmill testing and myocardial perfusion imaging have received a class III indication (no justification for their use) for screening asymptomatic individuals.[105,106]

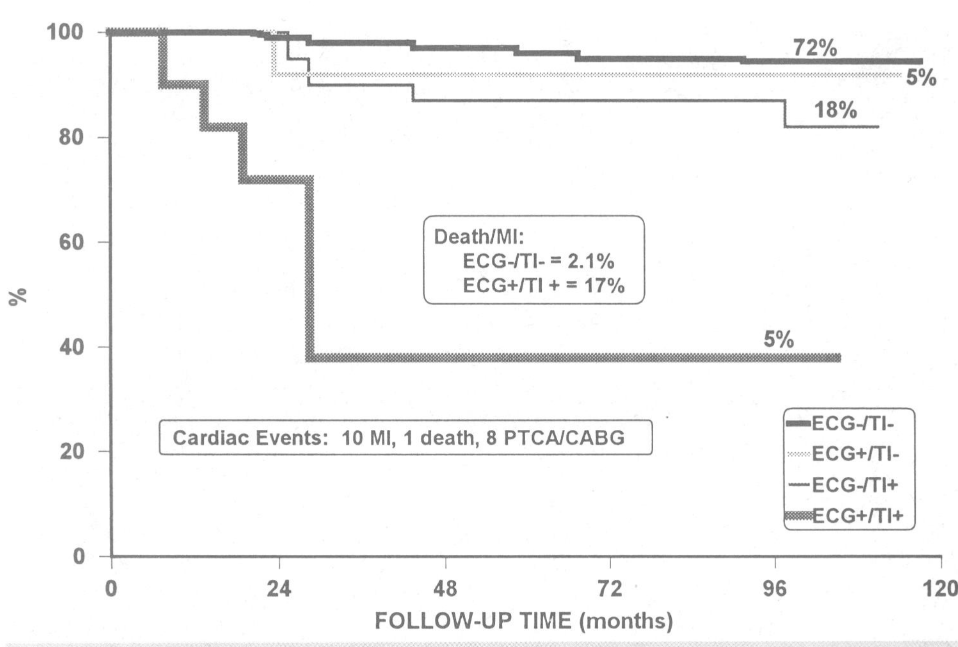


FIGURE 20-20 Kaplan-Meier survival curves based on exercise ECG and thallium-201 ($^{201}Tl$) scan results. The highest event rate is observed in patients with ischemia (+) by both tests. The percentage of patients with each test combination are shown above the curves. CABG = coronary artery bypass surgery; MI = myocardial infarction; PTCA = coronary angioplasty. (From Blumenthal et al.[63] Reproduced with permission from the publisher and authors.)

## EBCT

One of the most novel applications of EBCT may be as a screening test for identifying subjects with subclinical CAD based on the presence and severity of coronary artery calcification. EBCT is a simple and rapid technique that requires no patient preparation and is highly specific for detecting early coronary atherosclerosis. The growing wealth of prognostic information further supports the role of EBCT as an initial screening test beyond risk-factor analysis alone.[76–88] Recent studies emphasize the effectiveness of selectively combining stress myocardial perfusion imaging with EBCT in the anticipated small (10 percent) number of asymptomatic subjects who will have a high (≥400) CACS so as to specifically identify those with silent myocardial ischemia[62,69] (Fig. 20-21). This testing strategy may prove to be optimal based on the known prognostic value of perfusion imaging and the superior sensitivity of EBCT over the former for detecting preclinical CAD. Although the cost-effectiveness of using EBCT as a screening test requires further clinical investigation, it has been proposed that the CACS might be used to guide therapeutics and recommend the need for additional diagnostic testing.[107] This approach was not yet sanctioned by the last ACC/AHA expert consensus document on EBCT for the diagnosis and prognosis of CAD (see also Chap. 43 and 57).[108]

### Tracking Changes in Coronary Artery Calcification

Sequential testing with EBCT may be useful in determining the rate of progression of coronary atherosclerosis.[109,110] or in identifying treatment effects based on lack of progression and/or regression of coronary artery calcification.[110–112] In order for sequential testing to have any clinical relevance, the biological changes being studied need to be greater than the intrinsic variability of the test result and the temporal variability in the test result must be well defined in individual patients.

## EBCT REPRODUCIBILITY

The reproducibility of EBCT has been evaluated using the traditional Agatston scoring system and more recent volumetric and area methods. With the Agatston method, good inter- and intraobserver reproducibility is reported for recalculating the CACS on a single scan.[42,113] However, early studies showed significant variability when the results of two separate studies on the same patient were compared.[28,30,114–119] Devries et al. studied 91 subjects who had two EBCT scans performed within 24 h using an identical acquisition protocol.[114] The variability in CACS observed in the 42 subjects who were abnormal on both scans was 49 ± 45 percent. Variability was inversely related to the absolute value of the CACS, being particularly great when the initial score was <10 (72 ± 54 percent). Bielak et al. studied 256 patients who had two EBCT studies performed minutes apart.[115] The mean CACS was 73 ± 233 (scan 1) versus 75 ± 242 (scan 2). Linear regression analysis showed that the two scores were highly correlated ($r = 0.962$, $p = 0.0001$). The greatest CACS variability occurred in patients with low scores.

Over the years, technical advances and improvements in calcium scoring methodologies have reduced interscan variability. Aschenbach et al., using "state-of-the-art" EBCT imaging, reported an interscan variability of only 19.9 ± 36 percent with a median Agatston score variability of 7.8 percent.[118] As in previous studies, there was a strong inverse relationship between the initial CACS value and interscan reproducibility, with the largest percent variation occurring in patients with the lowest CACS (Table 20-6). The variability for a CACS ≥100 was minimal at 10.5 ± 10.4 percent, with a median variability of only 7.1 percent.

The traditional Agatston scoring system has been challenged by more recently proposed area[118–120] and volumetric scoring methods.[121] The volumetric method uses isotropic interpolation to calculate the volume of calcified plaque area with a density of ≥130 HU,[121] rather than generating a CACS based on an arbitrary

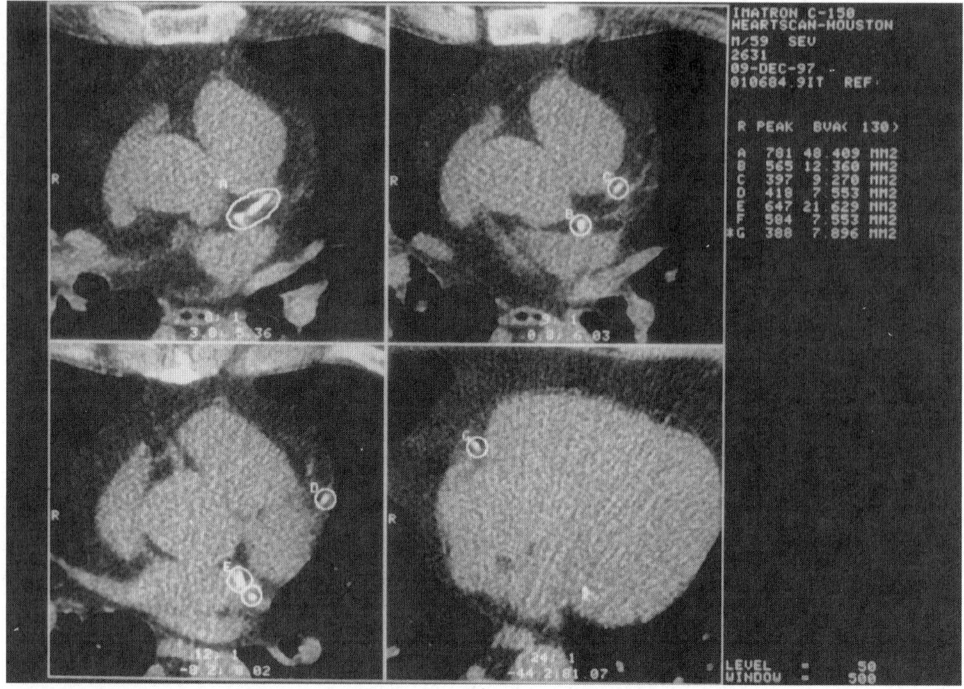


A



B

FIGURE 20-21 EBCT (*top*) and SPECT (*bottom*) images of asymptomatic subject who had a high-risk CACS of 937. Circles define regions of coronary calcification. The treadmill test was terminated at 9.0 min due to patient fatigue. SPECT demonstrated a large, reversible 48 percent perfusion defect within the distribution of all three major coronary arteries (COMP-SC) (*bottom*). This patient had severe three-vessel disease on angiography and underwent CABG. PDS indicates perfusion defect size. (From He et al.[62] Reproduced with permission from the publisher and authors.)

maximal plaque attenuation coefficient (i.e., Agatston method).[42] The calcified-area method directly measures and sums the area (in mm$^2$) of all coronary artery lesions. The volumetric and calcified-area methods are more reproducible than the Agatston method,[118,120,121] probably due to a reduction in partial volume effects and image noise on scan results.

In the largest series to date, Bielak et al. defined the reproducibility of sequential EBCT imaging in 1376 patients where scanning was performed minutes apart.[119] The total-calcified-area method was used to define scan reproducibility. The mean calcified area was 60.6 ± 154.1 mm$^2$ on scan 1 versus 59.8 ± 149.1 mm$^2$ on scan 2, with a correlation coefficient between scans of 0.98 ($p < 0.001$). The absolute difference in calcified area between scans was greatest at higher scores, whereas the relative percent difference was most pronounced at low scores. This large data set is the first to allow calculation of 95 percent confidence intervals for individual changes in sequential scores for calcified areas ranging as low as 5 mm$^2$ to over 1000 mm$^2$ (Table 20-7).

Despite improvements in image acquisition and processing, cardiac motion still remains an important source of scan variability. The optimization of ECG triggering when cardiac motion is at a nadir may further improve reproducibility.[120] The use of a variable ECG trigger based on resting heart rate[2] may significantly reduce interscan variability as compared to image acquisition triggered at the standard 80 percent RR interval, and particularly in patients with small (2 to 10 mm$^2$) calcium burdens (15.3 vs. 23.2 percent, respectively; $p < 0.01$).[120] To date, there are no studies evaluating the reproducibility of sequential imaging with mechanical CT scanning.

## TRACKING CALCIUM PROGRESSION

The reproducibility of EBCT with the area or volumetric methods appears adequate to track temporal changes in coronary atherosclerosis and assess the effects of pharmacologic therapy on plaque progression. In asymptomatic subjects with an abnormal EBCT, CACS progression is approximately 30 percent per year, which is significantly greater than the inherent variability in EBCT calcium score measurements.[110,122] However, patients without detectable calcium have a very low likelihood of further progression. In the series by Budoff et al., only 11 of 81 patients (14 percent) with a normal EBCT study developed calcification over 1 to 6 years of follow-up, and 82 percent had a subsequent score of <10.[110] Repeat scanning in patients with a normal EBCT study is probably not warranted for at least 3 to 5 years after the baseline study.

TABLE 20-6 Comparison of Interscan Variability for the Agatston and Volumetric Scores Depending on Severity of Initial Coronary Artery Calcium Score

| Agatston Score | Number of Patients | Agatston Score Variability (%) | Volumetric Score Variability (%) |
|---|---|---|---|
| ≥0 | 120 | 19.9 ± 36.0 (7.8) | 16.2 ± 29.6 (5.7) |
| ≥0.1 | 102 | 23.5 ± 39.5 (10.3) | 19.9 ± 31.2 (8.3) |
| ≥10 | 87 | 16.5 ± 22.7 (8.8) | 18.0 ± 24.6 (9.1) |
| ≥50 | 70 | 11.5 ± 11.1 (7.5) | 11.6 ± 11.2 (6.6) |
| ≥100 | 62 | 10.5 ± 10.4 (7.1) | 11.4 ± 11.0 (6.6) |
| ≥400 | 31 | 9.5 ± 9.1[a] (7.3) | 7.3 ± 8.0[a] (4.9) |
| ≥1000 | 11 | 8.3 ± 6.9 (6.2) | 6.1 ± 4.9 (5.9) |

[a]Volumetric score variability significantly lower than Agatston score variability. Values are expressed as mean ± SD (median).
SOURCE: From Achenbach,[118] with permission.

Retrospective studies indicate that the progression of coronary artery calcification can be significantly reduced with lipid-lowering therapy. Budoff et al. performed repeat imaging in 299 patients 2.2 ± 11 years after baseline EBCT. The rate of progression in the Agatston-derived CACS was significantly less in treated (15 ± 8 percent per year) versus untreated (39 ± 12 percent per year) subjects with hyperlipidemia $p < 0.001$.[110] Callister et al. studied 149 asymptomatic hyperlipidemic patients who had no history of prior CAD or treatment of hyperlipidemia and who underwent a baseline screening EBCT followed by repeat imaging at 13.7 ± 0.6 months.[111] After the baseline scan, patients were treated with a statin drug at the discretion of their referring physician. Serial measurements of LDL cholesterol were obtained and correlated with the change in calcified plaque volume. Sixty-five treated patients achieved an LDL cholesterol <120 mg/dL (mean 100 ± 17 mg/dL), whereas 40 did not (mean 139 ± 18 mg/dL). In the 44 untreated patients, the mean LDL cholesterol was 147 ± 22 mg/dL. Importantly, in the 44 untreated patients and in the 40 treated patients with an LDL cholesterol >120 mg/dL, the calcium score increased by 52 ± 36 percent and 25 ± 22 percent, respectively. However, in the treated patients who achieved an LDL cholesterol <120 mg/dL, the calcium score decreased by 7 ± 23 percent. Sixty-three percent of the patients in this group had a net decrease in their calcium volume score, whereas none of the other patients had a reduction in calcium score.

These results were confirmed in a prospective study where 66 untreated hyperlipidemic subjects (LDL cholesterol >130 mg/dL) had a baseline EBCT repeated at 14 ± 2.4 months.[112] A third EBCT was then performed after 12 months of cerivastatin (0.3 mg/day). The calcium score was calculated on all three studies using both the volumetric and Agatston methods. Cerivastatin significantly decreased total (244 ± 32 vs. 188 ± 78 mg/dL) and LDL (164 ± 30 vs. 107 ± 21 mg/dL) cholesterol, with a subsequent reduction in calcium progression (Fig. 20-22). This was most dramatic in patients who maintained an LDL cholesterol <100 mg/dL, where the rate of calcium progression was effectively halted (median change 3.4 percent volume score; 0 percent Agatston score).

These studies suggest that aggressive treatment with lipid-lowering medications can reduce calcified plaque burden as assessed by serial EBCT imaging. The reduction in calcified plaque burden presumably indicates a reduction in total atherosclerotic plaque, which is consistent with prior angiographic studies showing a small albeit significant reduction in the severity of coronary artery stenosis with long-term statin therapy.[123,124]

TABLE 20-7 Predicted Calcific Area in 1376 Asymptomatic Patients

| Mean Calcific Area in Dual-Scan Runs | Calcific Area at Limit of Agreement[a] Upper 95% | Lower 95% |
|---|---|---|
| 5 | 8 | 1 |
| 10 | 14 | 5 |
| 20 | 25 | 14 |
| 50 | 60 | 41 |
| 75 | 88 | 63 |
| 100 | 117 | 85 |
| 150 | 174 | 130 |
| 200 | 231 | 174 |
| 250 | 288 | 219 |
| 300 | 346 | 263 |
| 400 | 460 | 352 |
| 500 | 575 | 441 |
| 750 | 861 | 663 |
| 1000 | 1147 | 885 |

[a]Data are rounded to nearest whole number.
SOURCE: From Bielak et al.,[119] with permission.

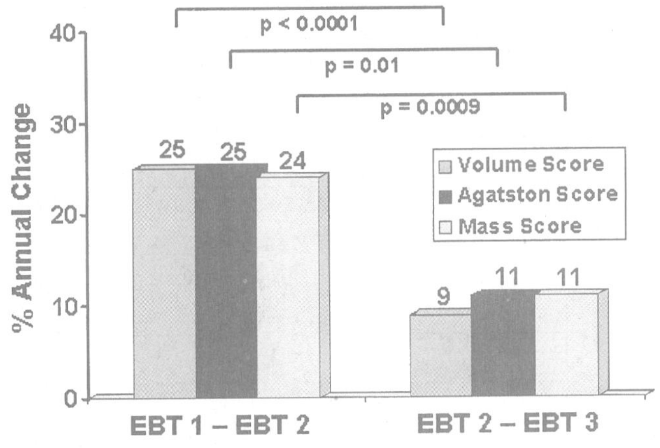

FIGURE 20-22 Median annualized relative increase in volume, Agatston and mass scores during the untreated period (EBT1 to EBT2) and following statin treatment (EBT2 to EBT3). (Redrawn from Achenbach et al.[112])

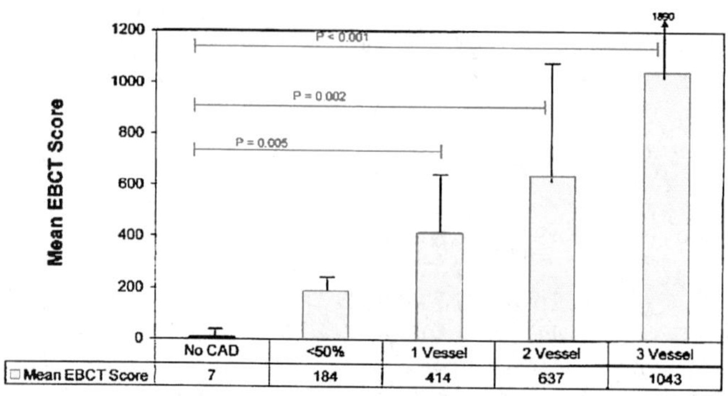


FIGURE 20-23 Mean EBCT CACS based on the presence and extent of angiographic coronary artery disease in patients with cardiomyopathy. (From Budoff et al.[126] Reproduced with permission from the publisher and authors.)

It is conceivable that sequential EBCT imaging may be able to track subsequent individual patient risk for cardiac events based on either the annual rate of calcium progression or upon reaching a certain "threshold" of CACS. Ongoing large prospective trials, such as the Multi-Ethnic Study of Atherosclerosis, will better define the role of sequential EBCT imaging in assessing therapeutics and subsequent outcome.[125]

## Distinguishing Ischemic from Nonischemic Conditions with CT

The presence or absence of coronary artery calcification by EBCT may help to distinguish patients with ischemic versus nonischemic dilated cardiomyopathy.[126,127] In one study, 44 of 53 patients (83 percent) without significant (>50 percent stenosis) CAD had a CACS of 0, whereas 71 of 72 (99 percent) with CAD had an abnormal EBCT study.[126] Importantly, 44 of 45 patients with a normal EBCT had nonischemic dilated cardiomyopathy (98 percent negative predictive value). The total CACS increased with the extent and severity of underlying CAD (Fig. 20-23). The differentiation of ischemic from nonischemic dilated cardiomyopathy has also been demonstrated with spiral CT.[127]

EBCT may be able to distinguish ischemic from nonischemic chest pain in patients presenting to the emergency department with nondiagnostic ECGs and also predict subsequent cardiac risk for future events.[128–130] Two recent series comprising 239 patients showed a 0 percent cardiac event rate over 1[128] and 4[129] months in those with a normal EBCT. A third study in 192 patients showed 100 percent infarct-free survival over 50 ± 10 months of follow-up in patients with a normal EBCT.[130] The cardiac event rate increased significantly with the CACS (Fig. 20-24). By multivariate analysis—combining age, gender, and cardiac risk factors—an abnormal EBCT was the best single predictor of subsequent cardiac events (RR 27.8, 1.88 to 815, $p < 0.02$).[126] The high negative predictive value of EBCT may improve triage of patients with questionable ischemic symptoms.

Lack of coronary calcification by EBCT predicts patients at low likelihood for acute myocardial infarction. In three recent reports, most asymptomatic patients who had a subsequent first acute myocardial infarction had coronary calcification by EBCT (96 percent).[74,85,131] Since many acute myocardial infarctions occur following rupture of nonobstructive plaques, it is not surprising that the CACS will be mild (<100) in a large percentage (34 percent) of patients and severe (>400) in relatively few (27 percent).[85] In one study evaluating survivors of a first myocardial infarction with spiral CT, 19 percent lacked coronary artery calcification.[132] This higher percentage of normal studies may reflect the lower sensitivity of spiral CT as compared to EBCT for detecting calcium. Patients without calcium are generally younger in age and tend to be active smokers.[85,133] With the exception of young smokers, a normal EBCT defines a population at low likelihood for significant CAD and subsequent acute cardiac events. Larger prospective trials in patients with acute coronary syndromes are needed to further delineate the role of EBCT in this population.

## Contrast Angiography of Bypass Grafts and Native Coronary Arteries

### BYPASS GRAFTS

Contrast-enhanced EBCT can be used to visualize coronary artery bypass grafts and assess their patency.[134–136] Initial studies using conventional CT angiography reported a sensitivity and specificity of 93 and 95 percent, respectively, for detecting graft patency when compared to coronary angiography.[137] More recently, single[138] and multislice[139] spiral CT has also been studied for identifying bypass graft patency. The sensitivity, specificity, and diagnostic accuracy for detecting graft patency were 92, 97, and 93 percent, respectively for single-slice spiral CT[138] but the figure may be somewhat higher for multislice CT due to relatively faster imaging speeds.[139] Positive predictive accuracy for graft closure was 78 percent and the negative predictive accuracy for graft patency was 99 percent. The accurate detection of internal mammary artery grafts was somewhat lower than that for vein grafts, as was the detection of distal anastomotic sites. Studies using EBCT have likewise reported high sensitivity (89 percent),

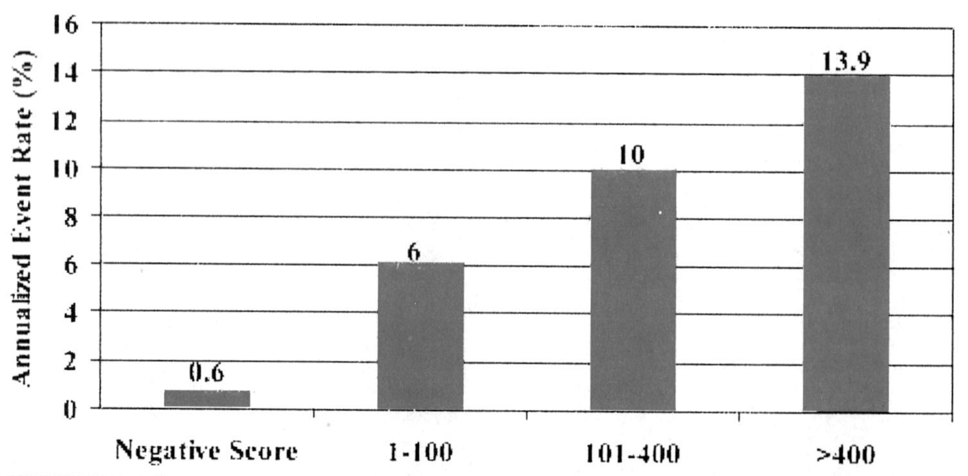


FIGURE 20-24 Annualized rates for future cardiovascular events by Cox proportional hazards regression. Patients with scores >400 had a significantly higher annualized event rate (13.9 percent) than those with scores of zero (0.6 percent) ($p < 0.001$). (From Georgiou et al.[130] Reproduced with permission from the publisher and authors.)

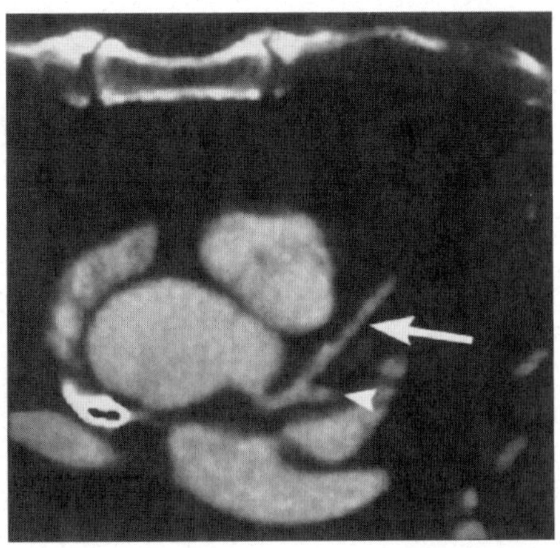
A

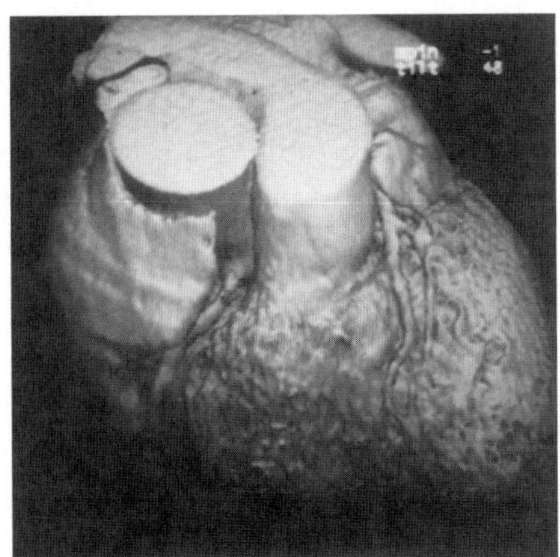
B

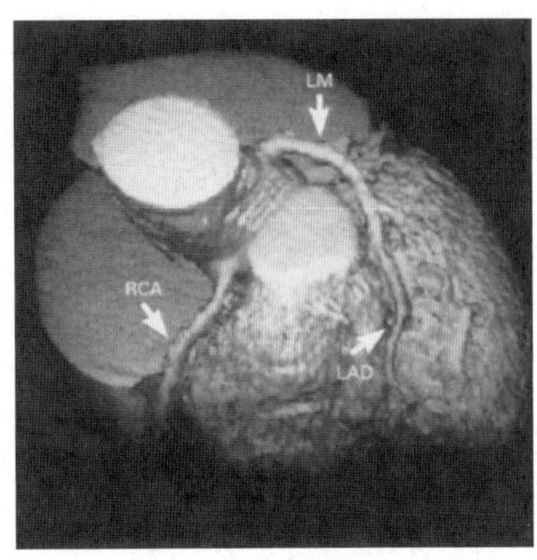

C

FIGURE 20-25 EBCT images of the heart. *A.* A cross section of the heart at the level of the aortic root depicting the origin of the left main (LM), proximal left anterior descending (LAD) (*arrow*), and left circumflex (*arrowhead*) coronary arteries. *B.* A contrast enhanced three-dimensional reconstruction of the entire heart. *C.* The main stem of the pulmonary artery and the atrial appendages have been removed to show the LM, LAD and right (RCA) coronary arteries. (From Achenbach et al.[144] Reproduced with permission from the publisher and authors.)

specificity (93 percent), and overall diagnostic accuracy (92 percent) for detecting bypass graft patency[134] However, as with spiral CT, EBCT cannot quantify stenosis severity, and the accuracy for assessing graft patency is worse for the right and circumflex arteries as compared to the left anterior descending coronary artery.

## NATIVE CORONARY ARTERIES

Both EBCT[140–148] and multislice spiral CT[149–155] can be used as noninvasive techniques to visualize the epicardial coronary arteries. The imaging technique is similar to that used for scanning for coronary artery calcification, but it requires the injection of intravenous contrast material. A scout scan is first performed to localize the position of the heart in the chest. The time from contrast material injection to peak contrast enhancement of the aortic root is then determined. Contrast material is administered at a rate of 4 mL/s and the amount of dye given is based on the heart rate and the number of slices desired. Some 40 to 50 contrast-enhanced cross-sectional images of the heart of 3-mm thickness are then obtained during full inspiration at an acquisition rate of 100 ms per image (1 image per cardiac cycle). Image acquisition is gated to the ECG in a standard fashion. Using the above parameters and depending on the heart rate, the total imaging time is between 30 and 50 s (Fig. 20-25). A similar procedure is used to acquire images with multislice CT. The spatial resolution of EBCT (0.7 mm) is generally less than that of multislice CT (0.5 mm), but this is offset by the improved temporal resolution of EBCT. Due to the worse temporal resolution of multislice CT, patients must routinely be given beta blockers prior to scanning so as to decrease heart rate to <60 beats per minute. The radiation exposure with multislice CT angiography is three- to sixfold higher than with EBCT, which increases further with greater tube currents.[139,141,147,148,156]

Several studies have compared EBCT to standard coronary angiography for detecting CAD (Table 20-8).[140–148] The overall sensitivity of EBCT for detecting significant (>50 percent) stenosis is 83 percent; it increases to 92 percent for detecting high-grade (>75 percent) stenosis (Fig. 20-26). Specificity is also comparably high at 91 percent, with a negative predictive accuracy of 96 percent. Similar results have been reported for multislice CT[149–155] (Table 20-9). Only one study directly compared EBCT to multislice CT angiography, and this was in patients without significant coronary artery stenosis by invasive angiography.[156] Multislice CT images had more motion and noise related artifacts than those generated by EBCT (Fig. 20-27).

EBCT can detect high-grade restenosis after previous coronary artery angioplasty with high sensitivity (94 percent) and specificity (82 percent).[157] Most patients (96 percent) without restenosis by EBCT have comparable normal angiographic findings (Fig. 20-28). A recent study indicates that EBCT can also assess in-stent restenosis (sensitivity 78 percent, specificity 98 percent) with successful imaging of most arteries (94 percent).[158] Coronary anomalies can also be detected and adequately visualized in most (97 percent) patients.[159]

These reports are encouraging; however, several points must be emphasized. EBCT and MSCT cannot assess approximately 20 percent of all coronary arteries due to technical factors, such as respiration artifact, the presence of severe coronary calcification, and motion artifacts. Respiration artifacts can be avoided by instructing patients about proper breathholding techniques. Motion artifacts are clearly more common with multislice CT than with EBCT and occur predominantly in the right and circumflex coronary arteries, since they lie in close proximity to the atria, which contract at end-diastole. The right and circumflex arteries also lie perpendicular to the imaging plane, limiting spatial resolution. Imaging at a different time in diastole (to avoid atrial contraction), shortening acquisition time, and imaging in different cardiac planes might obviate these problems.

Finally, EBCT and multislice CT generally best assess the proximal and middle segments of the epicardial coronary arteries. Due to limited spatial resolution, distal segments and side branches, which are <2 mm in diameter, cannot be adequately visualized.

# EVALUATION OF PERICARDIAL DISEASE

CT scanning provides excellent visualization of the pericardium and associated mediastinal structures[160–163] (Fig. 20-29). Although echocardiography remains the primary diagnostic technique for assessing pericardial abnormalities, CT scanning can be useful particularly when visualization of the pericardium is suboptimal with echocardiography. CT scanning can readily detect pericardial effusion and can help determine the characteristics of the fluid based on CT density.[164]

TABLE 20-8 Diagnostic Accuracy of Contrast Enhanced EBCT as Defined by Coronary Angiography

| | Year | Number of Patients | CAD Definition | ARI | Sensitivity | Specificity | PPA | NPA | OV ACC |
|---|---|---|---|---|---|---|---|---|---|
| Reddy et al.[140] | 1997 | 23 | >50% | 92% (64/69) | 88% (23/26) | 79% (34/43) | 72% (23/32) | 92% (34/37) | 83% (57/69) |
| Nakanishi et al.[141] | 1997 | 37 | >50% | (NA) | 74% (23/31) | 91% (106/117) | 68% (23/34) | 91% (106/117) | 85% (129/151) |
| Schmermund et al.[142] | 1998 | 28 | >50% | 88% (194/221) | 82% (31/38) | 88% (176/199) | 57% (31/54) | 96% (176/183) | 87% (207/237) |
| Rensing et al.[143] | 1998 | 37 | >50% | 81% (211/259) | 76% (25/33) | 94% (168/178) | 71% (25/35) | 95% (168/176) | 91% (193/211) |
| Achenbach et al.[144] | 1998 | 125 | >75% | 75% (376/500) | 92% (69/75) | 94% (282/301) | 78% (69/88) | 98% (282/288) | 93% (351/376) |
| Budoff et al.[145] | 1999 | 52 | >50% | 89% (185/208) | 78% (43/55) | 91% (118/130) | 78% (43/55) | 91% (118/130) | 87% (161/185) |
| Achenbach et al.[146] | 2000 | 36 | >75% | 80% (115/144) | 92% (33/36) | 92% (73/79) | 85% (33/39) | 96% (73/76) | 92% (106/115) |
| Leber et al.[147] | 2001 | 87 | >50% | 76% (581/767) | 78% (55/70) | 93% (489/524) | 65% (55/90) | 97% (489/504) | 92% (544/594) |
| Ropers et al.[148] | 2002 | 118 | >70% | 76% (90/118) | 90% (17/19) | 66% (47/71) | 42% (17/41) | 96% (47/49) | 71% (64/90) |
| Total | | 543 | | 79% (1816/2286) | 83% (319/383) | 91% (1493/1642) | 68% (319/468) | 96% (1493/1560) | 89% (1812/2028) |

ABBREVIATIONS: ARI = arteries (segments) interpretable by EBCT; NPA = negative predictive accuracy; OV ACC = overall accuracy; PPA = positive predictive accuracy.

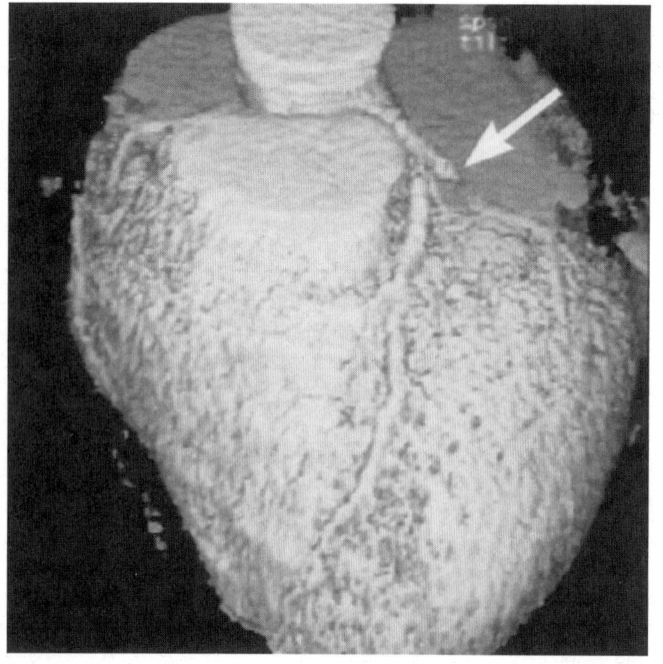

A

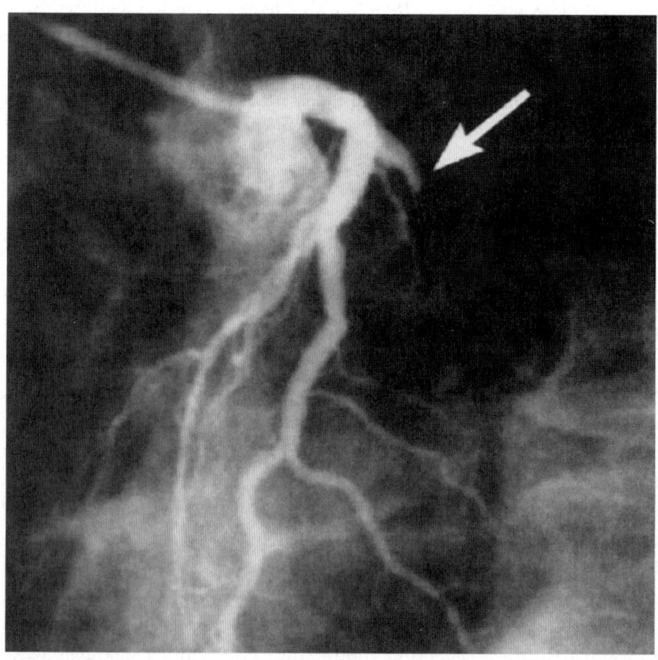

B

FIGURE 20-26 EBCT (*A*) and coronary angiography (*B*) of a patient with complete occlusion of the left circumflex coronary artery (*arrow*). (From Achenbach et al.[144] Reproduced with permission from the publisher and authors.)

TABLE 20-9 Diagnostic Accuracy of Contrast-Enhanced Multislice CT as Defined by Coronary Angiography

| | Year | Stenosis | Technique | Gating | Number of Patients | ARI | Sensitivity | Specificity | PPA | NPA | OV ACC |
|---|---|---|---|---|---|---|---|---|---|---|---|
| Knez et al.[149] | 2001 | ≥50% | MSCT | R | 43 | 94% (358/387) | 78% (39/59) | 98% (301/308) | 84% (39/46) | 96% (301/321) | 93% (340/367) |
| Achenbach et al.[150] | 2001 | >50% | MSCT | R | 64 | 68% (174/256) | 85% (40/47) | 76% (99/130) | 56% (40/71) | 93% (99/106) | 78% (139/177) |
| | | >70% | MSCT | R | | | 91% (32/35) | 84% (117/139) | 59% (32/54) | 98% (117/120) | 86% (149/174) |
| Nieman et al.[151] | 2002 | ≥50% | MSCT | R | 53 | 70% (358/513) | 82% (47/51) | 93% (276/307) | 66% (47/78) | 97% (276/280) | 90% (323/358) |
| Vogl et al.[152] | 2002 | >50% | MSCT | R | 64 | 72% (688/959) | 73% (58/79) | 99% (955/960) | 92% (58/63) | 98% (955/976) | 97% (1013/1039) |
| Giesler et al.[153] | 2002 | >70% | MSCT | R | 100 | 71%* (285/400) | 91% (51/56) | 89% (223/229) | 89% (51/57) | 98% (223/228) | 96% (274/285) |
| Nieman et al.[154] | 2002 | ≥50% | MSCT | R | 59 | 93% (214/231) | 95% (82/86) | 86% (125/145) | 97% (125/129) | 80% (82/102) | 90% (207/231) |
| Ropers et al.[155] | 2003 | >50% | MSCT | R | 77 | 88% (270/308) | 92% (57/62) | 93% (194/208) | 80% (57/71) | 97% (194/199) | 93% (251/270) |
| Total | | | | | 460 | 77% (2347/3054) | 85% (406/475) | 94% (2290/2426) | 79% (449/569) | 96% (2247/2332) | 93% (2696/2901) |

ABBREVIATIONS: ARI = arteries (segments) interpretable by multislice (MS) CT; NPA = negative predictive accuracy; OV ACC = overall accuracy; PPA = positive predictive accuracy; R = retrospective.

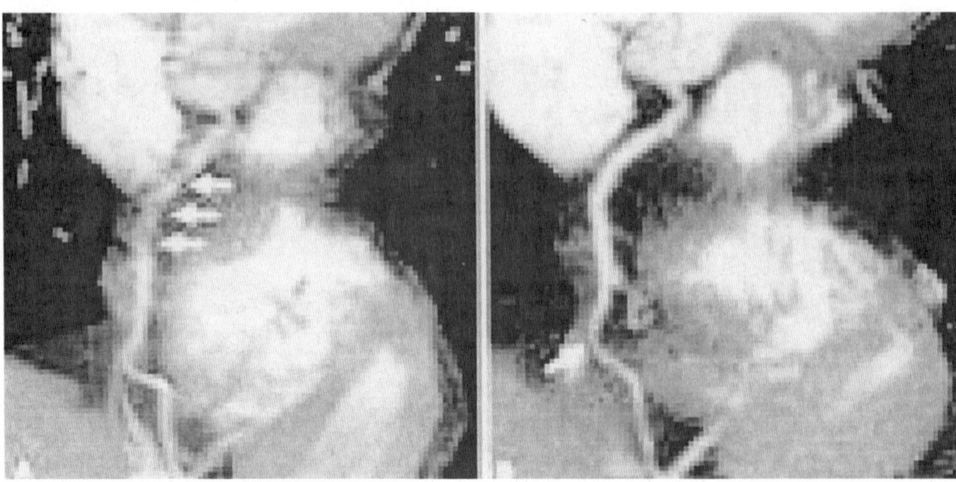

FIGURE 20-27 Comparison of multislice computed tomography (MSCT) (*left*) and EBCT (*right*) in the same patient (heart rate: 75 beats per minute). Multiplanar reconstruction of the right coronary artery. Overall visualized length in MSCT, 132 mm; in EBCT, 127 mm. Blurring of the vessel contours due to motion is clearly visible in the MSCT reconstruction (*arrows*). Only slight blurring by motion is seen in the EBT reconstruction (*arrow*). Percentage of vessel length visualized free of motion artifacts in MSCT, 75 percent; in EBT, 96 percent. (From Achenbach et al.[156] Reproduced with permission from the publisher and authors.)

CT scanning is useful in accurately diagnosing constrictive pericarditis and distinguishing it from similar conditions, such as restrictive myopathy.[161] Based on the presence of pericardial thickening (Fig. 20-30) or calcification (Fig. 20-31), cine EBCT can assess both the anatomic and functional abnormalities associated with pericardial constriction.[162] A pericardial thickness of more than 4 mm in a patient with typical abnormal rapid early left ventricular diastolic filling is diagnostic of pericardial constriction.

CT scanning can assess congenital abnormalities such as absence of the pericardium[165] or pericardial cyst.[166] CT scanning is currently one of the best techniques for defining the location and extent of mediastinal tumors and in diagnosing metastatic involvement of the pericardium.[166,167]

## EVALUATION OF CONGENITAL HEART DISEASE

Standard CT and EBCT are both useful techniques in the evaluation of patients with congenital heart disease. Anomalies of the aortic arch, septal defects, tetralogy of Fallot, Ebstein's anomaly, and abnormal arteriovenous connections can all be carefully evaluated with CT techniques.[168,169] (Fig. 20-32). EBCT, due to its high spatial resolution, can also evaluate the atrioventricular valves in conditions such as tricuspid and mitral valve atresia[170,171] and detect congenital abnormalities of the coronary arteries.[172] Beyond identifying structural abnormalities, EBCT can be used to accurately quantify intracardiac shunts,[173,174] assess right and left ventricular function,[10,12] measure myocardial mass,[6–8]

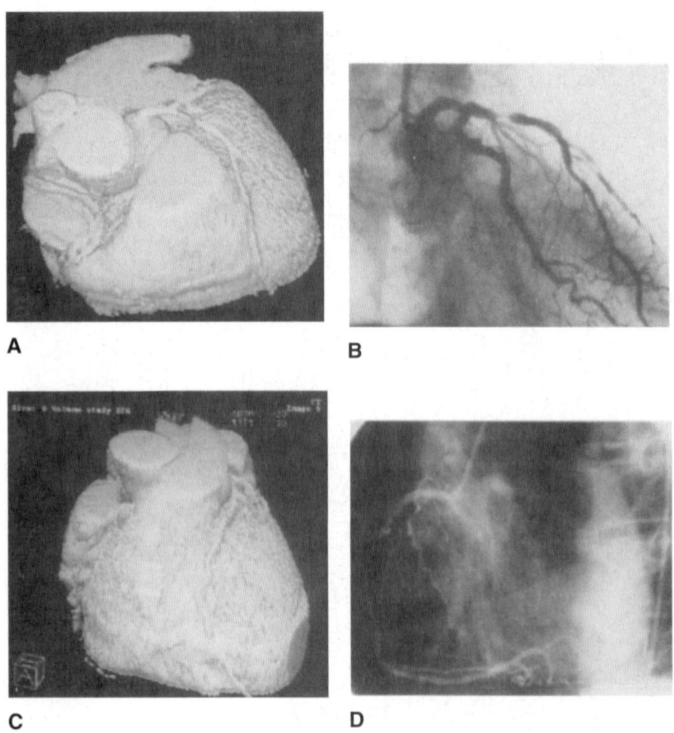


FIGURE 20-28 Three-dimensional EBCT reconstruction and coronary angiography depicting high-grade restenosis after coronary angioplasty of the proximal left anterior descending coronary artery (*A*, *B*) and right coronary artery (*C*, *D*). (From Achenbach et al.[157] Reproduced with permission from the publisher and authors.)

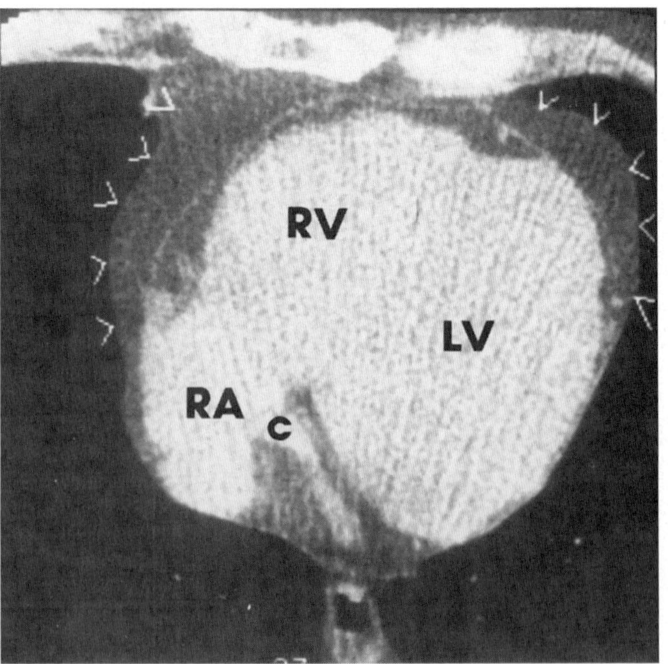


FIGURE 20-29 The fat that resides both inside and outside (*arrowheads*) the pericardium provides sufficient contrast to outline the normal pericardium, which is only 1 to 2 mm thick. Contrast enhancement with iodine agents is unnecessary. c = coronary sinus; LV = left ventricle; RA = right atrium; RV = right ventricle. (From Brundage BH, Mao SS. In: Schlant RC et al, eds. *Diagnostic Atlas of the Heart*. New York: McGraw-Hill; 1996:243. Reproduced with permission from the publisher and authors.)

and evaluate valvular function. Despite the application of CT in evaluating congenital heart disease, magnetic resonance imaging is the modality of choice, since it does not require x-ray exposure or the need for intravenous contrast for both structural and functional delineation.

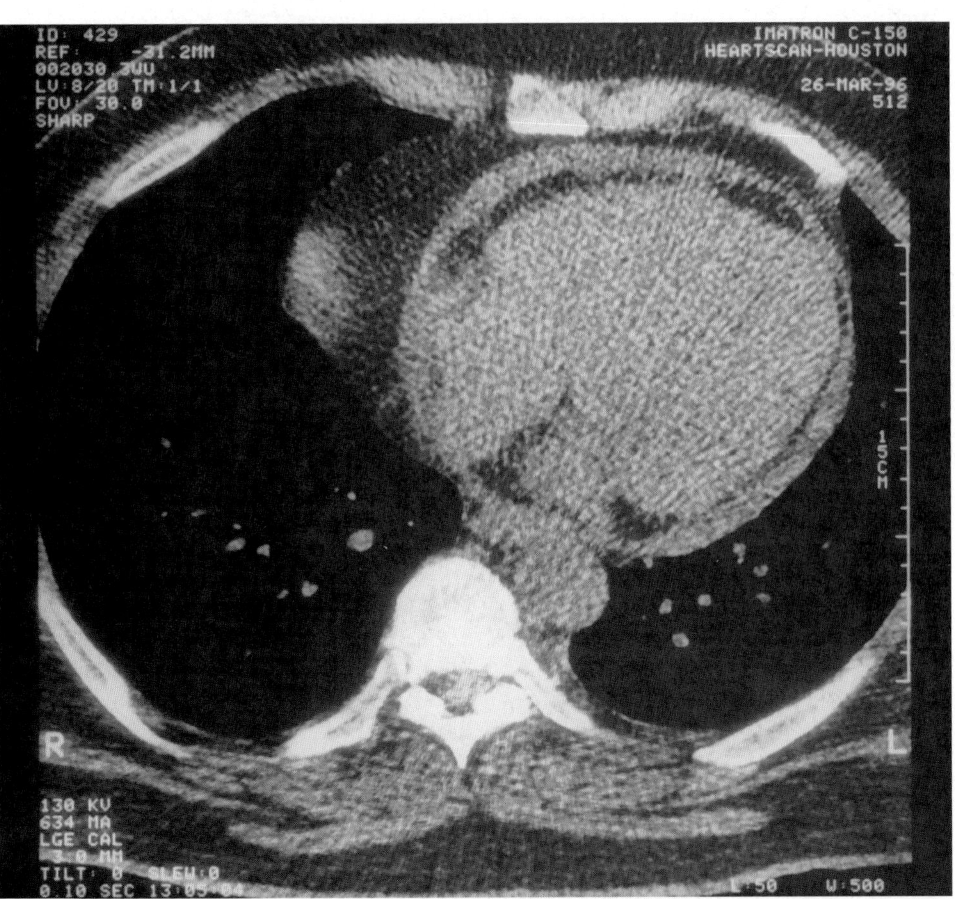


FIGURE 20-30 Diffuse pericardial thickening surrounding the entire heart in a patient with pericardial constriction.

## EVALUATION OF CARDIAC TUMORS

The presence and extent of intracardiac tumors can be well defined with either conventional CT or EBCT. CT scanning can also delineate metastatic tumor within the myocardial wall. Intracardiac tumors are readily detected by noninvasive two-dimensional echocardiography. Tumors such as myxomas, however, are also well visualized by EBCT, particularly when imaging is performed following intravenous contrast enhancement[175] (Fig. 20-33).

## DISEASES OF THE GREAT VESSELS

Conventional CT scanning is widely utilized for diagnosing thoracic aortic aneurysms and dissections.[176–178] With the introduction of spiral CT scanners, up to 60 images of approximately 2- to 3-mm thickness can be acquired within a single 30-s breathhold. A complete study of the thoracic aorta can be completed in only a few minutes. Following scan acquisition, three-dimensional reconstructions are readily produced, which can be rotated and viewed from multiple angulations to facilitate diagnosis. EBCT can also acquire rapid CT images with elimination of aortic pulsation as a cause of potential artifact.[179]

Aortic dissection is readily diagnosed with CT angiography with greater than 90 percent accuracy. In a recent study comparing spiral CT, magnetic resonance imaging, and two-dimensional echocardiography, CT and magnetic resonance imaging were shown to be superior to echocardiography in diagnostic accuracy.[178] Similar comparisons with EBCT are not available, but the increased imaging speed with EBCT over spiral CT would appear to be an advantage. Excellent definition of the intimal flap, false and true lumens, and the amount of intraaneurysmal thrombus can be determined.

CT scanning is also an effective method for diagnosing aortic aneurysm, defining its maximal diameter, and monitoring its expansion over time[179] (Fig. 20-34). CT scanning can diagnose traumatic aneurysms of the thoracic aorta,[177] sinus of Valsalva aneurysms, and coarctation of the aorta (Fig. 20-35). In patients undergoing "redo" coronary artery bypass surgery, CT scanning may guide the surgical approach by defining the position of the sternum to the right ventricle and aorta and thereby avoid unnecessary bleeding.[180]

Both spiral CT[181,182] and EBCT[183] can diagnose acute and chronic pulmonary thromboembolism (Fig. 20-36). CT scanning may be particularly useful in confirming the diagnosis of acute pulmonary embolism in patients with an intermediate nuclear ventilation perfusion scan.[182]

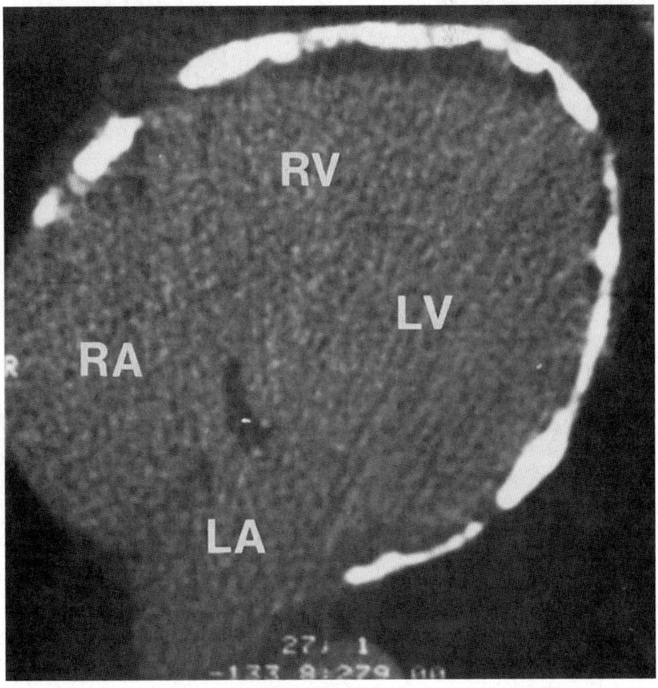


FIGURE 20-31 Densely calcified pericardium is easily identified in this scan of the mid-heart. LA = left atrium; LV = left ventricle; RA = right atrium; RV = right ventricle. (From Brundage BH, Mao SS. In: Schlant RC et al, eds. *Diagnostic Atlas of the Heart*. New York: McGraw-Hill; 1996:243. Reproduced with permission from the publisher and authors.)

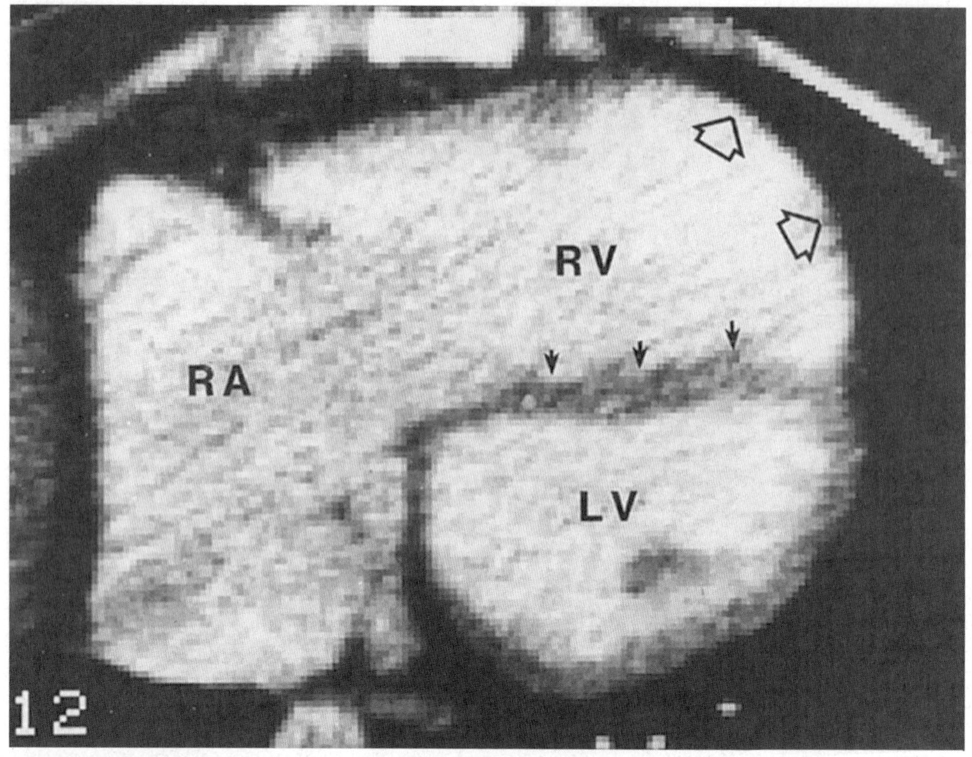


A

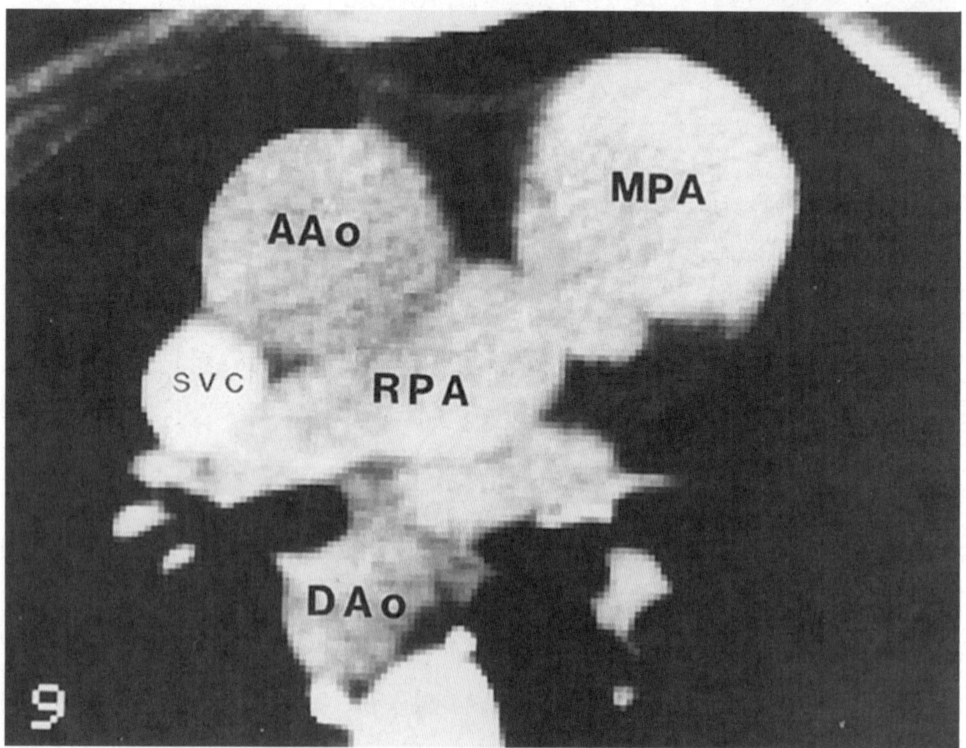


B

FIGURE 20-32 Postoperative EBCT study of a patient operated for tetralogy of Fallot demonstrates (*A*) right ventricular dilation and aneurysm (*open arrows*) with paradoxical diastolic flattening of the interventricular septum due to severe tricuspid regurgitation. The same study (*B*) revealed residual stenosis of the right pulmonary artery (RPA). AAo = ascending aorta; DAo = descending aorta; LV = left ventricle; MPA = main pulmonary artery; RA = right atrium; SVC = superior vena cava.

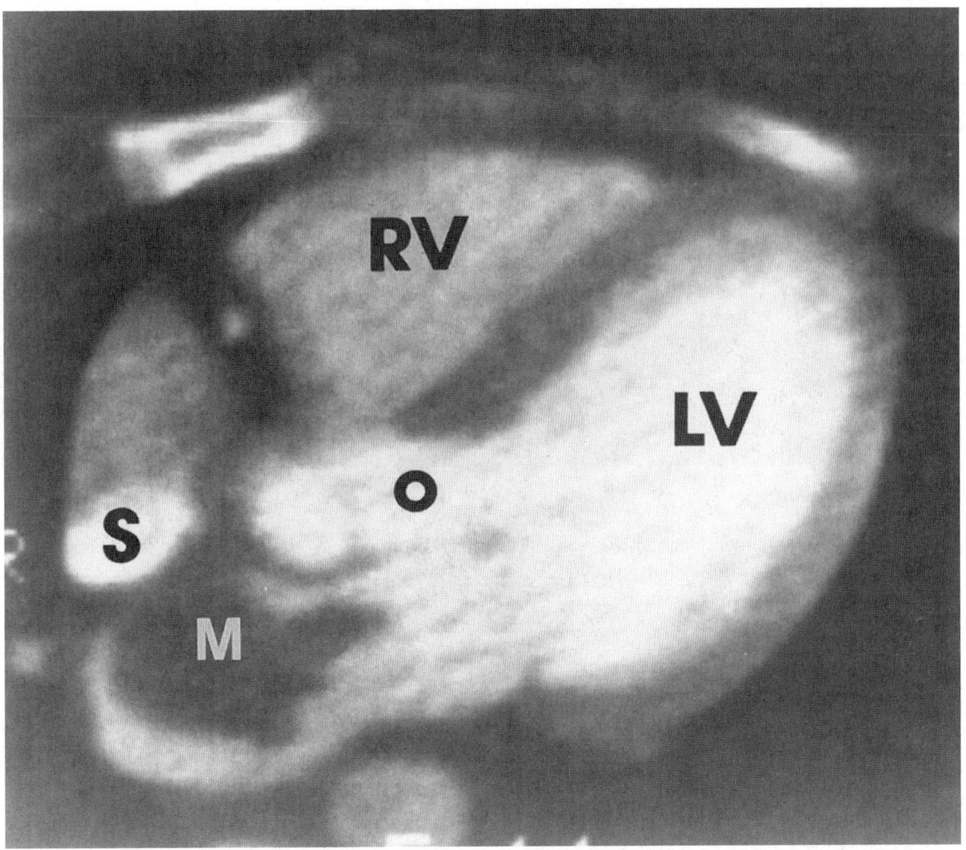


FIGURE 20-33 A single diastolic frame from a contrast-enhanced cine CT defines the left atrial septal attachment of a myxoma (M). The frond-like excrescences are characteristic of this tumor. LV = left ventricle; O = left ventricular outflow tract; RV = right ventricle; S = superior vena cava. (From Brundage BH, Mao SS. In: Schlant RC et al, eds. *Diagnostic Atlas of the Heart*. New York: McGraw-Hill; 1996:244. Reproduced with permission from the publisher and authors.)

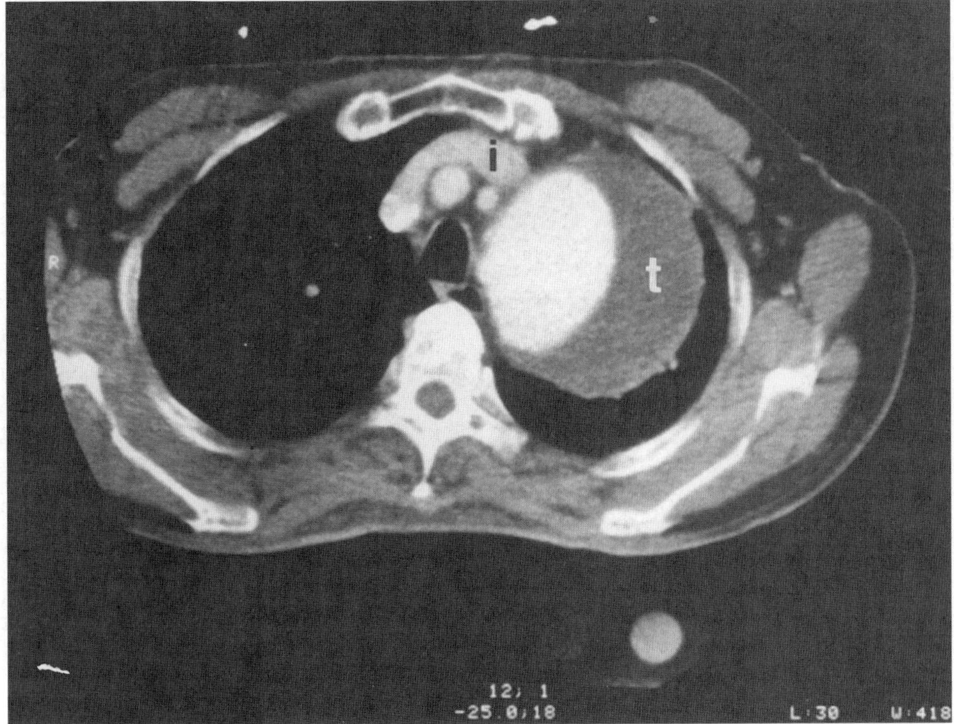


FIGURE 20-34 A large thrombus (t)-filled aneurysm of the aortic arch occupies most of the upper left thoracic cavity. The innominate vein (i) courses anterior to the innominate and left common carotid artery.

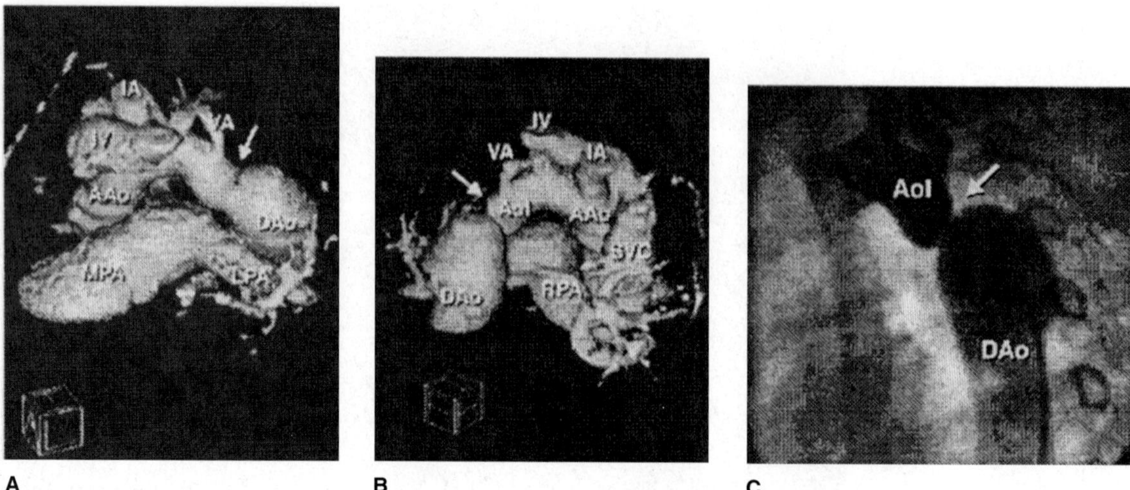


FIGURE 20-35 Three-dimensional EBCT reconstructions of aortic arch, innominate vein (IV), main (MPA), left pulmonary artery (LPA), and right pulmonary artery (RPA) in a patient with recurrent coarctation of the aorta. The upper panel (*A*) shows a possible web along the upper surface of the aortic isthmus (AoI) (*arrow*) with aneurysmal dilation of the descending aorta (DAo) below the coarctation site. The middle panel (*B*) shows a well-defined web (*arrow*). The corresponding aortogram (*C*) shows a discrete web below AoI with a DAo aneurysm. AAo = ascending aorta; IA = innominate artery; SVC = superior vena cava; VA = vertebral artery. (From Pitlick PT, Anthony CL, Moore P, et al. Three-dimensional visualization of recurrent coarctation of the aorta by electron-beam tomography and MRI. *Circulation* 1999;99:3086–3087. Reproduced with permission from the publisher and authors.)

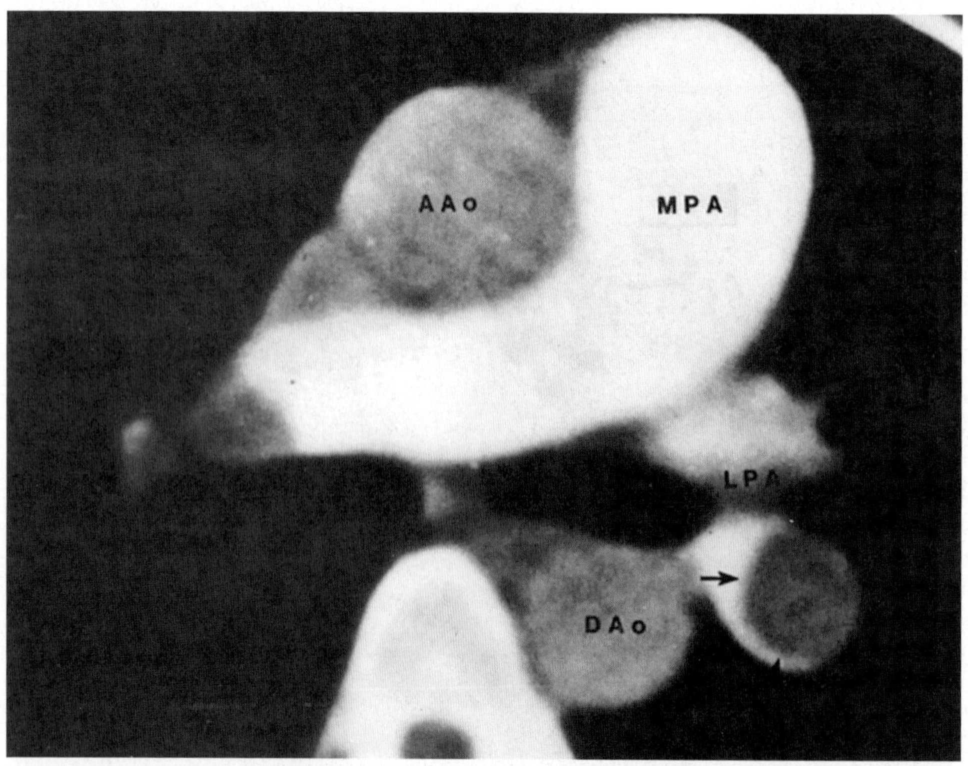


FIGURE 20-36 Large left pulmonary artery (LPA) chronic thrombus (*arrows*) is outlined by contrast medium on this high-resolution ultrafast CT scan. AAo = ascending aorta; DAo = descending aorta; MPA = main pulmonary artery.

## References


1. Boyd DP, Lipton MJ. Cardiac computed tomography. *Proc IEEE Nucl Sci* 1983;71:298–307.
2. Lu B, Mao SS, Zhuang N, et al. Coronary artery motion during the cardiac cycle and optimal ECG triggering for coronary artery imaging. *Invest Radiol* 2001;36:250–256.
3. Achenbach S, Ropers D, Holle J, et al. In-plane coronary arterial motion velocity. Measurement with electron-beam CT. *Radiology* 2000; 216:457–463.
4. McCollough CH, Zink FE, Morin RL. Radiation dosimetry for electron beam CT. *Radiology* 1994;192:637–642.
5. Horiguchi J, Nakanishi T, Ito K. Quantification of coronary artery calcium using multidetector CT and a retrospective ECG-gating reconstruction algorithm. *AJR* 2001;177:1429–1435.
6. Feiring AJ, Rumberger JA, Reiter SJ, et al. Determination of left ventricular mass in dogs with rapid-acquisition cardiac computed tomographic scanning. *Circulation* 1985;72:1355–1364.
7. Hajduczok ZD, Weiss RM, Stanford W, et al. Determination of right ventricular mass in humans and dogs with ultrafast cardiac computed tomography. *Circulation* 1990;82:202–212.
8. Roig E, Deorgiou D, Chomka EV, et al. Reproducibility of left ventricular myocardial volume and mass measurements by ultrafast computed tomography. *J Am Coll Cardiol* 1991;18:990–996.
9. Tada H, Shimizu W, Ohe T, et al. Usefulness of electron-beam computed tomography in arrhythmogenic right ventricular dysplasia. Relationship to electrophysiological abnormalities and left ventricular involvement. *Circulation* 1996;94:437–444.
10. Reiter SJ, Rumberger JA, Feiring AJ, et al. Precision of measurements of right and left ventricular volume by cine computed tomography. *Circulation* 1986;74:890–900.
11. Roig E , Chomka EV, Castaner A, et al. Exercise ultrafast computed tomography for the detection of coronary artery disease. *J Am Coll Cardiol* 1989;13:1073–1081.
12. Budoff MJ, Gillespie R, Georgiou D, et al. Comparison of exercise electron beam computed tomography and sestamibi in the evaluation of coronary artery disease. *Am J Cardiol* 1998;81:682–687.
13. Feiring AJ, Rumberger JA, Reiter SJ, et al. Sectional and segmental variability of left ventricular function: Experimental and clinical studies using ultrafast computed tomography. *J Am Coll Cardiol* 1988;12: 415–425.
14. Gerber TC, Behrenbeck T, Allison T, et al. Comparison of measurement of left ventricular ejection fraction by Tc-99m sestamibi first-pass angiography with electron beam computed tomography in patients with anterior wall acute myocardial infarction. *Am J Cardiol* 1999;83:1022–1026.
15. Hirose K, Reed JE, Rumberger JA. Serial changes in left and right ventricular systolic and diastolic dynamics during the first year after an index left ventricular Q wave myocardial infarction. *J Am Coll Cardiol* 1995;25:1097–1104.
16. Hirose K, Reed JE, Rumberger JA. Serial changes in regional right ventricular free wall and left ventricular septal wall lengths during the first 4 to 5 years after index anterior wall myocardial infarction. *J Am Coll Cardiol* 1995;26:394–400.
17. Chareonthaitawee P, Christian TF, Hirose K, et al. Relation of initial infarct size to extent of left ventricular remodeling in the year after acute myocardial infarction. *J Am Coll Cardiol* 1995;25:567–573.
18. Konstam MA, Rousseau MF, Kronenberg MW, et al. Effects of the angiotensin converting enzyme inhibitor enalapril on the long-term progression of left ventricular dysfunction in patients with heart failure. *Circulation* 1992;86:431–438.
19. Mahmarian JJ, Moye LA, Chinoy DA, et al. Transdermal nitroglycerin patch therapy improves left ventricular function and prevents remodeling after acute myocardial infarction: Results of a multicenter prospective randomized double-blind placebo controlled trial. *Circulation* 1998;97:2017–2024.
20. St. John Sutton M, Pfeffer MA, Plappert T, et al. Quantitative two-dimensional echocardiographic measurements are major predictors of adverse cardiovascular events after acute myocardial infarction. The protective effects of captopril. *Circulation* 1994;89:68–75.
21. Lipton MJ, Farmer DW, Killebrew EJ, et al. Regional myocardial dysfunction: Evaluation of patients with prior myocardial infarction with fast CT. *Radiology* 1985;157:735–740.
22. Tomoda H, Hoshiai M, Furuya H, et al. Evaluation of intracardiac thrombus with computed tomography. *Am J Cardiol* 1983;51: 843–852.
23. Lessick J, Sideman S, Azhari H, et al. Regional three-dimensional geometric ventricle with fibrous aneurysms: A cine computed tomography study. *Circulation* 1991;84:1072–1086.
24. Reiter SJ, Rumberger JA, Stanford W, et al. Quantitative determination of aortic regurgitant volume in dogs by ultrafast computed tomography. *Circulation* 1987;76:728–735.
25. Helgason CM, Chomka E, Louie E, et al. The potential role for ultrafast cardiac computed tomography in patients with stroke. *Stroke* 1989;20:465–472.
26. Mautner GC, Mautner SL, Froehlich J, et al. Coronary artery calcification: Assessment with electron beam CT and histomorphometric correlation. *Radiology* 1994;192:619–623.
27. Becker CR, Knez A, Jakobs TF, et al. Detection and quantification of coronary artery calcification with electron-beam and conventional CT. *Eur Radiol* 1999;9:620–624.
28. Budoff MJ, Mao S, Zalace CP, et al. Comparison of spiral and electron beam tomography in the evaluation of coronary calcification in asymptomatic persons. *Int J Cardiol* 2001;77:181–188.
29. Becker CR, Jakobs TF, Aydemir S, et al. Helical and single-slice conventional CT versus electron beam CT for the quantification of coronary artery calcification. *AJR* 2000;174:543–547.
30. Carr JJ, Crouse JR III, Goff DC Jr, et al. Evaluation of subsecond gated helical CT for quantification of coronary artery calcium and comparison with electron beam CT. *AJR* 2000;174:915–921.
31. Goldin JG, Yoon HC, Greaser III LE, et al. Spiral versus electron-beam CT for coronary artery calcium scoring. *Radiology* 2001;221:213–221.
32. Becker CR, Kleffel T, Crispin A, et al. Coronary artery calcium measurement: Agreement of multirow detector and electron beam CT. *AJR* 2001;176:1295–1298.
33. Knez A, Becker C, Becker A, et al. Determination of coronary calcium with multi-slice spiral computed tomography: A comparative study with electron-beam CT. *Int J Cardiovasc Imaging* 2002;18:295–303.
34. Rumberger JA, Simons DB, Fitzpatrick LA, et al. Coronary artery calcium area by electron-beam computed tomography and coronary atherosclerotic plaque area: A histopathologic correlative study. *Circulation* 1995;92:2157–2162.
35. Sangiorgi G, Rumberger JA, Severson A, et al. Arterial calcification and not lumen stenosis is highly correlated with atherosclerotic plaque burden in humans: A histologic study of 723 coronary artery segments using nondecalcifying methodology. *J Am Coll Cardiol* 1998;31: 126–133.
36. Janowitz WR, Agatston AS, Kaplan G, et al. Differences in prevalence and extent of coronary artery calcium detected by ultrafast computed tomography in asymptomatic men and women: Relation to age and risk factors. *Am J Cardiol* 1993;72:247–254.
37. Ikeda T Shirasawa T, Esaki Y, et al. Osteopontin mRNA is expressed by smooth muscle-derived foam cells in human atherosclerotic lesions of the aorta. *J Clin Invest* 1993;92:2814–2820.
38. Fitzpatrick LA, Severson A, Edwards WD, et al. Diffuse calcification in human coronary arteries: Association of osteopontin with atherosclerosis. *J Clin Invest* 1994;94:1597–1604.
39. Hirota S, Imakita M, Kohri K, et al. Expression of osteopontin messenger RNA by macrophages in atherosclerotic plaques: A possible association with calcification. *Am J Pathol* 1993;143:1003–1008.
40. Glagov S, Weisenberg BA, Zarins CK, et al. Compensatory enlargement of human atherosclerotic coronary arteries. *N Engl J Med* 1987;316:1371–1375.
41. Clarkson TB, Prichard RW, Morgan TM, et al. Remodeling of coronary arteries in human and non human primates. *JAMA* 1994;271: 289–294.

42. Agatston AS, Janowitz WR, Hildner FJ, et al. Quantification of coronary artery calcium using ultrafast computed tomography. *J Am Coll Cardiol* 1990;15:827–832.
43. Breen JF, Sheedy PF, Schwartz RS, et al. Coronary artery calcification detected with ultrafast CT as an indication of coronary artery disease. *Radiology* 1992;185:435–439.
44. Bielak LW, Kaufmann RB, Moll PP, et al. Small lesions in the heart identified at electron beam CT: Calcification or noise? *Radiology* 1994;192:631–636.
45. Kaufmann RB, Sheedy PF, Maher JE, et al. Quantity of coronary artery calcium detected by electron beam computed tomography in asymptomatic subjects and angiographically studied patients. *Mayo Clin Proc* 1995;70:223–232.
46. Rumberger JA, Sheedy PF, Breen JF, et al. Coronary calcium, as determined by electron beam computed tomography, and coronary disease on arteriogram. Effect of patient's sex on diagnosis. *Circulation* 1995; 91:1363–1367.
47. Braun J, Oldendorf M, Moshage W, et al. Electron beam computed tomography in the evaluation of cardiac calcification in chronic dialysis patients. *Am J Kidney Dis* 1996;27:394–401.
48. Budoff MJ, Georgiou D, Brody A, et al. Ultrafast computed tomography as a diagnostic modality in the detection of coronary artery disease. A multicenter study. *Circulation* 1996;93:898–904.
49. Detrano R, Hsiai T, Wang S, et al. Prognostic value of coronary calcification and angiographic stenoses in patients undergoing coronary angiography. *J Am Coll Cardiol* 1996;27:285–290.
50. Fallavollita JA, Brody AS, Bunnell IL, et al. Fast computed tomography detection of coronary calcification in the diagnosis of coronary artery disease. Comparison with angiography in patients <50 years old. *Circulation* 1994;89:285–290.
51. Baumgart D, Schmermund A, George G, et al. Comparison of electron beam computed tomography with intracoronary ultrasound and coronary angiography for detection of coronary atherosclerosis. *J Am Coll Cardiol* 1997;30:57–64.
52. Schmermund A, Baumgart D, Gorge D, et al. Coronary artery calcium in acute coronary syndromes: A comparative study of electron-beam computed tomography, coronary angiography, and intracoronary ultrasound in survivors of acute myocardial infarction and unstable angina. *Circulation* 1997;96:1461–1469.
53. Kennedy J, Shavelle R, Wang S, et al. Coronary calcium and standard risk factors in symptomatic patients referred for coronary angiography. *Am Heart J* 1998;135:696–702.
54. Bielak LF, Rumberger JA, Sheedy PF, et al. Probabilistic model for prediction of angiographically defined obstructive coronary artery disease using electron beam computed tomography calcium score strata. *Circulation* 2000;102:380–385.
55. Shavelle DM, Budoff MJ, LaMont DH, et al. Exercise testing and electron beam computed tomography in the evaluation of coronary artery disease. *J Am Coll Cardiol* 2000;36:32–38.
56. Haberl R, Becker A, Leber A, et al. Correlation of coronary calcification and angiographically documented stenoses in patients with suspected coronary artery disease: Results of 1,764 patients. *J Am Coll Cardiol* 2001;37:451–457.
57. Knollmann FD, Bocksch W, Spiegelsberger S, et al. Electron-beam computed tomography in the assessment of coronary artery disease after heart transplantation. *Circulation* 2000;101:2078–2082.
58. Rumberger JA, Sheedy PF, Breen JF, et al. Electron beam computed tomographic coronary calcium score cutpoints and severity of associated angiographic lumen stenosis. *J Am Coll Cardiol* 1997;29:1542–1548.
59. Guerci AD, Spadaro LA, Goodman KJ, et al. Comparison of electron beam computed tomography scanning and conventional risk factor assessment for the prediction of angiographic coronary artery disease. *J Am Coll Cardiol* 1998;32:673–679.
60. Budoff MJ, Diamond GA, Raggi P, et al. Continuous probabilistic prediction of angiographically significant coronary artery disease using electron beam tomography. *Circulation* 2002;105:1791–1796.
61. Schmermund A, Bailey KR, Rumberger JA, et al. An algorithm for noninvasive identification of angiographic three-vessel and/or left main coronary artery disease in symptomatic patients on the basis of cardiac risk and electron-beam computed tomographic calcium scores. *J Am Coll Cardiol* 1999;33:444–452.
62. He ZX, Hedrick TD, Pratt CM, et al. Severity of coronary artery calcification by electron beam computed tomography predicts silent myocardial ischemia. *Circulation* 2000;101:244–251.
63. Blumenthal RS, Becker DM, Moy TF, et al. Exercise thallium tomography predicts future clinically manifest coronary heart disease in a high-risk asymptomatic population. *Circulation* 1996;93: 915–923.
64. Fleg JL, Gerstenblith G, Zonderman AB, et al. Prevalence and prognostic significance of exercise-induced silent myocardial ischemia detected by thallium scintigraphy and electrocardiography in asymptomatic volunteers. *Circulation* 1990;81:428–436.
65. Iskandrian AS, Chae SC, Heo J, et al. Independent and incremental prognostic value of exercise single-photon emission computed tomographic (SPECT) thallium imaging in coronary artery disease. *J Am Coll Cardiol* 1993;22:665–670.
66. Hachamovitch R, Berman DS, Kiat H, et al. Exercise myocardial perfusion SPECT in patients without known coronary artery disease. Incremental prognostic value and use in risk stratification. *Circulation* 1996;93:905–914.
67. Olmos LI, Dakik H, Gordon R, et al. Long-term prognostic value of exercise echocardiography compared with exercise Tl-201, ECG, and clinical variables in patients evaluated for coronary artery disease. *Circulation* 1998; 98:2679–2686.
68. Iskander S, Iskandrian AE Risk assessment using single-photon emission computed tomographic technetium-99m sestamibi imaging. *J Am Coll Cardiol* 1998;32:57–62.
69. Miranda RS, Schisterman EF, Gallagher AM, et al. The extent of coronary calcium by electron beam computed tomography discriminates the likelihood of abnormal myocardial perfusion SPECT (abstr). *Circulation* 2000;102 (suppl II):II-543.
70. Ringqvist I, Fisher LD, Mock M, et al. Prognostic value of angiographic indices of coronary artery disease from the Coronary Artery Surgery Study (CASS). *J Clin Invest* 1983;71:1854–1866.
71. Emond M, Mock MB, David KR, et al. Long-term survival of medically treated patients in the Coronary Artery Surgery Study (CASS) Registry. *Circulation* 1994;90:2645–2657.
72. Goldstein JA, Demetriou D, Grines CL, et al. Multiple complex coronary plaques in patients with acute myocardial infarction. *N Engl J Med* 2000;343:915–922.
73. Huang H, Virmani R, Younis H, et al. The impact of calcification on the biomechanical stability of atherosclerotic plaques. *Circulation* 2001; 103:1051–1056.
74. Mascola A, Ko J, Bakhsheshi H, et al. Electron beam tomography comparison of culprit and non-culprit coronary arteries in patients with acute myocardial infarction. *Am J Cardiol* 2000;85:1357–1359.
75. Weiner DA, Ryan TJ, McCabe CH, et al. Significance of silent myocardial ischemia during exercise testing in patients with coronary artery disease. *Am J Cardiol* 1987;59:725–279.
76. Ekelund L-G, Suchindran CM, McMahon RP, et al. Coronary heart disease morbidity and mortality in hypercholesterolemic men predicted from an exercise test: The Lipid Research Clinics Coronary Primary Prevention Trial. *J Am Coll Cardiol* 1989;14:556–563.
77. Heller LI, Tresgallo M, Sciacca RR, et al. Prognostic significance of silent myocardial ischemia on a thallium stress test. *Am J Cardiol* 1990;65:718–721.
78. Detrano R, Hsiai T, Wang S, et al. Prognostic value of coronary calcification and angiographic stenoses in patients undergoing coronary angiography. *J Am Coll Cardiol* 1996;27:285–290.
79. Keelan PC, Bielak LF, Ashai K, et al. Long-term prognostic value of coronary calcification detected by electron-beam computed tomography in patients undergoing coronary angiography. *Circulation* 2001;104:412–417.
80. Secci A, Wong N, Tang W, et al. Electron beam computed tomographic coronary calcium as a predictor of coronary events: comparison of two protocols. *Circulation* 1997;96:1122–1129.

81. Detrano RC, Wong ND, Doherty TM. Coronary calcium does not accurately predict near-term future coronary events in high-risk adults. *Circulation* 1999;99:2633–2638.
82. Arad Y, Spadaro LA, Goodman K, et al. Predictive value of electron beam computed tomography of the coronary arteries. 19-month follow-up of 1173 asymptomatic subjects. *Circulation* 1996;93: 1951–1953.
83. Arad Y, Spadaro LA, Goodman K, et al. Prediction of coronary events with electron beam computed tomography. *J Am Coll Cardiol* 2000; 36:1253–1260.
84. Wong ND, Hsu JC, Detrano RC, et al. Coronary artery calcium evaluation by electron beam computed tomography and its relation to new cardiovascular events. *Am J Cardiol* 2000;86:495–498.
85. Raggi P, Callister TQ, Cooil B, et al. Identification of patients at increased risk of first unheralded acute myocardial infarction by electron-beam computed tomography. *Circulation* 2000;101:850–855.
86. Raggi P. Introduction. *Am J Cardiol* 2001;88(suppl):IE–3E.
87. Wayhs R, Zelinger A, Raggi P. High coronary artery calcium scores pose an extremely elevated risk for hard events. *J Am Coll Cardiol* 2002;39:225–230.
88. Callister TQ, Schisterman EF, Berman D, et al. Risk-adjusted mortality by extent of coronary calcification (abstr). *J Am Coll Cardiol* 2002; 39:447A.
89. Taylor AJ, Burke AP, O'Malley PG, et al. A comparison of the Framingham risk index, coronary artery calcification, and culprit plaque morphology in sudden cardiac death. *Circulation* 2000;101:1243–1248.
90. Park R, Detrano R, Xiang M, et al. Combined use of computed tomography coronary calcium scores and C-reactive protein levels in predicting cardiovascular events in nondiabetic individuals. *Circulation* 2002; 106:2073–2077.
91. Shepherd J, Cobbe SM, Ford I, et al. Prevention of coronary heart disease with pravastatin in men with hypercholesterolemia. *N Engl J Med* 1995;333:1301–1307.
92. Gordon DJ, Ekelund L-G, Karon JM, et al. Predictive value of the exercise tolerance test for mortality in North American men: The Lipid Research Clinics Mortality Follow-Up Study. *Circulation* 1986;74: 252–261.
93. Detrano RC, Wong ND, Tang W, et al. Prognostic significance of cardiac cinefluoroscopy for coronary calcific deposits in asymptomatic high risk subjects. *J Am Coll Cardiol* 1994;24:354–358.
94. Multiple Risk Factor Intervention Trial Research Group. Coronary heart disease death, nonfatal acute myocardial infarction and other clinical outcomes in the Multiple Risk Factor Intervention Trial. *Am J Cardiol* 1986;58:1–13.
95. Doherty TM, Tang W, Detrano RC. Racial differences in the significance of coronary calcium in asymptomatic black and white subjects with coronary risk factors. *J Am Coll Cardiol* 1999;34:787–794.
96. Budoff MJ, Yang TP, Shavelle RM, et al. Ethnic differences in coronary atherosclerosis. *J Am Coll Cardiol* 2002;39:408–412.
97. Downs JR, Clearfield M, Weis S, et al. Primary prevention of acute coronary events with lovastatin in men and women with average cholesterol levels: Results of AFCAPS/TexCAPS. Air Force/Texas Coronary Atherosclerosis Prevention Study. *JAMA* 1998;279;1615–1622.
98. Califf RM, Armstrong PW, Carver JR, et al. Task Force 5. Stratification of patients into high, medium and low risk subgroups for purposes of risk factor management. *J Am Coll Cardiol* 1996;27:1007–1019.
99. Wilson PWF, D'Agostino RB, Levy D, et al. Prediction of coronary heart disease using risk factor categories. *Circulation* 1998;97: 1837–1847.
100. Wong ND, Kouwabunpat D, Vo AN, et al. Coronary calcium and atherosclerosis by ultrafast computed tomography in asymptomatic men and women: Relation to age and risk factors. *Am Heart J* 1994;127: 422–430.
101. Newman AB, Naydeck BL, Sutton-Tyrrell K, et al. Coronary artery calcification in older adults to age 99. Prevalence and risk factors. *Circulation* 2001;104:2679–2684.
102. Hecht HS, Superko HR, Smith LK, et al. Relation of coronary artery calcium identified by electron beam tomography to serum lipoprotein levels and implications for treatment. *Am J Cardiol* 2001;87:406–412.
103. Kuller LH, Matthews KA, Sutton-Tyrrell K, et al. Coronary and aortic calcification among women 8 years after menopause and their premenopausal risk factors: The healthy women study. *Arterioscler Thromb Vasc Biol* 1999;19:2189–2198.
104. Hecht HS, Superko HR. Electron beam tomography and national cholesterol education program guidelines in asymptomatic women. *J Am Coll Cardiol* 2001;37:1506–1511.
105. Gibbons RJ, Balady GJ, Beasley JW, et al. ACC/AHA guidelines for exercise testing: A report of the American College of Cardiology/ American Heart Association Task Force on Practice Guidelines (Committee on Exercise Testing). *J Am Coll Cardiol* 1997;30:260–311.
106. Ritchie JL, Cheitlin MD, Garson A Jr, et al. Guidelines for clinical use of cardiac radionuclide imaging. Report of the American College of Cardiology/American Heart Association Task Force on Assessment of Diagnostic and Therapeutic Cardiovascular Procedures (Committee on Radionuclide Imaging), developed in collaboration with the American Society of Nuclear Cardiology. *J Am Coll Cardiol* 1995;25:521–547.
107. Rumberger JA, Brundage BH, Rader DJ, et al. Electron beam computed tomographic coronary calcium scanning: A review and guidelines for use in asymptomatic persons. *Mayo Clin Proc* 1999;74: 243–252.
108. O'Rourke RA, Brundage BH, Froelicher VF, et al. American College of Cardiology/American Heart Association Expert Consensus Document on electron-beam computed tomography for the diagnosis and prognosis of coronary artery disease. *J Am Coll Cardiol* 2000;36: 326–40.
109. Janowitz WR, Agatston AS, Viamonte M Jr. Comparison of serial quantitative evaluation of calcified coronary artery plaque by ultrafast computed tomography in persons with and without obstructive coronary artery disease. *Am J Cardiol* 1991;68:1–6.
110. Budoff MJ, Lane KL, Bakhsheshi H, et al. Rates of progression of coronary calcium by electron beam tomography. *Am J Cardiol* 2000; 86:8–11.
111. Callister TQ, Raggi P, Cooil B, et al. Effect of HMG-CoA reductase inhibitors on coronary artery disease as assessed by electron-beam computed tomography. *N Engl J Med* 1998;339:1972–1978.
112. Achenbach S, Ropers D, Pohle K, et al. Influence of lipid-lowering therapy on the progression of coronary artery calcification: A prospective evaluation. *Circulation* 2002;106:1077–1082.
113. Kajinami K, Seki H, Takekoshi N, et al. Quantification of coronary artery calcification using ultrafast computed tomography: Reproducibility of measurements. *Coron Artery Dis* 1993;4:1103–1108.
114. Devries S, Wolfkiel C, Shah V, et al. Reproducibility of the measurement of coronary calcium with ultrafast computed tomography. *Am J Cardiol* 1995;75:973–975.
115. Bielak LF, Kaufmann RB, Moll PP, et al. Small lesions in the heart identified at electron beam CT: Calcification or noise? *Radiology* 1994;192:631–636.
116. Yoon HC, Goldin JG, Greaser LE 3rd, et al. Interscan variation in coronary artery calcium quantification in a large asymptomatic patient population. *AJR* 2000;174:803–809.
117. Wang S, Detrano RC, Secci A, et al. Detection of coronary calcification with electron-beam computed tomography: Evaluation of interexamination reproducibility and comparison of three image-acquisition protocols. *Am Heart J* 1996;132:550–558.
118. Achenbach S, Ropers D, Mohlenkamp S, et al. Variability of repeated coronary artery calcium measurements by electron beam tomography. *Am J Cardiol* 2001;87:210–213.
119. Bielak LF, Sheedy PF, Peyser PA. Coronary artery calcification measured at electron-beam CT: Agreement in dual scan runs and change over time. *Radiology* 2001;218:224–229.
120. Mao S, Budoff MJ, Bakhsheshi H, et al. Improved reproducibility of coronary artery calcium scoring by electron beam tomography with a new electrocardiographic trigger method. *Invest Radiol* 2001;36: 363–367.
121. Callister TQ, Cooil B, Raya SP, et al. Coronary artery disease: Improved reproducibility of calcium scoring with an electron-beam CT volumetric method. *Radiology* 1998;208:807–814.

122. Maher JE, Bielak LF, Raz JA, et al. Progression of coronary artery calcification: A pilot study. *Mayo Clin Proc* 1999;74:347–355.
123. Blankenhorn DH, Azen SP, Kramasch DM, et al. Coronary angiographic changes with lovastatin therapy: The Monitored Atherosclerosis Regression Study (MARS). *Ann Intern Med* 1993;119:969–976.
124. Jukema JW, Bruschke AVG, van Boven AJ, et al. Effects of lipid lowering by pravastatin on progression and regression of coronary artery disease in symptomatic men with normal to moderately elevated serum cholesterol levels: The Regression Growth Evaluation Statin Study (REGRESS). *Circulation* 1995;91:2528–2540.
125. Bild DE, Bluemke DA, Burke GL, et al. Multi-ethnic study of atherosclerosis: Objectives and design. *Am J Epidemiol* 2002;156:871–881.
126. Budoff MJ, Shavelle DM, Lamont DH, et al. Usefulness of electron beam computed tomography scanning for distinguishing ischemic from nonischemic cardiomyopathy. *J Am Coll Cardiol* 1998;32:1173–1178.
127. Shemesh J, Tenenbaum A, Fisman EZ, et al. Coronary calcium as a reliable tool for differentiating ischemic from nonischemic cardiomyopathy. *Am J Cardiol* 1996;77:191–194.
128. McLaughlin VV, Balogh T, Rich S. Utility of electron beam computed tomography to stratify patients presenting to the emergency room with chest pain. *Am J Cardiol* 1999;84:327–328.
129. Laudon DA, Vukov LF, Breen JF, et al. Use of electron-beam computed tomography in the evaluation of chest pain patients in the emergency department. *Ann Emerg Med* 1999;33:15–21.
130. Georgiou D, Budoff MJ, Kaufer E, et al. Screening patients with chest pain in the emergency department using electron beam tomography: A follow-up study. *J Am Coll Cardiol* 2001;38:105–110.
131. Schmermund A, Baumgart D, Gorge D, et al. Coronary artery calcium in acute coronary syndromes: A comparative study of electron-beam computed tomography, coronary angiography, and intracoronary ultrasound in survivors of acute myocardial infarction and unstable angina. *Circulation* 1997;96:1461–1469.
132. Shemesh J, Stroh CI, Tenenbaum A, et al. Comparison of coronary calcium in stable angina pectoris and in first acute myocardial infarction utilizing double helical computerized tomography. *Am J Cardiol* 1998;81:271–275.
133. Schmermund A, Baumgart D, Adamzik M, et al. Comparison of electron-beam computed tomography and intracoronary ultrasound in detecting calcified and noncalcified plaques in patients with acute coronary syndromes and no or minimal to moderate angiographic coronary artery disease. *Am J Cardiol* 1998;81:141–146.
134. Stanford W, Brundage BH, MacMillan R, et al. Sensitivity and specificity of assessing coronary bypass graft patency with ultrafast computed tomography: Results of a multicenter study. *J Am Coll Cardiol* 1988;12:1–7.
135. Bateman TM, Gray RJ, Whiting JS, et al. Ultrafast computed tomographic evaluation of aortocoronary bypass graft patency. *J Am Coll Cardiol* 1986;8:693–698.
136. Bateman TM, Gray RJ, Whiting JS, et al. Prospective evaluation of ultrafast CT for determination of coronary bypass graft patency. *Circulation* 1987;75:1018–1024.
137. Brundage B, Lipton MJ, Herfkens RJ, et al. Detection of patent coronary artery bypass grafts by computed tomography: A preliminary report. *Circulation* 1980;61:826–831.
138. Tello R, Costello P, Ecker C, et al. Spiral CT evaluation of coronary artery bypass graft patency. *J Comput Assist Tomogr* 1993;17:253–259.
139. Ropers D, Ulzheimer S, Wenkel E, et al. Investigation of aortocoronary artery bypass grafts by multislice spiral computed tomography with electrocardiographic-gated image reconstruction. *Am J Cardiol* 2001; 88:792–795.
140. Reddy GP, Chernoff DM, Adams JR, et al. Coronary artery stenoses: Assessment with contrast-enhanced electron-beam CT and axial reconstructions. *Radiology* 1998;208:167–172.
141. Nakanishi T, Ito K, Imazu M, et al. Evaluation of coronary artery stenoses using electron-beam CT and multiplanar reformation. *J Comp Assist Tomog* 1997;21:121–127.
142. Schmermund A, Rensing BJ, Sheedy PF, et al. Intravenous electron-beam computed tomographic coronary angiography for segmental analysis of coronary artery stenoses. *J Am Coll Cardiol* 1998;31: 1547–1554.
143. Rensing BJ, Bongaerts A, van Geuns RJ, et al. Intravenous coronary angiography by electron beam computed tomography: A clinical evaluation. *Circulation* 1998;98:2509–2512.
144. Achenbach S, Moshage W, Ropers D, et al. Value of electron-beam computed tomography for the noninvasive detection of high-grade coronary-artery stenoses and occlusions. *N Engl J Med* 1998;339: 1964–1971.
145. Budoff MJ, Oudiz RJ, Zalace CP, et al. Intravenous three-dimensional coronary angiography using contrast enhanced electron beam computed tomography. *Am J Cardiol* 1999;83:840–845.
146. Achenbach S, Ropers D, Regenfus M, et al. Contrast enhanced electron beam computed tomography to analyse the coronary arteries in patients after acute myocardial infarction. *Heart* 2000;84: 489–493.
147. Leber AW, Knez W, Mukherjee R, White C, et al. Usefulness of calcium scoring using electron beam computed tomography and noninvasive coronary angiography in patients with suspected coronary artery disease. *Am J Cardiol* 2001;88:219–223.
148. Ropers D, Regenfus M, Stilianakis N, et al. A direct comparison of noninvasive coronary angiography by electron beam tomography and navigator-echo-based magnetic resonance imaging for the detection of restenosis following coronary angioplasty. *Invest Radiology* 2002;37: 386–392.
149. Knez A, Becker CR, Leber A, et al. Usefulness of multislice spiral computed tomography angiography for determination of coronary artery stenoses. *Am J Cardiol* 2001:88:1191–1194.
150. Achenbach S, Giesler T, Ropers D, et al. Detection of coronary artery stenoses by contrast-enhanced, retrospectively electrocardiographically-gated, multislice spiral computed tomography. *Circulation* 2001; 103:2535–2538.
151. Nieman K, Rensing BJ, vanGeuns R-JM, et al. Usefulness of multislice computed tomography for detecting obstructive coronary artery disease. *Am J Cardiol* 2002;89:913–918.
152. Vogl TJ, Abolmaali ND, Diebold T, et al. Techniques for the detection of coronary atherosclerosis: Multi-detector row CT coronary angiography. *Radiology* 2002;223:212–220.
153. Giesler T, Baum U, Ropers D, et al. Noninvasive visualization of coronary arteries using contrast-enhanced multidetector CT: Influence of Herat rate on image quality and stenosis detection. *AJR* 2002;179: 911–916.
154. Nieman K, Cademartiri F, Lemos PA, et al. Reliable noninvasive coronary angiography with fase submillimeter multislice spiral computed tomography. *Circulation* 2002;106:2051–2054.
155. Ropers D, Baum U, Pohle K, et al. Detection of coronary artery stenoses with thin-slice multi-detector row spiral computed tomography and multiplanar reconstruction. *Circulation* 2003;107:664–666.
156. Achenbach S, Giesler T, Ropers D et al. Comparison of image quality in contrast-enhanced coronary-artery visualization by electron beam tomography and retrospectively electrocardiogram-gated multislice spiral computed tomography. *Invest Radiol* 2003;38:119–128.
157. Achenbach S, Moshage W, Bachmann K. Detection of high-grade restenosis after PTCA using contrast-enhanced electron beam CT. *Circulation* 1997;96:2785–2788.
158. Pump H, Mohlenkamp S, Sehnert CA, et al. Coronary arterial stent patency: Assessment with electron-beam CT. *Radiology* 2000;214: 447–452.
159. Ropers D, Moshage W, et al. Visualization of coronary artery anomalies and their anatomic course by contrast-enhanced electron beam tomography and three-dimensional reconstruction. *Am J Cardiol* 2001; 87:193–197.
160. Ling LH, Oh JK, Tei C, et al. Pericardial thickness measured with transesophageal echocardiography: Feasibility and potential clinical usefulness. *J Am Coll Cardiol* 1997;29:1317–1323.
161. Isner JM, Carter BL, Bankoff MS, et al. Differentiation of constrictive pericarditis from restrictive cardiomyopathy by computed tomographic imaging. *Am Heart J* 1983;105:1019–1025.

162. Oren RM, Grover-McKay M, Stanford W, et al. Accurate preoperative diagnosis of pericardial constriction using cine computed tomography. *J Am Coll Cardiol* 1993;22:832–838.
163. Doppman JL, Rienmuller R, Lissner J, et al. Computed tomography in constrictive pericardial disease. *J Comput Assist Tomgr* 1981;5:1–11.
164. Tomoda H, Hoshiai M, Furuya H, et al. Evaluation of pericardial effusion with computed tomography. *Am Heart J* 1980;99:701–706.
165. Baim RS, MacDonald IL, Wise DJ, et al. Computed tomography of absent left pericardium. *Radiology* 1980;135:127–128.
166. Moncada R, Baker M, Salinas M, et al. Diagnostic role of computed tomography in pericardial heart disease: Congenital defects, thickening, neoplasms and effusions. *Am Heart J* 1982;103:263–282.
167. Glazer GM, Gross BH, Oringer MB, et al. Computed tomography of pericardial masses. *J Comput Assist Tomogr* 1984;8:895–899.
168. Farmer DW, Lipton MJ, Webb WR, et al. Computed tomography in congenital heart disease. *J Comput Assist Tomogr* 1984;8:677–687.
169. Webb WR, Gansu G, Speckman G, et al. CT demonstration of mediastinal aortic arch anomalies. *J Comput Assist Tomogr* 1982;6:445–451.
170. Eldridge WJ. Comprehensive evaluation of congenital heart disease using ultrafast computed tomography. In: Marcus ML, Schelbert HR, Skorton DJ, et al, eds. *Cardiac Imaging*. Philadelphia: Saunders; 1991:714.
171. Eldridge WJ, Flicker S, Steiner RM. Cine CT in the anatomical evaluation of congenital heart disease. In: Pohost G, Higgins CB, Morgenroth J, et al, eds. *New Concepts in Cardiac Imaging:* Vol 3. Chicago: Year Book; 1987:265.
172. MacMillan RM, Shakriari A, Sumithisena F, et a.: Contrast enhanced cine computed tomography for the diagnosis of right coronary to coronary sinus arteriovenous fistulae. *Am J Cardiol* 1985;56:997–998.
173. MacMillan RM , Rees MR, Eldredge WJ, et al. Quantitation of shunting at the atrial level using rapid acquisition computed tomography with comparison to cardiac catheterization. *J Am Coll Cardiol* 1986;7:946–948.
174. Skotvicki R , Maranhao V, Clark D, et al. Detection of atrial septal defect by cine CT scanning. *Catheter Cardiovasc Diagn* 1986;12:103–106.
175. Bateman TM, Sethna DH, Whiting JS, et al. Comprehensive noninvasive evaluation of left atrial myxoma using cardiac cine-computed tomography. *J Am Coll Cardiol* 1987;9:1180–1183.
176. Nienaber CA, von Kodolitsch Y, Nicolas V. The diagnosis of thoracic aortic dissection by noninvasive imaging procedures. *N Engl J Med* 1993;328:1–9.
177. Reardon MJ, Hedrick TD, Letsou GV, et al. CT reconstruction of an unusual chronic posttraumatic aneurysm of the thoracic aorta. *Ann Thorac Surg* 1997;64:1480–1482.
178. Sommer T, Fehske W, Holzknecht N, et al. Aortic dissection: A comparative study of diagnosis with spiral CT, multiplanar transesophageal echocardiography, and MR imaging. *Radiology* 1996;199:347–352.
179. Stanford W. Ultrafast computed tomography in the diagnosis of aortic aneurysms and dissections. *J Thorac Imaging* 1990;5:32–39.
180. Cremer J, Teebken OE, Simon A, et al. Thoracic computed tomography prior to redo coronary surgery. *Eur J Cardiothorac Surg* 1998;13:650–654.
181. Remy-Jardin M, Remy J, Deschildre F, et al. Diagnosis of pulmonary embolism with spiral CT: Comparison with pulmonary angiography and scintigraphy. *Radiology* 1996;200:699–706.
182. Mayo JR, Remy-Jardin M, Muller NL, et al. Pulmonary embolism: Prospective comparison of spiral CT with ventilation perfusion scintigraphy. *Radiology* 1997;205:447–452.
183. Teigen CL, Maus TP, Sheedy PF, et al. Pulmonary embolism diagnosis with contrast-enhanced electron-beam CT and comparison with pulmonary angiography. *Radiology* 1995;194:313–319.

C H A P T E R 21

# MAGNETIC RESONANCE IMAGING OF THE HEART

Michael Poon / Howard V. Dinh / Valentin Fuster



In 1945, Bloch and Purcell separately developed the technique of nuclear magnetic resonance (NMR) spectroscopy to analyze the composition of different chemical compounds.[1] This Nobel Prize–winning concept was introduced into the medical and pharmaceutical communities during the 60s and 70s through the contributions of Damadian and Lauterbur and other researchers.[2] The transition from the single dimension of NMR spectroscopy to the second dimension of spatial orientation formed the foundation of today's magnetic resonance imaging (MRI).

In the past two decades, advances in technology—such as the superconducting magnet and faster computers and software—have enabled this highly sophisticated tool to be used as a routine, noninvasive clinical instrument in many medical centers. In fact, MRI has become the imaging tool of choice when detailed morphologic assessment is required for the clinical decision-making process in areas such as brain, orthopedic, and spinal imaging. An important addition to this growing list has been the clinical application of MRI in the evaluation of cardiovascular diseases. More specifically, MRI has been developed to assess various facets of cardiovascular abnormalities, including but not limited to morphology, function, perfusion, and viability with ongoing clinical investigation into potential areas such as coronary, plaque, and interventional imaging. Given that the leading cause of death in the United States is related to atherosclerosis and that the "baby boomer" generation is fast approaching the age when ischemic heart disease may manifest itself silently, it is not surprising that noninvasive cardiovascular imaging has become one of the most important medical innovations of the past century.

This chapter focuses mainly on the clinical applications of cardiac magnetic resonance (CMR) today in a tertiary cardiac referral center and offers a brief review of the basic principles of magnetic resonance (MR) physics, image acquisition, and common CMR pulse sequences. The more inquisitive readers are encouraged to seek in-depth discussions on MR physics and pulse sequence analyses in specialized journals and dedicated textbooks. In addition, this chapter also touches on the practical aspects of patient care, including gating techniques, patient comfort, and contraindications to MRI.

## BASIC PRINCIPLES OF MRI

### MRI Physics

The physics of generating MRI depends on the random distribution of water and fat protons ($^1$H) within the body and the spin of those protons. Hydrogen is the most prevalent charged element in living tissues. The magnetic field created by a spinning proton is known as the magnetic dipole moment and is in the direction perpendicular to the rotation of the spin (Fig. 21-1). In the body, all the hydrogen protons normally spin in a random fashion and the sum of all the magnetic dipole moments cancel each other out. When an external magnetic field (Bo) is applied, the axes of the magnetic dipole moments will align in one of two energy states based on quantum mechanics. A dipole moment is considered parallel if it is aligned along the direction of Bo and antiparallel if opposite to the direction of Bo (Fig.

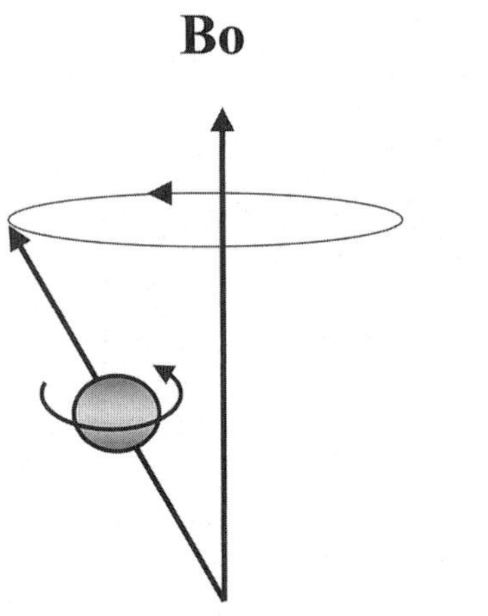


FIGURE 21-1 A spinning proton with its own magnetic dipole moment circling around an external magnet field (Bo).

21-2). The longitudinal magnetization created by placing protons in an external magnetic field cannot be detected by the receiving MR coils. In order to detect the physical presence of the protons in a given body of tissue, the longitudinal magnetization (aligned along the z axis) of the protons must be forced into the x-y plane. This is accomplished by the introduction of a weak electromagnetic wave, the radiofrequency (RF) pulse. The frequency of the RF pulse must match the precessional frequency of the spinning protons [i.e., Larmour frequency ($\omega$)], in order for the longitudinal magnetization to be "flipped." The flip angle ($\theta$), an MRI parameter, is the degree from the z axis that the longitudinal magnetization has been tipped. Its magnitude is dependent on both the frequency and duration of the RF pulse and typically ranges between <90 and 180 degrees, depending on the clinical application. After the RF pulse is given, the longitudinal magnetization is diminished and a new magnetization, called *transverse magnetization,* is generated by the precession of the protons in the x-y plane. Immediately after the transient RF pulse is

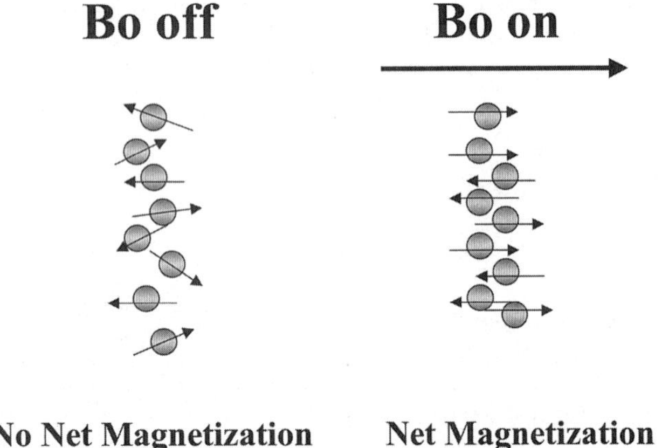


FIGURE 21-2 In the body, all the hydrogen protons are normally spinning in a random fashion and all the magnetic dipole moments, in sum, cancel each other out, resulting in no net magnetization (Bo off). When an external magnetic field (Bo on) is applied, the axes of the magnetic dipole moments will align in one of two energy states, either parallel or antiparallel, based on quantum mechanics.

turned off, exponential recovery and decay of the longitudinal and transverse magnetizations, respectively, occurs. The precession of protons in the x-y plane produces an MR signal, known as the *free-induction decay* (FID), which also decomposes exponentially. The frequency of these signals is then determined using a Fourier transform, and the amplitude in relation with time is calculated. MRI pulse sequences are programmed to sample, store, and process the FID signal so as to eventually reconstruct the MR image.

## Relaxation Time and MR Contrast

The recovery of longitudinal magnetization and the decay of transverse magnetization after the application of the RF pulse are commonly referred to as "relaxation" times—i.e., the time it takes for spins to return to their lowest energy states. The longitudinal relaxation time (T1) is the time it takes for spins to realign along the z axis (recovery of the longitudinal magnetization) or to give up the energy gained from the RF pulse excitation to the surrounding environment. T1 is thus dependent on interactions between the spins and the surrounding environment, also known as *the lattice*. T1 relaxation is also known as *spin-lattice relaxation*. For myocardium, the T1 is approximately 900 ms at 1.5-T field strength (and is less in a weaker magnetic field). The time it takes for the decay of the transverse magnetization is denoted by T2 relaxation (transverse relaxation). T2 relaxation is an exponential decay process caused by dephasing of spins in the x-y plane or the randomization of the phase of the spinning protons. This is secondary to the interactions between neighboring spins themselves (also known as *spin-spin relaxation*). The T2 for myocardium is about 80 ms. In reality, the FID (decay of the transverse magnetization) occurs at a much faster rate than that represented by the T2 time. This is the result of additional factors contributing to dephasing of the spins—namely, the fixed inhomogeneity of the external magnetic field and cardiac and respiratory motions. Therefore T2* (T2 "star") is the relaxation time that takes into account the T2 effect, the field inhomogeneity, and other environment factors; thus representing a more accurate measure of the FID. Different tissues have unique T1, T2, and T2* relaxations (Fig. 21-3). These unique physical properties of various tissues are used by the MRI technology to generate image contrasts, and the various pulse sequences are optimized to aid tissue characterization by focusing on the specific relaxation property of the tissue of interest, giving rise to the terms "T1 or T2 weighting."

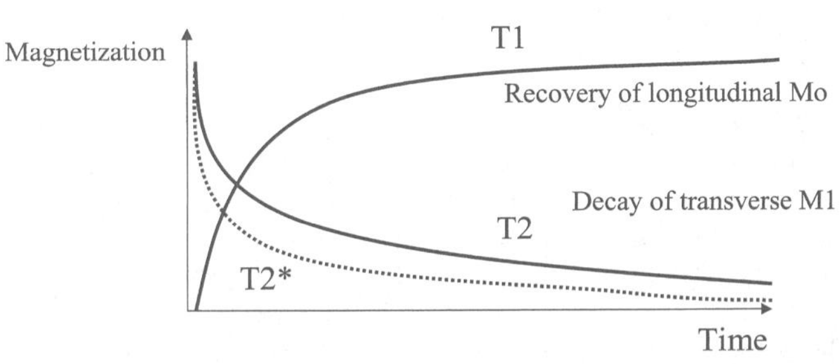


FIGURE 21-3 Three types of relaxation time (T1, T2, and T2*). T1 relaxation is the time it takes for spins to realign along the z axis (recovery of the longitudinal magnetization) or to give up the energy gained from the RF pulse excitation to the surrounding environment. T2 relaxation is an exponential decay process caused by dephasing of spins in the x-y plane or the randomization of the phase of the spinning protons. T2* relaxation is the relaxation time that takes into account both the T2 effect, the field inhomogeneity, and other environment factors.

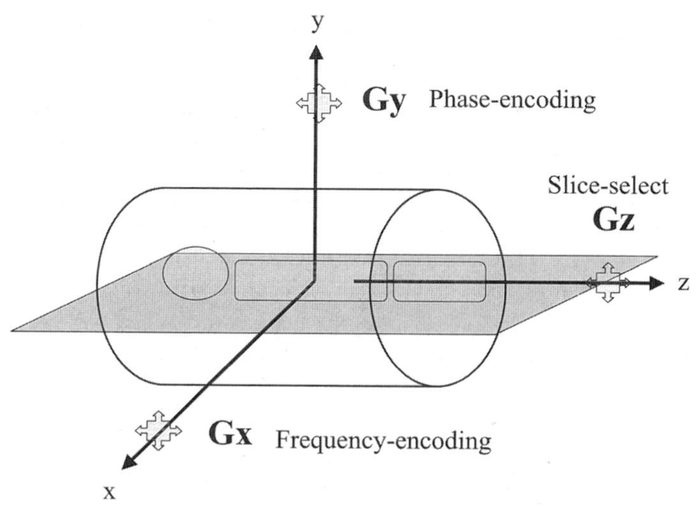


FIGURE 21-4 Three gradients are created by embedding the gradient coils in the main magnet bore. The gradients are arranged in the x, y, and z directions and are referred to as the Gx, Gy, and Gz. Gz, which runs in the craniocaudal direction, is referred to as the slice-select gradient, as MRI slices are based on the selection of the appropriate bandwidth that correlates to the frequency associated along the Gz gradient. Gx, which runs in the left-right direction, is known as the frequency-encoding gradient and is usually turned on during the readout of the echo (also known as "readout" gradient). Gy, which runs in the anteroposterior direction, is known as the phase-encoding gradient.

## Image Acquisition and Signal Processing

The sampled FID is the electromagnetic signal emanating from the entire body while in the magnet and does not contain any information regarding the specific position in the body from which the signal is coming. For an image to be created, signals must go through a series of complicated spatial encoding steps and signal processing. The first important step is the use of gradients to encode MR signals spatially. A *gradient* is a magnetic field that has a nonuniform distribution and shows a linear increase in field strength from one end to the other. The gradient is generated by gradient coils embedded in the main magnet bore. Typically, three gradients are created in the x, y, and z directions; they are referred to as the Gx, Gy, and Gz (Fig. 21-4). Gz, which runs in the craniocaudal direction, is referred to as the *slice-select gradient,* as MRI slices are based on the selection of the appropriate bandwidth that correlates to the frequency associated along the Gz gradient. Gx, which runs along the left-right direction, is known as the *frequency-encoding gradient* and is usually turned on during the readout of the echo. For this reason, it is sometimes referred to as the readout gradient. Gy, which runs along the anteroposterior direction, is known as the phase-encoding gradient. The three gradients are turned on and off at specific times to properly encode MR signals spatially. The assignments above are commonly used today, but in reality they are arbitrary and may be altered depending on the patient's orientation.

Once the MR signals are read, they are placed in a data matrix known as k-space. The stored data or signals are in the frequency domain and thus, they do not correlate to the actual MR image itself. In order to reconstruct the actual image, the Fourier transformation is applied to data in k-space in order to form the resultant MR image for clinical use.

## BASIC CARDIAC SEQUENCES

A pulse sequence is a series of computer instructions and algorithms that prepare and generate a MR signal. Pulse sequences utilizes a series of RF pulses and various applications of magnetic gradients to enhance or suppress tissue signals in order to obtain images with the desired contrast. There are many pulse sequences, of which spin-echo (SE) and gradient recall echo (GRE) sequences are the most commonly utilized in cardiac imaging.

### Spin Echo ("Dark Blood" Sequence)

The basic SE pulse sequence consists of a 90-degree excitation RF pulse followed by one or more 180-degree refocusing pulses. Recall that after the RF pulse is turned off, the FID (the MR signal) rapidly decomposes due to T2* effects (Fig. 21-5). The purpose of the 180-degree pulse is to allow the spins in the transverse plane (which are actively dephasing) to rephase and reform the signal, thus the term *echo*. The time between the 90-degree excitation RF pulse and the echo is denoted as *time of echo* (TE). This dual pair of excitation and rephasing pulses may be repeated as further spatial encoding is applied (via gradients). The time between one 90-degree RF to the next 90-degree RF is known as the *time to repetition* (TR). TE and TR times may be set by the computer and enhance important contrast

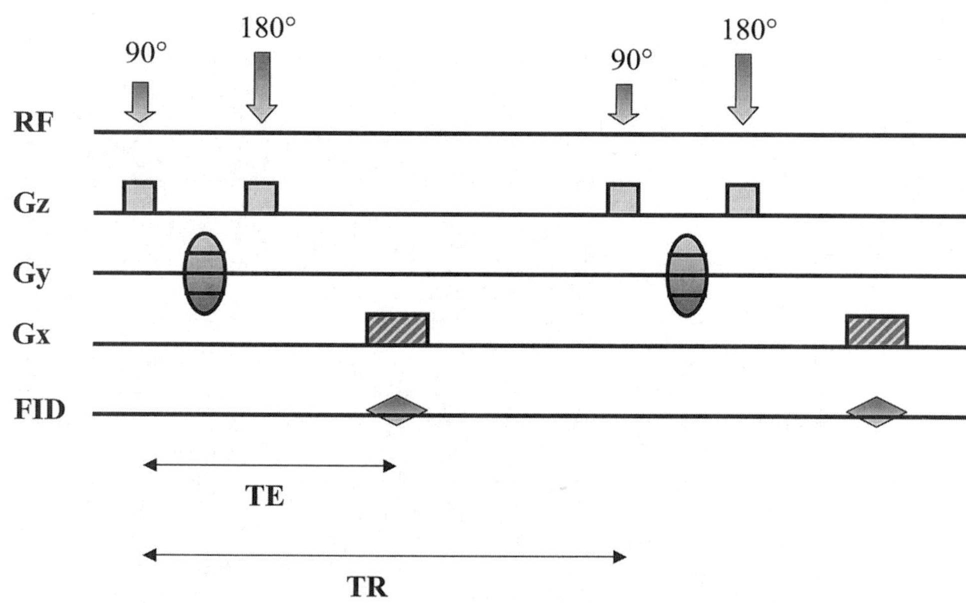


FIGURE 21-5 Diagrammatic representation of a typical spin-echo (SE) pulse sequence with its 90-degree excitation RF pulse followed by one or more 180-degree refocusing pulses. The time between the 90-degree excitation RF pulse and the echo is denoted as TE (time of echo). The time between one 90-degree RF to the next 90-degree RF is known as the TR (time to repetition).

characteristics between tissues being imaged based on the tissues' T1 and T2 characteristics (i.e., T1 and T2 weighting). In general, in SE sequences, short TE and TR times favor T1 weighting, whereas long TE and TR times favor T2 weighting.

SE sequences are also referred to as "dark blood" imaging because rapidly flowing blood moves out of the slice being excited and thus does not receive the 180-degree refocusing pulse. Therefore no echo is formed and the moving-blood signal void is represented as a dark image. In that regard, SE sequences provide great contrast between the blood pool and the surrounding tissues; as a result, they are commonly used in assessing cardiovascular morphology such as the pericardium, mediastinum, myocardium, and great vessels.

## Gradient Recall Echo ("Bright Blood" Sequence)

GRE sequences utilize a series of slice-selective RF pulses that have flip angles $\alpha$ (usually much less than the 90 degrees used in SE sequences) (Fig. 21-6). Because of the smaller flip angles, the recovery of longitudinal magnetization is faster and thus allows for much shorter TR and scanning times. In addition, no 180-degree refocusing pulses are used; instead, active dephasings and rephasings of the transverse magnetization are accomplished by the use of dual-polarity readout gradients to regenerate the FID. Because of the repeated use of multiple small flip-angled RF pulses that are slice-selective, flowing blood, which was initially outside of the imaging plane and thus has not been affected by the excitation, will have a higher longitudinal magnetization component to be flipped in the subsequent RF pulse. Compared to the stationary surrounding environment, which has been experiencing multiple flip-angle excitation, blood will carry a higher signal intensity; thus, GRE sequences produce images that display flowing blood as bright (i.e., "bright blood").

The shorter scanning time afforded by GRE sequences makes them ideal for imaging protocols where temporal resolution is of paramount importance. A variant of the basic GRE sequence is known as *echo-planar imaging* (EPI). In this sequence, instead of just one echo being recalled, a full set of rapid phase-encoded GREs are recalled through the use of a series of oscillating frequency-encoding gradients. EPI allows for a greater signal-to-noise ratio (SNR) and can dramatically reduce the imaging time (or better temporal resolution) depending on the length of the echo train. Currently, GRE sequences are utilized routinely in assessing ventricular function, cardiac perfusion, coronary artery imaging, valvular motion, and turbulent flow.

Other pulse sequences that are employed in cardiac imaging are not discussed in this chapter. Suffice to say that a good number of these sequences are simply variations of the SE and GRE sequences that allow for a greater reduction in scan time or that selectively enhance or null specific tissues of interest in order to achieve better contrast.

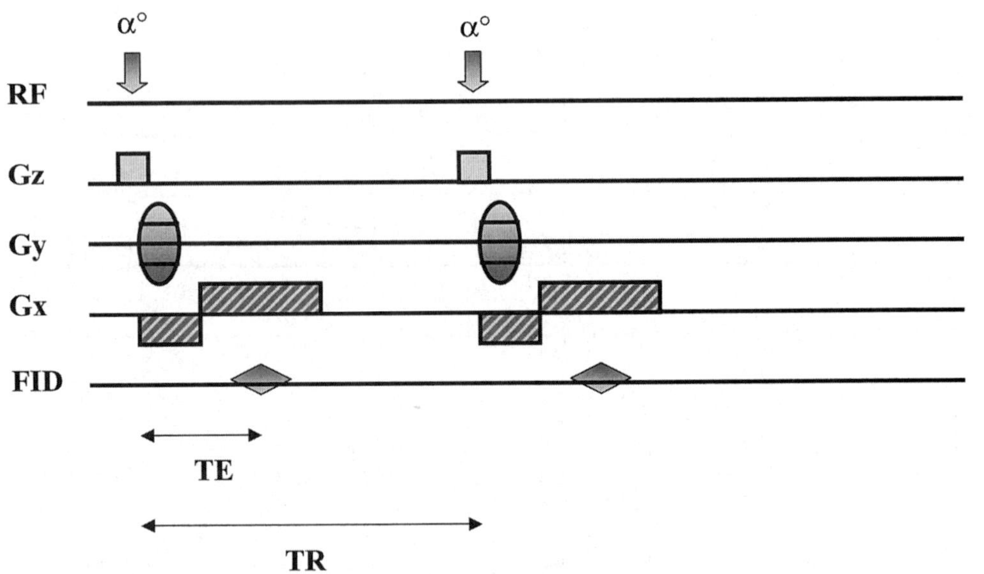


FIGURE 21-6 Diagrammatic representation of a typical GRE pulse sequence utilizing a series of slice-selective RF pulses that have a flip angle of $\alpha$ degrees (usually much less than the 90 degrees used in SE sequences).

# TECHNICAL ISSUES AND PATIENT SAFETY

Unlike other organs in the body, the heart is constantly in motion due to a combination of its own pulsation and the patient's respiratory activity. It is difficult to image such a rapidly moving target; however, various methods have been developed to do so. Cardiac motion can be "frozen" in time, to be imaged by using electrocardiography (ECG) for gating a specific point during the cardiac cycle. Furthermore, the acquisition of data for a specific image spans many cardiac cycles. This method, known as ECG-gated k-space segmentation, is commonly used. ECG gating is at times ineffective due to arrhythmia and artifacts, such as the so-called magnetohydrodynamic effects. In these situations, vector ECG or, more commonly, peripheral pulse gating may be used, with the caveat that in the latter method, the images are not acquired at the same time in the cardiac cycle as in ECG gating because of the delay between the R wave and the transmitted pulse.

Various methods are used to suppress respiratory motion artifacts. Of these, the most commonly used is breathholding, usually at end-expiration. However, many patients with respiratory problems, pulmonary hypertension, or heart failure may find it difficult to hold their breaths long enough for the image to be acquired; in such cases, respiratory bellows gating may be used. This technique involves placement of air-filled bellows between the chest wall and a rigid structure. A circumferential belt detects pressure changes due to chest wall movement, enabling acquisitions to be timed to a specific part of the pressure curve. A more advanced respiratory gating system involves navigator echoes. In this technique, RF excitations in high-contrast interfaces, such as the liver/lung or cardiac/lung borders, are used to gauge respiratory motion. Acquisition of images is then timed to a specific reference value in a manner similar to the technique of respiratory bellows gating outlined above.

Patient safety is particular important in an MR environment. Powerful magnetic fields can be hazardous due to their potential to move and/or dislodge metallic objects. RF fields can generate heat in metallic electrodes, wires, or devices. Cardiac patients with cardiac pacemakers, thermodilution catheters, and/or automatic implantable cardioverter defibrillators (AICDs) cannot be exposed to an MR

TABLE 21-1 Common Absolute and Relative Contraindications to the Use of MRI

- Absolute contraindications
  - Central nervous system aneurysm clips
  - Implantable electronic devices (automatic implantable cardioverter defibrillator, artificial pacemakers)
  - Pacer wires
  - Metallic inner ear implants
  - Ocular metallic fragments/chips
  - Metallic insulin pumps
  - Metal shrapnel or bullet
  - Hemodynamically unstable patients
- Relative contraindications
  - Claustrophobia
  - Pregnant women
  - Patients requiring cumbersome life-support equipment (depends on institution and accommodation of MRI suite)
  - Patients unable to cooperate or having excessive movement disorders (who cannot be sedated)

environment. On the other hand, patients with sternal wires, modern mechanical prosthetic heart valves, or coronary stents are not contraindicated. Table 21-1 is a list of absolute and relative contraindications to MR.

## BASIC CARDIAC EVALUATION

### Cardiac Function

At present, CMR is a highly accurate and effective imaging modality in the assessments of global and regional cardiac function and is being increasingly recognized as the "gold standard" for the noninvasive evaluation of cardiac function.[3,4] Already hailed as the gold standard for the assessment of left ventricular end-diastolic (EDV) and end-systolic volumes (ESV) and ejection fraction (EF), CMR provides accurate and reproducible tomographic, static, and cine images of high spatial and temporal resolution in any desired plane without exposing patients to ionizing radiation or nephrotoxic contrast agents.[5,6]

In order to achieve adequate resolution images of cardiac function, 7 to 10 separate cine GRE acquisitions in the short-axis and 2 or 3 in the long-axis are usually required.[7] The segmented fast low-angle shot (FLASH) technique is part of the routine protocol for evaluating left and right ventricular dimensions and function. Patients are required to hold their breaths in 15- to 20-s intervals with at least 10 to 12 breathholds.[7,8] However, with recent advances in MRI technology, spoiled GRE FLASH images have fallen out of favor due to their relatively low image quality. Decreased minimum repetition times and greater gradient performance have led to more successful implementations of fast imaging with steady-state precession (FISP).[9,10] While GRE FLASH imaging relies on inflow enhancement for image contrast, true FISP sequences depend on the ratio of T2 to T1 and thus offer higher contrast-to-noise ratios and superior image quality (Fig. 21-7). Lee et al. have developed a real-time true FISP imaging technique that is configured to acquire cine images at a series of section positions in one breathhold that will enable cardiac function, mass, and volume to be measured with greater speed and clarity.[7]

### Cardiac Anatomy

A unique feature of SE "black blood" images is that rapidly flowing blood appears dark while stagnant tissues appear brighter. The SE sequence is also relatively insensitive to magnetic field inhomogeneities produced by small metallic implants like vascular stents and clips. Compared with GRE, a SE sequence offers greater tissue contrast but a lower imaging speed. Its main clinical application is in the anatomic delineation of the pericardium and cardiac mediastinum, along with vessel structures, and the assessment of infiltrative heart diseases and cardiac tumors.[11]

## VALVULAR HEART DISEASE

The ideal assessment of valvular heart disease includes the following critical goals. First, the morphology of the valvular apparatus and associated cardiac structures must be clearly defined. Second, valvular stenosis or regurgitation must be detected and preferably quantified. Third, the structural changes of the various cardiac chambers and great vessels as well as the functional changes of the ventricular chambers must be accurately determined. To those ends, CMR has emerged as a highly useful and comprehensive diagnostic tool. Cardiac valvular dysfunction may be evaluated via the use of SE, GRE, and phase-contrast (velocity mapping) sequences. SE and GRE images provide a reasonable approach for determining the number of leaflets, the degree of excursion, and approximate leaflet thickness as well as overall chamber size and cardiac function. Furthermore, GRE and phase-contrast sequences are highly sensitive for the detection of

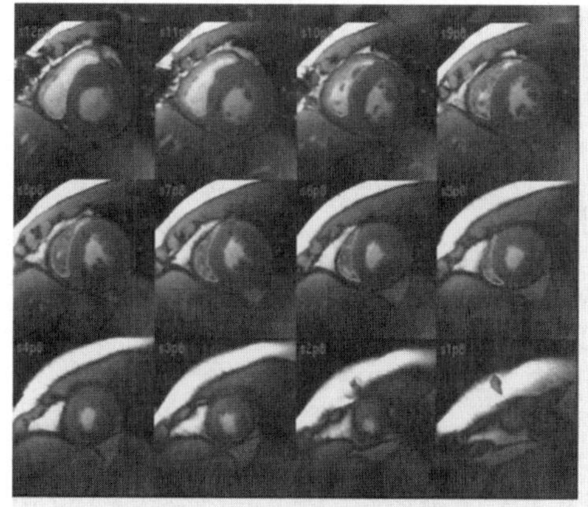

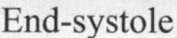

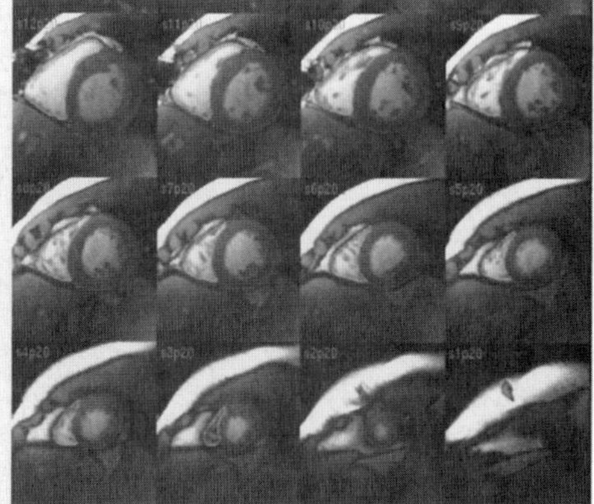


FIGURE 21-7 Determination of LV and RV ejection fraction by CMR. Twelve separate cine GRE acquisitions in the short axis of the end-systole and end-diastole were taken for the calculation of the ejection fraction based on the modified Simpson rule.

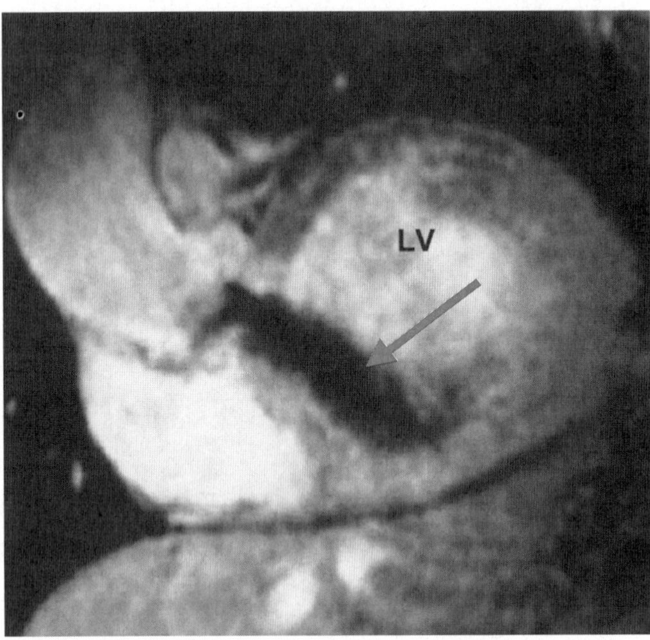


FIGURE 21-8 GRE sequence showing signal void due to high-velocity turbulent regurgitant flow (*blue arrow*) into the left ventricle (LV) as a result of severe aortic regurgitation.

stenotic and regurgitant jets and allow for the calculation of flow velocity through valvular orifices. From these data, major clinical parameters may be derived, such as flow volume, regurgitant fraction, pressure gradients, and estimates of valvular area.

## Valvular Regurgitation

Regurgitant valves allow backflow of blood, leading to volume overload and resulting in dilatation of the involved cardiac chambers. Chronic severe regurgitation involving either the aortic and/or mitral valves leads to left ventricular dilatation and dysfunction. The deterioration of cardiac function may occur insidiously; thus timely detection and accurate quantification of the severity of regurgitation, the resultant strain on the heart, and the effects on its dimensions is critical in the medical management and timing of surgical treatment. The severity of valvular dysfunction can be assessed by two MR methods: GRE and phase-contrast imaging. Using GRE technique, the chaotic motion of turbulent regurgitant flow results in dephasing and consequently in a reduction of MR signal within a high-intensity blood pool (bright blood) (Fig. 21-8). The territory of MR signal void corresponds to the area of color Doppler signal by echocardiography.[12,13] The degree and extent of the signal void is dependent on many factors, including the severity of the turbulent flow, direction of regurgitation, and acquisition parameters such as TE, TR, sampling size of the imaged volume element (voxel), and/or orientation of the imaging plane relative to the flow jet.[14,15] Thus, signal voids caused by valvular turbulent blood flow are indicative of the presence of regurgitation but may not be representative of its true severity. Regurgitant volumes and regurgitant fraction can be determined by measuring right ventricular (RV) and left ventricular (LV) stroke volumes and thus determining the severity of regurgitation—assuming that regurgitant lesions involve only one side (RV or LV).[16,17] In such a situation, the ventricle with the regurgitant valve will have to pump an excessive volume of blood per cardiac cycle.

Phase-contrast imaging can be used to assess the severity of regurgitation as well. In this imaging method, flow direction is encoded by varying the magnetic phases of the blood either in or through an image plane. Thus, information regarding velocity and flow of jets may be calculated based on the differences in the magnetic phase of flowing blood (Fig. 21-9). With phase contrast, there are two ways of assessing the regurgitant volume and fraction. The first calculates the difference in the stroke volume (derived from phase contrast) through the great vessels and that derived from volumetric calculations based on the MR modified Simpson method. This difference is the regurgitant volume. Note that this works only if there is a single regurgitant source (valve) for the ventricle of interest. Alternatively, phase contrast can be used to assess both forward and reverse flow, with the latter giving rise to the regurgitant volume, from which the regurgitant fraction may be derived as a percentage of the total systolic forward flow.

## Valvular Stenosis

GRE imaging can be used to approximate the degree of aortic stenosis by observing the extent of turbulent flow (signal loss) in the ascending aorta.[18] However, this method provides only a cursory assessment. A more accurate method involves the use of GRE sequences with a small field of view and slices selected axially through the aortic valve (with slice thickness reduced to about 2 to 4 mm). In this way, the end-systolic valve opening area may be quantified directly by commonly available software (Fig. 21-10).

The severity of a stenotic aortic valve can also be assessed using phase-contrast imaging for flow velocities up to 5 m/s.[18] In this way, the severity of aortic stenosis can be assessed more reliably, as the pressure gradient across the valve can be computed from the velocity of flow (modified Bernoulli equation).

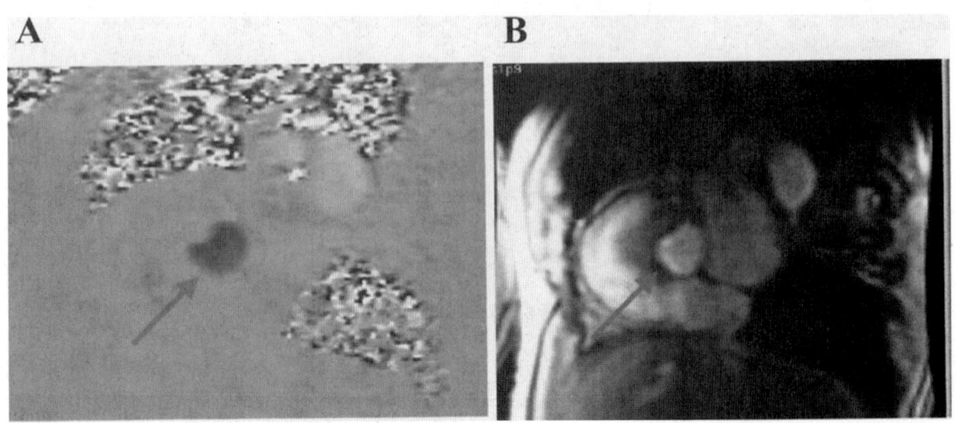


FIGURE 21-9 *A.* Phase-contrast imaging of severe aortic regurgitation in a short-axis view. The arrow points to the velocity-encoded cine image during diastole, demonstrating regurgitant flow into the left ventricle. *B.* Magnitude image of showing bright regurgitant blood flow (*arrow*) in the same short-axis view at the level of the aortic valve.

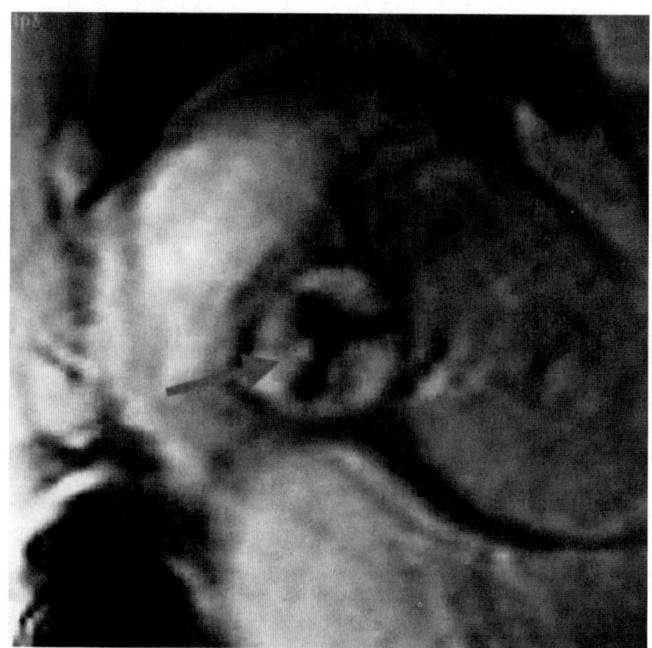

FIGURE 21-10 Visualization of a stenotic aortic valve using a small field-of-view GRE sequence in a short axial slice across the valve. Signal drop-off (*arrow*) occurs due to high turbulent flow along the leaflets of the stenotic trileaflet aortic valve.

## ISCHEMIC HEART DISEASE

Myocardial dysfunction, more commonly known as heart failure, is a common clinical problem affecting over 4.5 million patients in the United States. This number is expected to increase continuously as the average age of the general population continues to rise. Ischemic heart disease is a major cause of myocardial dysfunction. Over the past 30 years, many noninvasive cardiac imaging modalities have been developed to detect this common cause of sudden death and disability in the United States. Current noninvasive imaging techniques focusing on various important surrogate markers of ischemic myocardium—such as abnormalities in microvascular blood flow, contractile or perfusion reserve, and metabolic activity—have become an important part of diagnostic evaluation in clinical cardiology. Recent advancements in both MR hardware and software development have allowed CMR to emerge as an efficient, versatile imaging tool for the assessment of ischemic heart disease.

### Rest Cine Images of Cardiac Function

An essential feature of normal myocardium includes the preservation of normal contractile function. Viable myocardium may appear dysfunctional as a result of either acute reversible ischemic insults (myocardial stunning) or a chronic, gradual decrease in blood supply (hibernating myocardium). Thinning of the myocardial wall at rest is a reliable feature of scarred tissue resulting from extensive myocardial injury and remodeling. Systolic wall thickening at rest or during dobutamine stress of greater than 2 mm, as determined by ECG-gated breathhold MR cine sequences, is considered a reliable marker of viability.[19] Measuring wall thickness during end-diastole, Baer et al. reported a cutoff value of 5.5 mm as the lower limit of myocardial wall thickness for the presence of viable myocardium.[20] A similar relationship between wall thickness as determined by CMR and viability was noted using improvement in postrevascularization functional wall motion or thallium-201 uptake as markers of viability.[21–23] Thus, significant myocardial thinning or lack of endocardial thickening are reliable indicators of nonviable myocardial tissue.

### Stress Cine Imaging with Dobutamine

Like dobutamine stress echocardiography (DSE), dobutamine stress CMR evaluates an important parameter of muscle viability, i.e., contractile reserve. Low- and high-dose DSE images are useful for the assessment of myocardial viability. A biphasic response in which myocardial contractility is increased at low dose and decreased at high dose is considered a good predictor of recovery of cardiac function following revascularization.[24,25] Compared to echocardiography, cine CMR provides greater accuracy in the assessment of wall thickening due to its superior spatial and contrast resolution (Fig. 21-11).[26–29] Low-dose dobutamine stimulation with the infusion of 5 to 10 μg/kg/min together with cine CMR has been shown to be a reliable means of differentiating viable from nonviable myocardium. Higher doses of dobutamine (up to 40 μg/kg/min), with or without the addition of atropine at the peak dose of dobutamine, are used mainly to evaluate patients for coronary stenosis or cardiac ischemia. Using the results of coronary angiography as a reference standard, Nagel et al. reported both a sensitivity and specificity of 86 percent with high-dose dobutamine in detecting significant coronary artery disease.[30] When dobutamine cine CMR was combined with first-pass and late contrast enhancement, the sensitivity and specificity of the combined CMR modality increased further to 97 and 96 percent, respectively.[19] Failure of myocardial contractile augmentation in response to low-dose dobutamine stimulation does not necessarily exclude the presence of viable myocardial tissue, because a larger quantity of viable myocytes is needed to maintain contractile reserve than to achieve significant uptake of radionuclide tracer.[31]

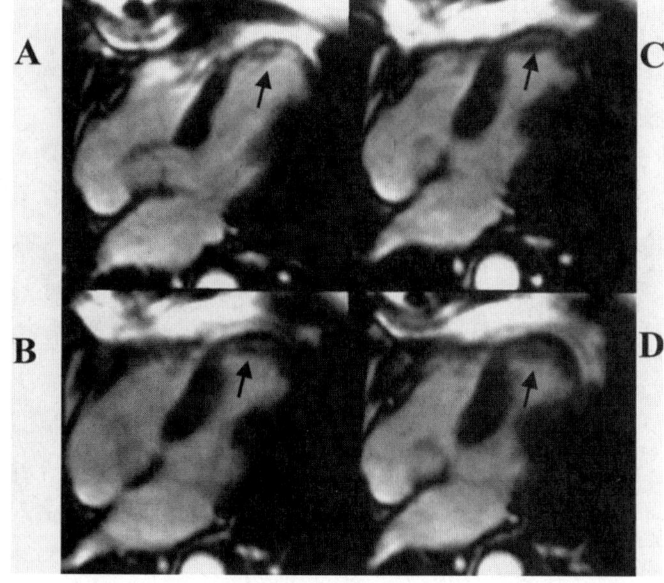


FIGURE 21-11 Dobutamine stress MR with escalating doses of intravenous dobutamine (A, B, C, and D = 5, 10, 20, and 40 μg/kg/min, respectively) showing apical hypokinesis and augmentation of septal and lateral wall thickening at high doses of dobutamine.

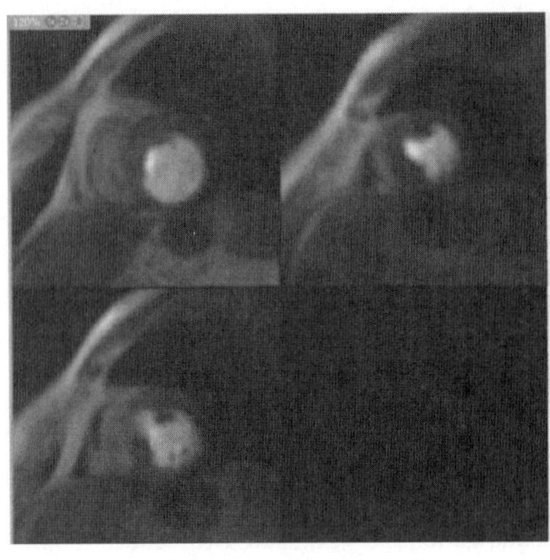


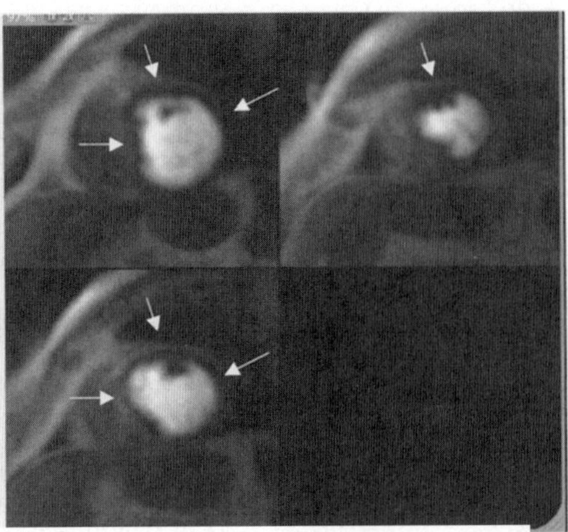


FIGURE 21-12 Rest and stress perfusion study with adenosine showing hypoperfusion (*white arrows*) involving the anteroseptal, anterolateral, and anteroapical walls in response to adenosine infusion.

## Adenosine Stress MR for Evaluation of Perfusion Reserve

Gadolinium (Gd-DTPA) is useful as a contrast and perfusion agent. Gd-DTPA containing extracellular contrast is administered through a peripheral vein. The functional significance of any coronary artery lesion can be evaluated based on the effect on blood flow at rest and during stress testing using standard vasodilator agents. Viable myocardium exhibits gradual signal enhancement and washout with the passage of the T1-enhancing contrast agent (Fig. 21-12). New or old infarcted myocardium exhibits decreased signal enhancement (hypoenhancement) on the first-pass images and hyperenhancement on the delayed images (5 to 15 min after injection of Gd-DTPA).[32] The addition of adenosine stress further accentuates the baseline perfusion defect in hibernating myocardium and helps differentiate normal from near-normal regions in stunned myocardium. Analogous to the detection of contractile reserve with low-dose dobutamine, vasodilator-induced perfusion defects detect myocardial perfusion reserve. Currently, the assessment of cardiac stress perfusion using CMR is mostly limited to specialized centers with the latest MR hardware and software, which offer very high temporal and spatial resolution for the routine clinical evaluation of cardiac stress and rest perfusion in a consistent and reproducible fashion. Furthermore, the lack of user-friendly post-processing software and tools for quantitative analysis of cardiac perfusion have also limited the popularity and everyday clinical application of CMR in the assessment of stress cardiac perfusion.

## Evaluation of Cardiac viability Using CMR

T1 weighted images acquired 5 to 30 min after the administration of an intravenous bolus of gadopentate dimeglumine (Gd-DTPA) demonstrate the presence of necrosis as areas with increased signal intensity, a phenomenon that has been termed *delayed hyperenhancement*. Retention of contrast agent in the myocardium indicates the presence of nonviable myocardium regardless of the age of the infarct (Fig. 21-13). In an experimental model, the presence of either early hypoenhancement or delayed hyperenhancement transmurally closely correlated with the loss of contractile reserve in response to low-dose dobutamine challenge.[33] Kim et al. correlated the percent transmural extent of late enhancement with the recovery of systolic wall thickening after surgical or percutaneous revascularization.[34] The smaller the area of late enhancement, the higher the probability of mechanical improvement. All the current conventional ultrasound- and radionuclide-based imaging modalities for the assessment of cardiac viability share one major limitation in that none can assess the transmural extent of viability in a damaged myocardium.

## "One-Stop-Shop" Comprehensive Evaluation of Myocardial Perfusion and Function

MRI as a single imaging modality is capable of assessing cardiac function, perfusion, and viability—a task that, in the past, usually required both scintigraphy and echocardiology. In a study comparing MRI with fluorodeoxyglucose positron emission tomography (FDG-PET) in the assessment of cardiac viability, Lauerma et al. reported that the combination of dobutamine stress, first-pass perfusion, and late contrast enhancement was the best approach for detecting cardiac viability in patients with multivessel coronary artery disease.[19] Poon et al. have recently proposed a combined "one-stop-shop" approach in the assessment of global and regional wall motion as well as the presence and extent of viable myocardium and perfusion at rest

FIGURE 21-13 Delayed hyperenhancement showing transmural (*A*) and subendocardial (*B*) scarring involving the inferorlateral (*A*) and inferior (*B*) walls.

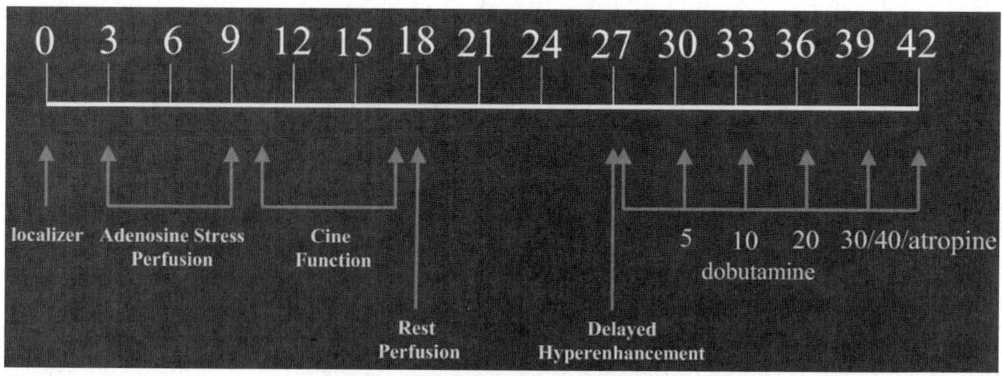


FIGURE 21-14 "A one-stop-shop" comprehensive evaluation of myocardial perfusion, viability, and function by CMR.

with pharmacologic stress in patients with ischemic heart disease (Fig. 21-14).[35]

## PULMONARY HYPERTENSION

The clinical workup of pulmonary hypertension (PH) can be enormously costly and time-consuming. Pulmonary artery pressures can be estimated with echocardiography by measuring the velocities of regurgitant jets through either the tricuspid or pulmonic valve, but there is wide variation in the literature in the reported accuracy of this method, ranging from 53 to 97 percent.[36,37] Problems with geometric assumptions and subsequent magnification of imaging errors, operator variability, and difficult acoustic windows have made echo less than optimal for use in this group of patients.[38] CMR is particularly useful in the evaluation of patients with severe PH as a result of its high-resolution imaging of RV morphology and function. Quantitative changes in the chamber size, the presence of cardiac mass, pericardial or pleural effusion, and septal deformity can be identified and may explain the cause and severity of PH and RV failure (Fig. 21-15). Furthermore, MRI can be an important diagnostic modality in ruling out secondary causes of PH such as valvular heart diseases, coexisting pulmonary parenchymal disorders, pericardial and infiltrative myocardial diseases, cardiac tumors or extracardiac masses, and various congenital and structural heart diseases (most of these entities are discussed elsewhere in this chapter). Finally, time-resolved contrast-enhanced magnetic resonance angiography (MRA) is extremely valuable in the functional assessment of pulmonary vascular abnormalities and cardiac shunts, which are also important causes of PH (Fig. 21-16). Patients with chronic PH show pathologic changes in the pulmonary vasculature, most commonly central pulmonary artery dilatation and peripheral pulmonary artery pruning (Fig. 21-17).

Accurate assessment of RV morphology can be obtained with ECG-gated SE sequences and ECG-gated, breathhold GRE sequences. Quantitative analysis of RV function is performed from dynamic cine images in the short-axis views using Simpson's rule (similar to the method described above for LV function assessment). Quantitative MR parameters such as RV mass and stroke volume in patients with PH have been studied in small populations and shown good correlation with the severity of pulmonary artery pressure. In an animal study, Katz et al. showed that MRI was able to quantify the mass of excised calf RV with a high degree of accuracy as compared to direct weighing (correlation coefficient of 0.97).[39] Patients with PH ($n = 13$) have a mean RV mass more than twice that of normal subjects ($p < 0.01$); furthermore, these mass measurements correlate positively with mean pulmonary artery pressures ($r = 0.75$, $p < 0.01$) as measured by right heart catheterization. Marcus et al. found that, in eight patients with PH secondary to chronic obstructive pulmonary disease (COPD), the mean RV mass was 17 percent greater ($p < 0.005$) than that in age-match normal controls.[40] In addition, there were statistically significant increases in RV wall thickness and decreases in RV stroke volume, indicative of the physiologic burden on RV function exerted by elevated pulmonary artery pressures. The differences in the MR volumetric parameters between normal and PH patients are summarized in Table 21-2.

The position of the ventricular septum at end-diastole is an important marker of ventricular function and biventricular interplay.[41] Normally, the septum is slightly convex (or "bowed") toward the RV in end-diastole. However, with severe PH, the bowing of the septum reverses toward the LV. This so-called leftward ventricular septal bowing (LVSB) (Fig. 21-15) was assessed in human patients with PH. Abnormal septal deformity is a noninvasive parameter that may

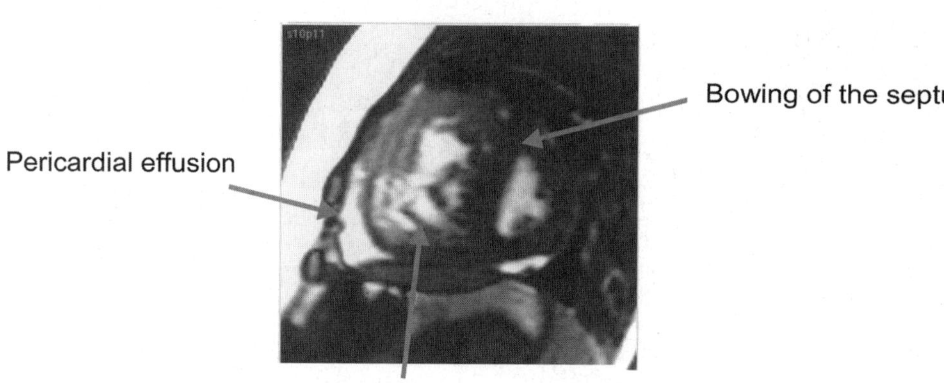


FIGURE 21-15 Poor prognosticators of severe pulmonary hypertension shown on CMR: Bowing of the interventricular septum, right ventricular hypertrophy, and the presence of pericardial effusion.

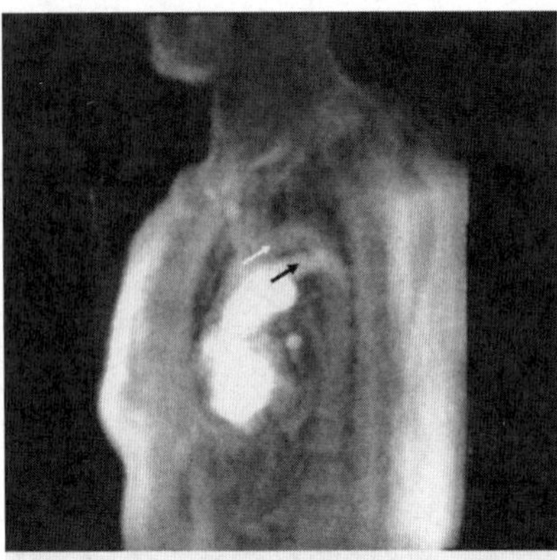


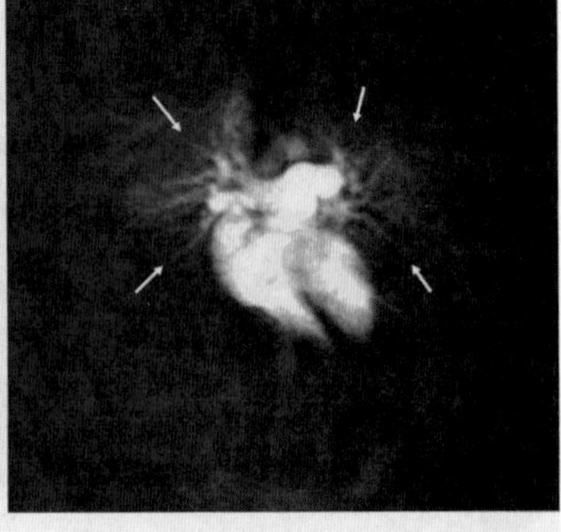


FIGURE 21-16 Time-resolved contrast-enhanced MRA of the thorax *A.* LAO projection of a patient with severe pulmonary hypertension due to an unrestricted ventricular septal defect resulting in Eisenmanger's syndrome. The picture shows the presence of a right-to-left shunt with filling of the aorta (*white arrow*) and the main pulmonary artery (*black arrow*) with contrast simultaneously. *B.* Coronal projection of a patient with a history of multiple pulmonary embolisms with multiple filling defects (*white arrows*).

be an important surrogate marker of severe PH and may prove useful in following patients' responses to various treatments.[42]

Interstitial and chronic obstructive lung diseases are an important cause of secondary PH. At present, the imaging of the lung parenchyma is performed using conventional x-ray–based modalities (chest roentgenograms and computed tomography). A few MR centers have been exploring the use of inhaled or aerosolized contrast agents such as oxygen, gadolinium chelates, sulfur hexaflouride, perfluorcarbons, helium-3, and xenon-129 to demonstrate lung morphology, gas exchange, and ventilation abnormalities.[43] This technology has advanced tremendously and it is anticipated that it will play a role in the clinical diagnosis of ventilation defects.

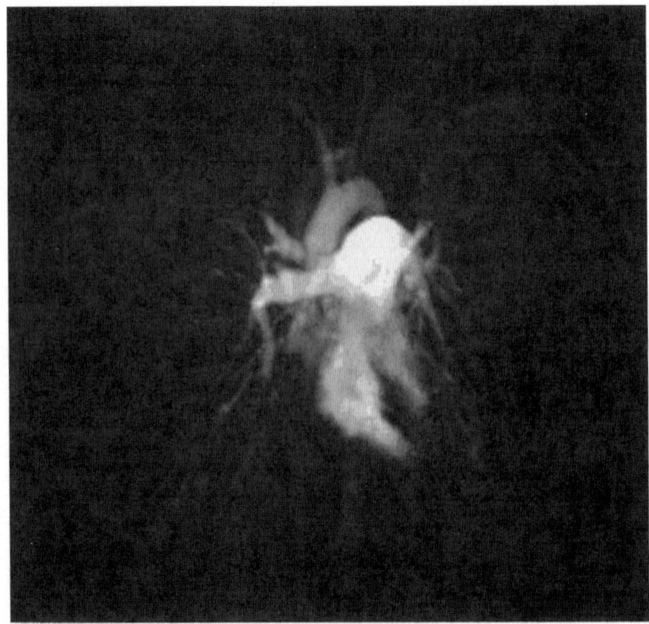

FIGURE 21-17 Time-resolved contrast-enhanced MRA of the thorax. Coronal projection of a patient with severe primary pulmonary hypertension showing enlarged main pulmonary artery, pruning of the peripheral pulmonary vessels, and hypoperfusion of the lung parenchyma.

## CARDIOMYOPATHY

MRI is a valuable tool in the assessment of cardiomyopathy because of its superior spatial and contrast resolution and large and unlimited field of view, which can help to determine the underlying cause of this common medical problem. Furthermore, its excellent reproducibility and non-operator-dependent image quality confer important advantages over more conventional noninvasive methods.

### Hypertrophic Cardiomyopathy

CMR allows an unobstructed view of the entire myocardium and its surrounding structures and correlates well with echocardiography and x-ray cine-ventriculography in delineating the precise site and extent of hypertrophy (Fig. 21-18).[44,45] CMR's unique ability to distinguish various tissue types based on their particular magnetic properties makes it possible to distinguish cardiac infiltrative disease from normal hypertrophy of the heart (Fig. 21-19). Apical hypertrophy, for example, may be difficult to visualize by conventional echocardiography but is readily distinguished by MRI.[46,47]

Functional MRI with GRE sequences [four-chamber and LV outflow tract views) may be used to assess the extent of turbulent flow (signal loss) in the LV outflow tract and the presence of systolic anterior motion of the anterior mitral valve leaflet, which signify the presence of dynamic LV outflow tract obstruction. Furthermore, quantitative assessment of the extent of the outflow tract obstruction and the thickness of the asymmetric septal hypertrophy can be determined using the short-axis SE sequences performed in end-systole across the outflow tract.

### Dilated Cardiomyopathy

Dilated cardiomyopathy can result from a myriad of disease processes and is typically characterized by biventricular and often biatrial enlargement with depressed global systolic function. MRI provides a noninvasive method for accurately determining RV and/or LV end-systolic and end-diastolic volumes, stroke volume, ejection fraction, thrombus, and/or valve dysfunction. Segmental wall thinning and regional dysfunction suggest a coronary artery disease etiology, whereas diffuse myocardial hypocontractility and dilatation are more likely infectious in origin.

Dilated cardiomyopathy may be a result of myocardial inflammation, whether infectious or toxic, or the progressive replacement of normal myocytes with fibrotic tissue. Both acute inflammation and fibrosis can be detected by contrast (gadolinium) enhanced MRI, presumably due to a combination of increased diffusion into necrotic cells, delayed contrast washin and washout kinetics, and increased vascularity (in the setting of acute inflammation). Studies have shown that contrast-enhanced SE sequences were able to detect patients with significant inflammation such as acute and Chagas myocarditis. Delayed hyperenhancement technique is also being utilized to detect chronic fibrosis and scarring.

TABLE 21-2 MR Characteristics Suggestive of Severe Pulmonary Hypertension

| | Normal [68] | Severe Pulmonary Hypertension[39,40,69] |
|---|---|---|
| Volumetric parameters | | |
| Mean RV ejection fraction | 61 ± 7% | 34 ± 10% |
| Mean RV mass | 46 ± 11 g | 109.6 ± 27 g |
| Anatomic parameters | | |
| RV wall thickness | Normal | Hypertrophied |
| End-diastolic septal bowing | Toward the RV | Toward the LV |
| Pulmonary artery (PA) | Normal | Dilated main PA, pruning of the peripheral pulmonary vessels |
| Functional parameters | | |
| MR angiography | Normal | In situ pulmonary artery thrombus or peripheral perfusion defect |

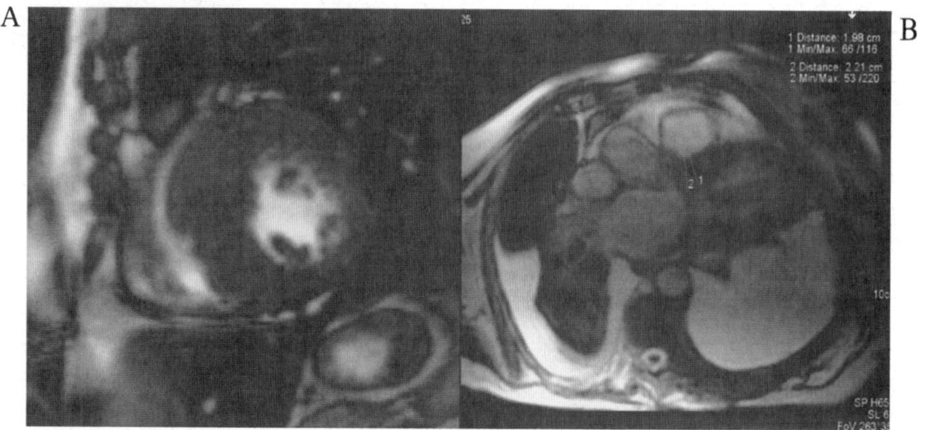


FIGURE 21-18 CMR of hypertrophic cardiomyopathy showing asymmetrical hypertrophy of the interventricular septum on the short-axis view (*A*) and the left ventricular outflow tract view (*B*).

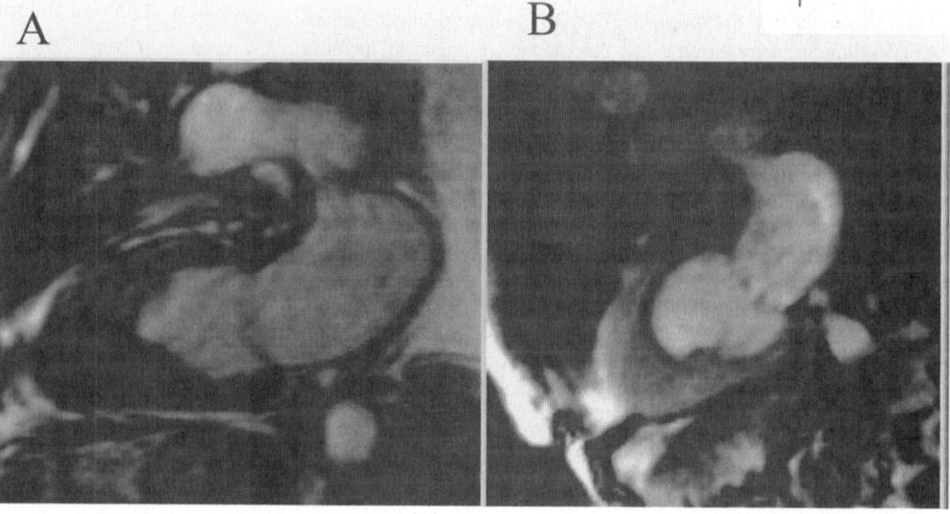


FIGURE 21-19 CMR of a case of restrictive cardiomyopathy due to eosinophilic endomyocardial disease (Löffler's syndrome) involving the apex. Cine image of a left ventricular two-chamber view showing the apical abnormality (*A*) and perfusion image showing abnormal perfusion of the apical myocardium (*B*).

## Restrictive Cardiomyopathy

Restrictive cardiomyopathy is characterized by myocardial thickening with normal to reduced chamber volumes and frequently depressed LV systolic function. In addition, because of restricted diastolic ventricular filling, the atria and vena cavae commonly are dilated.[48] Both SE and GRE MRI sequences may be used to assess cardiac chamber size, volume, and function. In patients with restrictive/constrictive hemodynamics, MRI can frequently distinguish between restrictive cardiomyopathy, which is often managed medically, and constrictive pericarditis, which in some cases must be treated surgically. The pericardium is thickened or may be calcified in constrictive pericarditis but is usually not thickened in restrictive cardiomyopathy.

Occasionally, restrictive cardiomyopathy may be the result of infiltrative myocaridal diseases such as hemochromatosis, sarcoidosis, or amyloidosis. Due to the excess deposition of iron, organs such as the liver, spleen, and heart may be involved. In cardiac hemochromatosis, the iron deposits tend to occur in the subepicardial regions. Iron deposits show low signal intensities on T1- and T2-weighted SE sequences. With treatment, serial MRI studies may be used to follow the zones of infiltration and their effect on ventricular function. Cardiac sarcoidosis is characterized by the appearance of intramyocardial granulomas. Typically, with gadolinum contrast, lesions hyperenhance on SE sequences. This pattern is similar to that of any fibrotic or scarred tissue and may, in fact, be a result of the subsequent myocardial scarring that occurs in chronic cardiac sarcoid (Fig. 21-20).[63] Diagnosing cardiac amyloidosis by CMR is often difficult and requires further investigation using a combination of SE, GRE, cardiac perfusion, and delayed hyperenhancement sequences.[64]

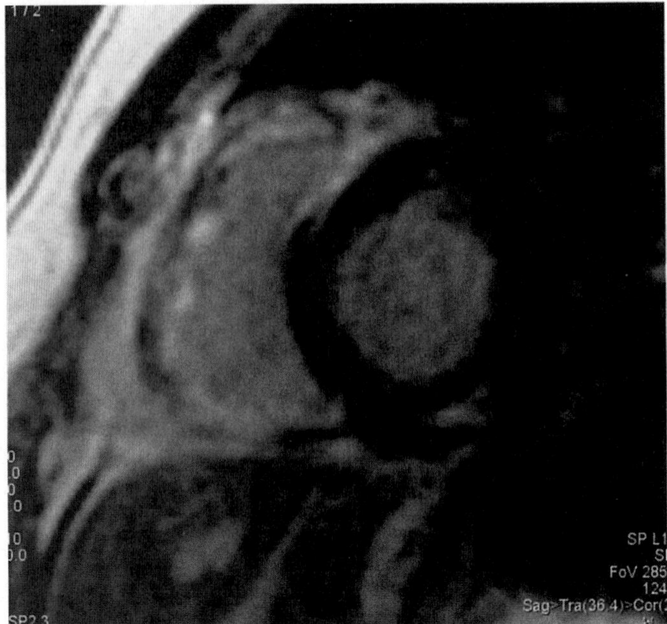


FIGURE 21-20 Delayed hyperenhancement image of the heart in a patient with history of sarcoidosis and arrhythmia. Patchy areas of hyperenhancement in the right ventricular free wall are consistent with fibrosis or scarring of the right ventricle due to cardiac sarcoid.

## ARRYTHMOGENIC RIGHT VENTRICULAR DYSPLASIA

Arrythmogenic right ventricular dysplasia (ARVD) is a condition of unclear etiology in which the myocardium is replaced by fibrofatty tissue. It has prevalence of about 0.4 percent. About 30 percent of the cases have a familial link. The fibrofatty transformation occurs most commonly but not exclusively in the RV free wall and may lead to RV dysfunction and failure, ventricular tachyarrythmias, and sudden death. The definitive diagnosis of ARVD is achieved via the histologic finding of a transmural RV fibrofatty replacement, usually obtained at autopsy or surgery. Diagnostic criteria for ARVD were established by the 1994 Task Force Report.[49] In order to make a diagnosis, 2 major criteria or 1 major criterion plus 2 minor criteria or 4 minor criteria were required (Table 21-3).

TABLE 21-3 Criteria for Diagnosis of Arrythmogenic Right Ventricular Dysplasia

| Major | Minor |
|---|---|
| Fibrofatty replacement | Regional right ventricular hypokinesis |
| Severe right ventricular dilatation | Mild right ventricular dilatation |
| Focal right ventricular aneurysms | Inverted T-waves ($V_1$ to $V_3$) |
| Epsilon waves on ECG ($V_1$ to $V_3$) | Late potentials |
| Widening of QRS complex >10 ms | Left bundle branch block |
| Familial disease (based on tissue examination from surgery or autopsy) | Ventricular extrasystoles |
| | Family history |

SOURCE: Modified from McKenna et al.[49] With permission.

Due to its high spatial resolution, unlimited and large field of view, and ability to distinguish fat or fibrosis from normal myocardium, CMR is by far the most sensitive noninvasive diagnostic modality for the diagnosis of ARVD.[65] MRI findings suggestive of ARVD include RV and/or RA dilatation, RV aneurysms or dyskinetic wall regions, myocardial thinning (suggesting fibrofatty transformation), high signal intensity in the RV intramyocardial regions (suggesting presence of fat), and ectasia of the RV outflow tract.. Intramyocardial fat may be observed by T1-weighted SE sequences and confirmed with a subsequent "fat-saturation" protocol to suppress the signal of fat from the regions of interest. SE sequences are also valuable in assessing the morphology of the RV wall. GRE or EPI may be used to assess for the presence of RV dysfunction and regional wall motion abnormalities.[66,67]

## ADULT CONGENITAL HEART DISEASE

With the medical and surgical advances of the past decade, it has been estimated that more than 90 percent of patients with congenital heart disease live for more than 10 years after surgical repair.[50] Although MRI may be used initially as a diagnostic procedure when such conditions are suspected during clinical examination in childhood, its usefulness in the adult population lies in the postoperative follow-up and the assessment of potential long-term complications of the corrective procedures.[51] A combination of both SE and GRE pulse sequences together with contrast-enhanced MRA allow for detailed morphologic assessment of the precise location of anatomic abnormalities, surgically altered anatomy, cardiac shunts, associated valvular abnormalities, vascular flow, and the physiologic impact of such abnormalities.[51,52] Common congenital conditions amenable to assessment by MRI include atrial septal defect, ventricular septal defect, patent ductus arteriosus, valvular heart disease, transposition of the great vessels, and tetralogy of Fallot.

MRI may be useful in the noninvasive assessment of these patients in a number of ways. First, the anatomic abnormality may be visualized and the area of the defect quantified (Fig. 21-21). If a surgical correction is contemplated, visualization of surrounding structures such as the great vessels, outflow tracts, and coexisting valvular abnormalities may be assessed. Second, the clinical impact of the congenital abnormality may be calculated (via measurement of volumetric parameters such as ejection fraction, stroke volume, diastolic and systolic volumes, as well as ventricular mass). Abnormalities in these parameters may precede the onset of symptoms and thus may signal the need for further hemodynamic investigation or early intervention. Third, by using phase-contrast MR, measurement of flow across a septal defect allows for the quantification of the shunt direction, shunt volume, and $\dot{Q}_p/\dot{Q}_s$ ratio.[53]

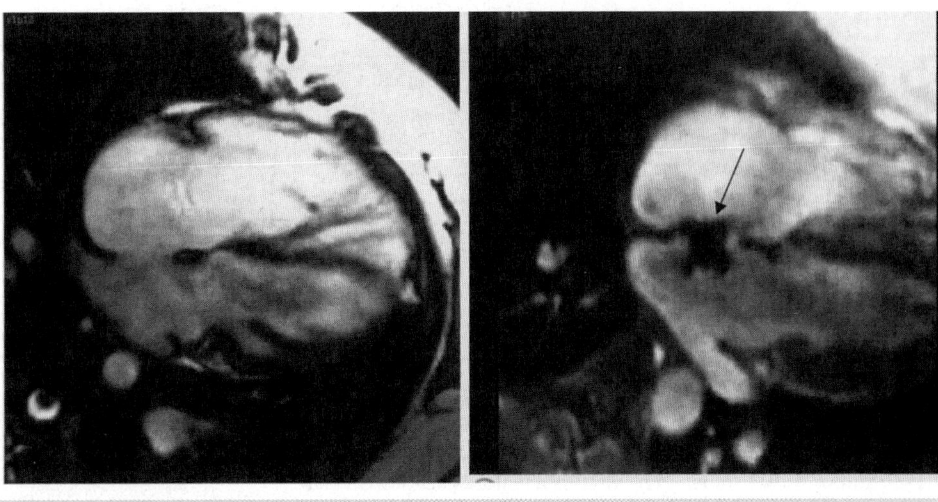

FIGURE 21-21 CMR of a case of large secundum atrial septal defect (*A*) and closure with a percutaneous ("angel wing") closure device (*B*).

Transposition of the great vessels accounts for 4.5 percent of all congenital cardiac malformations.[54] Uncorrected, this condition may be fatal. The transposition is corrected by redirecting systemic venous blood return directly to the morphologic left ventricle and pulmonary venous blood return to the morphologic right ventricle (Mustard or Senning techniques) Fig. 21-22. Currently, the Jatene (or arterial switch) procedure is the surgery of choice. Postoperative long-term complications are seen with either technique. With the arterial switch procedure, pulmonary stenosis is a serious complication and has been estimated to occur at an incidence up to 1 percent per year.[55] Complications seen after the Senning or Mustard procedures include severe RV hypertrophy and failure, which may occur in as many as 10 percent of patients. Other sequelae include baffle leaks and venous pathway obstructions. MRI is ideal for following these patients. Assessments of RV function and mass as well as baffle patency and leakage may be obtained without the need for an invasive procedure. Valvular stenosis or insufficiency may be qualitatively assessed with GRE MR. The regurgitant blood volume and maximum velocity of blood flow in valvular stenosis may be assessed quantitatively by phase-contrast and reconstruction of flow curves.[56]

Tetralogy of Fallot is another congenital heart condition that affects the pulmonary artery and RV. Tetrology accounts for about 5.5 percent of all congenital heart conditions and consists of ventricular septal defect (VSD), overriding aorta, RV outflow tract obstruction, and right ventricular hypertrophy (RVH).[54] Surgical treatment of this syndrome involves the correction of the VSD and transannular patch placement to relieve the RV outflow tract obstruction. Postoperative complications in these patients consist of pulmonary valve insufficiency Fig. 21-23, pulmonary valve stenosis, and persisting or recurrent

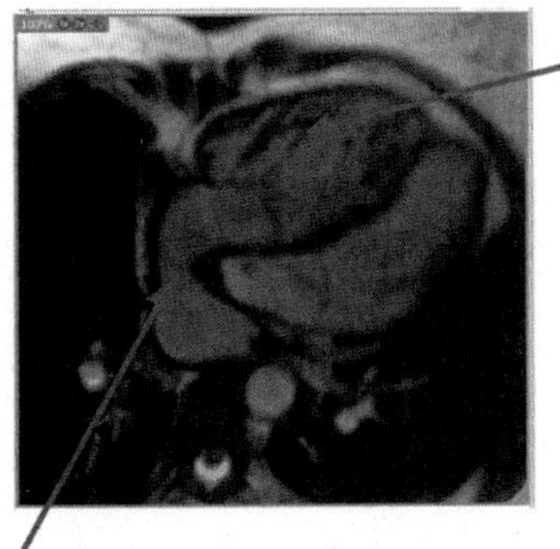


FIGURE 21-22 Transposition of the great vessels with a baffle (Mustard technique) shunting pulmonary venous blood to the systemic ventricle.

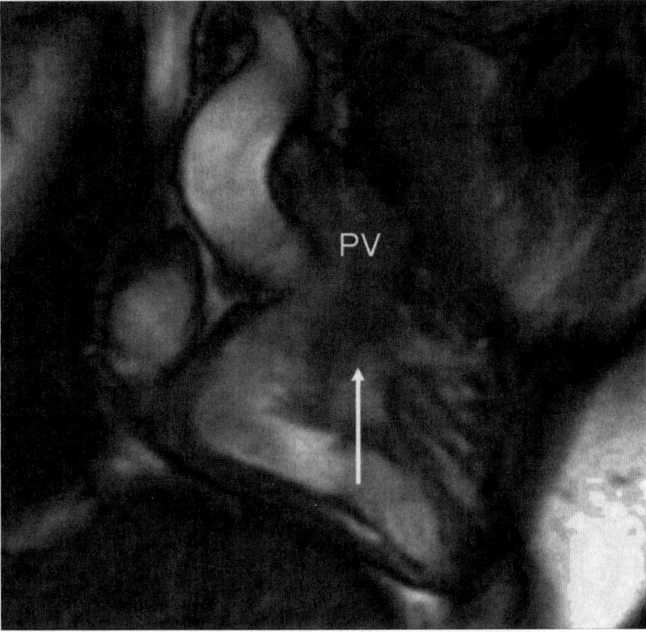


FIGURE 21-23 Postrepair of tetralogy of Fallot with pulmonary insufficiency (PV) as shown in this view of the right ventricular outflow tract with a regurgitant jet (*white arrow*) due to significant pulmonary insufficiency.

VSD. Pulmonary valve regurgitation may lead to RV dilation due to volume overload, whereas pulmonary stenosis may further increase RV hypertrophy. The consequences of a clinically significant VSD, as discussed above, include stress to the RV and pulmonary arterial system as well as cardiac shunting. Using standard GRE MR as well as phase-contrast MR, anatomic and functional assessment of biventricular function and valvular defects may be obtained.

## INTRACARDIAC MASSES AND THROMBI

The goals of MRI in assessing cardiac masses include the confirmation of the presence and number of masses, the spatial localization of the masses in relation to vital structures in the heart, and the tissue characterization of the mass to narrow the differential diagnosis. Masses within a heart chamber can be subdivided into two major classes: tumor versus "other"; thrombus is a major concern in the latter category. Cardiac tumors may be either benign or malignant and are classified according to whether they are primary or secondary (metastasis). Although primary tumors of the heart are rare, myxoma is the most common primary benign cardiac tumor in the adult population. Myxomas tend to originate in the left atrium (although they may be found in the right atrium) and are often pedunculated. Clinically, they may cause embolic phenomena or obstruct the mitral valve if they are large enough. On MRI, myxomas are diagnosed based on their typical location and morphology as well as their characteristic appearance in various pulse sequences (see also Chap. 85). Myxomas have low to very low signal intensity on GRE and T2-weighted SE sequences and intermediate signal intensity on T1-weighted SE. With the administration of gadolinium contrast, myxomas show moderate enhancement due to their hypervascularity. Other important benign tumors include lipomas, rhabdomyomas (most common in pediatric population), fibromas, hemangiomas, and leiomyomas. Their characteristic appearances in various MR sequences are summarized in Table 21-4.

Malignant cardiac tumors can be primary, though such tumors are less common than those secondary to metastasis. The differential diagnosis of malignant cardiac tumors is discussed elsewhere in this text. Because the same malignant tumor may differ in the amount of vascularity, calcification, necrosis, and tissue heterogeneity, a consistent delineation of characteristics on MRI may not be achievable. However, MRI certainly has a role in its detection or confirmation (Fig. 21-24).

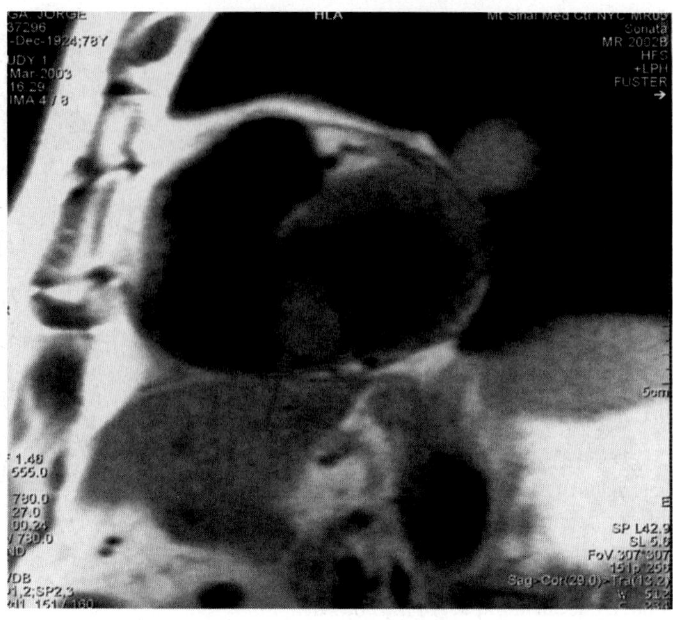


FIGURE 21-24 T1-weighted SE image of a cardiac mass in the interventricular septum in a man with a history of metastatic renal cell carcinoma.

The distinction between thrombus and cardiac masses is of great importance because of its clinical and therapeutic implications. To make this distinction, the addition of contrast (gadolinium) is key, because thrombus should not perfuse whereas tumors will enhance—with the one caveat that an organized thrombus may have recruited

TABLE 21-4 MR Characteristics of Selected Benign Tumors of the Heart

| | General Features | T1-Weighted SE | T2-Weighted SE | GRE | Gd Enhancement |
|---|---|---|---|---|---|
| Myxomas | Pedunculated, jelly-like, mobile | Intermediate SI (variable) | Intermediate SI (variable) | Very low SI | Hyperenhancement |
| Lipoma | Commonly arise from interatrial wall (right atrial side) | High SI | Intermediate SI (equivalent to subcutaneous fat) | | |
| Fibroma | Typically intramyocardial (LV septum) | Iso-hyperintense | Decreased SI compared to T1-weighted SE | | |
| Rhabdomyoma | Typically multiple lesions in ventricular myocardium | Hypointense compared to myocardium | Hyperintense | | |
| Cardiac hemangioma | Predominantly in ventricles | Higher SI compared to myocardium | | | Hyperenhancement |
| Intravenous leiomyomatosis | Usually noted as mobile mass in right atrium (but arises from uterine or venous wall) | Same SI as myocardium | Same SI as myocardium | | |

enough vasculature to possibly confuse this distinction. Without contrast, a fresh thrombus has high signal intensity on T1-weighted SE sequences. A chronic thrombus (>2 weeks) will have even higher signal intensity, as deoxyhemoglobin and methemoglobin are released within the thrombus. On GRE sequences, thrombus has low signal intensity.

## PERICARDIAL DISEASE

It has been postulated that the appearance is dark because of the nonlaminar flow of fluid within the pericardial sac as a consequence of cardiac motion. Such nonlaminar flow changes the spin phase and causes MR signal loss (Fig. 21-25). In GRE images, the pericardial fluid appears bright as a result of this flow, clearly separating the parietal pericardium from the myocardium.[57,58] The lower signal intensity of the normal pericardium results from the amount of fibrous tissue (with long T1 and short T2 relaxation times). Due to the relatively thin wall of the RV, the pericardium adjacent to the right ventricle is visualizable by MRI in nearly all individuals, whereas the pericardium along the lateral wall of the LV is visualized in only 61 percent.[59]

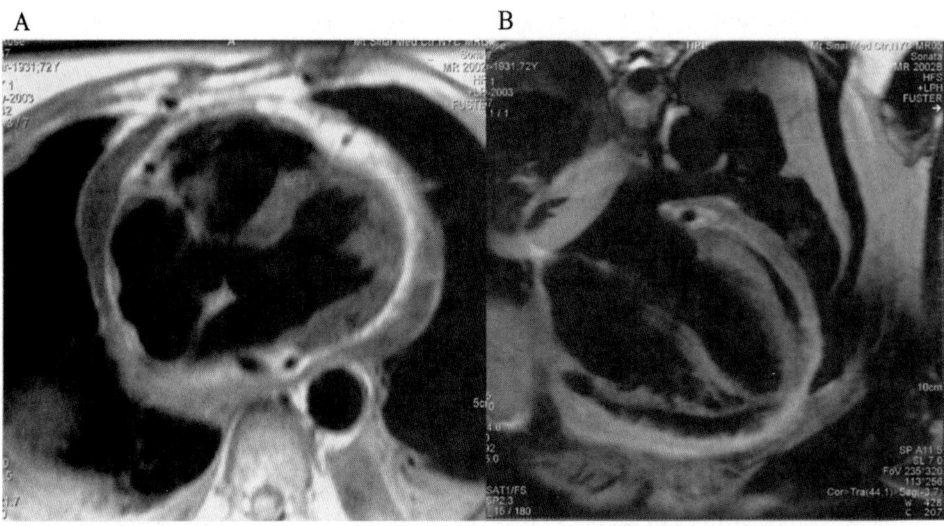


FIGURE 21-25 T2-weighted SE images of the heart with (*B*) and without (*A*) fat saturation, showing the pericardial fat separately from the myocardium, with isotense thickened pericardial fluid due to infected pericardial effusion.

MRI is better than echocardiography in detecting small fluid collections, especially in areas at the medial border of the right atrium or posterior to the LV apex.[60] Because of its lower cost and portability, echocardiography should be used as the first-line approach in assessing patients for pericardial effusion; however, MRI should be performed when a clinically suspected pericardial effusion is not detected on echocardiography. MRI is also useful for demonstrating loculated pericardial effusions.

In both MRI and computed x-ray tomography, a pericardial thickness of more than 4 mm is considered abnormal.[61] Pericardium visualized by MRI varies in thickness in different regions of the heart; thus, a standard imaging plane must be established. For this reason, transverse imaging at the levels of the right atrium and the RV and LV is recommended.

By demonstrating the presence or absence of a thickened pericardium, MRI can help distinguish between constrictive pericarditis and restrictive cardiomyopathy. Patients examined by MRI who had proven constrictive pericarditis had a pericardial thickening greater than 5 mm.[62] In addition, calcification of the pericardium, which demonstrates reduced signal intensity, also aids in the diagnosis of a pericardial rather than cardiomyopathic restrictive disease.

## THE FUTURE OF CMR

Cardiac MRI is an exciting and evolving field of noninvasive cardiac imaging. It can also be extremely helpful in the precise localization of cardiac structure and pathologic processes. MRI-guided interventions—such as cardiac biopsy, ablation, and coronary interventions including placement of MR-compatible coronary stents—are currently being investigated. Improved coil design and pulse sequences (e.g., parallel, spiral, and real-time imaging and partial Fourier analysis) are just some of the exciting new, currently available developments that will provide clinicians with greater flexibility with this technique, which was once considered an extremely cumbersome and user-unfriendly imaging modality. Stronger field magnets (magnets of 3 T or more) are currently being explored for potentially even greater spatial and temporal resolution for better and faster in vivo and ex vivo imaging.

## References


1. Sem DS, Pellecchia M. NMR in the acceleration of drug discovery *Curr Opin Drug Disc Dev* 2001;4:479.
2. Damadian R. Field focusing NMR (FONAR) and the formation of chemical images in man. *Philos Trans R Soc Lond B Biol Sci* 1980; 289:489.
3. Peshock RM, Franco F, Chwialkowski M, et al. Normal cardiac anatomy, orientation, and function. In: Manning WJ, Pennell DJ, eds. *Cardiovascular Magnetic Resonance.* New York: Churchill Livingstone; 2002.
4. Peshock RM, Willet D, Sayad D, et al. Quantitation of cardiac function by MRI. *MRI Clin North Am* 1996;4:287–306.
5. Ioannidis JPA, Trikalinos TA, Danias PG. Electrocardiogram-gated single photon emission computed tomography versus cardiac magnetic resonance imaging for the assessment of left ventricular volumes and ejection fraction. *J Am Coll Cardiol* 2002;39:2059.
6. Bellenger NG, Dudley JP. Assessment of cardiac function. In: Manning WJ, Pennell DJ, eds. *Cardiovascular Magnetic Resonance.* New York: Churchill Livingstone; 2002.
7. Lee VS, Resnick D, Bundy JM, et al. Cardiac function: MR evaluation in one breath hold with real-time true fast imaging with steady-state precession. *Radiology* 2002;222:853.
8. Schulen V, Schick F, Loichat J, et al. Evaluation of K-space segmented cine sequences for fast functional cardiac imaging. *Invest Radiol* 1996; 31:512.
9. Duerk JL, Lewin JS, Wendt M, et al. Remember true FISP? A high SNR, near 1-second imaging method for T2-like contrast in interventional MRI at .2 T. *J Magn Reson Imaging* 1998;8:203.
10. Chung YC, Merkle EM, Lewin JS, et al. "Fast T2-weighted imaging by PSIP at 0.2 T for interventional MRI. *Magn Reson Med* 1999;42:335.
11. Sodickson, Daniel K. Clinical cardiovascular magnetic resonance imaging techniques. In: Manning WJ, Pennell DJ, eds. *Cardiovascular Magnetic Resonance.* New York: Churchill Livingstone; 2002.
12. Schiebler N, Axel L, Reichek N, et al. Correlation of cine MR imaging with two-dimensional pulse Doppler echocardiography in valvular insufficiency. *J Comput Assist Tomogr* 1987;11:627–632.

13. Underwood SR, Klepstein RH, Firmin DN, et al. Magnetic resonance assessment of aortic and mitral regurgitation. *Br Heart J* 1986;56: 455–462.
14. Bryant DJ, Payne JA, Firman DN, Longmore DB. Measurement of flow with NMR imaging using a gradient pulse and phase difference technique. *J Comput Assist Tomogr* 1984;8:588.
15. Podolak MJ, Hedlund LW, Evans AJ, Herfkens RJ. Evaluation of flow through simulated vascular stenosis with gradient echo magnetic resonance imaging. *Invest Radiol* 1989;24:184.
16. Hundley WG, Li HF, Willard JE, et al. Magnetic resonance imaging assessment of the severity of mitral regurgitation: Comparison with invasive techniques. *Circulation* 1995;92:1151–1158.
17. Sechtem U, Pflugfelder PW, Cassidy MM, et al. Mitral and aortic regurgitation: Quantification of regurgitant volumes with cine MR imaging. *Radiology* 1988;167:425–430.
18. De Roos A, Reichek N, Axel L, Kressel HY. Cine MR imaging in aortic stenosis. *J Comput Assist Tomogr* 1989;13:421–425.
19. Lauerma K, Niemi P, Hanninen H, et al. Multimodality MR imaging assessment of myocardial viability: Combination of first-pass and late contrast enhancement to wall motion dynamics and comparison with FDG PET—Initial experience. *Radiology* 2000;217(3):729–736.
20. Baer FM, Voth E, Schneider CA, et al. Comparison of low-dose dobutamine-gradient-echo magnetic resonance imaging and positron emission tomography with [18F]fluorodeoxyglucose in patients with chronic coronary artery disease. A functional and morphological approach to the detection of residual myocardial viability. *Circulation* 1995;91(4):1006–1015.
21. Lawson MA, Johnson LL, Coghlan L, et al. Correlation of thallium uptake with left ventricular wall thickness by cine magnetic resonance imaging in patients with acute and healed myocardial infarcts. *Am J Cardiol* 1997;80(4):434–441.
22. Baer FM, Erdmann E. Methods of assessment and clinical relevance of myocardial hibernation and stunning. Assessment of myocardial viability. *Thorac Cardiovasc Surg* 1998;46(suppl 2):264–269.
23. Baer FM, Theissen P, Schneider CA, et al. Dobutamine magnetic resonance imaging predicts contractile recovery of chronically dysfunctional myocardium after successful revascularization. *J Am Coll Cardiol* 1998;31(5):1040–1048.
24. Cornel JH, Bax JJ, Elhendy A, et al. Biphasic response to dobutamine predicts improvement of global left ventricular function after surgical revascularization in patients with stable coronary artery disease: Implications of time course of recovery on diagnostic accuracy. *J Am Coll Cardiol* 1998;31(5):1002–1010.
25. Afridi I, Grayburn PA, Panza JA, et al. Myocardial viability during dobutamine echocardiography predicts survival in patients with coronary artery disease and severe left ventricular systolic dysfunction. *J Am Coll Cardiol* 1998;32(4):921–926.
26. Grothues F, Smith GC, Moon JC, et al. Comparison of interstudy reproducibility of cardiovascular magnetic resonance with two-dimensional echocardiography in normal subjects and in patients with heart failure or left ventricular hypertrophy. *Am J Cardiol* 2002;90(1):29–34.
27. Bellenger NG, Marcus NJ, Rajappan K, et al. Comparison of techniques for the measurement of left ventricular function following cardiac transplantation. *J Cardiovasc Magn Reson* 2002;4(2):255–263.
28. Myerson SG, Bellenger NG, Pennell DJ. Assessment of left ventricular mass by cardiovascular magnetic resonance. *Hypertension* 2002;39(3): 750–755.
29. Bellenger NG, Grothues F, Smith GC, Pennell DJ. Quantification of right and left ventricular function by cardiovascular magnetic resonance. *Herz* 2000;25(4):392–399.
30. Nagel E, Lehmkuhl HB, Bocksch W, et al. Noninvasive diagnosis of ischemia-induced wall motion abnormalities with the use of high-dose dobutamine stress MRI: Comparison with dobutamine stress echocardiography. *Circulation* 1999;99(6):763–770.
31. Gunning MG, Kaprielian RR, Pepper J, et al. The histology of viable and hibernating myocardium in relation to imaging characteristics. *J Am Coll Cardiol* 2002;39(3):428–435.
32. de Roos A, Matheijssen NA, Doornbos J, et al. Myocardial infarct size after reperfusion therapy: Assessment with Gd-DTPA–enhanced MR imaging. *Radiology* 1990;176(2):517–521.
33. Gerber BL, Rochitte CE, Bluemke DA, et al. Relation between Gd-DTPA contrast enhancement and regional inotropic response in the periphery and center of myocardial infarction. *Circulation* 2001;104(9): 998–1004.
34. Kim RJ, Wu E, Rafael A, et al. The use of contrast-enhanced magnetic resonance imaging to identify reversible myocardial dysfunction. *N Engl J Med* 2000;343(20):1445–1453.
35. Poon M, Fuster V, Fayad Z. Cardiac magnetic resonance imaging: A "one-stop-shop" evaluation of myocardial dysfunction. *Curr Opin Cardiol* 2002;17(6):663–670.
36. Abramson SV, Burke JB, Pauletto FJ, Kelly JJ Jr. Use of multiple views in the echocardiographic assessment of pulmonary artery systolic pressure. *J Am Soc Echocardiogr* 1995;8(1):55–60.
37. Borgeson DD, Seward JB, Miller FA, et al. Frequency of Doppler measurable pulmonary artery pressures. *J Am Soc Echocardiogr* 1996; 9(6):832–837.
38. Nicholas G. Bellenger DJP. Assessment of cardiac function. In: Warren J, Manning DJP, eds. *Cardiovascular Magnetic Resonance.* Philadelphia: Churchill Livingstone; 2002:99–111.
39. Katz J, Whang J, Boxt LM, Barst RJ. Estimation of right ventricular mass in normal subjects and in patients with primary pulmonary hypertension by nuclear magnetic resonance imaging. *J Am Coll Cardiol* 1993;21(6):1475–1481.
40. Marcus JT, Vonk Noordegraaf A, De Vries PM, et al. MRI evaluation of right ventricular pressure overload in chronic obstructive pulmonary disease. *J Magn Reson Imaging* 1998;8(5):999–1005.
41. Nelson GS, Sayed-Ahmed EY, Kroeker CA, et al. Compression of interventricular septum during right ventricular pressure loading. *Am J Physiol Heart Circ Physiol* 2001;280(6):H2639–H2648.
42. Sulica R, Boxt L, DePalo L, et al. A novel MRI-index of pulmonary hypertension, *Am J Respir Crit Care Med* 2002(suppl):2002.
43. Kauczor HU, Kreitner KF. Contrast-enhanced MRI of the lung. *Eur J Radiol* 2000;34(3):196–207.
44. Thompson RC, Lavine RA, Mille S, Dinsmore RE. Magnetic resonance imaging along the left ventricular axis in hypertrophic heart disease: Accurate characterization of cardiac hypertrophy. *Circulation* 1985; 72(suppl III):122.
45. Higgins CB, Byrd BF III, Stark D, et al. Magnetic resonance imaging in hypertrophic cardiomyopathy. *Am J Cardiol* 1985;55:1121–1126.
46. Webb JG, Sasson Z, Rakowski H, et al. Apical hypertrophic cardiomyopathy: Clinical follow-up and diagnostic correlates. *J Am Coll Cardiol* 1990;15:83–90.
47. Guado C, Pelliccia FTA, Nzilli G, et al. Magnetic resonance imaging for assessment of apical hypertrophy in hypertrophic cardiomyopathy. *Clin Cardiol* 1992;15:164–168.
48. Sechtem U, Higgins CB, Summerhoff BA, et al. Magnetic resonance imaging of restrictive cardiomyopathy. *Am J Cardiol* 1987;59: 480–482.
49. McKenna WJ, Thiene G, Nava A, et al. Diagnosis of arrhythmogenic right venticular dysplasia/cardiomyopathy. *Br Heart J* 1994;71:215–218.
50. Joyce L. Mended hearts grow up. *Stanford Med* 1994;11:18–25.
51. Perloff JK, Warnes CA. Challenges posed by adults with repaired congenital heart disease. *Circulation* 2001;103(21):2637–2643.
52. Wimpfheimer O, Boxt LM. MR imaging of adult patients with congenital heart disease. *Radiol Clin North Am* 1999;37(2):421–438, vii.
53. Roest AA, Helbing WA, van der Wall EE, de Roos A. Postoperative evaluation of congenital heart disease by magnetic resonance imaging. *J Magn Reson Imaging* 1999;10(5):656–666.
54. Hoffman JI. Incidence of congenital heart disease: I. Postnatal incidence. *Pediatr Cardiol* 1995;16(3):103–113.
55. Wyttenbach RJB, Higgins CB. Cardiovascular magnetic resonance of complex congenital heart disease in the adult. In: Warren J, Manning DJP, eds. *Cardiovascular Magnetic Resonance.* Philadelphia: Churchill Livingstone; 2002:311–323.

56. Arno AW, Roest RAN, Groenik M,, et al. Cardiovascular magnetic resonance of simple congenital cardiovascular defects. In: Warren J, Manning DJP, eds. *Cardiovascular Magnetic Resonance.* Philadelphia: Churchill Livingstone; 2002:295–310.
57. Stark DD, Higgins CB, Lanzer P, et al. Magnetic resonance imaging of the pericardium: Normal and pathologic findings. *Radiology* 1984;151: 469–474.
58. White CS. MR evaluation of the pericardium. *Top Magn Reson Imaging* 1995;7(4):258–266.
59. Sechtem U, Tscholakoff D, Higgins CB. MRI of the normal pericardium. *AJR* 1986;147:239.
60. Mulvagh SL, Rokey R, Vick GW, Johnston DL. Usefulness of nuclear magnetic resonance imaging for evaluation of pericardial effusions, in comparison with two-dimensional echocardiography. *J Am Coll Cardiol* 1989;64:1002–1009.
61. Sechtem U, Tscholakoff D, Higgins CB. MRI of the abnormal pericardium. *AJR* 1986;147:245.
62. Soulen RL, Stark DD, Higgins CB. Magnetic resonance imaging of constrictive pericardial disease. *Am J Cardiol* 1995;55:480–484.
63. Matsuki M, Matsuo M. MR findings of myocardial sarcoidosis. *Clin Radiol* 2000;55(4):323–325.
64. Asaumi J, Yanagi Y, Hisatomi M, et al. CT and MR imaging of localized amyloidosis. *Eur J Radiol* 2001;39(2):83–87.
65. van der Wall EE, Kayser HW, Bootsma MM, et al. Arrhythmogenic right ventricular dysplasia: MRI findings. *Herz* 2000;25(4):356–364.
66. Auffermann W, Wichter T, Breithardt G, et al. Arrhythmogenic right ventricular disease: MR imaging vs angiography. *AJR* 1993;161(3): 549–555.
67. Midiri M, Finazzo M, Brancato M, et al., Arrhythmogenic right ventricular dysplasia: MR features. *Eur Radiol* 1997;7(3):307–312.
68. Lorenz CH, Walker ES, Morgan VL, et al. Normal human right and left ventricular mass, systolic function, and gender differences by cine magnetic resonance imaging. *J Cardiovasc Magn Reson* 1999;1(1): 7–21.
69. Hoeper MM, Tongers J, Leppert A, et al. Evaluation of right ventricular performance with a right ventricular ejection fraction thermodilution catheter and MRI in patients with pulmonary hypertension. *Chest* 2001;120(2):502–507.

CHAPTER 22

# MAGNETIC RESONANCE IMAGING AND COMPUTED TOMOGRAPHY OF THE VASCULAR SYSTEM

Konstantin Nikolaou / Michael Poon / Valentin Fuster / Zahi A. Fayad



## IMAGING OF THE VASCULATURE WITH MRI AND CT

Imaging of the vasculature has evolved greatly in the past decade. Although the current "gold standard" is the time-honored but invasive method of x-ray angiography, noninvasive modalities such as magnetic resonance imaging (MRI) and computed tomography (CT) are becoming routine in the diagnostic examination of patients with vascular diseases. In many instances, either MRI or CT has replaced x-ray angiography as the imaging modality of choice, owing to the ever-increasing quality of the images, the noninvasive application of these modalities, the ease and comfort of the patients, and the clinical versatility of both CT and MRI. This chapter gives a comprehensive and state-of-the-art overview of the clinical utilities of MRI and CT in the evaluation of the major vascular systems.

### MR Angiography

Magnetic resonance angiography (MRA) has evolved rapidly since its introduction more than 15 years ago. Initially, non-contrast-enhanced MRA techniques found their way into clinical routine for imaging vascular morphology. These early approaches can in principle be divided into two subgroups, i.e., "black blood" and "bright blood" sequences. While black-blood techniques based on signal voids within vessels containing flowing spins can confirm vessel patency, they remain of limited use in the assessment of vascular morphology. They are currently gaining acceptance, however, for the evaluation of vascular walls.[1] Bright-blood MRA techniques are generally divided into those influenced by the effect of blood flow onto the signal amplitude (time of flight, or TOF) and those based on the flow effect onto phase (phase contrast, or PC). PC angiography derives image contrast from the differences in the phases accumulated by stationary and moving spins in a magnetic field gradient. The amount of phase accumulated is directly proportional to the flow velocity, allowing quantitative measurement of flow velocities and the discrimination of flow direction. Spins moving in the direction of a magnetic field gradient accumulate positive phase, while spins moving in the opposite direction accumulate negative phase. Hence, the magnitude of the phase determines the velocity, while the sign of the accumulated phase determines flow direction. The flow dependence and associated artifacts inherent to these techniques have restricted the clinical use of these MRA techniques primarily to the extra- and intracranial arterial system and the portal venous system. With the advent of high-performance gradient systems, a new, promising MRA strategy has been developed: contrast-enhanced MRA (CE-MRA) using gadolinium chelates. It is based on the combination of rapid three-dimensional (3D) imaging and the T1-shortening effect of intravenously infused paramagnetic contrast.[2] These techniques have been proven to give an extensive and diagnostically accurate evaluation of extracranial, thoracic, abdominal, and peripheral vessels. In many centers, contrast-enhanced 3D MRA has widely replaced conventional x-ray angiography for the clarification of pathologies in arterial vessels.[3]

### CT Angiography

Since spiral (i.e., helical) CT (SCT) became part of the routine diagnostic imaging in the early 1990s, CT as a whole has matured into a volume-scanning modality. Three-dimensional postprocessing methods like volume-rendering techniques (VRT) were clinically successful due to the availability of continuous volume data from spiral scanning.[4] However, in practice, the spiral data sets suffered from a considerable mismatch between the transverse (in-plane) and the longitudinal (out-of-plane) spatial resolution. Similarly, a number of practical limitations still remained that prevented the scanning protocol from being fully adapted to the diagnostic needs of routine practice. The recent advent of multi-detector-row CT (MDCT) systems is the first real quantum leap in CT since the introduction of SCT.[5] In general, the capabilities of SCT can be expanded in several ways: to scan anatomic volumes with standard techniques at significantly reduced scan times; to scan larger volumes previously not feasible within the practical limits of scan time, or to scan anatomic volumes with high axial resolution (narrow collimation) to closely approach the isotropic voxel of high-quality data sets for excellent three-dimensional postprocessing and diagnosis.

In addition, the faster gantry rotation time of the new MDCT systems of 500 ms or less revolutionized the CT application for diagnosis of moving organs. Particularly attractive is the cardiac-CT application to freeze heart motion by combining rapid "partial scan" techniques with ECG triggering.[6] Multislice spiral scans of the heart with ECG gating provide continuous 3D data sets during diastole. In combination with dedicated spiral reconstruction algorithms, which are optimized for a temporal resolution of 210 to 250 ms, significant advances have been reported for the diagnosis of coronary anatomy.[7,8] Besides cardiac CT, the advantages of MDCT for assessing the vasculature in general are substantial. MDCT allows reduction of iodinated contrast utilization, improves spatial resolution, and shows less pulsation artifacts and greater coverage than SCT. MDCT technology has substantially improved CT angiography of extracranial, thoracic, abdominal, pulmonary, and peripheral vasculature.

Another promising technique specially designed for cardiac imaging is electron-beam CT (EBCT) (see Chap. 20). EBCT has mainly been used for accurate quantification of coronary artery calcium, scanning the entire heart in a single breathhold from rapid (50 to 100 ms) tomographic scans done in synchrony with the heart cycle.[9] Additional indications for this burgeoning technique include noninvasive coronary artery imaging and assessment of coronary artery bypass grafts. However, the overall role of EBCT in other vascular territories is limited.

## CAROTID ARTERIES

### Background

Atherosclerosis of the carotid arteries results in significant morbidity and mortality. The multicenter North American Symptomatic Carotid Endarterectomy Trial (NASCET) has shown the benefit of carotid endarterectomy for patients with significant[10] and nonsignificant carotid artery stenoses[11] (see Chap. 99). Other studies have also provided convincing evidence that a decision regarding therapy should be based on the degree of stenosis.[12] Accurate measurement of stenosis severity is a clinically important parameter in determining the need for surgery in these patients. X-ray angiography has been the gold standard for diagnosis of carotid bulb disease. However, this modality provides projection images of the carotid bulb, which leads to variation in the measurement of the percent stenosis depending on the observer or the projection. Also, the associated direct and indirect costs and increased procedural risk have prompted the development of other less invasive imaging techniques. Noninvasive imaging tools of extracranial carotid disease include Doppler ultrasound, MRA, and CT angiography (CTA). In many centers, these modalities have become standard in the preoperative evaluation of carotid artery stenosis. MRA and CTA allow the rapid acquisition of data that can be reconstructed into 2- and 3D images. High-resolution axial images can provide a cross-sectional view of the carotid vessel and atherosclerotic plaques. Maximal intensity projection (MIP) allows data to be reconstructed into images that closely resemble conventional x-ray angiograms and can be rotated 360 degrees to be viewed from any angle. With both modalities, by utilizing both axial and MIP images, extensive information regarding the carotid bifurcation and plaque characteristics can be obtained.

### MR Angiography of the Carotid Arteries

MRA of the carotid arteries was initially implemented using 2- and 3D time-of-flight techniques, and good results for the detection of extracerebral arterial disease were reported.[13] Yet time-of-flight imaging involves long acquisition times and can result in overestimation of stenosis.[14] More recently, contrast-enhanced MRA has become the state-of-the-art technique for imaging the carotid circulation. Several studies have shown contrast-enhanced MRA have high sensitivities and specificities in revealing carotid artery stenosis (Table 22-1). It is now feasible to visualize the entire carotid circulation, including the circle of Willis and aortic branch vessels, on a single study (Fig. 22-1). In addition, breathholding has been used variably in MRA of the carotid arteries and arch vessels, the implication being that these vessels are unaffected by respiratory motion.[15]

It has been reported that differentiation of high-grade stenoses and total vessel occlusions can be difficult on MRAs of the carotid arteries, as the flow characteristics of high-grade stenoses may lead to a signal void in the area of stenoses and might mimic total vessel occlusion.[16] Also, early venous enhancement in the carotid circulation can interfere with visualization of the arterial system unless the contrast bolus is accurately timed to the arterial phase, as the timing window for a true arterial phase is only 6 to 8 s long.[17] Introduction of new MR acquisition strategies that can significantly shorten the total acquisition time of a high-resolution angiography has been used to overcome this problem—namely, parallel imaging techniques.[18] Another approach is the use of time-resolved techniques. This way, multiple short acquisitions of the carotid vasculature are performed, providing true arterial

TABLE 22-1 MRA and CTA of the Carotid Arteries[a]

| Reference | Technique | Carotids (*n*) | Sensitivity (%) | Specificity (%) |
|---|---|---|---|---|
| Johnson et al., 2000[134] | MRA | 76 | 94 | 95 |
| Serfaty et al., 2000[135] | MRA | 63 | 94 | 85 |
| Sardanelli et al., 1999[136] | MRA | 56 | 100 | 100 |
| Scarabino et al., 1998[14] | MRA | 46 | 100 | 100 |
| Leclerc et al., 1998[137] | MRA | 54 | 100 | 98 |
| Anderson et al., 2000[138] | CTA | 80 | 77 | 92 |
| Leclerc et al., 1999[139] | CTA | 44 | 100 | 97 |
| Marcus et al., 1999[140] | CTA | 46 | 93 | 97 |
| Verhoek et al., 1999[141] | CTA | 38 | 100 | 100 |
| Margarelli et al., 1998[142] | CTA | 40 | 92 | 98 |

[a]Sensitivity and specificity of magnetic resonance angiography (MRA) and computed tomography angiography (CTA) for the detection of significant carotid artery stenoses (>75 percent). Results of a selection of clinical trials as compared to conventional angiography.

phased images and the additional information of flow dynamics,[19,20] yet at the cost of decreased spatial resolution. Other new acquisition techniques alter the method of selecting the information from k space to enhance spatial resolution while suppressing venous overlap at the same time. Elliptic centric acquisition, a recently developed technique, acquires the high-contrast elements within k space prior to venous enhancement, which results in a relative suppression of venous signal intensity.[17] Using the modern imaging approaches described above, isotropic submillimeter voxel sizes can be achieved, covering the complete carotid vasculature in a short acquisition time for true arterial contrast.

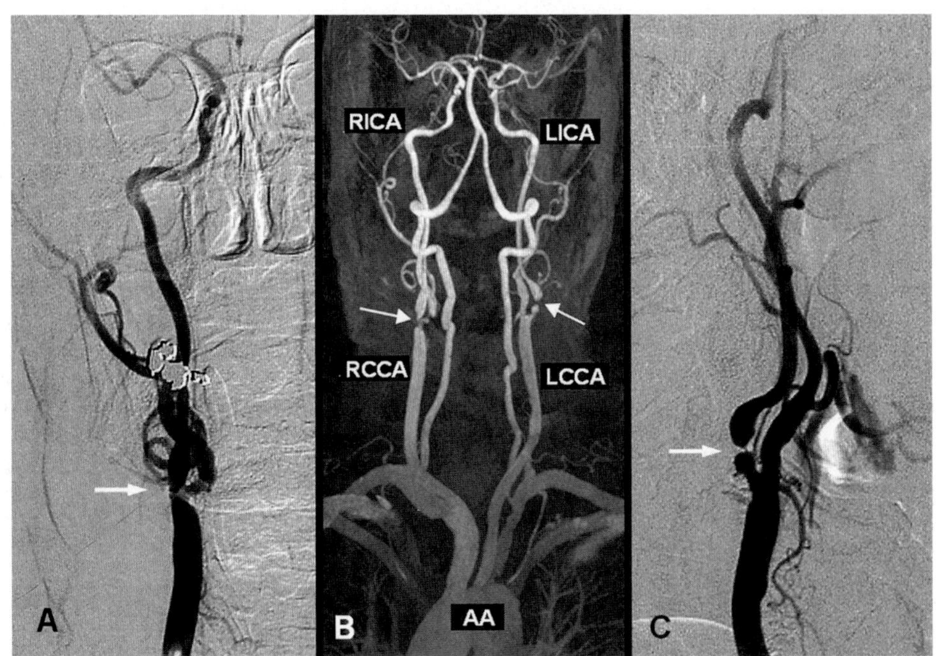


FIGURE 22-1 X-ray angiogram of the right (*A*) and left (*C*) carotid artery and 3D contrast-enhanced magnetic resonance angiogram of the supraaortic vessels (*B*). A complex stenosis of the right carotid bifurcation and a high-grade stenosis of the proximal left internal carotid artery are revealed by both modalities (*arrows*). Artifacts from teeth seen in the conventional angiogram of the right carotid artery (*arrowhead*). (AA = aortic arch, RCCA/LCCA = right/left common carotid artery, RICA/LICA = right/left internal carotid artery.) (Courtesy of B.J. Wintersperger, Ludwig-Maximilians-University, Munich, Germany.[179])

## CT Angiography of the Carotid Arteries

Besides MRA, CTA has been introduced as a noninvasive imaging procedure for the detection of significant carotid artery stenoses. Intravenous application of iodine contrast is required and imaging is not dependent on flow characteristics. Thus, severely stenotic but patent vessels can be visualized accurately. Axial images can be magnified to examine plaque morphology and avoid artifacts created by dense calcifications. Using single-slice helical CT systems, CTA has previously been reported to have a diagnostic accuracy approaching 90 percent.[21] Nevertheless single-slice scanners were limited in temporal and spatial resolution. The advantages of 4-DCT were significant.[22] Recent studies on the newest generation of 16-DCT systems have reported further improvements. A scan range of 30 cm can now be covered in an acquisition time of just 9 s, allowing for imaging the whole length of the carotid artery from the aortic arch to the circle of Willis in a true arterial phase (Fig. 22-2). The voxel size can be reduced to 0.3 $mm^3$ (0.6 × 0.6 × 0.75 mm). Preliminary results have demonstrated the potential of this technique to replace conventional x-ray angiography of the carotid arteries.[23] Using adapted contrast injection protocols, a comprehensive evaluation of the extra- and intracranial arterial system and of the intracerebral veins is feasible in a single CT scan.[24] Calcifications of the

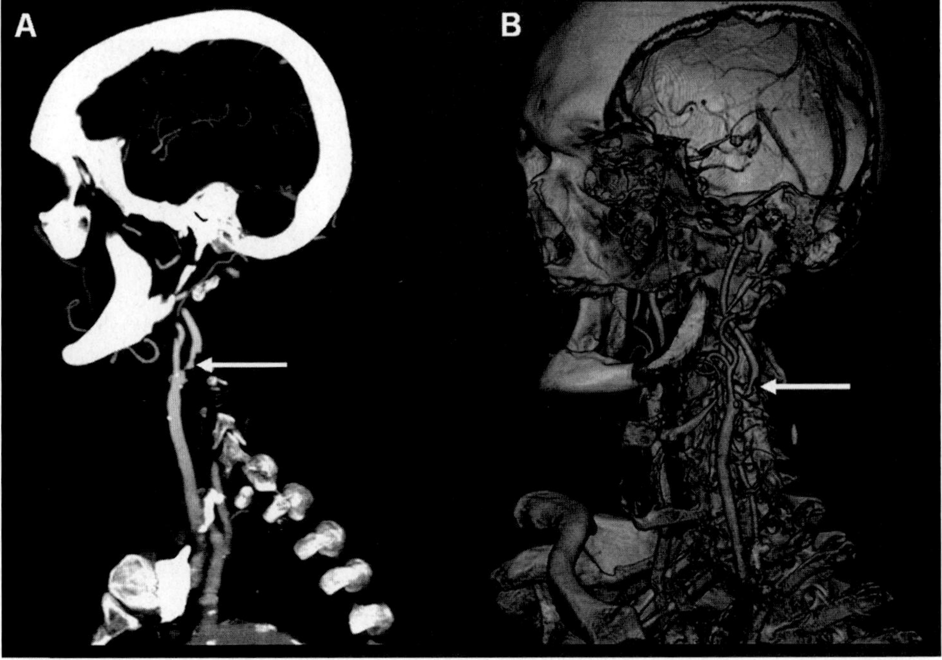


FIGURE 22-2 Contrast-enhanced 16-detector-row computed tomogram of the supraaortal and intracranial vessels, acquiring a caudocranial scan range of 30 cm in a total of just 12-s acquisition time with 0.75-mm slice thickness. Maximum-intensity projection (MIP) (*A*) and volume-rendering-technique (VRT) (*B*) both reveal a complex ulcerated plaque in the proximal right internal carotid artery associated with a high-grade stenosis (*arrows*). (Courtesy of B. Ertl-Wagner, Ludwig-Maximilians-University, Munich, Germany.[180])

carotids, especially in the region of the carotid bulb, may be a limitation of CTA due to overestimation of calcifications inherent in the CT technique. Some authors suggest manual segmentation or multiplanar reformatting for assessment of the true arterial lumen in the area of heavy calcifications.[25] The improvements in spatial resolution using 16-DCT systems will further improve the delineation of calcified plaques. Table 22-1 gives an overview over recent clinical studies on the value of CTA for the detection of significant stenoses of the carotid arteries.

### MR and CT Plaque Imaging of the Carotid Arteries

Other factors besides the degree of stenosis alone are also important in determining whether a carotid lesion will remain clinically silent. Plaques that are more prone to disruption, fracture, or fissuring may be associated with a higher risk of embolization, occlusion, and consequent ischemic neurologic events.[26] In contrast to vulnerable plaques in the coronary arteries, which are often characterized by high lipid content and a thin fibrous cap, high-risk plaques in carotid arteries are typically severely stenotic. Currently the term *high-risk* is used rather than the classic term *vulnerable,* which only implies the presence of a lipid-rich core. High-risk carotid plaques are heterogeneous, very fibrous, and not necessarily lipid-rich.[27] That is why increasing emphasis is put on tissue characterization of the carotid artery wall, using MRI[27,28] (Fig. 22-3) as well as contrast-enhanced MDCT.[29–31] These study findings indicate the importance of accurate delineation of the morphology of the carotid bifurcation as well as the degree of stenosis. The inability of conventional x-ray angiography to depict plaque ulceration is well documented[32] because it depicts only the vessel lumen, and a limited number of views are typically obtained. MRI reliably identifies plaque composition in the carotid artery vessel wall by using multicontrast high-resolution spin-echo–based MR sequences.[27,28] For black-blood sequences, the signal from the blood flow is rendered black by the use of preparatory pulses to better visualize the adjacent vessel wall. Hatsukami et al.[33] introduced the use of bright-blood time-of-flight imaging for the visualization of the fibrous cap's thickness and morphologic integrity. This sequence provides enhancement of the signal from flowing blood and a mixture of T1 and proton-density contrast weighting that highlights the fibrous cap. MRA and high-resolution black-blood imaging of the vessel wall can be combined. MRA demonstrates the severity of stenotic lesions and their spatial distribution, whereas the high-resolution wall-characterization techniques may show the composition of the plaques and facilitate risk stratification and selection of the treatment modality. Improvements in spatial resolution have been possible with the design of new phased-array coils tailored for carotid imaging and new imaging sequences, such as long-echo-train fast spin-echo imaging with "velocity-selective" flow suppression.[34] CT, on the other hand, has also been shown to differentiate various tissue types in the carotid artery wall[29,30] and to reliably assess vessel wall thickness.[31] Contrast-enhanced MDCT was able to differentiate between calcified, fibrous, and lipid plaque components with moderate to high sensitivity and specificity.[30] Yet it does not reach the potential of tissue characterization that is inherent to MRI, and in-plane spatial resolution requires improvement for a more reliable assessment of plaque components and for identifying plaques at risk.

## AORTA

### Aortic Dissection

Acute aortic dissection is a challenging clinical emergency that may have catastrophic consequences if it is not diagnosed and treated promptly (see Chap. 99). There are 10 to 20 cases per million population per year; if they are not treated, 36 to 72 percent of patients die within 48 h of diagnosis and 62 to 91 percent within a week.[35] However, recent technical advances in noninvasive imaging have greatly improved early diagnosis and treatment planning. Gadolinium-enhanced MRA has become established as a safe and reliable technique for evaluation of stenoses in the thoracic and abdominal aorta and major aortic branch arteries.[36] However, aortic dissection is potentially life-threatening and has routinely been evaluated with x-ray angiography and more recently with spiral CT. Both modalities have typically been chosen because of their availability and rapid examination times. In the past, emergency MR evaluation for aortic injury or disease was impractical and unsafe due to prolonged examination times. The choice of imaging technique still remains controversial. Each imaging modality has certain advantages and disadvantages with respect to accuracy, speed, convenience, risk, and cost, but no single modality is superior over all others in all situations. Single- or even multislice spiral CT is now available in most hospitals, usually on an emergency basis. It is both sensitive and

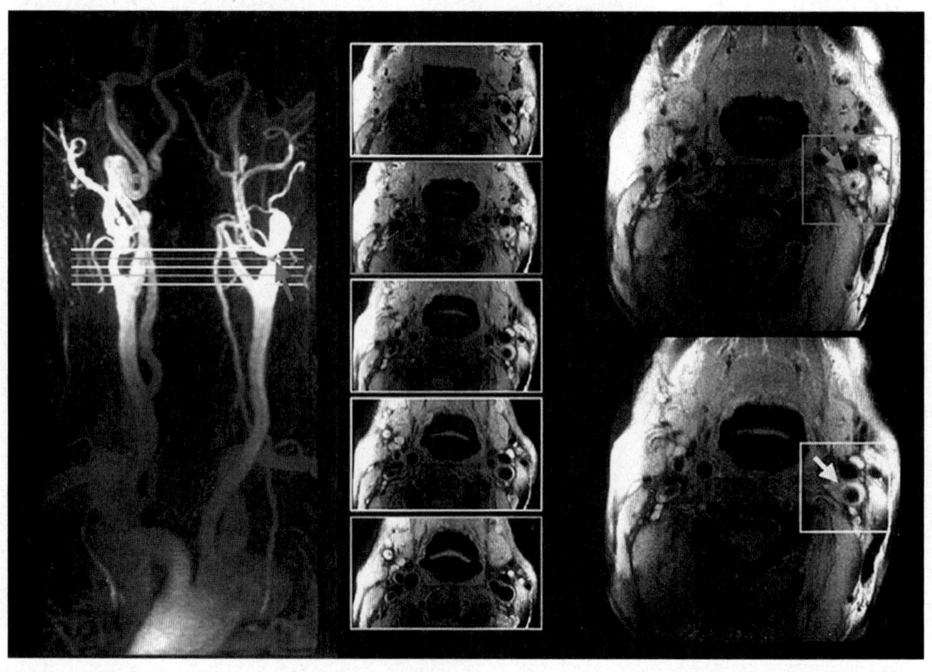

FIGURE 22-3 Carotid MR angiogram (*left panel*) showing severe stenosis in the left internal carotid artery (*arrow, left panel*). MR angiogram was obtained with a contrast-enhanced 3D fast gradient–echo and carotid–aortic arch phased-array coil. Cross-sectional MR black-blood images of carotid arteries are shown in the middle and right panels. Display of MR slice positions are shown in left panel (*lines*). Magnified views of some carotid plaques are shown in right panel. Arrows indicate carotid plaques. (Courtesy of Z. Fayad, Mount Sinai School of Medicine, New York.[109])

specific in the diagnosis of aortic dissection, and its accuracy has been improved by the recent availability of ultrafast scanning and 3D reconstruction.[37] However, it is unable to provide hemodynamic information and relies on the use of nephrotoxic contrast agents. On the other hand, MRI offers improved anatomic delineation of the aorta and can provide high-quality images in several planes, including a left anterior oblique view that displays the entire thoracic aorta (Fig. 22-4). It does not require the use of nephrotoxic contrast agents but is relatively expensive and not as readily available as conventional CT. Furthermore, MRI is contraindicated in patients with pacemakers and certain metallic prosthetic heart valves; moreover, it can be inappropriate in hemodynamically unstable patients, who may be intubated and receiving intravenous medication with continuous arterial pressure monitoring. Total examination time for a complete diagnostic MR evaluation of the aorta has been reported to be between 10 and 45 min; it is therefore suitable only for medically stable patients. With the recent combination of steady-state gradient-echo techniques and advanced gradient hardware, a family of high-speed pulse sequences with very favorable vascular imaging properties has been introduced. Imaging of the aorta can be achieved in a significantly shorter time with adequate diagnostic quality and the imaging time can be reduced to 10 min or less.[38] In cases where endoluminal repair or fenestration is considered, x-ray angiography is still a preferred imaging modality, which allows assessment of the access arteries (usually the iliacs), measurement of the aorta to permit selection of the correct device length and diameter, confirmation of branch-vessel involvement, and assessment of bilateral luminal manometry prior to fenestration.[39]

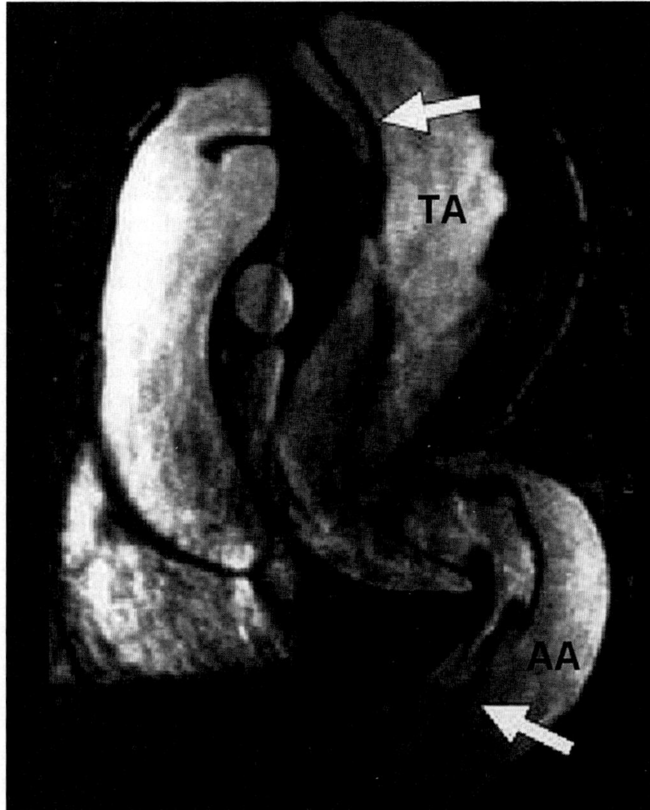


FIGURE 22-4 Contrast-enhanced magnetic resonance angiogram of a 32-year-old patient suffering from Marfan's syndrome. The oblique multiplanar reconstruction (MPR) shows an aneurysm of the aorta, extending from the thoracic to the abdominal aorta (TA = thoracic aorta, AA = abdominal aorta) with extensive elongation and kinking in the course of the complete descending aorta. A dissecting membrane extending from the aortic arch to the distal abdominal aorta (*arrows*) can be depicted. (Courtesy of A. Huber, Ludwig-Maximilians-University, Munich, Germany.[181])

## Aortic Aneurysm

### THORACIC AORTIC ANEURYSM

Although thoracic aortic aneurysms expand at a slower rate than abdominal aortic aneurysms, surgical repair is contemplated when thoracic aneurysms reach a diameter of 5 to 6 cm, depending on their shape and etiology (see Chap. 98). Aneurysms of the thoracic aorta may be classified according to their localization (sinus of Valsalva, ascending aorta, aortic arch, descending aorta), their etiology (congenital, atherosclerotic, luetic, mycotic, traumatic, inflammatory), or their shape (saccular, fusiform, dissecting). For the thoracic aorta, a diameter exceeding 4 cm is generally considered aneurysmal. When a fusiform aneurysm exceeds 6 cm in diameter, the risk of rupture is increased and surgical repair is recommended for patients who can tolerate major surgery. For those who cannot tolerate surgery, endoluminal stenting may be considered. Saccular aneurysms, mycotic aneurysms, and aneurysms that are rapidly increasing in size at a rate exceeding 1 cm/year are also thought to be at increased risk for rupture.[40]

***MR Angiography of Thoracic Aneurysms*** Three-dimensional contrast-enhanced MRA provides a comprehensive overview of the thoracic vascular anatomy, particularly the relationship of aortic aneurysms to branch vessel origins.[41] Both true and false aneurysms are equally well depicted. A study correlating 3D contrast-enhanced MRA with conventional angiography and surgical exploration demonstrated a diagnostic accuracy of 100 percent for assessing the size and extent of the aneurysm and its relationship to aortic branches.[42] By evaluating the entire aorta, 3D MRA clearly delineates the number of aneurysms present. Arterial-phase MRA, however, contains little information about the morphology of the aortic wall. It displays the lumen but may fail to show the full extent of an aneurysm, such as an area that is partially thrombosed. 3D MRA should therefore be complemented by postcontrast acquisitions. The remaining contrast within the blood permits easy differentiation between flowing blood and thrombus. The aortic wall can also be assessed. Enhancement of the aortic wall and surrounding soft tissues is indicative of an inflammatory process, as found in mycotic aneurysms or aortitis.[43] Involvement of the aortic valve should always be considered in the presence of an aneurysm affecting the ascending aorta. Here, the acquisition of cine steady state free procession (SSFP) sequences in a plane along the axis of the aortic outflow tract can determine whether aortic stenosis and/or regurgitation is present.

***CT Angiography of Thoracic Aneurysms*** CTA is also a useful tool for diagnosing thoracic aortic aneurysms, determining their extent, and predicting appropriate management. While the diagnosis of aortic aneurysm is readily made from transverse sections, an assessment of the extent of the lesion, particularly when the brachiocephalic branches are involved, is facilitated by an assessment of reconstruction techniques such as maximum-intensity projections, multiplanar reconstructions, or volume rendering. Spiral CT can facilitate surgical planning by delineating the extent of the aneurysm and the involvement of aortic branches. Due to the tortuosity and curvature of the thoracic aorta, aneurysm sizing is performed most accurately when double-oblique images are generated perpendicular to the aortic flow lumen. The major challenge of this approach is that data concerning the risk of aneurysm rupture and expansion rate are based on measurements made from transverse sections, where true diameters can be overestimated. MDCT provides the same information regarding aneurysmal size and extent of mural thrombus as that available with conventional, single-slice spiral CT; however, the volumetric acquisition of thinner slices allows multiplanar and 3D renderings to be generated perpendicular to the long axis of the aneurysm, resulting in greater accuracy of the aneurysmal size measurements.[44]

## ABDOMINAL AORTIC ANEURYSM

Abdominal aortic aneurysms (AAAs) are characteristically fusiform in configuration, although occasionally a saccular aneurysm may be seen.[45] Evaluation of patients with abdominal aortic aneurysm should include a systematic description of the following morphologic details: (1) the relationship of the aneurysm to the main and accessory renal, iliac, superior, and inferior mesenteric arteries; (2) the extension of the aneurysm into the common, external, or internal iliac arteries to determine the type and length of prosthetic graft utilized; and (3) evaluation of coexistent iliac or renal occlusive disease. Conventional x-ray aortography has traditionally been the imaging modality of choice prior to resection of AAAs. Yet, advantages of cross-sectional imaging provided by MR or CT over x-ray angiography are well established. CT angiography has been the preferred modality for cross-sectional imaging of the abdominal aorta. Three-dimensional contrast-enhanced MRA, however, has overcome limitations inherent to conventional MR techniques including long imaging times and reduced vessel-to-background contrast in regions of slow flow.

***MR Angiography of Abdominal Aortic Aneurysms*** Previously, the use of MRI in the assessment of patients with AAAs has been limited. Non-contrast-enhanced bright blood and black blood, gradient-echo and spin-echo MRA techniques depend on flow effects to create contrast between vessels and background tissue. The complex and frequently slow-flow patterns typically seen within AAAs result in signal loss and may lead to difficulties in distinguishing between slow flow and thrombus. To prevent saturation effects, images must be acquired in a plane perpendicular to the vessels, resulting in long imaging times with consequent image degradation due to respiratory artifacts and patient motion. Contrast-enhanced MRA techniques are essentially flow-independent. Imaging can be performed in any plane, allowing rapid acquisitions covering a large field of view during a single breathhold. Analysis of an aneurysmal aorta should always be based on both the arterial phase 3D contrast-enhanced MRA, displaying the aortic lumen, in combination with delayed postcontrast scans, depicting the thrombosed portion of the lumen.[46] These delayed scans also evaluate enhancement of the aortic wall and surrounding tissues in inflammatory or mycotic aneurysms. With contrast-enhanced MRA, all details of the aneurysmal morphology are well depicted. The large coronal field-of-view reveals extension of the aneurysm into the iliac arteries. Multiplanar reformations help unfold even highly tortuous vascular morphology. Based on subvolume MIPs as well as multiplanar reformations, the exact dimensions of the aneurysm can be determined prior to any surgical or percutaneous intervention. MRA is also effective in demonstrating the status of renal arterial origins and their relationship to the aortic aneurysm. High diagnostic accuracy of 3D CE-MRA regarding morphologic analysis of AAAs has been confirmed by several clinical studies.[47,48]

***CT Angiography of Abdominal Aortic Aneurysms*** CT has been advocated in the preoperative evaluation of AAAs.[49] It is noninvasive, more accurate than conventional angiography for predicting the size of an AAA, and is superior to angiography in its ability to demonstrate mural thrombus within an aneurysm, inflammatory aneurysms, perianeurysmal blood due to contained rupture, and coexistent nonvascular abdominal disease. Single-slice spiral CT has been shown to enable an accurate depiction of the aneurysmal neck relative to aortic branch vessels as well as an evaluation of the aortic branch vessels themselves.[50] Juxta- and suprarenal extension of an AAA can be missed on x-ray angiography due to the presence of mural thrombus and atheroma at the proximal neck. The ability of CTA to identify renal artery stenoses in the presence of AAAs has been reported with a 94 percent sensitivity and 96 percent specificity for significant stenoses (>50 percent).[50] The introduction of MDCT with adapted contrast-injection protocols has further increased image quality and diagnostic accuracy.[51] MDCT provides the same information regarding aneurysmal size and extent of mural thrombus available with single-slice helical CT; however, the volumetric acquisition of thinner slices allows multiplanar and 3D renderings to be generated perpendicular to the long axis of the aneurysm, resulting in greater accuracy of the aneurysmal size measurements.[44] Additionally, the improved quality of the data set available for 3D image reconstruction and manipulation makes possible the routine display, in considerable detail, of the mesenteric vasculature (Fig. 22-5).

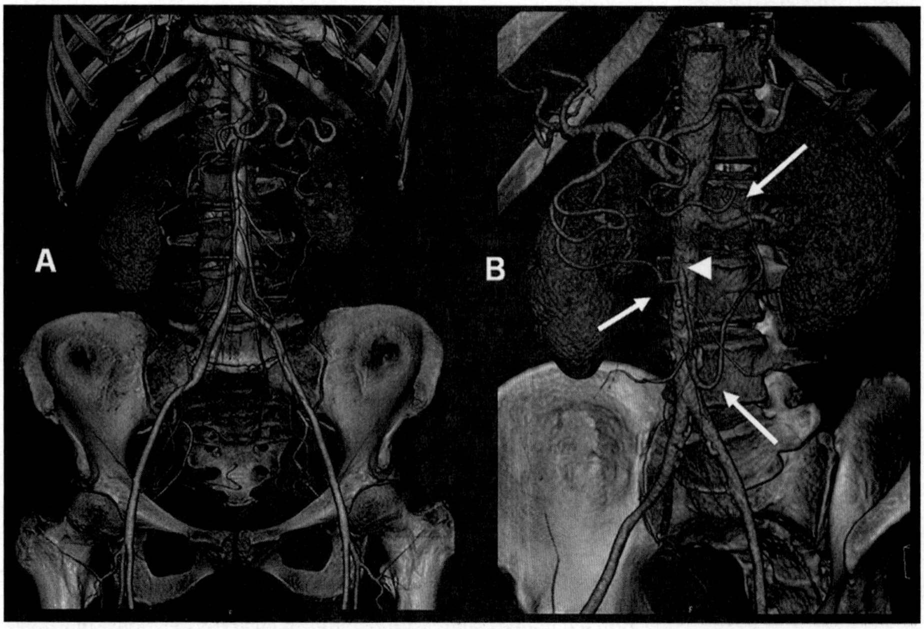

FIGURE 22-5 *A.* Three-dimensional volume-rendering reconstruction of an abdominal 16-DCT angiogram from a healthy volunteer, acquired in a single breathhold with 0.75-mm slice thickness. The mesenteric vasculature is depicted in great detail, with assessable mesenteric vessel branches up to fourth-order branches. *B.* 16-DCT angiogram of a patient with a proximal occlusion of the superior mesenteric artery (SMA). A collateral refilling is demonstrated with an arch of collateral vessels originating from the inferior mesenteric artery (IMA) and the arcarde of Riolan (*arrows*). (Courtesy of B.J. Wintersperger, Ludwig-Maximilians-University, Munich, Germany.[182])

## PERIPHERAL VESSELS

### MR Angiography of the Peripheral Vessels

Successful surgical and endovascular arterial revascularization depends on accurate and detailed imaging of the location and degree of the occlusive arterial lesions (see Chaps. 100 and 101). X-ray angiography has been considered the imaging standard in evaluating peripheral arteries and planning treatment of lower limb ischemia. However, x-ray angiography has been questioned as the gold standard because it may fail to reveal patent infrapopliteal vessels in patients with multisegmental occlusive lesions and low inflow pressure.[52] Furthermore, a noninvasive alternative to x-ray angiography is attractive due to a small but significant risk of serious complications of 2 to 3 percent using the transfemoral technique.[53]

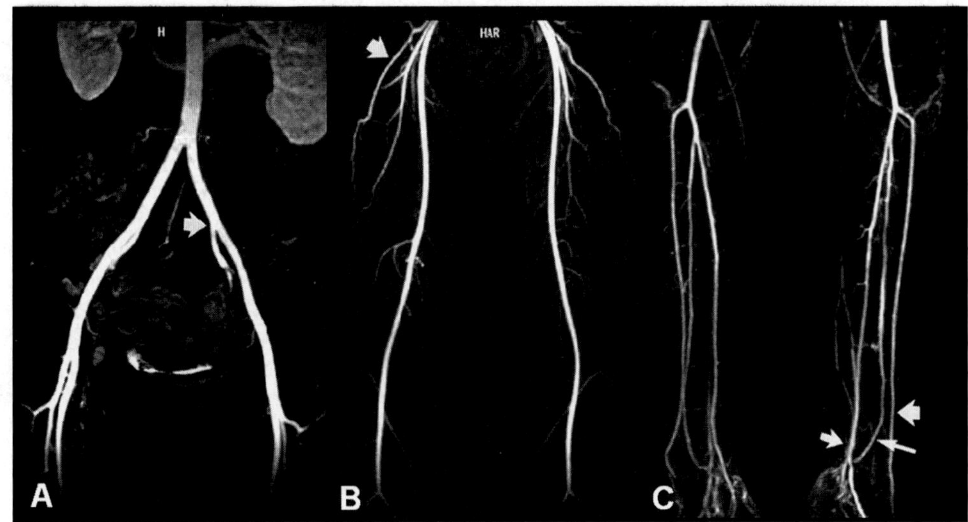


FIGURE 22-6 Maximal-intensity-projection reconstructions of subtracted MR angiography data sets of the peripheral vessels from the distal aorta to the ankle joint in a 26-year-old healthy male volunteer. *A.* Maximal-intensity-projection reconstruction shows distal aorta, common iliac arteries, proximal parts of internal iliac arteries, external iliac arteries, and proximal parts of common femoral arteries. Note branching to internal iliac artery (*arrow*). *B.* Maximal-intensity-projection reconstruction at the upper leg level shows superficial femoral arteries, proximal popliteal arteries, and branches of deep femoral arteries (*arrow*). *C.* Maximal-intensity-projection reconstruction at lower leg level shows distal parts of popliteal arteries and three major arteries of the lower leg down to the ankle. Note the anterior tibial artery (*large short arrow*), posterior tibial artery (*small short arrow*), and peroneal artery (*long arrow*). (Courtesy of A. Huber, Ludwig-Maximilians-University, Munich, Germany.[144])

Several studies concerning MRA prior to surgical and endovascular treatment have been reported using non-contrast-enhanced time-of-flight MRA (TOF-MRA).[54,55] Yet TOF-MRA faces several drawbacks. Imaging of the iliac arteries is complicated by their curved course relative to the acquisition plane, causing in-plane saturation effects that can lead to false-positive diagnosis of stenoses and occlusions. Misreadings caused by pulsation artifacts have been reported. TOF-MRA requires an acquisition time of approximately 60 to 120 min for a full lower limb examination. Therefore the TOF-MRA technique has never become a common alternative to x-ray angiography except in a few highly experienced centers. The introduction of contrast-enhanced MRA has overcome many of these limitations.[56] In CE-MRA, the inflow pressure is not as essential as in TOF-MRA or conventional contrast arteriography. Due to short echo times, CE-MRA reduces the examination time, minimizing both clip artifacts and artifacts caused by movements. The total examination time is now less than 30 min for a full lower limb examination. A standard 1.5-T MR system is satisfactory and special coils are not obligatory; however, a dedicated lower extremity coil is beneficial in imaging small distal vessels.[57] CE-MRA can be performed as a multistation examination, using a single infusion of contrast followed by series of MRA images at three stations using special moving-table techniques[58,59] (Fig. 22-6). Alternatively, MRA can be performed as one to three series of separate contrast injections and image acquisitions, using image subtraction to eliminate the effect of the preceding contrast injection.[60] Using only one station, selective images with a minimum of venous or tissue signal can be performed—i.e., visualizing distal runoff.[57] At present, no single method has emerged as the preferred option, each having different strengths and weaknesses.[61] In various clinical studies, CE-MRA was found to be superior to duplex ultrasound and highly accurate compared to conventional arteriography, with pooled values of sensitivity of 81 to 100 percent and specificities of 83 to 99 percent (Table 22-2).

In conclusion, in reviewing the literature, the agreement between x-ray angiography and CE-MRA in patients facing vascular reconstruction is good, and CE-MRA is proving to be a promising noninvasive alternative to x-ray angiography in presurgical evaluation. Contrast-enhanced MRA is currently the "state-of-the-art" MRA

TABLE 22-2 MRA and CTA of the Peripheral Arteries[a]

| Reference | Technique | Patients (*n*) | Sensitivity (%) | Specificity (%) |
|---|---|---|---|---|
| Ruehm et al., 2000[143] | MRA | 61 | 92 | 98 |
| Huber et al., 2000[144] | MRA | 24 | 100 | 98 |
| Meaney et al., 1999[145] | MRA | 20 | 81 | 91 |
| Sueyoshi et al., 1999[146] | MRA | 23 | 97 | 99 |
| Yamashita et al., 1998[147] | MRA | 20 | 96 | 83 |
| Martin et al., 2003[65] | MDCTA (4) | 41 | 98 | 97 |
| Ofer et al., 2003[148] | MDCTA (4) | 18 | 91 | 92 |
| Rieker et al., 1997[149] | SCTA | 30 | 93 | 99 |
| Raptopoulos et al., 1996[150] | SCTA | 39 | 93 | 96 |
| Lawrence et al., 1995[151] | SCTA | 6 | 93 | 96 |

[a]Sensitivity and specificity of magnetic resonance angiography (MRA) and computed tomography angiography (CTA) for the detection of significant stenoses of peripheral arteries (>75 percent). Results of a selection of clinical trials as compared to conventional angiography. (SCTA = spiral CTA, MDCTA = multidetector CTA, (4) = four detector rows.)

technique, overcoming the troublesome aorto-iliac region, reducing the examination time, and increasing the accuracy compared to the TOF-MRA technique. In selected patients, both CE-MRA and TOF-MRA can demonstrate patent runoff vessels not seen on x-ray angiography, possibly increasing the limb salvage rate. It is expected, in the foreseeable future, that the clinical demand for CE-MRA will gradually be increasing. New MR imaging techniques such as parallel imaging acquisitions are likely to further refine peripheral MRA techniques.[62]

### CT Angiography of the Peripheral Vessels

Until the recent introduction of MDCT, CT angiography was limited to not more than 40 cm of craniocaudal coverage during a single intravenous contrast injection. While this distance was sufficient for imaging the majority of systemic arteries, it was insufficient for studying the arterial inflow and runoff of the lower extremities. MDCT with four channels of simultaneous acquisition has eliminated this limitation. This modality is now able to assess lower extremity arterial inflow and runoff while offering shorter acquisition times, lower doses of contrast medium, and improved spatial resolution for assessing smaller arterial branches.[63] The newest 16-DCT systems are able to cover a range of up to 150 cm in less than 40 s with a 0.75-mm slice thickness, acquiring about 1500 axial images in total[64] (Fig. 22-7). Several clinical studies on the implementation of spiral and MDCT for the assessment of peripheral arterial disease have been published, reporting sensitivities of 91 to 98 percent and specificities of 92 to 99 percent for significant stenoses >75 percent (Table 22-2). Severe diffuse calcifications may lead to misinterpretations by CT, leading to both false-positive and false-negative results.[44] The inability of conventional angiography to show calf vessels in patients with proximal occlusions is well documented, and it has been indicated that MDCT angiography may allow better visualization of calf vessels in these patients, because a systemic contrast bolus is used and because image quality is largely unaffected by patient motion.[65] The high level of interobserver agreement in the published clinical trials so far indicates that the results as determined by MDCT angiography are highly reproducible. With the 16-DCT scanners, lower extremity MDCT angiography can now be performed with thinner collimation. Imaging protocols on 4-DCT scanners must use high table speed to cover the full range of the peripheral runoff, which in some cases can lead to insufficient opacification of distal calf vessels. Slowing table speed by using a narrower slice thickness on the 16-DCT systems reduces this problem of 4-DCT scanners. An important consideration in the implementation of CT is that of radiation dose. In the first clinical study on peripheral MDCT angiography, the calculated radiation dose was 3.9 times lower than that with x-ray angiography.[63] Clearly, radiation doses will vary greatly depending on the technique used and the patient's body habitus. As MDCT angiography continues to improve, techniques must be refined further to minimize radiation exposure without compromising image quality. Nevertheless, MDCT angiography at its relatively early stage of development has a clear advantage over x-ray angiography with regard to radiation dose. MDCT angiography may be more sensitive than x-ray angiography in identifying patent vessels distal to severe occlusions, but this difference in sensitivity will have to be evaluated by comparing these two techniques with a more sensitive reference standard, such as MR angiography or intraoperative angiography. The validation of MDCT angiography will require further investigation regarding its effect on clinical decision making, patient outcomes, and cost-effectiveness. However, MDCT angiography of the lower extremities appears to be a promising new diagnostic test that will likely have an important role in the investigation of peripheral vascular disease.

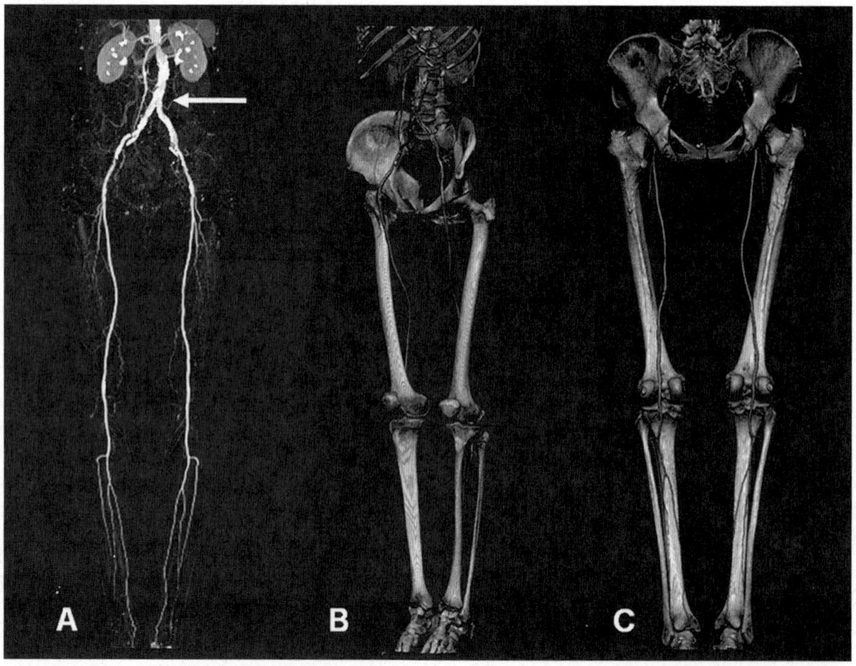

FIGURE 22-7 A 16-DCT angiogram of the peripheral vasculature in a 74-year-old male patient, acquiring 1500 images in an acquisition time of under 40 s; 0.75-mm slice thickness. For maximum-intensity projections (MIP) (*A*), bony structures have to be segmented manually for a clear visualization of the peripheral vessels. Significant calcifications are demonstrated in the abdominal aorta (*arrow*), but patent arteries are depicted down to the ankle joints on both sides. Using volume-rendering techniques (VRT) (*B,C*), 3D reconstruction is fast and easy, but bony structures are still visible, so various rotational views have to be obtained for full delineation of the peripheral vessels. (Courtesy of B.J. Wintersperger, Ludwig-Maximilians-University, Munich, Germany.[64])

## PULMONARY ARTERIES

### Background

The diagnosis of pulmonary embolism (PE) remains difficult in clinical practice, because clinical findings are nonspecific and all available objective tests have practical or clinical limitations[66] (see Chap. 63). Pulmonary x-ray angiography remains the gold-standard diagnostic test, but it is invasive, can give false-negative results, and is not readily available in many centers.[67] Various combinations of noninvasive aids to diagnosis, including assessment of clinical probability of PE, plasma D-dimer concentrations, ventilation/perfusion ($\dot{V}/\dot{Q}$) lung scanning, and venous compression ultrasonography of the legs have been developed and validated to reduce the need for pulmonary angiography. Nevertheless, this procedure is still necessary in a significant percentage of patients with regard to whom the clinical suspicion for PE is high, even after a combina-

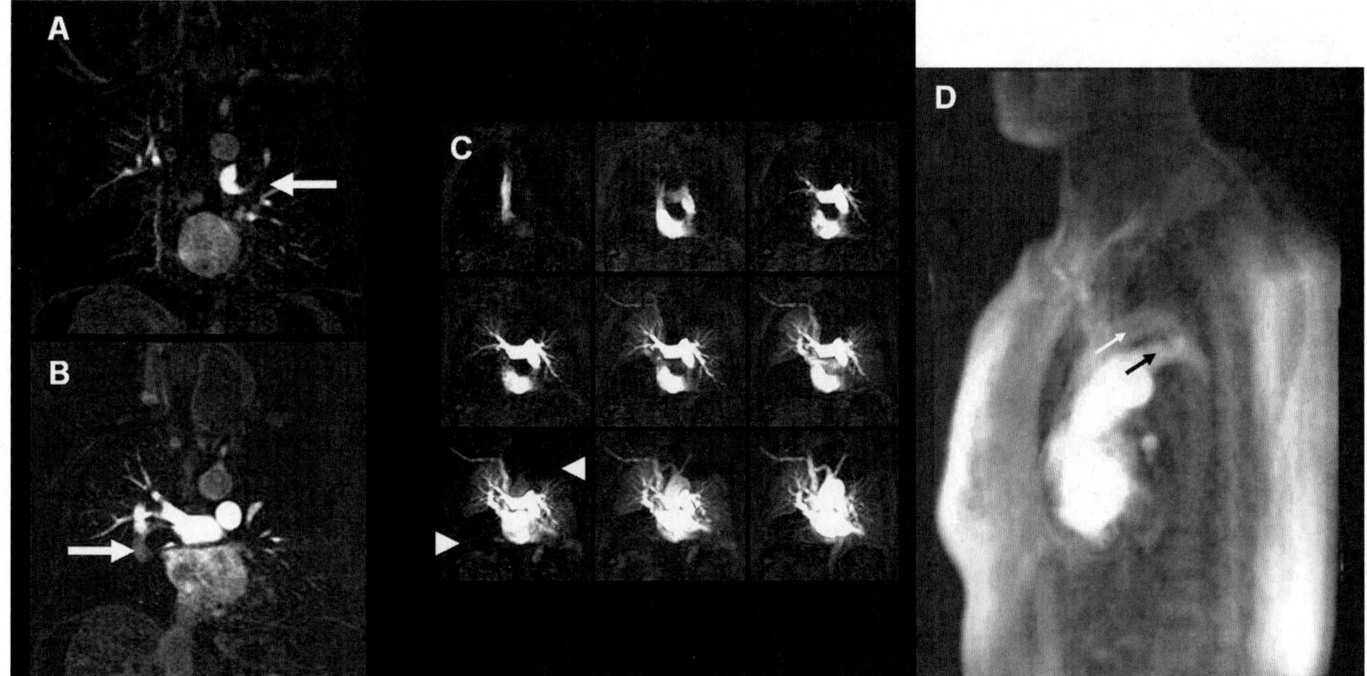


FIGURE 22-8 Three-dimensional contrast-enhanced high-resolution MRA of the pulmonary vasculature in a 55-year-old patient (*A,B*) revealing large thomboembolic clots in the central pulmonary artery tree on both sides (*arrows*). Using time-resolved MRA perfusion techniques and acquiring one data set every 1.1 s, significant perfusion defects in the left upper and right lower lobe become visible (*arrowheads*) (*C*). (Courtesy of K. Nikolaou, Ludwig-Maximilians-University, Munich, Germany.[183]) *D*. Time-resolved, contrast-enhanced high-resolution MRA of the pulmonary vasculature in a 33-year-old patient with Eisenmenger's syndrome due to a large membranous ventricular septal defect. The left anterior oblique view of the MRA shows spontaneous contrast filling of both the main pulmonary artery (*black arrow*) and the aorta (*white arrow*) as a result of the right-to-left shunt. (Courtesy of M. Poon, Mount Sinai Medical Center, New York, NY.)

tion of all the available noninvasive diagnostic tests has been used.[67] In addition to being an invasive test, conventional x-ray angiography carries a risk of major complications of 1 percent and a mortality risk of 0.5 percent.[68] In the last decade, spiral CT and MRA have become viable alternatives to conventional angiography in the diagnosis of acute and chronic pulmonary embolism.[69]

## MR Angiography of the Pulmonary Arteries

Contrast-enhanced MR imaging uses even safer contrast agents (i.e., gadolinium chelates) than CT and does not involve radiation exposure. In addition, MRI allows for the depiction of functional aspects such as perfusion and ventilation, which may further aid in the (differential) diagnosis of PE and thus appropriate patient care and treatment[70,71] (Fig. 22-8*A*–*C*). This diagnostic technique is improving constantly, and by using contrast-enhanced breathhold techniques, pulmonary vessels can be visualized effectively in most cases.[72] A number of clinical studies have reported high sensitivities and specificities for the detection of pulmonary emboli as compared to conventional pulmonary angiography (Table 22-3). However, MRA is still time-consuming and patients with acute pulmonary embolism might not be stable enough to undergo this examination. Although faster scanning techniques have permitted MRA to be performed in shorter time periods than before, MRA does not yield optimal image quality in people who are unable to hold their breath. Motion-compensated or real-time techniques with radial k-space scanning may offer potential in these patients and has been tested with satisfying diagnostic accuracy.[69] In conclusion, MRI is a promising diagnostic tool, but to date it has not had a widespread clinical utility in emergency medicine and in critically ill patients, mainly because of the long examination time required, difficulties in patient monitoring, higher costs, and the limited availability of MR in most community-based medical centers. It has a role in the assessment of stable patients with chronic lung disease in the diagnostic workup of pulmonary hypertension and in ruling out right-to-left cardiac shunt (Fig. 22-8*D*).

TABLE 22-3 MRA and CTA of the Pulmonary Arteries[a]

| Reference | Technique | Patients (*n*) | Sensitivity (%) | Specificity (%) |
|---|---|---|---|---|
| Oudkerk et al., 2002[152] | MRA | 118 | 77 | 98 |
| Goyen et al., 2001[153] | MRA | 8 | 100 | 75 |
| Kruger et al., 2001[154] | MRA | 50 | 100 | N/A |
| Kreitner et al., 2000[155] | MRA | 20 | 87 | 100 |
| Gupta et al., 1999[156] | MRA | 36 | 85 | 96 |
| Perrier et al., 2001[157] | CTA | 299 | 70 | 91 |
| Blachere et al., 2000[158] | CTA | 179 | 94 | 95 |
| Qanadli et al., 2000[159] | CTA | 158 | 90 | 94 |
| Remy-Jardin et al., 2000[160] | CTA | 370 | 96 | 100 |
| Kim et al., 1999[161] | CTA | 110 | 92 | 96 |

[a]Sensitivity and specificity of magnetic resonance angiography (MRA) and computed tomography angiography (CTA) for the detection of thromboembolic events in the pulmonary vasculature. Results of a selection of clinical trials as compared to conventional angiography.

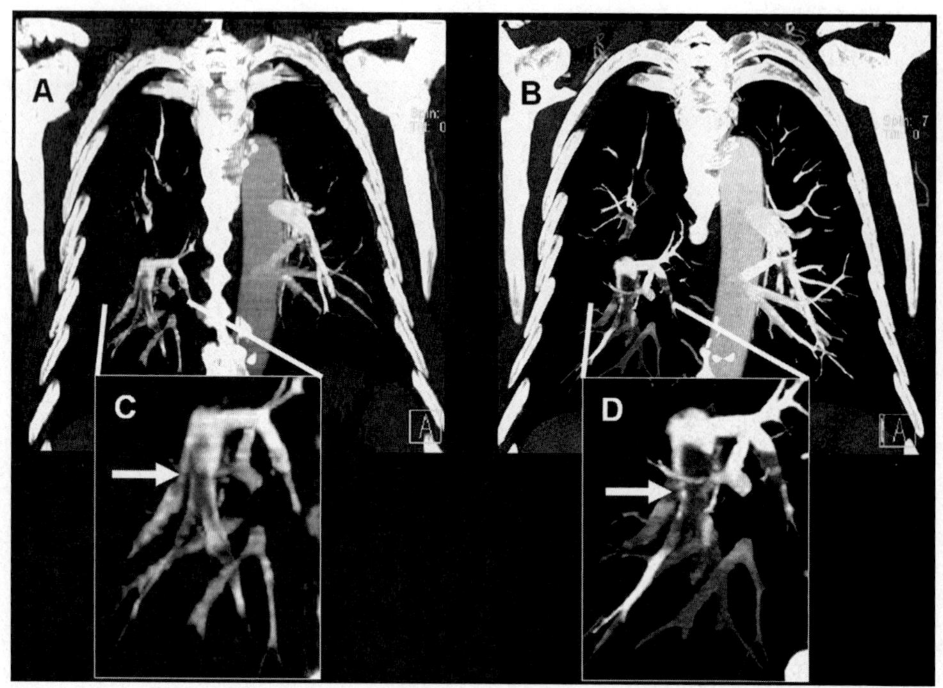


FIGURE 22-9 Contrast-enhanced pulmonary angiogram obtained on a 4-DCT system (*A*) and a 16-DCT system (*B*) in the same patient with a large thromboembolic clot in the right lower pulmonary artery. The enlarged images (*C,D*) clearly demonstrate the advance in image quality and the sharper delineation of the clot (*arrows*) in the 16-DCT image (*D*) due to thinner slices and shorter acquisition (i.e., shorter breathhold) time. (Courtesy of C. Becker, Ludwig-Maximilians-University, Munich, Germany.)

## CT Angiography of the Pulmonary Arteries

Conventional x-ray angiography has in many institutions been replaced by spiral CT, which is more readily available and yields lower procedure-associated risks. The sensitivity of spiral CT is on the order of 90 percent for central, lobar, or segmental pulmonary emboli (Table 22-3). CTA has been proven to be an accurate, safe, noninvasive, easily and rapidly performed, widely accepted, and cost-effective technique for direct detection and demonstration of intraluminal PE.[73] Depending on the patient's clinical status and the CT technology available, a 4- to 40-s breathhold is required to scan the entire pulmonary vasculature. The ability to accurately rule out the presence of PE is an undisputed advantage of CT. Examination of the leg veins may be indicated in negative CT. The widespread use of MDCT is expected to increase the acquisition speed, image quality, and overall accuracy of the test (Fig. 22-9). Follow-up studies of patients without anticoagulation are mandatory. Spiral CT pulmonary angiography should be considered the initial imaging modality of choice, particularly in subgroups known for a high rate of nondiagnostic $V/\dot{Q}$ scans, such as hospitalized patients, patients with a history of cardiopulmonary disease, or those with abnormal chest x-rays.

# CORONARY ARTERIES

## Noninvasive Coronary Angiography

### BACKGROUND

The small size and fast motion of the coronary arteries puts any noninvasive diagnostic imaging modality to the test. So far, no cross-sectional imaging modality has proven to be capable of depicting the coronary arteries with a sufficiently high temporal and spatial resolution for a consistent and adequate image quality as good as that of x-ray angiography. Alternative modalities like EBCT, MRI, and 4-DCT systems have all been tested for their ability to reliably detect significant coronary artery stenoses, with varying results and conclusions.[74,75] In some studies, good diagnostic results have been reported. However, in most reports, the number of vessel segments or patients excluded—due to nonassessability as a direct result of the limitations in image quality—were quite high (ranging from 5 to 30 percent).[76,77] In addition, the assessment was usually limited to the proximal and middle segments of the vessels. Active research and development to overcome the technical barriers of EBCT and MRI is ongoing. At the time this is being written, both MR and EBCT appear to be outperformed by 16-DCT. For the first time, 16-DCT has arrived as a robust and reliable noninvasive imaging modality that is capable of producing consistent, high-quality images of the coronary arteries in most patients.

### MR ANGIOGRAPHY OF THE CORONARY ARTERIES

Although several noninvasive imaging modalities have been tested clinically for the detection of coronary artery lesions, MRI deserves special attention. MRI can deliver high-resolution images with superb contrast characteristics in any desired orientation; it is therefore especially suited to studies of the coronary anatomy. Additionally, functional parameters like myocardial function or perfusion under rest and pharmacologic stress can be used to complement the evaluation of suspected coronary artery lesions. Coronary arteries are surrounded by epicardial fat; thus, using bright-blood techniques, fat suppression is essential for adequate visualization of the vessel. Further improvements to enhance contrast from the coronary artery to the myocardium include additional preparatory pulses such as magnetization transfer and T2 preparation,[78] which are likely to improve the image quality overall.

Since the publication of first clinical results in 1993,[79] noninvasive coronary MRA has undergone numerous technical improvements and innovations. Three major groups or "generations" of coronary MRA techniques have been proposed by several authors.[80,81] Of all the imaging techniques available, 2D breathhold coronary MRA scans,[82] 3D respiratory-gated coronary MRA[83,84] (Fig. 22-10), and breathhold 3D coronary MRA[85,86] have been evaluated most extensively. Recently, a multicenter study using a 3D prospective respiratory navigator approach has been presented, reporting an acceptable overall sensitivity of 82 percent for significant stenoses (≥50 percent) in proximal and middle vessel segments and a diagnostic accuracy of 75 percent for diagnosing coronary artery disease (CAD).[87] Still, after 10 years of preclinical trials using these different coronary MRA techniques, no technique has yet emerged as superior and able to provide a sensitivity and specificity for coronary lesion detection that can compare with that of traditional x-ray coronary angiography (Table 22-4).

To date, MRI methods continue to improve. Advanced second-generation coronary MRA techniques using navigator pulse feedback, 3D k-space reordering,[88] or adaptive prospective correction of slice position with signal averaging[89] improve both reliability and image quality and thus increase the sensitivity of the technique. The third-generation non-contrast-enhanced[86] and contrast-enhanced[90,91] 3D breathhold techniques appear to be fast and easy to use. These and other various new coronary MRA techniques await further clinical trials to determine their effectiveness. Recent studies of 2D fast spin-echo black-blood techniques report maximized signal for coronary MRA at no loss in image spatial resolution. This suggests that the extension of black-blood coronary MRA with a 3D imaging technique would allow for a further increase in signal.[92] Segmented 3D steady-state free precession sequences were also described as a promising technique, with substantially increased signal-to-noise and contrast-to noise ratios for coronary artery imaging compared to conventional 3D gradient-echo techniques with the same imaging time.[93] New intravascular contrast agents may provide the long-awaited boost for reliable MR coronary angiography. First studies on animals[94] and in healthy volunteers[95] have shown promising results. Additionally, the majority of manufacturers now offer dedicated MRI cardiac scanners with strong imaging gradients (>30 mT/m) and fast rise times (>150 mT/m/ms) optimized for a smaller effective imaging field of view to provide higher speed and a better signal-to-noise ratio. Introduction of parallel MRI acquisition techniques, such as simultaneous acquisition of spatial harmonics (SMASH)[96] and sensitivity encoding (SENSE)[97] may provide additional speed enhancement required to shorten imaging time.

Today, established clinical applications include the evaluation of the patency of coronary artery bypass grafts (see "Noninvasive Imaging of Bypass Grafts," below) and the imaging of anomalous coronary arteries.[98] The capability to reliably detect significant coronary artery stenoses in proximal and middle-vessel segments with an acceptable sensitivity using any of the techniques available today is still being discussed, with significant differences of opinion. As the MR techniques continue to improve, the long-term value of coronary MRA cannot be underestimated in spite of the advent of MDCT coronary angiography.

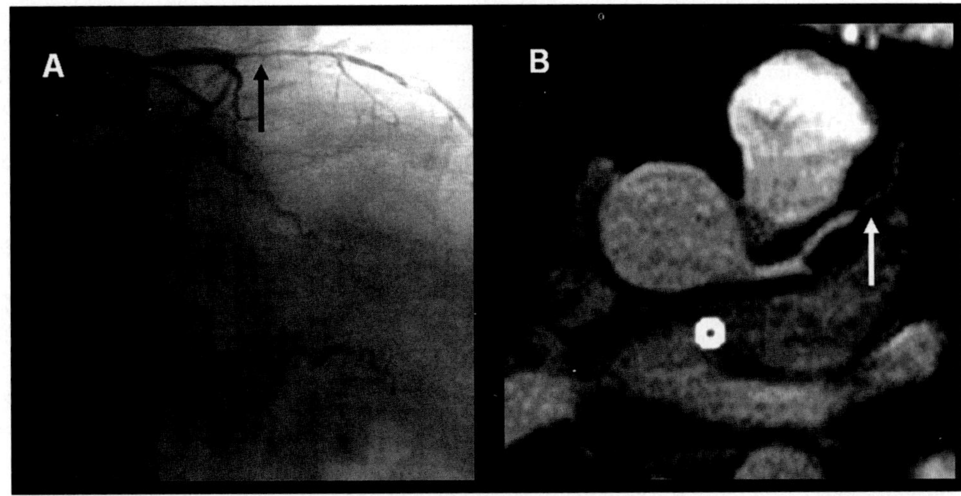


FIGURE 22-10 Conventional coronary x-ray angiogram of a 60-year-old male patient shows a high-grade extended stenosis beginning in the proximal left anterior descending coronary artery (LAD) (*black arrow*) (*A*). A maximum-intensity projection (MIP) of a 3D non-contrast-enhanced navigator-gated time-of-flight magnetic resonance coronary angiogram shows a signal loss in the corresponding vessel segment (*white arrow*) (*B*). (Courtesy of K. Nikolaou, Ludwig-Maximilians-University, Munich, Germany.[77])

## CT ANGIOGRAPHY OF THE CORONARY ARTERIES

The introduction of 4-DCT scanner systems in 1998 had a major impact on noninvasive imaging of the coronary arteries.[99] The introduction of its immediate successor, the 16-DCT system in 2002 has extended the dominant role of CT in noninvasive coronary imaging today. The 16-DCT scanner offers several advantages for angiographic examinations in general and especially for the coronary arteries.[100] First, the gantry rotation time in 16-DCT for cardiac investigations is 420 ms, allowing for 210-ms exposure time up to a heart rate of 65 beats per minute. This is a 20 percent gain in temporal resolution over that of a 4-channel detector system. With higher

TABLE 22-4 MRA, MDCTA, and EBCTA Coronary Arteries[a]

| Reference | Technique | Patients (*n*) | Sensitivity (%) | Specificity (%) |
|---|---|---|---|---|
| Regenfus et al., 2003[162] | MRA | 61 | 85 | 90 |
| Plein et al., 2003[163] | MRA | 40 | 74 | 88 |
| Watanabe et al., 2002[164] | MRA | 22 | 80 | 85 |
| Kim et al., 2002[165] | MRA | 109 | 93 | 42 |
| Nikolaou et al., 2001[84] | MRA | 40 | 72 | 60 |
| Ropers et al., 2003[131] | MDCTA (16) | 77 | 92 | 93 |
| Nieman et al., 2002[166] | MDCTA (16) | 59 | 95 | 86 |
| Knez et al., 2001[167] | MDCTA (4) | 44 | 78 | 98 |
| Nieman et al., 2001[99] | MDCTA (4) | 35 | 81 | 97 |
| Achenbach et al., 2001[76] | MDCTA (4) | 64 | 85 | 76 |
| Nikolaou et al., 2002[77] | EBCTA | 20 | 85 | 77 |
| Achenbach et al., 2000[168] | EBCTA | 36 | 92 | 94 |
| Budoff et al., 1999[169] | EBCTA | 52 | 78 | 91 |
| Schmermund et al., 1998[170] | EBCTA | 28 | 82 | 88 |
| Nakanishi et al., 1997[171] | EBCTA | 37 | 74 | 94 |

[a]Sensitivity and specificity of magnetic resonance angiography (MRA) and computed tomography angiography for the detection of significant coronary artery stenoses (>75 percent). Results of a selection of clinical trials as compared to conventional angiography. (MDCTA = multidetector-row computed tomography angiography, 16 = 16 detector rows, 4 = 4 detector rows, EBCTA = electron-beam computed tomography angiography.)

heart rates and multisegment reconstruction algorithms, the exposure time varies from 105 to 210 ms, depending on the heart rate. Second, the spatial resolution along the Z axis improves by 25 percent, now being 0.75 mm, or above the 1.0 mm acquired previously on a 4-DCT system. In-plane resolution has remained the same, but still, using 16-DCT, almost isotropic voxels can now be acquired with a voxel size of about 0.6 × 0.6 × 0.75 mm. Thereby, beam-hardening artifacts of stents or of calcium deposits in the vessel wall might be reduced because of reduced partial volume effects. Thus, depiction and delineation of calcified and noncalcified plaques is improved. Third and probably most important, the complete heart can now be depicted in a significantly shorter breathhold time of less than 20 s, compared to the 35- to 40-s breathhold time on a 4-DCT. This results in a considerable reduction in motion artifacts. Additional advantages of this shorter scan time are less venous contrast enhancement and a lower contrast dose. The well-tolerated examination can be performed within 15 min and requires no hospital admission. Concerning radiation exposure, the increase in dosage comparing 4-DCT to 16-DCT coronary angiography is not significant, being around 4 milli-sieverts (mSv) for 4-DCT and 5 mSv for 16-DCT if prospective tube current modulation is used. Using this technique, the tube current is decreased during systole. In doing so, radiation exposure can be reduced by half at low heart rates.[101] Beta-blocker preparation in patients with heart rates >65 beats per minute is mandatory to ensure motion-free image quality. Using 16-DCT with short acquisition times, contrast timing should be more accurate, so that less contrast agent is needed. For contrast enhancement of the coronaries, the amount of contrast can be reduced significantly using 16-DCT, being now 80 mL of contrast in comparison to 120 mL for 4-DCT, according to a previously published protocol.[102] The continuous data acquisition of a coronary MDCT data set allows slice reconstruction at different time positions within the cardiac cycle. These scans are typically reviewed on the basis of the cross-sectional images in combination with 3D reconstructions.[103]

Clinical studies using 4-DCT scanners have reported sensitivities and specificities for significant coronary artery stenoses (>75 percent) of 78 to 85 percent and 76 to 98 percent, respectively (Table 22-4). These reports showed promising results but were not robust enough to consistently produce reliable coronary imaging. Up to 30 percent of the proximal and middle coronary segments were uninterpretable because of insufficient image quality. The first clinical studies on 16-DCT coronary angiography report high sensitivities and specificities of 92 to 95 percent and 86 to 93 percent, respectively (Table 22-4). Most remarkably, the number of poorly assessable segments was very low, indicating the robustness of this technique. Figure 22-11 shows a correct identification of a large thrombus formation in the left anterior descending (LAD) artery using a contrast-enhanced MDCT technique, with good correlation to conventional angiography.

Despite the promising initial experiences with 16-DCT coronary angiography, there are still certain limitations to the technique. Currently, MDCT coronary angiography is not reliable in patients with arrhythmias, moderate to high heart rates not amenable to beta blockade, or severely calcified vessels. Severe calcifications are still causing partial volume and beam-hardening artifacts in spite of the improvement in spatial resolution, producing false-negative results compared to cardiac x-ray angiography. In segments with extensive calcifications, significant coronary artery stenoses can neither be concluded nor ruled out. Although 16-DCT has outstandingly high spatial resolution among noninvasive imaging modalities, small-caliber vessels can still produce false-positive findings compared to x-ray coronary angiography. Coronary stents can now be well visualized using 16-DCT. Insight into the patency of the stent lumen is not only plausible but, in most patients with adequately slow heart rates, it can be confirmed or excluded. However, the degree of in-stent stenosis is not assessable at this juncture.

In conclusion, the main advantage of 16- over 4-DCT angiography of the coronary arteries seems to be the increased number of investigations with sufficiently good image quality. This robustness of its clinical application can also be ascertained by the shorter breath-holding time, 20 percent improved temporal resolution, and the decreasing need of beta blocker for heart rate control. However, MSCT has yet to achieve the quantitative accuracy of x-ray-based imaging techniques. Nevertheless it does allow noninvasive detection and exclusion of significant coronary obstructions. From the published studies on coronary MDCT so far, the negative predictive value compared to coronary x-ray angiography was in the range of 96 to 98 percent. This high negative predictive value indicates that MDCT may be an ideal tool to rule out CAD in low-prevalence populations, as in symptomatic patients with atypical chest pain. However, MSCT currently appears not to be suited to determine disease severity or progression in CAD patients with typical angina or positive evidence of significant myocardial ischemia on exercise testing or after coronary intervention. These patients would still best be approached by conventional x-ray angiography, which would also allow percutaneous coronary interventions in the same session.

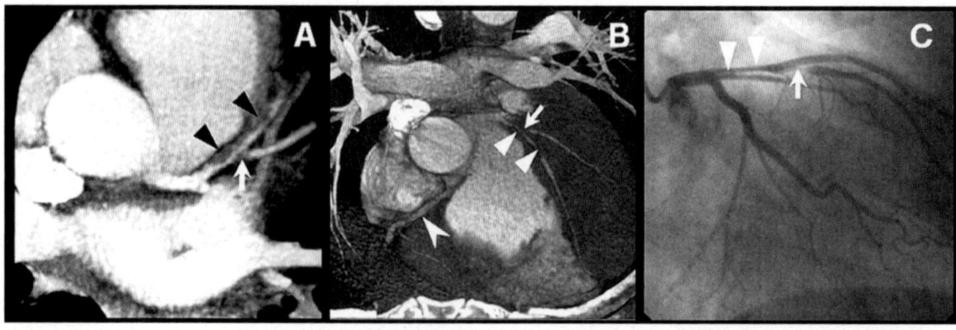


FIGURE 22-11 Images of a 41-year-old man with atypical chest pain. The maximum-intensity projection of a contrast-enhanced helical 4-DCT scan reveals a luminal obstruction in the left anterior descending coronary artery (*arrowheads*) and first diagonal branch (*arrow*) (*A*). The 3D volume-rendering reconstruction of the same CT data set again shows a luminal reduction of the proximal left anterior descending coronary artery (*arrowheads*) with involvement of the first diagonal branch (*arrow*) (*B*). The right coronary artery (*spearhead*) shows normal luminal diameters (*B*). The conventional angiogram confirms the findings of the CT scan and also reveals a high-grade stenosis of the left anterior descending coronary artery (*arrowheads*) and first diagonal branch (*arrow*) (*C*). (Courtesy of C. Becker, Ludwig-Maximilians-University, Munich, Germany.[184])

Another promising CT technique for cardiac imaging and coronary angiography is EBCT. EBCT has mainly been used for accurate quantification of coronary artery calcium, scanning the entire heart in a single breathhold from rapid (100-ms) tomographic scans done in synchrony with the heart cycle.[104] In various clinical studies, the sensitivity and specificity reported for the detection of significant coronary artery stenoses was 74 to 92 percent and 77 to 94 percent, respectively (Table 22-4) (see also

Chap. 57). Next-generation ECBT scanners will combine a higher temporal resolution of up to 50 ms with reduced slice thicknesses (i.e., higher spatial resolution), but so far no reports on the potential clinical advantages of these new scanners have become available.

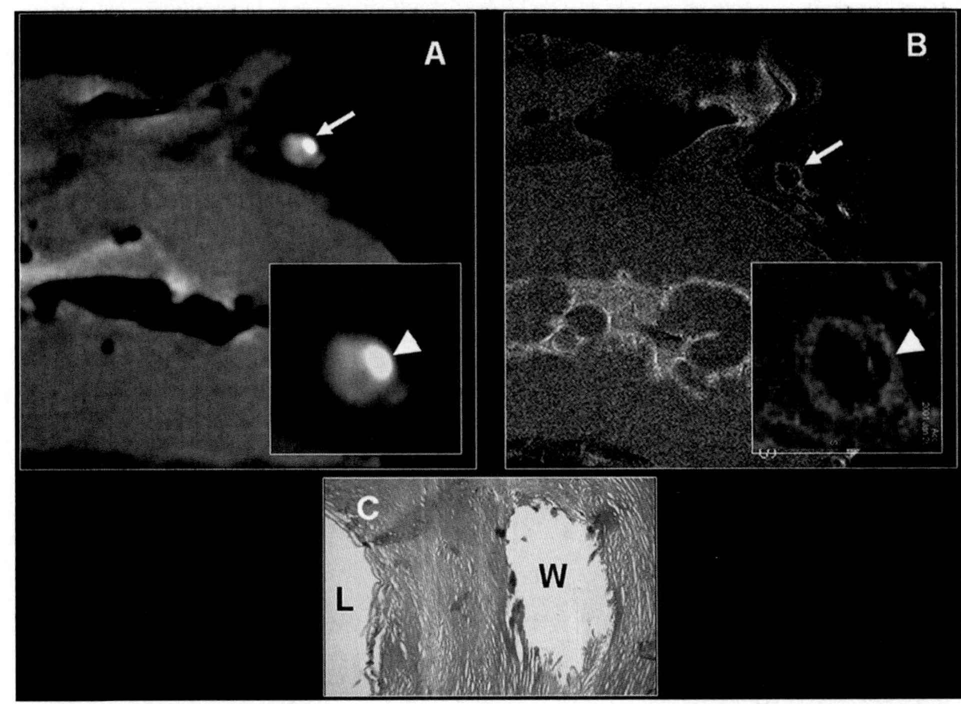


FIGURE 22-12 Ex vivo images of a human heart, with a fibrocalcified left anterior descending coronary artery (LAD), corresponding to a type Vb atherosclerotic lesion according to the classification of the American Heart Association (AHA). MDCT (*A*, with magnified inlet of the LAD) show a cross-sectional image of the vessel with a high-density lesion and typical blooming artifacts caused by the calcifications (*arrow, arrowhead*). MRI (*B*, with magnified inlet; T2-weighted fast spin-echo technique) shows vessel wall thickening and complete signal loss in the area of the calcification (*arrow, arrowhead*). On a corresponding histopathologic section (*C*) with a calcification in the area of the media, calcium is washed out (W) during the preparation process (L = lumen of the coronary artery). (Courtesy of K. Nikolaou, Ludwig-Maximilians-University Munich, Germany.[186])

## Coronary Plaque Imaging

### BACKGROUND

Currently available imaging techniques for the diagnosis of CAD are subject to several limitations. Conventional coronary angiography, widely accepted as the gold-standard for the detection of CAD, demonstrates the degree of luminal narrowing but fails to visualize the coronary artery wall. It has been shown that plaque composition rather than the severity of an actual stenosis predicts the risk of plaque rupture and acute clinical complications of CAD.[105–107] Thus, new imaging techniques that can image the arterial wall and characterize different lesion types may allow for identification and follow-up of patients at risk and for selecting appropriate therapeutic strategies.[108]

Presently, several imaging modalities are employed to study atherosclerosis and to assess luminal diameter, wall thickness, and plaque volume.[109] Two noninvasive imaging modalities, CT and MRI, have been introduced to the study of atherothrombosis. Both have been shown to be capable of imaging vessel wall structures and differentiating various stages of atherosclerotic wall changes. The latest generation of MDCT scanners allow for quantitative measurement of atherosclerotic burden, including calcified and noncalcified plaques[110] and characterization of the plaque components.[111] MRI has been applied in various in vivo human studies to image atherosclerotic plaques in carotid[28] and aortic[112] atherosclerotic disease. Initial in vivo studies in human coronary arteries have used noninvasive black-blood spin-echo techniques with breathholding[113] or a real-time navigator for respiratory gating.[114]

By possibly combining the advantages of both techniques, detecting significant coronary artery stenoses, and describing the plaque composition at the same time, information could be provided that may predict cardiovascular risk, facilitate further study of atherothrombosis progression and its response to therapy, and provide an important parameter for the assessment of subclinical disease.

### MR PLAQUE IMAGING OF THE CORONARY ARTERIES

High-resolution MR has emerged as the potential leading noninvasive in vivo imaging modality for atherosclerotic plaque characterization. MR differentiates plaque components on the basis of biophysical and biochemical parameters such as chemical composition and concentration, water content, physical state, molecular motion, and diffusion.[115] With a combination of multicontrast MRI sequences, differentiation of fibrocellular, lipid-rich, and calcified regions of the atherosclerotic coronary plaque is feasible, as shown in an ex vivo study on human coronary arteries in correlation to histopathology[116] (Fig. 22-12). In vivo studies of coronary artery plaques are obviously more challenging. Preliminary studies in a pig model showed that the difficulties of coronary wall imaging result from a combination of cardiac and respiratory motion artifacts, nonlinear course, small size, and location.[117] A human in vivo coronary MR plaque imaging study conducted by Fayad et al.[118] was performed during breathholding to minimize respiratory motion with a resolution of $0.46 \times 0.46 \times 2.0$ mm$^3$. Figure 22-13 shows in vivo MR coronary plaque images. To eliminate the need for breathholding, Botnar et al.[119] have combined the black-blood fast spin echo (FSE) method and a real-time navigator for respiratory gating and correction of real-time slice position. A near isotropic spatial resolution ($0.7 \times 0.7 \times 0.8$ mm$^3$) was achieved with the use of a 2D local inversion and black-blood preparatory pulses.[119] This method provided a quick way to image a long segment of the coronary artery wall and may be useful for rapid coronary plaque burden measurements. Future studies are needed to further explore these advanced imaging techniques.

### CT PLAQUE IMAGING OF THE CORONARY ARTERIES

Primary requisites for the assessment of atherosclerotic calcified and noncalcified coronary plaques are similar to the requirements for a high-quality CTA of the coronaries—i.e., achieving both high spatial and high temporal resolution at the same time. Compared to low-pressure arterial systems, such as the pulmonary arteries where calcifications are absent and the injection rate can be increased to visualize the smallest arterial branches, in coronary arteries the opacification must not exceed about 300 Hounsfield units (HU) for a reliable depiction and judgment of calcifications. Optimization of the vessel

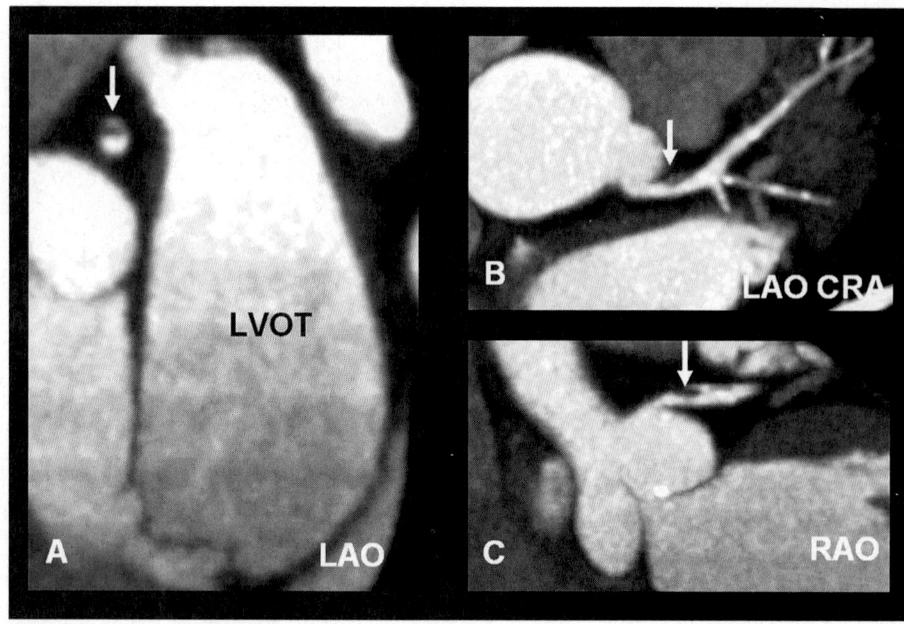


FIGURE 22-13 Contrast-enhanced 16-DCT angiography of the coronary arteries. Maximum-intensity projections (MIPs) are performed in three predefined orientations to resemble projection techniques used in conventional coronary angiography. *A.* LAO = left anterior oblique view shows a cross-sectional image of the left main coronary artery (LM) (*arrow*) with a significant luminal obstruction due to a fibrocalcified plaque (density: 90 Hounsfield units, HU). *B.* LAO CRA = left anterior oblique cranial view displays the course of the LM and the left anterior descending coronary artery (LAD), again with the fibrocalcified plaque in the distal area of the LM (*arrow*). C. RAO = right anterior oblique view of the LM with the same plaque (*arrow*). (Courtesy of K. Nikolaou, Ludwig-Maximilians-University Munich, Germany.[110])

contrast-to-noise ratio is also mandatory for sufficient visualization of noncalcified plaques. Methods to enhance the contrast-to-noise ratio in the vessel wall include either the use of a test bolus setting (20 mL + 50mL NaCl) or bolus tracking. Because nonenhanced blood and noncalcified plaques have a similar attenuation on CT (50 to 70 HU), this type of lesion can be detected only after the administration of contrast media. Therefore a vessel enhancement significantly above the CT values of noncalcified lesions (150 HU) must be achieved to allow for reliable detection of noncalcified plaques. A target attenuation of 200 HU seems best suited to fulfill this requirement. With this vessel enhancement, calcified coronary lesions remain detectable because their attenuation is significantly higher.[120]

CT has become an established method for the noninvasive and highly sensitive detection of coronary artery calcifications.[121] Recently, it was shown that CT has the potential to identify early, noncalcified plaques in vivo in the coronary arteries (Fig. 22-14).[122,123] Various imaging features of noncalcified and calcified plaques depicted with CT correlate with histopathologic stages of atherosclerosis defined by the American Heart Association,[124] as demonstrated in a recent ex vivo study on human hearts[116] (Fig. 22-12). Intravascular ultrasound (IVUS) is the reference standard for detecting and evaluating atherosclerotic plaques in vivo (see Chap. 18). For plaques with and without signs of calcification detected on intravascular ultrasound, EBCT without contrast enhancement yielded a sensitivity of 97 and 47 percent and a specificity of 80 and 75 percent, respectively.[125] In an in vivo study on contrast-enhanced MDCT versus IVUS for accuracy in determining coronary lesion configuration, Schroeder et al.[120] reported a good correlation of these two modalities. MDCT was able to differentiate between soft, intermediate, and calcified plaques as compared to IVUS, with significant differences in CT attenuation values. In recent studies on MDCT of ex vivo coronary arteries versus histopathology as the gold standard, a good correlation was again found. Lipid-rich, fibrous, and calcified plaques were differentiated reliably.[126] Acute intravascular thrombi can also be detected in vivo; the appearance of the irregular thrombus was typical, with low attenuation numbers in the range of 20 to 30 HU (Fig. 22-11). Additionally, new software applications may make possible the quantification of noncalcified atherosclerotic lesions in vivo.[110]

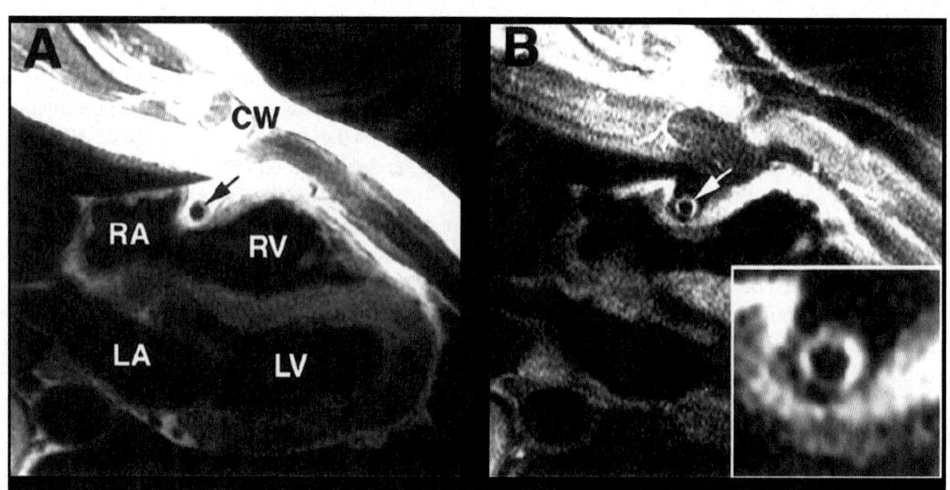


FIGURE 22-14 In vivo cross-sectional black-blood MRIs of lumen (*A*) and wall (*B*) of the right coronary artery (RCA) from a 45-year-old male patient with ectatic atherosclerotic coronary arteries and a thickened coronary wall. The luminal image (*A*) is obtained without fat saturation; the wall image (*B*) is obtained with fat saturation to better delineate the coronary artery wall. Blood flow in the coronary artery lumen is suppressed with velocity-selective inversion preparatory pulses. Maximum wall thickness is 3.3 mm. The BB-MR cross-sectional luminal image reveals a circular lumen and anterior plaque (*arrow*) (*A*). The cross-sectional image of the wall clearly reveals a variably thick proximal RCA, with the wall being thinner around the 6 o'clock position and thicker in other sectors (*B*). B, Inset, Magnified view. (LA = left atrium; RA = right atrium; LV = left ventricle, RV = right ventricle.) (Courtesy of Z. Fayad, Mount Sinai School of Medicine, New York, NY.[113])

## Noninvasive Imaging of Bypass Grafts

### BACKGROUND

Coronary artery bypass graft surgery is a frequently performed revascularization procedure in patients with multivessel CAD. The clinical outcome after bypass surgery depends on the status of the grafts postoperatively. Initially most patients are free of angina, but patients may develop chest pain as a result of acute occlusion early after surgery or gradual progression of atherosclerosis in the long term. Coronary angiography is the gold standard to evaluate the status of graft patency, but this is an invasive procedure, which includes x-ray exposure, a brief hospitalization after the procedure to monitor any vascular complications, and a small risk of potentially serious complications. These disadvantages make the use of coronary angiography less attractive as a diagnostic screening tool for patients with bypass grafts who present with postoperative angina. The need for alternative noninvasive diagnostic methods is apparent.[127]

TABLE 22-5 MRA and CTA for Coronary Bypass Grafts[a]

| Reference | Technique | Patients ($n$) | Sensitivity (%) | Specificity (%) |
|---|---|---|---|---|
| Vetter et al., 2001[172] | MRA | 30 | 96 | 67 |
| Engelmann et al., 2000[173] | MRA | 40 | 76–100 | n./a. |
| Molinari et al., 2000[174] | MRA | 51 | 91 | 97 |
| Brenner et al., 1999[175] | MRA | 85 | 90 | 94 |
| Wintersperger et al., 1998[176] | MRA | 27 | 96 | 67 |
| Enzweiler et al., 2003[132] | EBCTA | 37 | 92 | 96 |
| Tello et al., 2002[133] | SCTA | 26 | 96 | 100 |
| Ropers et al., 2001[131] | MDCTA | 65 | 97 | 98 |
| Achenbach et al., 1997[177] | EBCT | 25 | 100 | 97 |
| Knez et al., 1996[178] | EBCT | 30 | 95 | 89 |

[a]Sensitivity and specificity of magnetic resonance angiography (MRA) and computed tomography angiography for the detection of bypass occlusion. Results of a selection of clinical trials as compared to conventional angiography. [EBCTA = electron-beam computed tomography angiography, MDCTA = multidetector-row computed tomography angiography, SCTA = spiral (single-slice) computed tomography angiography.]

### MR IMAGING OF BYPASS GRAFTS

Magnetic resonance imaging is a noninvasive alternative method that allows direct visualization of coronary bypass grafts. Previously, 2D spin-echo and gradient-echo MR techniques and 3D breathhold contrast-enhanced MR angiography techniques have enabled the evaluation of graft patency, but these techniques as a whole could only differentiate between graft patency and occlusion (Table 22-5). Visualization of different graft segments and detection of graft stenosis remains difficult.[128] Future approaches, such as navigator-gated fast MR techniques, resulting in high-resolution angiography in combination with breathhold MR flow mapping with high temporal resolution, might allow a comprehensive evaluation of bypass graft stenosis and function.[129] The assessment of bypass graft morphology as well as function makes possible complete evaluation of the graft status. Navigator-gated 3D MRA may be the best approach to achieve high-resolution volume images of grafts, as image time is not limited by the duration of a breathhold. For an optimal assessment of graft function during pharmacologic stress, an MR sequence with short acquisition time may be preferable. This would allow subsequent flow reserve measurements in different grafts and in different graft segments with minimal patient discomfort.[130]

### CT IMAGING OF BYPASS GRAFTS

Two alternative CT techniques are considered useful in the noninvasive evaluation of coronary artery bypass grafts—i.e., MDCT and EBCT. With the faster speed of 16-DCT systems, CTA of bypasses can now be performed with thin collimations. Depicting a range from the aortic arch to the base of the heart with a 0.75-mm collimation now takes 25 to 30 s. Using ECG triggering, a high-quality angiogram—even of small-caliber arterial bypasses, with motion-free depiction of the insertion of the bypass vessel to the grafted coronary artery—now becomes feasible (Fig. 22-15). Thus far only few clinical studies on the assessment of bypass grafts have been published using MDCT. A study reporting a sensitivity and specificity of 97 and 98 percent, respectively, for the evaluation of graft patency was recently published.[131] More extensive experience has been gathered using EBCT for this indication.[132] CT makes possible functional analysis of the bypass graft in addition to flow measurements in the grafted vessels.[133] Table 22-5 gives a comprehensive overview of the recent clinical CT studies on the assessment of coronary bypass grafts using different CT techniques.

## CONCLUSION

In conclusion, in the very near future and for most vascular territories, it will be possible to perform diagnostic angiography using noninvasive methods such as MRA or CTA. Both modalities offer significant advantages for certain vascular territories but with significant drawbacks inherent to both. In the peripheral circulation, MRA

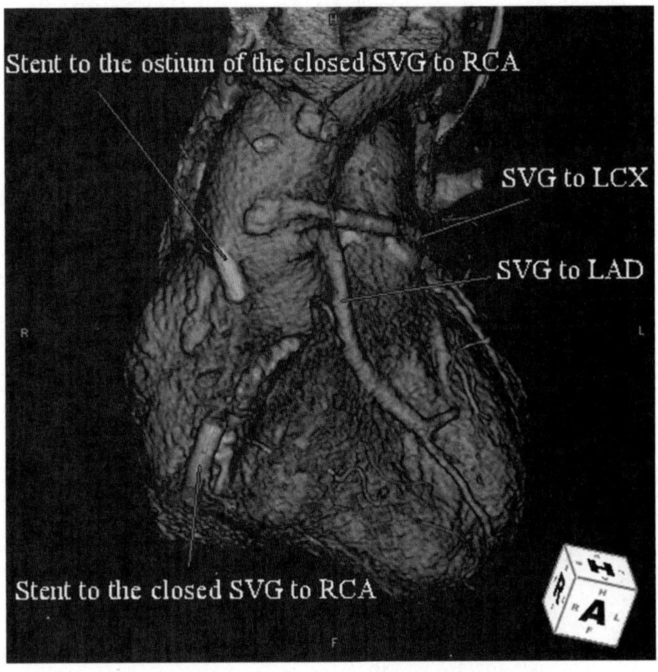


FIGURE 22-15 Three-dimensional volume-rendering MDCT image of the heart performed on a Sensation 16 (Siemens Medical Solutions, Forchheim, Germany) showing two patent saphenous vein grafts (SVGs) to the left anterior descending artery and obtuse marginal artery and one occluded SVG to the distal right coronary artery. One of the two patent SVGs has a proximal stent and the occluded SVG has two stents. (Courtesy of M. Poon, Mount Sinai Medical Center, New York, NY.)

might be the imaging modality of choice. CTA plays an important role in pulmonary and coronary imaging. MRA is more suited for elective diagnosis rather than clinical emergencies. Both noninvasive imaging technologies are improving by leaps and bounds. Thus it is difficult to predict which will dominate the future clinical applications and indications, as both are undergoing rapid evolution in hardware, principal acquisition techniques, postprocessing tools, and specific contrast agents. It is rather safe to conclude that the future of catheter-based x-ray angiography will generally be downgraded to an adjunctive role in the diagnosis of various vascular disease or primarily as a conduit to the rising number of catheter-based cardiovascular interventions.

## References


1. Quick HH, Debatin JF, Ladd ME. MR imaging of the vessel wall. *Eur Radiol* 2002;12(4):889–900.
2. Prince MR. Gadolinium-enhanced MR aortography. *Radiology* 1994; 191(1):155–164.
3. Carroll TJ, Grist TM. Technical developments in MR angiography. *Radiol Clin North Am* 2002;40(4):921–951.
4. Kalender WA, Seissler W, Klotz E, Vock P. Spiral volumetric CT with single-breath-hold technique, continuous transport, and continuous scanner rotation. *Radiology* 1990;176(1):181–183.
5. Klingenbeck-Regn K, Schaller S, Flohr T, et al. Subsecond multi-slice computed tomography: Basics and applications. *Eur J Radiol* 1999; 31(2):110–24.
6. Kachelriess M, Ulzheimer S, Kalender WA. ECG-correlated imaging of the heart with subsecond multislice spiral CT. *IEEE Trans Med Imaging* 2000;19(9):888–901.
7. Becker CR, Knez A, Leber A, et al. Detection of coronary artery stenoses with multislice helical CT angiography. *J Comput Assist Tomogr* 2002;26(5):750–755.
8. Nieman K, Oudkerk M, Rensing BJ, et al. Coronary angiography with multi-slice computed tomography. *Lancet* 2001;357(9256):599–603.
9. Rumberger JA, Behrenbeck T, Breen JF, Sheedy PF. 2. Coronary calcification by electron beam computed tomography and obstructive coronary artery disease: A model for costs and effectiveness of diagnosis as compared with conventional cardiac testing methods. *J Am Coll Cardiol* 1999;33(2):453–462.
10. Clinical alert: Benefit of carotid endarterectomy for patients with high-grade stenosis of the internal carotid artery. National Institute of Neurological Disorders and Stroke, Stroke and Trauma Division. North American Symptomatic Carotid Endarterectomy Trial (NASCET) investigators. *Stroke* 1991;22(6):816–817.
11. Hallett JW Jr, Pietropaoli JA Jr, Ilstrup DM, et al. Comparison of North American Symptomatic Carotid Endarterectomy Trial and population-based outcomes for carotid endarterectomy. *J Vasc Surg* 1998;27(5): 845–850.
12. Rothwell PM, Gutnikov SA, Warlow CP. Reanalysis of the final results of the European Carotid Surgery Trial. *Stroke* 2003;34(2):514–523.
13. Carriero A, Scarabino T, Magarelli N, et al. High-resolution magnetic resonance angiography of the internal carotid artery: 2D vs 3D TOF in stenotic disease. *Eur Radiol* 1998;8(8):1370–1372.
14. Scarabino T, Carriero A, Magarelli N, et al. MR angiography in carotid stenosis: a comparison of three techniques. *Eur J Radiol* 1998;28(2): 117–125.
15. Carr JC, Ma J, Desphande V, et al. High-resolution breath-hold contrast-enhanced MR angiography of the entire carotid circulation. AJR 2002;178(3):543–549.
16. Remonda L, Senn P, Barth A, et al. Contrast-enhanced 3D MR angiography of the carotid artery: Comparison with conventional digital subtraction angiography. AJNR 2002;23(2):213–219.
17. Huston J, Fain SB, Wald JT, et al. Carotid artery: Elliptic centric contrast-enhanced MR angiography compared with conventional angiography. *Radiology* 2001;218(1):138–43.
18. Sodickson DK, McKenzie CA, Li W, et al. Contrast-enhanced 3D MR angiography with simultaneous acquisition of spatial harmonics: A pilot study. *Radiology* 2000;217(1):284–289.
19. Golay X, Brown SJ, Itoh R, Melhem ER. Time-resolved contrast-enhanced carotid MR angiography using sensitivity encoding (SENSE). *AJNR* 2001;22(8):1615–1619.
20. Lenhart M, Framme N, Volk M, et al. Time-resolved contrast-enhanced magnetic resonance angiography of the carotid arteries: Diagnostic accuracy and inter-observer variability compared with selective catheter angiography. *Invest Radiol* 2002;37(10):535–541.
21. Schwartz RB, Jones KM, Chernoff DM, et al. Common carotid artery bifurcation: Evaluation with spiral CT. Work in progress. *Radiology* 1992;185(2):513–519.
22. Jones TR, Kaplan RT, Lane B, et al. Single- versus multi-detector row CT of the brain: Quality assessment. *Radiology* 2001;219(3):750–755.
23. Lell M, Wildberger JE, Heuschmid M, et al. CT-angiography of the carotid artery: First results with a novel 16-slice-spiral-CT scanner. *Rofo Fortschr Geb Rontgenstr Neuen Bildgeb Verfahr* 2002;174(9): 1165–1169.
24. Ertl-Wagner B, Hoffmann RT, Bruning R, Reiser MF. CT-angiographic evaluation of intracranial aneurysms—a review of the literature and first experiences with 4- and 16-slice multi detector CT scanners. *Radiologe* 2002;42(11):892–897.
25. Magarelli N, Scarabino T, Simeone AL, et al. Carotid stenosis: a comparison between MR and spiral CT angiography. *Neuroradiology* 1998;40(6):367–373.
26. Hatsukami TS, Ferguson MS, Beach KW, et al. Carotid plaque morphology and clinical events. *Stroke* 1997;28(1):95–100.
27. Fayad ZA, Fuster V. Clinical imaging of the high-risk or vulnerable atherosclerotic plaque. *Circ Res* 2001;89(4):305–316.
28. Yuan C, Mitsumori LM, Beach KW, Maravilla KR. Carotid atherosclerotic plaque: Noninvasive MR characterization and identification of vulnerable lesions. *Radiology* 2001;221(2):285–299.
29. Estes JM, Quist WC, Lo Gerfo FW, Costello P. Noninvasive characterization of plaque morphology using helical computed tomography. *J Cardiovasc Surg (Torino)* 1998;39(5):527–534.
30. Oliver TB, Lammie GA, Wright AR, et al. Atherosclerotic plaque at the carotid bifurcation: CT angiographic appearance with histopathologic correlation. *AJNR* 1999;20(5):897–901.
31. Porsche C, Walker L, Mendelow AD, Birchall D. Assessment of vessel wall thickness in carotid atherosclerosis using spiral CT angiography. *Eur J Vasc Endovasc Surg* 2002;23(5):437–440.
32. Comerota AJ, Katz ML, White JV, Grosh JD. The preoperative diagnosis of the ulcerated carotid atheroma. *J Vasc Surg* 1990;11(4):505–510.
33. Hatsukami TS, Ross R, Polissar NL, Yuan C. Visualization of fibrous cap thickness and rupture in human atherosclerotic carotid plaque in vivo with high-resolution magnetic resonance imaging. *Circulation* 2000;102(9):959–964.
34. Fayad ZA, Nahar T, Fallon JT, et al. In vivo magnetic resonance evaluation of atherosclerotic plaques in the human thoracic aorta: A comparison with transesophageal echocardiography. *Circulation* 2000; 101(21):2503–2509.
35. Prendergast BD, Boon NA, Buckenham T. Aortic dissection: Advances in imaging and endoluminal repair. *Cardiovasc Intervent Radiol* 2002; 25(2):85–97.
36. Ho VB, Prince MR. Thoracic MR aortography: Imaging techniques and strategies. *Radiographics* 1998;18(2):287–309.
37. LePage MA, Quint LE, Sonnad SS, et al. Aortic dissection: CT features that distinguish true lumen from false lumen. *AJR* 2001; 177(1):207–211.
38. Pereles FS, McCarthy RM, Baskaran V, et al. Thoracic aortic dissection and aneurysm: Evaluation with nonenhanced true FISP MR angiography in less than 4 minutes. *Radiology* 2002;223(1):270–274.
39. Moore AG, Eagle KA, Bruckman D, et al. Choice of computed tomography, transesophageal echocardiography, magnetic resonance imaging, and aortography in acute aortic dissection: International Registry of Acute Aortic Dissection (IRAD). *Am J Cardiol* 2002; 89(10):1235–1238.

40. Elefteriades JA. Natural history of thoracic aortic aneurysms: Indications for surgery, and surgical versus nonsurgical risks. *Ann Thorac Surg* 2002;74(5):S1877–S1880.
41. Krinsky GA, Rofsky NM, DeCorato DR, et al. Thoracic aorta: Comparison of gadolinium-enhanced three-dimensional MR angiography with conventional MR imaging. *Radiology* 1997;202(1):183–193.
42. Prince MR, Narasimham DL, Jacoby WT, et al. Three-dimensional gadolinium-enhanced MR angiography of the thoracic aorta. *AJR* 1996;166(6):1387–1397.
43. Anbarasu A, Harris PL, McWilliams RG. The role of gadolinium-enhanced MR imaging in the preoperative evaluation of inflammatory abdominal aortic aneurysm. *Eur Radiol* 2002;(12 suppl 4): S192–S195.
44. Rubin GD. MDCT imaging of the aorta and peripheral vessels. *Eur J Radiol* 2003;45 (suppl 1):S42–S49.
45. Coselli JS, Conklin LD, LeMaire SA. Thoracoabdominal aortic aneurysm repair: Review and update of current strategies. *Ann Thorac Surg* 2002;74(5):S1881–S1884.
46. Ludman CN, Yusuf SW, Whitaker SC. Feasibility of using dynamic contrast-enhanced magnetic resonance angiography as the sole imaging modality prior to endovascular repair of abdominal aortic aneurysms. *Eur J Vasc Endovasc Surg* 2000;19(5):524–530.
47. Hany TF, Debatin JF, Leung DA, Pfammatter T. Evaluation of the aortoiliac and renal arteries: Comparison of breath-hold, contrast-enhanced, three-dimensional MR angiography with conventional catheter angiography. *Radiology* 1997;204(2):357–362.
48. Prince MR, Narasimham DL, Stanley JC, et al. Breath-hold gadolinium-enhanced MR angiography of the abdominal aorta and its major branches. *Radiology* 1995;197(3):785–792.
49. Papanicolaou N, Wittenberg J, Ferrucci JT Jr, et al. Preoperative evaluation of abdominal aortic aneurysms by computed tomography. *AJR* 1986;146(4):711–715.
50. Van Hoe L, Baert AL, Gryspeerdt S, et al. Supra- and juxtarenal aneurysms of the abdominal aorta: preoperative assessment with thin-section spiral CT. *Radiology* 1996;198(2):443–448.
51. Fleischmann D, Rubin GD, Bankier AA, Hittmair K. Improved uniformity of aortic enhancement with customized contrast medium injection protocols at CT angiography. *Radiology* 2000;214(2):363–371.
52. Koelemay MJ, Lijmer JG, Stoker J. Magnetic resonance angiography for the evaluation of lower extremity arterial disease: A meta-analysis. *JAMA* 2001;285(10):1338–1345.
53. Egglin TK, O'Moore PV, Feinstein AR, Waltman AC. Complications of peripheral arteriography: A new system to identify patients at increased risk. *J Vasc Surg* 1995;22(6):787–794.
54. Ho KY, de Haan MW, Oei TK, et al. MR angiography of the iliac and upper femoral arteries using four different inflow techniques. *AJR* 1997;169(1):45–53.
55. Huber TS, Back MR, Ballinger RJ, et al. Utility of magnetic resonance arteriography for distal lower extremity revascularization. *J Vasc Surg* 1997;26(3):415–423.
56. Eiberg JP, Lundorf E, Thomsen C, Schroeder TV. Peripheral vascular surgery and magnetic resonance arteriography—A review. *Eur J Vasc Endovasc Surg* 2001;22(5):396–402.
57. Sharafuddin MJ, Stolpen AH, Sun S, et al. High-resolution multiphase contrast-enhanced three-dimensional MR angiography compared with two-dimensional time-of-flight MR angiography for the identification of pedal vessels. *J Vasc Interv Radiol* 2002;13(7):695–702.
58. Ruehm SG, Goyen M, Barkhausen J, et al. Rapid magnetic resonance angiography for detection of atherosclerosis. *Lancet* 2001;357(9262): 1086–1091.
59. Shetty AN, Bis KG, Duerinckx AJ, Narra VR. Lower extremity MR angiography: Universal retrofitting of high-field-strength systems with stepping kinematic imaging platforms—initial experience. *Radiology* 2002;222(1):284–291.
60. Hany TF, Carroll TJ, Omary RA, et al. Aorta and runoff vessels: Single-injection MR angiography with automated table movement compared with multi-injection time-resolved MR angiography—Initial results. *Radiology* 2001;221(1):266–272.
61. Prince MR, Grist TM, Debatin JF. *3D Contrast MR Angiography,* 3d ed. Berlin: Springer-Verlag; 2003.
62. Maki JH, Wilson GJ, Eubank WB, Hoogeveen RM. Utilizing SENSE to achieve lower station sub-millimeter isotropic resolution and minimal venous enhancement in peripheral MR angiography. *J Magn Reson Imaging* 2002;15(4):484–491.
63. Rubin GD, Schmidt AJ, Logan LJ, Sofilos MC. Multi-detector row CT angiography of lower extremity arterial inflow and runoff: Initial experience. *Radiology* 2001;221(1):146–158.
64. Wintersperger BJ, Herzog P, Jakobs TF, et al. Initial experience with the clinical use of a 16 detector row CT system. *Crit Rev Comput Tomogr* 2002;43:283–316.
65. Martin ML, Tay KH, Flak B, et al. Multidetector CT angiography of the aortoiliac system and lower extremities: A prospective comparison with digital subtraction angiography. *AJR* 2003;180(4):1085–1091.
66. Hyers TM. Venous thromboembolism. *Am J Respir Crit Care Med* 1999;159(1):1–14.
67. Perrier A, Desmarais S, Miron MJ, et al. Non-invasive diagnosis of venous thromboembolism in outpatients. *Lancet* 1999;353(9148): 190–195.
68. Stein PD, Athanasoulis C, Alavi A, et al. Complications and validity of pulmonary angiography in acute pulmonary embolism. *Circulation* 1992;85(2):462–468.
69. Haage P, Piroth W, Krombach G, et al. Pulmonary embolism: Comparison of angiography with spiral computed tomography, magnetic resonance angiography, and real-time magnetic resonance imaging. *Am J Respir Crit Care Med* 2003;167(5):729–734.
70. Mai VM, Bankier AA, Prasad PV, et al. MR ventilation-perfusion imaging of human lung using oxygen-enhanced and arterial spin labeling techniques. *J Magn Reson Imaging* 2001;14(5):574–579.
71. Kauczor HU, Hanke A, van Beek EJ. Assessment of lung ventilation by MR imaging: current status and future perspectives. *Eur Radiol* 2002;12(8):1962–1970.
72. Meaney JF, Johansson LO, Ahlstrom H, Prince MR. Pulmonary magnetic resonance angiography. *J Magn Reson Imaging* 1999;10(3):326–338.
73. Ghaye B, Remy J, Remy-Jardin M. Non-traumatic thoracic emergencies: CT diagnosis of acute pulmonary embolism: The first 10 years. *Eur Radiol* 2002;12(8):1886–1905.
74. Bunce NH, Lorenz CH, Pennell DJ. MR coronary angiography: 2001 update. *Rays* 2001;26(1):61–69.
75. Gaylord GM. Computed tomographic and magnetic resonance coronary angiography: Are you ready? *Radiol Mgt* 2002;24(4):16–20.
76. Achenbach S, Giesler T, Ropers D, et al. Detection of coronary artery stenoses by contrast-enhanced, retrospectively electrocardiographically-gated, multislice spiral computed tomography. *Circulation* 2001; 103(21):2535–2538.
77. Nikolaou K, Huber A, Knez A, et al. Intraindividual comparison of contrast-enhanced electron-beam computed tomography and navigator-echo-based magnetic resonance imaging for noninvasive coronary artery angiography. *Eur Radiol* 2002;12(7):1663–1671.
78. Botnar RM, Stuber M, Danias PG, et al. Improved coronary artery definition with T2-weighted, free-breathing, three-dimensional coronary MRA. *Circulation* 1999;99(24):3139–3148.
79. Manning WJ, Li W, Edelman RR. A preliminary report comparing magnetic resonance coronary angiography with conventional angiography (see comments). *N Engl J Med* 1993;328(12):828–832.
80. Duerinckx AJ. Imaging of coronary artery disease—MR. *J Thorac Imaging* 2001;16(1):25–34.
81. Wielopolski PA, van Geuns RJ, de Feyter PJ, Oudkerk M. Coronary arteries. *Eur Radiol* 2000;10(1):12–35.
82. Duerinckx A, Urman MK. Two-dimensional coronary MR angiography: Analysis of initial clinical results. *Radiology* 1996;193:731–738.
83. Huber A, Nikolaou K, Gonschior P, et al. Navigator echo-based respiratory gating for three-dimensional MR coronary angiography: Results from healthy volunteers and patients with proximal coronary artery stenoses. *AJR* 1999;173(1):95–101.
84. Nikolaou K, Huber A, Knez A, et al. Navigator echo-based respiratory gating for 3D-MR coronary angiography: Reduction of scan time

using a slice-interpolation technique. *J Comput Assist Tomogr* 2001;25(3):378–387.
85. Regenfus M, Ropers D, Achenbach S, et al. Noninvasive detection of coronary artery stenosis using contrast-enhanced three-dimensional breath-hold magnetic resonance coronary angiography. *J Am Coll Cardiol* 2000;36(1):44–50.
86. van Geuns RJ, Wielopolski PA, de Bruin HG, et al. MR coronary angiography with breath-hold targeted volumes: Preliminary clinical results. *Radiology* 2000;217(1):270–277.
87. Manning WJ, Kim YK, Danias PG, et al. Comparison of 3D coronary MRA with x-ray angiography for detection of coronary stenoses: A prospective international multicenter study. *Circulation* 2001;104(17):II-374.
88. Huber ME, Hengesbach D, Botnar RM, et al. Motion artifact reduction and vessel enhancement for free-breathing navigator-gated coronary MRA using 3D k-space reordering. *Magn Reson Med* 2001;45(4):645–652.
89. Hardy CJ, Saranathan M, Zhu Y, Darrow RD. Coronary angiography by real-time MRI with adaptive averaging. *Magn Reson Med* 2000;44(6):940–946.
90. Kessler W, Laub G, Achenbach S, et al. Coronary arteries: MR angiography with fast contrast-enhanced three-dimensional breath-hold imaging—Initial experience. *Radiology* 1999;210(2):566–572.
91. Li D, Carr JC, Shea SM, et al. Coronary arteries: Magnetization-prepared contrast-enhanced three-dimensional volume-targeted breath-hold MR angiography. *Radiology* 2001;219(1):270–277.
92. Stuber M, Botnar RM, Kissinger KV, Manning WJ. Free-breathing black-blood coronary MR angiography: Initial results. *Radiology* 2001;219(1):278–283.
93. Deshpande VS, Shea SM, Laub G, et al. 3D magnetization-prepared true-FISP: A new technique for imaging coronary arteries. *Magn Reson Med* 2001;46(3):494–502.
94. Li D, Zheng J, Weinmann HJ. Contrast-enhanced MR imaging of coronary arteries: Comparison of intra- and extravascular contrast agents in swine. *Radiology* 2001;218(3):670–678.
95. Sandstede JJ, Pabst T, Wacker C, et al. Breath-hold 3D MR coronary angiography with a new intravascular contrast agent (feruglose)—First clinical experiences. *Magn Reson Imaging* 2001;19(2):201–205.
96. Sodickson DK, McKenzie CA, Li W, et al. Contrast-enhanced 3D MR angiography with simultaneous acquisition of spatial harmonics: A pilot study. *Radiology* 2000;217(1):284–289.
97. Pruessmann KP, Weiger M, Scheidegger MB, Boesiger P. SENSE: Sensitivity encoding for fast MRI. *Magn Reson Med* 1999;42(5):952–962.
98. Taylor AM, Thorne SA, Rubens MB, et al. Coronary artery imaging in grown-up congenital heart disease: Complementary role of magnetic resonance and x-ray coronary angiography. *Circulation* 2000;101(14):1670–1678.
99. Nieman K, Oudkerk M, Rensing BJ, et al. Coronary angiography with multi-slice computed tomography. *Lancet* 2001;357:599–603.
100. Wintersperger BJ, Nikolaou K, Jakobs TF, et al. Cardiac multidetector-row computed tomography: Initial experience using 16 detector-row systems. *Crit Rev Comput Tomogr* 2003;44(1):27–45.
101. Jakobs TF, Becker CR, Ohnesorge B, et al. Multislice helical CT of the heart with retrospective ECG gating: Reduction of radiation exposure by ECG-controlled tube current modulation. *Eur Radiol* 2002;12(5):1081–1086.
102. Becker CR, Ohnesorge BM, Schoepf UJ, Reiser MF. Current development of cardiac imaging with multidetector-row CT. *Eur J Radiol* 2000;36(2):97–103.
103. Vogl TJ, Abolmaali ND, Diebold T, S et al. Techniques for the detection of coronary atherosclerosis: Multi-detector row CT coronary angiography. *Radiology* 2002;223(1):212–220.
104. Rumberger JA. Tomographic (plaque) imaging: State of the art. *Am J Cardiol* 2001;88(2A):66E–69E.
105. Virmani R, Kolodgie FD, Burke AP, et al. Lessons from sudden coronary death: A comprehensive morphological classification scheme for atherosclerotic lesions. *Arterioscler Thromb Vasc Biol* 2000;20(5):1262–1275.
106. Fuster V, Badimon L, Badimon JJ, Chesebro JH. The pathogenesis of coronary artery disease and the acute coronary syndromes (1). *N Engl J Med* 1992;326(4):242–250.
107. Fuster V, Badimon L, Badimon JJ, Chesebro JH. The pathogenesis of coronary artery disease and the acute coronary syndromes (2). *N Engl J Med* 1992;326(5):310–318.
108. Pasterkamp G, Falk E, Woutman H, Borst C. Techniques characterizing the coronary atherosclerotic plaque: Influence on clinical decision making? *J Am Coll Cardiol* 2000;36(1):13–21.
109. Fayad ZA, Fuster V. Clinical imaging of the high-risk or vulnerable atherosclerotic plaque. *Circ Res* 2001;89(4):305–316.
110. Nikolaou K, Becker CR, Wintersperger BJ, et al. Multidetector-row computed tomography of the coronary arteries: Predictive value and quantitative assessment of non-calcified vessel-wall changes. *Radiology* 2002;225:632.
111. Fayad ZA, Fuster V, Nikolaou K, Becker C. Computed tomography and magnetic resonance imaging for noninvasive coronary angiography and plaque imaging: Current and potential future concepts. *Circulation* 2002;106(15):2026–2034.
112. Fayad ZA, Nahar T, Fallon JT, et al. In vivo magnetic resonance evaluation of atherosclerotic plaques in the human thoracic aorta: A comparison with transesophageal echocardiography. *Circulation* 2000;101(21):2503–2509.
113. Fayad ZA, Fuster V, Fallon JT, et al. Noninvasive in vivo human coronary artery lumen and wall imaging using black-blood magnetic resonance imaging. *Circulation* 2000;102(5):506–510.
114. Botnar R, Stuber M, Kissinger K, et al. Noninvasive coronary vessel wall and plaque imaging with magnetic resonance imaging. *Circulation* 2000;102:2582–2587.
115. Toussaint JF, LaMuraglia GM, Southern JF, et al. Magnetic resonance images lipid, fibrous, calcified, hemorrhagic, and thrombotic components of human atherosclerosis in vivo. *Circulation* 1996;94(5):932–938.
116. Nikolaou K, Becker CR, Muders M. High-resolution magnetic resonance and multi-slice CT imaging of coronary artery plaques in human ex vivo coronary arteries. *Radiology* 2001;221:503.
117. Worthley SG, Helft G, Fuster V, et al. Noninvasive in vivo magnetic resonance imaging of experimental coronary artery lesions in a porcine model. *Circulation* 2000;101(25):2956–2961.
118. Fayad ZA, Fuster V, Fallon JT, et al. Noninvasive in vivo human coronary artery lumen and wall imaging using black-blood magnetic resonance imaging. *Circulation* 2000;102(5):506–510.
119. Botnar RM, Kim WY, Bornert P, et al. 3D coronary vessel wall imaging utilizing a local inversion technique with spiral image acquisition. *Magn Reson Med* 2001;46(5):848–854.
120. Schroeder S, Kopp AF, Baumbach A, et al. Noninvasive detection and evaluation of atherosclerotic coronary plaques with multislice computed tomography. *J Am Coll Cardiol* 2001;37(5):1430–1435.
121. Becker CR, Knez A, Jakobs TF, et al. Detection and quantification of coronary artery calcification with electron-beam and conventional CT. *Eur Radiol* 1999;9(4):620–624.
122. Becker CR, Knez A, Leber A, et al. Angiography with multi-slice spiral CT. Detecting plaque, before it causes symptoms. *MMW Fortschr Med* 2001;143(16):30–32.
123. Becker CR, Knez A, Ohnesorge B, et al. Imaging of noncalcified coronary plaques using helical CT with retrospective ECG gating. *AJR* 2000;175(2):423–424.
124. Stary HC. Natural history and histological classification of atherosclerotic lesions: an update. *Arterioscler Thromb Vasc Biol* 2000;20(5):1177–1178.
125. Baumgart D, Schmermund A, Goerge G, et al. Comparison of electron beam computed tomography with intracoronary ultrasound and coronary angiography for detection of coronary atherosclerosis. *J Am Coll Cardiol* 1997;30(1):57–64.
126. Becker CR, Schoepf UJ, Reiser MF. Coronary artery calcium scoring: Medicine and politics. *Eur Radiol* 2003;13(3):445–447.
127. Sarjeant JM, Rabinovitch M. Understanding and treating vein graft atherosclerosis. *Cardiovasc Pathol* 2002;11(5):263–271.

128. Langerak SE, Kunz P, De Roos A, et al. Evaluation of coronary artery bypass grafts by magnetic resonance imaging. *J Magn Reson Imaging* 1999;10(3):434–441.
129. Langerak SE, Vliegen HW, De Roos A, et al. Detection of vein graft disease using high-resolution magnetic resonance angiography. *Circulation* 2002;105(3):328–333.
130. Wittlinger T, Voigtlander T, Kreitner KF. Non-invasive magnetic resonance imaging of coronary bypass grafts. Comparison of the HASTE- and navigator techniques with conventional coronary angiography. *Int J Cardiovasc Imaging* 2002;18(6):469–477.
131. Ropers D, Ulzheimer S, Wenkel E, et al. Investigation of aortocoronary artery bypass grafts by multislice spiral computed tomography with electrocardiographic-gated image reconstruction. *Am J Cardiol* 2001; 88(7):792–795.
132. Enzweiler CN, Wiese TH, Petersein J, et al. Diameter changes of occluded venous coronary artery bypass grafts in electron beam tomography: Preliminary findings. *Eur J Cardiothorac Surg* 2003; 23(3):347–353.
133. Tello R, Hartnell GG, Costello P, Ecker CP. Coronary artery bypass graft flow: qualitative evaluation with cine single-detector row CT and comparison with findings at angiography. *Radiology* 2002;224(3): 913–918.
134. Johnson MB, Wilkinson ID, Wattam J, et al. Comparison of Doppler ultrasound, magnetic resonance angiographic techniques and catheter angiography in evaluation of carotid stenosis. *Clin Radiol* 2000; 55(12):912–920.
135. Serfaty JM, Chirossel P, Chevallier JM, et al. Accuracy of three-dimensional gadolinium-enhanced MR angiography in the assessment of extracranial carotid artery disease. *AJR* 2000;175(2):455–463.
136. Sardanelli F, Zandrino F, Parodi RC, De Caro G. MR angiography of internal carotid arteries: Breath-hold Gd-enhanced 3D fast imaging with steady-state precession versus unenhanced 2D and 3D time-of-flight techniques. *J Comput Assist Tomogr* 1999;23(2):208–215.
137. Leclerc X, Martinat P, Godefroy O, et al. Contrast-enhanced three-dimensional fast imaging with steady-state precession (FISP) MR angiography of supraaortic vessels: preliminary results. *AJNR* 1998; 19(8):1405–1413.
138. Anderson GB, Ashforth R, Steinke DE, et al. CT angiography for the detection and characterization of carotid artery bifurcation disease. *Stroke* 2000;31(9):2168–2174.
139. Leclerc X, Godefroy O, Lucas C, et al. Internal carotid arterial stenosis: CT angiography with volume rendering. *Radiology* 1999; 210(3):673–682.
140. Marcus CD, Ladam-Marcus VJ, Bigot JL, et al. Carotid arterial stenosis: evaluation at CT angiography with the volume-rendering technique. *Radiology* 1999;211(3):775–780.
141. Verhoek G, Costello P, Khoo EW, et al. Carotid bifurcation CT angiography: Assessment of interactive volume rendering. *J Comput Assist Tomogr* 1999;23(4):590–596.
142. Magarelli N, Scarabino T, Simeone AL, et al. Carotid stenosis: A comparison between MR and spiral CT angiography. *Neuroradiology* 1998;40(6):367–373.
143. Ruehm SG, Hany TF, Pfammatter T, et al. Pelvic and lower extremity arterial imaging: Diagnostic performance of three-dimensional contrast-enhanced MR angiography. *AJR* 2000;174(4):1127–1135.
144. Huber A, Heuck A, Baur A, et al. Dynamic contrast-enhanced MR angiography from the distal aorta to the ankle joint with a step-by-step technique. *AJR* 2000;175(5):1291–1298.
145. Meaney JF, Ridgway JP, Chakraverty S, et al. Stepping-table gadolinium-enhanced digital subtraction MR angiography of the aorta and lower extremity arteries: Preliminary experience. *Radiology* 1999; 211(1):59–67.
146. Sueyoshi E, Sakamoto I, Matsuoka Y, et al. Aortoiliac and lower extremity arteries: comparison of three-dimensional dynamic contrast-enhanced subtraction MR angiography and conventional angiography. *Radiology* 1999;210(3):683–688.
147. Yamashita Y, Mitsuzaki K, Ogata I, et al. Three-dimensional high-resolution dynamic contrast-enhanced MR angiography of the pelvis and lower extremities with use of a phased array coil and subtraction: Diagnostic accuracy. *J Magn Reson Imaging* 1998;8(5):1066–1072.
148. Ofer A, Nitecki SS, Linn S, et al. Multidetector CT angiography of peripheral vascular disease: A prospective comparison with intraarterial digital subtraction angiography. *AJR* 2003;180(3):719–724.
149. Rieker O, Duber C, Neufang A, et al. CT angiography versus intraarterial digital subtraction angiography for assessment of aortoiliac occlusive disease. *AJR* 1997;169(4):1133–1138.
150. Raptopoulos V, Rosen MP, Kent KC, et al. Sequential helical CT angiography of aortoiliac disease. *AJR* 1996;166(6):1347–1354.
151. Lawrence JA, Kim D, Kent KC, et al. Lower extremity spiral CT angiography versus catheter angiography. *Radiology* 1995;194(3):903–908.
152. Oudkerk M, van Beek EJ, Wielopolski P, et al. Comparison of contrast-enhanced magnetic resonance angiography and conventional pulmonary angiography for the diagnosis of pulmonary embolism: A prospective study. *Lancet* 2002;359(9318):1643–1647.
153. Goyen M, Ruehm SG, Jagenburg A, et al. Pulmonary arteriovenous malformation: Characterization with time-resolved ultrafast 3D MR angiography. *J Magn Reson Imaging* 2001;13(3):458–460.
154. Kruger S, Haage P, Hoffmann R, et al. Diagnosis of pulmonary arterial hypertension and pulmonary embolism with magnetic resonance angiography. *Chest* 2001;120(5):1556–1561.
155. Kreitner KF, Ley S, Kauczor HU, et al. Contrast media enhanced three dimensional MR angiography of the pulmonary arteries in patients with chronic recurrent pulmonary embolism—comparison with selective intra-arterial DSA. *Rofo Fortschr Geb Rontgenstr Neuen Bildgeb Verfahr* 2000;172(2):122–128.
156. Gupta A, Frazer CK, Ferguson JM, et al. Acute pulmonary embolism: Diagnosis with MR angiography. *Radiology* 1999;210(2):353–359.
157. Perrier A, Howarth N, Didier D, et al. Performance of helical computed tomography in unselected outpatients with suspected pulmonary embolism. *Ann Intern Med* 2001;135(2):88–97.
158. Blachere H, Latrabe V, Montaudon M, et al. Pulmonary embolism revealed on helical CT angiography: Comparison with ventilation-perfusion radionuclide lung scanning. *AJR* 2000;174(4):1041–1047.
159. Qanadli SD, Hajjam ME, Mesurolle B, et al. Pulmonary embolism detection: prospective evaluation of dual-section helical CT versus selective pulmonary arteriography in 157 patients. *Radiology* 2000; 217(2):447–455.
160. Remy-Jardin M, Remy J, Baghaie F, et al. Clinical value of thin collimation in the diagnostic workup of pulmonary embolism. *AJR* 2000;175(2):407–411.
161. Kim KI, Muller NL, Mayo JR. Clinically suspected pulmonary embolism: Utility of spiral CT. *Radiology* 1999;210(3):693–697.
162. Regenfus M, Ropers D, Achenbach S, et al. Diagnostic value of maximum intensity projections versus source images for assessment of contrast-enhanced three-dimensional breath-hold magnetic resonance coronary angiography. *Invest Radiol* 2003;38(4):200–206.
163. Plein S, Jones TR, Ridgway JP, Sivananthan MU. Three-dimensional coronary MR angiography performed with subject-specific cardiac acquisition windows and motion-adapted respiratory gating. *AJR* 2003;180(2):505–512.
164. Watanabe Y, Nagayama M, Amoh Y, et al. High-resolution selective three-dimensional magnetic resonance coronary angiography with navigator-echo technique: Segment-by-segment evaluation of coronary artery stenosis. *J Magn Reson Imaging* 2002;16(3):238–245.
165. Kim WY, Danias PG, Stuber M, et al. Coronary magnetic resonance angiography for the detection of coronary stenoses. *N Engl J Med* 2001;345(26):1863–1869.
166. Nieman K, Cademartiri F, Lemos P, et al. Reliable noninvasive coronary angiography with fast submillimeter multislice spiral computed tomography. *Circulation* 2002;106:2051–2054.
167. Knez A, Becker CR, Leber A, et al. Usefulness of multislice spiral computed tomography angiography for determination of coronary artery stenoses. *Am J Cardiol* 2001;88(10):1191–1194.
168. Achenbach S, Ropers D, Regenfus M, et al. Contrast enhanced electron beam computed tomography to analyze the coronary arteries in patients after acute myocardial infarction. *Heart* 2000;84(5):489–493.

169. Budoff MJ, Oudiz RJ, Zalace CP, et al. Intravenous three-dimensional coronary angiography using contrast enhanced electron beam computed tomography. *Am J Cardiol* 1999;83(6):840–845.
170. Schmermund A, Rensing BJ, Sheedy PF, et al. Intravenous electron-beam computed tomographic coronary angiography for segmental analysis of coronary artery stenoses. *J Am Coll Cardiol* 1998;31:1547–1554.
171. Nakanishi T, Ito K, Imazu M, Yamakido M. Evaluation of coronary artery stenoses using electron-beam CT and multiplanar reformation. *J Comput Assist Tomogr* 1997;21(1):121–127.
172. Vetter HO, Driever R, Mertens H, et al. Contrast-enhanced magnetic resonance angiography of mammary artery grafts after minimally invasive coronary bypass surgery. *Ann Thorac Surg* 2001;71(4): 1229–1232.
173. Engelmann MG, Knez A, von Smekal A, et al. Non-invasive coronary bypass graft imaging after multivessel revascularisation. *Int J Cardiol* 2000;76(1):65–74.
174. Molinari G, Sardanelli F, Zandrino F, et al. Value of navigator echo magnetic resonance angiography in detecting occlusion/patency of arterial and venous, single and sequential coronary bypass grafts. *Int J Cardiovasc Imaging* 2000;16(3):149–160.
175. Brenner P, Wintersperger B, von Smekal A, et al. Detection of coronary artery bypass graft patency by contrast enhanced magnetic resonance angiography. *Eur J Cardiothorac Surg* 1999;15(4):389–393.
176. Wintersperger BJ, Engelmann MG, von Smekal A, et al. Patency of coronary bypass grafts: Assessment with breath-hold contrast-enhanced MR angiography—Value of a non-electrocardiographically triggered technique. *Radiology* 1998;208(2):345–351.
177. Achenbach S, Moshage W, Ropers D, et al. Noninvasive, three-dimensional visualization of coronary artery bypass grafts by electron beam tomography. *Am J Cardiol* 1997;79(7):856–861.
178. Knez A, von Smekal A, Haberl R, et al. The value of ultrafast computerized tomography in detection of the patency of coronary bypasses. *Z Kardiol* 1996;85(9):629–634.
179. Wintersperger BJ, Huber A, Preissler G, et al. MR angiography of the supraaortic vessels. *Radiologe* 2000;40(9):785–791.
180. Ertl-Wagner B, Hoffmann RT, Bruning R, et al. Diagnostic evaluation of the craniocervical vascular system with a 16-slice multi-detector row spiral CT. Protocols and first experiences. *Radiologe* 2002; 42(9):728–732.
181. Huber A, Matzko M, Wintersperger BJ, Reiser M. Reconstruction methods in postprocessing of CT- and MR-angiography of the aorta. *Radiologe* 2001;41(8):689–694.
182. Wintersperger BJ, Helmberger TK, Herzog P, et al. New abdominal CT angiography protocol on a 16 detector-row CT scanner—first results. *Radiologe* 2002;42(9):722–727.
183. Nikolaou K, Schoenberg SO, Nittka M, et al. Magnetic resonance imaging in the diagnosis of pulmonary arterial hypertension: High resolution angiography and fast perfusion imaging using intelligent parallel acquisition techniques (IPAT). *Radiology* 2002;225:473.
184. Becker CR, Knez A, Ohnesorge B, et al. Imaging of noncalcified coronary plaques using helical CT with retrospective ECG gating. *AJR* 2000;175(2):423–424.
185. Nikolaou K, Becker CR, Wintersperger BJ, et al. Assessment of non-calcified vessel-wall changes in the coronary arteries using contrast-enhanced multirow-detector computed tomography. *Radiology* 2002; 225, 632.
186. Nikolaou K, Becker CR, Muders M, et al. High resolution magnetic resonance and multi-slice CT imaging of coronary artery plaques in human ex vivo coronary arteries. *Radiology* 2001;221(P):503.

CHAPTER 23

# POSITRON EMISSION TOMOGRAPHY

Heinrich R. Schelbert / John O. Prior



The study of the human heart with conventional radionuclide techniques, including single photon emission computed tomography (SPECT), is confined to assessments of the relative distributions of regional myocardial blood flow (MBF) and of global and regional myocardial contractile function. Positron emission tomography (PET) exceeds these capabilities because it offers assays for probing and defining regional functional processes in absolute units that span from blood flow to biochemical reaction rates, substrate fluxes, and neuronal activity. The many positron-emitting, biologically active tracers; the quantitative imaging capability; and the in vivo application of tracer kinetic principles are unique to PET and account for this capability. Aspects of the human heart's physiology and pathophysiology can thus be characterized more comprehensively. Also, novel insights into the function of the human heart can be gained while, at the same time, PET can decisively impact patient diagnosis and management. This chapter reviews the key ingredients of PET and describes the tools for the evaluation and/or quantification of local functional processes in the human heart. It continues by examining how these tools can be applied to the diagnosis and characterization of coronary artery disease and its consequences for regional myocardial tissue function and discusses the impact of PET findings on patient management.

## TOOLS FOR PROBING MYOCARDIAL TISSUE FUNCTION

Fundamental to the uniqueness of PET are (1) the quantitative imaging and high temporal resolution capability, (2) the in vivo application of tracer kinetic principles, and (3) the large number of physiologically active radiotracers.

### Imaging with Positron-Emitting Radiopharmaceuticals

#### DEDICATED PET SYSTEMS

The quantitative imaging capability of PET results from physical properties unique to positrons. After losing its kinetic energy, the positron combines with an electron and is "annihilated." This "annihilation" represents the conversion of mass into energy; that is, the combined mass of the positron and the electron is converted into two 511-keV photons that leave the site of the annihilation in diametrically opposed directions. If both, at the same time, strike two scintillation detectors connected by a coincidence circuitry, an annihilation event is registered. Its location in space can be defined by circular arrays of scintillation detectors. The nearly simultaneous arrival of two 511-keV photons at the two scintillation detectors positioned in opposite directions allows the use of tomographic reconstruction algorithms analogous to those used with x-ray CT. Accordingly, the spatial resolution throughout the image plane is rather homogeneous; this differs from that obtainable with conventional SPECT approaches, where the spatial resolution declines as the distance of the imaged object from the scintillation detectors increases. Further, by acquiring "transmission" images with external rotating or circular sources of positron-emitting isotopes and thus measuring the photon attenuation, the images of the tracer tissue concentrations ("emission images") are corrected for photon attenuation, so that the resulting tomographic images accurately represent the true regional radioactivity concentrations (mCi or $MBq/cm^3$). State-of-the-art PET systems offer spatial resolutions as high as 4- to 5-mm full-width half-maximum (FWHM). Further, because the imaging gantry is a stationary circular device, unlike the rotating detectors in SPECT, serial images can be acquired at sampling rates in the range of seconds. With PET, it is therefore possible to measure rapidly changing radiotracer concentrations in tissues.

***PET Combined with CT*** A more recent instrumentation-related development entails the fusion of PET with CT as a combined imaging device referred to as PET/CT. Designed primarily for oncologic applications, the CT component of the system measures the photon attenuation and its anatomic distribution and, thus, shortens total imaging times. In addition, the CT component visualizes the anatomy, so that combined PET and CT imaging systems are ideally suited for fusing functional with structural information (Fig. 23-1). Examination of the cardiovascular system has not yet taken advantage of this combination imaging approach, which holds promise not only for facilitating the correction of photon attenuation but also for merging functional information (i.e., myocardial blood flow) with structural information (i.e., coronary calcifications or even coronary angiography).

***Combined SPECT and PET*** Several institutions use SPECT and PET for the evaluation of cardiovascular disease. For example, the distribution of MBF is determined with thallium 201 ($^{201}Tl$)- or

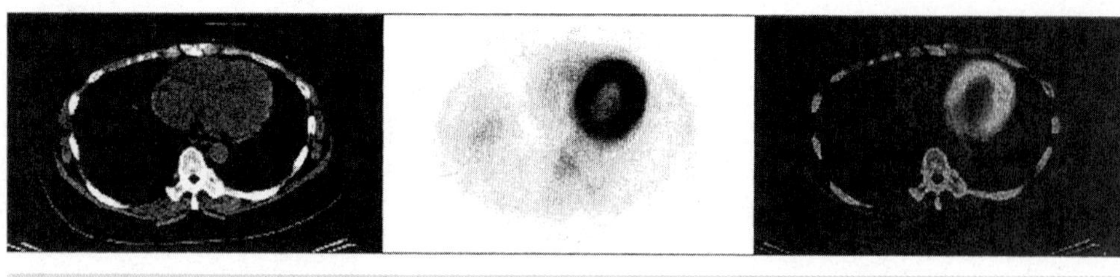

FIGURE 23-1 CT of the chest and PET FDG of the chest and CT-PET fusion images.

technetium 99m ($^{99m}Tc$)-labeled tracers of blood flow and then compared to the distribution of myocardial glucose utilization by imaging fluorine 18 ($^{18}F$)-deoxyglucose with dedicated PET systems.[1–4] While this particular approach yields a diagnostic accuracy that is comparable to that achieved with dedicated PET systems, diagnostic difficulties can arise due to differences in the geometry of the heart and spatial resolution on SPECT and PET images as well as photon attenuation–related artifacts on the SPECT images. This applies especially to the inferior wall and the interventricular septum, as pointed out in several publications.[5,6]

## Tracer Kinetic Principles

Positron-emitting isotopes of elements that constitute major parts of living matter—like carbon 11 ($^{11}C$), nitrogen 13 ($^{13}N$), and oxygen 15 ($^{15}O$)—can be inserted into biomolecules without disturbing their physiologic properties. Their high specific activity (radioactivity per mass) permits administration of such minute and, thus, true tracer quantities that they do not exert a mass effect and perturb the very process to be studied. As their physiologic half-life is short, functional processes can be measured repeatedly or different aspects of the myocardial tissue function be explored within the same study session. The radioactivity concentrations of these tracers in tissues like arterial blood and myocardium and their changes over time can be determined noninvasively. Time-activity curves derived from serially acquired tomographic images at sampling rates of 1 to 10 s are fitted with operational equations derived from tracer kinetic models; they thus yield quantitative estimates of regional functional processes.

Tracer compartment models describe the distribution of the tracer radiolabel in tissue and its time-dependent changes. Because only the activity concentration of the tracer radiolabel can be measured externally, these models relate the externally derived signal to the metabolic fate of the tracer label and its relationship to the functional process under study. Such tracer kinetic models typically consist of functional rather than anatomic compartments that contain the radiotracer or its metabolites (Fig. 23-2). Exchange of radiotracers between compartments is described typically by first-order rate constants. Flux of a radiotracer through a given compartment depends on the flux rate of tracer or of its metabolite as well as on the size of the compartment. Tracer compartment models provide the base for developing operational equations; applied to the externally derived radioactivity signal—as, for example, tissue time-activity curves—estimates of regional functional processes are derived in absolute units.

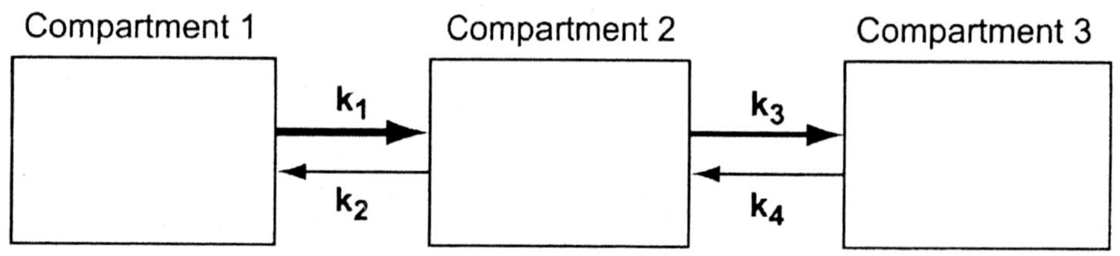


FIGURE 23-2 The activity in the vascular space (*left*), the tracer activity in tissue (*center*), and a pool of metabolically trapped tracer (*right*). The exchange between these three compartments is described by first-order rate constants (k; in this particular configuration $k_1$ describes the rate of exchange from blood into tissue and $k_2$ a return of tracer from the extravascular space into blood, while $k_3$ describes the rate constant for the metabolic reaction that traps the radiotracer).

## Positron-Emitting Tracers of Myocardial Tissue Function

### BLOOD VOLUME AND TISSUE CHARACTERIZATION

Blood can readily be radiolabeled with minute quantities of either oxygen 15 ($^{15}O$) or carbon 11 ($^{11}C$)-labeled carbon monoxide (CO). Once inhaled, the radiolabeled CO binds to hemoglobin, thereby tagging red blood cells. This serves to define the components of the myocardium in terms of vascular space, viable and normal myocytes, and scar tissue. One such characterization assumes that only living myocytes exchange water rapidly.[7] The approach employs transmission images representing the densities of the various tissues in the chest. They resemble low-spatial-resolution x-ray CT images and delineate, for example, the volume of the myocardium together with the blood in its cavities. The true extravascular volume can then be obtained by subtracting blood-pool images from the transmission images. The fraction of the extravascular volume that exchanges water rapidly is estimated with $^{15}O$-labeled water and is referred to as the *water-perfusable tissue index* (PTI). If all of the extravascular volume does indeed exchange water rapidly, then the PTI approaches unity.[7] If, on the other hand—as is the case in patients with prior myocardial infarction—a portion of the myocardium has been injured irreversibly and scar tissue has formed, this fraction becomes less than unity.[8,9] In fact, in animal experimental studies, the PTI was found to be inversely correlated with the fractional amount of fibrosis and scar tissue.[10] The PTI will also be reduced in instances of diffuse interstitial fibrosis. Clinical investigations have demonstrated that the fraction of irreversibly injured myocardium or of regional scar tissue formation can be measured and predicts whether an impairment in regional contractile function is irreversible or whether a postrevascularization improvement is likely.[9] In this regard, the PTI provides information analogous to that obtained with contrast magnetic resonance imaging (MRI).[11,12] If, however, functionally compromised but viable myocardium exchanges water as rapidly as normal myocardium, this might limit the predictive value of the PTI, for it does not distinguish between normal and "ischemically compromised" myocardium. Accordingly, a reduced PTI was found to be highly predictive of the irreversibility of contractile function, while a near-normal PTI was less accurate than $^{18}F$-deoxyglucose in predicting a postrevascularization improvement in contractile function.[13]

As another aspect of the PTI, the sum of viable and normal myocytes in a given myocardial segment can be used as a reference to which transmural estimates of blood flow or substrate metabolism can be related.[14]

## MYOCARDIAL BLOOD FLOW

Several approaches exist for the evaluation of the relative distribution of MBF and, in particular, of regional MBF in absolute units. Tracers like rubidium 82 ($^{82}$Rb) or nitrogen 13 ($^{13}$N)-ammonia are retained in myocardium in proportion to blood flow.[15,16] Images of their regional activity concentrations in the myocardium depict the relative distribution of blood flow at the time of tracer injection. Each tracer offers advantages and disadvantages. For example, because $^{82}$Rb is available through a generator-based pushbutton-operated infusion system, it is easy to use clinically.[17] Its physical half-life of only 75 s affords repeat studies at only 10-min time intervals and thus makes possible the evaluation of changes in regional blood flow in response to physiologic or pharmacologic interventions. This short physical half-life may produce low-count and thus statistically noisy images. Modern three-dimensional (3D) PET systems can overcome this limitation and even allow gated acquisition of $^{82}$Rb perfusion images. The longer physical half-life of $^{13}$N-ammonia (10 min), by contrast, produces images of higher count rates and thus of higher diagnostic quality, but an interval of 40 to 50 min between studies is required.[16]

Common to most flow tracers is the nonlinear uptake in response to increasing flows as a function of the curvilinear decline of the first-pass extraction fraction. Tracer compartment models compensate for this nonlinear tissue response, so that the noninvasive estimates of blood flow linearly trace changes in blood flow. Such compensation is not needed for $^{15}$O-water because capillary and sarcolemmal membranes exert little if any barrier effect on the exchange of $^{15}$O-water, so that the extraction fraction is largely independent of blood flow and the tracer net uptake increases linearly with flow. Hence, $^{15}$O-water, at least in theory, is most ideally suited for measurements of blood flow.[18] The tracer is also metabolically inert, while uptake and retention of $^{13}$N-ammonia or of $^{82}$Rb are potentially susceptible to alterations in regional myocardial metabolism. Animal experiments, however, failed to demonstrate significant effects of metabolism.[19,20]

Both the $^{13}$N-ammonia and the $^{15}$O-water technique yield comparable estimates of blood flow in human myocardium at rest and during pharmacologically induced hyperemia.[21–27] Myocardial blood flow can also be estimated with $^{82}$Rb, although the tracer underestimates hyperemic myocardial blood flows.[28] Some variability between studies probably derives from methodologic differences but also from intergroup differences in the hemodynamic state, for blood flow in normal myocardium depends largely on oxygen demand and thus on cardiac work.[29] Estimated from the rate-pressure product, MBF correlates closely with cardiac work. Thus, individual flow measurements should be interpreted within the context of the rate-pressure product.[30] Finally, there also appear to be gender-related differences in MBF, both at rest and during adenosine-induced hyperemia. Compared to an age-matched group of males, women demonstrated higher blood flows both at rest and during hyperemia, which the authors attributed to higher HDL cholesterol and lower triglyceride plasma levels in females.[31]

Important for studying effects of interventions is the reproducibility of blood flow measurements. Repeat studies in the same normal volunteers report a 10 ± 11 percent reproducibility (average percent difference of flows normalized to the rate-pressure product) for rest blood flow and of 12 ± 9 percent for hyperemic blood flows.[32] Other studies report similar values for both $^{13}$N-ammonia and $^{15}$O-water.[33–35] Furthermore, the validity of the noninvasive measurements of blood flow has been extensively established in animal experiments using the microsphere technique[21,23,36–38] and in humans using intracoronary flow-velocity probes.[39]

## MYOCARDIAL SUBSTRATE METABOLISM

The major components of the myocardial substrate metabolism are illustrated in Fig. 23-3. According to this highly simplified depiction, the myocardium chooses between various substrates; foremost are free fatty acid, glucose, lactate, and ketone bodies. Selection of a fuel substrate depends largely on its concentration in plasma and the overall hormonal milieu.[40,41] These, in turn, are governed by the dietary state, level of physical activity, and further, plasma concentrations of catecholamine, insulin, and glucagon. In the fasting state, for example, circulating free fatty acid levels are high and insulin levels are low, so that as much as 70 to 80 percent of the myocardium's oxygen consumption can be accounted for by oxidation of free fatty acid.[42] Conversely, oral glucose raises plasma glucose and, in response, also insulin levels, and it lowers free fatty acid levels, so that myocardium shifts its fuel selection to glucose.[41] Strenuous physical exercise increases release of lactate from skeletal muscle. Plasma levels therefore rise and lactate becomes the major fuel substrate.[43,44] In fact, as much as 60 percent of the oxygen consumption has been accounted for by oxidation of lactate during strenuous exercise. Other determinants of substrate selection include catecholamines, which accelerate lipolysis, so that circulating free fatty acid levels increase, in association with a shift in the heart's substrate selection to free fatty acid.

Glucose enters the cell via facilitated transport systems, the largely insulin-independent glucose transporter GLUT 1 and the insulin-dependent glucose transporter GLUT 4. The hexokinase reaction phosphorylates glucose to glucose-6-phosphate. The reaction product may be synthesized to glycogen or, alternatively, enters glycolysis with pyruvate as the end product. Converted to lactate, it may leave the myocardium or, if activated to acetyl-CoA, enter the tricarboxylic acid (TCA) cycle as the final oxidative pathway shared by most fuel substrates. Exogenous lactate can be converted via NAD$^+$ to pyruvate, which, after esterification to acyl-CoA, enters the TCA cycle. Free fatty acid may, like glucose, enter two different metabolic pathways. Upon entering the cells, it is esterified by the thiokinase reaction

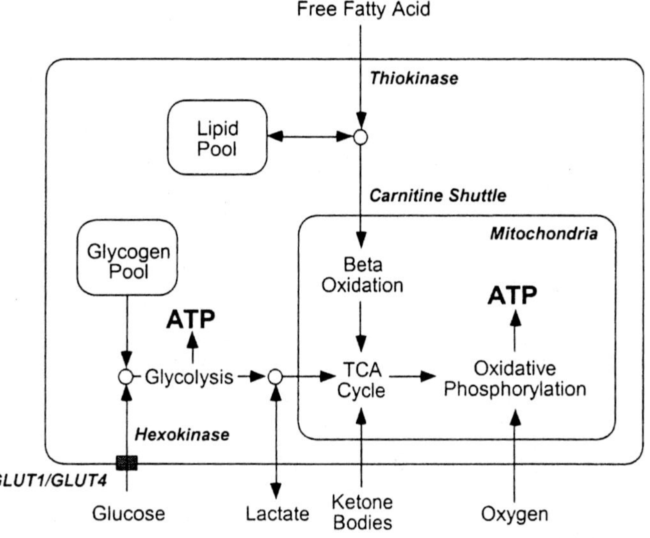


FIGURE 23-3 Highly simplified depiction of the myocardium's substrate metabolism. (TCA = tricarboxylic acid; ATP = adenosine triphosphate; GLUT1 and GLUT4 = glucose transporters 1 and 4).

to acetyl-CoA. This compound may then enter an endogenous lipid pool consisting mostly of glycerides and phospholipids or proceed via the carnitine shuttle to the inner mitochondrial membrane. It is there where $\beta$-oxidation cleaves off the long-chain acyl-CoA units into two-carbon fragments, which then engage in the TCA cycle. The TCA cycle metabolizes the two-carbon units into $CO_2$ and $H_2O$. The rate of flux through the TCA cycle is coupled closely to oxidative phosphorylation, where the energy resulting from the synthesis of oxygen and hydrogen ions is stored in the high-energy phosphate bonds of adenosine triphosphate (ATP). The latter is shuttled into the cytosol, with transfer of energy to the high-energy phosphate bond of creatine phosphate as a readily available source of energy. Other sites of high energy production include glycolysis. Energy yields in terms of ATP relative to oxygen differ between the various substrates. For example, for 1 mole of oxygen, glucose yields 6.3 moles of ATP; lactate, 6 moles ATP; and free fatty acid, 5.7 moles ATP.[45]

***Myocardial Glucose Utilization*** As shown schematically in Fig. 23-3, the initial metabolic step of exogenous glucose metabolism can be evaluated and quantitated with $^{18}$F-deoxyglucose. This radiolabeled glucose analogue exchanges across the capillary and sarcolemmal membranes in proportion to glucose, with which it then competes for hexokinase for phosphorylation to $^{18}$F-deoxyglucose-6-phosphate (see also Fig. 23-2).[46,47] Unlike its natural counterpart, the phosphorylated glucose analogue is a poor substrate for glycogen formation, glycolysis, and the fructose-pentose shunt; its rate of dephosphorylation is low in myocardium and it is relatively impermeable to the cell membrane. The phosphorylated tracer thus becomes trapped in the cells, so that images of the myocardial $^{18}$F activity concentrations, acquired about 40 to 60 min after tracer injection, reflect the relative distribution of exogenous glucose utilization rates. Because the compound traces only the initial steps of glucose utilization (up to the branch point between glycogen synthesis and glycolysis; Fig. 23-3), it offers no direct information on glycolytic rates, glucose oxidation, or glycogen synthesis. Yet in states of glycogen depletion—as, for example, during ischemia—exogenous glucose serves as the major source of glycolytic flux, so that $^{18}$F-deoxyglucose may offer an estimate of the rate of glycolysis.

The tissue kinetics of $^{18}$F-deoxyglucose are described by a unidirectional transport model,[46,47] which affords the quantification of regional rates of myocardial glucose utilization through relatively simple, rapid, and computationally efficient analysis.[48–50] Typical values for exogenous glucose utilization under different dietary conditions and as reported from several laboratories are about 0.10 to 0.24 $\mu$mol $\cdot$ min$^{-1}$ $\cdot$ g$^{-1}$ in the fasting state, about 0.69 $\mu$mol $\cdot$ min$^{-1}$ $\cdot$ g$^{-1}$ after oral glucose loading, and about 74 $\mu$mol $\cdot$ min$^{-1}$ $\cdot$ g$^{-1}$ during hyperinsulinemic-euglycemic clamping.[51–53] In order to adjust for differences in the affinity of glucose and the glucose analogue tracer for the hexokinase reaction and for differences in the transmembrane exchange, a "lumped constant" (LC) is used. The value used most frequently is 0.7, as derived for canine myocardium.[47] However, the LC may not truly be constant but can depend on study conditions.[54–56] This may be related to changes in the affinity of $^{18}$F-deoxyglucose for transmembrane exchange in hexokinase and hence in the LC, but, at the same time, it suggests that the LC can be derived individually from the morphology of the myocardial $^{18}$F time-activity curve.[57]

A more recent approach to measurements of myocardial glucose metabolism entails the use of $^{11}$C-glucose. The accumulation and clearance of radiotracer in the myocardium are estimated from serially acquired PET images. Using estimates of the myocardial extraction of $^{11}$C-glucose, of MBF as determined with $^{15}$O-water, and the arterial blood glucose concentration, the myocardial consumption of glucose can be measured.[58–61] Different from the $^{18}$F-deoxyglucose approach, the $^{11}$C-glucose method also offers estimates of the fraction of glucose that is oxidized.

***Myocardial Fatty Acid Metabolism*** This particular substrate pathway can be evaluated with 1-[$^{11}$C]-palmitate. The labeled long-chain fatty acid participates fully in the metabolic fate of its natural counterpart (Fig. 23-3). Once esterified to acyl-CoA, a fraction of tracer label proceeds via the carnitine shuttle into mitochondria, where $\beta$-oxidation catabolizes the long-chain fatty acid into two-carbon fragments that are then oxidized via the tricarboxylic acid (TCA) cycle. The label is released from the myocardium in the form of $^{11}CO_2$. The remaining fraction of the initially extracted and activated tracer enters intracellular lipid pools, consisting mostly of di- and triglycerides and phospholipids. The biexponential morphology of the myocardial tissue time-activity curve reflects the metabolic fate of the tracer. The slow turnover rate of the intracellular lipid pools accounts for the slow clearance phase, while the relative size and slope of the rapid clearance curve component correspond to the fraction of tracer that has entered oxidative pathways and its rate of oxidation. Ischemia reduces the rate of fatty acid oxidation and of TCA cycle activity. Accordingly, the size and rate of the rapid clearance curve component on the $^{11}$C myocardial time-activity curve typically decline.[62,63] A disproportionately greater fraction of tracer label is then shunted into slow turnover, endogenous lipid pools. However, enhanced backdiffusion of nonmetabolized tracer may complicate the evaluation of fatty acid oxidation in acutely ischemic myocardium, as demonstrated in dog experiments. Used mostly as a tracer for the qualitative evaluation of regional myocardial fatty acid metabolism, recent studies indicate the possibility of quantitating myocardial fatty acid oxidation in milliequivalents of free fatty acid per gram myocardium per minute.[58,61]

Another, more recently introduced approach for estimating the myocardial uptake of free fatty acid entails a radiofluorinated fatty acid analogue, $^{18}$F-fluoro-6-thia-heptadecanoic acid ($^{18}$FTHA). The compound is thought to selectively trace $\beta$-oxidation and, analogous to $^{18}$F-deoxyglucose, becomes metabolically trapped in the myocardium. Rates of myocardial free fatty acid utilization derived from serially acquired PET images after intravenous administration of $^{18}$FTHA are comparable to those obtained invasively with the Fick method and, further, are similar to those derived with $^{11}$C-palmitate.[64–66]

Preferential utilization of a fuel substrate—as, for example, glucose, lactate, or free fatty acid—depends on its concentration in arterial blood, which, in turn, depends on the dietary state, serum levels, insulin resistance, or physical stress.[67] Changes in the myocardium's preferential substrate utilization can be demonstrated with either $^{11}$C-palmitate or $^{18}$F-deoxyglucose or both radiotracers.[50,67,68] In the presence of high free fatty acid and low glucose and insulin levels, use of free fatty acid as the preferred substrate is reflected on the $^{11}$C-palmitate curve by the large relative size of the rapid clearance phase and its steep slope (both corresponding to increased fatty acid oxidation) and the low or even undetectable $^{18}$F-deoxyglucose uptake (Fig. 23-4). Carbohydrate ingestion raises plasma glucose levels, stimulates insulin secretion, and depresses free fatty acid levels. The corresponding shift in myocardial glucose utilization is reflected by a decline in the size and slope of the rapid clearance phase of $^{11}$C-palmitate and by an increase in myocardial $^{18}$F-deoxyglucose uptake.

***Myocardial Oxygen Consumption*** Molecular $^{15}$O-oxygen, administered by inhalation, affords measurements of myocardial oxygen consumption. The myocardial extraction of labeled oxygen is determined by PET first; when multiplied by MBF,[69,70] the mass of oxygen con-

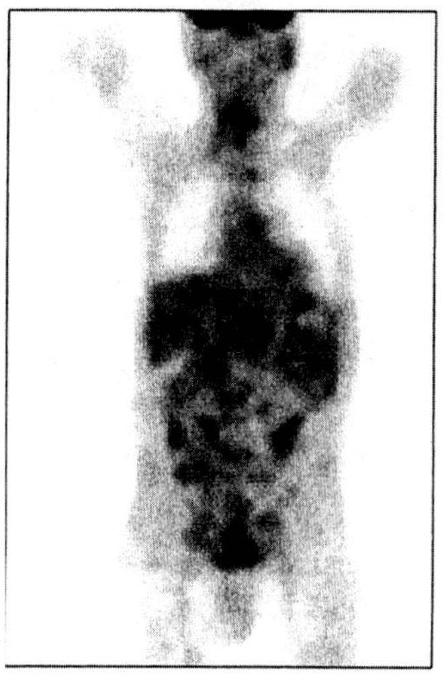


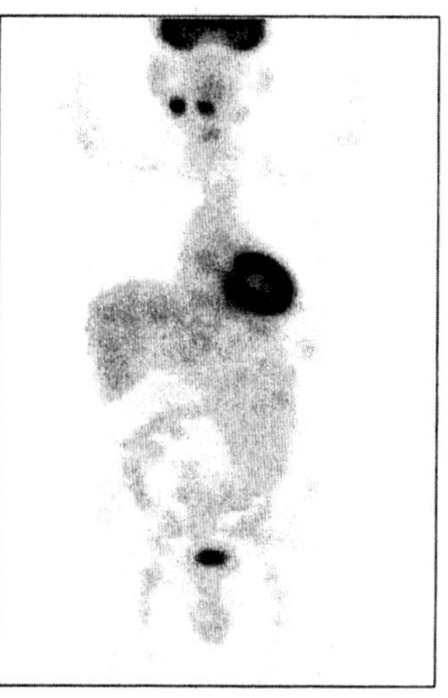


FIGURE 23-4 Whole-body images of $^{18}$F-deoxyglucose uptake obtained in a patient after overnight fasting (*left*) and 1 h after oral glucose loading (*right*). Note the $^{18}$F-deoxyglucose uptake by brain under both conditions and the absence of $^{18}$F-deoxyglucose uptake by the myocardium after an overnight fast, implicating free fatty acid as a preferred fuel substrate with little glucose utilization. However, in response to oral glucose loading, there is a marked increase in $^{18}$F-deoxyglucose uptake by the myocardium, suggesting a change in the substrate metabolism and utilization of glucose.

sumed per minute per gram myocardium can be estimated. A more widely applied means for estimating myocardial oxidative metabolism and thus of oxygen is rapid serial PET imaging with $^{11}$C-labeled acetate. The radiotracer clears rapidly from blood into the myocardium and produces high signal-to-background images.[71–74] It directly traces the rate of substrate flux through the TCA cycle as the final oxidative pathway common to most fuel substrates. The rate of clearance of $^{11}$C activity from the myocardium, as derived from serially acquired images, corresponds to the TCA cycle activity and, because of its close coupling to oxidative phosphorylation, to oxidative metabolism and myocardial oxygen consumption. It should be emphasized, however, that the tracer does not yield mass fluxes but only rate constants that can be converted into units of $O_2$ per minute per gram of myocardium. Unlike that of $^{11}$C-palmitate or $^{18}$F-deoxyglucose, the clearance rate of $^{11}$C-acetate from myocardium is relatively insensitive to changes in myocardial preferential substrate utilization.[72] A tracer compartment model, based on biochemical assays of the tracer tissue kinetics of $^{14}$C-acetate in isolated rat hearts,[75] forms the base for estimating in the human heart myocardial oxygen consumption in absolute units and, at the same time, of regional MBFs.[76,77] Both the $^{15}$O-oxygen and the $^{11}$C-acetate technique yield similar estimates of the myocardial oxygen consumption in the normal human myocardium.[78] However, values in regions with reduced blood flow have been found to differ, mostly because of methodologic differences, where the $^{11}$C-acetate approach yields average transmural values while the $^{15}$O-water approach renders estimates selectively for the water-perfusable tissue fraction.

## CLINICAL APPLICATIONS

A broader clinical acceptance of PET and of imaging of positron-emitting radionuclides have gained considerable momentum because investigational studies have demonstrated the potential of the technique in the diagnosis, characterization, and treatment monitoring of disease. It is especially the use of PET in oncology coupled with reimbursement that has also accelerated further instrumentation-related developments, as for example, of PET/CT and the dissemination of PET imaging devices. Major applications in cardiology have been (1) the identification and characterization of coronary artery disease (CAD) and (2) the detection of myocardial viability.

### Identification and Characterization of Coronary Artery Disease

#### GENERAL CONSIDERATIONS

Most studies with PET—for example, as performed with $^{13}$N-ammonia or $^{82}$Rb—evaluate the relative distribution of MBF from the retention of tracer in the myocardium. Recent investigations utilize PET's quantitative capability for estimating regional MBF in milliliters of blood per minute per gram myocardium in order to demonstrate abnormalities in vasomotion of the human coronary circulation during the early stages of coronary atherosclerosis.

Unlike the more conventional radionuclide approaches, PET has employed almost exclusively pharmacologic stress for the detection of CAD and for assessing its extent and functional significance. This is because the transmission images, essential for correction of photon attenuation, must be acquired with the patient in exactly the same position as during the emission images. Most commonly used as pharmacologic stress agents are dipyridamole and adenosine. Both afford an assessment of the myocardial flow reserve as the ratio of hyperemic to resting blood flows. The now classic studies by Gould[79] demonstrated a curvilinear, inverse correlation between stenosis severity and hyperemic flows or flow reserve. Thus, the magnitude of an attenuated response of blood flow during dipyridamole-induced hyperemia depends on the hemodynamic stenosis severity. As demonstrated by flow measurements with either $^{15}$O-water or $^{13}$N-ammonia, the vascular smooth muscle dilators dipyridamole and adenosine evoke interindividually variable hyperemic responses but induce, on average, a four- to fivefold increase in blood flow in normal myocardium.[21,24,25,80] The magnitude of the hyperemic flow response is similar for dipyridamole (at a dose of $0.56\ \text{mg} \cdot \text{kg}^{-1}$ over 4 min) and for adenosine (at $140\ \mu\text{g} \cdot \text{min}^{-1} \cdot \text{kg}^{-1}$, using a standard infusion time of 6 min).[26] Increases in the dipyridamole dose by 50 percent do not produce higher flows, nor do they reduce the interpatient variability in flow responses.[81] Additionally, the values of the normal flow reserve were derived from studies in young normal volunteers with an average age of 34 ± 16 years. This is important because the flow reserve has been reported to decline progressively with age (Fig. 23-5).[82–84] Possible contributing factors include an age-dependent decline in the vasodilator capacity as well as an age-dependent rise in baseline blood flow in response to a progressive increase in the rate-pressure product as a major determinant of blood flow at rest. A progressive decline in vascular compliance serves as another possible explanation. Because of the importance of the arterial blood pressure as the coronary driving pressure during pharmacologically induced hyperemia, increases in the mean arterial blood pressure, either due to isometric handgrip exercise or due to supine bicycle exercise, were anticipated to augment the hyperemic response. However, both interventions attenuated the maximum flow response, most likely because of increased vascular resistance due to greater extravascular resistive forces.[81,85] These factors may also contribute to lesser flow increases during physical exercise, when flow increases in proportion to oxygen demand. These observations may also suggest that pharmacologically induced hyperemia might not necessarily prove to be more accurate in identifying functionally

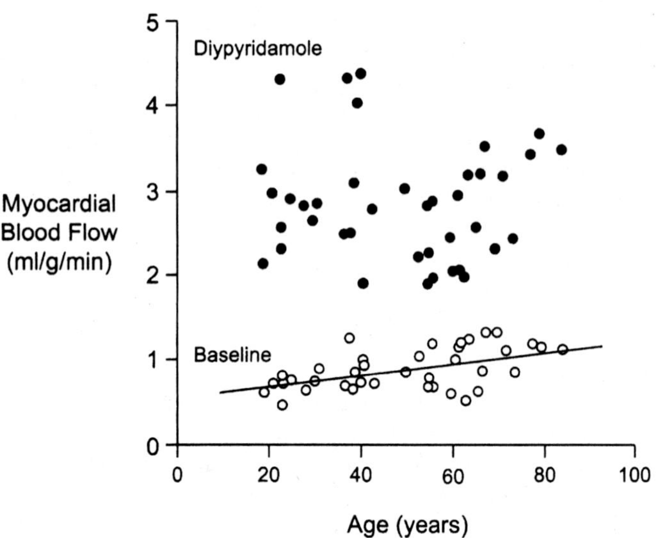


FIGURE 23-5 Age and myocardial blood flow at rest and during dipyridamole-induced hyperemia. Notice the progressive increase in resting myocardial blood flow, which occurred in response to a progressive increase in the rate-pressure product. However, no definitive trend is observed for the magnitude of dipyridamole-induced hyperemia.

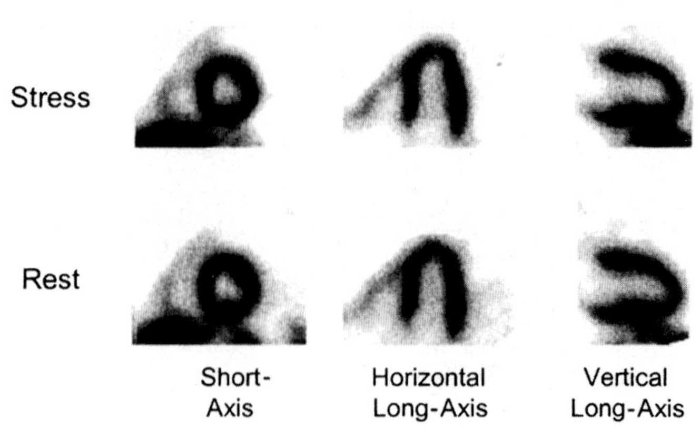


FIGURE 23-6 $^{13}N$-ammonia images of myocardial perfusion in a normal volunteer obtained during adenosine stress (*top*) and at rest (*bottom*). Note the homogenous distribution of tracer throughout the myocardium as seen on the short-axis, horizontal, and vertical long-axis images.

significant coronary stenosis. Even though flows in remote myocardium may rise less with exercise, depending on the level of cardiac work achieved, higher intracavitary left ventricular (LV) pressures and regional wall stresses in ischemic or dysfunctional myocardium might enhance extravascular resistive forces, so that flow responses in stenosis-dependent myocardium may in fact become more attenuated or suppressed. Finally, given the differences between ischemia produced by pharmacologic versus physical stress, the vasodilator reserve as determined pharmacologically may not necessarily truly reflect the myocardium's ability to raise flow during physical exercise. An example is that of patients with hypertrophic cardiomyopathy, where MBF during supine exercise failed to increase or even declined despite some residual flow reserve as demonstrated with dipyridamole.[86]

Another important consideration in regard to pharmacologic stress is the variability of the hyperemic response. In normal volunteers, responses may range from about two- to sixfold increases in flow. Several factors may account for this variability. Among these are (1) the coronary driving pressure, best reflected by the mean arterial blood pressure; (2) extravascular resistive forces as a function of wall tension and tension development, which in turn depend on the diastolic volume and the myocardium's contractile state; (3) $\beta$- and especially $\alpha$-adrenergic control of the basal vasomotor tone[87]; (4) endothelium-dependent vasomotion [88]; and (5) pharmacologic effects on smooth muscle relaxation. Importantly, the variability of estimates of the myocardial flow reserve as observed with pharmacologic vasodilation is unrelated to exercise capacity in normal volunteers.[89] Pharmacologic effects of dipyridamole and adenosine may be altered by antagonists like caffeine or theophylline-containing agents,[90] so that it is imperative for patients to refrain from these substances for at least 24 h prior to a pharmacologic stress study.

Positive inotropic agents like dobutamine are also employed for stress interventions. This predominantly $\beta_1$-adrenoreceptor agonist increases MBF in proportion to increases in cardiac work as measured by increases in the rate-pressure product.[91] In one study, for example, intravenous infusion of dobutamine in normal volunteers at a rate of 40 $\mu g \cdot min^{-1} \cdot kg^{-1}$ body weight increased the rate-pressure product by about 200 percent and was paralleled by a 225 percent increase in MBF.[91] To augment the flow response to dobutamine, mostly through further increases in heart rate, some laboratories supplement the infusion of dobutamine with intravenous atropine (typically 0.5 mg).[92]

## ASSESSMENT OF CORONARY ARTERY DISEASE

For the detection of CAD, the relative distribution of MBF is initially examined at rest and then during pharmacologic vasodilation. Either $^{82}Rb$ or $^{13}N$-ammonia is used. Both radiotracers are retained in myocardium in proportion to blood flow, so that the resulting images depict the distribution of MBF at rest and during hyperemia. This approach identifies true resting flow defects as well as attenuated responses of regional blood flow to hyperemia as a consequence of a coronary stenosis (Figs. 23-6 and 23-7). Images of rest and hyperemic perfusion are analyzed by visual inspection and by circumferential activity profile techniques or polar map approaches. While most investigations have relied on visual analysis, several laboratories routinely employ quantitative image analysis. All com-

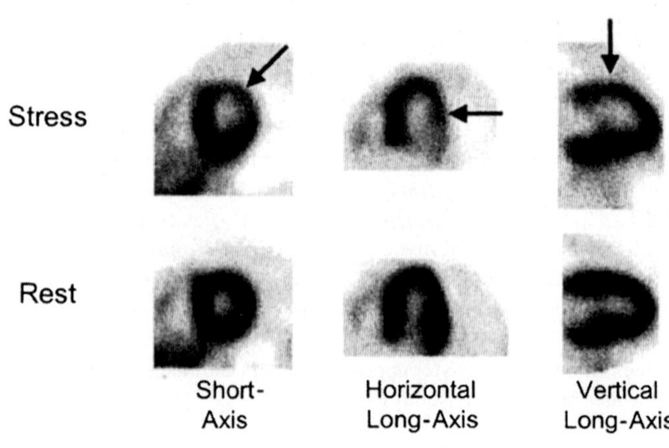


FIGURE 23-7 Myocardial perfusion images obtained with $^{13}N$- ammonia during adenosine stress and at rest in a patient with coronary artery disease. Note the extensive perfusion defect in the stress images (*arrows*) with normalization of myocardial perfusion during rest.

pare the regional tracer activity concentrations in a patient against databases of normal and display the relative distributions of tracer in the myocardium in various forms of cartographic displays—as, for example, in the polar (or azimuthal) or cylindrical (Mercator-like) projections or, in order to reduce geometric distortions, as surface-rendered three-dimensional displays of the LV myocardium.[93–96]

Clinical investigations have confirmed PET's excellent diagnostic performance for the detection of CAD.[97–103] Sensitivities range from 87 to 97 percent and specificities from 78 to 100 percent. Most studies compared rest or stress-induced flow defects to arteriographic findings by visual analysis, and most defined narrowing of 50 to 70 percent of the luminal diameter as significant stenosis. Given the well-known limitation of visual analysis, Gould et al.[104] and, subsequently, Demer et al.[99] graded the severity of stenosis by estimates of coronary flow reserve using quantitative arteriography. Coronary arteries were classified as moderately to severely stenosed if the predicted coronary flow reserve was less than 3, as intermediate if the coronary flow reserve ranged from 3 to 4, and as minimal for coronary flow reserve values greater than 4. According to this classification, 94 percent of vessels with moderate to severe, 49 percent of vessels with intermediate, and 5 percent of vessels with minimal stenosis were accurately identified in these studies with PET and pharmacologic vasodilator stress.

## COMPARISON OF PET TO CONVENTIONAL MYOCARDIAL PERFUSION IMAGING

The diagnostic accuracy of PET has been compared to that of more conventional approaches in order to more clearly define the diagnostic gain. Demer et al.[99] indirectly compared their findings to those of another laboratory using thallium-201 ($^{201}$Tl) SPECT but an identical angiographic approach for defining stenosis severity.[105] In this comparison, PET outperformed SPECT. Both studies defined stenosis severity by the angiographically predicted coronary flow reserve. Moderate to severe coronary stenoses were detected with 95 percent sensitivity by PET and 72 percent sensitivity by $^{201}$Tl SPECT, and intermediate stenoses with a 49 percent sensitivity by PET while none was detected by SPECT.

Other studies compared PET to SPECT in the same patients. An early study used supine bicycle stress and $^{13}$N-ammonia in 48 patients with CAD and reported comparable diagnostic performances for PET and SPECT.[98] Another investigation examined the relative merits of PET and SPECT in 202 patients during the same pharmacologic stress.[100] Myocardial blood flow was evaluated with $^{82}$Rb at rest and again 4 min after dipyridamole infusion. About 8 to 9 min later, or after a total of 12 to 13 min beyond the end of the 4-min dipyridamole infusion, $^{201}$Tl was injected and SPECT imaging performed within 10 min. PET and SPECT exhibited comparable specificities, while PET demonstrated a significantly higher sensitivity than SPECT. The results were similar when only 132 of the 202 patients without prior cardiac events such as angioplasty or bypass grafting were analyzed. A third study reported somewhat different findings in 81 patients.[101] Again, all patients underwent rest and dipyridamole stress imaging with $^{82}$Rb and PET; for the $^{201}$Tl SPECT study, 38 (or 47 percent) of the patients underwent treadmill stress and the remaining 43 (or 53 percent) pharmacologic stress with dipyridamole. In that study, PET and SPECT exhibited comparable sensitivities; however, the specificity was higher for PET than for SPECT. The diagnostic accuracies were similar for patients submitted to treadmill stress testing and patients with pharmacologically induced hyperemia for SPECT imaging with $^{201}$Tl. Thus, both studies support the high diagnostic accuracy of PET but differ in terms of higher sensitivities and specificities. While it might be argued that in the study by Go et al.[100] the hyperemic effect of dipyridamole had dissipated at the time of the $^{201}$Tl injection and thus accounted for the lower sensitivity of SPECT, continuous coronary sinus flow measurements have demonstrated an average decay half-time of 33 min for the hyperemic response. This suggests that the hyperemic response over a 4-min period had declined by only about 10 percent,[106] which is unlikely to fully explain the significantly lower sensitivity of SPECT $^{201}$Tl imaging. More plausible is the gain in specificity in the study by Stewart et al.[101] It most likely resulted from the adequate correction of photon attenuation and thus a reduction of false-positive findings. Although the reasons for the observed differences between both studies remain unclear, image analysis at different points of the receiver operating curve (ROC) might be one possible explanation. Further, the absence of a significant difference between PET and SPECT findings in the first study[98] might be attributed to the use of first-generation PET imaging instrumentation.

Larger clinical trials, especially in previously undiagnosed patients with normal blood flow and normal wall motion at baseline, are needed to define the diagnostic gain more clearly. Current information nevertheless indicates a substantial improvement in diagnostic accuracy, which might eliminate additional diagnostic procedures like coronary arteriography. This seems confirmed by a study that compared the effect of PET and of SPECT on subsequent referral to coronary angiography in 1490 and 102 patients, respectively.[107] Pretest likelihoods for CAD were similar for both patient groups. However, the rate of angiography was significantly less (16.7 percent) after PET than after SPECT (31.4 percent), which produced a cost saving of about 23 percent per patient.

## PROGNOSTIC IMPLICATIONS FOR REST/STRESS PET PERFUSION IMAGING

Only few investigations have explored the prognostic value of PET stress and rest perfusion imaging. One preliminary survey of 108 patients with a relatively low pretest likelihood of CAD found no cardiac morbidity or mortality for 2 years after a normal PET study.[108] When PET was employed in a population with strongly suspected or known CAD, the prognostic value of PET was maintained.[109] By following 685 patients for an average period of 41 months, a normal PET study was associated with a 0.9 percent annual cardiac mortality, as compared to a 4.3 percent annual mortality rate in patients with rest and/or stress-induced perfusion defects. Moreover, PET's value for assessing the preoperative risk in patients scheduled for aortic, carotid, and femoral artery surgery has been explored.[110] A normal PET study had a 92 percent negative predictive accuracy for a cardiac event. Conversely, extensive ischemic defects involving at least 5 of 24 myocardial segments were 64 percent accurate in predicting a perioperative cardiac event.

Specific criteria remain to be established to determine whether PET is preferable to SPECT for myocardial perfusion imaging in particular patients and under which clinical conditions. PET's advantage of accurate correction for photon attenuation, leading to fewer image artifacts, has largely been offset by gated SPECT, where assessment of regional contractile function aids in distinguishing between artifactual and true perfusion defects. Gated PET acquisition of perfusion or metabolism imaging, although feasible, has remained incompletely explored and its value is therefore not known.[111,112] Because of its higher spatial and contrast resolution, PET for myocardial perfusion imaging would seem to be preferable (1) in obese patients or females, both with a greater likelihood of producing image artifacts; (2) in patients suspected to have only mild coronary artery disease or to be at high risk for CAD; and (3) for assessing effects of risk-factor modification on regional myocardial perfusion. In asymptomatic first-degree relatives of patients with clinically established CAD, PET rest and stress imaging revealed perfusion defects in 50 percent of all patients and thus evidence of flow-limiting coronary stenosis.[113] Further, repeat perfusion imaging with PET in patients with CAD participating in risk-factor modification programs with a low-fat vegetarian diet, stress management, group support, and mild to moderate exercise demonstrated a moderate though statistically significant 5.1 ± 4.8 percent reduction in stress defect sizes. In contrast, defect sizes had increased by 10.3 ± 5.6 percent in a control group of patients managed mostly with antianginal treatment.[114] A subsequent investigation in 409 patients with CAD reported similar improvements in PET stress perfusion defects in patients on maximum risk-factor modification treatment when reexamined at 2.6 years after the baseline PET study. Again, a statistically significant improvement in stress-induced flow defects was observed. In contrast, stress perfusion defects worsened in the control group of CAD patients not on lipid-lowering diets or medications.[115] When followed over an additional 5 years, intense lifestyle modification plus pharmacologic lipid lowering and changes in the perfusion defect proved to be independent predictors of cardiac events.

## EFFECT OF CORONARY STENOSES ON REGIONAL MYOCARDIAL BLOOD FLOW

PET's quantitative capability for measurements of MBF has been utilized to explore the relationship between angiographic stenosis severity, hyperemic flow responses, and vasodilator capacity.[116–118] Statistically significant correlations between anatomic stenosis severity and attenuation of the hyperemic response to pharmacologic vasodilation have been found. Similar correlations between MBF and coronary stenosis severity were noted when blood flow was raised with dobutamine rather than with adenosine or dipyridamole.[119]

The inverse, nonlinear correlation between the reduction in cross-sectional area of the stenosis and flow reserve in the stenosis-dependent myocardium as reported in one of these investigations (Fig. 23-8)[118] resembles Gould's now classic nonlinear flow–stenosis relationship in experimental animals.[79] The flow-stenosis correlation in patients was observed only after confounding factors—such as stenosis in series or stenosis-dependent myocardium, supplied also by collateral vessels—were excluded from the analysis.[118] Nevertheless, there was considerable scatter of the data about the regression line. Several factors may account for this scatter. They include possible inaccuracies in regional flow measurements, the variability of the hyperemic response to pharmacologic stimulation, as well as differences in the patients' ages and in the baseline hemodynamic state. The scatter of the data may further point to disparities between anatomic and functional properties of human coronary artery stenosis. Different from the experimentally controlled idealized coronary stenosis in the animal experimental setting,[79] human coronary stenoses are of remarkably greater morphologic complexity, including eccentricity, variable stenosis inflow and outflow angles, and different lengths and irregular surfaces, all of which may not be fully appreciated by angiographic criteria or be adequately accounted for by assumptions underlying model-based estimates of stenosis severity. This, then, might suggest that evaluation of flow, either semiquantitatively or quantitatively, renders more accurate functional information on stenosis severity and, more broadly, on CAD. Moreover, estimates of an attenuated flow reserve obtained from static images of the relative distribution of MBF during hyperemic stress clearly offer invaluable information on the functional significance of coronary stenosis. However, given the nonlinear response in radiotracer uptake to increases in MBF, such "semiquantitative" estimates would tend to be less accurate indices of stenosis severity than those available through true measurements of MBF.

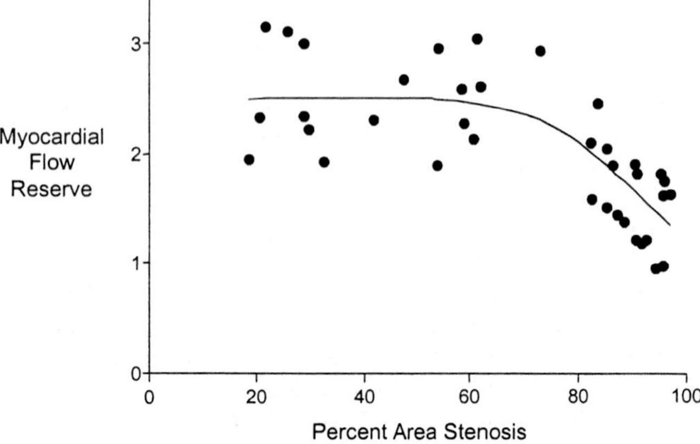


FIGURE 23-8 Myocardial flow reserve and severity of coronary artery stenosis by quantitative angiography. Note the curvilinear relationship between the myocardial flow reserve as determined quantitatively from hyperemic and rest myocardial blood flow (MBF) measurements with $^{13}$N- ammonia. (Reproduced from Di Carli et al.[118] with permission of the American Heart Association.)

## ASSESSMENT OF CORONARY VASOMOTION AND PRECLINICAL CORONARY ARTERY DISEASE

Noninvasive measurements of regional MBF offer the intriguing possibility of uncovering functional abnormalities of the human coronary circulation. If such alterations already exist during the early stages of coronary atherosclerosis, detection of disease during its evolutionary and preclinical stage may become possible. Such measurements further offer the prospect of monitoring disease progression as well as the responses to interventions aiming at regression of disease or slowing or halting its progression. Several lines of evidence support the possibility of early disease detection through PET measurements of MBF.

***Attenuation of the Myocardial Flow Reserve*** The now well-established beneficial effects of cholesterol lowering—and especially of HMG-CoA reductase inhibitors—have emphasized the importance of assessing functional rather than anatomic or structural alterations of the human coronary circulation. This is because dietary and/or pharmacologic cholesterol lowering causes relatively little change in the anatomic severity of stenosis, at least over the time periods studied, but it lowers cardiac morbidity and mortality strikingly.[120] Hence, these beneficial effects have been attributed to plaque stabilization and improvements in endothelial function.[121]

Invasive studies of the human coronary circulation—performed during cardiac catheterization with intracoronary administration of predominantly direct vascular smooth muscle dilator agents like adenosine or papavarine, together with intracoronary administration of acetylcholine as a pharmacologic probe of predominantly endothelium-mediated coronary vasomotion—have emphasized the central role of endothelial dysfunction early in the atherosclerotic process. For example, in human coronary arteries with minimal atherosclerotic changes (with irregular intraluminal surfaces but without flow-limiting stenosis or even any angiographic findings), normal, predominantly vascular smooth muscle–mediated vasodilator flow responses were present but attenuated or even highly abnormal endothelium-mediated flow responses occurred.[122–124] These invasive approaches probe endothelial function at two sites of the coronary circulation, the large epicardial conduit and the coronary resistance vessels.[122–124] Endothelium-dependent control mechanisms in concert with vascular smooth muscle–mediated vasomotion at both sites regulate changes in coronary and, thus, in MBF in response to physiologic or pharmacologic stimuli. Therefore, if MBF or its changes can be measured in absolute units, as is now possible with PET, it should be possible to derive information on coronary circulatory function noninvasively. Several lines of evidence indicate that this may indeed be possible.

PET-based measurements of MBF in asymptomatic patients with hypercholesterolemia revealed an about 32 percent reduction in myocardial perfusion reserve or an about 18 percent reduction in hyperemic flow during the administration of adenosine.[125–130] Some studies reported correlations between the myocardial flow reserve and the ratio of plasma total cholesterol over HDL cholesterol[125] or LDL cholesterol concentrations.[131] Other investigations extended these observations but also noted that elevated plasma triglycerides or, in young males, a family history of CAD alone or of hypertension was associated with diminished vasodilator capacities and myocardial flow reserves.[132–134] Other studies again observed diminished hyperemic responses in patients with diabetes,[134–137] and one study found a correlation between the hyperemic blood flow response and therapeutic control of the diabetic state.[138] Other factors found to modulate the myocardial perfusion reserve or flow responses to pharmacologic vasodilation included oxidized LDL and homocysteine,[139] asymmetric dimethyl arginine (ADMA),[140] and obesity.[141]

These observations differ from those made by invasive techniques, where frequently the predominantly vascular smooth muscle–mediated vasodilator response to, for example, intracoronary papavarine or adenosine was preserved even in the presence of coronary risk factors, while primarily endothelium-mediated responses were markedly abnormal.[142] On the other hand, as pointed out by Bache,[143] the major resistance to flow through the coronary circulation resides at vessels 100 to 400 $\mu$m in diameter. If increases in flow exert shear stresses on the endothelium of the 400-$\mu$m vessels, then primarily flow (endothelium)-dependent mechanisms augment the flow response to predominantly vascular smooth muscle vasodilators. Consistent with such augmentation are observations with measurements of forearm blood flow and with PET of MBF.[88,144] In both investigations in healthy volunteers, inhibition of endothelial nitric oxide synthase (eNOS) with L-$N^G$-monomethyl arginine (L-NMMA) or $N^G$-nitro-L-arginine-methyl ester (L-NAME) significantly reduced the adenosine-stimulated hyperemic flow (forearm blood flow by 30 percent and MBF by 21 percent). It is thus possible that coronary risk factors such as elevated LDL cholesterol, triglyceridemia, and diabetes known to reduce the bioavailability of NO or to impair the eNOS activity account for the attenuation of the hyperemic response to adenosine or dipyridamole. Responses of MBF to pharmacologic stress with predominantly vascular smooth muscle relaxants therefore represent a measure of the integrated, flow-independent and flow-dependent total coronary vasodilator capacity.

***Longitudinal Base-to-Apex Myocardial Perfusion Gradient*** Another attractive approach for noninvasively identifying functional alterations of the coronary circulation affecting predominantly the epicardial conduit vessels is the concept of the "longitudinal, base-to-apex myocardial perfusion gradient."[145] This concept explains the observed progressive decline in myocardial perfusion from the base to the apex of the left ventricle. The normal epicardial conduit vessel exerts little if any resistance to flow, so that the intracoronary pressure is fully maintained over the length of the conduit vessel and myocardial perfusion is homogenous. Diffuse luminal narrowing of the epicardial coronary arteries, however, even in the absence of discrete coronary stenosis, causes resistance to flow, so that intracoronary perfusion pressures progressively decline from the proximal to the distal coronary arterial tree. This decline is associated with a progressive base-to-apex decline in tissue perfusion. Because resistance to flow is also a function of the flow velocity, the intracoronary pressure decline—and thus, the base-to-apex perfusion gradient—is most prominent during adenosine- or dipyridamole-induced hyperemia. Intracoronary pressure measurements have confirmed the validity of this concept.[146] In coronary vessels free of angiographic disease in patients with CAD, intracoronary pressures were found to decrease from proximal to distal by about 5 mmHg at rest and 10 mmHg during pharmacologically induced hyperemia. This decrease in intracoronary pressure was significantly greater than that observed in normals. Further, in 8 percent of coronary arteries free of angiographic disease in patients with CAD, the intracoronary pressure gradient decline exceeded 25 percent, thus reaching ischemic levels.

A similar though less prominent perfusion gradient was also observed in patients without clinical evidence of CAD and with normal stress myocardial perfusion images but with coronary risk factors. This perfusion gradient was noted only during pharmacologically induced hyperemia and was identified only through quantitative measurements of MBF by PET.[147] Because coronary angiography had not been performed in these patients, diffuse luminal narrowing of the epicardial conduit vessels cannot be ruled out as a possible explanation. Even if diffuse luminal narrowing were absent, structural alterations—as, for example, increases in the intima-media thickness as identifiable by intracoronary vascular ultrasound[148]—might serve as another explanation, because it could reduce the bioavailability of NO to the vascular smooth muscle even if the endothelium responded appropriately to increases in shear stress. Moreover, a thickened intima-media might also be associated with increased vessel wall stiffness, which could mechanically restrict the dilation of conduit vessels. Finally, it is also possible that the flow-mediated vasodilator function would have been altered as a consequence of endothelial dysfunction.

***Sympathetic Stimulation through Cold Pressor Testing*** This approach offers a means of identifying alterations of the coronary circulatory function possibly related directly to endothelial function. As demonstrated with invasive studies of the coronary circulation, cold pressor testing evoked in non-flow-limiting CAD or in the presence of coronary risk factors only paradoxical narrowing of the epicardial conduit vessels. These cold-induced changes in vessel diameter correlated with flow-dependent diameter changes in response to downstream, intracoronary administration of vascular smooth muscle relaxants.[122,149,150] Furthermore, changes at the level of the resistance vessels were found to correlate with changes in response to intracoronary acetylcholine stimulation.[122,151,152] Although a causal relationship remains to be established, these observations imply by association the possibility of deriving information on coronary vasomotor control and, to some extent, on endothelial function through noninvasive measurements of MBF responses to cold pressor testing. Observations with PET measurements of MBF seem to support such possibility.

In young long-term smokers without other risk factors for CAD, the hyperemic flow response to intravenous dipyridamole was fully preserved when compared to an age-matched group of nonsmokers

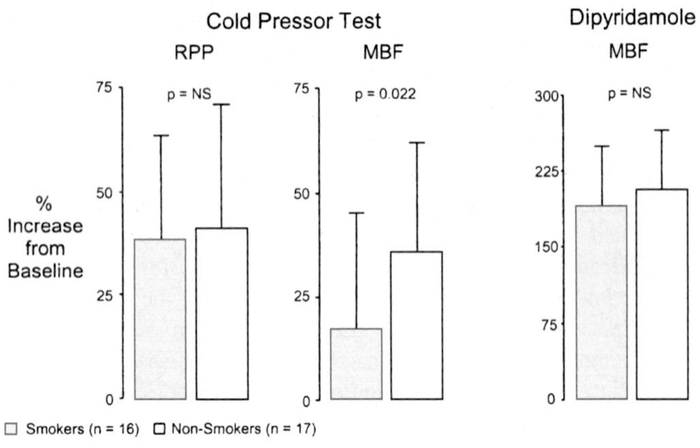


FIGURE 23-9 Increases in myocardial blood flow (MBF) in response to cold pressor testing and to IV dipyridamole in nonsmokers and long-term smokers (*shaded bars*). Note the comparable increases in MBF in response to dipyridamole in both groups. Also, cold pressor testing produced comparable increases in the rate-pressure product (RPP), while the increase in blood flow in long-term smokers was markedly attenuated as compared to normals. (Data from Campisi et al.[153])

(Fig. 23-9).[153] Cold pressor testing, however, produced in smokers only modest, statistically insignificant increases in MBF that were significantly different from those in a control group of nonsmokers. Consistent with observations through invasive techniques,[122,149,150] the cold-induced increases in rate-pressure product were associated with proportional increases in MBF in nonsmokers but not in the smokers. A similar uncoupling of flow responses from cardiac work has also been observed previously in patients with risk factors for CAD or with type 2 diabetes.[122,149,150] Mechanisms accounting for such uncoupling remain to be explored, although existing explanations point to endothelial dysfunction or reduced bioavailability of NO. The increase in cardiac work in response to sympathetic stimulation and as reflected by an increase in heart rate and systolic blood pressure is associated with an increase in MBF, possibly through metabolic control mechanisms, $\beta$-stimulation, or both. Local release of norepinephrine leads to stimulation of $\alpha$-adrenergic receptors and vascular smooth muscle contraction, which are offset by flow-mediated and endothelial $\alpha$-receptor–stimulated NO release. When the bioavailability of NO is diminished or endothelial dysfunction is present, the compensatory vasodilator effect is diminished or absent, so that the vasoconstrictor effect prevails.

That the abnormal flow response to cold pressor testing in smokers reflects a functional rather than structural alteration of vasomotor control appears confirmed by responses to acute administration of L-arginine as the substrate for NO.[154] L-Arginine restored the flow response to cold pressor testing, so that it was similar to the flow responses in nonsmokers (Fig. 23-10). The underlying mechanism for this improvement remains unclear, but, as mentioned below, could entail a direct effect on eNOS, competitive displacement of the eNOS inhibitor ADMA, or an insulin-mediated effect, especially because intravenous L-arginine infusion was associated with a significant rise in plasma insulin concentrations.

The utility of cold pressor testing combined with PET measurements of MBF for identifying coronary vasomotor abnormalities has been explored in a number of different conditions. In postmenopausal women, for example, MBF responses were found to be significantly diminished in comparison to young women studied at mid-menstrual cycle.[155] The abnormal flow response was noted in postmenopausal women with and without risk factors for CAD (Fig. 23-11). Postmenopausal women on hormone replacement therapy (HRT) but without coronary risk factors, by contrast, revealed normal flow responses to cold pressor testing, while flow responses to cold remained abnormal in women with risk factors despite HRT. The findings thus might imply a beneficial effect of HRT on coronary vasomotion in postmenopausal women, but only in the absence of risk factors. Other studies again report abnormal flow responses to cold in patients with type 2 diabetes.[137,156] These noninvasively observed changes are similar to those observed through invasive measurements and suggest a spectrum of coronary functional alterations associated with type 2 diabetes.[150]

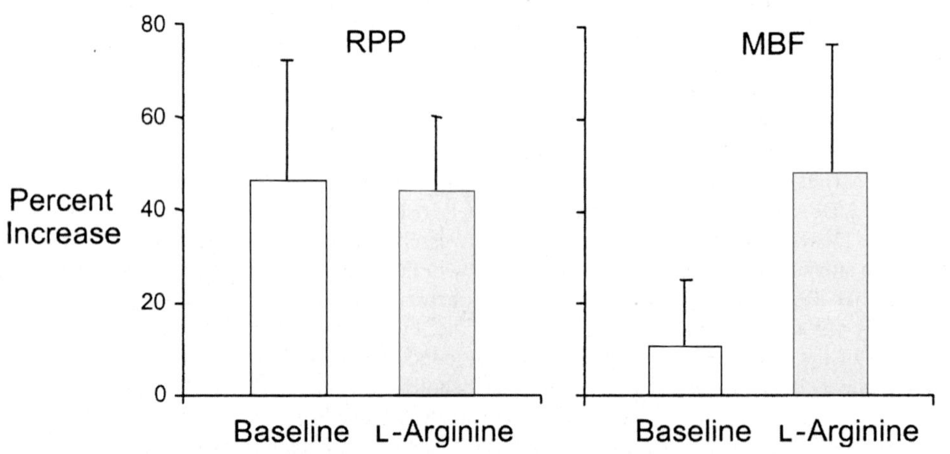


FIGURE 23-10 Effect of intravenous L-arginine on the myocardial flow response to cold pressor testing in long-term smokers. The panel on the left shows the percent increases in the rate-pressure product (RPP) and the panel on the right the increases in myocardial blood flow (MBF). At baseline, cold pressor testing increases the rate-pressure product by 46 percent and produces a small and statistically insignificant increase in myocardial blood flow. Following intravenous L-arginine, the response in the rate-pressure product remains unchanged, while the response of myocardial blood flow markedly improves and in fact no longer differs from flow responses observed in nonsmokers. (From Campisi et al.,[154] with permission.)

## MONITORING RESPONSES TO RISK-FACTOR MODIFICATION

PET measurements of MBF are equally suited for monitoring responses in coronary vasomotion to pharmacologic interventions as well as to risk-factor modification, as initially demonstrated in patients participating in a short (6-week) cardiovascular conditioning program.[157] The program consisted of dietary changes, regular exercise, and lifestyle modification and was associated with weight loss, decreases in heart rate and blood pressure at rest, and significant lowering of plasma total and LDL cholesterol. The observed 12 percent decline in MBF at rest was proportionate to the decrease in resting cardiac work as estimated by the rate-pressure product. Cardiovascular conditioning also produced a 9 percent increase in hyperemic flow and thus in vasodilator capacity, so that MBF reserve increased by a total of 20 percent.

Rigorous lifestyle and risk-factor modification had previously been shown with PET to result in smaller and less severe stress-induced perfusion defects.[114,158] More recent studies with PET-based measurements of MBF have demonstrated beneficial effects of cholesterol lowering by HMG-CoA reductase inhibitors.[159,160] In one study, a 6-month course of fluvastatin produced a 26 percent increase in hyperemic flows and thus in vasodilator capacity.[159] Of interest was a delayed improvement in vasodilator capacity in one study (Fig. 23-12). Despite a significant reduction in total and LDL cholesterol levels at 2 months, MBF remained essentially unchanged, but it had markedly improved when reexamined at 6 months. In these patients with CAD, the cumulative coronary function improved in myocardial territories subtended by both diseased and by nondiseased coronary arteries. These observations are at odds with those of another study that demonstrated a significant improvement in vasodilator capacity only in territories with stress-induced perfusion defects (an about 47 percent increase in hyperemic flows in response to 140 $\mu$g adenosine $\cdot$ min$^{-1}$ $\cdot$ kg$^{-1}$) but not in apparently normal myocardium,[161] whereas a third study demonstrated again an improvement of about 20 percent in hyperemic flows in remote myocardium.[160] In contrast to the delayed improvement in coronary vasomotion, other studies report immediate (within 24 h) improvements in hyperemic blood flows following LDL cholesterol plasmapheresis.[162] The reasons for these disparate observations are not entirely clear. In the latter study, however, plasma LDL apheresis reduced total cholesterol by 42 percent and LDL cholesterol by 58 percent, which was greater than in the fluvastatin study, with total and LDL cholesterol reductions of 29 and 37 percent, respectively.[159] Hence, possible explanations may include the markedly lower LDL cholesterol levels after LDL apheresis and/or significant changes in blood viscosity.

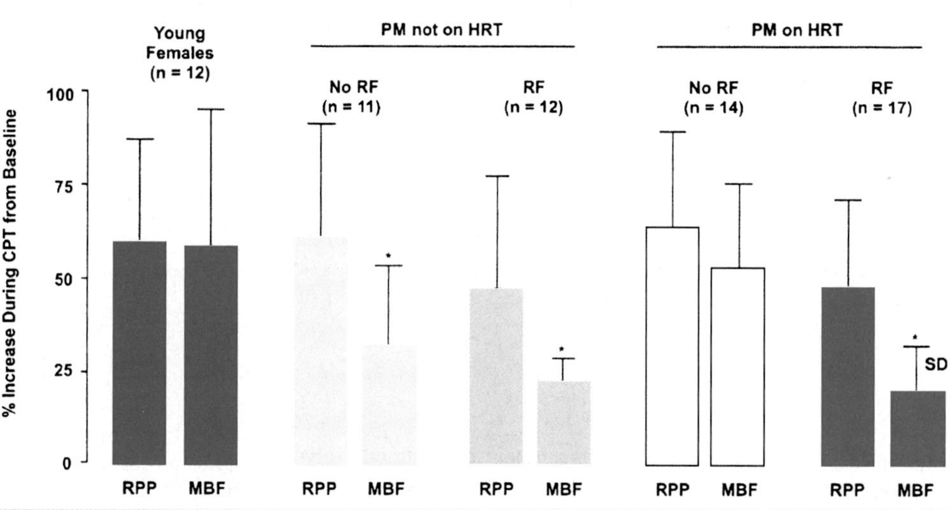


FIGURE 23-11 Cold pressor test–induced changes in rate-pressure product (RPP) and in myocardial blood flow (MBF) in postmenopausal women (PM): Each pair of bars represents the change in rate-pressure product and in myocardial blood flow as induced with cold pressor testing. Different from the findings in young females, the flow response to cold pressor testing is significantly attenuated in postmenopausal women with and without cardiac risk factors. In comparison, and as shown by the two pairs of bars on the right, the flow response to cold pressor testing remains abnormal in women with risk factors despite hormone replacement therapy (HRT), while in postmenopausal women without risk factors, the flow response to cold pressor testing no longer differs significantly from that in young, normal females. (From Campisi et al.,[155] with permission.)

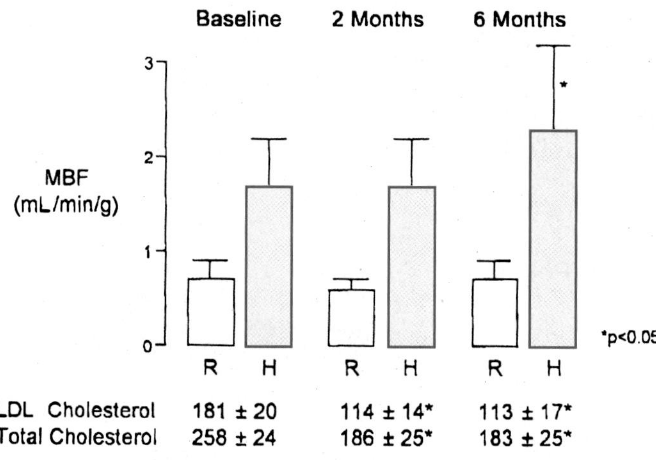


FIGURE 23-12 Changes in coronary artery vasodilator function in patients with CAD on a 6-month course of fluvastatin. Mean values of myocardial blood flow (MBF) at rest (R) and during adenosine stimulated hyperemia (H) are shown at baseline and after 2 months and 6 months fluvastatin treatment. Corresponding plasma levels of total and LDL cholesterol in mg per dL are indicated below. Note the delayed improvement of hyperemic MBF despite the significant decline in plasma total and LDL cholesterol at 2 months (*$p < 0.05$ versus baseline). Data after Guethlin et al.[159]

These studies evaluated the integrated response of the coronary circulation to a predominantly vascular smooth muscle–mediated vasodilator effect. Other investigations explored pharmacologic effects on predominantly endothelium-dependent coronary vasomotion. For example, intravenous L-arginine (30 g) as the substrate of eNOS in long-term smokers normalized the blood flow response to cold pressor testing, suggesting that endothelial function—or, at least, the bioactivity of NO—had normalized (see also Fig. 23-10).[154] Whether increases in the substrate for eNOS accelerates production of NO remains uncertain, especially in view of the low $K_m$, which renders the reaction relatively substrate-independent.[163] One possibility could be a nonspecific effect, perhaps on oxidative stress, as recently demonstrated with cold pressor testing in response to acute administration of vitamin C.[164] Other possible mechanisms include a competitive displacement of ADMA, an inhibitor of eNOS with known elevated plasma concentrations in hypercholesterolemic patients.[165] An insulin-dependent mechanism is also possible, especially because L-arginine infusions prompted three- to fourfold increases in plasma insulin concentrations.[154]

Irrespective of the underlying mechanisms, these observations confirm that effects of therapy on coronary vasomotion, either cumulative or confined to the endothelium, can be demonstrated noninvasively with PET. This capability therefore offers an opportunity to identify changes in coronary vasomotion during the early evolution of coronary atherosclerosis and CAD. Thus it might become possible to identify those individuals with a high likelihood of developing CAD and, further, whether dietary and/or pharmacologic cholesterol lowering in such patients would be effective in halting the progression of disease or even reversing it. Finally, for measurements of coronary vasoreactivity with PET to become clinically useful, it will be important to determine whether (1) abnormalities in coronary vasomotor function as identified with PET predict future cardiac events and (2) restoration or improvements in vasomotor function are predictive of a reduction of coronary risk. At present, direct evidence in support of either possibility is still lacking. However, invasively measured indices of flow-dependent coronary vasomotion in response to sympathetic stimulation or to intracoronary administration of vascular smooth muscle relaxants or acetylcholine have indeed been found to be independent predictors of cardiac death.[166–168]

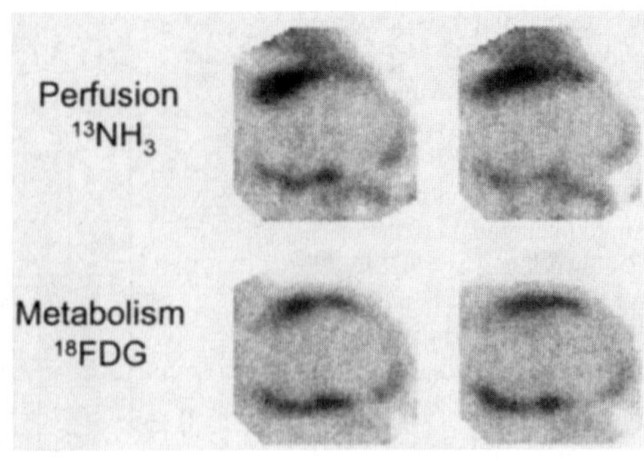


FIGURE 23-14 Myocardial blood flow metabolism match. The upper panel depicts two contiguous vertical long-axis images of myocardial perfusion obtained with $^{13}$N-ammonia, and the lower panel shows the corresponding vertical long-axis cuts on the $^{18}$F-deoxyglucose images. Note that the distribution of the $^{18}$F-deoxyglucose uptake parallels that of myocardial perfusion, consistent with the pattern of a perfusion metabolism match.

## Assessment of Myocardial Viability

Myocardial viability pertains to an impairment of contractile myocardial function that is potentially reversible. Distinguishing such a potentially reversible condition from an irreversible impairment of contractile function is of considerable clinical importance but remains diagnostically challenging. This is because both types of tissue injury share several features—as, for example, abnormal systolic wall motion, reduced blood flow, and electrocardiographic abnormalities. Specific to viable myocardium is, however, persistence of metabolic activity for sustaining vital, energy-requiring processes including cellular homeostasis. Residual metabolic activity depends on some residual blood flow for removal of inhibitory metabolites as well as for supply of fuel substrates. Hence, key features of viable myocardium include the following:

- Impairment of systolic wall motion at rest
- Normal or reduced but not absent blood flow
- Preservation of cellular homeostasis
- Persistent metabolic activity for high-energy phosphate production
- Recruitable contractile reserve

### GENERAL CONSIDERATIONS

Findings in experimental animals have provided the basis for the detection of myocardial viability. Initial investigations had indicated that known alterations in substrate metabolism during acute myocardial ischemia could indeed be demonstrated noninvasively with positron-emitting tracers of myocardial substrate metabolism.[169] Consistent with an impaired fatty acid oxidation was the diminished initial uptake of $^{11}$C-palmitate and its delayed subsequent rate of clearance from the myocardium.[62,63] Additionally, the known increase in glucose extraction and utilization was reflected by a regional increase in $^{18}$F-deoxyglucose uptake.[170] Initial studies in patients with clinical evidence of acute myocardial ischemia revealed patterns of blood flow and glucose metabolism that were virtually identical to those found in animals—e.g., enhanced $^{18}$F-deoxyglucose uptake in hypoperfused dysfunctional myocardial regions. Unexpected, however, was the existence of the same pattern in patients with chronic CAD but without clinical signs of acute ischemia (Fig. 23-13). This, then, raised the question of whether the pattern of blood-flow metabolism observed on PET was indeed unique to acute ischemia or whether it represented a more general metabolic pattern in chronically dysfunctional and hypoperfused myocardium. No less intriguing were observations in other CAD patients with a segmentally reduced $^{18}$F-deoxyglucose uptake, which paralleled the reduction in regional MBF (Figs. 23-14 and 23-15).[171] A more systematic exploration of these findings in patients scheduled for coronary artery bypass grafting confirmed the working hypothesis that the regionally enhanced $^{18}$F-deoxyglucose uptake, in contrast to a reduction, reflected sustained glucose utilization and, thus, metabolic activity as evidence of viability in myocardium with complete

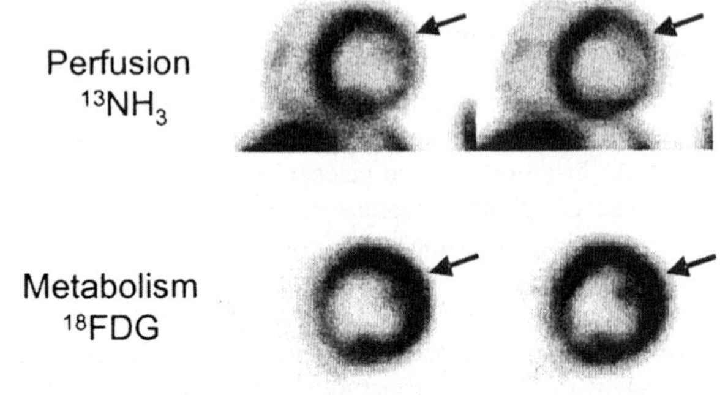


FIGURE 23-13 Myocardial blood flow metabolism mismatch (*arrows*): The upper panel demonstrates two contiguous short-axis myocardial perfusion images with a moderate decrease in perfusion in the anterior and anterolateral wall. On the $^{18}$F-deoxyglucose metabolism images, as shown in the bottom panel, glucose utilization is enhanced in the hypoperfused myocardium, consistent with a perfusion metabolism mismatch.

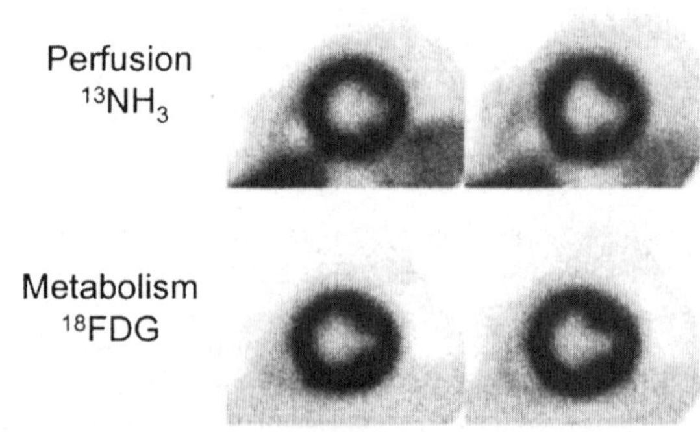


FIGURE 23-15 Normal pattern of myocardial blood flow and metabolism. Note the homogenous distribution of myocardial perfusion and of metabolism as seen on the two contiguous short-axis views of myocardial blood flow ($^{13}$N-ammonia) and of metabolism ($^{18}$FDG).

or partial loss of contractile function.[172] Restoration of tissue perfusion was followed by an improvement of contractile function in myocardium with persistent glucose metabolic activity.

## POSSIBLE MECHANISMS OF THE BLOOD-FLOW METABOLISM PATTERN

The above-described observations established the clinical utility of these PET findings, although the underlying mechanisms remained uncertain. Patients with CAD undergoing supine bicycle exercise revealed in myocardium with stress-induced flow defects an augmented $^{18}$F-deoxyglucose uptake when the radiotracer was administered 20 to 30 min after exercise and after the stress-induced flow defect had resolved.[173] This, then, implied that the enhanced tracer uptake might indeed represent "stunned myocardium," a possibility supported by observations in experimental animals and in patients with either collaterized myocardium or unstable angina.[174–176] These studies also demonstrated the evolution of a blood-flow metabolism pattern in chronically reperfused myocardium: an immediate postreperfusion decrease in glucose uptake was followed by an increase that subsequently declined to normal as contractile function returned.[174] The enhanced $^{18}$F-deoxyglucose uptake was attributed to increased lactate release and thus to anaerobic glycolysis, which persisted even after blood flow had been restored.[177] The evolution of such a metabolic pattern might pertain also to early postinfarction patients[178] but does not fully explain the flow metabolism observations in patients with chronic CAD. Another possibility is "repetitive stunning"[179] as an explanation of the persistent increase in $^{18}$F-deoxyglucose uptake in dysfunctional myocardium. An impairment in contractile function associated with enhanced glucose utilization was noted in collateral-dependent myocardium only if the flow reserve was markedly restricted.[175] The coronary circulation is then unable to respond appropriately to increases in oxygen demand during daily life, leading to transient ischemic episodes, each followed by stunning and preventing recovery of contractile function. Consistent with this concept are findings during dobutamine stimulation where development of wall motion abnormalities depended on the residual perfusion reserve and, in turn, on the angiographic severity of coronary stenosis.[180,181]

Myocardial hibernation serves as another possible explanation.[182] The postulated downregulation of contractile function in response to diminished resting blood flow is thought to be associated with an alteration of the myocardium's substrate metabolism, with a dominant role for the more oxygen-efficient glucose. Hibernation in its truest sense then implies that the downregulated energy requirements match the available energy supply. A new supply-demand imbalance is established, but at a lower level. Such a new balance would, however, be a precarious one, because even moderate increases in demand or decreases in supply could disturb the steady state and cause ischemia. It is thus possible and likely that both "hibernation" and "stunning" coexist to varying extents in many patients. Observations in experimental animals suggest that sustained reductions in both blood flow and contractile function can be maintained for some time without significant necrosis, although structural alterations develop that resemble those in patients with chronic CAD[183–187] and that provide an animal experimental underpinning for the concept of "hibernation."

Both concepts, repetitive "stunning" and "hibernation," may, in their purest form, represent the two ends of a spectrum. This spectrum begins with a reduction in myocardial flow reserve when increases in demand can no longer be fully met by appropriate increases in supply and ends with a complete loss of the myocardial flow reserve and a reduction in regional MBF at rest, associated with a downregulation of contractile function and adaptation of substrate metabolism. The spectrum could also represent a temporal progression in coronary stenosis severity. Recent findings in chronically instrumented animals with a progressive decline and ultimately loss of regional flow reserve associated with a decrease in resting blood flow support such a scenario.[188–190] On the other hand, reductions in flow may also occur rapidly in view of the high incidence of blood-flow metabolism mismatches in early postinfarction patients.[171,178,191] As acute animal experimental studies have demonstrated, sudden moderate reductions of regional blood flow are initially associated with evidence of acute ischemia—as, for example, release of lactate and enhanced glucose uptake. An apparent "resetting" or "adjustment" of demand occurs thereafter, when lactate release converts to uptake, high-energy phosphate stores are replenished, and a new supply-demand balance seems to have appeared.[183,192,193] Some debate has focused on the issue ofwhether blood flow at rest can indeed be chronically reduced.[194] This was because hibernating myocardium no longer demonstrated the postulated perfusion-contraction match. To some extent, this may be because of the admixture or coexistence of scar tissue or replacement fibrosis but also because of ultrastructural changes of myocytes, including loss of contractile proteins (see below), that is specific neither to repetitive stunning nor to myocardial hibernation. Nevertheless, findings in chronic animal experiments as well as substantial improvements in resting blood flow following surgical revascularization argue in favor of the possibility of a true chronic regional hypoperfusion.[187,189,190,195,196]

## ULTRASTRUCTURAL AND HISTOCHEMICAL OBSERVATIONS

Other attempts to gain mechanistic insights into the enhanced $^{18}$F-deoxyglucose uptake include morphometric and histochemical analyses of biopsy specimens harvested from dysfunctional human myocardium during surgical revascularization. It had already been known from autopsy studies that there existed a general correlation between the degree of myocardial fibrosis and the severity of the impairment of regional contractile function. Yet, there were exceptions.[197] In some instances, dyskinetic myocardium was free of fibrosis on autopsy or, conversely, some normally contracting myocardium contained as much as 40 percent fibrosis.[198] It was also known that "abnormal" myocytes (Fig. 23-16) existed in chronically dysfunctional myocardium.[199] More recent investigations noted correlations between the externally determined relative blood flows and relative $^{18}$F-deoxyglucose concentrations on the one hand and the morphometrically determined fractions of fibrosis, abnormal myocytes, and normal myocardium on the other.[175,200,201] The various studies agree on a general correlation between relative blood flow and the percentage of tissue fibrosis (Fig. 23-17) yet differ in regard to the fraction of "abnormal myocytes." In one study, this fraction is virtually the same in reversibly and irreversibly dysfunctional myocardium,[200] while a second study notes a significantly greater fraction in reversibly than in irreversibly dysfunctional myocardium.[201] Because of centrally located glycogen granules as one of the key features of such "abnormal myocytes" and a statistically significant correlation between the fraction of such abnormal myocytes and the relative $^{18}$F-deoxyglucose uptake, these abnormal myocytes have been thought of as the ultrastructural correlate of the enhanced $^{18}$F-deoxyglucose uptake in chronically dysfunctional myocardium. Other observations argue against such an explanation. Again, electron microscopy and histochemistry of biopsy samples retrieved during surgical bypass grafting from the center of the dysfunctional myocardial wall demonstrate considerable differences

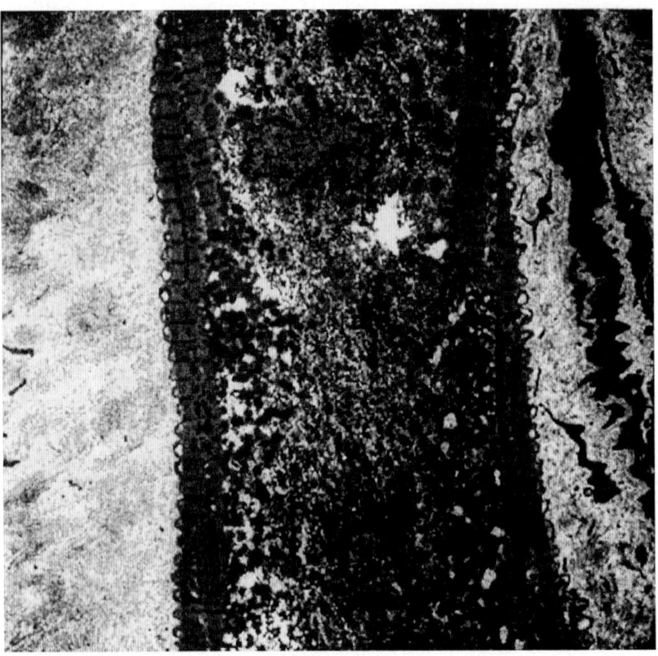

FIGURE 23-16 Abnormal myocyte in chronically dysfunctional human myocardium. Note the irregularly shaped nucleus, the loss of sarcomeres in the center of the myocyte, and the extensive deposition of glycogen. (Courtesy of M. Borgers, Maastricht, The Netherlands.)

in the severity of morphologic alterations in myocardial regions with comparable blood-flow metabolism mismatches.[202] Despite identical flow metabolism findings on PET imaging, nearly half of the patients in this study exhibited minimal if any significant morphologic changes, while the other half demonstrated the structural abnormalities as described above. Such variability of morphologic alterations argues against the "structurally abnormal myocyte" and especially the glycogen granules as an explanation of the enhanced $^{18}$F-deoxyglucose uptake. More likely explanations include (1) translocation and possibly upregulation of the relatively insulin-independent glucose transporter GLUT1[203] as a flux-generating step, (2) uncoupling of glycolysis from glucose oxidation regulated probably by malonyl-CoA and carnitine palmitate transferase I,[204,205] and (3) possibly an ischemia-related loss of adrenergic innervation or function,[206] shown to be associated with increased exogeneous glucose utilization. As recently demonstrated in partially reinnervated cardiac allografts, for example, glucose utilization in denervated myocardium was about 7 percent higher than in reinnervated myocardium.[207]

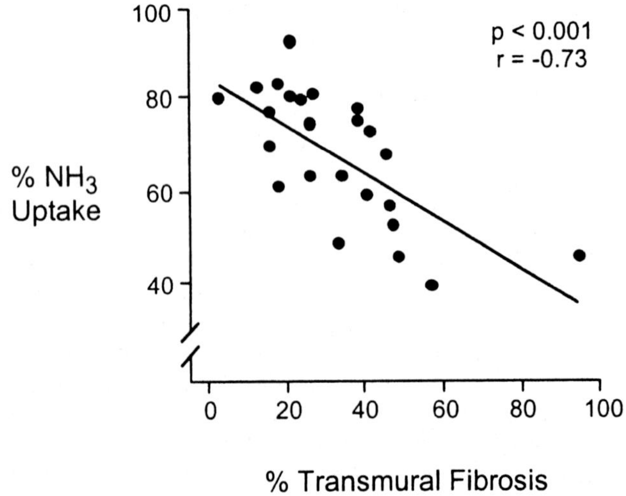


FIGURE 23-17 Inverse correlation between the fractional amount of tissue fibrosis by morphometry and MBF by relative $^{13}$N-ammonia tissue concentration ( percent $NH_3$ uptake). (From Depré at al.,[201] with permission of the American Heart Association.)

***Abnormal Myocytes in Chronically Dysfunctional Myocardium***
Whether "abnormal" myocytes as described initially by Flameng and colleagues[199] and subsequently observed in biopsy material from "mismatched" myocardium are specific for mechanism of contractlie dysfunction or are a more general feature of reversibly impaired contractile function remains uncertain. Two schools of thought exist. One holds that the morphologic alterations result from (1) contractile unloading; (2) increased wall stress (stretch); and (3) a metabolic substrate switch to preferential glucose utilization.[208] In fact, contractile unloading has recently been demonstrated to result in virtually identical structural changes.[209,210] The expression and distribution patterns of other features, as of $\alpha$-smooth muscle actin, cardiotin, and titin[208] as well as the increased expression of GLUT1 mRNA,[203] are features that resemble those seen in embryonic and/or neonatal myocytes and suggest that the changes of abnormal myocytes may represent "dedifferentiation."[208] Histochemical analysis has further uncovered alterations in the extracellular matrix, with increased amounts of collagen and fibronectin surrounding the abnormal myocytes.[208] Finally, like neonatal myocytes, these "abnormal myocytes" have been found to be relatively tolerant of ischemia.[211] The absence of true degenerative changes has further been claimed to support this possibility.

The other school of thought emphasizes a progressive deterioration rather than a stable state of the cell's morphology, and therefore referred to hibernation, as "incomplete adaptation to ischemia."[212] The process begins with few if any structural changes but a switch in substrate selection to glucose, either because of its greater oxygen efficiency or, alternatively, loss of enzymes essential for fatty acid oxidation, followed by loss of contractile protein and accumulation of glycogen and mitochondrial and nuclear alterations, ultimately leading to cell death and scar tissue formation.[202] Other studies again report reduced expression of contractile and cytoskeletal proteins associated with increased expression of extracellular matrix proteins,[212] implying a progressive loss of contractile protein and of the cell structure that is paralleled by accelerated formation of tissue fibrosis and hence a progressive loss of viability, which was further found to be associated with apoptosis and replacement fibrosis. Clinical observations lend further support to such a downhill course. Biopsies from patients with preoperatively viable myocardium but without a postrevascularization improvement in contractile function demonstrated an about threefold increase in mRNA of caspase-3, a promoter of apoptosis, together with an about 50 percent reduction in the expression of the antideath genes *Bcl-2* and *p53,* again consistent with continued cell death and replacement fibrosis.[213] Chronic animal experimental studies similarly have demonstrated significant increases in apoptotic myocytes in hibernating myocardium with reduced resting blood flow and critically reduced or absent flow reserve.[189] The fact that myocyte apoptosis in these studies occurred scattered and not in clusters raises the question of whether apoptosis is indeed the endpoint of the progressively deteriorating abnormal myocyte or whether such apoptosis represents a process that occurs in parallel. To some extent this may depend on the duration and severity of the ischemic compromise. For instance, other animal studies with more sudden reductions in flow and shorter time periods report higher rates of myocyte apoptosis occurring in clusters.[214]

A progressive deterioration of reversibly dysfunctional myocardium is also consistent with clinical observations (Fig. 23-18). Studies point to the high prevalence of mismatch patterns in patients with prior myocardial infarctions[171,215] but note a declining incidence of blood-flow metabolism mismatches as a function of time after an acute myocardial infarction.[191] Moreover, the potential for an improvement in global LV function is lost if revascularization is delayed by more than 6 months.[216] Finally, the increase in tissue fibrosis and lack of functional recovery after revascularization as a function of the duration of clinical symptoms[217] all seem all to support such progression and raise the question whether a new supply-demand balance rest at a lower level can in fact be sustained permanently. If not, then the blood-flow metabolism mismatch represents a transient rather than a permanent state of reversibly dysfunctional myocardium. The divergent opinions may also stem from the possibility that reversibility can be maintained up to a certain degree of functional alterations. Once this critical point has been reached, myocytes become committed to irreversibility and cell death.

In the clinical setting, prompt restoration of adequate tissue perfusion through interventional revascularization will therefore be essential, regardless whether abnormal myocytes represent "dedifferentiation" or "degeneration." As it remains uncertain at what stage the structural alterations become irreversible, it would seem that

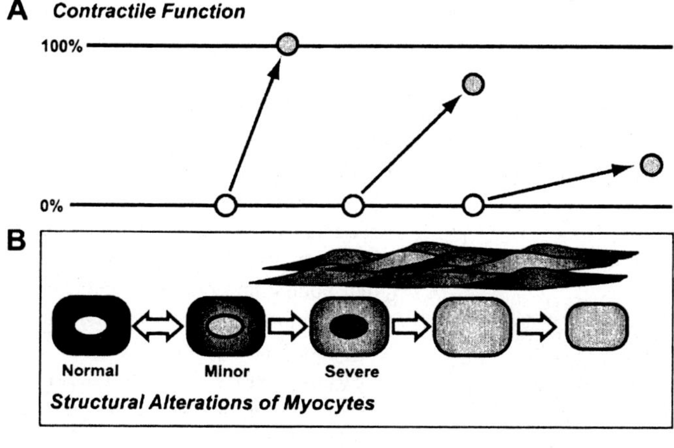


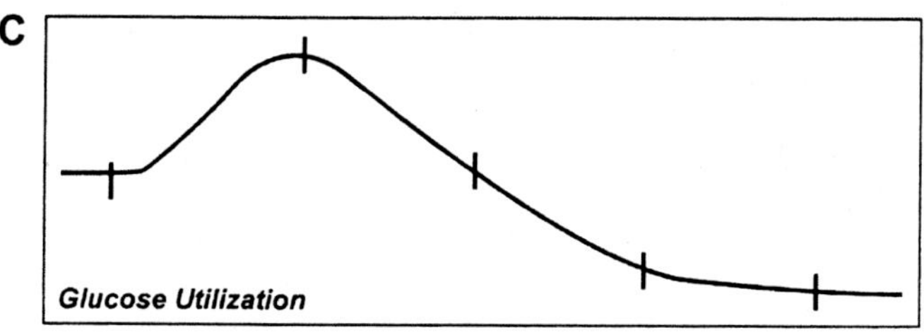


FIGURE 23-18 *A* to *C*. Schematic representation of the progressive deterioration of structure and function in dysfunctional myocardium. *B*. Progressive loss of myocytes with increasing amounts of tissue fibrosis. *C*. This is associated initially with a marked increase in $^{18}$F-deoxyglucose uptake, especially when structural alterations of the myocytes are still mild, followed by a progressive decrease and finally absence of $^{18}$F-deoxyglucose uptake. The upper panel (*A*) depicts the recovery of contractile function (in both total amount and rate of recovery) for revascularization performed at each stage. When only minor structured alterations are present, function presumably recovers completely and rapidly as compared with the right. The amount of functional recovery will be only small and delayed when extensive structural alterations are present.

ultimately the return of contractile function will depend upon the amount of connective tissue. Once fibrosis and scar tissue occupy more than 35 to 40 percent of the myocardium, dysfunction has been shown to be irreversible.[8,9] As another clinical implication, the presence of structural changes in viable myocardium, as demonstrated with blood-flow metabolism imaging, implies that if the contractile machinery in "abnormal" or "dedifferentiated" myocytes can be reconstructed, the recovery of contractile function will not be immediate but slow, as animal experimental[218] and clinical investigations have indeed demonstrated.[219,220] As observed clinically, rates and completeness of recovery of contractile function are related to regional MBF at baseline.[221,222] Diminished perfusion at baseline was associated with slow and incomplete recovery and thus may reflect more severe structural abnormalities, including alterations of myocytes and of extracellular tissue. The delay in cell repair may also explain the persistence of increased $^{18}$F-deoxyglucose uptake after successful revascularization.[223]

## VIABILITY ASSESSMENT IN THE CLINICAL SETTING

The classic and now most widely applied approach entails evaluation of the relative distribution of blood flow and of exogenous glucose utilization with $^{18}$F-deoxyglucose with dedicated PET systems. Initial studies uncovered three distinct patterns:

- Normal blood flow and normal or enhanced glucose uptake;
- Reduced blood flow but normal and glucose uptake in excess of blood flow ("mismatch")
- Reduced blood flow and proportionately reduced glucose uptake ("match")[172]

While the above listed terms are purely operational, they imply, at least to some extent, the underlying pathophysiology accounting for the contractile dysfunction. Normal flow and/or metabolism might represent "stunned," while the classic "mismatch" might be consistent with "hibernating" myocardium. Both patterns predict a postrevascularization improvement in contractile function whereas the concordant reduction blood flow and metabolism predicts that function will not improve.[172,224,225] It should be emphasized that the reduction in regional flow for both matches and mismatches may vary considerably between patients. Modest concordant reductions in both blood flow and $^{18}$F-deoxyglucose uptake would indicate a prior nontransmural infarction as compared to a more severe reduction or even absence of both in transmural infarctions. Also, flow reductions in mismatches may vary considerably as a reflection of varying degrees of transmural involvement.

The observed correlations between tissue fibrosis and relative flow tracer uptake indicate that regional MBF can serve as a measure of reversible contractile dysfunction.[201] Severe reductions to less than 25 percent of normal or complete absence of blood flow reflect complete or nearly complete transmural scar tissue formation and hence nonreversibility.[226] According to another study, flow reductions of more than 60 percent were highly accurate in predicting nonreversibility of contractile dysfunction.[227] Conversely, normal or only mildly reduced (<20 percent) flow in dysfunctional myocardium argues against the presence of significant amounts of tissue fibrosis; it possibly reflects myocardial stunning and thus indicates functional reversibility.[221,222] Intermediate flow reductions are less reliable discriminators; for example, a nontransmural infarction may result in a mild flow reduction; if the remainder of the myocardial wall consists of normal myocardium, then revascularization is unlikely to improve contractile function. If combined with a metabolic study, the $^{18}$F-deoxyglucose uptake in this case would be reduced in proportion to blood flow.[228] Conversely, an increase in glucose uptake would indicate the coexistence of reversibly dysfunctional myocardium with scar tissue and predict an improvement in contractile function.

Another, again limited approach for identifying reversible contractile dysfunction is the use of $^{18}$F-deoxyglucose alone. This approach derives from comparative studies with gated MRI and PET and assumes that regional reductions in $^{18}$F-deoxyglucose greater than 50 percent relative to remote myocardium represent irreversible contractile function, whereas mildly reduced or normal uptake indicates the presence of reversible dysfunction.[229,230] While used for some time as a benchmark or measure for defining the accuracy of $^{201}$Tl-based techniques for assessing myocardial viability,[229] only recent studies have tested the validity of this particular approach against the postrevascularization outcome in regional contractile function.[231] ECG-gated image acquisition affords simultaneous evaluation of regional function and metabolism and thus can further augment the predictive accuracy of the $^{18}$F-deoxyglucose stand-alone approach.[232,233] The utility of measurements of exogenous glucose utilization in absolute units has also been explored. A threshold value of 0.25 $\mu$mol · min$^{-1}$ · g$^{-1}$ yielded a 93 percent positive and a 95 percent negative predictive accuracy for the improvement of contractile dysfunction.[234] Nevertheless, limitations with this approach remain, especially when glucose utilization and, hence, $^{18}$F-deoxyglucose uptake cannot be sufficiently controlled. Because of this, another study pointed out the limited value of quantitative glucose uptake measurements for identifying myocardial viability.[235] Further, use of $^{18}$F-deoxyglucose alone may prove unreliable for identifying normal myocardium. $^{18}$F-deoxyglucose uptake may be markedly diminished or even absent when myocardium preferentially utilizes free fatty acid, so that normal myocardium will be difficult to distinguish from scar tissue. However, scar tissue can readily be identified and distinguished from scar tissue by evaluating the distribution of regional MBF.[236]

A clinically more difficult issue is the pattern of normal regional blood flow and glucose metabolism associated with mild to severe hypokinesis in severely dysfunctional left ventricles. One study reports that of 32 such myocardial regions, only 8, or 25 percent, improved following surgical revascularization.[237] Such regions may therefore represent remodeled LV myocardium. On the other hand, a postrevascularization improvement in wall motion may have been consistent with prior myocardial stunning. If this is suspected, careful evaluation of the coronary anatomy, or, if unavailable, the addition of a pharmacologic stress study can aid in distinguishing between stunned and remodeled LV myocardium.

## ALTERNATE APPROACHES TO BLOOD-FLOW AND GLUCOSE METABOLISM IMAGING

Several institutions successfully use SPECT myocardial perfusion imaging with either $^{201}$Tl or $^{99m}$Tc-sestamibi and metabolic imaging with $^{18}$F-deoxyglucose with dedicated PET systems (Fig. 23-19). These institutions report predictive accuracies for changes in segmental and global LV function that approach those obtained with dedicated PET systems.[2] Nevertheless, such combined PET/SPECT approaches present at times with diagnostic limitations, especially because of considerable differences in contrast and spatial resolutions as well as artifactual reductions in tracer concentrations due to photon attenuation.[5,6] This, then, can limit the ability to accurately estimate the extent of a blood-flow metabolism mismatch which, as discussed below, may be useful for predicting the magnitude of changes in global LV function and symptoms related to congestive heart failure. Other approaches rely solely on the use of multipurpose SPECT-like systems, equipped with ultrahigh photon energy general purpose collimators. Studies with SPECT $^{201}$Tl- or $^{99m}$Tc-labeled flow tracers and with SPECT $^{18}$F-deoxyglucose imaging report predictive accuracies comparable to those reported with dedicated PET systems.[238,239]

Further, $^{201}$Tl rest-redistribution imaging has been useful for identifying myocardial viability and for predicting the postsurgical outcome of ischemic cardiomyopathy, although with a somewhat lower predictive accuracy. While the concept of $^{201}$Tl redistribution for evaluation of blood flow and the myocardial potassium pool as an indicator of cell membrane integrity is clearly a scientifically sound one, it suffers from instrumentation-related shortcomings, especially in patients with poor LV function and consequently poor signal-to-noise ratios. $^{201}$Tl offers a negative signal (reduced tracer uptake) as compared to $^{18}$F-deoxyglucose with a positive signal (enhanced tracer uptake), which is more readily accessible to visual analysis.[236] Consistent with this are findings in patients with severely depressed LV function. One study, for example, reports that $^{18}$F-deoxyglucose and PET identified myocardial viability in 18 of 20 patients with an average ejection fraction of 23 percent and only fixed $^{201}$Tl defects on SPECT,[240] which is similar to a more recent report of viability by $^{18}$F-deoxyglucose in 17 of 33 patients (LVEF <35 percent) with fixed or minimally redistributing $^{201}$Tl defects.[241] Further, in a comparison study of $^{201}$Tl and

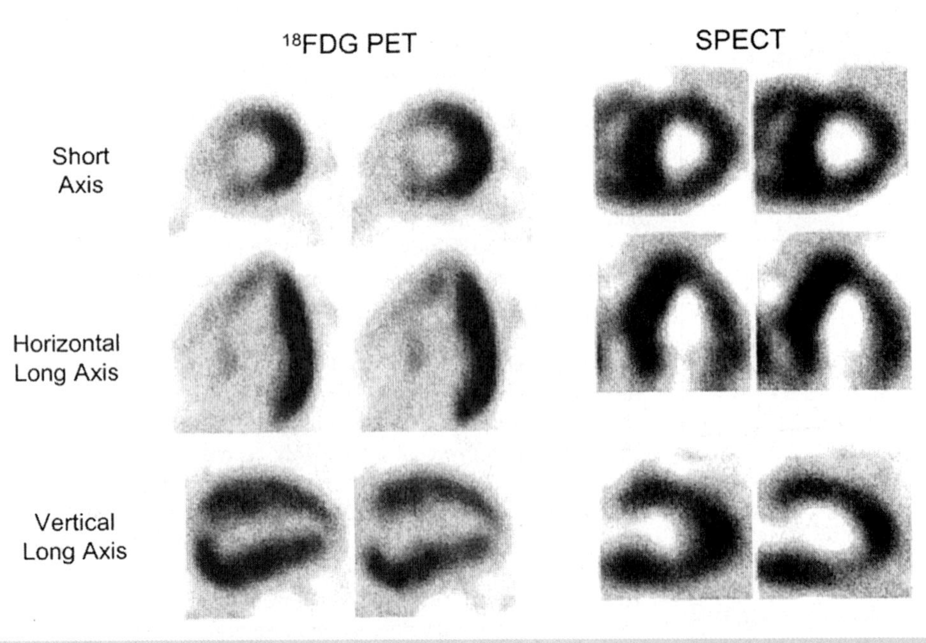


FIGURE 23-19 Myocardial perfusion imaging with SPECT (*right panel*) combined with metabolism imaging with PET (*left panel*). The $^{18}$F-deoxyglucose images demonstrate enhanced tracer accumulation in the lateral, anterolateral, and inferolateral wall, while tracer uptake is low in the interventricular septum. The SPECT perfusion images identify perfusion in the septum to be normal, while the moderate reduction in perfusion in the lateral wall is associated with the marked $^{18}$F-deoxyglucose uptake.

$^{18}$F-deoxyglucose SPECT, there was generally an excellent agreement between both approaches.[242] However, disparities occurred in patients with severely depressed LV function, where $^{18}$F-deoxyglucose revealed more viable myocardial segments than $^{201}$Tl SPECT.

In synthesizing the currently available information, it appears that ultimately the total fraction of scar tissue in a given myocardial segment determines largely whether or not contractile function will improve. Because of the linear correlation between scar tissue and relative blood-flow,[175,200,201] evaluation or even quantitation of regional blood flow offers information on potential reversibility. On the other hand, if, in viable though functionally compromised myocardium, blood flow is also reduced, then the augmented glucose utilization as evidenced by the enhanced $^{18}$F-deoxyglucose uptake offers additional and critical information. This has prompted some investigators to predict the ultimate functional outcome from a combined assessment of blood flow and $^{18}$F-deoxyglucose uptake.[243,244] Further, the temporal recovery of contractile function after revascularization appears to depend on the degree of ultrastructural changes of myocytes as well as the fractional distribution between myocytes with only mild and with severe ultrastructural changes.[244] If, as postulated, only mild structural changes are associated with a full functional recovery within 3 months, more severe structural changes may require substantially longer time periods and, further, may account for the persistence of increased $^{18}$F-deoxyglucose uptake even for many months following revascularization.[223]

## CLINICAL ROLE OF PET VIABILITY ASSESSMENT

Conclusions reached from a metanalysis of 24 clinical investigations, including 3088 patients with CAD, reduced LV ejection fraction (average 32 ± 8 percent), and congestive heart failure systems [average New York Heart Association (NYHA) functional class 2.8], highlight the importance of myocardial viability.[245] All patients had been examined for the presence of viable myocardium, using either low-dose dobutamine stress (8 investigations), $^{201}$Tl rest-redistribution scintigraphy (6 investigations), or blood-flow metabolism imaging with $^{18}$F-deoxyglucose (11 investigations). During the 25 ± 10 months follow-up period, 375 cardiac deaths occurred. Grouping of patients by presence or absence of myocardial viability and further by treatment (medically and revascularization) revealed significant intergroup differences in cardiac mortality. Patients without myocardial viability revealed an annual mortality rate of 6.2 percent on medical treatment as compared to 7.7 percent ($p = 0.23$, not significant) when treated by revascularization. Importantly, the annual mortality for patients with myocardial viability was 16 percent on medical treatment but only 3.2 percent when treated surgically ($p < 0.0001$). While these findings need to be interpreted with caution, given the retrospective nature of the investigations and possible interstudy differences in patient selection and diagnosis of viability, they nevertheless suggest that the search for viable myocardium can identify patients at an especially high risk of cardiac death and, further, that such risk can be substantially modified by means of revascularization. Thus, in addition to identifying patients with ischemic cardiomyopathy who are likely to benefit most from therapeutic revascularization, the assessment of myocardial viability might also provide prospective information on other clinically relevant questions, including the amount of viable myocardium or the extent of scar tissue needed for a postrevascularization change in LV function and possibly congestive heart failure–related symptoms as well as an assessment of the risk-benefit ratio of the surgical procedure. Finally, the assessment of myocardial viability may also aid in identifying the leading cause of poor LV function and thus distinguish between an intrinsic myopathic process and CAD.

## ISCHEMIC VERSUS IDIOPATHIC DILATED CARDIOMYOPATHY

In addition to heart failure symptoms, ischemic cardiomyopathy shares several other features with idiopathic dilated cardiomyopathy—such as, for example, the LV enlargement, frequently diffuse hypokinesis, low LV ejection fraction, and, frequently, mitral regurgitation. Biventricular enlargement has been thought of as a feature characteristic of idiopathic dilated cardiomyopathy but can also be present in ischemic cardiomyopathy. Conduction abnormalities often limit the accuracy of ECG criteria to distinguish between both entities. Additionally, an intrinsic myopathic process including LV remodeling may also exist in patients with CAD, so that the leading cause of the poor LV function may remain unknown or difficult to elucidate. Importantly, however, the therapeutic approach to both disease entities will strikingly differ.

Both disease entities reveal remarkably different patterns of blood flow and substrate metabolism on PET. A comparison study in patients with ischemic cardiomyopathy and with idiopathic dilated cardiomyopathy found the distribution of MBF to be characteristically homogeneous in idiopathic cardiomyopathy as compared to distinct flow reductions clearly corresponding in ischemic cardiomyopathy to the coronary vascular territories.[246] Similarly, uptake of $^{18}$F-deoxyglucose was noted to be homogeneous in dilated cardiomyopathy, while matches and/or mismatches between blood flow and $^{18}$F-deoxyglucose uptake were present in ischemic cardiomyopathy (Fig. 23-20). Combined imaging of blood flow and glucose metabolism distinguished with an overall accuracy of 85 percent between both disease entities. This value exceeded the diagnostic accuracy of ECG criteria, regional wall motion abnormalities, and right ventricular enlargement.

## PREDICTION OF THE OUTCOME IN GLOBAL LEFT VENTRICULAR FUNCTION

Numerous clinical investigations report the high accuracy of $^{18}$F-deoxyglucose imaging with PET in predicting postrevascularization outcome in regional LV wall motion.[2,172,224,225,230,231,247–249] Even though some of these investigations employed permutations of the

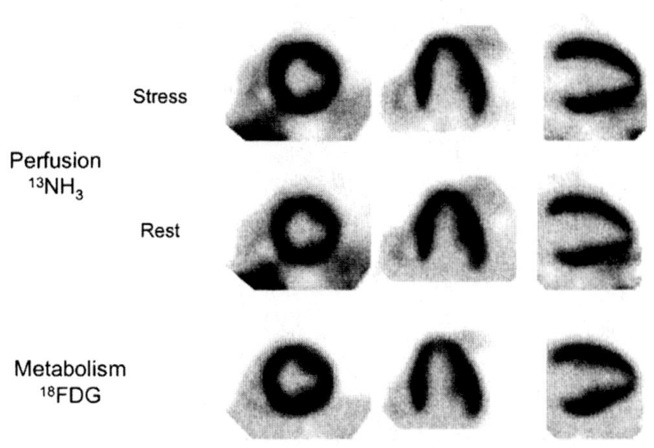


FIGURE 23-20 Perfusion and metabolism imaging in idiopathic dilated cardiomyopathy. Short axis and vertical and horizontal long-axis slices of myocardial perfusion during stress and at rest obtained with $^{13}$N ammonia and of metabolism obtained with $^{18}$F-deoxyglucose are shown. Note moderate enlargement of the left ventricular chamber. Importantly, perfusion is homogenous at rest and remains homogenous during exercise. Similarly, there is homogenous uptake of $^{18}$F-deoxyglucose.

initially described blood-flow metabolism approach or relied only on the evaluation of regional $^{18}$F-deoxyglucose uptake in dysfunctional myocardium,[230,231] the predictive accuracy, both positive and negative, remained high. Such studies examining contractile function in myocardial regions have been important because they prove the concept of patterns of blood-flow metabolism as accurate predictors of the outcome of regional wall motion after restoration of MBF. More relevant in the clinical setting is, however, whether patterns of blood-flow metabolism can predict the postrevascularization outcome in global LV function.

Initial semiquantitative studies demonstrated some correlation between the extent of the blood-flow metabolism mismatch and the postrevascularization gain in LV ejection fraction.[172] Patients with blood-flow metabolism mismatches that occupied at least two or more of a total of seven myocardial segments revealed a statistically significant increase in the LV ejection fraction following coronary artery bypass grafting.[172] No such improvement was observed in patients with only one mismatch segment or in patients with only matches. Subsequent studies confirmed these initial observations and reported significant gains in LV function in patients with blood-flow metabolism mismatches as compared to no improvement in those patients without metabolic evidence of viability.[2,3,195,200–202,216,223,225,237,239,241,250–257] Several investigations report statistically significant correlations between the percentage of the LV with a blood-flow metabolism mismatch and the postrevascularization increase in the LV ejection fraction. This, then, implies that the extent of a blood-flow metabolism mismatch has value in predicting the postsurgical gain in global LV performance (Fig. 23-21).[237,255,258] A mismatch of at least 20 to 25 percent of the LV myocardium appears necessary for achieving a significant postrevascularization gain in LV ejection fraction (≥5 percent).

One series of investigations fails to report a significant postrevascularization improvement in the LV ejection fraction at rest, despite the presence of "blood-flow metabolism mismatches." It appears, however, that this difference is related to the laboratory-unique image and analysis approach.[223,248] MBF is evaluated with $^{82}$Rb at rest and during pharmacologic stress. The distribution of MBF during stress is compared to the myocardial glucose uptake at rest. The approach therefore identifies both stress-induced ischemia and "viable myocardium" at rest. Hence, blood flow and, possibly, wall motion at rest may be normal in some patients, so that revascularization predominately improves the capacity of the LV to respond to exercise more appropriately[248,259] and thus to improve quality of life even though no significant correlations between mismatch size and changes in congestive heart failure (CHF) functional class were observed.[258,260]

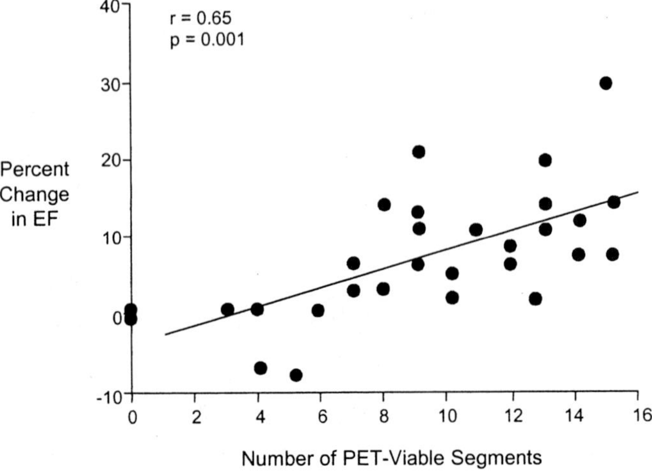


FIGURE 23-21 Postrevascularization improvement in LVEF as a function of the number of viable myocardial segments as determined by PET. (From Pagano et al.,[255] with permission.)

The magnitude of an improvement in LV function following surgical revascularization depends further on the fraction of irreversibly injured myocardium or scar tissue. In evaluating the outcome of LV function following coronary artery bypass grafting in 82 patients with an LV ejection fraction of <35 percent, the fraction of scar as identified at baseline by PET $^{18}$F-deoxyglucose and by PET $^{13}$N-ammonia or SPECT $^{99m}$tetrofosmin rest perfusion imaging was found to be an independent predictor of a change in the LV ejection fraction.[261] Other predictors included time from PET to revascularization and diabetes, which raises the intriguing question of the extent to which diabetes itself influenced the perfusion metabolism pattern. A mismatch between MBF and metabolism was also found to be predictive, but only after adjustments were made for differences in the approach to myocardial perfusion imaging (by PET and by SPECT).

The improvement in regional and especially global LV function may not occur immediately but rather occurs slowly though progressively following revascularization. In a highly selected patient group, blood flow had been shown to recover promptly following revascularization by angioplasty, while contractile function remained initially unchanged.[219] On reexamination 67 ± 19 days later, no further improvements in regional blood flow were noted, while systolic wall motion had now significantly improved. Clinical observations suggest a correlation between severity of the mismatch and the rate and completeness of recovery of contractile function. Wall motion recovered faster and more completely in segments with normal blood flow as compared to segments with reduced flow and, possibly, more severe structural alterations.[221,222] For example, 13.4 and 27.2 percent of severely dysfunctional myocardial regions but with normal blood flow at rest were found to have fully restored function at 14 weeks and at more than 1 year, respectively. In contrast, corresponding full recovery rates were only 2.6 and 13.2 percent for myocardial regions with reduced blood flow at baseline. The slow recovery of contractile function may be related to rebuilding of the contractile machinery, as suggested by observations indicating that contractile function appears to recover or improve more promptly in myocardial regions without marked ultrastructural abnormalities or with a lesser fraction of "abnormal" myocytes.[244] Finally, in addition to a slow recovery of contractile function in reversibly dysfunctional myocardium, other studies describe an associated decline in end-diastolic and end-systolic volumes suggesting the possibility of a reversal of LV remodeling.[262]

## EFFECT ON CONGESTIVE HEART FAILURE–RELATED SYMPTOMS

A related question is whether such functional improvement is also associated with relief or amelioration of CHF symptoms. Several retrospective studies do in fact indicate such possible symptomatic improvement. For example, two investigations concluded that patients with blood-flow metabolism mismatches undergoing surgical revascularization demonstrated a significantly higher incidence of improvement in functional class (NYHA CHF class) as compared to patients without mismatches or with matches but not submitted to revascularization.[263,264] Among the 52 patients with mismatches and CHF class III or IV, 81 percent of the 26 patients undergoing revas-

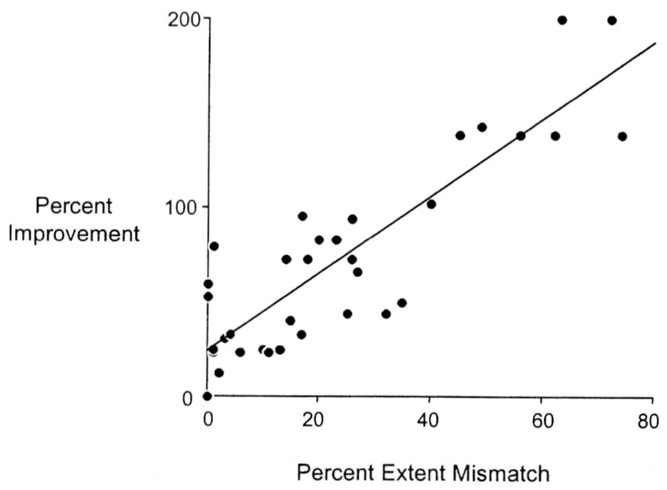


FIGURE 23-22 Correlation between the presurgical extent of a blood-flow metabolism mismatch and postsurgical improvement in the ability to perform physical work as defined on a specific activity scale (SAS) and expressed in percent movement of metabolic units (METS). (From Di Carli et al.,[276] with permission.)

cularization revealed a significant improvement in CHF class (by at least one class) as compared to only 23 percent of 26 patients treated conservatively.[264]

The amount of viable myocardium as determined through blood flow and $^{18}$F-deoxyglucose imaging with PET appears to contain information on the magnitude of the postrevascularization improvement in CHF symptoms.[265] The level of physical activity that patients were able to perform prior to and 24 ± 14 months following coronary artery bypass grafting was graded on a specific activity scale and expressed in metabolic equivalents.[266] Among the 36 patients in this study with an average LV ejection fraction of only 28 ± 6 percent prior to revascularization, the extent of the blood-flow metabolism mismatch ranged from 0 to 74 percent (mean 23 ± 22 percent) on polar map analysis. When patients were grouped according to the extent of the mismatch, 11 patients with a mismatch occupying less than 5 percent of the LV myocardium revealed a statistically significant but only mild improvement in functional status (34 percent increase in metabolic equivalents). Intermediate-size mismatches (5 to 17 percent) in 8 patients were associated with a 42 percent increase in metabolic equivalents whereas large mismatches, that is greater than 18 percent, in 17 patients were followed after revascularization by an average increase of 107 percent in metabolic equivalents. Furthermore, as seen in Fig. 23-22, there was a statistically significant correlation between the improvement in functional status and the anatomic extent of the blood-flow metabolism mismatch. Last, blood-flow metabolism mismatches equal to or greater than 18 percent were 70 percent sensitive and 78 percent specific in predicting an improvement in physical activity or functional status following successful surgical revascularization.

## IMPACT ON LONG-TERM SURVIVAL

Several studies examined the long-term fate of patients after being evaluated for MBF and metabolism with PET.[257,263,264,267–270] These studies presented compelling evidence for the notion of an increased incidence of cardiac events in patients with blood-flow metabolism mismatches and on medical treatment. They also implied that revascularization of blood-flow metabolism mismatches might avert future nonfatal and fatal cardiac events.

Despite this general agreement, important differences emerged from these studies. One study in 129 chronic CAD patients followed clinically for an average time period of 17 ± 19 months found the presence of mismatches in the absence of revascularization to be independent predictors of the 17 nonfatal ischemic events.[269] Nevertheless, the LV ejection fraction and the patient's age contained the highest predictive values for the 13 cardiac deaths in this patient group. Given a wide range of functional compromise in the patients of this study, the high predictive value of the ejection fraction does not surprise. In patient series with more homogeneously depressed LV function, the predictive value of a low ejection fraction applied equally to all groups. This then affords an analysis of other factors as prognosticators of cardiac mortality. As shown in Fig. 23-23, the cumulative long-term survival was lowest in the patient subgroup with blood-flow metabolism mismatches who were on medical treatment. Of note, all four subgroups were similar in regards to age, clinical and hemodynamic findings. There were no significant intergroup differences in LV ejection fraction, which for the entire patient group averaged 25 ± 7 percent. Of note, patients with mismatches submitted to revascularization demonstrated higher cumulative survival, which was similar to that in the groups without mismatches. Further, LV ejection fraction was without significant predictive value, while by Cox model analysis, the extent of a mismatch had a significant negative effect on survival ($p < 0.02$) and revascularization of mismatch patients a significant positive effect on survival ($p < 0.04$).[264] While submitted to a less rigorous statistical analysis, a second study in patients with a similar uniform depression of LV ejection fractions reached similar conclusions.[263] Among the patient groups with and without mismatches, the subgroup of patients with mismatches demonstrated a 33 percent incidence of cardiac death during the 12-month follow-up period as compared to an only 4 percent mortality in patients with mismatches undergoing revascularization.

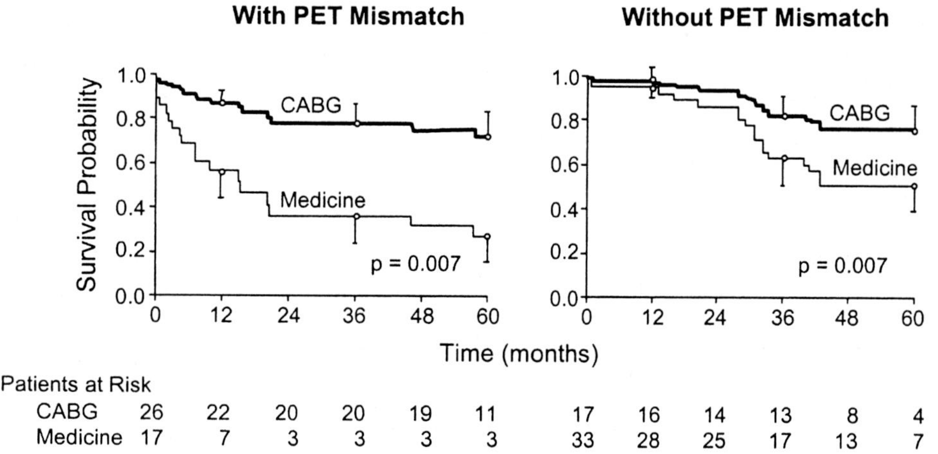


FIGURE 23-23 Estimated survival probabilities by Kaplan-Meyer analysis for patients with LV function treated medically (*medicine*) and with surgical revascularization (*CABG*) based on the absence or presence of viability as determined by PET blood flow-metabolism imaging. (From Di Carli et al.,[270] with permission.)

## ASSESSMENT OF PERIOPERATIVE RISK

Critical for planning surgical revascularization of patients with ischemic cardiomyopathy is the high perioperative mortality and morbidity. This then raises the question whether imaging of blood flow and glucose metabolism with PET can contribute to predicting the surgical risk. Two investigations have explored the contribution of PET to the surgical risk assessment.[253,271] Both studies include a total of 317 patients with ischemic cardiomyopathy and LV ejection fractions of less than 35 percent. The patients were categorized into two groups. Patients in group 1 (35 and 88 patients, respectively, in each study) underwent coronary artery bypass grafting based on standard clinical criteria including LV size or ejection fraction, suitability of the coronary anatomy for surgical revascularization, and presence of comorbidities. The same criteria were applied also to patients in the second group (41 and 153 patients per study), which in addition underwent blood-flow metabolism imaging with PET. Of 41 patients, 34 (83 percent) in one and 110 of 153 patients (72 percent) in the other group demonstrated evidence of reversibly dysfunctional myocardium involving at least 20 to 30 percent of the LV and subsequently underwent bypass grafting. Both studies report lower perioperative mortalities in patients studied with PET imaging (30-day mortalities of 0 and 0.9 percent) as compared to mortalities of 11.4 and 19.8 percent in patients not evaluated by PET. Further, 1-year cardiac mortalities were lower for patients evaluated with PET (3 and 10 percent, respectively) as compared to patients without PET (21 and 30 percent, respectively). Patients with PET-demonstrated viability required less inotropic support or intraaortic balloon pumping; they had better cardiac output and shorter intensive care unit stays. While these reports include relatively few patients or are retrospective, further confirmation of such short-term benefits seems warranted. If confirmed, PET evaluations of patients with ischemic cardiomyopathies would then offer important and possibly critical prognostic information on the immediate and long-term risks of cardiovascular surgery in patients with severe ischemic cardiomyopathy.

In summary, these observations imply that the presence of blood-flow metabolism mismatches identifies patients who are at high risk for a nonfatal cardiac event and, in instances of severely depressed LV function, for sudden cardiac death. The observations further suggest that revascularization may significantly lower the cardiac risk and improve long-term survival. If large enough, a mismatch further contains predictive information on the postrevascularization improvement in CHF-related symptoms and, further, on the outcome in global LV function. Blood-flow metabolism imaging therefore can decisively impact the risk-benefit ratio of surgical revascularization and thus more generally affect therapeutic strategies. The absence of viability can affirm the decision to proceed with medical management or cardiac transplantation. Conversely, in the presence of large amounts of viable myocardium, interventional revascularization represents a true and effective alternative. In fact, the prevalence of significant amounts of reversibly dysfunctional myocardium is substantial. A survey of 283 patients with ischemic cardiomyopathy revealed a 55 percent prevalence of blood flow and glucose metabolism mismatches.[272] Half of these mismatches involved 25 percent or more of the LV myocardium and thus would lead to significant gains in LV function and clinical symptoms after revascularization. The remainder of mismatches were smaller but, if not revascularized, might be associated with an increased long-term cardiac morbidity and mortality. Indeed, in the setting of ischemic cardiomyopathy, inclusion of PET in the diagnostic algorithm can be cost-effective and, at the same time, cost-saving.[273,274] Clinical criteria for deciding on coronary artery bypass grafting in patients with ischemic cardiomyopathy have already been developed.[275] In addition to the diastolic dimension, the LV ejection fraction, and suitable target vessels, the criteria include the presence of viable myocardium affecting at least 15 to 20 percent of the LV myocardium.

## SUMMARY AND CONCLUSIONS

Imaging with positron-emitting tracers has provided novel and important information on the cardiovascular physiology and, specifically, on functional alterations of the human coronary circulation associated with evolving or established CAD as well as on consequences of severe and end-stage CAD, especially in patients with ischemic cardiomyopathy. Observations with PET have raised numerous mechanistic questions in regard to "hibernation" and "stunning." At the same time, assessment of these entities in the clinical setting with radiotracers of blood flow and of glucose metabolism has emerged as a "gold standard" for determining myocardial viability. Other radiotracers again have remained investigational and await future clinical applications. Importantly, instrumentation-related developments and wider availability of radiotracers of metabolism have rapidly expanded the clinical availability of positron-emitting radiotracers for imaging. This, in turn, has resulted in a rapid dissemination of this new technology into the clinical setting. While the now more widespread use of positron imaging focuses mostly on diagnostic and management issues in oncology, it is likely to be associated with a greater use for cardiovascular diseases in the clinical setting.

## ACKNOWLEDGMENTS

This work was supported in part by the Laboratory of Structural Biology & Molecular Medicine, which is operated for the U.S. Department of Energy by the University of California under Contract #DE-AC03-76-SF00012. This work was also supported in part by the Director of the Office of Energy Research, Office of Health and Environmental Research, Washington D.C.; by Research Grants #HL 29845 and #HL 33177, National Institutes of Health, Bethesda, MD; and by an Investigative Group Award by the Greater Los Angeles Affiliate of the American Heart Association, Los Angeles, CA. The authors thank Jane Espitia for her assistance in preparing this manuscript and Luke Deltricci for preparing the figures.

## References

1. Altehoefer C, Kaiser H-J, Dörr R, et al. Fluorine-18 deoxyglucose PET for assessment of viable myocardium in perfusion defects in 99mTc-MIBI SPET: A comparative study in patients with coronary artery disease. *Eur J Nucl Med* 1992;19:334–342.
2. Lucignani G, Paolini G, Landoni C, et al. Presurgical identification of hibernating myocardium by combined use of technetium-99m hexakis 2-methoxyisobutylisonitrile single photon emission tomography and fluorine-18 fluoro-2-deoxy-D-glucose positron emission tomography in patients with coronary artery disease. *Eur J Nucl Med* 1992;19:874–881.
3. vom Dahl J, Eitzman D, Al-Aouar A, et al. Relation of regional function, perfusion, and metabolism in patients with advanced coronary artery disease undergoing surgical revascularization. *Circulation* 1994;90:2356–2366.
4. Bax JJ, Visser FC, Poldermans D, et al. Prognostic value of perfusion-FDG mismatch in ischemic cardiomyopathy. *J Nucl Cardiol* 2002;9:675–677.
5. Sawada S, Allman K, Muzik O, et al. Positron emission tomography detects evidence of viability in rest technetium-99m sestamibi defects. *J Am Coll Cardiol* 1994;23:92–98.

6. Sand NP, Böttcher M, Madsen MM, et al. Evaluation of regional myocardial perfusion in patients with severe left ventricular dysfunction: Comparison of 13N-ammonia PET and 99mTc sestamibi SPECT. *J Nucl Cardiol* 1998;5:4–13.
7. Iida H, Rhodes C, de Silva R, et al. Myocardial tissue fraction—Correction for partial volume effects and measure of tissue viability. *J Nucl Med* 1991;32:2169–2175.
8. de Silva R, Yamamoto Y, Rhodes CG, et al. Preoperative prediction of the outcome of coronary revascularization using positron emission tomography. *Circulation* 1992;86:1738–1742.
9. Yamamoto Y, De Silva R, Rhodes C, et al. A new strategy for the assessment of viable myocardium and regional myocardial blood flow using $^{15}$O-water and dynamic positron emission tomography. *Circulation* 1992;86:167–178.
10. Iida H, Tamura Y, Kitamura K, et al. Histochemical correlates of (15)O-water-perfusable tissue fraction in experimental canine studies of old myocardial infarction. *J Nucl Med* 2000;41:1737–1745.
11. Kim RJ, Wu E, Rafael A, et al. The use of contrast-enhanced magnetic resonance imaging to identify reversible myocardial dysfunction. *N Engl J Med* 2000;343:1445–1453.
12. Wagner A, Mahrholdt H, Holly TA, et al. Contrast-enhanced MRI and routine single photon emission computed tomography (SPECT) perfusion imaging for detection of subendocardial myocardial infarcts: an imaging study. *Lancet* 2003;361:374–379.
13. Bax JJ, Fath-Ordoubadi F, Wijns W, Camici PG. Water-perfusable tissue fraction for the assessment of myocardial viability: Comparison with F18-Fluorodeoxyglucose. *Circulation* 1999;100:(suppl I):I-865.
14. Marinho N, Keogh B, Costa D, et al. Pathophysiology of chronic left ventricular dysfunction. *Circulation* 1996;93:737–744.
15. Budinger TF, Yano Y, Derenzo SE, et al. Rb-82 myocardial positron emission tomography. *J Nucl Med.* 1979;20:P603.
16. Schelbert HR, Phelps ME, Hoffman EJ, et al. Regional myocardial perfusion assessed with N-13 labeled ammonia and positron emission computerized axial tomography. *Am J Cardiol* 1979;43:209–218.
17. Gould KL. Identifying and measuring severity of coronary artery stenosis. Quantitative coronary arteriography and positron emission tomography. *Circulation* 1988;78:237–245.
18. Bergmann SR, Fox KAA, Rand AL, et al. Quantification of regional myocardial blood flow in vivo with $H_2{}^{15}O$. *Circulation* 1984;70: 724–733.
19. Schelbert HR, Phelps ME, Huang SC, et al. N-13 ammonia as an indicator of myocardial blood flow. *Circulation* 1981;63:1259–1272.
20. Goldstein RA, Mullani NA, Marani SK, et al. Perfusion imaging with rubidium-82: II. Effects of pharmacologic interventions on flow and extraction. *J Nucl Med* 1983;24:907–915.
21. Bergmann SR, Herrero P, Markham J, et al. Noninvasive quantitation of myocardial blood flow in human subjects with oxygen-15-labeled water and positron emission tomography. *J Am Coll Cardiol* 1989;14: 639–652.
22. Krivokapich J, Smith GT, Huang SC, et al. N-13 ammonia myocardial imaging at rest and with exercise in normal volunteers: Quantification of absolute myocardial perfusion with dynamic positron emission tomography. *Circulation* 1989;80:1328–1337.
23. Bellina C, Parodi O, Camici P, et al. Simultaneous in vitro and in vivo validation of nitrogen-13-ammonia for the assessment of regional myocardial blood flow. *J Nucl Med* 1990;31:1335–1343.
24. Hutchins G, Schwaiger M, Rosenspire K, et al. Noninvasive quantification of regional blood flow in the human heart using N-13 ammonia and dynamic positron emission tomographic imaging. *J Am Coll Cardiol* 1990;15:1032–1042.
25. Araujo L, Lammertsma A, Rhodes C, et al. Noninvasive quantification of regional myocardial blood flow in coronary artery disease with oxygen-15-labeled carbon dioxide inhalation and positron emission tomography. *Circulation* 1991;83:875–885.
26. Chan S, Brunken R, Czernin J, et al. Comparison of maximal myocardial blood flow during adenosine infusion with that of intravenous dipyridamole in normal men. *J Am Coll Cardiol* 1992; 20: 979–985.
27. Nitzsche E, Choi Y, Czernin J, et al. Noninvasive quantification of myocardial blood flow in humans. A direct comparison of the [$^{13}$N] ammonia and the [$^{15}$O] water techniques. *Circulation* 1996;93: 2000–2006.
28. Lin JW, Sciacca RR, Chou RL, et al. Quantification of myocardial perfusion in human subjects using 82Rb and wavelet-based noise reduction. *Am J Nucl Med* 2001;42:201–208.
29. Holmberg S, Serzysko W, Varnauskas E. Coronary circulation during heavy exercise in control subjects and patients with coronary heart disease. *Acta Med Scand* 1971;190:465–480.
30. Brunken R, Czernin J, Chan S, et al. Can the myocardial blood flow response to pharmacologic vasodilation be predicted by systemic hemodynamic changes? *J Am Coll Cardiol* 1993;21:57A.
31. Duvernoy CS, Meyer C, Seifert-Klauss V, et al. Gender differences in myocardial blood flow dynamics: lipid profile and hemodynamic effects. *J Am Coll Cardiol* 1999;33:463–470.
32. Nagamachi S, Czernin J, Kim AS, et al. Reproducibility of measurements of regional resting and hyperemic myocardial blood flow assessed with PET. *Am J Nucl Med* 1996;37:1626–1631.
33. Sawada S, Muzik O, Beanlands RS, et al. Interobserver and interstudy variability of myocardial blood flow and flow-reserve measurements with nitrogen 13 ammonia-labeled positron emission tomography. *J Nucl Cardiol* 1995;2:413–422.
34. Kaufmann PA, Gnecchi-Ruscone T, Yap JT, et al. Assessment of the reproducibility of baseline and hyperemic myocardial blood flow measurements with 15O-labeled water and PET. *Am J Nucl Med* 1999; 40:1848–1856.
35. Wyss CA, Koepfli P, Mikolajczyk K, et al. Bicycle exercise stress in PET for assessment of coronary flow reserve: Repeatability and Comparison with Adenosine Stress. *J Nucl Med.* 2003;44:146–154.
36. Kuhle WG, Porenta G, Huang SC, et al. Quantification of regional myocardial blood flow using 13N-ammonia and reoriented dynamic positron emission tomographic imaging. *Circulation* 1992;86: 1004–1017.
37. Bol A, Melin JA, Vanoverschelde J-L, et al. Direct comparison of [$^{13}$N] ammonia and [$^{15}$O] water estimates of perfusion with quantification of regional myocardial blood flow by microspheres. *Circulation* 1993;87: 512–525.
38. Muzik O, Beanlands RSB, Hutchins GD, et al. Validation of nitrogen-13-ammonia tracer kinetic model for quantification of myocardial blood flow using PET. *J Nucl Med* 1993;34:83–91.
39. Merlet P, Mazoyer B, Hittinger L, et al. Assessment of coronary reserve in man: Comparison between positron emission tomography with oxygen-15-labeled water and intracoronary Doppler technique. *J Nucl Med* 1993;34:1899–1904.
40. Opie LH. Metabolism of the heart in health and disease. *Am Heart J* 1968;76:685–698.
41. Liedtke AJ. Alterations of carbohydrate and lipid metabolism in the acutely ischemic heart. *Progr Cardiovasc Dis* 1981;23:321–336.
42. Bing RJ. The metabolism of the heart. In: *Harvey Lecture Series*. New York: Academic Press; 1954:27–70.
43. Keul J, Doll E, Steim H, et al. Über den Stoffwechsel des menschlichen Herzens. III. Der oxidative Stoffwechsel des menschlichen Herzens unter verschiedened Arbeitsbedingungen II. *Pfluegers Arch* 1965;282:43–53.
44. Keul J, Doll E, Steim H, et al. Uber den Stoffwechsel des menschlichen Herzens. I. Substratversorgung des gesunden Herzens in Ruhe, während und nach körperlicher Arbeit. *Pfluegers Arch* 1965;282:1–27.
45. Taegtmeyer H. Myocardial metabolism. In: Phelps M, Mazziotta J, Schelbert H, eds. *Positron Emission Tomography and Autoradiography: Principles and Applications for the Brain and Heart.* New York: Raven Press; 1986:149–195.
46. Sokoloff L, Reivich M, Kennedy C, et al. The [14C]-deoxyglucose method for the measurement of local cerebral glucose utilization: Theory, procedure and normal values in the conscious and anesthetized albino rat. *J Neurochem* 1977;28:897–916.
47. Ratib O, Phelps ME, Huang SC, et al. Positron tomography with deoxyglucose for estimating local myocardial glucose metabolism. *Am J Nucl Med* 1982;23:577–586.

48. Gambhir SS, Schwaiger M, Huang SC, et al. Simple noninvasive quantification method for measuring myocardial glucose utilization in humans employing positron emission tomography and fluorine-18 deoxyglucose. *Am J Nucl Med* 1989;30:359–366.
49. Choi Y, Hawkins R, Brunken R, et al. Evaluation of regional heterogeneity of myocardial glucose metabolism in normal humans using dynamic FDG-PET. *J Nucl Med* 1991;32:938.
50. Choi Y, Brunken R, Hawkins R, et al. Factors affecting myocardial 2-[F-18]fluoro-2-deoxy-D-glucose uptake in positron emission tomography studies of normal humans. *Eur J Nucl Med* 1993;20: 308–318.
51. Hicks R, von Dahl J, Lee K, et al. Insulin-glucose clamp for standardization of metabolic conditions during F-18 fluoro-deoxyglucose PET imaging. *J Am Coll Cardiol* 1991;17:381A.
52. vom Dahl J, Hicks R, Hermann W, et al. Insulin substitution significantly improves the quality of myocardial tissue viability studies with FDG-PET in patients with diabetes mellitus. *J Nucl Med* 1991;32:988.
53. Knuuti M, Nuutila P, Ruotsalainen U, et al. Euglycemic hyperinsulinemic clamp and oral glucose load in stimulating myocardial glucose utilization during positron emission tomography. *J Nucl Med* 1992;33:1255–1262.
54. Hariharan R, Bray M, Ganim R, et al. Fundamental limitations of [18F]2-deoxy-2-fluoro-D-glucose for assessing myocardial glucose uptake (see comments). *Circulation* 1995;91:2435–2444.
55. Doenst T, Taegtmeyer H. Complexities underlying the quantitative determination of myocardial glucose uptake with 2-deoxyglucose. *J Mol Cell Cardiol* 1998;30:1595–1604.
56. Depré C, Vanoverschelde JL, Taegtmeyer H. Glucose for the heart. *Circulation* 1999;99:578–588.
57. Bøtker HE, Goodwin GW, Holden JE, et al. Myocardial glucose uptake measured with fluorodeoxyglucose: A proposed method to account for variable lumped constants. *Am J Nucl Med* 1999;40: 1186–1196.
58. Davila-Roman VG, Vedala G, Herrero P, et al. Altered myocardial fatty acid and glucose metabolism in idiopathic dilated cardiomyopathy. *J Am Coll Cardiol* 2002;40:271–277.
59. Herrero P, Sharp TL, Dence C, et al. Comparison of 1-(11)C-glucose and (18)F-FDG for quantifying myocardial glucose use with PET. *J Nucl Med* 2002;43:1530–1541.
60. Herrero P, Weinheimer CJ, Dence C, et al. Quantification of myocardial glucose utilization by PET and 1-carbon-11-glucose. *J Nucl Cardiol* 2002;9:5–14.
61. de las Fuentes L, Herrero P, Peterson LR, et al. Myocardial fatty acid metabolism: Independent predictor of left ventricular mass in hypertensive heart disease. *Hypertension.* 2003;41:83–87.
62. Schön HR, Schelbert HR, Najafi A, et al. C-11-labeled palmitic acid for the noninvasive evaluation of regional myocardial fatty acid metabolism with positron computed tomography. II. Kinetics of C-11 palmitic acid in acutely ischemic myocardium. *Am Heart J.* 1982;103: 548–561.
63. Schelbert HR, Henze E, Schön HR, et al. C-11 palmitic acid for the noninvasive evaluation of regional myocardial fatty acid metabolism with positron computed tomography. IV. In vivo demonstration of impaired fatty acid oxidation in acute myocardial ischemia. *Am Heart J* 1983;106:736–750.
64. Mäki MT, Haaparanta M, Nuutila P, et al. Free fatty acid uptake in the myocardium and skeletal muscle using fluorine-18-fluoro-6-thia-heptadecanoic acid. *J Nucl Med* 1998;39:1320–1327.
65. Stone CK, Pooley RA, DeGrado TR, et al. Myocardial uptake of the fatty acid analog 14-fluorine-18-fluoro-6-thia-heptadecanoic acid in comparison to beta-oxidation rates by tritiated palmitate. *J Nucl Med* 1998;39:1690–1696.
66. Takala TO, Nuutila P, Pulkki K, et al. 14(*R, S*)-[(18)F]Fluoro-6-thia-heptadecanoic acid as a tracer of free fatty acid uptake and oxidation in myocardium and skeletal muscle. *Eur J Nucl Med Mol Imaging* 2002;29:1617–1522.
67. Schelbert HR, Henze E, Schön HR, et al. C-11 palmitate for the noninvasive evaluation of regional myocardial fatty acid metabolism with positron computed tomography. III. In vivo demonstration of the effects of substrate availability on myocardial metabolism. *Am Heart J* 1983;105:492–504.
68. Cohen MB. Synthesis and utilization of 13N compounds for positron scanning. *Int J Nucl Med Biol* 1978;5:201.
69. Iida H, Rhodes C, Araujo L, et al. Noninvasive quantification of regional myocardial metabolic rate for oxygen by use of $^{15}O_2$ inhalation and positron emission tomography: Theory, error analysis, and application in humans. *Circulation* 1996;94:792–807.
70. Yamamoto Y, de Silva R, Rhodes C, et al. Noninvasive quantification of regional myocardial metabolic rate of oxygen by $^{15}O_2$ inhalation and positron emission tomography: Experimental validation. *Circulation* 1996;94:808–816.
71. Armbrecht JJ, Buxton DB, Brunken RC, et al. Regional myocardial oxygen consumption determined noninvasively in humans with [1-$^{11}$C] acetate and dynamic positron tomography. *Circulation* 1989;80:863–872.
72. Buxton DB, Nienaber CA, Luxen A, et al. Noninvasive quantitation of regional myocardial oxygen consumption in vivo with [1-$^{11}$C] acetate and dynamic positron emission tomography. *Circulation* 1989;79: 134–142.
73. Henes C, Bergmann S, Walsh M, et al. Noninvasive quantification of myocardial metabolic reserve by positron emission tomography (PET) with C-11 acetate and dobutamine. *Circulation* 1989;80:II-312.
74. Armbrecht JJ, Buxton DB, Schelbert HR. Validation of [1-$^{11}$C] acetate as a tracer for noninvasive assessment of oxidative metabolism with positron emission tomography in normal, ischemic, post-ischemic and hyperemic canine myocardium. *Circulation* 1991;81:1594–1605.
75. Ng NCK, Huang SC, Schelbert HR, Buxton DB. Validation of a model for [1-11C]acetate as a tracer of cardiac oxidative metabolism. *Am J Physiol* 1994;266:H1304–1315.
76. Sun K, Chen K, Huang S-C, et al. Compartment model for measuring myocardial oxygen consumption using [1-$^{11}$C] acetate. *J Nucl Med* 1997;38:459–466.
77. Sun KT, Yeatman LA, Buxton DB, et al. Simultaneous measurement of myocardial oxygen consumption and blood flow using [1-carbon-11]acetate. *Am J Nucl Med* 1998;39:272–280.
78. Ukkonen H, Knuuti J, Katoh C, et al. Use of [11C]acetate and [15O]$O_2$ PET for the assessment of myocardial oxygen utilization in patients with chronic myocardial infarction. *Eur J Nucl Med.* 2001;28: 334–339.
79. Gould KL, Lipscomb K, Hamilton GW. Physiologic basis for assessing critical coronary stenosis. Instantaneous flow response and regional distribution during coronary hyperemia as measures of coronary flow reserve. *Am J Cardiol* 1974;33:87–94.
80. Chan S, Kobashigawa J, Stevenson L, et al. Myocardial blood flow at rest and during pharmacologic vasodilation in cardiac transplants during and after successful treatment of rejection. *Circulation* 1994; 90:204–212.
81. Czernin J, Auerbach M, Sun K, et al. Effects of modified pharmacologic stress approaches on hyperemic myocardial blood flow. *J Nucl Med* 1995;36:575–580.
82. Senneff M, Geltman E, Bergmann S, Hartman J. Noninvasive delineation of the effects of moderate aging on myocardial perfusion. *J Nucl Med* 1991;32:2037–2042.
83. Czernin J, Muller P, Chan S, et al. Influence of age and hemodynamics on myocardial blood flow and flow reserve. *Circulation* 1993;88: 62–69.
84. Uren N, Camici P, Melin J, et al. Effect of aging on myocardial perfusion reserve. *J Nucl Med* 1995;36:2032–2036.
85. Müller P, Czernin J, Choi Y, et al. Effect of exercise supplementation during adenosine infusion on hyperemic blood flow and flow reserve. *Am Heart J* 1994;128:52–60.
86. Nienaber CA, Gambhir SS, Mody FV, et al. Regional myocardial blood flow and glucose utilization in symptomatic patients with hypertrophic cardiomyopathy. *Circulation* 1993;87:1580–1590.
87. Czernin J, Sun K, Brunken R, et al. Effect of acute and long-term smoking on myocardial blood flow and flow reserve. *Circulation* 1995;91:2891–2897.

88. Buus NH, Bottcher M, Hermansen F, et al. Influence of nitric oxide synthase and adrenergic inhibition on adenosine-induced myocardial hyperemia. *Circulation* 2001;104:2305–2310.
89. Raitakari OT, Toikka JO, Laine H, et al. Reduced myocardial flow reserve relates to increased carotid intima-media thickness in healthy young men. *Atherosclerosis* 2001;156:469–475.
90. Böttcher M, Czernin J, Sun K, et al. Effect of caffeine on myocardial blood flow at rest and during pharmacological vasodilation. *J Nucl Med* 1995;36:2016–2021.
91. Krivokapich J, Huang S-C, Schelbert H. Assessment of the effects of dobutamine on myocardial blood flow and oxidative metabolism in normal human subjects using nitrogen-13 ammonia and carbon-11 acetate. *Am J Cardiol* 1993;71:1351–1356.
92. Tadamura E, Iida H, Matsumoto K, et al. Comparison of myocardial blood flow during dobutamine-atropine infusion with that after dipyridamole administration in normal men. *J Am Coll Cardiol* 2001; 37:130–136.
93. Gould K. *Coronary Artery Stenosis*. New York: Elsevier; 1990.
94. Porenta G, Kuhle W, Czernin J, et al. Semiquantitative assessment of myocardial viability and perfusion utilizing polar map displays of cardiac PET images. *J Nucl Med* 1992;33:1623–1631.
95. Laubenbacher C, Rothley J, Sitomer J, et al. An automated analysis program for the evaluation of cardiac PET studies: Initial results in the detection and localization of coronary artery disease using nitrogen-13-ammonia. *J Nucl Med* 1993;34:968–978.
96. Nekolla SG, Miethaner C, Nguyen N, et al. Reproducibility of polar map generation and assessment of defect severity and extent assessment in myocardial perfusion imaging using positron emission tomography. *Eur J Nucl Med* 1998;25:1313–1321.
97. Schelbert HR, Wisenberg G, Phelps ME, et al. Noninvasive assessment of coronary stenoses by myocardial imaging during pharmacologic coronary vasodilation. VI. Detection of coronary artery disease in man with intravenous N-13 ammonia and positron computed tomography. *Am J Cardiol* 1982;49:1197–1207.
98. Tamaki N, Yonekura Y, Senda M, et al. Value and limitation of stress thallium-201 single photon emission computed tomography: Comparison with nitrogen-13 ammonia positron tomography. *J Nucl Med* 1988;29:1181–1188.
99. Demer LL, Gould KL, Goldstein RA, et al. Assessment of coronary artery disease severity by positron emission tomography. Comparison with quantitative arteriography in 193 patients. *Circulation* 1989;79: 825–835.
100. Go R, Marwick T, MacIntyre W, et al. A prospective comparison of rubidium-82 PET and thallium-201 SPECT myocardial perfusion imaging utilizing a single dipyridamole stress in the diagnosis of coronary artery disease. *J Nucl Med* 1990;31:1899–1905.
101. Stewart R, Schwaiger M, Molina E, et al. Comparison of rubidium-82 positron emission tomography and thallium-201 SPECT imaging for detection of coronary artery disease. *Am J Cardiol.* 1991;67:1303–1310.
102. Simone G, Mullani N, Page D, Anderson B Sr. Utilization statistics and diagnostic accuracy of a nonhospital-based positron emission tomography center for the detection of coronary artery disease using rubidium-82. *Am J Physiol Imaging* 1992;7:203–209.
103. Williams B, Millani N, Jansen D, Anderson B. A retrospective study of the diagnostic accuracy of a community hospital-based PET center for the detection of coronary artery disease using rubidium-82. *J Nucl Med* 1994;35:1586–1592.
104. Gould KL, Goldstein RA, Mullani NA, et al. Noninvasive assessment of coronary stenoses by myocardial perfusion imaging during pharmacologic coronary vasodilation VIII. Clinical feasibility of positron cardiac imaging without a cyclotron using generator-produced rubidium-82. *J Am Coll Cardiol* 1986;7:775–789.
105. Zijlstra F, Fioretti P, Reiber J, Serruys P. Which cineangiographically assessed anatomical variable correlates best with functional measurements of stenosis severity? A comparison of quantitative analysis of the coronary cineangiogram with measured coronary flow reserve and exercise/redistribution thallium-201 scintigraphy. *J Am Coll Cardiol* 1988;12:686–691.
106. Brown BG, Josephson MA, Peterson RB, et al. Intravenous dipyridamole combined with isometric handgrip for near maximal acute increase in coronary flow in patients with coronary artery disease. *Am J Cardiol* 1981;48:1077–1085.
107. Merhige ME, Houston T, Shalton V, et al. PET myocardial perfusion imaging reduces the cost of coronary disease management by eliminating unnecessary invasive diagnostic and therapeutic procedures. *Circulation* 1999;100:(suppl I):I-26.
108. Flamm S, Khanna S, DiCarli M, et al. Prognostic significance of normal adenosine stress myocardial perfusion PET study in patients presenting with chest pain. *J Nucl Med* 1994;35:60P.
109. Marwick TH, Shan K, Patel S, et al. Incremental value of rubidium-82 positron emission tomography for prognostic assessment of known or suspected coronary artery disease. *Am J Cardiol* 1997;80:865–870.
110. Marwick TH, Shan K, Go RT, et al. Use of positron emission tomography for prediction of perioperative and late cardiac events before vascular surgery. *Am Heart J* 1995;130:1196–1202.
111. Boyd HL, Rosen SD, Rimoldi O, et al. Normal values for left ventricular volumes obtained using gated PET. *G Ital Cardiol* 1998;28: 1207–1214.
112. Hattori N, Bengel FM, Mehilli J, et al. Global and regional functional measurements with gated FDG PET in comparison with left ventriculography. *Eur J Nucl Med* 2001;28:221–229.
113. Sdringola S, Patel D, Gould KL. High prevalence of myocardial perfusion abnormalities on positron emission tomography in asymptomatic persons with a parent or sibling with coronary artery disease. *Circulation* 2001;103:496–501.
114. Gould K, Ornish D, Scherwitz L, et al. Changes in myocardial perfusion abnormalities by positron emission tomography after long-term, intense risk factor modification. *JAMA* 1995;274:894–901.
115. Sdringola S, Nakagawa K, Nakagawa Y, et al. Combined intense lifestyle and pharmacologic lipid treatment further reduce coronary events and myocardial perfusion abnormalities compared with usual-care cholesterol-lowering drugs in coronary artery disease. *J Am Coll Cardiol* 2003;41:263–272.
116. Uren N, Melin J, De Bruyne B, et al. Relation between myocardial blood flow and the severity of coronary-artery stenosis. *N Engl J Med* 1994;330:1782–1788.
117. Beanlands R, Schwaiger M. Changes in myocardial oxygen consumption and efficiency with heart failure therapy measured by $^{11}$C acetate PET. *Can J Cardiol* 1995;11:293–300.
118. Di Carli M, Czernin J, Hoh C, et al. Relation among stenosis severity, myocardial blood flow, and flow reserve in patients with coronary artery disease. *Circulation* 1995;91:1944–1951.
119. Krivokapich J, Czernin J, Schelbert HR. Dobutamine positron emission tomography: Absolute quantitation of rest and dobutamine myocardial blood flow and correlation with cardiac work and percent diameter stenosis in patients with and without coronary artery disease. *J Am Coll Cardiol* 1996;28:565–572.
120. Smith SC Jr. Risk-reduction therapy: The challenge to change. Presented at the 68th scientific sessions of the American Heart Association November 13, 1995 Anaheim, California. *Circulation* 1996;93: 2205–2211.
121. Libby P. Molecular bases of the acute coronary syndromes. *Circulation* 1995;91:2844–2850.
122. Zeiher S, Drexler H, Wollschläger H, Just H. Modulation of coronary vasomotor tone: Progressive endothelial dysfunction with different early stages of coronary atherosclerosis. *Circulation* 1991; 83:391–401.
123. Egashira K, Inou T, Hirooka Y, et al. Impaired coronary blood flow response to acetylcholine in patients with coronary risk factors and proximal atherosclerotic lesions. *J Clin Invest* 1993;91:29–37.
124. Zeiher A, Drexler H, Saurbier B, Just H. Endothelium-mediated coronary blood flow modulation in humans. Effects of age, atherosclerosis, hypercholesterolemia, and hypertension. *J Clin Invest* 1993;92: 652–662.
125. Dayanikli F, Grambow D, Muzik O, et al. Early detection of abnormal coronary flow reserve in asymptomatic men at high risk for coronary

artery disease using positron emission tomography. *Circulation* 1994;90:808–817.

126. Pitkänen O, Raitakari O, Niinikoski H, et al. Coronary flow reserve is impaired in young men with familial hypercholesterolemia. *J Am Coll Cardiol* 1996;28:1705–1711.
127. Yokoyama I, Murakami T, Ohtake T, et al. Reduced coronary flow reserve in familial hypercholesterolemia. *J Nucl Med* 1996;37:1937–1942.
128. Yokoyama I, Ohtake T, Momomura S, et al. Reduced coronary flow reserve in hypercholesterolemic patients without overt coronary stenosis. *Circulation* 1996;94:3232–3238.
129. Raitakari OT, Pitkeanen OP, Lehtimeaki T, et al. In vivo low density lipoprotein oxidation relates to coronary reactivity in young men. *J Am Coll Cardiol* 1997;30:97–102.
130. Rönnemaa T, Viikari J, Taskinen MR, et al. Coronary flow reserve in young men with familial combined hyperlipidemia. *Circulation* 1999;99:1678–1684.
131. Kaufmann PA, Gnecchi-Ruscone T, Schäfers KP, et al. Low density lipoprotein cholesterol and coronary microvascular dysfunction in hypercholesterolemia. *J Am Coll Cardiol* 2000;36:103–109.
132. Pitkanen OP, Raitakari OT, Ronnemaa T, et al. Influence of cardiovascular risk status on coronary flow reserve in healthy young men. *Am J Cardiol* 1997;79:1690–1692.
133. Yokoyama I, Ohtake T, Momomura S, et al. Altered myocardial vasodilatation in patients with hypertriglyceridemia in anatomically normal coronary arteries. *Arterioscler Thromb Vasc Biol* 1998;18: 294–299.
134. Yokoyama I, Ohtake T, Momomura S, et al. Impaired myocardial vasodilation during hyperemic stress with dipyridamole in hypertriglyceridemia. *J Am Coll Cardiol* 1998;31:1568–1574.
135. Yokoyama I, Momomura S, Ohtake T, et al. Reduced myocardial flow reserve in non-insulin-dependent diabetes mellitus (see comments). *J Am Coll Cardiol* 1997;30:1472–1477.
136. Pitkänen OP, Nuutila P, Raitakari OT, et al. Coronary flow reserve is reduced in young men with IDDM. *Diabetes* 1998;47:248–254.
137. Di Carli MF, Bianco-Batlles D, Landa ME, et al. Effects of autonomic neuropathy on coronary blood flow in patients with diabetes mellitus. *Circulation* 1999;100:813–819.
138. Yokoyama I, Ohtake T, Momomura S, et al. Hyperglycemia rather than insulin resistance is related to reduced coronary flow reserve in NIDDM. *Diabetes* 1998;47:119–124.
139. Laaksonen R, Janatuinen T, Vesalainen R, et al. High oxidized LDL and elevated plasma homocysteine contribute to the early reduction of myocardial flow reserve in healthy adults. *Eur J Clin Invest* 2002;32: 795–802.
140. Paiva H, Laakso J, Laine H, et al. Plasma asymmetric dimethylarginine and hyperemic myocardial blood flow in young subjects with borderline hypertension or familial hypercholesterolemia. *J Am Coll Cardiol* 2002;40:1241–1247.
141. Sundell J, Laine H, Luotolahti M, et al. Obesity affects myocardial vasoreactivity and coronary flow response to insulin. *Obes Res* 2002; 10:617–624.
142. Reddy K, Nair R, Sheehan H, Hodgson JM. Evidence that selective endothelial dysfunction may occur in the absence of angiographic or ultrasound atherosclerosis in patients with risk factors for atherosclerosis. *J Am Coll Cardiol* 1994;23:833–843.
143. Bache RJ. Vasodilator reserve: A functional assessment of coronary health (editorial; comment). *Circulation*. 1998;98:1257–1260.
144. Smits P, Williams S, Lipson D, et al. Endothelial release of nitric oxide contributes to the vasodilator effect of adenosine in humans. *Circulation* 1995;92:2135–2141.
145. Gould KL, Nakagawa Y, Nakagawa K, et al. Frequency and clinical implications of fluid dynamically significant diffuse coronary artery disease manifest as graded, longitudinal, base to apex, myocardial perfusion abnormalities by noninvasive positron emission tomography. *Circulation*. 2000;101:1931–1939.
146. De Bruyne B, Hersbach F, Pijls NH, et al. Abnormal epicardial coronary resistance in patients with diffuse atherosclerosis but "normal" coronary angiography. *Circulation* 2001;104:2401–2406.
147. Hernandez-Pampaloni M, Keng FY, Kudo T, et al. Abnormal longitudinal, base-to-apex myocardial perfusion gradient by quantitative blood flow measurements in patients with coronary risk factors. *Circulation* 2001;104:527–532.
148. Tuzcu EM, Kapadia SR, Tutar E, et al. High prevalence of coronary atherosclerosis in asymptomatic teenagers and young adults: evidence from intravascular ultrasound. *Circulation* 2001;103:2705–2710.
149. Zeiher AM. Endothelial modulation of coronary vasomotor tone in humans. Effects of atherosclerosis and risk factors for coronary artery disease. *Arzneimittelforschung* 1994;44:439–442.
150. Nitenberg A, Ledoux S, Valensi P, et al. Impairment of coronary microvascular dilation in response to cold pressor–induced sympathetic stimulation in type 2 diabetic patients with abnormal stress thallium imaging. *Diabetes*. 2001;50:1180–1185.
151. Nabel E, Ganz P, Gordon J, et al. Dilation of normal and constriction of atherosclerotic coronary arteries caused by the cold pressor test. *Circulation*. 1988;77:43–52.
152. Zeiher AM, Drexler H, Wollschlaeger H, et al. Coronary vasomotion in response to sympathetic stimulation in humans: Importance of the functional integrity of the endothelium (see comments). *J Am Coll Cardiol* 1989;14:1181–1190.
153. Campisi R, Czernin J, Schöder H, et al. Effects of long-term smoking on myocardial blood flow, coronary vasomotion, and vasodilator capacity. *Circulation* 1998;98:119–125.
154. Campisi R, Czernin J, Schöder H, et al. L-Arginine normalizes coronary vasomotion in long-term smokers. *Circulation* 1999;99: 491–497.
155. Campisi R, Nathan L, Pampaloni MH, et al. Noninvasive assessment of coronary microcirculatory function in postmenopausal women and effects of short-term and long-term estrogen administration. *Circulation* 2002;105:425–430.
156. Momose M, Abletshauser C, Neverve J, et al. Dysregulation of coronary microvascular reactivity in asymptomatic patients with type 2 diabetes mellitus. *Eur J Nucl Med Mol Imaging* 2002;29: 1675–1679.
157. Czernin J, Barnard J, Sun K, et al. Effect of short term cardiovascular conditioning and low fat diet on myocardial blood flow and flow reserve. *Circulation* 1995;92:197–204.
158. Gould K, Martucci J, Goldberg D, et al. Short-term cholesterol lowering decreases size and severity of perfusion abnormalities by positron emission tomography after dipyridamole in patients with coronary artery disease. A potential noninvasive marker of healing coronary endothelium. *Circulation* 1994;89:1530–1538.
159. Guethlin M, Kasel AM, Coppenrath K, et al. Delayed response of myocardial flow reserve to lipid-lowering therapy with fluvastatin. *Circulation* 1999;99:475–481.
160. Yokoyama I, Momomura S, Ohtake T, et al. Improvement of impaired myocardial vasodilatation due to diffuse coronary atherosclerosis in hypercholesterolemics after lipid-lowering therapy. *Circulation* 1999; 100:117–122.
161. Huggins GS, Pasternak RC, Alpert NM, et al. Effects of short-term treatment of hyperlipidemia on coronary vasodilator function and myocardial perfusion in regions having substantial impairment of baseline dilator reverse (see comments). *Circulation* 1998;98: 1291–1296.
162. Mellwig KP, Baller D, Gleichmann U, et al. Improvement of coronary vasodilatation capacity through single LDL apheresis. *Atherosclerosis* 1998;139:173–178.
163. Harrison DG. Endothelial control of vasomotion and nitric oxide production: A potential target for risk factor management. *Cardiol Clin* 1996;14:1–15.
164. Jeserich M, Schindler T, Olscheski M, et al. Vitamin C improves endothelial function of epicardial coronary arteries in patients with hypercholestaemia or essental hypertension: Assessed by cold pressor testing. *Eur Heart J* 1999;20:1676–1680.
165. Böger RH, Bode-Böger SM, Szuba A. Asymmetric dimethylarginine (ADMA): A novel risk factor for endothelial dysfunction: its role in hypercholesterolemia. *Circulation* 1998;98:1842–1847.

166. Schachinger V, Britten MB, Zeiher AM. Prognostic impact of coronary vasodilator dysfunction on adverse long-term outcome of coronary heart disease. *Circulation* 2000;101:1899–1906.
167. Suwaidi JA, Hamasaki S, Higano ST, et al. Long-term follow-up of patients with mild coronary artery disease and endothelial dysfunction. *Circulation* 2000;101:948–954.
168. Schindler TH, Hornig B, Buser PT, et al. Prognostic value of abnormal vasoreactivity of epicardial coronary arteries to sympathetic stimulation in patients with normal coronary angiograms. *Arterioscler Thromb Vasc Biol.* 2003;23:495–501.
169. Opie LH. Myocardial ischemia: Metabolic pathways and implications of increased glycolysis. *Cardiol Drugs Ther* 1990;4:777–790.
170. Schelbert HR, Phelps ME, Selin C, et al. Regional myocardial ischemia assessed by $^{18}$fluoro-2-deoxyglucose and positron emission computed tomography. In: Kreuzer H, Parmley W, Rentrop P, Heiss H, eds. *Quantification of Myocardial Ischemia*. New York: Gehard Witzstrock; 1980:437–447.
171. Marshall RC, Tillisch JH, Phelps ME, et al. Identification and differentiation of resting myocardial ischemia and infarction in man with positron computed tomography 18F-labeled fluorodeoxyglucose and N-13 ammonia. *Circulation* 1983;67:766–778.
172. Tillisch J, Brunken R, Marshall R, et al. Reversibility of cardiac wall motion abnormalities predicted by positron tomography. *N Engl J Med* 1986;314:884–888.
173. Camici P, Araujo LI, Spinks T, et al. Increased uptake of $^{18}$F-fluorodeoxyglucose in postischemic myocardium of patients with exercise-induced angina. *Circulation* 1986;74:81–88.
174. Schwaiger M, Schelbert HR, Ellison D, et al. Sustained regional abnormalities in cardiac metabolism after transient ischemia in the chronic dog model. *J Am Coll Cardiol* 1985;6:336–347.
175. Vanoverschelde J-L, Wijns W, Depré C, et al. Mechanisms of chronic regional postischemic dysfunction in humans: New insights from the study of noninfarcted collateral-dependent myocardium. *Circulation* 1993;87:1513–1523.
176. Gerber BL, Wijns W, Vanoverschelde JJ, et al. Myocardial perfusion and oxygen consumption in reperfused noninfarcted dysfunctional myocardium after unstable angina: Direct evidence for myocardial stunning in humans. *J Am Coll Cardiol* 1999;34:1939–1946.
177. Schwaiger M, Neese RA, Araujo L, et al. Sustained nonoxidative glucose utilization and depletion of glycogen in reperfused canine myocardium. *J Am Coll Cardiol* 1989;13:745–754.
178. Schwaiger M, Brunken R, Grover-McKay M, et al. Regional myocardial metabolism in patients with acute myocardial infarction assessed by positron emission tomography. *J Am Coll Cardiol* 1986;8: 800–808.
179. Bolli R, Triana F, Jeroudi MO. Postischemic mechanical and vascular dysfunction (myocardial "stunning" and microvascular "stunning") and the effects of calcium-channel blockers on ischemia/reperfusion injury. *Clin Cardiol* 1989;12:III-16–III-25.
180. Barnes E, Dutka DP, Khan M, et al. Effect of repeated episodes of reversible myocardial ischemia on myocardial blood flow and function in humans. *Am J Physiol Heart Circ Physiol* 2002;282:H1603–1608.
181. Barnes E, Hall RJ, Dutka DP, Camici PG. Absolute blood flow and oxygen consumption in stunned myocardium in patients with coronary artery disease. *J Am Coll Cardiol* 2002;39:420–427.
182. Rahimtoola SH. The hibernating myocardium. *Am Heart J* 1989;117: 211–221.
183. Schulz R, Rose J, Martin C, et al. Development of short-term myocardial hibernation: Its limitation by the severity of ischemia and inotropic stimulation. *Circulation* 1993;88:684–695.
184. Chen C, Gillam L, Chen L, et al. Temporal hierarchy in functional and ultrastructural recoveries between short-term and chronic hibernating myocardium after reperfusion. *Circulation* 1995;92:I-552.
185. Chen C, Chen L, Fallon J, et al. Functional and structural alterations with 24-hour myocardial hibernation and recovery after reperfusion. *Circulation* 1996;94:507–516.
186. Fallavollita J, Bryan P, Canty J. $^{18}$F-2-deoxyglucose deposition and regional flow in pigs with chronically dysfunctional myocardium: Evidence for transmural variations in chronic hibernating myocardium. *Circulation* 1997;95:1900–1909.
187. Fallavollita JA, Canty JM Jr. Differential 18F-2-deoxyglucose uptake in viable dysfunctional myocardium with normal resting perfusion: evidence for chronic stunning in pigs. *Circulation* 1999;99:2798–2805.
188. Fallavollita JA, Perry BJ, Canty JM Jr. 18F-2-deoxyglucose deposition and regional flow in pigs with chronically dysfunctional myocardium. Evidence for transmural variations in chronic hibernating myocardium. *Circulation* 1997;95:1900–1909.
189. Lim H, Fallavollita JA, Hard R, et al. Profound apoptosis-mediated regional myocyte loss and compensatory hypertrophy in pigs with hibernating myocardium. *Circulation* 1999;100:2380–2386.
190. Shivalkar B, Flameng W, Szilard M, et al. Repeated stunning precedes myocardial hibernation in progressive multiple coronary artery obstruction. *J Am Coll Cardiol* 1999;34:2126–2136.
191. Fragasso G, Chierchia S, Lucignani G, et al. Time dependence of residual tissue viability after myocardial infarction assessed by [18F] fluorodeoxyglucose and positron emission tomography. *Am J Cardiol* 1993;72:131G–139G.
192. Fedele FA, Gewortz J, Capone RJ, et al. Metabolic response to prolonged reduction of myocardial blood flow distal to a severe coronary artery stenosis. *Circulation* 1988;78:729–735.
193. Schaefer S, Schwartz G, Wisneski J, et al. Response of high-energy phosphates and lactate release during prolonged regional ischemia in vivo. *Circulation* 1992;85:342–349.
194. Camici P, Wijns W, Borgers M, et al. Pathophysiological mechanisms of chronic reversible left ventricular dysfunction due to coronary artery disease (hibernating myocardium). *Circulation* 1997;96: 3205–3214.
195. Maes A, Vlameng W, Borgers M, et al. Regional myocardial blood flow, glucose utilization and contractile function before and after revascularization and ultrastructural findings in patients with chronic coronary artery disease. *Eur J Nucl Med* 1995;22:1299–1305.
196. Wolpers H, Burchert W, van den Hoff J, et al. Assessment of myocardial viability by use of $^{11}$C-acetate and positron emission tomography. *Circulation* 1997;95:1417–1424.
197. Stinson EB, Griepp RB, Bieber CP, Shumway NE. Changes in coronary blood flow during rejection of the orthotopically transplanted canine heart. *J Thorac Cardiovasc Surg* 1972;63:854–864.
198. Cabin HS, Clubbs KS, Vita N, Zaret BL. Regional dysfunction by equilibrium radionuclide angiography: A clinicopathologic study evaluating the relation of degree of dysfunction to the presence and extent of myocardial infarction. *J Am Coll Cardiol* 1987;10:743–747.
199. Flameng W, Suy R, Schwarz F, et al. Ultrastructural correlates of left ventricular contraction abnormalities in patients with chronic ischemic heart disease: Determinants of reversible segmental asynergy post-revascularization surgery. *Am Heart J* 1981;102:846–857.
200. Maes A, Flameng W, Nuyts J, et al. Histological alterations in chronically hypoperfused myocardium: Correlation with PET findings. *Circulation* 1994;90:735–745.
201. Depré C, Vanoverschelde J-LJ, Melin J, et al. Structural and metabolic correlates of the reversibility of chronic left ventricular ischemic dysfunction in humans. *Am J Physiol* 1995;268:H1265–H1275.
202. Schwarz E, Schaper J, vom Dahl J, et al. Myocyte degeneration and cell death in hibernating human myocardium. *J Am Coll Cardiol* 1996; 27:1577–1585.
203. Schwaiger M, Sun D, Deeb G, et al. Expression of myocardial glucose transporter (GLUT) mRNAs in patients with advanced coronary artery disease (CAD). *Circulation* 1994;90:I-113.
204. Lopaschuk G, Stanley W. Glucose metabolism in the ischemic heart. *Circulation* 1997;95:313–315.
205. Lopaschuk GD. Treating ischemic heart disease by pharmacologically improving cardiac energy metabolism. *Am J Cardiol* 1998;82: 14K–17K.
206. Allman K, Wieland D, Muzik O, et al. Carbon-11 hydroxyephedrine with positron emission tomography for serial assessment of cardiac adrenergic neuronal function after acute myocardial infarction in humans. *J Am Coll Cardiol* 1993;22:368–375.

207. Bengel F, Ueberfuhr P, Ziegler SI, et al. Effect of cardiac sympathetic innervation on metabolism of the human heart by positron emission tomography. *Circulation* 1999;100(suppl I):I-201.
208. Borgers M, Ausma J. Structural aspects of the chronic hibernating myocardium in man. *Basic Res Cardiol* 1995;90:44–46.
209. Ausma J, Wijffels M, van Eys G, Koide M, et al. Dedifferentiation of atrial cardiomyocytes as a result of chronic atrial fibrillation. *Am J Pathol* 1997;151:985–997.
210. Depré C, Shipley GL, Chen W, et al. Unloaded heart in vivo replicates fetal gene expression of cardiac hypertrophy. *Nat Med* 1998;4: 1269–1275.
211. Ausma J, Thonae F, Dispersyn GD, et al. Dedifferentiated cardiomyocytes from chronic hibernating myocardium are ischemia-tolerant. *Mol Cell Biochem* 1998;186:159–168.
212. Elsässer A, Schlepper M, Klövekorn W-P, et al. Hibernating myocardium: An incomplete adaptation to ischemia. *Circulation* 1997;96: 2920–2931.
213. Elsaesser A, Greiber S, Hein S, et al. Hibernating myocardium: Upregulation of caspase-3 gene and reduction of bcl-2. *Circulation* 1999;100(suppl I):I-758.
214. Chen C, Lijie M, Linfert D, et al. Myocardial cell death and apoptosis in hibernating myocardium. *J Am Coll Cardiol* 1997;30:1407–1412.
215. Brunken R, Mody F, Hawkins R, et al. Metabolic imaging with positron emission tomography detects viable tissue in myocardial segments with persistent defects on twenty-four hour tomographic thallium-201 scintigraphy. *Circulation* 1992;86:1357–1369.
216. Beanlands RS, Hendry PJ, Masters RG, et al. Delay in revascularization is associated with increased mortality rate in patients with severe left ventricular dysfunction and viable myocardium on fluorine 18-fluorodeoxyglucose positron emission tomography imaging. *Circulation* 1998;98:II51–II56.
217. Schwarz E, Schoendube F, Kostin S, et al. Prolonged myocardial hibernation exacerbates cardiomyocyte degeneration and impairs recovery of function after revascularization. *J Am Coll Cardiol* 1998; 31:1018–1026.
218. Ausma J, Duimel H, Wouters L, et al. Structural atrial remodeling in the goat by 16 weeks of atrial fibrillation is not reversed 8 weeks after cardioversion. *Circulation* 1999;100(suppl I):I-10.
219. Nienaber C, Brunken R, Sherman C, et al. Metabolic and functional recovery of ischemic human myocardium after coronary angioplasty. *J Am Coll Cardiol* 1991;18:966–978.
220. Vanoverschelde JL, Depre C, Gerber BL, et al. Time course of functional recovery after coronary artery bypass graft surgery in patients with chronic left ventricular ischemic dysfunction. *Am J Cardiol* 2000;85:1432–1439.
221. Haas F, Augustin N, Holper K, et al. Time course and extent of improvement of dysfunctioning myocardium in patients with coronary artery disease and severely depressed left ventricular function after revascularization: Correlation with positron emission tomographic findings. *J Am Coll Cardiol* 2000;36:1927–1934.
222. Haas F, Jennen L, Heinzmann U, et al. Ischemically compromised myocardium displays different time-courses of functional recovery: correlation with morphological alterations? *Eur J Cardiothorac Surg* 2001;20:290–298.
223. Marwick T, MacIntyre W, Lafont A, et al. Metabolic responses of hibernating and infarcted myocardium to revascularization: A follow-up study of regional perfusion, function, and metabolism. *Circulation* 1992;85:1347–1353.
224. Tamaki N, Yonekura Y, Yamashita K, et al. Positron emission tomography using fluorine-18 deoxyglucose in evaluation of coronary artery bypass grafting. *Am J Cardiol* 1989;64:860–865.
225. Carrel T, Jenni R, Haubold-Reuter S, et al. Improvement of severely reduced left ventricular function after surgical revascularization in patients with preoperative myocardial infarction. *Eur J Cardiothorac Surg* 1992;6:479–484.
226. Gewirtz H, Fischman A, Abraham S, et al. Positron emission tomographic measurements of absolute regional myocardial blood flow permits identification of nonviable myocardium in patients with chronic myocardial infarction. *J Am Coll Cardiol* 1994;23:851–859.
227. Duvernoy CS, vom Dahl J, Laubenbacher C, Schwaiger M. The role of nitrogen 13 ammonia positron emission tomography in predicting functional outcome after coronary revascularization. *J Nucl Cardiol* 1995;2:499–506.
228. Bax JJ, Poldermans D, Elhendy A, et al. Improvement of left ventricular ejection fraction, heart failure symptoms and prognosis after revascularization in patients with chronic coronary artery disease and viable myocardium detected by dobutamine stress echocardiography. *J Am Coll Cardiol* 1999;34:163–169.
229. Bonow R, Dilsizian V, Cuocolo A, Bacharach S. Identification of viable myocardium in patients with chronic coronary artery disease and left ventricular dysfunction: Comparison of thallium scintigraphy with reinjection and PET imaging with F-18-fluorodeoxyglucose. *Circulation* 1991;83:26–37.
230. Knuuti M, Saraste M, Nuutila P, et al. Myocardial viability: Fluorine-18-deoxyglucose positron emission tomography in prediction of wall motion recovery after revascularization. *Circulation* 1994;90: 2356–2366.
231. Baer F, Voth E, Deutsch H, et al. Predictive value of low dose dobutamine transesophageal echocardiography and fluorine-18 fluorodeoxyglucose positron emission tomography for recovery of regional left ventricular function after successful revascularization. *J Am Coll Cardiol* 1996;28:60–69.
232. Buvat I, Bartlett M, Srinivasan G, et al. Can gated FDG PET assess LV function as well as gated bloodpool SPECT? *J Nucl Med* 1996;37:39P.
233. Buvat I, Kitsiou A, Srinivasan G, et al. Relationship between metabolism and function in CAD patients using gated FDG PET. *J Nucl Med* 1996;37:161P.
234. Fath-Ordoubadi F, Beatt KJ, Spyrou N, Camici PG. Efficacy of coronary angioplasty for the treatment of hibernating myocardium. *Heart* 1999;82:210–216.
235. Gerber BL, Ordoubadi FF, Wijns W, et al. Positron emission tomography using(18)F-fluoro-deoxyglucose and euglycaemic hyperinsulinaemic glucose clamp: optimal criteria for the prediction of recovery of post-ischaemic left ventricular dysfunction. Results from the European Community Concerted Action Multicenter study on use of (18)F-fluoro-deoxyglucose positron emission tomography for the detection of myocardial viability. *Eur Heart J* 2001;22: 1691–701.
236. DePuey EG, Ghesani M, Schwartz M, et al. Comparative performance of gated perfusion SPECT wall thickening, delayed thallium uptake, and F-18 fluorodeoxyglucose SPECT in detecting myocardial viability. *J Nucl Cardiol* 1999;6:418–428.
237. Schöder H, Campisi R, Ohtake T, et al. Blood flow-metabolism imaging with positron emission tomography in patients with diabetes mellitus for the assessment of reversible left ventricular contractile dysfunction. *J Am Coll Cardiol* 1999;33:1328–1337.
238. Bax J, Cornel J, Visser F, et al. Prediction of improvement of contractile function in patients with ischemic ventricular dysfunction after revascularization by fluorine-18 fluorodeoxyglucose single-photon emission computed tomography. *J Am Coll Cardiol* 1997;30: 377–383.
239. Bax J, Cornel J, Visser F, et al. Prediction of improvement of global function after revascularization in patients with ischemic left ventricular dysfunction: Detection by F18-fluorodeoxyglucose SPECT. *J Am Coll Cardiol* 1997;29:377A.
240. Dreyfus G, Duboc D, Blasco A, et al. Myocardial viability assessment in ischemic cardiomyopathy: Benefits of coronary revascularization. *Ann Thorac Surg*. 1994;57:1402–1408.
241. Akinboboye OO, Idris O, Cannon PJ, Bergmann SR. Usefulness of positron emission tomography in defining myocardial viability in patients referred for cardiac transplantation. *Am J Cardiol.* 1999;83: 1271–1274, A9.
242. Srinivasan G, Kitsiou AN, Bacharach SL, et al. [18F]fluorodeoxyglucose single photon emission computed tomography: Can it replace

PET and thallium SPECT for the assessment of myocardial viability? (see comments). *Circulation* 1998;97:843–850.

243. Grandin C, Wijns W, Melin J, et al. Delineation of myocardial viability with PET. *J Nucl Med* 1995;36:1543–1552.

244. Shivalkar B, Maes A, Borgers M, et al. Only hibernating myocardium invariably shows early recovery after coronary revascularization. *Circulation* 1996;94:308–315.

245. Allman KC, Shaw LJ, Hachamovitch R, Udelson JE. Myocardial viability testing and impact of revascularization on prognosis in patients with coronary artery disease and left ventricular dysfunction: a meta-analysis. *J Am Coll Cardiol* 2002;39:1151–1158.

246. Vaghaiwalla MR, Mody F, Brunken R, et al. Differentiating cardiomyopathy of coronary artery disease from non-ischemic dilated cardiomyopathy utilizing positron tomography. *J Am Coll Cardiol* 1991;17:373–383.

247. Tamaki N, Ohtani H, Yamashita K, et al. Metabolic activity in the areas of new fill-in after thallium-201 reinjection: comparison with positron emission tomography using fluorine-18-deoxyglucose. *J Nucl Med* 1991;32:673–678.

248. Marwick T, Nemec J, Lafont A, et al. Prediction by postexercise fluoro-18 deoxyglucose positron emission tomography of improvement in exercise capacity after revascularization. *Am J Cardiol* 1992; 69:854–859.

249. Gropler RJ, Geltman EM, Sampathkumaran K, et al. Comparison of carbon-11-acetate with fluorine-18-fluorodeoxyglucose for delineating viable myocardium by positron emission tomography. *J Am Coll Cardiol* 1993;22:1587–1597.

250. Paolini G, Lucignani G, Zuccari M, et al. Identification and revascularization of hibernating myocardium in angina-free patients with left ventricular dysfunction. *Eur J Cardiothorac Surg* 1994;8: 139–144.

251. vom Dahl J, Altehoefer C, Büchin P, et al. Effect of myocardial viability and coronary revascularization on clinical outcome and prognosis: A follow-up study of 161 patients with coronary heart disease. *Zeitschr Kardiol* 1996;85:868–881.

252. Flameng WJ, Shivalkar B, Spiessens B, et al. PET scan predicts recovery of left ventricular function after coronary artery bypass operation. *Ann Thorac Surg* 1997;64:1694–1701.

253. Haas F, Haehnel C, Picker W, et al. Preoperative positron emission tomographic viability assessment and perioperative and postoperative risk in patients with advanced ischemic heart disease. *J Am Coll Cardiol* 1997;30:1693–1700.

254. Fath-Ordoubadi F, Pagano D, Marinho NV, et al. Coronary revascularization in the treatment of moderate and severe postischemic left ventricular dysfunction. *Am J Cardiol* 1998;82:26–31.

255. Pagano D, Townend JN, Littler WA, et al. Coronary artery bypass surgery as treatment for ischemic heart failure: The predictive value of viability assessment with quantitative positron emission tomography for symptomatic and functional outcome. *J Thorac Cardiovasc Surg* 1998;115:791–799.

256. Bax JJ, Visser FC, Poldermans D, et al. Relationship between preoperative viability and postoperative improvement in LVEF and heart failure symptoms. *J Nucl Med* 2001;42:79–86.

257. Zhang X, Liu XJ, Wu Q, et al. Clinical outcome of patients with previous myocardial infarction and left ventricular dysfunction assessed with myocardial (99m)Tc-MIBI SPECT and (18)F-FDG PET. *J Nucl Med* 2001;42:1166–1173.

258. Pasquet A, Lauer MS, Williams MJ, et al. Prediction of global left ventricular function after bypass surgery in patients with severe left ventricular dysfunction. Impact of preoperative myocardial function, perfusion, and metabolism. *Eur Heart J* 2000;21:125–136.

259. Marwick TH, Zuchowski C, Lauer MS, et al. Functional status and quality of life in patients with heart failure undergoing coronary bypass surgery after assessment of myocardial viability. *J Am Coll Cardiol* 1999;33:750–758.

260. Pasquet A, Williams MJ, Secknus MA, et al. Correlation of preoperative myocardial function, perfusion, and metabolism with postoperative function at rest and stress after bypass surgery in severe left ventricular dysfunction. *Am J Cardiol.* 1999;84:58–64.

261. Beanlands RS, Ruddy TD, deKemp RA, et al. Positron emission tomography and recovery following revascularization (PARR-1): The importance of scar and the development of a prediction rule for the degree of recovery of left ventricular function. *J Am Coll Cardiol* 2002;40:1735–1743.

262. Vanoverschelde J, Melin J, Depré C, et al. Time-course of functional recovery of hibernating myocardium after coronary revascularization. *Circulation* 1994;90:I-378.

263. Eitzman D, Al-Aouar Z, Vom Dahl J, et al. Clinical outcome of patients with advanced coronary artery disease after viability studies with positron emission tomography. *J Am Coll Cardiol* 1992;20:559–565.

264. Di Carli M, Davidson M, Little R, et al. Value of metabolic imaging with positron emission tomography for evaluating prognosis in patients with coronary artery disease and left ventricular dysfunction. *Am J Cardiol* 1994;73:527–533.

265. Di Carli M, Asgarzadie F, Phelps M, Schelbert H. Can myocardial viability be assessed by quantitative measurements of myocardial perfusion at rest and during pharmacologic stress. *J Nucl Med* 1995; 36:66P.

266. Goldman L, Hashimoto B, Cook E, Loscalzo A. Comparative reproducibility and validity of systems for assessing cardiovascular functional class: advantages of a new specific activity scale. *Circulation* 1981;64:1227–1234.

267. Tamaki N, Kawamoto M, Takahashi N, et al. Prognostic value of an increase in fluorine-18 deoxyglucose uptake in patients with myocardial infarction: Comparison with stress thallium imaging. *J Am Coll Cardiol* 1993;22:1621–1627.

268. Di Carli M, Sherman T, Khanna S, et al. Myocardial viability in asynergic regions subtended by occluded coronary arteries: Relation to the status of collateral flow in patients with chronic coronary artery disease. *J Am Coll Cardiol* 1994;23:860–868.

269. Lee K, Marwick T, Cook S, et al. Prognosis of patients with left ventricular dysfunction, with and without viable myocardium after myocardial infarction. *Circulation* 1994;90:2687–2694.

270. Di Carli MF, Maddahi J, Rokhsar S, et al. Long-term survival of patients with coronary artery disease and left ventricular dysfunction: Implications for the role of myocardial viability assessment in management decisions. *J Thorac Cardiovasc Surg* 1998;116:997–1004.

271. Landoni C, Lucignani G, Paolini G, et al. Assessment of CABG-related risk in patients with CAD and LVD. Contribution of PET with [18F]FDG to the assessment of myocardial viability. *J Cardiovasc Surg* 1999;40:363–372.

272. Auerbach MA, Scheoder H, Hoh C, et al. Prevalence of myocardial viability as detected by positron emission tomography in patients with ischemic cardiomyopathy. *Circulation* 1999;99:2921–2926.

273. Duong T, Hendi P, Fonarow G, et al. Role of positron emission tomographic assessment of myocardial viability in the management of patients who are referred for cardiac transplantation. *Circulation* 1995; 92:I-123.

274. Duong T, Fonarow G, Laks H, et al. Cost-effectiveness of positron emission tomography (PET) in the management of ischemic cardiomyopathy patients who are referred for cardiac transplantation. *J Am Coll Cardiol* 1996;27:144A.

275. Louie H, Laks H, Milgalter E, et al. Ischemic cardiomyopathy: criteria for coronary revascularization and cardiac transplantation. *Circulation* 1991;84:III-290–III-295.

276. Di Carli M, Farbod A, Schelbert H, et al. Quantitative relation between myocardial viability and improvement in heart failure symptoms after revascularization in patients with ischemic cardiomyopathy. *Circulation* 1995;92:3436–3444.

P A R T T H R E E

# HEART FAILURE

CHAPTER 24

# PATHOPHYSIOLOGY OF HEART FAILURE

Gary S. Francis / W. H. Wilson Tang / Edmund H. Sonnenblick



## DEFINITION OF TERMS AND CLASSIFICATION

### Heart Failure

Heart failure, a complex clinical syndrome, arises from a process of ventricular dysfunction (acute or chronic), where the venous return to the heart is normal but the heart is unable to pump sufficient blood to meet the body's metabolic needs at normal filling pressures. Ventricular systolic dysfunction is characterized by a loss of contractile strength of the myocardium accompanied by "compensatory" ventricular hypertrophy and/or dilatation (ventricular remodeling). Systolic ventricular dysfunction due to focal loss of contraction can be dynamic and transient, as may occur with acute ischemia. With restoration of metabolic requirements of an ischemic segment of myocardium, either from restoring adequate coronary flow or reducing oxygen requirements, myocardial contraction may be restored. Sometimes restoration is delayed, so-called *stunning*. Chronically reduced coronary flow may be inadequate to preserve contraction but adequate for myocardial survival. Such persistent depression of the myocardium has been termed *hibernation;* with reperfusion, contractility may recover over time.

As ventricular dysfunction proceeds, there is activation of the sympathetic and renin-angiotensin-aldosterone systems; this, although meant to physiologically augment contractility and heart rate in the former system and to preserve salt and water balance in the latter, contributes to further cardiac remodeling, peripheral vasoconstriction with sodium retention, and progressive cardiomegaly. Heart failure is also generally associated with a very poor prognosis, even when symptoms are mild.[1,2] *Systolic left ventricular (LV) dysfunction* or *failure* reflects a decrease in normal emptying capacity [usually with an ejection fraction (EF) of 45 percent or less] that is usually associated with a compensatory increase in diastolic volume. *Isolated diastolic ventricular dysfunction* or *failure* is present when the filling of one or both ventricles is impaired while the emptying capacity is normal. It may be due to a thickened (hypertrophied) ventricular wall, restrictive or infiltrative cardiomyopathies, and/or tachycardia that limits time for diastolic filling, resulting in increased ventricular filling pressures and eventually pulmonary edema.

*Congestive heart failure* denotes a clinical syndrome with complex and variable signs and symptoms, including dyspnea, increased fatigability, and fluid accumulation (edema). In most patients with clinical congestive heart failure due to mechanical or myocardial abnormalities, the heart (pump) failure is preceded by a substantial period of *myocardial* dysfunction, during which cardiac *pump* function and cardiac output (at least while at rest) may be maintained by compensatory mechanisms that include myocardial hypertrophy and ventricular dilatation. For this reason, in the early stages, patients may have little or no limitations or symptoms. Initially, the cardiac output may be within the normal range at rest, but it fails to increase or may even decline during exercise or stress. Ultimately, the cardiac output is decreased even at rest. Associated changes include an increase in systemic vascular resistance (SVR) at rest and a failure of the SVR to decrease with increased metabolic needs.

When the intravascular circulatory congestion is present for any length of time with elevation of LV diastolic and pulmonary venous pressures, fluid transudation occurs from the pulmonary capillaries into the interstitial spaces. Pulmonary edema develops if the rate of transudation exceeds the rate of lymphatic drainage. Pulmonary edema is often detected initially by x-ray examination, and there may be a time lag before audible rales are detected on physical examination. Elevated jugular venous pressure is often visible and may be accompanied by dependent peripheral edema and hepatomegaly. In the majority of patients, congestive heart failure develops chronically and is associated with the retention of sodium and water by the kidneys.

*Acute or decompensated heart failure* can develop during acute ischemia of the ventricle (i.e., a myocardial infarction), incessant tachycardia, or the rupture of a cardiac valve. An acute shift of blood from the systemic to the pulmonary circulation can occur before the retention of significant $Na^+$ or water. The term *congestive heart failure* should not be used unless there is congestion of cardiac origin. When the cause of the pulmonary or peripheral congestion is not clear, however, it is usually preferable to describe the symptoms or signs, which are nonspecific, and to avoid improperly diagnosing heart failure.

TABLE 24-1 Classifications and Definitions of Some Common Types of Heart Failure

*Heart failure* A clinical syndrome with classic symptoms of breathlessness, fatigue, and exercise intolerance that are attributable to impaired myocardial function.

*Congestive heart failure* Similar to the preceding but with features of circulatory congestion such as jugular venous distention, rales, peripheral edema, and ascites.

*Noncardiac circulatory congestion* A syndrome that is clinically indistinguishable from congestive heart failure where there is no reason to ascribe the condition to structural heart disease. There must be a noncardiac cause such as acute renal failure.

*Systolic heart failure* A clinical syndrome with classic symptoms of breathlessness, fatigue, and exercise intolerance whereby the dominant cardiac feature is a large, dilated heart and impaired systolic performance. There may or may not be concomitant valvular disease.

*Heart failure with normal systolic function* Sometimes referred to as *diastolic heart failure,* this is a clinical syndrome characterized by breathlessness, fatigue, and exercise intolerance whereby the dominant cardiac feature is impaired diastolic function (usually diagnosed by echo) and normal or near-normal ejection phase indices. There is often LV hypertrophy and impaired filling of the heart due to altered LV stiffness or other evidence of diastolic dysfunction. Often, severe systemic hypertension is present. There may or may not be concomitant valvular disease, such as mitral insufficiency. This form of heart failure may coexist with systolic heart failure.

*Right-sided heart failure* A clinical syndrome characterized by tissue congestion including jugular venous distention, peripheral edema, ascites, and abdominal organ engorgement. There is marked impairment of right ventricular systolic performance, usually with right ventricular dilatation and severe tricuspid regurgitation. There are multiple causes of this syndrome, including severe left-sided heart failure, severe lung disease with chronic hypoxemia and pulmonary hypertension (so-called cor pulmonale), right ventricular myocardial infarction, and primary pulmonary hypertension.

## CLASSIFICATION AND STAGES OF HEART FAILURE

Numerous classification schemes and definitions have evolved over the years (Table 24-1), including the antiquated "forward heart failure" and "backward heart failure," concepts that are no longer very useful. Even the New York Heart Association classification system, though widely used, lacks precision (see also Chap. 12).

### *New York Heart Association Functional Classification*

I. Patients with cardiac disease but without resulting limitations of physical activity. Ordinary physical activity does not cause undue fatigue, palpitation, dyspnea, or anginal pain.
II. *Patients with cardiac disease resulting in slight limitation of physical activity.* These patients are comfortable at rest. Ordinary physical activity results in fatigue, palpitation, dyspnea, or anginal pain.
III. *Patients with cardiac disease resulting in marked limitation of physical activity.* These patients are comfortable at rest. Less than ordinary physical activity causes fatigue, palpitation, dyspnea, or anginal pain.
IV. *Patients with cardiac disease resulting in inability to carry on any physical activity without discomfort.* Symptoms of cardiac insufficiency or of the anginal syndrome may be present even at rest. If any physical activity is undertaken, discomfort is increased.

A more recent and useful "staging" scheme of heart failure is now being used more commonly by guideline committees and regulatory agencies and is more closely intertwined with prevention and therapy.[3] It is outlined below.

### *Stages in the Evolution of Heart Failure (2001 ACC/AHA Guidelines)*

*Stage A.* Patients at risk of developing heart failure because of comorbid conditions that are strongly associated with the development of HF. Such patients have no signs or symptoms of HF and have never manifested signs or symptoms of HF. There are no structural or functional abnormalities of the valves or ventricles. Examples: systemic hypertension, coronary artery disease, diabetes mellitus.

*Stage B.* Patients who have developed structural heart disease that is strongly associated with the development of HF but have no symptoms of HF and have never manifested signs or symptoms of HF. Examples: left ventricular hypertrophy (LVH); enlarged, dilated ventricles asymptomatic valvular heart disease; previous myocardial infarction.

*Stage C.* Patients who have current or prior symptoms of HF associated with underlying structural heart disease. This represents the largest group of patients with clinical evidence of heart failure.

*Stage D.* Patients with marked symptoms of heart failure at rest despite maximal medical therapy and who require specialized interventions. Examples include patients who cannot be safely discharged from the hospital, who are repeatedly hospitalized, who are in the hospital awaiting heart transplantation, who are residing in a hospice setting, who are living at home and receiving continuous intravenous support for symptom relief, or who are being supported with a mechanical circulatory assist device.

This newer staging scheme is very clinically oriented and allows physicians to target therapy in a more focused manner toward specific subsets of patients. It is recognized that stages A and B do not represent true heart failure but rather comprise patients at risk for developing heart failure. Problems can arise because of our inability to quantitate the degree of physical disability by simple history and physical examination as well as the lack of correlation of shortness of breath and fatigue with ventricular dysfunction.

## Systolic and Diastolic Dysfunction

A useful contemporary distinction in heart failure is that between systolic and diastolic dysfunction (Table 24-2 and Fig. 24-1). These labels, however, are most appropriately defined in terms of altered ventricular architecture rather than systemic hemodynamics. *Systolic dysfunction* describes a large, dilated ventricle whose output is limited by impaired ejection, whereas *diastolic dysfunction* refers to a thickened, small-cavity ventricle in which filling is limited. It is appropriate to reserve the term *systolic dysfunction* for a dilated, often eccentrically hypertrophied ventricle and *diastolic dysfunction* for a thick-walled, concentrically hypertrophied ventricle with a normal or small cavity, highlighting the important architectural differences between these two entities. Both may manifest dyspnea due to elevated filling pressures.

Diastolic heart failure (or heart failure with preserved LV systolic function) is increasingly recognized as a major and growing epidemiologic clinical problem.[4–6] As many as 40 percent of patients presenting with heart failure have preserved LV systolic function, and the proportion may be even higher in hospitals caring for elderly and inner-city patients. Diastolic heart failure often coexists with poorly controlled systemic hypertension and the systolic hypertension found commonly in the elderly. Factors contributing to altered LV diastolic function include myocardial fibrosis, hypertrophy, ischemia, and increased afterload, all of which tend to increase with aging.[7] Myocardial ischemia is an especially important mechanism to identify[8] because, like hypertension, it is usually treatable.

TABLE 24-2 The Differential Diagnosis of Systolic Heart Failure and Heart Failure with Normal Systolic Function (Diastolic Heart Failure)

| Systolic Heart Failure | Diastolic Heart Failure |
|---|---|
| Large, dilated heart | Small LV cavity, concentric LV hypertrophy |
| Normal or low blood pressure | Systemic hypertension |
| Broad age group; more common in men | Elderly women more common |
| Low ejection fraction | Normal or increased ejection fraction |
| $S_3$ gallop | $S_4$ gallop |
| Systolic and diastolic impairment by echo | Diastolic impairment by various echo measurements |
| Treatment well established | Treatment not well established |
| Poor prognosis | Prognosis not as poor |
| Role of myocardial ischemia important in selected cases | Myocardial ischemia common |

It is clear that systolic and diastolic dysfunction frequently coexist in patients with heart failure and that systolic events can influence diastolic function.[9,10] The diagnosis of diastolic dysfunction can be challenging, but advancing echocardiographic techniques have improved substantially, revealing altered patterns of ventricular filling and left atrial enlargement. Limitations imparted by loading

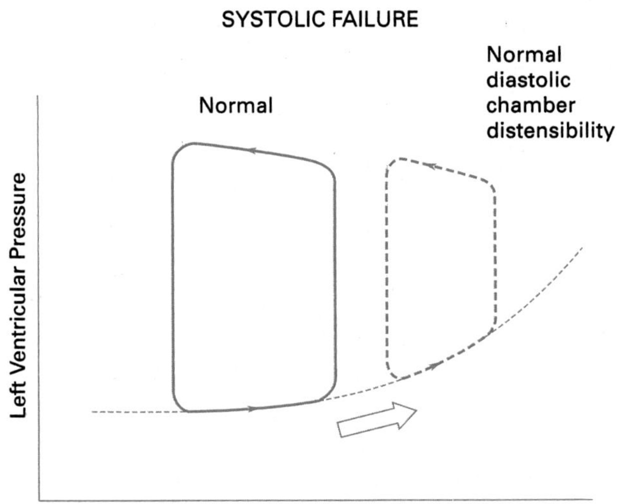


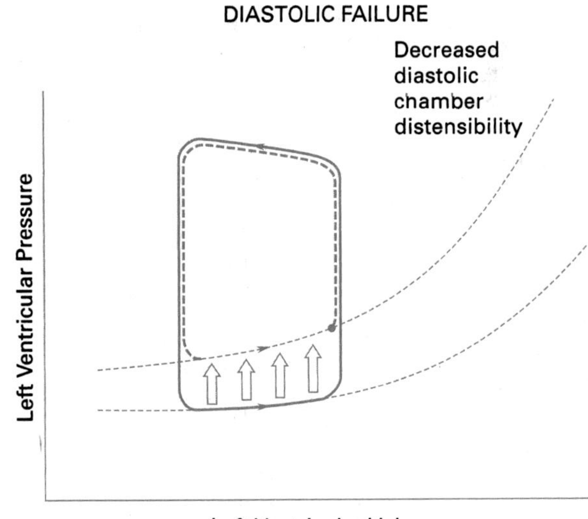


FIGURE 24-1 The left panel shows a schematized left ventricular (LV) pressure-volume loop from a patient with primary systolic failure. A normal LV pressure-volume loop (*solid loop*) is shown on the left portion of the curve; the transition to inotropic failure (*dashed loop*) is shown on the right. Systolic failure is manifest as an increase in LV end-systolic volume and as a reduction in the extent of shortening (stroke volume). LV end-diastolic pressure (LVEDP) is increased because LV volume is increased. As indicated by the arrow, the diastolic portion of the pressure-volume loop has simply shifted to the right, along the same diastolic pressure-volume relationship; thus no change in the distensibility of the left ventricle has occurred. The right panel shows an LV pressure-volume loop from a patient with primary diastolic failure (*dashed loop*). Note that the LVEDP is the same as that in the patient with primary inotropic failure, as denoted by the heavy dot on both pressure-volume loops. In the right panel, however, this is caused by an upward shift of the LV diastolic pressure-volume relationship (*arrows*), which indicates a decrease in LV diastolic distensibility such that a higher diastolic pressure is required to achieve the same diastolic volume. In this patient, no change in end-diastolic volume or systolic shortening has occurred. (From Lorell BH: Left ventricular diastolic pressure-volume relations: Understanding and managing congestive heart failure. *Heart Failure* 1988;4:206–223. Reproduced with permission from the publisher and author.)

conditions, heart rate, and age have to some extent been overcome by new applications of continuous-wave Doppler, color Doppler M-mode, and tissue Doppler imaging.[11–13]

Women seem to be overrepresented in the category of diastolic heart failure,[14] especially elderly women with hypertension, diabetes mellitus, and LV hypertrophy. For any given afterload stress, women seem to develop more hypertrophy than men. Women with diabetes mellitus also have more myocardial mass than men. Patients with heart failure and normal systolic function have a somewhat lower mortality risk than patients with a reduced EF,[15] but they still have a fourfold mortality risk compared with control subjects who are free of heart failure.[16] It is important to assess LV architecture and function by echocardiography before initiating therapy in a patient with heart failure, since the natural history and treatment of systolic and diastolic heart failure may be different. Knowledge of renal function and renal vasculature may also be important, especially in patients with severe hypertension. For example, many elderly patients with heart failure and severe hypertension have associated renal artery stenosis,[17] and treating them with angiotensin-converting enzyme (ACE) inhibitors could further worsen their renal function. Likewise, prolonged, aggressive use of diuretics in patients with severe LV hypertrophy and a small LV cavity may lead to a reduced stroke volume and hypotension. It is important, therefore, to have knowledge of myocardial architecture, anatomy, and function in planning therapy and in determining prognosis.

Generally, systolic ventricular dysfunction is characterized by an increase in end-diastolic volume (EDV) and a normal or somewhat reduced stroke volume (SV), resulting in a decrease in EF. This relationship of SV to EDV is normally described by the Frank-Starling relationship (Fig. 24-2). The increase in EDV is associated with an increase in ventricular end-diastolic pressure (EDP) in consonance with the resting pressure-volume curve. The filling pressure may be further elevated for a given EDV by concentric hypertrophy or myocardial fibrosis. Conversely, this hypertrophy and fibrosis actually may be decreased by chronic overdistention (eccentric hypertrophy). The relation between LV wall force and fiber length is depicted in Fig. 24-3.

In patients with mild heart failure, the ventricular EDP and the cardiac output may be normal at rest, but the former may become elevated to abnormal levels during stress, such as exercise or an increase in afterload. The ability to increase the cardiac output in response to the increase in oxygen consumption is also reduced (see below and Chap. 4). In patients with more severe systolic dysfunction, both the early pressure and the EDP may be elevated even at rest. As diastolic volume is increased, so is end-systolic volume. This results in reduced elastic recoil of the ventricle during relaxation and is reflected in loss of rapid early diastolic ventricular filling (as revealed by a reduced E wave of the echocardiogram). This helps increase the mean diastolic pressure further. The elevated LV diastolic pressure increases pulmonary venous and capillary pressures and contributes to increased dyspnea as a result of changes in pulmonary

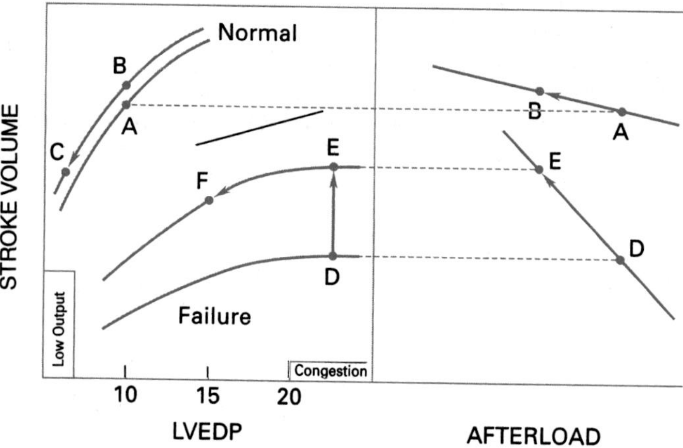


FIGURE 24-2 Relationship between stroke volume and left ventricular (LV) end-diastolic pressure (LVEDP) (*left*) and afterload (*right*). Normally, the ventricle operates on a sharply rising Frank-Starling curve with an LVEDP less than 12 mmHg (point *A*), where small changes in filling pressure yield large changes in stroke volume. Further, stroke volume is largely independent of the afterload. When failure occurs, ventricular function is characterized by a shift of the curve relating stroke volume to LVEDP to the right and downward. Low output may ensue if the curve is sufficiently depressed, while pulmonary congestion occurs as the LVEDP is increased. At the same time, this failing ventricle is now highly afterload-dependent, in that small changes in afterload produce large changes in stroke volume. When afterload is reduced in the normal heart (point A to point B, *right*), stroke volume rises very slightly. If, at the same time, venodilation reduces filling pressure, stroke volume falls to point C (*left*). The net result is a decrease in cardiac output. On the contrary, when afterload is reduced in the presence of severe ventricular failure, stroke volume is increased (point D to point E, *right*). Since the Frank-Starling curve is relatively flattened, a simultaneous decrease in filling pressure leads to a decrease in LVEDP with only a small decrease in stroke volume (point E to point F, *left*). The net result of these opposing consequences can be an increase in stroke volume. These results are observed clinically when a vasodilator is administered along with a diuretic in treating the failing ventricle.

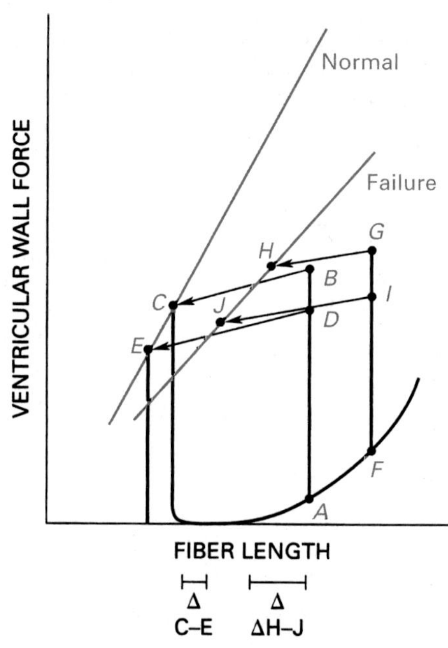


FIGURE 24-3 Relationship between LV wall force and fiber length. Hypothetical contractile cycles have been portrayed for the normal and the failing ventricle. In the normal heart, contraction starts at point A, LV pressure rises until the aortic valve is opened (point B), the ventricle empties (points B to C), and relaxation ensues. When arterial pressure (afterload) is reduced (e.g., to point D), ejection starts at point D and proceeds to point E, which increases stroke volume. When the ventricle fails, the fiber length in diastole is increased, and ventricular contraction starts at point F. With systolic contraction, ventricular pressure rises to point G, and with ventricular emptying, fiber length decreases to point H. With a similar decrease in the afterload, wall force only needs to reach point I when ventricular emptying occurs to point J. As a result, for the same relative change in afterload, the increase in shortening is greater in the failing ventricle (ΔH–J) than in the normal heart (ΔC–E).

compliance due to pulmonary congestion and edema. It is also apparent that before this stage of clinical heart failure is reached, the body has used many compensatory mechanisms after the onset of the initial abnormality or stress and that these compensatory mechanisms eventually have failed to maintain the needs for cardiac output (see below).

## Causes of Pump Failure

The causes of overall heart pump failure may be classified into four main categories: (1) failure primarily related to work overload or mechanical abnormalities, (2) failure mostly related to primary myocardial abnormalities, (3) failure related to abnormal cardiac rhythm or conduction disturbances, and (4) myocardial ischemia/infarction. Myocardial infarction resulting in a quantitative loss of myocardium creates a special type of work overload. During the acute infarction, the EF falls as the EDV is sometimes increased to sustain a falling SV. The fall in EF is approximately proportional to the amount of myocardium lost. With time, the EF tends to remain at this reduced level. With healing of the infarction, the akinetic infarcted region becomes a scar that not only cannot contribute to ventricular emptying but may even contribute to the load. Thus the entire load falls on the remaining nonischemic myocardium. This load is further increased by the increased diastolic volume itself, which causes wall tension to be increased for any given pressure. This is consistent with the Laplace relation, where wall tension is directly related to the product of the radius and pressure and inversely related to ventricular wall thickness. Wall tension increases even though the nonischemic myocardium hypertrophies in proportion to the amount of myocardium that is lost. Heart failure may emerge months or years later as a so-called ischemic cardiomyopathy resulting from progressive ventricular dilatation and reactive hypertrophy.

## Cardiomyopathy

Virtually any form of heart disease can lead to heart failure, and there are many causes of both "primary" and "secondary" heart failure. However, these distinctions are quite arbitrary and of little clinical value. *Primary heart failure* usually refers to so-called *cardiomyopathy,* a vague term that can include idiopathic dilated cardiomyopathy, familial dilated cardiomyopathy (an increasingly recognized cause of dilated cardiomyopathy), or hypertrophic cardiomyopathy. It simply depends on how one defines the term *cardiomyopathy*. Idiopathic dilated cardiomyopathy denotes cardiac dilation, commonly biventricular, without known etiology—i.e., without inflammation or positive family history and with normal coronaries. Pathologically, it is characterized by myocyte loss and patchy fibrosis. Familial dilated cardiomyopathy is more common than previously believed.[18] It cannot be predicted by clinical or phenotypic techniques and requires family screening for identification. It is important always to consider familial dilated cardiomyopathy in evaluating patients with "idiopathic dilated cardiomyopathy," because it may have a more virulent natural history. It can be associated with a very rapid downhill course, necessitating early referral to a heart transplant center.[19] Cardiac abnormalities are common in asymptomatic relatives of patients with dilated cardiomyopathy.[20] As many as 30 percent or more of patients with dilated cardiomyopathy may have an inherited disorder,[21] the molecular genetic basis of which is under intense study.[22]

Hypertrophic obstructive cardiomyopathy (HOCM) and nonobstructive hypertrophic cardiomyopathy are also often familial, affecting about 1 in 500 people in the general population (see Chap. 77). Most cases are inherited in an autosomal dominant manner with variable clinical penetrance and expression. Many different mutations have been described for at least seven abnormal sarcomeric proteins. Late-onset expression of HOCM may be a distinct clinical entity. Unfortunately, the genetic heterogeneity of this disease has made routine genetic testing impractical. Clinical screening may be warranted for members of families characterized by hypertrophic cardiomyopathy.

Unlike familial dilated or hypertrophic cardiomyopathy, alcoholic cardiomyopathy and "viral" cardiomyopathy (e.g., secondary to inflammatory myocarditis) may be overdiagnosed by clinicians. There are no specific clinical markers for so-called alcoholic cardiomyopathy, and there is no good evidence indicating an alcohol dose-response relationship. Apparently, a broad segment of the alcoholic population remains somehow immune to this complication. Nevertheless, patients believed to be "heavy" users of alcohol who present with dilated cardiomyopathy and in whom heart failure resolves on cessation of alcohol use probably have an "alcoholic cardiomyopathy."

*Viral myocarditis* can be diagnosed only by examining myocardial tissue (e.g., myocardial biopsy), since we now know that the "clinical" diagnosis of viral myocarditis is notoriously inaccurate. Only 5 to 10 percent of biopsies taken from the hearts of patients suspected clinically of having inflammatory myocarditis are actually "positive." Physicians should refrain from telling patients that their heart failure is due to a virus unless there is tissue verification. There are, of course, patients with mild or subclinical acute myocarditis who progress to heart failure and present with "dilated cardiomyopathy." The prognosis of patients with proven inflammatory myocarditis may be somewhat better than that of patients with idiopathic dilated cardiomyopathy, since spontaneous improvement in EF is not uncommon.[23] However, others have found no difference in the 5-year survival between patients with myocarditis and those with idiopathic dilated cardiomyopathy (56 versus 54 percent, respectively).[24] Patients with active inflammatory myocarditis may suffer severe rejection earlier after heart transplantation. Idiopathic giant-cell myocarditis is important to distinguish from inflammatory lymphocytic myocarditis because it has a worse survival rate and may respond better to immunotherapy and heart transplantation.[25]

Anthracycline-induced heart failure is now increasingly recognized as a form of "toxic" heart failure.[26] It is clearly a dose-related phenomenon and may present as a "cardiomyopathy." A rapidly growing number of persons, including a fraction of the 150,000 adults in the United States who have survived childhood cancers, will develop anthracycline-induced cardiomyopathy.[27,28] There may be a long latency period (years) between treatment and onset of symptoms. Recently, herceptin (recombinant humanized anti-HER2 antibody) has been approved for the treatment of breast cancer. About 27 percent of patients receiving both herceptin and doxorubicin or paclitaxel experience cardiac dysfunction,[29] which is a far greater percentage than those receiving anthracycline or paclitaxel alone. Cardiac toxicity should be a major concern for patients receiving herceptin, which is often used in conjunction with an anthracycline. Heart failure induced by these drugs is not a simple complication that can be "managed" by drug therapy but rather a potentially lethal complication that requires skillful care. Other causes of toxic cardiomyopathy include cocaine, other cytostatic agents, interferons, interleukin-2, anabolic steroids, and a host of miscellaneous agents.[29] Spontaneous improvement can occur with anthracycline-induced cardiomyopathy, and such patients may respond to beta-adrenergic blockers.

The cause of LV systolic dysfunction in patients with chronic obstructive lung disease is unknown, although the combination of hypoxia and hypercapnia may be important. LV diastolic dysfunction in such patients is in part secondary to the pronounced right ventricular hypertrophy and dilatation with secondary elevation of LV diastolic pressure due to ventricular interdependence. The latter phenomenon is also important in the pathophysiology of the acute pulmonary edema occasionally encountered in patients with acute pulmonary embolus.

## Myocardial "Overload"

Myocardial failure may develop from many causes of "overload." It may evolve from pressure overload in which myocytes hypertrophy to meet the demands of the load. Hypertrophied cells contract and relax more slowly[30] and may be subject to metabolic limitations. In addition, hypertrophied myocardial cells may have a shortened life span.[31,32] This is of considerable prognostic importance because cardiac myocytes appear to have a reduced capacity to proliferate. When age-related myocyte loss is added to the picture, particularly in association with a late decrease in myocyte contractile activity, diastolic failure may ensue. As the process continues, ventricular dilatation may occur, with systolic failure as well. Loss of myocytes—whether segmental, as in acute myocardial infarction, or diffuse, as in myocarditis—sets up a vicious cycle that leads to reactive hypertrophy in remaining myocytes. As compensatory hypertrophy becomes more marked in some disease states, the contractility unit of the myocardium often declines because of molecular changes in the heart's contractile proteins and activation system. This is especially likely to occur in response to pressure overload, as in systemic arterial hypertension or aortic stenosis, but also ensues when myocytes are lost from any mechanism.

Ultimately, myocardial failure (plus mechanical abnormalities that may be present) leads to a decrease in systolic pump function that is sufficient to produce pump failure. In most patients, significant dysfunction and failure of the myocardium occur long before the clinical syndrome of congestive heart failure becomes apparent.

## High-Output Failure

Some patients with high-output states or primary noncardiac circulatory overload may develop pulmonary congestion and edema secondary to an abnormal elevation of ventricular diastolic pressure at a time when the total cardiac output (systolic, or pump, function) and EF of the left ventricle are normal or even increased. The latter syndrome also can occur in conditions associated with an increase in blood volume from the accumulation of excess salt and water due to salt-retaining steroids, excess blood or fluid administration, acute glomerulonephritis, oliguria, or anuria. In other patients, it may occur with an abnormally increased venous return and/or decreased peripheral resistance, as might be seen in patients with arteriovenous fistulas, beriberi, hyperthyroidism, cirrhosis, severe anemia, and large vascular tumors. Under such conditions, the chronic volume and/or pressure overload on the ventricle eventually may lead to ventricular dilatation, functional mitral regurgitation (resulting from dilatation), and finally systolic failure. When symptoms of pulmonary congestion or pulmonary edema secondary to elevated diastolic pressure occur while the cardiac output is still normal or elevated, the syndrome is sometimes referred to as *high-output failure*.

High-output heart failure is rare in the United States. For example, to have high-output heart failure from chronic anemia, a hematocrit of about 13 percent (9 to16 percent) would typically be necessary.[33] However, this condition may be found in areas of the world where chronic parasite infestation can lead to severe, chronic anemia. As with low-output heart failure, patients with high-output heart failure have salt and water retention, reduced renal blood flow, and neuroendocrine activation.[33] A low concentration of hemoglobin in patients with anemia may lead to reduced ability to degrade nitric oxide (NO), leading to the vasodilation that is so typical of high-output heart failure. Low blood pressure may, in turn, activate neuroendocrine activity. Various conditions that increase cardiac output are depicted in Table 24-3.

TABLE 24-3 Conditions That Increase Cardiac Output

| | |
|---|---|
| Bacteremia/sepsis | Fibrous dysplasia (Albright's syndrome) |
| Anemia (acquired or congenital) | Renal disease (acute or chronic) |
| Hyperthyroidism | Hepatic disease |
| Beriberi | Environmental temperature extremes |
| Arteriovenous fistulas (acquired or congenital) | Polycythemia vera |
| Pregnancy | Carcinoid syndrome |
| Paget's disease | Dermatologic abnormalities |
| Hyperdynamic heart syndrome | Erythroderma syndrome |
| Arterial hypertension | Kaposi's sarcoma |

## Left and Right Heart Failure

*Left heart* (*left-sided*) *failure* and *right heart* (*right-sided*) *failure* are clinical terms for conditions in which the primary impairment is of the left side of the heart or of the right side of the heart, respectively. Since both sides of the heart are in a circuit, it is apparent that one side cannot pump significantly more blood than the other side for any length of time in the absence of abnormal shunts, communications, or regurgitation. Furthermore, experimentally produced failure of one ventricle may produce significant hemodynamic and biochemical abnormalities of the other ventricle, even without the usual hemodynamic manifestations of ventricular failure. Abnormal function of the left ventricle not only overloads the right ventricle from augmented pulmonary pressures but also may affect the right ventricle via the shared septum and the phenomenon of ventricular interdependence or interaction (see below). Altered elastic recoil of the left ventricle in diastole also may affect the right ventricle. Accordingly, when the pumping ability of one ventricle is primarily impaired, the output of the contralateral ventricle can be secondarily decreased; the biochemistry and hemodynamics of the contralateral ventricle also can be abnormal even in "pure" one-sided failure.

Right-sided heart failure commonly follows left-sided heart failure. In most situations, the expression *left-sided heart failure* is used clinically in reference to symptoms and signs of elevated pressure and congestion in the pulmonary veins and capillaries, whereas the term *right-sided heart failure* is used clinically in reference to symptoms and signs of elevated pressure and congestion in the systemic veins and capillaries. Actually, significant amounts of sodium and water retention, with subsequent peripheral edema formation, may occur with pure left-sided heart failure without hemodynamic evidence of right-sided heart failure. As noted previously, an increase in the diastolic pressure in either ventricle can increase the diastolic pressure or decrease the distensibility of the contralateral ventricle, especially if the pericardium is intact.

## Compensated Heart Failure

*Compensated heart failure* is that condition in which the symptoms of heart failure are relieved by therapy or compensatory mechanisms (Table 24-4), although the EDV and EDP often remain elevated and the EF reduced. The term *compensated heart failure* is frequently used in reference to patients with heart failure whose symptoms and signs of pulmonary or peripheral congestion have been relieved by therapy. In many such patients, reduced myocardial function and low cardiac output persist, as does an increased rate of death.

TABLE 24-4 Compensatory Mechanisms Initiated by Low Cardiac Output[a]

| Mechanism | Short-Term Adaptive Response | Long-Term Maladaptive Response |
|---|---|---|
| Salt and water retention | ⇑ Preload<br>⇑ Cardiac output[b] | Edema, anasarca, pulmonary congestion |
| Vasoconstriction | ⇑ Afterload<br>Maintained blood pressure | ⇓ Cardiac output, ⇑ ardiac energy expenditure<br>Cell death[b] |
| ⇑ Cardiac, adrenergic drive | ⇑ Contractility, ⇑ relaxation, ⇑ heart rate<br>⇑ Cardiac output[b] | Arrhythmias, ⇑ cardiac energy expenditure<br>Cell death[b] |
| Transcription factor activation, cell growth | Adaptive hypertrophy<br>⇑ Sarcomere number<br>⇑ Cardiac output[b] | Maladaptive hypertrophy<br>Apoptosis, mitochondrial DNA abnormalities<br>Cell death[b] |

[a]The compensatory mechanisms initiated by a short-term fall in cardiac output, as occurs following hemorrhage, generate an adaptive response. However, when sustained, as in the chronically over-loaded heart, these same mechanisms cause maladaptive responses that further reduce cardiac output, exacerbate symptoms, and appear to accelerate cell death.

[b]Secondary responses.

SOURCE: Adapted with permission from Katz AM.[31]

## MECHANISMS OF HEART FAILURE

Since virtually any form of heart disease can lead to heart failure, there can be no single causative mechanism. At the organ and the cellular level, there is likewise no single mechanism that is consistently operative. Identification of fundamental mechanisms remains an area of very active investigation (Table 24-5). Multiple alterations in organ and cellular physiology may contribute to heart failure under various circumstances and at different points in time. Adaptive processes occur that can adversely affect the myocardium, kidneys, smooth and skeletal muscles, endothelium, peripheral vasculature, and multiple reflex control mechanisms, adding to the complexity of the syndrome (Tables 24-6 and 24-7).

TABLE 24-5 Possible Mechanisms of Myocardial Failure

- Loss of myocytes
- Hypertrophy of remaining myocytes
- Energy production and utilization
  - Oxygen and energy supply
  - Substrate utilization and energy storage
  - Inadequate mitochondria mass and function
- Ventricular remodeling
- Contractile proteins
  - Abnormal myofibrillar or myosin ATPase
  - Abnormal myocardial proteins
  - Defective protein synthesis
  - Nonuniformity of contraction and function
- Activation of contractile elements
  - Membrane $Na^+,K^+$-ATPase defects
  - Abnormal sarcoplasmic reticulum function
    - Abnormal $Ca^{2+}$ release
    - Abnormal $Ca^{2+}$ uptake
- Abnormal myocardial receptor function
  - Downregulation of beta adrenoreceptors
  - Decreased $\beta_1$ receptors
  - Decreased $G_s$ protein
  - Increased $G_1$ protein
- Autonomic nervous system
  - Abnormal myocardial norepinephrine function or kinetics
  - Abnormal baroreceptor function
- Increased myocardial fibroblast growth and collagen synthesis
- Aging changes, presbycardia
- Sustained tachycardia
- Miscellaneous

TABLE 24-6 Compensatory Mechanisms in Heart Failure

- Autonomic nervous system
  - Heart
    - Increased heart rate
    - Increased myocardial contractile stimulation
    - Increased rate of relaxation
  - Peripheral circulation
    - Arterial vasoconstriction (increased afterload)
    - Venous vasoconstriction (increased preload)
- Kidney (renin-angiotensin-aldosterone)
  - Arterial vasoconstriction (increased afterload)
  - Venous vasconstriction (increased preload)
  - Sodium and water retention (increased preload and afterload)
  - Increased myocardial contractile stimulation
- Endothelin-1 (increased preload and afterload)
- Arginine vasopressin (increased preload and afterload)
- Atrial and brain natriuretic peptides (decreased afterload)
- Prostaglandins
- Peptides
- Frank-Starling law of the heart
  - Increased end-diastolic fiber length, volume, and pressure (increased preload)
- Hypertrophy
- Peripheral oxygen delivery
  - Redistribution of cardiac output
  - Altered oxygen-hemoglobin dissociation
  - Increased oxygen extraction by tissues
- Anaerobic metabolism

TABLE 24-7 Neurohormonal Changes in Heart Failure

Increased sympathetic nervous system activity (increased norepinephrine, epinephrine)
Increased endothelin
Increased arginine vasopressin
Increased renin and angiotensin II
Increased aldosterone
Increased neuropeptide Y
Increased atrial and B-type natriuretic peptides
Increased
- Insulin
- Cortisol
- Growth hormone [decreased insulin-like growth factor 1 (IGF-1)]
- Tumor necrosis factor $\alpha$ (TNF-$\alpha$)
- Interleukin-6
- Vasoactive intestinal peptide (VIP)
- Adrenomedullin
- Urodilantin
- Urotensin-II
- Cardiotropin-I

Increased dopamine
Increased prostaglandins ($PGI_2$, $PGE_2$)
Increased vasodilator peptides (e.g., bradykinin)

NOTE: Measurements in individual patients vary significantly and changes may not always be present.

The schema of the sequence of events in heart failure is daunting (Fig. 24-4). Distinguishing primary etiologic forces from secondary epiphenomena has been very difficult. Identification of the precise mechanisms whereby heart failure evolves and quantifying the contributions of individual components (e.g., apoptosis) have remained elusive. What triggers the early activation of the sympathetic nervous system and withdrawal of vagal tone or how spontaneous resolution of heart failure occurs remains unclear. Nevertheless, enough information has accrued to construct a reasonably coherent working hypothesis.

To understand heart failure, it is useful to think in terms of evolutionary theory.[34] The cell, the organ, and the organism each have evolved adaptive responses to offset hostile environments, thus allowing a survival advantage. In many cases, heart failure may begin as an acute injury to the heart, such as an acute myocardial infarction or severe inflammatory myocarditis. In other cases, there may be a phenotypically silent mutation that is finally expressed (perhaps due to environmental influences), leading to structural and functional perturbations of such magnitude that the heart eventually fails. Valvular heart disease may lead to unusual loading conditions, forcing the myocytes to adapt by increasing their size (hypertrophy). In essence, there is an *index* or *initial event* that in many cases is not clinically visible or may occur secondary to unknown toxins or an unusual mechanical load on the heart. The heart and its circulatory physiology must somehow "adapt" to this "hostile" new environment. Physiologic adaptations can become pathologic, in some instances enhancing and inducing progression of heart failure.

In response to increased load, whether created by increased pressure or loss of myocytes, hypertrophy occurs and tends to normalize the load per cell. With an increased volume load, myocytes elongate and to a small extent may undergo division.[35,36] Hyperplasia and apoptosis of myocytes occur with abnormal loading, but this involves less than 1 percent of the cardiac myocytes. Reprogramming of the cardiac myocytes occurs, resulting in a more fetal-like state. More B-type natriuretic peptide is synthesized. Metabolism begins to favor glucose over free fatty acids. The myocytes enlarge, presumably rendering a short-term structural and functional advantage.[37,38] The reprogramming requires altered signals, both mechanical and "chemical," to reach the nucleus of the cardiac myocyte in order to set into motion "new" gene transcription.[39] Contractile proteins are altered and gain an economic advantage. Ultimately, there is a transition from hypertrophy to heart failure,[40] which has been recognized for more than 100 years but is still not well understood.[32] In a sense, this "unnatural growth response" of myocyte hypertrophy leads to the structural changes of LV remodeling, thus creating a large, dilated, and poorly functioning heart. The processes of cellular remodeling and subsequent architectural changes in cell and chamber size as well as shape are highly complex[39] and include many components other than myocardial cell hypertrophy. Myocardial fibrosis and cell dropout occurs and perhaps also myocyte slippage, thus increasing dilatation. As cardiac output falls, multiple neurohormones, including renin and norepinephrine, are released in order to protect blood pressure and organ perfusion,[41] while atavistic counterregulatory natriuretic peptides are released so as to offset vasoconstriction, hypertrophy, and volume conservation.[42] The story is undoubtedly much more complex than this[43] and includes a myriad of molecular mechanisms,[39,44] some of which primarily affect the cardiac interstitium and others the cardiac myocytes. The pathophysiologic changes observed in heart failure are partially depicted in Table 24-6 and Fig. 24-5.

Maladaptive remodeling of cardiac myocyte size and shape begins long before the onset of clinical heart failure.[45–48] Alterations in myocyte proteins and mitochondrial size and as well as changes in myocardial interstitium and collagen content/architecture are seen in response to a variety of "injuries," including pressure overload,[49–51] volume overload,[52] and myocardial ischemia.[53,54] Additional phenotypic changes in heart failure include apoptosis[55,56] and possibly side-to-side slippage of myocytes.[57] It is important to recognize that much of the neuroendocrine activation that occurs in a primordial attempt to conserve organ perfusion appears to facilitate this myriad of pathologic changes in the heart at the cellular level,[41] thereby possibly contributing to the success of neuroendocrine blockers as therapy for heart failure. Last, there is no single phenotypic change, protein expression, or signal-transduction pathway that is dominant. Rather, there is extraordinary redundancy in these mechanisms. This observation has important implications for therapy. For example, blocking of one neuroendocrine system may lead to enhanced overactivity of other neuroendocrine systems. Blocking of one signal-transduction pathway may lead the cell to hypertrophy through alternative pathways. Thus it is likely that polypharmacy will always be necessary in the treatment of heart failure.

In summary, heart failure often begins with an index event that results in loss of myocardium (e.g., acute myocardial infarction) or excessive overload (e.g., valvular heart disease, acute myocardial infarction, mutation leading to dilated or hypertrophic cardiomyopathy, etc.). Where hypertrophy cannot sustain the increased load, ventricular dilatation occurs, and the ventricle assumes a more globular shape (i.e., eccentric hypertrophy), thus allowing for maintenance of stroke volume despite a reduced EF. This provides short-term benefit. Absence of some dilatation probably would lead to shock and early death. Neuroendocrine activation presumably occurs in response to a perceived need to protect perfusion pressure and circulating volume, but neurohormones also facilitate the LV remodeling process, thus contributing importantly to the pathogenesis and progression of heart

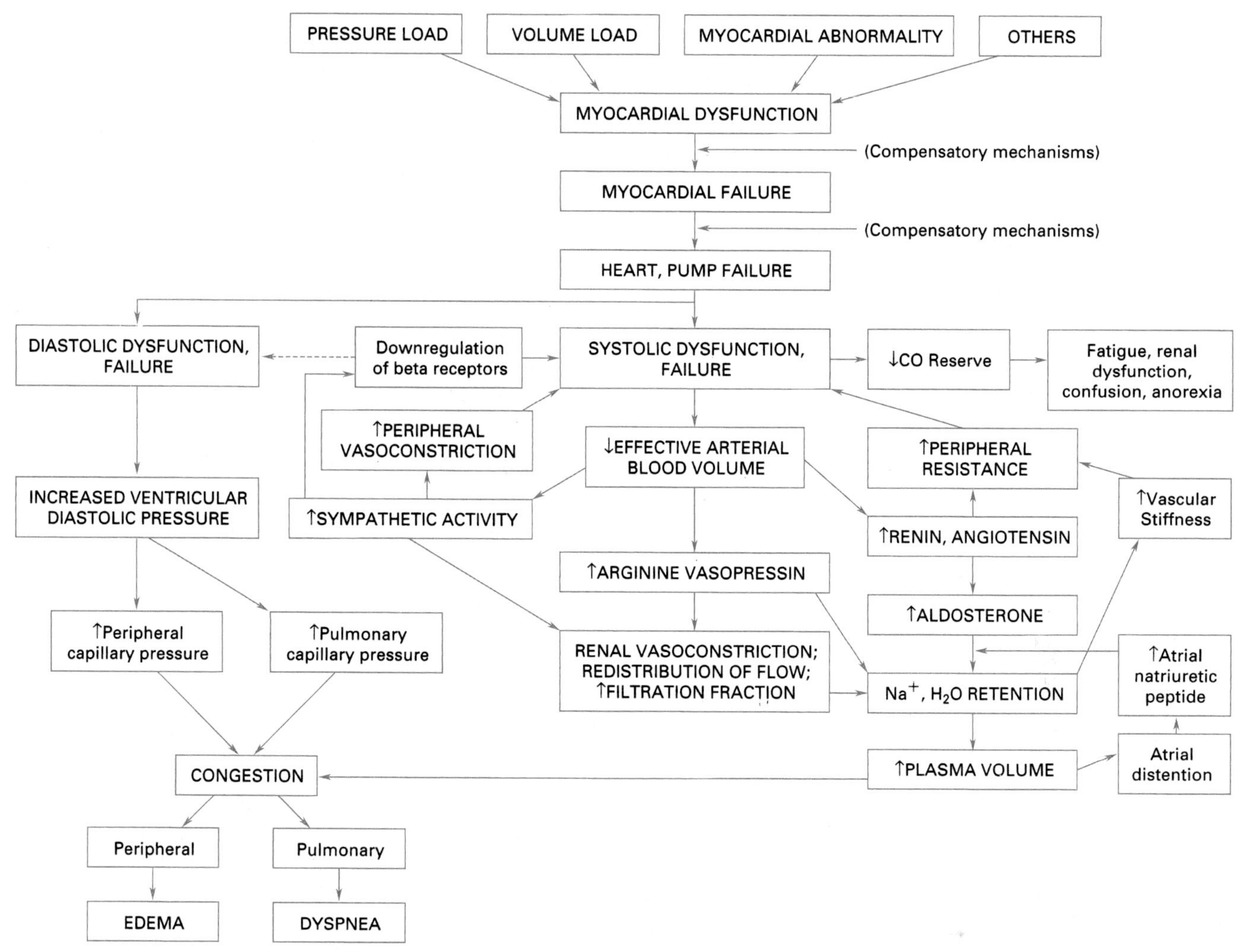


FIGURE 24-4 Schema of the sequence of events in heart failure. An increased load or myocardial abnormality leads to myocardial failure and eventually to heart failure. This results in increased sympathetic activity; increased levels of renin, angiotensin II, and aldosterone; pulmonary and peripheral congestion and edema; and decreased cardiac output reserve. Endothelial dysfunction also occurs, with decreased endothelium-dependent vasodilatation and with increased plasma levels of endothelin-1, a very strong vasoconstrictor. See text for details.

failure. Despite the presumed coherence of this oversimplified working hypothesis, many gaps in our knowledge remain to be filled in, particularly with regard to the quantitative contribution that each phenotypic change makes toward the progression of heart failure. Moreover, matching the genotype change to the phenotype change in dilated cardiomyopathy has been a daunting task.[58,59]

## Molecular, Physiologic, and Biochemical Alterations Occurring with Hypertrophy and the Progression to Heart Failure

In the failing heart, alterations are found in numerous contractile proteins, especially in heredity-based idiopathic dilated cardiomyopathies. In the latter situation, these alterations can interact with the environment (e.g., abnormal loading condition) to cause heart failure. Such alterations have been found in the cytoskeleton, myosin, troponin T, and actin and likely contribute to diminished myocardial performance. Findings in animal models of overload-produced heart failure may vary from model to model, and observations made in human failing hearts may be different from those made in animal models. Many changes in gene expression at the mRNA or protein level have been found in human failing hearts harvested at the time of cardiac transplantation. However, these are often hearts with end-stage myocardial disease in which many factors (such as receiving multiple inotropic drugs) may obscure pathogenesis. Despite these caveats, we have learned much from such studies, only some of which are discussed here.

### β-MYOSIN HEAVY CHAIN

Two myosin heavy-chain (MHC) isoforms are present in mammalian heart, α- and β-MHC. The α-MHC is cardiac-specific and is more enzymatically active. The less active β-MHC is present in heart and also in slow-twitch skeletal muscle. The distribution of α- and β-MHC is developmentally and hormonally regulated. Mechanical stress, such as pressure overload, induces a transition of α- to β-MHC in the ventricles of experimental animals, thus imparting a slower but more economical type of work for the overloaded heart. Either way, myosin remains the principal structural and contractile

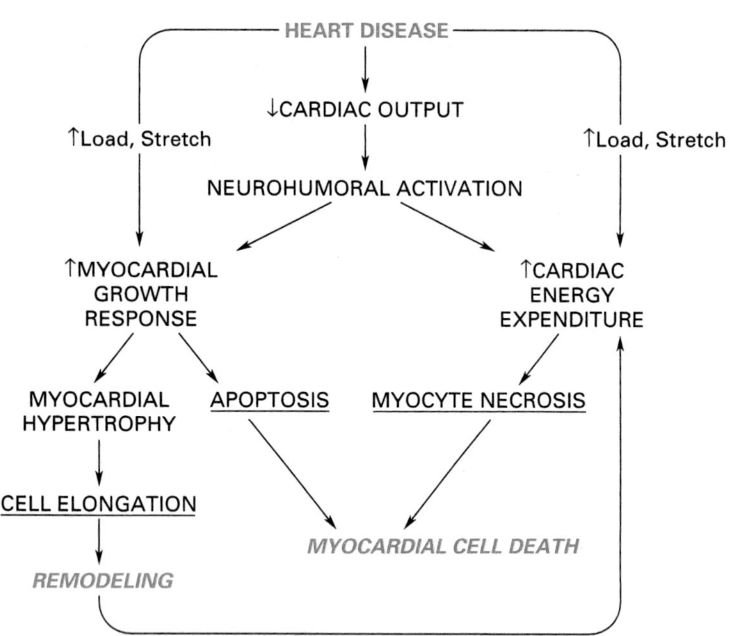


FIGURE 24-5 Possible mechanisms by which overloading can cause progressive deterioration of the heart ("cardiomyopathy of overload"). Several mechanisms, including myocyte stretch, activate a growth response that initiates myocardial hypertrophy in the overloaded heart (*left*). The same growth response may also activate signal transduction systems that cause programmed cell death (apoptosis). The hypertrophic response to overload, by causing sarcomeres to be added in series, can also lead to cell elongation and so accelerate remodeling; the resulting increase in wall tension, along with the overload itself (*right*), increases cardiac energy expenditure that, in the overloaded heart, can accelerate myocyte necrosis. Reduced cardiac output activates neurohumoral responses (*center*), which, by increasing afterload and $\beta$-adrenergic stimulation of the heart, also increase cardiac energy expenditure. Because many mediators of the neurohumoral response to a fall in cardiac output promote myocardial cell growth, neurohumoral activation can also accelerate both apoptosis and remodeling.

unit of muscle fiber. Lowes et al.[60] have demonstrated downregulation of $\alpha$-MHC and upregulation of $\beta$-MHC using mRNA measurements from right ventricular endomyocardial biopsies from nonfailing hearts and failing human hearts. This alteration, if translated into protein expression, would decrease myosin ATPase enzyme velocity and slow the speed of contraction. Although such adaptive changes could be viewed to have an "economical" survival advantage in the face of increased load, slower contraction and relaxation could contribute to diastolic dysfunction. Moreover, the extent of this phenomenon in humans is unclear and controversial.

## SARCOPLASMIC RETICULUM FUNCTION

The basic mechanism of cardiac excitation-contraction coupling involves calcium ($Ca^{2+}$) entry from the extracellular fluid via the voltage-dependent L-type calcium channel to produce a trigger in increasing $[Ca^{2+}]_i$ and opening of the intracellular sarcoplasmic reticulum (SR) $Ca^{2+}$ release channel or "ryanodine receptor" (RyR).[61] There is substantial evidence that defects in sarcolemmal $Ca^{2+}$ uptake (sarcolemmal transport via $Na^+$,$K^+$-ATPase) and release by the SR are present in heart failure, especially at later stages.[62–64] Alternatively, uptake of calcium by the SR may remain intact.[65] These alterations in calcium transport may be secondary to quantitative alterations of gene expression of SR calcium transport proteins, especially the sarco(endo)plasmic reticulum $Ca^{2+}$-ATPase (SERCA)[66] and phospholamban,[67] a reversible inhibitor of cardiac SR $Ca^{2+}$-ATPase activity. Other calcium cycling proteins, such as $Na^+$-$Ca^{2+}$ exchanger proteins,[68] may also be altered in heart failure. Phosphokinase A hyperphosphorylation of RyR has recently been shown to alter calcium signaling from the SR by depleting calcium stores and reducing calcium transients that may impair contractility in the failing myocardium.[69,70] Several of these alterations may occur concurrently, and results may vary from model to model and may not always be relative to failing human hearts. Nevertheless, it is likely that heart failure is characterized by reduced myofilament activation and decreased calcium available for activation as well as heightened cytosolar calcium levels in diastole. Some studies have shown increased myofibrillar calcium sensitivity[71] and altered calcium kinetics.[72] These abnormalities of calcium metabolism may be of primary importance in some types of heart failure and secondary or epiphenomenal in other types. Most abnormalities of myocardial contractile activation have been demonstrated only in the late stages of heart failure and therefore may be the result of maladaptive hypertrophy rather than a primary cause of ventricular dysfunction.

## FORCE-FREQUENCY RESPONSE IN HEART FAILURE

The failing human myocardium is characterized by an abnormal force-frequency response that parallels the severity of heart failure. Normally, an increase in frequency of stimulation is accompanied by an increased rate of force development, a decrease duration of contraction, and an enhanced rate of relaxation, thereby increasing the force of contraction (Bowditch effect). This tends to preserve or increase contractile force while preserving diastolic time. The latter effect is important in the tachycardic intact heart in preserving time in diastole to prevent ventricular filling and coronary blood flow.[72] In isolated failing heart muscle, an increase in heart rate has been accompanied by a decrease in myocardial performance.[72] Some impairment of systolic function in response to increased heart rate may also be related to impaired LV filling, although a negative inotropic effect, as shown in isolated muscle, has been related to alterations in intracellular $Ca^{2+}$ handling.[72] A reduced force of contraction and lack of shortening of contractile activity may contribute importantly to impairment of cardiac function during exercise.[73,74]

## ENERGY PRODUCTION AND USE

Oxygen deprivation, which is most often due to coronary artery disease, results in impaired relaxation and weakened contraction, as may be seen in angina pectoris. When transient, these are readily reversible. With prolonged ischemia, decreased contraction (dyskinesis) may persist for hours beyond return of blood flow (stunning). If coronary blood flow is chronically reduced, myocardium may fail to contract normally (hibernation), even if necrosis does not ensue. With more serious loss of flow, infarction can occur. All these stages may produce substantial dyskinesia, and the remaining myocardium must sustain this load. The result is hypertrophy of the nonischemic portion of the ventricle; if this is inadequate, an increase in ventricular volume occurs using the Frank-Starling mechanism to sustain stroke volume. Whether there is a limitation of energy supply or its utilization in the failing myocardium remains controversial.

In patients with heart failure, the total oxygen requirement of the heart may be increased significantly because of the increased total mass, the increase in myocardial systolic wall tension due to the Laplace relationship, and perhaps some wasted contractile energy. This increase may result in the extraction of a greater amount of oxygen from each unit of coronary blood flow and a widening of the coronary arteriovenous oxygen difference. Many patients with heart failure are able to increase coronary blood flow during exercise; however, some patients with a dilated ventricle that increases in diameter during exercise may have a further widening of the coronary arteriovenous oxygen difference during exercise and a decrease in coronary blood flow reserve (see Chaps. 4 and 46). In the presence of severe LV hypertrophy, coronary blood flow per unit mass of myocardium is usually normal at rest. On the other hand, the capacity of the coronary vascular bed to dilate during reactive hyperemia, which is normally four- to fivefold, is reduced. In the presence of severe hypertrophy where filling pressures are elevated, tachycardia, such as may occur with atrial fibrillation, may reduce diastolic coronary perfusion, producing ischemic ventricular failure. While reduced perfusion is probably common in end-stage heart failure, a deficit in coronary blood flow or oxygen delivery has not been clearly demonstrated to be a primary cause of heart failure associated with hypertrophy except in the presence of obstructive coronary disease (see below).

## SUBSTRATE USE AND ENERGY STORAGE

Although the myocardial uptake of fatty acids and glucose per 100 g of myocardium is normal in heart failure,[75] there is conflicting evidence on whether or not there is a primary decrease in energy liberation by mitochondrial oxidative phosphorylation.[31,32,75–79] The reductions in stores of myocardial high-energy phosphate, creatine phosphate, and/or adenosine triphosphate (ATP) generally found in heart failure usually are thought to be secondary and to be the consequence of the failure rather than the primary cause of the failure.[75–84] There may also be reduced levels of creatine kinase and changes in the isoenzymes of creatine kinase in heart failure.[84]

The major consequences of the state of energy starvation that are probably seen in many or most failing hearts are due to attenuation of important allosteric (regulatory) effects of ATP rather than reduction in the supply of substrate for the many energy-consuming reactions involved in contraction, relaxation, and excitation-contraction coupling. By facilitating the many calcium fluxes involved in excitation-contraction coupling and relaxation, these allosteric effects of ATP exert both inotropic and lusitropic effects.[79]

## MITOCHONDRIAL MASS AND FUNCTION

There are conflicting data on whether or not there is a significant decrease in the mass of mitochondria relative to the mass of myofibrils that occurs in experimental cardiac hypertrophy.[82–84] It is possible that this is one of the limitations of severe hypertrophy. Defects in mitochondrial oxidative phosphorylation and mitochondrial calcium metabolism may also be associated with myocardial failure.[85] Except in circumstances where coronary flow is limited, as with large vessel obstructive disease (see Chap. 57) or purported microvascular obstructive or vasospastic disease, a primary role of energy limitation in the evolution of heart failure has yet to be demonstrated.[76] It is possible that it may play a role during periods of higher metabolic demand, such as tachycardia,[78] as noted previously.[86,87]

## VENTRICULAR REMODELING (HYPERTROPHY AND DILATATION)

When one portion of the ventricle is disabled, an increase in intraventricular volume slowly occurs. This involves increased myocyte length, with the limit being at the level of the sarcomere at 2.2 $\mu$m. With systolic overload, compensatory hypertrophy occurs with the addition of sarcomeres in parallel, leading to a lateral thickening of the myocyte while sarcomere length does not change.

Acute dilatation is also limited by the sarcomere, which at 2.2 $\mu$m attains maximum force. Beyond this point, stiffness of the sarcomere and the myocardium becomes very large and resting tension rises to high levels. Such acute dilatation may lead to relative "side to side" slippage of myocytes. When distending forces become chronic, the addition of new sarcomeres occurs in series. Dilatation of the ventricle also adds to the load by the Laplace relation. Tension in the wall rises with increased volume at the same pressure. This results in some lateral growth of myocytes, although elongation is the major alteration. In addition, functional mitral regurgitation may result from excessive ventricular volume, and this adds to the volume overload. When increased systolic tension occurs, myocyte hypertrophy due to the laying down of sarcomeres in parallel is accomplished by biochemical alterations in both the contractile proteins and activating membrane systems (see Chap. 6). The regulation of sarcomere assembly is not well understood, but clearly mechanical forces must be sensed that, in turn, alter gene transcription via complex stretch-activated pathways.[88]

In addition to the synthesis of sarcomeres in series with preexisting sarcomeres, "slippage" of myofibrils and myocardial fibers and rearrangement of myocardial fibers along cleavage planes of the left ventricle may occur.[57] Thus, although overstretch of sarcomeres may rarely be present very transiently, it does not appear to be an important primary mechanism of chronic heart failure. There is evidence, however, that excessive stretch of myocytes can lead to myocyte death, apparently by the process of apoptosis (programmed cell death), which may lead to further heart failure.[55,89] The effects of the law of Laplace with ventricular dilatation were noted earlier. Nonuniformity of myocardial contraction and functional mitral regurgitation also contribute to heart failure. The discoordinated contraction is particularly troublesome for patients with underlying cardiac dysfunction. Resynchronization by pacing the left ventricle improves mechanoenergetic efficiency and systolic function and reduces systolic wall stress (see Chap. 27).[90,91]

## MYOCARDIAL RECEPTOR FUNCTION

One of the hallmarks of heart failure is a decreased response to inotropic stimuli. Although no single mechanism accounts for this, reduction in myocardial $\beta$-adrenergic receptors and its subsequent second messenger cAMP may play an important role.[92] $\beta$-Adrenergic stimulation contributes importantly to the cardiac response to exercise,[93] and $\beta$-adrenergic desensitization and uncoupling may be at least partially responsible for the reduced chronotropic and inotropic response to peak exercise commonly found in patients with heart failure.[93] The $\beta$-adrenergic receptor abnormalities in heart failure appear to be due to desensitization and uncoupling of the $\beta_1$ receptor produced by local and not systemic alterations in catecholamines.[94] In severe heart failure, the norepinephrine (NE) stores in sympathetic nerve endings are depleted. In a sense, the failing myocardium becomes functionally denervated. cAMP responses are reduced by about 30 to 35 percent, leading to further contractile dysfunction.[81] Despite downregulation of the $\beta_1$ receptor, a relatively high proportion of $\beta_2$ receptors remain to mediate chronotropic and inotropic responses.[95] However, there is some uncoupling of the $\beta_2$ receptor from its G protein and a modest upregulation of the $G_{\alpha i}$ subunit, further contributing to a depressed response to chronotropic and inotropic stimuli.[96–98] There is also a profound decrease in cardiac $\beta$-adrenergic responsiveness with aging,[99] which has clinical implications because heart failure is heavily concentrated in the aging population.

The desensitization and uncoupling of $\beta$-adrenergic receptors occurs early, with mild to moderate ventricular dysfunction. It is related to the degree of heart failure and is associated with a very reduced response to $\beta$-adrenergic stimulation with drugs such as dobutamine.[100] Long-term stimulation of $\beta$-adrenergic receptors may enhance myocardial $\beta$-adrenergic receptor kinase ($\beta$-ARK) activity,[101] leading to further desensitization and uncoupling of the $\beta$-adrenergic receptor.

Of some interest, $\beta$-adrenergic blockade with metoprolol, a relatively cardioselective $\beta_1$ blocker, upregulates the $\beta_1$ receptor, whereas carvedilol, a nonselective $\beta_1$ and $\beta_2$ blocker with additional $\alpha_1$ blocking activity, does not increase $\beta_1$ receptor density.[102] Both drugs can improve LV function substantially. The improvement in cardiac function seen with chronic $\beta$-blocker use may not be due to upregulation of $\beta$-adrenergic receptors, and the beneficial effects of $\beta$-adrenergic receptor blockade in heart failure remains unexplained. Moreover, high plasma norepinephrine levels do not predict benefit from carvedilol,[103] suggesting that there is not a simple relation between activation of the sympathetic nervous system and response to $\beta$-adrenergic blocking drugs in patients with heart failure.

### AUTONOMIC NERVOUS SYSTEM DYSFUNCTION

Heart failure is characterized by many abnormal reflex control mechanisms. Peripheral vascular resistance is increased, there is defective cardiac parasympathetic control,[104] an abnormal response to upright tilt,[105] altered baroreceptor function,[106–109] and reduced cardiac sympathetic activity in response to a variety of stimuli.[110–112] Indeed, an early sign of heart failure is increased sympathetic tone accompanied by reduced vagal tone, resulting in an increased heart rate even at rest.

An increase in systemic vascular resistance is generally observed in well-established heart failure. It is likely due to a combination of locally active heightened vasoconstrictors (norepinephrine, angiotensin II, endothelin, vasopressin, neuropeptide Y) and to structural changes in blood vessels from fluid retention and reduced endothelium-dependent vasodilation. Early in heart failure there may be a fall in cardiac output, arterial pressure, and baroreceptor activity, leading to an "adaptive" increase in excessive neuroendocrine drive. The sympathetic nervous system is activated early, followed by the renin-angiotensin-aldosterone system (RAAS). Arginine vasopressin is released. Sodium and water retention occur, hypervolemia restores cardiac output and arterial pressure, and neuroendocrine activity may reach a steady state. However, as heart failure progresses, there is impaired cardiosensory activity that fails to reduce neuroendocrine drive. For unclear reasons, cardiac afferent activity to the central nervous system is reduced, leading to unhindered, efferent excitatory responses from the brain to the periphery. Reflex vasoconstrictor responses to unloading the heart are paradoxically blunted.[105,112] There are abnormal vascular responses to postural change.[113] Some of these changes lead to the alterations in regional blood flow that accompany heart failure.[114] Parasympathetic (vagal) tone is decreased and heart rate variability is markedly reduced, a hallmark of congestive failure. Further, decreased heart rate variability may provide independent prognostic value in the identification of patients at risk for premature death.[115]

Although the genesis of these abnormal reflex control mechanisms is *poorly* understood, the changes may be more functional than structural. Heart transplantation reverses cardiopulmonary baroreflex control mechanisms to some extent,[116,117] but this is inconsistent.[118,119] The role that abnormal reflex control mechanisms play in the progression of heart failure, like other neuroendocrine alterations, has been difficult to quantitate. Nevertheless, it is now increasingly clear that the sympathetic nervous system and the RAAS greatly influence the progression and natural history of heart failure. The therapeutic implications derived from these observations have proven to be very important.[120,121]

## MECHANICAL AND HEMODYNAMIC FEATURES OF HEART FAILURE

The term *heart failure* implies structural heart disease, and the central problem of heart failure remains impaired cardiac performance, although many of the secondary "adaptive" responses become maladaptive and contribute substantially to progression of heart failure. An understanding of how these changes occur can provide insight into the pathophysiology of the syndrome.

As ventricular function becomes impaired, the Frank-Starling law of the heart becomes operative (see Fig. 24-2). Inadequate emptying of the ventricle leads to increased EDVs. This is referred to as *increased preload,* and it produces an increase in SV during the next contraction. The Frank-Starling law simply states that the increase in contractile force (i.e., contractility) is related to sarcomere lengthening (up to 2.2 $\mu$m). For any given amount of $Ca^{2+}$ released into the myocyte, there is increased cross-bridge formation and enhanced sensitivity of the myofilament to $Ca^{2+}$ as the sarcomeres lengthen.

In the failing ventricle, the extent of shortening for a given diastolic fiber length and load (afterload) is reduced. The ventricle can maintain a normal or near-normal SV with an increased EDV and thus maintain end-diastolic fiber length for a period of time. Eventually, the filling pressure rises inordinately, limiting this compensation (see Fig. 24-1). Further, the clinically dilated ventricle tends to "give," like an overstretched elastic band, and end-diastolic volume may increase somewhat with no increase in LV end-diastolic pressure, reflecting a shift in the passive pressure-volume curve to the right. An obligatory reduction in EF occurs when SV is maintained in the face of a large EDV (EF = SV/EDV; normal EF = 0.62 + 0.12). Eventually, further increases in EDP produce little change in EDV, thus flattening the SV-EDP curve (see Fig. 24-1). There is no true descending limb to Starling curve because increasing preload indefinitely will ultimately lead to mitral regurgitation.[122,123] As the heart dilates, the increase in wall stress according to the Laplace relationship also will increase afterload, which may account for any observed reduction in SV as the heart dilates further (i.e., the perception of a descending limb). It is important to keep in mind that LV performance depends not only on systolic pump function but also on active relaxation, diastolic elastic recoil, passive diastolic properties, and vascular loading conditions. It is likely that at high LV end-diastolic pressure, valvular incompetence (mitral regurgitation) is a major cause of a decrease in cardiac output. Thus, in end-stage heart failure in the intact circulation, the Starling curve flattens out. It is possible under certain experimental conditions that the severely failing heart is able to utilize the Frank-Starling mechanism,[124] but a hallmark of heart failure is the inability of the chamber to respond robustly to an increase in preload.

### Afterload and the Concept of the Laplace Relation

A characteristic feature of the dilated, failing heart is that it gradually becomes less sensitive to preload (EDV and fiber length) and more sensitive to afterload stress. At very high LV filling pressures (>30 mmHg) when the sarcomeres are fully extended and the preload reserve is exhausted, the SV becomes exquisitely sensitive to alterations in the afterload.[125] The impedance to ejection includes blood viscosity, vascular resistance, vascular distensibility, and myocardial wall tension. The afterload is the total load that the heart must work against during contraction. Much of the afterload is made up of ventricular myocardial wall tension. In the ventricle, the tension on the walls increases as ventricular chamber volume increases, even if intraventricular pressure remains constant. As the ventricle empties, tension is reduced even as pressure rises. Calculations of myocardial wall tension are defined by the Laplace equation and are expressed in terms of tension $T$ per unit of cross-sectional area (dynes per centimeter).

Within a cylinder, the law of Laplace states that wall tension is equal to the pressure within the cylinder times the radius of curvature of the wall:

$$T = P \times R$$

where $T$ is wall tension (dyn/cm), $P$ is pressure (dyn/cm$^2$), and $R$ is the radius (cm). Basically, wall tension is proportional to radius. Because the heart has thick ventricular walls, wall tension is distributed over a large number of muscle fibers, thereby reducing tension on each. The equation for a thick-walled cylinder such as the heart is as follows:

$$T = (P \times R)/h$$

where $h$ is wall thickness. The equation is sometimes stated as

$$T = \frac{P \times R}{2\,h}$$

Since the geometry of a ventricle is more complex than that of a cylinder, ventricular wall tension cannot be measured with precision. Wall stress, the force distributed across an area, is actually more correct but is seldom measured.

Two fundamental principles stem from the relationship between the geometry of the ventricular cavity and the tension on its muscular walls:

1. *Dilation of the ventricles leads directly to an increase in tension on each muscle fiber.*
2. *An increase in wall thickness reduces the tension on any individual muscle fiber. Therefore, ventricular hypertrophy reduces afterload by distributing tension among more muscle fibers.*

The wall tension is highest in the inner surface of the heart. The endocardial surfaces must do more work and therefore are also more vulnerable to reductions in coronary blood flow. Dilatation of the heart decreases cardiac efficiency unless hypertrophy is sufficient to normalize wall stress. In heart failure, wall tension (or stress) is high; thus afterload is increased. The energetic consequences of the law of Laplace may have some role in progressive deterioration of energy-starved cardiac myocytes in the failing heart.

Another major disadvantage of the dilated ventricle is the inability to decrease the average radius during contraction. In the normal heart, wall tension falls during ventricular ejection as the volume decreases, even though pressure is rising. In heart failure, given the dilated heart with reduced ejection, the average tension in the myocardial fibers actually may continue to increase from the beginning of the ejection until peak systolic pressure is reached,[126–128] adding additional afterload during ejection. The rate of myocardial fiber shortening is reduced, further contributing to diminished myocardial performance. It is difficult to overstate the importance of the law of Laplace in considering the syndrome of heart failure. This contrast is apparent in mitral insufficiency. With preserved contractility and a relatively small EDV, mitral insufficiency leads to rapid unloading of volume and reduced tension. When ventricular dilatation occurs with decreased ventricular contractility, ejection is reduced and tension remains high during systole, leading to an unsteady state that cannot be maintained for long.

Ventricular dilatation, though initially adaptive as an attempt to sustain SV, eventually becomes a substantial disadvantage and contributes importantly to impaired myocardial performance. As the left and right ventricles dilate, functional mitral and tricuspid regurgitation can occur, adding to circulatory congestion. Stretched myocardial cells can induce programmed cell death (apoptosis), thereby contributing to further disease progression.[129] Any treatment that slows progressive dilatation of the heart, such as the use of ACE inhibitors or $\beta$-adrenergic blockers, will likely have a powerful role in the treatment of heart failure. The plasticity of the process of progressive dilatation is now more apparent, with remarkable reversal of dilatation observed under specific circumstances, as due to the action of ACE inhibitors and $\beta$-adrenergic blockers, cessation of alcohol use in patients with alcoholic cardiomyopathy, and spontaneous improvement in patients with inflammatory myocarditis.

## Myocardial Hypertrophy

Hypertrophy of myocardial myocytes occurs to meet the demand of increased rate of use of mechanical energy. It is basically a response to sustained hemodynamic overloading of the heart, be it a volume or pressure overload or a combination of the two. Ischemic heart disease leads to a reduction of contractile tissue, ventricular dilatation, and a volume overload on the remaining viable myocytes. In this sense, it is a form of volume overload hypertrophy. Up to a point, the increased mass of cardiac muscle is beneficial in terms of normalizing wall stress and providing for a larger number of contractile elements (sarcomeres).

The heart demonstrates remarkable plasticity in response to a variety of growth factors and hemodynamic loads.[39] Isolated cell deformation is a sufficient stimulus for the induction of hypertrophic growth, but the modulating role of angiotensin II, norepinephrine, altered membrane ion channels, and numerous growth factors is of obvious importance. Changing loading conditions appear to be the primary driving force behind myocardial hypertrophy in heart failure, and other factors likely act as modulators or facilitators of the process. Hyperplasia, or an increase in new myocardial cells, may occur to some extent under conditions of excessive loading or myocyte loss.[130,131] However, the capacity for new cardiac myocytes to form is limited, and whether they are functionally useful is unknown. Rather, the primary response to altered load is the assembly of new working units or sarcomeres per myocardial cell. In general, pressure overload results in replication of sarcomeres in parallel, whereas volume overload leads to new sarcomeres both in parallel and in series.[132] There is hyperplasia of fibroblasts,[117,133–139] which outnumber cardiac myocytes by 3 : 1 to 4 : 1. It is the fibroblasts that are the major source of the reparative and replacement collagen when myocytes are lost in the evolution of heart failure.

Of course, other changes in the myocardium are occurring simultaneously, and hypertrophy is only one important factor. Biochemical changes, phenotypic changes in protein synthesis, altered excitation-contraction, slower velocity of shortening due to a slower myosin, and reduced $\beta$-adrenergic receptor density are all occurring simultaneously. Reduced velocity of contraction, delayed time to peak tension, and slower relaxation are observed in the myocardium of failing hearts. All these factors likely converge to produce clinical decompensation. Delayed ventricular relaxation may limit filling, leading to heightened filling pressure, pulmonary congestion, and shortness of breath. Force development and shortening capacity remain intact in the face of hypertrophy, and only in very late failure does contractility or contractile force decline. What ultimately happens to the patient may depend on the acuteness or chronicity of the load, the extent of hypertrophy and fibrosis, the amount of myocyte loss, the heart rate synchrony of atrioventricular contraction, and a host of invisible perturbations occurring at the level of the cell (Fig. 24-6).

## Diastolic Heart Failure

Diastolic heart failure is often present when there is limitation of exercise tolerance and dyspnea that cannot be explained by lung disease or the extent of underlying LV systolic dysfunction. Diastole is usually divided into several mechanical phases (Fig. 24-7). Investigation of patients with heart failure and normal systolic function, usually by echocardiography, often indicates LV hypertrophy and abnormal diastolic function, with concomitant left atrial enlargement. However, there is no agreement as to what constitutes abnormal diastolic function. Disturbances include alterations in relaxation (reduced rate of decline in wall tension), an upward shift of the LV diastolic pressure-volume relationship (a decrease in LV diastolic distensibility) (see Fig. 24-1), discoordinate wall motion during isovolumic relaxation, and altered ventricular inflow velocity. These measurements are influenced by loading conditions, ischemia, heart rate, and age, making it difficult to determine the actual contribution of diastolic dysfunction to heart failure. This is why some prefer the phrase "heart failure with intact or normal systolic function." Nevertheless, disturbances in diastolic function are common in patients with heart failure and are multifactorial. Diastolic impairment is frequently symptomatic in patients with LV hypertrophy, coronary artery disease, and diabetes mellitus. There also may be impairment of diastolic function due to an infiltrative process such as amyloid or restrictive cardiomyopathy. For any given EDV, there is often a higher LV end-diastolic pressure, indicating increased chamber stiffness and a smaller cavity size.

As the population ages, one can expect to see more diastolic heart failure.[140] With atrial dilatation, atrial fibrillation may develop, resulting in reduced diastolic ventricular filling time and resultant acute pulmonary edema in such patients. Although not as lethal as heart failure with a reduced EF, the prognosis of diastolic heart failure is poor. Diastolic abnormalities usually coexist with alterations in systolic function in patients with dilated cardiomyopathy.[141] The recognition, evaluation, and treatment of diastolic heart failure remain an obvious challenge,[142,143] but diastolic heart failure is an important component of the syndrome of heart failure and must be considered by all who care for patients with heart failure.

## Hibernating and Stunned Myocardium

There is now a considerable body of evidence indicating that the myocardium can adapt its activity successfully to prevailing energetic circumstances.[144,145] *Hibernating* myocardium is a condition of reduced myocardial blood flow and impaired myocardial function that improves with revascularization. Myocardial *stunning* is the mechanical dysfunction that persists after reperfusion despite the absence of irreversible damage. Hibernation is particularly important to recognize, diagnose, and treat because revascularization may be associated with a lower cardiovascular event rate.[146] The most commonly used tests for diagnosing hibernating myocardium are dobutamine echocardiography, thallium and sestamibi single-photon-emission computed tomographic (SPECT) myocardial perfusion imaging, positron-emission tomography (PET), and magnetic resonance imaging (MRI) with gadolinium (see Chaps. 19, 21–23). Essentially, these imaging techniques are used to define myocardial viability.[147] Many large referral centers have developed their preferred method of assessment. LV function often improves or normalizes with revascularization when there is a "significant" amount of hibernating but viable myocardium as the major cause of LV dysfunction. When hibernating myocardium is documented, revascularization rather than heart transplantation is the appropriate therapy provided that the coronary arteries are suitable for revascularization.

The precise mechanism of hibernating myocardium has not been determined. It is as though the heart downgrades its myocardial function so that blood flow and function are once again in equilibrium. It seems likely that the heart can adapt to chronically low myocardial blood flow and that a new steady state between perfusion and contraction can be achieved and maintained. The pathophysiology is undoubtedly highly complex and is accompanied by phenotypic changes and morphologic alterations.[148] Hibernating myocardium appears to represent a precarious though reversible state, and failure to revascularize may lead to an increased rate of adverse events and a poor prognosis. Hibernating myocardium may also be the end result of repetitive myocardial stunning, perpetuated by renewed episodes of ischemia.

## The Cardiac Interstitium

Collagen and the interstitium are normally in a steady state but increase during hypertrophy and following loss of myocytes due to myocardial injury. In heart failure, the interstitial space includes reparative and interstitial fibrosis. Contrary to previous concepts, the interstitium is a very dynamic structure, with both matrix removal and synthesis occurring simultaneously. Connective tissue remodeling, either physiologic or pathologic, is in most cases a homeostasis between collagen synthesis and collagen degradation by matrix metalloproteases (MMPs). The matrix of the heart is a very complex scaffolding composed of fibrillar and ground substance proteins (collagen) that appear around and between myocytes in a very precise and organized pattern. The matrix likely plays a very important role in maintaining an ideal ventricular shape.[149] Changes in the cardiac "skeleton" can contribute to impairment of both diastolic and systolic function.[136] In the failing human heart with advanced coronary disease (so-called ischemic cardiomyopathy), fibrosis is the major force of LV remodeling. Infarct scars may account for 30 percent of fibrosis, whereas microscopic fibrosis remote from the infarct may account for 70 percent of the total fibrous tissue found in the ventricles.[150] In general, interstitial loci of fibrosis are the "tombstones" of lost myocytes. It is likely that increased MMPs contribute to ventricular dilatation in heart failure.[151] Tissue inhibitors of MMPs (TIMPS) exist in the myocardium and are regulated independently of MMPs,[151] an observation with potentially important therapeutic implications. Enhanced protease activity in heart failure contributes to fibrillar collagen degradation, setting the stage for weakened connective tissue and disrupted organ integrity, myocyte slippage, and ventricular remodeling.

The growth of the interstitium in response to pressure and volume overload is highly complex and involves fibroblasts and their ability to sense altered mechanical forces. Hormones, including the RAAS[137] and endothelin,[152] also facilitate the production of collagen via their interaction with fibroblasts. Once abnormal loading conditions are removed, connective tissue hypertrophy regresses more slowly than myocyte hypertrophy. The importance of this ground substance, once considered inert, has emerged over the past 15 years, and it is now clear that the cardiac interstitium is very important in the syndrome of heart failure, contributing in many ways to the structural and functional alterations.

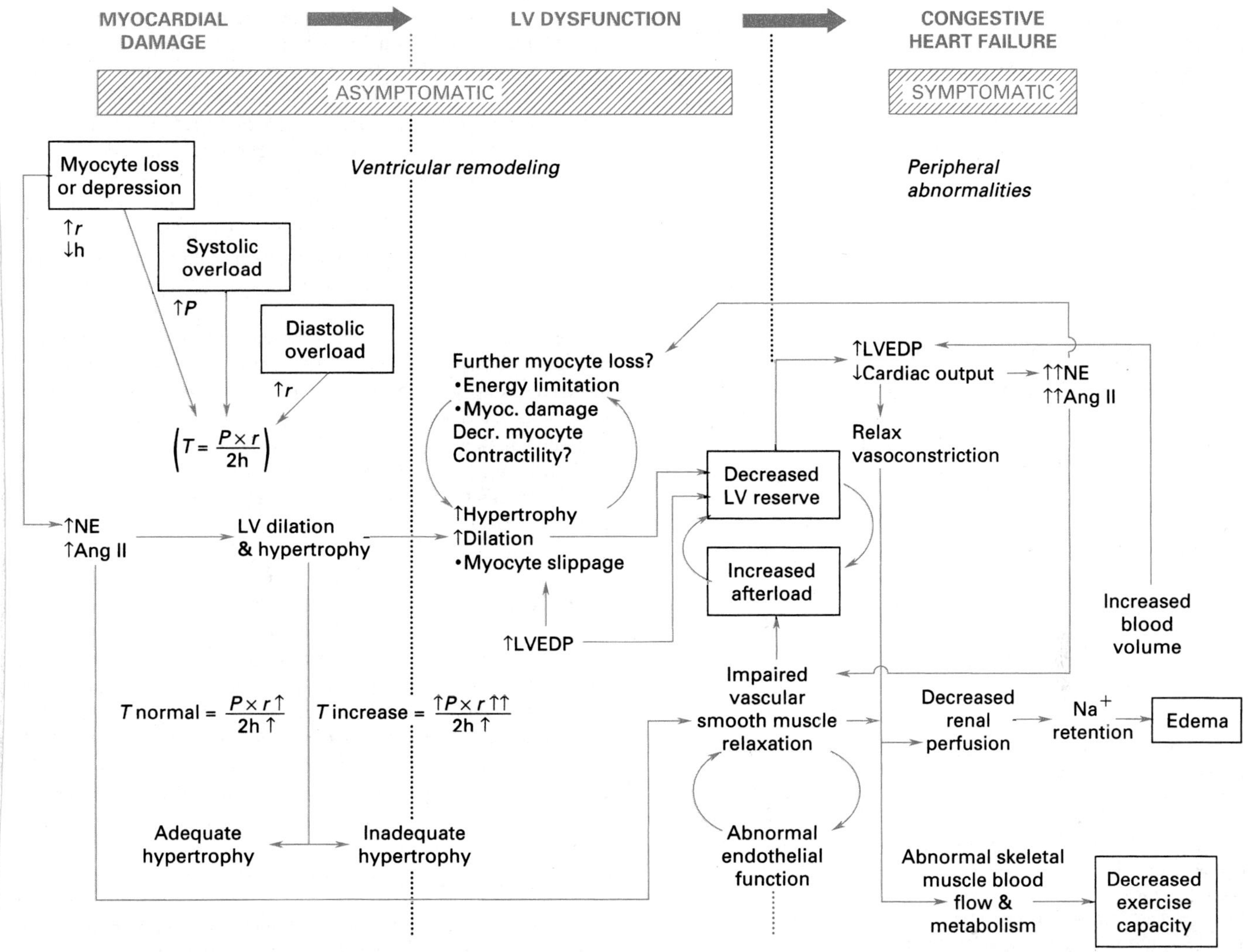


FIGURE 24-6 Evolution of myocardial damage to left ventricular function and ultimate congestive heart failure. The syndrome of congestive heart failure is the end result of processes that evolve in response to initial myocardial damage and/or cardiac overloads. The initiating event may be myocyte loss, either segmental, as with acute myocardial infarction, or diffuse, as with idiopathic cardiomyopathies and myocarditis; systolic overload, such as hypertension or aortic stenosis; or diastolic overload, such as mitral regurgitation or aortic regurgitation. Major loss of myocytes may also stimulate the renin-angiotensin-aldosterone and adrenergic systems, which may contribute to ventricular and vascular remodeling. All of these overloads create an increased workload for the heart, as characterized by the Laplace relationship, where tension ($T$) is equal to the product of pressure ($P$) and ventricular radius ($r$) divided by twice the wall thickness (h). The initial adaptation to these overloads, termed *ventricular remodeling*, comprises an increase in both myocyte length and diameter as well as an increase in ventricular volume to maintain adequate stroke volume and hence cardiac output. If hypertrophy is adequate to normalize the tension load, a relatively steady state may be maintained. Myocytes continue to be lost as a function of aging per se, however, and this tends to lead to further myocyte hypertrophy and cardiac dilatation. Moreover, the aging process may be amplified by hypertrophy. Should there be a sudden increase in end-diastolic pressure within the ventricle, an added factor of relative myocyte slippage within the wall tends to occur, which may lead to a further decrease in myocytes across the ventricular wall, further increasing ventricular wall tension. This may create a downward spiral in which progressive cell loss leads to further ventricular remodeling and continued ventricular dilation. As noted above, the entire process of ventricular remodeling may occur asymptomatically, and myocardial damage progresses to LV dysfunction, which is characterized by an increasing diastolic volume and thus a reduced ventricular EF. Symptoms associated with congestive heart failure occur when decreased left ventricular reserve limits cardiac output response to exercise. As the process of heart failure evolves, abnormalities of endothelial function in the peripheral arterioles lead to reduced ability of the peripheral vasculature to dilate in response to metabolic need. As these abnormalities occur, abnormal skeletal muscle blood flow occurs in response to exercise and decreased exercise tolerance. In addition, decreased renal perfusion leads to further activation of the renin-angiotensin-aldosterone system (RAAS), with increased aldosterone secretion and sodium retention. The combination of these two events leads to decreased exercise capacity and peripheral edema, important components of the symptom complex of congestive heart failure. Decreased cardiac performance promotes neurohumoral responses characterized by activation of the sympathetic nervous system and the RAAS, leading to peripheral vasoconstriction and sodium accumulation. These factors feed back to increase the ventricular remodeling process and to amplify cardiac damage. Thus, initial myocardial damage progresses to ventricular dysfunction and ultimately to congestive heart failure. It is important to note that the myocardial damage and LV dysfunction are often asymptomatic; by the time symptomatic heart failure ensues, the disease process is far advanced. (Revised from LeJemtel TH, Sonnenblick EH. Heart failure and maladaptive processes: Introduction. *Circulation* 1993;87(suppl VII):VII1–VII4. Reproduced with permission from the American Heart Association and the authors.)

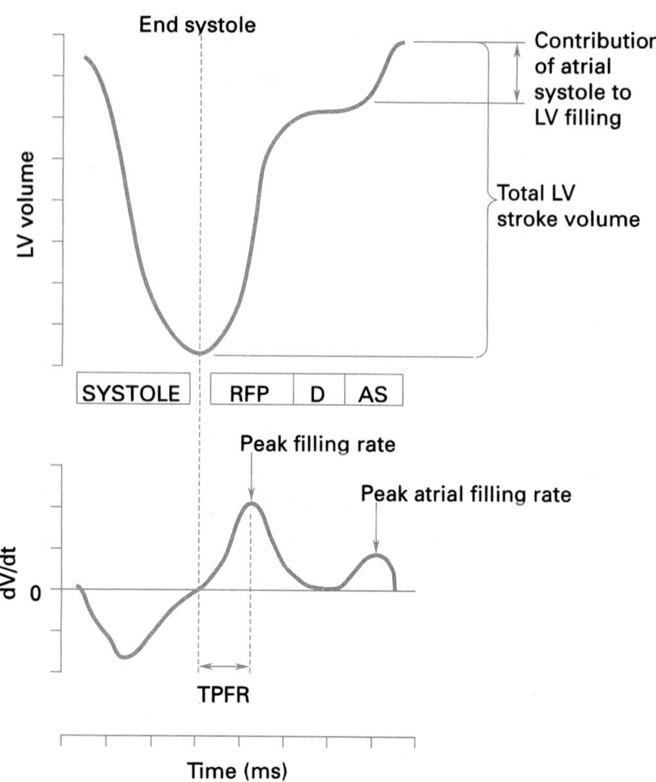


FIGURE 24-7 Idealized plot of LV volume versus time (*top*) and the rate of change of volume (dV/dt) versus time (*bottom*), such as might be obtained from contrast or radionuclide ventriculographic studies. The representative cardiac cycle begins at end-diastole. Subsequent events, as depicted by the bars in the center of the figure, are (1) systole, during which left ventricular volume decreases to a minimum and dV/dt reaches its maximum, and (2) diastole, the beginning of which is signaled by the opening of the mitral valve and the onset of LV filling. Diastole has three distinct phases in normal individuals: (1) the rapid filling phase (RFP), during which the left ventricle fills rapidly but passively and the peak filling rate occurs; (2) diastasis (D), during which relatively little left ventricular volume change occurs; and (3) atrial systole (AS), in which active atrial contraction fills the left ventricle to its end-diastolic volume. The diastolic parameters that have been derived from such analysis are the peak filling rate, the time to peak filling rate (TPFR), the percent contribution of atrial systole, and the first third filling fraction. (From Labovitz AJ, Pearson AC. Evaluation of left ventricular diastolic function: Clinical relevance and recent Doppler echocardiographic insights. *Am Heart J* 1987;114:836–849. Reproduced with permission from the publisher and authors.)

## NONCARDIAC "ADAPTATIONS" IN HEART FAILURE

### The Neurohumoral Hypothesis

A large number of neurohormones have been found to circulate in abnormal quantities in heart failure (Table 24-7). The natriuretic peptides—atrial natriuretic peptide (ANP), BNP, and C-type natriuretic peptide (CNP)—are considered counterregulatory because they tend to reduce right atrial pressure, systemic vascular resistance, aldosterone secretion, sympathetic nerve stimulation, and hypertrophy of cells and can enhance sodium excretion.[153,154] The predominant consequence of most neurohormone "release" in heart failure, however, is vasoconstriction coupled with salt and water retention. The regulation of body fluid volume is very complex but has a primitive relation to many of the neurohormones and their propensity to facilitate retention of sodium and water while at the same time protecting perfusion pressure. The integrity of the arterial circulation as a function of cardiac output and SVR is also determined by flexibility in renal sodium and water excretion.[155] Underfilling of the arterial bed by low cardiac output or vasodilation activates neuroendocrine reflexes that stimulate sodium and water retention. Sodium and water retention cease to be major problems after heart transplantation, indicating that there is no intrinsic renal dysfunction in heart failure. The kidney responds to a perceived reduction in arterial filling in an appropriate manner by retaining volume. Decreases in blood pressure, stroke volume (pulse pressure), and perfusion (flow) in heart failure are sensed by mechanoreceptors in the left ventricle, carotid sinus, aortic arch, and renal afferent arterioles. When there is diminished activation of these receptors, as in heart failure, there is augmentation of sympathetic outflow, activation of the RAAS, and nonosmotic release of arginine vasopressin (AVP).[155] Heightened peripheral vasoconstriction occurs along with increased blood volume, thereby "restoring" circulatory integrity and perfusion pressure. Of course, neuroendocrine activation has many important actions at the cellular level, including facilitation of myocyte hypertrophy[39] and collagen synthesis.[137] Activation of the sympathetic nervous system contributes to tachycardia and arrhythmias and may be directly toxic to the myocardium.[156,157] Cardiac myocyte necrosis also occurs in response to low levels of angiotensin II.[158] Although neuroendocrine responses are not the primary cause of heart failure under most circumstances, they clearly contribute to the progression of the syndrome[159] (Fig. 24-8). The overly simplistic view that neurohormones in heart failure are a response to perceived "hypovolemia" is clearly incorrect.[160] Neuroendocrine mechanisms are now the targets of several important and successful therapeutic interventions in heart failure and hypertension[161] and have a key role in determining prognosis.[162] ACE inhibitors, $\beta$-adrenergic blockers, and aldosterone antagonists now have a prominent role in the treatment of heart failure, and new, more innovative neuroendocrine-blocking agents are being developed rapidly, adding strong support to the neurohumoral hypothesis.[159]

### Norepinephrine

It has long been recognized that patients with heart failure manifest signs of a hyperadrenergic state. Vascular constriction, tachycardia, diaphoresis, and oliguria are clear signs of increased sympathetic drive. Starling's observations in 1897,[163] amplified in the early 1960s, predicted increased plasma norepinephrine (NE) levels in patients with heart failure.[164] Myocardial stores of NE were found to be depleted,[165] but later studies by various investigators using the more sensitive radioenzymatic technique of plasma NE described a correlation with functional class[166] and extent of hemodynamic dysfunction.[167]

Norepinephrine synthesis begins in the body of the neuron with the synthesis of enzymes necessary to change from tyrosine to NE. The enzymes are transported down the neuron to the dendrites of the cell, where the actual synthetic steps take place. Dopamine is synthesized and transported into storage vesicles, where the final synthetic steps occur. These storage vesicles are both large and small, the large vesicles containing additional peptides such as neuropeptide Y. Following discharge of an axonal action potential, exocytosis occurs, allowing the vesicle contents to be released into the synaptic cleft. The vast majority of the NE is then taken back up into the cell for storage and rerelease (uptake 1). Some NE is taken up by effector organs and metabolized (uptake 2), and only a small quantity is released into the plasma ($\cong$5 percent), where it circulates as plasma

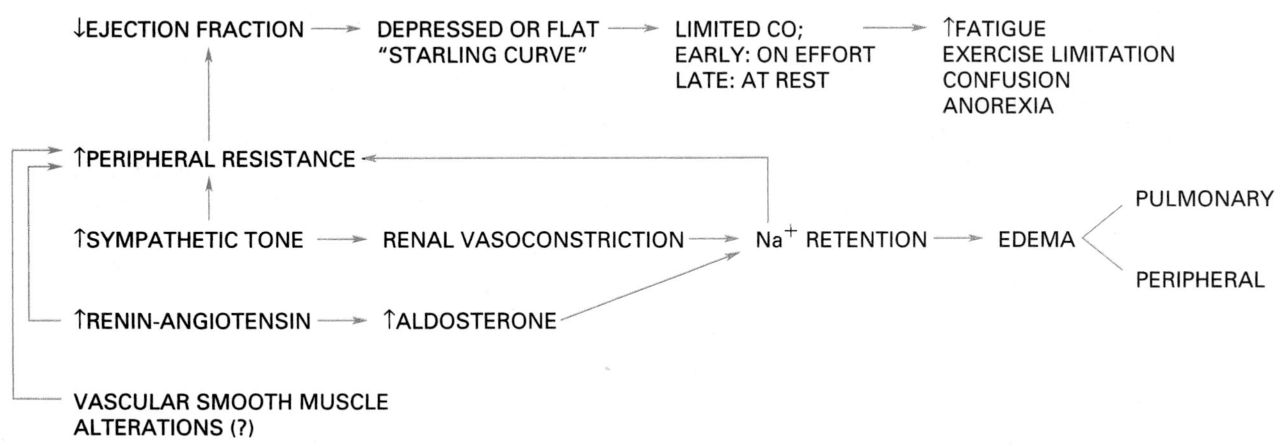


FIGURE 24-8 Schema of events in congestive heart failure leading to symptoms. Note that fatigue and other symptoms of limited cardiac output are primarily related to decreased ejection, whereas peripheral and pulmonary edema are related to sodium and water retention from increased sympathetic tone and increased renin-angiotensin-aldosterone. See text for details.

NE. There are now microneurographic techniques than can be used to directly measure sympathetic traffic direction[168] and "spillover" techniques using tritiated norepinephrine, that can measure specific organ sympathetic activity.[169] In the course of heart failure, increased cardiac sympathetic traffic precedes more generalized sympathetic activation.[170] Plasma NE level has served as a useful research and prognostic guide for the study of patients with heart failure.[171]

It is overly simplistic to consider NE to be "good" or "bad" for patients with heart failure. Those with severe New York Heart Association (NYHA) class IV heart failure may be quite dependent on catecholamine support[171] and sometimes require a continuous dobutamine infusion to maintain suitable organ perfusion prior to heart transplantation. However, there is no question that NE is toxic to the myocardium and is responsible in part for progressive LV remodeling.[172,173] The favorable and detrimental effects of sympathetic drive are depicted in Table 24-8. These observations imply that blocking the sympathetic nervous system effects are most likely to benefit NYHA class I to III patients, whereas such action potentially could worsen the condition of class IV patients who manifest congestion.

TABLE 24-8 Favorable and Detrimental Effects of Sympathetic Drive in Patients with Heart Failure

| Effects | NYHA class |
|---|---|
| **Favorable** | |
| ↑ HR, improved cardiac output<br>↑ contractility, improved cardiac output maintenance of perfusion pressure | NYHA class IV |
| **Detrimental** | |
| Progressive LV remodeling<br>LV hypertrophy → failure<br>↑ myocardial $\dot{M}V_{O_2}$, arrhythmias<br>↑ SVR → ↑ afterload<br>$Na^+$ and $H_2O$ retention, facilitation of renin release, oliguria | NYHA class I-III |

Yet, $\beta$-adrenergic blockers are equally effective in patients with advanced heart failure.[174]

## The Renin-Angiotensin-Aldosterone System

The RAAS plays an important role in the pathogenesis of heart failure (Fig. 24-8), and consistent benefit has been derived from ACE-inhibitor therapy in patients with heart failure. The mechanisms responsible for the release of renin from the renal cortex have been exhaustively studied[175] and include sympathetic drive to the kidneys, hyponatremic perfusate to the macula densa of the kidney, and use of diuretics and a low-sodium diet, which tends to promote a relative volume contraction. Renin proteolytic enzyme has little biologic activity, but it interacts with angiotensinogen to split off two amino acids to form angiotensin I, which is then cleaved by ACE, which is distributed widely in the vascular system, especially the lungs, to produce angiotensin II, a peptide with a vast range of biological activities. Angiotensin II in turn stimulates release of aldosterone from the adrenal cortex, which also has an array of biological effects, including sodium and water retention, kaliuresis, and enhanced collagen turnover and organ remodeling.

There now are at least four recognized angiotensin II (AT) receptors, but much of the activity is subserved by the $AT_1$ receptor. The $AT_1$ actions include arterial vasoconstriction, cell growth (hypertrophy), apoptosis in myocytes, polydypsia, NE release, sensitization of blood vessels to NE, AVP release, and aldosterone release. The $AT_2$ receptor appears to subserve somewhat counterregulatory effects, including antigrowth/antiremodeling, apoptosis, vasodilation, and activation of the kinin–nitric oxide–cGMP system.[176] Since $AT_1$ receptor–blocking drugs (so-called ARBs) increase angiotensin II levels, they may indirectly activate unoccupied $AT_2$ receptor activity. Angiotensin II levels tend to "escape" the pharmacologic effects of chronic ACE inhibition irrespective of dosage,[177] and may stimulate $AT_2$ and $AT_2$ receptor activity. It is also now clear that the RAAS is not solely a classic endocrine system but has autocrine and paracrine activity that may be particularly important in cardiovascular, brain, and renal tissue. With our current knowledge that ACE inhibitors remarkably reduce all cardiovascular events and even limit the onset of new diabetes mellitus in patients with cardiovascular disease,[178] it is difficult to overstate the role of the RAAS in the pathogenesis of heart and vascular disease, including progressive heart failure.[179–181]

## Arginine Vasopressin

Patients with heart failure sometimes have water retention in excess of sodium retention, leading to hyponatremia. The hyponatremia is due in part to nonosmotic release of AVP, which acts on the kidney to reduce free water clearance. Release of AVP in heart failure probably occurs via activation of carotid baroreceptors.[155] Plasma AVP levels are often but not always increased in patients with LV dysfunction[182] and heart failure.[113] AVP acts on the $V_2$ receptors in the collecting duct of the kidney via adenylate cyclase to translocate aquaporin-2 water channels from cytoplasmic vesicles to the apical surface of the collecting duct. AVP also increases aquaporin-2 channel synthesis. Activation of $V_1$ receptors in vascular tissue contributes to heightened vascular resistance and myocardial dysfunction in heart failure.[183] Recognition of the role of AVP in the pathogenesis of heart failure has led to the development and investigation of selective $V_2$ and dual $V_1$-$V_2$ receptor blockers (such as conivaptan and tolvaptan) as potential adjunctive treatment.

## Natriuretic Peptides

A family of natriuretic peptides—including ANP, BNP, and CNP—is encoded by separate genes, each with a tissue-specific distribution, regulation, and biological activity.[153] These natriuretic peptides are often increased in patients with heart failure, and BNP has been used as a marker for asymptomatic LV dysfunction or early heart failure.[184,185] ANP is a 28–amino acid peptide that is normally synthesized and stored in the atria and to some extent in the ventricles. It is released into the circulation during atrial distention. BNP is synthesized mainly by the ventricles and is released in LV dysfunction or early heart failure. For the most part, these peptides act via guanylate cyclase receptors to promote vasodilation (ANP, BNP, CNP) and natriuresis (ANP, BNP). They also may attenuate NE release, RAAS activity, and the growth/hypertrophy of target cells—hence the term *counterregulatory hormones*.

Patients with heart failure are relatively resistant to the natriuretic effects of these peptides when they are administered exogenously, perhaps due to decreased sodium delivery to the collecting duct as a result of diminished glomerular filtration or increased sodium reabsorption in the proximal tubule.[155] Nevertheless, BNP infusion has a beneficial hemodynamic effect in heart failure,[186,187] and drugs designed to inhibit degradation of natriuretic peptides (so-called neutral endopeptidase inhibitors, or vasopeptidase inhibitors such as omapatrilat) have been combined with ACE-inhibitor activity as potential therapy for hypertension and heart failure. The role of natriuretic peptides as potential therapy is evolving, though a recent randomized controlled trial of omapatrilat indicated no survival benefit.[188]

## Endothelin

Endothelins are a family of vasoconstrictor peptides produced by vascular endothelial cells.[189,190] Their physiologic function is as yet unclear. Although blood levels are increased in patients with heart failure,[191,192] endothelin-1 (ET-1) is more of a paracrine than an endocrine hormone. In heart failure, myocardial tissue ET-1 levels are increased, possibly more due to decreased clearance by the lungs than to increased synthesis.[193] Endothelial cells synthesize ET-1 rapidly and convert "big" endothelin-1 into endothelin by an endothelin-converting enzyme. The synthesis of ET-1 is enhanced by angiotensin II, NE, growth factors, insulin, hypoxia, oxidized low-density lipoproteins (ox-LDLs), shear stress, and thrombin.[189] Its synthesis is antagonized by ANP and prostaglandins.

Endothelin acts on at least two types of G protein–coupled receptors, A and B. The ET-A receptor subserves smooth muscle vasoconstriction and cell proliferation/hypertrophy and mainly resides on vascular smooth muscle cells. The ET-B receptor, which is mainly endothelial, subserves vasodilation that is probably mediated by a variety of mechanisms, including increased production of nitric oxide and prostaglandins and activation of potassium channels. ET-1 also can act on the heart to cause hypertrophy, on the adrenal gland to release aldosterone, and on the kidney to promote sodium and water retention.[189] The importance of ET-1 in the pathogenesis of heart failure is highlighted by the development and clinical testing of several new endothelin antagonists.[194] Bosentan, a dual $ET_A$-$ET_B$–receptor blocker, failed to demonstrate a survival benefit in patients with heart failure but is marketed for the treatment of primary pulmonary hypertension.

## Additional Neurohormones

Other neurohormones that may play a role in the pathogenesis of heart failure include neuropeptide Y, vasointestinal peptide, bradykinin, prostaglandins, adrenomedullin, urodilantin, cardiotropin-1, and urotensin-II; some of these may emerge as "systems" to block or enhance in heart failure, depending on their primary function.

## Cytokines

Circulating tumor necrosis factor alpha (TNF-$\alpha$), a proinflammatory cytokine, is increased in cachetic patients with chronic heart failure.[195] Proinflammatory cytokines such as TNF-$\alpha$ may play an important role in modulating abnormal myocardial structure and function in late stages of heart failure.[196–198] This group of proinflammatory cytokines also includes interleukin 1 (IL-1) and interleukin 6 (IL-6), proteins that are largely products of macrophages and lymphocytes and may, under some circumstances, be expressed by myocardial tissue. Each of these cytokines can influence the expression of the other two, and each can modulate cardiovascular performance when expressed in sufficiently high levels. A continuous infusion of TNF-$\alpha$ leads to time-dependent depression in LV function in an animal model[199] and provokes a hypertrophic growth response in adult cardiac myocytes.[200] When synthesized in large quantities, TNF-$\alpha$ spills over into the circulation and acts as an endocrine "hormone" leading to metabolic wasting and cachexia.[201,202] Overexpression of TNF-$\alpha$ in a transgenic mouse model leads to a phenotype consistent with cardiomyopathy.[203] TNF-$\alpha$ acts via two different membrane receptors. The transduction signal pathways are not fully understood, but in the heart they may mediate cell growth, negative inotropy, and apoptosis. These observations have led to two clinical trials with etanercept, a fusion molecule that binds circulating TNF-$\alpha$, and a trial of infliximab, a monoclonal antibody against TNF-$\alpha$, for the treatment of patients with late-stage heart failure. However, these trials (RENEWAL and ATTACH, respectively) failed to demonstrate a survival benefit for either of these drugs.[204]

## Renal Retention of Salt and Water

Renal retention of sodium and water, resulting in signs and symptoms of fluid retention, has long been a hallmark of heart failure. The precise mechanism whereby the heart signals the kidney in the early stages of heart failure to retain sodium and water is still unknown, although in the late stages reduced cardiac output and impaired renal blood flow are likely playing a major role. In early heart failure, when normal cardiac output is maintained via compensatory mechanisms and renal blood flow is not reduced, some sodium retention still occurs. Curiously, some patients with advanced heart failure may not demonstrate peripheral edema or ascites. This suggests that in some cases, counterregulatory natriuretic peptides may be acting to maintain natriuresis. Perhaps release of ANP and BNP in the early stages of heart failure may offset the tendency to retain sodium. Salt and water retention usually becomes evident in heart failure as peripheral vasoconstriction occurs in the face of a falling cardiac output.[205] This is associated with activation of the RAAS.[206] Angiotensin II preserves glomerular filtration rate in patients with heart failure even when renal perfusion is severely compromised, independent of its propensity to support systemic blood pressure.[207] Intraglomerular hydraulic pressure and therefore glomerular filtration are preserved by the constriction of glomerular efferent arterioles via angiotensin II.[208] Increased intrarenal formation of angiotensin II during a reduction in renal artery pressure maintains efferent arteriolar tone and, consequently, the effective filtration pressure.[209] The resulting high level of filtration fraction favors changes in the postglomerular circulation that promote avid proximal fluid reabsorption via elevated peritubular capillary oncotic pressure.[210] Increased aldosterone acts principally on the cortical collecting tubules to conserve sodium, with a concomitant loss of potassium. Because the plasma volume and blood pressure vary considerably from day to day, there is no consistent relation between the RAAS and fluid retention.

The mechanisms of sodium and water retention in heart failure are multiple and complex. Sympathetic nervous system traffic to the kidney favors sodium retention. Increased AVP activity diminishes the clearance of free water. The prostaglandins normally dilate afferent glomerular arterioles to enhance intraglomerular flow and pressure, and their inhibition by nonsteroidal anti-inflammatory agents may lead to a marked reduction in filtration and sodium retention. Enhanced sodium reabsorption of heart failure also occurs in the ascending loop of Henle as well as in the cortical and medullary collecting ducts. Eventually, plasma volume expansion occurs, but at the expense of circulatory and tissue congestion.

## Endothelial Dysfunction, Insulin Resistance, Nitric Oxide, Exercise Intolerance, and Sleep Disorders

Animal and human studies indicate that endothelium-dependent vasodilation is abnormal in a number of disease states, including atherosclerosis, hypertension, heart failure, hyperhomocysteinemia, insulin resistance, and hypercholesterolemia. Endothelial dysfunction has been demonstrated in experimental animals[211] and in patients with heart failure.[212–214] Such endothelial dysfunction in heart failure (i.e., failure to vasodilate in response to a specific endothelium-dependent vasodilator) may be due to a reduced release of nitric oxide during stimulation.[212,215] The basal release of nitric oxide may be preserved or even enhanced in heart failure[216] and may be compensatory by antagonizing neuroendocrine vasoconstrictor forces. However, impairment of endothelium-dependent peripheral vasodilation may be a factor contributing to exercise intolerance in patients with chronic heart failure, perhaps by limiting nutritive skeletal muscle flow during exercise.[217] This dysfunction of the endothelium may be related to deconditioning in later stages of heart failure; with training, it is largely reversible. Further, abnormal endothelium-dependent responses in heart failure are reversible following heart transplantation.[218] Several recent studies also observed a high prevalence of insulin resistance in patients with heart failure in the absence of overt diabetes.[219,220] The role of insulin resistance in heart failure is unclear, although subclinical ischemia due to endothelial dysfunction may play an important role, which may explain why the presence of insulin resistance has found to be an independent prognostic factor.[221]

The roles of nitric oxide and nitric oxide synthase in the failing heart are much more complex.[222,223] Nitric oxide inhibits the positive inotropic response to $\beta$-adrenergic stimulation in the failing heart, while smaller physiologic amounts of constitutive nitric oxide (cNOS, or NOS3) are necessary for normal function and have an antioxidant effect to protect cells. High levels of nitric oxide in the heart may exert proapoptotic and cytotoxic effects. The inducible isoform of nitric oxide synthase (iNOS, or NOS2) is overexpressed in human heart failure[224] and therefore may contribute to worsening heart failure. On the other hand, there is decreased myocardial nitric oxide synthesis during decompensation of experimental heart failure.[225] Thus the roles of nitric oxide may also differ at different stages in the evolution of heart failure.

Many factors limit increased cardiac output during exercise in patients with heart failure, including a reduced myocardial force-frequency response, inability to fully use the Starling effect, and chronotropic incompetence. When combined with endothelial dysfunction, reduced nutritive skeletal muscle blood flow, and disuse atrophy of skeletal muscles, exercise tolerance is reduced. The latter effects appear to be excessively dependent on a glycolytic metabolism,[226] in part due to reduced metabolic efficiency in performing external work. Additional mechanisms include changes in muscle fiber recruitment, selective atrophy of oxidative fibers, and physical deconditioning. The mitochondrial content of skeletal muscle is reduced[227] in heart failure. Increased expression of the inducible isoform of nitric oxide synthase in skeletal muscle is correlated with reduced mitochondrial creatine kinase expression and exercise intolerance.[228] Apoptosis is frequently found in skeletal muscle of patients with heart failure and is also associated with exercise impairment.[229] Of importance, exercise capacity and EF are very poorly correlated in heart failure, suggesting that impairment in limited cardiac output is not the dominant reason for exercise intolerance.

Pulmonary dysfunction is common in patients with heart failure and may contribute to exercise intolerance. The amount of intrathoracic space available for ventilation may be decreased by alveolar and interstitial edema, pleural effusions, or an increase in blood volume. Increased pulmonary vascular congestion decreases lung compliance and increases the work of breathing. Excessive ventilation including an increased $V_E/\dot{V}O_2$ slope during exercise is a hallmark of heart failure, and has important prognostic implications.[230] Acute reduction in pulmonary capillary wedge pressure has no effect on the augmented ventilatory response, and the extent of excessive ventilation does not relate to either resting or exercise pulmonary capillary wedge pressure.

In summary, potential mechanisms responsible for exercise intolerance in heart failure are numerous (Table 24-9). Exercise intolerance is clearly multifactorial and is a potent prognostic indicator used to help determine the optimal timing of heart transplantation (e.g., peak $\dot{V}O_2$ of less than 50 percent predicted for size and age). Exertional symptoms generally correlate with reduced maximal exercise capacity,[231] although exertional symptoms frequently underestimate the severity of functional disability. It is important to note that EF does not correlate well with exercise tolerance, which may be better related to blood flow to the muscles. A peak $\dot{V}O_2$ of $\leq$ 14 mL/kg/min or $V_E/\dot{V}O_2$ slope $\geq$ 45 during exercise indicates a very poor prognosis, to the point where heart transplantation should be considered. Cardiopulmonary exercise testing should be done in patients with heart failure to assess functional capacity and prognosis. Importantly, exercise tolerance can improve with training, which should be encouraged in patients with classes I to III heart failure symptoms.[232]

TABLE 24-9 Mechanisms of Exercise Intolerance in Heart Failure

| |
|---|
| Inability of endothelium to respond to vasodilator stimulus |
| Reduced nutritive blood flow to skeletal muscle |
| Inability to increase stroke volume in response to exercise |
| Chronotropic incompetence |
| Reduced myocardial force-frequency response |
| Diminished myocardial $\beta$-adrenergic receptor density |
| Skeletal muscle atrophy |
| Shift from slow- to fast-twitch fiber types |
| Atrophy of fast-twitch type II fibers |
| Reduced level of skeletal muscle mitochondrial enzymes |
| Reduced skeletal muscle mitochondrial size |
| Increased skeletal muscle apoptosis |
| Reduced lung compliance |
| Excessive ventilatory response to exercise |
| Generalized deconditioning |

Periodic breathing (Cheyne-Stokes) is common in patients with severe heart failure and is associated with a poor prognosis.[233] It can be caused by lung edema, which can excite carbon dioxide responses through vagal reflexes. Enhanced sensitivity to carbon dioxide may predispose some patients with heart failure to the development of central sleep apnea.[234] Successful treatment of Cheyne-Stokes respiration with nocturnal nasal oxygen improves sleep, exercise tolerance, and cognitive function in patients with heart failure.[235] Severe untreated sleep-disordered breathing can further impair LV function, leading to arterial oxyhemoglobin desaturation and arrhythmias.[236] Central sleep apnea may occur in as many as 40 percent of patients with heart failure, and 10 percent suffer from obstructive sleep apnea.[237] Obstructive sleep apnea increases afterload and heart rate during sleep but is responsive to continuous positive airway pressure.[238]

## CONCLUSIONS

Heart failure is a complex clinical syndrome that is growing in magnitude as the population ages. It is difficult to define but relatively straightforward to diagnose. Heart failure implies underlying structural and functional changes in the heart that contribute importantly to the clinical syndrome. There is no single cause or unifying mechanism of heart failure. Although the molecular underpinnings of heart failure are still incompletely understood, the importance of pathophysiologic principles such as reduced preload reserve and enhanced sensitivity to afterload is now well recognized. Neuroendocrine and inflammatory responses are common in patients with heart failure and serve as important therapeutic targets.

## References


1. Ho KK, Anderson KM, Kannel WB, et al. Survival after the onset of congestive heart failure in Framingham Heart Study subjects. *Circulation* 1993;88:107–115.
2. Cowie MR, Mosterd A, Wood DA, et al. The epidemiology of heart failure. *Eur Heart J* 1997;18:208–225.
3. Hunt SA, Baker DW, Chin MH, et al. ACC/AHA guidelines for the evaluation and management of chronic heart failure in the adult: Executive summary. A report of the American College of Cardiology/American Heart Association Task Force on Practice Guidelines (Committee to revise the 1995 Guidelines for the Evaluation and Management of Heart Failure). *J Am Coll Cardiol* 2001;38:2101–2113.
4. Chen HH, Lainchbury JG, Senni M, et al. Diastolic heart failure in the community: Clinical profile, natural history, therapy, and impact of proposed diagnostic criteria. *J Card Fail* 2002;8:279–287.
5. Vasan RS, Benjamin EJ, Levy D. Congestive heart failure with normal left ventricular systolic function. Clinical approaches to the diagnosis and treatment of diastolic heart failure. *Arch Intern Med* 1996;156:146–157.
6. Vasan RS, Benjamin EJ, Levy D. Prevalence, clinical features and prognosis of diastolic heart failure: An epidemiologic perspective. *J Am Coll Cardiol* 1995;26:1565–1574.
7. Bonow RO, Udelson JE. Left ventricular diastolic dysfunction as a cause of congestive heart failure: Mechanisms and management. *Ann Intern Med* 1992;117:502–510.
8. Kunis R, Greenberg H, Yeoh CB, et al. Coronary revascularization for recurrent pulmonary edema in elderly patients with ischemic heart disease and preserved ventricular function. *N Engl J Med* 1985;313:1207–1210.
9. Rihal CS, Nishimura RA, Hatle LK, et al. Systolic and diastolic dysfunction in patients with clinical diagnosis of dilated cardiomyopathy: Relation to symptoms and prognosis. *Circulation* 1994;90:2772–2279.
10. Eichhorn EJ, Willard JE, Alvarez L, et al. Are contraction and relaxation coupled in patients with and without congestive heart failure? *Circulation* 1992;85:2132–2139.
11. Douglas PS. Diastolic dysfunction: Old dog, new tricks. *Am Heart J* 1999;137:777–778.
12. Cohen GI, Pietrolungo JF, Thomas JD, Klein AL. A practical guide to assessment of ventricular diastolic function using Doppler echocardiography. *J Am Coll Cardiol* 1996;27:1753–1760.
13. Nishimura RA, Tajik AJ. Evaluation of diastolic filling of left ventricle in health and disease: Doppler echocardiography is the clinician's Rosetta Stone. *J Am Coll Cardiol* 1997;30:8–18.
14. Lindenfeld J, Krause-Steinrauf H, Salerno J. Where are all the women with heart failure? *J Am Coll Cardiol* 1997;30:1417–1419.
15. Cohn JN, Johnson G. Heart failure with normal ejection fraction. The V-HeFT Study. Veterans Administration Cooperative Study Group. *Circulation* 1990;81:III48–III53.
16. Vasan RS, Larson MG, Benjamin EJ, et al. Congestive heart failure in subjects with normal versus reduced left ventricular ejection fraction: Prevalence and mortality in a population-based cohort. *J Am Coll Cardiol* 1999;33:1948–1955.
17. MacDowall P, Kalra PA, O'Donoghue DJ, et al. Risk of morbidity from renovascular disease in elderly patients with congestive cardiac failure. *Lancet* 1998;352:13–16.
18. Mestroni L, Rocco C, Gregori D, et al. Familial dilated cardiomyopathy: Evidence for genetic and phenotypic heterogeneity. Heart Muscle Disease Study Group. *J Am Coll Cardiol* 1999;34:181–190.
19. Valantine HA, Hunt SA, Fowler MB, et al. Frequency of familial nature of dilated cardiomyopathy and usefulness of cardiac transplantation in this subset. *Am J Cardiol* 1989;63:959–963.
20. Baig MK, Goldman JH, Caforio AL, et al. Familial dilated cardiomyopathy: Cardiac abnormalities are common in asymptomatic relatives and may represent early disease. *J Am Coll Cardiol* 1998;31:195–201.
21. Grunig E, Tasman JA, Kucherer H, et al. Frequency and phenotypes of familial dilated cardiomyopathy. *J Am Coll Cardiol* 1998;31:186–194.
22. Olson TM, Keating MT. Defining the molecular genetic basis of idiopathic dilated cardiomyopathy. *Trends Cardiovasc Med* 1997;7:60–63.
23. Mason JW, O'Connell JB, Herskowitz A, et al. A clinical trial of immunosuppressive therapy for myocarditis. The Myocarditis Treatment Trial Investigators. *N Engl J Med* 1995;333:269–275.
24. Grogan M, Redfield MM, Bailey KR, et al. Long-term outcome of patients with biopsy-proved myocarditis: Comparison with idiopathic dilated cardiomyopathy. *J Am Coll Cardiol* 1995;26:80–84.
25. Cooper LT Jr, Berry GJ, Shabetai R. Idiopathic giant-cell myocarditis—Natural history and treatment. Multicenter Giant Cell Myocarditis Study Group Investigators. *N Engl J Med* 1997;336:1860–1866.

26. Singal PK, Iliskovic N. Doxorubicin-induced cardiomyopathy. *N Engl J Med* 1998;339:900–905.
27. Shan K, Lincoff AM, Young JB. Anthracycline-induced cardiotoxicity. *Ann Intern Med* 1996;125:47–58.
28. Singal PK, Iliskovic N, Li T, Kumar D. Adriamycin cardiomyopathy: Pathophysiology and prevention. *FASEB J* 1997;11:931–936.
29. Feenstra J, Grobbee DE, Remme WJ, Stricker BH. Drug-induced heart failure. *J Am Coll Cardiol* 1999;33:1152–1162.
30. Skelton CL, Sonnenblick EH. Heterogeneity of contractile function in cardiac hypertrophy. *Circ Res* 1974;35:suppl II:83–96.
31. Katz AM. Cardiomyopathy of overload: A major determinant of prognosis in congestive heart failure. *N Engl J Med* 1990;322:100–110.
32. Katz AM. The cardiomyopathy of overload: An unnatural growth response in the hypertrophied heart. *Ann Intern Med* 1994;121:363–371.
33. Anand IS, Chandrashekhar Y, Ferrari R, et al. Pathogenesis of oedema in chronic severe anaemia: Studies of body water and sodium, renal function, haemodynamic variables, and plasma hormones. *Br Heart J* 1993;70:357–362.
34. Harris P. Evolution and the cardiac patient. *Cardiovasc Res* 1983;17: 313–319, 373–378, 437–445.
35. Kajstura J, Leri A, Finato N, et al. Myocyte proliferation in end-stage cardiac failure in humans. *Proc Natl Acad Sci USA* 1998;95:8801–8805.
36. Anversa P, Kajstura J. Ventricular myocytes are not terminally differentiated in the adult mammalian heart. *Circ Res* 1998;83:1–14.
37. Linzbach AJ. Heart failure from the point of view of quantitative anatomy. *Am J Cardiol* 1960;5:370–382.
38. Gerdes AM, Kellerman SE, Moore JA, et al. Structural remodeling of cardiac myocytes in patients with ischemic cardiomyopathy. *Circulation* 1992;86:426–430.
39. Hunter JJ, Chien KR. Signaling pathways for cardiac hypertrophy and failure. *N Engl J Med* 1999;341:1276–1283.
40. Lorell BH. Transition from hypertrophy to failure. *Circulation* 1997; 96:3824–3827.
41. Harris P. Congestive cardiac failure: Central role of the arterial blood pressure. *Br Heart J* 1987;58:190–203.
42. de Bold AJ. Atrial natriuretic factor: A hormone produced by the heart. *Science* 1985;230:767–770.
43. Francis GS. Changing the remodeling process in heart failure: Basic mechanisms and laboratory results. *Curr Opin Cardiol* 1998;13: 156–161.
44. Swynghedauw B. Molecular mechanisms of myocardial remodeling. *Physiol Rev* 1999;79:215–262.
45. Onodera T, Tamura T, Said S, et al. Maladaptive remodeling of cardiac myocyte shape begins long before failure in hypertension. *Hypertension* 1998;32:753–757.
46. Francis GS, McDonald KM. Left ventricular hypertrophy: An initial response to myocardial injury. *Am J Cardiol* 1992;69:3G–7G.
47. Francis GS, McDonald KM, Cohn JN. Neurohumoral activation in preclinical heart failure. Remodeling and the potential for intervention. *Circulation* 1993;87:IV90–IV96.
48. Francis GS, Carlyle WC. Hypothetical pathways of cardiac myocyte hypertrophy: response to myocardial injury. *Eur Heart J* 1993;14 Suppl J:49–56.
49. Tamura T, Onodera T, Said S, Gerdes AM. Correlation of myocyte lengthening to chamber dilation in the spontaneously hypertensive heart failure (SHHF) rat. *J Mol Cell Cardiol* 1998;30:2175–2181.
50. Gerdes AM, Onodera T, Wang X, McCune SA. Myocyte remodeling during the progression to failure in rats with hypertension. *Hypertension* 1996;28:609–614.
51. Wang X, Li F, Gerdes AM. Chronic pressure overload cardiac hypertrophy and failure in guinea pigs: I. Regional hemodynamics and myocyte remodeling. *J Mol Cell Cardiol* 1999;31:307–317.
52. Liu GS, Thornton J, Van Winkle DM, et al. Protection against infarction afforded by preconditioning is mediated by A1 adenosine receptors in rabbit heart. *Circulation* 1991;84:350–356.
53. Anversa P, Loud AV, Levicky V, Guideri G. Left ventricular failure induced by myocardial infarction. II. Tissue morphometry. *Am J Physiol* 1985;248:H883–889.
54. Anversa P, Li P, Zhang X, et al. Ischaemic myocardial injury and ventricular remodelling. *Cardiovasc Res* 1993;27:145–157.
55. Olivetti G, Abbi R, Quaini F, et al. Apoptosis in the failing human heart. *N Engl J Med* 1997;336:1131–1141.
56. Williams RS. Apoptosis and heart failure. *N Engl J Med* 1999;341: 759–760.
57. Olivetti G, Capasso JM, Sonnenblick EH, Anversa P. Side-to-side slippage of myocytes participates in ventricular wall remodeling acutely after myocardial infarction in rats. *Circ Res* 1990;67:23–34.
58. Chien KR. Genotype, phenotype: Upstairs, downstairs in the family of cardiomyopathies. *J Clin Invest* 2003;111:175–178.
59. Schonberger J, Seidman CE. Many roads lead to a broken heart: The genetics of dilated cardiomyopathy. *Am J Hum Genet* 2001;69: 249–260.
60. Lowes BD, Minobe W, Abraham WT, et al. Changes in gene expression in the intact human heart: Downregulation of alpha-myosin heavy chain in hypertrophied, failing ventricular myocardium. *J Clin Invest* 1997;100:2315–2324.
61. Brillantes AM, Allen P, Takahashi T, et al. Differences in cardiac calcium release channel (ryanodine receptor) expression in myocardium from patients with end-stage heart failure caused by ischemic versus dilated cardiomyopathy. *Circ Res* 1992;71:18–26.
62. Mercadier JJ, Lompre AM, Duc P, et al. Altered sarcoplasmic reticulum $Ca^{2+}$-ATPase gene expression in the human ventricle during end-stage heart failure. *J Clin Invest* 1990;85:305–309.
63. Gwathmey JK, Copelas L, MacKinnon R, et al. Abnormal intracellular calcium handling in myocardium from patients with end-stage heart failure. *Circ Res* 1987;61:70–76.
64. Meyer M, Schillinger W, Pieske B, et al. Alterations of sarcoplasmic reticulum proteins in failing human dilated cardiomyopathy. *Circulation* 1995;92:778–784.
65. Movsesian MA, Bristow MR, Krall J. $Ca^{2+}$ uptake by cardiac sarcoplasmic reticulum from patients with idiopathic dilated cardiomyopathy. *Circ Res* 1989;65:1141–1144.
66. Arai M, Matsui H, Periasamy M. Sarcoplasmic reticulum gene expression in cardiac hypertrophy and heart failure. *Circ Res* 1994;74: 555–564.
67. Kiss E, Ball NA, Kranias EG, Walsh RA. Differential changes in cardiac phospholamban and sarcoplasmic reticular $Ca^{2+}$-ATPase protein levels. Effects on $Ca^{2+}$ transport and mechanics in compensated pressure-overload hypertrophy and congestive heart failure. *Circ Res* 1995;77:759–764.
68. Hasenfuss G, Schillinger W, Lehnart SE, et al. Relationship between Na+-Ca2+-exchanger protein levels and diastolic function of failing human myocardium. *Circulation* 1999;99:641–648.
69. Marx SO, Reiken S, Hisamatsu Y, et al. PKA phosphorylation dissociates FKBP12.6 from the calcium release channel (ryanodine receptor): Defective regulation in failing hearts. *Cell* 2001;101: 365–376.
70. Reiken S, Gaburjakova M, Guatimosim S, et al. Protein kinase A phosphorylation of the cardiac calcium release channel (ryanodine receptor) in normal and failing hearts. *J Biol Chem* 2003;278:444–453.
71. Wolff MR, Buck SH, Stoker SW, et al. Myofibrillar calcium sensitivity of isometric tension is increased in human dilated cardiomyopathies: Role of altered beta-adrenergically mediated protein phosphorylation. *J Clin Invest* 1996;98:167–176.
72. Sonnenblick EH, Morrow AG, Williams JFJ. Effects of heart rate on the dynamics of force development in the intact human ventricle. *Circulation* 1966;33:945–951.
73. Bhargava V, Shabetai R, Mathiasen RA, et al. Loss of adrenergic control of the force-frequency relation in heart failure secondary to idiopathic or ischemic cardiomyopathy. *Am J Cardiol* 1998;81: 1130–1137.
74. Hajjar RJ, DiSalvo TG, Schmidt U, et al. Clinical correlates of the myocardial force-frequency relationship in patients with end-stage heart failure. *J Heart Lung Transplant* 1997;16:1157–1167.
75. Scheuer J. Metabolism of the heart in cardiac failure. *Prog Cardiovasc Dis* 1970;13:24–54.

76. Schwartz A, Sordahl LA, Entman ML. Abnormal biochemistry in myocardial failure. In: Mason DT, ed. *Congestive Heart Failure: Mechanisms, Evaluation and Treatment*. New York: Yorke Medical; 1976:25–44.
77. Badeer HS. *Cardiovascular Physiology*. Basel: Karger; 1984:1–276.
78. Katz AM. Is the failing heart an energy-starved organ? *J Card Fail* 1996;2:267–272.
79. Katz AM. *Physiology of the Heart*. New York: Raven Press; 1995.
80. Alpert NR, Hamrell BB. Cardiac hypertrophy: A compensatory and anticompensatory response to stress. In: Vassalle M, ed. *Cardiac Physiology For The Clinician*. New York: Academic Press; 1976: 174–201.
81. Feldman MD, Copelas L, Gwathmey JK, et al. Deficient production of cyclic AMP: Pharmacologic evidence of an important cause of contractile dysfunction in patients with end-stage heart failure. *Circulation* 1987;75:331–339.
82. Rabinowitz M, Zak R. Mitochondria and cardiac hypertrophy. *Circ Res* 1975;36:367–376.
83. Sievers R, Parmley WW, James T, Wikman-Coffelt J. Energy levels at systole vs. diastole in normal hamster hearts vs. myopathic hamster hearts. *Circ Res* 1983;53:759–766.
84. Ingwall JS, Kramer MF, Fifer MA, et al. The creatine kinase system in normal and diseased human myocardium. *N Engl J Med* 1985;313: 1050–1054.
85. Lentz RW, Harrison CE Jr, Dewey JD, et al. Functional evaluation of cardiac sarcoplasmic reticulum and mitochondria in human pathologic states. *J Mol Cell Cardiol* 1978;10:3–30.
86. Scheuer J. Metabolic factors in myocardial failure. *Circulation* 1993; 87:VII54–VII57.
87. Markiewicz W, Wu S, Sievers R, et al. Influence of heart rate on metabolic and hemodynamic parameters in the Syrian hamster cardiomyopathy. *Am Heart J* 1987;114:362–368.
88. Force T, Michael A, Kilter H, Haq S. Stretch-activated pathways in left ventricular remodeling. *J Card Fail* 2002;8:S351–S358.
89. Steenbergen C, Afshari CA, Petranka JG, et al. Alterations in apoptotic signaling in human idiopathic cardiomyopathic hearts in failure. *Am J Physiol Heart Circ Physiol* 2003;284:H268–H276.
90. Ukkonen H, Beanlands RS, Burwash IG, et al. Effect of cardiac resynchronization on myocardial efficiency and regional oxidative metabolism. *Circulation* 2003;107:28–31.
91. Auricchio A, Spinelli JC, Trautmann SI, Kloss M. Effect of cardiac resynchronization therapy on ventricular remodeling. *J Card Fail* 2002;8:S549–S555.
92. Bristow MR, Ginsburg R, Minobe W, et al. Decreased catecholamine sensitivity and beta-adrenergic-receptor density in failing human hearts. *N Engl J Med* 1982;307:205–211.
93. White M, Yanowitz F, Gilbert EM, et al. Role of beta-adrenergic receptor downregulation in the peak exercise response in patients with heart failure due to idiopathic dilated cardiomyopathy. *Am J Cardiol* 1995;76:1271–1276.
94. Bristow MR, Minobe W, Rasmussen R, et al. Beta-adrenergic neuroeffector abnormalities in the failing human heart are produced by local rather than systemic mechanisms. *J Clin Invest* 1992;89: 803–815.
95. Bristow MR, Ginsburg R, Umans V, et al. Beta 1- and beta 2-adrenergic-receptor subpopulations in nonfailing and failing human ventricular myocardium: Coupling of both receptor subtypes to muscle contraction and selective beta 1-receptor down-regulation in heart failure. *Circ Res* 1986;59:297–309.
96. Feldman AM, Cates AE, Bristow MR, Van Dop C. Altered expression of alpha-subunits of G proteins in failing human hearts. *J Mol Cell Cardiol* 1989;21:359–365.
97. Vatner DE, Sato N, Galper JB, Vatner SF. Physiological and biochemical evidence for coordinate increases in muscarinic receptors and Gi during pacing-induced heart failure. *Circulation* 1996;94:102–107.
98. Feldman AM, Cates AE, Veazey WB, et al. Increase of the 40,000-mol wt pertussis toxin substrate (G protein) in the failing human heart. *J Clin Invest* 1988;82:189–197.
99. White M, Roden R, Minobe W, et al. Age-related changes in beta-adrenergic neuroeffector systems in the human heart. *Circulation* 1994;90:1225–1238.
100. Fowler MB, Laser JA, Hopkins GL, et al. Assessment of the beta-adrenergic receptor pathway in the intact failing human heart: Progressive receptor down-regulation and subsensitivity to agonist response. *Circulation* 1986;74:1290–1302.
101. Iaccarino G, Tomhave ED, Lefkowitz RJ, Koch WJ. Reciprocal in vivo regulation of myocardial G protein-coupled receptor kinase expression by beta-adrenergic receptor stimulation and blockade. *Circulation* 1998;98:1783–1789.
102. Gilbert EM, Abraham WT, Olsen S, et al. Comparative hemodynamic, left ventricular functional, and antiadrenergic effects of chronic treatment with metoprolol versus carvedilol in the failing heart. *Circulation* 1996;94:2817–2825.
103. Richards AM, Doughty R, Nicholls MG, et al. Neurohumoral prediction of benefit from carvedilol in ischemic left ventricular dysfunction. Australia–New Zealand Heart Failure Group. *Circulation* 1999;99:786–792.
104. Eckberg DL, Drabinsky M, Braunwald E. Defective cardiac parasympathetic control in patients with heart disease. *N Engl J Med* 1971;285:877–883.
105. Levine TB, Francis GS, Goldsmith SR, Cohn JN. The neurohumoral and hemodynamic response to orthostatic tilt in patients with congestive heart failure. *Circulation* 1983;67:1070–1075.
106. Hirsch AT, Dzau VJ, Creager MA. Baroreceptor function in congestive heart failure: Effect on neurohumoral activation and regional vascular resistance. *Circulation* 1987;75:IV36–IV48.
107. Zucker H, Wang W, Brandle M. Baroreflex abnormalities in congestive heart failure. *NIPS* 1993;8:87–90.
108. Thames MD, Kinugawa T, Smith ML, Dibner-Dunlap ME. Abnormalities of baroreflex control in heart failure. *J Am Coll Cardiol* 1993;22: 56A–60A.
109. Mortara A, La Rovere MT, Pinna GD, et al. Arterial baroreflex modulation of heart rate in chronic heart failure: Clinical and hemodynamic correlates and prognostic implications. *Circulation* 1997;96:3450–3458.
110. Dibner-Dunlap ME, Thames MD. Control of sympathetic nerve activity by vagal mechanoreflexes is blunted in heart failure. *Circulation* 1992;86:1929–1934.
111. Grassi G, Seravalle G, Cattaneo BM, et al. Sympathetic activation and loss of reflex sympathetic control in mild congestive heart failure. *Circulation* 1995;92:3206–3211.
112. Newton GE, Parker JD. Cardiac sympathetic responses to acute vasodilation: Normal ventricular function versus congestive heart failure. *Circulation* 1996;94:3161–3167.
113. Goldsmith SR, Francis GS, Cowley AW Jr, et al. Increased plasma arginine vasopressin levels in patients with congestive heart failure. *J Am Coll Cardiol* 1983;1:1385–1390.
114. Zelis R, Nellis SH, Longhurst J, et al. Abnormalities in the regional circulations accompanying congestive heart failure. *Prog Cardiovasc Dis* 1975;18:181–199.
115. Brouwer J, van Veldhuisen DJ, Man in 't Veld AJ, et al. Prognostic value of heart rate variability during long-term follow-up in patients with mild to moderate heart failure. The Dutch Ibopamine Multicenter Trial Study Group. *J Am Coll Cardiol* 1996;28:1183–1189.
116. Levine TB, Olivari MT, Cohn JN. Effects of orthotopic heart transplantation on sympathetic control mechanisms in congestive heart failure. *Am J Cardiol* 1986;58:1035–1040.
117. Ellenbogen KA, Mohanty PK, Szentpetery S, Thames MD. Arterial baroreflex abnormalities in heart failure: Reversal after orthotopic cardiac transplantation. *Circulation* 1989;79:51–58.
118. Mohanty PK, Thames MD, Arrowood JA. Impairment of cardiopulmonary baroreflex after cardiac transplantation in humans. *Circulation* 1987;75:914–921.
119. Sinoway LI, Minotti JR, Davis D, et al. Delayed reversal of impaired vasodilation in congestive heart failure after heart transplantation. *Am J Cardiol* 1988;61:1076–1079.

120. Ferguson DW, Abboud FM, Mark AL. Selective impairment of baroreflex-mediated vasoconstrictor responses in patients with ventricular dysfunction. *Circulation* 1984;69:451–460.
121. Francis GS, Cohn JN. The autonomic nervous system in congestive heart failure. *Annu Rev Med* 1986;37:235–247.
122. Katz AM. The descending limb of the Starling curve and the failing heart. *Circulation* 1965;32:871–875.
123. MacGregor DC, Covell JW, Mahler F, et al. Relations between afterload, stroke volume, and descending limb of Starling's curve. *Am J Physiol* 1974;227:884–890.
124. Holubarsch C, Ruf T, Goldstein DJ, et al. Existence of the Frank-Starling mechanism in the failing human heart: Investigations on the organ, tissue, and sarcomere levels. *Circulation* 1996;94:683–689.
125. Ross J Jr. Afterload mismatch and preload reserve: A conceptual framework for the analysis of ventricular function. *Prog Cardiovasc Dis* 1976;18:255–264.
126. Badeer HS. Contractile tension in the myocardium. *Am Heart J* 1963;66:432–434.
127. Lakatta EG. Starling's law of the heart is explained by an intimate interaction of muscle length and myofilament calcium activation. *J Am Coll Cardiol* 1987;10:1157–1164.
128. Hoh JF, Rossmanith GH, Kwan LJ, Hamilton AM. Adrenaline increases the rate of cycling of crossbridges in rat cardiac muscle as measured by pseudo-random binary noise-modulated perturbation analysis. *Circ Res* 1988;62:452–461.
129. Cheng W, Li B, Kajstura J, et al. Stretch-induced programmed myocyte cell death. *J Clin Invest* 1995;96:2247–2259.
130. Anversa P, Ricci R, Olivetti G. Quantitative structural analysis of the myocardium during physiologic growth and induced cardiac hypertrophy: A review. *J Am Coll Cardiol* 1986;7:1140–1149.
131. Anversa P, Capasso JM, Olivetti G, Sonnenblick EH. Cellular basis of ventricular remodeling in hypertensive cardiomyopathy. *Am J Hypertens* 1992;5:758–770.
132. Grossman W, Jones D, McLaurin LP. Wall stress and patterns of hypertrophy in the human left ventricle. *J Clin Invest* 1975;56:56–64.
133. Weber KT, Clark WA, Janicki JS, Shroff SG. Physiologic versus pathologic hypertrophy and the pressure-overloaded myocardium. *J Cardiovasc Pharmacol* 1987;10:S37–S50.
134. Weber KT, Janicki JS, Shroff SG. Collagen compartment remodeling in the pressure overloaded left ventricle. *J Appl Cardiol* 1988;3: 37–46.
135. Weber KT, Janicki JS, Shroff SG, et al. Collagen remodeling of the pressure-overloaded, hypertrophied nonhuman primate myocardium. *Circ Res* 1988;62:757–765.
136. Weber KT. Cardiac interstitium in health and disease: The fibrillar collagen network. *J Am Coll Cardiol* 1989;13:1637–1652.
137. Weber KT, Brilla CG. Pathological hypertrophy and cardiac interstitium. Fibrosis and renin- angiotensin-aldosterone system. *Circulation* 1991;83:1849–1865.
138. Weber KT, Pick R, Silver MA, et al. Fibrillar collagen and remodeling of dilated canine left ventricle. *Circulation* 1990;82:1387–1401.
139. Zhao MJ, Zhang H, Robinson TF, et al. Profound structural alterations of the extracellular collagen matrix in postischemic dysfunctional ("stunned") but viable myocardium. *J Am Coll Cardiol* 1987;10: 1322–1334.
140. Kelly DT. Paul Dudley White International Lecture. Our future society: A global challenge. *Circulation* 1997;95:2459–2464.
141. Grossman W, McLaurin LP, Rolett EL. Alterations in left ventricular relaxation and diastolic compliance in congestive cardiomyopathy. *Cardiovasc Res* 1979;13:514–522.
142. Little WC, Downes TR. Clinical evaluation of left ventricular diastolic performance. *Prog Cardiovasc Dis* 1990;32:273–290.
143. Stauffer JC, Gaasch WH. Recognition and treatment of left ventricular diastolic dysfunction. *Prog Cardiovasc Dis* 1990;32:319–332.
144. Bolli R. Mechanism of myocardial "stunning". *Circulation* 1990;82: 723–738.
145. Marban E. Myocardial stunning and hibernation: The physiology behind the colloquialisms. *Circulation* 1991;83:681–688.
146. Rahimtoola SH. Importance of diagnosing hibernating myocardium: How and in whom? *J Am Coll Cardiol* 1997;30:1701–1706.
147. Marwick TH. The viable myocardium: Epidemiology, detection, and clinical implications. *Lancet* 1998;351:815–819.
148. Vanoverschelde JL, Wijns W, Borgers M, et al. Chronic myocardial hibernation in humans: From bedside to bench. *Circulation* 1997;95: 1961–1971.
149. Weber KT, Brilla CG, Janicki JS. Myocardial fibrosis: Functional significance and regulatory factors. *Cardiovasc Res* 1993;27: 341–348.
150. Weber KT. Monitoring tissue repair and fibrosis from a distance. *Circulation* 1997;96:2488–2492.
151. Thomas CV, Coker ML, Zellner JL, et al. Increased matrix metalloproteinase activity and selective upregulation in LV myocardium from patients with end-stage dilated cardiomyopathy. *Circulation* 1998;97:1708–1715.
152. Harada M, Itoh H, Nakagawa O, et al. Significance of ventricular myocytes and nonmyocytes interaction during cardiocyte hypertrophy: Evidence for endothelin-1 as a paracrine hypertrophic factor from cardiac nonmyocytes. *Circulation* 1997;96:3737–3744.
153. Levin ER, Gardner DG, Samson WK. Natriuretic peptides. *N Engl J Med* 1998;339:321–328.
154. Cowie MR, Mendez GF. BNP and congestive heart failure. *Prog Cardiovasc Dis* 2002;44:293–321.
155. Schrier RW, Abraham WT. Hormones and hemodynamics in heart failure. *N Engl J Med* 1999;341:577–585.
156. Rona G. Catecholamine cardiotoxicity. *J Mol Cell Cardiol* 1985;17: 291–306.
157. Mann DL, Kent RL, Parsons B, Cooper GT. Adrenergic effects on the biology of the adult mammalian cardiocyte. *Circulation* 1992;85: 790–804.
158. Tan LB, Jalil JE, Pick R, et al. Cardiac myocyte necrosis induced by angiotensin II. *Circ Res* 1991;69:1185–1195.
159. Francis GS, Goldsmith SR, Levine TB, et al. The neurohumoral axis in congestive heart failure. *Ann Intern Med* 1984;101:370–377.
160. Packer M. Neurohormonal interactions and adaptations in congestive heart failure. *Circulation* 1988;77:721–730.
161. Packer M. The neurohormonal hypothesis: A theory to explain the mechanism of disease progression in heart failure. *J Am Coll Cardiol* 1992;20:248–254.
162. Packer M, Lee WH, Kessler PD, et al. Role of neurohormonal mechanisms in determining survival in patients with severe chronic heart failure. *Circulation* 1987;75:IV80–IV92.
163. Starling EH. Points on pathology of heart disease. *Lancet* 1897;1: 569–572.
164. Chidsey CA, Harrison DC, Braunwald E. Augmentation of the plasma norepinephrine response to exercise in patients with congestive heart failure. *N Engl J Med* 1962;267:650–654.
165. Braunwald E, Chidsey CA, Pool PE. Congestive heart failure: Biochemical and physiological considerations. *Ann Intern Med* 1966; 64:904–941.
166. Thomas JA, Marks BH. Plasma norepinephrine in congestive heart failure. *Am J Cardiol* 1978;41:233–243.
167. Levine TB, Francis GS, Goldsmith SR, et al. Activity of the sympathetic nervous system and renin-angiotensin system assessed by plasma hormone levels and their relation to hemodynamic abnormalities in congestive heart failure. *Am J Cardiol* 1982;49: 1659–1666.
168. Leimbach WN Jr, Wallin BG, Victor RG, et al. Direct evidence from intraneural recordings for increased central sympathetic outflow in patients with heart failure. *Circulation* 1986;73:913–919.
169. Hasking GJ, Esler MD, Jennings GL, et al. Norepinephrine spillover to plasma in patients with congestive heart failure: Evidence of increased overall and cardiorenal sympathetic nervous activity. *Circulation* 1986;73:615–621.
170. Rundqvist B, Elam M, Bergmann-Sverrisdottir Y, et al. Increased cardiac adrenergic drive precedes generalized sympathetic activation in human heart failure. *Circulation* 1997;95:169–175.

171. Gafney TE, Braunwald E. Importance of the adrenergic nervous system in the support of circulatory function in patients with congestive heart failure. *Am J Med* 1963;34:320–324.
172. Hall SA, Cigarroa CG, Marcoux L, et al. Time course of improvement in left ventricular function, mass and geometry in patients with congestive heart failure treated with beta-adrenergic blockade. *J Am Coll Cardiol* 1995;25:1154–1161.
173. Eichhorn EJ, Bristow MR. Medical therapy can improve the biological properties of the chronically failing heart. A new era in the treatment of heart failure. *Circulation* 1996;94:2285–2296.
174. Packer M, Coats AJC, Fowler MB, et al. Effect of carvedilol on survival in severe chronic heart failure. *N Engl J Med* 2001;344: 1651–1658.
175. Keeton TK, Campbell WB. The pharmacologic alteration of renin release. *Pharmacol Rev* 1981;31:81–227.
176. Matsubara H. Pathophysiological role of angiotensin II type 2 receptor in cardiovascular and renal diseases. *Circ Res* 1998;83:1182–1191.
177. Tang WHW, Vagelos RH, Yee YG, et al. Neurohormonal and clinical responses to high- versus low-dose enalapril therapy in chronic heart failure. *J Am Coll Cardiol* 2002;39:70–78.
178. Yusuf S, Sleight P, Pogue J, et al. Effects of an angiotensin-converting-enzyme inhibitor, ramipril, on cardiovascular events in high-risk patients. The Heart Outcomes Prevention Evaluation Study Investigators. *N Engl J Med* 2000;342:145–153.
179. Francis GS. The renin-angiotensin system. In: Parmley W, Chatterjee K, eds. *Cardiology*. New York: Lippincott-Raven; 1997:1–16.
180. Gibbons GH, Pfeffer MA. The role of angiotensin in cardiovascular disease: Pathophysiologic insights and therapeutic implications. In: Topol EJ, ed. *Textbook of Cardiovascular Medicine*. New York: Lippincott-Raven; 1998:1–12.
181. Pitt B, Zannad F, Remme WJ, Cody R, et al. The effect of spironolactone on morbidity and mortality in patients with severe heart failure. Randomized Aldactone Evaluation Study Investigators. *N Engl J Med* 1999;341:709–717.
182. Francis GS, Benedict C, Johnstone DE, et al. Comparison of neuroendocrine activation in patients with left ventricular dysfunction with and without congestive heart failure. A substudy of the Studies of Left Ventricular Dysfunction (SOLVD). *Circulation* 1990;82: 1724–1729.
183. Goldsmith SR, Francis GS, Cowley AW Jr, et al. Hemodynamic effects of infused arginine vasopressin in congestive heart failure. *J Am Coll Cardiol* 1986;8:779–783.
184. Cowie MR, Struthers AD, Wood DA, et al. Value of natriuretic peptides in assessment of patients with possible new heart failure in primary care. *Lancet* 1997;350:1349–1353.
185. Niinuma H, Nakamura M, Hiramori K. Plasma B-type natriuretic peptide measurement in a multiphasic health screening program. *Cardiology* 1998;90:89–94.
186. Mills RM, LeJemtel TH, Horton DP, et al. Sustained hemodynamic effects of an infusion of nesiritide (human b-type natriuretic peptide) in heart failure: A randomized, double-blind, placebo-controlled clinical trial. Natrecor Study Group. *J Am Coll Cardiol* 1999;34:155–162.
187. Intravenous nesiritide vs nitroglycerin for treatment of decompensated congestive heart failure: A randomized controlled trial. *JAMA* 2002; 287:1531–1540.
188. Packer M, Califf RM, Konstam MA, et al. Comparison of omapatrilat and enalapril in patients with chronic heart failure: The Omapatrilat Versus Enalapril Randomized Trial of Utility in Reducing Events (OVERTURE). *Circulation* 2002;106:920–926.
189. Levin ER. Endothelins. *N Engl J Med* 1995;333:356–363.
190. Yanagisawa M, Kurihara H, Kimura S, et al. A novel potent vasoconstrictor peptide produced by vascular endothelial cells. *Nature* 1988;332:411–415.
191. Rodeheffer RJ, Lerman A, Heublein DM, Burnett JC Jr. Increased plasma concentrations of endothelin in congestive heart failure in humans. *Mayo Clin Proc* 1992;67:719–724.
192. McMurray JJ, Ray SG, Abdullah I, et al. Plasma endothelin in chronic heart failure. *Circulation* 1992;85:1374–1379.
193. Zolk O, Quattek J, Sitzler G, et al. Expression of endothelin-1, endothelin-converting enzyme, and endothelin receptors in chronic heart failure. *Circulation* 1999;99:2118–2123.
194. Benigni A, Remuzzi G. Endothelin antagonists. *Lancet* 1999;353: 133–138.
195. Levine B, Kalman J, Mayer L, et al. Elevated circulating levels of tumor necrosis factor in severe chronic heart failure. *N Engl J Med* 1990;323:236–241.
196. Torre-Amione G, Kapadia S, Benedict C, et al. Proinflammatory cytokine levels in patients with depressed left ventricular ejection fraction: A report from the Studies of Left Ventricular Dysfunction (SOLVD). *J Am Coll Cardiol* 1996;27:1201–1206.
197. Torre-Amione G, Kapadia S, Lee J, et al. Tumor necrosis factor-alpha and tumor necrosis factor receptors in the failing human heart. *Circulation* 1996;93:704–711.
198. Bristow MR. Tumor necrosis factor-alpha and cardiomyopathy. *Circulation* 1998;97:1340–1341.
199. Bozkurt B, Kribbs SB, Clubb FJ Jr, et al. Pathophysiologically relevant concentrations of tumor necrosis factor-alpha promote progressive left ventricular dysfunction and remodeling in rats. *Circulation* 1998;97: 1382–1391.
200. Yokoyama T, Nakano M, Bednarczyk JL, et al. Tumor necrosis factor-alpha provokes a hypertrophic growth response in adult cardiac myocytes. *Circulation* 1997;95:1247–1252.
201. Anker SD, Chua TP, Ponikowski P, et al. Hormonal changes and catabolic/anabolic imbalance in chronic heart failure and their importance for cardiac cachexia. *Circulation* 1997;96:526–534.
202. Anker SD, Clark AL, Kemp M, et al. Tumor necrosis factor and steroid metabolism in chronic heart failure: Possible relation to muscle wasting. *J Am Coll Cardiol* 1997;30:997–1001.
203. Bryant D, Becker L, Richardson J, et al. Cardiac failure in transgenic mice with myocardial expression of tumor necrosis factor-alpha. *Circulation* 1998;97:1375–1381.
204. Krum H. Tumor necrosis factor-alpha blockade as a therapeutic strategy in heart failure (RENEWAL and ATTACH). Unsuccessful, to be specific. *J Card Fail* 2002;8:365–368.
205. Cannon PJ. The kidney in heart failure. *N Engl J Med* 1977;296:26–32.
206. Dzau VJ. Renal and circulatory mechanisms in congestive heart failure. *Kidney Int* 1987;31:1402–1415.
207. Packer M, Lee WH, Kessler PD. Preservation of glomerular filtration rate in human heart failure by activation of the renin-angiotensin system. *Circulation* 1986;74:766–774.
208. Ichikawa I, Yoshioka T, Fogo A, Kon V. Role of angiotensin II in altered glomerular hemodynamics in congestive heart failure. *Kidney Int Suppl* 1990;30:S123–S126.
209. Hall JE, Guyton AC, Jackson TE, et al. Control of glomerular filtration rate by renin-angiotensin system. *Am J Physiol* 1977;233: F366–F372.
210. Ichikawa I, Pfeffer JM, Pfeffer MA, et al. Role of angiotensin II in the altered renal function of congestive heart failure. *Circ Res* 1984;55: 669–675.
211. Drexler H, Lu W. Endothelial dysfunction of hindquarter resistance vessels in experimental heart failure. *Am J Physiol* 1992;262: H1640–H1645.
212. Drexler H, Hayoz D, Munzel T, et al. Endothelial function in chronic congestive heart failure. *Am J Cardiol* 1992;69:1596–1601.
213. Kubo SH, Rector TS, Bank AJ, et al. Endothelium-dependent vasodilation is attenuated in patients with heart failure. *Circulation* 1991;84:1589–1596.
214. Treasure CB, Vita JA, Cox DA, et al. Endothelium-dependent dilation of the coronary microvasculature is impaired in dilated cardiomyopathy. *Circulation* 1990;81:772-779.
215. Le Jemtel TH, Katz SD, Sonnenblick EH. Peripheral circulatory response in cardiac failure. *Hosp Pract (Off Ed)* 1991;26:75–82.
216. Winlaw DS, Smythe GA, Keogh AM, et al. Increased nitric oxide production in heart failure. *Lancet* 1994;344:373–374.
217. Katz SD, Schwarz M, Yuen J, LeJemtel TH. Impaired acetylcholine-mediated vasodilation in patients with congestive heart failure: Role of

endothelium-derived vasodilating and vasoconstrictive factors. *Circulation* 1993;88:55–61.
218. Kubo SH, Rector TS, Bank AJ, et al. Effects of cardiac transplantation on endothelium-dependent dilation of the peripheral vasculature in congestive heart failure. *Am J Cardiol* 1993;71:88–93.
219. Swan JW, Anker SD, Walton C, et al. Insulin resistance in chronic heart failure: Relation to severity and etiology of heart failure. *J Am Coll Cardiol* 1997;30:527–532.
220. Jamali AH, Witteles RM, Tang WHW, et al. High prevalence of impaired glucose metabolism in patients with idiopathic dilated cardiomyopathy (abstr). *J Am Coll Cardiol* 2002;39:181A.
221. Paolisso G, Tagliamonte MR, Rizzo MR, et al. Prognostic importance of insulin-mediated glucose uptake in aged patients with congestive heart failure secondary to mitral and/or aortic valve disease. *Am J Cardiol* 1999;83:1338–1344.
222. Kelly RA, Balligand JL, Smith TW. Nitric oxide and cardiac function. *Circ Res* 1996;79:363–380.
223. Drexler H. Nitric oxide synthases in the failing human heart: A doubled-edged sword? *Circulation* 1999;99:2972–2975.
224. Haywood GA, Tsao PS, von der Leyen HE, et al. Expression of inducible nitric oxide synthase in human heart failure. *Circulation* 1996;93:1087–1094.
225. Recchia FA, McConnell PI, Bernstein RD, et al. Reduced nitric oxide production and altered myocardial metabolism during the decompensation of pacing-induced heart failure in the conscious dog. *Circ Res* 1998;83:969–979.
226. Massie BM. Exercise tolerance in congestive heart failure: Role of cardiac function, peripheral blood flow, and muscle metabolism and effect of treatment. *Am J Med* 1988;84:75–82.
227. Massie BM, Simonini A, Sahgal P, et al. Relation of systemic and local muscle exercise capacity to skeletal muscle characteristics in men with congestive heart failure. *J Am Coll Cardiol* 1996;27:140–145.
228. Hambrecht R, Adams V, Gielen S, et al. Exercise intolerance in patients with chronic heart failure and increased expression of inducible nitric oxide synthase in the skeletal muscle. *J Am Coll Cardiol* 1999;33:174–179.
229. Adams V, Jiang H, Yu J, et al. Apoptosis in skeletal myocytes of patients with chronic heart failure is associated with exercise intolerance. *J Am Coll Cardiol* 1999;33:959–965.
230. Robbins M, Francis G, Pashkow FJ, et al. Ventilatory and heart rate responses to exercise: Better predictors of heart failure mortality than peak oxygen consumption. *Circulation* 1999;100:2411–2417.
231. Wilson JR, Hanamanthu S, Chomsky DB, Davis SF. Relationship between exertional symptoms and functional capacity in patients with heart failure. *J Am Coll Cardiol* 1999;33:1943–1947.
232. Recommendations for exercise training in chronic heart failure patients. *Eur Heart J* 2001;22:125–135.
233. Lanfranchi PA, Braghiroli A, Bosimini E, et al. Prognostic value of nocturnal Cheyne-Stokes respiration in chronic heart failure. *Circulation* 1999;99:1435–1440.
234. Javaheri S. A mechanism of central sleep apnea in patients with heart failure. *N Engl J Med* 1999;341:949–954.
235. Andreas S, Clemens C, Sandholzer H, et al. Improvement of exercise capacity with treatment of Cheyne-Stokes respiration in patients with congestive heart failure. *J Am Coll Cardiol* 1996;27:1486–1490.
236. Javaheri S, Parker TJ, Wexler L, et al. Occult sleep-disordered breathing in stable congestive heart failure. *Ann Intern Med* 1995;122: 487–492.
237. Javaheri S, Parker TJ, Liming JD, et al. Sleep apnea in 81 ambulatory male patients with stable heart failure: Types and their prevalences, consequences, and presentations. *Circulation* 1998;97:2154–2159.
238. Tkacova R, Rankin F, Fitzgerald FS, et al. Effects of continuous positive airway pressure on obstructive sleep apnea and left ventricular afterload in patients with heart failure. *Circulation* 1998;98:2269–2275.

C H A P T E R 25

# DIAGNOSIS AND MANAGEMENT OF HEART FAILURE

Thierry H. LeJemtel / Edmund H. Sonnenblick / William H. Frishman



The management of patients with congestive heart failure (CHF) has progressed in three directions. The first direction is the increased awareness that as patients age with systemic hypertension, type 2 diabetes, and the metabolic syndrome, they are likely to develop CHF despite preserved left ventricular systolic function as evidenced by a normal ejection fraction.[1,2] The presence of three or more of the following criteria characterize the highly prevalent metabolic syndrome: abdominal obesity, hypertriglyceridemia, low high-density lipoprotein (HDL) cholesterol, and a high blood pressure or elevated fasting blood glucose.[3] Large double-blind placebo-controlled trials conducted in patients with a reduced left ventricular (LV) systolic function have demonstrated the therapeutic efficacy of angiotensin-converting enzyme (ACE) inhibition, angiotensin receptor blockers (ARBs), and beta-adrenergic blockade (BAB). However, such trials have yet to be conducted with all these drug classes in patients with preserved LV systolic function. Nevertheless, in hypertensive and diabetic patients, studies have shown that physical activity, tighter control of blood pressure, blood sugar, and body weight are essential in prevention and treatment of CHF with preserved LV systolic function.

The second direction involves the use of nonpharmacologic approaches in the management of patients with CHF due to reduced LV systolic function. The pharmacologic management alone has remained essentially unchanged after the remarkable successes with long-term use of ACE inhibition, ARBs and BAB.[4] Cardiac resynchronization with biventricular pacing improves functional capacity and quality of life in symptomatic patients with CHF and intraventricular conduction defect despite optimal pharmacologic management.[5–12] Internal cardioverter defibrillators (ICDs) prolong life in patients with CHF resulting from obstructive coronary artery disease.[13] Left ventricular assist devices (LVADs) prolong life in some patients with end-stage CHF refractory to optimal medical therapy and ineligible for cardiac transplantation.[14] The LVADs are evolving with smaller units that only provide augmentation of the cardiac output. Improvement in power supplies and internalization of the entire device to avoid infection may enhance long-term efficacy.

The third direction relates to the use of stem cells to replace lost myocardium. Experimental studies demonstrate that all myocardial cells are not terminally differentiated and that stem cells can form new myocytes and blood vessels.[15] The feasibility and safety of using stem cells for cardiac repair are currently under investigation in humans.[16]

In view of the absence of controlled data in patients with CHF and preserved LV systolic function, the present chapter will mainly deal with the treatment of patients with CHF and reduced LV systolic function where therapeutic progress has been made.

## PATHOPHYSIOLOGY AND DIAGNOSIS OF CONGESTIVE HEART FAILURE

The dynamic process by which ventricular dysfunction evolves into CHF can be described in three phases[17] (Fig. 25-1). Each phase and its duration depend heavily on specific primary etiology. Myocardial damage with massive myocyte loss and fibrotic repair may be rapid, as occurs with an acute transmural myocardial infarction or a viral myocarditis, or may evolve over years, as occurs with overloads resulting from systemic hypertension or valvular disease.[18,19] Without overt clinical symptoms, such as chest pain with a myocardial infarction or sudden (flash) pulmonary edema, the initial damage may go on undiagnosed. The two-dimensional echocardiogram may indicate the presence and extent of LV dysfunction and segmental wall motion abnormalities, since ventricular dilatation is common in largely asymptomatic patients.

The second stage in the evolution of heart failure involves an adaptation to myocardial damage, termed *ventricular remodeling*. Myocardial hypertrophy occurs in response to myocardium that is lost or overloaded. Ventricular dilatation helps to sustain cardiac output (see Fig. 25-1). In a sense, loss of myocardium, whether segmental as occurs with myocardial infarction or diffuse as occurs with cardiomyopathies, creates an overload for the myocardium since less myocardium must maintain the work of the heart. The myocardium responds to this overload with changes in growth and architecture,

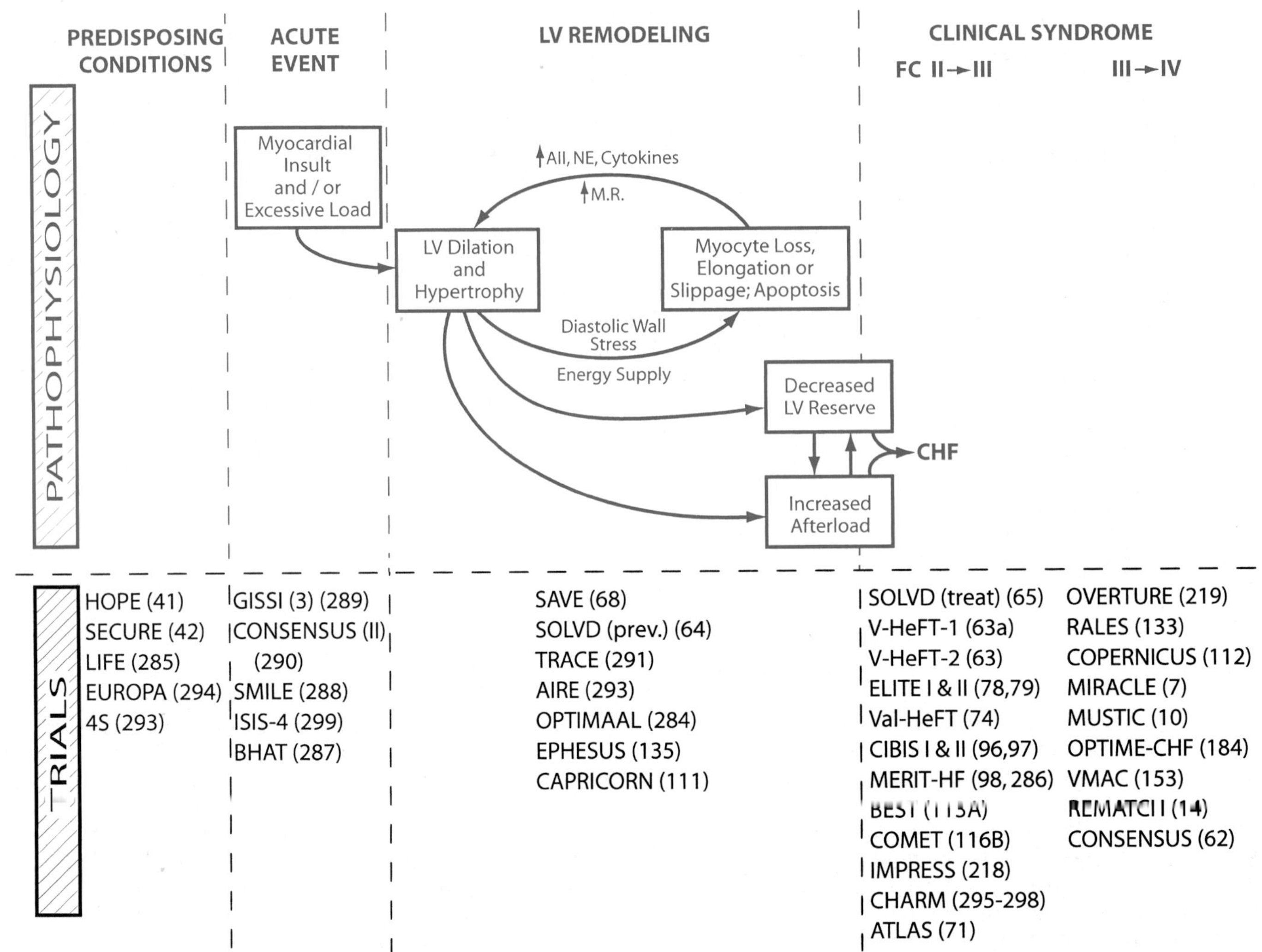


FIGURE 25-1 The pathophysiology of heart failure from predisposing conditions such as hypertension, atherosclerosis, coronary artery disease, and dyslipidemias to left ventricular (LV) remodeling after an acute event and to the clinical syndrome of heart failure that progresses from functional class (FC) II–III to III–IV according to the New York Heart Association criteria. In the majority of patients, symptoms become noticeable only when the LV remodeling process is nearly completed. The adaptive responses to cardiac myocyte loss/dysfunction and/or persistent overload include myocardial hypertrophy and LV chamber dilatation. Chamber dilatation augments diastolic wall stress that produces deformation of the LV wall and functional mitral regurgitation (MR), as well as further myocyte loss by apoptosis. Local neurohumoral systems become activated with increased norepinephrine (NE) and angiotensin II concentration. Parasympathetic tone is reduced. These structural and functional alterations constitute what is termed *ventricular remodeling*. With progression of these processes and with increasingly reduced capacity of the LV chamber to increase its output as required along with retention of sodium, central and peripheral edema ensue, with limitation of physical capacity. Thus, the clinical syndrome that follows the silent phase of LV remodeling finally becomes manifest. Shown at the bottom of the figure are the various trials addressing the predisposing conditions and the three phases of heart failure in terms of morbidity and mortality. These trials have shaped the present therapy of heart failure. They are referenced at the end of the chapter.

which comprise *ventricular remodeling*. This includes increases in myocyte length, as well as lateral dimension. With an increased pressure load, myocytes respond by laying down more contractile units in parallel, thus increasing the lateral dimensions of the myocyte and its force potential. This form of hypertrophy tends to normalize the tension in the ventricular wall. When volume is increased, whether due to increased flow from an insufficient valve or due to increased diastolic filling pressure that results as a compensation for lost myocardium, myocytes elongate in order to maintain force and shortening. Acutely, this occurs within the limits created by the physiologic lengthening of the sarcomere (i.e., the Frank Starling length-tension curve). With a sustained diastolic load, sarcomeres are added in series, resulting in increased myocyte length. Since augmented diastolic volume itself results in increased ventricular wall tension, lateral growth (hypertrophy) of myocytes commonly accompanies myocyte lengthening. In addition to hypertrophy of myocytes, other dynamic events are occurring in the myocardium.

Myocytes may be lost diffusely when excessive overloads occur through the process of apoptosis, and focal necrosis with replacement fibrosis. With sustained diastolic loads, ventricular dilatation proceeds with not only marked myocyte lengthening, but also apparent displacement of myocytes or groups of myocytes one to the other, a process labeled "myocyte slippage." While hypertrophy of myocytes is readily demonstrable, hyperplasia of myocytes have also been observed.[20,21] Taken together, hypertrophy, myocyte hypertrophy, further myocyte loss, and hyperplasia, along with ventricular wall restructuring, comprise *ventricular remodeling*.[15] With systolic overloads, it is generally characterized by an increased ventricular wall thickness with normal intraventricular volumes (e.g., normal ejection fraction). When the hypertrophy itself cannot sustain required systolic tension, whether due to a primary decrease in force production by a given myocyte,[22] or loss of myocytes, ventricular dilatation occurs with a resultant fall in the ejection fraction. Generally, ventricular remodeling proceeds silently unless it is heralded by clinical symptoms such as dyspnea or exertion that may reflect an increased diastolic filling pressure, or developing peripheral edema.

The factors that mediate progressive ventricular remodeling (hypertrophy) involve both physical forces as well as neurohumoral factors (e.g., angiotensin) that are activated.[23] Early on, activation of the sympathetic nervous system with parasympathetic withdrawal leads to tachycardia and peripheral vasoconstriction. Activation of the renin–angiotensin system causes further vasoconstriction and salt accumulation via stimulated aldosterone secretion. Both these latter factors, along with excessive stretch of the myocardium, can lead to further myocyte loss with fibrosis, along with further myocyte hypertrophy, while ventricular dilatation may induce functional mitral and/or tricuspid insufficiency, creating an additional hemodynamic load (Fig. 25-2).[24]

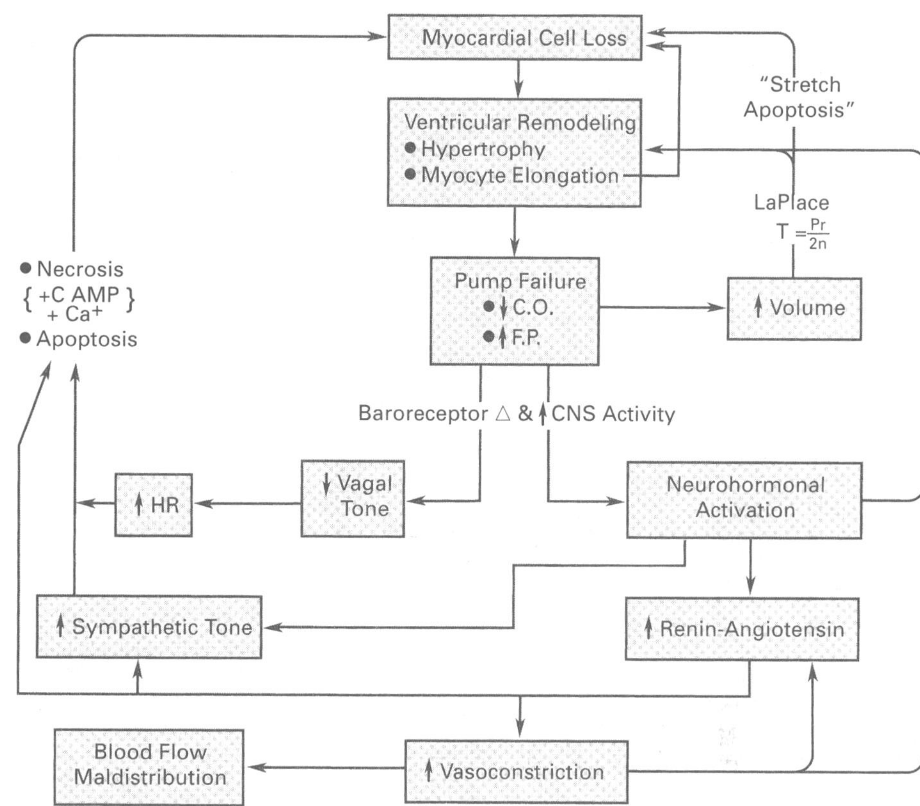


FIGURE 25-2 Ventricular remodeling and progression of ventricular dysfunction. Myocardial cell loss leads to ventricular remodeling, characterized by myocyte hypertrophy and elongation. An increase in ventricular volume (the Starling effect) helps to maintain cardiac output (CO) but at the cost of increasing ventricular filling pressures. The increase in diastolic stretch and pressure produces further damage, including stretch-induced myocyte death (apoptosis), which amplifies the process of remodeling. With inadequate pump function, neurohumoral activation occurs with decreased vagal tone and enhanced sympathetic tone. With activation of the renin–angiotensin system and increased sympathetic tone, arterial vasoconstriction occurs with resultant maldistribution of blood flow. Decreased vagal and increased sympathetic stimulation induce tachycardia, and the latter system along with the activated renin–angiotensin system via angiotensin II can produce further myocyte death. In this manner, the process is self-perpetuating, in that ventricular damage leads to remodeling, which, in turn, leads to further damage. These interrelated cycles thus provide therapeutic opportunities.

The third phase in the evolution of heart failure evolves from these adaptive changes, with development of the symptoms of CHF, characterized by decreased exercise tolerance, pulmonary and systemic congestion, and central and peripheral edema. The interval between initiation of ventricular dysfunction and the onset of symptoms, during which ventricular remodeling occurs, may extend over a long period following an acute myocardial infarction; this period can be very short. With more chronic processes, such as those that occur with hypertension or idiopathic cardiomyopathies, this period may extend over months or years. Indeed, when patients were first identified with asymptomatic LV dysfunction in the Studies of Left Ventricular Dysfunction (SOLVD) trial (discussed later), their average ejection fraction was already reduced to 28 percent, indicating that extensive ventricular damage had already occurred (Fig. 25-3). At this point, exercise performance, as represented by peak oxygen consumption, was moderately reduced but not to such an extent as to limit exercise performance or produce symptoms. Circulating norepinephrine was increased slightly, while plasma renin levels (slashed lines) were not, except when diuretics had been administered (open bars). Once symptoms occurred, there was a progressive increase in circulating norepinephrine and plasma renin. A progressive decline in exercise capacity was documented as patients progressed from New York Heart Association (NYHA) class I to class IV. The reduction in exercise performance was relatively greater than the decrease in the ejection fraction. Exercise performance and ejection fraction are poorly related. This reflects the finding that inactivity reduces the capacity for peripheral vasodilatation and thus limits skeletal muscle performance. Ventricular dysfunction may involve the left or right ventricles or both. In addition, such abnormalities may be amplified by overloads created by valvular insufficiency (e.g., mitral or tricuspid) or systolic overloads (e.g., aortic stenosis, arterial or pulmonary hypertension). Separating the effects of myocardial dysfunction from such imposed overloads is difficult. Moreover, functional mitral and/or tricuspid insufficiency resulting from ventricular dilatation imposes a further volume load on an already damaged ventricle.

Abnormalities of ventricular function can be usefully divided into problems of ventricular filling (diastole) and ventricular emptying (systole). Even in the presence of normal systolic ventricular performance, abnormalities of ventricular filling, termed *diastolic ventricular dysfunction,* may be observed (Fig. 25-4). This is characterized by an increased ventricular filling pressure for any end-diastolic volume (EDV) due to reduced compliance of the ventricle. Thus, with normal EDV and stroke volume (SV), filling pressures

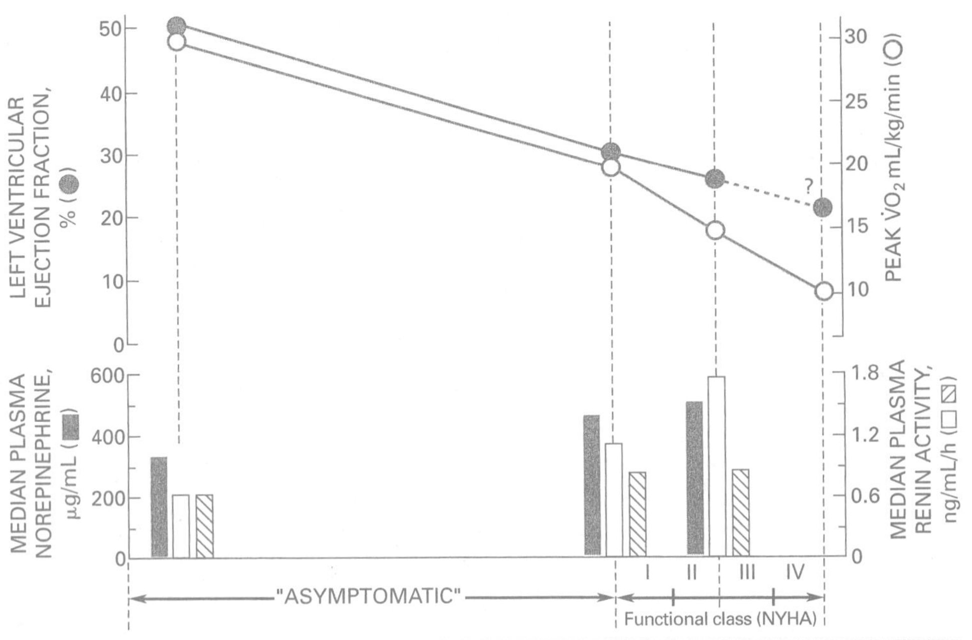


FIGURE 25-3 Progression of initial ventricular damage to sympathetic congestive heart failure. Data from the SOLVD trial of enalapril therapy; plotted in terms of LV ejection fraction and exercise capacity measured in terms of peak oxygen consumption ($\dot{V}O_2$). Also shown are median plasma norepinephrine and plasma renin activity. The latter is shown in terms of patients who did or did not receive diuretics.

may be markedly increased, leading to signs of pulmonary congestion despite a normal ejection fraction. Such a situation may occur with LV hypertrophy, especially when associated with a rapid heart rate, which further limits the time for ventricular filling. It can also be seen with aging, where diffuse myocyte loss with replacement fibrosis and reactive myocyte hypertrophy occurs.[25]

Systolic ventricular dysfunction is characterized by reduced ability to generate pressure isovolumically and decreased capacity to eject blood in systole. The SV depends on the EDV, as well as the afterload, which is directly related to the arterial pressure. If the afterload is reasonably normal, there is a linear relation between SV and EDV, and the resultant slope (SV/EDV) is termed the *ejection fraction*. Should the slope of the relation linking end-systolic pressure and LV volume be reduced, as occurs when the ventricle is depressed, the SV at any EDV is reduced, resulting in a decreased ejection fraction. If the afterload is approximately normal, this reduced ejection fraction can serve as a measure of *reduced systolic ventricular performance*. Since the extent of shortening of myocardium is reduced as afterload is increased, an increased systolic ventricular pressure can by itself reduce SV and hence tend to decrease ejection fraction, as can occur in severe aortic stenosis. Similarly, with severe mitral insufficiency, which decreases afterload via a low impedance pathway into the left atrium, an increased SV tends to occur, yielding an artificially increased ejection fraction. Thus, the ejection fraction provides a useful index of systolic ventricular performance.

Although complex indices of systolic ventricular function have been described on the basis of myocardial muscle function, the measurement of ejection fraction has served as the clinical standard, whether determined noninvasively by nuclear imaging techniques or invasively with angiography. In addition to an overall depression of myocardial function, focal abnormalities of ventricular wall motion, described in terms of hypokinesis and akinesis, may produce major alterations in overall LV function, as seen in coronary artery disease. While a segment of the LV wall may be replaced by fibrotic scar, focal abnormalities of contraction may occur in viable myocardium when coronary perfusion is transiently reduced, leading to prolonged decrease in contraction; this is termed *stunning*. Alternatively, with a sustained reduction in coronary blood flow that is still adequate to sustain viability, contraction can be persistently reduced or absent; this is termed *hibernation*.[26] These important alterations can occur simultaneously in a given patient and are hard to separate. Defining these abnormalities in coronary heart disease with heart failure is extremely important, since reversal of

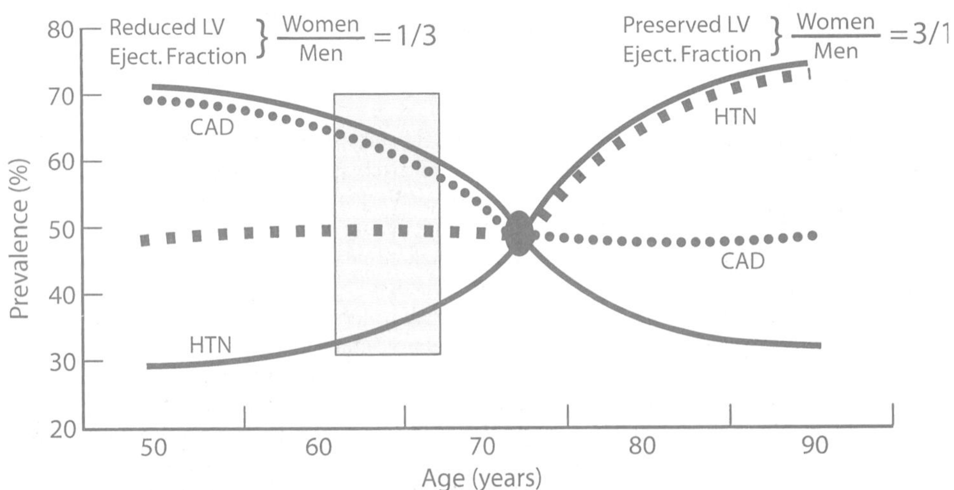


FIGURE 25-4 When chronic heart failure is associated with reduced left ventricular (LV) ejection fraction, patients are mostly men. Their age ranges from 55 to 70 years old. Coronary artery disease (CAD) is the preponderant etiology of chronic heart failure associated with reduced LV ejection fraction. When chronic heart failure is associated with preserved LV ejection fraction, patients are mostly women. Their age ranges from 65 to 90 years old. Hypertension (HTN) is the preponderant etiology of chronic heart failure associated with preserved LV ejection fraction. Except for CHARM,[295–298] randomized trials of new therapeutic modalities have mostly involved patients with chronic heart failure associated with reduced LV ejection fraction. These trials dealt with men aged 60 to 65 years old and LV systolic dysfunction, predominantly due to CAD (hatched rectangle).

transient or persistent ischemia with vascular reperfusion may be vital for restoring segmental contraction and improving overall ventricular function.[27] Various techniques have been employed to identify such tissue, including echocardiographic studies using catecholamine or exercise stress,[28–30] angiographic studies using nitroglycerin,[31] or extrasystolic potentiation following a premature ventricular contraction.[32]

Once ventricular dysfunction is manifest, abnormalities of reflex control of the circulation ensue. Decreased baroreceptor sensitivity occurs with augmented sympathetic tone and reduced parasympathetic tone (see Fig. 25-2).[33] This results in an increase in heart rate along with reduced beat-to-beat heart rate variability and loss of the Valsalva overshoot. These changes also help to establish the diagnosis of heart failure.

With reduced ventricular function, exercise performance tends to be reduced as measured by a reduced maximum $O_2$ uptake on a treadmill ($Vo_2$). However, this reduction in exercise performance does not always correlate with a reduced ejection fraction, since it also reflects the *training* state of the peripheral circulation.

## Clinical Assessment in Directing Therapy

Clinically, the initial diagnosis of heart failure is made by the patient's history, physical findings, and and serum B-type natriuretic peptide (BNP) levels.[34] The symptoms of shortness of breath and fatigue are initially related to exertion and later become permanent in the late stages of CHF. Physical exam often reveals a third heart sound and holosystolic murmur of functional mitral regurgitation and peripheral edema.[35] Pulmonary rales are often absent in patients with CHF due to increased lymphatic drainage. Overall, physical findings in heart failure are not sensitive for the detection of fluid retention, and the availability of serum BNP level greatly improves diagnostic accuracy of the physical exam.

Nuclear imaging techniques, computed tomography, and magnetic resonance imaging have been useful in assessing ventricular volume, shapes, and motion and have provided an excellent assessment of ventricular function. However, two-dimensional echocardiography will provide much of the necessary information in a practical and cost-effective manner and remains the clinical standard (Fig. 25-5). Its accuracy and usefulness depend on the care expended in performing the procedure and the professional oversight that is utilized in both detecting and interpreting the findings that are obtained. Echo-Doppler examination not only provides information about systolic and diastolic volumes, and thus ejection fraction, but also allows for the evaluation of valve structure and function, including regurgitation and stenosis. Reasonably accurate measurements of gradients, and thus valvular orifices, can be made, which can help direct therapy.

In defining the etiology of heart failure, segmental wall motion abnormalities with hypokinetic and contralateral hyperkinetic segments suggest an ischemic etiology. Indeed, following an acute myocardial infarction, a two-dimensional echocardiogram obtained within a few days is essential. The finding of ventricular dilatation within a few days of an acute anterior wall infarction tends to predict progressive LV dilatation with a falling ejection fraction. In patients sustaining an anterior wall infarction without initial ventricular dilatation, approximately one-third will show ventricular dilatation at 3 months. In contrast, ventricular dilatation rarely occurs following inferior wall infarctions, except when the region involved is large, extending from the base of the heart to the apex. After an acute myocardial infarction,[36] LV enlargement, as measured by two-dimensional echocardiography, is associated with an increased incidence of adverse cardiovascular events. When LV diastolic volumes

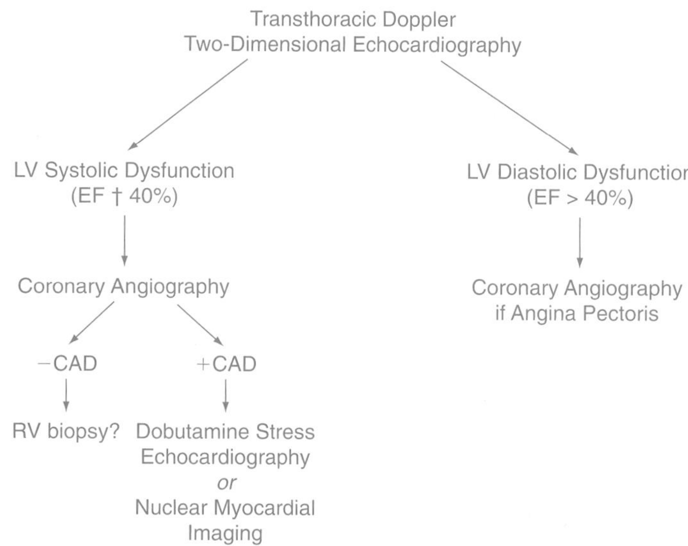


FIGURE 25-5 Evaluation of patients with congestive heart failure. Transthoracic Doppler and two-dimensional echocardiography provide a central modality to evaluate ventricular function and valvular abnormalities. Ventricular wall thickness and both end-diastolic and end-systolic volumes can be determined. With an ejection fraction (EF) >40 percent, coronary angiography is indicated in the presence of angina pectoris or evidence of significant ischemia. With an ejection fraction <40 percent, coronary arteriography is indicated since the underlying ischemic depression may be amenable to reperfusion by either angioplasty or coronary bypass surgery. Nuclear imaging techniques are used to define viable ischemic myocardium, while stimulation of such myocardium with dobutamine or extrasystolic potentiation may indicate recoverable hibernating myocardium. Right ventricular biopsy may be indicated in the absence of coronary artery disease to rule out processes such as amyloid or sarcoid abnormalities.

of patients with infarction are divided into quartiles, patients in the fourth quartile have a mortality rate of 45.5 percent, while patients in the third quartile have a mortality rate of 21.1 percent and patients in the first and second quartiles have the same mortality rate of 16.7 percent.[37] If LV dilatation occurs much later, however, two-dimensional echocardiography will not differentiate between the cause of heart failure (i.e., coronary artery disease or other etiologies). Moreover, patients with a primary cardiomyopathy may also exhibit segmental wall motion abnormalities. As noted earlier, stimuli that elicit latent contraction, such as low-dose dobutamine, stress, or premature ventricular contractions, may help identify patients with dilated left ventricles and severe coronary artery disease who also have *hibernating* or *stunned* myocardium.[26,38]

# TREATMENT OF CONGESTIVE HEART FAILURE

The management of the clinical syndrome of CHF has traditionally consisted of controlling fluid and sodium retention with the aim of alleviating exertional shortness of breath and fatigue. Current approach to the management of patients with CHF has evolved from control of fluid and sodium retention to prevention or reversal of structural and functional cardiac abnormalities that eventually lead to the clinical syndrome of CHF. When CHF is due to LV systolic dysfunction, the initial aims of interventions should be directed to prevention or reversal of LV dilatation while enhancing myocardial contractility. Symptomatic relief becomes later in time. When developing in patients with a normal LV ejection fraction, CHF is commonly attributed to LV diastolic dysfunction.[39] The initial therapeutic aims in patients with CHF and normal LV ejection are to reduce LV mass as may occur with control of hypertension while treating comorbid conditions such as diabetes.

Guidelines for the management of CHF have represented the progression of heart failure in stages A to D.[40] Stage A refers to patients at risk without structural cardiac abnormalities; stage B includes patients with structural abnormalities but no heart failure symptoms; stage C consists of structural abnormalities and symptoms; and, last, stage D refers to patients with end-stage CHF. By placing much emphasis on the presence or absence of cardiac structural abnormalities, this classification fails to recognize the seminal importance of vascular abnormalities in the initial genesis of LV systolic or diastolic dysfunction and later in the development of CHF. A history of systemic hypertension can be elicited in 75 to 85 percent of patients with LV systolic or diastolic dysfunction. Two-thirds and one-half of patients with CHF due to LV systolic and diastolic dysfunction, respectively, have coronary artery disease. Forty percent of patients with LV diastolic dysfunction and 30 percent of patients with LV systolic dysfunction also have diabetes mellitus. Thus, obstructive coronary disease, systemic hypertension, along with type 2 diabetes mellitus, are the overwhelming purveyors of the syndrome of CHF.

Consequently, therapeutic interventions that afford vascular protection such as ACE inhibition or angiotensin receptor blockade (ARB) are the first line of defense against structural cardiac abnormalities. In the Heart Outcomes Prevention Evaluation Study (HOPE),[41] patients at high risk for vascular events who were randomized to ramipril had significantly fewer hospitalizations for CHF than did patients randomized to placebo. The mechanisms by which ACE inhibition and ARBs mediate their clinical benefits in patients with vascular diseases are incompletely understood. Both ACE inhibition and ARBs inhibit the development of atherosclerosis in experimental preparations.[42,43] Enhancement of vascular endothelial function and nitric oxide production, reduction of plasminogen activator inhibitor-1 (PAI-1) and vascular oxidative stress, and regression of LV and vascular smooth muscle hypertrophy may also contribute to this vascular protection.

Therapeutic guidelines, experience and results of randomized trials are far more abundant in patients with CHF and reduced LV systolic function than they are in patients with CHF and preserved LV systolic function. The clinical profile of CHF patients with reduced and preserved LV systolic function differs, as illustrated in Fig. 25-1. Patients with CHF due to reduced LV systolic function are predominantly men aged 60 to 65 years old with a background of hypertension and coronary artery disease. Nearly all randomized trials involving patients with CHF have been conducted in patients with LV systolic dysfunction. In contrasts, CHF associated with preserved LV systolic dysfunction occurs predominantly in women. They are on average 8 to 10 years older than men with CHF due to reduced LV systolic function. The medical background of women with CHF and preserved LV systolic function commonly includes hypertension, diabetes mellitus, and obesity along with a low socioeconomic background. The exact mechanisms that are responsible for the syndrome of CHF in patients with preserved LV systolic function are poorly understood although hypertension plays an important role.[39] It is likely that functional and structural abnormalities involving heart, kidneys, or peripheral circulation may contribute importantly to CHF in the setting of preserved LV systolic function. Moreover with aging, systolic hypertension evolves in the majority of patients and leads to enhanced LV mass and diastolic dysfunction.

From a conceptual and practical standpoint, the prevention or reversal of vascular and cardiac remodeling is different than the management of fluid and sodium retention. In patients with minimal or no symptoms of heart failure the primary aim of therapy is to prevent or reverse vascular and cardiac remodeling. The therapeutic challenge is to convince minimally symptomatic patients to accept and be compliant with open-ended pharmacologic interventions aimed at preserving vascular and cardiac function and structure. Evidence indicates that compliance to such interventions may be better accepted when they are initiated during hospitalization for an acute event.[44] In contrast to long-term prevention of cardiac and vascular remodeling in ambulatory patients, control of fluid and sodium retention occurs in the setting of deteriorating symptoms that require a brief stay in the emergency room or hospitalization. The therapeutic challenge in patients hospitalized for clinical decompensation of heart failure is the return to a compensated state within the few days as allowed by third-party payment for this diagnosis.

The approach to BAB illustrates well the differences encountered in managing ambulatory and hospitalized patients with CHF. Current guidelines require increasing BAB toward maximally recommended doses in ambulatory patients. To the contrary, BAB may be reduced or even withheld in hospitalized patients for clinical decompensation. Accordingly, for the sake of clarity and practicality, management of patients with CHF in the outpatient setting will be reviewed first. The management of ambulatory patients becomes quite different from the care required for the hospitalized patient. In the former, as will be detailed, ACE inhibitors and BAB are central to therapy, and diuretics are administered as needed. Intravenous short-term administration of vasodilating and/or positive inotropic agents and vigorous diuresis are routinely recommended in hospitalized patients. The management of hospitalized patients will focus on the alterations required to the outpatient regimen and indications for transient intravenous afterload reduction or inotropic support.

As noted initially, the treatment of heart failure requires close attention to both the primary etiology and the relief of symptoms, while attempting to reduce the risk of death from the process. This includes vigorous control of hypertension, if present, and an evaluation for treatment of myocardial ischemia. As noted earlier and discussed further relative to surgical approaches to heart failure, noncontractile but viable myocardium, whether due to stunning or hibernation, requires definition with consideration of coronary reperfusion.[26,45] Valvular disease that imposes an excessive volume or pressure overload must be considered relative to the need for surgical correction. For example, critical aortic stenosis with heart failure is an urgent indication for aortic valve replacement, when possible, not medical therapy. To those ends, there is a multifactorial approach to therapy[46] depending on the etiology and stage of the heart failure process (Fig. 25-6).

## General Principles in the Pharmacologic Treatment of Congestive Heart Failure

Therapy is tailored to the phase of heart failure. In the initial phase where ventricular damage is a primary concern, identification of etiology is essential with appropriate therapy. This might be termed *treatment of ventricular dysfunction and its causes*. Hypertension must be controlled aggressively. Even mild hypertension should be treated in the presence of the diabetic state to hopefully prevent large and small vessel coronary disease. Overt or silent ischemia should be identified and treated. Early inhibition of the neurohumoral responses to initial cardiac damage with both beta-adrenergic blockade and inhibition of the activated renin–angiotensin–aldosterone system (RAAS) requires consideration. This is particularly the case as one moves into the phase of ventricular remodeling where inhibition of

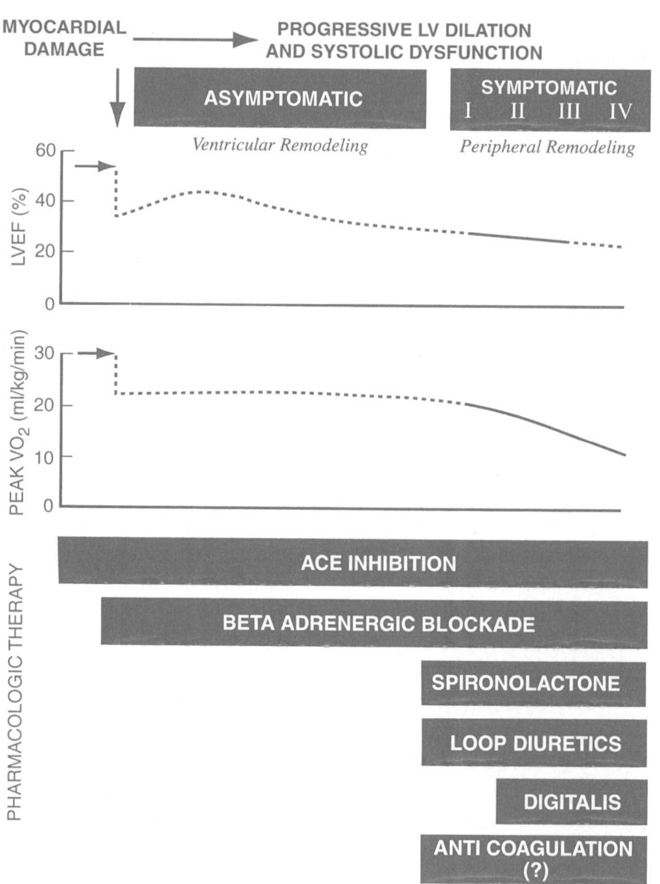


FIGURE 25-6 Staged use of therapeutic agents in heart failure. Initial approaches include control of the conditions that predispose to heart failure. Angiotensin-converting enzyme (ACE) inhibition is of paramount importance in patients with hypertension and vascular conditions who are at high risk of events. Unanticipated tachycardia may enhance myocardial oxygen demand while reducing the time in diastole for oxygen delivery. Shortened duration of diastole can lead to marked elevation of diastolic pressure and thereby to myocardial ischemia. Moreover, atrial fibrillation will deprive LV filling from the "atrial kick" and lead to further elevation of LV diastolic pressure. These considerations are of special importance with LV hypertrophy and resultant diastolic dysfunction. Beta-adrenergic blockade prolongs life expectancy and reduces morbidity during the acute event, the LV remodeling process, and the entire clinical syndrome of heart failure from functional class I to class IV. The therapeutic usefulness of loop diuretics is to control salt and water retention in symptomatic patients with central or peripheral edema. Although their effect on mortality is neutral, digitalis glycosides are safe and reduce morbidity in severely symptomatic men with chronic heart failure. Digitalis glycosides reduce sympathetic tone, and enhance parasympathetic tone while providing modest positive inotropic support. The therapeutic usefulness of anticoagulation with warfarin to prevent systemic embolic events is currently being investigated in patients with LV systolic dysfunction who are in sinus rhythm.

progressive ventricular damage is essential. It is important to remember that symptoms that bother the patient, such as edema and shortness of breath, are generally not life-threatening, while therapy that may reduce mortality, such as beta blockers, may do nothing to alleviate symptoms. Thus, both agendas must be addressed. In general, mortality has been used to measure efficacy. Improvement in symptoms has been difficult to assess and a combined endpoint of mortality and a need for hospitalization has been useful. As the syndrome of CHF ensues, pharmacologic treatment is directed to three demonstrable hemodynamic endpoints: (1) to reduce volume overloads and maintain a stable volume state, (2) to reduce preload and afterload to enhance ventricular performance, and (3) to improve ventricular contractility when necessary. An additional pharmacologic aim is to reduce heightened neurohumoral activity, which is seen in patients with heart failure, with the hope of limiting abnormal loading created by these systems and preventing the progression of the heart failure process. The ultimate aim is to reduce morbidity and perhaps extend life.

## Inactivation of the Renin–Angiotensin System and Alternative Therapies

Neurohumoral activation plays an important role in the progression of the syndrome of chronic LV systolic dysfunction and heart failure. Following initial increases in sympathetic tone and decreases in parasympathetic tone, the renin–angiotensin system (RAS) is activated.[47] This generally occurs when diuretics are initiated or, in their absence, with the onset of clinical symptoms of CHF. With release of renin from the kidneys, angiotensinogen, which is circulating in the blood, is converted to inactive angiotensin I, which in turn is converted to the highly active angiotensin II by a converting enzyme that is ubiquitously located along vascular walls.

Angiotensin II in turn stimulates aldosterone secretion by the adrenals, which results in sodium accumulation and also produces marked arteriolar constriction, which augments peripheral vascular resistance. Both phenomena, which increase ventricular preload (filling pressure) and afterload (systolic pressure), contribute to the clinical picture of CHF. In addition to these actions, angiotensin II serves as a growth factor, adding to myocardial hypertrophy and apparently fostering fibrosis. It may also contribute to subtle myocyte loss through enhancing apoptosis.[48]

## Outpatient Therapy of Congestive Heart Failure

A critical issue when dealing with patients with minimal or no symptoms of heart failure is to detect the presence of LV dilatation, reduced systolic function, or increased LV mass. As a rule LV dilatation, systolic dysfunction, or increased mass, if present, should be detected by two-dimensional Doppler echocardiography during hospitalization hastened by an acute cardiovascular event such a myocardial infarction, hypertension crisis, cerebrovascular accident, or arrhythmia. Ambulatory patients at risk of developing LV systolic dysfunction such as those with long-standing hypertension, coronary artery disease, relatives with dilated cardiomyopathy, or physical evidence of valvular regurgitation should also undergo two-dimensional Doppler echocardiography. In addition, patients with systemic conditions involving the heart and patients with chronic obstructive lung disease that often masks or mimics the signs and symptoms of heart failure should undergo two-dimensional Doppler echocardiography. The usefulness of BNP serum level in detecting asymptomatic patients with LV dilatation and reduced LV systolic function is conflicting.[49] Elderly women may have elevated serum BNP levels in the absence of LV dysfunction, and asymptomatic patients with a modestly reduced LV ejection fraction and near normal LV filling pressure are unlikely to have marked elevation of serum BNP level.[50] However, serum BNP levels are quite useful in distinguishing CHF decompensation from chronic obstructive pulmonary disease (COPD) exacerbating symptomatic patients with coexisting conditions. Marked elevation of serum BNP level orients toward CHF decompensation as it cannot be right ventricular overload alone.

## ANGIOTENSIN-CONVERTING ENZYME INHIBITORS

Independently from the presence or absence of LV dilatation, reduced systolic function, or increased LV mass, long-term ACE inhibition is indicated in all patients with vascular diseases who are at high risk to experience cardiovascular events (Table 25-1).[51] Vascular patients who carry a high risk of complications are those with a history of stroke, coronary or peripheral artery disease, or diabetes with one other cardiovascular risk factor.[41] In view of the determining role of angiotensin II in cardiac hypertrophy and fibrosis, vascular smooth cell hypertrophy and endothelial dysfunction, long-term ACE inhibition is most often favored as the intervention of choice to prevent or attenuate the progression of LV systolic or diastolic dysfunction in hypertensive patients.

The initial impetus toward the use of ACE inhibitors for the treatment of patients with CHF was to duplicate with one agent the hemodynamic effects produced by the combination of nitrate and hydralazine.[52] In the late 1970s, combined administration of nitrate and hydralazine was shown to enhance LV systolic performance and alleviate symptoms in patients with CHF. In severe heart failure this resulted from the combined action of nitrates to reduce diastolic filling pressures (preload) and hydralazine to reduce peripheral arterial resistance (afterload). The result was reduced filling pressures accompanied by an increased cardiac output. Initial hemodynamic studies with captopril demonstrated substantial lowering of ventricular filling pressures, a modest increase in cardiac output, and a reduction in systemic arterial pressure without tachycardia. In a landmark randomized, placebo-controlled study, administration of captopril for 3 months produced sustained improvement in LV performance, improved functional class, and increased duration of maximal exercise,[53] resulting in approval from the Food and Drug Administration (FDA) of captopril for the treatment of CHF. In the first weeks of the study, exercise duration improved in patients on placebo as well. This initial improvement in exercise duration on placebo is probably due to familiarization with exercise equipment and increased patient motivation.

Several aspects of long-term therapy with ACE inhibitors in patients with CHF are worthy of mention:

1. The magnitude of the initial hemodynamic change does not predict the long-term clinical response. Some of the beneficial effects of lower ventricular filling and systemic arterial pressures may relate to increased levels of kinins, resulting from decreased enzymatic destruction that is also mediated by ACE inhibitors.[52] Whether sustained elevation in kinin levels exerts long-term clinical benefits is still uncertain. The dissociation between acute hemodynamic effects and long-term clinical benefit suggests that mechanisms underlying the benefits of ACE inhibitors may be related to structural and functional changes occurring in the peripheral vasculature. Improvement in peak aerobic capacity ($VO_2$) has been directly related to enhanced perfusion of skeletal muscle at maximal exercise. The exact mechanisms that mediate the benefits of ACE inhibitors on the vasculature are still poorly understood. Improvement of vascular endothelial function, which is reversibly depressed in CHF, as by response to local administration of acetylcholine, is so far the best documented vascular effect of ACE inhibitors in patients with CHF. Improved vascular endothelial function during long-term ACE inhibition may be, in part, mediated via the kinin pathway. Whether lowering tissue levels of angiotensin II affects vascular smooth muscle structure and function is unknown. However, angiotensin II is a smooth muscle growth factor and its reduction may reduce smooth muscle mass and thereby affect vascular tone and compliance.
2. The impact of long-term ACE inhibition on LV systolic function appears to be modest.[52] Thus, the absolute increase in LV ejection fraction observed in large multicenter randomized trials ranged from 1 to 3 absolute units. With long-term use of ACE inhibitors, LV end-diastolic and systolic volumes are modestly altered. Initial reduction in LV EDV during long-term ACE inhibition appears largely related to decreased loading of the failing ventricle rather than structural cardiac alterations, since LV volume increases within a few days after withdrawal of ACE inhibition. However, persistent diastolic unloading with these agents may reduce progression of dilatation.
3. Long-term use of ACE inhibitors has significant natriuretic effects. From a hormonal point of view, a decrease in angiotensin II tends to reduce aldosterone secretion, with resultant lessening of sodium accumulation and reduced potassium loss. However, aldosterone synthesis is modulated by factors other than angiotensin II, such as potassium levels, corticotropin, and endothelin.[54] During long-term treatment with ACE inhibitors, levels of aldosterone remain elevated

TABLE 25-1 FDA Approved Indications for ACE Inhibitors

| ACE Inhibitor | Hypertension | CHF | Acute MI | LV Dysfunction | Diabetic Nephropathy |
|---|---|---|---|---|---|
| Benazepril | + | | | | |
| Captopril | + | + (post MI) | | +* | + |
| Enalapril | + | + | | +† | |
| Fosinopril | + | + | | | |
| Lisinopril | + | + (post MI) | + | | |
| Moexipril | + | | | | |
| Perindopril | + | | | | |
| Quinapril | + | + | | | |
| Ramipril | + + | +‡ | | | |
| Trandolapril | + | +§ | | +§ | |

*Captopril is indicated in clinically stable patients with left ventricular (LV) dysfunction (ejection fraction <40 percent) after myocardial infarction (MI), to improve survival and to reduce the incidence of overt heart failure.

†Enalapril is indicated in clinically stable asymptomatic patients with LV dysfunction (ejection fraction <35 percent) to decrease the rate of development of overt heart failure and to decrease the incidence of hospitalization due to congestive heart failure (CHF).

‡Ramipril is indicated in stable patients who have demonstrated clinical signs of CHF within the first few days after sustaining acute MI, to decrease mortality and progression to severe heart failure.

§Trandolapril is indicated for treatment of heart failure after MI and of LV dysfunction after MI.

SOURCE: Reproduced with permission from Cheng A, Frishman WH. Use of angiotensin converting enzyme inhibitors as monotherapy and in combination with diuretics and calcium channel blockers. *J Clin Pharm* 1998;38:477–491.

in up to 38 percent of patients with CHF.[55] Thus, one cannot assume that long-term ACE inhibition alone can reliably lower plasma aldosterone levels. Increased diuresis with the consequent reduction in the dose of loop diuretics has been reported during long-term therapy with captopril.[56] This natriuretic effect of captopril may be related to the increase in renal blood flow demonstrated after administration of captopril, despite the concomitant reduction in systemic arterial pressure.[57]

A major impetus that has led to an increasing use of ACE inhibitors in patients with LV systolic dysfunction and CHF derived from the experimental work of Pfeffer and other.[42,58–60]

In addition to the work of Pfeffer et al., several large survival trials in patients with heart failure were launched and completed.[61–66] An unexpected finding of these trials was the lower incidence of recurrent myocardial infarction in patients randomized to ACE inhibitors. Whether this reduction in the incidence of acute coronary events in patients with coronary artery disease is associated with long-term ACE inhibition or related to the improvement in endothelium vasomotor dysfunction, which was subsequently demonstrated with quinapril, another ACE inhibitor, is not known.[67] It is also possible that ACE inhibition plays a role in stabilizing atherosclerotic plaques, perhaps by reducing smooth muscle growth. Importantly, as noted later, the same considerations have been raised by the Survival and Ventricular Enlargement (SAVE) trial of ACE inhibition in the depressed heart following myocardial infarction.[68]

The impetus for an earlier use of an ACE inhibitor in patients with LV dysfunction and heart failure has also been provided by the results of the HOPE study.[41] Therapy with ACE inhibitors has been traditionally recommended in patients with CHF related to LV systolic dysfunction, as defined by an LV ejection fraction <40 percent (to 35 percent) in most clinical trials. By demonstrating that long-term administration of ramipril, a tissue-specific ACE inhibitor, improved life expectancy in patients with vascular disease or diabetes and one cardiovascular factor and no evidence of LV systolic dysfunction, the findings of the HOPE trial indirectly but strongly argued for the use of ACE inhibitor at a pre-LV dysfunction stage in patients with clinical conditions known to be associated with the development of congestive heart failure.[51] These results also emphasize the vascular benefits of ACE inhibitors since other morbid vascular events, such as stroke, were significantly reduced. Since the conditions that lead to LV systolic and diastolic dysfunction are similar, the early use of ACE inhibitors is warranted in patients with both LV systolic and diastolic dysfunction. Besides the effects of ACE inhibitors on skeletal muscle vasculature, and the prevention of subsequent acute coronary events by ACE inhibitors, the results of the HOPE trial point out the importance of the vascular effects of ACE inhibitors in mediating their clinical benefits. To a large extent, in the majority of patients with CHF, deterioration of LV function is related to progression of systemic and coronary vascular processes that now can be favorably altered by ACE inhibitors. The vascular benefits of ACE inhibitors appear to be additional to those provided by aspirin, BAB, and lipid-lowering agents.[41]

That ramipril exerted vascular benefits in patients who were receiving aspirin is of particular importance, as the attenuations of the hemodynamic effects of ACE inhibitors have been reported in patients receiving aspirin.[69] The negative interaction between ACE inhibitors and aspirin is presumably due to interference with kinin-mediated synthesis of prostaglandin. The loss of benefit from ACE inhibitors noted in patients treated with aspirin in some large trials contrasts with the findings of the HOPE trial and others.[70] In view of the importance of the kinin pathway in vascular biology, one would expect that if a negative interaction exists between ACE inhibitors and aspirin, it would have been observed in patients enrolled in the HOPE trial. Whether the use of ticlopidine or clopidogrel is preferable in a subset of patients with LV dysfunction, CHF, and renal insufficiency, who are treated with ACE inhibitors, is currently unknown.

By preventing events related to myocardial ischemia and progression of atherosclerosis, ACE inhibitors are now becoming the cornerstone of both treatment and prevention in patients with LV dysfunction, independent of the presence or absence of symptoms. Whether patients should be treated for vascular protection with ACE inhibitors other than those specifically approved for the treatment of LV systolic dysfunction and CHF is unclear. So far there is no study that has included clinical endpoints to show an advantage of one ACE inhibitor over another. Tissue-specific ACE inhibitors appear more apt to exert vascular benefits than do ACE inhibitors with low-tissue specificity. Tissue specificity is probably most relevant at low doses of ACE inhibitors. At maximally recommended doses of ACE inhibition, tissue specificity is less likely to be relevant. Overall, in several clinical trials and in daily practice, the dose of ACE inhibitors is strikingly low.[64,65] The patients randomized to ACE inhibition in the SOLVD trial were receiving only 11 mg of enalapril daily.[64] Several small studies and the Assessment of Treatment with Lisinopril and Survival (ATLAS) study have failed to show that high doses of ACE inhibitors produce clearly greater clinical benefits than do low doses.[71]

The RAS is composed of circulatory and tissue-bound components; the latter accounting for about 90 percent of RAS activity. One differentiates ACE inhibitors with high and low tissue affinity based on their lipophilic index and rate of dissociation from ACE in vitro. Whether low and high tissue affinity ACE inhibitors afford equal vascular protection remains unclear. Since the ACE inhibitor selected for the HOPE trial had high tissue affinity one might exclusively recommend the use of ACE inhibitors with high tissue affinity for vascular protection. However, either low or high tissue affinity ACE inhibitors enhance vascular endothelial function in patients with coronary artery disease or hypertension.[72] Moreover, the modest increment in clinical benefits resulting from high-dose compared to low-dose ACE inhibition argue that, independently from tissue affinity, even low doses of ACE inhibitors are sufficient to fully inhibit tissue ACE.[73] In summary, although the only trial that unequivocally demonstrated vascular protection in patients with normal LV systolic function was conducted with a high tissue affinity ACE inhibitor, a large body of data indicates that all ACE inhibitors achieve vascular protection independently of their level of affinity for tissue ACE.

Besides pregnancy and ACE inhibitor- or ARB-induced angioedema, bilateral renal artery stenosis or unilateral stenosis with a solitary kidney are the only other formal contraindications to ACE inhibition. Bilateral renal stenosis should be suspected in patients with "flash" pulmonary edema, abdominal bruit, or hypertension that is difficult to control especially when associated with renal insufficiency. Of note, rapid progression of renal insufficiency after initiation of ACE inhibitor therapy should also alert one to the presence of bilateral renal artery stenosis.

Patients who are unable to tolerate ACE inhibitors due to angioedema or cough should receive angiotensin II type 1-receptor antagonists. The Valsartan Heart Failure Trial (Val-HeFT) demonstrated a 33 percent reduction in mortality in patients who, not treated with ACE inhibitors, were randomized to valsartan, when compared to patients randomized to a placebo.[74] The overall benefit of adding angiotensin II type 1 receptor antagonists in a medical regimen that already includes an ACE inhibitor is extremely modest, especially if the patient is receiving an adequate dose of ACE inhibitors.[75] Moreover adding an ARB to a medical regimen that already includes ACE inhibition and BAB may hasten fatal events, especially in patients with severe CHF who cannot tolerate sympatholysis.[76]

The benefits of ACE inhibitors have not been looked for in patients with serum creatinine levels >2.5 mg/dL, since they have been excluded from clinical trials. The important effects of ACE inhibitors on cardiovascular protection that are independent from any renal effects argue in favor of a trial of ACE inhibitors in patients with CHF with severe chronic renal insufficiency as defined by a serum creatinine level >3.0 mg/dL. However, patients with serum levels of creatinine >3.0 mg/dL require careful follow-up, including daily monitoring of renal function after initiation of ACE inhibitors at the lowest possible dose. Since inhibition of angiotensin II production leads to dilatation of the efferent artery of the glomerulus, a decrease in glomerular perfusion pressure occurs and a modest rise in serum creatinine (0.5 to 1.9 mg/L) is anticipated. This poses no problem unless the creatinine continues to rise, when ACE inhibition needs to be reduced. Indeed, in the presence of diabetes, renal protection is afforded by ACE inhibition, and the rise in creatinine, which is reversible, does not reflect ACE-inhibitor-induced renal damage.[77] Moreover, ACE inhibitors that are, in part, excreted by the liver are preferable in this clinical situation. Overall, it is always recommended to avoid prescribing nonsteroidal anti-inflammatory drugs (NSAIDs) in patients with CHF, but this is particularly important in patients with decreased renal function. Renal function is likely to further deteriorate after initiation of ACE inhibitor therapy in patients treated with NSAIDs. Patients with plasma levels of potassium >5.0 mmol/L at baseline, particularly if they are diabetic with renal tubular acidosis, require daily measurement of electrolytes and renal function at initiation of ACE inhibitor therapy.

A potential drug–drug interaction with aspirin and ACE inhibitors has been described with a potential loss of ACE inhibition's protective effects on patient survival in heart failure. However, this finding has not been substantiated from analyses of large clinical data bases.[70]

In summary, the rationale for ACE inhibition in patients with CHF has evolved since their introduction in the late 1970s. Initially, the therapeutic usefulness of ACE inhibitors was to provide balanced arteriovenous dilatation and thereby replace the combination of hydralazine and nitrate. The following stage focused on attenuation of LV dilatation based on the seminal work of Pfeffer and colleagues in experimental and human myocardial infarction.[58–60] These investigators convincingly demonstrated the beneficial effects of ACE inhibitors on LV remodeling after a large myocardial infarction. Nowadays, the effects of ACE inhibition on enhancing endothelial function, lowering PAI-1 production, preventing coronary events, and delaying the spontaneous progression of the atherosclerotic process, thereby affording vascular protection, are well recognized.

## ALTERNATIVES TO ANGIOTENSIN-CONVERTING ENZYME INHIBITORS

***Angiotensin II Receptor Antagonists*** Several angiotensin II receptor antagonists (ARBs; Fig. 25-7) are approved by the FDA for the treatment of hypertension (losartan, valsartan, irbesartan, candesartan, telmisartan, and eprosartan). Although trials are in progress involving the use of ARBs alone or in combination with ACE inhibitors in heart failure, none, as yet, are approved for this purpose. The first comparison of ACE inhibition with captopril (150 mg daily) and ARB (losartan 50 mg daily) was undertaken in 722 patients with CHF older than 65 years. The results suggested that losartan may be preferable to captopril.[78] Death and hospitalization for heart failure was 9.4 percent in patients randomized to losartan and 13.2 percent in patients randomized to captopril [risk reduction was 32 percent; 955 confidence interval (CI) 4 to 55 percent, $p = 0.075$]. The results of ELITE I were not confirmed by a subsequent study of identical design, but that included over 3000 patients in ELITE II.[79] In fact, while the number of deaths or hospitalization was similar during the first 12 months of the study, thereafter fewer patients randomized to captopril died or were hospitalized for heart failure than were patients randomized to losartan. Thus, the results of ELITE II failed to confirm the hypothesis derived from ELITE I, suggesting that ARBs may be superior to ACE inhibition for the treatment of patients with CHF. Of note, the design of ELITE II and the number of patients studied do not allow the conclusion that the two interventions are equal, based on a lack of statistical difference between the number of events noted in patients randomized to captopril and in patients randomized to losartan. The ELITE II trial must also be viewed as inconclusive since there remains a question of adequate dosage and, as noted later, the potential for the concomitant use of ACE inhibition and ARBs.

The present use of ARBs for the treatment of CHF is limited to patients who experience intolerable cough or angioedema while receiving ACE inhibitors. Patients who cannot tolerate ACE inhibitors due to worsening renal function or hyperkalemia are likely to experience similar side effects with ARBs.

Another potential use of ARB for the management of CHF is to counteract the attenuation of the benefits of ACE inhibition that may occur with time, a phenomenon often referred to as "ACE escape." After long-term (1 year) ACE inhibition, plasma angiotensin II levels rise above initial

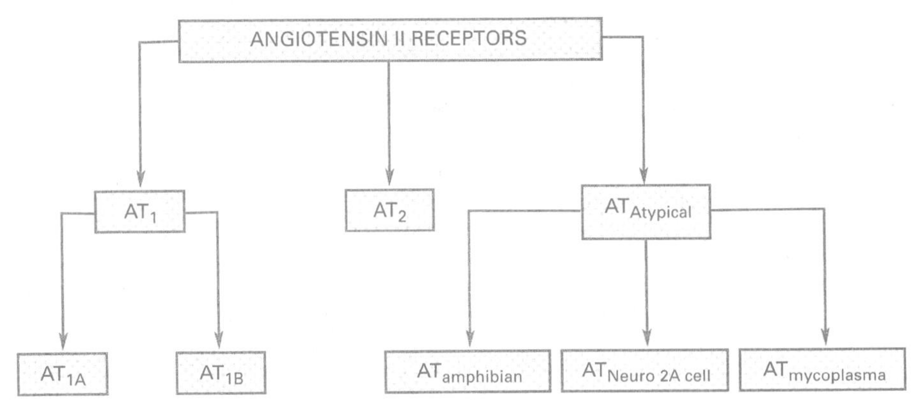


FIGURE 25-7 The classification and characteristics of angiotensin II receptors. DTT, dithiothreitol. (From Kang PM, Landau AJ, Eberhardt RT, Frishman WH. Angiotensin II receptor antagonists: a new approach to blockade of the renin-angiotensin system. *Am Heart J* 1994;127:1388–1401.)

values and LV antiremodeling and lowering norepinephrine effects attenuate.[68,80,81] Whether this is due to ACE inhibition becoming partial with time or whether angiotensin II is generated via other pathways than the converting enzyme is still controversial.[82] Independent of the underlying mechanisms that mediate ACE escape, the addition of ARB to ACE inhibition negates the detrimental effects of elevated levels of tissue and circulating angiotensin.[83,84]

Several experimental and small studies have clearly demonstrated the added benefits of combined ARB and ACE inhibition on LV performance, functional capacity, and safety.[85–89] The Val-HeFT demonstrated the safety of adding ARB to ACE inhibition in patients with CHF who were not receiving BAB.[74] Subgroup analysis suggested that ARBs may exert an adverse effect on mortality in patients with CHF, low LV ejection fraction, and symptoms compatible with functional class II to III who are treated with ACE inhibitors and BAB. The negative interaction between ARBs when combined with ACE and BAB, according to the subgroup analysis, may not occur in other clinical situations. Patients with hypertension or postmyocardial infarction do not seem to experience ill effects when receiving ARBs in addition to ACE and BAB. The beneficial effects of combined ARB and ACE inhibition on neurohumoral parameters were demonstrated in the Val-HeFT trial.[90] The impressive effects of valsartan on mortality in patients who were not receiving ACE inhibition have led to its approval in this patient population. However, ARBs are not superior to ACE inhibitors in reducing mortality in CHF.[91]

***Other Vasodilators*** Vasodilator agents may be used as adjunctive therapy in the management of heart failure. The combination of hydralazine and isosorbide dinitrate is an alternative therapy when ACE inhibitors are contraindicated or cannot be tolerated. Daily doses of hydralazine, up to 300 mg, in combination with isosorbide dinitrate, 160 mg, in the presence of cardiac glycosides and diuretics probably have some effect in reducing mortality of patients with CHF but not in reducing hospitalization for heart failure. At these doses, the combination caused greater increases in exercise performance than did enalapril.[63] The effects of hydralazine and nitrates, alone or in combination, when added to ACE inhibitors are unknown. There is no evidence of proven benefit when either nitrates or hydralazine are used alone, but nitrates are often prescribed without hydralazine. Nitrates also may be used effectively for the treatment of concomitant angina. Early development of hemodynamic tolerance (tachyphylaxis) to nitrates may occur with frequent dosing (every 4 to 6 h) but is less with intervals of 8 to 12 h or in conjunction with ACE inhibition. Also, hemodynamic tolerance may be less during coadministration with hydralazine.[92]

Prostacyclin, which is a potent systemic vasodilator used in the treatment of primary pulmonary hypertension, has not been shown to improve mortality outcome in patients with heart failure despite improvements in hemodynamics. Similarly, alpha blockers, despite their potent vasodilatory activity, have not shown benefit in patients with CHF, probably related to hemodynamic tolerance with prolonged drug treatment.

***Calcium Antagonists*** Calcium antagonists are not recommended for the treatment of CHF due to their negative inotropic effects. However, second-generation dihydropyridine-type calcium antagonists such as amlodipine and felodipine may be considered for the treatment of concomitant arterial hypertension or angina. Some second-generation calcium antagonists are still under investigation with respect to their long-term effect on mortality in CHF, in addition to baseline therapy including ACE inhibition. Preliminary data indicate either no effect or a positive outcome in restricted patient populations (i.e., in patients with idiopathic dilated cardiomyopathy).[93] Although in these studies the second-generation dihydropyridine agents evaluated appeared to be safe and not to increase mortality, there are as yet no reasons to recommend these agents for the treatment of heart failure due to systolic dysfunction. Rather they can be recommended as adjunctive medication for ischemia. Due to the potential benefits noted later, however, beta blockers should be preferable to the calcium blockers for patients with CHF and ischemia.

A study evaluated the dihydropyridine agent amlodipine as an adjunctive therapy for patients with congestive cardiomyopathy.[93] Similarly, the selective T-channel calcium antagonist mibefradil, a drug having no apparent effect on myocardial function has been studied. No beneficial effects of mibefradil on survival were demonstrated in patients with heart failure, and unfavorable drug–drug interactions, especially with amiodarone, led to mibefradil's withdrawal from the market.[94] The use of calcium blockers (e.g., verapamil) in patients with diastolic dysfunction has been reported, but there are no long-term outcome studies with this form of treatment. The use of verapamil in the treatment of patients with hypertrophic cardiomyopathy has been well defined.[93]

## BETA-ADRENERGIC BLOCKADE

In view of the marked benefits afforded by BAB in patients with heart failure after a myocardial infarction, BAB was advocated 30 years ago for the treatment of patients with dilated cardiomyopathies. In the BHAT trial, where propranolol was begun 7 to 21 days after an acute myocardial infarction and continued for 24 months, 5 lives per 100 were saved when heart failure was present, and only 2 lives when heart failure was absent.[95] Just as the use of ACE inhibitors in patients with CHF did not become widely accepted until the positive results of large survival trials were known, the use of BAB did not gain broad acceptance until large survival trials demonstrated their benefits on survival in patients with CHF.[96] The Cardiac Insufficiency Bisoprolol Study II (CIBIS II) evaluated the effects of bisoprolol, a $beta_1$-selective adrenergic blocker, on mortality from all causes in patients with CHF (NYHA class III to class IV and LV ejection fraction <40 percent) treated with standard medical regimens, including ACE inhibitors.[97] The trial was discontinued prematurely because mortality from all causes was significantly less in the bisoprolol group than it was in the placebo group. The most common dose of bisoprolol was 10 mg in 564 patients followed by 5 mg in 176 patients and 7.5 mg in 152 patients. Sudden death and hospitalization for worsening CHF were 42 and 32 percent fewer, respectively, in patients randomized to bisoprolol. In summary, in a trial that did not include a run-in period and thus did not select patients who tolerated BAB, bisoprolol lowered the risk of mortality from all causes by 32 percent. Bisoprolol was as efficacious in patients with ischemic cardiomyopathy and in patients with functional class II and class IV. However, in view of the overall low mortality rate of patients randomized to placebo, one may question how many patients were really in functional class IV prior to prerandomization.

In the Metoprolol CR/XL Randomised Intervention Trial (MERIT-HF), the effects of a controlled release and extended release formulation of metoprolol (CR/XL) on mortality was studied in patients with CHF (NYHA class II to class IV and LV ejection fraction <40 percent) treated with a standard medical regimen, including ACE inhibitors.[98] Patients were randomized to metoprolol (target dose 200 mg) for 2 months or to a placebo, after a 2-week single-blind placebo period. The study was terminated prematurely on the recommendation of the Safety Committee after a mean follow-up of 12 months.

Of the 1990 patients randomized to metoprolol, 145 died, and 217 of the 2001 patients randomized to placebo died ($p = 0.0062$). The mortality rates were 7.2 and 22 percent per patient-year of follow-up, respectively, with a relative risk of 0.66 (955 CI 0.53 to 0.81). Sudden death and death from aggravated heart failure were fewer among treated patients: 79 versus 132, 0.59 (0.45 to 0.78), $p < 0.0002$, and 30 versus 58, 0.51 (0.33-0.79), $p = 0.0023$. The mean daily dose of metoprolol was 159 mg, with 87 percent of patients receiving more than 100 mg and 64 percent receiving the target dose of 200 mg. As demonstrated with bisoprolol, metoprolol CR/XL lowered mortality from all causes by 34 percent in patients with CHF already treated with ACE inhibitors and diuretics. As noted in the CIBIS II trial, most of the patients enrolled in the MERIT-HF trial had moderate CHF as evidenced by the low mortality of patients in the placebo group. Few patients in functional class IV participated in MERIT-HF. Thus, too few patients in functional class IV were randomized to active therapy in both the CIBIS II and MERIT-HF trials to assess the safety and efficacy of bisoprolol and metoprolol in this population.

Both the CIBIS II and MERIT-HF trials demonstrated that mortality from all causes can be reduced by a selective $beta_1$-adrenergic agent in patients with mild to moderate CHF. Metoprolol is about 80-fold more selective for human $beta_1$ than $beta_2$ receptor, and bisoprolol is approximately 120-fold more selective.[99] Based on the MERIT-HF trial, metoprolol has been approved for clinical use in patients with class II to III heart failure.

While both $beta_1$ and $beta_2$ receptors are present in the normal human myocardium, $beta_2$ receptors predominate in the human failing myocardium, since $beta_1$ receptors are downregulated.[100] Thus, selection of a nonselective beta-blocking agent may seem preferable, when the therapeutic aim is to protect the heart from beta-adrenergic stimulation. Carvedilol is a nonselective beta-adrenergic blocker that also has alpha-blocking and antioxidant properties.[101]

Carvedilol is the only alpha-beta blocker currently approved by the FDA for the treatment of patients with NYHA class II to class IV CHF.[101] The United States Carvedilol Program, which led to the initial approval in class II to III CHF, was composed of four trials and was stopped prematurely by the Safety Committee due to a highly significant reduction in mortality in treated patients (65 percent, $p < .0001$) compared to the placebo.[101–106] The four trials were the Multicenter Oral Carvedilol in Heart Failure Assessment (MOCHA), Prospective Randomized Evaluation of Carvedilol in Symptoms and Exercise (PRECISE), and the "mild" and "severe" heart failure trials.[102–105] The intended duration of these trials was 6 months. The primary endpoints were submaximal exercise for the MOCHA and PRECISE trials, a composite endpoint of death, reduction in cardiovascular hospitalizations, a need to increase heart failure medications for the "mild" heart failure trial, and quality-of-life evaluation for the "severe" heart failure trial. The MOCHA and PRECISE trials had completed enrollment by the time the program was interrupted. Whereas primary endpoints were not reached except in the "mild" heart failure trial, average LV ejection fraction increased substantially in patients randomized to carvedilol in all trials. LV ejection fraction remained unaltered in patients randomized to the placebo.[102–105] The improvement in LV ejection fraction was noted in patients who were already receiving optimal standard therapy, including ACE inhibitors. A dose-related reduction in mortality and enhancement of LV ejection fraction was noted in the MOCHA trial.[102] Cardiovascular hospitalizations were fewer, and symptoms were alleviated in patients randomized to carvedilol in the PRECISE trials.[103] Last, global heart failure assessments were improved in patients randomized to carvedilol in the "severe" heart failure trial.[105] Thus, although the primary endpoints were different, the carvedilol trials demonstrated substantial reduction in mortality and dose-dependent improvement in ejection fraction. This improvement was present in both ischemic and nonischemic cardiomyopathies, although it was greater in the latter group.

The Australia-New Zealand (ANZ) trial included an initial phase of 6 months and a longer phase with an average follow-up of 19 months.[107] Submaximal exercise, the endpoint of the initial phase, remained unchanged in patients randomized to carvedilol. During the second phase of the ANZ trial, fewer patients randomized to carvedilol died or were hospitalized.

The effects of BAB on LV function and dimensions are unique. No other pharmacologic intervention has been shown to reverse LV remodeling and improve LV ejection fraction so consistently in patients with CHF due to LV systolic dysfunction. In all clinical trials where patients received BAB for at least 3 months, LV ejection fraction increased.[101] Long-term administration of selective and nonselective BAB increases LV ejection fraction consistently to a much greater extent than that achieved by vasodilator therapy. The long-term benefits of BAB on LV performance are in contrast with the deterioration that may be observed initially. The time course of the effects of BAB includes an initial reduction in LV ejection fraction during the first weeks of treatment, a return to initial ejection fraction at 4 weeks, and a substantial increase ranging from 5 to 10 absolute units at 3 months.[108] Thereafter, from 4 to 12 months, LV end-systolic and end-diastolic volumes and mass steadily decrease, a phenomenon often referred to as "reversed remodeling."[109] Reversal of LV remodeling has been documented with carvedilol at 12 months in a substudy of the ANZ trial.[110] At 1 year, LV ejection fraction was greater and LV end-diastolic volume index was 14 $mL/m^2$ smaller in patients randomized to carvedilol than it was in patients randomized to the placebo.

Carvedilol has been studied in symptomatic patients with a low ejection fraction after an acute myocardial infarction, and compared to a placebo; a benefit was shown on all-cause mortality and the rate of recurrent myocardial infarction.[111] Carvedilol has also been studied in patients with symptoms of heart failure at rest or with minimal exertion who were clinically euvolemic with an ejection fraction <25 percent. Compared to placebo, carvedilol caused a 27 percent reduction in the combined risk of death or hospitalization for a medical reason.[112] Carvedilol-treated patients were less likely than placebo-treated patients to experience a serious adverse effect, especially worsening heart failure, sudden death, cardiogenic shock, or ventricular tachycardia. Based on the results of this last study, the FDA approved carvedilol for the treatment of NYHA class IV patients, using doses of up to 25 mg twice daily.

Not every patient benefits from long-term adrenergic blockade. In those who benefit, the rise in ejection fraction averages 10 percent. Increases in LV ejection fraction up to 15 to 20 percent with a normalization of LV volumes have been observed in individual patients. Systolic blood pressure and myocardial contractility, as evaluated by LV $dp/dt$, are predictors of the response to long-term beta-adrenergic blockade in relation to LV ejection fraction.[113] The higher systolic blood pressure and LV $dp/dt$ are, the more likely is ejection fraction to increase during long-term BAB.

The Beta Blocker Estimation of Survival Trial (BEST),[113a] a large randomized, placebo-controlled study of the effect of bucindolol, a third-generation BAB with direct vasodilating properties, on survival of 2708 patients with NYHA functional class III and class IV, was stopped because of the futility of the lack of benefit seen. A preliminary report indicates that whereas bucindolol reduced mortality in patients in functional class III, it did not do so in patients in functional class IV.

The long-term and acute effects of BAB on LV performance have important therapeutic and pathophysiologic implications. First, the deterioration in LV performance that is routinely observed during the first weeks of therapy mandates that beta-adrenergic blockade be initiated at the lowest dose possible of a given agent in stable patients with CHF. Since BAB is aimed at altering the progression of the syndrome of CHF and not at providing acute relief of symptoms, effective beta blockade can be progressively reached by increasing doses of beta-blocker agents every 2 to 3 weeks. When CHF is associated with angina or excessive tachycardia, and effective beta blockade is needed for control of symptoms, the doses of beta blockers can be increased every few days under close in-hospital monitoring.

An important unresolved issue concerning BAB in CHF is the treatment of patients whose symptoms worsen to functional class IV while being treated with BAB. No data are presently available to provide guidelines to manage these patients. A pragmatic approach is to hospitalize patients who decompensate while receiving BAB and treat them with temporary inotropic support with a specific phosphodiesterase (PDE) inhibitor, such as milrinone, which does not require beta receptors for its activity. Patients who improve are kept on a BAB, and inotropic support is discontinued after a few days. BAB should be tapered off and withdrawn in patients who fail to improve. The pathophysiologic implications of successful BAB is that the process of LV dysfunction can be reversed by pharmacologic means even in patients with markedly reduced LV function. Thus, a certain amount of plasticity that was previously unrecognized remains in dilated fibrotic left ventricles. The cellular and molecular mechanisms that reverse myocyte dysfunction thereby enhancing global LV performance are poorly understood (Table 25-2).[99,114,115] Since patients with both ischemic and nonischemic cardiomyopathy benefit from long-term BAB, dysfunction of surviving myocytes is a common characteristic of CHF independent of its etiology.[116] Patients with nonischemic cardiomyopathy were initially thought to experience greater benefit from long-term BAB than were patients with ischemic cardiomyopathy. Since it is practically impossible to compare patients with different etiologies of CHF at a similar stage of their disease process, definite conclusions concerning the effects of long-term BAB as a function of the etiology should probably not be drawn.

It was recently shown that in patients with idiopathic dilated cardiomyopathy, functional improvement related to treatment with BABs is associated with changes in myocardial gene expression.[116a]

Both carvedilol and sustained-release metoprolol are approved for use in patients with CHF. The rationale for choosing a nonselective agent over a selective beta$_1$ antagonist has previously been mentioned. A large trial has been completed that compared the relative benefits of carvedilol and the nonsustained release formulation of metoprolol in patients with CHF [Carvedilol or Metoprolol Evaluation Trial (COMET)]. The preliminary results show a 17 percent reduction in mortality with carvedilol.[116b]

In summary, in the absence of an indication, such as reversible airways obstructive disease, advanced heart block, or episodic decompensation, all symptomatic patients with CHF should be treated with long-term BAB.[100,101,117] Treatment should be initiated at the lowest possible dose, and advanced to full BAB over 1 to 2 months as tolerated. Patients who do not tolerate the full dose should be kept on intermediate doses that still result in substantial improvement in LV function and a reduction in mortality.[101] BAB is the only pharmacologic intervention that reverses LV remodeling, whereas ACE inhibition is the only intervention that improves the vascular disease processes. Thus, BAB is not an exclusive intervention but a complementary intervention. Both ACE inhibition and BAB are essential interventions for the pharmacologic treatment of CHF.

TABLE 25-2 Possible Mechanisms by Which Beta-Adrenergic Blockers Improve Ventricular Function in Chronic Congestive Heart Failure

| |
|---|
| Upregulation of beta receptors |
| Direct myocardial protective action against catecholamine toxicity |
| Improved ability of noradrenergic sympathetic nerves to synthesize norepinephrine |
| Decreased release of norepinephrine from sympathetic nerve endings |
| Decreased stimulation of other vasoconstrictive systems including renin–angiotensin–aldosterone, vasopressin, and endothelin |
| Potentiation of kallikrein–kinin system and natural vasodilatation (increase in bradykinin) |
| Antiarrhythmic effects raising ventricular fibrillation threshold |
| Protection against catecholamine-induced hypokalemia |
| Increase in coronary blood flow by reducing heart rate and improving diastolic perfusion time; possible coronary dilation with vasodilator–beta blocker |
| Restoration of abnormal baroreflex function |
| Prevention of ventricular muscle hypertrophy and vascular remodeling |
| Antioxidant effects (carvedilol?) |
| Shift from free fatty acid to carbohydrate metabolism (improved metabolic efficiency) |
| Vasodilation (e.g., carvedilol) |
| Antiapoptosis effect, allowing myocardial cell regeneration to occur |
| Improved left atrial contribution to left ventricular filling |
| Modulation of postreceptor inhibitory G proteins |
| Normalization of myocyte $Ca^{2+}$ regulatory proteins and improved $Ca^{2+}$ handling |
| Increasing natriuretic peptide production |
| Attenuation of inflammatory cytokines |
| Restoring cardiac calcium release channel (ryanodine receptor) |
| Favorable changes in myocardial gene expression |

## DIURETICS

Sodium accumulation tends to occur in the early stages of CHF, with peripheral edema accompanied by weight gain. Diuretics, along with salt restriction, remain the best therapeutic tool for treating the edematous state in heart failure.[118] Despite the advent of new agents for treating symptomatic CHF, diuretics continue to be among the most commonly prescribed drugs in the world.

The mechanism for edema is generally multifactorial and includes renal vasoconstriction, increased aldosterone and vasopressin activity, and/or increased venous pressures. Increased sympathetic nervous system activity (tone) tends to occur early in the course of heart failure. Activation of the renin–angiotensin axis tends to occur somewhat later, commonly when diuretics are begun.[47] This leads to increased aldosterone, leading to sodium accumulation and potassium loss. Even with asymptomatic LV dysfunction, avidity of the kidneys for sodium and water is greatly enhanced, and peripheral edema comprises an early physical sign that brings the problem of CHF to the physician's attention. Salt and water retention lead to an expanded intravascular volume, with an increase in LV filling pressures in order to maintain cardiac output.[119] With continued worsening of LV function, progressive volume expansion continues and LV end-diastolic pressure rises along with venous hydrostatic pressure in both the systemic and pulmonary beds. This alteration in Starling forces favors transudation of intravascular fluid into the interstitial compartment, culminating in edema formation. Eventually a point is reached at which additional increases in LV filling pressure fail to augment cardiac output, and with progressive increases in peripheral arterial vasoconstriction, renal perfusion is reduced. By this time, overt heart failure is established, and the kidney's ability to excrete a salt load severely impaired.[119] Important mediators in this process are (1) activation of the renin–angiotensin–aldosterone axis; (2) stimulation of the sympathetic nervous system; (3) increased levels of antidiuretic hormone leading to water retention and hyponatremia; and (4) resistance to atrial natriuretic peptide (ANP), which is an endogenous hormonal vasodilator and diuretic.

The appropriate use of diuretics will depend on the stage of disease and severity. With mild fluid accumulation, characterized by peripheral edema, pulmonary rales, and weight gain, oral diuretics are indicated. Long-acting but less potent diuretics, such as hydrochlorothiazide and chlorthalidone, may be adequate. Intermittent use of more potent loop diuretics, such as furosemide, bumetanide, or torsemide, may allow one to regain dry weight more rapidly. Efficacy can be assessed by daily weights and diuretic regimens adjusted appropriately.

***Loop Diuretics*** The most potent diuretics are those whose action is in the medullary thick ascending limb of Henle, because of the percentage of filtrate reabsorption that occurs at this segment of the nephron. In the euvolemic state, about 20 percent of filtered sodium load is reabsorbed in the thick ascending limb, compared with only 7 percent in the distal tubule and 5 percent in the collecting duct.[120] Drugs in this diuretic class include furosemide, bumetanide, torsemide, and ethacrynic acid. The loop diuretics are more than 98 percent protein-bound and therefore not freely filtered by the glomerulus. Rather, they access the tubular lumen, where they act by secretion via an organic anion transporter. This secretion of loop diuretic may be impaired and their action limited by the presence of elevated levels of endogenous organic acids, such as occurs in renal failure, and by probenecid, salicylates, and NSAIDs. Once in the lumen of the tubule, the loop diuretics compete with chloride for binding to the Na+/K+/2Cl cotransporter situated on the apical membrane of cells of the medullary thick ascending limb, thereby inhibiting the reabsorption of both sodium and chloride. The urinary diuretic concentration best represents the fraction of drug delivered to the thick ascending limb and significantly correlates with the natriuretic response following diuretic administration.[121]

Furosemide is the most widely used loop diuretic. In normal patients, the oral bioavailability of furosemide is 50 percent. Following an oral dose, the onset of action occurs within 30 to 60 min, peaks at 1 to 2 h, and has a duration of action of 6 h, with a half-life of 50 min.[122] Furosemide may be given intravenously over 1 to 2 min; following intravenous administration; diuresis begins within 15 min and peaks at 30 to 60 min. The duration of action is up to 2 h when given intravenously. Sixty percent of furosemide is excreted unchanged in the urine; the rest is conjugated with glucuronic acid in the kidney.[122] In renal insufficiency [glomerular filtration rate (GFR) $<$30 mL/min)], the elimination half-life is prolonged, although the diuretic response is impaired, largely because of reduced drug delivery to its site of action within the tubule.[123]

In CHF, the pharmacokinetics of oral furosemide are also altered; furosemide absorption is delayed, which leads to a delay in the time at which peak concentration occurs.[121] Altered furosemide pharmacodynamic properties occur independent of the route of administration, due to adaptations within the glomerular microcirculation and renal tubule that are present during chronic diuretic administration.[121] Bumetanide is 40 times more potent than furosemide and is available in both oral and intravenous formulations. In normal patients, the bioavailability is 80 percent following an oral dose, and the onset of diuretic effects occurs within 30 min and peaks within 1 h. The duration of action of oral bumetanide is between 3 and 6 h, with a half-life between 1 and 3.5 h.[122] Similar to furosemide, the delayed absorption of oral bumetanide in heart failure results in lower peak concentrations as well as in a delayed time to peak concentration.

Torsemide is a loop diuretic that differs from others in its class in that 80 percent of a dose undergoes hepatic metabolism. Because only 20 percent of the drug is excreted unchanged in the urine, its half-life is minimally altered in renal failure.[121] Torsemide is rapidly absorbed and is 80 to 90 percent bioavailable. In patients with chronic renal insufficiency or with cirrhosis, the natriuretic response following a dose of torsemide is unaffected by route of administration.[124] Maximal sodium excretion occurs within the first 2 h after either routine. In healthy individuals, the half-life of torsemide is 3.3 h but is prolonged to 8 h in those with cirrhosis.[121,125] When selecting an oral agent in patients with heart failure, the physician may find oral torsemide to be advantageous since its absorption is unimpaired and is less variable than that with oral furosemide.[126] In fact, the pharmacokinetics of torsemide in those with CHF are comparable to those in healthy persons. As is the case with all loop diuretics, however, dose-response curves for torsemide in patients with CHF are shifted downward and to the right, suggesting altered drug pharmacodynamics and a diminished diuretic response. The efficacy of loop diuretics is often significantly reduced in decompensated heart failure. Impaired drug absorption has been implicated as one cause of variable efficacy. Reduced gastric and intestinal motility, edematous bowel wall, and decreased splanchnic blood flow may delay absorption. The total amount of furosemide absorbed over 24 h, however, is similar to that found in healthy individuals.[127]

In patients with stable, compensated heart failure given oral furosemide, the time to peak urinary excretion is prolonged to about 190 min (normal, 90 min) and peak urinary excretion rate is reduced by 50 percent.[121] Furosemide and bumetanide, when given in doses of equivalent potency, induce a similar natriuretic response in patients with heart failure.[121] The pharmacokinetic properties of intravenous furosemide are unaltered in heart failure patients compared with those in healthy individuals.[121] The effectiveness of loop diuretics is limited by two phenomena in patients with chronic heart failure and normal renal function. The *rebound phenomenon* consists of a decrease in sodium excretion below baseline after the effect of the loop diuretic has worn off. The *braking phenomenon* refers to an increase in tubular sodium reabsorption by the distal tubule, which occurs during long-term administration of loop diuretics.

In decompensated heart failure, the intravenous route of administration is preferable when possible, since the onset of diuresis is shorter and more predictable (Fig. 25-8). In patients with CHF refractory to standard doses of intravenous furosemide, higher doses may be efficacious. In patients with severe CHF previously resistant to lower intravenous doses of furosemide,[128] intravenous furosemide was administered at doses of $\geq$500 mg daily, with increased diuresis, weight reduction, and symptomatic improvement.

Continuous intravenous rather than intermittent administration of loop diuretics is an effective method of overcoming diuretic resistance in heart failure. In a randomized crossover study comparing continuous versus bolus bumetanide in patients with chronic renal failure (mean GFR of 17 mL/min), a greater net sodium excretion was observed during continuous infusion despite comparable drug excretion.[129] Only one prospective, randomized crossover study is available that compares the continuous infusion of furosemide (loading dose 30 to 40 mg followed by infusion at a rate of 2.5 to 3.3 mg/h for 48 h) with intermittent intravenous bolus administration (30 to 40 mg every 8 h for 48 h) in NYHA class III and class IV heart failure.[130] When infused continuously, furosemide's pattern of delivery produced more effective drug utilization, that is, sodium excretion relative to total furosemide excretion, whereas with intermittent bolus furosemide, wide fluctuations in urine output and sodium excretion were observed. Theoretically, an infusion of furosemide at a constant rate may be safer than using intermittent intravenous dosing, although a larger study is needed to confirm this.

In summary, loop diuretics with salt restriction monitored by weight measurement by scale remains the basis for treatment of edema. As CHF progresses, increasing oral doses of loop diuretics tend to be needed. In severe CHF with hospitalization, intravenous loop diuretics, commonly at higher doses, become essential. As will be discussed later, other agents, such as metolazone, may be required as well to increase and sustain sodium loss. Limitations to diuretic use remain hyponatremia and a progressive increase in serum creatinine, which may require careful dose reductions (Table 25-3).

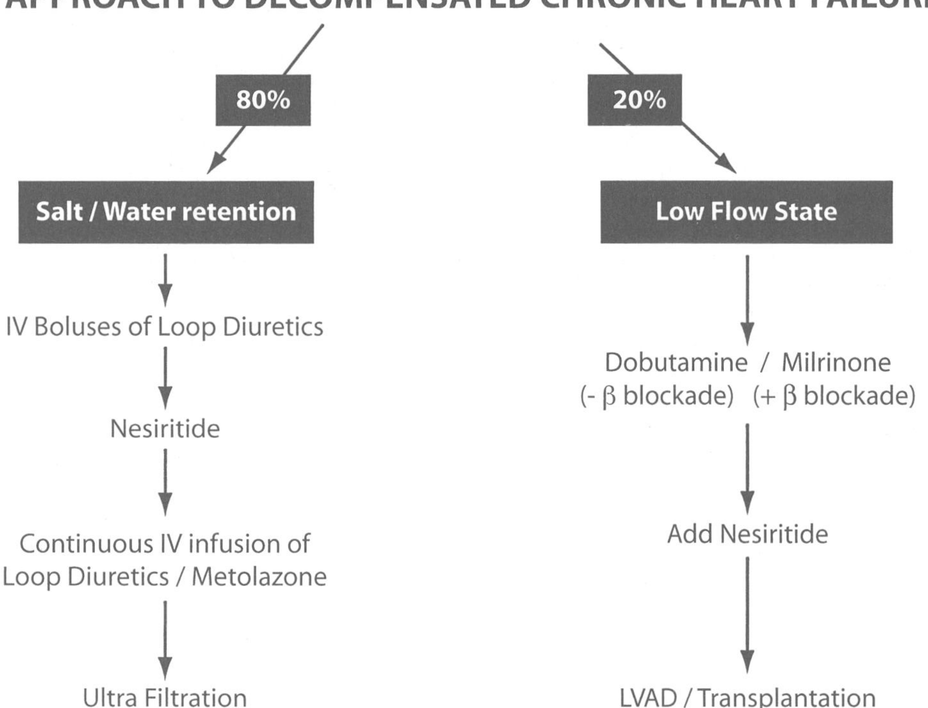


FIGURE 25-8 Clinical decompensation of heart failure. The treatment is directed toward controlling salt and water retention (central of peripheral edema) and/or relieving a low-flow state by increasing cardiac output while reducing very increased filling pressures. Dobutamine is useful to increase cardiac output except when β blockade is not present. Milrinone, a type III phosphodiesterase inhibitor that stimulates adenyl cyclase beyond the receptor, is preferable to dobutamine in patients still receiving β blockade. Patients with persistent marked elevation of filling pressures may benefit from addition of nesiritide when their systolic blood pressure may benefit from addition of nesiritide when their systolic blood pressure is >85–90 mmHg. When an adequate cardiac output can no longer be maintained, surgical implantation of left ventricular assist device (LVAD) may be used to pump blood from the LV to the aorta as destination therapy or bridge to cardiac transplantation. When salt and water retention is the overwhelming manifestation, treatment of clinical decompensation should be initiated with intravenous (IV) boluses of loop diuretics. If IV administration of loop diuretics fails to generate a negative balance, nesiritide is often of value in promoting substantial diuresis in patients with systolic blood pressure >90 mmHg. When loop diuretics fail to promote salt and water excretion, mechanical removal of water needs to be considered.

***Thiazides*** The thiazide diuretics may be reasonable first-line natriuretic agents in early LV dysfunction when renal perfusion is not yet significantly compromised. In overt ventricular failure, however, thiazides are usually ineffective or inadequate. Thiazides are 50 percent protein-bound, and more than 95 percent of the dose is excreted unchanged in the urine.[122] They gain access into the tubular lumen by both glomerular filtration and tubular secretion. In the kidney, they inhibit sodium chloride reabsorption in the early distal tubule where they compete for the chloride site on the apically located Na+/Cl cotransporter.

TABLE 25-3 Stepwise Approach to Loop Diuretic Resistance

1. Enforce strict low-sodium diet
2. Use effective doses of loop diuretics
3. Combination administration of long-acting thiazide with loop diuretic to offset the antinatriuretic rebound effect observed with administration of short-acting loop diuretics
4. Constant intravenous infusion of loop diuretic

Hydrochlorothiazide is the most widely prescribed drug in this class of diuretics. Seventy-one percent of an oral dose is absorbed. The onset of diuresis is within 2 h, peaks between 3 and 6 h, and continues for up to 12 h.[122] Hydrochlorothiazide's pharmacokinetics follow a two-compartment model of elimination ($\alpha$ phase, 5 h; $\beta$ phase, 6 to 15 h), and the half-life is prolonged in patients with decompensated heart failure and in those with renal insufficiency.

Metolazone is a quinazoline diuretic and is similar to the thiazides in structure and mechanism of action.[122] Although its major effect is in the cortical diluting segment, metolazone has a minor inhibitory effect on proximal tubular sodium reabsorption. Metolazone is lipid-soluble and easily accesses the tubular lumen during states of renal insufficiency, unlike the thiazides.[122] Another advantage of metolazone is its longer duration of action (12 to 24 h).[122]

***Potassium-Sparing Diuretics*** Aldosterone, an endogenous adrenal hormone, normally increases sodium reabsorption with the simultaneous excretion of potassium. Aldosterone levels are increased in heart failure, to some degree due to its augmented secretion induced by angiotensin II. In heart failure, an increase in aldosterone activity may cause significant sodium retention, potassium depletion, and magnesium depletion. Increased aldosterone activity can also be harmful by causing an augmentation of sympathetic stimulation and a decreased activity of the parasympathetic nervous system, thereby contributing to baroreflex dysfunction, a poor prognostic finding in patients with heart failure. Aldosterone may also promote formation of patchy myocardial fibrosis, leading to arrhythmias and further depression of LV dysfunction.

Spironolactone, a lipid-soluble potassium-sparing diuretic, competes with aldosterone for binding to its receptor in the principal cell of the collecting duct and thus leads to diuresis.[122] Spironolactone is particularly advantageous during states of reduced renal perfusion because the drug's delivery to its site of action is not dependent on GFR. Spironolactone may be a useful adjunct to hydrochlorothiazide in offsetting its effect to produce hypokalemia resulting from sodium–potassium exchange. Since the exchange of sodium for potassium is reduced, potassium loss is reduced and hypokalemia may be corrected. Indeed, potassium supplements given for hypokalemia should generally be stopped in order to avoid hyperkalemia. If the use of spironolactone is warranted in a severe heart failure patient receiving an ACE inhibitor, therapy may be initiated at a dose of 25 mg a day. Because of the risk of hyperkalemia, serum potassium concentration should be closely monitored not only during concomitant therapy with ACE inhibitors or ARBs, but also during periods of declining renal function.[130a] If the serum potassium concentration exceeds 5.5 meq/L, the spironolactone dose should be reduced to 25 mg every other day. Alternatively, after 8 weeks, the spironolactone dose may be increased to 50 mg/day in patients with stable serum potassium concentrations who are experiencing worsening heart failure symptoms. Maintenance doses of 50 mg/day or greater should be limited to patients with refractory or severe heart failure who have evidence of pulmonary or peripheral edema due to an increased incidence of hyperkalemia. In this particular patient population, however, doses as high as 200 mg/day may be necessary. However, once the patient's condition has stabilized, the dose of spironolactone should be decreased to the maintenance level (25 to 50 mg/day) used prior to the heart failure exacerbation.[131] The use of spironolactone has also been associated with reduced mortality in CHF, perhaps by helping to maintain potassium levels, thereby reducing the risk of arrhythmic death in patients with heart failure,[132] or by inhibiting other pathologic processes influenced by aldosterone.[133] Spironolactone has also been shown to improve endothelial dysfunction, increase nitric oxide bioactivity, and inhibit the conversion of angiotensin I to II, providing additional mechanisms for its beneficial effects on cardiovascular mortality.[134]

The benefits of aldosterone receptor blockade on mortality that had been reported in patients with CHF were also demonstrated in patients with recent myocardial infarction and depressed LV systolic function with symptoms of heart failure or diabetes mellitus.[135] While receiving optimal medical treatment, 6632 patients were randomized to aldosterone receptor blockade with eplerenone, a selective mineralocorticoid blocker, or placebo. The mean follow-up was 16 months. There were 487 deaths in the eplerenone group and 557 deaths in the placebo group (relative risk 0.85; 95 percent CI 0.75 to 0.96; $p = 0.008$). Although this trial was conducted in patients with recent myocardial infarction and not in patients with CHF, the substantial effects of aldosterone receptor blockade on mortality in patients undergoing LV remodeling indicate that one may not wait for functional class III to class IV to initiate this therapy in patients with CHF.[136] Recently, eplerenone was approved for use in CHF.

Amiloride and triamterene are similar to spironolactone in that they are potassium-sparing and act on the principal cell; however, they must be delivered intralumenally to be effective. More specifically, they reduce sodium flux into principal cells by blocking the apically located sodium channel.[122] When used alone, the potassium-sparing diuretics are relatively weak. In heart failure, they are of benefit when used in combination with a loop diuretic to overcome diuretic resistance and to reduce potassium wasting.[137]

***Combined Use of Diuretics*** Numerous reports have demonstrated a rapid, profound diuresis (1 to 2 L daily within 24 to 48 h), accompanied by clinical improvement, following the addition of metolazone to furosemide in patients with CHF (see Fig. 25-8) who were previously resistant to furosemide alone.[138–140] Metolazone, a thiazide-like diuretic, is particularly advantageous since it has a prolonged duration of action, is lipophilic, and remains effective in states of renal impairment. In a study comparing metolazone with a thiazide, however, when either was used in combination with a loop diuretic, no significant difference in sodium excretion or urine output was observed between the two drugs.[140] Spironolactone, when used in combination with a loop diuretic (see Fig. 25-8), has also been associated with an improvement in diuretic response in patients with CHF previously resistant to loop diuretics.[137]

In summary, thiazides, potassium-sparing diuretics, and aldosterone inhibitors (e.g., spironolactone, eplerenone), along with loop diuretics, provide potent tools to reduce salt accumulation in those with CHF. Early in CHF, their use is mainly to reduce or eliminate peripheral edema and help relieve pulmonary congestion. Once dry weight is approximated, intermittent and reduced diuretic use is advisable to avoid electrolyte problems. Daily weights are the best guide to adequacy of this therapy. Early in CHF, thiazides with potassium-sparing diuretics may be all that are necessary, although loop diuretics provide increased diuresis. Indeed, loop diuretics can be used intermittently on top of thiazides, when needed. It is possible that the early use of diuretics can hasten the evolution of CHF by increasing reflex neurohumoral responses that may have adverse consequences, such as activation of the renin–angiotensin system.[47] As CHF progresses, the loop diuretics in increasing amounts are generally required. Here again, a scale for weight provides guidance for dosage. With excessive diuresis in very severe CHF, increasing renal insufficiency may be induced by hypovolemia, and this, in itself, may increase loop diuretic dose, its use intravenously, and the need for concomitant use of thiazides (metolazone) or spironolactone.

## In-Hospital Therapy of Congestive Heart Failure

The factors that precipitate clinical deterioration in CHF are identifiable in less than 50 percent of patients hospitalized for clinical decompensation.[141] Inadequate adherence to a complex medical regimen or a low sodium diet often associated with depression, pulmonary infection or embolism, paroxysmal atrial fibrillation, chronic anemia, obstructive sleep apnea, and renal insufficiency are traditional events that lead to clinical deterioration. Anemia is common in elderly patients with CHF and its prevalence increases with severity of disease.[142] The presence of anemia also predicts a poor prognosis in patients with CHF, especially when anemia is due to hemodilution.[143] These complicating issues require close patient surveillance. Nevertheless, the transition from a compensated to a decompensated state of CHF often remains unexplained, especially in patients who are already markedly symptomatic even in a compensated state.

Rarely is the transition from a compensated to a decompensated state due to a further measurable reduction in myocardial contractility. Rather clinical decompensation is associated with a decrease in an already reduced cardiac output and an increase in LV filling pressure. Worsening of functional mitral regurgitation occurs, which may trigger the event. Indeed, a vicious cycle occurs wherein increasing diastolic filling pressures and volumes can increase the extent of an already present mitral insufficiency and increasing mitral insufficiency produces more mitral insufficiency. The increase in mitral regurgitant volume occurs largely at the expense of forward stroke volume. As the cardiac output falls, the patient loses the ability to redistribute an already limited cardiac output to essential organs. Even before decompensation, the cascade of events that allow preferential perfusion to essential organs as cardiac outputs falls in patients with severe CHF is poorly understood. Preferential redistribution of a reduced cardiac output to vital organs permits patients with severe CHF to remain functional; in the absence of redistribution, a shock-like state would be present. Thus, in severe but compensated CHF the patient can digest food, walk, and maintain a satisfactory cardiac output but may only be able to perform one of these functions at a time. When preferential distribution of blood flow is impaired, clinical decompensation occurs with increasing renal dysfunction.[144] As is observed in patients with septic shock and presumably related to localized inflammation, release of smooth muscle-relaxing substances may promote generalized vasodilatation that impairs preferential blood flow redistribution to specific organs in patients with CHF. Thus, clinical deterioration does not appear to be primarily due to a further depression in myocardial contractility in patients with CHF. Rather, clinical decompensation results from a fall in cardiac output that in turn leads to increased right ventricular (RV) and LV filling pressures with increasing functional mitral regurgitation. As cardiac output falls, preferential perfusion of essential organs is no longer maintained and generalized organ dysfunction ensues.

Measurements of serum BNP are useful in assessing the status of patients with decompensated CHF.[145,146] The predominant stimulus to production and release of BNP by the LV is filling pressure, and a rise in serum BNP level is an extremely sensitive and specific biomarker of clinical decompensation.[34] Monitoring of serum BNP level is particularly useful in evaluating therapeutic efficacy during a hospitalization for decompensated CHF.[147] Despite clinical improvement acknowledged by the patient, the likelihood of rehospitalization within 6 weeks from discharge is extremely high when the serum BNP level is not substantially lower than that noted on admission.[147]

The nature of events that lead to clinical deterioration affects the prognosis and approach to patients hospitalized for decompensated CHF. Documentation of an abundant response to a dose of diuretic equal to the regular outpatient dose or a low serum digoxin level can strengthen the suspicion of poor compliance to medications or diet. When bacterial pulmonary or urinary sepsis is suspected in patients with decompensated CHF, broad spectrum antibiotic therapy should be immediately initiated without waiting for results of cultures.

The hemodynamic status of patients with decompensated CHF can be classified in four profiles according the presence or absence of fluid overload and systemic poor perfusion.[148] An easier approach is to consider patients with prominent evidence of fluid overload and patients with overt manifestations of low cardiac output as two separate clinical entities (see Fig. 25-8).

## FLUID AND SODIUM RETENTION

Eighty percent of patients with CHF hospitalized for clinical decompensation present with overt fluid and sodium retention. Weight gain, inability to fit in clothes or shoes, and presence of lower limb edema are the best evidence of fluid retention. Indirect evaluation of right atrial pressure by examination of jugular venous distension is fraught with many limitations, the most glaring limitation being changes in venous compliance as the syndrome progresses. Physical examination is notoriously inaccurate for detection of pulmonary congestion. Pulmonary rales are often absent due to increased lymphatic drainage. Similarly, patients with marked elevation of pulmonary vascular resistance at late stages of CHF may no longer present with orthopnea. Pulmonary congestion is best assessed by roentgenographic findings, especially the presence of pleural effusions. However, when assessing the effects of acute therapy, one needs to keep in mind the lag between roentgenographic findings and LV filling pressure. The amount of fluid retention is the difference between the admitting weight and the dry weight, if known. Blood volume measurement based on the concept of the indicator dilution technique is not routinely performed in patients with CHF, although this technique may provide the most objective endpoint for assessing the need for diuretic therapy. The optimal rate of diuresis to prevent intravascular depletion varies from patient to patient, but overall it corresponds to a negative balance ranging from 2 to 3 L per 24 h when the serum albumin concentration is normal. The optimal rate of diuresis is obviously lower when low serum albumin concentration impedes fluid transport from the interstitial to the intravascular space. A stepwise approach to the care of patients hospitalized for decompensated CHF and presenting with clinical and x-rays findings compatible with fluid and sodium retention is depicted in Fig 25-8.

The first step is administration of an intravenous bolus of loop diuretics. The next step, when intravenous boluses of loop diuretics fail to generate a negative fluid balance, is continuous infusion of nesiritide with a loading bolus of 2 $\mu$g/kg and a maintenance rate of infusion ranging from 0.01 to 0.03 $\mu$g/kg/min. When nesiritide does not promote an adequate diuresis, one can add metolazone orally at a daily dose ranging from 2.5 to 10 mg and/or switch to continuous infusion of loop diuretics. Last, in the few cases where all pharmacologic interventions aimed at promoting diuresis have failed, hemofiltration should be considered.

## LOW FLOW STATE

The clinical profile of the syndrome of low flow state in patients with CHF hospitalized for clinical decompensation is dominated by two symptoms that distract the attention from the heart. The first symptom is extreme fatigue, often to the point of lethargy. The second symptom is nonspecific abdominal discomfort or pain. The severity of the abdominal discomfort often motivates a surgical consultation in the emergency room. Abdominal discomfort or pain is rapidly relieved by interventions that enhance the cardiac output. Physical examination reveals a blood pressure <90 mmHg with a narrow pulse pressure, the absence of overt signs of fluid overload, especially pulmonary rales, and of abdominal guarding or rebound, and the presence of cold extremities. A low body temperature of 95°F (35.0°C) is common in patients presenting in low flow state in the absence of coexisting infection. Therapy with ACE inhibitors and BAB has often been discontinued over the preceding days due to hypotension and increasing fatigue.

The management of patients in a low flow state is best guided by serial measurements of mixed venous oxygen saturation and pulmonary capillary wedge pressure obtained by right side of the heart catheterization. Determination of pulmonary capillary wedge pressure also allows avoidance of excessive diuresis. This may result in severe intravascular depletion and thereby low LV filling pressure, which can limit cardiac output and worsen the low flow state. If not already done, BAB therapy needs to be discontinued in patients with mixed venous saturation <50 percent. Due to the common presence of tricuspid regurgitation, the thermodilution technique often overestimates cardiac output in patients with end-stage CHF. Determination of mixed venous oxygen saturation is less subject to such bias and thus provides a more accurate method to estimate the lower range of cardiac output. The approach to management of patients hospitalized for decompensated CHF and presenting in low flow state is depicted in Fig 25-8.

When mixed venous oxygen saturation is >50 percent, BAB can be continued and therapy with milrinone initiated. Once the patient has symptomatically improved, one discontinues therapy with milrinone. When the patient does not improve, one may reduce the dose of BAB by half. When the patient fails to improve while receiving half the usual dose of BAB, BAB should be discontinued and milrinone continued for a few days. Severe pulmonary hypertension or evolving myocardial ischemia is the other indication for choosing milirinone over dobutamine for temporary positive inotropic support. In general, dobutamine is used to augment cardiac output. Dobutamine, as detailed later, increases cardiac output and lowers systemic vascular resistance with little alteration in blood pressure or heart rate. The response to dobutamine may be reduced with previous BAB. Milrinone, by inhibiting PDE type III, also enhances cardiac output and reduces LV filling pressure, but is more likely to produce hypotension.[149] Dobutamine is clearly the preferred agent in patients who are not receiving BAB and in patients with borderline systolic blood pressure. The vasodilating properties of dobutamine are substantially less potent than are those of milrinone. Once patients have been stabilized by dobutamine, the addition of nesiritide may lead to further improvement by reducing LV filling pressure and the amount of functional mitral regurgitation.

Patients in low output state who fail inotropic therapy are candidates for mechanical support with intraaortic balloon counterpulsation and LVAD as a bridge to cardiac transplantation, if eligible, or as destination therapy if they are not candidates for cardiac transplantation. When patients fail to respond to positive inotropic therapy and are not eligible for long-term mechanical cardiac support, palliation becomes a central issue and careful and open discussion with the family involved becomes essential.[150] An implanted defibrillator should be turned off. At this point, the "quality of death" is the issue and agents such as morphine may be useful in maintaining terminal comfort.

## NESIRITIDE

Nesiritide is a recombinant form of human BNP that dilates the arterial and venous circulation in a balanced manner. Nesiritide also has natriuretic and diuretic properties and is devoid of any positive inotropic action.[151] It is only available for parenteral administration. Nesiritide has a distribution half-life of about 2 min, and steady-state serum levels are reached after 90 min of continuous infusion at a rate ranging from 0.01 to 0.03 $\mu$g/kg/min. Nesiritide levels are then four- to sixfold greater than spontaneous endogenous BNP levels. Nesiritide has three major modes of elimination: binding to the cell surface receptor natriuretic peptide receptor C followed by internalization and degradation; hydrolysis by neutral endopeptidase; and renal elimination. Nesiritide has a main terminal half-life of about 20 min. The rate of infusion does not require dose adjustment in patients with renal insufficiency. After binding to the natriuretic peptide receptor A, and to a lesser extent to the natriuretic peptide receptor B, nesiritide activates an intracellular guanylyl cyclase domain that, in turn, increases production of the second messenger cyclic guanosine monophosphate (cGMP). In addition to its vasodilatory, natriuretic, and diuretic properties, nesiritide increases the permeability of the vascular endothelium, suppresses the RAAS, and inhibits sympathetic neurotransmission in the peripheral vasculature.[151,151a] The mechanisms that mediate these additional properties of nesiritide have not been elucidated. What is known is that cGMP is not involved.

The hemodynamic effects of nesiritide have been studied in patients with CHF primarily due to LV systolic dysfunction, in whom worsening of symptoms including dyspnea at rest had led to hospitalization.[152] Although they were in a decompensated state, patients were required by protocol to have a systolic blood pressure >90 mmHg. The largest randomized trial was the Vasodilatation in the Management of Acute Congestive Heart Failure (VMAC) study.[153] By protocol, a change in pulmonary capillary wedge pressure was the primary endpoint. Nesiritide reduced pulmonary capillary wedge pressure consistently with a mean reduction that was greater than that noted with nitroglycerin. Pulmonary capillary wedge pressure decreased within 15 min of nesiritide administration. Nesiritide also consistently reduced right atrial and pulmonary artery pressures while enhancing cardiac index significantly. The concomitant reduction in mean systemic blood pressure was significant but modest, indicating that systemic vascular resistances fell substantially. Heart rate did not change.

Nesiritide is the first agent shown to improve symptoms in patients who were symptomatic on presentation to the hospital, and receiving treatment in an intensive care unit or an electrocardiogram (ECG)-monitored setting. Dyspnea at rest was the symptom selected as the primary endpoint. Using a five-point scale, the change in the severity of dyspnea was assessed at 3 or 6 h after administration of nesiritide, intravenously administered nitroglycerin, or placebo.[153] When compared to patients randomized to placebo or nitroglycerin, a slightly greater percentage of patients randomized to nesiritide experienced symptomatic relief at 3 or 6 h after the onset of therapy (77 versus 65 percent, $p = 0.03$). Mortality was not a prespecified clinical endpoint of the nesiritide trials, and thus the collection of data was retrospective. When analyzed in this manner, observations regarding the effects of nitroglycerin, nesiritide, or dobutamine on mortality at 6 months remain speculative. The 6-month mortality was similar in patients who received nesiritide or nitroglycerin, and appears to be worse in patients who received dobutamine.[154] Moreover, statistical profiling cannot adequately account for the severity of CHF on admission, thereby further limiting analysis of the data at 6 months.

The Prospective Randomized Evaluation of Cardiac Ectopy with Dobutamine and Nesiritide Therapy (PRECEDENT) trial demonstrated that devoid of positive inotropic action and not affecting calcium transients, nesiritide is not proarrhythmic in contrast to dobutamine.[155] The clinical benefits of nesiritide in patients with decompensated CHF and preserved LV systolic function were documented in a small subset of subjects enrolled in the VMAC trial.[153] In contrast to nonspecific vasodilators, nesiritide does not increase but, to the contrary, decreases neurohumoral activity of the renin–angiotensin–aldosterone system and sympathetic nervous systems in patients with decompensated CHF. Such neurohormonal effects of nesiritide are concordant with the observation that tachycardia does not accompany observed decreases in blood pressure.

***Indications for Nesiritide Therapy*** Once they have failed intravenous diuretic therapy, patients with CHF who are hospitalized for severe fluid and sodium retention and have a systolic blood pressure >90 mmHg may benefit from nesiritide therapy. In contrast to nitroglycerin or nitroprusside that often requires close monitoring relative to dose initiation and optimization, nesiritide therapy is not time consuming. The dosing schedule involves only three rates of infusion, and the risk of hastening hypotension is minimal. In contrast to nitroglycerin, the hemodynamic effects of nesiritide are sustained without evidence of tachyphylaxis. The relative benefits of these agents in restabilizing a patient with decompensated CHF may be modest, especially when comparable endpoints of circulatory response are studied. However, nesiritide is easier to administer in efficacious doses than is nitroglycerin.

Nesiritide is equally useful in symptomatic patients with either preserved or reduced LV systolic function. Thus, nesiritide has a role in the treatment of patients hospitalized for overt fluid retention who have failed to improve after a single intravenous bolus of loop diuretic. Nesiritide therapy is of special interest in patients with severe functional mitral regurgitation and/or pulmonary hypertension where reduction of RV and LV diastolic and systolic pressures can be particularly beneficial.

## INOTROPIC AGENTS

The use of inotropic agents in the treatment of CHF is predicated on the finding that a major contributing factor in reducing ventricular performance results from depression of myocardial contractility and that this can be reversed, or at least improved, by inotropic drugs.[156] That there is reduced myocardial contractility in failing heart muscle, whether from a sustained work overload of pressure or in response to losing myocardium, has been well demonstrated and appears to be largely due to inadequate calcium availability for activation. All inotropic agents currently available act to increase calcium for activation in both normal and failing myocardium. This is the case whether the mechanism of action is via the cyclic adenosine monophosphate (cAMP) system excitation (e.g., catecholamines) or by sarcolemmal $Na^+$-$K^+$-ATPase (adenosine triphosphatase) inhibition (e.g., digitalis glycosides). The problem remains whether this increase in intracellular $Ca^{2+}$ will benefit pump function while doing no harm, such as enhancing the propensity for arrhythmia or theoretically producing further myocyte loss. Moreover, agents that reduce afterload may enhance ventricular emptying without these potential hazards. In end-stage, severely decompensated CHF, inotropic agents (e.g., dobutamine) may be temporarily lifesaving (see Fig. 25-6), and at somewhat earlier stages, they may reduce morbidity (e.g., digitalis glycosides). In earlier stages of CHF, benefits of inotropic agents may not outweigh risk, and their use is relegated to later stages in the disease process (see Fig. 25-6).

***Digitalis Glycosides*** Digitalis glycosides have had a long and venerable history in the treatment of *CHF* and are the only oral inotropic agents available currently for this purpose (Fig. 25-9). In 1785, William Withering[157] reported on his use of the digitalis leaf as a purported diuretic agent to treat anasarca, presumably due to CHF.

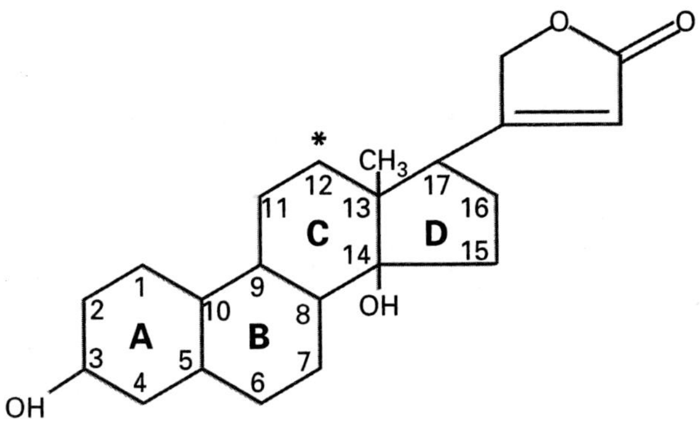

FIGURE 25-9 Structure of digitalis molecule. *Digitoxin becomes digoxin with OH placement at C12. (From Sonnenblick EH, LeJemtel TH, Frishman WH. Digitalis preparations and other inotropic agents. In: Frishman WH, Sonnenblick EH, eds. *Cardiovascular Pharmacotherapeutics*. New York: McGraw-Hill; 1997:241. Reproduced with permission from the publisher and authors.)

Indeed, the major effects of digitalis were initially thought to be on the kidneys, although important effects on heart rate were noted. Only during the latter part of the nineteenth century did it become apparent that there was a direct action of digitalis glycosides to increase cardiac contractility,[158] while in the earlier part of the twentieth century the effects of digitalis on the peripheral circulation and the autonomic nervous system were noted.[159] Despite this long history, the risks and benefits of digitalis administration on patients with sinus rhythm have remained controversial. The controversy has been partially addressed in a large randomized, placebo-controlled clinical trial of digoxin use in CHF.[160] Overall, digoxin was shown to be safe with a significant reduction in morbidity, expressed in terms of less need for hospitalization, but not in mortality. The benefit on hospitalization for heart failure appears greatest in those with lower ejection fractions. As discussed later, with serum digoxin levels below 1 $\mu$g/mL, the neurohumoral and autocrine effects of digoxin predominate over the inotropic effects. Digoxin therapy may be most effective when the serum digoxin level is maintained between 0.5 and 0.8 ng/mL.[161] Of note, a retrospective analysis of the Digitalis Investigation Group (DIG) trial found a 4.2 percent increase in mortality in men but not in women.[162]

Digitalis glycosides have important effects on multiple systems in addition to augmenting the contractility of the myocardium. Electrophysiologically, digitalis glycosides speed conduction in the atrium while inhibiting conduction at the atrioventricular node. This has made them useful in rate control in atrial fibrillation. In the normal circulation, digitalis glycosides also produce generalized arteriolar vasoconstriction, while affecting the central nervous system to enhance parasympathetic tone and reduce sympathetic nervous system activation. Digitalis glycosides sensitize baroreflexes to decrease efferent sympathetic activity, which acts to reduce sinus node activity and thus reduce heart rate. The precise mechanism for these effects is still unclear. The increase in baroreflex sensitization also increases parasympathetic tone, even in mild heart failure, while central vagal nuclei are also stimulated. The broad enhancement of parasympathetic activity with digitalis glycosides helps to explain the sinus heart rate slowing observed with digitalis glycosides even with sinus rhythm, as well as their therapeutic efficacy in control of supraventricular arrhythmias. As discussed later, in the failing state, the effects of sympathetic withdrawal may be dominant so as to reduce arterial vascular resistance, while in the normal circulation, arterial vasoconstriction may be dominant. Integration of these various actions adds to the inotropic activity and therapeutic usefulness of digitalis glycosides.

The positive inotropic action of digitalis glycosides to increase contractility and alter electrophysiology of heart muscle occurs through binding to and inhibition of the enzyme $Na^+$, $K^+$-ATPase on the surface membrane of myocardial cells, which results in an increase in the cytocyclic calcium concentration.[163] The $Na^+$, $K^+$-ATPase is an energy-requiring "sodium pump" that extrudes three sodium ions, which enter the cell during depolarization in exchange for two potassium ions, thus creating an electrical current and a negative resting potential.[164] Contraction is initiated with an action potential that depolarizes the surface membrane of the cell. This is created by a rapid inward current of sodium into the cell that opens sarcolemmal calcium channels, permitting calcium to enter the cell. This calcium releases substantially more calcium from stores in the sarcoplasmic reticulum within the cell, which in turn activates the contractile mechanism by binding to a component of the troponin-tropomyosin system that had been maintaining the resting state. With calcium bound to troponin, actin and myosin can interact to produce force and shortening. The greater the amount of activating calcium, the greater the force and shortening.[163,164] When calcium is released from troponin and taken up by the sarcoplasmic reticulum, relaxation occurs.[163] The relatively small amount of calcium that enters the cell with activation is ultimately removed by an electrogenic $Na^+/Ca^{2+}$ exchange, which extrudes 1 calcium for 3 sodium ions. When intracellular sodium is increased, less exchange occurs and the net amount of intracellular calcium is increased. Thus, by inhibiting the $Na^+$, $K^+$-ATPase, digitalis glycosides produce a decrease in intracellular potassium and an increase in intracellular sodium that increases intracellular calcium (Fig. 25-10).[163,164] In general, the main way in which all inotropic agents, including digitalis glycosides, increase contractility is by increasing the amount of calcium available for activation. This is the case in both normal and failing myocardium. In the failing heart, there is also a decrease in the calcium released into the cytosol with activation.[165] Digitalis glycosides increase this intracellular calcium that augments calcium stores in the sarcoplasmic reticulum, resulting in a subsequent increase in previously reduced myocyte contraction.

Although there are numerous digitalis glycosides with varying duration of action and metabolic fate, digoxin has relatively rapid onset and intermediate duration of action. Digoxin has its most beneficial hemodynamic actions when substantial ventricular depression is evident along with CHF. In this circumstance, it augments myocardial performance while reflexly reducing peripheral resistance.[166] Acutely, digoxin also reduces cardiac norepinephrine spillover and reduces efferent sympathetic nerve activity in skeletal muscles in the patient with CHF.[166] Slowing of the heart rate, whether via enhanced parasympathetic tone and reduced sympathetic activity to reduce sinus rate or via control of heart rate in atrial fibrillation (as discussed later), will greatly benefit ventricular filling and reduce pulmonary congestion.[167] In the treatment of CHF, digoxin is generally employed along with diuretics and vasodilator agents. Thus, by reducing peripheral resistance, digoxin and peripheral vasodilators act in a complementary manner.

In acute heart failure—either due to massive sudden loss of myocardium, as may occur with a myocardial infarction, or with increasing decompensation in severe CHF, characterized by acute pulmonary edema, severe limitations of cardiac output, and perhaps hypotension—rapidly acting inotropic agents such as intravenous dobutamine or milrinone (discussed later) may be required (see Fig. 25-8) together with loop diuretics and vasodilators. This situation may occur in the setting of rapid deterioration of the patient with more CHF or following a large myocardial infarction. In this circumstance, the main aim is to increase cardiac output and reduce filling pressures as a setting for longer term stabilization. While rapidly acting inotropic agents are used, digitalization may be begun cautiously for its longer-term effects. In the setting of myocardial infarction, the situation is more complex. Due to a fear that arrhythmias may be induced or oxygen consumption increased, which might be detrimental, digoxin is generally avoided in the first few days following infarction, although in a longer term treatment of CHF, digitalization, especially if dosing is carefully controlled, may be of value along with other agents, especially ACE inhibitors.

For chronic CHF, digoxin is of use over the long term when administered in association with loop diuretics and ACE inhibitors. Benefits are most evident in patients with NYHA class III or IV CHF.

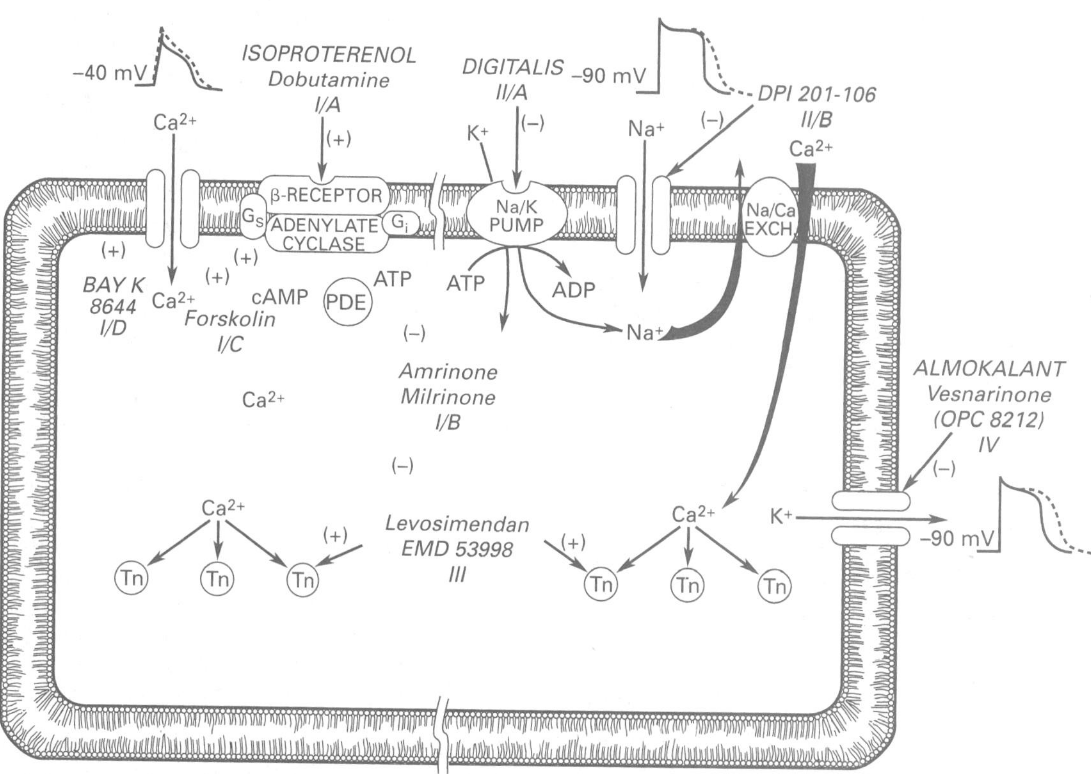


FIGURE 25-10 Diagram of various inotropic sites of action on and within the cardiac cell. While catecholamines act at cell surface receptors, agents such as amrinone and milrinone (phosphodiesterase III inhibitors) act within the cell to augment adenylate cyclase. Calcium sensitizers increase $Ca^{2+}$ sensitivity of troponin (Tn) in the contractile system itself. (From Varro A, Papp JG. Classification of positive inotropic actions based on electrophysiologic characteristics: Where should calcium sensitizers be placed? *J Cardiovasc Pharmacol* 1995;26 (suppl 1):S32. Reproduced with permission from the publisher and authors.)

In this circumstance, the response of the circulation is characterized by a decrease in venous pressures and ventricular filling pressures and an increase in cardiac output. Heart rate is slowed and EF tends to rise, while peripheral resistance falls with little or no change in arterial pressure. These salutary effects are attributed to a combination of augmented myocardial contractility and restoration of baroreceptor sensitivity, which results in enhanced parasympathetic and decreased sympathetic tone. Whereas myocardial oxygen consumption may increase in the heathy heart from the increased contractility, in heart failure it tends to be reduced due to a decrease in heart size and, thus, ventricular wall tension and a slowing of heart rate. Earlier concepts supported the view that digoxin was of greatest benefit when atrial fibrillation was present and controlled. It is now clear that efficacy is also present when the patient with heart failure is in sinus rhythm.[168] Withdrawal of digoxin from such patients has led to rapid deterioration, even when both diuretics and ACE inhibitors were used.[169,170] While digoxin has been associated with an increase in EF, vasodilators have been shown to cause more significant increments in exercise performance.[171] These considerations would justify the combined use of these agents. Whereas the use of ACE inhibitors may well be indicated when the ejection fraction is reduced and symptoms are limited (class I and class II), however, digoxin should probably be reserved for use with more overt symptoms (class III and class IV).

While digoxin can be given once a day without tolerance or tachyphylaxis, the dose is a matter of issue.[172] In general, a serum level of 0.5 to 0.8 ng/mL is felt to be therapeutic.[161] This level may vary from patient to patient, and a clear dose–response relation has not been established. Indeed, some of the greatest benefits may be gained from lower doses (e.g., 0.125 mg/day), which may induce the neurohumoral benefits of lower sympathetic and higher parasympathetic tone while reducing the incidence of possible toxic side effects[172] (as discussed later). There appear to be no adverse effects from digoxin usage in terms of mortality in patients with CHF,[160] and substantially increased morbidity noted when the drug is withdrawn[169,173] suggests such a result. It was shown that the effect of digoxin therapy differs between men and women, with an increased risk of death from any cause among women but not in men with heart failure and depressed systolic function.[162] Effects on mortality with digoxin are complicated because the nature and progression of the underlying process, which led to failure in the first place, may well be the ultimate determinant of mortality. If morbidity is reduced substantially with digoxin, as demonstrated,[160] a neutral effect on ultimate mortality would be acceptable.

Digoxin has been shown to be of limited value in treatment of right-sided heart failure, which can occur in cor pulmonale or with left-to-right shunts. Digoxin also has limited value in acute LV failure due to acute myocardial infarction, although it is useful in the subsequent treatment of ischemic-related CHF. Nevertheless, since mortality may be increased after infarction by digoxin, especially when clear evidence of heart failure is absent, its use is best reserved for patients with overt CHF.

Toxicities from digitalis glycosides can be numerous and are somewhat dependent on serum level. Central nervous symptoms include loss of appetite and nausea, and visual changes may be seen. Cardiac limitations include atrioventricular block, premature ventricular extrasystoles, and ultimately ventricular tachycardia and fibrillation. Monitoring serum levels may be useful in the patient with sinus rhythm, while the ventricular rate provides an adequate guide to dosing in the presence of atrial fibrillation. Except in dire circumstances, such as a suicide attempt, cessation of therapy is adequate. In the former circumstance, antibodies to digoxin may be indicated.

***Catecholamines*** As noted earlier, positive inotropism is based on enhancing the delivery of calcium to the contractile system so as to increase force and shortening. Increasing calcium in the serum will affect this transiently, while digitalis glycosides increase calcium for activation by inhibiting sarcolemmal $Na^+$-$K^+$-ATPase. Catecholamines increase activating calcium via beta-adrenergic receptors and the adenyl cyclase system (see Fig. 25-9).

Beta receptors are located in the sarcolemma and comprise a complex structure that spans the membrane. The beta receptor is connected with G proteins (see Fig. 25-10) that either activate (Gs) or inhibit (Gi) a secondary enzyme system, adenylate cyclase, which, when activated by Gs, induces the formation of cAMP. cAMP in turn activates certain protein kinases, which lead to intracellular phosphorylation of proteins that both enhance the entry and removal of intracellular calcium.[174] By providing more calcium to the troponin-tropomyosin system, a greater interaction between actin and myosin occurs, increasing force and shortening. Increasing the rate of calcium removal from the cytoplasm speeds the rate of relaxation.

In the healthy heart, norepinephrine is synthesized and stored in the sympathetic nerve endings that invest the entire heart, including atria, conduction system, and ventricle.[175] When these nerve endings are depolarized, norepinephrine is released from granules in nerve endings into myocardial clefts containing beta-adrenergic receptors, which, when activated, turn on the sequence of events noted earlier. Not only does this enhance calcium entry into the myocyte to augment contraction, but it also phosphorylates phospholamban, which enhances relaxation.[174] Subsequently, most of the released norepinephrine is returned and restored in the sympathetic nerve endings. Released norepinephrine is also inactivated by two enzymes, catechol *O*-methyltransferase and monoamine oxidase, and the products are excreted largely by the kidneys.[174]

In very severe heart failure, stores of norepinephrine in the ventricle are largely depleted and the sympathetic nerve endings fail to take up norepinephrine normally. Rapid turnover of whatever norepinephrine stores remain is suggested by increased cardiac norepinephrine spillover in CHF. At the same time, circulating norepinephrine released from peripheral sympathetic nerve endings may be increased, especially in severe failure. In less severe heart failure, the serum norepinephrine levels tend to be normal despite increased sympathetic nerve activity.[176]

In both the normal and failing myocardium, activation of the adenyl cyclase system can augment contractility. Agents that do this may be divided into two categories. The first comprises the catecholamines (e.g., norepinephrine, epinephrine) and their synthetic derivatives (e.g., dobutamine, isoproterenol), which act via cell-surface adrenergic receptors (see Fig. 25-10).[174] The second includes agents that inhibit the breakdown of cAMP by inhibition of PDE type III (e.g., amrinone, milrinone, and levosimendan), resulting in an increase in cAMP.[176] Some of these agents, such as levosimendan, may also increase myofibril sensitivity to calcium and then further augment contraction.[177]

Catecholamines constitute an endogenous hormonal system exerting reflex control of the heart and circulation. Their effects depend on localized, controlled neural release and receptor specificity in terms of action. Dopamine is the naturally occurring precursor of both norepinephrine and epinephrine (Fig. 25-11).[178] While epinephrine is released from the adrenal medulla, norepinephrine is the primary mediator in the heart and peripheral circulation.[174]

The actions of both endogenous and exogenous catecholamines depend on their activation of specific alpha- and beta-adrenergic receptors (Tables 25-4 and 25-5).[174] Alpha receptors include $alpha_1$ receptors, which are postsynaptic and are located in vascular smooth

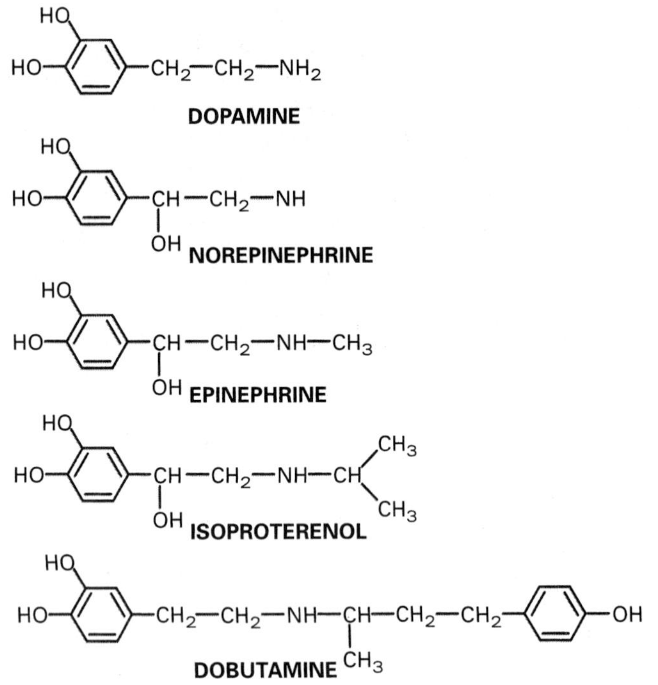

HO, HO–[ring]–$CH_2$–$CH_2$–$NH_2$
**DOPAMINE**

HO, HO–[ring]–CH(OH)–$CH_2$–NH
**NOREPINEPHRINE**

HO, HO–[ring]–CH(OH)–$CH_2$–NH–$CH_3$
**EPINEPHRINE**

HO, HO–[ring]–CH(OH)–$CH_2$–NH–CH($CH_3$)($CH_3$)
**ISOPROTERENOL**

HO, HO–[ring]–$CH_2$–$CH_2$–NH–CH($CH_3$)–$CH_2$–$CH_2$–[ring]–OH
**DOBUTAMINE**

FIGURE 25-11 Structure of catecholamines.

muscle and the myocardium. In smooth muscle, they mediate vasoconstriction; in the heart, they mediate weak positive inotropic and negative chronotropic effects. Alpha$_2$ receptors are presynaptic and, when stimulated, decrease norepinephrine release from peripheral nerve endings as well as sympathetic outflow from the central nervous system. Alpha$_2$ receptors may also mediate vasoconstriction in specific peripheral vascular beds.

Beta-adrenergic receptors can be divided into beta$_1$ and beta$_2$ subtypes. Beta$_1$ receptors are located in the myocardium where they mediate positive inotropic, chronotropic, and dromotropic effects.[176] Their activation occurs primarily by norepinephrine released from neurons in the heart. Beta$_2$ receptors are located in vascular smooth muscle, where they mediate vasodilatation, and in the sinoatrial node, where they are chronotropic. In general, beta$_2$ receptors are activated by circulating catecholamines released from peripheral sites such as the adrenal medulla.

Another type of receptor, which has been termed the *dopaminergic receptor,* is localized to the mesenteric and renal circulation and mediates arterial vasodilatation. The physiologic and pharmacologic action of various catecholamines depend on which receptor they activate, both in the heart and in the periphery (see Tables 25-4 and 25-5).

Norepinephrine has potent alpha$_1$ and beta$_1$ activity. When norepinephrine is released from cardiac nerve endings, as occurs in normal exercise, myocardial contractility and heart rate are augmented. When norepinephrine is administered exogenously, its major action is to stimulate alpha$_1$ receptors, leading to marked peripheral arterial vasoconstriction. Thus, norepinephrine has been used to increase arterial blood pressure in the presence of severe hypotension so as to maintain blood flow to vital organs. Long-term renal vasoconstriction from continued norepinephrine administration may produce ischemic renal damage, including acute tubular necrosis, so that prolonged use (i.e., more than 24 to 48 h) is usually untenable. For the failing heart, this peripheral vasoconstriction also provides an undesirable added pressure load (afterload), which tends to vitiate the potential benefits of beta$_1$ stimulation.

TABLE 25-4 Adrenergic Receptor Activity of Sympathomimetic Amines

| | $\geq\alpha_1$ | $\beta_1$ | $\beta_2$ | Dopaminergic | Dose |
|---|---|---|---|---|---|
| Dopamine | +++ | ++ | + | ++++ | <2 μg/kg/min—vasodilation effects on peripheral dopaminergic receptors<br>2–10 μg/kg/min—inotropic effects, $\beta_1$-receptor activation<br>5–20 μg/kg/min—peripheral vasoconstriction, α effects |
| Norepinephrine | ++++ | ++++ | 0 | 0 | Initiate with 8–12 μg/min; maintain 2–4 μg/min |
| Epinephrine | +++ | ++++ | ++ | 0 | |
| Isoproterenol | 0 | ++++ | ++++ | 0 | 0.5–5 μg/min |
| Dobutamine | +++ | ++++ | ++ | 0 | Start at 2–3 μg/kg/min and titrate upward |

SOURCE: From Sonnenblick EH, LeJemtel TH, Frishman WH. Inotropic agents. In: Frishman WH, Sonnenblick EH, Sica DA, eds. *Cardiovascular Pharmacotherapeutics,* 2nd ed. New York: McGraw Hill; 2003:191–202.

Dopamine[178] has both alpha$_1$ and beta$_1$ activity but also stimulates dopaminergic receptors in the renal vasculature to produce arterial dilation and increased renal blood flow. Its beta$_1$ effects in the heart occur largely through the release of endogenous norepinephrine, which may be largely depleted in the failing heart. As doses of dopamine are increased, conversion to norepinephrine also occurs, which tends to produce relatively more pressor effects than myocardial inotropic stimulation (see Table 25-4). As such, the benefits of dopamine administration, if any, are at low doses (e.g., 0.02 mg/kg/min), which may induce renal arterial vasodilatation. In general, dopamine is employed in association with more potent inotropic agents (e.g., dobutamine).

Dobutamine[179] is a synthetic variant of the catecholamines whose structure has been altered to optimize hemodynamic response in the dog, characterized by an increase in cardiac output and a decrease in ventricular filling pressure with little change in heart rate. Since arterial pressure also rises modestly, peripheral vascular resistance must of necessity fall. The positive inotropic activity of dobutamine is mediated by direct stimulation of beta$_1$-adrenergic receptors in the myocardium (see Table 25-8). It is unclear why a concomitant increase in heart rate does not always occur. One possibility is that an increase in cardiac output that increases arterial pressure serves to buffer any heart rate increase. Given its capacity to increase cardiac output and reduce filling pressures without substantial heart rate change, dobutamine has been widely used to treat severe acute LV failure in the absence of profound hypotension, which is poorly responsive to diuretics and vasodilators (see Fig. 25-8). This may be seen following a very large myocardial infarction or in acute decompensation in the course of chronic CHF. In the presence of severe hypotension, the $\text{beta}_2$ stimulation of dobutamine may be harmful, and administration of an $\text{alpha}_1$-stimulating vasoconstrictor, such as norepinephrine or higher dose dopamine, may also be necessary in order to increase arterial peripheral resistance.

TABLE 25-5 Physiologic and Pharmacologic Actions of Catecholamine Receptors

| Receptor | Receptor Activity | Primary Location |
|---|---|---|
| $\beta_1$ | Positive inotropic and chronotropic action; increased AV conduction | Heart (atria, ventricle AV node) |
| $\beta_2$ | Peripheral vasodilation | Arterioles, arteries, veins, bronchioles |
| $\alpha_1$ | Arteriolar vasoconstriction | Arterioles |
| $\alpha_2$ | Presynaptic inhibition of norepinephrine release | Sympathetic nerve endings, CNS |
| Dopaminergic | Renal and mesenteric vasodilation, natriuresis, diuresis | Kidneys |

ABBREVIATIONS: AV = atrioventericular; CNS = central nervous system.
SOURCE: From Sonnenblick EH, LeJemtel TH, Frishman WH. Inotropic agents. In: Frishman WH, Sonnenblick EH, Sica DA, eds. *Cardiovascular Pharmacotherapeutics,* 2nd ed. New York: McGraw Hill; 2003:191–202.

Dobutamine infusion is generally begun at 2 $\mu$g/kg/min and titrated to optimize cardiac output while reducing LV filling pressure. Tachycardia is carefully avoided so as not to increase myocardial oxygen demands and induce ischemia. The effects on myocardial oxygen consumption ($M\dot{V}O_2$) are complex.[179] While the increase in contractility will increase $M\dot{V}O_2$, a decrease in heart size will tend to reduce it. The end result is generally a modest increase in $M\dot{V}O_2$ induced by dobutamine. With a better maintained arterial pressure and reduced LV diastolic pressure in the absence of tachycardia, coronary perfusion pressure may also be increased. The major side effects of dobutamine are an excessive increase in heart rate with high doses and ventricular arrhythmias, both of which may mandate dose reduction and even drug discontinuation. Data have raised the possibility that short-term administration of dobutamine is associated with a poor outcome at 6 months.[154] However, patients who receive dobutamine are in a more precarious hemodynamic state than those who receive vasodilation. Definite assessment of the effect of short-term dobutamine administration on long-term outcome will require a true double-blind randomized trial of dobutamine versus vasodilator agents in patients with severe CHF.

***Phosphodiesterase Inhibitors and Other Agents*** The adenyl cyclase–cyclic AMP system can also be activated beyond the beta receptor. Hormones such as glucagon activate the system and can increase myocardial contractility acutely despite $\text{beta}_1$ blockade. While intravenous glucagon administration is useful in overcoming beta-adrenergic blockade when necessary, glucagon may induce gastric atony and nausea, and this has limited its more generalized use. Amrinone and milrinone are prototypes of cardiotonic agents that activate the adenyl cyclase system through inhibition of the enzyme that breaks down cAMP, PDE type III.[180,181] Type III PDE inhibitors decrease the breakdown of cAMP in the myocardium and increase cGMP in vascular smooth muscle, resulting in an increase in myocardial contractility as well as arterial and venous vasodilatation. Other members of this class of drugs include enoximone and pimobendan, although only intravenous amrinone and milrinone have been approved by the FDA for treatment of acute heart failure. The mechanisms by which vasodilatation occurs are not completely understood. Increased cGMP induces phosphorylation of myosin light-chain kinase, which decreases sensitivity to calcium and calmodulin.

In the heart, inotropism may relate not only to increased cAMP–mediated calcium availability for contraction and increased rates of its removal for relaxation but also to increased sensitivity of the contractile system for calcium.[182] Both amrinone and milrinone[181] have substantial ability to augment cardiac output while reducing both RV and LV filling pressures. The lowering of filling pressures is greater than that seen with dobutamine. Dilatation of the pulmonary arterial vasculature is also a very useful therapeutic effect. Arterial pressure tends to be reduced, while an increase in heart rate may occur. Since dobutamine increases cAMP and milrinone reduces its breakdown, the combination of these agents is substantially more potent than either agent alone.[181] When either dobutamine or milrinone is utilized, ectopic activity may be increased, which requires careful supervision in either drug's use. PDE type III inhibitors are also orally active and produce the same hemodynamic improvement as seen with intravenous use. In longer-term oral use, however, increased mortality was seen with the use of milrinone, especially in the presence of class IV heart failure.[183] This increased mortality may have been due to the relatively short action of this agent (90-min half-life), which leads to large peaks and valleys in dosing and concomitant arrhythmias.

Short-term use of milrinone in addition to standard therapy was shown to be detrimental in patients hospitalized with exacerbation of CHF who did not require inotropic support.[184] The absence of an indication for positive inotropic support may have biased the study against milrinone.

## NEWER INOTROPIC AGENTS

Agents under investigation include the inodilatory benzimidazoline PDE inhibitors, such as levosimendan, which acutely increase cardiac output and reduce filling pressure while improving exercise tolerance in patients with CHF.[185] Levosimendan, and other drugs in this class (MCI-154, EMD 53998, EMD 57033), may have additional effects to enhance calcium binding to troponin-C, a calcium-sensitizing action (see Fig. 25-9).[177,185,186] Theoretically, this could enhance contractile response for a given amount of cytolytic $Ca^{2+}$, which could lead to less arrhythmogenicity. This may be an important consideration since the activation of the cAMP system may be detrimental in inducing tachycardia and arrhythmias. Clinical trials evaluating the efficacy and safety of levosimendan are in progress. Preliminary results from one study that compared levosimendan to dobutamine [Levosimendan Infusion versus Dobutamine (LIDO)][187] demonstrated comparable hemodynamic activities with less chest pain and arrhythmia with levosimendan. The critical issues to be addressed, now that acute efficacy is apparent, are whether these agents will improve symptoms—that is, reduce morbidity—and/or improve mortality.

### ADJUNCTIVE THERAPIES

As mentioned earlier, patients with heart failure require treatment of underlying disease processes that may be aggravating the myopathic process. Systemic hypertension and anemia should be treated vigorously. In diabetic patients, hyperglycemia should be controlled. Aspirin prophylaxis, folic acid supplementation, and cholesterol-lowering drugs should be used in patients with coronary artery disease.[187a] It is not known if estrogen replacement therapy in postmenopausal women can modify the course of heart failure.[188]

Heart failure patients with mental depression have an increased morbidity and mortality risk.[189] The tricyclic antidepressant drugs have been associated with myocardial depression and are probably contraindicated in heart failure patients. However, the selective serotonin reuptake inhibitors have a favorable risk profile in cardiac patients and could be considered an adjunctive treatment for relieving mental depression.[189a] However, many of these drugs interfere with the hepatic cytochrome $P_{450}$ system, which may affect the metabolism of drugs used to treat heart failure (see chap. 90).

BAB should be considered in all patients who survive a myocardial infarction, with or without ventricular dysfunction. As described earlier, carvedilol, metoprolol, and bisoprolol should probably be the beta blockers of choice in patients with symptomatic mild-to-moderate CHF of ischemic and nonischemic origin. Propranolol, metoprolol, atenolol, or timolol should be used in myocardial infarction survivors who are asymptomatic, with and without LV dysfunction.

Patients with CHF are liable to develop venoembolic disease and systemic emboli from intracardiac mural thrombi. These embolic events are major causes of morbidity and mortality in CHF. In patients with atrial fibrillation and CHF, with and without mitral stenosis, anticoagulation is indicated. In patients with normal sinus rhythm and cardiomyopathy, the role of prophylactic anticoagulation with warfarin is not well defined.[117] A cohort analysis of the SOLVD population focused on the relation between warfarin use and the risk of all-cause mortality and found a beneficial effect with the anticoagulant.[190] Most of this benefit appeared to relate to reduced ischemic events. It is more difficult to anticoagulate patients with CHF because of drug–drug interactions, malabsorption of medications, varying perfusion of the liver, and malnutrition.[191] Patients with CHF who have developed a phlebothrombotic process or who have definite evidence of ventricular mural thrombi and systemic embolism should receive warfarin despite the potential problems with regulation of anticoagulation in these patients.

Patients with heart failure have a markedly increased prevalence of ventricular ectopy and incidence of sudden death. Patients should be assessed for hypokalemia, hypomagnesemia, hypoxia, infection, and use of antidepressant drugs. Many antiarrhythmic drug regimens have negative inotropic actions and may aggravate the heart failure process. Amiodarone and BABs have been used in patients with LV dysfunction with less risk involved and are probably the drugs of choice when treatment of ventricular ectopy is considered.[192,193] There is little evidence to show that antiarrhythmic drug therapy changes the natural history of advanced CHF.[193] Amiodarone can also be used to treat atrial arrhythmias, with and without digoxin and calcium channel blockers.

### DIASTOLIC DYSFUNCTION

Diastolic dysfunction of the LV and RV will often lead to all the signs and symptoms of systolic dysfunction, but the therapeutic approach varies for these two conditions. Often, there is significant LV hypertrophy present, and aggressive management of systemic hypertension is required.[4,192,194] These patients will develop significant congestion, so that diuretics are often necessary. With hypovolemia from other diseases, however, patients are prone to develop hypotension. The effects of diuretics in these patients should be carefully monitored. Digoxin is probably of no use unless the patient is in atrial fibrillation, and vasodilating drugs with peripheral venodilator actions may cause hypotension. The role of ACE inhibitors, ARBs, and other vasodilator drugs are not well defined in this condition, and they may cause hypotension. Large clinical trials have begun to include patients having diastolic dysfunction as their primary cause for clinical heart failure. A placebo-controlled study with the ARB candesartan demonstrated a moderate benefit in preventing admission for CHF among patients who had symptomatic CHF and left ventricular ejection fractions >40 percent. No mortality benefit of candesartan was observed in this study.[194a]

Tachycardia needs to be avoided. Rate-lowering calcium blockers (verapamil, diltiazem) are useful drugs of choice for reducing elevated blood pressure, keeping the heart rate under control, and improving ventricular compliance.[195] BABs are first-line therapy in maintaining relative bradycardia so as to maintain time for diastolic ventricular filling. However, their effects on ventricular compliance are not as well defined. Both verapamil and beta blockers can be used with caution in patients with heart failure due to hypertrophic cardiomyopathy.

## Surgical Treatment

### CARDIAC RESYNCHRONIZATION THERAPY

Cardiac resynchronization with biventricular pacing has been shown to improve functional class, LV ejection fraction, distance walked in 6 min, and quality of life in patients with severe CHF, reduced LV systolic function, and intraventricular conduction delay with a QRS interval >130 ms.[7,10] A meta-analysis of four randomized controlled trials suggest that cardiac resynchronization therapy can reduce death from progressive heart failure by 51 percent [odds ratio (OR), 0.49; 95 percent CI, 0.25 to 0.93], and hospitalization for heart failure by 29 percent (OR, 0.71; 95 percent CI, 0.53 to 0.96). Cardiac resynchronization does not significantly alter overall mortality, ventricular tachycardia, or ventricular fibrillation (OR, 0.92; 95 percent CI, 0.67 to 1.27). Cardiac resynchronization presumably enhances LV function by correcting the inhomogeneous and discordant LV contraction that results from intraventricular dysynchrony which is energy inefficient.[9] Regionally diminished myocardial function or disturbed temporal sequence of contraction further worsens systolic function in patients with dilated cardiomyopathy. Conversely biventricular pacing significantly decreased LV end-systolic and end-diastolic volumes and tended to increase ejection fraction in patients with a dilated cardiomyopathy accompanied by a prolonged QRS interval >130 ms and a NYHA functional class III.[11]

However, biventricular pacing is not a panacea for the treatment of patients with CHF due to reduced LV systolic function for several reasons. First, only 30 percent of patients with symptomatic CHF have intraventricular conduction delay evidenced by left or right bundle branch block leading to loss of coordinated cardiac contraction.[6] Second, the response to biventricular pacing is highly variable from patient to patient. A reasonable estimate is that less than one third of patients experience clinically meaningful benefits. The number of patients who experience clinical benefits may be even lower if one takes into account the possible placebo effect that results from implantation of a potentially helpful cardiac device. Such variability in the response to biventricular pacing is concordant with the disparate effects on exercise capacity and LV systolic function.[5,7] Last, implantation of a pacing lead into the coronary sinus is unsuccessful in 8 to 10 percent of patients and complicated by rupture or dissection of the coronary sinus in 5 percent of patients.[6]

In view of the wide variability of the clinical response to biventricular pacing and the substantial cost of the device and the procedure, the indications for biventricular pacing may become less inclusive than they are at present. Unpublished experience seems to indicate that patients with idiopathic or end-stage hypertensive cardiomyopathy, moderately severe functional mitral regurgitation, and relatively preserved right ventricular function are the most likely to clinically improve after cardiac resynchronization. Patients with severe RV failure, myocardial infarctions involving anterior and lateral walls, and severe functional mitral regurgitation are less likely to derive clinical benefits from this procedure.

## IMPLANTABLE CARDIOVERTER DEFIBRILLATORS

In patients with documented sustained ventricular tachycardia or ventricular fibrillation, the implantable cardioverter defibrillator (ICD) is highly effective in treating recurrences of these arrhythmias by antitachycardia pacing or cardioversion-defibrillation, thereby reducing morbidity and the need for rehospitalization. Insertion of an ICD significantly decreased mortality in patients with a previous myocardial infarction, LV ejection fraction $<$35 percent, and an ECG, QRS duration $>$120 msec, when compared to drug therapy alone.[196] Over a mean follow-up of 20 months there were 14.2 percent deaths in patients randomized to ICD and 19.8 percent deaths in patients receiving drug therapy alone (a 31 percent mortality reduction). Whether ICD also decreases mortality in patients with nonischemic cardiomyopathy is under investigation.

## MECHANICAL CARDIAC SUPPORT

In view of the longer-term survival of patients with refractory CHF randomized to an LVAD (Heartmate vented electric device, Thoratec, Pleasanton, CA) in the Randomized Evaluation of Mechanical Assistance for the Treatment of Congestive Heart Failure (REMATCH) trial, this device has been approved by the FDA for sustained use (i.e., destination therapy and not just a bridge to cardiac transplantation).[14] Patients eligible for the REMATCH trial had an LV ejection fraction $<$25 percent, a peak oxygen uptake $<$13 mL/kg/min (later increased to15 mL/kg/min), and symptoms compatible with NYHA functional class IV despite optimal medical therapy. Patients eligible for REMATCH were ineligible for cardiac transplantation due to age, diabetes with end-organ damage, or renal insufficiency. The rate of survival at 1 year was 52 percent with the device and 25 percent with medical therapy ($p = 0.002$). Survival at 2 years was 23 percent with the device and 8 percent with medical therapy ($p = 0.09$). The most frequent adverse events observed in patients randomized to the device were infection, bleeding, and device malfunction. The risk of infection is particularly high and can attain 1.88 episodes of infection per patient at 6 months.[197] A conservative estimate of the hospital cost for implantation of an LVAD is around $200,000. This estimate includes the device but excludes major complications and their substantial cost. Thus, an overriding problem with LVAD destination therapy is the cost to the health care system that is even now economically challenged. The dilemmas posed by this issue will depend on complex considerations of currently inadequate information.

Other indications of LVADs rest on temporary use either in patients awaiting cardiac transplantation who are hemodynamically unstable (cardiac index $<$2L/min/m$^2$, systolic blood pressure $<$80 mmHg and LV filling pressure $>$20 mmHg) despite optimal intravenous therapy (i.e., bridge to transplantation or in patients deemed likely to recover LV functional capacity (i.e., bridge to recovery). The data regarding the bridge to recovery are controversial.[198] A retrospective chart review of 111 who received an LVAD for intractable end-stage CHF predominantly due to obstructive coronary disease identified only 5 patients who, with significant myocardial recovery, could tolerate successful removal of the device.[199] A higher rate of myocardial recovery, as demonstrated by successful LVAD explantation, has been reported in patients with CHF due to idiopathic dilated cardiomyopathy.[200] Differences in the etiology of CHF may explain, in part, such disparate rates of myocardial recovery. Inflammation may play an important role in the pathogenesis of idiopathic dilated cardiomyopathy and is somewhat reversible while the recovery from end-stage CHF due to multiple ischemic insults is unlikely.

The Heartmate and the Novacor are the only two LVADs presently approved by the FDA for bridge to cardiac transplantation. Both devices are pulsatile pumps that can only be implanted in patients with a body surface area greater than 1.5 m$^2$. Both devices have drive lines through the skin that increase the risk of infection. They also have a portable controller and battery that allow patients to be discharged from the hospital, as well as excellent patient mobility. In contrast to the Novacor, the Heartmate does not require anticoagulation, but its mechanical durability is less than that of the Novacor.

While the Heartmate and the Novacor provide support only to the left ventricle, Thoratec can entirely support the RVs and LVs. The right and left pulsatile pumps remain extracorporeal. Thoratec is the only device available for long-term RV support. It requires strict anticoagulation and allows limited mobility to the patient. Thoratec is not approved for home use.

Continuous-flow pumps are under investigation. These are smaller and use axial flow like a turbine rather than compression to move blood.[197] They are designed to provide partial support to the LV, delivering flow of about 2 L/min. The small size of these continuous-flow pumps has made them attractive although they will require full anticoagulation. Should LVADs become a significant part of therapy for end-stage CHF, it is likely that this type of device will be utilized.

The indications for long-term mechanical cardiac support are expanding. Implantation of a LVAD was considered exclusively in patients who became hemodynamically unstable while awaiting a donor heart, as stated earlier. Implantation of a LVAD can now be considered independently of suitability for cardiac transplantation in patients with end-stage CHF who become hemodynamically unstable in the absence of precipitating factors. However, such an option is only available for patients who, late in their disease process, do not have severe pulmonary hypertension and have the emotional and financial resources to cope with a very demanding therapy.

## HEART TRANSPLANTATION

Heart transplantation is now an accepted mode of treatment for end-stage CHF. Transplantation significantly increases survival, exercise capacity, return to work, and quality of life compared to conventional treatment, provided proper selection criteria are applied. Results in patients on triple immunosuppressive therapy show a 5-year survival of approximately 70 to 80 percent[201] and return to full- or part-time work or seeking employment after 1 year in about two-thirds of the patients in the best series.[202]

Patients who should be considered for transplantation are those with severe CHF with no alternative form of treatment. Predictors of poor survival are taken into account. The patient must be willing and capable to undergo intensive medical treatment and be emotionally stable so as to withstand the many uncertainties likely to occur both before and after transplantation.

Besides shortage of donor hearts, the main problem of heart transplantation is rejection of the allograft, which is responsible for a considerable percentage of deaths in the first postoperative year. The long-term outcome is limited predominantly by the consequences of immunosuppression (infection, hypertension, renal failure, malignancy, and accelerated progression of atherosclerotic vascular disease) and by transplant coronary artery disease.

Experimental work is under way exploring xenotransplantation of myocardial cells and entire organs (pig hearts) as potential heart failure treatment. The humoral immune response of the recipient against the graft remains a preeminent hurdle. There is also limited information regarding the physiology of the pig heart as a replacement for the human heart.

### CORONARY REVASCULARIZATION SURGERY

A major and important surgical approach to ischemic cardiomyopathies is reperfusion of ischemic tissue by coronary bypass surgery.[203] This is based on the concept that transiently ischemic myocardium (stunning) and myocardium with reduced flow (hibernating) have reduced contractility, which may return to normal with restoration of an adequate coronary blood flow. Moreover, revascularization of ischemic regions of the ventricle may prevent recurrent infarction in this area, and so help prevent further deterioration of ventricular function. In such patients, it is necessary to establish that significant amounts of viable tissue remain in an akinetic or hypokinetic zone; this can be accomplished with nuclear techniques such as a 24-h thallium perfusion study or positron emission tomographic scanning.[204] If contractile activity can also be elicited, as shown in echo studies with low-dose dobutamine stimulation[26] or postextrasystolic potentiation, coronary bypass surgery provides a good chance to stabilize or improve ventricular function[205] and enhance survival.[206] In this era, every patient with an ischemic cardiomyopathy should be evaluated for possible revascularization and assumed to be a candidate until proven otherwise.[207]

### OTHER PROCEDURES

Other surgical approaches to the dilated heart have included the concept of removing a segment of the LV wall, the "Battista operation," so as to reduce LV volume and thus wall stress. The surgical risk is immense, and specific benefits have yet to be established.[208]

Autologous skeletal myoblasts have been injected into the myocardium of human beings with ischemic cardiomyopathy undergoing placement of an LVAD.[208a] Successful engraftment and differentiation of the myoblasts was observed. It remains to be seen if skeletal muscle transplantation will provide clinical benefit to patients with ischemic cardiomyopathy. The injection of autologous bone marrow stem cells have also been considered a treatment modality for patients with cardiomyopathy.[208b] Stem cells have long been regarded as undifferentiated cells capable of self renewal, the production of large numbers of different progeny, and the regeneration of tissues.[208c] Clinical studies are now in progress assessing this innovative treatment modality. There are also data to suggest that a population of cardiac stem cells exist which could be used as a source of tissue renewal. The possibility of mobilizing cardiac stem cells with various cytokines to treat patients with ischemic heart disease and cardiomyopathy is a promising new approach to cardiac treatment.[208d] Evidence exists that cardiac myocytes, which have an intrinsic ability to regenerate themselves in the face of heart failure, myocardial infarction, and heart transplantation,[208e,f,g] might provide an additional therapeutic approach if this process can be accelerated.

Enhanced external counterpulsation is a noninvasive therapy consisting of gated diastolic sequential leg compression, producing similar hemodynamic effects as an intraaortic balloon pump. The procedure has been shown to improve exercise capacity and LV failure in patients with heart failure already receiving medical therapy.[209]

Immunoabsorption procedures have been directed against beta$_1$-adrenergic receptor antibodies with clinical improvement found in patients with heart failure.[210]

## Drug Therapies under Investigation

### NEUTRAL ENDOPEPTIDASE INHIBITORS

Neutral endopeptidase inhibitor administration is associated with a rise in endogenous ANP levels due to the inhibition of ANP metabolism.[211–214] In a canine model of CHF, Cavero et al. reported that, at similar ANP levels, neutral endopeptidase inhibitor treatment was associated with a better diuretic and natriuretic effect than with an ANP infusion.[212] In human studies, however, the two modalities appear to have similar natriuretic and diuretic effects. In 1989, Northridge and colleagues were the first to report a diuresis following neutral endopeptidase inhibitor infusion in six patients with mild CHF (mean ejection fraction 37 percent).[213] A 60 percent increase in the 4-h urine sodium excretion was observed, associated with a three- to fivefold rise in ANP levels. The same investigators compared the renal and hemodynamic effects of neutral endopeptidase inhibitor administration to low-dose furosemide in mild CHF.[215] Eighteen patients were randomized to receive either a neutral endopeptidase inhibitor, candoxatrilat, 200 mg twice daily, candoxatrilat, 400 mg twice daily, or furosemide 20 mg twice daily. The administration of a neutral endopeptidase inhibitor was associated with a diuresis; however, the change in urine flow rate and sodium excretion from baseline was greater in the low-dose furosemide group. Although its diuretic effect was modest, the neutral endopeptidase inhibitor was associated with desirable hemodynamic effects, including marked preload reduction (pulmonary capillary wedge pressure decreased by 40 percent), and with no stimulation of plasma renin activity. In comparison, the group given furosemide experienced only a 15 percent reduction in pulmonary capillary wedge pressure and a threefold rise in plasma renin activity.

The natriuretic properties of neutral endopeptidase inhibitors are mediated by inhibition of sodium reabsorption within the renal tubule, since they do not significantly alter renal hemodynamics (GFR or renal plasma flow). This is supported by their association with an increased fractional excretion of lithium, a marker of proximal tubular reabsorption.[212] In addition to inhibiting ANP degradation, the neutral endopeptidase inhibitors inhibit the breakdown of bradykinin and BNP. They have also been shown to enhance prostacyclin synthesis, another mechanism by which they may exert a natriuretic effect.[216] In the most severe stages of CHF (NYHA class III to class IV; ejection fraction, 22 percent), an impaired renal response to neutral endopeptidase inhibitor treatment can be expected. Munzel and colleagues[217] reported an unpredictable natriuretic response to candoxatrilat in nine patients with severe CHF. Three patients had no diuresis, five had a minimal response, and one (cardiac index >2.5 L/min) had a good diuresis. The natriuretic response correlated closely with the cardiac output, which, theoretically, was most likely related to renal perfusion status.

It is believed that the attenuation of responsiveness to endogenous ANPs with endopeptidase inhibition is due to activation of the RAAS. This has prompted the development of agents that both augment the action of ANP and block the RAAS, the dual neutral endopeptidase-ACE inhibitor drugs (e.g., omapatrilat, sampatrilat), which have been examined in patients with systemic hypertension and CHF.[214]

In patients with heart failure, omapatrilat was initially shown to be more effective in improving symptoms and reducing the combined risk of death and hospitalization than has the ACE inhibitor lisinopril.[218] In addition, fewer omapatrilat-treated patients exhibited signs of renal dysfunction. Results from a substudy showed omapatrilat caused greater improvement in arterial compliance.[218] Omapatrilat was compared to enalapril in a long-term survival study [Omapatrilat versus Enalapril Randomized Trial of Utility in Reducing Events (OVERTURE)]—a double-blind, randomized trial including 5770 patients with severe heart failure (class II, III, or IV symptoms, LV ejection fraction <30 percent) and a hospitalization for heart failure within the last 12 months.[219] Patients received optimal therapies for heart failure (i.e., 50 percent on beta blockers, 40 percent on spironolactone, and 60 percent on digoxin). Subjects were randomized to enalapril, 10 mg bid, or omapatrilat, 40 mg once daily. The primary endpoint was all-cause mortality/CHF hospitalizations, which showed a 6 percent reduction with omapatrilat, but this did not reach statistical significance. Adverse events showed a lower incidence of impaired renal function with omapatrilat and only a slightly increased rate of angioedema compared to enalapril. The promising future for omapatrilat in CHF was not realized per se in this trial, and additional studies need to be performed with this compound or other such compounds if its development continues.

Another naturally occurring natriuretic peptide being evaluated for the treatment of patients with heart failure is adrenomedullin,[151a,220] a hypotensive peptide originally isolated from human pheochromocytoma.

## ENDOTHELIN INHIBITORS

Endothelin-1 exhibits potent inotropic activity in isolated hearts, cardiac muscle strips, isolated cells, and in instrumented intact animals.[221] High-affinity receptors for endothelin have been demonstrated in both the atria and ventricles. Intravenous endothelin-1 produces a delayed prolonged augmentation of LV performance in addition to its biphasic vasoactive effects of a transient vasodilation followed by a sustained vasoconstriction.

Endothelin is also a potent secretagogue of atrial natriuretic factor, which is a naturally occurring antagonist of endothelin that acts by inhibiting its release.[222] The endothelin-A receptor appears to mediate endothelin's actions of vasoconstriction and the stimulation of the ANP secretion, and the endothelin-B receptor mediates endothelin-induced vasodilatation and activation of the RAAS. Urinary water excretion is mediated through both receptors, but sodium excretion is mediated through the endothelin-A receptor.

Increased endothelin levels have been described in patients with CHF that are predictive of increased mortality risk.[221,223,224] It has also been suggested that increased endothelin levels may be playing an important role in the increased systemic vascular resistance observed in CHF.[225,226] Endothelin-1 levels decrease with therapy and have been found to correlate significantly with symptomatic improvement. It therefore appears that endothelin-1 is an independent, noninvasive predictor of functional and hemodynamic response to therapy in patients with CHF.[227] Increased endothelin levels have also been observed in the plasma and hearts of cardiomyopathic Syrian hamsters[228] and in the cells of endothelial cells infected with *Trypanosoma cruzi* in experimental Chagas' cardiomyopathy.[229]

Although selective endothelin-A-receptor blockers as well as nonselective endothelin antagonists have been studied in CHF,[230–232] the optimal agent class remains a subject of discussion and ongoing research. This is the case because of the possible adverse effects of blockade of endothelin B receptor–induced vasodilatation.[233–237]

A clinical trial (Research on Endothelin Antagonists in Chronic Heart Failure; REACH-1) investigated the long-term effects of bosentan, a nonselective endothelin receptor antagonist, on clinical events in CHF and showed an improvement in symptoms.[234] However, the trial had to be stopped prematurely because of elevated liver enzymes with active therapy. Bosentan can interact with bile excretion in larger oral doses. Lower dosages of bosentan were evaluated in the Endothelin Antagonist Bosentan for Lowering Cardiac Events in Heart Failure (ENABLE) trials.[238] ENABLE 1 and ENABLE 2 trials were conducted concurrently enrolling U.S. patients and patients from Europe and Australia, respectively. In these placebo-controlled, double-blind trials, patients assigned to bosentan were given an initial dose of 6.25 mg qid for 4 weeks, followed by 12.5 mg bid for the duration of follow-up. The trials were designed to determine if bosentan would have an effect on the primary outcome of death and heart failure hospitalizations or on the second outcome of all-cause death. Enrolled patients had severe heart failure (NYHA class III and class IV) and a mean LV ejection fraction of 25 percent. In these trials, bosentan failed to reduce mortality or hospitalizations and may have contributed to higher rates of adverse effects. The orally active selective ETA blockers darusentan (LU 135252) and BMS-192884 are also being evaluated in patients with heart failure.[237a] Tezosentan, the first intravenous endothelin A/B antagonist, has also been evaluated as treatment in acute and chronic heart failure, with no benefit seen.[236]

Enrasentan was also shown to be of no clinical benefit (ENCORE trial) in patients already receiving heart failure therapies including diuretics, ACE inhibitors, digoxin, and beta-blockers.[237b]

## VASOPRESSIN ANTAGONISTS

Elevated levels of vasopressin have been observed in patients with CHF, and these elevations correlate with both disease severity and the presence of hyponatremia. Increased vasopressin release can be precipitated by many factors including hypotension, a low output state, angiotensin, and catecholamines.[239]

All vasopressin receptors are coupled to G-proteins, and two have been characterized: the $V_1$ and $V_2$ receptors. $V_1$ receptors are found primarily in vascular smooth muscle and mediate vasoconstriction. The $V_2$ receptors are found primarily in the kidney and mediate reabsorption of free water and vasopressin's antidiuretic activity. Vasopressin elevations in heart failure can induce heightened vasoconstriction and volume overload.

The first peptide receptor selective vasopressin antagonists were introduced in the 1980s.[240] Recently, combined $V_1/V_2$ receptor antagonists have become available for clinical use in patients with CHF. These drugs have the ability to increase sodium free water excretion, reverse hyponatremia, increase cardiac output, and reduce peripheral vascular resistance.

Three orally active $V_2$-receptor antagonists (WAY-VPA985, SR49-059, and OPC41061) and a combined receptor antagonist (YM087) are currently being evaluated in clinical trials in patients with advanced heart failure who are already receiving standard treatment, including inotropic infusion.

The effects of WAY-VPA985 have been evaluated using a single oral dose in patients with symptomatic heart failure. Subsequently, 28 patients with chronic LV failure were assessed in a randomized, double-blind, placebo-controlled trial. All subjects had class III or IV CHF and either mild hypotremia or normotremia. Patients had their previous medications for heart failure discontinued, and they received a fixed sodium and potassium diet. The average levels of urine osmolality ranged from 400 to 600 mOsm/kg at baseline. Patients received doses of drug ranging from 30 to 250 mg. The study findings included a highly significant reduction in urinary osmolality; with the highest dose the minimal urinary osmolality was reduced to

<100 mOsm/kg. In addition, patients on active treatment had a significant dose-related increase in urinary volume excretion.

Studies have been carried out with tolvaptan (OPC41061) that were designed to assess the effects of the drug on the body weight of patients with NYHA class I to IV CHF, including those with volume overload. The secondary objectives of the study were to assess quantitative measures of edema and quality of life and urinary sodium excretion volume and osmolality. The subjects were patients with a history of heart failure, with evidence of volume overload, who were receiving stable doses of furosemide. Patients were randomized to receive three dosing regimens (30 mg, 45 mg, 60 mg) of oral tolvaptan once daily or placebo. All three doses of tolvaptan were associated with decreased body weight and the effect was maintained throughout the 25-day study period. The three doses of tolvaptan were also associated with improved edema score and an increase in mean 24 h urine sodium excretion. There were no effects of the drug on serum potassium, heart rate, or blood pressure. The rate of adverse effects tended to be lower with tolvaptan, which included a decrease in the need to be hospitalized for heart failure.[241]

Trials with YM087 also included NYHA class III and IV heart failure patients. Early open-label evaluation required patients to be hyponatremic with serum sodium ranging from 120 to 132 mmol/L with maximal background medical therapy, which included continuous IV inotropic infusions. In this dose-escalation study, 20, 40, 80 and 120 mg of YM087 were given in two divided doses. Compared to the observation period in which the average urinary osmolality was about 450 mOsm/kg, there was a prompt reduction in urinary osmolality during the administration of YM087, an effect which was sustained throughout the evaluation and maintenance phases of the study. This fall in urinary osmolality and increase in free water clearance resulted in a correction of the hyponatremia. There was no substantial increase in thirst during the period.[242]

## ADENOSINE RECEPTOR ANTAGONISM

Blockade of adenosine (A1) receptors in animals can induce a brisk natriuresis without a kaliuretic effect,[243,244] an observation that has been confirmed in humans in short-term studies using FK-4531, a selective A1 receptor antagonist.[244–246] The mechanism for this lack of kaliuretic action has not been elucidated, neither has the safety and efficacy of this drug class in long-term clinical trials.

## ORAL DOPAMINE RECEPTOR AGONISTS

The unique, selective vasodilatory and inotropic actions of intravenous dopamine are limited by the lack of oral formulation. This has led investigators to develop newer dopamine agonists that are orally effective. Unlike L-dopa, which has been used in heart failure, these new drugs do not cross the blood-brain barrier but maintain most of the pharmacologic activity of dopamine.[247]

Ibopamine, which is an orally active derivative of dopamine, has dopaminergic $D_1$ and $D_2$ activity with alpha- and beta-adrenergic actions. In therapeutic doses, it is a peripheral vasodilator and appears to have favorable cardiovascular and renovascular actions in patients with heart failure. The results of the Prospective Randomized Study of Ibopamine on Mortality and Efficacy in Heart Failure (PRIME-2), however, raised serious questions about the safety of ibopamine and agents of this class in patients with heart failure.[248] Fenoldopam is a selective $D_1$ agonist that has been used to treat patients with CHF and hypertension. Because of bioavailability problems with the oral formulation, only the intravenous form is available for patients with severe hypertension.[249] Dopexamine is an intravenous $D_1$ and $beta_2$-receptor agonist that is being studied in patients with CHF and low cardiac output states.

## INHIBITION OF IMMUNE ACTIVATION

Cytokines are small pleiotropic endogenous peptides produced by a variety of cell types in response to a variety of different stimuli. Tumor necrosis factor alpha (TNF-$\alpha$), interleukin (IL) 1$\alpha$ and 1$\beta$, and IL-6 are classified as "proinflammatory" cytokines. These substances are responsible for initiating the primary host response to bacterial infections as well as initiating the repair of injured tissues.[250]

Cytokines are involved in augmenting the expression of adhesion molecules and for enhanced cell-to-cell interactions involved in inflammation. In addition, the proinflammatory cytokines are able to affect cardiovascular functioning by promoting LV remodeling, causing ventricular dysfunction, and uncoupling myocardial beta receptors.[250] They are elevated in the serum in various cardiovascular disorders and are often a marker of the severity of disease.[251,252]

TNF-$\alpha$ was originally discovered in 1975 as a protein with necrotizing effects in certain transplantable mouse tumors. More recently, this cytokine has been shown to exert a spectrum of pleiotropic effects in many different cell types.[253] The major biologic role of TNF-$\alpha$ is thought to be a host response to systemic infections, most notably gram-negative sepsis.[254] In fact, TNF-$\alpha$ levels are considerably elevated in patients with septic shock, and TNF-$\alpha$ has been implicated as an important mediator in the lethal effect of endotoxin, possibly causing the symptoms characteristic of the "shock state."

Many experimental and clinical studies have shown there is an association between depressed myocardial function and elevated levels of TNF-$\alpha$.[255] The basis of this association is not yet clear; however, there are studies suggesting that elevated levels of TNF-$\alpha$ play a major role in causing myocardial depression, whereas other studies conclude that TNF-$\alpha$ is likely to play a part in the alleviation of this condition.[256] A third school of thought suggests that the elevated levels of TNF-$\alpha$ are merely a marker that may indicate the stage of progression of the disease. Thus, although it is clear there are elevated levels of TNF-$\alpha$ in various cardiac diseases, the reasons for these increased levels and the mechanisms of their effects are not agreed on. Since there is a strong association and possibly a causative relation exists between TNF-$\alpha$ and CHF, various drug trials were carried out looking at TNF-$\alpha$ and its possible metabolic pathways as a therapeutic target in the treatment of heart disease.[257]

A randomized, double-blind, placebo-controlled study assessed the long-term effects and efficacy of etanercept in the treatment of 47 patients with advanced heart failure. The results of this study showed that treatment with etanercept for 3 months was safe and well tolerated, and it resulted in a significant dose-dependent improvement in LV structure and ejection fraction, as well as functional status.[258] Multicenter trials have been carried out to assess whether the beneficial effects of etanercept can be sustained over longer periods and in larger patient populations. These trials are the Randomized Etanercept North American Strategy to Study Antagonism of Cytokines (RENAISSANCE), Research into Etanercept Cytokine Antagonism in Ventricular Dysfunction (RECOVER), and Randomized Etanercept Worldwide Evaluation (RENEWAL). The trial results have been disappointing.

The drugs thalidomide and pentoxifylline have been shown, in small studies, to suppress the production of TNF-$\alpha$ in patients having heart failure with favorable effects on hemodynamics being reported.

The enzyme that processes precursor TNF-$\alpha$ has been identified as a microsomal metalloproteinase called TNF-$\alpha$-converting enzyme (TACE). TACE presents a novel target for therapeutic intervention in that inhibitors of the enzyme block TNF-$\alpha$ production.

A clinical trial evaluated the use of the intravenous immunoglobulin IgG in patients with new onset of dilated cardiomyopathy with no apparent benefit when compared to placebo. In experimental studies, the cytokine IL-10 has been used successfully to treat viral myocarditis.[259,260]

Studies with prednisone and cyclosporine have shown no clinical benefit in treatment of patients with dilated cardiomyopathy and myocarditis.[261,262]

Other approaches under consideration for attenuating the heightened inflammatory responses observed in patients with heart failure include monoclonal antibodies that interfere with complement activation and those that interfere with neutrophil adhesion and migration.[263]

## NITRIC OXIDE

Inhaled nitric oxide, a vasodilator substance produced by the endothelium, has been investigated as a possible treatment for CHF.[264,265] Arginine, a nitric oxide precursor, and agents that potentiate nitric oxide synthesis, now present potential directions for new heart failure therapies. To date, results with L-arginine use in patients with heart failure have been inconclusive. Nitric oxide donor substances are also being evaluated.[266] Sildenafil, a drug approved for the treatment of male erectile dysfunction, increases cGMP, which mediates many of the biological effects of nitric oxide. The drug has been shown to be well tolerated and effective in patients with erectile dysfunction and CHF.[267]

## IMIDAZOLINE RECEPTOR AGONISTS

The drugs, rilmenidine and moxonidine, are centrally acting antihypertensive agents that decrease sympathetic outflow by stimulation of nonadrenergic imidazole-1 receptors found in the brain.[268] These drugs are similar to clonidine in their pharmacologic activities, but cause less sedation. Modulation of the sympathetic nervous system by decreasing central catecholamine release has been proposed as a therapeutic approach to prolonging life in patients with CHF. However, the results of a study using moxonidine in heart failure patients did not show any benefit on survival.[268]

## MATRIX METALLOPROTEINASE INHIBITORS

Matrix metalloproteinase and their inhibitors are biological proteins that are involved with the formation and breakdown of collagen and interstitial tissue.[269] Matrix metalloproteinase activity is elevated in patients with heart failure, suggesting that these proteins may be contributors to myocardial remodeling and worsening of symptoms. Natural and symthetic matrix metalloproteinase inhibitors are being considered as treatments for heart failure.[269]

## SUPPLEMENTARY HORMONES AND ANTIOXIDANTS

Increasing experimental evidence and preliminary clinical data suggest that growth hormones may have beneficial effects in the treatment of heart failure.[188] However, the mechanisms behind these favorable actions are not well understood.[188,270] Growth hormone exerts its effects either directly or indirectly via insulin growth factors.

In experimental studies, growth hormone has been shown to increase the force of contraction by increasing the number of myocardial cross-bridges and the amount of available calcium. Growth hormone can also enhance peripheral blood flow and increase skeletal muscle mass. Growth hormone has been shown to attenuate pathologic remodeling without inducing LV hypertrophy.

In patients with heart failure, growth hormone has been shown to improve LV systolic function and exercise tolerance, while normalizing plasma levels of BNP. Long-term morbidity and mortality studies in patients with heart failure remain to be done.

Anabolic steroids have been evaluated in patients with heart failure.[188] They have been shown to improve left myocardial performance, increase skeletal muscle, and a sense of well being. However, there is little long-term morbidity and mortality experience with this treatment.

## METABOLIC ENHANCERS AND ANTIMETABOLITES

Abnormalities of energy metabolism are often cited as key elements in the progression of worsening LV dysfunction that characterizes heart failure. Ranolazine is one of a class of partial inhibitors of fatty oxidation (pFOX inhibitors). By shifting ATP production away from fatty acid oxidation toward carbohydrate oxidation, ranolazine reduces oxygen demand without decreasing cardiac work and maintaining coupling of glycolysis to pyruvate oxidation, which minimizes lactate accumulation. Ranolazine may be useful as an antianginal drug, and in experimental heart failure studies the drug has been shown to improve LV performance.[271] It is now being evaluated as a treatment for heart failure in clinical trials (see also Chap. 57).

Carnitine is a biological substance that has an important role in the oxidation of long-chain fatty acids. It also allows for the removal of short- and medium-chain fatty acids from the cell. Carnitine has also been shown to facilitate the aerobic metabolism of carbohydrates.[272]

It has been demonstrated by investigators that myocardial carnitine levels are decreased in many pediatric and adult cardiomyopathies where myocardial fatty acid metabolism is impaired. It has been proposed that the restoration of normal carnitine levels through the administration of exogenous L-carnitine would be of therapeutic value in heart failure by its ability to stimulate fatty acid metabolism.

The usefulness of oral L-carnitine for the treatment of pediatric cardiomyopathy is well established.[271] A few small studies in patients with heart failure have examined the effects of L-carnitine and have demonstrated improvements in hemodynamics, functional capacity, and survival.[272] A large randomized, placebo-controlled trial is still required to adequately assess the usefulness of L-carnitine in heart failure.

Coenzyme Q10 (CoQ10), or ubiquinone, is an endogenous cellular membrane constituent that has been shown to have antioxidant properties. Its central physiologic role is in mediating electron transport between nicotinamide adenine dinucleotide and succinate dehydrogenases and the cytochrome system.

CoQ10 has been suggested as a treatment for CHF where low levels of the substance in the myocardium have been observed. Despite a theoretical benefit in patients with heart failure, trials with CoQ10 supplementation have not demonstrated any clinical effectiveness.[271,273]

Heart failure has also been associated with the accumulation of oxygen-free radicals, which can cause cellular damage in the heart.[274] At this juncture, treatments with various nutritive antioxidants (vitamins and minerals) and naturally occurring enzymatic free-radical scavengers have not been associated with efficacy in patients with heart failure.

## ANTIAPOPTOSIS THERAPY

Innovative approaches to preserving myocardial function are interventions that can interfere with programmed myocardial cell death (apoptosis), a natural process that is accelerated by aging, myocardial ischemia, hypertension, diabetes mellitus, and myocardial cell stretch (LV dilation).[274a] Utilization of angiotensin II receptor blockers and the infusion of insulin growth factor in rats can inhibit the amount of myocardial apoptosis by 50 percent, and suggests future therapeutic approaches in human beings. Caspase, an enzyme essential to the apoptotic process, can be inhibited pharmacologically, with evidence of enhanced myocardial preservation in experimental animals.[275]

**GENE THERAPY**

In experimental studies, gene therapy has been shown to improve failing human cardiac myocyte function.[276,277] It was demonstrated that the abnormal contraction, relaxation, and contraction amplitude-frequency relation of isolated myocytes obtained from patients with dilated cardiomyopathy could be normalized by transfection of the myocytes in vitro with an adenovirus expressing the sarcoplasmic reticulum $Ca^{2+}$-ATPase (SERCA2a); transfection increased $Ca^{2+}$ ATPase activity by 80 percent. The enhanced function of the myocytes was associated with corresponding improvements in the kinetics of the $Ca^{2+}$ transient. The isolated myocyte results confirm previous in vitro findings by Meyer et al. in normal rabbit myocytes that indicated that adenoviral transfection of SERCA2a can improve contraction and relaxation.[278]

## Nonpharmacologic Aspects of Treatment

Nonpharmacologic factors contribute to the overall efficacy of care. Weight reduction by dieting is generally advisable when obesity is present. Often, however, nutritional status is compromised and cachexia is present.[279] Limitation of salt intake is important and may delay the time when diuretics may be necessary as well as reduce the amount required. In advanced heart failure, strict salt limitation is essential, although it is difficult to maintain. A diet containing less than 20 g/day of salt is desirable. Intake of fluids should be reduced to 1 to 1.5 L every 24 h in patients with advanced heart failure, with or without hyponatremia, except in warm climates. As will be stressed in relation to the use of diuretics, a readable weight scale is essential, and daily weights are of great value in judging therapy.

Smoking should be strongly discouraged in all patients, especially in the presence of obstructive vascular disease. Alcohol is a cardiac depressant in general and should be forbidden if an alcoholic cardiomyopathy is suspected. In all other cases, daily intake of alcohol probably should not exceed 40 g/day in men and 30 g/day in women, although there are, as yet, insufficient data on the effects of alcohol in patients with mild heart failure to support these recommendations.[280]

Patients should routinely receive vaccinations against influenza and pneumococcal pneumonia. Deconditioning related to muscular inactivity in association with muscular atrophy and decreased metabolic vascular dilatation is a major factor in reducing exercise performance as heart failure progresses.[281] The 6-min walk test is a semiquantitative assessment tool for assessing functional capacity before and after treatment. Low-level exercise, such as walking, should be encouraged, whereas strenuous isometric activities should be discouraged. Specific exercise training needs to be tailored to the appropriate level of the patient's disease and always performed under medical guidance. Isometric exercise should be avoided. In patients with stable heart failure, there is evidence that appropriate physical exercise and exercise training can lead to improvements in both exer-

TABLE 25-6 Chronic Heart Failure—Choice of Pharmacologic Therapy

| | ACE Inhibitor | Diuretic | Potassium-Sparing Diuretic | Cardiac Glycosides | Vasodilator (Hydralazine/ ISDN) | Beta Blocker |
|---|---|---|---|---|---|---|
| Systolic dysfunction | | | | | | |
| Asymptomatic LV dysfunction | Indicated in some | Not indicated (unless ↑ BP) | Not indicated | Only with atrial fibrillation | Not indicated | After MI |
| Symptomatic HF (NYHA-II) | Indicated | | | (a) When atrial fibrillation is present or (b) when improved from more severe HF in sinus rhythm* | If ACE inhibitors are not tolerated | Indicated (under specialist care) |
| − Fluid retention | | Indicated in some | Not indicated | | | |
| + Fluid retention | | Indicated | Persisting hypokalemia | | | |
| Worsening/severe HF (NYHA III–IV) | Indicated | Indicated, combinations of diuretics | Persisting hypokalemia; spironolactone for efficacy | Indicated | If ACE inhibitors are not tolerated or insufficient | Indicated (under specialist care) |
| End-stage HF (persisting NHYA IV) | Indicated | Indicated, combinations of diuretics | Persisting hypokalemia; spironolactone for efficacy | Indicated | If ACE inhibitors are not tolerated or insufficient | Indicated (under specialist care) |

*Preliminary data from the DIG (Digitalis Investigation Group) trial suggest that digoxin also may be indicated in NYHA II heart failure and sinus rhythm.

ABBREVIATIONS: ACE = angiotensin-converting enzyme; BP = blood pressure; HF = heart failure; ISDN = isosorbide dinitrate; LV = left ventricular; MI = myocardial infarction; NYHA = New York Heart Association.

SOURCE: From Task Force of the Working Group on Heart Failure of the European Society of Cardiology. The treatment of heart failure. *Eur Heart J* 1997;18:748. Reproduced with permission from the publisher and authors.

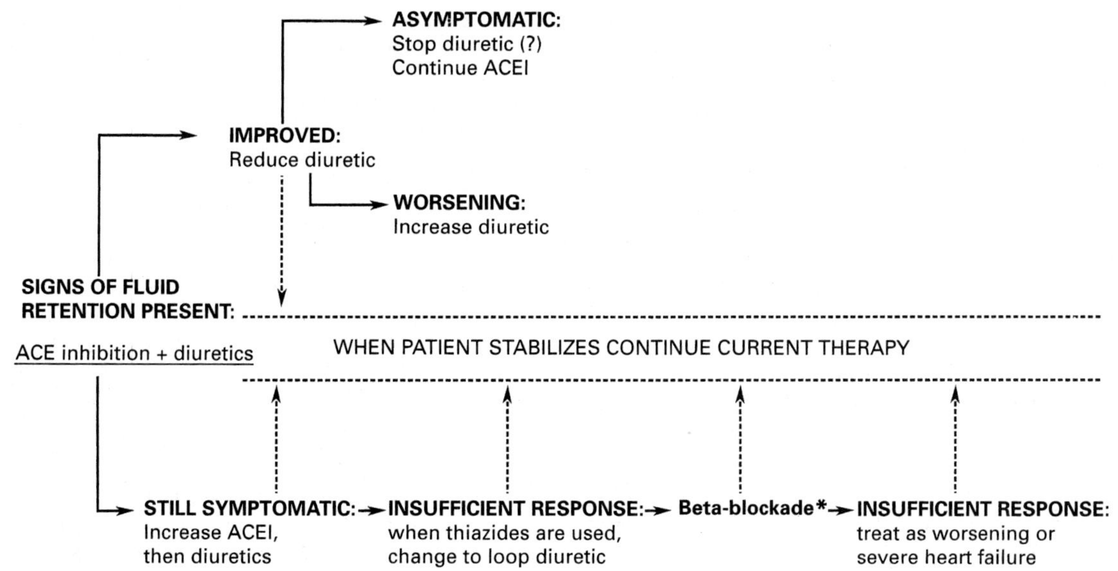


FIGURE 25-12 Flow chart of pharmacologic treatment of mild symptomatic systolic left ventricular (LV) dysfunction, New York Hear Association class II, and signs of fluid retention. *Data available only for carvedilol. (From Task Force of the Working Group on Heart Failure of the European Society of Cardiology. The treatment of heart failure. *Eur Heart J* 1997;18:746. Reproduced with permission from the publisher and authors.)

cise capacity and the quality of life of the patient, although the effect of this intervention on prognosis is unknown.[282,283,283a] Specific recommendations include dynamic aerobic exercise (walking) three to five times a week for 20 to 30 min, or cycling for 20 min at 70 to 80 percent of peak heart rate five times a week.[282]

In patients with acute heart failure or in those with exacerbations of CHF, bedrest is advisable. Prolonged rest, however, should not be encouraged in patients with stable CHF. Continuous nasal positive airway pressure has also been utilized as an adjunct therapy in patients with advanced heart failure.[283b]

## GENERAL APPROACH TO THERAPY IN CONGESTIVE HEART FAILURE

Appropriate therapy in CHF depends on the stage of the disease process (Table 25-6, Figs. 25-12 and 25-13). While one seeks to define and treat the factors that initiated the process, one also attempts to reduce symptoms and prolong life. Thus, with initial damage (e.g., following a large myocardial infarction) ACE inhibition or ARB is indicated. BABs are also indicated at this stage because of mortality

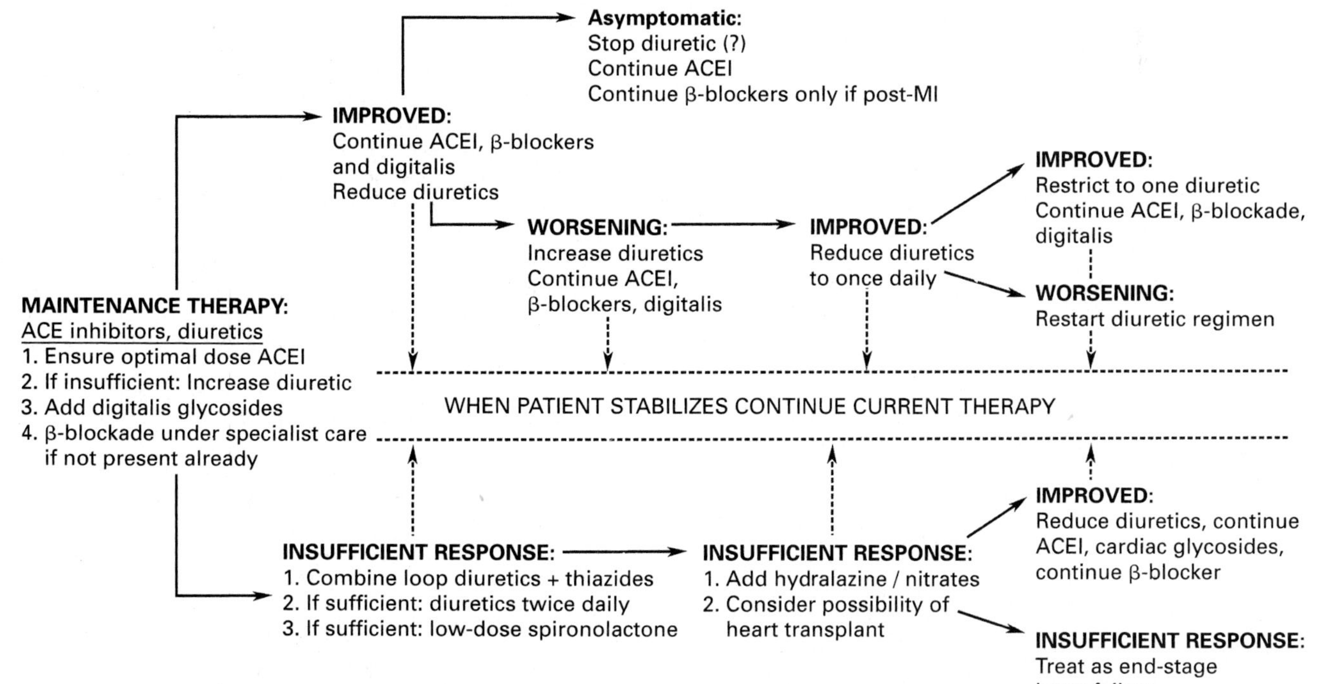


FIGURE 25-13 Flowchart of pharmacologic treatment of symptomatic left ventricular dysfunction and worsening heart failure (New York Heart Association class III to IV). (From Task Force of the Working Group on Heart Failure of the European Society of Cardiology. The Treatment of heart failure. *Eur Heart J* 1997;18:747. Reproduced with permission from the publisher and authors.)

reduction. As failure progresses to more symptomatic phases, beta blockers also appear indicated, along with ACE inhibition. Once symptoms increase and edema and central congestion occur, loop diuretics and spironolactone become useful to maintain dry weight. In order to prevent further ischemic tissue loss, other measures, such as cessation of smoking and appropriate lipid control, are essential. Digitalis glycosides, especially in modest doses, are indicated when class II to III symptoms occur.

In acute decompensation, such as may occur following a massive myocardial infarction or intermittently in class III to IV CHF, more aggressive therapy may be required, along with hospitalization for Swan-Ganz catheter monitoring. In this circumstance, short-term stimulation of the myocardium with dobutamine and/or milrinone, along with increasing amounts of intravenous diuretics, may be required for short periods to regain a stable state. At present there are no oral agents of this nature available to extend this care to the outpatient, and if dobutamine cannot be withdrawn, occasional administration by an external pump is required. Such therapy presents a short outcome of days or months.

In summary, the therapy of heart failure seeks the reversal or attenuation of the processes that initiated the syndrome while treating the patient to relieve symptoms and prolong life. The latter end is best achieved early in the disease process through prevention of further loss of myocardium (e.g., reperfusion) or reduction of loading (e.g., appropriate valve surgery or treatment of hypertension). In late stages of the disease, relief of symptoms can now be accomplished with modest gains in life expectancy.

## References


1. Redfield MM, Jacobsen SJ, Burnett JC Jr., et al. Burden of systolic and diastolic ventricular dysfunction in the community. Appreciating the scope of the heart failure epidemic. *JAMA* 2003;289:194–202.
2. Kitzman DW, Little WC, Brubaker PH, et al. Pathophysiological characterization of isolated diastolic heart failure in comparison to systolic heart failure. *JAMA* 2002;288:2144–2150.
3. Ford ES, Giles WH, Dietz WH. Prevalence of the metabolic syndrome among US adults. Findings from the Third National Health and Nutrition Examination Survey. *JAMA* 2002;287:356–359.
4. Jessup M, Brozena S. Heart failure. *N Engl J Med* 2003;348:2007–2018.
5. Young JB, Abraham WT, Smith AL, et al for the Multicenter InSync ICD Randomized Clinical Evaluation (MIRACLE ICD) Trial Investigators: Combined cardiac resynchronization and implantable cardioversion defibrillation in advanced chronic heart failure. The MIRACLE ICD Trial. *JAMA* 2003;289:2685–2694.
6. Hare JM. Cardiac resynchronization therapy for heart failure. *N Engl J Med* 2002;346:1902–1905.
7. Abraham WT, Fisher WG, Smith AL, et al for the MIRACLE Study Group. Cardiac resynchronization in chronic heart failure. *N Engl J Med* 2002;346:1845–1853.
8. Bradley DJ, Bradley EA, Baughman KL, et al. Cardiac resynchronization and death from progressive heart failure. A meta-analysis of randomized controlled trials. *JAMA* 2003;289:730–740.
9. Gerber TC, Nishimura RA, Holmes DR Jr., et al. Left ventricular and biventricular pacing in congestive heart failure. *Mayo Clin Proc* 2001;76:803–812.
10. Cazeau S, LeClercq C, Lavergne T, et al. for the Multisite Stimulation in Cardiomyopathies (MUSTIC) Study Investigators: Effects of multisite biventricular pacing in patients with heart failure and intraventricular conduction delay. *N Engl J Med* 2001;344:873–880.
11. Saxon LA, DeMarco T, Schafer J, et al for the VIGOR Congestive Heart Failure Investigators: Effects of long-term biventricular stimulation for resynchronization on echocardiographic measures of remodeling. *Circulation* 2002;105:1304–1310.
12. Leclercq C, Kass DA. Retiming the failing heart: principles and current clinical status of cardiac resynchronization. *J Am Coll Cardiol* 2002;39:194–201.
13. Moss AJ. MADIT-II and its implications. *Eur Heart J* 2003;24:16–18.
14. Rose EA, Gelijns AC, Moskowitz AJ, et al for the Randomized Evaluation of Mechanical Assistance for the Treatment of Congestive Heart Failure (REMATCH) Study Group: Long-term use of left ventricular assist device for endstage heart failure. *N Engl J Med* 2001;345:1435–1443.
15. Nadal-Ginard B, Kajstura J, Anversa P, Leri A. A matter of life and death: cardiac myocyte apoptosis and regeneration. *J Clin Invest* 2003;111:1457–1459.
16. Strauer BE, Kornowski R. Stem cell therapy in perspective. *Circulation* 2003;107:929–934.
17. LeJemtel TH, Sonnenblick EH. Heart failure: Adaptive and maladaptive processes. *Circulation* 1993;87(suppl VII):1–4.
18. Carabello BA, Crawford FA. Valvular heart disease. *N Engl J Med* 1997;337:32–41.
19. Vasan RS, Larson MG, Benjamin EJ, et al. Left ventricular dilatation and the risk of congestive heart failure in people without myocardial infarction. *N Engl J Med* 1997;336:1350–1355.
20. Olivetti G, Melissari M, Balbi T, et al. Myocyte nuclear and possible cellular hyperplasia contribute to ventricular remodeling in the hypertrophic senescent heart in humans. *J Am Coll Cardiol* 1994;24:140–149.
21. Anversa P. Myocyte death in the pathological heart. *Circ Res* 2000;86:121–124.
22. Hunter JJ, Chien KR. Signaling pathways for cardiac hypertrophy and failure. *N Engl J Med* 1999;341:1276–1283.
23. Schrier RW, Abraham WT. Hormones and hemodynamics in heart failure. *N Engl J Med* 1999;341:577–585.
24. Olivetti G, Abbi R, Quaini F, et al. Apoptosis in the failing human heart. *N Engl J Med* 1997;336:1131–1141.
25. LeJemtel TH, Sonnenblick EH. Heart failure in elderly patients. In: Aronow W, Tresch DD, eds. *Cardiovascular Disease in the Elderly Patient*. New York: Marcel Dekker;1993:473–484.
26. Bonow RO. Identification of viable myocardium. *Circulation* 1996;94:2674–2680.
27. Vanoverschelde J-LJ, Wijns W, Borgers M, et al. Chronic myocardial hibernation in humans. *Circulation* 1996;95:1961–1971.
28. Perrone-Filardi P, Pace L, Prastaro M, et al. Dobutamine echocardiography predicts improvement in hypoperfused dysfunctional myocardium after revascularization in patients with coronary artery disease. *Circulation* 1995;91:2556–2565.
29. Cigarroa CG, deFilippi CR, Bricker E, et al. Dobutamine stress echocardiography identifies hibernating myocardium and predicts recovery of left ventricular function after coronary revascularization. *Circulation* 1993;88:430–436.
30. Cornel JH, Bax JJ, Elhendy A, et al. Biphasic response to dobutamine predicts improvement of global left ventricular function after surgical revascularization in patients with stable coronary artery disease. Implications of time course of recovery on diagnostic accuracy. *J Am Coll Cardiol* 1998;31:1002–1010.
31. Helfant RH, Pine R, Meister SG, et al. Nitroglycerin to unmask reversible asynergy. Correlation with post coronary bypass ventriculography. *Circulation* 1974;50:108–113.
32. Rahimtoola SH. Hibernating myocardium has reduced blood flow at rest that increases with low-dose dobutamine. *Circulation* 1996;94:3055–3061.
33. Floras JS. Clinical aspects of sympathetic activation and parasympathetic withdrawal in heart failure. *J Am Coll Cardiol* 1993;22(suppl A):72A–84A.
34. Maisel AS, Krishnaswamy P, Nowak RM, et al. Rapid measurement of B-type natriuretic peptide in the emergency diagnosis of heart failure. *N Engl J Med* 2002;347:161–167.
35. Drazner MH, Rame JE, Stevenson LW, Dries DL. Prognostic importance of elevated jugular venous pressure and a third heart sound in patients with heart failure. *N Engl J Med* 2001;345:574–581.

36. Picard MH, Wilkins GT, Ray PA, Weyman AE. Natural history of left ventricular size and function after acute myocardial infarction. Assessment and prediction by echocardiographic endocardial surface mapping. *Circulation* 1990;82:484–494.
37. St. John Sutton M, Pfeffer MA, Plappert T, et al for the SAVE Investigators. Quantitative two-dimensional echocardiographic measurements are major predictors of adverse cardiovascular events after acute myocardial infarction. The protective effects of captopril. *Circulation* 1994;89:68–75.
38. Marmor A, Raphael T, Marmor M, Blondheim D. Evaluation of contractile reserve by dobutamine echocardiography: Noninvasive estimation of the severity of heart failure. *Am Heart J* 1996;132: 1195–1201.
39. Burkhoff D, Maurer MS, Packer M. Heart failure with a normal ejection fraction. Is it really a disorder of diastolic function? *Circulation* 2003;107:656–658.
40. Hunt SA, Baker DW, Chin MH, et al. ACC/AHA guidelines for the evaluation and management of chronic heart failure in the adult: executive summary. A Report of the American College of Cardiology/American Heart Association Task Force on Practice Guidelines. *J Am Coll Cardiol* 2001;38:2101–2113.
41. The Heart Outcomes Prevention Evaluation Study Investigators. Effects of an angiotensin-converting-enzyme inhibitor, ramipril, on cardiovascular events in high-risk patients. *N Engl J Med* 2000;342: 145–53.
42. Lonn EM, Yusuf S, Dzavik V, et al for the SECURE Investigators. Effects of ramipril and vitamin E on atherosclerosis. The study to evaluate carotid ultrasound changes in patients treated with ramipril and vitamin E (SECURE). *Circulation* 2001;103:919–925.
43. Schiffrin EL, Park JB, Intengan HD, Touyz RM. Correction of arterial structure and endothelial dysfunction in human essential hypertension by the angiotensin receptor antagonist losartan. *Circulation* 2000;101:1653–1659.
44. Butler J, Arbogast PG, BeLue R, et al. Outpatient adherence to beta blocker therapy after acute myocardial infarction. *J Am Coll Cardiol* 2002;40:1589–1595.
45. Gheorghiade M, Bonow RO. Chronic heart failure in the United States. A manifestation of coronary artery disease. *Circulation* 1998; 97:282–89.
46. Packer M, Cohn JN, on behalf of the Steering Committee and Membership of the Advisory Council to Improve Outcomes Nationwide in Heart Failure: Consensus Recommendations for the Management of Chronic Heart Failure. *Am J Cardiol* 1999;3(suppl 2A):1–38.
47. Francis GS, Benedict C, Johnstone DE, et al. Comparison of neuroendocrine activation in patients with left ventricular dysfunction with and without congestive heart failure. A Substudy of the Studies of Left Ventricular Dysfunction (SOLVD). *Circulation* 1990;82: 1724–1729.
48. Kajstura J, Cigola E, Malhotra A, et al. Angiotensin II induces apoptosis of adult ventricular myocytes in vitro. *J Mol Cell Cardiol* 1997; 29:859–870.
49. Shapiro BP, Chen HH, Burnett JC Jr., Redfield MM. Use of plasma brain natriuretic peptide concentration to aid in the diagnosis of heart failure. *Mayo Clin Proc* 2003;78:481–486
50. Redfield MM, Rodeheffer RJ, Jacobsen SJ, et al. Plasma brain natriuretic peptide concentration: impact of age and gender. *J Am Coll Cardiol* 2002;40:976–982.
51. Arnold JMO, Yusuf S, Young J, et al on behalf of the HOPE Investigators. Prevention of heart failure in patients in the Heart Outcomes Prevention Evaluation (HOPE) study. *Circulation* 2003;107:1284–1290.
52. Banerjee A, Talreja A, LeJemtel TH. Evolving rationale for angiotensin converting enzyme inhibitor therapy in chronic heart failure. *Mt. Sinai J Med* 2003;70:225–231.
53. Captopril Multicenter Research Group. A placebo-controlled trial of captopril in refractory chronic congestive heart failure. *J Am Coll Cardiol* 1983;2:755–763.
54. Zannad F. Aldosterone and heart failure. *Eur Heart J* 1995;16 (suppl N):98–102.
55. MacFadyen RJ, Lee AFC, Morton JJ, et al. How often are angiotensin II and aldosterone concentrations raised during chronic ACE inhibitor treatment in cardiac failure? *Heart* 1999;82:57–61.
56. Volpe M, Tritto C, DeLuca N, et al. Angiotensin converting enzyme inhibition restores cardiac and hormonal responses to volume overload in patients with dilated cardiomyopathy and mild heart failure. *Circulation* 1992;86:1800–1809.
57. LeJemtel TH, Maskin CS, Chadwick B. Effect of acute angiotensin converting enzyme inhibition on renal blood flow in patients with stable congestive heart failure. *Am J Med Sci* 1986;292:123–27.
58. Pfeffer MA, Braunwald E. Ventricular remodeling after myocardial infarction. Experimental observations and clinical implications. *Circulation* 1990;81:1161–1172.
59. Pfeffer MA, Lamas GA, Vaughan DE, et al. Effect of captopril on progressive ventricular dilatation after anterior myocardial infarction. *N Engl J Med* 1988;319:80–86.
60. Pfeffer MA, Braunwald E, Moye LA, et al. Effect of captopril on mortality and morbidity in patients with left ventricular dysfunction after myocardial infarction. *N Engl J Med* 1992;327:669–677.
61. ACE Inhibitor Myocardial Infarction Collaborative Group. Indications for ACE inhibitors in the early treatment of acute myocardial infarction. Systematic overview of individual data from 100,000 patients in randomized trials. *Circulation* 1998;97:2202–12.
62. The CONSENSUS Trial Study Group. Effect of enalapril on mortality in severe congestive heart failure: Results of the Cooperative North Scandinavian Enalapril Survival Study (CONSENSUS). *N Engl J Med* 1987;316:1429–1435.
63. Cohn JN, Johnson G, Ziesche S, et al. A comparison of enalapril with hydralazine-isosorbide dinitrate in the treatment of chronic congestive heart failure. *N Engl J Med* 1991;325:303–310.
64. The SOLVD Investigators. Effect of enalapril on survival in patients with reduced left ventricular ejection fraction and congestive heart failure. *N Engl J Med* 1991;325:293–302.
65. The SOLVD Investigators. Effect of enalapril on mortality and the development of heart failure in asymptomatic patients with reduced left ventricular ejection fractions. *N Engl J Med* 1992;327:685–691.
66. Yusuf S, Pepine CJ, Garces C, et al. Effect of enalapril on myocardial infarction and unstable angina in patients with low ejection fractions. *Lancet* 1992;340:1173–1178.
67. Mancini GBJ, Henry GC, Macaya C, et al. Angiotensin converting enzyme inhibition with quinapril improves endothelial vasomotor dysfunction in patients with coronary artery disease. The TREND (Trial on Reversing ENdothelial Dysfunction) Study. *Circulation* 1996;94:258–265.
68. St. John Sutton M, Pfeffer MA, Moye L, et al for the SAVE Investigators. Cardiovascular death and left ventricular remodeling two years after myocardial infarction. Baseline predictors and impact of long-term use of captopril: information from the Survival and Ventricular Enlargement (SAVE) trial. *Circulation* 1997;96: 3294–3299.
69. Hall D, Zeitler H, Rudolph W. Counteraction of the vasodilator effects of enalapril by aspirin in severe heart failure. *J Am Coll Cardiol* 1992;20:1549–1555.
70. Latini R, Santoro E, Masson S, et al on behalf of the GISSI-3 Investigators. Aspirin does not interact with ACE inhibitors when both are given early after acute myocardial infarction: results of the GISSI-3 trial. *Heart Disease* 2000;2:185–190.
71. Packer M, Poole-Wilson PA, Armstrong PW, et al on behalf of the ATLAS Study Group. Comparative effects of low and high doses of the angiotensin-converting inhibitor, lisinopril, on morbidity and mortality in chronic heart failure. *Circulation* 1999;100:2312–2318.
72. Drakos SG, Papamichael CM, Alexopoulos GP, et al. Effects of high doses versus standard doses of enalapril on endothelial cell function in patients with chronic congestive heart failure secondary to idiopathic dilated or ischemic cardiomyopathy. *Am J Cardiol* 2003;91: 885–887.
73. Giannatasio C, Achilli F, Grappiolo A, et al. Radial artery flow mediated dilatation in heart failure patients. *Hypertens* 2001;38:1451–1455.

74. Cohn JN, Tognoni G, for the Valsartan Heart Failure Trial Investigators. A randomized trial of the angiotensin-receptor blocker valsartan in chronic heart failure. *N Engl J Med* 2001;345:1667–1675.
75. Cohn JN. Angiotensin receptor blockers and clinical trials in heart failure. *Eur Heart J* 2003;24:125–126.
76. Bristow MR. β-Adrenergic receptor blockade in chronic heart failure. *Circulation* 2000;101:558–569.
77. Ruggenenti P, Perna A, Gherardi G, et al. Renal function and requirement for dialysis in chronic nephropathy patients on long-term ramipril: REIN follow-up trial. *Lancet* 1998;352:1252–1256.
78. Pitt B, Segal R, Martinez FA, et al on behalf of ELITE Study Investigators. Randomised trial of losartan versus captopril in patients over 65 with heart failure (Evaluation of Losartan in the Elderly Study, ELITE). *Lancet* 1997;349:747–52.
79. Pitt B, Poole-Wilson P, Segal R, et al. Effects of losartan versus captopril on mortality in patients with symptomatic heart failure: rationale, design, and baseline characteristics of patients in the Losartan Heart Failure Survival Study–ELITE II: *J Cardiac Fail* 1999;5:146–54.
80. Francis GS, Cohn JN, Johnson G, et al for the V-HeFT VA Cooperative Studies Group. Plasma norepinephrine, plasma renin activity, and congestive heart failure. Relations to survival and the effects of therapy in V-HeFT II. *Circulation* 1993;87 (suppl VI):VI-40–VI-48.
81. Rousseau MF, Konstam MA, Benedict CR, et al. Progression of left ventricular dysfunction secondary to coronary artery disease, sustained neurohormonal activation and effects of ibopamine therapy during long-term therapy with angiotensin-converting enzyme inhibitor. *Am J Cardiol* 1994;73:488–93.
82. Kokkonen JO, Saarinen J, Kovanen PT. Regulation of local angiotensin II formation in the human heart in the presence of interstitial fluid. Inhibition of chymase by protease inhibitors of interstitial fluid and of angiotensin-converting enzyme by Ang-(1-9) formed by heart carboxypeptidase A-like activity. *Circulation* 1997;95: 1455–1463.
83. Ménard J, Campbell DJ, Azizi M, Gonzales M-F. Synergistic effects of ACE inhibition and Ang II antagonism on blood pressure, cardiac weight, and renin in spontaneously hypertensive rats. *Circulation* 1997;96:3072–3078.
84. Sica DA, Gehr TWB, Frishman WH. The renin-angiotensin axis: angiotensin-converting enzyme inhibitos and angiotensin-receptor blockers. In: Frishman WH, Sonnenblick EH, Sica DA, eds. *Cardiovascular Pharmacotherapeutics,* 2nd ed. New York: McGraw Hill; 2003:131–156.
85. Spinale FG, Iannini JP, Mukherjee R, et al. Angiotensin AT1 receptor inhibition, angiotensin-converting enzyme inhibition, and combination therapy with developing heart failure: Cellular mechansims of action. *J Cardiac Fail* 1998;4:325–332.
86. Krombach RS, Clair MJ, Hendrick JW, et al. Angiotensin converting enzyme inhibition, AT1 receptor inhibition, and combination therapy with pacing induced heart failure: effects on left ventricular performance and regional blood flow patterns. *Cardiovasc Res* 1998;38: 631–645.
87. Hamroff G, Blaufarb I, Mancini D, et al. Angiotensin II receptor blockade further reduces afterload safely in patients maximally treated with angiotensin converting enzyme inhibitors for heart failure. *J Cardiovasc Pharmacol* 1997;30:533–536.
88. Baruch L, Anand I, Cohen IS, et al for the Vasodilator Heart Failure Trial (V-HeFT) Study Group augmented short- and long-term hemodynamic and hormonal effects of an angiotensin receptor blocker added to angiotensin converting enzyme inhibitor therapy in patients with heart failure. *Circulation* 1999;99:2658–2664.
89. Hamroff G, Katz SD, Mancini D, et al. Addition of angiotensin II receptor blockade to maximal angiotensin-converting enzyme inhibition improves exercise capacity in patients with severe congestive heart failure. *Circulation* 1999;99;990–992.
90. Latini R, Masson S, Anand I, et al for the Val-HeFT Investigators. Effects of valsartan on circulating brain natriuretic peptide and norepinephrine in symptomatic chronic heart failure. The Valsartan Heart Failure Trial (Val-HeFT). *Circulation* 2002;106:2454–2458.
91. Jong P, Demers C, McKelvie RS, Liu PP. Angiotensin receptor blockers in heart failure: Meta-analysis of randomized controlled trials. *J Am Coll Cardiol* 2002;39:463–470.
92. Gogia H, Mehra A, Parikh S, et al. Prevention of tolerance to hemodynamic effects of nitrates with concomitant use of hydralazine in patients with chronic heart failure. *J Am Coll Cardiol* 1995;26: 1575–1580.
93. Frishman WH, Sica DA: Calcium channel blockers. In: Frishman WH, Sonnenblick EH, Sica DA, eds. *Cardiovascular Pharmacotherapeutics,* 2nd ed. New York: McGraw-Hill; 2003:105–130.
94. Levine TB, Bernink PJLM, Caspi A, et al. Effect of mibefradil, a T-type channel blocker, on morbidity and mortality in moderate to severe congestive heart failure. The MACH-1 Study. *Circulation* 2000;101:758–64.
95. Frishman WH, Furberg CD, Friedewald WT. β-Adrenergic blockade in survivors of acute myocardial infarction. *N Engl J Med* 1984;310: 830–837.
96. Lechat P, Escolano S, Golmard JL, et al on behalf of the CIBIS Investigators. Prognostic value of bisoprolol-induced hemodynamic effects in heart failure during the Cardiac Insufficiency Bisoprolol Study (CIBIS). *Circulation* 1997;96:2197–2205.
97. CIBIS-II Investigators and Committees. The Cardiac Insufficiency Bisoprolol Study II (CIBIS-II): A randomised trial. *Lancet* 1999;353: 9–13.
98. MERIT-HF Study Group. Effect of metoprolol CR/XL in chronic heart failure: metoprolol CR/XL randomised intervention trial in congestive heart failure (MERIT-HF*). Lancet* 1999;353:2001–2007.
99. Frishman WH. Alpha- and beta-adrenergic blocking drugs. In: Frishman WH, Sonnenblick EH, Sica DA, eds: *Cardiovascular Pharmacotherapeutics,* 2nd ed. New York: McGraw Hill; 2003:67–97.
100. Bristow MR. β-Adrenergic receptor blockade in chronic heart failure. *Circulation* 2000;101:558–69.
101. Frishman WH. Carvedilol. *N Engl J Med* 1998;339:1759–1765.
102. Bristow MR, Gilbert EM, Abraham WT, et al for the MOCHA Investigators. Carvedilol produces dose-related improvements in left ventricular function and survival in subjects with chronic heart failure. *Circulation* 1996;94:2807–2816.
103. Packer M, Colucci WS, Sackner-Bernstein JD, et al. for the PRECISE Study Group. Double-blind, placebo-controlled study of the effects of carvedilol in patients with moderate to severe heart failure. The PRECISE trial. *Circulation* 1996;94:2793–2799.
104. Colucci WS, Packer M, Bristow MR, et al for the U.S. Carvedilol Heart Failure Study Group. Carvedilol inhibits clinical progression in patients with mild symptoms of heart failure. *Circulation* 1996;94: 2800–2806.
105. Cohn JN, Fowler MB, Bristow MR, et al. Safety and efficacy of carvedilol in severe heart failure. *J Cardiac Fail* 1997;3:173–179.
106. Packer M, Bristow MR, Cohn JN, et al for the U.S. Carvedilol Heart Failure Study Group. The effect of carvedilol on morbidity and mortality in patients with chronic heart failure. *N Engl J Med* 1996; 334:1349–1355.
107. Australia/New Zealand Heart Failure Research Collaborative Group. Randomised, placebo-controlled trial of carvedilol in patients with congestive heart failure due to ischaemic heart disease. *Lancet* 1997; 349:375–380.
108. Hall SA, Cigarroa CG, Marcoux L, et al. Time course of improvement in left ventricular function, mass and geometry in patients with congestive heart failure treated with beta-adrenergic blockade. *J Am Coll Cardiol* 1995;25:1154–1161.
109. LeJemtel TH, Galvao M, Sonnenblick EH. Beta-adrenergic blockade reverses, while ACE inhibition attenuates, left ventricular remodeling in patients with chronic heart failure. *Heart Failure* 1998;Spring: 57–63.
110. Doughty RN, Whalley GA, Gamble G, et al on behalf of the Australia-New Zealand Heart Failure Research Collaborative Group. Left ventricular remodeling with carvedilol in patients with congestive heart failure due to ischemic heart disease. *J Am Coll Cardiol* 1997;29: 1060–1066.

111. Dargie HJ. Effect of carvedilol on outcome after myocardial infarction in patients with left ventricular dysfunction: The CAPRICORN randomised trial. *Lancet* 2001;357:1385–1390.
112. Packer M, Fowler MB, Roecker EB, et al for the Carvedilol Prospective Randomized Cumulative Survival (COPERNICUS) Study Group. Effect of carvedilol on the morbidity of patients with severe chronic heart failure. Results of the Carvedilol Prospective Randomized Cumulative Survival (COPERNICUS) Study. *Circulation* 2002; 106:2194–2199.
113. Packer M. Effects of beta-adrenergic blockade on survival of patients with chronic heart failure. *Am J Cardiol* 1997;80 (11A):46L–54L.
113a. The Beta Blocker Evaluation of Survival Trial Investigators. A trial of the beta-blocker bucindolol in patients with advanced chronic heart failure. *N Engl J Med* 2001;344:1659–1667.
114. Barry WH, Gilbert EM. How do $\beta$ blockers improve ventricular function in patients with congestive heart failure? *Circulation* 2003;107: 2395–2397.
115. Reiken S, Wehrens XHT, Vest JA, et al. $\beta$ Blockers restore calcium release channel function and improve cardiac muscle performance in human heart failure. *Circulation* 2003;107:2459–2466.
116. Schmidt U, del Monte F, Miyamoto MI, et al. Restoration of diastolic function in senescent rat hearts through adenoviral gene transfer of sarcoplasmic reticulum $Ca^{2+}$-ATPase. *Circulation* 2000;101: 790–796.
116a. Lowes BD, Gilbert EM, Abraham WT, et al. Myocardial gene expression in dilated cardiomyopathy treated with beta-blocking agents. *N Engl J Med* 2002;346:1357–1365.
116b. Poole-Wilson PA, Swedberg K, Cleland JGF, et al, for the COMET Investigators: Comparison of carvedilol and metoprolol on clinical outcomes in patients with chronic heart failure in the Carvedilol or Metoprolol European Trial (COMET): randomized controlled trial. *Lancet* 2003;362:7–13.
117. HFSA Guidelines for the Management of Patients with Heart Failure due to Left Ventricular Systolic Dysfunction—Pharmacological Approaches. *Congestive Heart Fail* 2000;6:11–38.
118. Gehr TWB, Sica DA, Frishman WH. Diuretic therapy in cardiovascular disease. In Frishman WH, Sonnenblick EH, Sica DA (eds): *Cardiovascular Pharmacotherapeutics,* 2nd ed. New York: McGraw Hill; 2003;157–176.
119. Schlant RC, Sonnenblick EH. Pathophysiology of heart failure. In: Hurst JW, Schlant RC, Rackly CE, eds. *The Heart,* 7th ed. New York: McGraw-Hill;1990:387–397.
120. Koeppen B, Stanton B. Regulation of extracellular fluid volume. In: Koeppen BM, Stanton BA, eds. *Renal Physiology*. St. Louis: Mosby Year Book;1992:91–109.
121. Brater DC. Clinical pharmacology of loop diuretics in health and disease. *Eur Heart J* 1992;13(suppl G):10–14.
121a. Brater DC. Diuretic therapy. *N Engl J Med* 1998;339:387–395.
122. Knoben JE, Anderson PO, eds. Diuretics. In: *Clinical Drug Data,* 6th ed. Illinois: Drug Intelligence Publications;1988.
123. Voelker JR, Brown-Cartwright D, Anderson S, et al. Comparison of loop diuretics in patients with chronic renal insufficiency: Mechanism of difference in response. *Kidney Int* 1987;32:572–578.
124. Rudy DW, Gehr TWB, Matzke GR, et al. The pharmacodynamics of IV and oral torsemide in patients with chronic renal insufficiency. *Clin Pharmacol Ther* 1994;56:39–47.
125. Schwartz S, Brater C, Pound D, et al. Bioavailability, pharmacokinetics, and pharmacodynamics of torsemide in patients with cirrhosis. *Clin Pharmacol Ther* 1993;54:90–97.
126. Vargo DL, Kramer WG, Black PK, et al. Bioavailability, pharmacokinetics, and pharmacodynamics of torsemide and furosemide in patients with congestive heart failure. *Clin Pharmacol Ther* 1995;57:601–609.
127. Van Meyel JJM, Gerlag PGG, Smits P, et al. Absorption of high dose furosemide in congestive heart failure. *Clin Pharmacokinet* 1992;22: 308–318.
128. Marangoni E, Oddone A, Surian M, et al. Effect of high-dose furosemide in refractory congestive heart failure. *Angiology* 1990;41: 862–868.
129. Rudy DW, Voelker JR, Greene PK, et al. Loop diuretics for chronic renal insufficiency: A continuous infusion is more efficacious than bolus therapy. *Ann Intern Med* 1991;115:360–366.
130. Lahav M, Regev A, Ra'Anani P, Theodor E. Intermittent administration of furosemide vs continuous infusion preceded by a loading dose for congestive heart failure. *Chest* 1992;102:725–731.
130a. Bozkurt B, Agoston I, Knowlton AA. Complications of inappropriate use of spironolactone in heart failure: When an old medicine spirals out of new guidelines. *J Am Coll Cardiol* 2003;41:211–214.
131. Aull MJ, Sanoski CA. Optimizing inhibition of aldosterone: use of spironolactone in chronic heart failure. *Formulary* 1999;34:752–763.
132. Cooper HA, Dries DL, Davis CE, et al. Diuretics and risk of arrhythmic death in patients with left ventricular dysfunction. *Circulation* 1999;100:1311–1315.
133. Pitt B, Zannad F, Remme WJ, et al. The effect of spironolactone on morbidity and mortality in patients with severe heart failure. *N Engl J Med* 1999;341:709–717.
134. Farquharson CAJ, Struthers AD. Spironolactone increases nitric oxide bioactivity, improves endothelial vasodilator dysfunction, and suppresses vascular angiotensin I/Angiotensin II conversion in patients with chronic heart failure. *Circulation* 2000;101: 594–597.
135. Pitt B, Remme WJ, Zannad F, et al. Eplerenone, a selective aldosterone blocker in patients with left ventricular dysfunction after myocardial infarction. *N Engl J Med* 2003;348:1309–1321.
136. Stier CT Jr., Koenig S, Lee DY, et al. Aldosterone and aldosterone antagonism in cardiovascular disease: focus on eplerenone (Inspra). *Heart Dis* 2003;5:102–118.
137. Van Vliet AA, Donker AJM, Nauta JJP, Verheught FWA. Spironolactone in congestive heart failure refractory to high-dose loop diuretic and low-dose angiotensin converting enzyme inhibitor. *Am J Cardiol* 1993;71:21A–28A.
138. Channer KS, Richardson M, Crook R, Jones JV. Thiazides with loop diuretics for severe congestive heart failure. *Lancet* 1990;335: 922–923.
139. Kiyingi A, Field MJ, Pawsey CC, et al. Metolazone in treatment of severe refractory congestive cardiac failure. *Lancet* 1990;335:29–31.
140. Channer KS, McLean KA, Lawson-Matthew P, Richardson M. Combination diuretic treatment in severe heart failure: Randomized controlled trial. *Br Heart J* 1994;71:146–150.
141. Chin MH, Goldman L. Factors contributing to the hospitalization of patients with congestive heart failure. *Am J Pub Health* 1997;87: 643–648.
142. Mancini DM, Katz SD, Lang CC, et al. Effect of erythropoietin on exercise capacity in patients with moderate to severe chronic heart failure. *Circulation* 2003;107:294–299.
143. Androne A-S, Katz SD, Lund L, et al. Hemodilution is common in patients with advanced heart failure. *Circulation* 2003;107:226–229.
144. Hillege HL, Girbes ARJ, de Kam PJ, et al. Renal function, neurohormonal activation, and survival in patients with chronic heart failure. *Circulation* 2000;102:203–210.
145. Morrison LK, Harrison A, Krishnaswamy P, et al. Utility of rapid B-natriuretic peptide assay in differentiating congestive heart failure from lung disease in patients presenting with dyspnea. *J Am Coll Cardiol* 2002;39:202–209.
146. Dao Q, Krishnaswamy P, Kazanegra R, et al. Utility of B-type natriuretic peptide in the diagnosis of congestive heart failure in an urgent-care setting. *J Am Coll Cardiol* 2001;37:379–385.
147. Maisel A. B-type natriuretic peptide levels: Diagnostic and prognostic in congestive heart failure. What's next? (editorial) *Circulation* 2002;105:2328–2331.
148. Nohria A, Lewis E, Warner Stevenson L. Medical management of advanced heart failure. *JAMA* 2002;287:628–640.
149. Baruch L, Patacsil P, Hameed A, et al. Pharmacodynamic effects of milrinone with and without a bolus loading infusion. *Am Heart J* 2000;141:e6.
150. Albert NM, Davis M, Young J. Improving the care of patients dying of heart failure. *Cleveland Clin J Med* 2002;69:321–328.

151. Keating GM, Goa KL. Nesiritide: A review of its use in acute decompensated heart failure. *Drugs* 2003;63:47–70.
151a. Frishman WH, Sica DA, Cheng JWM, et al. Natriuretic peptides: Nesiritide. In, Frishman WH, Sonnenblick EH, Sica DA, eds. *Cardiovascular Pharmacotherapeutics Manual* 2nd ed. New York: McGraw Hill; 2004:412–420.
152. Colucci WS, Elkayam U, Horton DP, et al. Intravenous nesiritide, a natriuretic peptide, in the treatment of decompensated congestive heart failure. *N Engl J Med* 2000;343:246–253.
153. Publication Committee of the VMAC Investigators: Intravenous nesiritide vs nitroglycerin for treatment of decompensated congestive heart failure. A randomized controlled trial. *JAMA* 2002;287: 1531–1540.
154. Silver MA, Horton DP, Ghali JK, Elkayam U. Effect of nesiritide versus dobutamine on short-term outcomes in the treatment of patients with acutely decompensated heart failure. *J Am Coll Cardiol* 2002; 39:798–803.
155. Burger AJ, Elkayam U, Neibaur MT, et al. Comparison of the occurrence of ventricular arrhythmias in patients with acutely decompensated congestive heart failure receiving dobutamine versus nesiritide therapy. *Am J Cardiol* 2001;88:35–39.
156. Sonnenblick EH, LeJemtel TH, Frishman WH. Inotropic agents. In Frishman WH, Sonnenblick EH, Sica DA, eds. *Cardiovascular Pharmacotherapeutics,* 2nd ed. New York: McGraw Hill; 2003:191–202.
157. Withering W. *An Account of the Foxglove, and Some of Its Medical Uses: With Practical Remarks on Dropsy and Other Diseases*. London: G.G.J. and J. Robinson; 1785.
158. Fothergill JM. *Digitalis: Its Mode of Action*. London, 1871.
159. Dock W, Tainter ML. The circulatory changes after full therapeutic doses of digitalis, with critical discussion of views on cardiac output. *J Clin Invest* 1929;8:467–484.
160. The Digitalis Investigation Group. The effect of digoxin on mortality and morbidity in patients with heart failure. *N Engl J Med* 1997; 336:525–533.
161. Rathore SS, Curtis JP, Wang Y, et al. Association of serum digoxin concentration and outcomes in patients with heart failure. *JAMA* 2003;289:871–878.
162. Rathore SS, Wang Y, Krumholz HM. Sex-based differences in the effect of digoxin for the treatment of heart failure. *N Engl J Med* 2002;347:1403–1411.
163. Fozzard HA, Sheets MF. Cellular mechanism of action of cardiac glycosides. *J Am Coll Cardiol* 1985;5:10A–15A.
164. Charlemagne D. Molecular and cellular level of action of digitalis. *Herz* 1993;18:79.
165. Li P, Park C, Micheletti R, et al. Myocyte performance during evolution of myocardial infarction in rats: Effects of propionyl-*L*-carnitine. *Am J Physiol* 1995;268:H1702–1713.
166. Mason DT, Braunwald E, Karsh RB, Bullock FA. Studies on digitalis. X: Effects on ouabain on forearm vascular resistance and venous tone in normal subjects and in patients with heart failure. *J Clin Invest* 1964;43:532–543.
167. Van Veldhuisen DJ, de Graeff PA, Remme WJ, Lie KI. Value of digoxin in heart failure and sinus rhythm: New features of an old drug? *J Am Coll Cardiol* 1996;28:813–819.
168. Kraus F, Rudolph C, Rudolph W. Efficacy of digitalis in patients with chronic congestive heart failure and sinus rhythm: An overview of randomized, double-blind, placebo-controlled studies. *Herz* 1993; 18:95.
169. Packer M, Gheorghiade M, Young JB, et al. Withdrawal of digoxin from patients with chronic heart failure treated with angiotensin-converting-enzyme inhibitors. RADIANCE Study. *N Engl J Med* 1993;329:1–7.
170. Adams KF Jr., Gheorghiade M, Uretsky BF, et al. Patients with mild heart failure worsen during withdrawal from digoxin therapy. *J Am Coll Cardiol* 1997;30:42–48.
171. Captopril-Digoxin Multicenter Research Group. Comparative effects of therapy with captopril and digoxin in patients with mild to moderate heart failure. *JAMA* 1988;259:539–544.
172. Slatton ML, Irani WN, Hall SA, et al. Does digoxin provide additional hemodynamic and autonomic benefit at higher doses in patients with mild to moderate heart failure and normal sinus rhythm? *J Am Coll Cardiol* 1997;29:1206–1213.
173. Tauke J, Goldstein S, Gheorghiade M. Digoxin for chronic heart failure: A review of the randomized controlled trials with special attention to the PROVED and RADIANCE Trials. *Prog Cardiovasc Dis* 1994;37:49–58.
174. Hoffman BB, Taylor P. Neurotransmission: The autonomic and somatic motor nervous system. In Hardman JG, Limbird LE (eds): *Goodman & Gilman's The Pharmacological Basis of Therapeutics,* 10th ed. New York: McGraw-Hill; 2001:115–153.
175. Kelley RB. Storage and release of neurotransmitters. *Cell/Neuron* 1993;72/10 (suppl):43–53.
176. Insel PA. Adrenergic receptors—evolving concepts and clinical implications. *N Engl J Med* 1996;334:580–585.
177. Frishman WH. Advances in positive inotropic therapy: levosimendan (editorial). *Crit Care Med* 2003;31:2408–2409.
178. Goldberg LI, Raifer SI. Dopamine receptors: Applications in clinical cardiology. *Circulation* 1985;72:245–248.
179. Sonnenblick EH, Frishman WH, LeJemtel TH. Dobutamine: A new synthetic cardioactive sympathetic amine. *N Engl J Med* 1979;300: 17–22.
180. Braunwald E, Sonnenblick EH, Chakrin LW, et al (eds). *Milrinone Investigation: A New Inotropic Therapy for Congestive Heart Failure*. New York: Raven;1984.
181. Grose R, Strain J, Greenberg M, LeJemtel TH. Systemic and coronary effects of intravenous milrinone and dobutamine in congestive heart failure. *J Am Coll Cardiol* 1986;7:1107–1113.
182. Nielsen-Kudsk JE, Aldershville J. Will calcium sensitizers play a role in the treatment of heart failure? *J Cardiovasc Pharmacol* 1995; 26 (suppl 1):S77–S84.
183. Packer M, Carver JR, Rodeheffer RJ, et al for the PROMISE Study Research Group. Effect of oral milrinone on mortality in severe chronic heart failure. *N Engl J Med* 1991;325:1468–1475.
184. Cuffe MS, Califf RM, Adams KF Jr., et al for the Outcomes of a Prospective Trial of Intravenous Milrinone for Exacerbation of Chronic Heart Failure (OPTIME-CHF) Investigators: Short-term intravenous milrinone for acute exacerbation of chronic heart failure. A randomized controlled trial. *JAMA* 2002;287:1541–1547.
185. Rector TW, Cohn JN with the Pimobendan Multicenter Research Group. Assessment of patient outcome with the Minnesota Living with Heart Failure questionnaire: Reliability and validity during a randomized, double-blind, placebo-controlled trial of pimobendan. *Am Heart J* 1992;124:1017–1025.
186. Lilleberg J, Sundberg S, Nieminen MS. Dose-range study of a new calcium sensitizer, levosimendan, in patients with left ventricular dysfunction. *J Cardiovasc Pharmacol* 1995;26(suppl 1):S63–S69.
187. Follath F, Cleland JGF, Just H, et al. Efficacy and safety of intravenous levosimendan compared with dobutamine in severe low-output heart failure (LIDO study): A randomized double-blind trial. *Lancet* 2002; 360:196–202.
187a. Vasan RS, Beiser A, D'Agostino RB, et al. Plasma homocysteine and risk of congestive heart failure in adults without prior myocardial infarction. *JAMA* 2003;289:1251–1257.
188. Frishman WH, Gomberg-Maitland M, Freeman R, et al. Hormones as cardiovascular drugs: Estrogens, progestins, thyroxine, growth hormone, corticosteroids, and testosterone. In: Frishman WH, Sonnenblick EH, Sica DA eds. *Cardiovascular Pharmacotherapeutics,* 2nd ed. New York: McGraw-Hill; 2003:617–654.
189. Sullivan M, Simon G, Spertus J, Russo J. Depression-related costs in heart failure care. *Arch Intern Med* 2002;162:1860–1866.
189a. Khawaja IS, Feinstein RE. Cardiovascular effects of selective serotonin reuptake inhibitors and other novel antidepressants. *Heart Dis* 2003;5:153–160.
190. Al-Khadra AS, Salem DN, Rand WM, et al. Warfarin anticoagulation and survival: a cohort analysis from the Studies of Left Ventricular Dysfunction. *J Am Coll Cardiol* 1998;31:749–753.

191. Sokol SI, Cheng-Lai A, Frishman WH, Kaza CS. Cardiovascular drug therapy in patients with hepatic diseases and patients with congestive heart failure. *J Clin Pharmacol* 2000;40:11–30.
192. McAlister FA, Teo KT. The management of congestive heart failure. *Postgrad Med J* 1997;73:194–200.
193. Singh SN, Fletcher RD, Fisher SG, et al. Amiodarone in patients with congestive heart failure and asymptomatic ventricular arrhythmia. *N Engl J Med* 1995;333:77–82.
194. Gottdiener JS, Reda DJ, Massie BM, et al for the VA Cooperative Study Group of Antihypertensive Agents. Effect of single-drug therapy on reduction of left ventricular mass in mild to moderate hypertension comparison of six antihypertensive agents. The Department of Veterans Affairs Cooperative Study Group on Antihypertensive Agents. *Circulation* 1997;95:2007–2014.
194a. Yusuf S, Pfeffer MA, Swedberg K, et al, for the CHARM Investigators and Committees. Effects of candesartan in patients with chronic heart failure and preserved left ventricular ejection fraction: the CHARM-Preserved Trial. *Lancet* 2003;362:777–781.
195. Nul DR, Doval HC, Grancelli HO, et al. Heart rate is a marker of amiodarone mortality reduction in severe heart failure. *J Am Coll Cardiol* 1997;29:1199–1205.
196. Moss AJ, Zareba W, Hall WJ, et al, for the Multicenter Automatic Defibrillator Implantation Trial II Investigators. Prophylactic implantation of a defibrillator in patients with myocardial infarction and reduced ejection fraction. *N Engl J Med* 2002;346:877–883.
197. Nemeh HW, Smedira NG. Mechanical treatment of heart failure: the growing role of LVADs and artificial hearts. *Cleveland Clin J Med* 2003;70:223–233.
198. Mann DL, Willerson JT. Left ventricular assist devices and the failing heart. A bridge to recovery, a permanent assist device, or a bridge too far? (editorial) *Circulation* 1998;98:2367–2369.
199. Mancini DM, Beniaminovitz A, Levin H, et al. Low incidence of myocardial recovery after left ventricular assist device implantation in patients with chronic heart failure. *Circulation* 1998;98:2383–2389.
200. Hetzer R, Müller J, Weng Y, et al. Cardiac recovery in dilated cardiomyopathy by unloading with a left ventricular assist device. *Ann Thorac Surg* 1999;68:742–749.
201. The Registry of the International Society of Heart and Lung Transplantation. Ninth Official Report 1992. *J Heart Lung Transplant* 1992;11:599–606.
202. Paris W, Woodbury A, Thompson S, et al. Returning to work after heart transplantation. *J Heart Lung Transplant* 1993;12:46–54.
203. Mickleborough LL, Carson S, Tamariz M, Ivanov J. Results of revascularization in patients with severe left ventricular dysfunction. *J Thorac Cardiovasc Surg* 2000;119:550–557.
204. Maddahi J, Schelbert H, Brunken R, DiCarli M. Role of thallium-201 and PET imaging in evaluation of myocardial viability and management of patients with coronary artery disease and left ventricular dysfunction. *J Nucl Med* 1994;35:707–715.
205. Samady H, Elefteriades JA, Abbott BG, et al. Failure to improve left ventricular function after coronary revascularization for ischemic cardiomyopathy is not associated with worse outcome. *Circulation* 1999;100:1298–1304.
206. Elefteriades JA, Tolis G Jr, Levi E, et al. Coronary artery bypass grafting in severe left ventricular dysfunction: Excellent survival with improved ejection fraction and functional state. *J Am Coll Cardiol* 1993;22:1411–1417.
207. Pitt M, Lewis ME, Bonser RS. Coronary artery surgery for ischemic heart failure: risks, benefits and the importance of assessment of myocardial viability. *Prog Cardiovasc Dis* 2001;43:373–386.
208. Thomas B, Batista RJV. Left ventricular reduction surgery. *Heart Failure* 2000;2:248–253.
208a. Pagani FD, DerSimonian H, Zawadzka A, et al. Autologous skeletal myoblasts transplanted to ischemia-damaged myocardium in humans. *J Am Coll Cardiol* 2003;41:879–888.
208b. Frishman WH, Anversa P. Stem cell therapy for myocardial regeneration: The future is now (editorial). *Heart Dis* 2002;4:205.
208c. Toma C, Pittenger MF, Cahill KS, et al. Human mesenchymal stem cells differentiate to a cardiomyocyte phenotype in the adult murine heart. *Circulation* 2002;105:93–98.
208d. Orlic D, Kajstura J, Chimenti S, et al. Bone marrow cells regenerate infarcted myocardium. *Nature* 2001;410:710–705.
208e. Quaini F, Urbanek K, Beltrami AP, et al. Chimerism of the transplanted heart. *N Engl J Med* 2002;346:5–15.
208f. Beltrami AP, Urbanek K, Kajstura J, et al. Evidence that human cardiac myocytes divide after myocardial infarction. *N Engl J Med* 2001;344:1750–1757.
208g. Beltrami AP, Barlucci L, Torella D, et al. Adult cardiac stem cells are multipotent and support myocardial regeneration. *Cell* 2003;114:763–776.
209. Gorcsan III J, Crawford L, Soran O, et al. Improvement in left ventricular performance by enhanced external counterpulsation in patients with heart failure (abst). *J Am Coll Cardiol* 2000;35(suppl A):230A.
210. Dörffel WV, Felix SB, Wallukat G, et al. Short-term hemodynamic effects of immunoabsorption in dilated cardiomyopathy. *Circulation* 1997;95:1994–1997.
211. Frishman WH. Recent advances in cardiovascular pharmacology. *Curr Probl Cardiol* 2000;25(4):221–296.
212. Cavero PG, Margulies KB, Winaver J, et al. Cardiorenal actions of neutral endopeptidase inhibition in experimental congestive heart failure. *Circulation* 1990;82:196–201.
213. Northridge DB, Jardine AG, Alabaster CT, et al. Effects of UK 69 578: A novel atriopeptidase inhibitor. *Lancet* 1989;2:591–593.
214. Frishman WH, Nawarskas J, Rajan V, Sica DA. Vasopeptidase inhibitors: neutral endopeptidase inhibitors and dual inhibitors of angiotensin converting enzyme and neutral endopeptidase. In: Frishman WH, Sonnenblick EH, Sica DA, eds. *Cardiovascular Pharmacotherapeutics,* 2nd ed. New York: McGraw-Hill; 2003:813–820.
215. Northridge DB, Jackson NC, Metcalfe MJ, et al. Effects of candoxatril, a novel endopeptidase inhibitor, compared with frusemide in mild chronic heart failure. Proceedings of the British Pharmacological Society, University of Glasgow, July 10–12, 1991. *Br J Clin Pharmacol* 1991;32:645.
216. Lang CC, Motwani J, Coutie W, Struthers AD. Influence of candoxatril on plasma brain natriuretic peptide in heart failure. *Lancet* 1991;338:255.
217. Munzel T, Kurz S, Holtz J, et al. Neurohumoral inhibition and hemodynamic unloading during prolonged inhibition of ANP degradation in patients with severe chronic heart failure. *Circulation* 1992;86:1089–1098.
218. Rouleau JL, Pfeffer MA, Stewart DJ, et al, for the IMPRESS Investigators: Comparison of vasopeptidase inhibitor, omapatrilat, and lisinopril on exercise tolerance and morbidity in patients with heart failure: IMPRESS randomized trial. *Lancet* 2000;356:615–620.
219. Packer M, Califf RM, Konstam MV, et al for the OVERTURE Study Group. Comparison of omapatrilat and enalapril in patients with chronic heart failure. The Omapatrilat Versus Enalapril Randomized Trial of Utility in Reducing Events (OVERTURE). *Circulation* 2002;106:920–926.
220. Nagaya N, Satoh T, Nishikimi T, et al. Hemodynamic, renal and hormonal effects of adrenomedullin infusion in patients with congestive heart failure. *Circulation* 2000;101:498–503.
221. Frishman WH, Kaur S, Singh I, Tamirisa P. Endothelin as a therapeutic target in the treatment of cardiovascular disease. In Frishman WH, Sonnenblick EH, Sica DA (eds): *Cardiovascular Pharmacotherapeutics,* 2nd ed. New York: McGraw Hill; 2003;527–543.
222. Moe GW, Ferrazzi S, Naik G, Howard RJ. Endothelin in heart failure: Temporal evolution, source of production and interaction with atrial natriuretic peptide (abstr). *Circulation* 1994;90(4, pt 2):I-592.
223. Pacher R, Stanek B, Hulsmann M, et al. Prognostic impact of big endothelin-1 plasma concentrations compared with invasive hemodynamic evaluation in severe heart failure. *J Am Coll Cardiol* 1996;27:633–641.
224. Sakai S, Miyauchi T, Sakurai T, et al. Endogenous endothelin-1 participates in the maintenance of cardiac function in rats with congestive

heart failure. Marked increase in endothelin-1 production in the failing heart. *Circulation* 1996;93:1214–1222.

225. Webb DJ. Evidence for endothelin-1-mediated vasoconstriction in severe chronic heart failure. Endothelin antagonism in heart failure. *Circulation* 1995;92:3372.

226. Cannan CR, Burnett JC Jr, Lerman A. Enhanced coronary vasoconstriction to endothelin-B-receptor activation in experimental congestive heart failure. *Circulation* 1996;93:646–651.

227. Krum H, Gu A, Wilshire Clement M, et al. Changes in plasma endothelin-1 levels reflect clinical response to beta blockade in chronic heart failure. *Am Heart J* 1996;131:337–341.

228. Inada T, Tanaka M, Hasegawa K, et al. Increased levels of endothelin-1 in plasma and heart tissue of cardiomyopathic Syrian hamsters (abstr). *Circulation* 1994;90(4, pt 2):I-260.

229. Wittner M, Morris SA, Christ GJ, et al. Infection of cultured human endothelial cells increasesendothelin levels (abstr). *Circulation* 1994; 90(4, pt 2):I-293.

230. Givertz MM, Colucci WS, LeJemtel TH, et al. Acute endothelin A receptor blockade causes selective pulmonary vasodilation in patients with chronic heart failure. *Circulation* 2000;101:2922–2927.

231. Sakai S, Miyauchi T, Yamaguchi I. Long-term endothelin receptor antagonist administration improves alterations in expression of various cardiac genes in failing myocardium of rats with heart failure. *Circulation* 2000;101:2849.

232. Wada A, Tsutamoto T, Ohnishi M, et al. Effects of a specific endothelin-converting enzyme inhibitor on cardiac, renal, and neurohumoral functions in congestive heart failure. Comparison of effects with those of endothelin A receptor antagonism. *Circulation* 1999;99:570.

233. Wada A, Tsutamoto T, Fukai D, et al. Comparison of the effects of selective endothelin ETA and ETB receptor antagonists in congestive heart failure. *J Am Coll Cardiol* 1997:30(5):1385.

234. Packer M, Caspi A, Charlon V, et al. Multicenter, double-blind, placebo-controlled study of long-term endothelin blockade with bosentan in chronic heart failure—results of the REACH-1 trial. *Circulation* 1998;98 (suppl S):12.

235. Ruschitzka F, Noll G, Mitrovic V, et al. Clinical and hemodynamic effects of chronic selective ETA-receptor blockade in congestive heart failure (HEAT, Heart Failure ETA Receptor Blockade Trial). *Eur Heart J* 2000;71(suppl S):705.

236. Kaluski E, Kobrin I, Zimlichman R, et al, for the RITZ-5 Investigators. Randomized IV tezosentan (an endothelin A/B antagonist) for the treatment of pulmonary edema. A prospective, multicenter, double-blind, placebo-controlled study. *J Am Coll Cardiol* 2003;41: 204–210.

237. Ellahham SH, Charlon V, Abassi Z, et al. Bosentan and endothelin system in congestive heart failure. *Clin Cardiol* 2000;23:803.

237a. Philipp S, Monti J, Pagel I, et al. Treatment with darusentan over 21 days improved cGMP generation in patients with chronic heart failure. *Clin Sci (London)* 2002;103(Suppl 48):249s–253s.

237b. Cosenzi A. Enrasentan, an antagonist of endothelin receptors. *Cardiovasc Drug Rev* 2003;21:1–16.

238. Moore J. ENABLE 1, 2: Bosentan did not improve HF symptoms. *Today Cardiol* 2002;5:8.

239. Frishman WH, Klapholz M, Acharya N, Mayerson AB. Vasopressin and vasopressin receptor antagonists in cardiovascular disease. In: Frishman WH, Sonnenblick EH, Sica DA, eds. *Cardiovascular Pharmacotherapeutics,* 2nd ed. New York: McGraw-Hill; 2003:601–616.

240. Manning M, Sawyer WH. Discovery, development and some uses of vasopressin and oxytocin antagonists. *J Lab Clin Med* 1989;114: 617–632.

241. Gheorghiade M, Niazi I, Ouyang J, et al: Chronic Effects of Vasopressin Receptor Blockade with Tolvaptan in Congestive Heart Failure: A Randomized, Double-Blind Trial (abstr). *Circulation* 2000; 102:II-592.

242. Abraham WT, Suresh DP, Wagoner LE, et al. Pharmacotherapy for hyponatremia in heart failure: effects of a new dual $V_{1a}/V_2$ vasopressin antagonist YM087 (abstr). *Circulation* 1999;100:I-299.

243. Kuan CJ, Herzer WA, Jackson EK. Cardiovascular and renal effects of blocking A1 adenosine receptors. *J Cardiovasc Pharmacol* 1993; 21:822–828.

244. Frishman WH, Gianos E, Lee J, Somer BG. Adenosine receptor agonism and antagonism in cardiovascular disease. In: Frishman WH, Sonnenblick EH, Sica DA, eds. *Cardiovascular Pharmacotherapeutics,* 2nd ed. New York: McGraw-Hill; 2003:545–564.

245. Balakrishnan VS, Coles GA, Williams JD. A potential role for endogenous adenosine in control of human glomerular and tubular function. *Am J Physiol* 1993;265:F504–510.

246. VanBuren M, Bijlsma JA, Boer P, et al. Natriuretic and hypotensive effect of adenosine-1 blockade in essential hypertension. *Hypertension* 1993;22:728–734.

247. Frishman WH, Hotchkiss H. Selective and nonselective dopamine receptor agonists. In: Frishman WH, Sonnenblick EH, Sica DA, eds. *Cardiovascular Pharmacotherapeutics,* 2nd ed. New York: McGraw-Hill; 2003:443–449.

248. Hampton JR, Van Veldhuisen DJ, Kleber FX, et al. Randomised study of effect of ibopamine on survival in patients with advanced severe heart failure: Second Prospective Randomised Study of Ibopamine on Mortality and Efficacy (PRIME II) Investigators. *Lancet* 1997;349:971–977.

249. Post JB IV, Frishman WH. Fenoldopam: a new dopamine agonist for the treatment of hypertensive urgencies and emergencies. *J Clin Pharmacol* 1998;38:2–13.

250. Mann DL, Young JB. Basic mechanisms in congestive heart failure: Recognizing the role of proinflammatory cytokines. *Chest* 1994;105: 897–904.

251. Muray DR, Freeman GL. Proinflammatory cytokines. Predictors of a failing heart? *Circulation* 2003;107:1460–1462.

252. Raymond RJ, Dehmer GJ, Theoharides TC, et al. Elevated interleukin-6 levels in patients with asymptomatic left ventricular systolic dysfunction. *Am Heart J* 2001;141:435–438.

253. Yokoyama T, Vaca L, Rossen RD, et al. Cellular basis for the negative inotropic effects of tumor necrosis factor-alpha in the adult mammalian heart. *J Clin Invest* 1993;92:2303–2312.

254. Bazzoni F, Beutler B. The tumor necrosis factor ligand and receptor families. *N Engl J Med* 1996;334:1717–1725.

255. Frishman WH, Retter A, Mobati D, Fernandez M, et al. Innovative drug targets for treating cardiovascular disease: Adhesion molecules, cytokines, neuropeptide Y, calcineurin, bradykinin, urotensin, and heat shock protein. In: Frishman WH, Sonnenblick EH, Sica DA, eds. *Cardiovascular Pharmacotherapeutics,* 2nd ed. New York: McGraw-Hill; 2003:705–739.

256. Katz SD, Rao R, Berman JW, et al. Pathophysiological correlates of increased serum tumor necrosis factor in patients with congestive heart failure: Relation to nitric oxide dependant vasodilation in the forearm circulation. *Circulation* 1994;90:12–16.

257. Mohler ER III, Sorensen LC, Ghali JK, et al. Role of cytokines in the mechanism of action of amlodipine: The PRAISE Heart Failure Trial. *J Am Coll Cardiol* 1997;30:35–41.

258. Bozkurt B, Torre-Amione G, Warren MS, et al. Results of targeted anti-tumor necrosis factor therapy with etanercept (ENBREL) in patients with advanced heart failure. *Circulation* 2001;103:1044–1047.

259. Nishio R, Matsumori A, Shioi T, et al. Treatment of experimental viral myocarditis with interleukin-10. *Circulation* 1999;100:1102–08.

260. Frishman WH, O'Brien M, Naseer N, Anandasabapathy S: Innovative drug treatments for viral and autoimmune myocarditis. *Heart Dis* 2002;4:171–183.

261. Parrillo JE, Cunnion RE, Epstein SE, et al. A prospective, randomized, controlled trial of prednisone for dilated cardiomyopathy. *N Engl J Med* 1989;321:1061–1068.

262. Mason JW, O'Connell JB, Herskowitz A, et al. A clinical trial of immunosuppressive therapy for myocarditis. *N Engl J Med* 1995;333: 269–275.

263. Aukrust P, Gullestad L, Lappegard KT, et al. Complement activation of patients with congestive heart failure. Effect of high dose intravenous immunoglobulin treatment. *Circulation* 2001;104:1494–1500.

264. Matsumoto A, Momomura S, Sugiura S, et al. Effect of inhaled nitric oxide on gas exchange in patients with congestive heart failure: A randomized, controlled trial. *Ann Intern Med* 1999;130:40–44.

265. Natori S, Hasebe N, Jin YT, et al. Inhaled nitric oxide modifies left ventricular diastolic stress in the presence of vasoactive agents in heart failure. *Am J Respir Crit Care Med* 2003;167:895–901.

266. Frishman WH, Helisch A, Naseer N, et al. Nitric oxide donors in the treatment of cardiovascular disease. In: Frishman WH, Sonnenblick EH, Sica DA, eds. *Cardiovascular Pharmacotherapeutics,* 2nd ed. New York: McGraw-Hill; 2003:565–587.

267. Bocchi EA, Guimaraes G, Mocelin A, et al. Sildenafil effects on exercise, neurohormonal activation, and erectile dysfunction in congestive heart failure. A double-blind, placebo-controlled, randomized study followed by a prospective treatment for erectile dysfunction. *Circulation* 2002;106:1097–1103.

268. Frishman WH, Palkhiwala SA, Yu A, Rim F. Imidazoline receptor agonist drugs for treatment of systemic hypertension and congestive heart failure. In: Frishman WH, Sonnenblick EH, Sica DA, eds. *Cardiovascular Pharmacotherapeutics,* 2nd ed. New York: McGraw-Hill; 2003:515–525.

269. Frishman WH, Ahangar BA, Sinha S. Matrix metalloproteinases and their inhibitors in cardiovascular disease. In: Frishman WH, Sonnenblick EH, Sica DA, eds. *Cardiovascular Pharmacotherapeutics,* 2nd ed. New York: McGraw-Hill; 2003:797–811.

270. Gomberg-Maitland M, Frishman WH. Recombinant growth hormone: a new cardiovascular drug therapy. *Am Heart J* 1996;132: 1244–1262.

271. Frishman WH, Retter A, Misalidis J, et al. Innovative pharmacologic approaches for the treatment of myocardial ischemia. In: Frishman WH, Sonnenblick EH, Sica DA, eds. *Cardiovascular Pharmacotherapeutics,* 2nd ed. New York: McGraw-Hill; 2003:655–690.

272. Retter A. Carnitine and its role in cardiovascular disease. *Heart Disease* 1999;1:108–113.

273. Witte KKA, Clark AL, Cleland JGF. Chronic heart failure and micronutrients. *J Am Coll Cardiol* 2001;37:1765–1774.

274. Frishman WH, Kruger NA, Nayak DU, Vakili BA. Antioxidant vitamins and enzymatic and synthetic oxygen-derived free radical scavengers in the prevention and treatment of cardiovascular disease. In: Frishman WH, Sonnenblick EH, Sica DA, eds. *Cardiovascular Pharmacotherapeutics,* 2nd ed. New York: McGraw-Hill; 2003:407–427.

274a. Abbate A, Biondi-Zoccai GGL, Bussani R, et al. Increased myocardial apoptosis in patients with unfavorable left ventricular remodeling and early symptomatic post-infarction heart failure. *J Am Coll Cardiol* 2003;41:753–760.

275. Frishman WH, Guttenplan N, Leehealey C, et al. Inhibition of myocardial apoptosis as a therapeutic target: focus on caspase inhibition. In: Frishman WH, Sonnenblick EH, Sica DA, eds. *Cardiovascular Pharmacotherapeutics,* 2nd ed. New York: McGraw-Hill; 2003: 789–796.

276. del Monte F, Harding SE, Schmidt U, et al. Restoration of contractile function in isolated cardiomyocytes from failing human hearts by gene transfer of SERCA2a. *Circulation* 1999;100:2308–11.

277. Medin JA, Buttrick PM. Gene transfer in the cardiovascular system. In: Frishman WH, Sonnenblick EH, Sica DA, eds. *Cardiovascular Pharmacotherapeutics,* 2nd ed. New York: McGraw-Hill; 2003: 777–788.

278. Meyer M, Bluhm WF, He H, et al. Phospholamban-to-SERCA2 ratio controls the force-frequency relationship. *Am J Physiol* 1999;276: H779–85.

279. Ankers S, Ponikowski P, Varney S, et al. Wasting as an independent risk factor for mortality in chronic heart failure. *Lancet* 1997;349: 1050–1053.

280. Frishman WH, Del Vecchio A, Sanal S, Ismail A. Cardiovascular manifestations of substance abuse (Part 1 Cocaine;Part 2 Alcohol, amphetamines, heroin, cannabis, caffeine). *Heart Dis* 2003:5:187–201.

281. Mancini DM, Davis L, Wexler JP, et al. Dependence of enhanced maximal exercise performance on increased peak skeletal muscle perfusion during long-term captopril therapy in heart failure. *J Am Coll Cardiol* 1987;10:845–850.

282. Coats AJS, Adamopoulos S, Radeaelli A, et al. Controlled trial of physical training in chronic heart failure. Exercise performance, hemodynamics, ventilation and autonomic function. *Circulation* 1992; 85:2119–2131.

283. Hambrecht R, Niebauer J, Fiehn E, et al. Physical training in patients with stable chronic heart failure: Effects on cardiorespiratory fitness and ultra-structural abnormalities of leg muscles. *J Am Coll Cardiol* 1995;25:1239–1249.

283a. Monchamp T, Frishman WH. Exercise as a treatment modality for congestive heart failure. *Heart Dis* 2002;4:110–116.

283b. Midelton GT, Frishman WH, Passo SS. Congestive heart failure and continuous positive airway pressure therapy: Support of a new modality for improving the prognosis and survival of patients with advanced congestive heart failure. *Heart Dis* 2002;4:102–109.

284. Dickstein K, Kjekshus J, and the OPTIMAAL Steering Committee for the OPTIMAAL Study Group. Effects of losartan and captopril on mortality and morbidity in high-risk patients after acute myocardial infarction: The OPTIMAAL randomized trial. *Lancet* 2002;360: 752–760.

285. Dahlof B, Devereux RB, Kjeldsen SE, et al, for the LIFE study group. Cardiovascular morbidity and mortality in the Losartan Intervention for Endpoint reduction in hypertensive study (LIFE): A randomized trial against atenolol. *Lancet* 2002;359:995–1003.

286. Hjalmarson A, Goldstein S, Fagerberg B, et al, for the MERIT-HF Study Group. Effects of controlled-released metoprolol on total mortality, hospitalizations, and well-being in patients with heart failure. The Metoprolol CR/XL Randomized Intervention Trial in Congestive Heart Failure (MERIT-HF). *JAMA* 2000;283:1295–1302.

287. $\beta$-Blocker Heart Attack Trial Research Group. A randomized trial of propranolol in patients with acute myocardial infarction. 1. Mortality results. *JAMA* 1982;247:1707–1714.

288. Ambrosioni E, Borghi C, Magnani B, for the Survival of Myocardial Infarction Long-Term Evaluation (SMILE) Study Investigators. The effect of the angiotensin converting enzyme inhibitor zofenopril on mortality and morbidity after anterior myocardial infarction. *N Engl J Med* 1995;332:80–85.

289. Gruppo Italiano per lo Studio della Sopravvivenza nell-Infarto Miocardico: GISSI 3. Effects of lisinopril and transdermal glyceryl trinitrate singly and together on 6-week mortality and ventricular function after acute myocardial infarction. *Lancet* 1994;343:1115–1122.

290. Swedberg K, Held P, Kjekshus J, et al, on behalf of the CONSENSUS II Study Group. Effects of the early administration of enalapril on mortality in patients with acute myocardial infarction. *N Engl J Med* 1992;327:678–684.

291. Kober L, Torp-Pedersen C, Carlsen JE, et al, for the Trandolapril Cardiac Evaluation (TRACE) Study Group. A clinical trial of the angiotensin converting enzyme inhibitor trandolapril in patients with left ventricular dysfunction after myocardial infarction. *N Engl J Med* 1995;333:1670–1676.

292. The Acute Infarction Ramipril Efficacy (AIRE) Study Investigators. Effect of ramipril on mortality and morbidity of survivors of acute myocardial infarction with clinical evidence of heart failure. *Lancet* 1993;342:821–828.

293. Scandinavian Simvastatin Survival Study Group. Randomised trial of cholesterol lowering in 4444 patients with coronary heart disease: The Scandinavian Simvastatin Survival Study (4S). *Lancet* 1994;344: 1383–1389.

294. Efficacy of perindopril in reduction of cardiovascular events among patients with stable coronary artery disease: Randomised, double blind, placebo controlled, multicentre trial (the EUROPA study). *Lancet* 2003;362:782–785.

295. Pfeffer MA, Swedberg K, Granger CB, et al, for the CHARM Investigators and Committee. Effects of candesartan on mortality and morbidity in patients with chronic heart failure. The CHARM-Overall Programme. *Lancet* 2003;362:759–766.

296. McMurray JJV, Ostergren J, Swedberg K, et al, for the CHARM Investigators and Committees. Effects of candesartan in patients with chronic heart failure and reduced left ventricular systolic function taking angiotensin converting enzyme inhibitors: The CHARM-Added Trial. *Lancet* 2003;362:767–771.
297. Granger CB, McMurray JJV, Yusuf S, et al, for the CHARM Investigators and Committees. Effects of candesartan in patients with chronic heart failure and reduced left ventricular systolic function intolerant to angiotensin converting enzyme inhibitors: The CHARM-Alternative Trial. *Lancet* 2003;362:772–767.
298. ISIS Collaborative Group: ISIS-4. Randomized study of oral captopril in over 50,000 patients with suspected acute myocardial infarction (abst). *Circulation* 1993;88 Suppl I: I–394.
299. Cohn JN, Archibald DG, Ziesche S, et al. Effects of vasodilator therapy on mortality in chronic congestive heart failure: Results of a Veterans Administration Cooperative Study. *N Engl J Med* 1986;314: 1547–1552.
300. Pfeffer MA, McMurray JJV, Velazquez EJ, et al, for the Valsartan in Acute Myocardial Infarction Trial Investigators. Valsartan, captopril, or both in myocardial infarction complicated by heart failure, left ventricular dysfunction, or both. *N Engl J Med* 2003;349: 1893–1906.

CHAPTER 26

# SURGICAL TREATMENT OF HEART FAILURE, CARDIAC TRANSPLANTATION, AND MECHANICAL VENTRICULAR SUPPORT

John S. Schroeder / Susan D. Moffatt / Gerald J. Berry / Robert C. Robbins



## HISTORY AND OVERVIEW

Although several major advances in the treatment for progressive myocardial failure have saved or at least prolonged the lives of many patients with previously terminal myocardial dysfunction, a sizable number of young patients are fated to die or be severely disabled because of irreversible myocardial disease. In patients with such end-stage disease, biological replacement of the heart has become standard therapy; it is currently widely accepted as a modality for prolonging life and improving its quality in carefully selected patients. As technological and engineering advances occur, mechanical replacement of the heart and xenotransplantation (transplantation of animal organs) may become competitive or complementary modalities for the treatment of such patients; however biological replacement with human donor hearts is the current standard of therapy.

Interest in developing surgical techniques to interpose a functioning heart into a recipient's circulation dates back at least to the early part of the twentieth century. In 1905, Carrel and Guthrie[1] described the heterotopic transplantation of a functioning donor heart into the neck of a dog. The heart in that model functioned in sequence with the recipient's heart in the circulation and was not actually capable of supporting the circulation. Although the exact anatomic connections were not described in detail, this apparently nonworking model of heterotopic transplantation beat regularly for approximately 2 h before the blood clotted in all the chambers. Carrel and his colleague Guthrie developed innovative surgical techniques for vascular anastomoses at the University of Chicago, and those advances set the stage for anastomoses leading to organ transplantation.[2] This work was partially responsible for Carrel being awarded the Nobel Prize for medicine and physiology in 1912.

It was not until 1933 that Mann and coworkers from the Mayo Clinic published their seminal report of a technique for heterotopic heart transplantation with circulatory loading of the right ventricle.[3] Presumably because this was a working model, the chambers did not clot immediately, and the hearts in their dogs beat for a mean of 4 days. Mann perceived several important surgical points, including the importance of avoiding ventricular distention and air embolism and the prevention of thrombosis by heparin. His most incisive and critical observation was that failure of a transplanted heart was not always due to faulty surgical technique "but to some biologic factor which is probably identical to that which prevents survival of other homotransplanted tissues and organs." In what was undoubtedly the first description of acute allograft rejection, Mann recounts: "When the heart was removed just before it became quiescent . . . the surface of the heart was covered with mottled areas of ecchymoses . . . histologically the heart was completely infiltrated by large mononuclears and polymorphonuclears."[3] It took another 30 years to better understand and manipulate the "biologic factor" Mann described as limiting the survival of allografted organs. In 1960, Lower and Shumway performed orthotopic heart transplants in dogs using cardiopulmonary bypass and topical hypothermia for donor heart preservation.[4] The dogs survived between 6 and 21 days and died of rejection. Lower and Shumway also recognized that "if the immunologic mechanisms of the host were prevented from destroying the graft, in

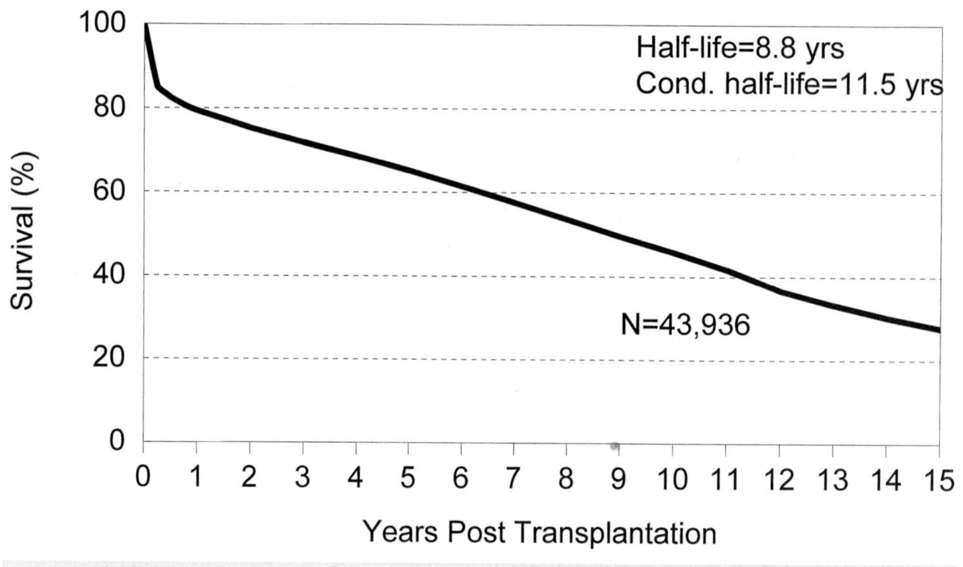


FIGURE 26-1 Data from the International Society for Heart and Lung Transplantation: overall cardiac transplant recipient postoperative survival rates. (From Hosenpud et al.,[11] with permission.)

all likelihood it would continue to function adequately for the normal lifespan of the animal." Their technique, involving anastomoses at the midatrial level and the supravalvular level in the great vessels, remained the basis of cardiac transplant technique in the 1990s.

In the early 1960s, the concept of pharmacologic immunosuppression was introduced; it ushered in the marriage of surgical and medical technology that is known today as the field of organ transplantation. Immunosuppression was, of course, seen as a means to mitigate the "biologic factor" that otherwise limited organ graft survival. The first clinical transplants were of the kidney, a logical choice since hemodialysis was then available as a backup system if the graft failed, and the field has flourished since the early 1960s.[5]

The first human heart allograft procedure was performed in South Africa in 1967,[6] followed shortly by the first U.S. transplant by Shumway at Stanford in 1968 and subsequently by a flurry of transplant activity in many centers.[7] This initial enthusiasm subsided as it became evident that postoperative survival was limited by a variety of complex medical problems, including opportunistic infections and graft rejection. Most major centers discontinued performing heart transplantation in the early 1970s, and it was not until the introduction of cyclosporine-based immunosuppression at Stanford in 1980 and the demonstration of the attendant improvement in survival rates[7] that the procedure reemerged as a widely accepted therapy for end-stage heart disease. In the 1990s, many tertiary care centers provided programs for heart transplantation, and most medical care payers in the United States, including the federal government, provided coverage for such care.

Cardiopulmonary transplantation was introduced at Stanford in 1981,[8] and subsequent experience with heart and lung and with both single- and double-lung transplantation in many centers has proved that these procedures are valid therapies for a wide variety of primary lung diseases and end-stage cardiopulmonary disorders.[9]

## Current Status

The most accurate data on volume and outcomes of thoracic organ transplantation are provided by the Registry of the International Society for Heart and Lung Transplantation and are updated yearly and published in the journal of that society. Since 1994, the Registry has been administered by the U.S. donor allocation organization, the United Network for Organ Sharing (UNOS), but it includes data on the vast majority of non-U.S. programs as well as all U.S. programs. As of the most recent Registry report,[9] there has been a plateau of heart transplant operations at approximately 2500 to 3500 procedures worldwide on an annual basis since the late 1980s, a level due to the limitations of donor availability. This report includes data on 61,533 transplant procedures reported since the Registry's inception in 1982 and documents overall patient survival rates of 79, 71, and 63 percent, at 1, 3, and 5 years, respectively (Fig. 26-1). After the first year, there is a linear attrition rate of 4 percent per year to a survival of about 40 to 50 percent at 10 years.

According to this Registry, there are currently 304 programs in clinical heart transplantation, of which 165 are in the United States. A large number of these U.S. programs have very low volume, and low volume is associated with inferior survival rates.[10,11]

# RECIPIENT SELECTION AND MANAGEMENT

As is the case with any surgical procedure, careful selection of patients for heart transplantation results in optimum postoperative survival rates. Decisions regarding candidacy for heart transplantation must take into consideration a limited donor supply and the necessity of following a highly complex medical regimen for the rest of the patient's posttransplant life. These considerations can make selecting recipients most difficult. Major guidelines for recipient selection have been developed and generally reflect experience with the selection of patients who are most likely to survive and benefit, with a return to a normal life after the transplant.

Some basic or general criteria can be described that are universally accepted; these criteria are summarized in Table 26-1. They include the most basic criterion: the existence of end-stage cardiac disease irremediable by other, more conventional forms of medical or surgical therapy. The increasingly long waiting times for a suitable

TABLE 26-1 Criteria for Acceptance of Cardiac Transplant Recipients

- Unacceptable heart failure that has not responded to an aggressive medical or surgical regimen
- Unacceptable prognosis for survival of 1–2 years
- Biological age less than 55–60 years
- Absence of irreversible pulmonary hypertension
- Absence of other systemic diseases that would limit long-term survival
- Medically compliant, with the ability to follow a complex medical regimen
- Adequate psychosocial support to assure compliance with medical directions and office visits
- Absence of self-abusive behavior that would interfere with postoperative course

TABLE 26-2 Typical Pharmacologic Regimen for Advanced Heart Failure Patients

| |
|---|
| ACE inhibitor/angiotensin II blocker |
| Loop diuretic |
| Triamterene/hydrochlorothiazide |
| Digoxin (low dose) |
| Coumadin |
| Enteric-coated aspirin if CAD |
| HMG-CoA reductase inhibitor if CAD |
| Beta-blocker trial |

ABBREVIATIONS: ACE = angiotensin-converting enzyme; CAD = coronary artery disease.

donor caused by increased patient numbers on the transplant waiting list now require the much more difficult task of estimating 1- to 2-year mortality in potential candidates. *With the recent major advances in heart failure therapy has come the realization that many transplant operations in patients referred for transplantation can be avoided by utilizing aggressive medical therapies.* Many transplant centers have found that as many as 30 to 50 percent of patients referred for heart transplants can be stabilized or even have their heart failure reversed by an aggressive, well-organized medical approach. Thus, most heart transplant centers have evolved into centers for heart failure management as well as transplantation. Table 26-2 lists a typical initial drug regimen for a patient with advanced heart failure who is waiting for a donor heart. The frequency of clinic visits for monitoring varies from every week to every 4 weeks, depending on the status of the patient. Furthermore, the introduction of transvenously placed antitachycardia and defibrillation devices and the increasing use of new beta blockers have improved the stabilization of patients in order to avoid or delay heart transplantation. Also, a small percentage of patients may have their left ventricular (LV) dysfunction reversed by high-risk percutaneous interventional procedures or coronary bypass surgery in order to restore blood flow to areas of "hibernating myocardium." It is also important to identify potentially reversible causes of cardiomyopathy as summarized in Table 26-3. Cessation of excessive alcohol intake or slowing of the ventricular rate with drugs or atrioventricular (AV) nodal ablation in patients with rapid heart rates occasionally results in a dramatic reversal of the heart failure.[12] Although it is more controversial, some centers continue to treat biopsy-proven acute lymphocytic myocarditis with high-dose steroids and giant-cell myocarditis with immunosuppression. This approach also is used for sarcoid cardiomyopathy.

Age limits for cardiac transplant recipients are a second criterion for acceptance, and those limits have been expanded considerably in both directions over the past several years. Since the advent of cyclosporine-based immunosuppression in 1980, it has become apparent that survival rates are no longer inferior in older age groups.[13] In the most recent year in which such data were analyzed in the Registry of the International Society for Heart Transplantation, the 30-day mortality rates according to age were identical (at 10 percent) for all ages between 10 and 69,[14] and in the current Registry data, 1- and 5-year mortality risk increases only slightly over age 65. Most centers have now advanced the official age of acceptability to 60 and may accept patients up to age 65 as well as highly selected patients over age 65.

TABLE 26-3 Identification of Potentially Reversible Causes of Congestive Heart Failure

| |
|---|
| Ischemic left ventricular dysfunction reversible with interventional or surgical reperfusion |
| Cardiomyopathy secondary to |
| Lymphocytic myocarditis |
| Sarcoidosis |
| Tachycardia |
| Ethanol |

Potential cardiac transplant recipients also are screened for the existence of any other systemic disease that independently is likely to limit their survival. The coexistence of an active malignancy and the potentially increased tendency for its advancement in the presence of immunosuppression are an obvious problem, and such patients are routinely excluded. How to deal with a patient with end-stage heart disease and a remote history of malignancy is a more difficult problem. Cautious acceptance of such patients may be justified.[15]

The coexistence of one other major systemic disease—insulin-requiring diabetes—had been considered a contraindication to cardiac transplantation in otherwise acceptable patients. As steroid requirements have become lower, this requirement generally has been relaxed to allow the inclusion of stable insulin-requiring diabetic patients, and in recent years several reports have attested to the safety and efficacy of heart transplantation in very carefully selected diabetic patients.[16–18]

*Human immunodeficiency virus (HIV)* positivity generally is considered an absolute contraindication to heart transplantation. Other comorbid conditions must be considered on an individual basis, but irreversible organ dysfunction such as emphysema, severe peripheral vascular disease, and hepatic or renal dysfunction out of proportion to that predictable as a consequence of severe congestive heart failure are strong relative contraindications. The presence of an active infection is an often temporary absolute contraindication to transplantation because of the mandatory posttransplant institution of immunosuppression. Early in the years of clinical experience with heart transplantation, it was found that a normal donor right ventricle (RV) is unable to increase its external workload acutely to overcome elevated *pulmonary vascular resistance (PVR)*. Because of this, patients who have end-stage heart disease with an elevated *PVR* often experience acute RV failure and cardiogenic shock after the transplantation of a healthy heart with a RV that has not been conditioned to pump against high resistance. This problem was a major cause of intraoperative deaths in the early years of transplantation and led to the setting of an upper limit of 4 Wood Units of *PVR* (approximately 320 dynes · s/cm$^5$) as the cutoff point, or fourth criterion, for suitability for cardiac transplantation. In recent years, the concept of reactivity of the pulmonary vasculature and the potential reversibility of elevated *PVR* has gained acceptance. Because of this, potential candidates with *PVR* greater than 4 Wood Units (320 dynes · s/cm$^5$) at baseline usually are subjected to pharmacologic maneuvers during hemodynamic monitoring, using nitroprusside and/or prostaglandin $E_1$ or inhaled nitric oxide to determine whether the elevated *PVR* is reversible; such patients are accepted as candidates for transplantation if the *PVR* can be reduced to acceptable levels while systemic arterial pressure remains adequate.

Experience has shown that *pulmonary infarcts* have a high probability of becoming pulmonary abscesses after the institution of immunosuppression. For this reason, waiting recipients who sustain a pulmonary infarction usually are removed temporarily from the waiting list until the infarct resolves radiographically. Unfortunately, such resolution can be quite slow.

On the basis of these criteria, a group of patients is selected who are believed to have the best chance of benefiting from the operation and the attendant substantial commitment of medical resources. The type of underlying heart disease in the adult population selected for the procedure is nearly evenly split between idiopathic cardiomyopathy and ischemic disease.

## DONOR SELECTION AND MANAGEMENT

Acceptance of the concept of brain death, both legally and medically, has been central to the emergence of organ transplantation in the modern era. The mandatory "warm ischemic time" that would be involved if cardiopulmonary death were the only accepted criterion of death would make heart transplantation impossible. Acceptance of the concept of irreversible brain death has been a perhaps surprisingly recent phenomenon. In 1970, Kansas became the first state in the United States to pass legislation recognizing the legal concept of brain death. The most recent and widely accepted set of guidelines was set out in the President's Commission Report in 1980.[19] It has been estimated that only 15 to 20 percent of persons who qualify as brain dead and have usable or transplantable organs become organ donors in the United States.[20] The reasons include a lack of public awareness of the potential to donate organs as well as reticence among medical staff to make a request for donation. Heart transplantation probably will be a donor-limited field for the foreseeable future.

To be considered suitable donors for cardiac transplantation, brain-dead individuals must meet certain minimum criteria. Age criteria vary, but most cardiac donors have been under age 40. The donor obviously should not have had any significant cardiac disease, malignant disease, or acute or chronic infection. Risk factors for cardiovascular disease such as diabetes and severe hypertension or hypercholesterolemia are relative exclusion factors. Donors routinely are screened serologically for human immunodeficiency virus (HIV) and hepatitis B and C. If there is any suspicion of cardiac disease in the donor, appropriate diagnostic studies (including echocardiography, cardiac catheterization, and coronary angiography) to assure the normality of the potential cardiac graft are pursued.

Once a potential donor is identified, the procurement process is initiated by contacting and referring to the local organ procurement organization (OPO), which maintains a registry of waiting recipients and coordinates equitable distribution of donor organs within a geographic area. Donor-recipient matching is fairly straightforward and requires ABO blood group compatibility as well as overall body size comparability, with $\pm 20$ percent body weight considered an acceptable discrepancy.

Most donor hearts currently are "harvested," or removed, from the donor by a transplant donor team from the transplantation center and transported back to the center for implantation. A "cold ischemic time" of 4 h in adult hearts generally is considered safe; this requirement leads to the rationale for geographic subdivision into OPOs for cardiac allografts despite the drive for a "national" list for other organs.

## SURGICAL TECHNIQUE

The surgical technique used in most centers today differs little from that described by Lower and Shumway in 1960.[4] With this procedure, both the donor and recipient hearts are removed by transecting the atria at the midatrial level, leaving the multiple pulmonary venous connections to the left atrium (LA) intact in the posterior wall of the LA, and then transecting the aorta and pulmonary artery just above their respective semilunar valves (Fig. 26-2).

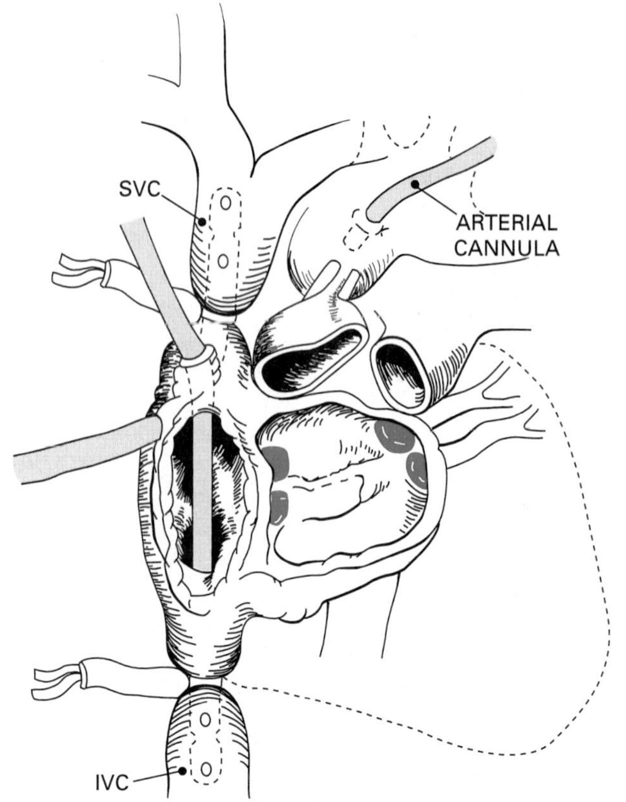

FIGURE 26-2 Diagram of recipient's mediastinum with heart resected and arterial and venous cannulas in place.

The donor heart usually is explanted, or harvested, by a surgical team at a hospital remote from the transplant center, and this surgery needs to be coordinated with the requirements of other surgical teams procuring nonthoracic organs for transplantation at other centers. The donor heart is arrested with cold crystalloid or blood cardioplegic solution, and the explanted heart then is cooled topically by being placed in an iced preservation solution; it then is placed in a secure container and transported expeditiously to the transplant center. Ischemic times average 3 to 4 h. Implantation of the heart in the orthotopic position begins with reanastomosis at the midatrial level, beginning with the atrial septum (Fig. 26-3). Efforts are made to include a generous cuff of donor right atrium so that the sinoatrial node will be included. The great vessels are reanastomosed just above the semilunar valves.

In recent years, there has been a move to alter the surgical technique "bicaval anastomosis" by leaving the donor atria intact and making anastomoses at the level of the superior and inferior venae cavae and pulmonary veins.[21–23] This technique is associated with a decreased requirement for pacemaker placement for donor sinus node malfunction with less AV valve regurgitation.[24,25]

Immediate postoperative care differs little from that after more routine heart surgery except for the institution of immunosuppression (described later) and the need for chronotropic support of the donor sinoatrial node for the first 2 to 3 postoperative days, usually with temporary pacemaker support but occasionally with infusion of isoproterenol. Uncomplicated patients may be discharged from the hospital 7 to 10 days postoperatively.

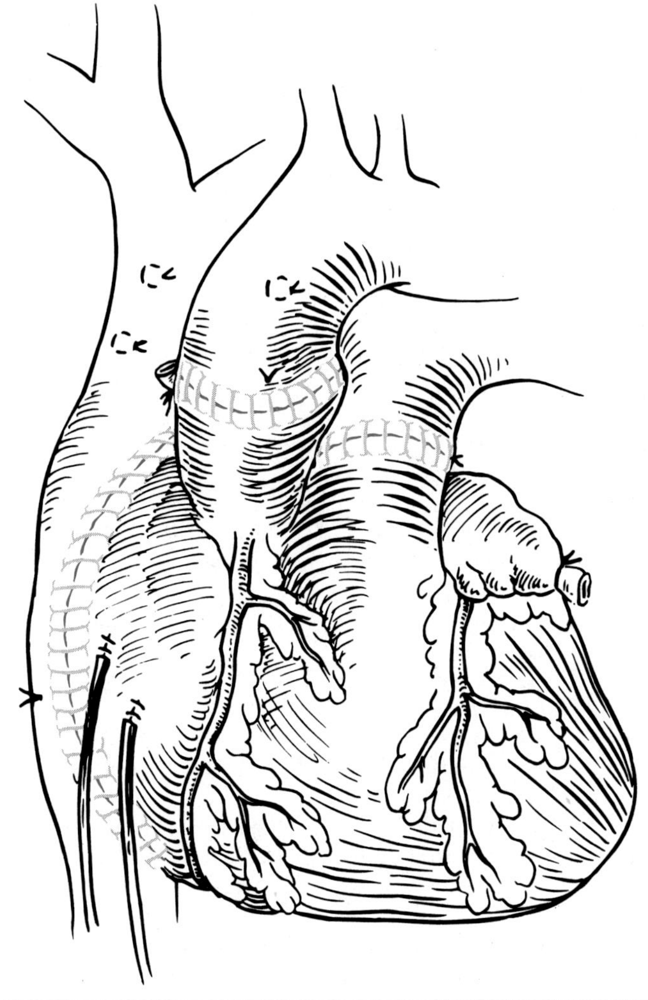

FIGURE 26-3 Diagram of donor heart anastomosed in the orthotopic position. Suture lines at the midatrial level and the aorta and pulmonary artery above semilunar valves.

## POSTOPERATIVE MANAGEMENT

### Immunosuppression

#### GENERAL

Historically, most clinically used immunosuppressive regimens have consisted of a combination of several agents used concurrently and sequentially. This multiple-drug approach continues to be considered the state of the art. The number of drugs and the timing of their administration vary from institution to institution, but utilize several general principles.

The first general principle is that immune reactivity and tendency toward graft rejection are highest early after graft implantation and decrease with time, although they probably never disappear entirely. Thus, most regimens employ the highest levels of immunosuppression immediately after surgery and decrease those levels later, eventually settling on the lowest maintenance levels of suppression that are compatible with preventing recurrent graft rejection. The second general principle is to use low doses of several drugs without overlapping toxicities in preference to higher (and more toxic) doses of fewer drugs whenever feasible. The third general principle is that too much or too intense immunosuppression is undesirable because it leads to a myriad of undesirable effects, such as susceptibility to infection and malignancy. Finding the right balance between over- and underimmunosuppression in an individual patient is truly an art that utilizes science. As newer immunosuppressive agents and modalities are developed, the possible array of drug regimens can be expected to multiply accordingly.

There is currently a relatively limited choice of approved agents for immunosuppression after organ transplantation, but their numbers are likely to increase. Most programs employ a long-term two- or three-drug regimen, and roughly half additionally use a brief early postoperative course of "induction" cytolytic therapy. Most programs employ glucocorticoids as one of the agents, usually in relatively high doses early postoperatively and then tapering to low doses or discontinuing the drug during the first postoperative year. The commonly used drugs and their toxicities are outlined in Table 26-4.

In managing patients on these drugs, it is most important to be aware of the potential for drug interactions when other agents are added to or deleted from the patient's regimen. A list of the most common and clinically important drug interactions is shown in Table 26-5. It is also important to keep in mind the potential for changing drug concentrations when intercurrent hepatic or renal dysfunction exist.

#### SURVEILLANCE AND THERAPY FOR REJECTION

Cardiac allograft rejection is diagnosed almost exclusively by examining histologic findings in surveillance RV endomyocardial biopsies. Many noninvasive methods to diagnose rejection have been investigated, but none has been determined to have sufficient sensitivity and specificity to replace the biopsy. Protocols for the timing of surveillance endomyocardial biopsies generally are chosen to match the observed frequency of rejection episodes, which is clearly highest in the early postoperative period. Most programs perform surveillance biopsies on a weekly basis for the first 4 to 6 postoperative

TABLE 26-4 Currently Available Immunosuppressive Agents

| Agent | Toxicities | Avoid Toxicity |
|---|---|---|
| Cyclosporine | Renal dysfunction | Follow blood levels |
| | Hypertension | Antihypertensive medication |
| | Neurotoxicity | ? |
| Tacrolimus (FK 506) | Renal dysfunction | Follow blood levels |
| | Neurotoxicity | ? |
| Mycophenolate mofetil | Gastrointestinal disturbances | Reduce dose |
| | Marrow toxicity (mild) | Follow CBC |
| Azathioprine | Marrow toxicity | Follow CBC |
| | Hepatotoxicity | Discontinue drug |
| Glucocorticoids | Cushingoid habitus | Minimize dose |
| | Glucose intolerance | |
| | Osteoporosis | |
| Methotrexate | Marrow toxicity | Follow CBC |

ABBREVIATIONS: CBC = complete blood count.

TABLE 26-5 Drug Interactions with Azathioprine and/or Cyclosporine

| Medication | Effects | Mechanism | Management | Onset | Severity |
|---|---|---|---|---|---|
| **Allopurinol** | Neutropenia 2° bone marrow suppression | Competitive inhibition of azathioprine metabolism | 1. *Don't use* allopurinol unless absolutely necessary<br>2. If used, monitor WBC count and adjust azathioprine dose accordingly | Delayed 2–3 weeks | Major |
| Amphotericin | Increased nephrotoxicity | Possible synergism with cyclosporine | Follow renal function; titrate dose accordingly | Delayed 1–2 weeks | Moderate |
| Barbiturates | Decreased cyclo levels | Increased hepatic metabolism | Follow cyclo levels carefully; increase cyclo doses PRN | Delayed 1 week | Moderate |
| Diltiazem (?? other $Ca^{2+}$ antagonists) | Increased cyclo levels | Unknown | Follow cyclo levels carefully; decrease cyclo doses PRN | Delayed 1–2 weeks | Moderate |
| Erythromycin | Increased cyclo levels | Decreased hepatic metabolism | Decrease cyclo dose by approximately *half;* follow levels carefully during and after therapy | Rapid | Major |
| Hydantoins | Decreased cyclo levels | Increased hepatic metabolism | Increase cyclo dose 25%; follow levels carefully | Rapid | Major |
| Imipenem | Increased CNS effects | Unknown | Avoid the antibiotic | Rapid | Moderate |
| Ketoconazole or itraconazole | Increased cyclo levels | Unknown | Follow levels carefully; decrease cyclo doses PRN | Delayed 1–2 weeks | Moderate |
| Metoclopramide | Increased cyclo levels | Increased cyclo bioavailability | Follow cyclo levels carefully; decrease cyclo doses PRN | Delayed 1–2 weeks | Moderate |
| Rifampin | Decreased cyclo levels | Increased hepatic metabolism | Increase cyclo dose by 100%; follow levels carefully | Delayed 1 week | Major |
| Sulfamethoxazole/ trimethoprim | Increased nephrotoxicity<br>Increased marrow suppression<br>Neutropenia | Unknown | Follow WBC count and renal function; adjust cyclo and azathioprine doses PRN | Delayed 2–3 weeks | Moderate |

ABBREVIATIONS: CNS = central nervous system; cyclo = cyclosporine; PRN = when necessary; 2° = secondary; WBC = white blood cells.

weeks and then with diminishing frequency in a stable patient but at a minimum every 3 months for the first postoperative year. The need for continued surveillance biopsies after the first year in clinically stable patients has been questioned[26,27] but most centers continue to do them every 4 to 6 months.

Rejection episodes are treated with augmented immunosuppression, the intensity of which is matched to the histologic, or occasionally clinical, severity of the episode. Early or first rejection episodes usually are treated with methylprednisolone given intravenously in a dose of 1 g daily for 3 days followed by a repeat biopsy in 7 to 10 days. Episodes after 3 months that are not clinically severe can be treated safely with an increase in the oral steroid dose.[28] More severe rejection is treated with glucocorticoids and the addition of cytolytic therapy with either polyclonal antithymocyte globulin (commonly of rabbit or equine origin) or the murine monoclonal anti-CD3 preparation OKT3. Such treatment is highly effective,[29] but sensitization can limit its use.[30]

Several strategies are employed as adjunctive therapy for repetitive or recalcitrant rejection episodes. They include the use of two modalities with proven efficacy in therapy for autoimmune disease: total lymphoid irradiation[31] and low-dose methotrexate.[32] Both have been shown to be of benefit in patients with frequent or difficult-to-treat cardiac allograft rejection.[33–36] Tacrolimus (FK506), when substituted for cyclosporine, has been reported to benefit several heart transplant recipients with resistant rejection,[37] as well as to be safe and effective as a primary agent in a cohort of patients.[38] Similar success has been reported with the use of mycophenolate mofetil in therapy for recalcitrant rejection.[39]

A new class of drugs, Target of Rapamycin (TOR) inhibitors, have been approved for use in renal transplantation. These drugs are used for prevention of acute rejection and management of recalcitrant rejection in heart transplant recipients. This new class of drugs, which include sirolimus (Rapamycin) and everolimus (Certican), block growth-factor-mediated IL-2 and IL-15-driven proliferation of human T-cells, B-cells, and vascular smooth muscle cells by inhibiting activation of p70S6 kinase and arresting the cell cycle at the G1 to S phase.[40] The propensity of calcineurinine antagonists to act at an earlier phase in the cellular immune response, suggested by their combinations with sirolimus (Rapamycin) or everolimus (Certican), should allow more effective abrogation of the cellular proliferative responses involved in both acute and chronic rejection. Indeed, in a phase II randomized double-blind trial conducted in heart transplant patients, treatment with sirolimus was shown to reverse acute rejection in 90 percent of patients.[41] Similarly, in a phase III randomized controlled study in 634 hearts transplant recipients, everolimus reduced the incidence of acute rejection in a dose-dependent fashion, compared to azathioprine.[42] Moreover, everolimus was shown to produce a significant decrease in the incidence of cardiac allograft vasculopathy (CAV), compared to azathioprine, and this effect occurred in a dose-dependent fashion, independent of stain use. Similar observations from smaller clinical trials have been reported with sirolimus.

If all these strategies fail and severe graft dysfunction supervenes, retransplantation is the only remaining option and is offered in many centers. The results of retransplantation in this setting are, however, disappointing, with only 33 percent 1-year survival in one registry and consistently inferior survival in the international registry.

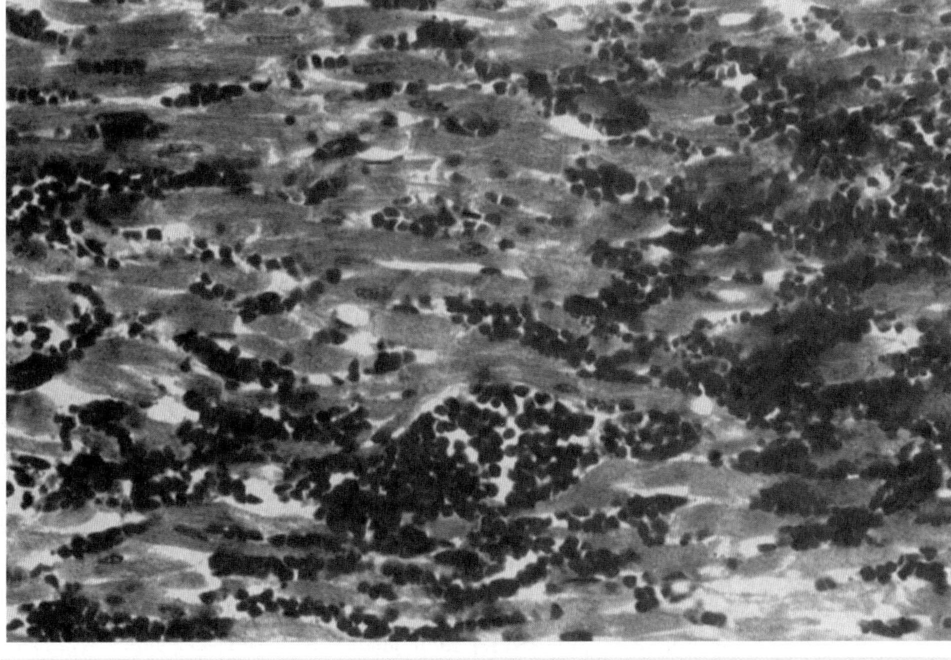

FIGURE 26-4 Hyperacute rejection is characterized by diffuse interstitial hemorrhage. (H&E ×400)

## PATHOLOGY OF ACUTE REJECTION

### Macroscopic Pathology

In advanced cardiac rejection, the heart is larger than normal, stiff, and noncompliant. In the early posttransplant period a fibrinous pericarditis may also be present. The heart appears edematous and hemorrhagic with a dark plum color. Along the atrial sutures, a sharp tinctorial delineation between the hemorrhagic myocardium of the donor and the pale tan myocardium of the recipient is characteristic of severe allograft rejection. Less commonly, the valves can be swollen and turgid. The trabecular muscles are prominent and often demonstrate subendocardial hemorrhages.

### Microscopic Pathology

#### HYPERACUTE REJECTION

This rare pattern of allograft rejection occurs in the setting of circulating preformed antibodies such as ABO blood group incompatibility, major histocompatibility antigens in the donor (e.g., anti-HLA class 1 antibodies) or donor endothelial antigens.[43] Possible risk factors include presensitization following multiple blood transfusions, multiparity, and previous cardiac surgical procedures.[44] The myocardium is globally edematous and hemorrhagic as a result of diffuse interstitial hemorrhages. Neutrophils and fibrin thrombi may be seen within the microvasculature (Fig. 26-4). Hyperacute rejection manifests as severe graft failure within the first few minutes or hours after transplantation. Without inotropic and mechanical cardiopulmonary support, plasmapheresis, and emergent retransplantation, the recipient usually does not survive.

#### ACUTE CELLULAR REJECTION

The principal histopathologic features of acute cellular rejection are the distribution and extent of inflammation and the presence or absence of myocyte damage. The severity of the rejection process reflects these features along a morphologic continuum. Since 1990 a uniform and standardized grading scheme has been used by most transplant centers.[45] The Working Formulation of the International Society of Heart and Lung Transplantation assigns a numerical and descriptive grade to each biopsy sample. This classification requires at least four pieces of myocardium using a standard bioptome, 50 percent of which must be evaluable myocardium (i.e., not a biopsy site or scar). If a smaller bioptome (7F or smaller) is used, at least six pieces of myocardium are required.

Six patterns of acute cellular rejection have been described (Table 26-6). Mild acute rejection is divided into two patterns on the basis of the cytoarchitectural features. Focal mild rejection (grade 1A) represents a circumscribed, usually perivascular arrangement of lymphocytes in one or more sites that is not associated with myocyte damage. In diffuse mild rejection (grade 1B), the infiltrates are arranged in an interstitial architectural pattern; myocyte damage is not found. Focal moderate rejection (grade II) is characterized by a solitary, sharply circumscribed inflammatory focus that is associated with myocyte damage or architectural disruption. The other biopsy pieces may be free of rejection or have a lower grade. In multifocal moderate rejection (grade IIIA), at least two foci of inflammatory infiltrate display myocyte damage. These foci are often in different pieces of myocardium. Diffuse moderate rejection (grade IIIB) is represented by diffuse interstitial infiltrates in most or all of the biopsy pieces. Myocyte damage is significant and the findings may be classified as

TABLE 26-6 Standardized Cardiac Biopsy Grading (Modified)

| "Old" Nomenclature | Grade | "New" Nomenclature |
|---|---|---|
| No rejection | 0 | No rejection |
| Mild rejection | I | A = Focal (perivascular or focal interstitial infiltrate without myocyte damage)<br>B = Sparse focal interstitial infiltrate without myocyte damage |
| "Focal" moderate rejection | II | One focus only with activated lymphocytes and myocyte damage |
| "Low" moderate rejection | III | A = Multifocal lymphocytic infiltrates with myocyte damage |
| "Borderline/severe" rejection | | B = Diffuse (sometimes polymorphous) inflammatory process |
| "Severe/acute" rejection | IV | Diffuse, polymorphous infiltrate with myocyte necrosis ± edema ± hemorrhage ± vasculitis |
| "Resolving" rejection | Denoted by a lower grade | Healing tissue with fibroblasts and pigmented macrophages |
| "Resolved" rejection | 0 | Mature scar tissue |

SOURCE: From Billingham ME, Carey NRB, Hammond EH, et al. A working formulation for the standardization of nomenclature in the diagnosis of heart and lung rejection: Heart rejection study group. *J Heart Transplant* 1990;9:587–592, with permission.

borderline severe rejection (Fig. 26-5). In severe rejection (grade IV), a dense polymorphous infiltrate that includes lymphocytes, neutrophils, and eosinophils is present diffusely in the interstitium. Myocyte damage, edema, and hemorrhage are conspicuous as a result of injury of the microvasculature. Resolved or resolving acute rejection is denoted by a lower grade on the biopsy than was observed on the previous biopsy.

## MORPHOLOGIC MIMICS OF ACUTE REJECTION

Inflammatory infiltrates and myocyte damage of the allograft can be found in conditions other than cellular rejection. The diagnosis of acute rejection should be made after the careful exclusion of these morphologic mimics (Table 26-7). Within the first 3 weeks after transplantation, endomyocardial biopsies often show evidence of ischemic or preservation injury. Reperfusion of the allograft contributes to myocyte damage. Likewise, the use of pressor agents for hemodynamic support either before harvesting or in the perioperative period can result in small circumscribed foci of myocyte damage. These infiltrates are composed of neutrophils in the initial stages and are replaced by granulation tissue in the healing phases. Sharply delineated endocardial infiltrates composed of lymphocytes and a delicate vascular stroma have been designated the "quilty effect" and can be confused with rejection when the infiltrate extends into the subadjacent myocardium. Infectious myocarditis, particularly toxoplasmic and cytomegalovirus (CMV) myocarditis can resemble acute rejection. The infiltrates are usually polymorphous (lymphocytes, histiocytes, neutrophils, and eosinophils), and the characteristic inclusions are found. Immunohistochemical or molecular techniques are useful in difficult cases.[46] The granulation tissue and inflammation associated with previous biopsy sites can also be confused with rejection. Posttransplant lymphoproliferative disease (PTLD) uncommonly involves the cardiac allograft. Both polyclonal and monoclonal lesions have been reported, and histopathologic analysis and clonality studies are essential for classification and prognosis.[47] The presence of atypical lymphocytes, abundant tissue necrosis, and frequent mitotic figures should suggest the possibility of PTLD.[48]

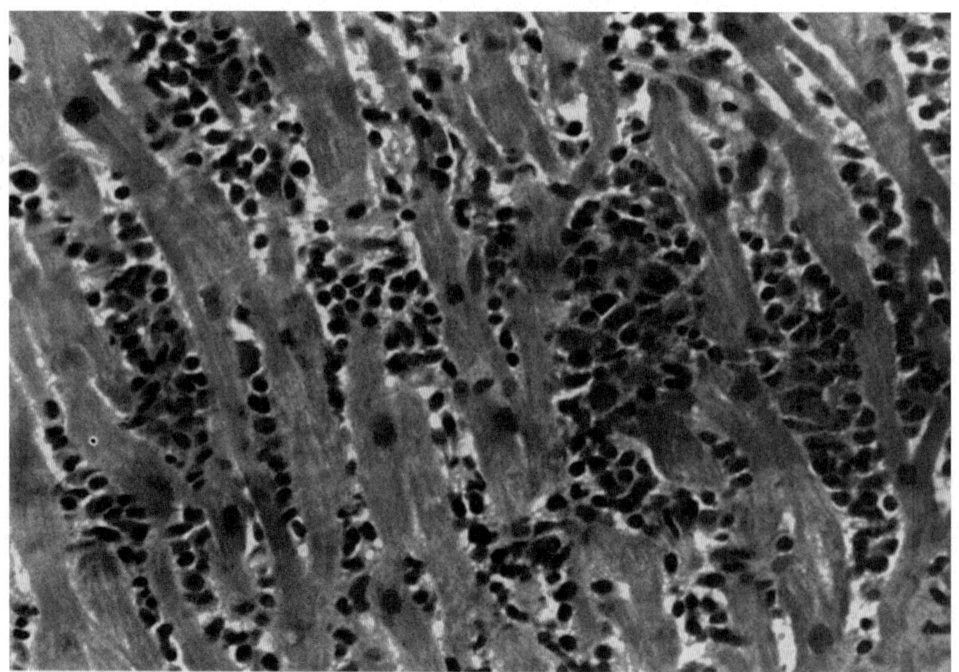

FIGURE 26-5 Diffuse moderate acute rejection (grade IIIB) showing activated lymphocytes within the interstitium and myocyte damage. (H&E ×400)

## ACUTE VASCULAR (HUMORAL) REJECTION

Most episodes of allograft rejection consist of a cytotoxic cell-mediated alloimmune mechanism directed at myocytes. Hammond and colleagues described cases of allograft dysfunction

TABLE 26-7 Histopathologic Mimics of Acute Rejection

Reperfusion/ischemic injury
Quilty effect
Infectious myocarditis (cytomegalovirus/toxoplasmic)
Previous biopsy site
Posttransplant lymphoproliferative disorder

occurring in the first 6 weeks after transplantation in which the classic features of cellular rejection were absent.[49] Immunofluorescence studies on fresh-frozen myocardial samples demonstrated deposition of immunoglobulin, complement, and fibrinogen suggesting a humoral immune response mediated by endothelial cells and B-cells, and the term *vascular, or humoral, rejection* was applied. The myocardium displays large prominent endothelial cells in venules, small arterioles and capillaries, perivascular and interstitial edema, and a paucity of inflammatory cells. Immunohistochemical studies have shown the swollen microvasculature to contain numerous intravascular histiocytes.[51] The diagnosis of acute vascular rejection requires both histologic and immunologic findings. Cases of mixed cellular and vascular rejection have been reported. Infection and ischemic injury must be excluded, as there is an overlap of immunologic findings. Possible risk factors include elevated panel reactive antibody screens (PRA), female recipients, CMV seropositive recipients, prior sensitization to OKT3, and a retrospective positive cross-match. A number of studies have suggested that patients with acute vascular rejection are at higher risk for the development of early accelerated graft coronary disease.[50]

## Infectious Complications

Although less frequent in the cyclosporine "era," infections are the major cause of death during the first postoperative year and remain a threat throughout the life of a chronically immunosuppressed patient. Effective therapy requires an extremely aggressive approach to obtaining a specific diagnosis and a background of experience in recognizing the more common clinical presentations of CMV, *Aspergillus,* and other opportunistic infectious agents. Several well-proven regimens for infection prophylaxis are commonly used and are outlined in Table 26-8. Infection surveillance is mainly clinical,

TABLE 26-8 Infection Prophylaxis Regimens

| Pathogen/Disease | Strategy |
|---|---|
| *Aspergillus* | ? Air filtration<br>? Prophylactic antifungals |
| Bacterial endocarditis | Standard subacute bacterial endocarditis prophylaxis |
| Cytomegalovirus | Blood product selection<br>Prophylactic ganciclovir<br>Prophylactic immunoglobulin |
| Influenza | None recommended |
| *Pneumococcus* | Preoperative vaccine |
| *Pneumocystis* | Sulfamethoxazole/trimethoprim<br>Inhaled pentamidine |
| *Toxoplasma* | Pyrimethamine if donor sero positive |

TABLE 26-9 Posttransplant Lymphoproliferative Disorder Incidence in Organ Transplantation

| Organ | Incidence, % |
|---|---|
| Kidney | 1.0 |
| Heart | 1.8 |
| Liver | 3.0 |
| Heart/lung | 4.6 |

SOURCE: Reproduced from Penn I. Roundtable report: Immunosuppression and lymphoproliferative disorders, 1992. (With permission of the author and Pro/Com International, Parsippany, NJ.)

but routine chest radiography often detects infections, especially fungal and mycobacterial ones, at an early and asymptomatic stage.

## Posttransplant Malignancy

Any program of chronic immunosuppression is associated with a subsequent increased risk of lymphoproliferative malignancy.[52] Organ transplantation has proved to be no exception, and the incidence of PTLD in heart transplant recipients is somewhat higher than that in kidney transplant recipients but not as high as that in liver recipients (Table 26-9).[53] According to the most recent registry report, malignancy occurs in 29 percent of patients by 7 years posttreatment, including a 16 percent incidence of skin malignancy and 4.4 percent incidence of lymphoma.

There is convincing evidence that most PTLDs are related to infection (either primary or reactivation) with the Epstein-Barr virus (EBV).[54–56] They frequently occur in unusual, extranodal locations and may respond to reduction in immunosuppression,[57] although such reduction is clearly a "double-edged sword" with a cardiac allograft for which there is no alternative system if the graft is rejected. PTLDs are usually quite radiosensitive, and both radiotherapy and surgical resection can play a major role in therapy when there is a single lesion.

There is anecdotal evidence that the use of the antiviral agent acyclovir may be useful in therapy for PTLD,[58] and most centers employ it as an adjunctive therapy. In recent years, there has been interest in the use of interferon for these malignancies,[59] and a multicenter oncology group protocol is in progress to evaluate its efficacy. There has been interest in the use of infusions of donor leukocytes[60] and donor-derived EBV-specific cytotoxic lymphocytes for this disease in bone marrow transplant recipients.[61] The technology may well be transferred to organ transplant recipients but would require the maintenance of donor tissue lines prospectively.

## Allograft Vasculopathy

### INCIDENCE

When clinical heart transplantation was introduced, the frequent development of diffuse and often rapidly progressive obliterative coronary artery disease in young donor hearts was not expected. It occurs angiographically in approximately 10 percent of cardiac transplant recipients by the first postoperative year and in 50 percent by 5 years postoperatively,[62,63] and its incidence did not decrease after the introduction of cyclosporine-based immunosuppression in the early 1980s.[64] *The ischemic sequelae of this vasculopathy account for the vast majority of late posttransplant deaths, and it is the main factor limiting long-term survival.*

TABLE 26-10 Angiographic Features of Cardiac Allograft Coronary Artery Disease

| |
|---|
| Distribution: diffuse distal, concentric, longitudinal obliterative lesions |
| May coexist with focal proximal lesions |
| Collateral vessel formation uncommon |

## MORPHOLOGY

The angiographic morphology of cardiac allograft vasculopathy (CAV) has been well described,[65,66] and its main features are summarized in (Table 26-10). The very diffuseness of the disease makes it easy to underestimate angiographically even when, as is usually recommended, similar angiographic views from serial angiograms are reviewed simultaneously with side-by-side projectors.

*In recent years, the use of intravascular ultrasound (Chap. 18) has gained acceptance as a sensitive and early detector of the intimal thickening that characterizes CAV.*[67–69] Intravascular ultrasound measurements of the extent of coronary intimal thickening serve as surrogate endpoints for the prevention of CAV in several trials of new immunosuppressive agents that have lessoned the incidence of CAV in animal models.

## PATHOLOGY

The morphologic features of accelerated transplant vasculopathy and the principal differences from conventional atherosclerosis have been described.[70–72] In transplant arteriopathy, the major epicardial vessels, their branches, and often the intramyocardial divisions display uniform, diffuse involvement extending along their entire length. The arteries are cordlike in texture, and cross-sections show uniform, concentric luminal narrowing (Fig. 26-6). The asymmetric and calcified plaques or lesions composed of cholesterol that are characteristic of conventional atherosclerosis are not found in uncomplicated lesions of vessels affected by transplant vasculopathy. Histopathologic sections show a thickened intimal layer composed of modified smooth muscle cells, foamy macrophages, and variable numbers of histiocytes and lymphocytes within a connective tissue matrix that ranges from loose, edematous, and myxoid in early lesions to densely hyalinized and fibrotic in older lesions (Fig. 26-7). The internal elastic membrane is usually preserved, with only focal interruptions and reduplications. The medial layer is generally intact but may show atrophy in advanced lesions. Intraluminal thrombosis is uncommon.

## CLINICAL PRESENTATION, SCREENING, AND PROGNOSIS

Because most cardiac transplant recipients have a persistent state of both afferent and efferent cardiac denervation, most are incapable of experiencing the subjective sensation of angina pectoris. Clinical presentations of ischemia in this patient population usually are related to sequelae of the ischemia, such as arrhythmias or left ventricular dysfunction. It has been convincingly shown, however, that some cardiac transplant recipients do have physiologic evidence of reinnervation[73–76] and may experience angina pectoris.[77]

The usual lack of angina and the diffuseness of the disease have made standard clinical and noninvasive screening for native coronary artery disease fairly insensitive in detecting this form of CAV.[78] Most of this technology is designed to detect uneven myocardial perfusion caused by focal lesions and is less effective in detecting the global ischemia of diffuse obliterative disease. Several reports suggest dobutamine stress echocardiography may be the one noninvasive technique that offers reasonable sensitivity and specificity, as well as prognostic value in screening for this disease,[79,81a] and it offers an attractive alternative to the usual annual coronary angiography performed in these patients.

The prognosis for survival once significant graft vasculopathy is detected angiographically is generally poor. In one study, the 1- and 2-year survival rates after the detection of any 40 percent coronary artery stenosis were 67 and 44 percent, respectively. After an ischemic event such as congestive heart failure or myocardial infarction, 1-year survival was only 18 to 20 percent in this study.

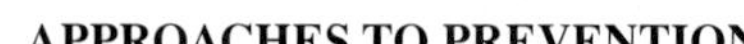

## APPROACHES TO PREVENTION

Several approaches to the prevention of CAV have been proposed, and some show promise. A decreased incidence of CAV is one of the desired endpoints in all preclinical and clinical trials of new immunosuppressive agents that are in progress. In addition, two randomized studies have shown some decrease in the incidence and sequelae of CAV with the use of other agents: one with a calcium channel blocker diltiazem added to the patient regimen early after surgery[82] and another with the lipid-lowering agent pravastatin added.[83] A study documented similar results with simvastatin, and this benefit is probably a class effect.[84]

The mechanism of action for either of these agents remains speculative. Since the etiology of CAV is most likely immunologic, improved methods of inducing specific graft tolerance may lead to the disappearance of this

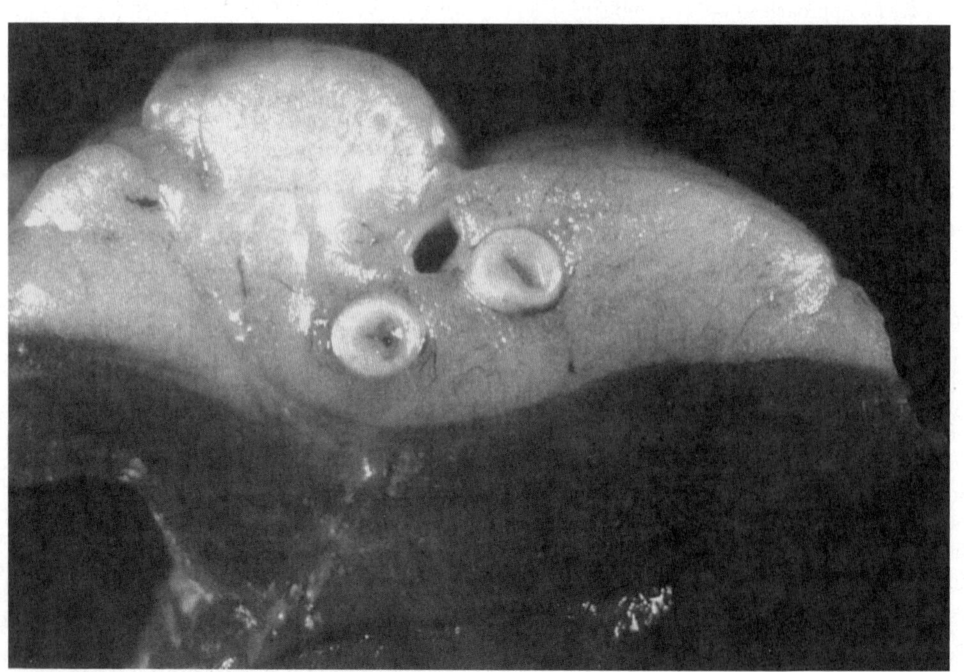

FIGURE 26-6 The mid-left anterior descending artery at autopsy in a 63-year-old man with advanced graft coronary disease.

disease and permit truly long-term survival rates after heart and other organ transplantation.

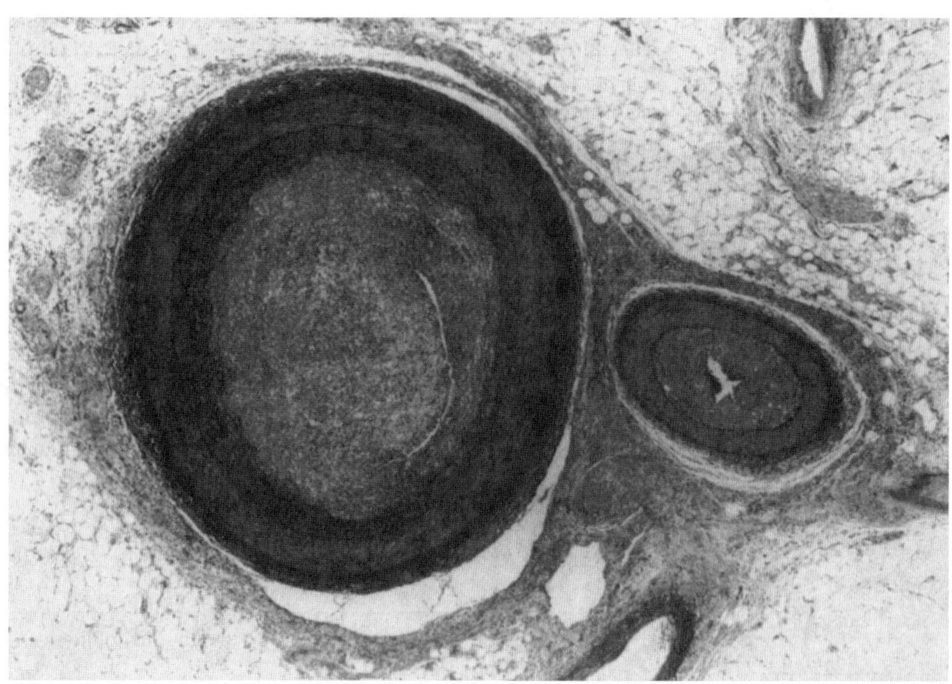

FIGURE 26-7 A main epicardial artery and division vessel showing occlusive graft coronary disease. Note the concentric intimal proliferation with a slitlike lumen. The internal elastica of both vessels is intact. (EUG ×10)

**APPROACHES TO THERAPY**

The choice of treatment for established CAV is often difficult and controversial. No agent or modality has been shown to reverse the process. Its very diffuseness makes the disease only infrequently amenable to otherwise standard revascularization procedures such as angioplasty and surgical bypass grafting. A registry of revascularization procedures performed on heart transplant recipients in 13 large transplant centers in the United States documented 97 balloon angioplasty procedures in 66 patients before November 1991.[85] There was an angiographic 94 percent success rate and an acceptable complication rate. There was, however, a 55 percent restenosis rate at a mean of 8 months after angioplasty, and 19 patients underwent 31 repeat angioplasty procedures for 24 restenoses and 30 new lesions. In the same registry, 12 surgical coronary bypass procedures were reported; 4 of these patients died in the hospital, a fifth died suddenly 2 months postoperatively, and a sixth has required further palliative angioplasty. Revascularization is clearly, at best, *short-term palliation* for this highly lethal disease.

The most definitive form of therapy for graft failure resulting from severe vasculopathy is obviously retransplantation for selected patients with advanced CAV, but otherwise good organ function. Survival rates after retransplantation, however, are clearly inferior to those after primary transplants, averaging only 52 percent at 1 year in the most recent registry data.[9] While this clearly represents an improvement in the individual patient's prognosis, these lower survival rates, along with the increased costs involved,[86] have led some to question the ethics of performing retransplantation.[87] Nevertheless, most large programs continue to offer the option to highly selected patients.

## SURGICAL TREATMENT FOR HEART FAILURE

Surgical management of heart failure has become one of the fastest growing aspects of cardiovascular surgery. Advances in cardiac surgical techniques, improved postoperative care, and better understanding of the pathophysiology have broadened the complexity of patients recommended for operative intervention. With experience, it has become evident that LV dysfunction is not a contraindication to surgery; but rather an invitation to consider one of the many surgical options.[88] An attempt has been made to delay cardiac transplantation, with its limited resources, whenever feasible and medical and surgical management that can improve quality of life are undertaken.[88,89]

### Left Ventricular Restoration

**ANATOMIC CONSIDERATIONS**

Understanding ventricular anatomy is critical in understanding ventricular remodeling and the onset and treatment of heart failure. Torrent-Guasp and associates have demonstrated through thousands of anatomic dissections that the heart, if properly unfolded and prepared, consists of a single myocardial muscle band that stretches from the pulmonary artery to the aorta.[90] It curls in a helical manner that is described by 2 spirals called the basal and apical loops. By folds and twists, the band forms the LV by a double helical loop and the RV by a transversely oriented segment of the band (Fig. 26-8). Normal physiologic states as well as pathologic states in the context of Torrent-Guasp et al.'s anatomic discoveries have been described.[91,92] It has demonstrated that cardiac ejection, isovolumetric contraction, and filling are all related to the individual contractions of different parts of the myocardial band. That is, the heart's ability to attain an ejection fraction (EF) of 60 percent in normal health is a result of the left ventricle's double helical shape.[92] In the failing heart, the double helical shape becomes more transverse as the overall shape of the heart becomes more spherical and less ellipsoid, thereby decreasing the EF.[93] By attempting to restore the normal helical geometry of the heart, a completely new class of cardiac procedures involving surgical resection of the ventricle has evolved. These procedures include the Dor procedure and the subsequent surgical anterior ventricular endocardial restoration procedure, referred to as the SAVER technique, and the partial left ventriculectomy, known as the Batista procedure. Although functional improvements after ventricular restoration procedures are due to geometric rearrangement, investigators have also demonstrated that mass reduction has a significant effect on the mechanical stress experienced by the myocardium.[94]

**ENDOVENTRICULAR PATCH PLASTY: THE DOR PROCEDURE/SURGICAL ANTERIOR VENTRICULAR ENDOCARDIAL RESTORATION (SAVER)**

A large anterior transmural myocardial infarction (MI) causes both early and late distortion of the heart. The adverse shape raises wall tension and produces mechanical disadvantages and adverse remodeling. Endoventricular patch plasty, referred to as the Dor procedure, uses a patch to exclude noncontracting segments of myocardium

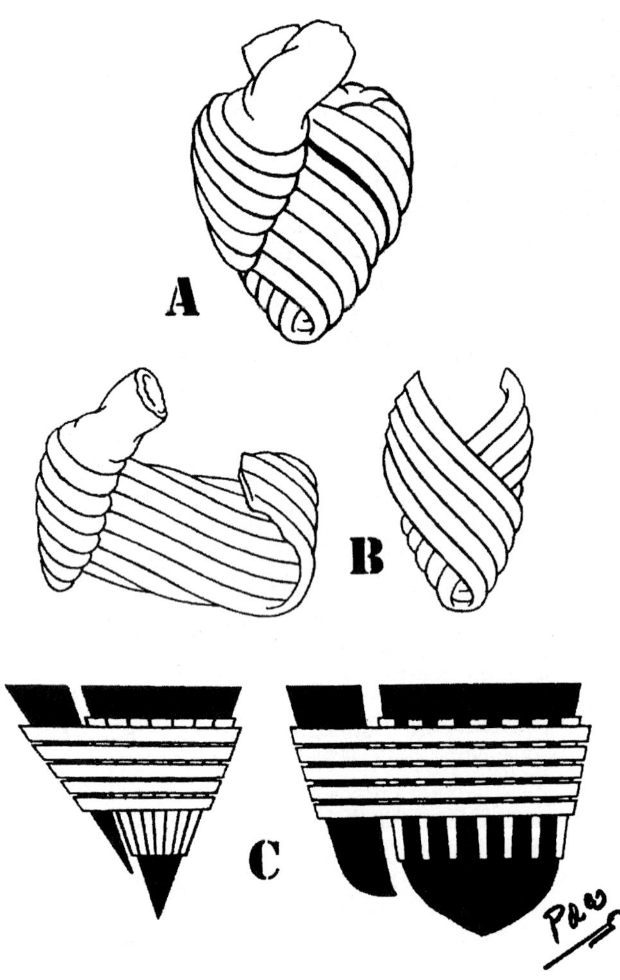


FIGURE 26-8 At the ventricular mass (*A*) the direction of the fibers is predominantly horizontal at the basal loop (*B*, left) and vertical at the apical loop (*B*, right). Schematic representation of the normal and a dilated myocardiomyopathic heart (*C*). (Reproduced with permission from Torrent-Guasp F, Buckberg GD, Clemente C, et al. The structure and function of the helical heart and its buttress wrapping. I. The normal macroscopic structure of the heart. *Sem Thorac Cardiovasc Surg* 2001;13:301–319.)

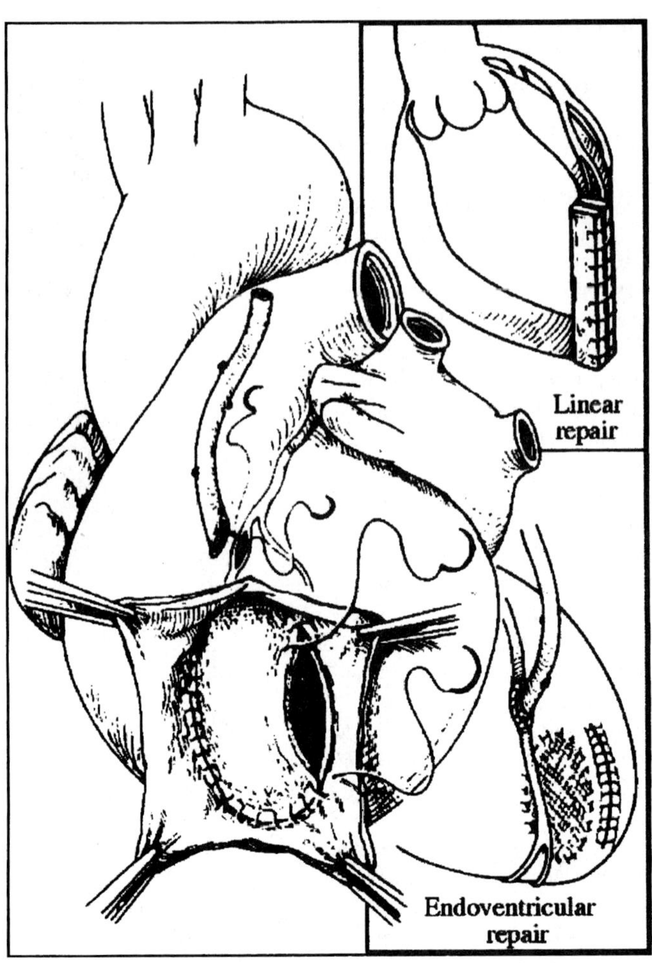


FIGURE 26-9 Endoventricular patch plasty: The Dor Procedure. Left ventricular remodeling for a large area of scarred post infarction anterior myocardium. (Reproduced with permission from Westaby S. Non-transplant surgery for heart failure. *Heart* 2000;83: 603–610.)

inside cardiomyopathic ventricles. Using cardiopulmonary bypass, the LV is opened through the infarct scar and a subtotal endocardectomy is performed over the septum and posterior wall. In the event of recurrent ventricular arrhythmias, cryotherapy is applied at the limits of the ventricular resection. The boundary between normal endocardium and scar is defined and a circumferential endoventricular (Fontan) circular suture is passed between 1 and 2 cm outside the limit of healthy muscle. This restores the "neck" of the contracting ventricle that is retained and provides a more normal oval curvature of the ventricle. The residual apical defect is then closed with a Dacron patch cut according to the circumference of the circular suture. Care must be taken to avoid restricting the LV cavity. Important to this methodology is the fact that akinesia is treated the same as dyskinesia in that both types of endocardium are excluded and the patch is used to redirect muscle fiber tension toward a normal helical arrangement[95,96] (Fig. 26-9).

An international group of cardiologists and surgeons from 13 centers on 4 continents, referred to as the RESTORE group, has assembled to investigate the surgical role of SAVER in the treatment of post infarction ventricular dilation. This procedure is essentially the Dor procedure with technical modifications and additional emphasis on revascularization and mitral valve repair and replacement.[97,98] The technical modifications include using a balloon catheter to measure the intraventricular volume by introducing a balloon that is inflated at the theoretical diastolic ventricular capacity of the patient (40 to 50 mL/m$^2$ of body surface area). Also, cardioplegia arrest is used during the revascularization and mitral valve component of the operation followed by open-beating technique during patch placement.[97] The RESTORE group has reported an approach to the mitral valve that involves reducing the mitral annulus through the ventricle with pledged sutures, rather than an annuloplasty ring.[98]

In over 1000 patients worldwide who have undergone ventricular reconstruction, Dor and the RESTORE group have revascularized 92 percent of patients (90 percent with left internal mammary arteries), repaired the mitral valve in 22 percent of patients, and replaced the mitral valve in 3 percent. Improved New York Heart Association (NYHA) functional class, as well as systolic and diastolic function, has resulted.[94–96] Of the patients classified as NYHA class II or III, 80 percent were alive at 10 years, whereas survival was only 50 percent in patients with NYHA class IV. Ventricular arrhythmias, either spontaneous or inducible, were controlled in 90 percent of patients and hospital mortality was reported as 8 percent.[99] When assessing the factors associated with mortality, patients who died had higher preoperative functional class of heart failure and had more clinical signs of heart failure than did survivors. Clinical variables of age, number of stenotic coronary vessels, spontaneous or inducible tachycardia, operative parameters, including bypass or clamp time or perioperative complications, did not affect overall survival.[100] Freedom from readmission to hospital for heart failure was 89 percent at 3 years. In general, the SAVER technique has a favorable result on survival in patients suffering from class III and IV heart failure post myocardial infarction.[96–101]

## LEFT VENTRICULAR REDUCTION: THE BATISTA PROCEDURE

Randas Batista of Brazil developed the procedure now referred to as partial left ventriculectomy, or more commonly termed the *Batista procedure*. This procedure was developed based on the premise that an increase in ventricular cavity radius leads to an increase in ventricular wall mass whereas, when the radius increases without an appropriate increase in mass, ventricular dilation leads to heart failure. Reducing the radius by excising part of the ventricular wall would diminish mural tension and thereby improve overall LV function. The primary etiologies of heart failure for which Batista operated were Chagas disease and ischemic and dilated cardiomyopathies. Batista originally reported on a 34-year-old patient whose EF rose from 17 to 44 percent at 2 months postoperatively.[102] He went on to describe 154 such cases, but follow-up was lacking. The procedure itself involves cardiopulmonary bypass and is performed on a beating heart. An incision is made in the apex of the LV and is extended to the base. The mitral valve is either repaired or replaced after a wedge of ventricular muscle is removed. The ventriculotomy is then closed with two layers and often buttressed with bovine pericardium. (Fig. 26-10)

In the United States, Batista and associates collaborated and reported the results of 120 patients.[103] The 30-day mortality was 22 percent and the 2-year mortality was 45 percent. Ten percent of patients had no improvement in NYHA functional class, and 57 percent of survivors were is class I. Difficulty arose because the patients deemed suitable in the United States were those that were otherwise not transplant candidates and the follow-up was again lacking for the Brazilian patients.[103]

Recognizing the potential benefit of Batista's procedure, McCarthy et al. undertook a prospective study to evaluate the benefits of partial left ventriculectomy.[104] Of 95 percent of patients who were transplant candidates, 62 underwent partial left ventriculectomy with concomitant mitral valve surgery. Batista's procedure was associated with significant early failure, and event-free survival at 3 years was only 26 percent. Overall survival at 3 years was 80 percent, but this was determined to be due to aggressive use of LV assist device support and transplantation after failure of the Batista procedure. The Society of Thoracic Surgeons deemed it inappropriate to perform the Batista procedure routinely until better documentation of long-term survival and evidence for prolonged benefit was demonstrated.[105] However, it was suggested that this procedure could be used in situations where transplantation was not possible or as a biologic bridge to transplantation.[104,105]

Other groups have similarly attempted using partial left ventriculectomy in heart failure with equally limited success. Despite their initial improvement, many patients who underwent partial left ventriculectomy required relisting for transplantation.[106] Moreira et al. performed Batista's procedure with mitral valve preservation and although LV dysfunction initially improved, the high incidence of heart failure progression and arrhythmia-related deaths precluded recommending the clinical application of this procedure.[107,108]

## SURGICAL TREATMENT FOR ISCHEMIC HEART FAILURE TRIAL

The Surgical Treatment for Ischemic Heart Failure (STICH) multicenter randomized trial was designed to address two hypotheses in patients with heart failure and LV dysfunction who have coronary artery disease amenable to revascularization. First, revascularization with intensive medical therapy improves long-term survival compared to medical therapy alone. Second, in patients with anterior LV dysfunction, ventricular restorative surgery improves survival for cardiac causes in comparison to revascularization alone.

Over 3 years, beginning in 2002, 50 clinical sites will recruit 2800 patients with heart failure, EFs less than 35 percent and coronary artery disease amenable to revascularization. The three treatment groups include intensive medical therapy for heart failure, medical therapy plus revascularization, and medical therapy plus revascularization and surgical ventricular restoration. The results of this important study will help to define the best therapy for patients with heart failure secondary to an ischemic cardiomyopathic process.

# MECHANICAL VENTRICULAR SUPPORT

When aggressive medical management fails to improve cardiac performance such that the heart can no longer provide adequate organ perfusion, the insertion of a mechanical support device must be entertained. These devices range from intraaortic balloon pumps

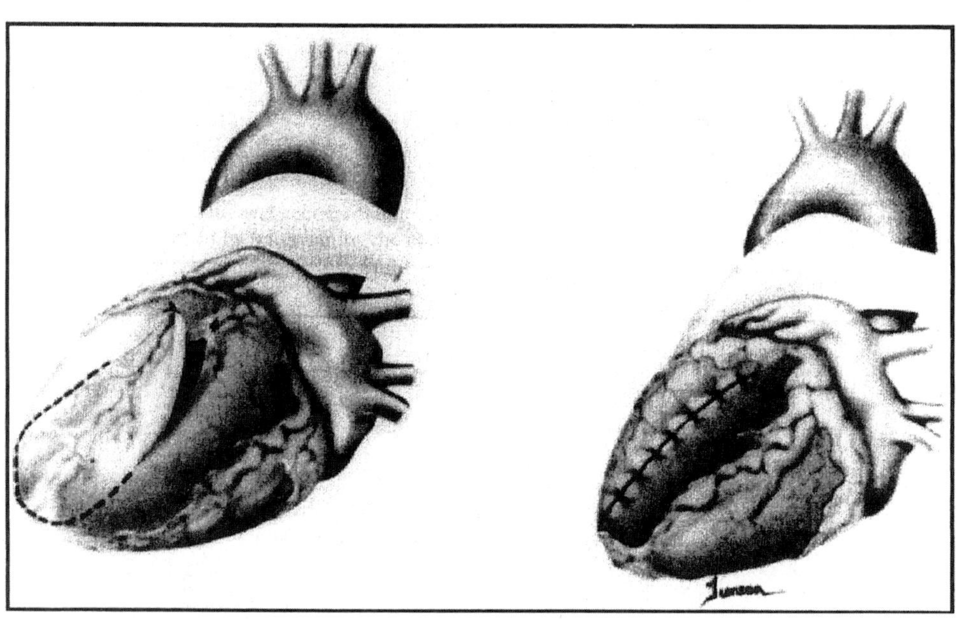

FIGURE 26-10 Left ventricular reduction: The Batista Procedure. (Reproduced with permission from Westaby S. Non-transplant surgery for heart failure. *Heart* 2000;83:603–610.)

(IABP) that can be inserted at the bedside, to LV assist devices of varying complexity, to the total artificial heart. The insertion and use of devices to support the failing heart necessitates an intensive care setting and a multidisciplinary team. As experience increases and technology improves, outpatient management of mechanically supported patients will become routine.

## Intraaortic Balloon Pump

The IABP was first used clinically in 1968 for supporting patients in cardiogenic shock after acute MI.[109] It was later expanded to postoperative support and weaning patients from cardiopulmonary bypass.[110,111] Most IABPs available are inserted surgically or percutaneously. Using the Salinger technique, a guidewire is used to access retrograde the descending aorta. The balloon is inserted over the guidewire and is placed just distal to the left subclavian artery under echocardiography guidance or external body measurement. If the femoral artery is difficult to access, a surgical cut-down is used to access the femoral artery safely. Rarely, the femoral arteries are not accessible due to severe aortoiliac disease and the IABP can then be inserted transthoracically into the descending thoracic aorta at the time of surgery. Proper timing of inflation and deflation of the balloon is necessary for IABP counterpulsation to provide effective cardiac assistance. The balloon is timed to open immediately after the aortic valve is closed and deflated at the onset of systole. If properly timed, the IABP will augment coronary blood flow by increasing the diastolic perfusion pressure and lessen the ventricular work by reducing afterload with rapid deflation in systole (Fig. 26-11).

Indications for use of the IABP include ongoing unstable angina refractory to medical management, acute myocardial infarction or ischemic postpercutaneous transluminal angioplasty, perioperative low cardiac output, cardiac shock postmyocardial infarction, heart failure refractory to medical management, bridge to transplant, ischemic ventricular septal defect, acute mitral regurgitation, and poorly controlled perioperative ventricular arrhythmias.[112]

The IABP has become the most widely used circulatory assist device, but it is not without complications. The reported incidence of complications varies greatly, with rates ranging between 6.5 and 15 percent reported.[113,114] In general, the incidence has decreased since the first implementation of this technology.[114] The complications include limb ischemia, aortic dissection, mesenteric and renal infarction, and infection.[114,115]

German investigators have introduced the concept of the IABP "score."[116] The IABP score can be used to predict death or survival early after IABP implantation.

$$\begin{aligned}\text{IABP score} &= \text{I (adrenaline dose} > 0.5\ \mu\text{g)} \times \text{kg body weight}^{-1} \times \text{min}^{-1}) \\ &\quad \times 2 + \text{I (urine output} < 100\ \text{mL/h)} + \text{I (SvO}_2 < 60\%) \\ &\quad + \text{I (LAP} > 15\ \text{mmHg)}\end{aligned}$$

I was equal to 1 if the parameter was clinically valid. Patients with IABP scores of 5 had 0 probability of living 30 days, whereas patients with a score of 1 had an 86 percent chance of living more than 30 days. Furthermore, they reported that the higher the IABP score, the more likely the patient would benefit from the placement of a ventricular assist device.[116]

Progress has been made to introduce the use of an ambulatory IABP[117] and a permanent implantable IABP.[118] This technology will allow heart failure patients to regain better cardiac performance in an outpatient setting.

## Ventricular Assist Devices

Ventricular assist devices (VADs) are mechanical support devices for the failing heart that has become refractory to inotropic support and IABP support. The first use of a VAD was in 1963 when DeBakey inserted one in the left thorax, connecting the left atrium and the descending thoracic aorta in a patient with postcardiotomy heart failure. Due to the increasing number of heart failure patients and the unmatched number of donor hearts, ventricular support will continue to be clinically important in managing patients with heart failure. In fact, the Institute of Medicine (Washington, DC) reported that 70,000 Americans could benefit from ventricular assistance yearly.[119]

The hemodynamic criteria for implantation of VAD are typically a cardiac index $< 2.0$ L/min/m$^2$, a systolic blood pressure $< 80$ mmHg despite inotropic support, pulmonary capillary artery pressure $> 20$ mmHg, and maximized medical therapy including inotropes and IABP.[120] There are two categories of VADs: (1) extracorporeal, with the pump chamber outside the body and (2) implantable. Furthermore, implantable devices can be pulsatile or consist of axial flow pumps. When a VAD is implanted, it is either

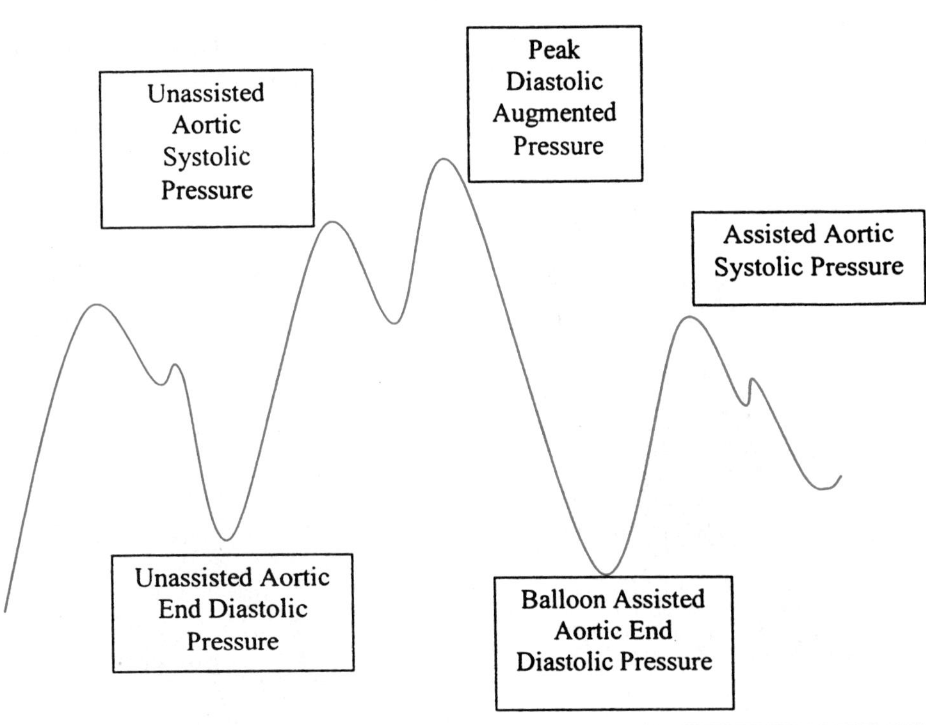


FIGURE 26-11 A diagram of intraaortic balloon pump (IABP). The IABP is timed to inflate in the diastolic phase of the cardiac cycle, after the closure of the aortic valve. The end result of IABP is elevated diastolic perfusion pressure and enhanced circulatory blood flow.

for the purpose of bridging to recovery or transplant or as destination therapy. Table 26-11 outlines which devices the Food and Drug Administration (FDA) have approved and for what indication. A consensus report concerning mechanical cardiac support has been published in the *Journal of the American College of Cardiology.*[119]

TABLE 26-11 FDA-Approved Mechanical Ventricular Support Devices

| Device | Ventricular Support | Indication | Type |
|---|---|---|---|
| AMBIOMED BVS 5000 | Biventricular | Bridge to recovery | Extracorporeal |
| BioMedicus Centrifugal Pump | Biventricular | Bridge to recovery<br>Bridge to transplant | Extracorporeal |
| Thoratec VAD | Biventricular | Bridge to transplant<br>Bridge to recovery | Extracorporeal |
| HeartMate IP LVAD | Left ventricular | Bridge to transplant | Implantable |
| Novacor LVAD | Left ventricular | Bridge to transplant | Implantable |
| HeartMate VE LVAD | Left ventricular | Bridge to transplant<br>Destination therapy | Implantable |

The extracorporeal VADs include the AMBIOMED BVS 5000 (AMBIOMED Cardiovascular, Inc., Danvers, MA), Thoratec VAD (Thoratec Laboratories, Pleasanton, CA), and the BioMedicus (Medtronic, Eden Prairie, MN). The AMBIOMED BVS 5000 is an external, pulsatile, mechanical support system that is designed for short-term support and can provide left, right, or biventricular support for up to 30 days. The advantages of this support device is its ease of use and availability. Thromboembolic, bleeding, and infectious complications, however, limit the support period.[120–122] As a bridge device, the AMBIOMED BVS 5000 allows time to assess the patient's cardiac function and recovery or, conversely, the suitability for heart transplantation.[119]

The Thoratec VAD can provide right, left, or biventricular support and has been approved as a bridge to recovery or transplantation.[123,124] The Thoratec paracorporeal pump is pneumatically driven and designed for long-term use. For LV support, the inflow cannula is placed either in the LV apex or the left atrium and the outflow cannula is placed in the ascending aorta. These cannula are connected to an external pump consisting of a rigid housing chamber containing a polyurethane blood sac.[120] For biventricular assistance, two pumps are used. An external drive console sends pressurized air to the pump, compressing the blood sac and ejecting blood through mechanical valves thereby necessitating anticoagulation. The extracorporeal position of this device facilitates exchange in cases of malfunction, thrombus, or infection; an intracorporeal version of this VAD is currently under development.[124]

Short-term ventricular support can be provided in most centers with the BioMedicus centrifugal pump.[125,126] This device can also be used for femoral–femoral bypass, cardiopulmonary bypass, and extracorporeal membrane oxygenation (ECMO). This device is relatively inexpensive compared to other short-term VADs. Temporary cardiopulmonary support with the BioMedicus pump is most commonly used for elective and emergency cardiac procedures requiring cardiopulmonary bypass. Cannulation is usually central into the right or left atrium, and the pulmonary artery or distal ascending aorta is cannulated for the pump arterial outflow. Femoral vein and artery cannulation is also possible but used less commonly. The BioMedicus is designed to support patients for no more than 2 to 3 weeks; if ventricular recovery is insufficient, then this device can be used as a bridge to another device or transplantation.

The implantable ventricular support devices that are clinically available include the Novacor LVAD (Novacor Corp. Oakland, CA), the HeartMate IP LVAD (Thoratec Laboratories, Pleasanton, CA), and the HeartMate XVE LVAD (Thoratec Laboratories, Pleasanton, CA). The Novacor is an implantable, electric, dual-pusher-plate device designed for long-term ventricular support as a bridge to transplantation. The device is implanted via a sternotomy with an inflow conduit to the LV apex and an outflow conduit to the ascending aorta. This device has porcine valves in the inflow and outflow positions to ensure unidirectional flow. The pump is positioned in the abdominal wall and a console or portable pack regulates the pump rate.[127,128] The current wearable model (N 100PC) was developed in 1991 and used clinically for the first time in 1993.[129] The worldwide clinical experience is in excess of 1200 recipients with the longest implant being 4.1 years.[130] The hospital discharge rate with this implantable device has increased with experience from a rate of 22 percent in 1994 to 90 percent in 1999. Anticoagulation is required with this device in order to reduce the incidence of thromboembolic events.[130]

The HeartMate LVAD consists of two types. The Implantable Pneumatic (IP) version is powered and controlled by an external pneumatic drive console. The Vented Electric (VE) version contains an electric motor within the blood pump housing. It receives external power and control signals from an external microprocessor using a vented driveline. Both systems have porcine valves and textured blood-containing surfaces that become covered by a "pseudoneointimal" layer.[131] This results in a very low incidence of thromboembolic events and is used for patients who cannot be anticoagulated. Like the Novacor LVAD, the HeartMate VE has an external drive system and a portable power pack option (Fig. 26-12). In a prospective, multicenter trial conducted at 24 centers in the United States, 280 transplant candidates unresponsive to inotropic drug and/or IABP therapy were treated with the HeartMate VE. Of the LV assist device supported patients 71 percent survived and 67 percent received a heart transplant.[132] Compared to a cohort of patients not supported with a VAD, the 1-year posttransplant survival rate was significantly better.[132]

Adverse events associated with the implantation of VADS are well known and include bleeding postimplantation, right-sided heart failure, sepsis, and thromboembolic events. Catastrophic mechanical failure of the device not amenable to backup measures has occurred in less than 1 percent of patients.[133] Overall infection remains a major impediment to long-term support, and it is now recognized that patient–pump interactions leading to changes in a patient's coagulation and immune system may ultimately affect outcomes. Once confidence in the benefits and reliability of VAD support grows, more patients will be discharged home with these devices. Heart failure patients will therefore be able to have an improved quality of life with minimal morbidity associated with device function and support.

## The Artificial Heart

The AbioCor implantable replacement heart has been developed as a potential alternative to heart transplantation. In a bovine model, the implantable device worked well, demonstrating excellent hemodynamics generating flows of 10 L/min and the maintenance of normal

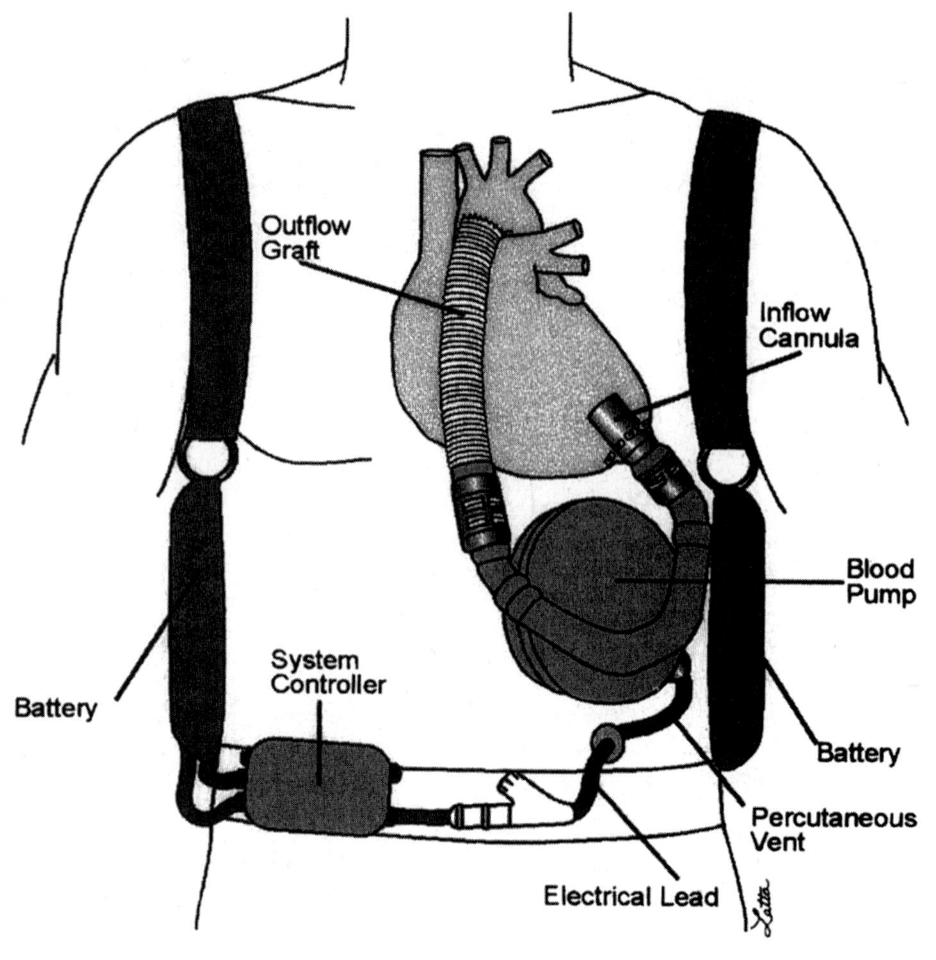


FIGURE 26-12 HeartMate VE left ventricular assist system with an implanted pump-drive unit, percutaneous connection, belt-clipped controller, and underarm battery packs.

pressures in the heart.[134] In July 2001, surgeons from the University of Louisville first implanted the AbioCor in a patient who had been rejected for transplantation.[135] The device consists of an internal thoracic unit, an internal rechargeable battery, an internal miniaturized electronics package and an external battery pack. The ventricles are excised at the time of implantation, leaving the mitral and tricuspid annula intact. The use of transcutaneous energy transmission eliminates the need for the patient to be immobilized permanently by tubes or wires connected to an external power source thereby reducing the rate of infection and facilitating out-of-hospital care.[136] The patients that have had the replacement heart implanted were ineligble for heart transplantation and were dependent on inotropes and/or intraaortic balloon counterpulsation with a greater than 70 percent risk of dying in 30 days or less. All potential candidates underwent computed tomography of the chest to ensure that the system fit. The most common complication causing death has been cerebrovascular accidents.

The CardioWest total artificial heart is approved for use in the United States under an FDA investigational device exemption. Its indication is for use as a bridge to transplantation in patients with biventricular failure. The inclusion criteria are: (1) patients must be listed for transplantation and in imminent danger of dying within 48 h or becoming ineligible for transplant; (2) cardiac index $< 2.0$ L/min/m$^2$ with either systolic blood pressure $< 90$ mmHg or central venous pressure $> 18$ mmHg and/or 2 inotropes; (3) pulmonary vascular resistance $< 8$ Wood Units; (4) absence of systemic infection; (5) absence of renal or hepatic failure, and (6) cytotoxic antibody level $< 10$ percent.[135–138] The CardioWest heart is pneumatically driven and is implanted in the orthotopic position following bilateral ventriculectomy.[137] The pump consists of a rigid pump housing that contains dual spherical polyurethane chambers; dual pneumatic drivelines exit transcutaneously to a console control system that monitors pump pressures and performance. Experience with the CardioWest heart has been favorable. The mean duration of implant was 34 days. Complications included bleeding, hepatic failure, renal failure, respiratory failure, neurologic events, infections, and thromboembolic events with a mean complication rate of 3 events per patient. A survival rate of 81 percent was reported for those patients surviving to transplantation and up to 90 percent of those transplanted surviving more than 5 years.[138–140]

## Future Endeavors in Mechanical Support

During the past decade, mechanical support has gained increased acceptance as a treatment for patients with severe heart failure who are unresponsive to conventional treatment. These devices have been shown to save lives and in some cases allow for long-term assistance out of hospital. However, the ideal mechanical support device has yet to be developed.[141]

The LionHeart LVAD 2000 (Arrow International, Reading, PA) is a totally implantable pulsatile LVAD system tested in human trials. In Europe this device has been shown to be clinically useful and is the first system to undergo clinical testing as a device exclusively designed for destination therapy.[142,143]

The HeartSaver ventricular assist device (World Heart Corporation, Ottawa, Canada) was designed as a portable system to be implanted in the thoracic cavity.[142,144] Its goals were to have a device that was thoracic in position, totally implantable without percutaneous connections, and controlled from remote locations.[145] The selection of the intrathoracic implant site for the system was based on the fact that the inflow cannula could be shorter compared to intraabdominal devices; shortened inflow cannula may improve inflow characteristics and the rib cage would provide a secure anchoring site to eliminate device migration.[145] HeartSaver VAD is undergoing final animal testing before regulatory approval and introduction to clinical application.

Alternatives to pulsatile systems are continuous nonpulsatile flow pumps of axial design. The LVAD systems of nonpulsatile, axial flow design undergoing experimental investigation in human trials include the Jarvik 2000 Heart (Jarvik Heart Inc., New York, NY), MicroMed

DeBakey VAD (MicroMed Technology Inc., Houston, TX), and HeartMate II (Thoratec Laboratories Inc., Pleasanton, CA).

The Jarvik 2000 is a miniature LVAD weighing only 90 g that can be implanted via a left lateral thoracotomy, off cardiopulmonary bypass, into the LV and the descending thoracic aorta.[146,147] It has been approved for use in the United States under an FDA investigational device exemption. The power cable is connected to a percutaneous retroauricular skull-mounted pedestal and the portable batteries and control unit only weigh 1.5 kg (Fig. 26-13). The Jarvik 2000 functions as a true assist device by partially unloading the LV and thereby optimizing the patient's hemodynamics. Experience in patients with class IV heart failure has shown that it is a valid option for long-term treatment for patients, including children, in a truly outpatient setting.[147–150]

The MicroMed DeBakey VAD is an externally powered axial-flow, nonpulsatible device based on technology used in NASA's space shuttle. The device is normally placed using a median sternotomy although in patients with previous sternotomies, the device has been successfully implanted via a left lateral thoracotomy. It was the first of the continuous flow LVADs to undergo clinical trials both in Europe and North America. The experience has been favorable although thromboembolic events may be limiting.[151–153]

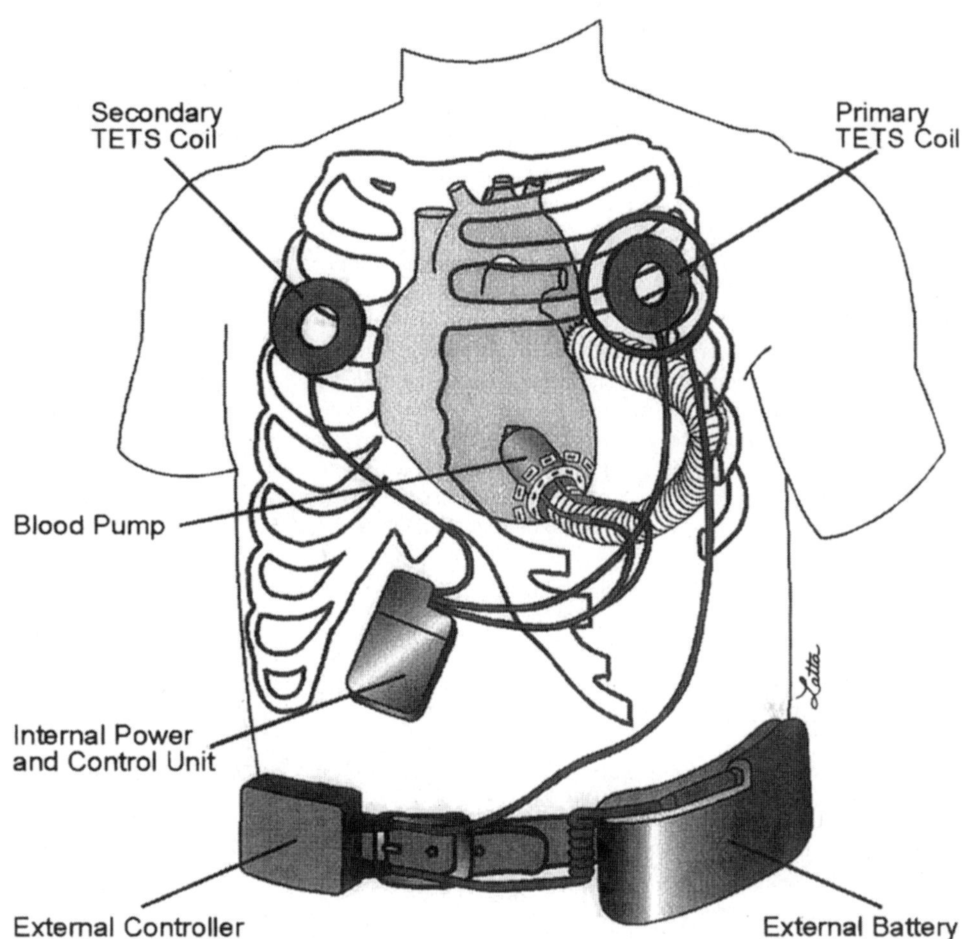


FIGURE 26-13 Jarvik 2000 heart. Fully implantable configuration with an intraventricular pump, internal controller, redundant transcutaneous energy transmission system, and wearable external controller and battery pack.

## Bridge to Transplantation

VADs have become well-accepted treatment modalities to bridge patients with severe heart failure to transplantation. The appropriate VAD patient has been defined as one that is considered a transplant candidate with hemodynamic variables including a cardiac index $< 2.0$ L/min$^{-1}$/m$^{-2}$, a systolic blood pressure $< 80$ mmHg, a pulmonary capillary wedge pressure $> 20$ mmHg, and taking maximal medical therapy.[154] Other considerations must also be taken into account, the most important of which is right heart status. Right heart failure is the most important cause of perioperative mortality in this selected population. The right heart may have to be supported prior to transplantation in order to improve end-organ perfusion. Decisions concerning bi- versus univentricular support will ultimately dictate which device is to be used. Evaluation of the patient's neurologic status is another important but difficult factor in deciding the appropriateness of VAD support. Infection is an important consideration because of the overall prevalence among patients in intensive care settings with invasive monitoring. Ideally patients are to have negative blood cultures for the week before implantation. Patients bridged to transplantation should not be dialysis dependent.[154] Liver function is also predictive of poor outcomes with decreasing survival correlating with increasing bilirubin. Coagulopathic states render VAD therapy difficult.[154]

Patients who undergo VAD insertion prior to transplantation have been found to have improvement in their functional class as well as experience improvement in end-organ function. Therefore, although VAD patients are more seriously ill prior to transplantation, VAD support may ultimately allow for healthier transplant candidates.[155] Which device provides the best outcomes is debatable, but most centers will use clinical experience and patient characteristics and goals to optimize outcomes of VAD support.

## Destination Therapy

VADs can be used when acute heart failure complicates cardiotomy and patients have difficulty weaning from cardiopulmonary bypass.[156,157] Survival rates for this group of patients ranges from 20 to 40 percent at 1 year. Fortunately, the use of VAD support for the goal of recovery in chronic heart failure patients is significantly better.[158–160] In these selected patients, mechanical unloading of the ventricle results in recovery of myocardial function. These patients then have their VAD removed and return to normal clinical function having avoided heart transplantation.

The largest group of patients who are started on VAD support are completely dependent on the device and, therefore, long-term support is an acceptable therapy as a bridge to transplantation. Transplantation, however, can never meet the ever-increasing numbers of patients with congestive heart failure. Recognizing that VAD therapy can successfully support the entire circulatory system, VAD support is therefore reasonable as destination therapy. The Randomized Evaluation of Mechanical Assistance for the Treatment of Congestive Heart Failure (REMATCH) trial was a multicenter study supported by the National Heart, Lung and Blood Institute to compare long-term implantation of LV assist devices with optimal medical management for patients with end-stage heart failure who would otherwise require, but did not qualify for, cardiac transplantation.[161,162] To qualify for the REMATCH trial, patients had to have symptoms of NYHA class IV heart failure and were ineligible for cardiac transplantation based on age > 65 years, presence of insulin-dependent diabetes with end-organ damage, and chronic renal failure or any major comorbidity, physical or psychiatric, that would make the patient ineligible. Patients randomized to assist devices received the HeartMate VE LVAD, whereas the medically managed patients were treated with digoxin, diuretics, and angiotensin-converting enzyme inhibitors. The trial revealed that the use of LVAD support in patients with heart failure resulted in clinically meaningful survival benefit and an improved quality of life compared to those treated medically. Rates of survival at 1 year were 52 percent in the device group, as compared to 25 percent in the medical-therapy group. Subsequent to this successful study, the HeartMate VE was approved by the FDA for destination therapy in heart failure patients.[161,162]

## References


1. Carrel A, Guthrie CC. The transplantation of veins and organs. *Am J Med* 1905;10:1101.
2. Edwards WS, Edwards PD. *Alexis Carrel: Visionary Surgeon.* Springfield, IL: Charles C Thomas; 1974.
3. Mann FC, Priestly JT, Markowitz J, Yater WM. Transplantation of the intact mammalian heart. *Arch Surg* 1933;26:219–224.
4. Lower RR, Shumway NE. Studies of orthotopic homotransplantation of the canine heart. *Surg Forum* 1960;11:18–19.
5. Starzl TE, Marchioro RI, Waddell WR. The reversal of rejection in human renal homografts with subsequent development of homograft tolerance. *Surg Gynecol Obstet* 1963;117:385–395.
6. Barnard CN. The operation. *S Afr Med J* 1967;41:1271–1274.
7. Oyer PE, Stinson EB, Jamieson SW, et al. Cyclosporine A in cardiac allografting: A preliminary experience. *Transplant Proc* 1983;15: 1247–1252.
8. Reitz BA, Wallwork JL, Hunt SA, et al. Heart-lung transplantation: Successful therapy for patients with pulmonary vascular disease. *N Engl J Med* 1982;306:557–564.
9. Hertz HI, Mohacsi PJ, Taylor DO, et al. The Registry of the International Society for Heart and Lung Transplantation: Introduction to the Twentieth Annual Report—2003. *J Heart Lung Transplant* 2003;22:610–615.
10. Laffel GL, Barrett AI, Finkelstein S, Kaye ML. The relation between experience and outcome in heart transplantation. *N Engl J Med* 1992;327:1220–1225.
11. Hosenpud JD, Breen TJ, Edwards EB, et al. The effect of transplant center volume on cardiac transplant outcome. A report of the United Network for Organ Sharing Scientific Registery. *JAMA* 1994;271:1844–1849.
12. Packer DL, Bardy GH, Worley SJ, et al. Tachycardia-induced cardiomyopathy: A reversible form of left ventricular dysfunction. *Am J Cardiol* 1986;57:563–570.
13. Bull DA, Karwande SV, Hawkins JA, et al. Older transplant recipients still do less well. *J Thorac Cardiovasc Surg* 1996;111:423–428.
14. Heck CF, Shumway SJ, Kaye MP. The Registry of the International Society for Heart Transplantation: Sixth official report, 1989. *J Heart Transplant* 1989;8:271–276.
15. Edwards BS, Hunt SA, Fowler MB, et al. Cardiac transplantation in patients with preexisting malignant disease. *Am J Cardiol* 1990;65: 501–504.
16. Rhenman MJ, Rhenman B, Icenogle T, et al. Diabetes and heart transplantation. *J Heart Transplant* 1988;7:356–358.
17. Badellino MM, Cavarocchi B, Narins M, et al. Cardiac transplantation in diabetic patients. *Transplant Proc* 1990;22:2384–2388.
18. Ladowski JS, Kormos RL, Uretsky BP, et al. Heart transplantation in diabetic patients. *Transplantation* 1990;49:303–305.
19. Report of the medical consultants on the diagnosis of death to the President's Commission for the study of Ethical Problems in Medicine and Biomedical and Behavioral Research: Guidelines for the determination of death. *JAMA* 1981;246:2184–2186.
20. Evans RW, Manninen DL, Garrison LP, Maier MA. Donor availability as the primary determinant of the future of heart transplantation. *JAMA* 1986;255:1892–1898.
21. Dreyfus G, Jebara V, Mihaileanu MD, Carpentier A. Total orthotopic heart transplantation: An alternative to the standard technique. *Ann Thorac Surg* 1991;52:1181–1184.
22. Yacoub M, Mankad P, Ledingham S. Donor procurement and surgical techniques for cardiac transplantation. *Semin Thorac Cardiovasc Surg* 1990;2:153–161.
23. El Gamel A, Yonan NA, Grant S, et al. Orthotopic cardiac transplantation: A comparison of standard and bicaval Wythenshawe techniques. *J Thorac Cardiovasc Surg* 1995;109:721–730.
24. Traversi E, Pozzoli M, Grande A, et al. The bicaval anastomosis technique for orthotopic heart transplantation yields better atrial function than the standard technique: An echocardiographic automatic boundary detection study. *J Heart Lung Transplant* 1998;17: 1065–1074.
25. Beniaminovitz A, Savoia MT, Oz M, et al. Improved atrial function in bicaval versus standard orthotopic techniques in cardiac transplantation. *Am J Cardiol* 1997;80:1631–1637.
26. Sethi GK, Kosaraju S, Arabia FA, et al. Is it necessary to perform surveillance endomyocardial biopsies in heart transplant recipients? *J Heart Lung Transplant* 1995;14:1047 1051.
27. White JA, Guiraudon C, Pflugfelder PW, Kostuk WJ. Routine surveillance myocardial biopsies are unnecessary beyond one year after heart transplantation. *J Heart Lung Transplant* 1995;14:1052–1056.
28. Michler RE, Smith CR, Drusin RE. Reversal of cardiac transplant rejection without massive immunosuppression. *Circulation* 1986;74 (suppl III):III68–III74.
29. Costanzo-Nordin MR, Silver MA, O'Connell JB. Successful reversal of cardiac allograft rejection with OKT3 monoclonal antibody. *Circulation* 1987;76(suppl V):V71–V79.
30. Macris MP, Frazier OH, Lammermeier D, et al. Clinical experience with Muromonab-CD3 monoclonal antibody (OKT3) in heart transplantation. *J Heart Transplant* 1989;8:281–287.
31. Strober S. Total lymphoid irradiation in alloimmunity and autoimmunity. *J Pediatr* 1987;111(6, part 2):1051–1055.
32. Weinblatt ME. Methotrexate for chronic diseases in adults. *N Engl J Med* 1995;332:330–331.
33. Hunt SA, Strober S, Hoppe RT, Stinson EB. Total lymphoid irradiation for treatment of intractable cardiac allograft rejection. *J Heart Lung Transplant* 1991;10:211–216.
34. Levin B, Bohannon L, Warvariv V, et al. Total lymphoid irradiation (TLI) in the cyclosporine era-use of TLI in resistant cardiac allograft rejection. *Transplant Proc* 1989;21:1793–1795.
35. Costanzo-Nordin MR, Grusk BB, Silver MA. Reversal of recalcitrant cardiac allograft rejection with methotrexate. *Circulation* 1988;78 (suppl III): III47–III57.
36. Bouchart F, Gundry SR, Van Schaack-Gonzales J, et al. Methotrexate as rescue/adjunctive immunotherapy in infant and adult heart transplantation. *J Heart Lung Transplant* 1993;12:427–433.
37. Armitage JM, Kormos RL, Griffith BL, et al. A clinical trial of FK506 as primary and rescue immunosuppression in cardiac transplantation. *Transplant Proc* 1991;23:1149–1152.
38. Pham SM, Kormos RL, Hattler BG, et al. A prospective trial of tacrolimus (FK506) in clinical heart transplantation: Intermediate term results. *J Thorac Cardiovasc Surg* 1996;111:1–9.
39. Renlund DG, Gopinathan SK, Kfoury AG, Taylor DO. Mycophenolate mofetil (MMF) in heart transplantation: Rejection prevention and treatment. *Clin Transplant* 1996;10(1, part 2):136–139.

40. Lorber MI, Basadonna GP, Friedman AL, et al. The evolving role of tor inhibitors for individualizing posttransplant immunosuppression. *Transplant Proc* 2001;33(7-8):3075–3077.
41. Miller L, Brozena S, Valantine HA, for the Rapamycin Investigators. Treatment of acute cardiac allograft rejection with rapamycin; a multicenter dose-ranging study. *J Heart Lung Transplant* 1997;16;(1):44.
42. Eisen HJ, Tuzcu EM, Dorent R, et al. Everolimus for the prevention of allograft rejection and vasculopathy in cardiac-transplant recipients. *N Engl J Med* 2003;349(9):847–858.
43. Trento A, Hardesty T, Griffith BP, et al. Role of the antibody to vascular endothelial cells in hyperacute rejection in patients undergoing cardiac transplantation. *J Thorac Cardiovasc Surg* 1988;95:37–41.
44. Kemnitz J, Cremer J, Restropo-Spectit I, et al. Hyperacute rejection in heart allografts. *Pathol Res Prac* 1991;187:23–29.
45. Billingham ME, Carey NRB, Hammond EH, et al. A working formulation for the standardization of nomenclature in the diagnosis of heart and lung rejection: Heart rejection study group. *J Heart Transplant* 1990;9:587–592.
46. Weiss LM, Movahed LA, Berry GJ, Billingham ME. In situ hybridization studies for CMV viral nucleic acids in heart and lung allograft biopsies. *Am J Clin Pathol* 1990;93:675–679.
47. Randhawa PS, Yousem SA, Paradis IL, et al. The clinical spectrum, pathology and clonal analysis of Epstein-Barr virus-associated lymphoproliferative disorders in heart-lung transplant recipients. *Am J Clin Pathol* 1989;92:177–185.
48. Chadburn A, Chen JM, Hsu DT, et al. The morphologic and molecular genetic categories of posttransplant lymphoproliferative disorders are clinically relevant. *Cancer* 1998;82:1978–1987.
49. Hammond EH, Hansen JK, Spenser LS, Ensley RD. Vascular rejection in cardiac transplantation: Histologic, immunopathologic and ultrastructural features. *Cardiovasc Pathol* 1993;2:21–34.
50. Hammond EH, Yowell RI, Price GD, et al. Vascular rejection of human cardiac allografts and the role of humoral immunity in chronic allograft rejection. *Transplant Proc* 1991;23(suppl 2):26–30.
51. Michaels PJ, Espejo ML, Kobashigawa J, et al. Humoral rejection in cardiac transplantation: RISK factors, hemodynamic consequences and relationship to transplant coronary artery disease. *J Heart Lung Transplant* 2003;22:58–69.
52. Silvergleid AJ, Schrier S. Acute myelogenous leukemia in two patients treated with azathioprine for non-malignant diseases. *Am J Med* 1974;57:885–888.
53. Penn I. Cancers after cyclosporine therapy. *Transplant Proc* 1988;20 (suppl I):276–279.
54. Young L, Alfieri C, Hennessy K, et al. Expression of Epstein-Barr virus transformation-associated genes in tissues of patients with EBV lymphoproliferative diseases. *N Engl J Med* 1989;321:1080–1085.
55. Hanto DW, Frizzera G, Gail-Peczalska KJ, et al. The Epstein-Barr virus (EBV) in the pathogenesis of post transplant lymphoma. *Transplant Proc* 1981;13:756–760.
56. Hanto DW. Classification of Epstein-Barr virus-associated post transplant lymphoproliferative diseases: Implications for understanding their pathogenesis and developing rational treatment strategies. *Annu Rev Med* 1995;46:381–394.
57. Starzl TE, Porter FA, Iwatsuki S, et al. Reversibility of lymphoma and lymphoproliferative lesions developing under cyclosporine-steroid therapy. *Lancet* 1984;1:583–587.
58. Hanto DW, Frizzera G, Gail-Peczalska KJ, et al. Epstein-Barr virus induced B-cell lymphoma after renal transplantation. *N Engl J Med* 1982;306:913–918.
59. Shapiro RS, Chauvenet A, McGuire W, et al. Treatment of B-cell lymphoproliferative disorders with interferon alpha and intravenous gamma globulin. *N Engl J Med* 1988;318:1334.
60. Papdopoulos EB, Ladanyi M, Emanuel D, et al. Infusions of donor leukocytes to treat Epstein-Barr virus-associated lymphoproliferative disorders after allogeneic bone marrow transplantation. *N Engl J Med* 1994;330:1185–1191.
61. Rooney CM, Smith CA, Ng CYC, et al. Use of gene-modified virus-specific T lymphocytes to control Epstein-Barr-virus related lymphoproliferation. *Lancet* 1995;345:9–13.
62. Gao SZ, Schroeder JS, Alderman EL, et al. Clinical and laboratory correlates of accelerated coronary artery disease in the cardiac transplant patient. *Circulation* 1987;76(suppl V):56–61.
63. Uretsky BF, Murali s, Reddy PS, et al. Development of coronary artery disease in cardiac transplant patients receiving immunosuppressive therapy with cyclosporine and prednisone. *Circulation* 1987;76:827–834.
64. Gao SZ, Schroeder JS, Alderman EL, et al. Prevalence of accelerated coronary artery disease in heart transplant survivors: Comparison of cyclosporine and azathioprine regimens. *Circulation* 1989;80(suppl III):III100–III105.
65. Gao SZ, Alderman EL, Schroeder JS, et al. Accelerated coronary vascular disease in the heart transplant patient: Coronary arteriographic findings. *J Am Coll Cardiol* 1988;12:334–340.
66. Newton M, Vetrovec G, Hastillo A. Coronary angiographic characteristics of chronic cardiac transplant rejection (abstract). *Circulation* 1984;70(suppl II):174.
67. St. Goar FG, Pinto FJ, Alderman EL. Intracoronary ultrasound in cardiac transplant recipients: In vivo evidence of "angiographically silent" intimal thickening. *Circulation* 1992;85:979–987.
68. Heroux AL, Silvermann P, Costanzo MR, et al. Intracoronary ultrasound assessment of morphological and functional abnormalities associated with cardiac allograft vasculopathy. *Circulation* 1994;89:272–277.
69. Rickenbacher PR, Pinto FJ, Lewis NP, et al. Prognostic importance of intimal thickness as measured by intracoronary ultrasound after cardiac transplantation. *Circulation* 1995;92:3445–3452.
70. Billingham ME. Cardiac transplant atherosclerosis. *Transplant Proc* 1987;(suppl 5):19–25.
71. Pucci AM, Forbes RDC, Billingham ME. Pathologic features in long-term cardiac allografts. *J Heart Lung Transplant* 1990;9:385–388.
72. Berry GJ, Rizeq MN, Weiss LM, Billingham ME. Graft coronary disease in pediatric heart and combined heart-lung transplant recipients: A study of 15 cases. *J Heart Lung Transplant* 1993;12:S309–S319.
73. Kaye DM, Esler M, Kingwell B, et al. Functional and neurochemical evidence for partial cardiac sympathetic reinnervation after cardiac transplantation in humans. *Circulation* 1993;88:1110–1118.
74. Bernardi L, Bianchini B, Spadacini G, et al. Demonstrable cardiac reinnervation after human heart transplantation by carotid baroreflex modulation of RR interval. *Circulation* 1995;92:2895–2903.
75. Givertz MM, Hartley LH, Collucci WS. Long-term sequential changes in exercise capacity and chronotropic responsiveness after cardiac transplantation. *Circulation* 1997;96:232–237.
76. Bengel FM, Ueberfuhr P, Ziegler SI, et al. Serial assessment of sympathetic reinnervation after orthotopic heart transplantation: A longitudinal study using PET and C-11 hydroxyephedrine. *Circulation* 1999;99:1866–1871.
77. Stark RP, McGinn AL, Wilson RF. Chest pain in cardiac transplant recipients: Evidence of sensory reinnervation after cardiac transplantation. *N Engl J Med* 1991;324:1791–1794.
78. Smart FW, Ballantyne CM, Cocanougher B, et al. Insensitivity of noninvasive tests to detect coronary artery vasculopathy after heart transplant. *Am J Cardiol* 1991;67:243–247.
79. Akosah KO, Mohanty PK, Funai JT. Noninvasive detection of transplant coronary artery disease by dobutamine stress echocardiography. *J Heart Lung Transplant* 1994;13:1024–1038.
80. Derumeaux G, Redonnet M, Mouton-Schliefer D. Dobutamine stress echocardiography in orthotopic heart transplant recipients. *J Am Coll Cardiol* 1995;25:1665–1672.
81. Spes CH, Klauss V, Mudra H, et al. Diagnostic and prognostic value of serial dobutamine stress echocardiography for noninvasive assessment of cardiac allograft vasculopathy: A comparison with coronary angiography and intravascular ultrasound. *Circulation* 1999;100:509–515.
81a. Keogh AM, Valantine HA, Hunt SA, et al. Impact of proximal or mid-vessel discrete coronary artery stenosis on survival after heart transplantation. *J Heart Lung Transplant* 1992;11:892–901.

82. Schroeder JS, Gao SZ, Alderman EL, et al. A preliminary study of diltiazem in the prevention of coronary artery disease in heart transplant recipients. *N Engl J Med* 1993;328:164–170.
83. Kobashigawa JA, Katznelson S, Laks H, et al. Effect of pravastatin on outcomes after cardiac transplantation. *N Engl J Med* 1995;333:621–627.
84. Wenke K, Meiser B, Thiery J, et al. Simvastatin reduces graft vessel disease and mortality after heart transplantation: A four-year randomized trial. *Circulation* 1997;96:1398–1402.
85. Halle AA, DiSciascio G, Massin EK, et al. Coronary angioplasty, atherectomy and bypass surgery in cardiac transplant recipients. *J Am Coll Cardiol* 1995;26:120–128.
86. Smith JA, Ribakove GH, Hunt SA, et al. Heart retransplantation: The 25 year experience at a single institution. *J Heart Lung Transplant* 1995;14:832–839.
87. Ubel PA, Arnold RM, Caplan AL. Rationing failure: The ethical issues of the retransplantation of scarce vital organs. *JAMA* 1993;270: 2469–2474.
88. Starling RC. Introduction: Cardiac Surgery for Heart Failure. *Semin Thorac Cardiovasc Surg* 2002;14(2):122–124.
89. Hertz MI, Taylor DO, Trulock EP, et al. The Registry of the International Society for Heart and Lung Transplantation: Nineteenth Official Report—2002. *JISHLT* 2002;21(9):950–970.
90. Torrent-Guasp F, Buckberg GD, Clemente C, et al. The structure and function of the helical heart and its buttress wrapping. I. The normal macroscopic structure of the heart. *Semin Thorac Cardiovasc Surg* 2001;13:301–319.
91. Buckberg GD, Clemente C, Cox JL, et al. The structure and function of the helical heart and its buttress wrapping. Part IV. Concepts of dynamic function from the normal macroscopic helical structure. *Semin Thorac Cardiovasc Surg* 2001;13:358–385.
92. Buckberg GD, Coghlan HC, Torrent-Guasp F. The structure and function of the helical heart and its buttress wrapping. Part V. Anatomic and physiologic considerations in the healthy and failing heart. *Semin Thorac Cardiovasc Surg* 2001;13:358–385.
93. Buckberg GD, Coghlan HC, Torrent-Guasp F. The structure and function of the helical heart and its buttress wrapping. Part VI. Geometric concepts of heart failure and use for structural correction. *Semin Thorac Cardiovasc Surg* 2001;13:386–401.
94. Dickstein ML, Spotnitz HM, Rose EA, Burkhoff D. Heart reduction surgery: An analysis of the impact on cardiac function. *J Thorac Cardiovasc Surg* 1997;113:1032–1040.
95. Dor V, Sabatier M, Di Donato M, et al. Efficacy of endoventricular patch plasty in large postinfarction akinetic scar and severe left ventricular dysfunction: Comparison with a series of large dyskinetic scars. *J Thorac Cardiovasc Surg* 1998;116:50–59.
96. Dor V, Di Donato M, Sabatier M, et al. Left ventricular reconstruction by endoventricular circular patch plasty repair: A 17-year experience. *Semin Thorac Cardiovasc Surg* 2001;13:435–447.
97. Athanasuleas CL, Stanley AWH, Buckberg GD, et al. Surgical anterior ventricular endocardial restoration (SAVER) for dilated ischemic cardiomyopathy. *Semin Thorac Cardiovasc Surg* 2001;13:448–458.
98. Athanasuleas CL, Stanley AWH, Buckberg GD, et al. Surgical anterior ventricular endocardial restoration (SAVER) in the dilated remodeled ventricle after anterior myocardial infarction. *J Am Coll Cardiol* 2001; 37:1199–1209.
99. Menicanti L, Di Donato M. Surgical ventricular reconstruction and mitral regurgitation: What have we learned from 10 years of experience? *Semin Thorac Cardiovasc Surg* 2001;13:496–503.
100. Di Donato M, Toso A, Maioli M, et al. Intermediate survival and predictors of death after surgical ventricular restoration. *Semin Thorac Cardiovasc Surg* 2001;13:468–475.
101. Suma H, Isomura T, Horii T, Hisatomi K. Left ventriculoplasty for ischemic cardiomyopathy. *Eur J Cardiothorac Surg* 2001;20:319–323.
102. Batista RJV, Santos JLV, Takeshita N, et al. Partial left ventriculectomy to improve left ventricular function in end-stage heart disease. *J Cardiovasc Surg* 1996;11:96–97.
103. Batista RJV, Verde J, Nery P, et al. Partial left ventriculectomy to treat end-state heart disease. *Ann Thorac Surg* 1997;64:634–638.
104. Franco-Cerecada A, McCarthy PM, Blackstone EH, et al. Partial left ventriculectomy for dilated cardiomyopathy: Is this an alternative to transplantation? *J Thorac Cardiovasc Surg* 2001;121:879–893.
105. Replogle RL, Kaiser GC, Cohn LH, et al. Left ventricular reduction surgery. *Ann Thorac Surg* 1997;63:909–911.
106. Etoch SW, Koenig SC, Laureano MA, et al. Results after partial left ventriculectomy versus heart transplantation for idiopathic cardiomyopathy. *J Thorac Cardiovasc Surg* 1999;117:952–959.
107. Moreira LFP, Stolf NAG, Bocchi EA, et al. Partial left ventriculectomy with mitral valve preservation in the treatment of patients with dilated cardiomyopathy. *J Thorac Cardiovasc Surg* 1998;115:800–807.
108. Moreira LFP, Stolf NAG, Higuchi M, et al. Current perspectives of partial left ventriculectomy in the treatment of dilated cardiomyopathy. *Eur J Cardiothorac Surg* 2001;19:54–60.
109. Kantrowitz A, Tjonneland S, Freed P, et al. Initial clinical experience with intra-aortic balloon pumping in cardiogenic shock. *JAMA* 1968; 203:113–118.
110. Buckley M, Craver J, Gold H, et al. Intra-aortic balloon pump assist for cardiogenic shock after cardiopulmonary bypass. *Circulation* 1973;67 (suppl III): III90–III93.
111. Christenson J, Badel P, Simonet F, Schmuziger M. Preoperative intraaortic balloon pump enhances cardiac performance and improves the outcome of redo CABG. *Ann Thorac Surg* 1997;64:1237–1244.
112. Baskett RJF, Ghali WA, Maitland A, Hirsch GM. The intraaortic balloon pump in cardiac surgery. *Ann Thorac Surg* 2002;74: 1276–1287.
113. Cohen M, Dawson M, Kopistansky C, McBride R. Sex and other predictors of intra-aortic balloon counterpulsation-related complications: Prospective study of 1119 consecutive patients. *Am Heart J* 2000; 139:282–287.
114. Christenson JT, Cohen M, Ferguson JJ, et al. Trends in intraaortic balloon counterpulsation complications and outcomes in cardiac surgery. *Ann Thorac Surg* 2002;74:1086–1091.
115. Meco M, Gramegna G, Yassini A, et al. Mortality and morbidity from intra-aortic balloon pumps. *J Cardiovasc Surg* 2002;43:17–23.
116. Hausmann H, Potapov EV, Koster A, et al. Prognosis after the implementation of an intra-aortic balloon pump in cardiac surgery calculated with a new score. *Circulation* 2002;106(suppl I):I-203–I-206.
117. Cochran RP, Starkey TD, Panos AL, Kunzelman KS. Ambulatory intraaortic balloon pump use as bridge to transplant. *Ann Thorac Surg* 2002;74:746–752.
118. Jeevanandam V, Kayakar D, Anderson AS, et al. Circulatory assistance with a permanent implantable IABP: Initial human experience. *Circulation* 2002;106(suppl I): I-183–I-188.
119. Stevenson LW, Kormos RL. Consensus conference report. Mechanical cardiac support 2002: Current application and future trial design. *J Am Coll Cardiol* 2001;37:340–370.
120. Delgado DH, Rao V, Ross HJ, et al. Mechanical circulatory assistance. State of the art. *Circulation* 2002;106:2046–2050.
121. Couper GS, Dekkers RJ, Adams DH. The logistics and cost-effectiveness of circulatory support: Advantages of the AMBIOMED BVS 5000. *Ann Thorac Surg* 1999;68:646–649.
122. Samuels LE, Holmes EC, Thomas MP, et al. Management of acute cardiac failure with mechanical assist: Experience with the AMBIOMED BVS 5000. *Ann Thorac Surg* 2001;71:S6–S72.
123. Pagani FD, Aaronson KD. LVAD therapy: The future is upon us. *ACC Curr J Rev* 2002;Sept/Oct:90–94.
124. Farrar DJ. The Thoratec ventricular assist device: A paracorporeal pump for treating acute and chronic heart failure. *Semin Thorac Cardiovasc Surg* 2002;12:243–250.
125. Noon GP, Lafuente JA, Irwin S. Acute and temporary ventricular support with BioMedicus centrifugal pump. *Ann Thorac Surg* 1999;68:650–654.
126. Curtis JJ, Walls JT, Wagner-Mann CC, et al. Centrifugal pumps: Description of devices and surgical techniques. *Ann Thorac Surg* 1999; 68:666–671.
127. Robbins RC, Kown MH, Portner PM, Oyer PE. The totally implantable Novacor left ventricular assist system. *Ann Thorac Surg* 2001;71:S162–S165.

128. Robbins RC, Oyer PE. Bridge to transplant with the Novacor left ventricular assist system. *Ann Thorac Surg* 1999;68:695–697.
129. Dagenais F, Portner PM, Robbins RC, Oyer PE. The Novacor left ventricular assist system: Clinical experience from the Novacor registry. *J Cardiovasc Surg* 2001;16:267–271.
130. El-Banayosy A, Arusogul L, Kizner L, et al. Novacor left ventricular assist system versus HeartMate vented electric left ventricular assist system as a long-term mechanical circulatory support device in bridging patient: A prospective study. *J Thorac Cardiovasc Surg* 2000; 119:581–587.
131. McCarthy PM, Smedira NO, Vargo RL, et al. One hundred patients with the HeartMate left ventricular assist device: Evolving concepts and technology. *J Thorac Cardiovasc Surg* 1998;115:904–912.
132. Frazier OH, Rose EA, Oz MC, et al. Multicenter clinical evaluation of the HeartMate vented electric left ventricular assist system in patients awaiting heart transplantation. *J Thorac Cardiovasc Surg* 2001;122: 1186–1195.
133. Kasirajan V, McCarthy PM, Hoercher KJ, et al. Clinical experience with long-term use of implantable left ventricular assist devices: Indications, implantation and outcomes. *Semin Thorac Cardiovasc Surg* 2000;12:229–237.
134. Dowling RD, Etoch SW, Stevens K, et al. Initial experience with the AbioCor implantable replacement heart at the University of Louisville. *American Society of Artificial Internal Organs* J 2000;46:579–581.
135. SoRelle R. Totally contained AbioCor artificial heart implanted July 3, 2001. *Circulation* 2001;104:9005.
136. Arabia FA. Update on the total artificial heart. *J Cardiovasc Surg* 2001;16:222–227.
137. Arabia FA, Copeland JG, Pavie A, Smith RG. Implantation technique for the CardioWest total artificial heart. *Ann Thorac Surg* 1999;68: 698–704.
138. Copeland JG, Smith RG, Arabia FA, et al. The CardioWest total artificial heart as a bridge to transplantation. *Semin Thorac Cardiovasc Surg* 2000;12:238–242.
139. Copeland JG, Arabia FA, Smith RG, et al. Arizona experience with CardioWest total artificial heart bridge to transplantation. *Ann Thorac Surg* 1999;68:756–760.
140. Copeland JG, Smith RG, Arabia FA, et al. The CardioWest total artificial heart as bridge to transplantation. *Semin Thorac Cardiovasc Surg* 2000;12:238–242.
141. Frazier OH. Future direction of cardiac assistance. *Semin Thorac Cardiovasc Surg* 2000;12:251–258.
142. McCarthy PM. Mechanical assist devices. *J Cardiovasc Surg* 2001;16: 178–192.
143. Mehta SM, Pae WE, Rosenberg G, et al. The LionHeart LVAD-2000: A completely implantable left ventricular assist device for chronic circulatory support. *Ann Thorac Surg* 2001;71:S156–S161.
144. Mussivand T, Hendry PJ, Masters RG, Keon WJ. Development of a ventricular assist device for out-of-hospital use. *J Heart Lung Transplant* 1999;18:166–171.
145. Mussivand T, Hendry PJ, Masters RG, et al. Progress with the HeartSaver ventricular assist device. *Ann Thorac Surg* 1999;68:785–789.
146. Westaby S, Banning AP, Jarvik R, et al. First permanent implant of the Jarvik 2000 heart. *Lancet* 2000;356:900–903.
147. Siegenthaler MP, Martin J, van de Loo A, et al. Implantation of the permanent Jarvik-2000 left ventricular assist device. *J Am Coll Cardiol* 2002;39:1764–1772.
148. Westaby S, Frazier OH, Beyersdorf F, et al. The Jarvik 2000 heart: Clinical validation of the intraventricular position. *Eur J Cardiothorac Surg* 2002;22:228–232.
149. Frazier OH, Myers TJ, Gregoric ID, et al. Initial clinical experience with the Jarvik 2000 implantable axial-flow left ventricular assist system. *Circulation* 2002;105:2855–2860.
150. Frazier OH, Myers TJ, Jarvik RK, et al. Research and development of an implantable, axial-flow left ventricular assist device: The Jarvik 2000 heart. *Ann Thorac Surg* 2001;71:S125–S132.
151. Noon GP, Morley DL, Irwin S, et al. Clinical experience with the MicroMed DeBakey ventricular assist device. *Ann Thorac Surg* 2001; 71:S133–S138.
152. Wieselthaler GM, Schima H, Lassnigg A, et al. The DeBakey VAD axial flow pump: First clinical experience with a new generation of implantable, nonpulsatile blood pumps for long-term support prior to transplantation. *Wien Klin Wochenschr* 1999;111:629–635.
153. Wieselthaler GM, Schima H, Hiesmayr M, et al. First clinical experience with the DeBakey VAD continuous-axial-flow pump for bridge to transplantation. *Circulation* 2000;101:356–359.
154. Williams MR, Oz MC. Indications and patient selection for mechanical ventricular assistance. *Ann Thorac Surg* 2001;71:S86–S91.
155. Burnett CM, Duncan JM, Frazier OH, et al. Improved multiorgan function after prolonged univentricular support. *Ann Thorac Surg* 1993;55: 65–71.
156. Smedira NG, Blackstone EH. Postcardiotomy mechanical support: Risk factors and outcomes. *Ann Thorac Surg* 2001;71:S60–S66.
157. Pennington DG, Smedira NG, Samuels LE, et al. Mechanical circulatory support for acute heart failure. *Ann Thorac Surg* 2001;71: S56–S59.
158. Farrar DJ, Holman WR, McBride LR, et al. Long-term follow up of Thoratec ventricular assist device bridge-to-recovery patients successfully removed from support after recovery of ventricular function. *J Heart Lung Transplant* 2002;21:516–521.
159. Frazier OH, Myers TJ. Left ventricular assist system as a bridge to myocardial recovery. *Ann Thorac Surg* 1999;68:734–741.
160. Kumpati GS, McCarthy PM, Hoercher KJ. Left ventricular assist device bridge to recovery: A review of the current status. *Ann Thorac Surg* 2001;71:S103–S108.
161. Rose EA, Moskowitz AJ, Packer M, et al. The REMATCH trial: Rationale, design and end points. *Ann Thorac Surg* 1999;67:723–730.
162. Rose EA, Gelijns AC, Moskowitz AJ, et al. Long-term use of a left ventricular assist device for end-stage heart failure. *N Engl J Med* 2001; 345:1435–1443.

PART FOUR

# RHYTHM AND CONDUCTION DISORDERS

C H A P T E R 27

# MECHANISMS OF CARDIAC ARRHYTHMIAS AND CONDUCTION DISTURBANCES

Albert L. Waldo / Andrew L. Wit



Because of the increasing availability of sophisticated electrophysiologic techniques for the study of cardiac tissues both in vivo and in vitro and the ability to study arrhythmias and conduction disturbances both in experimental models and in patients, knowledge about the mechanisms of arrhythmias and conduction disturbances has increased greatly. Although much is now known, much remains to be understood. Arrhythmias are due to normal or abnormal impulse generation, abnormal impulse conduction, or a combination of simultaneous abnormalities of impulse generation and conduction.[1–9] This chapter provides an overview of these mechanisms and identifies the clinical arrhythmias with which they are thought to be associated. The discussion requires that the reader have a rudimentary knowledge of the basic cellular electrophysiology of the heart, including the ionic channels and membrane currents causing the resting potential and the cardiac action potential, as well as the mechanisms for automaticity and conduction. However, much of this material is included in the discussion of the mechanisms of arrhythmias, since the chapter considers how alterations in normal electrophysiology lead to abnormal cardiac rhythms.

## ARRHYTHMIAS CAUSED BY IMPULSE INITIATION

The term *impulse initiation* is used to indicate that an electrical impulse can arise in a single cell or a group of closely coupled cells through depolarization of the cell membrane and, once initiated, can spread through the rest of the heart. Impulse initiation occurs because of localized changes in ionic currents that flow across the membranes of single cells. There are two major causes for the impulse initiation that may result in arrhythmias: automaticity and triggered activity. Each has its own unique cellular mechanism that results in membrane depolarization (Table 27-1).

### Automaticity

It is convenient to subdivide automaticity into two kinds: normal and abnormal. Normal automaticity is found in the primary pacemaker of the heart, the sinus node, as well as in certain subsidiary or latent pacemakers that can become the pacemaker under the conditions described below. Impulse initiation is a normal property of these latent pacemakers. By contrast, abnormal automaticity, whether the result of experimental interventions or of disease, occurs in cardiac cells only when there are major abnormal changes in their transmembrane potentials, in particular in steady-state depolarization of the membrane potential. This property of abnormal automaticity is not confined to any specific latent pacemaker cell type but may occur almost anywhere in the heart.

#### NORMAL AUTOMATICITY: PACEMAKER MECHANISMS

The normal site of impulse initiation is the sinus node. The cause of normal automaticity in the sinus node is a spontaneous decline in the transmembrane potential during diastole, referred to as the *pacemaker potential, phase 4,* or *diastolic depolarization* (the terms are interchangeable). Diastolic depolarization is the part of the sinus node membrane potential labeled *dd* in the top panel (*A*) of Fig. 27-1. When the depolarization reaches the threshold potential (dashed line labeled *TP*), the upstroke of the spontaneous action potential is initiated. In the case of the sinus node this upstroke is caused mainly by an inward-directed calcium current through L-type calcium channels. This fall in membrane potential during phase 4 reflects a gradual shift in the balance between inward and outward membrane

TABLE 27-1 Types of Tachycardias and Their Selected Characteristics and Documented or Presumed Mechanism

| Tachycardia | Mechanism | Origin | Rate Range, bpm | AV or VA Conduction |
|---|---|---|---|---|
| Sinus tachycardia | Automatic (normal) | Sinus node | ≥100 | 1:1 |
| Sinus node reentry | Reentry | Sinus node and right atrium | ?110–180 | 1:1 or variable |
| Atrial fibrillation | Reentry | Atria | 260–450 | Variable |
| | Fibrillatory conduction | Pulmonary veins, SVC | ? | Variable |
| Atrial flutter | Reentry | Right atrium, left atrium (infrequent) | 240–350, usually 300 ± 20 | 2:1 or variable |
| Atrial tachycardia | Reentry | Atria | 150–240 | 1:1, 2:1, or variable |
| | Automatic (normal or abnormal) | Atria | ? | ? |
| | Triggered (DADs) 2° to digitalis toxicity | Atria | 150–240 | 1:1, 2:1, or variable |
| AV nodal reentry tachycardia | Reentry | AV node with an atrial component | 120–250, usually 150–220 | 1:1 |
| AV reentry (WPW or concealed accessory AV connection) | Reentry | Circuit includes accessory AV connection, atria, AV node, His-Purkinje system, ventricles | 140–250, usually 150–220 | 1:1 |
| Accelerated AV junctional tachycardia | Automatic or ? triggered (? digitalis toxicity) | AV junction (AV node and His bundle) | 61–200, usually 80–130 | 1:1 or variable |
| Accelerated idioventricular rhythm | Abnormal automaticity | Purkinje fibers | >60–? | Variable, 1:1, or AV dissociation |
| Ventricular tachycardia | Reentry | Ventricles | 120–300, usually 140–240 | AV dissociation, variable |
| | Automatic (rare) (normal or abnormal) | Ventricles | ? | Variable, 1:1, or AV dissociation |
| Bundle branch reentrant tachycardia | Reentry | Bundle branches and ventricular septum | 160–250, usually 195–240 | AV dissociation, variable, or 1:1 |
| Right ventricular outflow tract | ? Triggered (DADs) | Right ventricular outflow tract | 120–200 | AV dissociation, variable, or 1:1 |
| Torsades de pointes tachycardia | ? Triggered (EADs) with reentry | Ventricles | >200 | AV dissociation |

ABBREVIATIONS: AV = atrioventricular; DAD = delayed afterdepolarization; WPW = Wolff-Parkinson-White syndrome; EAD = early afterdepolarization; bpm = beats per minute; SVC = superior vena cava.

currents in the direction of net inward (depolarizing) current. Studies have been done to elucidate and characterize the membrane currents that cause diastolic (phase 4) depolarization in the sinus node, using voltage clamp techniques. The cause of the pacemaker potential is still controversial. There is some evidence that diastolic depolarization results from the turning on of an inward current, called $i_f$, which is activated after repolarization of the sinus node action potential. The net inward $i_f$ current is carried largely by $Na^+$.[10] From the voltage clamp studies, it is known that the $i_f$ channels are inactivated at positive membrane potentials, begin to activate after hyperpolarization to around −40 mV, and are fully activated after hyperpolarization to around −100 mV.[11–13] Since the maximum diastolic potential of the sinus node pacemaker cells is between −60 and −70 mV, the $i_f$ current is turned on during repolarization to this level, although it is not fully activated at the maximum diastolic potential. Activation of the $i_f$ conductance also has a time dependency; therefore, the inward current continues to increase after complete repolarization, causing the progressive fall in the membrane potential during phase 4. Important roles for other membrane currents, including the potassium current $i_K$ and the T- and L-type $Ca^{2+}$ currents in causing spontaneous diastolic depolarization, also have been proposed.[14–22] Therefore, there may be no single pacemaker current in the sinus node; rather, a number of currents may contribute to the occurrence of automaticity.[18]

The intrinsic rate at which sinus node pacemaker cells initiate impulses is determined by the interplay of three factors[23]: (1) the maximum diastolic potential, (2) the threshold potential, and (3) the rate or slope of phase 4 depolarization. The third factor is related to the properties of the pacemaker current or currents. A change in any one of these factors will alter the time required for phase 4 depolarization to carry the membrane potential from its maximum diastolic level to threshold and thus alter the rate of impulse initiation. For example, if

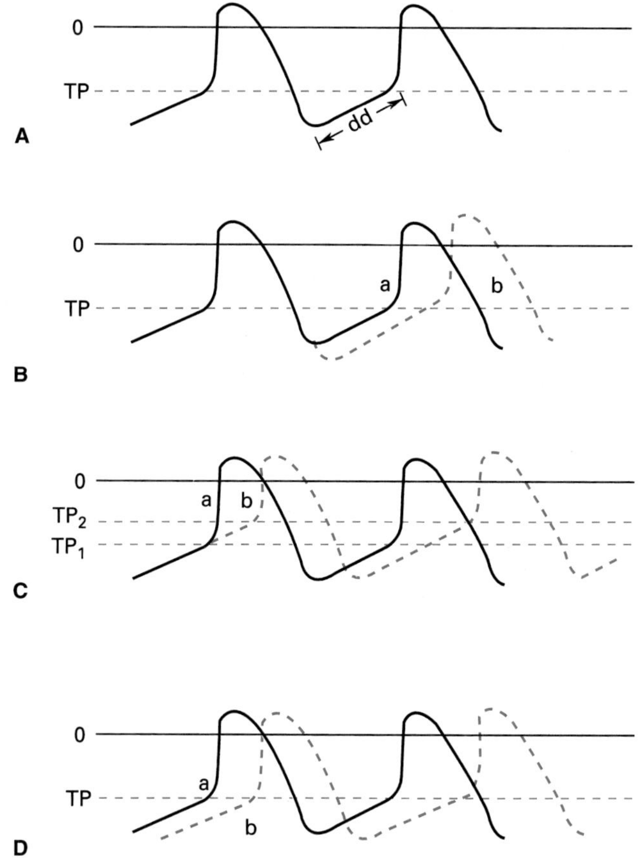


FIGURE 27-1 Diagrams of sinus node action potentials illustrating normal automaticity caused by spontaneous diastolic depolarization and the factors that change the rate of impulse initiation. *A*. Typical sinus node action potential with spontaneous diastolic depolarization (*dd*). *B*. Change in the rate when the maximum diastolic potential is shifted to a more negative level (from *a* to *b*). *C*. Change in rate caused by change in threshold potential to a less negative level (from $TP_1$ to $TP_2$). *D*. Change in rate that occurs when the slope of phase 4 depolarization is decreased (from *a* to *b*). (Modified after Wit AL, Janse MJ. *The Ventricular Arrhythmias of Ischemia and Infarction: The Electrophysiological Mechanisms*. Mount Kisco, NY: Futura; 1992:3. Reproduced with permission from the publisher and authors.)

the maximum diastolic potential increases (becomes more negative), going from the solid trace to the dashed trace in Fig. 27-1*B*, spontaneous depolarization to the threshold potential will take longer and the rate of impulse initiation will fall. Conversely, a decrease in the maximum diastolic potential will tend to increase the rate of impulse initiation (going from dashed trace to solid trace). Similarly, changes in threshold potential or changes in the slope of phase 4 depolarization will alter the rate of impulse initiation. In Fig. 27-1*C*, a change in threshold potential from $TP_1$ to the less negative $TP_2$ causes spontaneous diastolic depolarization to proceed for a longer time (dashed action potential trace) before an impulse is initiated, slowing the rate. In Fig. 27-1*D*, a decrease in the slope of spontaneous diastolic depolarization from *a* to *b* also results in a longer interval between action potentials (dashed trace) because of the longer time required for membrane potential to reach the threshold potential. In Fig. 27-1*C* and *D*, changes in the threshold potential or slope of diastolic depolarization in the opposite direction would speed up the rate.

The alterations in the rate of impulse initiation in the sinus node resulting from the factors discussed above may lead to arrhythmias. These arrhythmias are often a result of the actions of the autonomic nervous system on the sinus node. Parasympathetic stimulation and the resultant release of acetylcholine hyperpolarize the membrane potential through stimulation of muscarinic receptors and the activation of a K current (Fig. 27-1*B*).[24,25] Acetylcholine also decreases the inward $Ca^{2+}$ current and the $i_f$ pacemaker current.[26] A combination of these effects slows the rate. This is a primary mechanism of sinus bradycardia. Sympathetic stimulation and norepinephrine release increase the slope of diastolic depolarization and therefore sinus rate (sinus tachycardia; Table 27-1) by increasing L-type $Ca^{2+}$ current[27] and increasing activation of the inward $i_f$ current at the completion of action potential repolarization.[12,13,28] These effects are mediated through $beta_1$-receptor stimulation.

In addition to the sinus node, cells with pacemaking capability in the normal heart are located in some parts of the atria and ventricles, although they are not pacemakers while the sinus node is functioning normally. These are latent or subsidiary pacemakers. Since spontaneous diastolic depolarization is a normal property, the automaticity generated by these cells is classified as normal. In the atria, cells with well-polarized membrane potentials (resting potentials of around −80 mV) and action potentials characterized by fast upstrokes, a plateau phase of repolarization, and spontaneous diastolic depolarization are located along the crista terminalis (Fig. 27-2*A*).[29] Subsidiary atrial pacemakers with somewhat lower maximum diastolic potentials (−75 to −70 mV) and prominent phase 4 depolarization are located at the junction of the inferior right atrium and the inferior vena cava, near or on the eustachian ridge (a remnant of the eustachian valve of the inferior vena cava) (Fig. 27-2*B*).[30–32] Other

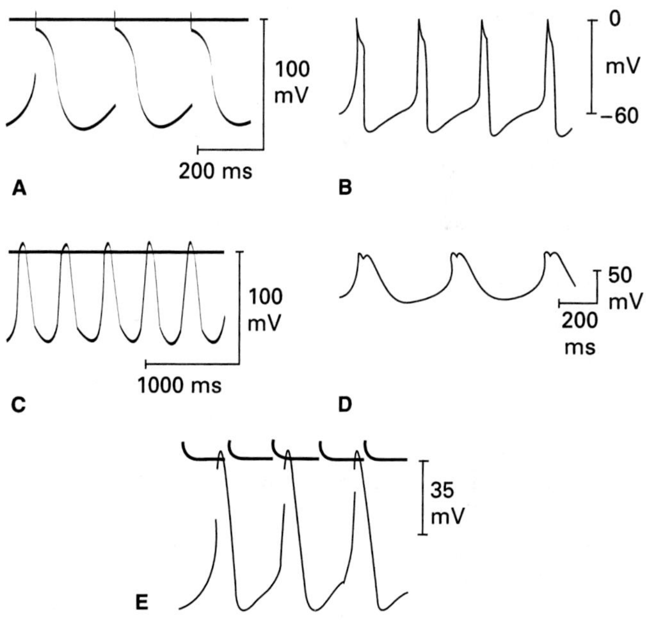


FIGURE 27-2 Transmembrane potentials recorded in isolated superfused preparations from some subsidiary pacemaker cells with the property of normal automaticity. Spontaneous diastolic depolarization that developed in the absence of overdrive suppression is shown in each panel. *A*. Atrial fiber in the crista terminalis in the presence of isoproterenol. *B*. Atrial fiber in the inferior right atrium. *C*. Atrial fiber in the ostium of the coronary sinus in the presence of norepinephrine. *D*. Atrial fiber in stretched mitral valve leaflet. *E*. Atrioventricular nodal fiber of the rabbit heart after the AV node was separated from the atrium. (From Wit AL, Janse MJ. *The Ventricular Arrhythmias of Ischemia and Infarction: The Electrophysiological Mechanisms*. Mount Kisco, NY: Futura; 1992:7. Reproduced with permission from the publisher and authors.)

potential atrial pacemakers are at the orifice of the coronary sinus (Fig. 27-2*C*)[33] and in the atrial muscle that extends into the tricuspid and mitral valves (Fig. 27-2*D*).[34–36] Action potentials of cells in the valves have slow upstrokes that probably are caused to a significant extent by L-type $Ca^{2+}$ current. The cardiac muscle sleeves that extend into the cardiac veins (vena cavae and pulmonary veins) may also have the property of normal automaticity.[36a,b,c] In the AV junction, AV nodal cells possess the intrinsic property of automaticity (Fig. 27-2*E*),[37] although there is still some uncertainty about the exact location of these pacemakers in the node.[38] The intrinsic rate of the atrial pacemakers is greater than that of AV junctional pacemakers.[39] Both atrial and AV junctional subsidiary pacemakers are under autonomic control, with the sympathetics enhancing pacemaker activity through beta$_1$-adrenergic stimulation and the parasympathetics inhibiting pacemaker activity through muscarinic receptor stimulation.[40–43] In the ventricles, latent or subsidiary pacemakers are found in the His-Purkinje system, where Purkinje fibers have the property of spontaneous diastolic depolarization (Fig. 27-3).[23,44] The intrinsic Purkinje fiber pacemaker rate in general is lower than the rate of atrial and AV junctional pacemakers and decreases from the His bundle to the distal Purkinje branches.[45] The spontaneous diastolic depolarization in this region is also under similar autonomic control. As in the atria, sympathetic activation enhances automaticity,[46] while parasympathetic activation can reduce it, mostly through inhibition of sympathetic influences.[47,48]

The membrane currents that cause the normal spontaneous diastolic depolarization at ectopic sites also have been studied. The most thorough analyses have been done on the pacemaker current in Purkinje's cells (Figure 27-3) using voltage clamp techniques. These studies have shown the presence of an $i_f$ pacemaker current, as in the sinus node.[28,49,50] The $i_f$ channels are deactivated during the action potential upstroke and the initial plateau phase of repolarization but begin to activate as repolarization brings the membrane potential to levels more negative than about −60 mV. Since the activation kinetics are slow, the channels continue to activate throughout diastole, leading to an increasing net inward current carried mostly by $Na^+$ and diastolic depolarization.[49,50] Other currents are also likely to contribute to the pacemaker potential in Purkinje's cells.[28,51–53] It is likely that the net increase in inward current during diastole that causes spontaneous diastolic depolarization in Purkinje fibers is a result of an increase in an inward current $i_f$ and a decrease in outward currents ($i_{K1}$ and $i_K$).[52]

## ABNORMAL AUTOMATICITY: PACEMAKER MECHANISMS

Working atrial and ventricular myocardial cells do not normally have spontaneous diastolic depolarization and do not initiate spontaneous impulses even when they are not excited for long periods of time by propagating impulses. When the resting potentials of working atrial or ventricular myocardial cells are reduced sufficiently, however, spontaneous diastolic depolarization may occur and cause repetitive impulse initiation, a phenomenon called *depolarization-induced automaticity* or *abnormal automaticity*. The level of membrane potential at which abnormal automaticity occurs is often in a range between −70 and −30 mV.[54] Likewise, cells in the Purkinje system, which are normally automatic at high levels of membrane potential, also show abnormal automaticity when the membrane potential is reduced.[55] As was discussed before, the $i_f$ channels that participate in normal pacemaker activity in Purkinje fibers have a gating mechanism controlling channel opening and closing that is dependent on the transmembrane voltage. At membrane potentials that are positive to about −60 mV, as occurs after the upstroke and during the early phases of repolarization, the channels are closed. In response to the negative potentials that occur after complete repolarization, the channels reopen, generating the inward pacemaker current.[49,50] For this reason, when the steady-state membrane potential of Purkinje fibers is reduced to around −60 mV or less, as sometimes may occur in ischemic regions of the heart, these normal pacemaker channels are not functional and automaticity is not caused by the normal pacemaker mechanism. It can, however, be caused by an "abnormal" mechanism (described below).

In Fig. 27-4, the transmembrane potential recorded from a spontaneously firing Purkinje fiber with normal automaticity is shown in panel *A*, and abnormal automatic activity occurring while the membrane potential is depolarized to progressively lower membrane potentials is shown in panel *B*, *1*, *2*, and *3*. The abnormal automatic rate increased as membrane potential became more positive. This is a general characteristic of abnormal automaticity in atrial and ventricular cells as well. A low level of membrane potential is not the only criterion for defining abnormal automaticity. If this were so, the automaticity of the sinus node would have to be considered abnormal. Therefore, an important distinction between abnormal and normal automaticity is that the membrane potentials of fibers showing the abnormal type of activity are reduced from their own normal level. For this reason, automaticity in the AV node or valves, where membrane potential is normally low, is not classified as abnormal automaticity. A likely cause of automaticity at depolarized membrane potentials in ventricular muscle is activation and deactivation of the delayed rectifier K current.[56,57] The conductance of this K channel is activated during the normal action potential plateau, and the outward current that flows through it normally contributes to repolarization. The channel then deactivates during

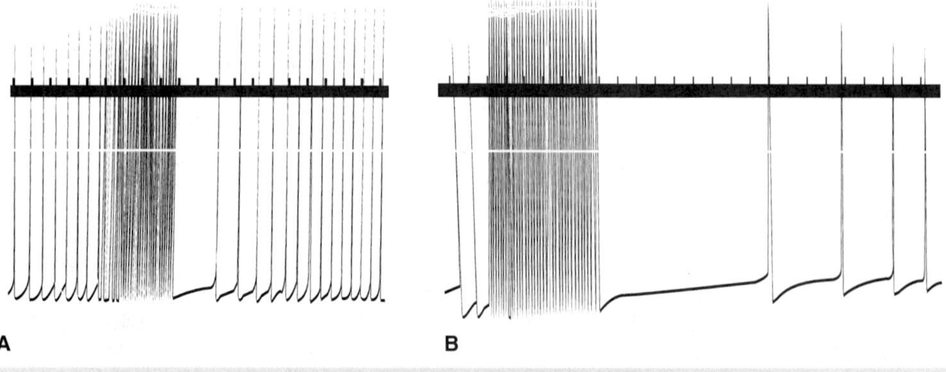


FIGURE 27-3 Overdrive suppression of normal automaticity in a canine Purkinje fiber. The action potentials are displayed at a slow oscilloscopic sweep speed, and so the time course of repolarization cannot be seen. Note the warmup of the spontaneous pacemaker after the termination of pacing. (From Cranefield PF. *The Conduction of the Cardiac Impulse: The Slow Response and Cardiac Arrhythmia*. Mount Kisco, NY: Futura; 1975. Reproduced with permisson from the publisher and author.)

diastole. No significant outward current flows through this channel at normal diastolic potentials, since the resting potential lies near the reversal potential and the driving force is negligible.[57] When the membrane potential is depolarized, however, an outward current flows through this channel, which is activated at the depolarized membrane potentials. This current hyperpolarizes the membrane potential. As the channel then deactivates at the hyperpolarized potentials, spontaneous diastolic depolarization occurs. If either Na or Ca channels have been reactivated since the preceding action potential, the spontaneous depolarization caused by K-channel deactivation may lead to an upstroke caused by current flowing through one of these channels (depending on the level of the membrane potential).[57] A similar mechanism may cause abnormal automaticity in partially depolarized Purkinje fibers.

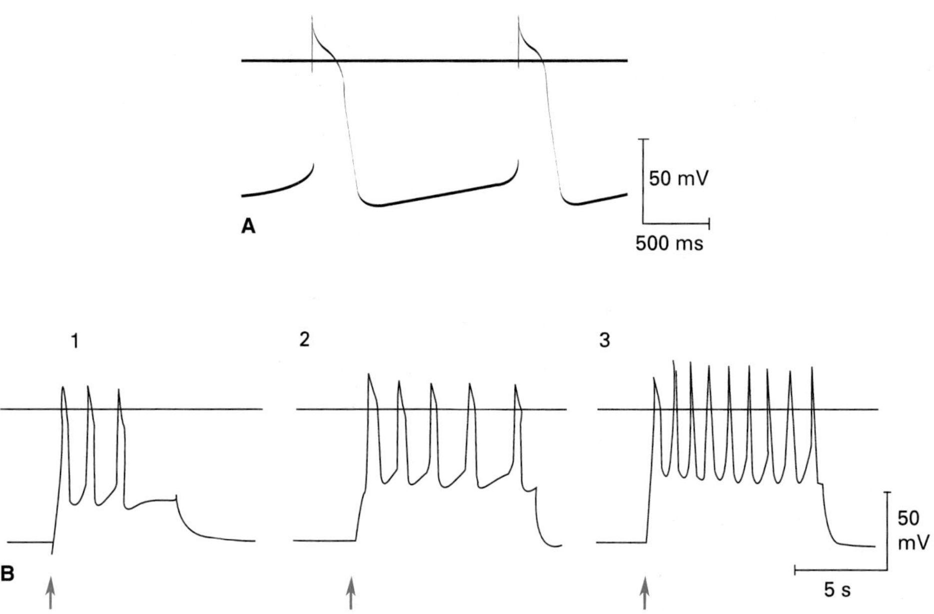


FIGURE 27-4 Normal and abnormal automaticity in a canine Purkinje fiber. *A.* Transmembrane potential recording from a Purkinje fiber with a normal maximum diastolic potential of −85 mV and spontaneous diastolic depolarization. *B.* Abnormal automaticity that occurred when membrane potential was decreased: (1) Fiber was depolarized (*at arrow*) to a membrane potential of −45 mV by the injection of a long-lasting current pulse through a microelectrode, (2) membrane potential was reduced to −40 mV (*at arrow*), (3) membrane potential was reduced to −30 mV (*at arrow*). (Reproduced from Wit AL, Friedman PF. Basis for ventricular arrhythmias accompanying myocardial infarction: Alterations in electrical activity of ventricular muscle and Purkinje fibers after coronary artery occlusion. *Arch Intern Med* 1975;135:459. Reproduced with permission from the publisher and author.)

Experiments on depolarized human atrial myocardium from dilated atria indicate that $Ca^{2+}$-dependent processes also may contribute to abnormal pacemaker activity at low membrane potentials.[58,59] It was proposed that intracellular $Ca^{2+}$ released from the sarcoplasmic reticulum (SR) controls membrane permeability to an inward current during diastole, leading to spontaneous diastolic depolarization and abnormal automaticity. The mechanism may be similar to the one that causes the transient inward current responsible for DADs (see "Triggered Rhythms," below). An increase in intracellular $Ca^{2+}$ also is expected to cause an inward $Na^+$ current through $Na^+$–$Ca^{2+}$ exchange. In summary, therefore, several different mechanisms probably cause abnormal automaticity, including activation and deactivation of $K^+$ currents, $Ca^{2+}$-dependent activation of an inward current, inward $Ca^{2+}$ currents, and even some contribution by the pacemaker current $i_f$. It has not been determined which of these mechanisms are operative in the different pathologic conditions in which abnormal automaticity may occur.

The upstrokes of the spontaneously occurring action potentials generated by abnormal automaticity may be caused by either $Na^+$ or $Ca^{2+}$ inward currents or possibly a mixture of the two. In the range of diastolic potentials between approximately −70 and −50 mV, repetitive activity is dependent on extracellular $Na^+$ concentration and can be decreased or abolished by the $Na^+$ channel blockers lidocaine and tetrodotoxin, indicating that the $Na^+$ inward current is involved. In a diastolic potential range of approximately −50 to −30 mV, repetitive activity depends on extracellular $Ca^{2+}$ concentration and is reduced by $Ca^{2+}$ channel blockers, $Mn^{2+}$, and verapamil, indicating a role for the L-type $Ca^{2+}$ inward current.[5,60] The decrease in the membrane potential of cardiac cells required for abnormal automaticity to occur may be induced by a variety of factors related to cardiac disease. Although an increase in the extracellular potassium concentration can reduce membrane potential, normal or abnormal automaticity in working atrial, ventricular, and Purkinje fibers usually does not occur when $[K]_o$ is elevated because of the increase in $K^+$ conductance (and hence net outward current) that results from an increase in $[K]_o$.[61,62] This argues against abnormal automaticity being responsible for arrhythmias arising in acutely ischemic myocardium, where cells are partially depolarized by increased extracellular $K^+$.[63–65] A decrease in $[K]_i$, which also causes a decreased membrane potential, has been shown to occur in the Purkinje fibers that survive on the endocardial surface of infarcts, and this decrease persists for at least 24 h after the coronary occlusion.[66] The reduction in $[K]_i$ contributes to the low membrane potential[67] and the accompanying abnormal automaticity.[68,69] Isolated preparations of diseased atrial and ventricular myocardium from human hearts superfused with Tyrode's solution show phase 4 depolarization and abnormal automaticity at membrane potentials in the range of −50 to −60 mV.[70–72] It has been proposed that a decrease in membrane potassium conductance is an important cause of the low membrane potentials in the atrial fibers.[71]

## SUPPRESSION OF NORMAL AND ABNORMAL AUTOMATIC SUBSIDIARY PACEMAKERS

During sinus rhythm in a normal heart, the intrinsic rate of impulse initiation resulting from automaticity of cells in the sinus node is higher than that of the other potentially automatic cells, and the latent pacemakers are excited by propagated impulses from the sinus node before they can depolarize spontaneously to threshold potential. Not only are latent pacemakers prevented from initiating an impulse because they are depolarized before they have a chance to fire, but the diastolic (phase 4) depolarization of the latent pacemaker cells with the property of normal automaticity is actually inhibited because they are repeatedly depolarized by the impulses from the sinus node.[73,74]

This inhibition can be demonstrated by suddenly stopping the sinus node, e.g., by vagal stimulation (vagal stimulation also inhibits subsidiary pacemakers in the atria and AV junction) or in the tissue bath after termination of overdrive pacing (Fig. 27-3). Impulses then usually arise from a subsidiary pacemaker in the ventricular Purkinje system, but that impulse initiation generally is preceded by a long period of quiescence.[75,76] Impulse initiation by the Purkinje fiber pacemaker then begins at a low rate and only gradually speeds up to a final steady rate that is, however, still slower than the original sinus rhythm. The quiescent period after abolition of the sinus rhythm reflects the inhibitory influence exerted on the subsidiary pacemaker by the dominant sinus node pacemaker. This inhibition is called *overdrive suppression*. Similarly, the sinus node also overdrive-suppresses subsidiary atrial pacemakers.[77]

The mechanism of overdrive suppression has been characterized in microelectrode studies of isolated Purkinje fiber bundles exhibiting pacemaker activity.[73] It is mediated mostly by enhanced activity of the $Na^+$,$K^+$ exchange pump that results from driving a pacemaker cell faster than its intrinsic spontaneous rate. During normal cardiac rhythm, the sinus node drives the latent pacemakers at a faster rate than their normal (intrinsic) automatic rate. As a result, the intracellular $Na^+$ of the latent pacemakers is increased to a higher level than would be the case if the pacemakers were firing at their own intrinsic rate. This is the result of $Na^+$ entering the cells during each action potential upstroke. The rate of activity of the $Na^+$ pump is determined largely by the level of intracellular $Na^+$ concentration,[78] so that pump activity is enhanced during high rates of stimulation.[73] The increased pump activity prevents intracellular $Na^+$ from rising to very high levels, although there is some increase in the steady-state $Na^+$ concentration at high rates of firing. Since the $Na^+$ pump moves more $Na^+$ outward than $K^+$ inward, it generates a net outward (hyperpolarizing) current across the cell membrane.[79] When subsidiary pacemaker cells are driven faster than their intrinsic rate by the sinus node, the enhanced outward pump current hyperpolarizes the membrane potential and suppresses spontaneous impulse initiation in these cells, which, as was described before, is dependent on the net inward current. When the dominant (overdrive) pacemaker is stopped, this suppression continues because the $Na^+$ pump continues to generate the outward current as it reduces the intracellular $Na^+$ levels toward normal. The continued $Na^+$ pump–generated outward current is responsible for the period of quiescence, which lasts until the intracellular $Na^+$ concentration, and hence the pump current, becomes small enough to allow subsidiary pacemaker cells to depolarize spontaneously to threshold. Intracellular $Na^+$ concentration decreases during the quiescent period because $Na^+$ is constantly being pumped out of the cell and little is entering.[60] Intracellular $Na^+$ and pump current continue to decline even after spontaneous firing begins because of the slow rate, causing a gradual increase in the discharge rate of the subsidiary pacemaker.

The higher the overdrive rate or the longer the duration of overdrive, the greater the enhancement of pump activity, so that the period of quiescence after the cessation of overdrive is directly related to the rate and duration of overdrive.[73] The sinus node itself also can be overdrive-suppressed if it is driven at a rate more rapid than its intrinsic rate. Thus, there may be a quiescent period after termination of either overdrive pacing or a rapid ectopic arrhythmia before the sinus rhythm resumes.[80–83] When overdrive suppression of the normal sinus node occurs, however, it is of lesser magnitude than that of subsidiary pacemakers overdriven at comparable rates.[30,80] The sinus node action potential upstroke is largely dependent on slow inward current carried by $Ca^{2+}$ through the L-type $Ca^{2+}$ channels, and far less $Na^+$ enters the fiber during the upstroke than occurs in latent pacemaker cells such as Purkinje fibers. As a result, the activity of the $Na^+$ pump probably is not increased to the same extent in sinus node cells after a period of overdrive; therefore, there is less overdrive suppression caused by enhanced $Na^+$ pump current. The relative resistance of the normal sinus node to overdrive suppression may be important in enabling it to remain the dominant pacemaker even when its rhythm is perturbed transiently by external influences such as transient shifts of the pacemaker to an ectopic site. The diseased sinus node, however, may be much more easily overdrive-suppressed.[84]

There is an important distinction between the effects of the dominant sinus pacemaker on the two kinds of automaticity, as abnormal automaticity at reduced levels of membrane potential is not overdrive-suppressed to the same extent as is the normal automaticity that occurs at high levels of membrane potential.[85–87] The amount of suppression of spontaneous diastolic depolarization that causes abnormal automaticity by overdrive is directly related to the level of membrane potential at which the automatic rhythm occurs.[86,87] For example, Purkinje fibers that show automaticity at moderately depolarized membrane potentials of $-60$ to $-70$ mV still manifest some overdrive suppression, although less than do fibers with automaticity at $-90$ mV. Automaticity in Purkinje fibers with membrane potentials less than $-60$ mV is suppressed only slightly by overdrive, if it is suppressed at all. These differences in the effects of overdrive may be related to the reduction in the amount of $Na^+$ entering the cell as the membrane potential decreases, as was described for overdrive of the sinus node. At low levels of membrane potential, $Na^+$ channels are inactivated, decreasing the fast inward $Na^+$ current; therefore, there is a reduction in the amount of $Na^+$ entering the cells during overdrive and the degree of stimulation of the sodium-potassium pump.[88]

In addition to overdrive suppression being of paramount importance for maintenance of normal rhythm, the characteristic response of automatic pacemakers to overdrive, as was discussed in the previous paragraphs, is often useful for identifying mechanisms of arrhythmias in the in situ heart, where arrhythmia mechanisms cannot be identified by recording transmembrane potentials because of the technical difficulties. Not all mechanisms of arrhythmogenesis respond in the same way to overdrive that automatic pacemakers do, and the differences in response sometimes can be used to distinguish among mechanisms. In addition to overdrive suppression, a mechanism that may suppress subsidiary pacemakers is the electrotonic interaction between the pacemaker cells and the nonpacemaker cells in the surrounding myocardium.[89] This mechanism may be particularly important in preventing AV nodal automaticity[90,91] or automaticity in the distal Purkinje system, where the pacemaking Purkinje fibers are in contact with nonpacemaking working ventricular muscle.[89,92,93]

## ARRHYTHMIAS CAUSED BY AUTOMATICITY

Arrhythmias caused by normal or abnormal automaticity of cardiac fibers may occur for several different reasons. Such arrhythmias may result simply from an alteration in the rate of impulse initiation by the normal sinus node pacemaker without a shift of impulse origin to a subsidiary pacemaker at an ectopic site. Sinus bradycardia and tachycardia are examples of these arrhythmias (Table 27-1). The cellular mechanisms that can change the rate of impulse initiation in the sinus node are described in Fig. 27-1. During alterations in sinus rate, there may be shifts of the pacemaker site within the sinus node.[23,94] A shift in the site of impulse initiation to one of the regions where normal or abnormal subsidiary pacemakers are located also results in arrhythmias. This would be expected to happen when any of the following occurs: (1) The rate at which the sinus node activates subsidiary pacemakers falls considerably below the intrinsic rate of the subsidiary pacemakers, (2) inhibitory electrotonic influences between nonpacemaker cells and pacemaker cells are interrupted, or (3) impulse initiation in subsidiary pacemakers is enhanced.

The rate at which the sinus node activates subsidiary pacemakers may be decreased in a number of situations. Impulse initiation by the sinus node may be slowed or inhibited altogether by heightened activity in the parasympathetic nervous system[95] or as a result of sinus node disease.[96] Alternatively, there may be block of impulse conduction from the sinus node to the atria or block of conduction from the atria to the ventricles. A latent pacemaker also may be protected from being overdriven by the sinus node if it is surrounded by a region in which impulses of sinus origin block (entrance block) before reaching the pacemaker cells. Such block, however, must be unidirectional, so that activity from the pacemaker can propagate into surrounding myocardium whenever the surrounding regions are excitable. Some possible mechanisms for unidirectional block are discussed later in this chapter. The protected pacemaker is said to be a *parasystolic focus*.[97] In general, under these conditions, a protected focus of automaticity of this type can fire at its own intrinsic frequency. Electronic current flow from surrounding regions also may influence the cycle length of a protected focus, either prolonging or abbreviating it, depending on whether the surrounding activity occurs during the early or late stage of diastolic depolarization.[98–100] Under any of the above conditions (sinus slowing, sinoatrial or AV block, parasystolic focus), there may be "escape" of a subsidiary pacemaker.

There is a natural hierarchy of intrinsic rates of subsidiary pacemakers that have normal automaticity, with atrial pacemakers having faster intrinsic rates than do AV junctional pacemakers and AV junctional pacemakers having faster rates than do ventricular pacemakers.[45,74] Once overdrive suppression is removed by sinus node inhibition, the pacemaker with the fastest rate becomes the site of impulse origin (Table 27-1).[74] Sometimes mechanisms responsible for the suppression of impulse initiation in the sinus node also suppress pacemaker activity in the atria. In experimental studies in which the sinus node is damaged or removed, the most prevalent atrial pacemaker site is at the junction of the inferior vena cava and the posterior wall of the right atrium.[30,101–103] These atrial pacemakers may cause atrial arrhythmias if the sinus node or its arterial supply is damaged.[104]

Ectopic impulse initiation may occur in the AV junction. In fact, an AV junctional pacemaker may become the dominant rhythm in the absence of normal sinus node function. Atrioventricular junctional pacemakers may be located either in the AV node or in the His bundle. These different sites have somewhat different properties, including their intrinsic rates (faster in the AV node than in the His bundle) and responses to autonomic nerve activity (parasympathetic activity suppresses AV nodal pacemakers to a greater extent than it does His bundle pacemakers). Atrioventricular junctional rhythms may occur during AV block, since the site of block is often proximal to the AV junctional pacemaker location.[38] If AV junctional pacemakers also are suppressed or if the site of disease causing AV block is in the His bundle or bundle branches, the subsidiary pacemaker location is in the His-Purkinje system. The His bundle at the proximal end of the specialized AV conduction system has a faster intrinsic rate than do the more distally located Purkinje fibers.[45] The electrocardiogram (ECG) during idioventricular rhythm in patients with complete heart block often is characterized by a wide, aberrant QRS complex, suggesting impulse initiation in the distal Purkinje system.[105] In acute myocardial ischemia, particularly when it occurs in the inferior wall, parasympathetic activity may be enhanced, depressing the sinus rate, AV conduction, or both.[106] Ectopic impulse initiation then may arise in the ventricular specialized conduction system.[107]

Any event that decreases intercellular coupling between latent subsidiary pacemaker cells and surrounding nonpacemaker cells may remove the inhibitory influence of electrotonic current flow on the latent pacemakers and allow them to fire at their intrinsic rate.[89] Coupling may be reduced by fibrosis, which can separate myocardial fibers. For example, fibrosis in the atrial aspect of the AV junctional region that results in heart block may release nodal pacemakers from electrotonic suppression by surrounding atrial cells and permit them to become the dominant pacemakers driving the ventricles. Uncoupling also may be caused by factors that increase intracellular $Ca^{2+}$,[108] since elevated intracellular $Ca^{2+}$ levels decrease coupling between myocardial cells by decreasing the conductance of gap junction channels (*connexons*). This may result, for example, from treatment with digitalis,[109] which inhibits $Na^+$ extrusion and thus increases $Ca^{2+}$ levels in the cell.[110] In myocardial infarction, Purkinje fiber pacemakers may be uncoupled from damaged ventricular muscle cells, allowing the Purkinje fibers to fire at their intrinsic rates. Some inhibition of the sinus node is still necessary for the site of impulse initiation to shift to an ectopic site that is no longer inhibited because of uncoupling from surrounding cells, since, as explained above, the intrinsic firing rate of subsidiary pacemakers is still slower than that of the sinus node.

Subsidiary pacemaker activity also may be enhanced, causing impulse initiation to shift to ectopic sites even when sinus node function is normal. One cause may be enhanced sympathetic nerve activity. Norepinephrine released locally from sympathetic nerves steepens the slope of diastolic depolarization of latent pacemaker cells[23,33,34,111,112] and diminishes the inhibitory effects of overdrive.[113] The increase in slope of spontaneous diastolic depolarization may result from effects of norepinephrine on the $i_f$ current, as was described above, as well as from an increase in inward $Ca^{2+}$ current in those cells in which this current participates in pacemaker activity. Localized effects on subsidiary pacemakers may occur in the absence of sinus node stimulation.[114] Therefore, sympathetic stimulation may enable the membrane potential of ectopic pacemakers to reach threshold before they are activated by an impulse from the sinus node, resulting in ectopic premature impulses or automatic rhythms. There is evidence that in the subacute phase of myocardial ischemia, increased activity of the sympathetic nervous system may enhance automaticity of Purkinje fibers, enabling them to escape from sinus node domination. Enhanced subsidiary pacemaker activity also may not require sympathetic stimulation. The flow of current between partially depolarized myocardium and normally polarized latent pacemaker cells may enhance automaticity.[115] This mechanism has been proposed to be a cause of some of the ectopic beats that arise at the borders of ischemic areas in the ventricle.[93]

Inhibition of the electrogenic sodium-potassium pump results in a net increase in inward current during diastole because of the decrease in outward current normally generated by the pump and therefore may increase automaticity in subsidiary pacemakers sufficiently to cause arrhythmias. This may occur after adenosine triphosphate (ATP) is depleted during prolonged hypoxia or ischemia or in the presence of toxic amounts of digitalis.[116,117] A decease in the extracellular potassium level also enhances normal automaticity,[75] as does acute stretch.[118] Stretch can induce rapid automatic rates in Purkinje fibers with normal maximum diastolic potentials.[119,120] Stretch of the ventricles also can induce arrhythmias in an intact heart,[121] although the site of origin of the ectopic impulses has not been localized. Stretch of the Purkinje system may occur in akinetic areas after acute ischemia or in ventricular aneurysms in hearts with healed infarcts. At normal sinus rates, there may be little overdrive suppression of pacemakers with abnormal automaticity. As a result of the lack of overdrive suppression, even transient sinus pauses or occasional long sinus cycle lengths may permit an ectopic focus with a slower rate than the sinus node to capture the heart for one or more beats. In contrast, ectopic pacemakers with normal automaticity probably would be quiescent during relatively short, transient sinus pauses because they are overdrive-suppressed.

It is also possible that the depolarized level of membrane potential at which abnormal automaticity occurs may cause entrance block into the focus and prevent it from being overdriven by the sinus node even when impulses initiated in the focus could leave it (unidirectional block).[122] This would lead to parasystole, an example of an arrhythmia caused by a combination of an abnormality of impulse conduction and initiation. All these features of abnormal automaticity are evident in the Purkinje fibers that survive in regions of transmural myocardial infarction and cause ventricular arrhythmias during the subacute phase.[68] The firing rate of an abnormally automatic focus also might be enhanced above that of the sinus node, leading to arrhythmias in the absence of sinus node suppression or conduction block between the focus and the surrounding myocardium. The automatic rate is a direct function of the level of membrane potential: the greater the depolarization, the faster the rate.[5,55,57,123,124] Experimental studies have shown firing rates in muscle and Purkinje fibers of 150 to 200/min at membrane potentials less than −50 mV, and these rates should be sufficiently rapid to enable these pacemakers sometimes to control the rhythm of the heart. Catecholamines also increase the rate of firing caused by abnormal automaticity[125] and therefore may contribute to a shift in the pacemaker site from the sinus node to a region with abnormal automaticity. Among the clinical arrhythmias that are likely to be caused by abnormal automaticity is accelerated idioventricular rhythm after myocardial infarction (see Chap. 52).

Normal or abnormal automaticity may also lead to arrhythmias caused by nonautomatic mechanisms. Premature beats, caused by automaticity, can initiate reentry. Rapid automatic activity in sites such as the cardiac veins can cause fibrillatory conduction, reentry, and atrial fibrillation[36a,b,c] (see below).

## Triggered Activity

*Triggered activity* is a term used to describe impulse initiation in cardiac fibers that is dependent on afterdepolarizations.[126–128] (For arrhythmias caused by triggered activity, see Table 27-1.) Afterdepolarizations are oscillations in membrane potential that follow the upstroke of an action potential. Two kinds of afterdepolarizations may cause triggered activity. One occurs early, i.e., during repolarization of the action potential (early afterdepolarizations, EADs), and the other is delayed until repolarization is complete or nearly complete (delayed afterdepolarizations, DADs). When either kind of afterdepolarization is large enough to reach the threshold potential for activation of a regenerative inward current, action potentials result that are referred to as "triggered." Therefore, a key characteristic of triggered activity, discriminating it from automaticity, is that for triggered activity to occur, at least one action potential must precede it (the trigger). Automatic rhythms can arise de novo in the absence of any prior electrical activity, such as after long periods of quiescence, whereas triggered activity cannot.[5,128] Triggered activity will cause arrhythmias when the site of impulse initiation shifts from the sinus node to the triggered focus. For this to occur, the rate of triggered impulses should be faster than the sinus rate either transiently or persistently. This may result when firing of the sinus node is slowed or inhibited, when there is block of sinus impulses, or when the rate of triggered activity is faster than normal sinus node impulse initiation. The factors causing the shift in the site of impulse initiation should be very similar to those described in the discussion of automaticity.

### DELAYED AFTERDEPOLARIZATIONS AND TRIGGERED ACTIVITY

Figure 27-5 shows an example of a DAD recorded with a microelectrode in a superfused preparation of atrial muscle exposed to catecholamines. The DAD is an oscillation in membrane potential that occurs after repolarization of the action potential (indicated in the figure by the unfilled arrow). The DAD is caused by events occurring during the action potential that are described below. Figure 27-5*A* also shows that a DAD may be preceded by an afterhyperpolarization (blue arrow), in which case the membrane potential transiently becomes more negative after the action potential than it was just before it. Afterhyperpolarizations, however, do not always precede DADs. The transient nature of the DAD clearly distinguishes it from normal spontaneous diastolic (pacemaker) depolarization, during which the membrane potential declines almost monotonically until the next action potential occurs (compare Fig. 27-5*A* with Fig. 27-1). In addition to microelectrode recordings such as the one shown in Fig. 27-5*A*, DADs can be identified by using techniques for recording extracellular potentials.[129–133] A triggered impulse is initiated when a DAD depolarizes the membrane potential to the threshold potential for activation of the inward current responsible for the upstroke of the action potential. Triggered impulses are shown in Fig. 27-5*B*. Afterdepolarizations do not always reach threshold, so that triggerable fibers sometimes may be stimulated at a regular rate without becoming rhythmically active, e.g., the stimulated action potential in Fig. 27-5*A*. Probably the most important influence that causes subthreshold DADs to reach threshold is a decrease in the cycle length (an increase in the rate) at which action potentials occur. Therefore, arrhythmias triggered by DADs can be expected to be initiated by either a spontaneous or a pacing-induced increase in the heart rate. A triggered action potential also is followed by an afterdepolarization that may or may not reach threshold. When it does not reach threshold, only one triggered action impulse occurs. Quite often, the first triggered action potential is followed by a short or long "train" of additional triggered action potentials, each arising from the afterdepolarization caused by the previous action potential (Fig. 27-5*B*).

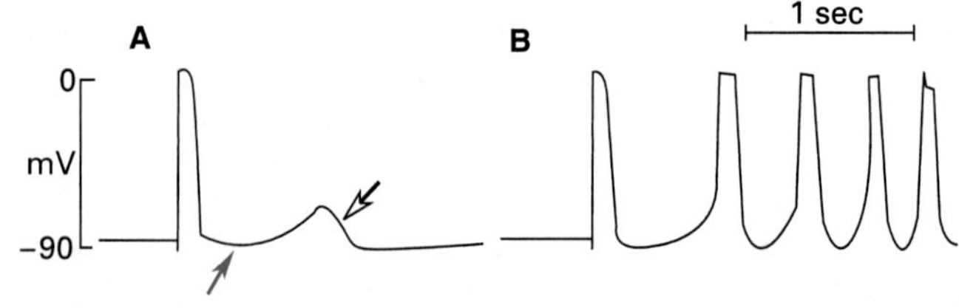


FIGURE 27-5 An example of a DAD (*unfilled arrow*) recorded with a microelectrode from an atrial fiber in the canine coronary sinus. The blue arrow indicates an afterhyperpolarization. *B*. The onset of triggered activity is shown. (From Wit AL, Rosen MR. Afterdepolarizations and triggered activity: Distinction from automaticity as an arrhythmogenic mechanism. In: Fozzard HA, Haber E, Jennings RB, et al., eds. *The Heart and Cardiovascular System. Scientific Foundations,* 2d ed. New York, Raven Press; 1991:2113. Reproduced with permission from the publisher and author.)

## Causes of Delayed Afterdepolarizations and Triggered Activity

Delayed afterdepolarizations usually occur under a variety of conditions in which there is an increase in $Ca^{2+}$ in the myoplasm and the SR above normal levels (sometimes referred to as *Ca overload*). Abnormalities in the sequestration and release of $Ca^{2+}$ by the SR also may contribute to their occurrence. On depolarization of the membrane during an action potential, the intracellular free $Ca^{2+}$ normally increases, primarily by $Ca^{2+}$ influx through the L-type $Ca^{2+}$ channels. Initially, this rapid rate of change of intracellular $Ca^{2+}$ triggers $Ca^{2+}$ release from the SR, causing a further rise in intracellular free $Ca^{2+}$ and contraction.[134] Repolarization then induces synchronous $Ca^{2+}$ uptake by the SR in the cell and relaxation. If intracellular $Ca^{2+}$ is very high or if catecholamines or cyclic adenosine monophosphate (AMP) is present, both of which enhance $Ca^{2+}$ uptake by the SR, the $Ca^{2+}$ in the SR may rise during repolarization to a critical level, at which time a secondary spontaneous release of $Ca^{2+}$ from the SR occurs after the action potential and relaxation of contraction.[134] This secondary release of $Ca^{2+}$ generates an aftercontraction as well as the transient inward (TI) current and the afterdepolarization. The TI current is an oscillatory membrane current that is distinct from the pacemaker currents.[135–142] After one or several afterdepolarizations, myoplasmic $Ca^{2+}$ may decrease because $Na^+$–$Ca^{2+}$ exchange extrudes $Ca^{2+}$ from the cell, and the membrane potential stops oscillating. The exact mechanism by which the secondary rise in myoplasmic $Ca^{2+}$ after repolarization causes the TI current is unclear. Two possibilities have been considered. The first is that the $Ca^{2+}$ released from the SR after repolarization acts on the sarcolemma to increase its conductance to ions (mainly $Na^+$) that flow into the cell down a concentration gradient through membrane channels. The second mechanism proposed for the origin of the TI current is that the rise in $Ca^{2+}$ causes the TI current through an electrogenic (rheogenic) exchange of $Ca^{2+}$ for $Na^+$.[143–145]

The most widely recognized cause of DAD-dependent triggered activity is digitalis toxicity.[116,117,145–151] Afterdepolarizations caused by digitalis sometimes may reach threshold to cause triggered action potentials, particularly if the rate of stimulation is sufficiently rapid. Ventricular arrhythmias (repetitive responses) caused by digitalis in the heart in situ also can be initiated by pacing at rapid rates.[152] As toxicity progresses, the duration of the trains of repetitive responses induced by pacing increases.[153–155] It is assumed that these arrhythmias are caused by DADs. In addition, spontaneously occurring accelerated ventricular rhythms and ventricular tachycardia that occur during digitalis toxicity are likely to be caused by DADs.

Cardiac glycosides cause DADs by inhibiting the $Na^+$,$K^+$ pump. In toxic amounts, this effect results in a measurable increase in intracellular $Na^+$.[156,157] An increase in intracellular $Na^+$ in turn causes an increase in intracellular $Ca^{2+}$.[158] When intracellular $Na^+$ is increased, the concentration-dependent driving force for $Na^+$ across the sarcolemma is decreased, and this, in turn, diminishes $Ca^{2+}$ extrusion from the cell by $Na^+$–$Ca^{2+}$ exchange. Hence, there is a net inward $Ca^{2+}$ movement.[44,159,160]

Catecholamines are probably the next most widely recognized cause of DADs. Delayed afterdepolarizations and triggered activity caused by catecholamines have been recorded with microelectrodes in atrial fibers of the mitral valve,[161] atrial fibers lining the coronary sinus,[33] atrial fibers in the inferior right atrium,[31] and atrial fibers from hearts with cardiomyopathy.[162] The DADs in Fig. 27-5 were caused by catecholamines in atrial fibers of the canine coronary sinus. Infusion of catecholamines through a catheter into the coronary sinus in the dog causes atrial tachycardia that has all the characteristics of triggered activity[163]; therefore, some naturally occurring atrial tachycardias caused by triggered activity probably are induced by the sympathetic nervous system. Ventricular muscle and Purkinje fibers also can develop DADs in the presence of catecholamines.[164,165] Sympathetic stimulation therefore may also cause triggered ventricular arrhythmias, possibly some of the ventricular arrhythmias that accompany exercise[166] and some ventricular arrhythmias that occur during ischemia and infarction.[167,168]

Catecholamines may cause DADs by increasing the slow inward L-type $Ca^{2+}$ current through stimulation of beta-adrenergic receptors.[169,170] The net effect is an increase in transsarcolemmal $Ca^{2+}$ entry into cardiac cells. In addition to increasing the inward $Ca^{2+}$ current, catecholamines enhance the uptake of $Ca^{2+}$ by the SR, leading to increased $Ca^{2+}$ stored in the SR and the subsequent release of an increased amount of $Ca^{2+}$ from the SR during contraction.[134,171,172] The increased $Ca^{2+}$ in the SR induced by catecholamines also may lead to the occurrence of DADs.

Delayed afterdepolarizations and triggered activity also may occur in the absence of pharmacologic agents, catecholamines, or an increase in extracellular $Ca^{2+}$. Triggerable fibers have been found in the upper pectinate muscles bordering the crista terminalis in the rabbit heart, branches of the sinoatrial ring bundle or transitional fibers between the ring bundle and ordinary pectinate muscle,[173] apparently normal fibers in human atrial myocardium,[174] human atrial fibers with very low membrane potentials (below −60 mV) and slow-response action potentials,[70,71,174] rat ventricular muscle that is hypertrophic secondary to renovascular hypertension,[175] and ventricular myocardium from diabetic rats.[176] Abnormal SR function, in which the ability of the SR to sequester calcium during diastole is compromised, may lead to DADs. Such abnormal SR function may result from genetically based alterations in SR proteins and may be the cause of certain inherited ventricular tachyarrhythmias.[176a]

## Properties of Delayed Afterdepolarizations

The TI current that causes DADs is maximal at around −60 mV and diminishes at more positive and more negative membrane potentials.[138,140,177] As a result of the dependence of the TI current on the level of membrane potential, the amplitude of DADs and therefore the possibility of triggered activity are influenced by the level of membrane potential at which the action potentials occur.[178–182] Delayed afterdepolarizations are influenced by the action potential duration, with longer action potential durations favoring the occurrence of DADs.[180] When the action potential duration is longer, more $Ca^{2+}$ is able to enter the cell. Drugs such as quinidine, which prolong action potential duration, may increase DAD amplitude,[183] while drugs such as lidocaine, which shorten action potential duration, may decrease DAD amplitude.[184] The amplitude of DADs is dependent on the number of action potentials that precede them; i.e., after a period of quiescence, the initiation of a single action potential may be followed by either no afterdepolarization or only a small one. With continued stimulation, the afterdepolarizations increase in amplitude, and triggered activity eventually may occur.[33,117,147,161,185] The amplitude of DADs and their coupling interval to the previous action potentials also are dependent on the cycle length at which action potentials are occurring, and triggered activity can be induced by a critical decrease in the drive cycle length.[117,147,161,168,173,175,176] This is illustrated by the effects of the stimulus cycle length on the amplitude of DADs recorded from an atrial fiber in the canine coronary sinus

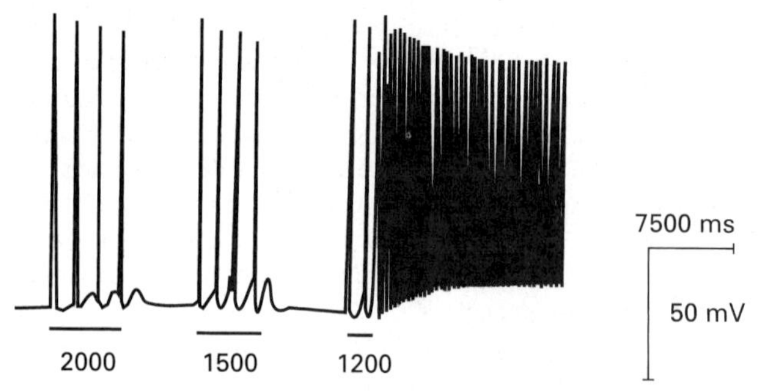


FIGURE 27-6 Effects of stimulation rate on DADs and triggered activity. Transmembrane action potentials were recorded from an atrial fiber in the canine coronary sinus superfused with Tyrode's solution containing norepinephrine. The stimulus cycle lengths and the periods of stimulation are indicated by the black bars. Sustained triggered activity occurred after stimulation at a cycle length of 1200 ms. The rate of triggered activity is so rapid that the individual action potentials cannot be seen at the slow oscilloscopic sweep speed. (From Wit AL, Cranefield PF. Triggered and automatic activity in the canine coronary sinus. *Circ Res* 1977;41:435. Reproduced with permission from the publisher and author.)

(Fig. 27-6). The transmembrane potentials at the left were recorded when the stimulus cycle length was 2000 ms; the afterdepolarization amplitude after the last stimulated impulse is 5 mV. In the center, the stimulus cycle length was 1500 ms, and the afterdepolarization amplitude after the last stimulated impulse is 15 mV. At the right, at a stimulus cycle length of 1200 ms, afterdepolarization amplitude reached 20 mV after the third stimulated action potential before triggered activity was initiated. A decrease in the length of even a single drive cycle (i.e., a premature impulse) also results in an increase in the amplitude of the DAD that follows the premature cycle.

The premature coupling interval at which triggered activity occurs is also dependent on the basic drive cycle length. As the basic drive cycle length decreases, the premature coupling interval needed to induce triggered activity increases.[186] Decreasing the drive cycle length, in addition to increasing amplitude, tends to decrease the coupling interval of DADs to the action potential upstroke or terminal phase of repolarization by increasing the rate of depolarization of the afterdepolarization.[33,117,147,173] As a result, there is a direct relation between the drive cycle length at which triggered impulses are initiated and the coupling interval between the first triggered impulse and the last stimulated impulse that induced them; i.e., as the drive cycle length is reduced, the first triggered impulse occurs earlier with respect to the last driven action potential. This characteristic property forms the basis for one of the indirect ways in which triggered activity induced by a decrease in the drive cycle length in the whole heart sometimes is distinguishable from reentrant activity induced by a decrease in the drive cycle length, since the relationship for reentrant impulses initiated by rapid stimulation is often the opposite; i.e., as drive cycle length is reduced, the first reentrant impulse occurs later with respect to the last driven action potential because of rate-dependent conduction slowing in the reentrant pathway (described in more detail further on in this chapter). The increased time during which the membrane is in the depolarized state at shorter stimulation cycle lengths or after premature impulses increases $Ca^{2+}$ in the myoplasm and the SR, thus increasing the TI current responsible for the increased afterdepolarization amplitude and causing the current to reach its maximum amplitude more rapidly, decreasing the coupling interval of triggered impulses. The repetitive depolarizations can increase intracellular $Ca^{2+}$ because of repeated activation of the inward $Ca^{2+}$ current that flows through L-type $Ca^{2+}$ channels.

How triggered activity caused by DADs is initiated by stimulation is described above. These characteristics may be of use in identifying triggered activity in the in situ heart (described below). Also of importance in identifying triggered arrhythmias in situ are the effects of electrical stimulation on established triggered activity. In general, triggered activity is influenced markedly by overdrive pacing (i.e., pacing at a rate faster than the rate of the triggered rhythm). These effects are dependent on both the rate and the duration of overdrive pacing.[186–190] When overdrive pacing is done for a critical duration of time and at a critical rate during a catecholamine-dependent triggered rhythm, the rate of triggered activity slows until the triggered rhythm stops. The slowing and termination of triggered activity after a period of overdrive pacing are caused by enhanced activity of the electrogenic $Na^+$ pump.[187] During a period of overdrive pacing, there is a transient increase in intracellular $Na^+$ because the increased number of action potentials stimulates the pump to generate increased outward current.[73,189]

When overdrive pacing is not rapid enough to terminate the triggered rhythm, it can cause overdrive acceleration. Premature stimuli also may terminate triggered rhythms,[166,186,188,191] although termination is much less common than it is by overdrive pacing.[190] It has not been demonstrated that the premature impulse must occur at a critical point in the cycle length of triggered activity.

## EARLY AFTERDEPOLARIZATIONS AND TRIGGERED ACTIVITY

Early afterdepolarizations are manifest as a sudden change in the time course of repolarization of an action potential such that the membrane potential does not follow the trajectory characteristic of normal repolarization but suddenly shifts in a depolarizing direction. This is illustrated in the example of an EAD recorded with an intracellular microelectrode in a superfused Purkinje fiber shown in Fig. 27-7. The normal time course of repolarization of the action potential is shown in panel *A*. The arrow in panel *B* shows the deviation in membrane potential that constitutes the EAD. Early afterdepolarizations may appear at the plateau level of membrane potential, which is usually more positive than −60 mV, as in Fig. 27-7*B*, or they may appear later, during phase 3 of repolarization. In Fig. 27-8*B*, trace 1 shows the normal time course of repolarization of a Purkinje fiber ac-

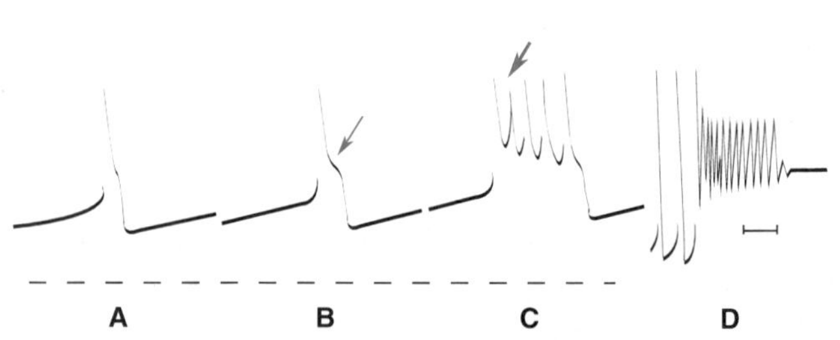


FIGURE 27-7 Early afterdepolarizations and triggered activity during repolarization in a Purkinje fiber. *A*. Transmembrane potential with normal repolarization of a spontaneously active Purkinje fiber. *B*. Early afterdepolarization (*arrow*) occurring during the plateau phase of the action potential. *C*. Triggered action potentials (*arrow*) during the plateau. *D*. Arrest of repolarization at a low level of membrane potential after a period of triggered activity. (From Cranefield PF. Action potentials, afterpotentials and arrhythmias. *Circ Res* 1977;41:415–425. Reproduced with permission from the publisher and author.)

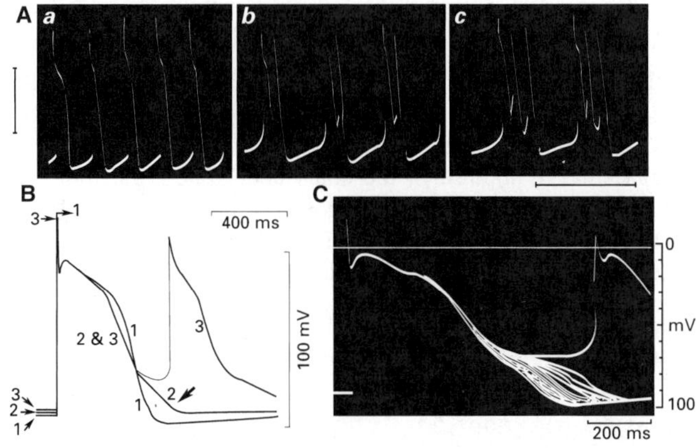


FIGURE 27-8 Early afterdepolarizations and triggered activity during late repolarization in a Purkinje fiber. *A*. Three panels are shown: (*a*) a spontaneously firing Purkinje fiber with prominent phase 4 depolarization, (*b*) occurrence of a single triggered action potential caused by an EAD, occurring during repolarization of each spontaneous action potential, (*c*) two triggered action potentials caused by an EAD occurring during repolarization of each spontaneous action potential. *B*. Development of an EAD and a triggered action potential in three superimposed traces: (1) normal Purkinje fiber action potential, (2) alteration in the time course of late repolarization leading to the occurrence of an EAD (*arrow*), (3) further alteration in late repolarization, leading to a triggered action potential. *C*. Superimposed traces recorded from a Purkinje fiber in the course of developing EADs and a triggered action potential. (From Coulombe A et al. Role of the "Na window" current and other ionic currents in triggering early after-depolarizations and re-excitation in Purkinje fibers. In: Zipes DP, Jalife J, ed. *Cardiac Electrophysiology and Arrhythmias*. New York: Grune & Stratton; 1985:43. Reproduced with permission from the publisher and author.)

tion potential, while trace 2 shows a deviation from this normal time course late during phase 3, which is the EAD. Early afterdepolarizations occurring late in repolarization occur at membrane potentials more negative than −60 mV in atrial, ventricular, or Purkinje cells that have normal resting potentials. Normally, a net outward membrane current shifts the membrane potential progressively in a negative direction during repolarization of the action potential. An EAD occurs when for some reason the current-voltage relation is altered to cause outward current during repolarization to approach or attain 0, at least transiently. Such a shift can be caused by any factors that either decrease outward current, mostly carried by $K^+$, or increase inward current, carried by $Na^+$ or $Ca^{2+}$. If the change in the current-voltage relation results in a region of net inward current during the plateau range of membrane potentials,[192] it can lead to a secondary depolarization (a triggered action potential) during the plateau or phase 3 by activating a regenerative inward current.

Under certain conditions, EADs can lead to "second upstrokes"[5,127] or action potentials; when an EAD is large enough, the decrease in membrane potential leads to an increase in net inward (depolarizing) current, and a second action potential occurs before complete repolarization of the first, as shown in panel *C* (arrow) of Fig. 27-7 and trace 3 in panel *B* of Fig. 27-8. The second action potential occurring during repolarization is triggered in the sense that it is evoked by an EAD, which in turn is induced by the preceding action potential. The second action potential also may be followed by other action potentials, all occurring at the low level of membrane potential characteristic of the plateau (Fig. 27-7*C*) or at the higher level of membrane potential of later phase 3 (Fig. 27-8, panels *Ab*, *Ac*, and *B*). Without the initiating action potential, there could be no triggered action potentials. The sustained rhythmic activity may continue for a variable number of impulses and terminates when repolarization of the initiating action potential returns membrane potential to a high level (Fig. 27-7*C*). As repolarization occurs, the rate of the triggered rhythm slows because the rate is dependent on the level of membrane potential in the same way that abnormal automaticity is. Sometimes repolarization to the high level of membrane potential may not occur, and membrane potential may remain at the plateau level or at a level intermediate between the plateau level and the resting potential[62] (Fig. 27-7*D*). The sustained rhythmic activity then may continue at the reduced level of membrane potential and assumes the characteristics of abnormal automaticity.[127]

The level of membrane potential at which the triggered action potentials occur determines both the rate of triggered activity and whether the triggered action potentials can propagate and excite adjacent normal regions.[193] At the more positive membrane potentials of the plateau, the rate of triggered activity is more rapid than it is late during phase 3. Triggered action potentials occurring at the plateau level have slow upstrokes; therefore, conduction of these action potentials sometimes may block,[194,195] while the faster upstrokes of triggered action potentials occurring later during phase 3 enable them to propagate more easily. The ionic current responsible for the upstrokes of the action potentials during triggered activity caused by EADs is determined by the level of membrane potential at which the action potentials occur. Triggered action potentials occurring during the plateau phase and early during phase 3, at a time when most fast $Na^+$ channels are still inactivated, most likely have upstrokes caused by the inward L-type $Ca^{2+}$ current.[5,196] At higher membrane potentials during late phase 3 of repolarization, where there is partial reactivation of the $Na^+$ channels, the upstrokes are caused by the fast inward $Na^+$ current. Current flowing through both L-type $Ca^{2+}$ channels and partially reactivated fast $Na^+$ channels may be involved over intermediate ranges of membrane potential.

## Causes of Early Afterdepolarizations and Triggered Activity

Early afterdepolarizations and triggered activity have been produced in experimental studies under a variety of conditions, some of which would never be expected to be associated with naturally occurring arrhythmias in the in situ heart. Most of these conditions somehow delay repolarization of the action potential by increasing inward current or decreasing outward current during the plateau and repolarization phases. Most often, EADs occur more readily in Purkinje fibers than in ventricular or atrial muscle, although EADs can readily occur in the so-called M cells, which are ventricular muscle cells with a prominent plateau phase.[197] Early afterdepolarizations may occur when the rate of stimulation is markedly slowed, reducing the outward current generated by the $Na^+$,$K^+$ pump, especially when $K^+$ in the extracellular environment is lower than normal, also reducing outward current.[128]

At a "physiologic range" of cycle lengths (a range that encompasses the normal sinus rhythm of the adult human heart: 1000 to 700 ms), EADs have rarely occurred in studies of isolated preparations of cardiac fibers. As cycle length is increased and repolarization is prolonged, EADs and triggered activity are more likely to occur.[198] The result is a bradycardia-induced tachycardia during which there may be very slow conduction. Another important characteristic is that the longer the basic drive cycle length, the greater the number of impulses that are triggered by EADs.[198] Once EADs have achieved a steady-state magnitude at a constant drive cycle length, any event that shortens drive cycle length tends to reduce their amplitude.[198] Hence, the initiation of a single premature depolarization, which is associated with an acceleration of repolarization, will reduce the magnitude of the EADs that accompany the premature action potential; as a result, triggered activity is not expected to follow premature stimulation. Polymorphic ventricular tachycardias that sometimes resemble torsades de pointes have been induced in dogs by the infusion of cesium, which blocks $i_{Ki}$ to cause EADs.[199] Occurrence of tachycardia is preceded by QT-interval prolongation, a consequence of delayed repolarization, as is characteristically seen in patients with torsades de pointes.[200] The initial beat of the tachycardia caused by cesium often occurs during repolarization, i.e., during the T wave.

Early depolarizations and triggered activity have been seen in monophasic action potentials recorded from the ventricles in dogs with cesium-induced ventricular tachycardia.[201,202] Because the experimental arrhythmias caused by agents such as cesium, which are known to induce EADs, resemble torsades de pointes, it has been proposed that clinically occurring torsades de pointes sometimes may be caused by EADs. Other agents that can cause EADs and triggered activity are used therapeutically, and therefore, arrhythmias associated with their use may result from triggered activity. Antiarrhythmic drugs that prolong the duration of the action potential of Purkinje fibers or ventricular muscle (e.g., sotalol,[203,204] *N*-acetylprocainamide,[205] and quinidine[206,207]) can cause EADs and triggered activity when administered to isolated preparations, particularly when the rate of stimulation is low and the extracellular $K^+$ concentration is lower than normal, e.g., <4 m*M*/L.

The mechanisms by which these effects are exerted have been studied in detail for only some of these drugs. Both the D (no beta-receptor blockade) and the L (beta-blocking) forms of sotalol prolong the action potential duration by inhibiting the repolarizing K current, $i_{Ki}$.[204] Similarly, the prolongation of the action potential by quinidine, which may lead to EADs, is related to the blocking effect of quinidine on the outward membrane repolarizing $K^+$ current, not to that drug's well-known blocking effect on the $Na^+$ channel.[208] It is known that quinidine may cause ventricular tachyarrhythmias in patients undergoing antiarrhythmic therapy with that drug. Interestingly, the arrhythmias may occur at low plasma quinidine concentrations that do not cause widening of the QRS complex in the ECG,[209] consistent with observations in superfused Purkinje fibers that afterdepolarizations caused by quinidine occur without depression of the action potential upstroke. Hypokalemia and bradycardia both predispose to the occurrence of quinidine-induced torsades de pointes,[200,210] and both have been shown to potentiate the induction of EADs in vitro by quinidine.[206,207] Torsades de pointes also has been associated with the administration to patients of *N*-acetylprocainamide[211] and sotalol[212] as well as other drugs with "class III" antiarrhythmic properties. Magnesium has been shown to abolish EAD-dependent triggered activity in experimental studies.[207,213] Magnesium also has been shown to provide effective therapy when used to treat some clinical cases of drug-induced torsades de pointes,[214,215] providing further evidence that this clinical arrhythmia may be a manifestation of triggered activity (see Chap. 31).

Recently, a great deal of attention has been focused on genetically induced changes in ion channel function in patients that might lead to the occurrence of early afterdepolarizations. A number of alterations in the principal repolarizing K channel ($I_K$) cause a decrease in function (decreased outward current), prolonging repolarization and resulting in EADs. An increase in function of the Na channel (increased inward current) has a similar effect. Patients with these abnormalities often have prolonged QT on their ECGs and ventricular tachycardia that may cause sudden death.[215a]

## ARRHYTHMIAS CAUSED BY REENTRY

The excitation wavefront originating in the sinus node normally activates the cardiac tissues in an orderly sequence and then dies out. Thus, during normal sinus rhythm, each heartbeat is generated by a new pacemaker impulse in the sinus node. There are, however, arrhythmias in which, in the presence of a requisite set of circumstances, an excitation wavefront does not die out but rather can propagate continuously and thus continue to excite the heart because it always encounters excitable tissue. Such an arrhythmia is called *reentrant* (see Table 27-1).

### Requisites for Reentrant Excitation

The earliest description of reentrant excitation was by Mayer[3] in 1906 in the excitable subumbrella ring of tissue of the Scyphomedusae (jellyfish), as is shown in Fig. 27-9. This example well illustrates the requisites for reentrant excitation. First, a substrate must be present that will support reentrant excitation, in this case the subumbrella ring of excitable tissue of the jellyfish. Second, the excitation wavefront propagating in this substrate must encounter unidirectional block (Fig. 27-9*B*). Unidirectional block must be present or the excitation wavefronts traveling around the ring will collide and extinguish each other (Fig. 27-9*A*). If the site of unidirectional block instead manifests bidirectional block, reentrant excitation will not occur because the circulating excitation wavefront will be unable to propagate through the area of block to reexcite the tissue that initially was excited. Third, there must be a central area of block around which the reentrant excitation wavefront can circulate. In this example, it is the hole in the center of the ring that clearly is inexcitable. Without a central area of block, the excitation wavefront will not necessarily be conducted around the ring of excitable tissue. Rather, it could take a shortcut, permitting the circulating excitation wavefront to arrive quite early at the site where it originated. If it arrives sufficiently early, the latter tissue will still be refractory, and reentrant excitation will not be possible. But even with the presence of a central area of block and without the presence of a shortcut, the circulating wavefront will manifest reentrant excitation only if the tissue it initially activated has had sufficient time to recover its excitability by the time the reentrant wavefront returns. Thus, conduction of the circulating excitation wavefront in the rest of the circuit must take long enough for this to happen, and there must always be a gap of excitable tissue (either fully or partially excitable) ahead of the cir-

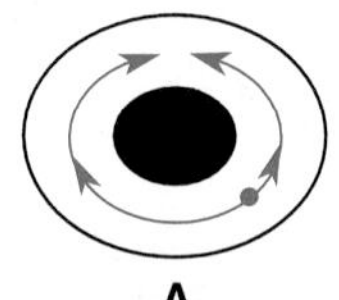

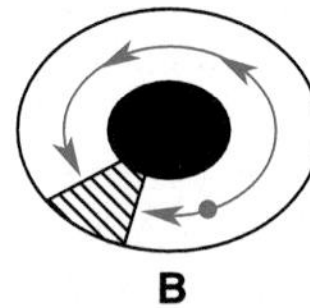

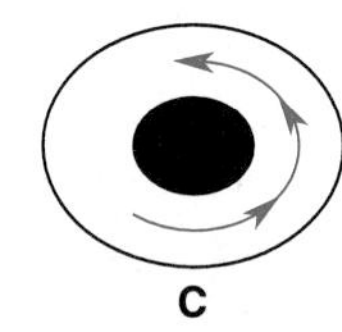


FIGURE 27-9 Schematic representation of reentry in a ring of excitable tissue. *A*. Ring was stimulated in the area indicated by the blue dot. Impulses propagated away from the point of stimulation in both directions (*arrows*) and collided; no reentry occurred. *B*. The striped area was compressed while the ring was stimulated, again at the blue dot. The impulse propagated around the ring in only one direction, having been blocked in the other direction by the area of compression. Then, immediately after stimulation, the compression was relieved. *C*. Circulating impulse is shown returning to its point of origin and then continuing around the ring. Identical reentry would occur if the striped area in *B* were a region of permanent unidirectional conduction block with block in the right-to-left direction.

culating wavefront (the so-called excitable gap). In the case of the experiment by Mayer on the subumbrella ring of excitable tissue of the jellyfish, conduction velocity was constant and the length of the ring was long enough that conduction time around the ring was longer than the effective refractory period of the excitable tissue constituting the ring, permitting reentry. If the length of the ring had been critically shorter or if the conduction velocity had been critically faster, the circulating excitation wavefront would have arrived at the site of initial excitation before sufficient recovery of excitability had occurred, preventing reexcitation.

From these sorts of observations grew the concept of the wavelength of the circulating impulse.[4,216,217] The wavelength is the product of the conduction velocity of the circulating excitation wavefront and the effective refractory period of the tissue in which the excitation wavefront is propagating. It quantifies how far the impulse travels relative to the duration of the refractory period. Thus, the wavelength of the reentrant excitation wavefront must be shorter than the length of the pathway of the potential reentrant circuit for reentrant excitation to occur; i.e., the impulse must travel a distance during the refractory period that is less than the complete reentrant path length to give myocardium ahead of it sufficient time to recover excitability.

For virtually all clinically important reentrant arrhythmias resulting from ordered reentry, however, in the presence of uniform, normal conduction velocity along the potential reentrant pathway, the wavelength would be too long to permit reentrant excitation. Thus, virtually all these arrhythmias must have, and in fact do have, one or more areas of slow conduction as a part of the reentrant circuit. The associated changes in conduction velocity (as well as associated changes in refractory periods) actually cause the wavelength to change in different parts of the circuit. However, the presence of one or more areas of slow conduction permits the average wavelength of reentrant activation to be shorter than the path length.

The fact that the reentrant circuit of virtually all clinically important reentrant arrhythmias has one or more areas of slow conduction serves to emphasize the fact that the electrophysiologic properties of the cardiac tissue making up the reentrant circuit are not uniform. In fact, there may be, and usually are, variations of conduction velocity and refractoriness along the course of the reentrant circuit. An additional requisite for random reentry is the necessity of a critical mass of tissue to sustain the one or usually more simultaneously circulating reentrant excitation wavefronts.[218] Thus, it is essentially not possible to achieve sustained fibrillation of ventricles of very small normal mammalian hearts and equally difficult to achieve sustained fibrillation of the normal atria of humans or smaller mammals.

Finally, another prerequisite for reentrant excitation to occur is often (but not always) the presence of an initiating trigger. The trigger, usually the occurrence of one or more premature beats, frequently is required because it elicits or brings to a critical state one or more of the conditions necessary to achieve reentrant excitation. Thus, a premature impulse initiating reentry may arrive at one site in the potential reentrant circuit sufficiently early that it encounters unidirectional block because that tissue has had insufficient time to recover excitability after excitation by the prior beat (Fig. 27-9). Furthermore, in the other limb of the potential reentrant circuit, the premature arrival of the excitation wavefront either causes slow conduction or results in further slowing of conduction of the excitation wavefront through an area of already slow conduction. The resulting increase in conduction time around this limb of the potential reentrant circuit serves to allow the region of unidirectional block in the tissue in the other limb activated initially by the premature beat to recover excitability. Thus, when the circulating excitation wavefront of the premature beat arrives at these tissue sites, the excitation wavefront can reexcite the tissue, thus manifesting reentrant excitation (Fig. 27-9).

It should be noted that the mechanism causing the premature beat may be different from the reentrant mechanism causing the tachycardia. Thus, the premature beat may be caused by automaticity or triggered activity. An example of the latter may be torsades de pointes, in which the initiating beat (or beats) is the result of triggered activity caused by early afterdepolarization, but the remainder of the beats in this rhythm (it is frequently nonsustained) are now thought to be due to reentry.[219] Another example may occur during cardiac catheterization, in which the premature beat may be due to the catheter forcefully hitting the heart wall, i.e., a mechanical cause. However, the trigger to initiate reentrant excitation need not be a premature beat. It may, rather, be the normal sinus beat. One example is the rhythm known as nonparoxysmal AV junctional reentrant tachycardia.[220,221] In this example, the potential reentrant circuit contains an area (an accessory AV connection) of permanent unidirectional block in an antegrade direction. Moreover, the potential reentrant circuit also has a relatively stable area of very slow retrograde VA conduction (the accessory AV connection), causing the wavelength of the propagating excitation wavefront to be shorter than the path length of the potential reentrant circuit. In this circumstance, the normal sinus beat propagates around the reentrant circuit with sufficient delay that when it arrives in a retrograde direction at the area of permanent antegrade unidirectional block, the tissue at that site has recovered excitability. Furthermore, the conduction time around the reentrant circuit is such that the excitation wavefront continually encounters excitable tissue in the direction in which it is propagating, resulting in continuous reentrant excitation and an incessant tachycardia. Another example where a premature beat is not necessary is when reentrant premature ventricular beats occur, as in ventricular bigeminy (see Chap. 31).

## Components of the Reentrant Circuit

### THE SUBSTRATE

The cardiac tissue that constitutes the substrate for reentrant excitation can be located almost anywhere in the heart. Furthermore, the reentrant circuit may be a variety of sizes and shapes and may include a number of different kinds of myocardial cells, e.g., atrial, ventricular, nodal, and Purkinje. The reentrant circuit may be an anatomic structure such as a loop of fiber bundles in the Purkinje system.[222] The reentrant circuit may be a functionally rather than an anatomically defined pathway, with its existence, size, and shape determined by the electrophysiologic properties of cardiac tissues in which the reentrant wavefront circulates, as has been shown in some patients with atypical atrial flutter.[223–224a] Or it may be an anatomic-functional combination, as for some intraatrial reentrant rhythms, such as atrial flutter.[224,224b]

### THE AREA(S) OF SLOW CONDUCTION

As has been discussed, a condition necessary for reentry is that the impulse be delayed sufficiently in the alternative pathway(s) to allow elements proximal to the site of unidirectional block to recover excitability. If reentry is to succeed, the impulse traveling around the reentrant circuit in one direction as a result of the unidirectional block must not return to this site of block before it and regions around it recover excitability. In the presence of normal conduction, sufficient time to allow recovery of excitability may occur if the alternative pathway is sufficiently long. Reentry is facilitated when conduction in all or a part of the alternative pathway is slow, since sufficiently long pathways are usually not present in the heart. The area(s) of slow conduction may be an anatomic structure normally expected to manifest slow conduction, such as the AV node. Thus, the AV node is the area of slow conduction in the usual form of AV reentrant tachycardia (a reentrant tachycardia in which the circuit involves the atria, the AV node, the His-Purkinje system, the ventricles, and an accessory AV connection). The area of slow conduction may be in cardiac tissue that normally does not manifest slow conduction. Such an area might not be present during sinus rhythm (in contrast to the AV node), but be functionally present during the tachycardia. These areas may develop as a result of premature excitation or may evolve during a rapid transitional rhythm as occurs during atrial flutter.[224,225] An example of a functionally determined area of slow conduction is found in the posteroinferior right atrium during atrial flutter in patients[226] or in the free wall of the right atrium of the canine sterile pericarditis model of atrial flutter.[224] The slow conduction might also be present during sinus rhythm such as in tissue that has been damaged, as after a myocardial infarct. Such tissue normally would not manifest slow conduction.[227] Slow conduction can be a consequence of active membrane properties determining the characteristics of inward currents depolarizing the membrane during the action potential, or it can be a consequence of passive properties governing the flow of current between cardiac cells.

## Depression of Resting Membrane Potential

An important feature of the transmembrane action potential of atrial, ventricular, and Purkinje fibers that governs the speed of propagation is the magnitude of the inward $Na^+$ current flowing through the fast $Na^+$ channels in the sarcolemma during the upstroke. The magnitude of this current flow is reflected in the rate at which the cell depolarizes ($\dot{V}_{max}$ of phase 0)[228] and the overshoot of the upstroke (the positive level of depolarization). The depolarization phase or upstroke of the action potential results from the opening of specific membrane channels (fast $Na^+$ channels) through which $Na^+$ ions rapidly pass from the extracellular fluid into the cell.

During conduction of the impulse, the inward transmembrane $Na^+$ current flowing during the depolarization phase (phase 0) of the action potential results in the flow of axial current along the cardiac fiber through the cytoplasm and the gap junctions of the intercalated disks that connect the cardiac cells. The current flows out of the cells through the membrane ahead as resistive and capacitive current. The conduction velocity depends on both how much capacitive current flows out of the cell at unexcited sites ahead of the propagating wavefront and the distance at which the capacitive current can bring membrane potential to threshold. One important factor that influences the amount of current flowing through the sarcoplasm of a muscle fiber (axial current), and therefore capacitive current, is the amount of fast inward current causing the propagating action potential. A reduction in this inward current, leading to a reduction in the rate or amplitude of depolarization during phase 0, may decrease axial current flow, slow conduction, and lead to conduction block. Such a reduction may result from inactivation of $Na^+$ channels. The intensity of the inward $Na^+$ current depends on the fraction of $Na^+$ channels that open when the cell is excited and the size of the $Na^+$ electrochemical potential gradient (relative concentration of $Na^+$ in the extracellular space compared with $Na^+$ concentration inside the cell[229]). The fraction of $Na^+$ channels available for opening is determined largely by the level of membrane potential at which an action potential is initiated.[229] The $Na^+$ channels are inactivated either after the upstroke of an action potential or if the steady-state resting membrane potential is reduced. Immediately after the upstroke, cardiac fibers are inexcitable because of $Na^+$ channel inactivation at the positive level of membrane potential.

During repolarization, progressive removal of inactivation allows increasingly large $Na^+$ currents to flow through the still partially inactivated $Na^+$ channels when the cells are excited. The inward $Na^+$ current, amplitude, and rate of rise of premature action potentials initiated during this relative refractory period are reduced because the $Na^+$ channels are only partly reactivated.[229] In Fig. 27-10*B*, premature action potentials *a, b,* and *c* have low amplitudes and slow rates of depolarization because they were initiated before full repolarization of the action potential. Hence, the conduction velocity of these premature action potentials is low. Premature activation of the heart therefore may induce reentry because premature impulses conduct slowly in regions of the heart where the cardiac fibers are not completely repolarized (where $Na^+$ channels are to some extent still inactivated).

Conduction slow enough to facilitate reentry also may occur in cardiac cells with persistently low levels of resting potential (which may be between −60 and −70 mV) caused by disease. At these resting potentials, a significant percentage of the $Na^+$ channels are inactivated[229]; therefore, they are unavailable for activation by a depolarizing stimulus. Also, at these resting membrane potentials, recovery from inactivation is markedly prolonged and extends beyond complete repolarization.[230] The magnitude of the inward current during phase 0 of the action potential is reduced; consequently, both the speed and the amplitude of the upstroke are dimin-

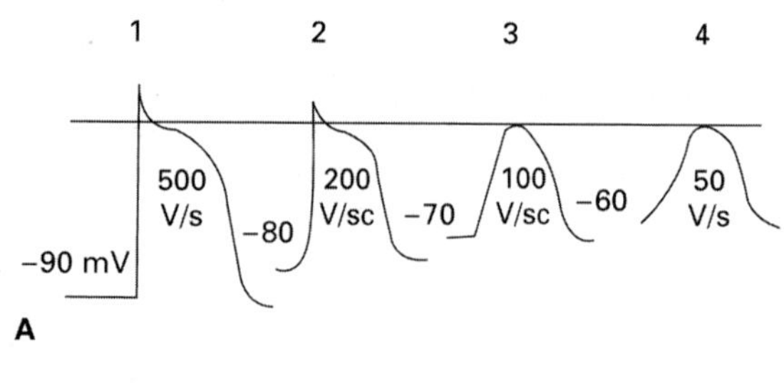


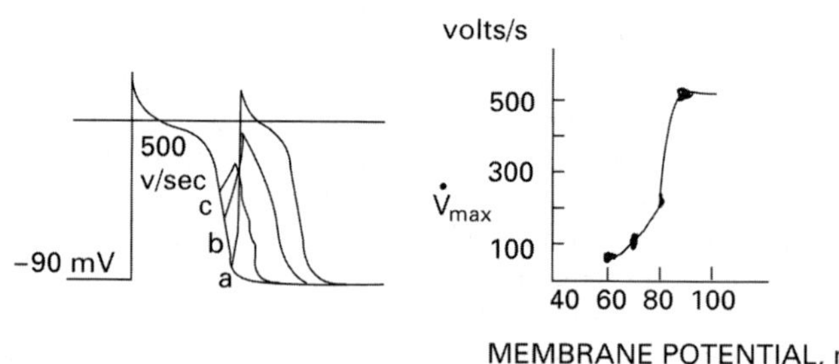


FIGURE 27-10 Diagrammatic representation of the relation between the level of membrane potential at the onset of phase 0 and the maximum rate of depolarization during phase 0 ($dv/dt_{max}$ or $\dot{V}_{max}$). *A*. Fiber has been depolarized by progressively increasing the extracellular potassium concentration. As resting membrane potential decreases, the rate of depolarization of the action potential upstroke decreases. *B*. Fiber is activated by premature stimuli that occur at different times during phase 3 (*a, b,* and *c*). The premature action potentials have reduced rates of depolarization because they arise at reduced membrane potentials. *C*. For both types of experiments, the general relationship between $\dot{V}_{max}$ and membrane potential is shown. As the membrane potential becomes smaller (less negative), the rate of phase 0 depolarization ($\dot{V}_{max}$) decreases and therefore conduction velocity decreases.

ished (Fig. 27-10*A*, action potentials 2, 3, and 4), decreasing axial current flow and slowing conduction significantly. Such action potentials with upstrokes dependent on inward current flowing via partially inactivated $Na^+$ channels sometimes are referred to as *depressed fast responses*. Further depolarization of the resting membrane potential and further inactivation of the $Na^+$ channel may decrease the excitability of cardiac fibers to such an extent that they may become a site of unidirectional conduction block.[231] Thus, in a diseased region with partially depolarized fibers, there may be some areas of slow conduction and some areas of conduction block, depending on the level of resting potential and the number of $Na^+$ channels that are inactivated. This combination may cause reentry. The chance for reentry in such fibers is even greater during premature activation or during rhythms at a rapid rate, because slow conduction or the possibility of block is increased even further owing to the prolonged time for the $Na^+$ channels to recover from inactivation when the resting potential is partially depolarized.

After the upstroke of the normal action potential of atrial, ventricular, or Purkinje cells, membrane potential begins to return to the resting level because the $Na^+$ channels are inactivated and the fast (depolarizing) $Na^+$ current ceases to flow. This return, however, is slowed by a second inward current that is smaller and slower than the fast $Na^+$ current and probably is carried by both $Na^+$ and $Ca^{2+}$ ions.[232] This secondary inward current flows through L-type $Ca^{2+}$ channels that are distinct from the fast $Na^+$ channels.[20] The threshold for activation of the L-type $Ca^{2+}$ current is in the range of −30 to −40 mV, compared with about −70 mV for the fast $Na^+$ current. This current inactivates much more slowly than does the fast $Na^+$ current and gradually diminishes as the cell repolarizes. It causes much of the plateau phase of the action potential. Under special conditions, this $Ca^{2+}$ current also may underlie the occurrence of the slow conduction that causes reentrant arrhythmias.[5] Although the fast $Na^+$ channel may be largely inactivated at membrane potentials near −50 mV, the L-type $Ca^{2+}$ channel is not inactivated and is still available for activation.[5,232]

Under certain conditions, when the resting potential is reduced to levels lower than −60 mV (as occurs when membrane conductance is very low or when catecholamines are present), this normally weak inward $Ca^{2+}$ current may give rise to regenerative action potentials that propagate very slowly and are prone to block. The propagated action potential, which is dependent on inward $Ca^{2+}$ current, is referred to as the *slow response*.[5] Slow-response action potentials can occur in diseased cardiac fibers with low resting potentials that normally have Na channel–dependent fast responses, but they also occur in some normal tissue of the heart, such as cells of the sinus and AV nodes, where the maximum diastolic potential is normally about −60 mV or less.[5,233] In fact, slow conduction is a normal property of both the sinus and the AV nodes. Thus, it should be of no surprise that either of these nodes may be a critical area of slow conduction in some reentrant circuits, e.g., the AV node in AV reentrant tachycardia involving an accessory AV connection.

## Anisotropy

The slow conduction that facilitates the occurrence of reentry also can be caused by factors other than a decrease in inward current during the upstroke of the transmembrane action potential. An increased resistance to axial current flow, which can be expressed as *effective axial resistance* (defined as resistance to current flow in the direction of propagation[234,235]), decreases the magnitude and spread of axial current of the propagating impulse among the myocardial fibers and may decrease conduction velocity. During conduction of the impulse, axial current flows from one myocardial cell to the adjacent cell through the gap junctions of the intercalated disks, which form a major source of intercellular resistance to current flow between fiber bundles.[228] Therefore the structure of the myocardium that governs the extent and distribution of these gap junctions has a profound influence on axial resistance and conduction.

The atria (crista terminalis) and certain regions of the ventricles (except for the subepicardial muscle) are composed of bundles of myocardial cells that have been called *unit bundles* by Sommer and Dolber.[236] Such bundles are made up of 2 to 30 cells surrounded by a connective tissue sheath. Within a unit bundle, cells are tightly connected or coupled to each other through intercalated disks that contain the gap junctions. All the cells of a unit bundle are connected to each other within the space of 30 to 50 μm down the length of a strand.[236] An individual cardiac myocyte may be connected to as many as nine other myocytes through one or more intercalated disks.[237] These connections are mainly at the ends of the myocytes rather than along their sides, but the overlapping nature of the junctions effectively connects myocytes within a bundle in the transverse direction as well as the longitudinal direction. Therefore, as a consequence of the many intercellular connections, the myocytes in a unit bundle are activated uniformly and synchronously as an impulse propagates along the bundle. The unit bundles also are connected to each other. Unit bundles lying parallel to each other in normal atrial and ventricular muscle are connected in a lateral (transverse) direction at intervals in the range of 100 to 150 μm.[236] As a consequence of this structure, the myocardium in regions in which unit bundles occur is better coupled in the direction of the long axis of its cells and bundles (because of the high frequency of the gap junctions within a unit bundle) than in the direction transverse to the long axis (because of the low frequency of interconnections between the unit bundles). This is reflected in a lower axial resistivity in the longitudinal direction than in the transverse direction in cardiac tissues that are composed of many unit bundles.[238,239]

The structure of the interconnections between muscle fibers is somewhat different in the subepicardial regions of the ventricles (and possibly other regions as well) but is still a cause of lower longitudinal axial resistance rather than transverse axial resistance. The subepicardial region is not made up of unit bundles.[240] Each ventricular muscle cell is connected to approximately 11 to 12 other muscle cells in three dimensions. The junctions that connect the cells occur at both the ends and the sides of cells in roughly equivalent numbers; approximately half of all connections are side to side, and half are end to end. Therefore, activation wavefronts can conduct equally well between individual cells in both the longitudinal and transverse directions because there are equal numbers of gap junctions. In the transverse direction, however, a wavefront encounters more gap junctions than it does over an equivalent distance in the longitudinal direction because cell diameter is much smaller than cell length; therefore the wavefront must traverse more cells transversely. Thus, there is a greater resistance transversely than longitudinally because of the increased number of gap junctions per unit distance traveled.[238]

As stated above, the effective axial resistivity is an important determinant of the conduction velocity; therefore conduction through atrial and ventricular myocardium is much more rapid in the longitudinal direction, owing to the lower resistivity, than it is in the transverse direction. Thus cardiac muscle is anisotropic; its conduction properties vary depending on the direction in which they are measured.

Spach and associates[234,235,241,242] classified anisotropy into two major subdivisions: uniform and nonuniform. Uniform anisotropy is

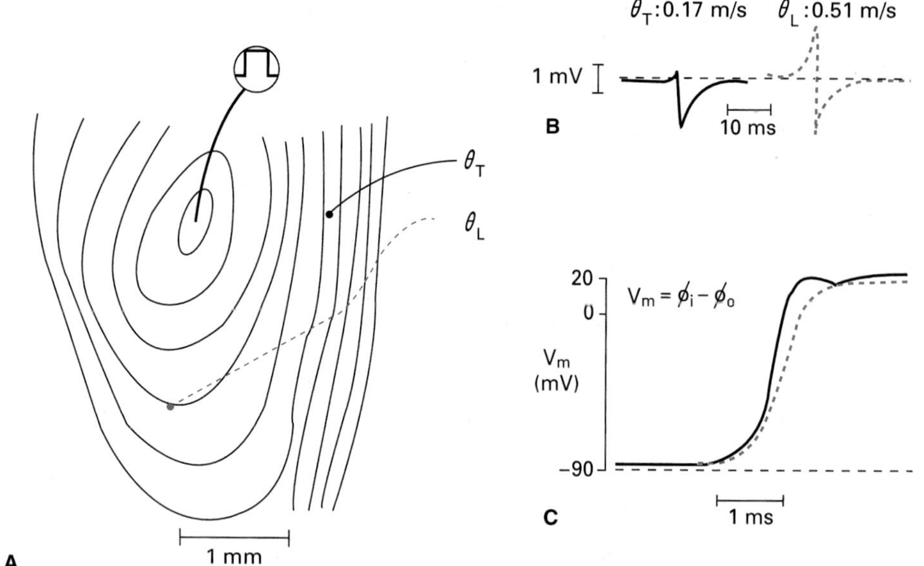


FIGURE 27-11 Relation between the spread of excitation in uniform anisotropic ventricular muscle (*A*) and extracellular (*B*) and transmembrane potential waveforms (*C*). The excitation sequence in *A* was constructed from the extracellular waveforms measured at 100 positions on the endocardial surface of the right ventricular septum. The extracellular waveforms in *B* were measured at the sites indicated by the solid dots superimposed on the isochrones of *A*. The direction of propagation at the single transmembrane recording site was altered by initiating propagation at different locations, one to produce propagation along the longitudinal axis of the impaled fiber and the other to produce propagation along the transverse axis. Panel *C* shows the effects of the different directions of propagation on the upstroke of the action potential. (From Spach MS, Dolber PC. The relation between discontinuous propagation in anisotropic cardiac muscle and the "vulnerable period" of reentry. In: Zipes DP, Jalife J, eds. *Cardiac Electrophysiology and Arrhythmias*. New York: Grune & Stratton, 1985:241. Reproduced with permission from the publisher and author.)

characterized by an advancing wavefront that is smooth in all directions (longitudinal and transverse to fiber orientation), indicating relatively tight coupling between groups of fibers in all directions. Uniform anisotropy is exemplified by the conduction properties of normal septal ventricular muscle, as shown in Fig. 27-11*A*. The muscle in the diagram was stimulated in the center (pulse symbol), and activation spread away from this site in all directions. In the direction of the longitudinal axis of the fibers (from top to bottom), the activation isochrones are widely spaced, indicating rapid conduction, in this case, 0.51 m/s. There is a relatively broad area of fast conduction with an elliptic shape of the isochrones that is characteristic of uniform anisotropy.[241] In the direction transverse to the long axis (to the right and to the left), the isochrones are spaced close together, indicating slower conduction: 0.17 m/s in this example. As the direction of propagation changes between these two axes, the apparent conduction velocity changes monotonically from fast to slow, another characteristic of uniform anisotropy.[234]

The slow conduction in the direction transverse to the longitudinal fiber axis occurs despite action potentials with normal resting potentials and upstroke velocities and is caused by the higher transverse axial resistance. Associated with the differences in conduction velocity that are based on the direction of propagation, however, are unexpected changes in the action potentials. Thus, when going from fast longitudinal conduction to slow transverse conduction, the rate of depolarization during the upstroke of the action potential ($\dot{V}_{max}$) increases and the time constant of the foot of the upstroke decreases without any change in the resting potential, as shown in Fig. 27-11*C;* the upstroke that is dashed was recorded from a cell during longitudinal propagation, while the upstroke indicated by the solid line was recorded from the same cell during transverse propagation.[234] These characteristics are opposite to the changes in the action potentials associated with slowing of conduction when the membrane currents are altered (e.g., by membrane depolarization).[243,244] Despite the increase in $\dot{V}_{max}$, when conduction is slowed in the transverse direction, the slowing of conduction is associated with a decrease in the amplitude of the extracellular electrogram, showing that there is a decrease in the extracellular current flow as a result of the increased axial resistivity.

In uniformly anisotropic tissue, the extracellular unipolar waveform has a large-amplitude, smooth biphasic, positive-negative, morphology during propagation in the fast longitudinal direction (Fig. 27-11*B,* dashed line) and a low-amplitude, smooth triphasic (negative-positive-negative) morphology in the transverse direction (Fig. 27-11*B*, solid line). The initial negativity of the electrogram in the transverse direction is a reflection of distant activity rapidly propagating along the longitudinal axis.[245]

Nonuniform anisotropy has been defined[235] as tight electrical coupling between cells in the longitudinal direction but recurrent areas in the transverse direction in which side-to-side electrical coupling of adjacent groups of parallel fibers is absent. Therefore, propagation of normal action potentials transverse to the long axis is interrupted so that adjacent bundles are excited in a markedly irregular sequence (*zigzag conduction*).[235,241] In nonuniformly anisotropic muscle, there also may be an abrupt transition in conduction velocity from the fast longitudinal direction to the slow transverse direction, unlike the case with uniform anisotropic muscle, in which intermediate velocities occur between the two directions. This pattern of excitation in nonuniform anisotropic atrial pectinate bundles from older patients is diagrammed in Fig. 27-12*A*. The white arrow on the outline of the preparation indicates the narrow region of fast conduction down the long axis of the fibers when the bundle was excited at the asterisk. The zigzag arrow indicates the irregular course of excitation across the fibers, which occurred all along the length of the zone of fast conduction. Conduction in the transverse direction in these nonuniformly anisotropic bundles was nearly as slow at the slowest conduction associated with membrane depolarization and slow-response action potentials.[5] In pectinate muscles from older patients, mean fast velocity was 0.69 m/s and slow velocity was 0.07 m/s, a ratio of almost 10,[241] despite the normal resting potential and the fast action potential upstroke of the atrial cells. As in uniform anisotropy, the upstroke velocity of the action potential is more rapid in the slow direction transverse to the long axis of the fibers than in the fast direction parallel to the long axis.

The morphologic basis for the nonuniform anisotropic properties in human atrial muscle is that the fascicles of muscle bundles are sep-

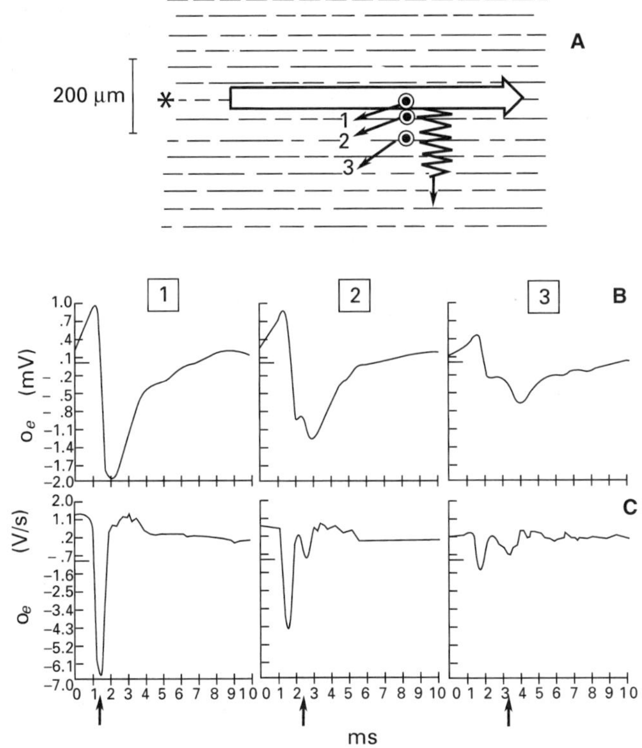


FIGURE 27-12 *A*. Diagram of a nonuniform anisotropic atrial muscle bundle with the long axis of the myocardial fibers indicated by the dashed lines. The bundle was stimulated at the asterisk. Propagation of the longitudinal wavefront is shown by the large white arrow. Transverse propagation occurred as diagrammed by the zigzag arrow. *B*. Electrograms recorded from sites 1, 2, and 3 on the diagram. *C*. The first derivative of these electrograms is shown. (From Spach MS, Dolber PC. Relating extracellular potentials and their derivatives to anisotropic propagation at a microscopic level in human cardiac muscle: Evidence for uncoupling of side-to-side fiber connections with increasing age. *Circ Res* 1986;58:356. Reproduced with permission from the publisher and author.)

arated in the transverse direction by fibrous tissue that proliferates with aging to form longitudinally oriented insulating boundaries. Intercellular connections cannot occur where the cardiac fibers are separated by connective tissue septa, and there is uncoupling between parallel-oriented groups of fibers.[235,241] Part of the reduction of the conduction velocity in this transverse direction may be a result of the tortuous path length necessary for the wavefront to propagate transversely from one bundle to another because of these septa, accounting for the zigzag activation pattern. Similar connective tissue septa cause nonuniform anisotropy in other normal cardiac tissues, such as the crista terminalis and the interatrial band in adult atria or ventricular papillary muscle, as well as pathologic situations such as chronic ischemia or a healing myocardial infarction, in which fibrosis in the myocardium occurs.

The irregular activation transversely is evident in the extracellular electrogram, which is characterized by a sequence of multiple deflections, each representing activation of a separate bundle of fibers, with the largest, most rapid intrinsic deflection produced by local excitation and less rapid and lower-amplitude deflections produced by excitation of adjacent fascicles.[235] In Fig. 27-12*B*, the multiple deflections can be seen in electrograms recorded from sites 2 and 3 in the atrial pectinate muscle and are even more prominent in the derivatives of these electrograms (Fig. 27-12*C*). A similarly fractionated electrogram also can be recorded from diseased regions of the ventricles. During longitudinal propagation, large biphasic electrograms are still evident (electrogram at site 1).

Anisotropy on a macroscopic scale also can influence conduction at sites where a bundle of cardiac fibers branches or where separate bundles coalesce. Marked slowing can occur when there is a sudden change in the fiber direction, causing an abrupt increase in the effective axial resistivity.[235] Figure 27-13 illustrates this point. The drawings show a small branch of an atrial pectinate muscle from the crista terminalis. The general direction of the fiber orientation is indicated by the thin broken lines, and the pattern of propagation is illustrated by the thick solid lines with arrows. In *A* (*1*) at the left, wavefronts initiated by stimulation at the top propagate throughout the crista and its branch along the longitudinal axis of the fibers throughout so that there is no conduction delay entering the branch. At the right in *A* (*2*), wavefronts initiated by stimulation at the bottom propagate up the crista and into the branch, but they encounter a marked change in the direction of the fibers from longitudinal to transverse while entering the branch, resulting in a slowing of conduction because of the sudden increase in axial resistance. Conduction block, which sometimes may be unidirectional, may occur at such junction sites, particularly when the inward current is decreased, described further on.

In addition to the structural features of the cellular interconnections influencing axial current flow and conduction as expressed in the anisotropic properties of cardiac muscle, the intercellular resistance may increase because of an increase in gap junctional resistance that results from a decrease in the conductance of the junctions, i.e., a decrease in the ease with which the ions that carry axial current move through the junctions. In a computer model, conduction velocity can be reduced by a factor of 20 by increasing disk resistance, and decremental conduction and block will result.[246,247]

Perhaps the most important influence on gap junctional resistance in pathologic situations is the level of intracellular $Ca^{2+}$. A significant rise increases resistance to current flow through the junctions and eventually leads to physiologic uncoupling of the cells.[248,249] Intracellular $Ca^{2+}$ increases during ischemia and may be a factor causing slow conduction and reentry.

Thus, there are several causes for slow conduction that may lead to reentry: (1) slow responses that are a normal property of some regions of the heart, such as the sinus and AV node, (2) depressed fast responses or slow responses caused by pathology-induced partial depolarization of the membrane potential, (3) anisotropy, and (4) changes in gap junctional resistance.

## UNIDIRECTIONAL BLOCK

Unidirectional block occurs when an impulse cannot conduct in one direction along a bundle of cardiac fibers but can conduct in the opposite direction. This condition is necessary for the occurrence of classic reentrant rhythms. Thus, unidirectional block in part of the circuit leaves a return pathway through which the impulse conducts to reenter previously excited areas. A number of mechanisms, involving both active and passive electrical properties of cardiac cells, may cause unidirectional block.

### Regional Differences in Recovery of Excitability

One cause of unidirectional block that allows the initiation of reentry is regional differences in recovery of excitability. When differences in the duration of the effective refractory period occur in adjacent areas, conduction of an appropriately timed premature impulse may be blocked in the region with the longest refractory period, which then becomes a site of unidirectional block, while conduction continues

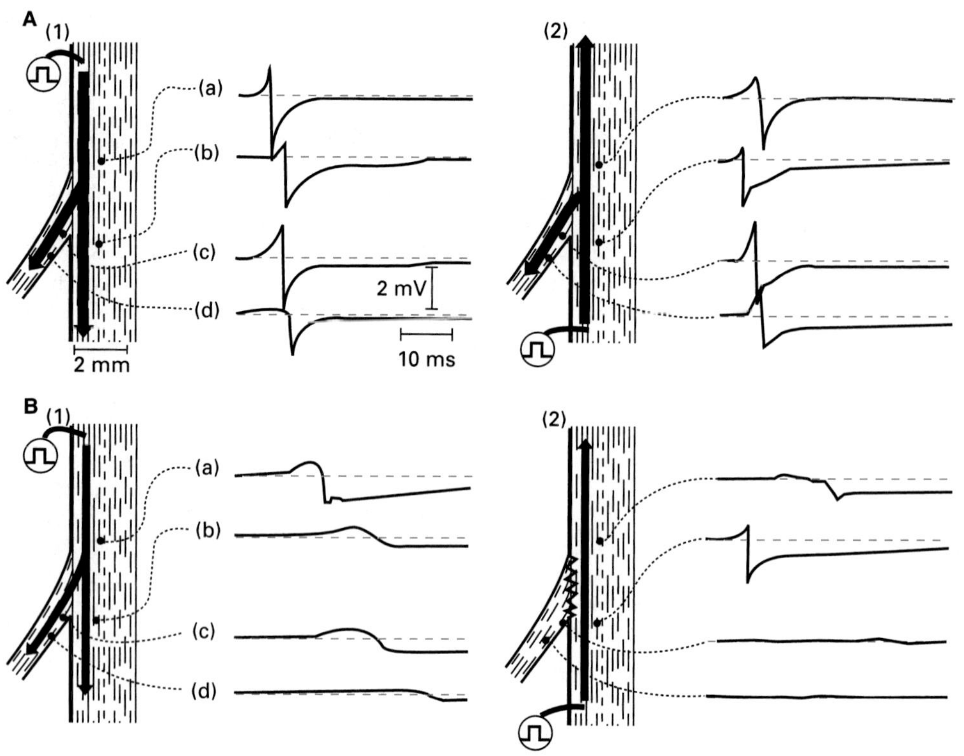


FIGURE 27-13 Conduction characteristics and unidirectional block at branch sites. The drawings represent a small branch formed by the origin of a pectinate muscle from the larger crista terminalis. The general direction of the fiber orientation is indicated by the broken lines. The patterns of propagation are shown by the solid arrows. Extracellular waveforms recorded at sites indicated by the dashed lines also are shown. (From Spach MS et al. The functional role of structural complexities in the propagation of depolarization in the atrium of the dog: Cardiac conduction disturbances due to discontinuities of effective axial resistivity. *Circ Res* 1982;50:175. Reproduced with permission from the publisher and authors.)

through regions with a shorter refractory period. Figure 27-14 is a schematic representation of the initiation and continuation of circus movement in an anatomically defined circuit, with differences in effective refractory period duration resulting from differences in the time course of action potential repolarization being the cause of unidirectional block in one of the pathways. The action potentials in various parts of the circuit are shown. In the upper panel (*A*), conduction of a premature impulse (extrasystole), which either can be induced by electrical stimulation or may occur "spontaneously," is blocked in the pathway with the long action potential duration and therefore long effective refractory period (to the left), referred to as the *blocked pathway*. The premature impulse, however, conducts in the other pathway with shorter action potential durations and refractory periods (to the right). This pattern of activation is indicated by the arrows. For block to occur, the premature impulse also must arise in a region with a short effective refractory period so that it occurs before repolarization of the action potentials in the left pathway occurs. In the lower panel (*B*), which shows the continuation of these events, the blocked pathway is invaded retrogradely by the impulse conducting from the right, thus causing the second action potential (arrow at the left). The proximal region where the premature impulse originated is then reexcited (reentry) as the impulse once again enters the right pathway and continues around the reentrant circuit, causing another action potential in the right pathway (large arrow). For successful reexcitation to occur in the region where the premature impulse was initiated, elements in the circuit at the region of block and proximal to it (toward the site of origin) must have regained their excitability by the time the cardiac impulse arrives there. Continuation of reentry induced by a premature impulse also is facilitated because the duration of the effective refractory period associated with conduction of the premature impulse is shortened. Therefore, on the next excursion of the reentrant impulse around the circuit, conduction occurs in a circuit with a shorter effective refractory period. Finally, the conduction velocity of premature impulses may be decreased, shortening the wavelength[250,251] and facilitating successful excitation of the region proximal to the unidirectional block.

Therefore, unidirectional block caused by regional differences in excitability is actually a result of transient block. Block occurs in the antegrade direction in the left pathway, while conduction is successful in the retrograde direction. This kind of unidirectional block can cause the initiation of reentry not only in anatomic circuits, as shown in Fig. 27-14, but also in functional circuits. For reentrant arrhythmias to arise because of regional differences in effective refractory periods, a premature impulse that initiates reentry is as necessary a requirement as are the conditions allowing the perpetuation of reentrant activation. Thus, both a "trigger" (the premature impulse) and a "substrate" (the reentrant circuit) are needed. The mechanism causing the premature impulse may be quite different from the arrhythmia it initiates. It may arise spontaneously by automaticity or result from triggered activity. The premature impulse also may be induced by an electrical stimulus during a programmed stimulation protocol. The degree of nonuniformity in effective refractory period duration necessary for a properly timed premature stimulus to cause unidirectional block may be quite small. This degree of nonuniformity often is referred to as the *dispersion in the refractory periods* or *dispersion in recovery of excitability,* meaning the difference between the shortest and longest refractory periods.

When stimuli were delivered in the region with the shortest refractory period at the border of two areas with different refractory periods in atrial tissue in the experiments of Allessie and coworkers,[252] the minimal difference in effective refractory period needed to cause block of an appropriately timed stimulated premature impulse was between 11 and 16 ms, well within the normal physiologic range of variation of effective refractory period durations. A properly timed single premature stimulus can initiate reentry in the atria because the differences in refractory period may cause unidirectional block.[252] In the ventricles, where refractory periods are much longer than they are in the atria, the physiologic differences between the longest and shortest refractory period durations is on the order of 40 ms.[253,254] Unlike the case in the atria, dispersion of refractory periods in normal ventricles is not sufficiently large to allow initiation of reentry by single premature impulses.

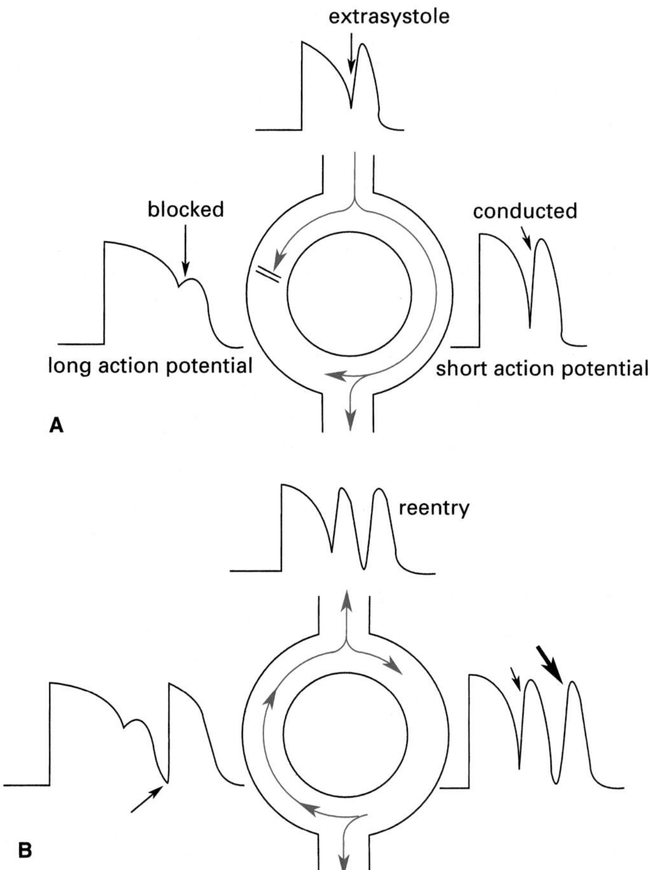


FIGURE 27-14 Diagram of reentry caused by dispersion in refractory periods. A ring of cardiac tissue is shown, and the pattern of conduction is indicated by the arrows. Action potentials with different durations located in different regions of the ring are diagrammed. (From Wit AL, Janse MJ. *The Ventricular Arrhythmia of Ischemia and Infarction: The Electrophysiological Mechanisms.* Mount Kisco, NY: Futura; 1992:86. Reproduced with permission from the publisher and authors.)

In experiments in which the dispersion of refractory periods was increased by local cooling of the ventricles and a critical difference between the shortest and longest effective refractory periods ranging from 95 to 145 ms was reached, premature stimuli delivered at the site with the shortest effective refractory period induced repetitive activity in the canine left ventricle, presumably because block of the premature impulses in the regions with a long effective refractory period created unidirectional block and permitted reentry.[255,256] Similarly, critical increases in the dispersion of refractory periods that are caused by acute or prolonged ischemia result in reentrant arrhythmias. The difference between the longest and shortest refractory periods is not the only factor that determines whether premature stimuli will induce reentry.[252] If the regions of long and short refractory periods are separated by a large distance, an early premature impulse arising in a region of short refractoriness may not be able to arrive in the region of long refractoriness sufficiently early to cause block because conduction between the regions may be slow. Regions of long refractory periods therefore must be relatively close to a region of shorter refractory periods where the premature impulse arises for block to occur. In addition, if block does occur, the size of the area of unidirectional block is of crucial importance, particularly in a functionally determined reentrant circuit. Even in the presence of large differences in effective refractory period duration, reentry may not occur when the area with long effective refractory periods resulting in unidirectional block is small. This is because the impulse can travel around the area of unidirectional block along an alternative pathway or pathways and will not be delayed sufficiently to allow reexcitation of the point of origin at the end of the latter's effective refractory period. This cannot occur in an anatomic circuit such as the one shown in Fig. 27-14.

Thus, *dispersion in recovery of excitability* is by itself not sufficient to describe the propensity for induction of reentrant arrhythmias. The regional differences in recovery of excitability that lead to unidirectional conduction block also may occur in the absence of regional differences in action potential duration. Computer models have shown that the activation sequence of a propagating impulse can lead to asynchronous repolarization and refractoriness even when membrane properties are homogeneous.[89,247] A stimulated premature impulse can block in a region that has been depolarized most recently by a prior wave of excitation and is therefore still refractory, but it may conduct into another region that was excited much earlier by the prior wave of excitation if it has had time to recover excitability. The conducting premature excitation wave then can later return to excite the area of block after it recovers, resulting in reentry.

## Asymmetric Depression of Excitability

Unidirectional conduction block in a reentrant circuit also can be persistent and independent of premature activation. Persistent unidirectional block often is associated with depression of the transmembrane potentials and excitability of cardiac fibers.[257] There are several possible mechanisms for the persistent unidirectional block in a region where action potentials are depressed. One mechanism is asymmetric depression of excitability. This asymmetric depression may occur because of asymmetric distribution of a pathologic event. As a simple example, the action potential upstrokes in a bundle of fibers may be diminished as a result of a reduction of perfusion after coronary occlusion, but the depression of the upstroke may be more severe toward one end of the bundle than toward the other. This situation is diagrammed in Fig. 27-15. A propagating impulse consisting of an action potential with a normal upstroke velocity (site 1) enters the poorly perfused region (stippled in the diagram) and propagates through this region with decrement (from left to right or from site 1

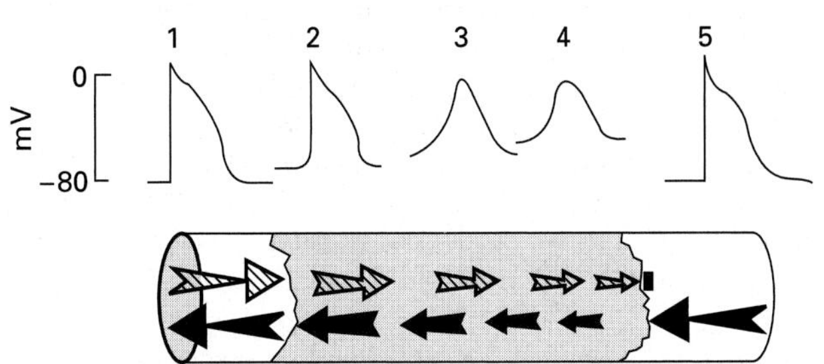


FIGURE 27-15 Asymmetric depression of excitability as a mechanism for unidirectional conduction block in a bundle of cardiac muscle fibers. The action potentials shown above were recorded from sites on the fiber bundle. The shaded part of the bundle is depressed. Conduction from left to right along the bundle is indicated by the striped arrows, conduction from right to left by the black arrows. (Modified from Wit AL, Rosen MR. Cellular electrophysiological mechanisms of cardiac arrhythmias. In: MacFarlane PW, Veitch Lawrie TD, eds. *Comprehensive Electrocardiology: Theory and Practice in Health and Disease*, vol. 2. New York: Pergamon Press; 1989:801. Reproduced with permission from the publisher and authors.)

to 4); i.e., as it conducts from the less depressed end (1) to the more severely depressed end (4), the action potential upstroke velocity and amplitude progressively decrease, as does the axial current flowing toward cells that will be excited by the upstroke (as indicated by the decreasing size of the striped arrows). When the impulse arrives at the opposite end of the depressed segment of the bundle, where there is suddenly a normally perfused bundle with normal action potentials (between action potentials 4 and 5), the action potential amplitude is markedly reduced and the weak axial current from site 4 is not sufficient to depolarize the normal membrane to threshold at site 5. Conduction therefore blocks in the left-to-right direction even though the normally perfused region is excitable. Conduction in the opposite direction (from right to left), however, still may succeed. The large axial current generated by the normal action potential at site 5 can flow for a considerable distance through the depressed region and may depolarize to threshold fibers at some distance from the most severely depressed region (perhaps as far as site 3). These cells in turn may be able to excite adjacent fibers in the direction of propagation (from right to left), and as a result, the impulse successfully propagates from site 3 to site 1, as indicated by the black arrows.

## Geometric Factors Causing Unidirectional Block

Geometric factors related to tissue architecture also may influence impulse conduction and under certain conditions lead to unidirectional block. An impulse can conduct rapidly in either direction along the length of a bundle of atrial, ventricular, or Purkinje fibers with normal electrophysiologic properties. There is usually some asymmetry in the conduction velocity, however, meaning that conduction in one direction may take slightly longer than it does in the other direction.[5,228,231] This is usually of no physiologic significance. The asymmetry of conduction can result from several factors. Bundles of cardiac muscle are composed of interconnecting myocardial fibers with different diameters packed in a connective tissue matrix. These bundles branch frequently (although the individual myocardial fibers do not branch). An impulse conducting in one direction encounters a different sequence of changes in fiber diameter, branching, and frequency and distribution of gap junctions than it does when traveling in the opposite direction. The configuration of pathways in each direction is not the same.[231] These structural features influence conduction by affecting the axial currents that flow ahead of the propagating wavefront.

The results of theoretical analyses indicate that the conduction velocity of an impulse passing abruptly from a fiber of small diameter to one of large diameter transiently slows at the junction because the larger cable results in a larger sink for the longitudinal axial current (there is more membrane for this current to depolarize to threshold if conduction of the impulse is to continue).[228,231,247,258,259] A similar slowing occurs when an impulse conducts into a region where there is an abrupt increase in branching of the myocardial syncytium; conduction transiently slows because of the larger current sink provided by the increased membrane area that must be depolarized.

In the opposite direction, it can be predicted that conduction will speed transiently as the impulse moves from a larger cable to a smaller cable because the small sink for axial current results in more rapid depolarization of the membrane to threshold.[228,258,259] Theoretically, if there is a large enough difference in the diameter of the two cables, an impulse conducting from the small cable to the large cable should block at the junction, while conduction in the opposite direction (from large cable to small cable) is maintained.

A probable example of unidirectional block based on this geometric factor in the normal heart occurs at the junctions between Purkinje's and muscle cells. At certain sites, propagation from muscle to Purkinje fibers is possible, while propagation from Purkinje fibers to muscle is not.[260] This asymmetry of conduction results from the difference in mass between the Purkinje and muscle layers. The smaller-mass Purkinje fiber bundle is the small-diameter cable, while the larger-mass muscle is the larger-diameter cable. It is unlikely that in normal circumstances these localized sites of unidirectional block predispose to reentry since the myocardium is quickly excited via the many other Purkinje-to-muscle junctions where the geometric differences are not sufficient to cause block. It is possible, however, when conduction in ischemic myocardium is slow and coupling resistance at the junction increases, that such sites of unidirectional block may become important in initiating reentry.[261–263]

It is doubtful that abrupt changes in geometric properties such as fiber diameter of the magnitude required to cause block of the *normal* action potential often exist (except at some Purkinje fiber–muscle junctions, as was described above) because the safety factor for conduction is large; i.e., there is a large excess of activating current over the amount required for propagation.[228] Dodge and Cranefield[231] pointed out that "only if an action potential is a relatively weak stimulus and the unexcited area is not easily excited will plausible changes in membrane resistance, cell diameter, or intercellular coupling produce block." There is a necessity for interaction of abnormal action potentials and decreased excitability with the preexisting anatomic impediments, as occurs in acute ischemia. When the resting potential of fibers in a muscle or Purkinje bundle is decreased, the reduced action potential upstroke results in a decreased axial current, and therefore, the action potential is a weak stimulus. The normal directional differences in conduction are then exaggerated.

At a critical degree of depression of the action potential upstroke, conduction may fail in one direction while being maintained in the other (although it may be slowed markedly). At this critical degree of depression, the reduced axial current may not be sufficient to depolarize the membrane to threshold where the current sink is increased because of the structural changes described above (increased fiber diameter), but the axial current is still more than adequate during conduction in the opposite direction. The anisotropic properties of cardiac muscle also represent a geometric factor that sometimes may contribute to the occurrence of unidirectional block. Spach and colleagues[234] have indicated that in anisotropic muscle, the safety factor for conduction is lower in the longitudinal direction of rapid conduction than it is in the transverse direction of slow conduction (the opposite of that predicted on the basis of continuous cable theory). The low safety factor longitudinally is a result of a large current load on the membrane associated with the low axial resistivity and large membrane capacitance in the longitudinal direction. This low safety factor may result in a preferential conduction block of premature impulses in the longitudinal direction relative to the transverse direction under certain conditions. In uniformly anisotropic muscle, a decrease in inward current during the depolarization phase of an action potential, as may result from premature activation, results in slowing of conduction in the longitudinal direction more than in the transverse direction, but propagation still continues as a spatially smooth process. Conduction block of early premature impulses occurs in both longitudinal and transverse directions nearly simultaneously in uniformly anisotropic muscle.[242]

In nonuniformly anisotropic muscle, however, premature activation can result in conduction block in the longitudinal direction even when the impulse is conducting from a region with a long refractory period into a region with a shorter refractory period while conduction in the transverse direction continues.[242] The site of block in the longitudinal direction can become a site of unidirectional block that

an increased electrical load; e.g., not only must a curved wavefront depolarize cells in front of it in the direction of propagation, but current also flows to cells on its sides. The slow activation by a rotor is not dependent on conduction in relatively refractory myocardium; therefore, there is an excitable gap despite the functional nature of reentry.[282] The location of the rotor can occur anywhere the second stimulated excitation encounters the wake of the first excitation with the appropriate characteristics.[287] Reentrant excitation that occurs during the initiation of ventricular fibrillation by strong electrical shocks[288,289] has characteristics consistent with spiral waves or rotors. These small circulating rotors are not stable and meet the criteria of random reentry. Spiral waves also may cause other kinds of arrhythmias. Even though nonuniform dispersions of refractoriness or anisotropy are not necessary for the initiation of reentrant excitation caused by rotors in excitable media, the myocardium, even when normal, is never homogeneous and the heterogeneities may modify the characteristics of the spiral waves.

## ARRHYTHMIAS CAUSED BY SIMULTANEOUS ABNORMALITIES OF IMPULSE GENERATION AND CONDUCTION (SEE TABLE 27-1)

### Parasystole

At times, an ectopic focus (automatic or reentrant) may be connected to the remainder of the heart through tissue or tissues in which there is unidirectional block. The unidirectional block prevents the dominant rhythm, usually a sinus rhythm, from entering the region where the ectopic focus is located. Thereby, the focus is protected. At the same time, because the block is unidirectional, impulses generated by the ectopic focus can be conducted out to other regions of the heart as long as they are not refractory. This kind of rhythm, called *parasystole,* may cause premature beats or even a tachycardia.

### Phase 4 Block

Block of an impulse may occur if the impulse arrives at a site, e.g., in the His bundle or one of the bundle branches, that is partially depolarized during spontaneous phase 4 depolarization but has not yet reached threshold. This spontaneous diastolic depolarization can depolarize the tissue sufficiently so that the fast $Na^+$ channels are inactivated enough to cause failure of propagation.[9]

#### FIBRILLATORY CONDUCTION

When cardiac impulses are continuously generated at a rapid rate from any source or due to any mechanism, they will activate the tissue of that cardiac chamber in a 1:1 manner up to a critical rate. However, when this critical rate is exceeded, so that not all the tissue of that cardiac chamber can respond 1:1, e.g., because the cycle length of the driver is shorter than the effective refractory period of those tissues, fibrillatory conduction will develop. Thus, fibrillatory conduction is characterized by activation of tissues at variable cycle lengths, all longer than the cycle length of the driver, because of variable conduction block. In that manner, activation is "fragmented." This is the mechanism of atrial fibrillation in several animal models[290–293] in which the driver consists of (1) a stable, abnormally automatic focus of very short cycle length[290]; (2) a stable reentrant circuit with very short cycle length[292,293]; or (3) unstable reentrant circuits with a very short cycle length.[291] It also appears to be the mechanism of atrial fibrillation in patients in whom activation of the atria at very short cycle lengths originates in one or more pulmonary veins. The impulses from the pulmonary vein(s) seem to precipitate and maintain atrial fibrillation.[293,294] It has also been suggested that fibrillatory conduction due to a reentrant "driver" may be the cause of ventricular fibrillation.[295]

## References


1. Hoffman BF, Rosen MR. Cellular mechanisms for cardiac arrhythmias. *Circ Res* 1981;49:1–15.
2. Waldo AL, Kaiser GA, Bowman OF Jr, Malm JR. Etiology of prolongation of the P-R interval in patients with an endocardial cushion defect: Further observations on internodal conduction and the polarity of the retrograde P wave. *Circulation* 1973;48:19–27.
3. Mayer AG. Rhythmical pulsation in *Scyphomedusae.* Publication no. 47. Washington, DC: Carnegie Institution of Washington; 1906:1.
4. Mines GR. On dynamic equilibrium in the heart. *J Physiol (Lond)* 1913;46:349–383.
5. Cranefield PF. *The Conduction of the Cardiac Impulse: The Slow Response and Cardiac Arrhythmia.* Mount Kisco, NY:Futura; 1975.
6. Schmitt OF, Erlanger J. Directional differences in the conduction of the impulse through the heart muscle and their possible relation to extrasystolic and fibrillary contractions. *Am J Physiol* 1928–1929; 87:326–347.
7. Wit AL, Hoffman BF, Cranefield PF. Slow conduction and reentry in the ventricular conduction system: I. Return extrasystole in canine Purkinje fibers. *Circ Res* 1972;30:1–10.
8. Cranefield PF, Wit AL, Hoffman BF. Genesis of cardiac arrhythmias. *Circulation* 1973;47;190–204.
9. Singer DH, Lazzara R, Hoffman BF. Interrelationships between automaticity and conduction in Purkinje fibers. *Circ Res* 1967;21: 537–558.
10. Di Francesco D. The hyperpolarization-activated current, $i_f$, and cardiac pacemaking. In: Rosen MR, Janse MJ, Wit AL, eds. *Cardiac Electrophysiology: A Textbook.* Mount Kisco, NY: Futura; 1990:117.
11. Yanagihara K, Irisawa H. Potassium current during the pacemaker depolarization in rabbit sinoatrial node cell. *Pflugers Arch* 1980;388: 255–260.
12. Di Francesco D. Characterization of single pacemaker channels in cardiac sinoatrial node cells. *Nature* 1986;324:470–473.
13. Di Francesco D, Ferroni A, Massanti M, Tromba C. Properties of the hyperpolarizing-activated current $i_f$ in cells isolated from the rabbit sino-atrial node. *J Physiol* 1986;37:61–88.
14. Brown HF. Electrophysiology of the sinoatrial node. *Physiol Rev* 1982;52:505–530.
15. Brown HF, Kimura K, Noble SJ. The relative contributions of various time-dependent membrane currents to pacemaker activity in the sino atrial node. In: Bouman LN, Jongsma HJ, eds. *Cardiac Rate and Rhythm: Physiological, Morphological and Developmental Aspects.* Boston: Martinus-Nijhoff; 1982:53.
16. Nakayama T, Kurachi Y, Noma A. Action potential and membrane currents of single pacemaker cells of the rabbit heart. *Pflugers Arch* 1984;402:248–257.
17. Shibasaki T. Conductance and kinetics of delayed rectifier potassium channels in nodal cells of the rabbit heart. *J Physiol* 1987;387: 227–250.
18. Irisawa H, Giles WR. Sinus and atrioventricular node cells: Cellular electrophysiology. In: Zipes DP, Jalife J, eds. *Cardiac Electrophysiology: From Cell to Bedside.* Philadelphia: Saunders; 1990:95.
19. Reuter H. Ion channels in cardiac cell membranes. *Annu Rev Physiol* 1984;46:473–484.
20. Bean BP. Two kinds of calcium channels in canine atrial cells. *J Gen Physiol* 1985;85:1–30.
21. Hagiwara N, Irisawa H, Kameyama M. Contribution of two types of calcium currents to the pacemaker potentials of rabbit sino-atrial node cells. *J Physiol* 1988;409:121–141.

22. Doerr T, Denger R, Trautwein W. Calcium currents in single SA nodal cells of the rabbit heart studied with action potential clamp. *Pflugers Arch* 1989;413:599–603.
23. Hoffman BF, Cranefield PF. *Electrophysiology of the Heart*. New York: McGraw-Hill; 1960.
24. Trautwein W. Effects of acetylcholine on the SA node of the heart. In: Carpenter O, ed. *Cellular Pacemakers: Mechanisms of Pacemaker Generation*. New York: Wiley; 1981:127.
25. Soejima M, Noma A. Mode of regulation of the ACh-sensitive K channel by the muscarinic receptor in rabbit atrial cells. *Pflugers Arch* 1984;400:424–431.
26. Di Francesco D, Tromba C. Inhibition of the hyperpolarizing-activated current, $i_f$, induced by acetylcholine in rabbit sino-atrial node myocytes. *J Physiol* 1988;405:477–491.
27. Noma A, Kotake H, Irisawa H. Slow inward current and its role mediating the chronotropic effect of epinephrine in the rabbit sinoatrial node. *Plfugers Arch* 1980;388:1–9.
28. Di Francesco D. The cardiac-hyperpolarizing activated current, $i_f$. Origins and developments. *Prog Biophys Mol Biol* 1985;46:163–183.
29. Hogan PM, David LD. Evidence for specialized fibers in the canine atrium. *Circ Res* 1968;23:387–396.
30. Jones SB, Euler DE, Hardie E, et al. Comparison of SA nodal and subsidiary pacemaker function and location in the dog. *Am J Physiol* 1978;234:H471–H476.
31. Rozanski GJ, Lipsius SL. Electrophysiology of functional subsidiary pacemakers in canine right atrium. *Am J Physiol* 1985;249: H594–H603.
32. Rozanski GJ, Lipsius SL, Randall WD. Functional characteristics of sinoatrial and subsidiary pacemaker activity in the canine right atrium. *Circulation* 1983;67:1378–1387.
33. Wit AL, Cranefield PF. Triggered and automatic activity in the canine coronary sinus. *Circ Res* 1977;41:435–445.
34. Wit AL, Fenoglio JJ Jr, Wagner BM, Bassett AL. Electrophysiological properties of cardiac muscle in the anterior mitral valve leaflet and the adjacent atrium in the dog: Possible implications for the genesis of atrial dysrhythmias. *Circ Res* 1973;32:731–745.
35. Bassett AL, Fenoglio JJ, Wit AL, et al. Electrophysiologic and ultrastructural characteristics of the canine tricuspid valve. *Am J Physiol* 1976;230:1366–1377.
36. Rozanski GJ. Electrophysiological properties of automatic fibers in rabbit atrioventricular valves. *Am J Physiol Heart Circ Physiol* 1987; 22:H720–H727.
36a. Chen Yi-Jen, Chen Shih-Ann, Chang M-S, Lin C-I. Arrhythmogenic activity of cardiac muscle in pulmonary veins of the dog: implication for the genesis of atrial fibrillation. *Cardiovasc Res* 2000;48:265–273.
36b. Chen Y-C, Chen S-A, Chen Y-C, et al. Effects of rapid atrial pacing on the arrhythmogenic activity of single cardiomyocytes from pulmonary veins. Implications for the initiation of atrial fibrillation. *Circulation* 2001;104:2849–2854.
36c. Chen Y-C, Chen Y-C, Yeh H-I, et al. Electrophysiology and arrhythmogenic activity of single cardiomyocytes from canine superior vena cava. *Circulation* 2002;105:2679–2685.
37. Kokobun S, Nishimura M, Noma A, Irisawa H. The spontaneous action potential of rabbit atrioventricular node cells. *Jpn J Physiol* 1980;30:529–540.
38. James TN, Isobe JH, Urthaler JH. Correlative electrophysiological and anatomical studies concerning the site of origin of escape rhythm during complete atrioventricular block in the dog. *Circ Res* 1979;45:108–119.
39. Jones SB, Euler DE, Randall WC, et al. Atrial ectopic foci in the canine heart: Hierarchy of pacemaker automaticity. *Am J Physiol Heart Circ Physiol* 1980;238:H788–H793.
40. Randall WC, Talano J, Kaye MP, et al. Cardiac pacemakers in the absence of the SA node: Responses to exercise and autonomic blockade. *Am J Physiol* 1978;234:H465–H470.
41. Wallick DW, Levy MN, Felder DS, Zieske H. Effects of repetitive bursts of vagal activity on atrioventricular junctional rate in dogs. *Am J Physiol* 1979;237:H275–H281.
42. Spear JF, Moore EN. Influence of brief vagal and stellate nerve stimulation on pacemaker activity and conduction within the atrioventricular conduction system of the dog. *Circ Res* 1973;2:27–40.
43. Rozanski GJ, Jalife J. Automaticity in atrioventricular valve leaflets of rabbit heart. *Am J Physiol Heart Circ Physiol* 1986;19:H397–H406.
44. Weidmann S. *Elektrophysiologie Der Herzmuskelfaser*. Bern and Stuttgart: Medizinischer Verlag Hans Huber; 1956.
45. Hope RR, Scherlag BJ, El-Sherif N, Lazzara R. Hierarchy of ventricular pacemakers. *Circ Res* 1976;39:883–888.
46. Vassalle M, Levine MJ, Stuckey JH. On the sympathetic control of ventricular automaticity: The effects of stellate ganglia stimulation. *Circ Res* 1968;23:249–258.
47. Levy MN. Sympathetic-parasympathetic interactions in the heart. *Circ Res* 1971;29:437–445.
48. Levy MN, Blattberg B. Effect of vagal stimulation on the overflow of norepinephrine into the coronary sinus during cardiac sympathetic nerve stimulation in the dog. *Circ Res* 1976;38:81–85.
49. Di Francesco D. A new interpretation of the pacemaker current in calf Purkinje fibers. *J Physiol* 1981;314:359–376.
50. Di Francesco D. A study of the ionic nature of the pacemaker current in calf Purkinje fibers. *J Physiol* 1981;314:377–393.
51. Noble D. The surprising heart: A review of recent progress in cardiac electrophysiology. *J Physiol* 1984;353:1–50.
52. Vasalle M, Yu H, Cohen IS. The pacemaker current in cardiac Purkinje myocytes. *J Gen Physiol* 1995;106:559–578.
53. Gintant GA, Cohen IS. Advances in cardiac cellular electrophysiology: Implications for automaticity and therapeutics. *Annu Rev Pharmacol Toxicol* 1988;28:61–81.
54. Hauswirth O, Noble D, Tsien RW. The mechanism of oscillatory activity at low membrane potentials in cardiac Purkinje fibers. *J Physiol* 1969;200:255–265.
55. Imanishi S. Calcium-sensitive discharge in canine Purkinje fibers. *Jpn J Physiol* 1971;21:443–463.
56. Noble D, Tsien RW. The kinetics and rectifier properties of the slow potassium current in cardiac Purkinje fibers. *J Physiol* 1968;195: 185–214.
57. Katzung BG, Morgenstern JA. Effects of extracellular potassium on ventricular automaticity and evidence for a pacemaker current in mammalian ventricular myocardium. *Circ Res* 1977;40:105–111.
58. Escande D, Coraboeuf E, Planche C. Abnormal pacemaking is modulated by sarcoplasmic reticulum in partially depolarized myocardium from dilated right atria in humans. *J Mol Cell Cardiol* 1987;19: 231–241.
59. Kimura T, Imanishi S, Atria M, et al. Two differential mechanisms of automaticity in diseased human atrial fibers. *Jpn J Physiol* 1988; 38:851–867.
60. January CT, Fozzard HA. The effects of membrane potential, extracellular potassium and tetrodotoxin on the intracellular sodium ion activity in sheep cardiac muscle. *Circ Res* 1984;54:652–665.
61. Carmeliet EE. *Chloride and Potassium in Cardiac Purkinje Fibers*. Thesis, Editions ARSCI, S.A. Brussels: Presses Academiques Europeennes; 1961.
62. Gadsby DC, Cranefield PF. Two levels of resting potential in cardiac Purkinje fibers. *J Gen Physiol* 1977;70:725–746.
63. Hill JL, Gettes LS. Effects of acute coronary artery occlusion on local myocardial extracellular $K^+$ activity in swine. *Circulation* 1980;61: 768–778.
64. Hirche HJ, Franz C, Bos L, et al. Myocardial extracellular $K^+$ and $H^+$ increase and noradrenaline release as possible cause of early arrhythmias following acute coronary artery occlusion in pigs. *J Mol Cell Cardiol* 1980;12:579–593.
65. Kleber AG. Resting membrane potential, extracellular potassium activity and intracellular sodium activity during acute global ischemia in isolated perfused guinea-pig hearts. *Circ Res* 1983;52: 442–450.
66. Dresdner KP, Kline R, Wit AL. Intracellular $K^+$ activity, intracellular Na activity and maximum diastolic potential of canine subendocardial Purkinje cells from one-day-old infarcts. *Circ Res* 1987;60: 122–132.

67. Dresdner KP, Kline RP, Wit AL. Cytoplasmic $K^+$ and $N^+$ activity in subendocardial canine Purkinje fibers from one-day-old infarcts using double-barrel ion sensitive electrodes. *Biophys J* 1985;47:463.
68. Friedman PL, Stewart JR, Wit AL. Spontaneous and induced cardiac arrhythmias in subendocardial Purkinje fibers surviving extensive myocardial infarction in dogs. *Circ Res* 1973;33:612–626.
69. Lazzara R, El-Sherif N, Scherlag BJ. Electrophysiological properties of canine Purkinje cells in one-day-old myocardial infarction. *Circ Res* 1973;33:722–734.
70. Hordof AJ, Edie R, Malm JR, et al. Electrophysiological properties and response to pharmacological agents of fibers from diseased human atria. *Circulation* 1976;54:774–779.
71. TenEick RE, Singer DH. Electrophysiological properties from diseased human atria: I. Low diastolic potential and altered cellular response to potassium. *Circ Res* 1979;44:545–557.
72. Singer DH, Baumgarten CM, TenEick RE. Cellular electrophysiology of ventricular and other dysrhythmias: Studies on diseased and ischemic hearts. *Progr Cardiovasc Dis* 1981;24:97–156.
73. Vassalle M. Electrogenic suppression of automaticity in sheep and dog Purkinje fibers. *Circ Res* 1970;27:361–377.
74. Vassalle M. The relationship among cardiac pacemakers: Overdrive suppression. *Circ Res* 1977;41:269–277.
75. Vassalle M. Cardiac pacemaker potentials at different extra- and intracellular K concentrations. *Am J Physiol* 1965;208:770–775.
76. Vassalle M, Caress DL, Slovin AJ, Stuckey JH. On the cause of ventricular asystole during vagal stimulation. *Circ Res* 1967;20: 228–241.
77. Randall WC, Rinkema LE, Jones SB, et al. Overdrive suppression of atrial pacemaker tissues in the alert, awake dog before and chronically after excision of the sinoatrial node. *Am J Cardiol* 1982;49: 1166–1175.
78. Glitsch HG. Characteristics of active Na transport in intact cardiac cells. *Am J Physiol* 1979;236:H189–H199.
79. Gadsby DC, Cranefield PF. Electrogenic sodium extrusion in cardiac Purkinje fibers. *J Gen Physiol* 1979;73:819–837.
80. Jordan JL, Yamaguchi I, Mandel WJ, McCullen AE. Comparative effects of overdrive on sinus and subsidiary pacemaker functions. *Am Heart J* 1977;93:367–374.
81. Kodama I, Goto J, Ando A, et al. Effects of rapid stimulation on the transmembrane action potentials of rabbit sinus node pacemaker cells. *Circ Res* 1980;46:90–99.
82. Greenberg YJ, Vassalle M. On the mechanism of overdrive suppression in the guinea pig sino-atrial node. *J Electrocardiol* 1990;37: 53–67.
83. Gang ES, Reiffel JA, Livelli FD Jr, Bigger JT Jr. Sinus node recovery times following the spontaneous termination of supraventricular tachycardia and following atrial overdrive pacing: A comparison. *Am Heart J* 1983;105:210–215.
84. Breithardt G, Seipel L, Loogen F. Sinus node recovery time and calculated sinoatrial conduction time in normal subjects and patients with sinus node dysfunction. *Circulation* 1977;56:43–50.
85. Carmeliet E. The slow inward current: Non-voltage clamp studies. In: Zipes DP, Bailey JC, Elharrar V, eds. *The Slow Inward Current and Cardiac Arrhythmias.* The Hague: Martinus Nijhoff; 1980:97.
86. Hoffman BF, Dangman KH. Are arrhythmias caused by automatic impulse generation? In: Paes de Carvalho A, Hoffman BF, Lieberman M, eds. *Normal and Abnormal Conduction in the Heart.* Mount Kisco, NY: Futura; 1982:429.
87. Dangman KH, Hoffman BF. Studies on overdrive stimulation of canine cardiac Purkinje fibers: Maximum diastolic potential as a determinant of the response. *J Am Coll Cardiol* 1983;2:1183–1191.
88. Falk RT, Cohen IS. Membrane current following activity in canine cardiac Purkinje fibers. *J Gen Physiol* 1984;83:771–799.
89. Van Capelle FJL, Durer D. Computer simulation of arrhythmias in a network of coupled excitable elements. *Circ Res* 1980;47:454–466.
90. Wit AL, Cranefield PF. Mechanism of impulse initiation in the atrioventricular junction and the effect of acetylstrophantidin (abstr). *Am J Cardiol* 1982;49:921.
91. Kirchhof CJ, Bonke FIM, Allessie MA. Evidence for the presence of electrotonic depression of pacemakers in the rabbit atrioventricular node: The effects of uncoupling from the surrounding myocardium. *Basic Res Cardiol* 1988;83:190–201.
92. Opthof T, van Ginneken ACG, Bouman LN, Jongsma HJ. The intrinsic cycle length in small pieces isolated from the rabbit sinoatrial node. *J Mol Cell Cardiol* 1987;19:923–934.
93. Janse MJ, Van Capelle FJL. Electrotonic interactions across an inexcitable region as a cause of ectopic activity in acute regional myocardial ischemia: A study in intact porcine and canine hearts and computer models. *Circ Res* 1982;50:527–537.
94. Boineau JP, Schuessler RB, Mooney CR, et al. Multicentric origin of the atrial depolarization waves: The pacemaker complex: Relation to dynamics of atrial conduction, P wave changes and heart rate control. *Circulation* 1978;58:1036–1048.
95. Toda N, West TC. Changes in sino-atrial node transmembrane potentials on vagal stimulation of the isolated rabbit atrium. *Nature* 1965;205:808–809.
96. Ferrer MI: *The Sick Sinus Syndrome*. Mount Kisco, NY: Futura; 1974.
97. Katz LN, Pick A. *Clinical Electrocardiography: The Arrhythmias.* Philadelphia: Lea & Febiger; 1956.
98. Jalife J, Moe GK. Effect of electrotonic potentials on pacemaker activity of canine Purkinje fibers in relation to parasystole. *Circ Res* 1976;39:801–808.
99. Jalife J, Moe GK. A biologic model of parasystole. *Am J Cardiol* 1979;43:761–772.
100. Moe GK, Jalife J, Mueller WJ, Moe B. A mathematical model of parasystole and its application to clinical arrhythmias. *Circulation* 1977;56:968–979.
101. Euler DE, Jones SB, Gunnar WP, et al. Cardiac arrhythmias in the conscious dog after excision of the sinus node and crista terminalis. *Circulation* 1979;59:468–475.
102. Loeb JM, Euler DE, Randall WC, et al. Cardiac arrhythmias after chronic embolization of the sinus node artery: Alterations in parasympathetic pacemaker control. *Circulation* 1980;61: 192–198.
103. Randall WC, Rinkema LE, Jones SB, et al. Functional characteristics of atrial pacemaker activity. *Am J Physiol* 1982;242:H98–H106.
104. Gillette PC, Kugler JD, Garson A Jr, et al. Mechanisms of cardiac arrhythmias after the Mustard operation for transposition of the great arteries. *Am J Cardiol* 1980;45:1225–1230.
105. Klein HO, Lebson R, Cranefield PF, Hoffman BF. Effect of extrasystoles on idioventricular rhythm: Clinical and electrophysiologic correlation. *Circulation* 1973;47:758–764.
106. Webb SW, Adgey AAJ, Pantridge JF. Autonomic disturbance of onset of acute myocardial infarction. *Br Med J* 1972;3:89–92.
107. Lie KI, Wellens HJJ, Schuilenburg RM. Mechanism and significance of widened QRS complexes during complete atrioventricular block in acute inferior myocardial infarction. *Am J Cardiol* 1974;33: 833–839.
108. Dahl G, Isenberg G. Decoupling of heart muscle cells: Correlation with increased cytoplasmic calcium activity and with changes of nexus ultrastructure. *J Membr Biol* 1980;53:63–75.
109. Weingart R. The actions of ouabain on intercellular coupling and conduction velocity in mammalian ventricular muscle. *J Physiol* 1977;264:341–365.
110. Ellis D. The effects of external cations and ouabain on the intracellular sodium activity of sheep heart Purkinje fibers. *J Physiol* 1977;273:211–240.
111. Davis LD. Effects of autonomic neurohumors on transmembrane potentials of atrial plateau fibers. *Am J Physiol* 1975;229:1351–1364.
112. Tsien RW. Effects of epinephrine on the pacemaker potassium current of cardiac Purkinje fibers. *J Gen Physiol* 1974;64:293–319.
113. Pliam MB, Krellenstein DJ, Vassalle M, Brooks CMcC. The influence of norepinephrine, reserpine and propranolol on overdrive suppression. *J Electrocardiol* 1975;8:17–24.
114. Armour JA, Hageman GR, Randall WC. Arrhythmias induced by local cardiac nerve stimulation. *Am J Physiol* 1972;223:1068–1075.

115. Katzung BG, Hondeghem LM, Grant AO. Cardiac ventricular automaticity induced by current of injury. *Pflugers Arch* 1975;360: 193–197.
116. Rosen MR, Gelband H, Hoffman BF. Correlation between the effects of ouabain on the canine electrocardiogram and transmembrane potentials of isolated Purkinje fibers. *Circulation* 1973;47:65–72.
117. Rosen MR, Gelband H, Merker C, Hoffman BF. Mechanisms of digitalis toxicity: Effects of ouabain on phase four of canine Purkinje fiber transmembrane potentials. *Circulation* 1973;47:681–689.
118. Deck KA. Aenderungen des Ruhepotentials und der Kabeleigenschaften von Purkinje-Faden bei der Dehnung. *Pflugers Arch* 1964; 280:131–140.
119. Dudel J, Trautwein W. Das Aktionspotential und Mechanogramm des Herzmuskels unter dem Einflusz der Dehnung. *Cardiologia* 1954;25: 344–362.
120. Kaufmann R, Theopile U. Automatie fördernde Dehnungseffekte am Purkinje Faden, Papillarmuskeln und Vorhoftrabekeln von Rhesusaffen. *Pflugers Arch* 1967;291:174–189.
121. Hansen DE, Craig CS, Hondeghem LM. Stretch-induced arrhythmias in the isolated canine ventricle: Evidence for the importance of mechanoelectrical feedback. *Circulation* 1990;81:1094–1105.
122. Ferrier GR, Rosenthal JE. Automaticity and entrance block induced by focal depolarization of mammalian ventricular tissues. *Circ Res* 1980;47:238–248.
123. Imanishi S, Surawicz B. Automatic activity in depolarized guinea-pig ventricular myocardium. *Circ Res* 1976;39:751–759.
124. Brown HF, Noble SJ. Membrane currents underlying delayed rectification and pacemaker activity in frog atrial muscle. *J Physiol* 1969;204:717–736.
125. Hume J, Katzung BG. Physiological role of endogenous amines in the modulation of ventricular automaticity in the guinea pig. *J Physiol* 1980;309:275–286.
126. Cranefield PF, Aronson RS. Initiation of sustained rhythmic activity by single propagated action potentials in canine cardiac Purkinje fibers exposed to sodium-free solution or to ouabain. *Circ Res* 1974; 34:477–481.
127. Cranefield PF. Action potentials, afterpotentials and arrhythmias. *Circ Res* 1977;41:415–425.
128. Cranefield PF, Aronson RS. *Cardiac Arrhythmias: The Role of Triggered Activity and Other Mechanisms*. Mount Kisco, NY: Futura; 1988.
129. Cramer M, Siegal M, Bigger JT Jr, Hoffman BF. Characteristics of extracellular potentials recorded from the sinoatrial pacemaker of the rabbit. *Circ Res* 1977;41:292–300.
130. Wit AL, Boyden PA, Gadsby CD, Cranefield PF. Triggered activity as a cause of atrial arrhythmias. In: Narula OS, ed. *Cardiac Arrhythmias: Electrophysiology, Diagnosis and Management*. Baltimore: Williams & Wilkins; 1979:14.
131. Olsson SB, Blomström-Lundqvist C, Wohlfart B. Endocardial monophasic action potentials: Correlations with intracellular electrical activity. *Ann NY Acad Sci* 1990;601:119–127.
132. Harriman RJ, Holzman R, Gough WB, et al. In vivo demonstration of delayed afterdepolarization as a cause of ventricular rhythms in one-day-old infarction. *J Am Coll Cardiol* 1984;3:478.
133. Priori SG, Mantica M, Schwartz PJ. Delayed afterdepolarizations elicited in vivo by left stellate ganglion stimulation. *Circulation* 1988; 78:178–185.
134. Fabiato A, Fabiato F. Contraction induced by a calcium-triggered release of calcium from the sarcoplasmic reticulum of single skinned cardiac cells. *J Physiol* 1975;249:469–495.
135. Aronson RS, Gelles JM, Hoffman BF. Effect of ouabain on the current underlying spontaneous diastolic depolarization in cardiac Purkinje fibers. *Nature New Biol* 1973;245:118–120.
136. Lederer WJ, Tsien RW. Transient inward current underlying arrhythmogenic effect of cardiotonic steroids in Purkinje fibers. *J Physiol* 1976;263:73–100.
137. Kass RS, Lederer WJ, Tsien RW, Weingart R. Role of calcium ions in transient inward currents and after contractions induced by strophantidin in cardiac Purkinje fibers. *J Physiol* 1978;281:187–208.
138. Kass RS, Tsien RW, Weingart R. Ionic basis of transient inward current induced by strophantidin in cardiac Purkinje fibers. *J Physiol* 1978;281:209–226.
139. Karagueuzian HS, Katzung BG. Voltage clamp studies of transient inward current and mechanical oscillations induced by ouabain in ferret papillary muscle. *J Physiol* 1982;327:255–271.
140. Vassalle M, Mugelli A. An oscillatory current in sheep cardiac Purkinje fibers. *Circ Res* 1981;48:618–631.
141. Lipsius SL, Gobbins WR. Membrane currents, contractions and aftercontractions in cardiac Purkinje fibers. *Am J Physiol* 1982;243: H77–H86.
142. Eisner DA, Lederer WJ. Inotropic and arrhythmogenic effects of potassium-depleted solutions on mammalian cardiac muscle. *J Physiol* 1979;294:255–277.
143. Baker PF, Blaustein MP, Hodgkin AL, Steinhardt RA. The influence of calcium on sodium efflux in squid axons. *J Physiol* 1969;200: 431–458.
144. Mullins LJ. The generation of electrical currents in cardiac fibers by Na/Ca exchange. *Am J Physiol* 1979;236:C103–C110.
145. Eisner DA, Lederer WJ. Na-Ca exchange: Stoichiometry and electrogenicity. *Am J Physiol* 1985;248:C189–C202.
146. Davis LD. Effect of changes in cycle length on diastolic depolarization produced by ouabain in canine Purkinje fibers. *Circ Res* 1973; 32:206–214.
147. Ferrier GR, Saunders JH, Mendez C. A cellular mechanism for the generation of ventricular arrhythmias by acetylstrophantidin. *Circ Res* 1973;32:600–609.
148. Ferrier GR, Moe GK. Effect of calcium on acetylstrophantidin-induced transient depolarizations in canine Purkinje tissue. *Circ Res* 1973;33:508–515.
149. Hashimoto K, Moe GK. Transient depolarizations induced by acetylstrophantidin in specialized tissue of dog atrium and ventricle. *Circ Res* 1973;32:618–624.
150. Hogan PM, Wittenberg SM, Kocke FJ. Relationship of stimulation frequency to automaticity in the canine Purkinje fiber during ouabain administration. *Circ Res* 1973;32:377–384.
151. Aronson RS, Cranefield PF. The effect of resting potential on the electrical activity of canine cardiac Purkinje fibers exposed to Na-free solution or to ouabain. *Pflugers Arch* 1974;347:101–116.
152. Zipes DP, Arbel E, Knope RF, Moe GK. Accelerated cardiac escape rhythms caused by ouabain intoxication. *Am J Cardiol* 1974;33: 248–253.
153. Lown B, Cannon RL, Rossi MA. Electrical stimulation and digitalis drugs: Repetitive response in diastole. *Proc Soc Exp Biol Med* 1967; 126:697–701.
154. Lown B. Electrical stimulation to estimate the degree of digitalization: II. Experimental studies. *Am J Cardiol* 1968;22:251–259.
155. Castellanos A, Lemberg L, Centurion MJ, Berkovits BV. Concealed digitalis-induced arrhythmias unmasked by electrical stimulation of the heart. *Am Heart J* 1967;73:484–490.
156. Deitmer JW, Ellis D. The intracellular sodium activity of cardiac Purkinje fibers during inhibition and re-activation of the Na-K pump. *J Physiol* 1978;284:241–259.
157. Lee CO, Dagostino M. Effect of strophantidin on intracellular Na ion activity and twitch tension of constantly driven cardiac Purkinje fibers. *Biophys J* 1982;40:185–198.
158. Lee CO, Kang DH, Sokol JH, Lee KS. Relation between intracellular Na ion activity and tension of sheep cardiac Purkinje fibers exposed to dihydro-ouabain. *Biophys J* 1980;29:315–330.
159. Reuter H, Seitz N. The dependence of calcium efflux from cardiac muscle on temperature and external ion composition. *J Physiol* 1968; 195:451–470.
160. Mullins JL. *Ion Transport in Heart*. New York: Raven Press; 1981.
161. Wit A, Cranefield PF. Triggered activity in cardiac muscle fibers of the simian mitral valve. *Circ Res* 1976;38:85–98.
162. Boyden PA, Tilley LP, Albala A, et al. Mechanisms for atrial arrhythmias associated with cardiomyopathy: A study of feline hearts with primary myocardial disease. *Circ Res* 1984;69:1036–1047.

163. Malfatto G, Rosen TS, Rosen MR. The response to overdrive pacing of triggered atrial and ventricular arrhythmias in the canine heart. *Circulation* 1988;77:1139–1148.
164. Belardinelli L, Isenberg G. Actions of adenosine and isoproterenol on isolated mammalian ventricular myocyte. *Circ Res* 1983;53: 287–297.
165. Lazzara R, Marchi S. Electrophysiological mechanisms for the generation of arrhythmias with adrenergic stimulation. In: Brachman J, Schomig A, eds. *Adrenergic System and Ventricular Arrhythmias in Myocardial Infarction*. Heidelberg: Springer Verlag; 1989:231.
166. Lerman BB, Belardinelli L, West A, et al. Adenosine-sensitive ventricular tachycardia: Evidence suggesting cyclic AMP-mediated triggered activity. *Circulation* 1986;74:270–280.
167. El-Sherif N, Zeiler R, Gough WB. Effects of catecholamine, verapamil, and tetrodotoxin on triggered automaticity in canine ischemic Purkinje fibers (abstr). *Circulation* 1980;62:281.
168. El-Sherif N, Gough WB, Zeiler RH, Mehra R. Triggered ventricular arrhythmias in one-day-old myocardial infarction in the dog. *Circ Res* 1983;52:566–579.
169. Reuter H. Localization of beta adrenergic receptors and effects of noradrenaline and cyclic nucleotides on action potentials, ionic currents and tension in mammalian cardiac muscle. *J Physiol* 1974; 242:429–451.
170. Horn EM, Johnson NJ, Bilezikian JP, Rosen MR. Developmental changes in the electrophysiological properties and the beta-adrenergic receptor-effector complex in atrial fibers of the canine coronary sinus. *Circ Res* 1989;65:325–333.
171. Morad M, Rolett E. Relaxing effect of catecholamine on mammalian heart. *J Physiol* 1972;224:537–558.
172. Fabiato A. Calcium-induced release of calcium from the cardiac sarcoplasmic reticulum. *Am J Physiol* 1983;245:C1–C14.
173. Saito T, Otoguro M, Matsubara T. Electrophysiological studies on the mechanism of electrically induced sustained rhythmic activity in the rabbit right atrium. *Circ Res* 1978;42:199–206.
174. Mary-Rabine L, Hordof AJ, Danilo P, et al. Mechanisms for impulse initiation in isolated human atrial fibers. *Circ Res* 1980;47:267–277.
175. Aronson RS. Afterpotentials and triggered activity in hypertrophied myocardium from rats with renal hypertension. *Circ Res* 1981;48: 720–727.
176. Nordin C, Gilat E, Aronson RS. Delayed afterdepolarizations and triggered activity in ventricular muscle from rats with streptozotocin-induced diabetes. *Circ Res* 1985;57:28–34.
176a. Priori SG, Napolitano C, Memmi M, et al. Clinical and molecular characterization of patients with catecholaminergic polymorphic ventricular tachycardia. *Circulation* 2002;106:69–74.
177. Arlock P, Katzung BG. Effects of sodium substitutes on transient inward current and tension in guinea-pig and ferret papillary muscle. *J Physiol* 1985;360:105–120.
178. Ferrier G. Effects of transmembrane potential on oscillatory afterpotentials induced by acetylstrophantidin in canine ventricular tissues. *J Pharmacol Exp Ther* 1981;215:332–341.
179. Wasserstrom JA, Ferrier GR. Voltage dependence of digitalis afterpotentials, aftercontractions, and inotropy. *Am J Physiol* 1981; 241:H646–H653.
180. Henning B, Wit AL. Action potential characteristics control afterdepolarization amplitude and triggered activity in canine coronary sinus. *Circulation* 1981;64:IV–50.
181. LeMarec H, Dangman KH, Danilo P, Rosen MR. An evaluation of automaticity and triggered activity in the canine heart one to four days after myocardial infarction. *Circulation* 1985;71:1224–1236.
182. Gough WB, El-Sherif N. Dependence of delayed afterdepolarizations on diastolic potentials in ischemic Purkinje fibers. *Am J Physiol* 1989; 257:H770–H777.
183. Wit AL, Tseng G-N, Henning B, Hanna MS. Arrhythmogenic effects of quinidine on catecholamine-induced delayed afterdepolarizations in canine atrial fibers. *J Cardiovasc Electrophysiol* 1990;1:15–30.
184. Sheu SS, Lederer WJ. Lidocaine's negative inotropic and antiarrhythmic actions: Dependence on shortening of action potential duration and reduction of intracellular sodium activity. *Circ Res* 1985;57:578–590.
185. Aronson RS. Characteristics of action potentials of hypertrophied myocardium from rats with renal hypertension. *Circ Res* 1980;47: 443–454.
186. Moak JP, Rosen MF. Induction and termination of triggered activity by pacing in isolated canine Purkinje fibers. *Circulation* 1984;69: 149–162.
187. Wit AL, Gadsby DC, Cranefield PF. Electrogenic sodium extrusion can stop triggered activity in the canine coronary sinus. *Circ Res* 1981;49:1029–1042.
188. Johnson N, Danilo P, Wit A, Rosen MR. Response to pacing of triggered activity occurring in catecholamine-treated canine coronary sinus. *Circulation* 1986;741:1168–1179.
189. Gadsby DC, Cranefield PF. Direct measurement of changes in sodium pump current in canine cardiac Purkinje fibers. *Proc Natl Acad Sci USA* 1979;76:1783–1787.
190. Johnson N, Rosen MR. The distinction between triggered activity and other cardiac arrhythmias. In: Brugada P, Wellens HJJ, eds. *Cardiac Arrhythmias: Where to Go from Here*. Mount Kisco, NY: Futura; 1987:129.
191. Dangman KH, Hoffman BF. The effects of single premature stimuli on automatic and triggered rhythms in isolated canine Purkinje fibers. *Circulation* 1985;71:813–822.
192. Trautwein W. Mechanisms of tachyarrhythmias and extrasystoles. In: Sandoe E, Flenstad-Jenson E, Olesen K, eds. *Symposium on Cardiac Arrhythmias*. Sodertalje, Sweden: AB Astra; 1970:53.
193. January CT, Shorofsky S. Early afterdepolarizations: Newer insights into cellular mechanisms. *J Cardiovasc Electrophysiol* 1990;1: 161–169.
194. Mendez C, Delmar M. Triggered activity: Its possible role in cardiac arrhythmias. In: Zipes DP, Jalife J, eds. *Cardiac Electrophysiology and Arrhythmias*. Orlando, FL: Grune & Stratton, 1985:311.
195. Kupersmith J, Hoff P. Occurrence and transmission of localized repolarization abnormalities in vitro. *J Am Coll Cardiol* 1985;6: 152–160.
196. Wit AL, Wiggins JR, Cranefield PF. Some effects of electrical stimulation on impulse initiation in cardiac fibers: Its relevance for the determination of the mechanisms of clinical cardiac arrhythmias. In: Wellens JH, Lie KI, Janse MJ, eds. *The Conduction System of the Heart*. Philadelphia: Lea & Febiger; 1976:163.
197. Antzelevitch C, Sicouri S. Clinical relevance of cardiac arrhythmias generated by afterdepolarizations: Role of M cells in the generation of U waves, triggered activity and torsade de pointes. *J Am Coll Cardiol* 1994;23:259–277.
198. Damiano BP, Rosen MR. Effects of pacing on triggered activity induced by early afterdepolarizations. *Circulation* 1984;69: 1013–1025.
199. Brachmann J, Scherlag BJ, Rosenshtraukh LV, Lazzara R. Bradycardia dependent triggered activity: Relevance to drug-induced multiform ventricular tachycardia. *Circulation* 1983;68:846–856.
200. Kay GN, Plumb VJ, Arciniegas JG, et al. Torsade de pointes: The long-short initiating sequence and other clinical features: Observations in 32 patients. *J Am Coll Cardiol* 1983;2:806–817.
201. Ben David J, Zipes DP. Differential response to right and left ansae subclaviae stimulation of early afterdepolarizations and ventricular tachycardia induced by cesium in dogs. *Circulation* 1988;78: 1241–1250.
202. Levine JH, Spear JF, Guarnieri T, et al. Cesium chloride–induced long QT syndrome: Demonstration of afterdepolarizations and triggered activity in vivo. *Circulation* 1985;72:1092–1104.
203. Strauss HC, Bigger JT Jr, Hoffman BF. Electrophysiological and beta-blocking effects of MJ 1999 on dog and rabbit cardiac tissue. *Circ Res* 1970;26:661–678.
204. Carmeliet E. Electrophysiologic and voltage clamp analyses of the effects of sotalol on isolated cardiac muscle and Purkinje fibers. *J Pharmacol Exp Ther* 1985;232:817–825.

205. Dangman KH, Hoffman BF. In vivo and in vitro antiarrhythmic and arrhythmogenic effects of *N*-acetylprocainamide. *J Pharmacol Exp Ther* 1981;217:851–862.
206. Roden DM, Hoffman BF. Action potential prolongation and induction of abnormal automaticity by low quinidine concentrations in canine Purkinje fibers: Relationship to potassium and cycle length. *Circ Res* 1985;56:857–867.
207. Davidenko JM, Cohen L, Goodrow R, Antzelevitch C. Quinidine-induced action potential prolongation, early afterdepolarizations, and triggered activity in canine Purkinje fibers: Effects of stimulation rate, potassium, and magnesium. *Circulation* 1989;79:674–686.
208. Colatsky T. Mechanisms of action of lidocaine and quinidine on action potential duration in rabbit cardiac Purkinje fibers: An effect on steady-state sodium currents. *Circ Res* 1982;50:17–27.
209. Selzer A, Wray HW. Quinidine syncope: Paroxysmal ventricular fibrillation occurring during treatment of chronic atrial arrhythmias. *Circulation* 1964;30:17–26.
210. Smith WM, Gallagher JJ. "Les torsades de pointes": An unusual ventricular arrhythmia. *Ann Intern Med* 1980;93:578–584.
211. Olshansky B, Martins J, Hunt S. *N*-acetyl procainamide causing torsades de pointes. *Am J Cardiol* 1982;50:1439–1441.
212. Kuck KH, Kunze DP, Roewer N, Bleifield W. Sotalol-induced torsades de pointes. *Am Heart J* 1984;107:179–180.
213. Bailie DS, Inoue H, Kaseda S, et al. Magnesium suppression of early afterdepolarizations and ventricular tachyarrhythmias induced by cesium in dogs. *Circulation* 1988;77:1395–1402.
214. Tzivoni D, Keren A, Cohen AM, et al. Magnesium therapy for torsades de pointes. *Am J Cardiol* 1984;53:528–530.
215. Perticone F, Adinolfi L, Bonaduce D. Efficacy of magnesium sulfate in the treatment of torsade de pointes. *Am Heart J* 1986;112:847–849.
215a. Priori SG, Barhanin J, Hauer RNW, et al. Genetic and molecular basis of cardiac arrhythmias: Impact on clinical management. Parts I and II. *Circulation* 1999;99:518–528
216. Lewis T. *The Mechanism and Graphic Registration of the Heart Beat*, 3d ed. London: Shaw Sons; 1925.
217. Smeets JLRM, Allessie MA, Lammers WJEP, et al. The wavelength of cardiac impulse and reentrant arrhythmias in isolated rabbit atrium: The role of heart rate, autonomic transmitters, temperature, and potassium. *Circ Res* 1986;58:96–108.
218. Garrey W. The nature of fibrillary contraction of the heart: Its relation to tissue mass and form. *Am J Physiol* 1914;33:397–414.
219. El Sherif N, Carel EB, Yin H, Restivo M. The electrophysiological mechanism of ventricular arrhythmias in the long-QT syndrome: Tridimensional mapping of activation and recovery patterns. *Circ Res* 1996;79:474–492.
220. Coumel P, Cabrol C, Fabiato A, et al. Tachycardie permanente par rhythme reciproque. *Arch Mal Coeur Vaiss* 1967; 60:1830–1864.
221. Critelli G, Gallagher JJ, Monda V, et al. Anatomic and electrophysiologic substrate of the permanent form of junctional reciprocating tachycardia. *J Am Coll Cardiol* 1984;4:601–610.
222. Wit AL, Cranefield PF, Hoffman BF. Slow conduction and reentry in the ventricular conducting system: II. Single and sustained circus movement in networks of canine and bovine Purkinje fibers. *Circ Res* 1972;30:11–22.
223. Kall JH, Rubenstein DS, Kopp DE, et al. Atypical atrial flutter originating in the right atrial free wall. *Circulation* 2000;101:270–279.
224. Uno K, Kumagai K, Khrestian C, Waldo AL. New insights regarding the atrial flutter reentrant circuit: Studies in the canine sterile pericarditis model. *Circulation* 1999;100:1354–1360.
224a. Scheinman MM, Cheng J, Yang Y. Mechanisms and clinical implications of atypical atrial flutter. *J Cardiovasc Electrophysiol* 1999;10: 1153–1157.
224b. Cheng J, Cabeen WR Jr, Scheinman MM. Right atrial flutter due to lower loop reentry: Mechanism and anatomic substrates. *Circulation* 1999;99:1700–1705.
225. Shimizu A, Nozaki A, Rudy Y, Waldo AL. Onset of induced atrial flutter in the canine pericarditis model. *J Am Coll Cardiol* 1991;17: 1223–1234.
226. Olshansky B, Okumura K, Hess PG, Waldo AL. Demonstration of an area of slow conduction in human atrial flutter. *J Am Coll Cardiol* 1990;16:1639–1648.
227. Klein H, Karp RB, Kouchoukus NT, et al. Intraoperative electrophysiological mapping of the ventricles during sinus rhythm in patients with a previous myocardial infarction: Identification of the electrophysiological substrate for the generation of ventricular arrhythmias. *Circulation* 1982;66:847–853.
228. Fozzard HA. Conduction of the action potential. In: Berne RM, ed. *The Cardiovascular System*. Bethesda, MD: American Physiological Society; 1979:335.
229. Weidmann S. The effect of the cardiac membrane potential on the rapid availability of the sodium carrying system. *J Physiol* 1955;127: 213–224.
230. Gettes LS, Reuter H. Slow recovery from inactivation of inward currents in mammalian myocardial fibers. *J Physiol* 1974;240: 703–724.
231. Dodge FA, Cranefield PF. Nonuniform conduction in cardiac Purkinje fibers. In: Paes de Carvalho A, Hoffman BF, Lieberman M, eds. *Normal and Abnormal Conduction in the Heart*. Mount Kisco, NY: Futura; 1982:379.
232. Tisen RW. Calcium channels in excitable cell membranes. *Annu Rev Physiol* 1983;45:341–358.
233. Zipes DP, Mendez C. Action of manganese ions and tetrodotoxin on atrioventricular nodal transmembrane potentials in isolated rabbit hearts. *Circ Res* 1973;32:447–454.
234. Spach MS, Miller WT, Geselowitz DB, et al. The discontinuous nature of propagation in normal canine cardiac muscle: Evidence for recurrent discontinuities of intracellular resistance that effect membrane currents. *Circ Res* 1981;48:39–54.
235. Spach MS, Miller WT, Dolber PC, et al. The functional role of structural complexities in the propagation of depolarization in the atrium of the dog: Cardiac conduction disturbances due to discontinuities of effective axial resistivity. *Circ Res* 1982;50: 175–191.
236. Sommer JR, Dolber PC. Cardiac muscle: The ultrastructure of its cells and bundles. In: Hoffman BF, Lieberman M, Paes de Carvallo A, eds. *Normal and Abnormal Conduction of the Heart Beat*. Mount Kisco, NY: Futura; 1982:1.
237. Hoyt RH, Cohen ML, Saffitz JE. Distribution and three-dimensional structure of intercellular junctions in canine myocardium. *Circ Res* 1989;64:563–574.
238. Roberts DE, Hersh LT, Scher AM. Influence of cardiac fiber orientation on wavefront voltage, conduction velocity and tissue resistivity in the dog. *Circ Res* 1979;44:701–712.
239. Clerc L. Directional differences of impulse spread in trabecular muscle from mammalian heart. *J Physiol* 1976;255:335–346.
240. Saffitz JE, Kanter HL, Green KG, et al. Tissue-specific determinants of anisotropic conduction velocity in canine atrial and ventricular myocardium. *Circ Res* 1994;74:1065–1070.
241. Spach MS, Dolber PC. Relating extracellular potentials and their derivatives to anisotropic propagation at a microscopic level in human cardiac muscle: Evidence for uncoupling of side-to-side fiber connections with increasing age. *Circ Res* 1986;58:356–371.
242. Spach MS, Dolber PC, Heidlage JF. Influence of the passive anisotropic properties on directional differences in propagation following modification of the sodium conductance in human atrial muscle: A model of reentry based on anisotropic discontinuous propagation. *Circ Res* 1988;62:811–832.
243. Hunter PJ, McNaughten PA, Noble D. Analytical models of propagation in excitable cells. *Prog Biophys Mol Biol* 1975;30: 99–144.
244. Dominguez C, Fozzard HA. Influence of extracellular $K^+$ concentration on cable properties and excitability of sheep cardiac Purkinje fibers. *Circ Res* 1970;26:565–574.
245. Spach MS, Miller WT, Miller-Jones E, et al. Extracellular potentials related to intracellular action potentials during impulse conduction in anisotropic canine cardiac muscle. *Circ Res* 1979;45:188–204.

246. Rudy Y, Quan W. A model study of the effects of the discrete cellular structure on electrical propagation in cardiac tissue. *Circ Res* 1987; 61:815–823.
247. Quan W, Rudy Y. Unidirectional block and reentry of cardiac excitation: A model study. *Circ Res* 1990;60:367–382.
248. DeMello WC. Effect of intracellular injection of calcium and strontium in cell communication in heart. *J Physiol* 1975;250:231–245.
249. Hess SP, Weingart R. Intracellular free calcium modified by pHi in sheep cardiac Purkinje fibres. *J Physiol* 1980;307:60P–61P.
250. Van Dam RTH. *Experimenteel Onderzoek Naar het Prikkelbaarhei-Dsverloop van de Hartspier*. Thesis. Amsterdam: University of Amsterdam, Klein Offsetdrukkerij Poortpers; 1960.
251. Rensma PL, Allessie MA, Lammers WJEP, et al. Length of excitation wave and susceptibility to reentrant atrial arrhythmias in normal conscious dogs. *Circ Res* 1988;62:395–410.
252. Allessie MA, Bonke FIM, Schopman FJG. Circus movement in rabbit atrial muscle as a mechanism of tachycardia: 2. The role of nonuniform recovery of excitability in the occurrence of unidirectional block as studied with multiple microelectrodes. *Circ Res* 1976;39:168–177.
253. Han J, Moe GK. Nonuniform recovery of excitability of ventricular muscle. *Circ Res* 1964;14:44–60.
254. Janse MJ. *The Effects of Changes in Heart Rate on the Refractory Period of the Heart*. Thesis. Amsterdam: University of Amsterdam, Mondeel-Offsetdrukkerij; 1971.
255. Wallace AG, Mignone RS. Physiologic evidence concerning the reentry hypothesis for ectopic beats. *Am Heart J* 1966;72:60–70.
256. Kuo C-S, Munakata K, Reddy CP, Surawicz B. Characteristics and possible mechanisms of ventricular arrhythmia dependent on the dispersion of action potential durations. *Circulation* 1983;67: 1356–1367.
257. Cranefield PK, Klein HO, Hoffman BF. Conduction of the cardiac impulse: 1. Delay, block and one-way block in the pressed Purkinje fibers. *Circ Res* 1971;28:199–219.
258. Joyner RW, Overholt ED, Ramza B, Veenstra RD. Propagation through electrically coupled cells: Two inhomogeneously coupled cardiac tissue layers. *Am J Physiol* 1984;247:H596–H609.
259. Goldstein SS, Rall W. Changes in action potential shape and velocity for changing core conductor geometry. *Biophys J* 1974;14:731–757.
260. Overholt ED, Joyner RW, Veenstra RD, et al. Unidirectional block between Purkinje and ventricular layers of papillary muscles. *Am J Physiol* 1984;247:H584–H595.
261. Janse MJ, Wilms-Schopman F, Wilensky RJ, Tranum-Jensen J. Role of the subendocardium in arrhythmogenesis during acute ischemia. In: Zipes DP, Jalife J, eds. *Cardiac Electrophysiology and Arrhythmias*. Orlando, FL: Grune & Stratton, 1985:353.
262. Gilmour RF, Evans JJ, Zipes DP. Purkinje-muscle coupling and endocardial response to hyperkalemia, hypoxia, and acidosis. *Am J Physiol* 1984;247:H303–H311.
263. Gilmour RF, Evans JJ, Zipes DP. Preferential interruption of impulse transmission across Purkinje-muscle junctions by interventions that depress conduction. In: Zipes DP, Jalife J, eds. *Cardiac Electrophysiology and Arrhythmias*. Orlando, FL: Grune & Stratton;1985:287.
264. Delmar M, Michaels DC, Johnson T, Jalife J. Effects of increasing intercellular resistance on transverse and longitudinal propagation in sheep epicardial muscle. *Circ Res* 1987;60:780–785.
265. Delgado C, Steinhaus B, Delmar M, et al. Directional differences in excitability and margin of safety for propagation in sheep ventricular epicardial muscle. *Circ Res* 1990;67:97–110.
266. Frame LH, Page RL, Boyden PA, et al. Circus movement in the canine atrium around the tricuspid ring during experimental atrial flutter and during reentry in vitro. *Circulation* 1987;76:1155–1175.
267. Moe GK. On the multiple wavelet hypothesis of atrial fibrillation. *Arch Int Pharmacodyn Ther* 1962;140:180–188.
268. Moe GK, Rheinboldt WC, Abildskov JA. A computer model of atrial fibrillation. *Am Heart J* 1964;67:200–220.
269. Coumel P. Role of the autonomic nervous system in paroxysmal atrial fibrillation. In: Touboul P, Waldo AL, eds. *Atrial Arrhythmias*. St Louis: Mosby–Year Book; 1990:248.
270. Allessie MA, Lammers WJEP, Bonke FIM, Hollen J. Experimental evaluation of Moe's multiple wavelet hypothesis of atrial fibrillation. In: Zipes DP, Jalife J, eds. *Cardiac Electrophysiology and Arrhythmias*. New York: Grune & Stratton, 1985:265.
271. Waldo AL. Mechanisms of atrial fibrillation, atrial flutter, and ectopic atrial tachycardia—A brief review. *Circulation* 1987;75: III37–40.
272. Allessie MA, Bonke FIM, Schopman FJG. Circus movement in rabbit atrial muscle as a mechanism of tachycardia: 3. The "leading circle" concept—A new model of circus movement in cardiac tissue without the involvement of an anatomical obstacle. *Circ Res* 1977;41: 9–18.
273. Allessie MA, Lammers WJEP, Bonke FIM, Hollen J. Intra-atrial reentry as a mechanism for atrial flutter by acetylcholine and rapid pacing in the dog. *Circulation* 1984;70:123–135.
274. Boyden PA. Activation sequence during atrial flutter in dogs with surgically induced right atrial enlargement: I. Observations during sustained rhythms. *Circ Res* 1988;62:596–608.
275. Cosio FG. Endocardial mapping of atrial flutter. In: Touboul P, Waldo AL, eds. *Atrial Arrhythmias: Current Concepts and Management*. St Louis: Mosby–Year Book; 1990:229.
275a. Chan DP, Van Hare GF, Mackall JA, et al. Role of functional block extension in lesion-related atrial flutter. *Circulation* 2001;103: 1025–1030.
275b. Tomita Y, Matsuo K, Sahadevan J, et al. Role of functional block extension in lesion-related atrial flutter. *Circulation*2001;103: 1025–1030.
276. Spinelli W, Hoffman BF. Mechanisms of termination of reentrant atrial arrhythmias by class I and class III antiarrhythmic agents. *Circ Res* 1989;65:1565–1579.
277. Wit AL, Dillon SM. Anisotropic reentry. In: Zipes DP, Jalife J, eds. *Cardiac Electrophysiology: From Cell to Bedside*. Philadelphia: Saunders; 1990:353.
278. Allessie MA, Bonke FIM, Schopman FJG. Circus movement in rabbit atrial muscle as a mechanism of tachycardia. *Circ Res* 1973;32: 54–62.
279. Dillon S, Allessie MA, Ursell PC, Wit AL. Influence of anisotropic tissue structure on reentrant circuits and the sub-epicardial border zone of subacute canine infarcts. *Circ Res* 1988;63:182–206.
280. Schalij MJ. *Anisotropic Conduction and Ventricular Tachycardia*. PhD thesis. Maastricht, the Netherlands: University of Limburg;1988.
281. Peters NS, Coromilas J, Hanna MS, et al. Characteristics of the temporal and spatial excitable gap in anisotropic reentrant circuits causing sustained ventricular tachycardia. *Circ Res* 1998;82:279–293.
282. Winfree AT. Electrical instability in cardiac muscle: Phase singularities and rotors. *J Theoret Biol* 1989;138:353–405.
283. Winfree AT. Ventricular reentry in three dimensions. In: Zipes DP, Jalife J, eds. *Cardiac Electrophysiology: From Cell to Bedside*. Philadelphia: Saunders; 1990:224.
284. Courtemanche M, Winfree AT. Re-entrant rotating waves in a Beeler-Reuter based model of two-dimensional cardiac electrical activity. *Int J Bifurc Chaos* 1991;1:431–444.
285. Davidenko JM, Kent PF, Chialvo DR, et al. Sustained vortex-like waves in normal isolated ventricular muscle. *Proc Natl Acad Sci USA* 1990;87:8785–8789.
286. Jalife J, Davidenko J, Michaels DC. A new perspective on the mechanisms of arrhythmias and sudden cardiac death: Spiral waves of excitation in heart muscle. *J Cardiovasc Electrophysiol* 1991; 2(suppl 3):S133–S152.
287. Winfree AT. Vortex action potentials in normal ventricular muscle. Mathematical approaches to cardiac arrhythmias. *Ann NY Acad Sci* 1990; 591:190–207.
288. Shibata N, Chen P-S, Dixon EG, et al. Influence of shock strength and timing on induction of ventricular arrhythmias in dogs. *Am J Physiol* 1988;225:H891–H901.
289. Chen P-S, Wolf PD, Dixon EG, et al. Mechanism of ventricular vulnerability to single premature stimuli in open-chest dogs. *Circ Res* 1988;62:1191–1209.

290. Scherf D, Romano FJ, Terranova R. Experimental studies in auricular flutter and auricular fibrillation. *Am Heart J* 1958;36:241–251.
291. Kumagai K, Khrestian C, Waldo AL. Simultaneous multisite mapping during atrial fibrillation in the canine sterile pericarditis model. Insights into self-sustaining mechanisms. *Circulation* 1997;95: 511–521.
292. Skanes A, Mandapati R, Verenfeld O, et al. Spatiotemporal periodicity during atrial fibrillation the isolated sheep heart. *Circulation* 1998; 98:1236–1248.
293. Matsuo H, Tomita Y, Khrestian CM, Waldo AL. A new mechanism of sustained atrial fibrillation: Studies in the sterile pericarditis model (abstr). *Circulation* 1998;98:209.
294. Haissaguerre M, Jais P, Shah DC, et al. Spontaneous initiation of atrial fibrillation by ectopic beats initiating in the pulmonary veins. *N Engl J Med* 1998;339:659–666.
295. Samie FH, Jalife J. Mechanisms underlying ventricular tachycardia and its transition to ventricular fibrillation in the structurally normal heart. *Cardiovasc Res* 2001;50:242–250.

CHAPTER 28

# APPROACH TO THE PATIENT WITH CARDIAC ARRHYTHMIAS

Eric N. Prystowsky / Richard I. Fogel



The diagnosis and management of specific cardiac arrhythmias are detailed in other chapters in this textbook. The purpose of this chapter is to provide the clinician with an approach to the overall evaluation of patients presumed to have a cardiac arrhythmia. Without a doubt, the two key elements in assessing patients are the history and, if available, the electrocardiogram (ECG) rhythm strip obtained at the time of their symptom. Findings on the physical examination and judicious use of noninvasive and invasive tests can be quite helpful in certain circumstances.

## HISTORY

It is imperative that a complete history of the patient's symptoms be obtained. Many elements must be sought for in this process, including: (1) documentation of initial onset of symptoms; (2) complete characterization of symptoms; (3) identifying conditions that appear to initiate symptoms; (4) duration of episodes; (5) frequency of episodes; (6) pattern of symptoms over time, for example, better or worse; (7) effect of any treatment; and (8) family history of a similar problem. It is also important to ascertain any pertinent past medical history that might be helpful in the diagnosis. This might include history of myocardial infarction, especially in a patient who presents with palpitations and syncope, or the recent initiation of an antihypertensive agent in a patient who now presents with dizzy spells. In our experience, careful and thorough attention to obtaining the preceding information typically results in an efficient and focused approach to the patient's problem.

## PHYSICAL EXAMINATION

Observations from the physical examination are helpful primarily to define whether cardiovascular disease is present. For example, in a patient who presents with dizzy spells or syncope, the presence of orthostatic hypotension, a carotid bruit, or decreased carotid pulses may be important findings that lead to a diagnosis. Likewise, identification of peripheral vascular disease suggests that the patient has atherosclerosis and may also have coronary artery disease. Auscultation of the lungs may reveal changes of chronic lung disease that are very important in certain arrhythmias, for example, atrial fibrillation (AF). Most importantly, the presence of specific cardiac murmurs or an $S_3$ or $S_4$ gallop may direct the clinician toward a cardiac cause for the patient's symptoms. One should also pay attention to the patient's gender, age, and physiognomy. Paroxysmal supraventricular tachycardia (PSVT) that occurs in a 12-year-old boy is more likely caused by atrioventricular reentry tachycardia (AVRT), whereas PSVT presenting in a 45-year-old woman more commonly is due to AV node reentry. A very obese person might be prone to sleep apnea, which has been linked to AF, and other features might suggest Marfan's syndrome or other similar problems that have an association with various cardiac arrhythmias.

## SYNCOPE, PRESYNCOPE, DIZZINESS

Patients with syncope, presyncope, or dizziness are often referred to the electrophysiologist for evaluation for fear that the symptoms are caused by an arrhythmia. Unless you are fortunate enough to record an ECG rhythm strip at the time of the patient's event, you can never positively eliminate an arrhythmic cause. Regardless, a detailed history typically points one in the correct direction (see Chap. 40). It is well established that syncope related to a cardiac cause is associated with a relatively high sudden death rate, and therefore it is very important that one establishes whether or not cardiac disease is present.[1–3] This includes a thorough history and physical examination as well as analysis of a 12-lead ECG and echocardiogram. The ECG may disclose many clues to the cause of syncope, including evidence for myocardial infarction, cardiac hypertrophy, sinus node dysfunction, conduction abnormality, Wolff-Parkinson-White syndrome, or long QT interval. If a long QT interval is discovered, it is important to determine whether there is a family history of syncope or sudden death, or the patient has been prescribed a drug that increases the QT interval. Evaluation of the echocardiogram may lead to a variety of cardiac diagnoses.

Certain historic features are typically associated with various forms of syncope. Neurally mediated syncope is very common and has a characteristic clinical presentation. The patient is typically in an upright position, either sitting or standing, and may recount a feeling of being hot or warm with or without concomitant nausea prior to loss of consciousness. Sweating is a common feature, although the patient may state that it occurred upon regaining consciousness rather than prior to syncope. Patients often recount being told by those witnessing the event that the patient was "white as a ghost" or pale in color. Normally the patient is alert upon regaining consciousness but may feel fatigued. While patients often state that their heart was "pounding" or faster than usual upon awakening, they do not give a history of a rapid regular pulse that persists for minutes after the event. This latter feature should direct one to a possible arrhythmic cause for syncope. "Church" syncope, that is, patients who have presyncope or syncope during church services is almost always vagally mediated in our experience.

Cardiac syncope is often sudden in onset and frequently unaccompanied by any prodrome. In some circumstances patients relate a feeling of rapid palpitations prior to loss of consciousness, and these individuals should be evaluated for a cardiac arrhythmia regardless of whether heart disease is present. One should remember that rapid PSVT as well as ventricular tachycardia can cause syncope. Unfortunately, a sudden loss of consciousness without prodrome is not specific for an arrhythmia, and patients with an arrhythmia can present with some features of a vasovagal syncope.

For patients who present with dizziness or presyncope, it is important to distinguish between vertigo and true light-headedness. Ask the patient whether she or he feels like the room or they are spinning compared with a sensation that "the lights are going out" or they are about to lose consciousness. This will often lead to the appropriate differentiation of these two problems. For all patients, but especially for older patients it is important to ascertain whether any new drugs have been started, especially antihypertensive agents. Not uncommonly, removal of these agents cures the problem.

Additional tests will depend on the results of the initial workup as described earlier. If a cardiac arrhythmia, in particular sustained ventricular tachycardia, is considered the cause of syncope then an electrophysiologic study should be performed (see Chap. 34). In a patient presumed to have neurally mediated syncope, one may or may not want to perform a head-up tilt table evaluation (see later). Event recorders may play a key role in identifying the etiology of syncope in some patients (see Chap. 33).

## PALPITATIONS

Few people have not experienced on some occasion a feeling that their heart is not beating right. For many patients palpitations often are correlated with sinus rhythm.[4] Palpitations are described by patients in many ways including skipped beats, a sudden thump, hard beating, fluttering in the chest, a jittery sensation, a rapid pulse, or as merely a vague feeling that their heart is irregular. These are only some of the characterizations related by patients, and many others exist. The authors have noted that many patients equate a "strong heart beat" as palpitations, and it is important to distinguish this from irregular heart beats. A premature atrial or ventricular complex often cannot be felt by the patient, and what they experience is the strong heart beat that follows the pause. In this situation they will often describe a sensation of an empty feeling or no heart beat ended by a thump. The authors find it useful to tap out various cadences for the patient. For example, to distinguish between AF and PSVT one can tap out a rapid irregular cadence compared with a rapid regular cadence—patients will often recognize one over the other. Similarly, one can tap out a cadence of extra beats with a pause. Palpitations are often more prominent at night, especially when patients lie on their left side. While these may be premature beats, often it is simply sinus rhythm.

Other historic features often tailor the initial workup. A rapid regular rhythm that occurs a few times per year and has been ongoing for many years is likely a form of PSVT. In the absence of a previous correlation with an ECG rhythm strip or 12-lead ECG, an electrophysiologic study will typically be required for diagnostic and/or therapeutic reasons. Noninvasive monitoring for such infrequent arrhythmias is usually futile, and, although one could prescribe an implantable loop recorder (see Chap. 34), an electrophysiologic study is preferred. In contrast, for patients with more frequent symptoms, noninvasive event recorder monitoring is often our choice, and a unique new form of technology using wireless outpatient continuous monitoring can even identify asymptomatic arrhythmic episodes (see Chap. 33). Even if sinus rhythm is identified as the cause of palpitations, the results will be valuable to the patient. Most patients want some diagnosis and will be reassured that their symptoms are not life-threatening, which in many cases is the reason that brought the patient to the physician.

Women might present with palpitations during the week prior to menstruation, and the diagnosis is often premature atrial or ventricular complexes that occur during a specific time of hormonal change. It is commonly believed that alcohol and caffeine are arrhythmogenic, and while this may be so in certain patients, it has been the authors' experience that these agents typically play a rather minor role in patients who have arrhythmias. Obviously, patients with AF might have episodes during heavy alcohol intake, but such is usually not the case for PSVT and sustained ventricular tachycardia. Regardless, it is very important to glean from the history any information that might help in the treatment of the patient's palpitations.

## FATIGUE, CHEST PAIN, AND DYSPNEA

On occasion, patients will present with symptoms such as fatigue, chest pain, or dyspnea that do not appear to be related to an arrhythmia. This particularly is true for those who have AF. It is surprising how many patients with AF do not experience palpitations, and will present with either fatigue or shortness of breath. Thus, while these symptoms typically direct the clinician toward another diagnostic road, one should remember that they might be caused by an arrhythmia. Of particular importance is a patient who presents with AF and symptoms of heart failure without palpitations. Often these individuals have tachycardia-mediated cardiomyopathy, and with appropriate control of the ventricular rate the ventricular function might even normalize. Since the patient does not experience palpitations, they typically present with symptoms of myocardial dysfunction secondary to the prolonged rapid ventricular rates experienced during AF.

## ADJUNCTIVE TESTS

### Electrocardiogram

A patient's symptoms captured on a 12-lead ECG is extremely helpful to the diagnosis. Analysis of the ECG in various situations is covered elsewhere (see Chaps. 13 and 53). Two specific findings on the 12-lead ECG during PSVT as noted in Figs. 28-1 and 28-2 should be emphasized. Figure 28-1 demonstrates a pseudo r′ in $V_1$ that is very typical for patients who present with AV node reentry. The pseudo r′ results from superimposition of the P-wave on the end of the QRS complex and is noted best in $V_1$. In contrast, the typical finding in patients with AV reentry due to retrograde conduction over an

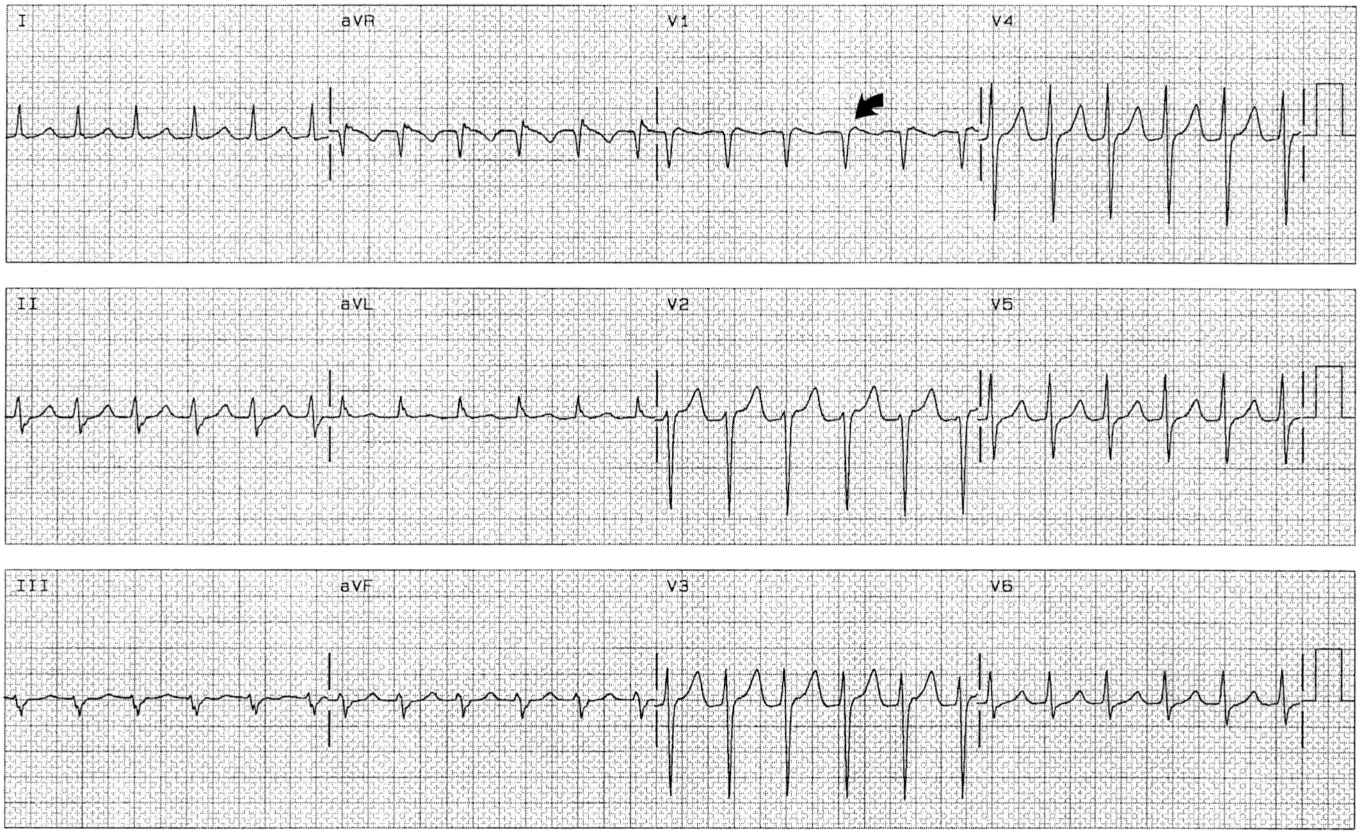

FIGURE 28-1 2-lead electrocardiogram of atrioventricular node reentry. The arrow points to the retrograde P-wave at the end of the QRS complex in $V_1$ and appears as a pseudo r-prime.

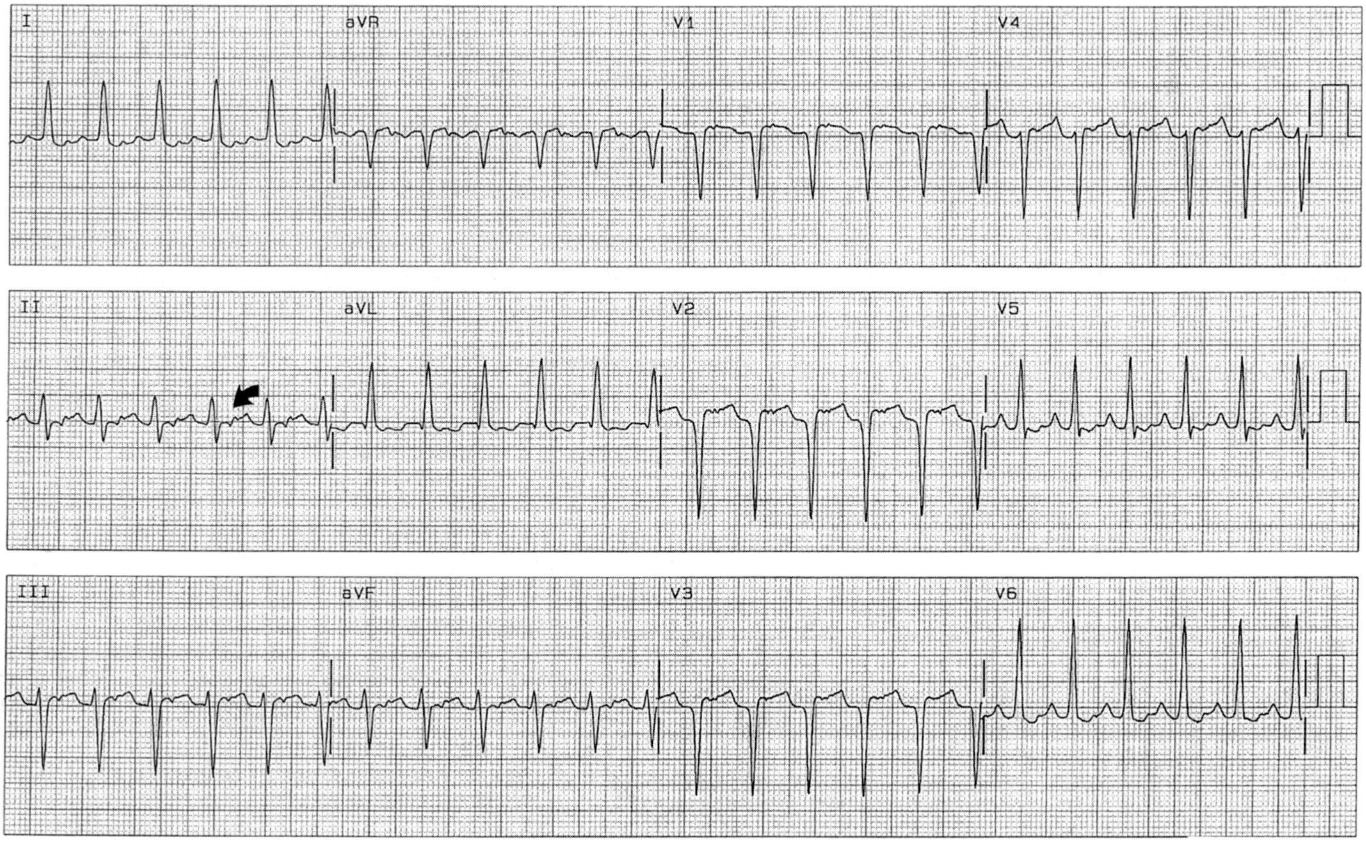

FIGURE 28-2 2-lead electrocardiogram of atrioventricular reentry. The arrow points to the retrograde P-wave in the early S-T segment of lead II.

accessory pathway (Wolff-Parkinson-White syndrome) is shown in Fig. 28-2. Note that the P-wave is positioned in the early ST segment.

## Head-Up Tilt Table Testing

Head-up tilt table testing (HUT) is a diagnostic technique to assess the susceptibility of an individual to neurally mediated syncope.[5] The classic features of neurally mediated syncope may be absent, and in these cases HUT may be diagnostic, especially when the symptoms on the tilt table reproduce the patient's clinical presentation.

The protocol[5] for HUT generally involves footrest supported head-up tilting at 70° to 80° for 30 to 45 min (Fig. 28-3). If HUT is negative, then the test may be repeated following pharmacologic provocation. Several agents including sublinqual nitroglycerin,[6] epinephrine,[7] and adenosine have been studied; however, most laboratories use isoproterenol at a dose of 1 to 3 $\mu$g/min. Repeat tilting is generally performed for 10 min after a steady state has been reached. Higher doses of isoproterenol, especially when coupled with longer durations of tilt, significantly decrease the specificity of the test.[7]

The pathophysiology of HUT is not completely understood.[8] Head-up tilting induces an orthostatic redistribution of circulating blood volume resulting in secondary sympathetic activation. The effect of aggressive ventricular contractility with a relatively under filled ventricle activates a central reflex, believed to be mediated by serotonin, that leads to a vagal efferent activation. In classic neurally mediated syncope, there is a mixed decrease in blood pressure and heart rate, although cases of predominant vasodepressor syncope without bradycardia are common. Factors that may sensitize an individual to neurally mediated syncope include volume depletion and high adrenergic states.

In control patients with no history of syncope, 70° head-up tilting has a specificity of approximately 90 percent.[9] In patients with unexplained syncope HUT can yield a diagnosis in 40 to 64 percent[10–13] particularly in the absence of other structural heart disease. In one study of 71 patients with recurrent unexplained syncope, the procedure reproduced symptoms in 53 patients (75 percent).[14] Forty patients had bradycardia, and 13 had a predominant vasodepressor response.[14] Although more controversial, serial tilt table testing has been used to predict the effectiveness of therapy for neurally mediated syncope.[10,11] Studies have demonstrated variable results, and there are a few randomized placebo-controlled trials.

At this point, the class 1 indications for HUT include the following:[5]

1. The evaluation of recurrent syncope or a single syncopal event with physical injury in patients with no evidence of structural heart disease.
2. Patients with syncope in whom organic heart disease is present but in whom other causes of syncope have been excluded.
3. Patients in whom syncope has been associated with a bradyarrhythmia but in whom the diagnosis of neurally mediated syncope may affect treatment.
4. The evaluation of patients with exercise-related syncope.

Several noninvasive techniques have been developed to assist clinicians in the assessment of risk stratification postmyocardial infarction. These tests may be divided into two categories. The first category includes techniques that evaluate subtle features not readily apparent in the standard ECG. These include signal-averaged electrocardiography (SAECG) to identify high-frequency potentials at the end of the QRS complex (late potentials) and microvolt changes in T-wave amplitude. The second category assesses autonomic tone by analyzing spontaneous and induced changes in heart rate and blood pressure.

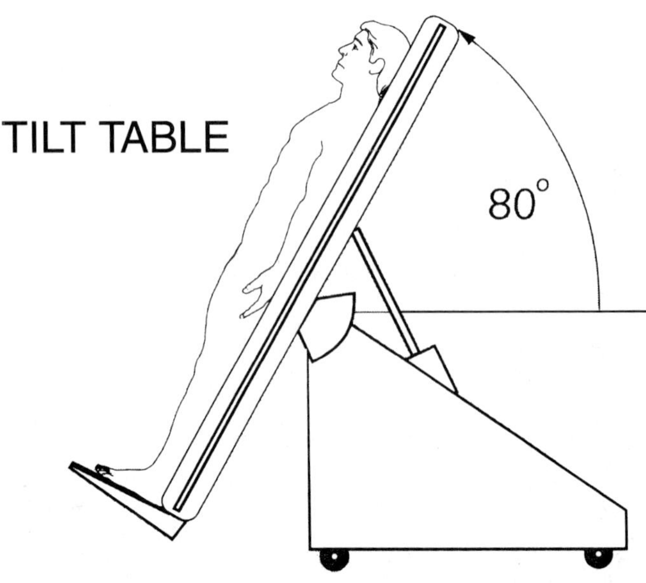


FIGURE 28-3 Tilt table with footboard support. (From Prystowsky EN, Klein GT. *Cardiac Arrhythmias: An Integrated Approach for the Clinician*. New York: McGraw-Hill, 1994, p 353. Reproduced with permission from McGraw-Hill.)

## Signal-Averaged Electrocardiography

SAECG allows the identification of small potentials in the surface ECG that are not seen because their amplitude is less than the noise intrinsic to the ECG signal.[15] The mathematical concept that underlies the SAECG is that the noise is random and by averaging many beats, the noise will be reduced.

A more detailed description of the technique may be found elsewhere.[16] In brief, orthogonal surface XYZ ECG leads are acquired for approximately 200 beats and digitally stored. High-pass filtering is used to minimize the contribution of low-frequency content. The X, Y, and Z leads are then combined into a vector magnitude referred to as the filtered QRS complex (Fig. 28-4).

Most commonly the SAECG has been used to identify late potentials appearing at the end of the QRS complex. These potentials correspond to fragmented electrical activity that is generated in areas of slow conduction either within or at the border zone of infarcts, which may be arrhythmogenic and prone to reentry.[17,18]

Three parameters have been identified to describe late potentials: filtered QRS duration (QRSd), root mean square voltage of the terminal 40 ms of the QRS complex (RMS40) and the duration of the low-amplitude signal (LAS) under 40 mV. The latter two parameters represent the amplitude and duration of the late potential, respectively. With 40 Hz filtering, a QRSd greater than 114 ms, RMS40 less than 20 mV, and LAS greater than 38 ms are considered abnormal.[15] The interpretation of the SAECG is problematic in the presence of a significant baseline intraventricular conduction defect.

The SAECG has been used most often in postmyocardial infarction risk stratification.[19–21] Late potentials were hypothesized to be associated with an increased incidence of ventricular arrhythmias and sudden death. In one of the earlier studies, Breithardt et at.[19]

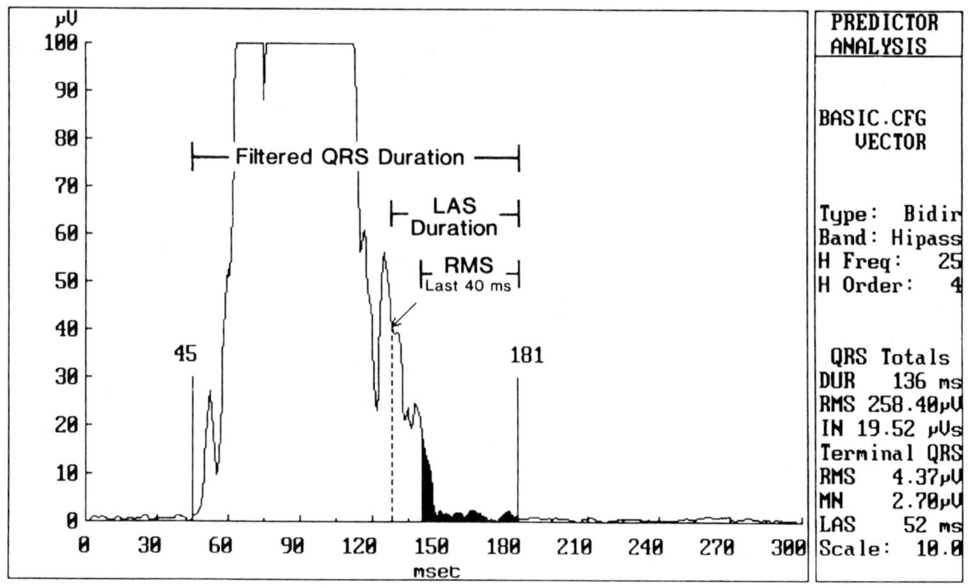


FIGURE 28-4 Positive signal-averaged electrocardiogram in a patient with sustained ventricular tachycardia. All three measured parameters are abnormal: Filtered QRS duration (DUR) is 136 ms; and the root-mean-square (RMS) voltage of the last 40 ms of the QS complex is 4.37 μV. (From Prystowsky EN, Klein GT. *Cardiac Arrhythmias: An Integrated Approach for the Clinician*. New York: McGraw-Hill, 1994, p 345. Reproduced with permission from McGraw-Hill.)

identified late potentials in 81 out of 160 (50.6 percent) patients after acute myocardial infarction. Sustained ventricular tachycardia occurred in 4 patients, all of whom had an abnormal SAECG. Sudden death occurred in 3 of 79 patients (3.8 percent) without late potentials, and in 11.1 percent in patients with a late potential greater than 40 ms. An arrhythmic event (ventricular tachycardia or sudden death) occurred in 21.7 percent of patients with late potentials and an anterior wall infarction, as compared with 5.4 percent with late potentials and an inferior wall infarction. In subsequent studies 26 to 44 percent of patients following a myocardial infarction had an abnormal SAECG. During follow-up the incidence of an arrhythmic event was 17 to 29 percent when late potentials were present.[21–23] When late potentials were absent, the incidence of sudden death was 3.5 to 5 percent. Other studies showed that late potentials were an independent risk factor when assessed along with left ventricular ejection fraction.[22,24,25] The combination of an abnormal SAECG and a reduced ejection fraction identified an arrhythmic risk of 30 percent of patients in one study of 102 patients.[22] The combination of an abnormal SAECG, reduced ejection fraction, and high-grade ectopy identified a population with a 50 percent risk in the same study.

It should be noted that most of the published data on the SAECG was derived in the prethrombolytic era. Since thrombolysis and percutaneous coronary interventions result in smaller infarcts and a reduced incidence of late potentials,[26,27] the predictive ability of the SAECG may not be as strong.

SAECG has been proposed as a screening tool for patients with syncope of unknown origin. Specifically, because of its high-negative predictive value it has been proposed as a screening test for ventricular arrhythmias. In general, the authors have recommended electrophysiology testing directly for patients with syncope who have either a prior myocardial infarction or reduced ejection fraction.[28] Thus, the authors have not found the SAECG useful in this setting. However, there is one specific application of SAECG that is notable. Patients with arrhythmogenic right ventricular dysplasia often have late potentials, and the SAECG can assist in the diagnosis.[29]

Finally, signal-averaged techniques have been applied to P-wave analysis in attempts to predict patients at risk for AF.[30,31] The clinical utility of signal averaging in this setting requires further study.

## Microvolt T-Wave Alternans

Microvolt T-wave alternans (TWA) is a technique that measures small changes in T-wave amplitude that occur on an alternating beat-to-beat basis. Visually apparent TWA is uncommon, but when identified has been associated with an increased risk of malignant ventricular arrhythmias.[32] It was hypothesized that TWA may be more prevalent in patients at risk of sudden death, but not usually detected because it occurred at the microvolt level. Several techniques[33] have now been developed to detect and quantify these subtle variations in T-wave amplitude. The most common method involves the spectral analysis of a large number of beats. Using this technique, an "alternans power" and "alternans voltage" can be determined. The alternans voltage represents the magnitude of the variation of the alternans T-wave amplitude from the mean T-wave amplitude. Rosenbaum et al.[34] reported the prospective assessment of microvolt TWA in the prediction of sudden death and inducibility at electrophysiologic study. Eighty-three consecutive patients had TWA assessed immediately prior to electrophysiology study. TWA was determined by atrial pacing at 100 beats/min. Sustained ventricular arrhythmias were induced in 32 patients. The presence of TWA was an independent predictor of inducibility at the electrophysiology study [relative risk (RR) 5.2]. Thirteen of 66 patients followed for up to 20 months had an arrhythmic event. The 20-month arrhythmic-free survival was 19 percent when microvolt TWA was present, and 94 percent when TWA was absent.

The most significant limitation of this technique is the requirement of atrial pacing to elevate heart rate. Because TWA was found to be heart rate dependent, other techniques that used exercise were developed.[35,36] Patients who developed TWA at lower heart rates had a higher risk. Patients who developed TWA only at high heart rates were felt to be a lower risk.[37]

Subsequent clinical studies identified exercise-induced microvolt T-wave alternans as a predictor of arrhythmic risk.[37,38] The test is considered positive if the onset of TWA occurs at <110 beats/min. The predictive power of microvolt TWA is independent of other risk-stratifying techniques including heart rate variability, SAECG, baroreceptor sensitivity testing, ejection fraction, and electrophysiologic testing.[38] Microvolt TWA is now commercially available; however, its most appropriate use has yet to be determined.

## Heart Rate Variability

Heart rate variability (HRV) analysis is based on subtle variations in sinus cycle length and has been used to assess cardiac autonomic status.[39] High levels of vagal tone have been reported to have a protective effect on the electrophysiologic characteristics of the ventricle and can increase the ventricular fibrillation threshold. Two different techniques have been developed to measure heart rate variability. In both techniques the ECG is digitally acquired, and the RR intervals identified. Time domain methods identify the RR-interval sequences and then apply statistical techniques to express the variance. The most commonly employed measure is the standard deviation of all RR intervals (SDNN); however, multiple other measures have been used.

Frequency domain methods apply the fast Fourier transform to the RR-interval sequence to develop a power spectral density that describes how the variance of the signal (i.e., power) is distributed as a function of frequency. Three main spectral components have been identified: a very-low-frequency component (<0.04 Hz), low-frequency component 0.04 to 0.15 Hz, and high-frequency component 0.15 to 0.40 Hz.[39,40]

In brief, heart rate variability provides a noninvasive method to assess sympathovagal balance.[41] The high-frequency component has been associated with vagal activity.[42,43] The low-frequency component is considered by some to represent sympathetic activity and by others to represent both sympathetic and vagal influences.[42,44,45] Over the course of 24-h there is an increase in low-frequency power during the day and an increase in high-frequency power at night.[42]

HRV has been used for postmyocardial risk stratification. Several studies have shown that decreased heart rate variability is associated with an increased risk of sudden death.[46–49] An SDNN <50 to 70 ms appears to identify patients at highest risk. Kleiger et al.[47] demonstrated that the relative risk of mortality was 5.3 times higher for a group of patients following myocardial infarction who had an SDNN <50 ms compared with a group with heart rate variability greater than 100 ms. Results from the GISSI-2 trial demonstrated that the predictive ability of HRV was preserved following thrombolytic therapy.[50] Additionally, heart rate variability increases with beta-blocker treatment[51] and is consistent with the protective effects of beta-adrenergic-blocking agents postmyocardial infarction. Of note, Katz et at.[49] showed that a simple test of heart rate variability done at the bedside predicted subsequent mortality after myocardial infarction.

### Baroreflex Sensitivity

Baroreflex sensitivity (BRS) testing is another technique to assess the cardiac autonomic nervous system. Typically, as carotid pressure rises, the RR interval is prolonged. The increase in carotid pressure is detected by the carotid sinus baroreceptors and results in vagal activation offsetting the rise in systemic blood pressure.[52] Under normal circumstances there is resting vagal predominance and sympathetic inhibition. The theory underlying BRS sensitivity testing is that decreased BRS may be present postmyocardial infarction and that a substantial reduction in BRS is a marker of increased risk for ventricular fibrillation.[53]

Most commonly, BRS is assessed by measuring the heart rate response following infusion of a vasoactive agent. Usually phenylephrine is given in doses to increase systolic blood pressure 20 to 40 mmHg. The changes in RR intervals are plotted against systolic blood pressure changes, and the slope is considered the BRS. In a group of normal controls, the average BRS was 14.8 ± 9 ms/mmHg.[54] Overall baroreceptor sensitivity decreases when the sympathetic nervous system is activated. An alternative technique employs neck collar suction to activate carotid baroreceptors.

Several studies[55,56] of postmyocardial patients demonstrated that patients who survived following myocardial infarction had a higher BRS than patients who died. A cut-off BRS <3 ms/mmHg identified patients at higher risk of death. Furthermore, these studies showed that the prognostic value of BRS was independent of LV function and heart rate variability.[57]

In the Autonomic Tone and Reflexes After Myocardial Infarction (ATRAMI) study,[58] the investigators followed 1284 patients after myocardial infarction and assessed BRS and HRV. Over an average of 21 months, there were 44 cardiac deaths and 5 nonfatal cardiac arrests. The multivariate risk of cardiac mortality was 2.8 when the BRS was <3 ms/mmHg, and 3.2 when the SDNN was <70 ms. In patients with BRS less than 3 ms/mmHg and SDNN <70 ms there was 17 percent mortality. In patients with BRS >3 and SDNN >70, the mortality was 2 percent. The ATRAMI investigators concluded that the analysis of vagal reflexes using BRS had prognostic value independent from left ventricular function and additive to the prognostic value of heart rate variability following myocardial infarction.

## CONCLUSION AND IMPLICATIONS

In the evaluation of patients following myocardial infarction, SAECG, TWA, heart rate variability, and BRS each confer independent prognostic information. The strength of these tests either alone or in combination is their relatively high-negative predictive value; the weakness is the rather low-positive predictive value. The population at risk is large, and these screening tests will identify only a small fraction of those who ultimately will sustain a cardiac arrest. Consequently, more data are needed to define their position in general patient care.

## References

1. Kapoor WN, Karpf M, Wieand S, et al. A prospective evaluation and follow-up of patients with syncope. *N Engl J Med* 1983;309:197–204.
2. Savage DD, Corwin L, McGee DL, et al. Epidemiologic features of isolated syncope: The Framingham Study. *Stroke* 1985;16(4):626–629.
3. Soteriades ES, Evans JC, Larson MG, et al. Incidence and prognosis of syncope. *N Engl J Med* 2002;347(12):878–885.
4. Fogel RI, Evans JJ, Prystowsky EN. Utility and cost of event recorders in the diagnosis of palpitations, presyncope and syncope. *Am J Cardiol* 1997;79:207–208.
5. Benditt DG, Ferguson DW, Grubb BP, et al. Tilt table testing for assessing syncope. An American College of Cardiology expert consensus document. *J Am Coll Cardiol* 1996;28:263–275.
6. Raviele A, Menozzi C, Brignole M, et al. Value of head-up tilt testing potentiated with sublingual nitroglycerin to assess the origin of unexplained syncope. *Am J Cardiol* 1995;76:267–272.
7. Calkins H, Kadish A, Sousa J, et al. Comparison of response to isoproterenol and epinephrine during head up tilt in suspected vasodepressor syncope. *Am J Cardiol* 1991;67:207–209.
8. Rea AF. Neurally mediated hypotension and bradycardia: Which nerves? How mediated? *J Am Coll Cardiol* 1989;14:1633.
9. Natale A, Akhtar M, Jazayeri M, et al. Provocation of hypotension during head-up tilt testing in subjects with no history of syncope or presyncope. *Circulation* 1995;92:54–58.
10. Raviele A, Gasparini G, DiPede F, et al. Usefulness of head-up tilt test in evaluating patients with syncope of unknown origin and negative electrophysiologic study. *Am J Cardiol* 1990;65:1322–1327.
11. Grubb BP, Temesy-Armos P, Hahn H, Elliot L. Utility of upright tilt table testing in the evaluation and management of syncope of unknown origin. *Am J Med* 1991;90:6–10.

12. Grubb BP, Wolfe D, Samoil D, et al. Recurrent unexplained syncope in the elderly: The use of head-upright tilt table testing in evaluation and management. *J Am Geriatric Soc* 1992;40:1123–1128.
13. Sra JS, Anderson AJ, Sheikh SH, et at. Unexplained syncope evaluated by electrophysiologic studies and head-up tilt testing. *Ann Intern Med* 1991;114:1013–1019.
14. Fitzpatrick A, Sutton R. Tilting towards a diagnosis in unexplained syncope. *Lancet* 1989;1:658–660.
15. Cain ME, Anderson JL, Arnsdorff MF, et al. American College of Cardiology expert consensus document: Signal averaged electrocardiography. *J Am Coll Cardiol* 1996;27:238–249.
16. Simson MB. Use of signals in the terminal QRS complex to identify patients with ventricular tachycardia after myocardial infarction. *Circulation* 1981;64:235.
17. Simson MB, Untereker WJ, Speilman SR, et al. Relation between late potentials on the body surface and directly recorded fragmented electrograms in patients with ventricular tachycardia. *Am J Cardiol* 1983;51:105–112.
18. El-Sherif N, Smith A, Evans K. Canine ventricular arrhythmias in the late myocardial infarction period: Epicardial mapping of reentrant circuits. *Circ Res* 1981;49:255.
19. Breithardt G, Schwarzmaier J, Boggrefe M, et al. Prognostic significance of late potentials after acute myocardial infarction. *Eur Heart J* 1983;4:487–495.
20. Savard P, Rouleau JL, Ferguson J, et al. Risk stratification after myocardial infarction using signal-averaged electrocardiographic criteria adjusted for sex, age, and myocardial infarction location. *Circulation* 1997;96:202–213.
21. Denniss AR, Richards DA, Cody DV, et al. Prognostic significance of ventricular tachycardia and fibrillation induced at programmed stimulation and delayed potentials detected on the signal-averaged electrocardiograms of survivors of acute myocardial infarction. *Circulation* 1986;74:731–745.
22. Gomes JA, Winters SL, Stewart D, et al. A new noninvasive index to predict sustained ventricular tachycardia in the first year after myocardial infarction: Bases on signal-averaged electrocardiogram, radionuclide ejection fraction and Holter monitoring. *J Am Coll Cardiol* 1987;10:349–357.
23. Kuchar DL, Thorburn CW, Sammel NL. Prediction of serious arrhythmic events after myocardial infarction: Signal averaged electrocardiogram, Holter monitoring and radionuclide ejection fraction. *J Am Coll Cardiol* 1987;9: 531–538.
24. Kanovsky MS, Falcone RA, Dresden DA, et al. Identification of patients with ventricular tachycardia after myocardial infarction: Signal averaged electrocardiogram, Holter monitoring and cardiac catheterization. *Circulation* 1984;70:264–270.
25. Buckingham TA, Ghosh S, Homan SM, et al. Independent value of signal-averaged electrocardiography and left ventricular function in identifying patients with sustained ventricular tachycardia with coronary artery diseases. *Am J Cardiol* 1987;59:568–572.
26. Denes P, El-Sherif N, Katz R, et al. Prognostic significance of signal averaged electrocardiogram after thrombolytic therapy and/or angioplasty during acute myocardial infarction (CAST substudy). *Am J Cardiol* 1994;74:216–220.
27. Gang ES, Les AS, Hong M, et al. Decrease incidence of ventricular late potentials after successful thrombolytic therapy for acute myocardial infarction. *N Engl J Med* 1989;321:712–716.
28. Prystowsky EN, Knilans TK, Evans JJ. Diagnostic evaluation and treatment strategies for patients at risk of serious cardiac arrhythmias: Part I. Syncope of unknown origin. *Mod Concepts Cardiovasc Dis* 1991;60: 49–54.
29. Kinoshita O, Fontaine G, Rosas Andrade F, et al. Time and frequency domain analyses if the signal averaged ECG in patients with arrhythmogenic right ventricular dysplasia. *Circulation* 1995;91:715–721.
30. Stafford PJ, Turner I, Vincent R. Quantitative analysis of signal averaged P waves in idiopathic paroxysmal atrial fibrillation. *Am J Cardiol* 1991;68:751–755.
31. Guidera SA, Steinberg JS. The signal averaged P wave duration: A rapid noninvasive marker of risk for atrial fibrillation. *J Am Coll Cardiol* 1993;21:1645–1651.
32. Schwartz P, Malliani A. Electrical alternation of the T wave: Clinical and experimental evidence of its relationship with the sympathetic nervous system with the long QT syndrome. *Am Heart Journal* 1975;89: 45–50.
33. Smith JM, Clancy EA, Valeri CR, et al. Electrical alternans and electrical instability. *Circulation* 1988;77:110–121.
34. Rosenbaum DS, Jackson LE, Smith JM, et al. Electrical alternans and vulnerability to ventricular arrhythmias. *N Engl J Med* 1994;330: 235–241.
35. Rosenbaum DS, Albrecht O, Cohen RJ. Predicting sudden cardiac death from T wave alternans: Promise and pitfalls. *J Cardiovasc Electrophysiol* 1996;7:1095–1111.
36. Hohnloser SH, Klinenheben T, Zabel M, et al. T wave alternans during exercise and atrial pacing in humans. *J Cardiovasc Electrophysiol* 1997;8:987–993.
37. Estes MNA, Michaud G, Zipes DP, et al: Electrical alternans during rest and exercise as predictors of vulnerability to ventricular arrhythmias. *Am J Cardiol* 1997;80:1314–1318.
38. Hohnloser SH, Klingenheben T, Yi-Gang L, et al. T wave alternans as a predictor of recurrent ventricular tachyarrhythmias in ICD recipients: Prospective comparison with conventional risk markers. *J Cardiovasc Electrophysiol* 1989;9:1258–1268.
39. Task force of the European Society of Cardiology and the North American Society of Pacing and Electrophysiology: Heart rate variability—standards of measurement, physiologic interpretation and clinical use. *Circulation* 1996;93:1043–1065.
40. Akselrod S, Gordon D, Ubel FA, et al. Power spectrum analysis of heart rate fluctuation: A quantitative probe of best to beat cardiovascular control. *Science* 1981;213:220–222.
41. Pagani M, Lombardi F, Guzzetti S, et al. Power spectral analysis of heart rate and arterial pressure variabilities as a marker of sympathovagal interaction in man and conscious dog. *Circ Res* 1986;59:178–193.
42. Malliani A, Pagani M, Lombardi F, Cerutti S. Cardiovascular neural regulation explored in the frequency domain. *Circulation* 1991;84: 1482–1492.
43. Pomeranz M, Macaulay RJB, Caudill MA, et al. Assessment of autonomic function in humans by heart rate spectral analysis. *Am J physiol* 1985;248:H151–H153.
44. Kamath MV, Fallen EL. Power spectral analysis of heart rate variability: A noninvasive signature of cardiac autonomic function. *Crit Rev Biomed Eng* 1993;21:245–311.
45. Appel ML, Berger RD, Saul JP, et al. Beat to beat variability in cardiovascular variables: Noise or music? *J Am Coll Cardiol* 1989;14: 1139–1148.
46. Farrell TG, Bashir Y, Gipps T, et al. Risk stratification for arrhythmic events in postinfarction patients based on heart rate variability, ambulatory electrocardiographic variables and signal averaged electrocardiogram. *J Am Coll Cardiol* 1991;18:687.
47. Kleiger RE, Miller JJP, Bigger JT, Moss AJ, and the Multicenter Post-Infarction Research Group. Decreased heart rate variability and its association with increased mortality after acute myocardial infarction. *Am J Cardiol* 1987;59:256–262.
48. Bigger JT, Fleiss JL, Steinmann RC, et al. Frequency domain measures of heart period variability and mortality and mortality after myocardial infarction. *Circulation* 1992;85:164–171.
49. Katz A, Liberty IF, Porath A, et al. A simple bedside test of 1-minute heart rate variability during deep breathing as a prognostic index after myocardial infarction. *Am Heart J* 1999;138:32–38.
50. Zuanetti G, Nelson JM; Lantini R, et al, on behalf of GISSI-2 Investigators. Prognostic significance of heart rate variability in post myocardial infarction patients in the fibrinolytic era. The GISSI-2 results. *Circulation* 1996;94:432–436.
51. Sandrone G, Mortara A, Torzillo D, et al. Effects of beta blockers (atenolol or metoprolol) on heart rate variability after acute myocardial infarction. *Am J Cardiol* 1994;74:340–345.

52. Kirchheim HR. Systemic arterial baroreceptor reflexes. *Physiologic Rev* 1976;56:100–176.
53. Schwartz PJ, Vanoli W, Stramba-Basiele M, et al: Autonomic mechanisms and sudden death: New insights from the analysis of baroreceptor reflexes in conscious dogs with and without a myocardial infarction. *Circulation* 1988;78:969–979.
54. Bristow JD, Honour AJ, Pickering JW, et al: Cardiovascular and respiratory changes during sleep in normal and hypertensive subjects. *Cardiovasc Res* 1969;3:476–485.
55. LaRovere MT, Speechia G, Motara A, Schwarz PJ. Baroreceptor sensitivity, clinical correlates and cardiovascular mortality among patients with a first myocardial infarction: A prospective study. *Circulation* 1988;78:816–824.
56. Farrell TG, Odemuyiwa O, Bashir Y, et al. prognostic value of baroreflex sensitivity testing after acute myocardial infarction. *Br Heart J* 1992;67:129–137.
57. Bigger JT, LaRovere MT, Steinman RC, et al. Comparison of baroreflex sensitivity and heart period variability after myocardial infarction. *J Am Coll Cardiol* 1989;14:1511–1518.
58. LaRovere MT, Bigger JT, Marcus FL, et al. for the ATRAMI (Autonomic Tone and Reflexes After Myocardial Infarction) Investigators. Baroreflex sensitivity and heart-rate variability in prediction of total cardiac mortality after myocardial infarction. *Lancet* 1998;351:478–484.

CHAPTER 29

# ATRIAL FIBRILLATION, ATRIAL FLUTTER, AND ATRIAL TACHYCARDIA

G. Neal Kay / Vance J. Plumb



Atrial fibrillation, atrial flutter, and atrial tachycardia are common arrhythmias that are associated with a variety of cardiac conditions. Indeed, atrial fibrillation is the most common sustained cardiac arrhythmia encountered in clinical practice and is increasing in prevalence.[1,2] These arrhythmias are associated with deterioration of hemodynamics, a wide spectrum of symptoms, and significant morbidity, mortality, and medical costs. Perhaps because no single therapy has been shown to be ideal for all patients, there are a variety of treatment strategies that may be applied to these arrhythmias, ranging from no treatment at all to such invasive therapies as cardiac surgery. Despite this wide range of potential treatments, consensus is gradually emerging as to how patients with these arrhythmias should be managed.[3] This chapter describes the epidemiology, electrophysiologic mechanisms, and approach to management of patients with atrial fibrillation, atrial flutter, and atrial tachycardia.

## ATRIAL FIBRILLATION

Atrial fibrillation is characterized by disorganized atrial electrical activation and uncoordinated atrial contraction. The surface electrocardiogram characteristically demonstrates rapid fibrillatory waves with changing morphology and a ventricular rhythm that is irregularly irregular (Fig. 29-1). Depending on the size of the left atrium and the underlying cardiac disease, fibrillatory waves can be of large or small amplitude. For example, patients with rheumatic mitral stenosis often demonstrate large-amplitude fibrillatory waves in the anterior precordial leads ($V_1$ and $V_2$) that can be confused with atrial flutter. However, careful examination of the fibrillatory waves reveals them to have a varying cycle length and morphology. The distinction between atrial fibrillation and atrial flutter can also be confusing in patients who demonstrate a transition between these arrhythmias. Thus, atrial fibrillation may organize to atrial flutter or atrial flutter may degenerate to atrial fibrillation. Intracardiac recordings demonstrate variability in the atrial electrogram morphology, amplitude, and cycle length from beat to beat. The cycle length during atrial fibrillation is characteristically shortest in the pulmonary veins, longer in the left atrium, and longest in the right atrium. The ventricular rate during atrial fibrillation can be quite variable, depending on autonomic tone, the electrophysiologic properties of the atrioventricular (AV) node, and the effects of medications that act on the AV conduction system. The ventricular rate may be very rapid (>300 beats per minute) in patients with the Wolff-Parkinson-White syndrome, with conduction over accessory pathways having short antegrade refractory periods. The ventricular rate in atrial fibrillation may become very rapid during exercise, with an increase in sympathetic and a decrease in parasympathetic tone. In contrast, a regular, slow ventricular rhythm during atrial fibrillation suggests a junctional rhythm, either as an escape mechanism with complete AV block or as an accelerated junctional pacemaker. Patients with severe underlying heart disease may develop the combination of atrial fibrillation and ventricular tachycardia, leading to a rapid, regular, wide-QRS-complex tachycardia.

### Classification

Atrial fibrillation has been described in a variety of ways, such as paroxysmal or chronic, lone, idiopathic, nonvalvular, valvular, self-terminating, etc. Each of these classifications has implications for the response to therapy, and the lack of a consistent nomenclature has led to difficulties in comparing one study with another.[4] For example, *chronic atrial fibrillation* could mean atrial fibrillation that does not terminate. The term *chronic paroxysmal atrial fibrillation* could also be applied to a long-standing condition of paroxysmal atrial fibrillation. In response to this confusion, the American Heart Association (AHA), American College of Cardiology (ACC), and the European Society of Cardiology (ESC) have proposed a standardized classification scheme to describe atrial fibrillation (Fig. 29-2).[3,5] At the initial detection of atrial fibrillation, it may be difficult to be certain of the subsequent pattern of duration and frequency of recurrences. Thus, a designation of *first detected* episode of atrial fibrillation is made on the initial diagnosis. When the patient has experienced two or more episodes, atrial fibrillation is classified as *recurrent*. After the termination of an episode of atrial fibrillation, the rhythm can be classified as *paroxysmal* or *persistent*. Paroxysmal atrial fibrillation is characterized by self-terminating episodes that generally last less than 7 days (most <24 h), while persistent atrial fibrillation generally lasts more than 7 days and often requires electrical or

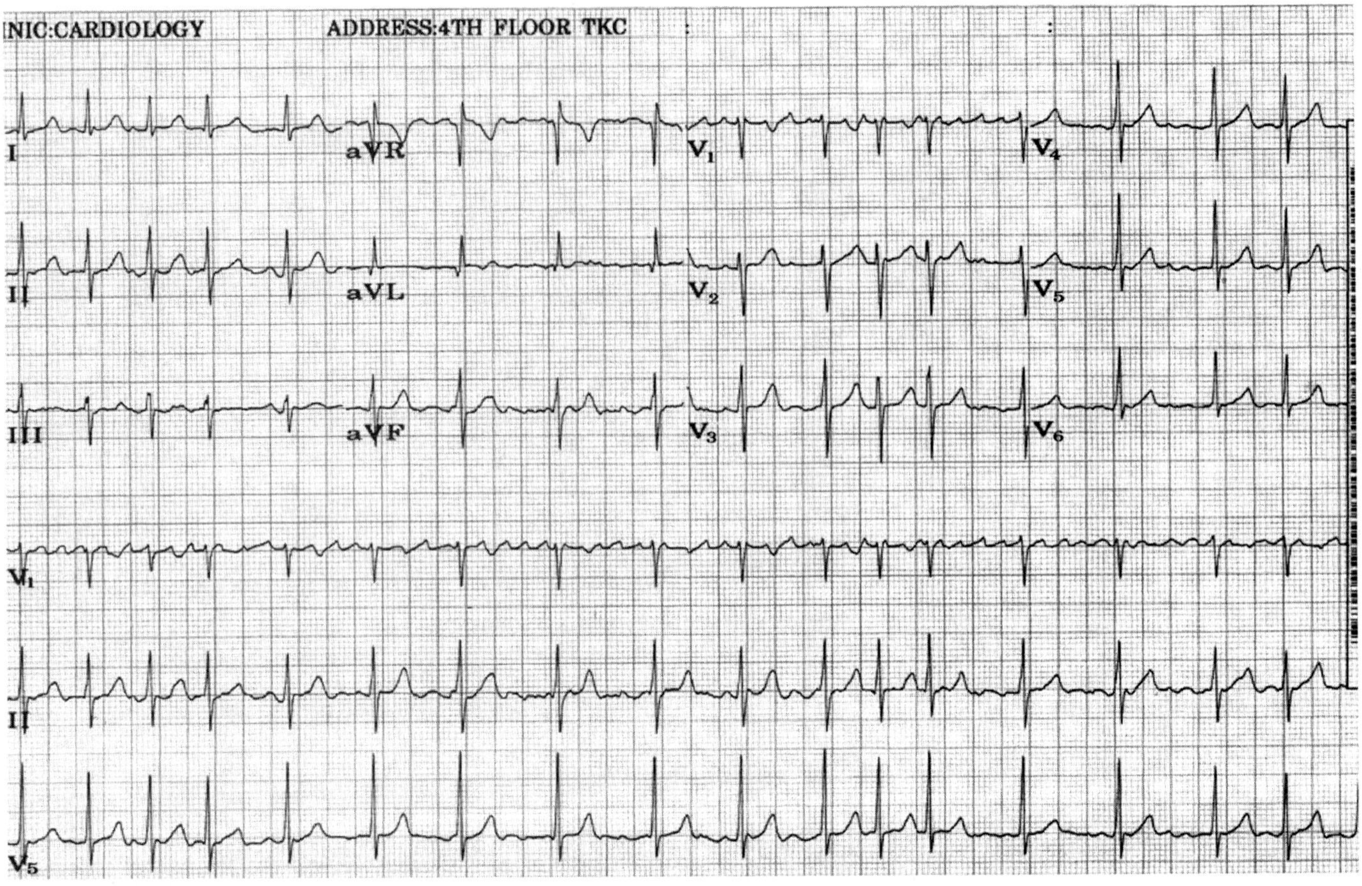

FIGURE 29-1 Twelve-lead electrocardiogram of atrial fibrillation. Note the rapid, irregular, changing, low-amplitude fibrillatory waves and an irregularly irregular ventricular response.

pharmacologic cardioversion. Atrial fibrillation is classified as *permanent* when it has failed cardioversion, has been sustained for more than a year, or when further attempts to terminate the arrhythmia are deemed futile. While this classification scheme is generally useful, the pattern of atrial fibrillation may change in response to treatment. Thus, atrial fibrillation that has been persistent may become paroxysmal during pharmacologic therapy with antiarrhythmic medications. On the other hand, atrial fibrillation that had been perma-

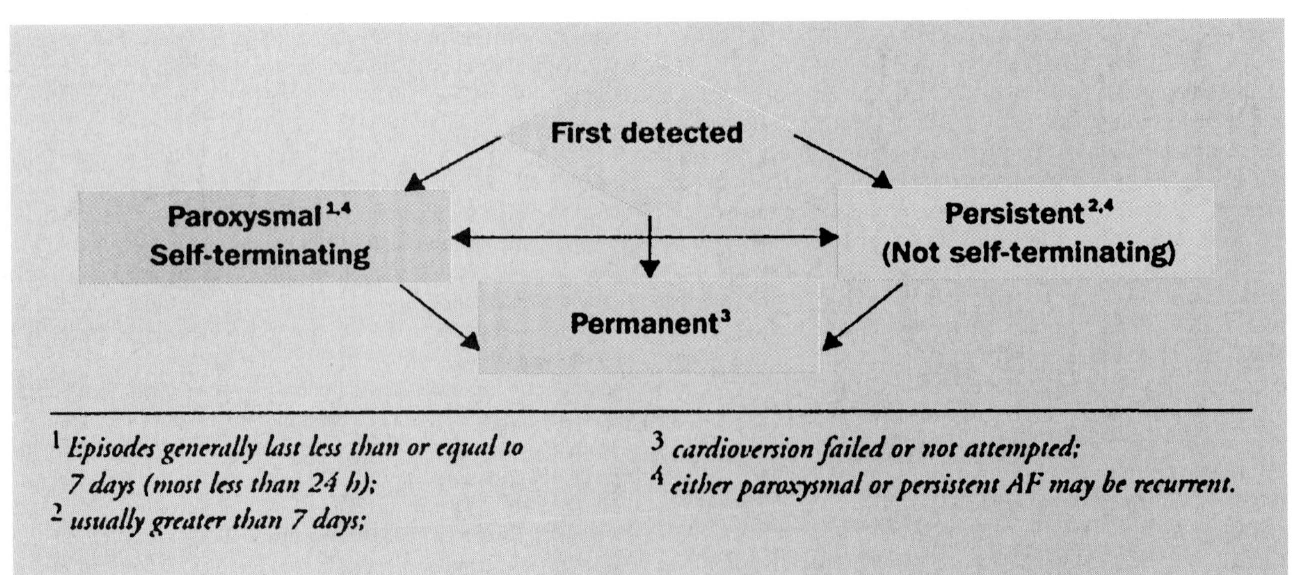


FIGURE 29-2 ACC/AHA/ESC classification of atrial fibrillation. Atrial fibrillation may be the first detected episode or may be paroxysmal (defined as episodes terminating in less than 7 days), persistent with episodes requiring medical intervention for termination, or permanent in which further attempts to restore sinus rhythm have been abandoned.

nent may be cured by nonpharmacologic therapies such as atrial fibrillation surgery or catheter ablation. The distinction between persistent and permanent atrial fibrillation is a function of the underlying arrhythmia as well as the clinical pragmatism of the patient and physician. Despite these caveats, the AHA/ACC/ESC classification allows better assessment of studies involving patients with atrial fibrillation and has been widely adopted. Atrial fibrillation that is related to a transient, reversible cause—such as thyrotoxicosis, acute myocardial infarction, acute pericarditis, recent cardiac surgery, or acute pulmonary disease—is considered separately. These causes of atrial fibrillation are generally eliminated by treatment of the underlying precipitating condition.

## Epidemiology

Atrial fibrillation is the most common arrhythmia requiring treatment, with approximately 2.2 million Americans experiencing paroxysmal or persistent atrial fibrillation.[1,6–9] The overall prevalence in the general population is estimated to be 0.4 percent.[10] The incidence and prevalence of atrial fibrillation steadily increase with age, such that this arrhythmia occurs in <0.5 percent of the population below 50 years of age and increases to approximately 2 percent at ages 60 to 69, 4.6 percent for ages 70 to 79, and 8.8 percent for ages 80 to 89.[7,11,12] The age-adjusted prevalence of atrial fibrillation is higher for men than women[7,8] and for whites than blacks.[9] The incidence of atrial fibrillation in the Framingham Study was 0.04 percent per year for men aged 30 to 39 and increased to 4.6 percent per year for men aged 80 to 89.[13] The Cardiovascular Health Study[7] found a prevalence of atrial fibrillation of 5 percent by 24-h ambulatory monitoring. Most cases of atrial fibrillation occur in patients with evidence of structural heart disease, though there may be no evidence of concomitant disease in over 50 percent of patients with paroxysmal atrial fibrillation.[14–16] In contrast, over 80 percent of patients with permanent atrial fibrillation have an identifiable underlying cause.[17] The cardiac factors predicting the development of atrial fibrillation in the Framingham Study were stroke, congestive heart failure, rheumatic heart disease, and hypertension.[9,18] Left atrial enlargement, increased left ventricular wall thickness, and reduced left ventricular fractional shortening predict an increased risk.[9,19] The left atrial dimension is a powerful predictor of the development of nonvalvular atrial fibrillation.[20] Electrocardiographic criteria for left ventricular hypertrophy and a clinical history of diabetes mellitus have also been associated with an increased risk of atrial fibrillation.[9]

Atrial fibrillation confers an increased relative risk of overall mortality ranging from 1.4 times controls in the Manitoba Study[21] to 2.3 times controls in the Whitehall study[12] (average 1.7 times controls)[3] and is predominantly due to stroke. The risk of stroke among patients with nonrheumatic atrial fibrillation is approximately 5 percent per year, with an average relative risk of stroke approximately 6 times that of age-matched controls.[11,12,16,20,22–24] In the absence of anticoagulation, the relative risk of stroke in patients with rheumatic atrial fibrillation is increased approximately 17-fold.[25] The Framingham Study demonstrated that the risk of stroke in atrial fibrillation is clearly related to age, with an annual risk of stroke of 1.5 percent in patients aged 50 to 59 years, which increased to 23.5 percent in patients aged 80 to 89 years.[11] The risk of stroke in nonvalvular atrial fibrillation has been estimated to be approximately 7 percent per year.[3,26–29] The development of atrial fibrillation is a strong predictor of increased mortality in cardiac conditions such as hypertrophic or restrictive cardiomyopathy.[30–33]

## Pathophysiology

Atrial fibrillation is associated with a wide variety of predisposing factors (Fig. 29-3). In the developed world, the most common clinical diagnoses associated with permanent atrial fibrillation are hypertension and coronary artery disease.[9] The presence of congestive heart failure markedly increases the risk of atrial fibrillation.[7–9] In developing countries, hypertension, rheumatic valvular heart disease, and congenital heart disease are the most commonly related conditions.[34,35]

Two concepts of the underlying mechanism of atrial fibrillation have received considerable attention: factors that *trigger* the onset and factors that *perpetuate* this arrhythmia. In general, patients with frequent, self-terminating episodes of atrial fibrillation are likely to have a predominance of factors that trigger atrial fibrillation, while patients with atrial fibrillation that does not terminate spontaneously are more likely to have a predominance of perpetuating factors. While such a gross generalization has clinical utility, there is often considerable overlap of these mechanisms. In addition, the presence of atrial fibrillation leads to functional and structural changes in the atrial myocardium that favor its maintenance.[35]

| Epidemiologic Indicators | Clinical States | Clinical Investigations |
|---|---|---|
| Old age | Cardiac failure | 12-Lead ECG |
| Male sex | Hypertension | 24-h Ambulatory ECG |
| Heart failure | Ischemic heart disease | Signal-averaged ECG |
| Left ventricular dysfunction | Myocardial infarction | Event ECG recording |
| Ischemic heart disease | Pulmonary disease | Echocardiography |
| Myocardial infarction | Valvular heart disease | Ventriculography |
| Hypertension | Cardiac or thoracic surgery | Coronary angiography |
| Left ventricular hypertrophy | Pericarditis | Chest radiography |
| Left atrial dilatation | Congenital heart disease | Clinical electrophysiologic study |
| Smoking | Rheumatic heart disease | Exercise ECG |
| Diabetes | Hyperthyroidism | Biochemical markers |
| Diuretic use | Alcohol poisoning | Autonomic assessment |
| Cardiac/thoracic surgery | Autonomic dysfunction | |
| CVA/TIA | Sick sinus syndrome | |
| | Supraventricular tachyarrhythmia | |

CVA/TIA indicates cerebrovascular accident/transient ischemic attack.

FIGURE 29-3 Factors that predispose to atrial fibrillation and means for clinical investigation. (From Allessie et al.[35] With permission.)

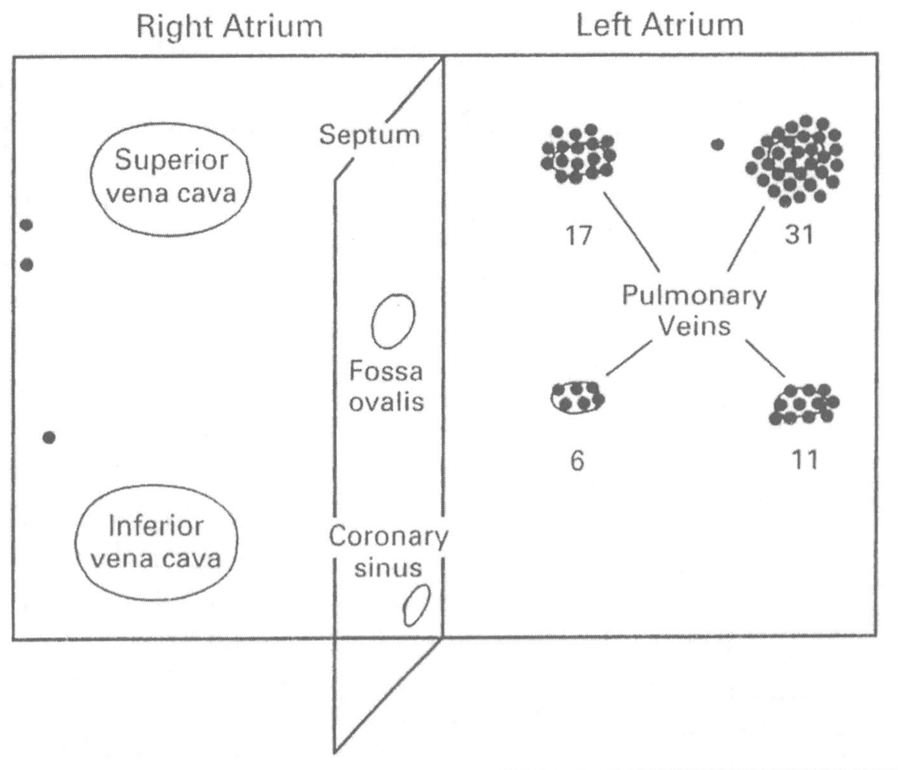


FIGURE 29-4 Anatomic distribution of focal triggers of atrial fibrillation in patient with paroxysmal atrial fibrillation. ABBREVIATION: ● = number and location of triggering foci. (From Haissaguerre et al.[37] With permission.)

Triggering foci of rapidly firing cells within the sleeve of atrial myocytes extending into the pulmonary veins have been clearly shown to be the underlying mechanism of most paroxysmal atrial fibrillation (Fig. 29-4).[36–38] In animal models, these pulmonary vein foci manifest delayed afterpotentials and triggered activity in response to catecholamine stimulation, rapid atrial pacing, or acute stretch.[35,39] The pulmonary veins of patients with paroxysmal atrial fibrillation demonstrate abnormal properties of conduction such that there is a markedly reduced effective refractory period within the pulmonary veins, progressive conduction delay within the pulmonary vein in response to rapid pacing or programmed stimulation, and often conduction block between the pulmonary vein and the left atrium (Fig. 29-5).[40] Such findings are much more common in patients with paroxysmal atrial fibrillation than in control subjects without this arrhythmia. Rapidly firing foci can often be recorded within the pulmonary veins

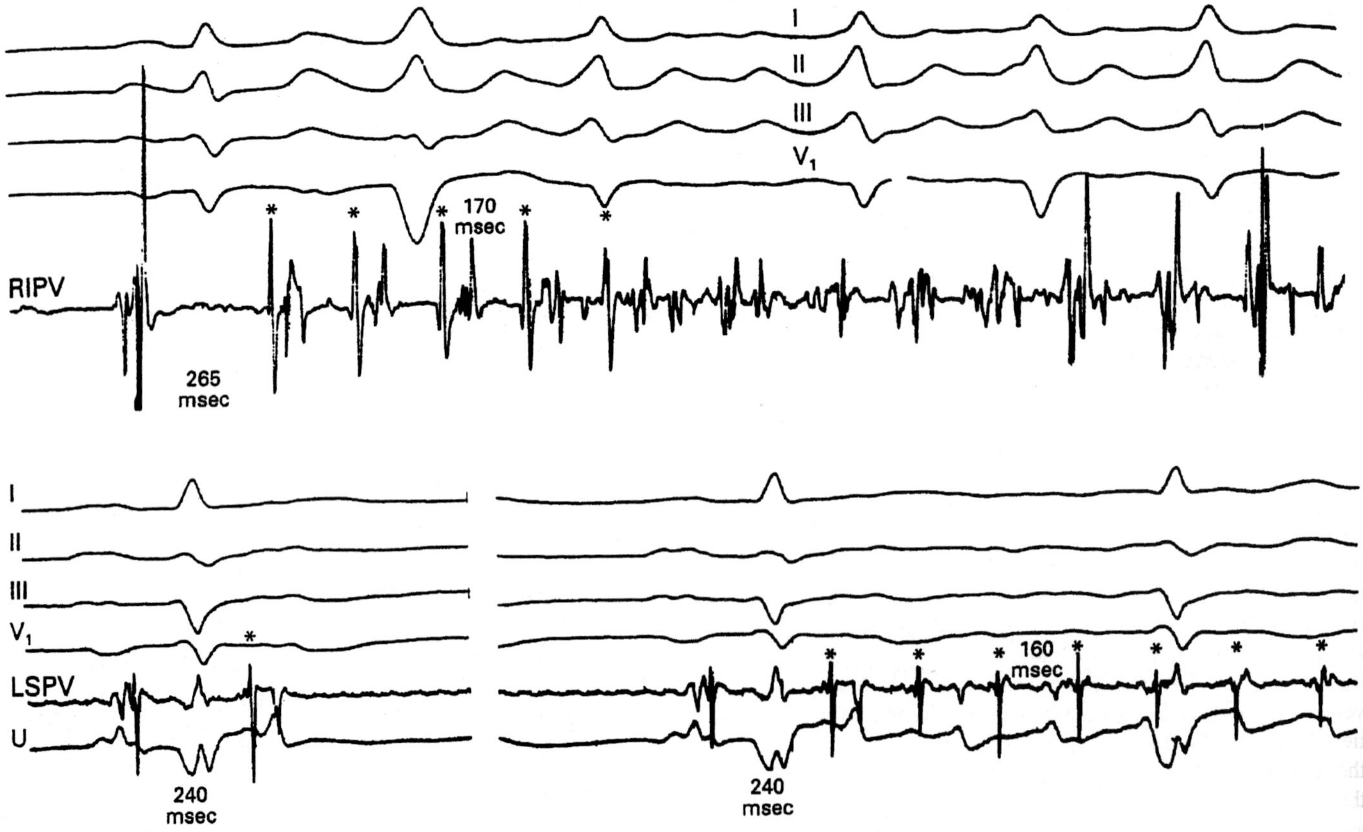

FIGURE 29-5 *Top:* Rapid firing in a pulmonary vein with the spontaneous onset of atrial fibrillation. *Bottom left:* Premature beats in a pulmonary vein (*asterisk*) with conduction block to the left atrium. *Bottom right:* Rapid firing at the same coupling interval conducts to the atrium with induction of atrial fibrillation. (From Haissaguerre et al.[37])

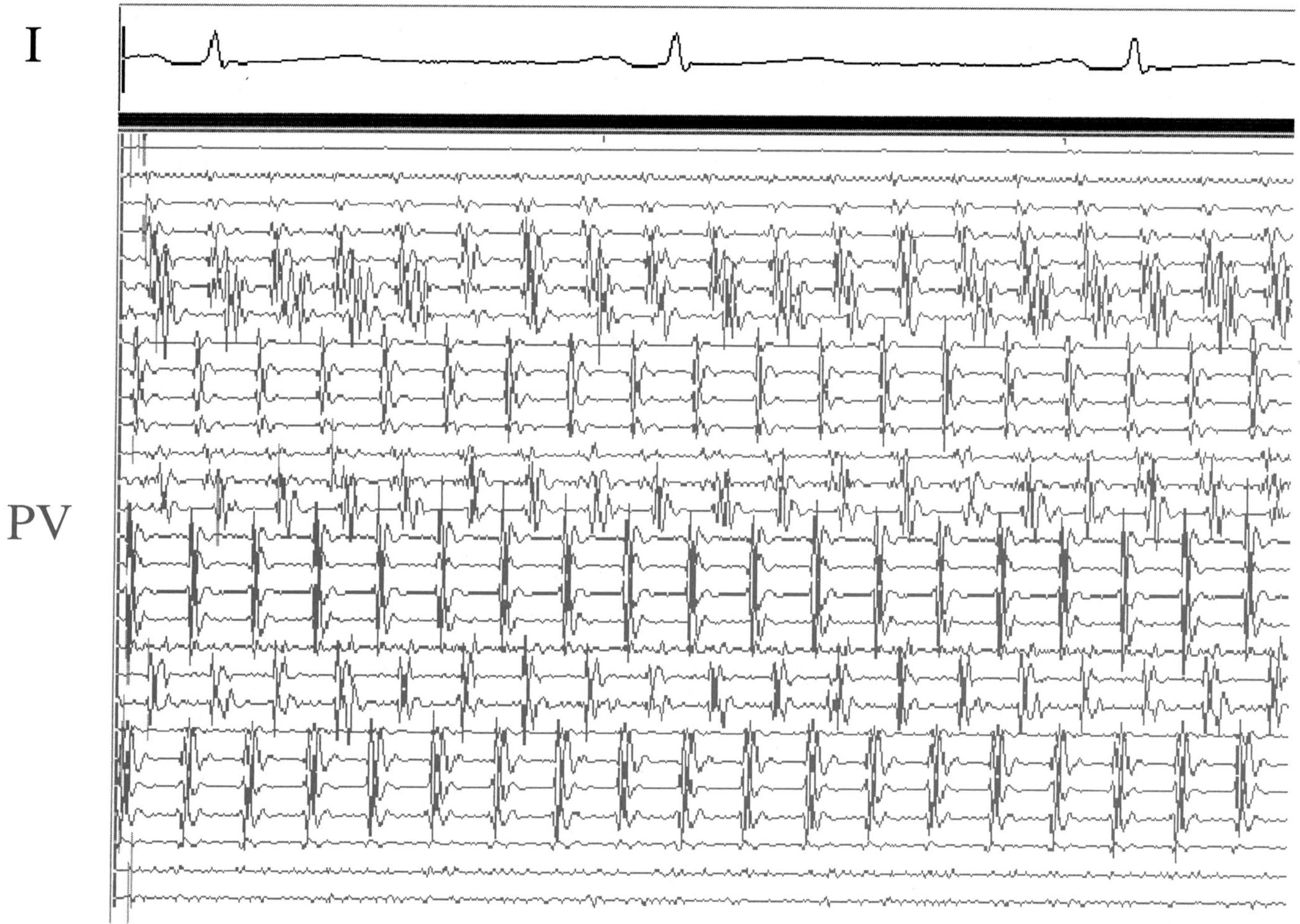


FIGURE 29-6 Simultaneous recordings of surface electrocardiographic lead I and bipolar electrograms from the right superior pulmonary vein of a patient after catheter ablation at the ostium of the vein had produced conduction block from the vein into the left atrium. Note the rapid, irregular electrical activity recorded with a 64-electrode basket catheter within the pulmonary vein, with sinus rhythm in the remainder of the atria as recorded on the surface electrocardiogram.

with conduction block to the left atrium.[37,38] Administration of catecholamines such as isoproterenol can lead to shortening of the left atrial refractory period, thereby allowing these foci to propagate to the left atrium with the induction of spontaneous atrial fibrillation.[37] These discontinuous properties of conduction within the pulmonary vein may also provide a substrate for reentry within the pulmonary vein itself, though this remains to be proven (Fig. 29-6). Although over 95 percent of triggering foci that are mapped during electrophysiologic studies occur in the pulmonary veins in patients with paroxysmal atrial fibrillation, foci within the superior vena cava,[41] the ligament of Marshall,[42] and the musculature of the coronary sinus[43] have been identified (Fig. 29-7). The ligament of Marshall is the vestigial remnant of the left cardinal vein that usually involutes to form a fibrous ligament extending from the coronary sinus and coursing superiorly anterior to the left inferior and left superior pulmonary veins.[44] While these locations of triggering foci are uncommon in patients with paroxysmal atrial fibrillation, the common factor is that the site of origin is often within a venous structure that connects to the atrium. Other sites of initiating foci may be recorded in the left atrial wall or along the crista terminalis in the right atrium.[45] While the typical patient with paroxysmal atrial fibrillation has identifiable ectopic foci initiating the arrhythmia, these triggers cannot be recorded in all patients. Conversely, occasional patients with persistent or permanent atrial fibrillation may be cured of their arrhythmia by ablation of a single triggering focus, suggesting that perpetual firing of the focus may be the mechanism sustaining this arrhythmia in some cases. Autonomic tone may play an important role in the triggering of atrial fibrillation. For patients with pulmonary vein foci, a primary increase in adrenergic tone followed by a marked vagal predominance has been reported just prior to the onset of paroxysmal atrial fibrillation.[46] A similar pattern of autonomic tone has been reported in an unselected group of patients with paroxysmal atrial fibrillation and a variety of cardiac conditions.[47] Vagal stimulation shortens the refractory period of atrial myocardium, though with a nonuniform distribution of effect. These factors support the importance of vagal stimulation in the induction of paroxysmal atrial fibrillation. Whereas vagal stimulation results in maintenance of atrial fibrillation, catheter ablation of the parasympathetic autonomic nerves entering the right atrium from the superior vena cava prevents vagally induced atrial fibrillation in animal models.[48] A variety of electrophysiologic and structural factors promote the perpetuation of atrial fibrillation. Moe and colleagues[49,50] proposed the multiple wavelet hypothesis as the mechanism of atrial fibrillation. Fractionation of wavefronts traversing the atria into daughter wavelets has been proposed as the mechanism by which this nonrepeating arrhythmia perpetuates. The number of wavelets on the heart at any

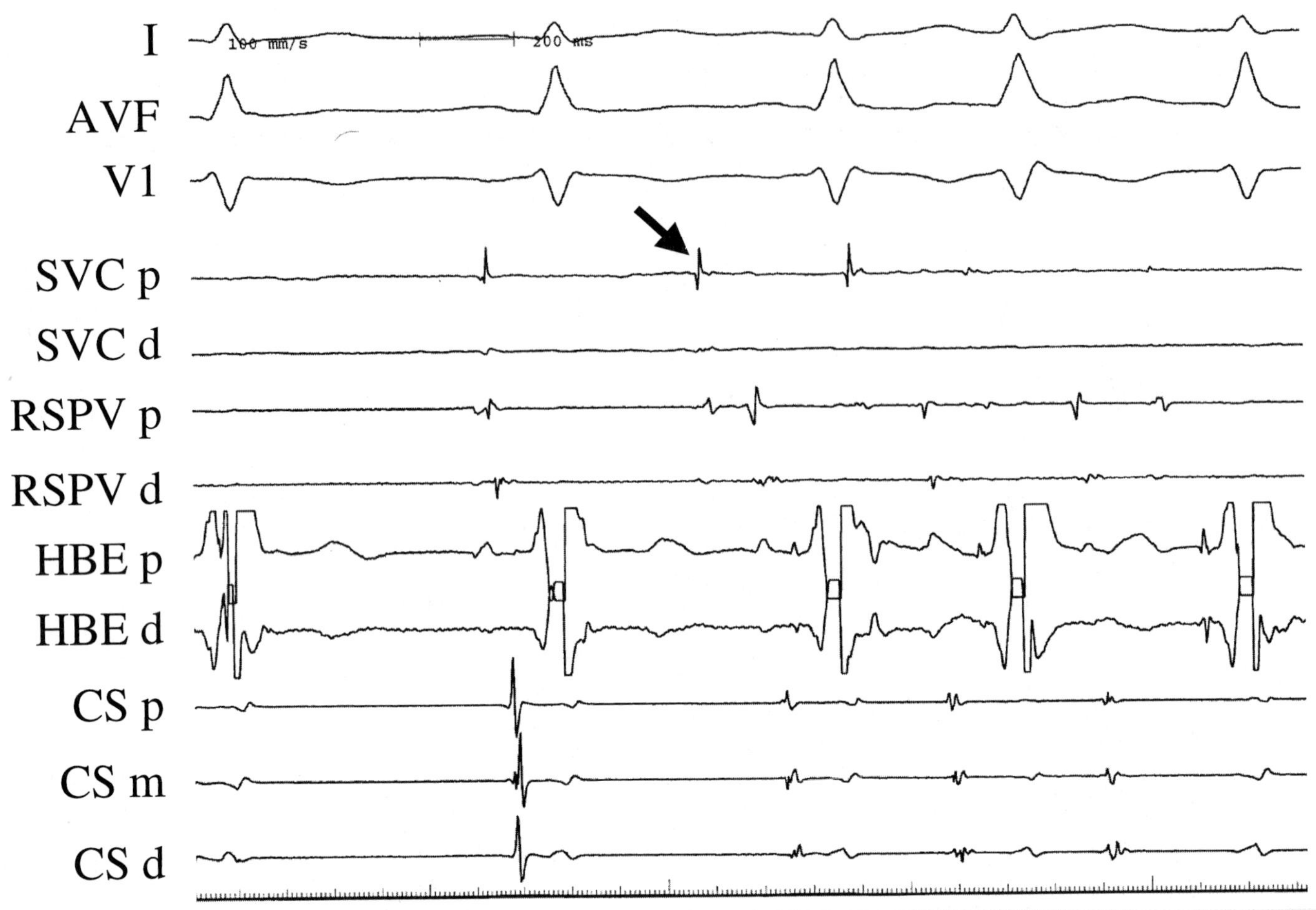


FIGURE 29-7 A rapidly firing focus in the superior vena cava (SVC) that induces atrial fibrillation. Surface leads I, aVF and $V_1$ are recorded simultaneously with intracardiac bipolar electrograms from the SVC proximal (SVC p) and distal (SVC d) pairs, right superior pulmonary vein (RSPV p and RSPV d), His bundle (HBE p and HBE d), and coronary sinus (CS p, CS m, CS d). The arrow indicates early activation in the superior vena cava.

moment depends on the refractory period, conduction velocity, and anatomic obstacles in different portions of the atria. Li and colleagues demonstrated in a canine model of heart failure that interstitial fibrosis predisposed to intraatrial reentry and atrial fibrillation.[51] The strong association of sinus node dysfunction and atrial fibrillation (the bradycardia-tachycardia syndrome) suggests that replacement of atrial myocytes by interstitial fibrosis may play an important part in the pathogenesis of atrial fibrillation in the elderly. Fibrosis of the atria may produce inhomogeneity of conduction within the atria, leading to conduction block and intraatrial reentry.[52] When combined with inhomogeneous dispersion of effective refractory periods within the atria, conduction block is an ideal substrate for reentry. The greater the slowing of conduction velocity in scarred myocardium, the shorter the anatomic circuit that can sustain a reentrant wavelet. Since antiarrhythmic drugs often slow conduction velocity as well as prolong the effective refractory period, these agents may have limited usefulness in atrial fibrillation due to atrial fibrosis, since the functional substrate for reentry would persist.[35] A variety of clinical studies have demonstrated that patients with atrial fibrillation have delayed interatrial conduction and inhomogeneous dispersion of atrial refractory periods.[53] Apoptosis has been identified in atrial biopsies of patients with atrial fibrillation undergoing cardiac surgery.[54] Such programmed cell death may be an important mechanism leading to replacement of atrial myocytes by interstitial fibrosis. Long-standing atrial fibrillation results in loss of myofibrils, accumulation of glycogen granules, disruption in cell-to-cell coupling at gap junctions,[55] and organelle aggregates.[56,57] ADAMS (a disintegrin and metalloproteinase), a family of membrane-bound glycoproteins that regulate cell-cell and cell-matrix interactions, have been reported to double in concentration during atrial fibrillation in human biopsies of atrial myocardium. This increased disintegrin and metalloproteinase activity may be one mechanism contributing to atrial dilatation in atrial fibrillation. Thus, atrial fibrillation itself seems to produce a variety of alterations of atrial architecture that further contribute to atrial remodeling, mechanical dysfunction, and perpetuation of fibrillation.

The structure of the dilated atria may have important electrophysiologic effects that are related to stretch of the atrial myocardium, which may affect both automaticity and reentry. In a population-based study of elderly patients without atrial fibrillation at baseline, Tsang and colleagues[20] demonstrated that atrial fibrillation developed in direct relation to the echocardiographic left atrial volume index. An even stronger predictor of the development of nonvalvular atrial fibrillation was a restrictive transmitral Doppler flow pattern ($p < 0.001$). Thus, clinical evidence for diastolic dysfunction strongly supports the concept that myocardial stretch is an important mechanism of atrial fibrillation in the elderly. Altered stretch on atrial myocytes results in opening of stretch-activated channels.[35] Force transmitted to stretch-activated channels in the membrane or via cytoskeletal integrins produces opening of these channels as well as increasing local production of angiotensin II (which in turn increases L-type $Ca^{2+}$ current and decreases the transient outward $K^+$ current). The antiarrhythmic effects of the angiotensin II receptor antagonist irbesartan have been demonstrated in patients undergoing electrical cardioversion.[58] Stretch-activated channels increase G protein–coupled pathways leading to increased protein kinase A and C activity and increased L-type $Ca^{2+}$ current through the cell membrane and release of $Ca^{2+}$ from the sarcoplasmic reticulum (promoting afterdepolarizations and triggered activity).[35]

Atrial fibrillation also produces electrical remodeling that promotes further atrial fibrillation. The electrophysiologic changes typical of atrial myocytes during atrial fibrillation are a decrease in effective refractory period, decrease in action potential duration, and reduction in the amplitude of the action potential plateau. The action potential of fibrillating atrial myocytes is also characterized by a loss of response of action potential duration to changes in rate (abnormal restitution). Whereas the normal atrial action potential duration shortens in response to pacing at shorter cycle lengths, atrial fibrillation results in loss of this rate dependence of the action potential.[59] These changes can be attenuated by the sarcoplasmic reticulum's release of the calcium antagonist ryanodine, suggesting the importance of increased intracellular calcium to the maladaptation of atrial myocardium during atrial fibrillation. The reduction in the atrial effective refractory periods produced by atrial fibrillation are not uniform throughout the atria.[60] Most studies have demonstrated a reduction in atrial conduction velocity in response to prolonged rapid atrial rates.[61–63] Reduction in $I_{to}$, $IK_{UR}$, have been reported in animals and humans with atrial fibrillation while the L-type $Ca^{2+}$ current decreases within 24 h. The outward currents $I_{K1}$ and $I_{K,Ach}$ increase in chronically fibrillating atria. The net result of increased outward current and decreased inward current during the plateau phase is a marked shortening of the action potential duration and effective refractory period of the atrial myocyte. The presence of underlying congestive heart failure may further interact with these electrophysiologic changes to promote atrial fibrillation. For example, Shinagawa and colleagues[60] reported that prolonged atrial fibrillation could be induced in 0 of 14 control dogs, 2 of 14 dogs with congestive heart failure (CHF), 4 of 12 dogs subjected to rapid atrial pacing at 400 beats per minute for 1 week, and 8 of 13 dogs with both CHF and rapid atrial pacing. These observations may help to explain why some patients with paroxysmal atrial fibrillation without apparent structural heart disease do not seem to progress to persistent or permanent atrial fibrillation over a period of many years. On the other hand, patients with significant structural heart disease may develop permanent atrial fibrillation with their first episode.

## Hemodynamic Effects

Atrial fibrillation produces several adverse hemodynamic effects, including loss of atrial contraction, a rapid ventricular rate, and an irregular ventricular rhythm. The loss of mechanical AV synchrony may have a dramatic impact on ventricular filling and cardiac output when there is reduced ventricular compliance, as with left ventricular hypertrophy from hypertension, restrictive cardiomyopathy, hypertrophic cardiomyopathy, or the increased ventricular stiffness associated with aging. In addition, patients with mitral stenosis, constrictive pericarditis, or right ventricular infarction typically experience marked hemodynamic deterioration at the onset of atrial fibrillation. The loss of AV synchrony results in a decrease in left ventricular end-diastolic pressure (LVEDP) as the loading effect of atrial contraction is lost, thereby reducing stroke volume and left ventricular contractility by the Frank-Starling mechanism. While there is a reduction in the LVEDP, there is an increase in the left atrial mean diastolic pressure. Patients with significant restrictive physiology may experience pulmonary edema and/or hypotension with the onset of atrial fibrillation. In contrast, patients with dilated cardiomyopathy and high left ventricular filling pressures may experience minimal hemodynamic compromise with atrial fibrillation if their left ventricular compliance is not significantly impaired. The inappropriately rapid ventricular rate during atrial fibrillation also limits the duration of diastole and reduces ventricular filling. In occasional patients, the first clinical manifestation of atrial fibrillation may be congestive heart failure related to a tachycardia-induced cardiomyopathy.[64–66] This clinical syndrome is generally limited to patients who experience minimal or no palpitations during atrial fibrillation with a sustained ventricular rate >120 beats per minute for more than 1 to 2 months. In these patients, control of the ventricular rate by cardioversion, AV nodal–blocking medications, or catheter ablation typically reverses the impaired left ventricular function within weeks. The irregular ventricular rhythm has adverse hemodynamic effects that are independent of the ventricular rate. Irregularity significantly reduces cardiac output[67] and coronary blood flow[68] as compared with a regular ventricular rhythm at the same average heart rate. The effect of ventricular irregularity on coronary blood flow may explain in part why some patients with atrial fibrillation experience precordial pain in the presence of normal coronary arteriography.

### THROMBOEMBOLISM

Stroke is the most feared consequence of atrial fibrillation, and its prevention is a major focus of the management of patients with this condition. While patients with atrial fibrillation have a dramatically increased risk of stroke, there does not appear to be an increased risk of carotid atherosclerosis in this population.[69] Nevertheless, up to 25 percent of strokes in patients with atrial fibrillation are related to carotid artery disease, ascending aortic atherosclerosis, or intrinsic cerebrovascular conditions.[70,71] Thus, patients with atrial fibrillation who experience symptoms of cerebral ischemia require careful evaluation of other causes, especially if they have been therapeutically anticoagulated.

Most thrombi associated with atrial fibrillation arise within the left atrial appendage.[72–74] Flow velocity within the left atrial appendage is reduced during atrial fibrillation due to the loss of organized mechanical contraction.[75,76] Although transthoracic echocardiography can provide useful information regarding left atrial size and compliance of the left ventricle,[77–81] it cannot be relied upon to exclude the presence of thrombi within the left atrium. The transesophageal echocardiogram offers a much more sensitive and specific means of assessing left atrial thrombi and spontaneous echo contrast, an indicator of reduced flow.[82–84] Although spontaneous echo contrast (caused by ultrasound backscatter from clumps of red blood cells and plasma proteins) is a predictor of increased risk of thromboemboli, this finding does not disappear with oral anticoagulation; it may also be identified in sinus rhythm, usually in the presence of an enlarged left atrium and lower left atrial appendage flow velocity.[85–89]

Several factors contribute to the enhanced thrombogenicity of atrial fibrillation. Since nitric oxide (NO) production is increased by cyclic shear stress during atrial contraction and reduced during low-flow states, the loss of effective atrial mechanical contraction during atrial fibrillation results in a downward regulation of NO production. NO production in the left atrial endocardium is reduced in experimental atrial fibrillation, with an increase in levels of the prothrombotic protein plasminogen activator inhibitor (PAI-1).[90] The lowest levels of NO and the highest levels of PAI-1 were recorded in the left atrial appendage during atrial fibrillation. Patients with atrial fibrillation have elevated levels of β-thromboglobulin and platelet factor 4[91,92]; elevated plasma levels of von Willebrand factor (vWF), soluble thrombomodulin, and fibrinogen have been reported in patients with permanent atrial fibrillation with no evidence of diurnal

ACC/AHA/ESC Task Force Recommendation

**Minimum evaluation**

1. History and physical examination, to define
   - The presence and nature of symptoms associated with AF
   - The clinical type of AF (first episode, paroxysmal, persistent, or permanent)
   - The onset of the first symptomatic attack or date of discovery of AF
   - The frequency, duration, precipitating factors, and modes of termination of AF
   - The response to any pharmacologic agents that have been administered
   - The presence of any underlying heart disease or other reversible conditions (eg, hyperthyroidism or alcohol consumption)
2. Electrocardiogram, to identify
   - Rhythm (verify AF)
   - LV hypertrophy
   - P-wave duration and morphology or fibrillatory waves
   - Preexcitation
   - Bundle branch block
   - Prior MI
   - Other atrial arrhythmias
   - To measure and follow the RR, QRS, and QT intervals in conjunction with antiarrhythmic drug therapy
3. Chest radiograph, to evaluate
   - The lung parenchyma, when clinical findings suggest an abnormality
   - The pulmonary vasculature, when clinical findings suggest an abnormality
4. Echocardiogram, to identify
   - Valvular heart disease
   - Left and right atrial size
   - LV size and function
   - Peak RV pressure (pulmonary hypertension)
   - LV hypertrophy
   - LA thrombus (low sensitivity)
   - Pericardial disease
5. Blood tests of thyroid function
   - For a first episode of AF, when the ventricular rate is difficult to control, or when AF recurs unexpectedly after cardioversion

**Additional testing**

- One or several tests may be necessary

1. Exercise testing
   - If the adequacy of rate control is in question (permanent AF)
   - To reproduce exercise-induced AF
   - To exclude ischemia before treatment of selected patients with a type IC antiarrhythmic drug
2. Holter monitoring or event recording
   - If diagnosis of the type of arrhythmia is in question
   - As a means of evaluating rate control
3. Transesophageal echocardiography
   - To identify LA thrombus (in the LA appendage)
   - To guide cardioversion
4. Electrophysiologic study
   - To clarify the mechanism of wide-QRS-complex tachycardia
   - To identify a predisposing arrhythmia such as atrial flutter or paroxysmal supraventricular tachycardia
   - Seeking sites for curative ablation or AV conduction block/modification

AF indicates atrial fibrillation; LV, left ventricular; MI, myocardial infarction; RV, right ventricular; LA, left atrial; and AV, atrioventricular. Type IC refers to the Vaughan Williams classification of antiarrhythmic drugs.

FIGURE 29-8 Suggested evaluation of patients with atrial fibrillation. (From Fuster et al.[3] With permission.)

variation in thrombogenicity.[93,94] In the SPAF-III study,[95] increased plasma levels of vWF were strongly correlated with the clinical predictors of stroke in atrial fibrillation (age, prior cerebral ischemia, CHF, diabetes, and body mass index). There was a stepwise increase in vWF with increasing clinical risk of stroke in this population. In contrast, plasma levels of soluble P selectin (a marker of arterial platelet activation) were associated with factors known to play a role in atherosclerosis but not with the clinical risk of thromboemboli.

## Clinical Manifestations

The clinical manifestations of atrial fibrillation range from no symptoms at all to profound hemodynamic deterioration with cardiogenic shock. Many patients experience minimal symptoms or may present with a vague sense of fatigue or effort intolerance. For others, the major symptom is palpitations, ranging from a vague sense of uneasiness in the chest to profound sense of impending doom. Although several studies have reported a marked reduction in quality of life in patients with atrial fibrillation who are referred for nonpharmacologic therapies,[96,97] these studies included subjects who were highly motivated to undergo invasive treatment of their arrhythmia. The much larger AFFIRM study[98] demonstrates that patients referred for randomization between rate-control and rhythm-control strategies have a reduced quality of life as compared with healthy controls. Perhaps because of the widely varying clinical manifestations of atrial fibrillation, there has been no clear consensus as to how the "average" patient should be managed. Nevertheless, the ACC/AHA/ESC task force on practice guidelines has recommended a minimal evaluation for patients with atrial fibrillation[3] (Fig. 29-8). This evaluation includes a history and physical examination, electrocardiogram, chest radiograph, echocardiogram, and thyroid function studies.

## Treatment

### ANTICOAGULATION

There is widespread consensus that all patients with rheumatic valvular heart disease and atrial fibrillation require anticoagulation with warfarin unless there is an absolute contraindication. The risk factors for ischemic stroke and systemic embolism in patients with nonvalvular atrial fibrillation are shown in Table 29-1.[33] Importantly, there is no difference in the risk of stroke between patients with intermittent or permanent atrial fibrillation. Patients can be risk-stratified as to their risk of stroke (Table 29-2), with the highest risk being in patients with a prior history of stroke or transient ischemic attack (10 to 12 percent per year).[3,99–108] Other independent risk factors include CHF, hypertension, increasing age, diabetes mellitus, and female gender. Nearly half of all strokes related to atrial fibrillation occur in patients over 75 years of age. Patients with thyrotoxicosis may be at especially high risk for thromboembolism and require anticoagulation with warfarin.[109–111] Analysis of the six randomized, controlled trials of warfarin versus placebo for the treatment of nonvalvular atrial fibrillation suggests that the risk of stroke is reduced by over 60 percent with anticoagulation[112–122] (Fig. 29-9). Although aspirin is associated with a 20 percent reduction in the risk of stroke in nonvalvular atrial fibrillation as compared with placebo, warfarin is clearly superior (Figs. 29-10, 29-11).[123,124] Although bleeding complications of warfarin increase with age, so does the relative benefit of anticoagulation therapy. Three risk-stratification schemes have been published which, though differing slightly, indicate which patients should receive warfarin anticoagulation.[3] There is general consensus that patients with nonvalvular atrial fibrillation who are less than 65 years of age and do not have a prior history of stroke or transient

TABLE 29-1 Risk Factors for Stroke in Atrial Fibrillation

| Risk Factors (Control Groups) | Relative Risk |
|---|---|
| Previous stroke or TIA[a] | 2.5 |
| History of hypertension | 1.6 |
| Congestive heart failure | 1.4 |
| Advanced age (continuous, per decade) | 1.4 |
| Diabetes mellitus | 1.7 |
| Coronary artery disease | 1.5 |

[a]Transient ischemic attack.

TABLE 29-2 Recommendations for Anticoagulation in Atrial Fibrillation

| Source | High Risk | Intermediate Risk | Low Risk |
|---|---|---|---|
| Atrial Fibrillation Investigators | Age greater than or equal to 65 years<br>History of hypertension<br>Coronary artery disease<br>Diabetes | | Age less than 65 years<br>No high-risk features |
| American College of Chest Physicians | Age greater than 75 years<br>History of hypertension<br>Left ventricular dysfunction[a]<br>More than 1 intermediate risk factor | Age 65–75 years<br>Diabetes<br>Coronary artery disease<br>Thyrotoxicosis | Age less than 65 years<br>No risk factors |
| Stroke Prevention in Atrial Fibrillation | Women greater than 75 years<br>Systolic BP[b] greater than 160 mmHg<br>Left ventricular dysfunction[c] | History of hypertension<br>No high-risk features | No high-risk features<br>No history of hypertension |

Patients with AF and prior thromboembolism are at high risk of stroke, and anticoagulation is indicated for secondary prevention in such cases.
[a]Left ventricular dysfunction refers to moderate to severe wall motion abnormality assessed globally by two-dimensional echocardiography, reduced ejection fraction, fractional shortening less than 0.25 by M-mode echocardiography, or clinical heart failure.
[b]BP indicates blood pressure. Patients are classified on the basis of the presence or absence of any risk factor.
[c]Did not distinguish high- from intermediate-risk patients.
SOURCE: From Pearce et al.[108]

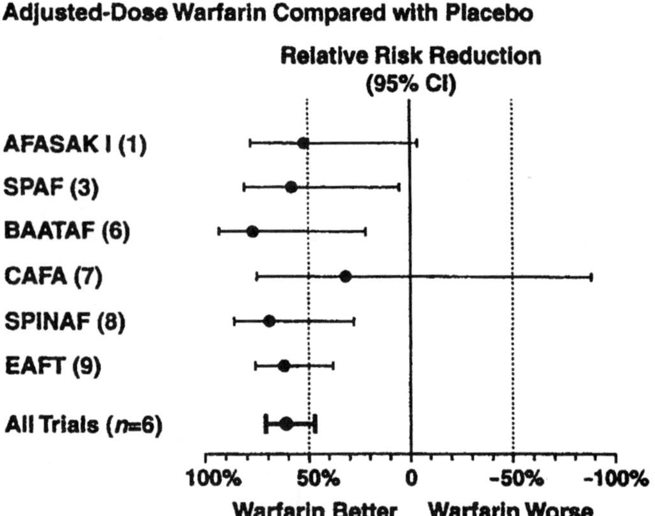


FIGURE 29-9 Effects of wafarin versus placebo on risk of stroke in six randomized, placebo-controlled clinical trials in nonvalvular atrial fibrillation. ABBREVIATIONS: AFASAK I (1) = The Copenhagen Atrial Fibrillation, Aspirin, and Anticoagulant Therapy Study; SPAF (3) = Stroke Prevention in Atrial Fibrillation; BAATAF (6) = Boston Area Anticoagulation Trial for Atrial Fibrillation; CAFA (7) = Canadian Atrial Fibrillation Anticoagulation; SPINAF (8) = Stroke Prevention in Atrial Fibrillation; EAFT (9) = European Atrial Fibrillation Trial. (Adapted from Hart and Halperin.[24] With permission.)

ischemic attack (TIA), hypertension, diabetes, coronary artery or other structural heart diseases, or thyrotoxicosis need not receive warfarin. Aspirin is indicated in this low-risk group. For patients who are not in the low-risk subgroup, it is prudent to consider therapy with warfarin. The target INR should be between 2.0 and 3.0, as this range offers the best trade-off between reduction in the risk of stroke and the occurrence of bleeding complications (Fig. 29-12). Despite these recommendations, there are some patients who have absolute contraindications to anticoagulation, such as prior intracerebral hemorrhage, recurrent massive gastrointestinal bleeding, or subdural hematoma while receiving anticoagulation. For these patients, surgical amputation of the left atrial appendage or investigational percutaneous occlusion of the left atrial appendage may be considered.

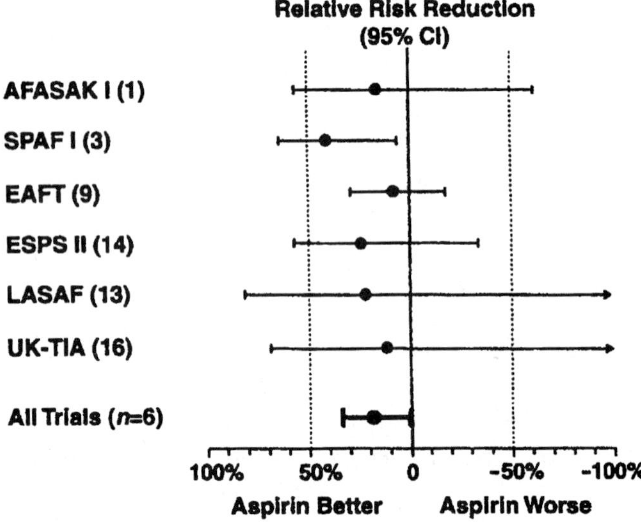


FIGURE 29-10 Effects of aspirin versus placebo on risk of stroke in five randomized, placebo-controlled trials in nonvalvular atrial fibrillation. ABBREVIATIONS: ESPS II (14) = European Stroke Prevention Study; LASAF (13) = Alternate-Day Dosing of Aspirin in Atrial Fibrillation Pilot Study Group; UK-TIA (16) = United Kingdom Transient Ischaemic Attack Study Group or Trial. (Adapted from Hart and Halperin.[24] With permission.)

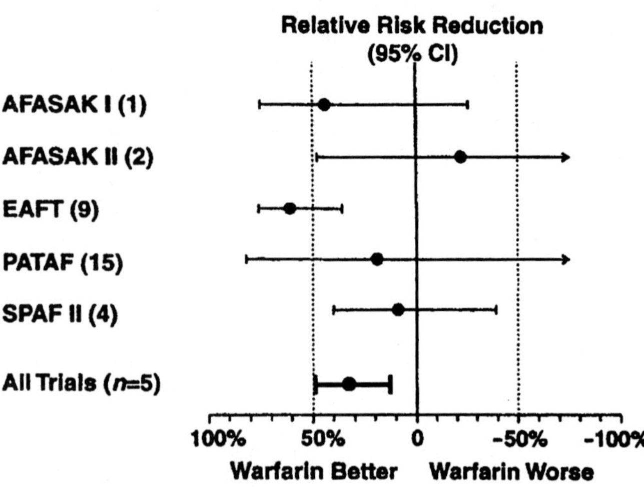


FIGURE 29-11 Effects of aspirin versus warfarin on risk of stroke in five randomized, controlled clinical trials in nonvalvular atrial fibrillation. ABBREVIATION: PATAF (15) = Primary Prevention of Arterial Thromboembolism in Nonrheumatic Atrial Fibrillation. (Adapted from Hart and Halperin.[24] With permission.)

## CARDIOVERSION

Although no randomized comparisons of anticoagulation versus placebo have been published for patients undergoing cardioversion, the standard of care requires anticoagulation to be addressed. There is general consensus, based on very little data, that atrial fibrillation that has been present for less than 48 h can be cardioverted without prior anticoagulation. In a retrospective analysis of cardioversion experience from nine European hospitals, Gallagher et al.[125] reported that confirmed or probable systemic emboli occurred in 2 of 198 patients cardioverted from atrial fibrillation of less than 48 h duration who were not anticoagulated. This was similar to 2 of 133 confirmed emboli that occurred in unanticoagulated patients with atrial fibrillation of greater than 2 days' duration. It should be recognized that thrombi can develop in a matter of hours and that the risk of stroke in paroxysmal atrial fibrillation is no different than that in persistent or permanent atrial fibrillation. These observations would suggest a cautious approach to cardioversion even when fibrillation has been present for <48 h. There are two basic strategies to deal with cardioversion: (1) oral warfarin with a therapeutic INR (2 to 3) for 3 to 4 weeks before cardioversion followed by continued anticoagulation thereafter or (2) transesophageal echocardiography (TEE) and heparin immediately before cardioversion followed by oral warfarin thereafter.[126] The ACUTE study randomized 1222 patients with atrial fibrillation undergoing direct-current cardioversion between these strategies and found no difference in the rate of embolic events (0.5 percent TEE vs. 0.8 percent conventional) but a lower risk of bleeding complications (2.9 vs. 5.5 percent) and a shorter interval to cardioversion (3.0 vs. 31 days) in the TEE-guided group.[127] The important point is that left atrial mechanical function is significantly impaired for up to several weeks following cardioversion from atrial fibrillation to sinus rhythm. This "stunning" effect may occur after either electrical or pharmacologic cardioversion[128–134] and is more marked the longer the duration of atrial fibrillation. While it has been common practice to discontinue anticoagulation 3 to 4 weeks following cardioversion, there is really very little evidence to justify this practice. Instead, if the patient had a standard indication for warfarin before cardioversion, anticoagulation should be continued indefinitely unless atrial fibrillation had been related to a transient, reversible cause. There is general consensus that electrical cardioversion should be commenced with at least 200 J (monophasic) or at least 100 J (biphasic), with the defibrillator synchronized to the R wave. Rather than use handheld paddles, adhesive gel electrodes should be placed anteriorly over the sternum (with the upper edge at the sternal angle) and posteriorly (just to the left of the spine).[135] Biphasic waveforms clearly improve defibrillation efficacy at all energy settings as compared with monophasic shocks.[136] For example, at 100 J, a biphasic shock restored sinus rhythm in 60 percent of patients with atrial fibrillation compared with 22 percent for a monophasic shock. At shock strengths of 200 and 360 J, the higher efficacy of biphasic shocks was also demonstrated (77 vs. 44 percent and 91 vs. 85 percent).[137] For resistant cases of atrial fibrillation, pretreatment with intravenous ibutilide has been demonstrated to improve the efficacy of defibrillation.[138] Elective cardioversion must be performed with the patient fasting for at least 6 h, with rapid-acting intravenous sedation using agents such as propofol or methohexital. Elective cardioversion can be safely performed in an outpatient setting. Consideration should be given for most patients undergoing electrical cardioversion to receive an antiarrhythmic drug (usually started before cardioversion), since the chances of maintaining sinus rhythm without drug therapy are less than 20 percent at 1-year follow-up.[139,140]

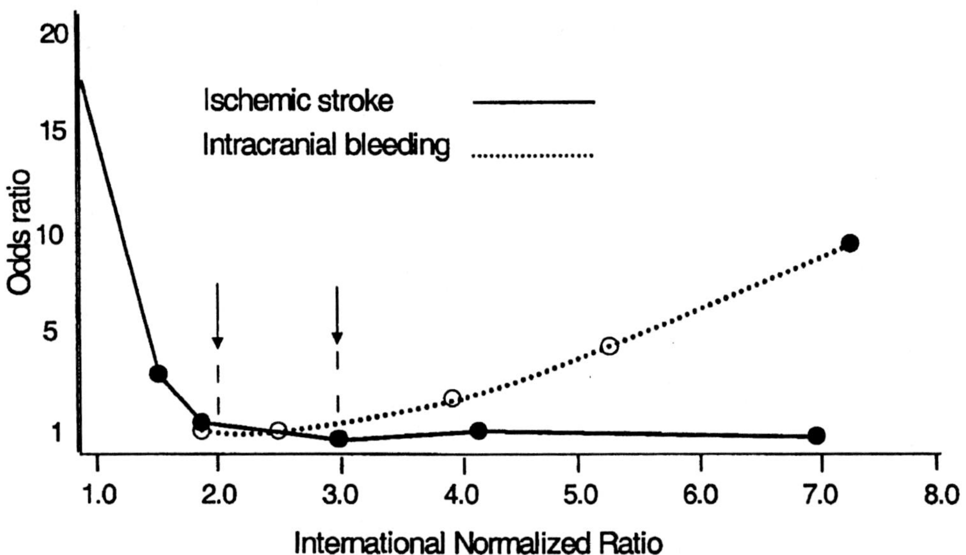


FIGURE 29-12 Odds ratios for ischemic stroke and intracranial bleeding as a function of the international normalized ratio (INR) for patients with atrial fibrillation. (Adapted from Hylek et al.[122] With permission.)

Cardioversion of atrial fibrillation can be accomplished either pharmacologically or by a synchronized direct-current shock. A single oral dose of propafenone converts recent-onset atrial fibrillation to sinus rhythm in 58 to 83 percent of patients, with lower efficacy for atrial fibrillation of longer duration.[141] A single 600-mg oral dose of propafenone converted atrial fibrillation of <1 week duration to sinus rhythm in 45 percent of patients at 3 h and 76 percent of patients at 8 h (compared with 18 and 37 percent after placebo), with no advantage from using the intravenous route.[142–144] In a randomized comparison of oral propafenone (600 mg), oral flecainide (300 mg), or placebo for recent-onset atrial fibrillation, the 8-h conversion rates were 72, 78, and 39 percent, respectively.[145] Since a type 1C drug may convert atrial fibrillation to atrial flutter, an AV nodal blocking agent should usually be administered concomitantly. At a dose of 500 $\mu$g bid, approximately 30 percent of patients converted to sinus rhythm on oral dofetilide, 91 percent of whom converted by 36 h.[146] Because of the risk of torsades de pointes, dofetilide must be initiated in a hospitalized, monitored setting.

Intravenous ibutilide has also been demonstrated to provide effective cardioversion of recent-onset atrial fibrillation or flutter.[147–151] At a dose of 0.025 mg/kg, intravenous ibutilide converted 46 percent of patients to sinus rhythm, with a mean time to conversion of 19 min.[148] The risk of nonsustained or sustained torsades de pointes ventricular tachycardia was 3.6 percent. Thus, while effective, intravenous ibutilide requires monitoring for at least 4 h after administration. Ibutilide is far more effective than intravenous procainamide (51 vs. 21 percent) for the acute termination of atrial fibrillation.[150] For termination of atrial flutter, ibutilide terminated 76 percent, while procainamide converted 14 percent. The simultaneous infusion of magnesium sulfate (2 g) may reduce the risk of torsades de pointes with ibutilide, though data are scant. Intravenous amiodarone, because of its long interval from administration to electrophysiologic effect in the atria, has been demonstrated to be only marginally more effective than placebo for the acute termination of atrial fibrillation (68 percent conversion to sinus with amiodarone vs. 60 percent with placebo at 24 h).[152]

## Postoperative Atrial Fibrillation

Atrial fibrillation may complicate the postoperative course of patients undergoing cardiac surgery, prolonging hospitalization and increasing costs. The mechanism may be related to pericarditis and high catecholamine concentrations in the myocardium. The most effective therapy to prevent atrial fibrillation is the routine use of beta blockers throughout the perioperative period. Beta blockers bring about a dramatic reduction in the incidence of postoperative atrial fibrillation with minimal adverse effects.[153] Postoperative amiodarone given for 1 week may also reduce the frequency of postoperative atrial fibrillation. For patients without a preoperative history of atrial fibrillation, this arrhythmia is generally an acute, transient phenomenon that does not require long-term treatment. Patients undergoing thoracic operations may also have transient postoperative atrial fibrillation. In these patients, rate control with diltiazem or verapamil may be quite effective. Patients with postoperative atrial fibrillation are at risk for systemic emboli and should be anticoagulated, like other patients with atrial fibrillation.

## Rate-Control versus Rhythm-Control Strategies

Two prospective, randomized trials have been published comparing the strategies of rate control and rhythm control in patients with atrial fibrillation.[154,155] The AFFIRM trial enrolled 4060 patients aged >65 years or with risk factors for stroke, randomizing them to rate versus rhythm control.[154] Over a mean follow-up period of 3.5 years, there was no significant difference in overall mortality

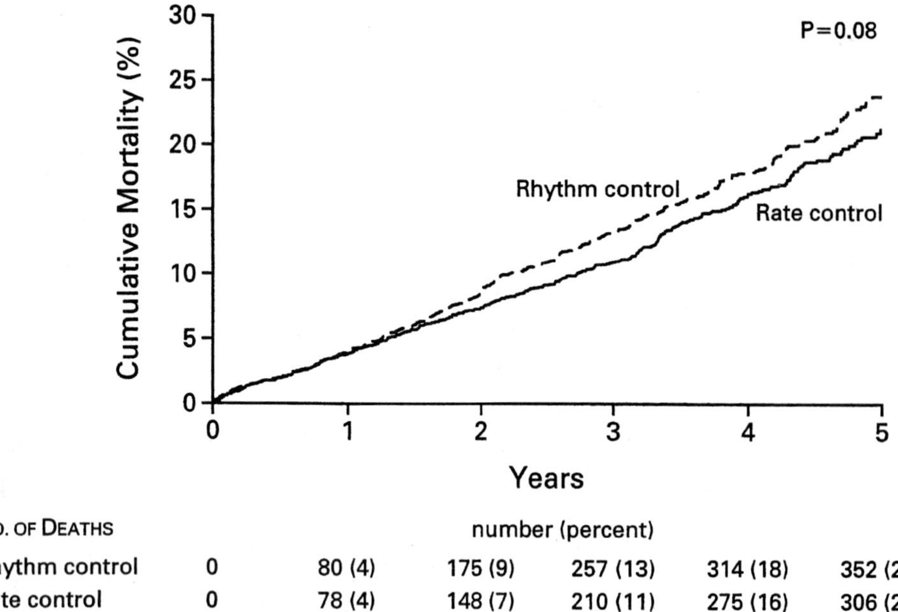


FIGURE 29-13 Results of rate control versus rhythm control on overall survival in the AFFIRM trial. (From Wyse et al.[154] With permission.)

between the two groups (Fig. 29-13), with 77 ischemic strokes in the rate-control arm and 80 ischemic strokes in the rhythm-control arm. Most strokes occurred in patients who were not receiving warfarin anticoagulation or were being given it in subtherapeutic dosages. At the 5-year follow-up evaluation, 35 percent of patients assigned to rate control were in sinus rhythm, compared with 63 percent assigned to rhythm control. Approximately two-thirds of patients assigned to rhythm control received amiodarone during the study. The RACE trial[155] randomly assigned 522 patients with persistent atrial fibrillation after electrical cardioversion to either a rate-control or a rhythm-control treatment. After a mean of 2.3 years, 39 percent of patients in the rhythm-control arm maintained sinus rhythm, as compared with 10 percent in the rate-control arm (Fig. 29-14). There was no difference in the primary endpoint of the study (a composite of cardiovascular death, CHF, thromboemboli, bleeding, need for pacemaker, or serious drug side effects) between the two strategies. Thus, these studies indicate that both approaches have similar clinical outcomes provided that appropriate anticoagulation is maintained.

In view of these randomized trials, how should an individual patient with atrial fibrillation be managed? The choice of strategy is primarily determined by the symptoms that the patient experiences while in atrial fibrillation. For patients who are discovered to have atrial fibrillation on routine examination with no or minimal symptoms, a rate-control strategy may be most appropriate. These individuals are more likely to be elderly and typical of the randomized trials. On the other hand, many patients are markedly troubled by palpitations, dyspnea, fatigue, and anxiety during atrial fibrillation (more common with paroxysmal than permanent atrial fibrillation). For these individuals attempts to maintain sinus rhythm are most appropriate (and appreciated). For some patients, such as those with restrictive ventricular physiology (e.g., hypertrophic or restrictive cardiomyopathy), maintenance of sinus rhythm is vital for the prevention of congestive heart failure.

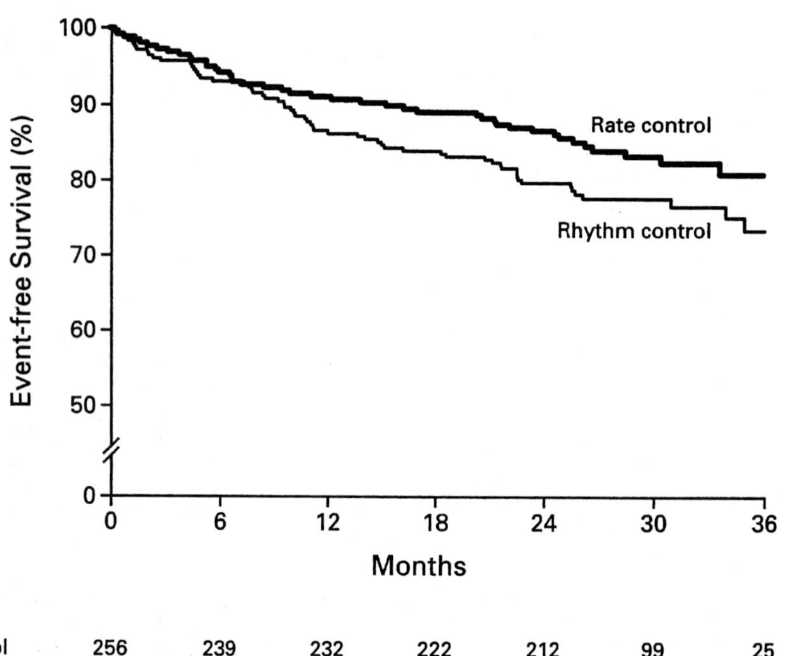


FIGURE 29-14 Comparison of rate-control and rhythm-control strategies on survival in the RACE trial. (Adapted from Van Gelder et al.[155] With permission.)

## Control of Ventricular Rate

Control of the ventricular rate involves both acute and chronic phases. In the acute phase, intravenous diltiazem, metoprolol, esmolol, or verapamil have all been demonstrated to provide slowing of AV nodal conduction within 5 min; these drugs are indicated for patients with severe symptoms related to a rapid ventricular rate.[156] Intravenous digoxin requires a longer duration to achieve rate control and is less useful. Not all patients require acute intravenous medications to slow the ventricular rate. For patients with only mild or moderate symptoms, oral medications that slow AV nodal conduction should be prescribed. After control of the resting ventricular rate has been achieved, attention is paid to the ambulatory heart rate. Some patients with depressed AV nodal function have relatively slow ventricular rates and may not require AV nodal blocking medications. The ventricular rate is considered to be well controlled when it is between 60 and 80 beats per minute at rest and less than 115 beats per minute during moderate exercise.[3] For patients in permanent atrial fibrillation, digoxin often provides effective control of the resting heart rate but is often ineffective during exertion. $\beta$-adrenergic blockers or calcium channel antagonists provide much better control of the ventricular rate during exercise and should be considered for most patients. Digoxin is most useful in the setting of impaired systolic function and can provide additional rate control for some patients who fail to respond to beta blockers or calcium antagonists. If a rhythm-control strategy is chosen, amiodarone or sotalol has the benefit of controlling ventricular rate as well. However, like AV nodal blocking agents, these drugs also depress sinus node function. Control of the ventricular rate can be especially challenging for patients with the tachycardia-bradycardia syndrome, who experience rapid ventricular rates during atrial fibrillation and sinus bradycardia or sinus pauses when atrial fibrillation terminates. Permanent pacemaker implantation is indicated for patients who experience significant sinus node dysfunction while receiving medications required to control the ventricular rate during atrial fibrillation.

## Ablation of the Atrioventricular Node

Despite the usefulness of medications to control the ventricular rate during atrial fibrillation, many patients may continue to experience significant symptoms from a rapid or irregular ventricular rhythm. In patients with a chronically elevated ventricular rate (usually >120 beats per minute) despite adequate trials of AV nodal blocking agents, tachycardia-induced cardiomyopathy may result.[64,65] Catheter ablation of the AV conduction system and permanent pacemaker implantation is a highly effective means of establishing permanent control of the ventricular rate during atrial fibrillation in selected patients.[157–160] AV nodal ablation improves quality of life, exercise capacity, symptom frequency and severity; it also reduces the need for antiarrhythmic or AV nodal blocking drugs.[96] For patients with impaired left ventricular systolic function related to a rapid ventricular rate, AV nodal ablation improves the left ventricular ejection fraction and the symptoms of congestive heart failure.[96,158] This technique has been associated with long-term survival similar to that of patients with atrial fibrillation who are treated medically.[96] Despite the many favorable effects of this procedure, there are several limitations. First, AV nodal ablation does not change the long-term need for anticoagulation. Second, although an adequate junctional escape rhythm is typically present after ablation, patients should be considered permanently pacemaker dependent. Third, because this procedure does not restore AV synchrony, patients who are highly dependent on mechanical atrial contraction often do not experience as much improvement as other patients. Fourth, right ventricular pacing produces an abnormal left ventricular contraction sequence, and acute worsening of hemodynamics has been observed in some patients. Finally, there is a small but real incidence of polymorphous ventricular tachycardia or fibrillation (<2 percent) in the first 2 weeks after AV nodal ablation and permanent pacemaker implantation.[158] Pacing with a lower programmed rate of 90 beats per minute for the first 2 weeks after AV nodal ablation may reduce the risk of sudden cardiac death. The lower pacing rate is then gradually decreased in follow-up, though rarely should the rate be programmed less than 70 beats per minute. The use of catheter ablation to modify the posterior inputs to the AV node (the slow AV nodal pathway) without the requirement for permanent pacemaker implantation has been reported to slow the ventricular rate in patients with atrial fibrillation.[161] However, this technique has several limitations, including inadvertent induction of complete AV block and a later increase in the ventricular rate over the first 6 months after ablation. Thus, AV nodal modification is only rarely used for patients with atrial fibrillation and rapid ventricular rates.

## Maintenance of Sinus Rhythm

When a rhythm control strategy is chosen for patients with paroxysmal or persistent atrial fibrillation, prophylactic treatment with antiarrhythmic drugs is usually needed to maintain sinus rhythm.[162–166] Although the ideal of pharmacologic therapy would be to prevent all recurrences of atrial fibrillation, this is unrealistic for many patients. Rather, marked reduction of the frequency, duration, and symptoms of atrial fibrillation may be a very acceptable clinical goal. In addition, the use of pharmacologic agents to prevent atrial fibrillation does not change the indication for anticoagulation. If a patient is in a low-risk category (less than 65 years of age without risk factors for stroke), aspirin may be combined with antiarrhythmic drugs.[3] However, if the patient has an indication for anticoagulation, warfarin is prescribed regardless of whether or not it is decided to use an antiarrhythmic drug. As compared with drug therapy for life-threatening arrhythmias, the choice of pharmacologic agent is largely determined by the potential side effects of a given drug in an individual patient. The first drug chosen is usually one associated with a low risk of serious side effects. For example, in paroxysmal atrial fibrillation, a drug with relatively low efficacy such as a beta blocker may be tried first because of the very low risk of serious toxicity with these agents. For patients with paroxysmal atrial fibrillation who are <65 years old and have no evidence of structural heart disease, a class IC drug such as flecainide or propafenone may be particularly effective.[167] Before prescribing these drugs, the physician must be quite confident that the patient does not have coronary artery disease; the minimum workup for such a patient would include a radionuclide stress perfusion scan. It is in young patients without structural heart disease that triggering foci from the pulmonary veins are most likely to be demonstrated. The class IC drugs seem to be quite effective for these patients and can be safely started in an outpatient setting. Since class IC drugs may suppress atrial fibrillation but promote atrial flutter, it is often prudent to combine them with a beta blocker to decrease the risk of rapid AV nodal conduction should atrial flutter occur. Monitoring of the QRS duration and PR interval is helpful during class IC therapy. If the QRS duration increases to 150 percent of the baseline value, the dosage should be reduced.

Sotalol may also be effective as initial therapy for paroxysmal atrial fibrillation but requires inpatient monitoring to exclude excessive QT prolongation. Amiodarone and dofetilide are recommended as alternatives to flecainide, propafenone, or sotalol.[3] While amiodarone can be started on an outpatient basis, dofetilide requires monitoring for at least the first 48 h. Although quinidine, procainamide, or disopyramide may be useful in some patients without significant structural heart disease, these class IA drugs are usually reserved for failure or intolerable side effects with the other agents. The class IA drugs always require inpatient initiation with monitoring of the QT interval. With the exception of amiodarone, monitoring of the QTc interval is useful for sotalol, dofetilide, or the class IA drugs. If the QTc exceeds 520 ms, the dose should be decreased or the patient switched to another agent. Amiodarone is a particularly effective antiarrhythmic drug for patients in whom factors that promote the maintenance of atrial fibrillation predominate. For elderly patients with paroxysmal or persistent atrial fibrillation, amiodarone appears to be especially effective, often in a dose as low as 100 mg per day.

In these patients, sinus bradycardia may limit the use of amiodarone or require permanent pacemaker implantation for its safe use.

## Antiarrhythmic Drugs: Special Considerations

Patients with congestive heart failure are particularly at risk for ventricular proarrhythmia with antiarrhythmic drugs[168] (Fig. 29-15). The only drugs with proven safety in patients with congestive heart failure are amiodarone and dofetilide.[169–172] The one exception to this may be the patient with an implantable cardioverter-defibrillator, in whom sotalol may be very useful, as it may suppress atrial fibrillation while decreasing the defibrillation threshold in the ventricles. As mentioned above, patients with coronary artery disease, even if asymptomatic, should not be treated with class IC antiarrhythmic drugs because of the risk of developing ventricular tachycardia or fibrillation.[173,174] Sotalol may be an excellent choice for patients with coronary artery disease and good left ventricular function, as it has less toxicity than amiodarone.[175] In addition, dofetilide has a proven record of safety after myocardial infarction and should be considered a second-line agent.[146] Amiodarone has been demonstrated to pose a very low risk of proarrhythmia in patients with coronary artery disease and is often effective for atrial fibrillation even in low dose.[176,177] Its chief limitation is the risk of side effects, though these are quite manageable when patients are carefully monitored.[178,179] Significant left ventricular hypertrophy increases the risk of drug-induced torsades de pointes ventricular tachycardia. Thus, when the free wall of the left ventricle exceeds 14 mm in thickness, drugs such as sotalol, dofetilide, or the class IA drugs should be avoided.[3,180] In the presence of significant left ventricular hypertrophy, amiodarone is the first-line agent. Patients with the Wolff-Parkinson-White syndrome may experience episodes of atrial fibrillation with very rapid antegrade conduction over the accessory pathway; this can be life-threatening. Although an initial pharmacologic cardioversion with procainamide or ibutilide can be used for stable patients, electrical cardioversion should be employed at the first sign of hemodynamic compromise. The definitive treatment of atrial fibrillation related to the Wolff-Parkinson-White syndrome is catheter ablation of the accessory pathway rather than antiarrhythmic drugs.

## Surgical Treatment

Based on the pioneering research of Cox et al., several surgical treatments (Fig. 29-16) for the prevention of atrial fibrillation have been developed.[181–187] For patients with atrial fibrillation who are undergoing open heart surgery, such as mitral valve replacement or repair or coronary artery bypass grafting, consideration should be given to concomitant atrial fibrillation surgery. Patients with profoundly symptomatic atrial fibrillation have also been treated with surgery as a primary indication. The standard indications for such surgery are atrial fibrillation that is markedly symptomatic and refractory to standard antiarrhythmic drugs, a history of recurrent systemic emboli despite therapeutic anticoagulation, or the requirement for concomitant open heart surgery. The surgical approaches to the cure of atrial fibrillation are based on electrical isolation of the pulmonary veins by incision, radiofrequency cautery, or cryoablation in combination with linear ablation in the left and right atria. These operations also amputate, ligate, or oversew the left atrial appendage as a means of decreasing the risk of systemic emboli. Although the exact mechanism by which these operations eliminate atrial fibrillation has not been clearly proven, they all have the potential to prevent triggering foci in the pulmonary veins from initiating atrial fibrillation. The linear ablation lines also prevent large macroreentrant wavefronts from sustaining, with most wavefronts self-extinguishing. The published data suggest that the more elaborate Cox-Maze III operation cures atrial fibrillation in over 90 percent of patients, with a low operative mortality (<1 percent) and low risk of inducing sinus node dysfunction requiring

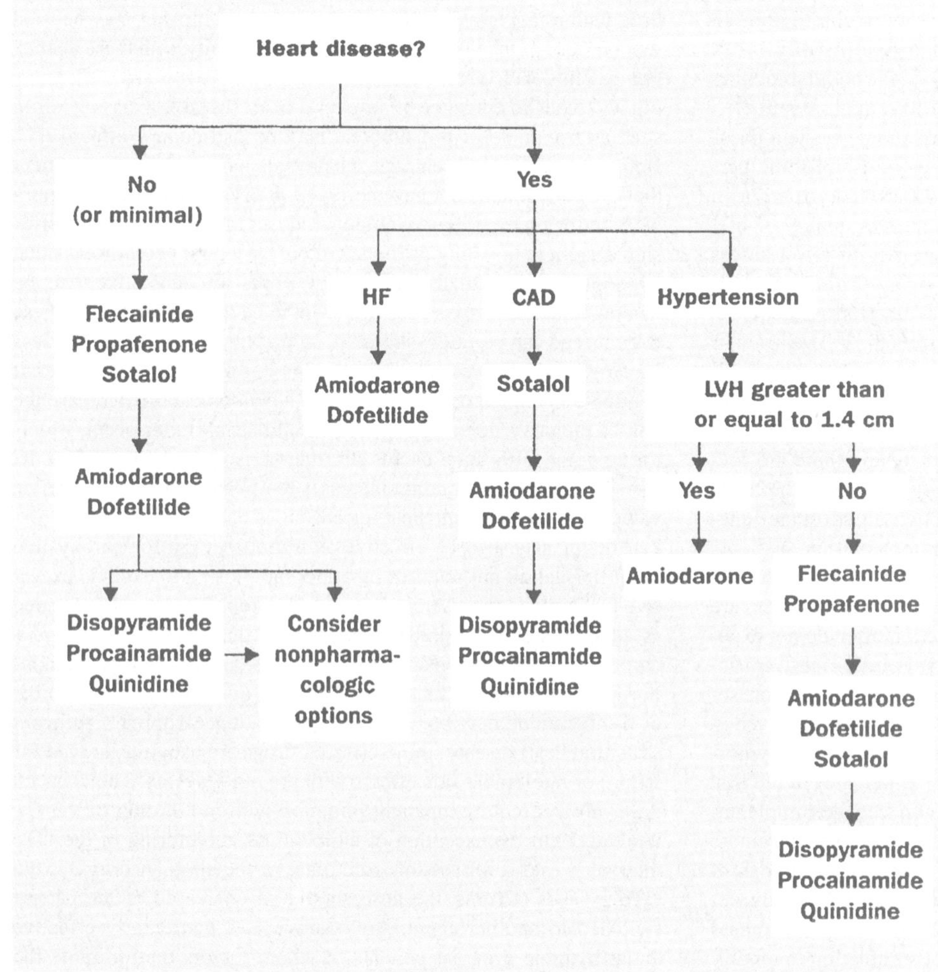


FIGURE 29-15 Proposed strategy for use of antiarrhythmic drugs to maintain sinus rhythm in patients with atrial fibrillation. (From Fuster et al.[3] With permission.)

permanent pacing (<10 percent).[184] More limited operations that only encircle the pulmonary veins may prevent atrial fibrillation in approximately 70 percent of cases. The major morbidity of these operations has been transient fluid retention that is likely due to a marked decline in atrial natriuretic peptide concentration over the first 6 weeks postoperatively. Thus virtually all patients must be treated with diuretics for the first 1 to 2 months after atrial fibrillation surgery. Although there has been concern about the mechanical function of the left atrium after atrial fibrillation surgery, most patients demonstrate return of atrial transport function toward the normal range by 6 months after operation and do not require long-term anticoagulation.

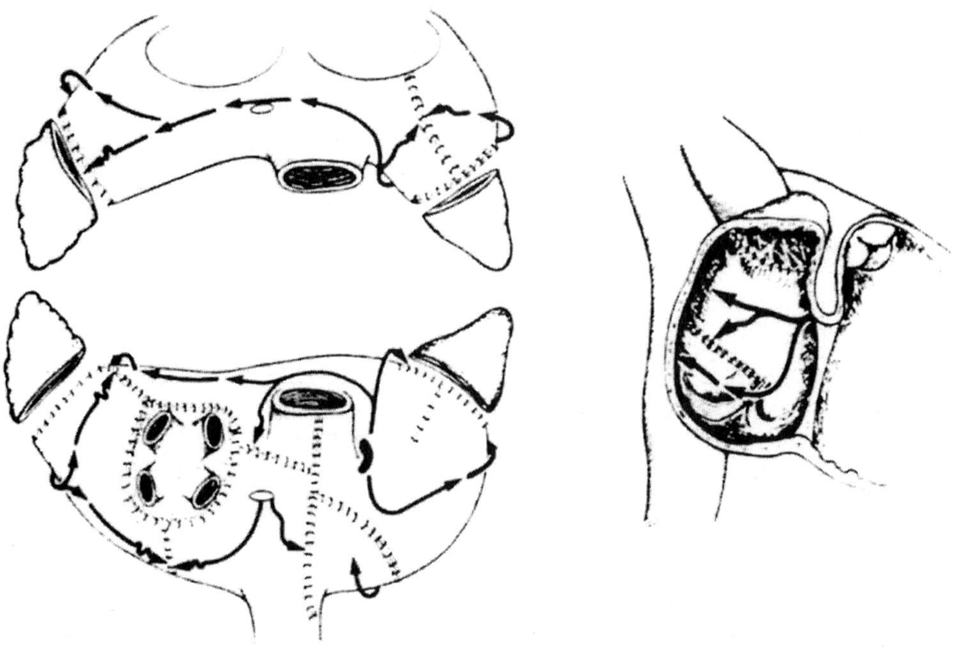

FIGURE 29-16 Diagram of surgical incisions and pathways for electrical propagation through the atria following the Cox-Maze III operation. (From Cox JL et al.[182] With permission.)

## Catheter Ablation

The initial efforts to treat atrial fibrillation by catheter ablation were modeled on atrial fibrillation surgery. The goal of these procedures was to create electrical barriers to propagation within the atria, thereby preventing macroreentrant wavefronts from sustaining. The initial trials demonstrated that even permanent atrial fibrillation could be terminated by catheter ablation and patients rendered free of recurrence. The initial observations were that ablation within the right atrium does not appear to be either necessary or sufficient to interrupt atrial fibrillation, whereas ablation in and around the pulmonary veins was most likely to be effective. Although these trials demonstrated the feasibility of linear catheter ablation to treat atrial fibrillation, the risks of adverse effects such as stroke, pericardial effusion, or pulmonary vein stenosis were recognized.

More recently, catheter ablation has been used to eliminate triggering foci, usually within the pulmonary veins.[37,38,41,45,188–197] Although the initial studies demonstrated the high prevalence of these foci within the pulmonary veins, mapping of triggering foci had the intrinsic limitation of requiring the observation of spontaneous onset of atrial fibrillation. The strategy of this technique has evolved so that the goal is the electrical isolation of all four pulmonary veins. These procedures require transseptal catheterization of the left atrium, followed by pulmonary venography to define the anatomy of the pulmonary veins and left atrium. Following definition of the pulmonary vein anatomy, a multielectrode circular mapping catheter (Fig. 29-17) or 64-electrode basket catheter is placed within the pulmonary vein to record left atrial and pulmonary vein potentials (Fig. 29-18). The site of earliest pulmonary vein electrical activation during sinus rhythm or left atrial pacing is recorded and used as the initial target for catheter ablation (Fig. 29-19). Catheter ablation is usually performed using radiofrequency current applied to the ostium of the pulmonary vein. Only sites recording electrical potentials with early activation are targeted for ablation. Ablation is performed in segments of the pulmonary vein–left atrial junction until there is electrical isolation of the pulmonary vein, characterized by elimination or dissociation of pulmonary vein potentials from the underlying atrial rhythm. Intracardiac ultrasound imaging has greatly assisted in the accurate placement of mapping and ablation catheters within the left atrium and pulmonary veins. An alternative approach to catheter ablation involves encircling the pulmonary vein ostia, with catheter ablation energy applied to the posterior left atrium. The goal of this strategy is to reduce the amplitude of the left atrial electrograms within the encircled region. Both approaches have similar efficacy, with most laboratories reporting that approximately 70 percent of patients with paroxysmal atrial fibrillation are rendered free of recurrence without the use of antiarrhythmic drugs (Fig. 29-20). Another 15 to 20 percent of patients may become responsive to previously ineffective antiarrhythmic medications. The efficacy appears to be significantly lower for patients with persistent or permanent atrial fibrillation. In these patients, more extensive left atrial ablation, including linear ablation, may be useful to prevent recurrences. Ideal candidates for pulmonary vein isolation are patients without significant structural heart disease with paroxysmal atrial fibrillation that remains symptomatic despite a trial of antiarrhythmic medications. Patients must have enough symptoms due to atrial fibrillation to justify the risks of the procedure. The risks of catheter ablation include those inherent to transseptal catheterization: pericardial tamponade, phrenic nerve injury, stroke, and pulmonary vein stenosis. Pulmonary vein stenosis is particularly important to consider when patients present with pulmonary symptoms such as cough, dyspnea, hemoptysis, chest discomfort, or localized pulmonary edema following pulmonary vein ablation.[198] These patients are often misdiagnosed as having primary pulmonary infections. The diagnosis is established by spiral computed tomography or magnetic resonance imaging of the pulmonary veins with high-resolution slices in the region of interest. Radionuclide ventilation/perfusion imaging may be a useful screening tool in patients suspected of having pulmonary vein stenosis. These images generally demonstrate marked reduction in pulmonary perfusion in the affected pulmonary lobe with no change in the ventilation image. The treatment of pulmonary vein stenosis involves balloon dilatation or stenting, though the rate of recurrent stenosis is very high after either of these treatments.

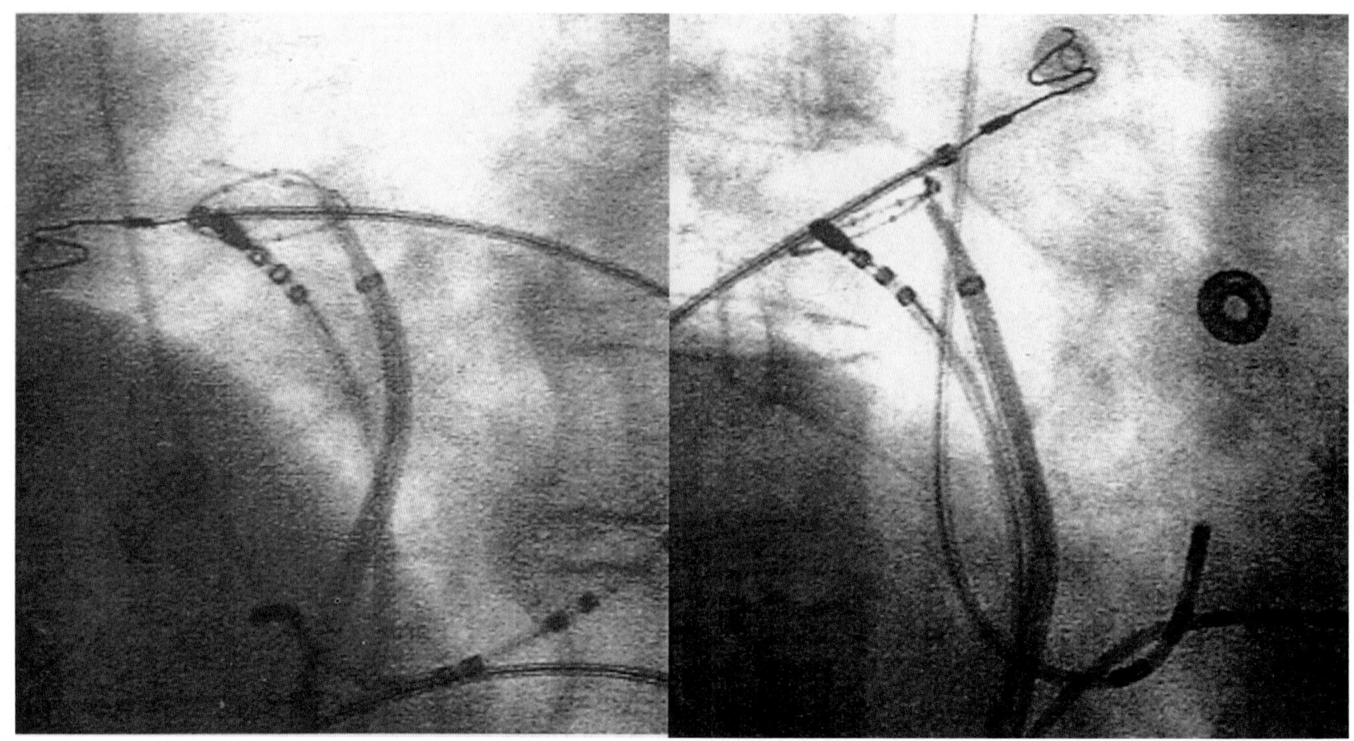


FIGURE 29-17 Left anterior oblique (*left*) and right anterior oblique fluoroscopic views of a circular mapping catheter placed in the right superior pulmonary vein of a patient with paroxysmal atrial fibrillation. A quadripolar ablation catheter is used to apply radiofrequency current to a site at the pulmonary vein ostium near the electrodes recording earliest activation of the pulmonary veins during sinus rhythm.

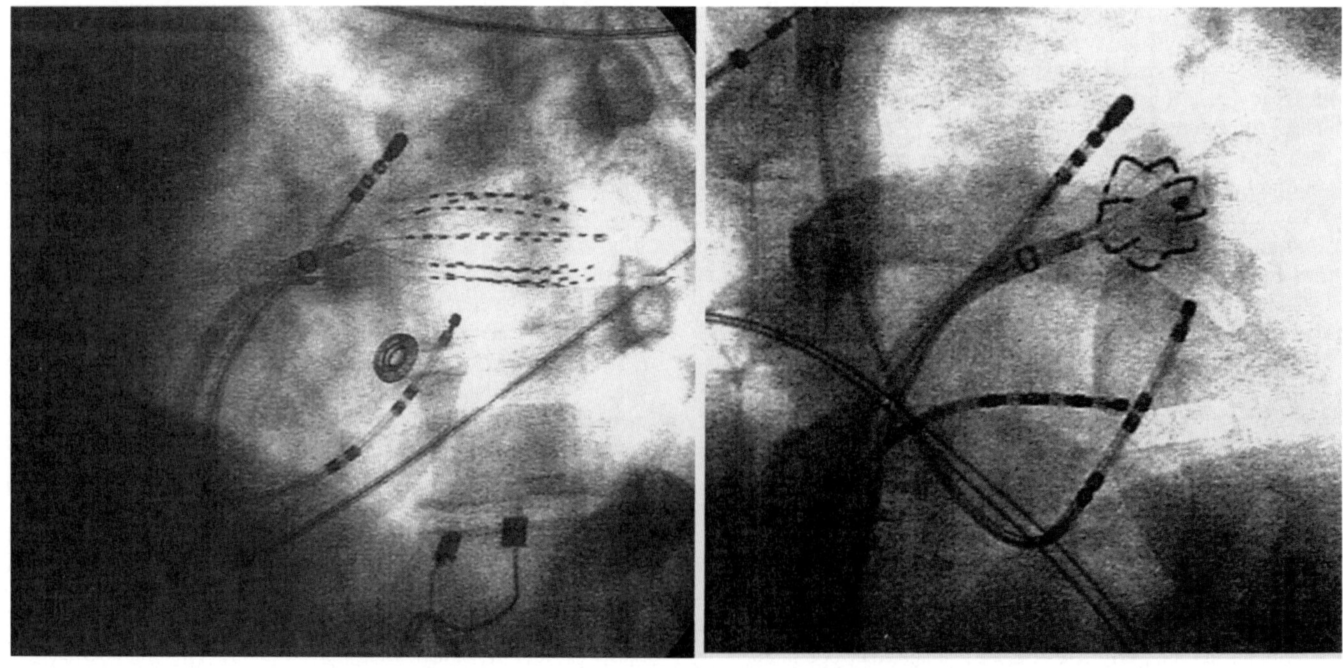


FIGURE 29-18 Left anterior oblique and right anterior oblique radiographic images of a 64-electrode basket catheter positioned in the left inferior pulmonary vein.

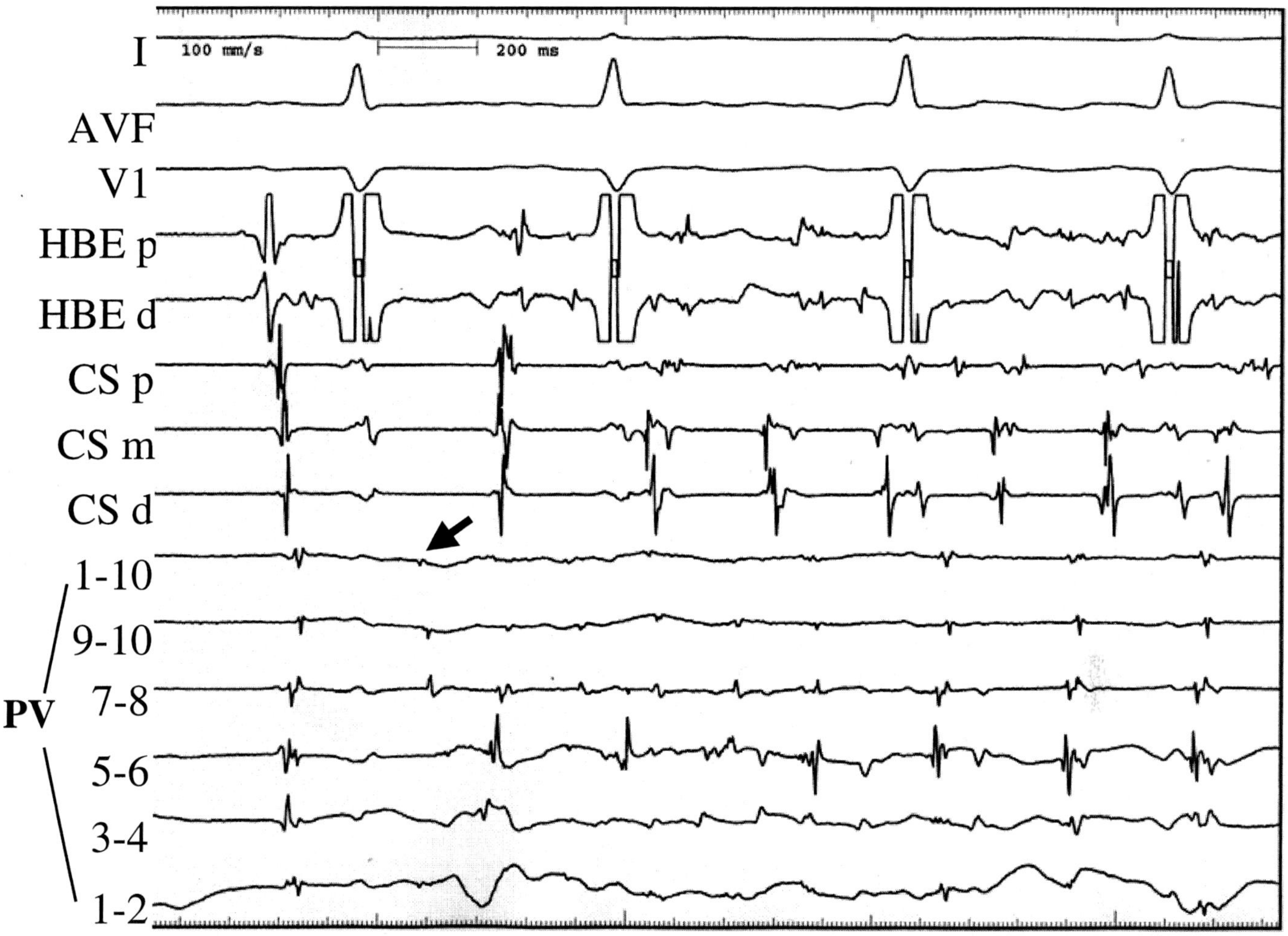


FIGURE 29-19 Spontaneous onset of atrial fibrillation by rapid firing from a pulmonary vein. The onset of atrial fibrillation (*arrow*) is produced by rapid firing from the pulmonary vein 1-10 electrode pair of a circular mapping catheter in the pulmonary vein (PV). Note that pulmonary vein activity occurs before the coronary sinus electrograms (CS). HBE p and HBE d represent His bundle electrograms.

## Pacing

It is clear from both retrospective and prospective studies of atrial-based versus ventricular-based pacing that there is a higher risk of developing atrial fibrillation and stroke in patients receiving single-chamber, ventricular-based pacemakers (VVI or VVIR). However, it remains to be proven whether this is an adverse effect of VVI(R) pacing or an antiarrhythmic effect of atrial-based pacing. Perhaps the most useful aspect of permanent pacemaker implantation for patients with paroxysmal or persistent atrial fibrillation is that atrial-based pacemakers often allow the use of higher doses of antiarrhythmic drugs to be prescribed since sinus node dysfunction is treated. Several small clinical trials suggest that algorithms designed to increase the atrial pacing rate in response to intrinsic atrial beats (dynamic atrial overdrive) may produce a statistically significant reduction in the frequency of symptomatic atrial fibrillation in patients undergoing pacemaker implantation. Whether this is a clinically significant reduction in the burden of atrial fibrillation has not been established. Dual-site right atrial pacing with placement of pacing leads in the right atrial appendage and near the coronary sinus ostium may have a modest beneficial effect to reduce the frequency of paroxysmal atrial fibrillation when combined with antiarrhythmic drugs.[199] Pacing from the interatrial septum or Bachmann's bundle may also reduce the frequency of atrial fibrillation in patients requiring permanent pacemaker implantation.[200] Thus, patients with paroxysmal or persistent atrial fibrillation who have a standard indication for permanent pacemaker implantation may benefit from atrial-based pacing with either dual-site right atrial pacing or interatrial septal pacing. The use of an algorithm for overdrive atrial stimulation may further help to decrease the frequency of atrial fibrillation.

# ATRIAL FLUTTER

## Electrocardiographic Characteristics

Atrial flutter is characterized by rapid regular atrial activation with an atrial rate that is usually >240 beats per minute unless slowed by antiarrhythmic medications. The ventricular response depends on the status of atrioventricular nodal conduction. Atrial flutter may be categorized as typical or atypical based on the morphology of the flutter waves. An older scheme divided atrial flutter into types I or II, based on atrial rate.[201] It is now known that the predominant mechanism of atrial flutter is right atrial macroreentry with circular activation

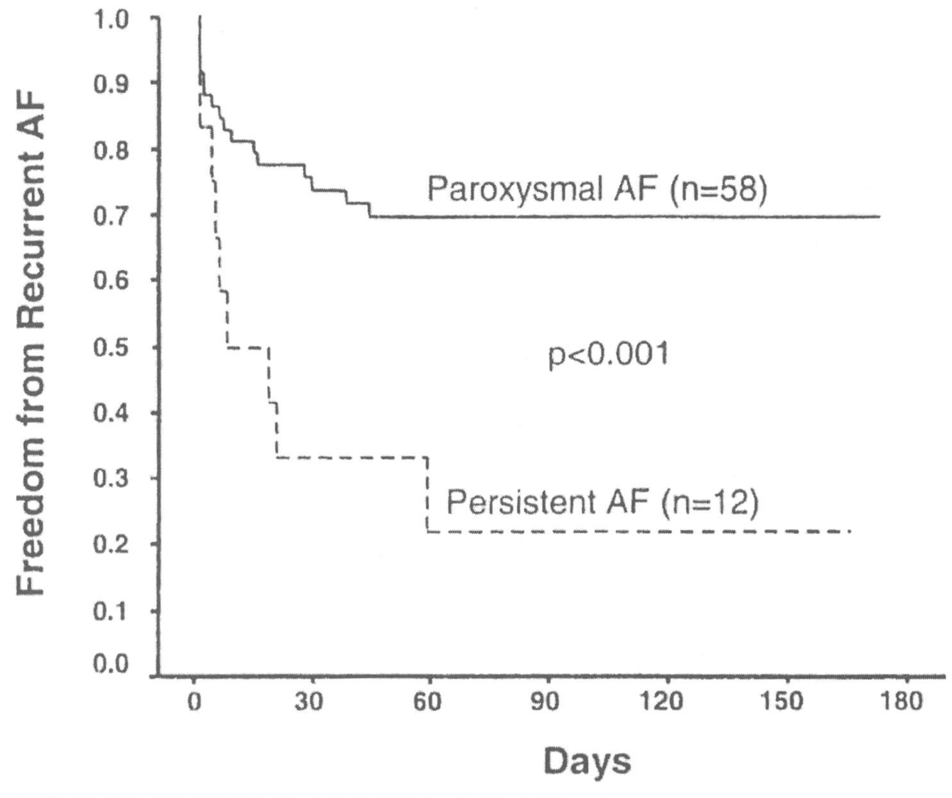


FIGURE 29-20 Freedom from recurrence of paroxysmal or persistent atrial fibrillation after segmental pulmonary vein isolation. (Adapted from Oral et al.[188] With permission.)

bounded by the tricuspid annulus anteriorly, the crista terminalis posteriorly, and the eustachian ridge inferiorly.[202] Reentry is produced by unidirectional block and slow conduction in the low right atrial isthmus between the inferior vena cava, eustachian ridge, coronary sinus ostium, and tricuspid valve.[203–206] It is more clinically relevant to divide flutter into isthmus-dependent and non-isthmus-dependent types. During typical isthmus-dependent atrial flutter, the rotation of right atrial activation is counterclockwise (as viewed from the left anterior oblique projection), producing sawtooth inverted flutter waves in electrocardiographic (ECG) leads II, III, and aVF and upright flutter waves in lead $V_1$ (Fig. 29-21). Reversal of the right atrial circuit with clockwise isthmus-dependent atrial flutter produces flutter waves that are upright in the inferior ECG leads and inverted in lead $V_1$. Other mechanisms of atrial flutter, such as reentry in the left atrium and reentry around surgical incisions in the atria, are seen less commonly and will also produce atypical flutter waves. In general, if the flutter waves have the same polarity in lead aVF and lead $V_1$, the mechanism is unlikely to be isthmus-dependent (Fig. 29-22).

## Epidemiology

The incidence of atrial flutter in the general population has been estimated to be 88 per 100,000.[207] Many patients with atrial flutter have also had atrial fibrillation, and the majority of cases occur in the setting of either a predisposing condition or structural heart disease. The risk of developing atrial flutter is also increased by a history of heart failure. Recent open heart surgery is a particularly common predisposing factor, especially in the elderly.[208] The prophylactic administration of beta-blocking agents reduces the occurrence of atrial flutter after coronary artery bypass surgery[209] and diltiazem reduces its incidence after major thoracic operations.[210] Atrial flutters due to mechanisms other than tricuspid annular reentry are most commonly associated with advanced atrial pathology such as a previous atrial incision for the repair of congential heart disease or as residua from catheter or surgical procedures for the ablation of atrial fibrillation.

## Pathophysiology

Animal models of atrial flutter[211–213] have shown the importance of anatomic obstacles in the formation of atrial flutter reentry circuits. Transient entrainment and interruption of atrial flutter by atrial pacing have shown that human atrial flutter is an intraatrial reentrant tachycardia with an excitable gap.[214] The reentrant circuit of typical atrial flutter is confined to the right atrium, with secondary activation of the left atrium.[215] As viewed from the left anterior oblique projection, the reentrant circuit during typical atrial flutter circulates counterclockwise in a caudocranial direction along the interatrial septum and in a craniocaudal direction along the right atrial free wall. The circuit can also be activated in a clockwise direction. An area of slow conduction and unidirectional block is present in an isthmus between the tricuspid annulus and the eustachian ridge.[216] Marked anisotropy due to transverse myocardial fiber orientation in the eustachian ridge is thought to be responsible for the conduction delay and block that occur in this isthmus.[217] The two functional boundaries that serve to maintain atrial flutter are the crista terminalis and the eustachian ridge. At rapid pacing rates, the crista terminalis becomes refractory to transverse conduction, thereby creating a protected corridor along the free wall of the right atrium bounded by the crista terminalis posteriorly and the tricuspid annulus anteriorly. The second functional barrier provided by the eustachian ridge forces the atrial flutter circuit between the coronary sinus ostium and the tricuspid annulus. Both of these functional barriers tend to permit conduction across themselves at slow rates but prevent conduction at high rates. This fact helps to explain why atrial flutter is virtually always induced by another tachyarrhythmia such as atrial tachycardia or atrial fibrillation and does not arise as a de novo arrhythmia. Antiarrhythmic drugs that slow atrial conduction, such as the class IC agents, tend to promote the development of atrial flutter by further contributing to the development of these functional barriers. And it is not uncommon for patients receiving these drugs for the treatment of atrial fibrillation to develop atrial flutter.

Atypical atrial flutters that do not depend on the cavotricuspid isthmus often involve reentry around surgical obstacles such as suture lines in the right atrium or around large sheets of scarred myocardium in either atrium related to diffuse atrial pathology. These are particularly common in patients with congenital heart disease such as those who have undergone the Fontan operation, after intraatrial baffle surgery (Senning or Mustard operations), after lung transplantation surgery, or after linear catheter ablation. In nearly all of these cases, an isthmus of conduction can be identified that is amenable to catheter ablation.

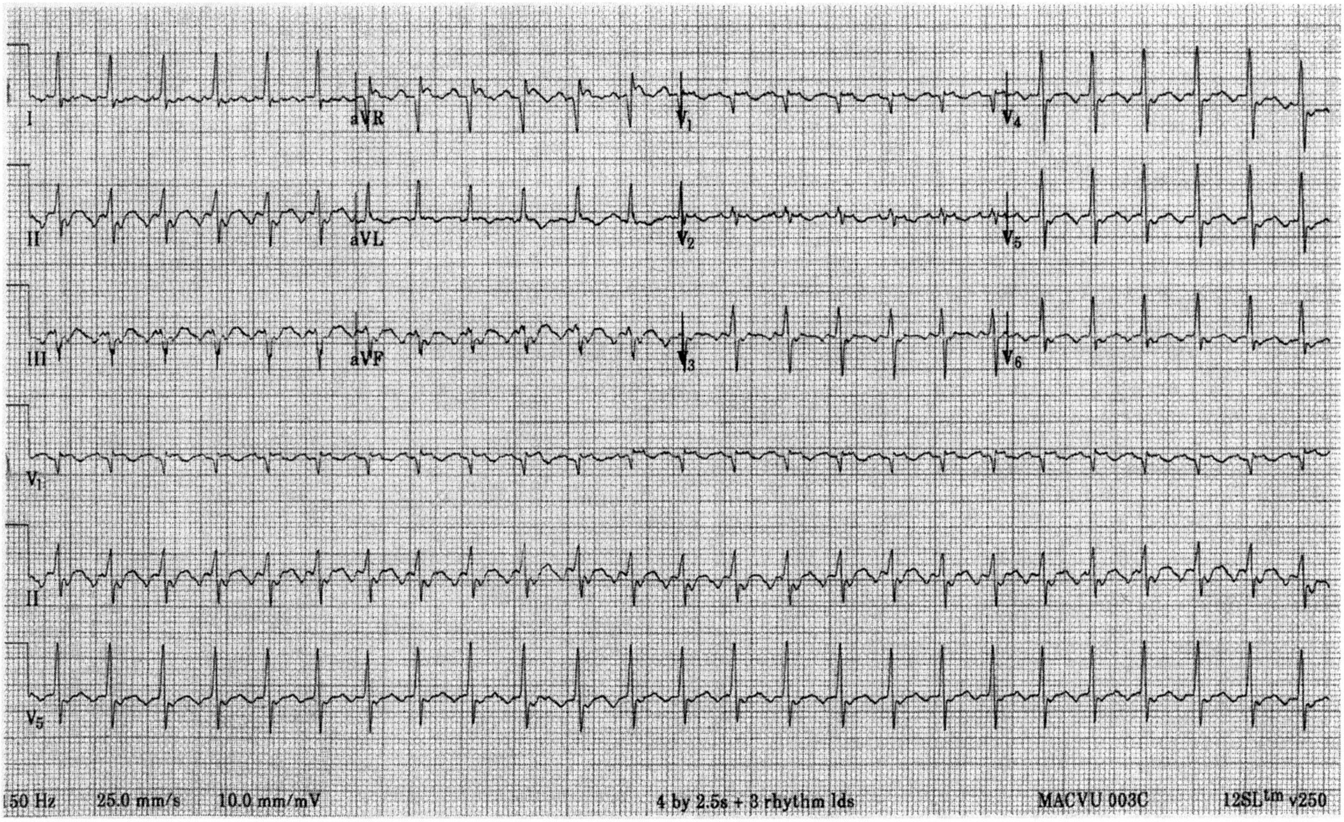

I aVR V1 V4

II aVL V2 V5

III aVF V3 V6

V1

II

V5

150 Hz 25.0 mm/s 10.0 mm/mV 4 by 2.5s + 3 rhythm lds MACVU 003C 12SL™ v250

FIGURE 29-21 Twelve-lead electrocardiogram of typical atrial flutter. Note the negative flutter waves in leads II, III, and aVF and the upright flutter waves in lead $V_1$. This is characteristic of counterclockwise, isthmus-dependent atrial flutter.

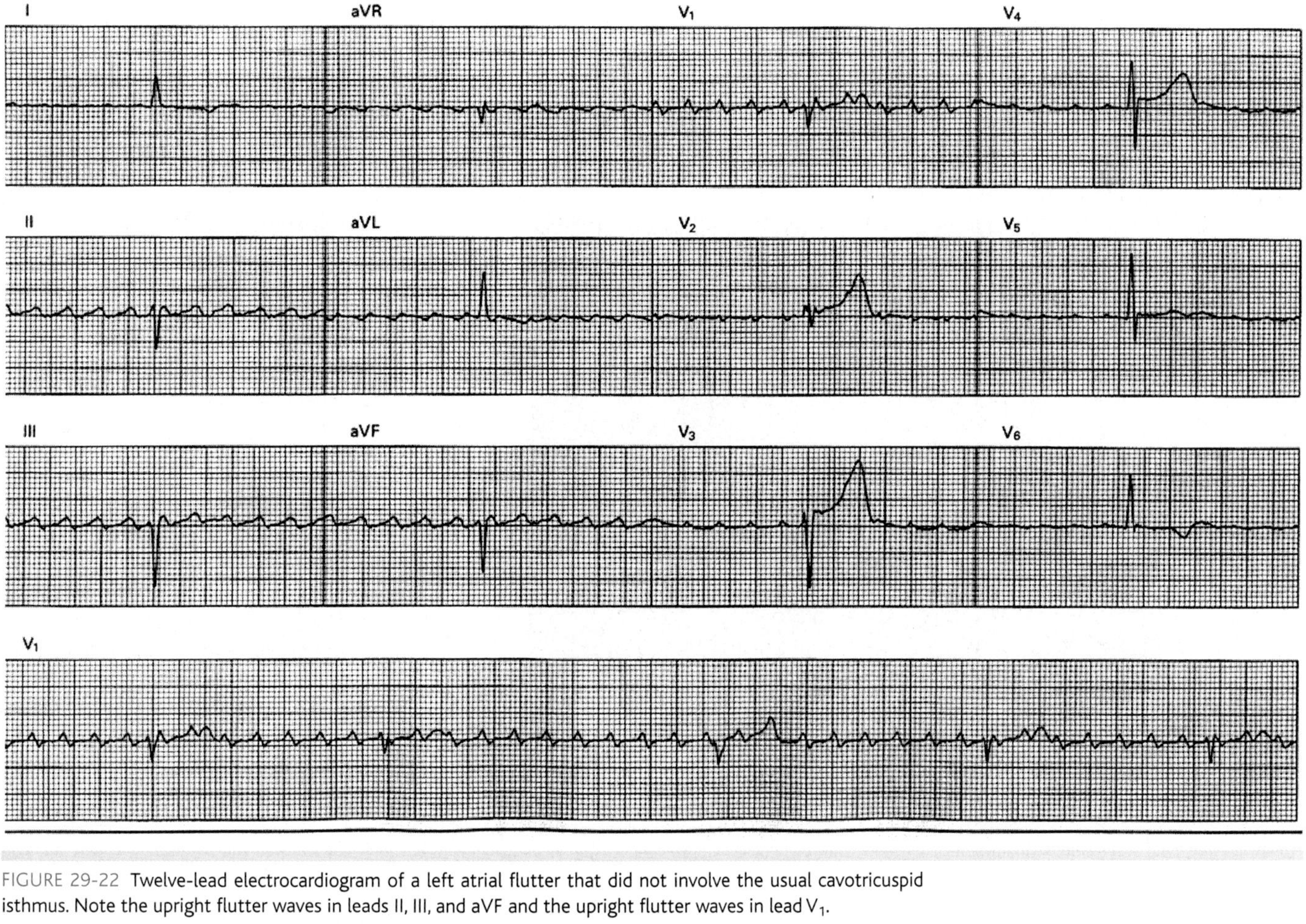

I aVR $V_1$ $V_4$

II aVL $V_2$ $V_5$

III aVF $V_3$ $V_6$

$V_1$

FIGURE 29-22 Twelve-lead electrocardiogram of a left atrial flutter that did not involve the usual cavotricuspid isthmus. Note the upright flutter waves in leads II, III, and aVF and the upright flutter waves in lead $V_1$.

## Management

Presenting symptoms in atrial flutter are largely related to the ventricular rate. Although some patients are asymptomatic, most are not. Symptoms of palpitations, dizziness, dyspnea, weakness, fatigue, angina, syncope, worsening heart failure, or even cardiogenic shock may be present. Even when patients are initally symptomatic, uncontrolled rapid rates can lead to progressive left ventricular dysfunction due to a tachycardia-mediated cardiomyopathy. The diagnosis of atrial flutter should be considered in the differential diagnosis of most supraventricular tachycardias. Since flutter waves can be difficult to identify on the ECG during a tachycardia and the atrial rate in atrial flutter may be slowed by antiarrhythmic therapy or advanced atrial pathology, atrial flutter may present with a wide range of atrial rates and ventricular responses yet have the same basic mechanism. Typically, atrial flutter presents with some degree of AV conduction block—i.e., 2 : 1 or 4 : 1 AV conduction (even conduction ratios are most common). The ventricular response may be regular, regularly irregular, or irregularly irregular. Atrial flutter with 1 : 1 AV conduction can rarely occur in otherwise normal hearts when AV conduction is enhanced and is a potentially life-threatening complication in the Wolff-Parkinson-White syndrome if an accessory pathway has a short antegrade refractory period and is capable of rapid antegrade conduction. AV conduction that is 1 : 1 can also develop as a complication of antiarrhythmic drug therapy, with slowing of the atrial rate, thereby allowing the AV node to conduct each of the circulating wavefronts. Class IC antiarrhythmic agents are particularly likely to cause this complication.[218] When there is antegrade conduction over an accessory pathway, the QRS is wide with marked ventricular preexcitation. Otherwise the QRS is narrow unless bundle branch block is present.

The flutter waves usually have a constant cycle length and intracardiac electrogram morphology with an isoelectric baseline between successive complexes. When the atrial activity cannot be clearly identified, carotid sinus massage or the parenteral administration of AV node blocking agents such as adenosine, esmolol, verapamil, or diltiazem can be used to increase the degree of AV block and expose the underlying flutter waves. If adenosine is used for this purpose, one must be aware that atrial fibrillation may be induced, because this drug shortens the atrial effective refractory period. There are also case reports of accelerated AV conduction following adenosine requiring emergency cardioversion.[219] When the diagnosis remains uncertain, the recording of an atrial electrogram from either the esophagus or from endocardial or epicardial electrodes will allow the diagnosis to be made.

### ACUTE TREATMENT

Treatment of atrial flutter requires control of the ventricular rate and interruption of the reentrant circuit. Intravenous calcium channel blockers (verapamil or diltiazem)[220,221] or beta blockers[222] can be titrated to achieve an acute slowing of the ventricular rate with later conversion to oral therapy. The acute termination of atrial flutter can be attempted by intravenous drug therapy, by rapid atrial pacing techniques, by direct-current cardioversion, or by acute catheter ablation. Ibutilide is successful in terminating most episodes of atrial flutter of recent onset, but it precipitates sustained or nonsustained polymorphic ventricular tachycardia in approximately 3.6 percent of patients.[223] Rapid atrial pacing can effectively terminate typical atrial flutter[224] and can be instituted via esophageal electrode, via transvenous electrode (permanent lead or temporary electrode), or by epicardial electrodes. A critical pacing rate is required, usually 115 to 125 percent of the spontaneous atrial rate. The conversion of atrial flutter to sinus rhythm by atrial pacing is enhanced by pretreatment with antiarrhythmic drug therapy using class 1A or 1C agents.[225–227] Synchronized electrical direct-current cardioversion is a highly effective method to terminate atrial flutter and usually requires lower energy than termination of atrial fibrillation.[228,229] Patients in distress with extremely rapid ventricular responses should be rapidly treated by direct-current cardioversion after intravenous sedation.[230] As with atrial fibrillation, patients with atrial flutter of more than 48 h duration should be anticoagulated before and after cardioversion. Transesophageal echocardiography may be very useful in allowing prompter cardioversion, though anticoagulation is indicated after the procedure, as with atrial fibrillation.

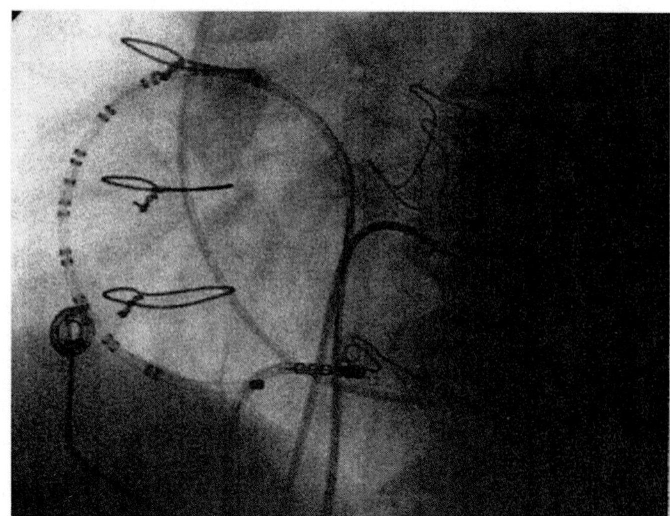


FIGURE 29-23 Left anterior oblique fluoroscopic view of a circular 20-electrode catheter placed in the right atrium to record electrical activation. A quadripolar ablation catheter is placed along the tricuspid valve annulus near the coronary sinus ostium.

### CHRONIC TREATMENT

Radiofrequency ablation of atrial flutter is the treatment of choice for patients with symptomatic atrial flutter without a clearly identifiable transient, reversible cause.[231–237] The strategy for ablation of atrial flutter is interruption of the critical isthmus between the inferior vena cava, the coronary sinus ostium, and the tricuspid annulus. The goal of atrial flutter ablation is to create bidirectional conduction block in this isthmus (Figs. 29-23 and 29-24). Failure to achieve complete conduction block in the low right atrial isthmus is associated with the recurrence of atrial flutter.[238,239] Paroxysmal atrial fibrillation coexists with atrial flutter in up to 30 percent of patients, and patients undergoing radiofrequency ablation of atrial flutter are at risk for the later development of atrial fibrillation.[240,241] In view of the high procedural success rate and a very low risk of complica-

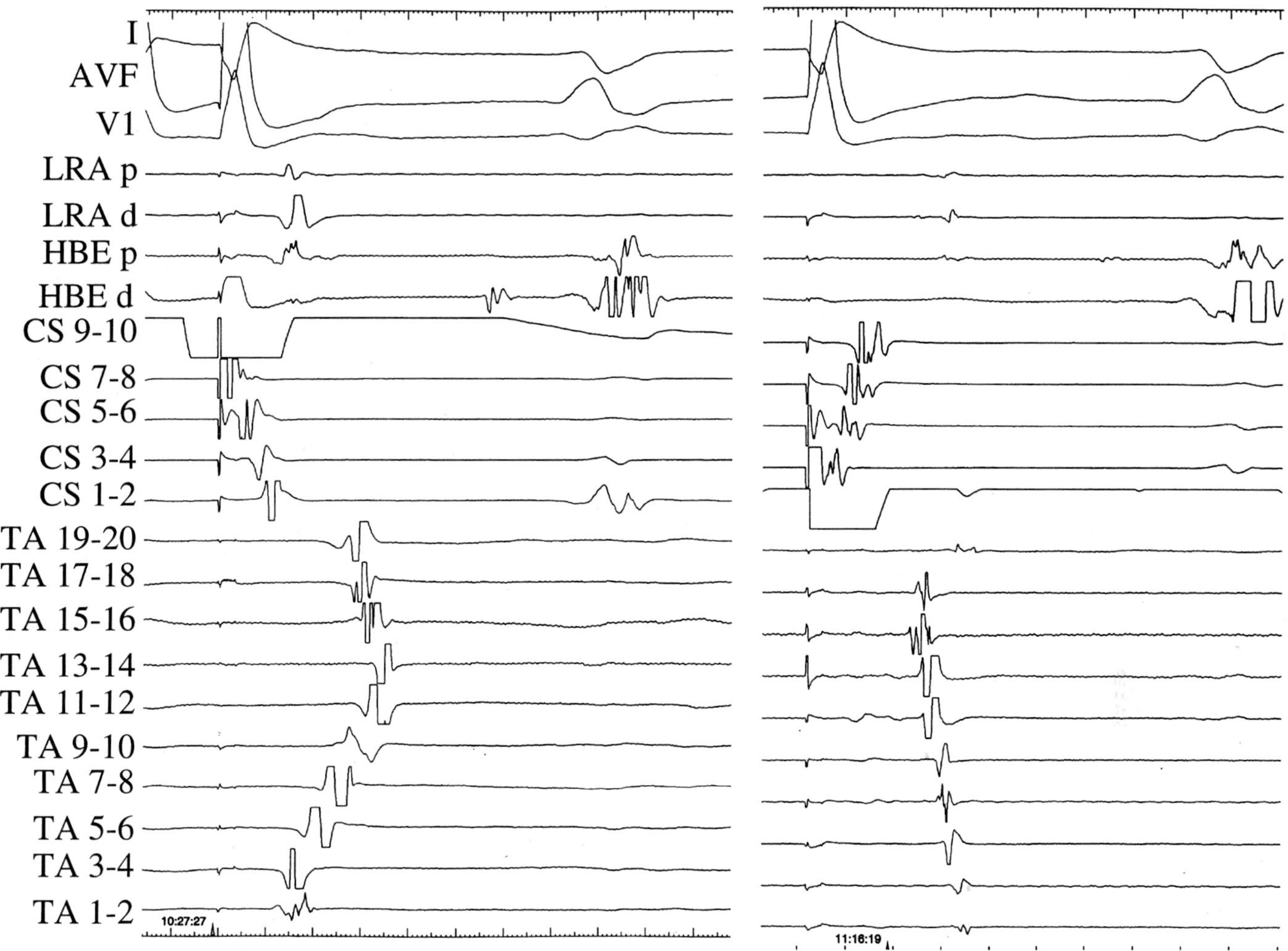


FIGURE 29-24 Intracardiac electrograms before (*left*) and after (*right*) catheter ablation of the cavotricuspid isthmus as recorded from a circular catheter around the tricuspid annulus (TA 19-20 through TA 1-2). Electrode pair 1-2 is located close to the coronary sinus ostium. During pacing from the coronary sinus 9-10 (CS 9-10) electrode pair, there are two wavefronts of activation around the tricuspid annulus, as noted by early activation of the tricuspid annulus catheter at electrode pairs 19-20 and 1-2 with collision of wavefronts at electrode pair TA 13-14. After ablation of the cavotricuspid isthmus, activation proceeds from electrode pair TA 19-20 progressively, later to finally activate electrode pair TA 1-2. This indicates conduction block within the isthmus.

tions, radiofrequency ablation of atrial flutter should be considered as the therapy of first choice for both acute and chronic cases in the absence of reversible causes such as pericarditis, hyperthyroidism, or recent cardiac surgery. The frequent coexistence of atrial flutter and atrial fibrillation makes concomitant ablation of atrial flutter advisable in many patients undergoing ablation of atrial fibrillation. A subset of patients with successful suppression of atrial fibrillation by antiarrhythmic therapy but with spontaneous atrial flutter should be considered for atrial flutter ablation and continued effective antiarrhythmic treatment of the atrial fibrillation.[242,243] Atrial flutter not due to macroreentry around the tricuspid annulus can also be ablated, but the success rate is lower.[244] Anticoagulation is advised for patients with chronic atrial flutter and standard coexisting risk factors such as advanced age, hypertension, diabetes mellitus, left atrial enlargement, or prior systemic embolism.[3] However, the risk of systemic emboli is probably less than for chronic atrial fibrillation.[245] The acute conversion of atrial flutter should usually be followed by systemic anticoagulation for a few weeks even in the absence of coexistent atrial fibrillation. Chronic anticoagulation is advised in the large proportion of patients with atrial fibrillation despite the successful ablation of atrial flutter.

## ATRIAL TACHYCARDIAS

Atrial tachycardias are less common than either atrial flutter or atrial fibrillation. They are not dependent on AV nodal conduction for their perpetuation and may involve variable degrees of AV block. The electrocardiographic diagnosis of atrial tachycardia is made by a supraventricular tachycardia that usually has sudden onset and offset, with a P-wave morphology that is typically different from that recorded during sinus rhythm (Fig. 29-25). However, the P wave may be similar or even identical to the sinus rhythm P wave if the site of origin of the tachycardia is near (or involves) the sinus node. The presence of AV block during the tachycardia is highly suggestive of an atrial tachycardia. While the P-wave morphology is typically constant during atrial tachycardias, a changing P-wave morphology and atrial rate are typical of multifocal atrial tachycardia. Differentiation of atrial tachycardias from atrial flutter can occasionally be problematic, though most atrial tachycardias have a distinct isoelectric segment on the surface electrocardiogram between P waves, whereas atrial flutters usually do not. In addition, the typically sawtooth flutter-wave morphology cannot be identified in atrial tachycardias.

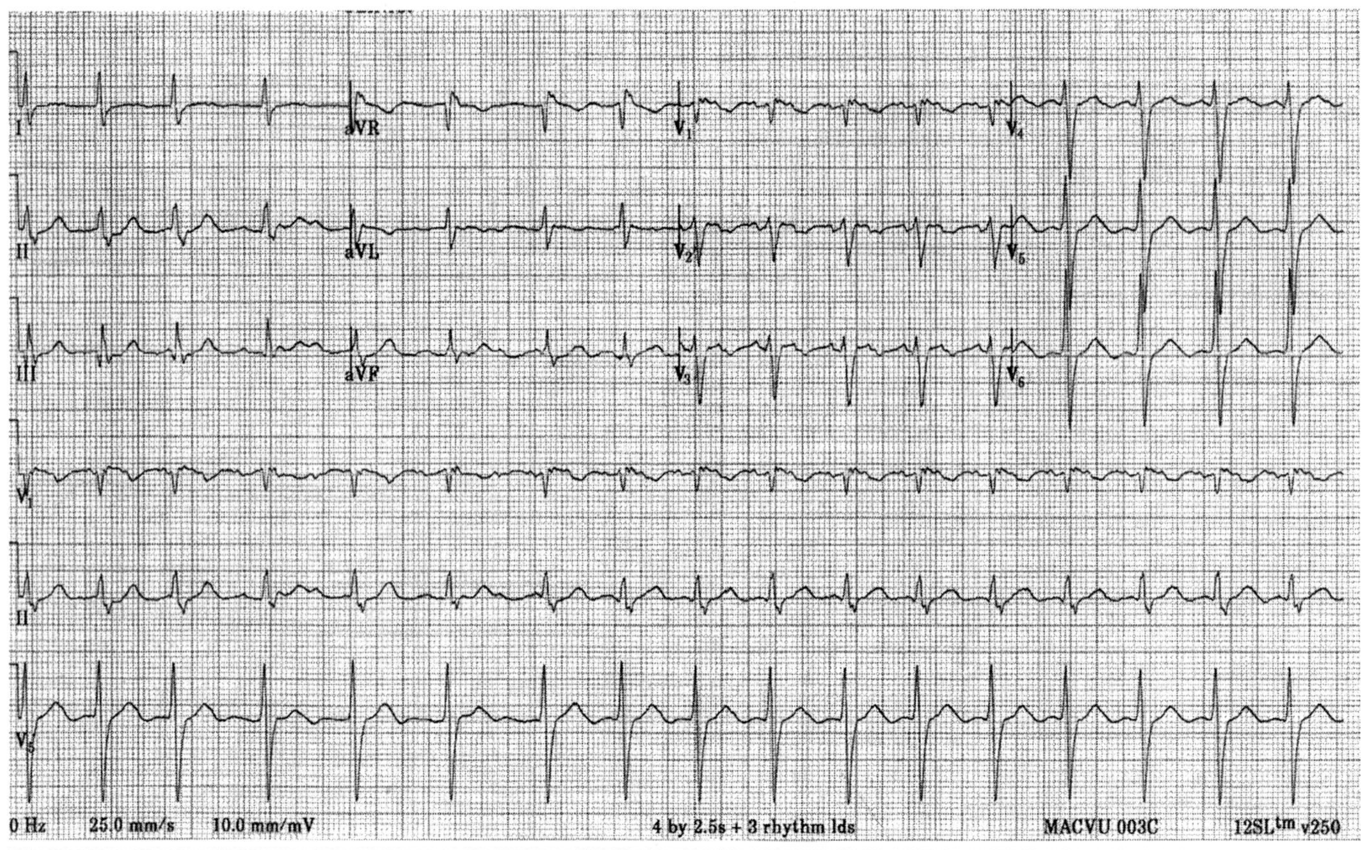


FIGURE 29-25 Surface electrocardiogram of an atrial tachycardia involving the right atrium. Note the discrete P waves with 2 : 1 AV conduction.

The mechanism of atrial tachycardia can be either intraatrial reentry, a focal firing related to abnormal automaticity, or triggered activity.[246–248] In patients without structural heart disease, a focal mechanism predominates. In patients with advanced atrial disease, such as after surgery for congenital heart disease, intraatrial reentry is a more common mechanism.[249–253] A relatively uncommon form of atrial tachycardia that mimics sinus tachycardia involves reentry within the region of the sinus node (sinus node reentrant tachycardia). This arrhythmia is more likely to occur in elderly patients and has a P-wave morphology closely resembling that of sinus tachycardia. Sinus node reentrant tachycardia can be distinguished from sinus tachycardia by its characteristic sudden onset and termination. Sinus node reentrant tachycardia can be induced and terminated by programmed atrial stimulation, whereas sinus tachycardia cannot. In addition, the PR interval typically lengthens during sinus node reentrant tachycardia but shortens during sinus tachycardia. The site of origin of focal atrial tachycardias is often along the crista terminalis within the right atrium.[254] Other common sites for focal atrial tachycardias are within the triangle of Koch near the AV node,[255,256] within the musculature of the coronary sinus,[257] within the pulmonary veins, or along the mitral valve annulus in the left atrium.[253] The P-wave morphology reflects the site of origin within the atria. Thus, if the origin is along the crista terminalis in the right atrium, the P wave is typically upright in leads I and aVL and inverted in lead aVR. If the P wave is inverted in lead I and aVL and upright in lead aVR, a left atrial origin is suggested. A coronary sinus origin may be suspected in the presence of a P wave that is strongly negative in leads II, III, and aVF while being biphasic in both aVL and aVR. An origin near the region of the AV node is suggested by a very short P-wave duration of low amplitude in the inferior leads with similar polarity in both aVL and aVR.

## Clinical Manifestations

Most atrial tachycardias produce symptoms of rapid palpitations, though patients may be asymptomatic if there is 2 : 1 AV conduction with a well-controlled ventricular rate or 1 : 1 AV conduction with a relatively slow atrial and ventricular rate. Atrial tachycardias may present as a tachycardia-induced cardiomyopathy if the ventricular rate exceeds 120 bears per minute for a period of several months. Tachycardia-induced cardiomyopathy is an especially common presentation in children and young adults with incessant atrial tachycardia. Focal mechanisms of atrial tachycardia often demonstrate considerable variability in the atrial rate, with slowing during periods of rest and acceleration during exercise.[258]

## Management

Atrial tachycardias that are symptomatic are initially treated by AV nodal blocking agents. However, if the atrial rate is less than 150 beats per minute, it may be difficult to achieve 2 : 1 AV conduction with AV nodal blocking drugs such as beta blockers or calcium channel antagonists. If the mechanism of an incessant atrial tachycardia is focal, treatment with antiarrhythmic drugs is notoriously ineffective. These tachycardias cannot be interrupted by overdrive pacing or cardioversion, and antiarrhythmic medications are usually ineffective. For patients with rapid ventricular rates that cannot be adequately controlled with drugs that block the AV node, catheter ablation is the treatment of choice. Catheter ablation involves mapping of the site of earliest atrial activation and pacing techniques to prove that intra-atrial reentry is not the underlying mechanism. After identification of the site of earliest atrial activation during a focal mechanism of atrial tachycardia, radiofrequency current is applied. The typical response to catheter ablation is an acceleration of the atrial tachycardia rate (due to heating of the focus), followed by abrupt termination.

Intraatrial reentrant tachycardias may respond to class I or III antiarrhythmic medications. These drugs typically slow the atrial rate or interrupt the tachycardia. Catheter ablation of intraatrial reentrant tachycardias is usually reserved for patients who fail antiarrhythmic drugs. When the mechanism of an atrial tachycardia is reentry within the atria, extensive mapping is required to identify an isthmus of atrial tissue within the circuit that can be targeted for ablation. Ablation involves the application of radiofrequency current within an isthmus of atrial tissue that is bounded by anatomic obstacles.[252,253] The typical response to the application of radiofrequency current within a protected isthmus that supports atrial tachycardia is gradual slowing followed by termination of the tachycardia.

## References


1. Chugh SS, Blackshear JL, Shen W-K, et al. Epidemiology and natural history of atrial fibrillation: clinical implications. *J Am Coll Cardiol* 2001;37:371–378.
2. Kopecky SL, Gersh BJ, McGoon MD, et al. The natural history of lone atrial fibrillation. A population-based study over three decades. *N Engl J Med* 1987;317:669–674.
3. Fuster V, Ryden LE, Asinger RW, et al. ACC/AHA/ESC Guidelines for the management of patients with atrial fibrillation: Executive summary. A report of the American College of Cardiology/American Heart Association Task Force of Practice Guidelines and the European Society of Cardiology Committee for Practice Guidelines and Policy Conferences (Committee to Develop Guidelines for the Management of Patients with Atrial Fibrillation. *Circulation* 2001;104: 2118–2150.
4. Levy S. Nomenclature of atrial fibrillation or the Tower of Babel. *J Cardiovasc Electrophysiol* 1998;9(8 suppl):S83–S85.
5. Levy S. Classification system of atrial fibrillation. *Curr Opin Cardiol* 2000;15:54–57.
6. Bialy D, Lehmann MH, Schumacher DN, et al. Hospitalization for arrhythmias in the United States: Importance of atrial fibrillation (abstr). *J Am Coll Cardiol* 1992;19:41A.
7. Furberg CD, Psaty BM, Manolio TA, et al. Prevalence of atrial fibrillation in elderly subjects (the Cardiovascular Health Study). *Am J Cardiol* 1994;74:236–241.
8. Kannel WB, Abbott RD, Savage DD, McNamara PM. Coronary heart disease and atrial fibrillation: The Framingham Study. *Am Heart J* 1983;106:389–396.
9. Psaty BM, Manolio TA, Kuller LH, et al. Incidence of and risk factors for atrial fibrillation in older adults. *Circulation* 1997;96:2455–2461.
10. Ostranderld JR, Brandt RL, Kjelsberg MO, Epstein FH. Electrocardiographic findings among the adult population of a total natural community, Tecumseh, Michigan. *Circulation* 1965;31:888–898.
11. Wolf PA, Abbott RD, Kannel WB. Atrial fibrillation as an independent risk factor for stroke: The Framingham Study. *Stroke* 1991;22: 983–988.
12. Flegel KM, Shipley MJ, Rose G. Risk of stroke in non-rheumatic atrial fibrillation. *Lancet* 1987;1:526–529.
13. Brand FN, Abbott RD, Kannel WB, Wolf PA. Characteristics and prognosis of lone atrial fibrillation. 30-year follow-up in the Framingham Study. *JAMA* 1985;254:3449–3453.
14. Levy S, Maarek M, Coumel P, et al. Characterization of different subsets of atrial fibrillation in general practice in France: the ALFA study. The College of French Cardiologists. *Circulation* 1999;99:3028–3035.
15. Murgatroyd FD, Gibson SM, Baiyan X, et al. Double-blind placebo-controlled trial of digoxin in symptomatic paroxysmal atrial fibrillation. *Circulation* 1999;99:2765–2770.
16. Evans W, Swann P. Lone auricular fibrillation. *Br Heart J* 1954;16: 189–194.
17. Benjamin EJ, Levy D, Vaziri SM, et al. Independent risk factors for atrial fibrillation in a population-based cohort: The Framingham Heart Study. *JAMA* 1994;271:840–844.
18. Benjamin EJ, Levy D, Vaziri SM, et al. Independent risk factors for atrial fibrillation in a population-based cohort. The Framingham Heart Study. *JAMA* 1994;271:840–844.
19. Vaziri SM, Larson MG, Benjamin EJ, Levy D. Echocardiographic predictors of nonrheumatic atrial fibrillation: the Framingham Heart study. *Circulation* 1994;89:724–730.
20. Tsang TSM, Gersch BJ, Appleton CP, et al. Left ventricular diastolic dysfunction as a predictor of the first diagnosed nonvalvular atrial fibrillation in 840 elderly men and women. *J Am Coll Cardiol* 2002; 40:1636–1644.
21. Krahn AD, Manfreda J, Tate RB, et al. The natural history of atrial fibrillation: Incidence, risk factors, and prognosis in the Manitoba follow-up study. *Am J Med* 1995;98:476–484.
22. Wolf PA, Abbott RD, Kannel WB. Atrial fibrillation: A major contributor to stroke in the elderly. The Framingham Study. *Arch Intern Med* 1987;147:1561–1564.
23. Risk factors for stroke and efficacy of antithrombotic therapy in atrial fibrillation. Analysis of pooled data from five randomized controlled trials [published erratum appears in *Arch Intern Med* 1994 Oct 10;154(19):2254]. *Arch Intern Med* 1994;154:1449–1457.
24. Hart RG, Halperin JL. Atrial fibrillation and thromboembolism: A decade of progress in stroke prevention. *Ann Intern Med* 1999;131: 688–695.
25. Wolf PA, Dawber TR, Thomas HE Jr, Kannel WB. Epidemiologic assessment of chronic atrial fibrillation and risk of stroke: the Framingham study. *Neurology* 1978;28:973–977.
26. Feinberg WM, Seeger JF, Carmody RF, et al. Epidemiologic features of asymptomatic cerebral infarction in patients with nonvalvular atrial fibrillation. *Arch Intern Med* 1990;150:2340–2344.
27. Kempster PA, Gerraty RP, Gates PC. Asymptomatic cerebral infarction in patients with chronic atrial fibrillation. *Stroke* 1988;19:955–957.
28. Stroke Prevention in Atrial Fibrillation Study. Final results. *Circulation* 1991;84:527–539.
29. Petersen P, Madsen EB, Brun B, et al. Silent cerebral infarction in chronic atrial fibrillation. *Stroke* 1987;18:1098–1100.
30. Savage DD, Seides SF, Maron BJ, et al. Prevalence of arrhythmias during 24-hour electrocardiographic monitoring and exercise testing in patients with obstructive and nonobstructive hypertrophic cardiomyopathy. *Circulation* 1979;59:866–875.
31. Russell JW, Biller J, Hajduczok ZD, et al. Ischemic cerebrovascular complications and risk factors in idiopathic hypertrophic subaortic stenosis. *Stroke* 1991;22:1143–1147.
32. Robinson K, Frenneaux MP, Stockins B, et al. Atrial fibrillation in hypertrophic cardiomyopathy: A longitudinal study. *J Am Coll Cardiol* 1990;15:1279–1285.
33. Higashikawa M, Nakamura Y, Yoshida M, Kinoshita M. Incidence of ischemic strokes in hypertrophic cardiomyopathy is markedly increased if complicated by atrial fibrillation. *Jpn Circ J* 1997;61:673–681.
34. Lip GY, Beevers DG. ABCs of atrial fibrillation: history, epidemiology and importance of atrial fibrillation. *Br Med J* 1995;311:1361–1363.
35. Allessie MA, Boyden PA, Camm AJ, et al. Pathophysiology and prevention of atrial fibrillation. *Circulation* 2001;103:769–777.
36. Jais P, Haissaguerre M, Shah DC, et al. A focal source of atrial fibrillation treated by discrete radiofrequency ablation. *Circulation* 1997;95:572–576.
37. Haissaguerre M, Jais P, Shah DC, et al. Spontaneous initiation of atrial fibrillation by ectopic beats originating in the pulmonary veins. *N Engl J Med* 1998;339:659–666.
38. Chen SA, Hseih MH, Tai CT, et al. Initiation of atrial fibrillation by ectopic beats originating from the pulmonary veins : electrophysiologic

characteristics, pharmacologic responses and effects of radiofrequency ablation. *Circulation* 1999;100:1879–1886.
39. Cranefield P, Aronson R. *Cardiac Arrhythmias: The Role of Triggered Activity and Other Mechanisms*. New York: Futura; 1988.
40. Tse HF, Lau CP, Kou W, et al. Prevalence and significance of exit block during arrhythmias arising in pulmonary veins. *J Cardiovasc Electrophysiol* 2000;11:379–386.
41. Tsai CF, Tai CT, Hsieh MH, et al. Initiation of atrial fibrillation by ectopic beats originating from the superior vena cava: Electrophysiological characteristics and results of radiofrequency ablation. *Circulation* 2000;102:67–74.
42. Doshi RN, Wu TJ, Yashima M, et al. Relation between ligament of Marshall and adrenergic atrial tachyarrhythmia. *Circulation* 1999; 100:876–883.
43. Chen PS. Chou CC. Coronary sinus as an arrhythmogenic structure. *J Cardiovasc Electrophysiol* 2002;13:863–864.
44. Kim DT, Lai AC, Hwang C, et al. The ligament of Marshall: A structural analysis in human hearts with implications for atrial arrhythmias. *J Am Coll Cardiol* 2000;36:1324–1327.
45. Chen SA, Tai CT, Yu WC, et al. Right atrial focal atrial fibrillation: electrophysiologic characteristics and radiofrequency catheter ablation. *J Cardiovasc Electrophysiol* 1999;10:328–335.
46. Zimmerman M, Kalusche D. Fluctuation in autonomic tone is a major determinant of sustained atrial arrhythmias in patients with focal ectopy originating from the pulmonary veins. *J Cardiovasc Electrophysiol* 2001;12:285–291.
47. Bettoni M, Zimmermann M. Autonomic tone variations before the onset of paroxysmal atrial fibrillation. *Circulation* 2002;105: 2753–2759.
48. Schauerte P, Scherlag BJ, Pitha J, et al. Catheter ablation of cardiac autonomic nerves for prevention of vagal atrial fibrillation. *Circulation* 2000;102:2774–2779.
49. Moe GK, Abildskov JA. Atrial fibrillation as a self sustaining arrhythmia independent of focal discharge. *Am Heart J* 1959;58:59–70.
50. Moe GK, Abildskov JA. Observations on the ventricular dysrhythmia associated with atrial fibrillation in the dog heart. *Circ Res* 1964;4: 447–460.
51. Li D, Fareh S, Leung TK, et al. Promotion of atrial fibrillation by heart failure in dogs: Remodeling of a different sort. *Circulation* 1999; 100:87–95.
52. Spach MS, Josephson ME. Initiating reentry: The role of nonuniform anisotropy in small circuits. *J Cardiovasc Electrophysiol* 1994;5: 182–209.
53. Tai C-T, Chen S-A, Tzeng J-W, et al. Prolonged fractionation of paced right atrial electrograms in patients with atrial flutter and fibrillation. *J Am Coll Cardiol* 2001;37:1651–1657.
54. Aime-Sempe C, Folliguet T, Rucker-Martin C, et al. Myocardial cell death in fibrillating and dilated human right atria. *J Am Coll Cardiol* 1999;34:1577–1586.
55. Polontchouk L, Haefliger J-A, Ebelt B, et al. Effects of chronic atrial fibrillation on gap junctions distribution in human and rat atria. *J Am Coll Cardiol* 2001;38:883–891.
56. Mary-Rabine L, Albert A, Pham TD, et al. The relationship of human atrial cellular electrophysiology to clinical function and ultrastructure. *Circ Res* 1983;52:188–199.
57. Ausma J, Wijffels M, Thoné F, et al. Structural changes of atrial myocardium due to sustained atrial fibrillation in the goat. *Circulation* 1997;96:3157–3163.
58. Madrid AH, Bueno MG, Rebollo JMG, et al. Use of irbesartan to maintain sinus rhythm in patients with long-lasting persistent atrial fibrillation. A prospective and randomized study. *Circulation* 2002;106: 331–336.
59. Kim B-S, Kim Y-H, Hwang G-S, et al. Action potential duration restitution kinetics in human atrial fibrillation. *J Am Coll Cardiol* 2002;39: 1329–1236.
60. Shinagawa K, Li D, Leung TK, Nattel S. Consequences of atrial tachycardia-induced remodeling depend on the preexisting atrial substrate. *Circulation* 2002;105:251–257.
61. Morillo CA, Klein GJ, Jones DL, et al. Chronic rapid atrial pacing: Structural, functional, and electrophysiological characteristics of a new model of sustained atrial fibrillation. *Circulation* 1995;91: 1588–1595.
62. Gaspo R, Bosch RF, Talajic M, et al. Functional mechanisms underlying tachycardia-induced sustained atrial fibrillation in a chronic dog model. *Circulation* 1997;96:4027–4035.
63. Elvan A, Wylie K, Zipes DP. Pacing-induced chronic atrial fibrillation impairs sinus node function in dogs: electrophysiological remodeling. *Circulation* 1996;94:2953–2960.
64. Packer DL, Bardy GH, Worley SJ, et al. Tachycardia-induced cardiomyopathy: A reversible form of left ventricular dysfunction. *Am J Cardiol* 1986;57:563–570.
65. Grogan M, Smith HC, Gersh BJ, Wood DL. Left ventricular dysfunction due to atrial fibrillation in patients initially believed to have idiopathic dilated cardiomyopathy. *Am J Cardiol* 1992;69: 1570–1573.
66. Kieny JR, Sacrez A, Facello A, et al. Increase in radionuclide left ventricular ejection fraction after cardioversion of chronic atrial fibrillation in idiopathic dilated cardiomyopathy. *Eur Heart J* 1992;13: 1290–1295.
67. Clark DM, Plumb VJ, Epstein AE, Kay GN. Hemodynamic effects of an irregular sequence of ventricular cycle lengths during atrial fibrillation. *J Am Coll Cardiol* 1997;30:1039–1045.
68. Kochiadakis GE, Skalidis EI, Kalebubas D, et al. Effect of acute atrial fibrillation on phasic coronary blood flow pattern and flow reserve in humans. *Eur Heart J* 2002;23:734–741.
69. Kanter MC, Tegeler CH, Pearce LA, et al. Carotid stenosis in patients with atrial fibrillation. Prevalence, risk factors, and relationship to stroke in the Stroke Prevention in Atrial Fibrillation Study. *Arch Intern Med* 1994;154:1372–1377.
70. Miller VT, Rothrock JF, Pearce LA, et al. Ischemic stroke in patients with atrial fibrillation: Effect of aspirin according to stroke mechanism. Stroke Prevention in Atrial Fibrillation Investigators. *Neurology* 1993;43:32–36.
71. Bogousslavsky J, Van Melle G, Regli F, Kappenberger L. Pathogenesis of anterior circulation stroke in patients with nonvalvular atrial fibrillation: The Lausanne Stroke Registry. *Neurology* 1990;40: 1046–1050.
72. Stoddard MF, Dawkins PR, Prince CR, Ammash NM. Left atrial appendage thrombus is not uncommon in patients with acute atrial fibrillation and a recent embolic event: A transesophageal echocardiographic study. *J Am Coll Cardiol* 1995;25:452–459.
73. Collins LJ, Silverman DI, Douglas PS, Manning WJ. Cardioversion of nonrheumatic atrial fibrillation. Reduced thromboembolic complications with 4 weeks of precardioversion anticoagulation are related to atrial thrombus resolution. *Circulation* 1995;92:160–163.
74. Manning WJ, Silverman DI, Waksmonski CA, et al. Prevalence of residual left atrial thrombi among patients with acute thromboembolism and newly recognized atrial fibrillation. *Arch Intern Med* 1995;155:2193–2198.
75. Manning WJ, Leeman DE, Gotch PJ, Come PC. Pulsed Doppler evaluation of atrial mechanical function after electrical cardioversion of atrial fibrillation. *J Am Coll Cardiol* 1989;13:617–623.
76. Grimm RA, Stewart WJ, Maloney JD, et al. Impact of electrical cardioversion for atrial fibrillation on left atrial appendage function and spontaneous echo contrast: Characterization by simultaneous transesophageal echocardiography. *J Am Coll Cardiol* 1993;22: 1359–1366.
77. Zabalgoitia M, Halperin JL, Pearce LA, et al. Transesophageal echocardiographic correlates of clinical risk of thromboembolism in nonvalvular atrial fibrillation. Stroke Prevention in Atrial Fibrillation III Investigators. *J Am Coll Cardiol* 1998;31:1622–1626.
78. The Stroke Prevention in Atrial Fibrillation Investigators. Predictors of thromboembolism in atrial fibrillation: I. Clinical features of patients at risk. *Ann Intern Med* 1992;116:1–5.
79. Echocardiographic predictors of stroke in patients with atrial fibrillation: A prospective study of 1066 patients from 3 clinical trials. *Arch Intern Med* 1998;158:1316–1320.

80. The Stroke Prevention in Atrial Fibrillation Investigators. Predictors of thromboembolism in atrial fibrillation: II. Echocardiographic features of patients at risk. *Ann Intern Med* 1992;116:6–12.
81. Dittrich HC, Pearce LA, Asinger RW, et al. Left atrial diameter in nonvalvular atrial fibrillation: An echocardiographic study. Stroke Prevention in Atrial Fibrillation Investigators. *Am Heart J* 1999;137: 494–499.
82. Aschenberg W, Schluter M, Kremer P, et al. Transesophageal two-dimensional echocardiography for the detection of left atrial appendage thrombus. *J Am Coll Cardiol* 1986;7:163–166.
83. Mugge A, Kuhn H, Nikutta P, et al. Assessment of left atrial appendage function by biplane transesophageal echocardiography in patients with nonrheumatic atrial fibrillation: Identification of a subgroup of patients at increased embolic risk. *J Am Coll Cardiol* 1994;23:599–607.
84. Mitusch R, Lange V, Stierle U, et al. Transesophageal echocardiographic determinants of embolism in nonrheumatic atrial fibrillation. *Int J Card Imaging* 1995;11:27–34.
85. Asinger RW, Koehler J, Pearce LA, et al. Pathophysiologic correlates of thromboembolism in nonvalvular atrial fibrillation: II. Dense spontaneous echocardiographic contrast (The Stroke Prevention in Atrial Fibrillation [SPAF-III] study). *J Am Soc Echocardiogr* 1999; 12:1088–1096.
86. Black IW, Chesterman CN, Hopkins AP, et al. Hematologic correlates of left atrial spontaneous echo contrast and thromboembolism in nonvalvular atrial fibrillation. *J Am Coll Cardiol* 1993;21:451–457.
87. Daniel WG, Nellessen U, Schroder E, et al. Left atrial spontaneous echo contrast in mitral valve disease: An indicator for an increased thromboembolic risk. *J Am Coll Cardiol* 1988;11:1204–1211.
88. Fatkin D, Kelly RP, Feneley MP. Relations between left atrial appendage blood flow velocity, spontaneous echocardiographic contrast and thromboembolic risk in vivo. *J Am Coll Cardiol* 1994;23:961–969.
89. Sadanandan S, Sherrid MV. Clinical and echocardiographic characteristics of left atrial spontaneous echo contrast in sinus rhythm. *J Am Coll Cardiol* 2000;35:1932–1938.
90. Cai H, Li Z, Goette A, et al. Downregulation of endocardial nitric oxide synthetase expression and nitric oxide production in atrial fibrillation. Potential mechanisms for atrial thrombosis and stroke. *Circulation* 2002;1062854–1062858.
91. Heppel RM, Berkin KE, McLenachan JM, et al. Haemostatic and haemodynamic abnormalities associated with left atrial thrombosis in non-rheumatic atrial fibrillation. *Heart* 1977;77:407–411.
92. Sohara H, Amitani S, Kurose M, et al. Atrial fibrillation activates platelets and coagulation in a time-dependent manner: A study in patients with paroxysmal atrial fibrillation. *J Am Coll Cardiol* 1997;29:106–112.
93. Li-Saw-Hee FL, Blann AD, Lip GY. A cross-sectional and diurnal study of thrombogenesis among patients with chronic atrial fibrillation. *J Am Coll Cardiol* 2000;35:1926–1931.
94. Li-Saw-Hee FL, Blann AD, Lip GY. Effect of blood pressure on the hypercoaguable state in chronic atrial fibrillation. *Am J Cardiol* 2000; 86:795–797.
95. Conway DSG, Pearce LA, Chin BSP, et al. Plasma von Willebrand factor and soluble P-selectin as indices of endothelial damage and platelet activation in 1321 patients with nonvalvular atrial fibrillation. Relationship to stroke risk factors. *Circulation* 2002;106:1962–1967.
96. Wood MA, Brown-Mahoney C, Kay GN, Ellenbogen KA. Clinical outcomes after ablation and pacing therapy for atrial fibrillation: a meta-analysis. *Circulation* 2000;101:1138–1144.
97. Dorian P, Jung W, Newman D, et al. The impairment of health-related quality of life in patients with intermittent atrial fibrillation: implications for the assessment of investigational therapy. *J Am Coll Cardiol* 2002;36:1303–1309.
98. Epstein AE, Vidaillet H, Greene HL, et al. Frequency of symptomatic atrial fibrillation in patients enrolled in the Atrial Fibrillation Follow-up Investigation of Rhythm Management (AFFIRM) study. *J Cardiovasc Electrophysiol* 2002;13:667–671.
99. Adjusted-dose warfarin versus low-intensity, fixed-dose warfarin plus aspirin for high-risk patients with atrial fibrillation: Stroke Prevention in Atrial Fibrillation III randomised clinical trial. *Lancet* 1996; 348:633–638.
100. Boysen G, Nyboe J, Appleyard M, et al. Stroke incidence and risk factors for stroke in Copenhagen, Denmark. *Stroke* 1988;19:1345–1353.
101. Stroke Prevention in Atrial Fibrillation Investigators. Risk factors for thromboembolism during aspirin therapy in patients with atrial fibrillation: the Stroke Prevention in Atrial Defibrillation Study. *J Stroke Cerebrovasc Dis* 1995;5:147–157.
102. EAFT (European Atrial Fibrillation Trial) Study Group. Secondary prevention in non-rheumatic atrial fibrillation after transient ischaemic attack or minor stroke. *Lancet* 1993;342:1255–1262.
103. Beyth RJ, Quinn L, Landefeld CS. A multicomponent intervention to prevent major bleeding complications in older patients receiving warfarin. A randomized, controlled trial. *Ann Intern Med* 2000;133: 687–695.
104. Hart RG, Pearce LA, McBride R, et al. Factors associated with ischemic stroke during aspirin therapy in atrial fibrillation: analysis of 2012 participants in the SPAF I-III clinical trials. The Stroke Prevention in Atrial Fibrillation (SPAF) Investigators. *Stroke* 1999;30:1223–1229.
105. Landefeld CS, Goldman L. Major bleeding in outpatients treated with warfarin: incidence and prediction by factors known at the start of outpatient therapy. *Am J Med* 1989;87:144–152.
106. Moulton AW, Singer DE, Haas JS. Risk factors for stroke in patients with nonrheumatic atrial fibrillation: A case-control study. *Am J Med* 1991;91:156–161.
107. Laupacis A, Albers G, Dalen J, et al. Antithrombotic therapy in atrial fibrillation. *Chest* 1998;114:579S–589S.
108. Pearce LA, Hart RG, Halperin JL. Assessment of three schemes for stratifying stroke risk in patients with nonvalvular atrial fibrillation. *Am J Med* 2000;109:45–51.
109. Hurley DM, Hunter AN, Hewett MJ, Stockigt JR. Atrial fibrillation and arterial embolism in hyperthyroidism. *Aust N Z J Med* 1981;11:391–393.
110. Yuen RW, Gutteridge DH, Thompson PL, Robinson JS. Embolism in thyrotoxic atrial fibrillation. *Med J Aus.* 1979;1:630–631.
111. Staffurth JS, Gibberd MC, Fui SN. Arterial embolism in thyrotoxicosis with atrial fibrillation. *Br Med J* 1977;2:688–690.
112. Hart RG, Halperin JL. Atrial fibrillation and thromboembolism: A decade of progress in stroke prevention. *Ann Intern Med* 1999;131:492–501.
113. Petersen P, Boysen G, Godtfredsen J, et al. Placebo-controlled, randomised trial of warfarin and aspirin for prevention of thromboembolic complications in chronic atrial fibrillation. The Copenhagen AFASAK study. *Lancet* 1989;1:175–179.
114. Ezekowitz MD, Bridgers SL, James KE, et al. Warfarin in the prevention of stroke associated with nonrheumatic atrial fibrillation. Veterans Affairs Stroke Prevention in Nonrheumatic Atrial Fibrillation Investigators [published erratum appears in *N Engl J Med* 1993 Jan 14;328(2): 148]. *N Engl J Med* 1992;327:1406–1412.
115. The Stroke Prevention in Atrial Fibrillation Investigators. Bleeding during antithrombotic therapy in patients with atrial fibrillation. *Arch Intern Med* 1996;156:409–416.
116. Gorter JW. Major bleeding during anticoagulation after cerebral ischemia: patterns and risk factors. Stroke Prevention In Reversible Ischemia Trial (SPIRIT). European Atrial Fibrillation Trial (EAFT) study groups. *Neurology* 1999;53:1319–1327.
117. Fihn SD, Callahan CM, Martin DC, et al. The risk for and severity of bleeding complications in elderly patients treated with warfarin. The National Consortium of Anticoagulation Clinics. *Ann Intern Med* 1996;124:970–979.
118. The Boston Area Anticoagulation Trial for Atrial Fibrillation Investigators. The effect of low-dose warfarin on the risk of stroke in patients with nonrheumatic atrial fibrillation. *N Engl J Med* 1990; 323:1505–1511.
119. Hart RG, Benavente O, McBride R, Pearce LA. Antithrombotic therapy to prevent stroke in patients with atrial fibrillation: a meta-analysis. *Ann Intern Med* 1999;131:492–501.
120. Sudlow M, Thomson R, Thwaites B, et al. Prevalence of atrial fibrillation and eligibility for anticoagulants in the community. *Lancet* 1998;352:1167–1171.

121. The European Atrial Fibrillation Trial Study Group. Optimal oral anticoagulant therapy in patients with nonrheumatic atrial fibrillation and recent cerebral ischemia. *N Engl J Med* 1995;333:5–10.
122. Hylek EM, Skates SJ, Sheehan MA, Singer DE. An analysis of the lowest effective intensity of prophylactic anticoagulation for patients with nonrheumatic atrial fibrillation. *N Engl J Med* 1996;335:540–546.
123. The Atrial Fibrillation Investigators. The efficacy of aspirin in patients with atrial fibrillation. Analysis of pooled data from 3 randomized trials. *Arch Intern Med* 1997;157:1237–1240.
124. Stroke Prevention in Atrial Fibrillation III Study. Patients with nonvalvular atrial fibrillation at low risk of stroke during treatment with aspirin: The SPAF III Writing Committee for the Stroke Prevention in Atrial Fibrillation Investigators. *JAMA* 1998;279:1273–1277.
125. Gallagher MM, Hennessy BJ, Edvardsson N, et al. Embolic complications of direct current cardioversion of atrial arrhythmias: association with low intensity of anticoagulation at the time of cardioversion. *J Am Coll Cardiol* 2002;40:926–933.
126. Klein EA. Assessment of Cardioversion Using Transesophageal Echocardiography (TEE) multicenter study (ACUTE I): Clinical outcomes at eight weeks. *J Am Coll Cardiol* 2000;36:324.
127. Klein AL, Grimm RA, Murray RD, et al. Assessment of Cardioversion Using Transesophageal Echocardiography Investigators. Use of transesophageal echocardiography to guide cardioversion in patients with atrial fibrillation. *N Engl J Med* 2001;344:1411–1420.
128. Antonielli E, Pizzuti A, Bassignana A, et al. Transesophageal echocardiographic evidence of more pronounced left atrial stunning after chemical (propafenone) rather than electrical attempts at cardioversion from atrial fibrillation. *Am J Cardiol* 1999;84:1092–1010.
129. Falcone RA, Morady F, Armstrong WF. Transesophageal echocardiographic evaluation of left atrial appendage function and spontaneous contrast formation after chemical or electrical cardioversion of atrial fibrillation. *Am J Cardiol* 1996;78:435–439.
130. Bellotti P, Spirito P, Lupi G, Vecchio C. Left atrial appendage function assessed by transesophageal echocardiography before and on the day after elective cardioversion for nonvalvular atrial fibrillation. *Am J Cardiol* 1998;81:1199–1202.
131. Harjai K, Mobarek S, Abi-Samra F, et al. Mechanical dysfunction of the left atrium and the left atrial appendage following cardioversion of atrial fibrillation and its relation to total electrical energy used for cardioversion. *Am J Cardiol* 1998;81:1125–1129.
132. Sparks PB, Jayaprakash S, Vohra JK, et al. Left atrial "stunning" following radiofrequency catheter ablation of chronic atrial flutter. *J Am Coll Cardiol* 1998;32:468–475.
133. Mitusch R, Garbe M, Schmucker G, et al. Relation of left atrial appendage function to the duration and reversibility of nonvalvular atrial fibrillation. *Am J Cardiol* 1995;75:944–947.
134. Grimm RA, Leung DY, Black IW, et al. Left atrial appendage "stunning" after spontaneous conversion of atrial fibrillation demonstrated by transesophageal Doppler echocardiography. *Am Heart J* 1995; 130:174–176.
135. Botto GL, Politi A, Bonini W, et al. External cardioversion of atrial fibrillation: role of paddle position on technical efficacy and energy requirements. *Heart* 1999;82:726–730.
136. Mittal S, Ayati S, Stein KM, et al. Transthoracic cardioversion of atrial fibrillation: Comparison of rectilinear biphasic versus damped sine wave monophasic shocks. *Circulation* 2000;101:1282–1287.
137. Page RL, Kerber RE, Russell JK, et al. Biphasic versus monophasic shock waveform for conversion of atrial fibrillation: the results of an international randomized, double-blind multicenter trial. *J Am Coll Cardiol* 2002;39:1956–1963.
138. Oral H, Souza JJ, Michaud GF, et al. Facilitating transthoracic cardioversion of atrial fibrillation with ibutilide pretreatment. *N Engl J Med* 1999;340:1849–1854.
139. Lundstrom T, Ryden L. Chronic atrial fibrillation. Long-term results of direct current conversion. *Acta Med Scand* 1988;223:53–59.
140. Van Gelder IC, Crijns HJ, Tieleman RG, et al. Chronic atrial fibrillation. Success of serial cardioversion therapy and safety of oral anticoagulation. *Arch Intern Med* 1996;156:2585–2592.
141. Khan IA. Single oral loading dose of propafenone for pharmacological cardioversion of recent-onset atrial fibrillation. *J Am Coll Cardiol* 2001;37:542–547.
142. Boriani G, Martignani C, Biffi M, et al. Oral loading with propafenone for conversion of recent-onset atrial fibrillation: A review on in-hospital treatment. *Drugs* 2002;62:415–423.
143. Boriani G, Biffi M, Capucci A, et al. Oral propafenone to convert recent-onset atrial fibrillation in patients with and without underlying heart disease: A randomized, controlled trial. *Ann Intern Med* 1997; 126:621–625.
144. Botto GL, Capucci A, Bonini W, et al. Conversion of recent-onset atrial fibrillation to sinus rhythm using a single loading oral dose of propafenone: Comparison of two regimens. *Int J Cardiol* 1997;58:55–61.
145. Capucci A, Boriani G, Botto GL, et al. Conversion of recent-onset atrial fibrillation by a single oral loading dose of propafenone or flecainide. *Am J Cardiol* 1994;74:503–505.
146. Singh S, Zoble RG, Yellen L, et al. Efficacy and safety of oral dofetilide in converting to and maintaining sinus rhythm in patients with chronic atrial fibrillation or atrial flutter. The Symptomatic Atrial Fibrillation Investigative Research of Dofetilide (SAFIRE-D) Study. *Circulation* 2000;102:2385–2390.
147. Stambler BS, Wood MA, Ellenbogen KA, et al. Efficacy and safety of repeated intravenous doses of ibutilide for rapid conversion of atrial flutter or fibrillation. Ibutilide Repeat Dose Study Investigators. *Circulation* 1996;94:1613–1621.
148. Ellenbogen KA, Stambler BS, Wood MA, et al. Efficacy of intravenous ibutilide for rapid termination of atrial fibrillation and atrial flutter: A dose-response study. *J Am Coll Cardiol* 1996;28:130–136.
149. Stambler BS, Wood MA, Ellenbogen KA. Antiarrhythmic actions of intravenous ibutilide compared with procainamide during human atrial flutter and fibrillation: Electrophysiological determinants of enhanced conversion efficacy. *Circulation* 1997;96:4298–4306.
150. Volgman AS, Carberry PA, Stambler B, et al. Conversion efficacy and safety of intravenous ibutilide compared with intravenous procainamide in patients with atrial flutter or fibrillation. *J Am Coll Cardiol* 1998;31:1414–1419.
151. Vos MA, Golitsyn SR, Stangl K, et al. Superiority of ibutilide (a new class III agent) over DL-sotalol in converting atrial flutter and atrial fibrillation. The Ibutilide/Sotalol Comparator Study Group. *Heart* 1998;79:568–575.
152. Galve E, Rius E, Ballester R, et al. Intravenous amiodarone in treatment of recent-onset atrial fibrillation: Results of a randomized, controlled study. *J Am Coll Cardiol* 1996;27:1079–1082.
153. Crystal E, Connolly SJ, Sleik K, et al. Interventions on prevention of postoperative atrial fibrillation in patients undergoing heart surgery. A meta-analysis. *Circulation* 2002;106:75–80.
154. Wyse DG, Waldo AL, DiMarco JP, et al. The Atrial Fibrillation Follow-up Investigation of Rhythm Management (AFFIRM) Investigators. A comparison of rate control and rhythm control in patients with atrial fibrillation. *N Engl J Med* 2002;347:1825–1833.
155. Van Gelder IC, Hagens VE, Bosker HA, et al. Rate Control versus Electrical Cardioversion for Persistent Atrial Fibrillation Study Group. A comparison of rate control and rhythm control in patients with recurrent persistent atrial fibrillation. *N Engl J Med* 2002;347: 1834–1840.
156. Prystowsky EN, Benson DW Jr, Fuster V, et al. Management of patients with atrial fibrillation. A statement for healthcare professionals. From the Subcommittee on Electrocardiography and Electrophysiology, American Heart Association. *Circulation* 1996;93: 1262–1277.
157. Marshall HJ, Harris ZI, Griffith MJ, et al. Prospective randomized study of ablation and pacing versus medical therapy for paroxysmal atrial fibrillation: effects of pacing mode and mode-switch algorithm. *Circulation* 1999;99:1587–1592.
158. Kay GN, Ellenbogen KA, Giudici M, et al. The Ablate and Pace Trial: A prospective study of catheter ablation of the AV conduction system and permanent pacemaker implantation for treatment of atrial fibrillation. APT Investigators. *J Intervent Cardiol Electrophysiol* 1998;2:121–135.

159. Brignole M, Gianfranchi L, Menozzi C, et al. Assessment of atrioventricular junction ablation and DDDR mode-switching pacemaker versus pharmacological treatment in patients with severely symptomatic paroxysmal atrial fibrillation: A randomized controlled study. *Circulation* 1997;96:2617–2624.
160. Marshall HJ, Harris ZI, Griffith MJ, Gammage MD. Atrioventricular nodal ablation and implantation of mode-switching dual-chamber pacemakers: Effective treatment for drug refractory paroxysmal atrial fibrillation. *Heart* 1998;79:543–547.
161. Williamson BD, Man KC, Daoud E, et al. Radiofrequency catheter modification of atrioventricular conduction to control the ventricular rate during atrial fibrillation. *N Engl J Med* 1994;331:910–917.
162. Anderson JL, Gilbert EM, Alpert BL, et al. Prevention of symptomatic recurrences of paroxysmal atrial fibrillation in patients initially tolerating antiarrhythmic therapy. A multicenter, double-blind, crossover study of flecainide and placebo with transtelephonic monitoring. Flecainide Supraventricular Tachycardia Study Group. *Circulation* 1989;80:1557–1570.
163. Clementy J, Dulhoste MN, Laiter C, et al. Flecainide acetate in the prevention of paroxysmal atrial fibrillation: A nine-month follow-up of more than 500 patients. *Am J Cardiol* 1992;70:44A–49A.
164. Suttorp MJ, Kingma JH, Koomen EM, et al. Recurrence of paroxysmal atrial fibrillation or flutter after successful cardioversion in patients with normal left ventricular function. *Am J Cardiol* 1993;71:710–713.
165. Feld GK. Atrial fibrillation. Is there a safe and highly effective pharmacological treatment? (editorial; comment). *Circulation* 1990;82: 2248–2250.
166. Coumel P, Thomas O, Leenhardt A. Drug therapy for prevention of atrial fibrillation. *Am J Cardiol* 1996;77:3A–9A.
167. Van Gelder IC, Crijns HJ, van Gilst WH, et al. Efficacy and safety of flecainide acetate in the maintenance of sinus rhythm after electrical cardioversion of chronic atrial fibrillation or atrial flutter. *Am J Cardiol* 1989;64:1317–1321.
168. Coplen SE, Antman EM, Berlin JA, et al. Efficacy and safety of quinidine therapy for maintenance of sinus rhythm after cardioversion. A meta-analysis of randomized control trials. *Circulation* 1990;82: 1106–1116.
169. Pedersen OD, Bagger H, Keller N, et al. Efficacy of dofetilide in the treatment of atrial fibrillation-flutter in patients with reduced left ventricular function: A Danish investigation of arrhythmia and mortality on dofetilide (DIAMOND) substudy. *Circulation* 2001;104:292–296.
170. Kober L, Bloch Thomsen PE, Moller M, et al. Danish Investigations of Arrhythmia and Mortality on Dofetilide (DIAMOND) Study Group. Effect of dofetilide in patients with recent myocardial infarction and left-ventricular dysfunction: A randomised trial. *Lancet* 2000;356: 2052–2058.
171. Torp-Pedersen C, Moller M, Bloch-Thomsen PE, et al. Dofetilide in patients with congestive heart failure and left ventricular dysfunction. Danish Investigations of Arrhythmia and Mortality on Dofetilide Study Group. *N Engl J Med* 1999;341:857–865.
172. Chun SH, Sager PT, Stevenson WG, et al. Long-term efficacy of amiodarone for the maintenance of normal sinus rhythm in patients with refractory atrial fibrillation or flutter. *Am J Cardiol* 1995;76:47–50.
173. Akiyama T, Pawitan Y, Greenberg H, et al. Increased risk of death and cardiac arrest from encainide and flecainide in patients after non-Q-wave acute myocardial infarction in the Cardiac Arrhythmia Suppression Trial. CAST Investigators. *Am J Cardiol* 1991;68:1551–1555.
174. Echt DS, Liebson PR, Mitchell LB, et al. Mortality and morbidity in patients receiving encainide, flecainide, or placebo. The Cardiac Arrhythmia Suppression Trial. *N Engl J Med* 1991;324:781–788.
175. Waldo AL, Camm AJ, deRuyter H, et al. Effect of D-sotalol on mortality in patients with left ventricular dysfunction after recent and remote myocardial infarction. The SWORD Investigators. Survival With Oral D-Sotalol. *Lancet* 1996;348:7–12.
176. Julian DG, Camm AJ, Frangin G, et al. Randomised trial of effect of amiodarone on mortality in patients with left-ventricular dysfunction after recent myocardial infarction: EMIAT. European Myocardial Infarct Amiodarone Trial Investigators *Lancet* 1997;349:667–674.
177. Cairns JA, Connolly SJ, Roberts R, Gent M. Randomised trial of outcome after myocardial infarction in patients with frequent or repetitive ventricular premature depolarisations: CAMIAT. Canadian Amiodarone Myocardial Infarction Arrhythmia Trial Investigators. *Lancet* 1997;349:675–682.
178. Gosselink AT, Crijns HJ, Van Gelder IC, et al. Low-dose amiodarone for maintenance of sinus rhythm after cardioversion of atrial fibrillation or flutter. *JAMA* 1992;267:3289–3293.
179. Opolski G, Stanislawska J, Gorecki A, et al. Amiodarone in restoration and maintenance of sinus rhythm in patients with chronic atrial fibrillation after unsuccessful direct-current cardioversion. *Clin Cardiol* 1997;20:337–340.
180. Ben David J, Zipes DP, Ayers GM, Pride HP. Canine left ventricular hypertrophy predisposes to ventricular tachycardia induction by phase 2 early afterdepolarizations after administration of BAY K 8644. *J Am Coll Cardiol* 1992;20:1576–1584.
181. Cox JL, Canavan TE, Schuessler RB, et al. The surgical treatment of atrial fibrillation: II. Intraoperative electrophysiologic mapping and description of the electrophysiologic basis of atrial flutter and atrial fibrillation. *J Thorac Cardiovasc Surg* 1991;101:406–426.
182. Cox JL, Boineau JP, Schuessler RB, et al. Modification of the maze procedure for atrial flutter and atrial fibrillation: I. Rationale and surgical results. *J Thorac Cardiovasc Surg* 1995;110:473–484.
183. Nitta T, Lee R, Schuessler RB, et al. Radial approach: a new concept in surgical treatment for atrial fibrillation: I. Concept, anatomic and physiologic bases and development of a procedure. *Ann Thorac Surg* 1999;67:27–35.
184. Cox JL, Schuessler RB, D'Agostino HJ Jr, et al. The surgical treatment of atrial fibrillation: III. Development of a definitive surgical procedure. *J Thorac Cardiovasc Surg* 1991;101:569–583.
185. Melo J, Adragao P, Neves J, et al. Surgery for atrial fibrillation using radiofrequency catheter ablation: assessment of results at one year. *Eur J Cardiothorac Surg* 1999;15:851–854.
186. Hioki M, Ikeshita M, Iedokoro Y, et al. Successful combined operation for mitral stenosis and atrial fibrillation. *Ann Thorac Surg* 1993;55: 776–778.
187. Williams MR, Stewart JR, Bolling SF, et al. Surgical treatment of atrial fibrillation using radiofrequency energy. *Ann Thorac Surg* 2001; 71:1939–1944.
188. Oral H, Knight BP, Ozaydin M, et al. Segmental ostial ablation to isolate the pulmonary veins during atrial fibrillation. Feasiblity and mechanistic insights. *Circulation* 2002;106:1256–1262.
189. Haissaguerre M, Shah DC, Jais P, et al. Electrophysiological breakthroughs from the left atrium to the pulmonary veins. *Circulation* 2000;102:2463–2465.
190. Shah DC, Haissaguerre M, Jais P, et al. Curative catheter ablation of paroxysmal atrial fibrillation in 200 patients: Strategy for presentations ranging from sustained atrial fibrillation to no arrhythmias. *Pacing Clin Electrophysiol* 2001;24:1541–1558.
191. Tada H, Oral H, Wasmer K, et al. Pulmonary vein isolation: Comparison of bipolar and unipolar electrograms at successful and unsuccessful ostial ablation sites. *J Cardiovasc Electrophysiol* 2002;13:13–19.
192. Pappone C, Rosanio S, Oreto G, et al. Circumferential radiofrequency ablation of pulmonary vein ostia: a new anatomic approach for curing atrial fibrillation. *Circulation* 2000;102:2619–2628.
193. Oral H, Knight BP, Tada H, et al. Pulmonary vein isolation for paroxysmal and persistent atrial fibrillation. *Circulation* 2002;105: 1077–1081.
194. Chen P, Wu T, Hwang C, et al. Thoracic veins and the mechanisms of non-paroxysmal atrial fibrillation. *Cardiovasc Res* 2002;54:295–301.
195. Oral H, Ozaydin M, Tada H, et al. Mechanistic significance of intermittent pulmonary vein tachycardia in patients with atrial fibrillation. *J Cardiovasc Electrophysiol* 2002;13:645–650.
196. Wu TJ, Ong JJ, Chang CM, et al. Pulmonary veins and ligament of Marshall as sources of rapid activations in a canine model of sustained atrial fibrillation. *Circulation* 2001;103:1157–1163.
197. O'Donnell D, Furniss SS, Bourke JP. Paroxysmal cycle length shortening in the pulmonary veins during atrial fibrillation correlates with

arrhythmogenic triggering foci in sinus rhythm. *J Cardiovasc Electrophysiol* 2002;13:124–128.
198. Robbins IM, Colvin EV, Doyle TP, et al. Pulmonary vein stenosis after catheter ablation of atrial fibrillation. *Circulation* 1998;98:1769–1775.
199. Saksena S, Prakash A, Ziegler P, et al. DAPPAF Investigators. Improved suppression of recurrent atrial fibrillation with dual-site right atrial pacing and antiarrhythmic drug therapy. *J Am Coll Cardiol* 2002;40:1140–1150.
200. Bailin SJ, Adler S, Giudici M. Prevention of chronic atrial fibrillation by pacing in the region of Bachmann's bundle: Results of a multicenter randomized trial. *J Cardiovasc Electrophysiol* 2001;12:912–917.
201. Wells JL, MacLean WAH, James TN, Waldo AL. Characterization of atrial flutter. *Circulation* 1979;60:665–673.
202. Olgin JE, Kalman JM, Fitzpatrick AP, Lesh MD. Role of right atrial structures as barriers to conduction during human type 1 atrial flutter. Activation and entrainment mapping guided by intracardiac echocardiography. *Circulation* 1995;92:1839–1848.
203. Feld GK, Fleck RP, Chen P-S, et al. Radiofrequency catheter ablation for the treatment of human type I atrial flutter. Identification of the critical zone in the reentrant circuit by endocardial mapping techniques. *Circulation* 1992;86:1233–1240.
204. Cosio FG, Lope-Gil M, Goicolea A, et al. Radiofrequency ablation of the inferior vena cava–triscuspid valve isthmus in common atrial flutter. *Am J Cardiol* 1993;71:705–709.
205. Fischer B, Haissaquerre M, Garrigues S, et al. Radiofrequency catheter ablation of common atrial flutter in 80 patients. *J Am Coll Cardiol* 1995;25:1365–1372.
206. Olgin JE, Kalman JM, Fitzpatrick AP, et al. Role of right atrial endocardial structures as barriers to conduction during human type I atrial flutter: Activation and entrainment mapping guided by echocardiography. *Circulation* 1995;92:1839–1848.
207. Granada J, Uribe W, Chyou P-H, et al. Incidence and predictors of atrial flutter in the general population. *J Am Coll Cardiol* 2000;36:2242–2246.
208. Leitch JW, Thomson D, Baird DK, et al. The importance of age as a predictor of atrial fibrilation and flutter after coronary artery bypass grafting. *J Thorac Cardiovasc Surg* 1990;100:338–342.
209. Andrews TC, Reimold SC, Berlin JA, et al. Prevention of supraventricular arrhythmias after coronary artery bypass surgery. *Circulation* 1991;84[suppl III]:III236–III244.
210. Amar D, Roistacher N, Rusch VW, et al. Effects of diltiazem prophylaxis on the incidence and clinical outcome of atrial arrhythmias after thoracic surgery. *J Thorac Cardiovasc Surg* 2000;120:790–798.
211. Rosenblueth A, Garcia-Ramos J. Studies on flutter and fibrillation: II. The influence of artificial obstacles on experimental auricular flutter. *Am Heart J* 1947;33:677–684.
212. Frame LH, Page RL, Hoffman FB. Atrial reentry around an anatomic barrier with a partially refractory excitable gap. A canine model of atrial flutter. *Circ Res* 1986;58:495–511.
213. Page P, Plumb VJ, Okumura K, et al. A new model of atrial flutter. *J Am Coll Cardiol* 1986;8:872–879.
214. Waldo A, MacLean WAH, Karp RB, et al. Entrainment and interruption of atrial flutter with atrial pacing. *Circulation* 1977;56:737–745.
215. Puech P, Latour H, Grolleau R. Le flutter et ses limites. *Arch Mal Coeur* 1970;63:116–144.
216. Olshansky B, Okumura K, Hess PG, et al. Demonstration of an area of slow conduction in human atrial flutter. *J Am Coll Cardiol* 1990;16:1639–1648.
217. Racker DK, Ursell PC, Hoffman BF. Anatomy of the tricuspid annulus: Circumferential myofibers as the structural basis for atrial flutter in a canine model. *Circulation* 1991;84:841–851.
218. Randazzo DN, Schweitzer P, Stein E, et al. Flecainide induced atrial tachycardia with 1:1 ventricular conduction during exercise testing. *PACE* 1994;17:1509–1514.
219. Brodsky MA, Hwang C, Hunter D, et al. Life-threatening alterations in heart rate after the use of adenosine in atrial flutter. *Am Heart J* 1995;130:564–571.
220. Plumb VJ, Karp RB, Kouchoukos NT, et al. Verapamil therapy of atrial fibrillation and atrial flutter following cardiac operation. *J Thorac Cardiovasc Surg* 1982;83:590–596.
221. Ellenbogen KA, Dias VC, Plumb VJ, et al. A placebo-controlled trial of continuous intravenous diltiazem infusion for 24-hour heart rate control during atrial fibrillation and atrial flutter: A multicenter study. *J Am Coll Cardiol* 1991;18:891–897.
222. Platia EV, Michelson EL, Porterfield JK, et al. Esmolol versus verapamil in the acute treatment of atrial fibrillation or atrial flutter. *Am J Cardiol* 1989;63:925–929.
223. Ellenbogen KA, Stambler BS, Wood MA, et al. Efficacy of intravenous ibutilide for rapid termination of atrial fibrillation and atrial flutter: A dose-response study. *J Am Coll Cardiol* 1996;28:130–136.
224. Waldo A, MacLean WAH, Karp RB, et al. Entrainment and interruption of atrial flutter with atrial pacing. *Circulation* 1977;56:737–745.
225. Heldal M, Orning OM. Effects of flecainide on termination of atrial flutter by rapid atrial pacing. *Eur Heart J* 1993;14:421–424.
226. Doni F, Della Bella P, Kheir A, et al. Atrial flutter termination by overdrive transesophageal pacing and the facilitating effect of oral propafenone. *Am J Cardiol* 1995;76:1242–1246.
227. Crawford W, Plumb VJ, Epstein AE, et al. Prospective evaluation of transesophageal pacing for the interruption of atrial flutter. *Am J Med* 1989;86:663–667.
228. Elhendy A, Gentile F, Khandheria BK, et al. Thromboembolic complications after electrical cardioversion in patients with atrial flutter. *Am J Med* 2001;111:433–438.
229. Crijns HJ, Van Gelder IC, Tieleman RG, et al. Long-term outcome of electrical cardioversion in patients with chronic atrial flutter. *Heart* 1997;77:56–61.
230. Schmidt C, Alt E, Plewan A, et al. Low energy intracardiac cardioversion after failed conventional external cardioversion of atrial fibrillation. *J Am Coll Cardiol* 1996;28:994–999.
231. Feld GK, Fleck RP, Chen PS, et al. Radiofrequency catheter ablation for the treatment of human type 1 atrial flutter. *Circulation* 1992;86:1233–1240.
232. Cosio FG, Lopez-Gil M, Goicolea A, et al. Radiofrequency ablation of the inferior vena cava–tricuspid valve isthmus in common atrial flutter. *Am J Cardiol* 1993;71:705–709.
233. Calkins H, Leon A, Deam G, et al. Catheter ablation of atrial flutter using radiofrequency energy. *Am J Cardiol* 1994;73;353–356.
234. Lesh MD, Van Hare GF, Epstein LM, et al. Radiofrequency catheter ablation of atrial arrhythmias. *Circulation* 1994;89:1074–1089.
235. Kirkorian G, Moncada E, Chevalier P, et al. Radiofrequency ablation of atrial flutter. *Circulation* 1994;90:2804–2814.
236. Steinberg JS, Prasher S, Zelekofske S, et al. Radiofrequency catheter ablation of atrial flutter: Procedural success and log-term outcome. *Am Heart J* 1995;130:85–92.
237. Cosio FG, Arribas F, Lopez-Gil M, et al. Radiofrequency ablation of atrial flutter. *J Cardovasc Electrophysiol* 1996;7:60–70.
238. Schumacher B, Pfeiffer D, Tebbenjohanns J, et al. Acute and long-term effects of consecutive radiofrequency applications on conduction properties of the subeustachian isthmus in type I atrial flutter. *J Cardiovasc Electrophysiol* 1998;9:152–163.
239. Mangat I, Yang Y, Cheng J, et al. Optimizing the detection of bidirectional block across the flutter isthmus for patients with typical isthmus-dependent atrial flutter. *Am J Cardiol* 2003;91:559–564.
240. Philippon F, Plumb VJ, Epstein AE, et al. The risk of atrial fibrillation following radiofrequency catheter ablation of atrial flutter. *Circulation* 1995;92:430–435.
241. Paydak H, Kall JF, Burke MC, et al. Atrial fibrillation after radiofrequency ablation of type I atrial flutter: Time to onset, determinants, and clinical course. *Circulation* 1998;98:315–322.
242. Nabar A, Rodriguez LM, Timmermans C, et al. Radiofrequency ablation of "class IC atrial flutter" in patients with resistant atrial fibrillation. *Am J Cardiol* 1999;83:785–787.
243. Schumacher B, Jung W, Lewalter T, et al. Radiofrequency ablation of atrial flutter due to administration of class IC antiarrhythmic drugs for atrial fibrillation. *Am J Cardiol* 1999;83:710–713.

244. Bogun F, Bender B, Li YG, Hohnloser SH. Ablation of atypical atrial flutter guided by the use of concealed entrainment in patients without prior cardiac surgery. *J Cardiovasc Electrophysiol* 2000;11:136–145.
245. Wood KA, Eisenberg SJ, Kalman JM., et al. Risk of thromboembolism in chronic atrial flutter. *Am J Cardiol* 1997;79:1043–1047.
246. Iwai S, Markowitz SM, Stein KM, et al. Response to adenosine differentiates focal from macroreentrant atrial tachycardia: Validation using three-dimensional electroanatomic mapping. *Circulation* 2002; 106:2793–2799.
247. Knight BP, Ebinger M, Oral H, et al. Diagnostic value of tachycardia features and pacing maneuvers during paroxysmal supraventricular tachycardia. *J Am Coll Cardiol* 2000;36:574–582.
248. Saoudi N, Cosio F, Waldo A, et al. Classification of atrial flutter and regular atrial tachycardia according to electrophysiologic mechanism and anatomic bases: A statement from a joint expert group from the Working Group of Arrhythmias of the European Society of Cardiology and the North American Society of Pacing and Electrophysiology. *J Cardiovasc Electrophysiol* 2001;12:852–866.
249. Nakagawa H, Shah N, Matsudaira K, et al. Characterization of reentrant circuit in macroreentrant right atrial tachycardia after surgical repair of congenital heart disease: Isolated channels between scars allow "focal" ablation. *Circulation* 2001;103:699–709.
250. Rosales AM, Walsh EP, Wessel DL, Triedman JK. Postoperative ectopic atrial tachycardia in children with congenital heart disease. *Am J Cardiol* 2001;88:1169–1172.
251. Markowitz SM, Brodman RF, Stein KM, et al. Lesional tachycardias related to mitral valve surgery. *J Am Coll Cardiol* 2002;39:1973–1983.
252. Nakagawa H, Jackman WM. Catheter ablation of macroreentrant atrial tachycardia in patients following atriotomy. *Eur Heart J* 2002;23: 1566–1568.
253. Ouyang F, Ernst S, Vogtmann T, et al. Characterization of reentrant circuits in left atrial macroreentrant tachycardia: Critical isthmus block can prevent atrial tachycardia recurrence. *Circulation* 2002;105: 1934–1942.
254. Kalman JM, Olgin JE, Karch MR, et al. "Cristal tachycardias." Origin of right atrial tachycardias from the crista terminalis identified by intracardiac echocardiography. *J Am Coll Cardiol* 1998;31:451–459.
255. Frey B, Kreiner G, Gwechenberger M, Gossinger HD. Ablation of atrial tachycardia originating from the vicinity of the atrioventricular node: Significance of mapping both sides of the interatrial septum. *J Am Coll Cardiol* 2001;38:394–400.
256. Weiss C, Ventura R, Meinertz T, Willems S. Subthreshold stimulation at the focal origin of para-Hisian-located ectopic atrial tachycardia. *Pacing Clin Electrophysiol* 2001;24:1430–1432.
257. Volkmer M, Antz M, Hebe J, Kuck KH. Focal atrial tachycardia originating from the musculature of the coronary sinus. *J Cardiovasc Electrophysiol* 2002;13:68–71.
258. Takatsuki S, Mitamura H, Miyoshi S, Ogawa S. Respiratory cycle-dependent left atrial tachycardia. *J Cardiovasc Electrophysiol* 2001; 12:1202.

CHAPTER 30

# SUPRAVENTRICULAR TACHYCARDIA: AV NODAL REENTRY AND WOLFF-PARKINSON-WHITE SYNDROME

Vinod K. S. Jayam / Hugh Calkins



Supraventricular tachycardias (SVTs) include all tachyarrhythmias that either originate from or incorporate supraventricular tissue in a reentrant circuit. The ventricular rate may be the same or less than the atrial rate, depending on the AV nodal conduction. The term *paroxysmal supraventricular tachycardia* (PSVT) refers to a clinical syndrome characterized by a rapid, regular tachycardia with abrupt onset and termination. Approximately two-thirds of cases of PSVT result from (AV) nodal reentrant tachycardia (AVNRT). Orthodromic AV reciprocating tachycardia (AVRT), which involves an accessory pathway, is the second most common cause of PSVT, accounting for approximately one-third of cases. The term *Wolff-Parkinson-White syndrome* designates a condition comprising both preexcitation and tachyarrhythmias. Atrial tachycardias, which arise exclusively from atrial tissue, account for approximately 5 percent of all cases of PSVT.[1–3] The purpose of this chapter is to review the mechanism, clinical features, and approach to diagnosis and treatment of AVNRT and accessory pathway–mediated tachycardias (including the Wolff-Parkinson-White syndrome).

## AV NODAL REENTRANT TACHYCARDIA

AVNRT is an important arrhythmia for several reasons. First, AVNRT is extremely common. Studies have reported that AVNRT occurs in approximately 10 percent of the general population and accounts for up to two-thirds of all cases of PSVT.[4] Although AVNRT can occur at any age, it is extremely uncommon prior to the age of 5 years. The usual age of onset is beyond the fourth decade and is later than the usual age of onset of accessory pathway-mediated tachycardias.[4–10] Women are affected twice as often as men.[6–10] A second reason for the importance of AVNRT is the fact that it can result in significant debility and decreased quality of life.[11] And a third reason for the importance of AVNRT is that, in very rare circumstances, AVNRT may be life-threatening.[12]

### Pathophysiologic Basis of AVNRT

#### ANATOMICAL CONSIDERATIONS OF THE AV NODE

Early descriptions of the AV nodal tissue came from Albert Kent over a century ago.[13] The AV node is located epicardially, just underlying the right atrial epicardium, anterior to the nodal artery and between the coronary sinus and medial tricuspid valve leaflet, posterosuperior to the membranous septum. It comprises three different components: the transitional cell zone, the compact node, and the penetrating bundle of His (Fig. 30-1). The "compact" AV node refers to the most easily histologically distinguishable tissue located at the apex of the triangle of Koch (TOK), which is delineated leftward by the intersection of the eustachian valve and the tricuspid valve annulus, forming the apex, and the rightward ostium of the coronary sinus forming the base. A zone of transitional cells is interposed between the compact node and the atrial myocardium. Transitional cells enter the TOK to join the compact node superiorly, inferiorly, posteriorly, and from the left. At its distal extent, the AV node is distinguished from the penetrating bundle not so much by cellular characteristics as by the presence of a fibrous collar surrounding the specialized cells. Systematic anatomic investigation of the AV node in patients with AVNRT is lacking. No obvious histologic abnormalities have been identified among patients with AVNRT versus patients without AVNRT.[14] Several recent autopsy studies have reported that the sites of successful slow pathway ablation were clearly away from the histologic compact AV node, about 1 or 2 cm inferior and posterior to it.[15–17]

#### CONCEPT OF DUAL PATHWAYS

The concept of dual AV nodal physiology was introduced by Moe et al. in the 1950s in an effort to explain AVNRT.[18] It was proposed that dual AV node physiology results from functional dissociation within the compact node into fast and slow pathways. Moe et al. went on to propose that AVNRT resulted from reentry within the AV node involving the fast and slow pathways. The condition was hence initially considered incurable without causing AV block. However, a case report of inadvertent cure of AVNRT by Pritchett et al., after a failed attempt at surgical cryoablation of the AV node., paved the way for a new understanding.[19] This surgical experience made it clear that the fast and slow pathways are anatomically distinct and that AVNRT can be permanently cured by surgical procedures confined to perinodal tissue around the TOK, in the low right atrial septum and away from the compact AV node.[20–22] On the basis of this experience, several investigators developed a catheter-based ablative technique that used direct current shocks[23,24] or radiofrequency energy[25–27] to eliminate the fast AV pathway and permanently eliminate AVNRT.

Despite the excellent results of this procedure, it was complicated by a small but definite risk of AV block, requiring permanent pacemaker implantation. A technique to interrupt slow-pathway conduction without affecting normal AV conduction through the fast pathway by ablating small segments of myocardium in the posterior septum near the coronary sinus ostium was subsequently described.[5] This experience paved the way for the current approach using catheter ablation of this arrhythmia.[28–33]

TABLE 30-1 Differential Diagnosis for Types of SVT Based on ECG Characteristics

I. Long-RP tachycardia: RP >= PR
   i. Atypical AV nodal reentrant tachycardia
   ii. Atrial tachycardia
   iii. AVRT with a slowly conducting pathway (e.g., PJRT)
   iv. Sinus node reentry
   v. Sinus tachycardia
II. Short-RP tachycardia RP < PR
   i. Typical AVNRT
   ii. AV reentry

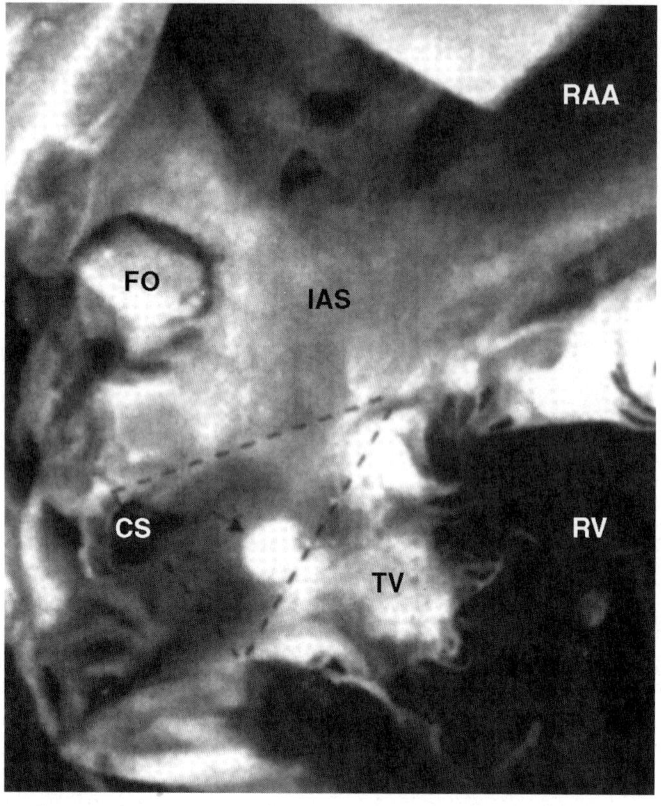


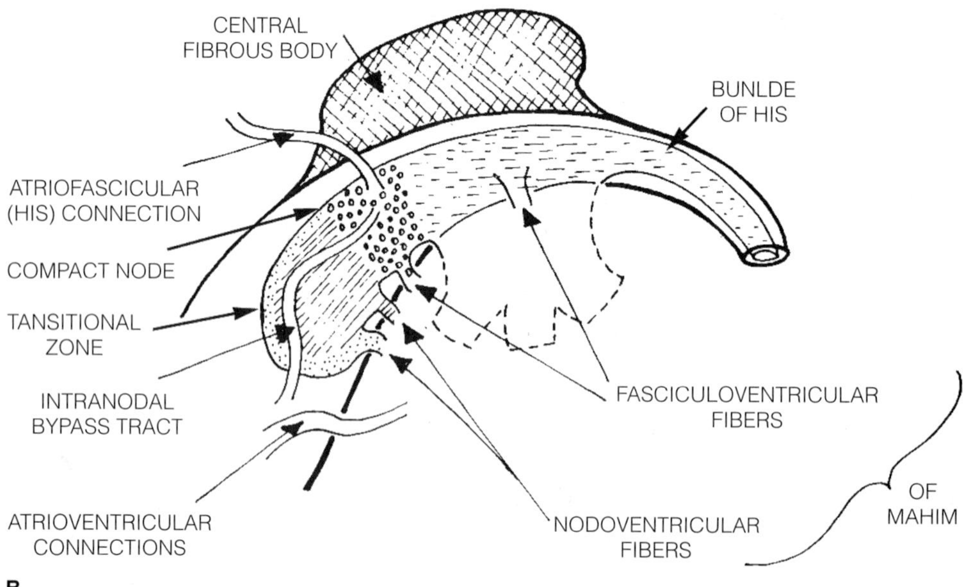


FIGURE 30-1 Structure of the AV node. *A.* Heart specimen from patient with AVNRT. Koch's triangle is formed by tendon of Todaro, coronary sinus (CS), ostium, and septal attachment of tricuspid valve (TV). Arrow represents site of successful ablation. IAS = interatrial septum, RV = right ventricle, FO = fossa ovalis, RAA = right atrial appendage. (From Olgin et al.[16] With permission) *B.* Schematic drawing depicting the three zones of the AV node and various types of perinodal and atrioventricular bypass tracts. (From McManus BM, Harji S, Wood SM. Morphologic features of normal and abnormal conductions systems. In: Singer I, ed. *Interventional Electrophysiology*, 2d ed. New York: Lippincott Williams & Wilkins; 2001:23. With permission.)

**TYPES OF AVNRT**

Three types of AVNRT have been described (Table 30-1). Typical or slow/fast AVNRT is the most prevalent type, accounting for 85 to 90 percent of cases. Atypical AVNRT, which represents the other 10 to 15 percent of cases, can be further differentiated into fast/slow and slow/slow (or intermediate) AVNRT. Induction of typical and atypical AVNRT in the same patient is possible but unusual. The typical or slow/fast AVNRT is thought to use the slow pathway for antegrade conduction and the fast pathway for retrograde conduction (Fig. 30-2). When an atrial premature complex APC blocks the fast pathway and proceeds slowly along the slow pathway, the fast pathway has enough time to recover from its refractoriness. This allows the impulse to activate the fast pathway retrogradely and return to the atrium, giving rise to an AV nodal reentrant echo beat. The impulse then travels down along the slow pathway again. Continuation of this gives rise to AVNRT. It has been proposed that the fast/slow AVNRT uses the fast pathway for anterograde conduction and the slow pathway for retrograde conduction. The slow/slow AVNRT, on the other hand, requires presence of two or more slow pathways with different conduction properties and refractory periods; one slow pathway is used for antegrade conduction and the other slow pathway for retrograde conduction.

## Diagnosis

**CLINICAL FEATURES**

Patients with AVNRT typically present with the clinical syndrome of paroxysmal supraventricular tachycardia. This is characterized as a regular rapid tachycardia of abrupt onset and termination. Patients also commonly describe palpitations and dizziness.[34] Rapid ventricular rates may be associated with complaints of

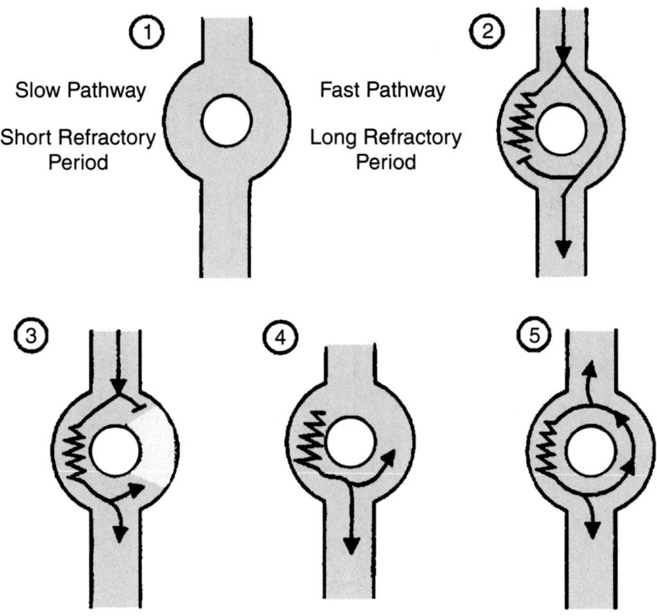


FIGURE 30-2 Schematic drawing showing dual AV nodal conduction. (1) The two AV nodal pathways, one with fast conduction and a relatively long refractory period and a second with slower conduction and shorter refractory period. (2) During sinus rhythm, impulses are conducted over both pathways but reach the bundle of His through the fast pathway. (3) A premature atrial impulse finds the fast pathway still refractory and is conducted over the slow pathway. (4 and 5) If the fast pathway has enough time to recover excitability, the impulse may reenter the fast pathway retrogradely and establish reentry. (Modified from Fogel RI, Prystowsky EN. Atrioventricular nodal reentry. In: Podrid PJ, Kowey PR, eds. *Cardiac Arrhythmia: Mechanisms, Diagnosis and Management.* New York: Lippincott Williams & Wilkins; 2001:436. With permission.)

dyspnea, weakness, angina, or even frank syncope and can at times be quite disabling.[35] Neck pounding during tachycardia in patients with AVNRT is due to simultaneous contraction of both atria and ventricles against closed mitral and tricuspid valves.[36,37] This clinical feature has been reported to be in distinguishing PSVT resulting from AVNRT from that due to orthodromic AV reciprocating tachycardia. Episodes may last from seconds to several hours. Patients often learn to use certain maneuvers such as carotid sinus massage or the Valsalva maneuver to terminate the arrhythmia, although many require pharmacologic treatment to achieve this. There is no significant association of AVNRT with other types of structural heart disease. The physical examination is usually remarkable only for a rapid, regular heart rate. At times, because of the simultaneous contraction of atria and ventricles, cannon A waves can be seen in the jugular venous waveform.

## ELECTROCARDIOGRAPHIC CHARACTERISTICS

AVNRT is characterized by a tachycardia with a narrow QRS complex with sudden onset and termination generally at regular rates between 120 and 200 beats per minute. Uncommonly, the rate can be as low as 110 beats per minute and, occasionally, especially in children, it may exceed 200 beats per minute. The rate of tachycardia may vary from episode to episode. In typical or slow/fast AVNRT, anterograde AV node conduction usually exceeds 200 ms. As the retrograde conduction is through the fast pathway, the VA interval is short, resulting in superimposition of the P wave onto the QRS complex on the surface electrocardiogram (ECG). Usually, the P wave is obscured by the QRS or may be seen slightly before or after the QRS complex. The presence of a pseudo r' wave in lead $V_1$ or pseudo s wave in leads II, III, and aVF suggests typical AVNRT (Fig. 30-3). Due to fast retrograde conduction, the RP interval is shorter than the PR interval.

In atypical fast/slow or slow/slow AVNRT, the AH interval is relatively short and the HA interval long. The P wave on surface ECG hence can be well delineated and is inverted in II, III, and aVF. The RP interval is equal to or longer than the PR interval (Fig. 30-4). This is one of the causes of "long RP" tachycardia (Table 30-1).

Functional bundle branch block may develop, producing a wide QRS tachycardia. However, functional bundle branch block should not affect the rate of tachycardia. Less commonly, dual pathways can be manifest on the ECG during sinus rhythm by sudden prolongation

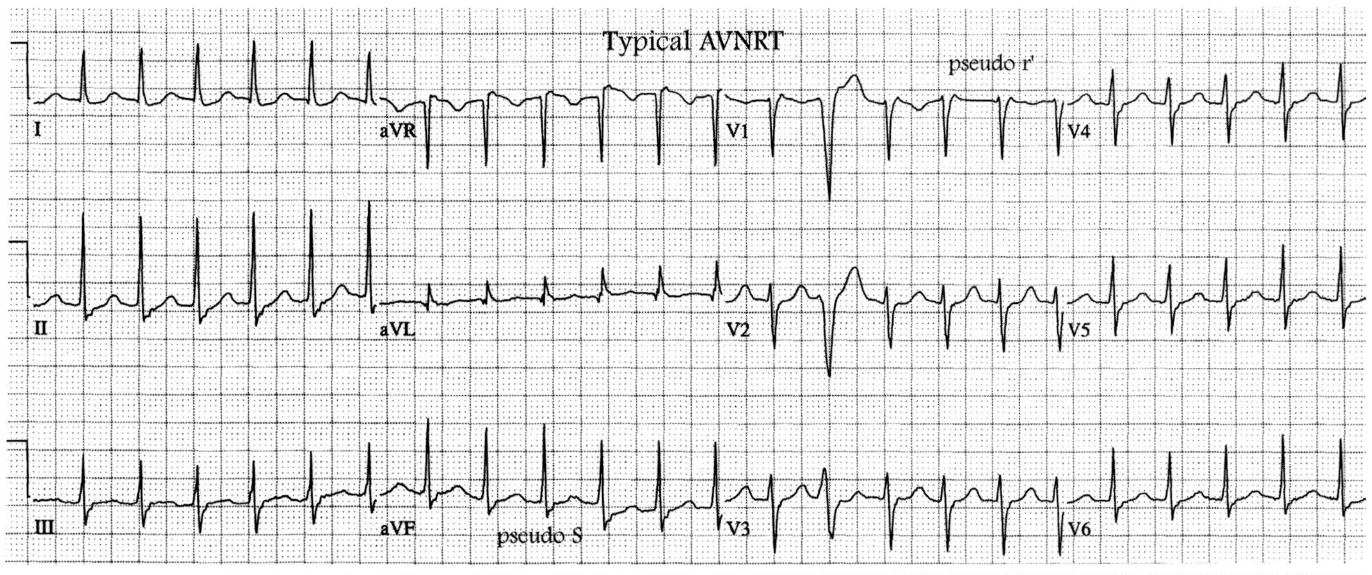


FIGURE 30-3 Twelve-lead ECG of a patient with typical AVNRT. Note the pseudo r' and pseudo S waves, very typical of this arrhythmia.

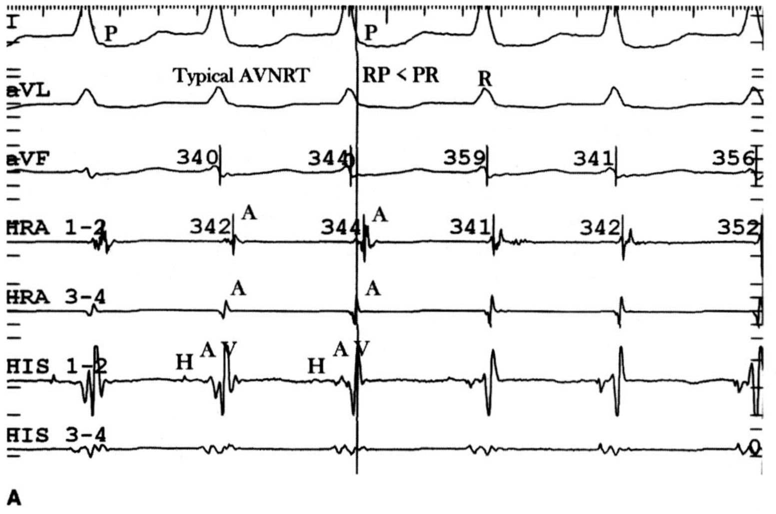


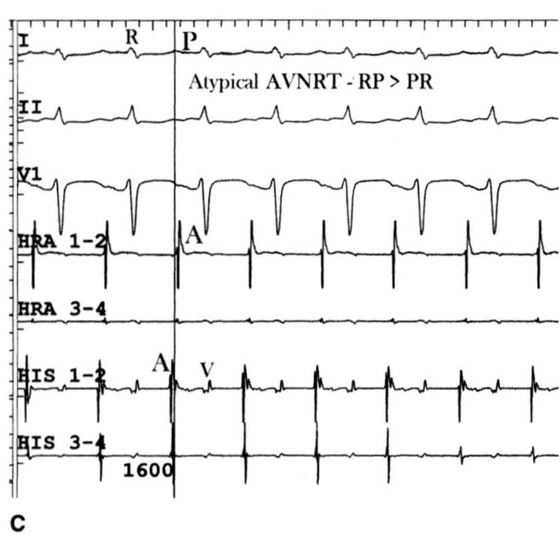


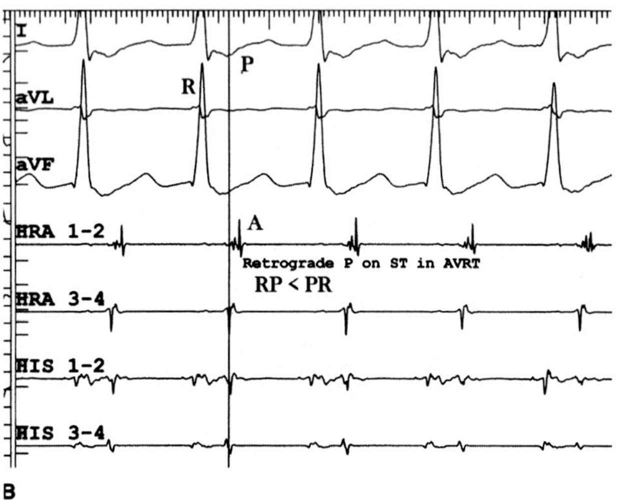


FIGURE 30-4 Surface ECG and intracardiac electrograms shown simultaneously in three different PSVTs. The vertical line in each of the panels shows the onset of atrial depolarization to indicate the timing of the P wave relative to the QRS. *A*. Typical AVNRT. *B*. AVRT involving an accessory pathway. *C*. Atypical AVNRT. R and P denote the corresponding waves on the surface ECG. A = atrial and V = ventricular deflection.

of the PR interval, PR alternans, and two QRS complexes in response to a single P wave[38] (Fig. 30-5).

Other ECG changes may be seen during or after the termination of AVNRT. Significant ST-segment depressions can be observed during tachycardia in nearly 25 to 50 percent of patients with AVNRT, and this is not predictive of ischemia.[39–43] There is no correlation between the rate of tachycardia and the presence and extent of ST-segment changes. However, one study found that 33 percent of patients with AVNRT above age 45 did have coronary artery disease, even though the symptoms were absent.[40]

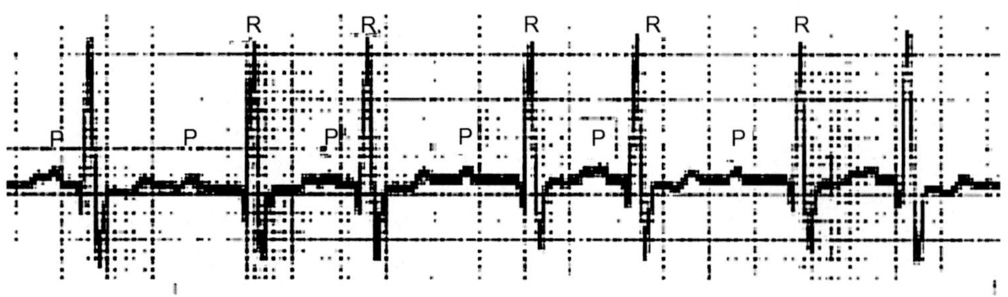

FIGURE 30-5 Rhythm strip of a patient during sinus rhythm. Note the sudden alternation of the PR interval from beat to beat. PR alternans is a manifestation of dual AV node physiology.

Newly acquired T-wave inversions after termination of AVNRT, commonly in anterior or inferior leads, can be seen in nearly 40 percent of patients.[44] They may be seen immediately after termination of tachycardia or may develop within 6 h, and they can persist for a variable duration. This occurrence is also not related to rate or duration of tachycardia. This is also not the result of coronary artery disease but due to repoloarization abnormalities, probably because of ionic current alterations resulting from the rapid rate.

A beat-to-beat oscillation in the QRS amplitude (i.e., QRS alternans) can be observed, although uncommonly, during episodes of AVNRT. Studies have reported that QRS alternans is observed more frequently in association with accessory pathway–mediated tachycardias than during AVNRT.[45] Morady et al. reported that QRS alternans is largely a rate-related phenomenon, being observed more commonly when the rate of tachycardia exceeds 200 beats per minute.[46]

## ELECTROPHYSIOLOGIC TESTING

Dual AV nodal physiology can be demonstrated by two pacing tech-

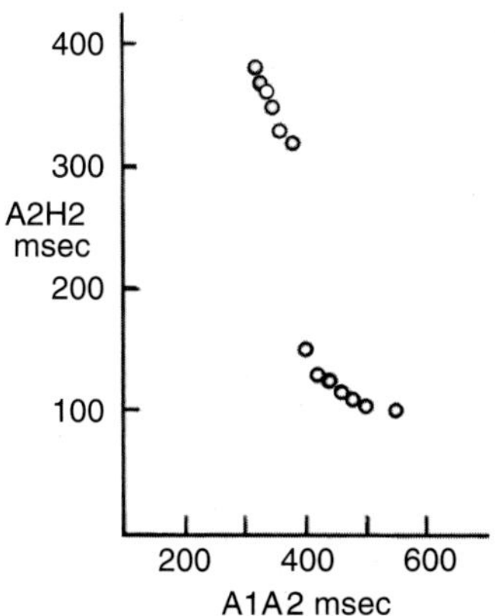


FIGURE 30-6 AV nodal function curve in a patient with dual AV nodal physiology. As the coupling interval of $A_1A_2$ is progressively decreased, there is a progressive prolongation of $A_2H_2$ intervals. At a coupling interval of around 360 ms, there is a large jump in the $A_2H_2$ interval. This is due to the fast pathway effectively reaching refractoriness at 360 ms and conduction proceeding over the slow pathway, which has a shorter refractory period but slower conduction. (Modified with permission from: Josephson M. Supraventricular tachycardias. In: Josephson M, ed. *Clinical Cardiac Electrophysiology: Technique and Interpretation,* 3d ed. Lippincott Williams & Wilkins, 2002:173.)

niques. Atrial pacing with introduction of PACs with increasing prematurity shows a gradual and progressive conduction delay in the AH interval. At a critical atrial coupling interval, a 10-ms decrement in the $A_1A_2$ results in a marked (>50-ms) prolongation of the $A_2H_2$ interval. It is a well-accepted convention that a 50-ms or greater increase in the AH interval in response to a 10-ms shortening of the $A_1A_2$ is considered evidence of dual AV node physiology. A plot of the $A_1A_2$ versus the $A_2H_2$ or the $A_2H_2$ versus the $H_1H_2$ shows a discontinuous curve (Fig. 30-6). The fast pathway has a shorter conduction time and longer refractory period and that the slow pathway has a longer conduction time and shorter refractory period. The abrupt increase in AV nodal conduction time is due to block in the conduction of fast pathway with a selective conduction over the slow pathway (Fig. 30-7). Some patients with AVNRT may not have discontinuous refractory period curves and some patients without AVNRT can exhibit discontinuous refractory period curves. It has been estimated that "dual AV node physiology" is present in approximately 10 percent of the general population. Such existence in the latter patients is a benign finding. Multiple AV nodal pathways can be demonstrated in occasional patients. More than one pathway may be involved in clinical tachycardia. The development of a PR interval that is greater than the atrial pacing cycle length during stable 1:1 AV conduction is a quite specific sign of slow AV nodal conduction.

Curtis et al. have recently demonstrated the differential effect of adenosine on the slow and the fast pathways.[47] The fast pathway is usually more sensitive to adenosine; when this is given during sinus rhythm, it can cause an abrupt prolongation of PR interval due to conduction proceeding over the slow pathway. This effect can be exploited to determine whether patients with SVT are likely to have a diagnosis of AVNRT.[48] Typical AVNRT is usually not inducible with ventricular pacing, while this is the rule with atypical AVNRT. Lack of reproducible arrhythmia induction is most often due to block in retrograde fast pathway. Other causes include slow-pathway block

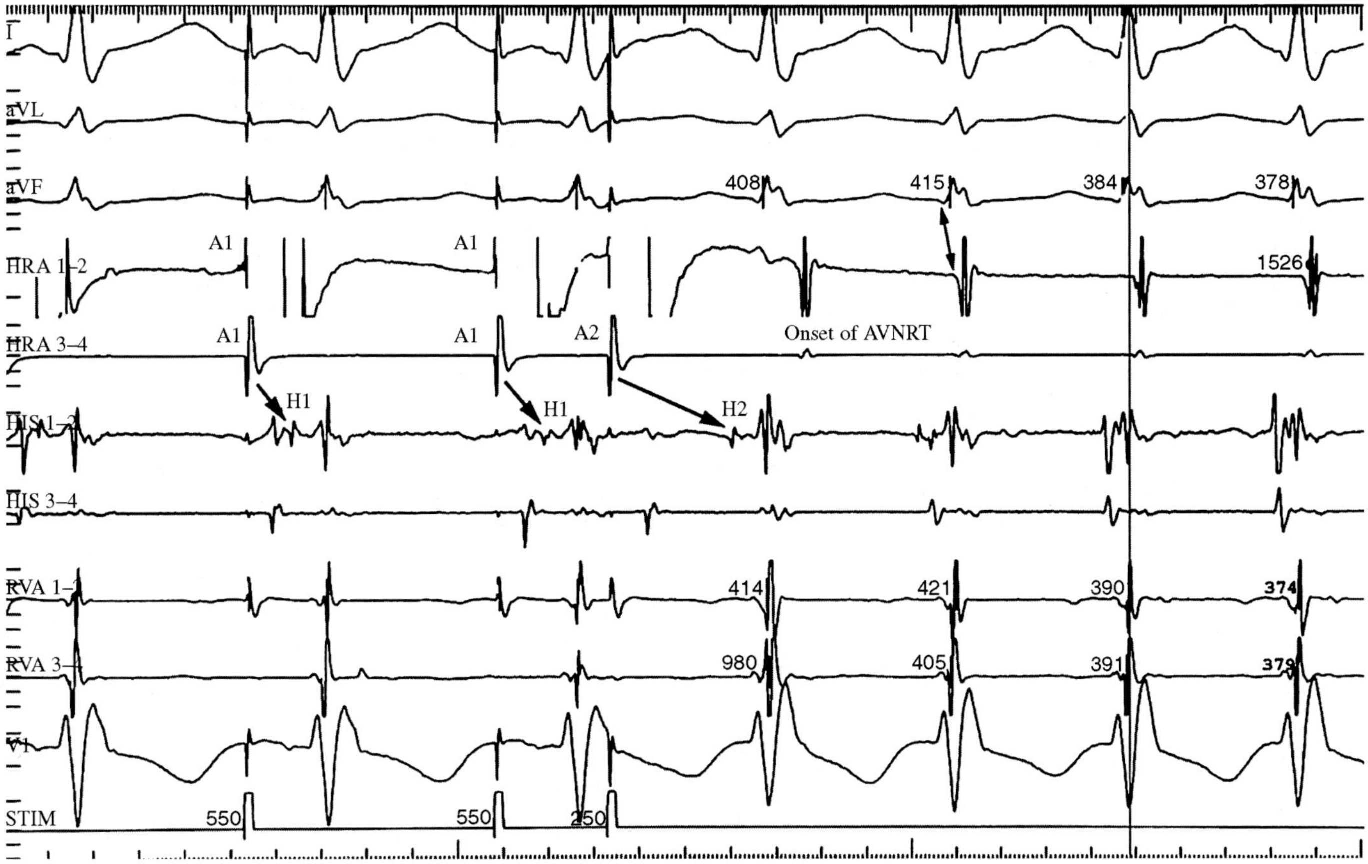

FIGURE 30-7 Electrophysiologic demonstration of dual AV nodal physiology and initiation of AVNRT. At an $A_1A_2$ coupling interval of 350 ms, there is a jump in the $A_2H_2$ interval (*arrows*). This is followed by initiation of tachycardia. Note the very short VA conduction time.

and inability to achieve a critical delay in the AH interval. Esmolol has been shown to prolong the effective refractory period of the fast pathway more than the slow pathway.[49] Increased vagal tone has also recently been shown to have differential effects on the fast and slow pathways.[50]

During typical AVNRT, the atrial and ventricular activation is nearly simultaneous, hence causing short HA intervals. An HA interval of <70 ms is virtually diagnostic of AVNRT[50] (Fig. 30-7). Differentiation of AVNRT, particularly of the atypical type, from other forms of SVT can be challenging, requiring the use of several maneuvers at electrophysiologic study (EPS).[51]

## Management

Since AVNRT is generally a benign arrhythmia that does not influence survival, the main reason for treating it is to alleviate symptoms. The threshold for initiation of therapy will vary based on patient preference and also on the frequency and duration of the episodes of tachycardia as well as the associated symptoms. The threshold for treatment will also reflect whether the patient is a competitive athlete, a woman considering pregnancy, or someone with a high-risk occupation such as scuba diving. The North American Society for Pacing and Electrophysiology has recently developed a policy statement on catheter ablation. The recommendations made by this task force are reviewed at the end of this section.

### ACUTE MANAGEMENT

The dependence of AVNRT on AV nodal conduction has important therapeutic implications. Because of the known influence of autonomic tone on AV nodal conduction, maneuvers that increase vagal tone, such as the Valsalva and Mueller maneuvers, gagging, carotid sinus massage, and occasionally exposing the face to ice water can been used to terminate the tachycardia. The effect of vagal maneuvers is most pronounced on the slow pathway.[50] Hence, in the slow/fast form of AVNRT, the tachycardia typically terminates in the anterograde direction; in the fast/slow type of AVNRT, the block is in the retrograde limb of the tachycardia circuit.

Adenosine, a purinergic blocking agent that causes acute and transient AV nodal blockade, is the drug of choice for acute termination of AVNRT. Multiple studies have shown that adenosine is nearly 100 percent effective in terminating AVNRT.[54,55] It has a rapid onset of action (seconds) and a short half life (<10 s); moreover, it does not impair contractility. When used for termination of a narrow-complex tachycardia, an initial dose of 6 mg may be followed by 12 mg if the first dose is ineffective. Because of its short duration of action, it is essential that adenosine be administered as a rapid bolus. This is best achieved by having a syringe with adenosine and a 5 mL flush attached to the patient using a stopcock. In this fashion, the dose of adenosine can be followed immediately by a saline flush to ensure rapid delivery of the drug. Minor side effects, including transient dyspnea or chest pain, are common with adenosine. Sinus arrest or bradycardia may occur but resolve quickly if appropriate upward dosing is used. With termination of PSVT, atrial and ventricular premature beats are frequently seen; a few patients with adenosine-induced polymorphic ventricular tachycardia have been reported.[54] These patients had long baseline QT intervals and long pauses during adenosine-induced AV block. Adenosine shortens the atrial refractory period, and atrial ectopy may induce atrial fibrillation. This may be dangerous if the patient has an accessory pathway capable of rapid antegrade conduction. Because adenosine is cleared so rapidly, reinitiation of tachycardia after initial termination may occur. Either repeat administration of the same dose of adenosine or substitution of a calcium channel blocker will be effective. Adenosine mediates its effects via a specific cell surface receptor, the $A_1$ receptor. Theophylline and other methylxanthines block the $A_1$ receptor. Caffeine levels achieved after beverage ingestion may be overcome by the doses of adenosine used to treat PSVT.[56] Dipyridamole blocks adenosine elimination, thereby potentiating and prolonging its effects. Adenosine is also shown to produce faster termination of SVT in the presence of isoproterenol.[55] Cardiac transplant recipients are also unusually sensitive to adenosine. If adenosine is chosen in these latter situations, much lower starting doses (i.e., 1 mg) should be selected. Adenosine should also be used with great caution in patients with a history of asthma, as it may trigger bronchospasm.

Several other drugs that affect the AV node can also be used for acute termination of AVNRT. Verapamil, a calcium channel blocker, can terminate AVNRT and prevent induction.[53] It slows conduction both in the slow and fast pathways, and termination is usually caused by anterograde block. A 5-mg bolus of verapamil may be followed by one or two additional 5-mg boluses 10 min apart if the initial dose does not terminate the tachycardia; this has been an effective regimen in up to 90 percent of patients.[55] Drugs that enhance vagal tone, such as digoxin, or that block the sympathetic effect, like beta blockers, can also be used to terminate AVNRT.[57,58] Digoxin, which has a slower onset of action than the other AV nodal blockers, is not favored for the acute termination of AVNRT except if there are relative contraindications to the other agents. Class Ia and IC sodium-channel blockers can also be employed in treating an acute event of AVNRT—a strategy that is rarely used when other regimens have failed. Unlike the other agents, the sodium channel blocking agents depress retrograde fast-pathway conduction. If a patient's tachycardia cannot be terminated with intravenous drugs, direct-current (DC) shock cardioversion can always be used. Energies in the range of 10 to 50 J are usually adequate.

### LONG-TERM MANAGEMENT

***Catheter Ablation*** Catheter ablation of AVNRT is performed by ablating the slowly conducting portion of the AV node using the "posterior approach." Once the diagnosis of AVNRT is established and the endpoint for ablation defined (either the presence of dual AV node physiology or reproducibly inducible AVNRT), the ablation catheter is positioned across the tricuspid valve at the level of the coronary sinus (CS) ostium (Fig. 30-8). The ablation catheter is then slowly withdrawn with clockwise catheter torque until a small multicomponent atrial electrogram is observed together with a large ventricular electrogram. The most common site of successful ablation is at the level of the superior aspect of the CS ostium.[4,59] (Fig. 30-8). In patients with unusual forms of AVNRT, the site of successful ablation is slightly inferior to the CS ostium or, at times, within the floor of the CS. Once an appropriate site is identified, radiofrequency (RF) energy is applied. The development of a junctional rhythm during RF application is a marker for a successful ablation site. If a junctional rhythm develops, VA conduction should be monitored carefully; if VA or AV conduction block is observed, RF energy should immediately be discontinued.

Successful ablation of AVNRT with the posterior approach is usually characterized by an increase in the AV block cycle length and in the AV nodal effective refractory period; a normal PR interval on ECG and lack of inducibility of AVNRT both at baseline and during isoproterenol infusion are also seen. Retrograde conduction is generally not affected. The presence of more than one AV nodal echo beat or a PR prolongation that exceeds the paced atrial cycle length during stable 1:1 AV conduction suggest that the AVNRT is likely to recur and will require further RF applications.

This technique was initially described by Jackman et al.[5] nearly a decade ago and has since been widely accepted as the standard approach. Calkins et al.[10] reported the largest multicenter experience with the posterior approach. In this trial of over 1000 patients with AV tachycardias, 373 patients had AVNRT. The overall success rate of ablation was 97 percent. AV block is the most common complication, occurring in 0.5 to 1 percent of patients. The incidence of recurrence after successful ablation is approximately 3 percent. Because of the higher efficacy and lower incidence of AV block and arrhythmia recurrence and the greater likelihood of maintaining a normal PR interval during sinus rhythm, the posterior approach is now considered the preferred approach to ablation of AVNRT.[28–33,60–63]

***Medical Therapy*** Most pharmacologic agents that depess AV nodal conduction may be demonstrated to reduce the frequency of recurrences of AVNRT. These pharmacologic agents include beta blockers, calcium channel blockers, class 1a antiarrhythmic agents such as procainamide and disopyramide, class 1c antiarrhythmic agents such as flecainide and propafenone, and class 3 antiarrhythmic agents such as betapace and amiodarone. The best-studied among these have been the class Ic antiarrhythmic agents.[64–71]

Henthorn et al.[64] studied 34 patients with PSVT, many of whom had documented or suspected AVNRT. Flecainide in doses up to 200 mg twice a day prevented recurrent tachycardia in 79 percent at 60 days, compared to 15 percent in the placebo arm ($p < 0.001$). The median time to the first recurrence of tachycardia increased from 11 days in the placebo arm to 55 days in the treated patients ($p < 0.001$). In dose-ranging studies, flecainide was effective in preventing SVT over a 1-month period in almost 60 percent of patients at a dose of 50 mg twice a day and 86 percent of patients at a dose of 150 mg twice a day.[65] The real advantage of flecainide is the minimal occurrence of extracardiac side effects, which are lower than with other antiarrhythmic drugs. In some cases of coexistent atrial tachycardia, flecainide can increase conduction through the AV node, resulting in rapid ventricular rates. Use of AV nodal blocking agents in such circumstances is highly advisable.

Pritchett et al.[69] reported similar efficacy with propafenone, the other currently available class Ic agent. They studied 33 patients with PSVT. The time to first recurrence of tachycardia was prolonged with propafenone ($p = 0.004$). Recurrence of tachycardia with treatment was decreased to one-fifth of the recurrence rate with placebo. The effective dose of propafenone is 150 to 300 mg three times a day for the long-term treatment of PSVT.

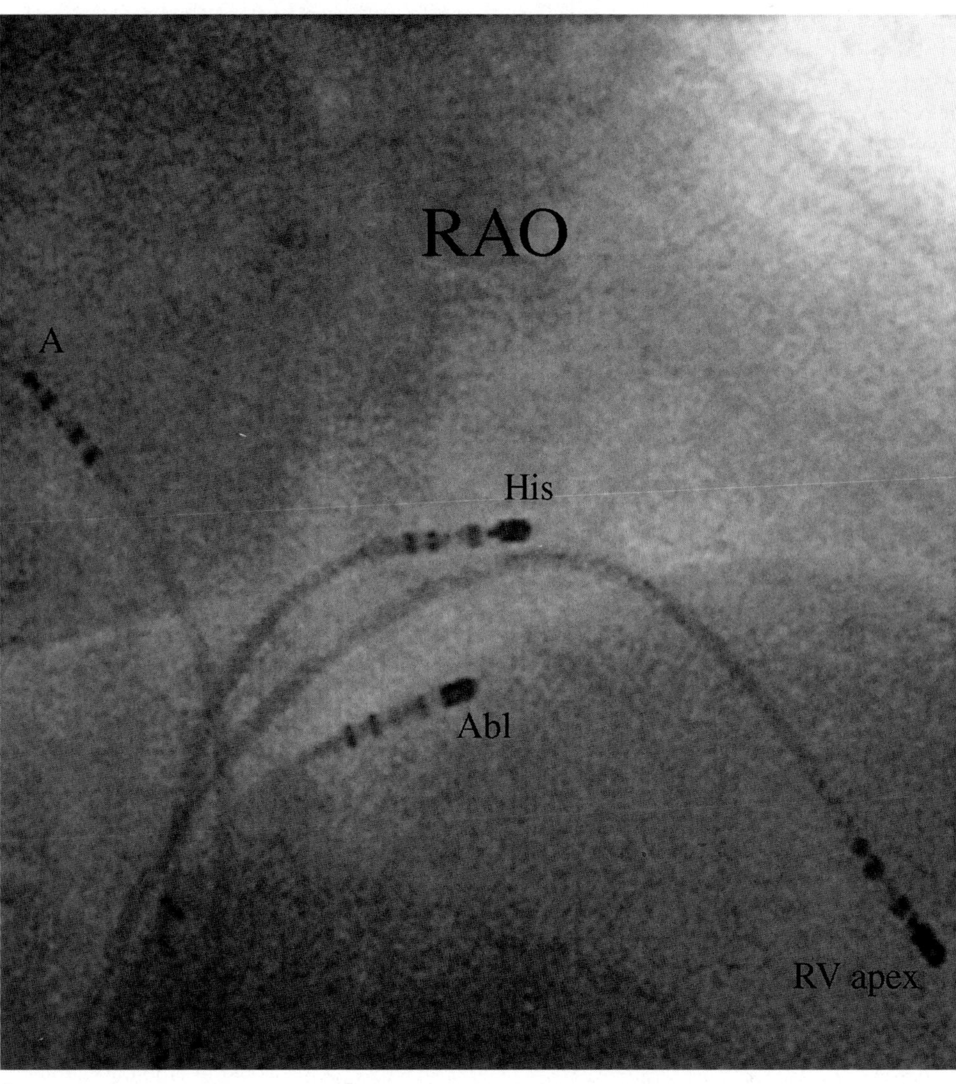


A

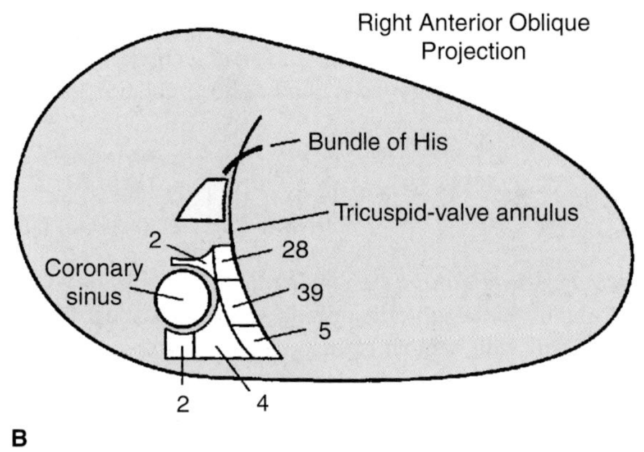


B

FIGURE 30-8 Site of slow-pathway ablation for AVNRT. *A.* Fluoroscopic images showing the alignment of the catheters during slow-pathway ablation. Note that the site of the slow pathway is a considerable distance from the site of the His bundle or compact AV node. *B.* Schematic showing the orientation of heart during corresponding fluoroscopic projection. RAO = right anterior oblique. The numbers represent the sites of successful slow-pathway ablation in corresponding patients. (Modified from Jackman et al.[5] With permission.)

Sotalol, a class III agent, has been studied for long-term suppression of AVNRT. Hikuri et al. reported in a study that sotalol in a dose of 0.1 mg/kg prevented induction of AVNRT in 8 of 8 patients.[70] Sotalol in oral doses of 160 to 480 mg/day prevented long-term recurrence of SVT in all patients who took it chronically. Wanless et al.[71] observed, in a multicenter study, that the time to recurrence of PSVT was significantly less compared with placebo when patients were receiving sotalol 80 mg ($p = 0.018$) and sotalol 160 mg ($p = 0.0009$). Because of a higher incidence of side effects associated with amiodarone, it is rarely indicated for the treatment of AVNRT.

## Management Strategy

Patients with AVNRT typically present with the clinical syndrome of PSVT. The diagnosis of PSVT can be made with a high degree of certainty based on the clinical history alone, even if the tachycardia has never been documented by an ECG. Physicians may try to document the tachycardia with an ECG using either a 30-day event monitor or by instructing the patient to go to an emergency room or physician's office if another episode of tachycardia occurs. Since AVNRT is not a life-threatening arrhythmia, the primary indication for its treatment relates to its impact on a patient's quality of life. Patients who develop a highly symptomatic episode of PSVT, particularly if it requires an emergency room visit for termination, may elect to initiate therapy after a single episode. In contrast, a patient who presents with minimally symptomatic episodes of PSVT that terminate spontaneously or with a Valsalva maneuver may elect to be followed clinically without specific therapy.

Once it is decided to initiate treatment for AVNRT, the question arises of whether to initiate pharmacologic therapy or to use catheter ablation. Because of its greater than 95 percent efficacy and low incidence of complications, catheter ablation is now considered first-line therapy. The recently published NASPE Policy Statement on Catheter Ablation includes catheter ablation of AVNRT using the posterior approach as a class 1 indication for catheter ablation. According to this statement, "for those patients in whom treatment of AVNRT is deemed necessary, ablation can be offered as an initial therapy option."[52] It is therefore reasonable to discuss catheter ablation with all patients suspected of having AVNRT. Depending on the frequency and severity of tachycardia episodes, the patient's lifestyle, and his or her preferences, an individual may elect to be followed clinically without specific therapy, to begin a trial of pharmacologic therapy with a beta blocker or calcium channel blocker, or to undergo electrophysiology testing and catheter ablation.

# AV REENTRANT TACHYCARDIA AND WOLFF-PARKINSON-WHITE SYNDROME

Accessory pathways (APs) are important because they provide a substrate for antidromic and orthodromic AV reciprocating tachycardia, are associated with sudden cardiac death, and may be detected in asymptomatic patients on a routine screening ECG. The sections that follow cover the pathophysiology, diagnosis, and management of this fascinating clinical entity.

## Pathophysiology

The Wolff-Parkinson-White syndrome was first described in 1930 in an article by Louis Wolff, Sir John Parkinson, and Paul Dudley White. The authors described 11 patients with recurrent tachycardia associated with an ECG pattern of "bundle branch block with short PR interval." Since publication of this initial report, our understanding of the anatomic and pathophysiologic features of preexcitation syndromes has improved enormously.[72]

TABLE 30-2 Types of Accessory Pathway

I. Based on site of origin and insertion:
   a. Atrioventricular
      i. Right-sided: anteroseptal, RV free wall, posteroseptal
      ii. Left-sided: anteroseptal, LV free wall, posteroseptal
   b. Atriofasicular (Brechenmacher fibers)
   c. Nodofasicular (Mahaim fibers)
II. Based on direction of conduction:
   a. Antegrade
   b. Retrograde (concealed)
   c. Bidirectional
III. Based on conduction property:
   a. Slow, decremental
   b. Fast, nondecremental
IV. Based on number:
   a. Single
   b. Multiple

Accessory pathways are anomalous, typically extranodal connections that connect the epicardial surfaces of the atrium and ventricle along the AV groove. Accessory bypass tracts, which conduct antegrade from the atrium to the ventricle and therefore are detectable on an ECG, have been reported to be present in 0.15 to 0.25 percent of the general population.[73,74] A higher prevalence of 0.55 percent has been reported in first-degree relatives of patients with WPW syndrome.[75]

### CLASSIFICATION

Accessory pathways can be classified based on their site of origin and insertion, location along the mitral or tricuspid annulus, type of conduction (antegrade or retrograde conduction or both), and properties of conduction (decremental or nondecremental) (Table 30-2). Accessory pathways usually exhibit rapid, nondecremental conduction, similar to that which is present in normal His-Purkinje tissue and atrial or ventricular myocardium. Approximately 8 percent of accessory pathways display decremental antegrade or retrograde conduction.[76] Accessory pathways, which are capable only of retrograde conduction, are referred to as "concealed," whereas those capable of antegrade conduction are referred to as "manifest," demonstrating preexcitation on a standard ECG (Fig. 30-9). Accessory

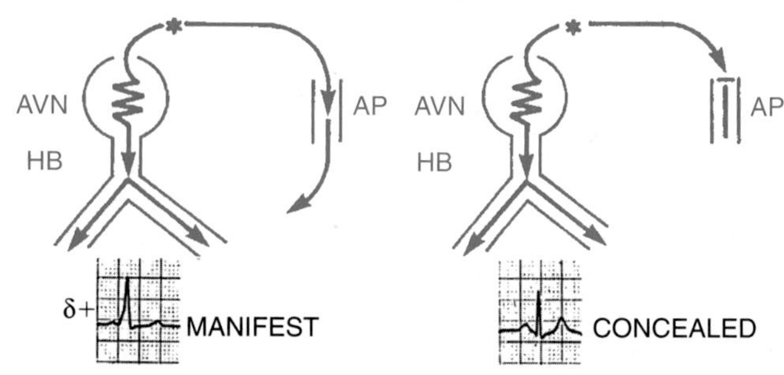


FIGURE 30-9 Atrioventricular conduction patterns and QRS morphologies during sinus rhythm for manifest and concealed accessory pathways. AVN = atrioventricular node, HB = His bundle, AP = accessory pathway. (Modified with permission from: Cain et al.[82] With permission.)

pathways usually conduct both antegrade and retrograde. Antegrade-only accessory pathways are particularly uncommon. When present, they are usually right-sided and frequently demonstrate decremental conduction (Mahaim fiber). Concealed accessory pathways are less common, accounting for approximately 15 percent of all accessory pathways.[77] Patients with Ebstein's anomaly who also have WPW syndrome frequently have more than one accessory pathway.

Variant accessory pathways include those that connect the atrium to the distal or compact AV node (James fibers), the atrium to the His bundle (the Brechenmacher fiber) and the AV node or His bundle to the distal Purkinje fibers or ventricular myocardium (the Mahaim fibers)[78] (Fig. 30-1*B*).

## CONCEPT OF PREEXCITATION

The hallmark of an accessory pathway function during sinus rhythm is depolarization of all or part of the ventricles earlier than expected if conduction has occurred only over the normal AV conduction system, resulting in preexcitation. The intraventricular conduction delay begins with the onset of the QRS complex, in contrast to intraventricular conduction defects such as left or right BBB, in which the delay occurs throughout or during the terminal portion of the QRS complex. The resultant slurred upstroke or downstroke comprising the initial part of the preexcited QRS complex is known as "delta wave" (Fig. 30-10).

The degree of shortening of the PR interval and the extent of ventricular preexcitation depend on several factors, including location of the accessory pathway, the relationship between antegrade conduction times and refractory periods of the AV bypass tract, and the normal AV conduction system. A bypass tract that crosses the AV groove in the left lateral region may also result in inapparent preexcitation and minimal PR-interval shortening during sinus rhythm due to greater interatrial distance for impulse propagation from the sinus node to this site of atrial input into the AP. On the other hand, an AP on the right side is more likely to demonstrate marked preexcitation. Preexcitation may be less apparent during sinus tachycardia, when sympathetic tone is high and vagal tone low, resulting in faster AV node conduction time than that in the AP. On the other extreme, during conditions of slowed conduction through the AV node either by intrinsic nodal factors, withdrawal of sympathetic tone, or increased vagal tone, the amount of preexcitation apparent on the 12-lead ECG is maximized due to relatively greater conduction through the AP. Rapid intravenous administration of adenosine causing blocking or slowing of AV node conduction and exposing the anterograde AP conduction has been used as a diagnostic maneuver.[79,80] The degree of preexcitation can also be enhanced with atrial pacing directly over the AP, eliminating the intraatrial conduction delay from the sinus node to the atrial insertion site of AP (Fig. 30-11).

Intermittent preexcitation is characterized by abrupt loss of delta wave, normalization of the QRS duration, and an increase in the PR interval during a continuous ECG recording, often despite only minor variations in resting sinus rhythm heart rate. This should be distinguished from day-to-day variability in preexcitation or inapparent preexcitation due to factors described above. The presence of intermittent preexcitation has been considered to suggest that the refractory period in the AP is long, making them very unlikely to mediate a rapid, preexcited ventricular response during atrial fibrillation.[81]

## TACHYCARDIAS ASSOCIATED WITH ACCESSORY PATHWAYS

Tachycardias associated with APs can be subdivided into those in which the AP is necessary for initiation and maintenance of tachycardia and those in whom the AP acts as a bystander.

AV reentrant tachycardia (AVRT) is a macroreentrant tachycardia involving the atrium, the AP, the AV node, and the ventricle. AVRT is further subclassified into orthodromic and antidromic AVRT (Fig. 30-12). During orthodromic AVRT, the reentrant impulse utilizes the AV node and specialized conduction system for conduction from the atrium to the ventricle and utilizes the AP for conduction from

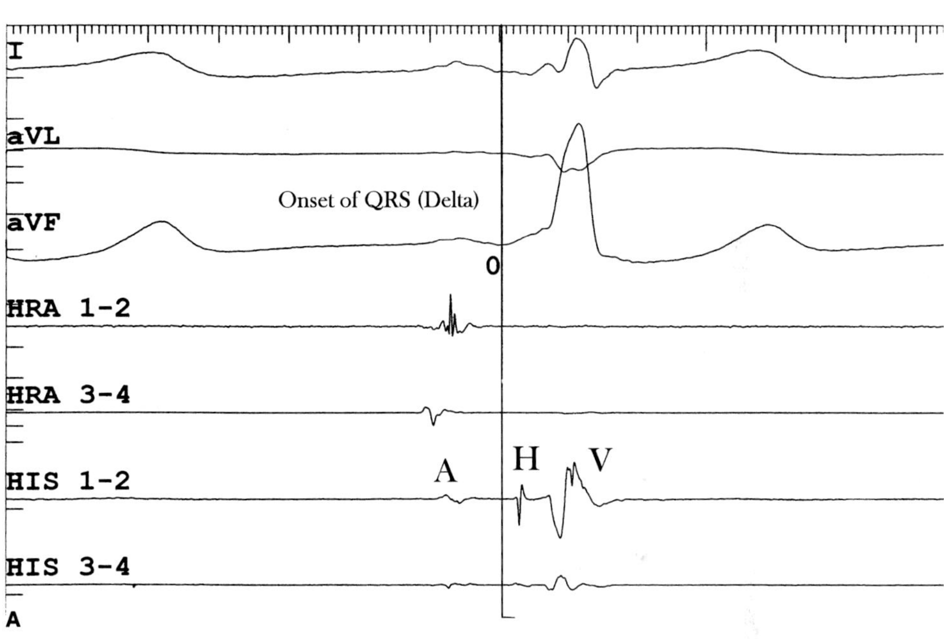


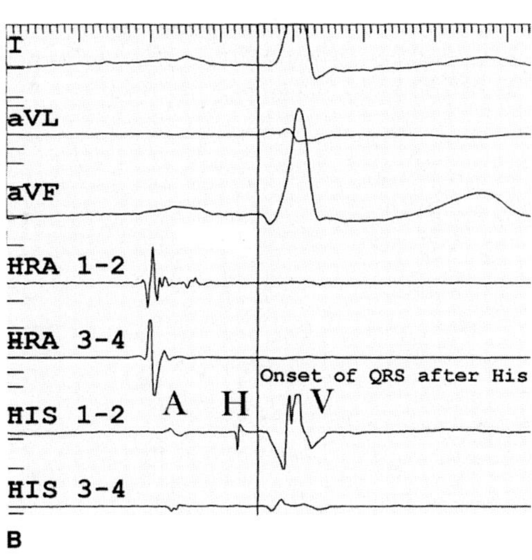


FIGURE 30-10 Electrophysiologic confirmation of preexcitation. *A.* Preexcited QRS complex in WPW syndrome. Onset of QRS or delta wave is clearly before the His electrogram before ablation. *B.* Loss of preexcitation and shift of onset of QRS to after His deflection postablation. HRA = high right atrium, HIS = His bundle electrogram, A, H, V = atrial, His, and ventricular electrograms.

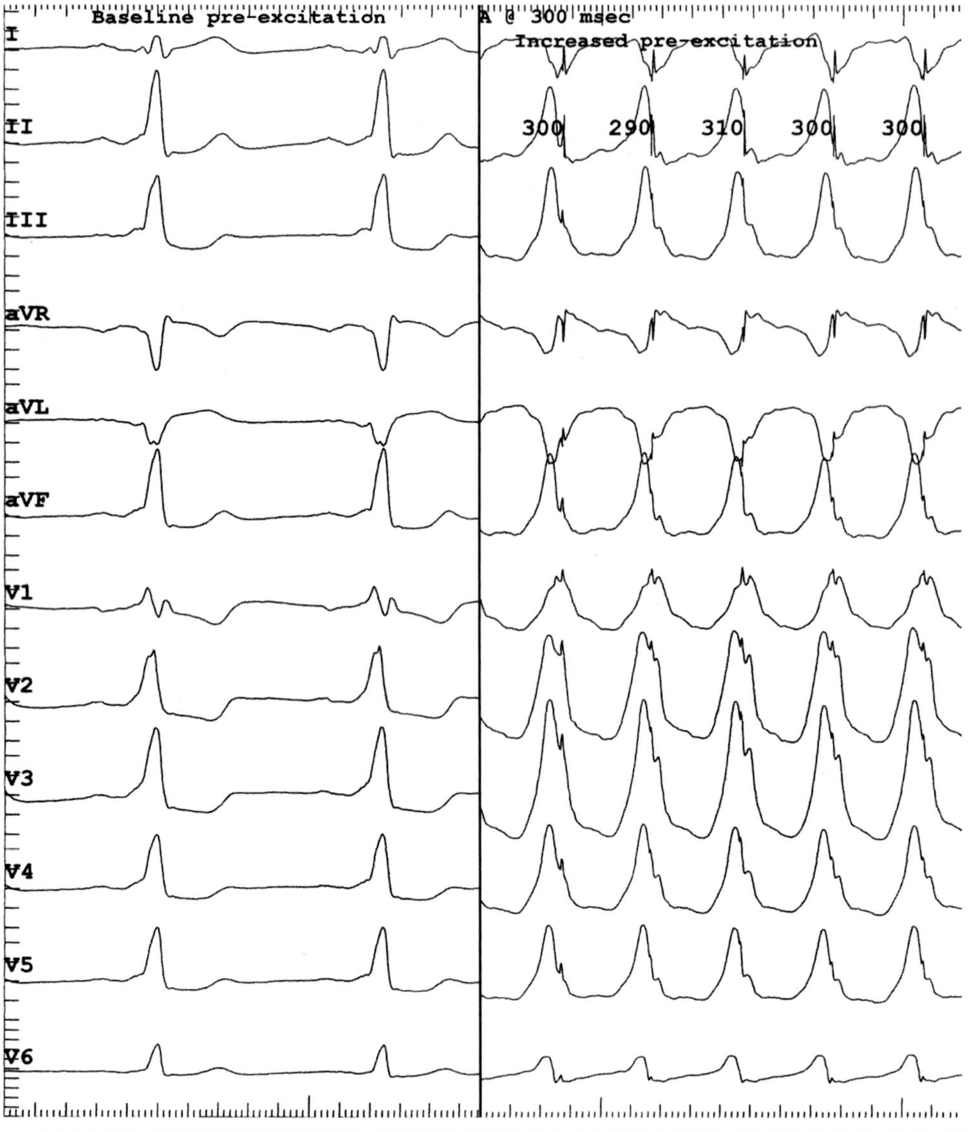

FIGURE 30-11 Increase in degree of preexcitation with atrial pacing. Left panel shows 12-lead ECG during sinus rhythm. Note the obvious increase in preexcitation in the right panel with atrial pacing at a cycle length of 300 ms (200 beats per minute). Increase in atrial input causes decremental conduction in the AV node, resulting in increased conduction over the accessory pathway.

the ventricle to the atrium. Orthodromic AVRT can be initiated by atrial or ventricular premature depolarizations (APD or VPD). APDs initiating the tachycardia block antegradely in the AP and conduct relatively slowly over the AV nodal tissue to the ventricles. The impulse then retrogradely conducts over the AP reentering the atria at the atrial insertion site of the pathway, thus completing the reentrant loop (Fig. 30-13). A VPD, on the other hand, blocks in the His Purkinje system and retrogradely reaches the atria through retrogradely conducting AP. The impulse then conducts antegradely through the AV nodal tissue, completing the circuit. The QRS complex during orthodromic AVRT hence is not preexcited.

During antidromic AVRT, on the other hand, the reentrant impulse travels in the reverse direction, with conduction from the atrium to the ventricle occurring via the AP. Antidromic AV reciprocating tachycardia is rare, occurring in only 5 to 10 percent of patients with the WPW syndrome. APDs that occur at a coupling interval that is longer than the refractory period of the AP and shorter than the AV nodal refractory period can initiate the antidromic AVRT; the converse is true with a VPD. Susceptibility of antidromic AVRT appears to depend on the existence of adequate separation between the AP and the AV nodal tissue. Hence, most of the antidromic AVRTs seem to occur only with left-sided bypass tracts.[82]

Other forms of SVTs—like atrial tachycardia, junctional tachycardia, AVNRT, and even ventricular tachycardia—can occur in patients with bypass tracts. Dual AV nodal physiology has been noted in nearly 12 percent of patients with WPW syndrome.[83] Coexisting ventricular tachycardia is less likely, as patients with WPW tend to present at a younger age and have less structural heart disease.

Atrial fibrillation is a less common but potentially more serious arrhythmia in patients with the WPW syndrome. If an AP has a short antegrade refractory period, atrial fibrillation can result in a rapid ventricular response with subsequent degeneration to ventricular fibrillation.[84–86] The risk of sudden death has been shown to be higher if the shortest RR interval is less than 250 ms during spontaneous or induced atrial fibrillation.[84] It has been estimated that one-third of patients with WPW syndrome also have atrial fibrillation.[87] APs appear to play a pathophysiologic role in the development of atrial fibrillation in these patients, as most are young and do not have structural heart disease. Furthermore, surgical or catheter ablation of APs usually results in elimination of atrial fibrillation as well.[88,89]

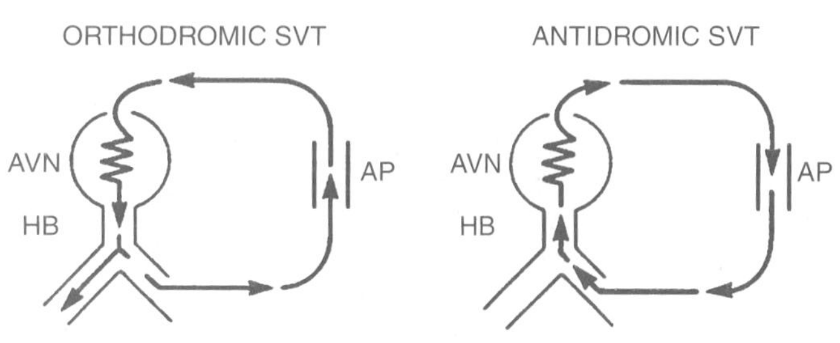


FIGURE 30-12 Schematic representation of the patterns of conduction through an accessory pathway (AP) and the normal conduction system (AVN-HB) during orthodromic AVRT and antidromic AVRT. (Modified from Cain et al.[82] With permission.)

## Diagnosis

### CLINICAL FEATURES

Preexcitation occurs in the general population at a frequency of around 1.5 per 1000. Of these 50 to 60 percent of patients become symptomatic. Approximately one-third of all patients with PSVT are diagnosed as having an AP-mediated tachycardia. Patients with AP-mediated tachycardias most commonly present with the syndrome of PSVT. Population-based studies have demonstrated a bimodal distribution of symptoms for patients with preexcitation, with a peak in early childhood, followed by a second peak in young adulthood. Nearly 25 percent of patients will become asymptomatic over time. More than half the patients with an episode will suffer a recurrence.[90]

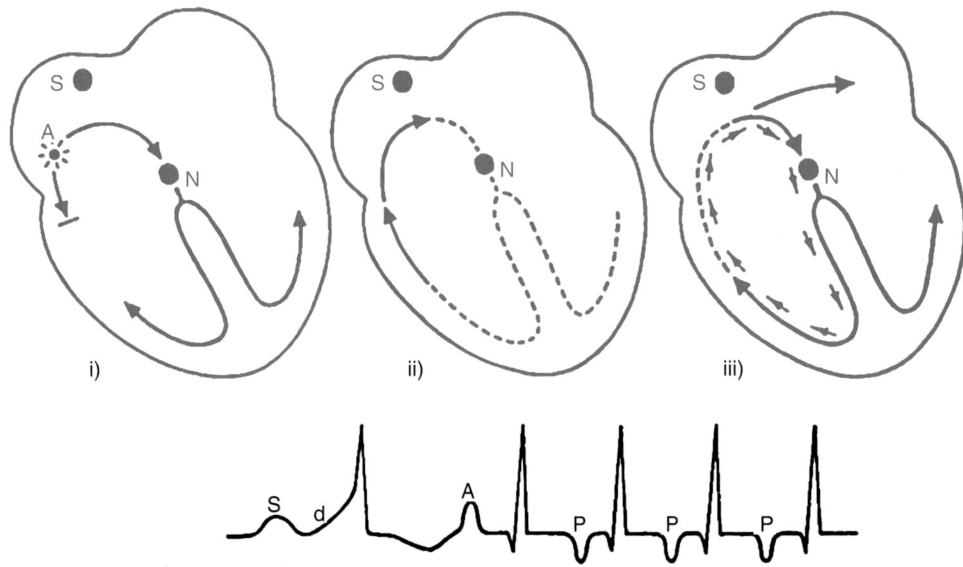


FIGURE 30-13 Schematic of initiation of orthodromic atrioventricular reentrant tachycardia. A diagrammatic ECG recording shows the first P wave of sinus-node (S) origin yielding a preexcited QRS complex with a delta wave (d) and short PR interval. (i) An ectopic atrial impulse (A) blocks antegradely in the bypass tract but still conducts over the AV node (N) and His-Purkinje system to the ventricles. This causes the second QRS complex to appear nonpreexcited. (ii) The premature impulse continues to conduct retrogradely over the bypass tract, as the latter had time recover excitability while the impulse was conducting over the node. (iii) The retrogradely conducted impulse has activated the atria from the bypass tracts' atrial insertion point and generated the first retrograde P wave (P) of AVRT. Reentrance of impulse through the node then occurs, causing AVRT to perpetuate. (Modified from Chung EK. Wolff-Parkinson-White syndrome: Current views. *Am J Med* 1977;62:261. With permission.)

Symptoms range from palpitations to syncope.[90] As in AVNRT, episodes of tachycardia may be associated with dyspnea, chest pain, decreased exercise tolerance, anxiety, dizziness, or syncope. Although syncope is often considered a bad prognostic sign, the evidence is not clear. Auricchio et al. evaluated 101 consecutive patients with WPW syndrome, 36 of who had syncope. Although a higher percentage of patients who had syncope had a history of aborted sudden death (28 vs. 18 percent), the difference was not significant.[91] Leitch et al. investigated the mechanism of syncope in patients with PSVT and found that most had AVRT. Leitch et al. reported that syncope during SVT might, in fact, be due to a vasodepressor mechanism and not to a rapid rate of tachycardia.[92] Physical examination demonstrates a fast, regular pulse with a constant-intensity first heart sound. The jugular venous pressure waveform is usually constant, although it can sometimes be elevated. The incidence of sudden cardiac death in patients with the WPW syndrome has been estimated to range from 0.15 to 0.39 percent.[90,93–95] It is distinctly unusual for cardiac arrest to be the first symptomatic manifestation of the WPW syndrome.[96,149] Given the high prevalence of atrial fibrillation among patients with WPW syndrome and the concern for sudden cardiac death resulting from rapid preexcited atrial fibrillation, the low annual incidence of sudden death among patients with the WPW syndrome is reassuring.

Patients with functioning AV bypass tracts tend to have certain congenital abnormalities, particularly Ebstein's anomaly of the tricuspid valve. Nearly 10 percent of patients with Ebstein's anomaly have preexcitation.[97,98] APs also commonly occur in patients with corrected transposition of great vessels. In this case, the Ebstein's anomaly of the left (tricuspid) valve is associated with APs to the functioning systemic ventricle (anatomic right ventricle). In addition, multiple bypass tracts are frequently seen in Ebstein's anomaly. Conversely, of patients with WPW syndrome presenting with SVT early in childhood, only 5 percent have Ebstein's anomaly, despite the fact that it is the most common from of congenital heart disease associated with WPW syndrome. Interestingly, Deal et al. found that organic heart disease is less likely in patients with left-sided APs than in those with right-sided pathways (5 vs. 45 percent). In this study, organic heart disease was present in only 20 percent of the patients presenting with the WPW syndrome in the first 4 months of life.[98]

### ECG CHARACTERISTICS

The ECG hallmark of an antegradely conducting AP is the delta wave, along with a shorter than usual PR interval. On the other hand, the presence of retrograde conduction only in an AP will not be apparent on a surface ECG during sinus rhythm. ECG during orthodromic AVRT has a normal QRS complex with retrogradely conducting P wave after the completion of the QRS complex in the ST segment or early in the T wave (Fig. 30-4), whereas the QRS during antidromic AVRT is fully preexcited.

Numerous algorithms have been described to localize the site of the AP using the axis of the delta wave and QRS morphology.[99–111] The location of the AP along the AV ring is classified variously into 5 or 10 regions, which can be broadly divided into those on the left and the right of the AV groove. Distribution along these lines is not homogenous. Some 46 to 60 percent of the pathways are found on the left free wall space. Nearly 25 percent are within the posteroseptal and midseptal spaces, 15 to 20 percent in the right free wall space, and 2 percent in the anteroseptal space.[99,100] The positive predictive value of these algorithms is better when the delta wave polarity is included and when algorithms involve less than six locations.[111] A simple algorithm that includes both the delta wave axis and the QRS axis is shown in Fig. 30-14.

QRS alternans may be present in nearly 38 percent of patients with circus-movement tachycardia involving an AP.[112] Green et al reported a series of 161 patients with SVT of who 36 had QRS alternans.[45] Of these 36 patients, 33 had AVRT (92 percent), 2 had AVNRT, and 1 had atrial tachycardia. The mechanism for this is not clear. Morady et al. proposed that it could be a rate-related

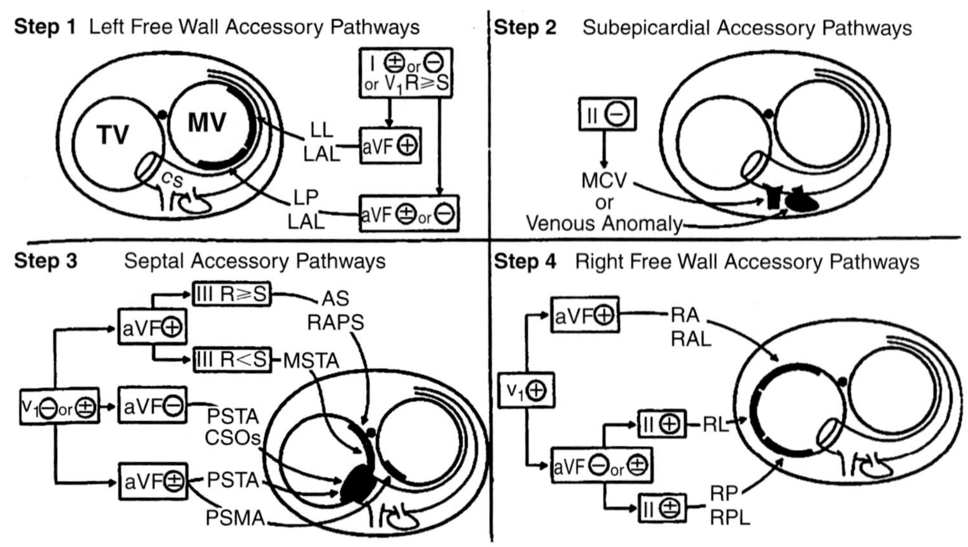


FIGURE 30-14 Localization of accessory pathways in patients with WPW syndrome. The line drawings illustrate the anatomic relationships between the tricuspid (TV) and mitral valves (MV), the coronary sinus (CS), AV conducting system, and accessory pathways. For each accessory pathway location indicated, the combination of QRS vectors most likely to result are shown, based on upright (+) or inverted (−) QRS waveforms. These vectorial guidelines are generally useful but not necessarily precise, since activation patterns from specific sites may vary in individual patients. Nomenclature for accessory pathway location: RA, anterior; RAL, right anterolateral; RL, right lateral; RPL, right posterolateral; RP, right posterior; PSTA, posteroseptal tricuspid annulus; CSOs, coronary sinus ostium; MSTA, mid-septal tricuspid annulus; AS, anteroseptal; RAPS, right anterior paraseptal; MCV, middle cardiac vein (coronary vein); CS, coronary sinus; venous anomaly (coronary sinus diverticulum); PSMA, posteroseptal mitral annulus; LP, left posterior; LPL, left posterolateral; LL, left lateral; LAL, left anterolateral. (From Arruda et al.[101] With permission.)

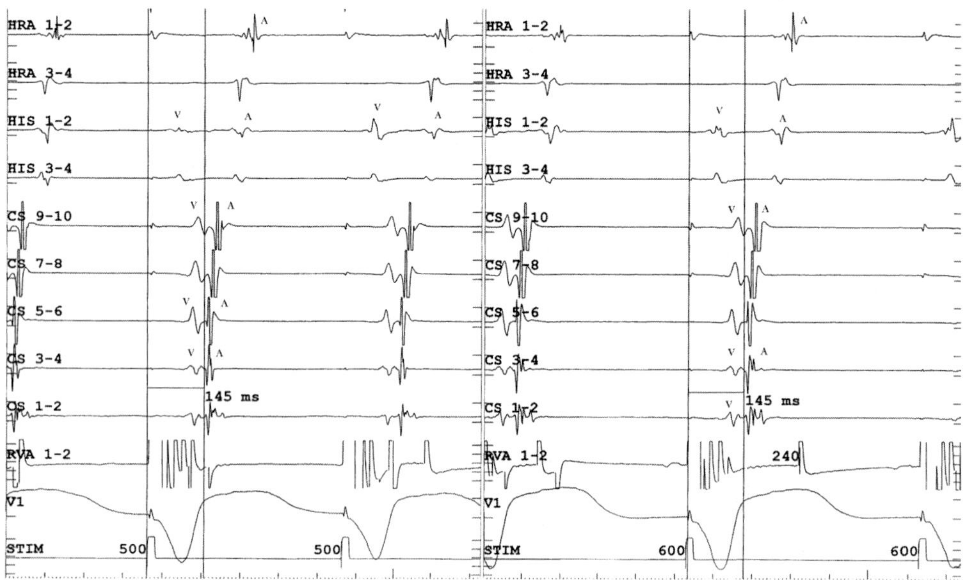


FIGURE 30-15 Nondecremental retrograde conduction in the accessory pathway. Note the eccentric activation of the atrium with pacing from the ventricle, with earliest atrial depolarization at the distal CS lead (CS 1-2). The left panel shows right ventricular pacing at a 120 beats per minute (cycle length of 500 ms) and the right panel shows the same at 100 beats per minute (cycle length of 600 ms). Note that the VA conduction time shown between the vertical lines remains the same with varying pacing rates. HRA = high right atrium, HIS = His bundle electrogram, CS = coronary sinus, RVA = right ventricular apex. 1-2 represent distal electrodes and 3-4 represent the proximal electrodes in each catheter. CS 9-20 is the most proximal electrode in the CS catheter. V and A represent ventricular and atrial electrograms.

phenomenon.[46] It could also be due to oscillations in the relative refractory period of the His-Purkinje system.[113]

ST-segment depression may also occur during orthodromic AVRT. It may occur even in the young, who are unlikely to have coronary artery disease. The location of the ST-segment depression may vary with location of the AP. ST-segment depression in $V_3$ to $V_6$ is almost invariably seen with a left lateral pathway; a negative T wave in the inferior leads is associated with a posteroseptal or posterior pathway; while a negative or notched T wave in $V_2$ or $V_3$ with a positive retrograde P wave in at least two inferior leads suggest an anteroseptal pathway.[39–41] However, ST-segment depression occurring during orthodromic AVRT episodes in older patients or associated with symptoms of ischemia mandate the consideration of coexisting coronary artery disease.

## ELECTROPHYSIOLOGIC TESTING

EP study in patients with AVRT is done to not only confirm the presence of an AP and to differentiate this condition from other forms of SVT but also to find the pathway participating in the tachycardia and aid in ablative therapy.

By definition, if an AP is present and conducting antegradely, some part of the ventricle begins activation earlier than expected, so that the HV interval is less than normal at rest (Fig. 30-10). As the QRS complex is a fusion complex of conduction down both the AV node and the AP, slowing of conduction down the normal pathway results in an increasing degree of preexcitation.

Eccentric atrial activation with ventricular pacing makes it easy to identify the presence of an AP (Fig. 30-15). Retrograde conduction over most APs is nondecremental. Hence, in the absence of intraventricular conduction delay or presence of multiple bypass tracts, the VA conduction time is the same over a range of pace cycle lengths (Fig. 30-15). The exception to this is the slowly conducting decremental posteroseptal pathway found in the permanent form of junctional reciprocating tachycardia, in which the VA conduction time increases with increasing ventricular pacing rate.

It is important and often challenging to differentiate retrograde conduction over septal pathway from conduction over the normal AV system. One maneuver that can make this differentiation is "differential pacing"—i.e., pacing both from the right ventricular apex and the RV base—and measuring the VA conduction time. Retrograde conduction over the normal AV conduction system is fastest when pacing from the apex, since conduction can occur rapidly over the His-Purkinje system. VA intervals are longer when the pacing site is moved from the apex to the base. The converse is true in the presence of an AP, with VA intervals shortest when pacing from the base, closer to the site of pathway insertion, than from the apex. The technique of "para-Hisian pacing" is useful in differentiating the anteroseptal pathway from AVNRT.

Development of BBB aberration during tachycardia can be useful in determining both presence of and participation of an AP in tachycardia (Fig. 30-16). An increase in tachycardia cycle length due to an increase in VA conduction time with functional BBB is consistent with the presence of an AP ipsilateral to the BBB.

## Management

### CATHETER ABLATION OF APs

Catheter ablation of APs is performed in conjunction with a diagnostic electrophysiology test. Once the AP is localized to a region of the heart, precise mapping and ablation is performed using a steerable electrode catheter. No prospective randomized clinical trials have evaluated the safety and efficacy of catheter ablation of APs. However, the results of catheter ablation of APs have been reported in a large number of other trials.[10,26,62,114–119] The largest prospective, multicenter clinical trial to evaluate the safety and efficacy of radiofrequency ablation was reported by Calkins et al.[10] This study involved analysis of 1050 patients, of whom 500 had APs. Overall success of catheter ablation in curing APs was 93 percent. The success rate for catheter ablation of left free wall APs is slightly higher than for catheter ablation of right-sided APs (95 vs. 90 percent, $p = 0.03$). Following an initially successful procedure, recurrence of AP conduction is found in approximately 5 percent of patients. The recurrence-free interval postablation was also best with left-sided pathways (Fig. 30-17). APs that recur can usually be successfully reablated. Complications associated with catheter ablation of APs may result from obtaining vascular access (hematomas, deep venous thrombosis, perforation of the aorta, arteriovenous fistula, pneumothorax), catheter manipulation (valvular damage, microemboli, perforation of the coronary sinus or myocardial wall, coronary dissection and/or thrombosis), or delivery of RF energy (AV block, myocardial perforation, coronary artery spasm or occlusion, transient ischemic attacks, or cerebrovascular accidents).

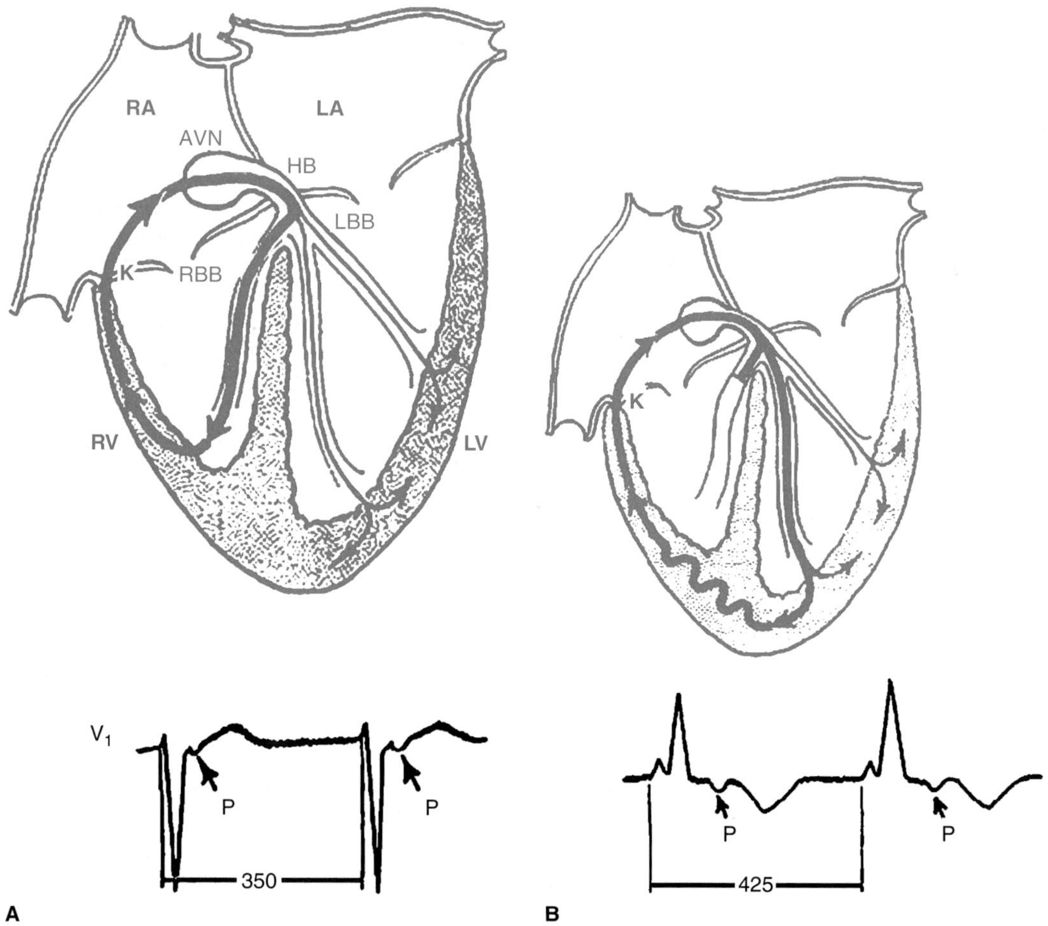


FIGURE 30-16 Effect of BBB on AVRT. *A*. AVRT involving a right-sided accessory pathway. Schematic at the bottom shows the ECG appearance of the tachycardia at a cycle length of 350 ms. *B*. Appearance of BBB on the same side leads to increase the cycle length of the tachycardia to 425 ms. See text for discussion. (Modified with permission from: Josephson M. Preexcitation syndromes. In: Josephson M, ed. *Clinical Cardiac Electrophysiology: Technique and Interpretation*, 3d ed. New York: Lippincott Williams & Wilkins; 2002:370. With permission.)

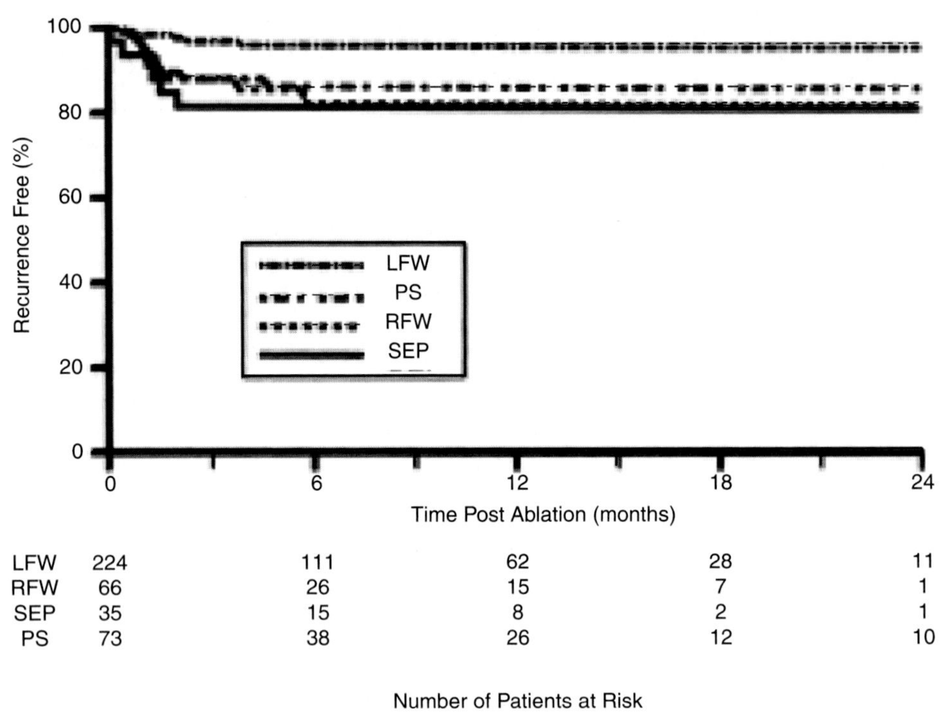


FIGURE 30-17 Kaplan-Meier curve showing freedom from arrhythmia recurrence among patients who underwent successful ablation of an AP subclassified by its location. This analysis was confined to those patients in whom successful ablation was achieved with the investigational ablation system. LFW = left free wall; RFW = right free wall; SEP = septal; PS = posteroseptal. (From Calkins H, Yong P, Miller JM, et al. Catheter ablation of accessory pathways, atrioventricular nodal reentrant tachycardia, and the atrioventricular junction: Final results of a prospective, multicenter clinical trial. The Atakr Multicenter Investigators Group. *Circulation* 1999;99:262–270. With permission.)

Calkins et al. reported the incidence of major complications in their trial to be 3 percent and of minor complications around 8 percent. The procedure-related mortality associated with catheter ablation of APs has ranged from 0 to 0.2 percent. The two most common types of major complications reported during catheter ablation of APs are inadvertent complete AV block and cardiac tamponade. The incidence of inadvertent complete AV block ranges from 0.17 to 1.0 percent. Most instances of complete AV block occur in the setting of the ablation of septal and posteroseptal APs. The frequency of cardiac tamponade as a result of the ablation of APs varies between 0.13 and 1.1 percent.

## MEDICAL THERAPY

Antiarrhythmic drugs represent one therapeutic option for management of AP-mediated arrhythmias. As AV reciprocating tachycardia involves conduction both through the AP and the AV node, antiarrhythmic drugs that modify the electrophysiologic characteristics of either of these critical components of the circuit may prove effective in treating these arrhythmias. Antiarrhythmic drugs that primarily modify conduction through the AV node include verapamil, beta blockers, and adenosine. In contrast, the antiarrhythmic drugs, which primarily modify conduction across the AP, consist of class 1 drugs such as procainaminde, disopyramide, propafenone, and flecainide as well class 3 antiarrhythmic drugs such as sotalol and amiodarone. The approach to acute termination of these arrhythmias generally differs from that used for long-term suppression and prevention of further episodes of SVT. In general, the approach employed does not vary based on the specific tachycardia mechanism, which generally is unknown when the patient first presents to an emergency room. Pharmacologic agents are in general more effective in terminating an acute episode of tachycardia than in preventing future recurrences. Verapamil or diltiazem should not be administered intravenously to patients with atrial fibrillation and preexcitation, as they may accelerate conduction through the AP and precipitate a cardiac arrest.

There have been no controlled trials of drug prophylaxis involving patients with AV reentry. However, a number of small, nonrandomized trials have been performed (each involving fewer than 50 patients), which have reported the safety and efficacy of drug prophylaxis for maintenance of sinus rhythm in patients with supraventricular arrhythmias. A subset of the patients in these studies had AV reentry as their underlying arrhythmia. Available data do not allow a comparison of the efficacy of these drugs.

Manolis et al. reported the largest published study evaluating the efficacy of propafenone in 11 adult patients, 9 of whom had a manifest AP. During 9 ± 6 months of follow-up, none of the 10 patients discharged on a combination of propafenone and a beta blocker experienced a recurrence. No major side effects were reported.[120] Other small trials have evaluated the efficacy of propafenone in the treatment of AV reentry in children.[121–124] The largest of these involved 26 young children (<10 years) with AV reentry.[121] Complete arrhythmia control was accomplished in 20 patients and partial control in one additional patient. The mean duration of follow-up was 14 months.

A number of studies have examined the acute and long-term efficacy of oral and intravenous flecainide in the treatment of patients with AV reentry. Helmy et al. reported the largest of these, involving 20 patients with AV reentry.[125] The oral administration of flecainide resulted in inability to induce sustained tachycardia in 17 of these 20 patients. During 15 ± 7 months of follow-up on oral flecainide treatment, 3 patients developed a recurrence of tachycardia. Other studies have reported similar findings.[125–132] The addition of a beta blocker results in greater efficacy, with >90 percent of patients achieving abolition of symptomatic tachycardia. In addition to studies that specifically focused on patients with a known AV reentry, there have been several randomized trials evaluating the efficacy of flecainide in the treatment of patients with paroxysmal SVT. The precise tachycardia mechanism in these patients was not determined. In one study by Henthorn et al., 34 patients with PSVT were randomized into a double-blind placebo-controlled trial with an 8-week crossover design. Flecainide was shown to be superior to placebo, demonstrating an actuarial 79 percent freedom from symptomatic PSVT events compared with a 15 percent freedom from events on placebo. Of the 34 patients studied, 8 had a recurrence during flecainide therapy as compared with 29 having a recurrence on placebo.

The efficacy of oral sotalol in the prevention of AV reentry has been reported in a single study involving 17 patients with an AP.[133] Of 15 patients with inducible sustained tachycardia during EPT, 14 continued to have inducible tachycardia after administration of intravenous sotalol. Thirteen of the 16 patients who were discharged on oral sotalol were free of symptomatic recurrences during a median of 36 months of follow-up.

Amiodarone has been evaluated in several trials for its efficacy in the treatment of patients with AP mediated tachycardias.[134–137] However, these studies do not demonstrate that amiodarone is superior to class 1C antiarrhythmic agents or sotalol. Acute studies have also revealed that amiodarone does not consistently prolong the AP refractory period and, as a result, cannot be considered to be protective against sudden death in all patients with WPW syndrome.[137] As a result of these findings—combined with the well-recognized organ toxicity associated with amiodarone and the high rate of discontinuation of this drug due to noncardiac adverse effects—amiodarone generally does not play an important role in the treatment of patients with APs.

Verapamil, although less studied, can be moderately effective in the prevention of AVRT.[138] No studies have been performed to determine the short- or long-term efficacy of procainamide or quinidine in the treatment of AV reentry.

## Management Considerations

### MANAGEMENT OF ASYMPTOMATIC PREEXCITATION

Most patients with asymptomatic preexcitation have a good prognosis. Because of the small but real risks associated with invasive procedures, EPT is not routinely recommended for risk stratification and/or ablative therapy. The recently published NASPE Policy Statement on Catheter Ablation states that catheter ablation is not indicated (class 3) for patients with asymptomatic preexcitation unless they fall into a high-risk group, such as school bus drivers, pilots, and scuba divers.[52,141,142] When screening studies are performed in patients with asymptomatic preexcitation, approximately 20 percent of those who are asymptomatic will demonstrate a rapid ventricular rate during atrial fibrillation induced at EPT.[139,140] More recent evidence makes a stronger case for use of EPT in risk stratifying all asymptomatic patients with preexcitation.[147] Pappone et al studied 212 consecutive asymptomatic WPW patients after a baseline EPT over 5 years.[148] After a mean follow-up of 37.7 months, 33 patients became symptomatic. Of these, 29 had inducible SVT on EPT and only 4 were not inducible. More importantly, there were 3 sudden deaths in the entire population, and all those occurred in patients in whom AVRT and atrial fibrillation were inducible during EPT. The electrophysiology community has not changed its clinical practice based on these findings and is awaiting confirmaiton of the results of this study prior to adopting a more aggressive approach to catheter ablation in patients with asymptomatic preexcitation.

Studies have identified markers that identify patients at increased risk.[81,87,143–146] These include (1) a short preexcited RR interval <250 ms during spontaneous or induced atrial fibrillation, (2) a history of symptomatic tachycardia, (3) multiple APs, and (4) Epstein's anomaly. A short preexcited RR interval during atrial fibrillation of >250 ms has been reported to have a negative predictive value of >95 percent.[91]

Several noninvasive and invasive tests have been proposed as useful in stratifying patients for the risk of sudden death. The detection of intermittent preexcitation—which is characterized by an abrupt loss of the delta wave, normalization of the QRS complex, and an increase in the PR interval during a continuous ECG recording—is evidence that an AP has a relatively long refractory period and is unlikely to precipitate ventricular fibrillation.[86] The loss of preexcitation after administration of antiarrhythmic drugs like procainaminde or ajmaline has also been used to indicate a low-risk subgroup.[146] These noninvasive tests are generally considered inferior to electrophysiologic testing in the assessment of risk of sudden cardiac death. Because of this, they play little role in patient management at present.

In an asymptomatic patient with a right-sided AP, consideration should be given to obtaining an echocardiogram to look for Ebstein's anomaly.

### MANAGEMENT OF SYMPTOMATIC WPW

The recently published NASPE Policy Statement on Catheter Ablation states that catheter ablation is considered first-line therapy (class 1) and the treatment of choice for patients with WPW syndrome—i.e., patients with manifest preexcitation along with symptoms.[149] It is curative in more than 95 percent of patients and has a low complication rate. It also obviates the unwanted side effects of antiarrhythmic agents. Catheter ablation is also considered first-line therapy (class 1) for patients with PSVT involving a concealed AP. However, since concealed APs are not associated with an increased risk of sudden cardiac death in these patients, catheter ablation can be presented as one of a number of potential therapeutic approaches including pharmacologic therapy and clinical follow-up alone (see discussion of management of AVNRT). When pharmacologic therapy is selected for patients with concealed APs, it is reasonable to consider a trial of beta blocker therapy, calcium channel blocker therapy, or a class 1C antiarrhythmic agent. It is important to note that beta blockers and calcium channel blockers generally are not recommended for the management of patients who have evidence of preexcitation.

## References


1. Wu D, Denes P, Amat-y-Leon F, Dhingra R, et al. Clinical, electrocardiographic and electrophysiologic observations in patients with paroxysmal supraventricular tachycardia. *Am J Cardiol* 1978;41: 1045–1051.
2. Josephson ME, Wellens HJ. Differential diagnosis of supraventricular tachycardia. *Cardiol Clin* 1990;8(3):411–442.
3. Rostagno C, Paladini B, Taddei T, et al. Out-of-hospital symptomatic supraventricular arrhythmias. Epidemiological aspects derived from 10 years experience of the Florence Mobile Coronary Care Unit. *G Ital Cardiol* 1993;23(6):549–562.
4. Denes P, Wu D, Dhingra RC, et al. Dual atrioventricular nodal pathways—A common electrophysiological response. *Br Heart J* 1975;37:1069–1076.
5. Jackman WM, Beckman KJ, McClelland JH, et al. Treatment of supraventricular tachycardia due to atrioventricular nodal reentry by radiofrequency catheter ablation of slow-pathway conduction. *N Engl J Med* 1992;327:313–318.
6. Haissaguerre M, Gaita F, Fischer B, et al. Elimination of atrioventricular nodal reentrant tachycardia using discrete slow potentials to guide application of radiofrequency energy. *Circulation* 1992;85: 2162–2175.
7. Kay GN, Epstein AE, Dailey SM, et al. Selective radiofrequency ablation of the slow pathway for the treatment of atrioventricular reentrant tachycardia: Evidence for involvement of perinodal myocardium within the reentrant circuit. *Circulation* 1992;85: 1675–1688.
8. Goyal R, Zivin A, Souza J, et al. Comparison of the ages of tachycardia onset in patients with atrioventricular nodal reentrant tachycardia and accessory pathway–mediated tachycardia. *Am Heart J* 1996;132: 765–767.
9. Clague JR, Dagres N, Kottkamp H, et al. Targeting the slow pathway for atrioventricular nodal reentrant tachycardia: Initial results and long-term follow-up in 379 consecutive patients. *Eur Heart J* 2001;22:82–88.

10. Calkins H, Yong P, Miller JM, Olshansky B, et al. Catheter ablation of accessory pathways, atrioventricular nodal reentrant tachycardia, and the atrioventricular junction: Final results of a prospective, multicenter clinical trial. The Atakr Multicenter Investigators Group. *Circulation* 1999; 99:262–270.
11. Bubien RS, Knotts-Dolson SM, Plumb VJ, Kay GN. Effect of radiofrequency catheter ablation on health-related quality of life and activities of daily living in patients with recurrent arrhythmias *Circulation* 1996;94:1585–1591.
12. Wang YS, Scheinman MM, Chien WW, et al. Patients with supraventricular tachycardia presenting with aborted sudden death: Incidence, mechanism and long-term follow-up. *J Am Coll Cardiol* 1991;18(7):1711–1719.
13. Kent AFS. Researches on the structure and function of the mammalian heart. *J Physiol* 1893;14:233–254.
14. Ho SW, McComb JH, Scott CD, et al. Morphology of the cardiac conduction system in patients with electrophysiologically proven dual atrioventricular nodal pathway. *J Cardiovasc Electrophysiol* 1993; 4(5):504–512.
15. Sanchez-Quintana D, Davies DW, Ho SY, et al. Architecture of the atrial musculature in and around the triangle of Koch: Its potential relevance to atrioventricular nodal reentry. *J Cardiovasc Electrophysiol* 1997;8:1396–1407.
16. Olgin JE, Ursell P, Kao AK, et al. Pathological findings following slow pathway ablation for AV nodal reentrant tachycardia. *J Cardiovasc Electrophysiol* 1996;7:625–631.
17. Inoue S, Becker AE. Posterior extensions of the human compact atrioventricular node: A neglected anatomic feature of potential clinical significance. *Circulation* 1998;97:188–193.
18. Moe GK, Preston JB, Burlington H. Physiologic evidence for a dual AV transmission system. *Cir Res* 1956;4:357–375.
19. Pritchett EL, Anderson RW, Benditt DG, et al. Reentry within the atrioventricular node; surgical cure with preservation of the atrioventricular conduction. *Circulation* 1979;60:440–446.
20. Holman VVL, Ikeshita M, Lease JG, et al. Alteration of anterograde atrioventricular conduction by cryoablation of per-AV nodal tissue. *J Thorac Cardiovasc Surg* 1984;88:67–75.
21. Cox JL, Holman WL, Cain ME. Cryosurgical treatment of atrioventricular node reentrant tachycardia. *Circulation* 1987;76:1329–1336.
22. Fujimura O, Guiraudon GM, Yee R, et al. Operative therapy of atrioventricular node reentry and results of an anatomically guided procedure. *Am J Cardiol* 1989;64:1327–1332.
23. Haissaguerre M, Warin JF, Lemetayer P, et al. Closed chest ablation of retrograde conduction in patients with atrioventricular nodal reentrant tachycardia. *N Engl J Med* 1989;320:426–433.
24. Epstein LM, Scheinman MM, Langberg JJ, et al. Percutaneous catheter modification of the atrioventricular node. *Circulation* 1989; 80:757–768.
25. Lee MA, Morady F, Kadish A, et al. Catheter modification of the atrioventricular junction with radiofrequency energy in patients with atrioventricular nodal reentry tachycardia. *Circulation* 1991;83: 827–835.
26. Calkins H, Sousa J, El-Atassi R, et al. Diagnosis and cure of the Wolff-Parkinson-White syndrome or paroxysmal supraventricular tachycardia during a single electrophysiologic test. *N Engl J Med* 1991;324:1612–1618.
27. Goy JJ, Fromer M, Schlaepfer J, et al. Clinical efficacy of radiofrequency current in the treatment of patients with atrioventricular node reentrant tachycardia. *J Am Coll Cardiol* 1990;16: 418–423.
28. Jazayeri MR, Hempe SL, Sra JS, et al. Selective transcatheter ablation of the fast and slow pathways using radiofrequency energy in patients with atrioventricular nodal reentrant tachycardia. *Circulation* 1992;85:1318–1328.
29. Kottkamp H, Hindricks G, Willems S, et al. An anatomically and electrogram-guided stepwise approach for effective and safe catheter ablation of the fast pathway for elimination of atrioventricular node reentrant tachycardia. *J Am Coll Cardiol* 1995;25:974–983.
30. Epstein LM, Lesh MD, Griffin JC, et al. A direct midseptal approach to slow atrioventricular nodal pathway ablation. *Pacing Clin Electrophysiol* 1995;18(Pt 1):57–64.
31. Kalbfleisch SJ, Strickberger SA, Williamson B, et al. Randomized comparison of anatomic and electrogram mapping approaches to ablation of the slow pathway of atrioventricular node reentrant tachycardia. *J Am Coll Cardiol* 1994;23:716–723.
32. Janse MJ, Anderson RH, McGuire MA, Ho SY. "AV nodal" reentry: Part I: AV nodal reentry revisited. *J Cardiovasc Electrophysiol* 1993;4: 561–572.
33. McGuire MA, Janse MJ, Ross DL. "AV nodal" reentry: Part II: AV nodal, AV junctional or atrionodal reentry? *J Cardiovasc Electrophysiol* 1993;4:573–586.
34. Josephson ME, Kastor JA. Paroxysmal supraventricular tachycardia: Is atrium a necessary link? *Circulation* 1976;54:430.
35. Wood KA, Drew BJ, Schieneman MM. Frequency of disabling symptoms in supraventricular tachycardia. *Am J Cardiol* 1997;79: 145–149.
36. Gürsoy S, Steurer G, Brugada J, et al. The homodynamic mechanism of pounding in the neck in atrioventricular nodal reentrant tachycardia. *N Engl J Med* 1992;327:772–774.
37. Geelen P, Primo J, Brugada J, et al. Neck pounding during sinus rhythm: A new clinical manifestation of dual atrioventricular nodal pathways. *Heart* 1998;79:490–492.
38. Fisch C, Mandrola JM, Rardon DR. Electrocardiographic manifestations of dual atrioventricular node conduction during sinus rhythm. *J Am Coll Cardiol* 1997;29:1015–1022.
39. Riva SI, Della Bella P, Fassini G, et al. Value of analysis of ST segment changes during tachycardia in determining type of narrow QRS complex tachycardia. *J Am Coll Cardiol* 1996;27:1480–1485.
40. Gulec S, Ertab F, Karaoouz R, et al. Value of ST-segment depression during paroxysmal supraventricular tachycardia in the diagnosis of coronary artery disease. *Am J Cardiol* 1999;83:458–460.
41. Nelson SD, Kou WH, Annesley T, et al. Significance of ST segment depression during paroxysmal supraventricular tachycardia. *J Am Coll Cardiol* 1988;12:383–387.
42. Petsas AA, Anastassiades LC, Anonopoulos AG. Exercise testing for assessment of the significance of ST segment depression observed during episodes of paroxysmal supraventricular tachycardia. *Eur Heart J* 1990;11:974–979.
43. Takayanagy K, Hoshi H, Shimizu M, et al. Pronounced ST-segment depression during paroxysmal supraventricular tachycardia. *Jpn Heart J* 1993;34:269–278.
44. Paparella N, Ouyang F, Fuca G, et al. Significance of newly acquired negative T waves after interruption of paroxysmal reentrant supraventricular tachycardia with narrow QRS complex. *Am J Cardiol* 2000;85:261–263.
45. Green M, Heddle B, Dassen W, et al. Value of QRS alternation in determining the site of origin of narrow QRS supraventricular tachycardia. *Circulation* 1983;68:368–373.
46. Morady F, DiCarlo LA Jr, Baerman JM, et al. Determinants of QRS alternans during narrow QRS tachycardia. *J Am Coll Cardiol* 1987; 9(3):489–499.
47. Curtis AB, Belardinelli L, Woodard DA, et al. Induction of atrioventricular node reentrant tachycardia with adenosine: Differential effect of adenosine on fast and slow atrioventricular node pathway. *J Am Coll Cardiol* 1997;30:1778–1784.
48. Tebbenjohanns J, Niehaus M, Korte T, et al. Noninvasive diagnosis in patients with undocumented tachycardias: Value of the adenosine test to predict AV nodal reentrant tachycardia. *J Cardiovasc Electrophysiol* 1999;10(7):916–923.
49. Philippon F, Plumb VJ, Kay GN. Differential effect of esmolol on the fast and slow AV nodal pathways in patients with AV nodal reentrant tachycardia. *J Cardiavasc Electrophysiol* 1994;5:810–817.
50. Chiou CW, Chen SA, Kung MH, et al. Effects of continuous enhanced vagal tone on dual atrioventricular node and accessory pathways. *Circulation* 2003;107(20):2583–2588.

51. Knight BP, Ebinger M, Oral H, Kim et al. Diagnostic value of tachycardia features and pacing maneuvers during paroxysmal supraventricular tachycardia. *J Am Coll Cardiol* 2000;36:574–582.
52. Scheinman M, Calkins H, Gillette P, et al. NASPE policy statement on catheter ablation: Personnel, policy, procedures, and therapeutic recommendations. *PACE* 2003;26:1–11.
53. Rinkinberger RL, Prystowsky EN, Heger JJ, et al. Effect of IV and chronic oral verapamil administration in patients with variety of supraventricular tachyarrhythmias. *Circulation* 1980;62:996–1010.
54. DiMarco JP, Miles W, Akhtar M, et al. Adenosine for paroxysmal supraventricular tachycardia: Dose ranging and comparison with verapamil. Assessment in placebo-controlled, multicenter trials. The adenosine for PSVT study group. *Ann Intern Med* 1990;113:104–110.
55. Donahue KJ, Orias D, Berger RB, et al. Comparison of adenosine effects on atrioventricular node reentry and atrioventricular reciprocating tachycardias. *Clin Cardiol* 1998;21:743–745.
56. Ferguson JD, DiMarco JP. Contemporary management of paroxysmal supraventricular tachycardia. *Circulation* 2003;107:1096.
57. Wellens HJJ, Durer DR, Liem KL, et al. Effect of digitalis in patients with paroxysmal atrioventricular nodal tachycardia. *Circulation* 1975; 52:779–788.
58. Wu D, Denes P, Dhingra RC, et al. The effects of propranolol on induction of AV nodal reentrant paroxysmal tachycardia. *Circulation* 1974;50:665–677.
59. Calkins H. Catheter ablation for cardiac arrhythmias. *Med Clin North Am* 2001;2:473–502.
60. Langberg JJ, Leon A, Borganelli M, et al. A randomized, prospective comparison of anterior and posterior approaches to radiofrequency catheter ablation of atrioventricular nodal reentry tachycardia. *Circulation* 1993;87(5):1551–1556.
61. Lickfett L, Pfeiffer D, Schimpf R, et al. Long-term follow-up of fast pathway radiofrequency ablation in atrioventricular nodal reentrant tachycardia. *Am J Cardiol* 2002;89(9):1124–1125.
62. Shieneman NM. NASPE survey on catheter ablation. *Pacing Clin Electrophysiol* 1995;18:1474.
63. Calkins H, Prsytowsky E, Berger R, et al. Recurrences of conduction following radiofrequency catheter ablation procedures: Relationship to ablation target and electrode temperature. *J Cardiovasc Electrophysiol* 1996;7:704.
64. Henthorn RW, Waldo AL, Anderson JL, et al. Flecainide acetate prevents recurrence of symptomatic paroxysmal supraventricular tachycardia. The Flecainide Supraventricular Tachycardia Study Group. *Circulation* 1991;83:119–125.
65. Falk RH, Fogel RI. Flecainide. *J Cardiovasc Electrophysiol* 1994;5: 964–981.
66. Anderson JL, Platt ML, Guarnieri T, et al. Flecainide acetate for paroxysmal supraventricular tachyarrhythmias. The flecainide supraventricular tachycardia study group. *Am J Cardiol* 1994;74:578–584.
67. Neuss H, Schlepper M. Long term efficacy and safety of flecainide of supraventricular tachycardia. *Am J Cardiol* 1988;62:56D–61D.
68. Musto B, Cavallaro C, Musto A, et al. Flecainide single oral dose for management of paroxysmal supraventricular tachycardia in children and young adults. *Am Heart J* 1992;124:110–115.
69. Pritchett EL, McCarthy EA, Wilkinson WE. Propafenone treatment of symptomatic paroxysmal supraventricular arrhythmias: A randomized, placebo-controlled, crossover trial in patients tolerating oral therapy. *Ann Intern Med* 1991;114:539–544.
70. Huikuri HV, Koistinen MJ, Takkunen JT. Efficacy of intravenous sotalol for suppressing inducibility of supraventricular tachycardias at rest and during isometric exercise. *Am J Cardiol* 1992;69(5):498–502.
71. Wanless RS, Anderson K, Joy M, et al. Multicenter comparative study of the efficacy and safety of sotalol in the prophylactic treatment of patients with paroxysmal supraventricular tachyarrhythmias. *Am Heart J* 1997;133(4):441–446.
72. Wolff L, Parkinson J, White PD. Bundle-branch block with short PR interval in healthy young people prone to paroxysmal tachycardia. *Am Heart J* 1930;5:685–704.
73. Krahn AD, Manfreda J, Tate RB, et al. The natural history of electrocardiographic preexcitation in men: The Manitoba follow-up study. *Ann Intern Med* 1992;116:456–460.
74. Sorbo MD, Buja GF, Miorelli M, et al. Prevalence of Wolff-Parkinson-White syndrome in a population of 116,452 young males. *G Ital Cardiol* 1995;25:681–687.
75. Vidaillet HJ Jr, Pressley JC, Henke E, et al. Familial occurrence of accessory atrioventricular pathways (preexcitation syndrome). *N Engl J Med* 1987;317:65–69.
76. Murdock CJ, Leitch JW, Teo WS, et al. Characteristics of accessory pathways exhibiting decremental conduction. *Am J Cardiol* 1991; 67:506–510.
77. Ross DL, Uther JB. Diagnosis of concealed accessory pathways in supraventricular tachycardia. *Pacing Clin Electrophysiol* 1984;7: 1069–1085.
78. Anderson RH, Becker AE, Brechenmacher C, et al. Ventricular preexcitation: A proposed nomenclature for its substrates. *Eur J Cardiol* 1975;3:27–36.
79. Cohen TJ, Tucker KJ, Abbott JA, et al. Usefulness of adenosine in augmenting ventricular preexcitation for noninvasive localization of accessory pathway. *Am J Cardiol* 1992;69:1178–1185.
80. Canby RC, Horton RP, Kessler DJ, et al. Use of transesophageal atrial pacing with adenosine infusion to evaluate ventricular preexcitation. *Am J Cardiol* 1995;75:548–550.
81. Klein GJ, Gulamhusien SS. Intermittent preexcitation in the Wolff-Parkinson-White syndrome. *Am J Cardiol* 1983;52:292–296.
82. Cain ME, Luke RA, Lindsay BD. Diagnosis and localization of accessory pathways. *Pacing Clin Electrophysiol* 1992;15:801–824.
83. Reyes W, Milstein S, Dunnigan A, et al. Indications for modification of coexisting dual atrioventricular node pathways in patients undergoing surgical ablation of accessory atrioventricular connections. *J Am Coll Cardiol* 1991;17:1561–1567.
84. Klein GJ, Bashore TM, Sellers TD, et al. Ventricular fibrillation in the Wolff-Parkinson-White syndrome. *N Engl J Med* 1979;301: 1080–1085.
85. Dreifus LS, Haiat R, Watanabe Y, et al. Ventricular fibrillation—A possible mechanism of sudden death in patients with Wolff-Parkinson-White syndrome. *Circulation* 1971;43:520–527.
86. Wellens HJJ, Durrer D. Wolff-Parkinson-White syndrome and atrial fibrillation. *Am J Cardiol* 1974;34:777–782.
87. Campbell RWF, Smith R, Gallagher JJ, et al. Atrial fibrillation in the preexcitation syndrome. *Am J Cardiol* 1977;40:514–520.
88. Sharma AD, Klein GJ, Guiraudon GM, et al. Atrial fibrillation in patients with Wolff-Parkinson-White syndrome: Incidence after surgical ablation of the accessory pathway. *Circulation* 1985;72:161–169.
89. Dagres N, Clague JR, Lottkamp H, et al. Impact of radiofrequency catheter ablation of accessory pathways on the frequency of atrial fibrillation during long-term follow-up: High recurrence rate of atrial fibrillation in patients older than 50 years of age. *Eur Heart J* 2001; 22(5):423–427.
90. Munger TM, Packer DL, Hammill SC, et al. A population study of the natural history of Wolff-Parkinson-White syndrome in Olmsted Country, Minnesota, 1953–1989. *Circulation* 1993;87:866–873.
91. Auricchio A, Klein H, Trappe HJ, et al. Lack of prognostic value of syncope in patients with Wolff-Parkinson-White syndrome. *J Am Coll Cardiol* 1991;17:152–158.
92. Leitch JW, Klein GJ, Yee R, et al. Syncope associated with supraventricular tachycardia. An expression of tachycardia rate or vasomotor response? *Circulation* 1992;85(3):1064–1071.
93. Smith RF. The Wolff-Parkinson-White syndrome as an aviation risk. *Circulation* 1990;82:1718–1723.
94. Timmermans C, Smeets JL, Rodriguez LM, et al. Aborted sudden death in the Wolff-Parkinson-White syndrome. *Am J Cardiol* 1995;76: 492–494.
95. Pappone C, Santinelli V, Rosanio S, et al. Usefulness of invasive electrophysiologic testing to stratify the risk of arrhythmic events in asymptomatic patients with Wolff-Parkinson-White pattern: Results

from a large prospective long-term follow-up study. *J Am Coll Cardiol* 2003;41(2):239–244.

96. Lundberg A. Paroxysmal atrial tachycardia in infancy: Long term follow-up study of 49 subjects. *Pediatrics* 1982;70:638.
97. Lev M, Givson S, Miller RA. Ebsteins' disease with Wolff-Parkinson-White syndrome. Am *Heart J* 1955;49:724.
98. Deal BJ, Keana JF, Gillette PC, et al. Wolff-Parkinson-White syndrome and supraventricular tachycardia during infancy: Management and follow-up. *J Am Coll Cardiol* 1985;5:130.
99. Gallager JJ, Pritchett ELC, Sealy WC, et al. The preexcitation syndromes. *Prog Cardiovasc Dis* 1978;20:285–327.
100. Ross DL, Uther JB. Diagnosis of concealed accessory pathways in supraventricular tachycardia. *Pacing Clin Electrophysiol* 1984;7: 1069–1085.
101. Arruda MS, McClelland JH, Wang X, et al. Development and validation of an ECG algorithm for identifying accessory pathway ablation site in Wolff-Parkinson-White syndrome. *J Cardiovasc Electrophysiol* 1998;9(1):2–12.
102. Fitzpatrick AP, Gonzales RP, Lesh MD, et al. New algorithm for the localization of accessory atrioventricular connections using a baseline electrocardiogram. *J Am Coll Cardiol* 1994;23(1):107–116.
103. Lindsay BD, Crossen KJ, Cain ME. Concordance of distinguishing electrocardiographic features during sinus rhythm with the location of accessory pathways in the Wolff-Parkinson-White syndrome. *Am J Cardiol* 1987;59(12):1093–1102.
104. Cain ME, Luke RA, Lindsay BD. Diagnosis and localization of accessory pathway. *Pacing Clin Electrophysiol* 1992;15:801–824.
105. d'Avila A, Brugada J, Skeberis V, et al. A fast and reliable algorithm to localize accessory pathways based on the polarity of the QRS complex on the surface ECG during sinus rhythm. *Pacing Clin Electrophysiol* 1995;18(9 Pt 1):1615–1627.
106. Milstein S, Sharma AD, Guiraudon GM, et al. An algorithm for the electrocardiographic localization of accessory pathways in the Wolff-Parkinson-White syndrome. *Pacing Clin Electrophysiol* 1987;10 (3 Pt 1):555–563.
107. Xie B, Heald SC, Bashir Y, et al. Localization of accessory pathways from the 12-lead electrocardiogram using a new algorithm. *Am J Cardiol* 1994;74(2):161–165.
108. Haissaguerre M, Marcus F, Poquet F, et al. Electrocardiographic characteristics and catheter ablation of parahissian accessory pathways. *Circulation* 1994;90(3):1124–1128.
109. Diker E, Ozdemir M, Tezcan UK, et al. QRS polarity on 12-lead surface ECG. A criterion for the differentiation of right and left posteroseptal accessory atrioventricular pathways. *Cardiology* 1997;88(4):328–332.
110. Boersma L, Garcia-Moran E, Mont L, et al. Accessory pathway localization by QRS polarity in children with Wolff-Parkinson-White syndrome. *J Cardiovasc Electrophysiol* 2002;13(12):1222–1260.
111. Basiouny T, de Chillou C, Fareh S, et al. Accuracy and limitations of published algorithms using the twelve-lead electrocardiogram to localize overt atrioventricular accessory pathways. *J Cardiovasc Electrophysiol* 1999;10(10):1340–1349.
112. Kappenberger LJ, Fromer MA, Steinbrunn W, et al. Efficacy of amiodarone in the Wolff-Parkinson-White syndrome with rapid ventricular response via accessory pathway during atrial fibrillation. *Am J Cardiol* 1984;54(3):330–335.
113. Lai W, Voon W, Yen H, et al. Comparison of the electrophysiologic effects of oral sustained-release and intravenous verapamil in patients with paroxysmal supraventricular tachycardia. *Am J Cardiol* 1993; 71:405–408.
114. Jackman WM, Wang X, Friday KJ, et al. Catheter ablation of accessory atrioventricular pathways (Wolff-Parkinson-White syndrome) by radiofrequency current. *N Engl J Med* 1991;324:1605–1611.
115. Kuck KH, Schluter M, Geiger M, et al. Radiofrequency current catheter ablation of accessory atrioventricular pathways. *Lancet* 1991; 337(8757):1557–1561.
116. Calkins H, Langberg J, Sousa J, et al. Radiofrequency catheter ablation of accessory atrioventricular connections in 250 patients: Abbreviated therapeutic approach to Wolff-Parkinson-White syndrome. *Circulation* 1992;85:1337–1346.
117. Lesh MD, Van Hare G, Scheinman MM, et al. Comparison of the retrograde and transseptal methods for ablation of left free-wall accessory pathways. *J Am Coll Cardiol* 1993,22:542–549.
118. Kay GN, Pressley JC, Packer DL, et al. Value of 12-lead electrocardiogram in discriminating atrioventricular nodal reciprocating tachycardia from circus movement atrioventricular utilizing a retrograde accessory pathway. *Am J Cardiol* 1987;59:296–300.
119. Tchou PJ, Lehmann MJ, Donga J, et al. Effect of sudden rate acceleration on the human His-Purkinje system: Adaptation of refractoriness in a damped oscillatory pattern. *Circulation* 1986;73:920–929.
120. Manolis AS, Katsaros C, Cokkinos DV. Electrophysiological and elctropharmacological studies in pre-excitation syndromes: Results with propafenone therapy and isoproterenol infusion testing. *Eur Heart J* 1992;13:1489–1495.
121. Janoušek J, Paul T, Reimer A, Kallfelz H. Usefulness of propafenone for supraventricular arrhythmias in infants and children. *Am J Cardiol* 1993;72:294–300.
122. Musto B, D'Onofrio A, Cavallaro C, Musto A. Electrophysiological effects and clinical efficacy of propafenone in children with recurrent paroxysmal supraventricular tachycardia. *Circulation* 1988;78:863–869.
123. Vignati G, Figini M, Figini A. The use of propafenone in the treatment of tachyarrhythmias in children. *Eur Heart J* 1993;14:546–550.
124. Vassiliadis, Papoutsakis P, Kallikazaros I, et al. Propafenone in the prevention of non-ventricular arrhythmias associated with the Wolff-Parkinson-White syndrome. *Int J Cardiol* 1990;27:63–70.
125. Helmy I, Scheinman MM, Herre JM, et al. Electrophysiologic effects of isoproterenol in patients with atrioventricular reentrant tachycardia treated with flecainide. *J Am Coll Cardiol* 1990;16:1649–1655.
126. Kim SS, Lal R, Ruffy R. Treatment of paroxysmal supraventricular tachycardia with flecainide acetate. *Am J Cardiol* 1986;58:80–85.
127. Cockrell J, Scheinman MM, Titus C, et al. Safety and efficacy of oral flecainide therapy in patients with atrioventricular reentrant tachycardia. *Ann Intern Med* 1991;114:189–194.
128. Hoff PI, Tronstad A, Oie B, Ohm OJ. Electrophysiologic and clinical effects of flecainide for recurrent paroxysmal supraventricular tachycardia. *Am J Cardiol* 1988;62:585–589.
129. Wiseman MN, Elstob JE, Camm AJ, et al. A study of the use of flecainide acetate in the long-term management of cardiac arrhythmias. *PACE* 1990;13:767–775.
130. Benditt DG, Dunnigan A, Buetikofer J, Milstein S. Flecainide acetate for long-term prevention of paroxysmal supraventricular tachyarrhythmias. *Circulation* 1991;83:345–349.
131. Pritchett ELC, DaTorre SD, Platt ML, et al. Flecainide acetate treatment of paroxysmal supraventricular tachycardia and paroxysmal atrial fibrillation. *J Am Coll Cardiol* 1991;17:297–303.
132. Manolis AS, Estes NAM. Reversal of electrophysiologic effects of flecainide on the accessory pathway by isoproterenol in the Wolff-Parkinson-White syndrome. *Am J Cardiol* 1989;64:194–198.
133. Kunze K, Schluter M, Kuck K. Sotalol in patients with Wolff-Parkinson-White syndrome. *Circulation* 1987;75:1050–1057.
134. Mason JW. Amiodarone. *N Engl J Med* 1987;316:455–466.
135. Rosenbaum MD, Chiale PA, Ryba D, et al. Control of tachyarrhythmias associated with Wolff-Parkinson-White syndrome by amiodarone hydrochloride. *Am J Cardiol* 1974;34:215–223.
136. Wellens HJJ, Lie KI, Bar FW, et al. Effect of amiodarone in the Wolff-Parkinson-White syndrome. *Am J Cardiol* 1976;38:189–194.
137. Hindricks G. The Multicenter European Radiofrequency Survey (MERFS): Complications of radiofrequency catheter ablation of arrhythmias. The Multicenter European Radiofrequency Survey (MERFS) investigators of the Working Group on Arrhythmias of the European Society of Cardiology. *Eur Heart J* 1993;14:1644–1653.
138. Scheinman MM, Huang S. The 1998 NASPE prospective catheter ablation registry. *Pacing Clin Electrophysiol* 2000;23:1020–1028.
139. Brembilla-Perrot B, Ghawi R. Electrophysiological characteristics of asymptomatic Wolff-Parkinson-White syndrome. *Eur Heart J* 1993; 14:511–515.

140. Leitch JW, Klein GJ, Yee R, Murdock C. Prognostic value of electrophysiology testing in asymptomatic patients with Wolff-Parkinson-White pattern. *Circulation* 1990;82:1718–1723.
141. Priori SG, Aliot E, Blomstrom-Lundqvist C, et al. Task force on sudden cardiac death of the European society of cardiology. *Eur Heart J* 2001;22:1374–1450.
142. Zipes DP, DiMarco JP, Gillette PC, et al. Guidelines for clinical intracardiac electrophysiological and catheter ablation procedures. A report of the American College of Cardiology/American Heart Association Task Force on Practice Guidelines (Committee on Clinical Intracardiac Electrophysiologic and Catheter Ablation Procedures), developed in collaboration with the North American Society of Pacing and Electrophysiology. *J Am Coll Cardiol* 1995;26:555–573.
143. Beckman KJ, Gallastegui JL, Bauman JL, et al. The predictive value of electrophysiologic studies in untreated patients with Wolff-Parkinson-White syndrome. *J Am Coll Cardiol* 1990;15:640–647.
144. Attoyan C, Haissaguerre M, Dartigues JF, et al. Ventricular fibrillation in Wolff-Parkinson-White syndrome. Predictive factors. *Arch Mal Coeur Vaiss* 1994;87:889–897.
145. Montoya PT, Brugada P, Smeets J, et al. Ventricular fibrillation in the Wolff-Parkinson-White syndrome. *Eur Heart J* 1991;12:144–150.
146. Wellens HJ, Bar FW, Gorgels AP, et al. Use of ajmaline in patients with the Wolff-Parkinson-White syndrome to disclose short refractory period of the accessory pathway. *Am J Cardiol* 1980;45:130–133.
147. Fitzsimmons PJ, McWhirter PD, Peterson DW, et al. The natural history of Wolff-Parkinson-White syndrome in 228 military aviators: A long-term follow-up of 22 years. *Am Heart J* 2001;142(3):530–536.
148. Pappone C, Santinelli V, Rosanio S. Usefulness of invasive electrophysiology testing to stratify the risk of arrhythmic events in asymptomatic patients with Wolff-Parkinson-White pattern. Results from a large prospective long-term follow-up study. *J Am Coll Cardiol* 2003;41:239–244.
149. Blomström-Lundqvist C, Scheinman MM, Aliot EM, et al. ACC/AHA/ESC Guidelines for the Management of Patients with Supraventricular Arrhythmias—Executive Summary: A Report of the American College of Cardiology/American Heart Association Task Force on Practice Guidelines and the European Society of Cardiology Committee for Practice Guidelines (Writing Committee to Develop Guidelines for the Management of Patients with Supraventricular Arrhythmias). *Circulation* 2003;108(15):1871–1909.

CHAPTER 31

# VENTRICULAR ARRHYTHMIAS

Robert W. Rho / Richard L. Page



Ventricular arrhythmias are observed commonly in clinical practice and vary from the more benign (such as asymptomatic premature ventricular complexes and nonsustained ventricular tachycardia) to potentially fatal (as with sustained monomorphic ventricular tachycardia or ventricular fibrillation). Appropriate management depends on the associated symptoms, hemodynamic consequences, and associated long-term prognosis. Initial management, risk stratification, and treatment of ventricular arrhythmias pose a significant challenge to clinicians caring for such patients. This chapter provides an overview of the clinical significance, diagnosis, and therapeutic options for the ventricular arrhythmias encountered in clinical practice (Table 31-1).

## DEFINITIONS

Premature ventricular complexes (PVCs) are defined as ectopic beats originating from the ventricles occurring before the next anticipated beat of supraventricular origin. Two successive PVCs are designated as a couplet. In ventricular bigeminy, PVCs occur with a relatively fixed coupling interval after every conducted sinus beat.

*Nonsustained ventricular tachycardia* is defined as a run of three or more beats but less than 30 s (an arbitrary duration), at a rate greater than 120 beats per minute. *Sustained ventricular tachycardia* is defined at electrophysiologic study as a run that is longer than 30 s or if the run results in hemodynamic compromise requiring termination even if it does not last 30 s. Spontaneous sustained ventricular tachycardia (VT) is variously defined and there is no accepted standard definition for it. *Ventricular fibrillation* is a rapid irregular ventricular arrhythmia with no discernable QRS complex. *Torsades de pointes* is a rapid, irregular polymorphic VT that appears to twist around a central axis and is associated with prolongation of the QT interval on the electrocardiogram.

## PREMATURE VENTRICULAR COMPLEXES

PVCs are seen commonly in clinical practice. They may occur in patients with and without structural heart disease. In general, PVCs detected in clinical practice do not require specific therapy. The significance of PVCs depends on their frequency, the presence and severity of structural heart disease, and the presence of associated symptoms.

### Premature Ventricular Complexes in the Absence of Organic Heart Disease

PVCs occur frequently in the general population.[1] In general, PVCs that occur in patients without structural heart disease are not associated with excess risk of sudden death. Kennedy et al. described 73 patients with frequent ventricular ectopy on a 24-h ambulatory (Holter) monitor who were followed for an average of 6.5 years, and no excess in mortality was reported. This study excluded patients

TABLE 31-1 Ventricular Arrhythmias: Mechanisms and Clinical Features

| Ventricular arrhythmia | ECG features | Mechanism | Clinical features |
|---|---|---|---|
| PVCs | Variable:<br>CAD: RBBB morphology<br>RVOT PVCs: LBBB morphology | Reentry<br>Focal<br>Triggered | Significance depends on structural heart disease |
| Monomorphic ventricular tachycardia | Variable:<br>Usually RBBB morphology | Reentry most common | Significance depends on etiology/ hemodynamic consequences/EF |
| VT in ARVD | LBBB VT morphology | Reentry most common | Multiple morphologies<br>Progressive disease |
| VT in cardiac sarcoid | Usually RBBB VT morphology | Reentry most common | Associated with conduction abnormalities |
| VT in Chagas' disease | Variable:<br>Usually RBBB VT morphology | Reentry most common<br>Often epicardial | LV dysfunction/aneurysm<br>South American Protozoa: *T. Cruzi* |
| BBR VT | Usually LBBB pattern but may be RBBB pattern (in ischemic cardiomyopathy) | Reentry | A sustained monomophic VT in dilated cardiomyopathy<br>Ammenable to RF ablation |
| RVOT VT | LBBB VT with left inferior axis | Triggered activity<br>Increased automaticity | Benign. Treat symptoms or tachycardiomyopathy |
| Idiopathic LVT | RBBB VT with left superior axis | Probably reentry involving left anterior/ posterior fascicles | Benign. Treat symptoms or tachycardiomyopathy<br>Sensitive to verapamil |
| AIVR | Variable morphology | Increased automaticity | Usually a benign arrhythmia |
| Ventricular fibrillation | Rapid and irregular<br>No discernable QRS complex | Functional reentry | Fatal unless immediate defibrillation<br>Associated with ischemia |
| Torsade de pointes | Polymorphic VT twisting around central axis | Triggered activity initiates and functional reentry maintains VT | Associated with long QT syndrome<br>Drugs prolonging QT must be identified and discontinued |

ABBREVIATIONS: ECG = electrocardiograph; PVC = premature ventricular complex; CAD = coronary artery disease; RBBB = right bundle branch block; LBBB = left bundle branch block; RVOT = right ventricular outflow tract; EF = ejection fraction; VT = ventricular tachycardia; ARVD = arrhythmogenic right ventricular dysplasia; LV = left ventricular; BBR = bundle branch reentry; RF = radiofrequency; LVT = left ventricular tachycardia; AIVR = accelerated idioventricular rhythm.

with mitral valve prolapse, minimal left ventricular (LV) dysfunction, and a family history of sudden death.[2] PVCs that occur in patients with a structurally normal heart warrant no therapy unless significant symptoms are present.

## Premature Ventricular Complexes after Myocardial Infarction

The relationship between PVCs following myocardial infarction and sudden death has been studied extensively. In general, the presence of PVCs after a myocardial infarction is associated with an increased risk of sudden death when the frequency of PVCs exceeds > 10 per hour. This risk is greater in patients with larger myocardial infarctions and lower LV ejection fractions. Ruberman et al.[3,4] reported a threefold increase in sudden death in 1739 men with ventricular bigeminy, couplets, multiform ventricular premature beats (VPBs), or couplets in comparison to men without ventricular ectopy recorded on a 1-h electrocardiographic (ECG) monitoring session. The mean follow-up of this study was 2 years. In the European Infarction Study Group, patients with more than 10 PVCs per hour had a 4 percent 2-year mortality. Patients with nonsustained VT (more than three consecutive ventricular beats) had a 14.8 percent 2-year mortality in this study.[5]

Both the Multicenter Investigation of the Limitation of Infarct Size (MILIS)[6] and the Multicenter Postinfarction Study Group[7] reported frequent PVCs (more than 10 PVCs per hour) to be an independent risk factor for sudden death.

The previously referenced studies were performed before the thrombolytic era. Data from trials of thrombolytic therapy also show an association between PVCs and sudden death. GISSI-2 confirmed the prognostic importance of PVCs in patients with acute myocardial infarction receiving thrombolytic therapy. In an analysis of GISSI-2, Statters et al.[8] compared the prognostic value of PVCs among 680 patients who received or did not receive thrombolytics. They reported the greatest risk of sudden death among the patients who had greater than 10 PVCs per hour and did not receive thrombolytics. In contrast, PVCs did not predict sudden death in patients who received thrombolytics until the frequency of PVCs was greater than 25 per hour. These observations reflect the contribution of infarct size and, by association, ejection fraction to the prognosis of patients who have experienced a myocardial infarction.

## Treatment of Premature Ventricular Complexes Associated with an Acute Myocardial Infarction

The association of PVCs with sudden death led to the routine use of intravenous lidocaine in patients suffering myocardial infarctions (MIs). MacMahon et al. [9] reported that lidocaine use in patients experiencing an MI reduced the incidence of primary ventricular fibrillation (VF) by one-third. The Cardiac Arrhythmia Suppression Trial

(CAST) was a randomized, placebo-controlled study testing the hypothesis that suppression of PVCs after an MI would reduce arrhythmic death. PVC suppression was achieved with encainide, flecainide, and moricizine. This study was stopped because of an increased number of arrhythmic deaths in patients treated with encainide and flecainide despite marked suppression of PVCs. The relative risk of arrhythmic death was 3.6 (4.5 percent for drug treated patients and 1.2 percent for placebo). Total mortality was also greater with encainide or flecainide (7.7 percent) compared with placebo (3.0 percent) (relative risk = 2.5).[10] The Survival With Oral D-Sotalol (SWORD) study, which tested the use of d-sotalol (a pure class III antiarrhythmic) in patients who had MI and depressed LV function was terminated early because of a significant increase in mortality in patients receiving treatment with d-sotalol versus placebo.[11] Based on these findings, the routine prophylactic use of antiarrhythmic agents for patients following an MI was largely abandoned.

The use of amiodarone in this population is debated. Amiodarone has unique pharmacologic properties beyond its effects on the cardiac sodium and potassium channels. It is also a beta-adrenergic receptor blocker and calcium channel blocker with anti-ischemic effects.[12] The European Myocardial Infarction Amiodarone Trial (EMIAT) and Canadian Myocardial Infarction Amiodarone Trial (CAMIAT) both evaluated the empiric use of amiodarone in patients with MI. EMIAT randomized 1486 patients with an ejection fraction of $<$ 40 percent and prior MI to amiodarone or placebo. No difference in total mortality was observed in either group after a mean follow-up of 21 months.[13] In CAMIAT, on the other hand, 1202 patients with prior MI and frequent ventricular ectopy ($>$ 10 PVCs per hour) were randomized to amiodarone or placebo. The primary endpoint (combined arrhythmic death and resuscitated VF) was observed in 0.6 percent of the amiodarone group and 3.3 percent of the placebo group ($p = 0.016$). Most of the benefit was in patients who were treated concomitantly with beta-adrenergic blockers. Although a significant benefit in arrhythmic death was observed in the amiodarone group, no significant difference in total mortality was seen in this study.[14] A recent metanalysis of 13 trials of amiodarone after myocardial infarction or congestive heart failure reported a reduction in mortality and arrhythmic death in those patients treated with amiodarone.[15] This metanalysis also included studies of amiodarone in patients with no history of MI. Based on the available information on amiodarone after MI, the prophylactic use of amiodarone in this case has not been shown to improve survival and therefore is not recommended. However, the use of amiodarone for the treatment of other types of arrhythmia, such as atrial fibrillation, in the postinfarct setting appears to be safe, including patients with depressed LV ejection fraction.

## Premature Ventricular Complexes and Nonsustained Ventricular Tachycardia in Nonischemic Cardiomyopathy

PVCs that occur in patients with nonischemic cardiomyopathy do not appear to be associated with an increase in sudden death or total mortality. Von Olshausen et al.[16] followed 73 patients for 3 years with nonischemic cardiomyopathy and frequent PVCs on baseline ambulatory monitoring. Multivariate analysis found only the presence of left bundle branch block and depressed LV ejection to be predictive of sudden death. Several large trials, including GESICA and the V-HEFT study, have found that nonsustained VT is a risk factor for sudden death.[17,18] In another study of ambulatory monitors performed in 674 patients with dilated cardiomyopathy, nonsustained VT was not associated with a worse survival rate.[19] Therefore the clinical significance of nonsustained VT in patients with dilated cardiomyopathy remains unclear.

## Outflow-Tract Premature Ventricular Complexes

PVCs originating from the right ventricular (RV) outflow tract (RVOT) are characterized on the 12-lead electrocardiogram to have a left bundle branch block pattern in $V_1$ and monophasic tall R waves in the inferior leads (Fig. 31-1). RVOT PVCs occur in patients with structurally normal hearts and are not associated with a poor prognosis. They may manifest as frequent single PVCs or as repetitive salvos of monomorphic VT. The frequency of RVOT PVCs is often augmented by exercise. Symptomatic RVOT PVCs may respond to beta-adrenergic blocking agents and calcium channel blockers. Radiofrequency catheter ablation can be a curative treatment option for patients with symptomatic PVCs from the RVOT when drug therapy has proven ineffective. Before referring a patient for ablation therapy, it is important to rule out other causes of RVOT ectopy, such as arrhythmogenic RV dysplasia.

## Exercise-Induced Premature Ventricular Complexes

The significance of PVCs in patients that occur during or in the recovery phase of exercise stress testing has been controversial, especially in those patients with structurally normal hearts. A recent report from the Paris Prospective Study of 6101 asymptomatic men who underwent exercise stress testing stated that ventricular ectopy during exercise was associated with a relative risk of death from cardiovascular causes of 2.63 (95 percent confidence interval, 1.93 to 3.59) when patients were followed for an average of 23 years.[20] In another study of 29,244 patients (70 percent men) without a history of heart failure, valve disease, or arrhythmia, frequent ventricular ectopy (defined by $>$ 7 PVCs/min, ventricular bigeminy or trigeminy, VT, ventricular flutter, torsades de pointes, or VF), the presence of frequent ventricular ectopy during recovery predicted an increased risk of death with an adjusted hazard ratio of 1.5 (95 percent confidence interval 1.1 to 1.9; $p = 0.003$), but frequent ventricular ectopy during exercise did not predict increased risk of death. The mean follow-up of this study was 5.3 years.[21] Specific treatment recommendations cannot be derived on the basis of these observational studies. Further research is necessary to define the mechanism of exercise-induced PVCs and to determine the optimal method for the follow-up and treatment of patients with this finding.

## Management of Patients with Premature Ventricular Complexes

Patients with structurally normal hearts and frequent PVCs have no increased risk of sudden death; therefore no specific therapy is indicated. In patients with significantly symptomatic PVCs, therapy aimed at alleviating symptoms may be necessary. Initial treatment should include reassurance and the avoidance of exogenous stimulants (caffeinated beverages and other stimulants, environmental stress). If these measures fail, trial of a low-dose beta blocker may be sufficient to alleviate symptoms. Although the response to beta-adrenergic blockers is likely a pharmacologic class effect, acebutolol is approved by the U.S. Food and Drug Administration (FDA) for treatment of PVCs and may be better tolerated due to its intrinsic sympathomimetic properties.

Patients with PVCs associated with structural heart disease should be evaluated carefully, as they may be at increased risk of sudden death. Patients with ischemic cardiomyopathy and frequent PVCs are a high-risk subgroup. These patients should be approached with a heightened vigilance to further risk stratification for sudden death. Patients with an LV ejection fraction $<$ 40 percent should receive an ambulatory electrocardiographic (ECG) (Holter) monitor.

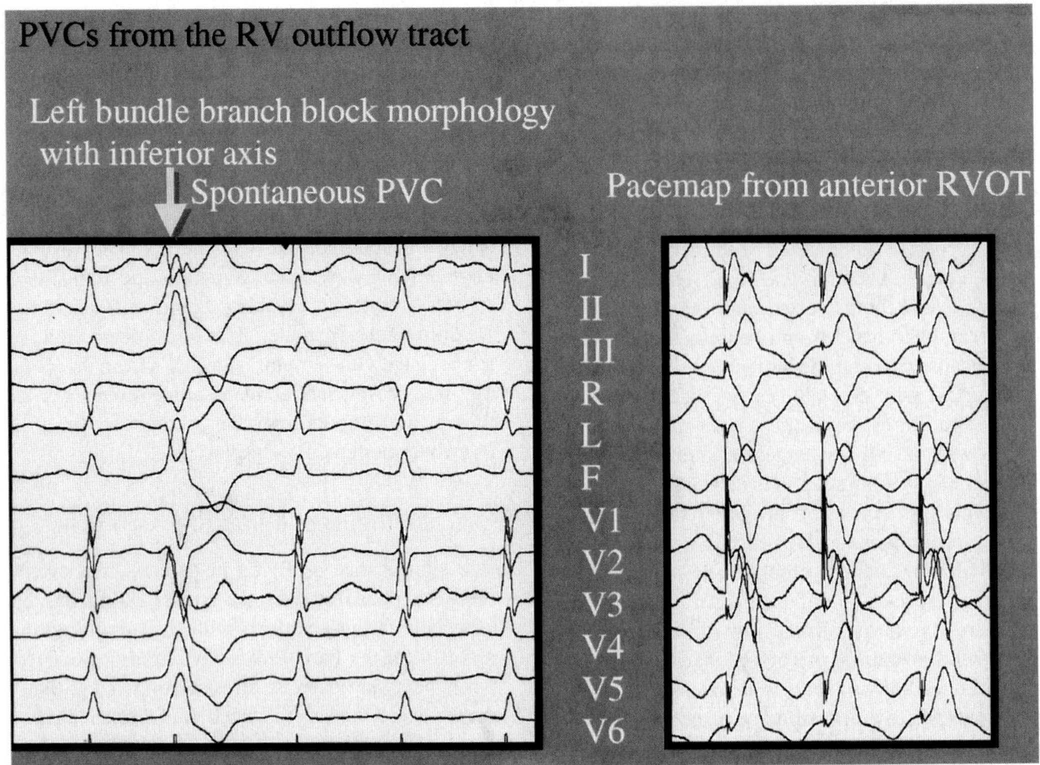


FIGURE 31-1 The electrocardiogram on the right reveals a typical right ventricular outflow tract premature ventricular complex (PVC). Note the tall monophasic R waves in the inferior leads (II,III,a$V_F$) and the left bundle branch block (LBBB) morphology in $V_1$. These PVCs were highly symptomatic in this 32-year-old woman with frequent palpitations that increased with exercise. She was brought to the electrophysiology laboratory. A mapping catheter was placed in the right ventricular outflow tract immediately below the pulmonary valve. Pacing was performed at the site of origin of this PVC, (electrocardiogram on the left) and the morphology of all 12 leads matches the spontaneous PVC, electrocardiogram on the right. A single radiofrequency lesion was applied to this region, with successful elimination of the PVCs clinically.

If nonsustained VT (three or more successive ventricular beats) is detected, the patient should undergo invasive electrophysiology study and, if the study is positive, should be offered an implantable cardioverter/defibrillator (ICD). Independent of the presence of PVCs or NSVT, patients with chronic ischemic cardiomyopathy and severely depressed ejection fraction (EF $< 30$ percent) should be considered for an ICD.[22] Patients with PVCs associated with nonischemic cardiomyopathy require no specific treatment other than aggressive heart failure management.

## VENTRICULAR TACHYCARDIA IN PATIENTS WITH CORONARY ARTERY DISEASE

VT in patients with coronary disease ranges from asymptomatic nonsustained VT (NSVT) to sustained VT that leads to hemodynamic compromise and sudden death. The understanding of the pathophysiology of VT in patients with coronary artery disease has been greatly enhanced by animal studies, electrophysiologic studies in humans, and the results of recent multicenter randomized trials.

FIGURE 31-2 *A.* Utility of QRS morphology during ventricular tachycardia (VT) to identify the location of the exit site of VT. *Step 1:* look at the QRS configuration of lead $V_1$. The pattern of right bundle branch block (RBBB) suggests that the exit site of the VT is originating from the left ventricle (LV). (Some left ventricular septal VTs may have a LBBB pattern.) *Step 2 for LBBB pattern VT:* the site of origin is from the right ventricle (or LV septum in patients with prior myocardial infarction; see below). *Step 2 for RBBB pattern VT:* the site of origin is from the LV. To distinguish basal (near mitral valve) versus apical exit sites, the mid- to lateral precordial leads are helpful. VT exit sites from the base will be (+) in $V_3$ to $V_6$. *Step 3 for RBBB pattern VT:* to distinguish anterior wall from posterior wall exit sites, look at leads II, III, and a$V_F$. VT exiting from the anterior wall will be positive in II, III, and a$V_F$ and VT exiting the posterior wall will be negative in II, III, and a$V_F$. *Step 4 for RBBB pattern VT:* to distinguish between septal and lateral wall exit sites, look at leads I and a$V_L$. VT exiting from the septum will be positive in I and a$V_L$, whereas VT exiting from the lateral wall will be negative in leads I and a$V_L$. *Step 2 for LBBB pattern VT* suggests VT from the right ventricle. Look at leads II, III, and a$V_F$. If tall monophasic R waves are present in these leads, only one morphology of VT is present and the patient has a structurally normal heart; think of right ventricular outflow tract (RVOT) VT. In patients with ischemic cardiomyopathy, think of VT from the LV septum. Multiple morphologies of monomorphic VT should raise the suspicion of VT associated with arrhythmogenic RV dysplasia. *B.* An example of a patient with ischemic cardiomyopathy who has had a large inferior posterior myocardial infarction. He presented with a clinical VT that resulted in multiple shocks from his implantable cardioverter/defibrillator despite the initiation of amiodarone. He was brought to the electrophysiology laboratory for mapping and ablation of his VT. $V_1$ shows a right bundle configuration. This places the exit site in the left ventricle. Base versus apex: Use $V_3$ to $V_6$. $V_3$ to $V_6$ in this VT is (+), placing the exit site in the base of the LV. Anterior versus posterior: Use II, III, and a$V_F$. II, III, and a$V_F$ in the VT are (−), placing the exit site in the posterior wall of the LV. Septal versus lateral: Use I and a$V_L$. I and a$V_L$ are (+) in this VT, placing the exit site near the septum. The panel on the right shows a pacemap with a near match of the clinical VT. The site of pacing is in the inferior septum of the LV near the mitral valve.

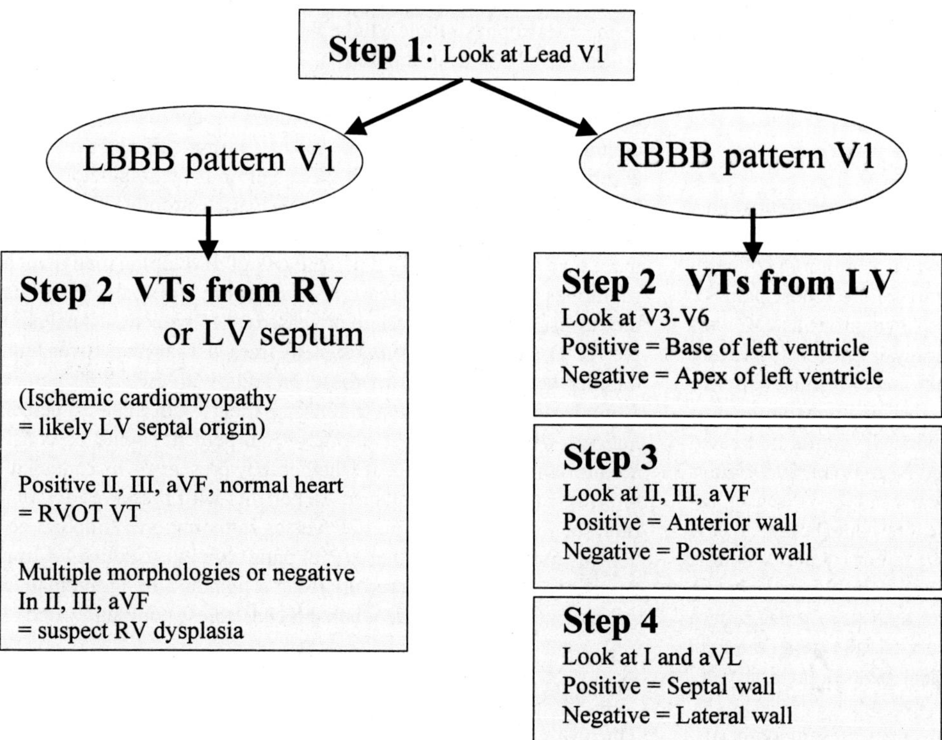
12 Lead localization of the exit site of ventricular tachycardia
Step 1: Look at Lead V1
LBBB pattern V1
RBBB pattern V1
Step 2 VTs from RV or LV septum
(Ischemic cardiomyopathy = likely LV septal origin)
Positive II, III, aVF, normal heart = RVOT VT
Multiple morphologies or negative In II, III, aVF = suspect RV dysplasia
Step 2 VTs from LV
Look at V3-V6
Positive = Base of left ventricle
Negative = Apex of left ventricle
Step 3
Look at II, III, aVF
Positive = Anterior wall
Negative = Posterior wall
Step 4
Look at I and aVL
Positive = Septal wall
Negative = Lateral wall

A

Ventricular tachycardia

Pacemap from inferior septum near the mitral valve of the left ventricle.

I II III aVR aVL aVF V1 V2 V3 V4 V5 V6

B

## Pathophysiology

The anatomic substrate from which sustained monomorphic VT originates usually involves an extensive healed scar following an acute MI. This substrate of healthy and damaged myocardium interlaced with fibrous scar is found primarily at the border zone of the scar (transition between scar and healthy tissue) and serves as a basis for slowed conduction and reentry.[23–25] Evolution of the electrophysiologic substrate occurs over 2 weeks after an index MI and then remains indefinitely.[26] The substrate may be modified by subsequent ischemic insults and by late ventricular remodeling or worsening pump function. These changes may lead to neurohormonal activation, progressive LV dilatation, and regional and global elevations in wall tension, all of which may contribute to proarrhythmia. Patients with VT have a high risk of recurrence of VT even when heart failure and coronary ischemia are controlled.[27] The risk of VT is highest during the first year (3 to 5 percent) after a MI, but new onset of VT may occur many years later.[6] Patients with larger infarctions and lower ejection fractions are at highest risk.

## Mechanism

The mechanism of VT in the majority of cases is reentry. Ischemic VT is usually initiated, terminated, and reset with programmed electrical stimulation in the electrophysiology laboratory; this response to programmed electrical stimulation supports reentry as the mechanism for this form of VT.[28] In contrast, arrhythmias caused by enhanced automaticity are not induced with programmed stimulation. The reentry circuit most frequently exists within the border zone of the scar.[23] VT exits the scar into healthy myocardium and depolarizes the myocardium at a region proximate to the location of the reentry circuit. The exit site can be identified, based on the QRS configuration on a 12-lead surface ECG (Fig. 31-2).

## Clinical Presentation and Management

As mentioned above, the symptoms associated with ischemic VT are quite variable. The main determinants of hemodynamic tolerance are the rate of the VT[29] and the degree of LV dysfunction.[30] The clinical presentation of sustained VT may not be prognostic of the presentation of subsequent events. In the AVID (Antiarrhythmics Versus Implantable Defibrillators) registry, patients with hemodynamically tolerated VT at presentation had similar mortality as patients with syncopal VT (mean follow-up 11.7 ± 8.6 months).[31]

## Management of Sustained Ventricular Tachycardia

Patients who present in clinical stable VT may be treated with antiarrhythmic drugs, antitachycardia pacing when available, or synchronous direct current (DC) cardioversion. Patients in VT with hemodynamic compromise, congestive heart failure, chest pain, or ischemia should be treated promptly with synchronous DC cardioversion. When antiarrhythmic drug therapy is chosen to prevent recurrence, amiodarone is the treatment of choice in most patients. The efficacy of amiodarone is superior to that of lidocaine or procainamide in this setting.[32,33] All patients with VT should be treated with a beta blocker unless this is prohibited by hypotension, bradycardia, or other clinical factors (e.g., reactive airway disease, vasospastic coronary disease). Reversible factors contributing to VT, such as the exacerbation of congestive heart failure, acute ischemia, or electrolyte abnormalities should be diagnosed rapidly and treated. In patients who have refractory VT despite aggressive treatment, a subset of selected patients may be treated successfully with emergent radiofrequency catheter ablation, mechanical ventricular assist devices, and cardiac transplantation.[34,35]

The long-term management of patients who present with sustained VT begins with the assessment of LV function, as this is a well-established independent risk factor for sudden cardiac death in patients with ventricular arrhythmias.[36,37] In a retrospective analysis of the Electrophysiologic Study Versus Electrocardiographic Monitoring (ESVEM) trial population, 285 of the 486 patients enrolled had an arrhythmia occurrence. For enrollment in ESVEM, patients had to have a history of (1) resuscitated sudden cardiac death, (2) documented sustained VT, or (3) history of unmonitored syncope; in addition, all patients had > 10 PVCs per hour on ambulatory monitoring and inducible sustained VT or VF at electrophysiologic study. Over a 6-year follow-up, patients with an ejection fraction (EF) of more than 40 percent had a 5 percent risk of developing malignant arrhythmias. With each decrease of 5 percent in LVEF, the risk of cardiac arrest or arrhythmic death increased by 15 percent.[38] Analysis of the AVID study revealed that benefit from ICD therapy over amiodarone therapy occurred in those patients with EF < 30 percent. Amiodarone was equivalent to ICD in patients with EF > 30 percent. Patients with sustained VT and EF < 30 percent should be considered for an ICD regardless of whether they present asymptomatically or with hemodynamic collapse. In patients with preserved LV function, the implantation of an ICD versus initiating oral amiodarone is controversial. Therefore therapy for patients with sustained VT or resuscitated VF and preserved LV function should be individualized. All patients should receive a beta blocker unless contraindicated.

## Management of Nonsustained Ventricular Tachycardia

The evaluation and management of patients with asymptomatic NSVT begins with the evaluation of LVEF. Patients with low EF and NSVT are at risk of sudden death. In patients with an LVEF of less than 40 percent, the annual mortality post-MI is estimated to be 8 to 10 percent).[39,40] The importance of treating these patients with an angiotensin-converting enzyme (ACE) inhibitor, aspirin, and a beta-adrenergic receptor blocker cannot be overemphasized. A diagnostic electrophysiologic study with programmed stimulation in the right ventricle may be helpful in further risk stratification of asymptomatic postinfarct patients with NSVT. In patients with LVEF ≤ 40 percent, inducibility of sustained monomorphic VT with programmed electrical stimulation is associated with a 2-year actuarial risk of sudden death or cardiac arrest of 50 percent, compared with 11 percent in patients who did not have reproducibly inducible VT.[41] An example of monomorphic VT induced during programmed electrical stimulation is shown in Fig. 31-3. In the Multicenter UnSustained Tachycardia Trial (MUSTT), 704 patients with prior MI, EF of ≤ 40 percent, and NSVT were randomized to no antiarrhythmic therapy versus a strategy of eletrophysiologically guided antiarrhythmic drug ad-

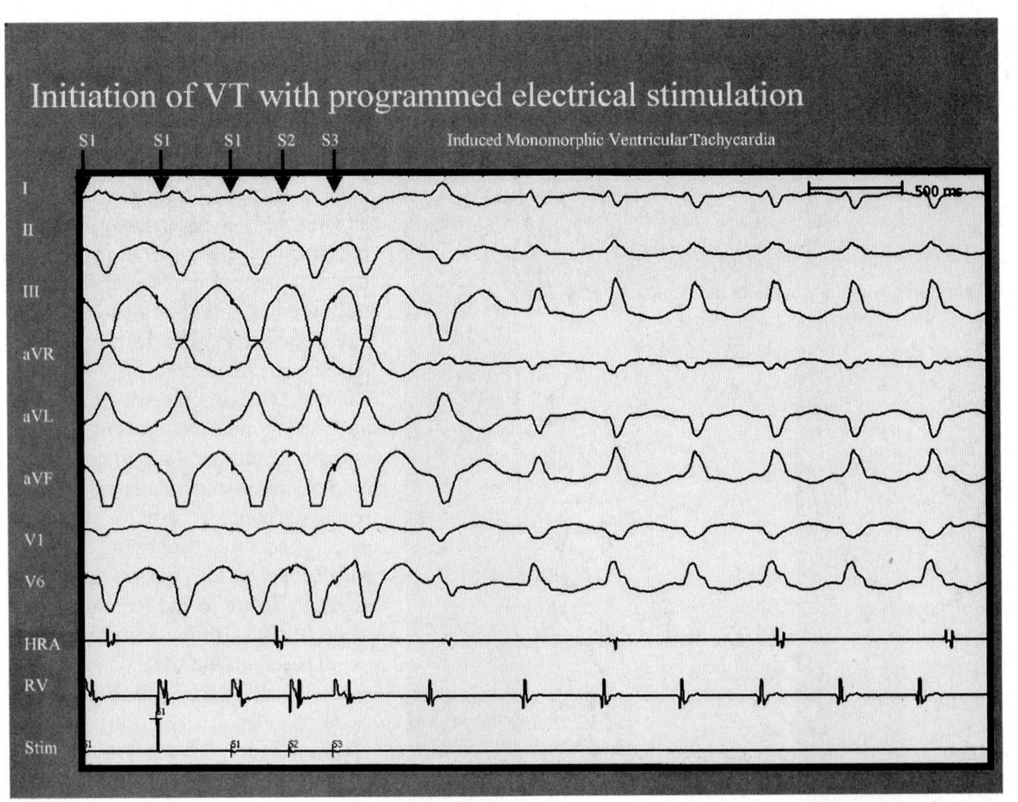


FIGURE 31-3 Programmed electrical stimulation (PES) is performed by pacing with a stable drive of eight pulses (S1) followed by up to three premature beats induced by pacing (S2, S3, S4). This is performed at two sites in the right ventricle. In susceptible patients, inducible monomorphic ventricular tachycardia (VT) may be induced, as depicted in this example, where PES with two extra stimuli induce monomorphic VT. Note the dissociation in the electrograms recorded in the HRA catheter and the RV catheter. The patient subsequently had a cardiac defibrillator implanted. HRA = high right atrium, RV = RV apical catheter, Stim = stimulation channel.

ministration or implantation of an ICD if drug therapy proved unsuccessful. A significant improvement occurred in the treatment arm, although the benefit was seen only in those patients who received the ICD. Notable in the study was the high mortality rate of patients followed in a registry who were excluded from the study because they were not inducible at electrophysiologic (EP) study. The incidence of arrhythmic death at 24-month follow-up in the registry was 12 percent. In general, patients with EF ≤ 40 percent should be considered for electrophysiologically guided treatment with an ICD.[42] Patients with severe LV dysfunction (EF ≤ 30 percent) may benefit from a defibrillator even in the absence of NSVT or a positive EP study. The MADIT II study randomized 1232 patients with ischemic cardiomyopathy on the basis of LV function alone (LVEF ≤ 30 percent), with no requirement for the documentation of NSVT. After an average follow-up of 20 months, a significant reduction in all-cause mortality was observed in patients who received an ICD. Based on the results of this trial, the prophylactic implantation of an ICD in patients with severe LV dysfunction (EF ≤ 30 percent) has a class IIa indication under the guidelines of the American College of Cardiology/American Heart Association/North American Society of Pacing and Electrophysiology (ACC/AHA/NASPE) guidelines for implantation of an ICD[22] (Table 31-2).

TABLE 31-2 Indications for Implantation of an Implantable Defibrillator

Class I Indications

1. Cardiac arrest due to VF or VT not due to a transient or reversible cause.
2. Spontaneous sustained VT in association with structural heart disease.
3. Syncope of undetermined origin with clinically relevant, hemodynamically significant sustained VT or VF induced at electrophysiologic study when drug therapy is ineffective, not tolerated, or not preferred.
4. Nonsustained VT in patients with coronary disease, prior MI, LV dysfunction, and inducible VF or sustained VT at electrophysiologic study that is not suppressible by a Class I antiarrhythmic drug.
5. Spontaneous sustained VT in patients without structural heart disease not amenable to other treatments.

Class IIa Indications

1. Patients with left ventricular ejection fraction of less than or equal to 30% at least 1 month post myocardial infarction and 3 months post coronary artery revascularization surgery.

Class IIb Indications

1. Cardiac arrest presumed to be due to VF when electrophysiologic testing is precluded by other medical conditions.
2. Severe symptoms (e.g. syncope) attributable to ventricular tachyarrhythmias in patients awaiting heart transplant.
3. Familial or inherited conditions with a high risk for life-threatening ventricular tachyarrhythmias such as long-QT syndrome or hypertrophic cardiomyopathy.
4. Nonsustained VT with coronary artery disease, prior MI, LV dysfunction, and inducible sustained VT or VF at electrophysiologic study.
5. Recurrent syncope of undetermined origin in the presence of ventricular dysfunction and inducible ventricular arrhythmias at electrophysiologic study when other causes of syncope are excluded.
6. Syncope of unexplained origin or family history of unexplained sudden cardiac death in association with typical or atypical right bundle branch block and ST-segment elevations (Brugada's syndrome).
7. Syncope in patients with advanced structural heart disease in which thorough invasive and noninvasive investigation has failed to define a cause.

ABBREVIATIONS: VF = ventricular fibrillation; VT = ventricular tachycardia; MI = myocardial infarction; LV = left ventricular.

In summary, according to the available literature guiding the primary prevention of sudden death in patients with coronary artery disease and depressed LV function, patients with ischemic cardiomyopathy and severely depressed LV function (EF ≤ 30 percent) should be offered an ICD regardless of the presence or absence of NSVT. Patients with a LV ejection fraction of 30 to 40 percent should be monitored for the presence of NSVT, usually with a 24-h ambulatory recording. Those patients with NSVT should undergo an EP study with programmed electrical stimulation. If the EP study is positive, the patient should be offered implantation of an ICD. Patients with no inducible monomorphic VT should be treated with optimal medical management for heart failure and coronary disease, although the significant mortality rate in the noninducible patients followed in the MUSTT registry necessitates careful follow-up of these individuals.

Patients who receive ICDs may require adjunctive therapy with an antiarrhythmic drug (usually amiodarone). Care must be taken in programming the ICD, as antiarrhythmic medications can have varying effects on defibrillation thresholds and may slow the rate of the VT.

Those patients with persistent VT refractory to medications can be successfully treated with radiofrequency catheter ablation. The central common pathways or exit sites of these reentry circuits are mapped using classic entrainment techniques. A radiofrequency lesion delivered to these regions of reentry results in termination of VT during the application of the lesion. The initial success rate for this procedure is approximately 75 percent in selected patients and approximately two-thirds of patients remain arrhythmia-free at 12-year follow-up. In general, the ideal candidate for this procedure is a patient with hemodynamically tolerated VT. However, "unmappable" VTs that result in hemodynamic collapse can be successfully ablated using pacemapping and entrainment mapping techniques coupled with strategically placed linear lesions[43,44] (see Chap. 36).

## VENTRICULAR TACHYCARDIA IN PATIENTS WITH NONISCHEMIC CARDIOMYOPATHY

Dilated cardiomyopathy is due to a heterogeneous group of etiologies resulting in LV and/or RV dilatation. Causes of dilated cardiomyopathy include valvular heart disease, ethanol ingestion, viral infections, and cardiac sarcoidosis, among others. Sudden death in dilated cardiomyopathy is usually due to a ventricular tachyarrhythmia.

The contribution of bradyarrhythmias to the etiology of sudden death in patients with dilated cardiomyopathy may also be important. Significant conduction abnormalities manifesting as a left bundle branch block, right bundle branch block (with or without concomitant left anterior or posterior hemiblock), and significant PR prolongation in patients with dilated congestive heart failure are common. In a report of 157 cases of sudden death in idiopathic cardiomyopathy in which the rhythm preceding death was available from ambulatory monitoring, 62 percent of patients had organized VT that progressed to VF, 13 percent had primary VF, but 17 percent had bradyarrhythmia.[45] In another report of 20 patients with dilated cardiomyopathy, the cause of death was electromechanical dissociation/bradycardia in 13 of 20 patients and only 7 of 20 died of a ventricular arrhythmia.[46] Although ventricular arrhythmias are frequent causes of sudden death, bradyarrhythmias may also play a significant role in the etiology of sudden death in patients with severe dilated cardiomyopathy.[45–47]

## Pathophysiology

The pathogenesis of ventricular arrhythmias in dilated cardiomyopathy is not well understood and may reflect a variety of mechanisms. In a study of the autopsy findings in 152 patients with idiopathic dilated cardiomyopathy, subendocardial scarring was present in 33 percent of patients. Histologic sectioning revealed multiple patchy areas of fibrosis in 57 percent of patients. These patchy areas of fibrosis, intermingled with viable myocardium, may serve as the substrate for reentry.[48] Changes in ventricular mechanics and geometry may alter regional refractoriness within the ventricle and also predispose to reentry, enhanced automaticity, or triggered activity.[49] Furthermore, the conduction system may also serve as a substrate for reentry in patients with dilated cardiomyopathy. Bundle branch reentry is a type of reentry VT that utilizes the left and right bundle branches and a portion of the ventricular myocardium as its circuit. Bundle branch reentry is a common cause of sustained monomorphic VT in patients with dilated cardiomyopathy (DCM) and may represent up to 41 percent of VTs present in this subgroup.[50] In another series of 26 patients with monomorphic VT and nonischemic cardiomyopathy, the etiology of VT was scar-related reentry in 62 percent, an ectopic focus in 27 percent, and bundle branch reentry in 19 percent of patients.[51] The identification of bundle branch reentry is important in patients with dilated cardiomyopathy because bundle branch reentry is easily treated with radiofrequency catheter ablation (see below).

## Clinical Presentation and Management

NSVT is common in patients with dilated cardiomyopathy. NSVT is seen on 24-h ambulatory and telemetry monitoring in 50 to 60 percent of these patients. The significance of NSVT as an independent predictor of sudden death in this setting is unclear. Sustained VT or VF is thought to be the cause of death in 8 to 50 percent of deaths.[52–54] The prevalence of NSVT increases with worsening heart failure symptoms. In patients with class I to II congestive heart failure, the prevalence of NSVT is 15 to 20 percent; in class IV heart failure, the prevalence is 50 to 70 percent.[55]

Patients with dilated cardiomyopathy should be treated with an ACE inhibitor and beta blocker. The role of amiodarone in patients with nonischemic cardiomyopathy is controversial. The GESICA trial examined whether low-dose amiodarone (300 mg/day) would improve survival in patients with severe congestive heart failure (CHF) (class II to IV and EF $<$ 35 percent). Although GESICA included patients with both ischemic and nonischemic VT, this South American trial had a high representation of nonischemic etiology (62 percent nonischemic, 10 percent with Chagas' disease). A total of 516 patients were randomized to amiodarone versus placebo and followed for a mean of 2 years. Amiodarone was associated with a 28 percent reduction in mortality in comparison to placebo (33.5 percent vs. 41.6 percent deaths, $p = 0.024$).[56] CHF-STAT, a placebo-controlled, randomized trial of amiodarone conducted in North America, failed to show benefit to amiodarone, although the subgroup analysis of patients with nonischemic cardiomyopathy showed a trend toward lower mortality ($p = 0.07$).[57]

Currently the role of ICDs in the primary prevention of sudden death in patients with DCM is not clear. Bansch et al.[58] randomized 104 patients with IDCM and LVEF $\leq$ 30 percent with no prior history of VT or VF to ICD or no ICD. After a mean follow-up of 5.5 years, no significant difference in survival was observed between patients with and without an ICD. Several other trials are currently under way to shed light on the role of amiodarone and ICDs in the primary prevention of sudden death in patients with dilated cardiomyopathy. SCD-HEFT (Sudden Cardiac Death–Heart Failure Trial) is a randomized, prospective, three-arm trial comparing ICD therapy, amiodarone, and placebo in patients with either ischemic or nonischemic cardiomyopathy (EF $<$ 35 percent, class II to III CHF). The ongoing DEFINITE trial will look at the role of ICD in patients with nonischemic cardiomyopathy (EF $<$ 35 percent and symptomatic CHF). Until the results of these trials of amiodarone and ICD in the primary prevention of sudden death in nonischemic cardiomyopathy are available, the routine use of amiodarone and ICD implantation will remain controversial.

Radiofrequency catheter ablation of VT in patients with drug-refractory VT may serve as an adjunctive treatment option for patients suffering multiple recurrences of VT or frequent ICD therapies. In one series of 29 patients with monomorphic VT referred for ablation, radiofrequency ablation was successful in 60 percent of scar-related VTs and 86 percent of patients with VTs caused by focal automaticity.[51] Successful ablation of scar-related VTs in patients with sarcoidosis, scleroderma, and Chagas' disease has been reported; however, experience is limited.

## Bundle Branch Reentry Ventricular Tachycardia

The clinical recognition of bundle branch reentry (BBR) VT is essential because this arrhythmia can potentially be cured by radiofrequency catheter ablation.[50,51] The rate of BBR is usually rapid and may be associated with syncope. The sinus rhythm 12-lead ECG usually demonstrates an intraventricular conduction delay or a left bundle branch block (LBBB). The 12-lead ECG during VT has an LBBB configuration and may be indistinguishable from a supraventricular tachycardia conducting with an LBBB. These two arrhythmias can easily be distinguished in the electrophysiology laboratory. The treatment of choice for this arrhythmia is radiofrequency catheter ablation of the right bundle branch. Antiarrhythmic drugs for BBR are associated with a high recurrence rate. A controversial issue is whether patients with BBR should receive an ICD after successful ablation of the right bundle, as they remain at risk for other lethal ventricular arrhythmias. An example of the typical ECG features of BBR as well as a graphic of the mechanism of BBR is provided in Fig. 31-4.

## Ventricular Tachycardia in Arrhythmogenic Right Ventricular Dysplasia

Arrhythmogenic right ventricular dysplasia (ARVD) is characterized by fatty infiltration, fibrosis, and thinning of the right ventricle. The most frequently involved areas of the right ventricle are the posterior base, apex, and the infundibulum. These areas are collectively called the *triangle of dysplasia*. Diagnosis of ARVD can be difficult. Magnetic resonance imaging, echocardiography, ECG, and signal-averaged ECG may be helpful in the diagnosis of ARVD. A family history is present in 30 to 50 percent of cases[59] (see Chap. 10).

The sinus rhythm ECG in ARVD has some distinctive features. T-wave inversion may be present ECG leads $V_1$ to $V_3$. The prevalence of T-wave inversion increases over time. In patients with ARVD who present with VT, the prevalence of T-wave inversion in $V_1$ to $V_3$ increased from 50 to 98 percent during a follow-up period of 9.5 ± 3.2 years.[60] An increased QRS duration > 110 ms in $V_1$ may be seen as a manifestation of delayed conduction in the Purkinje system in the free wall of the right ventricle. Finally, epsilon waves, or small high-frequency deflections immediately beyond the QRS complex in leads $V_1$ to $V_3$, may be present.[60]

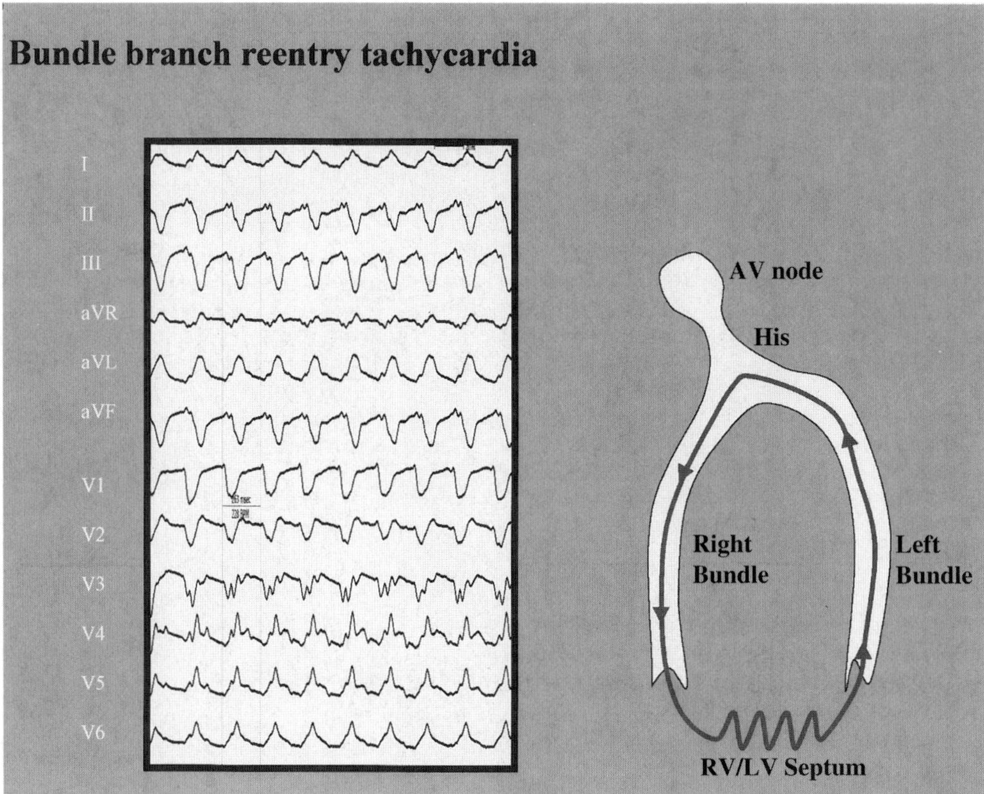


FIGURE 31-4 Bundle branch reentry ventricular tachycardia (VT). Note the left bundle branch pattern and left superior axis. The reentry circuit involves the right bundle branch as the anterograde limb and the left bundle branch as the retrograde limb, as depicted schematically on the right.

Patients with ARVD may present with stable monomorphic VT or with sudden death due to VF. VT is characterized by an LBBB pattern in $V_1$. Multiple morphologies of VT are often present in a given individual. VT that originates from the infundibulum, or right ventricular outflow tract (RVOT), may be difficult to distinguish from RVOT VT, which is a benign disease in patients with structurally normal hearts. The presence of multiple morphologies of VT with a superior QRS axis (negative in leads II, III, and $AV_F$) favors ARVD as the etiology.

Treatment of ventricular arrhythmias arising from ARVD is aimed at preventing sudden death and palliation of the clinical burden of VT. Clinical data on the efficacy of antiarrhythmic drugs and patient selection for implantable defibrillators are lacking. Treatment of sustained VT may include amiodarone, beta blockers, and sotalol as first-line choices. Patients who have had unstable VT or a history of cardiac arrest from VF should receive an ICD. Recurrent VT not responsive to antiarrhythmic medications can be successfully ablated by mapping guided by classic entrainment techniques. An example of successful ablation of VT in patients with ARVD is provided in Fig. 31-5, Plate 75. Although ablation of one clinical VT may be successful, an ICD is often implanted due to the finding of multiple VT morphologies that occur with the progression of disease. An ongoing United States registry has been established to provide further insight about the diagnosis, prognosis, and best management strategies for patients with ARVD.[61]

## Ventricular Tachycardia in Cardiac Sarcoidosis

Sarcoidosis is a granulomatous disease involving multiple organ systems. The incidence of cardiac symptoms in patients with sarcoidosis is relatively low.[62] However, 20 to 30 percent of patients with sarcoidosis are found to have evidence of cardiac involvement. Myocardial involvement may be diffuse but is frequently focal or patchy, with a propensity for the basal free wall and the anteroapical septum.[62–64] Ventricular arrhythmias are common in cardiac sarcoidosis, with reentry facilitated by the patchy fibrosis, scarring, and granulomatous involvement of the myocardium. Consistent with the reentrant mechanism, monomorphic VT in sarcoidosis can be induced with programmed stimulation. Also, local abnormal fractionated electrograms and middiastolic potentials can be recorded during the mapping of VT, lending further support to reentry as the mechanism of arrhythmia.

Currently there are insufficient data on the efficacy of specific treatment strategies in patients with ventricular arrhythmias due to cardiac sarcoidosis. Until such data are available, patients with symptomatic VT may be treated initially with amiodarone; implantation of a cardiac defibrillator should be considered in survivors of cardiac arrest, especially those with depressed LV function. Catheter ablation of VT is a reasonable option for those patients with VT refractory to antiarrhythmic medications. However, multiple morphologies of VT are common and ablation should be directed toward the most clinically relevant VT.

## Ventricular Arrhythmias in Chagas' Cardiomyopathy

Chagas' disease is the major cause of VT in Central and South America. The protozoan *Trypanosoma cruzi* is transmitted to humans via the reduviid bug. The etiology of chronic Chagas' cardiomyopathy is unknown but may be related to a cell-mediated autoimmune reaction. Recurrent monomorphic VT is common in chronic Chagas' cardiomyopathy. The majority of the VTs can be induced with

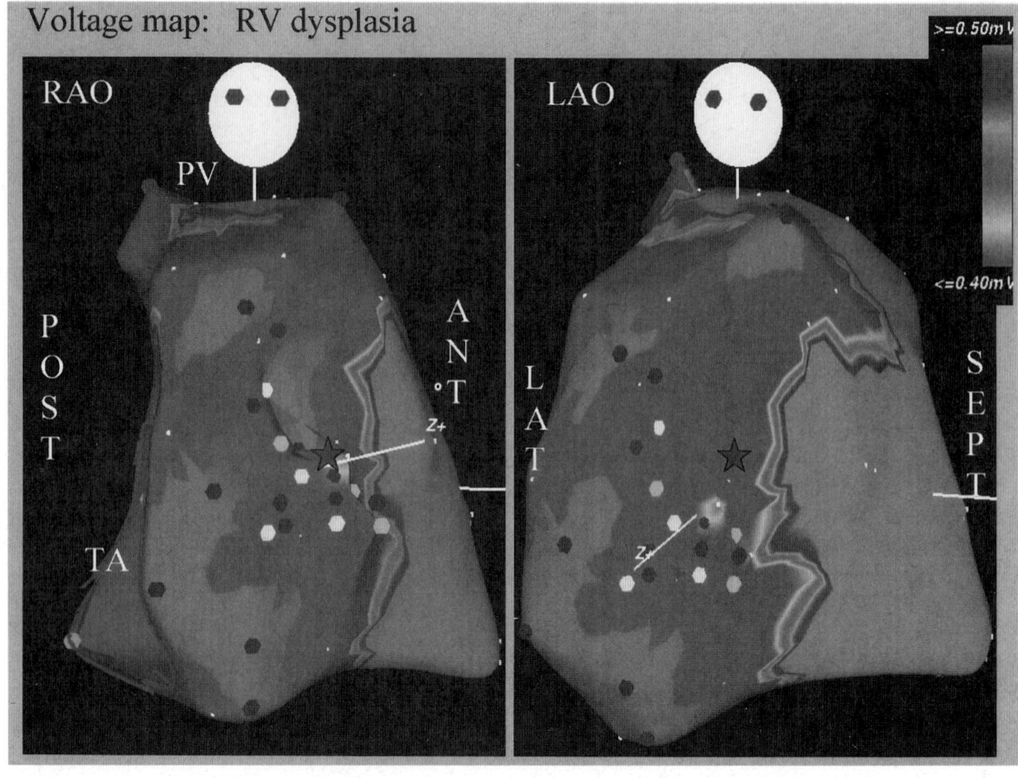


**A**

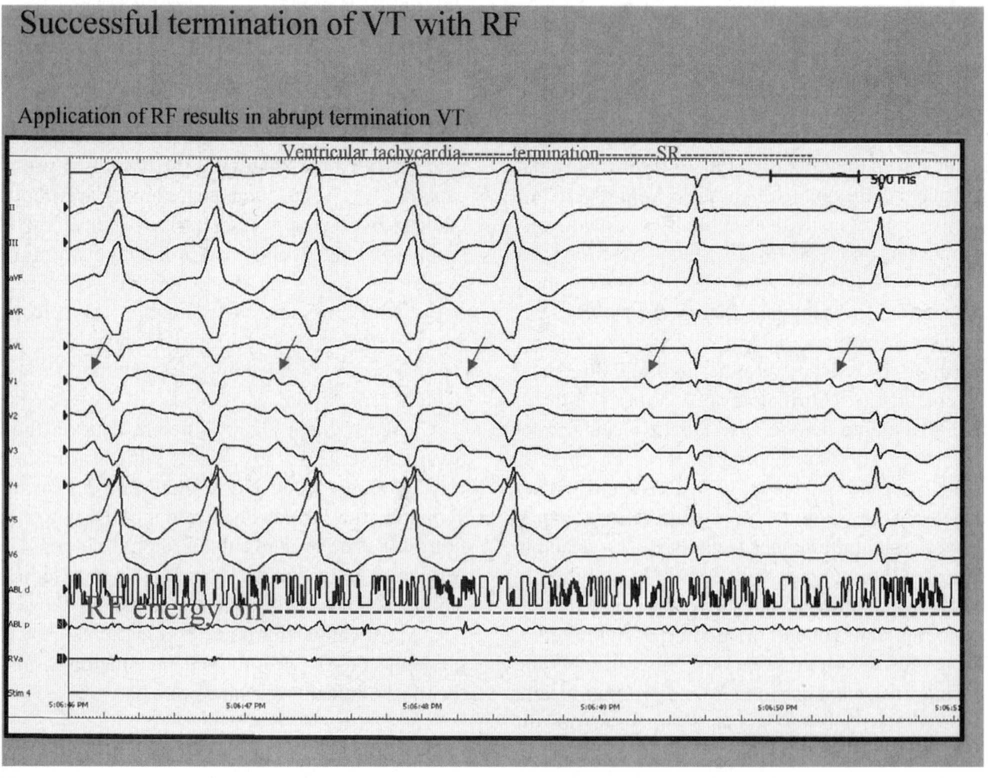


**B**

FIGURE 31-5 (Plate 75) *A*. Voltage map of the right ventricle, acquired using the Biosense Webster Carto, the three-dimensional electroanatomic mapping system. The red and gray areas indicate scar (low-voltage intracardiac electrograms) and the purple area represents healthy tissue (>0.5 mV intracardiac electrogram amplitude). The right anterior oblique (RAO) and left anterior oblique (LAO) projections are shown. A large basal free wall scar is present, extending from the base to beyond the midcavity of the right ventricle. TA = tricuspid annulus; Post = posterior; Ant = anterior; Lat = lateral; Sept = septal. The blue star represents the site where the vulnerable isthmus of the ventricular tachycardia (VT) circuit is mapped and where application of a radiofrequency lesion terminates VT (*B*).

programmed stimulation and entrained during VT favoring reentry as the mechanism.

Histologic examination of patients with Chagas' disease reveals focal and diffuse fibrosis of the myocardium, predominantly in the subepicardium and interspersed with surviving myocardial fibers. Regional wall motion abnormalities are present, often in the inferolateral wall of the LV. Apical septal and apical inferior aneurysms have also been described.[65] Mapping of VT in Chagas' disease reveals a high prevalence of circuits located in the epicardium. During mapping, middiastolic potentials and early activation are observed more frequently on the epicardium than on the endocardium, correlating with the histologic findings of predominantly epicardial involvement. Finally, the acute success rate and long-term efficacy of epicardial radiofrequency catheter ablation of VT is superior to an endocardial approach.[65–67] No significant data on the long-term efficacy and safety of epicardial radiofrequency catheter ablation and pharmacologic treatment of ventricular arrhythmias in Chagas' disease are currently available.

## IDIOPATHIC VENTRICULAR TACHYCARDIA

Idiopathic VT, by definition, occurs in patients with structurally normal hearts and represented approximately 10 percent of patients referred for evaluation of VT in one center.[68] The two main clinical entities of idiopathic VT include repetitive monomorphic VT (RVOT) and idiopathic left ventricular tachycardia (LVT; fascicular or verapamil-sensitive VT). The differentiation of these VTs from VTs associated with structural heart disease is important because they often respond well to drug therapies, are associated with an excellent prognosis, and can be cured with radiofrequency catheter ablation.

### Repetitive Monomorphic Ventricular Tachycardia

Repetitive monomorphic VT (RMVT), also referred to as right ventricular outflow tract VT (RVOT VT), was first described by Gallavardin in 1922 and is characterized by repetitive salvos of monomorphic nonsustained VT.[69] It occurs frequently in young middle-aged patients without structural heart disease. Men and women are affected equally.[70] This arrhythmia is usually provoked by exercise and emotional stress. Recurrence may be associated with exercise, stress, or caffeine; in women, it occurs more frequently during premenstrual, perimenopausal, and gestational periods.[71]

RMVT typically arises from the anterior septum of the RVOT immediately inferior to the pulmonary valve. Sites of origin of this VT have also been mapped to the free wall of the RVOT, LVOT, and aortic sinus of Valsalva.[72–74] The cellular mechanism of the tachycardia is thought to be cAMP-mediated triggered activity from delayed afterdepolarizations. This mechanism is confirmed by the sensitivity of the arrhythmia to adenosine infusion, which often (but not always) terminates the arrhythmia.[75] It is a recent observation that RMVT can originate not only in the RVOT but also from the LV epicardium, LVOT, and aortic sinus of Valsalva; this pattern is not surprising, as myocardial cells of these regions of the heart share a common embryologic origin.[76]

RMVT has a characteristic pattern on the 12-lead ECG, with a LBBB morphology and inferior axis, consistent with a RVOT tract site of origin[70] (Fig. 31-6). Most patients have a single VT morphology; the presence of multiple VT morphologies should alert the clinician to the possibility of arrhythmogenic RV dysplasia.[77]

Evaluation of patients with suspected RMVT includes an echocardiogram to confirm the absence of structural heart disease, ambulatory ECG monitoring, and exercise stress testing. In patients with RMVT, an exercise stress test will induce the arrhythmia either during exercise or during recovery. An LBB inferior axis VT in the setting of a structurally normal heart should confirm the diagnosis.

RMVT is associated with an excellent prognosis; therefore treatment is aimed at the alleviation of symptoms. Beta blockers and calcium channel antagonists are usually the first choice for the treatment of symptomatic VT, although their efficacy in preventing arrhythmia recurrence is modest. Verapamil was found to eliminate exercise-induced RMVT in 56 percent ($n = 29$) of patients who had RMVT induced during stress testing.[78] In general, beta blockers are effective in approximately 25 to 50 percent of patients, while calcium channel blockers are effective in approximately 25 to 30 percent.[79] Catheter ablation strategies utilizing pace mapping has emerged as an attractive option for the treatment of RMVT. This procedure has a low complication rate and success rates ranging from 80 to 100 percent.[80,81]

### Idiopathic Left Ventricular Tachycardia

Idiopathic LVT (fascicular VT) is another ventricular arrhythmia found in patients with structurally normal hearts. An RBB pattern left- superior-axis VT characterizes the appearance of this VT on a 12-lead ECG. Belhassen was the first to describe the sensitivity of this tachycardia to verapamil.[82] Approximately 70 percent of patients with this form of VT are men. The resting ECG is usually normal. Patients usually have a structurally normal heart but may present with incessant fascicular VT. A reversible tachycardia–mediated cardiomyopathy has been described.[83] The site of origin of the

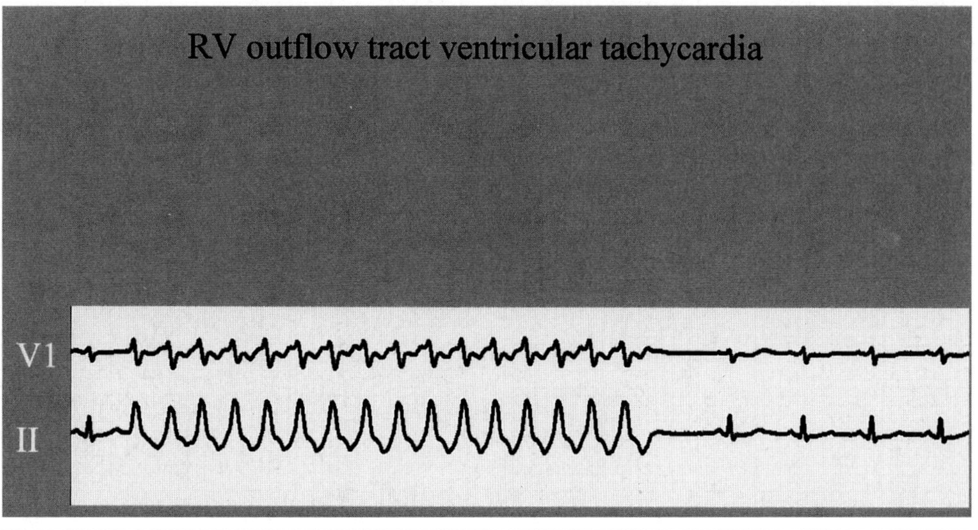


FIGURE 31-6 Repetitive monomorphic ventricular tachycardia (VT) (right ventricular outflow tract VT) is characterized by a left bundle branch block pattern in $V_1$ and an inferior axis (tall monophasic R waves in II, III, and $aV_F$). Repetitive salvos of VT characterize the clinical presentation of this arrhythmia.

tachycardia is usually in the region of the left posterior fascicle (inferoposterior LV septum). The ability to induce idiopathic LVT using programmed stimulation and the ability to entrain this tachycardia supports reentry as the its mechanism.[84,85] The mechanism appears to be reentry around the distal Purkinje network of the left posterior fascicle, accounting for the relatively narrow QRS.[86]

The clinical features of this VT include (1) a structurally normal heart, (2) an RBB pattern left-superior-axis VT with a relatively narrow QRS (<140) (Fig. 31-7), (3) sensitivity to verapamil, (4) and induction with atrial pacing.[87] The arrhythmia usually presents in patients between 15 and 40 years of age. Patients usually have no evidence of coronary disease and typically have a normal echocardiogram. False tendons are found in a high percentage of patients with idiopathic LVT. The precise anatomic and functional significance of these false tendons is not known.[88,89] Patients with idiopathic LVT may have symptoms ranging from palpitations to presyncope and syncope. This clinical syndrome is not associated with an increased incidence of sudden death in individuals affected.[79]

Idiopathic LVT responds well to verapamil for acute termination of VT as well as for long-term arrhythmia control.[83,90–92] Antiarrhythmic medications are rarely indicated in the treatment of this arrhythmia and are usually ineffective.[93] In patients with poor control on verapamil or who desire potential cure, radiofrequency catheter ablation is performed with acute success rates ranging from 85 to 100 percent.[94–97]

## ACCELERATED IDIOVENTRICULAR RHYTHM

Accelerated idioventricular rhythm (AIVR) is an automatic rhythm originating in the ventricle with rates between 40 and 120 beats per minute (Fig. 31-8) It is often seen gradually accelerating beyond the sinus rate, resulting in isoarrhythmic atrioventricular dissociation.[98] Fusion beats may be seen at the onset and termination of the arrhythmia. AIVR may be associated with ischemic cardiomyopathy, acute coronary syndromes, rheumatic heart disease, dilated cardiomyopathy, and acute myocarditis.[99–102] Furthermore, AIVR has been described in patients with no apparent heart disease.[103]

In the setting of acute coronary syndromes, AIVR is considered to be a noninvasive marker for successful reperfusion after thrombolytic therapy. The incidence of AIVR is not affected by the location of MI or the infarct size. Finally, the presence of AIVR after a MI is not associated with an increase in mortality.[104]

The mechanism of AIVR is thought to be increased automaticity in a region of the ventricle; however, in some instances, as in myocardial ischemia and in digitalis toxicity, the mechanism may be triggered activity.[105]

AIVR is a benign rhythm and no specific treatment is necessary. In the acute setting when loss of atrioventricular synchrony results in hemodynamic compromise, atrial overdrive pacing or atropine may reestablish AV synchrony when the two rhythms are competing.

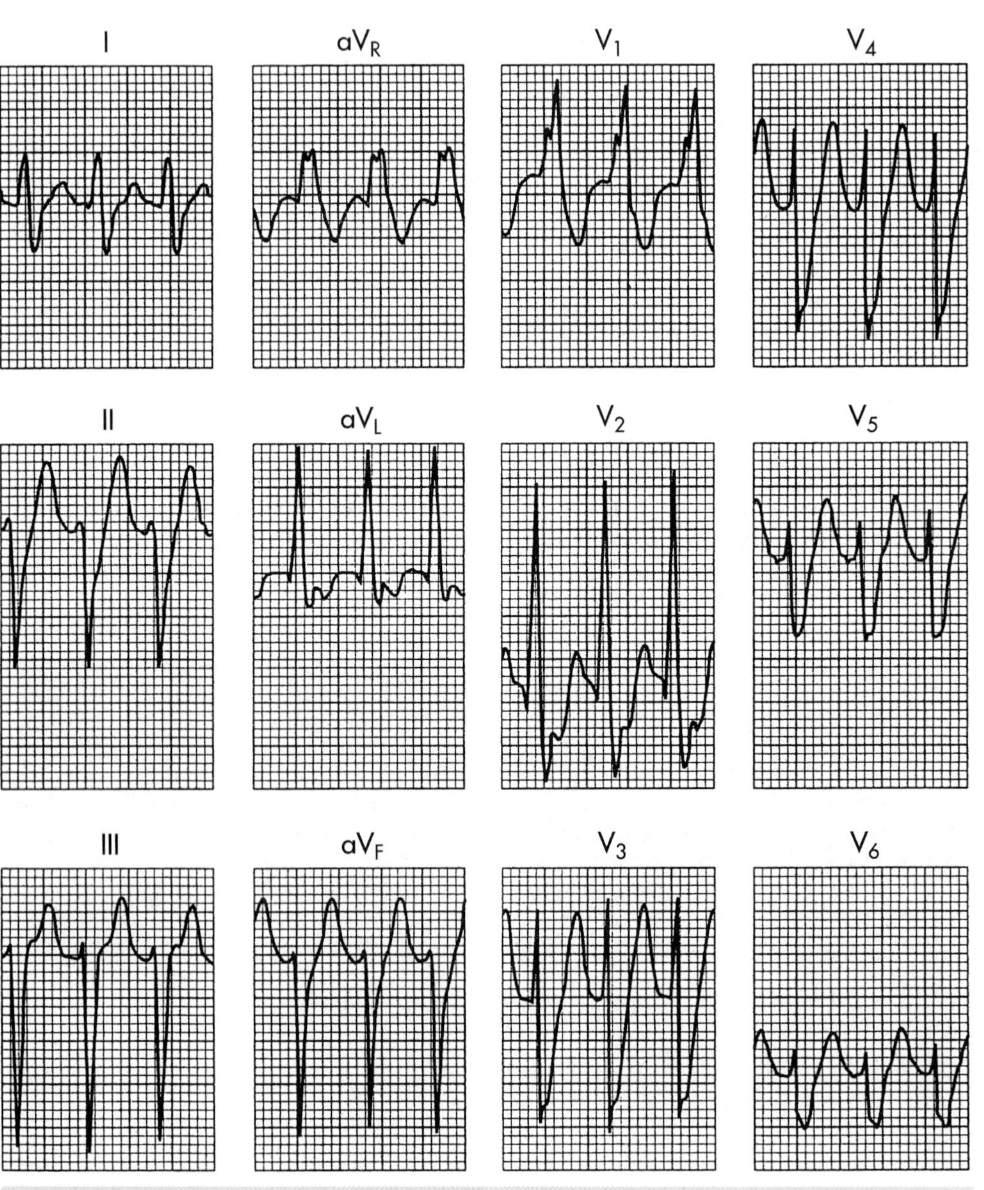


FIGURE 31-7 Idiopathic left ventricular tachycardia. The distinctive features are a right bundle branch morphology in $V_1$ and a left superior axis in the limb leads. Note the RBB left anterior fascicular block pattern and relatively narrow QRS complex in this example. (From Marriott HJL, ed. *Advanced Concepts in Arrhythmias*, 1998. Permission from Mosby, Inc.)

## VENTRICULAR FIBRILLATION

VF (see Chap. 41) is characterized by rapid, chaotic, and asynchronous contraction of the left ventricle. The surface electrogram of VF reveals a rapid, irregular, dysmorphic, pattern

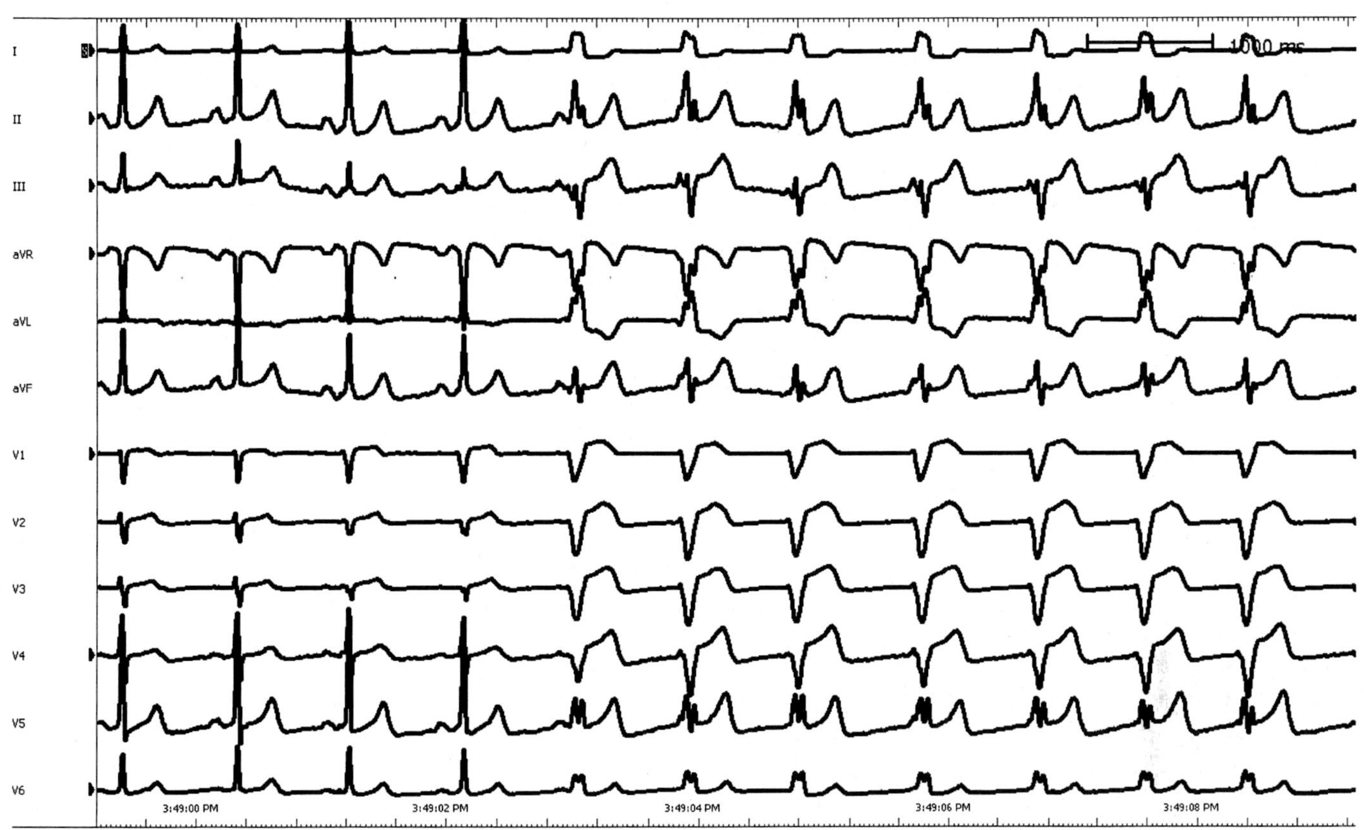


FIGURE 31-8 Accelerated idioventricular rhythm. This rhythm is typically regular with a wide QRS complex of ventricular origin < 120 beats per minute. In this example, an accelerated idioventricular rhythm competes with sinus rhythm.

with no clearly defined QRS complex. VF is associated with rapid hemodynamic collapse and is the most common arrhythmia resulting in out-of-hospital cardiac arrest. Furthermore, patients who suffer a cardiac arrest have significant risk of subsequent arrest.[106]

## Mechanism

Our understanding of the mechanism of VF has been enhanced through animal studies and computer-simulation models. Moe et al. found that multiple wavelets of functional reentry could occur to sustain atrial fibrillation in the setting of significant dispersion of refractory periods.[107] Experimental studies in VF suggest functional reentry as the mechanism of propagation. These functional reentry wavelets have the appearance of nonstationary rotating spiral waves in mathematical models.[108–110] The ever-changing pathways of these wavelets through the complex three-dimensional geometry of the ventricle accounts for the chaotic appearance of this rhythm on a rhythm strip or 12-lead ECG (Fig. 31-9).

Coronary artery disease and resultant MI is the most common etiology of VF and cardiac arrest.[111] Other causes of VF include dilated cardiomyopathies,[112] hypertrophic cardiomyopathy,[113] myocarditis,[114] valvular heart disease,[115] congenital heart disease,[116] proarrhythmia from drugs,[117] acid-base and electrolyte abnormalities,[118,119] long-QT syndrome (LQTS),[120] and atrial fibrillation in a patient with Wolff-Parkinson-White (WPW) syndrome with an anterogradely conducting bypass tract.[121]

Identification of the etiology of VF may be helpful in the risk stratification and prevention of further bouts of this arrhythmia. Revascularization of patients with myocardial ischemia due to coronary disease, ablation of a bypass tract in a patient with VF due to WPW syndrome or elimination of proarrhythmic drugs should minimize the risk of future VF episodes. However, patients with "reversible" causes of arrest may continue to be at risk for further bouts of VF. In an analysis of the AVID trial, Wyse et al. reported a similar mortality rate in patients with reversible cause of arrest compared with those considered to have a nonreversible cause of their VT or VF.[122]

## Clinical Presentation and Management

Patients with VF require immediate defibrillation. Early defibrillation is an essential part of the "chain of survival," and patient survival and morbidity are closely linked to the delay in conversion of the heart rhythm.[123] Successful defibrillation depends on time to defibrillation, energy delivered, defibrillation waveform, transthoracic impedance, shock electrode placement, surface area of the shock electrodes, and the patient's metabolic status (acid-base and electrolytes).[124]

Excessive energy and current may potentially cause irreversible myocardial necrosis and functional damage to the ventricular myocardium and conduction system,[125,126] although evidence of clinical importance of this postshock injury in humans has been difficult to demonstrate. For the traditional monophasic shock waveform, the recommended first shock energy is 200 J followed by 300 and then 360 J. Biphasic waveforms appear to have an advantage over monophasic waveforms in that less energy is required for defibrillation and that the lower-energy biphasic shocks result in less postshock ST-segment abnormalities.[127]

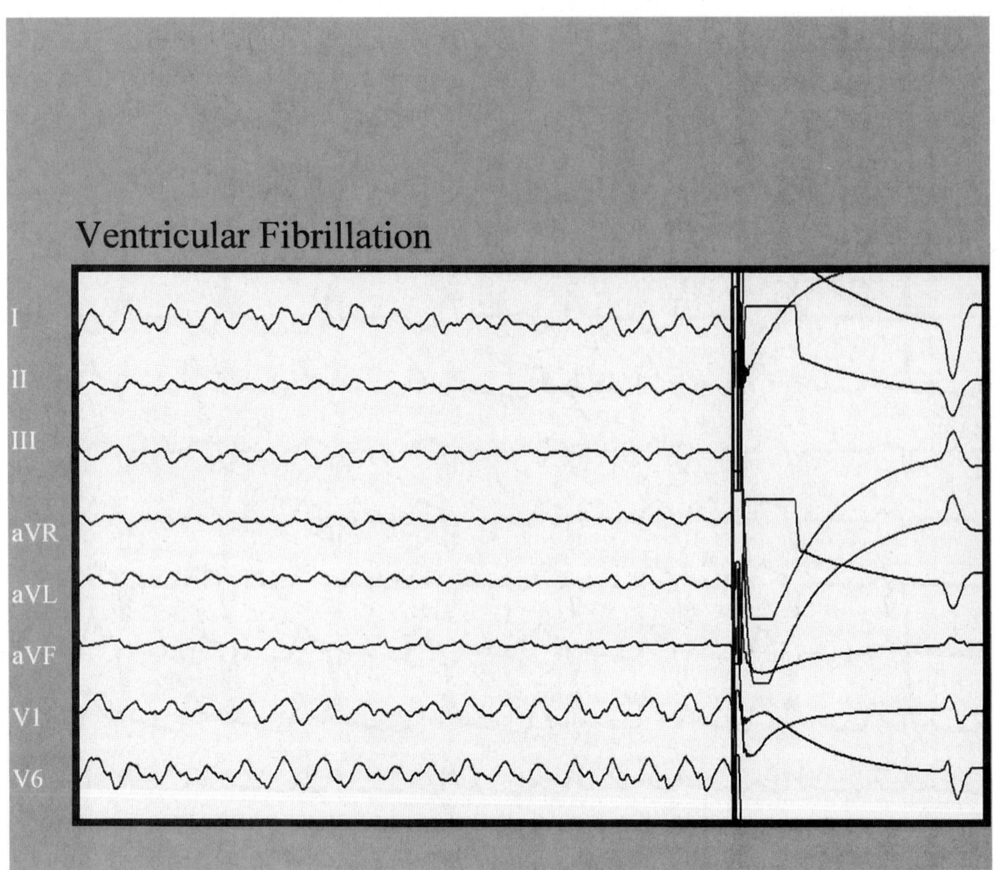


FIGURE 31-9 Ventricular fibrillation. This rhythm is characterized by a rapid irregular wide complex tachycardia with no discrete QRS complex. In this example, prompt defibrillation results in successful termination of this lethal arrhythmia.

Recognizing that early defibrillation is critical to survival in patients suffering VF arrest, significant technologic advances have improved survival among patients suffering from VF arrest. One of these, the automated external defibrillator (AED), has the potential to significantly affect survival after out-of-hospital arrests. The AED has been proven to be safe, accurate, and effective even in the hands of nontraditional first responders.[128]

The chronic management of patients suffering VF arrest is aimed at determining its cause and treating potential recurrence. All patients should have an assessment of the presence or absence of epicardial coronary artery disease with a 12-lead ECG and coronary angiography. In addition, serial cardiac enzymes should be evaluated and an echocardiogram should be performed to assess LV function. In patients with structurally normal-appearing hearts without evidence of ischemia or MI, other etiologies of VF should be considered, including WPW syndrome, proarrhythmia from medications, LQTS, Brugada's syndrome, and hypertrophic cardiomyopathy.

When it occurs in the setting of an acute MI, VF usually occurs in the first 4 h. In GISSI-2, the incidence of early VF (occurring in the first 4 h after presentation) was 3.1 percent, whereas the incidence of late VF (occurring in the subsequent 4 to 48 h) was only 0.6 percent. Patients with early VF had a more complicated in-hospital course than matched controls. Both early [odds ratio (OR) 2.47, 95 percent confidence interval (CI) 1.48 to 4.13] and late VF (OR 3.97, 95 percent CI 1.51 to 10.48) were independent predictors of in-hospital mortality. Death rates from discharge to 6-month follow-up were similar for both VF subgroups and controls. VF, independent of its timing, was an independent predictor of in-hospital mortality. Prognosis from discharge to 6-month follow-up was unaffected by the occurrence of either early or late VF.[129] Other studies have shown that VF with a Q-wave MI is associated with an increased in-hospital mortality but does not predict long-term survival.[123,124] Based on these findings, patients with VF associated with a Q-wave MI are not treated with an ICD. It is important to emphasize that all patients suffering an acute MI should undergo revascularization (if appropriate) and be treated with an aspirin, beta blocker, statin, and ACE inhibitor.

In patients who present with VF arrest due to chronic ischemic or nonischemic cardiomyopathy, the recurrence rate of VF arrest is high and aggressive therapy is indicated. One-year survival of sudden death ranges between 70 to 84 percent.[130–132] Identification and treatment of reversible causes of VF, such as removal of proarrhythmic medications and correction of electrolyte abnormalities, should be performed without delay. Patients with LQTS should be treated with a beta blocker and temporary pacing should be considered if significant bradycardia is playing a role in arrhythmia recurrence (see below). When the patient's workup is complete and all reversible causes or contributions to VF are corrected, most patients suffering VF arrest should undergo implantation of an ICD. Defibrillator implantation has become the mainstay of therapy for cardiac arrest survivors (see also Chap. 38).

The ICD has significantly affected outcomes from the primary and secondary treatment of patients suffering from ventricular arrhythmias. Currently three general treatment options exist for patients with VT or VF: (1) antiarrhythmic drug therapy, (2) radiofrequency catheter ablation (VT), and (3) and an ICD. Currently, most patients with life-threatening ventricular arrhythmias receive an ICD with antiarrhythmic drug therapy and radiofrequency catheter ablation as adjunctive treatment options. The indications for ICD therapy taken from the 2002 ACC/AHA/NASPE for Practice Guidelines are shown in Table 31-2.[133]

## LONG-QT SYNDROME AND TORSADES DE POINTES

The LQTSs (see also Chap. 10) are a heterogeneous group of disorders resulting from congenital or acquired defects in the ion currents underlying repolarization. Iatrogenic (drug-induced) causes are by far more common than congenital LQTS. The prolongation of repolarization in LQTS is associated with significant regional dispersion of refractory periods within the ventricular myocardium. Early afterdepolarizations occur as a result of the abnormality in repolarization and result in triggered ventricular premature beats.[134] Under the right circumstances, triggered ventricular beats occurring in a substrate of inhomogeneous areas of repolarization may initiate multiple scroll waves of functional reentry manifesting clinically as polymorphic VT or torsades de pointes[134] (Fig. 31-10).

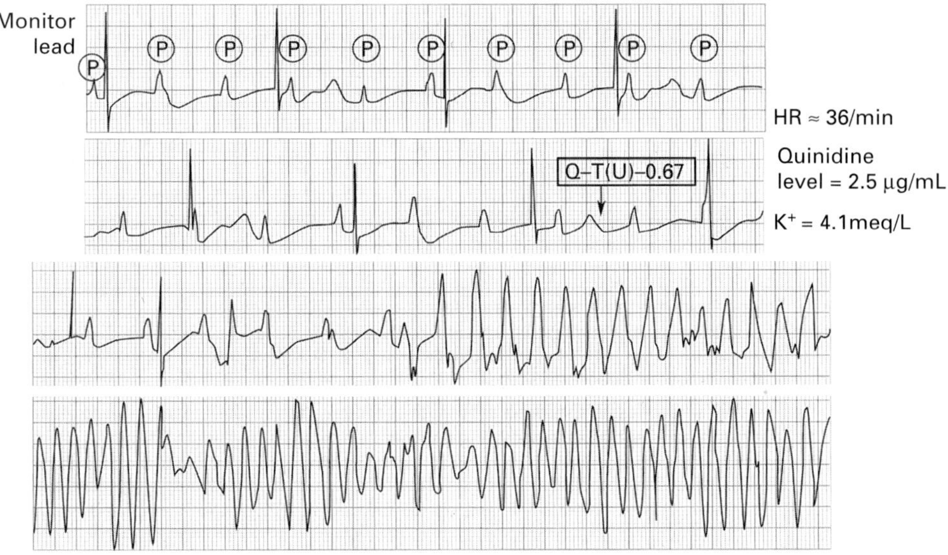


FIGURE 31-10 Torsades de pointes. The patient, a 49-year-old female, has complete heart block and was receiving quinldine sulfate for a ventricular arrhythmia. The rhythm shown in the bottom two strips occured shortly after institution of therapy. Note the prolonged QT(U) interval (0.67 s) and the onset of classical torsades de pointes.

Torsades de pointes (TdP) is the hallmark arrhythmia in the LQTS. TdP is characterized by a rapid polymorphic VT that constantly changes (cycle length, axis, morphology) in a pattern that appears to twist around a central axis. TdP may be repetitive, nonsustained, or sustained and may degenerate into VF. Patients with long repetitive salvos of TdP or sustained polymorphic VT/VF may manifest with presyncope or syncope. Although LQTS is most commonly associated with TdP, other conditions such as hypokalemia, hypomagnesemia, severely altered nutritional states, and neurologic catastrophe have been associated with TdP.[135]

## Treatment of Long-QT Syndrome

In the assessment of patients presenting with TdP and LQTS, electrolyte abnormalities (especially K and Mg) should be corrected. Drugs associated with QT prolongation should be identified and discontinued. Additional treatment options for LQTS include (1) beta blockers, (2) cardiac pacing, and (3) implantation of an ICD.

Beta blockers are effective in the prevention of ventricular arrhythmias in long-QT syndrome. The 10-year mortality rate among symptomatic patients with congenital LQTS decreased from 50 percent (untreated patients) to less than 5 percent (treated with a beta-adrenergic receptor blocker).[136,137] In another study, although beta blockers are associated with a significant reduction in cardiac events in LQTS patients, it was found that syncope, aborted cardiac arrest, and LQTS-related death continued to occur while patients were on prescribed beta blockers. The chance of having a recurrent cardiac event within 5 years after starting a beta blocker was 32 percent in probands. Fourteen percent of patients who had aborted sudden death prior to taking beta blockers had recurrent cardiac arrest within 5 years despite therapy.[138] This study highlights the limitations of beta-blocker therapy in preventing sudden death. Furthermore, beta blockers are not effective in patients with LQT3 (sodium channel mutation).[139]

Cardiac pacing has been advocated because TdP in patients with congenital LQTS has been associated with bradycardia or pauses. Programming of the pacemaker should include pacing at a higher lower-rate limit and the instigation of pause-prevention algorithms such as rate smoothing.[140] Pacing should be used as an adjunct to beta-blocker therapy in patients with significant sinus bradycardia or AV conduction abnormalities. In recent years many physicians have elected to offer ICD when a pacemaker is considered. ICDs may be lifesaving in patients with recurrent symptoms despite optimal beta-blocker and pacing therapies, and many physicians consider the ICD as the therapy of choice when initial therapy is unsuccessful in suppressing recurrent TdP.

## References

1. Horan MJ, Kennedy HL. Ventricular ectopy. History, epidemiology, and clinical implications. *JAMA* 1984;251(3):380–386.
2. Kennedy HL, Whitlock JA, Sprague MK, et al. Long-term follow-up of asymptomatic healthy subjects with frequent and complex ventricular ectopy. *N Engl J Med* 1985;312:193–197.
3. Ruberman W, Weinblatt E, Frank CW, et al. Ventricular premature beats and mortality after myocardial infarction. *N Engl J Med* 1977;297:750–757.
4. Ruberman W, Weinblatt E, Goldberg JD, et al. Ventricular premature complexes and sudden death after myocardial infarction. *Circulation* 1981;64(2):297–305.
5. Andreson D, Bethge KP, Boissel JP, et al. Importance of quantitative analysis of ventricular arrhythmias for predicting the prognosis in low-risk postmyocardial infarction patients. European Infarction Study Group. *Eur Heart J* 1990:11(6):529–536.
6. Mukharji J, Rude RE, Poole WK, et al. Risk factors for sudden death after acute myocardial infarction: Two-year follow-up. *Am J Cardiol* 1984;54(1):31–36.
7. Bigger JT Jr, Fleiss JL, Kleiger R, et al. The relationships among ventricular arrhythmias, left ventricular dysfunction, and mortality in the 2 years after myocardial infarction. *Circulation* 1984;69:250–258.
8. Statters DJ, Malik M, Redwood S, et al. Use of ventricular premature complexes for risk stratification after acute myocardial infarction in the thrombolytic era. *Am J Cardiol* 1996;77:133–138.
9. MacMahon S. Effects of prophylactic lidocaine in suspected acute myocardial infarction. An overview of results from the randomized, controlled trials. *JAMA* 1988;260:1910–1916.
10. Echt DS, Liebson PR, Mitchell LB, et al. Mortality and morbidity in patients receiving encainide, flecainide, or placebo. The Cardiac Arrhythmia Suppression Trial. *N Engl J Med* 1991;324:781–788.
11. Waldo A, Camm A, deRyuter H, et al. For the survival with oral d-sotalol (SWORD) investigators. Effect of d-sotalol on mortality in patients with left ventricular dysfunction after recent and remote myocardial infarction. *Lancet* 1996;348:7–12.
12. Singh SN, Fletcher RD, Fisher SG, et al. Amiodarone in patients with congestive heart failure and asymptomatic ventricular arrhythmias. *N Engl J Med* 1995;333:77–82.
13. Julian D, Camm A, Frangin G, et al. for the European Myocardial Infarct Amiodarone Trial (EMIAT) investigators. Randomized trial of

the effect of amiodarone on mortality in patients with left ventricular dysfunction after recent myocardial infarction: EMIAT. *Lancet* 1997;349:667–674.

14. Cairns J, Connolly S, Roberts R, et al. for the Canadian Amiodarone Myocardial Infarction Arrhythmia Trial (CAMIAT) Investigators. *Lancet* 1997;349:675–682.
15. Connoly SJ. Meta-analysis of antiarrhythmic drug trials. *Am J Cardiol* 1999;84(9A);90R–93R.
16. Von Olshausen K, Stienen U, Schwarz F, et al. Long term prognostic significance of ventricular arrhythmias in idiopathic dilated cardiomyopathy. *Am J Cardiol* 1988;61:146–151.
17. Fletcher RD, Cintron GB, Johnson G, et al. Enalapril decreases prevalence of ventricular tachycardia in patients with chronic congestive heart failure. The V-HeFT II VA Cooperative Studies Group. *Circulation* 1993;87(6 suppl):VI49–VI55.
18. Doval HC, Nul DR, Grancelli HO, et al. Nonsustained ventricular tachycardia in severe heart failure. Independent marker of increased mortality due to sudden death. GESICA-GEMA Investigators. *Circulation* 1996;94:3198–3203.
19. Singh SN, Fisher SG, Carson PE, et al. Prevelence and significance of non-sustained ventricular tachycardia in patients with premature ventricular contractions and heart failure treated with vasodilator therapy. *Am J Cardiol* 1998;32(4):942–947.
20. Jouven X., Zureikm J, Desnos M, et al. Long-term outcome in asymptomatic men with exercise-induced premature ventricular depolarizations. *N Engl J Med* 2000;343(12):826–833.
21. Frolkis JP, Pothier CE, Blackstone EH, et al. Frequent ventricular ectopy after exercise as a predictor of death. *N Engl J Med* 2003;348:781–790.
22. Moss AJ, Zareba W, Hall J, et al. Prophylactic implantation of a defibrillator in patients with myocardial infarction and reduced ejection fraction. *N Engl J Med* 2002;346:877–883.
23. DeBakker JM, van Cappele F, Janse MJ, et al. Reentry as a cause of ventricular tachycardia in patients with chronic ischemic heart disease: Electrophysiologic and anatomic correlation. *Circulation* 1988;77: 589–606.
24. Josephson ME, Horowitz LN, Farshidi A, et al. Recurrent sustained ventricular tachycardia. 2. Endocardial mapping. *Circulation* 1978;57: 440–447.
25. Josephson ME, Horowitz LN, Farshidi A, et al. Continuous local electrical activity: A mechanism of recurrent ventricular tachycardia. *Circulation* 1978;57:659–665.
26. McGuire M, Kuchar D, Ganis J, et al. Natural history of late potentials in the first ten days after acute myocardial infarction and relation to early ventricular arrhythmias. *Am J Cardiol* 1988;61:1187–1190.
27. A comparison of antiarrhythmic-drug therapy with implantable defibrillators in patients resuscitated from near-fatal ventricular arrhythmias. The Antiarrhythmics Versus Implantable Defibrillators (AVID) Investigators. *N Engl J Med* 1997;337:1576–1584.
28. Josephson ME, Almendral JM, Buxton AE, et al. Mechanism of ventricular tachycardia. *Circulation* 1987;75:III41–III47.
29. Hamer AWF, Rubin SA, Peter CT, et al. Factors that predict syncope during ventricular tachycardia in patients. *Am Heart J* 1984;107: 997–1005.
30. Lima JA, Weiss L, Guzman PA, et al. Incomplete filling and incoordinate contraction as mechanisms of hypotension during ventricular tachycardia in man. *Circulation* 1983;68:928–930.
31. Anderson JL. Long-term survival in the Antiarrhythmics Versus Implantable Defibrillators (AVID) Registry. *J Am Coll Cardiol* 1998; 31:160A.
32. Levine JH, Massumi A, Scheinman MM, et al. Intravenous amiodarone for recurrent sustained hypotensive ventricular tachyarrhythmias. *J Am Coll Cardiol* 1996;27:67–75.
33. Gorgels AP, Van den Dool A, Hofs A, et al. Comparison of procainamide and lidocaine in terminating sustained monomorphic ventricular tachycardia. *Am J Cardiol* 1996;78:43–46.
34. Schwartzman D, Jadonath R., Callans DJ, et al. Radiofrequency catheter ablation for control of frequent ventricular tachycardia with healed myocardial infarction. *Am J Cardiol* 1995;75:297–299.
35. Iqbal I, Ventura HO, Smart FW, et al. Difficult cases in heart failure: Left ventricular assist device implantation for the treatment of recurrent ventricular tachycardia in end stage heart failure. *Congest Heart Fail* 1999;5:129–130.
36. Wilber DJ, Garan H, Finkelstein D, et al. Out of hospital cardiac arrest. Use of electrophysiologic testing in the prediction of long term outcome. *N Engl J Med* 1988;318:19–24.
37. Kim SG, Fischer J, Choue CW, et al. The influence of left ventricular function on the outcome of patients treated with implantable defibrillators. *Circulation* 1992;85:1304–1310.
38. Caruso AC, Marcus FI, Hahn EA, et al and the ESVEM investigators. Predictors of arrhythmic death in the ESVEM trial. *Circulation* 1997;96:1888–1892.
39. Friedman PL, Stevenson W. Unsustained ventricular tachycardia: To treat or not to treat? *N Engl J Med* 1996;335:1984–1985.
40. Waldo AL, Camm A, deRuyter H, et al. Effect of d-sotalol on mortality in patients with left ventricular dysfunction after recent and remote myocardial infarction. *Lancet* 1996;348:7–12.
41. Wilber DJ, Olshansky B, Moran JF, et al. Electrophysiologic testing and nonsustained ventricular tachycardia: Use and limitation in patients with coronary artery disease and impaired ventricular function. *Circulation* 1990;82:350–358.
42. Buxton AE, Lee K, DiCarlo L, et al. Nonsustained ventricular tachycardia in coronary artery disease: Relation to inducible sustained ventricular tachycardia. *Ann Intern Med* 1996;125:35–39.
43. Soejima K, Suzuki M, Maisel WH, et al. Catheter ablation in patients with multiple and unstable ventricular tachycardias after myocardial infarction: Short ablation lines guided by reentry circuit isthmuses and sinus rhythm mapping. *Circulation* 2001;104:664–669.
44. Marchlinski FE, Callans D, Gottlieb CD, et al. Linear ablation lesions for control of unmappable ventricular tachycardia in patients with ischemic and nonischemic cardiomyopathy. *Circulation* 2000;101:1288–1296.
45. Bayes de Luna A, Coumel P, Leclercq JF, et al. Ambulatory sudden cardiac death: Mechanisms of production of fatal arrhythmia on the basis of data from 157 cases. *Am Heart J* 1989;117:115–159.
46. Luu M, Stevenson WG, Stevenson LW, et al. Diverse mechanisms of unexpected cardiac arrest in advanced heart failure. *Circulation* 1989;80:1675–1680.
47. Tamburro P, Wilber D. Sudden death in idiopathic dilated cardiomyopathy. *Am Heart J* 1992;124:1035–1045.
48. Franz MR, Burkoiff D, Yue DT, et al. Mechanically induced action potential changes and arrhythmia in isolated in situ canine hearts. *Cardiovasc Res* 1989;23:213–223.
49. Tchou P, Blanck Z, McKinnie J, et al. Mechanism of inducible ventricular tachycardia in patients with idiopathic dilated cardiomyopathy (abstr). *Circulation* 1983;67:674.
50. Chien WW, Scheinman M., Cohen TJ, et al. Importance of recording the right bundle branch deflection in the diagnosis of bundle branch reentrant ventricular tachycardia. *Pacing Clin Electrophysiol* 1992;15: 1015–1024.
51. Delacretaz E, Stevenson W, Ellison K, et al. Mapping and radiofrequency catheter ablation of the three types of sustained monomorphic ventricular tachycardia in nonischemic cardiomyopathy. *Heart* 2000;11:11–17.
52. Stevenson LW, Fowler MB., Shroeder JS, et al. Poor survival in patients with idiopathic cardiomyopathy considered too well for transplantation. *Am J Med* 1987;83:871–876.
53. DeMaria R, Gavazzi A, Caroli A, et al. Ventricular arrhythmias in dilated cardiomyopathy as an independent prognostic hallmark. *Am J Cardiol* 1992;69:1451–1457.
54. Huang SK, Medsser JV, Denes P. Significance of ventricular tachycardia in idiopathic dilated cardiomyopathy: Observations in 35 patients. *Am J Cardiol* 1983;51:507–512.
55. Kjekshus, J. Arrhythmias and mortality in congestive heart failure. *Am J Cardiol* 1990;65:42I–48I.
56. Doval H, Nul DR, Grancelli H, et al, for the Grupo de Estudio de la Sobrevida en la Insuficiencia congestive heart failure. *Lancet* 1994; 344:493–498.

57. Singh, Fletcher R, Fisher S, et al, for the Survival Trial of Antiarrhythmic Therapy in Congestive Heart Failure (CHF-STAT) Investigators. Amiodarone in patients with congestive heart failure and asymptomatic ventricular arrhythmia. *N Engl J Med* 1995;333:77–82.
58. Bansch D, Antz M, Boczar M, et al. Primary prevention of sudden cardiac death in idiopathic dilated cardiomyopathy. The Cardiomyopathy Trial (CAT). *Circulation* 2002;105:1453–1458.
59. Marcus FI. Update of arrhythmogenic right ventricular dysplasia. *Cardiac Electrophysiol Rev* 2002;6:54–56.
60. Jaoude SA, Leckercq HF, Coumel P. Progressive ECG changes in arrhythmogenic right ventricular disease. *Eur Heart J* 1996;17: 1717–1722.
61. Marcus F, Calkins H, Towbin J, et al. North American Arrhythmogenic RV dysplasia registry. http://www.arvd.org.
62. Silverman KJ, Hutchins GM, Bulkley BH, et al. Cardiac sarcoid: A clinicopathologic study of 84 unselected patients with systemic sarcoidosis. *Circulation* 1978;58:1204–1211.
63. Valantine H, McKenna WJ, Nihoyannopoulos P, et al. Sarcoidosis: A pattern of clinical and morphological presentation. *Br Heart J* 1987;57:256–263.
64. Roberts WC, McAllister HA Jr, Ferrans VJ. Sarcoidosis of the heart. A clinicopathologic study of 35 necropsy patients (group 1) and review of 78 previously described necropsy patients (group 11). *Am J Med* 1977;63:86–108.
65. Sosa E, Scanhavacca M, D'Avila A, et al. Endocardial and epicardial ablation guided by nonsurgical transthoracic epicardial mapping to treat recurrent ventricular tachycardia. *J Cardiovasc Electrophysiol* 1998;9:229–239.
66. Sosa E, Scanhavacca M, D'Avila A, et al. Radiofrequency catheter ablation of ventricular tachycardia guided by nonsurgical epicardial mapping in chronic Chagasic heart disease. *Pacing Clin Electrophysiol* 1999;22:128–130.
67. Sosa E, Scanavacca M, D'Avila A, et al. Transthoracic epicardial catheter ablation to treat recurrent ventricular tachycardia. *Curr Cardiol Rep* 2001;3:451–458.
68. Brooks R, Burgess JH. Idiopathic ventricular tachycardia: A review. *Medicine* 1988;67:271.
69. Gallavardin L. Extrasystolie ventriculaire a paroxysmes tachycardiques prolonges. *Arch Mal Coeur* 1922;15:298.
70. Deal BJ, Miller SM, Scagliotti D, et al. Ventricular tachycardia in a young population without overt heart disease. *Circulation* 1986;73:1111.
71. Marchlinski FE, Deely MP, Zado ES. Sex-specific triggers for right ventricular outflow tract tachycardia. *Am Heart J* 2000;139:1009.
72. Calkins H, Kalbfleisch S, El-Atassi R. Relation between efficacy of radiofrequency catheter ablation and site of origin of idiopathic ventricular tachycardia. *Am J Cardiol* 1993;71:827.
73. Wilber D, Baerman J, Olshansky B. Adenosine-sensitive ventricular tachycardia: Clinical characteristics and response to catheter ablation. *Circulation* 1993;126–134.
74. Hachiya H, Aonuma K, Yamauchi Y, et al. How to diagnose, locate, and ablate coronary cusp ventricular tachycardia. *J Cardiovasc Electrophysiol* 2002;13(6):551–556.
75. Lerman, BB, Stein K, Engelstein ED, et al. Mechanism of repetitive monomorphic ventricular tachycardia. *Circulation* 1995;92(3):421–429.
76. Kochilas L, Merscher-Gomez S, Lu MM, et al. The role of neural crest during cardiac development in a mouse model of DiGeorge syndrome. *Dev Biol* 2002;251(1):157–166.
77. Marcus FI, Fontaine G, Guiraudon G. Right ventricular dysplasia: A report of 24 adult cases. *Circulation* 1982;65:384.
78. Gill JS, Blaszyk K, Ward De, et al. Verapamil for the suppression of idiopathic ventricular tachycardia of left bundle branch block–like morphology. *Am Heart J* 1993;126(5):1126–1133.
79. Lerman B, Stein K, Markowitz S. Ventricular tachycardia in patients with structurally normal hearts. In: Zipes D, Jalife J, eds. *Cardiac Electrophysiology: From Cell to Bedside*, 3d ed. Philadelphia: Saunders; 2000.
80. Callans D. Repetitive monomorphic idiopathic ventricular tachycardia. *J Am Coll Cardiol* 1997;29:1023–1027.
81. Globits S, Kreiner G, Frank H. Significance of morphological abnormalities detected by MRI in patients undergoing successful ablation of right ventricular outflow tract tachycardia. *Circulation* 1997;96:2633–2640.
82. Belhassen B, Laniado S. Response of recurrent sustained ventricular tachycardia to verapamil. *Br Heart J* 1981;46:679–682.
83. Ward D, Nathan A, Camm A. Fascicular tachycardia sensitive to calcium antagonists. *Eur Heart J* 1984;5:896–905.
84. Okumura K, Yamahe H, Tsuchiya T, et al. Characteristics of slow conduction zone demonstrated during entrainment of idiopathic ventricular tachycardia of left ventricular origin. *Am J Cardiol* 1996; 77(5):379–383.
85. Okumura K, Matsuyama K, Miyagi H, et al. Entrainment of idiopathic ventricular tachycardia of left ventricular origin with evidence for reentry with an area of slow conduction and effect of verapamil. *Am J Cardiol* 1988;62(10 Pt 1):727–732.
86. Andrade F, Eslami M, Elias J. Diagnostic clues from the surface ECG to identify idiopathic (fascicular) ventricular tachcyardia: Correlation with electrophysiologic findings. *J Cardiovasc Electrophysiol* 1996;7:2–8.
87. Zipes D, Foster P. Atrial induction of ventricular tachycardia: Reentry versus triggered activity. *Am J Cardiol* 1979;44:1–8.
88. Lin FC, Wen MS, Wang CC, et al. Left ventricular fibromuscular band is not a specific substrate for idiopathic left ventricular tachycardia. *Circulation* 1996;93(3):525–528.
89. Thakur RK, Klein GJ, Sivaram CA, et al. Anatomic substrate for idiopathic left ventricular tachycardia. *Circulation* 1996;93(3): 497–501.
90. Ohe T. Idiopathic verapamil-sensitive sustained left ventricular tachycardia. *Clin Cardiol* 1993;16(2):139–141.
91. Ohe T, Shimomura K, Aihara N, et al. Idiopathic sustained left ventricular tachycardia: Clinical and electrophysiologic characteristics. *Circulation* 1988;77(3):560–568.
92. Ohe T, Aihara N, Kamakura S, et al. Long-term outcome of verapamil-sensitive sustained left ventricular tachycardia in patients without structural heart disease. *J Am Coll Cardiol* 1995;25(1):54–58.
93. Mont L, Seixas T, Brugada P. The electrocardiographic, clinical and electrophysiologic spectrum of idiopathic monomorphic ventricular tachycardia. *Am Heart J* 1992;124(3):746–753.
94. Nakagawa H, Beckman KJ, McClelland JH, et al. Radiofrequency catheter ablation of idiopathic left ventricular tachycardia guided by a Purkinje potential. *Circulation* 1993;88(6):2607–2617.
95. Klein LS, Miles WM. Ablative therapy for ventricular arrhythmias. *Prog Cardiovasc Dis* 1995;37(4):225–242.
96. Coggins DL, Lee RJ, Swenney J, et al. Radiofrequency catheter ablation as a cure for idiopathic tachycardia of both left and right ventricular origin. *J Am Coll Cardiol* 1994;23(6):1333–1341.
97. Page RL, Shenasa H, Evans JJ, et al. Radiofrequency catheter ablation of idiopathic recurrent ventricular tachycardia with right bundle branch block, left axis morphology. *Pacing Clin Electrophysiol* 1993;16(2):327–336.
98. Gallagher JJ, Damato AN, Lau SH. Electrophysiologic studies during accelerated idioventricular rhythms. *Circulation* 1971;44(4):671–677.
99. Gressin V, Louvari D, Pezaano M, et al. Holter recording of ventricular arrhythmias during intravenous thrombolysis for acute myocardial infarction. *Am J Cardiol* 1992;69(3):152–159.
100. Rothfeld EL, Zucker IR, Leff NA, et al. Coexisting paroxysmal ventricular tachycardia and idioventricular rhythm in acute myocardial infarction. *J Electrocardiol* 1973;6(2):149–152.
101. Abreau P, Fernandes A, Ventosa A. Unsustained ventricular tachycardia and accelerated idioventricular rhythm-clinical and electrocardiographic features. *Rev Port Cardiol* 1992;11:641–648.
102. Nakagawa M, Hamaoka K, Okano S. Multiform accelerated idioventricular rhythm in a child with acute myocarditis. *Clin Cardiol* 1988;11:853–855.
103. Massumi RA, Ali N. Accelerated isorhythmic ventricular rhythms. *Am J Cardiol* 1970;26(2):170–185.
104. Norris R. Significance of idioventricular rhythms in acute myocardial infarction. *Am J Cardiol* 1974;34:667–670.

105. Sclarovsky S, Strasberg B, Fuchs J, et al. Multiform accelerated idioventricular rhythm in acute myocardial infarction: Electrocardiographic characteristics and response to verapamil. *Am J Cardiol* 1983;52(1).43–47.
106. Eisenberg MS, Hallstrom A, Bergner L. Long-term survival after out-of-hospital cardiac arrest. *N Engl J Med* 1982;306(22):1340–1343.
107. Moe G, Rehinbolt W, Abildskov J. A computer model of atrial fibrillation. *Am Heart J* 1964;67:200–220.
108. Gray R, Jalife J, Panfilov A. Mechanisms of cardiac fibrillation. *Science* 1995;270:1222–1223.
109. Winfree A. Electrical turbulence in three-dimensional heart muscle. *Science* 1994;266:1003–1006.
110. Persov A, Davidenko R, Salomontsz J. Spiral waves of excitation underlie reentrant activity in isolated cardiac muscle. *Circ Res* 1993;72:631–650.
111. Davies M, Thomas A. Thrombosis and acute coronary artery lesions in sudden cardiac ischemic death. *N Engl J Med* 1984;310:1137
112. Packer M. Sudden unexpected death in patients with congestive heart failure: A second frontier. *Circulation* 1985;72:681.
113. Kowey P, Eisenberg R, Engel T. Sustained arrhythmias in hypertrophic obstructive cardiomyopathy. *N Engl J Med* 1984;310:1566.
114. Strain J, Grose R, Factor S. Results of endomyocardial biopsy in patients with spontaneous ventricular tachycardia but without apparent structural heart disease. *Circulation* 1983;68:1171.
115. Schwartz L, Goldfischer J, Sprague G. Syncope and sudden death in aortic stenosis. *Am J Cardiol* 1969;23:647.
116. Downar E, Harris L, Kimber S. Ventricular tachycardia after surgical repair of tetralogy of Fallot: Results of intraoperative mapping studies. *J Am Coll Cardiol* 1992;20:648.
117. Roden D. Mechanisms and management of proarrhythmia. *Am J Cardiol* 1998;82:47I–57I.
118. Surawicz B. Ventricular fibrillation. *J Am Coll Cardiol* 1985; 5(6suppl):43B–54B.
119. Gerst P, Fleming W, Malm J. Increased susceptibility of the heart to ventricular fibrillation during metabolic acidosis. *Circ Res* 1966;19:63.
120. Jackman WM, Friday K, Anderson J. The long QT syndromes: A critical review, new clinical observations and a unifying hypothesis. *Prog Cardiovasc Dis* 1988;31:115.
121. Klein G, Bashore T, Sellers T. Ventricular fibrillation in the Wolff-Parkinson-White syndrome. *N Engl J Med* 1979;301(1080).
122. Wyse DG, Friedman PL, Brodsky MA, et al. Life-threatening ventricular arrhythmias due to transient or correctable causes: High risk for death in follow-up. *J Am Coll Cardiol* 2001;38(6):1718–1724.
123. Cummins R, Ornato JP, Thies WH, et al. Improving survival from sudden cardiac arrest: The "chain of survival" concept. *Circulation* 1991;83:1832–1847.
124. Creed J, Packard JM, Lambrew CT, et al. Defibrillation and synchronized cardioversion. In: McIntyre K, Lewis A, eds. *Textbook of Advanced Cardiac Life Support*. Vol 89. Dallas: *American Heart Association,* 1983.
125. Warner E, Dahl C, Ewy G. Myocardial injury from transthoracic defibrillator countershock. *Arch Pathol* 1975;99:55–59.
126. Weaver W, Copass M, Holstrom A. Ventricular defibrillation: Comparative trial using 175 joule and 320 joule shocks. *N Engl J Med* 1982;307:1101–1106.
127. Bardy GH, Marchlinski FE, Sharma AD, et al. Multicenter comparison of truncated biphasic shocks and standard damped sine wave monophasic shocks for transthoracic ventricular defibrillation. Transthoracic Investigators. *Circulation* 1996;94(10):2507–2514.
128. Page RL, Joglar JA, Kowal RC, et al. Use of automated external defibrillators by a U.S. airline. *N Engl J Med* 2000;343(17):1210–1216.
129. Volpi A, Cavalli A, Santaro L, et al. Incidence and prognosis of early primary ventricular fibrillation in acute myocardial infarction—Results of the Gruppo Italiano per lo Studio della Sopravvivenza nell'Infarto Miocardico (GISSI-2) database. *Am J Cardiol* 1998; 82(3):265–271.
130. Tofler GH, Stone PH, Muller JE, et al. Prognosis after cardiac arrest due to ventricular tachycardia or ventricular fibrillation associated with acute myocardial infarction (the MILIS Study). Multicenter Investigation of the Limitation of Infarct Size. *Am J Cardiol* 1987; 60(10):755–761.
131. Nicod P, Gilpin E, Dittrich H, et al. Late clinical outcome in patients with early ventricular fibrillation after myocardial infarction. *J Am Coll Cardiol* 1988;11(3):464–470.
132. Cobbe S, Dalziel K, Ford I, et al. Survival of 1476 patients initially resuscitated from out of hospital cardiac arrest. *BMJ* 1996;312: 1633–1637.
133. Gregoratos G, Abrams J, Epstein AE, et al. ACC/AHA/NASPE 2002 Guideline Update for Implantation of Cardiac Pacemakers and Antiarrhythmia Devices. *Circulation* 2002;106:2145–2161.
134. El-Sherif N, Chinushi M, Caref EB, et al. Electrophysiological mechanism of the characteristic electrocardiographic morphology of torsade de pointes tachyarrhythmias in the long-QT syndrome: Detailed analysis of ventricular tridimensional activation patterns. *Circulation* 1997;96(12):4392–4399.
135. Goldschlager N, Epstein AE, Grubb BP, et al. Etiologic considerations in the patient with syncope and an apparently normal heart. *Arch Intern Med* 2003;163(2):151–162.
136. Moss AJ, Schwartz PJ, Crampton RS, et al. The long QT syndrome: A prospective international study. *Circulation* 1985;71(1):17–21.
137. Moss AJ, Schwartz PJ, Crampton RS, et al. The long QT syndrome. Prospective longitudinal study of 328 families. *Circulation* 1991; 84(3):1136–1144.
138. Moss AJ, Zareba W, Hall WJ, et al. Effectiveness and limitations of beta-blocker therapy in congenital long-QT syndrome. *Circulation* 2000;101(6):616–623.
139. Schwartz PJ. The long QT syndrome. *Curr Probl Cardiol* 1997; 22(6):297–351.
140. Viskin S. Cardiac pacing in the long QT syndrome: Review of available data and practical recommendations. *J Cardiovasc Electrophysiol* 2000;11(5):593–600.

CHAPTER 32

# BRADYARRHYTHMIAS AND PACEMAKERS

Pugazhendhi Vijayaraman / Kenneth A. Ellenbogen



## BRADYARRHYTHMIAS

Bradyarrhythmias are most commonly due to failure of impulse formation (sinus node dysfunction) or to failure of impulse conduction across the atrioventricular (AV) node/His-Purkinje system. Bradyarrhythmias may be caused by disease processes that directly alter the structural and functional integrity of the sinus node, atria, AV node, and His-Purkinje system or by extrinsic factors (autonomic disturbances, drugs, etc.) without causing structural abnormalities (Table 32-1).

### Anatomy of the Sinus Node and Conduction System

#### SINOATRIAL NODE

Normal electrical activation of the heart arises from the principal pacemaker cells that spontaneously depolarize, located laterally in the epicardial grove of the sulcus terminalis,[1] near the junction of the right atrium and the superior vena cava (Fig. 32-1). The sinus node in adults measures approximately 1 to 2 cm long and 0.5 mm wide. The central zone of the sinus node containing the principal pacemaker cells (P cells based on their pale appearance on electron microscopy) is small and located within a fibrous tissue matrix. In the periphery of the node along the crista terminalis, transitional cells with pacemaker function are also present. Experimental and clinical evidence now suggest that the sinus node region is less well defined than previously appreciated. The principal pacemaker site within this region may migrate resulting in subtle alterations in P-wave morphology.[2] The conduction velocities within the sinus node are very slow (2 to 5 cm/s). Once the impulse exits the sinus node and the perinodal tissues, it traverses the atrium to the AV node. Although it has been claimed that anatomic evidence shows the presence of three internodal pathways connecting the sinus node to the AV node, the existence of such pathways is still controversial. The anterior internodal pathway runs from the sinus node anteriorly around the superior vena cava to join Bachmann's bundle and continues to the left atrium joining the superior end of the AV node. The conduction of impulses from right to left atrium has been postulated to occur preferentially via Bachmann's bundle. The posterior internodal pathway runs from the posterior margin of the sinus node along the crista terminalis and eustachian ridge and around the coronary sinus ostium into the posterior margin of the AV node. A middle internodal tract has also been described. Preferential internodal conduction between the sinus and AV nodes has been well established and may be due to the geometric orientation of the muscle bundles rather than specialized tracts.

#### ATRIOVENTRICULAR NODE

Once the sinus node impulse activates the atrium, electrical activation continues through the AV node with a conduction delay ensuring complete atrial contraction before the initiation of ventricular conduction. The AV nodal complex is considered to have three related regions: the transitional cell zone, the compact AV node, and the penetrating AV bundle.[3] The transitional zone consists of the main atrial approaches to the compact AV node—the anterior and posterior approaches have been implicated in dual AV nodal conduction. The compact AV node is shaped like a half oval, measuring approximately $1 \times 3 \times 5$ mm, located beneath the right atrial endocardium at the apex of the triangle of Koch. The triangle of Koch is formed by the base of the septal leaflet of the tricuspid valve and the tendon of Todaro (formed by the extension of the eustachian valve into the central fibrous body). The coronary sinus ostium is located at the base of this triangle. The distal end of the compact AV node enters the central fibrous body to become the penetrating bundle and continues in the membranous septum as the bundle of His. The speed of conduction through the AV nodal complex is at 0.03 m/s, while the His-Purkinje fibers conduct at 2.4 m/s.

#### HIS-PURKINJE SYSTEM

The penetrating part of the AV bundle continues through the annulus fibrosis into the membranous septum, along the crest of the left side of the interventricular septum for 1 to 2 cm and then divides into the right and left bundle branches. The right bundle branch continues intramyocardially along the right side of the interventricular septum and emerges subendocardially beneath the anterior papillary muscle of the right ventricle. The left bundle begins as a sheet of fascicles and runs along the left side of the interventricular septum, and soon separates into anterior and posterior sheets corresponding to the papillary muscles. In many hearts, the left bundle may appear more as a network rather than a well-defined bifascicular system. The terminal

TABLE 32-1 Classification of Bradyarrhythmias

**Sinus Node Dysfunction**
- Sinus bradycardia
- Sinus pauses, sinus arrest
- Sinoatrial exit block
- Tachycardia-bradycardia syndrome
- Chronotropic incompetence

**AV Conduction Abnormalities**
- First-degree heart block
- Second-degree heart block
  - Mobitz type I (Wenckebach)
  - Mobitz type II
  - 2:1 atrioventricular block
- High-grade atrioventricular block
- Third-degree (complete) heart block
- Atrioventricular dissociation

**Bundle Branch Block**
- Left bundle branch block
- Right bundle branch block
- Left anterior hemiblock
- Left posterior hemiblock
- Bifascicular block/trifascicular block
- Nonspecific intraventricular conduction defect

Purkinje fibers arising from the bundle branches form interweaving networks on the endocardial surface of both the right and left ventricles. The rapid conduction of electrical impulses across this network results in near simultaneous activation of both right and left ventricles.

### BLOOD SUPPLY

The sinus node receives its blood supply from the sinoatrial (SA) nodal artery arising from the right coronary artery in 59 percent of the patients, from the left circumflex artery in 38, and from both arteries with a dual blood supply in 3 percent.[4] The AV node is supplied by the AV nodal artery arising from the right coronary artery in 90 percent of patients, while the left circumflex artery provides it in the remaining 10 percent of patients. The bundle of His is supplied by both the AV nodal artery and branches of the left anterior descending artery. The left bundle has a rich blood supply from the AV nodal artery, posterior descending artery, and branches of the left anterior descending artery.[5]

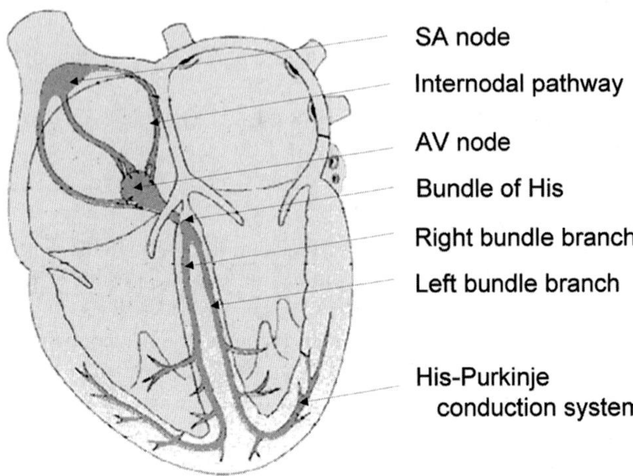


FIGURE 32-1 Schematic representation of the cardiac conduction system. AV, atrioventricular; SA, sinoatrial.

### INNERVATION

The conduction system of the heart is significantly influenced by both the parasympathetic and sympathetic nervous system. The sinus node is richly innervated with postganglionic adrenergic and cholinergic nerve terminals. Vagal stimulation slows the sinus node discharge rate and increases the intranodal conduction time, occasionally to the point of sinus node exit block. Adrenergic stimulation increases the sinus node discharge rate. Parasympathetic tone predominates at rest in healthy individuals, and parasympathetic withdrawal occurs with increased sympathetic discharge during exercise and emotion. The effects of sympathetic and parasympathetic stimulation on the AV node are more pronounced than they are on the His-Purkinje system. While sympathetic stimulation shortens AV-nodal conduction time and refractoriness, vagal stimulation prolongs AV-nodal conduction time and refractoriness. Both sympathetic and vagal stimulation have minimal effect on normal conduction in the His bundle.

## Sinus Node Dysfunction

Sinus node dysfunction is a common clinical syndrome, comprising a wide range of electrophysiologic abnormalities from failure of impulse generation, failure of impulse transmission into the atria, inadequate subsidiary pacemaker activity, and increased susceptibility to atrial tachyarrhythmias.[6,7] This disorder has also been variably termed the *sick sinus syndrome*, *tachycardia-bradycardia syndrome*, *SA disease*, and *SA dysfunction*.

### PATHOPHYSIOLOGY

Disorders of sinus node dysfunction may be caused by intrinsic (processes that directly affect the anatomy and physiology of the sinus node and/or the surrounding atrial tissue) or extrinsic factors (processes that affect sinus node function in the absence of structural abnormalities) (Table 32-2). However, in some patients a combination of intrinsic and extrinsic factors may be responsible for sinus node dysfunction. In patients with sinus node dysfunction, histopathologic evaluation has revealed the following patterns:[8,9]

- Significant loss of nodal cells, with replacement fibrosis
- Amyloid deposition in the nodal region
- Hypoplastic or atrophic sinus node
- No detectable morphologic abnormality

While an idiopathic degenerative disorder of the sinus node is the most common cause for intrinsic sinus node dysfunction, ischemic heart disease is responsible in a significant number of patients. Chronic ischemia from sinus node artery disease[8] or acute myocardial infarction (MI),[10] especially inferior wall MI may result in sinus bradycardia, sinus arrest, and atrial tachyarrhythmias. Other potential causes include long-standing hypertension, cardiomyopathy (especially infiltrative disorders such as amyloidosis and sarcoidosis), inflammation, and inherited neuromuscular disorders. In some cases, the condition appears to be familial in origin.[11] Rare cases of sinus node dysfunction requiring pacemaker therapy have been reported with Lyme disease (Borrelia burgdorferi infection).[12] In children and young adults, damage to the sinus node during atrial surgery (closure of atrial septal defects of the sinus-venosus-type, mustard procedure for transposition of great arteries)[13] has been commonly associated with sinus node dysfunction. Sinus node dysfunction is also not uncommon in the donor hearts of patients with orthotopic cardiac transplantation.[14] Such dysfunction is quite prominent early after transplantation and most show significant improvement within 3 to 6 months after surgery. The need for pacemaker implantation has decreased significantly to approximately 2 percent with improvement in surgical techniques and reduction of ischemic times of the donor heart.[2]

The most important causes of sinus node dysfunction in patients without structural abnormalities are drugs and autonomic nervous system influences (Table 32-2). Drugs may alter sinus node function by direct pharmacologic effects on nodal tissue or indirectly by neurally mediated effects.[15] Antiarrhythmic drugs used to maintain sinus rhythm in patients with atrial fibrillation may cause significant sinus node dysfunction especially in patients with underlying asymptomatic sinus node dysfunction. Other causes for sinus node dysfunction include electrolyte abnormalities such as hyperkalemia, hypothermia, intracranial hypertension, hypoxia, hypercapnia, and hypothyrodism.

TABLE 32-2 Etiology of Sinus Node Dysfunction

| Intrinsic | Extrinsic |
|---|---|
| Idiopathic degenerative disorder | Drugs |
| Ischemic heart disease | Antiarrhythmic agents |
| Chronic ischemia | Class IA—quinidine, procainamide |
| Acute myocardial infarction | Class IC—propafenone, flecainide |
| Hypertensive heart disease | Class II—beta blockers |
| Cardiomyopathy | Class III—sotalol, amiodarone, dronedarone |
| Trauma | Class IV—diltiazem, verapamil |
| Surgery for congenital heart disease | Cardiac glycosides |
| Heart transplant | Antihypertensive agents |
| Inflammation | Clonidine, reserpine, methyldopa |
| Collagen vascular disease | Antipsychotic agents |
| Rheumatic fever | Lithium, phenothiazines, amitriptyline |
| Pericarditis | Autonomically mediated |
| Infection | Vasovagal syncope (cardioinhibitory) |
| Viral myocarditis | Carotid sinus hypersensitivity |
| Lyme disease (*Borrelia burgdorferi*) | Hypothyroidism |
| Neuromuscular disorder | Intracranial hypertension |
| Friedreich's ataxia | Hypothermia |
| X-linked muscular dystrophy | Hyperkalemia |
| Familial disorder | Hypoxia |

## ELECTROCARDIOGRAPHIC MANIFESTATIONS

A variety of electrocardiogram (ECG) abnormalities have been described in patients with sinus node dysfunction. Many of the ECG abnormalities that define sinus node dysfunction may be asymptomatic, and these abnormalities by themselves do not warrant therapy.

***Sinus Bradycardia*** Sinus bradycardia is defined as sinus rate below 60 bpm. In most instances sinus bradycardia is a benign arrhythmia. In healthy young adults and trained athletes, resting sinus bradycardia may be a normal phenomenon due to increased vagal tone. Also sinus bradycardia during sleep in elderly individuals is common. Inability to increase sinus rates adequately during exercise is considered abnormal. Sinus bradycardia less than 40 bpm (not associated with sleep or physical conditioning) is generally considered abnormal. Correlation of symptoms with sinus bradycardia is critical in the evaluation of these patients.

***Sinus Pause and Sinus Arrest*** Sinus pause or arrest means failure of sinus node discharge with lack of atrial activation of sinus origin. This results in absence of P waves and periods of ventricular asystole if lower pacemakers (junctional or ventricular) do not initiate escape beats (Fig. 32-2). The resulting pause in sinus activity should not be in multiples of preceding sinus cycle length (P-P interval). Asymptomatic sinus pauses of up to 3 s in duration are not uncommon in trained athletes.[15] Pauses longer than 3 s need careful clinical correlation with symptoms and warrant further evaluation.

***Sinoatrial Exit Block*** In SA exit block, as the name implies, the impulse is formed in the sinus node but fails to conduct to the atria, unlike sinus arrest. This particular arrhythmia is recognized on ECG by pauses resulting from the absence of normal P waves and the duration of the pause measuring an exact multiple of the preceding P-P interval (Fig. 32-3). SA block can also be described in the same way as AV block. In first-degree SA block, there is significant prolongation of the time for the sinus impulse to exit into the atria (SA conduction time). This cannot be identified clinically or electrocardiographically. Similar to AV block, second-degree SA block can be type I (Wenckebach) or type II. In type I there is progressive

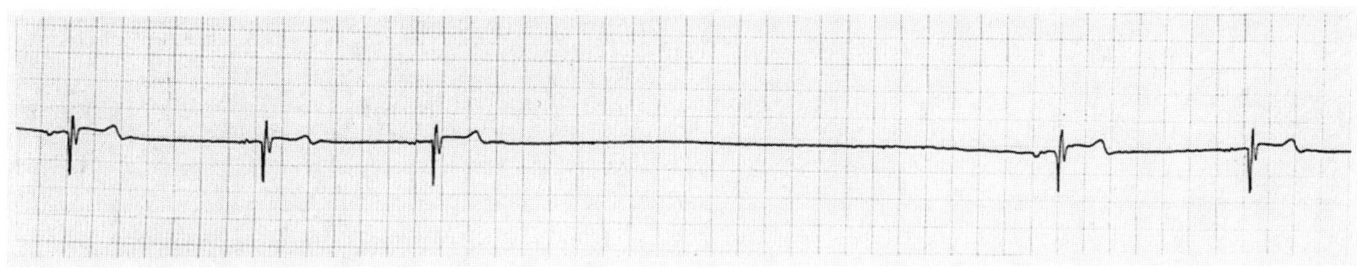

FIGURE 32-2 Telemetry strip demonstrating sinus bradycardia followed by 4.6-s sinus pause.

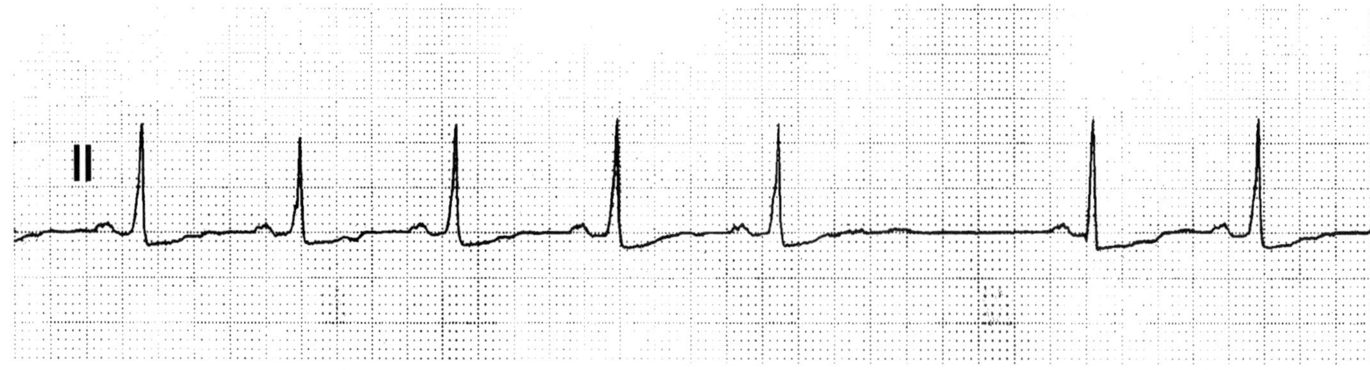


FIGURE 32-3 Telemetry strip demonstrating a sinus pause twice the length of the preceding P-P interval suggesting sinoatrial exit block.

prolongation of SA conduction, manifested on surface ECG as progressive shortening of P-P interval, prior to the pause created by loss of a P wave. In type II SA exit block, the P-P intervals remain constant before the pause. Third-degree or complete SA block will manifest as absence of P waves, with long pauses resulting in lower pacemaker escape rhythm; it is impossible to diagnose with certainty without invasive sinus node recordings.

***Tachycardia-Bradycardia Syndrome*** Sinus bradycardia interspersed with periods of atrial tachyarrhythmias is a common manifestation of sinus node dysfunction. The atrial tachyarrhythmias usually range from paroxysmal atrial tachycardia to atrial flutter to atrial fibrillation and occasionally AV nodal or AV reentrant tachycardias. Apart from underlying sinus bradycardia of varying severity, these patients often experience prolonged sinus arrest and asystole upon termination of the atrial tachyarrhythmias, resulting from suppression of sinus node and secondary pacemakers (Fig. 32-4). Long sinus pauses that occur following electrical cardioversion of atrial fibrillation are another manifestation of sinus node dysfunction. Therapeutic strategies to control tachyarrhythmias often result in the need for pacemaker therapy. These patients are at increased risk for thromboembolism[16] and the issue of long-term anticoagulation should be addressed to prevent strokes.

Chronic atrial fibrillation with a slow ventricular response in the absence of AV nodal blocking drugs may also be a manifestation of sinus node dysfunction. These patients may demonstrate very slow ventricular rates at rest or during sleep and occasionally have long pauses. They may also conduct rapidly and develop symptoms due to tachycardia during exercise. Occasionally they may develop complete AV block with a junctional or ventricular escape rhythm.

***Persistent Atrial Standstill*** Atrial standstill is a rare clinical syndrome in which there is no spontaneous atrial activity and the atria cannot be electrically stimulated.[17] The surface ECG usually reveals junctional bradycardia without atrial activity. This has to be differentiated from fine atrial fibrillation with complete heart block. Intracardiac electrograms do not show any atrial activity. Atria are generally fibrotic and without any functional myocardium. Myocarditis, amyloidosis, and familial etiology have been recognized as causes in some cases. Lack of mechanical atrial contraction poses a high risk for thromboembolism in these patients.

***Chronotropic Incompetence*** Chronotropic incompetence is the inability of the sinus node to achieve at least 80 percent of the age predicted heart rate. It is estimated to be present in 20 to 60 percent of patients with sinus node dysfunction.[18] While the resting heart rates may be normal, these patients may have either the inability to increase their heart rate during exercise or have unpredictable fluctuations in heart rate during activity. Some patients may initially experience a normal increase in heart rate with exercise, which then plateaus or decreases inappropriately. Chronotropic incompetence may be secondary to intrinsic sinus node dysfunction or secondary to drugs with negative chronotropic effects.

## CLINICAL PRESENTATION

Even though sinus node dysfunction can occur in any age group, more than half the patients affected are older than 50 years of age at the time of diagnosis. The incidence of sinus node dysfunction is equal in both men and women. Patients with sinus node dysfunction commonly present with symptoms of syncope, near syncope, or dizzy spells, predominantly related to prolonged sinus pauses. Patients with sinus bradycardia or chronotropic incompetence, however, may present with decreased exercise capacity or fatigue. Patients with atrial fibrillation may also present with palpitations or congestive heart failure. Elderly individuals may have unexplained confusion or memory loss. Occasionally, stroke may be the first man-

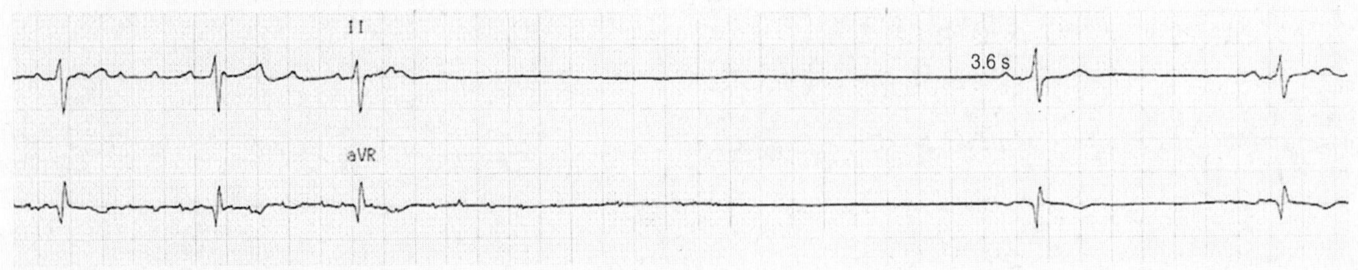


FIGURE 32-4 An example of atrial tachyarrhythmia terminating with 3.6-s sinus pause.

ifestation of sinus node dysfunction in patients presenting with paroxysmal atrial fibrillation and thromboembolism.

## DIAGNOSTIC EVALUATION

The diagnosis of sinus node dysfunction in patients who present with typical symptoms and ECG findings is straightforward. However, due to the intermittent nature of the symptoms and rhythm manifestations, the diagnosis can be time-consuming and frustrating. A number of noninvasive and invasive tests are available to assist in the evaluation.

***Electrocardiographic Recordings*** Documentation of the various arrhythmias associated with sinus node dysfunction can be obtained with routine telemetric monitoring during hospitalization or with outpatient ambulatory 24- to 48-h Holter recordings. If the symptoms are infrequent in nature, then event recorders capable of intermittent or continuous monitoring can be used. If other noninvasive and invasive tests are inconclusive, patients may benefit from an implantable loop recorder, which has the ability to record both patient-triggered and automatic device-triggered events over a period of 18 to 24 months. Exercise testing to assess chronotropic incompetence can be valuable in select patients. Many patients with sinus node dysfunction may achieve peak heart rates similar to matched controls during specific exercise protocols, however the time course of heart rate acceleration during activity and deceleration after activity may be markedly abnormal.[19]

***Autonomic Testing*** Abnormalities of autonomic control of sinus node alone or in association with intrinsic sinus node disease can result in clinical symptoms and electrocardiographic findings of sinus node dysfunction. This can be assessed by observing the response of heart rate and rhythm with carotid sinus massage, head-up tilt testing, and Valsalva maneuver. Pharmacologic evaluation of the sinus node can be performed with atropine, isoproterenol, and propranolol. Following injection of atropine 0.04 mg/kg intravenously, the heart rate increases by 15 percent and to more than 90 bpm. Isoproterenol infusion at 1 to 3 $\mu$g/min increases heart rate by 25 percent. Patients with sinus node dysfunction show blunted heart rate responses to the preceding infusions. Another method to assess sinus node function is to measure the intrinsic heart rate (IHR) of the sinus node when the autonomic influence is negated by both atropine (0.04 mg/kg) and propranolol (0.2 mg/kg), using the following equation:[20]

$$\text{IHR} = 117.2 - (0.53 \times \text{age}) \text{ bpm}$$

Patients with sinus node dysfunction demonstrate a decreased intrinsic heart rate.

***Electrophysiology Study*** Invasive electrophysiology study, in addition to assessing sinus node function, offers insight into other potential etiologies for symptoms of syncope and palpitations (AV block, supraventricular tachycardia, ventricular tachycardia). The sinus node recovery time (SNRT) is a measure of sinus node automaticity and is measured as the longest pause after atrial overdrive pacing.[22] SA conduction time (SACT) is a measure of the interval from sinus node depolarization to activation of atrial muscle.

## MANAGEMENT

***Pharmacologic Treatment*** Theophylline and beta-adrenergic agonists have been used to treat symptomatic bradycardia. Although they have been shown to increase the heart rate and reduce the duration of sinus pauses, they do not prevent recurrent syncope.[21,22] In patients with extrinsic causes for sinus node dysfunction, treatment should be directed toward the underlying etiology. Drugs known to depress sinus node function can be switched to other agents that lack effects on the cardiac conduction system. This is not possible, however, in many patients. Patients with paroxysmal atrial tachyarrhythmias either require drugs to maintain sinus rhythm or agents to control ventricular rate, both of which may have significant depressant effects on sinus node function. In many of these patients pacemaker therapy becomes essential. At the time of diagnosis of sinus node dysfunction, the incidence of atrial fibrillation is reported to be about 8 percent and the likelihood of developing new atrial fibrillation in this group of patients is 5 percent per year.[23] The prevalence of thromboembolism was reported to be 15.2 percent in this group. This underscores the importance of monitoring for atrial fibrillation and the need for oral anticoagulation in intermediate to high-risk patients.

***Pacing Therapy in Sinus Node Dysfunction*** The current indications for pacing in the setting of sinus node dysfunction are shown in Table 32-3. In this and subsequent tables, the format used for American Heart Association (AHA)/American College of Cardiology (ACC) guidelines is used, with class I-III indications denoting the

TABLE 32-3 Indications for Pacing in Sinus Node Dysfunction (ACC/AHA/NASPE 2002 revised guidelines)

**Class I**

1. Sinus node dysfunction with documented symptomatic bradycardia or sinus pauses. Sinus node dysfunction as a result of essential long-term drug therapy of a type and dose, for which there are no acceptable alternatives. (Level of evidence: C)
2. Symptomatic chronotropic incompetence. (Level of evidence: C)

**Class IIa**

1. Sinus node dysfunction occurring spontaneously or as a result of necessary drug therapy, with heart rates less than 40 bpm when a clear association between significant symptoms consistent with bradycardia and the actual presence of bradycardia has not been documented. (Level of evidence: C)
2. Syncope of unexplained origin when major abnormalities of sinus node function are discovered or provoked in electrophysiologic studies. (Level of evidence: C)

**Class IIb**

1. In minimally symptomatic patients, chronic heart rates less than 40 bpm while awake. (Level of evidence: C)

**Class III**

1. Sinus node dysfunction in asymptomatic patients, including those in whom substantial sinus bradycardia (heart rate less than 40 bpm) is a consequence of long-term drug treatment.
2. Sinus node dysfunction in patients with symptoms suggestive of bradycardia that are clearly documented as not associated with a slow heart rate.
3. Sinus node dysfunction with symptomatic bradycardia due to nonessential drug therapy.

degree of agreement for a given procedure or treatment that is useful and effective (class I indicates a highly effective procedure with a high degree of agreement to class III, which indicates that the procedure is *not* useful or effective). The weight of evidence is ranked highest (A) when data are derived from multiple randomized clinical trials to lowest (C) for evidence that is based on nonrandomized studies or registries. Sinus node dysfunction is the most common indication for permanent pacemaker implantation in North America, accounting for 40 to 60 percent of new pacer implants.[24] The optimal pacemaker choice is influenced by a number of factors. At the time of diagnosis of sinus node dysfunction, 17 percent of patients have been reported to have AV conduction abnormalities in the form of a PR interval >240 ms, bundle branch block, H-V interval prolongation, AV Wenckebach rates <120 bpm, and second- or third-degree AV block. The incidence of new AV block developing over time was reported to be less than 2.7 percent per year.[23] Generally, if the patient has persistent atrial fibrillation, a single chamber ventricular pacemaker (VVIR) is recommended. In all other situations a rate-responsive dual-chamber pacemaker (DDDR) is used, while a single-chamber atrial pacemaker (AAIR) can be implanted if no evidence of AV conduction disease is present.

Clinical Trials and Pacing Mode Many nonprospective, nonrandomized studies have suggested significant survival benefit with physiologic pacing compared to ventricular pacing (VVI mode) in patients with sinus node dysfunction. This led to randomized, large-scale prospective trials, the results of which are summarized in Table 32-4. The first randomized trial comparing atrial to ventricular pacing in 225 patients with sick sinus syndrome demonstrated significant reduction in the incidence of atrial fibrillation, thromboembolism, and cardiovascular mortality in the atrial pacing group.[25] Subsequent large-scale trials have not confirmed these mortality or stroke prevention benefits. The Canadian Trial of Physiologic Pacing (CTOPP)[26] randomized 2568 patients with symptomatic bradycardia without chronic atrial fibrillation to receive either a physiologic (atrial or dual-chamber) pacemaker or a ventricular pacemaker and followed them for an average of 3 years. The primary outcome of stroke or cardiovascular mortality was not different among the two groups (4.9 vs 5.5 percent), while the annual rate of atrial fibrillation was significantly less in the physiologic pacing group (5.3 percent) than it was in the ventricular pacing group (6.6 percent) for a relative risk reduction of 18 percent. Another large randomized trial of dual-chamber pacing versus ventricular pacing was MOST (MOde Selection Trial in sinus node dysfunction),[27] which involved 2010 patients. It also confirmed the benefit of reducing the risk for atrial fibrillation in dual-chamber-paced patients without significant reduction in mortality or nonfatal stroke.

## Carotid Sinus Hypersensitivity and Vasovagal Syncope

The pathophysiology, diagnosis, and specific management of these disorders are discussed separately in Chap. 40. A hypersensitive response to carotid sinus stimulation of 5 to 10 s is defined as asystole due to sinus arrest or AV block of more than 3 s (cardioinhibitory), a substantial symptomatic decrease in systolic blood pressure of 50 mmHg or more, (vasodepressor) or both (mixed; Fig. 32-5). The pathophysiology of carotid sinus syncope is complex and poorly understood and is hypothesized to result from abnormalities of neuromuscular structures surrounding the carotid sinus mechanoreceptors, a central defect of the autonomic nervous system and association with atherosclerotic disease. Carotid sinus syncope predominantly occurs in elderly males with associated coronary artery disease. While carotid sinus hypersensitivity is not uncommon, carotid sinus syncope is relatively rare accounting for 11 to 19 percent of patients with syncope of undetermined cause.[28] Initial management of patients with carotid sinus syncope should consist of simple elimination of any recognized provocative activities (tight collars, shaving, head turning, looking up, Valsalva maneuver) that precipitate an

TABLE 32-4 Randomized Trials of Pacing Modes in Patients with Sinus Node Dysfunction

| Trial | Indication | Mode comparison | No. of Patients | Follow-up | Endpoints | Results |
|---|---|---|---|---|---|---|
| **Danish**[27] | SSS | AAI vs VVI | 225 | 8 years | Total mortality, AF, thromboembolism | Atrial pacing significantly reduced mortality (RR 0.66), AF (RR 0.54), and stroke (RR 0.47). |
| **PASE**[50] | SSS and AVB | DDDR vs VVIR | 407 | 30 months | Primary: QOL<br>Secondary: Total mortality, stroke, AF, HF | No change in QOL, mortality, stroke or AF. Improved QOL in SSS pts with physiologic pacing |
| **CTOPP**[28] | SSS and AVB | DDDR/AAIR vs VVIR | 2568 | 3 years | Primary: Stroke, CV mortality<br>Secondary: Total mortality, AF, hospitalization for HF | No reduction in mortality or stroke. Relative risk reduction of 18% for AF with physiologic pacing |
| **MOST**[29] | SSS | DDDR vs VVIR | 2010 | 33 months | Primary: Total mortality, stroke<br>Secondary: Composite of death, stroke or hosp for HF; AF; QOL; HF score | No difference in primary or secondary endpoint except for AF. Lower incidence of AF with DDD pacing (Hazard ratio of 0.79) |

Abbreviations: AF = Atrial fibrillation; AVB = Atrioventricular block; CTOPP = Canadian trial of physiologic pacing; CV = Cardiovascular; HF = Heart failure; MOST = Mode selection trial; PASE = Pacemaker selection in the elderly; QOL = quality of life; RR = Relative risk; SSS = Sick sinus syndrome.

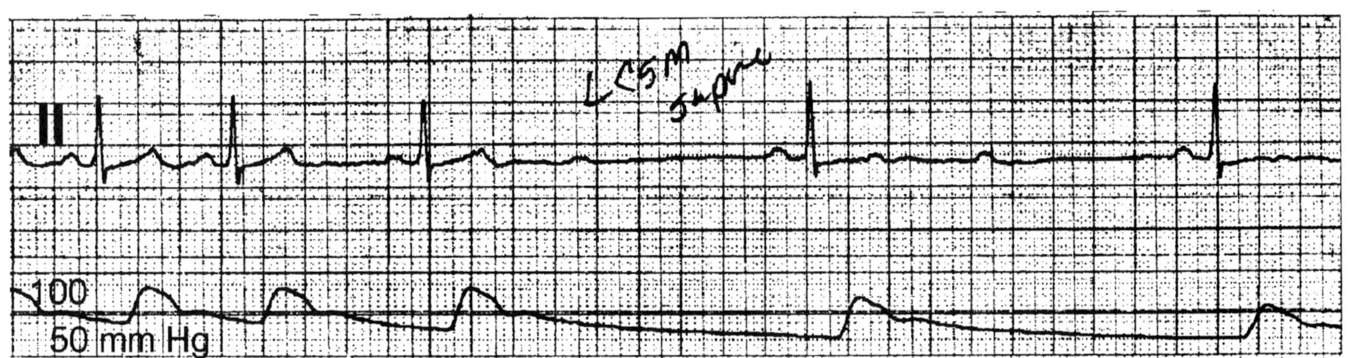


FIGURE 32-5 Carotid sinus hypersensitivity. Left carotid sinus massage results in slowing of the sinus rate and 2:1 atrioventricular block with symptoms of near syncope. Note that the systolic blood pressure decreases significantly from 90 mmHg to about 50 mmHg as evidenced by finger plethysmography.

event. For patients with recurrent or severe carotid sinus syncope of the cardioinhibitory type, permanent pacemaker implantation is the accepted and proven modality of treatment as evidenced by many small randomized trials.[29] DDI or DDD pacemakers are generally the accepted mode of pacing for patients with carotid sinus syncope, while AAI pacing is contraindicated because many patients may demonstrate associated AV block. The current indications for pacing in hypersensitive carotid sinus syndrome and neurocardiogenic syncope are shown in Table 32-5.

Vasovagal syncope is a common condition caused by inappropriate reflex vasodilation and bradycardia, and occasionally even asystole. Tilt-table testing in patients with vasovagal syncope may reveal a cardioinhibitory, vasodepressor or a mixed response. Many pharmacologic agents (atenolol, midodrine, paroxetine) have shown efficacy in prevention of vasovagal syncope in uncontrolled clinical trials. Dual-chamber pacemakers with "rate-drop response" or "rate hysteresis" feature are currently a treatment option in a select group of patients with recurrent syncope and cardioinhibitory response on tilt-table testing. Three randomized but nonplacebo controlled trials have assessed the role of permanent pacemakers in patients with vasovagal syncope and cardioinhibitory response during tilt-table testing (Table 32-6). The North American Vasovagal Pacemaker Study (VPS) showed 85 percent relative-risk reduction for recurrent syncope in the pacemaker-treated patients compared with patients receiving no therapy, but no difference in the number of presyncopal spells.[30] In the Vasovagal Syncope International Study, 5 percent of patients with pacemakers had recurrent syncope as compared with 61 percent in the no-pacemaker arm during a mean follow-up of 3.7 years.[31] The Syncope Diagnosis and Treatment Study[32] compared pacing therapy to treatment with atenolol and showed a significant reduction in recurrence of syncope in patients with pacemakers (4.3 percent) than there was in patients treated with atenolol (25.5 percent). However, the Vasovagal Pacemaker Study II, in which all patients received permanent pacemakers and were randomized to either DDD mode with rate-drop response or ODO mode, did not show a significant reduction in the risk of recurrent syncope in patients with DDD pacing.[33]

TABLE 32-5 Recommendations for Permanent Pacing in Hypersensitive Carotid Sinus Syndrome and Neurocardiogenic Syncope

**Class I**

1. Recurrent syncope caused by carotid sinus stimulation; minimal carotid sinus pressure induces ventricular asystole of more than 3-s duration in the absence of any medication that depresses the sinus node or AV conduction. (Level of evidence: C)

**Class IIa**

1. Recurrent syncope without clear, provocative events and with a hypersensitive cardioinhibitory response. (Level of evidence: C)
2. Significantly symptomatic and recurrent neurocardiogenic syncope associated with bradycardia documented spontaneously or at the time of tilt-table testing. (Level of evidence: C)

**Class III**

1. A hyperactive cardioinhibitory response to carotid sinus stimulation in the absence of symptoms or in the presence of vague symptoms such as dizziness, light-headedness or both.
2. Recurrent syncope, light-headedness or dizziness in the absence of a hyperactive cardioinhibitory response.
3. Situational vasovagal syncope in which avoidance behavior is effective.

## Disorders of Atrioventricular Conduction

AV block occurs when atrial conduction to the ventricle is blocked at a time when the AV junction is not physiologically refractory. This can be due to conduction block in the atrium, AV node, and/or His-Purkinje system. Using His-bundle electrogram recordings, three anatomic sites of AV block can be identified: AV nodal, intra-Hisian, or infra-Hisian. Block at the AV nodal level implies a favorable prognosis while block at or below the His-bundle level implies an unfavorable prognosis. Surface ECGs will very often provide adequate information to make a diagnosis regarding the site of the block, while occasionally intracardiac recordings are necessary to confirm the level of the block.

### PATHOPHYSIOLOGY OF ATRIOVENTRICULAR BLOCK

Transient or persistent AV block of varying degrees can occur in a variety of clinical situations (Table 32-7). Heightened vagal tone in athletes or during sleep may be associated with first-degree or type I second-degree AV block and occasionally even complete heart block. The AV block in these situations is usually preceded by slowing of the heart rate. Vagally mediated AV block may occur in response to

TABLE 32-6 Randomized Trials of Permanent Pacing In Patients with Recurrent Vasovagal Syncope

| Trial | Inclusion criteria | Treatment groups | No. of patients | Follow-up | Endpoints | Results |
|---|---|---|---|---|---|---|
| **VPS**[33] | Syncope × 6, Positive tilt-table test with relative bradycardia | DDD pacer with RDR vs no pacer | 54 | 15 months | First recurrence of syncope | 85% relative risk reduction for recurrent syncope (22% in pacemaker vs 70% in no pacemaker arm) |
| **VASIS**[34] | >3 syncope in last 2 years, Positive tilt-table test with HR < 40 or asystole >3 s, Age >40 years | DDI pacer with rate hysteresis vs no pacer | 42 | 3.7 years (mean) | First recurrence of syncope | Significant reduction in recurrent syncope, 5% in pacemaker arm vs 61% in no pacer arm |
| **SYDIT**[35] | >3 syncope in last 2 years, Positive tilt-table test with relative bradycardia, Age >35 years | DDD pacer with RDR vs atenolol | 93 | 17 months (mean) | First recurrence of syncope | Significant reduction in recurrent syncope, 4.3% in pacer group vs 25.5% in atenolol group |
| **VPS II**[36] | >5 syncope/lifetime or >2 syncope/2 years, Positive tilt-table test with relative bradycardia, Age >19 years | DDD pacer with RDR vs pacer in ODO mode | 100 | 6 months | First recurrence of syncope | Nonsignificant reduction in recurrent syncope (DDD paced patients 30 vs 40% in ODO). |

ABBREVIATIONS: HR = heart rate; RDR = rate drop response; SYDIT = Syncope Diagnosis and Treatment study; VASIS = Vasovagal Syncope International Study; VPS = Vasovagal Pacemaker Study.

various stimuli such as carotid sinus hypersensitivity, coughing, swallowing, or micturition.[34] Varying degrees of heart block have been described in a large variety of infectious diseases (viral, bacterial, rickettsial, and protozoal). Heart block associated with endocarditis may be transient or permanent. In patients with endocarditis and ring abscess, heart block may not resolve and pacing may be required. With Lyme disease, cardiac involvement may occur in 8 to 10 percent of patients. More than 50 percent of patients with cardiac involvement may develop advanced heart block requiring temporary pacing.[35] Even complete AV block generally resolves in 1 to 2 weeks, and permanent pacing is seldom necessary. Chagas' cardiomyopathy may be associated with persistent AV block. Other causes of transient or reversible AV block include metabolic disturbances such as hyperkalemia, hypermagnesemia, hypothyroidism, Addison's disease, and drugs (see Table 32-7).

Idiopathic progressive fibrosis of the conduction system is a common cause of acquired AV block. Lev's disease, also known as idiopathic bilateral bundle branch fibrosis, is characterized by progressive replacement of the proximal bundle branches by fibrosis as a result of the aging process exaggerated by hypertension and arteriosclerosis.[36] Lenegre's disease is a variant of idiopathic conduction disorder involving young patients and the peripheral parts of the bundle branches.[37] Some cases of Lenegre's disease may be due to mutations in the sodium channel gene SCN5a, causing a hereditary form of AV conduction disease.[38]

AV block occurs in 12 to 25 percent of all patients with acute MI; first-degree AV block occurs in 2 to 12 percent, second-degree AV block in 3 to 10 percent; and third-degree AV block in 3 to 7 percent.[39] Ischemic injury can produce conduction block at any level of the AV or intraventricular conduction system. Second-degree type I AV block occurs more commonly in inferior than anterior MIs. Inferior infarctions are often associated early on with increased vagal tone causing sinus bradycardia and AV block. AV block occurring late in the course of the infarct may be caused by ischemia to the AV node or ischemic metabolites such as potassium and adenosine. Most patients are asymptomatic, and rarely type I AV block may progress to complete AV block. Second-degree type II AV block occurs in 1 percent of patients with acute MI and predominantly occurs in patients with anterior infarctions. The risk of progression to complete AV block is high in these patients. Complete AV block can occur in both inferior and anterior infarctions. In inferior MIs, the block is at the level of the AV node and the escape rhythm typically arises from the AV junction, with a narrow QRS and an escape rate of 40 to 60 bpm. The prognosis in these patients is generally good as the AV block resolves in the vast majority of patients within a few days. Complete AV block resulting from anterior infarction is usually at the His or infra-Hisian level, and the escape rhythm is from the distal Purkinje fibers or the ventricle, with a wide QRS interval and a rate of 20 to 40 bpm. Because of the coexisting extensive infarction and pump failure, AV block resulting from anterior infarctions are associated with high mortality. In patients with acute MI, temporary pacing is generally indicated in patients with complete AV block at any level, type II second-degree AV block, and in patients with type I second-degree AV block if associated with symptomatic bradycardia. Although the incidence of complete AV block in acute MIs has decreased following thrombolytic therapy, the mortality still remains high.[40] The indications for permanent pacing in patients with acute MI are listed in Table 32-8. Patients with coronary artery disease and ischemic cardiomyopathy may develop persistent AV block. AV nodal block can occur transiently during episodes of ischemia especially with Prinzmetal's angina.

A variety of uncommon autoimmune, oncologic, infectious, and iatrogenic disorders can also lead to heart block and are listed in Table 32-7. Certain neuromuscular disorders (myotonic dystrophy,

Kearns-Sayre syndrome, peroneal muscular atrophy, Erb's limb-girdle dystrophy, and X-linked muscular dystrophies) may give rise to progressive and insidiously developing conduction disorders of the His-Purkinje system. Myotonic dystrophy and Kearns-Sayre syndrome are associated with high incidence of unpredictable and rapidly progressive conduction system disease.[41] Complete heart block may occur after aortic or mitral valve replacement surgery, and rarely after coronary artery bypass surgery. Preoperative right bundle branch block and multivalve surgery involving the tricuspid valve were shown to be strong independent predictors of postoperative heart block requiring permanent pacemaker implantation.[42] Complete AV block is more common after surgical procedures to correct ventricular septal defects, tetralogy of Fallot, AV canal defects, or myectomy for hypertrophic obstructive cardiomyopathy. Congenital heart diseases such as corrected transposition of great arteries, ostium primum atrial septal defects, and ventricular septal defects may be associated with complete heart block. Congenital complete AV block is a rare anomaly that results from abnormal embryonic development of the AV node and is not associated with structural heart disease in 50 percent of cases. Congenital complete heart block is also associated with maternal lupus erythematosus. Most of the children with isolated congenital complete AV block have a stable escape rhythm with a narrow complex. Pacing is generally indicated in children with complete heart block if the heart rate in the awake child is <50 bpm or if associated with left ventricular systolic dysfunction or ventricular arrhythmias. The indications for pacing in children, adolescents, and patients with congenital heart disease are outlined in Table 32-9.

TABLE 32-7 Etiology of Atrioventricular Block

| Reversible | Permanent |
|---|---|
| Physiologic | Idiopathic fibrosis |
| Heightened vagal tone (athletes, sleep apnea) | Lev's disease |
| Autonomic mediated | Lenegre's disease |
| Carotid sinus hypersensitivity | Congenital |
| Neurocardiogenic syncope | Congenital heart disease |
| Coronary artery disease | Maternal systemic lupus erythematosus |
| Acute myocardial infarction | Coronary artery disease |
| Angina (Prinzmetal's) | Acute myocardial infarction |
| Infectious disease | Ischemic cardiomyopathy |
| Infective endocarditis | Cardiomyopathy |
| Myocarditis | Infiltrative disease |
| Viral, rickettsial, Lyme disease, | Amyloidosis |
| Rheumatic fever | Sarcoidosis |
| Metabolic | Hemochromatosis |
| Hyperkalemia | Infectious disease |
| Hypermagnesemia | Endocarditis |
| Addison's disease | Syphilis |
| Traumatic | Tuberculosis |
| Catheter induced | Chagas' disease |
| Radiofrequency energy | Collagen vascular disease |
| Surgery | Systemic lupus erythematosus |
| Drug induced | Rheumatoid arthritis |
| Digitalis | Scleroderma |
| Beta blockers | Trumatic |
| Calcium channel blockers | Surgery |
| Class III antiarrhythmic agents | Radiofrequency ablation |
| Class I antiarrhythmic agents | Radiation |
| Adenosine | Tumors |
| Lithium | Mesothelioma |
| | Rhabdomyoma |
| | Hodgkin's lymphoma |
| | Melanoma |
| | Neuromuscular disease |
| | Myotonic dystrophy |
| | Kearns-Sayre Syndrome |
| | Erb's dystrophy |
| | X-linked muscular dystrophy |
| | Peroneal muscular atrophy |

## ELECTROCARDIOGRAPHIC MANIFESTATIONS

***First-Degree Atrioventricular Block*** Prolongation of the PR interval to more than 200 ms constitutes first-degree AV block. It is most commonly due to conduction delay within the AV node and occasionally due to intraatrial or infra-Hisian conduction delay. If the QRS duration is normal, the site of conduction delay is almost always within the AV node. If first-degree AV block occurs in the presence of bundle branch block, the conduction delay can be in the AV node (60 percent of cases), His-Purkinje system, or both. Patients with first-degree AV block have an excellent prognosis even when associated with chronic bifascicular block as the rate of progression to third-degree AV block is low, and no specific therapy is indicated.[43]

***Second-Degree Atrioventricular Block*** Second-degree AV block is characterized by intermittent failure of conduction from the atria to the ventricles. If the AV block occurs with the atrial rate in the physiologic range, then it is considered a primary arrhythmia. AV block in the setting of atrial tachyarrhythmias is generally a normal response. Based on the electrocardiographic patterns, second-degree AV block is classified into Mobitz type I and type II.

*Second-degree AV block of the Wenckebach type (Mobitz type I)* is characterized by the following features: (1) progressive prolongation of the P-R interval prior to a nonconducted P wave; (2) P-R interval prolongation at progressively decreasing increments; (3) progressive shortening of R-R intervals; (4) pause encompassing the blocked P wave shorter than the sum of two P-P cycles; and (5) the last conducted P-R interval prior to the blocked P wave longer than the next conducted P-R interval (Fig. 32-6). Type I second-degree AV block often occurs with regularity leading to patterns of "group beating."

TABLE 32-8 Indications for Pacing in Atrioventricular Block Associated with Acute Myocardial Infarction

**Class I**

1. Persistent second-degree atrioventricular (AV) block in the His-Purkinje system with bilateral bundle branch block or third-degree AV block within or below the His-Purkinje system after AMI. (Level of evidence:B)
2. Transient advanced (second- or third-degree) infranodal AV block and associated bundle-branch block. If the site of block is uncertain, an electrophysiology study may be necessary. (Level of evidence: B)
3. Persistent and symptomatic second- or third-degree AV block. (Level of evidence: C)

**Class IIb**

1. Persistent second- or third-degree AV block at the AV node level. (Level of evidence: B)

**Class III**

1. Transient AV block in the absence of intraventricular conduction defects. (Level of evidence: B)
2. Transient AV block in the presence of isolated left anterior fascicular block. (Level of evidence: B)
3. Acquired left anterior fascicular block in the absence of AV block. (Level of evidence: B)
4. Persistent first-degree AV block in the presence of bundle-branch block that is old or age indeterminate. (Level of evidence: B)

TABLE 32-9 Indications for Pacing in Children, Adolescents, and Patients with Congenital Heart Disease

**Class I**

1. Advanced second- or third-degree atrioventricular (AV) block associated with symptomatic bradycardia, ventricular dysfunction, or low cardiac output. (Level of evidence: C)
2. Sinus node dysfunction with correlation of symptoms during age-inappropriate bradycardia. The definition of bradycardia varies with the patient's age and expected heart rate. (Level of evidence: B)
3. Postoperative advanced second- or third-degree AV block that is not expected to resolve or persists at least 7 days after cardiac surgery. (Level of evidence: B,C)
4. Congenital third-degree AV block with a wide QRS escape rhythm, complex ventricular ectopy, or ventricular dysfunction. (Level of evidence: B)
5. Congenital third-degree AV block in the infant with the ventricular rate less than 50 to 55 bpm or with congenital heart disease and a ventricular rate less than 70 bpm. (Level of evidence: B,C)
6. Sustained pause-dependent VT, with or without prolonged QT, in which the efficacy of pacing is thoroughly documented. (Level of evidence: B)

**Class IIa**

1. Bradycardia-tachycardia syndrome with the need for long-term antiarrhythmic treatment other than digitalis. (Level of evidence: C)
2. Congenital third-degree AV block beyond the first year of life with an average heart rate less than 50 bpm, abrupt pauses in ventricular rate that are two or three times the basic cycle length, or associated with symptoms due to chronotropic incompetence. (Level of evidence: B)
3. Long-QT syndrome with 2:1 AV or third-degree AV block. (Level of evidence: B)
4. Asymptomatic sinus bradycardia in the child with complex congenital heart disease with resting heart rate less than 40 bpm or pauses in ventricular rate more than 3 s. (Level of evidence: C)
5. Patients with congenital heart disease and impaired hemodynamics due to sinus bradycardia or loss of AV synchrony. (Level of evidence: C)

**Class IIb**

1. Transient postoperative third-degree AV block that reverts to sinus rhythm with residual bifascicular block. (Level of evidence: C)
2. Congenital third-degree AV block in the asymptomatic infant, child, adolescent, or young adult with an acceptable rate, narrow QRS complex, and normal ventricular function. (Level of evidence: B)
3. Asymptomatic sinus bradycardia in the adolescent with congenital heart disease with resting heart rate less than 40 bpm or pauses in ventricular rate more than 3 s. (Level of evidence: C)
4. Neuromuscular diseases with any degree of AV block (including first-degree AV block), with or without symptoms, because there may be unpredictable progression of AV conduction disease.

**Class III**

1. Transient postoperative AV block with return of normal AV conduction. (Level of evidence: B)
2. Asymptomatic postoperative bifascicular block with or without first-degree AV block. (Level of evidence: C)
3. Asymptomatic type I second-degree AV block. (Level of evidence: C)
4. Asymptomatic sinus bradycardia in the adolescent with longest R-R interval less than 3 s and minimum heart rate more than 40 bpm. (Level of evidence: C)

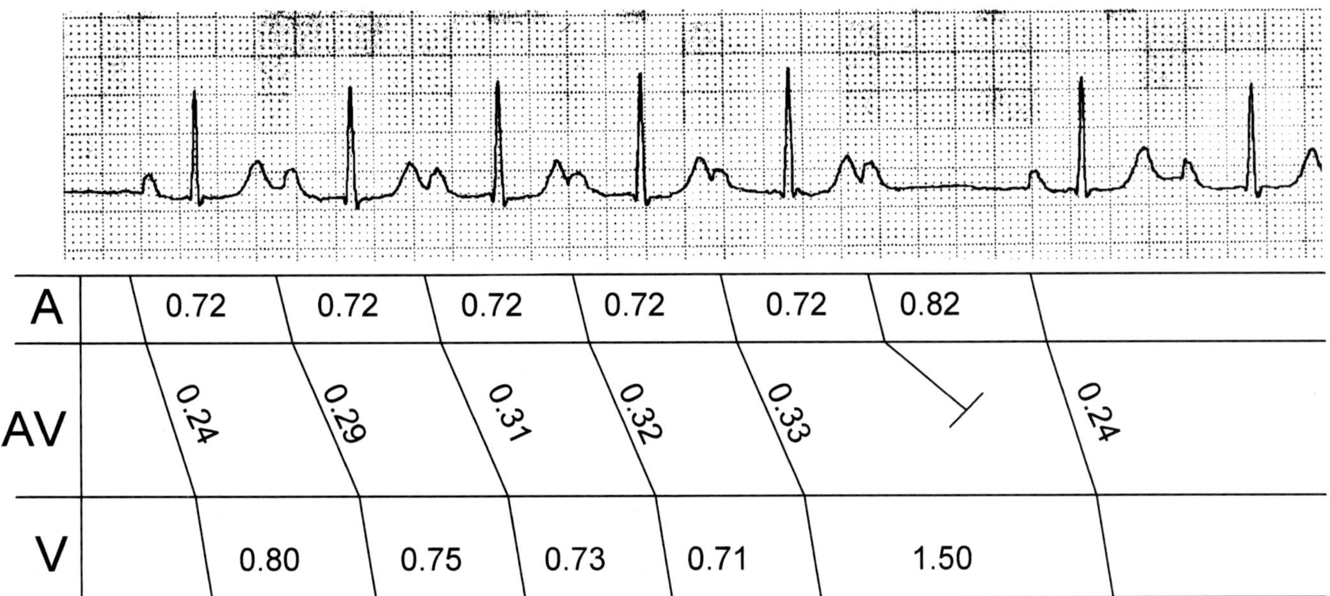


FIGURE 32-6 Type I second-degree atrioventricular (AV) block. A 6:5 AV Wenckebach periodicity is shown. Note that the P-R interval progressively lengthens with a decreasing increment. This results in shortening of R-R intervals. The last conducted P-R interval (0.33 s) is significantly longer than the next conducted P-R interval (0.24 s).

When type I second-degree AV block occurs in association with a normal QRS interval, block is almost always in the AV node. In the presence of a prolonged QRS interval, block may be in the AV node, His-Purkinje (rare), or both. Very long P-R intervals are usually due to a block in the AV node. Type I second-degree AV block occurs in a small percentage of normal people and not uncommonly in well-trained athletes. Most patients are asymptomatic while some develop symptomatic bradycardia, near syncope, or occasionally syncope due to progression to complete AV block.

*Mobitz type II second-degree* AV block is characterized by (1) constant P-P intervals and R-R intervals; (2) constant P-R intervals prior to a nonconducted P wave; and (3) pause encompassing the nonconducted P wave equal to two P-P cycles. Type II AV block usually occurs in the presence of bundle branch block and is almost always due to a block in the His-Purkinje system (Fig. 32-7). Rarely type II AV block can occur in patients with normal QRS duration. Type II AV block frequently progresses to a complete AV block and may result in syncopal attacks.

***2:1 Atrioventricular Block*** In this form of second-degree AV block, every other P wave is not conducted making it difficult to diagnose the level of AV block (Fig. 32-8). A 2:1 AV block with normal QRS duration or with a very long P-R interval generally suggests a block in the AV node. A 2:1 AV block in the presence of bundle branch block favors a block below the AV node, but is not diagnostic. A prolonged electrocardiographic recording may sometimes reveal a transition to varying degrees of AV block (3:2 or 4:3), with type I or type II features that aids in the diagnosis. Intracardiac recordings with a His-bundle catheter is sometimes necessary to determine the site of the block. In patients with a 2:1 AV block, vagal maneuvers are helpful in diagnosing the level of AV block. Carotid sinus stimulation may worsen the degree of block if it is in the AV node, while slowing of

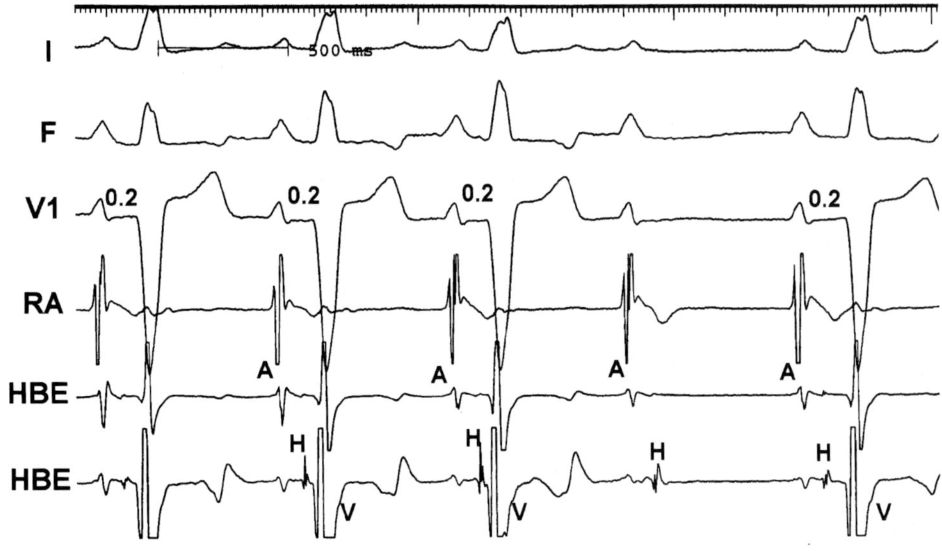


FIGURE 32-7 Type II second-degree atrioventricular block. Surface electrocardiogram (ECG); leads I, aVF, and $V_1$ and intracardiac electrograms from the right atrial (RA), proximal, and distal His bundle (HBE) catheters are shown. Surface ECGs show that the P-R intervals are constant at 0.2 s with a left bundle branch block morphology of the QRS complex, and the fourth P wave is not followed by a QRS complex. The His-bundle electrograms reveal that the site of block of the fourth P wave is below the His bundle.

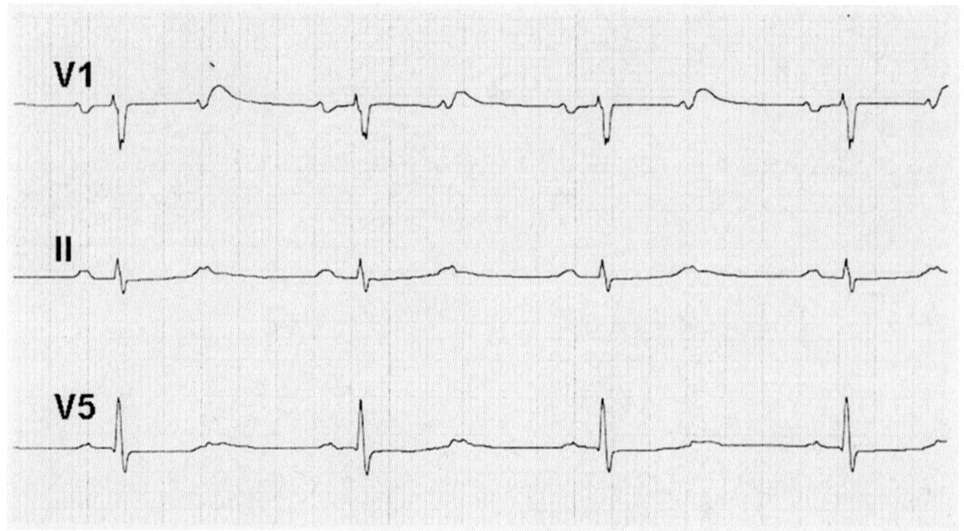


FIGURE 32-8 *A.* Surface electrocardiogram from leads $V_1$, II, and $V_5$ demonstrating 2:1 atrioventricular (AV) block with narrow QRS complexes. Although a definite diagnosis of type I or type II AV block cannot be made, longer rhythm strip recordings might reveal Wenckebach periodicity. Vagal maneuvers or exercise might assist further in the final diagnosis. *B.* Surface leads $V_1$ and II showing 2:1 AV block. The first QRS has normal morphology, the next two QRS complexes have incomplete left bundle branch block morphology and the last three QRS complexes have right bundle branch block morphology. This alternating bundle branch block pattern is highly suggestive of Mobitz II second-degree AV block.

the sinus rate may paradoxically improve the ratio of AV conduction and increase ventricular rate if the block is located in the His-Purkinje system. Similarly, atropine improves AV nodal conduction, but the increased sinus rate may worsen the ratio of AV conduction in patients with His-Purkinje block, resulting in worsened bradycardia. Hence, atropine should be used with caution in patients with a 2:1 AV block and bundle branch block where His-Purkinje disease is strongly suspected.

***High-Grade Atrioventricular Block*** When two or more consecutive atrial impulses do not conduct to the ventricle, it is defined as high-grade AV block. It may be associated with a junctional or ventricular escape rhythm. Occasionally, runs of consecutive atrial impulses may fail to conduct to the ventricles for up to 10 to 20 s with or without an escape rhythm resulting in ventricular asystole and syncope. The block is usually initiated by a conducted or blocked atrial or ventricular premature beat. The block persists until terminated by an escape beat. Unless a clearly defined reversible etiology is identified, permanent pacing is indicated.

***Third-Degree Atrioventricular Block*** Complete or third-degree AV block is characterized by failure of all P waves to conduct to the ventricle. This results in complete dissociation of P waves and QRS complexes. Complete AV block may occur as a result of block in the AV node or at the His-Purkinje level. In patients with block at the AV nodal level, the escape rhythm is usually junctional, with a narrow QRS complex (unless associated with preexisting bundle branch block), at rates of 40 to 60 bpm (Fig. 32-9). In complete heart block resulting from His-Purkinje disease, the escape rhythm is ventricular in origin, with a wide QRS interval and at rates of 20 to 40 bpm.

***Atrioventricular Dissociation*** It is characterized by atrial and ventricular activity independent of each other. AV dissociation may be secondary to AV block (complete heart block) or physiological refractoriness. AV dissociation can occur when the sinus rate is slower than the secondary junctional or ventricular pacemaker as in patients with sinus bradycardia. In contrast, AV dissociation can also occur in the presence of normal sinus rhythm and accelerated junctional (junctional tachycardia) or ventricular (ventricular tachycardia)

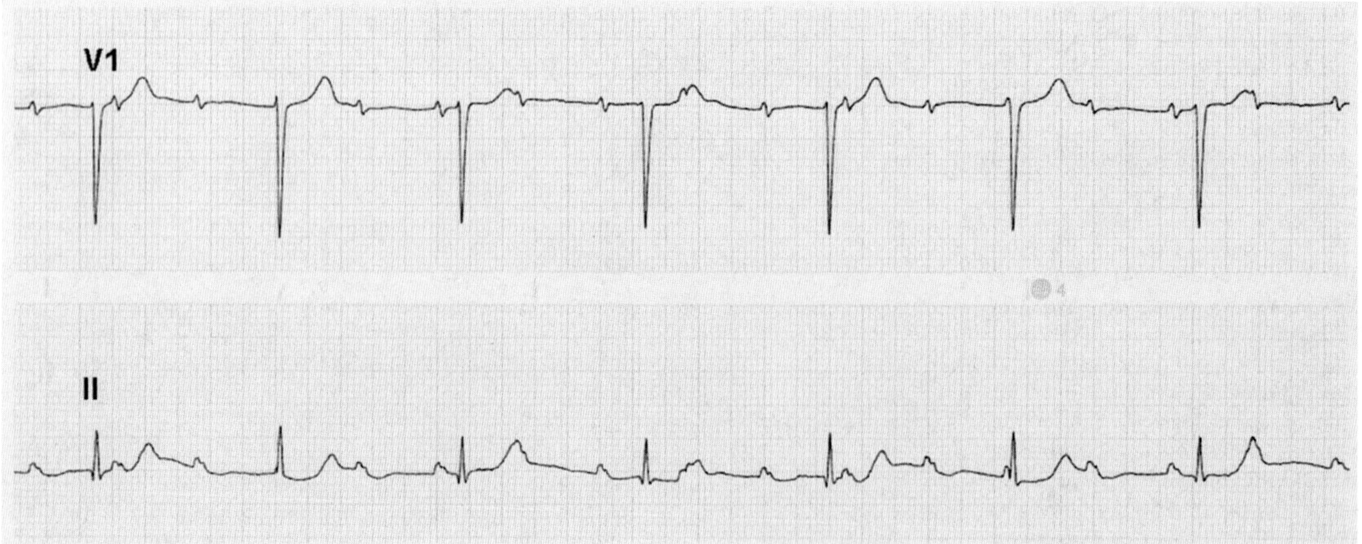


FIGURE 32-9 Complete heart block. Surface leads $V_1$ and II shows sinus tachycardia at 120 bpm and is completely dissociated from a regular junctional (narrow QRS complexes) escape rhythm at 54 bpm. The site of atrioventricular (AV) block is most likely within the AV node.

rhythm with retrograde conduction block. In patients with complete heart block the atrial rate is faster than is the ventricular rate, while in AV dissociation the ventricular rate is faster than is the atrial rate. While AV dissociation is present in complete heart block, it is not synonymous. AV dissociation is usually a manifestation of another rhythm abnormality such as complete heart block, sinus bradycardia, or ventricular tachycardia. Treatment is usually directed toward the underlying cause.

## CLINICAL PRESENTATION

Symptoms in patients with AV conduction abnormalities are generally due to bradycardia and loss of AV synchrony. Patients with significantly prolonged P-R intervals may behave in a similar fashion to patients with pacemaker syndrome due to loss of AV synchrony. In patients with structural heart disease and LV dysfunction, this may result in worsening of heart failure. Symptoms due to more advanced AV block may range from exercise intolerance, easy fatigability, dyspnea on exertion, dizzy spells, and near syncope to frank syncope. In patients with paroxysmal or intermittent complete heart block, these symptoms are episodic and routine ECGs may not be diagnostic. Children and adolescents with isolated complete heart block may be generally asymptomatic, while some may develop symptoms later as adults due to chronotropic incompetence. Children with complete heart block associated with structural heart disease are symptomatic very early on and have an increased risk for sudden death.[44]

## DIAGNOSTIC EVALUATION

The prognosis and treatment of AV block depends on its association with symptoms and the level of AV block. Routine 12-lead surface ECGs are adequate to establish the diagnosis of varying degrees of AV block in many patients. Analyzing the P-R interval, QRS duration, Wenckebach phenomenon, and ventricular rates on the surface ECG provides important clues to the level of AV block. In certain situations such as 2:1 AV block, additional maneuvers may be necessary to establish the level of AV block. Responses to carotid sinus massage, atropine, and exercise are often very helpful. In patients with complete heart block at the level of the AV node, the resultant junctional escape rhythm usually accelerates with exercise in contrast to the ventricular escape rhythm with infranodal block, which usually remains unchanged.

In patients with paroxysmal symptoms of near syncope or syncope and no significant conduction abnormalities on the surface ECG, prolonged electrocardiographic monitoring with 24- to 48-h Holter recordings or 30-day event monitors may be helpful. Occasionally an implantable loop recorder may be necessary to establish the diagnosis. Electrophysiology study is indicated in patients with syncope or near syncope in whom high-grade AV block is suspected as the cause. In patients with structural heart disease, in addition to AV conduction disease, ventricular tachycardia can also be a major etiology for syncope, and electrophysiology study can be very useful in establishing the diagnosis.

## MANAGEMENT

Identifying transient or reversible causes for AV conduction disturbances is the first step in management. Withdrawal of any offending drugs such as digoxin, calcium channel blockers, or beta blockers, correction of any electrolyte abnormalities, or treatment of any infectious processes should be considered prior to permanent pacing therapy. If the drugs causing AV block are essential for treatment of other medical conditions, then permanent pacing may be considered. In patients with advanced AV block and hemodynamic decompensation unresponsive to drug therapy such as atropine or isoprenaline, as in digitalis toxicity, hyperkalemia, acute anterior MI, or Lyme's myocarditis, temporary pacing should be instituted until AV block resolves or permanent pacing can be initiated. Temporary pacing can be accomplished by transcutaneous pacing systems in those patients at low to moderate risk for developing complete heart block or in patients with complete heart block and hemodynamically stable escape rhythms. Transcutaneous pacing for prolonged periods is very uncomfortable and transvenous pacing should be performed in patients with need for continuous active pacing.

Permanent pacemaker implantation is indicated in most patients with advanced heart block associated with symptoms. Permanent pacemakers are also indicated in asymptomatic patients with complete heart block and infra-Hisian second-degree AV block. Permanent pacing has clearly been shown to decrease mortality in patients with advanced heart block and syncope.[45] The indications for pacing in children with AV block and in adults with acquired heart block are described in Tables 32-9 and 32-10, respectively.

Most patients with AV block require dual-chamber pacemakers, as this mode of pacing maintains AV synchrony and prevents development of pacemaker syndrome. In patients with associated sinus node dysfunction, dual-chamber pacemakers with rate-responsive function (DDDR) are the preferred mode of choice. In patients with normal sinus node function and AV block, VDD pacing using a single lead with a series of electrodes for atrial sensing and ventricular pacing and sensing is an ideal mode of pacing, as it provides AV synchrony and rate-responsiveness, and is superior to single-chamber VVI pacing. In patients with chronic atrial fibrillation and bradycardia, rate-responsive single-chamber ventricular pacing (VVIR) is adequate. Early studies of comparison of pacing modes in a small number of patients with AV block had shown that physiologic pacing (DDD or VDD) enhanced survival compared to VVI pacing.[46,47] However, prospective, randomized, large-scale trials showed that dual-chamber pacing provided little benefit over ventricular pacing for the prevention of death (see Table 32-4).[26] The incidence of pacemaker syndrome was as high as 26 percent in patients with ventricular pacing necessitating crossover to dual-chamber pacing in the Pacemaker Selection in the Elderly trial.[48]

## BUNDLE BRANCH BLOCK

Conduction disturbances that occur at various levels of the branches of the His-Purkinje system are described as bundle branch block or intraventricular conduction defects (IVCD). In patients with isolated chronic right or left bundle branch block, the progression to advanced AV block is rare. Patients with bifascicular block (right bundle branch block and left anterior or posterior fascicular block) or left bundle branch block and left axis deviation have a 6 percent incidence of progression to complete heart block.[49,50] In patients with acute MI, the development of new bifascicular block and first-degree AV block is associated with a very high risk (40 percent) for progression to high-grade AV block. These patients are generally recommended to undergo prophylactic temporary pacing.[39] Alternating bundle branch block, even in asymptomatic patients, is a sign of advanced conduction disturbance in the His-Purkinje system and is considered a class I indication for permanent pacing. In patients with bundle branch block, His-bundle ECGs can occasionally be helpful in identifying patients at high risk for progression to high-grade AV block. The incidental findings of markedly prolonged H-V interval ($\geq$100 ms) or atrial-pacing-induced infra-Hisian block[51] that is not physiologic during an electrophysiology study are considered to indicate high risk for progression to advanced AV block, and prophylactic permanent pacing is recommended (Table 32-11). Intraventricular conduction disturbances are usually associated with significant

TABLE 32-10 Indications for Pacing in Acquired Atrioventricular Block in Adults

**Class I**

1. Third-degree and advanced second-degree atrioventricular (AV) block at any anatomic level, associated with any one of the following conditions:
   a. Bradycardia with symptoms (including heart failure) presumed to be due to AV block. (Level of evidence: C)
   b. Arrhythmias and other medical conditions requiring drugs that result in symptomatic bradycardia. (Level of evidence: C)
   c. Documented periods of asystole greater than or equal to 3.0 s or any escape rate less than 40 bpm in awake, symptom free patients. (Levels of evidence: B,C)
   d. After catheter ablation of the AV junction. (Levels of evidence: B,C) There are no trials to assess outcome without pacing, and pacing is virtually always planned in this situation unless the operative procedure is AV junction modification.
   e. Postoperative AV block that is not expected to resolve after cardiac surgery. (Level of evidence: C)
   f. Neuromuscular diseases with AV block, such as myotonic muscular dystrophy, Kearns-Sayre syndrome, Erb's dystrophy, and peroneal muscular atrophy, with or without symptoms, because there may be unpredictable progression of AV conduction disease. (Level of evidence: B)
2. Second-degree AV block regardless of type or site of block, with associated symptomatic bradycardia. (Level of evidence: B)

**Class IIa**

1. Asymptomatic third-degree AV block at any anatomic site with average awake ventricular rates of 40 bpm or faster especially if cardiomegaly or left ventricular dysfunction is present. (Levels of evidence: B,C)
2. Asymptomatic type II second-degree AV block with a narrow QRS. When type II second-degree AV block occurs with a wide QRS, pacing becomes a class I recommendation. (Level of evidence: B)
3. Asymptomatic type I second-degree AV block at intra- or infra-His levels found at electrophysiology study performed for other indications. (Level of evidence: B)
4. First- or second-degree AV block with symptoms similar to those of pacemaker syndrome. (Level of evidence: B)

**Class IIb**

1. Marked first-degree AV block (more than 0.30 s) in patients with LV dysfunction and symptoms of congestive heart failure in whom a shorter AV interval results in hemodynamic improvement, presumably by decreasing left atrial filling pressure. (Level of evidence: C)
2. Neuromuscular diseases such as myotonic muscular dystrophy, Kearns-Sayre syndrome, Erb's dystrophy, and peroneal muscular atrophy with any degree of AV block (including first-degree AV block) with or without symptoms, because there may be unpredictable progression of AV conduction disease. (Level of evidence: B)

**Class III**

1. Asymptomatic first-degree AV block. (Level of evidence: B)
2. Asymptomatic type I second-degree AV block at the AV nodal level or not known to be intra- or infra-Hisian. (Levels of evidence: B, C)
3. AV block expected to resolve and/or unlikely to recur (e.g., drug toxicity, Lyme disease, or during hypoxia in sleep apnea syndrome in absence of symptoms). (Level of evidence: B)

TABLE 32-11 Indications for Pacing in Chronic Bifascicular and Trifascicular Block

**Class I**

1. Intermittent third-degree atrioventricular (AV) block. (Level of evidence: B)
2. Type II second-degree AV block. (Level of evidence: B)
3. Alternating bundle branch block. (Level of evidence: C)

**Class IIa**

1. Syncope not demonstrated to be due to AV block when other likely causes have been excluded, specifically ventricular tachycardia. (Level of evidence: B)
2. Incidental finding at electrophysiology study of markedly prolonged HV interval (greater than or equal to 100 ms) in asymptomatic patients. (Level of evidence: B)
3. Incidental finding at electrophysiology study of pacing induced infra-His block that is not physiologic. (Level of evidence: B)

**Class IIb**

1. Neuromuscular diseases such as myotonic muscular dystrophy, Kearns-Sayre syndrome, Erb's dystrophy, and peroneal muscular atrophy with any degree of fascicular block with or without symptoms, because there may be unpredictable progression of AV conduction disease. (Level of evidence: C)

**Class III**

1. Fascicular block without AV block or symptoms. (Level of evidence: B)
2. Fascicular block with first-degree AV block without symptoms.

structural heart disease, especially dilated (ischemic or idiopathic) cardiomyopathies and are a marker of poor prognosis both in terms of advanced heart failure and increased mortality in these patients (discussed later in this chapter).

## PACEMAKERS

The science of cardiac pacing is only about 50 years old and has seen tremendous growth and evolution. Since the introduction of transvenous pacing in 1958,[52] the field of cardiac pacing has benefited greatly from advances made in electronics, computer technology, power sources, and miniaturization. The initial mercury-zinc powered, asynchronous, fixed rate and fixed output, large-sized, single-chamber pacemakers implanted via thoracotomy have evolved into the current lithium-iodine powered, AV sequential, rate-responsive, multiprogrammable, miniature, biventricular devices capable of treating bradycardia and tachyarrhythmias and heart failure. The rapid growth in pacemaker design and functions has made the understanding of these devices more complex and difficult. As the potential indications for pacing had expanded, prospective, randomized trials to assess the efficacy of these devices have become an integral part of the discipline. Several prospective clinical trials have been initiated and completed during the last several years and have answered many important clinical questions.

### Pacemaker System

#### PACEMAKER

A permanent pacemaker system consists of an implanted pulse generator and the leads through which it delivers electrical stimuli in the various chambers of the heart. The pacemaker is composed of the pulse generator, housing the complex electronic circuitry and the battery, the power source. The pulse generator contains an output circuit, sensing circuit, timing circuit, and telemetry coil that sends and receives programming instructions and diagnostic information. Most of the current devices also have another circuit for the rate-adaptive sensor. Modern pacemakers almost exclusively use lithium-iodine batteries as their power source. The advantages of the lithium-iodine battery is that it has a high-energy density, long shelf-life, low interval loss due to internal self-discharge, and predictable characteristics that allow early warning of battery depletion. Most single-chamber pacemakers have an expected battery longevity of 7 to 12 years, while dual-chamber pacemakers have an expected longevity of 5 to 10 years. Most pacemakers generate 2.8 V at the beginning of life. When the voltage nears the end of life (2.1 to 2.4 V), several elective replacement indicators in the pacemaker are activated. The common indicators of elective replacement of the pacemaker are:

1. Percent or fixed decrease in pacing rate on magnet application or free running rate
2. Increase in pulse-width duration
3. Change to a simpler pacing mode (DDDR to VVI; VVIR to VOO)
4. Reduced battery voltage
5. Elevated battery impedance
6. Restricted programmability

Once the elective replacement indicators are activated, the pacemaker is generally replaced within weeks to months, earlier if the patient is pacemaker dependent. When the battery reaches the end of life (EOL, $<2.1$ V), the pacemaker changes to the simplest mode (VOO), fails to communicate or reprogram, fails to pace or sense, and may function erratically. If the pacemaker reaches the end of life, it should be replaced immediately.

#### PACEMAKER LEADS

Permanent pacing leads have 5 major components: electrodes, conductors, insulation, connector pin, and fixation mechanism. The pacing leads may be unipolar or bipolar. Although most of the leads used are bipolar in configuration, it is essential to understand both lead systems. In unipolar leads, only a single electrode is present at the lead tip (cathode) in contact with the myocardial tissue and the surface of the pacemaker-can acts as the anodal terminal. Bipolar lead systems have a cathodal tip electrode and an anodal ring electrode, 10 to 20 mm proximal to the tip electrode. Unipolar leads have a simple structural design and excellent durability but may infrequently exhibit skeletal myopotential oversensing, far-field sensing, crosstalk (atrial stimulus sensed by ventricular lead), and skeletal muscle stimulation. The newer pacemakers and bipolar leads allow a change in configuration of the pacing/sensing to unipolar or bipolar, as the situation warrants. Contemporary electrodes have a small tip surface area with a porous or roughened surface and steroid-eluting capability that reduces stimulation thresholds, decreases current drain, and improves sensing. The electrodes are connected to the connecter pin at the proximal end of the leads by the conductor wires that are usually made of Elgiloy (alloy of nickel). The materials used for insulation of the pacing leads are of 2 varieties, silicone rubber and polyurethane. Polyurethane insulation has the advantage of having high tear strength, low friction, and smaller diameter and are relatively nonthrombogenic compared to silicone-insulated leads.

The most commonly used transvenous endocardial leads have either a passive or an active fixation mechanism to avoid early dislodgement. The passive fixation mechanisms include tines, fins, or wings that are entrapped within the trabeculae of the right side of the heart chambers and are subsequently covered by fibrous tissue. Although several different fixation mechanisms such as screws, barbs, or hooks have been developed, most contemporary active fixation leads use an extendable/retractable screw mechanism. The active fixation leads allow precise positioning of the pacing lead in locations other than the right atrial appendage or right ventricular apex. They reduce the acute dislodgement rates of the right atrial leads and are also easier to extract compared to the passive fixation leads.

#### PACEMAKER IMPLANTATION

Almost all pacemaker implantations are performed transvenously under local anesthesia and conscious sedation using the cephalic, subclavian, or axillary vein. Axillary vein access avoids the potential complication of compression damage to the leads inserted via medial subclavian puncture in the tight costoclavicular angle. It also provides easy access to the introduction of two or more leads compared to the cephalic vein or the subclavian vein approach. The pulse generator is usually placed in the upper pectoral region subcutaneously, and occasionally the pacemaker is implanted behind the pectoral muscle or behind the breast via an inframammary approach, especially in young women.

***Pacing Site*** The atrial lead is generally placed in the right atrial appendage, however, in patients with prior cardiac surgery, the atrial septum or the lateral wall is preferred. Atrial septal pacing and Bachmann's bundle pacing[53] have been tested in an attempt to reduce the frequency of episodes of atrial fibrillation. Similarly, dual-site atrial pacing with one atrial lead placed in the atrial appendage and a second atrial lead placed in or around the coronary sinus ostium has been shown to decrease the number of episodes of paroxysmal atrial fibrillation and increase the interval to recurrence.[54] The ventricular lead is typically placed in the right ventricular apex. However, attempts to maintain the normal sequence of ventricular activation by high septal pacing near the His-bundle and right ventricular outflow

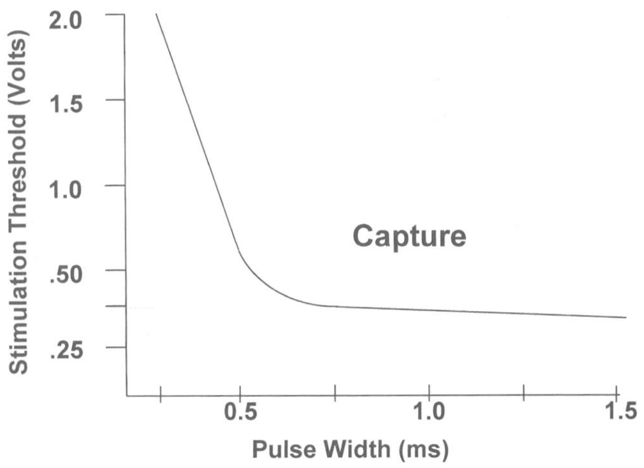


FIGURE 32-10 Strength-duration curve. This curve is obtained by plotting the voltage threshold obtained at various pulse widths. When programming the pacemaker output, this curve should be considered to ensure at least two times the safety margin. Increasing the pulse width beyond 0.6 ms generally does not decrease the voltage threshold.

tract, especially in patients with cardiomyopathies, have suggested hemodynamic benefits by improving cardiac output compared to right ventricular apical pacing.[55] With the advent of biventricular pacing for hemodynamic improvement in patients with advanced heart failure and intraventricular conduction disturbances, the left ventricular lead is placed in the posterior or lateral vein of the left ventricle through the coronary sinus. Epicardial pacing via thoracotomy has to be considered in occasional patients with inadequate venous access or mechanical prosthetic tricuspid valve, in patients undergoing cardiac surgery, in patients with right to left shunting, and in patients who have failed transvenous left ventricular lead placement.

***Pacing Threshold and Sensing*** Atrial and ventricular leads are placed into the appropriate chambers after ensuring adequate pacing and sensing thresholds. The basic premise in obtaining acute pacing and sensing thresholds during implant is that these thresholds may degenerate over time, and adequate safety margins need to be maintained to ensure safe long-term pacing and sensing. Pacing threshold is obtained by fixing the pulse width at 0.5 ms and reducing the voltage until the lowest voltage that achieves constant pacing. Alternatively, the voltage can be fixed and the pulse width decreased gradually to obtain the lowest pulse width that maintains constant pacing. It is essential to understand the strength-duration curve (Fig. 32-10). The strength-duration curve for stimulation is the quantity of voltage required to stimulate the heart at a series of pulse widths. As shown in the figure, increasing the pulse width beyond 0.6 ms usually does not decrease the voltage threshold. At implant, an atrial pacing threshold of <1.5 V and ventricular threshold of <1 V should be obtained. The threshold commonly rises over the next 2 to 4 weeks, reaches a peak, and then decreases to a chronic threshold level after 6 to 8 weeks. With steroid-eluting leads, the acute rise in threshold is ameliorated and the chronic threshold is significantly lower than is the nonsteroid-eluting leads.[56] During initial programming, the pacing output is programmed at 3 to 5 times the threshold voltage with a pulse width of 0.4 to 0.5 ms. At the 2- to 3-month follow-up visit, the output is decreased to no less than twice the threshold in order to maintain an adequate safety margin and to prevent battery drain. Some newer pacemakers have the ability to confirm capture on a beat-by-beat basis.[57] Using algorithms to automatically check pacing-capture thresholds, these pacers adjust pacing voltages to just above the pacing threshold in order to reduce current drain and prolong battery longevity.

Sensing is usually measured as the peak-to-peak or base-to-peak amplitude of the intracardiac electrogram in millivolts. The ventricular electrograms should measure at least 5 mV and frequently measure in excess of 10 to 20 mV. Ventricular sensitivity (the level in millivolts that the intracardiac electrogram has to exceed in order to be sensed by the device) is generally programmed between 2 to 3 mV so that an adequate safety margin exists for sensing intrinsic ventricular depolarization without the risk of oversensing T waves or other artifacts. Atrial electrograms are lower in amplitude than ventricular electrograms; however, a minimum atrial electrogram of 1 to 2 mV should be obtained. In patients with paroxysmal atrial fibrillation or flutter, the atrial electrogram during tachycardia might be smaller than during sinus rhythm. The atrial sensitivity is usually programmed at 0.5 mV, however, the sensitivity may have to be adjusted depending on the size of the far-field ventricular electrogram and associated atrial arrhythmias.

***Impedance*** Lead impedance is the resistance to the flow of current from the generator to the myocardial tissue through the lead. Although there is a wide variability of normal lead impedances (250 to 1200 Ω), chronic lead impedances should not vary widely between outpatient follow-up visits. A fractured lead exhibits markedly elevated lead impedance. Insulation breaks manifest by reduced lead impedances. Lead fractures or insulation breaks often are intermittent problems. Therefore, normal lead impedances and pacing and sensing thresholds do not rule out these problems. The leads can be stressed by having the patient change position and do various provocative arm movements (e.g., isometric exercise) to facilitate diagnosis of lead-related problems that are not otherwise observed.

## PACEMAKER NOMENCLATURE

The North American Society of Pacing and Electrophysiology (NASPE) and the British Pacing and Electrophysiology Group (BPEG) have established a 5-letter pacemaker code to describe the basic pacemaker mode and function (Table 32-12).[58] The first letter

TABLE 32-12 The Pacemaker Code

| I<br>Chamber-Paced | II<br>Chamber-Sensed | III<br>Response to Sensing | IV<br>Programmability/Rate Response | V<br>Antitachycardia Function(s) |
|---|---|---|---|---|
| O (None) | O (None) | O (None) | O (None) | O (None) |
| A (Atrium) | A (Atrium) | I (Inhibit) | R (Rate responsive) | P (Antitachycardia pacing) |
| V (Ventricle) | V (Ventricle) | T (Triggered) | P (simple programmable) | S (Shock) |
| D (Dual) | D (Dual) | D (I + T) | M (Multiprogrammable) | D (P + S) |
| S (Single Chamber) | S (Single Chamber) | | C (Communicating) | |

represents the chamber being paced: *A* for atrium, *V* for ventricle, and *D* for both atrium and ventricle. The second letter refers to the chamber in which sensing occurs: codes are similar to the first position. The third position describes the response of the pacemaker to a sensed event: *I* for inhibition, *T* for triggered, and *D* for both inhibition and triggering. The pacemaker can either inhibit (I) pacing output from one or both of its leads, or it can trigger (T) pacing after the sensed event. In a DDD pacemaker, a sensed atrial event inhibits the atrial pacing channel and triggers ventricular pacing after a programmable AV delay. The fourth position refers to the programmability of the device: *R* for rate-responsive pacing; the letters *C* (communicating), *P* (simple programmable), and *M* (multiprogrammable) are obsolete as all current devices are fully programmable. The fifth position refers to antitachycardia function; with the evolution of implantable defibrillators this position is rarely used. With the evolution of biventricular pacemakers, the pacemaker code currently in practice needs to be revised.

## Pacing Modes

### VVI MODE

As the pacemaker code indicates, the ventricle is the chamber sensed and paced, with inhibition of ventricular pacing in response to a sensed ventricular event. A sensed or paced ventricular event initiates two timing cycles:

1. A refractory period that is programmable (ventricular refractory period) during which period no ventricular sensing occurs in order to prevent inappropriate sensing of T waves. Any ventricular event occurring during this interval will also not reset the timing cycle.
2. A lower rate interval (LRI), which corresponds to the programmed pacing rate. If there is no sensed ventricular event following the end of the ventricular refractory period and this interval expires, the pacemaker initiates a paced ventricular event. If a ventricular event is sensed following the ventricular refractory period, the pacemaker resets the timing cycle to begin a new LRI and VRP (see Fig. 32-11).

Hysteresis is a programmable function in which the ventricular escape interval is longer after a sensed ventricular event than it is after a paced ventricular event. This feature can be used in patients with sinus rhythm so that VVI pacing would not initiate until the sinus rate drops below the hysteresis rate, which is lower than the pacemaker rate.

VVI pacing is the most commonly used pacing mode. Although it is a simple pacing mode and offers protection against bradyarrhythmias, loss of AV synchrony is not well tolerated in many patients and may lead to pacemaker syndrome (discussed later in the chapter). In patients with chronic atrial fibrillation, this is an ideal pacing mode, especially if rate-responsiveness is available.

### AAI MODE

Similar to VVI mode, sensing and pacing occurs in the atrium, with the atrial pacing channel inhibited in response to a sensed atrial activity. An atrial refractory period (ARP) and an LRI are initiated in response to a sensed or paced atrial event. AAIR pacing with rate-responsiveness is an excellent pacing mode in patients with sinus node dysfunction and normal AV conduction. Atrial pacing has been shown to be superior to ventricular pacing in terms of reducing the future incidence of atrial fibrillation.[25] Patients with sinus node dysfunction may develop AV block, which may be a source of concern when using AAI pacing. However, with careful selection of patients, including normal P-R intervals, absence of bundle branch block, and AV Wenckebach phenomenon occurring at atrial pacing rates of more than 120 bpm, the risk of development of second- or third-degree AV block is less than 0.6 percent per year.[59] Another concern with AAI pacing mode is that if the far-field ventricular signal is large enough, it may inhibit the atrial channel. This can be overcome by decreasing the atrial sensitivity or by prolonging the atrial refractory period.

### VOO/AOO MODES

In these asynchronous pacing modes, there is no sensing. The chamber is paced asynchronously at the lower rate limit. The timing cycle consists of only an LRI and will not be reset by any intrinsic activity. Since there is no sensing, there are no refractory periods. This mode is rarely used except during procedures utilizing constant electrocautery in order to avoid inhibition of pacing caused by sensing of the high-frequency impulses of electrocautery. When a magnet is applied over the pulse generator, the pacemaker switches to an asynchronous mode (VVI to VOO, DDD to DOO). The obvious disadvantage of this pacing mode is the possibility of asynchronous pacing during the vulnerable period and initiation of either atrial or ventricular fibrillation (extremely rare).

### DDI MODE

This mode behaves as both AAI and VVI modes combined. In this mode, although sensing and pacing occur in both chambers, the response to sensing is inhibition only, as a result of which there will not be ventricular tracking of P waves. Atrial sensing will not initiate an AV interval (AVI). Atrial pacing at the lower rate limit will initiate an AVI and AV sequential pacing. In patients with atrial tachyarrhythmias, this mode will prevent rapid ventricular pacing as there will be no ventricular tracking of atrial arrhythmias at the upper rate limit as in DDD mode. This mode is rarely programmed as the primary mode of choice, but can be used as the fallback mode during the mode switch for atrial tachyarrhythmias.

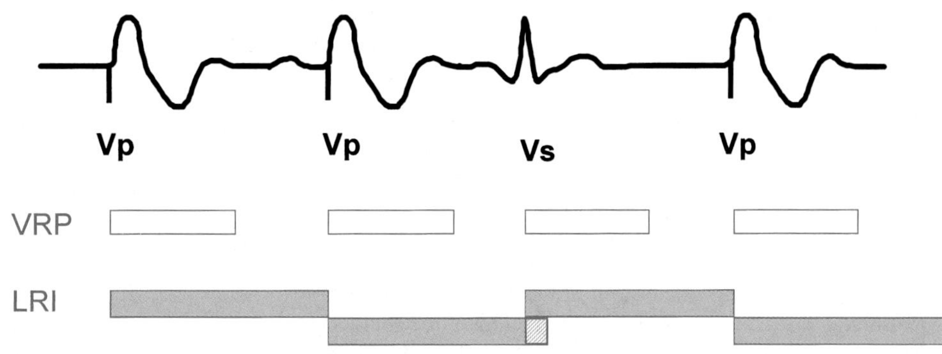


FIGURE 32-11 Single-chamber ventricular inhibited pacing mode. The first two beats are ventricular-paced (Vp) events. The third beat is a ventricular-sensed (Vs) event. A Vs or Vp event starts a lower rate interval (LRI) at the end of which ventricular pacing is initiated. A sensed- or paced-event also initiates a ventricular refractory period (VRP) during which no sensing will occur. The LRI following a sensed-event can be separately programmed at a longer interval to allow for native rhythm. This is called *hysteresis*.

**VDD MODE**

In this mode, the pacemaker paces only the ventricle, senses in both the atrium and the ventricle, and responds to atrial sensing with ventricular pacing. The ventricular channel will also be inhibited by spontaneous ventricular activity. A sensed atrial event will start an AVI followed by ventricular pacing. If spontaneous AV conduction occurs before the termination of the AVI, ventricular pacing will be inhibited. If there is no spontaneous atrial activity, ventricular pacing will occur at the lower rate limit as in a VVI pacemaker. However, as there is no atrial pacing, this mode should not be used in patients with sinus node dysfunction. In patients with normal sinus node function and AV block, this is an excellent mode choice. A single lead with two distal electrodes capable of bipolar ventricular sensing and pacing and a floating proximal electrode for atrial sensing is currently available for VDD pacing systems.

**DDD MODE**

A DDD pacemaker senses and paces in both the atrium and the ventricle, and the response to sensing involves both inhibition and triggered output. The DDD pacemaker utilizes numerous timing cycles, and it is essential to understand the following intervals. Most timing cycles are ventricular based and are explained as such.

The LRI starts with a sensed or paced ventricular event and ends with a paced ventricular event, and consists of two portions. The ventricular event initiates an atrial escape interval (AEI) or VA interval at the end of which atrial pacing is initiated. The atrial paced or sensed event initiates the AVI at the end of which ventricular pacing is initiated. So, LRI = VA + AVI. A sensed atrial event occurring before the completion of the VA interval terminates this interval and starts the AVI. A sensed ventricular event occurring before the completion of the AVI will terminate this interval and the lower rate interval and reinitiate the LRI. A sensed or paced ventricular event will also initiate the ventricular refractory period (VRP) to avoid T wave oversensing and simultaneously initiates the postventricular atrial refractory period (PVARP). The postventricular atrial refractory period helps prevent the sensing and tracking of any retrograde P waves. This refractory period is programmable and is essential to the prevention of pacemaker mediated, endless-loop tachycardia, which is an arrhythmia where the dual chamber pacemaker serves as the antegrade limb and the patient's retrograde conduction as the retrograde limb. The AVI and the PVARP together constitute the total atrial refractory period (TARP) during which period the atrial channel remains refractory and will not be tracked. This in essence determines the upper rate interval (URI) or the maximal tracking rate interval (MTRI) in a DDD pacemaker.

In patients with DDD pacemakers, four different rhythm scenarios are possible, and many patients exhibit more than one scenario:

1. Normal sinus rhythm with no atrial or ventricular pacing: Here the patient's rate is faster than the programmed lower rate of the pacemaker and the native PR interval is shorter than the programmed AVI as a result of which both the atrial and ventricular channels are inhibited (Fig. 32-12A).
2. Atrial sensed, ventricular pacing: The patient's atrial rate is faster than the lower rate limit and the AV conduction interval is longer than the programmed AVI or there is no AV conduction resulting in sensing of P waves and triggering of the ventricular channel after the programmed AVI. In this situation the patient is ventricularly paced at the patient's sinus rate until the upper rate limit (Fig. 32-12B).
3. Atrial paced and ventricular sensed: In this situation the patient's atrial rate is slower than the programmed lower rate and the patient's AV conduction interval shorter than the programmed AVI. Here the patient is atrially paced at the lower rate limit (Fig. 32-12C).
4. Atrial and ventricular pacing: Here the sinus rate is slower than the lower rate limit and AV conduction is longer or absent resulting in atrial and ventricular pacing at the lower rate limit (Fig. 32-12D).

## Atrioventricular Interval

The AVI following a sensed atrial event is usually programmed to a shorter value than the AVI following a paced atrial event and is termed *differential AVI*. Some DDD pacemakers also have the added capability of shortening the AVI with increase in heart rates and is called *dynamic, or rate-adaptive, AVI*. Another available feature in modern pacemakers is AV hysteresis, in which the device periodically increases the AVI to allow native AV conduction and intrinsic ventricular activation. The paced AVI is considered as a single interval with two subportions. The initial interval is the blanking period (12 to 50 ms, programmable) during which the ventricular channel is blanked in order to avoid ventricular sensing of the atrial pacing artifact. If a spontaneous ventricular event occurs in this period it will not be sensed. The second portion of the AVI is the crosstalk sensing window during which a ventricular event will be sensed if it occurs and will lead to ventricular safety pacing with a shorter AVI of 100 to 110 ms. This is to avoid "cross talk" or inhibition of the ventricular channel by sensing of the atrial pacing artifact (Fig. 32-13).

## Upper Rate Behavior

In VDD and DDD modes, in addition to the programmed lower rate limit, there is an upper rate limit beyond which ventricular tracking of atrial events will not occur. When the atrial rate exceeds the programmed upper rate limit the pacemaker will exhibit either Wenckebach or 2:1 AV block behavior. When the patient with complete heart block exercises to a sinus rate beyond the upper rate limit of the pacemaker, the P wave that is sensed will be followed by ventricular pacing with prolongation of the AVI beyond the programmed value, in order to not violate the upper rate limit for pacing. When one of the subsequent P waves falls in the postventricular atrial refractory period, it will not be tracked resulting in *pacemaker* Wenckebach behavior (Fig. 32-14). When the atrial rate increases further such that every other P wave falls in the total atrial refractory period (TARP), 2:1 pacemaker AV block pattern occurs. The TARP should be programmed shorter than the upper rate interval to prevent sudden development of 2:1 pacemaker AV block.

In young patients with complete heart block, the upper rate of the pacemaker should be programmed to faster rates corrected for the patient's age to prevent Wenckebach behavior of the pacemaker during exercise. Programming dynamic AVI and dynamic PVARP will allow the TARP to be shorter at higher pacing rates and avoid sudden slowing of ventricular pacing rates. Another option is rate-responsive features where a separately programmable sensor rate will allow the pacemaker to continue to pace at the sensor-driven rate during exercise.

## Mode Switch

When pacemaker patients with AV block (in DDD or VDD mode) develop atrial tachyarrhythmias (atrial tachycardia, flutter or fibrillation), many of the atrial events will be sensed and ventricular tracking will occur up to the programmed upper rate of the device. The surface ECG typically shows an irregular ventricular paced rhythm at

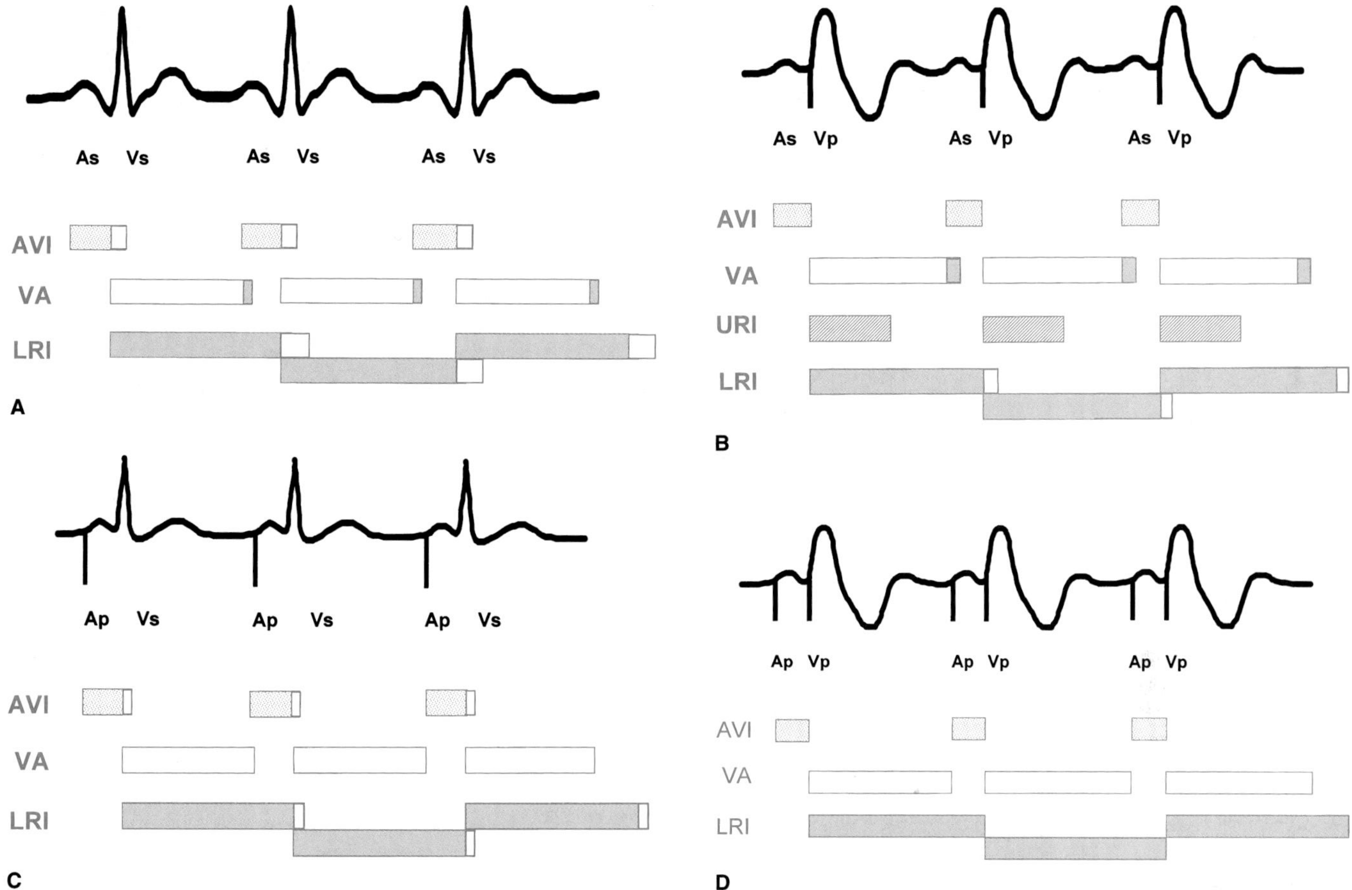


FIGURE 32-12 *A*. DDD pacing mode: atrial- and ventricular-sensed. In this example, atrial-sensed activity (As) initiates an atrioventricular interval (AVI) and normal conduction results in a ventricular-sensed (Vs) event that terminates the AV interval and the lower rate interval (LRI) and initiates an LRI and the atrial escape interval (VA). Spontaneous atrial activity (As) again terminates the VA interval and starts a new AV interval. *B*. DDD pacing mode: atrial-sensed ventricular pacing. In this example, the atrial-sensed (As) event leads to ventricular pacing (Vp) at the completion of the programmed AV interval (AVI), as there is no native AV conduction to the ventricle. The Vp event starts the VA interval, the lower rate interval (LRI), and the upper rate interval (URI). The VA and the LRIs are terminated by the spontaneous atrial activity that starts a new AV interval. *C*. DDD pacing mode: atrial-paced–ventricular-sensed. In this example, atrial pacing (Ap) starts the AV interval (AVI), but is terminated by the ventricular event that occurs prior to the completion of the AV interval. The Vs event initiates the atrial escape interval (VA) and the lower rate interval (LRI). If there is no spontaneous atrial activity, the VA interval times out and atrial pacing occurs. *D*. DDD pacing mode: atrial- and ventricular-paced. The atrial-paced (Ap) event starts the AV interval (AVI), at the completion of which the ventricle is paced (Vp) since there is no spontaneous ventricular activity. The Vp event initiates the atrial escape interval (VA) and results in atrial pacing as there is no spontaneous atrial activity. Both Ap and Vp occur at the lower rate limit (LRI).

rates close to the upper rate limit of the device. Occasionally in patients with slower atrial flutter, every other atrial electrogram may fall in the PVARP resulting in 2:1 AV block. In patients with intact conduction, the ventricular rates will be determined by the patient's intrinsic AV conduction.

In patients with persistent atrial tachyarrhythmias, reprogramming the pacemaker to DDI(R) or VVI(R) mode will avoid rapid ventricular tracking of the atrial arrhythmias. Automatic mode switching is a programmable option in all current generation pacemakers for patients with paroxysmal atrial tachyarrhythmias (Fig. 32-15). When the atrial rate exceeds the programmed mode switch rate, the device automatically changes its mode to either the VVI or DDI mode in which ventricular tracking of atrial sensed events will not occur. Current devices can also provide a complete history of mode switch episodes with regard to the duration and frequency of these episodes and provide electrograms to confirm their nature. Arrhythmia logs from the device provide a very efficient way of assessing the effects of various drug therapies in patients with atrial fibrillation.

## Rate-Responsive Pacing

Rate-responsive pacing refers to the ability of the pacemaker to increase their lower rate in response to physiologic stimuli. Simple VVI and AAI pacemakers do not have the ability to increase their pacing rates in response to exercise. In patients with normal sinus node function and DDD pacemakers, the ventricular pacing rate increases in response to an increase in sinus rate and is physiologic. However, in the presence of sinus node dysfunction, the pacing rate will not increase commensurate with the increase in physiologic need. Rate-responsive pacemakers provide the ability to increase pacing rates through special sensors incorporated in the pacing system that monitor various physiologic processes. Based on information from the sensors, the lower rate of the pacemakers constantly varies up to the upper sensor rate. At any point in time the sensor rate overrides the programmed lower rate of the pacemaker. Rate-responsive pacing is available in most current pacemakers in VVIR, AAIR, DDIR, and DDDR modes. In patients with sinus node dysfunction, rate-responsive pacing in AAIR, DDIR, or DDDR mode is

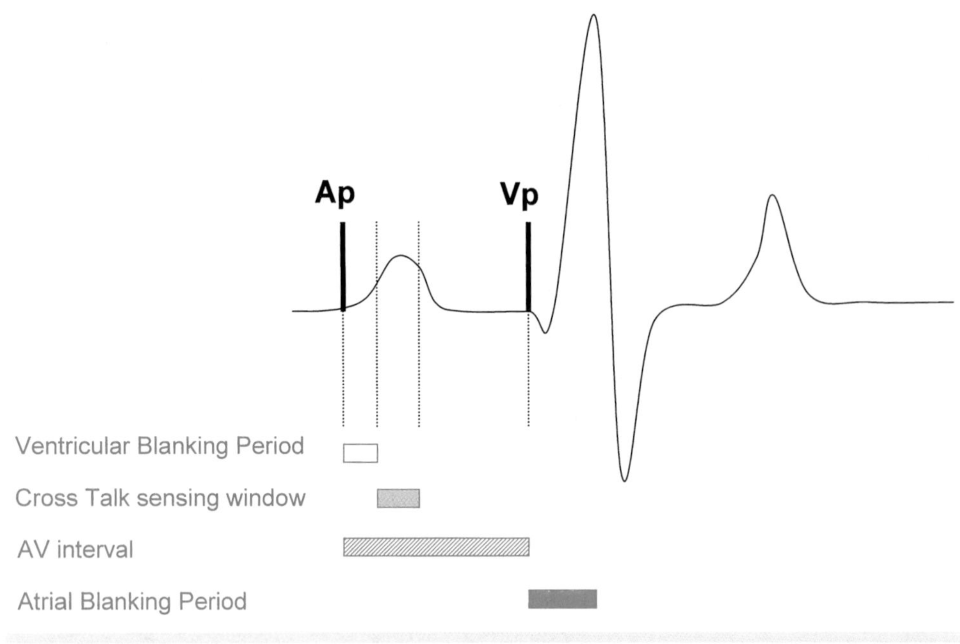


FIGURE 32-13 Atrioventricular (AV) interval and blanking periods. The AV interval following atrial pacing has two subportions. During the initial ventricular blanking period, sensing is suspended to avoid ventricular sensing of the leading edge of the atrial pacing artifact. During the second portion (crosstalk sensing window), if ventricular activity is sensed, ventricular pacing will occur with a shorter AV delay. The purpose of this safety feature (ventricular safety pacing) is to avoid inhibition of the ventricular channel by sensing of the atrial pacing artifact during this time window. Similar to the ventricular blanking period, there is an atrial blanking period following ventricular pacing, during which sensing is suspended in the atrial channel to avoid atrial oversensing of the far-field ventricular pacing artifact.

preferable to non-sensor-driven pacing. Also in patients with chronic atrial fibrillation and heart block, VVIR pacing is preferable to VVI pacing. In patients with severe coronary artery disease, it may be necessary to limit the programmed upper rate limit. The ideal mode for pacing is decided based on information regarding sinus node function, AV nodal function, atrial arrhythmias, and heart rate response to exercise (Fig. 32-16).

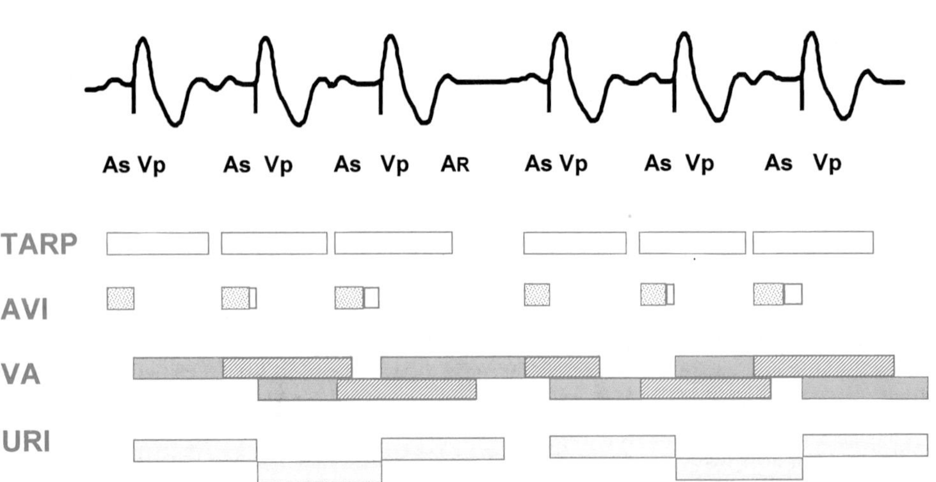


FIGURE 32-14 DDD pacemaker: Wenckebach behavior at upper rate limit. The first beat shows the ventricular paced (Vp) event synchronized to the atrial-sensed (As) event at the programmed AV interval (AVI). The next atrial event initiates an AVI, but when the AVI times out, the upper rate limit has not been satisfied so the AVI is prolonged. When the upper rate limit is satisfied, ventricular pacing occurs. Due to the delayed ventricular pacing, the next P wave falls even earlier into the next cardiac cycle and the AVI extension is even greater. The next P wave falls within the total atrial refractory period (TARP) and is not sensed. This atrial event is labeled AR and is not followed by ventricular pacing. The following P wave occurs before the VA interval expires and tracking occurs at the programmed AV delay since the upper rate limit cannot be exceeded.

## RATE-RESPONSIVE SENSORS

An ideal rate-responsive pacing system should provide rate response that is appropriate for the metabolic demand during a wide range of activities. The optimal sensor should provide the following:

- Proportionate increase in heart rate to match increase in metabolic demand
- Appropriate rapid change in heart rate with exercise onset
- High sensitivity and specificity
- Appropriate slowing of heart rate following exercise

Sensors available or under development can be classified using a physiologic or technical classification system. In physiologic classification,[60] the sensors are classified according to the physiologic level at which they sense (Table 32-13). A primary sensor detects a physiologic factor that modulates sinus node function such as catecholamine levels or autonomic nervous system activity. A secondary sensor detects physiologic factors such as QT interval, minute ventilation, venous temperature, and pH, which are the consequences of exercise. A tertiary sensor detects the external changes such as vibration or acceleration that result from exercise.

***Activity Sensors*** Activity-based sensors using piezoelectric crystals or accelerometers to detect vibration are the most widely used sensors. While the piezoelectric crystal senses vibration associated with up–down motion, the accelerometer detects anteroposterior motion of the body. Accelerometer-based sensors provide adequate and quick increases in heart rate during treadmill exercise as compared to that of piezoelectric crystals. While both sensors have been shown to provide excellent rate-responsiveness, direct manual pressure, walking down stairs, horseback riding, or riding on a bumpy street can cause an inappropriate increase in heart rate with the piezoelectric crystal-based sensor. These activity-based sensors do not provide adequate heart rate response with emotional stress or isometric exercises.

***Minute-Ventilation Sensor*** The specificity and sensitivity of minute-ventilation sensing pacemakers for changes in metabolic workload are excellent. Current pulses (1-mA at 15-$\mu s$ duration) are emitted from the pacemaker can, and the proximal ring electrode of the right ventricular lead and

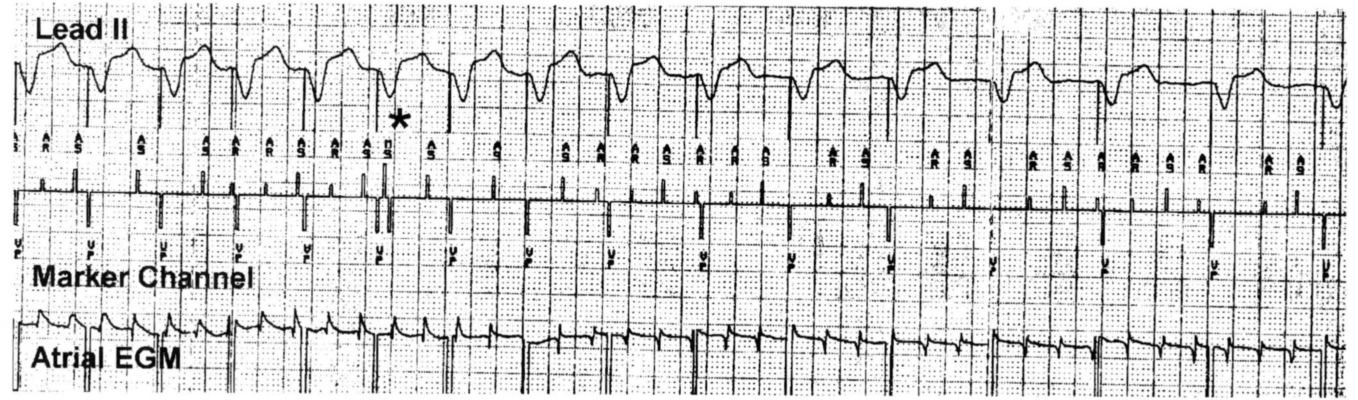


FIGURE 32-15 Mode switch behavior of DDD pacemaker during atrial flutter. Surface lead II, marker channel, and atrial electrograms (EGMs) are shown. In the beginning of the tracing, atrial flutter is sensed and the ventricle is paced at, but does not exceed the upper rate limit of 110 bpm. Once atrial tachyarrhythmia detection criteria are met, mode switch occurs (*). Pacemaker switches mode to DDI (no atrial tracking) at 70 bpm with rate-smoothing function to avoid an abrupt change in pacing rate.

transthoracic impedances are measured every 50 ms. Measurement of phasic impedance changes provides respiratory rate and tidal volume information and thus the minute ventilation is determined. The minute ventilation changes are used to calculate the pacing rate and have excellent correlation with exercise. Minute-ventilation sensing pacemakers can increase inappropriately pacing rates with hyperventilation, coughing, and mechanical ventilation and in patients with chronic obstructive pulmonary disease exacerbations.

***QT-Interval Sensors*** This sensor measures the interval from the onset of a paced QRS complex to the end of the T wave, which is affected by autonomic activity and heart rate. The device uses the change in stimulus-T interval to calculate the sensor rate. This sensor has been used for many years and has proven to be an excellent sensor providing appropriate and specific heart rate response. The QT sensor does not respond well to emotion or non-exercise-related stress.

A number of other sensors are available or under development. Physiologic parameters such as central venous temperature, venous pH, mixed venous $O_2$ saturation, stroke volume, and change in right ventricular pressure (dP/dt) have been utilized as sensors. Most of these sensors require a special lead capable of measuring these parameters. Although these sensors have shown clinical potential, they have not achieved popularity.

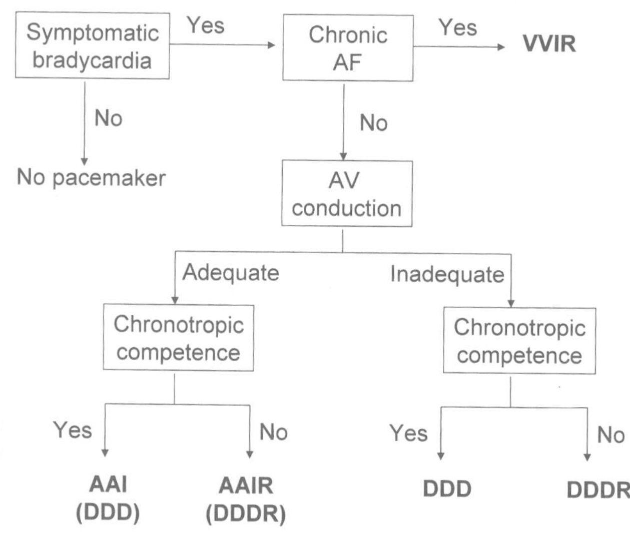


FIGURE 32-16 Pacemaker mode selection. AF, atrial fibrillation; AV, atrioventricular.

***Dual Sensors*** Most of the currently available sensors have an excellent track record, although they may occasionally respond to nonphysiologic stimuli. A multisensor rate-responsive pacemaker can improve specificity by having one sensor verify the other sensor (e.g., sensor cross-checking). A combination of two sensors can better simulate the normal sinus node response. Both sensors have to indicate a need for rate-response to allow an increase in sensor-driven heart rate. Some sensors systems provide the advantage of more physiologic pacing during steady state but have a slow response time during initiation of exercise. Other sensors, particularly activity sensors, have faster response times at initiation of activity but may not produce physiologic responses during peak or steady-state activity. Pacers with dual sensors can provide patients with rapid responses during the start of exercise to augment the heart rate and then use a more physiologic sensor (QT, minute ventilation) to provide more proportional heart rate responses during steady state (e.g., sensor blending).[61] Dual-sensor rate-responsive pacemakers are increasingly used now, with the most common combinations being the minute ventilation with activity or the QT interval with activity sensor.

***Programming Rate-Responsive Parameters*** Every patient who is programmed to a rate-responsive mode must be functionally assessed to determine whether the rate-response to the sensors is appropriate. Most patients who cannot perform standard treadmill exercise testing are asked to walk in the corridor at a casual pace for 2 min on the morning after the implant. The rate-response should be reassessed in the outpatient clinic in 3 months and as needed. Different pacemakers have different algorithms that can automate the adjustments of the rate-responsiveness.

## Indications for Pacing

The guidelines of the ACC and the AHA and the North American Society of Pacing and Electrophysiology for the implantation of pacemakers were revised and updated on 2002. The indications for permanent pacing can be considered in categories of bradyarrhythmia and nonbradyarrhythmia. The bradyarrhythmic indications were discussed in the earlier part of this chapter.

TABLE 32-13 Physiologic Classification of Sensors

| Type | Description | Physiologic Parameters |
|---|---|---|
| **Primary** | Physiologic factors that modulate sinus function | Catecholamine level<br>Autonomic nervous system activity |
| **Secondary** | Physiologic parameters that are the consequence of exercise | QT,* respiratory rate*<br>Minute ventilation,* temperature*<br>pH, stroke volume<br>Preejection interval, $Sv_{O_2}$<br>Peak endocardial acceleration |
| **Tertiary** | External changes that result from exercise | Vibration*<br>Acceleration* |

*Available clinically.

## Pacing for Nonbradyarrhythmic Indications

### PACING TO PREVENT OR TERMINATE TACHYARRHYTHMIAS

Pacing can be useful in preventing and terminating tachyarrhythmias. The long QT syndrome is characterized by abnormally prolonged ventricular repolarization with the tendency to develop pause dependent ventricular arrhythmias (torsades de pointes), syncope, and sudden death. In patients with long QT syndrome, recurrent pause-dependent VT may be prevented by continuous pacing and pacing, in addition to beta blockade has been shown to shorten QT interval and prevent sudden death in high-risk patients.[62]

Reentrant supraventricular arrhythmias such as AV node reentrant tachycardia, AV reentrant tachycardia, and atrial flutter may be terminated by a variety of pacing methods that include programmed stimulation and short bursts of rapid overdrive pacing.[63] These antitachycardia pacemakers must detect a tachyarrhythmia and then spontaneously initiate an antitachycardia pacing algorithm, or they can be programmed to respond to external magnet application. With significant advancement and success with catheter ablation techniques, the need for pacemaker therapy to treat supraventricular arrhythmias has virtually vanished.

For patients with sick sinus syndrome and heart block, atrial pacing has been shown to be more effective than ventricular pacing to prevent atrial fibrillation[25,27,64] The Canadian Trial of Physiologic Pacing prospectively followed 2568 patients with symptomatic bradycardia who had either dual-chamber or ventricular pacemaker implantations. Dual-chamber pacing significantly decreased the incidence of atrial fibrillation and progression to chronic atrial fibrillation.[26,65] There are several studies showing pacing from the interatrial septum[66] or from Bachman's bundle[67] decreases the incidence of paroxysmal and chronic atrial fibrillation. Atrial overdrive pacing has been shown in several studies to decrease the incidence and duration of episodes of atrial fibrillation,[68,69] while other investigators have been unable to show a benefit to atrial overdrive pacing.[70] Dual-site right atrial or biatrial pacing (right atrial appendage or interatrial septum and coronary sinus) have been used to prevent atrial fibrillation in drug refractory patients. Dual site pacing probably decreases dispersion of atrial refractoriness, preexcites the abnormal atrial substrate, enhances atrial repolarization and recovery of atrial excitability, and thus theoretically reduces the window of opportunity for atrial fibrillation initiation. Saksena et al.[54] have shown in a crossover study of 120 patients with atrial fibrillation, long-term dual-site atrial pacing combined with antiarrhythmic drugs reduced the incidence of atrial fibrillation by 34 percent. Further trials are ongoing to determine the best pacing approach for the prevention of atrial fibrillation. The indications for pacemaker therapy to prevent or treat tachyarrhythmias are shown in Table 32-14.

### PACING IN DILATED CARDIOMYOPATHY

Permanent dual-chamber pacing with a short AV delay and a conventional pacemaker (ventricular lead in the right ventricular apex) was initially proposed a decade ago as adjuvant treatment of advanced heart failure.[71] However, initially encouraging results were not confirmed in several subsequent, small randomized, prospective studies.[72,73,74] Bakker and colleagues first suggested a clinical benefit from biventricular pacing in heart failure patients with intraventricular conduction disorder.[75] Thereafter, biventricular pacing has been studied in a number of acute and short-term studies followed by many prospective, randomized trials,[76,77,78] the results of which are summarized in Table 32-15. Approximately 30 percent of the patients with chronic heart failure

TABLE 32-14 Indications for Pacing to Prevent or Terminate Tachycardias

**Class I**

1. Sustained pause-dependent ventricular tachycardia, with or without prolonged QT, in which the efficacy of pacing is thoroughly documented. (Level of evidence: C)

**Class IIa**

1. High-risk patients with congenital long-QT syndrome. (Level of evidence: C)
2. Symptomatic recurrent supraventricular tachycardia that is reproducibly terminated by pacing in the unlikely event that catheter ablation and/or drugs fail to control the arrhythmia or produce intolerable side effects. (Level of evidence: C)

**Class IIb**

1. Recurrent SVT or atrial flutter that is reproducibly terminated by pacing as an alternative to drug therapy or ablation. (Level of evidence: C)
2. AV reentrant or AV node-reentrant supraventricular tachycardia not responsive to medical or ablative therapy. (Level of evidence: C)
3. Prevention of symptomatic, drug refractory recurrent atrial fibrillation in patients with coexisting sinus node dysfunction. (Level of evidence: B)

**Class III**

1. Tachycardias frequently accelerated or converted to fibrillation by pacing.
2. The presence of accessory pathways with the capacity for rapid anterograde conduction whether or not the pathways participate in the mechanism of the tachycardia.
3. Frequent or complex ventricular ectopic activity without sustained VT in the absence of the long QT syndrome.
4. Torsade de pointes VT due to reversible causes.

TABLE 32-15 Trials of Biventricular Pacing for Heart Failure (Completed)

| Study | Inclusion Criteria | Design | Endpoints | Results |
|---|---|---|---|---|
| **PATH-CHF**[78] Pacing therapies in congestive heart failure | NYHA class II-IV QRS > 120 ms Sinus rate > 55 bpm | Longitudinal study with second placebo control phase. First and third period are crossover between BiV and LV pacing ($n$ = 42) | Primary: Peak $VO_2$, Peak $VO_2$ at anaerobic threshold, 6-min walk; secondary: QOL, hospitalization, NYHA class | CRT improved functional capacity, QOL and functional status |
| **InSync**[79] | NYHA class III-IV, LVEF < 35% QRS >150 ms, LVEDD > 60 mm Pacing indication allowed | Prospective longitudinal trial ($n$ = 103) | Primary: 6-min walk, ORS width; secondary: QOL, NYHA class | CRT improved functional class, QOL and 6-min walk |
| **MUSTIC SR**[84] Multisite Stimulation in Cardiomyopathy Sinus Rhythm | NYHA class III, LVEF < 35% LVEDD > 60 mm, QRS > 150 ms 6-min walk < 450 m, NSR | Prospective, randomized, single-blind crossover study ($n$ = 67) | Primary: 6-min walk, QOL, NYHA class; secondary: Hospitalization, peak $VO_2$ | Improved 6-min walk, QOL, peak $VO_2$ and reduced hospitalizations. Patients preferred biventricular pacing |
| **MUSTIC AF**[80] Multisite Stimulation in Cardiomyopathy Atrial Fibrillation | NYHA class III, LVEF < 35% LVEDD > 60 mm, QRS > 150 ms 6-min walk <450 m, AF | Prospective, randomized, single-blind crossover study ($n$ = 64) | Primary: 6-min walk, QOL, NYHA class; secondary: Hospitalization, peak $VO_2$ | Improved 6-min walk, QOL, peak $VO_2$ and reduced hospitalizations. Patients preferred biventricular pacing |
| **MIRACLE**[86] Multicenter InSync Randomized Clinical Evaluation | NYHA class III, LVEF < 35% LVEDD > 55 mm, QRS > 130 ms Stable 3-month regimen of BB and ACEI | Prospective, randomized, double-blind, parallel, controlled trial for 6 months ($n$ = 300) | Primary: 6-min walk, QOL, NYHA class, device and lead safety; secondary: Neurohormone levels, echo indices, peak $VO_2$ | Improved NYHA class, 6-min walk, QOL, LVEF, Ventricular volumes and mitral regurgitation |
| **InSync III**[92] | NYHA class III-IV, LVEDD > 55 mm, LVEF < 35%, QRS > 130 ms | Prospective, nonrandomized trial to evaluate safety and efficacy of InSync III device, OTW lead and programmable RV-LV timing | Safety and efficacy of InSync III device and over the wire (OTW) lead performance QOL, functional capacity | Device and lead safety confirmed. QOL, functional capacity and 6-min walk improved compared to historic control from MIRACLE |
| **VENTAK CHF/ CONTAK CD**[89] | NYHA class II-IV, LVEF < 35% QRS > 120 ms, ICD indication Normal sinus node | 6-month parallel, double-blind trial between CRT and no CRT, beginning 1 month after implant ($n$ = 581) | Primary: Effectiveness and safety of ICD + CRT Secondary: NYHA class, QOL, 6-min walk, peak $VO_2$ | Device safety confirmed; peak $VO_2$ improved; Class III and IV patients without RBBB showed QOL improvement |
| **InSync ICD**[88] | NYHA class II-IV, LVEF < 35% LVEDD > 55 mm, QRS > 130 ms ICD indication | Prospective, longitudinal trial to evaluate safety and efficacy of CRT in CHF patients with ICD indication ($n$ = 84) | Primary: 6-min walk, effectiveness and safety of ICD + CRT; Secondary: NYHA class, QOL | CRT − ICD safe to use; Improvement in endpoints for NYHA class III and IV only |
| **COMPANION**[90] Comparison of Medical Therapy Pacing and Defibrillation in Heart Failure | NYHA class III-IV, EF < 35% QRS > 120 ms, PR > 150 ms, no indication for pacer or ICD | Randomized, open-label, 3-arm study of optimal drug therapy, CRT and CRT-ICD ($n$ = 2200) | Combined all cause mortality and hospitalization, QOL, functional capacity, peak exercise performance | Terminated early after 1520 patients, with 40% reduction in mortality with CRT-ICD. Significant reduction in hospitalization in CRT and CRT-ICD groups |

ABBREVIATIONS: ACEI = angiotensin-converting enzyme inhibitor; AF = atrial fibrillation; BB = beta blocker; BiV = biventricular; CHF = congestive heart failure; CRT = cardiac resynchronization therapy; EF = ejection fraction; HF = heart failure; ICD = implantable cardioverter defibrillator; LV = left ventricle; LVEDD = left ventricle end diastolic diameter; NYHA = New York Heart Association; NSR = normal sinus rhythm; QOL = quality of life; RV = right ventricle; RBBB = right bundle branch block; $VO_2$ = oxygen uptake.

manifest intraventricular conduction disorder with QRS intervals longer than 130 ms.[79] Intraventricular conduction disturbances of the left bundle branch block type lead to delay in the activation of left ventricular free wall as compared to the septum and right ventricle resulting in intra- and interventricular mechanical dyssynchrony. Ventricular dyssynchrony is associated with paradoxical septal motion, decreased diastolic filling times, prolonged mitral regurgitation, and reduced left ventricular stroke volume. Biventricular pacing by simultaneous pacing of the right and left ventricle has been shown to coordinate the septal and the left ventricular free-wall contraction and decrease right and left atrial filling pressures and mitral regurgitation, as well as improve diastolic filling, cardiac output, and left ventricular ejection fraction in patients with severe left ventricular systolic dysfunction and prolonged IVCD.[80] Biventricular pacing also has been shown to reduce myocardial oxygen consumption with improvement in ventricular contraction.[81,82,83]

***Clinical Trials (Table 32-15)*** The Multisite Stimulation in Cardiomyopathy (MUSTIC) trial was the first randomized, prospective study of biventricular pacing.[84] There was a significant improvement in the 6-min walk distance, quality of life, and reduction in hospitalizations in the pacing group as compared to the nonpacing group.[84] In a long-term open-label follow-up of these patients, these significant clinical benefits were maintained at 24 months.[85] The Multicenter InSync Randomized Clinical Evaluation (MIRACLE) study was a prospective, randomized, placebo-controlled, double-blind trial involving 453 patients with class III–IV heart failure, left ventricular ejection fraction of 35 percent or less, and QRS duration of 130 ms or longer.[86] Patients who received biventricular pacing experienced significant improvement in the 6-min distance walked (+39 m vs +10 m, $p = 0.005$), functional class, quality of life, and ejection fraction (+4.6 vs −0.2 percent, $p < 0.001$). Both these trials showed significant clinical improvement in patients with biventricular pacing despite maximal medical therapy for congestive heart failure with beta blockers, diuretics, digoxin, and angiotensin-converting enzyme inhibitors.

Metanalysis pooling data from 4 studies showed that cardiac resynchronization therapy (CRT) reduced death from progressive heart failure by 51 percent compared to control (odds ratio, 0.49; 95 percent confidence interval, 0.25 to 0.93), and reduced heart failure hospitalization by 29 percent (odds ratio, 0.71; confidence interval, 0.53 to 0.96). CRT was not associated with a statistically significant effect on nonheart failure mortality or a reduction in the number of patients experiencing ventricular tachycardia or ventricular fibrillation.[87] Preliminary experience with a biventricular pacemaker in combination with an implantable cardioverter defibrillator (ICD) has been published.[88,89] The early termination of the COMPANION (*COMP*arison of Medic*A*l, Resynchronizatio*N*, and Defibrillat*ION* Therapies in Heart Failure) trial has answered the question regarding the mortality benefit of ICD therapy combined with biventricular pacing in this patient group.[90] The trial was terminated prematurely after enrolling almost 1600 patients, as initial results demonstrated that combined biventricular pacemaker-ICDs reduced mortality by 40 percent (from 19 to 11 percent) compared to optimal medical therapy, while biventricular pacemakers alone showed only a 15-percent reduction in mortality.

***Biventricular Pacemaker System*** In addition to the usual right atrial and right ventricular lead, the biventricular pacing system uses an additional lead to pace the left ventricle. A specifically designed lead with a lumen to allow for passage of the lead over a guidewire is placed in the coronary venous system and manipulated through the vein branches until an adequate site with acceptable pacing and sensing thresholds is located on the left ventricular epicardium. Acute data indicate that optimal hemodynamic response in most patients is obtained if the left ventricular lead is placed via the coronary sinus in a posterolateral, lateral, or anterolateral vein to provide resynchronization therapy.[76] Figure 32-17 demonstrates an occlusive venogram of the coronary sinus, showing great cardiac vein and branch vein anatomy. Chest x-rays in posteroanterior and lateral views of a patient with a biventricular pacemaker is shown in Fig. 32-18. Figure 32-19 demonstrates the ECGs of this patient in sinus rhythm with left bundle branch block and with biventricular stimulation, respectively. The preferred pacing mode is VDD, in which both ventricles are paced simultaneously following sensed atrial activity with a short AVI. The InSync III trial suggested a possible increased hemodynamic benefit with sequential biventricular pacing by varying the interventricular activation sequence compared to simultaneous biventricular pacing.[82] In order for this therapy to be effective, the patients have to maintain predominant ventricular pacing. Biventricular pacing has also been shown to improve functional status and heart failure symptoms in patients with chronic atrial fibrillation and AV-node ablation.[78,83] The current indications for pacing in patients with dilated cardiomyopathy are shown in Table 32-16.

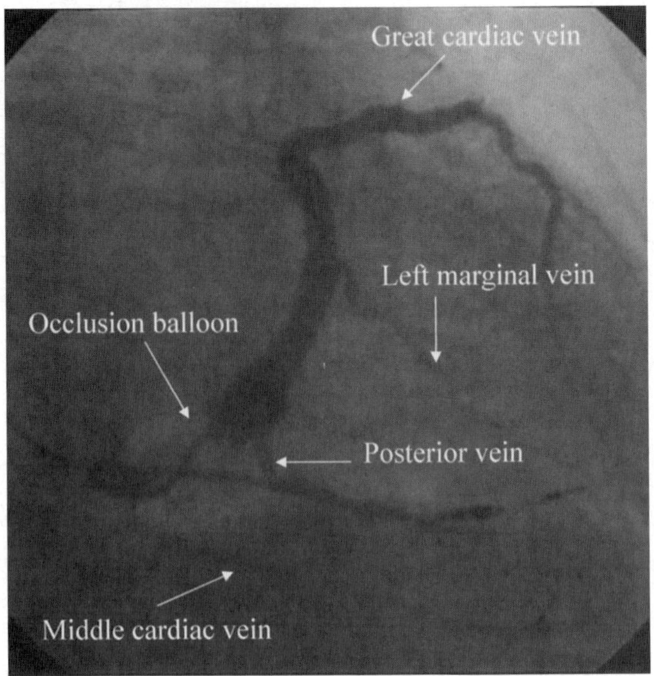


FIGURE 32-17 Right anterior oblique view of an occlusive venogram of the great cardiac vein and the other branch veins of the coronary sinus (left marginal vein, left posterior vein, and the middle cardiac vein).

***Future Directions*** One of the most basic questions in CRT that remains unanswered is how to identify or refine currently used electrical and mechanical markers of dyssynchrony. Careful analysis of clinical trials shows that up to 30 percent of patients receiving a CRT device may not benefit from this therapy. While QRS duration is a good marker, it has not been shown that the extent of QRS narrowing by biventricular pacing predicts the magnitude of clinical response. Several studies have shown that the degree of left ventricular dyssynchrony measured by a variety of techniques, tagged magnetic resonance imaging (MRI), echocardiographic and echo-contrast imaging, and color tissue Doppler imaging have shown that the degree of

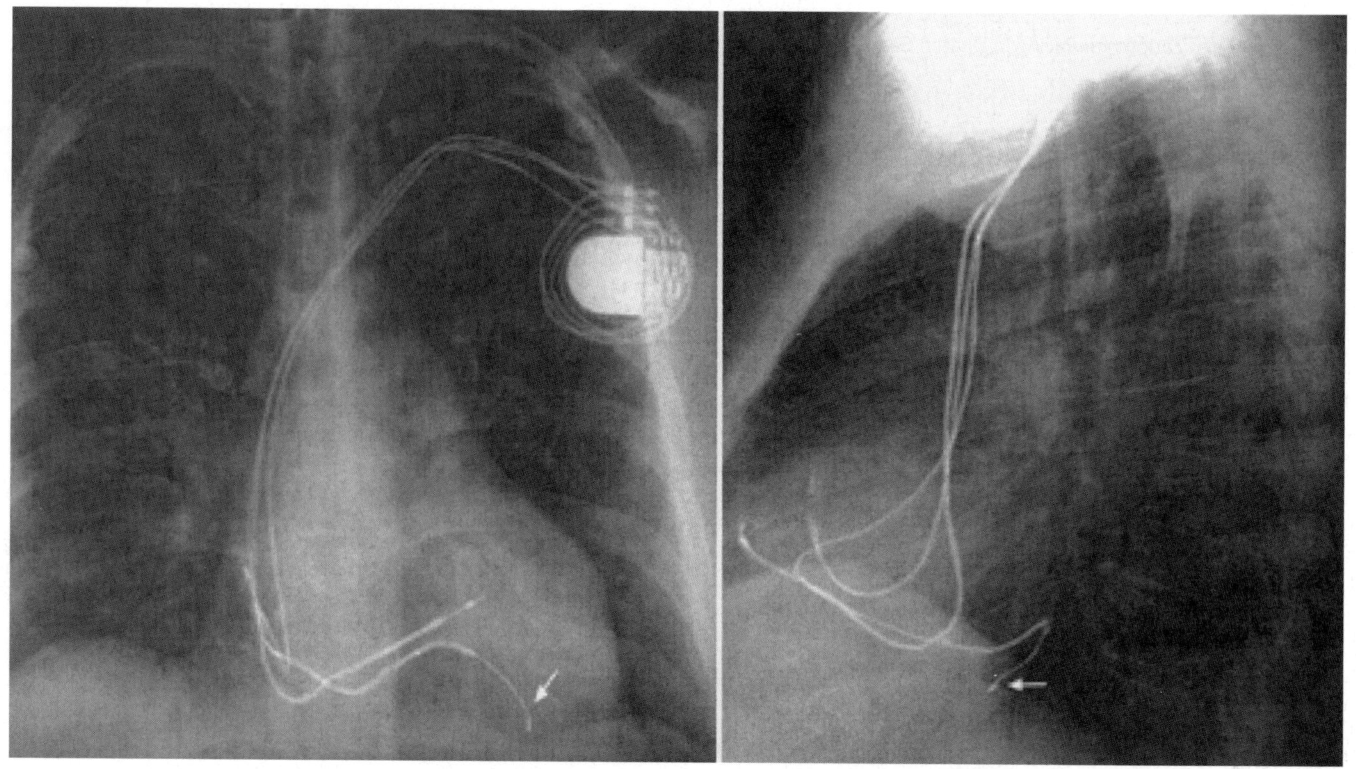

FIGURE 32-18 Posteroanterior and lateral chest x-rays demonstrating the right atrial, right ventricular (RV), and the left ventricular (LV) leads in a patient with a biventricular pacemaker. The LV lead (arrow) is placed in the posterolateral vein branch of the coronary sinus allowing for simultaneous activation of the septum and the LV free wall.

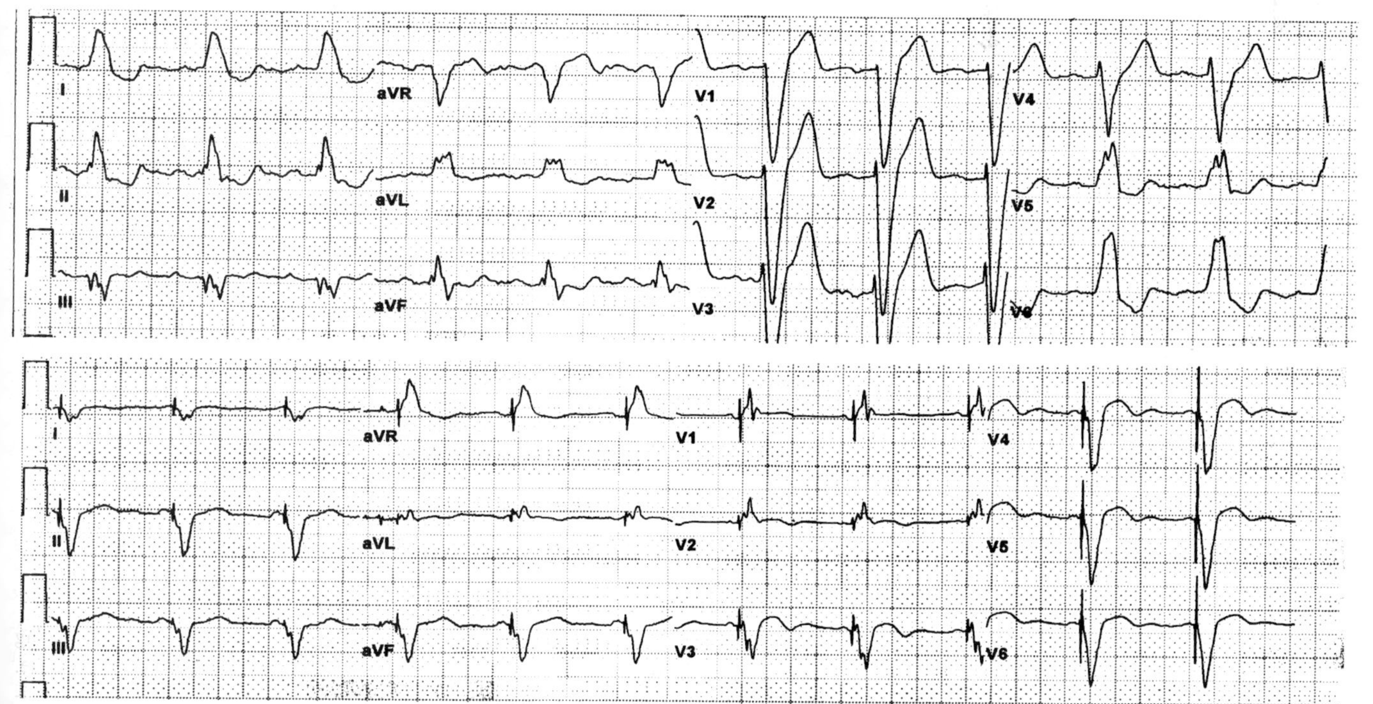


FIGURE 32-19 Electrocardiograms of the patient shown in Figure 32-27. Top: Normal sinus rhythm with left bundle branch block and QRS width of 200 ms. Bottom: Atrial-sensed biventricular stimulation; note how the paced QRS complex has narrowed significantly from the baseline.

TABLE 32-16 Indications for Pacing in Dilated Cardiomyopathy

**Class I**

1. Class I indications for sinus node dysfunction or atrioventricular (AV) block as previously described. (Level of evidence: C)

**Class IIa**

1. Biventricular pacing in medically refractory, symptomatic New York Heart Association class III or IV patients with idiopathic dilated or ischemic cardiomyopathy, prolonged QRS interval (≥ 130 ms), LV end-diastolic diameter ≥ 55 mm, and ejection fraction ≤ 35%. (Level of evidence: A)

**Class III**

1. Asymptomatic dilated cardiomyopathy.
2. Symptomatic dilated cardiomyopathy when patients are rendered asymptomatic by drug therapy.
3. Symptomatic ischemic cardiomyopathy when the ischemia is amenable to intervention.

left ventricular dyssynchrony can successfully predict responders to resynchronization therapy. However, these measures have not been prospectively tested in large, prospective clinical trials. Additional questions regarding optimization of AV delay or interventricular delay to optimize the CRT device function and how best to measure the benefit of these changes remain largely unanswered.

## PACING IN HYPERTROPHIC CARDIOMYOPATHY

Dynamic left ventricular outflow tract obstruction is present in approximately 25 percent of patients with hypertrophic cardiomyopathy. Symptoms such as dyspnea, angina, palpitations, and syncope may coexist in patients with left ventricular outflow obstruction. Obstruction occurs in hypertrophic cardiomyopathy because of two main hemodynamic events: abnormal orientation of the papillary muscle and the leaflet leading to systolic anterior motion causing outflow obstruction; and asymmetric septal hypertrophy and narrowing of the left ventricular outflow tract, resulting in the generation of Venturi forces and causing a systolic gradient. Although the severity of symptoms does not correlate well with the severity of obstruction, reduction or elimination of the outflow gradient seems to correlate with clinical improvement. Right ventricular apical pacing results in preexcitation of interventricular septum and reverses the ventricular activation sequence leading to an increase in the outflow tract diameter and reduction of the outflow gradient. While gradient reduction may reduce effective cardiac workload, abnormal ventricular activation from pacing may cause impaired relaxation and may be more detrimental in patients with preexisting diastolic abnormalities. Hassenstein and Wolter first reported in 1967 that right ventricular pacing resulted in significant reduction of the left ventricular outflow gradient in patients with hypertrophic cardiomyopathy.[91] Subsequent to this and few other such reports, many small and large observational studies suggested reduction of the outflow tract gradient, modest improvement in exercise tolerance, and favorable changes in the degree of angina, syncope, and functional class following dual-chamber pacemaker implantation.[92] Subsequent placebo-controlled, blinded, randomized studies have shown only modest benefit with pacemaker therapy. For example, the Pacing in Hypertrophic Cardiomyopathy (PIC) trial examined 83 patients with hypertrophic cardiomyopathy and randomized to DDD pacing or AAI pacing for 12 weeks and then crossed over. DDD pacing was associated with 51-percent reduction in the left ventricular outflow gradient and 63 percent improvement in functional class. DDD pacing, however, did not improve exercise tolerance. At the end of 6 months, 76 patients preferred the active DDD pacing mode.[93]

TABLE 32-17 Indications for Pacing in Hypertrophic Obstructive Cardiomyopathy

**Class I**

1. Class I indications for sinus node dysfunction or AV block as previously described. (Level of evidence: C)

**Class IIb**

1. Medically refractory, symptomatic hypertrophic cardiomyopathy with significant resting or provoked left ventricular outflow tract obstruction. (Level of evidence: A)

**Class III**

1. Patients who are asymptomatic or medically controlled.
2. Symptomatic patients without evidence of left ventricular outflow tract obstruction.

Dual-chamber pacing is considered only for patients who are not surgical candidates or who cannot tolerate medical therapy (Table 32-17). Surgery with septal myectomy remains the gold standard therapy for patients with hypertrophic obstructive cardiomyopathy and refractory symptoms.

TABLE 32-18 Pacemaker Complications

| Acute | Subacute or Chronic |
|---|---|
| Pneumothorax | Venous occlusion |
| Hemothorax | Infection |
| Air embolism | Pacemaker allergy |
| Cardiac perforation and tamponade | Twiddler's syndrome |
| Coronary sinus dissection | Pacemaker syndrome |
| Coronary vein perforation | Pacemaker-mediated arrhythmias |
| Pocket hematoma | Pacemaker-mediated tachycardia |
| Venous thrombosis | Runaway pacemaker |
| Lead dislodgement | Lead Failure |
| Infection (pocket, sepsis) | Pacemaker malfunction |
| Loose setscrews | Electromagnetic interference |
| Diaphragmatic stimulation | |

### Pacemaker Complications

Patients undergoing a new pacemaker system implantation are generally monitored in the hospital for a day in anticipation of any untoward complications. The various complications associated with pacemakers are outlined in Table 32-18.

## PNEUMOTHORAX

At the time of implantation, subclavian or axillary venous access can rarely result in pneumothorax, hemothorax, or hemopneumothorax. This can occur from inadvertent puncture and laceration of the subclavian vein or the subclavian artery or the lung. The use of venograms to locate the venous system in difficult cases and the routine use of axillary venous access have reduced these complications significantly. Occasionally air embolism may occur during cephalic vein or subclavian vein cannulation. The use of "safe sheaths" with one-way valve mechanism has minimized this risk.

## CARDIAC PERFORATION

Cardiac perforation resulting in pericardial effusion and occasionally cardiac tamponade is a rare but potentially life-threatening complication of pacemaker lead insertion. This may be recognized at the time of lead insertion by fluoroscopic position of the lead, right bundle branch block morphology of the paced QRS complex, diaphragmatic stimulation, or hypotension resulting from cardiac tamponade. If identified at the time of implantation, lead withdrawal and repositioning is usually not associated with tamponade. In patients with chest pain, friction rub, and a small pericardial effusion, serial echocardiograms may be performed to assess for hemodynamic deterioration. Cardiac perforation and pericarditis may also develop as a late complication and occasionally lead to tamponade weeks to months after the pacemaker implantation, especially with active fixation leads.[94]

## HEMATOMAS

Hematomas occurring at the pacemaker pocket site can vary from a small ecchymosis to large and tense swelling. Most small hematomas can be managed conservatively with cold compresses and withdrawal of antiplatelet or antithrombotic agents. Occasionally large hematomas that compromise the suture line or skin integrity may have to be surgically evacuated. In patients who require therapeutic anticoagulation, heparin should be delayed for at least 24 to 48 h after implantation to avoid bleeding complications.

## VENOUS OCCLUSION

Venous occlusion may result from acute subclavian or axillary vein thrombosis and lead to ipsilateral arm edema and thrombosis. Venous thrombosis is generally treated with heparin and 3 to 6 months of warfarin. Rarely invasive surgical interventions may be required. Up to 30 to 40 percent of patients undergoing pacemaker implantation may develop partial to complete venous occlusion over time and may remain asymptomatic due to the development of venous collaterals.[95] Occasionally superior vena caval occlusion leading to superior vena cava syndrome may result from pacemaker lead implantation.[96]

## INFECTION

The use of prophylactic antibiotics and pocket irrigation with antibiotic solutions has decreased the rate of acute infections following pacemaker implantations to less than 1 to 2 percent in most series. While early infections are generally caused by *Staphylococcus aureus* and may be aggressive, late infections associated with pacemakers are usually due to *S. epidermidis* and their course tends to be indolent. The signs of infection include local inflammation and abscess formation, erosion of the pacer, and fever with positive blood cultures without an identifiable focus of infection. Occasionally the infected pacemaker tends to erode through the skin. Transesophageal echocardiography helps to determine whether vegetations are present on the pacemaker leads. Removal of the pacemaker leads and generator is usually required to completely eliminate pacemaker infections.[97]

## LEAD DISLODGEMENT

Leads may dislodge from the initial implant site in the first few days to few weeks following the implantation. Active and passive fixation mechanisms of leads help prevent this complication. Atrial lead dislodgement is slightly more common than it is for ventricular leads. While passive fixation leads are stable in the atrial appendage, active fixation leads are necessary to prevent dislodgment in patients with prior cardiac surgery. Lead dislodgment may result in an increase in pacing thresholds, failure to capture, or failure to sense. Lead dislodgment may be radiographically visible or it may be a "microdislodgment," where there is no radiographic change in position, but there is significant increase in pacing threshold and/or decline in the electrogram amplitude.

## DIAPHRAGMATIC/PHRENIC NERVE STIMULATION

Diaphragmatic/phrenic nerve stimulation may lead to significant discomfort. This phenomenon may be observed in patients with atrial leads placed in the lateral wall or more commonly in patients with left ventricular coronary vein branch lead placement for biventricular stimulation. During implant, high-output pacing at maximal voltage and pulse width should be tested routinely to avoid diaphragmatic stimulation. Since this testing is performed in the supine position, diaphragmatic stimulation may only be noticed postimplant, when the patient is in upright position.

## PACEMAKER ALLERGY

Pacemaker allergy is a rare complication and is suspected when there is evidence of chronic inflammation in the absence of any infection. Allergy can occur with any component of the pacemaker system, including the pacemaker can (titanium) or the lead insulation (silicone rubber or polyurethane) and, if proven, may require removal of the offending component and possibly replacement with another system.

## TWIDDLER'S SYNDROME

*Twiddler's syndrome* is a term applied to patients who intentionally or unintentionally manipulate their pulse generator, causing twisting of the entire pacemaker system. This leads to lead dislodgment or fracture. This may also result from an excessively large pacemaker pocket allowing rotation of the pacemaker.

## PACEMAKER SYNDROME

The constellation of neurologic and cardiovascular signs and symptoms resulting from deleterious hemodynamics induced by ventricular pacing has been termed *pacemaker syndrome*. The variety of symptoms and signs associated with pacemaker syndrome are listed in Table 32-19. They are attributable to a decrease in cardiac output and arterial pressure due to loss of AV synchrony or to cardiovascular or humoral reflexes elicited by increases in pulmonary venous or right atrial pressures. The basis for pacemaker syndrome is not only loss of AV synchrony but also the presence of ventriculoatrial conduction. Atrial contraction against closed AV valves leads to increases in jugular and pulmonary venous pressure causing cough and malaise in patients with intact cardiac function and congestive heart failure in other patients with structural heart disease. The symptoms may vary from mild to severe and the onset of symptoms range from acute to chronic.

The exact incidence of pacemaker syndrome is unknown, but severe manifestations are expected to occur in 5 to 7 percent of ventricularly paced patients. Milder symptoms or significant drops in

TABLE 32-19 Symptoms and Signs of Pacemaker Syndrome

| Symptoms | Signs |
|---|---|
| Neck pulsations | Cannon A waves |
| Fatigue | Elevated jugular venous pressure |
| Palpitations | Palpable liver pulsations |
| Cough | Peripheral edema |
| Apprehension | $S_3$ gallop |
| Chest fullness | Pulmonary rales |
| Choking sensation | Drop in systolic blood pressure > 20 mmHg during ventricular pacing |
| Orthopnea | |
| Exertional dyspnea | |
| Dizziness, near syncope or syncope | |
| Confusion, altered mental state | |

systolic blood pressure and cardiac output during ventricular pacing occur in more than 20 percent of patients.[98] In the Pacemaker Selection in the Elderly trial, 26 percent of the patients in the ventricular pacing arm crossed over to the DDD pacing mode because of symptoms due to pacemaker syndrome.[50]

Pacemaker syndrome is not specific to VVI pacing mode alone, as AV dyssynchrony can occur with other pacing modes. If the AV conduction is significantly prolonged, AAI or AAIR pacing can result in pacemaker syndrome. Similarly during DDI pacing, when the atrial rate exceeds the lower rate limit, it may also result in pacemaker syndrome. Rarely, during DDD pacing, significant interatrial conduction delay, if present, may result in left atrial and left ventricular dyssynchrony.

The management of pacemaker syndrome usually requires restoration of AV synchrony. In many patients, an upgrade to a dual-chamber pacer is indicated. In some patients with intact sinus and AV conduction, lowering the pacing rate in VVI mode and using the hysteresis mode may promote sinus rhythm, lessening the symptoms associated with pacemaker syndrome.

## PACEMAKER-MEDIATED ARRHYTHMIAS

***Pacemaker-Mediated Tachycardia*** Pacemaker-mediated tachycardia (PMT), or "endless-loop tachycardia," is a well-recognized arrhythmia mediated by the pacemaker in patients with atrial-sensed ventricular pacing systems. In patients with intact ventriculoatrial conduction, a premature ventricular contraction may result in retrograde conduction to the atria, which, if outside the PVARP, will be sensed and followed by ventricular pacing after the programmed AVI. The paced ventricular event will again be followed by VA conduction resulting in endless-loop tachycardia. PMT can be prevented by programming the PVARP to be longer than the native VA conduction time. However, if the VA interval is very long, the PVARP cannot be lengthened as this will limit the upper rate. Modern pacemakers have several options to prevent or terminate PMT. One such feature is automatic extension of PVARP following a sensed premature ventricular beat to prevent tracking of retrogradely conducted P waves. If PMT is established (atrial-sensed ventricular pacing close to the upper rate limit with stable VA intervals), the PVARP is automatically extended to a longer interval of 500 ms for one cycle, usually terminating the tachycardia (Fig. 32-20).

***Runaway Pacemaker*** Runaway pacemaker is an uncommon, potentially lethal, circuit malfunction characterized by sudden onset of erratic pacing at rapid nonphysiologic rates.[99] Pacemakers may fail unpredictably due to component failure or battery depletion. Runaway pacemakers due to neutron beam radiation and use of electrocautery have been reported. Runaway pacemaker remains a rare but serious complication and, if a patient develops rapid arrhythmias due to pacing, the device should be disabled as quickly as possible, including emergency explantation of the pacemaker.

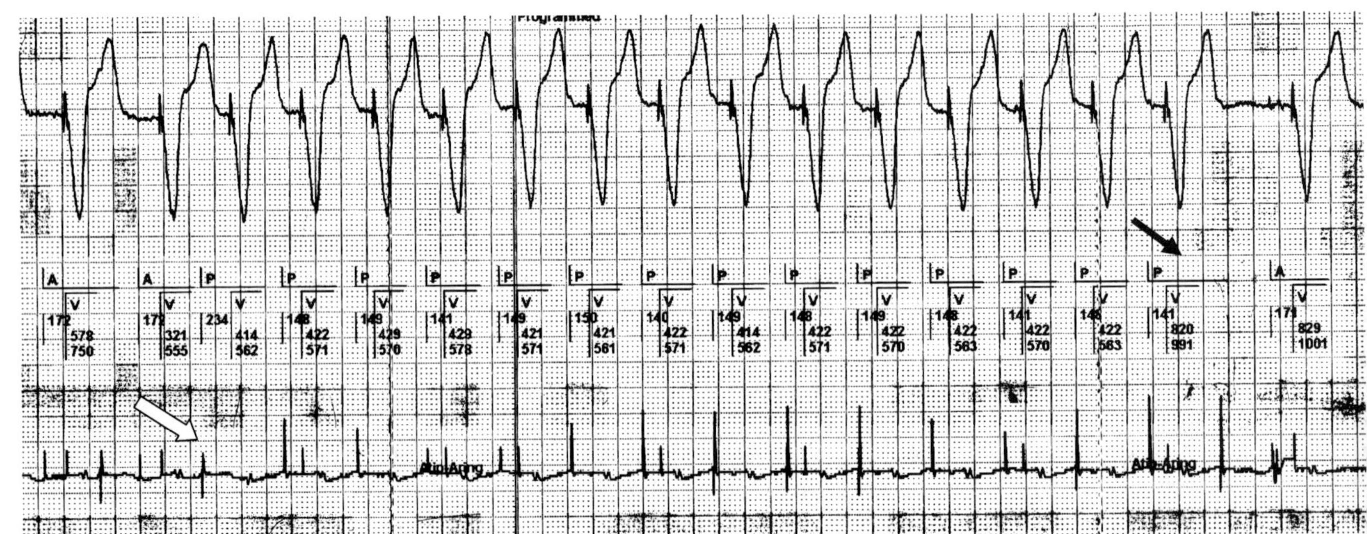

FIGURE 32-20 Pacemaker-mediated tachycardia. Surface electrocardiogram; marker channel with AV, VA, and VV intervals; and intracardiac atrial electrograms are displayed. The atrium is paced (A) at subthreshold output leading to noncapture resulting in atrioventricular dissociation. The second-paced ventricular event is followed by a native P wave with a VA interval of 320 ms [postventricular atrial refractory period (PVARP) 275 ms] and is sensed leading to ventricular pacing. This is followed by a retrogradely conducted P wave (open arrow) with a VA interval of 420 ms and sets up the endless-loop tachycardia. As the ventricular pacing rate is above the programmed pacemaker-mediated tachycardia rate of 100 bpm, the device automatically extends the PVARP on the second-to-last ventricular paced beat to 500 ms (arrow), resulting in nonsensing of the retrograde P wave terminating the tachycardia.

### LEAD FAILURE

The pacemaker leads are subject to long-term complications. The insulation of the leads may break, leading to problems with oversensing (due to electrical noise), undersensing, and failure to capture (due to current leak). This problem often manifests intermittently and may be difficult to detect during a routine pacer check. The patient may complain of pectoral muscle stimulation due to current leakage around an insulation break. An abnormally low impedance with demonstrable lead malfunction is diagnostic for insulation break. Subtle insulation breaks may be detected by having the patient perform provocative maneuvers while monitoring an ECG (and marker channels) and/or measuring lead impedances. Leads may also fracture over time. Early lead fractures lead to increased impedances associated with failure to capture, oversensing, and undersensing. Lead damage can occur at the site of venous access (subclavian vein) in the costoclavicular space causing the crush syndrome.

## Pacemaker System Malfunction: Troubleshooting

Pacemaker system malfunction can be secondary to pacemaker circuitry failure or to lead dysfunction. Not uncommonly what appears to be pacemaker malfunction may actually represent normal functioning of the pacemaker: A pacing artifact may be delivered in the middle of the normal QRS and may represent pseudofusion (due to late sensing) and not undersensing; Unexplained longer pauses after sensed, but not paced, complexes might suggest oversensing, while it may represent normal function due to hysteresis. Major electrocardiographic abnormalities of pacemaker system malfunction can broadly be categorized into the following: failure to capture, failure to output, undersensing, and oversensing.

### FAILURE TO CAPTURE

The loss of pacemaker capture occurs when there is a visible pacing stimulus and no atrial or ventricular depolarization. The differential diagnosis of failure to capture is outlined in Table 32-20. Failure to capture may be intermittent or persistent. Lead dislodgment can

TABLE 32-20 Differential Diagnosis of Failure to Capture

| Etiology | Pacing Threshold | Impedance |
|---|---|---|
| Lead dislodgement | Elevated | Normal |
| Lead insulator failure | Elevated | Decreased |
| Lead conductor fracture | Elevated | Increased |
| Loose setscrew | Elevated | Increased |
| Battery depletion | Normal | Normal |
| Functional noncapture | Normal | Normal |

cause obvious failure to capture. An increase in the pacing threshold above the programmed pacing output can occur as a result of the rise of the threshold within a few weeks following lead placement because of drug therapy, electrolytes, MI, or ischemia. Fracture of the lead, insulation breaks, and loose setscrews are mechanical problems that can cause failure to capture (Fig. 32-21). Last, battery depletion may cause the pacing output to decline sufficiently such that pacing failure occurs. Loss of capture requires a check of the pacing threshold and of pacing lead impedance and a chest x-ray. For instance, if the problem is an elevated pacing threshold, pacing outputs must be increased. Abnormal lead impedances may confirm a lead failure and the need for lead replacement. Functional noncapture occurs, when a stimulus falls during the physiologic refractory period of a native depolarization. It may be secondary to undersensing or as a function of the pacing mode (AOO, VOO).

### FAILURE TO OUTPUT

Another pacing system malfunction is the absence of pacing stimuli and hence no capture. In bipolar systems, the pacing artifact is diminutive especially if isoelectric in some surface leads. It is important to record multiple leads simultaneously. Failure to output is often due to oversensing and inhibition of pacing output and less commonly due to circuitry failure (Table 32-21). Oversensing may

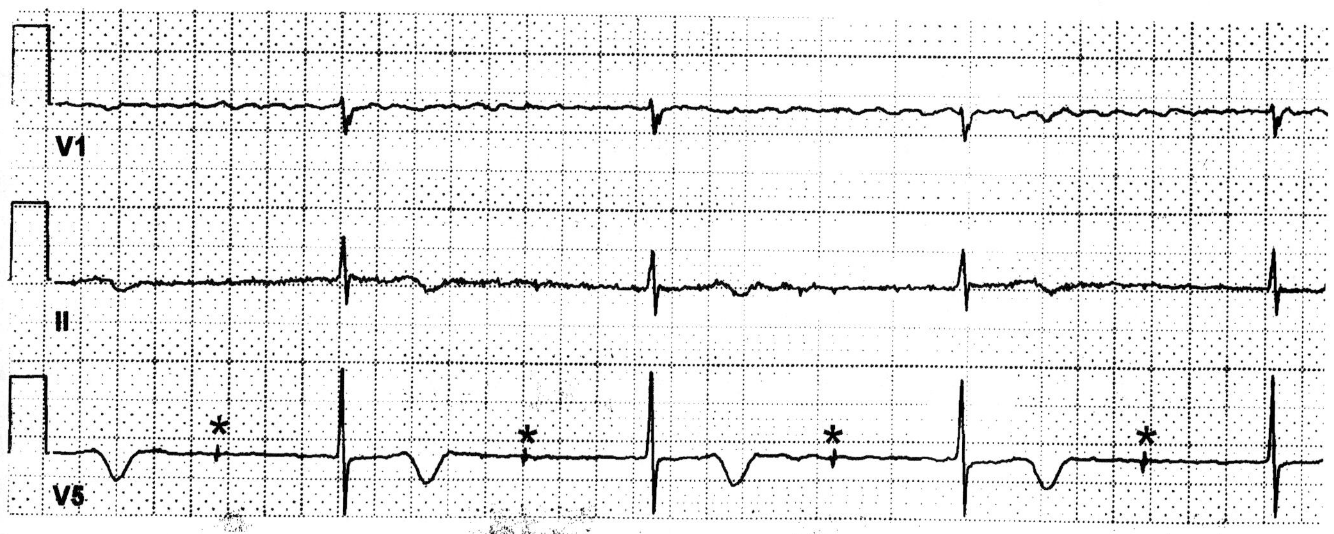


FIGURE 32-21 Failure to capture. Surface electrocardiogram of a patient with VVI pacemaker at a lower rate limit of 60 ppm is shown at the bottom. The pacemaker spikes (*) are not followed by ventricular depolarization (no capture). Patient has spontaneous ventricular activity at 35 bpm. The device clearly senses the ventricular event as the pacemaker spike appears 1000 ms (60 ppm) after the sensed event. On interrogation of the device his lead impedance was significantly lower (300 Ω) than the implant values, and his pacing threshold had increased significantly. These findings are consistent with lead failure secondary to insulation break. Chest x-ray revealed evidence of insulation break at the subclavian venous access site.

TABLE 32-21 Differential Diagnosis of Failure to Output

| Etiology | Diagnosis/Management |
|---|---|
| Oversensing | Application of magnet eliminates pauses |
| T wave, P wave, R wave | Reduce sensitivity |
| Myopotential/diaphragmatic | Change unipolar to bipolar sensing |
| Electromagnetic interference | |
| Crosstalk | |
| Make–break potential | |
| Insulation failure | Pauses persist despite magnet application |
| | Impedance low; replace lead |
| Open circuit | Pauses persist despite magnet application |
| Conductor fracture | Impedance high |
| Loose setscrew | Chest x-ray may show conductor deformity |
| | Loosely seated lead pin |
| Component malfunction | Pauses persist despite magnet application |
| | Replace pulse generator |
| Pseudomalfunction | Pauses follow only sensed beats |
| Hysteresis | Reassurance |
| Mode switching | |
| Pacemaker-mediated tachycardia intervention | |

be due to T waves, P waves, or far-field R waves and may cause inhibition of pacing output. In unipolar systems, oversensing of myopotentials is not uncommon. A loose setscrew may cause noise and oversensing leading to inhibition of pacing output (Fig. 32-22). Electromagnetic signals from arc welding and electrocautery may be sensed by the pacemaker. Occasionally, the ventricular channel may be inhibited by oversensing the atrial channel output (crosstalk). If the absence of pacing output is due to oversensing, then a magnet application will change the pacemaker to an asynchronous mode and this will eliminate the pauses. In generator component malfunction, there is no delivery of pacing output by the device. Magnet application in the preceding scenarios will not restore pacing output. Systematic analysis of the pacing parameters, evaluation of lead impedances at rest, and provocative isometric exercises and chest x-ray may help identify the cause.

## OVERSENSING

In a single-chamber pacemaker, oversensing leads to inhibition of the pacing channel and causes inappropriate pauses. However, in dual-chamber pacemakers, oversensing will elicit either inappropriate inhibition or triggering, depending on the channel in which oversensing occurs and the programmed pacing mode. Oversensing in the ventricular channel in the DDD or DDI mode will result in inhibition of both atrial and ventricular outputs and resetting of timing cycles. In patients with complete heart block, this may result in ventricular asystole (Fig. 32-23). Oversensing in the atrial channel can lead to inappropriate triggering of ventricular output. The various etiologies of oversensing were discussed in the previous section. One example of oversensing peculiar to dual-chamber pacemakers is crosstalk. The atrial channel output can be sensed in the ventricular channel as a far-field signal and inhibit the ventricular pacing output. In patients with complete heart block this can result in ventricular asystole. Although far more common with unipolar systems, crosstalk can also occur in bipolar pacing systems. To prevent this phenomenon, there is a programmable ventricular blanking period (51 to 150 ms) following atrial pacing during which the ventricular channel is refractory. Additionally, there is a crosstalk sensing window following the blanking period during which a ventricular event, if sensed, will lead to ventricular pacing with a shorter AVI. Oversensing due to lead fracture, insulation break, or other electrode problems will usually be random and erratic. With early lead problems, the malfunction is typically intermittent and may be exacerbated by certain body positions or motions. In later stages, the combination of oversensing, undersensing, and failure to capture is almost always diagnostic of a lead-related problem. Programming to an asynchronous mode may temporarily control this problem while awaiting lead replacement, which should be carried out as promptly as possible.

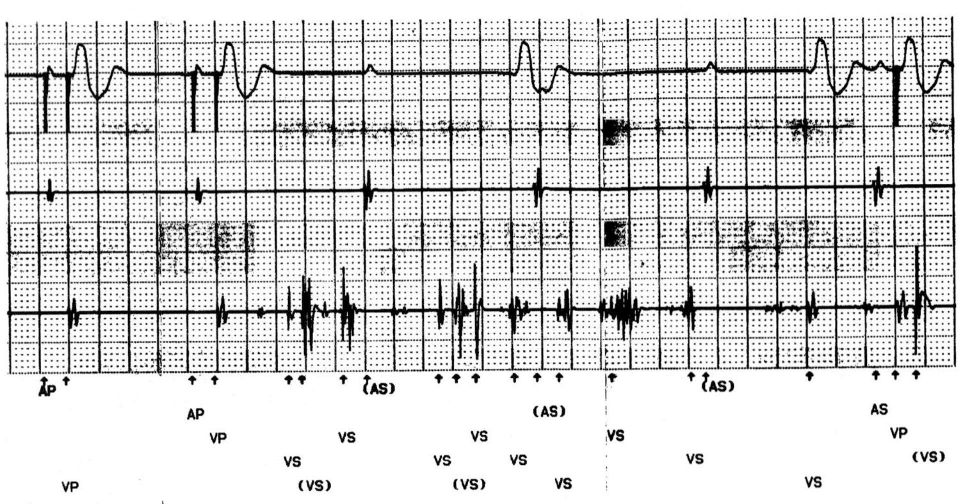


FIGURE 32-22 Failure to ouput. Surface electrocardiogram and atrial and ventricular electrograms with pacemaker event markers are shown. In this patient with dual-chamber pacemaker, loose setscrew resulted in noise on the ventricular channel leading to oversensing and inhibition of the ventricular output.

## UNDERSENSING

An inadequate intracardiac signal can lead to undersensing (see Table 32-22). The intracardiac electrograms can deteriorate due to inflammation or scar formation at the tissue lead interface. Additionally, some drugs, electrolyte abnormalities, infarction, ischemia, lead fracture, or insulation breaks can all lead to undersensing. Cardioversion or defibrillation can

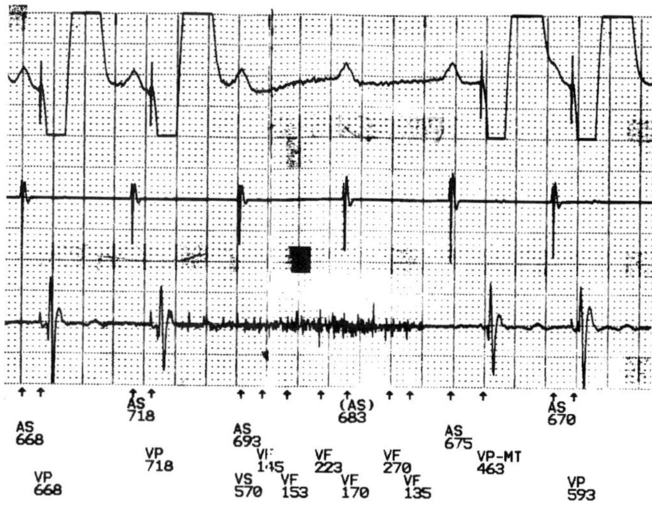


FIGURE 32-23 Oversensing of diaphragmatic myopotentials. Surface electrocardiogram and atrial and ventricular electrograms with event markers are shown. In this patient with a dual-chamber defibrillator, deep respiration reproduced the diaphragmatic myopotentials resulting in inhibition of ventricular output. The patient developed dizzy spells due to underlying complete heart block. The ventricular lead was repositioned in the right ventricular outflow tract eliminating the diaphragmatic oversensing.

also cause attenuation of intracardiac electrograms. Usually, undersensing is a greater problem in the atrium than it is in the ventricle. The atrial electrograms are typically significantly lower in amplitude during atrial fibrillation than they are during sinus rhythm. The optimal solution is to program an enhanced sensitivity (decrease sensing level). With bipolar systems, the programmed sensitivity can usually be reduced to 0.18 mV in the atrium, without oversensing of myopotentials or other extraneous signals. Other etiologies for undersensing occur when intrinsic atrial or ventricular complexes fall within one of the programmed refractory periods. Undersensing can also result when a pacemaker is inadvertently programmed to an asynchronous mode (occasionally occurring with battery depletion or pacemaker generator reset).

TABLE 32-22 Etiology of Undersensing

- Lead dislodgement
- Decrease in electrogram amplitude/slew rate
  - Local inflammation
  - Infarction
  - Ischemia
  - Electrolyte abnormalities
  - Drug effect (quinidine, procainamide, amiodarone)
  - Postcardioversion/defibrillation
  - Atrial fibrillation (atrial undersensing)
- Lead insulation failure
- Lead fracture
- Component failure
- Battery depletion
- Electromagnetic interference (mode reset to VOO)
- Functional undersensing (events occurring in refractory periods)

TABLE 32-23 Sources of Electromagnetic Interference

| Hospital | Daily Life/Work |
|---|---|
| Magnetic resonance imaging | Cellular telephones |
| Electrocautery | Electronic article surveillance devices |
| Cardioversion/defibrillation | Metal detectors |
| Spinal cord stimulator | Improperly grounded appliances |
| Transcutaneous electric nerve stimulator | High-voltage power lines |
| Radiofrequency ablation | Arc welding |
| Diathermy | Transformers |
| Lithotripsy | |
| Radiation therapy | |

## Electromagnetic Interference

Electromagnetic interference (EMI) is defined as any nonphysiologic electrical signal that interferes with pacemaker function. EMI can originate from a variety of sources both within the hospital environment and outside (Table 32-23). EMI can result in the inhibition of the pacemaker, inappropriate triggering, noise reversion, resetting of the pacemaker parameters, and occasionally damage to the circuitry or electrode–myocardial interface.[100] Unipolar pacemakers are more susceptible to EMI than are bipolar pacemakers.

In the hospital environment, the most common sources of EMI include electrocautery and defibrillation. Electrocautery can cause inhibition of the pacemaker, and, in a pacemaker-dependent patient, this may result in severe bradycardia or asystole. Use of electrocautery should be entirely avoided near a pacemaker. It is preferable to program the pacemaker to an asynchronous mode to avoid oversensing of the electrical signals. In addition, short bursts of cautery and use of bipolar cautery are recommended. Both electrocautery and defibrillation can cause irreversible damage to the pacemaker. They may also cause resetting of the pacemaker to a backup or noise reversion mode. Cardioversion or defibrillation should be performed with pads in the anteroposterior position rather than the anteroapical location to prevent damage to the pacemaker. Transient undersensing and increase in pacing threshold may occur following cardioversion. Pacemaker interrogation with pacing and sensing thresholds should be performed before and after any procedure with a potential for EMI.

Other potential sources of EMI in the hospital include extracorporeal lithotripsy, radiation therapy, and MRI. MRI should generally be avoided in patients with pacemakers as this can potentially be hazardous, most commonly by causing rapid pacing triggered by the pulsing of the magnetic field. Lithotripsy can also result in inappropriate inhibition or oversensing especially in rate-responsive pacemakers with piezoelectric crystals. The pacemaker should generally be programmed to VVI or VOO mode with the rate-responsive feature turned off prior to lithotripsy. Radiation therapy should be avoided directly over the field of the pacemaker. If shielding of the pacemaker and limiting the field of radiation cannot be performed with safety, then repositioning of the pacemaker prior to radiotherapy should be considered. Other possible EMI sources in the hospital include therapeutic diathermy, radiofrequency catheter ablation, transcutaneous electric nerve stimulator (TENS) units, and spinal cord stimulators.

Daily sources of EMI include digital cellular phones, electronic article surveillance devices, metal detectors, and electric razors, and work or industrial environment sources include high-voltage power lines, transformers, welding, and electric motors. Activated digital cell phones should not be placed in the breast pocket ipsilateral to the pacemaker, and the phone should be held to the ear contralateral to the pacemaker. Electronic surveillance devices or antitheft devices present in most stores and libraries can cause transient asynchronous pacing, atrial oversensing with tracking, and ventricular oversensing and inhibition. Patients with pacemakers should quickly walk through these devices and avoid lingering near them. Common household appliances such as electric can openers, stereos, televisions, video recorders, power tools, electric blankets, electric shavers, microwave ovens, and electric lawnmowers do not cause any pacemaker interference.

## References


1. Katz LN, Pick A. *Clinical Electrocardiography. Part I: The Arrhythmias*. Philadelphia: Lea & Febiger; 1956:20.
2. Benditt DG, Sakaguchi S, Goldstein MA, et al. Sinus node dysfunction, pathophysiology, clinical features, evaluation, and treatment. In: Zipes DP, Jaliffe J, eds. *Cardiac Electrophysiolgy: From Cell to Bedside*, 2nd ed. Philadelphia: Saunders; 1995:1215–1247.
3. Hecht HH, Kossmann CE, Childers RW, et al. Atrioventricular and intraventricular conduction: Revised nomenclature and concepts. *Am J Cardiol* 1973;31:232–244.
4. Kyrialikdis MK, Kouraouklis CB, Papaioannou JT, et al. Sinus node coronary arteries studied with angiography. *Am J Cardiol* 1983;51: 749–750.
5. Frink RJ, James TN. Normal blood supply to the human His bundle and proximal bundle branches. *Circulation* 1973;43:491–502.
6. Ferrer MI: The sick sinus syndrome. *Circulation* 1973;47:635.
7. Moss AJ, Davis RJ. Brady-tachy syndrome. *Prog Cardiovasc Dis* 1974;16:439–454.
8. Evans R, Shaw D. Pathological studies in sinoatrial disorder (sick sinus syndrome). *Br Heart J* 1977;39:778.
9. Thery C, Gosselin B, Lekieffre J, et al. Pathology of the sino atrial node: Correlation with electrophysiological findings in 111 patients. *Am Heart J* 1977;93:735.
10. Adgey AAJ, Geddes JS, Mulho JF. Incidence, significance and management of early bradyarrhythmia complicating acute myocardial infarction. *Lancet* 1968;2:1097–1101.
11. Barak M, Herschkowitz S, Shapiro I, et al. Familial combined sinus node and atrioventricular conduction dysfunctions. *Int J Cardiol* 1987; 15:231–239.
12. Bartunek P, Nemec J, Mrazek V, et al. Borrelia burgdorferi as a cause of sick sinus syndrome. *Cas Lek Cesk* 1996;135:729–731.
13. Greenwood RD, Rosenthal A, Sloss LJ, et al. Sick sinus syndrome after surgery for congenital heart disease. *Circulation* 1975;52:208–213.
14. Bexton RS, Nathan AW, Hellerstrand KJ, et al. Sinoatrial function after cardiac transplantation. *J Am Coll Cardiol* 1984;3:712–723.
15. Talan DA, Bauernfeind RA, Ashley WW, et al. Twenty-four hour continuous ECG recordings in long distance runners. *Chest* 1982;82:19–24.
16. Fairfax AJ, Lambert CD, Leatham A. Systemic embolism in chronic sinoatrial disorder. *N Engl J Med* 1976;295:190–192.
17. Talwar KK, Dev V, Chopra P, et al. Persistent atrial standstill: Clinical, electrophysiological and morphological study. *Pacing Clin Electrophysiol* 1991;14:1274–1280.
18. Gwynn N, Leman R, Kratz, et al. Chronotropic incompetence: A common and progressive finding in pacemaker patients. *Am Heart J* 1992; 123:1216.
19. Forbath P, Darling DS, Quimet S. Adapting the rate modulation to the type of chronotropic incompetence. *PACE* 1991;14:685.
20. Jose AD, Collison D. The normal range and determinants of intrinsic heart rate in man. *Cardiovasc Res* 1970;4:160.
21. Alboni P, Menozzi C, Brignole M, et al. Effect of permanent pacemaker and oral theopylline in sick sinus syndrome, the THEOPACE study: A randomized controlled trial. *Circulation* 1997;96(1):260–266.
22. Avery P, Small J, Shaw DB. Xamoterol in sinus node disease. *Int J Cardiol* 1993;40:45.
23. Sutton R, Kenny RA. The natural history of sick sinus syndrome. *PACE* 1986;9:1110.
24. Bernstein AD, Parsonnet V. Survey of cardiac pacing and implanted defibrillator practice patterns in the United States in 1997. *Pacing Clin Electrophysiol* 2001;24(5):842–855.
25. Andersen HR, Nielsen JC, Thomsen PEB, et al. Long-term follow up of patients from a randomized trial of atrial versus ventricular pacing for sick sinus syndrome. *Lancet* 1997;350:1210–1216.
26. Connolly SJ, Kerr CR, Gent M, et al. Effects of physiologic pacing versus ventricular pacing on the risk of stroke and death due to cardiovascular causes. *N Engl J Med* 2000;342:1385–1391.
27. Lamas GA, Lee KL, Sweeney M, et al. Ventricular pacing or dual chamber pacing for sinus node dysfunction. *N Engl J Med* 2002; 346: 1854–1862.
28. Teichman SL, Felder SD, Matos JA. The value of electrophysiologic studies in syncope of undetermined origin: Report of 150 cases. *Am Heart J* 1985;110:469.
29. Katritsis D, Ward DE, Camm AJ. Can we treat carotid sinus syndrome? *PACE* 1991;14:1367.
30. Connolly SJ, Sheldon R, Roberts R, et al. The North American Vasovagal Pacemaker Study: A randomized trial of permanent cardiac pacing for the prevention of vasovagal syncope. *J Am Coll Cardiol* 1999;33:16–20.
31. Sutton R, Brignole M, Menozzi C, et al. Dual-chamber pacing in the treatment of neurally mediated tilt-positive cardioinhibitory syncope. Pacemaker versus no therapy: A multicenter randomized study. *Circulation* 2000;102:294–299.
32. Ammirati F, Colivicchi F, Santini M, et al. Permanent cardiac pacing versus medical treatment for the prevention of recurrent vasovagal syncope: A multicenter, randomized, controlled trial. *Circulation* 2001;104:52–57.
33. Connolly SJ, Sheldon R, Thorpe KE, et al. Pacemaker therapy for prevention of syncope in patients with recurrent severe vasovagal syncope. Second Vasovagal Pacemaker Study (VPS II): A Randomized Trial. *JAMA* 2003;289:2224–2229.
34. Strasberg B, Lam W, Swiryn S, et al. Symptomatic spontaneous paroxysmal AV nodal block due to localized hyperresponsiveness of the AV node to vagotonic reflexes. *Am Heart J* 1982;103:79.
35. Steere AC, Batsford WP, Weinberg M, et al. Lyme carditis: Cardiac abnormalities of Lyme disease. *Ann Intern Med* 1980;93(1):8.
36. Lev M. The pathology of complete AV block. *Prog Cardiovasc Dis* 1964;6:317.
37. Lenegre J. Etiology and pathology of bilateral bundle branch fibrosis in relation to complete heart block. *Prog Cardiovasc Dis* 1964;6:409.
38. Probst V, Kyndt F, Potet F, et al. Haploinsufficiency in combination with aging causes SCN5A-linked hereditary Lenégre disease. *J Am Coll Cardiol* 2003;41:643–652.
39. Ellenbogen KA, de Guzman M, Kawanishi DT, et al. Pacing for acute and chronic AV conduction system disease. In: Ellenbogen KA, Kay GN, Wilkoff BL (eds): *Clinical Cardiac Pacing and Defibrillation*. Philadelphia: Saunders; 2000:426–454.
40. Harpaz, D, Behar S, Gottileb S, et al. Complete atrioventricular block complicating acute myocardial infarction in the thrombolytic era. *J Am Coll Cardiol* 1999;34:1721–1728.
41. Perloff JK. The heart in neuromuscular disease. In: O'Rourke RA (ed): *Current Problems in Cardiology*. Chicago: Year book; 1986:513–517.
42. Koplan BA, Stevenson WG, Epstein LM, et al. Development and validation of a simple risk score to predict the need for permanent pacing after cardiac valve surgery. *J Am Coll Cardiol* 2003;41:795–801.
43. McAnulty JH, Rahimtoola SH, Murphy E, et al. Natural history of 'high risk' bundle-branch block: Final report of a prospective study. *N Engl J Med* 1982;307:137–143.
44. Camm AJ, Bexton RS. Congenital complete heart block. *Eur Heart J* 1984;5:115–117.
45. Donmoyer TL, DeSanctis RW, Austen WG. Experience with implantable pacemakers using myocardial electrodes in the management of heart block. *Ann Thorac Surg* 1967;3:218–227.

46. Alpert MA, Curtiss JJ, Sanfelippo JF, et al. Comparative survival after permanent ventricular and dual chamber pacing for patients with chronic high-degree atrioventricular block with and without preexistent congestive heart failure. *J Am Coll Cardiol* 1986;7:925.
47. Linde-Edelstam C, Gulberg B, Norlander R, et al. Longevity in patients with high degree atrioventricular block paced in the atrial synchronous mode or the fixed rate ventricular inhibited mode. *PACE* 1992;15:304.
48. Lamas GA, Orav EJ, Stambler BS, et al. Quality of life and clinical outcomes in elderly patients treated with ventricular pacing as compared with dual chamber pacing. *N Engl J Med* 1998;338:1097–1104.
49. Dhingra RC, Amat-Y-Leon F, Wyndham C, et al. Significance of left axis deviation in patients with left bundle branch block. *Am J Cardiol* 1978;42:551–556.
50. Smith RF, Jackson DH, Harthorne JW, et al. Acquired bundle branch block in a healthy population. *Am Heart J* 1970;80:746–751.
51. Scheinman MM, Peters RW, Suave MJ, et al. Value of the H-Q interval in patients with bundle branch block and the role of prophylactic permanent pacing. *Am J Cardiol* 1982;50:1316–1322.
52. Furman S, Schwedel JB. An intracardiac pacemaker for Stoakes-Adams seizures. *N Engl J Med* 1959;261:943–948.
53. Bailin SJ, Johnson WB, Hoyt R. A prospective randomized trial of Bachmann's bundle pacing for the prevention of atrial fibrillation (abstract). *J Am Coll Cardiol* 1997;29:74A.
54. Saksena S, Prakash A, Ziegler P, et al. Improved suppression of recurrent atrial fibrillation with dual-site right atrial pacing and antiarrhythmic drug therapy. *J Am Coll Cardiol* 2002;40(6):1140–1150.
55. de Cock CC, Meyer A, Kamp O, et al. Hemodynamic benefits of right ventricular outflow tract pacing: Comparison with right ventricular apex pacing. *Pacing Clin Electrophysiol* 1998;21(3):536–541.
56. Ellenbogen KA, Wood MA, Gilligan DM, et al. Steroid eluting high impedance pacing leads decrease short and long-term current drain: Results from a multicenter clinical trial of CapSure Z investigators. *PACE* 1999;22:39–48.
57. Clarke M, Liu B, Schuller H, et al. Automatic adjustment of pacemaker stimulation output correlated with continuously monitored capture thresholds: A multicenter study. *PACE* 1998;21:1567–1575.
58. Bernstein AD, Camm AJ, Fletcher R, et al. The NASPE/BPEG generic pacemaker code for antibradyarrhythmia and adaptive rate pacing and antitachyarrhythmia devices. *PACE* 1987;10:794–799.
59. Andersen HR, Nielsen JC, Thomsen PEB, et al. Atrioventricular conduction during long-term follow-up of patients with sick sinus syndrome. *Circulation* 1998;98:1315–1321.
60. Rickards AF, Donaldson RM. Rate-responsive pacing. *Clin Prog Pacing Electrophysiol* 1983;1:12–19.
61. Leung SK, Lau CP, Tng MO. Cardiac output is a sensitive indicator of difference in exercise performance between single and dual sensor pacemakers. *PACE* 1998;21:35–41.
62. Eldar M, Griffin JC, Van Hare GF, et al. Combined use of beta-adrenergic blocking agents and long-term cardiac pacing for patients with the long-QT syndrome. *J Am Coll Cardiol* 1992;20:830–837.
63. Ward DE, Camm AJ, Spurrell RA. The response of regular supraventricular tachycardia to right heart stimulation. *PACE* 1979;2:586–595.
64. Andersen HR, Thussen L, Bagger JP, et al. Prospective randomized trial of atrial versus ventricular pacing in sick sinus syndrome. *Lancet* 1994;344:1523–1528.
65. Skanes AC, Krahn AD, Yee R, et al. Progression to chronic atrial fibrillation after pacing: The Canadian Trial of Physiologic Pacing. *J Am Coll Cardiol* 2001;38:167–172.
66. Padeletti L, Pieragnoli P, Ciapetti C, et al. Randomized crossover comparison of right atrial appendage pacing versus interatrial septum pacing for prevention of paroxysmal atrial fibrillation in patients with sinus bradycardia. *Am Heart J* 2001;142:1047–1055.
67. Bailin SJ, Adler S, Giudici M. Prevention of chronic atrial fibrillation by pacing in the region of Bachmann's bundle: Results of a multicenter randomized trial. *J Cardiovasc Electrophysiol* 2001;12:912–917.
68. Garrigue S, Barold SS, Cazeau S, et al. Prevention of atrial arrhythmias during DDD pacing by atrial overdrive. *Pacing Clin Electrophysiol* 1998;21:1751–1759.
69. Defaye P, Dournaux F, Mouton E. Prevalence of Supraventricular arrhythmias from the automated analysis of data stored in the DDD pacemakers of 617 patients: The AIDA study. *Pacing Clin Electrophysiol* 1998;21:250–255.
70. Levy T, Walker S, Rex S, Paul V. Does atrial overdrive pacing prevent paroxysmal atrial fibrillation in paced patients? *Int J Cardiol* 2000;75: 91–97.
71. Hochleitner H, Hortnagl H, Ng CK, et al. Usefulness of physiologic dual chamber pacing in drug resistant idiopathic dilated cardiomyopathy. *Am J Cardiol* 1990;66:198–202.
72. Linde C, Gadler F, Edner M, et al. Results of atrioventricular synchronous pacing with optimized delay in patients with severe congestive heart failure. *Am J Cardiol* 1995;75:919–923.
73. Gold MR, Feliciano Z, Gottileb SS, et al. Dual chamber pacing with a short atrioventricular delay in congestive heart failure: A randomized study. *J Am Coll Cardiol* 1995;26:967–973.
74. Innes D, Leitch JW, Fletcher PJ. VDD pacing at short atrioventricular intervals does not improve cardiac output in patients with dilated heart failure. *PACE* 1994;17:959–965.
75. Bakker P, Chin K, Sen A, et al. Biventricular pacing improves functional capacity in patients with end stage heart failure (abstract). *PACE* 1995;18:825.
76. Auricchio A, Stellbrink C, Block M, et al. Effect of pacing chamber and atrioventricular delay on acute systolic function of paced patients with congestive heart failure. The Pacing Therapies for Congestive Heart Failure Study Group. The Guidant Congestive Heart Failure Research Group. *Circulation* 1999;99:2993–3001.
77. Gras D, Mabo P, Tang T, et al. Multisite pacing as a supplemental treatment of congestive heart failure: Preliminary results of the Medtronic Inc. InSync Study. *Pacing Clin Electrophysiol* 1998;2:2249–2255.
78. Daubert JC, Linde C, Cazeau S, et al. Clinical effects of biventricular pacing in patients with severe heart failure and chronic atrial fibrillation: Results from the Multisite Stimulation in Cardiomyopathy-MUSTIC-study group II (Abstract). *Circulation* 2000;102(suppl II):693.
79. Farwell D, Patel NR, Hall A, et al. How many people with heart failure are appropriate for biventricular resynchronization? *Eur Heart J* 2000; 21:1246–1250.
80. Auricchio A, Stellbrink C, Block M, et al. Effect of pacing chamber and atrioventricular delay on acute systolic function of paced patients with congestive heart failure. *Circulation* 1999;99:2993–3001.
81. Nelson G, Berger RD, Feltics BJ, et al. Left or biventricular pacing improves cardiac function at diminished energy cost in patients with dilated cardiomyopathy and left bundle branch block. *Circulation* 2000; 102:3053–3059.
82. Leon A, Brozena S, Liang CS, et al. Effect of cardiac resynchronization therapy with sequential biventricular pacing in Doppler derived left ventricular stroke volume, functional status and exercise capacity in patients with ventricular dysfunction and conduction delay: The US InSync III trial (abstract). *PACE* 2002;24:141.
83. Leon AR, Greenberg JM, Kanuru N, et al. Cardiac resynchronization in patients with congestive heart failure and chronic atrial fibrillation. *J Am Coll Cardiol* 2002;39:1258–1263.
84. Cazeau S, LeClerq C, Lavergne T, et al. Effects of multisite biventricular pacing in patients with heart failure and intraventricular conduction delay. *N Engl J Med* 2001;344:873–880.
85. Linde C, Leclercq C, Rex S, et al. Long-Term benefits of biventricular pacing in congestive heart failure: Results from the Multisite Stimulation In Cardiomyopathy (MUSTIC) Study. *J Am Coll Cardiol* 2002; 40:111–118.
86. Abraham WT, Fisher WG, Smith AL, et al. Cardiac resynchronization in chronic heart failure. *N Engl J Med* 2002;346:1845–1853.
87. Bradley DJ, Bradley EA, Baughman KL, et al. Cardiac resynchronization and death from progressive heart failure: A meta-analysis of randomized controlled trials. *JAMA* 2003;289:730–740.
88. Kuhlkamp V. Initial experience with an implantable cardioverter-defibrillator incorporating cardiac resynchronization therapy. *J Am Coll Cardiol* 2002;39:790–797.

89. Higgins SL, Young P, Scheck D, et al. Biventricular pacing diminishes the need for implantable cardioverter defibrillator therapy. *J Am Coll Cardiol* 2000;36:824–827.
90. Salukhe TV, Francis DP, Sutton R. Comparison of medical therapy, pacing and defibrillation in heart failure (COMPANION) trial terminated early; combined biventricular pacemaker-defibrillators reduce all-cause mortality and hospitalization. *Int J Cardiol* 2003;87: 119–120.
91. Hassenstein VP, Wolter HH. Therapeutische beherrschung einer bedrohmichen situation bei der idiopathischen hypertrophischen subaortenstenose. *Verh Dtsch Ges Kreislaufforsch* 1967;33:242–246.
92. Sorajja P, Elliott PM, McKenna WJ. Pacing in hypertrophic cardiomyopathy. *Cardiol Clin* 2000;18:67–79.
93. Appenberger L, Linde C, Daubert C, et al. Pacing in hypertrophic cardiomyopathy. A randomized crossover study. PIC study group. *Eur Heart J* 1997;18:1249–1256.
94. Ellenbogen KA, Wood MA, Shepard RK. Delayed complications following pacemaker implantation. *Pacing Clin Electrophysiol* 2002;25: 1155–1158.
95. Oginosawa Y, Abe H, Nakashima Y. The incidence and risk factors for venous obstruction after implantation of transvenous pacing leads. *Pacing Clin Electrophysiol* 2002;25:1605–1611.
96. Mazzetti H, Dussaut A, Tentori C, et al. Superior vena cava occlusion and/or syndrome related to pacemaker leads. *Am Heart J* 1993;125: 831–837.
97. Smith HJ, Fernot NE, Byrd CL, et al. Five-years experience with intravascular lead extraction. *Pacing Clin Electrophysiol* 1994;17:2016.
98. Travill CM, Sutton R, Pacemaker syndrome: An iatrogenic condition. *Br Heart J* 1992;68:163.
99. Vijayaraman P, Vaidya K, Kim SG, et al. Runaway pulse genertor malfunction resulting from undetected battery depletion. *Pacing Clin Electrophysiol* 2002;25:220–222.
100. Pinski SI, Trohman RG. Interference in implanted cardiac devices. *Pacing Clin Electrophysiol* 2002;25:1367–1381.

CHAPTER 33

# LONG-TERM CONTINUOUS ELECTROCARDIOGRAPHIC RECORDING

R. Joe Noble / Eric N. Prystowsky



Long-term electrocardiographic recording is a method of recording the ECG over an extended time period.[1] Technological advances in the past few years have provided a diversity of recording, transmitting, and analysis systems.

## INDICATIONS

Ambulatory ECG (AECG) recording may be helpful in diagnosing and, less frequently, quantitating arrhythmias in patients with symptoms potentially related to an arrhythmia. The recording of a rhythm disturbance simultaneous with a patient's symptoms may be the only means of diagnosis, particularly when the symptoms and arrhythmia are relatively infrequent (Fig. 33-1). Importantly, the recording of a normal rhythm when the patient is symptomatic may prove equally valuable in excluding a rhythm disturbance as the cause for the patient's symptoms.[2]

AECG recordings used to detect asymptomatic arrhythmias—for example, nonsustained ventricular tachycardia—may be indicated in certain patients to assess risk for future cardiac events. Such patients include those with idiopathic hypertrophic cardiomyopathy and those who have survived myocardial infarction with substantial left ventricular (LV) dysfunction.[3] However, the value of AECG in predicting risk is compromised by low sensitivity and specificity.

Patients who undergo treatment for arrhythmias, such as atrial fibrillation (AF) or ventricular tachycardia, may benefit from AECG recordings in order to assess the efficacy of therapy. An example may be determination of rate control over 24 h in patients with persistent AF.[4] Similarly, patients in whom pacemakers have been implanted who have symptoms consistent with pacemaker malfunction or require evaluation of their rate-responsive physiologic pacing function may require long-term AECG recording.

Other potential uses of AECG are detection of myocardial ischemia and measurement of heart rate variability and QT dispersion. Correlation of symptoms that occur during normal daily activity with demonstration of significant ST segment–T-wave alterations that cannot be reproduced by hyperventilation or by change in position, particularly when reinforced by documentation in the patient's diary of simultaneous symptoms of angina, proves highly suggestive of ischemic heart disease. The reader is referred to *Guidelines for Ambulatory Electrocardiography,* published jointly by the American College of Cardiology and the American Heart Association, for a more complete consideration of clinical indications for ambulatory AECG recordings.[3]

## RECORDING TECHNIQUES

Four general types of devices for acquiring data are currently available: continuous recorders, intermittent or event recorders, instruments for real-time recording and transmission of ECGs, and implantable recorders (Table 33-1).

### Continuous Recorders

The ECG can be recorded continuously on cassette tape or digitally in solid-state memory. The tape recorder is a battery-powered, miniature device with a very slow tape speed that is small enough to be suspended by a strap over the shoulder or around the waist.

All digital recording systems amplify, digitize, and store the ECG in solid-state memory. Two types of digital recorders are available. In the first, each QRS complex is recorded, similar in this sense to the continuous tape recording. "Full disclosure" of the ECG is provided by enhanced storage capacity on a memory card the size of a credit card. With the second, microcomputers and microelectronic circuits sample the cardiac rhythm in real time as it is being recorded, convert the analogue signal into a digital signal, and analyze the data in terms of maximal and minimal rates, RR intervals, and changes in RR

Rapid Heartbeat Symptom

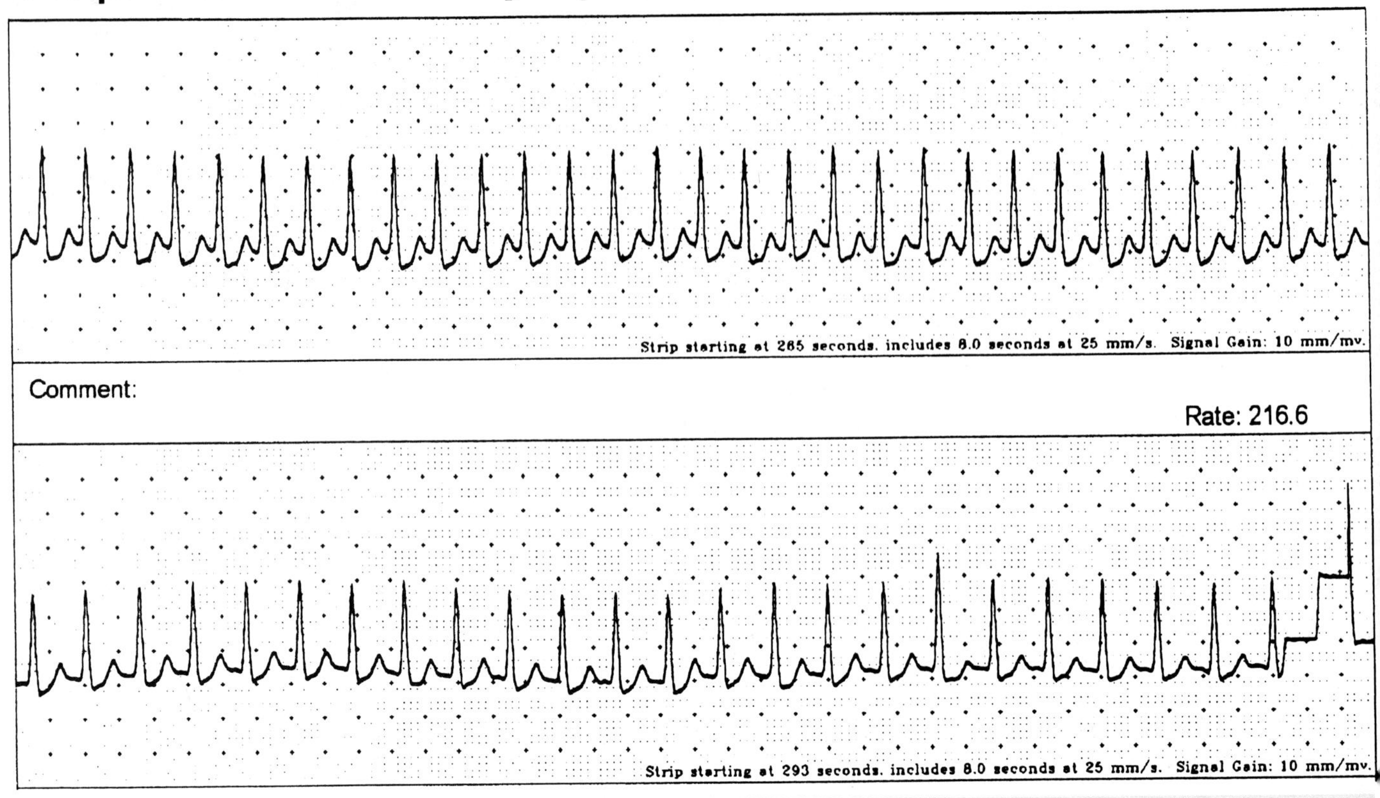


FIGURE 33-1 An episode of rapid paroxysmal supraventricular tachycardia captured with a handheld event recorder during a typical period of symptoms.

intervals. Within minutes of the instrument's disconnection from the patient, the information can be retrieved in the form of a histogram covering the entire recording period, and a printout of selected segments in real time can be obtained. This instrument is different from those used to make continuous tape or digital recordings in that the actual ECG has not been recorded on tape; only the histogram has been stored. Selected brief segments of the patient's ECG—e.g., 6- to 10-s intervals—can also be stored, however. Microcomputers that can analyze electronic data over prolonged periods, even several days, have been developed.

The lead systems on recorders vary from one manufacturer to another. Meticulous attention must be paid to placing the electrodes on the patient's chest, since poor electrode contact will produce technically inadequate recordings.

## Event Recorders

An alternative method records not continuously but only when the patient senses symptoms or an event. Of the numerous event recorders available, traditionally there have been two basic types, which are differentiated on the basis of memory.

In the *postevent recorder,* without memory, the unit may continuously monitor the ECG via attached leads. Typically, the patient wears the recorder continuously, activating it when symptoms appear; this device does not record the ECG until it is activated. Alternatively, the patient may carry a miniature solid-state recorder with which the rhythm can be recorded whenever the symptoms appear simply by placing the unit on the precordium or, in some cases, on the wrist. The recorded data are stored in memory until the patient submits the information either directly or transtelephonically to an ECG receiver, where it is recorded.

With a *preevent recorder,* employing a memory loop, the rhythm is monitored continuously via leads, either at the extremities or over the precordium, connected to a recorder typically worn on a belt. Patients activate the unit when they experience symptoms, so that an abnormal rhythm or an ECG synchronous with the symptoms can be recorded. The loop recorder is capable of recording information several seconds or minutes before or after a recognized event; the number of events that can be recorded and the allotment of recording time prior to and after activation of the unit are programmable and are different for various models.

Preevent and postevent recorders have several limitations: (1) inability to record asymptomatic arrhythmias, (2) no method for the patient to transmit specific symptoms with each event, and (3) frequent missed events due to patient error in using the device.[2] A new event recorder has been developed to address these concerns. Kowey et al.[5] recently reported preliminary data on a mobile cardiac outpatient telemetry system that consists of a three-electrode, two-channel sensor transmitting wirelessly to a portable monitor, which analyzes and stores ECG data. Significant arrhythmias, whether symptomatic or asymptomatic, are transmitted by the wireless net-

TABLE 33-1 Types of Electrocardiographic Recording Instruments

| Type | Recording | Scanning | Transmitting |
|---|---|---|---|
| | | **CONTINUOUS** | |
| Analogue | All ECG complexes, "full disclosure" | Technician with computer assistance, templating, area determination, and superimposition | None |
| Digital—continuous recording | All ECG complexes, "full disclosure" | Technician with computer assistance, templating, area determination, and superimposition | Transtelephonic |
| Digital—real-time analysis | Computer analysis of ECG and selected ECG printouts | Real time by microprocessor with retrospective technician editing | None |
| | | **EVENT RECORDER** | |
| "Postevent," nonlooping, without memory Handheld or worn | ECG, selected by patient activation | Direct visualization | Transtelephonic |
| "Preevent," looping, with memory, monitor worn with attached electrodes | ECG, selected by patient activation, with memory of preevent | Direct visualization | Transtelephonic |
| Continuous mobile outpatient telemetry system | ECG, selected by patient or automatic | Direct visualization; technician with computer assistance | Transtelephonic |
| | | **IMPLANTABLE DEVICES** | |
| Subcutaneous, implanted digital recorder | ECG, selected by patient activation with memory of preevent or automatic | Direct visualization | Direct telemetry |
| Automatic electronic sensor in ICD or pacemaker | ECG, when activated by ICD discharge or recognized by sensor in pacemaker, with memory | Direct visualization of analysis or ECG | Direct telemetry |
| | | **REAL TIME** | |
| Real-time transtelephonic monitoring | ECG at central monitoring station—no recording at device | Direct visualization | Transtelephonic |

work to a monitoring station and analyzed by trained personnel. Serious arrhythmias are dealt with promptly. Patient-activated events are sent together with a choice of symptoms and activity at the time of the event. Of the initial 28 monitored patients, 15 had previously gone undiagnosed by other ambulatory monitoring techniques and 6 (40%) were found to have a significant arrhythmia.

## Implantable Recorders

A miniaturized *event recorder* has been developed that can be implanted subcutaneously to be mechanically activated by the patient to record an ECG when the patient suffers serious symptoms such as syncope. Preset high and low heart rate parameters are selected and will automatically record events if the rate threshold is met. These devices are particularly useful to capture events that occur relatively infrequently—for example, a few times per year[6] (Fig. 33-2).

Event recording is also provided by some newer-generation pacemakers and implantable cardioverter/defibrillators (Fig. 33-3). These instruments automatically recognize abnormal rhythms, such as tachycardia, and provide, via telemetric transmission, either actual ECG records or an analysis of the number, rate, and duration of recognized arrhythmias.

## Real-Time Monitoring

As another variation, the device that acquires data can transmit the ECG information directly and transtelephonically, in real time, without recording the data in the unit. With such a device, for instance,

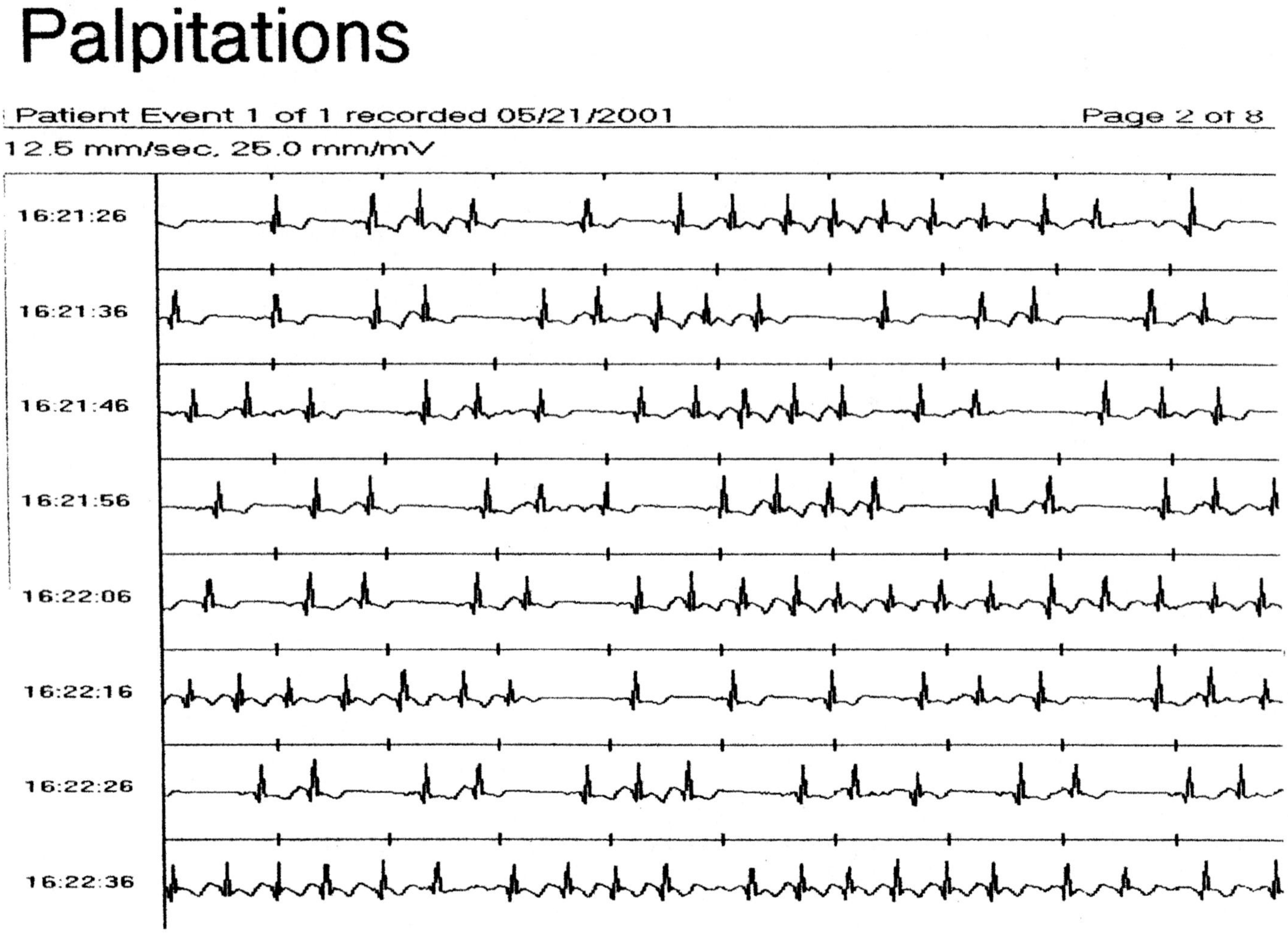

# Palpitations

Patient Event 1 of 1 recorded 05/21/2001 Page 2 of 8

12.5 mm/sec, 25.0 mm/mV

FIGURE 33-2 ECG tracing from implantable loop recorder at time of palpitations. Note the intermittent episodes of supraventricular tachycardia.

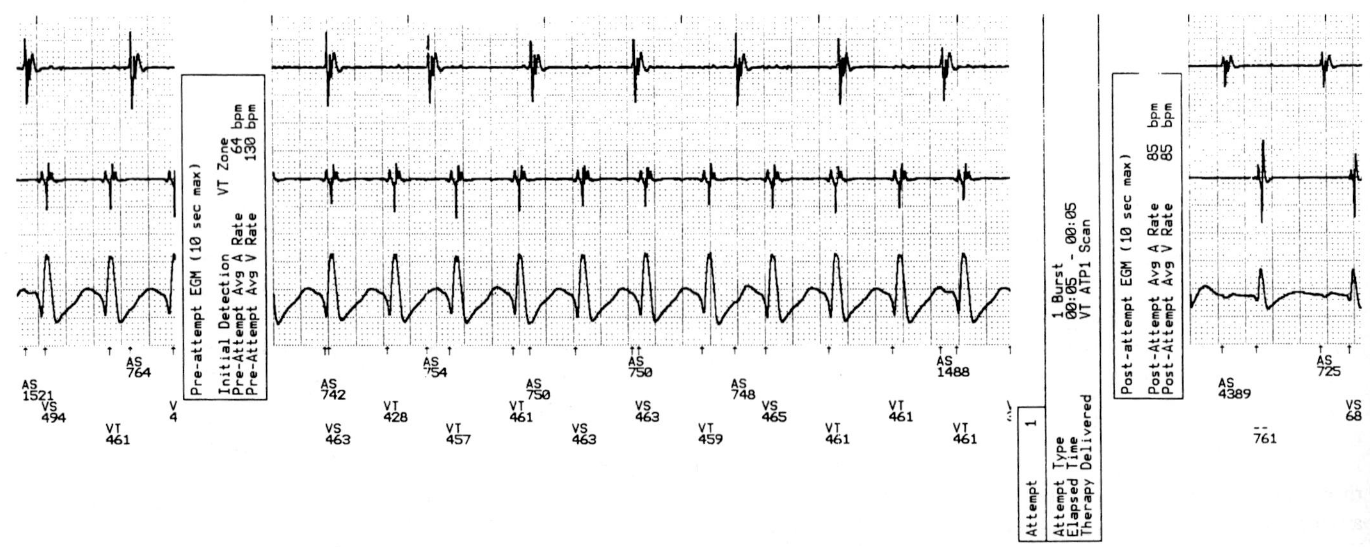


FIGURE 33-3 Intracardiac electrograms from a dual-chamber implantable cardioverter defibrillator (ICD) for an episode of ventricular tachycardia. The simultaneous tracings are the atrial electrogram and ventricular electrogram far-field ECG. Note atrioventricular dissociation during ventricular tachycardia (*left* and *center*) and normal sinus rhythm after termination of ventricular tachycardia by antitachycardia pacing (*right*).

the patient can transmit his or her ECG daily or even multiple times each day, with or without symptoms, at some distance from the medical institution to the recording station. Routine pacemaker evaluations use such systems.

### Recordings of ST Segments and T Waves

For several reasons, both technical and physiologic, long-term ECG recording devices do not provide the same degree of reliability in interpretation of the pattern of the ST segment and T wave as in the detection of rhythm disturbances. Technical limitations include certain characteristics of the patient's ECG: normal sinus rhythm, an isoelectric ST segment and absence of broad Q waves, intraventricular conduction delays, and LV hypertrophy are prerequisites. Even more important than these technical considerations, however, are certain physiologic limitations. For instance, standing, hyperventilation, eating, anxiety, use of drugs, and change in heart rate or autonomic tone are all daily events that may result in depression of the ST segment or inversion of the T wave to simulate ischemic changes. Striking ST-segment elevation has been recorded during prolonged recording in patients without organic heart disease.[7]

## SCANNING AND ANALYSIS TECHNIQUES

The recording can be analyzed by scanning the tape or digital record at high speed, by printing it out directly, or—as in the case of microcomputers—by processing during the recording and printing out the analysis at the end of sampling.

Scanning techniques include technician-dependent analysis, in which a technician interprets the cardiac rhythm as it is played back at high speed on an oscilloscope at 30 to 240 times the speed of the actual event. One commonly used method of scanning superimposes each QRS complex on the immediately preceding complex so that identical QRS contours present as a stationary image. Variations in QRS contour then become readily apparent. Simultaneously displayed on the oscilloscope for each cardiac cycle is a vertical bar graph, the height of which is directly proportional to each RR interval and QRS morphology. Thus the occurrence of a premature ventricular extrasystole would alter the stationary image by producing a variation in the QRS contour, alter the pitch and sound of the audio signal, and shorten the vertical bar reflecting cycle lengths. When such an abnormal event is noted, the tape can be played at a normal rate of speed for analysis on a standard ECG machine.

To minimize the human factor and provide accurate quantitative data, the tape can be analyzed by a semiautomated electronic analyzer, which quantitates the number of abnormalities it recognizes. The accuracy of the system depends on the system's ability to distinguish abnormal from normal.

A computer can be interfaced with the scanner to quantitate the data even more accurately. The playback analysis can occur at up to 240 times the normal rate. Electronic analyzers and computers, as well as the scanner, can be programmed to recognize the patient's own QRS complex template and then to recognize any deviation from normal. The computer program can provide summaries of heart rates, heart rate variability, frequency of premature atrial or ventricular extrasystoles, coupling intervals, runs of tachycardia or other arrhythmias, and variations in QRS, ST, QT, or T-wave pattern during any time period. Hard copies can be printed out for verification. When arrhythmias or pattern changes are detected, an automatic ECG printout can be triggered by the event marker or by the computer. An alternative to scanning is the direct printout of the entire record.

## SELECTION OF DEVICE FOR PROLONGED ECG RECORDING

The ultimate selection of a long-term ECG recording system depends on the individual patient's needs (Table 33-1).[2,3,5,6,8] If a precise count of ectopy is required, a continuous recorder with computer-based analysis is essential. These devices are also very useful to evaluate daily ventricular rate control in atrial fibrillation. On the other hand, if the purpose of the recording is to detect episodic arrhythmic events such as ventricular tachycardia or AF, an event recorder would be an excellent choice. An event recorder provides an opportunity to monitor over prolonged periods of time and is of benefit to the patient whose symptoms do not occur on a daily basis. When the goal is to correlate the patient's rhythm or ECG pattern with symptoms that are very infrequent—for example, every few months—an implantable loop recorder appears to be the best choice. The choice between preevent and postevent recorder depends on the duration and type of patient symptoms. A preevent loop recorder is needed for patients with syncope or symptoms of brief duration.

## DURATION OF RECORDING

Arrhythmias are often evanescent, occurring only rarely. In such patients, 24-h ECG recordings are unlikely to detect the abnormal rhythm. Even when arrhythmias are frequent, marked variation in the frequency and complexity of the rhythm disturbance is expected, with variations occurring during and between days.

The ideal duration of recording varies from patient to patient, depending on the physician's goals. If the objective is to correlate the cardiac rhythm or pattern with a symptom such as syncope, palpitations, or chest pain, the monitoring period must be extended sufficiently to incorporate a symptomatic period, whether these intervals occur with a frequency of hours or months. The actual recording period, however, may be only seconds. For assessment of rate control for a patient with AF, a 24-h ECG monitoring period is sufficient.

## ARTIFACTS AND ERRORS

Artifacts registered during prolonged ECG recording have mimicked virtually every variety of supraventricular and ventricular bradycardia and tachycardia and have led to misdiagnosis and inappropriate and unnecessary treatment.[9,10]

Most of these artifacts are identical to those plaguing the standard 12-lead ECG but are simply detected more frequently due to the length of the recording; however, many are unique to extended recording by virtue of the magnetic tape recorder.

Probably the most common artifact is that resulting from a loose electrode (Fig. 33-4) or mechanical "stimulation" of the electrode. Failure of either the battery or the motor of the recorder generally results in a slowing of the tape speed as the ECG is recorded. When played back, the heart rate will appear fast; i.e., it will mimic a tachycardia (Fig. 33-5). The interpreter may be alerted to the artifact by the concomitant shortening of all ECG intervals (PR, QRS, QT, and RR) and decrease in QRS voltage. Conversely, transient slowing or sticking of the tape during playback will suggest bradycardia or atrioventricular (AV) or intraventricular conduction disturbances (Fig. 33-6). Recording an ECG on a previously used tape that is incompletely erased results in the simultaneous registration of two ECGs and potentially the misinterpretation of a "parasystolic" ectopic rhythm (Fig. 33-7). Digital recording in solid-state memory eliminates these various mechanical failures of tape recordings.

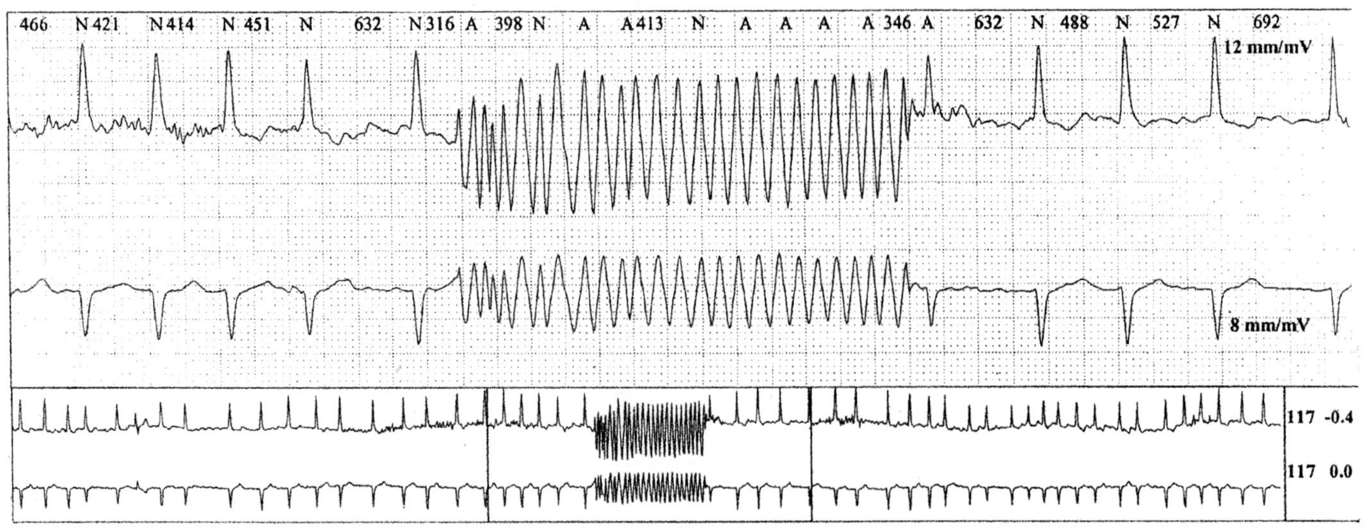


FIGURE 33-4 Artifact recorded from a Holter monitor. A loose electrode was responsible for the artifactual tracing mimicking ventricular flutter/fibrillation recorded by the monitor.

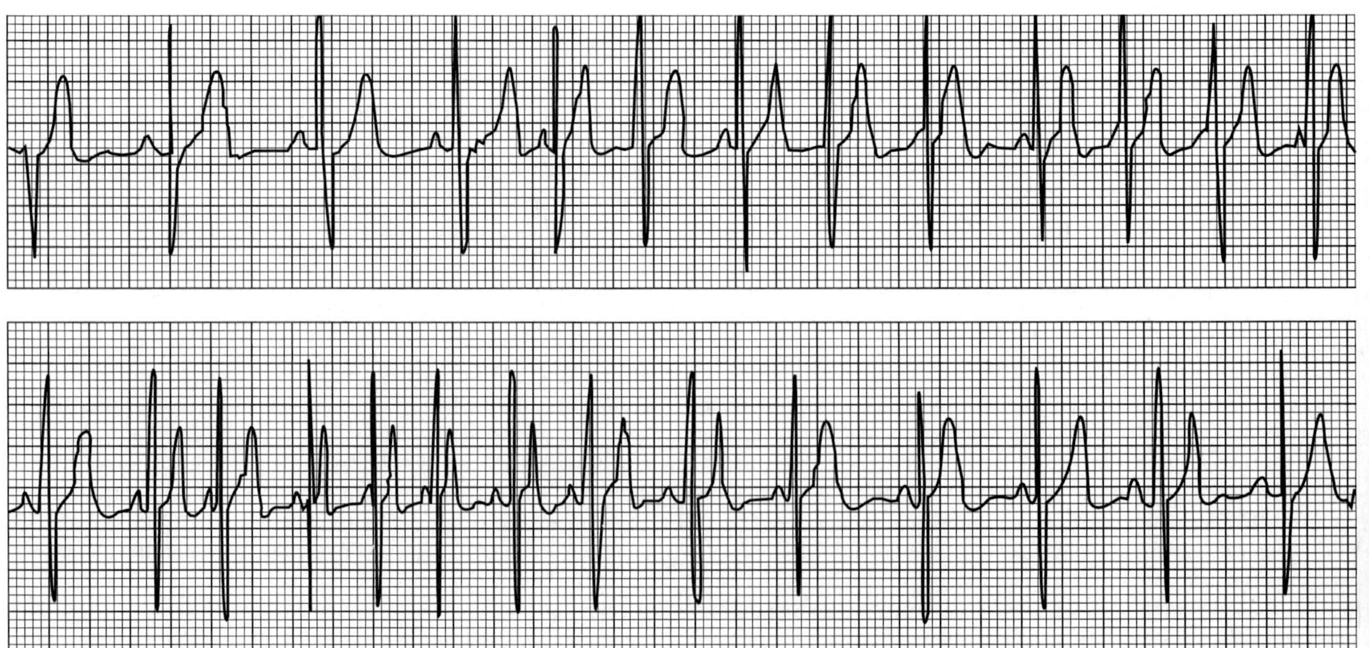

FIGURE 33-5 Deceleration of tape during recording. Supraventricular tachycardia is simulated toward the end of the top and beginning of the second trace as the tape, which transiently slowed as a result of battery failure during recording, was played back on recording paper at proper speed. Note the foreshortening of the duration of the P wave, PR interval, QRS complex, and QT interval.

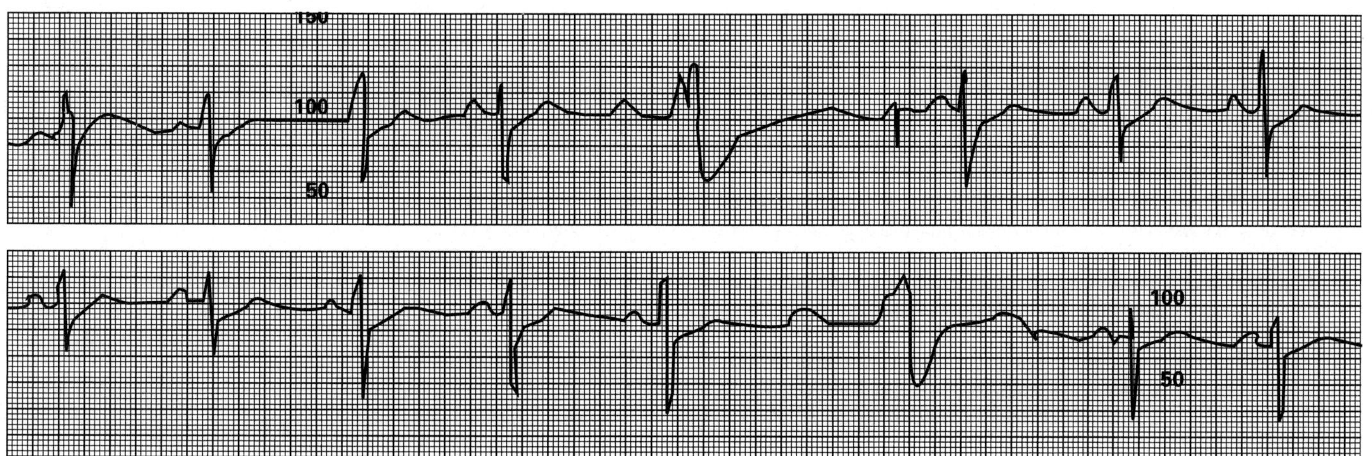


FIGURE 33-6 Deceleration of tape during playback. Slowing or sticking of the tape during playback spreads out the P wave, PR interval, and QRS complex to resemble sinus deceleration or transient atrioventricular or intraventricular conduction delay (fifth complex in top trace; sixth complex in bottom trace).

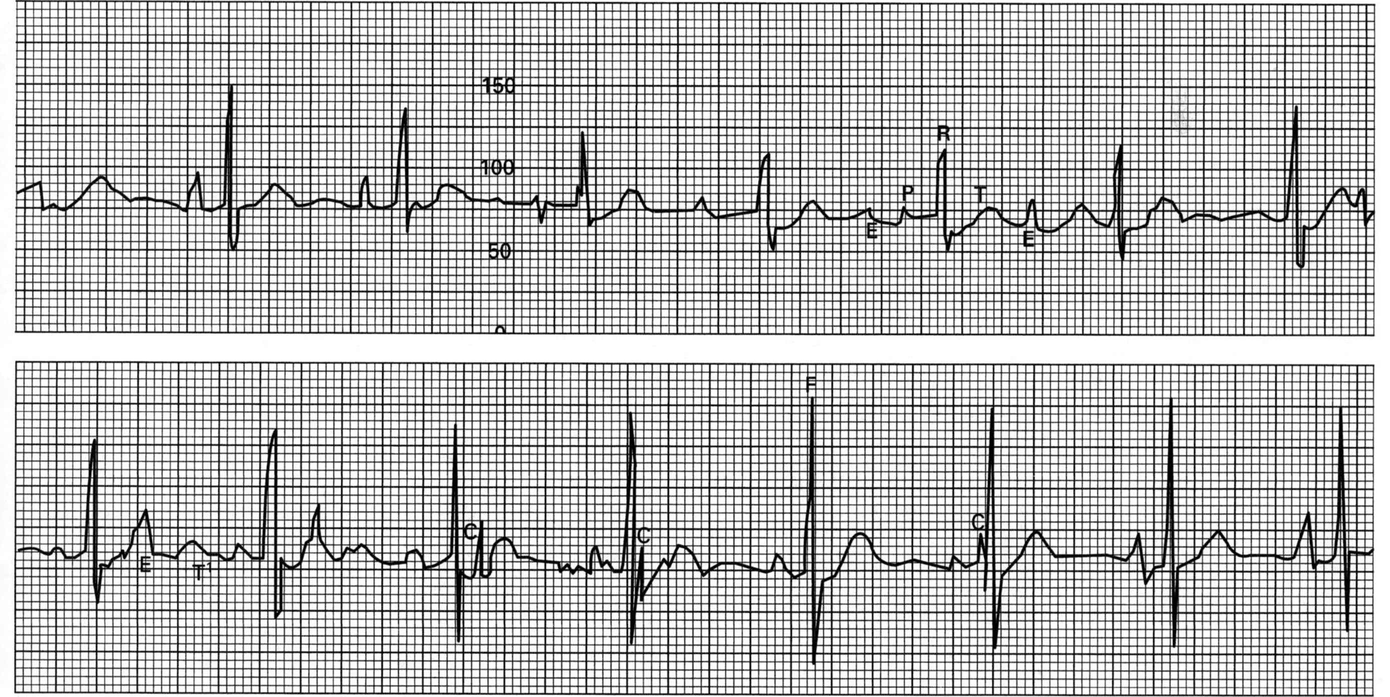


FIGURE 33-7 Incomplete erasure of tape. Two independent ventricular rhythms are identified: a larger QRS, labeled R, whose P wave and T wave are also labeled, and a smaller QRS, considered "ectopic" and labeled E; its T wave is labeled T. The sequence could be recorded with a piggyback heart transplant or in Siamese twins. Alternatively, ectopic complex E may be misinterpreted to represent a parasystolic rhythm even fusing with complex R at F. The very short coupling intervals (C) preclude this possibility and indicate that the ECG record of one patient is superimposed on that of another.

The technician and/or physician who interprets prolonged ECG recordings must have a working knowledge of these and other potential artifacts in order to interpret the records properly.

## References


1. Holter NJ. New method for heart studies: Continuous electrocardiography of active subjects over long periods is now practical. *Science* 1961; 134:1214–1220.
2. Fogel R, Evans J, Prystowsky E. Utility and cost of event recorders in the diagnosis of palpitations, presyncope and syncope. *Am J Cardiol* 1997;79:207–208.
3. ACC/AHA. Guidelines for Ambulatory electrocardiography: A report of the American College of Cardiology/American Heart Association Task Force on Practice Guidelines. *J Am Coll Cardiol* 1999;34:(3)917–948.
4. Prystowsky EN, Katz A. Atrial Fibrillation. In: Topol EJ, ed. *Textbook of Cardiovascular Medicine,* 2d ed. Philadelphia: Lippincott-Raven; 2002: 1403–1428.
5. Kowey PR, Joshi A, Prystowsky EN, et al. First experience with a mobile cardiac outpatient telemetry system for the diagnosis and management of cardiac arrhythmias. *PACE* 2003;26:(II)1090.
6. Krahn A, Klein G, Yee R, Takle-Newhouse T: Use of an extended monitoring strategy in patients with problematic syncope. *Circulation* 1999; 99(3):406–410.
7. Golding B, Wolf E, Tzivoni D, Stern S. Transient S-T elevation detected by 24-hour ECG monitoring during normal daily activity. *Am Heart J* 1973;86:501–507.
8. Kinlay S, Leitch J, Neil A, et al. Event recorders yield more diagnoses and are more cost-effective than 48-hour Holter monitoring in patients with palpitations. *Ann Intern Med* 1996;124(1 pt 1):16–20.
9. Krasnow AZ, Bloomfield DK. Artifacts in portable electrocardiographic monitoring. *Am Heart J* 1976;91:349–357.
10. Knight BP, Pelosi F, Michaud GF, et al. Clinical consequences of electrocardiographic artifact mimicking ventricular tachycardia. *N Engl J Med* 1999;341:1270–1274.

C H A P T E R 34

# TECHNIQUES OF ELECTROPHYSIOLOGIC EVALUATION

Masood Akhtar



The recording of intracavitary electrocardiographic signals and various forms of pacing programs have experienced enormous growth during the past three decades. Recordings of intracardiac signals from the region of the His bundle, initially made by Scherlag et al.,[1] were rapidly applied to clinical problems including atrioventricular (AV) blocks and supraventricular and ventricular tachyarrhythmias.[1–10] Such recordings were then complemented by pacing to unmask sinus node dysfunction and AV conduction abnormalities as well as to initiate supraventricular tachycardias (SVTs).[3–8] Intracardiac electrophysiologic studies (EPSs) have since found utility in a variety of cardiac arrhythmias, including sinus node dysfunction, intraventricular and AV conduction disturbances, SVTs, ventricular tachycardias (VTs), preexcitation syndromes, and atrial and ventricular fibrillation (VF). Such studies are now also employed as a prelude to correction of various arrhythmias and conduction defects. This chapter addresses recording and pacing techniques and their clinical utility.[9–12]

## TECHNIQUES OF INTRACARDIAC ELECTROPHYSIOLOGIC STUDIES

The exact type of electrical signal recordings, specific equipment used, and pacing protocol depend on the nature of the clinical problem, the type of electrophysiologic assessment, and the anticipated course of action. Routine cardiac EPSs are performed while patients are in a nonsedated postabsorptive state.[13] Although some degree of sedation is advisable in apprehensive patients, the use of drugs that may alter the properties of the cardiac conduction system should be avoided. Antiarrhythmic drugs are usually but not always stopped prior to these studies. In selected cases, antiarrhythmic drugs may be continued if a clinical event occurred while the patient was on a specific agent.

The typical electrode catheters used for both recording and cardiac stimulation are multipolar (sizes varying from 4 to 8F). Catheters can be inserted via peripheral veins such as the antecubital, femoral, subclavian, or internal jugular veins. When a catheter is intended to be left in place for several days, subclavian and internal jugular veins are preferable. For most electrophysiologic testing, the catheter is placed in the high right atrium, at the His bundle, or at the right bundle branch region across the tricuspid valve and right ventricular apex or outflow. For accessory pathways or AV junctional tachycardias, a catheter is placed in the region of the coronary sinus. Heparin may be given at approximately 1000 U/h. For His bundle and right bundle branch recording, the catheter is introduced via the femoral vein, advanced across the tricuspid valve, and gradually withdrawn until an appropriate recording from the right bundle and/or the His bundle is obtained (Fig. 34-1). For a routine study, left-sided heart catheterization is seldom necessary. In patients with VT and/or left-sided accessory pathways, however, this is performed for diagnostic or therapeutic purposes. Continuous heparinization is desirable for left heart catheterization to avoid thromboembolic complications.

### Electrophysiologic Recordings

Once the electrode catheters are placed appropriately, the connections are made via a junction box and isolation units to prevent excess current in the event of random electrical surges. All of the electrograms are displayed simultaneously on a multichannel oscilloscopic recorder. In addition to the intracardiac signals, several unfiltered surface electrocardiographic leads (i.e., X, Y, and Z or leads I, II, or aVF and $V_1$) are recorded. Although appropriately placed electrode catheters will record desired signals at any filtering frequency, filter settings between 30 to 40 and 500 Hz are best suited for

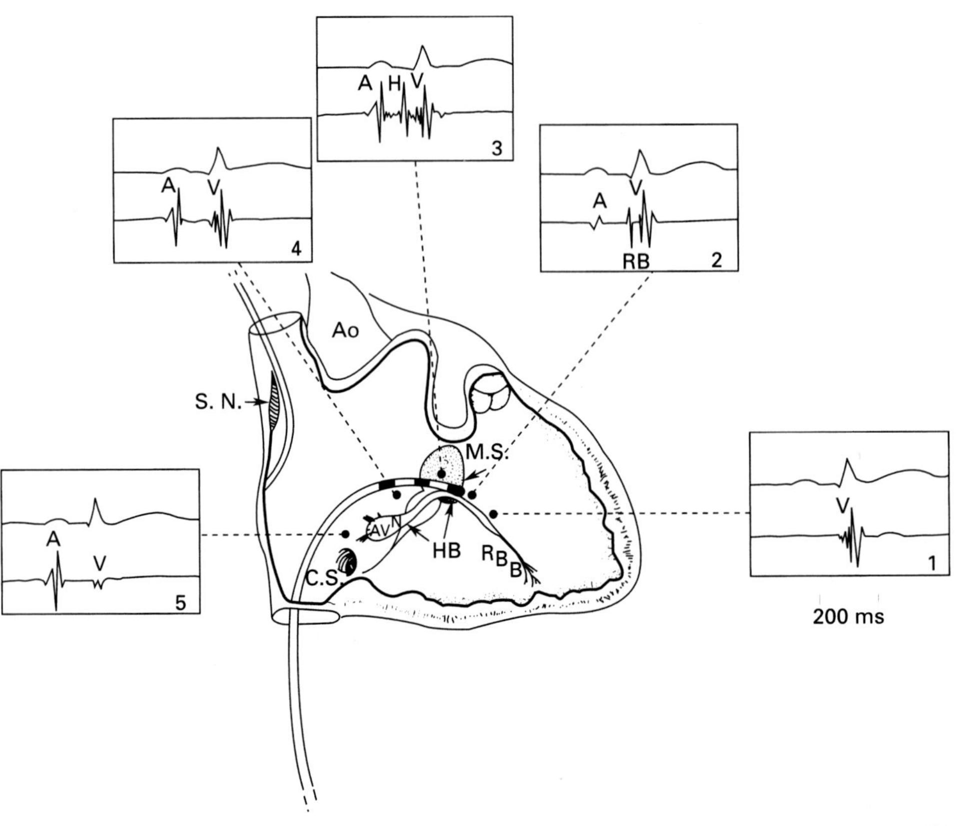


FIGURE 34-1 Intracardiac recordings from the specialized conduction system in the atrioventricular (AV) junction. The recording of various electrograms along the right side of the interventricular septum with gradual withdrawal of the catheter across the tricuspid valve is shown. The intracardiac recordings are labeled. Numbers 1 through 5 refer to intracardiac location of catheters along with corresponding electrogram. CS = coronary sinus; SN = sinus node; Ao = aorta; MS = membranous septum; AVN = atrioventricular node; HB = His bundle; RBB = right bundle branch; A = atrial deflection; H and RB = His and right bundle potentials; V = ventricular deflection. (From Gallagher and Damato.[57] Reproduced with permission from the publisher and authors.)

sharp intracardiac signals such as those from the His bundle and accessory pathways (Fig. 34-2). Undesirable low-frequency signals can be reduced by a high-pass filter setting of more than 50 to 100 Hz. On the other hand, 60-cycle interference can be eliminated with a low-pass filter setting at 50 Hz.

The main value of intracardiac/electrocardiographic tracings is the timing of electrical events and determining the direction of impulse propagation. To acquire true local electrical activity, a bipolar electrogram with an interelectrode distance of less than 1 cm is desirable. When unipolar electrograms are obtained, a rapid intrinsic deflection will identify a point of local activation. For routine intracardiac electrocardiographic studies, unipolar electrograms provide a relatively limited advantage over bipolar signals, and therefore the latter are more often utilized. For patients with atrial fibrillation, which seems primarily a left atrial arrhythmia originating in the pulmonary veins, left atrial catheterization is necessary. A sleeve of atrial myocardium that enters the pulmonary veins to a variable distance has recordable electrical activity and may very well be the source of atrial fibrillation in many cases, particularly those labeled as having lone atrial fibrillation. Cannulation of the pulmonary veins is done via a conventional electrode catheter that has been placed there either via patent foramen, transseptal procedure, or retrograde techniques.

The foregoing description relates to the standard diagnostic invasive EPS. In other clinical situations, different types of diagnostic methods are employed. For instance, during intraoperative mapping, direct placement of electrodes over the epicardium or endocardium is necessary to get appropriate signals for identifying the precise origin and route of impulse propagation.[14] These electrodes can be in the form of either handheld probes or plaques that can be placed or sutured over the myocardium. Socks and balloons incorporating several electrodes can also be used for epicardial and endocardial mapping techniques, respectively.[15,16] All electrical signals can be recorded on either a disk or frequency-modulated tape for permanent storage.

More recently, several other types of mapping and recording equipment have emerged to locate the origin of cardiac arrhythmias more accurately. Two of the systems likely to find clinical utility in the mapping of arrhythmic origins are (1) nonfluoroscopic electromagnetic endocardial mapping [CARTO, Biosense (Cordis Webster) Marlton, NJ] and (2) noncontact mapping (EnSite, Endocardial Solutions, Saint Paul, MN).

## THE CARTO SYSTEM

The CARTO system consists of a magnetic field generator locator pad placed under the patient table, a sensor-mounted catheter and a reference catheter placed intracardially, a mapping system, and a graphic computer.[17] The catheter tip allows orientation in relation to the reference signal. The accuracy of catheter tip position is within a millimeter of arrhythmia location in this low magnetic field. By moving the sensor sequentially, one can generate a three-dimensional (3D) activation map. By color coding, both the earliest and the latest directions of electrical activation can be recorded. Once the initial fluoroscopy-guided placement of reference catheter and other catheters is satisfactory, several points are acquired. A 3D map is generated, and sensor-mounted catheters are manipulated further without the help of fluoroscopy.

Aside from creation of an accurate map guiding the origin and activation sequence, the CARTO system is also helpful in separating micro- from macroreentry circuits. For example, in atrial flutter, by virtue of its large circuit, the impulse propagation along the entire route can be outlined. Due to the nature of reentry, the leading propagation front is found nearest to the trailing end and can be easily identified by color coding. The atrial focal tachycardia, on the other hand, can be distinguished by its radial spread from an atrial focus. A typical map generated during this technique is shown in Fig. 34-3, Plate 76.

## THE ENSITE 3000 SYSTEM

Noncontact mapping can be done using the Endocardial Solutions EnSite 3000 system.[18] This is a relatively new endocardial 3D map-

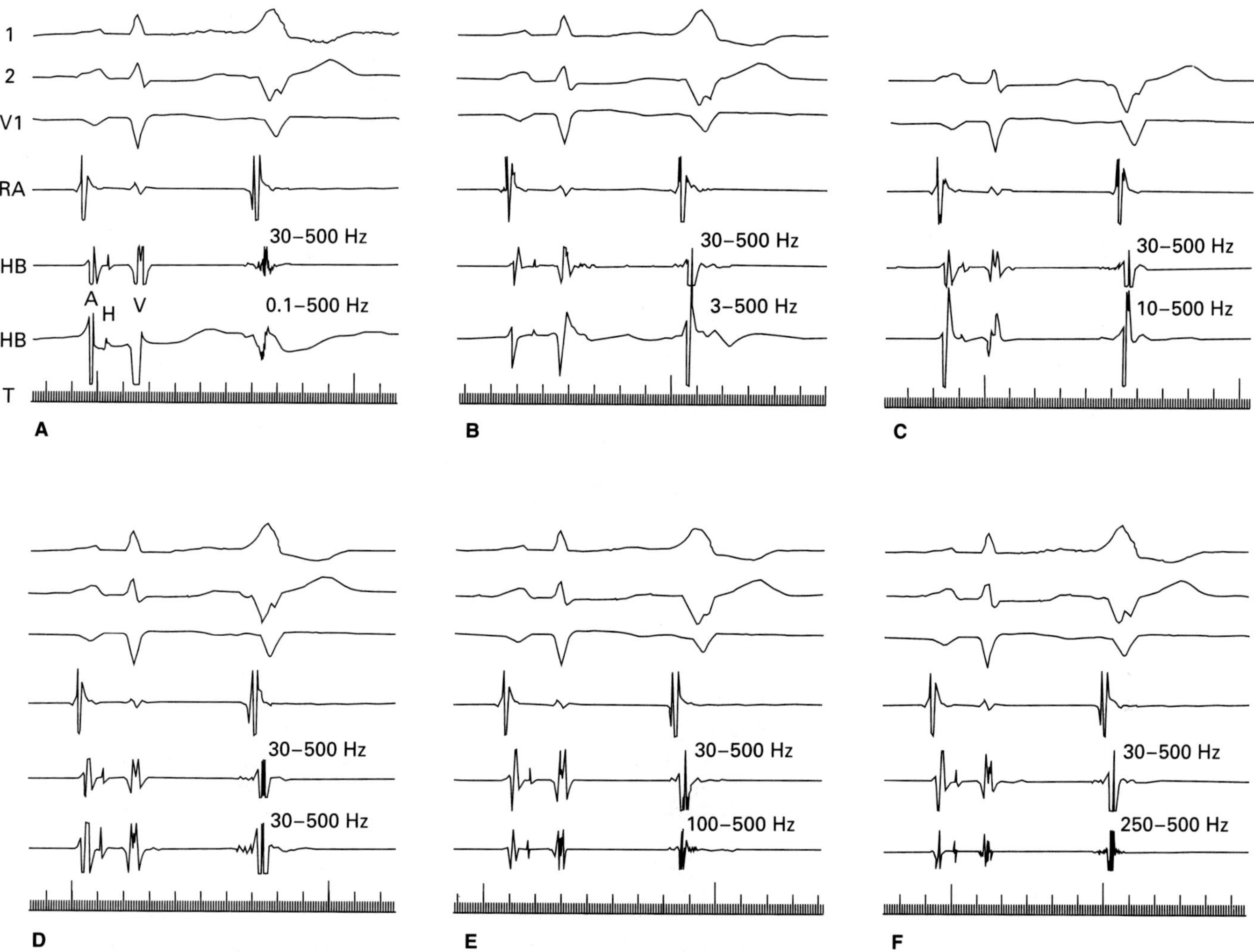


FIGURE 34-2 Effects of various filtering frequencies on the morphologic appearance of intracardiac electrograms *A* through *F*. The tracings from top to bottom are electrocardiographic leads I, II, $V_1$, right atrial (RA), two His bundle (HB) electrograms, and time (T) line. Similar abbreviations are used in subsequent figures and tracings. In each panel, the first beat is of sinus origin and is followed by a spontaneous ventricular premature beat. The top HB, RA, and RV are filtered at 30 to 500 Hz (i.e., the usual filtering frequencies). The bottom HB tracing shows the effect of various filtering frequencies on the appearance. The low-frequency signals are mostly eliminated at high-bandpass filter frequency settings above 10 Hz (*C*). The low-bandpass filter settings above 500 Hz generally do not have a significant effect on the intracardiac electrogram appearance. It should be pointed out that the high-bandpass setting reduces the overall magnitude of the electrogram, necessitating an increase in amplification. It should also be noted that, at all frequencies depicted, the HB deflection can be clearly identified. (From Akhtar.[13] Reproduced with permission from the publisher and authors.)

ping system that takes a different approach to such mapping (Fig. 34-4, Plate 77). Like the CARTO system, the EnSite 3000 system also makes use of an amplifier and computer system with custom software. The EnSite catheter uses a balloon design with a 64-electrode array arranged over the outside of the balloon. This balloon is positioned in the center of the chamber and does not come in contact with the walls of the chamber being mapped. Employing data from the 64-electrode-array catheter, the computer uses sophisticated algorithms to compute an *inverse solution* to determine the activation sequence on the endocardial surface. Data from all points in the chamber are acquired simultaneously.

To create a map, the balloon catheter is positioned in the chamber and deployed. A conventional (roving) deflectable catheter is also positioned in the chamber and used to collect geometry information. A 5-kHz signal is emitted from the tip electrode of the conventional catheter, and the computer analyzes this signal to determine the position of the roving catheter relative to the position of the balloon. The roving catheter is moved throughout the chamber, and the location information is collected by the system. Using this information, the computer creates a model, called a *convex hull,* of the chamber during diastole. After the chamber geometry is determined, mapping in sinus rhythm of the arrhythmia can begin. The data acquisition process is performed automatically by the system, and all data for the entire chamber are acquired simultaneously. Following this, the segment must be analyzed by the operator to find the early activation or vulnerable region of the reentry circuit. The locator technology that was used to collect the geometry information for the convex hull can then be used to guide an ablation catheter to the proper location in the heart.

Because data from the entire chamber are collected simultaneously with the EnSite 3000 system, it can be used to map nonsustained rhythms such as premature atrial complexes, irregular rhythms

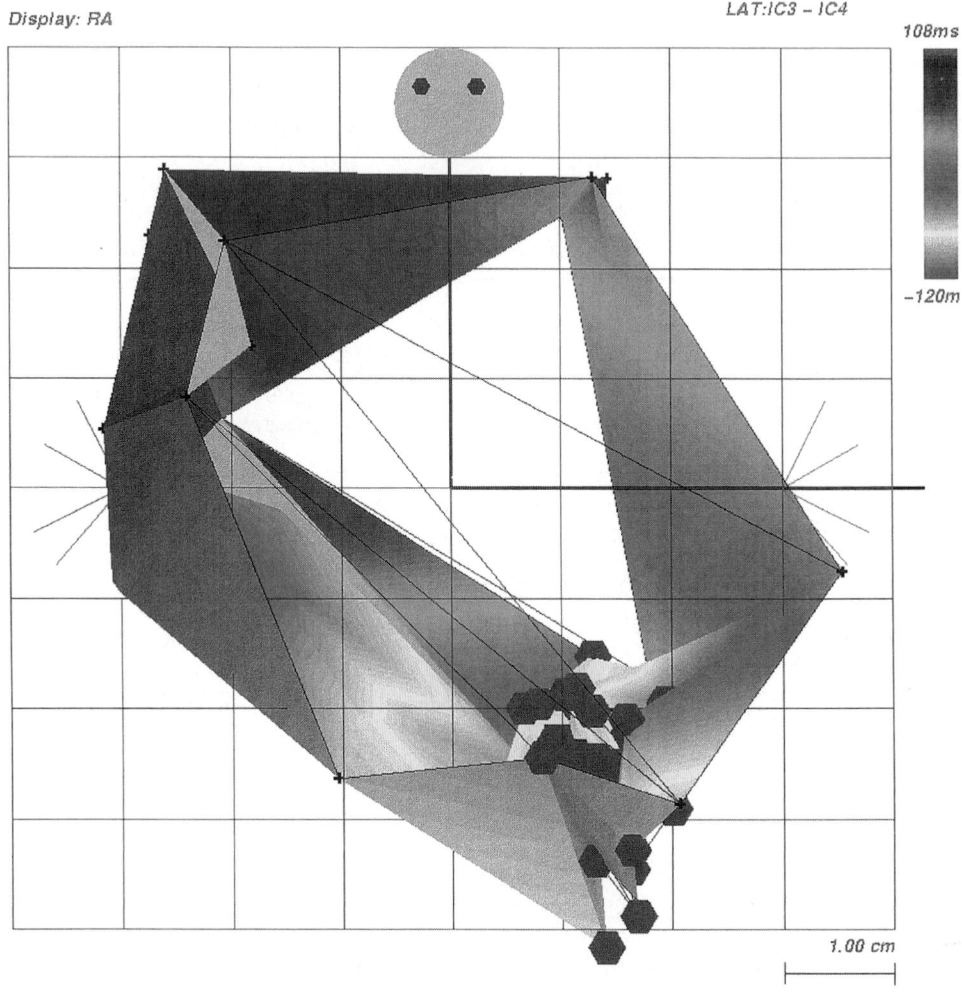


FIGURE 34-3 (Plate 76) Anterior-posterior view of the right atrium during typical, inferior vena cava (IVC)-tricuspid valve annulus isthmus-dependent atrial flutter using the Biosense CARTO system. The red shows the earliest activation with respect to the timing reference (typically the proximal coronary sinus recording), and the blue and the violet represent areas of late activation. The gray areas are where early activation meets late activation, a characteristic of reentrant tachycardias. The brown hexagons mark the location of radiofrequency lesions positioned on the isthmus to ablate the atrial flutter. RA = right atria.

such as atrial fibrillation or polymorphic VT, and rhythms that are not hemodynamically stable. The system is highly useful for identifying focal arrhythmias (Fig. 34-4) and atrial flutter. Currently approved indications, however, are for the right atrium only. Left atrial mapping can also be accomplished via transseptal catheterization. The other significant limitation of the system results from its reliance on the large-diameter balloon catheter with its current 9.5F lumen.

These mapping systems, both of which are relatively new, provide electrophysiologists with new tools for diagnosing and treating what are often complex arrhythmias.

## THE NAVEX SYSTEM

Further improvements in technology will enable the operator an anatomic view of the cardiac chambers noninvasively. Navex is a step in the right direction. Navex (Endocardial Solutions, St. Paul, MN) is a method for catheter tracking and location, recording ablation lesion location, and cardiac chamber anatomy reconstruction.[19–21] Based on the LocaLisa (Medtronic Inc., Minneapolis, MN) technology, this system combines catheter location and tracking features of LocaLisa with the ability to create an anatomic model of the cardiac chamber using only a single, conventional EP catheter and skin patches (Fig. 34-5). This approach may be useful in treating certain types of arrhythmias where the ablation strategy is primarily anatomically based; it could possibly be combined with other technologies for treating complex arrhythmias.

### Programmed Electrical Stimulation

After satisfactory placement of the electrode catheters, patches, or other forms of recording equipment, baseline recordings are made and programmed stimulation is initiated from the right and left atria and right ventricle. For ventricular stimulation, the pacing sites are the right ventricular apex, outflow tract, and rarely some other right ventricular site. In recent years left ventricular (LV) pacing in patients with congestive heart failure is being done increasingly via some branch of the coronary sinus. Endocardial LV pacing is seldom used, but when it is done, it is used for tachycardia induction. A variety of pacing programs can be utilized, depending on the nature of the underlying arrhythmic problem under investigation. At least two formats of pacing protocol are common. The first is incremental atrial or ventricular pacing, which is pacing at a constant cycle length with gradual shortening until the occurrence of a desirable event, such as induction of a tachycardia or production of AV or VA block. Bursts of pacing at a constant cycle length are occasionally used to induce SVT, VT, or VF or for study of sinus node function and integrity of subsidiary pacemakers.

The second pacing format is premature (or extra) stimulation from atrial or ventricular sites. For the study of a physiologic phenomenon, refractory periods, and conduction characteristics, a single extra stimulus is usually applied after a series of beats with a constant cycle length (Fig. 34-6). The scanning is initiated late during electrical diastole, and the coupling interval is progressively decreased until the atrial and/or ventricular muscle is refractory. For induction of SVTs, single, double, or more extra stimuli are delivered (Fig. 34-7). For the induction of VT, up to three ventricular extra stimuli are employed. The sensitivity of pacing protocols seems to be directly related to the number of extra stimuli utilized.[17] This occurs, however, at the expense of specificity when polymorphic VT/VF can be induced at very short coupling intervals by using multiple extra stimuli. Regardless of the pacing protocol, the induction of sustained monomorphic VT constitutes a specific response and is seldom induced in patients not prone to such arrhythmias clinically. In contrast, the induction of polymorphic VT/VF with three extra stimuli at short coupling intervals can be nonspecific and does not provide a reliable guide for serial drug testing. Both polymorphic VT and VF can be avoided to a great extent at short coupling intervals (<200 ms) if the induction of latency between the stimulus artifact and the local ventricular electrograms is avoided.[22–24]

During routine EPSs, a variety of electrophysiologic parameters are measured, including sinus node function and intraatrial, AV nodal, and His-Purkinje system conduction. Initiation of SVT and VT is attempted to determine the mechanisms, the site of origin (by pacing and mapping techniques), and the potential of overdrive termination as a therapy option. After baseline studies, intravenous drugs may be administered to facilitate either induction of tachycardias, aggravation of sinus node function, or production of AV block (Fig. 34-8), or to determine drug efficacy.[22–24] The role of EPSs in patient management has evolved over the past decades from a purely diagnostic method to a frequently applied therapeutic tool. A brief outline of the value of clinical EPSs in various arrhythmia settings is outlined separately under diagnostic and therapeutic categories, below.

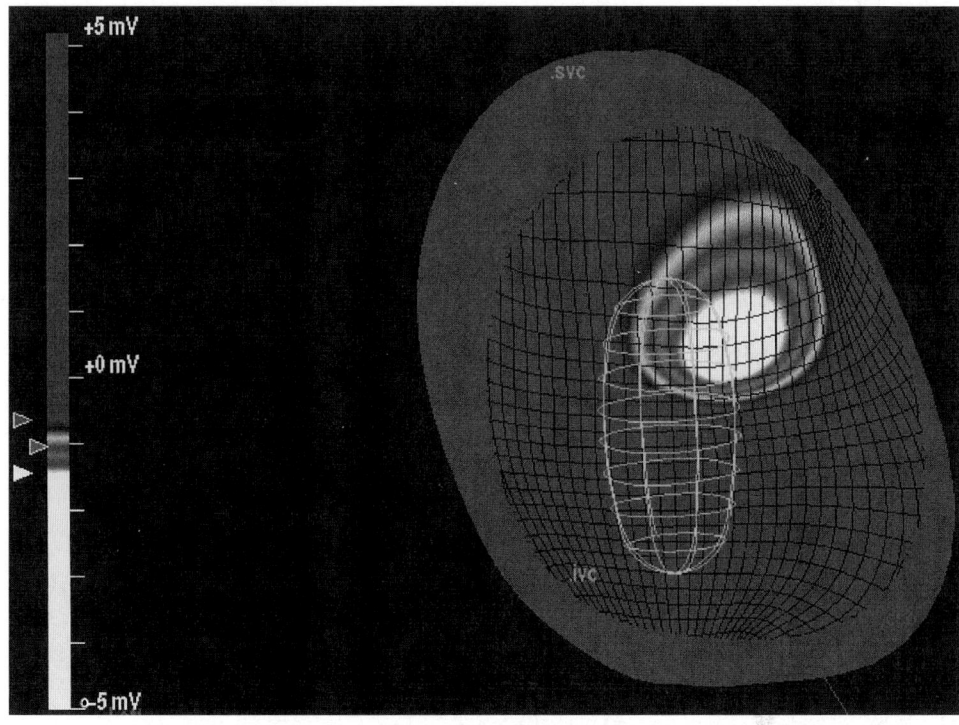

FIGURE 34-4 (Plate 77) Activation of the right atrium during focal atrial tachycardia, mapped with the Endocardial Solutions EnSite 3000 system. The white represents tissue that is fully activated, and purple is tissue that is not yet activated. SVC = superior vena cava; IVC = inferior vena cava.

## INVASIVE ELECTROPHYSIOLOGIC STUDIES FOR DIAGNOSIS

### Sinus Node Dysfunction[3,4,25,26]

EPSs are performed to detect suspected sinus node dysfunction in patients with dizziness, presyncope, syncope, etc., in whom the diagnosis cannot be made noninvasively. The most frequently performed test is that of sinus node suppression by using overdrive atrial pacing. After pacing at several basic cycle lengths for a period of approximately 30 s or longer, the pacing is interrupted. The resultant escape interval, which is called *sinus node recovery time,* is measured. By deducting the predominant sinus cycle length from this interval, one can obtain the so-called corrected sinus node recovery time. In one study,[3] sinus node recovery time in patients with sinus node disease averaged 3087 ms; it averaged 1073 ms in normal individuals. In another series,[6] the value for corrected sinus node recovery time was less than 525 ms in normal individuals and exceeded those values in patients with overt sinus node dysfunction.

In the vast majority of patients with true sinus node disease, sinoatrial conduction abnormalities are the predominant reason for sinus node dysfunction. The sinoatrial conduction time in the absence of obvious sinus node disease is less than 100 ms. The sensitivity of sinus node recovery time for the detection of sinus node dysfunction is 54 percent, whereas that of sinoatrial conduction time is 51 percent, with a combined sensitivity of the two tests of around 64 percent. Poor sensitivity of such testing relates in part to the fact

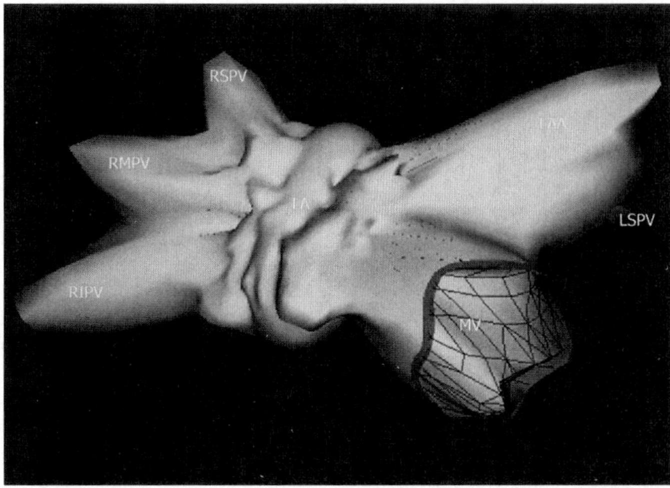


FIGURE 34-5 Anatomic reconstruction of the left atrium in a patient using Navex, anterior-posterior projection. A cutout is shown at the location of the mitral valve. RSPV = right superior pulmonary vein, RMPV = right middle pulmonary vein emptying directly into the left atrium, RIPV = right inferior pulmonary vein, LSPV = left superior pulmonary vein, LA = left atrium, LAA = left atrial appendage, MV = mitral valve.

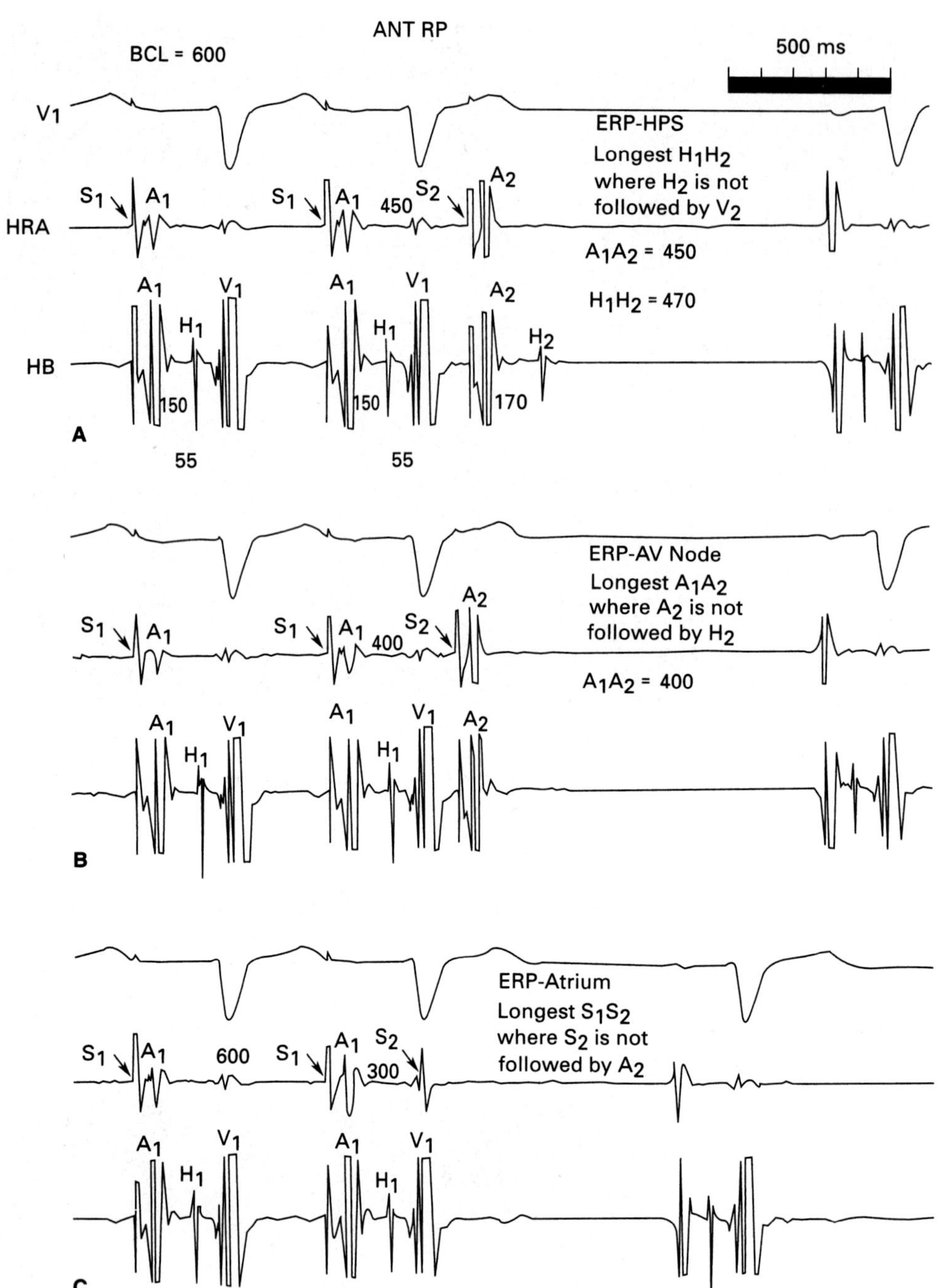


FIGURE 34-6 Determination of cardiac refractory periods during atrial pacing (*A* through *C*). During a basic cycle-length pacing at 600 ms ($S_1S_1$ or $A_1A_1$), atrial premature stimulation ($S_2$ or $A_2$) at progressively shorter coupling intervals ($S_1S_2$ or $A_1A_2$) is depicted. The definition of the effective refractory period (ERP) of the His-Purkinje system (HPS), atrioventricular node, and atrium are labeled. ANT RP = antegrade refractory period. (From Akhtar.[13] Reproduced with permission from the publisher and authors.)

that, in previous studies, documented episodes of sinus bradycardia or sinus arrest due to neurocardiogenic mechanisms may have been included as examples of sinus node dysfunction.[27] The specificity of the two tests combined is approximately 88 percent. It is important to test the AV conduction in patients with sinus node dysfunction, since the former is also frequently abnormal. In patients with bradycardia/tachycardia syndrome, tachycardias are frequent, particularly those arising in the atrium, and testing may also be necessary for the proper diagnosis and therapy of the concomitant tachyarrhythmia.

## Atrioventricular Block

In asymptomatic patients with first-degree AV block (prolonged PR interval), electrophysiologic assessment is unnecessary, regardless of

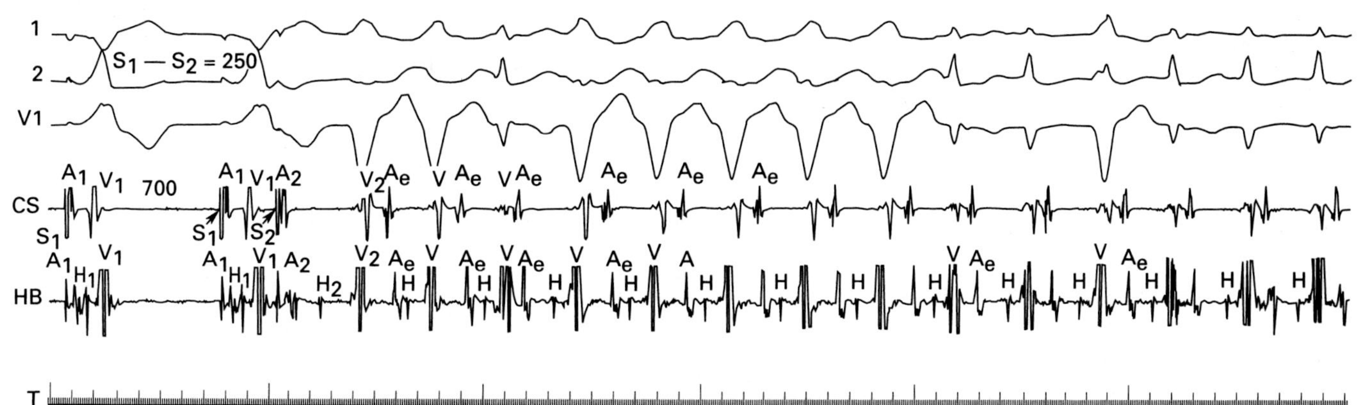


FIGURE 34-7 Induction of supraventricular tachycardia (SVT) in Wolff-Parkinson-White syndrome. The tracings are labeled. Atrial pacing from coronary sinus (CS) is done at a 700-ms basic cycle. During the basic drive pacing, left free wall accessory pathway conduction to the ventricle produces ventricular preexcitation. A single premature beat ($S_2$) blocks in the accessory pathway (AP) and conducts over the normal pathway with a left bundle branch block morphology, and the SVT is initiated. Note the intermittent normalization of the QRS complex during this SVT. (From Jazayeri et al.[58] Reproduced with permission from the publisher and authors.)

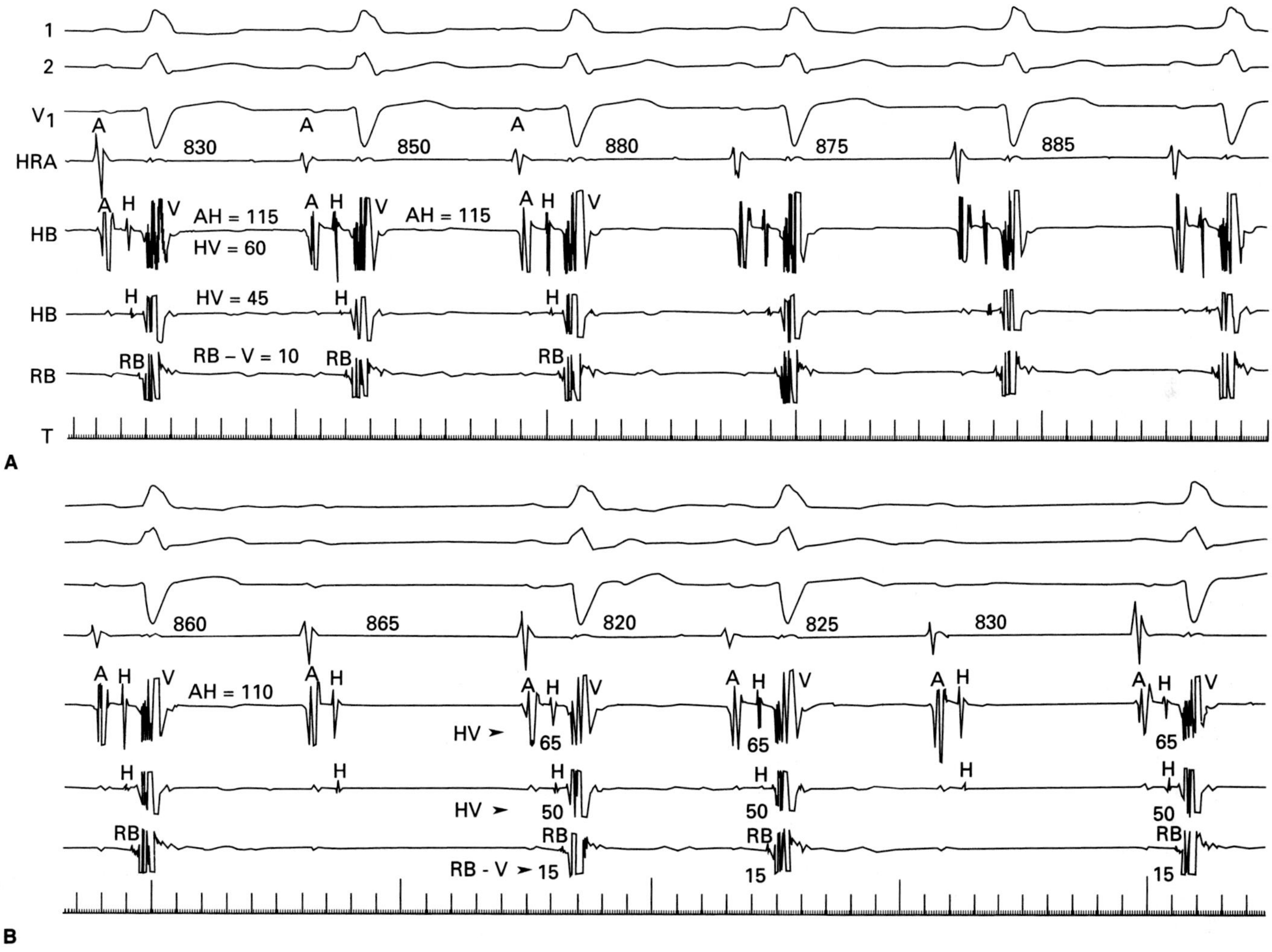

FIGURE 34-8 Atrioventricular (AV) block in the His-Purkinje system (HPS). *A*. Control. A 1:1 AV conduction is depicted in a patient with unexplained syncope. Following 150 mg of intravenous procainamide (*B*), a second-degree AV block in the HPS is noted (i.e., His bundle potential is not followed by a QRS complex), an abnormal response to a small dose of procainamide suggesting AV block in the HPS as a potential cause of syncope.

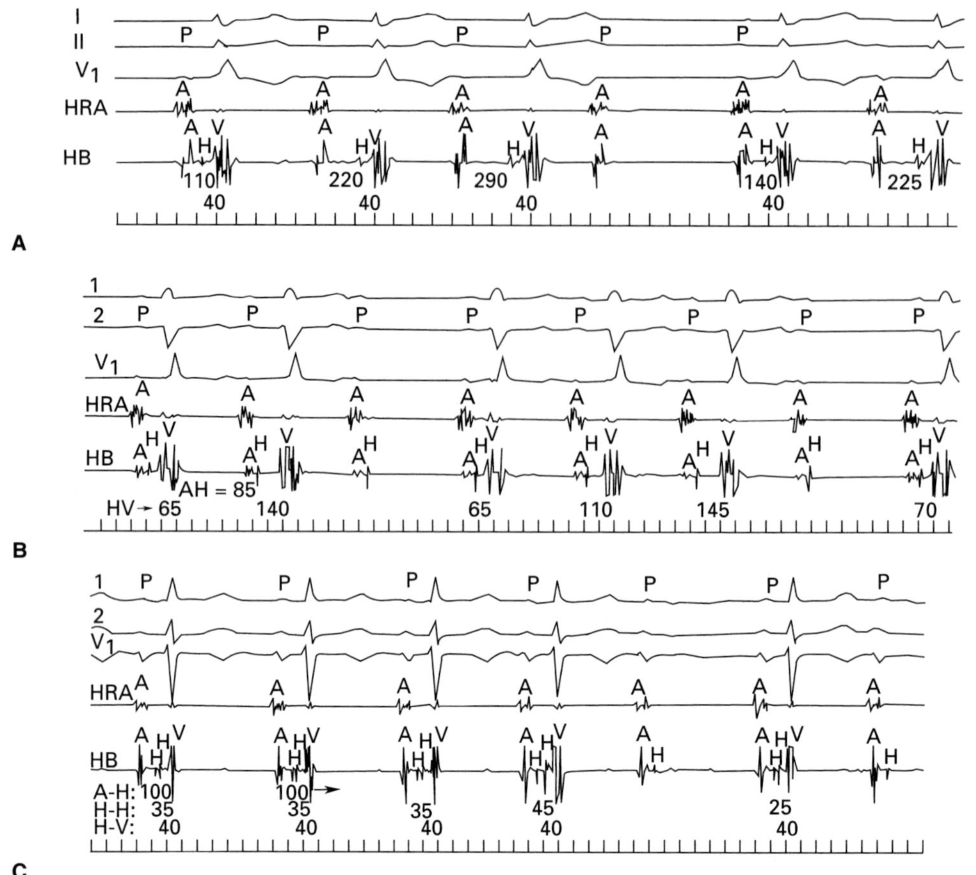

FIGURE 34-9 His bundle (HB) electrograms in atrioventricular (AV) block. The tracings are from three different patients with second-degree AV block. In *A* and *B*, the conducted QRS complexes are wide and associated with bundle branch block. In *A*, the block is within the AV node (i.e., the A wave on the HB is not followed by an HB deflection). In *B*, it can be appreciated that the block is distal to the HB even though the surface electrocardiogram (ECG) demonstrates a Wenckebach phenomenon. The latter can obviously occur in the His-Purkinje system as well, as depicted in this figure. *C*. The site of the block is within the HB. This is suggested by split HB potentials (labeled H and $H^+$), and the block is distal to the H but proximal to the $H^+$. Intra-His block is difficult to diagnose from the surface ECG but can be suspected when a Mobitz type II occurs in association with a normal PR interval and a narrow QRS complex. (From Akhtar.[13] Reproduced with permission from the publisher and author.)

the QRS morphology of the conducted beats. In asymptomatic individuals with second-degree AV block, electrophysiologic assessment is used to find the site of the block (Fig. 34-9). Patients with intra- or infra-Hisian block tend to have a more unpredictable course, and permanent pacing is desirable.[28] On the other hand, asymptomatic patients with AV nodal block generally do not require permanent pacing. Even though the intranodal block usually presents as Wenckebach's phenomenon or Mobitz type I, it is not uncommon to see Wenckebach phenomena within the His-Purkinje system or within the His bundle. There is no difference in prognosis regardless of how the infra- or intra-Hisian second-degree block manifests itself, i.e., type I versus type II (Fig. 34-9). On occasion, intranodal blocks are preceded by no discernible change in PR interval and, from a surface electrocardiogram, may appear as forms of Mobitz type II. The absolute length of the PR interval is usually quite diagnostic in that it is markedly prolonged (i.e., >300 ms), and there is a PR shortening exceeding 100 ms following the block beat (Fig. 34-9). In symptomatic patients with second-degree AV block, the role of EPS is limited because permanent pacing is the appropriate intervention. On the other hand, if the patient's symptoms cannot be explained on the basis of AV block and may be related to another arrhythmia, such as VT, EPS should be considered. In patients with third-degree or complete AV block, EPSs are seldom required; permanent pacing is the obvious option in symptomatic patients.

A discernible His bundle recording enables one to determine the exact site of AV conduction abnormality, i.e., proximal to, within, or distal to the His bundle region. This, in combination with surface electrocardiographic morphology of conducted beats, enables one to identify precisely the location of conduction abnormality.

If 1:1 AV conduction is noted during EPS in patients suspected of intermittent AV block, incremental atrial pacing should be done to see whether AV block can be reproduced. AV block in the His-Purkinje system is abnormal during incremental atrial pacing but may be a physiologic response during atrial extrastimulation (see Fig. 34-6*A*). First- and second-degree blocks in the AV node are considered physiologic responses during incremental atrial pacing or atrial extrastimulation (see Fig. 34-6*B*).

## Wide QRS Tachycardia

Wide QRS tachycardia occurs due to a variety of electrophysiologic mechanisms, both from supraventricular and ventricular origins in the presence or absence of accessory pathways (Fig. 34-10).[29] The underlying nature of the wide QRS tachycardia is critical for both prognosis and therapy. EPSs have proven invaluable for distinguishing the various etiologies (Fig. 34-11). With few exceptions, when the nature of the arrhythmic problem is not known and the direction of therapy is not clear, patients with wide QRS tachycardia should undergo EPS. This is particularly true in situations where nonpharmacologic therapy is the desired goal.

## Unexplained Syncope[23,28]

Unexplained syncope may be due to cardiovascular mechanisms. The most common reason for cardiovascular syncope is cardiac arrhythmia. Electrophysiologic evaluation constitutes an integral part of the evaluation of patients with unexplained syncope, especially those with heart disease. During such studies, all arrhythmic possibilities—such as sinus node dysfunction, AV conduction abnormalities, SVT, and VT—should be excluded. Neurocardiogenic mechanisms constitute the most common causes of syncope in patients without structural heart disease, and incomplete assessment of these patients may lead to inappropriate therapy (Fig. 34-12).[27,30] The possibility of neurocardiogenic dysfunction should always be considered in younger patients (<50 years of age) with syncope and

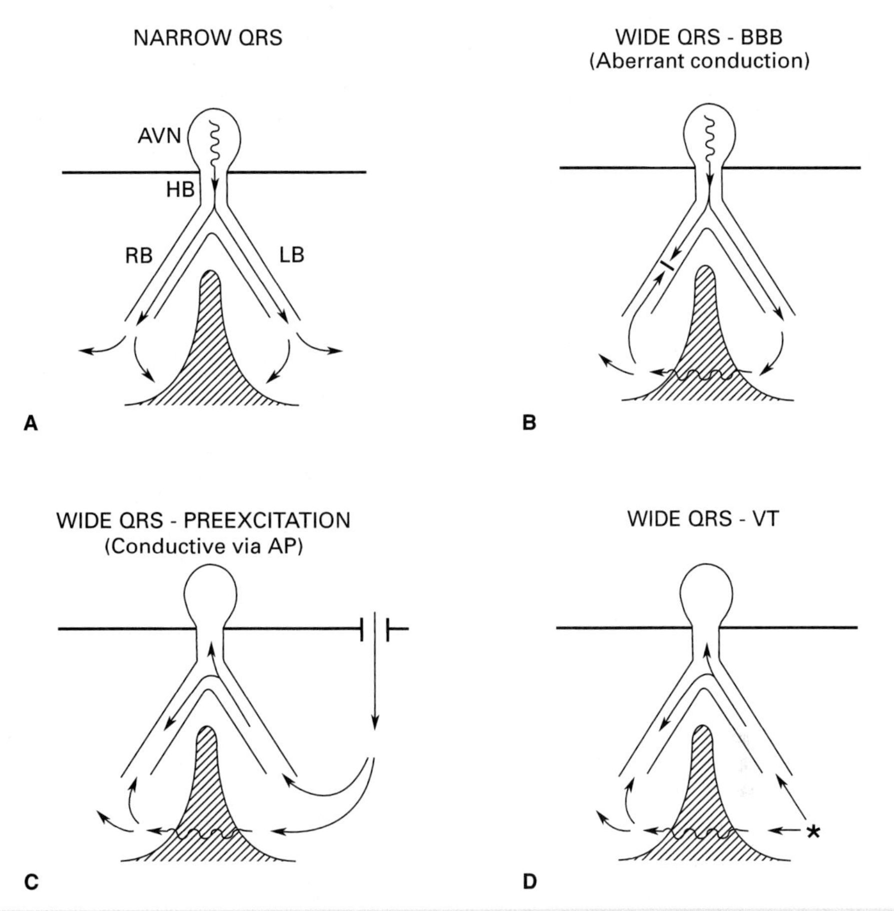


FIGURE 34-10 Wide QRS tachycardia. Routes of impulse propagation during a wide QRS tachycardia in various settings are depicted. It should be noted that only in *A* and *B* is His bundle activation expected to precede ventricular activation. This helps the delineation from other causes of wide QRS tachycardia shown in *C* and *D*.

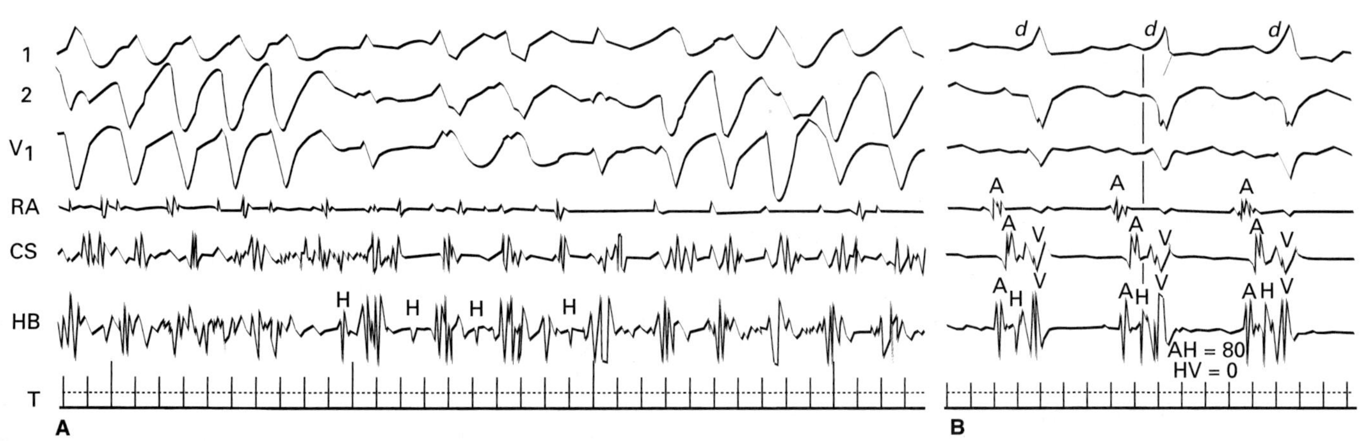


FIGURE 34-11 Wide QRS tachycardia. *A*. Wide QRS complexes of at least two varieties are seen. Those showing a left bundle branch block pattern are due to conduction over an accessory pathway, while those with a right bundle branch pattern are aberrant in nature. Note the His bundle activation prior to both narrow and aberrant complexes but not before preexcited complexes. A right posteroseptal preexcitation can be appreciated in *B*, with a short PR, a delta wave (*d*), a His to ventricle (HV) of zero, and negative delta wave in lead $V_1$.

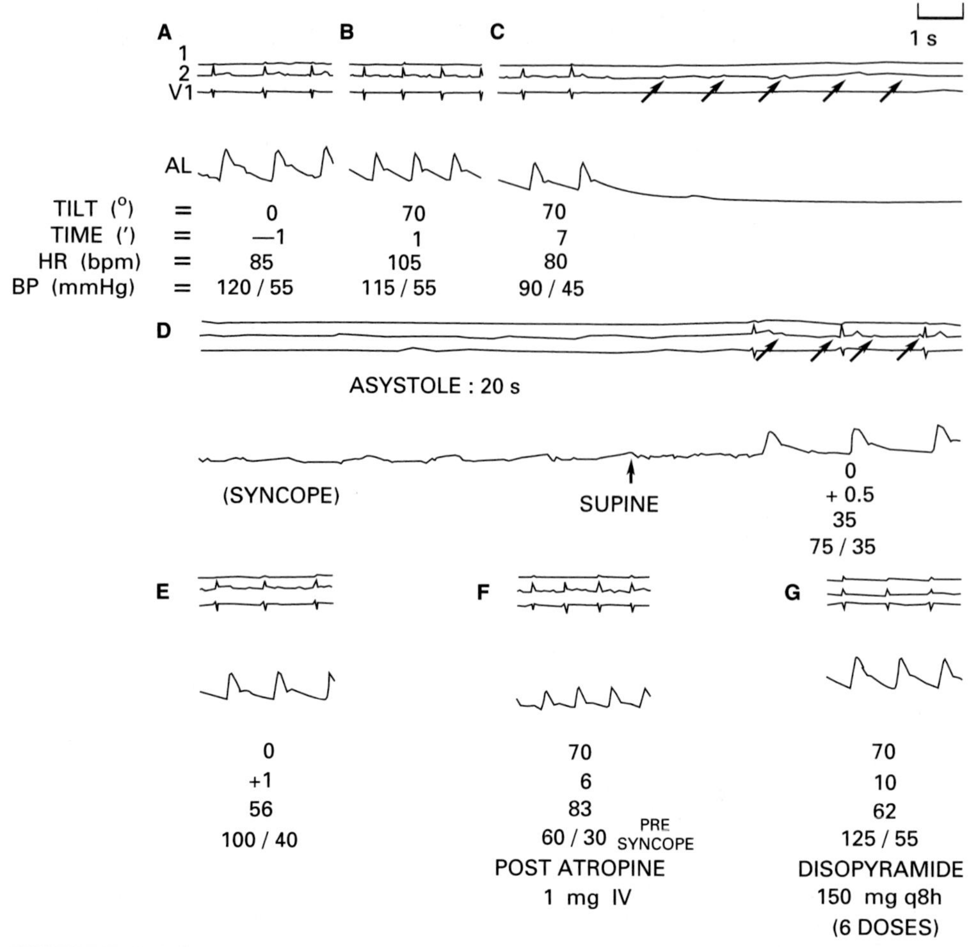


FIGURE 34-12 Asystole in neurocardiogenic syncope. Note the normal heart rate (HR) and blood pressure (BP) in supine position. At the beginning of head-up tilt at 70 degrees (*B*), some degree of tachycardia is noted. Seven minutes after the onset of tilt (*C*), an episode of atrioventricular block occurs and is followed by sinus arrest and a total asystole of 20 s. Syncopal episodes follow. Presyncope is still present when asystole is prevented by atropine (*F*). Findings in *C* might tempt one to prescribe permanent pacing, an inappropriate choice of therapy. In this patient with neurocardiogenic syncope, disopyramide (*G*) prevented hypotension and syncope without the need for a permanent pacemaker. This patient has remained asymptomatic on this therapy for more than 6 years now. (From Sra et al.[27] Reproduced with permission from the publisher and authors.)

documented bradycardia (sinus arrest or AV block) and can be unmasked on a tilt table. The triage of patients toward one or the other, i.e., electrophysiologic testing versus head-up tilt, is fairly simple and predicted by clinical history and the presence or absence of structural heart disease.[30–35] Patients with underlying structural heart disease—such as old myocardial infarction, primary myocardial disease, or poor LV function—generally have underlying VT to explain the symptoms of syncope (Fig. 34-13). When arrhythmias occur in patients without overt structural heart disease, sinus node dysfunction, AV block (particularly intra-Hisian block), or SVTs are likely. Less frequently, VT can occur in the absence of an overt structural heart disease.

### Survivors of Sudden Cardiac Arrest

In many patients with documented episodes of cardiac arrest from the onset, VF can be documented as the initial cause. Patients dying suddenly usually have underlying structural heart disease (usually coronary artery disease or primary myocardial disease) and are prone to VT/VF due to electrical instability. It seems prudent to investigate both the nature and extent of organic heart disease and also to assess vulnerability to recurrent VT/VF. At present, EPS is considered a routine part of the overall patient assessment in this group of individuals.[36,37]

EPSs in survivors of VT/VF are desirable for a variety of reasons. Some are listed here:

1. Occasionally the underlying VT leading to cardiac arrest is bundle branch reentry or BBR (Fig. 34-14). In our experience almost 40 percent of patients with monomorphic VT in association with idiopathic dilated cardiomyopathy and valvular heart disease have BBR as the underlying mechanism. We feel this arrhythmia is preferably managed with bundle branch ablation, which is curative, rather than with an implantable cardioverter defibrillator (ICD) alone.
2. Several VT morphologies or other types of tachycardia may be induced in addition to VT. Lack of awareness of such arrhythmias may complicate patient management. For example, the coexistence of rapid SVT may require separate attention to prevent unnecessary ICD shocks.
3. In some cases, supraventricular arrhythmia may trigger VT/VF. This may happen in patients with severe coronary artery disease, congestive heart failure, Wolff-Parkinson-White syndrome, etc. Elimination of the underlying causes is a more rational therapeutic approach in such cases.
4. Patients with VT/VF often have underlying sick sinus syndrome or AV block, which can be further aggravated with antiarrhythmic drugs and may require permanent pacing. Assessment for this eventuality can be done during the conduct of an EPS and may help selection of a particular device. Because of the increasing flexibility of these devices, this need for EPS may be less relevant in the future.

## INVASIVE CARDIAC ELECTROPHYSIOLOGIC STUDIES FOR THERAPEUTIC INTERVENTION

Because of the episodic nature of most cardiac arrhythmias, the efficacy of any therapeutic intervention is difficult to assess unless the arrhythmia in question can be replicated. Diagnostic EPS provides that opportunity, and it seems logical to use the same tool to assess therapeutic interventions.[38–41] This method to assess efficacy can be applied for both pharmacologic and nonpharmacologic therapy.

### Pharmacologic Therapy

It is arguable whether the assessment of pharmacologic intervention is essential in patients with relatively benign cardiac arrhythmias.

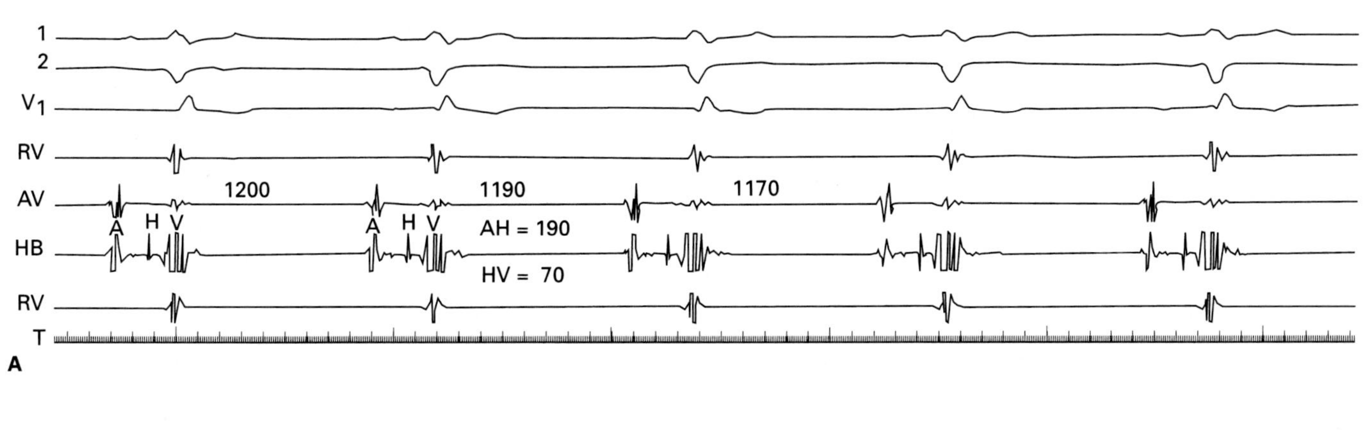


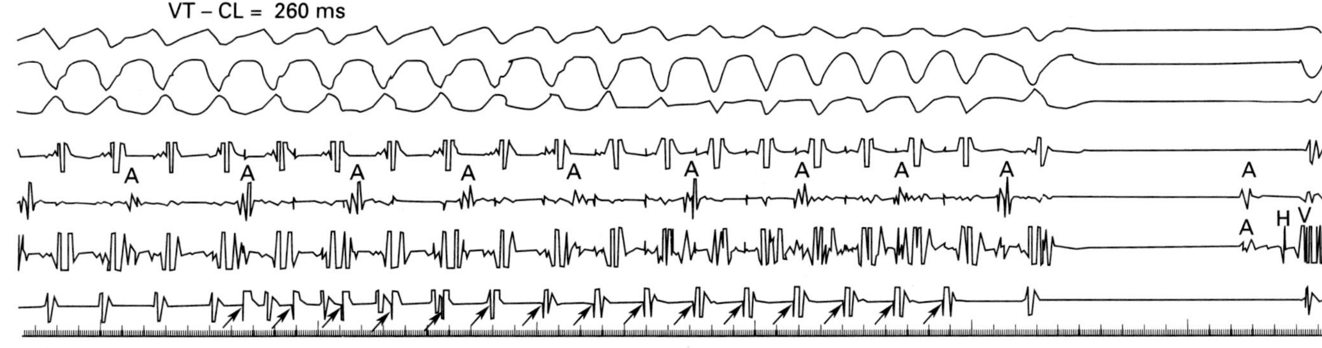


FIGURE 34-13 Arrhythmic causes of syncope. *A*. Sinus rhythm in a patient with unexplained syncope. Sinus bradycardia, bifascicular block, and a long PR interval from surface electrocardiogram suggest possible bradycardia etiology. In this patient, however, ventricular tachycardia (*B*) was inducible with ventricular extrastimulation and was the actual cause of syncope. Control of ventricular tachycardia (VT) without a pacemaker was sufficient to prevent syncope in this patient. Termination of tachycardia and restoration of sinus rhythm are shown in *B*.

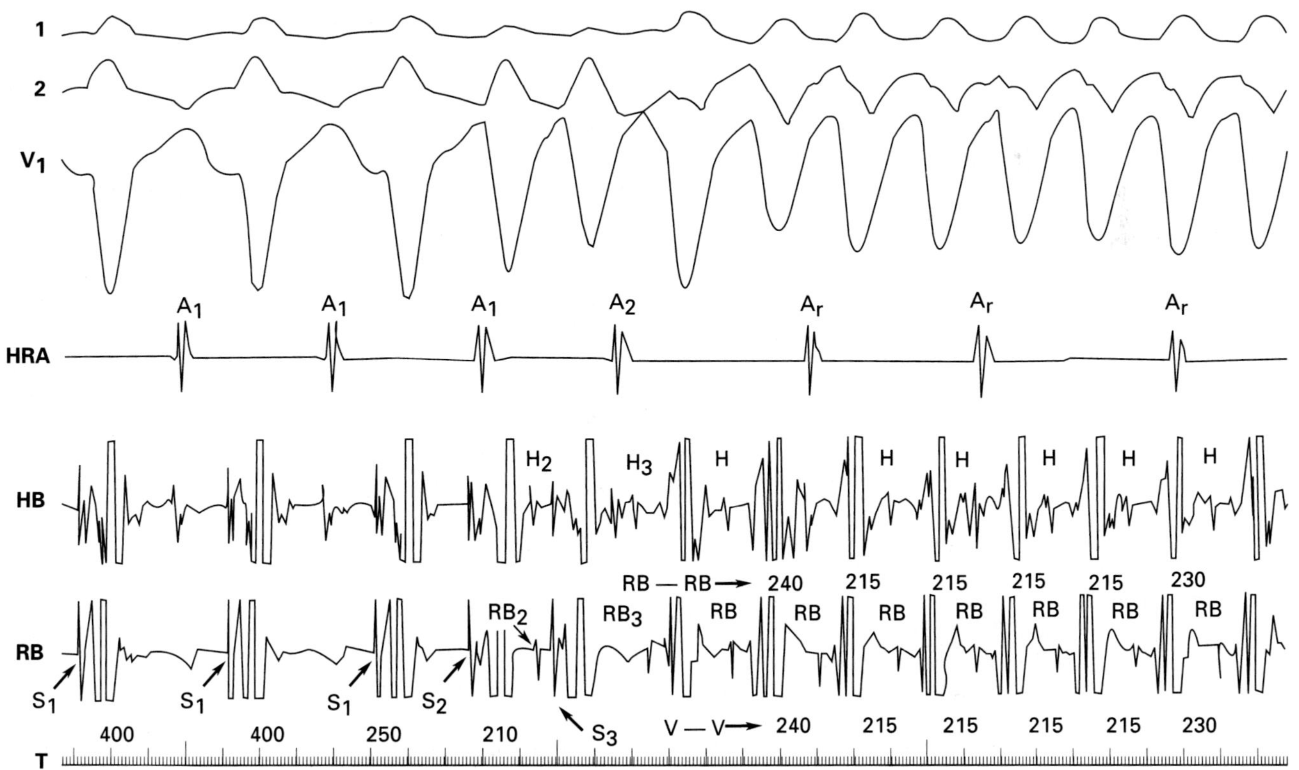


FIGURE 34-14 Induction of sustained ventricular tachycardia due to bundle branch reentry (BBR). The surface electrocardiogram and intracardiac tracings are labeled. Basic cycle length ($S_1S_1$) is 400 ms during ventricular pacing. Sustained BBR is induced with two extra stimuli ($S_2S_3$). Note that the His bundle and right bundle (RB) deflections precede the QRS, suggesting supraventricular tachycardia with aberrant conduction. However, there is 2:1 ventricular atrial (VA) block, indicating the ventricular nature of this tachycardia. Without His bundle/right bundle (HB/RB) recordings, the diagnosis can be difficult and, consequently, the likelihood of inappropriate therapy will be high. RB-RB and V-V (ventricular) intervals are labeled. (From Jazayeri et al.[59] Reproduced with permission from the publisher and authors.)

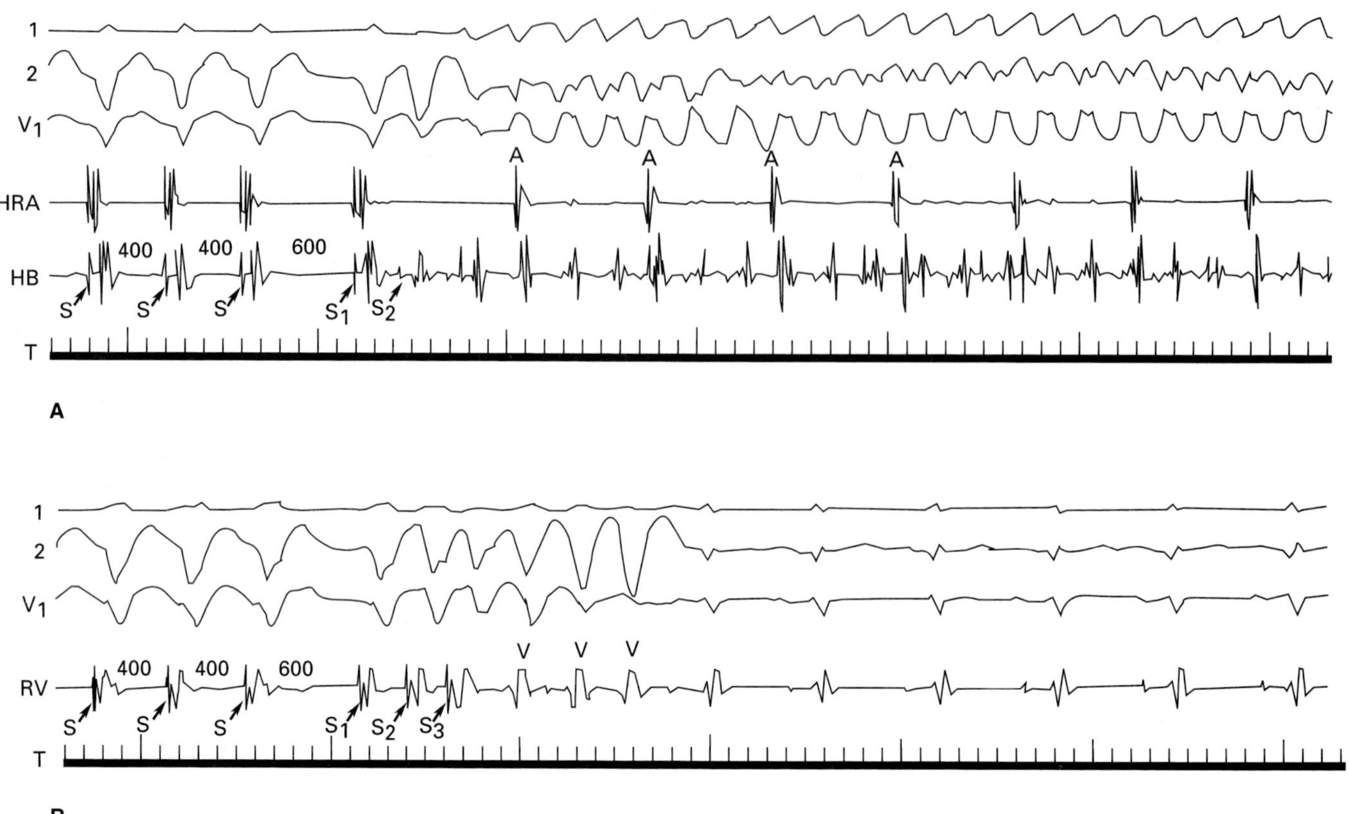


FIGURE 34-15 *A.* Control. *B.* Post-procainamide (PA) + mexiletine. Initiation of sustained monomorphic ventricular tachycardia (VT) of myocardial origin is shown in *A.* After oral procainamide and mexiletine, the sustained VT could not be induced despite using a more aggressive pacing protocol.

The clinical course can be observed to determine whether control has been achieved. With life-threatening tachycardias, such as VT/VF, or with severe manifestations of cardiac arrhythmias, such as syncope or presyncope, it is desirable to assess efficacy of pharmacologic intervention (Fig. 34-15).[40,41] A technique of drug testing has been developed whereby the elimination of inducibility of a given tachycardia is assessed following a drug administration. Both the drug's efficacy or inefficacy can be evaluated by this method. When drug therapy does eliminate induction of a previously inducible tachycardia, the addition of isoproterenol will frequently demonstrate reversal of therapeutic drug effect.[42,43] This is helpful in considering additional beta-blocker therapy. The latter can be accomplished with ease in patients with good LV function, whereas the addition of beta blockers may pose a problem in patients with VT and poor LV function. Failure of serial drug testing is associated with a significant recurrence rate and is a strong indication for nonpharmacologic intervention.

Some controversy has arisen regarding the value of EPS for the prediction of drug efficacy in comparison to ambulatory monitoring.[39] However, because of the infrequency of spontaneous VT/VF in most patients with life-threatening ventricular arrhythmias, ambulatory monitoring is an impractical approach. At present, serial drug studies with multiple oral antiarrhythmic agents are seldom carried out for SVT or VT.

## Nonpharmacologic Therapy

Nonpharmacologic intervention has become an integral part of patient management in cardiac arrhythmias. With documented cardiac arrest from VF, implantation of an automatic ICD is fairly common and electrophysiologic assessment before such therapy is routine.[45] Both preoperative and postimplant electrophysiologic evaluation can be done through permanent leads of an ICD through a wand and programmer. Pacing, antitachycardia function, low-energy cardioversion, and cardiac defibrillation can all be programmed with newer devices. When problems are encountered following discharge of a patient with an ICD, electrophysiologic reassessment via ICD is frequently necessary, both for reprogramming and for troubleshooting. For assessment of certain other electrophysiologic parameters (e.g., AV conduction and mechanism of SVTs), however, transvenous catheterization may be necessary.

Patients with coronary artery disease and mappable VT are also candidates for VT surgery when it cannot be managed with an ICD, antiarrhythmic drugs, and/or catheter ablation.[46–48] Preoperative EPS assessment for this possibility is important. Surgery for VT in the form of endocardial resection or cryoablation can be performed very effectively and relatively safely in patients with an LV ejection fraction greater than 20 percent. This curative procedure provides effective control in approximately 75 percent of the patients who have monomorphic VT that can be appropriately mapped; it may be considered when other forms of therapies are ineffective.

Surgery for SVT has gone through a significant evolution. The introduction of catheter ablative techniques has made it rare for patients to undergo surgery for Wolff-Parkinson-White syndrome and/or AV nodal reentrant tachycardia. Some individuals with resistant atrial fibrillation and flutter and those who fail catheter ablative therapy may still be considered candidates for such a procedure, but this is now becoming exceedingly less frequent.

## CATHETER ABLATION TECHNIQUES[49–53]

The realization that the origin of VT and SVT can be effectively mapped has made the catheter ablative technique a rational approach. The radiofrequency form of energy delivered through a catheter has permitted controlled trauma to cardiac tissue to abolish or modify reentrant circuits. This is true for both SVT and VT. Unifocal atrial tachycardia, AV nodal reentry of all varieties, and accessory pathways including atriofascicular fibers can be cured in over 90 percent of patients with radiofrequency catheter ablation. Among the VTs, BBR tachycardia seen in association with dilated cardiomyopathy (both ischemic and nonischemic) and valvular disease is an ideal substrate for catheter ablation. Patients with monomorphic VT associated with myocardial scarring or other substrates can also be considered candidates, particularly when they are not suitable for VT surgery and have failed drug therapy. Additionally, in patients with incessant VT or frequency VT with inadequate control despite ICD therapy, VT ablation should be considered. By using electromagnetic mapping, the scarred area can be mapped during sinus rhythm and ablation of this substrate can effectively eliminate VT.[52] The noncontact mapping techniques outlined above are likely to further help improve the ablation success rate with unifocal or possibly multifocal tachycardias.[53]

## IATROGENIC PROBLEMS ENCOUNTERED DURING ELECTROPHYSIOLOGIC STUDIES

Mechanical irritation from catheters during placement, even when they are not being manipulated, can cause a variety of arrhythmias and conduction disturbances.[54] These include induction of atrial, junctional, and ventricular ectopic beats and right bundle branch block and thus AV block in the His-Purkinje system in patients with preexisting left bundle branch block during right ventricular catheterization.[54] Obviously, AV block in the His-Purkinje system can occur in patients with preexisting right bundle branch block during LV catheterization. Ventricular stimulation can also occur from physical movement of the ventricular catheter coincident with atrial contraction, producing electrocardiographic patterns of ventricular preexcitation. Recognition of all these iatrogenic patterns is important for avoiding misinterpretation of electrophysiologic phenomena and the significance of findings in the laboratory.

Certain types of arrhythmias must be avoided at all costs, such as atrial fibrillation and VF. Atrial fibrillation will obviously not permit study of any other form of SVT, and VF will require prompt cardioversion, making it difficult to continue the EPS. If atrial fibrillation must be initiated for diagnostic purposes (i.e., to assess ventricular response over the accessory pathway in Wolff- Parkinson-White syndrome), it should be done at the end of the study. Patients with a prior history of atrial fibrillation are more prone to the occurrence of sustained atrial fibrillation in the laboratory. Frequently, this will occur during initial placement of catheters; excessive manipulation of catheters in the atria should therefore be avoided. Catheter trauma resulting in abolition of accessory pathway conduction or the reentrant pathway may make the curative ablation difficult or impossible.

### Risks and Complications

The complication rate is relatively low when only right heart catheterization is done, with almost negligible mortality.[55,56] Other complications include deep venous thrombosis, pulmonary embolism, infection at catheter sites, systemic infection, pneumothorax, and perforation of a cardiac chamber or coronary sinus. Potentially lethal arrhythmias such as rapid VT or VF are common in the laboratory. These are not necessarily counted as complications, however, but are often expected and anticipated. Nonetheless, their common occurrence makes the electrophysiology laboratory a place for only highly trained personnel equipped to handle such problems.

## References


1. Scherlag BJ, Lau SH, Helfant RH, et al. Catheter technique for recording His bundle activity in man. *Circulation* 1969;39:13–18.
2. Goldreyer BN, Bigger JT. Spontaneous and induced reentrant tachycardia. *Ann Intern Med* 1969;70:87–98.
3. Mandel WJ, Hayakawa H, Danzig R, Marcus HS. Evaluation of sinoatrial node function in man by overdrive suppression. *Circulation* 1971;44:59–66.
4. Narula OS, Samet P, Javier RP. Significance of the sinus node recovery time. *Circulation* 1972;45:140–158.
5. Damato AN, Lau SH, Helfant RH, et al. A study of heart block in man using His bundle recordings. *Circulation* 1969;39:297–305.
6. Narula OS, Scherlag BJ, Samet P, Javier RP. Atrioventricular block: Localization and classification by His bundle recordings. *Am J Med* 1971;50:146–165.
7. Goldreyer BN, Damato AN. The essential role of atrioventricular conduction delay in the initiation of paroxysmal supraventricular tachycardia. *Circulation* 1971;43:679–687.
8. Wellens HJJ, Schuilenberg RM, Durrer D. Electrical stimulation of the heart in patients with the Wolff-Parkinson-White syndrome type A. *Circulation* 1971;43:99–114.
9. Mason JW, Winkel RA. Electrode catheter arrhythmia induction in the selection and assessment of antiarrhythmic drug therapy for recurrent ventricular tachycardia. *Circulation* 1978;58:971–985.
10. Ruskin JN, DiMarco JP, Garan H. Out of hospital cardiac arrest: Electrophysiologic observations in selection of long-term antiarrhythmic therapy. *N Engl J Med* 1980;303:607–613.
11. Nelson GS, Berger RD, Fetics BJ, et al. Left ventricular or biventricular pacing improves cardiac function at diminished energy cost in patients with dilated cardiomyopathy and left bundle-branch block. *Circulation* 2000;102:3053–3059.
12. Auricchio A, Kloss M, Trautmann SI, et al. Exercise performance following cardiac resynchronization therapy in patients with heart failure and ventricular conduction delay. *Am J Cardiol* 2002;89:198–203.
13. Akhtar M. Invasive cardiac electrophysiologic studies: An introduction. In: Parmley WW, Chatterjee K, eds. *Cardiology,* vol 1: *Physiology, Pharmacology, Diagnosis*. Philadelphia: Lippincott; 1991.
14. Josephson ME, Harken PH, Horowitz LN. Endocardial excision: A new surgical technique for the treatment of recurrent ventricular tachycardia. *Circulation* 1979;60:1430–1439.
15. Fann JI, Loeb JM, LoCicero J III, et al. Endocardial activation mapping and endocardial pace-mapping using a balloon apparatus. *Am J Cardiol* 1985;55:1076.
16. Mickleborough LL, Harris L, Downar E, et al. A new intraoperative approach for endocardial mapping of ventricular tachycardia. *J Thorac Cardiovasc Surg* 1988;95:271.
17. Gepstein L, Hayam G, Ben-Haim SA. A novel method for nonfluoroscopic catheter-based electroanatomical mapping of the heart. *Circulation* 1997; 95:1611–1622.
18. Schilling RJ, Peters NS, Davies DW. A non-contact catheter for simultaneous endocardial mapping in the human left ventricle: Comparison of contact and reconstructed electrograms during sinus rhythm. *Circulation* 1998;98:887–898.
19. Wittkampf F, Wever E, Derksen R, et al. LocaLisa new technique for real-time 3-dimensional localization of regular intracardiac electrodes. *Circulation* 1999;99:1312–1317.
20. Wittkampf F, Wever E, Derksen R, et al. Accuracy of the LocaLisa system in catheter ablation procedures. *J Electrocardiol* 1999;32(suppl):7–12.

21. Wittkampf F, Loh P, Derksen R, et al. Real-time, three-dimensional, nonfluoroscopic localization of the lasso catheter. *J Cardiovasc Electrophysiol* 2002;13:630.
22. Brugada P, Green M, Abdollah H, Wellens HJ. Significance of ventricular arrhythmias initiated by programmed ventricular stimulation: The importance of the type of ventricular arrhythmia induced and the number of premature stimuli required. *Circulation* 1984;69:87–92.
23. Avitall B, McKinnie J, Jazayeri M, et al. Induction of ventricular fibrillation versus monomorphic ventricular tachycardia during programmed stimulation: Role of premature beat conduction delay. *Circulation* 1992;85:1271–1278.
24. Akhtar M. Clinical application of electrophysiologic studies in the management of patients requiring pacemaker therapy. In: Barold S, ed. *Modern Cardiac Pacing*. Mount Kisco, NY: Futura; 1985:3.
25. Hariman RJ, Krongrad E, Boxer RA, et al. Method for recording electrical activity of the sinoatrial node and automatic atrial foci during cardiac catheterization in human subjects. *Am J Cardiol* 1980;45: 775–781.
26. Gomes JA. The sick sinus syndrome and evaluation of the patient with sinus node disorders. In: Parmley WW, Chatterjee K, eds. *Cardiology*, vol 1: *Physiology, Pharmacology, Diagnosis*. Philadelphia: Lippincott; 1991.
27. Sra JS, Jazayeri MR, Avitall B, et al. Comparison of cardiac pacing with drug therapy in the treatment of neurocardiogenic (vasovagal) syncope with bradycardia or asystole. *N Engl J Med* 1993;328:1085–1090.
28. Dhingra RC, Wyndham CRC, Bauernfiend R, et al. Significance of block distal to the His bundle induced by atrial pacing in patients with chronic bifascicular block. *Circulation* 1979;60:1455–1464.
29. Akhtar M, Jazayeri M, Avitall B, et al. Electrophysiologic spectrum of wide QRS complex tachycardia. In: Zipes DP, Jalife J, eds. *Cardiac Electrophysiology: From Cell to Bedside*. Orlando, FL: Saunders; 1990: 635.
30. Sra J, Anderson A, Sheikh S, et al. Unexplained syncope evaluated by electrophysiologic studies and head-up tilt testing. *Ann Intern Med* 1991;114:1013–1019.
31. DiMarco JP, Garan H, Ruskin JN. Cardiac electrophysiologic techniques in recurrent syncope of unknown cause. *Ann Intern Med* 1981; 95:542–548.
32. Akhtar M, Shenasa M, Denker S, et al. Role of cardiac electrophysiologic studies in patients with unexplained recurrent syncope. *Pacing Clin Electrophysiol* 1983;6:192–201.
33. Morady F, Scheinman MM. The role and limitations of electrophysiologic testing in patients with unexplained syncope. *Int J Cardiol* 1983;4:229–234.
34. Teichman SL, Felder DS, Matos JA, et al. The value of electrophysiologic studies in syncope of undetermined origin: Report of 150 cases. *Am Heart J* 1985;110:469–479.
35 Moazez F, Peter T, Simonson J, et al. Syncope of unknown origin: Clinical noninvasive and electrophysiologic determinants of arrhythmia induction and symptom recurrence during long-term follow-up. *Am Heart J* 1991;121:81–88.
36. Akhtar M, Garan H, Lehmann MH, Troup PJ. Sudden cardiac death: Management of high-risk patients. *Ann Intern Med* 1991;114:499–512.
37. Ruskin JN, DiMarco JP, Garan H. Out-of-hospital cardiac arrest: Electrophysiologic observations and selection of long-term antiarrhythmic therapy. *N Engl J Med* 1980;303:607–612.
38. Morady F, Scheinman MM, Hess DS, et al. Electrophysiologic testing in the management of survivors of out-of-hospital arrest. *Am J Cardiol* 1983;51:85–89.
39. Wu D, Wyndham CR, Denes P, et al. Chronic electrophysiological study in patients with recurrent paroxysmal tachycardia: A new method for developing successful oral antiarrhythmic therapy. In: Kulbertus HE, ed. *Reentrant Arrhythmias*. Baltimore: University Park Press; 1976:294.
40. Horowitz LN, Josephson ME, Farshidi A, et al. Recurrent sustained ventricular tachycardia: Role of the electrophysiologic study in selection of antiarrhythmic regimens. *Circulation* 1978;58:986–997.
41. Mason JW, Winkle RA. Accuracy of ventricular tachycardia induction study for predicting long-term efficacy and inefficacy of antiarrhythmic drugs. *N Engl J Med* 1980;303:1073–1077.
42. Niazi I, Naccarelli G, Dougherty A, et al. Treatment of atrioventricular node reentrant tachycardia with encainide: Reversal of drug effect with isoproterenol. *J Am Coll Cardiol* 1989;13:904–910.
43. Jazayeri M, Van Wyhe G, Avitall B, et al. Isoproterenol reversal of antiarrhythmic effects in patients with inducible sustained ventricular tachyarrhythmias. *J Am Coll Cardiol* 1989;14:705–711.
44. Mason JW. A comparison of electrophysiologic testing with Holter monitoring to predict antiarrhythmic-drug efficacy for ventricular tachyarrhythmias. *N Engl J Med* 1993;329:445–451.
45. Akhtar M, Avitall B, Jazayeri M, et al. Role of implantable cardioverter defibrillator therapy in the management of high risk patients. *Circulation* 1992;85(suppl I):I131–I139.
46. Josephson ME, Harken AH, Horowitz LN. Long-term results of endocardial resection from sustained ventricular tachycardia in coronary disease patients. *Am Heart J* 1982;104:51–57.
47. Caceres J, Werner P, Jazayeri M, et al. Efficacy of cryosurgery alone for refractory monomorphic sustained ventricular tachycardia due to inferior wall infarct. *J Am Coll Cardiol* 1988;11:1254–1259.
48. Caceres J, Akhtar M, Werner P, et al. Cryoablation of refractory sustained ventricular tachycardia due to coronary artery disease. *Am J Cardiol* 1989;63:296–300.
49. Jackman WM, Wang X, Friday KJ, et al. Catheter ablation of accessory atrioventricular pathways (Wolff-Parkinson-White syndrome) by radiofrequency current. *N Engl J Med* 1991;324:1605–1611.
50. Calkins H, Sousa J, El-Atassi R, et al. Diagnosis and cure of the Wolff-Parkinson-White syndrome or paroxysmal supraventricular tachycardias during a single electrophysiologic test. *N Engl J Med* 1991;324:1612–1618.
51. Jazayeri M, Hempe SL, Sra JS, et al. Selective transcatheter ablation of the fast and slow pathways using radiofrequency energy in patients with atrioventricular nodal reentrant tachycardia. *Circulation* 1992;85: 1318–1328.
52. Saoudi N, Atallah G, Kirkorian G, Touboul P. Catheter ablation of the atrial myocardium in human type I atrial flutter. *Circulation* 1990;81: 762–771.
53. Klein LS, Shih HT, Hackett FK, et al. Radiofrequency catheter ablation of ventricular tachycardia in patients without structural heart disease. *Circulation* 1992;85:1666–1674.
54. Akhtar M, Damato AN, Gilbert-Leeds CJ, et al. Induction of iatrogenic electrocardiographic patterns during electrophysiologic studies. *Circulation* 1977;56:60–65.
55. Di Marco JP, Garan H, Ruskin JN. Complications in patients undergoing cardiac electrophysiologic procedures. *Ann Intern Med* 1982;97: 490–493.
56. Horowitz L. Risks and complications of clinical cardiac electrophysiologic studies: A prospective analysis of 1000 consecutive patients. *J Am Coll Cardiol* 1987;9:1261–1268.
57. Gallagher JJ, Damato AN. Technique of recording His bundle activity in man. In: Grossman W, ed. *Cardiac Catheterization and Angiography*. Philadelphia: Lea & Febiger; 1980:283.
58. Jazayeri M, Caceres J, Tchou P, et al. Electrophysiologic characteristics of sudden QRS axis deviation during orthodromic tachycardia. *J Clin Invest* 1989; 83:952–959.
59. Jazayeri M, Sra J, Akhtar M. Wide QRS complexes: Electrophysiologic basis of a common electrocardiographic diagnosis. *J Cardiovasc Electrophysiol* 1992;3:36–39.

CHAPTER 35

# ANTIARRHYTHMIC DRUGS

Raymond L. Woosley / Julia H. Indik



Antiarrhythmic drugs were developed with the expectation that they would extend and improve life for many patients with cardiovascular disease and those with a history of life-threatening arrhythmias. Their usefulness, however, has been limited by ineffectiveness and/or toxicity. In mortality trials, benefit has not been clearly demonstrated, and worsened mortality rates have been observed with several drugs. In a study of the treatment of atrial fibrillation, the Atrial Fibrillation Follow-up Investigation of Rhythm Management (AFFIRM) trial[1] could not detect a survival benefit in a comparison of patients randomized to arrhythmia conversion or rate control. Strokes occurred in both treatment groups and were related to either discontinuation of warfarin or a subtherapeutic international normalized ratio (INR). Care must be taken, therefore, in deciding on the mode of antiarrhythmic treatment or, in fact, whether to treat at all.

Many antiarrhythmic agents are available today and more are under development. So many are needed because no agent is completely effective for all patients, and every agent has the potential for inducing serious adverse effects. Drug selection is often empiric. In fact, the side-effect profiles of the available drugs are very different and are often the determining factor in drug selection. Known side effects may completely eliminate the use of certain classes of drugs for a specific patient. Because of the narrow margin between effective and potentially toxic dosages, it is essential that physicians be thoroughly familiar with the clinical pharmacology, dosage, and adverse effects of all these agents.

The use of antiarrhythmic drugs has been dramatically altered by the findings of the Cardiac Arrhythmia Suppression Trial (CAST).[2] This landmark study was designed to test the hypothesis that suppression of asymptomatic ventricular arrhythmias in patients with recent myocardial infarction would reduce mortality rates due to cardiac arrest and/or arrhythmic sudden death. Prior to the CAST, antiarrhythmic drugs were prescribed for these patients to suppress asymptomatic arrhythmias and thus improve mortality rates. Based on the results of a feasibility and planning trial, the Cardiac Arrhythmia Pilot Study (CAPS), the CAST evaluated encainide, flecainide, and moricizine. These drugs were chosen because they were all tolerated and had reasonable ability to suppress symptomatic ventricular arrhythmias. In April 1989, the CAST was interrupted by the Data Safety and Monitoring Committee, and encainide and flecainide were removed because they had been found to increase mortality rates two- to threefold. The CAST II continued to evaluate the remaining drug, moricizine. However, the CAST II was also terminated prematurely in August 1991, when it became apparent that moricizine was producing a similar trend toward harm and there was no reasonable chance that a beneficial effect on the mortality rate could be detected.[3] These results shocked the medical community but have influenced thinking in this and many other areas of medicine. Hine et al.[4] reported a metanalysis of the CAST and similar studies with sodium channel–blocking antiarrhythmic drugs and found overall support for the conclusion of the CAST. The CAST has also led to recommendations by the U.S. Food and Drug Administration (FDA) for more restrictive labeling for all sodium channel–blocking antiarrhythmic drugs. In 1991, these drugs were given class labeling with indications for the treatment of documented ventricular arrhythmias that, in the judgment of the physician, are life-threatening. Exceptions among the sodium channel–blocking drugs are quinidine, propafenone, and flecainide, which have an additional indication for supraventricular arrhythmias. Because of discouraging results with sodium channel–blocking drugs, drugs that prolong the action potential (often termed *class III*) have been studied. Developers had been encouraged, since one drug with this action, amiodarone, may improve or at least not worsen mortality rates in patients with cardiac disease.[5,6] Dofetilide, ibutilide, and the *d*-isomer of sotalol all prolong the action potential duration and were developed in the hope that they would have the efficacy of amiodarone but without its propensity to cause serious side effects. However, the first of these drugs to be evaluated in a mortality trial, *d*-sotalol, was found to increase mortality rates after myocardial infarction.[7] Development of *d*-sotalol was halted, but the other two have been marketed with restrictions placed on their indications and/or clinical use. Clearly, antiarrhythmic drugs are the most complex drugs in clinical use today and must be administered with care.

## CLASSIFICATION OF ANTIARRHYTHMIC DRUGS

Antiarrhythmic drugs are often classified according to their electrophysiologic effects.[8] The scheme most often employed was originally proposed by Vaughan Williams as a classification of drug actions that should be antiarrhythmic, not a classification of drugs.[8] This is a subtle but important distinction that is made for the following reasons: Most antiarrhythmic drugs have multiple actions; hence their pharmacology is more complex than indicated by a simple drug classification scheme. The actions of a given drug differ in different cardiac tissues. Many antiarrhythmic agents have pharmacologically active metabolites whose activity may be quite different from—and in a class other than—that of the parent compound. The relative amounts of these metabolites produced are genetically determined for several of these drugs and often vary extensively within the population.

Drugs having class I action possess "local anesthetic" or "membrane-stabilizing" activity. Their predominant action is to block the fast inward sodium channel. This produces a decrease in the maximum depolarization rate, $\dot{V}_{max}$, of the action potential (phase 0) and slows intracardiac conduction. These agents have been further subclassified as belonging to class IA, IB, or IC on the basis of their effects on specific aspects of intracardiac conduction and refractoriness.[9] Drugs having class IA action include quinidine, procainamide, and disopyramide. These agents also produce measurable increases in ventricular refractoriness and prolongation of the QT interval. Lidocaine, mexiletine, and tocainide have actions belonging to class IB. Their potency for blocking sodium channels is only moderate, and in isolated tissues they shorten the action potential duration (APD) and refractoriness. They generally exert little effect on the PR, QRS, or QT intervals. Drugs with class IC actions are the more potent agents: flecainide and propafenone. Because these are potent sodium channel inhibitors, slowing conduction velocity while having little effect on repolarization, they increase the PR and QRS intervals but cause little change in QT. *Class II action* refers to beta-adrenergic antagonism, possessed by agents such as propranolol, carvedilol, atenolol, and metoprolol. These drugs are effective for the treatment of supraventricular arrhythmias and tachyarrhythmias secondary to excessive sympathetic activity. Although the mechanism is unknown, they are the only antiarrhythmic drugs found clearly effective in preventing sudden cardiac death in patients with prior myocardial infarction. Furthermore, in a study of patients with "electrical storm," that is, recurrent cardiac arrest due to sustained ventricular tachyarrhythmias following myocardial infarction, there was an 82 percent mortality with therapy guided by standard Advanced Cardiac Life Support (ACLS), which used lidocaine as first-line antiarrhythmic therapy, compared to 22 percent with sympathetic blockade, which was achieved with either beta blockers or left stellate ganglionic blockade.[10] Beta blockers are also effective in reducing total mortality in patients with heart failure,[11] which may in part be due to a decrease in sudden death.[12]

Drugs whose predominant effect is to prolong the duration of the cardiac action potential and refractoriness have class III action. These drugs include amiodarone, sotalol, ibutilide, dofetilide, and *N*-acetylprocainamide (NAPA), the major metabolite of procainamide.

Class IV action is calcium channel antagonism. Antiarrhythmic drugs with this action include verapamil, bepridil, diltiazem, and nifedipine.

Because of the many limitations of the Vaughan Williams classification of antiarrhythmic drugs, a new approach has been proposed,[13] termed the *Sicilian gambit*. This classification system is based on the differential effects of antiarrhythmic drugs on (1) channels, (2) receptors, and (3) transmembrane pumps. The grouping is based primarily on the predominant action of drugs, but it also considers the other ancillary actions that may be clinically relevant. As shown in Fig. 35-1, because of the sequence of drugs listed, the symbols for these primary actions are generally aligned diagonally. For example, in this system, quinidine is a sodium channel antagonist with potassium channel–and alpha-blocking activity. This provides a more complete and accurate description of the pharmacologic actions of the drugs than simply designating it class IA. When combined with an understanding of the electrophysiologic role of these actions, one can predict the effects likely to occur in vivo. In this case one would expect slowing of conduction, increased APD (and refractoriness), and vasodilation to result from these three actions of quinidine.

The Sicilian gambit also creates a framework in which newly discovered actions of drugs can readily be added. It emphasizes the multiple actions of drugs and the subtle differences and similarities that exist, and it is more complete. At present, our understanding of the pharmacology of these drugs has progressed to the point that oversimplification can be misleading. The increased detail of the new system reflects the current state of our knowledge at a level necessary for optimal use of these drugs.

Owing to the low efficacy of any one agent, the treatment of acute or chronic ventricular arrhythmias frequently necessitates the use of multiple drugs, sequentially or in combination. One may produce increased sodium channel blockade and, it is hoped, increase drug efficacy by using combinations of drugs with different kinetics of interaction with the sodium channel. Basic to these considerations is an understanding of the regulation of sodium channel function. Hodgkin and Huxley[14] proposed that sodium channels exist in three distinct states: open, closed, and inactivated. According to the modulated receptor theory of cardiac sodium channel regulation proposed by Hille[14a] and by Hondeghem and Katzung,[15] sodium channels in each of these states have differing affinities for a given local anesthetic drug (Fig. 35-2).

The theory also provides a potential explanation for the phenomenon of "frequency-" or "use-" dependence. Use-dependence is the increase in conduction block observed at an increasing rate of stimulation in response to sodium channel–blocking antiarrhythmic agents. Since an increase in the rate of stimulation increases the number of sodium channels in the open and inactivated states, antiarrhythmic agents having greater affinity for activated (open) or inactivated channels (as opposed to rested channels) would have a greater opportunity to bind to the receptor and slow conduction. Therefore greater block will occur during tachycardia, leaving less drug action at normal heart rates. Also, antiarrhythmic drugs have different affinities for the different states of the sodium channel, and this is manifest as different rates for onset or recovery from block. Drugs that slowly associate with the receptor will cause block to accumulate over the first few cardiac cycles, as is shown for procainamide in Fig. 35-3. Drugs that associate more rapidly, such as lidocaine, produce little additional block after the first beat in a train of stimuli. This effect is compared to that of procainamide in Fig. 35-3. Likewise, drugs dissociate from the sodium channel at different rates, leading to differences in rates of recovery from block. The rate of onset of block of sodium channels has been proposed as a means of subclassifying antiarrhythmic drugs.[16] This is the electrophysiologic correlate of the subclassification of sodium channel blockers proposed by Harrison, which was based on differences in clinical effects of the drugs.[9]

*Reverse use-dependence*—i.e., greater drug effect at slower rates—refers to the effect of potassium channel blockade on cardiac repolarization. The delayed rectifier potassium channels are classified according to their activation properties. The rapidly activating, inwardly rectifying potassium channel, $I_{Kr}$, is blocked by the drugs with class III actions. The slowly activating and deactivating channel, $I_{Ks}$, is not blocked by these drugs; thus, in the presence of $I_{Kr}$ blockade, it is the activation/deactivation kinetics of the $I_{Ks}$ channel that determine repolarization. At fast heart rates, the $I_{Ks}$ channel is mostly in an active state and allows for repolarization. At slow heart rates,

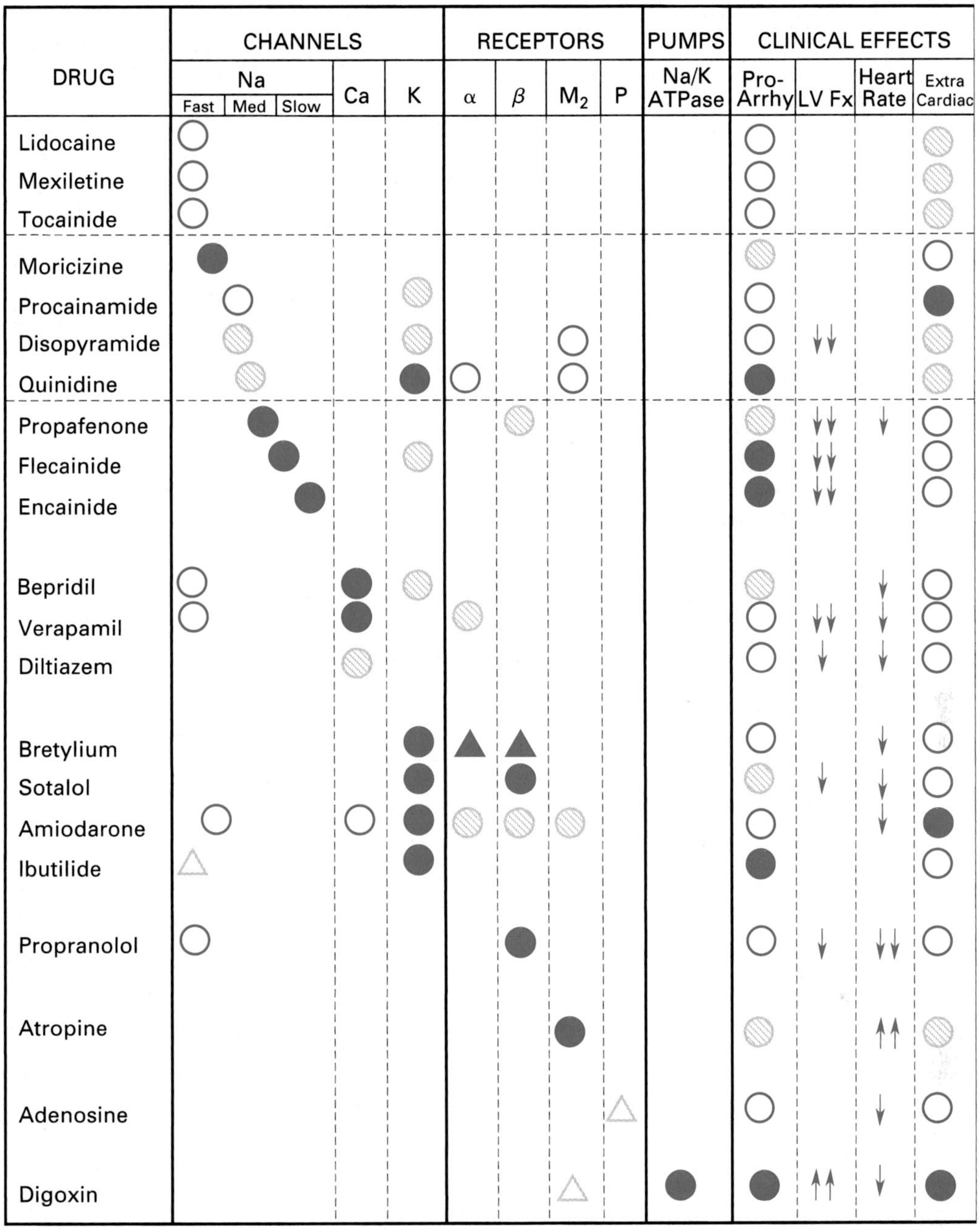

| DRUG | CHANNELS | | | | | RECEPTORS | | | | PUMPS | CLINICAL EFFECTS | | | |
|---|---|---|---|---|---|---|---|---|---|---|---|---|---|---|
| | Na | | | Ca | K | α | β | $M_2$ | P | Na/K ATPase | Pro-Arrhy | LV Fx | Heart Rate | Extra Cardiac |
| | Fast | Med | Slow | | | | | | | | | | | |
| Lidocaine | ○ | | | | | | | | | | ○ | | | ◍ |
| Mexiletine | ○ | | | | | | | | | | ○ | | | ◍ |
| Tocainide | ○ | | | | | | | | | | ○ | | | ◍ |
| Moricizine | ● | | | | | | | | | | ◍ | | | ○ |
| Procainamide | | ○ | | | ◍ | | | | | | ○ | | | ● |
| Disopyramide | | ◍ | | | ◍ | | | ○ | | | ○ | ↓↓ | | ◍ |
| Quinidine | | ◍ | | | ● | ○ | | ○ | | | ● | | | ◍ |
| Propafenone | | ● | | | | | ◍ | | | | ◍ | ↓↓ | ↓ | ○ |
| Flecainide | | | ● | | ◍ | | | | | | ● | ↓↓ | | ○ |
| Encainide | | | ● | | | | | | | | ● | ↓↓ | | ○ |
| Bepridil | ○ | | | ● | ◍ | | | | | | ◍ | | ↓ | ○ |
| Verapamil | ○ | | | ● | | ◍ | | | | | ○ | ↓↓ | ↓ | ○ |
| Diltiazem | | | | ◍ | | | | | | | ○ | ↓ | ↓ | ○ |
| Bretylium | | | | | ● | ▲ | ▲ | | | | ○ | | ↓ | ○ |
| Sotalol | | | | | ● | | ● | | | | ◍ | ↓ | ↓ | ○ |
| Amiodarone | ○ | | | ○ | ● | ◍ | ◍ | ◍ | | | ○ | | ↓ | ● |
| Ibutilide | △ | | | | ● | | | | | | ● | | | ○ |
| Propranolol | ○ | | | | | | ● | | | | ○ | ↓ | ↓↓ | ○ |
| Atropine | | | | | | | | ● | | | ◍ | | ↑↑ | ◍ |
| Adenosine | | | | | | | | | △ | | ○ | | ↓ | ○ |
| Digoxin | | | | | | | | △ | | ● | ● | ↑↑ | ↓ | ● |

FIGURE 35-1 Summary of the potentially most important actions of drugs on membrane channels, receptors, and ionic pumps in the heart. Listed are drugs used to modify cardiac rhythm. Most are marketed as antiarrhythmic agents. The drugs (rows) are ordered in a fashion similar to the columns, so that generally the darker symbols for their predominant action or actions form a diagonal. Drugs with multiple actions (e.g., amiodarone) depart strikingly from the diagonal trend. The actions of drugs on the sodium, calcium, and potassium channels are indicated. Sodium channel blockade is subdivided into three groups of actions characterized by fast (300 ms), medium (med; 300–1500 ms), and slow (greater than or equal to 1500 ms) time constants for recovery from block. This parameter is a measure of "use dependence" and predicts the likelihood that a drug will decrease conduction velocity of normal sodium-dependent tissues in the heart and perhaps the propensity of a drug for causing bundle branch block or proarrhythmia. Drug interactions with receptors alpha, beta, $M_2$, and P (alpha- and beta-adrenergic, muscarinic subtype, and $A_1$ purinergic) and drug effects on the sodium-potassium pump ($Na^+$, $K^+$-ATPase) are indicated. Symbols indicate the types of action at receptors or channels. (Antagonist relative potency: ○ low; moderate; ● high; △ agonist; ▲ agonist/antagonist.) Filled triangles for bretylium indicate its biphasic action to initially stimulate alpha and beta receptors by release of norepinephrine, followed by blocking of norepinephrine release and indirect antagonism of these receptors. (Adapted from the Task Force of the Working Group on Arrhythmias of the European Society of Cardiology.[9] With permission.)

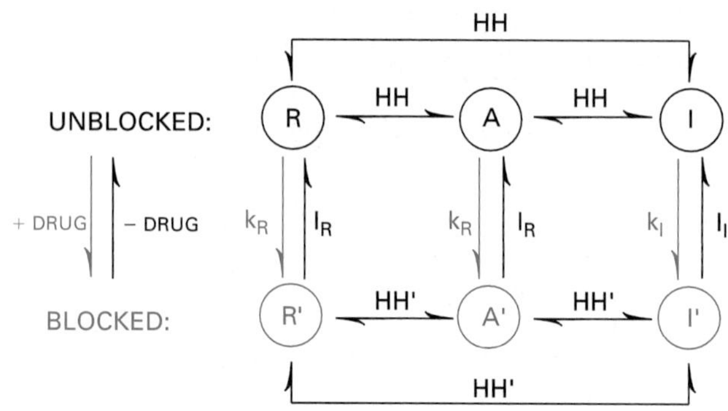


FIGURE 35-2 Diagram of the modulated receptor mechanism for antiarrhythmic drug action. The three fractions of the sodium channel population proposed by Hodgkin and Huxley are represented in the upper part of the figure in the drug-free condition and in the lower part of the figure blocked by an antiarrhythmic agent ($R^+$, $A^+$, and $I^+$, respectively). HH-standard Hodgkin-Huxley rate constants; $HH^+$-HH with voltage dependence altered by drug binding; $k_R$, $k_A$, and $k_I$-association rate constants; $l_R$, $l_A$, and $l_I$-dissociation rate constants for the respective channel fractions. (From Hondeghem and Katzung.[11] Reproduced with permission from the authors and the American Heart Association.)

there is sufficient time for $I_{Ks}$ deactivation to occur. Hence, in the presence of $I_{Kr}$ blockade, repolarization is impaired. Thus, drugs that block $I_{Kr}$ lead to greater prolongation of the QT interval at slow heart rates, where $I_{Ks}$ is relatively deactivated, but less at fast heart rates, where $I_{Ks}$ remains activated.

This chapter reviews the clinical pharmacology and applications of the currently available antiarrhythmic drugs excluding digoxin, beta-receptor antagonists, and calcium channel blockers, which are addressed in other chapters. The drugs reappear in the same order as listed in Fig. 35-1, an updated revision of the Sicilian gambit classification. The pharmacokinetics, usual dosages, and ranges of plasma concentration for the major drugs are listed in Tables 35-1 and 35-2.

## DRUGS

### Lidocaine (Xylocaine)

#### CLINICAL APPLICATIONS

Lidocaine, introduced as a local anesthetic, was first used as an antiarrhythmic agent in the 1950s for the treatment of arrhythmias arising during cardiac catheterization.[17] It is still a commonly used intravenous antiarrhythmic drug. Since extensive first-pass metabolism makes it unsatisfactory for oral use, congeners such as mexiletine were developed that would possess similar sodium channel-blocking actions and be active when taken orally.

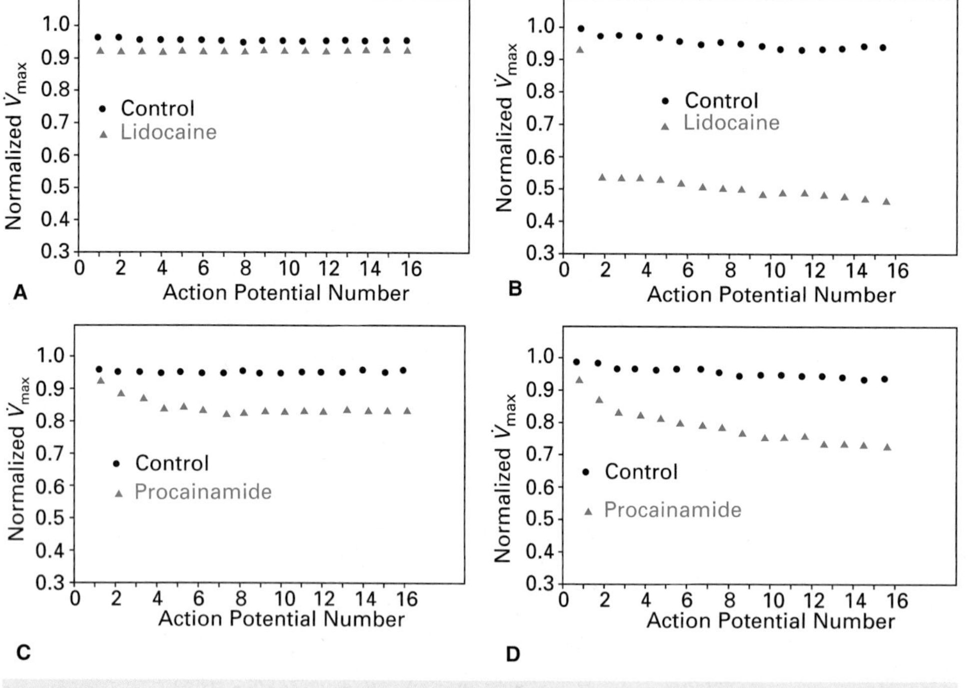


FIGURE 35-3 Rate- (interval-) dependent depression of $\dot{V}_{max}$ by lidocaine and procainamide. Following a 20-s rest period, a train of 16 action potentials was elicited using interstimulus intervals (ISIs) of 1 s or 200 ms in the presence (*triangles*) or absence (*circles*) of lidocaine or procainamide. For the duration of the train, $\dot{V}_{max}$ was relatively constant when measured at either ISI in the absence of drug. *A.* In the presence of lidocaine (22 $\mu M$), stimulation at an ISI of 1 s produced no use-dependent block. *B.* However, stimulation at 200 ms produced a 50 percent reduction in $\dot{V}_{max}$ from baseline, which was first observed for the second action potential and was constant thereafter. *C.* A different pattern is seen in the presence of 276 $\mu M$ procainamide, which produced a significant depression of $\dot{V}_{max}$ at an ISI of 1 s. *D.* This depression was more pronounced when the ISI was shortened to 200 ms. Unlike the case for lidocaine, the use-dependent depression of $\dot{V}_{max}$ due to procainamide required multiple action potentials to approach steady-state values. (From Ehring BR, Moyer JW, Hondeghem LM. Quantitative structure activity studies of antiarrhythmic properties in a series of lidocaine and procainamide derivatives. *J Pharmacol Exp Ther* 1989;244:479–492. Reproduced with permission from the publisher and authors.)

Lidocaine is very often the drug of first choice for the acute suppression of ventricular arrhythmias. Although such therapy does not reduce total mortality rates, it is effective in decreasing the incidence of primary ventricular fibrillation in patients with documented acute myocardial infarction.[18,19] However, lidocaine is not recommended for routine use to prevent ventricular arrhythmias during acute myocardial infarction. Recently the utility of lidocaine for shock resistant ventricular fibrillation has been questioned.[20] A study of out-of-hospital cardiac arrest resistant to defibrillation, the Amiodarone versus Lidocaine in Prehospital Ventricular Fibrillation Evaluation (ALIVE) trial,[20] found that amiodarone improved survival to hospital admission more effectively than lidocaine. The "Guidelines 2000 for Cardiopulmonary Resuscitation and Emergency Cardiovascular Care" (ACLS 2000)[21] consider the benefit of lidocaine for shock refractory ventricular fibrillation (VF) to be indeterminate. Because of the complex pharmacokinetics of lidocaine, a monitored environment is desirable to permit evaluation of the patient's response and detection of toxicity.

TABLE 35-1 Pharmacokinetics of Antiarrhythmic Drugs

| Agent | Inactivation or Elimination,[a] % | Protein Binding, % | $V_D$, L/kg | Elimination Half-life, h | Bioavailability, % | Apparent Oral Clearance, mL/min |
|---|---|---|---|---|---|---|
| Quinidine | Hepatic, 50–90<br>Renal, 10–30 | 80–90 | 2.5 | 3–19 | 70 | 200–400 |
| Procainamide | Hepatic, 40–70[b]<br>Renal, 30–60 | 15 | 2 | 2–4 | 100 | 400–700 |
| Disopyramide | Hepatic, 20–30<br>Renal, 40–50 | 20–50 | 0.6 | 6–8 | 80–90 | 90 |
| Lidocaine | Hepatic, 90 | 40–70 | 1.1 | 1.5–4 | 35[c] | 700–1000[c] |
| Tocainide | Hepatic, 30–40<br>Renal, 40 | 10 | 1.5–3 | 8–20 | 90 | 150–200 |
| Mexiletine | Hepatic, 85–90[b]<br>Renal, 10–15 | 70 | 5.5–9.5 | 8–20 | 90 | 400–700 |
| Flecainide | Hepatic, 70[b]<br>Renal, 30 | 40 | 7–10 | 7–26 | 90–95 | 200–800 |
| Propafenone | Hepatic, 99[b] | 90 | 3–4 | 2–24[b] | 10–50[b] | 800–5000[b] |
| Amiodarone | Hepatic, 99 | 95 | 20–200 | 13–103 days | 20–80 | 6500–11,000 |
| Bretylium | Renal, 90 | Low | 3–4 | 4–16 | 25[c] | 1300 |
| Ibutilide | Hepatic, 93 | 40 | 11 | 2–12 | — | — |
| Dofetilide | Renal, 80 | 60–70 | 3 | 10 | >90 | — |

[a]Renal elimination of unchanged drug.
[b]Dependent on metabolic phenotype (see text).
[c]Not recommended for oral administration.

TABLE 35-2 Dosage and Plasma Concentration Ranges for Antiarrhythmic Agents[a]

| Agent | Usual Initial Dosage[b] | Modification of Dosage in Disease | Dosage Range | Maximum Single Dose | Therapeutic Range,[c] μg/mL |
|---|---|---|---|---|---|
| Quinidine (sulfate) | 200 mg q 6 h | None | 800–2400 mg/day | 600 | 0.7–5.5 |
| Procainamide (sustained release) | 500 mg q 6 h | ↓ CHF<br>↓ RI | 2000–6000 mg/day | 1500 | 4–8 |
| Disopyramide | 100 mg q 6 h | ↓ CHF<br>↓ HI<br>↓ RI | 300–1200 mg/day | 300 | 2–5 |
| Lidocaine | See text | ↓ CHF<br>↓ HI | 1–4 mg/min IV | — | 1.5–5 |
| Tocainide | 400 mg q 8 h | ↓ HI<br>↓ RI | 1200–2400 mg/day | 800 | 4–10 |
| Mexiletine | 200 mg q 8 h | ↓ CHF<br>↓ HI? | 600–1200 mg/day | 400 | 0.7–2 |
| Flecainide | 50–100 mg q 12 h | ↓ CHF<br>↓ RI<br>↓ HI? | 200–400 mg/day | 200 | 0.2–1 |
| Propafenone | 150 mg q 8 h | See text | 300–900 mg/day | 300 | 0.5–3? |
| Amiodarone | 600–1400 mg/day (load) | None | 200–600 mg/day | 600 | 1–2 |
| Bretylium | See text | ↓ RI | 1–4 mg/min IV | — | — |
| Ibutilide | 1 mg, repeat after 10 min | — | 0.01 mg/kg–1 mg × 2 | 1 mg | — |
| Dofetilide | 500 mcg bid | ↓ RI | 125–1000 mcg/d | 500 mcg | 0.001–0.003 |

[a]These are general guidelines only. Dosage should be determined for each patient based on clinical presentation, disease states, clinical response, and tolerance to the drug.
[b]Dosage usually recommended in absence of significant cardiac, renal, or hepatic failure.
[c]The range of therapeutic plasma concentrations is a statistical range that should be considered only a guideline to therapy.
ABBREVIATIONS: CHF = congestive heart failure; HI = hepatic insufficiency; RI = renal insufficiency. See text for details.

Lidocaine has little effect on atrial tissue in vitro,[22] consistent with the clinical observation that it has no value in treating supraventricular tachyarrhythmias. Although lidocaine has been used to decrease the ventricular response during atrial fibrillation in patients whose atrioventricular (AV) conduction occurs over an accessory pathway,[23] some workers have reported accelerated conduction,[24] and other drugs, such as procainamide and amiodarone, are preferred in this situation.

## MECHANISM OF ACTION

In concentrations similar to those attained during clinical use, lidocaine reduces $\dot{V}_{max}$ and produces shortening or no change in APD and the effective refractory period of normal Purkinje fibers. This contrasts with quinidine and procainamide, which additionally block potassium channels and produce lengthening of APD.[25,26] Lidocaine has little effect on the electrophysiology of the normal conduction system, but it has produced variable effects in patients with conduction system abnormalities. Some studies have failed to detect significant changes in conduction,[27,28] while others have found slowing of ventricular rate or potentiation of infranodal block in patients with conduction system defects.[29,30] Variability in dosage and pharmacokinetics may explain some of these discrepancies.

## CLINICAL PHARMACOLOGY

Orally administered lidocaine is well absorbed, but it has poor oral bioavailability because it undergoes extensive first-pass hepatic metabolism. Lidocaine clearance is well approximated by measurement of liver blood flow.[31,32] The two desethyl metabolites, which are excreted by the kidneys, have less antiarrhythmic potency than the parent drug and may contribute to the production of central nervous system side effects occurring with lidocaine.[33,34] Following intravenous administration, lidocaine's biphasic disposition is well represented by a two-compartment pharmacokinetic model.[35] Since antiarrhythmic activity is correlated with lidocaine's concentration in the central compartment and the half-life of distribution out of this compartment is rapid (8 min), regimens employing a series of multiple loading doses and a maintenance infusion should be used to achieve and then maintain a therapeutic concentration in plasma and myocardial tissue. Regardless of the initial regimen employed, the lidocaine concentration during prolonged constant infusion eventually reaches steady state, dependent only on the drug's infusion rate and clearance. The time required to reach steady-state conditions is approximately 8 to 10 h in normal individuals and up to 20 to 24 h in some patients with heart failure and/or liver disease. This is longer than often anticipated because of the failure to recognize the relatively long elimination half-life (1.5 to 2 h in normal subjects and longer in patients with heart failure or hepatic disease).

## DOSAGE AND ADMINISTRATION

The primary use of lidocaine is for acute, rapid suppression of highly symptomatic ventricular arrhythmias. Single intravenous boluses will achieve only transient therapeutic effects because the drug is rapidly distributed out of the plasma and myocardium; therefore multiple loading doses should be used in order to achieve more sustained therapeutic plasma levels of lidocaine rapidly. Based on pharmacokinetic models validated in clinical studies, several regimens have been designed to maintain a relatively constant therapeutic level. For a stable patient, a total loading dose of lidocaine should be approximately 3 to 4 mg/kg body weight administered over 20 to 30 min. After injection of an initial dose of 1 mg/kg over 2 min, a series of three loading boluses can be administered slowly (approximately 50 mg each over 2 min) 8 to 10 min apart, while the patient is continuously observed for the development of side effects. Loading should be stopped should the transient, usually mild, central nervous system side effects persist or serious unwanted effects occur.

Another effective and well-tolerated loading regimen was suggested by Wyman et al.[36] For a 75-kg person, an initial bolus of 75 mg is recommended, followed by 50 mg every 5 min repeated three times to a total dose of 225 mg. This regimen usually achieves and maintains plasma concentrations within usual therapeutic guidelines (1.5 to 5 $\mu$g/mL). A priming dose of 75 mg followed by a loading infusion of 150 mg over 18 min has also been used successfully.[37] At the time of initiation of the loading regimen, a maintenance infusion—designed to replace ongoing losses due to drug elimination—should be started. This may be calculated as the product of the desired plasma concentration (about 3 $\mu$g/mL) and the expected clearance. This calculation usually yields a dosage in the range of 20 to 60 $\mu$g/kg/min.

Even in normal individuals, there is great variability in the peak plasma concentration and consequently in the calculated size of the central compartment for lidocaine. During loading, therefore, the patient's electrocardiogram (ECG), blood pressure, and mental status should be monitored; the process should be stopped at the first sign of lidocaine excess. When symptomatic arrhythmias persist in the presence of documented adequate dosage (defined by side effects or plasma concentration in excess of 5 to 7 $\mu$g/mL), another agent should be used. If the maintenance infusion has reached steady state but the concentration is below the level needed to prevent recurrence and the arrhythmia reappears while side effects are absent, the appropriate actions are as follows: (1) obtain a plasma sample for measurement of lidocaine concentration for future reference, (2) administer a small bolus of lidocaine (25 to 50 mg over 2 min), and (3) increase the maintenance infusion rate proportionally. The plasma concentration can be used to estimate clearance for calculation of the final maintenance infusion (i.e., maintenance dosage = clearance × desired plasma concentration, and clearance = infusion rate ÷ plasma concentration measured at steady state). Little therapeutic effect is evident at lidocaine plasma concentrations below 1.5 $\mu$g/mL, while the risk of toxicity increases above 5 $\mu$g/mL. In some patients, however, concentrations in the range of 5 to 9 $\mu$g/mL may be required for arrhythmia suppression and can safely be achieved with cautious drug administration.[38]

Once steady-state conditions have been achieved, simply terminating a lidocaine infusion will result in a gradual decline in plasma levels over the next 8 to 10 h, as elimination occurs. Not only is there no reason to taper lidocaine infusions, but it may be dangerous if oral antiarrhythmic therapy is initiated too early, since unpredictable additive effects may occur between lidocaine and newly started oral therapy. If a patient has reached steady-state equilibrium, it is possible to estimate when the plasma lidocaine concentration will fall below usually therapeutic levels. The plasma lidocaine concentration should be determined at the time the infusion is terminated, and the number of half-lives needed for that level to reach approximately 1.5 $\mu$g/mL can be estimated. The half-life of lidocaine for an individual patient can be estimated from the following equation: $t_{1/2}$ = plasma concentration × $V_D$ × 0.693 infusion rate, where $V_D$ is the final volume of distribution. The measured plasma concentration and the infusion rate are known components of the equation. $V_D$ is usually 1.1 L/kg, but it may be reduced by 50 percent or more in patients with heart failure.

## MODIFICATION OF DOSAGE IN DISEASE STATES

Initial loading regimens require no adjustment in patients with renal or liver disease[35]; however, maintenance infusions must be decreased in liver disease and heart failure to compensate for decreased clearance. Since clearance alone is altered in liver disease, with little change in the volume of distribution, the half-life of elimination is prolonged greatly (as much as 5 h), and steady-state conditions may not be achieved until 20 to 25 h following the institution of an intravenous infusion. Despite the fact that lidocaine metabolites are excreted by the kidneys, renal disease has not been reported to exert any significant effect on lidocaine dosing regimens. With mechanical ventilation, there is often a decrease in cardiac output and hepatic blood flow; in that case, a decrease in lidocaine dosage may be required.[39] Patients with congestive heart failure achieve lidocaine levels that are almost double those in normal individuals given the same dose.[35] Since the central volume of distribution is generally halved in heart failure, loading doses should be reduced by 50 percent; since clearance is also approximately halved, maintenance doses should be reduced proportionately from an infusion rate of 30 $\mu$g/kg/min used for usual patients to about half that figure. The time required to achieve steady-state conditions following the institution of a maintenance infusion is still 8 to 10 h in many patients with heart failure because of concomitant changes in $V_D$ and clearance, resulting in a half-life similar to that seen in patients without heart failure.

In summary, general recommendations for initial lidocaine dosage selection should be adjusted for each patient based on clinical presentation, clinical response, and the results of plasma level monitoring. Some patients with congestive heart failure may experience toxicity when given an infusion as low as 0.5 mg/mL; thus, blood level monitoring is essential for proper dosage adjustment. In post–myocardial infarction patients receiving lidocaine infusions for more than 24 h, plasma lidocaine levels can increase, and the elimination phase half-life can increase up to 50 percent.[40] This increase is due in part to changes occurring in protein binding of lidocaine during the first few days of therapy. Assays for plasma lidocaine measure the sum of both protein-bound and free lidocaine as total lidocaine and thus do not give a true picture of the amount of free drug available. An increase in plasma lidocaine occurring at this time often reflects an elevation in plasma levels of alpha$_1$-acid glycoprotein (AAG), to which it binds,[41] and does not always indicate an increase in free, active drug. In this case, the lidocaine dosage should not be reduced to compensate for the higher total plasma concentration as long as the patient displays no adverse effects. Subsequent decreases in AAG concentrations will result in an apparent decrease in plasma lidocaine, which may reflect a drop in only that fraction bound to AAG.

### ADVERSE REACTIONS

Central nervous system symptoms are the most frequent side effects of lidocaine administration. A rapid bolus can induce tinnitus or seizures. With more gradual attainment of excessive levels, drowsiness, dysarthria, confusion, hallucinations, and dysesthesia may occur. Excessive lidocaine can also cause coma, which should be a consideration in patients after cardiac arrest. Lidocaine can depress cardiac function, which decreases its clearance and produces an even greater increase in lidocaine concentrations. Advanced degrees of sinus node dysfunction have been reported in isolated instances.[42,43] In patients with known conduction abnormalities below the AV node, lidocaine should be administered cautiously if at all unless a temporary pacemaker is readily available.

### DRUG INTERACTIONS

An additive or synergistic depression of myocardial function or conduction may occur when lidocaine is used in combination with other antiarrhythmic agents,[44] especially during conversion from lidocaine to another antiarrhythmic agent. A pharmacokinetic drug interaction between propranolol and lidocaine has been described experimentally and in humans in which beta-adrenergic blockade caused decreases in cardiac output and liver blood flow, with a resultant decreased lidocaine clearance.[45]

Cimetidine has been reported to decrease lidocaine's volume of distribution, decrease splanchnic (and hence liver) blood flow, and inhibit the enzymes responsible for lidocaine metabolism. This may raise plasma concentrations of lidocaine, and both loading and maintenance dosages may require downward adjustment in patients receiving cimetidine.[46]

## Mexiletine (Mexitil)

### CLINICAL APPLICATIONS

Mexiletine is used in the treatment of ventricular arrhythmias and has, on occasion, been effective in treating arrhythmias that were refractory to other agents. Success rates vary between 6 and 60 percent, and more than half of the studies suggest limited efficacy (less than 20 percent).[47] Mexiletine does not prolong the QT interval and therefore can be useful for patients with a history of drug-induced torsades de pointes or long-QT syndrome when quinidine, sotalol, procainamide, or disopyramide are contraindicated. While the rate of response to mexiletine used alone is low, it has been combined successfully with quinidine,[48] propranolol,[49] or procainamide[50] and is also commonly combined with amiodarone. This mode of therapy takes advantage of the additive and perhaps synergistic antiarrhythmic response produced by the combination of these agents. Since lower than usual dosages of both agents can be used, dosage-related adverse effects are reduced concomitantly. Mexiletine exerts minimal effects on both hemodynamics and myocardial contractility, even in patients with severe congestive heart failure.[51]

### MECHANISM OF ACTION

Mexiletine is an orally active lidocaine congener with class IB sodium channel–blocking activity and structural similarity to tocainide. It was originally developed as an anorexiant and anticonvulsant agent; its antiarrhythmic properties were only later recognized. Mexiletine blocks fast sodium channels, decreasing $\dot{V}_{max}$ and shortening the repolarization phase of ventricular myocardium.[52]

### CLINICAL PHARMACOLOGY

The systemic bioavailability of mexiletine approximates 90 percent,[53] with a large volume of distribution (5.5 to 9.5 L/kg) reflecting extensive tissue uptake. About 1 percent of the total body content of mexiletine is in the plasma compartment, with approximately 70 percent of this bound to serum proteins. Mexiletine has little first-pass metabolism but is eliminated primarily by hepatic metabolism, with only 10 to 15 percent being excreted unchanged in the urine. Its half-life of elimination is between 8 and 20 h (9 and 12 h for healthy subjects), with the time needed to reach steady state ranging between 1 and 3 days.[54] Mexiletine undergoes extensive hepatic metabolism by cytochrome P450 2D6 (CYP2D6)[55,56]; consequently clearance is extremely variable (see below).[57]

### DOSAGE AND ADMINISTRATION

Mexiletine therapy should be initiated with a low dosage, which is increased at 2- to 3-day intervals until efficacy or intolerable side effects, such as tremor or other central nervous system symptoms, develop. With normal renal function, the recommended initial oral mexiletine dosage is 200 mg every 8 h. As with most drugs having extensive liver metabolism, clearance will be widely variable within the population. This is especially true for mexiletine because CYP2D6, responsible for its metabolism, is absent in 7 percent of the Caucasian population. Also, consideration of dosage adjustment to compensate for the action of agents (discussed below) that induce or inhibit hepatic mexiletine metabolism is required.

### MODIFICATION OF DOSAGE IN DISEASE STATES

Patients with renal failure who also inherit a deficiency of hepatic CYP2D6 are likely to have extremely slow elimination for mexiletine[58]; for this reason, all patients with renal failure should be given low initial doses. Elimination half-life and clearance may be prolonged by overt congestive heart failure[59] and hepatic failure[60]; dosage reduction is required in such cases.

### ADVERSE REACTIONS

Adverse reactions to mexiletine are dose-related and neurologic. They include tremor, visual blurring, dizziness, dysphoria, and nausea. Thrombocytopenia has been reported to occur infrequently with mexiletine therapy,[61,62] and a positive antinuclear antibody test result occurs rarely. Severe bradycardia and abnormal prolongation of sinus node recovery time have been reported in patients with the sick-sinus syndrome.[63] At high concentrations, worsening of heart block has been reported.[64] Oral mexiletine does not depress ventricular function or induce increased heart failure,[65] although intravenous mexiletine, which is not available in the United States, has been noted to increase congestive heart failure.[66]

### DRUG INTERACTIONS

The hepatic metabolism of mexiletine can be increased by phenobarbital, phenytoin (Dilantin), or rifampicin, which reduce the half-life of mexiletine, possibly changing an effective dose to an ineffective one.[47,54,67] Conversely, if treatment with an inducing agent is stopped, an effective dose may become toxic. In one study, mexiletine decreased the clearance and increased the plasma concentrations of theophylline.[68] Quinidine inhibits the CYP2D6 enzyme primarily responsible for the metabolic clearance of mexiletine, and plasma concentration of mexiletine may increase in those individuals who express the enzyme (93 percent of Caucasians).

## Procainamide (Pronestyl-SR, Procan-SR)

### CLINICAL APPLICATIONS

Procainamide, like quinidine, is effective against both supraventricular and ventricular arrhythmias.[69] Although the two drugs have similar electrophysiologic effects, they are clinically different, and one agent may be effective for a patient when the other is not. Procainamide is useful in the acute management of patients with reentrant supraventricular tachycardia and atrial fibrillation and flutter associated with Wolff-Parkinson-White syndrome.[70] In the current ACLS guidelines, amiodarone and procainamide are recommended before lidocaine or adenosine for the initial treatment of hemodynamically stable wide-complex tachycardia.[21]

The active metabolite of procainamide, *N*-acetylprocainamide (NAPA), produces class III antiarrhythmic activity in some patients, although not always those who respond to procainamide.[71] This is most likely due to the very different electrophysiologic actions of procainamide and NAPA.[72] NAPA was investigated as an antiarrhythmic drug and was shown to be effective in the treatment of ventricular arrhythmias, but since its use was limited by a narrow therapeutic index, development was halted.[71]

The development of procainamide as an antiarrhythmic agent resulted from a systematic search for a useful congener of procaine, whose use was precluded by adverse reactions.[73] Since procainamide is an effective agent but is not without adverse effects, it has served as a prototype for the development of several of the newer antiarrhythmic agents.

### MECHANISM OF ACTION

Like other agents demonstrating class I activity, procainamide slows conduction and decreases the automaticity and excitability of atrial and ventricular myocardium and Purkinje fibers.[74] Because of its effect on potassium channels, it also prolongs APD and refractoriness. Compared to quinidine, procainamide has very little vagolytic activity and does not prolong the QT interval to as great an extent.[69] NAPA has predominantly class III antiarrhythmic activity; it prolongs APD and refractoriness in both atrial and ventricular myocardium and prolongs the QT interval.[75,76] It has little or no effect on $\dot{V}_{max}$ in either Purkinje fibers or ventricular cells and does not alter His-Purkinje conduction velocity because of its very low potency as a sodium channel antagonist.

### CLINICAL PHARMACOLOGY

Procainamide is rapidly absorbed and 100 percent orally bioavailable. About 15 percent of procainamide is bound to serum proteins. Its short half-life of elimination, 2 to 4 h in patients with normal renal function, necessitates dosing every 3 to 6 h. Dosing every 6, 8, or 12 h is possible with sustained-release preparations; the frequency depends on the formulation. The varied formulations and their very different dosing requirements often create confusion and can lead to dangerous mistakes in dosing.

Slightly more than half of the general population are phenotypically rapid acetylators of procainamide and quickly convert it to NAPA, a metabolite with very pure class III antiarrhythmic action.[71] As would be expected, however, the response to one agent does not predict response to the other. When each is given as the sole agent, the usually effective plasma concentration is 4 to 8 $\mu$g/mL for procainamide and 7 to 15 $\mu$g/mL for NAPA.[71] During oral procainamide therapy, both agents are present in variable amounts, and there is no way to determine readily the contribution of NAPA to arrhythmia suppression under these conditions. Consequently, because of this variable hepatic conversion to NAPA, the utility of measuring plasma levels of procainamide during chronic therapy is limited. Monitoring of plasma concentrations for determination of compliance or prevention of toxicity is feasible and recommended (see below).

### DOSAGE AND ADMINISTRATION

Procainamide is available for either intravenous or oral use. With normal renal and cardiac function, the initial recommended oral maintenance dose is 50 mg/kg/day. Frequent administration is required for oral procainamide, which is inconvenient and makes compliance difficult. Sustained-release forms of procainamide are available, which permits dosing every 6, 8, or 12 h, depending on the formulation. During chronic therapy, levels of NAPA may accumulate to effective or toxic levels in some individuals, resulting in achievement of maximum pharmacologic effect long after the time procainamide has reached steady state.[71,77] Therefore the elimination half-life of 2 to 4 h for procainamide may be misleading as a predictor of time to the occurrence of stable pharmacologic action. Thus dosage should be initiated at conservative levels, and the patient should be monitored carefully until both procainamide and its metabolite have reached steady state. Patients with ventricular tachycardia may need higher dosages,[71,72] although such dosages often lead to adverse effects. Since the electrophysiologic effects of procainamide and NAPA are quite different, monitoring of patients receiving procainamide should at some point include measurement of plasma concentrations of both agents to determine their relative concentrations. Patients who are rapid acetylators or who have impaired renal function usually have plasma concentrations of NAPA higher than those of procainamide at steady state. These individuals should be monitored for excessive accumulation of NAPA during dose titration to maintain plasma levels of NAPA below 20 μg/mL. The practice of using the sum of the plasma concentration of procainamide and NAPA is not recommended.

When administered intravenously, procainamide can be given as a constant 25-min loading infusion of 275 μg/min/kg or by a series of doses (100 mg delivered over 3 min) given every 5 min, up to a total dose of 1 g.[78,79] If the loading infusion is well tolerated with no hypotension and less than 25 percent QRS or QT widening, a maintenance intravenous infusion of 20 to 60 μg/kg/min can then be given. Larger and more rapid loading infusions of 1 g over 15 to 20 min have been given in the electrophysiology laboratory to prevent induction of ventricular tachycardia by programmed ventricular stimulation. A second loading infusion of 0.5 to 1 g has been given in some instances where an initial loading infusion was well tolerated but ineffective. These large dosages are accompanied by a higher incidence of hypotension and conduction disturbance and often result in the attainment of unacceptably high plasma concentrations.

### MODIFICATION OF DOSAGE IN DISEASE STATES

With renal dysfunction or a low cardiac output, both procainamide and NAPA in usual doses may accumulate to potentially toxic levels, and the dose should be reduced.[80] Increased plasma levels of procainamide and/or NAPA may occur with congestive heart failure because of decreased urinary excretion and hydrolysis of procainamide.[81] On the other hand, one study of procainamide pharmacokinetics following a single intravenous bolus revealed no difference in volume of distribution, clearance, elimination half-life, unbound drug fraction, or peak procainamide concentrations between patients with congestive heart failure and normal individuals.[82] Although intravenous procainamide does depress myocardial contractility and lower blood pressure, worsening of heart failure is uncommon during oral therapy when the usual dosages and plasma concentrations are maintained.

### ADVERSE REACTIONS

Side effects associated with long-term procainamide therapy limit its usefulness. Up to 40 percent of patients discontinue therapy in the first 6 months due to adverse reactions. The potential exists for the aggravation of arrhythmia, including the development of torsades de pointes due to procainamide or, more often, NAPA.[83] Therefore, just as with all agents possessing class IA activity, procainamide should not be used in patients with a long-QT syndrome, a history of torsades de pointes, or hypokalemia.[84] In order to reduce the occurrence of proarrhythmia, potassium levels should be maintained above 4 meq/L in those taking procainamide. Heart block and sinus node dysfunction can occur in patients with preexisting conduction system abnormalities.[85]

Between 15 and 20 percent of patients receiving chronic oral procainamide therapy develop a lupus-like syndrome, which is often difficult to recognize but regresses with discontinuation of treatment. The syndrome usually begins insidiously as mild arthralgia but progresses to frank arthritis, fever, malar erythematous rash, and pleural and or pericardial effusions, with serum antibodies against nucleoprotein (histone) appearing as antinuclear antibodies with a "smooth" or "diffuse" pattern. These symptoms abate if procainamide is discontinued and generally resolve at a rate proportional to their duration. Almost all patients treated chronically develop detectable antinuclear antibodies, only 15 to 20 percent develop symptoms of the lupus syndrome. It is therefore unnecessary to discontinue therapy solely because of the positive antinuclear antibody titer. The patient should be fully informed of the symptoms, which should be reported, so that therapy can be discontinued at the earliest symptoms or signs of the lupus syndrome. Continuing procainamide after symptoms of the lupus syndrome have appeared is dangerous because of the above-noted possibility of pleural effusion and potentially lethal pericardial tamponade.[86]

More recently, procainamide therapy has been associated with the development of agranulocytosis. It has been suggested but not proven that the sustained-release form of the drug may be especially capable of inducing this toxicity.[87] The manufacturer recommends that a white blood cell count be obtained every 2 weeks for the first 3 months.

### DRUG INTERACTIONS

Unlike quinidine, procainamide does not cause an increase in digoxin levels. There are few reports of interactions between procainamide and other drugs. Its clearance is reduced between 30 and 50 percent by cimetidine, which blocks the renal tubular secretion of procainamide.[88,89] A similar competition has been found between procainamide and its predominant metabolite, NAPA.[90] Ranitidine affects procainamide pharmacokinetics by reducing both its renal clearance and its absorption, the former by 14 to 23 percent and the latter by 10 to 24 percent, depending on the dose.[91]

## Disopyramide (Norpace)

### CLINICAL APPLICATIONS

Disopyramide is effective against a broad range of supraventricular and ventricular arrhythmias, its antiarrhythmic profile being similar to that of quinidine and procainamide. Disopyramide, in contrast to quinidine and procainamide, is better suited for long-term therapy, having relatively little associated chronic toxicity. While newer than quinidine or procainamide, disopyramide is still one of the older antiarrhythmic agents, having been in use in the United States since 1977. Its negative inotropic and anticholinergic actions occur frequently and limit its usefulness.

### MECHANISMS OF ACTION

The class IA antiarrhythmic effects of disopyramide are predominantly those associated with sodium and potassium channel blockade. Its effects are similar to those of quinidine and procainamide on automaticity, conduction, and refractoriness in atrial and ventricular tissue.[92]

### CLINICAL PHARMACOLOGY

The oral bioavailability of disopyramide is 80 to 90 percent.[93] Its half-life of elimination, usually 6 to 8 h, is lengthened to as much as 15 h in cardiac patients.[94] About half of the compound is eliminated by the kidneys unchanged and the remainder as an active metabolite resulting from hepatic *N*-dealkylation.[95] Protein binding of disopyramide is complex, with between 20 and 50 percent of disopyramide being bound to plasma proteins. For most drugs, the percentage bound to plasma protein is a constant over the usual range of therapeutic concentrations. The saturation of disopyramide-binding sites on plasma proteins at usual doses means that there are disproportionate increases in levels of free drug in plasma compared to the magnitude of dosage increment.[96]

### DOSAGE AND ADMINISTRATION

Loading doses are not recommended with disopyramide. The usually effective dosage for disopyramide is 100 to 400 mg three to four times daily, to a maximal dose of 800 mg/day. Therapy should be very carefully titrated, beginning with low doses and allowing ample time for the achievement of steady-state equilibrium. While rapid fluctuations in plasma concentration are undesirable, they are difficult to avoid because of disopyramide's saturable protein binding. The controlled-release form of disopyramide may be useful in reducing adverse effects by decreasing fluctuations in the concentration of free disopyramide in plasma.[97] Because of saturable protein binding,[22] the generally accepted therapeutic range for total disopyramide in plasma, 2 to 5 μg/mL, should not be strictly relied on. While monitoring of the plasma concentrations of free disopyramide has been recommended,[98] the range of concentrations associated with arrhythmia suppression has not been clearly delineated and overlaps with that causing adverse effects.

### MODIFICATION OF DOSAGE IN DISEASE STATES

The patient's response to disopyramide should be monitored especially closely following acute myocardial infarction because both the absorption and elimination of disopyramide are decreased at this time.[99] In fact, in view of the negative inotropic actions of disopyramide and changes in levels of binding proteins in plasma following a myocardial infarction, other antiarrhythmic agents should be considered first. Disopyramide is contraindicated in patients with uncompensated heart failure because it can worsen failure.[100] The initial dosage of disopyramide should be reduced to 50 to 100 mg every 12 h in patients with renal insufficiency[101] or decreased hepatic function.[102]

### ADVERSE REACTIONS

The predominant side effects of disopyramide include new or worsened congestive heart failure and symptoms resulting from dose-related anticholinergic actions, including urinary retention, constipation, dry mouth, and esophageal reflux. Because of this anticholinergic action, patients with obstructive uropathy or glaucoma should not receive this agent.[103] For some patients, the anticholinergic side effects can be prevented or alleviated by concomitant use of cholinesterase inhibitors, such as physostigmine and neostigmine, without reduction in antiarrhythmic efficacy.[104] As with all agents that prolong repolarization, disopyramide should not be used in patients with long-QT syndrome, hypokalemia, or a history of torsades de pointes[105] because of its potential for aggravating arrhythmia. Direct actions of disopyramide on the sinus node can lead to excessive bradycardia in patients with sinus nodal dysfunction[106]; this may contribute to the development of torsades de pointes in patients with hypokalemia.[107]

### DRUG INTERACTIONS

Disopyramide does not increase digoxin levels,[108] and the effects of warfarin are not potentiated by disopyramide.[109] Phenytoin, rifampicin, and phenobarbital induce hepatic metabolism of disopyramide, thus increasing its elimination and potentially leading to loss of antiarrhythmic effect.[110] Significant depression of myocardial contractility may result from the combined administration of disopyramide with beta-adrenergic or calcium channel antagonists and should be avoided in patients with impairment of ventricular function.[111]

## Quinidine (Quinaglute, Quinadex, Others)

### CLINICAL APPLICATIONS

Quinidine has been used successfully for a variety of supraventricular and ventricular arrhythmias, including conversion of atrial fibrillation or flutter,[112,113] supraventricular tachycardia,[112,113] ventricular extrasystoles,[114] and ventricular tachycardia and fibrillation.[115,116] Digitalis is used in the treatment of atrial fibrillation, atrial flutter, and other arrhythmias. This important drug is discussed in Chap. 23.

A grouped analysis of six small placebo-controlled trials in patients with atrial fibrillation showed a statistically significant increase in mortality rate for the patients treated with quinidine.[117] Because of the similar negative effects on mortality rate seen in the CAST and CAST II, one must assume—until a definitive prospective study is available—that the results of this metanalysis are valid.

### MECHANISM OF ACTION

Quinidine has multiple actions, but the action thought by many to be primarily responsible for its efficacy is block of the rapid inward sodium channel. This results in a decrease in $\dot{V}_{max}$ of the action potential upstroke and slowed conduction, more marked in the His-Purkinje system than in the atria. The effects of quinidine on sodium channels are greatest at increased heart rate and less negative membrane potential; that is, they are pH-, rate-, and voltage-dependent. Dose-related changes in the electrocardiogram (ECG) are increases in the PR, QRS, and $QT_c$ intervals, which reflect the multiple actions of quinidine.[118] Quinidine also inhibits the transient-outward current, $I_{to}$, responsible for phase 1 of the action potential. Small studies have suggested that this effect may prevent recurrences of ventricular fibrillation in patients with Brugada syndrome,[119] where ST-segment elevation in the right precordial leads is thought to represent voltage gradients between the epicardial action potential, which has a prominent $I_{to}$ notch, and the endocardial action potential.[120]

### CLINICAL PHARMACOLOGY

The effective dosage of quinidine varies among individuals because of several factors. Although quinidine sulfate is usually administered every 6 h, there are wide interindividual differences in its elimination half-life, which varies from 3 to 19 h.[121] Plasma protein binding also varies widely, ranging from 50 to 95 percent.[121] Oral bioavailability is approximately 70 percent, and clearance after oral administration ranges from 200 to 400 mL/min. Quinidine is inactivated or eliminated by both hepatic metabolism (50 to 90 percent) and renal elimination (10 to 30 percent). Several potentially active metabolites are formed in amounts that vary among individuals,[122] but the clinical role for most has not been determined. One of the metabolites of quinidine, 3-hydroxyquinidine, has been shown to possess antiarrhythmic activity when given to humans.[122] Experimental data indicate some contribution by metabolites of quinidine to its antiarrhythmic action.[123–125]

### DOSAGE AND ADMINISTRATION

Quinidine therapy (as the sulfate) is usually initiated with an oral dosage of 200 mg every 6 h, and the dosage is carefully titrated every

3 or more days. Elderly patients often require lower dosages of quinidine because of both reduced clearance and volume of distribution. Quinidine is available commercially in at least three different forms: quinidine sulfate, gluconate, and polygalacturonate. Since the quinidine content varies among these at 83, 62, and 60 percent, respectively, the need for dosage adjustment should be considered if one form is substituted for another. The usually effective dosage of quinidine sulfate ranges from 800 to 2400 mg day, with the maximum recommended single dose being 600 mg. Because the half-life varies from 3 to 19 h, one should wait 4 days between dosage increases to prevent unexpected drug accumulation. The range of therapeutic plasma concentrations measured with assays that differentiate quinidine from its metabolites is 0.7 to 5.5 μg/mL.[126,127] Rapid escalation in quinidine dosage has been used to convert atrial fibrillation, but this therapy is no longer recommended because of unnecessary toxicity.

Intravenous therapy with quinidine is usually avoided if alternatives are feasible. Vasodilation and hypotension result from quinidine-induced alpha-adrenergic blockade. If quinidine is given intravenously (as quinidine gluconate), the patient should be carefully monitored and the infusion rate should be no greater than 16 mg/min. This should be discontinued if hypotension is observed or the QRS is prolonged by more than 30 percent.

## MODIFICATION OF DOSAGE IN DISEASE STATES

No adjustment in initial dosage is usually needed for patients with renal or hepatic disease,[128,129] although, due to decreased protein binding in patients with hepatic failure, a lower than usual total plasma concentration can produce toxicity.[130] Slower dose titration is advisable to permit attainment of steady state and complete accumulation of active metabolites; however, because the usual range of effective dosages is wide, dosage for these patients is not markedly different. Patients with rapid quinidine elimination may require higher dosages (up to 600 mg every 6 h). This is often due to induction of hepatic metabolism caused by other drugs.

Patients with congenital long-QT syndrome, hypokalemia, or a history of torsades de pointes[131] should not be given quinidine because of their increased risk for this form of proarrhythmic event. For patients with congestive heart failure, problems associated with the use of quinidine are proarrhythmia and digitalis (either digitoxin or digoxin) toxicity. Prudent use of quinidine in individuals taking digitalis requires the following: (1) that titration begin at a reduced dosage, (2) that dosage of any cardiac glycoside being administered concomitantly be reduced, and (3) that plasma electrolyte levels, especially potassium levels, be maintained above 4 meq/L.

Although quinidine does possess some direct negative inotropic effects, they are usually counteracted by its vasodilatory effect; therefore oral quinidine is well tolerated hemodynamically when given at dosages producing usual plasma concentrations, even in patients with reduced ventricular function.[132] In a study of over 650 patients, 35 percent of whom had congestive heart failure, quinidine therapy resulted in no induction or worsening of congestive heart failure.[133] On the other hand, a significant problem for patients with congestive heart failure receiving quinidine therapy is proarrhythmia, with quinidine-induced torsades de pointes being potentiated in the setting of bradycardia and low serum levels of magnesium or potassium.[107,134]

## ADVERSE REACTIONS

Marked prolongation of the QT interval has been seen in some patients receiving low or usual dosages of quinidine, and the risk of torsades de pointes is markedly increased. This arrhythmia may be responsible for quinidine syncope, which occurs in as many as 5 to 10 percent of patients within the first days of quinidine treatment, and for quinidine-induced sudden death.[135] Torsades de pointes usually occurs in patients (more often women than men) with low serum concentrations of quinidine, hypokalemia, poor ventricular function, and bradycardia.[135,136] In a study by Drici et al., dihydrotestosterone reduced the sensitivity to the effects of quinidine on the QT interval in animals.[137] This study[137] and a subsequent study by Benton et al.,[138] in which women were shown to be more sensitive to the effects of quinidine on the QT interval, provide evidence that sex hormones have direct effects on cardiac tissue that may be responsible for the difference in the incidence of torsades de pointes in men and women.[136]

For patients who develop torsades de pointes, treatment with pacing or isoproterenol is very effective. Magnesium sulfate injection is often recommended as initial therapy for torsades de pointes, although controlled trials are not available. These measures should also include correction of hypokalemia. Clinically, it is essential to distinguish torsades de pointes from polymorphic ventricular tachycardia occurring in the setting of a normal QT interval, because the latter should be treated with local anesthetic antiarrhythmic drugs and may be worsened by the above-mentioned treatment for torsades de pointes.

Since quinidine acts via alpha-adrenergic blockade to produce vasodilatation,[139] hypotension may occur, especially in patients concomitantly receiving nitrates or other vasodilators. Other adverse effects include a high incidence of diarrhea and vomiting, tinnitus at high plasma levels, rare thrombocytopenia,[140] and, in unusual cases, conduction block in patients with existing conduction system disease.[133] In patients treated with quinidine for atrial flutter without prior AV nodal blockade by digitalis, there have been reports of sudden increases in AV conduction and rapid ventricular rates.[139] This results from a slight reduction of the flutter rate and enhanced AV nodal conduction due to the anticholinergic effects of quinidine. This permits 1:1 conduction through the AV node, often at 200 to 250 beats per minute, which may be of particular concern for patients receiving other drugs that increase conduction time through the AV node, such as beta-adrenergic agonists.

## DRUG INTERACTIONS

Quinidine metabolism is inhibited by cimetidine[141] and induced by phenytoin, phenobarbital,[142] and rifampicin,[140] with the latter agents leading to reduced, often subtherapeutic quinidine concentrations. Clinical digoxin toxicity has been described in 20 to 40 percent of patients receiving quinidine and digoxin concurrently.[141] The magnitude of this interaction is dependent on quinidine dosage, and in some patients it may not appear until the dosage is increased to higher levels.[143,144] The rise in digoxin levels appears with the first dose of quinidine; it is therefore suggested that digoxin dosage be halved when quinidine therapy is initiated. A similar interaction has been reported for quinidine and digitoxin.

Quinidine is a potent inhibitor of the hepatic cytochrome P450 (CYP) specific for debrisoquine metabolism (CYP2D6),[145,146] although it is not metabolized by this specific P450 isozyme.[147,148] Thus, it may interfere with the biotransformation and actions of pharmacologic agents dependent on this cytochrome for their metabolism, which include propafenone, mexiletine, flecainide, metoprolol, timolol, sparteine, and bufuralol.[149] Quinidine worsens neuromuscular blockade in patients with myasthenia gravis[150] and may prolong the effects of succinylcholine.[151]

## Propafenone (Rythmol)

### CLINICAL APPLICATIONS

Propafenone was developed in Germany, where it has been marketed since 1977. It is similar to other antiarrhythmic agents in overall efficacy and tolerance by patients. It has a role in the treatment of many types of arrhythmias, including supraventricular arrhythmias.[152] For atrial fibrillation without structural heart disease, propafenone, along with flecainide and sotalol, are recommended as first-line choices for antiarrhythmic therapy.[153]

### CLINICAL PHARMACOLOGY

Propafenone has been described as having class IC antiarrhythmic activity because of its potent ability to slow conduction velocity with little change in APD.[154,155] It has a marked structural similarity to propranolol, and studies have shown that propafenone can accumulate during continued administration to levels capable of producing clinically significant beta-adrenergic inhibition.[156]

Propafenone, like mexiletine and flecainide, is eliminated by a metabolic pathway that has a polymorphic pattern of inheritance. Patients deficient in CYP2D6 activity have very slow elimination of propafenone and fail to form measurable quantities of the potentially active metabolite, 5-hydroxypropafenone.[157] The accumulation of high concentrations of propafenone leads to significant beta-receptor antagonism at both low and high dosages in poor metabolizers but only at high dosages in extensive metabolizers of propafenone.[158] Although metabolic phenotype does not seem to dramatically influence the antiarrhythmic response to propafenone in many patients,[157] it clearly influences the degree of beta blockade occurring during therapy.

### DOSAGE AND ADMINISTRATION

Effective dosages range from 300 to 900 mg day in two to four divided dosages. In order to prevent unexpected accumulation of pharmacologic action, propafenone dosage should not be changed more frequently than every 3 days; there is slow elimination of the parent drug in poor metabolizers, and there is slow accumulation of the metabolite or metabolites in extensive metabolizers. Propafenone has also been successfully used to achieve pharmacologic cardioversion of atrial fibrillation with a single oral dose of 450 to 600 mg in placebo controlled trials.[153,159] Propafenone should be used with caution, if at all, in patients with reduced ventricular function, with careful monitoring for deterioration in ventricular function, which may result from beta-adrenergic receptor antagonism and or the direct negative inotropic effect.[160]

### MODIFICATION OF DOSAGE IN DISEASE STATES

The manufacturer's label recommends that dosage be decreased by 70 to 80 percent in patients with hepatic dysfunction. There are no specific recommendations for patients with renal insufficiency, but such patients should be monitored closely.

### DRUG INTERACTIONS

It is very likely that there will be drug interactions between propafenone and other agents that utilize or inhibit cytochrome CYP2D6 for their metabolism. Such an interaction has already been documented between propafenone and metoprolol[161] and should be expected with timolol, many antidepressants, many neuroleptics, and perhaps other agents. Quinidine, which inhibits this cytochrome, inhibits the formation of 5-hydroxypropafenone in extensive metabolizers[162]; however, the clinical consequence of such inhibition is unknown and difficult to predict. One would expect greater beta blockade to occur after combining quinidine with propafenone therapy because of the resulting higher propafenone concentrations.

## Flecainide (Tambocor)

### CLINICAL APPLICATIONS

Flecainide is very effective in suppressing a variety of ventricular and supraventricular tachycardias.[163,164] The finding of increased mortality rates when flecainide is given to patients with ischemic heart disease has led to restricted usage (see above); however, there has been no evidence to indicate that this increase in mortality rate is seen when flecainide is given to treat supraventricular arrhythmias in patients without known coronary artery disease.[165] Overall, the antiarrhythmic response to flecainide in patients with symptomatic life-threatening ventricular arrhythmias is not markedly better than with older agents, such as quinidine or procainamide.[163,166] Although it is far better tolerated than older agents, the negative inotropic actions of flecainide restrict its use to patients having moderately well preserved ventricular function. Likewise, its potential to increase mortality rates in patients with ischemic heart disease limits its usefulness to patients without structural heart disease.

### MECHANISM OF ACTION

Flecainide has sodium channel-blocking activity and is considered to have class IC actions. It has also been found to block the delayed rectifier potassium channel in feline ventricular myocytes, and this action may be clinically relevant.[167]

Flecainide slows intraventricular conduction velocity more than it prolongs effective refractory periods.[168] It prolongs AH and HV intervals and measurably increases PR and QRS intervals on the surface ECG at therapeutic doses. The $QT_c$ interval is slightly increased, primarily due to prolongation of the QRS, but its ability to block the delayed rectifier potassium channel may contribute to QT changes.

### CLINICAL PHARMACOLOGY

The systemic bioavailability of oral flecainide is 90 to 95 percent,[169] and flecainide is predominantly metabolized in the liver to compounds that are not pharmacologically active at the concentrations usually found in plasma.[163] Flecainide, like many other antiarrhythmic agents, is metabolized by CYP2D6.[170] Because flecainide is also eliminated by the kidneys to a considerable extent, the enzyme deficiency has little effect on the pharmacokinetics of flecainide. If, however, those patients without the enzyme develop renal insufficiency or if renal patients are given a drug that blocks the metabolism of flecainide, extremely high plasma concentrations are likely to occur.[171] A potential advantage of flecainide is its very slow elimination, with half-life ranging from 7 to 23 h in normal individuals and tending to be even longer (14 to 26 h) in patients with cardiac disease, even in the absence of heart failure.[169,172]

### DOSAGE AND ADMINISTRATION

The usual dosage of flecainide for ventricular arrhythmias is 100 to 150 mg every 12 h in patients without cardiac or renal failure. A total daily dosage of more than 400 mg may sometimes be used under close medical monitoring (see below). Patients with supraventricular tachycardia are recommended to receive 50 mg every 12 h as a starting dose. The range of therapeutic plasma concentrations of flecainide is reported to be between 200 and 1000 ng/mL, although adverse effects may occur in some patients at concentrations within this range,[173,174] and many patients tolerate concentrations well above this range. To reduce the incidence of adverse effects, flecainide therapy should start with a low dosage that is maintained until steady state has been reached (at least 4 days) and altered relative to clinical response.

### MODIFICATION OF DOSAGE IN DISEASE STATES

Although flecainide is not recommended in heart failure, it has been used as adjunctive therapy, usually with amiodarone, for refractory ventricular tachycardia, particularly in patients who already have intracardiac defibrillators. The usual starting dose in this situation is 25 to 50 mg every 12 h. Since 7 percent of Caucasian patients with renal failure will not have the CYP2D6 enzyme and because flecainide is usually eliminated by both metabolism and renal excretion, all patients with renal failure should be given very low dosages and titrated very carefully. Monitoring of plasma concentration will be essential in patients with renal disease or cardiac or hepatic dysfunction. Any significant reduction in ejection fraction should be expected to lengthen elimination half-life and hence the time needed to attain steady-state equilibrium, while reductions in clearance may occur in renal or hepatic dysfunction and lead to higher plasma concentrations at steady state.

### ADVERSE REACTIONS

Although aggravation of arrhythmias seen in the early days of the evaluation of flecainide was often due to excessive initial doses and frequent dose increments, flecainide has a potential to induce proarrhythmic events, even when prescribed as recommended. This is especially true in patients with severe heart disease and if flecainide is given in higher dosages.[175] Because of its negative inotropic effects at dosages necessary to suppress arrhythmias, flecainide produces a measurable decrease in left ventricular function in most patients.[176,177] The increased mortality rate seen in the CAST seemed to be confined to patients with structural heart disease.[165] A retrospective study of five multiple-dose efficacy trials showed that, of patients with a history of congestive heart failure, oral flecainide precipitated heart failure in 15 percent. A dose-related depression of myocardial performance was found after rapid (1 to 2 mg/kg) intravenous injections.[178]

Other side effects of flecainide include depression of sinus node activity in patients with preexisting sinus node dysfunction[179] and prolongation of QRS and PR intervals on the surface ECG. If below 25 percent, these effects do not necessarily indicate excessive dosage.

Flecainide increases pacing thresholds by as much as 200 percent and should therefore be used with caution in patients dependent on pacemakers.[180,181] Since it also increases the threshold for electrical defibrillation, patients with implanted devices should be evaluated carefully.[182]

### DRUG INTERACTIONS

Cimetidine reduces flecainide clearance and prolongs flecainide elimination half-life.[183] Studies in normal volunteers have demonstrated an increase in the plasma concentrations of digoxin and propranolol when flecainide is coadministered.[184,185] Not unexpectedly, propranolol and flecainide have been found to have additive negative inotropic effects. An interaction with amiodarone, resulting in elevation of plasma flecainide concentration and necessitating reduction of flecainide dosage, has been described.[186]

## Calcium Channel Blockers

Some calcium channel blockers are also used as antiarrhythmic agents.[187,188] Verapamil and diltiazem are useful in the management of supraventricular tachycardia, where they are administered to slow the ventricular rate in patients with atrial fibrillation or flutter and to treat and prevent AV nodal reentrant tachycardia. Intravenous diltiazem is useful for the temporary control of rapid ventricular rate during atrial fibrillation and flutter. In controlled clinical trials, conversion to sinus rhythm occurred with diltiazem and placebo with equal frequency. Calcium channel blockers may prevent atrial electrical remodeling, including shortening of the atrial refractory period, which predisposes to early recurrence of atrial fibrillation.[189]

## Sotalol (Betapace)

### CLINICAL APPLICATIONS

Sotalol has been used for up to 20 years in many countries for angina and hypertension, and it was in this setting that its value as an antiarrhythmic agent was first observed. Sotalol is unlike other beta-adrenergic antagonists in that it prolongs the action potential, producing a dose-related increase in refractoriness of cardiac tissues.[190] This unique combination of properties makes sotalol effective in a variety of supraventricular and ventricular arrhythmias. It has been found to be effective in patients with sustained ventricular tachycardia evaluated by programmed ventricular stimulation. In a controlled comparison to procainamide, sotalol was effective in 30 percent of patients with inducible sustained ventricular tachycardia, whereas only 20 percent responded to procainamide ($p < 0.2$).[191] This is consistent with the response rate for sotalol (31 percent) in the Electrophysiology Study Versus ECG Monitoring (ESVEM) trial sponsored by the National Institutes of Health, which compared therapy guided by programmed electrical stimulation with therapy guided by ambulatory monitoring.[192] In this study, a mean of only 12 percent of patients responded to the other antiarrhythmic drugs evaluated.

### MECHANISM OF ACTION

Sotalol has two main actions, each of which can contribute to its antiarrhythmic efficacy.[193] The drug was originally synthesized for its actions as a beta-adrenergic receptor antagonist. Unlike other beta-receptor antagonists, it markedly prolongs refractoriness in atrial and ventricular tissues, a class III antiarrhythmic action. These actions slow heart rate, decrease AV nodal conduction, and increase refractoriness of atrial, ventricular, AV-nodal, and AV accessory pathways in both the anterograde and retrograde directions.[194] When given in dosages between 160 and 640 mg day, there are increases of 40 to 100 ms in the QT interval and 10 to 40 ms in $QT_c$.[195]

### CLINICAL PHARMACOLOGY

Oral bioavailability of sotalol is greater than 90 percent, and peak concentrations are seen 2.5 to 4 h after a dose. It is not bound to plasma proteins and is eliminated by the kidneys unchanged, with an elimination half-life of approximately 12 h. Because of the relatively long half-life and twice daily dosing regimen, it is recommended that testing for efficacy be conducted near the end of the dosing interval at steady state. The age of the patient per se does not influence the pharmacokinetics of sotalol other than in terms of the natural decline in renal function that occurs with age.

### DOSAGE AND ADMINISTRATION

Sotalol is available only in the oral form in the United States. The recommended initial dose of sotalol is 80 mg every 12 h. In patients with relatively normal renal function, steady state is reached in 2 to 3 days. If evaluation at this dosage indicates a lack of response without evidence of excessive effects on repolarization (QT below 500 ms), the dosage may be increased to 160 mg twice daily and, if necessary, to 240 mg twice daily. Some patients with life-threatening arrhythmias have required dosages of 640 mg/day. Accelerated titration regimens have been used with close monitoring and without apparent increase in the frequency of adverse events.[196]

### MODIFICATION OF DOSAGE IN DISEASE STATES

Because sotalol is mainly eliminated unchanged in the urine, the dosage must be adjusted for altered renal function. For patients with a creatinine clearance greater than 60 mL/min, the usual dosing interval is every 12 h. If the creatinine clearance ($CL_{CR}$) is between 30 and 60 mL/min, the recommended interval between doses is 24 h. For patients with $CL_{CR}$ between 10 and 30 mL/min, the interval should be every 36 to 48 h or the usual dose halved and given every 24 h. The dosage for patients with $CL_{CR}$ below 10 mL/min should be individualized. Because of the increased risk of proarrhythmia and congestive heart failure, patients with reduced cardiac output should be given lower doses and monitored carefully.

### ADVERSE REACTIONS

A major concern with sotalol treatment has been the occurrence of torsades de pointes. Reports of this syndrome have predominantly been cases of suicidal overdoses or involved patients who were receiving concomitant diuretics and inadequate potassium replacement. Clearly, hypokalemia and bradycardia are predisposing factors for the development of this arrhythmia during sotalol therapy, as they are with quinidine, disopyramide, and procainamide. The manufacturer observed an overall incidence of torsades de pointes of 2 percent, broken down to 4 percent of patients with sustained ventricular tachycardia and 1.5 percent of patients with supraventricular arrhythmias. It is more common in women and patients with congestive heart failure and those with a history of sustained ventricular tachycardia (7 percent). The incidence of torsades de pointes should be minimized by careful screening and consideration of predisposing factors, such as gender, bradycardia, baseline prolongation of the QT interval, and electrolyte disturbances, (especially hypokalemia); careful dose escalation beginning at 160 mg/day; and limitation of the maximum QT-interval prolongation to less than 550 ms.

The incidence of new or worsened congestive heart failure is only about 3 percent. This may be attenuated because of the increased inotropy produced by its action to prolong repolarization. Other side effects typical of beta blockers are to be expected, including bronchospasm in asthmatic patients, masking of the signs and symptoms of hypoglycemia in diabetic patients, and catecholamine hypersensitivity withdrawal syndrome.

### DRUG INTERACTIONS

Concomitant use of sotalol with agents that prolong repolarization has the potential to increase the likelihood of torsades de pointes. No pharmacokinetic interactions have been seen with sotalol and or warfarin, digoxin, cholestyramine, or hydrochlorothiazide. Because of the beta-blocking actions of sotalol, it is likely that there would be increased pharmacologic effect if the drug is combined with amiodarone, calcium channel blockers, antihypertensive agents, or antiarrhythmic agents.

## Amiodarone (Cordarone)

### CLINICAL APPLICATIONS

Although amiodarone has been reported to have efficacy in a wide range of arrhythmias, the FDA has recommended it only for life-threatening ventricular arrhythmias refractory to other available forms of therapy. Nevertheless, there are now numerous trials in the literature describing the efficacy of amiodarone in the conversion and slowing of atrial fibrillation, AV-nodal reentrant tachycardia, and tachycardias associated with the Wolff-Parkinson-White syndrome.[197,198] The reasons for the limited labeling of amiodarone are (1) the documented potentially lethal complications of chronic amiodarone therapy, (2) the complications associated with its variable onset of action, and (3) multiple dangerous drug interactions.

After the results of the CAST appeared, antiarrhythmic drugs were examined for their effects on mortality rate. After several small or uncontrolled trials seemed to indicate that amiodarone could have a beneficial effect on mortality rate,[5,199] adequate trials were undertaken. The Veteran's Administration trial, Congestive Heart Failure Survival Trial of Antiarrhythmic Therapy (CHF STAT),[6] examined the effects of amiodarone on total mortality rate in patients with a history of congestive heart failure, more than 10 premature ventricular contractions per hour on ambulatory monitoring, and an ejection fraction below 40 percent. The study found no difference in the placebo- and amiodarone-treated arms. Two other major trials have evaluated amiodarone in patients with recent myocardial infarction: The Canadian Myocardial Infarction Amiodarone Trial (CAMIAT)[200] and the European Myocardial Infarction Amiodarone Trial (EMIAT).[201] The results of these trials are mixed, in that neither found amiodarone to reduce overall mortality rate, but the Canadian trial reported a reduced incidence of ventricular fibrillation or arrhythmic death among survivors of myocardial infarction with ventricular ectopy. It is important to note that there was no increase in mortality rate, as has been seen with other antiarrhythmic drugs. In recent years, there have been attempts to perform metanalyses of the many trials with amiodarone.[202,203] They have generally confirmed a modest reduction in mortality rate in cardiac patients. One study concluded that the benefit could be extended to patients with congestive heart failure,[203] but another did not.[202] The Antiarrhythmics versus Implantable Defibrillators (AVID) trial sponsored by the National Institutes of Health (NIH) found that the devices were superior to amiodarone in reducing mortality rates in patients who had been resuscitated from sudden death or who had sustained ventricular tachycardia. This conclusion was confirmed by the Canadian Implantable Defibrillator Study (CIDS) trial,[204] which compared the intracardiac defibrillator to amiodarone therapy for patients resuscitated from ventricular tachycardia/ventricular fibrillation (VT/VF). CIDS found that patients most likely to benefit from the defibrillator were elderly or those with a low left ventricular ejection fraction or advanced heart failure symptoms New York Heart Association (NYHA) class III/IV.

In 1993, an intravenous formulation of amiodarone became available in the United States. Although it had been used extensively in most countries for many years, controlled trials became available only recently. Three completed controlled trials demonstrated the value of amiodarone in patients with recurrent life-threatening ventricular tachycardia or fibrillation. A comparison of three dosages found that the recurrence of arrhythmia decreased with increasing dosages of 125, 500, and 1000 mg/24 h.[204a] Hypotension was the major side effect seen, but it occurred equally in all groups, about 26 percent. The second study in a similar group of patients was a comparison of bretylium to two doses of amiodarone.[205] The arrhythmia event rate for the first 48 h of therapy was equivalent for the high dose of amiodarone and bretylium, and both were more effective than the low dose of amiodarone. Hypotension was common in all groups but significantly higher in the bretylium group. Hypotension has been attributed to the solvent in the intravenous formulation. However, a new aqueous preparation appears to avoid these hypotensive effects.[206] Amiodarone was approved for intravenous therapy of ventricular arrhythmia by the U.S. Food and Drug Administration (FDA) in 1995 and is considered first-line antiarrhythmic therapy for VT or VF resistant to defibrillation. In patients with out-of-hospital cardiac arrest due to resistant VF or pulseless VT, amiodarone therapy resulted in a higher survival to time of hospital admission compared to placebo[207] and lidocaine.[20] No trial, however, has yet shown an improvement to hospital discharge with any antiarrhythmic drug. Although not yet approved in labeling, intravenous amiodarone was effective for the prevention of postoperative atrial fibrillation.[208]

## MECHANISM OF ACTION

Amiodarone is an iodinated benzofuran that has structural similarity to thyroxine and procainamide and was originally developed as an antianginal agent. It was incidentally noted to suppress a wide variety of ventricular and supraventricular arrhythmias. This efficacy has been assumed to be due to its prolongation of refractoriness and APD in myocardial tissue (Vaughan Williams class III antiarrhythmic activity), although amiodarone has been found to have many diverse pharmacologic actions (see Table 35-1); the action or actions responsible for its high degree of antiarrhythmic efficacy remain unidentified. In intracellular recordings of rabbit cardiac myocytes, amiodarone prolongs APD and increases refractoriness of both atrial and ventricular myocardium, Purkinje fibers, and sinus and AV nodal tissues. Amiodarone decreases phase 3 depolarization of myocardial cells, blocks sodium channels that are in the inactivated state, and slows phase 4 depolarization of the sinus node as well as conduction through the AV node.[209,210] The electrophysiologic actions of the major metabolite of amiodarone, desethylamiodarone (DEA), differ from those of amiodarone, with the metabolite having greater effects on sodium channels and hence on conduction.[211] Intracoronary injection of amiodarone has shown little cardiac effect compared to the ability of DEA to prolong cardiac refractoriness.[212]

Electrophysiologic changes in humans depend on the route of administration and the duration of therapy. Following acute intravenous amiodarone administration, prolongation of the AH interval and an increase in the refractory periods of the AV node and bypass tracts are seen, but this may be due to the presence of the solubilizing agent polysorbate 80 (Tween 80) in the intravenous formulation. No acute changes occur in either sinus rate or atrial or ventricular refractoriness, which are prolonged during chronic oral therapy. Chronic amiodarone therapy also prolongs the AH and HV intervals and the PR and QT intervals of the surface ECG. Data conflict on the time course of these changes and how they may relate to antiarrhythmic efficacy.

Changes in APD and refractoriness are seen in hypothyroidism that are similar to changes resulting from oral amiodarone therapy.[213] Since these changes can be prevented in animals by coadministration of thyroid hormone with amiodarone,[214] some have concluded that the antiarrhythmic efficacy of amiodarone is due to production of "cardiac hypothyroidism." This is supported by the observation that the major metabolite of amiodarone causes noncompetitive inhibition of thyroid hormone binding to nuclear receptors.[215] On the other hand, amiodarone also causes noncompetitive blockade of alpha and beta receptors[216] and muscarinic receptors[217] as well as both calcium and sodium channel blockade, any combination of which may contribute to its antiarrhythmic efficacy.

## CLINICAL PHARMACOLOGY

Amiodarone is a highly lipid-soluble compound with extremely variable and complex pharmacokinetics. It is slowly absorbed from the gastrointestinal tract, and bioavailability varies over a fourfold range.[218] Amiodarone is extensively metabolized to DEA, and little if any is excreted unchanged in the urine. Concentrations of DEA in plasma vary from 0.4 to 2.0 times that of amiodarone during chronic therapy.[219] This metabolite has antiarrhythmic potency equal to or greater than that of amiodarone in in vitro and animal models.[220] Amiodarone is rapidly concentrated in some tissues, including myocardium, but accumulates more slowly in others, such as adipose tissue. It redistributes out of myocardial tissue while still accumulating in adipose and other tissues.[219,221] Until all tissues are saturated, rapid redistribution out of the myocardium may be responsible for early recurrence of arrhythmias after discontinuation of therapy or rapid reduction of dosage. Because of drug accumulation in tissues, the volume of distribution for amiodarone is very large, 20 to 200 L/kg.[221] After intravenous administration, the measured half-life in plasma is from 4.8 to 68.2 h,[222] with tissue uptake being the primary factor responsible for the decline in plasma concentration. As tissues become saturated, however, the decline in plasma levels is slow, reflecting mainly elimination and slow redistribution of the drug out of adipose and muscle tissues. This leads to slow and extremely variable elimination from plasma, with half-lives ranging from 13 to 103 days at steady state.[221] It is also possible that amiodarone inhibits its own elimination after chronic therapy, contributing to the differences between half-life early in therapy to that after prolonged therapy.

## DOSAGE AND ADMINISTRATION

Without a loading-dose regimen, amiodarone requires several weeks to months before producing its antiarrhythmic action. Large intravenous dosages or oral loading dosages can hasten the onset of therapeutic effects. From small prospective studies, loading dosages have varied from 600 to 1400 mg/day for 2 to 21 days.[223] Recent large clinical trials have utilized a lower loading dose, of 600 to 800 mg daily for 14 days.[6,224] Because of relatively rapid redistribution out of myocardial tissue, the dosage should be tapered over a period of several weeks. The usual maintenance dose varies from 200 to 600 mg/day; because of the severe nature of adverse reactions, the lowest effective dosage should be prescribed. Patients with supraventricular arrhythmias may respond to lower dosages than those with ventricular arrhythmias, but there are many exceptions. Because of the variable pharmacokinetics and oral bioavailability, such generalizations may be unreliable. Some patients with extensive absorption (approximately 80 to 90 percent bioavailability) of even low doses may have the same drug exposure as a person with limited bioavailability given a high dose.

For intravenous administration, the manufacturer recommends a three-phase infusion over the first 24 h: 150 mg over 10 min, followed by 360 mg over the next 6 h (or 1 mg/min), followed by 0.5 mg/min. The drug can be continued at this rate, but monitoring of plasma concentrations is recommended. An additional 150 mg can be infused over 10 min for those patients who continue to have recurrent ventricular tachycardia or fibrillation or whose arrhythmia recurs during downward titration of the infusion. Concentrations of drug greater than 3 mg/mL should be infused through a central catheter to prevent phlebitis. Also, the surfactant properties of the drug alter the size of a drop of infusate, and pumps that count drops will give approximately 30 percent less drug than intended. In patients with pulseless VT and VF, ACLS guidelines[21] recommend a rapid bolus infusion of 300 mg diluted in 20 to 30 mL of saline or dextrose in water supplemented by additional doses of 150 mg if VT/VF recurs.

Amiodarone concentrations are usually between 1 and 2 μg/mL during effective oral therapy.[225,226] Similar concentrations of DEA accumulate during therapy and, although this is unproven, are likely to contribute to antiarrhythmic efficacy. Because of extensive overlap between the range of concentrations required for arrhythmia suppression and those associated with toxicity, monitoring of plasma concentrations is of limited value. Clearly, levels of amiodarone above 3 to 4 $\mu$g/mL for prolonged periods of time are associated with a higher incidence of adverse effects.[227]

### MODIFICATION OF DOSAGE IN DISEASE STATES

Long-term oral therapy with amiodarone appears to be well tolerated hemodynamically in patients with congestive heart failure. In the CHF STAT study, discussed above, amiodarone failed to prolong life for patients with congestive heart failure and arrhythmias but was associated with improved ventricular function as measured by radionuclide ejection fraction.[6]

### ADVERSE REACTIONS

Intravenous amiodarone at dosages greater than 5 mg/kg decreases cardiac contractility and peripheral vascular resistance, producing severe hypotension in some instances. Some of this effect, like the electrophysiologic effects described earlier, may be due to the effects of polysorbate 80 or benzyl alcohol, since oral administration at usual dosages improves myocardial contractility. Aqueous intravenous formulations of amiodarone are currently being studied and appear to avoid hypotension.[207] A small randomized comparison of aqueous amiodarone compared to lidocaine demonstrated effectiveness in treating shock-resistant VT.[228]

The safety of amiodarone is controversial. The early reports found it to be very well tolerated and described it as the "ideal antiarrhythmic drug." Some studies continue to find that it is relatively safe and effective, even in the treatment of arrhythmias in children.[229] The early experience with amiodarone in the United States, with a very high incidence of intolerable and sometimes lethal reactions, may have been the result of the high dosages required to control life-threatening arrhythmias. In less urgent conditions, lower dosages are given and are much better tolerated. Determination of the incidence of adverse reactions is difficult because of highly variable dosages and durations of treatment.[209,230]

The most serious adverse reaction is lethal interstitial pneumonitis,[209,231] which may be more common in patients with preexisting lung disease. Monitoring is essential, since the pneumonitis is reversible if detected early. A chest x-ray every 3 months may be useful, but serial pulmonary function tests are of little value for follow-up. Hyper- or hypothyroidism is seen in about 4 percent of patients treated chronically.[213]

Accumulation of corneal microdeposits is almost uniform during long-term therapy and in many cases can progress to the point of interfering with vision.[232] Some Caucasian patients develop a slate-gray or bluish discoloration of sun-exposed areas of the skin.[233] Many also complain of photosensitivity, which can sometimes be prevented or alleviated with sunscreens and protective garments. Thirty percent or more of patients have abnormally elevated serum hepatic enzyme levels, and progression to jaundice and cirrhosis has been reported.[234,235] Serial laboratory tests to screen for amiodarone toxicity can be costly and generally are of limited value; however, it is wise to obtain a reliable assessment of baseline test results—including complete blood count, blood chemistry, tests of thyroid and pulmonary function, a slit-lamp examination, and measurement of blood levels of other drugs—whenever possible.

### DRUG INTERACTIONS

Amiodarone interferes with the clearance of many drugs. This may involve the formation of a metabolically inactive cytochrome P450 Fe(II)–metabolite complex, which has been described in animals treated with amiodarone,[236] and may explain the reduced metabolism and unexpected accumulation of warfarin,[237] quinidine, procainamide, disopyramide, mexiletine, and propafenone[238] and the resulting bleeding, heart block, or torsades de pointes. It does not, however, explain interaction with drugs eliminated predominantly by the kidneys, such as digoxin.[239] The elimination of other drugs may be impaired by amiodarone; therefore the lowest effective dosage should be sought.

## Ibutilide (Corvert)

### CLINICAL APPLICATIONS

In 1995, ibutilide was given FDA approval for the rapid conversion of recent-onset atrial fibrillation or flutter.[240,241] It has completed testing in other arrhythmias and in patients with atrial fibrillation or flutter of long duration (greater than 90 days). It should not be given to patients who have hypokalemia, hypomagnesemia, or $QT_c$ prolongation at baseline greater than 440 ms. In placebo-controlled studies summarized in the manufacturer's labeling, the placebo conversion rate for atrial fibrillation or flutter was approximately 2 percent. Ibutilide terminated the arrhythmia in approximately 44 percent of patients treated with 1 mg followed by either 0.5 or 1 mg. Approximately 20 percent of patients responded to the first infusion, and approximately 25 percent of those not responding to the first infusion responded to the second infusion. Response usually occurred at 20 to 30 min, ranging from 5 to 88 min after infusion. The response in patients with atrial fibrillation and atrial flutter was not significantly different in the early trials performed. However, in patients with post-operative arrhythmias, there was a greater response in patients with atrial flutter, with an overall conversion rate of 57 percent compared to 15 percent with placebo.[242] Ibutilide may have value in conversion of atrial fibrillation in patients with Wolff-Parkinson-White syndrome.[242] Ibutilide can also be used to improve the success of electrical cardioversion.[243]

### MECHANISM OF ACTION

Ibutilide is a remarkably potent methanesulfonamide analogue of sotalol that has class III action to prolong cardiac refractoriness and action potential duration.

The mechanism of action of ibutilide is unclear. The manufacturer's data indicate that the class III action of the drug is due to an increase in inward sodium current, as observed in guinea pig ventricular myocytes at $10^{-7}$ *M* concentrations. They observed that higher concentrations ($10^{-5}$ *M*) increase an outward potassium current to shorten action potential duration.[244] Other investigators reported that—as has been seen with dofetilide, sotalol, and other methanesulfonamides—$10^{-8}$ *M* concentrations of ibutilide block the rapid component of the delayed rectifier potassium current, $I_{Kr}$, in mouse and human cardiac cells.[245]

### CLINICAL PHARMACOLOGY

Ibutilide is available only for intravenous administration. When given over 10 min, it distributes rapidly in a multiexponential fashion, with the relevant component having a half-life from 2 to 12 h (mean 6 h). The plasma concentration and pharmacokinetics are highly variable, and dosing is recommended on the basis of weight. The drug is mainly eliminated by oxidative hepatic metabolism, and systemic clearance is rapid (about 29 mL/min/kg). Since formal drug interaction studies have not been performed, it is not possible to anticipate which enzymes are likely responsible for its elimination.

**DOSAGE AND ADMINISTRATION**

Ibutilide is given undiluted or diluted in saline as an infusion over 10 min. The recommended dose for a patient over 60 kg is 1 mg and for a patient under 60 kg, 0.01 mg/kg. For patients whose arrhythmias have not converted by 10 min after completion of the first dose, a second dose of equal size may be administered. Since conversion of the arrhythmias is usually associated with peak levels, slower infusion rates are not likely to be as effective.

It is essential that patients receiving ibutilide be treated in a carefully monitored environment during and at least 4 h subsequent to treatment. The FDA-approved labeling recommends that skilled personnel, facilities, and medication for defibrillation or resuscitation be readily available.

**MODIFICATION OF DOSAGE IN DISEASE STATES**

Although specific studies with heart failure and renal or hepatic disease have not been conducted, current information does not indicate that any dosage adjustments should be necessary in these conditions. Patients with severe left ventricular dysfunction, however, have a higher risk of developing ventricular arrhythmias, including torsades de pointes. Since the duration of drug effect is determined by distribution, it is very possible that patients with severe congestive heart failure will have decreased volumes of distribution and hence an exaggerated and prolonged duration of effect.

**ADVERSE REACTIONS**

The most serious adverse reaction to ibutilide is torsades de pointes. There were, however, only 586 patients participating in trials before marketing, and patients with a $QT_c$ greater than 440 ms or potassium concentrations less than 4 meq/L were excluded. In spite of these precautions, the incidence of sustained polymorphic VT requiring cardioversion was 1.7 percent. Another 2.7 percent developed nonsustained polymorphic VT, 4.9 percent had nonsustained monomorphic VT, 1.5 percent had AV block, and 1.9 percent had bundle branch block. The risk of polymorphic VT was highest in women and or those who had evidence of reduced ventricular performance. The incidence of these adverse effects may well be higher in general clinical use, where electrolyte disorders and concomitant therapies may be more common. Bradycardia and multiple episodes of sinus arrest have been reported.[242,246] A single case of acute renal failure has been reported with ibutilide.[247]

**DRUG INTERACTIONS**

No specific drug interaction studies have been performed. Concomitant beta-receptor or calcium channel antagonists do not apparently interact, although data are limited. The manufacturer's labeling warns against combining ibutilide with other drugs that prolong the QT interval. During the development of ibutilide, such drugs were discontinued for at least five half-lives prior to administration of ibutilide and were not allowed until at least 4 h after administration.

## Dofetilide (Tikosyn)

**CLINICAL APPLICATIONS**

Dofetilide was approved and marketed in 2000 for oral therapy of atrial fibrillation and flutter. In controlled trials comprising approximately 1000 patients, about 30 percent of patients with atrial fibrillation given a dosage of 500 $\mu$g bid converted to normal sinus rhythm, compared to 6 percent in the control group treated with sotalol and 1 percent of patients given placebo. Prevention of recurrence was demonstrated, with 62 to 71 percent remaining in sinus rhythm after 6 months, compared to 59 percent for sotalol and 26 to 37 percent for placebo (personal communication, S. Singh, Washington, DC). A large mortality trial (the Danish Investigators of Arrhythmia and Mortality on Dofetilide trial, or DIAMOND) in 1518 patients with reduced ejection fraction and symptoms of heart failure examined the effects of dofetilide on mortality rate and atrial fibrillation. A decrease in the incidence of hospitalization for heart failure was observed. Although the antiarrhythmic efficacy of dofetilide was confirmed in the lower incidence of atrial fibrillation, a positive effect on mortality rate was not observed. However, because of the previously observed increases in mortality rate with sodium channel blockers (CAST[2,248] and CAST II[3]) and with *d*-sotalol (SWORD[7]), the lack of harm in the DIAMOND trial with dofetilide[249] was interpreted as a positive indication of the safety of the drug. A caveat to this safety was the potentially important role of extensive screening and monitoring for potential harm. Even with these efforts, 3.3 percent of patients in this trial developed torsades de pointes. Because of the risk of torsades de pointes, the manufacturer will require physicians to receive special training prior to prescribing dofetilide, and the FDA has required that labeling include a warning that therapy should be initiated in the hospital, with continuous ECG monitoring for at least 3 days.

**MECHANISM OF ACTION**

Dofetilide is one of the most potent $I_{Kr}$ blockers of the rapid component of the delayed rectifier potassium current ($I_{Kr}$) ever synthesized. Perhaps an additional advantage is the twofold greater ability to prolong action potential duration in atrial compared to ventricular tissue.[250] It does not depress cardiac function at usual dosages, even in patients with reduced ejection fraction.

**CLINICAL PHARMACOLOGY**

Dofetilide is well absorbed after oral administration and is partially metabolized by cytochrome P450 3A4[251] to inactive metabolites; it is excreted predominantly in urine. In most patients, the elimination half-life ranges from 8 to 10 h, but it is prolonged, and clearance is reduced in patients with renal failure. Dofetilide is susceptible to several drug interactions because it is metabolized by CYP3A4 (see below). It is very likely that these interactions increase the risk of torsades de pointes.

**DOSAGE AND ADMINISTRATION**

The recommended dosage of dofetilide is 500 $\mu$g bid. Lower dosages are recommended for patients who develop excessive $QT_c$ prolongation on 500 $\mu$g bid. In the largest clinical trial, *excessive* was defined as greater than 550 ms or greater than 20 percent longer than baseline.

**MODIFICATION OF DOSAGE IN DISEASE STATES**

Dosage should be reduced in patients with renal disease (250 mg bid for creatinine clearance 60 to 40 mL/min and 250 mg daily for creatinine clearance 40 to 20 mL/min). Data are not available for adjustment of dosage in patients with liver disease. It is not clear whether the greater risk of torsades de pointes in women is influenced by a pharmacokinetic difference between sexes.

**ADVERSE DRUG REACTIONS**

The major adverse effect of dofetilide is torsades de pointes. The overall incidence during clinical development was 0.9 percent. In the DIAMOND trial, 3.3 percent of patients with a history of heart failure developed torsades de pointes.

### DRUG INTERACTIONS

Concomitant administration of dofetilide with verapamil, ketoconazole, megestrol, prochlorperazine, or cimetidine (but not ranitidine) results in increased plasma concentrations of dofetilide, especially in patients with reduced renal function.[252] Recently, hydrochlorothiazide, with or without triamterene, has also been demonstrated to increase dofetilide levels as well as the QT interval; therefore it is contraindicated as well. Because it is known to be a substrate for CYP3A4, there may be other important interactions with erythromycin, other macrolides, or antifungals. No interactions have been seen between dofetilide and digoxin or warfarin.

## Beta-Receptor Antagonists

See Chap. 57 for a discussion of beta-receptor antagonists.

## Adenosine (Adenocard)

### CLINICAL APPLICATIONS

Adenosine is very effective for the acute conversion of paroxysmal supraventricular tachycardia (PSVT) due to reentry involving the AV node. Sixty percent of patients respond at a dose of 6 mg, and an additional 32 percent respond when given a higher dose of 12 mg. Because of the fleeting and relatively selective action of adenosine on the AV node, some have suggested that it be used as a diagnostic tool in patients with narrow- and wide-complex tachycardia.[253] However, it is preferable, when possible, to make the correct diagnosis before giving any drugs because of their risk of adverse effects.

### MECHANISM OF ACTION

Adenosine is a nucleoside formed in the body by serial dephosphorylation of adenosine triphosphate (ATP), from cyclic adenosine monophosphate, or from hydrolysis of *S*-adenosylhomocysteine. It is formed both intra- and extracellularly, and its actions are rapidly terminated by active transport into cells followed by metabolism. The actions of adenosine are highly dependent on the rate and route of administration. A rapid intravenous injection into a central venous line is thought to activate carotid body chemoreceptors and usually produces an initial increase in blood pressure of 10 to 15 mmHg, followed by a small and transient decrease. These reflexes are attenuated during surgery, and in this setting adenosine decreases peripheral vascular resistance, increases cardiac output, and increases heart rate moderately. Bolus injections also produce biphasic effects on heart rate. Approximately 20 s after injection, sinus bradycardia occurs for 10 to 15 s, followed by sinus tachycardia thought to be due to chemoreceptor activation. Activation of the carotid chemoreceptors stimulates respiration and causes secondary activation of pulmonary stretch receptors. Adenosine has a direct effect of slowing AV-nodal conduction, which can result in transient AV block. Although adenosine has no direct effect on the His-Purkinje system, it does attenuate the effects of catecholamine stimulation and, in patients with heart block, can block acceleration of the ventricular escape rate by isoproterenol. Adenosine usually has no effect on anterograde or retrograde accessory pathway conduction. Pathways that demonstrate decremental conduction often respond to adenosine, probably because they are partially depolarized and can be hyperpolarized by adenosine. Slow injections into a peripheral line often produce no clinical benefit or changes in blood pressure or heart rate.

The development of synthetic agonists and antagonists of adenosine receptors has made possible the subclassification of $A_1$ and $A_2$ receptor subtypes. The $A_1$ receptors are present in myocardial cells and mediate the negative inotropic, dromotropic, and chronotropic actions of adenosine. The $A_2$ receptors are present in the endothelium and vascular smooth muscle cells and cause coronary vasodilatation when activated. The efficacy of adenosine in PVST is most likely due to the following actions in atrial myocardium and the AV node: (1) hyperpolarization of sinoatrial nodal cells and slowing of rate of firing, (2) shortening of the action potential of atrial cells, and (3) depression of conduction velocity in the AV node. These actions are due to activation of $A_1$ adenosine-receptor subtypes, which leads to activation of the cyclic AMP–independent, acetylcholine adenosine–regulated potassium current $IK_{ACh,Ado}$.

### CLINICAL PHARMACOLOGY

After intravenous injection, adenosine is rapidly transported into red blood cells and endothelial cells. A half-life of elimination has ranged from 1.5 to 10 s. The drug is rapidly metabolized in the plasma and in cells to form inosine and adenosine monophosphate. Maximal pharmacologic effects are seen within 30 s after injection into a peripheral intravenous line but occur within 10 to 20 s when given into a central line.

### DOSAGE AND ADMINISTRATION

Adenosine should be injected intravenously into a proximal tubing site and flushed quickly with saline solution. For adults, the initial dose is 6 mg injected over 1 to 2 s. If the arrhythmia persists, a 12-mg dose can be injected 1 to 2 min later. This can be repeated, but doses larger than 12 mg are not recommended by the manufacturer. A dosage regimen based on body weight has been proposed, with an initial dose of 50 $\mu$g/kg incremented by 50 $\mu$g/kg until the PSVT is terminated or side effects become intolerable.[245] Higher doses may be required for patients who have received caffeine or theophylline because of their antagonistic effects at $A_1$ receptors. Lower doses are recommended if the patients are receiving dipyridamole or carbamazepine.

### MODIFICATION OF DOSAGE IN DISEASE STATES

Although the pharmacokinetics of adenosine are unlikely to be altered in patients with renal or hepatic disease, these patients often have electrolyte imbalances that could alter the clinical response. Although patients with congestive heart failure have not been reported to respond abnormally, cardiac transplant patients appear to require one-third to one-fifth of the usual dose because of denervation hypersensitivity.[254]

### ADVERSE REACTIONS

Adenosine is contraindicated in patients with sick-sinus syndrome or second- or third-degree heart block unless the patient has a functioning artificial pacemaker. Because of the rapid clearance of adenosine, side effects such as facial flushing, dyspnea, or chest pressure last less than 60 s. Although intrapulmonary administration of adenosine has precipitated bronchospasm in asthmatic patients, this has not been reported with intravenous administration. Other less frequent side effects include nausea, light-headedness, headache, sweating, palpitations, hypotension, and blurred vision. Intravenous theophylline, which has been recommended to reverse the effects of adenosine, should be prepared and ready for injection in high-risk patients.

### DRUG INTERACTIONS

Several proven interactions can increase or decrease the activity of adenosine. Dipyridamole pretreatment increases the potency of adenosine, probably because it blocks cellular uptake of adenosine.[255]

On the other hand, caffeine and theophylline antagonize the actions of adenosine.[256] The manufacturer cautions that carbamazepine may potentiate the actions of adenosine.

## INVESTIGATIONAL DRUGS

Only a few new antiarrhythmic agents are currently under development in the United States. Dronedarone (previously labeled SR33589)[257–259] is a noniodinated benzofuran analogue of amiodarone. Dronedarone is currently in phase III trials, including EURIDIS and ADONIS, for the maintenance of sinus rhythm in patients with atrial fibrillation. However, the phase III trial ANDROMEDA, a placebo-controlled trial in heart failure patients with ventricular dysfunction, was recently halted after an interim safety analysis suggested that there was an increase in mortality in the treatment group. Other amiodarone analogues with an alkyl ester group at position 2 of the benzofurane moiety (e.g., ATI-2001) have also been studied in animal models.[260,261] The impetus for the development of these agents lies in the hope that they will have the efficacy of amiodarone without its complex pharmacokinetics and/or toxicity.

Azimilide is another drug with class III action that was initially believed to be a highly selective blocker of the slow component of the delayed rectifier ($I_{Ks}$), but studies suggest that azimilide also blocks $I_{Kr}$. It is unclear whether the effects on $I_{Ks}$ contribute any novel aspects to its actions or safety. $I_{Ks}$ blockade is thought to be desirable because the effect is resistant to antagonism by isoproterenol. In the Azimilide Post-Infarct Survival Evaluation (ALIVE), no significant difference was seen in the primary endpoint of total mortality in high-risk patients with reduced ventricular function treated with azimilide or placebo. Ongoing phase III trials include A-COMET, which is a study of the efficacy and safety in patients with atrial fibrillation who require electrical cardioversion. A-STAR is a study of the efficacy and safety of azimilide in patients with paroxysmal atrial fibrillation with or without ischemic heart disease or heart failure.

A new class of drugs that act as adenosine $A_1$-receptor agonists are being investigated to terminate AV nodal–dependent tachycardia such as AV node and AV reentry and to control the heart rate in atrial fibrillation. Activation of this receptor results in slowing of conduction through the AV node by activating the inhibitory $G_1$-protein pathway. These agents also activate an adenosine- or acetylcholine-sensitive potassium current that leads to hyperpolarization of the atrial membrane potential and decreased firing frequency of the atrial action potential.[189,262]

Ambasilide is a class III drug in development that does not show reverse use dependence. Chromanol 293B and HMR 1556 are in preclinical testing as potent blockers of $I_{Ks}$. Other novel drugs that are being investigated include NIP-142, which inhibits the Kv1.5 channel and is responsible for the ultrarapid potassium channel $I_{Kur}$, which is present only in atrial tissue.[263]

## References


1. The AFFIRM Investigators. A comparison of rate control and rhythm control in patients with atrial fibrillation. *N Engl J Med* 2002;347:1825–1833.
2. CAST investigators. Preliminary report: Effect of encainide and flecainide on mortality in a randomized trial of arrhythmia suppression after myocardial infarction. *N Engl J Med* 1989;321:406–412.
3. CAST-II investigators. Effect of the antiarrhythmic agent moricizine on survival after myocardial infarction. *N Engl J Med* 1992;327:227–233.
4. Hine LK, Laird NM, Hewitt P, Chalmers TC. Meta-analysis of empirical long-term antiarrhythmic therapy after myocardial infarction. *JAMA* 1989;262:3037–3040.
5. Pfisterer ME, Kiowski W, Brunner H, et al. Long-term benefit of 1-year amiodarone treatment for persistent complex ventricular arrhythmias after myocardial infarction. *Circulation* 1993;87:309–311.
6. Singh SN, Fletcher RD, Fisher SG, et al. Amiodarone in patients with congestive heart failure and asymptomatic ventricular arrhythmia: Survival Trial of Antiarrhythmic Therapy in Congestive Heart Failure. *N Engl J Med* 1995;333:77–82.
7. Waldo AL, Camm AJ, deRuyter H, et al. Effect of D-sotalol on mortality in patients with left ventricular dysfunction after recent and remote myocardial infarction. The SWORD Investigators. Survival With Oral D-Sotalol. *Lancet* 1996;348:7–12.
8. Vaughan Williams EM. A classification of antiarrhythmic actions reassessed after a decade of new drugs. *J Clin Pharmacol* 1984;24:129–147.
9. Harrison DC. Antiarrhythmic drug classification: New science and practical applications. *Am J Cardiol* 1985;56:185–187.
10. Nademanee K, Taylor R, Bailey WE. Rieders DE. Kosar EM. Treating electrical storm: Sympathetic blockade versus advanced cardiac life support-guided therapy. *Circulation* 2000;102:742–747.
11. Lechat P, Packer M, Chalon S, et al. Clinical effects of beta adrenergic blockade in chronic heart failure. A meta-analysis of double-blind, placebo-controlled, randomized trials. *Circulation* 1998;98:1184–1191.
12. MERIT-HF Study Group. Effect of metoprolol CR/XL in chronic heart failure: Metoprolol CR/XL randomized intervention trial in congestive heart failure (MERIT-HF). *Lancet* 1999;353:2001–2007.
13. Task Force of the Working Group on Arrhythmias of the European Society of Cardiology. The Sicilian gambit: A new approach to the classification of antiarrhythmic drugs based on their actions on arrhythmogenic mechanisms. *Circulation* 1991;84:1831–1851.
14. Hodgkin AL, Huxley AF. A quantitative description of membrane current and its application to conduction and excitation in nerve. *J Physiol* 1952;117:500–544.

14a. Hille B. Local anesthetics: Hydrophilic and hydrophobic pathways for the drug-receptor reaction. *J Gen Physiol* 1977;69:497–515.

15. Hondeghem LM, Katzung BG. Test of a model of antiarrhythmic drug action: Effects of quinidine and lidocaine on myocardial conduction. *Circulation* 1980;61:1217–1224.
16. Campbell TJ. Kinetics of onset of rate-dependent effects of class I antiarrhythmic drugs are important in determining their effects on refractoriness in guinea-pig ventricle, and provide a theoretical basis for their subclassification. *Cardiovasc Res* 1983;17:344–352.
17. Southworth JL, McKusick VA, Pierce EC II, Rawson FL Jr. Ventricular fibrillation precipitated by cardiac catheterization. *JAMA* 1950;143:717–720.
18. Lie KI, Wellens HJ, van Capelle FJ, Durrer D. Lidocaine in the prevention of primary ventricular fibrillation: A double-blind, randomized study of 212 consecutive patients. *N Engl J Med* 1974;291:1324–1326.
19. MacMahon S, Collins R, Peto R, et al. Effects of prophylactic lidocaine in suspected acute myocardial infarction. *JAMA* 1988;260:1910–1916.
20. Dorian, P, Cass, D, Schwartz B, et al. Amiodarone as compared with lidocaine for shock-resistant ventricular fibrillation. *N Engl J Med* 2002;346:884–890.
21. Guidelines 2000 for Cardiopulmonary Resuscitation and Emergency Cardiovascular Care: An international consensus on science. 5. Pharmacology I: agents for arrhythmias. *Circulation* 2000;102:Suppl I:I-112–I-128.
22. Pedersen LE, Bonde J, Graudal NA, et al. Quantitative and qualitative binding characteristics of disopyramide in serum from patients with decreased renal and hepatic function. *Br J Clin Pharmacol* 1987;23:41–46.
23. Josephson ME, Kastor JA, Kitchen JG III. Lidocaine in Wolff-Parkinson-White syndrome with atrial fibrillation. *Ann Intern Med* 1976;84:44–45.

24. Akhtar M, Gilbert CJ, Shenasa M. Effect of lidocaine on atrioveritricular response via the accessory pathway in patients with Wolff-Parkinson-White syndrome. *Circulation* 1981;63:435–441.
25. Davis LD, Temte JV. Electrophysiological actions of lidocaine on canine ventricular muscle and Purkinje fibers. *Circ Res* 1969;24:639–655.
26. Bigger JT Jr, Mandel WJ. Effect of lidocaine on the electrophysiological properties of ventricular muscle and Purkinje fibers. *J Clin Invest* 1970;49:63–77.
27. Kunkel F, Rowland M, Scheinman MM. The electrophysiologic effects of lidocaine in patients with intraventricular conduction defects. *Circulation* 1974;49:894–899.
28. Bekheit S, Murtagh JG, Morton P, Fletcher E. Effect of lidocaine on conducting system of human heart. *Br Heart J* 1973;35:305–311.
29. Gupta PK, Lichstein E, Chadda KD. Lidocaine-induced heart block in patients with bundle branch block. *Am J Cardiol* 1974; 33:487–492.
30. Aravindakshan V, Kuo C-S, Gettes LS. Effect of lidocaine on escape rate in patients with complete atrioventricular block: A. Distal His block. *Am J Cardiol* 1977;40:177–183.
31. Stenson RE, Constantino RT, Harrison DC. Interrelationships of hepatic blood flow, cardiac output, and blood levels of lidocaine in man. *Circulation* 1971;43:205–211.
32. Zito RA, Reid PR. Lidocaine kinetics predicted by indocyanine green clearance. *N Engl J Med* 1978;298:1160–1163.
33. Blumer J, Strong JM, Atkinson AJ Jr. The convulsant potency of lidocaine and its *N*-dealkylated metabolites. *J Pharmacol Exp Ther* 1973;186:31–36.
34. Narang PK, Crouthamel WG, Carliner NH, Fisher ML. Lidocaine and its active metabolites. *Clin Pharmacol Ther* 1978;24:654–662.
35. Thomson PD, Melmon KL, Richardson JA, et al. Lidocaine pharmacokinetics in advanced heart failure, liver disease and renal failure in humans. *Ann Intern Med* 1973;78:499–508.
36. Wyman MG, Slaughter RL, Farolino DA, et al. Multiple bolus technique for lidocaine administration in acute ischemic heart disease: II. Treatment of refractory ventricular arrhythmias and the pharmacokinetic significance of severe left ventricular failure. *J Am Coll Cardiol* 1983;2:764–769.
37. Stargel WW, Shand DG, Routledge PA, et al. Clinical comparison of rapid infusion and multiple injection methods for lidocaine loading. *Am Heart J* 1981;102:872–876.
38. Alderman EL, Kerber RE, Harrison DC. Evaluation of lidocaine resistance in man using intermittent large-dose infusion techniques. *Am J Cardiol* 1974;34:342–349.
39. Richard C, Berdeaux A, Delion F, et al. Effect of mechanical ventilation on hepatic drug pharmacokinetics. *Chest* 1986;90:837–841.
40. LeLorier J, Grenon D, Latour Y, et al. Pharmacokinetics of lidocaine after prolonged intravenous infusions in uncomplicated myocardial infarction. *Ann Intern Med* 1977;87:700–702.
41. Routledge PA, Shand DG, Barchowsky A, et al. Relationship between alpha$_1$-acid glycoprotein and lidocaine disposition in myocardial infarction. *Clin Pharmacol Ther* 1981;30:154–157.
42. Cheng TO, Wadhwa K. Sinus standstill following intravenous lidocaine administration. *JAMA* 1973;223:790–792.
43. Marriott HJL, Phillips K. Profound hypotension and bradycardia after a single bolus of lidocaine. *J Electrocardiol* 1974;7:79–82.
44. Cote P, Harrison DC, Basile J, Schroeder JS. Hemodynamic interaction of procainamide and lidocaine after experimental myocardial infarction. *Am J Cardiol* 1973;32:937–942.
45. Ochs HR, Carstens G, Greenblatt DJ. Reduction in lidocaine clearance during continuous infusion and by coadministration of propranolol. *N Engl J Med* 1980;303:373–377.
46. Feeley J, Wilkinson GR, McAllister CB, Wood AJJ. Increased toxicity and reduced clearance of lidocaine by cimetidine. *Ann Intern Med* 1982;96:592–593.
47. Campbell RWF. Mexiletine. *N Engl J Med* 1987;316:29–34.
48. Duff HJ, Kolodgie FD, Roden DM, Woosley RL. Electropharmacologic synergism with mexiletine and quinidine. *J Cardiovasc Pharmacol* 1986;8:840–846.
49. Leahey EB Jr, Heissenbuttel RH, Giardina E-GV, Bigger, JT Jr. Combined mexiletine and propranolol treatment of refractory ventricular arrhythmia. *Br Med J* 1980;281:357–358.
50. Ruskin JN, DiMarco JP, Garan H. Out-of-hospital cardiac arrest: Electrophysiologic observations and selection of long-term antiarrhythmic therapy. *N Engl J Med* 1980;303:607–613.
51. Stein J, Podrid P, Lown B. Effects of oral mexiletine on left and right ventricular function. *Am J Cardiol* 1984;54:575–578.
52. Yamaguchi I, Singh BN, Mandel WJ. Electrophysiological effects of mexiletine on isolated rabbit atria and canine ventricular muscle Purkinje fiber. *Cardiovasc Res* 1979;13:288–296.
53. Prescott LF, Clements JA, Pottage A. Absorption, distribution, and elimination of mexiletine. *Postgrad Med J* 1977;53(suppl 1):50–55.
54. Woosley RL, Wang T, Stone W, et al. Pharmacology, electrophysiology, and pharmacokinetics of mexiletine. *Am Heart J* 1984;107: 1058–1065.
55. Brown JE, Shand DG. Therapeutic drug monitoring of antiarrhythmic agents. *Clin Pharmacokinet* 1982;7:125–148.
56. Beckett AH, Chidomere EC. The distribution, metabolism and excretion of mexiletine in man. *Postgrad Med J* 1977;53(suppl 1):60–66.
57. Campbell NPS, Kelley JG, Adgey AAJ, Shanks RG. The clinical pharmacology of mexiletine. *Br J Clin Pharmacol* 1978;6:103–108.
58. el Allaf D, Henrard L, Crochelet L, et al. Pharmacokinetics of mexiletine in renal insufficiency. *Br J Clin Pharmacol* 1982;14:431–435.
59. Leahey EB Jr, Giardina E-GV, Bigger JT Jr. Effect of ventricular failure on steady state kinetics of mexiletine. *Clin Res* 1980;26:239A.
60. Pentikainen PJ, Hietakorpi S, Halinen MO, Lampinen LM. Cirrhosis of the liver markedly impairs the elimination of mexiletine. *Eur J Clin Pharmacol* 1986;30:83–88.
61. Fasola GP, D'Osualdo F, de Pangher V, Barducci E. Thrombocytopenia and mexiletine. *Ann Intern Med* 1984;100:162.
62. Girmann G, Pees H, Scheurlen PG. Pseudothrombocytopenia and mexiletine. *Ann Intern Med* 1984;100:767.
63. Roos JC, Paalman ACA, Dunning AJ. Electrophysiological effects of mexiletine in man. *Br Heart J* 1976;38:1262–1271.
64. Campbell RWF, Dolder MA, Prescott LF, et al. Comparison of procainamide and mexiletine in prevention of ventricular arrhythmias after acute myocardial infarction. *Lancet* 1975;l:1257–1259.
65. Stein J, Podrid PJ, Lampert S, et al. Long-term mexiletine for ventricular arrhythmia. *Am Heart J* 1984;107:1091–1098.
66. Saunamaki KI. Hemodynamic effects of a new anti-arrhythmic agent mexiletine (Ko 1173) in ischaemic heart disease. *Cardiovasc Res* 1975;9:788–792.
67. Pentikainen PJ, Koivula IH, Hiltunen HA. Effect of rifampicin treatment on the kinetics of mexiletine. *Eur J Clin Pharmacol* 1982;23: 261–266.
68. Bigger JT Jr. The interaction of mexiletine with other cardiovascular drugs. *Am Heart J* 1984;107:1079–1085.
69. Hoffman BF, Rosen MR, Wit AL. Electrophysiology and pharmacology of cardiac arrhythmias: VII. Cardiac effects of quinidine and procainamide. *Am Heart J* 1975;90:117–122.
70. Wellens HJ, Braat S, Brugada P, et al. Use of procainamide in patients with the Wolff-Parkinson-White syndrome to disclose a short refractory period of the accessory pathway. *Am J Cardiol* 1982;50: 1087–1089.
71. Roden DM, Reele SB, Higgins SB, et al. Antiarrhythmic efficacy, pharmacokinetics and safety of *N*-acetylprocainamide in human subjects: Comparison with procainamide. *Am J Cardiol* 1980;46: 463–468.
72. Jaillon P, Winkle RA. Electrophysiologic comparative study of procainamide and *N*-acetylprocainamide in anesthetized dogs: Concentration-response relationships. *Circulation* 1979;60:1385–1394.
73. Mark LC, Kayden HJ, Steele JM, et al. The physiologic disposition and cardiac effects of procainamide. *J Pharmacol Exp Ther* 1951; 102:5–15.
74. Komeichi K, Tohse N, Nakaya H, et al. Effects of *N*-acetylprocainamide and sotalol on ion currents in isolated guinea-pig ventricular myocytes. *Eur J Pharmacol* 1990;187:313–322.

75. Dangman KH, Hoffman BF. In vivo and in vitro antiarrhythmic and arrhythmogenic effects of *N*-acetylprocainamide. *J Pharmacol Exp Ther* 1981;217:851–862.
76. Jaillon P, Rubenson D, Peters F, et al. Electrophysiologic effects of *N*-acetylprocainamide in human beings. *Am J Cardiol* 1981;47: 1134–1140.
77. Funck-Brentano C, Lineberry MD, Light RT, et al. Pharmacokinetic and pharmacodynamic interaction on *N*-acetylprocainamide and procainamide in man. *J Cardiovasc Pharmacol* 1989;14:364–373.
78. Giardina E-GV, Heissenbuttel RH, Bigger JT Jr. Intermittent intravenous procainamide to treat ventricular arrhythmias: Correlation of plasma concentration with effect on arrhythmia, electrocardiogram and blood pressure. *Ann Intern Med* 1973;78:183–193.
79. Lima JJ, Goldfarb AL, Conti DR, et al. Safety and efficacy of procainamide infusions. *Am J Cardiol* 1979;43:98–105.
80. Karlsson, E. Clinical pharmacokinetics of procainamide. *Clin Pharmacokinet* 1978;3:97–107.
81. du Souich P, Erill S. Metabolism of procainamide in patients with chronic heart failure, chronic respiratory failure and chronic renal failure. *Eur J Clin Pharmacol* 1978;14:21–27.
82. Kessler KM, Kayden DS, Estes DM, et al. Procainamide pharmacokinetics in patients with acute myocardial infarction or congestive heart failure. *J Am Coll Cardiol* 1986;7:1131–1139.
83. Olshansky B, Martins J, Hunt S. *N*-acetyl procainamide causing torsades de pointes. *Am J Cardiol* 1982;50:1439–1441.
84. Brachmann J, Scherlag BJ, Rosenshtraukh LV, Lazzara R. Bradycardia-dependent triggered activity: Relevance to drug-induced multiform ventricular tachycardia. *Circulation* 1983;68:846–856.
85. Wyse DG, McAnulty JH, Rahimtoola SH. Influence of plasma drug level and the presence of conduction disease on the electrophysiologic effects of procainamide. *Am J Cardiol* 1979;43:619–626.
86. Kosowsky BD, Taylor J, Lown B, Ritchie RF. Long-term use of procaine amide following acute myocardial infarction. *Circulation* 1973;47:1204–1210.
87. Ellrodt AG, Murata GH, Riedinger MS, et al. Severe neutropenia associated with sustained-release procainamide. *Ann Intern Med* 1984;100:197–201.
88. Somogyi A, McLean A, Heinzow B. Cimetidine-procainamide pharmacokinetic interaction in man: Evidence of competition for tubular secretion of basic drugs. *Eur J Clin Pharmacol* 1983;25: 339–345.
89. Christian CD Jr, Meredith CG, Speeg KV Jr. Cimetidine inhibits renal procainamide clearance. *Clin Pharmacol Ther* 1984;36:221–227.
90. Funck-Brentano C, Jared LL, Roden DM, Woosley RL. Interaction of procainamide and *N*-acetylprocainamide in man. *Circulation* 1987;76 (suppl):IV-520.
91. Somogyi A, Bochner F. Dose and concentration dependent effect of ranitidine on procainamide disposition and renal clearance in man. *Br J Clin Pharmacol* 1984;18:175–181.
92. Mirro MJ, Watanabe AM, Bailey JC. Electrophysiological effects of disopyramide and quinidine on guinea pig atria and canine Purkinje fibers. *Circ Res* 1980;46:660–668.
93. Dubetz DK, Brown NN, Hooper WD, et al. Disopyramide pharmacokinetics and bioavailability. *Br J Clin Pharmacol* 1978;6:279–281.
94. Rangno RE, Warnica W, Ogilvie RI, et al. Correlation of disopyramide pharmacokinetics with efficacy in ventricular tachyarrhythmia. *J Int Med Res* 1976;4(suppl 1):54–58.
95. Hinderling PH, Garrett ER. Pharmacodynamics of the antiarrhythmic disopyramide in healthy humans: Correlation of the kinetics of the drug and its effect. *J Pharmacokinet Biopharm* 1976;4:231–242.
96. Meffin PJ, Robert EW, Winkle RA, et al. The role of concentration-dependent plasma protein binding in disopyramide disposition. *J Pharmacokinet Biopharm* 1979;7:29–46.
97. Davies RF, Siddoway LA, Shaw L, et al. Immediate- versus controlled-release disopyramide: Importance of saturable binding. *Clin Pharmacol Ther* 1993;54:16–22.
98. Edvardsson N, Olsson SB. Clinical value of plasma concentrations of antiarrhythmic drugs. *Eur Heart J* 1987;8 (suppl A):83–89.
99. Kumana CR, Rambihar VS, Tanser PH, et al. A placebo-controlled study to determine the efficacy of oral disopyramide phosphate for the prophylaxis of ventricular dysrhythmias after acute myocardial infarction. *Br J Clin Pharmacol* 1982;14:519–527.
100. Podrid PJ, Schoenberger A, Lown B. Congestive heart failure caused by oral disopyramide. *N Engl J Med* 1980;302:614–617.
101. Johnston A, Henry JA, Warrington SJ, Hamer NAJ. Pharmacokinetics of oral disopyramide phosphate in patients with renal impairment. *Br J Clin Pharmacol* 1980;10:245–248.
102. Bonde J, Gradual NA, Pedersen LE, et al. Kinetics of disopyramide in decreased hepatic function. *Eur J Clin Pharmacol* 1986;31:73–77.
103. Mokler CM, Hillman RA. Nature of the anticholinergic action of some antiarrhythmic drugs. *Pharmacol Res Commun* 1972;4:171–178.
104. Teichman SL, Ferrick A, Kim SG, et al. Disopyramide-pyridostigmine interaction: Selective reversal of anticholinergic symptoms with preservation of antiarrhythmic effect. *J Am Coll Cardiol* 1987;10:633–641.
105. Schweitzer P, Mark H. Torsades de pointes caused by disopyramide and hypokalemia. *Mt Sinai J Med* 1982;49:110–114.
106. LaBarre A, Strauss HC, Scheinman MM, et al. Electrophysiologic effects of disopyramide phosphate on sinus node function in patients with sinus node dysfunction. *Circulation* 1979;59:226–235.
107. Roden DM, Hoffman BF. Action potential prolongation and induction of abnormal automaticity by low quinidine concentrations in canine Purkinje fibers: Relationship to potassium and cycle length. *Circ Res* 1985;56:857–867.
108. Risler T, Burk M, Peters U, et al. On the interaction between digoxin and disopyramide. *Clin Pharmacol Ther* 1983;34:176–180.
109. Sylven C, Anderson P. Evidence that disopyramide does not interact with warfarin. *Br Med J* 1983;286:1181.
110. Kessler JM, Keys PW, Stattford RW. Disopyramide and phenytoin interaction. *Clin Pharm* 1982;1:263–264.
111. Cumming AD, Robertson C. Interaction between disopyramide and practolol. *Br Med J* 1979;2:1264.
112. Sodermark T, Edhag O, Sjogren A, et al. Effect of quinidine on maintaining sinus rhythm after conversion of atrial fibrillation or flutter: A multicenter study from Stockholm. *Br Heart J* 1975;37:486–492.
113. Levi GF, Proto C. Combined treatment of atrial fibrillation with quinidine and beta-blockers. *Br Heart J* 1972;34:911–914.
114. Bloomfield SS, Romhilt DW, Chou T-C, Fowler NO. Natural history of cardiac arrhythmias and their prevention with quinidine in patients with acute coronary insufficiency. *Circulation* 1973;47:967–973.
115. Carliner NH, Crouthamel WG, Fisher ML, et al. Quinidine therapy in hospitalized patients with ventricular arrhythmias. *Am Heart J* 1979; 98:708–715.
116. Winkle RA, Gradman AH, Fitzgerald JW. Antiarrhythmic drug effect assessed from ventricular arrhythmia reduction in the ambulatory electrocardiogram and treadmill test: Comparison of propranolol, procainamide and quinidine. *Am J Cardiol* 1978;42:473–480.
117. Coplen SE, Antman EM, Berlin JA, et al. Efficacy and safety of quinidine therapy for maintenance of sinus rhythm after cardioversion: A meta-analysis of randomized control trials. *Circulation* 1990;82: 1106–1114.
118. Denes P, Gabster A, Huang SK. Clinical, electrocardiographic and follow-up observations in patients having ventricular fibrillation during Holter monitoring: Role of quinidine therapy. *Am J Cardiol* 1981;48: 9–16.
119. Belhassen B. Viskin S. Fish R, et al. Effects of electrophysiologic-guided therapy with class IA antiarrhythmic drugs on the long-term outcome of patients with idiopathic ventricular fibrillation with or without the Brugada syndrome. *J Cardiovasc Electrophysiol* 1999;10:1301–1312.
120. Yan G-X, Antzelevitch C. Cellular basis for the Brugada syndrome and other mechanisms of arrhythmogenesis associated with ST-segment elevation. *Circulation* 1999;100:1660–1666.
121. Sokolow M, Edgar AL. Blood quinidine concentrations as a guide in the treatment of cardiac arrhythmias. *Circulation* 1950;1:576–592.
122. Vozeh S, Oti-Amoako K, Uematsu T, Follath F. Antiarrhythmic activity of two quinidine metabolites in experimental reperfusion arrythmia:

Relative potency and pharmacodynamic interaction with the parent drug. *J Pharmacol Exp Ther* 1987;43:297–301.

123. Vozeh S, Bindschedler M, Huy-Riem HA, et al. Pharmacodynamics of 3-hydroxyquinidine alone and in combination with quinidine in healthy persons. *Am J Cardiol* 1987;59:681–684.
124. Kavanagh KM, Wyse DG, Mitchell LB, et al. Contribution of quinidine metabolites to electrophysiologic responses in human subjects. *Clin Pharmacol Ther* 1989;46:352–358.
125. Thompson KA, Blair IA, Woosley RL, Roden DM. Comparative in vitro electrophysiology of quinidine, its major metabolites and dihydroxyquinidine. *J Pharmacol Exp Ther* 1987;241:84–90.
126. Drayer DE, Lorenzo B, Reidenberg MM. Liquid chromatography and fluorescence spectroscopy compared with a homogeneous enzyme immunoassay technique for determining quinidine in serum. *Clin Chem* 1981;27:308–310.
127. Lehmann CR, Boran KJ, Pierson WP, et al. Quinidine assays: Enzyme immunoassay versus high performance liquid chromatography. *Ther Drug Monit* 1986;8:336–339.
128. Drayer DE, Lowenthal DT, Restivo KM, et al. Steady-state serum levels of quinidine and active metabolites in cardiac patients with varying degrees of renal function. *Clin Pharmacol Ther* 1978;24:31–39.
129. Kessler KM, Humphries WC, Black M, Spann JF. Quinidine pharmacokinetics in patients with cirrhosis or receiving propranolol. *Am Heart J* 1978;96:627–635.
130. Ochs HR, Greenblatt DJ, Woo E. Clinical pharmacokinetics of quinidine. *Clin Pharmacokinet* 1980;5:150–168.
131. Kay GN, Plumb VJ, Arciniegas JG, et al. Torsades de pointes: The long-short initiating sequence and other clinical features: Observations in 32 patients. *J Am Coll Cardiol* 1983;2:806–817.
132. Gottlieb SS, Weinberg M. Hemodynamic and neurohormonal effects of quinidine in patients with severe left ventricular dysfunction secondary to coronary artery disease or idiopathic dilated cardiomyopathy. *Am J Cardiol* 1991;67:728–731.
133. Cohen IS, Jick H, Cohen SI. Adverse reactions to quinidine in hospitalized patients: Findings based on data from the Boston Collaborative Drug Surveillance Programs. *Prog Cardiovasc Dis* 1977;20:151–163.
134. Dargie HJ, Cleland JGF, Leckie BJ, et al. Relation of arrhythmias and electrolyte abnormalities to survival in patients with severe chronic heart failure. *Circulation* 1987;75(suppl IV):IV-98–IV-107.
135. Roden DM, Woosley RL, Primm RK. Incidence and clinical features of the quinidine-associated long-QT syndrome: Implications for patient care. *Am Heart J* 1986;111:1088–1093.
136. Makkar RR, Fromm BS, Steinman RT, et al. Female gender as a risk factor for torsades de pointes associated with cardiovascular drugs. *JAMA* 1993;270:2590–2597.
137. Drici MD, Burklow TR, Haridasse V, et al. Sex hormones prolong the QT interval and down-regulate potassium channel expression in the rabbit heart. *Circulation* 1996;94:1471–1474.
138. Benton RE, Sale M, Flockhart DA, Woosley RL. Greater quinidine induced $QT_c$ interval prolongation in women. *Clin Pharmacol Ther* 2000;67:413–418.
139. Schmid PG, Nelson LD, Mark AL, et al. Inhibition of adrenergic vasoconstriction by quinidine. *J Pharmacol Exp Ther* 1974;188: 124–134.
140. Nair MR, Duvernoy WF, Leichtman DA. Severe leukopenia and thrombocytopenia secondary to quinidine. *Clin Cardiol* 1981;4:247–257.
141. Polish LB, Branch RA, Fitzgerald GA. Digitoxin-quinidine interaction: Potentiation during administration of cimetidine *South Med J* 1981;74:633–634.
142. Data JL, Wilkinson GR, Nies AS. Interaction of quinidine with anticonvulsant drugs. *N Engl J Med* 1976;294:699–702.
143. Leahey EB Jr, Reiffel JA, Drusin RE, et al. Interactions between quinidine and digoxin. *JAMA* 1978;240:533–534.
144. Bussey HI. The influence of quinidine and other agents on digitalis glycosides. *Am Heart J* 1982;104:289–302.
145. Brinn R, Brosen K, Gram LF, et al. Spartine oxidation is practically abolished in quinidine-treated patients. *Br J Clin Pharmacol* 1986;22:194–197.
146. Spiers CJ, Murray S, Boobis AR, et al. Quinidine and the identification of drugs whose elimination is impaired in subjects classified as poor metabolizers of debrisoquine. *Br J Clin Pharmacol* 1986; 22:739–743.
147. Guengerich FP, Muller-Enoch D, Blair IA. Oxidation of quinidine by human liver cytochrome P-450. *Mol Pharmacol* 1986;30:287–295.
148. Mikus G, Ha HR, Vozeh S, et al. Pharmacokinetics and metabolism of quinidine in extensive and poor metabolizers of spartine. *Eur J Clin Pharmacol* 1986;31:69–72.
149. Brosen K, Gram LF, Haghfelt T, Bertilsson L. Extensive metabolizers of debrisoquin become poor metabolizers during quinidine treatment. *Pharmacol Toxicol* 1987;60:312–314.
150. Kornfeld P, Horowitz SH, Genkins G, Papatestas AE. Myasthenia gravis unmasked by antiarrhythmic agents. *Mt Sinai J Med* 1976;43: 10–14.
151. Grogono AW. Anesthesia for atrial fibrillation: Effect of quinidine on muscle relaxation. *Lancet* 1963;2:1039–1040.
152. Connolly SJ, Mulji AS, Hoffert DL, et al. Randomized placebo controlled trial of propafenone for treatment of atrial tachyarrhythmias after cardiac surgery. *J Am Coll Cardiol* 1987;10:1145–1148.
153. Fuster V, Ryden LE, Asinger RW et al. ACC/AHA/ESC guidelines for the management of patients with atrial fibrillation: Executive summary. *J Am Coll Cardiol* 2001;38:1231–1265.
154. von Philipsborn G, Gries J, Hofmann HP, et al. Pharmacological studies on propafenone and its main metabolite 5-hydroxypropafenone. *Arzneimittelforschung* 1984;34:1489–1497.
155. Valenzuela C, Delgado C, Tamargo J. Electrophysiological effects of 5-hydroxypropafenone on guinea pig ventricular muscle fibers. *J Cardiovasc Pharmacol* 1987;10:523–529.
156. McLeod AA, Stiles GL, Shand DG. Demonstration of beta adrenoceptor blockade by propafenone hydrochloride: Clinical pharmacologic, radioligand binding, and adenylate cyclase activation studies. *J Pharmacol Exp Ther* 1984;228:461–466.
157. Siddoway LA, Thompson KA, McAllister CB, et al. Polymorphism of propafenone metabolism and disposition in man: Clinical and pharmacokinetic consequences. *Circulation* 1987;75:785–791.
158. Lee JT, Kroemer HK, Silberstein DJ, et al. The role of genetically determined polymorphic drug metabolism in the beta-block produced by propafenone. *N Engl J Med* 1990;322:1764–1768.
159. Botto GL, Capucci A, Bonini W, et al. Conversion of recent onset atrial fibrillation to sinus rhythms using a single oral loading dose of propafenone: Comparison of two regimens. *Int J Cardiol* 1997;58: 55–61.
160. Baker BJ, Dinh H, Kroskey D, et al. Effect of propafenone on left ventricular ejection fraction. *Am J Cardiol* 1984;54 (suppl):20D–22D.
161. Wagner F, Kalusche D, Trenk D, et al. Drug interaction between propafenone and metoprolol. *Br J Clin Pharmacol* 1987;24:213–220.
162. Funck-Brentano C, Kroemer HK, Pavlou H, et al. Genetically determined interaction between propafenone and low dose quinidine: Role of active metabolites in modulating net drug effect. *Br J Clin Pharmacol* 1989;27:435–444.
163. Roden DM, Woosley RL. Flecainide. *N Engl J Med* 1986;315:36–41.
164. Hellestrand KJ, Nathan AW, Bexton RS, et al. Cardiac electrophysiologic effects of flecainide acetate for paroxysmal reentrant junctional tachycardias. *Am J Cardiol* 1983;51:770–776
165. Pritchett EL, Wilkinson WE. Mortality in patients treated with flecainide and encainide for supraventricular arrhythmias. *Am J Cardiol* 1991;67:976–980.
166. The Flecainide-Quinidine Research Group. Flecainide versus quinidine for treatment of chronic ventricular arrhythmias: A multicenter clinical trial. *Circulation* 1983;67:1117–1123.
167. Follmer CH, Colatsky TJ. Block of delayed rectifier potassium current, $I_K$, by flecainide and E-4031 in cat ventricular myocytes. *Circulation* 1990;82:289–293.
168. Estes NAM III, Garan H, Ruskin JN. Electrophysiological properties of flecainide acetate. *Am J Cardiol* 1984;53(suppl):26B–29B.
169. Conard GJ, Ober RE. Metabolism of flecainide. *Am J Cardiol* 1984; 53(suppl):41B–51B.

170. Haefeli WE, Bargetzi MJ, Follath F, et al. Potent inhibition of cytochrome p450IID6 (debrisoquin 4-hydroxylase) by flecainide in vitro and in vivo. *J Cardiovasc Pharmacol* 1990;15:776–779.
171. Johnston A, Warrington S, Turner P. Flecainide pharmacokinetics in healthy volunteers: The influence of urinary pH. *Br J Clin Pharmacol* 1985;20:333–338.
172. Franciosa JA, Wilen M, Weeks CE, et al. Pharmacokinetics and hemodynamic effects of flecainide in patients with chronic low output heart failure. *J Am Coll Cardiol* 1983;1:699.
173. Winkelman BR, Leinberger H. Life-threatening flecainide toxicity: A pharmacodynamic approach. *Ann Intern Med* 1987;106:807–814.
174. Salerno DM, Granrud GA, Sharkey P, et al. Pharmacodynamics and side effects of flecainide acetate. *Clin Pharmacol Ther* 1986;40:101–107.
175. Morganroth J, Horowitz LN. Flecainide: Its proarrhythmic effect and expected changes on the surface electrocardiogram. *Am J Cardiol* 1984;53(suppl):89B–94B.
176. Josephson MA, Kaul S, Hopkins J, et al. Hemodynamic effects of intravenous flecainide relative to the level of ventricular function in patients with coronary artery disease. *Am Heart J* 1985;109:41–45.
177. Muhiddin KA, Turner P, Blackett A. Effect of flecainide on cardiac output. *Clin Pharmacol Ther* 1985;37:260–263.
178. Josephson MA, Ikeda N, Singh BN. Effects of flecainide on ventricular function: Clinical and experimental correlations. *Am J Cardiol* 1984;53:95B–100B.
179. Vik-Mo H, Ohm O-J, Lund-Johansen P, Electrophysiological effects of flecainide acetate in patients with sinus nodal dysfunction. *Am J Cardiol* 1982;50:1090–1094.
180. Hellestrand KJ, Nathan AW, Bexton RS, Camm AJ. Electrophysiologic effects of flecainide acetate on sinus node function, anomalous atrioventricular connections and pacemaker thresholds. *Am J Cardiol* 1984;53(suppl):30B–38B.
181. Hellestrand KJ, Burnett PJ, Milne JR, et al. The effect of the antiarrhythmic agent flecainide on acute and chronic pacing thresholds. *PACE* 1983;6:892–899.
182. Hernandez R, Mann DE, Breckinridge S, et al. Effects of flecainide on defibrillation thresholds in the anesthetized dog. *J Am Coll Cardiol* 1989;14:777–781.
183. Tjandra-Maga TB, van Hecken A, van Melle P, et al. Altered pharmacokinetics of oral flecainide by cimetidine. *Br J Clin Pharmacol* 1986;22:108–110.
184. Weeks CE, Conard GJ, Kvam DC, et al. The effect of flecainide acetate, a new antiarrhythmic, on plasma digoxin levels. *J Clin Pharmacol* 1986;26:27–31.
185. Lewis GP, Holtzman JL. Interaction of flecainide with digoxin and propranolol. *Am J Cardiol* 1984;53(suppl):52B–57B.
186. Shea P, Lal R, Kim SS, et al. Flecainide and amiodarone interaction. *J Am Coll Cardiol* 1986;7:1127–1130.
187. Rowland E. Antiarrhythmic drugs: Class IV. *Eur Heart J* 1987; 8(suppl A):61–63.
188. Singh BN, Nademanee K, Baky SH. Calcium antagonists: Clinical use in the treatment of arrhythmias. *Drugs* 1983;25:125–153.
189. Bril A. Recent advances in arrhythmia therapy: Treatment and prevention of atrial fibrillation. *Curr Opin Pharmacol* 2002;2:154–159.
190. Singh BN, Nademanee K. Sotalol: A beta-blocker with unique antiarrhythmic properties. *Am Heart J* 1987;114:121–139.
191. Singh BN, Kehoe R, Woosley RL, et al. Multicenter trial of sotalol compared with procainamide in the suppression of inducible ventricular tachycardia: A double-blind, randomized parallel evaluation. Sotalol Multicenter Study Group. *Am Heart J* 1995;129:87–97.
192. Mason JW, ESVEM Investigators. A comparison of seven antiarrhythmic drugs in patients with ventricular tachyarrhythmias. *N Engl J Med* 1993;329:452–458.
193. Wang T, Bergstrand RH, Thompson KA, et al. Concentration-dependent pharmacologic properties of sotalol. *Am J Cardiol* 1986;57: 1160–1165.
194. Kopleman HA, Woosley RL, Lee JT, et al. Electrophysiologic effects of intravenous and oral sotalol for sustained ventricular tachycardia secondary to coronary artery disease. *Am J Cardiol* 1988;61:1006–1011.
195. Hohnloser SH, Woosley RL. Sotalol. *N Engl J Med* 1994;331:31–38.
196. Barbey JT, Sale ME, Woosley RL, et al. Pharmacokinetic, pharmacodynamic, and safety evaluation of an accelerated dose titration regimen of sotalol in healthy middle-aged subjects. *Clin Pharmacol Ther* 1999;66:91–99.
197. Graboys TB, Podrid PJ, Lown B. Efficacy of amiodarone for refractory supraventricular tachyarrhythmias. *Am Heart J* 1983;106:870–876.
198. Horowitz LN, Spielman SR, Greenspan AM, et al. Use of amiodarone in the treatment of persistent and paroxysmal atrial fibrillation resistant to quinidine therapy. *J Am Coll Cardiol* 1985;6:1402–1407.
199. Peters RW, Fisher ML. Use of amiodarone. *Choices Cardiol* 1994;8: 57–60.
200. Cairns JA, Connolly SJ, Roberts R, et al. Randomized trial of outcome after myocardial infarction in patients with frequent or repetitive ventricular premature depolarizations: CAMIAT. *Lancet* 1997;349:675–682.
201. Julian DG, Camm AJ, Frangin G, et al. Randomized trial of effect of amiodarone on mortality in patients with left-ventricular dysfunction after recent myocardial infarction: EMIAT. *Lancet* 1997;349: 667–674.
202. Connolly SJ. Meta-analysis of antiarrhythmic drug trials. *Am J Cardiol* 1999;84:90R–93R.
203. Piepoli M, Villani GQ, Ponikowski P, et al. Overview and meta-analysis of randomised trials of amiodarone in chronic heart failure. *Int J Cardiol* 1998;66:1–10.
204. Connolly SJ. Gent M. Roberts RS. Dorian P. Roy D. Sheldon RS. Mitchell LB. Green MS. Klein GJ. O'Brien B. Canadian implantable defibrillator study (CIDS): A randomized trial of the implantable cardioverter defibrillator against amiodarone (comment). *Circulation* 2000;101:1297–1302.
204a. Scheinman MM, Levine JH, Cannom DS, et al. Dose-ranging study of intravenous amiodarone in patients with life-threatening ventricular tachyarrhythmias. *Circulation* 1995;92:3264–3272.
205. Kowey PR, Levine JH, Herre JM, et al. Randomized, double-blind comparison of intravenous amiodarone and bretylium in the treatment of patients with recurrent, hemodynamically destabilizing ventricular tachycardia or fibrillation. *Circulation* 1995;92:3255–3263.
206. Gallik DM, Singer I, Meissner MD, et al. Hemodynamic and surface electrocardiographic effects of a new aqueous formulation of intravenous amiodarone. *Am J Cardiol* 2002;90:964–968.
207. Kodenchuk PJ, Cobb LA, Copass MK, et al. Amiodarone for resuscitation after out-of-hospital cardiac arrest due to ventricular fibrillation. *N Engl J Med* 1999;341:871–878.
208. Guarnieri T, Nolan S, Gottlieb SO, et al. Intravenous amiodarone for the prevention of atrial fibrillation after open heart surgery: The amiodarone reduction in coronary heart (ARCH) trial. *J Am Coll Cardiol* 1999;34:343–347.
209. Mason JW. Amiodarone. *N Engl J Med* 1987;316:455–466.
210. Mason JW, Hondeghem LM, Katzung BG. Amiodarone blocks inactivated cardiac sodium channels. *Pflugers Arch* 1983;396:79–81.
211. Talajic M, DeRoode MR, Nattel S. Comparative electrophysiologic effects of intravenous amiodarone and desmethylamiodarone in dogs: Evidence for clinically relevant activity of the metabolite. *Circulation* 1987;75:265–271.
212. Nanas JN, Mason JW. Pharmacokinetics and regional electrophysiological effects of intracoronary amiodarone administration. *Circulation* 1995;91:451–461.
213. Albert SG, Alves LE, Rose EP. Thyroid dysfunction during chronic amiodarone therapy. *J Am Coll Cardiol* 1987;9:175–183.
214. Singh BN, Nademanee K. Amiodarone and thyroid function: Clinical implications during antiarrhythmic therapy. *Am Heart J* 1983;106: 857–869.
215. Singh BN, Nademanee K. Amiodarone and thyroid function: Clinical implications during antiarrhythmic therapy. *Am Heart J* 1983;106: 857–869.
216. Charlier R, Deltour G, Baudine A, Chaillet F. Pharmacology of amiodarone, and anti-anginal drug with a new biological profile. *Arzneimittelforschung* 1968;18:1408–1417.

38. Page RL, Kerber RE, Russell JK, et al. Biphasic versus monophasic shock waveform for conversion of atrial fibrillation. *J Am Coll Cardiol* 2002;39:1956–1963.
39. American Heart Association Guidelines 2000 for Cardiopulmonary Resuscitation and Emergency Cardiac Care. *Circulation* 2000;102: I-1–I-284.
40. Yamanouchi Y, Brewer JE, Mowrey KA. Sawtooth first phase biphasic defibrillation waveforms: A comparison with standard waveform in clinical devices. *J Cardiovasc Electrophysiol* 1997;8:517–528.
41. Pagan-Carlo LA, Allan JJ, Spencer KT, et al. Encircling overlapping multipulse shock waveforms for transthoracic defibrillation. *J Am Coll Cardiol* 1998;32:2065–2071.
42. Jones JL, Jones RE. Improved safety factor for triphasic deflbrillator waveforms. *Circ Res* 1989;64:1172–1177.
43. Zhang Y, Ramabadran R, Boddicker K, et al. Triphasic shocks are superior to biphasic shocks for transthoracic defibrillation: Experimental studies. *J Am Coll Cardiol* 2003;42:568–575.
44. Warner ED, Dahl C, Ewy GA. Myocardial injury from transthoracic defibrillator countershock. *Arch Pathol* 1975;99:55–59.
45. Weaver WD, Copass MK, Holstrom AP. Ventricular defibrillation: Comparative trial using 175 joule and 320 joule shocks. *N Engl J Med* 1982;307:1101–1106.
46. Trouton PG, Allen JD, Yong LK, et al. Metabolic changes in mitochondrial dysfunction early following transthoracic countershocks in dogs. *Pacing Clin Electrophysiol* 1989;12:1827–1834.
47. Caterine MR, Spencer KT, Pagan Carlo LA, et al. Direct current shocks to the heart generate free radicals: An electron paramagnetic resonance study. *J Am Coll Cardiol* 1996;28:1598–1609.
48. Clark CB, Zhang Y, Martin SM, et al. The nitric oxide synthase inhibitor $N^G$-nitro-L-arginine decreases defibrillation-induced free radical generation. *Resuscitation* 2003;57:101–108.
49. Tang W, Weil MH, Sun S, et al. The effects of biphasic and conventional monophasic defibrillation post-resuscitation myocardial function. *J Am Coll Cardiol* 1999;34:815–822.
50. Kerber RE, Becker LB, Bourland JD, et al. Automatic external defibrillators for public access defibrillation: Recommendations for specifying and reporting arrhythmia analysis algorithm performance, incorporating new waveforms, and enhancing safety. *Circulation* 1997; 95:1677–1682.
51. Page RL, Joglar J, Kowal RC, et al. Use of automated defibrillators by a U.S. airline. *N Engl J Med* 2000;343:1210–1216.
52. Valenzuela T, Roe DJ, Nichol G, et al. Outcomes of rapid defibrillation by security officers after cardiac arrest in casinos. *N Engl J Med* 2000;343:1206–1209.
53. Caffrey SL, Willoughy P, Pepe PE, et al. Public use of automated external defibrillators. *N Engl J Med* 2002;347:1242–1247.
54. White RD, Asplin BR, Bugliosi TF, et al. High discharge survival rate after out-of-hospital ventricular fibrillation with rapid defibrillation by police and paramedics. *Ann Emerg Med* 1996;28:480–485.
55. Weaver DL, Peberdy MA. Defibrillation in public places—One step closer to home. *N Engl J Med* 2002;347:1223–1224.
56. Weisfeldt ML, Kerber RE, McGoldrick RP, et al. American Heart Association report on Public Access Defibrillation Conference, December 8–10, 1994: Automatic External Defibrillation Task Force. *Circulation* 1995;92:684–692.
57. Eisenberg MS, Moore J, Cummins RO, et al. Use of the automatic external defibrillator in homes of survivors of out-of-hospital ventricular fibrillation. *Am J Cardiol* 1989;63:443–446.
58. Aurrichio A, Klein H, Geller C, et al. Clinical efficacy of the wearable cardioverter defibrillator in acutely terminating episodes of ventricular fibrillation. *Am J Cardiol* 1998;81:1253–1257.
59. Feldman A, Klein H, Tchou P. New therapeutic option for patients with time-dependent risk of sudden cardiac arrest: Application of novel wearable defibrillator (abstr). *J Am Coll Cardiol* 2002;39:101A.

CHAPTER 38

# THE IMPLANTABLE CARDIOVERTER DEFIBRILLATOR

Robert A. Bleasdale / Jeremy N. Ruskin / Peter A. O'Callaghan



## HISTORICAL PERSPECTIVE

Sudden and unexpected cardiac death (SCD) is estimated to claim 200,000 to 400,000 lives annually in the United States.[1] Despite a significant reduction in total cardiac mortality rates in recent years, the proportion of deaths that are sudden has remained unchanged. Electrocardiographic (ECG) monitoring at the scene of an out-of-hospital cardiac arrest has demonstrated that the principal cause of SCD is ventricular fibrillation (VF).[2] Automated external defibrillators (AEDs) applied within 1 min of the collapse documents VF in 70 to 90 percent of cardiac arrest victims.[2,3] Since self-termination of VF is exceedingly rare, the single most important factor determining survival is the time between event onset and first defibrillation attempt.[4] Overall mortality rates associated with out-of-hospital cardiac arrest remain high, mainly because of the delay in providing defibrillation therapy.[5] In witnessed cardiac arrests due to VF, in whom the time to first defibrillation is less than three minutes, the survival rates reach 74 percent.[2] As originally conceived by Mirowski, the implantable cardioverter defibrillator (ICD) was designed to circumvent the delay in providing definitive therapy to ambulatory individuals with life-threatening ventricular tachyarrhythmia.[6] The ICD responds by delivering an internal electrical shock within 10 to 15 s of arrhythmia onset, a time frame in which the potential for arrhythmia reversal approaches 100 percent. The first experimental canine model was successfully tested in 1969.[7] After 10 years of research and development, Mirowski and coworkers implanted the first ICD in a human at the Johns Hopkins University Medical Center in 1980.[8] In the original article, the authors state, "It is intended to protect patients at particularly high risk of sudden death whenever and wherever they are stricken by these lethal arrhythmias. . . . The only purpose of this device is to achieve defibrillation automatically, before the victim of a lethal arrhythmia can be reached by a cardiac resuscitation team." In 1985, the ICD received approval from the U.S. Food and Drug Administration for market release. Since then, the indications for ICD implantation have greatly expanded, and the number of devices implanted annually has steadily increased, reaching 80,000 new implants worldwide in 2000.[9]

## FUNCTIONAL CHARACTERISTICS

The ICD system consists of a pulse generator and a lead electrode for arrhythmia detection and therapy delivery. In addition to internal defibrillation, an ICD can also deliver pacing (antitachycardia and antibradycardia) and synchronized cardioversion. Detailed diagnostic data (intracardiac electrograms, event markers, etc.) relating to therapy delivery are stored for retrieval and analysis. The pulse generator is essentially a self-powered computer within a hermetically sealed titanium can. Lithium batteries and defibrillator capacitors occupy the bulk of the space. The ICD lead incorporates both pacing electrodes and large-surface-area defibrillation coils. The defibrillation circuit is completed by the titanium case of the pulse generator, which also acts as a defibrillation electrode.

### Tachyarrhythmia Detection

Reliable sensing of ventricular depolarization is essential for proper functioning of the ICD. Sensing electrodes transmit unfiltered electrograms to the sense amplifier of the ICD. The sense amplifier amplifies, filters, and rectifies the incoming signals. It then compares them to a sensing threshold and produces a set of RR intervals for the detection algorithm to use[10] (Fig. 38-1*A*). Intracardiac electrogram amplitude can vary markedly during ventricular fibrillation. Fixed gain and sensitivity, as used in pacemakers, would result in either under- or oversensing, depending on the settings chosen. Therefore all ICDs utilize some form of automatically adjusting signal amplifier (Fig. 38-1*B*). Automatic gain control continuously varies the gain so that the amplitude of the processed signal is constant. Autoadjusting sensitivity threshold sets the sensitivity to a proportion of the

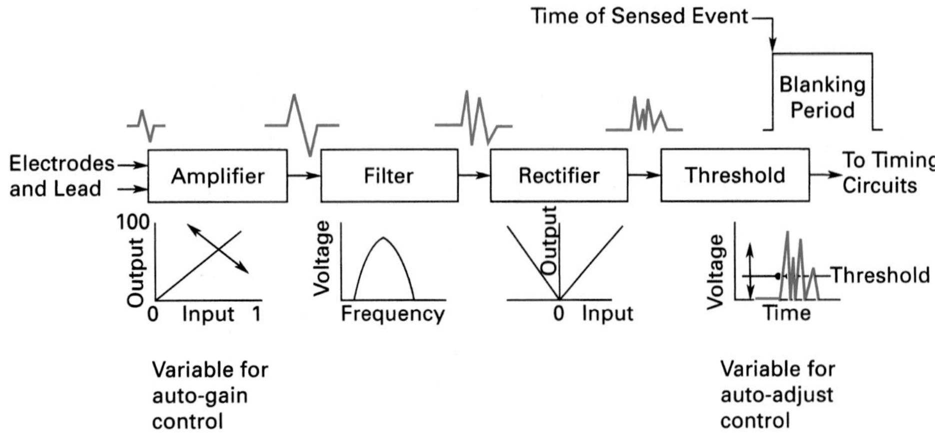


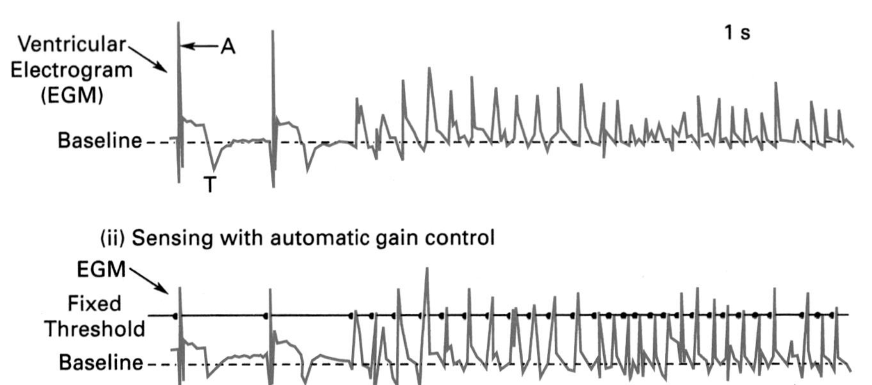


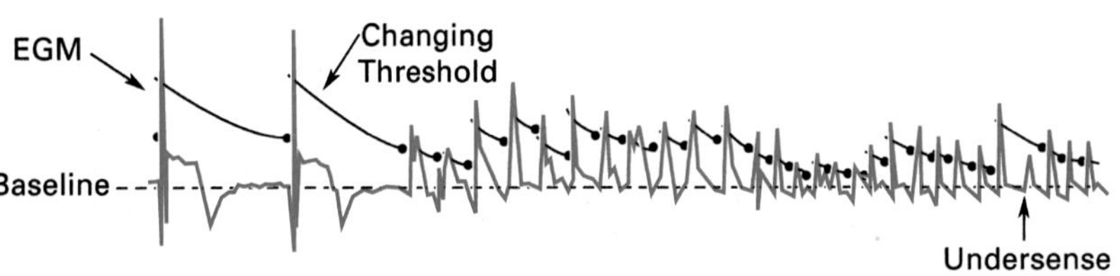


FIGURE 38-1 Sensing of electrogram signals by implantable cardioverter-defibrillators. *A.* A functional block diagram for an ICD sense amplifier consists of an amplifier that may be fixed or have automatic gain control, a bandpass filter to reject low-frequency T waves and high-frequency noise, a rectifier to eliminate polarity dependency, and a threshold detector that may be fixed or autoadjusting. The net result is a single pulse for each ventricular depolarization that is used by timing circuits to determine a series of cycle lengths. The effects of each block on a biphasic electrogram are shown above the blocks, and each functional operation is shown below each block. *B.* Sinus rhythm and ventricular fibrillation signals are shown for the raw electrogram in panel *(i)*, for automatic gain control in panel *(ii)*, and for automatic adjusting threshold in panel *(iii)*. With automatic gain control, the small electrograms are amplified compared to panel *(i)*, and sensing is shown by the dots where the signal crosses the fixed threshold. With automatic adjusting threshold, the electrograms are the same as in panel *(i)*, and the threshold varies according to the amplitude of the electrogram; sensing is again shown by the dots where the signal crosses the variable threshold. (From Olson,[10] with permission.)

amplitude of the last sensed event, and the sensitivity then gradually increases until the next event is sensed. Sensed events are then analyzed using a detection algorithm.

The range of all possible ventricular cycle lengths is divided into rate zones that do not overlap, including a VF zone, ventricular tachycardia (VT) zones, a normal rate zone, and a bradycardia zone.

Devices employ rate criteria as the sole method of detecting VF. An X/Y detector triggers when X out of the previous Y-sensed intervals (typical setting, 8/12 intervals) are shorter than the VF detection interval. This approach is very good at ignoring the effect of a small number of undersensed events due to small-amplitude signals during VF. The utilization of rate detection in an X/Y detection algorithm results in maximal sensitivity at the expense of specificity. Any tachycardia with a cycle length less than the tachycardia detection interval will be detected as VF by the device, and VF therapy will be initiated. During capacitor charging and prior to therapy delivery, a reconfirmation algorithm must be fulfilled. This prevents inappropriate shock therapy for self-terminating events, such as nonsustained VT.

The VT detection algorithm is different from that in the VF zone. VT detection algorithms require a programmable number of consecutive intervals shorter than the VT detection interval. An interval longer than the detection interval (e.g., due to RR variability in atrial fibrillation) would reset the counters. In certain patients, both ventricular and supraventricular tachycardias (e.g., sinus tachycardia, atrial fibrillation, or atrial flutter) may result in ventricular rates within the VT zone. Up to 25 percent of ICD discharges are inappropriate when rate is employed as the sole criterion for VT therapy.[11] To increase specificity, optional VT detection enhancements are programmable. Single-chamber ICD detection enhancements include sudden onset, rate stability, and electrogram morphologic (QRS width) criteria. These programmable options are not available in the VF zone, where maximal sensitivity is required. The onset criterion is intended to distinguish sinus tachycardia with a gradual rate increase from VT characterized by a sudden rate increase. The rate stability criterion is used to differentiate sustained monomorphic VT with a small variation in cycle length from atrial fibrillation with large cycle length variability. The electrogram morphologic criterion measures the width of the intracardiac electrogram to differentiate ventricular from supraventricular tachycardias with normal conduction. In one study, programming stability and onset criteria significantly reduced inappropriate therapies to 13 percent, compared to 28 percent in patients using the rate criterion only.[12]

Dual-chamber defibrillators, requiring an additional atrial lead, provide not only dual-chamber pacing but also dual-chamber detection algorithms.[13] These employ a stepwise analysis of rate, stability, atrioventricular (AV) association, and onset (ventricular acceleration, atrial acceleration, or nonaccelerated).[14] Although sophisticated VT detection improves specificity, it does so at the risk of prolonging detection times or of failure to detect an episode of VT; it should therefore be used judiciously, especially at tachycardia rates that are not hemodynamically tolerated by the patient.

### Device Therapy

ICDs employ electrical defibrillation as the sole therapy option for the treatment of VF. In contrast to bradycardia pacing, which requires depolarization during diastole of a small number of cells located close to the electrode, defibrillation requires depolarization of the majority of ventricular cells, many of which are relatively refractory and can be up to 10 cm away. Successful defibrillation may require voltages up to 100 times greater than the voltage of the ICD battery (approximately 6.4 V). A capacitor is used to store charge immediately prior to therapy delivery. This energy is then delivered in a biphasic defibrillation pulse between the high-voltage electrodes and depolarizes the intervening myocardium, restoring baseline rhythm (Fig. 38-2). The time interval between VF onset and delivery of defibrillation energy is usually 10 to 15 s, with capacitor charge time accounting for most of the delay. During this time, the subject may experience presyncope or syncope, with restoration of consciousness after successful defibrillation and restoration of cardiac output. One study of ICD recipients found that 16 percent of patients who received device therapy experienced syncope. In comparison, 65 percent of these patients had experienced syncope during tachyarrhythmia prior to device implantation.[15]

In contrast to VF therapy, treatment options in the VT zones include antitachycardia pacing (ATP), cardioversion, and defibrillation. Therapy progresses through a programmable sequence of responses until the episode is terminated. Most sustained monomorphic VTs, particularly in patients with coronary artery disease, are due to reentry and can be terminated by a critical pacing sequence.[16] Pacing at faster rates increases the probability of VT termination but also increases the risk of tachycardia acceleration. ATP, with backup defibrillation if acceleration occurs, is an attractive, well-tolerated treatment that avoids high-energy shock therapy, which is painful and diminishes battery life (Fig. 38-3). The most common form of ATP is adaptive-burst pacing, which delivers a train of stimuli at a fixed percentage of the tachycardia cycle length. Repeated and more aggressive pacing trains can be administered, resulting in either termination of the tachycardia or progression to the next treatment modality (cardioversion or defibrillation). ATP is extremely effective, with over 90 percent successful termination of spontaneous VTs.[17] Cardioversion, in contrast to defibrillation, is a synchronized shock, usually of low energy. Compared to high-energy defibrillation, low-energy cardioversion reduces the time to therapy and conserves battery life. Efficacy rates and acceleration rates are similar for these two treatment modalities.[18]

All ICDs provide backup bradycardia pacing. Approximately 20 percent of ICD recipients need antibradycardia pacing, and most of them would benefit from a dual-chamber device.[19] However, it has been argued that dual-chamber ICDs confer advantages over single-chamber ICDs, including dual-chamber tachyarrhythmia sensing, atrioventricular synchrony, and the ability to optimize heart failure medications. As a result, in some centers, the majority of ICD implants are the dual-chamber type. A prospective randomized trial comparing dual-chamber with ventricular backup pacing in ICD patients with an ejection fraction ≤40 percent but without indications for antibradycardia pacing concluded that dual-chamber pacing was detrimental and significantly increased the combined primary endpoint of death or hospitalization for heart failure (27 versus 14 percent, $p < 0.05$).[20] Results from this trial and also from MADIT II[21] suggest that right ventricular (RV) stimulation promotes heart failure progression by the mechanism of ventricular desynchronization. As a result, consideration should be given to maintaining ventricular synchronization, either by implanting a single-chamber ICD with backup bradycardia pacing only or, in select patients with symptomatic heart failure, considering a dual-chamber biventricular ICD.

## DEVICE IMPLANTATION

ICDs are implanted using techniques similar to those for permanent pacemaker implantation (Fig. 38-4). An integrated lead—consisting of pace-sense electrodes and either one (right ventricular) or two (right ventricular and superior vena cava) high-energy defibrillation coils—is inserted, preferably via the cephalic vein to avoid the risks of subclavian puncture and possibly future subclavian crush syndrome.[22] In patients requiring a dual-chamber device, a separate atrial lead is inserted; in select patients with severe left ventricular dysfunction, cardiac resynchronization therapy may be delivered via an additional coronary sinus lead (Fig. 38-4).

Local anesthesia in conjunction with intravenous sedation is now the most frequently applied method of anesthesia.[23] The pulse generator is usually implanted into a subcutaneous pocket; however, patients with a thin layer of subcutaneous tissue may still require subpectoral implantation. As outlined above, the position of the pulse generator affects the defibrillation wavefront; the generator should, when possible, be implanted in the left pectoral region. Right-sided implantation results in significantly higher defibrillation thresholds (DFTs) than left-sided implantation.[24] Correct lead positioning involves advancing its tip as close as possible to the apex of the right ventricle. During sinus rhythm, R-wave amplitude, rate of change of the signal voltage (slew rate), pacing threshold, and lead impedances are assessed. The minimum acceptable R-wave amplitude is greater than 5 mV, so as to ensure satisfactory sensing during both sinus rhythm and VF.

Safety margin testing is carried out at 10 J below the maximum output for the particular device. The device induces VF either by a critically timed T-wave shock or by very rapid burst (50-Hz) ventricular pacing. The relationship between defibrillation energy and success is best described as a sigmoid dose-response curve, the probability of success increasing steadily with each increase in energy until a 100 percent success plateau is reached.[25] Two successive successful defibrillations with a 10-J safety margin are required to satisfy implant criteria and to ensure future efficacy. Today it is relatively uncommon not to achieve an adequate safety margin at implantation. Boriani et al. achieved a safety margin of greater than or equal to 10 J and successfully implanted a single-lead unipolar system with a maximum energy output of only 29 J in 54 of 55 patients (98 percent).[26] If the safety margin test is failed at implantation, repeat testing can be performed after repositioning the lead (usually by attempting to get as close to the right ventricular apex as possible); changing the lead polarity, pulse duration, or waveform; adding additional defibrillation electrodes; taking the SVC coil out of the circuit; or changing to a higher-energy-output device. In addition, in unipolar systems, a pneumothorax can greatly increase the defibrillation energy requirement. In patients taking amiodarone, if an

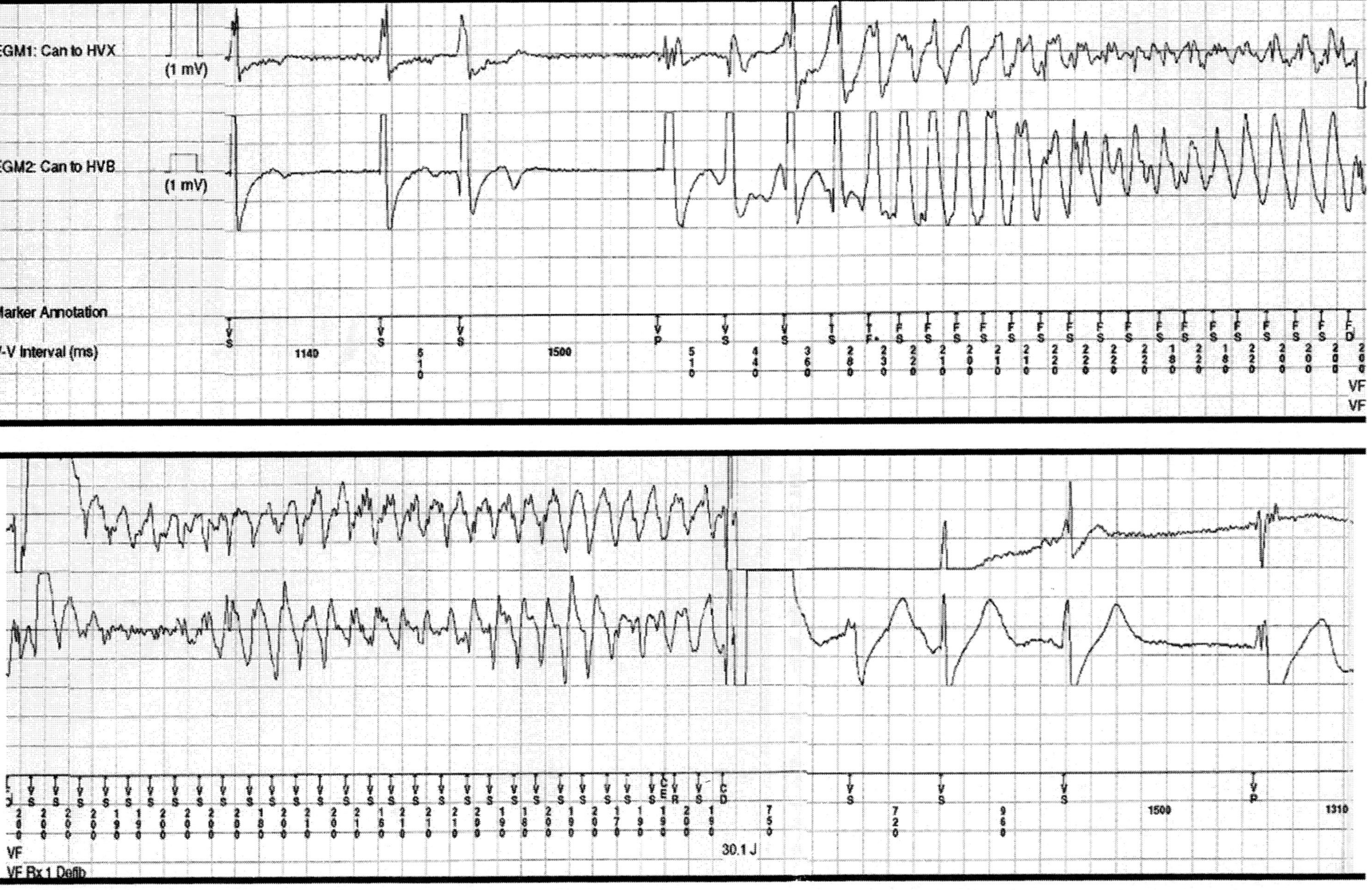


FIGURE 38-2 Stored electrogram of successful defibrillation of ventricular fibrillation. The recording is a continuous strip from a single chamber defibrillator. The output consists of two ventricular electrocardiogram channels (EGM 1 and EGM 2), a marker annotation channel, and a V-V interval (cycle length) channel. Two sinus beats are followed by a premature ventricular complex [all marked "ventricular sense" (VS)]. The subsequent pause is interrupted by a ventricular paced beat (VP), which is followed by an abrupt reduction in the cycle length. The reduction in the cycle length and change in QRS morphology is recognized as a tachycardia and the rhythmn is marked TF*. A period of rhythm confirmation is marked "fibrillation sense" (FS), after which VF is diagnosed (FD). While the device charges, it carries out a further confirmation of the diagnosis and ensures that the rhythm is sustained. A high-voltage, 30.1-J shock is delivered (CD), denoted by a full-scale positive rectangular marker in both the waveform and status channels. This restores sinus rhythm (VS) with restoration of the normal cycle length. Total duration of VF is approximately 11 s. Information regarding the device, date and time of the episode, duration, and the reason the event was stored is located on a separate printout

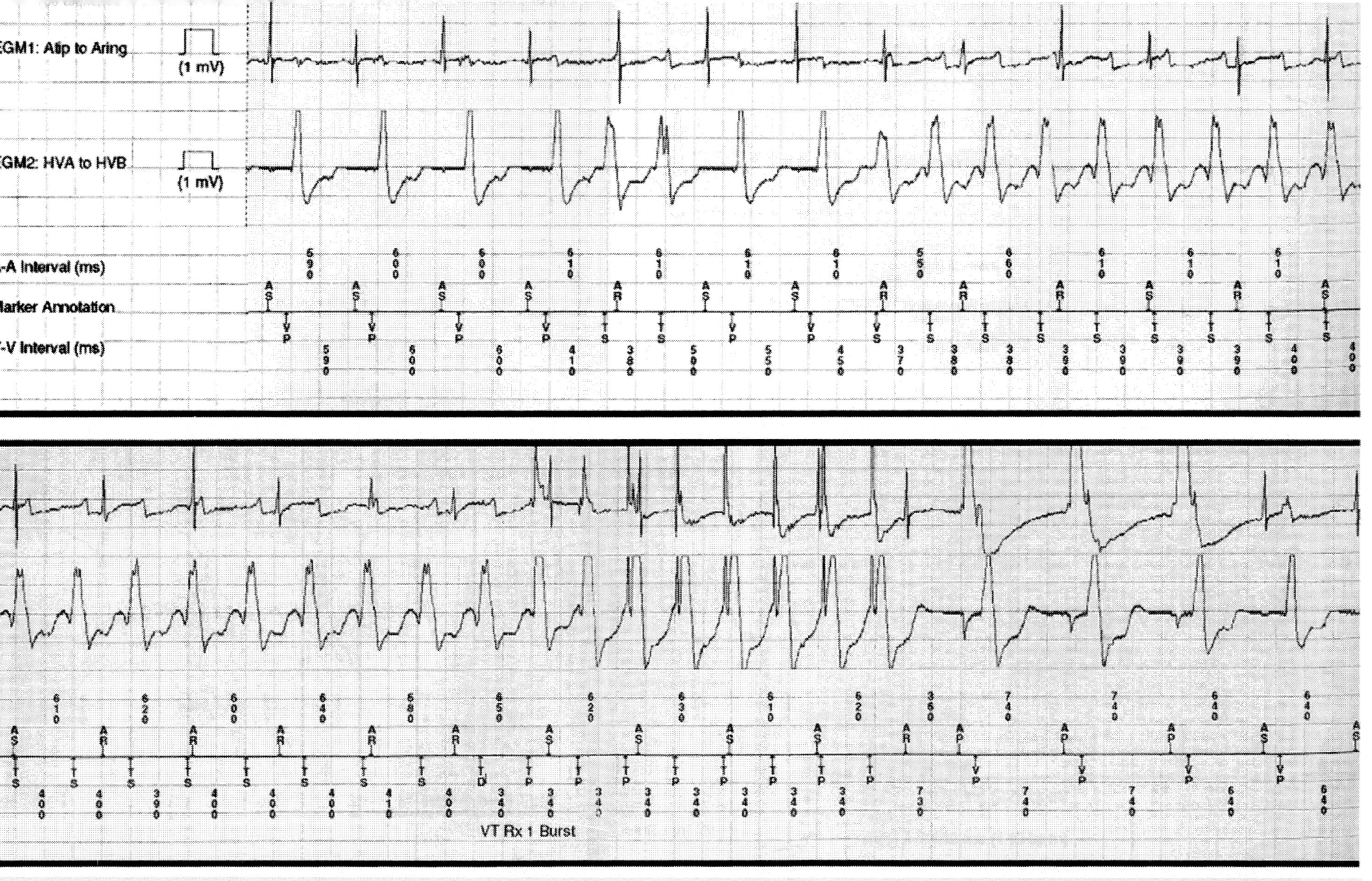


FIGURE 38-3 Stored electrogram of successful antitachycardia pacing of VT. The recording is a continuous strip recorded from a dual-chamber defibrillator. It consists of an atrial electrocardiogram channel (EGM 1), a ventricular electrocardiogram channel (EGM 2), an atrial cycle length channel (A-A interval), a "marker annotation" channel, and a ventricular cycle length channel (V-V interval). The initial four beats are atrial sense (AS) and ventricular pace (VP). This period is followed by a premature ventricular complex (TS), which is recognized by a reduction in cycle length and a change in QRS morphology, after which an atrial event is sensed and marked "atrial refractory" (AR). The device then detects a further premature beat (TS) before the cycle length normalizes. This is followed by two atrial sense (AS) and ventricular paced (VP) beats. Subsequently the cycle length abruptly changes, as does the QRS morphology. There then follows a period of sustained tachycardia sensing (TS), during which the atrial and ventricular channels demonstrate atrioventricular dissociation. Once the detection criteria for VT are met, the marker annotation channel shows TD and the device delivers eight rapid antitachycardia pacing beats (TP), which terminate the VT, resulting initially in atrial and ventricular pacing, which then returns to the original atrial sensing and ventricular pacing. Successful antitachycardia pacing (ATP) in this patient avoided high-energy shock delivery. (Courtesy of Medtronic Inc.)

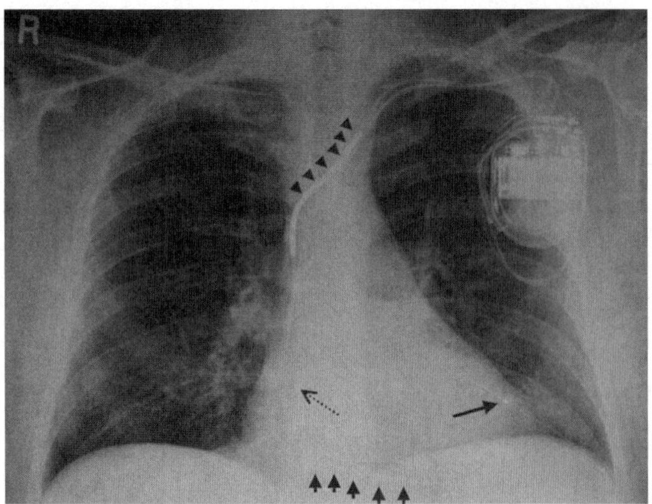

FIGURE 38-4 Posteroanterior chest x-ray of a pectoral dual-chamber biventricular ICD device. An integrated lead is inserted via the cephalic vein and positioned at the right ventricular apex (*arrowheads*). A left ventricular pacing electrode, introduced via a subclavian vein puncture, is positioned on the left ventricular free wall via a posterior coronary sinus branch vein (*solid arrow*). An atrial electrode is introduced via the cephalic vein and positioned in the right atrial appendage (*broken arrow*). These are attached to a pulse generator implanted in the left pectoral region. The integrated lead consists of right ventricular and superior vena cava defibrillation coils (*arrowheads*) and a tip electrode. In addition to the defibrillation coils, the titanium case of the pulse generator acts as a large-surface-area defibrillation electrode (*active can*). The defibrillation pathway in this patient is right ventricular coil to both superior vena cava coil and active can.

unacceptable safety margin is encountered at implantation, it is our practice to complete the procedure and retest the safety margin with intravenous sedation after a 4- to 6-week washout period.

Prior to discharge, the pace-sense characteristics of the ICD system are assessed in all patients and posteroanterior and lateral chest x-rays are reviewed to rule out lead dislodgment. Changes in lead position that can potentially result in failure to detect or terminate VF invariably result in a change in pace-sense variables relative to implant values. The characteristics of induced VT correlate poorly with those of subsequent spontaneous VT episodes due to the frequent induction of faster, "nonclinical" VT.[27] Fortunately, empirically programmed ATP successfully terminates VT in over 90 percent of cases.[17] As the most common tachyarrhythmia recorded during follow-up, even in VF survivors, is monomorphic VT,[28] empiric programming of a VT zone should be considered prior to discharge in the majority of ICD recipients.

A multicenter study of 473 patients implanted with a pectoral unipolar device reported successful device implantation in 98 percent of patients. In 7 percent, implant criteria either were not met or were not fully assessed. No patient died within 24 h of the procedure, and the 1-month (perioperative) mortality rate was 0.9 percent.[29] Patients were followed for a mean of 6 months. Twenty-nine patients (6 percent) had serious procedure- or device-related complications requiring surgical intervention. However, the complication rate depends on the definitions used and the duration of follow-up. If one includes mild device-related complications (e.g., inappropriate therapy delivery), approximately 50 percent of patients experience an adverse event within the first year of ICD implantation.[30] This must be considered when device implantation in high-risk asymptomatic patients is being recommended.

Lead-related problems—such as dislodgment, insulation defects, or conductor fracture, which can result in failure to sense, failure to pace, and either inappropriate defibrillation shocks or inability to defibrillate VF—remain significant despite the enormous advances in lead technology.[30]

One of the most devastating complications is infection of the ICD system. Among 950 patients who had a transvenous system implanted, the infection rate was 0.6 percent.[31] Infection resembles that observed with permanent pacemaker implantation. In general, explantation of the entire ICD system is required. If all clinical evidence of infection is resolved after a regimen of intense antibiotic therapy, reimplantation at a different site may be performed, but the risk of reinfection is higher than following a primary implant.

## LONG-TERM FOLLOW-UP

### Routine Patient Follow-up

Patients are reviewed routinely every 3 months to assess the pace-sense and impedance characteristics of the ICD system, to assess the charge times, and to diagnose the cause of any delivered therapy. Radiographs of the ICD system are obtained annually. Fortunately careful, regular follow-up will identify the majority of asymptomatic problems. If routine assessment reveals a significant alteration in the pace-sense or impedance characteristics of the system and if no defibrillation shock was recently administered, the safety margin is rechecked noninvasively under intravenous sedation. Medium-term follow-up has shown that by 1 year, 2.3 percent of systems have undergone a clinically significant rise in defibrillation threshold (DFT). This figure rises to 6.5 percent after 1 year.[32] However, one large series has shown an incidence of DFT rise of only 0.4 percent, with all but one of these cases being predicted by a change in pace-sense characteristics or the introduction of a new class I/III antiarrhythmic agent.[33]

Accurate diagnosis of the cause of an ICD shock is an essential part of the long-term management of ICD patients. Analysis of stored intracardiac electrograms recorded during the time interval preceding and following ICD therapy, in addition to marker channels that annotate each sensed event, results in a confident diagnosis of the causes of most ICD therapies (Figs. 38-2 and 38-3). If this analysis reveals inappropriate device function, real-time measurements (sensing, pacing, and impedance measurements) can be obtained, the ICD system can be x-rayed, and VF may be induced under intravenous sedation in order to determine the cause. Occasionally, problems such as loose connections become obvious only by device manipulation or a patient's movement during real-time telemetry. Accurate diagnosis is essential in order to institute the appropriate action, which may include device reprogramming, activation of VT-detection enhancement algorithms, alteration of antiarrhythmic drug therapy, or surgical revision of the ICD system.

All patients with an ICD should be considered for pulse generator replacement when there is evidence of battery depletion, since late shocks occurring many years after primary implantation appear to define a continuing need for this therapy in many patients. At the time of elective pulse generator replacement, the pace-sense characteristics of the ICD system are reassessed, and VF is induced in order to confirm satisfactory sensing and ability to defibrillate VF with a safety margin of 10 J or more. Occasionally, a patient's defibrillation energy requirements may be unexpectedly elevated at the time of generator replacement; appropriate revision of the system or implantation of a new integrated lead is then required.

### Psychosocial Issues

The ICD is generally well tolerated in the vast majority of patients for whom it is recommended. Large prospective trials comparing ICD and antiarrhythmic drug therapy have shown a similar effect on quality of life.[34] Furthermore, participants showed a significant improvement in quality of life in association with ICD implantation; however, amiodarone produced either no change in the quality of life or worsened it.[35] Depression, anxiety, and reduced sexual function may occur after device implantation. Factors that adversely affect quality of life include frequent or inappropriate shocks, device malfunction, or product recall. Since shock delivery has a major impact on quality of life, it is appropriate to consider measures such as concomitant drug therapy, empiric programming of ATP for VT, and use of detection enhancement algorithms to minimize the risk of both appropriate and inappropriate shock delivery during long-term follow-up. In a prospective, multicenter trial of ICD patients randomized to receive either sotalol or placebo, sotalol significantly reduced the mean annual number of shocks (1.4 shocks) compared to placebo (3.9 shocks) and significantly prolonged the time interval to first shock.[36] Also regular communication between health care providers (cardiologist/ICD specialist nurse/ICD technician) and ICD recipients about psychosocial issues can facilitate patient adjustment and identify patients who would benefit from more intensive support.

### Automobile Driving

A major concern among ICD patients is driving restrictions. Because of the risk of an arrhythmia recurrence or the delivery of high-energy shocks, restrictions on driving should be considered and discussed with all patients prior to device implantation. The period for greatest risk of ICD discharge is within the first 6 months after implantation. Patients receiving implantable defibrillators comprise a heterogeneous population. At one end of the spectrum is the patient with drug-refractory recurrent sustained ventricular tachyarrhythmia causing syncope or cardiac arrest, which is likely to receive more frequent device discharges. At the other end of the spectrum is the asymptomatic high-risk patient who has never experienced a spontaneous episode of life-threatening ventricular tachyarrhythmia. A more restrictive approach to the issue of driving seems appropriate for the former group of patients but is inappropriate for the latter and may make such patients unwilling to accept ICD therapy. The ACC/AHA/NASPE guidelines recommend that patients who receive an ICD because of a previously documented episode of VT or VF should be prohibited from all driving for the first 6 months after ICD implantation.[37] After 6 months, if an ICD discharge has not occurred, patients may resume driving. Patients who have a prophylactic ICD implant and who have never had a documented episode of spontaneous ventricular tachyarrhythmia should not be prohibited from noncommercial driving. The recommendations make no distinction between patients whose primary treatment is antiarrhythmic drug therapy rather than ICD therapy. In prospective comparative studies, patients with an ICD resumed driving no later than those treated with antiarrhythmic drugs.[38] Interestingly an anonymous questionnaire showed that 57 percent of ICD patients have resumed driving by 3 months against advice.[39]

## THE EVIDENCE BASE FOR ICD THERAPY

As a therapeutic modality, the ICD is unsurpassed in its ability to prevent SCD. Nevertheless, despite a marked reduction in SCD rates, overall mortality rates in ICD recipients remain high, with almost 20 percent 2-year mortality rates in most series.[40] The degree of survival benefit conferred by the defibrillator in a given patient population is dependent on the sudden arrhythmic death rate relative to the nonarrhythmic death rate. Patients with heart failure constitute a large proportion of ICD recipients. There was concern that implantable defibrillators may have little effect on overall survival rates in this population of patients for several reasons. First, as New York Heart Association (NYHA) functional class deteriorates, the proportion of deaths that are sudden and unexpected decreases. Second, successfully terminating an episode of VT or VF will have little effect on overall survival if the patient dies shortly thereafter of progressive pump failure. Because of these concerns, prospective randomized trials were conducted to test the hypothesis that ICDs significantly improve total survival rates.

### Secondary Prevention of Sudden Cardiac Death

Aborted SCD is, in the majority of cases, caused by life-threatening ventricular tachyarrhythmia (VF and hypotensive VT). Structural heart disease is almost invariably present, which, in adult populations, is most frequently coronary artery disease (see Chap. 41). Survivors of cardiac arrest, in the absence of an acute myocardial infarction (first 48 h), are at high risk of future recurrence. Data from the 1970s, which today reflect the natural history of this condition, show a 36 percent 1-year mortality rate in patients who were successfully resuscitated, hospitalized, and discharged home following an out-of-hospital VF arrest.[41]

The role of ischemia in the pathogenesis of SCD is not clearly defined. Only a small proportion of cardiac arrest survivors have clinical evidence of an acute myocardial infarction. Nonetheless, since the majority of cardiac arrest survivors have evidence of significant chronic coronary atherosclerosis, transient ischemia is suspected as one trigger factor for life-threatening ventricular tachyarrhythmia. Cardiac catheterization identifies those survivors of SCD who have critical obstructive coronary artery disease. It is our practice to revascularize these patients whenever feasible. Cardiac arrest occurring in the setting of acute clinical ischemia or within 48 h of an acute myocardial infarction is, with rare exception, treated in the conventional manner without electrophysiologic workup or ICD implantation. In addition, select patients with significant multivessel coronary artery disease, reversible ischemia on functional assessment, and no obvious arrhythmic substrate (no prior Q-wave infarction, preserved left ventricular function, and negative signal-averaged ECG) usually require revascularization rather than ICD implantation. In this group, we perform an electrophysiologic study following revascularization, and those with no inducible arrhythmias are considered to be a low-risk group; treatment usually consists of beta blockade.[42] These two groups (patients with acute clinical ischemia and those with significant multivessel coronary artery disease, reversible ischemia, and no obvious arrhythmic substrate) account for only a minority of cardiac arrest survivors. The majority of cardiac arrest survivors have an obvious arrhythmic substrate (prior Q-wave infarction, depressed left ventricular ejection fraction (LVEF), positive signal-averaged ECG, or inducible sustained monomorphic VT); in such patients, in addition to revascularization, we advise ICD implantation.

The results of three large prospective ICD trials comparing implantable defibrillators to antiarrhythmic drug therapy (mainly amiodarone) in patients with life-threatening ventricular tachyarrhythmia have consistently shown that the ICD improves overall survival. In the Antiarrhythmic Versus Implantable Defibrillator (AVID) trial of over 1000 patients, ICDs resulted in a 31 percent reduction in total mortality rate at 3 years compared to the antiarrhythmic drug therapy group (25 vs. 36 percent; $p < 0.02$).[43] The Canadian Implantable Defibrillator Study (CIDS) randomized over 600 patients to treatment with either the implantable defibrillator or amiodarone. After 3 years of follow-up, patients randomized to receive the implantable defibrillator had a 20 percent reduction in total mortality rate compared to amiodarone-treated patients (25 vs. 30 percent; $p = 0.07$).[44] The Cardiac Arrest Study–Hamburg (CASH) randomized 346 cardiac arrest survivors. During follow-up, patients randomized to receive the ICD had a 37 percent reduction in total mortality rate compared to antiarrhythmic treated patients (12 vs. 20 percent; $p = 0.047$).[45] Although each of these three large studies found lower total mortality rates in ICD recipients, only the AVID trial reached clear statistical significance. A metanalysis of these three trials found that the ICD reduced the total mortality rate by 27 percent compared to amiodarone ($p < 0.05$).[46] All three studies followed patients for a relatively short time (3 years). Follow-up of a subgroup of 120 patients from the CIDS study found that intention-to-treat survival curves for the amiodarone versus ICD patients continued to diverge up to 11 years after randomization.[47] As a result of evidence from these clinical trials, the ICD is now accepted as the therapy of first choice in survivors of symptomatic sustained ventricular tachyarrhythmia.

When a cardiac arrest is due to a transient or reversible disorder, correction of the underlying cause reduces the risk of recurrence and, according to the latest guidelines, ICD therapy is contraindicated.[37] This advice must be accepted with caution in light of recent analysis of the AVID trial registry of screened nonrandomized patients, which reported that the overall mortality rate in these patients remains unacceptably high.[48] Determining whether this high mortality rate is due to sudden arrhythmic death or progressive pump failure requires further study and may significantly affect our management of these patients.

## Primary Prevention of Sudden Cardiac Death

The majority of patients at risk of SCD have not previously experienced a sustained ventricular tachyarrhythmia. Because the prognosis associated with a first cardiac arrest is so poor, an effective primary prevention strategy is required to identify and treat high-risk patients who have not yet experienced a spontaneous episode of life-threatening ventricular tachyarrhythmia. Defining populations of patients who are at sufficiently high risk that primary ICD implantation is justified has been the focus of several prospective clinical trials (Table 38-1). Included are select patients with left ventricular dysfunction and nonsustained ventricular tachycardia (NSVT), high-risk coronary artery disease, patients who have undergone surgical revascularization, and patients with either ischemic or nonischemic dilated cardiomyopathy.

NSVT in the setting of a previous myocardial infarction and left ventricular dysfunction is associated with a 2-year mortality rate of approximately 20 to 30 percent.[49] The Multicenter Automatic Defibrillator Implantation Trial (MADIT) was designed to determine whether prophylactic ICD implantation in patients with prior myocardial infarction, left ventricular ejection fraction (LVEF) less than or equal to 35 percent, NSVT, and inducible, nonsuppressible VT or VF would improve survival rates compared to conventional medical therapy.[50] Total mortality rates in the ICD group were significantly less than in the conventional treatment group. The Multicenter Unsustained Tachycardia Trial (MUSTT) was designed to determine whether electrophysiologically guided antiarrhythmic therapy would reduce the risk of sudden death among patients with coronary artery disease, LVEF less than or equal to 40 percent, NSVT, and inducible VT or VF compared to no antiarrhythmic therapy.[51] Patients randomized to antiarrhythmic therapy (ICD or electrophysiologically guided drug therapy) had a significantly reduced arrhythmic mortality rate compared to the conservative treatment group. It is noteworthy that the improvement in outcome was entirely due to the ICD patients; electrophysiologically guided drug therapy (mostly class I agents) did not improve and may have worsened outcome. Therefore the results of the MADIT and MUSTT trials confirm that, in patients with coronary artery disease, depressed LVEF, NSVT, and inducible sustained ventricular tachyarrhythmias who have never had a spontaneous episode of sustained VT or VF, the ICD is effective in significantly reducing the risk of SCD and prolonging overall survival. In clinical practice, however, these patients are common and there is at present no consensus as to which patients should proceed to invasive electrophysiologic study and possible ICD implantation. Within the population of patients with prior myocardial infarction (MI), LVEF is the most powerful predictor of overall survival.[52] The Multicenter Automatic Defibrillator Implantation Trial II (MADIT-II) tested the hypothesis that ICD therapy improves survival compared to conventional medical therapy in patients with prior MI and LVEF <30 percent regardless of the presence or absence of arrhythmia markers. The results showed a clear survival advantage in subjects given an ICD.[21] At 3 years follow-up, total actuarial mortality in the ICD group was significantly less than in the conventional group (22 vs 31 percent, $p = 0.007$) (Fig. 38-5). The role of surgical revascularization in MADIT II–type patients must not be overlooked. The Coronary Artery Bypass Graft (CABG) Patch trial randomized patients with LVEF less than 36 percent and a positive signal-averaged ECG who were undergoing coronary artery bypass surgery to a prophylactic ICD or no specific antiarrhythmic therapy. There was no survival benefit from prophylactic ICD implantation, probably due to the beneficial effects of revascularization in the conventional treatment group.[53] Nonetheless, the results of MADIT II suggest that patients who have experienced a prior myocardial infarction who still have an LVEF <30 percent 3 months post-CABG remain better protected with an ICD.

The results of negative ICD trials emphasize the fact that ICD therapy prolongs survival in a population of patients only if that population has a sufficiently high incidence of life-threatening ventricular tachyarrhythmia and a sufficiently low incidence of death from all other causes. The cost-effectiveness of screening large numbers of these patients has not been assessed, but the challenge over the next few years will be developing means of accurately identifying patients at sufficiently high risk of life-threatening ventricular tachyarrhythmia and sufficiently low risk of death from all other causes in whom ICD therapy is both efficacious and cost-effective.

## Cost-Effectiveness

The cost of ICD therapy compared to alternative therapies has been the focus of much study and discussion in recent years. In addition to hardware costs (approximately $30,000), there are implantation costs, hospital admission charges, and the cost of routine follow-up and pulse generator replacement. Long-term costs must be compared with outcome measures, including total mortality rate and quality of life, in order to assess cost-effectiveness. When the results of pooled clinical trial data are added to a model to project the full gain in life expectancy, the cost-effectiveness of the ICD was $31,500 per life year added.[37] This compares favorably to surgical coronary revascularization ($18,200) and peritoneal dialysis ($57,300). Patient selection largely determines the cost-effectiveness of ICD therapy; the most cost-effective use of the ICD is in patients at high risk of death due to ventricular tachyarrhythmia and at low risk of death from

TABLE 38-1 Multicenter Primary Prevention ICD Trials

| Trial | Study Population | Treatment Groups | Sample Size | Primary Endpoint | Study Period | Outcome |
|---|---|---|---|---|---|---|
| **MADIT** (Multicenter Automatic Defibrillator Implantation Trial) | Prior MI with EF ≤ 35%, NSVT and inducible, nonsuppressible VT/VF | ICD vs. conventional medical therapy | 196 patients | Total mortality | 1990–1996 | Total mortality in ICD group significantly less than in conventional group (16 vs. 39%, $p < 0.01$) |
| **MUSTT** (Multicenter Unsustained Tachycardia Trial) | CAD with EF ≤ 40%, NSVT and inducible VT or VF | Antiarrhythmic therapy (ICD or EP-guided antiarrhythmic drug) vs. no antiarrhythmic therapy | 704 patients | Cardiac arrest or death from arrhythmia | 1990–1998 | 5-year incidence of cardiac arrest or death from arrhythmia significantly less among "antiarrhythmic therapy" compared to "no antiarrhythmic therapy" patients (25 vs. 32%, $p = 0.04$) |
| **CABG Patch** (Coronary Artery Bypass Graft Patch Trial) | CABG with EF > 36% and positive SAECG | ICD + CABG vs. CABG only | 900 patients | Total mortality | 1990–1997 | At 4 years follow-up, total actuarial mortality in ICD group no different than in control group (27 vs. 32%, $p = 0.7$) |
| **SCD-HeFT** (Sudden Cardiac Death in Heart Failure Trial) | Ischemic or dilated cardiomyopathy with CHF (NYHA II–III) and EF < 35% | ICD vs. amiodarone vs. conventional group | ~2500 | Total mortality | 1996–Present | Ongoing |
| **MADIT II** (2d Multicenter Automatic Defibrillator Implantation Trial) | Prior myocardial infarction with EF ≤ 30% | ICD vs. conventional group | 1232 | Total mortality | 1998–2002 | At 3 years follow-up, total actuarial mortality in the ICD group was significantly less than in the conventional group (22 vs. 31%, $p = 0.007$) |

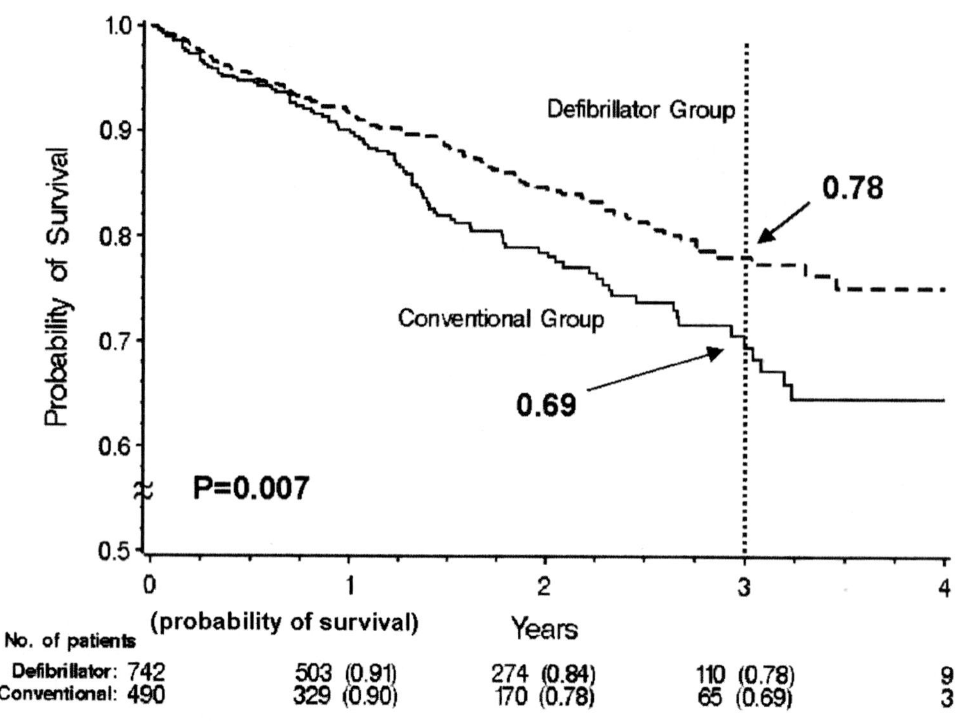


FIGURE 38-5 A Kaplan-Meier survival plot from the MADIT II trial showing that at 3 years follow-up, there was a significant survival gain in the ICD arm. Probability of survival 78 versus 69 percent, $p = 0.007$ (From the MADIT II investigators,[21] with permission.)

all other causes. More accurate risk stratification is necessary to ensure that ICD therapy is applied in an optimally efficient and cost-effective manner.

## ICD THERAPY IN SPECIFIC CLINICAL SETTINGS

### Sustained Monomorphic Ventricular Tachycardia

In patients with sustained momomorphic ventricular tachycardia (SMVT) that has resulted in a cardiac arrest or syncope, the ICD is usually employed as first-line therapy (Table 38-2). In patients with SMVT that is tolerated hemodynamically, other potential therapeutic options include empiric amiodarone therapy, electrophysiologically guided antiarrhythmic drug therapy, transcatheter radiofrequency ablation, and arrhythmia surgery. Empiric amiodarone therapy is associated with high rates of drug discontinuation due to adverse side effects. "Guided" drug therapy using either invasive electrophysiologic study or noninvasive Holter monitoring has failed to adequately protect against arrhythmia recurrence and has largely been abandoned. Catheter ablation, the treatment of choice in patients with VT and structurally normal hearts, is usually employed only as adjunctive therapy in patients with underlying structural heart disease, typically in those with implanted devices.[54] Catheter ablation is suitable in only about 10 percent of patients with spontaneous sustained ventricular tachycardia.[55] Arrhythmia surgery is the only therapy with SCD rates similar to those for ICD therapy.[56,57] Although this approach can be curative, perioperative mortality rates are much higher than those associated with ICD implantation, ranging from 9 to 15 percent. Combined aneurysmectomy and intraoperative map-guided subendocardial resection yields a low rate of arrhythmia recurrence and is indicated only in highly selected patients who have a discrete left ventricular aneurysm.

In summary, compared to the other available treatments, ICD therapy is widely applicable, well tolerated, and associated with good short- and long-term results. Today it is the preferred mode of therapy in the vast majority of patients with structural heart disease and SMVT. The various therapeutic options available should be considered as complementary rather than competing therapies. In managing individual patients, more than one therapy or even all therapies may be employed over a period of time.

### Inherited Arrhythmogenic Ion Channel Syndromes

#### CONGENITAL LONG-QT SYNDROME

Congenital long-QT syndrome is characterized by syncope and sudden cardiac death due to malignant ventricular arrhythmias associated with congenital prolongation of ventricular repolarization. Patients usually present in childhood or early adulthood. The initial therapy of choice in the majority of cases is beta-blocker therapy. Long-term follow-up of patients on beta-blocker therapy reveals a 4 percent overall risk of cardiac arrest in patients with the more common forms of long-QT syndrome (LQT1 and LQT2) and a 17 percent risk of cardiac arrest in the small subgroup of LQT3 patients.[58] The comorbidity and long-term problems associated with device therapy must be carefully assessed when ICD therapy is being considered, especially in patients who have yet to reach adult size. ICD implantation is recommended for select patients in whom recurrent syncope, sustained ventricular arrhythmias, or recurrent cardiac arrest occurs despite drug therapy. Furthermore, ICD therapy should be considered in patients in whom a cardiac arrest is the initial presentation, those with a strong family history of sudden death, or when compliance with or tolerance of drug therapy is poor.[37] In addition, primary ICD therapy should be considered in patients with the LQT3 genotype.

#### BRUGADA SYNDROME

Five to ten percent of out-of-hospital cardiac arrests occur in individuals with apparently normal hearts (idiopathic ventricular fibrillation). The Brugada syndrome represents one distinctive subgroup of idiopathic VF characterized by right bundle branch block, persistent ST-segment elevation in precordial leads $V_1$ to $V_3$, and a history of syncope or aborted sudden death. In contrast to the congenital long-QT syndrome, there is no effective drug therapy and the lethality rate associated with each arrhythmic event is substantially greater. As a result, the ICD is recommended as first-line therapy.[37] The role of ICD therapy in asymptomatic relatives with normal resting ECGs who exhibit the Brugada pattern following a pharmacologic chal-

TABLE 38-2 ACC/AHA/NASPE Guidelines for ICD Implantation

**Class I: ICD Indicated**
1. Cardiac arrest due to VF or VT not due to a transient or reversible cause
2. Spontaneous sustained VT in association with structural heart disease
3. Syncope of undetermined origin (SUO) with clinically relevant, hemodynamically significant sustained VT or VF induced at electrophysiologic study (EPS) when drug therapy is ineffective, not tolerated, or not preferred
4. Nonsustained VT in patients with coronary disease, prior MI, reduced LVEF, and inducible VF or sustained VT at EPS that is not suppressible by class I agents (patients who fulfill MADIT I criteria)
5. Spontaneous sustained VT in patients without structural heart disease not amenable to other treatments

**Class IIa: ICD Probably recommended**
1. Patients with LVEF $\leq$ 30% at least 1 month post-MI and 3 months post-CABG (MADIT II patients)

**Class IIb: ICD efficacy less well established**
1. Cardiac arrest presumed due to VF when EPS is precluded by other medical conditions
2. Severe symptoms attributable to ventricular tachyarrhythmia in patients awaiting cardiac transplantation
3. Inherited conditions with a high risk of life-threatening ventricular tachyarrhythmia such as long-QT syndrome, Brugada syndrome, or hypertrophic cardiomyopathy
4. Nonsustained VT with coronary artery disease, prior MI, reduced LVEF, and inducible sustained VT or VF at EPS (screened MADIT I individuals rather than patients)
5. Recurrent syncope of undetermined origin, SUO in the presence of a reduced LVEF, and inducible ventricular arrhythmia at EPS when other causes of syncope have been excluded
6. Syncope in patients with advanced structural heart disease in whom thorough invasive and noninvasive investigations have failed to define a cause

**Class III: ICD Not recommended**
1. SUO in a patient without inducible ventricular tachyarrhythmia and without structural heart disease
2. Incessant VT or VF
3. VF or VT resulting from arrhythmia amenable to surgical or catheter ablation
4. Ventricular tachyarrhythmia due to a transient or reversible disorder when correction of the disorder is considered feasible and likely to substantially reduce the risk of recurrent arrhythmia
5. Significant psychiatric illness that may be aggravated by device implantation or may preclude systematic follow-up
6. Terminal illness with projected life expectancy less than 6 months
7. Patients with coronary artery disease with a reduced LVEF and prolonged QRS duration in the absence of spontaneous or inducible sustained or nonsustained VT who are undergoing CABG
8. NYHA class IV drug-refractory congestive heart failure in patients who are not candidates for transplantation

SOURCE: Adapted from Gregoratos et al.,[37] with permission.

lenge with a sodium-channel blocking drug or in asymptomatic individuals in whom the Brugada pattern ECG is diagnosed as an incidental finding remains to be clarified, as does the role of diagnostic electrophysiologic testing in the risk stratification of such individuals.

## Hypertrophic Cardiomyopathy

Ventricular tachyarrhythmia is a common mechanism of sudden cardiac death in patients with hypertrophic cardiomyopathy. Well-established risk factors for SCD in this population include a family history of SCD in more than two primary relatives, a clear history of recurrent syncope, a flat blood pressure response (a less than 20-mmHg rise) during exercise, evidence of NSVT on ECG monitoring, and left ventricular wall thickness greater that 30 mm.[59] If any risk factors are present, amiodarone is recommended. If two or more risk factors are identified, ICD is recommended, as the risk of SCD rises substantially and ventricular tachyarrhythmia appears to be the principal mechanism of SCD in this subpopulation.[60]

## Syncope of Undetermined Origin

Syncope is a common, usually benign condition. However, when associated with structural heart disease and inducible VT at electrophysiologic study, it carries a high risk of SCD. One representative study reported a survival rate of 45 percent at 2 years in patients with syncope of undetermined origin and inducible sustained VT, compared to 16 percent in patients with negative electrophysiologic study results.[61] The risk of death in patients presenting with syncope plus inducible ventricular tachyarrhythmia on electrophysiologic study is similar to that in patients presenting with documented spontaneous VT or VF.[62] The ACC/AHA/ NASPE guidelines recommend ICD therapy in patients with syncope of undetermined origin, structural heart disease, and inducible hypotensive ventricular tachycardia (Table 38-2).

Patients with idiopathic dilated cardiomyopathy who present with syncope have a high mortality rate, and, in contrast to patients with coronary artery disease, the role of electrophysiologic study is ill defined. According to the latest guidelines, ICD therapy is contraindicated in patients with syncope of undetermined origin and no inducible ventricular tachyarrhythmia. Knight et al. reported on 14 consecutive patients with nonischemic cardiomyopathy, unexplained syncope, and a negative electrophysiologic test result who underwent defibrillator implantation.[63] Fifty percent of patients received appropriate shocks during 2 years of follow-up, supporting the use of ICD therapy in these patients. Prospective studies are needed to identify which patients with dilated cardiomyopathy and undetermined syncope may benefit from ICD implantation. Meanwhile, these patients need careful clinical assessment; surgical implantation of a continuous loop recorder (Reveal device, Medtronic Inc.) may be required to establish the diagnosis.

### Severe Left Ventricular Dysfunction

Prior to the publication of secondary prevention ICD trials, it was argued that preventing sudden death in patients with severe left ventricular dysfunction would not improve overall survival due to "conversion" of sudden death into a refractory heart failure death shortly thereafter. In contrast, subgroup analysis of both the AVID and CIDS trials has found that patients with an LVEF less than or equal to 35 percent derive the greatest survival benefit from defibrillator therapy.[64,65] Patients who describe NYHA class III/ IV limitation despite maximal tolerated medical therapy—with a QRS duration >130 ms and an LVEF <35 percent as well as a left ventricular end-diastolic diameter >55 mm—derive significant benefit from biventricular pacing.[37] A significant proportion of these patients are at high risk of ventricular arrhythmia. The Comparison of Medical Therapy, Pacing, and Defibrillation in Chronic Heart Failure (COMPANION) trial was designed to evaluate three treatment strategies: biventricular ICD therapy, biventricular pacemaker therapy, and maximal tolerated medical therapy. The data and safety monitoring board terminated this study early when it achieved its primary endpoint, a significant reduction in mortality and hospitalization. Although the full results are yet to be published, there was a 20 percent reduction in mortality and all-cause hospitalization in both device arms. Furthermore, there was a 40 percent reduction in all-cause mortality in the biventricular ICD arm.[66] One could speculate that the biventricular pacing reduced the number of heart failure deaths, whereas the ICD reduced the incidence of SCD. At present ICD therapy is contraindicated in patients with drug-refractory NYHA class IV heart failure unless they are awaiting cardiac transplantation based on the prediction that they are more likely to experience a heart failure death than an SCD.[37] This may no longer be appropriate for patients fulfilling the criteria for biventricular pacemaker implantation. One observation from both MADIT II and DAVID trials was a significant increase in hospitalizations for heart failure therapy in patients with severe left ventricular dysfunction receiving an ICD (see "Device Therapy," above). In a carefully selected subgroup, these undesirable hemodynamic consequences may be avoided by offering biventricular pacing.[67] It would therefore now seem appropriate to offer patients with severe left ventricular dysfunction and an indication for ICD implantation a device capable of both ICD and biventricular pacing therapy.

## FUTURE DIRECTIONS

It is anticipated that the number of ICD implants worldwide will continue to grow rapidly in the next few years, with significant implications for healthcare providers. Technological advances may assist this increased growth: more automated follow-up using systems such as continuous home monitoring will alert physicians to significant changes in pacing, sensing, or impedance parameters and allow remote interrogation following shock therapy; improvements in battery longevity should greatly increase the intervals between pulse generator changes and improve the cost-effectiveness of ICD therapy; sophisticated software may enable companies to sell a basic ICD package at a reduced price, and patients or their healthcare providers may later purchase programmable options if and when indicated.

The role of ICD therapy in the primary prevention of SCD will continue to grow. The greatest challenge will be delivering therapy to patients fulfilling the MADIT II entry criteria. In the short-term, therapy should be targeted at subgroups at greatest risk, such as MADIT II individuals with prolonged QRS durations. In addition, a significant proportion of patients requiring prophylactic ICD therapy will have symptomatic heart failure and an indication for biventricular pacing, greatly increasing the number of biventricular ICD implants. Preliminary data suggest that shock therapy can be safely delivered via an integrated lead inserted in the coronary sinus.[68] Advances in coronary sinus lead technology, resulting in a decreased rate of lead displacement, may in the future result in the development of a single-lead, left ventricle–based pacing-defibrillation system that is safe and reliable and incorporates the hemodynamic advantages of biventricular pacing.

Finally, research is required to more accurately risk-stratify patients at future risk of sudden cardiac death. Although primary prevention trials have identified clearly defined groups whose risk of death is reduced by ICD therapy, a substantial proportion of these ICD recipients never use their device yet are subjected to the morbidities and risks associated with long-term device therapy. Defining which subgroups of patients will not require ICD implantation or benefit from it is a major challenge for the future.

## References

1. Poole JE, Bardy GH. Sudden cardiac death. In: Zipes DP, Jalife J, eds. *Cardiac Electrophysiology: From Cell to Bedside.* Philadelphia: Saunders; 2000:615–640.
2. Valenzuela TD, Roe DJ, Nichol G, et al. Outcomes of rapid defibrillation by security officers after cardiac arrest in casinos. *N Engl J Med* 2000; 343:1206–1209.
3. Colquhoun MC. Defibrillation by general practitioners. *Resuscitation* 2002;52:143–148.
4. Cummins RO, Ornato JP, Thies WH, et al. Improving survival from sudden cardiac arrest: the "chain of survival" concept. A statement for health professionals from the Advanced Cardiac Life Support Subcommittee and the Emergency Cardiac Care Committee, American Heart Association. *Circulation* 1991;83:1832–1847.
5. Weaver WD, Cobb LA, Hallstrom AP, et al. Factors influencing survival after out-of-hospital cardiac arrest. *J Am Coll Cardiol* 1986;7:752–757.
6. Mirowski M. The automatic implantable cardioverter-defibrillator: an overview. *J Am Coll Cardiol* 1985;6:461–466.
7. Mirowski M, Mower MM, Staewen WS, et al. Standby automatic defibrillator. An approach to prevention of sudden coronary death. *Arch Intern Med* 1970;126:158–161.
8. Mirowski M, Reid PR, Mower MM, et al. Termination of malignant ventricular arrhythmias with an implanted automatic defibrillator in human beings. *N Engl J Med* 1980;303:322–324.
9. Investors Guide to ICD 2000. New York: Morgan Stanley Dean Witter and Co.
10. Olson WH. Tachyarrhythmia sensing and detection. In: Singer I, ed. *Implantable Carioverter Defibrillator.* New York: Futura; 1994:71.
11. Marchlinski FE, Callans DJ, Gottlieb CD, et al. Benefits and lessons learned from stored electrogram information in implantable defibrillators. *J Cardiovasc Electrophysiol* 1995;6:832–851.
12. Weber M, Bocker D, Bansch D, et al. Efficacy and safety of the initial use of stability and onset criteria in implantable cardioverter defibrillators. *J Cardiovasc Electrophysiol* 1999;10:145–153.

13. Nair M, Saoudi N, Kroiss D, et al. Automatic arrhythmia identification using analysis of the atrioventricular association. Application to a new generation of implantable defibrillators. Participating Centers of the Automatic Recognition of Arrhythmia Study Group. *Circulation* 1997;95:967–973.
14. Hintringer F, Schwarzacher S, Eibl G, et al. Inappropriate detection of supraventricular arrhythmias by implantable dual chamber defibrillators: a comparison of four different algorithms. *Pacing Clin Electrophysiol* 2001;24:835–841.
15. Olatidoye AG, Verroneau J, Kluger J. Mechanisms of syncope in implantable cardioverter-defibrillator recipients who receive device therapies. *Am J Cardiol* 1998;82:1372–1376.
16. Almendral J, Arenal A, Villacastin JP, et al. The importance of antitachycardia pacing for patients presenting with ventricular tachycardia. *Pacing Clin Electrophysiol* 1993;16:535–539.
17. Grosse-Meininghaus D, Siebels J, Wolpert C, et al. Efficacy of antitachycardia pacing confirmed by stored electrograms. A retrospective analysis of 613 stored electrograms in implantable defibrillators. *Z Kardiol* 2002;91:396–403.
18. Bardy GH, Poole JE, Kudenchuk PJ, et al. A prospective randomized repeat-crossover comparison of antitachycardia pacing with low-energy cardioversion. *Circulation* 1993;87:1889–1896.
19. Geelen P, Lorga FA, Chauvin M, et al. The value of DDD pacing in patients with an implantable cardioverter defibrillator. *Pacing Clin Electrophysiol* 1997;20:177–181.
20. Wilkoff BL, Cook JR, Epstein AE, et al. Dual-chamber pacing or ventricular backup pacing in patients with an implantable defibrillator: The Dual Chamber and VVI Implantable Defibrillator (DAVID) Trial. *JAMA* 2002;288:3115–3123.
21. Moss AJ, Zareba W, Hall WJ, et al. Prophylactic implantation of a defibrillator in patients with myocardial infarction and reduced ejection fraction. *N Engl J Med* 2002;346:877–883.
22. Roelke M, O'Nunain SS, Osswald S, et al. Subclavian crush syndrome complicating transvenous cardioverter defibrillator systems. *Pacing Clin Electrophysiol* 1995;18:973–979.
23. Manolis AS, Maounis T, Vassilikos V, et al. Electrophysiologist-implanted transvenous cardioverter defibrillators using local versus general anesthesia. *Pacing Clin Electrophysiol* 2000;23:96–105.
24. Friedman PA, Rasmussen MJ, Grice S, et al. Defibrillation thresholds are increased by right-sided implantation of totally transvenous implantable cardioverter defibrillators. *Pacing Clin Electrophysiol* 1999; 22:1186–1192.
25. Singer I, Lang D. Defibrillation threshold: Clinical utility and therapeutic implications. *Pacing Clin Electrophysiol* 1992;15:932–949.
26. Boriani G, Frabetti L, Biffi M, et al. Clinical experience with downsized lower energy output implantable cardioverter defibrillators. Ventak Mini II Clinical Investigators. *Int J Cardiol* 1998;66:261–266.
27. Monahan KM, Hadjis T, Hallett N, et al. Relation of induced to spontaneous ventricular tachycardia from analysis of stored far-field implantable defibrillator electrograms. *Am J Cardiol* 1999;83:349–353.
28. Ruppel R, Schluter CA, Boczor S, et al. Ventricular tachycardia during follow-up in patients resuscitated from ventricular fibrillation: Experience from stored electrograms of implantable cardioverter-defibrillators. *J Am Coll Cardiol* 1998;32:1724–1730.
29. Bardy GH, Yee R, Jung W. Multicenter experience with a pectoral unipolar implantable cardioverter-defibrillator. Active Can Investigators. *J Am Coll Cardiol* 1996;28:400–410.
30. Rosenqvist M, Beyer T, Block M, et al. Adverse events with transvenous implantable cardioverter-defibrillators: A prospective multicenter study. European 7219 Jewel ICD investigators. *Circulation* 1998;98:663–670.
31. Smith PN, Vidaillet HJ, Hayes JJ, et al. Infections with nonthoracotomy implantable cardioverter defibrillators: can these be prevented? Endotak Lead Clinical Investigators. *Pacing Clin Electrophysiol* 1998;21:42–55.
32. Brodsky CM, Chang F, Vlay SC. Multicenter evaluation of implantable cardioverter defibrillator testing after implant: The Post Implant Testing Study (PITS). *Pacing Clin Electrophysiol* 1999;22:1769–1776.
33. Brunn J, Bocker D, Weber M, et al. Is there a need for routine testing of ICD defibrillation capacity? Results from more than 1000 studies. *Eur Heart J* 2000;21:162–169.
34. Schron EB, Exner DV, Yao Q, et al. Quality of life in the antiarrhythmics versus implantable defibrillators trial: impact of therapy and influence of adverse symptoms and defibrillator shocks. *Circulation* 2002;105: 589–594.
35. Irvine J, Dorian P, Baker B, et al. Quality of life in the Canadian Implantable Defibrillator Study (CIDS). *Am Heart J* 2002;144:282–289.
36. Pacifico A, Hohnloser SH, Williams JH, et al. Prevention of implantable-defibrillator shocks by treatment with sotalol. *d,l*-Sotalol Implantable Cardioverter-Defibrillator Study Group. *N Engl J Med* 1999;340: 1855–1862.
37. Gregoratos G, Abrams J, Epstein AE, et al. ACC/AHA/NASPE 2002 guideline update for implantation of cardiac pacemakers and antiarrhythmia devices: Summary article: A report of the American College of Cardiology/American Heart Association Task Force on Practice Guidelines. *Circulation* 2002;106:2145–2161.
38. Hickey K, Curtis AB, Lancaster S, et al. Baseline factors predicting early resumption of driving after life-threatening arrhythmias in the Antiarrhythmics Versus Implantable Defibrillators (AVID) Trial. *Am Heart J* 2001;142:99–104.
39. Akiyama T, Powell JL, Mitchell LB, et al. Resumption of driving after life-threatening ventricular tachyarrhythmia. *N Engl J Med* 2001;345: 391–397.
40. Block M, Breithardt G. Long-term follow-up and clinical results of implantable cardioverter-defibrillators. In: Zipes DP, Jalife J, eds. *Cardiac Electrophysiology: From Cell to Bedside.* Philadelphia: Saunders; 1995: 1412.
41. Cobb LA, Baum RS, Alvarez H III, et al. Resuscitation from out-of-hospital ventricular fibrillation: 4 years follow-up. *Circulation* 1975;52: III223–III235.
42. Kelly P, Ruskin JN, Vlahakes GJ, et al. Surgical coronary revascularization in survivors of prehospital cardiac arrest: Its effect on inducible ventricular arrhythmias and long-term survival. *J Am Coll Cardiol* 1990;15:267–273.
43. The Antiarrhythmics versus Implantable Defibrillators (AVID) Investigators. A comparison of antiarrhythmic-drug therapy with implantable defibrillators in patients resuscitated from near-fatal ventricular arrhythmias. *N Engl J Med* 1997;337:1576–1583.
44. Connolly SJ, Gent M, Roberts RS, et al. Canadian Implantable Defibrillator Study (CIDS): A randomized trial of the implantable cardioverter defibrillator against amiodarone. *Circulation* 2000;101:1297–1302.
45. Kuck KH, Cappato R, Siebels J, et al. Randomized comparison of antiarrhythmic drug therapy with implantable defibrillators in patients resuscitated from cardiac arrest: The Cardiac Arrest Study Hamburg (CASH). *Circulation* 2000;102:748–754.
46. Connolly SJ, Hallstrom AP, Cappato R, et al. Meta-analysis of the implantable cardioverter defibrillator secondary prevention trials. AVID, CASH and CIDS studies. Antiarrhythmics vs Implantable Defibrillator study. Cardiac Arrest Study Hamburg. Canadian Implantable Defibrillator Study. *Eur Heart J* 2000;21:2071–2078.
47. Bokhari FA, Newman D, Korley V, et al. Implantable cardioverter defibrillator versus amiodarone: Eleven years follow-up of the Canadian Implantable Defibrillator Study. *Circulation* 2002;106:19.
48. Anderson JL, Hallstrom AP, Epstein AE, et al. Design and results of the antiarrhythmics vs implantable defibrillators (AVID) registry. The AVID Investigators. *Circulation* 1999;99:1692–1699.
49. Bigger JT Jr, Fleiss JL, Kleiger R, et al. The relationships among ventricular arrhythmias, left ventricular dysfunction, and mortality in the 2 years after myocardial infarction. *Circulation* 1984;69:250–258.
50. Moss AJ, Hall WJ, Cannom DS, et al. Improved survival with an implanted defibrillator in patients with coronary disease at high risk for ventricular arrhythmia. Multicenter Automatic Defibrillator Implantation Trial Investigators. *N Engl J Med* 1996;335:1933–1940.
51. Buxton AE, Lee KL, Fisher JD, et al. A randomized study of the prevention of sudden death in patients with coronary artery disease. Multicenter Unsustained Tachycardia Trial Investigators. *N Engl J Med* 1999;341:1882–1890.
52. Shah PK, Maddahi J, Staniloff HM, et al. Variable spectrum and prognostic implications of left and right ventricular ejection fractions in

patients with and without clinical heart failure after acute myocardial infarction. *Am J Cardiol* 1986;58:387–393.

53. Bigger JT Jr. Prophylactic use of implanted cardiac defibrillators in patients at high risk for ventricular arrhythmias after coronary-artery bypass graft surgery. Coronary Artery Bypass Graft (CABG) Patch Trial Investigators. *N Engl J Med* 1997;337:1569–1575.
54. O'Callaghan PA, Poloniecki J, Sosa-Suarez G, et al. Long-term clinical outcome of patients with prior myocardial infarction after palliative radiofrequency catheter ablation for frequent ventricular tachycardia. *Am J Cardiol* 2001;87:975–979.
55. Kim YH, Sosa-Suarez G, Trouton TG, et al. Treatment of ventricular tachycardia by transcatheter radiofrequency ablation in patients with ischemic heart disease. *Circulation* 1994;89:1094–1102.
56. Hargrove WC III, Josephson ME, Marchlinski FE, et al. Surgical decisions in the management of sudden cardiac death and malignant ventricular arrhythmias. Subendocardial resection, the automatic internal defibrillator, or both. *J Thorac Cardiovasc Surg* 1989;97:923–928.
57. Geha AS, Elefteriades JA, Hsu J, et al. Strategies in the surgical treatment of malignant ventricular arrhythmias. An 8-year experience. *Ann Surg* 1992;216:309–316.
58. Schwartz PJ, Priori SG, Spazzolini C, et al. Genotype-phenotype correlation in the long-QT syndrome: gene-specific triggers for life-threatening arrhythmias. *Circulation* 2001;103:89–95.
59. Elliott PM, Poloniecki J, Dickie S, et al. Sudden death in hypertrophic cardiomyopathy: Identification of high risk patients. *J Am Coll Cardiol* 2000;36:2212–2218.
60. Maron BJ, Shen WK, Link MS, et al. Efficacy of implantable cardioverter-defibrillators for the prevention of sudden death in patients with hypertrophic cardiomyopathy. *N Engl J Med* 2000;342:365–373.
61. Mittal S, Iwai S, Stein KM, et al. Long-term outcome of patients with unexplained syncope treated with an electrophysiologic-guided approach in the implantable cardioverter-defibrillator era. *J Am Coll Cardiol* 1999;34:1082–1089.
62. Olshansky B, Hahn EA, Hartz VL, et al. Clinical significance of syncope in the electrophysiologic study versus electrocardiographic monitoring (ESVEM) trial. The ESVEM Investigators. *Am Heart J* 1999; 137:878–886.
63. Knight BP, Goyal R, Pelosi F, et al. Outcome of patients with nonischemic dilated cardiomyopathy and unexplained syncope treated with an implantable defibrillator. *J Am Coll Cardiol* 1999;33:1964–1970.
64. Domanski MJ, Sakseena S, Epstein AE, et al. Relative effectiveness of the implantable cardioverter-defibrillator and antiarrhythmic drugs in patients with varying degrees of left ventricular dysfunction who have survived malignant ventricular arrhythmias. AVID Investigators. Antiarrhythmics Versus Implantable Defibrillators. *J Am Coll Cardiol* 1999; 34:1090–1095.
65. O'Brien BJ, Connolly SJ, Goeree R, et al. Cost-effectiveness of the implantable cardioverter-defibrillator: results from the Canadian Implantable Defibrillator Study (CIDS). *Circulation* 2001;103:1416–1421.
66. http://www.guidant.com/webcast/. Guidant. Companion trial results. 2002.
67. Abraham WT, Fisher WG, Smith AL, et al. Cardiac resynchronization in chronic heart failure. *N Engl J Med* 2002;346:1845–1853.
68. Butter C, Meisel E, Tebbenjohanns J, et al. Transvenous biventricular defibrillation halves energy requirements in patients. *Circulation* 2001; 104:2533–2538.

C H A P T E R 39

# PEDIATRIC ARRHYTHMIAS

Ronald J. Kanter / Timothy Knilans



The physiology, natural history, and treatment options of arrhythmias in the fetus, infant, child, and teenager are influenced by developmental changes in cardiac dimensions and hemodynamics, pharmacokinetics and pharmacodynamics of antiarrhythmic drugs, and specific electrophysiologic features of the maturing heart. Furthermore, a growing understanding of the developmental changes in myocyte ion channels, intercellular connections, and autonomic nervous system influences is helping to unravel our knowledge of the gross changes that occur during maturation. Finally, cardiac arrhythmias in the young are relatively more likely to be related to structural congenital heart disease, compared with arrhythmias in adults.

This chapter will focus on arrhythmia substrates in patients having congenital heart disease, arrhythmias exclusive to the pediatric age range, and pharmacologic and nonpharmacologic treatment of these arrhythmias in children.

## CONGENITAL ABNORMALITIES OF THE SPECIALIZED CONDUCTION SYSTEM

Although there is not yet consensus regarding the precise embryogenesis of the specialized conduction system in the human heart, it clearly is derived from specialized tissue in the intersegmental zones of the primitive heart tube. The prevailing theories of this development appear in Fig. 39-1. Currently, the favored concept involves a single ring of tissue that arises in the primary junction between the primitive ventricle and the bulbus cordis, and that stains with antibodies to chicken ganglion nodosum.[1] As the rightward portion of the primitive atrium forms a connection with the bulbus cordis, and the outflow tracts form and septate, a portion of this encircling ring of specialized conduction tissue is carried rightward and superiorly to create relationships with the right atrioventricular (AV) ring and the aortic valve annulus. Normally, the majority of this tissue involutes, leaving only those portions associated with the lower interatrial septum, the central fibrous body, and the crest of the muscular septum to become the compact AV node and the penetrating bundle. Reports of dissections of the specialized conduction systems from malformed hearts have proved complementary and have resulted in the accurate prediction of the anatomy of the conduction system in many forms of complex congenital heart disease.

Combined efforts by the congenital heart surgeon, cardiac pathologist, and clinician have helped elucidate the anatomy and functional importance of the specialized conduction systems in all forms of congenital heart disease. Particularly noteworthy over the last half century have been the contributions by Jesse Edwards, LHS VanMierop, Anton Becker, Robert Anderson, Maurice Lev, Saroja Bharati, and Richard and Stella Van Praagh. The most important of these cardiac malformations are discussed later.

### 1-Transposition of the Great Arteries

In levo transposition of the great arteries (1-TGA), also known as congenitally corrected transposition, there are both AV and ventriculoarterial discordance. Therefore, systemic venous return enters the pulmonary arteries, and pulmonary venous return is directed to the aorta, as they should. The majority have associated structural defects, most commonly ventricular septal defect (VSD) and/or pulmonic stenosis. The specialized AV conduction system is also structurally different, usually giving a QS or qR pattern in $V_1$ and an rS or RS pattern $V_6$ on standard electrocardiogram (ECG; Fig. 39-2). In Anderson's series of hearts having 1-TGA,[2] the AV node was located anteriorly in the right atrium near the mitral-pulmonary junction. The

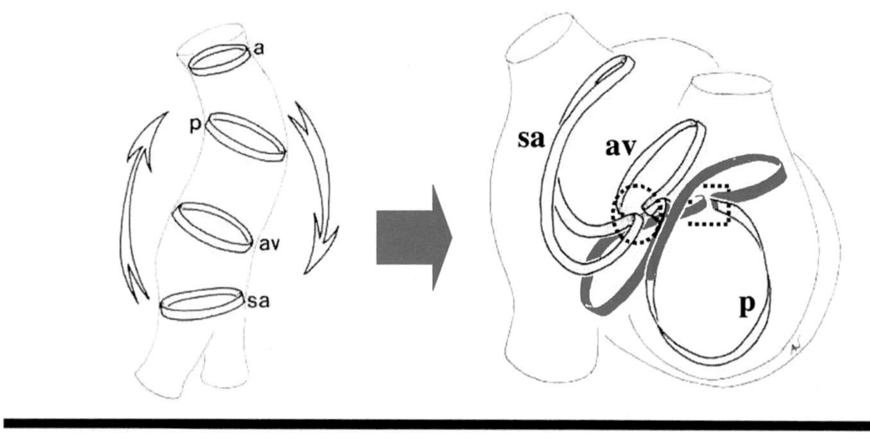


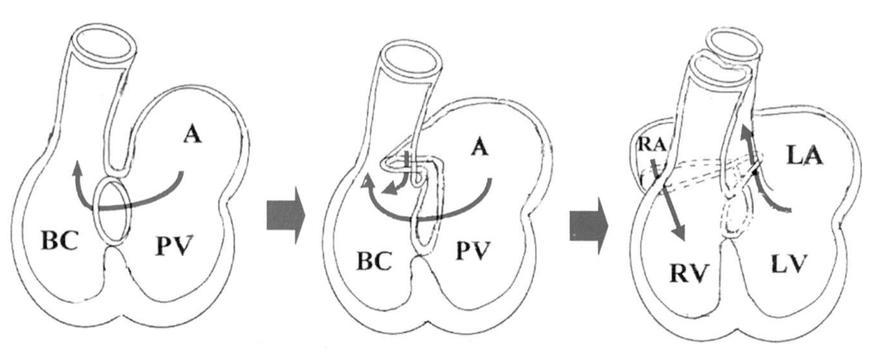


FIGURE 39-1 Two prevailing models of development of the specialized cardiac conduction system in the human. In the older model (*top*), the specialized conduction system derives from specialized tissue within the intersegmental zones of the sinoatrial junction (sa), atrioventricular junction (av), and the primary junction (p) between the primitive ventricle and bulbus cordis. These early relationships are depicted on the *left* when the heart tube is still straight. In the mature heart (*right*), the sa ring includes tissue of the sinus node, crista terminalis, Thebesian valve, and Eustachian valve. The AV junction forms from basal extension of the sa ring (to form part of the AV node), anterior invagination of the av ring (AV node), posterior invagination of av ring (AV node and penetrating bundle), and the p ring (distal penetrating bundle). The region of the AV node is identified by a dotted circle and the penetrating bundle by a dotted square. More recently, the concept that the specialized AV conduction system develops only from a ring of tissue encircling the primary interventricular junction (equivalent to "p" in the former model) (*bottom, left*) has been promoted. This tissue persists into the rightward expansion of the atrioventricular junction (*middle* and *right*) and accounts for the entire AV node and penetrating bundle. A = atrial mass; BC = bulbus cordis; LA = left atrium; LV = left ventricle; PV = primitive ventricle; RA = right atrium. (*Top* figures are adapted with permission from Wenink ACG. Embryology of the heart. In : Anderson RH, Baker EJ, Macartney FJ, et al. (eds). *Paediatric Cardiology,* 2nd ed. London: Churchill Livingstone; 2002:646.)

His bundle is relatively elongated as it crosses anterior to the pulmonary valve annulus before bifurcating on the anterior ventricular septum. When a VSD was also present, the His bundle bordered the anterosuperior quadrant of the defect. In most cases, a second, hypoplastic posterior AV node was also present just anterior to the coronary sinus, but only rarely did it connect with the ventricular mass via a posterior penetrating bundle. In specimens from older patients, the elongated penetrating bundle was typically infiltrated with fibrous tissue or completely disrupted. Congenital interruption of the penetrating bundle (and clinical AV block) in patients with 1-TGA has also been reported.[2]

Among 107 patients with 1-TGA, reported by Huhta et al.,[3] 22 percent had complete AV block, four congenitally. Data analysis showed an approximately 2 percent per year risk of developing AV block after diagnosis. The clinicians concluded that prophylactic pacemaker placement was not necessary in children, if their heart rates were greater than 50 beats/min. In patients also having a VSD requiring surgical closure, the risk of intraoperative AV block is higher than it is in patients not having 1-TGA. Special surgical handling of the superior portion of the defect is required to avoid this complication. In such cases, if AV block is avoided, the risk of late AV block is not increased.

Patients having 1-TGA have a higher than expected incidence of paroxysmal supraventricular tachycardia (PSVT)[4,5]—usually, AV reciprocating tachycardia (AVRT), utilizing one or more accessory AV connections associated with the left-sided tricuspid valve.[5] As a separate concern, because patients with 1-TGA have a high incidence of structural tricuspid valve (systemic AV valve) abnormalities, atrial fibrillation also occurs commonly, later in life.[6] Tricuspid regurgitation is associated with increased mortality at 20 years follow-up.[7] Finally, symptomatic ventricular tachycardia (VT) has been reported in 2 unoperated older patients (31 and 61 years old) having 1-TGA.[6,8]

## Tricuspid Atresia

Tricuspid atresia (TA) is a congenital abnormality of alignment in which there is no connection between the atrial mass and the morphologically right ventricle.[9] The right atrium ends in a muscular floor, and its only outlet is an atrial septal communication. The atrial and ventricular septa form normally (usually with a VSD). This causes the AV node to be located posterolateral to the blind-ending dimple in the muscular floor of the right atrium, maintaining a normal relationship with the tendon of Todaro and coronary sinus.[10]

The surface ECG reflects hemodynamic and anatomic influences, with right atrial enlargement in almost all, left axis deviation in about three fourths,[11] and a short PR interval ($<0.10$ s) in up to 12 percent[12] (see Fig. 39-2). Preexcitation occurs in between 0.29 percent[13] and 0.51 percent.[12] However, when Zellers and associates systematically evaluated 183 patients with TA, only 1 of 9 having preexcitation by ECG criteria actually had an accessory pathway,[12] prompting the use of the term *pseudopreexcitation* in the others.[13] Hence, clinical arrhythmias secondary to structural conduction system abnormalities are uncommon in patients having TA.

## Other Single Ventricles

This section will consider other congenital heart defects in which there is only one functional ventricle. "Hypoplastic left heart syndrome" is the most common of these but is associated with a normal specialized conduction system and does not merit further comment. The remainder of these complex congenital heart defects usually have abnormalities of the specialized conduction system. From the perspective of AV conduction, it is useful to consider these hearts according to whether there is left ventricular dominance or right ventricular dominance and according to whether there is ventricular dextro (d)-looping or l-looping. For example, when the ventricle is l-looped, there may be two AV nodes, one posteriorly located and the other along the anterolateral margin of the right AV orifice.

In the case of "double-inlet left ventricle," there is connection of anatomic right and left atria to the morphologically left ventricle, which, in turn, connects to the vestigial right ventricular outflow chamber via a VSD. There is transposition of the great arteries in 90 percent of cases, meaning that this outflow chamber is the systemic outlet. This may occur with d- or l-ventricular looping, but in all cases the ventricular septum does not extend to the crux of the heart but contacts the AV ring anteriorly. The primary ring of conduction tissue forms to the right of the interatrial septum, causing the AV node to from anterior and lateral to the atrial septum where it connects to the trabecular septum.[10] When there is ventricular l-looping and double-inlet left ventricle, the penetrating bundle has an elongated course, coursing anterosuperior to the VSD, and encircling the pulmonary valve annulus. It is prone to fibrous degeneration and complete AV block, as in hearts with two ventricles and l-TGA. If there is ventricular d-looping, the penetrating bundle is inferoposterior to the VSD. These anatomic considerations are critical, if surgical enlargement of the ventricular septal defect is necessary.

In single right ventricle, the ventricular septum always contacts the crux of the heart. In the presence of ventricular d-looping, the AV node is normally positioned with respect to atrial landmarks, and the penetrating bundle directly enters the ventricular septum.[14] In patients with ventricular l-looping, and "double-inlet right ventricle," or "straddling of the right AV valve," there may be an additional "sling" of conduction tissue[15] connecting two AV nodes.

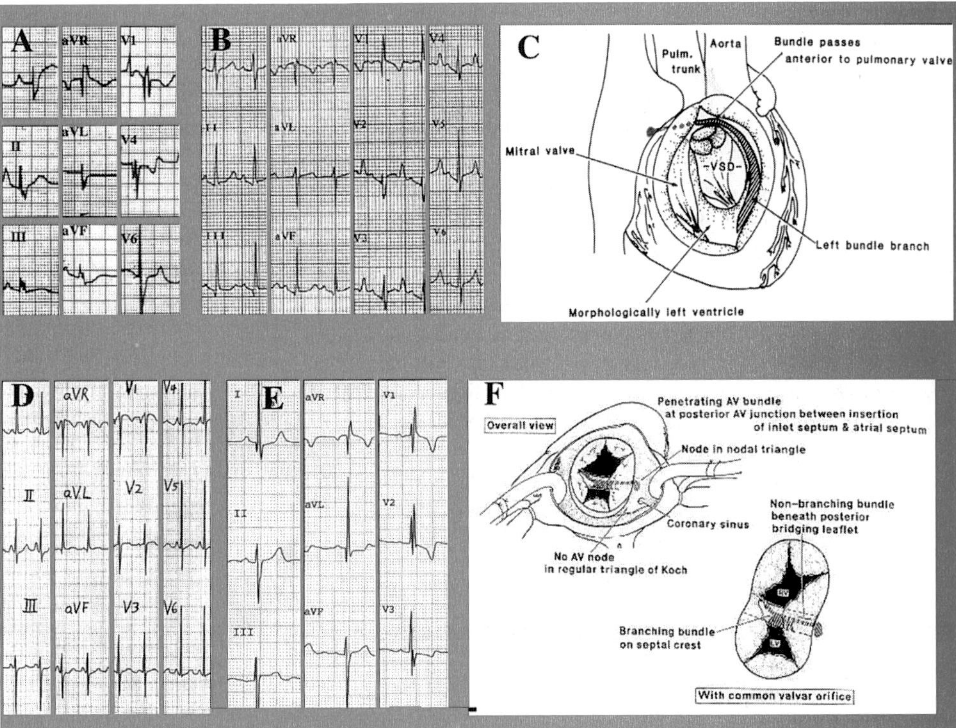


FIGURE 39-2 Examples of electrocardiograms from patients with congenital heart disease, who have both structural abnormalities of the specialized conduction system and abnormalities of cardiac chamber size due to the hemodynamic alterations. *A.* An 8-year-old with severe Ebstein's anomaly of the tricuspid valve, showing marked right atrial enlargement and incomplete right bundle branch block. *B.* A 3-year-old with l-TGA and pulmonic stenosis, showing a septal q in $V_1$ and RS in $V_6$, as well as right ventricular hypertrophy. *C.* The cardiac anatomy of l-TGA, showing the specialized conduction system and its relationships to a VSD. *D.* A 6-month-old with tricuspid atresia, illustrating left axis deviation, right atrial enlargement, and paucity of right-sided forces (abnormal R:S ratio in $V_1$). *E.* A 3-year-old with AV septal defect, demonstrating left axis deviation and right ventricular hypertrophy (RSR′ in $V_1$). *F.* Anatomic location of the AV conduction system in hearts with AV septal defect, from the surgeon's perspective (*top*) and in isolation (*bottom*). (*F* is reproduced with permission from Ebels T, Anderson RH. Atrioventricular septal defects. In: Anderson RH, Baker EJ, Macartney FJ, et al. (eds). *Paediatric Cardiology*, 2nd ed. London: Churchill Livingstone; 2002;955.)

## Ebstein's Anomaly of the Tricuspid Valve

In this disease, the tricuspid valve does not differentiate properly from the right ventricle, resulting in distal displacement of the tricuspid valve leaflets into the right ventricle. There may be significant tricuspid regurgitation into that thin-walled, hypocontractile portion of the right ventricle between the tricuspid valve leaflet coaptation plane and the normally positioned annulus. In moderate or severe cases, there may be chronic cyanosis, severe volume overload of both atria, and sometimes right ventricular outflow tract obstruction. Abnormalities of the right bundle branch and accessory AV connections are intrinsic malformations that are variably present. This combination of physiologic and anatomic abnormalities results in a patient group with a high incidence of arrhythmias. Even from early childhood the ECG from moderately or severely affected patients shows marked right atrial enlargement and—if Wolff-Parkinson-White (WPW) syndrome is not present—right ventricular conduction delay (see Fig. 39-2).

WPW syndrome occurs in 10 to 21 percent of patients[16–19] having Ebstein's anomaly. Paroxysmal supraventricular tachycardia contributes to morbidity but not to risk of sudden death,[16–18,20] and its incidence increases with age at presentation.[18,20,21] In Celermajer and associates' report of 220 cases of Ebstein's anomaly, arrhythmia was the most common presenting symptom (42 percent) in the adolescent and adult age group,[20] but not in children. Actuarial survival was 59 percent at 10 years, but sudden death accounted for only 14 percent of deaths. In Gentles et al.'s retrospective analysis of predictors of long-term survival in 48 patients,[19] 17 patients presented in the first week of life. Seven (14 percent) died by 5 months, none of whom had WPW syndrome. Of the 41 surviving patients, 10 (24 percent) had WPW syndrome, and there were 28 long-term (about 11 years mean follow-up) survivors (68 percent). Although atrial fibrillation was associated with nonsurvival ($p$ = 0.03), WPW syndrome did not appear to play a role in any deaths. Of 8 older patients having experienced sudden cardiac death, ventricular fibrillation related to severe cardiomegaly was thought to be the cause.

Most tachycardias associated with accessory pathways can now be treated nonpharmacologically. However, due to the abnormal anatomy, presence of multiple accessory pathways, and difficult accessory pathway potential mapping, radiofrequency catheter ablation of PSVT substrates has been especially challenging. Data from 65 Ebstein's patients undergoing catheter ablation were reported by Reich et al.[22] There were 82 nondecremental accessory pathways: 62 percent right freewall, 34 percent right septal, and 4 percent left-sided. There were 17 other supraventricular tachycardias: 1 atrial ectopic tachycardia, 7 AV node reentry tachycardias, 5 Mahaim fiber-related tachycardias, and 4 intraatrial reentry tachycardias (IART). Acute ablation success rates ranged from 75 percent for those not involving accessory pathways to 89 percent for septal accessory pathways. The overall recurrence rate was 30 percent. Smaller patient size and lesser degrees of tricuspid regurgitation predicted better acute and long-term success rates.

## Atrioventricular Septal Defect

In all forms of AV septal defect (AVSD), there are predictable abnormalities of the specialized AV conduction system. Embryologically, the AV node always forms at the insertion of the inlet ventricular septum and the atrial septum.[10] Due to the location of the AV septal deficiency in this disease, there is posteroinferior displacement of the AV node toward the ostium of the coronary sinus[23] (see Fig. 39-2). There is also a longer than normal penetrating bundle[10] and relative hypoplasia of the anterior portion of the left bundle branch,[23] resulting in the characteristic ECG findings: left axis deviation of the QRS complex with a superior counterclockwise vector loop in the frontal plane (see Fig. 39-2). Accessory AV connections may also exist in patients with AVSD, and they tend to be posteroseptal in location.

In Fournier and associates' small series of pre- and postoperative electrophysiology studies in 14 children (median age 3 years) with AVSDs,[24] sinus node dysfunction or first-degree AV block were common findings before surgery, but AV node dysfunction (in 4) and right bundle branch block (RBBB; in 13) were present postoperatively. Postoperative complete AV block is now uncommon following repair of this lesion, related to modifications in surgical technique. Arrhythmias related to postoperative hemodynamic status based upon Holter monitoring was reported by Daliento et al.[25] Among 106 patients, there was a 33 percent incidence of ventricular and a 10 percent incidence of atrial arrhythmias—highest in patients who were larger (and therefore older); who had a larger postoperative right ventricular end-diastolic dimension; who had had a large VSD; or who had postoperative RBBB. There were no episodes of sudden death.

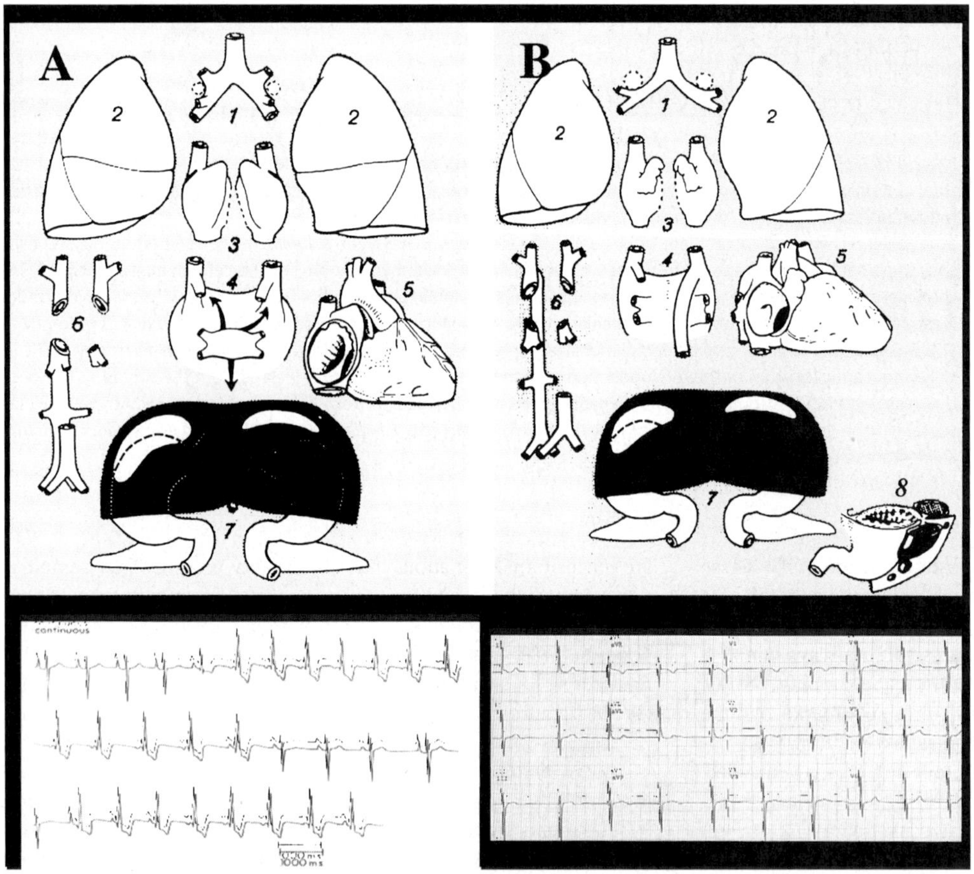

FIGURE 39-3 The heterotaxies. Characteristic gross organ abnormalities (*top*) and typical ECG findings (*bottom*) in *A*. Right atrial isomerism ("asplenia"). *B*. Left atrial isomerism ("polysplenia"). *A* depicts epiarterial bronchi (1), trilobed lungs (2), mirror-image right atrial appendages (3), and total anomalous pulmonary venous return (4). The rhythm strip shows evidence of duplicated conduction systems, with QRS axis changes following P-wave morphology and PR-segment changes. *B* shows hyparterial bronchi (1), bilobed lungs (2), mirror-image left atrial appendages (3), ipsilateral pulmonary venous return and azygos continuation of lower body venous return due to interrupted inferior vena cave (4), and multiple small spleens (8). The 12-lead electrocardiogram shows junctional rhythm. Common to both entities are common atrium, AV septal defect, and outflow tract obstructions (5); abnormalities in systemic venous return (6); and midline liver with gut malrotation (7). (The anatomic figures are adapted with permission from Van Mierop LHS, Gessner IH, Schiebler GL, Asplenia and polysplenia syndromes. *Birth Defects* 1972;8:36–43.)

## Heterotaxies

The heterotaxy syndromes are patterns of malformation involving multiple organs and thought to occur due to failure of lateralization of thoracic and abdominal viscera into either a normal pattern (situs solitus) or inverted pattern (situs inversus). They usually involve the cardiovascular system, often with severe congenital malformations. They are categorized as either right atrial isomerism (RAI) or left atrial isomerism (LAI), although there is great variability within each group (Fig. 39-3). The cardiac conduction system may be structurally abnormal, and congenital or acquired AV block is the most important clinical conduction defect.

Among patients having RAI (also known as "asplenia"), histopathologic studies have demonstrated bilateral sinus node-like structures, each at the superior vena caval–right atrial junction when bilateral cavae are present.[26,27] As might be expected, the P-wave axis tends to be inferior[28] and may vary, although the sinus rate tends to remain stable over time. The authors have observed two P-wave axes at different times in 2 patients each with RAI (see Fig. 39-3).

Patients with LAI (also known as "polysplenia") have hypoplastic or absent sinus node tissue in the lateral atrial walls.[27] Clinical correlates have included superior and unstable P-wave axis in 49 percent of patients,[29] and there is a tendency toward atrial rate slowing over time. By age 15 years, two thirds of children with LAI have been shown to evolve slow atrial or junctional rhythms[29](see Fig. 39-3).

Congenital or acquired complete AV block is frequent in patients with LAI, compared with those having RAI. In a series by Wren et al., 11 percent had AV block at presentation.[29] Histopathologic descriptions of the AV conduction systems in patients with LAI have frequently shown both anterior and posterior AV nodes, but often with discontinuity of both nodes with the ventricles.[27] This finding is most common in those having LAI and ventricular l-looping. Among those having two AV nodes/His bundles in continuity with the ventricular mass, a connecting sling of conduction tissue between the anterior and posterior penetrating bundles may be identified. Macroreentry tachycardias utilizing one specialized conduction system antegradedly and the other retrogradedly may occur and may be treated with catheter ablation of the retrogradedly conducting system.[30] However, the clinical relevance of most tachyarrhythmias in patients with heterotaxy is more related to the associated hemodynamic abnormalities imposed by the structural defects. Tachycardia suppression and support of unduly slow rate with artificial pacing are of great importance and may be technically challenging.

## ARRHYTHMIAS ASSOCIATED WITH COMMON CONGENITAL HEART DEFECTS

Among the most prevalent congenital heart defects are the VSD, the atrial septal defect (ASD), pulmonary valve stenosis, and aortic valve stenosis. Data regarding arrhythmia risk in patients having one or more of these lesions is available in natural history studies that have been reported in the last 15 years. The common general mechanisms of arrhythmogenesis include cumulative effects of hemodynamic abnormalities on myocardial tissue and specialized conduction tissue, plus the effects of surgical scar.

### Atrial Septal Defect

Clinically significant sinoatrial node dysfunction (SAND) may occur in some children and young adults with sinus venosus ASDs but not in those having ostium secundum ASDs. Since chronic left-to-right shunting results in dilatation of the right atrium and right ventricle in both lesions, the relatively proximate location of sinus venosus defects with respect to the sinoatrial node may play a role in this observation.[31] When considering adults having ASDs, however, the incidence of SAND has been reported to be 22 to 65 percent. Starting in early childhood and probably due to right ventricular stretch, right ventricular conduction delay is ubiquitous. Atrial flutter and/or fibrillation are increasingly prevalent in ASD patients with increasing age at presentation,[32–36] increasing pulmonary-to-systemic flow ratio,[31] and increasing pulmonary artery pressure.[33,34] This prevalence approaches 50 percent in patients >50 years old and 80 percent in octagenarians.[36] Surgical repair later in life may not protect these patients from atrial tachyarrhythmias. In a report by Murphy and associates of 123 patients who had undergone repair of ostium secundum or sinus venosus ASDs at the Mayo Clinic,[37] late follow-up (27 to 32 years) revealed that the incidence of atrial flutter or fibrillation increased directly with age at repair: 4 percent if operated on at ≤11 years old, 17 percent if at 12 to 24 years, 41 percent if at 25 to 41 years, and 59 percent if at >41 years. Pacemaker requirement was low for all groups (4 percent of total, including 2 with AV block). A more recent report showed additional risk factors for late postoperative atrial flutter or fibrillation: the presence of preoperative atrial flutter or fibrillation and the occurrence of immediate postoperative atrial flutter or fibrillation or junctional rhythm, as well as older age at surgery (>40 years).[38]

The First Natural History Study of patients having VSD, pulmonic stenosis, and/or aortic stenosis was based upon data from 2408 patients entered from 1958 to 1969. Upon original entry, 93 percent were less than 18 years of age. The following section is from The Second Natural History Study, which was published in 1993,[39] and is derived from late follow-up of those original patients. Of those patients having each of these defects, 87 percent were still less than 40 years old.

### Ventricular Septal Defect

Patients having a VSD develop chronic volume overload in the right ventricle, left atrium, and left ventricle proportionate to the size of the left-to-right shunt. In patients having large defects, pulmonary and right ventricular hypertension may also occur. Ambulatory ECG (Holter) data from 419 patients having a VSD demonstrated that 15.3 percent had supraventricular arrhythmias versus 5 percent of controls ($p < 0.0001$). Compared with age-appropriate controls, premature ventricular beats were more frequent in 11 to 17 percent of patients less that 40 years old (> 4/h) and in 22 to 39 percent of those greater than 40 years old (> 8/h). These incidences related to disease severity, occurring in 12 percent of those medically managed, in 20 percent of those surgically managed, and in 80 percent of those having Eisenmenger's physiology. The presence of *serious ventricular arrhythmias* (defined as the presence of ventricular couplets, multiform premature ventricular beats, or ventricular tachycardia) was determined from some combination of ECG, Holter, and exercise testing in all 1252 patients having a VSD. The incidences of and independent risk factors for having serious ventricular arrhythmias appear in Table 39-1. Again, these incidences increase with lesion severity. Clearly, arrhythmia risk is related to severity of hemodynamic alterations.

### Pulmonic Stenosis

Pulmonic stenosis results in right ventricular hypertension and hypertrophy proportionate to the degree of outflow tract obstruction. Treatment with surgical or balloon valvotomy can cause right ventricular volume overload from valve insufficiency. Among 182 patients having Holter data, 18.9 percent had supraventricular arrhythmias versus 5 percent of controls ($p < 0.001$), although this incidence was not influenced by prior valvotomy. However, only those having prior valvotomy had more premature ventricular beats than controls ($p < 0.0001$), suggesting a role for volume loading from pulmonary valve insufficiency. The incidence of "serious" ventricular arrhythmia appear in Table 39-1. The incidence did not increase with lesion severity, and the overall incidence of ventricular tachycardia (2 percent) was not greater than that of control patients. However, the severity of hemodynamic abnormality as represented by

TABLE 39-1 Serious Ventricular Arrhythmias in Patients Having Ventricular Septal Defect, Pulmonic Stenosis, or Aortic Stenosis[39]

| | Serious Ventricular Arrhythmias* | | | Sudden Unexplained Death |
|---|---|---|---|---|
| Congenital Heart Defect | Incidence (%) | Independent Risk Factors | Odds Ratio | Incidence (%) |
| Ventricular septal defect | 31.4 | Main pulmonary artery pressure (1) | 1.49 | 4.0 |
| | | Age (2) | 1.51 | |
| | | NYHA class (2) | 8.53 | |
| | | Cardiomegaly (2) | 2.79 | |
| Pulmonic stenosis | 29.7 | Age (1) | 1.05 | 0.5 |
| | | Age (2) | 1.04 | |
| | | NYHA Class (2) | 7.93 | |
| | | Cardiomegaly (2) | 3.21 | |
| Aortic stenosis | 44.8 | Left ventricular end-diastolic pressure (1) | 2.02 | 5.4 |
| | | Aortic regurgitation (2) | 11.70 | |
| | | Gender (2) | 4.10 | |
| | | Prior aortic valve replacement (2) | 4.80 | |

*Defined as ventricular couplets, multiform ventricular premature beats, or ventricular tachycardia; (1) = upon entry into First Natural History Study; (2) = upon entry into Second Natural History Study (See text for details.)
ABBREVIATION: NYHA = New York Heart Association.

New York Heart Association class and by the presence of cardiomegaly was related to the likelihood of serious ventricular arrhythmia.

### Aortic Stenosis

Aortic stenosis results in left ventricular hypertension and hypertrophy proportionate to the severity of obstruction. Aortic valve insufficiency may be associated naturally or occur following surgical or balloon valvotomy. As ventricular compliance worsens, subendocardial ischemia eventually results from a decreasing diastolic transmural coronary perfusion gradient. Among 134 patients having Holter data, 24.8 percent had supraventricular arrhythmias versus 5 percent of controls ($p < 0.001$), unrelated to prior valvotomy. As in the case of pulmonic stenosis, 13 percent of patients having undergone prior valvotomy had premature ventricular beats at a rate exceeding normal for age ($p < 0.0001$ versus controls). The incidences of serious ventricular arrhythmias were high in these patients, as depicted in Table 39-1, with an overall incidence of VT (13 percent) much greater than in controls. This incidence increased with increasing lesion severity, unlike that in patients with pulmonic stenosis. Independent predictors of risk of serious ventricular arrhythmias were identified only in patients having undergone valvotomy or valve surgery (see Table 39-1) and included hemodynamic, demographic, and surgical procedure characteristics.

Among patients having all types of congenital heart diseases, the relationship of serious ventricular arrhythmia (from noninvasive monitoring) to symptoms or to sudden cardiac death is tenuous, at best. This relationship is also unclear in patients having VSD, pulmonic stenosis, or aortic stenosis, as seen in Table 39-1. Although the incidence of serious ventricular arrhythmia is similar among the three groups, the risk of unexpected sudden death is significantly higher among VSD (4 percent) and aortic stenosis (5.4 percent) patients, as compared with controls. Patients with aortic stenosis or VSD and severe hemodynamic alterations do require close surveillance.

## ARRHYTHMIAS LONG-TERM FOLLOWING CONGENITAL HEART SURGERY

This section will consider four categories of arrhythmias that are of clinical concern long-term following congenital heart surgery: (1) sinoatrial node dysfunction (SAND) and (2) intraatrial reentry tachycardia following complex atrial surgery, especially atrial redirection procedures (Mustard and Senning operations) and atriopulmonary connections in patients with a single functional ventricle (Fontan operation); (3) AV block following VSD closure; and (4) ventricular tachyarrhythmias following ventricular outflow tract surgeries, such as tetralogy of Fallot.

### Sinoatrial Node Dysfunction and Intraatrial Reentry Tachycardia

The longest experience with arrhythmias following atrial surgery is with the Mustard and Senning operations for d-TGA. These operations are intended to direct the systemic venous return to the mitral valve and pulmonary venous return to the tricuspid valve and involve creation of an intraatrial baffle with prosthetic material or pericardium (Mustard operation) or atrial wall, itself (Senning). These suture lines may damage the sinus node, perinodal structures, and their blood supplies. Symptomatic bradycardia presents as exercise intolerance, fatigue, or presyncope and syncope. IART (referred to as "atrial flutter" in older literature) may rarely predispose to sudden death. (*IART* and *atrial flutter* will be used interchangably in this section.)

It is pertinent to this discussion to note that most babies born today with simple d-TGA undergo the arterial switch operation instead of atrial redirection procedures. Among 250 patients who had undergone the arterial switch operation at two centers, 24-h rhythm monitoring failed to demonstrate significant arrhythmias at 24 to 29 months follow-up.[40,41]

All variations of the Fontan operation are designed to direct systemic venous return to the pulmonary arteries in patients with a functionally single ventricle. These operations originally required that all or part of the right atrium have an elevated mean pressure. Hence, hemodynamic factors in addition to surgical scars likely account for the atrial tachycardias observed in these patients.

## INCIDENCE AND "NATURAL HISTORY"

When evaluated by ambulatory ECG monitoring 5 to 10 years postoperatively, between 20 and 40 percent of patients having Mustard procedures are still in sinus rhythm[42–45]; between 7 and 35 percent are in junctional rhythm,[42,44,45] up to 40 percent are in slow ectopic atrial rhythm,[45] and 10 percent have atrial flutter.[42,44,46,47] In their series of 249 patients, Gewillig et al. reported a 2.4 percent per year loss of sinus rhythm, and the presence of junctional rhythm carried a 2.1-fold increased risk of developing atrial flutter ($p < 0.05$).[44] At 23 years median follow-up of 86 adults who had undergone the Mustard operation, Puley et al. reported 48 percent with supraventricular tachycardia (mostly IART) and 22 percent had pacemakers.[48] Risk factors for supraventricular tachycardia included pulmonary hypertension, right ventricular dysfunction, and junctional rhythm. Sinoatrial node dysfunction appears to be more common following the Mustard procedure than following the Senning operation.[49]

Sudden death occurs late after these operations in between 3 and 15 percent of patients,[42,44,48,50] and the presence of atrial flutter increases this risk up to 4.7-fold ($p < 0.01$). The mechanism of sudden death has been thought to be 1:1 AV conduction during atrial flutter either directly causing ventricular fibrillation or followed by marked overdrive suppression of all subsidiary pacemakers with resultant asystole. However, primary ventricular tachycardia in those having depressed right ventricular function may also contribute to this risk.

Among Fontan patients, Driscoll et al. found 20 percent of 352 patients required antiarrhythmic drugs and/or pacemaker implantation at 5 to 15 years follow-up.[51] They attributed right atrial stretch, impaired ventricular function, and AV valve insufficiency as potential causes for the "tachy–brady" syndrome. Gewillig et al. found an 18 percent incidence of arrhythmias at 8-year follow-up, based upon 78 long-term modified Fontan survivors.[52] Multivariate analysis disclosed older age, increased right atrial size, and elevated pulmonary artery pressures as risk factors for arrhythmia development ($p < 0.001$). The most sobering report comes from the National Heart Hospital in London, England, where the actuarial arrhythmia-free survival for hospital survivors was only 60 percent at 10 years.[53] Again, these patients tended to have higher mean right atrial pressures and lower ejection fractions.

It is becoming clear that in Fontan patients, the specific surgical technique plays a role in the incidences of atrial arrhythmias. Animal studies have suggested that the total cavopulmonary connection (TCPC) is less arrhythmogenic acutely than the atriopulmonary connection (ACP), especially if the anterior suture line does not involve the crista terminalis.[54] Clinical reports have shown a lower incidence of immediate and medium-term (2 to 8 years) postoperative atrial tachycardias in TCPC patients,[55–58] especially when the crista is not violated.[57] The 5-year arrhythmia-free survival rate is as high as 78 percent.[55] The logic of reducing the portion of the right atrium included in the higher pressure, systemic venous part of the circuit has been furthered by use of a complete extracardiac conduit. Amodeo et al.[59] reported late tachyarrhythmias in only 4 of 54 such patients, with a 5-year arrhythmia-free survival rate of 92 percent.

The incidence of pacemaker requirement in patients following the modified Fontan operation ranges from 5 to 15 percent.[51,60,61] The indications include tachy–brady syndrome, congenital AV block, or postoperative AV block. The reported incidence of late arrhythmic death overall is 2 to 3 percent.[51,60,62] These data will also be influenced by newer surgical techniques.

## NONINVASIVE EVALUATION

Even if there are no symptoms, signs of sinus node dysfunction following atrial surgery requires aggressive patient surveillance. Otherwise, 24-h ambulatory ECGs are sufficient every 2 to 5 years. In patients having chronic fatigue and in those having syncope or dizziness at rest or with exercise, a 24-h ECG and exercise test should be performed. Hesslein et al. performed treadmill tests on 25 children following the Mustard operation at an average age of 10.2 years.[63] Using a modified Bruce protocol, patients performed to exhaustion in 90 percent of tests. In 70.4 percent of tests, the maximum attained heart rates were more than two standard deviations below predicted ($p < 0.001$), and in 59.3 percent of tests, heart rates 5 min following exercise were more than two standard deviations below predicted ($p < 0.001$). This relatively sudden drop in heart rate immediately following exercise may correlate with the frequently observed fatigue and dizziness that many patients experience immediately following exercise. Of the patients tested, 47 percent had abnormally low exercise capacity.

For patients having less frequent paroxysmal episodes of syncope, dizziness, or palpitations, ambulatory electrocardiographic monitoring systems having memory are useful.

## ELECTROPHYSIOLOGIC TESTING

Prolongation of the sinus node or pacemaker recovery times has been reported in greater than 50 percent, prolongation of the sinoatrial conduction time in greater than 33 to 50 percent, intraatrial conduction delay in 76 to 90 percent, and increased atrial effective refractory period in 40 to 45 percent[64–66] of patients following Mustard or Fontan operations. In one report of Mustard patients, sustained atrial reentry tachycardia was inducible in 51 percent of patients, half of whom later developed spontaneous atrial flutter.[45] AV conduction is usually normal.

Following atrial surgery, electrophysiologic study is indicated for any patient who has experienced syncope, presyncope, or palpitations suggestive of a tachyarrhythmia; or who has documented non-sinus tachycardia. (If atrial flutter is the cause of symptoms, it can be argued that electrophysiologic study can be deferred unless catheter ablation is to be performed.) Even if noninvasive monitoring shows bradycardia as the source for syncope, cardiac catheterization and electrophysiologic study may be useful prior to pacemaker implantation for several reasons: (1) evaluation of AV nodal function; (2) identification and possible ablation of coexisting tachyarrhythmias; and (3) demonstration of venous and atrial anatomy pertinent to permanent lead implantation.

## MANAGEMENT

The recommendations of the American Heart Association (AHA)/American College of Cardiology (ACC)/North American Society of Pacing and Electrophysiology Joint Committee on Pacing as they relate to patients who have undergone atrial surgery[67] are to insert a pacemaker in any patient with (1) "symptomatic" bradycardia (dizziness, light-headedness, and near or frank syncope) correlated with sudden severe bradycardia; marked exercise intolerance and chronotropic incompetence; or congestive heart failure and chronic bradycardia; (class I indication); (2) tachy–brady syndrome requiring treatment with an antiarrhythmic drug (other than digitalis) that could suppress the sinus node (class IIa indication); or (3) a resting heart rate <33 beats/min or pauses exceeding 3 s (class IIa indication in a child, class IIb in a teenager). These recommendations are only guidelines; the authors have offered permanent pacing in children having less defined symptoms of fatigue, morning headaches, or daytime somnolence and only moderate bradycardia while awake. The interplay with hemodynamic function is also not well defined by these recommendations. For example, a Fontan patient with an adequate rate but chronically junctional rhythm may benefit greatly from atrial pacing. A small series has also described the value of atrial pacing in Fontan patients having protein-losing enteropathy.[68]

In these patients, the technical aspects of atrial pacing frequently requires novel approaches to lead placement.[69–71] Advances in interventional catheterization have benefited some patients when superior vena caval baffle obstruction is present. Catheter-delivered stents not only relieve hemodynamic abnormalities, but may permit placement of intravenous pacing systems. The most contemporary iteration of the Fontan operation involves a completely extracardiac conduit, placing the entire atrial mass in the pulmonary venous circulation. In these patients eventually requiring atrial pacing, epicardial pacing will be required. The ideal epicardial lead would then have to be *active* fixation due to extensive epicardial scarring and would have a low chronic pacing threshold and high impedance. Dual-chamber pacing is necessary if AV conduction is inadequate. AV synchrony is especially important in Fontan patients, and ventricular pacing alone—even with rate adaptiveness—may not be acceptable.[72] Dual-chamber epicardial lead systems or novel transvenous atrial and epicardial ventricular lead systems are required in these instances.

Since sudden death in patients having the Mustard and Senning operations is most likely linked to *tachy*arrhythmias, complete arrhythmia suppression is often the goal of therapy. Occasionally, patients having impaired AV conduction remain asymptomatic with atrial flutter, due to 2–4:1 AV conduction and may not require aggressive treatment. Patients who present with atrial flutter (with or without symptoms) should undergo transvenous or transesophageal overdrive pacing termination or direct current cardioversion. Chronic treatment with an AV node-blocking agent alone following a first episode is reasonable until a timeline of recurrences is established, especially if that event is not associated with syncope or other evidence for severe cardiovascular decompensation. Following recurrences, three options are available: Antitachycardia pacing (with AV node blocking drug); class I (with AV node blocking drug and bradycardia pacing) or class III agents (with bradycardia pacing); or radiofrequency catheter ablation. Implantation of an antiachycardia pacemaker may obviate the need for potentially proarrhythmic drugs, but safety and efficacy of this modality must be demonstrated by electrophysiologic testing in the drug-free state. Radiofrequency ablation of IART can now be performed with success rates at long-term follow-up of 70 to 80 percent.[73,74] This is now the authors' preferred approach in patients with recurrent IART (Fig. 39-4).

Pharmacologic suppression of atrial tachycardias is more difficult following the Fontan-type operations. The importance of AV synchrony and adequate diastolic filling time makes arrhythmia control especially crucial.[75] Combinations of antiarrhythmic drugs, often including amiodarone, is often necessary. Antitachycardia pacing is occasionally helpful,[71] but may result in dangerous rhythm acceleration. Radiofrequency catheter ablation of IART is more difficult in these patients, due to the frequent presence of multiple tachycardia circuits and the increased atrial wall thickness compared with atria after other heart operations. In the large series of patients undergoing catheter ablation for IART after surgery for congenital heart disease by Triedman et al.,[76] 63 patients had undergone the Fontan operation. Multivariate factors relating to acute success included use of an irrigated ablation catheter (odd ratio = 3.8) and, in-

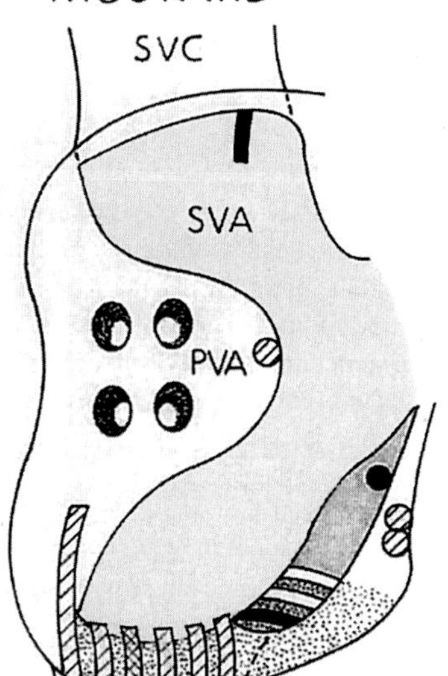


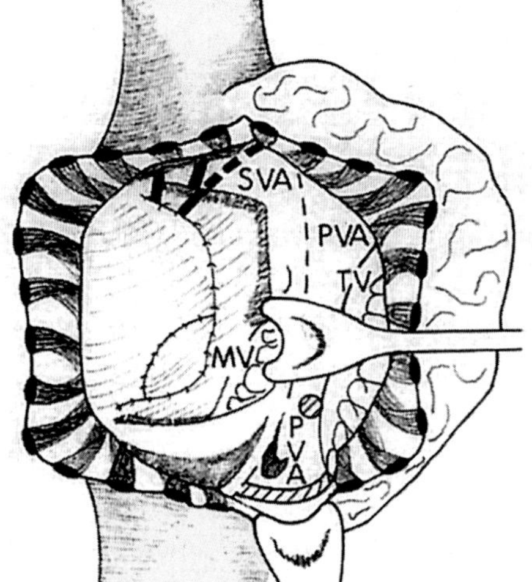


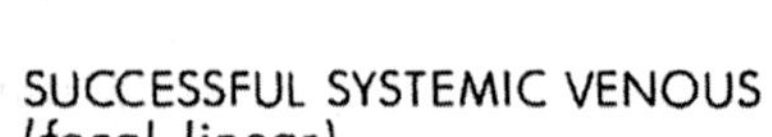


SUCCESSFUL PULM. VENOUS (focal, linear)

UNSUCCESSFUL PULM. VENOUS LINEAR

FIGURE 39-4 Successful and unsuccessful radiofrequency catheter ablation sites from patients having undergone the Mustard or Senning operations for *d*-TGA. Rectangular sites represent linear lesions for intraatrial reentry tachycardia, and circular sites represent focal lesions for "focal atrial tachycardia." In the figure depicting the Mustard operation, the gray region represents the systemic venous atrium, and the stippled zone represents the subtricuspid isthmus. In figure showing the Senning operation, the lightly shaded area is a part of the systemic venous atrium, whose roof (atrial freewall flap to the viewer's left) has been removed from its attachment to the atrial septal remnant (vertical dashed line); and a portion of the pulmonary venous atrium adjacent to the tricuspid valve is visible to the viewer's right of the vertical dashed line. IVC = inferior vena cava; MV = mitral valve; PVA = pulmonary venous atrium; SVA = systemic venous atrium; SVC = superior vena cava; TV = tricuspid valve. (Reproduced with permission from Kanter RJ, Papagiannis J, Carboni MP, et al. Radiofrequency catheter ablation of supraventricular tachycardia substrates after Mustard and Senning operations for d-transposition of the great arteries. *J Am Coll Cardiol* 2000;35:428–441.)

versely, a history of atrial fibrillation (odds ratio = 0.43). Favorable outcome at medium-term follow-up was related to complete procedural success (odds ratio = 3.9), the use of an electroanatomic mapping technique (odds ratio = 2.4); and, inversely, the number of IART circuits (odds ratio = 0.58).[76] Following the atriopulmonary connection-type of Fontan procedure, corridors of conduction critical to IART circuits and amenable to ablation seem to be clustered in the posterolateral right atrium associated with the atriotomy scar, in the subtricuspid isthmus (when present), and related to the atriopulmonary connection, itself (Fig. 39-5). Successful ablation of > 70 percent of these circuits is now being achieved,[77–79] although the recurrence rates remain high. Even better results can be expected with the use of larger tip and irrigated-tip ablation catheters, novel energy sources, and stereotactic catheter manipulation.

In 1998, Mavroudis and associates reported a surgical approach for IART treatment following the atriopulmonary-type Fontan patients, involving conversion to an extracardiac conduit with concomitant intraoperative mapping and a right atrial maze procedure (plus left atrial, if history of atrial fibrillation), using a linear cryoprobe.[80] These patients experienced improvement in hemodynamic status as well as arrhythmia control. The maze procedure may be tailored to the specific congenital anatomic substrate. Only 2 of their original 12 patients undergoing cryoablation still required antiarrhythmic drugs at 25 months median follow-up.[81]

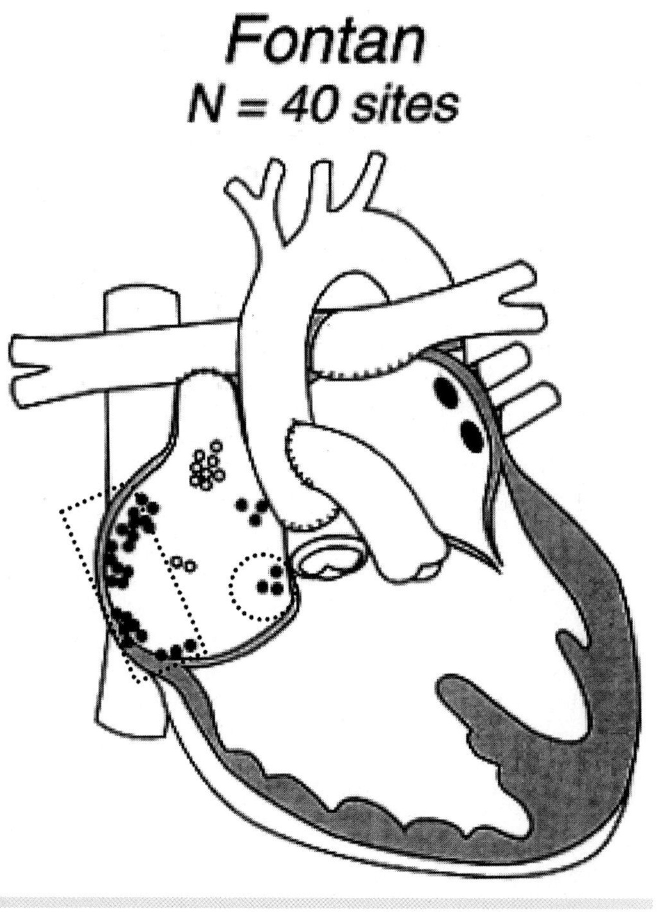

Fontan
N = 40 sites

FIGURE 39-5 Successful radiofrequency catheter ablation sites in patients having had Fontan operation (predominantly atriopulmonary connection) and intraatrial reentry tachycardia. Open circles are anterior, mostly associated with the right atrial appendage-to-pulmonary artery anastamosis; closed circles within the dotted rectangle are in the region of the right atriotomy; and closed circles within the dotted circle are in the region of the sub-tricuspid isthmus (when present). (Adapted with permission from Collins KK, Love BA, Walsh EP, et al. Location of acutely successful radiofrequency catheter ablation of intraatrial reentrant tachycardia in patients with congenital heart disease. *Am J Cardiol* 2000;86:969–974.)

## Arrhythmias following Ventricular Surgery

Postoperative AV block and ventricular tachyarrhythmias are the major clinical concerns in patients having undergone ventricular surgery. Based upon patients having undergone repair of tetralogy of Fallot, it was once believed that the occurrence of sudden death was related to sudden AV block; but it is now understood that ventricular tachycardia and fibrillation are the main etiologies. In general, complexity of the congenital lesion relates to the potential for residual hemodynamic abnormalities and risk of sudden death. For example, late sudden death ranges in incidence from approximately 4 percent of patients who have had VSD repair [24,82] to 18 percent of those who have had surgery for truncus arteriosus with single pulmonary artery.[83] This section will consider conduction disturbances and ventricular tachyarrhythmias separately. Most data are based upon patients having tetralogy of Fallot due to the high natural incidence of this defect.

### CONDUCTION DISTURBANCE

***Incidence and Clinical Significance*** Repair of tetralogy of Fallot requires closure of a perimembranous VSD and enlargement of the right ventricular outflow tract ("infundibulectomy"). Using this repair as a model for conduction system damage, approximately 80 percent of patients have complete RBBB, an additional 11 percent have the combination of RBBB with left axis deviation, and 3 percent have the combination of RBBB, left axis deviation, and first-degree AV block.[84] Accordingly, the presence of a prolonged HV interval or AV block at a slow atrial paced rate in any such patient having syncope may help guide clinical decision-making (see later). However, isolated RBBB rarely causes symptoms, irrespective of whether it resulted from proximal damage to the bundle itself, or from the right ventriculotomy and interruption of the distal Purkinje fibers in the right ventricular free wall. Nevertheless, patients having RBBB have issues, which—long-term—may be significant: (1) It will never be possible to identify progressive ventricular dilatation or hypertrophy from the ECG; (2) We are now learning that the dysynchronous ventricular activation, which always results from bundle branch block, may be deleterious to overall myocardial performance; and (3) In the presence of proximal RBBB, the development of left bundle branch block, which occasionally occurs later in life, will place these patients at risk for complete AV block.

***Evaluation*** Based upon the report by Friedli and Bolens, the ECG findings of RBBB and left axis deviation is usually associated with normal Q-wave to right ventricular apex activation times; and RBBB, left axis deviation, and first-degree AV block is usually associated with normal HV intervals in these patients.[85] Hence, the terms *bifascicular* and *trifascicular* block may not be appropriate, unless there are intracardiac conduction interval abnormalities. In the absence of symptoms, even "true" bifascicular or trifascicular block requires intervention in only certain circumstances: type II second-degree AV block during sinus rhythm; complete AV block; or marked HV interval prolongation (>100 ms). In the presence of syncope (and no inducible tachyarrhythmias), there is concern with any HV interval prolongation or block below the His bundle at atrial paced rates below 120/min.[85] In the presence of transient postoperative second-degree AV block or complete AV block (lasting less than 10 days postoperatively), 24-h ECG monitoring should be performed prior to discharge and then regularly. All patients following ventricular surgery involving the ventricular septum should have 24-h ECG monitoring every 2 to 5 years. The value of exercise testing to determine the maximum conducted sinus rate is unproved.

In the patient who has had an operation on the ventricles and has had syncope or presyncope, documentation of that patient's rhythm during symptoms is mandatory. The authors have seen syncope secondary to AV block, ventricular arrhythmias, atrial flutter with rapid AV conduction, and supraventricular tachycardia in this patient group. Although diagnostic techniques such as attached ambulatory event recorders ("loop recorders") or insertable loop recorders are reasonable first approaches, there is a tendency toward invasive electrophysiologic testing very early in that patient's course.

***Management*** Based upon the AHA/ACC/North American Society of Pacing and Electrophysiology Joint Committee on Pacing, a pacemaker should be implanted in any child with type II second-degree or complete AV block lasting more than 10 days postoperatively following heart surgery (class I indication).[67] In our opinion, similar consideration should be given to the patient with syncope and either a prolonged HV interval or AV block below the His at atrial paced rates below the 120 per minute. If ventricular tachycardia is also inducible, therapy must be individualized and ambulatory ECG event recording may be useful. Asymptomatic patients with prolonged HV interval or AV block below the His at atrial paced rates below 120 per minute should be followed closely with 24-h ambulatory ECG monitoring and exercise testing.

Occasional patients undergo pacemaker insertion in the postoperative period but later regain AV conduction. Data are not available to predict their risk of recurring AV block, but the question of pulse generator replacement inevitably is raised once the original unit reaches sufficient voltage depletion. In such instances, the authors use stringent criteria from 24-h ECG monitoring and electrophysiologic testing. Normal AV Wenckebach rate is required during incremental atrial pacing and a normal HV interval before considering discontinuation of permanent pacing. Even isolated marked first-degree AV block can cause symptoms analagous to pacemaker syndrome in some patients.

## VENTRICULAR TACHYARRHYTHMIAS

***Incidence and Risk Factors*** There are more data regarding ventricular arrhythmias from tetralogy of Fallot patients than from any other congenital heart defect. Therefore, most of the following comments are derived from that data. During 5 to 10 years mean follow-up after repair, ventricular arrhythmias were evident in approximately 5 to 10 percent of patients on routine ECG,[84,86,87] 20 to 40 percent on treadmill testing,[84,86,87] and 40 to 60 percent by 24-h ECG monitoring.[84,86–88] The presence and severity (using Lown grade) of ectopy has been historically related to older age at repair,[88–90] elevation of right ventricular systolic pressure (usually ≥ 60 mmHg),[84,86,88,90] and longer period of follow-up following surgery.[86,88,90] In contrast, Walsh et al. reported on 184 late survivors of tetralogy of Fallot repair, all of whom had been repaired before 18 months of age.[91] At mean follow-up of 60 months, there were no late arrhythmic deaths; and among 41 patients who had 24-h ECG data, only 1 patient had greater than Lown grade I ventricular ectopy. It was postulated that, compared with earlier series, the earlier age of repair may protect the heart from deleterious changes accrued from long-standing right ventricular hypertension, left ventricular volume overloading, and systemic desaturation.

The incidence of late sudden cardiac death following repair of tetralogy of Fallot ranges from 1.5 to 5 percent,[84,88,89,92] and most reports have implicated ventricular arrhythmias to be the etiology.[84,86,88,89,92] However, the association of that risk with asymptomatic ventricular arrhythmias of all Lown grades in questionable. It now appears that myocardial and global hemodynamic function are the critical determinants of arrhythmic risk. The paradigms of risk stratification are now requiring more sophisticated evaluation of myocardial metabolism, using magnetic resonance imaging and nuclear scanning technique but also relying upon new applications of old tests, such as the QRS duration and QT dispersion from the ECG (see later).

In summary, the preoperative milieu of chronic right ventricular hypertension and systemic desaturation, intraoperative myocardial preservation, and postoperative right ventricular hypertension and volume-overloading likely combine to influence risk of clinically important ventricular tachyarrhythmias. Earlier age of repair is now standard practice.

***Evaluation*** One of the main goals of routine evaluation of patients following ventricular surgery is to identify individuals who are at risk for symptoms or death from ventricular arrhythmias. The 12-lead ECG, chest radiograph, 24-h ECG, exercise tests, and echocardiogram all have roles in routine patient surveillance. Routine application of magnetic resonance imaging to quantify pulmonary valve regurgitant volume, radionuclide scanning to determine myocardial function, and signal averaged ECGs to identify late potentials are newer modalities being investigated. In patients with poor hemodynamics, follow-up is stricter than it is in those with excellent hemodynamics. Equivocal or minor symptoms may be evaluated with event recorders, but paroxysmal palpitations or syncope merit invasive electrophysiologic testing.

The 12-lead ECG may prove to be a valuable screen for patients at risk of having dangerous ventricular arrhythmias. An increased QRS duration appears to be sensitive and perhaps specific for such risk, with a cutoff value of ≥180 ms providing the greatest accuracy.[93,94] The coexistence of increased JT-interval dispersion may enhance the predictive value, suggesting that both repolarization and depolarization abnormalities are important.[94] There is also a correlation between an increased cardiothoracic ratio by chest radiograph and QRS prolongation.[93] Among correctable etiologies, cardiomegaly may result from either pressure or volume overloading. This new paradigm of risk stratification will soon incorporate measures of pulmonary valve insufficiency to help identify patients who will benefit from early valve replacement.

Despite the evolution in our knowledge of risk stratification in this patient group, Holter monitoring is commonly performed. Supporting its application from the older literature, the finding of complex ventricular arrhythmias [ventricular couplets, multiform ventricular premature beats (VPBs), or VT] on 24-h ECG monitoring was shown to reliably identify patients who subsequently have inducible ventricular tachycardia by electrophysiologic testing[88]; and Garson and associates showed that 7 of 21 patients having high-grade ventricular ectopy versus 0 of 421 having no ventricular ectopy eventually died.[95] However, the value of Holter monitoring has been called into question by Cullen's report of 47 patients prospectively followed for 12 years after an original postoperative Holter monitoring.[96] Those originally having high-grade ventricular ectopy (including 7 with nonsustained VT) were no more likely to later have clinical VT or to die suddenly than were those not originally having ventricular ectopy. The hemodynamic status was similar in patients of both groups. In conclusion, in this patient group, the presence of high-grade ventricular arrhythmias by ambulatory monitoring in a patient with poor ventricular function and/or the patient having a QRS duration ≥ 180 ms appears to be at high risk of clinical VT or sudden death.

The authors recommend invasive electrophysiologic testing following ventricular surgery in patients having sustained palpitations or syncope. The demonstration of symptomatic sustained monomorphic VT by noninvasive means is an indication for electrophysiologic testing only if catheter ablation is anticipated. In the era of implantable cardioverter-defibrillators, electrophysiologic testing as a guide for antiarrhythmic drug selection is becoming antiquated. In the absence of symptoms, ventricular programmed stimulation should also be considered if a patient has echocardiographic or catheterization-proven impairment of hemodynamics, significant cardiomegaly, or markedly prolonged QRS duration (see earlier), *plus* either Lown grade III ectopy or greater by 24-h ECG or during exercise testing.

Interpretation of data from patients having undergone programmed ventricular stimulation in this patient group has been obscured by a lack of uniformity in pacing protocol between institutions and heterogeneity in cardiac defects in patients studied. Chandar et al., in a multicenter study, noted that VT was not inducible in the presence of a negative 24-h ECG and normal right ventricular systolic pressure, but was inducible in 45 percent of patients having syncope, in 27 percent of those having high-grade ventricular ectopy, and in 47 percent of those having ventricular tachycardia by Holter monitoring.[88] Of 5 late deaths, none had inducible ventricular tachycardia with double extrastimuli, but all had at least one risk factor as defined earlier. More recently, Alexander and coworkers applied sophisticated statistical methods to a group of 130 patients who underwent programmed ventricular stimulation; 33 percent had tetralogy of Fallot, 25 percent d-TGA, and 12 percent left ventricular outflow tract obstructive lesions.[97] By univariate analysis, a positive study was associated with a sixfold risk of decreased survival. However, there was a 33 percent false-negative rate in 21 patients having documented clinical VT, and the positive predictive value of sudden cardiac death was only 20 percent. The entire group of patients had a 3 percent *annual* mortality and event risk, much higher than any previous reports. Thus, simply the subjective decision to perform ventricular programmed stimulation identified a group with a high prevalence of poor outcome. Contemporary diagnostic stimulation protocols add very little to the ability to assess risk in these patients.

SVT may also be the etiology of symptoms following ventricular surgery.[97,98] Among 53 tetralogy patients at 23 years median age, Roos-Hesselink et al. demonstrated atrial flutter or fibrillation in 23 percent and other supraventricular tachycardia in 11 percent.[98] The authors have ablated AV node reentry in several postoperative tetralogy patients. SVTs tend to be more poorly tolerated in these patients than they are in patients with healthy hearts. In summary, among patients having undergone ventricular surgery and who have tachycardias, electrophysiologic testing appears to be most useful to diagnose and treat supraventricular tachycardias and hemodynamically tolerated monomorphic macroreentry ventricular tachycardia.

***Management*** Symptomatic VT requires treatment. In the current era of device and ablation therapy, antiarrhythmic drug therapy has become less popular. Nevertheless, medium-term efficacy of phenytoin[99] and propranolol[100] has been reported, using serial electrophysiology studies and clinical follow-up. Amiodarone and sotalol are also potentially efficacious drugs. Class Ia drugs are not very useful for sustained VT in these patients, and class IC agents may be especially proarrhythmic.[101] Due to potential drug side-effects, suboptimal efficacy, and difficulty in proving efficacy, nonpharmacologic therapies are now favored. Following complete tachycardia circuit mapping in the electrophysiology laboratory, surgical resection, cryoablation,[102] and argon photoablation have all met with variable success. Radiofrequency catheter ablation has been used to successfully interrupt macroreentry VT circuits in several patients,[103,104] even when there are multiple VT circuits and when VT is poorly hemodynamically tolerated.[104] Newer electroanatomic mapping systems are very helpful in these patients. Programmed ventricular stimulation prior to hospital discharge and again at several months postablation is recommended to ensure successful elimination of VT substrate, unless an implantable cardioverter-defibrillator is also used. The implantable cardioverter-defibrillator is an excellent primary treatment modality for infrequent sustained monomorphic VT and is mandatory for patients having resuscitated sudden death. They provide antitachycardia pacing as well as the safety net of cardioversion or defibrillation, if necessary.[105]

Less clear are the indications for treating asymptomatic patients with high-grade ventricular ectopy by ambulatory monitoring. If their hemodynamics are acceptable, the authors would only follow these patients closely. In those with poor hemodynamics, options include ventricular programmed stimulation to *help* identify patients with inducible sustained tachycardia; surgical correction of hemodynamic abnormality when possible; or empiric implantation of implantable cardioverter-defibrillators. Until there are randomized clinical trials involving treatment and nontreatment of such patients, the best approach will remain unclear.

In summary, in patients who have undergone ventricular surgery, the authors recommend consideration of treatment for those who fall into the following categories: Asymptomatic patients with poor hemodynamics and high-grade ventricular ectopy by 24-h ECG monitoring or prolonged QRS duration; asymptomatic patients with poor hemodynamics and inducible sustained VT during electrophysiologic testing; and any patients with clinical sustained VT.

## SPECIFIC ARRHYTHMIAS IN THE YOUNG

This section will discuss arrhythmias specific to or requiring special considerations in this age group.

### Fetal Arrhythmias

Fetal arrhythmias are identified in as many as 3 percent of all pregnancies. Most arrhythmias are detected by auscultation during routine evaluation by the obstetrician. Less frequently, they are identified by ultrasound surveillance performed for routine evaluation of fetal development. Fetal echocardiography may be used to discriminate arrhythmia types, by using M-mode analysis of atrial and ventricular wall motion or of valve opening and closure; and by using Doppler flow across valves or in the aorta. More recently, fetal magnetocardiography has been employed to provide additional information about the mechanisms of arrhythmias and conduction abnormalities which are, otherwise, impossible to ascertain with conventional ultrasound techniques.[106–109] Newer Doppler tissue echocardiography helps evaluate the onset and pattern of propagation of ventricular activation and may provide additional information about the mechanisms of arrhythmias and conduction abnormalities.[110] The conventional ultrasound examination provides information about the physiologic response of the fetus to arrhythmias, including heart failure. Specifically, signs of fetal heart failure (hydrops fetalis) include ascites, pleural and pericardial effusions, and increased thickness of fetal scalp tissue from edema. Using current techniques, fetal arrhythmias may be detected as early as 6 weeks gestation.[111]

The vast majority of fetal arrhythmias are isolated atrial or ventricular extrasystoles and are usually benign.[112] They constitute about 70 percent of fetal arrhythmias in reported series.[113–116] Over 90 percent of these patients have atrial premature beats; the remainder being ventricular. Virtually all cases resolve at or shortly following birth.

Nonsinus fetal tachycardia represents about 15 to 20 percent of reported fetal arrhythmias.[113–116] Most of these patients have AV reentrant tachycardia, followed in frequency by atrial flutter. Other supraventricular and ventricular tachycardias are rarely seen. AV reentrant tachycardia typically has a rate of 250 to 300 beats/min and always has 1:1 relationship between atrial and ventricular mechanical events. It is most commonly initiated in the fetus by premature atrial contractions and terminated by AV nodal block and probably influenced by autonomic factors.[109] Atrial flutter has an atrial rate of 350 to 500 beats/min, typically with a ventricular rate one-half that of the atrial rate due to 2:1 AV conduction, but other conduction patterns are seen. It is rarely seen before 27 weeks of gestation, probably because the critical atrial size required to maintain macroreentry is not achieved until that age. Junctional and ventricular tachycardia may present with a ventricular rate faster than the atrial rate, but 1:1 retrograde conduction during these tachycardias make their diagnosis difficult using conventional ultrasound techniques. Again, magnetocardiography and Doppler tissue echocardiography may be helpful in prenatal diagnosis of these arrhythmias.[110]

Persistent regular fetal bradycardia constitutes about 10 percent of fetal arrhythmia and is usually caused by complete AV block.[113–116] Fetal ultrasound shows a regular pattern of ventricular contractions, which is slower and dissociated from the rate of atrial contractions. A minority of patients has associated congenital heart disease, usually severe. Patients with associated structural heart disease and those diagnosed in the first trimester have an extraordinarily high rate of fetal demise.[111] Nonconducted atrial bigeminy results in a regular ventricular bradycardia that must be discriminated from complete AV block. Ultrasound demonstrates an alternating long-short sequence of atrial mechanical events with a ventricular contraction sandwiched within the shorter interval of atrial events.

Treatment decisions for fetal tachycardia are based upon the duration and rate of tachycardia, the fetal response (signs of fetal hydrops, diminished fetal activity), and gestational age. Maternal administration of digoxin (load with 0.5 mg q 8 h × 3, attempting to achieve maternal level of 2 ng/mL) currently represents first-line therapy, but has a poor response rate when the fetus has hydrops.[117] Second-line therapy may include verapamil, sotalol, procainamide, quinidine, flecainide, or amiodarone. Maternal administration of flecainide (usually about 150 mg q 8 h) is especially efficacious, probably in part due to its excellent transplacental transfer, but proarrhythmic risk to the mother and negative inotropic effects on the fetus must be considered. Despite these risks to the hydropic fetus, flecainide may be considered first-line treatment. Atrial flutter is generally more difficult to control than AV reentrant tachycardia. Sotalol has been shown to be effective for treatment of fetal atrial flutter[118] and seems to be more effective for control of atrial flutter than it is for AV reentrant tachycardia.[119] Amiodarone may be required, despite the potential for causing fetal hypothyroidism. Maternal administration of amiodarone is generally well tolerated, but its longer administration course and poor transplacental transfer may delay treatment to the fetus. Direct fetal application of amiodarone (5mg/kg) using the umbilical vein, peritoneal cavity,[120] or intramuscular sites may result in a more rapid fetal response while limiting maternal effects. The long half-line of elimination is a benefit when this form of therapy is utilized.

## Congenital Heart Block

Congenital complete AV block occurs in about 1 of 22,000 live births and represents the most common cause of persistent pathologic bradycardia in the young. One quarter to one third of the involved infants have associated structural heart disease, most commonly l-transposition of the great arteries with ventricular inversion. In the majority of the remainder of patients, AV block is related to transplacental transfer of maternal autoantibodies of the anti-SSA/Ro or anti-SSB/La types. These IgG class proteins cross the placental barrier starting at 16 to 23 weeks gestation[121,122] and remain in the infant's circulation for up to 3 months postterm. Boutjdir and colleagues showed that perfusion of rat hearts with purified IgG, isolated from the serum of a mother with anti-Ro and anti-La antibodies (and whose child had complete AV block), resulted in inhibition of calcium current and no effect on the transient outward or inward rectifier potassium currents or sodium currents. This is consistent with the observation that inhibition of calcium channels is a factor contributing to congenital AV block;[123,124] however, other as yet unidentified factors appear to be involved. The pathology of the specialized conduction system in affected infants is variable but usually involves disruption and fibrosis of the compact node near its atrial inputs, while in other hearts, the disruption is closer to the penetrating bundle. About 75 percent of asymptomatic mothers having an infant with congenital heart block have anti-Ro antibodies.[125] Among women having clinical lupus or Sjogren's syndrome and anti-Ro or anti-La antibodies, the incidence of having an infant with congenital complete AV block is only about 2 percent.[126] The incidence of AV conduction abnormalities in individuals who themselves have these autoantibodies is low. Subsequent progression of less advanced degrees of AV block has been documented in infants whose mothers have autoantibodies, so an ECG should be performed at the time of birth on all such neonates.[127] Other children with congenital AV block and without structural heart disease or maternal autoantibodies have been shown to carry underlying genetic mutations known to be associated with AV block, such as mutations in NKX2.5, a homeobox transcription factor.[128,129] This same genetic mutation has been associated with structural heart disease in other members of the same families.

Once the diagnosis of congenital heart block has been made by fetal ultrasound, frequent follow-up is required. Efforts to reverse the destructive process occurring in the fetal conduction system by transplacental or umbilical venous administration of immunomodulatory agents are of unproven efficacy. Dexamethasone has been shown to improve some cases of intrauterine antibody mediated second-degree AV block, only to have it progress later to complete AV block.[127] Successful experiments in animals to artificially pace the fetal heart are fraught with ethical dilemmas when applying such a technology to humans.

Evidence for hydrops fetalis, irrespective of the escape heart rate, should prompt swift delivery, if the fetus' biophysical profile is favorable for extrauterine survival. Otherwise, measures to accelerate fetal lung maturity should be considered, so that delivery can be accomplished as soon as feasible. After delivery of the infant having congenital heart block, temporary transvenous, transesophageal, or transcutaneous pacing is necessary in the hydropic infant or in the presence of new onset of cardiovascular collapse. Permanent epicardial pacing may then be provided following a period of cardiopulmonary stabilzation. Deloof et al. reported success in treating two premature hydropic infants with this type of staged approach.[130] A fetus who is well compensated may decompensate after delivery due to increased oxygen consumption, increased work of breathing, and need for temperature self-regulation; but most nonhydropic neonates with complete AV block will be stable immediately after delivery.

Specific indications to permanently pace children with congenital complete AV block appear in Table 39-2.[67] In addition, it is becoming increasingly apparent that virtually all patients having congenital heart block should receive a pacemaker by early adulthood. This notion is supported by a longitudinal study from Sweden, which showed a disturbing incidence of sudden death among previously asymptomatic individuals with congenital heart block who had not been paced.[131] The authors recommend permanent pacing for all patients with complete AV block over the age of 15 years.[131]

TABLE 39-2 Recommendations for Permanent Pacing in Children, Adolescents, and Patients with Congenital Heart Disease

Class I: Conditions for which there is evidence and/or general agreement that cardiac pacing is beneficial, useful, and effective.

1. Advanced second- or third-degree atrioventricular (AV) block associated with symptomatic bradycardia, ventricular dysfunction or low cardiac output. (Level of evidence: C)
2. Sinus node dysfunction with correlation of symptoms during age-inappropriate bradycardia. The definition of bradycardia varies with the patient's age and expected heart rate. (Level of evidence: B)
3. Postoperative advanced second- or third-degree AV block that is not expected to resolve or persists at least 7 days after cardiac surgery. (Level of evidence: B, C)
4. Congenital third-degree AV block with a wide QRS escape rhythm, complex ventricular ectopy, or ventricular dysfunction. (Level of evidence: B)
5. Congenital third-degree AV block in the infant with a ventricular rate less than 50 to 55 beats/min or with congenital heart disease and a ventricular rate less than 70 beats/min. (Level of evidence: B, C)
6. Sustained pause-dependent VT, with or without prolonged QT, in which the efficacy of pacing is thoroughly documented. (Level of evidence: B)

Class IIa: Conditions for which there is conflicting evidence and/or a divergence of opinion about the usefulness/efficacy of cardiac pacing. Weight of evidence/opinion is in favor of usefulness/efficacy.

1. Bradycardia-tachycardia syndrome with the need for long-term antiarrhythmic treatment other than digitalis. (Level of evidence: C)
2. Congenital third-degree AV block beyond the first year of life with an average heart rate less than 50 beats/min, abrupt pauses in ventricular rate that are two or three times the basic cycle length, or associated with symptoms due to chronotropic incompetence. (Level of evidence: B)
3. Long-QT syndrome with 2:1 AV or third-degree AV block. (Level of evidence: B)
4. Asymptomatic sinus bradycardia in the child with complex congenital heart disease with resting heart rate less than 40 beats/min or pauses in ventricular rate more than 3 s. (Level of evidence: C)
5. Patients with congenital heart disease and impaired hemodynamics due to sinus bradycardia or loss of AV synchrony. (Level of evidence: C)

Class IIb: Usefulness/efficacy is less well established by evidence/opinion.

1. Transient postoperative third-degree AV block that reverts to sinus rhythm with residual bifascicular block. (Level of evidence: C)
2. Congenital third-degree AV block in the asymptomatic infant, child, adolescent, or young adult with an acceptable rate, narrow QRS complex, and normal ventricular function. (Level of evidence: B)
3. Asymptomatic sinus bradycardia in the adolescent with congenital heart disease with resting heart rate less than 40 beats/min or pauses in ventricular rate more than 3 s. (Level of evidence: C)
4. Neuromuscular diseases with any degree of AV block (including first-degree AV block), with or without symptoms, because there may be unpredictable progression of AV conduction disease.

Class III: Conditions for which there is evidence and/or general agreement that cardiac pacing is not useful/effective and in some cases may be harmful.

1. Transient postoperative AV block with return of normal AV conduction. (Level of evidence: B)
2. Asymptomatic postoperative bifascicular block with or without first-degree AV block. (Level of evidence: C)
3. Asymptomatic type I second-degree AV block. (Level of evidence: C)
4. Asymptomatic sinus bradycardia in the adolescent with longest RR interval less than 3 seconds and minimum heart rate more than 40 beats/min. (Level of evidence: C)

Level of evidence:
A: If the data were derived from multiple *randomized* clinical trials involving a large number of individuals. B: If the data were derived from a limited number of trials involving a comparatively small number of patients or from well-designed data analyses of *nonrandomized* studies or *observational* data registries.
C: If the consensus of experts was the primary source of the recommendation.

## Supraventricular Tachycardia and Wolff-Parkinson-White Syndrome

The age distribution of different types of PSVT in the pediatric age range has been estimated by esophageal electrophysiology studies,[132] by measuring the ventricular-atrial (V-A) interval from the esophageal catheter electrograms. AV reentrant tachycardia (in which the V-A interval > 70 ms) is thought to represent about 80 percent of supraventricular tachycardia in infancy. This may underestimate the frequency of AV nodal reentrant tachycardia in this age group which, in our experience, may be atypical in form. Ventricular stimulation, which is rarely performed in infants is required to differentiate these diagnoses. AV nodal reentry tachycardia is at least as frequent as AV reentry in older teenagers. Among neonates having WPW syndrome, about 25 to 35 percent will experience disappearance of the delta wave,[133,134] often by 1 year of age. The recurrence rate of PSVT following neonatal presentation has been reported to occur late in only 31 to 43 percent of cases.[133–135] However, older children experiencing their first episode of PSVT are far less likely to experience spontaneous resolution of their arrhythmia substrate. After the neonatal period, the peak age for the initial episode of PSVT is about 8 years of age.[134] This may be related to cardiac dimensional changes, functional changes of the conduction system and the accessory connection, maturation of the autonomic nervous system, and/or the influences of increased physical activity and caffeine use.

A single natural history study in children having WPW syndrome revealed 0 percent risk of sudden death at 3.4 years mean follow-up.[136] A prospective study in children and adults reported that 3 of 212 patients having asymptomatic ventricular preexcitation went on to have cardiac arrest at 5-year follow-up.[137] The 3 patients were 21 to 25 years of age, and all had multiple accessory AV connections and a short preexcited R-R interval during induced atrial fibrillation of 230 ms or less. This risk for catastrophic events in patients with ventricular preexcitation may increase in the presence of digoxin[133] and seems to be related to heightened adrenergic state. This combination of facts and impressions has directed most experts to recommend that no children having WPW syndrome and PSVT receive digoxin, and that nonpharmacologic therapy be considered first-line treatment for the combination of WPW syndrome and PSVT when beta-blocker therapy is contraindicated beyond 2 to 5 years of age. It is further recommended that children over the age of 5 years having asymptomatic ventricular preexcitation and wishing to participate in sports or requiring stimulant therapy undergo risk assessment for sudden death. This can be accomplished noninvasively with the demonstration of intermittent ventricular preexcitation on routine ECGs, Holter monitors, or exercise tests due to "phase 3" accessory pathway block. Care must be taken to evaluate the specific cause of intermittency of ventricular preexcitation.[138] If ventricular preexcitation is persistent, the authors will attempt to induce atrial fibrillation by esophageal pacing and measure both the average cycle length and the shortest R-R interval between preexcited beats.[139] If the results predict increased risk of sudden death, or if this information is obtained by intracardiac electrophysiologic study and there is additional potential for PSVT (even if the atrial fibrillation data does not predict increased risk), the authors will usually proceed to radiofrequency catheter ablation.

Approximately 10 percent of supraventricular tachycardia in children of all ages is primary atrial; either incessant automatic atrial tachycardia or a paroxysmal form, using a nonspecified but usually reentrant mechanism.[132] When incessant atrial tachycardia occurs in infancy and early childhood, pharmacologic control (usually sotalol or amiodarone) may be advisable, because there is a possibility that the tachycardia will spontaneously resolve. Even in adult patients, incessant atrial tachycardia is documented to resolve spontaneously without surgical or catheter ablation intervention in one third of patients.[140] The anatomic distribution of atrial tachycardia foci in children is similar to that reported in adults: the ostia of the pulmonary veins, along the crista terminalis from the sinus node to the coronary sinus ostium, and, less commonly, along the AV valve annuli. Atrial tachycardia foci from the pulmonary vein ostia and chaotic atrial tachycardia of infancy may involve similar substrates to that causing focal atrial fibrillation in adults (see later).

Tachycardia-induced cardiomyopathy in childhood most commonly results from incessant atrial tachycardia or the permanent form of junctional reciprocating tachycardia (a type of orthodromic AV reentrant tachycardia). Much less commonly, incessant ventricular tachycardia[141] or junctional ectopic tachycardia may be the etiology. Since children less than 3 years of age are preverbal, they are more likely to present with advanced signs of congestive heart failure than are older children. Management consists of aggressive pharmacologic treatment of congestive heart failure (including digoxin) and either antiarrhythmic drug therapy or radiofrequency ablation. When multiple foci of atrial tachycardia are suspected, radiofrequency ablation is less likely to be successful, and drug management may be preferable until ventricular function improves, and the child is better able to tolerate a prolonged procedure. The permanent form of junctional reciprocating tachycardia is very amenable to radiofrequency ablation, although risk of damage to the AV node may be a concern in young infants, depending upon the location of accessory pathway.

## Neonatal Atrial Flutter

The mechanism of atrial flutter in the fetus and newborn infant is likely similar to that in adults, although definitive invasive studies have not been performed. It is likely to be a macroreentrant tachycardia in the atrium, probably around the tricuspid valve. The atrial rate is typically 350 to 500 beats/min and, as in the fetus, the ventricular rate is typically one half the atrial rate due to 2:1 AV conduction, although variable AV conduction patterns may be seen. When the newborn infant is hydropic, there is the potential for significant morbidity and even mortality. In the nonhydropic newborn, conversion with either esophageal pacing, electrical cardioversion, or antiarrhythmic drug therapy is usually acutely successful and recurrence is rare, even in the absence of prophylactic treatment.[142–147] Nevertheless, treatment with digoxin for 6 to 12 months is still recommended by some practitioners.

## Chaotic Atrial Tachycardia

This uncommon tachycardia was first described in children in 1977[148] and seems to occur mostly in infants less than 1 year of age.[149–151] Unlike adults, in whom it is mostly associated with chronic obstructive pulmonary disease and theophylline use (and is usually referred to as "multifocal atrial tachycardia"), it is usually an isolated phenomenon in the child. Coexisting respiratory infections are present in about 35 percent of infants,[149–151] and structural heart defects are only occasionally present. The diagnosis is based upon the ECG and requires (1) ≥ 3 ectopic P waves in any single lead; (2) varying PP, PR, and RR intervals; (3) atrial rate greater than 100 beats/min; and (4) no dominant atrial pacemaker.[152,153] The atrial rate is typically between 250 and 600 beats/min,[150] and the ventricular response rate may be sufficiently fast to result in echocardiographic evidence of tachycardia-induced cardiomyopathy. Less commonly, overt congestive heart failure may occur. The mechanism of chaotic atrial tachycardia is not primary reentry, because it is unresponsive to adenosine, direct current cardioversion, and overdrive pacing. It has been theorized to use a triggered mechanism, although calcium channel blockers are also not efficacious. A rapid automatic mechanism with variable exit points seems to be the most plausible mechanism. Thus chaotic atrial tachycardia in infancy could be analogous to focal atrial fibrillation in adults (i.e., multiple reentry wavelets generated by a single nonreentry generator). This is supported by a single case report describing successful treatment of chaotic atrial tachycardia by ablating a single atrial focus.[154]

Infants having chaotic atrial tachycardia generally have an excellent outcome, typically with complete resolution by 1 year of age.[151] Sudden death has been reported in older series and may have been related to digitalis toxicity and factors not directly related to the arrhythmia.[155,156] If the ventricular response rate cannot be reliably controlled with digoxin, an oral beta blocker or calcium channel blocker may be added; or pharmacologic cardioversion to sinus rhythm may be accomplished with oral amiodarone,[157] flecainide,[158] or propafenone.[150,159] Once sinus rhythm is established and ventricular function returns to normal, the antiarrhythmic drug is generally empirically discontinued after 6 months of treatment or 1 year of age. Close follow-up including ambulatory ECGs is then required.

## Congenital Automatic Junctional Tachycardia

Automatic junctional tachycardia that presents in the first year of life is usually considered "congenital." It is defined as a regular narrow QRS tachycardia with AV dissociation and a ventricular rate faster than the atrial rate. It is not terminable with overdrive atrial pacing, adenosine, or cardioversion, proving the mechanism to be enhanced automaticity of a portion of the AV junction, below the atrial myocardium, and above the bundle branches—most likely the His bundle.[160]

Most cases present in the first months of life and are sporadic, although a familial predisposition is well known.[161] Due to its incessant nature, affected infants usually present with signs of congestive heart failure secondary to tachycardia-induced cardiomyopathy. In Villain's large series of 26 infants with congenital junctional ectopic tachycardia, the ventricular rate ranged from 140 to 370 beats/min (mean, 230 beats/min), and 16 patients had congestive heart failure.[162]

It is widely believed that congenital automatic junctional tachycardia is not self-limited, although cases of spontaneous and permanent resolution have been reported.[162–164] Unfortunately, sudden death[162] and evolution into complete AV block[165] may also occur. The possibilities that drug-induced proarrhythmia or sudden AV block caused those sudden deaths have been postulated. The primary goal of therapy is to reduce the ventricular rate to $<150$ beats/min in young infants in order to allow recovery of ventricular function. Amiodarone has been shown to be most efficacious,[162,164,166,167] although sotalol,[163] propranolol,[162] and propafenone [168] may also be used. Digoxin alone is not effective. If pharmacologic treatment fails, radiofrequency ablation of the junctional focus with preservation of normal AV conduction may be successful,[169–173] even in neonates.[174] Reports of the technical aspects of catheter ablation suggest the use of low energy "test" applications to regions of the proximal His bundle until acceleration occurs, followed by slightly higher energy until the arrhythmia disappears.[172] Atrial overdrive pacing will allow monitoring of AV conduction during energy delivery.[170] Some experts advocate pacemaker implantation in all such patients due to the unpredictable long-term stability of the AV junction,[162,165] although this issue is still unsettled.

## Postoperative Automatic Junctional Tachycardia

Postoperative automatic junctional tachycardia generally occurs within 24 h of congenital heart operations. It has been reported to occur in up to 8 percent of open heart operations,[175] most commonly following tetralogy of Fallot repair, Mustard operation for d-TGA, VSD closure, AVSD repair, repair of total anomalous pulmonary venous return, and following the Fontan operation.[175–177] These operations have in common the placement of suture lines near the penetrating bundle of His, which may result in a transient period of injury, and edema of the bundle; or, when it occurs following procedures remote from this structure, there may be pressure on the bundle, as may occur with postoperative pulmonary artery hypertension. Postoperative automatic junctional tachycardia has previously had a reported mortality rate of up to 50 percent caused by the adverse effect of both rate-related reduction in ventricular filling and AV asynchrony. Less severe forms of postoperative automatic junctional rhythm are seen. A review of pediatric patients (ages 1 day to 10.5 years) monitored following cardiac surgery at the Children's Hospital of Philadelphia showed an incidence of this rhythm of 5.6 percent in all patients operated during the study period. Of the patients with postoperative automatic junctional tachycardia, only 39 percent received therapeutic intervention.[178]

Similar to congenital automatic junctional tachycardia, the postoperative form is a regular tachycardia with a rate usually greater than 200 per minute and a QRS morphology identical to that seen during sinus rhythm. There is usually ventriculoatrial dissociation, with a ventricular rate faster than the atrial rate, and with occasional sinus capture beats. This can be best demonstrated by epicardial wire electrograms. Occasionally there is ventriculoatrial conduction, with a short- or intermediate-RP relationship. In those instances, automatic junctional tachycardia may be confused with atrial tachycardia and first-degree AV block. If epicardial wires are available, atrial pacing at a rate slightly faster than the intrinsic rhythm can differentiate these diagnoses, but as in the congenital form, postoperative automatic junctional tachycardia cannot be terminated by atrial or ventricular overdrive pacing or by direct current cardioversion. Pacing may result in overdrive suppression, which may last a few seconds prior to a gradual "warm up" to the previous rate.[160]

If the patient's hemodynamic status can be improved, given time, postoperative automatic junctional tachycardia generally resolves. Unfortunately, the agents used to improve inotropic function tend to increase the rate of this tachycardia. One study showed an association between postoperative dopamine use and the occurrence of postoperative junctional tachycardia.[178] The goals of therapy are to reduce the ventricular rate to less than 180 per minute in infants and less than 150 per minute in older children. Successful reduction in rate has been reported in a small series of patients using a variety of antiarrhythmiac agents, including digoxin,[175] flecainide,[177] amiodarone,[179] moricizine, and propafenone.[180] Hypotension, especially during the intravenous administration of intravenous propafenone[180] or amiodarone[179] is a definite risk. Walsh et al. used a more systematic approach in evaluating treatment options in 71 consecutive children having postoperative junctional tachycardia.[181] They proceeded in the following order: reduction in exogenous catecholamines; correction of fever; atrial pacing; digoxin; phenytoin, propranolol, or verapamil; procainamide or hypothermia; and, finally, procainamide *plus* hypothermia. Only correction of fever and combined procainamide plus hypothermia appeared to be efficacious. Amiodarone was not used in this study. Moderate hypothermia [32° to 34° C (89.6° to 93.2° F)][182] usually requires pharmacologic paralysis and may result in metabolic acidosis. Once the heart rate has been reduced by drugs or hypothermia, atrial pacing at a rate faster than that of the junctional tachycardia should be employed to achieve AV association. Till and Rowland used moderate hypothermia and atrial pacing to successfully treat 8 of 11 patients.[177] Success seemed to be related to early intervention, generally within 1 h of tachycardia onset. Survivors returned to sinus rhythm from 2 to 10 days posttherapy.

Patients refractory to all measures may be considered for transcatheter[183–186] or surgical His bundle ablation and dual-chamber pacemaker implantation. With early intervention, the use of atrial pacing and antiarrhythmic agents such as intravenous amiodarone, and occasionally with aggressive hemodynamic support using extracorporeal circulation or ventricular assist, this irreversible and unappealing therapy can nearly always be avoided.

## THERAPIES FOR PEDIATRIC ARRHYTHMIAS

This section will address treatment concepts in children with special attention to those differences from treating adults with arrhythmias.

### Antiarrhythmic Drugs

Drug therapy remains a necessary part of the armamentarium for treating arrhythmias in children for several reasons: Fetal tachycardia does not currently have alternate therapies; control of tachycardia in the infant with medications likely carries less risk than ablative therapies, and, in this population, the natural history of the disease may favor spontaneous resolution. In older children, drugs are useful in acute treatment of tachycardias and in chronic treatment of tachycardias that are not amenable to curative treatments. Basic concepts of antiarrhythmic drug pharmacology, classification, and specific applications will be presented in this section and in Table 39-3.

Children differ from adults in that the disposition and cellular electrophysiologic effects of antiarrhythmic drugs change throughout development. In early infancy, the volume of distribution of all antiarrhythmic drugs is greater due to greater total body water. This increases the central compartment, which more than offsets the decreased volume of the peripheral compartment. Although this requires larger loading doses, chronic dosing requirements may not be as high (on a per kilogram basis) due to lower protein binding, secondary to reduced plasma protein concentrations, reduced binding capability of fetal hemoglobin, competition for binding sites by free fatty acids and bilirubin, and lower blood pH.

Bioavailability of antiarrhythmic drugs after oral administration is reduced in young infants due to relative achlorhydria (until about 3 years of age; e.g., this reduces phenytoin absorption), delayed gastric emptying (until 6 to 8 months of age), and immature gut motility (until about 4 years of age). "First-pass" elimination of propranolol, lidocaine, and verapamil is similar in children and adults. Likewise, the effects of coexisting congestive heart failure, intestinal mucosal edema, and other drugs on bioavailability of these agents are similar to those in adults.

Drugs are eliminated by some combination of hepatic or red blood cell biotransformation, renal excretion, pulmonary exhalation, and fecal excretion. The volume of blood totally "cleared" of a drug (so-called "clearance") is reduced in the presence of renal or hepatic dysfunction, reduced blood flow to that organ, elevated plasma protein binding, and in the presence of immature organ function. Hepatic biotransformation of most drugs is markedly reduced in young infants until enzyme maturation occurs by about 6 months. Hence, drug half-lives are longer until that age. Most antiarrhythmic drug excretion occurs in the kidneys as a result of a combination of glomerular filtration, tubular secretion, and tubular reabsorption. At birth, these three processes are 20 to 30 percent that of an adult, reaching maturity by 1 year (filtration), 1 year (secretion), and 6 months (reabsorption).[187] Renal parenchymal disease and decreased renal perfusion, as in cases of congestive heart failure, obviously prolong the elimination half-life.

The clinical importance of drug metabolities (e.g. procainamide and propafenone), drug–drug interactions (e.g., amiodarone), pharmacokinetic interactions with nonantiarrhythmic drugs (e.g., alteration of gastric pH with antacids; enhancement of biotransformation with phenobarbital; inhibition of transformation with cimetidine; urinary acidification or alkalinization), and pharmacodynamic interactions (e.g., increased myocardial sensitivity to digoxin from diuretic-induced hypokalemia) is similar to that in adults and will not be further discussed.

Commonly available antiarrhythmic drugs (including digoxin) are presented in Table 39-3 and are organized according to the Vaughan-Williams classification. Important considerations regarding drug use in the pediatric age range which are different from adults (half-life, intravenous dosing, oral dosing) or which are specific to infants (transplacental passage, safety to the fetus, and passage in breast milk), are also included.

### Radiofrequency Catheter Ablation

Transcatheter delivery of radiofrequency energy to arrhythmia foci was shown to be efficacious in children initially through small series in the early 1990s.[188] Kugler et al. and the Pediatric Radiofrequency Registry of North America subsequently provided the first large experience with this treatment.[189] This section will focus on radiofrequency catheter ablation in children and how its application is different from that in adults.

#### PATIENT SIZE AND PHYSIOLOGY: EFFECTS ON RADIOFREQUENCY ABLATION TECHNIQUE

Catheter design and the electronics of radiofrequency energy delivery has heretofore limited the size of the catheter tip to no smaller than 3 mm in length of the distal electrode and no smaller than 5 F in circumference. Hence, lesion size cannot be focused any smaller than about 3 mm in diameter and depth. By delivering epicardial radiofrequency lesions in a newborn lamb model and allowing animals to mature, Saul et al.[190] demonstrated substantial growth of scar depth and width at the ventricular level; increase of scar width only at the atrial level; and only minimal scar growth when lesions were delivered at the annulus fibrosis. The potential for "collateral damage" is of greatest concern in the region of the AV node. Considering that in children less than 3 years of age, the base of Koch's triangle is only 3 to 5 mm and the length is only 3 to 6 mm,[191] the use of radiofrequency ablation is electively limited to patients greater than 20 kg (about 5 years old) for AV node reentry tachycardia, but for other supraventricular tachycardias it is limited to those greater than 12 kg. Younger children whose arrhythmias cannot be controlled with antiarrhythmic drugs may be considered for radiofrequency ablation with reportedly good outcomes.[192]

The physics of radiofrequency energy delivery from an internal catheter to an external dispersion pad is also different from that in adults. Unlike adults, among patients $< 1.5\ m^2$ body surface area, there is no correlation between patient size and impedance load.[193]

TABLE 39-3 Use of Antiarrhythmic Drugs in Children

| Drug | Half-Life | Intravenous Dosing | Oral Dosing | Transplacental Passage (%) | Pregnancy Category/ Safety for Fetus | Passage in Breast Milk | Indications |
|---|---|---|---|---|---|---|---|
| | | | CLASS IA | | | | |
| Disopyramide | 4.5–7.8 h | Not available | 10–30 mg/kg/d (infants); 10–20 mg/kg/d (children); 6–15 mg/kg/d (adolescents); 400–800 mg/d (adults) q 6h (regular), q 12 h (sustained release); maximum: 1600 mg/d) | 39 | C | 50–90% maternal blood level; safe for infant | PSVT; AF1; AF; VT in CHD with good ventricular function |
| Quinidine | 30–90 min (sulfate); 3.4–4.0 h (gluconate) | Not recommended | 30–60 mg/kg/d (450–900 mg/m$^2$); q 4–6 h; 10 mg/kg/d (adult); 20% higher if gluconate | 24–94 | C | Reported to occur; safe for infant | Rarely used due to "quinidine syncope"; PSVT; AFI; AF; VT in CHD |
| Procainamide | 1.7 h (children); 2.5–4.7 h (adults) (short acting) 6–7 h (slow release); shorter in children; longer in neonates | 10–15 mg/kg over 20 min; maintenance: 30–80 μg/kg/min | 50–100 mg/kg/d | 25–100 | C | Reported to occur; safe for infant | PSVT; AF1; AF; AET; VT in CHD; postoperative JET |
| | | | CLASS IB | | | | |
| Moricizine | 1.5–3.5 h; biologic T 1/2 48 h | Not available | 200 mg/m$^2$/d (initial) increase to 600 mg/m$^2$/d; q 8 h | Not known | B | Not known | AET; VT; PSVT |
| Lidocaine | 3.2 h (neonate); 1.5–2 h (children and adults) | 1 mg/kg, may repeat twice; maintenance: 20–50 μg/kg/min | Not effective | 50 | B (Fetal bradycardia reported; generally safe for fetus) | 40% maternal blood level; safe for infant | VT, especially ischemic |
| Mexiletine | 6.3–11.8 h | Not available | Infants: 8–25 mg/kg/d; children: 4.5–15 mg/kg/d; max: 600–1200 mg/d; q 8 h | 100 (equivalent to maternal blood level) | C | 100% maternal blood level; safe for infant | VT |

(Continued)

TABLE 39-3 Use of Antiarrhythmic Drugs in Children (*Continued*)

| Drug | Half-Life | Intravenous Dosing | Oral Dosing | Transplacental Passage (%) | Pregnancy Category/ Safety for Fetus | Passage in Breast Milk | Indications |
|---|---|---|---|---|---|---|---|
| Phenytoin | 75 ± 64 h (premature); 21 ± 12 h (term); 8 ± 4 h (1 mo); 22 ± 7 h (child-adult) | 10–15 mg/kg over 1 h | Load: 15 mg/kg ÷ q 6 h (day 1), 7.5 mg/kg ÷ q 6 h (day 2); maintenance: 0–2 wks: 4–8 mg/kg/d q 12 h; 2 wks–2 yrs: 8–12 mg/kg/d q 8 h; 3–12 yrs: 5–6 mg/kg/d q 12 h; >12 yrs: 4.5 mg/kg/d q 12 h | Excellent | D (11% have "fetal hydantoin syndrome"; 31% have lesser manifestations) | Safe for infant | VT |
| Tocainide | 15 h (adult) | Not available | Children: 350–700 mg/m²/d | Not known | C | Not known | VT |
| | | | CLASS 1C | | | | |
| Flecainide | 29 h (newborn); 11–12 h (infant); 8 h (children) 12– 27 h (adult) | 1–2 mg/kg over 5–10 min | 1–6 mg/kg/d or 50–150 mg/m²/d q 8 h (children) & q 12 h (newborn, infant and adult); maximum : 400 mg/d; avoid administration with milk-based formulas in infants | 100 (equivalent to maternal blood level) | C | Concentrated (2.3–3.7:1); safe for infant | PSVT; AF1; AF; PJRT; VT; fetal tachycardias; JET |
| Propafenone | 4.7 ± 1.3 h (extensive metabolizer); 16.8 ± 10.6 h (slow = 10% population); ↑ with time in both groups | 0.2 mg/kg q 10 min to effect (max = 2 mg/kg); maint: 4–7 μg/kg/min) | 200–600 mg/m²/d q 6–8 h; maximum: 900 mg/d | Not known | C | Not known | PSVT; AF1; AF; PJRT; VT; infantile CAT; JET |
| | | | CLASS II | | | | |
| Atenolol | 16–35 h (newborn); 3.5–7 h (children); 6–9 h (adults) | No pediatric data | 0.8–1.5 mg/kg/d q 12–24 h; when used for potentially life-threatening arrhythmia (LQTS), q 12 h recommended | 100 maternal blood level | D | Concentrated (1.5–6:8:1); fetal bradycardia | PSVT; rate control in AF1 and AF; VT in normal heart; LQTS |

(Continued)

TABLE 39-3 Use of Antiarrhythmic Drugs in Children (*Continued*)

| Drug | Half-Life | Intravenous Dosing | Oral Dosing | Transplacental Passage (%) | Pregnancy Category/ Safety for Fetus | Passage in Breast Milk | Indications |
|---|---|---|---|---|---|---|---|
| Esmolol | 4.5 ± 2.1 min (children); 9 min (adults) | Load: 500 μg/kg over 1 min; maint.: 50–600 μg/kg/min | Not applicable | Not known | C | Not known | PSVT; rate control in AF1 and AF |
| Nadolol | 20–24 h (adults); shorter in infants and children | Not available | 1–2 mg/kg/d q day | Some passage occurs | C (Hypoglycemia; symptomatic bradycardia) | Concentrated (3:1); fetal bradycardia | PSVT; rate control in AF1 and AF; VT in normal heart; LQTS |
| Propranolol | 3.9–6.4 h (children); 4–6 h (adults) | 0.01–0.15 mg/kg over 5 min | 1–5 mg/kg/d q 6–8 h (short acting); q 12–24 h (time release); when used for potentially life-threatening arrhythmia (LQTS), q 12 h recommended | 100 maternal blood level | C (IUGR; hypoglycemia; respiratory depression) | 64% maternal plasma level; safe for infant | PSVT; rate control in AF1 and AF; VT in normal heart; LQTS |
| Class III | | | | | | | |
| Amiodarone | 8–107 d; biphasic elimination (plasma level 50% after 10 d; rebounds days 12–21; falls again) | Load: 2–5 mg/kg over 5–30 min (repeat as needed: then 0.4–1.0 mg/kg/h | Load: 10 mg/kg/d q 8–12 h (up to 60 mg/kg/d x ≤ 3 d, if necessary); then, 5 mg/kg/d × 2 mos; then, wean to 2.5 mg/kg/d | 10–25 maternal blood level | D (Prematurity 12%; IUGR 21%; hypothyroidism 9%) | Exceeds maternal plasma level; safe for infant | PSVT; AF1; AF; VT; JET; AET |
| Sotalol | 9.5 h (children); 7–18 h (adult); beta-blocking effect longer | Not available | 2–8 mg/kg/d or 40–250 mg/m²/d q 8–12 h; maximum dose 640 mg/d; usual adult starting dose: 160 mg/d | 5–100 maternal blood level | B (Asymptomatic bradycardia) | Concentrated (5:4:1); may not be important | PSVT; AF1; AF; VT |
| Class IV | | | | | | | |
| Verapamil | 2.5–7 h (infancy); 5–12 h with chronic use | 0.1 mg/kg over 2 min (max: 10 mg); infusion: 5 μ/kg/min; not < 1 yr of age | 3–10 mg/kg/d q 8 h (short acting); q day (time release) | 15–50 maternal level | C | 23–100% maternal blood level; safe for infant | PSVT; rate control in AF1 and AF; fetal PSVT; occasional forms of VT in normal heart |

(Continued)

TABLE 39-3 Use of Antiarrhythmic Drugs in Children (*Continued*)

| Drug | Half-Life | Intravenous Dosing | Oral Dosing | Transplacental Passage (%) | Pregnancy Category/ Safety for Fetus | Passage in Breast Milk | Indications |
|---|---|---|---|---|---|---|---|
| | | | DIGOXIN | | | | |
| Digoxin | 61–170 h (premature); 35–45 h (term); 18–25 h (infant); 35 h (child); 38–48 h (adult) | Oral load (3 doses/16–24 h): 30 μg/kg (premature), 35 (term), 40–50 (<2 yrs), 30–40 (>2 yrs); maintenance: ¼ load ÷ q 12 h; Intravenous dose: 75–80% oral | | Similar to maternal level | C | Similar to maternal blood level; safe for infant | PSVT; fetal PSVT |

ABBREVIATIONS: AET = atrial ectopic tachycardia; AF = atrial fibrillation; AFl = atrial flutter; CAT = chaotic atrial tachycardia; CHD = congenital heart disease; JET = junctional ectopic tachycardia; LQTS = long QT syndrome; PJRT = permanent form of junctional reciprocating tachycardia; PSVT = paroxysmal supraventricular tachycardia; VT = ventricular tachycardia; United States FDA Pregnancy Categories: A = Controlled studies in women fail to demonstrate a risk to the fetus in the first trimester, and the possibility of fetal harm appears remote. B = Animal studies do not indicate a risk to the fetus and there are no controlled human studies, or animal studies do show an adverse effect on the fetus but well-controlled studies in pregnant women have failed to demonstrate a risk to the fetus. C = Studies have shown that the drug exerts animal teratogenic or embryocidal effects, but there are no controlled studies in women, or no studies are available in either animals or women. D = Positive evidence of human fetal risk exists, but benefits in certain situations (e.g., life-threatening situations or serious diseases for which safer drugs cannot be used or are ineffective) may make use of the drug acceptable despite its risks. X = Studies in animals or humans have demonstrated fetal abnormalities or there is evidence of fetal risk based on human experience, or both, and the risk clearly outweighs any possible benefit.

Therefore, applied power is similar to that for adults. It appears that thermistor- and thermocouple-linked closed-loop systems are as safe in children as they are in adults. Experience with irrigated tipped catheters in children is limited, but it is a promising modality in patients having complex atrial arrhythmias following Fontan operation in whom increased atrial wall thickness is a limiting factor for standard ablation catheters.

Complete electrophysiologic testing and radiofrequency ablation can, if necessary, be performed in even the smallest patients, despite limited venous capacity by using creative catheter combinations. For example, atrial sensing and pacing can be performed from an esophageal electrode catheter; 2 F quadripolar electrode catheters are now commercially available, and three of these fit through a single 7 F triple-lumen sheath; and a single catheter may be used for both right ventricular apical pacing and sensing and His bundle recording.[194] The normal femoral vein can easily accommodate up to 5-mm net circumference (5 F) in children weighing > 2.0 kg, 6 F if > 3.0 kg, 7 F if > 5 kg, 9 F if > 10 kg, 11 F if > 25 kg, and 14 F for larger patients. Venous obstruction has been reported when a total of 18 F (5 + 6 + 7) catheters were placed in children 8 to 21 years of age.[195] Arterial damage is of greater concern and is largely preventable with the widespread use of the transseptal approach to the left side of the heart.

The coexistence of congenital heart defects presents additional concerns. Femoral venous access may be obviated by iliofemoral vein thrombosis due to prior catheterizations, or there may be congenital interruption of the suprarenal inferior vena cava. In these instances, inferior access to the atria by transhepatic cannulation of a hepatic vein has become reasonably standard in some institutions.[74,196] In patients having complex congenital heart disease, complete knowledge of the cardiac anatomy is mandatory. This requires availability of prior echocardiograms and surgical reports, use of biplane fluoroscopy, and capacity to perform venography, atriography, and ventriculography during elecrophysiologic testing. The location of accessory pathways and AV nodes/His bundles may be predicted by knowledge of the anatomy (especially in Ebstein's anomaly, l-transposition of the great arteries, heterotaxies, straddling tricuspid valve, and double inlet left ventricle), but the operator should be prepared to perform meticulous mapping. Intracardiac ultrasound and electroanatomic mapping techniques are emerging technologies whose utility in congenital heart disease is just becoming realized.

## OTHER CONSIDERATIONS FOR PEDIATRIC CATHETER ABLATIONS

Technical considerations aside, developmentally, children have varying degrees of comprehension of the procedure that they are about to undergo. Age-appropriate reading material (including coloring books), play therapy, and opportunities to speak with same-age patients who had undergone ablations are useful techniques to help children have an atraumatic experience. General anesthesia or deep sedation are usually used for the procedure. Sedation is preferred in cases of highly sensitive arrhythmias, such as atrial tachycardia. When general anesthesia is used, propofol and isofluorane are equally useful, and neither suppresses arrhythmia inducibility.[197]

Propofol may slow AV node conduction velocity, and isofluorane increases the corrected QT interval.[197] An advantage of general anesthesia is that it permits muscle relaxation during the period of radiofrequency energy delivery, thus helping to prevent catheter dislodgement as may occur during spontaneous respiration.[198] The selection of sedation versus anesthesia should be individualized, but, in general, patients who are younger, or who have structural heart disease, coexisting medical problems, or potential airway obstruction are at higher risk for sedation and are better candidates for anesthesia.

## INDICATIONS FOR CATHETER ABLATION IN CHILDREN

In May 2000, an Expert Consensus Conference was held by the North American Society for Pacing and Electrophysiology. The report from this conference was published in 2002 and established consensus recommendations for the performance of radiofrequency catheter ablation in pediatric patients.[199] The recommendations are summarized in Table 39-4.

## RESULTS OF CATHETER ABLATION IN THE YOUNG

The Pediatric Radiofrequency Catheter Ablation Registry was established by the Pediatric Electrophysiology Society (of North America) in November of 1990 in order to collect and analyze data from patients 21 years of age and under who underwent radiofrequency ablation by a participating member. Kugler and coworkers initially published the Registry's early findings in 1994, after data from 652 patients from 24 centers had been submitted.[189] The following results are based upon subsequent updates presented at annual Pediatric Electrophysiology Society meetings. These results were compiled and analyzed by Kugler and Danford at the University of Nebraska, United States.

From January 1991 to February 1999, 7305 procedures were performed on 6604 patients in 49 institutions. The patients ranged in age from 0.1 to 20.9 years. Congenital heart disease was present in 10 percent of patients and cardiomyopathy in 2 percent. Indications for procedures were patient choice (49 percent), medically refractory tachycardia (31 percent), life-threatening symptoms (8 percent), adverse drug effect (5 percent), tachycardia-induced cardiomyopathy (3 percent), and pending surgery (1 percent).

There were 5235 accessory pathways that underwent attempted ablation, with an acute success rate of 91.2 percent, ranging from 96.1 percent in the left lateral location to 79.5 percent in the right anteroseptal location. Other acute success rates were AV node reentry tachycardia, 97 percent; atrial ectopic tachycardia, 88 percent; junctional ectopic tachycardia, 84 percent; atrial flutter, 75 percent; and ventricular tachycardia, 68 percent. Using multivariate analysis,

TABLE 39-4 Indications for Radiofrequency Catheter Ablation in Pediatric Patients

Class I: There is consistent agreement and/or supportive data that catheter ablation is likely to be medically beneficial or helpful for the patient.

1. Wolff-Parkinson-White (WPW) syndrome following an episode of aborted sudden cardiac death.
2. The presence of WPW syndrome associated with syncope when there is a short preexcited R-R interval during atrial fibrillation (preexcited R-R interval, 250 ms) or the antegrade effective refractory period of the AP measured during programmed electrical stimulation is $<$250 ms.
3. Chronic or recurrent supraventricular tachycardia (SVT) associated with ventricular dysfunction.
4. Recurrent VT that is associated with hemodynamic compromise and is amenable to catheter ablation.

Class II A: There is a divergence of opinion regarding the benefit or medical necessity of catheter ablation, the majority of opinions/data are in favor of the procedure.

1. Recurrent and/or symptomatic SVT refractory to conventional medical therapy and age $>$ 4 years.
2. Impending congenital heart surgery when vascular or chamber access may be restricted following surgery.
3. Chronic (occurring for $>$ 6 to 12 months following an initial event) or incessant SVT in the presence of normal ventricular function.
4. Chronic or frequent recurrences of intraatrial reentrant tachycardia (IART).
5. Palpitations with inducible sustained SVT during electrophysiological testing.

Class II B: There is clear divergence of opinion regarding the need for the procedure.

1. Asymptomatic preexcitation (WPW pattern on an electrocardiograph), age $>$ 5 years, with no recognized tachycardia, when the risks and benefits of the procedure and arrhythmia have been clearly explained.
2. SVT, age $>$ 5 years, as an alternative to chronic antiarrhythmic therapy which has been effective in control of the arrhythmia.
3. SVT, age $<$ 5 years (including infants), when antiarrhythmic medications, including sotalol and amiodarone, are not effective or associated with intolerable side effects.
4. IART, one to three episodes per year, requiring medical intervention.
5. AVN ablation and pacemaker insertion as an alternative therapy for recurrent or intractable IART.
6. One episode of VT associated with hemodynamic compromise and which is amenable to catheter ablation.

Class III: There is agreement that catheter ablation is not medically indicated and/or the risk of the procedure may be greater than the benefit for the patient.

1. Asymptomatic WPW syndrome, age $<$ 5 years.
2. SVT controlled with conventional antiarrhythmic medications, age $<$ 5 years.
3. Nonsustained, paroxysmal VT, which is not considered incessant (i.e., present on monitoring for hours at a time or on nearly all strips recorded during any 1-h period) and where no concomitant ventricular dysfunction exists.
4. Episodes of nonsustained SVT that do not require other therapy and/or are minimally symptomatic.

predictors of successful ablation included the presence of a left freewall accessory pathway, the presence of AV node reentry tachycardia, and greater procedural experience by the operator. Predictors of failure included coexisting congenital heart disease; extreme weight; or the presence of an anteroseptal accessory pathway, atrial flutter, or ventricular tachycardia. Not surprisingly, procedural durations and fluoroscopy times trended downward over the 8-year period, and the mean fluoroscopy time was 31 min in 1999.

Complications were classified as minor, such as groin hematoma, or major. Major complications occurred in 210 (2.9 percent) procedures, including 56 second-degree or third-degree AV blocks (27 percent of all major complications), 46 cardiac perforations (22 percent), 15 embolic events (7 percent), 13 brachial plexus injuries (6 percent), and pneumothoraces (5 percent). Predictors of AV block included the presence of an anteroseptal accessory pathway, presence of AV node reentry tachycardia, and smaller patient size. Other complications were more likely in children less than 4 years of age and were less likely with right freewall accessory pathways and with increased operator experience.

Schaffer et al. reported on mortality from this procedure from the first 4651 patients submitted to the Pediatric Radiofrequency Catheter Ablation Registry.[200] There were 10 deaths, including 5 of 4000 having healthy hearts (0.12 percent; ages 0.1 to 13.3 years) and 5 of 559 children having structural heart disease (0.89 percent; ages 1.5 to 17.4 years; $p = 0.01$ vs healthy patients). In those having healthy hearts, death was related to traumatic injury, myocardial perforation and hemopericardium, coronary or cerebral thromboembolism, and ventricular arrhythmias. All cases involved left-sided arrhythmia foci, and all ablations had been considered successful. Those with structurally healthy hearts were smaller and had received more radiofrequency lesions than did a matched control group. Hence, mortalities are rare in this procedure, but they are more frequent in the presence of underlying heart disease, among smaller patients who had received more radiofrequency lesions, and in patients undergoing left-sided procedures. Operator experience did not appear to be a factor.

## Pacemakers and Implantable Cardioverter-Defibrillators in Children

Technological advances in implanted antiarrhythmia devices and lead hardware has benefited children greatly, especially due to significant downsizing of pulse generators and lead bodies. Therefore, pediatric electrophysiologists have shifted investigative efforts to other areas: cellular, tissue, and whole organ responses to artificial pacing of the immature heart; optimization of pacing modes in children with congenital heart disease; and development of low-threshold, high-impedance epicardial leads for infants and for children with intracardiac shunts or single ventricle physiology. This section will consider pediatric pacing and how it differs from that in adults.

### CELLULAR AND WHOLE ORGAN BIOLOGY OF PACING

Using a puppy model of complete AV block, Karpawich et al. demonstrated undesirable ultrastructural myocyte changes and hemodynamic abnormalities after artificial pacing from the right ventricular apex compared with pacing from the ventricular septal summit.[201] Subtle abnormalities in left ventricular function also occur long term after right ventricular apical pacing in human children and appear to be related to the QRS duration.[202] When combined with our new knowledge regarding the efficacy of biventricular synchronous pacing in adults with cardiomyopathy and prolonged QRS duration, these observations in children may influence lead implantation practices in the future.

### INDICATIONS FOR PACING IN CHILDREN

Indications for permanent pacing in children, adolescents, and patients with congenital heart disease appear in the ACC/AHA/North American Society for Pacing and Electrophysiology 2002 Guideline Update for Implantation of Cardiac Pacemakers and Antiarrhythmia Devices.[67] These indications are categorized according to consensus of opinion, and each recommendation is annotated to indicate degree of support in the scientific literature. These recommendations appear as Table 39-2.

### TECHNICAL ASPECTS OF PACING IN CHILDREN

The primary differences between permanent pacing in children and in adults are (1) size limitation as relates to venous access; (2) somatic growth of the heart and great vessels; and (3) coexistence of congenital heart defects.

Most children and teenagers having hearts with separated circulations may be paced using transvenous systems, similar to adults. Although standard leads, which are passed through a 7 F introducer, may even be placed in infants, concern over long-term risk of venous thrombosis seems to be well-founded.[203] Figa et al. reviewed their patients who had undergone transvenous pacing, and they determined a relationship between risk of subclavian venous thrombosis and net cross-sectional area of leads in relation to the patient's body surface area.[203] The maximum total lead capacity [cross-sectional areas in millimeters squared divided by the body surface area (in meters squared)] should be $< 6.6$. This formula is applied to determine the advisability of transvenous versus epicardial pacing and in the selection of lead types.

It is common practice to introduce an extra length of lead into the right atrium of immature patients with the expectation that as the distance between the points of lead fixation separate due to growth, there will remain ample lead length so that the system does not need to be replaced. The size of the so-called "growth loop" may even be calculated based upon the child's height and age.[204] However, the introduction of a complete "loop" of lead in the right atrium is not without hazard, including spontaneous advancement into the right ventricle and across the pulmonary valve. Other techniques that may permit progressive release of excess lead from the pulse generator pocket include the use of absorbable suture for the lead sleeve and "packaging" the excess lead in an envelope of inert material. Unfortunately, the tendency for the lead to become fixed to the innominate vein or the superior vena cava due to fibrosis may render these other techniques useless.

Nearly all transvenous systems may include an infraclavicular pocket, considering the small size of current pulse generators. Subpectoral pockets (versus subcutanous) are preferred in thin children and in those who engage in sports activities. Although they are somewhat more challenging to reenter for pulse generator "change-outs," such pockets are also esthetically preferable to subcutaneous pockets. Unipolar systems may often not be used in a submuscular pocket without the risk of muscle pacing and myopotential sensing.

Epicardial pacing systems are generally used for infants and in patients having intracardiac shunts. Steroid-eluting plaque electrodes, such as the Medtronic model 4695, appears to ensure long-term, low-threshold pacing; although, like most epicardial leads, these have a high current drain due to low-lead impedance. Furthermore, finding a suitable pacing site may be challenging in children who have undergone prior heart surgery and have epicardial fibrosis. The diaphragmatic surface of the right ventricle or the lateral left ventricle may afford unused ventricular sites, and the left atrial appendage may be used for atrial pacing. Careful avoidance of the phrenic nerves must be kept in mind. There remains a great need to develop an active fixation, low-threshold, high-impedance, bipolar epicardial lead system.

Children who have undergone the Fontan procedure for single ventricle physiology present unique problems. If they have isolated SAND, a transvenous atrial lead may be placed, but chronic anticoagulation is recommended in nearly all such cases due to the higher than usual risk of atrial thrombosis. If they have AV block, an exclusive epicardial system may be placed, or a hybrid system, consisting of a transvenous atrial and epicardial ventricular lead system, may be constructed. In the latter instance, one of the leads must be tunneled to the pulse generator pocket. Even more problematic, patients who have undergone the more recent "extracardiac" Fontan connection do not have any means of venous access to the heart, even for an atrial lead.

### PSYCHOLOGIC AND SOCIAL ASPECTS OF PACING IN THE YOUNG

The need for a permanent pacemaker may be viewed as a chronic disease by a child or teenager. When compared to a group of children having undergone congenital heart surgery, but not requiring pacemaker implantation, and a group of healthy controls, Alpern et al. showed that children with pacemakers demonstrated healthy psychosocial adaptation, using denial and intellectualization to deal with stresses.[205] Although they largely maintained a healthy self-image, they were sensitive to very real negative peer responses. In a group of 15 paced patients less than 19 years of age who were followed for a mean of 6.7 years following pacemaker implantation, Andersen et al. discovered increased requirement for psychiatric treatment related to disturbed family dynamics as well as abnormal body images, compared with controls.[206] Furthermore, compared with adults, children and teenagers had greater difficulty incorporating their pacemaker into their body image. These studies underscore the importance of normalization of the other aspects of the lifestyle of a child with a pacemaker, at least within the constraints of safety considerations. Interest in sports participation among school-aged children has increased dramatically since the 1960s. There is general agreement that contact sports, such as wrestling, American football, and rugby, are forbidden in children with pacemakers. The authors view high-endurance activities, such as basketball, soccer, track, and swimming, as permissible in children who are not "pacemaker-dependent." This may be defined by the clinical demonstration that a stable escape rate compatible with life will not occur following interruption of pacing. (The authors expect a 1 to 5 s pause following abrupt loss of capture, due to overdrive suppression, and do not consider that observation, alone, as life-threatening.) All families must be informed of the increased risk of transvenous lead damage by activities that require excessive movement about the shoulders, such as swimming, basketball, and gymnastics.

### IMPLANTABLE CARDIOVERTER/DEFIBRILLATORS IN CHILDREN

The treatment of conditions predisposing to sudden cardiac death is discussed elsewhere in this text, according to disease type. Treatment algorithms for conditions in which life-threatening ventricular tachyarrhythmias exist have changed due to the advances in implantable cardioverter/defibrillator technology. It has been clearly shown that these devices permit greater longevity among affected adults who have acceptable cardiac function.[207,208] Silka et al. reported on the efficacy of implantable cardioverter/defibrillator use among 125 patients less than 20 years of age (1.9 to 19.9 years and weighing down to 9.7 kg).[209] The diagnoses included cardiomyopathy in 54 percent, primary electrical disease in 26 percent and congenital heart defects in 18 percent. At 31 months of mean follow-up, 59 percent had experienced at least one appropriate implantable cardioverter/defibrillator discharge and 20 percent at least one inappropriate discharge. Actuarial analysis estimated an overall postimplantable cardioverter/defibrillator survival rate of 85 percent at 5 years and sudden death-free survival rate of 90 percent. Because of these advances, implantable cardioverter/defibrillators are now considered first- or second-line therapy for children and teenagers who are clearly at risk for sudden cardiac death based upon the occurrence of resuscitated events in the presence of certain chronic cardiac conditions. These include dilated or hypertrophic cardiomyopathy, primary ventricular fibrillation, unstable ventricular tachycardia and congenital heart disease, and the long QT syndrome. The role of the implantable cardioverter/defibrillator in combination with antiarrhythmic drugs is an area of ongoing investigation.

Technically, active can devices may be placed in a subpectoral position in children as small as 25-kg body weight. In smaller children, adequate defibrillation thresholds have been demonstrated when the defibrillator is placed subcutaneously in the left upper quadrant, and the lead is tunneled to the left subclavian vein.[210] For infants and toddlers, creative patch placement subcutaneously and/or superficial to the pericardium is efficacious and avoids complications associated with epicardial patch placement. Leads having coils designed for transvenous use may also be used in an epicardial or extracardiac thoracic position and may provide adequate defibrillation thresholds.

## References


1. Wessels A, Vermaulen JL, Verbeck FJ, et al. Spatial distribution of tissue specific antigens in the developing human heart and skeletal muscle: An immunohistochemical analysis of the distribution of the neural tissue antigen GLN in the embryonic heart: Implications for the development of the atrioventricular conduction system. *Anat Rec* 1992; 232:97–111.
2. Anderson RH, Becker AE, Arnold R, et al. The conducting tissues in congenitally corrected transposition. *Circulation* 1974;50:911–923.
3. Huhta JC, Maloney JD, Ritter DG, et al. Complete atrioventricular block in patients with atrioventricular discordance. *Circulation* 1983;67:1374–1377.
4. Daliento L, Corrado D, Buja G, et al. Rhythm and conduction disturbances in isolated, congenitally corrected transposition of the great arteries. *Am J Cardiol* 1986;58:314–318.
5. Kanter RJ, Pressley JC, Packer DL, et al. Impact of coexisting heart disease on outcome of surgery for the Wolff-Parkinson-White syndrome in children. *J Amer Coll Cardiol* 1989;13:138A.
6. Presbitero P, Somerville J, Rabajoli F, et al. Corrected transposition of the great arteries without associated defects in adult patients: Clinical profile and follow up. *Br Heart J* 1995;74:57–59.
7. Prieto LR, Hordof AJ, Secic M, et al. Progressive tricuspid valve disease in patients with congenitally corrected transposition of the great arteries. *Circulation* 1998;98:997–1005.
8. Fontaine JM, Kamal BM, Sokil AB, et al. Ventricular tachycardia: A life-threatening arrhythmia in a patient with congenitally corrected transposition of the great arteries. *J Cardiovasc Electrophysiol* 1998;9: 517–522.
9. Rao PS. *Tricuspid Atresia.* Mt. Kisco, NY: Futura; 1992.
10. Anderson RH, Ho SY. The morphologic substrates for pediatric arrhythmias. *Cardiol Young* 1991;1:159–176.
11. Dick M, Fyler DC, Nadas AS. Tricuspid atresia: Clinical course in 101 patients. *Am J Cardiol* 1975;36:327–337.
12. Zellers TM, Porter C, Driscoll DJ. Pseudo-preexcitation in tricuspid atresia. *Tx Heart Inst J* 1991;18:124–126.

13. Dick M, Behrendt DM, Byrum CJ, et al. Tricuspid atresia and the Wolff-Parkinson-White syndrome: Evaluation methodology and successful surgical treatment of the combined disorders. *Am Heart J* 101; 1981:496–500.
14. Wilkinson JL, Dickinson D, Smith A, et al. Conducting tissues in univentricular heart of right ventricular type with double or common inlet. *J Thorac Cardiovasc Surg* 1979;77:691–698.
15. Becker AE, Wilkinson JL, Anderson RH. Atrioventricular conduction tissues: A guide in understanding the morphogenesis of the univentricular heart. In: Van Praagh R, Takao A (eds). *Etiology and Morphogenesis of Congenital Heart Disease.* Mount Kisco, NY: Futura; 1980.
16. Kumar AE, Fyler DC, Miettinen OS, et al. Ebstein's anomaly: Clinical profile and natural history. *Am J Cardiol* 1971;28:84–95.
17. Watson H. Natural history of Ebstein's anomaly of tricuspid valve in childhood and adolescence. *Br Heart J* 1974;36:417–427.
18. Oh JK, Holmes DR, Hayes DL, et al. Cardiac arrhythmias in patients with surgical repair of Ebstein's anomaly. *J Am Coll Cardiol* 1985;6: 1351–1357.
19. Gentles TL, Calder AL, Clarkson PM, et al. Predictors of long-term survival with Ebstein's anomaly of the tricuspid valve. *Am J Cardiol* 1992;69:377–381.
20. Celermajer DS, Bull C, Cullen S, et al. Ebstein's anomaly: Presentation and outcome from fetus to adult. *J Am Coll Cardiol* 1994;23: 170–176.
21. Radford DJ, Graff RF, Neilson GH. Diagnosis and natural history of Ebstein's anomaly. *Br Heart J* 1985;54:517–522.
22. Reich JD, Auld D, Hulse E, et al. The Pediatric Radiofrequency Ablation Registry's experience with Ebstein's anomaly. *J Cardiovasc Electrophysiol* 1998;9:1370–1377.
23. Feldt RH, DuShane JW, Titus JL. The atrioventricular conduction system in persistent common atrioventricular canal defect. *Circulation* 1970;42:437–444.
24. Fournier A, Young M-L, Garcia OL, et al. Electrophysiologic cardiac function before and after surgery in children with AV canal. *Am J Cardiol* 1986;57:1137–1141.
25. Daliento L, Rizzoli G, Marchiori MC, et al. Electrical instability in patients undergoing surgery for atrioventricular septal defect. *Intern J Cardiol* 1991;30:15–21.
26. Rossi L, Montella S, Frescura C, et al. Congenital atrioventricular block in right atrial isomerism (asplenia). *Chest* 1984;85:578–580.
27. Dickinson DF, Wilkinson JL, Anderson KR, et al. The cardiac conduction system in situs ambiguus. *Circulation* 1979;59:879–886.
28. Momma K, Takao A, Shibata T. Characteristics and natural history of abnormal atrial rhythms in left isomerism. *Am J Cardiol* 1990;65:231–236.
29. Wren C, MacCartney FJ, Deanfield JE. Cardiorhythm in atrial isomerism. *Am J Cardiol* 1987;59:1156–1158.
30. Epstein MR, Saul JP, Weindling SN, et al. Atrioventricular reciprocating tachycardia involving twin atrioventricular nodes in patients with complex congenital heart disease. *J Cardiovasc Electrophysiol* 2001; 12:671–679.
31. Kyger ER, Frazier H, Cooley DA, et al. Sinus venosus atrial septal defect: Early and late results following closure in 109 patients. *Ann Thorac Surg* 1978;25:44–50.
32. Sealy WC, Farmer JC, Young G, et al. Atrial dysfunction and atrial secundum defects. *J Thorac Cardiovasc Surg* 1969;57:245–250.
33. Hamilton WT, Haffajee CI, Dalen JE, et al. Atrial septal defect secundum: Clinical profile with physiologic correlates in children and adults. *Cardiovasc Clin* 1979;10:267–277.
34. Gatzoulis MA, Feeman MA, Siu SC, et al. Atrial arrhythmia after surgical closure of atrial septal defects in adults. *N Engl J Med* 1999; 340:839–846.
35. Rokseth R. Congenital heart disease in middle-aged adults. *Acta Med Scand* 1968;183:131–138.
36. Paolillo V, Dawkins KD, Miller GAH. Atrial septal defect in patients over the age of 50. *Int J Cardiol* 1985;9:139–147.
37. Murphy JG, Gersh BJ, McGoon MD, et al. Long-term outcome after surgical repair of isolated atrial septal defect. *N Engl J Med* 1990;323: 1645–1650.
38. Gatzoulis MA, Freeman MA, Siu SC, et al. Atrial arrhythmia after surgical closure of atrial septal defects in adults. *N Engl J Med* 1999; 340:839–846.
39. Wolfe RR, Driscoll DJ, Gersony WM, et al. Arrhythmias in patients with valvar aortic stenosis, velvar pulmonary stenosis, and ventricular septal defect. *Circulation* 1993;87:I-89–I-101.
40. Wernovsky G, Hougen TJ, Walsh EP, et al. Midterm results after the arterial switch operation for transposition of the great arteries with intact ventricular septum: Clinical, hemodynamic, echocardiographic, and electrophysiologic data. *Circulation* 1988;77:1333–1344.
41. Kramer H-H, Rammos S, Krogmann O, et al. Cardiac rhythm after Mustard repair and after arterial switch operation for complete transposition. *Int J Cardiol* 1991;32:5–12.
42. Hayes CJ, Gersony WM. Arrhythmias after the Mustard operation for transposition of the great arteries: A long-term study. *J Am Coll Cardiol* 1986;7:133–137.
43. Warnes CA, Somerville J. Transposition of the great arteries: Late results in adolescents and adults after the Mustard procedure. *Br Heart J* 1987;58:148–155.
44. Gewillig M, Cullen S, Mertens B, et al. Risk factors for arrhythmia and death after Mustard operation for simple transposition of the great arteries. *Circulation* 1991;84:III-187–III-192.
45. Vetter VL, Tanner CS, Horowitz LN. Electrophysiologic consequences of the Mustard repair of d-transposition of the great arteries. *J Am Coll Cardiol* 1987;10:1265–1273.
46. Garson A, Bink-Boelkens M, Hesslein PS, et al. Atrial flutter in the young: A collaborative study of 380 cases. *J Am Coll Cardiol* 1985;6: 871–878.
47. Flinn CJ, Wolff GS, Campbell RM, et al. Natural history of supraventricular rhythms in 182 children following the Mustard operation. *J Am Coll Cardiol* 1983;1:613–618.
48. Puley G, Siu S, Connelly M, et al. Arrhythmia and survival in patients >18 years of age after the Mustard procedure for complete transposition of the great arteries. *Am J Cardiol* 1999;83:1080–1084.
49. Helbing WA, Hansen B, Ottenkamp J, et al. Long-term results of atrial correction for transposition of the great arteries. *J Thorac Cardiovasc Surg* 1994;108:363–372.
50. Vetter VL, Tanner CS, Horowitz LN. Inducible atrial flutter after the Mustard repair of complete transposition of the great arteries. *Am J Cardiol* 1988;91:428–435.
51. Driscoll DJ, Offord KP, Feldt RH, et al. Five- to fifteen-year follow-up after Fontan operation. *Circulation* 1992;85:469–496.
52. Gewillig M, Wyse RK, DeLeval MR, et al. Early and late arrhythmias after the Fontan operation: Predisposing factors and clinical consequences. *Br Heart J* 1992;67:72–79.
53. Peters NS, Somerville J. Arrhythmias after the Fontan procedure. *Br Heart J* 1992;68:199–204.
54. Rodefeld MD, Bromberg BI, Schuessler RB, et al. Atrial flutter after lateral tunnel construction in the modified Fontan procedure: A canine model. *J Thorac Cardiovasc Surg* 1996;111:514–526.
55. Gardiner HM, Dhillon R, Bull C, et al. Prospective study of the incidence and determinants of arrhythmia after total cavopulmonary connection. *Circulation* 1996;94:(9 suppl):II17–II21.
56. Viullo DA, DeLeon SY, Berry TE, et al. Clinical improvement after revision in Fontan patients. *Ann Thorac Surg* 1996;61:1797–1804.
57. Hashimoto K, Kurosawa H, Tanaka A, et al. Total cavopulmonary connection without the use of prosthetic material: Technical considerations and hemodynamic consequences. *J Thorac Cardiovasc Surg* 1995;110:625–632.
58. Pearl JM, Laks H, Stein DG, et al. Total cavopulmonary anastamosis versus conventional modified Fontan procedure. *Ann Thorac Surg* 1991;52:189–196.
59. Amodeo A, Galletti L, Marianeschi S, et al. Extracardiac Fontan operation for complex cardiac anomalies: Seven year's experience. *J Thorac Cardiovasc Surg* 1997;114:1020–1030.
60. Weber HS, Hellenbrand WE, Kleinman CS, et al. Predictors of rhythm disturbances and subsequent morbidity after the Fontan operation. *Am J Cardiol* 1989;64:762–767.

61. Mair DD, Hagler DJ, Julsrud PR, et al. Early and late results of the modified Fontan procedure for double-inlet left ventricle: The Mayo Clinic experience. *J Am Coll Cardiaol* 1991;18:1727–1732.
62. Taliercio CP, Vlietstra RE, McGoon MD, et al. Permanent cardiac pacing after the Fontan procedure. *J Thorac Cardiovasc Surg* 1985;90: 414–419.
63. Hesslein PS, Gutgesell HP, Gillette PC. Exercise assessment of sinoatrial node function in children after Mustard's operation. *Pediatr Res* 1980;14:445.
64. Saalouke MG, Rios J, Perry LW, et al. Electrophysiologic studies after Mustard's operation for d-transposition of the great vessels. *Am J Cardiol* 1978;41:1104–1109.
65. Gillette PC, Kugler JD, Garson A, et al. Mechanisms of cardiac arrhythmias after the Mustard operation for transposition of the great arteries. *Am J Cardiol* 1980;45:1225–1230.
66. Kurer CC, Tanner CS, Vetter VL. Electrophysiologic findings after Fontan repair of functional single ventricle. *J Am Coll Cardiol* 1991; 17:174–181.
67. Gregoratos G, Abrams J, Epstein AE, et al. ACC/AHA/NASPE 2002 Guideline Update for Implantation of Cardiac Pacemakers and Antiarrhythmia Devices—Summary article: A report of the American College of Cardiology/American Heart Association Task Force on Practice Guidelines (ACC/AHA/NASPE Committee to Update the 1998 Pacemaker Guidelines). *J Am Coll Cardiol* 2002;40: 1703–1719.
68. Cohen MI, Rhodes LA, Wernovsky G, et al. Atrial pacing: An alternative treatment for protein-losing enteropathy after the Fontan operation. *J Thorac Cardiovasc Surg* 2001;121:582–583.
69. Gillette PC, Wampler DG, Shannon C, et al. Use of cardiac pacing after the Mustard operation for transposition of the great arteries. *J Am Coll Cardiol* 1986;7:138–141.
70. Gillette PC, Zeigler V, Case CL, et al. Atrial antitachycardia pacing in children and young adults. *Am Heart J* 1991;122:844–849.
71. Porter CJ, Fukushige J, Hayes DL, et al. Permanent antitachycardia pacing for chronic atrial tachyarrhythmias in postoperative pediatric patients. *Pacing Clin Electrophysiol* 1991;14:2056–2057.
72. Karpawich PP, Paridon SM, Pinsky WW. Failure of rate-responsive ventricular pairing to improve physiological performance in the univentricular heart. *Pacing Clin Electrophysiol* 1991;14:2058–2061.
73. Van Hare GF, Lesh MD, Ross BA, et al. Mapping and radiofrequency ablation of intraatrial reentrant tachycardia after the Senning or Mustard procedures for transposition of the great arteries. *Am J Cardiol* 1996;77:985–991.
74. Kanter RJ, Papagiannis J, Carboni MP, et al. Radiofrequency catheter ablation of supraventricular tachycardia substrates after Mustard and Senning operations for d-transposition of the great arteries. *J Am Coll Cardiol* 2000;35:428–441.
75. Fishberger SB, Wernovsky G, Gentles TL, et al. Long-term outcome in patients with pacemakers following the Fontan operation. *Am J Cardiol* 1996;77:887–889.
76. Triedman JK, Alexander ME, Love BA. Influence of patient factors and ablative technologies on outcomes of radiofrequency catheter ablation of intaatrial reentrant tachycardia in patients with congenital heart disease. *J Am Coll Cardiol* 2002;39:1827–1835.
77. Kalman JM, Van Hare GF, Olgin JE, et al. Ablation of 'incisional' reentrant atrial tachycardia complicating surgery for congenital heart disease; use of entrainment to define critical isthmus of conduction. *Circulation* 1996;93:502–512.
78. Triedman JK, Saul JP, Weindling SN, et al. Radiofrequency ablation of intraatrial reentrant tachycardia after surgical palliation of congenital heart disease. *Circulation* 1995;91:707–714.
79. Baker BM, Lindsay BD, Bromberg BI, et al. Catheter ablation of clinical intraatrial reentrant tachycardias resulting from previous atrial surgery: Localizing and transecting the critical isthmus. *J Am Coll Cardiol* 1996;28:411–417.
80. Mavroudis C, Backer CL, Deal BJ, et al. Fontan conversion to cavopulmonary connection and arrhythmia circuit cryoablation. *J Thorac Cardiovasc Surg* 1998;115:547–556.
81. Deal BJ, Mavroudis C, Backer CL, et al. Impact of arrhythmia circuit cryoablation during Fontan conversion for refractory atrial tachycardia. *Am J Cardiol* 1999;83:563–568.
82. Moller JH, Patton C, Varco RL, et al. Postoperative ventricular septal defect: 24–30 years follow-up of 232 patients. Proceedings of the Second World Congress of Pediatric Cardiology. New York: Springer-Verlag; 1985:20.
83. Fyfe DA, Driscoll DJ, DiDonato RM, et al. Truncus arteriosus with single pulmonary artery: Influence of pulmonary vascular obstructive disease on early and late operative results. *J Am Coll Cardiol* 1985; 5:1168–1172.
84. Garson A, Nihill MR, McNamara DG, et al. Status of the adult and adolescent after repair of tetralogy of Fallot. *Circulation* 1979;59: 1232–1240.
85. Friedli B, Bolens M. Intraventricular conduction disturbances after correction of tetralogy of Fallot: Can bifascicular and trifascicular block be diagnosed from the surface ECG. *Pediatr Cardiol* 1985;6: 133–136.
86. Garson A Jr, Gillette PC, Gutgesell HP, et al. Stress-induced ventricular arrhythmia after repair of tetralogy of Fallot. *Am J Cardiol* 1980; 46:1006–1012.
87. Deanfield JE, McKenna WJ, Hallidie-Smith KA. Detection of late arrhythmia and conduction disturbance after correction to tetralogy of Fallot. *Br Heart J* 1980;44:248–253.
88. Chandar JS, Wolff GS, Garson A, et al. Ventricular arrhythmias in postoperative tetralogy of Fallot. *Am J Cardiol* 1990;65:655–661.
89. Katz NM, Blackstone EH, Kirklin JW, et al. Late survival and symptoms after repair of tetralogy of Fallot. *Circulation* 1982;65:403–410.
90. Kobayashi J, Hirose H, Nakano S, et al. Ambulatory electrocardiographic study of the frequency and cause of ventricular arrhythmia after correction of tetralogy of Fallot. *Am J Cardiol* 1984;54:1310–1313.
91. Walsh EP, Rockenmacher S, Keane JF, et al. Late results in patients with tetralogy of Fallot repaired during infancy. *Circulation* 1988;77: 1062–1067.
92. Quattlebaum TG, Varghese PJ, Neill CA, et al. Sudden death among postoperative patients with tetralogy of Fallot. A follow-up study of 243 patients for an average of twelve years. *Circulation* 1975;54: 289–293.
93. Gatzoulis MA, Till JA, Somerville J, et al. Mechanoelectrical interaction in tetralogy of Fallot: QRS prolongation relates to right ventricular size and predicts malignant ventricular arrhythmias and sudden death. *Circulation* 1995;92:231–237.
94. Berul CI, Hill SL, Geggel RL, et al. Electrocardiographic markers of late sudden death risk in postoperative tetralogy of Fallot children. *J Cardiovasc Electrophysiol* 1997;8:1349–1356.
95. Gerson A, Randall DC, Gillette PC, et al. Prevention of sudden death after repair of tetralogy of Fallot: Treatment of ventricular arrhythmias. *J Am Coll Cardiol* 1985;6:221–227.
96. Cullen S, Celermajer DS, Franklin RCG, et al. Prognostic significance of ventricular arrhythmia after repair of tetralogy of Fallot: A 12-year prospective study. *J Am Coll Cardiol* 1994;23:1151–1155.
97. Alexander ME, Walsh EP, Saul JP, et al. Value of programmed ventricular stimulation in patients with congenital heart disease. *J Cardiovasc Electrophysiol* 1999;10:1033–1044.
98. Ross-Hesselink J, Perlroth MG, McGhie J, et al. Atrial arrhythmias in adults after repair of tetralogy of Fallot: Correlations with clinical, exercise, and echocardiographic findings. *Circulation* 1995;91: 2214–2219.
99. Kugler JD, Cheatham JP, Gumbiner CH, et al. Results of phenytoin and propranolol drug electrophysiology studies for ventricular tachycardia in patients having repaired lesions with tetralogy of Fallot physiology. *Circulation* 1985;72:III-341.
100. Deal BJ, Scagliotti D, Miller SM, et al. Electrophysiologic drug testing in symptomatic ventricular arrhythmias after repair of tetralogy of Fallot. *Am J Cardiol* 1987;59:1380–1385.
101. Reimer A, Paul T, Kallfelz HC. Efficacy and safety of intravenous and oral propafenone in pediatric cardiac dysrhythmias. *Am J Cardiol* 1991;68:741–744.

102. Downar E, Harris L, Kimber S, et al. Ventricular tachycardia after surgical repair of tetralogy of Fallot: Results of intraoperative mapping studies. *J Am Coll Cardiol* 1992;20:648–655.
103. Horton RP, Canby RC, Kessler DJ, et al. Ablation of ventricular tachycardia associated with tetralogy of Fallot: Demonstration of bidirectional block. *J Cardiovasc Electrophysiol* 1997;8:432–435.
104. Papagiannis J, Kanter RJ, Wharton JM. Radiofrequency catheter ablation of multiple haemodynamically unstable ventricular tachycardias in a patient with surgically repaired tetralogy of Fallot. *Cardiol Young* 1998;8:379–382.
105. Silka MJ, Kron J, Dunnigan A, et al. Sudden cardiac death and the use of implantable cardioverter/defibrillators in pediatric patients. *Circulation* 1993;87:800–807.
106. Menendez T, Achenbach S, Beinder E, et al. Usefulness of magnetocardiography for the investigation of fetal arrhythmias. *Am J Cardiol* 2001;88:334–336.
107. Kahler C, Grimm B, Schleussner E, et al. The application of fetal magnetocardiography (FMCG) to investigate fetal arrhythmias and congenital heart defects (CHD). *Prenat Diagn* 2001;21:176–182.
108. van Leeuwen P, Hailer B, Bader W, et al. Magnetocardiography in the diagnosis of fetal arrhythmia. *Br J Obstet Gynaecol* 1999;106:1200–1208.
109. Wakai RT, Strasburger JF, Li Z, et al. Magnetocardiographic rhythm patterns at initiation and termination of fetal supraventricular tachycardia. *Circulation* 2003;107:307–312.
110. Rein AJ, Levine JC, Nir A. Use of high-frame rate imaging and doppler tissue echocardiography in the diagnosis of fetal ventricular tachycardia. *J Am Soc Echocardiogr* 2001;14:149–151.
111. Vaccaro H, Amor F, Leyton M, et al. Arrhythmia in early pregnancy: A predictor of first-trimester pregnancy loss. *Ultrasound Obstet Gynecol* 1998;12:248–251.
112. Copal JA, Liang RI, Demasio K, et al. The clinical significance of the irregular fetal heart rhythm. *Am J Obstet Gynecol* 2000;182:813–817.
113. Maeno Y, Kiyomatsu Y, Rikitake N, et al. Fetal arrhythmias: Intrauterine diagnosis, treatment, and prognosis. *Acta Paediatrica Japonica* 1995;37:431–436.
114. Rane HS, Purandare HM, Chakraverty A. Type and significance of fetal arrhythmias. *Indian Heart J* 1996;48:40–44.
115. Kleinman CS. Prenatal diagnosis and management of intrauterine arrhythmias. *Fetal Therapy* 1986;1:92–95.
116. Silverman NH, Enderlein MA, Stanger P, et al. Recognition of fetal arrhythmia by echocardiography. *J Clin Ultrasound* 1985;13:255–263.
117. Simpson JM, Sharland GK. Fetal tachycardias: Management and outcome of 127 consecutive cases. *Heart* 1998;79:576–581.
118. Lisowski LA, Verheijen PM, Benatar AA, et al. Atrial flutter in the perinatal age group: Diagnosis, management and outcome. *J Am Coll Cardiol* 2000;35:771–777.
119. Oudijk MA, Michon MM, Kleinman CS, et al. Sotalol in the treatment of fetal dysrhythmias. *Circulation* 2000;101:2721–2726.
120. Flack NJ, Zosmer N, Bennett PR, et al. Amiodarone given by three routes to terminate fetal atrial flutter associated with severe hydrops. *Obstet Gynecol* 1993;82:714–716.
121. Lee LA, Weston WL. New findings in neonatal lupus syndrome. *Am J Dis Child* 1984;138:233–236.
122. Scott JS, Maddison PJ, Taylor PV, et al. Connective tissue disease, antibodies to ribonucleoprotein, and congenital heart block. *N Engl J Med* 1983;309:209–212.
123. Boutjdir M, Chen L, Zhang ZH, et al. Serum and immunoglobulin G from the mother of a child with congenital heart block induce conduction abnormalities and inhibit L-type calcium channels in a rat heart model. *Pediatr Res* 1998;44:11–19.
124. Boutjdir M. Molecular and ionic basis of congenital complete heart block. *Trends Cardiovasc Med* 2000;10:114–122.
125. Scott JS, Maddison PJ, Taylor PV, et al. Connective tissue disease, antibodies to ribonucleoprotein, and congenital heart block. *N Engl J Med* 1983;309:209–212.
126. Brucato A, Frassi M, Franceschini F, et al. Risk of congenital complete heart block in newborns of mothers with anti-Ro/SSA antibodies detected by counterimmunoelectrophoresis: A prospective study of 100 women. *Arthritis Rheumatol* 2001;44:1832–1835.
127. Askanase AD, Friedman DM, Copel J, et al. Spectrum and progression of conduction abnormalities in infants born to mothers with anti-SSA/Ro-SSB/La antibodies. *Lupus* 2002;11:145–151.
128. Benson DW, Silberbach GM, Kavanaugh-McHugh A, et al. Mutations in the cardiac transcription factor NKX2.5 affect diverse cardiac developmental pathways. *J Clin Invest* 1999;104:1567–1573.
129. Gutierrez-Roelens I, Sluysmans T, Gewillig M, et al. Progressive AV-block and anomalous venous return among cardiac anomalies associated with two novel missense mutations in the CSX/NKX2-5 gene. *Hum Mutat* 2002;20:75–76.
130. Deloof E, Devlieger H, Van Hoestenberghe R, et al. Management with a staged approach of the premature hydropic fetus due to complete congenital heart block. *Eur J Pediatr* 1997;156:521–523.
131. Michaelsson M, Riesenfeld T, Jonzon A. Natural history of congenital complete atrioventricular block. *Pacing Clin Electrophysiol* 1997;20(8 pt 2):2098–2101.
132. Ko JK, Deal BJ, Strasburger JF, Benson DW Jr. Supraventricular tachycardia mechanisms and their age distribution in pediatric patients. *Am J Cardiol* 1992;69:1028–1032.
133. Deal BJ, Keane JF, Gillette PC, et al. Wolff-Parkinson-White syndrome and supraventricular tachycardia during infancy: Management and follow-up. *J Am Coll Cardiol* 1985;5:130–135.
134. Perry JC, Garson A Jr. Supraventricular tachycardia due to Wolff-Parkinson-White syndrome in children: Early disappearance and late recurrence. *J Am Coll Cardiol* 1990;16:1215–1220.
135. Lundberg A. Paroxysmal atrial tachycardia in infancy: Long-term follow-up study of 49 subjects. *Pediatrics* 1982;70:638–642.
136. Hashino K, Ishii M, Toyoda O, et al. Natural history of asymptomatic Wolff-Parkinson-White syndrome in children [abstract]. *Circulation* 1999;18:I-322.
137. Pappone C, Santinelli V, Rosanio S, et al. Usefulness of invasive electrophysiologic testing to stratify the risk of arrhythmic events in asymptomatic patients with Wolff-Parkinson-White pattern: Results from a large prospective long-term follow-up study. *J Am Coll Cardiol* 2003;41:239–244.
138. Cnota JF, Ross JE, Knilans TK, et al. Does intermittent accessory pathway block during slow sinus rhythm always imply a low risk for rapid AV conduction of preexcited atrial fibrillation? *Cardiology* 2002;98:106–108.
139. Kanter RJ, Raines KJH, Wharton JM, et al. Characterization of sudden cardiac death risk in pediatric patients with the Wolff-Parkinson-White syndrome [abstract]. *J Am Coll Cardiol* 1990;15:212A.
140. Klersy C, Chimienti M, Marangoni E, et al. Factors that predict spontaneous remission of ectopic atrial tachycardia. *Eur Heart J* 1993;14:1654–1656.
141. Garson A, Smith RT, Moak JP, et al. Incessant ventricular tachycardia in infants: Myocardial hamartomas and surgical cure. *J Am Coll Cardiol* 1987;10:619–626.
142. Casey FA, McCrindle BW, Hamilton RM, et al. Neonatal atrial flutter: Significant early morbidity and excellent long-term prognosis. *Am Heart J* 1997;133:302–306.
143. Peng CC, Chen MR, Hou CJ, et al. Atrial flutter in the neonate and infancy. *Jpn Heart J* 1998;39:287–295.
144. Drago F, Mazza A, Garibaldi S, et al. Isolated neonatal atrial flutter: Clinical features, prognosis and therapy. *G Ital Cardiol* 1998;28:365–368.
145. Lisowski LA, Verheijen PM, Benatar AA, et al. Atrial flutter in the perinatal age group: Diagnosis, management and outcome. *J Am Coll Cardiol* 200;35:771–777.
146. Jaeggi E, Fouron JC, Drblik SP. Fetal atrial flutter: Diagnosis, clinical features, treatment, and outcome. *J Pediatr* 1998;132:335–339.
147. Uerpairojkit B, Tanawattanacharoen S, Manotaya S, et al. Intrauterine therapy of fetal atrial flutter. *J Obstet Gynaecol Res* 1998;24:135–139.
148. Farooki ZQ, Green EW. Multifocal atrial tachycardia in two neonates. *Br Heart J* 1977;39:872–874.
149. Salim MA, Case CL, Gillette PC. Chaotic atrial tachycardia in children. *Am Heart J* 1995;129:831–833.

150. Fish FA, Mehta AV, Johns JA. Characteristics and management of chaotic atrial tachycardia of infancy. *Am J Cardiol* 1996;78: 1052–1055.
151. Bradley DJ, Fischbach PS, Law IH, et al. The clinical course of multifocal atrial tachycardia in infants and children. *J Am Coll Cardiol* 2001;38:401–408.
152. Bisset GS III, Seigal SF, Gauw WE, et al. Chaotic atrial tachycardia in childhood. *Am Heart J* 1981;101:268–272.
153. Liberthson RR, Colan SD. Multifocal or chaotic atrial rhythm: Report of nine infants, delineation of clinical course and management and review of literature. *Pediatr Cardiol* 1982;2:179–184.
154. Brevilacqua LM, Rhee EK, Epstein MR, et al. Focal ablation of chaotic atrial rhythm in an infant with cardiomyopathy. *J Cardiovasc Electrophysiol* 2000;11:577–581.
155. Dodo H, Gow RM, Hamilton RM, et al. Chaotic atrial rhythm in children. *Am Heart J* 1995;129:990–995.
156. Yeager SB, Hougen TJ, Levy AM. Sudden death in infants with chaotic atrial tachycardia. *Am J Dis Child* 1984;138:689–692.
157. Celiker A, Kocak G, Lenk MK, et al. Short- and intermediate-term efficacy of amiodarone in infants and children with cardiac arrhythmia. *Turkish Heart J* 1997;39:219–225.
158. Houyel L, Fournier A, Davignon A. Successful treatment of chaotic atrial tachycardia with oral flecainide. *Intern J Cardiol* 1990;27:27–29.
159. Reimer A, Paul T, Kallfelz HC. Efficacy and safety of intravenous and oral propafenone in pediatric cardiac dysrhythmias. *Am J Cardiol* 1991;68:741–744.
160. Garson A, Gillette PC. Junctional ectopic tachycardia in children: electrocardiography, electrophysiology, and pharmacologic response. *Am J Cardiol* 1979;44:298–302.
161. Sarubbi B, Musto B, Ducceschi V, et al. Congenital junctional ectopic tachycardia in children and adolescents: A 20 year experience based study. *Heart* 2002;88:188–190.
162. Villain E, Vetter VL, Garcia JM, et al. Evolving concepts in the management of congenital junctional ectopic tachycardia. A multicenter study. *Circulation* 1990;81:1544–1549.
163. Maragnes P, Fournier A, Davignon A. Usefulness of oral sotalol for the treatment of junctional ectopic tachycardia. *Intern J Cardiol* 1992;35: 165–167.
164. Wu JM, Young ML, Wu MH, et al. Junctional ectopic tachycardia in infancy: Report of two cases. *J Formosan Med Assoc* 1991;90:517–519.
165. Henneveld H, Hutter P, Bink-Boelkens M, et al. Junctional ectopic tachycardia evolving into complete heart block. *Heart* 1998;80: 627–628.
166. Lupoglazoff JM, Denjoy I, Luton D, et al. Prenatal diagnosis of a familial form of junctional ectopic tachycardia. *Prenat Diagn* 1999;19: 767–770.
167. Celiker A, Ceviz N, Ozme S, Effectiveness and safety of intravenous amiodarone in drug-resistant tachyarrhythmias of children. *Acta Paediatrica Japonica* 1998;40:567–572.
168. Paul T, Reimer A, Janousek J, et al. Efficacy and safety of propafenone in congenital junctional ectopic tachycardia. *J Am Coll Cardiol* 1992; 20:911–914.
169. Van Hare GF, Velvis H, Langberg JJ. Successful transcatheter ablation of congenital junctional ectopic tachycardia in a ten-month-old infant using radiofrequency energy. *Pacing Clin Electrophysiol* 1990;13: 730–735.
170. Fukuhara H, Nakamura Y, Ohnishi T. Atrial pacing during radiofrequency ablation of junctional ectopic tachycardia—A useful technique for avoiding atrioventricular block. *Jpn Circulat J* 2001;65:242–244.
171. Fishberger SB, Rossi AF, Messina JJ, et al. Successful radiofrequency catheter ablation of congenital junctional ectopic tachycardia with preservation of atrioventricular conduction in a 9-month-old infant. *Pacing Clin Electrophysiol* 1998;21:2132–2135.
172. Wu MH, Lin JL, Chang YC. Catheter ablation of junctional ectopic tachycardia by guarded low dose radiofrequency energy application. *Pacing Clin Electrophysiol* 1996;19:1655–1658.
173. Young ML, Mehta MB, Martinez RM, et al. Combined alpha-adrenergic blockade and radiofrequency ablation to treat junctional ectopic tachycardia successfully without atrioventricular block. *Am J Cardiol* 1993;71:883–885.
174. Rychik J, Marchlinski FE, Sweeten TL, et al. Transcatheter radiofrequency abaltion for congenital junctional ectopic tachycardia in infancy. *Pediatr Cardiol* 1997;18:447–450.
175. Grant JW, Serwer GA, Armstrong BE, et al. Junctional tachycardia in infants and children after open heart surgery for congenital heart disease. *Am J Cardiol* 1987;59:1216–1218.
176. Bach SE, Shah JJ, Albers WH, et al. Hypothermia for the treatment of postsurgical greatly accelerated junctional ectopic tachycardia. *J Am Coll Cardiol* 1987;10:1095–1099.
177. Till JA, Rowland E. Atrial pacing as an adjunct to the management of post-surgical His bundle tachycardia. *Br Heart J* 1991;66:225–229.
178. Hoffman TM, Bush DM, Wernovsky G, et al. Postoperative junctional ectopic tachycardia in children: Incidence, risk factors, and treatment. *Ann Thorac Surg* 2002;74:1607–1611.
179. Perry JC, Fenrich AL, Hulse JE, et al. Pediatric use of intravenous amiodarone: Efficacy and safety in critically ill patients from a multicenter protocol. *J Am Coll Cardiol* 1996;27:1246–1250.
180. Vignati G, Mauri L, Figini A. The use of propafenone in the treatment of tachyarrhythmias in children. *Eur Heart J* 1993;14:546–550.
181. Walsh EP, Saul JP, Sholler GF, et al. Evaluation of a staged treatment protocol for rapid automatic junctional tachycardia after operation for congenital heart disease. *J Am Coll Cardiol* 1997;29:1046–1053.
182. Pfammatter JP, Paul T, Ziemer G, et al. Successful management of junctional tachycardia by hypothermia after cardiac operations in infants. *Ann Thorac Surg* 1995;60:556–560.
183. Hamdan M, Van Hare GF, Fisher W, et al. Selective catheter ablation of the tachycardia focus in patients with nonreentrant junctional tachycardia. *Am J Cardiol* 1996;78:1292–1297.
184. Ehlert FA, Goldberger JJ, Deal BJ, et al. Successful radiofrequency energy ablation of automatic juctional tachycardia preserving normal atrioventricular nodal conduction. *Pacing Clin Electrophysiol* 1993; 16:54–61.
185. Van Hare GF, Velvis H, Langberg JJ. Successful transcatheter ablation of congenital junctional ectopic tachycardia in a ten-month-old infant using radiofrequency energy. *Pacing Clin Electrophysiol* 1990;13:730–735.
186. Gillette PC, Garson A, Porter CJ, et al. Junctional automatic ectopic tachycardia: New proposed treatment by transcatheter His bundle ablation. *Am Heart J* 1983;106:619–623.
187. Moak JP, Pharmacology and electrophysiology of antiarrhythmic drugs. In: Gillette PC, Garson A Jr (eds). *Pediatric Arrhythmias: Electrophysiology and Pacing*. Philadelphia: Saunders; 1990:37–115.
188. Van Hare GF, Witherell CL, Lesh MD. Follow-up of radiofrequency catheter ablation in children: Results in 100 consecutive patients. *J Am Coll Cardiol* 1994;23:1651–1659.
189. Kugler JD, Danford DA, Deal BJ, et al. Radiofrequency catheter ablation for tachyarrhythmias in children and adolescents. The Pediatric Electrophysiology Society. *N Engl J Med* 1994;330:1481–1487.
190. Saul JP, Hulse JE, Papagiannis J, et al. Late enlargement of radiofrequency lesions in infant lambs: Implications for ablation procedures in small children. *Circulation* 1994;90:492–499.
191. Goldberg CS, Caplan MJ, Heidelberger KP, et al. The dimensions of the triangle of Koch in children. *Am J Cardiol* 1999;83:117–120.
192. Case CL, Gillette PC, Oslizlok PC, et al. Radiofrequency catheter ablation of incessant, medically resistant supraventricular tachycardia in infants and small children. *J Am Coll Cardiol* 1992;20:1405–1410.
193. Park JK, Halperin BD, Kron J, et al. Analysis of body surface area as a determinant of impedance during radiofrequency catheter ablation in adults and children. *J Electrocardiol* 1994;27:329–332.
194. Dick M, Law IH, Dorostkar PC, et al. Use of the His/RVA electrode catheter in children. *J Electrocardiol* 1996;29(suppl):227–233.
195. Miga DE, McKeller LF, Denslow S, et al. Incidence of femoral vein occlusion after catheter ablation in children: Evaluation with magnetic resonance angiography. *Pediatr Cardiol* 1997;18:204–207.
196. Fischbach P, Campbell RM, Hulse E, et al. Transhepatic access to the atrioventricular ring for delivery of radiofrequency energy. *J Cardiovasc Electrophysiol* 1997;8:512–516.

197. Erb TO, Kanter RJ, Hall JM, et al. A randomized comparison of electrophysiologic effects of propofol and isoflurane based anesthetics in children and adolescents undergoing radiofrequency catheter ablation for supraventricular tachycardia. *Anesthesiology* 2002;96:1386–1394.
198. Vazir-Marino F, Young ML, Kohli V, et al Controlled ventilation enhances catheter stability during radiofrequency ablation. *Pacing Clin Electrophysiol* 1999;22:86–90.
199. Friedman RA, Walsh EP, Silka MJ, et al. NASPE Expert Consensus Conference: Radiofrequency catheter ablation in children with and without congenital heart disease. Report of the writing committee. North American Society of Pacing and Electrophysiology. *Pacing Clin Electrophysiol* 2002;25:1000–1017.
200. Schaffer MS, Gow RM, Moak JP, et al. Mortality following radiofrequency ablation (from the Pediatric Radiofrequency Ablation Registry). *Am J Cardiol* 2000;86:639–643.
201. Karpawich PP, Justice CD, Cavitt DL, et al. Developmental sequelae of fixed-rate ventricular pacing in the immature canine heart: An electrophysiologic, hemodynamic, and histopathologic evaluation. *Am Heart J* 1990;119:1077–1083.
202. Tangengco MV, Thomas RL, Karpawich PP. Left ventricular dysfunction after long-term right ventricular apical pacing in the young. *J Am Coll Cardiol* 2001;37:2093–2100.
203. Figa FH, McCrindle BW, Bigras JL, et al. Risk factors for venous obstruction in children with transvenous pacing leads. *Pacing Clin Electrophysiol* 1997;20:1902–1909.
204. O'Sullivan JJ, Jameson S, Gold RG, et al. Endocardial pacemakers in children: Lead length and allowance for growth. *Pacing Clin Electrophysiol* 1993;16:267–271.
205. Alpern D, Uzark K, Dick M II. Psychosocial responses of children to cardiac pacemakers. *J Pediatr* 1989;114:494–501.
206. Andersen C, Horder K, Kristensen L, et al. Psychosocial aspects and mental health in children after permanent pacemaker implantation. *Acta Cardiol* 1994;49:405–418.
207. Meissner MD, Lehman MH, Steinman RT, et al. Ventricular fibrillation in patients without significant structural heart disease: A multicenter experience with implantable cardioverter-defibrillator therapy. *J Am Coll Cardiol* 1993;21:1406–1412.
208. Bocker D, Block M, Isbruck F, et al. Do patients with an implantable defibrillator live longer? *J Am Coll Cardiol* 1993;21:1638–1644.
209. Silka MJ, Kron J, Dunnigan A, et al. Sudden cardiac death and the use of implantable cardioverter-defibrillators in pediatric patients. *Circulation* 1993;87:800–807.
210. Fischbach PS, Law IH, Dick M II, et al. Use of single coil transvenous electrode with an abdominally placed implantable cardioverter defibrillator in children. *Pacing Clin Electrophysiol* 2000;23:884–887.

PART FIVE

# SYNCOPE, SUDDEN DEATH, AND CARDIOPULMONARY RESUSCITATION

CHAPTER 40

# DIAGNOSIS AND MANAGEMENT OF SYNCOPE

Steven D. Nelson / Harisios Boudoulas / Stephen F. Schaal / Richard P. Lewis



*Syncope* is a sudden and transient loss of consciousness. The occurrence of syncope in the general population, as reflected in the 26-year surveillance of the Framingham Study, is 3.0 percent in men and 3.5 percent in women in the general population. As a general rule, the incidence of syncope increases with age.[1]

As an initial presentation, syncope denotes a diversity of disorders ranging from a benign episode to potentially lethal cardiac arrhythmias. Studies in recent years have documented the multiple causes and the widely divergent mortality risks associated with an episode of syncope.[2] On the basis of these studies, patients with a transient episode of altered consciousness (presyncope) and those with complete loss of consciousness (syncope) can be classified into three broad categories, *cardiac syncope, noncardiac syncope,* and *syncope of undetermined cause.* The relative incidence of these categories varies with the clinical site from which the patients are selected. In the emergency room, noncardiac syncope is most common. For patients admitted to the hospital, cardiac syncope is the most common diagnosis.[3]

Clearly, the highest mortality occurs among those with cardiac syncope.[2] Among all patients with syncope associated with cardiac disease, the incidence of sudden death is extremely high.[2]

## NONCARDIAC SYNCOPE

Sudden transient loss or impairment of consciousness occurs under a wide variety of circumstances. The pathophysiologic mechanisms, diagnostic features, and therapy for these disorders are discussed below (Table 40-1).

### Neurocardiogenic Syncope

The syndrome of neurocardiogenic syncope, the common faint (also referred to as neurally mediated hypotension, neurocardiogenic syncope, vasovagal syncope, and vasodepressor syncope), is one of the most common causes of syncope. This disorder is considered to be an abnormality in the complex neurocardiovascular interactions responsible for maintaining systemic and cerebral perfusion during upright posture (Fig. 40-1).[4–10]

#### PATHOPHYSIOLOGY

The pathophysiology of neurocardiogenic syncope is quite complex and incompletely understood. Under normal circumstances, upright posture causes venous pooling and a transient decrease in arterial pressure, resulting in an unloading of baroreceptors. Reflex augmentation of sympathetic activity and parasympathetic withdrawal result in peripheral arterial vasoconstriction, venoconstriction, and an increase in heart rate and contractility. These adaptive mechanisms serve to maintain normal systemic and cerebral perfusion. Neuroendocrine systems (e.g., renin-angiotensin and vasopressin) may be important modulators of homeostasis during prolonged periods of orthostatic stress.[11] Cerebral blood flow velocity declines before arterial pressure.[12]

Individuals susceptible to neurocardiogenic syncope are unable to maintain the adaptive neurocardiovascular responses to upright posture for prolonged periods. These patients tend to have a modest reduction in central blood volume, which is aggravated by upright posture. Increases in circulating catecholamines and cardiac adrenergic tone in response to orthostatic stress result in increased myocardial contractility.[13] Studies in animal models suggest that, under these conditions, cardiopulmonary mechanoreceptors are activated, resulting in increased neural traffic across afferent C fibers leading to the central nervous system vasomotor center; this, in turn, results in reflex paradoxical vasodilation (vasodepressor response) and bradycardia (cardioinhibitory response).[14] The final result is hypotension, cerebral hypoperfusion, cerebral hypoxia, and syncope. This paradoxical reflex is believed to be a variant of the Bezold-Jarisch reflex and has also been documented during nitrate therapy for acute myocardial ischemia and during acute hemorrhagic syndromes.[15,16] In addition, vasomotor center activation is believed to cause several of the prodromal symptoms of diaphoresis, nausea, vomiting, and dyspnea that frequently accompany neurocardiogenic syncope. Recent

TABLE 40-1 Classification of Noncardiac Syncope

- Neurocardiogenic
- Orthostatic
- Cerebrovascular
- Seizure disorders
- Carotid sinus hypersensitivity
- Situational
  - Cough
  - Swallowing
  - Valsalva
  - Micturition
  - Defecation
  - Diver's
  - Postprandial
- Metabolic, drugs
  - Hypoxia
  - Hypoglycemia
  - Hyperventilation, panic attacks
  - Ethanol, other drugs
- Other forms of syncope or conditions mimicking syncope
  - Vertigo
  - Migraine
  - Psychiatric

evidence from patients with denervated hearts (i.e., cardiac transplantation patients) and those with neurocardiogenic syncope raises the possibility that other neurohumoral mechanisms, primarily involving the peripheral circulation, may play an important role.[17]

The mechanism of paradoxical vasodilation observed during neurocardiogenic syncope is incompletely understood. Clinical studies have shown that serum epinephrine concentrations surge prior to the syncopal event, with resultant intense $\beta_2$ activation, which may cause inappropriate vasodilation and syncope. Withdrawal of peripheral sympathetic neural activity at the time of neurocardiogenic syncope has also been demonstrated by direct recordings of sympathetic neural activity.[18]

The paradoxical bradycardia (cardioinhibitory response) during neurocardiogenic syncope is due to a surge in cardiac parasympathetic tone and usually lags vasodilation by several seconds.[19] The cardioinhibitory response is highly variable, ranging from a relative bradycardia with heart rates in the range of 40 to 60 beats per minute to profound periods of asystole. Variable degrees of atrioventricular (AV) block and junctional escape rhythms are observed as well. *Bradycardia aggravates hypotension during neurocardiogenic syncope but is not its principal cause.* Maintaining heart rate with atropine or cardiac pacing will often reduce but not prevent symptomatic hypotension during neurocardiogenic syncope. Elderly patients with neurocardiogenic syncope are likely to have a predominant vasodepressor response without a significant cardioinhibitory component.

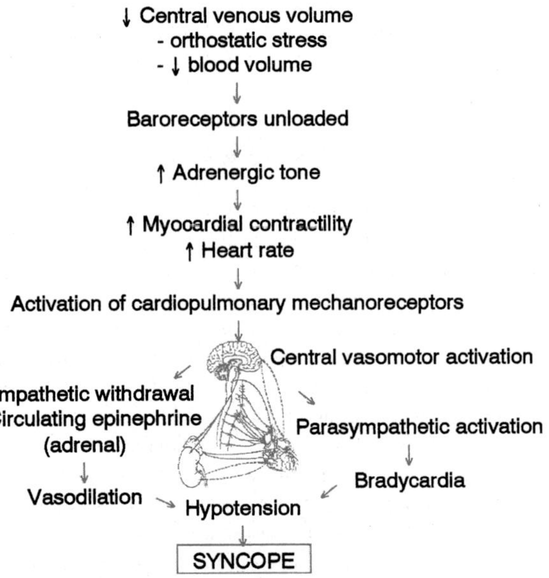

## CLINICAL CHARACTERISTICS

Predisposition to neurocardiogenic syncope occurs under a wide variety of clinical circumstances. Indeed, the neurocardiogenic reaction per se may be the ultimate cause of most types of syncope. Neurocardiogenic syncope may occur in individuals with transient reductions in blood volume, such as occur following a brisk diuresis or blood donation. Neurocardiogenic syncope complicates acute febrile infections and may occur after prolonged recumbency in chronic illness. Normal individuals at prolonged bed rest have a propensity for fainting, particularly when they arise abruptly from a sitting or recumbent position. Neurocardiogenic syncope is probably the most frequent cause of cardiovascular collapse during dental manipulations (dental syncope).[20] Neurocardiogenic syncope has been rarely noted to follow strenuous exercise. Neurocardiogenic syncope of an unusual type may occur in pregnancy, being precipitated when the patient is supine and reversed when the patient assumes a lateral decubitus or upright posture (see Chap. 82).

The identification of aggravating factors (*triggers*) is important not only for the diagnosis but also for the prevention of syncope. Situations that decrease central venous volume or increase cardiovascular adrenergic tone are particularly important in the aggravation of neurocardiogenic syncope. The postprandial state, exertion in warm environments, prolonged upright posture, sodium restriction or diuretic use, and emotional or stressful situations are but a few important triggers to consider. Evidence suggests a relationship between chronic fatigue syndrome and neurocardiogenic syncope.[21]

The classic syncopal spell is often preceded by a constellation of prodromal symptoms occurring several seconds prior to the syncopal event. The prodrome may include symptoms of nausea, headache, diaphoresis, dizziness, chest pain, palpitations, dyspnea, and paresthesia. These symptoms may also persist for several minutes to several hours after the syncopal episode has resolved. Patients with sudden loss of consciousness may not report prodromal symptoms. Usually the spell occurs when the patient is upright; it is less likely while the patient is seated. *Syncope while supine should prompt the search for etiologies other than neurocardiogenic syncope.*

During the syncopal episode, patients typically appear pale and diaphoretic, with a slow, diminished pulse. Occasionally, seizure-like activity may occur during asystolic periods. The syncopal spell classically resolves spontaneously once the patient is in the supine position, but it may recur if the patient stands or sits upright soon after the initial spell. The observations of a bystander are particularly helpful.

***Natural History*** The frequency and clinical significance of neurocardiogenic syncope are highly variable. Neurocardiogenic syncope



FIGURE 40-1 Presumed mechanisms of neurocardiogenic syncope. Schematic presentation. ↑ = increase; ↓ = decrease.

may occur as a single isolated event or as a cluster of spells over weeks to months or may be a recurrent lifetime problem. The overall prognosis in patients with neurocardiogenic syncope is quite favorable compared with arrhythmic or cardiac obstructive forms of syncope.[2] A very small subset of patients has been described as having *malignant* neurocardiogenic syncope.[22,23] This form of syncope is characterized by profound periods of asystole with sudden loss of consciousness, potentially leading to severe trauma and a theoretically increased risk of ischemia-mediated ventricular tachyarrhythmias. This risk is greatest in patients with underlying structural heart disease.

## DIAGNOSTIC EVALUATION

Head-up tilt (HUT) testing has become a useful diagnostic study for the identification of patients with neurocardiogenic syncope.[24–27] The sensitivity, specificity, and reproducibility of HUT testing depend on the patient population studied and the HUT protocol employed.[24–32] HUT at an angle of 60 to 90 degrees for a time period of 20 to 60 min has been found to yield a sensitivity ranging from 20 to 74 percent. Longer durations of HUT (45 to 60 min) lead to improved sensitivity without a significant increase in false-positive responses. Recent studies suggest that the optimal HUT angle should be between 60 and 80 degrees. Tilt angles less than 45 degrees sacrifice sensitivity, whereas angles greater than 80 degrees can result in more false-positive results.[25] An average of 63 percent of patients studied with HUT after a negative electrophysiologic study were found to have a positive HUT response, suggesting that a significant proportion of patients with unexplained syncope have neurocardiogenic syncope. Isoproterenol infusion during HUT testing has been shown to improve sensitivity.[24] Low-dose isoproterenol infusion (<2 $\mu$g min) has been shown to nearly double the number of positive responses compared with baseline (short-duration HUT), with an acceptable specificity of 93 percent and reproducibility of 83 percent.[30] High doses of isoproterenol, especially at HUT angles of greater than 80 degrees, markedly increase the incidence of false-positive responses.[31] High-dose intravenous isoproterenol, intravenous adenosine, and sublingual nitroglycerin during HUT have all been shown to increase sensitivity with some reduction in specificity and significant reduction in the time required to perform the test.[33–35]

## MANAGEMENT

The management of recurrent neurocardiogenic syncope is challenging and sometimes unsatisfactory. The choice of therapy should be based on an understanding of the neurocardiovascular cascade that eventually culminates in neurocardiogenic syncope. General measures include counseling the patient to avoid dehydration, prolonged periods of standing motionless, and situations known to trigger syncope. Avoiding medications that may aggravate neurocardiogenic syncope (i.e., vasodilators, diuretics) is advised.[36] Recent randomized studies have shown that the angiotensin-converting enzyme (ACE) inhibitor enalapril may actually prevent neurocardiogenic syncope by inhibition of reflex sympathethic system activiation.[37,38] Alcohol may also potentiate orthostatic hypotension. Increased salt and fluid intake is usually beneficial.[39,40] Patients should be educated to recognize premonitory symptoms and, if present, to assume a recumbent position and cough in order to maintain cerebral perfusion. Data suggest that tilt and exercise training may improve outcome.[41–43] In addition, isometric arm or leg counterpressure maneuvers may abort impending vasovagal syncope.[44,45]

The severity and frequency of recurrence of neurocardiogenic syncope are highly variable; therefore pharmacologic management must be highly individualized. Patients with infrequent near-syncopal spells may respond to general measures alone. Frequent syncopal spells, especially if trauma occurs, usually necessitate pharmacologic interventions.

Therapeutic options include volume expansion, beta-adrenergic receptor blockade, anticholinergic agents, serotonin reuptake inhibitors, methylxanthines, alpha agonists, and dual-chamber cardiac pacing. A stepped approach to pharmacologic therapy is advisable, starting with low initial doses, as these patients seem to be more prone to adverse reactions than the general population. The dose can be gradually titrated upward until the frequency and severity of spells are diminished. If one class of drug is ineffective, a combination of drugs, each acting on different limbs responsible for the neurocardiogenic syncope, may be beneficial. The reproducibility of HUT is variable; therefore repeated tilt testing may not accurately predict clinical response to therapy.[46,47] Few prospective randomized controlled trials of various therapies are available to support the superiority of any specific approach.

***Volume Expansion*** A significant proportion of patients with neurocardiogenic syncope have evidence of mild reduction in central plasma volume, and plasma volume expansion can prevent recurrence. Simple measures such as liberalizing salt and fluid intake may suffice.[48,49] Custom-fitted counterpressure support garments that extend from the ankle to the waist may be of benefit in highly motivated individuals. In some instances, fludrocortisone acetate may be helpful in augmenting salt retention and volume expansion. The initial dose is 0.1 mg daily; this may be increased by increments of 0.1 mg every 5 to 7 days. The maintenance dose varies from 0.1 to 1.0 mg daily.[50] Potential side effects include recumbent hypertension, marked fluid retention, congestive heart failure, and hypokalemia.

***Beta Blockers*** Increased adrenergic stimulation with resultant activation of cardiac mechanoreceptors is believed to be an important mechanism in the pathophysiologic cascade that culminates in neurocardiogenic syncope. The negative inotropic effect of beta blockers may theoretically prevent activation of the ventricular mechanoreceptors or block the peripheral vasodilator effects of beta-adrenergic receptor stimulation. Earlier nonrandomized trials have shown that metoprolol prevents symptom recurrence and neurocardiogenic syncope during tilt testing. Beta blockers may be more effective in patients who have abnormal tilt tests during isoproterenol infusion. Randomized trials suggest that not all beta blockers are equally effective compared to placebo controls.[51–53]

***Anticholinergic Agents*** During neurocardiogenic syncope, certain subsets of patients experience profound bradycardia that can aggravate the hypotension associated with vasodilation. This subset is believed to have a sudden surge in vagal activity because the bradyarrhythmia, but not the vasodilation, can be prevented by intravenous atropine. The profound bradyarrhythmias are primarily observed in the young and presumably healthy age group. Despite the unimpressive response of neurocardiogenic syncope to atropine, certain other anticholinergic drugs may be of benefit if tolerated. The anticholinergic activity of propantheline bromide may make this an effective treatment in nonrandomized trials.[54]

Transdermal scopolamine has been shown to be a useful preventive agent in certain subsets of patients with recurrent neurocardiogenic syncope. Its mechanism of action is poorly understood but is probably related to its peripheral anticholinergic actions as well as a depressant effect on central nervous system transmission to the autonomic nervous system. These central actions of scopolamine are believed to be important for the prevention of the nausea of motion sickness, which may incidentally involve neuropathways common to the vasovagal pathways.[55]

The class 1A antiarrhythmic drug disopyramide has known anticholinergic and negative inotropic properties. These properties, which are considered undesirable effects of disopyramide in the therapy of tachyarrhythmias, theoretically may prevent the activation of cardiopulmonary mechanoreceptors and the neurogenic reflex observed in neurocardiogenic syncope. However, data are conflicting regarding the efficacy of disopyramide. One randomized trial showed disopyramide and placebo to be equally effective.[46] Disopyramide is not a first-line therapy and must be used with caution because of its potential to cause proarrhythmia. In addition, the noncardiovascular anticholinergic side effects of disopyramide may be intolerable for some patients.

***Serotonin Reuptake Inhibitors*** Serotonin may be an important mediator of inappropriate vasodilation and bradycardia in animal models of hemorrhagic shock. Blockade of serotonin receptors with methysergide can block this event. Nonrandomized studies suggest that the serotonin reuptake inhibitors fluoxetine hydrochloride (Prozac) and sertraline hydrochloride (Zoloft) may both be beneficial in the prevention of neurocardiogenic syncope after 4 to 6 weeks of therapy in approximately 55 percent of patients with severe, recurrent neurocardiogenic syncope.[56] A randomized, double-blinded trial showed that paroxetine hydrochloride–treated patients had an 18 percent incidence of recurrence versus a 53 percent recurrence rate in the placebo group.[57] More recent data, however, show that paroxetine hydrochloride did not prevent the vasovagal reaction during lower body negative pressure in a small cohort of normal volunteers.[58]

***Methylxanthines*** In one nonrandomized trial, oral theophylline therapy was associated with a reduction in the frequency of neurocardiogenic syncope.[59] Even low doses of theophylline (6 to 12 mg/kg per day) appear to have benefit. In low concentrations, methylxanthines are potent adenosine receptor antagonists. Endogenous adenosine may be a modulator for tilt-induced syncope.[60] Unfortunately, side effects such as nervousness, anxiety, and gastrointestinal abnormalities limit the usefulness of theophylline in this setting.

***Alpha Agonists*** Nonrandomized studies in a small number of patients have suggested that alpha agonists may prevent neurocardiogenic syncope due to a potent vasoconstrictor effect that may reduce venous pooling and concomitant reflex arteriolar vasodilation. However, two double-blinded, randomized, placebo-controlled trials have yielded mixed results. Etilefrine was no better than placebo in the prevention of syncope. In contrast, the alpha agonist midodrine reduced the incidence of HUT-induced syncope and improved quality of life compared with placebo control.[61–63]

***Cardiac Pacing*** The indication for cardiac pacing in neurocardiogenic syncope is unclear. The vast majority of patients do not require pacing. Pacing may be of value in preventing the component of hypotension that is due to asystole; however, peripheral vasodilation may still occur despite heart rate control, as noted. *Cardiac pacing should be reserved for those rare patients who have "malignant" neurocardiogenic syncope with documented episodes of prolonged asystole associated with recurrent syncopal spells who fail medical management.*[64,65] These patients typically require pharmacologic therapy in addition to cardiac pacing to prevent the vasodepressor component. Dual-chamber pacing with rate-drop response is the preferred mode of pacing. The North American Vasovagal Pacemaker Study was the first randomized trial to demonstrate improvement with pacing in selected patients.[66] However, newer studies are ongoing to confirm these results.

## Orthostatic Syncope (Orthostatic Hypotension)

Orthostatic hypotension is a disorder in which assumption of the upright posture is associated with a fall in arterial pressure; this, in turn, is associated with light-headedness, blurring of vision, and a sense of weakness and unsteadiness.[2,67–73] Hypotension is progressive over a period of seconds to minutes, depending on the degree of loss in reflex adaptation. If the fall in perfusion pressure to the brain is profound, syncope occurs. If the individual assumes the recumbent posture, arterial pressure rapidly normalizes and consciousness is restored. Abnormal baroreflex responses and selective norepinephrine reuptake inhibition have been reported in patients with orthostatic hypotension.[74]

From the diagnostic viewpoint, orthostatic hypotension is conveniently classified in terms of three major causes[2]: *venous pooling and/or blood volume depletion, pharmacologic agents,* and *neurogenic causes* (Table 40-2). In certain cases, circulating endogenous vasodilators may cause orthostatic hypotension and syncope.

TABLE 40-2 Causes of Orthostatic Syncope

| Cause | |
|---|---|
| Venous pooling or volume depletion | |
| | Prolonged bed rest |
| | Prolonged standing |
| | Pregnancy |
| | Venous varicosities |
| | Blood loss |
| | Dehydration |
| Pharmacologic agents | |
| | Antihypertensive |
| | Sympathetic blocking agents |
| | Calcium-channel blockers |
| | Converting enzyme inhibitors |
| | Nitrates |
| | Diuretics |
| | Antidepressants, antipsychotics |
| | Phenothiazines |
| | Tranquilizers |
| | Antiparkinsonian drugs |
| | Central nervous system depressants |
| Neurogenic | |
| | Diabetes mellitus |
| | Alcoholic neuropathy |
| | Spinal cord disease |
| | Amyloidosis |
| | Multiple sclerosis |
| | Multiple cerebral infarcts |
| | Parkinsonism |
| | Tabes dorsalis |
| | Syringomyelia |
| | Idiopathic orthostatic hypotension |
| | Shy-Drager syndrome (multiple system atrophy) |
| Circulating endogenous vasodilators | |
| | Hyperbradykininism |
| | Mastocytosis |
| | Carcinoid syndrome |

### VENOUS POOLING AND/OR BLOOD VOLUME DEPLETION

Excessive venous pooling accounts for the postural hypotension accompanying sustained bed rest, prolonged standing, pregnancy, and marked venous varicosities. Deconditioning of normal autonomic reflex vasoconstriction may contribute to the orthostatic hypotension associated with prolonged bed rest and following extended periods of weightlessness in astronauts.[2] Blood volume depletion accounts for the orthostatic hypotension associated with dehydration, excessive diuresis, anemia, hemorrhage, excessive gastrointestinal fluid loss, third-space sequestration, prolonged fever, renal dialysis, excessive perspiration, adrenal insufficiency, pheochromocytoma, and diabetes insipidus.[75–79]

### PHARMACOLOGIC AGENTS

Pharmacologically induced postural hypotension is a side effect in the administration of several classes of drugs, including antihypertensives, sympathetic blocking agents, diuretics, nitrates, calcium-channel blockers, ACE inhibitors, antidepressants, phenothiazines, tranquilizers, antipsychotic drugs, antiparkinsonian drugs, and central nervous system depressants.

### NEUROGENIC CAUSES

Neurogenic postural hypotension has been observed in a wide variety of diseases affecting the autonomic nervous system. Specific entities include diabetes mellitus, alcoholic neuropathy, spinal cord injury, idiopathic orthostatic hypotension, and Shy-Drager syndrome (Table 40-2).[76–81] Administration of adrenergic blocking drugs and vasodilators may accentuate the predisposition to orthostatic hypotension in patients with primary neurogenic postural hypotension.

In the idiopathic form of orthostatic hypotension, postural hypotension is accompanied by relatively fixed heart rate, heat intolerance, anhidrosis, nocturnal polyuria, urinary and anal sphincter dysfunction, and impotence.[78,79] In the Shy-Drager syndrome, orthostatic hypotension is accompanied by multiple central nervous system manifestations and is referred to as *multiple system atrophy.*[76,80]

The central nervous system manifestations in multiple system atrophy may be indistinguishable from those of idiopathic Parkinson's disease and may precede or follow the onset of orthostatic hypotension. The prognosis appears to be worse in patients with multiple system atrophy than in those with idiopathic orthostatic hypotension, with death often resulting from general debilitation and its complications. Severe supine hypertension may complicate the presence of orthostatic hypotension.

When the total or central blood volume is depleted in the presence of an intact autonomic nervous system, associations including pallor, coldness of the extremities, tachycardia, and sweating are evident. Relative bradycardia may occur at the time of syncope, and the clinical presentation may be identical to that of neurocardiogenic syncope. When orthostatic hypotension is due to loss or severe impairment of autonomic reflexes, the syncope is associated with little or no change in heart rate, and there is an absence of the pallor, sweating, and other manifestations observed in patients with intact autonomic reflexes.

### THERAPY

Effective therapy in postural hypotension is closely linked to an accurate diagnosis. Primary emphasis must be placed on treatable causes, in particular, pharmacologically induced postural hypotension, blood volume loss, venous pooling, and reversible disease entities. A summary of treatment modalities currently applied among patients with chronic orthostatic hypotension is presented in Table 40-3. The wide variety of recommended approaches reflects the frequently disappointing therapeutic response to each of these modalities. Commonly, multiple maneuvers are necessary to achieve optimum control of postural hypotension. Of singular importance is the need to have the patient avoid experiences such as dehydration, which accentuate postural hypotension, and to restrict the use of pharmacologic agents that induce blood volume depletion, vasodilation, and sympathetic blockade. *Patients should be instructed about simple adaptive maneuvers, including slow rising from a recumbent or sitting position, flexing of the calf muscles during assumption of the upright posture, and avoidance of prolonged immobility during standing.*[82,83] Erythropoietin administration to expand red blood cell mass and blood volume has been used to maintain pressure in the upright posture in certain cases of orthostatic hypotension.[84]

TABLE 40-3 Treatment of Chronic Orthostatic Hypotension

Evaluation for reversible and accentuating disease entities
Specific modalities for irreversible orthostatic hypotension
- Mechanical measures
  - Head-up position of bed
  - Lower body compression garment
  - Slow motion and calf muscle flexing on arising
- Volume expansion
  - High-salt diet
  - Fludrocortisone acetate
- Pharmacologic agents
  - Sympathomimetics
  - Vasoconstrictors

## Cerebrovascular Syncope

In patients with extensive occlusive disease of the origins of the brachiocephalic vessels, such as pulseless disease (e.g., aortic arch syndrome and Takayasu's arteritis), syncope is not uncommon.[2,85] With lesser degrees of cerebral occlusive disease, as with atherosclerotic narrowing, transient lowering of arterial pressure such as that immediately following assumption of the upright posture may be followed by vague symptoms suggesting impaired cerebral blood flow. In patients with cerebrovascular occlusive disease, a transient decrease in cardiac output and arterial pressure may provoke syncope at levels of arterial pressure that would otherwise be tolerated (see "Multifactorial Syncope," below).

Impairment or loss of consciousness in relation to changing positions of the head, particularly hyperextension and lateral rotation, has been attributed to mechanical narrowing of the vertebral arteries by skeletal deformities of the cervical spine. Such symptoms have been observed in patients with Klippel-Feil deformity, cervical spondylosis, and severe cervical osteoarthritis. Altered consciousness is often preceded by vestibular symptoms. When vertigo is a predominant symptom, the syndrome of benign postural vertigo must be considered.

Among patients with major occlusive disease of the carotid-vertebrobasilar arterial system, manual compression of the carotid artery as a test for carotid sinus hypersensitivity may induce syncope, at times associated with focal neurologic signs. The occurrence of syncope under such circumstances may be misdiagnosed as carotid sinus syndrome. The occurrence of a cerebrovascular accident following manual compression of the carotid sinus has been reported in patients with carotid disease; therefore *carotid sinus massage should be avoided in patients with symptomatic or suspected occlusive carotid vascular disease.*

Syncope in the *subclavian steal syndrome* is caused by major occlusive disease of the subclavian artery proximal to the origin of the vertebral artery. During upper extremity exercise, blood flow is shunted retrograde, by the circle of Willis, to the distal subclavian artery. The consequent decrease in cerebral circulation induces cerebral ischemia.[85] This syndrome is suggested by the findings of diminished brachial arterial pressure on the affected side, a bruit that is maximal over the supraclavicular area adjacent to the origin of the vertebral artery, and the induction of symptoms by exercise of the involved extremity.

Although focal neurologic symptoms and signs are the usual neurologic manifestations of cerebral emboli, transient loss of consciousness can be a primary presenting symptom. *Syncopal episodes are more likely to occur when atherosclerotic occlusive disease involves the vertebrobasilar system, with compromised perfusion to the medullary arousal center.* In vertebrobasilar vascular insufficiency, syncope or presyncope is nearly always preceded by symptoms of vertigo, diplopia, dysarthria, and ataxia. The episodes are generally attributed to microemboli arising from an atherosclerotic plaque, although vasospasm or postural hypotension may contribute (see Chap. 89).

#### THERAPY

The treatment of recurrent syncope in cerebrovascular disease is predicated on an accurate diagnosis. In this regard, it is essential to segregate the potential contribution of cardiac and vascular factors and their interplay. Anticoagulants and/or platelet antiaggregant agents are recommended for the prevention of embolic disease from the heart or central vessels (see Chap. 44). Endarterectomy or percutaneous dilatation should be considered in carotid arterial occlusive disease.

### Seizure Disorders

The various types of syncope resulting from the loss of consciousness during a seizure are often differentiated on the basis of history alone.[86–88] Grand mal epilepsy as a cause of sudden loss of consciousness is suggested by the dramatic nature of the onset of the attack, which is often preceded by an aura. Other observations that aid in distinguishing epilepsy are the absence of hypotension and cardiac arrhythmia (other than sinus tachycardia); tongue biting; loss of consciousness with stress; the presence of sustained tonic-clonic convulsive movements with upturning of the eyes; head turning and posturing; prolonged unconsciousness; urinary incontinence; prodromal déjà vu; and postictal drowsiness, headache, and confusion. While any of these findings may occasionally occur in episodes of syncope, the frequent association of these several events generally allows differentiation of epilepsy as its cause. In fact, it is not uncommon for patients with true syncope to be incorrectly diagnosed as having a seizure disorder. Akinetic seizures and absence (petite mal) seizures may be difficult to differentiate from syncope. Their occurrence in childhood, a past history of recurrent episodes, and the absence of pallor in witnessed episodes are helpful diagnostic findings. Of note, the long-QT syndrome is often misdiagnosed as a seizure disorder in childhood; an electrocardiogram (ECG) should be obtained in selected individuals. *Temporal lobe seizures are the most likely form of epilepsy to masquerade as syncope.*

An abnormal electroencephalogram (EEG) between episodes of altered consciousness can aid in distinguishing a seizure disorder when clinical observations are not definitive, and in some instances continuous EEG and ECG monitoring are required. Careful history taking can distinguish syncope from seizures.[88]

### Carotid Sinus Hypersensitivity

Compression of the carotid sinus in normal persons is often associated with transient slowing of the heart rate and mild hypotension. In some patients, such stimulation is followed by a profound slowing of the heart rate and/or a marked diminution of arterial pressure. This disorder is referred to as *carotid sinus hypersensitivity.* It should be considered in all older adults who have nonaccidental falls.[89] There are three forms of carotid sinus syncope, as originally described by Weiss and Baker[90]: cardioinhibitory, vasodepressor, and mixed type.

#### CARDIOINHIBITORY TYPE

The cardioinhibitory type of carotid sinus syncope, which is the most common, is associated with slowing of the heart rate secondary to marked sinus bradycardia, sinoatrial block, and/or high-degree AV block. Syncope in this instance is related to the prolonged asystole rather than to a fall in peripheral vascular resistance.

#### VASODEPRESSOR TYPE

The vasodepressor type of carotid sinus syncope is that form of the syndrome in which syncope occurs as a result of a primary decrease in arterial pressure in the absence of profound bradycardia. Presyncopal signs—such as nausea, sweating, and pallor—are usually not observed, and the fall in arterial pressure may be precipitous.

#### MIXED FORM

In the mixed form of carotid sinus syncope with bradycardia and hypotension, the vasodepressor component may not be evident until after atropine blockade or during cardiac pacing. Under such circumstances, carotid sinus massage uncovers the hypotension in the absence of bradycardia.

Carotid sinus syncope and presyncope are commonly found in elderly patients in whom symptoms of light-headedness and impaired consciousness may be initiated by relatively minor stimulation of the carotid sinus.[2] Carotid sinus hypersensitivity in the elderly is often associated with generalized atherosclerosis.

Manual carotid sinus compression in elderly persons requires caution whenever this maneuver is attempted. Digital carotid massage should first be attempted with a very gentle and brief (2- to 4-s) compression, always when the patient is supine and with monitoring of the heart rate and blood pressure.[91–94] *The presence of carotid artery bruits is a relative contraindication to carotid massage.*

Carotid sinus syncope has been observed in patients with neoplasms, inflammatory masses, sternocleidomastoid muscle receptor dysfunction, and lymph nodes in the neck adjacent to the carotid sinus.[95] Carotid sinus syncope is well established as a complication of carotid body and parotid tumors. In certain patients, carotid sinus hypersensitivity may be documented only when carotid sinus massage is performed in the upright position or during HUT studies, with careful attention to the blood pressure response.

#### THERAPY

Thorough patient education concerning avoidance of carotid sinus pressure may be effective in preventing syncopal episodes. Anticholinergic and sympathomimetic agents may be tried, but the inadequacy of drug therapy and the occurrence of side effects usually necessitate pacemaker therapy. AV sequential pacing appears to minimize the hypotensive effect of cardiac pacing and is therefore the preferred form of pacemaker therapy in the mixed form of carotid sinus syncope. It is important that pacemaker effectiveness be verified objectively through observation of the effect of carotid sinus stimulation on cardiac rhythm and arterial pressure following pacemaker insertion.

## Situational Syncope

The term *situational syncope* has been applied to a group of syndromes defined by the circumstances that precipitate the event. In the past, the syncope in these disorders has been attributed mainly to mechanical factors. Recent observations suggest that, at least in part, neurocardiogenic factors contribute to the syncope.[96]

### COUGH SYNCOPE

Also called laryngeal vertigo, tussive syncope, and posttussive syncope, cough syncope is associated with loss of consciousness following a paroxysm of vigorous coughing. It is often seen in robust men and children but rarely in women. Cerebral blood flow is impaired by the marked increase in cerebrospinal fluid pressure during coughing, which increases cerebrovascular resistance. There is also a *concussive effect* transmitted via the cerebrospinal fluid. Reflex-induced sinus bradycardia, sinus arrest, and AV block have been observed in patients with cough syncope.[97]

In the treatment of cough syncope, the patient should be informed of the deleterious effects of vigorous coughing. Cessation of smoking and initiation of bronchodilator and anti-inflammatory therapy for associated bronchitis are mandatory for the prevention of cough-induced syncope.

### SWALLOWING, OR DEGLUTITION, SYNCOPE

Deglutition syncope has been reported in association with tumor, diverticulum, achalasia, stricture, and spasm of the esophagus. In some patients, no abnormality can be identified radiologically or endoscopically. This type of syncope is usually associated with AV block.[98]

Similar mechanisms have been implicated in syncope following distention of the viscera, glossopharyngeal neuralgia, fainting associated with irritation of the pleura or peritoneum, and cardiac asystole associated with esophagoscopy or bronchoscopy.[99]

### VALSALVA SYNCOPE

Valsalva syncope is related to the prolonged increases in intrathoracic pressure that may be observed during a sustained Valsalva maneuver. With prolonged exhalation against a closed glottis, there is a progressive fall in venous return, arterial pressure, and cardiac output.[2] These hemodynamic changes may be sufficient to impair cerebral circulation. An episode of Valsalva syncope may be the first indication of the presence of a disorder predisposing an individual to syncope (e.g., cerebrovascular occlusive disease or sick sinus syndrome). Instruction to the patient regarding avoidance of sustained Valsalva maneuvers is essential in preventing recurring episodes.

### MICTURITION SYNCOPE

Micturition syncope is often seen in adult men with nocturia. During or immediately following voiding, there is a loss of consciousness, often without premonitory symptoms. The ingestion of large quantities of alcoholic beverages before retiring is common.[2,100] A similar type of syncope may be observed following drainage of the distended bladder or after removal of large quantities of ascitic fluid. The loss of consciousness in these circumstances may be related to bradycardia and a sudden reflex decrease in peripheral arterial resistance induced by the precipitous fall of intraabdominal volume. The loss of consciousness of typical micturition syncope is precipitated by such factors as the Valsalva maneuver in the upright posture and the peripheral vasodilation associated with a warm bed and recent alcohol consumption.

### DEFECATION SYNCOPE

Defecation syncope occurs most commonly in the elderly, usually after arising from bed at night or during manual disimpaction of the rectum.[2,101] It has been attributed to sudden decompression of the rectum. Valsalva-related syncope could also explain some instances of this form of syncope. Many patients with defecation syncope have underlying gastrointestinal or cardiovascular disease.

### DIVER'S SYNCOPE

Diver's syncope is an unusual and poorly understood form of loss of consciousness or even sudden death that may occur in underwater diving. In some instances, diver's syncope may represent a form of neurocardiogenic syncope. Hypoxia and bradycardia of the diving reflex may be contributing factors.

### POSTPRANDIAL SYNCOPE

Hypotension postprandially may result in presyncope and/or syncope and is most common in the elderly. Tilt testing after meals showed 22 percent symptomic hypotension in functionally independent elders.[102] The mechanisms of postprandial hypotension and syncope are not fully understood. Possible contributing factors include inadequate sympathetic nervous system compensation for meal-induced splanchnic blood pooling, impairments in baroreflex function, inadequate postprandial increase in cardiac output, impairment of peripheral vasoconstriction, and release of gastrointestinal peptides.[103,104]

### TREATMENT

Therapy of situational syncope should be individualized and should be addressed to the specific circumstance associated with it. Episodes of syncope may be prevented by anticholinergic drugs such as atropine if they are administered prior to a procedure. Other measures include avoidance of vasodilators before meals and/or resting in a supine position after meals for patients with postprandial hypotension and sitting while urinating for men with micturition syncope. Octreotide, a somatostatin analogue, has been shown to be effective in patients with postprandial hypotension, but it is expensive and must be given parenterally.[103,104]

## Metabolic Syncope

### HYPOXIA-RELATED SYNCOPE

Hypoxia may induce syncope that is related directly to a lack of oxygen or to an episode of neurocardiogenic syncope initiated during a period of oxygen lack. In the presence of cardiovascular disease, pulmonary insufficiency, and anemia, symptoms of hypoxia occur at lesser levels of oxygen deprivation. The impairment of consciousness due to hypoxia is accompanied by sinus tachycardia, while arterial pressure is usually normal. Short-term exposure to moderate altitude may be related to otherwise unexplained syncope in healthy young adults. The environmental setting in which impaired consciousness due to hypoxia occurs usually leaves little difficulty in its differentiation from other forms of syncope.

#### HYPOGLYCEMIA-RELATED SYNCOPE

This form of syncope may be associated with weakness, sweating, a sensation of hunger, confusion, and altered consciousness. The symptoms are unrelated to posture and usually respond promptly to food ingestion or intravenous glucose administration. Impaired consciousness is usually associated with sinus tachycardia and is rarely accompanied by hypotension. In contrast to syncope of circulatory origin, it is gradual in onset. Hypoglycemia has been implicated as a factor that may possibly trigger neurocardiogenic syncope.

#### HYPERVENTILATION, PANIC ATTACKS, AND SYNCOPE

In normal persons, anxiety is accompanied by varying degrees of hyperventilation. In the hyperventilation syndrome or in a panic episode, anxiety is associated with an inordinate degree of hyperventilation. Symptoms of hypocapnia and alkalosis may dominate the clinical picture. During the episode, the patient may complain of a tightness in the chest and a feeling of suffocation. These symptoms may be followed by confusion, a sense of unreality, bewilderment, light-headedness, and a feeling of panic. Symptoms of palpitation, precordial oppression, and dyspnea may suggest an acute cardiac or pulmonary catastrophe. Digital and circumoral paresthesias may develop and, in severe cases, may be accompanied by carpopedal spasm, which is probably related to alkalosis-induced decreases in serum ionized calcium. The symptoms may be protracted and can persist while the subject is sitting or recumbent. During hyperventilation, there is slight hypotension but no profound fall in arterial pressure, while the heart rate is rapid. Although mentation is impaired, complete loss of consciousness rarely occurs. Typical neurocardiogenic syncope may be superimposed, making identification of the syndrome more difficult. *The induction of a typical episode by voluntary hyperventilation is helpful in distinguishing this syndrome and aids in educating the patient regarding the prevention and control of attacks.*

### Other Forms of Syncope or Conditions Mimicking Syncope

#### MIGRAINE-RELATED SYNCOPE

Symptoms suggesting syncope are unusual in ordinary types of migraine. In rare instances in which the basilar arterial system is involved (as opposed to the more usually affected carotid system), the premonitory aura of migraine terminates in a period of unconsciousness of several minutes' duration. The unconsciousness is slow in onset and may be preceded by a dreamlike state. When the patient awakens, there is severe headache, typically in the occipital area. This form of migraine usually afflicts young women and has a strong association with the menstrual cycle. The symptoms in syncopal migraine may suggest hyperventilation and/or hysterical syncope.

#### HYSTERICAL SYNCOPE

Altered consciousness of circulatory origin may be mimicked by hysteria. Hysterical episodes occur most frequently in young adults, often with severe emotional illness and generally in the presence of an audience.[105] The individual slumps gently, even gracefully, to the floor or in a convenient chair or sofa, typically without injury or awkwardness. The patient may be motionless or may exhibit symbolic restrictive movements. Episodes are of varying duration and may last an hour or more. Although the patient is unresponsive to verbal stimulation, there is evidence, such as eyelid movement, that consciousness is well preserved, and no abnormalities in pulse, arterial pressure, or skin color are evident.

## CARDIAC SYNCOPE

Either severe obstruction of cardiac output or disturbances of cardiac rhythm can produce syncope of cardiac origin.[2,106–118] Obstructive lesions and arrhythmias frequently coexist; indeed, one abnormality may accentuate the other. Common disorders associated with cardiac syncope are listed in Table 40-4.

### Syncope Related to Obstruction of Cardiac Output

Obstruction to cardiac output sufficient to cause syncope may occur in the left or right side of the heart. Syncope, particularly that occurring with effort, is a major symptom of aortic stenosis and is often the initial presentation. The mechanisms are unclear, but studies suggest a reflex fall in peripheral vascular resistance as the usual cause. Failure of cardiac output to increase adequately during exercise, while peripheral resistance decreases, may play a role (see also Chap. 56). Transient arrhythmias can also induce syncope in aortic stenosis. Syncope associated with effort (often occurring immediately after effort) is observed in patients with hypertrophic cardiomyopathy as well. Nonexertional syncope related to acute decreases in preload or afterload, to inotropic stimulation, or to transient arrhythmias may also occur in hypertrophic cardiomyopathy (see also Chap. 67). Left-sided malfunction of a prosthetic heart valve can produce transient and at times profound obstruction to blood flow with syncope (see Chap. 60). A left atrial myxoma may obstruct left ventricular filling, leading to low cardiac output and syncope. The obstruction of left ventricular inflow in atrial myxoma may be posturally induced (see also Chap. 77). Mitral stenosis can produce cardiac syncope but usually does so only when tachycardia or other arrhythmias supervene (see also Chap. 57).

Primary pulmonary hypertension and pulmonary hypertension secondary to congenital heart disease may both be complicated by

TABLE 40-4 Common Disorders Associated with Cardiac Syncope

- Left-sided heart
  - Aortic stenosis
  - Hypertrophic cardiomyopathy
  - Prosthetic valve malfunction
  - Mitral stenosis
  - Left atrial myxoma (rare)
- Right-sided heart
  - Eisenmenger syndrome
  - Tetralogy of Fallot
  - Pulmonary embolism
  - Pulmonary stenosis
  - Primary pulmonary hypertension
  - Cardiac tamponade
- Cardiac arrhythmia
  - Sinoatrial disease
  - Atrioventricular block
  - Supraventricular tachycardia
  - Ventricular tachycardia/fibrillation
- Pacemaker-related disorders

syncope, particularly effort-related syncope. In these conditions, limitation of right ventricular outflow markedly inhibits the cardiac output during increased peripheral demand. The fall in peripheral resistance in the presence of an inability to increase cardiac output may result in profound hypotension.[119] A reflex fall in peripheral resistance similar to that which occurs with aortic stenosis may play a role. In a young patient without a cardiac murmur who presents with syncope during or shortly after exertion, primary pulmonary hypertension should be considered (see also Chap. 52). In pulmonary stenosis and pulmonary embolism, similar mechanisms may account for syncope. Pulmonary embolism as a cause of syncope should also be suspected in paraplegic patients.[120] In tetralogy of Fallot, the magnitude of flow through the right-to-left shunt increases when systemic resistance falls with effort, since the right ventricular outflow obstruction is usually fixed. This shunting results in marked arterial hypoxia, which may precipitate a syncopal episode (see also Chap. 63).

Cardiac tamponade, which affects both the right and the left sides of the heart, can produce syncope, but this is extremely rare. The likelihood of syncope is increased by concomitant arrhythmias.

## Syncope Related to Cardiac Arrhythmia

Arrhythmias are a common cause of syncope and must be considered in any patient, particularly when cardiac disease is present. Either extreme of ventricular rate (bradycardia or tachycardia) can depress cardiac output to the point of critical hypotension, with cerebral hypoperfusion and syncope. As noted earlier for other forms of syncope, a neurocardiogenic reaction may be precipitated by the hemodynamic effects of arrhythmias[121] (see also Chaps. 23 and 24). The most common arrhythmias producing syncope or presyncope are profound sinus bradycardia, sinoatrial exit block or sinus pause, high-grade AV block, supraventricular tachycardia, and ventricular tachycardia. Although arrhythmias occur in the absence of demonstrable cardiac disease, they are usually secondary to such disorders as ischemic heart disease, cardiomyopathy, valvular heart disease (including marked mitral valve prolapse), and primary conduction system disease.

Primary degenerative disease of the sinus node and the specialized conduction tissue is the most common cause of sinoatrial disease (*sick sinus syndrome;* see Chap. 24). The sick sinus syndrome may be manifested by persistent or episodic sinus bradycardia or sinoatrial exit block, often with impaired junctional escape rhythm. The presence of alternating sinus bradycardia or sinoatrial block with paroxysmal supraventricular tachycardia of diverse types is quite common and is referred to as the *bradycardia-tachycardia syndrome. Syncope often occurs with asystole or bradycardia at the termination of tachycardia, when overdrive suppression of the sinoatrial or junctional pacemakers is present.*[122] A high incidence of associated AV and intraventricular conduction defects occurs in the sick sinus syndrome. AV block, impaired junctional escape rhythm, or ventricular arrhythmias may actually be responsible for syncope in the setting of sick sinus syndrome.[115]

High-grade AV block may be due to disease of either the AV node or the His-Purkinje system. Block of the AV node is usually associated with a junctional pacemaker and a normal QRS complex, whereas AV block due to disease of the His-Purkinje system is usually associated with a wide complex idioventricular escape rhythm, which may be quite slow. Bifascicular block in the presence of a prolonged PR interval is associated with a substantial risk of developing high-grade AV block and syncope. Progression to high-grade AV block in patients with bifascicular block and a normal PR interval is less common. Ventricular tachycardia can cause syncope in patients with AV block or other bradycardic rhythms (see Chap. 24).

Sinus bradycardia, AV block, or cardiac asystole may be mediated by reflex vagal mechanisms and have been observed in a variety of disease states or during diagnostic procedures. Ventricular asystole (usually sinus arrest, although AV block can occasionally be noted) is most commonly due to neurocardiogenic syncope. Transient sinus bradycardia or AV block can also occur in apparently healthy young individuals; certain of these patients may have mitral valve prolapse.[116] Paroxysmal supraventricular tachycardias is not a consistent cause of syncope in young individuals. Syncope, however, may occur in individuals who have accessory AV pathways due to the Wolff-Parkinson-White (WPW) syndrome, wherein supraventricular tachycardia or preexcited atrial fibrillation is associated with a very rapid ventricular response. Studies have shown, though, that syncope during supraventricular tachycardia may be related to vasomotor factors and not be due solely to heart rate.[121,122] Atrial fibrillation or atrial flutter with a rapid ventricular rate may result in syncope, especially in patients with cardiac disease, particularly obstructive outflow disorders, and older individuals may more commonly have hypotension significant enough to cause cerebral hypoperfusion and syncope.

Paroxysmal ventricular tachycardia may produce syncope at any age. The tachycardia often occurs in the setting of cardiac disease in which structural abnormalities and/or ischemia exists. Syncopal ventricular tachycardias may occur in patients with normal LV function [i.e., long-QT syndrome, Brugada's syndrome, arrhythmogenic right ventricular cardiomyopathy (ARVC), and idiopathic left ventricular tachycardia].[123–126] Ventricular tachycardia is the most common arrhythmic cause of syncope in most reported series. In some patients, ventricular and supraventricular tachycardia may coexist (see Chap. 24).

Syncope may occur with torsades de pointes ventricular tachycardia in the setting of the long-QT syndrome, which may be congenital or acquired (see Chaps. 11 and 24). The recognition of the long-QT syndrome depends on demonstration of QT prolongation, family history of syncope or sudden death, and history of recurrent syncope. However, a normal QT interval does not exclude this diagnosis, since this interval can be intermittently prolonged. Ventricular tachycardia in the heritable long-QT syndromes is often triggered by exercise or stress reaction.[127,128]

It is particularly important to recognize the polymorphic ventricular tachycardia associated with acquired long-QT syndromes because it is a potentially life-threatening side effect of many drugs and metabolic abnormalities. The most frequent causes of acquired long-QT syndromes are antiarrhythmic drugs and electrolyte disorders (hypokalemia and hypomagnesemia). A pause preceding the onset of tachycardia is common, since the early afterdepolarizations thought responsible for torsades are bradycardia-dependent.[117,128,129]

A variety of other drugs may produce or aggravate arrhythmias, resulting in syncope or presyncope. Beta-blocking drugs, calcium-channel blockers, sotalol, and amiodarone are some of the more common agents that may cause significant sinus bradycardia or AV block. Digitalis may occasionally cause sinoatrial exit block or AV block, particularly in patients with sinoatrial or AV nodal disease. Supraventricular and ventricular tachycardias can be a result of digitalis therapy, particularly in patients with organic heart disease and hypokalemia. Theophylline and beta agonists, used for therapy of chronic obstructive pulmonary disease, may precipitate ventricular or supraventricular arrhythmias. Therapy with diuretics often causes hypokalemia and hypomagnesemia, which predispose individuals to supraventricular and ventricular arrhythmias. Both caffeine and alcohol may precipitate either atrial or ventricular tachycardia.

In the patient with an artificial ventricular pacemaker, near syncope or syncope may be secondary to pacemaker malfunction or to the pacemaker syndrome (see Chap. 31). Dual-chamber pacemakers can produce pacemaker-mediated tachycardias when there is retrograde conduction of the ventricular impulse to the atria. Improvements in technology have reduced the incidence of this complication.[130,131]

## DIAGNOSTIC EVALUATION OF SYNCOPE ASSOCIATED WITH CARDIAC DISEASE

While the history and physical examination often establish the diagnosis of obstructive cardiac syncope, laboratory studies are usually required to determine the severity of the disorder. Cardiac catheterization is required when corrective cardiac surgery is contemplated.

By far the most challenging diagnostic evaluation occurs when arrhythmic cardiac syncope is suspected. Such patients often have evidence of underlying cardiovascular disease, which, when present, portends a poor prognosis. Thus, diagnostic studies directed to the nature and severity of the underlying cardiac disease must be pursued in addition to the arrhythmia evaluation.[132]

The various diagnostic tests used for the evaluation of arrhythmic syncope are listed in Fig. 40-2. Because of the transient nature of most arrhythmias, the routine ECG is generally of limited value. It is, however, very useful in identifying patients with abnormalities that may predispose individuals to syncope, such as prior infarction, a WPW pattern, AV or bundle branch block, long QT interval, incomplete right bundle branch block (RBBB) with right precordial ST-segment elevation suggestive of Brugada's syndrome, epsilon waves, or right precordial T-wave inversion suggestive of ARVC.

The signal-averaged ECG, for detecting late potentials, can be used as a noninvasive screening test to risk-stratify postinfarction patients.[134–137] Patients with right ventricular dysplasia may also have an abnormal signal-averaged ECG.[133] Exercise testing can directly provoke arrhythmias in patients with a history suggesting exercise-induced arrhythmias. Exercise should be performed when exertional arrhythmias are suspected but not documented by ambulatory monitoring or when ischemia is suspected (see also Chap. 14).[138,139] Continuous ECG monitoring is a widely used screening test for suspected arrhythmic syncope. It has a low yield in unselected patients. *It is important to recognize that one 24-h monitoring period may not be sufficient for detecting transient rhythm disturbances. The diagnostic yield, moreover, increases only slightly with more prolonged monitoring* (see also Chap. 25).[138–140]

When ambulatory monitoring does not document an arrhythmia, a patient-activated ECG device (event recorder) may prove efficacious. This type of monitoring is effective in documenting infrequent arrhythmia. It should not be used in patients with suspected life-threatening arrhythmias.[141–143] Extended monitoring with an implantable loop recorder has been demonstrated to provide diagnostic information in approximately two-thirds of patients with syncope of undetermined cause.[144,145]

When noninvasive testing is inconclusive for the diagnosis of suspected arrhythmic syncope, an electrophysiologic study may be useful in high-risk patients (i.e., those with underlying heart disease, suspicious arrhythmia by ECG monitoring, or recurrent syncope). Electrophysiologic testing should be considered early in the workup. Patients without identifiable heart disease are less likely to have the cause of syncope identified by electrophysiologic study. The cause of syncope most commonly identified by electrophysiologic study is ventricular tachycardia.

Electrophysiologic studies are useful in stratifying risk among symptomatic patients with bundle branch block or those with bifascicular block. Patients with normal electrophysiologic study results have a favorable prognosis even without treatment. Patients undergoing permanent pacing on the basis of electrophysiologic testing also have a favorable prognosis, with a low rate of symptom recurrence.[146–151]

The prognosis in patients with syncope due to supraventricular tachycardia is usually good, since therapeutic approaches are available (i.e., drugs and radiofrequency ablation). The prognosis in patients with inducible sustained ventricular tachycardia is less favorable but is improved with the use of an implantable cardioverter-defibrillator.[152,153]

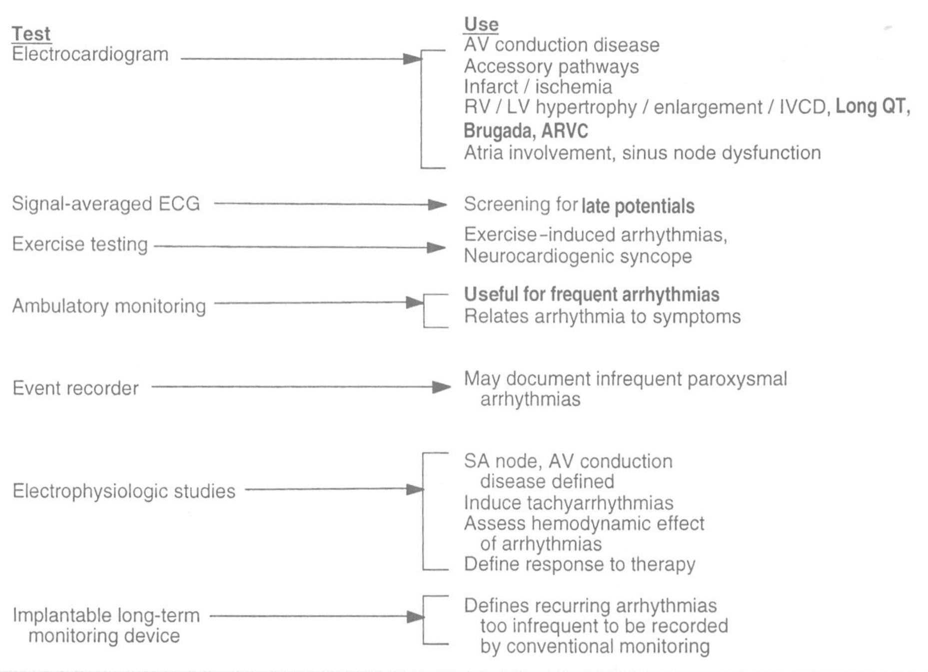


FIGURE 40-2 Diagnostic tests that can be used for the evaluation of arrhythmic syncope. ARVC = arrhythmogenic right ventricular cardiomyopathy; AV = atrioventricular; RV/LV = right ventricular/left ventricular; IVCD = intraventricular conduction defect; SA = sinoatrial.

## TREATMENT OF CARDIAC SYNCOPE

***Obstructive Heart Disease*** Cardiac surgery is often the treatment of choice for patients with syncope caused by obstructive heart disease. Patients with hypertrophic cardiomyopathy and syncope may respond well to pharmacologic therapy. Studies have suggested that an AV sequential pacemaker may control symptoms in certain patients with hypertrophic cardiomyopathy.[154–162] In patients with severe obstruction and persistent symptoms, surgery should be considered (see Chap. 67). Among all patients with obstructive heart disease and recurrent syncope, the diagnosis of fixed pulmonary hypertension is most difficult to treat because effective therapeutic options are limited (see Chap. 52).

***Arrhythmic Syncope*** A detailed discussion of therapy for cardiac arrhythmias is presented in Chap. 24. General principles of arrhythmia management as they apply to patients with syncope are summarized here. Treatment of arrhythmic syncope requires accurate definition of the arrhythmia associated with syncope or presyncope.

The bradycardic rhythm disturbances responsible for syncope, primarily AV and sinoatrial pauses or exit block, usually require the implantation of a pacemaker.[163] Patients receiving drugs that cause or contribute to the bradyarrhythmia, however, may benefit from withdrawal or substitution of the offending agent. Patients with bradycardia-tachycardia syndrome usually require pacemaker therapy, because the antiarrhythmic agents required for control of the tachycardia will often further suppress sinoatrial function. A select group of patients with symptomatic sick sinus syndrome may benefit from oral theophylline.[164]

Implicit in the approach to the tachycardias causing syncope is the accurate diagnosis of a specific tachycardia. The definition of the tachycardia and the response to antiarrhythmic therapy are often best achieved in the electrophysiologic laboratory. Patients with syncope due to supraventricular tachycardia associated with an accessory pathway are most often approached with catheter ablation of the accessory pathway.[165,166] Catheter ablation is also a successful mode of therapy in patients with AV nodal reentry supraventricular tachycardia or other supraventricular tachycardias associated with a rapid heart rate (see Chap. 28). Implantable cardioverter/defibrillators (ICDs) are the first-line treatment for syncopal ventricular tachycardia in the setting of structural heart disease. Many patients require additional antiarrhythmic drugs to reduce the frequency of shocks from the ICD. Ventricular tachycardia ablation may be palliative for slower ventricular tachycardia, which requires frequent ICD shocks. Right ventricular outflow tract tachycardia or idiopathic left ventricular tachycardia can be treated medically or with catheter ablation (see Chaps. 28 and 30).

Polymorphic ventricular tachycardia in the setting of a long-QT interval (torsades de pointes) is often secondary to drug therapy, particularly the use of antiarrhythmic drugs. The potential offending drug(s) should be stopped. Acute therapy includes intravenous magnesium and measures to increase the heart rate and shorten electrical diastole (i.e., cardiac pacing). Treatment of polymorphic ventricular tachycardia associated with a congenitally prolonged QT interval is discussed in Chap. 24.

Pacemaker-induced hypotension and syncope are rectified by changing from ventricular pacing to AV sequential pacing when hypotension due to loss of atrial transport or neurocardiogenic response is responsible for symptoms. Identification of pacemaker-mediated tachycardia usually requires only changes in pacemaker programming. Pacemaker malfunction or myopotential inhibition requires a change in programming or replacement of the defective part of the system.

## SYNCOPE OF UNDETERMINED CAUSE

Despite careful diagnostic evaluation, the cause of syncope often cannot be defined.[2] Unexplained syncope has a broad spectrum of etiologies. The varying mortality rate among patients with syncope of undetermined cause likely reflects the varying incidence of undetected cardiac syncope. A certain number of these patients have probably experienced syncope of multiple causes.[167,168]

## SPECIAL PROBLEMS IN SYNCOPE

### Syncope in the Elderly

Elderly persons are particularly prone to develop syncope or presyncope. The aging process can result in diminished cerebral oxygen delivery by a variety of physiologic mechanisms, including decreased cerebral blood flow from low cardiac output, cerebral vascular disease, decreased hemoglobin, and lower arterial $Po_2$. In addition, cerebral arteriolar sclerosis may be present, impairing autoregulation of cerebral perfusion. Thus, many older patients have only marginal cerebral oxygen delivery at rest.[169–172] Physiologic defenses against a fall in blood pressure may also be impaired, as discussed above.

The aged may also suffer from multiple sensory deficits (e.g., in vision, vestibular function, and peripheral sensory nerve function), variable degrees of dementia, bradykinesis, arthritis, and muscle weakness, all of which enhance the likelihood of a fall when cerebral perfusion is marginal. *Drop* attacks, in which muscle tone in the lower extremities is lost, are frequent in the elderly and must be distinguished from syncope. Carotid sinus hypersensitivity also is relatively common in the elderly, as is postprandial syncope; these entities should be evaluated as discussed previously. *The elderly frequently have multisystem disease and are likely to be taking several medications, which may aggravate the tendency to syncope (e.g., antihypertensive drugs, diuretics, vasodilators, antiarrhythmic drugs, psychoactive drugs).*

Arrhythmias are common in elderly individuals, especially in those presenting with syncope. Syncope is a significant contributor to unexplained automobile accidents among the elderly and should be suspected when external causes are not apparent.[173–175] In the elderly, syncope may be the presenting complaint for common disorders such as pneumonia, viral illness, acute myocardial infarction, or occult hemorrhage. Thus, the management of syncope in the aged often requires initial management of underlying diseases, with subsequent evaluation to determine whether such therapy controls syncope. Lower standing blood pressure is a predictor of falls in the elderly.[176]

### Multifactorial Syncope

In many instances, syncope requires that a constellation of events occur, either simultaneously or in sequence. Without the full complex, the patient may note only light-headedness or perhaps no definable symptoms. A carefully recorded history is required to elucidate such complex presentations.

Transient abnormalities such as fever, fatigue, hypoglycemia, or drug ingestion may increase the likelihood of syncope. Coexisting diseases may decrease the patient's physiologic defenses for maintaining adequate cerebral perfusion to sustain consciousness. A cardiac arrhythmia that ordinarily would not produce syncope with the patient supine may become a contributory factor when other predisposing factors are present and the patient is upright. With respect to combined causes of syncope, it is notable that, in the original description of Adams-Stokes syncope, the patients exhibited a permanently slow pulse rate accompanied by aortic stenosis.

The development of the neurocardiogenic reaction may determine whether a given stimulus initiates syncope. This relationship has been shown in such diverse causes of syncope as aortic stenosis, vasodilator drug therapy, volume loss, pulmonary embolism, tachyarrhythmias, pacemaker syndrome, postprandial state in the elderly, and after exercise.

## Syncope and Sudden Death

The risk of sudden death is increased among those with known cardiac syncope (both obstructive and arrhythmic), but occasionally sudden death may also occur in presumptive noncardiac syncope and syncope of unknown cause. It would appear, therefore, that in some patients syncope is a harbinger of sudden death. Patients with advanced heart failure and syncope are at especially high risk for sudden death regardless of the etiology.[177,178] Syncope is also associated with an increased mortality rate in patients with hypertrophic cardiomyopathy.[179] It is not always clear to what extent the occurrence of syncope per se is a risk factor for sudden death or whether the risk is more related to the underlying disease.

## Recurrent Syncope

In up to one-third of all patients with syncope, the event is recurrent. For most patients, the persistence of syncope increases morbidity from trauma but does not increase mortality. Such recurrences most often reflect a lack of effective therapy and/or a failure to establish the correct diagnosis.

Unexplained syncope in patients with negative initial diagnostic studies has a broad spectrum of etiologies, the most common of which is bradycardia. An implantable long-term monitoring device is useful for establishing a diagnosis when symptoms are recurrent but too infrequent for conventional monitoring techniques.[144,145,180] Recurrent syncope is particularly common in a subset of patients with mitral valve prolapse in whom dysautonomia, arrhythmia, and hypovolemia all play a role.[116] In certain patients with unexplained recurrent syncope, especially in individuals with multiple physical symptoms, screening for psychiatric disorder may be necessary. In patients with recurrent syncope, advice regarding the avoidance of certain activities, such as working with dangerous equipment, is needed and, in some cases in which public safety is involved, a change in jobs is required (e.g., airplane pilots or bus drivers).[181,182]

## Exercise and Syncope

Individuals with a history of syncope associated with activity and who participate in physical activities or competitive athletics constitute a special problem. Since exercise syncope may be a manifestation of serious underlying cardiac disease, complete evaluation is indicated to define the cause of syncope prior to recommendation for participation in sports. *Identification of myocardial or electrophysiologic abnormalities is paramount to the prevention of potential sudden cardiac death.*[183–191]

Syncope may occur during or immediately after exercise. The most common causes of exercise-induced syncope are shown in Fig. 40-3. Exercise-associated neurocardiogenic syncope is uncommon in highly trained individuals with high resting vagal tone; caution should be exercised in making this diagnosis without first excluding underlying structural myocardial abnormality. HUT studies can be used to assess patients at risk for neurocardiogenic syncope, but this test may lack sensitivity and specificity in highly trained individuals. Exercise testing is mandatory, especially if the syncope is exercise-induced. Exercise-induced ventricular ectopy, sustained ventricular tachycardia, or rapid supraventricular tachycardia requires electrophysiologic and general cardiologic evaluation. Cardiac stress testing does not accurately screen for anomalous origin coronary arteries.[192] Cardiac catheterization or magnetic resonance imaging may be required if the index of suspicion is high.

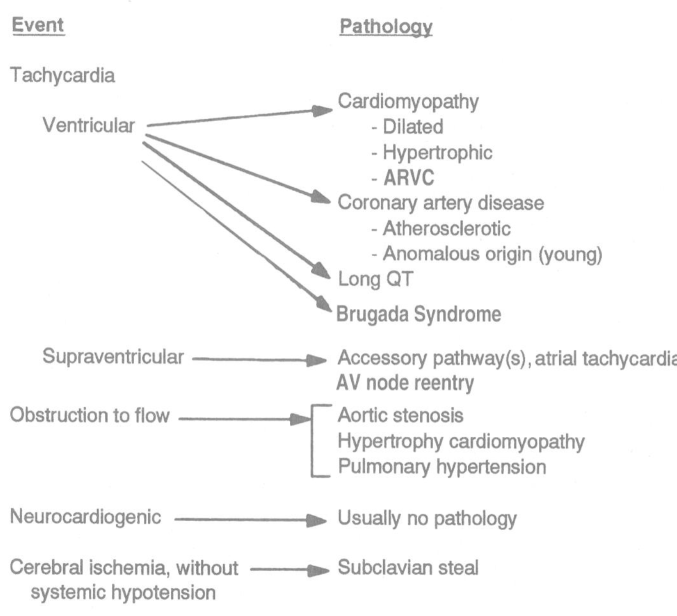


FIGURE 40-3 Exercise-induced syncope. Events and underlying pathology. ARVC = arrhythmogenic right ventricular cardiomyopathy.

The final recommendation and advice to participate in sports with high, moderate, or low intensity should be individualized. Recommendations should be balanced between restricting activity unduly and reducing the chance of death or injury from participation in sports.

## DIAGNOSTIC EVALUATION OF SYNCOPE: AN OVERVIEW

In the initial approach to the diagnosis of syncope, it is essential to distinguish the underlying cause in terms of the three basic categories—cardiac syncope, noncardiac syncope, and syncope of undetermined cause. This differentiation is accomplished in a majority of patients by a history (Fig. 40-4), physical examination (Fig. 40-5), and ECG (Fig. 40-6) and is supplemented by routine laboratory studies, including echocardiography (Fig. 40-7).[193–201]

The extent of evaluation should initially be predicated on the estimation of mortality and morbidity risk, which is high in cardiac syncope or syncope associated with cardiac disease and low in syncope without structural heart disease. Although cost-effectiveness in diagnostic testing should be kept in mind, the need for an assiduous search should not be dismissed when lethal disease is suspected.

Complete evaluation of syncope is required for the elderly and for patients with suspected arrhythmic syncope. When patients in such a selected group undergo a thorough evaluation, including an electrophysiologic study, an arrhythmic basis for syncope can be found in most. *Negative results are often as important as actual identification of an arrhythmia, since the negative evaluation usually denotes a favorable long-term prognosis.*

The diagnostic evaluation of patients with syncope of unknown cause presents a perplexing problem, particularly when syncope occurs repeatedly and because it may be a harbinger of sudden death. As our understanding of the mechanisms and the breadth of causes of syncope improves (particularly the role of multiple causes), it is reasonable to suspect that the number of patients with syncope of un-

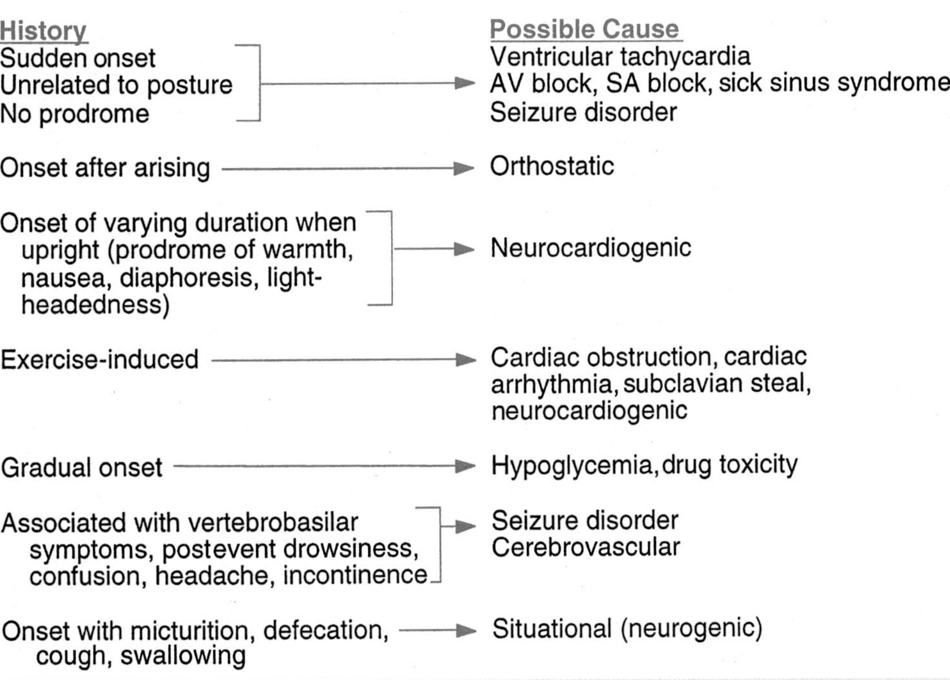


FIGURE 40-4 Differential diagnosis of syncope based on history. AV = atrioventricular; SA = sinoatrial.

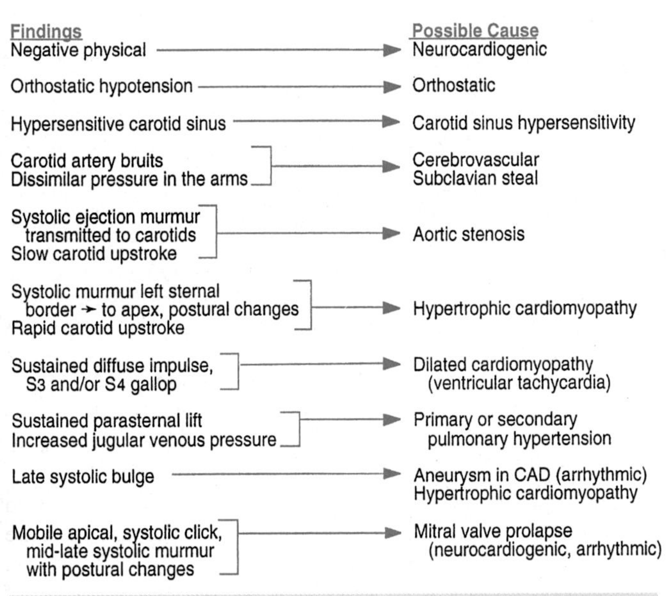


FIGURE 40-5 Differential diagnosis of syncope based on physical examination. CAD = coronary artery disease.

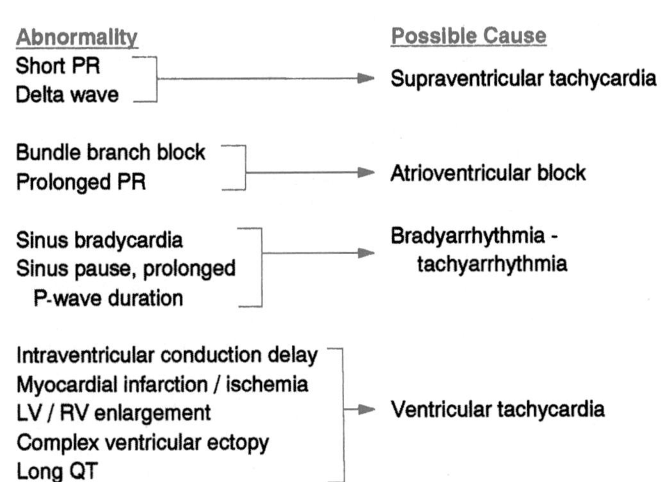


FIGURE 40-6 Differential diagnosis of syncope based on the electrocardiogram. LV/RV = left ventricular/right ventricular.

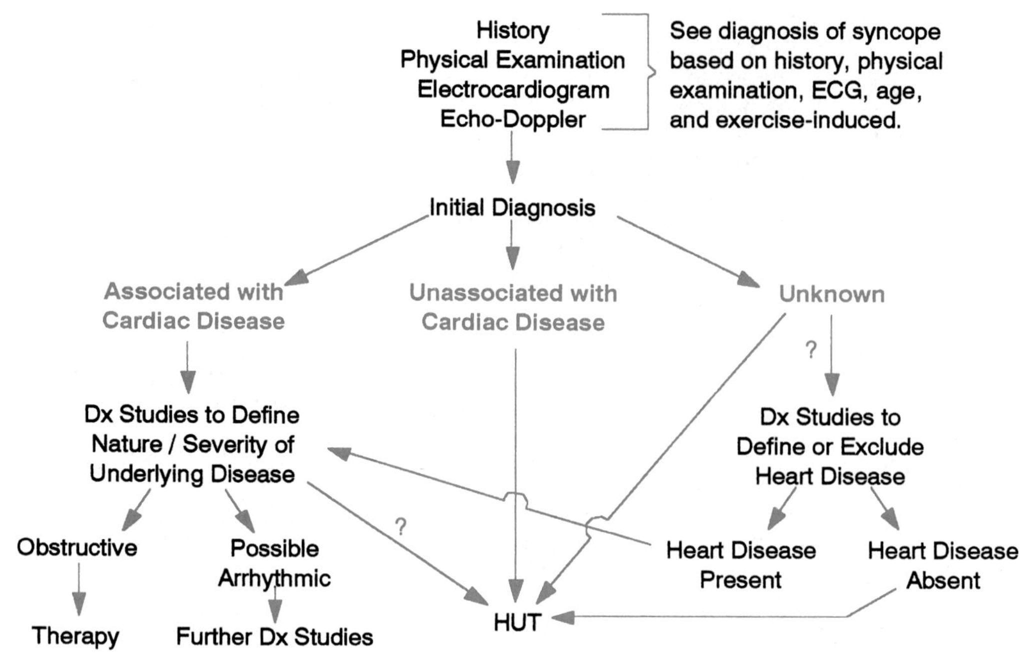


FIGURE 40-7 Basic schema for diagnostic evaluation of syncope. ECG = electrocardiogram; Dx = diagnostic; HUT = head-up tilt.

known cause will be further diminished in the future. In selected cases, devices with extended monitoring capabilities can be used.

## References


1. Savage DD, Corwin L, McGee DL, et al. Epidemiologic features of isolated syncope: The Framingham Study. *Stroke* 1985;16:626–629.
2. Soteriades ES, Evans JC, Larson MG, et al. Incidence and prognosis of syncope. *N Engl J Med* 2002;347:878.
3. Kapoor WN, Karpf M, Wieland S, et al. A prospective evaluation and follow-up of patients with syncope. *N Engl J Med* 1983;309:197–204.
4. Abbond F. Neurocardiogenic syncope. *N Engl J Med* 1993;328: 1117–1120.
5. Rea R, Thomas MD. Neural control and vasovagal syncope mechanisms. *J Cardiovasc Electrophysiol* 1993;4:587–595.
6. Burklow TR, Moak JP, Bailey JJ, et al. Neurally mediated cardiac syncope: Autonomic modulation after normal saline infusion. *J Am Coll Cardiol* 1999; 33:2059–2066.
7. Furlan R, Piazza S, Dell'Orto S, et al. Cardiac autonomic patterns preceding occasional vasovagal reactions in healthy humans. *Circulation* 1998;98:1756–1761.
8. White M, Cernacek P, Courtemanche M, et al. Impaired endothelin-1 release in tilt-induced syncope. *Am J Cardiol* 1998;81:460–464.
9. Kikushima S, Kobayashi Y, Nakagawa H, et al. Triggering mechanism for neurally mediated syncope induced by head-up tilt test. *J Am Coll Cardiol* 1999;33:350–357.
10. Theodorakis GN, Markianos M, Livanis EG, et al. Central serotonergic responsiveness in neurocardiogenic syncope: A clomipramine test challenge. *Circulation* 1998;98:2724–2730.
11. Van Lieshout JJ, Wouter W, Karemaker JM, et al. The vasovagal response. *Clin Sci* 1991;81:575–586.
12. Dan D, Hoag JB, Ellenbogen KA, et al. Cerebral blood flow velocity declines before arterial pressure in patients with orthostatic vasovagal presyncope. *J Am Coll Cardiol* 2002;39:1039–1045.
13. Shalev Y, Gal R, Tchou P, et al. Echocardiographic demonstration of decreased left ventricular dimension and vigorous myocardial contraction during syncope induced by head-up tilt. *J Am Coll Cardiol* 1991; 18:748–751.
14. Thoren P. Role of cardiac vagal C-fibers in cardiovascular control. *Rev Physiol Biochem Pharmacol* 1979;86:1–94.
15. Mark A. The Bezold-Jarisch reflex revisited: Clinical implications of inhibitory reflexes originating in the heart. *J Am Coll Cardiol* 1983; 1:90–102.
16. Rosoff MH, Cohen MV. Profound bradycardia after amyl nitrate in patients with a tendency to vasovagal episodes. *Br Heart J* 1986;55:97–100.
17. Fitzpatrick AP, Banner N, Cheng A, et al. Vasovagal reactions may occur after orthotopic heart transplantation. *J Am Coll Cardiol* 1993;21: 1132–1137.
18. Sra JS, Murthy V, Natale A, et al. Circulatory and catecholamine changes during head-up tilt testing in neurocardiogenic (vasovagal) syncope. *Am J Cardiol* 1994;73:33–37.
19. Chen MY, Goldenberg IF, Milstein S, et al. Cardiac electrophysiologic and hemodynamic correlates of neurally-mediated syncope. *Am J Cardiol* 1989;63:66–72.
20. Boorin MR. Anxiety: Its manifestation and role in the dental patient. *Dent Clin North Am* 1995;39:523–539.
21. Bou-Holagah I, Rowe PC, Kan J, et al. The relationship between neurally mediated hypotension and the chronic fatigue syndrome. *JAMA* 1995;274:961–967.
22. Milstein S, Buetikofer J, Lesser J, et al. Cardiac asystole: A manifestation of neurally-mediated hypotension-bradycardia. *J Am Coll Cardiol* 1989;14:1626–1632.
23. Folino AF, Buja GF, Martini B, et al. Prolonged cardiac arrest and complete AV block during upright tilt test in young patients with syncope of unknown origin: Prognostic and therapeutic implications. *Eur Heart J* 1992;13:1416–1421.
24. Almquist A, Goldenberg IF, Milstein S, et al. Provocation of bradycardia and hypotension by isoproterenol and upright posture in patients with unexplained syncope. *N Engl J Med* 1989;320:346–351.
25. Fitzpatrick AP, Theodorakis G, Vardas P, et al. Methodology of head-up tilt testing in patients with unexplained syncope. *J Am Coll Cardiol* 1991;17:125–130.
26. Bloomfield D, Maurer M, Bigger JT. Effects of age on outcome of tilt-table testing. *Am J Cardiol* 1999;83:1055–1058.
27. Moya A, Brignole M, Menozzi C, et al. Mechanism of syncope in patients with isolated syncope and in patients with tilt-positive syncope. *Circulation* 2001;104:1261–1267.

28. Sneddon JF, Slade A, Seo H, et al. Assessment of the diagnostic value of head-up tilt testing in the evaluation of syncope in hypertrophic cardiomyopathy. *Am J Cardiol* 1994;73:601–604.
29. Kenny RA, Bayliss J, Ingram A, et al. Head-up tilt: A useful test for investigating unexplained syncope. *Lancet* 1986;1:1352–1355.
30. Morello CA, Klein GJ, Zandri S, et al. Diagnostic accuracy of a low-dose isoproterenol head-up tilt protocol. *Am Heart J* 1995;129:901–906.
31. Natale A, Akhtar M, Jazayeri M, et al. Provocation of hypotension during head-up tilt testing in subjects with no history of syncope or presyncope. *Circulation* 1995;92:54–58.
32. Sheldon R, Rose S, Flanagan P, et al. Risk factors for syncope recurrence after a positive tilt-table test in patients with syncope. *Circulation* 1996;93:973–981.
33. Shen WK, Jahangir A, Beinborn D, et al. Utility of a single-stage isoproterenol tilt table test in adults: A randomized comparison with passive head-up tilt. *J Am Coll Cardiol* 1999;33:985–990.
34. Zeng C, Zhu Z, Hu W, et al. Value of sublingual isosorbide dinitrate before isoproterenol tilt test for diagnosis of neurally mediated syncope. *Am J Cardiol* 1999;83:1059–1063.
35. Mittal S, Stein KM, Markowitz SM, et al. Induction of neurally mediated syncope with adenosine. *Circulation* 1999;99:1318–1324.
36. Gaggioli G, Bottoni N, Mureddu R, et al. Effects on chronic vasodilator therapy to enhance susceptibility to vasovagal syncope during upright tilt testing. *Am J Cardiol* 1997;80:1092–1094.
37. Zeng C, Zhu Z, Liu G, et al. Randomized double-blind, placebo-controlled trial of oral enalapril in patients with neurally mediated syncope. *Am Heart J* 1998;136:852–858.
38. Zeng CY, Zhu Z, Liu G, et al. Inhibitory effect of enalapril on neurally mediated syncope in elderly patients. *J Cardiovasc Pharmacol* 1998; 31:638–642.
39. Schroeder C, Bush VE, Norcliffe LJ, et al. Water drinking acutely improves orthostatic tolerance in healthy subjects. *Circulation* 2002;106: 2806–2811.
40. Cooper VI, Hainsworth R. Effects of dietary salt on orthostatic tolerance, blood pressure and baroreceptor sensitivity in patients with syncope. *Clin Auton Res* 2002;12:236–241.
41. Di Girolamo E, Di Iorio C, Leonzio L, et al. Usefulness of a tilt training program for the prevention of refractory neurocardiogenic syncope in adolescents: A controlled study. *Circulation* 1999;100:1798–1801.
42. Mtinangi BL, Hainsworth R. Increased orthostatic tolerance following moderate exercise training in patients with unexplained syncope. *Heart* 1998;80:596–600.
43. Abe H, Kondo S, Kohshi K, Nakashima Y. Usefulness of orthostatic self-training for the prevention of neurocardiogenic syncope. *Pacing Clin Electrophysiol* 2002;25:1454–1458.
44. Brignole M, Croci F, Menozzi C, et al. Isometric arm counter-pressure maneuvers to abort impending vasovagal syncope. *J Am Coll Cardiol* 2002;40:2053–2059.
45. Krediet CT, Van Dijk N, Linzer M, et al. Management of vasovagal syncope: Controlling or aborting faints by leg crossing and muscle tensing. *Circulation* 2002;106:1684–1689.
46. Morillo CA, Leitch JW, Yee R, et al. A placebo-controlled trial of intravenous and oral disopyramide for prevention of neurally mediated syncope induced by head-up tilt. *J Am Coll Cardiol* 1993;22:1843–1848.
47. Moya A, Permanyer-Miralda G, Sagrista-Sauleda J, et al. Limitations of head-up tilt test for evaluating the efficacy of therapeutic interventions in patients with vasovagal syncope: Results of a controlled study of etilefrine versus placebo. *J Am Coll Cardiol* 1995;25:65–69.
48. Younoszai AK, Franklin WH, Chan DP, et al. Oral fluid therapy: A promising treatment for vasodepressor syncope. *Arch Pediatr Adolesc Med* 1998;152:165–168.
49. Mtinangi BL, Hainsworth R. Early effects of oral salt on plasma volume, orthostatic tolerance, and barorecptor sensitivity in patients with syncope. *Clin Auton Res* 1998;8:231–235.
50. Schatz IJ. Management of orthostatic hypotension. In: Schatz IJ, ed. *Orthostatic Hypotension.* Philadelphia: FA Davis; 1986:98.
51. Flevari P, Livanis EG, Theodorakis GN, et al. Vasovagal syncope: A prospective, randomized, crossover evaluation of the effect of propranolol, nadolol and placebo on syncope recurrence and patients' well-being. *J Am Coll Cardiol* 2002;40:499–504.
52. Ventura R, Maas R, Zeidler D, et al. A randomized and controlled pilot trial of beta-blockers for the treatment of recurrent syncope in patients with a positive or negative response to head-up tilt test. *Pacing Clin Electrophysiol* 2002;25:816–821.
53. Mahanonda N, Bhuripanyo K, Kangkagate C, et al. Randomized double-blind, placebo-controlled trial of oral atenolol in patients with unexplained syncope and positive upright tilt table test results. *Am Heart J* 1995;130:1250–1253.
54. Yu SC, Sung RJ. Clinical efficacy of propantheline bromide in neurocardiogenic syncope: Pharmacodynamic implications. *Cardiovasc Drugs Ther* 1997;10:687–692.
55. Kosinski D, Grubb BP, Temesy-Armos P. Pathophysiological aspects of neurocardiogenic syncope: Current concepts and new perspectives. *PACE* 1995;18:716–724.
56. Grubb BP, Samoil D, Kosinski D, et al. Use of sertraline hydrochloride in the treatment of refractory neurocardiogenic syncope in children and adolescents. *J Am Coll Cardiol* 1994;24:490–495.
57. Di Girolamo E, Di Lorio C, Sabatini P, et al. Effects of paroxetine hydrochloride, a selective serotonin reuptake inhibitor, on refractory vasovagal syncope: A randomized, double-blind, placebo-controlled study. *J Am Coll Cardiol* 1999;33:1227–1230.
58. Takata TS, Wasmund SL, Smith ML, et al. Serotonin reuptake inhibitor (Paxil) does not prevent the vasovagal reaction associated with carotid sinus massage and/or lower body negative pressure in healthy volunteers. *Circulation* 2002;106:1500–1504.
59. Nelson SD, Stanley M, Love CJ, et al. The autonomic and hemodynamic effects of oral theophylline in patients with vasodepressor syncope. *Arch Intern Med* 1991;151:2425–2429.
60. Saadjian AY, Levy S, Franceschi F, et al. Role of endogenous adenosine as a modulator of syncope induced during tilt testing. *Circulation* 2002;106:569–574.
61. Ward CR, Gray JC, Gilroy JJ, et al. Midodrine: A role in the management of neurocardiogenic syncope. *Heart* 1998;79:45–49.
62. Low PA, Gilden JL, Freeman R, et al. Efficacy of midodrine vs placebo in neurogenic orthostatic hypotension. A randomized, double-blind multicenter study. Midodrine Study Group. *JAMA* 1997;278:388.
63. Raviele A, Brignole M, Sutton R, et al. Effect of etilefrine in preventing syncopal recurrence in patients with vasovagal syncope: A double-blind, randomized, placebo-controlled trial—The Vasovagal Syncope International Study. *Circulation* 1999;99:1452–1457.
64. Sheldon R, Koshman ML, Wilson W, et al. Effect of dual-chamber pacing with automatic rate-drop sensing on recurrent neurally medicated syncope. *Am J Cardiol* 1998;81:158–162.
65. Ammirati F, Colivicchi F, Toscano S, et al. DDD pacing with rate drop response function versus DDI with rate hysteresis pacing for cardioinhibitory vasovagal syncope. *Pacing Clin Electrophysiol* 1998;21: 2178–2181.
66. Connolly SJ, Sheldon R, Roberts RS, et al. The North American Vasovagal Pacemaker Study (VPS): A randomized trial of permanent cardiac pacing for the prevention of vasovagal syncope. *J Am Coll Cardiol* 1999;33:16–20.
67. Schatz IJ. Orthostatic hypotension: Functional and neurogenic causes. *Arch Intern Med* 1984;144:773–777.
68. Ziegler MG. Postural hypotension. *Annu Rev Med* 1980;31:239–245.
69. Levine BD, Giller CA, Lane LD, et al. Cerebral versus systemic hemodynamics during graded orthostatic stress in humans. *Circulation* 1994;90:298–306.
70. Jacob G, Shannon JR, Costa F, et al. Abnormal norepinephrine clearance and adrenergic receptor sensitivity in idiopathic orthostatic intolerance. *Circulation* 1999;99:1706–1712.
71. Jacob G, Shannon JR, Black B, et al. Effects of volume loading and pressor agents in idiopathic orthostatic tachycarda. *Circulation* 1997; 96:575–580.
72. Furlan R, Jacob G, Snell M, et al. Chronic orthostatic intolerance: A disorder with discordant cardiac and vascular sympathetic control. *Circulation* 1998;98:2154–2159.

73. Masaki KH, Schatz IJ, Burchfiel CM, et al. Orthostatic hypotension predicts mortality in elderly men: The Honolulu Heart Program. *Circulation* 1998;98:2290–2295.
74. Farquhar WB, Taylor JA, Darling SE, et al. Abnormal baroreflex responses in patients with idiopathic orthostatic intolerance. *Circulation* 2000;102:3086–3091.
75. Leier CV, Boudoulas H. *Cardiorenal Disorders and Diseases,* 2d ed. New York: Futura; 1992.
76. Shy GM, Drager GA. A neurologic syndrome associated with orthostatic hypotension. *Arch Neurol* 1960;2:511–527.
77. Kontos HA, Richardson DW, Norvell JE. Norepinephrine depletion in idiopathic orthostatic hypotension. *Ann Intern Med* 1975; 82:336–341.
78. Ziegler MG, Lake CR, Kopin IJ. The sympathetic-nervous-system defect in primary orthostatic hypotension. *N Engl J Med* 1977;96: 293–297.
79. Kopin IJ, Polinsky RJ, Oliver JA, et al. Urinary catecholamine metabolites distinguish different types of sympathetic neuronal dysfunction in patients with orthostatic hypotension. *J Clin Endocrinol Metab* 1983; 57:632–637.
80. Khurana RK, Nelson E, Azzarelli B, et al. Shy-Drager syndrome: Diagnosis and treatment of cholinergic dysfunction. *Neurology* 1980; 30:805–809.
81. Cryer PE, Silverberg AB, Santiago JV, et al. Plasma catecholamines in diabetes: The syndromes of hypoadrenergic and hyperadrenergic postural hypotension. *Am J Med* 1978;64:407–416.
82. Henry R, Rowe J, O'Mahony D. Haemodynamic analysis of efficacy of compression hosiery in elderly fallers with orthostatic hypotension. *Lancet* 1999;354:45–46.
83. Ector H, Reybrouck T, Heidbuchel H, et al. Tilt training: A new treatment for recurrent neurocardiogenic syncope and severe orthostatic intolerance. *Pacing Clin Electrophysiol* 1998;21:193–196.
84. Hoeldtke RD, Streeten DHP, Phil D. Treatment of orthostatic hypotension with erythropoietin. *N Engl J Med* 1993;329:611–615.
85. Bousser MG, Dubois B, Castaigne P. Transient loss of consciousness in ischemic cerebral events: A study of 557 ischemic strokes and transient ischemic attacks. *Ann Intern Med* 1980;132:300–307.
86. Benbadis SR, Wolgamuth BR, Goren H, et al. Value of tongue biting in the diagnosis of seizures. *Arch Intern Med* 1995;155:2346–2349.
87. Delanty N, Vaughan CJ, French JA. Medical causes of seizures. *Lancet* 1998;352:383–390.
88. Sheldon R, Rose S, Ritchie D, et al. Historical criteria that distinguish syncope from seizures. *J Am Coll Cardiol* 2002;40:142–148.
89. Kenny RAM, Richardsohn DA, Steen N, et al. Carotid sinus syndrome: A modifiable risk factor for nonaccidental falls in older adults (SAFE PACE). *J Am Coll Cardiol* 2001;38:1491–1496.
90. Weiss S, Baker JP. The carotid sinus reflex in health and disease: Its role in the causation of fainting and convulsions. *Medicine (Baltimore)* 1933;12:297–354.
91. Graux P, Carlioz R, Guyomar Y, et al. Characteristics and influence of different clinical forms on the development and prognosis of carotid sinus syndrome. *Arch Mal Coeur* 1995;88:999–1006.
92. El-Sayed H, Hainsworth R. Relationship between plasma volume, carotic baroreceptor sensitivity and orthostatic tolerance. *Clin Sci* 1995;88:463–470.
93. Nishizaki M, Arita M, Sakurada H, et al. Long-term follow-up of the reproducibility of carotid sinus hypersensitivity in patients with carotid sinus syndrome. *Jpn Circ J* 1995;59:33–39.
94. Tea SH, Mansourati J, L'Heveder G, et al. New insights into the pathophysiology of carotid sinus syndrome. *Circulation* 1996;93:1411–1416.
95. Cicogna R, Bonomi FG, Curnis A, et al. Peripharyngeal space lesions syncope-syndrome: A newly proposed reflexogenic cardiovascular syndrome. *Eur Heart J* 1993;14:1476–1483.
96. Sumiyoshi M, Nakata Y, Mineda Y, et al. Response to head-up tilt testing in patients with situational syncope. *Am J Cardiol* 1998;82:1117–1118.
97. Mattle HP, Nirkko AC, Baumgartner RW, et al. Transient cerebral circulatory arrest coincides with fainting in cough syncope. *Neurology* 1995;45:498–501.
98. Bortolotti M, Cirignotta F, Labo G. Atrioventricular block induced by swallowing in a patient with diffuse esophageal spasm. *JAMA* 1982; 248:2297–2299.
99. Ferrante L, Artico M, Nardacci B, et al. Glossopharyngeal neuralgia with cardiac syncope. *Neurosurgery* 1995;36:58–63.
100. Godec CJ, Cass AS. Micturition syncope. *J Urol* 1981;126:551–556.
101. Kapoor WN, Peterson J, Karpf M. Defecation syncope: A symptom with multiple etiologies. *Arch Intern Med* 1986;146:2377–2382.
102. Maurer M, Karmally W, Rivadeneira H, et al. Upright posture and postprandial hypotension in elderly persons. *Ann Intern Med* 2000; 133:533–536.
103. Jansen RW, Connelly CM, Kelley-Gagnon M, et al. Postprandial hypotension in elderly patients with unexplained syncope. *Arch Intern Med* 1995;155:945–952.
104. Jansen RWMM, Lipsitz LA. Postprandial hypotension: Epidemiology, pathophysiology, and clinical management. *Ann Intern Med* 1995; 122:286–295.
105. Kapoor WN, Fortunato M, Hanusa BH, et al. Psychiatric illnesses in patients with syncope. *Am J Med* 1995;99:505–512.
106. Aminoff MJ, Scheimman MM, Griffin JC, et al. Electrocerebral accompaniments of syncope associated with malignant ventricular arrhythmias. *Ann Intern Med* 1988;108:791–796.
107. Constantin L, Martins JB, Fincham RW, et al. Bradycardia and syncope as manifestations of partial epilepsy. *J Am Coll Cardiol* 1990;15: 900–905.
108. Grech ED, Ramsdale DR. Exertional syncope in aortic stenosis: Evidence to support inappropriate left ventricular baroreceptor response. *Am Heart J* 1991;121:603–606.
109. Schwartz LS, Goldfisher J, Sprague GJ, et al. Syncope and sudden death in aortic stenosis. *Am J Cardiol* 1969;23:647–658.
110. Nienaber CA, Hiller S, Spielmann RP, et al. Syncope in hypertrophic cardiomyopathy: Multivariate analysis of prognostic determinants. *J Am Coll Cardiol* 1990;15:948–955.
111. Dressler W. Effort syncope as an early manifestation of primary pulmonary hypertension. *Am J Med Sci* 1952;223:131–143.
112. Scarpa WJ. The sick sinus syndrome. *Am Heart J* 1983;92:648–651.
113. Talwar KK, Edvardsson N, Varnauskas E. Paroxysmal vagally mediated AV block with recurrent syncope. *Clin Cardiol* 1985;8: 337–340.
114. Beder SD, Cohen MH, Riemenschneider TA. Occult arrhythmias as the etiology of unexplained syncope in children with structurally normal hearts. *Am Heart J* 1985;109:309–313.
115. Brignole M, Menozzi C, Moya A, et al. Mechanism of syncope in patients with bundle branch block and negative electrophysiological test. *Circulation* 2001:104:2045–2050.
116. Boudoulas H, Wooley CF. *Mitral Valve: Floppy Mitral Valve, Mitral Valve Prolapse, Mitral Valvular Regurgitation,* 2d ed. Armonk, NY: Futura; 2000.
117. Moss AJ, Schwartz PJ, Crampton RS, et al. The long QT syndrome: Prospective longitudinal study of 328 families. *Circulation* 1991;84: 1136–1144.
118. Menozzi C, Brignole M, Alboni P, et al. The natural course of untreated sick sinus syndrome and identification of the variables predictive of unfavorable outcome. *Am J Cardiol* 1998;82:1205–1209.
119. Mikhail GW, Gibbs JSR, Yacoub MH. Pulmonary and systemic arterial pressure changes during syncope in primary pulmonary hypertension. *Circulation* 2001;104:1326–1327.
120. Chen SY, Wang YH, Hwang JJ, et al. Pulmonary embolism presenting as syncope in paraplegia: A case report. *Arch Phys Med Rehabil* 1995; 76:387–390.
121. Leitch JW, Klein GJ, Yee R, et al. Syncope associated with supraventricular tachycardia. *Circulation* 1992;85:1064–1071.
122. Brignole M, Gianfranchi L, Menozzi C, et al. Role of autonomic reflexes in syncope associated with paroxysmal atrial fibrillation. *J Am Coll Cardiol* 1993;22:1123–1129.
123. Antzelevitch C, Brugada P, Brugada J, et al. Brugada syndrome: A decade of progress. *Circ Res* 2002;91:1114–1118.

124. Wilde AA, Antzelevitch C, Borggrefe M, et al. Proposed diagnostic criteria for the Brugada syndrome: Consensus report. *Circulation* 2002;106:2514–2519.
125. Priori SG, Napolitano C, Gasparini M, et al. Natural history of Brugada syndrome: Insights for risk stratification and management. *Circulation* 2002;105:1342–1347.
126. Gemayel C, Pelliccia A, Thompson P. Arrhythmogenic right ventricular cardiomyopathy. *J Am Coll Cardiol* 2001;38:1773–1781.
127. Splawski I, Shen J, Timothy KW, Lehmann MH, et al. Spectrum of mutations in long-QT syndrome genes. *KVLQT1, HERG, SCN5A, KCNE1*, and *KCNE2*. *Circulation* 2000;102:1178–1185.
128. Zareba W, Moss AJ, Schwartz PJ, et al. Influence of the genotype on the clinical course of the long-QT syndrome. *N Engl J Med* 1998; 339:960–965.
129. Menozzi C, Brignole M, Garcia-Civera R, et al. Mechanism of syncope in patients with heart disease and negative electrophysiologic test. *Circulation* 2002;105:2741–2745.
130. Ausubel K, Boal BH, Furmen S. Pacemaker syndrome: Definition and evaluation. *Cardiol Clin* 1985;3:587–589.
131. Lamas GA, Orav EJ, Stambler BS, et al. Quality of life and clinical outcomes in elderly patients treated with ventricular pacing as compared with dual-chamber pacing. *N Engl J Med* 1998;338:1097–1104.
132. Oh JH, Hanusa BH, Kapoor WN. Do symptoms predict cardiac arrhythmias and mortality in patients with syncope? *Arch Intern Med* 1999;159:375–380.
133. Corrado D, Basso C, Thiene G, et al. Spectrum of clinicopathologic manifestations of arrhythmogenic right ventricular cardiomyopathy dysplasia: A multicenter study. *J Am Coll Cardiol* 1997;30:1512–1520.
134. Winters SL, Stewart D, Gomes JA. Signal averaging of the surface QRS complex predicts inducibility of ventricular tachycardia in patients with syncope of unknown origin: A prospective study. *J Am Coll Cardiol* 1987;10:775–781.
135. Nalos PC, Gang ES, Mandel WJ, et al. The signal-averaged electrocardiogram as a screening test for inducibility of sustained ventricular tachycardia in high-risk patients: A prospective study. *J Am Coll Cardiol* 1987;9:539–548.
136. Cain ME, Anderson JL, Arnsdorf MF, et al. ACC Expert Consensus Document: Signal-averaged electrocardiography. *J Am Coll Cardiol* 1996;27:238–249.
137. Steinberg JS, Prystowsky E, Freedman RA, et al. Use of the signal-averaged electrocardiogram for predicting inducible ventricular tachycardia in patients with unexplained syncope: Relation to clinical variables in a multivariate analysis. *J Am Coll Cardiol* 1994;23:99–106.
138. Boudoulas H, Schaal SF, Lewis RP, et al. Superiority of 24-hour outpatient monitoring over multi-stage exercise testing for the evaluation of syncope. *J Electrocardiol* 1979;12:103–108.
139. Boudoulas H, Geleris P, Schaal SF, et al. Comparison between electrophysiologic studies and ambulatory monitoring in patients with syncope. *J Electrocardiol* 1983;16:91–96.
140. Dewey RC, Capeless MA, Levy AM. Use of ambulatory electrocardiographic monitoring to identify high-risk patients with congenital complete heart block. *N Engl J Med* 1987;316:835–839.
141. Linzer M, Prystowsky EN, Brunetti LL, et al. Recurrent syncope of unknown origin diagnosed by ambulatory continuous loop ECG recording. *Am Heart J* 1988;116:1632–1634.
142. Fetter JG, Stanton MS, Benditt DG, et al. Transtelephonic monitoring and transmission of stored arrhythmia detection and therapy data from an implantable cardioverter defibrillator. *Pacing Clin Electrophysiol* 1995;18:1531–1539.
143. Kinlay S, Leitch JW, Neil A, et al. Cardiac event recorders yield more diagnoses and are more cost-effective than 48-hour Holter monitoring in patients with palpitations. *Ann Intern Med* 1996;24:16–20.
144. Krahn AD, Klein GJ, Yee R, et al. Use of an extended monitoring strategy in patients with problematic syncope. *Circulation* 1999;99:406–410.
145. Zimetbaum PJ, Kim KY, Josephson ME, et al. Diagnostic yield and optimal duration of continuous-loop event monitoring for the diagnosis of palpitations. *Ann Intern Med* 1998;128:890–895.
146. Kushner JA, Kou WH, Kadish AM, et al. Natural history of patients with unexplained syncope and a nondiagnostic electrophysiologic study. *J Am Coll Cardiol* 1989;74:391–396.
147. Boudoulas H, Schaal SF, Lewis RP. Electrophysiologic risk factors in syncope. *J Electrocardiol* 1978;11:339–342.
148. Englund A, Bergfeldt L, Rehnqvist N, et al. Diagnostic value of programmed ventricular stimulation in patients with bifascicular block: A prospective study of patients with and without syncope. *J Am Coll Cardiol* 1995;26:1508–1515.
149. Bellinder G, Nordlander R, Pehrsson SK, et al. Atrial pacing in the management of sick sinus syndrome: Long-term observation for conduction disturbances and supraventricular tachyarrhythmias. *Eur Heart J* 1986;7:105–109.
150. Moss AJ, Liu JE, Gottlieb S, et al. Efficacy of permanent pacing in the management of high-risk patients with long QT syndrome. *Circulation* 1991;84:1524–1529.
151. Link MS, Kim KMS, Homoud MK, et al. Long-term outcome of patients with syncope associated with coronary artery disease and a nondiagnostic electrophysiologic evaluation. *Am J Cardiol* 1999;83: 1334–1337.
152. Moss AJ, Hall WJ, Cannom DS, et al. Improved survival with an implanted defibrillator in patients with coronary disease at high risk for ventricular arrhythmia. *N Engl J Med* 1996;335:1933–1940.
153. Buxton AE, Lee KL, Fisher JD, et al. A randomized study of the prevention of sudden death in patients with coronary artery disease. Multicenter Unsustained Tachycardia Trial Investigators. *N Engl J Med* 1999;341:1882–1890.
154. Nishimura RA, Giuliani ER, Brandenburg RO, et al. Hypertrophic cardiomyopathy. In: Giuliani ER, Gersh BJ, McGoon MD, eds. *Mayo Clinic Practice of Cardiology,* 3d ed. St. Louis: Mosby; 1996:689.
155. Henein MY, O'Sullivan CA, Ramzy IS, et al. Electromechanical left ventricular behavior after nonsurgical septal reduction in patients with hypertrophic obstructive cardiomyopathy. *J Am Coll Cardiol* 1999;34: 1117–1122.
156. Ommen SR, Nishimura RA, Squires RW, et al. Comparison of dual-chamber pacing versus septal myectomy for the treatment of patients with hypertrophic obstructive cardiomyopathy. *J Am Coll Cardiol* 1999;34:191–196.
157. Fananapazir L. Advances in molecular genetics and management of hypertrophic cardiomyopathy. *JAMA* 1999;281:1746–1747.
158. Henein MY, O'Sullivan C, Sutton GC, et al. Stress-induced left ventricular outflow tract obstruction: A potential cause of dyspnea in the elderly. *J Am Coll Cardiol* 1997;30:1301–1307.
159. Spirito P, Maton BJ. Perspectives on the role of new treatment strategies in hypertrophic obstructive cardiomyopathy. *J Am Coll Cardiol* 1999;33:1071–1075.
160. Kappenberger L, Linde C, McKenna DW, et al. Pacing in hypertrophic obstructive cardiomyopathy: A randomized crossover study. *Eur Heart J* 1997;18:1249–1256.
161. Suda K, Kohl T, Kovalchin JP, et al. Echocardiographic predictors of poor outcome in infants with hypertrophic cardiomyopathy. *Am J Cardiol* 1997;80:595–600.
162. Knight C, Kurbaan AS, Seggewiss H, et al. Nonsurgical septal reduction for hypertrophic obstructive cardiomyopathy: Outcome in the first series of patients. *Circulation* 1997;95:2075–2081.
163. Gregoratos G, Abrams J, Epstein AE, et al. ACC/AHA/NASPE 2002 Guideline update for implantation of cardiac pacemakers and antiarrhythmia devices—Summary article: A report of the American College of Cardiology/American Heart Association Task Force on Practice Guidelines (ACC/AHA/NASPE Committee to Update the 1998 Pacemaker Guidelines). *J Am Coll Cardiol* 2002;40:1703–1719.
164. Alboni P, Menozzi C, Brignole M, et al. Effects of permanent pacemaker and oral theophylline in sick sinus syndrome the THEOPACE study: A randomized controlled trial. *Circulation* 1997;96:260–266.
165. Jackman WM, Xunzhang W, Friday K, et al. Catheter ablation of accessory atrioventricular pathways (Wolff-Parkinson-White syndrome) by radio-frequency current. *N Engl J Med* 1991;324:1605–1611.

166. Calkins H, Sousa J, El-Atassi R, et al. Diagnosis and cure of the Wolff-White-Parkinson syndrome or paroxysmal supraventricular tachycardia during a single electrophysiologic test. *N Engl J Med* 1991;324:1612–1618.
167. Menozzi C, Brignole M, Garcia-Civera R, et al. International study on syncope of uncertain etiology investigators. Mechanism of syncope in patients with heart disease and negative electrophysiologic test. *Circulation* 2002;105:2741–2745.
168. Krahn AD, Klein GJ, Fitzpatrick A, et al. Predicting the outcome of patients with unexplained syncope undergoing prolonged monitoring. *Pacing Clin Electrophysiol* 2002;25:37–41.
169. Lipsitz LA. Syncope in the elderly. *Ann Intern Med* 1983; 99:92–105.
170. Jonsson PV, Lipsitz LA, Kelley M, et al. Hypotensive responses to common daily activities in institutionalized elderly. *Arch Intern Med* 1990;150:1518–1524.
171. Lipsitz LA, Nyquist RP Jr, Wei JY, et al. Postprandial reduction in blood pressure in the elderly. *N Engl J Med* 1983;309:81–83.
172. O'Mahony D. Pathophysiology of carotid sinus hypersensitivity in elderly patients. *Lancet* 1995;346:950–952.
173. Rehm CG, Ross SE. Syncope as etiology of road crashes involving elderly drivers. *Am Surg* 1995;61:1006–1008.
174. Rehm CG, Ross SE. Elderly drivers involved in road crashes: A profile. *Am Surg* 1995;61:435–437.
175. Lurie KG, Iskos D, Sakaguchi S, et al. Resumption of motor vehicle operation in vasovagal fainters. *Am J Cardiol* 1999;83:604–606.
176. Kario K, Tobin JN, Wolfson LI, et al. Lower standing systolic blood pressure as a predictor of falls in the elderly: A community-based prospective study. *J Am Coll Cardiol* 2001;38:246–252.
177. Middlekauff HR, Stevenson WG, Stevenson LW, et al. Syncope in advanced heart failure: High risk of sudden death regardless of origin of syncope. *J Am Coll Cardiol* 1993;21:110–116.
178. Kapoor WN, Hanusa BH. Is syncope a risk factor for poor outcomes? Comparison of patients with and without syncope. *Am J Med* 1996; 100:646–655.
179. Elliott PM, Poloniecki J, Dickie S,. Sudden death in hypertrophic cardiomyopathy: Identification of high-risk patients. *J Am Coll Cardiol* 2000;36:2212–2218.
180. Lascault G, Barnay C, Cazeau S, et al. Etude preliminaire d'un stimulateur double chambre a fonction diagnostique. *Arch Mal Coeur* 1995; 88:451–457.
181. Epstein AE, Miles WM, Benditt DG, et al. Personal and public safety issues related to arrhythmias that may affect consciousness: implications for regulation and physician recommendations. A medical/scientific statement from the American Heart Association and the North American Society of Pacing and Electrophysiology. *Circulation* 1996;94:1147–1166.
182. Akiyama T, Powell JL, Mitchell LB, et al. Antiarrhythmics versus implantable defibrillators investigators. *N Engl J Med* 2001;345:391–397.
183. Leenhardt A, Lucet V, Denjoy I, et al. Catecholaminergic polymorphic ventricular tachycardia in children: A 7-year follow-up of 21 patients. *Circulation* 1995;91:1512–1519.
184. Salim MA, DiSessa TG. QT interval response to exercise in children with syncope. *Am J Cardiol* 1994;73:976–978.
185. Noh CI, Song JY, Kim HS, et al. Ventricular tachycardia and exercise related syncope in children with structurally normal hearts: Emphasis on repolarization abnormality. *Br Heart J* 1995;73:544–547.
186. Sinkovec M, Rakovec P, Zorman D, et al. Exertional syncope in a patient with aortic stenosis and right coronary artery disease. *Eur Heart J* 1995;16:276–278.
187. Williams CC, Bernhardt DT. Syncope in athletes. *Sports Med* 1995; 19:223–234.
188. Thomson HL, Atherton JJ, Khafagi FA, et al. Failure of reflex venoconstriction during exercise in patients with vasovagal syncope. *Circulation* 1996;93:953–959.
189. Balaji S, Oslizlok PC, Allen MC, et al. Neurocardiogenic syncope in children with a normal heart. *J Am Coll Cardiol* 1994;23:779–785.
190. Liberthson RR. Sudden death from cardiac causes in children and young adults. *N Engl J Med* 1996;334:1039–1044.
191. Colivicchi F, Ammirati F, Biffi A, et al. Exercised-related syncope in young competitive athletes without evidence of structural heart disease. *Eur Heart J* 2002;23:1080–1082.
192. Basso C, Maron BJ, Corrado D, Thiene G. Clinical profile of congenital coronary artery anomalies with origin from the wrong aortic sinus leading to sudden death in young competitive athletes. *J Am Coll Cardiol* 2000;35:1493–1501.
193. Boudoulas H, Lewis RP. Cardiac syncope: Diagnosis, mechanism, and management. In: Hurst JW, ed. *The Heart,* 6th ed. New York: McGraw-Hill; 1986:321.
194. Calkins H, Shyr Y, Frumin H, et al. The value of the clinical history in the differentiation of syncope due to ventricular tachycardia, atrioventricular block, and neurocardiogenic syncope. *Am J Med* 1995;98: 365–373.
195. Kapoor WN. Current evaluation and management of syncope. *Circulation* 2002;106:1606–1609.
196. Gilman JK. Syncope in the emergency department. *Emerg Med Clin North Am* 1995;13:955–971.
197. Kroenke K, Lucas CA, Rosenberg ML, et al. Causes of persistent dizziness: A prospective study of 100 patients in ambulatory care. *Ann Intern Med* 1992;117:898–904.
198. Krahn AD, Klein GJ, Norris C, et al. The etiology of syncope in patients with negative tilt table and electrophysiological testing. *Circulation* 1995;92:1819–1824.
199. Schaal SF, Nelson SD, Boudoulas H, Lewis RP. Syncope. *Curr Probl Cardiol* 1992;14:211–264.
200. Alboni P, Brignole M, Menozzi C, et al. Diagnostic value of history in patients with syncope with or without heart disease. *J Am Coll Cardiol* 2001;37:1921–1928.
201. Brignole M, Alboni P, Benditt D, et al. Guidelines on management (diagnosis and treatment) of syncope. European Task Force on Syncope. European Society of Cardiology. *Eur Heart J* 2001;22:1256–1306.

CHAPTER 41

# SUDDEN CARDIAC DEATH

Duane S. Pinto / Mark E. Josephson



## DEFINITION OF SUDDEN CARDIAC DEATH

*Sudden cardiac death* (SCD) describes the unexpected natural death due to a cardiac cause within a short time period from the onset of symptoms in a person without any prior condition that would appear fatal. It is most often due to a sustained ventricular tachyarrhythmia. Although many cardiovascular disorders increase the risk of SCD, the presence or absence of preexisting cardiovascular disease is not necessary.[1,2] Prodromal symptoms such as palpitations, chest pain, and dyspnea may suggest a cardiovascular etiology such as arrhythmia, ischemia, or congestive heart failure, but they are not specific.[3,4] The definition of SCD includes the time interval from onset of the symptoms leading to collapse and then to death, the unexpected nature of the event, and the specific cause of death. More recent definitions have focused on time intervals of 1 h or less, which normally identify SCD populations having a 90 percent or more proportion of arrhythmic death.[5,6] Since 80 percent occur in the home environment and up to 40 percent of sudden deaths are not witnessed, the information necessary to establish a diagnosis of SCD is frequently lacking.[7–9]

Advances in emergency medical services, technological advances such as automated external defibrillators, and community-based interventions have resulted in a contradiction in terms. Biological death is an absolute and irreversible event, but patients can survive a cardiac arrest that would lead to SCD if left untreated. Processes such as malignant arrhythmias, pump failure, and coronary ischemia—which initiate the cascade of events leading to cardiovascular collapse—can be modified and the episode of SCD averted. Ultimately, though, the distinction between SCD, non-SCD, and noncardiac death is relevant more from a historical perspective. Total mortality rate is a more definitive endpoint in assessing the efficacy of an intervention aimed at improving survival.

## EPIDEMIOLOGY

### Incidence

SCD accounts for approximately 400,000 deaths yearly in the United States, depending on the definition used.[1,2] When the definition was restricted to death less than 2 h from onset of symptoms, 12 percent of all natural deaths were sudden and 88 percent of these were due to cardiac disease. In autopsy-based studies, a cardiac etiology of sudden death has been reported in 60 to 70 percent of sudden death victims.[8,9] SCD is the most common, and often the first, manifestation of coronary heart disease (CHD) and is responsible for half the mortality from cardiovascular disease,[1] the main cause of death in this country. The Framingham Study showed that 13 percent of all natural deaths were sudden in subjects without evidence of cardiac disease at entry, and 50 percent of SCDs in men and 64 percent in women occurred in people without known CHD. SCD was the first symptom of CHD in approximately 10 percent of all coronary events. The proportion of SCD was lower (20 to 34 percent) in patients with known coronary heart disease.[1]

The overall annual incidence of SCD in the United States is estimated using data derived from the National Center for Health

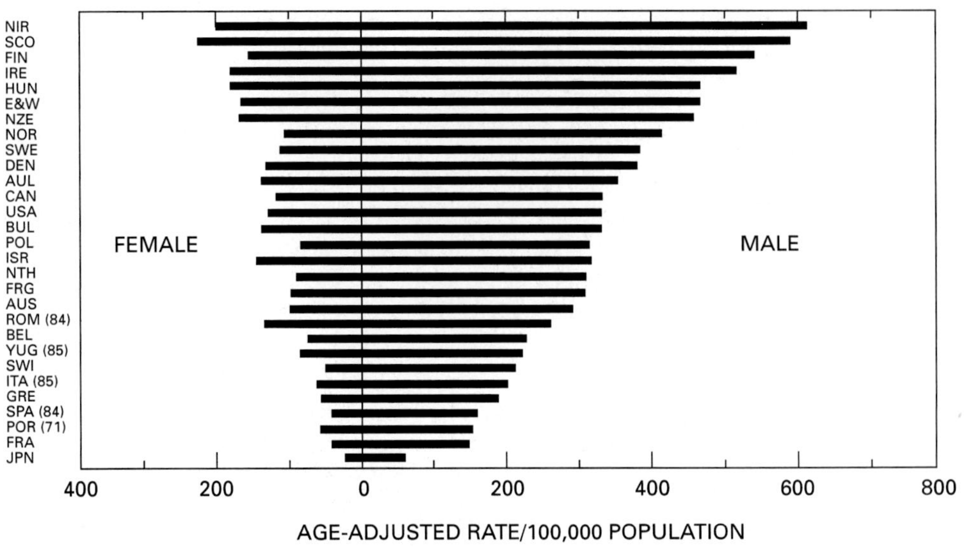


FIGURE 41-1 Sudden cardiac death rates by gender and country, ages 35 to 74 years, compiled from death certificates by the World Health Organization, Geneva, 1986. (From Manolio TA, Furberg CD. Epidemiology of sudden cardiac death. In: Akhtar M, Myerburg RJ, Ruskin JN, eds. *Sudden Cardiac Death*. Baltimore: Williams & Wilkins; 1994:3. Reproduced with permission from the publisher and authors.)

Statistics at the Centers for Disease Control and Prevention. These data estimate the SCD incidence per 1000 persons in 1999 to be 2.1 in men and 1.1 in women, resulting in 462,340 deaths of a total of 728,743 deaths from cardiac disease.[10] The average age of cardiac arrest victims is around 65 years, and 70 to 80 percent are men.[11] In the United States, several population-based studies have documented an age-adjusted decline in SCD rates of more than 8 percent over the last 15 years.[2] SCD rates in other developed countries are comparable to those inside the United States. The World Health Organization reported an annual incidence of SCD of 1.9 per 1000 persons in men and 0.6 in women, again accounting for nearly half the deaths from CHD.[3] SCD rates in developing countries are considerably lower, paralleling the rates of ischemic heart disease as a whole (Fig. 41-1).

## Influence of Age, Race, and Gender

### AGE

The incidence of SCD increases with age in men and women as well as whites and nonwhites because of the higher prevalence of ischemic heart disease at older ages (Fig. 41-2).[1,12] Among sudden natural deaths, the proportion of cardiac causes increases with advancing age. Among patients with CHD, however, the proportion of coronary deaths that are sudden decreases from over 74 percent of deaths in those aged 35 to 44 years to <60 percent of those aged 75 to 84 years.[1,2]

SCD accounts for approximately 20 percent of all sudden deaths in patients below age 20.[13] The overall incidence is low in the United States, accounting for about 600 cases per year. Structural cardiac abnormalities can be identified in over 90 percent of young victims of SCD, with the most common pathologic findings being myocarditis, hypertrophic cardiomyopathy, congenital coronary artery anomalies, atherosclerotic coronary heart disease, conduction system abnormalities, congenital arrhythmogenic disorders, arrhythmias associated with mitral valve prolapse, and aortic dissection.[14,15] Many SCDs in the pediatric population occur in patients with surgically treated congenital cardiac abnormalities, but in most, SCD is the first manifestation of underlying cardiac disease in otherwise healthy-appearing individuals (see Chap. 39).

Among young people with sudden death, aortic stenosis and primary or secondary pulmonary vascular obstruction have been shown to be the most common in patients without prior cardiac surgery, while tetralogy of Fallot and transposition of the great vessels were more common in postoperative patients. Ventricular arrhythmias and early transient heart block may play roles in tetralogy of Fallot,[16] while supraventricular rhythms, especially atrial flutter, may be important in transposition of the great vessels.[17] The presence of a QRS duration of 180 ms or more and severe left ventricular systolic function appears to identify a group at higher risk for sudden death after repair for tetralogy of Fallot[18] (see Chaps. 39 and 74).

### RACIAL DIFFERENCES

The annual incidence of SCD has been shown to be higher in African Americans than whites in numerous studies.[2,19] An analysis of cardiac death rates in the United States between 1989 and 1998 showed that the age-adjusted rates of SCD per 1000 persons were 5.0 for black men, 4.1 for white men, and 2.1 for Asians. In spite of the limitations of these studies, it is clear from these and other data that

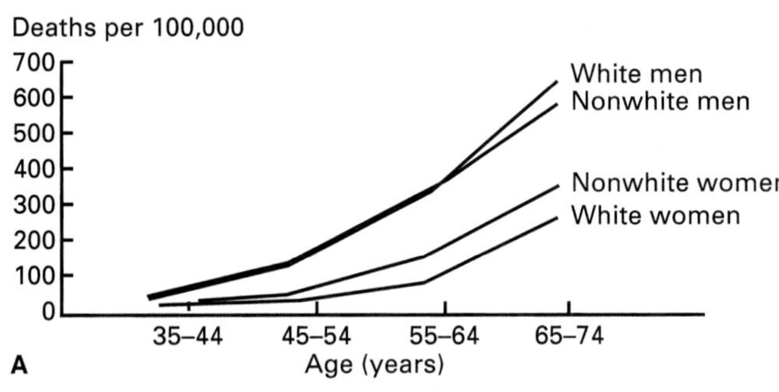


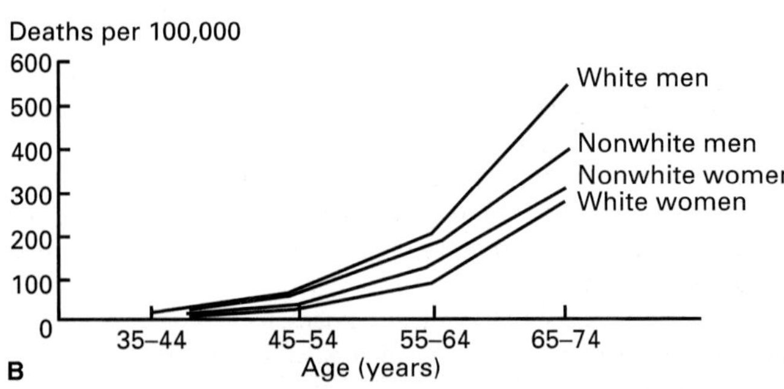


FIGURE 41-2 Plots of mortality rates (deaths per 100,000) for ischemic heart disease occurring (*A*) out-of-hospital or in emergency room (an estimate for sudden cardiac death rate) and (*B*) occurring in the hospital, by age, gender, and race in 40 states during 1985. (From the National Center for Health Statistics. Reproduced from Gillum.[12] With permission)

African Americans have the highest overall mortality rate from CHD of any ethnic group in the United States, with an increased proportion of sudden death.[20] The reasons for these findings are unclear. Postmortem analysis shows that differences in rates of sudden death may be due to an increased prevalence of hypertension, left ventricular hypertrophy, diabetes, and tobacco use.[21,22] Other factors that must be considered include limitations in access to preventive care, prehospital delays in patient activation of emergency medical services, and denial or self-treatment of prodromal symptoms. In one study, blacks were less likely to receive bystander cardiopulmonary resuscitation (CPR); however, differences in outcome could not be accounted for by differences in emergency medical team response time or administration of advanced cardiac life support.[19] These issues warrant further investigation.

**GENDER**

SCD has a much higher incidence in men than in women, reflecting gender differences in the incidence of CHD.[1,2] Between 70 and 89 percent of SCDs occur in men, and the annual incidence of SCD in men is overall three to four times higher than that in women. As is the case with coronary disease, however, this disparity decreases with advancing age, with a male:female ratio for SCD of 7:1 in 45- to 64-year-olds and a 2:1 ratio in 65- to 74-year-olds.

A higher percentage of SCD in women than in men (64 versus 50 percent) occurs in patients without prior evidence of coronary heart disease.[1] Among survivors of cardiac arrest, women are more likely than men to have other forms of structural heart disease (valvular heart disease, dilated cardiomyopathy) or a "normal" heart.[23] A greater percentage of sudden deaths occur outside of the hospital in women, and the aforementioned decline in sudden death rates has been noted to be lower in women (6 percent) than in men (12 percent). In fact, the rate of sudden death has increased by 21 percent in women aged 35 to 44 years. The reasons for these findings are myriad and include less aggressive treatment[24,25] or patients' lack of awareness of the importance of cardiovascular signs and symptoms. In fact, less than 10 percent of women consider heart disease their greatest health concern.[26] Strategies to modify the attitudes and behaviors of both physicians and patients are necessary to reverse these worrisome trends.

## Risk Factors for Sudden Cardiac Death

Only a fraction of patients survive a cardiac arrest, and there has been considerable interest in identifying the population at risk for sustained ventricular arrhythmias. More than 80 percent of SCDs occur in patients with underlying coronary disease. The risk factors for SCD largely reflect those for CHD, and most strategies aimed at preventing sudden death target these factors (see Chap. 43). Left ventricular dysfunction and CHD confer the highest risk for SCD.[27] In the Framingham Study, a multivariate model based on various risk factors found that 53 percent of men and 42 percent of women who were at risk for sudden death were in the upper decile of this analysis (Fig. 41-3).[1]

Despite the fact that numerous population-based studies have shown a strong relationship between risk factors for CHD and SCD, none of them has identified a single set of risk factors that are specific for SCD (Table 41-1).[27–32] The inability to determine risk factors specific for SCD reflects the fact that these factors are manifestations of chronic disease processes that create the structural basis for sustained arrhythmia. These structural abnormalities may be necessary but are not sufficient to cause an episode of SCD. To date, primary prevention of sudden death has mainly focused on modifying athero-

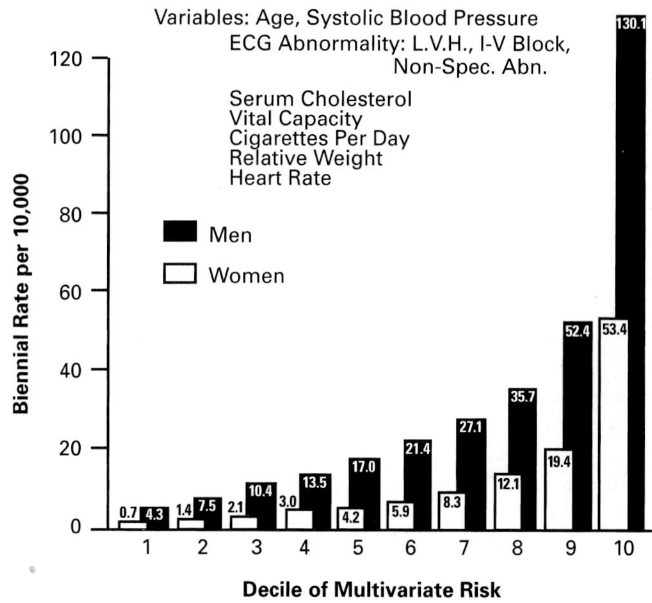


FIGURE 41-3 Risk of sudden cardiac death by decile of multivariate risk: 26-year follow-up, the Framingham Study. ECG = electrocardiographic; I-V = intraventricular; LVH = left ventricular hypertrophy; Non-Spec. Abn. = nonspecific abnormality. (From Kannel and Schatzkin.[29] With permission.)

sclerotic risk factors and heart failure, but individuals with these disorders represent only a small fraction of those who will experience sudden arrhythmic death. In the future, genotypic stratification of patients at risk for sudden death may prove useful in identifying those who are more likely to die. Novel markers to assess risk of sudden death are currently under investigation. Autoantibodies,[33] hemostatic factors,[34] homocysteine,[35] and inflammatory markers such as C-reactive protein[36] show promise. Clarification of the triggers of sudden death will lead to new therapies that may alter myocardial vulnerability to ventricular fibrillation. A challenge for the future will be to use knowledge of these indicators to further elucidate the mechanisms of sudden death as well as the interplay of environmental and genetic predispositions, so that patients at high risk for malignant arrhythmias can be targeted for intervention (see below).

**LIFESTYLE FACTORS**

Observations suggest that changes in lifestyle factors such as alcohol consumption, cigarette smoking, exercise, and stress can be of potential importance in modifying the risk of dying suddenly.[28,29,37–42] Individuals who consume large amounts of alcohol (more than five drinks per day) have increased risks of ventricular arrhythmia and SCD.[43,44] The relationship is less clear for drinkers of light to moderate amounts. A prospective analysis of 21,537 males in the Physicians' Health Study demonstrated a decreased risk of SCD. Men who consumed light to moderate amounts of alcohol (two to six drinks per week) had a significantly reduced risk of SCD compared with those who rarely or never consumed alcohol.[37,38]

Cigarette smoking is one of the few coronary risk factors that has been associated with a disproportionate number of sudden deaths as compared to coronary deaths. Smoking has been shown to induce physiologic changes that predispose to SCD, such as increased platelet adhesiveness and catecholamine release, decreased ventricular fibrillation threshold, acceleration of heart rate, increased blood pressure, coronary spasm, reduced oxygen-carrying capacity by accumulation of carboxyhemoglobin, and impairment of myoglobin utilization.[45]

TABLE 41-1 Risk Factors for Sudden Cardiac Death in Population-Based Studies

| Study | Study Population | Risk Factors for SCD |
|---|---|---|
| Kannel et al.[28,29] (Framingham Study) | 5128 men and women, age 30–62, no CHD at entry: 546 CHD deaths over 26 years, 46% (men) and 35% (women) SCD | Men<br>LVH (by ECG)<br>Cholesterol<br>Systolic blood pressure<br>Relative body weight<br>Cigarette smoking<br>Women<br>Vital capacity<br>Cholesterol<br>Hematocrit<br>Serum glucose |
| Hinkle et al.[27] | 269,755 men, age 20–65: 1839 CHD deaths over 5 years, 60% SCD | Hypertension<br>Cigarette smoking<br>Alcohol<br>History of CHD<br>LVH (by ECG)<br>Enlarged heart (CXR)<br>CHF<br>PVCs |
| Demirovic[30] (Yugoslavia Cardiovascular Disease study) | 6614 men, age 35–62, no CHD at entry: 143 CHD deaths over 15 years, 75% SCD | Age<br>Blood pressure<br>Cigarette smoking |
| Beaglehole et al.,[31] Aukland, New Zealand | 300 cases of SCD, age <70 | Cigarette smoking<br>Low-level HDL |
| Kagan et al.,[32] Hawaii | 7591 middle-aged Japanese men living in Hawaii | Blood pressure<br>Cholesterol<br>Cigarette smoking<br>Positive family history<br>LVH (by ECG) |

ABBREVIATIONS: CHD = coronary heart disease; CHF = congestive heart failure; CXR = chest x-ray; HDL = high-density lipoproteins; LVH = left ventricular hypertrophy; PVC = premature ventricular contraction; SCD = sudden cardiac death.

A postmortem study linked smoking and the presence of acute coronary thrombus. Fresh thrombus was found in over 50 percent of men who died suddenly, and cigarette smoking was a risk factor in 75 percent of these men, compared with 41 percent of the men with stable plaques ($p < 0.001$).[39] In the Framingham Study, the annual incidence of SCD increased from 13 per 1000 in nonsmokers to 31 per 1000 in those smoking more than 20 cigarettes per day.[28,29,45] Those who stop smoking have a prompt reduction in CHD mortality rate irrespective of the duration of previous smoking habits.[46]

There are many reports linking stress, particularly emotional stress, to SCD.[40,41] Patients experiencing intense anger tend to have higher rates of implantable cardioverter/defibrillator (ICD) discharge,[40] with an estimated seven times greater relative risk of appropriate discharge during mental stress.[47] In the hours following the 1994 earthquake in Northridge, California, there was a more than fourfold increase in SCD, illustrating the role of emotional stress as a trigger for SCD. Based on the difference of average and actual daily SCD rates in that period, it was estimated that as many as 40 percent of SCDs are precipitated by emotional stress.[42]

Socioeconomic factors can also contribute to SCD. For instance, a more than threefold increase of SCD following myocardial infarction was reported in men with low levels of education and complex ventricular ectopy compared with better-educated men with the same arrhythmias.[48] In a study of SCD in women, those who died suddenly were less often married, had fewer children, and had greater educational discrepancies with their spouses than did age-matched controls in the same neighborhood[49] (see Chap. 91).

There is increasing evidence that regular physical activity may help prevent CHD and its complications; however, the benefits of vigorous exercise in patients with known CHD is controversial. Several clinical and autopsy-based studies have reported triggering of SCD with exercise.[21,50–52] Data supporting the concept that vigorous physical activity can trigger ventricular fibrillation come from emergency medical records showing that 11 to 17 percent of adults collapsed during or immediately after exertion, but the amount of exertion is rarely quantified.[53] The increased risk of cardiac arrest due to ventricular fibrillation during or after exercise is also evident from cardiac rehabilitation programs and from exercise stress testing of patients with heart disease. Cardiac arrest rates of 1 in 12,000 to 15,000 (rehabilitation) and 1 per 2000 (stress testing) have been reported. Though these studies are of selected patients with known heart disease who are already at risk for sudden death, the rates are at least six times higher than those for patients not known to have heart disease.[53] These reported cases of cardiac arrest have rarely been fatal because of immediate and successful defibrillation. While the absolute risk of sudden death during any particular episode of vigourous exertion is low (1 sudden death per 1.51 million episodes of exertion), data from the Physicians' Health Study showed that the risk of sudden death increases over 16-fold in the first 30 min of vigorous activity. Nevertheless, there is ample experimental evidence that regular exercise may prevent ischemia-induced ventricular fibrillation and death,[51] and habitual vigorous exercise attenuates the relative risk of sudden death associated with vigorous exertion.[52] It appears that regular participation in moderate-intensity activities is associated with reduced rates of cardiovascular morbidity and mortality, while the risks of SCD and myocardial infarction are transiently increased during acute bouts of high-intensity activity.

SCD in competitive athletes is extremely rare. Between 10 and 25 sports-related sudden deaths from cardiac causes occur annually in the United States.[54] The annual incidence of SCD during exercise is 1 per 200,000 in competitive high school athletes.[14] Collapse usually occurs during or shortly after exercise, either in training or during competition. Unfortunately, SCD is often the first manifestation of the underlying cardiac disease that is present in the majority of these patients.[55–58] Age has been shown to be the most useful variable in predicting the type of underlying cardiac disease (Fig. 41-4). In athletes below 35 years of age, the vast majority of SCDs arise from a variety of congenital cardiovascular diseases, most commonly hypertrophic cardiomyopathy (48 percent) and congenital coronary artery anomalies (14 percent).[57] Myocarditis, arrhythmias associated with mitral valve prolapse, the Wolff-Parkinson-White syndrome, and aortic dissection are infrequent, but other disorders such as arrhythmogenic right ventricular dysplasia (ARVD) may be more frequent in endemic areas.[59] Coronary artery disease is present in 10 percent, compared with 80 percent in those older than 35 years.[56]

Screening programs for identifying relatively rare cardiac abnormalities in a large population of asymptomatic athletes are often costly and inefficient.[60] Guidelines for such screening have therefore been published; they are based mainly on detailed personal and family history, physical examination, and electrocardiography (ECG), with echocardiography and other noninvasive tests reserved for those with any positive finding during the initial evaluation. Guidelines have also been published outlining which athletes with cardiac arrhythmias can participate in competitive athletics[61] (see Chap. 95).

Blunt, nonpenetrating, and usually innocent-appearing chest blows leading to ventricular arrhythmia and sudden death have also been reported as causes of SCD in young persons. Termed *commotio cordis,* such an event often occurs during organized sports but can also occur in unstructured, informal settings. Most deaths occur with low-energy and low-velocity projectiles striking the chest. The majority of patients die as a result of the event, but bystander cardiopulmonary resuscitation (CPR) followed by prompt defibrillation can be lifesaving.[62]

## FAMILIAL AND GENETIC FACTORS

Studies showing that family history is an independent predictor of primary cardiac arrest suggest a role for inherited factors in the predisposition for SCD. There is an approximately twofold increase in the relative risk of sudden death associated with parental sudden death.[63,64] In most cases, an underlying condition associated with familial or genetic predispositions cannot be identified; however, genetic abnormalities have been identified in some diseases associated with sudden death. Genetic variations that facilitate the development of ischemic heart disease and subsequent sudden arrhythmic death include those that mediate atherosclerotic plaque growth and vulnerability, platelet function, and vasospasm.[65] Other genetic associations have been found among the cardiomyopathies associated with SCD, such as ARVD, idiopathic dilated cardiomyopathy, and hypertrophic cardiomyopathy. Mutations associated with the primary electrical disorders—such as catecholaminergic ventricular tachycardia (VT), the long-QT syndrome (LQTS), and Brugada syndrome—have also been identified.[65] It is likely that further knowledge of the arrhythmic risk of various genotypes and the interplay with environmental factors will lead to an improved understanding of the mechanisms of sudden death and to new diagnostic and therapeutic strategies that will improve patient care.

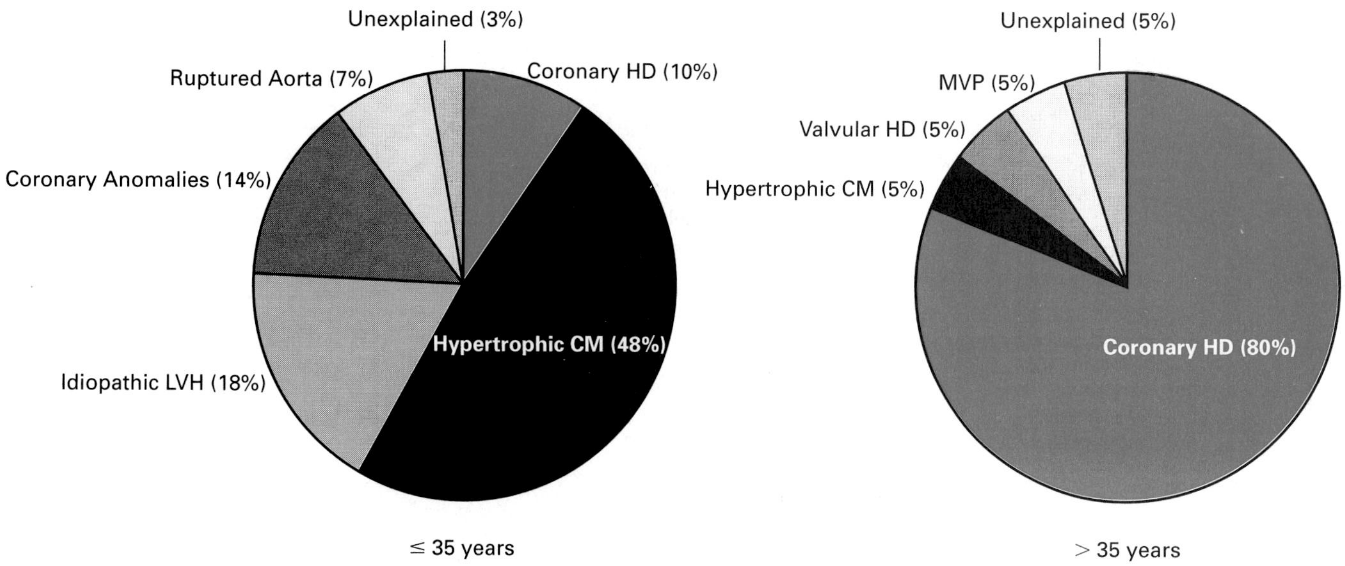


FIGURE 41-4 Causes of sudden cardiac death in competitive athletes by age group. There is evidence for structural heart disease in nearly all athletes who die suddenly of cardiac causes. In athletes younger than 35 years, hypertrophic cardiomyopathy is more prevalent, whereas in those older than 35 years, coronary heart disease is the most frequent cause. CM = cardiomyopathy; HD = heart disease; LVH = left ventricular hypertrophy; MVP = mitral valve prolapse. (From Maron et al.[57] With permission.)

# MECHANISM OF SUDDEN CARDIAC DEATH

## Relationship between Structure and Function in Sudden Cardiac Death

A vast majority of patients who have experienced SCD have cardiac structural abnormalities. In the adult population, these consist predominantly of CHD, cardiomyopathies, valvular heart disease, and abnormalities of the conduction system. These structural changes provide the substrate for ventricular tachyarrhythmias, which represent the cause of SCD in most cases. It is important to recognize the role of triggering factors—such as ischemia, hemodynamic changes, fluctuations in the autonomic nervous system, electrolyte abnormalities, and proarrhythmic effects of drugs—in the initiation of ventricular arrhythmias resulting in SCD (Fig. 41-5).[66,67] Strategies aimed at eliminating or reducing the triggers of arrhythmias may prove to be efficient short- and medium-term solutions, since most structural abnormalities cannot be cured or require long-term risk-factor modification to prevent their development.

## Tachyarrhythmias versus Bradyarrhythmias in Sudden Cardiac Death

Ventricular fibrillation is the first recorded rhythm in approximately 75 percent of patients who have cardiac arrest.[68] Sustained VT is only rarely (in less than 2 percent of patients) documented as the initial rhythm, but it is unknown how often it precedes and precipitates ventricular fibrillation. In a series of 157 ambulatory patients who were wearing an ECG monitor at the time of their cardiac arrest, primary ventricular fibrillation was documented in 8 percent, VT degenerating into ventricular fibrillation in 62 percent, and torsades de pointes in 13 percent.[69]

Electromechanical dissociation and asystole are found in about 30 percent of patients experiencing cardiac arrest; this finding is usually related to the time interval from collapse to first monitoring of the rhythm, suggesting that it is a later manifestation of cardiac arrest.[68] The incidence of bradycardia as the first documented rhythm varies according to the population studied. In patients who have died suddenly while wearing an ambulatory ECG monitor, bradyarrhythmias as the initial rhythm were documented infrequently, and ventricular tachyarrhythmias are most often the mode of cardiac arrest, even in patients with preexisting atrioventricular or intraventricular conduction defects.[69] In a small group of patients with severe congestive heart failure awaiting cardiac transplantation, bradycardia or electromechanical dissociation at the time of death was more frequent than ventricular arrhythmia.[70] We believe that in this population, bradycardia reflects the unrelenting failure of the severely impaired heart and is not a primary cause of sudden death unless the bradyarrhythmia allows for the development of a tachyarrhythmia. Therefore treatment of bradycardia may prevent the onset of tachyarrhythmias and is an important consideration in the prevention of SCD. An understanding of the mechanisms responsible for ventricular arrhythmia is essential in its prevention and treatment, but a complete discussion is beyond the scope of this chapter (see Chaps. 27 and 28).

## Electrophysiologic Effects of Ischemia

The electrophysiologic effects of acute ischemia lead to intercellular acidosis; loss of membrane integrity with efflux of potassium, influx

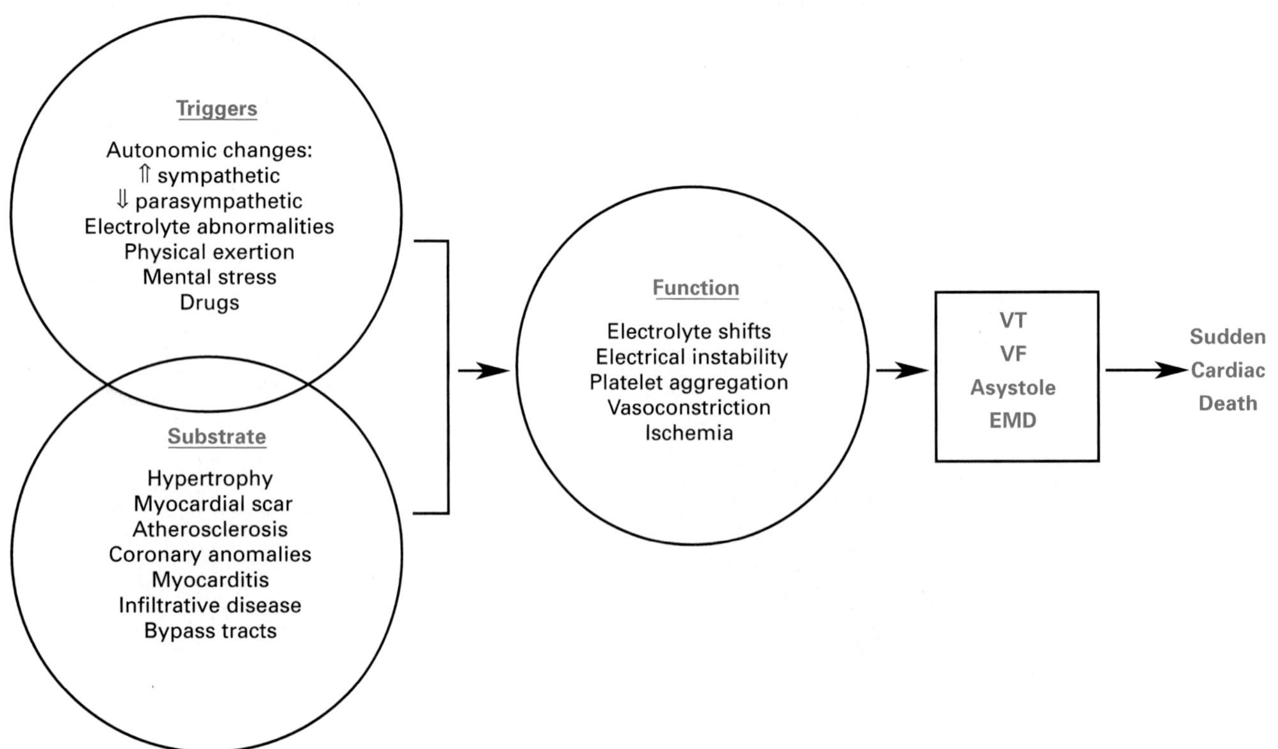


FIGURE 41-5 Interaction between structural cardiac abnormalities, functional changes, and triggering factors in the pathophysiology of sudden cardiac death. The role of triggering factors, such as changes in autonomic tone or reflexes, is increasingly being recognized. EMD = electromechanical dissociation; VF = ventricular fibrillation; VT = ventricular tachycardia.

of calcium; decrease in amplitude and upstroke velocity of the cardiac action potential; inhomogeneous depolarization of the resting membrane potential; and shortening of action potential duration.[71] Fast sodium and slow calcium channels in partially depolarized fibers may remain inactive, thereby prolonging refractoriness even after completion of repolarization. This postrepolarization refractoriness may further contribute to inhomogeneities in the electrophysiologic properties within and around the ischemic zone, causing significant conduction delays, unidirectional block, and reentrant arrhythmias.[72]

Ventricular arrhythmias during experimental coronary occlusion occur in two peaks, one between 2 and 10 min and a second at 15 to 20 min. Rapid polymorphic VT and fibrillation are the characteristic arrhythmias during the early stages of ischemia.[73] Activation mapping during ventricular fibrillation has demonstrated that the initial arrhythmias are due to reentry, which is facilitated by the inhomogeneous conduction velocities and refractory periods in and around the ischemic zone. The second peak of ventricular arrhythmias coincides with a peak in catecholamine release. Automatic and triggered rhythms have also been implicated in these arrhythmias.

Within the first 3 days of myocardial infarction, SCD may occur due to ventricular fibrillation initiated by early, frequent premature ventricular complexes (PVCs). Such PVCs have been shown, in experimental models, to be predominantly due to abnormal impulse initiation consistent with abnormal automaticity. Other manifestations of abnormal automaticity are the accelerated idioventricular rhythms and idiopathic VTs signifying reperfusion after thrombolysis, percutaneous revascularization, or spontaneous reperfusion. These arrhythmias appear to arise, for the most part, from surviving Purkinje fibers in the subendocardial border zone of a transmural infarction. They have no prognostic significance for development of late arrhythmias and usually subside after 2 to 3 days at about the same time that the resting membrane potential and action potential duration of Purkinje fibers normalize.[71]

In the late phases following myocardial infarction, when the infarction is healed, reentrant excitation appears to be the principal mechanism of ventricular arrhythmias. Critical areas of the reentrant circuit are formed by surviving myocardial cells in the epicardial and endocardial border zone of a healed infarction as well as surviving intramural fibers within the infarct zone.[73] It appears that the rate, time, and degree of myocardial reperfusion influence the incidence, rate, and duration of these arrhythmias. More work is needed to further define these relationships (see Chap. 27).

## Mechanoelectrical Feedback

Left ventricular dysfunction has been identified as the strongest independent predictor of SCD. Despite the clinical recognition that acute heart failure can precipitate ventricular tachyarrhythmias, the mechanism by which this occurs is incompletely understood. Besides mechanisms related to acute and chronic ischemia, it has been shown that acute changes in the mechanical state of the heart related to altered preload and contractility can have direct electrophysiologic effects that may precipitate arrhythmias; this relationship is usually referred to as *mechanoelectrical feedback*. An increase in right ventricular pressure has been shown to shorten action potential duration in humans.[74] An increase in both left ventricular preload and contractility has been shown to shorten action potential duration and refractoriness in the canine ventricle.[75] There is some evidence that these changes may be mediated through the beta-adrenergic receptor. Downstream effects leading to fluctuation of intracellular calcium levels or to an increase in a cyclic AMP–mediated potassium current, such as the slowly activating delayed rectifier, may serve as the cellular mechanism by which this phenomenon occurs.[75]

# CARDIAC DISEASES ASSOCIATED WITH SUDDEN CARDIAC DEATH

Table 41-2 summarizes cardiac abnormalities associated with sudden death.

## Ischemic Heart Disease

### CORONARY ATHEROSCLEROSIS

CHD is present in 40 to 86 percent of survivors of cardiac arrest, depending on the age and gender of the population.[76] Although the majority of patients who suffer SCD have severe multivessel coronary disease, fewer than half of the patients resuscitated from ventricular fibrillation evolve evidence of myocardial infarction by elevated cardiac enzymes, and less than 20 percent have Q-wave myocardial infarction.[68] Holter monitoring at the time of arrest has infrequently shown evidence of ischemic ECG changes before the event.[66,77] In postmortem examinations and catheterization studies, there was a significant (75 to 85 percent) stenosis in at least two major coronary arteries in as many as 76 percent of patients. Detailed pathologic studies have confirmed the presence of acute coronary arterial lesions (plaque fissure, plaque hemorrhage, and thrombosis) in up to 95 percent of patients dying suddenly, but only a fraction had total occlusion.[39,66,78,79] Thus, the important observation is that SCD can occur in the absence of infarction but is usually in the presence of diffuse coronary disease.

Coronary collateralization may play an important role in the presentation of coronary artery disease as SCD. It has been hypothesized that chronic ischemia may be a stimulus for the development of coronary collaterals, which in turn could have a protective effect during acute coronary occlusion. The mitigating effect of coronary collateralization is supported by a study of exercise testing in 894 healthy men followed for a mean of 12.7 years. In this study, the initial coronary event was acute myocardial infarction or SCD in 73 percent of those with a normal stress test result, as opposed to 20 percent of those with an abnormal stress test result.[80] It should be noted that patients with silent ischemia during exercise testing have the same likelihood of developing an acute myocardial infarction or SCD as do symptomatic patients.[81]

Since coronary artery disease is the major substrate of SCD, risk stratification following myocardial infarction is an important step in the prevention of SCD (see below). The incidence of SCD in the first 2 years after myocardial infarction ranges from 11 to 18 percent in various studies.[82,83] The variables identified to predict SCD following myocardial infarction in these studies are better in selecting a low-risk population for SCD than in predicting who will go on to die suddenly. It is hoped that further development of other noninvasive methods of assessing such triggers of SCD (e.g., heart rate variability, baroreflex sensitivity, nonlinear dynamics, T-wave alternans, and imaging of the cardiac autonomic innervation) will lead to more accurate models that can predict who will die suddenly better than the currently employed clinical variables or invasive electrophysiology study (see Chaps. 51 and 52).

### NONATHEROSCLEROTIC DISEASE OF THE CORONARY ARTERIES

Several nonatherosclerotic diseases of the coronary arteries are associated with an increased risk of SCD precipitated by cardiac ischemia.

TABLE 41-2 Cardiac Abnormalities Associated with Sudden Cardiac Death

| Ischemic Heart Disease | |
|---|---|
| Coronary atherosclerosis | Coronary artery spasm |
| Acute myocardial infarction | Coronary artery dissection |
| Chronic ischemic cardiomyopathy | Coronary arteritis |
| Anomalous origin of coronary arteries | Small vessel disease |
| Hypoplastic coronary artery | |
| **Nonischemic Heart Disease** | |
| Cardiomyopathies | Drug-induced and other toxic agents |
| Idiopathic dilated cardiomyopathy | Antiarrhythmic drugs (class Ia, Ic, and III) |
| Hypertrophic cardiomyopathy | Erythromycin |
| Hypertensive cardiomyopathy | Clarithromycin |
| Right ventricular cardiomyopathy | Astemizole |
| Infiltrative and inflammatory heart disease | Terfenadine |
| Sarcoidosis | Pentamidine |
| Amyloidosis | Ketoconazole |
| Hemochromatosis | Trimethoprim-sulfamethoxazole |
| Myocarditis | Psychotropic drugs (tricyclic antidepressants, haloperidol, phenothiazines, chloral hydrate) |
| Valvular heart disease | |
| Aortic stenosis | |
| Aortic regurgitation | Probucol |
| Mitral valve prolapse | Cisapride |
| Infective endocarditis | Cocaine |
| Congenital heart disease | Chloroquine |
| Tetralogy of Fallot | Alcohol |
| Transposition of the great vessels (post–Mustard-Senning) | Phosphodiesterase inhibitors |
| | Organophosphates |
| Ebstein's anomaly | Electrolyte abnormalities |
| Pulmonary vascular obstructive disease | Hypokalemia |
| Congenital aortic stenosis | Hypomagnesemia |
| Primary electrical abnormalities | Hypocalcemia |
| Long-QT syndrome | Anorexia nervosa and bulimia |
| Wolff-Parkinson-White syndrome | Liquid protein dieting |
| Congenital heart block | Diuretics |
| Idiopathic ventricular tachycardia | |
| Idiopathic ventricular fibrillation | |
| Syndrome of right bundle branch block, ST elevation, and sudden death (Brugada syndrome) | |
| Nocturnal death in Southeast Asian men | |

Congenital coronary artery anomalies, found in approximately 1 percent of all patients undergoing angiography and in 0.3 percent of patients undergoing autopsy, have been complicated by SCD, often exercise-related, in up to about 30 percent of patients.[84] Origin of the left main coronary artery from the right aortic sinus or origin of the right coronary artery from the left coronary sinus was most frequently the cause. It has been postulated that acute ischemia is due to compression of the anomalous coronary artery between the pulmonary artery and aorta during exercise-induced expansion of these vessels and to diminished coronary flow reserve due to the slitlike orifice and acute takeoff angle of the anomalous vessel.[84]

Life-threatening ventricular arrhythmias and SCD have been described in patients with coronary artery spasm (Prinzmetal's angina or variant angina). Significant arrhythmias during attacks of variant angina have been documented in these patients and appear to be associated with a higher risk of SCD.[85] Calcium-channel blockers are effective in many patients in preventing coronary spasm and appear also to protect from malignant ventricular arrhythmias if the attacks can be completely abolished.[86] The major predictors of major coronary events in this population include systemic hypertension, minor luminal irregularities on the initial coronary arteriogram, and QT dispersion.[85,87]

SCD has been described as a rare complication of coronary artery dissection in Marfan's syndrome, after labor and delivery, secondary to trauma or coronary catheterization, as a consequence of syphilitic aortitis, or as an extension of aortic dissection. Myocardial bridges have been reported in association with SCD during exercise, but they are also an incidental finding at autopsy in up to 25 percent of patients dying of other causes.[88] Coronary arteritis and subsequent infarction have been reported in Kawasaki's disease, giant-cell arteritis, Behçet's disease, systemic lupus erythematosus, and Churg-Strauss syndrome[89–94] (see Chap. 17).

## Cardiomyopathies

### IDIOPATHIC DILATED CARDIOMYOPATHY

Idiopathic dilated cardiomyopathy is the substrate for approximately 10 percent of SCDs in the adult population. The mortality rate for idiopathic dilated cardiomyopathy is high, reaching 10 to 50 percent annually, and seems most closely tied to the severity of pump dysfunction.[95] Mortality rates are higher among patients with advanced heart failure, but the proportion of SCDs is not increased.[96] In an overview of 14 studies including 1432 patients with idiopathic dilated cardiomyopathy, the mean mortality rate after a follow-up of 4 years was 42 percent, with 28 percent of deaths classified as sudden.[95] SCD in idiopathic dilated cardiomyopathy is usually attributed to both polymorphic and monomorphic ventricular tachyarrhythmias occurring in the setting of a high frequency of complex ventricular ectopy.[97] The terminal event may, however, also be due to simple pump failure with asystole or electromechanical dissociation, especially in patients with advanced left ventricular dysfunction.[70]

Risk stratification of patients with idiopathic dilated cardiomyopathy is difficult because there are few clinical predictors specific for SCD. The only clinical variable that identifies patients with a higher risk of SCD is unexplained syncope, and these patients should undergo further evaluation. One study looked at patients with implantable defibrillators, nonischemic dilated cardiomyopathy, and unexplained syncope with negative electrophysiologic testing results and found that appropriate shocks for ventricular arrhythmias were frequent.[98] The prognostic value of simple and complex PVCs as well as nonsustained VT (NSVT) is limited by the extremely high prevalence of these arrhythmias in patients with idiopathic dilated cardiomyopathy.[97] The prognostic value of intraventricular conduction delay on ECG, associated with decreased survival rates, is not specific for SCD, and other noninvasive tests lack significant sensitivity in patients with idiopathic dilated cardiomyopathy to be clinically useful.[99] The induction of polymorphic VT or fibrillation during electrophysiologic testing is nonspecific, and the absence of inducible ventricular tachyarrhythmias in this population does not accurately predict a low risk for SCD.[100] In up to 40 percent of patients with nonischemic dilated cardiomyopathy, inducible monomorphic VT can be due to a macroreentry circuit, such as bundle branch reentry, that is readily amenable to catheter ablation[101] (see Chaps. 76 and 79).

### HYPERTROPHIC CARDIOMYOPATHY

The incidence of SCD in patients with hypertrophic cardiomyopathy (HCM) is 2 to 4 percent per year in adults and 4 to 6 percent per year in children and adolescents.[102] Patients with HCM who die suddenly or are able to survive a cardiac arrest episode tend to be younger than 30 years of age and to have no previous functional limitation. Assessment of autonomic function in patients with HCM reveals abnormal responses of heart rate and hypotensive response to exercise in two-thirds, which is associated with a more malignant clinical course,[103] but most commonly these patients are performing sedentary or minimal physical activity at the time of cardiac arrest.[104] The presence of repeated bursts of NSVT on ambulatory monitoring also has been reported to be of value in identifying patients at increased risk.[104,105]

It should be emphasized that atrial arrhythmias can lead to ischemia and hemodynamic compromise and thus to sudden death in these patients. While hemodynamic events that diminish stroke volume, environmental variables, and/or ischemia have been implicated, no specific hemodynamic and echocardiographic variables such as the presence or absence of outflow tract obstruction have been shown to be useful in identifying patients at high risk for SCD.[106] A relationship between the maximum left ventricular wall thickness and sudden death has been noted in various series,[105,107,108] but other data do not support left ventricular wall thickness as a single predictor of sudden death.[109,110] While it is likely that patients with profoundly increased wall thickness (3.0 cm or more) have an increased risk of dying suddenly, the vast majority of patients with hypertrophic cardiomyopathy who die suddenly do not have such hypertrophy.

A clinical history of spontaneous, sustained monomorphic VT or sudden death in family members indicates a worse prognosis, as does onset of symptoms in childhood.[104,105] Syncope or near-syncope, especially when exertional or recurrent and unrelated to neurocardiogenic mechanisms, implies a worse prognosis.[104,105] The prognostic value of electrophysiologic study in the absence of spontaneous, sustained VT is limited, and the study itself may be dangerous. Sustained ventricular tachyarrhythmias, predominantly rapid polymorphic VT, can be induced in from 27 to 43 percent of patients with hypertrophic cardiomyopathy (HCM) at electrophysiologic study, but the prognostic significance is controversial.[111] Paced electrogram fractionation in HCM may be helpful in determining which patients are at risk for ventricular fibrillation.[112]

Patients without NSVT on ambulatory monitoring, syncope, hypotensive response to exercise, family history of sudden death, or markedly increased left ventricular wall thickness comprise a substantial subset (55 percent) of patients with HCM who have a less than 5 percent risk of SCD.[105] High-risk patients who have received ICDs—such as those with multiple clinical risk factors, prior cardiac arrest, or spontaneous VT—have a rate of appropriate device interventions as high as 11 percent annually.[113] The decision of whether to implant an ICD in the patient with only one risk factor is uncertain and should be based on clinician and patient tolerance for risk.

Numerous mutations in genes coding for various components of the cardiac sarcomere have been associated with HCM. Genotype-phenotype correlation studies have shown that mutations carry prognostic significance. Some mutations of the beta-myosin heavy chain are associated with a benign prognosis, while others are associated with a high incidence of SCD. Mutations in cardiac troponin T are associated with a mild degree of hypertrophy but a high incidence of SCD.[114,115] As with most genetic disorders, the phenotypic expression of the same genetic abnormality is highly variable, and clinical decisions cannot be reliably made based simply on genotype (see Chaps. 72 and 77).

### HYPERTENSIVE CARDIOMYOPATHY

Left ventricular hypertrophy has been identified as one of the strongest blood pressure–independent risk factors for sudden death, acute myocardial infarction, congestive heart failure, and other cardiovascular disease and death.[116–118] Hypertensive patients with left ventricular hypertrophy have a significantly greater prevalence of PVCs and complex ventricular arrhythmias than do patients without left ventricular hypertrophy or normotensive patients. In the Framingham Study, ECG evidence of left ventricular hypertrophy doubled the risk of SCD. Echocardiographic studies showed an incremental risk for cardiovascular deaths of 1.73 in men and 2.12 in women for each 50-g increment in the index of left ventricular mass.[119] A possible mechanism for the increased mortality rates in patients with left ventricular hypertrophy is ventricular tachyarrhythmia.[116] Decreased coronary blood flow, flow reserve, and endothelial dysfunction may all be factors favoring the development of transient ischemia,[118] and long-term, repeated transient ischemic episodes can lead to interstitial fibrosis, which may underlie the arrhythmias in this population.[120] Other potential contributing factors to the increased risk of SCD in hypertensive cardiomyopathy are the electrolyte disturbances associated with diuretic therapy of hypertension.[121,122] It remains to be shown that the reduction of hypertrophy or concomitant ventricular ectopy confers a clinical benefit that exceeds the one from the reduction of arterial pressure alone.[118,123]

### ARRHYTHMOGENIC RIGHT VENTRICULAR DYSPLASIA

Arrhythmogenic right ventricular dysplasia (ARVD) is predominantly right ventricular cardiomyopathy characterized by fatty or fibrofatty replacement of myocardium. It is a rare cause of SCD except in a few endemic regions and is a familial disorder in approximately 30 percent of cases. A locus on chromosome 1 has been physically mapped to the cardiac ryanodine receptor (*Ry*R2), the major calcium release channel on the sarcoplasmic reticulum in cardiomyocytes.[124] Mutation in this same receptor has been linked to catecholaminergic polymorphic VT (see Chap. 79).

Recurrent VT with multiple left bundle branch block morphologies typifies this disorder. In the fibrofatty variety, patchy myocarditis, programmed cell death, and/or congenital abnormalities of development appear to lead to myocardial atrophy and repair by fibrofatty replacement, which may become the basis for ventricular reentry. The left ventricle and ventricular septum can be involved in 50 to 67 percent of cases, especially later in the course of the disease, and such involvement confers a poor prognosis.[125,126]

The ECG manifestations in sinus rhythm include T-wave inversion in $V_1$ to $V_3$ or complete or incomplete right bundle branch block. Intraventricular conduction delay may produce a terminal notch on the QRS complex called an epsilon wave in approximately 50 percent of patients. The ventricular ectopy is usually of a left bundle branch pattern with a QRS axis between −90 and +110 degrees and generally arises from one of three sites of fatty degeneration. Called the triangle of dysplasia, these sites comprise the right ventricular outflow and inflow tract and apex. Any patient with frequent premature beats of a left bundle branch morphology and left axis deviation should be evaluated for this disorder, which must be differentiated from the usually benign right ventricular outflow-tract tachycardia. Diagnostic critieria for this disorder have been proposed.[127]

In patients with ARVD, particularly at early stages of the disease, VT is often precipitated by exercise, and its induction is usually found to be catecholamine-sensitive at electrophysiologic study.[15,128] The course and prognosis of ARVD are highly variable and difficult to predict even in patients with overt disease and significant ventricular arrhythmias. Patients with tolerated, non-life-threatening arrhythmias are usually treated with ICDs, but in our opinion, some cases can be treated medically or with ablative therapy. ICDs are often the primary therapy in those with sustained VT with hemodynamic compromise or ventricular fibrillation. While ICDs remain the most effective therapy in preventing sudden death, more data are required to define which asymptomatic patients with ARVD benefit from this therapy[127](see Chap. 79).

## Valvular Heart Disease

The risk of SCD in asymptomatic patients with aortic stenosis or regurgitation appears to be low.[129,130] In contrast, in the presurgical era, SCD was one of the three most common types of death in symptomatic patients with aortic stenosis, the other two being bacterial endocarditis and congestive heart failure.[131] There appears to be an increased risk of SCD following aortic valve replacement for aortic stenosis or regurgitation.[132,133] In 831 patients receiving a Bjork-Shiley prosthesis in the aortic (341 patients), mitral (345 patients), or double-valve (145 patients) position, the incidence of SCD in the subgroups was 1.8, 3.5, and 4 percent, respectively, over a follow-up period of 7 years.[133] Malignant tachyarrhythmias have been suggested as the cause of SCD in such patients, since PVCs are more frequent in patients who die suddenly than in those who die of other causes. Transient complete heart block is relatively common following both aortic (17.6 percent) and mitral (13 percent) valve replacement, pointing to bradyarrhythmias as the potential precipitating factor for SCD[134] (see Chap. 66).

## Mitral Valve Prolapse

Whether or not mitral valve prolapse (MVP) is a cause of SCD is controversial. The prevalence of MVP is so high that its presence may just be a coincidental finding in victims of SCD.[135,136] A prospective 8-year study of 237 asymptomatic or minimally symptomatic patients with echocardiographically documented MVP was not significantly different from that for a matched control population.[136] On the other hand, MVP may not always be benign. MVP associated with mitral regurgitation and left ventricular dysfunction clearly poses a higher risk for such complications as infective endocarditis, cerebroembolic events, and SCD.[137,138] MVP is the only structural cardiac disease found in a significant number of victims of SCD, especially in the young female population.[139,140] Several echocardiographic risk factors for SCD have been identified in asymptomatic or mildly symptomatic MVP patients without significant mitral regurgitation, including mitral valve annular circumference, thickness of the anterior and posterior mitral valve leaflets, presence and extent of endocardial plaque, and presence or absence of redundant mitral valve leaflets on M-mode echocardiography[136,141] The most important prognostic indicators for sudden death in MVP are probably a history of syncope and a family history of sudden death at a young age, as well as significant mitral regurgitation, abnormal left ventricular function, and a long QT interval[141] (see Chap. 68).

## Inflammatory and Infiltrative Myocardial Disease

Any inflammatory disease can cause SCD due to either ventricular tachyarrhythmias or complete heart block. Histologic findings suggestive of myocarditis have been reported in 10 to 44 percent of young victims of SCD.[54] In adults, the diagnosis of myocarditis is made much less frequently, perhaps because of concurrent structural heart disease or because the late manifestations of the disease are indistinguishable from idiopathic dilated cardiomyopathy (see Chap. 79). In South America, however, myocarditis due to specific pathogens, such as Chagas' disease, is the most frequent cause of cardiomyopathy and related SCD.[142] Patients with infective endocarditis may also be at risk for SCD due to acute coronary emboli from valvular vegetations. More often, SCD is caused by acute hemodynamic deterioration due to valvular failure. Intramyocardial abscesses can also precipitate VT and lead to SCD.

Infiltrative cardiomyopathies, such as primary or secondary amyloidosis, hemochromatosis, or sarcoidosis, have been associated with not only predominantly cardiac conduction defects but also ventricular tachyarrhythmias and SCD. VT is sometimes the mode of presentation of sarcoidosis, can usually be reproduced by programmed electrical stimulation, and is associated with a high rate of recurrent arrhythmia and SCD[143] (see Chap. 79).

## Congenital Heart Disease

A 25- to 100-fold increased risk of SCD due to an arrhythmia, increasing primarily in the second postoperative decade, has been found predominantly in four congenital conditions: tetralogy of Fallot, transposition of the great vessels, aortic stenosis, and pulmonary vascular obstruction.[144] In 793 adult patients who had undergone reparative surgery for tetralogy of Fallot, a QRS duration of 180 ms or more was found to be the most sensitive predictor of SCD and ventricular tachyarrhythmias and was correlated with other parameters of right ventricular volume overload. Older age at repair and increasing QRS duration also increased the risk of arrhythmia.[145] In those patients with previous repair and chronic pulmonary regurgitation, valve replacement seems to lead to stabilization of QRS duration and, in conjunction with intraoperative cryoablation, to a decrease in the incidence of preexisting atrial and ventricular tachyarrhythmia.[146] Transposition of the great vessels (post–Mustard-Senning) is associated with at least a 6 percent risk of late SCD, which is due in some cases to sinus node dysfunction and in others to ventricular tachyarrhythmias[147] (see Chaps. 73 and 74). SCD is often (45 to 60 percent) the mode of death in patients with primary or secondary pulmonary hypertension (see Chap. 62). Death is often precipitated by general anesthesia, dehydration, exertion, or pregnancy. Any process that decreases systemic vascular resistance increases right-to-left shunting and decreases pulmonary flow. The resultant peripheral desaturation may trigger lethal arrhythmias and SCD.[148] The SCD risk in congenital aortic stenosis is estimated to be 1 percent and occurs predominantly in symptomatic patients with severe left ventricular hypertrophy. Ebstein's anomaly is frequently (up to

25 percent) associated with the presence of accessory pathways and the Wolff-Parkinson-White syndrome, which carries a small risk of SCD (see below). Congenital heart block without associated structural heart disease occurs in 1 of 20,000 infants, and a moderate decrease in heart rate is usually well tolerated. A maternal risk factor is systemic lupus erythematosus. As previously noted, patients with severe bradycardia, however, have a tendency to develop ventricular arrhythmias. Pacemaker therapy has virtually eliminated the risk of SCD in this population.[148]

## Primary Electrical Abnormalities

### LONG-QT SYNDROME

SCD is one of the hallmarks of the idiopathic long-QT syndrome (LQTS), a group of genetically distinct disorders each resulting from a mutation in genes encoding cardiac ion channels or auxiliary ion-channel subunits.[149–152] The prolonged QT interval reflects abnormal prolongation of repolarization, and defects in outward currents (potassium) or impaired inactivation of inward currents (sodium) can cause abnormal prolongation of the action potential repolarization, enhancing the propensity to develop early afterdepolarizations (EADs), leading to triggered activity that is the initating mechanism for torsades de pointes[151] (see Chap. 27). Further data suggest that reentry due to transventricular heterogeneity may be responsible for sustaining the arrhythmia.[153] Over 90 percent of the congenital forms of LQTS have been linked to specific chromosomal defects, resulting in a genetically based classification: LQTS1–7.[151]

Several mutations have been identified in each gene, and this locus heterogeneity appears to be important prognostically. Carriers of the LQTS gene have been reported to have a 5 percent incidence of aborted SCD and a 63 percent incidence of recurrent syncope.[150] In a series of 196 patients enrolled in an international registry, the mean age at presentation was 24 years, and the annual incidences of SCD and recurrent syncope were 1.3 percent and 8.6 percent, respectively.[149] Multivariate analysis in the registry population identified female gender, congenital deafness, history of syncope, and a documented episode of torsades de pointes or ventricular fibrillation as independent risk factors for postenrollment syncope or SCD.[149] Echocardiographic studies have also been reported to reveal specific wall motion abnormalities associated with an increased risk (relative risk, 2.75) of syncope and SCD.[154]

Associations with certain triggers have been made with certain mutations. Cardiac events associated with exercise, especially with swimming, dominate the clinical picture of LQTS1, and auditory stimuli tend to be a trigger for arrhythmic events in LQTS2.[155] QT-interval prolongation and ventricular arrhythmias, particularly in LQTS2, are exacerbated by hypokalemia and can improve with normalization of the plasma potassium level. Although ventricular arrhythmias are common in this disorder, deterioration into a hemodynamically compromising rhythm or ventricular fibrillation is rare. The various genetic mutations seem to respond to therapy differently. Beta blockers are beneficial in LQTS1 and LQTS2. Pacing may be helpful in LQTS3 to avoid tachyarrhythmias induced by bradycardia, while pacing is of little benefit in LQTS2. Genetic typing in the future may facilitate risk stratification, providing valuable information not only about the underlying abnormality but also about the expected severity of the disease and preferred therapy[151] (see Chap. 72).

### IDIOPATHIC POLYMORPHIC VENTRICULAR TACHYCARDIAS AND VENTRICULAR FIBRILLATION

Several types of idiopathic polymorphic VTs have been described and are associated with an unfavorable prognosis. These arrhythmias include idiopathic ventricular fibrillation, torsades de pointes with a short coupling interval, and catecholaminergic polymorphic VT. The last disorder has been associated with mutation in the *RyR2* gene coding for the human cardiac ryanodin 2–receptor protein, and mutation in this gene is associated with events at a younger age.[156] This protein is a sarcoplasmic reticulum calcium release channel.[156] The *CASQ2* gene has also been implicated in the autosomal recessive form of catecholaminergic polymorphic VT. This gene encodes the calsequestrin protein, which serves as the major reservoir of calcium in the sarcoplasmic reticulum and is part of the complex that contains the ryanodine receptor.[157] Some patients with catecholaminergic polymorphous VT have a favorable response to beta-blocker therapy, but in many cases an ICD is necessary[156] (see Chap. 72).

Although the list of potential causes of SCD continues to grow, a definite cause of SCD cannot be established in approximately 1 percent of patients dying suddenly or after successful resuscitation from cardiac arrest.[158] These instances of SCD without evident cause are presumed to be due to idiopathic ventricular fibrillation. The incidence of idiopathic ventricular fibrillation is higher in selected populations, such as younger patients (up to 14 percent in patients below 40 years of age) who had experienced SCD [159] or female survivors of SCD unrelated to myocardial infarction (10 percent[23]). The risk of recurrent ventricular fibrillation in this young and otherwise healthy patient population ranges between 22 and 37 percent at 2 to 4 years.[158,160,161] In survivors of cardiac arrest due to idiopathic ventricular fibrillation, the diagnosis is made by exclusion if extensive cardiac workup (including physical examination, laboratory tests for acute myocardial infarction and electrolyte abnormalities, ECG, exercise test, echocardiographic study, cardiac catheterization, and electrophysiologic study to exclude significant conduction system abnormalities or accessory pathways) reveals no abnormality that is thought to account for the ventricular fibrillation episode. Noninvasive evaluation may help confirm the diagnosis of idiopathic ventricular fibrillation in selected patients, but such markers are present in fewer than half the patients with this disorder.[158,162] The prognostic role of electrophysiologic evaluation in these patients is controversial: sustained rapid polymorphic VT or ventricular fibrillation is inducible in 38 to 75 percent of patients studied[158,161–163]; however, these arrhythmias are generally considered a nonspecific finding,[164, 165] and noninducibility of ventricular fibrillation in this patient population did not predict a more favorable outcome.[161]

The syndrome of SCD associated with right bundle branch block and persistent ST-segment elevation in $V_1$ to $V_3$ in patients without demonstrable structural heart disease is known as the Brugada syndrome.[166] Diagnostic criteria for the Brugada syndrome have been proposed. The type 1 ECG pattern is characterized by a prominent coved ST-segment elevation displaying J-wave amplitude or ST-segment elevation 2 mm or greater or 0.2 mV at its peak followed by a negative T wave, with little or no isoelectric separation. This pattern without other factor(s) that could account for the ECG abnormality (Table 41-3) as well as clinical findings suggest the diagnosis of the Brugada synrdome.[167] The appearance of only typical ECG changes without clinical findings is considered to represent an idiopathic Brugada ECG pattern but not the Brugada syndrome. Clinical criteria include documented ventricular fibrillation, self-terminating polymorphic VT, a family history of sudden death (<45 years), coved-type ECGs in family members, electrophysiologic inducibility, syncope, or nocturnal agonal respiration. The diagnosis is also suggested in patients with clinical predictors and type 2 or 3 ECG patterns that convert to type 1 after administration of sodium-channel blockade. Even if strict criteria are not fulfilled, patients with intermediate ECG findings and clinical predictors should be considered for further evaluation with drug or electrophysiologic study.

TABLE 41-3 Abnormalities That Can Lead to ST-Segment Elevation in the Right Precordial Leads[a]

| |
|---|
| Right or left bundle branch block, left ventricular hypertrophy |
| Acute myocardial ischemia or infarction |
| Acute myocarditis |
| Right ventricular ischemia or infarction |
| Dissecting aortic aneurysm |
| Acute pulmonary thromboemboli |
| Various central and autonomic nervous system abnormalities |
| Heterocyclic antidepressant overdose |
| Duchenne muscular dystrophy |
| Friedreich's ataxia |
| Thiamine deficiency |
| Hypercalcemia |
| Hyperkalemia |
| Cocaine intoxication |
| Mediastinal tumor compressing the right ventricular outflow tract |
| Arrhythmogenic right ventricular dysplasia/cardiomyopathy |
| Long-QT syndrome type 3 |
| Early repolarization syndrome |
| Other normal variants (particularly in men) |

[a]The final two conditions that can lead to ST-segment elevation are more likely to give rise to type 2 and type 3 ECGs. Most conditions mentioned in this table can give rise to type 1 ECG.

SOURCE: Modified from Wilde et al.,[155] with permission.

A sudden unexpected nocturnal death syndrome described before the findings of Brugada et al.[166] appeared is believed to be identical to the Brugada syndrome and has been described in young, apparently healthy males from Southeast Asia; it is known among Asian-Pacific populations by several names.[168] The Thai describe it as *Lai Tai* (death during sleep). In the Philippines, it is known as *Bangungut* (to rise and moan in sleep followed by death); the Japanese call it *Pokkuri* (unexpected sudden death at night).[169–171] A majority of these patients have been found to have the ECG manifestations and many have the genetic mutations of the *SC5NA* gene on chromosomes that are associated with the Brugada syndrome. Of 163 patients who met the criteria for Brugada syndrome, 58 percent were of Asian origin in one review.[172]

Dozens of mutations of the gene for the sodium-channel SCN5A have been associated with the Brugada syndrome, but various other ion channels and proteins have been implicated because only about 20 percent of Brugada syndrome cases have been linked to SC5NA. The mutations associated with Brugada syndrome are distinct from those identified in right ventricular dysplasia, but some mutations have linked the long-QT syndrome and Brugada syndrome.[173,174] Some patients with the long-QT syndrome have been noted to both shorten the QT interval in response to flecainide and manifest the ECG abnormalities of the Brugada syndrome, further supporting a link.[175]

The mutations in the Brugada syndrome are not associated with structural heart disease and seem to lead to an acceleration of recovery of the sodium channel or nonfunctional sodium channels. There is a transmural and epicardial dispersion of repolarization and refractoriness. Local reexcitation via a phase 2 reentry mechanism can occur, leading to the development of very closely coupled premature ventricular contractions that can trigger VT and fibrillation through circus movement reentry.[176–178]

Symptomatic patients have a high incidence of SCD; those who have syncope, VT, and a prior history of cardiac arrest should be treated with ICD implantation. Studies have shown a lower risk of sudden death in asymptomatic patients who are not inducible at electrophysiologic study, and most agree that ICD placement is not beneficial in this setting.[179] The benefit of ICD is also not well established in asymptomatic patients who are inducible at the time of electrophysiologic study. In one series of 200 patients, inducibility at electrophysiologic study did not predict arrhythmic events. The same study also showed that the incidence of sudden death in aysmptomatic patients with a diagnositc ECG only after provocative testing was low[180] (see Chap. 72).

### WOLFF-PARKINSON-WHITE SYNDROME

The risk of SCD in patients with Wolff-Parkinson-White syndrome is less than 1 per 1000 patient-years of follow-up.[181] Although a rare event, it is an important one to consider, since it usually occurs in otherwise healthy individuals and, in the era of catheter ablation of accessory pathways, is a curable cause of SCD.[182] The mechanism of SCD in most patients with this syndrome is presumably the development of atrial fibrillation with rapid ventricular rates due to conduction over an accessory pathway and subsequent degeneration into ventricular fibrillation. There are no good predictors during sinus rhythm for the development of sudden death in these patients. The best predictor for development of ventricular fibrillation during atrial fibrillation is the spontaneous occurrence of a rapid ventricular response over the accessory pathway, with the shortest interval between preexcited ventricular beats (i.e., those conducted over the accessory pathway) being less than 220 ms, but the specificity of this finding is low.[182–186] Spontaneous or exercise-induced intermittent loss of preexcitation is helpful in identifying patients who will have a slower ventricular response in atrial fibrillation and may be at lower risk for sudden death. In symptomatic patients, an electrophysiologic study offers the opportunity to assess conduction properties of the accessory pathways, the propensity to develop tachyarrhythmias, and the possibility of cure at minimal risk with catheter ablation.

## Drugs and Other Toxic Agents

### PROARRHYTHMIA

The apparent paradox that antiarrhythmic agents can cause arrhythmias has been recognized since the introduction of quinidine in 1918.[187] The Cardiac Arrhythmia Suppression Trial (CAST) showed an increased mortality rate in postinfarction patients treated with encainide or flecainide compared with placebo, despite effective antiarrhythmic efficacy as documented by the suppression of PVCs.[188] In these cases, the initiation of the arrhythmia is often triggered by bradycardia or a characteristic "long-short" coupling interval that initiates a pause-dependent prolongation of the QT interval. The VT in this setting is usually of a typical torsades de pointes morphology. This form of proarrhythmia may be facilitated by electrolyte abnormalities such as hypokalemia or hypomagnesemia. It is usually an early event during drug therapy (within 3 days), and concomitant therapy with digitalis and diuretic agents may predispose patients to this complication.[189] Since it is not possible to predict who will develop proarrhythmic effects, we recommend initiation of antiarrhythmic therapy for ventricular arrhythmias in a telemetry unit. Outpatient initiation of antiarrhythmic therapy can be safely performed in patients with atrial fibrillation who have reverted to normal sinus rhythm by using transtelephonic monitoring or other ECG surveillance to follow PR interval, rhythm, QRS duration, and QT interval[190,191] (see Chap. 27).

Besides antiarrhythmic drugs, many other agents with diverse actions have been implicated in the induction of tachyarrhythmias. Other commonly used medications, such as haloperidol and erythromycin, have been implicated in prolonging ventricular refractoriness, leading to prolongation of the QT interval of the ECG and to the development of fatal torsades de pointes. The list of medications reported to cause this complication is constantly growing (Table 41-2), and a registry of drugs associated with it has been developed. An updated list of these drugs can be found online at *www.torsades.org.*

Proarrhythmia, predominantly with class IC antiarrhythmic drugs such as flecainide and propafenone, has been associated with acute ischemic events and occurs more frequently in patients with ischemic cardiomyopathy.[192] It is believed that the antiarrhythmic drug exacerbates ischemia-induced myocardial conduction delays in a heterogeneous fashion and promotes reentrant VTs.[192] Antiarrhythmic agents such as flecainide and propafenone also lead to proarrhythmia by converting atrial fibrillation to atrial flutter and allowing one-to-one conduction of the flutter waves. For this reason, nodal blocking agents are often administered with these medications. Phosphodiesterase inhibitors and other positive inotropic agents may promote arrhythmias via another mechanism. Possibly by increasing the intracellular calcium level, these medications have been shown to be proarrhythmic and to increase the risk of SCD, despite their beneficial effects on hemodynamic parameters.[193]

### COCAINE AND ALCOHOL

The increasingly widespread use of cocaine in the United States has led to the realization that this drug can precipitate life-threatening cardiac events, including SCD. In a series of 41 survivors of cardiac arrest due to ventricular fibrillation in patients 18 to 35 years of age, one-third had ingested alcohol or drugs (cocaine, heroin, or tricyclic agents).[194] The combination of alcohol and cocaine is especially dangerous due to the generation of a unique metabolite, cocaethylene, that has enhanced cardiotoxicity.[195] Cocaine causes coronary vasoconstriction, increases cardiac sympathetic effects, increases action potential duration, and precipitates cardiac arrhythmias irrespective of the amount ingested, prior use, or whether there is an underlying cardiac abnormality.[196] The combination of increased oxygen demand due to sympathetic stimulation and diminished coronary flow due to vasoconstriction may precipitate ischemia-induced arrhythmias and SCD (see Chap. 89).

### ELECTROLYTE ABNORMALITIES

Hypokalemia is often found in patients during and following resuscitation from a cardiac arrest. Although this is often a secondary phenomenon due to catecholamine-induced potassium shift into the cells, primary hypokalemia can also be arrhythmogenic. There is an almost linear inverse relationship between serum potassium concentration and the probability of VT in patients with acute myocardial infarction.[197] Electrolyte abnormalities are thought to play a role in the sudden death of patients treated with non-potassium-sparing diuretics[198] and in those with severe eating disorders, such as anorexia nervosa and bulimia, or those who abuse diuretics or are on liquid protein diets.

A decrease in the extracellular potassium level hypopolarizes the resting membrane potential, shortens the plateau duration, prolongs the phase of rapid repolarization in ventricular fibers, and causes an increase in pacemaker activity in Purkinje cells, triggering ventricular arrhythmias.[199] These changes in repolarization may increase the dispersion of the recovery of excitability and facilitate reentrant ventricular arrhythmias.[199] Many of the electrophysiologic effects of hypokalemia are similar to those caused by digitalis and catecholamine stimulation, explaining the high risk of ventricular arrhythmias when a combination of these factors is present.

Magnesium deficiency and changes in intracellular concentration of calcium may also be arrhythmogenic.[199,200] Increased intracellular calcium is believed to play a significant role in arrhythmias associated with digitalis glycosides, catecholamine-induced VT, reperfusion arrhythmias, and the proarrhythmic effect seen with phosphodiesterase inhibitors and other positive inotropic agents (see Chap. 27).

## CLINICAL PRESENTATION AND MANAGEMENT OF THE PATIENT WITH CARDIAC ARREST

### Out-of-Hospital Cardiac Arrest

About 75 percent of cardiac arrests occur at home, and about two-thirds are witnessed.[7,11,201] Individuals who live alone and women appear more likely to have unwitnessed deaths.[202] The most important determinant of successful resuscitation is the time interval from cardiovascular collapse to initial intervention. Since most patients are found in ventricular fibrillation, the time to successful defibrillation is a key element in the acute management of the cardiac arrest victim (see Chap. 42). The importance of early intervention is reflected in the "chain of survival" concept of emergency cardiac care systems: early access, early CPR, early defibrillation, and early advanced cardiac life support.[203] This concept has led to the development of tiered medical emergency systems in most urban areas. Following activation of the emergency call (911) system, the first response consists of the nearest emergency medical technicians or fire departments who are trained to provide basic CPR and defibrillation. The second response is by paramedics who are trained in advanced cardiac life support, including endotracheal intubation, intravenous medications, and additional defibrillation if necessary.

Initiation of bystander CPR is another important element of early intervention and improves the chances of successful resuscitation. In an overview of 17 controlled studies of survival from out-of-hospital cardiac arrest, bystander CPR was associated with a greater than twofold odds ratio of survival.[203] The earlier CPR is performed, the greater the proportion of patients who are found in ventricular fibrillation as opposed to bradycardia or asystole,[204] and there is an increased rate of successful defibrillation in these patients. Modification of the protocol for use of automated external defibrillators (see below) by emergency medical technicians in Seattle to include 90 s of preshock CPR led to improved survival when response times were greater than 4 min.[205] Community-based CPR training programs, such as those implemented in Seattle and Minneapolis, result in a higher likelihood of bystander CPR being administered in out-of-hospital cardiac arrest. It has been suggested that CPR should be taught as a mandatory course in high school, much like learning how to drive a car. A more efficient approach may be targeted CPR training for persons who have an increased likelihood of having to perform CPR.

In order to improve the time to initial defibrillation, early defibrillation by nonmedical personnel has been advocated. The widespread use of automated external defibrillators has the potential to improve significantly the availability of early defibrillation. These are relatively simple and inexpensive devices that have an automatic detection and treatment algorithm for ventricular tachyarrhythmias. One study evaluating the use of these devices in casinos demonstrated a remarkable 74 percent survival rate for those who received their first defibrillation no later than 3 min after a witnessed collapse and 49 percent for those who received their first defibrillation after more than 3 min.[206] Improvements in other settings have also been noted, but survival rates were markedly lower. When CPR was administered by police officers in the community setting, survival rates to hospital discharge improved from 9 to 17 percent in patients whose initial rhythm was ventricular fibrillation or pulseless VT. However, only 61 percent of patients had an initial shockable rhythm, reducing the absolute survival benefit to only 1.6 percent in the overall cohort.[207] In the Piacenza region of Italy, 173,114 persons were instructed in the use of these devices, and survival to hospital discharge improved from 3.3 to 10.5 percent.[208] These devices seem to reduce time to defibrillation, but the overall survival in these patients remains low and the effects on quality of life and long-term survival remain to be identified.

Although duration of arrest is the most important determinant of successful ventricular defibrillation, other factors should be kept in mind. To improve defibrillation efficacy, especially in individuals with large chests and expected high transthoracic impedance, the operator should use a gel, cream, or saline-soaked gauze between the paddles and the skin and press firmly on the largest handheld paddles available; several successive shocks may be necessary.[209] Recent experimental evidence suggests that ischemia-triggered release of endogenous adenosine may have deleterious effects on the success of defibrillation.[210] Development of specific adenosine antagonists and their administration during CPR in patients found in ventricular fibrillation might further improve the effectiveness of defibrillation.

## SURVIVAL AND PROGNOSIS AFTER CARDIAC ARREST

Survival to hospital discharge after cardiac arrest varies from 1.4 to 29 percent. Marked differences in survival rates following out-of-hospital cardiac arrest have been reported in different communities. Survival rates are lowest in large cities such as New York (1.4 percent) and Chicago (4 percent)[211] and highest in Seattle (29 percent), a midsized urban community where many of the early intervention concepts were pioneered.[212] The in-hospital mortality rate following successful resuscitation outside the hospital remains as high as 90 percent in some populations[212,213] (Fig. 41-6). Important factors associated with increased in-hospital mortality rates after out-of-hospital cardiac arrest are cardiogenic shock after defibrillation, age 60 years or greater, requirement of four or more shocks for defibrillation, absence of an acute myocardial infarction, and coma on admission to the hospital.[68,214]

Survival depends largely on the initial recorded rhythm. Some 40 to 60 percent of patients who are found in ventricular fibrillation are successfully resuscitated, but only a fraction will survive to be discharged from the hospital. The outcome is much better in the smaller (less than 7 percent) group of patients where VT is the initial documented rhythm. The survival rate is more than 85 percent to the hospital and over 75 percent of patients are discharged alive. Many of those discharged alive after treatment and lengthy resuscitation can resume independent living activities.[213] Bradycardias and electromechanical dissociation as the presenting rhythms are associated with the worst prognosis, and very few (less than 5 percent) of these patients survive to discharge from the hospital.[204] Other factors associated with improved survival include a low "comorbidity index," reflecting chronic conditions such as history of heart failure, diabetes, hypertension, and gastrointestinal disorders as well as recent symptoms prior to the event.[215]

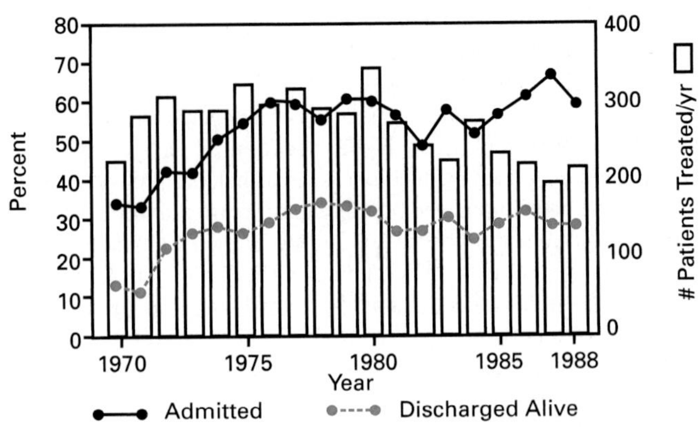


FIGURE 41-6 Percentage of out-of-hospital cardiac arrest victims admitted to the hospital by emergency medical service personnel and subsequently discharged alive during the period from 1970 to 1988. (From Cobb LA et al. Community-based interventions for sudden cardiac death: Impact, limitations, and changes. *Circulation* 1992;85:I98–I102. With permission.)

An important consideration in the treatment of the cardiac arrest victim is the appropriateness of CPR and the use of life-sustaining therapies in patients with a low likelihood of survival, such as chronically ill people found in asystole or electromechanical dissociation. Their chances of surviving until hospital discharge are less than 1 percent. Further, many older people prefer to die suddenly rather than experience chronic suffering.[216] Advance directives, when available, and consultation with family members and personal physicians might aid in the difficult decision process of when to administer supportive care rather than aggressive management.

## MANAGEMENT OF CARDIAC ARREST SURVIVORS AND RISK STRATIFICATION FOR SUDDEN CARDIAC DEATH

### Establishing the Underlying Cardiac Pathology

The initial management following successful resuscitation from cardiac arrest consists of allowing a period of hemodynamic and respiratory stabilization, after which every effort should be made to establish the cause of cardiac arrest and likelihood of recurrence. For this, the underlying cardiac disease should first be determined. History and physical examination may provide the first clues. Myocardial infarction must be excluded by serial enzyme measurements and ECG. Echocardiographic studies can determine left ventricular function, regional wall motion abnormalities, valvular heart disease, or cardiomyopathies. Stress-imaging studies can demonstrate inducible ischemia. Cardiac catheterization is often recommended to evaluate the coronary anatomy and right and left ventricular hemodynamic parameters. Other tests—such as radionuclide studies, magnetic resonance imaging, or cardiac biopsy—may be necessary in selected patients. As discussed above, an underlying cardiac disease can be found in nearly all patients.

#### PRIMARY VERSUS SECONDARY CARDIAC ARREST

One of the important questions following cardiac arrest is whether it was primarily due to acute circulatory or respiratory failure or to a arrhythmia. Although all these events are usually present during the arrest, it is important to distinguish whether the arrhythmia preceded or followed the hemodynamic collapse. While several clinical and historical clues help to answer this question (Table 41-4), the distinction sometimes cannot be made with certainty. Separating primary from secondary cardiac arrest has important prognostic and therapeutic implications. In 142 survivors of cardiac arrest with coronary artery disease, the 1-year survival rate was 89 percent, 80 percent, and 71 percent in the patients classified as having had cardiac arrest secondary to acute myocardial infarction (44 percent of patients), secondary to an ischemic event (34 percent), or due to a primary arrhythmic event (22 percent), respectively.[217] Patients who present with cardiac arrest secondary (and within 48 h) to an acute transmural myocardial infarction have a prognosis similar to that of patients who have an acute myocardial infarction without an arrhythmia.[68] Specific antiarrhythmic therapy is therefore usually not recommended if cardiac arrest occurs during or within 2 days of an acute Q-wave myocardial infarction. In contrast, if the arrhythmia is the primary event and myocardial infarction developed secondary to the acute hemodynamic deterioration during the arrhythmia, then antiarrhythmic therapy with a drug or device is recommended unless a transient or reversible cause is identified.

TABLE 41-4 Differences in Clinical Status Immediately before Death in Patients Dying Primarily of Arrhythmia versus Circulatory Failure

| Clinical Status Immediately before Death | Arrhythmic Deaths $n = 82$ | Circulatory Failure Deaths $n = 59$ |
|---|---|---|
| Comatose | 0/82 (0%) | 56/59 (95%) |
| Standing or actively moving | 39/82 (48%) | 0/59 (0%) |
| Terminal arrhythmia | | |
| Ventricular fibrillation | 15/18 (83%) | 3/9 (33%) |
| Asystole | 3/18 (17%) | 6/9 (67%) |
| Duration of terminal illness | | |
| <1 h | 53/82 (65%) | 4/59 (7%) |
| >24 h | 17/82 (21%) | 48/59 (81%) |
| Nature of terminal illness | | |
| Acute cardiac events | 80/82 (98%) | 8/59 (14%) |
| Noncardiac events | 1/82 (1%) | 51/59 (86%) |

SOURCE: Modified from Hinkle and Thaler,[6] with permission.

Every effort should be made to exclude potentially reversible causes of SCD (Table 41-5), including transient ischemic episodes in patients who are candidates for complete revascularization and in whom the onset of the arrhythmia is clearly preceded by ischemic ECG changes or symptoms. Other reversible etiologies for cardiac arrest include transient severe electrolyte disturbances and proarrhythmic effects of antiarrhythmic drugs and other pharmacologic agents. It can be difficult to establish a causal relationship between the proarrhythmic agent and the malignant ventricular arrhythmia as opposed to its being a coincidental finding. A pathologic prolongation of the QTc interval preceding initiation of the arrhythmia and return of the QTc interval to normal following discontinuation of the presumed proarrhythmic agent is strongly suggestive of a cause-and-effect relationship. Occasionally, especially when type IA agents are implicated in the cardiac arrest event, electrophysiologic evaluation, with programmed stimulation after washout and following reexposure to these agents, is necessary to confirm proarrhythmia as the sole cause of the episode of cardiac arrest. Another setting in which a reversible etiology for cardiac arrest is often present is in the hemodynamically unstable patient in the early postoperative period following cardiac surgery. Infusion of positive inotropic agents, electrolyte imbalances, and hypoxia are often precipitating factors. Nevertheless, one should be cautious in assigning, as the primary cause of arrest, a functional trigger such as ischemia or electrolyte imbalance. In the patient with structural heart disease, especially myocardial infarction, the underlying anatomic substrate should be considered the primary disorder, and the elimination of transient preturbations such as drug effects, hypoxia, and ischemia may not be sufficient in eliminating the risk for recurrent arrest. In fact, patients in the Amiodarone versus Implantable Defibrillator (AVID) trial who were thought to have arrested from a transient or correctable cause were excluded and followed in the AVID registry. These patients had a mortality rate that was similar to that in the general population of patients with ventricular fibrillatory arrest.[218]

TABLE 41-5 Potentially Reversible Causes of Cardiac Arrest Due to Ventricular Fibrillation

| | |
|---|---|
| Myocardial ischemia | Electrolyte abnormalities |
| Prinzmetal's angina | Hypoxia |
| Proarrhythmia | Acute congestive heart failure |
| Antiarrhythmic agents | |
| Other drugs | |

## Risk Stratification for Sudden Cardiac Death

Several clinical, noninvasive, and invasive strategies can aid in the risk stratification of patients for SCD. The underlying cardiac disease largely determines the choice of appropriate testing.

### CLINICAL HISTORY

There are several prognostic variables for SCD that are related to clinical history. The AVID registry showed that these included age >65 years, reduced ejection fraction, history of congestive heart failure, atrial fibrillation, pacemaker or diabetes, and smoking.[219] Interestingly, the hemodynamic impact of the qualifying arrhythmia was not a predictor of outcome in this study. Syncope in patients with a left ventricular ejection fraction below 30 percent is associated with increased risk of SCD (about 50 percent at 3 years) irrespective of finding an arrhythmic cause.[220] Patients with a history of myocardial infarction and impairment of left ventricular systolic function (LVEF <40 percent) should be considered for further evaluation and risk stratification for sudden death. Those with a history of unexplained impaired consciousness, especially if associated with congestive heart failure or other structural heart disease, should also be considered at high risk for sudden death and warrant further therapy or risk stratification.

## LEFT VENTRICULAR FUNCTION

Left ventricular dysfunction is a major independent predictor of total and sudden cardiac mortality rates in patients with ischemic as well as nonischemic cardiomyopathy. In survivors of cardiac arrest who have a left ventricular ejection fraction below 30 percent, the risk of SCD exceeds 30 percent over 1 to 3 years if they do not have inducible VT; it ranges between 15 and 50 percent in those who have inducible ventricular tachyarrhythmias despite therapy with drugs that suppressed the inducible arrhythmias or with empiric amiodarone.[221–223] Assessment of left ventricular function by clinical history (e.g., a history of congestive heart failure) and other noninvasive methods (echocardiographic or radionuclide studies) or invasive means (angiography) is therefore essential in the evaluation of a patient at risk for SCD.[224] Unfortunately, detection of severe left ventricular dysfunction serves to predict the total cardiac mortality rate but does not distinguish patients who will die suddenly from those who will die of progressive congestive heart failure.[224–226]

## ELECTROCARDIOGRAPHIC ABNORMALITIES

In survivors of out-of-hospital cardiac arrest, the presence of atrioventricular block or intraventricular conduction defects on ambulatory ECG (72 h) is associated with a higher recurrence rate of cardiac arrest (10 of 14 patients versus 1 of 28 patients without).[204] Other ECG parameters that have been reported to be associated independently with an increased risk of SCD are prolongation of the QT interval (in the absence of inherited or acquired LQTS),[227] increased dispersion of the QT interval,[228, 229] and an increase in resting heart rate above 90, particularly in men without a history of coronary artery disease.[230]

Detection of NSVT by ambulatory ECG monitoring has been reported to be of value in the risk stratification of patients for SCD.[231–235] The incidence of SCD in the 2 years following myocardial infarction in 766 patients enrolled in the Multicenter Post-Infarction Research Group increased with the frequency of PVCs detected during 24-h ECG monitoring from 3 percent for less than 1 per hour to 14 percent for greater than 30 per hour; similarly, patients with NSVT runs had a higher (17 percent) incidence of SCD than did those with single PVCs (6 percent).[231] The prognostic value of ambulatory ECG monitoring in patients with congestive heart failure is limited by the high incidence of these arrhythmias (up to 88 percent) in this population, resulting in a low specificity of this parameter.[236]

## MARKERS OF REDUCED VAGAL ACTIVITY

There is increasing evidence that cardiac abnormalities associated with a high risk of SCD are accompanied by changes in autonomic innervation of the heart. Myocardial infarction, for instance, has been shown to cause regional cardiac sympathetic and parasympathetic denervation.[237] This autonomic heterogeneity may predispose to arrhythmia development by creating dispersion of refractoriness and/or conduction. Sensitivity to sympathetic activation favors the onset of life-threatening cardiac arrhythmias, while vagal activation has been shown to have a protective effect in the presence of tonic sympathetic stimulation.[238]

Reduced baroreflex sensitivity (BRS) and heart rate variability (HRV) reflect an impairment in the vagal efferent component of the autonomic nervous system and may help to predict cardiovascular mortality rates and arrhythmic events, particularly in patients following myocardial infarction. In two prospective studies including a total of 200 patients following myocardial infarction, BRS was significantly reduced in the 14 patients with SCD or life-threatening arrhythmias compared to those without.[77,239] Studies show that the sensitivity of depressed BRS is approximately 70 to 80 percent and the specificity of BRS about 70 percent.[240–242]

Another noninvasive measure of sympathovagal balance is HRV, or beat-to-beat variations of RR intervals. Several measures of heart rate variability have been reported to be associated with an increased risk of sudden and total cardiac death following myocardial infarction.[240–243] In a prospective study of 6693 nonselected and consecutive patients who underwent 24-h ECG monitoring, those with reduced heart rate variability had a fourfold higher risk of SCD than patients with higher variability.[243]

One study compared the relative utility of these measures alone and in combination by measuring BRS, heart rate variability, 24-h ECG recording, and left ventricular ejection fraction in over 1000 patients after myocardial infarction.[241] NSVT, abnormal HRV, and BRS each were independently predictive of worse outcomes. The combination of all three risk factors signified a 22-fold increased risk of death, but the positive predictive value was only approximately 20 percent. These findings underscore the utility of identifying patients at low risk for events with negative test findings as well as the limitations of predicting events based on positive results.

## T-WAVE ALTERNANS

Macroscopic T-wave changes with an alternating pattern have been observed in patients with LQTS prior to onset of ventricular fibrillation as well as in the setting of mechanical alternans, which is sometimes present during cardiac tamponade. Recent studies have indicated that T-wave alternans that is discernible only by computer-averaging techniques may be a more ubiquitous phenomenon that can identify patients at risk for ventricular arrhythmias.[244] Techniques for computer-assisted analysis of T-wave alternans are being developed and may provide a quantitative, noninvasive method for assessing susceptibility to ventricular fibrillation. T-wave alternans assessed by computer analysis has been shown to predict arrhythmia-free survival over 20 months, with a nearly 90 percent sensitivity and specificity in a small cohort of 66 patients.[245] The positive predictive accuracy of this test appears to be similar to that of others with a very high negative predictive value.

## LATE POTENTIALS

Late potentials, microvolt waveforms extending the duration of a filtered QRS complex detected by signal-averaging ECG (SAECG), have been shown to be helpful in the risk stratification of patients following myocardial infarction. The prognostic significance of late potentials has been demonstrated in several studies, which reported a 17 to 29 percent incidence of SCD, ventricular fibrillation, or sustained VT in patients with an abnormal SAECG, in contrast to 0.8 to 3.5 percent in those without.[246] Although the negative predictive value of a normal SAECG is good, the application of SAECG in risk stratification for SCD is limited by a low positive predictive value in patients following myocardial infarction as well as by its low sensitivity in patients with nonischemic cardiomyopathies.[247] The sensitivity, specificity, and positive predictive value of SAECG are all improved when used in patients with known left ventricular dysfunction after myocardial infarction and/or NSVT[233] (see Chap. 34).

## ELECTROPHYSIOLOGIC STUDIES

Electrophysiologic studies have advanced our understanding of life-threatening ventricular arrhythmias and facilitated the development of new therapies for their prevention and treatment. Induction of sustained monomorphic VT is the generally accepted endpoint for programmed stimulation, while induction of NSVT, polymorphic VT, or ventricular fibrillation may be a nonspecific finding, depending on the aggressiveness of the stimulation protocol.[165,248] Information obtained during the electrophysiologic study—such as VT rate, morphology, origin, mechanism, and hemodynamic stability—is crucial to determining whether the patient is a candidate for serial drug testing, catheter ablation therapy, surgical therapy, or an implantable defibrillator. In patients who present with sustained monomorphic VT, VT is reproducibly inducible in the vast majority, especially in those with coronary artery disease.[248] Electrophysiologic testing is also useful in patients with structural heart disease presenting with unexplained syncope. VT is the most common abnormal finding in these patients, but demonstration of His-Purkinje conduction disease or hemodynamically unstable supraventricular tachycardia can also be important.

In survivors of cardiac arrest due to ventricular fibrillation, the prognostic value of electrophysiologic testing is less clear. For those who are candidates for CABG, preoperative electrophysiologic testing does not reliably identify who will have further arrhythmias after revascularization.[249] Postoperative testing in patients at high risk (e.g., advanced age, impaired left ventricular function) may reveal the mechanism of arrest, have prognostic significance, and help select an appropriate therapy; but since sustained VT or ventricular fibrillation is inducible in fewer than half the patients, suppression of induction of ventricular fibrillation by antiarrhythmic therapy is an unreliable endpoint. Controversy exists regarding the prognostic significance of a negative electrophysiologic study after cardiac arrest; some have shown that patients with no inducible ventricular arrhythmias remain at a high risk for recurrent cardiac arrest,[250,251] while others have shown that noninducibility after CABG in patients surviving cardiac arrest confers an excellent prognosis[252] (see Chap. 34).

## TREATMENT OPTIONS FOR PATIENTS AT RISK FOR SUDDEN CARDIAC DEATH

### General Considerations

There are few direct and randomized comparisons of various treatment strategies to prevent SCD. Since reduction of SCD rates does not necessarily parallel a reduction in total mortality rate, reduction in total mortality is a more appropriate endpoint in assessing antiarrhythmic efficacy. Patient selection affects the outcome of different treatment strategies. For example, in patients at low risk of SCD, proarrhythmia or surgical mortality rates may outweigh the benefits achieved with an antiarrhythmic intervention. On the other hand, in patients at high risk for recurrent cardiac arrest, the risk-benefit profile of antiarrhythmic treatment strategies may be more favorable. Selection of therapy is further limited by the patient's baseline characteristics. For instance, radiofrequency ablation of VT is an option only in patients with hemodynamically stable monomorphic VT or bundle branch reentry. In an era of limited health care resources, the cost-effectiveness of different treatment strategies is another element to be considered in choosing therapy. Last but not least, quality of life is an important aspect in the selection of the most appropriate therapy.

### Pharmacologic Therapy

Several medications have been shown to reduce the risk of SCD in patients known to have cardiac disease. Some, such as the statins and aspirin, reduce sudden death by reducing the incidence of coronary plaque rupture or platelet aggregation and thrombosis (see Chaps. 44 and 54). Beta blockers stabilize autonomic balance, improve pump function, and help reduce ischemia, while angiotensin-converting enzyme (ACE) inhibitors reduce the incidence of sudden death through similar and other complex mechanisms (see Chaps. 25 and 43).

#### BETA BLOCKERS

Of all the therapies currently available for the prevention of SCD, none are more established or more effective in patients with coronary heart disease than beta blockers.[253,254] In a review of 19,000 post–myocardial infarction patients who were randomized to beta blockers or placebo, active treatment was associated with a decrease in total mortality rate of 20 percent, of SCD rate of 30 percent, and of reinfarction of 35 to 40 percent.[255] The benefits of beta blockade are additive to those of standard treatment for congestive heart failure. The Metoprolol CR/XL Randomized Intervention Trial in Congestive Heart Failure (MERIT-HF) demonstrated a 34 percent decrease in the all-cause mortality rate, 38 percent decrease in the cardiovascular mortality rate, and a 41 percent decrease in the sudden death rate in 3991 patients who were randomized to metoprolol while being treated with standard medical therapy, including ACE inhibition, digitalis, and diuretics.[256] It is important to note that the beneficial effects of beta blockers on cardiac mortality are most pronounced in patients who are at higher risk for SCD, such as those with congestive heart failure, atrial and ventricular arrhythmias, post–myocardial infarction, and diabetes[253] (see Chap. 28).

#### ANGIOTENSIN-CONVERTING ENZYME INHIBITORS

Reduced mortality rates are well known with ACE inhibitors in patients with impaired ejection fraction with or without mild heart failure symptoms after myocardial infarction[257–260] and with established heart failure,[261–263] but data supporting a specific effect on SCD rates are mixed. Vasodilator therapy is an effective treatment in patients with congestive heart failure and has been shown to reduce mortality rates by up to 40 percent in the first year, but studies of patients with New York Heart Association class I through IV congestive heart failure treated with enalapril showed no significant difference in sudden death mortality rate compared to those treated with placebo, and approximately 20 percent of patients died suddenly.[261–263]

A metanalysis analyzed 15 trials that included 15,104 post–myocardial infarction patients treated with ACE inhibitors and found that there were 900 SCDs in these studies and a significant trend toward reduction in SCD in all of the larger ($n > 500$) trials.[264] One trial in patients with preserved ventricular function who were 55 years of age or older and had vascular disease or diabetes and one other coronary risk factor found significantly fewer patients treated with ramipril had a cardiac arrest (relative risk, 0.62; $p = 0.02$).[265] A distinct effect of ACE inhibitors in reducing sudden arrhythmic death that is independent of improvements in circulatory function will likely never be proven, but the survival advantage of these medications in those with impaired ventricular function and/or established vascular disease cannot be overlooked.

#### CLASS I ANTIARRHYTHMIC AGENTS

The role of antiarrhythmic drug therapy in the prevention of SCD has changed considerably since placebo-controlled trials such as the Cardiac Arrhythmia Suppression trial (CAST) demonstrated that suppression of spontaneous NSVT with certain drugs does not necessarily result in improved survival[188] (Table 41-6). There is no evidence that other class I antiarrhythmic drugs can prolong survival in any

TABLE 41-6 Trials for Primary Prevention of Sudden Cardiac Death

| | *N* | CAD | Low EF | PVCs | NSVT | Therapy | Follow-up (months) | Findings | Comments |
|---|---|---|---|---|---|---|---|---|---|
| | | | | | | CORONARY ARTERY DISEASE | | | |
| Class IC: | | | | | | | | | |
| CAST, 1989 | 1498 | + | + | + | − | Encainide or flecainide vs. placebo | 10 | 7.7% mortality (treatment) vs. 3.0% (placebo) | Terminated prematurely due to excess mortality in treatment group |
| Amiodarone: | | | | | | | | | |
| BASIS, 1990 | 312 | + | − | + | − | Amio vs. mexiletine or quinidine vs. placebo | 72 | 5% mortality (amio) vs. 10% (class I) vs. 13% (placebo) | Amio improved survival, nonsignificant trend with Holter-guided PVC supression |
| EMIAT, 1997 | 1486 | + | + | − | − | Amio vs. placebo | 21 | 7.2% mortality (both groups), 35% RR in arrhythmic death | Amio reduced arrhythmic death rate without affecting total survival |
| CAMIAT, 1997 | 1202 | + | − | + | − | Amio vs. placebo | 21 | 3.3% VF/SCD (amio) vs. 6.0% (placebo), RR 21.2% | Prophylactic amio improved survival for frequent/repetitive PVCs |
| ICD: | | | | | | | | | |
| MADIT, 1996 | 196 | + | − | + | + | ICD vs. conventional therapy | 27 | 15.7% mortality (ICD) vs. 38.6% (no ICD), RR 46% | Terminated prematurely because of significant ICD benefit |
| CABG-Patch, 1997 | 900 | + | + | − | − | ICD vs. no ICD | 36 | No difference in all-cause mortality | All patients had abnormal SAECG; no benefit of prophylactic ICD |
| MUSTT, 1999 | 704 | + | + | + | + | EP-guided or ICD vs. no antiarrhythmic therapy | 60 | 25% mortality (EP-guided or ICD) vs. 32% (no therapy) | EP-guided therapy with ICDs, but not with antiarrhythmic drugs, reduces the risk of SCD in high-risk patients with CAD |
| MADIT-2, 2002 | 1232 | + | + | − | − | ICD vs. conventional therapy | 20 | 15.7% mortality (ICD) vs. 19.8% (no-ICD), RR 31% | Cost-effectiveness remains to be determined. Patients on average were 3 years post-infarction |
| Sotalol: | | | | | | | | | |
| Julian et al., 1982 | 1456 | + | − | − | − | *d,l*-Sotalol vs. placebo | 12 | 7.3% mortality (sotalol) vs. 8.9% (placebo), RR 18% | *d,l*-Sotalol may reduce mortality by up to 25% |
| SWORD, 1996 | 3121 | + | + | − | − | *d*-Sotalol vs. placebo | 5 | 5.0% mortality (sotalol) vs. 3.1% (placebo) | Trial terminated due to excess mortality in the treatment group |
| | | | | | | CHF AMIODARONE TRIALS | | | |
| GESICA, 1994 | 516 | ~1/3 | + | − | − | Amio vs. standard therapy | 24 | 33.5% mortality (amio) vs. 41.4% (control) | Amio improved survival in symptomatic heart failure |
| CHF-STAT, 1995 | 674 | ~2/3 | + | − | − | Amio vs. placebo | 45 | 30.6% mortality (amio) vs. 29.2% (placebo) | No survival benefit with amio; trend to improved survival in DCM |

ABBREVIATIONS: + = Inclusion criterion; − = not inclusion criterion; amio = amiodarone; CAD = coronary artery disease; CHF = congestive heart failure; DCM = dilated cardiomyopathy; EF = ejection fraction; ICD = implantable cardioverter/defibrillator; NSVT = nonsustained ventricular tachycardia; PVCs = premature ventricular contractions; RR = risk reduction; SCD = sudden cardiac death; VF = ventricular fibrillation. See text for clinical trial abbreviations.

SOURCE: Modified with permission from: Welch PJ, Page RL, Hamdan MH. Management of ventricular arrhythmias: A trial-based approach. *J Am Coll Cardiol* 1999;34:621–630.

patient group studied. Results of a metanalysis of empiric long-term antiarrhythmic therapy after myocardial infarction demonstrated a higher mortality rate among those treated with class I agents.[266]

A metanalysis of lidocaine in acute myocardial infarction suggested an increase in in-hospital mortality rate despite a reduction in the prevalence of ventricular fibrillation.[267] Empiric use of these drugs in patients with sustained ventricular arrhythmias has been associated with a very high rate of SCD, between 30 and 70 percent at 2 years.[268] The propafenone arm was stopped early in the Cardiac Arrest Study Hamburg (CASH) because of excess mortality rates in cardiac arrest survivors compared with amiodarone, beta blockers, and implantable defibrillators (see also Chap. 28).[268a]

### SOTALOL

Sotalol, in the currently marketed form of a racemic mixture of the *d*- and *l*-stereoisomers, is a potent class III antiarrhythmic agent with nonselective beta-blocking effects.[269] Sotalol has been reported to suppress inducible VT in 30 to 40 percent of patients who present with sustained ventricular arrhythmias. In a randomized trial of sotalol and other antiarrhythmic agents in patients with sustained VT, the arrhythmia recurrence rate (21 percent at 1 year) and the arrhythmic death rate (12 percent at 4 years) was half of that achieved with class I agents.[270] However, since most patients receiving sotalol had failed other antiarrhythmic agents, the results were biased in favor of sotalol. The beta-blocking effect of sotalol seems to be essential for its benefit. The Survival with Oral *d*-Sotalol (SWORD) trial of the *d*-isomer (class III antiarrhythmic effect only, devoid of beta-blocking effect) in patients with prior myocardial infarction was associated with increased mortality rates[271] (Table 41-6). The most serious side effect encountered with sotalol is proarrhythmia (mostly torsades de pointes), which has been reported to occur in up to 8 percent of treated patients.[272] Sotalol therapy was less effective than ICDs in a group of patients with VT or ventricular fibrillation.[273]

### AMIODARONE

Amiodarone is widely considered the most effective antiarrhythmic agent for therapy of supraventricular and ventricular arrhythmias[274] (see Chap. 35). Uncontrolled trials in patients with sustained VT or ventricular fibrillation demonstrated a relatively low incidence of SCD in those treated with amiodarone despite a high recurrence rate of ventricular arrhythmias.[222,223] The most important predictor of SCD in patients treated with amiodarone for sustained VT or ventricular fibrillation is left ventricular ejection fraction. In a series of 122 such patients with mostly coronary artery disease, the actuarial probability of SCD at 5 years was 5 percent when the ejection fraction was greater than or equal to 40 percent and 49 percent when the ejection fraction was less than 40 percent.[275]

Amiodarone has been shown to reduce significantly SCD rates following myocardial infarction in several placebo-controlled randomized studies, but its effects on the total mortality rate are inconsistent.[276] The Basel Antiarrhythmic Study of Infarct Survival (BASIS)—a prospective randomized trial of empiric amiodarone, ambulatory ECG-guided conventional antiarrhythmic therapy, or placebo in 312 patients with complex ventricular ectopy following myocardial infarction—showed that amiodarone significantly reduced the total mortality rate at 1 year from 13 percent in the placebo group to 5 percent in amiodarone-treated patients ($p < 0.05$).[277] On the other hand, amiodarone therapy did not reduce the total mortality rate compared with placebo in nearly 2700 post–myocardial infarction patients enrolled in the Canadian Amiodarone Myocardial Infarction Arrhythmia Trial (CAMIAT)[278] and the European Myocardial Infarction Amiodarone Trial (EMIAT)[279] despite a 50 percent risk reduction in the arrhythmic mortality rate (Table 41-6). Concomitant use of beta blockers and amiodarone resulted in a significant reduction in total mortality rate and sudden death in subgroup analysis.

In patients with congestive heart failure, prophylactic therapy with amiodarone was shown to decrease the mortality rate (by 28 percent) in the Argentinean Grupo de Estudio de la Sobrevida en la Insuficiencia Cardiaca en Argentina (GESICA) trial[280] but not in the Survival Trial of Antiarrhythmic Therapy in Congestive Heart Failure (CHF-STAT).[281] Comparison of the two patient populations suggested that prophylactic amiodarone may be more beneficial in patients with nonischemic cardiomyopathy, found in greater number in the GESICA study (Table 41-6). The consequence of these amiodarone trials is that this drug can be used safely in patients with left ventricular dysfunction. Therefore, in our opinion, amiodarone is the drug of choice when antiarrhythmic drug treatment is indicated in patients with left ventricular dysfunction and congestive heart failure. Sotalol may be considered in those with left ventricular systolic dysfunction without congestive symptoms.

The efficacy of amiodarone in reducing total mortality rates in patients with ventricular fibrillation or hemodynamically unstable VT compared to ICD treatment has been evaluated prospectively in the randomized AVID study, which reported a survival benefit in the patients randomized to ICD therapy.[282] Prospective, randomized trials addressed a similar question in cardiac arrest survivors in the Canadian Implantable Defibrillator Study (CIDS)[283] and CASH[284] (see below).

The use of intravenous amiodarone in out-of-hospital cardiac arrest was studied. Intravenous amiodarone was compared to placebo in 504 patients suffering out-of-hospital cardiac arrest that was refractory to three or more precordial shocks. Patients receiving 300 mg of intravenous amiodarone had an improved rate of survival to admission to the hospital as compared to placebo, but only a small proportion survived to hospital discharge.[213] Another study of patients with out-of-hospital cardiac arrest compared lidocaine to amiodarone. More patients treated with amiodarone survived to hospital admission, but discharge rates from the hospital remained poor.[285] The relative efficacy of intravenous amiodarone compared to lidocaine in patients with longer arrest times or with presenting rhythms other than ventricular fibrillation is not certain. Whether use of intravenous amiodarone confers a survival benefit remains to be determined.

## Device Therapy

### AUTOMATIC IMPLANTABLE CARDIOVERTER/DEFIBRILLATOR

The ICD was initially developed to recognize ventricular fibrillation or rapid VT and terminate it automatically by delivering one or more high-energy shocks.[286] Newer-generation defibrillators have the additional ability to deliver low-energy cardioversion, antitachycardia pacing for VT, and antibradycardia pacing. The first generation of epicardial defibrillators required a thoracotomy to place the sensing and defibrillator leads epicardially and the generator size mandated implantation of the device in an abdominal pocket. The reduced size of defibrillators now allows for a subpectoral, transvenous endocardial lead system that integrates pacing, sensing, and high-voltage defibrillation abilities.[287]

To investigate the potential benefit of ICD therapy compared with antiarrhythmic drug treatment in secondary prevention, the AVID study, CASH, and CIDS studies randomized patients with documented sustained ventricular arrhythmia to one of these two treatment strategies. AVID and CIDS enrolled patients with ventricular fibrillation or poorly tolerated VT and left ventricular dysfunction. In the AVID trial, which enrolled 1016 such patients, the ICD group had 38 and 25 percent reductions in the overall mortality rate at 1 and 3 years, respectively, compared to the group of patients taking amiodarone or sotalol.[282] CIDS enrolled 659 patients. Results after 5 years of follow-up reported a 20 percent reduction in mortality with ICD.[283] CASH enrolled patients with cardiac arrest secondary to a ventricular arrhythmia regardless of the underlying disease or ventricular function. A nonsignificant 23 percent reduction of all-cause mortality in the ICD arm was found when compared with the drug arm (metoprolol or amiodarone).[284] These studies show that, compared to the best currently available antiarrhythmic drug therapy, ICDs improve survival rates in patients with a history of ventricular fibrillation or VT (Table 41-6).

Several studies looking at primary prevention or the prophylactic use of defibrillators in high-risk populations have been completed (Table 41-6). The Multicenter Automatic Defibrillator Implantation Trial (MADIT)[288] demonstrated a survival benefit of defibrillator therapy compared with conventional therapy in patients after myocardial infarction who have NSVT, left ventricular dysfunction, and inducible sustained VT not suppressed by procainamide. The Multicenter Unsustained Tachycardia Trial (MUSTT) was a randomized, controlled trial to test the hypothesis that electrophysiologically guided antiarrhythmic therapy would reduce the risk of sudden death among patients with coronary artery disease, a left ventricular ejection fraction of 40 percent or less, and asymptomatic NSVT. Patients in whom sustained ventricular tachyarrhythmias were induced by programmed stimulation were assigned to receive no antiarrhythmic therapy or antiarrhythmic therapy, including drugs and ICDs, as indicated by the results of electrophysiologic testing. Electrophysiologically guided antiarrhythmic therapy with ICDs, but not with antiarrhythmic drugs, reduced the risk of sudden death in high-risk patients with coronary disease[289] (Fig. 41-7).

The Multicenter Automatic Defibrillator Implantation Trial (MADIT) II was a follow-up study to the MADIT trial and questioned the need for risk stratification using electrophysiologic study. Patients with coronary artery disease, a left ventricular ejection fraction of 30 percent or less, and at least one myocardial infarction were randomized without further risk stratification to ICD implantation or conventional medical therapy. Patients were followed for a mean of 20 months and were matched with regard to baseline characteristics and use of aspirin, ACE inhibitors, and beta blockers. The trial was terminated early when interim analysis showed a 5.6 percent absolute and a 31 percent relative risk reduction in mortality rate in the ICD group that became evident at 9 months of follow-up.[290] Significant limitations of this trial were that the patients had a lower mortality than the noninducible group in MUSTT, were followed for 2 years in less than one-third, and were an average of 3 years postinfarction. One question is whether increased use of amiodarone in the conventional-therapy group would have narrowed difference in mortality rates in this cohort. Only 10 to 13 percent of patients in MADIT II were treated with amiodarone, which, as mentioned, has been shown to reduce arrhythmic mortality in those with impaired ventricular function after myocardial infarction.[278,279]

Another primary prevention trial addressed the routine use of ICD implantation at the time of surgical revacularization. The Coronary Artery Bypass Grafting (CABG)-Patch trial enrolled patients with coronary artery disease scheduled for elective CABG who also had a left ventricular ejection fraction of less than 30 percent and an abnormal SAECG. A total of 900 patients were randomized to receive either an ICD at the time of CABG or usual care. This study found no significant difference in the primary endpoint of total mortality at 30 days and a mean follow-up of 32 months.[291] The findings were not surprising in view of the known benefit of revascularization in preventing SCD (see below) and the poor positive predictive value of the SAECG (Table 41-6).

Since ICD therapy is therapeutic rather than preventive, these devices might effectively be combined with other antiarrhythmic strategies, such as drugs or catheter ablation, to prevent frequent recurrences of tachyarrhythmias. Despite the undisputed efficacy of implantable defibrillators in preventing SCD, several major questions remain to be answered: (1) Which patients will benefit most from defibrillator therapy? (2) Do ICDs improve quality of life? (3) Are ICDs cost-effective compared with antiarrhythmic drug therapy? and (4) Will adjunctive antiarrhythmic drug therapy add to the efficacy of ICDs? (see Chaps. 38 and 104 ).

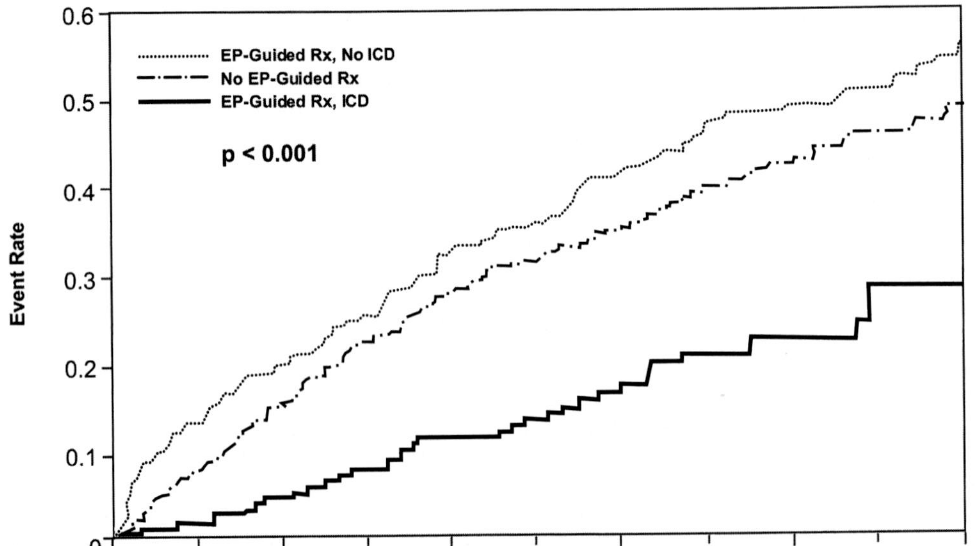

FIGURE 41-7 Kaplan-Meier estimates of the rates of overall mortality in a randomized trial between electrophysiologically guided (EPG) therapy versus no antiarrhythmic therapy (MUSTT Trial). The *P* value refers to two comparisons: between the patients in the group assigned to EPG therapy who received treatment with a defibrillator and those who did not receive such treatment and between the patients assigned to electrophysiologically guided therapy who received treatment with a defibrillator and those assigned to no antiarrhythmic therapy. (From the MUSTT Investigators.[289] With permission.)

## Role of Surgery

### REVASCULARIZATION

There is a reduced prevalence of SCD after coronary artery bypass grafting (CABG),[292] and attempts should b made to identify and revascularize ischemic myocardium in order to mitigate arrhythmic risk. While it is accepted that CABG reduces ventricular arrhythmias, the effect is unpredictable.[293] Among the 13,476 patients in the Coronary Artery Surgery Study (CASS) registry, all of whom had significant coronary artery disease, operable vessels, and no significant valvular disease, the mean incidence of SCD during the 4.6-year average follow-up was 5.2 percent in patients treated medically and 1.8 percent in those treated surgically.[292] The beneficial effect of CABG was even more pronounced in the subgroup of patients with reduced left ventricular ejection fraction and multivessel disease, where the survival rate free from SCD at 5 years was 91 percent for the surgical group versus 69 percent in the medical group.

The failure of ICDs in the CABG-Patch trial to save lives in patients with impaired ventricular function and abnormal signal-averaged ECGs who underwent CABG suggests that revascularization reduced the risk of sudden death to such a degree that no incremental advantage of ICD therapy could be detected.[291,294] Importantly, patients with a preexisting history of ventricular fibrillation or VT were excluded in this trial, but there are data to suggest that CABG is adequate in some but not all patients to reduce the risk of recurrent arrest. In an uncontrolled study of 265 survivors of cardiac arrest, 32 percent underwent CABG and 68 percent were treated medically; CABG was associated with a more than 50 percent risk reduction in recurrent cardiac arrest rate after adjusting for baseline differences.[295] Further analysis from the AVID trial showed that revascularization after the index arrhythmia conferred a survival advantage compared to those who did not undergo this procedure. Nevertheless, independent of revascularization, ICD implantation offered a similar survival advantage to those patients in the AVID registry with coronary artery disease.[296]

The protective effect of CABG against recurrent cardiac arrest appears to be best in patients with reversible ischemia as the major pathophysiologic factor in SCD. These patients are characterized by critical coronary artery disease, significant regions of myocardium at risk for ischemia, and no inducible monomorphic ventricular arrhythmias at electrophysiologic study.[221,295] Despite the encouraging results of CABG in survivors of cardiac arrest, it should be noted that only a minority of these patients are candidates for operative revascularization and that scar-mediated, monomorphic VT is often not controlled by myocardial revascularization alone.[249] The relative benefits of partial or complete percutaneous revascularization compared to CABG in this setting are also unclear.

## CATHETER ABLATION THERAPY

Catheter ablation of arrhythmias has emerged as a curative approach for many supraventricular arrhythmias and a few specific forms of VTs.[182] The role of catheter ablation in the prevention of SCD is less well established, but this form of therapy has been successfully employed in selected cases. Rarely, supraventricular tachycardias with a rapid ventricular response may degenerate into fatal ventricular tachyarrhythmias and cardiac arrest.[297] Radiofrequency catheter ablation can eliminate the risk of a rapid ventricular response by abolishing conduction over an accessory pathway in patients with Wolff-Parkinson-White syndrome, or it can slow or completely block conduction over the atrioventricular node in patients with atrial arrhythmias and rapid, medically uncontrolled atrioventricular conduction. Radiofrequency catheter ablation can potentially prevent SCD in patients with documented and inducible bundle branch reentrant VT as the only mechanism of cardiac arrest.[298] Improved mapping techniques of the VT circuit, better catheters, and perhaps other energy sources may help improve the efficacy of catheter ablation for VT and potentially expand its role in the prevention of SCD (see Chaps. 28 and 36).

## References

1. Kannel WB, Cupples LA, D'Agostino RB. Sudden death risk in overt coronary heart disease: the Framingham Study. *Am Heart J* 1987; 113:799–804.
2. Zheng ZJ, Croft JB, Giles WH, Mensah GA. Sudden cardiac death in the United States, 1989 to 1998. *Circulation* 2001;104:2158–2163.
3. Registers MIC. *Public Health in Europe 5.* Copenhagen: Regional Office for Europe, World Health Organization; 1976.
4. Madsen JK. Ischaemic heart disease and prodromes of sudden cardiac death. Is it possible to identify high risk groups for sudden cardiac death? *Br Heart J* 1985; 54:27–32.
5. Goldstein S. The necessity of a uniform definition of sudden coronary death: witnessed death within 1 hour of the onset of acute symptoms. *Am Heart J* 1982;103:156–159.
6. Hinkle LE Jr, Thaler HT. Clinical classification of cardiac deaths. *Circulation* 1982;65:457–464.
7. de Vreede-Swagemakers JJ, Gorgels AP, Dubois-Arbouw WI, et al. Out-of-hospital cardiac arrest in the 1990's: A population-based study in the Maastricht area on incidence, characteristics and survival. *J Am Coll Cardiol* 1997;30:1500–1505.
8. Leach IH, Blundell JW, Rowley JM, Turner DR. Acute ischaemic lesions in death due to ischaemic heart disease. An autopsy study of 333 cases of out-of-hospital death. *Eur Heart J* 1995; 16:1181–1185.
9. Matoba R, Shikata I, Iwai K, et al. An epidemiologic and histopathological study of sudden cardiac death in Osaka Medical Examiner's Office. *Jpn Circ J* 1989;53:1581–1588.
10. State-specific mortality from sudden cardiac death—United States, 1999. *MMWR Morb Mortal Wkly Rep* 2002;51:123–126.
11. Eisenberg MS, Horwood BT, Cummins RO, et al. Cardiac arrest and resuscitation: A tale of 29 cities. *Ann Emerg Med* 1990;19:179–186.
12. Gillum RF. Sudden coronary death in the United States: 1980–1985. *Circulation* 1989;79:756–765.
13. Wren C, O'Sullivan JJ, Wright C. Sudden death in children and adolescents. *Heart* 2000;83:410–413.
14. Maron BJ, Gohman TE, Aeppli D. Prevalence of sudden cardiac death during competitive sports activities in Minnesota high school athletes. *J Am Coll Cardiol* 1998;32:1881–1884.
15. Thiene G, Nava A, Corrado D, et al. Right ventricular cardiomyopathy and sudden death in young people. *N Engl J Med* 1988;318:129–133.
16. Hokanson JS, Moller JH. Significance of early transient complete heart block as a predictor of sudden death late after operative correction of tetralogy of Fallot. *Am J Cardiol* 2001;87:1271–1277.
17. Puley G, Siu S, Connelly M, et al. Arrhythmia and survival in patients >18 years of age after the mustard procedure for complete transposition of the great arteries. *Am J Cardiol* 1999;83:1080–1084.
18. Ghai A, Silversides C, Harris L, et al. Left ventricular dysfunction is a risk factor for sudden cardiac death in adults late after repair of tetralogy of Fallot. *J Am Coll Cardiol* 2002;40:1675–1680.
19. Becker LB, Han BH, Meyer PM, et al. Racial differences in the incidence of cardiac arrest and subsequent survival. The CPR Chicago Project [see comments]. *N Engl J Med* 1993;329:600–606.
20. Clark LT, Ferdinand KC, Flack JM, et al. Coronary heart disease in African Americans. *Heart Dis* 2001;3:97–108.
21. Burke AP, Farb A, Malcom GT, et al. Plaque rupture and sudden death related to exertion in men with coronary artery disease. *JAMA* 1999; 281:921–926.
22. Asher CR, Topol EJ, Moliterno DJ. Insights into the pathophysiology of atherosclerosis and prognosis of black Americans with acute coronary syndromes. *Am Heart J* 1999;138:1073–1081.
23. Albert CM, McGovern BA, Newell JB, Ruskin JN. Sex differences in cardiac arrest survivors. *Circulation* 1996;93:1170–1176.
24. Roger VL, Farkouh ME, Weston SA, et al. Sex differences in evaluation and outcome of unstable angina. *JAMA* 2000;283:646–652.

25. Schulman KA, Berlin JA, Harless W, et al. The effect of race and sex on physicians' recommendations for cardiac catheterization. *N Engl J Med* 1999;340:618–626.
26. Mosca L, Jones WK, King KB, et al. Awareness, perception, and knowledge of heart disease risk and prevention among women in the United States. American Heart Association Women's Heart Disease and Stroke Campaign Task Force. *Arch Fam Med* 2000;9:506–915.
27. Hinkle LE Jr. Short-term risk factors for sudden death. *Ann N Y Acad Sci* 1982;382:22–38.
28. Kannel WB, Thomas HE Jr. Sudden coronary death: The Framingham Study. *Ann NY Acad Sci* 1982;382:3–21.
29. Kannel WB, Schatzkin A. Sudden death: Lessons from subsets in population studies. *J Am Coll Cardiol* 1985;5:141B–149B.
30. Demirovic J. *Risk Factors and Incidence of Sudden Cardiac Death and Possibilities for Its Prevention.* Belgrade: University of Belgrade; 1985.
31. Beaglehole R, Stewart AW, Bonita R, et al. Myocardial infarction and sudden death in Auckland. *N Z Med J* 1984;97:715–718.
32. Kagan A, Yano K, Reed DM, MacLean CJ. Predictors of sudden cardiac death among Hawaiian-Japanese men (see comments). *Am J Epidemiol* 1989;130:268–277.
33. Baba A, Yoshikawa T, Ogawa S. Autoantibodies produced against sarcolemmal Na-K-ATPase: Possible upstream targets of arrhythmias and sudden death in patients with dilated cardiomyopathy. *J Am Coll Cardiol* 2002;40:1153–1159.
34. Soeki T, Tamura Y, Shinohara H, et al. Plasma concentrations of fibrinolytic factors in the subacute phase of myocardial infarction predict recurrent myocardial infarction or sudden cardiac death. *Int J Cardiol* 2002;85:277–283.
35. Burke AP, Fonseca V, Kolodgie F, et al. Increased serum homocysteine and sudden death resulting from coronary atherosclerosis with fibrous plaques. *Arterioscler Thromb Vasc Biol* 2002;22:1936–1941.
36. Albert CM, Campos H, Stampfer MJ, et al. Blood levels of long-chain n-3 fatty acids and the risk of sudden death. *N Engl J Med* 2002;346: 1113–1118.
37. Albert CM, Manson JE, Cook NR, et al. Moderate alcohol consumption and the risk of sudden cardiac death among US male physicians. *Circulation* 1999;100:944–950.
38. de Vreede-Swagemakers JJ, Gorgels AP, Weijenberg MP, et al. Risk indicators for out-of-hospital cardiac arrest in patients with coronary artery disease. *J Clin Epidemiol* 1999;52:601–607.
39. Burke AP, Farb A, Malcom GT, et al. Coronary risk factors and plaque morphology in men with coronary disease who died suddenly (see comments). *N Engl J Med* 1997;336:1276–1282.
40. Lampert R, Joska T, Burg MM, et al. Emotional and physical precipitants of ventricular arrhythmia. *Circulation* 2002;106:1800–1805.
41. Lampert R, Jain D, Burg MM, et al. Destabilizing effects of mental stress on ventricular arrhythmias in patients with implantable cardioverter-defibrillators. *Circulation* 2000;101:158–164.
42. Leor J, Poole WK, Kloner RA. Sudden cardiac death triggered by an earthquake (see comments). *N Engl J Med* 1996;334:413–419.
43. McElduff P, Dobson AJ. Case fatality after an acute cardiac event: The effect of smoking and alcohol consumption. *J Clin Epidemiol* 2001;54: 58–67.
44. Wannamethee G, Shaper AG. Alcohol and sudden cardiac death. *Br Heart J* 1992;68:443–448.
45. Kannel WB. Update on the role of cigarette smoking in coronary artery disease. *Am Heart J* 1981;101:319–328.
46. Hallstrom AP, Cobb LA, Ray R. Smoking as a risk factor for recurrence of sudden cardiac arrest. *N Engl J Med* 1986;314:271–275.
47. Fries R, Konig J, Schafers HJ, Bohm M. Triggering effect of physical and mental stress on spontaneous ventricular tachyarrhythmias in patients with implantable cardioverter-defibrillators. *Clin Cardiol* 2002;25:474–478.
48. Weinblatt E, Ruberman W, Goldberg JD, et al. Relation of education to sudden death after myocardial infarction. *N Engl J Med* 1978;299: 60–65.
49. Talbott E, Kuller LH, Detre K, Perper J. Biologic and psychosocial risk factors of sudden death from coronary disease in white women. *Am J Cardiol* 1977;39:858–864.
50. Mittleman MA, Maclure M, Tofler GH, et al. Triggering of acute myocardial infarction by heavy physical exertion. Protection against triggering by regular exertion. Determinants of Myocardial Infarction Onset Study Investigators (see comments). *N Engl J Med* 1993;329: 1677–1683.
51. Lemaitre RN, Siscovick DS, Raghunathan TE, et al. Leisure-time physical activity and the risk of primary cardiac arrest. *Arch Intern Med* 1999;159:686–690.
52. Albert CM, Mittleman MA, Chae CU, et al. Triggering of sudden death from cardiac causes by vigorous exertion. *N Engl J Med* 2000; 343:1355–1361.
53. Cobb LA, Weaver WD. Exercise: A risk for sudden death in patients with coronary heart disease. *J Am Coll Cardiol* 1986;7:215–219.
54. Liberthson RR. Sudden death from cardiac causes in children and young adults. *N Engl J Med* 1996;334:1039–1044.
55. Burke AP, Farb A, Virmani R, et al. Sports-related and non-sports-related sudden cardiac death in young adults. *Am Heart J* 1991;121: 568–575.
56. Maron BJ, Shirani J, Poliac LC, et al. Sudden death in young competitive athletes. Clinical, demographic, and pathological profiles (see comments). *JAMA* 1996;276:199–204.
57. Maron BJ, Roberts WC, McAllister HA, et al. Sudden death in young athletes. *Circulation* 1980;62:218–229.
58. Jensen-Urstad M. Sudden death and physical activity in athletes and nonathletes. *Scand J Med Sci Sports* 1995;5:279–284.
59. Corrado D, Thiene G, Nava A, et al. Sudden death in young competitive athletes: Clinicopathologic correlations in 22 cases (see comments). *Am J Med* 1990;89:588–596.
60. Maron BJ, Bodison SA, Wesley YE, et al. Results of screening a large group of intercollegiate competitive athletes for cardiovascular disease. *J Am Coll Cardiol* 1987;10:1214–1221.
61. Estes NA III, Link MS, Cannom D, et al. Report of the NASPE policy conference on arrhythmias and the athlete. *J Cardiovasc Electrophysiol* 2001;12:1208–1219.
62. Maron BJ, Gohman TE, Kyle SB, et al. Clinical profile and spectrum of commotio cordis. *JAMA* 2002;287:1142–1146.
63. Jouven X, Desnos M, Guerot C, Ducimetiere P. Predicting sudden death in the population: The Paris Prospective Study I. *Circulation* 1999;99:1978–1983.
64. Friedlander Y, Siscovick DS, Arbogast P, et al. Sudden death and myocardial infarction in first degree relatives as predictors of primary cardiac arrest. *Atherosclerosis* 2002;162:211–216.
65. Spooner PM, Albert C, Benjamin EJ, et al. Sudden cardiac death, genes, and arrhythmogenesis: Consideration of new population and mechanistic approaches from a national heart, lung, and blood institute workshop, part I. *Circulation* 2001;103:2361–2364.
66. Myerburg RJ, Kessler KM, Bassett AL, Castellanos A. A biological approach to sudden cardiac death: structure, function and cause. *Am J Cardiol* 1989;63:1512–1516.
67. Willich SN, Maclure M, Mittleman M, et al. Sudden cardiac death. Support for a role of triggering in causation. *Circulation* 1993;87: 1442–1450.
68. Greene HL. Sudden arrhythmic cardiac death—Mechanisms, resuscitation and classification: The Seattle perspective. *Am J Cardiol* 1990; 65:4B–12B.
69. Bayes de Luna A, Coumel P, Leclercq JF. Ambulatory sudden cardiac death: Mechanisms of production of fatal arrhythmia on the basis of data from 157 cases. *Am Heart J* 1989;117:151–159.
70. Luu M, Stevenson WG, Stevenson LW, et al. Diverse mechanisms of unexpected cardiac arrest in advanced heart failure. *Circulation* 1989; 80:1675–1680.
71. Janse MJ, Wit AL. Electrophysiological mechanisms of ventricular arrhythmias resulting from myocardial ischemia and infarction. *Physiol Rev* 1989;69:1049–1169.

72. Dillon SM, Allessie MA, Ursell PC, Wit AL. Influences of anisotropic tissue structure on reentrant circuits in the epicardial border zone of subacute canine infarcts. *Circ Res* 1988;63:182–206.
73. Pogwizd SM, Corr PB. Mechanisms underlying the development of ventricular fibrillation during early myocardial ischemia. *Circ Res* 1990;66:672–695.
74. Levine JH, Guarnieri T, Kadish AH, et al. Changes in myocardial repolarization in patients undergoing balloon valvuloplasty for congenital pulmonary stenosis: Evidence for contraction-excitation feedback in humans. *Circulation* 1988;77:70–77.
75. Lerman BB, Engelstein ED, Burkhoff D. Mechanoelectrical feedback: Role of beta-adrenergic receptor activation in mediating load-dependent shortening of ventricular action potential and refractoriness. *Circulation* 2001;104:486–490.
76. Goldstein S, Landis JR, Leighton R, et al. Characteristics of the resuscitated out-of-hospital cardiac arrest victim with coronary heart disease. *Circulation* 1981;64:977–984.
77. Bigger JT Jr. Patients with malignant or potentially malignant ventricular arrhythmias: Opportunities and limitations of drug therapy in prevention of sudden death. *J Am Coll Cardiol* 1985;5:23B–26B.
78. Davies MJ. Anatomic features in victims of sudden coronary death. Coronary artery pathology. *Circulation* 1992;85:I19–I24.
79. Roberts WC, Kragel AH, Gertz SD, Roberts CS. Coronary arteries in unstable angina pectoris, acute myocardial infarction, and sudden coronary death. *Am Heart J* 1994;127:1588–1593.
80. McHenry PL, O'Donnell J, Morris SN, Jordan JJ. The abnormal exercise electrocardiogram in apparently healthy men: A predictor of angina pectoris as an initial coronary event during long-term follow-up. *Circulation* 1984;70:547–551.
81. Weiner DA, Ryan TJ, McCabe CH, et al. Risk of developing an acute myocardial infarction or sudden coronary death in patients with exercise-induced silent myocardial ischemia. A report from the Coronary Artery Surgery Study (CASS) registry. *Am J Cardiol* 1988; 62:1155–1158.
82. Marcus FI, Cobb LA, Edwards JE, et al. Mechanism of death and prevalence of myocardial ischemic symptoms in the terminal event after acute myocardial infarction. *Am J Cardiol* 1988;61:8–15.
83. Holmes DR Jr, Davis K, Gersh BJ, et al. Risk factor profiles of patients with sudden cardiac death and death from other cardiac causes: A report from the Coronary Artery Surgery Study (CASS). *J Am Coll Cardiol* 1989;13:524–530.
84. Taylor AJ, Rogan KM, Virmani R. Sudden cardiac death associated with isolated congenital coronary artery anomalies. *J Am Coll Cardiol* 1992;20:640–647.
85. Parchure N, Batchvarov V, Malik M, et al. Increased QT dispersion in patients with Prinzmetal's variant angina and cardiac arrest. *Cardiovasc Res* 2001;50:379–385.
86. Myerburg RJ, Kessler KM, Mallon SM, et al. Life-threatening ventricular arrhythmias in patients with silent myocardial ischemia due to coronary-artery spasm (see comments). *N Engl J Med* 1992;326:1451–1455.
87. Bory M, Pierron F, Panagides D, et al. Coronary artery spasm in patients with normal or near normal coronary arteries. Long-term follow-up of 277 patients. *Eur Heart J* 1996;17:1015–1021.
88. Roberts WC, Dicicco BS, Waller BF, et al. Origin of the left main from the right coronary artery or from the right aortic sinus with intramyocardial tunneling to the left side of the heart via the ventricular septum. The case against clinical significance of myocardial bridge or coronary tunnel. *Am Heart J* 1982;104:303–305.
89. Corrado D, Thiene G, Cocco P, Frescura C. Non-atherosclerotic coronary artery disease and sudden death in the young. *Br Heart J* 1992;68:601–607.
90. Hunsaker JCD, O'Connor WN, Lie JT. Spontaneous coronary arterial dissection and isolated eosinophilic coronary arteritis: sudden cardiac death in a patient with a limited variant of Churg-Strauss syndrome. *Mayo Clin Proc* 1992;67:761–766.
91. Goldeli O, Ural D, Komsuoglu B, et al. Abnormal QT dispersion in Behcet's disease. *Int J Cardiol* 1997;61:55–59.
92. Tanaka N, Naoe S, Masuda H, Ueno T. Pathological study of sequelae of Kawasaki disease (MCLS). With special reference to the heart and coronary arterial lesions. *Acta Pathol Jpn* 1986;36:1513–1527.
93. Cohle SD, Titus JL, Espinola A, Jachimczyk JA. Sudden unexpected death due to coronary giant cell arteritis. *Arch Pathol Lab Med* 1982; 106:171–172.
94. Mandell BF. Cardiovascular involvement in systemic lupus erythematosus. *Semin Arthritis Rheum* 1987;17:126–141.
95. Tamburro P, Wilber D. Sudden death in idiopathic dilated cardiomyopathy. *Am Heart J* 1992;124:1035–1045.
96. Packer M. Lack of relation between ventricular arrhythmias and sudden death in patients with chronic heart failure. *Circulation* 1992; 85:I50–I56.
97. Larsen L, Markham J, Haffajee CI. Sudden death in idiopathic dilated cardiomyopathy: Role of ventricular arrhythmias. *Pacing Clin Electrophysiol* 1993;16:1051–1059.
98. Knight BP, Goyal R, Pelosi F, et al. Outcome of patients with nonischemic dilated cardiomyopathy and unexplained syncope treated with an implantable defibrillator (see comments). *J Am Coll Cardiol* 1999;33:1964–1970.
99. Middlekauff HR, Stevenson WG, Woo MA, et al. Comparison of frequency of late potentials in idiopathic dilated cardiomyopathy and ischemic cardiomyopathy with advanced congestive heart failure and their usefulness in predicting sudden death. *Am J Cardiol* 1990;66: 1113–1117.
100. Naccarelli GV, Prystowsky EN, Jackman WM, et al. Role of electrophysiologic testing in managing patients who have ventricular tachycardia unrelated to coronary artery disease. *Am J Cardiol* 1982; 50:165–171.
101. Caceres J, Jazayeri M, McKinnie J, et al. Sustained bundle branch reentry as a mechanism of clinical tachycardia. *Circulation* 1989;79: 256–270.
102. McKenna WJ, Camm AJ. Sudden death in hypertrophic cardiomyopathy. Assessment of patients at high risk (comment). *Circulation* 1989;80:1489–1492.
103. Counihan PJ, Fei L, Bashir Y, et al. Assessment of heart rate variability in hypertrophic cardiomyopathy. Association with clinical and prognostic features. *Circulation* 1993;8:1682–1690.
104. Maron BJ. Hypertrophic cardiomyopathy: A systematic review. *JAMA* 2002;287:1308–1320.
105. Elliott PM, Poloniecki J, Dickie S, et al. Sudden death in hypertrophic cardiomyopathy: identification of high-risk patients. *J Am Coll Cardiol* 2000;36:2212–2218.
106. Romeo F, Pelliccia F, Cristofani R, et al. Hypertrophic cardiomyopathy: Is a left ventricular outflow tract gradient a major prognostic determinant? *Eur Heart J* 1990;11:233–240.
107. Spirito P, Maron BJ. Relation between extent of left ventricular hypertrophy and occurrence of sudden cardiac death in hypertrophic cardiomyopathy. *J Am Coll Cardiol* 1990;15:1521–1526.
108. Spirito P, Rapezzi C, Autore C, et al. Prognosis of asymptomatic patients with hypertrophic cardiomyopathy and nonsustained ventricular tachycardia (see comments). *Circulation* 1994;90:2743–2747.
109. Elliott PM, Gimeno Blanes JR, Mahon NG, et al. Relation between severity of left-ventricular hypertrophy and prognosis in patients with hypertrophic cardiomyopathy. *Lancet* 2001;357:420–424.
110. Olivotto I, Gistri R, Petrone P, et al. Maximum left ventricular thickness and risk of sudden death in patients with hypertrophic cardiomyopathy. *J Am Coll Cardiol* 2003;41:315–321.
111. Fananapazir L, Chang AC, Epstein SE, McAreavey D. Prognostic determinants in hypertrophic cardiomyopathy. Prospective evaluation of a therapeutic strategy based on clinical, Holter, hemodynamic, and electrophysiological findings. *Circulation* 1992;86:730–740.
112. Saumarez RC, Heald S, Gill J, et al. Primary ventricular fibrillation is associated with increased paced right ventricular electrogram fractionation. *Circulation* 1995;92:2565–2571.
113. Maron BJ, Shen W-K, Link MS, et al. Efficacy of implantable cardioverter-defibrillators for the prevention of sudden death in

patients with hypertrophic cardiomyopathy. *N Engl J Med* 2000;342: 365–373.
114. Marian AJ, Roberts R. Molecular genetic basis of hypertrophic cardiomyopathy: genetic markers for sudden cardiac death. *J Cardiovasc Electrophysiol* 1998;9:88–99.
115. Moolman JC, Corfield VA, Posen B, et al. Sudden death due to troponin T mutations. *J Am Coll Cardiol* 1997;29:549–555.
116. Zehender M, Faber T, Koscheck U, et al. Ventricular tachyarrhythmias, myocardial ischemia, and sudden cardiac death in patients with hypertensive heart disease. *Clin Cardiol* 1995;18:377–383.
117. Frohlich ED. State of the art lecture. Risk mechanisms in hypertensive heart disease. *Hypertension* 1999;34:782–789.
118. Messerli FH. Hypertension and sudden cardiac death. *Am J Hypertens* 1999;12:181S–188S.
119. Levy D, Garrison RJ, Savage DD, et al. Prognostic implications of echocardiographically determined left ventricular mass in the Framingham Heart Study (see comments). *N Engl J Med* 1990;322: 1561–1566.
120. Tanaka M, Fujiwara H, Onodera T, et al. Quantitative analysis of myocardial fibrosis in normals, hypertensive hearts, and hypertrophic cardiomyopathy. *Br Heart J* 1986;55:575–581.
121. Siscovick DS, Raghunathan TE, Psaty BM, et al. Diuretic therapy for hypertension and the risk of primary cardiac arrest (see comments). *N Engl J Med* 1994;330:1852–1857.
122. Hoes AW, Grobbee DE, Lubsen J, et al. Diuretics, beta-blockers, and the risk for sudden cardiac death in hypertensive patients (see comments). *Ann Intern Med* 1995;123:481–487.
123. O'Kelly BF, Massie BM, Tubau JF, Szlachcic J. Coronary morbidity and mortality, pre-existing silent coronary artery disease, and mild hypertension. *Ann Intern Med* 1989;110:1017–1026.
124. Tiso N, Stephan DA, Nava A, et al. Identification of mutations in the cardiac ryanodine receptor gene in families affected with arrhythmogenic right ventricular cardiomyopathy type 2 (ARVD2). *Hum Mol Genet* 2001;10:189–194.
125. Zipes DP, Wellens HJ. Sudden cardiac death (see comments). *Circulation* 1998;98:2334–2351.
126. Corrado D, Basso C, Thiene G, et al. Spectrum of clinicopathologic manifestations of arrhythmogenic right ventricular cardiomyopathy/dysplasia: A multicenter study. *J Am Coll Cardiol* 1997;30: 1512–1520.
127. Corrado D, Fontaine G, Marcus FI, et al. Arrhythmogenic right ventricular dysplasia/cardiomyopathy: Need for an international registry. *Circulation* 2000;101:101–106.
128. Haissaguerre M, Le Metayer P, D'Ivernois C, et al. Distinctive response of arrhythmogenic right ventricular disease to high-dose isoproterenol. *Pacing Clin Electrophysiol* 1990;13:2119–2126.
129. Pellikka PA, Nishimura RA, Bailey KR, Tajik AJ. The natural history of adults with asymptomatic, hemodynamically significant aortic stenosis (see comments). *J Am Coll Cardiol* 1990;15:1012–1017.
130. Bonow RO, Lakatos E, Maron BJ, Epstein SE. Serial long-term assessment of the natural history of asymptomatic patients with chronic aortic regurgitation and normal left ventricular systolic function. *Circulation* 1991;84:1625–1635.
131. Braunwald E. On the natural history of severe aortic stenosis (comment). *J Am Coll Cardiol* 1990;15:1018–1020.
132. Foppl M, Hoffmann A, Amann FW, et al. Sudden cardiac death after aortic valve surgery: Incidence and concomitant factors. *Clin Cardiol* 1989;12:202–207.
133. Alvarez L, Escudero C, Figuera D, Castillo-Olivares JL. Late sudden cardiac death in the follow-up of patients having a heart valve prosthesis. *J Thorac Cardiovasc Surg* 1992;104:502–510.
134. Keefe DL, Griffin JC, Harrison DC, Stinson EB. Atrioventricular conduction abnormalities in patients undergoing isolated aortic or mitral valve replacement. *Pacing Clin Electrophysiol* 1985;8:393–398.
135. Farb A, Tang AL, Atkinson JB, et al. Comparison of cardiac findings in patients with mitral valve prolapse who die suddenly to those who have congestive heart failure from mitral regurgitation and to those with fatal noncardiac conditions. *Am J Cardiol* 1992;70:234–239.
136. Nishimura RA, McGoon MD, Shub C, et al. Echocardiographically documented mitral-valve prolapse. Long-term follow-up of 237 patients. *N Engl J Med* 1985;313:1305–1309.
137. Marks AR, Choong CY, Sanfilippo AJ, et al. Identification of high-risk and low-risk subgroups of patients with mitral-valve prolapse. *N Engl J Med* 1989;320:1031–1036.
138. Devereux RB. Diagnosis and prognosis of mitral-valve prolapse (editorial). *N Engl J Med* 1989;320:1077–1079.
139. Topaz O, Edwards JE. Pathologic features of sudden death in children, adolescents, and young adults. *Chest* 1985;87:476–482.
140. Vohra J, Sathe S, Warren R, Malignant ventricular arrhythmias in patients with mitral valve prolapse and mild mitral regurgitation. *Pacing Clin Electrophysiol* 1993;16:387–393.
141. Puddu PE, Pasternac A, Tubau JF, et al. QT interval prolongation and increased plasma catecholamine levels in patients with mitral valve prolapse. *Am Heart J* 1983;105:422–428.
142. Ramos SG, Matturri L, Rossi L, Rossi MA. Lesions of mediastinal paraganglia in chronic chagasic cardiomyopathy: cause of sudden death? (editorial). *Am Heart J* 1996;131:417–420.
143. Winters SL, Cohen M, Greenberg S, et al. Sustained ventricular tachycardia associated with sarcoidosis: Assessment of the underlying cardiac anatomy and the prospective utility of programmed ventricular stimulation, drug therapy and an implantable antitachycardia device. *J Am Coll Cardiol* 1991;18:937–943.
144. Silka MJ, Hardy BG, Menashe VD, Morris CD. A population-based prospective evaluation of risk of sudden cardiac death after operation for common congenital heart defects. *J Am Coll Cardiol* 1998;32: 245–251.
145. Gatzoulis MA, Balaji S, Webber SA, et al. Risk factors for arrhythmia and sudden cardiac death late after repair of tetralogy of Fallot: a multicentre study. *Lancet* 2000;356:975–981.
146. Therrien J, Siu SC, Harris L, et al. Impact of pulmonary valve replacement on arrhythmia propensity late after repair of tetralogy of Fallot. *Circulation* 2001;103:2489–2494.
147. Gelatt M, Hamilton RM, McCrindle BW, et al. Arrhythmia and mortality after the Mustard procedure: A 30-year single-center experience. *J Am Coll Cardiol* 1997;29:194–201.
148. Krongrad E. Syncope and sudden death. In: Emmanouilides GC, ed. *Moss and Adams' Heart Disease in Infants, Children, and Adolescents: Including the Fetus and Young Adult,* 5th ed. Vol 2. Baltimore: Williams & Wilkins; 1995:1610.
149. Moss AJ, Schwartz PJ, Crampton RS, et al. The long QT syndrome: A prospective international study. *Circulation* 1985;71:17–21.
150. Vincent GM, Timothy KW, Leppert M, Keating M. The spectrum of symptoms and QT intervals in carriers of the gene for the long-QT syndrome (see comments). *N Engl J Med* 1992;327:846–852.
151. Roden DM, Lazzara R, Rosen M, et al. Multiple mechanisms in the long-QT syndrome. Current knowledge, gaps, and future directions. The SADS Foundation Task Force on LQTS. *Circulation* 1996;94: 1996–2012.
152. Schwartz PJ, Locati EH, Moss AJ, et al. Left cardiac sympathetic denervation in the therapy of congenital long QT syndrome. A worldwide report (see comments). *Circulation* 1991;84:503–511.
153. Antzelevitch C, Shimizu W, Yan GX, et al. The M cell: Its contribution to the ECG and to normal and abnormal electrical function of the heart (see comments). *J Cardiovasc Electrophysiol* 1999;10:1124–1152.
154. Nador F, Beria G, De Ferrari GM, et al. Unsuspected echocardiographic abnormality in the long QT syndrome. Diagnostic, prognostic, and pathogenetic implications. *Circulation* 1991;84:1530–1542.
155. Wilde AA, Jongbloed RJ, Doevendans PA, et al. Auditory stimuli as a trigger for arrhythmic events differentiate HERG-related (LQTS2) patients from KVLQT1-related patients (LQTS1). *J Am Coll Cardiol* 1999;33:327–332.
156. Priori SG, Napolitano C, Memmi M, et al. Clinical and molecular characterization of patients with catecholaminergic polymorphic ventricular tachycardia. *Circulation* 2002;106:69–74.
157. Lahat H, Pras E, Olender T, et al. A missense mutation in a highly conserved region of CASQ2 is associated with autosomal recessive

catecholamine-induced polymorphic ventricular tachycardia in Bedouin families from Israel. *Am J Hum Genet* 2001;69:1378–1384.

158. Viskin S, Belhassen B. Idiopathic ventricular fibrillation. *Am Heart J* 1990;120:661–671.
159. Morady F, Scheinman MM, Hess DS, et al. Clinical characteristics and results of electrophysiologic testing in young adults with ventricular tachycardia or ventricular fibrillation. *Am Heart J* 1983;106: 1306–1314.
160. Siebels J, Schneider M, Geiger M. Unexpected recurrences in survivors of cardiac arrest without organic heart disease (abstr). *Eur Heart J* 1991;12(suppl):86.
161. Wever EF, Hauer RN, Oomen A, et al. Unfavorable outcome in patients with primary electrical disease who survived an episode of ventricular fibrillation (see comments). *Circulation* 1993;88:1021–1029.
162. Wellens HJ, Lemery R, Smeets JL, et al. Sudden arrhythmic death without overt heart disease. *Circulation* 1992;85:I92–I97.
163. Aizawa Y, Naitoh N, Washizuka T, et al. Electrophysiological findings in idiopathic recurrent ventricular fibrillation: Special reference to mode of induction, drug testing, and long-term outcomes. *Pacing Clin Electrophysiol* 1996;19:929–939.
164. Brugada P, Abdollah H, Heddle B, Wellens HJ. Results of a ventricular stimulation protocol using a maximum of 4 premature stimuli in patients without documented or suspected ventricular arrhythmias. *Am J Cardiol* 1983;52:1214–1218.
165. DiCarlo LA Jr, Morady F, Schwartz AB, et al. Clinical significance of ventricular fibrillation-flutter induced by ventricular programmed stimulation. *Am Heart J* 1985;109:959–963.
166. Brugada P, Brugada J. Right bundle branch block, persistent ST-segment elevation and sudden cardiac death: A distinct clinical and electrocardiographic syndrome. A multicenter report (see comments). *J Am Coll Cardiol* 1992;20:1391–1396.
167. Wilde AAM, Antzelevitch C, Borggrefe M, et al. Proposed diagnostic criteria for the Brugada syndrome: Consensus report. *Circulation* 2002;106:2514–2519.
168. Kirschner RH, Eckner FA, Baron RC. The cardiac pathology of sudden, unexplained nocturnal death in Southeast Asian refugees. *JAMA* 1986;256:2700–2705.
169. Gotoh K. A histopathological study on the conduction system of the so-called "Pokkuri disease" (sudden unexpected cardiac death of unknown origin in Japan). *Jpn Circ J* 1976;40:753–768.
170. Nademanee K, Veerakul G, Nimmannit S, et al. Arrhythmogenic marker for the sudden unexplained death syndrome in Thai men. *Circulation* 1997;96:2595–2600.
171. Corrado D, Nava A, Buja G, et al. Familial cardiomyopathy underlies syndrome of right bundle branch block, ST-segment elevation and sudden death (see comments). *J Am Coll Cardiol* 1996;27:443–448.
172. Alings M, Wilde A. "Brugada" syndrome: clinical data and suggested pathophysiological mechanism. *Circulation* 1999;99:666–673.
173. Clancy CE, Rudy Y. $Na^+$ channel mutation that causes both Brugada and long-QT syndrome phenotypes: A simulation study of mechanism. *Circulation* 2002;105:1208–1213.
174. Bezzina C, Veldkamp MW, van Den Berg MP, et al. A single $Na^+$ channel mutation causing both long-QT and Brugada syndromes. *Circ Res* 1999;85:1206–1213.
175. Priori SG, Napolitano C, Schwartz PJ, et al. The elusive link between LQT3 and Brugada syndrome: The role of flecainide challenge. *Circulation* 2000;102:945–947.
176. Yan G-X, Antzelevitch C. Cellular basis for the Brugada syndrome and other mechanisms of arrhythmogenesis associated with ST-segment elevation. *Circulation* 1999;100:1660–1666.
177. Antzelevitch C, Brugada P, Brugada J, et al. Brugada syndrome: A decade of progress. *Circ Res* 2002;91:1114–1118.
178. Lukas A, Antzelevitch C. Phase 2 reentry as a mechanism of initiation of circus movement reentry in canine epicardium exposed to simulated ischemia. *Cardiovasc Res* 1996;32:593–603.
179. Priori SG, Aliot E, Blomstrom-Lundqvist C, et al. Task Force on Sudden Cardiac Death of the European Society of Cardiology. *Eur Heart J* 2001;22:1374–1450.
180. Priori SG, Napolitano C, Gasparini M, et al. Natural history of Brugada syndrome: Insights for risk stratification and management. *Circulation* 2002;105:1342–1347.
181. Munger TM, Packer DL, Hammill SC, et al. A population study of the natural history of Wolff-Parkinson-White syndrome in Olmsted County, Minnesota, 1953–1989. *Circulation* 1993;87:866–873.
182. Jackman WM, Wang XZ, Friday KJ, et al. Catheter ablation of accessory atrioventricular pathways (Wolff-Parkinson-White syndrome) by radiofrequency current (see comments). *N Engl J Med* 1991;324:1605–1611.
183. Leitch JW, Klein GJ, Yee R, Murdock C. Prognostic value of electrophysiology testing in asymptomatic patients with Wolff-Parkinson-White pattern [published erratum appears in *Circulation* 1991 Mar;83(3):1124] (see comments). *Circulation* 1990;82:1718–1723.
184. Zardini M, Yee R, Thakur RK, Klein GJ. Risk of sudden arrhythmic death in the Wolff-Parkinson-White syndrome: Current perspectives. *Pacing Clin Electrophysiol* 1994;17:966–975.
185. Klein GJ, Bashore TM, Sellers TD, et al. Ventricular fibrillation in the Wolff-Parkinson-White syndrome. *N Engl J Med* 1979;301:1080–1085.
186. Chen SA, Chiang CE, Tai CT, et al. Longitudinal clinical and electrophysiological assessment of patients with symptomatic Wolff-Parkinson-White syndrome and atrioventricular node reentrant tachycardia. *Circulation* 1996;93:2023–2032.
187. Frey W. Weitere Erfahrungen mit Chinidin bei absoluter Herzunregelma bigkeit. *Wien Klin Wochenschr* 1918;55:849–853.
188. Echt DS, Liebson PR, Mitchell LB, et al. Mortality and morbidity in patients receiving encainide, flecainide, or placebo. The Cardiac Arrhythmia Suppression Trial (see comments). *N Engl J Med* 1991; 324:781–788.
189. Minardo JD, Heger JJ, Miles WM, et al. Clinical characteristics of patients with ventricular fibrillation during antiarrhythmic drug therapy. *N Engl J Med* 1988;319:257–262.
190. Zimetbaum PJ, Schreckengost VE, Cohen DJ, et al. Evaluation of outpatient initiation of antiarrhythmic drug therapy in patients reverting to sinus rhythm after an episode of atrial fibrillation. *Am J Cardiol* 1999;83:450–452, A9.
191. Fuster V, Ryden LE, Asinger RW, et al. ACC/AHA/ESC Guidelines for the Management of Patients with Atrial Fibrillation: Executive Summary Report of the American College of Cardiology/American Heart Association Task Force on Practice Guidelines and the European Society of Cardiology Committee for Practice Guidelines and Policy Conferences (Committee to Develop Guidelines for the Management of Patients with Atrial Fibrillation) Developed in Collaboration with the North American Society of Pacing and Electrophysiology. *Circulation* 2001;104:2118–2150.
192. Nattel S, Pedersen DH, Zipes DP. Alterations in regional myocardial distribution and arrhythmogenic effects of aprindine produced by coronary artery occlusion in the dog. *Cardiovasc Res* 1981;15:80–85.
193. Packer M, Medina N, Yushak M. Hemodynamic and clinical limitations of long-term inotropic therapy with amrinone in patients with severe chronic heart failure. *Circulation* 1984;70:1038–1047.
194. Raymond JR, van den Berg EK Jr, Knapp MJ. Nontraumatic prehospital sudden death in young adults. *Arch Intern Med* 1988;148: 303–308.
195. Hearn WL, Flynn DD, Hime GW, et al. Cocaethylene: A unique cocaine metabolite displays high affinity for the dopamine transporter. *J Neurochem* 1991;56:698–701.
196. Isner JM, Estes NAD, Thompson PD, et al. Acute cardiac events temporally related to cocaine abuse. *N Engl J Med* 1986;315: 1438–1443.
197. Nordrehaug JE, Johannessen KA, von der Lippe G. Serum potassium concentration as a risk factor of ventricular arrhythmias early in acute myocardial infarction. *Circulation* 1985;71:645–649.
198. Hoes AW, Grobbee DE, Peet TM, Lubsen J. Do non-potassium-sparing diuretics increase the risk of sudden cardiac death in hypertensive patients? Recent evidence. *Drugs* 1994;47:711–733.
199. Gettes LS. Electrolyte abnormalities underlying lethal and ventricular arrhythmias. *Circulation* 1992;85:I70–I76.

200. Eisenberg MJ. Magnesium deficiency and sudden death (editorial). *Am Heart J* 1992;124:544–549.
201. Litwin PE, Eisenberg MS, Hallstrom AP, Cummins RO. The location of collapse and its effect on survival from cardiac arrest. *Ann Emerg Med* 1987;16:787–791.
202. Kuller LH, Perper JA, Cooper MC. Sudden and unexpected death due to arteriosclerotic heart disease. *Mod Trends Cardiol* 1974;3:292–332.
203. Cummins RO, Ornato JP, Thies WH, Pepe PE. Improving survival from sudden cardiac arrest: the "chain of survival" concept. A statement for health professionals from the Advanced Cardiac Life Support Subcommittee and the Emergency Cardiac Care Committee, American Heart Association. *Circulation* 1991;83:1832–1847.
204. Myerburg RJ, Conde CA, Sung RJ, et al. Clinical, electrophysiologic and hemodynamic profile of patients resuscitated from prehospital cardiac arrest. *Am J Med* 1980;68:568–576.
205. Cobb LA, Fahrenbruch CE, Walsh TR, et al. Influence of cardiopulmonary resuscitation prior to defibrillation in patients with out-of-hospital ventricular fibrillation. *JAMA* 1999;281:1182–1188.
206. Valenzuela TD, Roe DJ, Nichol G, et al. Outcomes of rapid defibrillation by security officers after cardiac arrest in casinos. *N Engl J Med* 2000;343:1206–1209.
207. Myerburg RJ, Fenster J, Velez M, et al. Impact of community-wide police car deployment of automated external defibrillators on survival from out-of-hospital cardiac arrest. *Circulation* 2002;106:1058–1064.
208. Capucci A, Aschieri D, Piepoli MF, et al. Tripling survival from sudden cardiac arrest via early defibrillation without traditional education in cardiopulmonary resuscitation. *Circulation* 2002;106:1065–1070.
209. Guidelines for cardiopulmonary resuscitation and emergency cardiac care. Emergency Cardiac Care Committee and Subcommittees, American Heart Association. Part I. Introduction (see comments). *JAMA* 1992;268:2171–2183.
210. Lerman BB, Engelstein ED. Metabolic determinants of defibrillation. Role of adenosine. *Circulation* 1995;91:838–844.
211. Leenhardt A, Glaser E, Burguera M, et al. Short-coupled variant of torsades de pointes. A new electrocardiographic entity in the spectrum of idiopathic ventricular tachyarrhythmias. *Circulation* 1994;89:206–215.
212. Cobb LA, Weaver WD, Fahrenbruch CE, et al. Community-based interventions for sudden cardiac death. Impact, limitations, and changes. *Circulation* 1992;85:I98–I102.
213. Kudenchuk PJ, Cobb LA, Copass MK, et al. Amiodarone for resuscitation after out-of-hospital cardiac arrest due to ventricular fibrillation (see comments). *N Engl J Med* 1999;341:871–878.
214. Dickey W, Adgey AA. Mortality within hospital after resuscitation from ventricular fibrillation outside hospital. *Br Heart J* 1992;67:334–338.
215. Hallstrom AP, Cobb LA, Yu BH. Influence of comorbidity on the outcome of patients treated for out-of-hospital ventricular fibrillation. *Circulation* 1996;93:2019–2022.
216. Longstreth WT Jr, Cobb LA, Fahrenbruch CE, Copass MK. Does age affect outcomes of out-of-hospital cardiopulmonary resuscitation? (see comments). *JAMA* 1990;264:2109–2110.
217. Kempf FC Jr, Josephson ME. Cardiac arrest recorded on ambulatory electrocardiograms. *Am J Cardiol* 1984;53:1577–1582.
218. Wyse DG, Friedman PL, Brodsky MA, et al. Life-threatening ventricular arrhythmias due to transient or correctable causes: High risk for death in follow-up. *J Am Coll Cardiol* 2001;38:1718–1724.
219. Pinski SL, Yao Q, Epstein AE, et al. Determinants of outcome in patients with sustained ventricular tachyarrhythmias: The Antiarrhythmics Versus Implantable Defibrillators (AVID) study registry. *Am Heart J* 2000;139:804–813.
220. Middlekauff HR, Stevenson WG, Saxon LA. Prognosis after syncope: Impact of left ventricular function. *Am Heart J* 1993;125:121–127.
221. Wilber DJ, Garan H, Finkelstein D, et al. Out-of-hospital cardiac arrest. Use of electrophysiologic testing in the prediction of long-term outcome. *N Engl J Med* 1988;318:19–24.
222. Herre JM, Sauve MJ, Malone P, et al. Long-term results of amiodarone therapy in patients with recurrent sustained ventricular tachycardia or ventricular fibrillation. *J Am Coll Cardiol* 1989;13:442–449.
223. Weinberg BA, Miles WM, Klein LS, et al. Five-year follow-up of 589 patients treated with amiodarone. *Am Heart J* 1993;125:109–120.
224. Greenberg H, McMaster P, Dwyer EM Jr. Left ventricular dysfunction after acute myocardial infarction: results of a prospective multicenter study. *J Am Coll Cardiol* 1984;4:867–874.
225. Tomaselli GF, Beuckelmann DJ, Calkins HG, et al. Sudden cardiac death in heart failure. The role of abnormal repolarization (see comments). *Circulation* 1994;90:2534–2539.
226. Wilson JR, Schwartz JS, Sutton MS, et al. Prognosis in severe heart failure: Relation to hemodynamic measurements and ventricular ectopic activity. *J Am Coll Cardiol* 1983;2:403–410.
227. Algra A, Tijssen JG, Roelandt JR, et al. QTc prolongation measured by standard 12-lead electrocardiography is an independent risk factor for sudden death due to cardiac arrest. *Circulation* 1991;83:1888–1894.
228. Day CP, McComb JM, Campbell RW. QT dispersion: An indication of arrhythmia risk in patients with long QT intervals. *Br Heart J* 1990;63:342–344.
229. Barr CS, Naas A, Freeman M, et al. QT dispersion and sudden unexpected death in chronic heart failure (see comments). *Lancet* 1994;343:327–329.
230. Shaper AG, Wannamethee G, Macfarlane PW, Walker M. Heart rate, ischaemic heart disease, and sudden cardiac death in middle-aged British men. *Br Heart J* 1993;70:49–55.
231. Bigger JT Jr, Fleiss JL, Kleiger R, et al. The relationships among ventricular arrhythmias, left ventricular dysfunction, and mortality in the 2 years after myocardial infarction. *Circulation* 1984;69:250–258.
232. Holmes J, Kubo SH, Cody RJ, Kligfield P. Arrhythmias in ischemic and nonischemic dilated cardiomyopathy: Prediction of mortality by ambulatory electrocardiography. *Am J Cardiol* 1985;55:146–151.
233. Gomes JA, Winters SL, Stewart D, et al. A new noninvasive index to predict sustained ventricular tachycardia and sudden death in the first year after myocardial infarction: Based on signal-averaged electrocardiogram, radionuclide ejection fraction and Holter monitoring. *J Am Coll Cardiol* 1987;10:349–357.
234. Kuchar DL, Thorburn CW, Sammel NL. Prediction of serious arrhythmic events after myocardial infarction: Signal-averaged electrocardiogram, Holter monitoring and radionuclide ventriculography. *J Am Coll Cardiol* 1987;9:531–538.
235. Farrell TG, Bashir Y, Cripps T, et al. Risk stratification for arrhythmic events in postinfarction patients based on heart rate variability, ambulatory electrocardiographic variables and the signal-averaged electrocardiogram (see comments). *J Am Coll Cardiol* 1991;18:687–697.
236. Chakko CS, Gheorghiade M. Ventricular arrhythmias in severe heart failure: Incidence, significance, and effectiveness of antiarrhythmic therapy. *Am Heart J* 1985;109:497–504.
237. Barber MJ, Mueller TM, Henry DP, et al. Transmural myocardial infarction in the dog produces sympathectomy in noninfarcted myocardium. *Circulation* 1983;67:787–796.
238. Takahashi N, Zipes DP. Vagal modulation of adrenergic effects on canine sinus and atrioventricular nodes. *Am J Physiol* 1983;244:H775–H781.
239. Hull SS Jr, Vanoli E, Adamson PB, et al. Exercise training confers anticipatory protection from sudden death during acute myocardial ischemia (see comments). *Circulation* 1994;89:548–552.
240. Barron HV, Lesh MD. Autonomic nervous system and sudden cardiac death [published erratum appears in *J Am Coll Cardiol* 1996 Jul;28(1):286]. *J Am Coll Cardiol* 1996;27:1053–1060.
241. La Rovere MT, Pinna GD, Hohnloser SH, et al. Baroreflex sensitivity and heart rate variability in the identification of patients at risk for life-threatening arrhythmias: Implications for clinical trials. *Circulation* 2001;103:2072–2077.
242. Farrell TG, Odemuyiwa O, Bashir Y, et al. Prognostic value of baroreflex sensitivity testing after acute myocardial infarction. *Br Heart J* 1992;67:129–137.
243. Algra A, Tijssen JG, Roelandt JR, et al. Heart rate variability from 24-hour electrocardiography and the 2-year risk for sudden death. *Circulation* 1993;88:180–185.

244. Rosenbaum DS, He B, Cohen RJ. New approaches for evaluating cardiac electrical activity: Repolarization alternans and body surface mapping. In: Zipes DP, Jalife J, eds. *Cardiac Electrophysiology: From Cell to Bedside.* Philadelphia: Saunders; 1995.
245. Rosenbaum DS, Jackson LE, Smith JM, et al. Electrical alternans and vulnerability to ventricular arrhythmias. *N Engl J Med* 1994;330: 235–241.
246. Simson MB. Noninvasive identification of patients at high risk for sudden cardiac death. Signal-averaged electrocardiography. *Circulation* 1992;85:I145–I151.
247. Mancini DM, Wong KL, Simson MB. Prognostic value of an abnormal signal-averaged electrocardiogram in patients with nonischemic congestive cardiomyopathy (see comments). *Circulation* 1993;87:1083–1092.
248. Ruskin JN. Role of invasive electrophysiological testing in the evaluation and treatment of patients at high risk for sudden cardiac death. *Circulation* 1992;85:I152–I159.
249. Kelly P, Ruskin JN, Vlahakes GJ, et al. Surgical coronary revascularization in survivors of prehospital cardiac arrest: Its effect on inducible ventricular arrhythmias and long-term survival (see comments). *J Am Coll Cardiol* 1990;15:267–273.
250. Andresen D, Steinbeck G, Bruggemann T, et al. Prognosis of patients with sustained ventricular tachycardia and of survivors of cardiac arrest not inducible by programmed stimulation. *Am J Cardiol* 1992; 70:1250–1254.
251. Poole JE, Mathisen TL, Kudenchuk PJ, et al. Long-term outcome in patients who survive out-of-hospital ventricular fibrillation and undergo electrophysiologic studies: Evaluation by electrophysiologic subgroups (see comments). *J Am Coll Cardiol* 1990;16:657–665.
252. Mangi AA, Boeve TJ, Vlahakes GJ, et al. Surgical coronary revascularization and antiarrhythmic therapy in survivors of out-of-hospital cardiac arrest. *Ann Thorac Surg* 2002;74:1510–1516.
253. Kendall MJ, Lynch KP, Hjalmarson A, Kjekshus J. Beta-blockers and sudden cardiac death (see comments). *Ann Intern Med* 1995;123: 358–367.
254. Yusuf S, Peto R, Lewis J, et al. Beta blockade during and after myocardial infarction: An overview of the randomized trials. *Prog Cardiovasc Dis* 1985;27:335–371.
255. Singh BN. Advantages of beta blockers versus antiarrhythmic agents and calcium antagonists in secondary prevention after myocardial infarction. *Am J Cardiol* 1990;66:9C–20C.
256. Goldstein S, Hjalmarson A. The mortality effect of metoprolol CR/XL in patients with heart failure: Results of the MERIT-HF Trial. *Clin Cardiol* 1999;22(suppl 5):V30–V35.
257. Pfeffer MA, Braunwald E, Moye LA, et al. Effect of captopril on mortality and morbidity in patients with left ventricular dysfunction after myocardial infarction. Results of the Survival and Ventricular Enlargement trial. The SAVE Investigators (see comments). *N Engl J Med* 1992;327:669–677.
258. Ambrosioni E, Borghi C, Magnani B. The effect of the angiotensin-converting-enzyme inhibitor zofenopril on mortality and morbidity after anterior myocardial infarction. The Survival of Myocardial Infarction Long-Term Evaluation (SMILE) Study Investigators (see comments). *N Engl J Med* 1995;332:80–85.
259. Kober L, Torp-Pedersen C, Carlsen JE, et al. A clinical trial of the angiotensin-converting-enzyme inhibitor trandolapril in patients with left ventricular dysfunction after myocardial infarction. Trandolapril Cardiac Evaluation (TRACE) Study Group (see comments). *N Engl J Med* 1995;333:1670–1676.
260. Cohn JN, Johnson G, Ziesche S, et al. A comparison of enalapril with hydralazine-isosorbide dinitrate in the treatment of chronic congestive heart failure (see comments). *N Engl J Med* 1991;325:303–310.
261. Effects of enalapril on mortality in severe congestive heart failure. Results of the Cooperative North Scandinavian Enalapril Survival Study (CONSENSUS). The CONSENSUS Trial Study Group. *N Engl J Med* 1987;316:1429–1435.
262. Effect of enalapril on survival in patients with reduced left ventricular ejection fractions and congestive heart failure. The SOLVD Investigators (see comments). *N Engl J Med* 1991;325:293–302.
263. Effect of enalapril on mortality and the development of heart failure in asymptomatic patients with reduced left ventricular ejection fractions. The SOLVD Investigators [published erratum appears in *N Engl J Med* 1992 Dec 10;327(24):1768] (see comments). *N Engl J Med* 1992;327: 685–691.
264. Domanski MJ, Exner DV, Borkowf CB, et al. Effect of angiotensin converting enzyme inhibition on sudden cardiac death in patients following acute myocardial infarction. A meta-analysis of randomized clinical trials. *J Am Coll Cardiol* 1999;33:598–604.
265. The Heart Outcomes Prevention Evaluation Study Investigators. Effects of an angiotensin-converting-enzyme inhibitor, ramipril, on cardiovascular events in high-risk patients. *N Engl J Med* 2000;342: 145–153.
266. Teo KK, Yusuf S, Furberg CD. Effects of prophylactic antiarrhythmic drug therapy in acute myocardial infarction. An overview of results from randomized controlled trials (see comments). *JAMA* 1993;270: 1589–1595.
267. Hine LK, Laird N, Hewitt P, Chalmers TC. Meta-analytic evidence against prophylactic use of lidocaine in acute myocardial infarction. *Arch Intern Med* 1989;149:2694–2698.
268. Moosvi AR, Goldstein S, VanderBrug Medendorp S, et al. Effect of empiric antiarrhythmic therapy in resuscitated out-of-hospital cardiac arrest victims with coronary artery disease. *Am J Cardiol* 1990;65: 1192–1197.
268a. Kuck KH, Cappato R, Siebels J, Ruppel R. Randomized comparison of antiarrhythmic drug therapy with implantable defibrillators in patients resuscitated from cardiac arrest: The Cardiac Arrest Study Hamburg (CASH). *Circulation* 2000;102:748–754.
269. Hohnloser SH, Woosley RL. Sotalol. *N Engl J Med* 1994;331:31–38.
270. Mason JW. A comparison of electrophysiologic testing with Holter monitoring to predict antiarrhythmic-drug efficacy for ventricular tachyarrhythmias. Electrophysiologic Study versus Electrocardiographic Monitoring Investigators (see comments). *N Engl J Med* 1993;329:445–451.
271. Waldo AL, Camm AJ, deRuyter H, et al. Effect of *d*-sotalol on mortality in patients with left ventricular dysfunction after recent and remote myocardial infarction. The SWORD Investigators. Survival With Oral *d*-Sotalol (see comments) [published erratum appears in *Lancet* 1996 Aug 10;348(9024):416]. *Lancet* 1996;348:7–12.
272. Siebels J, Kuck KH. Implantable cardioverter defibrillator compared with antiarrhythmic drug treatment in cardiac arrest survivors (the Cardiac Arrest Study Hamburg). *Am Heart J* 1994;127:1139–1144.
273. Bocker D, Haverkamp W, Block M, et al. Comparison of *d,l*-sotalol and implantable defibrillators for treatment of sustained ventricular tachycardia or fibrillation in patients with coronary artery disease. *Circulation* 1996;94:151–157.
274. Zipes DP, Prystowsky EN, Heger JJ. Amiodarone: Electrophysiologic actions, pharmacokinetics and clinical effects. *J Am Coll Cardiol* 1984;3:1059–1071.
275. Olson PJ, Woelfel A, Simpson RJ Jr, Foster JR. Stratification of sudden death risk in patients receiving long-term amiodarone treatment for sustained ventricular tachycardia or ventricular fibrillation. *Am J Cardiol* 1993;71:823–826.
276. Nademanee K, Singh BN, Stevenson WG, Weiss JN. Amiodarone and post-MI patients. *Circulation* 1993;88:764–774.
277. Burkart F, Pfisterer M, Kiowski W, et al. Effect of antiarrhythmic therapy on mortality in survivors of myocardial infarction with asymptomatic complex ventricular arrhythmias: Basel Antiarrhythmic Study of Infarct Survival (BASIS) (see comments). *J Am Coll Cardiol* 1990;16:1711–1718.
278. Cairns JA, Connolly SJ, Roberts R, Gent M. Randomised trial of outcome after myocardial infarction in patients with frequent or repetitive ventricular premature depolarisations: CAMIAT. Canadian Amiodarone Myocardial Infarction Arrhythmia Trial Investigators [published erratum appears in *Lancet* 1997 Jun 14;349(9067):1776] (see comments). *Lancet* 1997;349:675–682.
279. Julian DG, Camm AJ, Frangin G, et al. Randomised trial of effect of amiodarone on mortality in patients with left-ventricular dysfunction

after recent myocardial infarction: EMIAT. European Myocardial Infarct Amiodarone Trial Investigators [published errata appear in *Lancet* 1997 Apr 19;349(9059):1180 and 1997 Jun 14;349(9067): 1776] (see comments). *Lancet* 1997;349:667–674.

280. Doval HC, Nul DR, Grancelli HO, et al. Randomised trial of low-dose amiodarone in severe congestive heart failure. Grupo de Estudio de la Sobrevida en la Insuficiencia Cardiaca en Argentina (GESICA) (see comments). *Lancet* 1994;344:493–498.
281. Singh SN, Fletcher RD, Fisher SG, et al. Amiodarone in patients with congestive heart failure and asymptomatic ventricular arrhythmia. Survival Trial of Antiarrhythmic Therapy in Congestive Heart Failure (see comments). *N Engl J Med* 1995;333:77–82.
282. A comparison of antiarrhythmic-drug therapy with implantable defibrillators in patients resuscitated from near-fatal ventricular arrhythmias. The Antiarrhythmics versus Implantable Defibrillators (AVID) Investigators (see comments). *N Engl J Med* 1997;337: 1576–1583.
283. Connolly SJ, Gent M, Roberts RS, et al. Canadian implantable defibrillator study (CIDS): A randomized trial of the implantable cardioverter defibrillator against amiodarone (see comments). *Circulation* 2000;101:1297–1302.
284. Kuck KH, Cappato R, Siebels J, Ruppel R. Randomized comparison of antiarrhythmic drug therapy with implantable defibrillators in patients resuscitated from cardiac arrest: The Cardiac Arrest Study Hamburg (CASH). *Circulation* 2000;102:748–754.
285. Dorian P, Cass D, Schwartz B, et al. Amiodarone as compared with lidocaine for shock-resistant ventricular fibrillation. *N Engl J Med* 2002;346:884–890.
286. Mirowski M, Reid PR, Mower MM, et al. Termination of malignant ventricular arrhythmias with an implanted automatic defibrillator in human beings. *N Engl J Med* 1980;303:322–324.
287. Zipes DP, Roberts D. Results of the international study of the implantable pacemaker cardioverter-defibrillator. A comparison of epicardial and endocardial lead systems. The Pacemaker-Cardioverter-Defibrillator Investigators. *Circulation* 1995;92:59–65.
288. Moss AJ, Hall WJ, Cannom DS, et al. Improved survival with an implanted defibrillator in patients with coronary disease at high risk for ventricular arrhythmia. Multicenter Automatic Defibrillator Implantation Trial Investigators (see comments). *N Engl J Med* 1996;335: 1933–1940.
289. Buxton AE, Lee KL, Fisher JD, et al. A randomized study of the prevention of sudden death in patients with coronary artery disease. Multicenter Unsustained Tachycardia Trial Investigators (see comments) [published erratum appears in *N Engl J Med* 2000 Apr 27;342(17):1300]. *N Engl J Med* 1999;341:1882–1890.
290. Moss AJ, Zareba W, Hall WJ, et al. Prophylactic implantation of a defibrillator in patients with myocardial infarction and reduced ejection fraction. *N Engl J Med* 2002;346:877–883.
291. Bigger JT Jr. Prophylactic use of implanted cardiac defibrillators in patients at high risk for ventricular arrhythmias after coronary-artery bypass graft surgery. Coronary Artery Bypass Graft (CABG) Patch Trial Investigators (see comments). *N Engl J Med* 1997;337: 1569–1575.
292. Holmes DR Jr, Davis KB, Mock MB, et al. The effect of medical and surgical treatment on subsequent sudden cardiac death in patients with coronary artery disease: A report from the Coronary Artery Surgery Study. *Circulation* 1986;73:1254–1263.
293. Garan H, Ruskin JN, DiMarco JP, et al. Electrophysiologic studies before and after myocardial revascularization in patients with life-threatening ventricular arrhythmias. *Am J Cardiol* 1983;51:519–524.
294. Veenhuyzen GD, Singh SN, McAreavey D, et al. Prior coronary artery bypass surgery and risk of death among patients with ischemic left ventricular dysfunction. *Circulation* 2001;104:1489–1493.
295. Every NR, Fahrenbruch CE, Hallstrom AP, et al. Influence of coronary bypass surgery on subsequent outcome of patients resuscitated from out of hospital cardiac arrest. *J Am Coll Cardiol* 1992;19:1435–1439.
296. Cook JR, Rizo-Patron C, Curtis AB, et al. Effect of surgical revascularization in patients with coronary artery disease and ventricular tachycardia or fibrillation in the Antiarrhythmics Versus Implantable Defibrillators (AVID) Registry. *Am Heart J* 2002;143:821–826.
297. Wang YS, Scheinman MM, Chien WW, et al. Patients with supraventricular tachycardia presenting with aborted sudden death: Incidence, mechanism and long-term follow-up (see comments). *J Am Coll Cardiol* 1991;18:1711–1719.
298. Langberg JJ, Desai J, Dullet N, Scheinman MM. Treatment of macroreentrant ventricular tachycardia with radiofrequency ablation of the right bundle branch. *Am J Cardiol* 1989;63:1010–1013.

CHAPTER 42

# CARDIOPULMONARY RESUSCITATION AND THE SUBSEQUENT MANAGEMENT OF THE PATIENT

Nisha Chandra-Strobos / Myron L. Weisfeldt



## INTRODUCTION: HISTORICAL ISSUES

Since biblical times, humans have attempted to restore life to the dead or nearly dead individual. The modern era of resuscitation began in 1940, when Wiggers pioneered the study of the mechanisms and treatment of ventricular fibrillation.[1] Major developments occurred in 1954, when Elam and colleagues showed that mouth-to-mouth or mouth-to-nose resuscitation was superior to the Schafer prone method of resuscitation in terms of efficacy of ventilation.[2,3] The importance of the circulation of blood was also recognized, and direct or internal cardiac massage became an accepted technique as early as 1916. Largely due to its complication rates and limited practical usefulness, it was replaced by noninvasive techniques of resuscitation.[4,5] In 1960, Kouwenhoven and coworkers developed the present technique of external chest compression in the supine position and coupled this with artificial respiration.[6] This technique of cardiopulmonary resuscitation (CPR) gained rapid popularity and was shown to be effective.[7] Only recently has the importance of prompt defibrillation taken a primary position in resuscitation efforts. Studies in large populations have confirmed that survival from prehospital cardiac arrest depends on both prompt CPR and prompt defibrillation.

## MECHANISMS OF MOVEMENT OF BLOOD DURING CARDIOPULMONARY RESUSCITATION

The original hypothesis suggested that blood flow to the periphery during external chest compression resulted from direct compression of the heart between the sternum and the vertebral column.[6] According to this concept, chest compression ("systole"), similar to internal cardiac massage, resulted in blood being squeezed from both ventricles into the great arteries as the pulmonary and aortic valves opened.

Retrograde flow of blood was prevented by closure of the mitral and tricuspid valves. During the release phase of chest compression ("diastole"), the ventricles recoiled to their original shape and filled by a suction effect, while elevated arterial pressure was thought to close both the pulmonic and aortic valves.

This widely held concept is not, however, consistent with a number of observations in animal models[8] and humans[9]; these suggest a correlation between the rise in intrathoracic pressure during chest compression and the apparent magnitude of carotid flow and pressure. The importance of fluctuations in intrathoracic pressure as a means for generating blood flow is further supported by the observations of Criley et al. that, by the continuous and early initiation of coughing, patients in ventricular fibrillation can maintain consciousness as long as cough is continued.[10] The critical ingredient of the cough is clearly a rise in intrathoracic pressure, probably with no cardiac compression. Criley's observations strongly suggest that following cardiac arrest, a rise in intrathoracic pressure is a potent mechanism for the movement of blood to the brain in humans.[10]

## EXPERIMENTAL OBSERVATIONS

For brain blood flow to occur during CPR, a carotid arterial-to-jugular pressure gradient must be present during chest compression. In large animals, chest compression during CPR results in an essentially equal rise in central venous, right atrial, pulmonary artery, aortic, esophageal, and lateral pleural space pressures with no transcardiac gradient being developed (Fig. 42-1).[11]

In large animals, aortic pressure is transmitted directly to the carotid arteries, but retrograde transmission of intrathoracic venous pressure into the jugular veins is prevented by valves at the thoracic inlet. Thus, during chest compression (systole), a peripheral arteriovenous pressure gradient appears, and blood flow occurs consequent to this gradient. During compression, there is no pressure gradient across the heart, therefore, the heart cannot be the pump responsible for generating blood flow during CPR. In fact, the heart functions merely as a passive conduit.

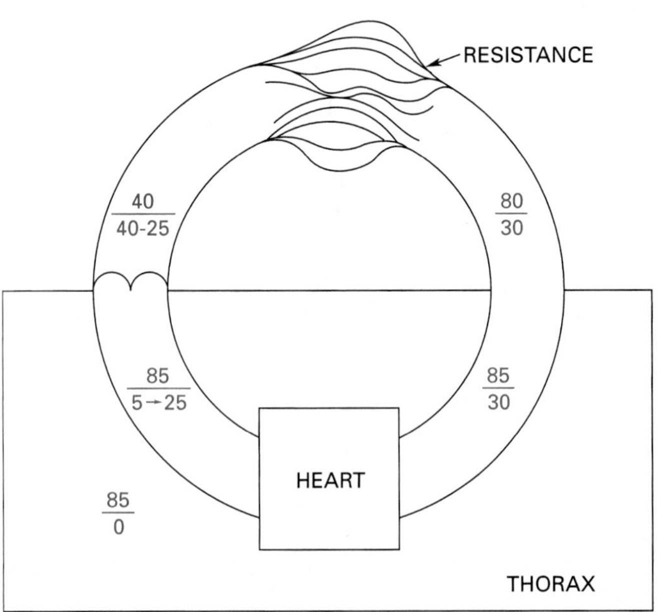


FIGURE 42-1 Representative pressures recorded during conventional cardiopulmonary resuscitation with forward carotid flow. Pressures are those recorded during compression. Intrathoracic pressures were indexed from esophageal pressures. There is no significant pressure gradient across the heart. The extrathoracic arterial pressure is similar to the intrathoracic aortic pressure. The extrathoracic venous pressure is markedly lower than the intrathoracic venous (right atrial) pressure. There is an extrathoracic arteriovenous pressure gradient that results in forward flow.

During diastole, a modest gradient also develops between the intrathoracic aorta and the right atrium and determines myocardial flow. Limited retrograde flow occurs into the aorta from extrathoracic arteries, raising aortic diastolic pressure and increasing coronary flow. The rise in intrathoracic pressure during chest compression is likely a consequence of airway collapse, which occurs at the level of the small bronchioles and results in air trapping. With the release of chest compression, this airway collapse is relieved.[12]

Unlike the hemodynamic pattern described above, in some animals intrathoracic vascular pressures during vigorous chest compression are much higher than pleural pressure.[13] In such animals, the rise in vascular pressures probably results from compression of the heart during chest compression, and the classic mechanism of direct cardiac compression is probably operating in these animals. Even during cardiac compression, however, venous valves at the thoracic inlet remain essential for establishing a peripheral arteriovenous pressure gradient, which facilitates peripheral flow. It is likely that flow produced by the two mechanisms operating simultaneously can occur, and in such situations the resultant flow is additive.

The position of the mitral valve during chest compression came to be regarded as a marker for the mechanism of blood flow during CPR, with mitral valve closure suggesting direct cardiac compression.[14] Some investigators, using transesophageal echocardiography, have demonstrated mitral valve closure during CPR in humans.[15] Others have reported that the mitral valve remains open during chest compression.[16] Animal studies have demonstrated that mitral valve closure or position cannot be used to identify the primary mechanism for blood flow during CPR.[17]

Studies of the perfusion of vital organs indicate that during CPR (irrespective of the primary mechanism for blood flow) cerebral flow is dependent on the gradient between the carotid artery and the intracranial pressure during systole, with myocardial flow being dependent on the gradient between the aorta and right atrium during diastole.[18] Recent data confirm that stopping chest compression for ventilation during CPR significantly decreases coronary perfusion pressures.

## OBSERVATIONS IN HUMANS

Unfortunately, at this point we can draw no final conclusion as to the frequency or importance of the two mechanisms (cardiac compression or generalized increase in intrathoracic pressure) during conventional cardiopulmonary resuscitation in humans. Published studies, however, suggest that manipulation of intrathoracic pressure is probably the dominant mechanism.[19] In a number of patients, comparable arterial and right atrial pressures have been observed as well as the presence of a pressure gradient at the thoracic inlet upon withdrawing an intravascular catheter from the superior vena cava to the extrathoracic internal jugular vein.[11,20,21] This hemodynamic pattern favors the concept of forward flow of blood through manipulation of intrathoracic pressure. This concept is further strengthened by the observation that maneuvers designed to increase intrathoracic pressure during chest compression—such as prolonged compression or vest CPR—are rewarded by a significant increase in peripheral arterial pressure. Recent studies have also shown increased peripheral arterial pressures in humans during CPR with the use of an inspiratory airflow resistance valve. Inspiratory resistance is designed to reduce diastolic intrathoracic pressure (during the release phase of chest compression) and thereby increase net intrathoracic pressure fluctuations.[23] Perhaps the strongest evidence supporting the theory of manipulation of intrathoracic pressure as a mechanism for blood flow in humans is found in the documented efficacy of "cough CPR."[10] In some patients, who are usually thin-chested, with cardiomegaly, extremely high arterial pressures are generated with conventional CPR. In a few of these patients, central venous pressure was found to be lower than arterial pressure. This hemodynamic picture suggests cardiac compression. In other patients, however, this higher arterial pressure may reflect higher generalized intrathoracic pressure during chest compression. This may be a result of functional airway obstruction due to airway collapse, pulmonary congestion, and/or bronchospasm.[12] In the majority of the patients in whom radial artery pressure has been measured during CPR, the arterial pressure has been relatively low and similar to that seen in the dog during conventional CPR.[19,20]

In human beings (and also in animals), it is not essential to think about the mechanisms of blood flow during CPR in an exclusive fashion. As the force of chest compression changes or as chest wall anatomy and chest compliance change during prolonged resuscitation, the dominant mechanism for blood flow (during resuscitation) may also change.

Building on these concepts, several experimental maneuvers and techniques have been developed to increase arterial pressure during chest compression. Following clinical evaluation, some are now being considered for limited clinical use. Some of these techniques require special equipment, whereas others can be performed by unequipped health care providers.

## EXPERIMENTAL AND ALTERNATIVE TECHNIQUES OF CARDIOPULMONARY RESUSCITATION

"High-impulse CPR" requires no special equipment and has been shown to improve vascular pressures.[13] It incorporates high-force, rapid down-thrust chest compression. However, clinical experience with this technique is limited.

*Interposed abdominal compression* (IAC) CPR can be performed by three unequipped health care providers. In this technique, the upper abdomen is compressed when the chest is released. The mechanism of benefit with IAC CPR in humans is unclear but may relate to improved venous return, decreased arterial runoff, or greater rise in intrathoracic pressure (with the diaphragm pushed up before chest compression). This technique increases carotid flow and improves survival in animals. Human clinical trials during in-hospital IAC CPR have also shown improved survival as compared with conventional CPR.[24] Based on these results, the 2000 American Heart Association (AHA) Guidelines for CPR suggest that IAC CPR be considered an alternative to conventional in-hospital CPR (class 2A recommendation).[25] The clinical value of this technique in the prehospital arrest patient, however, remains unproven.

The technique of phased chest and abdominal compression-decompression has also undergone animal and limited clinical testing. This technique is a mechanized IAC CPR in which the rescuer uses a special chest-abdomen manual compression device (the Lifestick Resuscitator); the chest and abdomen are thus compressed alternately. Its originators suggest that this technique, although similar to IAC CPR, is safer and more effective. Clinical studies are presently ongoing.[26]

The technique of perithoracic high-pressure vest inflation without airway manipulation (vest CPR) requires special equipment and allows cyclic increments in intrathoracic pressure to 100 to 150 mmHg during external chest compression. It has been shown to significantly increase cerebral and myocardial blood flow during CPR in animals. This technique employs a special computer-controlled pneumatic vest device positioned around the chest. Initial human data confirm higher vascular pressures during vest CPR as compared with conventional resuscitation.[22] Survival studies are lacking. A multicenter randomized survival trial was terminated prior to target patient enrollment. Data suggest that this technique may be of value as an alternative to standard CPR for short-term hemodynamic support.[26] Building on the technique of vest CPR, "Autopulse" CPR was developed and recently approved by the FDA. It consists of an electromechanical band, which is used for compression, with an air-filled cushion positioned between the band and the chest to distribute chest compression forces. It has had limited clinical testing.

*Active compression-decompression CPR* (ACD CPR) requires a special suction-cup plunger-type device that can be readily deployed by first responders. It incorporates a negative pressure "pull" on the thorax during the release phase of chest compression and slightly improves vascular pressures and air exchange during CPR.[27] The mechanism of benefit from this technique of resuscitation may relate to improved venous return and/or increased intrathoracic pressure. Except for one 500-patient French study, all other recent, large, in-hospital and out-of-hospital studies in cardiac arrest patients have shown no survival benefit of ACD CPR.[28,29] It may, however, be of some value in improving short-term resuscitation outcomes. Lurie et al. have reported on the hemodynamic benefits of an inspiratory impedance valve attached to the endotracheal tube during resuscitation. Preliminary human data suggest that this device, coupled with ACD CPR, increases coronary perfusion pressures and improves end-tidal $CO_2$ and increased return of spontaneous circulation.[23] Larger clinical studies and FDA approval are necessary before the clinical usefulness of this technique is assessed.

The clinical experience of hypothermia, following return of spontaneous circulation in patients with out-of-hospital, primarily witnessed ventricular fibrillation, is extremely promising and was reported in two separate clinical trials.[29a,29b] In such patients hypothermia to 33°C (91.4°F) was induced, maintained for 12 to 24 h, and resulted in a near doubling of survival to discharge and a significant increase in favorable neurologic outcomes. Based on these studies, it is now a recommended strategy of care for such patients, i.e., patients with out-of-hospital ventricular fibrillation arrest and successful resuscitation. In summary, data suggest that several experimental CPR techniques may offer short-term survival benefit—i.e., survival to hospital admission—but the data on long-term improved outcome as compared to conventional CPR are less compelling for all strategies studied.

Although such experimental techniques lend themselves to limited clinical use, their study has resulted in a better understanding of physiology, which, in turn, allows several aspects of conventional external chest compression to be manipulated in order to optimize vital organ perfusion pressures.[30] At higher rates of chest compression, more time per minute is spent in chest compression. Based on these data, changes in the AHA recommendations regarding chest compression rate have evolved. The 2000 standards recommend that chest compressions be performed at a rate of approximately 100/min.[25]

## DIAGNOSIS AND IDENTIFICATION OF CARDIAC ARREST

Cardiac arrest is defined as the sudden cessation of effective cardiac pumping function as a result of either ventricular asystole (electrical or mechanical) or ventricular fibrillation. Rapid diagnosis and treatment are essential because (1) more than a few minutes of total cardiac arrest result in permanent cerebral anoxic damage and (2) the success of resuscitative measures is related to the rapidity with which they are instituted following arrest. Based on these and other observations, the concept of early activation of emergency medical systems (EMS) has evolved for victims of out-of-hospital cardiac arrest[25] (see also Chap. 41).

## Preliminary Patient Evaluation and Triage

Cardiac arrest should be considered in the differential diagnosis of sudden collapse in any patient. It can be clinically confirmed by pulseless major vessels and absent heart sounds.

Although respirations (agonal respirations) may continue for a minute or two, the patient with cardiac arrest rapidly becomes cyanotic and unconscious.

Once the diagnosis of cardiac arrest is made and no trauma is suspected, the unconscious patient should be positioned supine on a firm surface and the airway opened using the head tilt–chin lift technique or alternative strategies, as described below (in the discussion of ventilation during CPR). The patient should receive rescue breathing either with a bag valve-mask device or with mouth-to-mouth breathing. Simple airway barrier devices, which are easily deployed, can be used to minimize direct patient contact and are perceived as being more hygienic during mouth-to-mouth resuscitation. Following airway opening and rescue breathing, chest compressions should be promptly initiated at approximately 100/min. Animal data suggest that ventilation can be deferred for several minutes in witnessed cardiac arrest without changing survival if chest compressions are initiated promptly. In addition, a recent study that randomized patients receiving dispatcher-assisted CPR to ventilation or no ventilation failed to demonstrate any benefit of early ventilation.[31] Pausing chest compressions for ventilation clearly compromises coronary perfusion pressures. These and other data have raised several questions regarding the need and benefit for early ventilation in patients in cardiac arrest. Nevertheless, the AHA continues to recommend early ventilation for all patients.[25]

If available, an electrocardiogram (ECG) can confirm the diagnosis and identify asystole, ventricular fibrillation, or electromechanical dissociation as the mechanism of arrest. However, CPR should be initiated immediately, as described above, once the clinical diagnosis is made without delaying to obtain this information. Prehospital CPR studies in several patients have confirmed that, early in cardiac arrest, the mechanism of arrest is usually ventricular fibrillation and that survival is critically dependent on the time to defibrillation.[32] Most hospitals and paramedics are now equipped with defibrillators with "quick look" paddles that simultaneously allow the ECG rhythm to be analyzed. On the basis of the rhythm, an etiology for the arrest can then be explored in a more focused way and appropriate therapy initiated. A recent debate has emerged prompted by animal data from Niemann et al. showing that animals receiving CPR prior to early defibrillation did better than those in whom no CPR preceded defibrillation.[33] This observation is further supported by recent data from Cobb et al. showing that 90 s of "high-quality" CPR prior to defibrillation improved outcome in patients receiving bystander CPR.[34] A recent randomized study of 200 patients in cardiac arrest with ventricular fibrillation compared immediate defibrillation to defibrillation preceded by 3 min of CPR and demonstrated no difference in survival. However, in patients with response times of >5 min, the group with prior CPR appeared to have better outcomes.[34a] The current recommendation is that if defibrillation is delayed, CPR should be performed immediately. However, if a defibrillator is available, the value of "predefibrillation CPR" is unclear. Clearly, if defibrillation fails to restore circulation, CPR should be performed immediately. Also, if collapse time without CPR is known to be more than 2 to 4 min, 90 s of initial CPR will likely be of value.

## AUTOMATED EXTERNAL DEFIBRILLATORS

Given the value of early defibrillation, automated external defibrillators (AEDs) were developed for use by first (minimally trained) professional responders and were shown to dramatically improve survival after prehospital arrest.[35,36] AEDs have an approximately 90 percent sensitivity and specificity for successfully recognized ventricular fibrillation. They are designed for use by first responders or persons with little medical training (e.g., fire fighters, EMS technicians). These devices have varying degrees of automation and can deliver several successive defibrillatory shocks via two self-adhesive electrodes placed by the user directly on the left anterior and left lateral chest. Most manual physician- or paramedic-operated waveform defibrillators deliver monophasic shocks. In recent years commercially available AEDs deliver a biphasic waveform shock. Recent research has focused on the relative efficacy of these two waveforms. Data suggest that biphasic waveform defibrillation using shocks <200 J are safe and as effective (if not more so) as higher-energy monophasic shocks. Also, animal data suggest less postshock myocardial dysfunction following biphasic waveform defibrillation. Various modifications of the biphasic waveform (sawtooth pattern, etc.) are being evaluated. Current recommendations do not clearly rank one defibrillatory waveform over the other; both are acceptable.

AEDs have been successfully used by nontraditional health care professionals (airline crews, police, and security guards) with dramatic improvement in patient survival. This program has been termed *public-access defibrillation.* All such AED defibrillation programs have been under strict physician-guided training and supervision. Perhaps the most compelling results of this strategy of emergency care were reported recently by White et al. in Rochester, Minnesota, where police-initiated AED defibrillation and resuscitation resulted in a survival to hospital discharge of approximately 50 percent (Fig. 42-2).[35] The value of training the on-site nontraditional health care provider was further tested and ratified when Valenzuela et al. trained casino security guards and demonstrated significant increases in resuscitation rates. They have demonstrated the compelling benefit of early defibrillation (Fig. 42-3).[37] AEDs were also used on a U.S. airline and had 100 percent specificity and sensitivity.[37a] There was an excellent rate of survival to discharge in patients so treated. Recently the Public Access Defibrillation Trial assessed the value of equipping lay rescuers with AEDs in select areas. This randomized trial demonstrated a near 50 percent greater survival to discharge in patients treated at AED-equipped sites. Some authors have questioned the cost-effectiveness of deploying first-responder AEDs. A treatment should be considered economically attractive if it is associated with an incremental cost-effectiveness ratio of less than twice the average annual income per life-year (i.e., approximately $50,000 per life-year). Modeling studies and clinical trials have demonstrated that the cost-effectiveness of first-responder AED programs is well within the cost of programs deemed to be clinically appropriate if achieved by a low-intensity intervention such as police or lay responder defibrillation (estimated cost, $29,000 to $46,700 per year). Available data suggest that time to defibrillation is not cost-effectively reduced by adding to existing EMS systems.[38] In a dramatic move to test the value of early AED deployment, several AEDs have been prominently positioned at Chicago's O'Hare Airport and have been successfully used by airport patrons. Recent state and federal legislation that endorses early AED deployment by trained, supervised persons and indemnifies users, trainers, and other owners of AEDs has paved the way to evaluate public-access defibrillation.

It is highly recommended that all first-responder EMS units be equipped with AEDs. Several agencies have developed training programs that incorporate AEDs and basic CPR training. However, the duration of training needed to correctly teach the use of an AED is likely much less than that currently used by most training agencies (i.e., only 3 h or less appear to be needed).

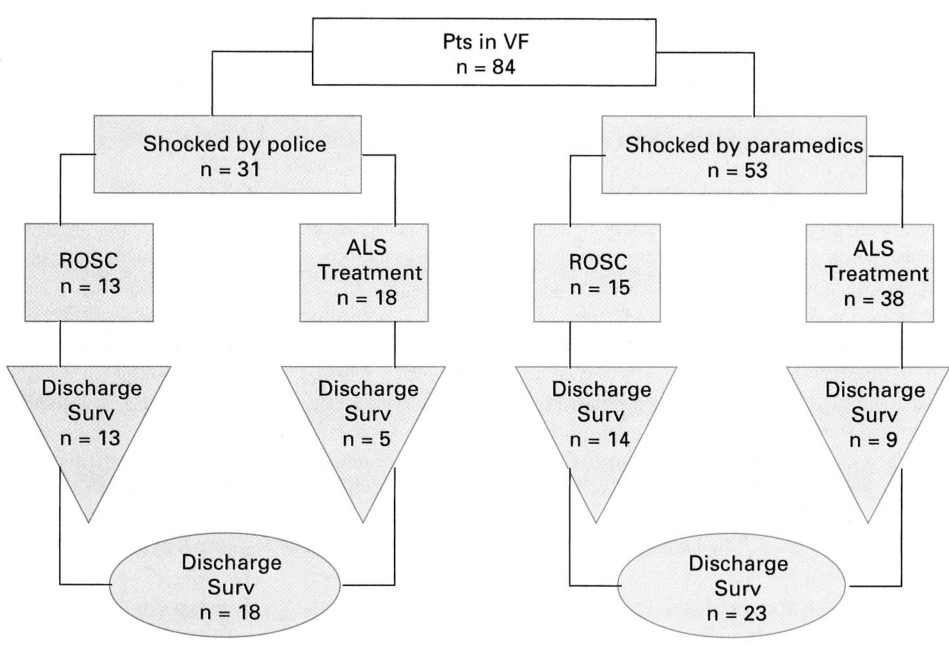


FIGURE 42-2 Police and paramedic treatment groups and patient outcome. VF = ventricular fibrillation; ROSC = restoration of spontaneous circulation; ALS = advanced life support. (From White et al.,[35] with permission.)

## RESPIRATORY ARREST

Respiratory arrest is the cessation of effective respiratory effort. It can result from airway obstruction (due to a foreign body or other causes), drowning, smoke inhalation, drug overdose, head trauma, cerebrovascular accident, or suffocation. When respiratory arrest occurs suddenly (as with foreign-body obstruction), the patient rapidly becomes cyanotic, though a palpable pulse with blood pressure, consciousness, and ineffective respiratory efforts may be maintained for several minutes. Opening of the airway and/or rescue breathing may be all that is necessary to resuscitate such a patient.

The Heimlich maneuver is recommended for relieving foreign-body airway obstruction. It is implemented by standing behind the victim and delivering a series of sharp thrusts to the upper abdomen with a closed fist.[39] Abdominal thrusts can also be used directly in the unconscious, supine patient by the trained health care provider to help dislodge a foreign body mechanically. The Heimlich maneuver can also be self-administered by placing the fist between the navel and the xiphoid process and delivering a series of quick upward thrusts. If incorrectly administered, this maneuver can lead to visceral damage.[40] When properly used, however, the technique is both safe and effective.

Manual removal of a foreign body in the unconscious victim should be done only by trained health care providers. This can be achieved by opening the victim's mouth and attempting to dislodge any obvious foreign body with a finger. As a single method, back blows may not be as effective as the Heimlich maneuver in adults.

## VENTILATION AND CHEST COMPRESSION DURING CARDIOPULMONARY RESUSCITATION

The 1980s defined the physiology of circulation during CPR. Thereafter, several investigators focused on understanding the physiology of ventilation during CPR (see below). Although several questions remain unanswered, recent research has served to challenge several "dogmas," as discussed below.

Clearing the airway is of the utmost importance. Foreign bodies, loose dentures, or any other oral obstruction should be removed. Next, the head tilt–chin lift technique, which causes the tongue to move anteriorly, is used to open the airway. The chin is lifted forward, with the fingers of one hand supporting the jaw, and the head is tilted back by the other hand, which rests on the patient's forehead.[35] The head tilt–neck lift method of opening the airway is also commonly employed and is an acceptable technique for use by the skilled rescuer. Here, the rescuer tilts the head back with one hand on the patient's forehead; the other hand is placed behind the patient's neck, lifting it upward to open the airway. If no spontaneous respirations are present, mouth-to-mouth (or mouth-to-nose) ventilation is immediately initiated, with adequacy being judged by the rise and fall of the patient's chest with each breath. To minimize gastric distention, it is necessary to deliver slow (2-s) ventilatory breaths.

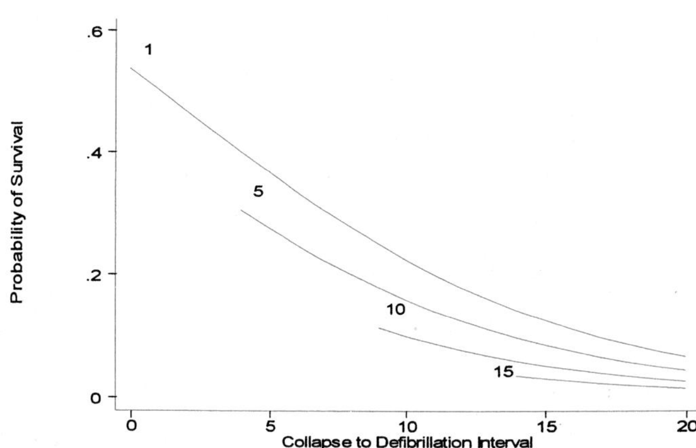


FIGURE 42-3 Relationship of collapse to CPR and defibrillation to survival: simplified model. Graphical representation of simplified (includes collapse to CPR and collapse to defibrillation only) predictive model of survival after witnessed out-of-hospital cardiac arrest due to VF. Each curve represents change in probability of survival as delay (minutes) to defibrillation increases fo a given collapse-to-CPR interval (minutes). (From Valenzuela et al.,[37] wit permission.)

Equipped rescuers will use a barrier device or a bag valve-mask technique of ventilation together with a small plastic oral "airway," which moves the tongue anteriorly. Adequate ventilation is difficult with the bag-valve-mask technique, since a single rescuer often has difficulty maintaining an adequate seal on the face, and rapid bag deflation commonly results in gastric distention and aspiration. Slow (2-s) ventilation must be employed if this technique is used.

Several invasive airway adjuncts have also been developed for use by nonphysician health care providers in prehospital situations, and several newer devices have been shown to be superior to the bag valve-mask technique of ventilation.[41] The esophageal obturator airway (EOA), esophageal gastric tube airway (EGTA), the Combitube, the laryngeal tracheal mask airway (LMA), and the pharyngotracheal lumen airway are among those that have been used in the prehospital setting. Considerable training and skill are needed in placing and using these devices properly. Serious, life-threatening complications have been reported following the use of the EOA or EGTA. As a consequence, their use has generally been abandoned in favor of other more safe and effective devices. Recent data suggest that the Combitube and LMA are attractive alternatives to endotracheal intubation with proven field success and ease of training.[42] Although endotracheal intubation remains a class I recommendation by the AHA (to achieve ventilation and secure the airway), these other devices do have a clinical role and are considered to be class IIA alternatives when compared to bag-valve-mask ventilation.

Endotracheal intubation is considered the ideal technique for ensuring adequate ventilation during CPR. Whenever possible, a nasogastric tube should be inserted following intubation to drain the stomach and thus decrease the chances of aspiration. Intubation can be rapidly implemented, but much valuable time can be wasted by repeated unskilled attempts at intubation. If this technique is used, CPR should be discontinued for no more than 20 to 30 s while the tube is being passed into the airway. If more than 20 to 30 s elapse without successful intubation, the laryngoscope should be withdrawn and CPR reinstituted. The concern of delaying resuscitation during intubation was supported by a recent study in a pediatric population that compared bag-valve-mask ventilation to endotracheal intubation and failed to demonstrate any benefit of endotracheal intubation, likely due to the delay in intubating patients.

The optimal requirements for ventilation during CPR in human beings remain unknown. No study has clearly identified the optimal timing, sequence in relation to chest compression, or tidal volume needed during CPR. During the first few minutes of cardiac arrest without prior hypoxia, as noted above, animal studies suggest that ventilation is less important relative to chest compression and defibrillation. Airflow from chest compression alone and air in the lungs at the time of arrest may be initially sufficient to sustain ventilation.[43,44] Recent human data from Seattle tend to support this observation, since dispatcher-assisted CPR with or without ventilation resulted in similar outcomes.[31] The value of expired air ventilation has further been called into question based on animal studies that show that expired air, when used for ventilation, actually worsens outcome in a ventricular fibrillation cardiac arrest model. The value of immediate expired air ventilation for victims of witnessed cardiac arrest has thus clearly been called into question. There are few data on the value (or lack thereof) of ventilation in the victim of an unwitnessed arrest. Based on these data, the new AHA guidelines for resuscitation recommend 100 chest compressions per minute with a 15:2 compression-ventilation ratio (for both single- and two-rescuer CPR) and ventilation with two breaths slowly delivered over 2 s with a tidal volume sufficient to achieve obvious chest rise (10 to 12 mL/kg) or, if a bag-valve-mask is used, 400 to 600 mL per breath.

In addition to these recommendations, it is critical, in performing chest compression, to use sufficient force to depress the sternum by approximately 2 in. (5 to 6 cm). As this is usually difficult to gauge, sufficient chest compression force should be used to generate a palpable femoral or carotid arterial pulse.

Airway, breathing, and chest compression (ABC) is the specific sequence used to initiate CPR in the United States, with survival rates as high as 35 percent in cities with advanced EMS systems[32,36] (see Chap. 41). ABC is also used in many other countries. However, in the Netherlands, CAB (chest compression first, followed by airway opening and breathing) is the common technique for CPR implementation, with resuscitation outcomes similar to those reported for ABC in the United States. Despite its proven efficacy, the recently perceived risk of infectious disease transmission during CPR has reduced the willingness of both lay and medical personnel to initiate mouth-to-mouth ventilation and CPR in unknown victims of cardiac arrest. In an effort to respond to these concerns and encourage the lay administration of CPR, some cities have mandated the public availability and use of barrier devices during mouth-to-mouth ventilation. The effectiveness of such barrier devices is, however, unknown. To overcome this limitation, potential rescuers who are reluctant to initiate CPR because of the perceived risk of infection should be encouraged to activate the EMS system immediately, open the victim's airway, and then initiate and continue chest compressions only until paramedics arrive (i.e., A and C). The paramedics can then initiate ventilation with the necessary protective equipment. It is important to note that a randomized comparison with CAB (chest compression, airway, breathing) or CAD (chest compression, airway opening, defibrillation) has never been done.

## DEFINITIVE THERAPY

*The AHA's 2000 Guidelines for Cardiopulmonary Resuscitation and Emergency Cardiac Care* adopted a new classification for therapeutic recommendations.[25] This classification allows a relative therapeutic value to be assigned to a given strategy of treatment based on scientific data. It is as follows:

1. Class I: Definitely helpful
2. Class IIA: Acceptable, probably helpful
3. Class IIB: Acceptable, possibly helpful, probably not harmful
4. Class III: Not indicated, may be harmful
5. Indeterminate: Clinical data too preliminary or insufficient to allow classification into the other four categories

During cardiac arrest, the ECG will usually show rapid ventricular tachycardia or fibrillation, asystole, or heart block—or it may be near normal.

### Ventricular Tachycardia or Fibrillation

With ventricular fibrillation, an attempt at electrical defibrillation should be made as quickly as possible. Successful defibrillation is accomplished by the passage of adequate electrical current (amperes) through the heart (see also Chap. 37). Current flow is dependent on the energy chosen (joules) and the transthoracic impedance (ohms), or resistance to current flow. Factors that affect transthoracic impedance include the energy selected, electrode size, skin-paddle coupling material, the number and time interval of previous shocks, the distance between the electrodes (size of the chest), phase of ventilation, and paddle electrode pressure.[45] Human transthoracic impedance ranges from 15 to 150 ohms, with the average adult impedance being 70 to 80 ohms. If transthoracic impedance is high, low-energy shocks are ineffective in generating enough current to achieve successful defibrillation. Transthoracic impedance can be reduced by firm pressure on handheld electrode paddles and a gel/cream or saline-soaked gauze pads between the electrode and the skin.[45] In addition, proper electrode/paddle placement is essential; one electrode should be placed to the right of the upper sternum below the clavicle and the other to the left of the nipple, with the center of the electrode in the midaxillary line. An acceptable alternative is one electrode anteriorly over the left precordium and the other posteriorly behind the heart in the right infrascapular location. The latter positioning is best achieved by using preadhesive rather than handheld electrodes. In female patients with large breasts, the electrodes are best placed to the right of the upper sternum and either under or lateral to the left breast. Direct current is employed during defibrillation. The paddles, coated with low-resistance gel, are applied firmly to the chest and then for monophasic defibrillations discharged with 200 J, which is repeated at 200 to 300 J if the first shock is unsuccessful. The current AHA standards suggest that a third 360-J shock should be delivered if ventricular fibrillation persists.[25] These three shocks should be delivered in rapid succession. Prospective studies by Adgey and others have shown 85 to 90 percent successful defibrillation using only 200 J in patients weighing up to 90 kg.[46,47] Some advocate higher-energy defibrillation, but few currently use more than 400 J.[48] High-energy defibrillation likely causes more cardiac injury, and increases postshock myocardial dysfunction; there is no clear evidence that it increases the frequency of successful resuscitation.[49] As mentioned above, several defibrillators have biphasic defibrillatory shock waveforms. Most conventional manual defibrillators use the monophasic exponential waveform, whereas several AEDs deliver a biphasic defibrillatory shock wave at lower energy levels with equal if not greater success.

When the ECG shows fine fibrillation waves, defibrillation efforts are often unsuccessful. Although commonly practiced, the early use of epinephrine in such situations is not supported by improved survival in clinical trials. Nevertheless, it is suggested that the administration of epinephrine (5 to 10 mL of 1:10,000) intravenously may result in a more vigorous and coarse fibrillation that is more responsive to defibrillation. This effect is possibly due to improved coronary flow following epinephrine administration (see below), although recent data raise the question of epinephrine-induced deleterious myocardial effects, especially at higher doses.[50] If defibrillation fails, it is likely that marked acidosis or hypoxemia is present. Emphasis should be on modest hyperventilation with supplemental oxygen to correct both hypoxemia and metabolic acidosis.[51] Sodium bicarbonate might then be administered (1 meq/kg) to aid in the management of acidosis, and defibrillation should be repeated with 360 J. By using instantaneous Fourier transformation analysis, Brown et al. have demonstrated that the coarseness of the waveform of ventricular fibrillation may be highly predictive of subsequent survival and appears to correlate with coronary flow.[52] Preliminary human data to confirm these observations are limited.

The value of intravenous amiodarone in shock-refractory ventricular fibrillation/ventricular tachycardia (VF/VT) has been tested in patients who had experienced prehospital cardiac arrest. Although it improved survival to hospital admission, there was no difference in survival to hospital discharge between those who did and did not receive amiodarone.[53] Although often given, there are few data to support the use of lidocaine, bretylium, procainamide, or magnesium in such patients—i.e., those with shock-refractory VF/VT (class of recommendation indeterminate).[54–56] Based on these data, it appears that amiodarone may be of some short-term benefit in patients with recurrent VT/VF (class IIB). Amiodarone is usually dosed as a bolus of 150 to 300 mg over 10 min, 1.0 to 2.0 mg/min for 6 h, then 0.5 to 1.0 mg/min for 6 to 24 h. For recurrent VF in the setting of ischemia, intravenous propranolol or other intravenous beta blockers or amiodarone may be effective.[54] Beta blockers seem particularly helpful in the setting of primary ventricular fibrillation complicating acute myocardial infarction.[54] In fact, the early benefit of amiodarone has been ascribed by some to its beta-blocking properties.

Hyperkalemia is a readily treated condition that can cause atrioventricular (AV) block, impaired intraatrial and intraventricular conduction, and occasionally ventricular fibrillation or, less commonly, asystole. It can be recognized by the development of tall, peaked T waves with a normal QT interval and sine wave–like ventricular tachycardia. Life-threatening hyperkalemia responds most readily to calcium infusion; 10 to 30 mL of 10% calcium gluconate is infused intravenously over 1 to 5 min under constant ECG monitoring. Calcium counteracts the adverse effects of potassium on the neuromuscular membranes but does not alter plasma potassium. Its effect, though immediate, is transient. Hyperkalemia should subsequently be treated by glucose-insulin or ion-exchange resins. Sodium bicarbonate is also used as an agent to lower potassium.

With VT in an alert and responsive patient, cough may reverse the arrhythmia without defibrillation, and repeated cough may maintain the conscious state as a result of the rise in intrathoracic pressure.[10,57] It is an appropriate strategy for immediate use pending more definitive drug or electrical intervention. It is commonly used during electrophysiology testing or in monitored patients. The efficacy of the precordial thump (precordial chest blows) has been variably reported in patients with VT. A thump is generally ineffective for terminating prehospital VF. Hence, it should never be used in the patient with VT and a pulse unless a defibrillator is immediately available.

## Asystole or Heart Block

For patients with prehospital cardiac arrest, asystole has been shown to be an ominous rhythm with a very low likelihood of successful resuscitation.[32] On the other hand, asystole due to vagal stimulation is the most common cause of cardiac arrest associated with anesthesia induction and surgical procedures. Asystole also occurs as a result of heart block or sinus node disease (see Chap. 32). Atropine (0.5 mg) given intravenously and repeated in 5 min can be used acutely to prevent or reverse severe bradycardia in many of these settings.

If asystole is witnessed or of short duration, vigorous blows to the precordium may sometimes restart the heart. Rhythmic chest blows may maintain limited perfusion and can be continued if needed while palpating the femoral or carotid pulse until other treatment is available. If the chest blow fails, CPR should be initiated and intravenous epinephrine (5 to 10 mL of 1:10,000) administered. Possible treatable causes of asystole—such as acidosis, hypoxemia, hyper- or hypokalemia, and hypothermia—should be considered and treated appropriately if suspected. If an overdose of calcium channel blocker is suspected, calcium chloride, 1 g given as an intravenous bolus, may be very effective (class IIA recommendation). Resuscitation measures may result in the return of a slow ventricular rhythm, which can subsequently be supported with atropine (1 to 2 mg IV) until a temporary pacemaker is placed. Temporary pacing is the optimal treatment for true asystole or profound bradycardia. Obviously, considerable skill and training are required for temporary transvenous pacemaker placement (see Chap. 32). Transcutaneous pacing has been developed as a noninvasive and simple technique that can be implemented rapidly. It uses external surface electrodes with a high-voltage pacing source. Higher voltages are required to overcome transthoracic resistance, but they are painful and are therefore used mainly on unconscious patients. The energy delivered to the heart by this technique is variable, as is its efficacy. Pacing sources with longer pacing stimulus duration have been developed and may offer less painful and more effective pacing. Prehospital studies of transcutaneous pacing for asystole have not confirmed an improvement in survival.[58] It may, however, be of some benefit for patients early in asystole (class IIB intervention). Clinical evidence does not support its routine use in all patients with asystole.

In rare instances, very fine VF may result in an almost straight line on a single-lead ECG and thus be mistaken for asystole. In such cases, where the diagnosis of asystole is in question, it is suggested that a perpendicular ECG lead be viewed. Rotation of "quick look" ECG paddles by 90 degrees easily achieves this. If ventricular fibrillation is present, the perpendicular ECG lead will demonstrate a typical fibrillation pattern; whereas in true asystole, a straight line will be seen in all ECG leads. If VF is diagnosed, the initial treatment should be according to the outline above—i.e, three successive countershocks. There is little value in defibrillating true asystole.

### Electromechanical Dissociation

In *electromechanical dissociation* (EMD), there is evidence of organized electrical activity on the ECG at a reasonable rate but failure of effective perfusion (no pulse or blood pressure). The most treatable causes of this condition are hypovolemia due to severe hemorrhage, pericardial tamponade, tension pneumothorax, hypoxia, hypothermia, acidosis, hyperkalemia, and massive pulmonary embolism. Signs of these problems should be sought and definitive therapy undertaken with fluids and/or blood replacement, pericardiocentesis, placement of a pleural needle or tube, endotracheal intubation, and other maneuvers as deemed necessary. These conditions should also be strongly considered if CPR results in no palpable pulse or evidence of perfusion. Unfortunately, many patients with electromechanical dissociation have primary myocardial failure. Following diagnosis, ventilation should be optimized and epinephrine administered. Calcium chloride has been used for EMD, but prospective studies have not shown it to improve survival.[59] In acute myocardial infarction, sudden electromechanical dissociation is a sign of myocardial rupture. In such cases, pericardiocentesis and surgical repair can rarely result in survival.

## ESTABLISHMENT OF AN INTRAVENOUS ROUTE

While external chest compression and artificial ventilation are continued, a plastic catheter should be inserted into a large peripheral vein. Drug administration during CPR should be preferentially accomplished only from a source above the diaphragm, since there is little cephalad flow from veins below the diaphragm. If a peripheral vein cannot be cannulated, a cutdown should be attempted or a central venous line placed by a percutaneous route. If CPR is properly performed, drugs administered through a peripheral line will often reach the arterial circulation within 15 to 30 s.[51] Data suggest that a 20-mL fluid bolus significantly improves peripheral drug delivery to the central compartment. Larger amounts of fluids should be used if drugs are given via a femoral line. Intracardiac injections are unnecessary except when there is no intravenous access. If an intravenous route is unavailable, epinephrine (1 to 2 mg in 10 mL of sterile distilled water) and lidocaine (50 to 100 mg in 10 mL of sterile distilled water) can be administered by way of the endotracheal tube into the bronchial tree. The drug should be injected through a long catheter passed beyond the tip of the endotracheal tube. Cardiac compression should be withheld, and several insufflations with an Ambu bag should immediately follow drug administration to aid drug absorption through aerosolization.

## MAJOR DRUGS USED DURING CARDIOPULMONARY RESUSCITATION

Drugs that are used for the treatment of various arrhythmias are mentioned above. Catecholamines are used in cardiac arrest to (1) increase arterial and coronary perfusion during and following CPR, (2) stimulate spontaneous contraction during asystole, (3) make fine VF more responsive to defibrillation, and (4) act as an inotropic agent.

Epinephrine was among the earliest pressors evaluated during resuscitation. It is effective in achieving several of these goals, although recent data have highlighted its possible deleterious effects on postresuscitation left ventricular function. Both animal and clinical studies have extensively evaluated the hemodynamic effects of epinephrine during resuscitation. Animal studies show that during conventional CPR, cerebral and myocardial perfusion pressures are low. Epinephrine increases brain and heart flow by two mechanisms: (1) It prevents carotid artery collapse and raises arterial pressure during both chest compression and the release phase of chest compression (i.e., systole and diastole, respectively). This results in higher carotid arterial systolic and aortic diastolic pressures, which, in turn, are reflected in higher cerebral perfusion and myocardial perfusion pressures and flow. (2) It preferentially reduces blood flow to the external carotid, renal, and splanchnic beds, thereby redirecting flow toward the brain and heart.[60,61]

Arterial collapse at the thoracic inlet has been shown to be the critical limiting factor for cerebral perfusion pressure and flow during prolonged CPR. Arterial collapse results from high extravascular intrathoracic pressures, low intravascular volumes, and loss of arterial tone. Collapse results in a precipitous fall in carotid arterial and hence cerebral perfusion pressure. Epinephrine during CPR can not only reverse arterial collapse but also prevent it from developing. With the administration of epinephrine during conventional manual CPR in the dog, cerebral blood flow can be maintained at approximately 15 percent and myocardial flow at approximately 5 percent of prearrest values for 20 min.

These data strongly support the early and frequent use of epinephrine during CPR in an effort to optimize the perfusion of vital organs. The recommended dose of epinephrine (1 mg IV every 3 to 5 min) is comparable to a 0.007- to 0.014-mg/kg dose in a 70-kg person. This dose has been questioned, since animal studies using higher doses of epinephrine have shown improved blood flow to vital organs and improved survival.[61] Other studies of higher doses of epinephrine, however, have shown increased myocardial oxygen demand despite this improved blood flow.[62] Higher than recommended doses of epinephrine have been reported to increase arterial pressure and coronary perfusion pressure in a small number of human studies. These studies spawned an intense interest in the use of higher doses of epinephrine during CPR. Results from several prospective randomized out-of-hospital clinical trials of more than 2400 adult cardiac arrest victims, however, have shown no statistically significant improvement in survival to hospital admission or discharge or improved neurologic survival when higher doses of epinephrine (0.1 to 0.2 mg/kg) were compared with standard doses.[63,64] On the other hand, these trials did not demonstrate any obvious deleterious effect of the higher doses of epinephrine.

Retrospective studies suggest that higher cumulative doses of epinephrine are associated with worse hemodynamic and neurologic outcome even when duration of cardiac arrest are accounted for. Hence, most experts would use 1 mg IV uniformly. Higher doses worsen postresuscitation myocardial dysfunction, hence its use is not routinely recommended.[25] The recommended dose is 0.5 to 1 mg IV, and this dose should be repeated at approximately 3- to 5-min intervals unless effective cardiac activity is restored. If an intravenous route is not available, epinephrine can be administered down the endotracheal tube; 10 mL of a 1:10,000 solution should be used, and this can also be repeated every 3 to 5 min.

The benefits of epinephrine are principally due to the alpha vasoconstriction induced by this agent. The inotropic effects of the drug may not be helpful, since these effects increase myocardial oxygen demand, even during ventricular fibrillation, when supply or blood flow is limited.[62] Consequently, there is some interest in using a pure vasoconstrictor during CPR rather than epinephrine. Animal studies of vital organ perfusion and human survival studies comparing epinephrine and phenylepinephrine (a pure alpha vasoconstrictor) have yielded similar results. Vasopressin has recently been evaluated as an alternative pressor agent, with promising results.[64a] Animal studies have demonstrated it to be as effective as a pressor but with less resultant myocardial dysfunction as compared to epinephrine. Initial human data has been encouraging. However, a large prospective randomized out-of-hospital study of vasopressin versus epinephrine failed to confirm any survival benefit of this agent.[64b] It may be considered an alternative pressor to epinephrine for patients in shock-refractory VF (class IIB).

Norepinephrine is a potent vasoconstrictor and generally produces a rise in blood pressure; it is also an inotropic agent. Its disadvantage is renal and mesenteric vasoconstriction, and it should not be used in the initial phase of resuscitation. This agent is most useful where severe hypotension is present but where the chronotropic effects of epinephrine are not desirable (as in acute myocardial infarction or severe ischemia). This agent should be administered cautiously, since severe tissue injury results from extravasation around an intravenous site. A large prehospital trial failed to identify any differences in survival following treatments with norepinephrine, high-dose epinephrine, or standard epinephrine.[63]

Similarly, dopamine (a chemical precursor of norepinephrine) and dobutamine (a synthetic catecholamine) are preferred for use as inotropic agents because of their lesser chronotropic effect. Animal data suggest that dobutamine may be particularly effective in reducing postresuscitation left ventricular dysfunction. Isoproterenol (a synthetic catecholamine) is a pure adrenergic agonist and effective vasodilator. Therefore, its use during CPR is contraindicated since it can significantly decrease vital organ perfusion pressures. In patients with a palpable pulse, however, it is useful for treatment of bradycardia due to heart block or asystole until a temporary pacemaker is placed.

### Sodium Bicarbonate

The AHA recommendations deemphasize the role of sodium bicarbonate and suggest that much less sodium bicarbonate should be used than previously advocated for acid-base control during cardiac arrest. As with other types of metabolic acidosis, if adequate alveolar ventilation is achieved, the metabolic acidosis of arrest is partially corrected through $CO_2$ excretion.[51] Recent clinical trials failed to demonstrate improved outcome from cardiac arrest with buffer therapy.[65] Rather, several deleterious effects of bicarbonate administration including respiratory acidosis, hypernatremia, and hyperosmolality have been reported. Ideally, sodium bicarbonate should be given according to the results of measurement of arterial blood pH, $CO_2$ determination, and calculation of the base deficit. Bicarbonate should be used, if at all, only after more established interventions such as defibrillation, ventilation with endotracheal intubation, and pharmacologic therapies (epinephrine and antiarrhythmic drugs) have been tried.[25] If needed, 1 meq/kg of sodium bicarbonate should be administered; then no more than half this dose may be repeated every 15 min. Excessive use of sodium bicarbonate can result in metabolic alkalosis, hypernatremia, and hyperosmolality. Some benefit of the usual bicarbonate solution (7.2%) may occur as a result of the hyperosmolality of the solution temporarily drawing fluid into the intravascular compartment.

On the other hand, bicarbonate may be most useful during the immediate postresuscitation period, when a profound metabolic acidosis occurs. In most instances during CPR, its use should be considered as a class IIB recommendation.[30]

### Calcium Chloride

Calcium chloride (5 to 7 mg/kg) enhances the contractile state of the heart and is indicated in treating severe hypotension due to an overdose of calcium channel blocker or hyperkalemia. It is no longer recommended for use in asystole or electromechanical dissociation.

## TERMINATION OF CARDIOPULMONARY RESUSCITATION

Despite resuscitative efforts, the patient in cardiac arrest may not regain spontaneous circulation. The decision to end (or even initiate) CPR should be based on a physician's assessment of the patient's prior advance directives (if known) and the cerebral, cardiovascular, and general status of the patient.[66,67] Recent prospective and retrospective data confirm that survival is unlikely in patients who have no return of spontaneous circulation after 30 min of advanced cardiac life support (ACLS) care.[68] Studies have demonstrated that continued in-hospital CPR efforts (in patients failing prehospital advanced cardiac life support) are not only common but also expensive and unsuccessful.[69] Persistent deep unconsciousness and absence of respiration, reflex response, or pupillary reaction suggest cerebral death, and resuscitative efforts are usually unproductive. These guidelines, however, should be altered in patients with hypothermia, barbiturate overdose, and perhaps following electrocution, where recovery has been seen even after hours of resuscitation.[70]

## POSTARREST CARE

Patients who have been successfully resuscitated usually require monitoring in an intensive care setting. These patients are prone to develop cardiac arrhythmias, hemodynamic and ventilatory instability, and ischemic encephalopathy. Ventilatory support with a respirator may well be necessary initially. Serial arterial blood gas determinations should be made to identify hypoxemia and assess the rapidly changing acid-base status. Commonly, hyperventilation was employed postresuscitation to not only treat acidosis but also help reduce central nervous system edema. Recent studies raise the possibility of worsening cerebral ischemia with low $P_{CO_2}$ levels after brain ischemia. Based on these observations, normal ventilation is preferred in the comatose postresuscitation patient.

Several therapeutic strategies have been employed in animal models to help reduce hypoxic encephalopathy after cardiac arrest.

Recent studies have confirmed the neuroprotective efficacy of prompt, moderate hypothermia to 33°C (91.4°F) for 12 to 24 h postresuscitation. It is now a recommended standard of care.

The treatment of encephalopathy after cardiac arrest involves the prevention of further hypoxia and hypotension. For cerebral edema after cardiac arrest, methylprednisolone (60 to 100 mg) or dexamethasone sodium phosphate (12 to 20 mg IV every 6 h) has been recommended, but there is no conclusive evidence that these agents are beneficial. The value of high-dose barbiturates or lidoflazine in human beings is negligible. The prognosis of the patient with anoxic encephalopathy is related to the depth and continued duration of cerebral dysfunction (see also Chap. 99). Failure to exhibit neurologic improvement 24 to 72 h following resuscitation is usually an ominous sign. Clinical and laboratory evaluations (electroencephalography, sensory evoked potentials) are often employed to help define prognosis and thus guide further care in such individuals.

Other potential life-threatening problems in the postarrest period include acute renal failure, bowel infarction, infection, adult respiratory distress syndrome, and sepsis. Patients regaining consciousness may have postarrest amnesia or may develop psychotic behavior.

## OUTCOME OF RESUSCITATION

In their initial study, Kouwenhoven and colleagues reported a 24 percent successful resuscitation and discharge rate from the hospital.[6] Studies have shown that with a paramedical response system, a near 40 percent successful out-of-hospital resuscitation rate can be achieved.[32,71] Many of these patients die in hospital, however, with the dominant cause of death being anoxic encephalopathy. Data suggest that somatosensory evoked potentials may be useful and highly predictive in identifying patients who are likely to have irreversible brain injury.[72] The critical factors for successful out-of-hospital resuscitation include approximately 7 min total duration of CPR, approximately 4 min from collapse to the initiation of CPR, and approximately 10 min to successful delivery of the first countershock. Given the benefit of hypothermia therapy postresuscitation, these parameters will likely need to be revisited.

It is important to point out, however, that the quality of life for patients surviving to hospital discharge is often quite good, with most discharged patients being able to return to gainful employment.

## CHAIN OF SURVIVAL

The concept of a "chain of survival" has been adopted by several agencies and underscores the importance of an integrated public education and health care system if outcome from prehospital cardiac arrest is to be optimized.[25] Early access (to EMS systems), early CPR (to include bystander CPR), early defibrillation (to include the use of AEDs), and early ACLS care are the major links in the chain, and any one weak link weakens the whole chain of survival.

This is best exemplified in two publications that reported on prehospital cardiac arrest outcomes in New York and Chicago, where survival rates were only 1 to 2 percent. Despite a mature EMS system and considerable public training in CPR, delayed defibrillation—due to traffic, elevators, and other factors—contributed significantly to the poor outcome in these studies.[73,74] Other cities, where prompt defibrillation has been possible, have reported a 20 to 30 percent survival rate.[75] To overcome this tragic limitation, AEDs were developed and have been shown to facilitate prompt defibrillation and thereby improve survival (Fig. 42-3). Hence, the American Heart Association and American College of Cardiology have jointly recommended that all professional first-responder units (especially in rural areas where long transport times are common) be equipped with AEDs. Based on recent studies, the U.S. government may soon mandate AEDs in large public buildings.

If mortality from out-of-hospital arrest is to be reduced, public education programs to increase awareness of the warning signs of a heart attack and teach CPR are critical (Fig. 42-3). Despite many years of public education, the incidence of bystander CPR nationwide remains low.[73,74] This may have several explanations, including a lack of training in high-risk populations, poor performance or lack of retention despite training, unnecessarily complex training programs, or a fear of communicable disease during mouth-to-mouth resuscitation. Family members of patients with heart disease should be taught to at least activate EMS ("call") and start chest compressions ("pump"). Ventilation ("blow") could then be started by suitably equipped trained EMS rescuers. Present data indicate that a refocusing of basic life support (BLS) training programs is essential, with efforts being targeted at simplification of training, with specific education and training penetration into high-risk patient groups (older patients and minority groups). The CPR message must be kept simple (for example, "call-pump-blow"). These goals must be achieved if the first two links in the chain of survival (early access and early CPR) are to be strengthened. Universal 911 would facilitate early and easy access and should be encouraged in all communities. Minimal standards of performance and excellence for EMS systems should be established and monitored. Dispatcher-assisted CPR teaches CPR on the telephone to the person who is calling to report the arrest (while professional help is in transit) and has been shown to be effective. The Seattle-King County EMS system is proof that such efforts directly improve outcome (Fig. 42-3).[75] On the other hand, the Chicago-New York experience is a chilling reminder of the consequence of one weak link in the chain of survival. The outcome from prehospital arrest can be improved only if each community strives to optimize its own chain of survival.

## References


1. Wiggers CJ. The physiologic basis for cardiac resuscitation from ventricular fibrillation method of serial defibrillation. *Am Heart J* 1940;20:413–422.
2. Comroe JH. Retrospectroscope: In comes the good air. *Am Rev Respir Dis* 1979;119:803–809.
3. Elam JO, Brown ES, Elder JD. Artificial respiration by mouth-to-mask method. *N Engl J Med* 1954;250:749–754.
4. Sanders AB, Kern KB, Ewy GA. Open chest massage for resuscitation from cardiac arrest. *Resuscitation* 1988;16:153–154.
5. Eldor J, Frankel DZN, Davidson JT. Open chest cardiac massage: A review. *Resuscitation* 1988;l6:155–162.
6. Kouwenhoven WB, Jude JR, Knickerbocker GG. Closed chest cardiac massage. *JAMA* 1960;173:1064–1067.
7. Jude JR, Kouwenhoven WB, Knickerbocker GG. Cardiac arrest: Report of application of external cardiac massage on 118 patients. *JAMA* 1961;178:1063–1071.
8. Weale FE, Rothwell-Jackson RL. The efficiency of cardiac massage. *Lancet* 1962;1:990–992.
9. MacKenzie GJ, Taylor SH, McDonald AH, Donald KW. Hemodynamic effects of external cardiac compression. *Lancet* 1964;1: 1342–1345.
10. Criley JM, Blaufuss AN, Kissel GL. Cough-induced cardiac compression. *JAMA* 1976;236:1246–1250.
11. Rudikoff MT, Maughan WL, Effron M, et al. Mechanisms of flow during cardiopulmonary resuscitation. *Circulation* 1980;61:345–351.
12. Halperin H, Brower R, Weisfeldt ML, et al. Air trapping in the lungs during cardiopulmonary resuscitation in dogs: A mechanism for

generating changes in intrathoracic pressure. *Circ Res* 1989;65: 946–954.

13. Maier GW, Tyson GS, Olsen CO, et al. The physiology of external cardiac massage: High impulse cardiopulmonary resuscitation. *Circulation* 1984;70:86–101.
14. Feneley MP, Maier GW, Gaynor JW, et al. Sequence of mitral valve motion and transmitral blood flow during manual cardiopulmonary resuscitation in dogs. *Circulation* 1987;76:363–375.
15. Deshmukh HG, Weil MH, Gudipati CV, et al. Mechanism of blood flow generated by precordial compression during CPR: I. Studies on closed chest precordial compression. *Chest* 1989;95:1092–1099.
16. Werner JA, Greene HL, Janko CL, Cobb LA. Visualization of cardiac valve motion in man during external chest compression using two-dimensional echocardiography: Implications regarding the mechanism of blood flow. *Circulation* 1981;63:1417–1421.
17. Halperin HR, Weiss JL, Guerci AD, et al. Cyclic elevation of intrathoracic pressure can close the mitral valve during cardiac arrest in dogs. *Circulation* 1988;78:754–760.
18. Koehler RC, Chandra N, Guerci AD, et al. Augmentation of cerebral perfusion by simultaneous chest compression and lung inflation with abdominal binding following cardiac arrest in dogs. *Circulation* 1983; 67:266–275.
19. Swenson RD, Weaver WD, Nisaken RA, et al. Hemodynamics in humans during conventional and experimental methods of cardiopulmonary resuscitation. *Circulation* 1988;78:630–639.
20. Chandra NC, Tsitlik JE, Halperin HR, et al. Observations of hemodynamics during cardiopulmonary resuscitation. *Crit Care Med* 1990;18:929–934.
21. Paradis N, Martin G, Goetting M, et al. Simultaneous aortic, jugular bulb, and right atrial pressures during cardiopulmonary resuscitation in humans: Insights into mechanisms. *Circulation* 1989;80: 361–368.
22. Halperin HR, Tsitlik JE, Gelfand N, et al. A preliminary study of cardiopulmonary resuscitation with circumferential compression of the chest with use of a pneumatic vest. *N Engl J Med* 1993;329: 762–768.
23. Plaisance P, Lurie KG, Payen D. Inspiratory impedance during ACD-CPR. *Circulation* 2000;101:989–994.
24. Sack J, Kesselbrenner M, Bergman D. Survival from in-hospital arrest with interposed abdominal counterpulsation during cardiopulmonary resuscitation. *JAMA* 1992;276:379–385.
25. Guidelines 2000 for cardiopulmonary resuscitation and emergency cardiovascular care: International Consensus on Science. *Circulation* 2000;102:I1–I384.
26. Tang W, Weil MH, Schock RB, et al. Phased chest and abdominal compression-decompression. *Circulation* 1997;95:1335–1340.
27. Cohen TJ, Tucker KJ, Lurie KG, et al. Active compression-decompression resuscitation: A new method of cardiopulmonary resuscitation. *JAMA* 1992;267:2916–2923.
28. Stiell IG, Hébert PC, Wells GA, et al. The Ontario trial of active compression-decompression cardiopulmonary resuscitation for in-hospital and prehospital cardiac arrest. *JAMA* 1996;275:1417–1423.
29. Gueugniaud P, Mols P, Goldstein P, et al. A comparison of repeated high doses and repeated standard doses of epinephrine for cardiac arrest outside the hospital. *N Engl J Med* 1998;339:1595–1601.

29a. Bernard SA, Gray TW, Buist MD, et al. Treatment of comatose survivors of out-of-hospital cardiac arrest with induced hypothermia. *N Engl J Med* 2002;346(8):557–563.

29b. Mild therapeutic hypothermia to improve the neurologic outcome after cardiac arrest. *N Engl J Med* 2002;346(8):549–556.

30. Halperin HR, Tsitlik JE, Guerci AD, et al. Determinants of blood flow to vital organs during cardiopulmonary resuscitation in dogs. *Circulation* 1986;73:539–551.
31. Hallstrom A, Cobb L, Johnson E, Copass M. Cardiopulmonary resuscitation by chest compression alone or with mouth to mouth ventilation. *N Engl J Med* 2000;342:1546–1553.
32. Eisenberg MS, Horwood BT, Cummins RO, et al. Cardiac arrest after resuscitation: A tale of 29 cities. *Ann Emerg Med* 1990;19:179–186.
33. Niemann JT, Cairns CB, Sharma J, Lewis RJ. Treatment of prolonged ventricular fibrillation: Immediate countershock versus high dose epinephrine and CPR preceding countershock. *Circulation* 1992;85(l): 281–287.
34. Cobb LA, Fahrenbruch CE, Walsh TR. Influence of cardiopulmonary resuscitation prior to defibrillation in patients with out-of-hospital ventricular fibrillation. *JAMA* 1999;281:1182–1188.

34a. Wik L, Hansen TB, Fylling F, et al. Delaying defibrillation to give basic cardiopulmonary resuscitation to patients with out-of-hospital ventricular fibrillation: A randomized trial. *JAMA* 2003;289: 1434–1436.

35. White RD, Asplin BR, Bugliosi TF, Hankins DG. High release survival from out-of-hospital ventricular fibrillation with rapid defibrillation by both police and paramedics. *Acad Emerg Med* 1996;3:422.
36. Weaver WD, Hill D, Fahrenbruch CE, et al. Use of the automatic external defibrillation in the management of out-of-hospital cardiac arrest. *N Engl J Med* 1988;319:661–666.
37. Valenzuela TD, Roe DJ, Cretin S, et al. Estimating effectiveness of cardiac arrest interventions. A logistic regression survival model. *Circulation* 1997;96:3308–3313.

37a. Page RL, Joglar JA, Kowal RC, et al. Use of automated external defibrillators by a U.S. airline. *N Engl J Med* 2000;343:1210–1216.

38. Nichol G, Hallstrom A, Ornato JP, et al. Potential cost-effectiveness of public access defibrillation in the United States. *Circulation* 1998; 97(13):1315–1320.
39. Heimlich HJ. A lifesaving maneuver to prevent from choking. *JAMA* 1975;234:398–401.
40. Visintine RE, Baick CH. Ruptured stomach after Heimlich maneuver. *JAMA* 1975;234:415.
41. Pepe PE, Zacharich BS, Chandra NC. Update on invasive airway techniques in resuscitation. *Ann Emerg Med* 1993;22:393–403.
42. Rumball CJ, MacDonald D. The PTL, Combitube, laryngeal mask, and oral airway. A randomized prehospital comparative study of ventilatory device effectiveness and cost-effectiveness in 470 cases of cardiorespiratory arrest. *Prehosp Emerg Care* 1997;1:1–10.
43. Chandra NC, Gruben KG, Tsitlik JE, et al. Observations of ventilation during resuscitation of a canine model. *Circulation* 1994;90: 3070–3075.
44. Locke CJ, Berg RA, Sanders AB, et al. Bystander cardiopulmonary resuscitation: Concerns about mouth to mouth contact. *Arch Intern Med* 1995;155:938–943.
45. Sirna SJ, Fergusson DW, Charbonnier F, Kerber RE. Electrical cardioversion in humans: Factors affecting transthoracic impedance. *Am J Cardiol* 1988;62:1048–1052.
46. Adgey AAJ, Patton JN, Campbell NPS, Webb SW. Ventricular defibrillation: Appropriate energy levels. *Circulation* 1979;60:219–223.
47. Gascho JA, Crampton RS, Cherwek ML, et al. Determinants of ventricular defibrillation in adults. *Circulation* 1979;60:231–240.
48. Tacker WA, Ewy GA. Emergency defibrillation dose, recommendation and rationale. *Circulation* 1979;60:223–225.
49. Weaver WD, Cobb LA, Copass MK, Hallstrom AP. Ventricular defibrillation: A comparative trial using 175-J and 320-J shocks. *N Engl J Med* 1982;307:1101–1106.
50. Tang W, Weil MH, Sun S, et al. Epinephrine increases the severity of postresuscitation myocardial dysfunction. *Circulation* 1995;92: 3089–3093.
51. Bishop RL, Weisfeldt ML. Sodium bicarbonate administration during cardiac arrest: Effect of arterial pH, $P_{CO_2}$ and osmolality. *JAMA* 1976; 235:506–509.
52. Brown CG, Dzwoncyk R, Martin DR. Physiologic measurement of the ventricular fibrillation ECG signal: Estimating the duration of ventricular fibrillation. *Circulation* 1993;22:70–74.
53. Kudenchuk PJ, Cobb LA, Copass MK, et al. Amiodarone for resuscitation after out-of-hospital cardiac arrest due to ventricular fibrillation. *N Engl J Med* 1999;341:871–878.
54. Levine JH, Massumi A, Scheinman MM, et al. Intravenous amiodarone for recurrent sustained hypotensive ventricular tachyarrhythmias. *J Am Coll Cardiol* 1996;27:67–75.

55. Kowey PR, Levine JH, Herre JM, et al. Randomized, double-blind comparison of intravenous amiodarone and bretylium in the treatment of patients with recurrent, hemodynamically destabilizing ventricular tachycardia and fibrillation. *Circulation* 1995;92:3255–3263.

56. Haynes RE, Copass MK, Chinn TL, Cobb LA. Comparison of bretylium tosylate and lidocaine in management of out-of-hospital ventricular fibrillation: A randomized clinical trial. *Am J Cardiol* 1981;48:353–356.

57. Wei JY, Greene HL, Weisfeldt ML. Cough-facilitated conversion of ventricular tachycardia. *Am J Cardiol* 1980;45:174–176.

58. Cummins RO, Grave JR, Larsen MP, et al. Out-of-hospital transcutaneous pacing by emergency medical technicians in patients with asystolic cardiac arrest. *N Engl J Med* 1993;328:1377–1382.

59. Stueven HA, Thompson BM, Aprahamian C, Tonsfeldt DJ. Calcium chloride: Reassessment of use in asystole. *Ann Emerg Med* 1984; 13:820–822.

60. Michael JR, Guerci AD, Koehler RC, et al. Mechanisms by which epinephrine augments cerebral and myocardial perfusion during cardiopulmonary resuscitation in dogs. *Circulation* 1984;69:822–835.

61. Brown CG, Wermn HA, Davis EA, et al. The effects of graded doses of epinephrine on regional myocardial blood flow during cardiopulmonary resuscitation in swine. *Circulation* 1987;75: 491–497.

62. Ditchey RV, Lindenfeld J. Failure of epinephrine to improve the balance between myocardial oxygen supply and demand during closed chest resuscitation in dogs. *Circulation* 1988;78:382–389.

63. Callaham M, Madsen CD, Barton CW, et al. A randomized clinical trial of high-dose epinephrine and norepinephrine vs standard dose epinephrine in prehospital cardiac arrest. *JAMA* 1992;268:2667–2672.

64. Brown CG, Martin DR, Pepe PE, et al. A comparison of standard-dose and high-dose epinephrine in cardiac arrest outside the hospital. *N Engl J Med* 1992;327:1051–1055.

64a. Lindner KH, Prengel AW, Brinkmann A, et al. Vasopressin administration in refractory cardiac arrest. *Ann Intern Med* 1996;124: 1061–1064.

64b. Stiell IG et al. Randomized, double blind controlled study of vasopressin vs epinephrine adult cardiac arrest. *Lancet.* In press.

65. Dybvik T, Strand T, Steen PA. Buffer therapy during out-of-hospital cardiopulmonary resuscitation. *Resuscitation* 1995;29:89–95.

66. Luce JM, Raffin TA. Withholding and withdrawal of life support from critically ill patients. *Chest* 1988;94:621–626.

67. Niemann JT. Cardiopulmonary resuscitation. *N Engl J Med* 1992;327: 1075–1080.

68. Pepe PE, Brown CG, Bonnin MJ, et al. Prospective validation criteria for on-scene termination of resuscitation after out-of hospital cardiac arrest (abstr). *Ann Emerg Med* 1993;22:884–885.

69. Gray WA, Capone RJ, Most AS: Unsuccessful emergency medical resuscitation—Are continued efforts in the emergency department justified? *N Engl J Med* 1991;325:1393–1398.

70. Ravitch MM, Lane R, Safar P, et al. Lightning stroke: Report of a case with recovery after cardiac massage and prolonged artificial respiration. *N Engl J Med* 1961;264:36–38.

71. Eisenberg MS, Hallstrom A, Bergner L. Long-term survival after out-of-hospital cardiac arrest. *N Engl J Med* 1982;306:1340–1343.

72. Berek K, Lechleitner P, Luef G, et al. Early determination of neurological outcome after prehospital cardiopulmonary resuscitation. *Stroke* 1995;26:543–549.

73. Lombardi G, Gallagher J, Gennis P. Outcome of out-of-hospital cardiac arrest in New York City: The pre-hospital arrest survival evaluation (PHASE) study. *JAMA* 1994;271:678–683.

74. Becker LB, Ostrander MP, Barrett J, Kondos GT. Outcome of CPR in a large metropolitan area—Where are the survivors? *Ann Emerg Med* 1991;20:355–361.

75. Cummins RO. From concept to standard-of-care? Review of the clinical experience with automated external defibrillators. *Ann Emerg Med* 1989;12;1269–1275.

P A R T S I X

# CORONARY HEART DISEASE

CHAPTER 43

# DYSLIPIDEMIA, OTHER RISK FACTORS, AND THE PREVENTION OF CORONARY HEART DISEASE

David J. Maron / Scott M. Grundy / Paul M. Ridker / Thomas A. Pearson



It is essential to identify and manage risk factors for coronary heart disease (CHD) in order to prevent its development in asymptomatic individuals (*primary prevention*) as well as to avoid its recurrence in patients with established disease (*secondary prevention*). *Risk factor management should be conceived as prevention of coronary atherosclerosis itself and, as such, should be included as an integral part of any management plan for the many acute or chronic manifestations of this disease.* The intensity of risk-factor intervention should correspond to the patient's level of absolute risk.[1] The presence of unmodifiable risk factors may necessitate more intense management of modifiable risk factors. This chapter reviews risk assessment for primary prevention, reviews CHD risk factors, discusses the efficacy of managing risk factors, and provides practical recommendations for preventive cardiology practice. The approach to risk assessment and management outlined in this chapter have been adapted from the American Heart Association (AHA) guidelines for primary prevention of cardiovascular disease,[2] the American Heart Association/American College of Cardiology (AHA/ACC) guidelines for secondary prevention,[3] and the recommendations of the National Cholesterol Education Program (NCEP) Adult Treatment Panel III (ATP III).[4]

## RISK ASSESSMENT BASED ON CLINICAL CONDITIONS AND RISK-FACTOR EVALUATION

### Categories of Absolute Risk

For the sake of simplicity, absolute risk can be divided into three categories: high, intermediate, and lower risk.[4] Patients at high risk deserve intensive risk-reduction therapy. Those at intermediate risk are also candidates for clinical intervention to the extent that therapy is effective, safe, and cost-effective. Finally, most lower-risk persons

TABLE 43-1 Risk Categories

| Risk Category | 10-Year Absolute Risk for Myocardial Infarction (nonfatal + fatal) |
|---|---|
| High | > 20% |
| Intermediate | 10–20% |
| Low | < 10% |

should be encouraged by their physicians to follow public health recommendations for primary prevention of CHD. A minority of these persons, however, may benefit from risk-reducing drug therapy.[4] Each category of absolute risk can be expressed in quantitative terms (Table 43-1).

## Identification of High-Risk Patients

### CLINICAL CORONARY HEART DISEASE

Patients at high risk are those whose absolute risk for CHD equals that of patients who already manifest clinical CHD.[4,5] Included in the category of clinical CHD are a history of acute coronary syndromes, stable angina, and coronary revascularization procedures. Evidence from clinical trials of cholesterol-lowering therapy indicates that patients with a prior history of myocardial infarction (MI) have a 10-year risk for recurrent nonfatal or fatal MI of about 26 percent.[6,7] Patients with stable angina pectoris have a 10-year risk for acute MI of about 20 percent.[8,9] Thus, it is reasonable to say that *patients without manifest CHD who have a 10-year risk for MI of greater than 20 percent are at high risk.* These patients also can be said to have a *CHD risk equivalent,* as discussed below.

### NONCORONARY FORMS OF CLINICAL ATHEROSCLEROTIC DISEASE

Patients in this group include those with peripheral arterial disease, abdominal aortic aneurysm, and symptomatic carotid artery disease.[4] Moreover, there is considerable evidence that asymptomatic patients with carotid narrowing ≥ 50 percent fall into the high-risk category.[4] The absolute risk for MI in patients with noncoronary atherosclerosis equals that for recurrent MI in patients with established CHD.[4]

### DIABETES

Patients with diabetes, particularly middle-aged and older patients with type 2 diabetes, who do not manifest CHD commonly carry a risk for major coronary events equivalent to that of nondiabetic patients with established CHD.[4,10] Moreover, many patients with type 2 diabetes have had a silent MI, and many others have silent ischemia. Thus, most patients with diabetes can be placed in the high-risk category, and ATP III has designated diabetes as a CHD equivalent.

### HIGH-RISK PATIENTS WITH MULTIPLE RISK FACTORS

The category of CHD risk equivalents includes persons without clinical manifestations of atherosclerosis who have multiple risk factors (other than diabetes). The absolute risk for the development of CHD over the next decade can be estimated for men and women by Framingham risk tables[4] (Tables 43-2 and 43-3). These tables show absolute risk for *hard CHD* (nonfatal and fatal MI) and exclude *soft CHD* (stable and unstable angina). *Hard* CHD is a better endpoint for defining CHD risk equivalency because risk-reduction therapy is aimed primarily at reducing risk for MI. *When absolute 10-year risk for hard CHD exceeds 20 percent, a CHD risk equivalent is identified.*

***Selection of Patients for Advanced Risk Assessment Using Emerging Risk Factors*** When patients without known atherosclerotic disease have a 10-year risk for hard CHD between 10 and 20 percent, they are potential candidates for advanced risk assessment. There has been intensive research to identify new risk factors that will improve the accuracy of prognosis. These *emerging risk factors* are divided into three categories: lipid risk factors, nonlipid risk factors, and subclinical atherosclerotic disease (see Table 43-4).[4] ATP III does not recommend routine measurement of any of these factors. However, evidence is accumulating to justify the measurement of certain factors to (1) elevate persons with multiple risk factors and intermediate risk to the category of CHD risk equivalent and (2) guide a decision about use of drugs to lower low-density-lipoprotein (LDL) cholesterol in persons with no or a single risk factor who have LDL cholesterol in the range of 160 to 189 mg/dL. Several of these tests are not commercially available, not well standardized, and are expensive. The NCEP recommends that they be considered as optional modifiers of therapy, but they should be used only as an adjunct to adjust the estimate of absolute risk status obtained with the major risk factors.[4]

If such testing is done, it should always be preceded by determination of Framingham risk scoring, which will provide greater perspective on a person's absolute risk than will advanced measures.

***High-Risk Patients Identified by Major Risk Factors Plus Subclinical Atherosclerosis*** Many patients will be found to have an absolute 10-year risk < 20 percent but will still have multiple CHD risk factors. Some of these patients undoubtedly will be at higher risk because of advanced subclinical coronary atherosclerosis. If the latter can be identified noninvasively, the projected risk level can be raised to that of a CHD risk equivalent. The potential utility of noninvasive testing for this purpose was reviewed in the American Heart Association's Prevention V Conference.[11] In the past, noninvasive testing in asymptomatic patients has been contentious.[12] Many investigators are concerned that asymptomatic patients with advanced subclinical atherosclerosis will be labeled as having CHD; if so, patients receiving this label might be referred inappropriately for invasive procedures. *Only if noninvasive techniques are used for risk assessment (prognosis) and not for diagnosis of "coronary artery disease" can noninvasive testing be justified for asymptomatic patients.* The goal of such testing is to add to the accuracy of risk prediction from conventional risk factors and thus to identify persons who will benefit most from intensive medical therapy for risk reduction. The goal is not case finding for invasive coronary interventions. Some authorities question whether the scientific evidence supporting noninvasive testing in asymptomatic patients is adequate to justify its recommendation[13] and believe that Framingham risk scoring is sufficient for risk stratification. Various techniques for noninvasive testing and their utility in risk assessment are reviewed briefly below.

***Exercise Treadmill Testing*** Exercise treadmill testing identifies patients whose coronary atherosclerosis has advanced sufficiently to produce myocardial ischemia with exercise (see also Chap. 16). A considerable body of data exists on risk prognostication for men of ages 45 to 70 years.[14] Exercise testing has reduced predictive value when the pretest probability for CHD is low. In middle-aged men, the combination of multiple risk factors and an abnormal exercise ECG

TABLE 43-2 **Estimate of 10-Year Risk for Men (Framingham Point Scores)**

| Age | Points |
|---|---|
| 20–34 | −9 |
| 35–39 | −4 |
| 40–44 | 0 |
| 45–49 | 3 |
| 50–54 | 6 |
| 55–59 | 8 |
| 60–64 | 10 |
| 65–69 | 11 |
| 70–74 | 12 |
| 75–79 | 13 |

| Total Cholesterol | Points at Ages 20–39 | Points at Ages 40–49 | Points at Ages 50–59 | Points at Ages 60–69 | Points at Ages 70–79 |
|---|---|---|---|---|---|
| <160 | 0 | 0 | 0 | 0 | 0 |
| 160–199 | 4 | 3 | 2 | 1 | 0 |
| 200–239 | 7 | 5 | 3 | 1 | 0 |
| 240–279 | 9 | 6 | 4 | 2 | 1 |
| ≥280 | 11 | 8 | 5 | 3 | 1 |

| | Points at Ages 20–39 | Points at Ages 40–49 | Points at Ages 50–59 | Points at Ages 60–69 | Points at Ages 70–79 |
|---|---|---|---|---|---|
| Nonsmoker | 0 | 0 | 0 | 0 | 0 |
| Smoker | 8 | 5 | 3 | 1 | 1 |

| HDL | Points |
|---|---|
| ≥60 | −1 |
| 50–59 | 0 |
| 40–49 | 1 |
| <40 | 2 |

| Systolic BP | If Untreated | If Treated |
|---|---|---|
| <120 | 0 | 0 |
| 120–129 | 0 | 1 |
| 130–139 | 1 | 2 |
| 140–159 | 1 | 2 |
| ≥160 | 2 | 3 |

| Point Total | 10-Year Risk | Point Total | 10-Year Risk |
|---|---|---|---|
| <0 | <1% | 11 | 8% |
| 0 | 1% | 12 | 10% |
| 1 | 1% | 13 | 12% |
| 2 | 1% | 14 | 16% |
| 3 | 1% | 15 | 20% |
| 4 | 1% | 16 | 25% |
| 5 | 2% | ≥17 | ≥30% |
| 6 | 2% | | |
| 7 | 3% | | |
| 8 | 4% | | |
| 9 | 5% | | |
| 10 | 6% | | |

SOURCE: From Third Report of the NCEP.[4] With permission.

TABLE 43-3 10-Year Risk Estimates for Women (Framingham Point Scores)

| Age | Points |
|---|---|
| 20–34 | −7 |
| 35–39 | −3 |
| 40–44 | 0 |
| 45–49 | 3 |
| 50–54 | 6 |
| 55–59 | 8 |
| 60–64 | 10 |
| 65–69 | 12 |
| 70–74 | 14 |
| 75–79 | 16 |

| Total Cholesterol | Points at Ages 20–39 | Points at Ages 40–49 | Points at Ages 50–59 | Points at Ages 60–69 | Points at Ages 70–79 |
|---|---|---|---|---|---|
| <160 | 0 | 0 | 0 | 0 | 0 |
| 160–199 | 4 | 3 | 2 | 1 | 1 |
| 200–239 | 8 | 6 | 4 | 2 | 1 |
| 240–279 | 11 | 8 | 5 | 3 | 2 |
| ≥280 | 13 | 10 | 7 | 4 | 2 |

| | Points at Ages 20–39 | Points at Ages 40–49 | Points at Ages 50–59 | Points at Ages 60–69 | Points at Ages 70–79 |
|---|---|---|---|---|---|
| Nonsmoker | 0 | 0 | 0 | 0 | 0 |
| Smoker | 9 | 7 | 4 | 2 | 1 |

| HDL | Points |
|---|---|
| ≥60 | −1 |
| 50–59 | 0 |
| 40–49 | 1 |
| <40 | 2 |

| Systolic BP | If Untreated | If Treated |
|---|---|---|
| <120 | 0 | 0 |
| 120–129 | 1 | 3 |
| 130–139 | 2 | 4 |
| 140–159 | 3 | 5 |
| ≥160 | 4 | 6 |

| Point Total | 10-Year Risk | Point Total | 10-Year Risk |
|---|---|---|---|
| <9 | <1% | 20 | 11% |
| 9 | 1% | 21 | 14% |
| 10 | 1% | 22 | 17% |
| 11 | 1% | 23 | 22% |
| 12 | 1% | 24 | 27% |
| 13 | 2% | ≥25 | ≥30% |
| 14 | 2% | | |
| 15 | 3% | | |
| 16 | 4% | | |
| 17 | 5% | | |
| 18 | 6% | | |
| 19 | 8% | | |

SOURCE: From Third Report of the NCEP.[4] With permission.

TABLE 43-4 Emerging Risk Factors

Lipid
- Triglycerides
- Lipoprotein remnant particles
- Lipoprotein(a)
- Small LDL particles
- HDL subspecies
- Apolipoprotein B
- Apolipoprotein A-I
- Total cholesterol/HDL cholesterol ratio

Nonlipid
- Homocysteine
- Thrombogenic/hemostatic factors
- Inflammatory markers
- Impaired fasting glucose

Detection of subclinical atherosclerosis
- Ankle brachial index
- Tests for myocardial ischemia
- Tests for atherosclerotic plaque burden (e.g., coronary calcium scanning, carotid sonography)

denotes a high risk for developing clinical CHD. Risk for angina pectoris is 12-fold elevated above that of men with a normal test result, and risk for MI is elevated fourfold.[14] These extremely high risk ratios are sufficient to elevate a patient's risk from intermediate risk to the level of CHD risk equivalent.

***Coronary Artery Calcium Scanning*** Electron-beam computed tomography (EBCT) and multidetector CT can be used to identify coronary calcification, which is a close correlate of coronary atherosclerosis.[15–18] Coronary calcification increases progressively with advancing age in parallel with coronary atherosclerosis. The finding of a high coronary calcium score by EBCT may provide a means to improve on the risk estimate beyond the Framingham algorithm. For example, patients with multiple risk factors plus a calcium score greater than the 75th percentile for age and gender may be reclassified through clinical judgment as having a CHD risk equivalent (see also Chap. 20).

***Carotid B-Mode Ultrasonography*** Carotid B-mode ultrasonography, which measures the intimal-medial thickness (IMT) of carotid arteries, provides an independent approximation of coronary atherosclerosis.[11] The extent of carotid atherosclerosis correlates with coronary atherosclerosis.[19,20] Recent reports indicate that carotid IMT carries independent predictive power for development of CHD.[21,22] Like coronary calcium scores, IMT scores could be used to elevate some patients with multiple risk factors to the level of CHD risk equivalent.[4]

***High-Risk Patients Identified by Major Risk Factors plus Inflammatory Markers*** In addition to noninvasive detection of subclinical atherosclerosis, the presence of inflammatory markers also may improve risk prognostication in intermediate-risk patients. Substantial evidence indicates that high-sensitivity C-reactive protein independently predicts coronary events.[23] The AHA and Centers for Disease Control and Prevention (CDC) recommend the optional use of C-reactive protein (CRP) in the evaluation of patients at intermediate risk (10 to 20 percent risk of CHD over 10 years) to help direct further evaluation and therapy (see "C-Reactive Protein," below).[23]

### Identification of Intermediate-Risk Patients

Patients at intermediate risk are those without known atherosclerosis but with two or more risk factors. Through Framingham risk scoring, three subcategories of risk can be identified[4]:

- 10-year risk for CHD > 20 percent (high risk)
- 10-year risk 10 to 20 percent (moderately high risk)
- 10-year risk < 10 percent (moderate risk)

Patients with a 10-year risk for CHD > 20 percent are considered by ATP III guidelines to have a CHD risk equivalent. Those with a 10-year risk of 10 to 20 percent are deemed potential candidates for treatment of major risk factors. For example, low-dose aspirin is recommended by the American Heart Association[2]; hypertension should be treated with anti-hypertensive agents to normalize blood pressure[24]; and cholesterol-lowering drugs are indicated if the goals of therapy are not achieved by lifestyle changes.[4] Finally, less intensive therapies are indicated for patients at moderate risk (10-year risk < 10 percent), although in some cases they must be considered to be at higher *long-term* risk and hence as potential candidates for risk reducing drugs.

### Risk Assessment In Elderly Patients

The predictive power of conventional risk factors declines in older patients, and age becomes the predominant risk factor. For these reasons, measures of myocardial ischemia, coronary plaque burden, or markers of inflammation may be especially useful in differentiating between high- and intermediate-risk elderly patients. The demonstration that aggressive medical therapy significantly reduces risk for CHD in the older population increases the need to define absolute risk in this population more accurately.

### Lower-Risk Patients

An important question is how to manage patients with a single categorical risk factor but who are otherwise at low risk. A fundamental principle of primary prevention is that *all categorical risk factors must be treated, regardless of absolute risk.*[25] For example, cigarette smoking can cause cancer and cardiovascular disease even in the absence of other risk factors. Hypertension alone can cause stroke, heart failure, and kidney failure. Therefore patients with categorical risk factors must not be ignored even if they are found to have a low absolute risk by Framingham scoring (Tables 43-2 and 43-3).

## RISK FACTORS FOR WHICH INTERVENTIONS HAVE PROVED TO LOWER RISK OF CORONARY HEART DISEASE

### Lipid Disorders

#### LOW-DENSITY-LIPOPROTEIN CHOLESTEROL

Evidence of several types supports the concept that low-density-lipoprotein cholesterol (LDL-C) is the primary atherogenic factor, and controlled clinical trials show that lowering LDL-C reduces risk for CHD. Accordingly, the NCEP has identified LDL-C as the primary target of lipid-lowering therapy.[4] Five decades of research on the role of LDL-C in the pathogenesis of CHD represents one of the major advances in modern medicine and public health.[4] This evidence is summarized briefly.

***Low-Density-Lipoprotein Cholesterol as the Primary Atherogenic Agent*** Many studies in laboratory animals indicate that raising serum levels of LDL-C and related lipoproteins will initiate and sustain atherogenesis.[26] Moreover, humans with genetic forms of severely elevated LDL-C exhibit premature atherosclerotic disease.[25] Both of these examples demonstrate that elevated LDL-C alone, without the need for other CHD risk factors, is independently atherogenic. For many years, it was believed that the major action of LDL was merely to deposit its cholesterol within the arterial wall. More recently, LDL has been found to be a proinflammatory agent,[27] setting into motion the chronic inflammatory response that is the hallmark of the atherosclerotic lesion. Elevated LDL appears to be involved with all stages of atherogenesis: endothelial dysfunction, plaque formation and growth, plaque instability and disruption, and thrombosis. Elevated levels of LDL-C in the plasma lead to increased retention of LDL particles in the arterial wall, their oxidation, and the secretion of various inflammatory mediators and chemoattractants (see Chap. 44). One sequela of this is the disruption of endothelial cell function by oxidized LDL,[28] with subsequent loss of production of nitric oxide. Treatment of elevated LDL-C levels has been shown to reestablish the normal coronary vasodilatory response to acetylcholine.[29,30] LDL is also a potent mitogen for smooth muscle cells.

The primacy of LDL as a pathogenic agent is supported by epidemiologic data of several types. In different populations, the risk for CHD is positively correlated with serum total cholesterol concentration,[31] which in turn is highly correlated with LDL-C.[4] The association between serum cholesterol levels and CHD risk is curvilinear (or long-linear).[31] Risk rises exponentially at higher cholesterol levels. In populations that have very low total (and LDL) cholesterol, risk for CHD likewise is low, even when other CHD risk factors (cigarette smoking, hypertension, and diabetes) are common.[25] This latter observation strongly suggests that an elevated LDL-C is the *primary* risk factor.

***Primary and Secondary Prevention*** There is a long history of clinical trials of cholesterol-lowering therapy that have included dietary and drug trials.[4] One trial also induced cholesterol lowering by intestinal surgery.[32] The aggregate results of early trials, both primary and secondary prevention, demonstrated that cholesterol-lowering therapy (or lipoprotein modification) reduces risk for CHD but failed to show an impact on total mortality.[33,34] This deficiency left many clinicians skeptical of the benefits of cholesterol-lowering therapy.

The introduction of HMG-CoA reductase inhibitors (statins),[35,36] which are powerful LDL-lowering drugs, made possible a more effective test of the cholesterol hypothesis.[37,38] Since 1993, seven major trials with statins have been published. The results of these studies are summarized in Table 43-5. All trials showed a marked reduction in major coronary events,[6,7,39–43] and some showed a reduction in

TABLE 43-5 Clinical Outcome Studies Using Statins

| Study *n* (% women) | Intervention | Baseline LDL (mg/dL) | % LDL Reduction | On-Trial LDL (mg/dL)[a] | % Reduction in Total Mortality | % Reduction in Coronary Events | % Reduction in CABG, PTCA |
|---|---|---|---|---|---|---|---|
| SECONDARY PREVENTION | | | | | | | |
| 4S[39] 4444 (19) | Simvastatin 20–40 mg/day | 188 | 35 | 120 | 30 ($p = 0.003$) | 34 ($p < 0.0001$) | 37 ($p < 0.0001$) |
| CARE[6] 4159 (14) | Pravastatin 40 mg/day | 139 | 32 | 95 | 9 (NS) | 24 ($p = 0.003$) | 27 ($p < 0.001$) |
| LIPID[7] 9014 (17) | Pravastatin 40 mg/day | 150 | 25 | 113 | 22 ($p < 0.0001$) | 24 ($p < 0.0001$) | 22[b] ($p < 0.001$) |
| HIGH-RISK PREVENTION | | | | | | | |
| HPS[41] 20,536 (25) | Simvastatin 40 mg/day | 131 | 29 | 92 | 18 ($p = 0.0003$) | 27 ($p < 0.0001$) | 24 ($p < 0.0001$) |
| PRIMARY PREVENTION | | | | | | | |
| WOSCOPS[40] 6595 (0) | Pravastatin 40 mg/day | 192 | 26 | 142 | 22 ($p = 0.051$) | 31 ($p < 0.001$) | 37 ($p = 0.009$) |
| AFCAPS/ TexCAPS[42] 6605 (15) | Lovastatin 20–40 mg/day | 150 | 25 | 113 | 0 (NS) | 37 ($p < 0.0001$) | 33 ($p = 0.001$) |
| ASCOT-LLA[43] 10,305 (19%) | Atorvastatin 10 mg/day | 134 | 33 | 90 | 13 ($p = 0.16$) | 29 ($p < 0.0005$) | NA[c] |

ABBREVIATIONS: 4S = Scandinavian Simvastatin Survival Study; CARE = Cholesterol and Recurrent Events trial; LIPID = Long-Term Intervention with Pravastatin in Ischaemic Disease trial; HPS = Heart Protection Study; WOSCOPS = West of Scotland Coronary Prevention Study; AFCAPS/TexCAPS = Air Force/Texas Coronary Atherosclerosis Prevention Study; ASCOT-LLA = Anglo-Scandinavian Cardiac Outcomes Trial-Lipid Lowering Arm; CABG = coronary artery bypass grafting; LDL = low-density lipoprotein; PTCA = percutaneous coronary angioplasty.

[a]On-trial LDL-C values are calculated from published data.

[b]Results for CABG; the need for PTCA was reduced by 19% ($p = 0.024$)

[c]Data not available.

SOURCE: Adapted from Maron et al.[37] With permission.

total mortality.[7,39,41] No increases in noncardiovascular mortality occurred in any of the trials. These trials documented convincingly that cholesterol-lowering therapy is both safe and effective for reducing CHD risk.

In this same time period, a series of angiographic trials was performed to determine whether reducing levels of LDL-C would decrease progression or promote regression of coronary atherosclerotic lesions. These trials typically employed aggressive cholesterol-lowering therapy, often with combined drug regimens. Indeed, most studies revealed that marked reductions of LDL levels will slow progression, and in some cases promote regression, of coronary lesions.[44,45] Although measurable angiographic changes in lesion size were small, the incidence of major coronary events was reduced strikingly. This observation engendered the concept that LDL reduction *stabilizes* coronary lesions rather than causing them to shrink markedly. Seemingly, lowering of LDL-C modifies lesion structure and composition more than it changes lesion size. Consequently, short-term cholesterol-lowering therapy appears to reduce the likelihood of coronary plaque rupture and thrombosis.

***Practice Recommendations for Lowering Low-Density Lipoprotein*** LDL lowering can be accomplished with nondrug and drug therapies (see Tables 43-6 and 43-7). *The importance of nondrug therapies must not be minimized.* Chief among them are reducing intake of cholesterol-raising fatty acids (saturated and *trans*-fatty acids) and dietary cholesterol.[4] The major sources of dietary saturated fatty acids are dairy fats (e.g., milk, butter, cream, cheese, and ice cream) and animal fats [e.g., fatty cuts of meat (especially hamburger), fatty processed meats, lard, and tallow]. *Trans*-fatty acids are present in shortening, hard margarine, and processed foods containing these forms of fat. Rich sources of dietary cholesterol are eggs, dairy fats, and other animal products. Current intake of cholesterol-raising fatty acids in the United States is in the range of 15 percent of total calories. For patients on cholesterol-lowering therapy, this should be reduced to less than 7 percent. Dietary cholesterol should be lowered to less than 200 mg/day. Achieving a desirable body weight will reduce LDL-cholesterol levels in most overweight patients and will decrease risk for CHD in several other ways.[46] There is growing interest in obtaining further risk reduction by use of dietary adjuncts. A daily intake of 3 g/day of plant stanols will reduce LDL-C concentrations 10 to 15 percent beyond that which can be achieved by reducing cholesterol-raising fatty acids and cholesterol in the diet.[47] High intakes of dietary fiber will produce another 3 to 5 percent decrease in LDL levels.[48] Unsaturated fatty acids (monounsaturated, *n*-6 polyunsaturated, and *n*-3 polyunsaturated fatty acids) will lower LDL and may reduce global risk for CHD via several other mechanisms.[49]

Statins head the list of cholesterol-lowering drugs. Table 43-8 compares the efficacy of the currently available statins in patients without hypertriglyceridemia.[37] Most patients tolerate statins with few side effects. Occasional patients will have a mild rise in liver transaminases, but this change is currently not believed to be an indication of hepatotoxicity. Statins can also produce myopathy, which is manifest by elevated creatine kinase. Rare patients have severe myopathy characterized by muscle weakness, myoglobinuria, and renal failure. Table 43-9 lists risk factors for severe myopathy.[50] For every doubling of the dose of a statin, the LDL-cholesterol level will fall by about 6 percent; a more efficacious way to enhance LDL lowering is to combine statins with ezetimibe or bile acid sequestrants. For patients with borderline elevated triglycerides (200 to 400 mg/dL) and high LDL, either a statin or nicotinic acid is an acceptable first-line drug provided that priority is given to achieving the LDL-C goal.[4] When triglycerides exceed 400 mg/dL, a fibrate or niacin is usually the most appropriate first-line agent; the purpose of therapy is to prevent acute pancreatitis. Table 43-10 summarizes the efficacy of different classes of lipid-altering medications.

***Goals of Therapy for LDL Cholesterol*** For *high-risk patients,* the NCEP recommends an LDL-C goal of $<$100 mg/dL.[4] This recommendation is based on the combined data from epidemiologic studies, angiographic trials, and endpoint trials. New clinical trials are in progress to define the optimal LDL-C goal for secondary prevention. However, the NCEP contends that multiple lines of evidence already converge to support an LDL-C target of $<$100 mg/dL.[4,51]

According to ATP III, a cholesterol-lowering drug should be started on all high-risk patients when the LDL-cholesterol level is $\geq$ 130 mg/dL. When the baseline LDL cholesterol is in the range of 100 to 129 mg/dL, several options are available. Certainly dietary therapy should be maximized, but a lipid-lowering drug is probably indicated. ATP III gives priority to therapy that will achieve the LDL-cholesterol goal of $<$100 mg/dL. The results of a recent clinical trial would support the initiation of a statin.[41] However, another clinical trial with a fibrate also showed efficacy in subjects with LDL levels in this range but with high triglycerides and low high-density-lipoprotein cholesterol (HDL-C).[52] If the LDL-C falls to the range of 100 to 130 mg/dL on statin therapy, several options again are available—e.g., increasing the dose of statin, adding a second LDL-lowering drug (e.g., bile acid sequestrant, niacin, or ezetimibe), or employing an alternative lipid-lowering drug (e.g., fibrate or nicotinic acid).[53] Finally, if the baseline LDL-C level is $<$ 100 mg/dL, options include still further LDL lowering, using either a statin,[41] another lipid-modifying drug,[52] or no lipid-altering drug therapy.

For patients with two or more risk factors (*intermediate risk*), a reasonable LDL-C goal is $<$ 130 mg/dL.[4] However, if a 10-year risk by Framingham scoring is $>$ 20 percent, the patient is considered to be at high risk and the goal is $<$ 100 mg/dL. For those whose risk is $<$ 20 percent, the intensity of therapy should be proportional to the level of risk. In such patients, first-line therapy is therapeutic lifestyle change. If the 10-year risk is 10 to 20 percent (moderately high risk), LDL-lowering drugs are indicated when LDL-C remains $>$ 130 mg/dL after lifestyle change. Moreover, low-dose aspirin therapy is recommended.[2] On the other hand, if 10-year risk $<$ 10 percent, LDL-lowering drugs are not indicated unless LDL cholesterol remains $\geq$ 160 mg/dL after lifestyle change, and long-term aspirin therapy is not recommended.

Finally, for persons with 0-1 risk factor (lower risk), the LDL-cholesterol goal is $<$ 160 mg/dL. Most lower-risk patients are not candidates for LDL-lowering drugs. However, if the LDL-cholesterol level is $\geq$ 190 mg/dL after lifestyle therapy, an LDL-lowering drug should be considered. Further, if the level is 160–189 mg/dL after lifestyle change, a drug can be considered under certain circumstances, as follows:

- A severe single risk factor (heavy cigarette smoking, poorly controlled hypertension, strong family history of premature CHD, or very low HDL cholesterol levels).
- Multiple life-habit risk factors
- High-risk levels of emerging risk factors, if measured (e.g., high-sensitivity C-reactive protein, coronary calcification)
- 10-year risk approaching 10 percent (if measured)

The majority of persons with baseline LDL-cholesterol levels in the range of 160 to 189 mg/dL should be able to attain an LDL-cholesterol goal of $<$ 160 mg/dL through therapeutic lifestyle change without the need for LDL-lowering drugs. The use of drugs for patients in this category depends on clinical judgment that is tailored to the individual patient.

TABLE 43-6 AHA Guide to Primary Prevention of Cardiovascular Disease: Risk Intervention

| Risk Intervention and Goals | Recommendations |
|---|---|
| Smoking<br>Goal: Complete cessation; no exposure to environmental tobacco smoke. | Ask about tobacco use status at every visit. Advise every tobacco user to quit. Assess the tobacco user's willingness to quit. Assist by counseling and developing a plan for quitting. Arrange follow-up, referral to special programs, or pharmacotherapy. Urge avoidance of exposure to secondhand smoke at work or home. |
| BP control<br>Goal: <140/90 mmHg; <130/85 mmHg if renal insufficiency or heart failure is present or <130/80 mmHg if diabetes is present. | Promote healthy lifestyle modification. Advocate weight reduction; reduction of sodium intake; consumption of fruits, vegetables, and low-fat dairy products; moderation of alcohol intake; and physical activity in persons with BP of ≥130 mmHg systolic or 80 mmHg diastolic. For persons with renal insufficiency or heart failure, initiate drug therapy if BP is ≥130 mmHg systolic or 85 mmHg diastolic (≥80 mmHg diastolic for patients with diabetes). Initiate drug therapy for those with BP ≥140/90 mmHg if 6 to 12 months of lifestyle modification is not effective, depending on the number of risk factors present. |
| Dietary intake<br>Goal: An overall healthy eating pattern. | Advocate consumption of a variety of fruits, vegetables, grains, low-fat or nonfat dairy products, fish, legumes, poultry, and lean meats. Match energy intake with energy needs. Reduce saturated fats (<10% of calories), cholesterol (<300 mg/day), and *trans*-fatty acids by substituting grains and unsaturated fatty acids from fish, vegetables, legumes, and nuts. Limit salt intake to <6 g/day. Limit alcohol intake (≤2 drinks/day in men, ≤1 drink/day in women) among those who drink. |
| Aspirin<br>Goal: Low-dose aspirin in persons at higher CHD risk (especially those with 10-year risk of CHD ≥ 10%). | Do not recommend for patients with aspirin intolerance. Do not use in persons at increased risk for gastrointestinal bleeding and hemorrhagic stroke. Consider 75–160 mg aspirin per day for persons at higher risk (especially those with 10-year risk of CHD of ≥10%). |
| Blood lipid management<br>Primary goal: LDL-C <160 mg/dL if ≤1 risk factor is present; LDL-C <130 mg/dL if ≥2 risk factors are present and 10-year CHD risk is <20%; or LDL-C <100 mg/dL if ≥2 risk factors are present and 10-year CHD risk is ≥ 20% or if patient has diabetes.<br>Secondary goals (if LDL-C is at goal range): If triglycerides are >200 mg/dL, then use non-HDL-C as a secondary goal: non-HDL-C <190 mg/dL for ≤1 risk factor; non-HDL-C <160 mg/dL for ≥2 risk factors and 10-year CHD risk ≤20%; non-HDL-C <130 mg/dL for diabetics or for ≥2 risk factors and 10-year CHD risk >20%.<br>Other targets for therapy: triglycerides >150 mg/dL; HDL-C <40 mg/dL in men and <50 mg/dL in women. | If LDL-C is above goal range, initiate additional therapeutic lifestyle changes consisting of dietary modifications to lower LDL-C: <7% of calories from saturated fat, cholesterol <200 mg/day, and, if further LDL-C lowering is required, dietary options [plant stanols/sterols not to exceed 2 g/day and/or increased viscous (soluble) fiber (10–25 g/day)], and additional emphasis on weight reduction and physical activity. If LDL-C is above goal range, rule out secondary causes (liver function test, thyroid-stimulating hormone level, urinalysis). After 12 weeks of therapeutic lifestyle change, consider LDL-lowering drug therapy if ≥2 risk factors are present, 10-year risk is >10%, and LDL-C is ≥130 mg/dL; ≥2 risk factors are present, 10-year risk is <10%, and LDL-C is ≥160 mg/dL; or ≤1 risk factor is present and LDL-C is ≥190 mg/dL. Start drugs and advance dose to bring LDL-C to goal range, usually a statin but also consider bile acid–binding resin or niacin. If LDL-C goal not achieved, consider combination therapy (statin+resin, statin+niacin). After LDL-C goal has been reached, consider triglyceride level: If 150–199 mg/dL, treat with therapeutic lifestyle changes. If 200–499 mg/dL, treat elevated non-HDL-C with therapeutic lifestyle changes and, if necessary, consider higher doses of statin or adding niacin or fibrate. If >500 mg/dL, treat with fibrate or niacin to reduce risk of pancreatitis. If HDL-C is <40 mg/dL in men and <50 |

(Continued)

TABLE 43-6 AHA Guide to Primary Prevention of Cardiovascular Disease: Risk Intervention (*Continued*)

| Risk Intervention and Goals | Recommendations |
|---|---|
| | mg/dL in women, initiate or intensify therapeutic lifestyle changes. For higher-risk patients, consider drugs that raise HDL-C (e.g., niacin, fibrates, statins). |
| Physical activity<br>Goal: At least 30 min of moderate-intensity physical activity on most (and preferably all) days of the week. | If cardiovascular, respiratory, metabolic, orthopedic, or neurologic disorders are suspected or if patient is middle-aged or older and is sedentary, consult physician before initiating vigorous exercise program. Moderate-intensity activities (40 to 60% of maximum capacity) are equivalent to a brisk walk (15–20 min per mile). Additional benefits are gained from vigorous-intensity activity (>60% of maximum capacity) for 20–40 min on 3–5 days per week. Recommend resistance training with 8–10 different exercises, 1–2 sets per exercise, and 10–15 repetitions at moderate intensity ≥2 days per week. Flexibility training and an increase in daily lifestyle activities should complement this regimen. |
| Weight management<br>Goal: Achieve and maintain desirable weight (body mass index 18.5–24.9 kg/m$^2$). When body mass index is ≥25 kg/m$^2$, waist circumference at iliac crest level ≤40 in. in men, ≤35 in. in women. | Initiate weight-management program through caloric restriction and increased caloric expenditure as appropriate. For overweight/obese persons, reduce body weight by 10% in first year of therapy. |
| Diabetes management<br>Goals: Normal fasting plasma glucose (<110 mg/dL) and near normal HbA1c (<7%). | Initiate appropriate hypoglycemic therapy to achieve near-normal fasting plasma glucose or as indicated by near-normal HbA1c. First step is diet and exercise. Second-step therapy is usually oral hypoglycemic drugs: sulfonylureas and/or metformin with ancillary use of acarbose and thiazolidinediones. Third-step therapy is insulin. Treat other risk factors more aggressively (e.g., change BP goal to <130/80 mmHg and LDL-C goal to <100 mg/dL). |

ABBREVIATIONS: BP = blood pressure; CHD, coronary heart disease; LDL-C = low-density-lipoprotein cholesterol; HDL-C = high-density-lipoprotein cholesterol.
SOURCE: From Pearson et al.[2] With permission.

## ATHEROGENIC DYSLIPIDEMIA: HYPERTRIGLYCERIDEMIA, LOW HIGH-DENSITY LIPOPROTEIN, AND SMALL, DENSE LOW-DENSITY LIPOPROTEIN

Although high LDL-C is the primary lipid risk factor, other lipid parameters increase the risk of CHD in persons with or without an elevated LDL-C. Specifically, the combination of elevated concentrations of triglycerides, small, dense LDL-C, and low levels of HDL-C is referred to as *atherogenic dyslipidemia.*[54] This is a complex dyslipidemia that usually results from a generalized metabolic derangement. Although an elevated LDL-C deserves primary emphasis for management, atherogenic dyslipidemia is assuming increasing importance as a contributor to CHD because of the growing prevalence of obesity in the United States and worldwide. Most patients with atherogenic dyslipidemia have a generalized metabolic disorder called *insulin resistance.* Patients with insulin resistance often have the metabolic syndrome (see below).

***Relation of Atherogenic Dyslipidemia to Coronary Heart Disease*** A long-standing debate is whether the individual components of atherogenic dyslipidemia are independent risk factors. This question has been difficult to resolve because each of the three lipid components is highly correlated with the other two. Nevertheless, there is growing evidence for independent atherogenicity of each component. For triglycerides, metanalyses of multiple prospective studies strongly suggest that elevated serum triglycerides are an independent risk factor for CHD.[55,56] Other prospective studies show that a low level of HDL-C is an independent risk factor.[57,58] Two important mechanisms by which HDL is thought to play a protective role against atherosclerosis are reverse cholesterol transport and inhibition of LDL oxidation. A lesser body of data also suggests that small, dense LDL particles are more atherogenic than normal-sized LDL.

***Prevention of CHD among Subjects with Atherogenic Dyslipidemia*** Clinical trials to support therapy of atherogenic dyslipidemia are less robust than those supporting therapy to lower LDL-C. Nonetheless, there is a growing body of evidence to support a moderate efficacy of drugs that target atherogenic dyslipidemia to reduce major coronary events. The drugs that most effectively modify atherogenic dyslipidemia are fibrates and nicotinic acid. A detailed summary of clinical trials with these agents is provided in the ATP III report.[4] Several trials with fibrates have shown a significant reduction of major coronary events. The largest of these include the World

TABLE 43-7 AHA/ACC Guidelines for Preventing Heart Attack and Death in Patients with Atherosclerotic Cardiovascular Diseases

<table>
<tr><th>Goals</th><th>Intervention Recommendations</th></tr>
<tr><td>Smoking<br>Goal<br>complete cessation</td><td>Assess tobacco use. Strongly encourage patient and family to stop smoking and to avoid secondhand smoke. Provide counseling, pharmacologic therapy, including nicotine replacement and bupropion, and formal smoking cessation programs as appropriate.</td></tr>
<tr><td>BP control<br>Goal<br><140/90 mmHg or <130/85 mmHg if heart failure or renal insufficiency<br><130/80 mmHg if diabetes</td><td>Initiate lifestyle modification (weight control, physical activity, alcohol moderation, moderate sodium restriction, and emphasis on fruits, vegetables, and low-fat dairy products) in all patients with blood pressure ≥130 mmHg systolic or 80 mmHg diastolic.<br>Add blood pressure medication, individualized to other patient requirements and characteristics (i.e., age, race, need for drugs with specific benefits) if blood pressure is not <140 mmHg systolic or 90 mmHg diastolic or if blood pressure is not <130 mmHg systolic or 85 mmHg diastolic for individuals with heart failure or renal insufficiency (<80 mmHg diastolic for individuals with diabetes).</td></tr>
<tr><td>Lipid management<br>Primary goal<br>LDL <100 mg/dL</td><td>Start dietary therapy in all patients (<7% saturated fat and <200 mg/day cholesterol) and promote physical activity and weight management. Encourage increased consumption of omega-3 fatty acids.<br>Assess fasting lipid profile in all patients, and within 24 hr of hospitalization for those with an acute event. If patients are hospitalized, consider adding drug therapy on discharge. Add drug therapy according to the following guide:
<table>
<tr><td>LDL <100mg/dL<br>(baseline or on-treatment)<br>Further LDL-lowering therapy not required<br>Consider fibrate or niacin (if low HDL or high TG)</td><td>LDL 100–129 mg/dL<br>(baseline or no-treatment)<br>Therapeutic options:<br>Intensity LDL-lowering therapy (statin or resin[a])<br>Fibrate or niacin (if low HDL or high TG)<br>Consider combined drug therapy (statin + fibrate or niacin) (if low HDL or high TG)</td><td>LDL ≥130 mg/dL<br>(baseline or no-treatment)<br>Intensity LDL-lowering therapy (statin or resin[a])<br>Add or increase drug therapy with lifestyle therapies</td></tr>
</table></td></tr>
<tr><td>Lipid management<br>Secondary goal<br>If TG ≥200 mg/dL, then non-HDL[b] should be <130 mg/dL</td><td>If TG ≥ 150 mg/dL or HDL <40 mg/dL: Emphasize weight management and physical activity. Advise smoking cessation.<br>If TG 200–499 mg/dL: Consider fibrate or niacin after LDL-lowering therapy[a]<br>If TG ≥500 mg/dL: Consider fibrate or niacin before LDL-lowering therapy[a]<br>Consider omega-3 fatty acids as adjunct for high TG</td></tr>
<tr><td>Physical activity<br>Minimum goal<br>30 minutes 3 to 4 days per week<br>Optimal daily</td><td>Assess risk, preferably with exercise test, to guide prescription.<br>Encourage minimum of 30 to 60 min of activity, preferably daily, or at least 3 or 4 times weekly (walking, jogging, cycling, or other aerobic activity) supplemented by an increase in daily lifestyle activities (e.g., walking breaks at work, gardening, household work). Advise medically supervised programs for moderate- to high-risk patients.</td></tr>
<tr><td>Weight management<br>Goal<br>BMI 18.5–24.9 kg/m$^2$</td><td>Calculate BMI and measure waist circumference as part of evaluation. Monitor response of BMI and waist circumference to therapy.<br>Start weight management and physical activity as appropriate. Desirable BMI range is 18.5–24.9 kg/m$^2$.<br>When BMI ≥25 kg/m$^2$, goal for waist circumference is ≤40 in. in men and ≤35 in. in women.</td></tr>
<tr><td>Diabetes management<br>Goal<br>$HbA1_c$ <7%</td><td>Appropriate hypoglycemic therapy to achieve near-normal fasting plasma glucose, as indicated by $HbA1_c$.<br>Treatment of other risks (e.g., physical activity, weight management, blood pressure, and cholesterol management).</td></tr>
</table>

(Continued)

TABLE 43-7 AHA/ACC Guidelines for Preventing Heart Attack and Death in Patients with Atherosclerotic Cardiovascular Diseases (*Continued*)

| Goals | Intervention Recommendations |
|---|---|
| Antiplatelet agents/anticoagulants | Start and continue indefinitely aspirin 75 to 325 mg/day if not contraindicated. Consider clopidogrel 75 mg/day or warfarin if aspirin contraindicated. Manage warfarin to international normalized ratio = 2.0 to 3.0 in post-MI patients when clinically indicated or for those not able to take aspirin or clopidogrel. |
| ACE inhibitors | Treat all patients indefinitely post MI: start early in stable high-risk patients [anterior MI, previous MI, Killip class II ($S_3$ gallop, rales, radiographic CHF)]. Consider chronic therapy for all other patients with coronary or other vascular disease unless contraindicated. |
| Beta Blockers | Start in all post-MI and acute ischemic syndrome patients. Continue indefinitely. Observe usual contraindications. Use as needed to manage angina, rhythm, or blood pressure in all other patients. |

ABBREVIATIONS: BP = blood pressure: TG = triglycerides; BMI = body mass index; $HbA1_c$ = major fraction of adult hemoglobin; MI = myocardial infarction; CHF = congestive heart failure.
[a]The use of resin is relatively contraindicated when TG >200 mg/dL.
[b]Non-HDL cholesterol = total cholesterol minus HDL cholesterol.
SOURCE: From Smith et al.[3] With permission.

Health Organization clofibrate trial,[59] the Helsinki Heart Study gemfibrozil trial,[60] and the Veterans Affairs HDL Intervention Trial (VA-HIT) with gemfibrozil.[52] Another trial, the Bezafibrate Infarction Prevention Study,[61] was negative overall but showed risk reduction in the subgroup with hypertriglyceridemia. Post hoc analyses of fibrate trials suggest that these drugs are most efficacious in patients with the metabolic syndrome.[62–64] Fibrates are not recommended as first-line drugs to reduce LDL-cholesterol levels.

Since LDL-lowering drugs have emerged as primary therapy in high-risk patients, the question can be asked whether fibrates might have a role as add-on therapy to a drug lowering LDL-C. Positive findings with fibrate therapy in clinical trials support this option. Although clinical trials with hard endpoints testing combined lipid-lowering drug therapy have not been conducted, the argument can be made that separate positive trials with drugs that act through different mechanisms may provide a sufficient rationale for combining these drugs in therapy. Smaller studies indicate that the overall lipoprotein pattern is markedly improved by therapy with statins and fibrates. There are reports of increased risk for severe myopathy in patients treated with statins and fibrates. The danger apparently is greatest when the fibrate is gemfibrozil. Recent data indicate that fenofibrate and bezafibrate are less likely to cause myopathy when used in combination with statins than is gemfibrozil.[65–67] At the present time, it is probably prudent to limit the use of statin and fibrate combination to higher-risk patients.

Another agent that favorably modifies atherogenic dyslipidemia is nicotinic acid. This drug favorably improves all of the lipid abnormalities of atherogenic dyslipidemia. It is especially efficacious for raising levels of HDL-C. In one clinical trial, the Coronary Drug Project,[68] nicotinic acid reduced major coronary events. Several other smaller trials were suggestive of benefit as well.[4] Nicotinic acid is attractive for combined drug therapy with statins because the combination has rarely been associated with severe myopathy. However, nicotinic acid does carry more side effects than fibrates; in fact, only about three-fourths of patients can remain on nicotinic acid in the long term. Common side effects of nicotinic acid include flushing, itching, skin rash, a rise in plasma glucose, uric acid, and liver transaminases, and in some patients, frank hepatotoxicity.

## LIPOPROTEIN(a)

Lp(a) consists of an LDL particle linked via a disulfide bond to an apolipoprotein(a) [apo(a)] polypeptide chain. Because of homology between apo(a) and plasminogen, Lp(a) has been hypothesized to serve as a competitive inhibitor for plasminogen binding and thus may inhibit endogenous fibrinolysis.[69] Lp(a) is largely genetically determined, and distributions differ between men and women, as well as between races.

Several retrospective case-control studies support the view that Lp(a) is an independent risk factor for thromboembolic disease. However, results of the major prospective studies evaluating baseline

TABLE 43-8 Comparative Efficacy of the Five Currently Available Statins on Lipids and Lipoproteins in Patients without Hypertriglyceridemia—Changes in Lipid and Lipoprotein Levels[a]

| Atorvastatin | Simvastatin | Lovastatin | Pravastatin | Fluvastatin | Total | LDL | HDL | Triglycerides |
|---|---|---|---|---|---|---|---|---|
| — | 10 | 20 | 20 | 40 | −22% | −27% | +4–8% | −10–15% |
| 10 | 20 | 40 | 40 | 80 | −27% | −34% | +4–8% | −10–20% |
| 20 | 40 | 80 | 80 | — | −32% | −41% | +4–8% | −15–25% |
| 40 | 80 | — | — | — | −37% | −48% | +4–8% | −20–30% |
| 80 | — | — | — | — | −42% | −55% | +4–8% | −25–35% |

[a]For the purpose of illustration, the lipid and lipoprotein responses are based on short-term clinical trials and are approximations of what might be observed in clinical practice.
SOURCE: Adapted from Maron et al.[37] With permission.

TABLE 43-9 Risk Factors for Severe Myopathy from Statin Therapy

- Very old patients (women > men)
- Small body frame and frailty
- Multisystem disease (e.g., chronic renal insufficiency, especially due to diabetes)
- Multiple medications
- Specific concomitant medications or consumptions (with various statins, check package insert for warnings)
  - Fibrates (especially gemfibrozil, but other fibrates too)
  - Nicotinic acid (rarely)
  - Cyclosporine
  - Azole antifungals
  - Itraconazole and ketoconazole
  - Macrolide antibiotics
  - Erythromycin and clarithromycin
  - HIV protease inhibitors
  - Nefazodone (antidepressant)
  - Verapamil
  - Large quantities of grapefruit juice (> 1 quart per day)
  - Alcohol abuse (independently predisposes to myopathy)
- Perioperative periods[a]
- Acute illnesses[a]

[a]In most patients admitted to the hospital for acute illnesses or surgery, statin therapy should be temporarily discontinued.
SOURCE: Adapted from Pasternak et al.[50] With permission.

Lp(a) concentration and future risks of MI and stroke have been inconsistent.[70] A possible explanation of these divergent results may be that Lp(a) adds to risk only among patients at high risk from other factors, such as high LDL-C, low HDL-C, or high fibrinogen.[71,72] Nevertheless, a metanalysis of prospective studies with at least 1 year of follow-up demonstrated a clear association between Lp(a) and CHD, but causality remains uncertain.[70]

***Primary and Secondary Prevention*** Although nicotinic acid and estrogen appear to reduce Lp(a) levels in some patients, no clinical trials have been conducted to test whether reducing plasma levels reduces risk.

PRACTICE RECOMMENDATIONS It is not yet clear whether Lp(a) provides information incremental to the conventional lipid profile, and no recommendation for screening can be made. If elevated levels prove clearly to increase risk among hypercholesterolemic individuals, it may be prudent to lower levels of LDL-C even more aggressively in such individuals than current guidelines dictate. Knowledge of Lp(a) levels may also be useful in the selection of agents to lower LDL-C (e.g., niacin) and may identify a possible treatable cause in the occasional patient with CHD and none of the major risk factors.

## Atherogenic Diet

An atherogenic diet (see Chap. 87) and a lack of physical activity are considered leading preventable causes of death, second only to tobacco use.[73] Considerable epidemiologic data indicate that populations with diets high in cholesterol and animal fats have high rates of CHD.[74,75] Conversely, those populations consuming large amounts of calories as vegetables, cereals, and fish have lower rates of CHD.[74] Countries that increased their animal fat consumption during the 1970s and 1980s increased their CHD mortality rates, while those that decreased their annual fat consumption showed CHD mortality reductions.[76] Similarly, populations consuming larger amounts of sodium in their diet have higher average blood pressures.[77] Caloric imbalance, in part due to excess calorie consumption, is related to the rising prevalence of obesity and diabetes. On an individual basis, clinical trials of modified diets have demonstrated reductions in angiographic progression[78] and in recurrence of clinical disease.[79]

It has been assumed that the harmful effects of the *western* diet have been mediated by saturated fats, *trans*-fatty acids, dietary cholesterol, and sodium via their effects on traditional risk factors such as LDL-C body weight, diabetes, and blood pressure. Part of the effect of a western diet appears to be attributable to these factors. However, there is evidence for other mechanisms. The Western Electric Study adjusted for traditional factors and continued to find an independent risk associated with dietary cholesterol.[80] The Lyon Diet Heart Study compared a Mediterranean-type diet high in alpha-linolenic acid with the AHA diet and showed a 65 percent reduction in recurrent coronary events despite no demonstrable change in any of the traditional risk factors.[79] Potential mechanisms responsible for these benefits include antioxidant, anti-inflammatory, and antiplatelet effects. Fish consumption and supplementation with omega-3 fatty acids appear to promote cardiovascular health and specifically to protect against sudden death through many possible mechanisms, including antiarrhythmic, antithrombotic, hypolipidemic, and anti-inflammatory effects.[81–84] This apparent independent benefit of a diet low in saturated fat, cholesterol, and sodium and high in monounsaturated fats, fruits, vegetables, and fish provides the rationale for inclusion of *atherogenic diet* as a separate, modifiable risk factor.

**PRIMARY PREVENTION**
Reduction in the dietary consumption of animal fat, cholesterol, and sodium should be the mainstay of populationwide coronary disease prevention. Populationwide cholesterol reductions observed in the United States from 1979 to 1991 are attributed solely to changes in dietary consumption patterns.[85] Two older clinical trials of long-term inpatients demonstrated reductions in coronary

TABLE 43-10 Efficacy of Different Classes of Lipid-Altering Medications

| | RANGE OF LIPID AND LIPOPROTEIN EFFECTS (% CHANGE) | | |
|---|---|---|---|
| Drug | LDL Cholesterol | HDL Cholesterol | Triglycerides |
| Statins | −20–55 | +5–15 | −10–20 |
| Niacin | −10–25 | +10–35 | −25–50 |
| Resins | −15–30 | +3–5 | [a] |
| Fibrates | −10–15[a] | +10–20 | −35–50 |
| Ezetimibe | −15–20 | +2–3 | −5–10 |
| Omega-3 fatty acids | +5–10 | +1–3 | −20–30 |

[a]May increase in patients with preexisting hypertriglyceridemia.

endpoints of 34 to 50 percent among patients on diets low in saturated fat and cholesterol.[86,87] Therefore *dietary interventions should be the initial step in the treatment of dyslipidemia, hypertension, diabetes, and obesity.*

### SECONDARY PREVENTION

Studies of low-fat diets, such as the STARS Trial[88] and the Lifestyle Heart Study,[78] used angiographic endpoints and showed a marked reduction in LDL-C and in new or progressive coronary stenoses. However, these studies were too small to test for clinical endpoint reduction. The Oslo Diet-Heart Study demonstrated a significant reduction in reinfarction rates with a diet low in saturated fat as well as a smoking cessation program.[89] As noted, the Lyon Diet Heart Study, with a Mediterranean-type diet enriched in alpha-linolenic acid, demonstrated a 65 percent reduction in recurrent cardiac events and death over a 4-year period of follow-up.[79] *The magnitude of benefit was similar to or greater than that shown in numerous trials of lipid-lowering drugs.*

### PRACTICE RECOMMENDATIONS

The current dietary recommendations emphasize a well-balanced diet low in saturated fat, cholesterol, and sodium while rich in fruits and vegetables. Very low fat diets are poorly complied with and have few long-term safety and efficacy data to support them.[90] A diet with less than 30 percent of calories from fat is generally recommended, but with caloric content compatible with the maintenance of ideal body weight. For patients with vascular disease or hyperlipidemia, less than 7 percent of calories from saturated fat and less than 200 mg of dietary cholesterol per day are suggested. Monounsaturated fats and omega-3 fatty acids from fish may be a beneficial source of calories, as compared with carbohydrates.[84,91] Consultation with a registered dietitian or other nutrition specialist can be recommended as part of a risk-modification program in high-risk patients.

## Cigarette Smoking

A strong dose-response relationship between cigarette smoking and CHD has been observed in both sexes, in the young, in the elderly, and in all racial groups.[92] Cigarette smoking increases risk two- to threefold and interacts with other risk factors to multiply risk. There is no evidence that filters or other modifications of the cigarette reduce risk.[93] Pipe smoking and cigar smoking, when the smoke is not inhaled, as well as oral tobacco use, whether chewing tobacco or snuff, carry rather small risks but are related to later resumption of cigarette smoking. Clearly, cigarette smoking remains a leading preventable cause of mortality, much of it due to cardiovascular disease.

Whereas active cigarette smoking has long been established as a cardiovascular risk factor, exposure to environmental tobacco smoke, or passive smoking, has increasingly been recognized as a modifiable risk factor.[94,95] In a metanalysis of 18 epidemiologic studies, exposure to tobacco smoke by nonsmokers was consistently associated with a 20 to 30 percent increase in risk.[96] This is in addition to an increased risk for respiratory tract cancers and other smoking-related diseases.

Pathophysiologic studies have identified a panoply of mechanisms through which cigarette smoking may cause CHD. Smokers have increased levels of oxidation products, including oxidized LDL.[97] Cigarette smoking also lowers the cardioprotective levels of HDL. These effects, along with direct effects of carbon monoxide and nicotine, produce endothelial damage. Possibly through these mechanisms, smokers have increased vascular reactivity.[97,98] The reduced capacity of the blood to carry oxygen also lowers the threshold for myocardial ischemia and increases the risk of coronary spasm. Cigarette smoking is also related to increased levels of fibrinogen and increased platelet aggregability.[99]

### PRIMARY PREVENTION

Cessation of smoking is associated with a precipitous fall in CHD events. *In a previous smoker, the relative risk declines nearly to that of a nonsmoker in a year or less.*[100] It is estimated that a 35-year-old who quits smoking extends his or her survival by 3 to 5 years,[101] with much of the improved life expectancy caused by a reduction in risk for CHD death.

### SECONDARY PREVENTION

The risk of a recurrent event in a patient surviving a myocardial infarction (MI) is strikingly reduced by smoking cessation. Compared with a patient who continues to smoke, the risk of recurrence can be reduced by 50 percent.[102,103] *The benefits of achieving complete abstinence from smoking for a patient with CHD compare favorably with the health benefits of any intervention in modern cardiology.*

### PRACTICE RECOMMENDATIONS

*Nothing less than complete cessation of smoking and other tobacco use should be acceptable in patients with cardiovascular disease. Moreover, the home and work environments to which patients return should be smoke-free, both to encourage cessation and to reduce the risk from passive smoking.* Cardiovascular specialists often have unique and time-limited opportunities to influence the behaviors of patients. After an acute event, the patient and his or her family members may be especially receptive to a smoking cessation intervention.

Smoking Cessation Clinical Practice Guidelines were first published by the Agency for Health Care Policy and Research in 1996 and form the basis for a successful smoking cessation program.[104] Those guidelines emphasize that tobacco use status be documented in every patient and that every smoker should be offered one or more of three effective treatment interventions. Even a brief intervention may be effective and should, at a minimum, be provided to every patient who uses tobacco[104,105] (Table 43-11). Three elements of a treatment program found to be effective include social support, skills training, problem solving, and nicotine replacement. More intense efforts by the care provider to achieve complete cessation will generally result in a greater success rate. The huge reduction in risk resulting from smoking cessation in the patient with cardiovascular disease provides a strong rationale for sustained and intense efforts to be expended.

Addiction to tobacco is a major barrier to cessation, and a number of pharmacologic agents can be recommended as an adjunct to a concurrent behavioral intervention on the basis of clinical trials demonstrating significantly increased rates of smoking cessation.[106] Sustained-release bupropion, nicotine gum, nicotine inhaler, nicotine nasal spray, and nicotine patch are all first-line drugs to prevent nicotine withdrawal; clonidine is reserved for second-line therapy. The safety of using of these agents in patients with coronary disease was initially a concern, but several studies have established a lack of association between the use of nicotine replacement agents and further cardiac events.[107–109]

## Hypertension

Several major prospective epidemiologic studies have found that both systolic and diastolic hypertension have a strong, positive, continuous, and graded relationship to CHD without evidence of a threshold risk level of blood pressure (see also Chap. 61).[110–113] A

TABLE 43-11 Strategies for Successful Cessation of Cigarette Smoking: The Four A's

Ask
- Systematically identify all tobacco users at every visit (e.g., include tobacco as a vital sign).
- Determine exposure to environmental tobacco smoke at home or at work.
- Identify patients with nicotine addiction.

Advise
- Provide a clear, strong, and personalized message urging every tobacco user to quit.
- Review benefits of quitting and risks of continuing.
- Assess patient's willingness to quit.

Assist
- Have the patient develop a quit plan, including setting a quit date, identifying sources of support for cessation for family and friends, and removing tobacco and other cues from the home and work environment.
- Provide counseling, information materials, and other behavioral interventions.
- Recommend use of pharmacotherapy including sustained-release bupropion, nicotine gum, nicotine inhaler, nicotine nasal spray, or nicotine patch.

Arrange
- Provide a reminder on the quit date.
- See the patient shortly after the quit date to assess success.
- If unsuccessful, identify barriers and methods for their removal.

SOURCE: From Pearson.[105] With permission.

widened pulse pressure, an indicator of arterial stiffness, is another blood pressure parameter that predicts CHD.[114,115] *Hypertension clusters with insulin resistance, hyperinsulinemia, glucose intolerance, dyslipidemia, left ventricular hypertrophy, and obesity and occurs in isolation in less than 20 percent of individuals.*[116] The potential mechanisms by which hypertension may cause coronary events include impaired endothelial function, increased endothelial permeability to lipoproteins, increased adherence of leukocytes, increased oxidative stress, hemodynamic stress triggering acute plaque rupture, and increased myocardial wall stress and oxygen demand.

## PRIMARY PREVENTION

A metanalysis of 17 randomized trials of antihypertensive drugs in over 47,000 men and women with mild to moderate hypertension found that stroke was reduced by 38 percent and CHD was reduced by 16 percent.[111] The mean difference in diastolic blood pressure over 5 years between treatment and control groups was only 5 to 6 mmHg. An important subset in whom events were reduced comprised elderly subjects with isolated systolic hypertension (systolic blood pressure ≥160 mmHg; diastolic blood pressure ≤90 mmHg).

The Antihypertensive and Lipid-Lowering Treatment to Prevent Heart Attack Trial (ALLHAT) was a 5-year, randomized, double-blind, actively controlled trial designed to establish optimal first-line antihypertensive therapy in 33,357 high-risk patients.[117] Subjects were randomized to an alpha-blocker (doxazosin), a diuretic (chlorthalidone), a calcium channel blocker (amlodipine), and an angiotensin-converting enzyme (ACE) inhibitor (lisinopril). The primary outcome was CHD death or nonfatal MI. A secondary outcome measure was combined cardiovascular disease (CVD), defined as the primary outcome, coronary revascularization, angina, stroke, heart failure, or peripheral artery disease. After 3 years, doxazosin was discontinued when it was found to carry twice the relative risk of congestive heart failure as chlorthalidone.[118] After 5 years, there was no difference between the remaining treatment groups in the primary outcome or all-cause mortality. In comparison with chlorthalidone, amlodipine was associated with a significantly higher rate of heart failure and lisinopril with significantly higher rates of combined CVD, stroke, and heart failure. Although chlorthalidone was equivalent to its comparators with regard to CHD death or nonfatal MI (the primary endpoint), the investigators concluded that thiazide-type diuretics are superior in preventing one or more major forms of cardiovascular disease, are less expensive, and should be the preferred initial therapy for hypertension.

The Second Australian National Blood Pressure Study compared outcomes with ACE inhibitors and diuretics for hypertension in 6083 subjects 65 to 84 years old using a prospective, randomized, open-label design.[119] After 4 years, despite similar reductions of blood pressure, treatment in older subjects with the ACE inhibitor (primarily enalapril) led to better outcomes than diuretic treatment (primarily with hydrochlorothiazide). The benefit was seen particularly in men. These results apparently contradict the findings of ALLHAT, but there were differences in study design, demographic and clinical characteristics, medications used, and endpoints measured, making a direct comparison between the two studies problematic.

The impact of the angiotensin II-receptor antagonist losartan was evaluated in a double-blind, randomized, actively controlled trial in 9193 subjects with hypertension and left ventricular hypertrophy (LVH) defined by electrocardiography (the Losartan Intervention for Endpoint reduction in hypertension study, or LIFE study).[120] Subjects were assigned to initial therapy with losartan or atenolol and followed for 4 years. The primary endpoint was cardiovascular death, MI, and stroke. There was no significant difference in the degree of blood pressure lowering achieved between groups. The primary endpoint occurred significantly less often in losartan than atenolol patients, but there was no significant difference between groups in the number of fatal and nonfatal MIs or cardiovascular deaths. The losartan group had significantly fewer fatal or nonfatal strokes. New-onset diabetes was less frequent with losartan.

Blood pressure can be lowered by weight loss, exercise, salt restriction, and avoidance of alcohol,[24] but the long-term utility of these measures to prevent CHD in hypertensives has not been tested in randomized controlled studies.

## SECONDARY PREVENTION

Clinical trials to test the effect of blood pressure lowering per se in CHD patients have not been performed.

## PRACTICE RECOMMENDATIONS

The Joint National Committee (JNC) on Detection, Evaluation, and Treatment of High Blood Pressure recommends a treatment goal of <140/90 mmHg.[24] A goal of <130/85 is appropriate for patients with renal insufficiency or congestive heart failure (CHF).[24] A goal of <130/80 is recommended for patients with diabetes.[3] Please refer to Chap. 61 for a complete discussion of the treatment of hypertension.

## Left Ventricular Hypertrophy

Left ventricular hypertrophy (LVH), defined either by electrocardiography or echocardiography, is a potent independent risk factor for CHD, roughly doubling the risk of cardiovascular death in both men and women.[121] LVH is the adaptive response of the heart to chronic pressure or volume overload (see Chap. 6). In addition to hypertension, LVH is associated with obesity, excessive salt intake, advanced age, and heredity.[122] Progressive LVH may lead to decreased left ventricular compliance, decreased coronary reserve, ventricular ectopy, and impaired systolic function. The Framingham Heart Study observed that electrocardiographic (ECG) evidence of LVH regression was associated with a reduction in cardiovascular disease morbidity and mortality.[123] Another observational, prospective evaluation of LVH using echocardiography indicated an improved prognosis among patients with a reduction of left ventricular mass on antihypertensive therapy.[124] Most antihypertensive drugs can reduce LVH, although not all drugs are equally effective in this regard despite their equipotent blood pressure–lowering capabilities. An analysis of several comparative studies and some metanalyses—including only double-blind, randomized, controlled studies with parallel group design—indicates that ACE inhibitors reduced left ventricular mass by 12 percent, calcium channel blockers by 11 percent, beta blockers by 5 percent, and diuretics by 8 percent.[125]

Two large trials provide insight into the clinical relevance of LVH regression. In the HOPE trial, ramipril resulted in more frequent prevention or regression of LVH compared with placebo. This effect of ramipril on LVH was independent of blood pressure changes and was associated with reduced risk of death, MI, stroke, and heart failure.[126] In the LIFE study, LVH was more significantly reduced in the losartan arm than in the atenolol arm ($p < 0.0001$) for a similar reduction in blood pressure, and the losartan arm had significantly fewer cardiovascular events.[127] Both the HOPE and the LIFE trials used ECG definitions of LVH.

# RISK FACTORS FOR WHICH INTERVENTIONS ARE LIKELY TO LOWER RISK OF CORONARY HEART DISEASE

## The Metabolic Syndrome: Multiple Metabolic Risk Factors

ATP III guidelines place increased emphasis on the metabolic syndrome, a condition characterized by multiple metabolic risk factors and increased risk for CHD.[4] The underlying causes of the metabolic syndrome are overweight/obesity, physical inactivity, and genetic factors. Metabolic changes with advancing age may contribute to development of the syndrome as well. Most patients with the metabolic syndrome have a generalized metabolic disorder called *insulin resistance;* this is characterized by impaired tissue responsiveness to insulin and hyperinsulinemia. In prospective epidemiologic studies, hyperinsulinemia is an independent risk factor for CHD in nondiabetic men after adjusting for body weight, blood pressure, and dyslipidemia.[128] There is considerable variation in inherent insulin resistance in the general population. The combination of obesity and genetic insulin resistance is commonly accompanied by the development of the metabolic syndrome.

ATP III views the metabolic syndrome primarily as a multiplex risk factor for the development of cardiovascular disease. However, persons with the metabolic syndrome also are at increased risk for developing type 2 diabetes. Five metabolic risk factors for cardiovascular disease were identified by ATP III:

- Atherogenic dyslipidemia
  - Elevated serum triglycerides [including remnants of very low density lipoprotein (VLDL)]
  - Small LDL particles
  - Low HDL-C
- Elevated blood pressure
- Insulin resistance ± elevated fasting glucose
- Proinflammatory state
- Prothrombotic state

The association between the risk factors of the metabolic syndrome and development of atherosclerotic disease is complex. There is growing evidence that each of the above risk factors independently promotes the development of atherosclerosis or predisposes to major coronary events.

One of the significant outcomes of the ATP III report was the development of criteria for the clinical diagnosis of the metabolic syndrome. According to ATP III, the metabolic syndrome can be said to be present when a person has three of the following five characteristics:

- Abdominal obesity [waist circumference > 40 in. (> 102 cm) in men and > 35 in. (> 88 cm) in women]
- Triglycerides ≥ 150 mg/dL
- HDL cholesterol < 40 mg/dL in men and < 50 mg/dL in women
- Blood pressure ≥ 130/85 mmHg
- Fasting glucose ≥ 110 mg/dL

Using these criteria, approximately one-fourth of U.S. adults, or 47 million U.S. residents, have the metabolic syndrome.[129] The prevalence increases with age, rising from roughly 7 percent in young adults to more than 40 percent in people ≥ 60 years.[129] The NCEP definition identified men with the metabolic syndrome as three to four times more likely to die over an 11-year follow-up period from CHD after adjusting for conventional risk factors compared to men without the metabolic syndrome.[130]

Although the ATP III definition for metabolic syndrome has the advantage of simplicity, it might be noted that it does not include all of the metabolic risk factors present in the syndrome. Several additional measures deserve comment and might be considered as either (1) alternatives to those listed in the ATP III clinical criteria or (2) measures that strengthen the clinical diagnosis. These measures include (1) elevated 2-h plasma glucose (≥ 140 mg/dL) during an oral glucose tolerance test (OGTT), (2) elevated fasting insulin, (3) a high level of high-sensitivity C-reactive protein (≥ 3 mg/dL), (4) increased serum levels of fibrinogen or PAI-1, and (5) the presence of small LDL particles, especially when combined with elevated apolipoprotein B (≥ 130 mg/dL). Measurements to identify these additional parameters can be considered optional; while they provide useful information, they are not essential for the clinical diagnosis of the metabolic syndrome.

Patients with the metabolic syndrome are candidates for intensified lifestyle changes, especially weight reduction and increased physical activity. Furthermore, in higher-risk patients with the metabolic syndrome, drug therapies directed toward the metabolic risk factors are indicated. For lipid risk factors, drugs to consider either alone or in combination include statins, fibrates, and nicotinic acid. These drugs also have been shown to reduce elevations of C-reactive protein. For elevated blood pressure, some ACE inhibitors may reduce insulin resistance as well as blood pressure.[131] Low-dose aspirin will help to mitigate the prothrombotic state.[2] Finally, glitazones and metformin are insulin-sensitizing agents that could be directed against a generalized insulin resistance. However, there is no evidence from controlled clinical trials that these latter agents will reduce risk for CHD in metabolic syndrome patients who do not have type 2 diabetes. Therefore their use for treatment of the metabolic syndrome per se cannot be recommended at present.

## Diabetes Mellitus

Diabetes mellitus is an independent risk factor for CHD, increasing risk for type 1 as well as type 2 patients by two to four times.[10,132,133] (See Chap. 86 for a complete discussion about diabetes and CHD.) Cardiovascular disease causes three-fourths of deaths among people with diabetes, most due to CHD.[134] Approximately 25 percent of MI survivors have diabetes.[132] *Diabetic patients without a history of MI have as high a risk of coronary mortality as nondiabetic patients with a history of MI.*[10] Once patients with type 2 diabetes suffer a myocardial infarction, their prognosis for recurrent MI and survival is much worse than that for CHD patients without diabetes.[10,135]

*Diabetes abolishes the usual protection from CHD afforded a premenopausal woman. Diabetic women have twice the risk of recurrent MI compared with diabetic men.*[136] The greater risk of CHD in type 2 diabetic women compared to diabetic men may be explained in part by the greater adverse effect of diabetes on lipoproteins in women.[137]

Potential mechanisms by which diabetes may cause atherosclerosis include low HDL-C, high triglycerides, increased lipoprotein remnant particles, increased small, dense LDL-C, elevated Lp(a) concentration, enhanced lipoprotein oxidation, glycation of LDL-C, increased fibrinogen, increased platelet aggregatability, increased PAI-1, impaired fibrinolysis, increased von Willebrand factor, hyperinsulinemia, and impaired endothelial function.

Diabetic dyslipidemia is present in approximately one-quarter to one-third of patients with type 2 diabetes.[138] Fifty percent of patients with type 1 diabetes and 80 percent of those with type 2 diabetes have hypertension.[139]

### PRIMARY AND SECONDARY PREVENTION

Tight glycemic control in patients with type 1 and type 2 diabetes prevents microvascular complications,[140,141] but the impact of glycemic control on macrovascular complications remains poorly defined. Prospective observational studies suggest that poor long-term glycemic control is associated independently with coronary atherosclerosis and CHD events,[142–145] but clinical trial evidence is inconclusive.[140,141,146] Pharmacologic interventions to control dyslipidemia and hypertension have been shown to have a clearly favorable effect on CHD events in type 2 diabetics.[146]

### PRACTICE RECOMMENDATIONS

Weight loss and exercise are key therapeutic interventions because they improve the constellation of metabolic abnormalities that accompany type 2 diabetes. Although the optimal proportion of dietary fat and carbohydrate is controversial, calorie restriction for obesity and avoidance of sugar and saturated fat are recommended. *Beta blockers should not be withheld from diabetic patients following MI unless strong contraindications exist, because diabetic MI survivors have fewer deaths if treated with a beta blocker.*[147] Although there is no consistent evidence to support chronic intensive glycemic control as a strategy to reduce macrovascular endpoints, fasting glucose and HbA1c should be reduced to near normal (HbA1c < 7 percent) to prevent microvascular complications.[2,3] The AHA, NCEP and American Diabetes Association guidelines recommend a more aggressive LDL-C goal (<100 mg/dL) in primary prevention of CHD in diabetics.[2,4,132] The blood pressure goal for patients with diabetes is <130/80 mmHg; antihypertensive agents with beneficial effects on CHD events are thiazide diuretics, beta blockers, ACE inhibitors, and angiotensin receptor blockers.[2,3,127,148,149]

## Physical Inactivity

*Physical inactivity is an independent risk factor for CHD and roughly doubles the risk.*[150] There is a dose-response relation between the amount of exercise performed weekly, from 700 to 2000 kcal of energy, and death from cardiovascular disease and all causes.[150] Data linking sedentary lifestyle with CHD derive from numerous lines of evidence, including animal studies, observational studies, and clinical trials. Moderate-intensity exercise reduces coronary atherosclerosis and widens coronary arteries in monkeys fed an atherogenic diet compared with monkeys fed the same diet but forced to be sedentary. Physical activity slows the progression of angiographically defined coronary atherosclerosis in humans.[151] Over 50 observational studies, primarily of men, have established that physical fitness, on-the-job physical activity, and leisure-time physical activity reduce the risk of CHD.[152] These studies of physical activity are subject to important potential biases, including self-selection and unmeasured confounding variables. An observational study of 73,743 postmenopausal women indicated that both walking and vigorous exercise are associated with substantial reductions in cardiovascular events, and that prolonged sitting predicts increased risk.[153] The risk of MI and sudden cardiac death is greatest during exercise, but the overall risk of sudden cardiac death is reduced among those who exercise regularly.[154] The greatest potential for reduced mortality is in sedentary individuals who become moderately active.[150] Moderate-intensity activity, as opposed to high-intensity activity, produces most of the beneficial effects of physical activity on cardiovascular mortality. A prospective study of more than 72,000 apparently healthy female nurses indicated that brisk walking and vigorous exercise are associated with substantial and similar reductions in coronary events.[155] Shorter exercise sessions can reduce CHD risk as effectively as longer sessions provided that the total energy expended is similar.[156] In addition to decreasing myocardial oxygen demand and increasing myocardial efficiency and electrical stability, other potential mechanisms of benefit include increasing HDL-C, lowering triglycerides, reducing blood pressure, reducing obesity, improving insulin sensitivity, decreasing platelet aggregation, and increasing fibrinolysis.[152]

### PRIMARY PREVENTION

A randomized, controlled trial of physical activity for primary prevention of CHD is not likely to be conducted because of cost and compliance issues.

### SECONDARY PREVENTION

Metanalyses of randomized trials of cardiac rehabilitation with exercise in over 4000 MI survivors demonstrated a 20 to 25 percent reduction in cardiovascular mortality, although there were no significant differences in nonfatal reinfarction (see Chap. 60 on cardiac rehabilitation).[157,158] Most of the studies combined exercise training with other risk-factor modification. The small number of trials with exercise as the only intervention does not permit definitive conclusions. The benefit of physical activity in female CHD patients is uncertain.

**PRACTICE RECOMMENDATIONS**

The American College of Sports Medicine and the Centers for Disease Control and Prevention recommend that every adult should accumulate 30 min or more of moderate-intensity physical activity on most, preferably all, days.[159] These are the same recommendations issued by the AHA for primary prevention.[2] Less than 25 percent of U.S. adults meet this goal.[160] The AHA recommends a minimal goal of 30 min of moderate-intensity activity three to four times a week for individuals with CHD.[3] Large-scale studies indicate that high-intensity physical activity is *not* required to achieve a mortality benefit, and that 200 calories expended daily in moderate-intensity physical activity will confer the majority of CHD risk reduction that exercise can provide. To accomplish this requires about 30 min of brisk walking; however, intermittent activity also provides substantial benefit. Therefore, the minimal goal of 30 min can be accumulated in short bouts of typical daily activities like walking, climbing stairs, housework, and gardening. Exercise testing should be recommended to apparently healthy men over 40 and women over 50 who are sedentary, as well as to younger adults with coronary risk factors, only if the individual plans to start a *vigorous* physical activity program (intensity > 60 percent individual maximum oxygen consumption).[161] For secondary prevention, exercise testing is recommended to guide exercise prescription, and high-risk patients should exercise in a medically supervised setting.[3] Structured exercise programs, whether on site or at home, help compliance with an exercise prescription.[162]

## Obesity

Obesity is defined by the AHA as a major risk factor for CHD.[163] Obesity is associated with insulin resistance; hyperinsulinemia; type 2 diabetes, hypertension; low HDL-C; hypertriglyceridemia; small, dense LDL; inflammation; thrombosis; diastolic dysfunction; and LVH.[24,164,165] Obesity accelerates the progression of coronary atherosclerosis in adolescent and young adult men[166] and it is associated with an increase in cardiovascular and all-cause mortality.[24,164,167,168] Body mass index (BMI) has been adopted widely as a measure of adiposity.[46] BMI is calculated as weight(kg)/height squared (m$^2$) and is estimated as [weight (pounds)/height (inches)$^2$] × 704.5. *Normal* weight is defined as a BMI of 18.5 to 24.9, *overweight* is defined as a BMI of 25 to 29.9, and *obesity* is defined as a BMI ≥ 30. The number of overweight and obese adults in the United States has increased dramatically over the past few decades. A survey conducted between 1999 and 2000 found that 34 percent of adults in the United States were overweight and an additional 30.5 percent were obese.[169] BMI correlates with total body fat content. Abdominal obesity adds to the health risks of obesity, and waist circumference correlates positively with abdominal fat content. In adults with a BMI between 25 and 35, increased relative risk is indicated in men with a waist circumference of >102 cm (>40 in.) and in women of >88 cm (>35 in.).[24]

*In univariate analysis, many observational studies have found obesity strongly and positively correlated with the risk of CHD.* In multivariate analysis—when controlling statistically for risk factors such as hypertension, diabetes, and dyslipidemia—obesity is not usually found to be an independent risk factor. This reflects the fact that many of the adverse consequences of obesity are mediated through resultant metabolic risk factors acting as pathogenetic links in the causal pathway. Nevertheless, some large prospective observational studies of long duration indicate that obesity is independently related to coronary and cardiovascular mortality in men and women.[170–172] Weight loss improves insulin sensitivity and glucose disposal, reduces HbA1c in patients with type 2 diabetes, reduces blood pressure and triglycerides, produces a modest reduction in LDL-C, and increases HDL-C.[24]

**PRIMARY AND SECONDARY PREVENTION**

Although weight loss leads to a number of favorable short-term changes in metabolism, it is unknown whether long-term weight loss results in reduced CHD events. No primary or secondary prevention trials of weight loss have been conducted.

**PRACTICE RECOMMENDATIONS**

BMI should be calculated and listed as a vital sign. Waist circumference should be measured in patients with a BMI ≥ 25.[2,3] Overweight and obese patients should be treated with diet and exercise and BMI and waist circumference should be monitored. The initial goal of weight-loss therapy is to reduce body weight by 10 percent from baseline in 12 months. The waist circumference goal is ≤ 40 inches in men and ≤ 35 inches in women. Lost weight is usually regained unless a program consisting of dietary therapy, physical activity, and behavior therapy is continued indefinitely.

Smoking cessation is associated with weight gain, on average 4.5 to 7 lb. The health hazards of smoking exceed the risks of moderate obesity; therefore cigarette smokers should be given the clear message that smoking cessation is of the highest priority even if it results in weight gain. Currently approved prescription medications for weight loss can help carefully selected obese patients lose weight and reduce the rate at which weight is regained.[173] Fenfluramine and dexfenfluramine were withdrawn from the market because of associated valvular heart disease. CHD endpoint trials with weight-loss drugs have not been conducted.

# RISK FACTORS FOR WHICH INTERVENTIONS MIGHT LOWER RISK OF CORONARY HEART DISEASE

## Psychosocial Factors

The role of personality, environment, social support, social contact, stress and lack of control at work, and depression have all been associated with increased risk for CHD. Acute emotional reactions have been implicated as triggers of acute coronary syndromes. See Chap. 91 for a discussion of these topics.

## Hyperhomocysteinemia

Homocysteine is a highly reactive sulfur-containing amino acid that is an intermediary product of methionine metabolism. B vitamins have a primary role as cofactors and substrates in homocysteine metabolism such that there is an inverse relationship between plasma homocysteine concentration and levels of folic acid, vitamin $B_6$, and vitamin $B_{12}$. Hyperhomocysteinemia is an independent risk factor for cardiovascular disease in several groups of high-risk subjects.[174] Homocysteine and its derivatives cause endothelial dysfunction, arterial intimal-medial thickening, oxidation of LDL-C, and a procoagulant state. The normal fasting levels of homocysteine are between 5 and 15 $\mu$mol/L. Hyperhomocysteinemia may be classified as moderate (16 to 30 $\mu$mol/L), intermediate (31 to 100 $\mu$mol/L), or severe (> 100 $\mu$mol/L).[174] The most important factor affecting plasma concentration is dietary intake of folate and vitamins $B_6$ and $B_{12}$. Other causes of hyperhomocysteinemia include increased age, male sex, menopause, smoking, heavy coffee intake, alcohol, and certain drugs (e.g., bile acid–binding resins, niacin, estrogen-containing oral contraceptives, cyclosporine, and metformin).

A series of cross-sectional and case-control studies and a met-analysis of 27 observational studies strongly support an independent association between total plasma homocysteine level and increased risk of CHD, cerebrovascular disease, and peripheral vascular disease.[174] Prospective cohort studies have been somewhat conflicting. A large cohort study from Norway reported a relative risk of CHD of 1.4 for every 4 $\mu$mol/L increase in plasma homocysteine.[174] Another study of patients with CHD found a strong, nearly linear dose-response relationship between plasma homocysteine levels and mortality, with a mortality ratio of 4.5 for patients with the highest levels compared with the lowest.[175] Other large studies have failed to show a relationship between homocysteine levels and CHD.[174]

Homocysteine lowering with vitamins has been shown in some studies to enhance endothelial function, and reduce arterial intimal-medial thickness, wall stiffness, and procoagulant activity.[174]

#### PRIMARY AND SECONDARY PREVENTION

Although folate and vitamins $B_6$ and $B_{12}$ reduce homocysteine concentration, no randomized trial data are yet available to indicate that reducing plasma levels reduces risk. One study has demonstrated that homocysteine lowering with these vitamins decreases the rate of restenosis and the need for revascularization after coronary angioplasty.[176]

#### PRACTICE RECOMMENDATIONS

Measurement of homocysteine may be useful in patients with CHD in the absence of major risk factors or with a history of recurrent arterial thromboses. Treatment with homocysteine-lowering vitamin therapy should be considered for patients undergoing coronary angioplasty.[176] Folic acid in daily doses of 0.5 to 5.7 mg for 4 weeks reduces homocysteine levels by 25 percent. Addition of vitamin $B_{12}$, up to 1 mg/day, will lower homocysteine an additional 7 percent. Vitamin $B_6$, in doses of 50 to 250 mg per day, is less effective in lowering homocysteine levels.[174]

### Oxidative Stress

Oxidative modification of LDL-C has been hypothesized to play a major role in the initiation and progression of atherosclerosis. Naturally occurring antioxidants such as vitamins E, C, and beta-carotene have been studied as agents for both primary and secondary prevention. A series of observational epidemiologic studies supports the hypothesis that increased dietary intake of antioxidants is associated with reduced cardiovascular risk, with the strongest evidence for vitamin E.[177–180] Unfortunately, it is impossible to conclude causation from observational studies, since individuals who take vitamins are also likely to employ other preventive lifestyle and dietary measures. This issue can be resolved only through large-scale, randomized clinical trials.

#### PRIMARY PREVENTION

In the Alpha-Tocopherol, Beta-Carotene Cancer Prevention Study, which enrolled 29,133 male smokers,[181] there was no evidence that vitamin E (given as 50 mg of alpha-tocopherol daily) reduced the subsequent risk of CHD or stroke, and a small increase in rates of cerebral hemorrhage was reported. In the same trial, beta-carotene was associated with a small increase in lung cancer and deaths due to CHD. In the Carotene and Retinol Efficacy Trial—conducted among 18,314 smokers, former smokers, and asbestos-exposed workers[182]—the combined use of 30 mg/day of beta-carotene plus 25,000 IU of retinol was associated with a small but statistically significant increase in lung cancer and all-cause mortality as well as a nonsignificant increase in cardiovascular mortality. In contrast, among 22,071 men participating in the Physicians' Health Study who were randomly allocated to 50 mg of beta-carotene on alternate days for a period of 12 years, supplementation resulted in no evidence of benefit or harm in terms of the incidence of cardiovascular disease or cancer.[183]

#### SECONDARY PREVENTION

In the Cambridge Heart Antioxidant Study,[184] higher doses of vitamin E were found to reduce rates of nonfatal MI substantially among a group of patients with known CHD. By contrast, in the large-scale Heart Outcomes Prevention Evaluation (HOPE) trial, no overall benefit was observed among those randomly allocated to vitamin E.[185] Subsequently, the Heart Protection Study of 20,536 high-risk individuals found no cardiovascular benefit over 5 years from antioxidant vitamin supplementation with 600 mg of vitamin E, 250 mg of vitamin C, and 20 mg of beta-carotene daily.[186] In a small, randomized, controlled angiographic trial, high-dose antioxidant vitamin supplementation (vitamin E 800 IU, vitamin C 1000 mg, beta carotene 25 mg, and selenium 100 μg daily) produced no angiographic benefits after 3 years and tended to diminish the benefits achieved with statin and niacin combination therapy.[187] Another, larger randomized controlled angiographic trial also found no favorable angiographic results from vitamin E 400 IU and vitamin C 1000 mg compared with placebo.[188]

#### PRACTICE RECOMMENDATIONS

Supplementation with beta-carotene, vitamin C, and vitamin E appears to offer no benefit for CHD prevention. Observational evidence supports the consumption of diets rich in fruits and vegetables.

### No Alcohol Consumption

Heavy alcohol intake is associated with increased risk of death from several causes and is a major public health concern. However, cross-sectional, case-control, and prospective cohort studies indicate that mild to moderate alcohol consumption is associated with reduced rates of CHD compared with no alcohol consumption.[189–192] These studies suggest a J-shaped relationship between the level of alcohol consumption and total mortality, such that a protective effect is apparent at low levels of consumption (one to two beverages daily) whereas there is substantial hazard among heavy consumers. In large part, this dose-dependent balance reflects summation of three effects (1) a positive association between alcohol use and cancer; (2) a U shaped relationship between alcohol use and total cardiovascular disease due to increased risks of cardiomyopathy, sudden death, and hemorrhagic stroke among heavy drinkers; and (3) a well-established L-shaped protective effect for coronary disease.[193]

Several mechanisms have been proposed for the cardioprotective effect of moderate alcohol use. Alcohol intake increases total HDL cholesterol levels as well as HDL2 and HDL3 subfractions.[194-19] Alcohol consumption also has potentially beneficial effects on fibrinolytic function,[198,199] platelet aggregation,[200,201] inflammation, oxidation, and endothelial function.[202]

#### PRIMARY AND SECONDARY PREVENTION

There have been no randomized trials of alcohol use for primary or secondary prevention.

**PRACTICE RECOMMENDATIONS**

How best to advise patients concerning the potential use of alcohol for cardiovascular protection is a complex process because of the potential for abuse.[202,203] Abstinence is advised for patients who are pregnant or who have hepatic disorders, pancreatic disease, congestive heart failure, idiopathic cardiomyopathy, or degenerative neurologic conditions. On the other hand, the recommendation to drink moderately (one drink per day for women and two drinks for men) may be safe when made on a case-by-case basis in the absence of a history of abuse or medical contraindication.[203] Whether specific beverage type matters in terms of cardiovascular protection is uncertain. Evidence indicating benefits for white wine, red wine, beer, and liquor suggest that alcohol content rather than type is the more important predictor of cardiovascular risk reduction.[190–192]

## UNMODIFIABLE RISK FACTORS

### Age and Sex as Risk Factors for Atherosclerotic Disease

The incidence and prevalence of CHD increase sharply with age, so that age might be considered one of the most potent cardiovascular risk factors. Atherosclerotic involvement of the coronary arteries is well established in men by young adulthood, as shown in Korean War and Vietnam War casualties.[204,205] CHD incidence rates in men are similar to those in women 10 years older.[206] Approximately 52 percent of women and 46 percent of men will eventually die of atherosclerotic disease.[207] The increased risk for men and older persons should trigger more intense management of modifiable risk factors. Persons at very advanced age should have the risks and benefits of preventive cardiology interventions weighed on an individual basis.

### Postmenopausal Status

CHD is relatively uncommon in premenopausal women. There is a dramatic rise in CHD incidence in women after age 55, coinciding with increasing age and a decline in endogenous estrogen levels. Early menopause (natural or surgical) is associated with increased CHD risk. These observations are consistent with the hypothesis that estrogen deficiency permits or promotes CHD and that estrogen reduces risk. Numerous observational studies show that postmenopausal users of estrogen replacement therapy (ERT) have a 40 to 50 percent lower risk of initial CHD events compared with nonusers.[208,209] Because of their observational design, these studies have been subject to selection bias and uncontrolled or unknown confounding variables. In most of these studies, ERT was unopposed by concomitant progestin therapy. One large prospective observational study found that combination estrogen and progestin therapy in healthy postmenopausal women was associated with a lower risk of CHD but a higher risk of stroke.[210] Estrogen raises HDL-C and lowers LDL-C, small, dense LDL-C, and Lp(a). Additional proposed mechanisms by which estrogen may confer benefit include favorable effects on fibrinogen, plasma viscosity, plasminogen activator inhibitor-1, tissue-type plasminogen activator, insulin sensitivity, homocysteine, and markers of platelet aggregation and endothelial cell activation. Furthermore, estrogen enhances endothelium-dependent and endothelium-independent coronary vasodilation and inhibits intimal hyperplasia and smooth muscle migration, promotes angiogenesis, and has antioxidant properties. On the other hand, hormone replacement therapy increases triglycerides, CRP levels, factor VII, and prothrombin fragments 1 and 2.[209,211] In contrast to oral estrogen, transdermal estrogen decreases plasma triglyceride concentration and produces larger LDL particles resistant to oxidation.

**PRIMARY PREVENTION**

The Women's Health Initiative (WHI) conducted the first randomized, controlled primary prevention trial of postmenopausal hormones in which 16,608 postmenopausal women aged 50 to 79 years with an intact uterus at baseline were randomized to conjugated equine estrogens, 0.625 mg/day plus medroxyprogesterone acetate, 2.5 mg/day or placebo.[208] The planned duration of the trial was 8.5 years. The primary outcome was nonfatal MI and CHD death. The primary adverse outcome was invasive breast cancer. The study was terminated prematurely because women in the active hormone group had an excess incidence of invasive breast cancer. Estimated hazard ratios [nominal 95 percent confidence intervals (CIs)] for other outcomes were as follows: CHD, 1.29 (1.02 to 1.63); stroke, 1.41 (1.07 to 1.85); pulmonary embolism, 2.13 (1.39 to 3.25); colorectal cancer, 0.63 (0.43 to 0.92); endometrial cancer, 0.83 (0.47 to 1.47); hip fracture, 0.66 (0.45 to 0.98); and death due to other causes, 0.92 (0.74 to 1.14). Absolute excess risks per 10,000 person-years attributable to estrogen plus progestin were 7 more CHD events, 8 more strokes, 8 more pulmonary emboli, and 8 more invasive breast cancers, while absolute risk reductions per 10,000 person-years were 6 fewer colorectal cancers and 5 fewer hip fractures. The absolute excess risk of events included in the global index was 19 per 10,000 person-years. All-cause mortality was not affected. The investigators concluded that the risk of estrogen plus progestin exceeded the benefit for the primary prevention of CHD and recommended that this regimen should not be initiated or continued for primary prevention of CHD.

**SECONDARY PREVENTION**

The Heart and Estrogen Progestin Replacement Study (HERS) investigated the impact of estrogen plus progestin on the risk of CHD in 2763 postmenopausal women with established coronary disease and an intact uterus.[212] Subjects were randomly assigned 0.625 mg of conjugated equine estrogens plus 2.5 mg of medroxyprogesterone daily or a placebo, with a mean follow-up of 4 years. There was no difference in the primary endpoint of nonfatal MI or CHD death. The lack of an overall effect occurred despite a net 11 percent lower LDL level and 10 percent higher HDL level in the hormone treatment group. Although there was no difference overall between groups, there was a statistically significant time trend, with more CHD events in the hormone group in year 1 and fewer events in years 4 and 5. More women in the hormone group suffered venous thromboembolic events and gallbladder disease. A report of the unblinded follow-up after an additional 2.7 years (HERS II) was completed in 2321 subjects.[213] There were no significant decreases in rates of any cardiovascular events among women assigned to hormone therapy compared with placebo in HERS, HERS II, or overall. The investigators concluded that postmenopausal hormone therapy should not be used to reduce risk for CHD in women with established CHD. Other large randomized trials of hormone replacement therapy for primary and secondary prevention are currently in progress. Angiographic trials of hormone replacement therapy in postmenopausal women with CAD have demonstrated no benefit on progression of atherosclerosis compared with placebo.[214,215]

**PRACTICE RECOMMENDATIONS**

On the basis of WHI and HERS, women with and without CHD who have not been on hormone replacement therapy should not be started on hormone therapy for primary or secondary prevention.[208,209,213]

The decision to continue or discontinue hormone therapy should be based on established noncardiovascular benefits and risks, and patient preference. In chronic users of hormone therapy, medication should be discontinued, at least temporarily, if a woman develops an acute coronary syndrome or is immobilized. Oral estrogen therapy is contraindicated in women with hypertriglyceridemia (e.g., serum triglycerides >400 mg/dL), but transdermal estrogen might be an appropriate substitute in such women for noncardiovascular indications.

### Socioeconomic Status: An Unmodifiable Coronary Risk Factor?

At any one point in time, markedly different CHD rates may be observed between socioeconomic subgroups of the population, as defined by occupation, education, income, and other measures. As a group becomes affluent, its members use their new wealth to purchase high-fat and high-salt foods, tobacco products, and automobiles. Less affluent groups lag behind this development, achieving access to these potentially deleterious products later. Affluent groups then learn about and adopt healthful lifestyles, reducing deleterious behaviors. Again, less affluent and less educated groups lag behind, eventually exceeding the rates of CHD in those educated groups whose CHD rates have begun to fall.

Currently, persons with low socioeconomic status are at high risk for CHD. A number of mechanisms may explain this.[216] First, risk factors for atherosclerosis—such as smoking, hypertension, obesity, and sedentary lifestyle—are higher in persons with low socioeconomic status. Second, some of these risk factors, as well as psychosocial responses to stressors, may increase exposure to CHD triggers in these groups. Finally, these groups may have less access to care.

### Family History of Early-Onset Coronary Heart Disease

*Over 35 case-control and prospective studies have consistently identified an association between CHD and a history of first-degree relatives with early-onset CHD.*[217] This risk generally persists even after adjustment for other risk factors. The family history most predictive of coronary disease is that of a first-degree relative developing CHD at an early age. Although CHD in a male relative with onset at age 55 or less or a female relative with onset at age 65 or less is defined as a positive family history, the larger the number of relatives with early-onset CHD or the younger the age of CHD onset in the relative, the stronger is the predictive value.[218,219]

*Although considered a nonmodifiable risk factor, a positive family history should result in the careful screening of individual risk factors known to aggregate in families. Such familial aggregations may represent monogenic factors with known phenotypic expressions and inheritance patterns, polygenic factors with less clear modes of expression and inheritance, or shared environments.* In early-CHD families, Williams et al. estimate that only 10 percent of families will not have a concordant risk factor,[219] most of which are amenable to intervention. Thus, family members of patients with CHD at a young age represent fruitful targets for risk factor assessment. *However, risk factor screening often does not extend beyond the coronary patient. A strong recommendation that siblings and children of early-CHD patients be screened for CHD risk factors should be delivered to each patient and their family members.*

## ADDITIONAL EMERGING RISK FACTORS

### Inflammatory Markers

#### FIBRINOGEN

Inflammation is involved in the initiation, growth, and complication of the atherosclerotic plaque.[23,220] This provides the rationale for the use of inflammatory markers as indicators of atherosclerosis and predictors of atherosclerotic complications. *Plasma fibrinogen level has been shown in several studies to predict the future risk of MI and stroke.*[71,221] When pooled, these studies indicate that individuals with fibrinogen concentrations in the upper third of the control distribution have a relative risk of future cardiovascular disease 2.0 to 2.5 times that of individuals with lower levels.[221] High fibrinogen levels result in increased whole blood viscosity and may play a direct role in atherogenesis and platelet aggregation. Fibrinogen levels increase with smoking, age, oral contraceptive use, and diabetes and decrease with physical activity.[222] This risk variable is poorly correlated with dyslipidemia and therefore may provide additional prognostic information beyond lipid and lipoprotein measurement.

#### C-REACTIVE PROTEIN

The desirable characteristics of a laboratory test to assess inflammation are stability of the analyte, the commercial availability of the assay, standardization of the assay to allow comparison of the results, and the precision of the assay as measured by the coefficient of variation.[23] Given these considerations, high-sensitivity C-reactive protein (CRP) is currently the best candidate assay to identify and monitor the inflammatory process. CRP is an acute-phase reactant derived from the liver. *CRP is increased with hypertension, obesity, cigarette smoking, metabolic syndrome, diabetes, low HDL-C/high triglycerides, postmenopausal hormone use, chronic infections, and chronic inflammation. CRP is decreased with moderate alcohol consumption, physical activity, weight loss, and treatment with statins, fibrates, niacin, and thiazolidinediones.*[23,223]

***Primary Prevention*** Several nested case-control studies as well as large-scale prospective studies have shown a single, nonfasting measure of CRP to be a potent predictor of first cardiovascular events among men, women, the elderly, those with metabolic syndrome or diabetes, and smokers.[23,223] Exercise frequency and body mass both correlate with CRP levels,[224,225] but CRP levels correlate minimally with lipid levels. CRP has an independent association with incident coronary events after adjusting for conventional risk factors using the Framingham Risk Score, including LDL cholesterol.[23,223] CRP is a stronger predictor of risk than LDL cholesterol or nuclear magnetic resonance–based evaluation of LDL-C particle size and concentration.[223] CRP can differentiate patients with the metabolic syndrome into relatively low, moderate, and high-risk groups. *Therefore CRP is an independent predictor of incident cardiovascular events that adds prognostic information to lipid screening,* to the metabolic syndrome, and to the Framingham Risk Score.

CRP does not correlate well with the extent of angiographically defined atherosclerosis.[23] There is currently no definitive evidence that lowering CRP will reduce cardiovascular event rates. However, weight loss, diet, exercise, and smoking cessation all reduce CRP levels.[223] Studies with all available statins show median CRP levels decline 15 percent to 25 percent as early as 6 weeks after initiation of therapy.[223] The magnitude of risk reduction with statin therapy appears to be greater in subjects with higher baseline CRP concentration.[223] Additionally, survival data from the Women's Health Study demonstrate event-free survival was worse for those with elevated CRP and low LDL compared with those with elevated LDL and low CRP.[223] The magnitude of relative risk reduction attributable to low-dose aspirin in reducing risk of first MI appears to be greatest among those with elevated CRP and declines proportionately in direct relation to CRP levels.[223]

***Secondary Prevention*** CRP consistently predicts recurrent coronary events in patients with a history of unstable angina and myocardial infarction.[23] The predictive capacity of CRP is independent of other risk factors. Thus, CRP may have a role in the risk stratification of patients with established CHD.

***Practice Recommendations*** The American Heart Association and Centers for Disease Control *endorse the optional use of CRP in primary prevention of patients at intermediate risk (10 to 20 percent risk of CHD over 10 years) to help direct further evaluation and therapy (class IIa, level of evidence B). In patients with stable coronary disease or acute coronary syndromes, CRP measurement may be useful as an independent marker for assessing probability of recurrent events. Measurement of CRP for widespread global screening of the adult population, to guide secondary preventive care or interventions for acute coronary syndromes, or to monitor therapy in patients with established CHD is not recommended.*[23] The guidelines recommend that the CRP test be performed in a person without obvious inflammatory or infectious conditions, and results should be expressed as mg/L.[23] If a level of $>$ 10 mg/L is obtained, a search should be made for an obvious source of inflammation or infection. Low risk is defined as $<$1.0 mg/L, average risk is 1.0 to 3.0 mg/L, and high risk is $>$3.0 mg/L. These risk categories correspond to tertiles of CRP in the adult population. The high risk tertile carries a twofold increase in relative risk compared with the low-risk tertile.[23]

## Infection

Viral and bacterial infections have been associated with atherosclerosis, leading to the hypothesis that certain infectious agents might trigger an inflammatory response that could initiate or exacerbate atherosclerosis. Among patients with vascular disease, the greater the number of pathogens for which an individual is seropositive, the greater the extent of atherosclerosis and cardiovascular mortality.[226] *Chlamydia pneumoniae* has received the most attention on the possible link between infection and CHD. Epidemiologic and pathology-based studies have indicated this prokaryote is associated with CHD. Antibiotic trials in patients with CHD and serologic evidence of *C. pneumoniae* infection have been inconsistent, with larger studies showing no benefit.[227]

## Endogenous Fibrinolysis: Tissue-Type Plasminogen Activator, PAI-1, and D-Dimer

The activity of the endogenous fibrinolytic system reflects a balance between plasma concentration of tissue-type plasminogen activator (t-PA) and its primary inhibitor, PAI-1. Prospective studies of initially healthy individuals[228,229] as well as patients with known CHD[230] indicate that elevated antigen levels of both enzymes are associated with increased risk of future MI. D-dimer and t-PA concentrations are elevated in relatives of patients with premature CHD compared with healthy controls.[231] Prospective data also indicate that t-PA antigen level is a potent marker of risk for stroke.[232]

Because both t-PA and PAI-1 contribute to the net fibrinolytic balance, it has been hypothesized that individuals at risk for future vascular occlusive events suffer from a net inhibition of fibrinolytic function, a finding supported in at least one prospective study.[233] Other data, however, indicate that elevations of D-dimer are also associated with increased risk of future MI[234] and peripheral vascular disease.[235,236] Since plasma D-dimer levels increase with fibrinogen turnover, these data raise the possibility that the endogenous fibrinolytic system is activated among individuals at risk.

Evidence is not available to support fibrinogen reduction as a measure to prevent CHD. Many factors affect endogenous fibrinolytic activity, including obesity, estrogen status, and exercise. In addition, pharmacologic interventions may soon be available that can favorably shift fibrinolytic function in an attempt to reduce vascular risk. To date, aspirin therapy, alcohol use, and ACE inhibitors have all shown promise in this regard.[237]

# OTHER PHARMACOLOGIC THERAPY

## Antiplatelet and Anticoagulant Therapy

See also Chap. 54.

### PRIMARY PREVENTION

Several prevention trials of aspirin have been completed in healthy men. The largest of these, the Physicians' Health Study, enrolled 22,071 apparently healthy male physicians aged 40 to 84 years of age and randomized them to 325 mg aspirin on alternate days or to placebo.[238] Aspirin resulted in a highly statistically significant 44 percent reduction in nonfatal MI. When the Physicians' Health Study data are combined with those of a similar trial among British men,[239] an overall 32 percent reduction in risk of first nonfatal MI appears to be associated with chronic aspirin prophylaxis.[240] In the Thrombosis Prevention Trial, low-dose aspirin (75 mg daily) and low-dose warfarin [target international normalized ratio (INR) = 1.5] were both effective, although combination therapy as compared with monotherapy remains controversial for primary prevention.[241]

### SECONDARY PREVENTION

The most recent metanalysis of randomized trials of antiplatelet therapy among high-risk patients with preexisting vascular disease reviewed 287 studies involving 135,000 patients in comparisons of antiplatelet therapy versus control and 77,000 in comparisons of different antiplatelet regimens.[242] Overall, allocation to antiplatelet therapy reduced serious vascular events by about one quarter. Aspirin was the most widely studied drug, with doses of 75 to 150 mg daily at least as effective as higher doses. Large-scale randomized comparisons of the effects of other antiplatelet drugs versus aspirin was available only for clopidogrel. Clopidogrel reduced serious vascular events by 10 percent compared with aspirin ($p$ = 0.03),[242] making that drug an appropriate alternative for patients with a contraindication to aspirin. Addition of dipyridamole to aspirin produced no additional benefit to that from aspirin alone.

A metanalysis of 31 trials evaluated the role of chronic oral anticoagulant therapy in the secondary prevention of coronary disease.[243] Moderate-intensity (INR 2 to 3) and high-intensity (INR 2.8 to 4.8) anticoagulation are effective in reducing MI and stroke but increase the risk of bleeding. In the presence of aspirin, low-intensity anticoagulation does not appear to be superior to aspirin alone, while moderate- to high-intensity anticoagulation and aspirin versus aspirin alone appears promising and the bleeding risk is modest.[243,244]

**PRACTICE RECOMMENDATIONS**

*The United States Preventive Services Task Force strongly recommends that the prescription of low-dose aspirin be considered in adults who are at increased risk for CHD, defined as those with a 5-year risk > 3 percent.*[245] For secondary prevention, 75 to 325 mg of aspirin daily is recommended, with treatment continued indefinitely. If aspirin is contraindicated, clopidogrel and then warfarin are recommended for secondary prevention, with an INR goal of 2 to 3.[3]

### Beta-Adrenergic Blocking Agents

Beta-adrenergic blocking agents reduce heart rate, systemic blood pressure, and ventricular contractility, all factors that decrease myocardial oxygen consumption. Beta blockers further have antiarrhythmic properties and appear to increase thresholds for ventricular fibrillation.[246]

**PRIMARY PREVENTION**

Few clinical trial data are available that directly test beta-blocking agents in the primary prevention of MI. The use of this class of agents in the treatment of hypertension, however, has been shown to be efficacious for CHD prevention,[247] and beta blockers have few long-term side effects.

**SECONDARY PREVENTION**

The utility of beta-blocking agents in the acute, subacute, and chronic phases following MI has been demonstrated in many clinical trials. Overview analyses indicate that therapy with beta blockers reduces mortality approximately 20 percent compared with placebo.[248,249] The mortality effect of long-term beta blockade results primarily from prevention of sudden death (pooled relative risk = 0.68), presumably due to a reduction in the incidence and complexity of ventricular arrhythmias. Beta blockers have also proven effective in reducing rates of nonfatal reinfarction (pooled relative risk = 0.74), an effect more likely to result from chronic reductions in heart rate, contractility, and vascular stress.

**PRACTICE RECOMMENDATIONS**

For primary prevention, beta blockers are recommended as first-line therapy for hypertension.[24] For secondary prevention, beta blockers are recommended in post-MI patients with arrhythmias, left ventricular dysfunction, and inducible ischemia.[3] Although specific studies of beta-blocker cessation are not available, it is commonly recommended that beta-blocker therapy be continued indefinitely as long as side effects are not present.[246]

### Angiotensin-Converting Enzyme Inhibitors

**PRIMARY PREVENTION**

The ALLHAT trial indicated that the ACE inhibitor lisinopril is not superior to the thiazide diuretic chlorthalidone in the primary prevention of fatal and nonfatal CHD events.[117] The Second Australian National Blood Pressure Study found that ACE inhibitor therapy (primarily with enalapril) was superior to the thiazide diuretic hydrochlorothiazide in the prespecified secondary endpoint of MI in a predominantly primary prevention elderly population.[119]

**SECONDARY PREVENTION**

ACE inhibitors were first recognized to reduce mortality in patients with heart failure and reduced left ventricular ejection fraction.[250] Subsequently, this class of agents was recognized as important adjunctive therapy following acute MI. The primary rationale for using these agents in this setting is based on the experimental observation that ACE inhibition slows the process of ventricular remodeling. This effect appears time-dependent in that the use of ACE inhibition after MI requires a sufficient length of therapy to result in detectable changes in ventricular volumes and size. The observation in several trials that rates of recurrent MI may also be reduced with ACE inhibition raises the possibility that these agents also result in enhanced endogenous fibrinolysis. The ability of ACE inhibition with ramipril to reduce risk of MI and cardiovascular mortality among high-risk patients without heart failure further demonstrates the efficacy of these agents.[185]

**PRACTICE RECOMMENDATION**

Based upon recent, large randomized controlled clinical trials it appears that ACE inhibitors are at least as effective as diuretics in the primary prevention of CHD death or nonfatal MI,[117,119] although national guidelines continue to recommend diuretics or beta blockers as first-line agents for the treatment of hypertension. ACE inhibitors are appropriate first line antihypertensive therapy in patients with diabetes and hypertension, and they are an excellent second step after diuretic therapy in hypertensive patients. For secondary prevention, ACE inhibitors should be prescribed indefinitely to all patients following MI and to patients with clinical evidence of congestive heart failure.[3] ACE inhibitors should be considered as chronic therapy for all other patients with coronary or other atherosclerotic vascular disease.[3]

## THE PRACTICE OF PREVENTIVE CARDIOLOGY

The evidence for a causal role of risk factors in the etiology of CHD and the feasibility and efficacy of risk factor modification in lowering CHD risk is among the most convincing in all of medicine. Despite this, there are both qualitative and quantitative gaps in our treatment of coronary risk factors and the application of evidence-based guidelines, even in patients at highest risk. Qualitative gaps entail the lack of any risk factor detection and management in many patients. Within 24 h of acute MI diagnosis, only 85 percent of patients receive aspirin, 53 percent receive beta blockers, and 24 percent receive ACE inhibitors.[251] Lipid-lowering therapy is also underutilized. An analysis of 138,001 patients from 1470 U.S. hospitals in the National Registry of Myocardial Infarction 3 revealed that only 32 percent of patients hospitalized with acute MI were discharged on lipid-lowering medication.[252] In another study, only 25 percent of 8515 patients hospitalized with an acute coronary syndrome were discharged on lipid-lowering therapy.[253]

The implementation of research findings in the outpatient setting is equally poor. Among 48,586 outpatients with CHD from 140 medical practices (80 percent cardiology), only 39 percent were treated with lipid-lowering medications and only 11 percent were documented to have LDL-C levels <100 mg/dL.[254] Only 11 percent of the population with CHD evaluated in the third National Health and Nutrition Examination Survey (NHANES III) were treated with lipid-lowering drugs.[255] In a study of 4888 patients receiving treatment for lipid disorders in the mid-1990s, only 17 percent of CHD patients reached their LDL-cholesterol goal of ≤100 mg dL, and only 37 percent of high-risk (2+ risk factors), non-CHD patients reached their goal of <130 mg dL.[256] Thus, preventive cardiology strategies backed by strong evidence for efficacy and cost-effectiveness are simply not being applied uniformly or widely, constituting a missed opportunity to reduce costs and improve prognosis.

## Barriers to Implementation of Preventive Cardiology Services

A number of barriers to the implementation of preventive services can be identified at the patient, physician, health care setting, and community society levels (Table 43-12).[257,258] The improved implementation of proven interventions therefore requires a variety of strategies targeted at patients, health care providers, inpatient care settings, ambulatory care settings, and health systems.

## Strategies to Improve Preventive Cardiology Services

### IMPROVING PATIENT COMPLIANCE

While there is a pervasive tendency to blame the patient, health care providers can take a number of actions to improve their patients' compliance with the treatment regimen.[259,260] These include (1) encouragement to engage in prevention and treatment behaviors essential to adherence with a regimen, such as acceptance and understanding of the need to control risk factors; (2) establishment of specific behavioral or physiological goals; (3) skills training of patients for adopting and maintaining the recommended behaviors; (4) recommending self-monitoring of progress toward the goals; and (5) helping patients anticipate and resolve problems that keep the goals from being realized. This will require regular communication between providers and patients about the goals and actions agreed upon.[259]

TABLE 43-12 Barriers to Implementation of Preventive Services

| |
|---|
| Patient |
| Lack of knowledge and motivation |
| Lack of access to care |
| Cultural factors |
| Social factors |
| Physician |
| Problem-based focus |
| Feedback on prevention is negative or neutral |
| Time constraints |
| Lack of incentives, including reimbursement |
| Lack of training |
| Poor knowledge of benefits |
| Perceived ineffectiveness |
| Lack of skills |
| Lack of specialist-generalist communication |
| Lack of perceived legitimacy |
| Health care settings (hospitals, practices, etc.) |
| Acute care priority |
| Lack of resources and facilities |
| Lack of systems for preventive services |
| Time and economic constraints |
| Poor communication between specialty and primary care providers |
| Lack of policies and standards |
| Community/society |
| Lack of policies and standards |
| Lack of reimbursement |

SOURCE: From Pearson et al.[258] With permission.

### IMPROVING PERFORMANCE BY HEALTH CARE PROVIDERS

Providers must foster effective communication with both their patients and other health professionals on the preventive cardiology team.[259] Strategies to improve this communication include verbal and written instructions, negotiation of goals and a plan with the patient, and anticipation of barriers to successful attainment of goals. There also must be documentation and monitoring of progress toward goals, with assessment of patient compliance at each visit and reminder systems (e.g., listing smoking status as a vital sign) to assure that risk factors are identified and attended to. One barrier to physician action in this area is a perceived lack of legitimacy by cardiovascular specialists for involvement in risk-factor management. *Professional societies counter this problem by strongly recommending that risk-factor management should be part of the optimal care of patients at high risk for cardiovascular disease and therefore be considered the responsibility of all health care providers.*[1]

### IMPROVING THE INPATIENT CARE SETTING

Admission to an inpatient unit provides an enormous opportunity for risk-factor modification and behavior change that should not be missed, for several reasons. First, the opportunity to reduce short-term risk in patients following infarction or revascularization has not been extensively studied, but several interventions such as antiplatelet therapy, ACE inhibitors, beta blockers, and even lipid management appear to provide benefit within days or weeks. Second, the patient and family are aroused to the risk of disability and death, and their receptivity to behavior-change messages is likely highest at this time. Finally, the message communicated to the patient and their primary care provider is that behavior change is an important, integral part of their postcoronary care, along with revascularization and pharmacotherapy.

The inpatient setting can be reorganized to provide efficient risk-factor assessment and management. The joint ACC/AHA guidelines for preventing MI and death in patients with atherosclerosis provide a convenient list of risk-factor goals and modification strategies (Table 43-7).[3] These can be transcribed onto a simple checklist or more elaborate care protocols. The cardiovascular specialist should confirm the diagnosis of prevalent risk factors, set goals for treatment, and integrate a treatment plan into the overall regimen of care. However, the physician is often not the best person to carry out the plan, due in part to time constraints and acute care focus. A better model is the multidisciplinary team approach, with nurses, nutritionists, and exercise physiologists assigned specific tasks for the patient's care. Factors associated with improved inpatient post-MI beta-blocker prescription are shared goals among clinical and administrative staff, substantial administrative support, strong physician leadership advocating beta-blocker use, and use of credible data feedback.[261] In one study, routine implementation of secondary prevention guidelines in all hospitalized CHD patients resulted in increased use of aspirin (68 to 92 percent), beta blockers (12 to 62 percent), ACE inhibitors (6 to 58 percent), and statins (6 to 86 percent), associated with a reduction in recurrent MI and 1-year mortality.[262] The AHA has developed a program called *Get with the Guidelines,* a hospital-based discharge program for CHD patients to ensure that they are discharged on appropriate medications and with risk-modification counseling.

## IMPROVING THE AMBULATORY CARE SETTING

The AHA guidelines for primary prevention of cardiovascular diseases (Table 43-6) and for comprehensive risk reduction for patients with coronary and other vascular disease (Table 43-7) provide clear risk-factor goals and risk-reduction strategies.[2,3] The office or clinic should strive to develop an environment supportive of risk factor management, including staff trained in behavior-modification skills, follow-up protocols, and tracking systems and reminders. A clear assignment of tasks and responsibilities is important, with defined roles for the physician, nurse, nutritionist, and even receptionist.

A number of specialty units might be convenient platforms for risk-factor management. Cardiac rehabilitation has been documented, in metanalyses of randomized clinical trials, to reduce coronary disease recurrence and death significantly, especially when the service includes risk-factor modification. The patients' extended exposure (after 12 weeks or longer) to a supportive environment provides the opportunity for behavior change, monitoring, and reinforcement. When compared with a contemporary cardiac rehabilitation program, a cardiovascular risk–reduction program supervised by a physician and case-managed by a nurse and a similar program administered by exercise physiologists and guided by a computerized participant management system produce similarly effective risk-factor change.[263]

## IMPROVING THE HEALTH SYSTEM

Supportive of this are a large number of guidelines from professional societies, expert bodies, and governmental agencies that support preventive cardiology practices. The joint ACC/AHA guidelines in risk reduction[3] are coordinated with more extensive guidelines for individual risk factors, including hyperlipidemia,[4] hypertension,[24] smoking,[264] cardiac rehabilitation,[265] and obesity.[46] These provide clear recommendations for health care providers as to the goals and scenarios required for optimal risk reduction. Increasingly, these guidelines are being used in quality assurance programs that use provision of preventive services and attainment of risk factor goals as quality-of-care indicators. The use of preventive cardiology services as such quality indicators has motivated health care systems to implement reorganization and reallocation of resources that have been shown to be effective in improving preventive cardiology care. In addition, the AHA has created a guide for community leaders to reduce the burden of cardiovascular disease at the community level.[266]

## References


1. Fuster V, Pearson TA. 27th Bethesda Conference: Matching the intensity of risk factor management. *J Am Coll Cardiol* 1996;27:957.
2. Pearson TA, Blair SN, Daniels SR, et al. AHA guidelines for primary prevention of cardiovascular disease and stroke: 2002 update: Consensus panel guide to comprehensive risk reduction for adult patients without coronary or other atherosclerotic vascular diseases. *Circulation* 2002;106:388–391.
3. Smith SC, Blair SN, Bonow RO, et al. AHA/ACC guidelines for preventing heart attack and death in patients with atherosclerotic cardiovascular disease: 2001 update: A statement for healthcare professionals from the American Heart Association and the American College of Cardiology. *Circulation* 2001;104:1577–1579.
4. Third Report of the National Cholesterol Education Program (NCEP) expert panel on detection, evaluation, and treatment of high blood cholesterol in adults (Adult Treatment Panel III). Final report. *Circulation* 2002;106:3143–3421.
5. Grundy SM. Primary prevention of coronary heart disease: Integrating risk assessment. *Circulation* 1999;100:988.
6. Sacks FM, Pfeffer MA, Moye LA, et al. The effect of pravastatin on coronary events after myocardial infarction in patients with average cholesterol levels. Cholesterol and Recurrent Events Trial Investigators. *N Engl J Med* 1996;335:1001.
7. Lipid Study Group. Prevention of cardiovascular events and death with pravastatin in patients with coronary heart disease and a broad range of initial cholesterol levels. The Long-Term Intervention with Pravastatin in Ischaemic Disease (LIPID) Study Group. *N Engl J Med* 1998;339:1349.
8. Cleland JG. Can improved quality of care reduce the costs of managing angina pectoris? *Eur Heart J* 1996;17:29.
9. Juul-Moller S, Edvardsson N, Jahnmatz B, et al. Double-blind trial of aspirin in primary prevention of myocardial infarction. *Lancet* 1992;340:1421.
10. Haffner SM, Lehto S, Ronnemaa T, et al. Mortality from coronary heart disease in subjects with type 2 diabetes and in nondiabetic subjects with and without prior myocardial infarction. *N Engl J Med* 1998;339:229–234.
11. Smith SC, Greenland P, Grundy SM: Beyond secondary prevention: Identifying the high-risk patient for primary prevention: Executive Summary: American Heart Association Prevention Conference. *Circulation* 2000;101:111–116.
12. O'Rourke RA, Brundage BH, Froelicher VF, et al. American College of Cardiology/American Heart Association expert consensus document on electron-beam computed tomography for the diagnosis and prognosis of coronary artery disease. *Circulation* 2000;102:126–140.
13. Pitt B, Rubenfire M. Risk stratification for the detection of preclinical coronary artery disease. *Circulation* 1999;99:2610.
14. Froelicher VF, Follansbee WP, Labovitz, AJ, et al. Special application: Screening apparently healthy individuals. In: Froelicher VF, Follansbee WP, Labovitz AJ, Myers J, eds. *Exercise and the Heart.* Boston: Mosby; 1993:208–229.
15. Rumberger JA, Schwartz RS, Simons DB, et al. Relation of coronary calcium determined by electron beam computed tomography and lumen narrowing determined by autopsy. *Am J Cardiol* 1994;73:1169.
16. Rumberger JA, Simons DB, Fitzpatrick LA, et al. Coronary artery calcium area by electron-beam computed tomography and coronary atherosclerotic plaque area: A histopathologic correlative study. *Circulation* 1995;92:2157.
17. Budoff MJ, Georgiou D, Brody A, et al. Ultrafast computed tomography as a diagnostic modality in the detection of coronary artery disease: A multicenter study. *Circulation* 1996;93:898.
18. Becker CR. Combined approach of contrast and non-contrast CT fo the assessment of coronary atherosclerosis. *Herz* 2003;28:32.
19. Crouse JR, Craven TE, Hagaman AP. Association of coronary disease with segment-specific intimal-medial thickening of the extracrania carotid artery. *Circulation* 1995;92:1141.
20. Visona A, Pesavento R, Lusiani L, et al. Intimal medial thickening o common carotid artery as indicator of coronary artery disease *Angiology* 1996;47:61.
21. Hodis HN, Mack WJ, LaBree L, et al. The role of carotid arteria intima-media thickness in predicting clinical coronary events. *An Intern Med* 1998;128:262.
22. O'Leary DH, Polak JF, Kronmal RA, et al. Carotid-artery intima an media thickness as a risk factor for myocardial infarction and stroke i older adults: Cardiovascular Health Study Collaborative Researc Group. *N Engl J Med* 1999;340:14.
23. Pearson TA, Mensah GA, Alexander RW, et al. Markers of in flammation and cardiovascular disease: Application to clinical an public health practice. A statement for healthcare professionals fror the Centers for Disease Control and Prevention and the America Heart Association. *Circulation* 2003;107:499–511.
24. Joint National Committee on Prevention, Evaluation, and Treatme of High Blood Pressure. *The Sixth Report of the Joint Nationa Committee on Prevention, Detection, Evaluation, and Treatment o High Blood Pressure.* Bethesda, MD: National Institutes of Healt National Heart, Lung, and Blood Institute; 1997.
25. Goldstein JL, Kita T, Brown MS. Defective lipoprotein receptors an atherosclerosis: Lessons from an animal counterpart of famili hypercholesterolemia. *N Engl J Med* 1983;309:288.

26. Babiak J, Rudel LL. Lipoproteins and atherosclerosis. *Baillieres Clin Endocrinol Metab* 1987;1:515.
27. Navab M, Berliner JA, Watson AD, et al. The Yin and Yang of oxidation in the development of the fatty streak: A review based on the 1994 George Lyman Duff Memorial Lecture. *Arterioscler Thromb Vasc Biol* 1996;16:831.
28. Flavahan NA. Atherosclerosis or lipoprotein-induced endothelial dysfunction: Potential mechanisms underlying reduction in EDRF nitric oxide activity. *Circulation* 1992;85:1927.
29. Treasure CB, Klein JL, Weintraub WS, et al. Beneficial effects of cholesterol-lowering therapy on the coronary endothelium in patients with coronary artery disease. *N Engl J Med* 1995;332:481.
30. Anderson TJ, Meredith IT, Yeung AC, et al. The effect of cholesterol-lowering and antioxidant therapy on endothelium-dependent coronary vasomotion. *N Engl J Med* 1995;332:488.
31. Law MR, Wald, NJ, Thompson SG. By how much and how quickly does reduction in serum cholesterol concentration lower risk of ischaemic heart disease? *BMJ* 1994;308:367.
32. Buchwald H. Program on the surgical control of hyperlipidemias (POSCH) trial: A pivotal 25-year study. In Grundy SM, ed. *Cholesterol Lowering Therapy: Evaluation of Clinical Trial Evidence.* New York: Marcel Dekker; 1999:117.
33. Gordon DJ. Cholesterol lowering and total mortality. In: Rifkind BM, ed. *Lowering Cholesterol in High Risk Individuals and Populations.* New York: Marcel Dekker; 1995:33.
34. Gordon DJ. Cholesterol and mortality: What can meta-analysis tell us? In: Gallo LL, ed. *Cardiovascular Disease,* 2d ed. New York: Plenum Press; 1995:333.
35. Endo AL. The discovery and development of HMG-CoA reductase inhibitors. *J Lipid Res* 1992;33:1569.
36. Grundy SM. HMG-CoA reductase inhibitors for treatment of hypercholesterolemia. *N Engl J Med* 1988;319:24.
37. Maron DJ, Fazio S, Linton MF. Current perspectives on statins. *Circulation* 2000;101:207.
38. Grundy SM. Cholesterol-lowering clinical trials: A historical perspective. In: Grundy SM, ed. *Cholesterol Lowering Therapy: Evaluation of Clinical Trial Evidence.* New York: Marcel Dekker; 1999:1.
39. Scandinavian Simvastatin Survival Study. Randomised trial of cholesterol lowering in 4444 patients with coronary heart disease: The Scandinavian Simvastatin Survival Study. *Lancet* 1994;344:1383.
40. Shepherd J, Cobbe SM, Ford L, et al. Prevention of coronary heart disease with pravastatin in men with hypercholesterolemia. West of Scotland Coronary Prevention Study Group. *N Engl J Med* 1995; 333:1301.
41. Heart Protection Study Collaborative Group. MRC/BHF heart protection study: Randomised placebo-controlled trial of cholesterol-lowering with simvastatin in 20,536 high-risk individuals. *Lancet* 2002;360(9326):7–22
42. Downs JR, Clearfield M, Weis S, et al. Primary prevention of acute coronary events with lovastatin in men and women with average cholesterol levels: Results of AFCAPS TexCAPS. Air Force Texas Coronary Atherosclerosis Prevention Study. *JAMA* 1998;279:1615.
43. Sever PS, Dahlof B, Poulter NR, et al for the ASCOT investigators. Prevention of coronary and stroke events with atorvastatin in hypertensive patients who have average or lower-than-average cholesterol concentrations, in the Anglo-Scandinavian Cardiac Outcomes Trial-Lipid Lowering Arm (ASCOT-LLA): A multicentre randomized controlled trial. *Lancet* 2003;361:1149–1158.
44. Brown BG, Zhao XQ, Sacco DE, et al. Lipid lowering and plaque regression: New insights into prevention of plaque disruption and clinical events in coronary disease. *Circulation* 1993;87:1781.
45. Holmes CL, Schulzer M, Mancini GBJ. Angiographic results of lipid-lowering trials: A systematic review and meta-analysis. In: Grundy SM, ed. *Cholesterol-Lowering Therapy: Evaluation of Clinical Trial Evidence.* New York: Marcel Dekker; 1999:191.
46. National Heart, Lung, and Blood Institute (NHLBI). *Clinical Guidelines on the Identification, Evaluation, and Treatment of Overweight and Obesity in Adults: The Evidence Report.* Bethesda; MD: National Institutes of Health, NHLBI; 1998.
47. Cater NB, Grundy SM. Lowering serum cholesterol with plant sterols and stanols: Historical perspectives. In: Nguyen TT, ed. *Postgraduate Medicine Special Report: New Developments in Dietary Management of High Cholesterol.* New York: McGraw-Hill; 1998:6.
48. Van Horn L. Fiber, lipids, and coronary heart disease: A statement for healthcare professionals from the Nutrition Committee, American Heart Association. *Circulation* 1997;95:2701.
49. Grundy SM, Denke MA. Dietary influences on serum lipids and lipoproteins. *J Lipid Res* 1990;31:1149–1172.
50. Pasternak RC, Smith SC Jr, Bairey-Merz CN, et al. ACC/AHA/NHLBI clinical advisory on the use and safety of statins. *J Am Coll Cardiol* 2002;40:567–572.
51. Lee TH, Cleeman JI, Grundy SM, et al. Clinical goals and performance measures for cholesterol management in secondary prevention of coronary heart disease. *JAMA* 2000;283:294.
52. Rubins HB, Robins SJ, Collins D, et al. Gemfibrozil for the secondary prevention of coronary heart disease in men with low levels of high-density lipoprotein cholesterol. Veterans Affairs High-Density Lipoprotein Cholesterol Intervention Trial Study Group. *N Engl J Med* 1999;341:410.
53. Grundy SM: Alternative approaches to cholesterol-lowering therapy. *Am J Cardiol* 2002;90:1135–1138.
54. Grundy SM. Hypertriglyceridemia, atherogenic dyslipidemia, and the metabolic syndrome. *Am J Cardiol* 1998;81:18B.
55. Hokanson JE, Austin MA. Plasma triglyceride level is a risk factor for cardiovascular disease independent of high-density lipoprotein cholesterol level: A meta-analysis of population-based prospective studies. *J Cardiovasc Risk* 1996;3:213.
56. Assmann G, Schulte H, Funke H, et al. The emergence of triglycerides as a significant independent risk factor in coronary artery disease. *Eur Heart J* 1998;19:M8.
57. Miller NE. High-density lipoprotein: A major risk factor for coronary atherosclerosis. *Baillieres Clin Endocrinol Metab* 1987;1:603.
58. Vega GL, Grundy SM. Hypoalphalipoproteinemia (low high density lipoprotein) as a risk factor for coronary heart disease. *Curr Opin Lipidol* 1996;7:209.
59. Committee of Principal Investigators. A co-operative trial in the primary prevention of ischaemic heart disease using clofibrate: Report from the Committee of Principal Investigators. *Br Heart J* 1978; 40:1069.
60. Frick MH, Elo O, Haapa K, et al. Helsinki Heart Study: Primary-prevention trial with gemfibrozil in middle-aged men with dyslipidemia—Safety of treatment, changes in risk factors, and incidence of coronary heart disease. *N Engl J Med* 1987;317:1237.
61. The BIP Study Group. Secondary prevention by raising HDL cholesterol and reducing triglycerides in patients with coronary artery disease: The Bezafibrate Infarction Prevention (BIP) study. *Circulation* 2000;102:21–27.
62. Tenkanen L, Manttari M, Manninen V. Some coronary risk factors related to the insulin resistance syndrome and treatment with gemfibrozil. Experience from the Helsinki Heart Study. *Circulation* 1995;92:1779–1785.
63. Bloomfield RH. High-density lipoprotein and coronary heart disease: Lessons from recent intervention trials. *Prev Cardiol* 2000;3:33–39.
64. Steinmetz A, Fenselau S, Schrezenmeir J. Treatment of dyslipoproteinemia in the metabolic syndrome. *Exp Clin Endocrinol Diabetes* 2001;109(4):S548–S559.
65. Kyrklund C, Backman JT, Kivisto KT, et al. Plasma concentrations of active lovastatin acid are markedly increased by gemfibrozil but not by bezafibrate. *Clin Pharmacol Ther* 2001;69:340–345.
66. Prueksaritanont T, Zhao JJ, Ma B, et al. Mechanistic studies on metabolic interactions between gemfibrozil and statins. *J Pharmacol Exp Ther* 2002;301:1042–1051.
67. Pan WJ, Gustavson LE, Achari R, et al. Lack of a clinically significant pharmacokinetic interaction between fenofibrate and pravastatin in healthy volunteers. *J Clin Pharmacol* 2000;40:316–323.

68. Berge KG, Canner PL. Coronary drug project: Experience with niacin. Coronary Drug Project Research Group. *Eur J Clin Pharmacol* 1991;40(suppl 1):S49–S51.
69. Scanu AM. Lipoprotein(a): A genetic risk factor for premature coronary heart disease. *JAMA* 1992;267:3326.
70. Danesh J, Collins R, Peto R. Lipoprotein(a) and coronary heart disease: Meta-analysis of prospective studies. *Circulation* 2000;102: 1082–1085.
71. Cantin B, Després J-P, Lamarch B, et al. Association of fibrinogen and lipoprotein(a) as a coronary heart disease risk factor in men (the Quebec Cardiovascular Study). *Am J Cardiol* 2002;89:662–666.
72. von Eckardstein A, Schulte H, Cullen P, et al. Lipoprotein(a) further increases the risk of coronary events in men with high global cardiovascular risk. *J Am Coll Cardiol* 2001;37:434–439.
73. McGinnis JM, Foege W. Actual causes of death in the United States. *JAMA* 1993;270:2207.
74. Kesteloot H, Joossens JV. Nutrition and international patterns of disease. In: Marmot M, Elliott P, eds. *Coronary Heart Disease Epidemiology: From Etiology to Public Health.* Oxford, UK: Oxford University Press; 1993:152.
75. Keys A. *Seven Countries: A Multivariate Analysis of Death and Coronary Heart Disease.* Cambridge, MA: Harvard University Press; 1980.
76. Epstein FH. The relationship of lifestyle to international trends in CHD. *Int J Epidemiol* 1989;18(3 suppl):S203.
77. INTERSALT Cooperative Research Group. Intersalt: An international study of electrolyte excretion and blood. *Br Med J* 1988;297:319.
78. Ornish D, Brown SE, Scherwitz LW, et al. Can lifestyle changes reverse coronary heart disease? The Lifestyle Heart. *Lancet* 1990; 336:129.
79. De Lorgeril M, Salen P, Martin JL, et al. Mediterranean diet, traditional risk factors, and the rate of cardiovascular complications after myocardial infarction: Final report of the Lyon Diet Heart Study. *Circulation* 1999;99:779.
80. Shekelle RB, Stamler J. Dietary cholesterol and ischaemic heart disease. *Lancet* 1989;1:1177.
81. Hu FB, Bronner L, Willett WC. Fish and omega-3 fatty acid intake and risk of coronary heart disease in women. *JAMA* 2002;287:1815–1821.
82. Albert CM, Campos H, Stampfer MJ, et al. Blood levels of long-chain n-3 fatty acids and the risk of sudden death. *N Engl J Med* 2002;346: 1113–1118.
83. Marchioli R, Barzi F, Bomba E, et al, on behalf of the GISSI-Prevenzione Investigators. Early protection against sudden death by n-3 polyunsaturated fatty acids after myocardial infarction: Time-course analysis of the results of the Gruppo Italiano per lo Studio della Sopravvivenza nell'Infarto Miocardico (GISSI)-Prevenzione. *Circulation* 2002;105:1897–1903.
84. Kris-Etherton PM, Harris WS, Appel LJ, for the Nutrition Committee. Fish consumption, fish oil, omega-3 fatty acids, and cardiovascular disease (AHA Scientific Statement). *Circulation* 2002;106:2747–2757.
85. Johnson CL, Rifkind BM, Sempos CT, et al. Declining serum total cholesterol levels among US adults. The National Health and Nutrition Examination Surveys. *JAMA* 1993;269:3002.
86. Dayton S, Pearce MC, Hashimoto S. A controlled trial of a diet high in unsaturated fat in preventing complications of atherosclerosis. *Circulation* 1969;39:1.
87. Turpeinen O. Effect of cholesterol-lowering diet on mortality from coronary heart disease. *Circulation* 1979;59:1.
88. Watts GF, Lewis B, Brunt JN, et al. Effects on coronary artery disease of lipid-lowering diet, or diet plus cholestyramine, in the St. Thomas' Atherosclerosis Regression Study (STARS). *Lancet* 1992;339:563.
89. Leren P. The Oslo diet-heart study: Eleven-year report. *Circulation* 1970;42:935.
90. Lichtenstein AH, Van Horn L. Very low fat diets. *Circulation* 1998; 98:935.
91. Kris-Etherton PM. AHA Science Advisory: Monounsaturated fatty acids and risk of cardiovascular disease. American Heart Association, Nutrition Committee. *Circulation* 1999;100:1253.
92. US Department of Health and Human Services. *The Health Consequences of Smoking: Cardiovascular Disease. A Report of the Surgeon General.* Washington, DC: Office of Smoking and Health, US Government Printing Office; 1983.
93. Castelli WP, Garrison RJ, Dawber TR, et al. The filter cigarette and coronary heart disease: The Framingham story. *Lancet* 1981;2:109.
94. Fielding JE, Phenow KJ. Health effects of involuntary smoking. *N Engl J Med* 1988;319:1452.
95. Glantz SA, Parmley WW. Passive smoking and heart disease: Mechanisms and risk. *JAMA* 1995;273:1047.
96. He J, Vupputuri S, Allen K, et al. Passive smoking and the risk of coronary heart disease: A meta-analysis of epidemiologic studies. *N Engl J Med* 1999;340:920.
97. Frei B, Forte TM, Ames BN, et al. Gas phase oxidants of cigarette smoke induce lipid peroxidation and changes in lipoprotein properties in human blood plasma: Protective effects of ascorbic acid. *Biochem J* 1991;277:133.
98. Celermajer DS, Sorensen KE, Georgakopoulos D, et al. Cigarette smoking is associated with dose-related and potentially reversible improvement of endothelium-dependent dilation in healthy young adults. *Circulation* 1993;88:2149.
99. Rival J, Riddle JM, Stein PD. Effects of chronic smoking on platelet function. *Thromb Res* 1987;45:75.
100. Gordon T, Kannel WB, McGee D, et al. Death and coronary attacks in men after giving up cigarette smoking: A report from the Framingham Study. *Lancet* 1974;2:1345.
101. Tsevat J, Weinstein MC, Williams LW, et al. Expected gains in life expectancy from various coronary heart disease risk factor modifications. *Circulation* 1991;83:1194.
102. Wilhelmsson C, Vedin JA, Elmfeldt D, et al. Smoking and myocardial infarction. *Lancet* 1975;1:415.
103. Hermanson B, Omenn GS, Kronmal RA, et al. Beneficial six-year outcome of smoking cessation in older men and women with coronary artery disease: Results from the CASS Registry. *N Engl J Med* 1988; 319:1365.
104. Fiore M, Bailey W, Cohen S, et al. *Smoking Cessation: Clinical Practice Guidelines No. 18.* Washington, DC: Agency for Healthcare Policy and Research, Public Health Service, US Department of Health and Human Services; 1996.
105. Pearson TA. Smoking cessation: Clinical evaluation and management of the cigarette smoker. In: Kelly WN, ed. *Textbook of Internal Medicine.* Philadelphia: Lippincott; 1992:1870.
106. Hughes JR, Goldstein MG, Hurt RD, et al. Recent advances in the pharmacotherapy of smoking. *JAMA* 1999;281:72.
107. Benowitz NL. The role of nicotine in smoking-related cardiovascular disease. *Prev Med* 1997;26:412.
108. Blann AD, Steele C, McCollum CN. The influence of smoking and of oral and transdermal nicotine on blood. *Thromb Haemost* 1997;78:1093.
109. Lucini D, Bertocchi F, Malliani A, et al. Autonomic effects of nicotine patch administration in habitual cigarette smokers: A double-blind, placebo-controlled study using spectral analysis of RR interval and systolic arterial pressure variabilities. *J Cardiovasc Pharmacol* 1998; 31:714.
110. MacMahon S, Peto R, Cutler J, et al. Blood pressure, stroke, and coronary heart disease: Part 1. Prolonged differences in blood pressure: Prospective observational studies corrected for the regression dilution bias. *Lancet* 1990;335:765.
111. Collins R, MacMahon S. Blood pressure, antihypertensive drug treatment and the risks of stroke and of coronary heart disease. *Br Med Bull* 1994;50:272.
112. Joint National Committee on Prevention, Evaluation, and Treatment of High Blood Pressure. *The Sixth Report of the Joint National Committee on Prevention, Detection, Evaluation, and Treatment of High Blood Pressure.* Bethesda, MD: National Institutes of Health, National Heart, Lung, and Blood Institute; 1997.
113. Vasan RS, Larson MG, Leip EP, et al. Impact of high-normal blood pressure on the risk of cardiovascular disease. *N Engl J Med* 2001;345:1291–1297.

114. Franklin SS, Khan SA, Wong ND, et al. Is pulse pressure useful in predicting risk for coronary heart disease? The Framingham Heart Study. *Circulation* 1999;100:354.

115. Vaccarino V, Holford TR, Krumholz HM. Pulse pressure and risk for myocardial infarction and heart failure in the elderly. *J Am Coll Cardiol* 2000;36:130–138.

116. Kannel WB. Blood pressure as a cardiovascular risk factor: Prevention and treatment. *JAMA* 1996;275:1571.

117. The ALLHAT Officers and Coordinators for the ALLHAT Collaborative Research Group. Major outcomes in high-risk hypertensive patients randomized to angiotensin-converting enzyme inhibitor or calcium channel blocker vs diuretic: The Antihypertensive and Lipid-Lowering Treatment to Prevent Heart Attack Trial (ALLHAT). *JAMA* 2002;288:2981–2997.

118. The ALLHAT Officers and Coordinators for the ALLHAT Collaborative Research Group. Major cardiovascular events in hypertensive patients randomized to doxazosin vs chlorthalidone: The Antihypertensive and Lipid-Lowering Treatment to Prevent Heart Attack Trial (ALLHAT). *JAMA* 2000;283:1967–1975.

119. Wing LMH, Reid CM, Ryan P, et al for the Second Australian National Blood Pressure Study Group. A comparison of outcomes with angiotensin-converting-enzyme inhibitors and diuretics for hypertension in the elderly. *N Engl J Med* 2003;348:583–592.

120. Dahlöf B, Devereux BR, Kjeldsen SE, et al for the LIFE Study Group. Cardiovascular morbidity and mortality in the Losartan Intervention For Endpoint reduction in hypertension study (LIFE): A randomised trial against atenolol. *Lancet* 2002;359:995–1003.

121. Levy D, Garrison RJ, Savage DD, et al. Prognostic implications of echocardiographically determined left ventricular mass in the Framingham Heart Study. *N Engl J Med* 1990;322:1561.

122. Harjai KJ. Potential new cardiovascular risk factors: Left ventricular hypertrophy. *Ann Intern Med* 1999;131:376.

123. Levy D, Salomon M, D'Agostino RB, et al. Prognostic implications of baseline electrocardiographic features and their serial changes in subjects with left ventricular hypertrophy. *Circulation* 1994;90:1786.

124. Verdecchia P, Schillaci G, Borgioni C, et al. Prognostic significance of serial changes in left ventricular mass in essential hypertension. *Circulation* 1998;97:48.

125. Schlaich MP, Schmieder RE. Left ventricular hypertrophy and its regression: Pathophysiology and therapeutic approach. Focus on treatment by antihypertensive agents. *Am J Hypertens* 1998;11:1394.

126. Matthew J, Sleight P, Lonn E, et al, for the Heart Outcomes Prevention Evaluation (HOPE) Investigators. Reduction of cardiovascular risk by regression of electrocardiographic markers of left ventricular hypertrophy by the angiotensin-converting enzyme inhibitor ramipril. *Circulation* 2001;104:1615–1621.

127. Lindholm LH, Ibsen H, Dahlöf B, et al for the LIFE Study Group. Cardiovascular morbidity and mortality in patients with diabetes in the Losartan Intervention For Endpoint reduction in hypertension study (LIFE): A randomised trial against atenolol. *Lancet* 2002;359:1004–1010.

128. Despres JP, Lamarche B, Mauriege P, et al. Hyperinsulinemia as an independent risk factor for ischemic heart disease. *N Engl J Med* 1996;334:952.

129. Ford ES, Giles WH, Dietz WH. Prevalence of the metabolic syndrome among US adults: Findings from the third National Health and Nutrition Examination Survey. *JAMA* 2002;287:356–359.

130. Lakka H-M, Laaksonen DE, Lakka TA, et al. The metabolic syndrome and total and cardiovascular disease mortality in middle-aged men. *JAMA* 2002;288:2709–2716.

131. Lithell HO: Hyperinsulinemia, insulin resistance, and the treatment of hypertension. *Am J Hypertens* 1996;9(11):150S–154S.

132. Grundy SM, Howard B, Smith S. Prevention conference VI: Diabetes and cardiovascular disease. Executive summary: Conference proceedings for healthcare professionals from a special writing group of the American Heart Association. *Circulation* 2002;105:2231–2239.

133. Krolewski AS, Kosinski EJ, Warram JH, et al. Magnitude and determinants of coronary artery disease in juvenile-onset, insulin-dependent diabetes mellitus. *Am J Cardiol* 1987;59:750–775.

134. Wingard DL, Barrett-Connor E. Heart disease and diabetes. In: Harris MI, ed. *Diabetes in America.* NIH Publication No. 95-1648. Washington, DC: US Government Printing Office; 1995:429–448.

135. Cho E, Rimm EB, Stampfer MJ, et al. The impact of diabetes mellitus and prior myocardial infarction on mortality from all causes and from coronary heart disease in men. *J Am Coll Cardiol* 2002;40:954–960.

136. Abbott RD, Donahue RP, Kannel WB, et al. The impact of diabetes on survival following myocardial infarction in men vs women: The Framingham Study. *JAMA* 1988;260:3456.

137. Walden CE, Knopp RH, Wahl PW, et al. Sex differences in the effect of diabetes mellitus on lipoprotein triglyceride and cholesterol concentrations. *N Engl J Med* 1984;311:953.

138. Garg A, Grundy SM. Management of dyslipidemia in NIDDM. *Diabetes Care* 1990;13:153–169.

139. Tarnow L, Rossing P, Gall MA, et al. Prevalence of arterial hypertension in diabetic patients before and after the JNC-V. *Diabetes Care* 1994;17:1247–1251.

140. DCCT Research Group: The effect of intensive diabetes treatment on the development and progression of long-term complications in insulin-dependent diabetes mellitus: The Diabetes Control and Complications Trial. *N Engl J Med* 1993;329:977.

141. UK Prospective Diabetes Study Group. Tight blood pressure control and risk of macrovascular and microvascular complications in type 2 diabetes: UKPDS 38. *BMJ* 1998;317:703–713.

142. Klein R. Hyperglycemia and microvascular and macrovascular disease in diabetes. *Diabetes Care* 1995;18:258–268.

143. Lehto S, Ronnemaa T, Pyorala K, et al. Poor glycemic control predicts coronary heart disease events in patients with type 1 diabetes without nephropathy. *Arterioscler Thromb Vasc Biol* 1999;19:1014–1019.

144. Larsen J, Brekke M, Dandvik L, et al. Silent coronary atheromatosis in type 1 diabetic patients and its relation to long-term glycemic control. *Diabetes* 2002;51:2637–2641.

145. Khaw K-T, Wareham N, Luben R, et al. Glycated haemoglobin, diabetes, and mortality in men in Norfolk cohort of European Prospective Investigation of Cancer and Nutrition (EPIC-Norfolk). *BMJ* 2001;322:1–6.

146. Libby P, Plutzky J. Diabetic macrovascular disease: The glucose paradox? *Circulation* 2002;106:2760–2763.

147. Gundersen T, Kjekshus J. Timolol treatment after myocardial infarction in diabetic patients. *Diabetes Care* 1983;6:285.

148. Arauz-Pacheco C, Parrott MA, Raskin P. The treatment of hypertension in adult patients with diabetes (TECHNICAL REVIEW). *Diabetes Care* 2002;25:134–147.

149. Heart Outcomes Prevention Evaluation (HOPE) Study Investigators. Effects of ramipril on cardiovascular and microvascular outcomes in people with diabetes mellitus: Results of the HOPE study and MICRO-HOPE substudy. *Lancet* 2000;355:253–259.

150. Fletcher GF, Balady G, Blair SN, et al. Statement on exercise: Benefits and recommendations for physical activity. *Circulation* 1996;94:857.

151. Hambrecht R, Niebauer J, Marburger C, et al. Various intensities of leisure time physical activity in patients with coronary artery disease: Effects on cardiorespiratory fitness and progression of coronary atherosclerotic lesions. *J Am Coll Cardiol* 1993;22:468.

152. Haskell WL. Sedentary lifestyle as a risk factor for coronary heart disease. In: Pearson TA, ed. *Primer in Preventive Cardiology.* Dallas: American Heart Association; 1994:173.

153. Manson JE, Greenland P, LaCroix AZ, et al. Walking compared with vigorous exercise for the prevention of cardiovascular events in women. *N Engl J Med* 2002;347:716–725.

154. Albert CM, Mittleman MA, Chae CU, et al. Triggering of sudden death from cardiac causes by vigorous exertion. *N Engl J Med* 2000;343:1355–1361.

155. Manson JE, Hu FB, Rich-Edwards JW, et al. A prospective study of walking as compared with vigorous exercise in the prevention of coronary heart disease in women. *N Engl J Med* 1999;341:650.

156. Lee I-M, Sesso HD, Paffenbarger RS. Physical activity and coronary heart disease risk in men: Does duration of exercise episodes predict risk? *Circulation* 2000;102:981–986.
157. Oldridge NB, Guyatt GH, Fischer ME, et al. Cardiac rehabilitation after myocardial infarction: Combined experience of randomized clinical trials. *JAMA* 1988;260:945.
158. O'Connor GT, Buring JE, Yusuf S, et al. An overview of randomized trials of rehabilitation with exercise after myocardial infarction. *Circulation* 1989;80:234.
159. Pate RR, Pratt M, Blair SN, et al. Physical activity and public health: A recommendation from the Centers for Disease Control and Prevention and the American College of Sports Medicine. *JAMA* 1995;273:402.
160. US Department of Health and Human Services. *Physical Activity and Health: A Report of the Surgeon General.* Atlanta: US Department of Health and Human Services, Centers for Disease Control and Prevention, National Center for Chronic Disease Prevention and Health Promotion; 1996.
161. Fletcher GF, Balady G, Froelicher VF, et al. Exercise standards: A statement for healthcare professionals from the American Heart Association. Writing Group. *Circulation* 1995;91:580.
162. King AC, Haskell WL, Taylor CB. Group- vs home-based exercise training in healthy older men and women. *JAMA* 1991;266:1535.
163. Eckel RH, Krauss RM. American Heart Association call to action: Obesity as a major risk factor. *Circulation* 1998;97:2099.
164. Mokdad AH, Ford ES, Bowman BA, et al. Prevalence of obesity, diabetes, and obesity-related health risk factors, 2001. JAMA 2003;289:76–79.
165. Eckel RH, Barouch WW, Ershow AG. Report of the National Heart, Lung, and Blood Institute—National Institute of Diabetes and Digestive and Kidney Diseases Working Group on the pathophysiology of obesity-related cardiovascular disease. *Circulation* 2002;105: 2923–2928.
166. McGill HC, McMahan CA, Herderick EE, et al, for the Pathobiological Determinants of Atherosclerosis in Youth (PDAY) Research Group. Obesity accelerates the progression of coronary atherosclerosis in young men. *Circulation* 2002;105:2712–2718.
167. Calle EE, Thun MJ, Petrilli JM, et al. Body-mass index and mortality in a prospective cohort of US adults. *N Engl J Med* 1999;341:1097.
168. Fontaine KR, Redden DT, Wang C, et al. Years of life lost due to obesity. *JAMA* 2003;289:187–193.
169. Flegal KM, Carroll MD, Ogden CL, et al. Prevalence and trends in obesity among US adults, 1999–2000. *JAMA* 2002;288:1723–1727.
170. Hubert HB, Feinleib M, McNamara PM, et al. Obesity as an independent risk factor for cardiovascular disease: A 26-year follow-up of participants in the Framingham Heart Study. *Circulation* 1983;67:968.
171. Manson JE, Willett WC, Stampfer MJ, et al. Body weight and mortality among women. *N Engl J Med* 1995;333:677.
172. Jousilahti P, Tuomilehto J, Vartiainen E, et al. Body weight, cardiovascular risk factors, and coronary mortality: 15-year follow-up of middle-aged men and women in eastern Finland. *Circulation* 1996;93: 1372.
173. Yanovski SZ, Yanovski JA. Obesity. *N Engl J Med* 2002;346:591–602.
174. Mangoni AA, Jackson SHD. Homocysteine and cardiovascular disease: Current evidence and future prospects. *Am J Med* 2002;112: 556–565.
175. Nygard O, Nordrehaug JE, Refsum H, et al. Plasma homocysteine levels and mortality in patients with coronary artery disease. *N Engl J Med* 1997;337:230.
176. Schnyder G, Roffi M, Pin R, et al. Decreased rate of coronary restenosis after lowering of plasma homocysteine levels. *N Engl J Med* 2001;345:1593–1600.
177. Stampfer MJ, Hennekens CH, Manson JE, et al. Vitamin E consumption and the risk of coronary disease in women. *N Engl J Med* 1993;328:1444.
178. Rimm EB, Stampfer A, Ascherio E, et al. Vitamin E consumption and the risk of coronary heart disease in men. *N Engl J Med* 1993; 328:1450.
179. Greenberg ER, Baron JA, Karagas MR, et al. Mortality associated with low plasma concentration of beta carotene and the effect of oral supplementation. *JAMA* 1996;275:699.
180. Jha P, Flather M, Lonn E, et al. The antioxidant vitamins and cardiovascular disease: A critical review of epidemiologic and clinical trial data. *Ann Intern Med* 1995;123:860.
181. The Alpha-Tocopherol, Beta Carotene Cancer Prevention Study Group. The effect of vitamin E and beta carotene on the incidence of lung cancer and other cancers in male smokers. *N Engl J Med* 1994;330:1029.
182. Omenn GS, Goodman GE, Thornquist MD, et al. Effects of a combination of beta carotene and vitamin A on lung cancer and cardiovascular disease. *N Engl J Med* 1996;334:1150.
183. Hennekens CH, Buring JE, Manson JE, et al. Lack of effect of long-term supplementation with beta carotene on the incidence of malignant neoplasms and cardiovascular disease. *N Engl J Med* 1996;334:1145.
184. Stephens NG, Parsons A, Schofield PM, et al. Randomised controlled trial of vitamin E in patients with coronary disease. *Lancet* 1996; 347:781.
185. Yusuf S, Sleight P, Pgue J, et al. Effects of an angiotensin-converting enzyme inhibitor, ramipril, on cardiovascular events in high-risk patients. The Heart Outcomes Prevention Evaluation Study Investigators. *N Engl J Med* 2000;342:145.
186. Heart Protection Study Collaborative Group. MRC/BHF Heart Protection Study of antioxidant vitamin supplementation in 20,536 high-risk individuals: A randomised placebo controlled trial. *Lancet* 2002;360:23–33.
187. Brown BG, Zhao XQ, Chait A, et al. Simvastatin and niacin, antioxidant vitamins, or the combination for the prevention of coronary disease. *N Engl J Med* 2001;345:1583–1592.
188. Waters DD, Alderman EL, Hsia J, et al. Effects of hormone replacement therapy and antioxidant vitamin supplements on coronary atherosclerosis in postmenopausal women: A randomized controlled trial. *JAMA* 2002;288:2432–2440.
189. Moore RD, Pearson TA. Moderate alcohol consumption and coronary artery disease: A review. *Medicine (Baltimore)* 1986;65:242.
190. Stampfer MJ, Colditz GA, Willett WC, et al. A prospective study of moderate alcohol consumption and the risk of coronary disease and stroke in women. *N Engl J Med* 1988;319:267.
191. Rimm EB, Giovannucci El, Willett WC, et al. Prospective study of alcohol consumption and risk of coronary disease in men. *Lancet* 1991;338:464.
192. Mukamal KJ, Conigrave KM, Mittleman MA, et al. Roles of drinking pattern and type of alcohol consumed in coronary heart disease in men. *N Engl J Med* 2003;348:109–118.
193. Maclure M. Demonstration of deductive meta-analysis: Ethanol intake and risk of myocardial infarction. *Epidemiol Rev* 1993;15:328.
194. Langer RD, Criqui MH, Reed DM. Lipoproteins and blood pressure as biological pathways for effect of moderate alcohol consumption on coronary heart disease. *Circulation* 1992;85:910.
195. Suh I, Shaten BJ, Cutler JA, et al. Alcohol use and mortality from coronary heart disease: The role of high-density lipoprotein cholesterol. The Multiple Risk Factor Intervention Trial Research Group. *Ann Intern Med* 1992;116:881.
196. Haskell WL, Camargo C Jr, Williams PT, et al. The effect of cessation and resumption of moderate alcohol intake on serum high-density lipoprotein subfractions. A controlled study. *N Engl J Med* 1984; 310:805.
197. Gaziano JM, Buring JE, Breslow JL, et al. Moderate alcohol intake, increased levels of high-density lipoprotein and its subfractions, and decreased risk of myocardial infarction. *N Engl J Med* 1993;329:1829.
198. Ridker PM, Vaughan DE, Stampfer MJ, et al. Association of moderate alcohol consumption and plasma concentration of endogenous tissue-type plasminogen activator. *JAMA* 1994;272:929.
199. Hendriks HF, Veenstra J, Velthuis-te Wierik EJ, et al. Effect of moderate dose of alcohol with evening meal on fibrinolytic factors. *BMJ* 1994;308:1003.

200. Deykin D, Janson P, McMahon L. Ethanol potentiation of aspirin-induced prolongation of the bleeding time. *N Engl J Med* 1982; 306:852.
201. Elmer O, Goransson G, Zoucas E. Impairment of primary hemostasis and platelet function after alcohol ingestion in man. *Haemostasis* 1984;14:223.
202. Goldberg IR. To drink or not to drink? *N Engl J Med* 2003;348: 163–164.
203. Pearson TA, Terry P. What to advise patients about drinking alcohol: The clinician's conundrum. *JAMA* 1994;272:967.
204. Enos WFJ, Beyer JC, Holmes RH. Pathogenesis of coronary disease in American soldiers killed in Korea. *JAMA* 1955;58:912.
205. McNamara JJ, Molot MA, Stemple JF, et al. Coronary artery disease in combat casualties in Vietnam. *JAMA* 1971;216:1185.
206. Castelli WP. Epidemiology of coronary heart disease: The Framingham Study. *Am J Med* 1984;76:4.
207. Thom TJ. Cardiovascular disease mortality among United States women. In: Eaker ED, ed. *Coronary Heart Disease in Women.* New York: Haymarket Doyma; 1987.
208. Writing Group for the Women's Health Initiative Investigators. Risks and benefits of estrogen plus progestin in healthy postmenopausal women: Principal results from the Women's Health Initiative randomized controlled trial. *JAMA* 2002;288:321–333.
209. Mosca L, Collins P, Herrington DM, et al. Hormone replacement therapy and cardiovascular disease: A statement for healthcare professionals from the American Heart Association. *Circulation* 2001;104:499–503.
210. Grodstein F, Manson JE, Colditz GA, et al. A prospective, observational study of postmenopausal hormone therapy and primary prevention of cardiovascular disease. *Ann Intern Med* 2000;133: 933–941.
211. Wakatsuki A, Okatani Y, Ikenoue N, et al. Different effects of oral conjugated equine estrogen and transdermal estrogen replacement therapy on size and oxidative susceptibility of low-density lipoprotein particles in postmenopausal women. *Circulation* 2002;106: 1771–1776.
212. Hulley SD, Grady D, Bush T, et al. Randomized trial of estrogen plus progestin for secondary prevention of coronary heart disease in postmenopausal women. Heart and Estrogen progestin Replacement Study (HERS) Research Group. *JAMA* 1998;280:605.
213. Grady D, Herrington D, Bittner V, et al for the HERS Research Group. Cardiovascular disease outcomes during 6.8 years of hormone therapy: Heart and Estrogen/Progestin Replacement Study follow-up (HERS II). *JAMA* 2002;288:49–57.
214. Herrington DM, Reboussin DM, Brosnihan KB, et al. Effects of estrogen replacement on the progression of coronary-artery atherosclerosis. *N Engl J Med* 2000;343:522–529.
215. Waters DD, Alderman EL, Hsia J, et al. Effects of hormone replacement therapy and antioxidant vitamin supplements on coronary atherosclerosis in postmenopausal women: A randomized controlled trial. *JAMA* 2002;288:2432–2440.
216. Kaplan GA, Keil JE. Socioeconomic factors and cardiovascular disease: A review of the literature. *Circulation* 1993;88:1973.
217. Hopkins PN, Williams RR. Human genetics and coronary heart disease: A public health perspective. *Annu Rev Nutr* 1989;9:303.
218. Rissanen AM. Familial aggregation of coronary heart disease in a high incidence area. *Br Heart J* 1979;42:294.
219. Williams RR, Hopkins PN, Wu LL, et al. Evaluating family history to prevent early coronary heart disease. In: Person TA, ed. *Primer in Preventive Cardiology.* Dallas: American Heart Association; 1994:93.
220. Libby P, Ridker PM, Meseri A. Inflammation and atherosclerosis. *Circulation* 2002;105:1135–1143.
221. Ernst E, Resch KL. Fibrinogen as a cardiovascular risk factor: A meta-analysis and review of the literature. *Ann Intern Med* 1993;118:956.
222. Abramson JL, Vaccarino V. Relationship between physical activity and inflammation among apparently healthy middle-aged and older US adults. *Arch Intern Med* 2002;162:1286–1292.
223. Ridker PM. Clinical application of C-reactive protein for cardiovascular disease detection and prevention. *Circulation* 2003;107:363–369.
224. Smith JK, Dykes R, Douglas JE, et al. Long-term exercise and atherogenic activity of blood mononuclear cells in persons at risk of developing ischemic heart disease. *JAMA* 1999;281:1722.
225. Visser M, Bouter LM, McQuillen GM, et al. Elevated C-reactive protein levels in overweight and obese adults. *JAMA* 1999;282:2131.
226. Espinola-Klein C, Rupprecht HJ, Blankenberg S, et al for the AtheroGene Investigators. Impact of infectious burden on extent and long-term prognosis of atherosclerosis. *Circulation* 2002;105:15–21.
227. Kalayoglu MV, Libby P, Byrne GI. *Chlamydia pneumoniae* as an emerging risk factor in cardiovascular disease. *JAMA* 2002;228: 2724–2731.
228. Ridker PM, Vaughan DE, Stampfer JE, et al. Endogenous tissue-type plasminogen activator and risk of myocardial infarction. *Lancet* 1993;341:1165.
229. Thogersen AM, Jansson JH, Boman K, et al. High plasminogen activator inhibitor and tissue plasminogen activator levels in plasma precede a first acute myocardial infarction in both men and women: Evidence for the fibrinolytic system as an independent primary risk factor. *Circulation* 1998;98:2241.
230. Thompson SG, Kienast J, Pyke SD, et al. Hemostatic factors and the risk of myocardial infarction or sudden death in patients with angina pectoris. European Concerted Action on Thrombosis and Disabilities Angina Pectoris Study Group. *N Engl J Med* 1995;332:635.
231. Mills JD, Mansfield MW, Grant PJ. Tissue plasminogen activator, fibrin D-dimer, and insulin resistance in the relatives of patients with premature coronary artery disease. *Ateriosc1er Thromb Vasc Biol* 2002;22:704–709.
232. Ridker PM, Hennekens CH, Stampfer MJ, et al. Prospective study of endogenous tissue plasminogen activator and risk of stroke. *Lancet* 1994;343:940.
233. Meade TW, Ruddock V, Stirling Y, et al. Fibrinolytic activity, clotting factors, and long-term incidence of ischaemic heart disease in the Northwick Park Heart Study. *Lancet* 1993;342:1076.
234. Ridker PM, Hennekens CH, Cerskus A, et al. Plasma concentration of cross-linked fibrin degradation product (D-dimer). *Circulation* 1994; 90:2236.
235. Fowkes FG, Lowe GD, Housley E, et al. Cross-linked fibrin degradation products, progression of peripheral arterial disease, and risk of coronary heart disease. *Lancet* 1993;342:84.
236. Lowe GD, Yamell JW, Sweetnam PM, et al. Fibrin D-dimer, tissue plasminogen activator, plasminogen activator inhibitor, and the risk of major ischaemic heart disease in the Caerphilly Study. *Thromb Haemost* 1998;79:129.
237. Vaughan DE, Rouleau JL, Ridker PM, et al. Effects of ramipril on plasma fibrinolytic balance in patients with acute anterior myocardial infarction. HEART Study Investigators. *Circulation* 1997;96:442.
238. Steering Committee of the Physicians' Health Study Research Group. Final report on the aspirin component of the ongoing Physicians' Health Study. *N Engl J Med* 1989;321:129.
239. Peto R, Gray R, Collins K, et al. Randomised trial of prophylactic daily aspirin in British male doctors. *Br Med J* 1988;296:313.
240. Hennekens CH, Peto R, Hutchison GB, et al. An overview of the British and American aspirin studies (letter). *N Engl J Med* 1988; 318:923.
241. Medical Research Council's General Practice Research Framework. Thrombosis prevention trial: Randomised trial of low-intensity oral anticoagulation with warfarin and low-dose aspirin in the primary prevention of ischaemic heart disease in men at increased risk. The Medical Research Council's General Practice Research Framework. *Lancet* 1998;351:233.
242. Antithrombotic Trialists' Collaboration. Collaborative meta-analysis of randomised trials of antiplatelet therapy for prevention of death, myocardial infarction, and stroke in high risk patients. *BMJ* 2002;324: 71–86.
243. Anand SS, Yusuf S. Oral anticoagulant therapy in patients with coronary artery disease: A meta-analysis. *JAMA* 1999;282:2058–2067.

244. Hurlen M, Abdelnoor M, Smith P, et al. Warfarin, aspirin, or both after myocardial infarction. *N Engl J Med* 2002;347:969–974.
245. U.S. Preventive Services Task Force. Aspirin for the primary prevention of cardiovascular events: Recommendations and rationale. *Ann Intern Med* 2002;136:157–160.
246. Stone PH, Sacks FM. Strategies for secondary prevention. In: Manson JE, ed. *Primary Prevention of Myocardial Infarction.* London: Oxford University Press; 1996.
247. Wikstrand J, Warnold I, Olsson G, et al. Primary prevention with metoprolol in patients with hypertension: Mortality. *JAMA* 1988; 259:1976.
248. Yusuf S, Peto R, Lewis J, et al. Beta blockade during and after myocardial infarction: An overview of the randomized trials. *Prog Cardiovasc Dis* 1985;27:335.
249. Lau J, Antman EM, Jimenez-Silva J, et al. Cumulative meta-analysis of therapeutic trials for myocardial infarction. *N Engl J Med* 1992;327:248.
250. Khalil ME, Basher AW, Brown EJ, et al. A remarkable story: Benefits of angiotensin-converting enzyme inhibitors in cardiac patients. *J Am Coll Cardiol* 2001;37:1757–1764.
251. French WJ. Trends in acute myocardial infarction management: Use of the National Registry of Myocardial Infarction in quality improvement. *Am J Cardiol* 2000;85:5B–9B, 10B–12B.
252. Fonarow GC, French WJ, Parsons LS, et al for the National Registry of Myocardial Infarction 3 Participants. Use of lipid-lowering medications at discharge in patients with acute myocardial infarction: Data from the National Registry of Myocardial Infarction 3. *Circulation* 2001;103:38–44.
253. Aronow HD, Topol EJ, Roe MT, et al. Effect of lipid-lowering therapy on early mortality after acute coronary syndromes: An observational study. *Lancet* 2001;357:1063–1068.
254. Sueta CA, Chowdhury M, Boccuzzi SJ, et al. Analysis of the degree of undertreatment of hyperlipidemia and congestive heart failure secondary to coronary artery disease. *Am J Cardiol* 1999;83: 1303–1307.
255. Jacobson TA, Griffiths GG, Varas C, et al. Impact of evidence-based "clinical judgment" on the number of American adults requiring lipid-lowering drug therapy based on updated NHANES III data. *Arch Intern Med* 2000;160:1361–1369.
256. Pearson TA. The Lipid Treatment Assessment Project (L-TAP): A multicenter survey to evaluate the percentages of dyslipidemic patients receiving lipid-lowering therapy and achieving low-density lipoprotein cholesterol goals. *Arch Intern Med* 2000;160:459.
257. Kottke TE, Blackburn H, Brekke ML, et al. The systematic practice of preventive cardiology. *Am J Cardiol* 1987;59:690.
258. Pearson TA, McBride PE, Miller NH, et al. 27th Bethesda Conference: Matching the intensity of risk factor management. *J Am Coll Cardiol* 1996;27:1039.
259. Houston-Miller N, Hill M, Kottke T, et al. The multilevel compliance challenge: Recommendations for a call to action. *Circulation* 1997;95:1085.
260. Levine DM. Behavioral and psychosocial factors, progress and strategies. In: Pearson TA, ed. *Primer in Preventive Cardiology.* Dallas: American Heart Association; 1994:214.
261. Bradley EH, Holmboe ES, Mattera JH, et al. A qualitative study of increasing beta blocker use after myocardial infarction. Why do some hospitals succeed? *JAMA* 2001;285:2604.
262. Fonarow GC, Gawlinski A, Moughrabi S, et al. Improved treatment of coronary heart disease by implementation of a Cardiac Hospitalization Atherosclerosis Management Program (CHAMP). *Am J Cardiol* 2001;87:819.
263. Gordon NF, English CD, Contractor AS, et al. Effectiveness of three models for comprehensive cardiovascular disease risk reduction. *Am J Cardiol* 2002;89:1263–1268.
264. US Department of Health and Human Services. *Treating Tobacco Use and Dependence: A Clinical Practice Guideline.* Washington, DC: US Department of Health and Human Services; 2000.
265. Wenger NK, Froelicher ES, Smith LK. *Cardiac Rehabilitation as Secondary Prevention.* Bethesda, MD: National Heart, Lung, and Blood Institute; 1995.
266. Pearson TA, Bazzarre TL, Daniels SR, et al. American Heart Association guide for improving cardiovascular health at the community level. *Circulation* 2003:107:645.

CHAPTER 44

# ATHEROTHROMBOSIS AND THROMBOSIS-PRONE PLAQUES

Erling Falk/Prediman K. Shah/Valentin Fuster



Coronary atherosclerosis is the underlying cause of nearly all cases of ischemic heart disease, and superimposed thrombosis is the proximate cause of the great majority of the life-threatening acute coronary syndromes (unstable angina, myocardial infarction, and sudden death).[1–3] The pathogenesis of peripheral arterial disease and, to a great extent, ischemic stroke is similar. Thus, atherosclerosis with superimposed thrombosis, ***atherothrombosis,*** is the leading cause of death and severe disability in the affluent countries, and it will soon be the same worldwide because of the pandemic growth of obesity, insulin resistance, and type 2 diabetes.[4,5]

Symptomatic coronary lesions (culprit lesions) contain a variable mix of chronic atherosclerosis and acute thrombosis. Atherosclerosis predominates in lesions responsible for chronic stable angina, whereas a critical component of thrombosis is usually present in culprit lesions responsible for acute coronary syndromes.[1–3] Because the exact nature of the mix is unknown in the individual patient, the term *atherothrombosis* is indeed appropriate.

## DEFINITIONS AND TERMINOLOGY

### Atherosclerosis

Atherosclerosis is a chronic immunoinflammatory, fibroproliferative disease fueled by lipids.[6] It affects primarily the intima of medium-sized and large arteries, resulting in intimal thickening, and may lead to luminal narrowing and inadequate blood supply. As the name implies, mature atherosclerotic plaques consist typically of two main components: one is lipid-rich and soft (*athére* is Greek for "gruel" or "porridge") and the other is collagen-rich and hard (*skleros* is Greek for "hard"). The flow-limiting potential of an intimal plaque may be modified by reactive changes in the underlying media and adventitia that may attenuate (positive remodeling) or accentuate (negative remodeling) luminal obstruction and consequent hemodynamic impact of the plaque.[7] Furthermore, enhanced vasoconstriction and reduced vasodilator capacity associated with atherosclerosis can further contribute an additional dynamic component to luminal obstruction.

### Thrombus-Related Plaque Features

The surface of atherosclerotic plaques begetting thrombosis is usually injured.[3,8,9] ***Plaque rupture*** is a deep injury that involves much more than just a missing or "disrupted" endothelium.[3,8,9] In plaque rupture, there is a real defect—a gap—in the fibrous cap that separates a lipid-rich atheromatous core from the flowing blood (Fig. 44-1, Plate 78). The thrombogenic core is exposed (risk of thrombosis), and blood may enter the soft core through the gap in the cap (rupture-related plaque hemorrhage). The size of such gaps varies greatly in width, length, and depth.[10]

In contrast to plaque rupture, ***plaque disruption*** is not a well-defined term. It has been used synonymously with *plaque rupture*[3,8] but also for all other kinds of plaque injuries found beneath thrombi, including superficial injuries in which only the endothelium is missing or "disrupted" (so-called plaque erosion).[9,11,12] Therefore, to avoid confusion, the term *disruption* should be used with great caution.

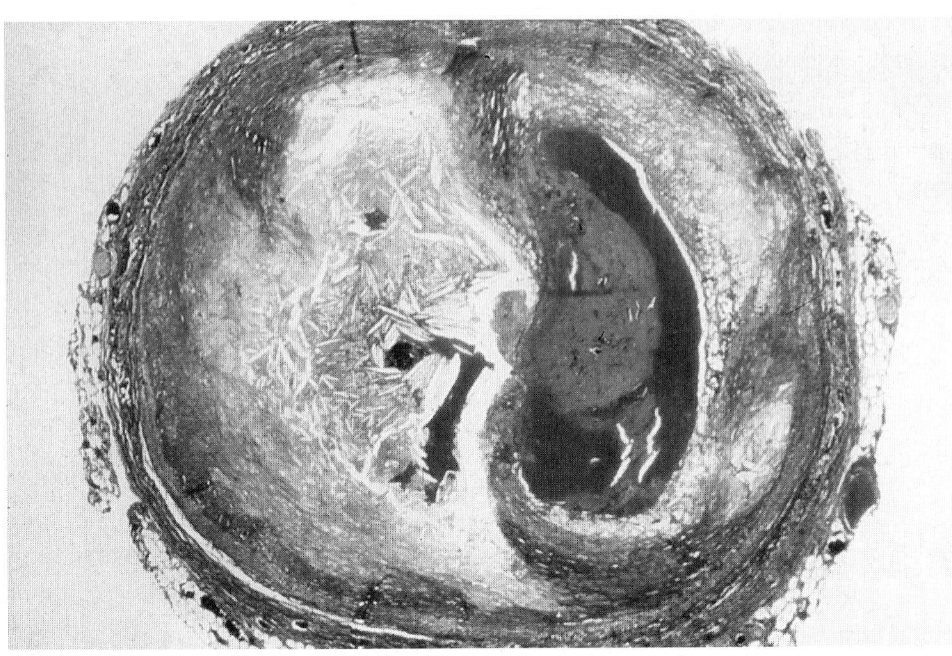

FIGURE 44-1 (Plate 78) Cross-sectioned coronary artery containing a ruptured plaque with a nonocclusive thrombosis superimposed. The actual defect in the fibrous cap is not seen in this section but is located nearby, documented by the presence of extravasated radiographic contrast medium (postmortem coronary angiography) in the soft, lipid-rich core just beneath the thin, inflamed fibrous cap. Trichrome stain, rendering thrombus red, collagen blue, and lipid colorless.

The term ***plaque fissuring*** has been used synonymously with *plaque rupture*[3] but also for superficial intimal tearing in the absence of a lipid-rich core.[13] Thus, *fissuring* is also a somewhat ambiguous term.

***Plaque erosion*** is an old nonspecific term with a new meaning. The term was revived by van der Wal et al.[14] and (re)defined by Virmani et al.[9] in the following way: "'Plaque erosion' is identified when serial sectioning of a thrombosed arterial segment fails to reveal fibrous cap rupture. Typically, the endothelium is absent at the erosion site." Thus it is the lack of plaque rupture rather than any specific pathoanatomic feature that "characterizes" these lesions (Fig. 44-2). According to this definition, rupture and erosion will together account for all plaque changes found at the plaque-thrombus interface.[14–16] A rare nonrupture type of plaque injury, the calcified nodule, was recently introduced as a peculiar subtype of plaque erosion.[9]

While *rupture, disruption, fissuring,* and *erosion* are terms used to describe plaque injuries seen beneath thrombi, the term ***vulnerable*** is generally used in a prospective way for plaques assumed to be at high risk of reaching this stage and/or becoming culprit for a future acute coronary event.[8,17–19] It has, however, most often been used only for rupture-prone plaques.[8,10,20] These different definitions focus on different aspects of plaques assumed to be dangerous. Regarding atherothrombosis and coronary artery disease, *vulnerable* is also an ambiguous term, characteristics of which need to be specified when it is used.

## Thrombosis

A ***thrombus*** is defined as any solid mass that arises in the bloodstream during life from components of the blood.[21] Thus, a thrombus may form not only within the heart and vessels but anywhere the blood is streaming—for example, in a false channel within the vessel wall (e.g., aortic dissection) or through a large gap in the surface of a ruptured plaque. Extravasation of blood is usually called a hemorrhage or bleeding, but Davies et al. introduced the term ***intraintimal thrombi*** for rupture-related hemorrhages into plaques because of their composition (often relatively rich in platelets and fibrin) and location (often next to a luminal thrombus).[22–24] However, many defects in ruptured caps are small, without significant potential for to-and-fro flow; consequently, the accumulated blood often looks more like a hemorrhage than a thrombus.

## EXPERIMENTAL ATHEROTHROMBOSIS

To reproduce in animals a vascular disease resembling human atherosclerosis, atherogenic lipoprotein concentrations need to be above a certain level. Normal wild-type mice do not develop hypercholesterolemia and are thus fundamentally resistant to atherosclerosis, even when fed a high-fat, high-cholesterol diet that induces the disease in other species, such as rabbits, pigs, birds, and nonhuman primates. Hypercholesterolemic atherosclerosis–prone mice have, however, been created by inactivating and/or overexpressing pertinent genes.[25–28] Over the past decade, remarkable progress has been made in our knowledge of vascular biology through the use of genetically engineered mice, and mice are

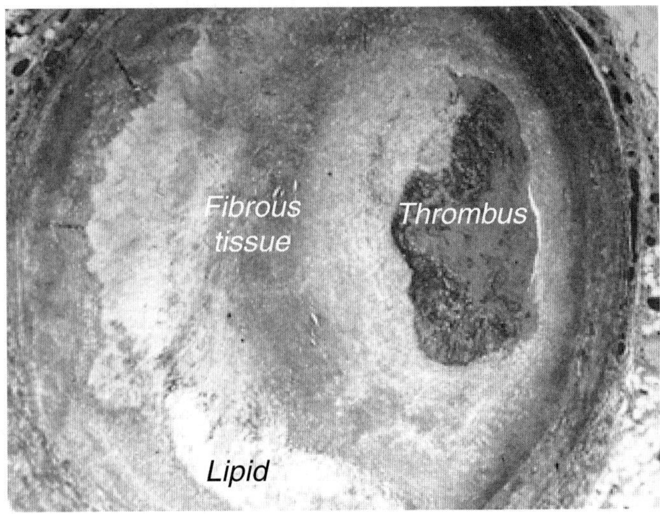


FIGURE 44-2 Cross section of a coronary artery containing a stenotic atherosclerotic plaque with an occlusive thrombosis superimposed. The endothelium is missing at the plaque-thrombus interface, but the plaque surface is otherwise intact (so-called plaque erosion). Thus there is no obvious local cause such as plaque rupture beneath the thrombus. Trichrome stain, rendering thrombus red, collagen blue, and lipid colorless.

being increasingly used as a model for the study of atherosclerosis and its risk factors.[25–28]

The most commonly used genetically altered murine models for studies of atherosclerosis are mice deficient in apolipoprotein E (apoE$^{-/-}$) and/or low-density lipoprotein receptor (LDLR$^{-/-}$). ApoE is a ligand for receptors that clear chylomicrons and very low density lipoprotein remnant particles. Consequently, apoE$^{-/-}$ mice develop severe hypercholesterolemia and atherosclerosis spontaneously on a normal chow diet, in contrast to LDLR$^{-/-}$ mice, which do so only when fed a high-fat, high-cholesterol diet.[29] The atherosclerotic lesions that develop in these atherosclerosis-prone mice are morphologically quite similar to those in humans, which is why the mouse has become the most common experimental animal model for atherosclerosis research.

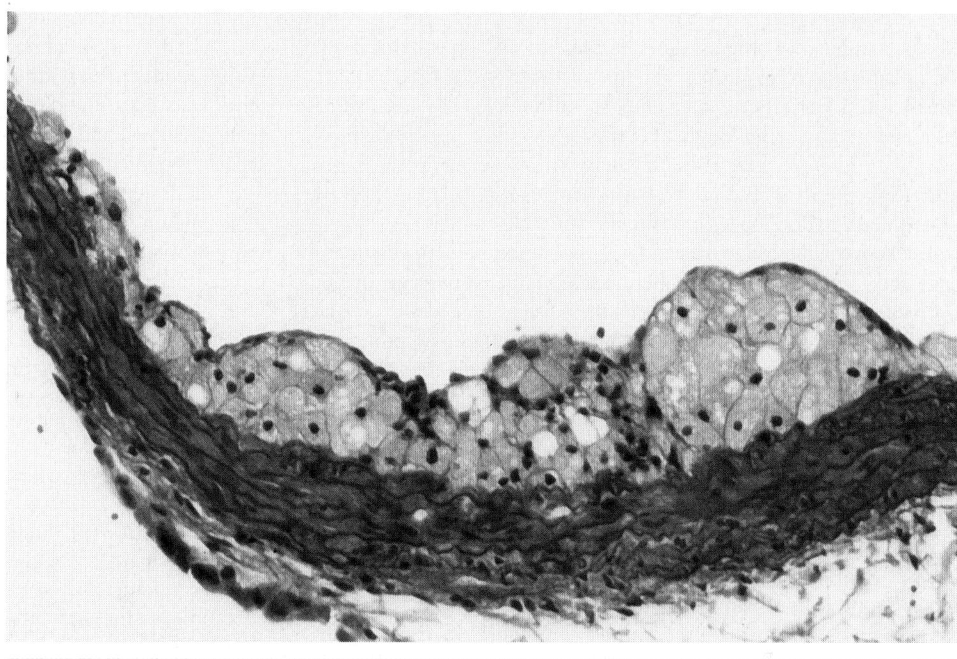

FIGURE 44-3 (Plate 79) An early atherosclerotic lesion (fatty streak) in the aortic root of a 3-month-old apolipoprotein E–deficient mouse fed a high-fat western-type diet for 6 weeks. The lesion consists of lipid-filled monocyte-derived macrophages (foam cells) and a few lymphocytes (T cells) beneath an intact endothelium. Elastin trichrome stain.

## Lesion-Prone Areas

In aortas of normocholesterolemic mice, VCAM-1 and ICAM-1 (vascular and intercellular adhesion molecule 1, respectively), but not E-selectin, are expressed by endothelial cells in regions predisposed to atherosclerotic lesion formation.[30] The complex hemodynamics in these lesion-prone areas may also increase the local transendothelial passage of lipoproteins and promote their retention and modification in the subendothelial space.[31] Oxidative modified LDL (oxLDL) has many proinflammatory properties, which may explain the local upregulation of these inducible endothelial cell adhesion molecules, even before lesion formation, in hypercholesterolemic atherosclerosis-prone animals.[30]

## Response to Retained Lipoproteins

The first event in the birth of a plaque is the transendothelial passage of atherogenic lipoproteins into the subendothelial space, where they are retained and modified.[6,32] In normal mice, the subendothelial space contains an acellular matrix of branching filaments (presumed to be mainly proteoglycans) and numerous collagen fibrils without any visible lipid deposition; normal mice do not spontaneously form an arterial intima.[33] The retention of lipoproteins in the subendothelial space provides a microenvironment where lipoprotein modification and aggregation can occur.[32] Modification—e.g., oxidation—of the retained lipoprotein makes it more atherogenic.[34,35] OxLDL is proinflammatory, cytotoxic, and recognized by the macrophage scavenger receptor promoting intracellular lipid accumulation and foam cell formation. In vitro studies suggest that lipoprotein retention involves interactions between apoB and matrix proteoglycans[36,37] and appears to be an important if not the key step in lesion development.

HDL and its major apolipoprotein, apoA-I, have powerful atheroprotective effects in hypercholesterolemic mice. Among other things, HDL/apoA-I prevents atherogenic modifications of LDL and promotes "reverse cholesterol transport" from the arterial wall, specifically from macrophage foam cells. In fact, recent observations in apoE$^{-/-}$ mice indicate that high-dose recombinant apoA-I$_{\text{Milano}}$ may rapidly "pacivate" lipid-rich and inflamed plaques.[38,39]

## Immunoinflammatory Response

One of the earliest detectable cellular responses in atherogenesis is the focal recruitment of circulating monocytes and, to a lesser extent, T cells into the arterial intima.[40] The persistence of this cellular response seems to underlie disease progression (Fig. 44-3, Plate 79).[41] A few B cells may also be present,[42] but granulocytes are rare in atherosclerosis. Atherosclerotic lesions develop initially beneath an intact but activated endothelium at lesion-prone sites, preferentially affecting the outer walls of bifurcations and the inner walls of curvatures. The local factors responsible for the focal development of lesions are not well understood, but hemodynamic shear stress, the frictional force acting on the endothelial cell surface as a result of blood flow, is weaker in the susceptible lesion-prone areas.[31,43] Hemodynamic shear stress is an important determinant of endothelial function and phenotype. High shear stress ($>$15 dyne/cm$^2$) induces endothelial quiescence and an atheroprotective gene expression profile, whereas low shear stress ($<$4 dyne/cm$^2$), which is prevalent at atherosclerosis-prone sites, stimulates an atherogenic phenotype.[31,43] The endothelium mediates the transendothelial trafficking of leukocytes into the intima by expressing specific and inducible adhesion molecules such as VCAM-1 and ICAM-1. These adhesion molecules are upregulated at lesion-prone sites in apoE$^{-/-}$ mice prior to lesion formation and thus probably play an important role in the recruitment of mononuclear cells during atherogenesis.[40] Sites of predilection for lesion development include the aortic root, the lesser curvature of the aortic arch, the principal branches of the aorta (in particular, the coronary arteries and the brachiocephalic trunk), the carotid bifurcations, the aortic bifurcation, the iliac arteries, and the pulmonary arteries. Adhesion of monocytes to the endothelial surface was seen already at 6 weeks, macrophage foam cell lesions (fatty streaks) developed as early as 8 weeks, and, as lesions continued to progress, smooth muscle cells appeared and advanced atherosclerotic plaques were present after 15 weeks. The latter consisted of a fibrous cap containing smooth muscle cells surrounded by connective tissue matrix that covered a necrotic core with numerous foamy macrophages. Thus, the apoE$^{-/-}$ mouse contains the entire spectrum of lesions observed during atherogenesis and was the first mouse model to develop lesions similar to those in humans.[44]

Leukocyte adhesion to the endothelium is not enough to get monocytes and T cells into the intima. For transendothelial passage, one or more chemokines (chemotactic cytokines) are also needed.[45,46] The proinflammatory chemokine monocyte chemoattractant protein 1 (MCP-1) attracts potently both monocytes and T cells but not neutrophils, eosinophils, and B cells, and it plays a fundamental role in the recruitment of these cells.[47] Endothelial cells, smooth muscle cells, and macrophages all contribute to overexpression of MCP-1 in atherosclerosis. Thus, once within the intima, monocytes recruit themselves by secreting MCP-1.[45,48–50] MCP-1 appears to be uniquely essential for monocyte recruitment in several inflammatory diseases,[51] including atherosclerosis.[49,50] Additionally, MCP-1 may induce tissue factor expression in plaque cells and thus increase the risk of atherosclerosis-mediated luminal thrombosis.[52] A prime candidate for upregulation of MCP-1 in the vessel wall is minimally oxidized LDL, linking hypercholesterolemia to fatty-streak formation, plaque progression, and tissue factor expression.[53]

Once within the intima and activated, macrophages may secrete a variety of potent cytokines that profoundly influence local cellular accumulation and function. Macrophages can both initiate the oxidation of LDL and take up oxLDL by specific scavenger receptors. Lesion size is reduced in atherosclerosis-prone mice lacking the macrophage-expressed oxygenating enzyme 12/15-lipoxygenase[54] and scavenger receptors, suggesting that lipoprotein oxidation and uptake are key events in atherogenesis.[35]

The humoral and cellular immune system modulates the development of atherosclerosis.[35,55] Plaque T cells and their products [e.g., interferon gamma (IFN-$\gamma$)] appear to promote atherosclerosis, whereas nonplaque B cells and their products (e.g., antibodies) are atheroprotective.[56,57] Hyperimmunization with oxLDL, resulting in high antibody titers, and polyclonal immunoglobulin therapy protect against atherosclerosis, whereas splenectomy (removal of a B cell–enriched immune organ) promotes atherosclerosis in apoE$^{-/-}$ mice.[57] In contrast, all proatherogenic activities of the immune system discovered until now have been associated with inflammatory responses elicited by macrophages and T cells within plaques.[57] Neither B nor T cells, however, are required for the development and growth of plaques, documented in apoE$^{-/-}$ $\times$ RAG mice lacking lymphocytes.[58,59] A variety of antigens are formed in developing plaques with immune activation and subsequent modulation, mediated by both cellular and humoral events, of the ongoing atherosclerotic process.[55] Further evidence of immune activation is the upregulated expression of the immune mediator CD40 and its ligand CD154 by all cell types present in advanced atherosclerotic lesions.[60] The interaction of CD40 with CD154 mediates both humoral and cellular immune responses, and blocking this interaction reduces lesion formation in atherosclerosis-prone mice.[61,62]

There are a number of candidate antigens in the lesion that could be responsible for immune activation, including modified LDL,[35] heat-shock proteins,[63–65] $\beta_2$-glycoprotein I,[66] and microbial antigens. Of these, the most extensive data support an important role for oxLDL, which is abundantly present in atherosclerotic plaques, where it is recognized by plaque T cells and gives rise to nonplaque B-cell stimulation.[55,57]

Inflammation, but not infection, plays a critical role in atherogenesis.[67] LDL$^{-/-}$ mice fed normal chow do not develop atherosclerosis, even when infected with *Chlamydia pneumoniae* (Cp), but if cholesterol is added to the diet, hypercholesterolemia-induced atherosclerosis develops, and Cp infection appears to accelerate its development.[68] Cp infection also appears to accelerate atherosclerosis in the hypercholesterolemic apoE$^{-/-}$ mice[69]; that is, Cp alone is not atherogenic, although it may be causally related to the development of atherosclerosis. Marek's disease in chickens (avian herpesvirus) is the only disease in which an infection alone causes an arterial disease with some morphologic similarities to human atherosclerosis, but full-blown human-like atherosclerosis develops only if the chickens concomitantly are fed a cholesterol-rich diet.[70] This infectious arterial disease in birds is preventable by vaccination.[71]

## Fibroproliferative Response

Only endothelial cells, monocyte-derived macrophages, and a few T cells participate in the early immunoinflammatory response, giving rise to early atherosclerotic lesions (fatty streaks) (Fig. 44-3). In disease progression, this immunoinflammatory response is accompanied by a fibroproliferative response in which the vascular smooth muscle cell plays a dominant role.[72] Smooth muscle cells are not normally present in the mouse intima, but they are, of course, present in the adjacent tunica media, from which they migrate into intima to become the matrix-synthesizing cell in the developing atherosclerotic plaque.[72] Macrophages and T cells continue to be present throughout plaque development and probably promote rather than retard progression.

Lipids begin to accumulate extracellularly, partly due to direct retention of atherogenic lipoproteins in the extracellular matrix and partly due to foam cell necrosis and apoptosis followed by the release of intracellular lipids to the extracellular space.[44] In such a way, a *necrotic* lipid-rich core with foamy macrophages and cholesterol crystals may form, covered by a fibrous cap containing both smooth muscle cells and inflammatory cells[44] (Fig. 44-4, Plate 80).

It has proved much easier to prevent and regress the early immunoinflammatory response than the subsequent fibroproliferative response[58,59,72–76]; consequently, much more is known about the molecular mechanisms controlling the former than the latter. All plaque cells, including smooth muscle cells, are capable of forming a large number of growth factors and cytokines, and T cell–derived IFN-$\gamma$ as well as responses mediated by CD40 ligation could play important roles in lesion progression.[56,60–62] The smooth muscle cell is the principal connective-tissue cell responsible for healing and repair of the arterial wall. It can elaborate all of the proteins of the matrix, including several forms of collagen (e.g., types I, III, and IV), elastic fiber proteins, and proteoglycans, which together create a complex, heterogeneous extracellular matrix.[72] Cartilaginous metaplasia[77] and calcification are frequently seen in advanced lesions, and both intimal calcification[78] and medial[79] calcification have been studied in atherosclerosis-prone mice.

## Thrombotic Response

It has been extremely difficult to reproduce in animals the most dangerous feature of human atherosclerosis: superimposed thrombosis. Human-like plaque rupture with superimposed thrombosis is rare in animal models of atherosclerosis (Fig. 44-5, Plate 81), but a few interesting models have been reported.[80–88] Their relevance for human atherothrombosis needs, however, to be clarified.

## HUMAN ATHEROSCLEROSIS

Following a series of review articles in which the normal arterial intima and its atherosclerosis-prone regions,[89] asymptomatic early lesions,[90] and advanced and potentially symptomatic lesions were described,[11] a practical histologic classification of human atherosclerotic lesions was published by the American Heart Association in 1995 (Fig. 44-6).[11] Subsequently, a modified classification was suggested by another group of investigators.[9] The following description is based on these excellent publications.

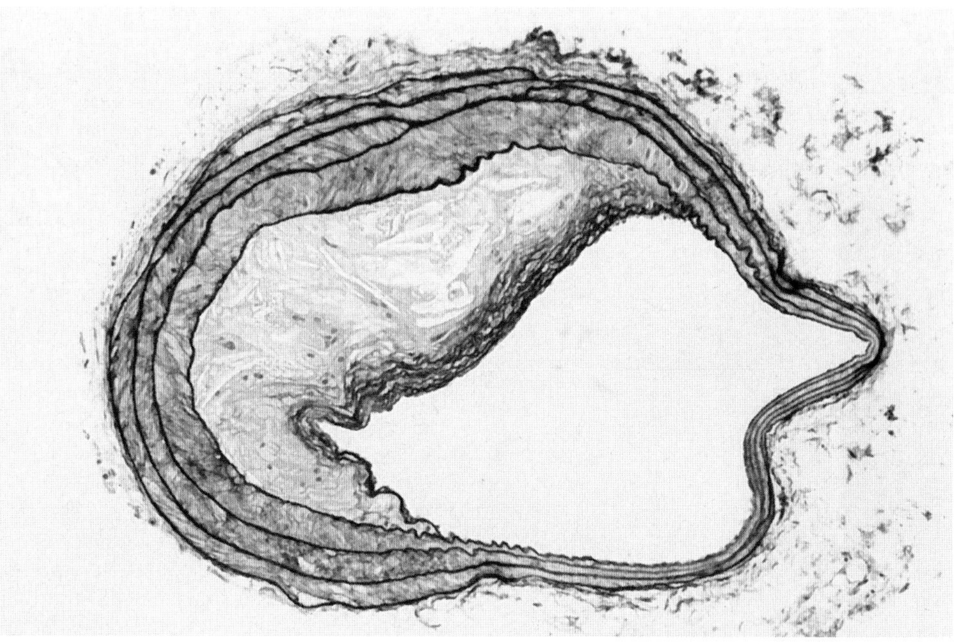

FIGURE 44-4 (Plate 80) An advanced atherosclerotic plaque in the brachiocephalic trunk of a 6-month-old apolipoprotein E–deficient mouse fed normal chow. The plaque appears vulnerable morphologically, consisting of a lipid-rich core with cholesterol crystals covered by a thin but intact fibrous cap. Orcein, staining elastic tissue black.

### Endothelial Dysfunction

Atherogenic stimuli may give rise to maldaptive changes in endothelial structure and function, such as enhanced permeability to plasma lipoproteins, hyperadhesiveness for blood leukocytes, and functional imbalances in local pro- and antithrombotic factors, growth stimulators and inhibitors, and vasoactive substances.[91] These manifestations, collectively termed *endothelial dysfunction,* play an important role in the initiation, progression, and clinical complications of atherosclerosis.[91] It is generally assumed but not proved that endothelial dysfunction as just defined equates with endothelial dysfunction as identified clinically as an impairment in endothelium-dependent vasodilation, largely mediated by the endogenous vasodilator nitric oxide and usually reversible. The mere presence of risk factors for ischemic heart disease—such as hypercholesterolemia, hypertension, cigarette smoking, diabetes mellitus, hyperhomocyst(e)inemia, and aging—is associated with endothelial dysfunction as defined clinically, even in the microcirculation and in arteries, such as the brachial artery, that are resistant to atherosclerosis.[92,93] Thus, clinically defined endothelial dysfunction is related to atherosclerosis but not necessarily causally.

### Atherosclerosis-Prone Areas

The normal human intima is covered by endothelial cells and contains, in contrast to intima of many laboratory animals (including mice), smooth muscle cells, isolated macrophages, occasional mast cells, and extracellular matrix.[90] The latter constitutes up to 60 percent of the volume and contains proteoglycans (predominantly chondroitin and dermatan sulfates), collagens (predominantly types I and III), elastin, and other components such as fibronectin, laminin, and plasma proteins.[90] Apparently, all plasma proteins are present in the lesion-free intima in concentrations related directly to the protein's plasma concentration and inversely to its molecular weight. In the normal artery, LDL is present in intima but is usually not detectable in media.[89]

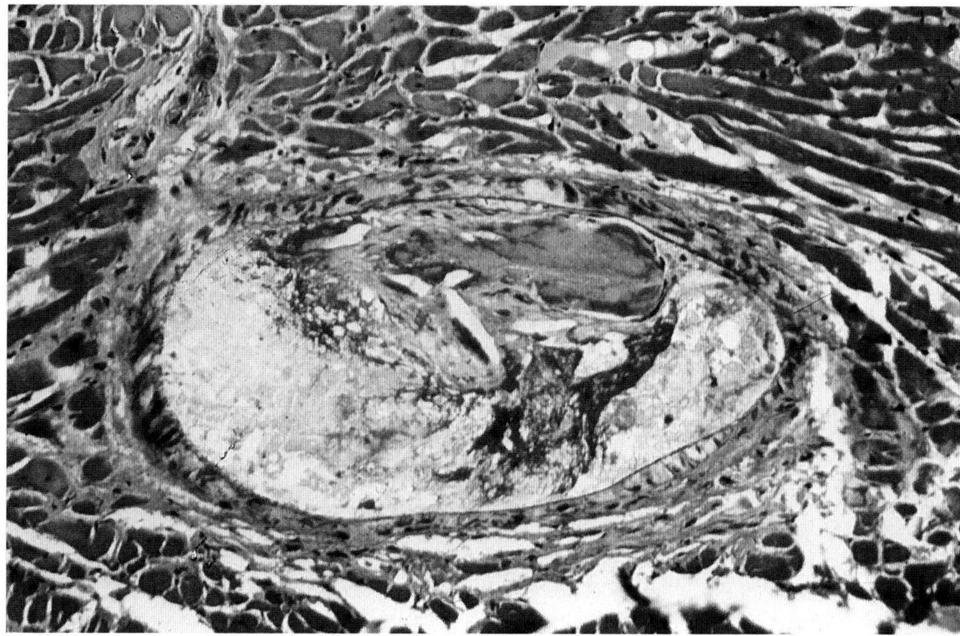

FIGURE 44-5 (Plate 81) Ruptured coronary plaque with occlusive thrombosis superimposed (natural death of a 21-month-old apolipoprotein E–deficient mouse). Spontaneous plaque rupture and/or luminal thrombosis are extremely rare in animal models of atherosclerosis. Elastin trichrome stain.

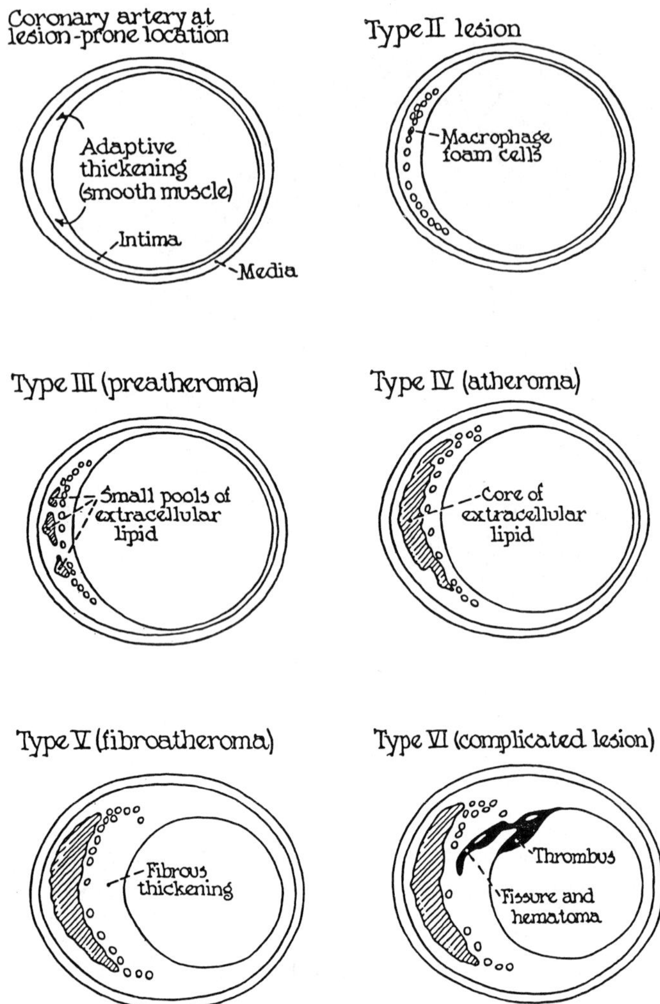


FIGURE 44-6 The 1995 American Heart Association classification of atherosclerotic lesions. The type I (initial) lesion, which consists of small, isolated groups of macrophages containing lipid droplets, is not shown in this figure. (Adapted from Stary et al.[11] Reproduced with permission from the publisher and authors.)

Regardless of atherogenic stimuli, nonobstructive intimal thickenings are present at constant locations in everyone from birth, particularly at bifurcations, and progress with time. Such adaptive intimal thickenings develop in response to mechanical forces such as pressure, circumferential stretch or tension, and shear stress.[89] Low shear stress and, probably more importantly, oscillatory flow and flow reversal may promote both adaptive intimal thickening and subsequent influx and accumulation of atherogenic lipoproteins.[31] Reduced wall shear stress (dilatation) and increased wall tensile stress (hypertension) promote adaptive intimal thickening, which tends to normalize shear and tension.[89] Eccentric intimal thickening is frequently seen near bifurcations and branch points where shear and tensile stresses are not uniformly distributed, and diffuse thickening may develop in relatively straight arterial segments with evenly distributed stresses.[89] Evidence suggests that the shape of a vessel, rather than the flow patterns, may determine the degree of adaptive intimal thickening and may ultimately constitute a risk factor for development of symptomatic lesions.[94]

In human arteries, there is no need for migration of smooth muscle cells into the intima from the media to initiate plaque formation, in contrast to many laboratory animals, where the intima does not normally contain smooth muscle cells. Under the influence of atherogenic stimuli, adaptive intimal thickenings appear to be good soil for the development of atherosclerosis.[33,95] The smooth muscle cells present early in preexisting intimal thickenings and later show "clonality" in superimposed atherosclerotic lesions, suggesting clonal expansion during lesion development.[96]

Although advanced lesions are not confined to regions with adaptive intimal thickenings, particularly not in hyperlipidemia-induced atherosclerosis in animals, lesions form earlier and more rapidly in these atherosclerosis-prone areas than elsewhere.[33] In humans, the topographic distribution of eccentric intimal thickening and of advanced atherosclerotic lesions is similar in the coronary arteries, the carotid bifurcation, the parasellar carotid artery, and the aorta.[89,94,97]

## Fatty Streaks

The earliest lesion of atherosclerosis, the ***fatty streak,*** is a pure immunoinflammatory reaction within intima, consisting of lipid-filled macrophages (foam cells) and T lymphocytes (Fig. 44-3).[6,90] Fatty streaks develop under an intact but activated and dysfunctioning endothelium, particularly in atherosclerosis-prone areas with preexisting intimal thickening. Extracellular lipid is hardly identifiable microscopically, and B lymphocytes and neutrophils are not seen. Fatty streaks are present in the aorta from early childhood and may, in fact, begin to develop during fetal life, particularly in fetuses of hypercholesterolemic mothers.[98] Fatty streaks do not protrude into the lumen; they are therefore asymptomatic.

Inflammation and immune responses play an important role in atherogenesis from its very beginning.[6,99–101] Hypercholesterolemia is associated with increased endothelial permeability, increased transcytosis and intimal retention of lipoproteins, and endothelial activation with focal expression of VCAM-1 leading to monocyte and T-lymphocyte recruitment. Within the intima, the monocyte-derived macrophages engulf the blood-derived LDLs, probably via their scavenger receptors after oxidative modification, and become lipid-filled foam cells. These inflammatory cells constitute by far the major part of the early fatty streak lesion, with a ratio of approximately 1:10 to 1:50 between T cells and macrophages, and they probably play a significant role in the progression of fatty streaks to mature atherosclerotic plaques.[99] The presence of activated macrophages and T cells strongly suggests that an immunologic reaction has taken place in the atherosclerotic plaque. The antigens that elicit this response are not yet known, and both autoantigens (e.g., oxidized LDL, beta microglobulin) and microorganisms (e.g., *C. pneumoniae*) have been proposed to play a role.[6,99–101]

The fate of fatty streaks remains controversial.[9,102] It is generally assumed that fatty streaks can progress to more advanced lesions because they occur at the same anatomical sites and because transitional stages have been observed.[90] A smaller subgroup of fatty streaks, those superimposed on preexisting intimal thickenings, appears to be particularly prone to progress to advanced symptomatic lesions, but the mode of progression and the factors controlling it are not clear.[90] Aortic fatty streaks are universally present in all populations around the world early in life, even in populations at low risk of symptomatic atherosclerosis later in life, such as the South African Bantu.[103] Females have more aortic fatty streaks than males early in life, despite the fact that males develop more advanced lesions than females later in life.[103,104] Blacks have more aortic fatty streaks than whites early in life, but the latter have more advanced lesions than the former later in life.[103,104] The thoracic aorta has more fatty streaks than the abdominal aorta early in life, but the opposite applies for advanced lesions later in life.[103] These contrasting relations seen in the human aorta, between asymptomatic fatty streaks in young persons and advanced and potentially symptomatic lesions in adults, may question the relevance of results obtained in short-term animal experiments, in which only the development of foam cell lesions (fatty streaks) in the aorta are studied (Fig. 44-3).

## Atherosclerotic Plaques

Advanced atherosclerotic lesions (plaques) may cause luminal narrowing and give rise to ischemic symptoms. When lipids begin to accumulate extracellularly, atherogenesis has passed beyond the fatty streak stage. Two different processes are responsible for the extracellular accumulation of lipids; blood-derived atherogenic lipoprotein particles may be trapped and retained directly within the proteoglycan-rich extracellular matrix, and/or lipid may be released from macrophage foam cells following their death.[105] Macrophages both proliferate and die within atherosclerotic plaques; the balance probably depends on whether the lesion is progressing, quiescent, or regressing. Later on, when a lipid-rich core has formed, erythrocytes and their lipid-rich membranes may contribute to the expansion of the core (hemorrhages caused by plaque rupture or rupture of microvessels within the plaque).[106]

Progression beyond the fatty streak stage is associated not only with lipid accumulation but also with accumulation of connective tissue, produced by smooth muscle cells and giving rise to very heterogenous atherosclerotic plaques (Fig. 44-7).[6] Some plaques are lipid-rich while others are lipid-poor, and morphologically dissimilar plaques may evolve next to each other. The endothelium is intact early during atherogenesis, but denuded areas, often related to superficial foam cell infiltration (inflammation) with adherent platelets, are later seen over mature plaques.[107–109] Then, growth factors released from adherent platelets and microthrombi may stimulate the smooth muscle cells within the plaque to produce more connective tissue matrix. Because of a leaky endothelium, not only lipoproteins but also many other blood-derived components, including albumin and fibrinogen, are present in evolving lesions.[110]

Endothelial cells and vascular smooth muscle cells are, according to conventional wisdom, presumed to be resident arterial cells. A recent series of investigations have, however, suggested a new paradigm in which smooth muscle cells and endothelial cells in atherosclerosis and neointimal lesions after vascular injury may derive, at least in part, from bone marrow or circulating blood cells.[111]

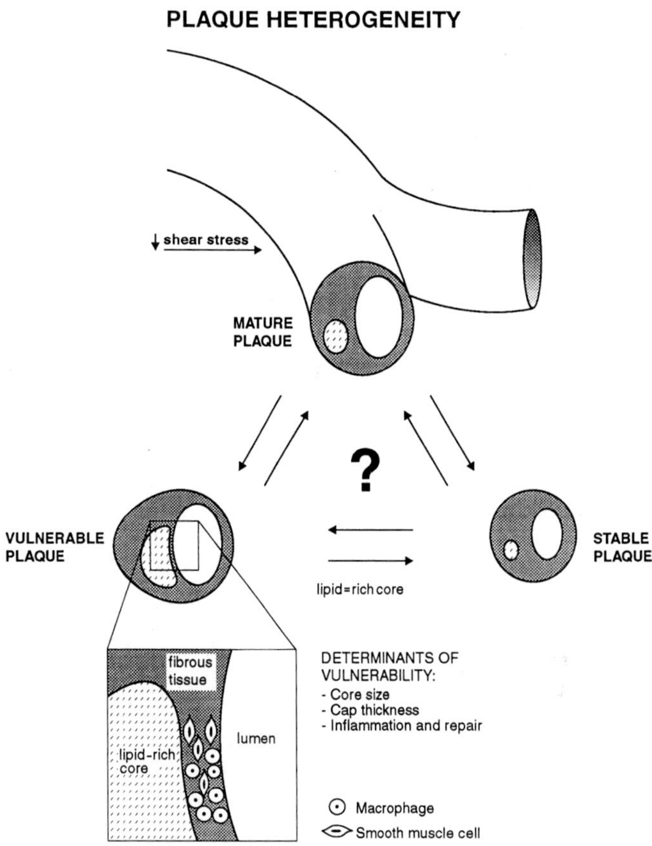


FIGURE 44-7 Advanced atherosclerotic plaques are extremely heterogeneous in composition. A subset of the advanced plaques are vulnerable (i.e., rupture-prone), with a high risk of becoming complicated by luminal thrombosis. The relation between vulnerable and stable plaques is not well defined. (Adapted from Ravn and Falk.[185] Reproduced with permission from the publisher and authors.)

## Calcification

Focal calcification in atherosclerotic plaques is very common and increases with age in both men and women.[112,113] Both lipid-rich and collagen-rich components may calcify, and the process may be active and controlled, resembling calcification in bone, rather than being passive and "dystrophic".[114] Coronary calcification in adults is almost always caused by atherothrombosis.[112] Medial calcification (Mönckeberg's calcinosis) is rare in coronary arteries, even in diabetic persons, where it frequently occurs in other arteries, particularly the muscular arteries of the legs.[115] Both autopsy and clinical data indicate that coronary calcification is a marker for the overall atherosclerotic plaque burden and correlates closely with it,[116–118] but calcification of a plaque does not correlate with its flow-limiting capacity (degree of stenosis)[116,117] or its risk of sudden occlusion (vulnerability).[19] If anything, heavily calcified plaques appear to be more stable than noncalcified plaques.[117,119] Vascular remodeling is a likely explanation for the poor correlation of plaque calcification with lumen narrowing and/or stenosis severity.[116]

Noninvasive detection of coronary calcification, rather than plaques, may identify patients at increased risk of a heart attack.[120] The greater the number of plaques present, the greater the likelihood that one of them will be vulnerable to rupture and thrombosis.

## Remodeling and Stenosis

Vascular remodeling is the ability of the vessel wall to reorganize its cellular and extracellular components in response to a chronic stimulus.[121] Remodeling is a bidirectional process.[122] Rupture-prone plaques (large lipid-rich core, thin cap, ongoing inflammation) and those responsible for the acute coronary syndromes are usually relatively large and associated with compensatory enlargement (positive remodeling), which tends to preserve a normal lumen despite the presence of significant and potentially dangerous vessel wall disease.[123–126] In contrast, plaques responsible for stable angina are usually smaller but, nevertheless, often cause more severe luminal narrowing because of concomitant local shrinkage of the artery (negative remodeling).[127] The reason for these different modes of remodeling is unknown, but processes in adventitia could play a critical role.

## Plaque Burden versus Stenosis as Predictor

The great majority of heart attacks and ischemic strokes originate from atherosclerotic lesions that, prior to the acute events, only were mildly to moderately stenotic—i.e., they were hemodynamically insignificant and probably asymptomatic (Fig. 44-8). Although the risk for occlusion, or myocardial infarction or stroke, increases with stenosis severity, the great majority of coronary occlusions (71 percent) in the Coronary Artery Surgery Study and myocardial infarctions (86 percent) in pooled studies originated from lesions that caused less than 70 to 80 percent angiographic stenosis prior to the acute events.[8] The reason is that stenotic lesions are markers of plaque burden, and lower-risk nonstenotic lesions will always by far outnumber the higher-risk stenotic ones and altogether increase the risk for an acute event much more than the few stenotic lesions at higher individual risk. And the same holds for ischemic stroke. Asymptomatic plaques at the carotid bifurcation, contralateral to symptomatic lesions, were evaluated and followed in the European Carotid Surgery Trial ($n = 2240$).[128] Only 13 (19 percent) of 67 new strokes were judged to have originated from initially asymptomatic lesions that at baseline caused more than 70 percent angiographic stenosis (Fig. 44-8). The reason: lower-risk nonstenotic carotid plaques ($n = 2113$) outnumbered by far the stenotic ones ($n = 127$) at higher risk. Furthermore, rupture-prone plaques and those responsible for acute ischemic events—at least in the coronary arteries—are usually associated with compensatory enlargement of the artery (positive remodeling), which tends to preserve a normal lumen.[illegible]

## Neovascularization

Neovasculature, often expressing leukocyte adhesion molecules such as VCAM-1 and ICAM-1 and associated with inflammatory cell infiltration, is frequenly present at the base of advanced plaques, and it has been suggested that these vasa vasorum–derived new vessels could play an active role in the recruitment of leukocytes into plaques and thus contribute to the progression of the disease.[129,130] Regardless of the integrity of the plaque surface, small low-pressure hemorrhages (extravasated erythrocytes) are also common in these neovascularized areas.[22] There is no convincing evidence that such low-pressure bleedings may precipitate rupture of the plaque surface and/or luminal thrombosis. Leaky microvessels in plaques may, however, contribute to plaque growth.[106,130]

# RUPTURE-PRONE PLAQUES

A subset of advanced but not necessarily stenotic plaques is particularly dangerous because of their vulnerability to rupture (and high thrombogenicity), which may precipitate a thrombus-mediated heart attack (Fig. 44-1). The risk of plaque rupture depends more on plaque composition than on the degree of stenosis produced by the plaque. Pathoanatomic studies have identified three major determinants of a plaque's vulnerability to rupture: (1) the size of the lipid-rich core, (2) inflammation with plaque degradation, and (3) lack of smooth muscle cells with impaired healing (Fig. 44-7).[8]

Lipid accumulation, macrophage infiltration, and lack of smooth muscle cells destabilize plaques, making them vulnerable to rupture. In contrast, smooth muscle cell–mediated healing and repair processes stabilize plaques, protecting them against disruption.[6,131] Plaque size or the severity of the associated stenosis do not predict a plaque's vulnerability to rupture.[20] Many rupture-prone plaques are

**Coronary stenosis: progression to occlusion**

**Serial angiography in 298 patients***

| Stenosis at baseline | Segments n | Occlusion, 5-year % | n | |
|---|---|---|---|---|
| < 5% | 2161 | .7 | 15 | |
| 5 - 49% | 430 | 2 | 10 | 51 |
| 50 - 80% | 258 | 10 | 26 | |
| 81 - 95% | 89 | 24 | 21 | |
| All | 2938 | | 72 | |

*Alderman EL et al. *J Am Coll Cardiol* 1993; 22:1141-54

**Coronary stenosis: progression to MI**

**Serial angiography in 239 patients#**

| Stenosis prior to MI | Segments n | Culprit for MI % | n | |
|---|---|---|---|---|
| 0% | 2674 | 0.3 | 8 | |
| 25% | 287 | 3.5 | 10 | 29 |
| 50% | 123 | 4.1 | 5 | |
| 75% | 76 | 7.9 | 6 | |
| 90 - 99% | 115 | 8.7 | 10 | |
| All | 3275 | | 39 | |

#Nobuyoshi M et al. *J Am Coll Cardiol* 1991; 18:904-10

**Carotid stenosis: progression to stroke**

**Angiography in 2240 patients¶**

| Stenosis at baseline | n | Ipsilateral stroke %, 3 y | n, 4.5 y | |
|---|---|---|---|---|
| 0 - 29% | 1270 | 1.8 | 28 | 54 |
| 30 - 69% | 843 | 2.1 | 26 | |
| 70 - 99% | 127 | 5.7 | 13 | |
| All | 2240 | | 67 | |

¶European Carotid Surgery Trial. *Lancet* 1995; 345:209-12

FIGURE 44-8 Most coronary occlusions (*top*) (51/72 = 71 percent), myocardial infarctions (*middle*) (29/39 = 74 percent), and ischemic strokes of carotid origin (*bottom*) (54/67 = 81 percent) are caused by acute thrombosis superimposed on atherosclerotic lesions that, prior to the acute events, were asymptomatic and only mildly to moderately stenotic. Overall, nonstenotic atherosclerotic lesions by far outnumber the stenotic ones at higher individual risk, which is why most acute clinical events originate from nonstenotic lesions at relative low individual risk. MI = myocardial infarction.

invisible angiographically (and also missed by stress testing) due to their small size and compensatory vascular remodeling.[123–126]

## Lipid Accumulation

The lipid-rich core of an atherosclerotic plaque is avascular, hypocellular, softlike gruel, and totally devoid of supporting collagen.[8] The size of such a soft core is, of course, critical for the stability of a plaque.[131] Recent studies have identified macrophage-specific antigens and apoptotic nuclear fragments within the gruel, indicating that lipid and other cell constituents released from dead macrophage foam cells could contribute significantly to the formation and growth of the lesion core, which is why it also has been referred to as the "graveyard of dead macrophages," emphasizing the inflammatory origin of this destabilizing core.[132,133]

## Inflammation

Ruptured fibrous caps are usually heavily infiltrated by macrophage foam cells,[8] and recent observations have revealed that such rupture-related macrophages are activated, indicating ongoing inflammation at the site of plaque disruption.[14] Van der Wal and coworkers found, utilizing immunohistochemical techniques, that macrophages and adjacent T lymphocytes (smooth muscle cells were usually lacking at rupture sites) were activated, indicating ongoing disease activity.[14] Further evidence of immune activation is the upregulated expression of CD40 receptor and its ligand by all cell types present in advanced atherosclerotic lesions.[134] Correspondingly, culprit lesions responsible for acute coronary syndromes contain significantly more macrophages than lesions responsible for stable angina.[135]

Macrophages are capable of degrading extracellular matrix by phagocytosis or by secreting proteolytic enzymes such as members of the matrix metalloproteinase (MMP) family (collagenases, gelatinases, and stromolysins), cysteine proteinases (e.g., elastolytic cathepsins S and K), and serine proteinases [mostly plasminogen and its activators, urokinase (uPA) and tissue-type plasminogen activator (tPA)], which may weaken the fibrous cap, predisposing it to rupture.[136] All of these proteinases have been identified in human plaques and have been implicated in plaque rupture, but the actual enzymatic culprits have not yet been conclusively identified.[137] The MMPs are secreted in a latent zymogen form requiring extracellular activation, after which they are capable of degrading virtually all components of the extracellular matrix. The MMPs and their cosecreted tissue inhibitors of metalloproteinases, TIMP-1 and TIMP-2, are critical for cell migration, tumor invasion and metastasis, and vascular remodeling. Besides macrophages, a wide variety of cells may produce MMPs. Activated mast cells may secrete powerful proteolytic enzymes such as tryptase and chymase that can activate pro-MMPs secreted by other cells (e.g., macrophages), and mast cells are actually present in shoulder regions of mature plaques and at sites of disruption, although at very low density.[138] Neutrophils are also capable of destroying tissue by secreting proteolytic enzymes, but they are rare in intact plaques.[14,99,139] However, contrary to conventional wisdom, recent data indicate that neutrophils are indeed present in culprit lesions responsible for acute coronary syndromes.[140] Regarding the role of MMPs in plaque rupture, their coexistence does not prove causality. For example, plaque rupture with superimposed thrombosis is rare in animal models of atherosclerosis, although MMPs are abundantly expressed in such lesions. Only a few exceptional cases have been reported.[80–88] Even overexpression of human MMP-1 (interstitial collagenase) has failed to induce plaque rupture in murine models.[141]

## Infection

Several infectious agents have been suggested to play an active role in the development of cardiovascular diseases, particularly *Chlamydia pneumoniae* but also herpesviruses (including cytomegalovirus) and *Helicobacter pylori.*[142–144] *Chlamydia* has been identified in atherosclerotic plaques[144]; it contains lipopolysaccharide and heat-shock protein 60, which are well-known strong inducers of many enzymes including MMPs.[145] Macrolide antibiotics (against *Chlamydia)* have been tested in the secondary prevention of cardiovascular disease, including patients with acute coronary syndromes.[146] No clear-cut benefit has emerged from these trials.[147] A recent case-control study by Naghavi et al.[148] and an influenza vaccine pilot study by Gurfinkel et al. (FLUVACS Study)[149] indicated, however, that influenza infection might play a role in triggering acute coronary events.

## Impaired Healing

Obviously, the thickness and collagen content of the fibrous cap is very important for its strength and stability: the thinner the cap, the weaker it is and the more vulnerable the plaque is to rupture.[8] Ruptured aortic caps contain fewer smooth muscle cells and less collagen than intact caps, and smooth muscle cells are usually missing at the actual site of disruption.[8,14,131] Collagen is responsible for the mechanical strength of the fibrous cap and is synthesized by intimal smooth muscle cells. It is important to realize that smooth muscle cell proliferation and matrix synthesis may, in fact, be good in protecting plaques against rupture, whereas local loss of smooth muscle cells or impaired smooth muscle cell function may be bad, leading to gradual plaque destabilization due to impaired healing and repair. It is unknown why smooth muscle cells are lacking at rupture sites, but apoptotic cell death could play an important role.[133]

## Calcification

Ruptured plaques have been reported to be calcified more frequently than nonruptured plaques (69 versus 23 percent).[15] This does not indicate, however, that calcification destabilizes plaques.[19] Clinical observations suggest that culprit lesions responsible for acute coronary syndromes generally are less calcified than plaques responsible for stable angina, indicating that calcium confers stability to plaques rather than the opposite.[117,119] The total amount of calcification—the calcium score—is a marker of plaque burden (and thus a marker of cardiovascular risk) rather than a marker of risk conferred by the individual calcified plaque.[19,120]

## Triggering

Sudden rupture of a thin and inflammed fibrous cap may occur spontaneously, but triggering could also play a role and thus help to explain the nonrandom onset of acute coronary syndromes.[12] For example, severe exertion is a potential trigger of rupture-mediated coronary thrombosis.[12,150] It should be remembered, however, that the great majority of heart attacks do not occur during strenuous exercise and that exercise appears to confer protection in the long run.[12]

## Vulnerability versus Triggers

In general, plaque rupture is probably the result of a dynamic interaction between *intrinsic* plaque changes (vulnerability) and *extrinsic* forces imposed on the plaque (triggers); the former predispose a plaque to rupture, whereas the latter may precipitate it.[8] As the presence of a vulnerable plaque is a prerequisite for plaque rupture, plaque vulnerability is probably more important than triggers of rupture in determining the risk of a future heart attack. If no vulnerable plaques are present in the coronary arteries, there is no rupture-prone substrate for a potential trigger to function on. Furthermore, the fact that exercise stress testing in individuals with advanced coronary artery disease rarely triggers an acute coronary event suggests that plaque vulnerability ultimately plays a more important role in plaque rupture than does physiologic stress or other potential triggers.

## PLAQUE RUPTURE PRECIPITATING THROMBOSIS

When a ruptured plaque is found beneath a thrombus, the question of which came first of course arises. The frequent finding of components from the lipid-rich core within the thrombus or downstream of the rupture site clearly indicates the sequence of events: plaque rupture precedes thrombus formation.[151,152] Furthermore, this sequence, rather than the opposite, makes sense, because the lipid-rich core is known to contain active tissue factor, which may generate thrombin and thus initiate platelet aggregation and fibrin formation when it is exposed.[153–157] Therefore if a ruptured plaque is found beneath a thrombus, it is generally considered a plausible precipitating cause. However, plaque rupture does not inevitably lead to significant luminal thrombosis.[24,151] The two other components of the triad of Virchow (blood and flow) are also decisive for the magnitude of the thrombotic response to plaque rupture.[158]

Plaque rupture is the major cause of coronary thrombosis worldwide, being responsible for approximately 76 percent of all fatal thrombotic events (Table 44-1).[152] Plaque rupture is a more frequent cause of coronary thrombosis in males (81 percent) than in females (59 percent). It is only rare in one extremely small subgroup of patients, namely premenopausal females, who constitute less than 1 percent of heart attack victims in the United States.[159] Except for gender and menopause, no particular risk factors have consistently been connected with a particular type of coronary plaque or mechanism of thrombosis.[152]

### Rapid Progression

Rupture of the plaque surface is followed by a variable amount of hemorrhage into the plaque and by luminal thrombosis (often small and nonobstructive), causing sudden and rapid but often clinically silent growth of the lesion.[8,160,161] It is probably the most important mechanism underlying the episodic (versus linear) progression of some coronary lesions observed by serial angiography. Plaque rupture is relatively frequent in diabetes and hypertension[162] and extremely common in fatal coronary artery disease.[22,151,163]

### Vasoconstriction

Plaque rupture, thrombosis, and vasospasm often coexist, and rupture/thrombosis most likely gives rise to vasospasm rather than the opposite.[8] Abnormal coronary vasoreactivity is common in acute coronary syndromes but *spasm* is usually confined to the culprit lesion, suggesting that it is caused by locally released vasoactive substances.[164] The plaque, particularly macrophages in ruptured plaques responsible for unstable angina, may contain potent vasoconstrictors such as endothelin 1,[165] and superimposed thrombosis may also contain or generate vasoconstrictors such as thrombin and platelet-derived serotonin and thromboxane $A_2$.[1]

TABLE 44-1 Worldwide, 1114 (76%) of 1460 Fatal Coronary Thrombi Precipitated by Plaque Rupture

| Patients | | Age, Years[a] | *n* | Rupture | Study |
|---|---|---|---|---|---|
| Hospital, | — | — | 19 | 19 = 100% | Chapman, 1965[186] |
| Hospital, | — | — | 17 | 17 = 100% | Constantinides, 1966[187] |
| Hospital, | AMI + SCD | 58 | 40 | 39 = 98% | Friedman et al., 1966[188] |
| Hospital, | AMI | 62 | 88 | 71 = 81% | Bouch et al., 1970[189] |
| Hospital, | AMI | 66 | 91 | 68 = 75% | Sinapius, 1972[190] |
| Coroner, | SCD | 53 | 20 | 19 = 95% | Friedman et al., 1973[191] |
| Hospital, | AMI | 67 | 76 | 69 = 91% | Horie et al., 1978[192] |
| Hospital, | AMI | 67 | 49 | 40 = 82% | Falk, 1983[151] |
| Coroner, | SCD | <65 | 32 | 26 = 81% | Tracy et al., 1985[193] |
| Med. exam, | SCD | <70 | 61 | 39 = 64% | El Fawal et al., 1987[194] |
| Hospital, | AMI | — | 83 | 52 = 63% | Yutani et al., 1987[195] |
| Coroner, | — | — | 85 | 71 = 84% | Richardson et al., 1989[13] |
| Hospital, | AMI | 63 | 20 | 12 = 60% | van der Wal et al., 1994[14] |
| Coroner, | SCD | — | 202 | 143 = 71% | Davies, 1997[b,196] |
| Hospital, | AMI | 69 | 291 | 218 = 75% | Arbustini et al., 1999[16] |
| Hospital, | AMI | 61 | 61 | 56 = 92% | Shi et al., 1999[197] |
| Hospital, | AMI | 69 | 100 | 81 = 81% | Kojima et al., 2000[198] |
| Med. exam, | SCD | 48 | 125 | 74 = 59% | Virmani et at., 2000[b,9] |
| AMI + SCD | | | 1460 | 1114 = 76% | Worldwide |

ABBREVIATIONS: — = not reported; AMI = acute myocardial infarction; SCD = sudden coronary death.

[a]Mean

[b]Davies[196] and Virmani et al.[9] are updated summaries, including previously published data.

## PLAQUE EROSION WITH SUPERIMPOSED THROMBOSIS

The term *plaque erosion* has gained popularity for the minority of thrombi not precipitated by plaque rupture (about 20 percent in males and 40 percent in females) (Fig. 44-2). Virmani et al. have published extensively on the role of these lesions in sudden coronary death, and they recently introduce the term *calcified nodule* for a rare subtype of plaque erosion.[9] It is a heterogeous group of atherothrombotic plaques where no deep injury is present to explain the overlying thrombus, only the endothelium is missing at the plaque-thrombus interface. The pathogenetic role of inflammation is controversial,[9,14] and although tissue factor immunoreactivity has been identified in some of these lesions,[166] its functionel role is unknown.

The precise mechanisms of thrombosis over eroded plaques are not known but probably reflect their heterogeneity. It is conceivable that systemic thrombogenic factors such as platelet hyperaggregability, hypercoagulability, circulating tissue factor, and/or depressed fibrinolysis play a major role in thrombosis over plaques that are only eroded (versus ruptured).[19,167] Recent studies have suggested that activated circulating leukocytes may transfer active tissue factor by shedding microparticles and transferring them onto adherent platelets.[168,169] It is possible that such circulating sources of tissue factor, rather than plaque-derived tissue factor, can contribute to thrombosis at sites of endothelial denudation, as in plaque erosion.

## THROMBOSIS

There are three major determinants of the thrombotic response to plaque rupture or the amount of thrombosis formed on top of an eroded plaque: (1) the local thrombogenic substrate, (2) local flow disturbances, and (3) the systemic thrombotic propensity (see Chap. 45).

### Local Thrombogenic Substrate

Ongoing inflammation, in particular macrophage infiltration and activation, and lipid accumulation are not only destabilize plaques, making them vulnerable to rupture, but these plaque components also appear to be highly thrombogenic when exposed to the flowing blood after plaque rupture. Activated macrophages express tissue factor, and the lipid-rich atheromatous core contains a lot of active tissue factor, probably originating from dead macrophages.[153–156] Culprit lesions responsible for the acute coronary syndromes contain more tissue factor than plaques responsible for stable angina.[157]

### Local Flow Disturbances

In contrast to venous thrombosis, rapid flow and high shear forces promote arterial thrombosis, probably via shear-induced platelet activation.[109,158] A platelet-rich thrombus may indeed form and grow within a severe stenosis, where the blood velocity and shear forces are highest. Irregularities of the exposed surface also increase platelet-mediated thrombus formation.[153]

### Systemic Thrombotic Propensity

The state (activation) of platelets, coagulation, and fibrinolysis is critical for the outcome of plaque rupture, documented by the protective effect of antiplatelet agents and anticoagulants in patients at risk of coronary thrombosis. Tissue factor probably plays an important prothrombotic role both locally (expressed by macrophages in the culprit lesion) and systemically (expressed by activated leukocytes in the peripheral blood).[168,169]

### Platelets and Fibrin

In coronary thrombosis, the initial flow obstruction is usually caused by platelet aggregation, but fibrin is important for the subsequent stabilization of the early and fragile platelet thrombus.[158] Thus, both platelets and fibrin are involved in the evolution of a stable and persisting coronary thrombus.

### Dynamic Thrombosis and Microembolization

The thrombotic response to plaque rupture is dynamic: thrombosis and thrombolysis, often associated with vasospasm,[164] tend to occur simultaneously, causing intermittent flow obstruction and distal embolization. The latter leads to microvascular obstruction, which may prevent myocardial reperfusion despite a "successfully" recanalized infarct-related artery.[170]

## MULTIPLE "ACTIVE" PLAQUES IN ACUTE CORONARY SYNDROMES

The risk of recurrent events is particularly high during the first month after an acute coronary syndrome. It has generally been assumed that the same atherothrombotic plaque, the culprit lesion, is responsible not only for the initial heart attack but also for early repeated events if they occur. Recent observations indicate, however, that not just one but multiple "active," complex, and rapidly progressing coronary lesions are often present in acute heart attack patients.[171–173]

### Pathoanatomic Evidence

Plaque rupture is not rare. Davies et al. found ruptured coronary plaques without luminal thrombosis in 9 percent of persons who died suddenly of noncardiac causes; this figure increased to 22 percent (including 5 percent with nonocclusive thrombosis) if an atheroma-related disease such as diabetes or hypertension was present.[162] And many more ruptured plaques are found in patients dying of coronary atherosclerosis rather than with it.[22,151,163] In 47 such patients, we identified at autopsy 103 ruptured coronary plaques (about 2.2 per patient) of which only 40 had obstructive and probably fatal luminal thrombosis superimposed, while the remaining 63 ruptures were without luminal thrombosis or covered only by a small nonobstructive and thus probably asymptomatic thrombus.[151] None of these ruptured plaques were healed, suggesting they had developed within a relatively short period of time before death, though not necessarily simultaneously. Frink identified 211 ulcerated plaques, of which many were judged to be chronic, in 83 cases of acute coronary death and concluded that ulcerated plaques without thrombosis are ubiquitous and multiple in such patients.[163] Finally, a special nonuniform pattern of dense (older) and loosely arranged (younger) collagen, judged to represent the healed stage of subclinical plaque disruption, has recently been identified in many coronary plaques, particularly in those causing chronic high-grade stenosis.[160,161] Therefore plaque rupture, causing episodic plaque growth, is not a rare event in the spontaneous progression of coronary atherosclerosis, and more than one ruptured plaque, with or without thrombosis superimposed, is usually present in persons dying of the disease. However, the temporal relation among multiple ruptured plaques, particularly whether they occurred simultaneously or not, remains, elusive, because exact dating of acute coronary lesions is difficult if not impossible.

Not only multiple ruptured plaques but even multiple thrombi are relatively frequent in those who die of an acute heart attack. We identified 51 recent coronary thrombi (and 29 old coronary occlusions) in 44 patients who died of coronary atherosclerosis.[151] In the landmark study by Davies and Thomas of sudden coronary death ($n = 100$), coronary thrombosis was present in 74 cases, of which 28 (38 percent) had more than one discontinuous segment with thrombosis.[22] In all, 115 separate thrombi were found, and major coronary thrombosis occluding more than 50 percent of the lumen was present in 44 of the 74 cases.[22] That is, many of the thrombi identified in this thorough autopsy study were small and nonobstructive and thus probably asymptomatic. Recently, Arbustini et al. reported their experience in a large autopsy series of 298 patients with acute myocardial infarction, finding multiple coronary thrombi in 29 (10 percent) of the cases, apparently unrelated to the integrity of the underlying plaque surface (whether it was ruptured or just eroded).[16] Hence multiple ruptured plaques, of which many are unhealed and probably recently ruptured, are frequently present in patients with an acute coronary syndrome, and multiple coronary thromboses are found in more than 10 percent of autopsied cases. It seems likely that patients with multiple coronary thromboses often have a rapid and fatal course, which may explain why this condition is rarely recognized clinically.[174]

### Clinical Evidence

Some years ago cardiologists were puzzled by the fact that the number and severity of coronary stenoses were similar in patients with stable and unstable angina, despite the worse short-term prognosis of the latter.[175] Ambrose et al. were the first to draw attention to the different angiographic morphology of culprit lesions,[176] and it was soon realized that the behavior of culprit lesions also differed in the two syndromes. In unstable angina, a typical culprit lesion is angiographically complex (ruptured plaque), intraluminal filling defects (nonocclusive thrombosis) and vasospasm are frequent in the acute phase, and rapid progression to total occlusion (occlusive thrombosis) is impending.[175] Later it was realized, primarily thanks to a series of provocative angiographic observations by Kaski's group,[177,178] that unstable patients often harbor multiple complex coronary lesions (about 2.6 per patient),[179] of which only one is usually pointed out as the main culprit. And importantly, the more complex plaques, the worse the prognosis.[175] Supportive evidence for the presence of multiple "active" lesions in unstable angina was recently provided by the demonstration of widespread (i.e., involvement of more than one major coronary artery) activation of neutrophils across the coronary vascular bed, regardless of the location of the culprit stenosis.[180] These findings have recently been extended to patients with myocardial infarction.[125,174,181–183] Goldstein et al. identified multiple complex coronary plaques in as many as 40 percent of infarct patients undergoing angiographic examination, and the presence of multiple (versus single) complex plaques was associated with adverse clinical outcomes.[182] This finding suggests multifocal disease activity with rapid progression of nonculprit lesions after myocardial infarction. Patients with single and multiple complex plaques did not differ significantly in age, sex ratio, or the frequency of coronary risk factors, including current smoking, diabetes mellitus, and hypercholesterolemia.[182] In non-Q-wave infarction, 423 complex lesions were identified in 274 patients,[184] but strangely, substantially fewer have also been reported for the same study population.[183] Although these figures for complex lesions are impressive, it should be remembered that angiography is able to identify only major plaque events and thus underestimates the real number of "active" coronary lesions. Overall, not only culprit lesions but also other complex, nonculprit lesions progress rapidly during and shortly after an acute heart attack, indicating that multiple plaque ruptures and/or thrombosis occur simultaneously or within a relatively short period of time in the coronary arteries of clinically unstable patients.

## CONCLUSION AND CLINICAL IMPLICATIONS

Coronary atherosclerosis is the underlying cause of nearly all cases of ischemic heart disease, and superimposed thrombosis is the usual proximate cause of the acute coronary syndromes. Coronary thrombosis is precipitated by plaque rupture in about 75 percent of the cases.

Atherothrombosis is a systemic immunoinflammatory disease fueled by lipid, and inflammation is particularly frequent and intense in ruptured plaques beneath coronary thrombi. In contrast, the role of inflammation in thrombosis not caused by plaque rupture (plaque erosion) is controversial. Many patients with acute coronary syndromes have signs of pancoronary inflammation with multiple "active," complex, and rapidly progressing coronary plaques rather than just a single culprit lesion.

The culprit lesion responsible for an acute coronary syndrome is frequently "dynamic," leading to intermittent flow obstruction and peripheral microembolization; the clinical presentation and the outcome depend on the location of the obstruction and the severity and duration of myocardial ischemia. A nonocclusive or transiently occlusive thrombus most frequently underlies acute coronary syndromes without ST-segment elevation, whereas a more stable and occlusive thrombus prevails in ST-segment-elevation myocardial infarction, overall modified by vascular tone and collateral flow. A critical thrombotic component is also frequent in culprit lesions responsible for out-of-hospital cardiac arrest and sudden coronary death.

## References


1. Fuster V, Fayad ZA, Badimon JJ. Acute coronary syndromes: Biology (review). *Lancet* 1999;353 (suppl 2):SH5–SH9.
2. Falk E. Stable versus unstable atherosclerosis: Clinical aspects (review). *Am Heart J* 1999;138(5 Pt 2):S421–S425.
3. Davies MJ. The pathophysiology of acute coronary syndromes (review). *Heart* 2000;83:361–366.
4. Fuster V. Epidemic of cardiovascular disease and stroke: The three main challenges. Presented at the 71st scientific sessions of the American Heart Association. Dallas, Texas. *Circulation* 1999;99: 1132–1137.
5. Grundy SM, Benjamin IJ, Burke GL, et al. Diabetes and cardiovascular disease: A statement for healthcare professionals from the American Heart Association (review). *Circulation* 1999;100:1134–1146.
6. Libby P. Inflammation in atherosclerosis (review). *Nature.* 2002;420: 868–874.
7. Vink A, Schoneveld AH, Richard W, et al. Plaque burden, arterial remodeling and plaque vulnerability: Determined by systemic factors? *J Am Coll Cardiol* 2001;38:718–723.
8. Falk E, Shah PK, Fuster V. Coronary plaque disruption (review). *Circulation* 1995;92:657–671.
9. Virmani R, Kolodgie FD, Burke AP, et al. Lessons from sudden coronary death: A comprehensive morphological classification scheme for atherosclerotic lesions (review). *Arterioscler Thromb Vasc Biol* 2000;20:1262–1275.

10. Falk E. Why do plaques rupture (review)? *Circulation* 1992;86(suppl): III30–III42.
11. Stary HC, Chandler AB, Dinsmore RE, et al. A definition of advanced types of atherosclerotic lesions and a histological classification of atherosclerosis. A report from the Committee on Vascular Lesions of the Council on Arteriosclerosis, American Heart Association (review). *Circulation* 1995;92:1355–1374.
12. Servoss SJ, Januzzi JL, Muller JE. Triggers of acute coronary syndromes (review). *Prog Cardiovasc Dis* 2002;44:369–380.
13. Richardson PD, Davies MJ, Born GV. Influence of plaque configuration and stress distribution on fissuring of coronary atherosclerotic plaques. *Lancet* 1989;2:941–944.
14. van der Wal AC, Becker AE, van der Loos CM, Das PK. Site of intimal rupture or erosion of thrombosed coronary atherosclerotic plaques is characterized by an inflammatory process irrespective of the dominant plaque morphology. *Circulation* 1994;89:36–44.
15. Farb A, Burke AP, Tang AL, et al. Coronary plaque erosion without rupture into a lipid core. A frequent cause of coronary thrombosis in sudden coronary death. *Circulation* 1996;93:1354–1363.
16. Arbustini E, Dal Bello B, Morbini P, et al. Plaque erosion is a major substrate for coronary thrombosis in acute myocardial infarction. *Heart* 1999;82:269–272.
17. Fayad ZA, Fuster V. Clinical imaging of the high-risk or vulnerable atherosclerotic plaque (review). *Circ Res* 2001;89:305–316.
18. Corti R, Badimon JJ. Biologic aspects of vulnerable plaque. *Curr Opin Cardiol* 2002;17:616–625.
19. Virmani R, Burke AP, Farb A, Kolodgie FD. Pathology of the unstable plaque. *Prog Cardiovasc Dis* 2002;44:349–356.
20. Mann JM, Davies MJ. Vulnerable plaque. Relation of characteristics to degree of stenosis in human coronary arteries. *Circulation* 1996;94: 928–931.
21. Majno G, Joris I. *Cells, Tissues, and Disease: Principles of General Pathology.* Cambridge, MA: Blackwell Science; 1996:646.
22. Davies MJ, Thomas A. Thrombosis and acute coronary-artery lesions in sudden cardiac ischemic death. *N Engl J Med* 1984;310:1137–1140.
23. Davies MJ, Thomas AC. Plaque fissuring—The cause of acute myocardial infarction, sudden ischaemic death, and crescendo angina (review). *Br Heart J* 1985;53:363–373.
24. Davies MJ. Going from immutable to mutable atherosclerotic plaques (review). *Am J Cardiol* 2001;88(suppl):2F–9F.
25. Lusis AJ. Atherosclerosis. *Nature* 2000;407:233–241.
26. Knowles JW, Maeda N. Genetic modifiers of atherosclerosis in mice. *Arterioscler Thromb Vasc Biol* 2000;20:2336–2345.
27. Wang X, Paigen B. Comparative genetics of atherosclerosis and restenosis: Exploration with mouse models. *Arterioscler Thromb Vasc Biol* 2002;22:884–886.
28. Svenson KL, Bogue MA, Peters LL. Genetic models in applied physiology: Invited review: Identifying new mouse models of cardiovascular disease: A review of high-throughput screens of mutagenized and inbred strains. *J Appl Physiol* 2003;94;1650–1659.
29. Lichtman AH, Clinton SK, Iiyama K, et al. Hyperlipidemia and atherosclerotic lesion development in LDL receptor–deficient mice fed defined semipurified diets with and without cholate. *Arterioscler Thromb Vasc Biol* 1999;19:1938–1944.
30. Iiyama K, Hajra L, Iiyama M, Li H, et al. Patterns of vascular cell adhesion molecule-1 and intercellular adhesion molecule-1 expression in rabbit and mouse atherosclerotic lesions and at sites predisposed to lesion formation. *Circ Res* 1999;85:199–207.
31. Traub O, Berk BC. Laminar shear stress: Mechanisms by which endothelial cells transduce an atheroprotective force. *Arterioscler Thromb Vasc Biol* 1998;18:677–685.
32. Skalen K, Gustafsson M, Rydberg EK, et al. Subendothelial retention of atherogenic lipoproteins in early atherosclerosis. *Nature* 2002;417: 750–754.
33. Schwartz SM. The intima: A new soil (editorial). *Circ Res* 1999;85: 877–879.
34. Steinberg D. Atherogenesis in perspective: Hypercholesterolemia and inflammation as partners in crime. *Nat Med* 2002;8:1211–1217.
35. Witztum JL, Palinski W. Are immunological mechanisms relevant for the development of atherosclerosis? (editorial). *Clin Immunopathol* 1999;90:153–156.
36. Camejo G, Hurt-Camejo E, Wiklund O, Bondjers G. Association of apo B lipoproteins with arterial proteoglycans: Pathological significance and molecular basis. *Atherosclerosis* 1998;139:205–222.
37. Kovanen PT, Pentikainen MO. Decorin links low-density lipoproteins (LDL) to collagen: A novel mechanism for retention of LDL in the atherosclerotic plaque. *Trends Cardiovasc Med* 1999;9:86–91.
38. Shah PK, Yano J, Reyes O, et al. High-dose recombinant apolipoprotein A-I(milano) mobilizes tissue cholesterol and rapidly reduces plaque lipid and macrophage content in apolipoprotein e-deficient mice. Potential implications for acute plaque stabilization. *Circulation* 2001;103:3047–3050.
39. Shah PK, Kaul S, Nilsson J, Cercek B. Exploiting the vascular protective effects of high-density lipoprotein and its apolipoproteins: An idea whose time for testing is coming, part I and II. *Circulation.* 2001;104:2376–2383 and 2498–2502.
40. Nakashima Y, Raines EW, Plump AS, et al. Upregulation of VCAM-1 and ICAM-1 at atherosclerosis-prone sites on the endothelium in the apoE-deficient mouse. *Arterioscler Thromb Vasc Biol* 1998;18: 842–851.
41. Patel SS, Thiagarajan R, Willerson JT, Yeh ET. Inhibition of alpha$_4$ integrin and ICAM-1 markedly attenuate macrophage homing to atherosclerotic plaques in ApoE-deficient mice. *Circulation* 1998;97: 75–81.
42. Zhou X, Hansson GK. Detection of B cells and proinflammatory cytokines in atherosclerotic plaques of hypercholesterolaemic apolipoprotein E knockout mice. *Scand J Immunol* 1999;50:25–30.
43. Malek AM, Alper SL, Izumo S. Hemodynamic shear stress and its role in atherosclerosis. *JAMA* 1999;282:2035–2042.
44. Nakashima Y, Plump AS, Raines EW, et al. ApoE-deficient mice develop lesions of all phases of atherosclerosis throughout the arterial tree. *Arterioscler Thromb* 1994:14:133–140.
45. Reckless J, Rubin EM, Verstuyft JB, et al. Monocyte chemoattractant protein-1 but not tumor necrosis factor-alpha is correlated with monocyte infiltration in mouse lipid lesions. *Circulation* 1999;99:2310–2316.
46. Reape TJ, Groot PHE. Chemokines and atherosclerosis. *Atherosclerosis* 1999;147:213–225.
47. Rollins BJ. Chemokines (review). *Blood* 1997:90:909–928.
48. Aiello RJ, Bourassa PA, Lindsey S, et al. Monocyte chemoattractant protein-1 accelerates atherosclerosis in apolipoprotein E–deficient mice. *Arterioscler Thromb Vasc Biol* 1999;19:1518–1525.
49. Gu L, Okada Y, Clinton SK, et al. Absence of monocyte chemoattractant protein-1 reduces atherosclerosis in low density lipoprotein receptor–deficient mice. *Mol Cell* 1998;2:275–281.
50. Gosling J, Slaymaker S, Gu L, Tseng S, et al. MCP-1 deficiency reduces susceptibility to atherosclerosis in mice that overexpress human apolipoprotein B. *J Clin Invest* 1999;103:773–778.
51. Lu B, Rutledge BJ, Gu L, et al. Abnormalities in monocyte recruitment and cytokine expression in monocyte chemoattractant protein 1–deficient mice. *J Exp Med* 1998;187:601–608.
52. Schecter AD, Rollins BJ, Zhang YJ, et al. Tissue factor is induced by monocyte chemoattractant protein-1 in human aortic smooth muscle and THP-1 cells. *J Biol Chem* 1997;272:28,568–528,573.
53. Boring L, Gosling J, Cleary M, Charo IF. Decreased lesion formation in CCR2$^{-/-}$ mice reveals a role for chemokines in the initiation of atherosclerosis. *Nature* 1998;394:894–897.
54. Cyrus T, Witztum JL, Rader DJ, et al. Disruption of the 12/15-lipoxygenase gene diminishes atherosclerosis in apo E–deficient mice. *J Clin Invest* 1999;103:1597–1604.
55. Zhou X, Paulsson G, Stemme S, Hansson GK. Hypercholesterolemia is associated with a T helper (Th) l/Th2 switch of the autoimmune response in atherosclerotic apo E-knockout mice. *J Clin Invest* 1998;101:1717–1725.
56. Gupta S, Pablo AM, Jiang XC, et al. IFN-gamma potentiates atherosclerosis in ApoE knockout mice. *J Clin Invest* 1997;99: 2752–2761.

57. Caligiuri G. *The Immune Response in Atherosclerosis and Acute Coronary Syndromes*. Thesis. Stockholm; Karolinska Institute; 1999.
58. Daugherty A, Pure E, Delfel-Butteiger D, et al. The effects of total lymphocyte deficiency on the extent of atherosclerosis in apolipoprotein $E^{-/-}$ mice. *J Clin Invest* 1997;100:1575–1580.
59. Dansky HM, Charlton SA, Harper MM, Smith JD. T and B lymphocytes play a minor role in atherosclerotic plaque formation in the apolipoprotein E–deficient mouse. *Proc Natl Acad Sci USA* 1997;94: 4642–4646.
60. Mach F, Schonbeck U, Bonnefoy JY, et al. Activation of monocyte/macrophage functions related to acute atheroma complication by ligation of CD40: Induction of collagenase, stromelysin, and tissue factor. *Circulation* 1997;96:396–399.
61. Mach F, Schonbeck U, Sukhova GK, et al. Reduction of atherosclerosis in mice by inhibition of CD40 signalling. *Nature* 1998;394: 200–203.
62. Lutgens E, Gorelik L, Daemen MJ, et al. Requirement for CD154 in the progression of atherosclerosis. *Nat Med* 1999;5:1313–1316.
63. Wick G, Schett G, Amberger A, et al. Is atherosclerosis an immunologically mediated disease? *Immunol Today* 1995;16:27–33.
64. Xu Q, Kiechl S, Mayr M, et al. Association of serum antibodies to heat-shock protein 65 with carotid atherosclerosis: Clinical significance determined in a follow-up study. *Circulation* 1999;100: 1169–1174.
65. Mayr M, Metzler B, Kiechl S, et al. Endothelial cytotoxicity mediated by serum antibodies to heat shock proteins of *Escherichia coli* and *Chlamydia pneumoniae:* Immune reactions to heat shock proteins as a possible link between infection and atherosclerosis. *Circulation* 1999;99:1560–1566.
66. George J, Harats D, Gilburd B, et al. Immunolocalization of $beta_2$-glycoprotein I (apolipoprotein H) to human atherosclerotic plaques: Potential implications for lesion progression. *Circulation* 1999;99: 2227–2230.
67. Ross R. Atherosclerosis: An inflammatory disease. *N Engl J Med* 1999;340:115–126.
68. Hu H, Pierce GN, Zhong G. The atherogenic effects of chlamydia are dependent on serum cholesterol and specific to *Chlamydia pneumoniae*. *J Clin Invest* 1999;103:747–753.
69. Moazed TC, Campbell LA, Rosenfeld ME, et al. *Chlamydia pneumoniae* infection accelerates the progression of atherosclerosis in apolipoprotein E–deficient mice. *J Infect Dis* 1999;180:238–241.
70. Fabricant CG, Fabricant J, Litrenta MM, et al. Virus-induced atherosclerosis. *J Exp Med* 1978;l48:335–340.
71. Fabricant C, Fabricant J, Minick CR, et al. Herpes virus induced atherosclerosis in chickens. *Fed Proc* 1983;42:2476–2479.
72. Ross R. The biology of atherosclerosis. In: Topol EJ, ed. *Comprehensive Cardiovascular Medicine*. Philadelphia: Lippincott-Raven; 1998:13.
73. Murayama T, Yokode M, Kataoka H, et al. Intraperitoneal administration of anti–c-fms monoclonal antibody prevents initial events of atherogenesis but does not reduce the size of advanced lesions in apolipoprotein E–deficient mice. *Circulation* 1999;99: 1740–1746.
74. Hasty AH, Linton MF, Brandt SJ, et al. Retroviral gene therapy in ApoE-deficient mice: ApoE expression in the artery wall reduces early foam cell lesion formation. *Circulation* 1999;99:2571–2576.
75. Xiao Q, Danton MJ, Witte DP, et al. Fibrinogen deficiency is compatible with the development of atherosclerosis in mice. *J Clin Invest* 1998;101:1184–1194.
76. Tangirala RK, Tsukamoto K, Chun SH, et al. Regression of atherosclerosis induced by liver-directed gene transfer of apolipoprotein A-I in mice. *Circulation* 1999;100:1816–1822.
77. Tse J, Martin-McNaulty B, Halks-Miller M, et al. Accelerated atherosclerosis and premature calcified cartilaginous metaplasia in the aorta of diabetic male Apo E knockout mice can be prevented by chronic treatment with 17 beta-estradiol. *Atherosclerosis* 1999;144: 303–313.
78. Qiao JH, Xie PZ, Fishbein MC, et al. Pathology of atheromatous lesions in inbred and genetically engineered mice: Genetic determination of arterial calcification. *Arterioscler Thromb* 1994;14: 1480–1497.
79. Towler DA, Bidder M, Latifi T, et al. Diet-induced diabetes activates an osteogenic gene regulatory program in the aortas of low density lipoprotein receptor–deficient mice. *J Biol Chem* 1998;273: 30,427–30,434.
80. Abela GS, Picon PD, Friedl SE, et al. Triggering of plaque disruption and arterial thrombosis in an atherosclerotic rabbit model. *Circulation* 1995;91:776–784.
81. Rekhter MD, Hicks GW, Brammer DW, et al. Animal model that mimics atherosclerotic plaque rupture. *Circ Res* 1998;83:705–713.
82. Rosenfeld ME, Polinsky P, Virmani R, et al. Advanced atherosclerotic lesions in the innominate artery of the ApoE knockout mouse. *Arterioscler Thromb Vasc Biol* 2000;20:2587–2592.
83. Johnson JL, Jackson CL. Atherosclerotic plaque rupture in the apolipoprotein E knockout mouse. *Atherosclerosis* 2001;154:399–406.
84. Zhou J, Moller J, Danielsen CC, et al. Dietary supplementation with methionine and homocysteine promotes early atherosclerosis but not plaque rupture in ApoE-deflcient mice. *Arterioscler Thromb Vasc Biol* 2001;21:1470–1476.
85. Calara F, Silvestre M, Casanada F, et al. Spontaneous plaque rupture and secondary thrombosis in apolipoprotein E-deficient and LDL receptor-deficient mice. *J Pathol* 2001;195:257–263.
86. Williams H, Johnson JL, Carson KG, Jackson CL. Characteristics of intact and ruptured atherosclerotic plaques in brachiocephalic arteries of apolipoprotein E knockout mice. *Arterioscler Thromb Vasc Biol* 2002;22:788–792.
87. von der Thüsen JH, van Vlijmen BJ, Hoeben RC, et al. Induction of atherosclerotic plaque rupture in apolipoprotein E-/- mice after adenovirus-mediated transfer of p53. *Circulation* 2002;105: 2064–2070.
88. Napoli C, Palinski W, Unraveling the mechanisms of plaque rupture in murine models (letters). *Circulation* 2002;106:el86.
89. Stary HC, Blankenhorn DH, Chandler AB, et al. A definition of the intima of human arteries and of its atherosclerosis-prone regions: A report from the Committee on Vascular Lesions of the Council on Arteriosclerosis, American Heart Association. *Circulation* 1992;85: 391–405.
90. Stary HC, Chandler AB, Glagov S, et al. A definition of initial, fatty streak, and intermediate lesions of atherosclerosis: A report from the Committee on Vascular Lesions of the Council on Arteriosclerosis, American Heart Association. *Circulation* 1994;89:2462–2478.
91. Verma S, Anderson TJ. Fundamentals of endothelial function for the clinical cardiologist. *Circulation* 2002;105:546–549.
92. Biegelsen ES, Loscalzo J. Endothelial function and atherosclerosis. *Coron Artery Dis* 1999;10:241–256.
93. Reddy KG, Nair RN, Sheehan HM, Hodgson JM. Evidence that selective endothelial dysfunction may occur in the absence of angiographic or ultrasound atherosclerosis in patients with risk factors for atherosclerosis. *Am Coll Cardiol* 1994;23:833–843.
94. Weninger WJ, Muller GB, Reiter C, et al. Intimal hyperplasia of the infant parasellar carotid artery: A potential developmental factor in atherosclerosis and SIDS. *Circ Res* 1999;85:970–975.
95. Schwartz SM, De Blois D, O'Brien ER. The intima: Soil for atherosclerosis and restenosis. *Circ Res* 1995;77:445–465.
96. Chung IM, Schwartz SM, Murry CE. Clonal architecture of normal and atherosclerotic aorta: Implications for atherogenesis and vascular development. *Am J Pathol* 1998;152:913–923.
97. Ikari Y, McManus BM, Kenyon J, Schwartz SM. Neonatal intima formation in the human coronary artery. *Arterioscler Thromb Vasc Biol* 1999;19:2036–2040.
98. Napoli C, Glass CK, Witztum JL, et al. Influence of maternal hypercholesterolaemia during pregnancy on progression of early atherosclerotic lesions in childhood: Fate of Early Lesions in Children (FELIC) study. *Lancet* 1999;354:1234–1241.

99. Hansson GK. Immune responses in atherosclerosis. In: Hansson GK, Libby P, eds. *Immune Functions of the Vessel Wall*. Amsterdam: Harwood Academic; 1996.
100. Hansson GK, Libby P, Schonbeck U, Yan ZQ. Innate and adaptive immunity in the pathogenesis of atherosclerosis (review). *Circ Res* 2002;91:281–291.
101. Binder CJ, Chang MK, Shaw PX, et al. Innate and acquired immunity in atherogenesis (review). *Nat Med* 2002;8:1218–1226.
102. Getz GS. When is atherosclerosis not atherosclerosis? *Arterioscler Thromb Vasc Biol* 2000;20:1694.
103. McGill HC Jr. George Lyman Duff memorial lecture. Persistent problems in the pathogenesis of atherosclerosis. *Arteriosclerosis* 1984; 4:443–451.
104. McGill HC Jr, McMahan CA, Malcom GT, et al. Effects of serum lipoproteins and smoking on atherosclerosis in young men and women. The PDAY Research Group. Pathobiological Determinants of Atherosclerosis in Youth. *Arterioscler Thromb Vasc Biol* 1997;17: 95–106.
105. Guyton JR. Phospholipid hydrolytic enzymes in a "cesspool" of arterial intimal lipoproteins: A mechanism for atherogenic lipid accumulation (editorial). *Arterioscler Thromb Vasc Biol* 2001;21: 884–886.
106. Pasterkamp G, Virmani R. The erythrocyte: A new player in atheromatous core formation. *Heart* 2002;88:115–116.
107. Davies MJ, Woolf N. Atherosclerosis: What is it and why does it occur? *Br Heart J* 1993;69(suppl):S3–S11.
108. Burrig K-F. The endothelium of advanced arteriosclerotic plaques in humans. *Arterioscler Thromb* 1991;11:1678–1689.
109. Ruggeri ZM. Platelets in atherothrombosis. *Nat Med* 2002;8: 1227–1234.
110. Falk E, Fernández-Ortiz A. Role of thrombosis in atherosclerosis and its complications. *Am J Cardiol* 1995;75:5B–11B.
111. Doherty TM, Shah PK, Rajavashisth TB. Cellular origins of atherosclerosis: Towards ontogenetic endgame? *FASEB J* 2003;17:592–597.
112. Blankenhorn DH. Coronary arterial calcification: A review. *Am J Med Sci* 1961;242:41–49.
113. Wexler L, Brundage B, Crouse J, et al. Coronary artery calcification: Pathophysiology, epidemiology, imaging methods, and clinical implications. A statement for health professionals from the American Heart Association. Writing Group. *Circulation* 1996;94:1175–1192.
114. Tintut Y, Demer LL. Recent advances in multifactorial regulation of vascular calcification (review). *Curr Opin Lipidol* 2001;12:555–560.
115. Lachman AS, Spray TL, Kerwin DM, et al. Medial calcinosis of Monckeberg. A review of the problem and a description of a patient with involvement of peripheral, visceral and coronary arteries. *Am J Med* 1977;63:615–622.
116. Sangiorgi G, Rumberger JA, Severson A, et al. Arterial calcification and not lumen stenosis is highly correlated with atherosclerotic plaque burden in humans: A histologic study of 723 coronary artery segments using nondecalcifying methodology. *J Am Coll Cardiol* 1998;31:126–133.
117. Mintz GS, Pichard AD, Popma JJ, et al. Determinants and correlates of target lesion calcium in coronary artery disease: A clinical, angiographic and intravascular ultrasound study. *J Am Coll Cardiol* 1997; 29:268–274.
118. Baumgart D, Schmermund A, Goerge G, et al. Comparison of electron beam computed tomography with intracoronary ultrasound and coronary angiography for detection of coronary atherosclerosis. *J Am Coll Cardiol* 1997;30:57–64.
119. Beckman JA, Ganz J, Creager MA, et al. Relationship of clinical presentation and calcification of culprit coronary artery stenoses. *Arterioscler Thromb Vasc Biol* 2001;21:1618–1622.
120. Keelan PC, Bielak LF, Ashai K, et al. Long-term prognostic value of coronary calcification detected by electron-beam computed tomography in patients undergoing coronary angiography. *Circulation* 2001; 104;412–417.
121. Gibbons GH, Dzau VJ. The emerging concept of vascular remodeling. *N Engl J Med* 1994;330:1431–1438.
122. Mintz GS, Kent KM, Pichard AD, et al. Contribution of inadequate arterial remodeling to the development of focal coronary artery stenoses. An intravascular ultrasound study. *Circulation* 1997;95:1791–1798.
123. Pasterkamp G, Schoneveld AH, van der Wal AC, et al. Relation of arterial geometry to luminal narrowing and histologic markers for plaque vulnerability: The remodeling paradox. *J Am Coll Cardiol* 1998;32:655–662.
124. Varnava AM, Mills PG, Davies MJ. Relationship between coronary artery remodeling and plaque vulnerability. *Circulation* 2002;105: 939–943.
125. Rioufol G, Finet G, Ginon I, et al. Multiple atherosclerotic plaque rupture in acute coronary syndrome: A three-vessel intravascular ultrasound study. *Circulation* 2002;106:804–808.
126. Schoenhagen P, Ziada KM, Kapadia SR, et al. Extent and direction of arterial remodeling in stable versus unstable coronary syndromes: An intravascular ultrasound study. *Circulation* 2000;101:598–603.
127. Smits PC, Pasterkamp G, Quarles van Ufford MA, et al. Coronary artery disease: Arterial remodelling and clinical presentation. *Heart* 1999;82:461–464.
128. European Carotid Surgery Trialists Collaborative Group. Risk of stroke in the distribution of an asymptomatic carotid artery. *Lancet* 1995;345:209–212.
129. O'Brien KD, McDonald TO, Chait A, et al. Neovascular expression of E-selectin, intercellular adhesion molecule-1, and vascular cell adhesion molecule-1 in human atherosclerosis and their relation to intimal leukocyte content. *Circulation* 1996;93:672–682.
130. Libby P. Current concepts of the pathogenesis of the acute coronary syndromes (review). *Circulation* 2001;104:365–372.
131. Davies MJ, Richardson PD, Woolf N, et al. Risk of thrombosis in human atherosclerotic plaques: Role of extracellular lipid, macrophage, and smooth muscle cell content. *Br Heart J* 1993;69: 377–381.
132. Ball RY, Stowers EC, Burton JH, et al. Evidence that the death of macrophage foam cells contributes to the lipid core of atheroma. *Atherosclerosis* 1995;114:45–54.
133. Björkerud S, Björkerud B, Apoptosis is abundant in human atherosclerotic lesions, especially in inflammatory cells (macrophages and T cells), and may contribute to the accumulation of gruel and plaque instability. *Am J Pathol* 1996;149:367–380.
134. Mach F, Schonbeck U, Bonnefoy JY, et al. Activation of monocyte/ macrophage functions related to acute atheroma complication by ligation of CD40: Induction of collagenase, stromelysin, and tissue factor. *Circulation* 1997;96:396–399.
135. Moreno PR, Falk E, Palacios IF, et al. Macrophage infiltration in acute coronary syndromes: Implications for plaque rupture. *Circulation* 1994;90:775–778.
136. Shah PK, Galis ZS. Matrix metalloproteinase hypothesis of plaque rupture: Players keep piling up but questions remain. *Circulation* 2001;104:1878–1880.
137. Parks WC. Who are the proteolytic culprits in vascular disease? *J Clin Invest* 1999;104:1167–1168.
138. Kaartinen M, van der Wal AC, van der Loos CM, et al. Mast cell infiltration in acute coronary syndromes: Implications for plaque rupture. *J Am Coll Cardiol* 1998;32:606–612.
139. Sugiyama S, Okada Y, Sukhova GK, et al. Macrophage myeloperoxidase regulation by granulocyte macrophage colony-stimulating factor in human atherosclerosis and implications in acute coronary syndromes. *Am J Pathol* 2001;158:879–891.
140. Naruko T, Ueda M, Haze K, et al. Neutrophil infiltration of culprit lesions in acute coronary syndromes. *Circulation* 2002;106: 2894–2900.
141. Lemaitre V, O'Byrne TK, Borczuk AC, et al. ApoE knockout mice expressing human matrix metalloproteinase-1 in macrophages have less advanced atherosclerosis. *J Clin Invest* 2001;107:1227–1234.
142. O'Connor S, Taylor C, Campbell LA, et al. Potential infectious etiologies of atherosclerosis: A multifactorial perspective (review). *Emerg Infect Dis* 2001;7:780–788.

143. Epstein SE. The multiple mechanisms by which infection may contribute to atherosclerosis development and course. *Circ Res* 2002; 90:2–4.
144. Ngeh J, Anand V, Gupta S. Chlamydia pneumoniae and atherosclerosis—What we know and what we don't (review). *Clin Microbiol Infect* 2002;8:2–13.
145. Kol A, Sukhova GK, Lichtman AH, Libby P. Chlamydial heat shock protein 60 localizes in human atheroma and regulates macrophage tumor necrosis factor-$\alpha$ and matrix metalloproteinase expression. *Circulation* 1998;98:300–307.
146. Cercek B, Shah PK, Noc M, et al. Effect of short-term treatment with azithromycin on recurrent ischaemic events in patients with acute coronary syndrome in the Azithromycin in Acute Coronary Syndrome (AZACS) trial: A randomised controlled trial. *Lancet* 2003;361: 809–813.
147. Neumann FJ. Chlamydia pneumoniae-atherosclerosis link: A sound concept in search for clinical relevance (editorial). *Circulation* 2002; 106:2414–2416.
148. Naghavi M, Barlas Z, Siadaty S, et al. Association of influenza vaccination and reduced risk of recurrent myocardial infarction. *Circulation* 2000;102:3039–3045.
149. Gurfinkel EP, de la Fuente RL, Mendiz O, Mautner B. Influenza vaccine pilot study in acute coronary syndromes and planned percutaneous coronary interventions: The FLU Vaccination Acute Coronary Syndromes (FLUVACS) Study. *Circulation* 2002;105: 2143–2147.
150. Burke AP, Farb A, Malcom GT, Liang Y, et al. Plaque rupture and sudden death related to exertion in men with coronary artery disease. *JAMA* 1999;281:921–926.
151. Falk E. Plaque rupture with severe pre-existing stenosis precipitating coronary thrombosis. Characteristics of coronary atherosclerotic plaques underlying fatal occlusive thrombi. *Br Heart J* 1983;50: 127–134.
152. Falk E, Plaque rupture underlies 76% of coronary thrombi. *Clin Cardiol.* In press.
153. Fernandez-Ortiz A, Babimon JJ, Falk E, et al. Characterization of the relative thrombogenicity of atherosclerotic plaque components: Implications for consequences of plaque rupture. *J Am Coll Cardiol* 1994;23:1562–1569.
154. Toschi V, Gallo R, Lettino M, et al. Tissue factor modulates the thrombogenicity of human atherosclerotic plaques. *Circulation* 1997; 95:594–599.
155. Badimon JJ, Lettino M, Toschi V, et al. Local inhibition of tissue factor reduces the thrombogenicity of disrupted human atherosclerotic plaques: Effects of tissue factor pathway inhibitor on plaque thrombogenicity under flow conditions. *Circulation* 1999;99: 1780–1787.
156. Mallat Z, Hugel B, Ohan J, et al. Shed membrane microparticles with procoagulant potential in human atherosclerotic plaques: A role for apoptosis in plaque thrombogenicity. *Circulation* 1999;99:348–353.
157. Ardissino D, Merlini PA, Ariens R, et al. Tissue-factor antigen and activity in human coronary atherosclerotic plaques. *Lancet* 1997; 349:769–771.
158. Falk E. Coronary thrombosis: Pathogenesis and clinical manifestations (review). *Am J Cardiol* 1991;68:28B–35B.
159. American Heart Association. *2002 Heart and Stroke Statistical Update.* Dallas: American Heart Association; 2001;12.
160. Mann J, Davies MJ. Mechanisms of progression in native coronary artery disease: Role of healed plaque disruption. *Heart* 1999;82: 265–268.
161. Burke AP, Kolodgie FD, Farb A, et al. Healed plaque ruptures and sudden coronary death: Evidence that subclinical rupture has a role in plaque progression. *Circulation* 2001;103:934–940.
162. Davies MJ, Bland JM, Hangartner JRW, et al. Factors influencing the presence or absence of acute coronary artery thrombi in sudden ischaemic death. *Eur Heart J* 1989;10:203–208.
163. Frink RJ. Chronic ulcerated plaques: New insights into the pathogenesis of acute coronary disease. *J Invasive Cardiol* 1994;6:173–185.
164. Bogaty P, Hackett D, Davies G, Maseri A. Vasoreactivity of the culprit lesion in unstable angina. *Circulation* 1994;90:5–11.
165. Zeiher AM, Goebel H, Schachinger V, Ihling C. Tissue endothelin-1 immunoreactivity in the active coronary atherosclerotic plaque: A clue to the mechanism of increased vasoreactivity of the culprit lesion in unstable angina. *Circulation* 1995;91:941–947.
166. Schonbeck U, Mach F, Sukhova GK, et al. CD40 ligation induces tissue factor expression in human vascular smooth muscle cells. *Am J Pathol* 2000;156:7–14.
167. Shah PK. Pathophysiology of coronary thrombosis: Role of plaque rupture and plaque erosion (review). *Prog Cardiovasc Dis* 2002;44: 357–368.
168. Rauch U, Nemerson Y. Circulating tissue factor and thrombosis. *Curr Opin Hematol* 2000;7:273–277.
169. Mallat Z, Benamer H, Hugel B, et al. Elevated levels of shed membrane microparticles with procoagulant potential in the peripheral circulating blood of patients with acute coronary syndromes. *Circulation* 2000;101:841–843.
170. Topol EJ, Yadav JS. Recognition of the importance of embolization in atherosclerotic vascular disease (review). *Circulation* 2000;101: 570–580.
171. Falk E. Multiple culprits in acute coronary syndromes: Systemic disease calling for systemic treatment (review). *Ital Heart J* 2000;1: 835–838.
172. Goldstein JA. Angiographic plaque complexity: The tip of the unstable plaque iceberg (editorial). *J Am Coll Cardiol* 2002;39:1464–1467.
173. Schoenhagen P, Tuzcu EM, Ellis SG, Plaque vulnerability, plaque rupture, and acute coronary syndromes: (Multi)-focal manifestation of a systemic disease process (editorial). *Circulation* 2002;106: 760–762.
174. Asakura M, Ueda Y, Yamaguchi O, et al. Extensive development of vulnerable plaques as a pan-coronary process in patients with myocardial infarction: An angioscopic study. *J Am Coll Cardiol* 2001; 37:1284–1288.
175. Falk E, Fuster V. Angina pectoris and disease progression (editorial). *Circulation* 1995;92:2033–2035.
176. Ambrose JA, Winters SL, Stern A, et al. Angiographic morphology and the pathogenesis of unstable angina pectoris. *J Am Coll Cardiol* 1985; 5:609–616.
177. Chen L, Chester MR, Redwood S, et al. Angiographic stenosis progression and coronary events in patients with "stabilized" unstable angina. *Circulation* 1995;91:2319–2324.
178. Kaski JC, Chester MR, Chen L, Katritsis D. Rapid angiographic progression of coronary artery disease in patients with angina pectoris. The role of complex stenosis morphology. *Circulation* 1995;92: 2058–2065.
179. Garcia-Moll X, Coccolo F, Cole D, Kaski JC. Serum neopterin and complex stenosis morphology in patients with unstable angina. *J Am Coll Cardiol* 2000;35:956–962.
180. Buffon A, Biasucci LM, Liuzzo G, et al. Widespread coronary inflammation in unstable angina. *N Engl J Med* 2002;347:5–12.
181. Guazzi MD, Bussotti M, Grancini L, et al. Evidence of multifocal activity of coronary disease in patients with acute myocardial infarction. *Circulation* 1997;96:1145–1151.
182. Goldstein JA, Demetriou D, Grines CL, et al. Multiple complex coronary plaques in patients with acute myocardial infarction. *N Engl J Med* 2000;343:915–922.
183. Kerensky RA, Wade M, Deedwania P, et al. Revisiting the culprit lesion in non-Q-wave myocardial infarction. Results from the VANQWISH trial angiographic core laboratory. *J Am Coll Cardiol* 2002;39:1456–1463.
184. Boden WE, Kerensky RA, Bertolet BD, et al. Coronary angiographic findings after non-Q-wave myocardial infarction: An analysis from the VANQWISH trial (abstr). *Eur Heart J* 1997;18(suppl):123.
185. Ravn HB, Falk E. Histopathology of plaque rupture. *Cardiol Clin* 1999;17(2):263–270.
186. Chapman I. Morphogenesis of occluding coronary artery thrombosis. *Arch Pathol* 1965;80:256–261.

187. Constantinides P. Plaque fissures in human coronary thrombosis. *J Atheroscler Res* 1966;6:1–17.
188. Friedman M, van den Bovenkamp GJ. The pathogenesis of a coronary thrombus. *Am J Pathol* 1966;48:19–44.
189. Bouch DC, Montgomery GL. Cardiac lesions in fatal cases of recent myocardial ischaemia from a coronary care unit. *Br Heart J* 1970;32:795–803.
190. Sinapius D. Beziehungen zwischen Koronarthrombosen und Myokardinfarkten. *Dtsch Med Wochenschr* 1972;97:443–448.
191. Friedman M, Manwaring JH, Rosenman RH, et al. Instantaneous and sudden deaths. Clinical and pathological differentiation in coronary artery disease. *JAMA* 1973;225:1319–1328.
192. Horie T, Sekiguchi M, Hirosawa K. Coronary thrombosis in pathogenesis of acute myocardial infarction. Histopathological study of coronary arteries in 108 necropsied cases using serial section. *Br Heart J* 1978;40:153–161.
193. Tracy RE, Devaney K, Kissling G. Characteristics of the plaque under a coronary thrombus. *Virchows Arch A Pathol Anat Histopathol* 1985;405:411–427.
194. el Fawal MA, Berg GA, Wheatley DJ, Harland WA. Sudden coronary death in Glasgow: Nature and frequency of acute coronary lesions. *Br Heart J* 1987;57:329–335.
195. Yutani C, Ishibashi-Ueda H, Konishi M, et al. Histopathological study of acute myocardial infarction and pathoetiology of coronary thrombosis: A comparative study in four districts in Japan. *Jpn Circ J* 1987;51:352–361.
196. Davies MJ. The composition of coronary-artery plaques (editorial). *N Engl J Med* 1997;336:1312–1314.
197. Shi H, Wei L, Yang T, et al. Morphometric and histological study of coronary plaques in stable angina and acute myocardial infarctions. *Chin Med J* 1999;112:1040–1043.
198. Kojima S, Nonogi H, Miyao Y, et al. Is preinfarction angina related to the presence or absence of coronary plaque rupture? *Heart* 2000;83:64–68.

C H A P T E R 45

# CORONARY THROMBOSIS: LOCAL AND SYSTEMIC FACTORS

Lina Badimon / Valentin Fuster / Roberto Corti / Juan Jose Badimon



The formation of a thrombus within a coronary artery—with obstruction of coronary blood flow and reduction in oxygen supply to the myocardium—produces several types of the acute coronary syndrome (ACS). These thrombotic episodes largely occur in response to atherosclerotic lesions that have progressed to a high-risk inflammatory/prothrombotic stage. Although they are distinct from one another, the atherosclerotic and thrombotic processes appear to be closely interrelated, causing ACS through a complex, multifactorial process called atherothrombosis. ACS represents a spectrum of ischemic myocardial events that share similar pathophysiology; they include unstable angina, non-Q-wave myocardial infarction, Q-wave myocardial infarction, and sudden death.

Atherosclerosis is a systemic disease involving the intima of large- and medium-sized arteries—including the aorta, carotids, coronaries, and peripheral arteries—that is characterized by intimal thickening due to the accumulation of cells and lipids (Fig. 45-1, Plate 82).[1,2] Lipid accumulation results from an imbalance between mechanisms responsible for lipid influx and efflux.[3] Secondary changes may occur in the underlying media and adventitia, particularly in advanced disease stages. The early atherosclerotic lesions might progress without compromising the lumen due to compensatory vascular enlargement (remodeling).[4] Importantly, the culprit lesions leading to acute coronary syndromes are usually mildly stenotic and therefore barely detected by angiography (Fig. 45-2).[5] These high-risk rupture-prone lesions usually have a large lipid core, a thin fibrous cap, and a high density of inflammatory cells (particularly at the shoulder region, where disruptions most often occur). A reliable, noninvasive imaging tool able to detect early atherosclerotic disease and characterize lesion composition would be clinically advantageous. Indeed, it would improve our understanding of the pathophysiologic mechanisms of atherothrombosis and help to stratify patients for risk.[6]

Growing thrombi on atherosclerotic vessels may occlude the lumen locally or embolize and be washed away by the blood flow to occlude distal vessels. However, thrombi may be physiologically and spontaneously lysed by mechanisms that block thrombus propagation. Thrombus size, location, and composition are regulated by hemodynamic forces (mechanical effects), thrombogenicity of exposed substrate (local molecular effects), relative concentration of fluid phase and cellular blood components (local cellular effects), and the efficiency of the physiologic mechanisms of control of the system, mainly fibrinolysis.[7]

## CELLULAR AND MOLECULAR MECHANISMS IN THROMBUS FORMATION

Endothelial dysfunction as well as a breach of the endothelial integrity triggers a series of biochemical and molecular reactions aimed at preventing excessive blood loss and repairing the vessel wall. Vasoconstriction and platelet adhesion at the site of injury cooperate to form a hemostatic aggregate as the first step in vessel wall repair and the hemostasis. A few scattered platelets may interact with subtly injured dysfunctional endothelium and contribute, by the release of growth factors, to intimal hyperplasia.[8] In contrast, platelets—from one to several layers—may be deposited on the lesion with mild injury, and this may or may not evolve to become a mural thrombus. The release of platelet growth factors may contribute significantly to an accelerated intimal hyperplasia, as occurs in the coronary vein grafts within the first postoperative year. In severe injury, with exposure of components of deeper layers of the vessel, as in spontaneous plaque rupture or in angioplasty, marked platelet aggregation with mural thrombus formation follows. Vascular injury of this magnitude also stimulates thrombin formation through both the intrinsic (surface-activated) and extrinsic (tissue factor–dependent) coagulation pathways, in which the platelet membrane facilitates interactions between clotting factors (Fig. 45-3, Plate 83).

### Platelets

After plaque rupture, some of the atherosclerotic plaque components exhibit a potent activating effect on platelets and coagulation. Our understanding of the biochemical events involved in platelet activation

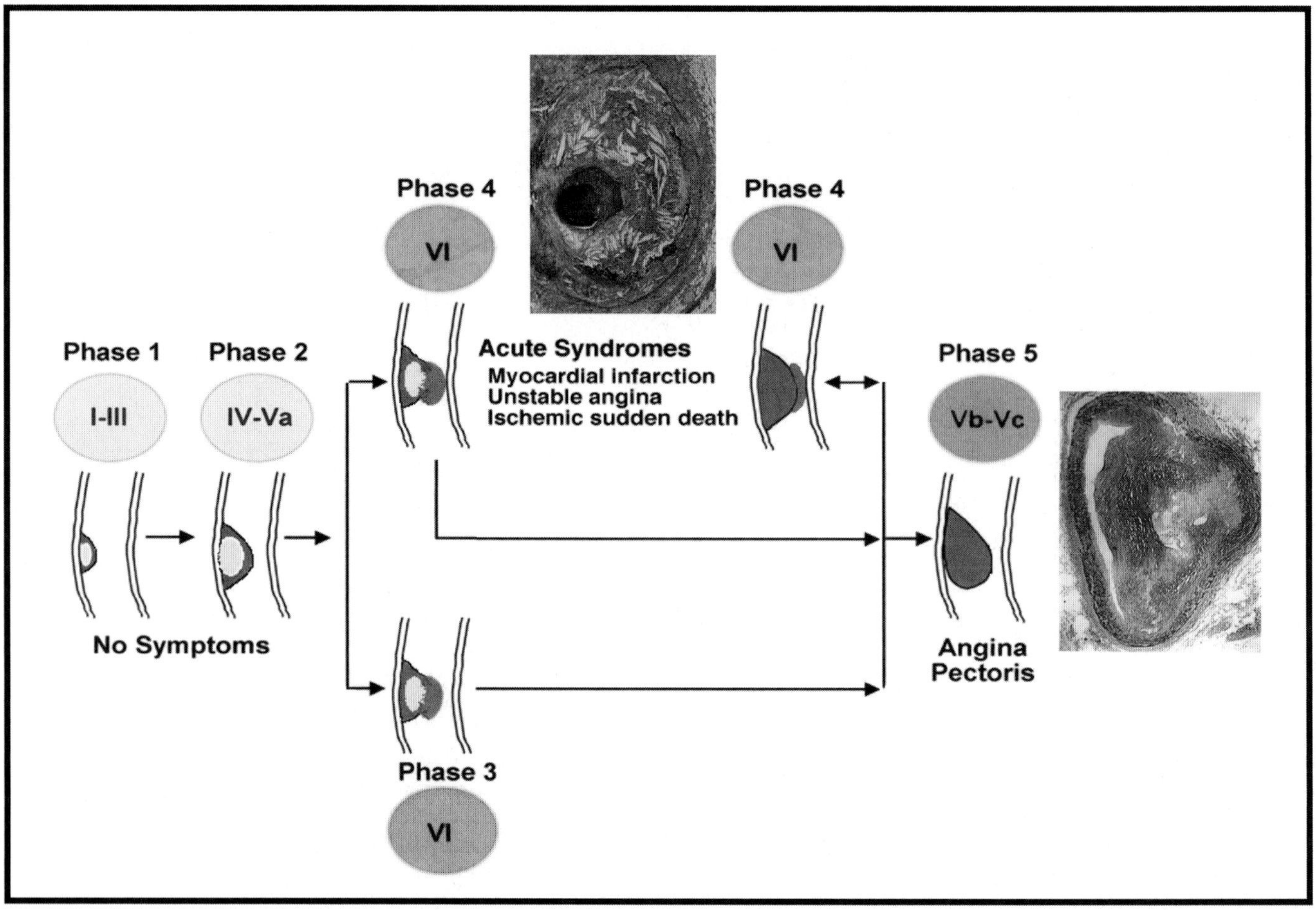

Phase 4
VI
Phase 4
VI
Phase 1
I-III
Phase 2
IV-Va
Acute Syndromes
Myocardial infarction
Unstable angina
Ischemic sudden death
Phase 5
Vb-Vc
No Symptoms
Angina
Pectoris
Phase 3
VI

FIGURE 45-1 (Plate 82) Simplified diagram of the evolution of coronary atherosclerosis. Phases and morphology of lesion progression.

Patients WITH ACS (%)
70
60
50
40
30
20
10
0
>70
50-70
<50
STENOSIS PRIOR TO ACS (%)
>70
50-70
<50

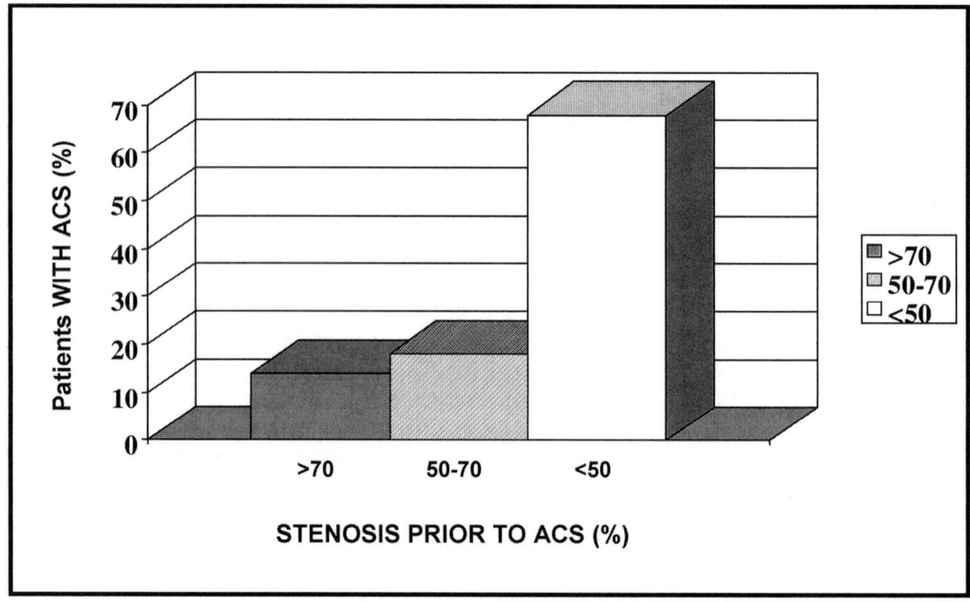

FIGURE 45-2 Relation of coronary stenosis severity (angiography) and presentation of acute coronary events from four studies with a total of 200 patients. (Modified from Falk E, Shah PK, Fuster V. Coronary plaque disruption. *Circulation* 1995;92:657–671.)

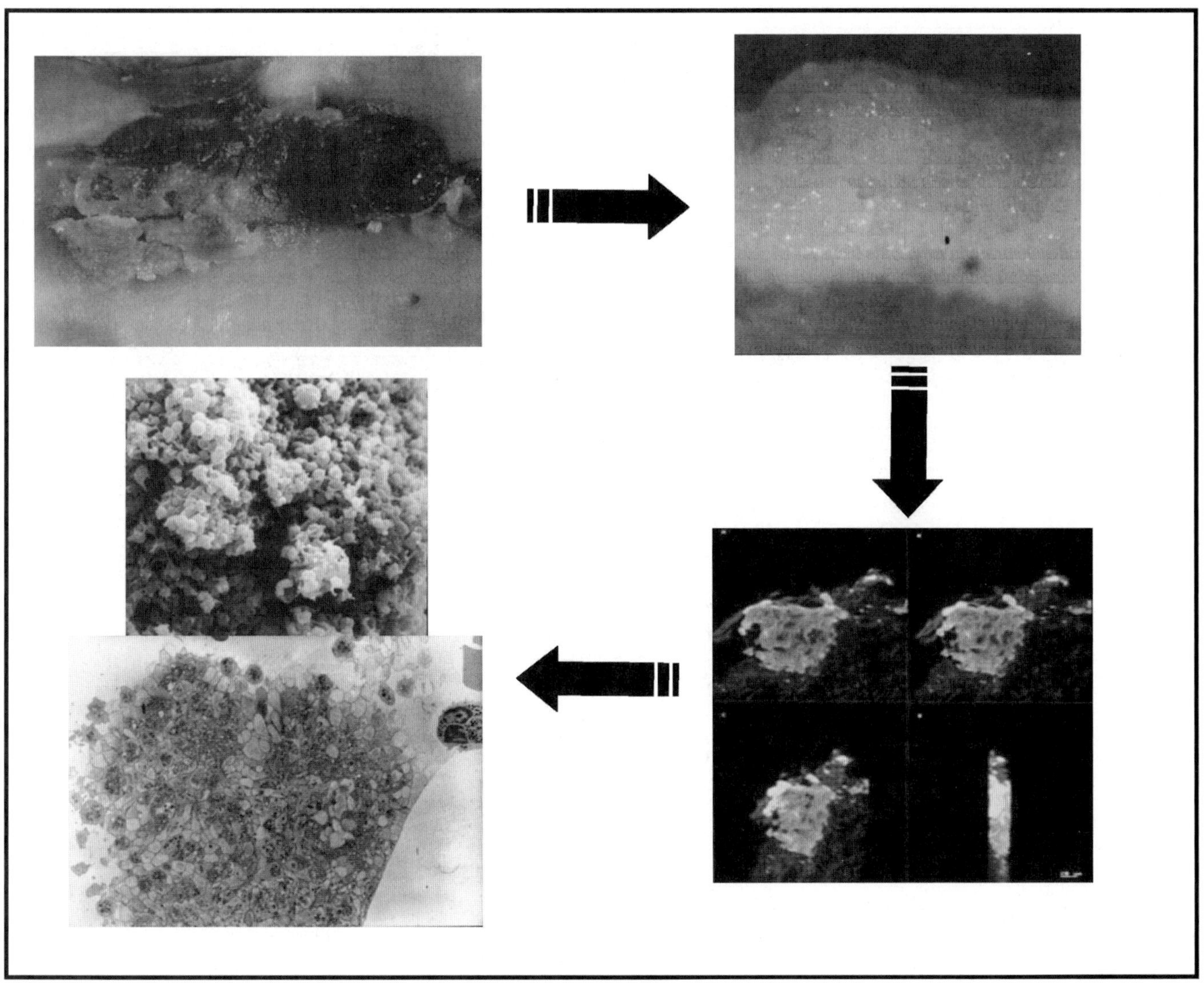

FIGURE 45-3 (Plate 83) Images of thrombosis. From naked eye observation to immunohistochemistry [green, platelets; red, fibrin(ogen)] and electronic microscopy (top, scanning; bottom, transmission).

has progressed significantly.[8–13] Exposed matrix from the vessel wall and thrombin generated by activation of the coagulation cascade, as well as epinephrine and adenosine diphosphate (ADP), are powerful platelet agonists. Each agonist stimulates the discharge of calcium and promotes the subsequent release of its granular content. Platelet-related ADP and 5-hydroxytryptamine (5-HT) stimulate adjacent platelets, further enhancing the process of platelet aggregation. Arachidonate, which is released from the platelet membrane by the stimulatory effect of collagen, thrombin, ADP, and 5-HT, promotes the synthesis of thromboxane $A_2$ by the sequential effects of cyclooxygenase and thromboxane synthetase. Thromboxane $A_2$ not only promotes further platelet aggregation but is also a potent vasoconstrictor[14] (Fig. 45-4). The initial recognition of damaged vessel wall by platelets involves (1) adhesion, activation, and adherence to recognition sites on the thromboactive substrate (extracellular matrix proteins such as von Willebrand factor, collagen, fibronectin, vitronectin, laminin); (2) spreading of the platelet on the surface; and (3) aggregation of platelets to form a platelet plug or white thrombus. The efficiency of platelet recruitment will depend on the underlying substrate and local geometry (local factors). A final step involving the recruitment of other blood cells also occurs; erythrocytes, neutrophils, and occasionally monocytes are found on evolving mixed thrombus.

Platelet function depends on adhesive interactions, and most of the glycoproteins on the platelet membrane surface are receptors for adhesive proteins. Many of these receptors have been identified, cloned, sequenced, and classified within large gene families that mediate a variety of cellular interactions[15,16] (Table 45-1). The most abundant is the integrin family, which includes, GP IIb/IIIa, GP Ic/IIa, the fibronectin receptor, and the vitronectin receptor, in decreasing order of magnitude. Another gene family present in the platelet membrane glycocalyx is the leucine-rich glycoprotein family represented by the GP Ib/IX complex, receptor for von Willebrand factor (vWF), on unstimulated platelets that mediates adhesion to subendothelium and GP V. Other gene families include the selectins (such as GMP-140) and the immunoglobulin domain protein [HLA

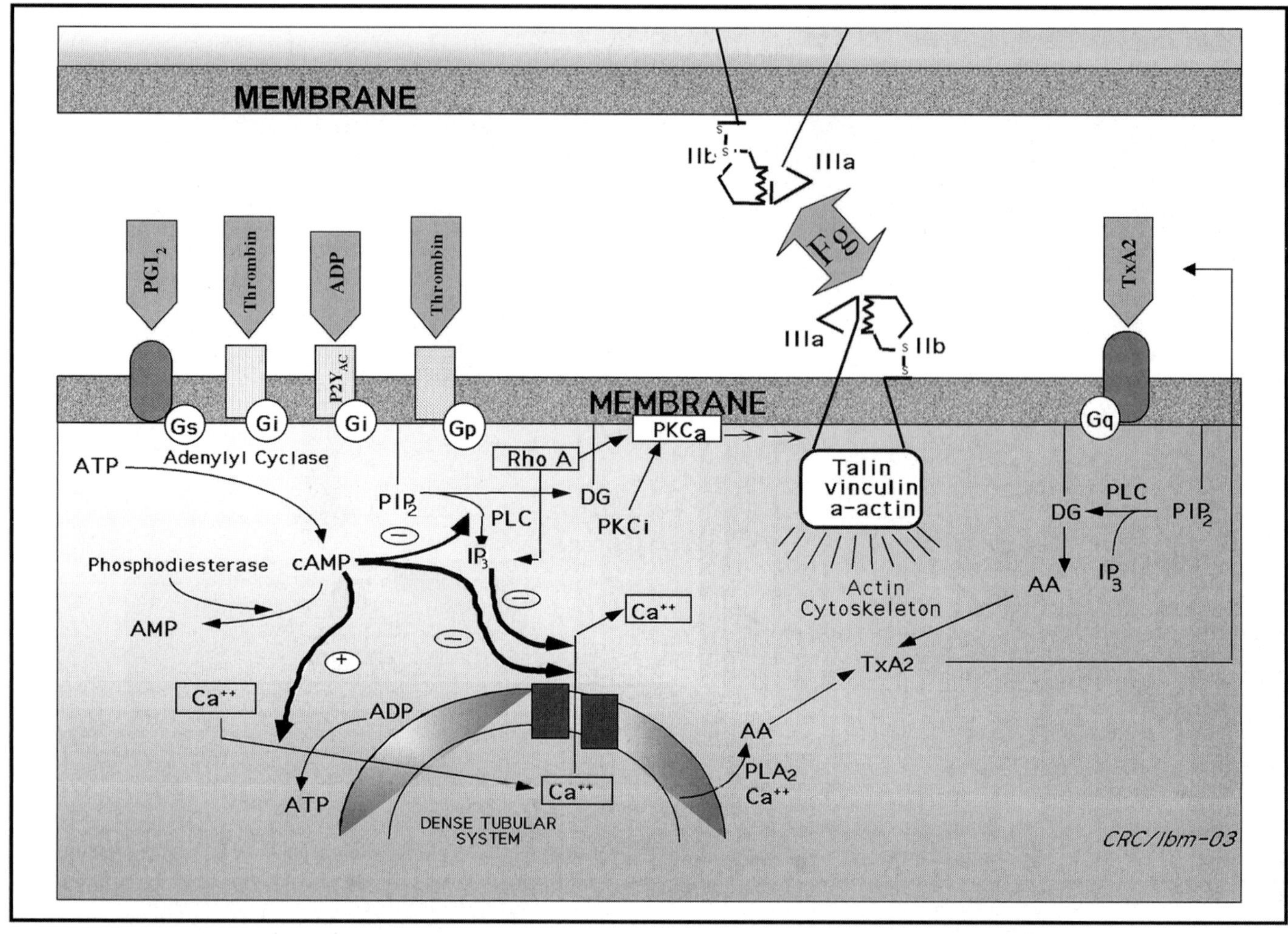


FIGURE 45-4 Signal transduction mechanisms of platelet activation and aggregation. $PGI_2$ = prostacyclin; $TxA_2$ = thromboxane $A_2$; $PIP_2$ = phosphoinositol diphosphate; PLC = phospholipase C; PKCi and PKCa = protein kinase C, inactivated and activated; DG = diacylglycerol; $IP_3$ = inositol 1,4,5-triphosphate; AA = arachidonic acid; $PLA_2$ = phospholipase $A_2$; Gs, Gi, Gp, Gq, guanine nucleotide-binding regulatory proteins; IIb/IIIa, receptor glycoprotein for adhesive protein ligands (mainly fibrinogen and vWF).

TABLE 45-1 Platelet Membrane Glycoprotein Receptors

| Glycoprotein Receptor | Function | Ligand |
|---|---|---|
| GP IIb/IIIa | Aggregation, adhesion at high shear rate | Fg, vWF, Fn, Ts, Vn |
| Receptor Vn | Adhesion | Vn, vWF, Fn, Fg, Ts |
| GP Ia/IIa | Adhesion | C |
| GP Ic/IIa | Adhesion | Fn |
| GP IcN/IIa | Adhesion | Ln |
| GP Ib/IX | Adhesion | vWF, T |
| GP V | Unknown | Substrate T |
| GP IV (GP IIIb) | Adhesion | Ts, C |
| GMP-140 (PADGEM) | Interaction with leukocytes | Unknown |
| PECAM-1 (GP IIa) | Unknown | Unknown |

ABBREVIATIONS: Fg = Fibrinogen; vW = von Willebrand factor; Fn = fibronectin; Ts = thrombospondin; Vn = vitronectin; C = collagen; Ln = laminin; T = thrombin; PECAM-1 = platelet/endothelial cell adhesion molecule 1.

class I antigen and platelet/endothelial cell adhesion molecule 1 (PECAM-1)]. Unrelated to any other gene family is the GP IV (IIIa)[15] (Table 45-1).

Randomly distributed on the surface of resting platelets are about 50,000 molecules of GP IIb/IIIa. The complex is composed of one molecule of GP IIb (disulfide-linked large and light chains) and one of GP IIIa (single polypeptide chain). It is a $Ca^{2+}$-dependent heterodimer, noncovalently associated on the platelet membrane.[17] Calcium is required for maintenance of the complex and for binding of adhesive proteins.[18,19] On activated platelets, the GP IIb/IIIa is a receptor for fibrinogen, fibronectin, vWF, vitronectin, and thrombospondin.[20] The receptor recognition sequences are localized to small peptide sequences [Arg/Gly/Asp (RGD)] in the adhesive proteins.[21] Fibrinogen contains two RGD sequences in its $\alpha$ chain, one near the N-terminus (residues 95 to 97) and a second near the C-terminus (residues 572 to 574).[22] Fibrinogen has a second site of recognition for GP IIb/IIIa: the 12–amino acid sequence located at the carboxyl terminus of the molecule's $\gamma$ chain.[23] This dodecapeptide is specific for fibrinogen and does not contain the RGD sequence but competes with RGD-containing peptides for binding to GP IIb/IIIa.[15,24,25]

The GP Ib/IX complex consists of two disulfide-linked subunits (GP Ib$\alpha$ and GP Ib$\beta$) tightly (not covalently) complexed with GP IX in a 1:1 heterodimer. GP Ib$\beta$ and GP IX are transmembrane glycoproteins and form the larger globular domain. The elongated, protruding part of the receptor corresponds to GP Ib$\alpha$. The major role of GP Ib/IX is to bind immobilized vWF on the exposed vascular subendothelium and initiate adhesion of platelets. GP Ib does not bind soluble vWF in plasma; apparently it undergoes a conformational change upon binding to the extracellular matrix and then exposes a recognition sequence for GP Ib/IX. The vWF-binding domain of GP Ib/IX has been narrowed to amino acids 251 to 279 on GP Ib$\alpha$.[26] The GPIb$\alpha$-binding domain of vWF resides in a tryptic fragment extending from residue 449 to 728 of the subunit that does not contain a RGD sequence.[27] The cytoplasmic domain of GP Ib/IX has a major function in linking the plasma membrane to the intracellular actin filaments of the cytoskeleton and functions to stabilize the membrane and to maintain the platelet shape.[28,29]

Thrombin plays an important role in the pathogenesis of arterial thrombosis. It is one of the most potent known agonists for platelet activation and recruitment. The thrombin receptor has 425 amino acids with seven transmembrane domains and a large $NH_2$-terminal extracellular extension that is cleaved by thrombin to produce a "tethered" ligand that activates the receptor to initiate signal transduction.[30,31] Thrombin is a critical enzyme in early thrombus formation, cleaving fibrinopeptides A and B from fibrinogen to yield insoluble fibrin, which effectively anchors the evolving thrombus. Both free and fibrin-bound thrombin are able to convert fibrinogen to fibrin, allowing propagation of thrombus at the site of injury.

Therefore platelet activation triggers intracellular signaling and expression of platelet membrane receptors for adhesion and initiation of cell contractile processes that induce shape change and secretion of the granular contents. The expression of the integrin IIb/IIa ($\alpha$IIb$\beta_3$) receptors for adhesive glycoprotein ligands (mainly fibrinogen and vWF) in the circulation initiates platelet-to-platelet interaction. The process is perpetuated by the arrival of platelets from the circulation. Most of the glycoproteins in the platelet membrane surface are receptors for adhesive proteins or mediate cellular interactions. Von Willebrand factor has been shown to bind to platelet membrane glycoproteins in both adhesion (platelet-substrate interaction) and aggregation (platelet-platelet interaction), leading to thrombus formation, as seen in perfusion studies conducted at high shear rates.[31–36] Ligand binding to the different membrane receptors triggers platelet activation with different relative potencies. Great interest in the platelet ADP receptors (P2Y, P2X) has recently been generated because of available pharmacologic inhibitors (see Chap. 54).

## Coagulation System

During plaque rupture, in addition to platelet deposition in the injured area, the clotting mechanism is activated by the exposure of the plaque contents. The activation of coagulation leads to the generation of thrombin, which is a powerful platelet agonist in addition to being an enzyme that catalyzes the formation and polymerization of fibrin. Fibrin is essential in the stabilization of the platelet thrombus and its ability to withstand removal forces by flow, shear, and high intravascular pressure. The efficacy of fibrinolytic agents pointedly demonstrates the importance of fibrin in thrombosis associated with myocardial infarction.

The blood coagulation system involves a sequence of reactions integrating zymogens (proteins susceptible to activation into enzymes via limited proteolysis) and cofactors (nonproteolytic enzyme activators) in three groups: (1) the contact activation (generation of factor XIa via the Hageman factor), (2) the conversion of factor X to factor Xa in a complex reaction requiring the participation of factors IX and VIII, and (3) the conversion of prothrombin to thrombin and fibrin formation[35] (Fig. 45-5).

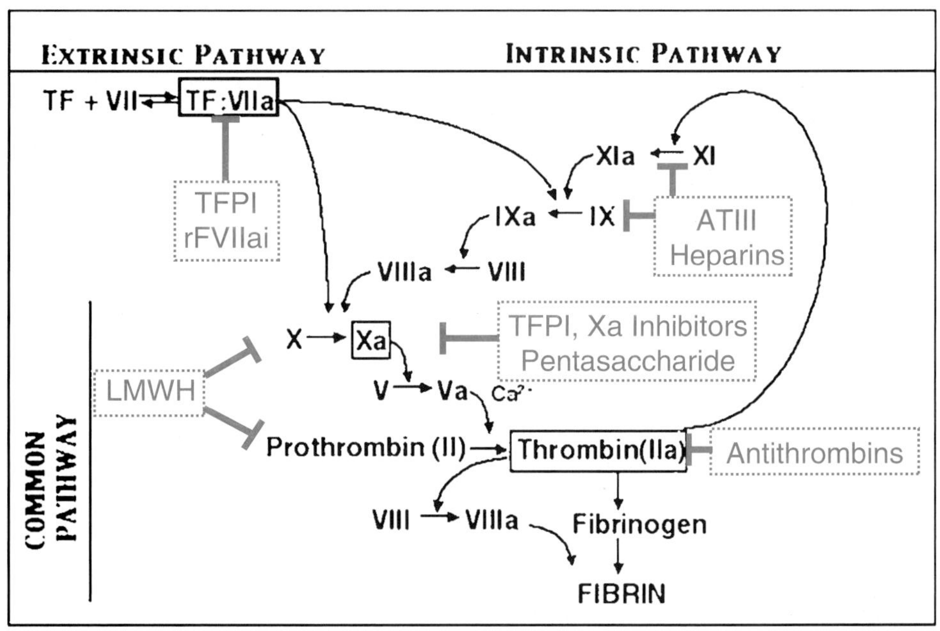


FIGURE 45-5 Simplified diagram of the coagulation cascade, with specific therapeutic targets for inhibitor drugs.

It has been suggested that glycosaminoglycans and sulfatides are the triggering surfaces for in vivo initiation of contact activation; however, the physiologic role of coagulation contact activation is unclear, since the absence of Hageman factor, prekallikrein, or high-molecular-weight kininogen does not induce a clinically apparent pathology. On the contrary, factor XI deficiency is associated with abnormal bleeding. Activated factor XI induces the activation of factor IX in the presence of $Ca^{2+}$. Factor IXa forms a catalytic complex with factor VIII on a membrane surface and efficiently activates factor X in the presence of $Ca^{2+}$. Factor IX is a vitamin K–dependent enzyme, as are factors VII and X, prothrombin, and protein C.

In citrated plasma, an anticoagulant is often used in studies of platelet–vessel wall interaction; these coagulation reactions do not proceed further than the activation of factor XI because of their dependence on $Ca^{2+}$. Platelets may provide the membrane requirements for the activation of factor X, although the participation of cells of the vessel wall (in exposed injured vessels) has not been excluded.[35] As such, endothelial cells in culture have been shown to support the activation of factor X.[36] Factor VIII forms a noncovalent complex with vWF in plasma, and its function in coagulation is the acceleration of the effects of IXa on the activation of X to Xa. Absence of factor VIII or IX produces the hemophilic syndromes[37] (Fig. 45-5).

The tissue factor (TF) pathway, previously known as the extrinsic coagulation pathway, through the TF–factor VIIa complex in the presence of $Ca^{2+}$, induces the formation of Xa. A second TF-dependent reaction catalyzes the transformation of IX into IXa. Tissue factor is an integral membrane protein that serves to initiate the activation of factors IX and X and to localize the reaction to cells on which TF is expressed. Other cofactors include factor VIIIa, which binds to platelets and forms the binding site for IXa, thereby forming the machinery for the activation of X; and factor Va, which binds to platelets and provides a binding site for Xa. The human genes for these cofactors have been cloned and sequenced. In physiologic conditions, no cells in contact with blood contain active TF, although cells such as monocytes and polymorphonuclear leukocytes can be induced to synthesize and express TF.[35]

Activated Xa converts prothrombin into thrombin. The complex that catalyzes the formation of thrombin consists of factors Xa and Va in a 1:1 complex. This activation results in the cleavage of fragment 1.2 and formation of thrombin from fragment 2. The interaction of the four components of the "prothrombinase complex" (Xa, Va, phospholipid, and $Ca^{2+}$) enhances the efficiency of the reaction.[38]

Activated platelets provide a procoagulant surface for the assembly and expression of both intrinsic Xase and prothrombinase enzymatic complexes.[39–41] These complexes respectively catalyze the activation of factor X to factor Xa and prothrombin to thrombin. The expression of activity is associated with the binding of both of the proteases, factor IXa and factor Xa, and the cofactors, VIIIa and Va, to procoagulant surfaces. The binding of IXa and Xa is promoted by VIIIa and Va, respectively, such that Va and likely VIIIa provide the equivalent of receptors for the proteolytic enzymes.[42,43] The surface of the platelet expresses the procoagulant phospholipids that bind coagulation factors and contribute to the procoagulant activity of the cell.[42]

Thrombin acts on multiple substrates, including fibrinogen, factor XIII, factors V and VIII, and protein C in addition to its effects on platelets. It plays a central role in hemostasis and thrombosis. The catalytic transformation of fibrinogen into fibrin is essential in the formation of the hemostatic plug and in the formation of arterial thrombi. Thrombin binds to the fibrinogen central domain and cleaves fibrinopeptides A and B, resulting in the formation of fibrin monomer and polymer formation.[44] The fibrin mesh holds the platelets together and contributes to the attachment of the thrombus to the vessel wall.

## Spontaneous Fibrinolysis

The control of the coagulation reactions occurs by diverse mechanisms, such as hemodilution and flow effects, proteolytic feedback by thrombin, inhibition by plasma proteins [such as antithrombin III (ATIII)] and endothelial cell–localized activation of an inhibitory enzyme (protein C), and fibrinolysis (Fig. 45-6). Although ATIII readily inactivates thrombin in solution, its catalytic site is inaccessible while bound to fibrin; it may still cleave fibrinopeptides even in the presence of heparin. Thrombin has a specific receptor in endothelial cell surfaces, thrombomodulin, which triggers a physiologic anticoagulation system.[45] The thrombin-thrombomodulin complex serves as a receptor for the vitamin K–dependent protein C, which is activated and released from the endothelial cell surface. In the presence of protein S, activated protein C inactivates factors Va and VIIIa and limits thrombin effects. Thrombin generated at the site of injury binds to thrombomodulin, an endothelial surface-membrane protein, initiating activation of protein C, which, in turn (in the presence of protein S), inactivates factors Va and VIIIa. Loss of Va decreases the role of throm-

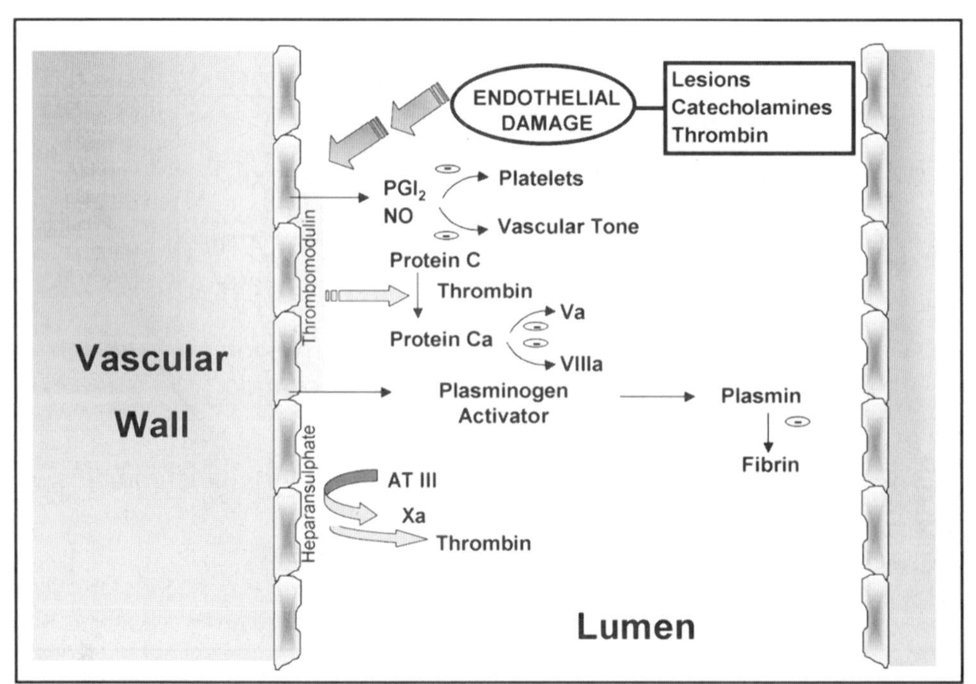


FIGURE 45-6 Simplified diagram of the physiologic anticoagulation system.

bin formation to negligible levels.[46] Thrombin stimulates successive release of both tissue plasminogen activator (t-PA) and plasminogen-activator inhibitor type 1 from endothelial cells, thus initiating endogenous lysis through plasmin generation from plasminogen by t-PA with subsequent modulation through plasminogen-activator inhibitor type 1. Thrombin therefore plays a pivotal role in maintaining the complex balance of initial prothrombotic reparative events and subsequent endogenous anticoagulant and fibrinolytic pathways.

Endogenous fibrinolysis, a repair mechanism, involves catalytic activation of zymogens, positive and negative feedback control, and inhibitor blockade[47,48] (Fig. 45-6). Blood clotting is blocked at the level of the prothrombinase complex by the physiologic anticoagulant-activated protein C and oral anticoagulants. Oral anticoagulants prevent posttranslational synthesis of $\gamma$-carboxyglutamic acid groups on the vitamin K–dependent clotting factors, preventing binding of prothrombin and Xa to the membrane surface. Activated protein C cleaves factor Va, rendering it functionally inactive.

## ROLE OF LOCAL FACTORS IN THE REGULATION OF CORONARY THROMBOSIS

The cellular and molecular mechanisms of platelet deposition and thrombus formation following vascular damage are modulated by the type of injury, the local geometry at the site damage (degree of stenosis) and local hemodynamic conditions.[49–52] Similarly, three major factors also determine the vulnerability of the fibrous cap: (1) circumferential wall stress, or cap "fatigue"; (2) lesion characteristics (location, size, and consistency); and (3) blood-flow characteristics.[3] A plaque is considered vulnerable when the lipid core accounts for more than 40 percent of the whole.

### Effects Derived from the Severity of Vessel Wall Damage

Exposure of de-endothelialized vessel wall, native fibrillar collagen type I bundles with a rough surface, or atherosclerotic plaque components at similar blood shear rate conditions leads to increasing degrees of platelet deposition.[49] Thromboplastin or tissue factor,[53,54] readily available in the atherosclerotic intimal space upon endothelial loss, contributes to the high thrombogenicity of atherosclerotic plaques. Overall, it is likely that when injury to the vessel wall is mild, the thrombogenic stimulus is relatively limited and the resulting thrombotic occlusion is transient, as occurs in unstable angina. On the other hand, deep vessel injury secondary to plaque rupture or ulceration results in exposure of collagen, tissue factor, and other elements of the vessel matrix, leading to relatively persistent thrombotic occlusion and myocardial infarction.[55]

It is likely that the nature of the substrate exposed after spontaneous or angioplasty-induced plaque rupture determines whether an unstable plaque proceeds rapidly to an occlusive thrombus or persists as nonocclusive mural thrombus. The analysis of the relative contribution of different components of human atherosclerotic plaques (fatty streaks, sclerotic plaques, fibrolipid plaques, atheromatous plaques, hyperplasic cellular plaque, and normal intima) to acute thrombus formation has shown that the atheromatous core is up to sixfold more active than the other substrates in triggering thrombosis.[56] The atheromatous core remained the most thrombogenic substrate when the various components were normalized by the degree of irregularity, as defined by the roughness index. Therefore ruptured plaques with a large atheromatous core are at high risk of leading to ACS.[56] The plaque TF content is directly related to its thrombogenicity.[57] As proof of concept, we showed that local tissue blockade of TF, by treatment with tissue factor pathway inhibitor (TFPI), significantly reduces thrombosis.[58] Recently the use of active site-inhibited recombinant FVIIa (FF-rFVIIa) has been shown to reduce thrombus growth on severely damaged vessels significantly.[59]

Monocytes/macrophages are key to the development of vulnerable plaques.[60,61] The vulnerable plaques (AHA type IV and Va), commonly composed of an abundant lipid core separated from the lumen by a thin fibrotic cap, are particularly soft and prone to disruption.[62] A high density of activated inflammatory cells has been detected in the disrupted areas of atherectomy specimens from patients with ACS.[63] These cells are capable of degrading extracellular matrix by secreting proteolytic enzymes, such as matrix metalloproteinases.[64] In addition, T cells isolated from rupture-prone sites can stimulate macrophages to produce metalloproteinases and may predispose to the disruption of lesions by weakening their fibrous caps.[65] Recently low-density lipoprotein (LDL) has been shown to downregulate the expression of lysil-oxidase (LOX) in vascular wall cells.[66] LOX is an enzyme that contributes to the maturation of the elastin and collagen fibrils of the extracellular matrix. Its decrease is associated with increased permeability of the vascular wall and hence may contribute to plaque destabilization. Recently, cell apoptosis and microparticles with procoagulant activity and postulated apoptotic origin have also been linked to inflammation and thrombosis.[67,68]

### Effects Derived From Geometry

Platelet deposition is directly related to the degree of stenosis in the presence of the same degree of injury, indicating a shear-induced platelet activation.[51,52] In addition, analysis of the axial distribution of platelet deposition indicates that the apex, and not the flow recirculation zone distal to the apex, is the segment of greatest platelet accumulation. These data suggest that the severity of the acute platelet response to plaque disruption depends in part on the sudden changes in geometry following rupture.[7] Interestingly, hemodynamic effects play a role in the regulation of the thrombotic response in different arteries. In the absence of atherosclerotic changes in the porcine normolipemic model, the dilatation of carotid and coronary arteries in the same animal produced significantly different levels of platelet deposition in the arterial beds, with the coronaries triggering a significantly greater deposition than the carotids.[69]

Spontaneous lysis of thrombus does occur, not only in unstable angina but also in acute myocardial infarction.[55] In these patients as well as in those undergoing thrombolysis for acute infarction, the presence of a residual mural thrombus predisposes to recurrent thrombotic vessel occlusion.[70–73] Two main contributing factors for the development of rethrombosis have been identified. First, because platelet deposition increases with increasing degrees of vessel stenosis, residual mural thrombus encroaching into the vessel lumen may result in an increased shear rate, which facilitates the activation and deposition of platelets on the lesion.[51,52] Second, a fragmented thrombus appears to present one of the most powerful thrombogenic surfaces. A gradual increase in platelet deposition in the area of maximal stenosis may be followed by an abrupt decrease in platelet deposition, probably due to spontaneous embolization of the thrombus or platelet deaggregation.[74] Such an episode can be immediately followed by a rapid increase in platelet deposition, suggesting that the remaining thrombus is markedly thrombogenic. In fact, platelet deposition is increased two to four times on residual thrombus compared with deeply injured arterial wall, and thrombus continues to grow during heparin therapy. However, it is inhibited by specific antithrombin treatment.[74]

A specific antithrombin such as r-hirudin (a recombinant molecule that blocks both the catalytic site and the anion-exosite of the thrombin molecule) (see Chap. 54) is capable of significantly inhibiting the secondary growth.[74] Thus, following lysis, thrombin becomes exposed to the circulating blood, leading to activation of the platelets, coagulation, and further thrombosis. The antithrombin activity of heparin is limited for three main reasons. First, a residual thrombus contains active thrombin bound to fibrin, which is thus poorly accessible to the large heparin–antithrombin III complexes; second, a platelet-rich arterial thrombus releases large amounts of platelet factor 4, which may inhibit heparin; third, fibrin II monomer, formed by the action of thrombin on fibrinogen, may also inhibit heparin. Conversely, molecules of hirudin and other specific antithrombins are at least ten times smaller than the heparin–antithrombin III complex, have no natural inhibitors, and therefore have greater access to thrombin bound to fibrin. These findings clarify the clinical observations in patients with acute myocardial infarction undergoing thrombolysis, which have shown that residual stenosis is in part related to residual nonlysed thrombus.[75] The effects of different antithrombotic treatment regimens on thrombus formation triggered by a residual mural thrombus have been evaluated, and specific thrombin inhibition has been shown to be the most effective method of slowing the progression of thrombus growth when compared to aspirin, heparin, or both.[76,77]

The fact that a clear predilection exists for lesion formation at arterial branch points strongly indicates the important influence of local hemodynamics and rheologic conditions on atherosclerosis. Furthermore, vascular-cell gene-expression profiles are also modulated by acute changes in flow profiles.[78]

## ROLE OF SYSTEMIC FACTORS IN THE REGULATION OF CORONARY THROMBOSIS

The severity of coronary thrombosis and associated ACS is modulated by the magnitude and/or stability of the formed thrombus.[3] In addition, successive events of plaque disruption and asymptomatic thrombus formation have been postulated to be responsible for the rapid progression of disease in certain patients.[3,79] Once a plaque ruptures, in addition to the local factors mentioned above, there are systemic factors that modulate, predispose, or lead to ACS.

One-third of ACS cases, particularly those involving sudden coronary death, develop without plaque disruption but just superficial erosion of a markedly stenotic and fibrotic plaque.[80] Under such conditions, thrombus formation seems to depend on the hyperthrombogenic state triggered by systemic factors (Table 45-2). Indeed, systemic factors—including elevated LDL, decreased high-density lipoprotein (HDL), cigarette smoking, diabetes, and disregulated hemostasis—are associated with increased thrombotic complications.[81–84] Our group has reported an increased blood thrombogenicity associated with hyperlipemia as well as diabetes[85,86]; more importantly, the effective management of these risk factors normalized this increased blood thrombogenicity.[85–87] Thrombogenic systemic factors can be modulated by controlling the cardiovascular risk factors and by dietary and pharmacologic strategies. The development of additional novel therapeutic approaches depends on the increasing knowledge of the pathogenesis of ACS.

The antithrombotic agents presently used in clinical practice can be subdivided into three categories, according to their mechanism of action: fibrinolytics, inhibitors of the intrinsic coagulation cascade, and antiplatelet agents. These are discussed in Chap. 54.

Among the novel antithrombotic strategies that are reaching clinical research are the inhibitors of the TF:FVIIa pathway. The newly generated understanding of the role of tissue factor in atherothrombosis has suggested the inhibition of its pathway as a new antithrombotic approach. The biochemistry of tissue factor and the clotting cascade has identified TF:VIIa, factor Xa, and thrombin as potential targets. Several direct and specific antagonists to each of these targets have been developed and are being investigated in the clinical arena. Specific anti–tissue factor antibodies, recombinant forms of endogenous tissue factor pathway inhibitors, inhibitors of factor VIIa,[88] and factor Xa inhibitors may afford at least a theoretical advantage over therapies that target more "downstream" components of the coagulation cascade.

Direct factor Xa inhibitors are also under investigation at the clinical level. The most advanced of this class of agents seems to be the indirect factor Xa inhibitor, fondaparinux. It inhibits thrombin generation, formation, and growth. This pentasaccharide provides potent antithrombotic activity through inhibition of factor Xa by high-affinity binding to antithrombin III. Superiority versus low-molecular-weight heparin was shown in the prevention of deep venous thrombosis after major orthopedic surgery.[89,90] In acute myocardial infarction, the PENTALYSE study found that pentasaccharide was as safe and effective as unfractionated-heparin in restoring coronary patency; it also showed a trend toward fewer complications.[91] The ongoing PENTUA trial is comparing fondaparinux with enoxaparin in patients with ACS with and without ST-segment elevation.[92]

Despite their potent anticoagulant effect and positive results in small clinical studies, the first-generation thrombin inhibitors (such as hirudin) have failed to provide remarkable beneficial outcomes compared with heparin in large randomized clinical trials and are presently approved by the U.S. Food and Drug Administration (FDA) only in the case of heparin-induced thrombocytopenia. In general, the administration of a thrombin

TABLE 45-2 Factors Modulating Thrombus Formation

| Local Fluid Dynamics | Nature of the Exposed Substrate | Systemic Thrombogenic Factors |
|---|---|---|
| Shear stress<br>Tensile stress | Degree of injury (mild vs. severe arterial injury)<br>Composition of atherosclerotic plaque<br>Residual mural thrombus | Hypercholesterolemia<br>Catecholamines (smoking, cocaine, stress, etc.)<br>Smoking<br>Diabetes<br>Homocysteine<br>Lipoprotein(a)<br>Infections (*Chlamydia pneumoniae*, *Helicobacter* cytomegalovirus)<br>Hypercoagulable state (Fg, vWF, TF, FVII)<br>Defective fibrinolytic state, etc. |

inhibitor shows a substantial effect during the period of administration, which is not maintained thereafter. Therefore oral forms of direct antithrombin that allow long-term treatment were considered a good option, and they have already been developed. Ximelagatran, one of the first of these agents to reach the clinical arena, has shown a reduction in the incidence of deep venous thrombosis and pulmonary embolism after total knee replacement.[93]

Other approaches, still in early preclinical phase, are inhibitors of GP Ib receptor (anti-vWF),[94] inhibitors of vWF-collagen binding (Saratin),[95] and inhibitors of the adenosine diphosphate receptor P2T,[96] among others.

## SUMMARY

The formation of a thrombus within a coronary artery with obstruction of coronary blood flow and reduction in oxygen supply to the myocardium produce the several types of ACS. These thrombotic episodes largely occur in response to atherosclerotic lesions that have progressed to a high risk–inflammatory/prothrombotic stage by a process modulated by local and systemic factors. Although distinct from one another, these atherosclerotic and thrombotic processes appear to be closely interrelated as the cause of ACS through a complex multifactorial process called atherothrombosis. The cellular and molecular mechanisms at play in the formation, growth, and stabilization of a coronary thrombus are being and have been thoroughly investigated, with many of the activation pathways and receptor-ligand interactions identified. Strategies combining dietary, pharmacologic-medical, and interventional-surgical therapies have enjoyed considerable success in the prevention and treatment of major cardiovascular events. These regimens focus on inhibiting the various pathways involved in thrombus generation. Novel strategies based on the knowledge generated in the biochemistry of platelet aggregation and the coagulation process as well as in the conditions encountered in the circulation are presently in different stages of development and in clinical trials. Advances in noninvasive imaging techniques will help to identify plaques at risk and reduce the clinical impact of atherothrombosis.

## ACKNOWLEDGMENTS

The work reported in this review has been partially supported by grants from PNS SAF2000/0174 (Spain) and FIS PI020361 (Spain) (LB), NIH SCOR HL54469 (USA) (JJB, VF).

## References


1. Stary HC, Chandler AB, Glagov S, et al. A definition of initial, fatty streak, and intermediate lesions of atherosclerosis. A report from the Committee on Vascular Lesions of the Council on Arteriosclerosis, American Heart Association. *Circulation* 1994;89:2462–2478.
2. Stary HC, Chandler AB, Dinsmore RE, et al. A definition of advanced types of atherosclerotic lesions and a histological classification of atherosclerosis. A report from the Committee on Vascular Lesions of the Council on Arteriosclerosis, American Heart Association. *Circulation* 1995;92:1355–1374.
3. Fuster V, Badimon L, Badimon JJ, et al. The pathogenesis of coronary artery disease and the acute coronary syndromes. (Part I) and (Part II). *N Engl J Med* 1992;326,242–250.
4. Glagov S, Weisenberg E, Zarins CK, et al. Compensatory enlargement of human atherosclerotic coronary arteries. *N Engl J Med* 1987;316: 1371–1375.
5. Ambrose JA, Weinrauch M. Thrombosis in ischemic heart disease. *Arch Intern Med* 1996;156:1382–1394.
6. Corti R, Fuster V, Badimon JJ, et al. New understanding of atherosclerosis (clinically and experimentally) with evolving MRI technology in vivo. *Ann N Y Acad Sci* 2001;947:181–195; discussion 195–198.
7. Badimon L, Chesebro JH, Badimon JJ. Thrombus formation on ruptured atherosclerotic plaques and rethrombosis on evolving thrombi. *Circulation* 1992;86:III-74–III-85.
8. Badimon JJ, Fuster V, Chesebro JH, et al. Coronary atherosclerosis. *Circulation* 1993;87:II-3–II-16.
9. Marcus A, Safier LB. Thromboregulation: Multicellular modulation of platelet reactivity in hemostasis and thrombosis. *FASEB J* 1993;7: 516–522.
10. Kroll MH, Schafer AI. Biochemical mechanisms of platelet activation. *Blood* 1989;74:1181–1195.
11. Brass LF. The biochemistry of platelet activation. In: Hoffman R, Benz EJ Jr, Shattil SJ, et al, eds. *Hematology: Basic Principles and Practice*. New York: Churchill Livingstone; 1991:1176–1197.
12. Colman RW, Walsh PN. Mechanisms of platelet aggregation. In: Colman RW, Hirsh J, Marder VJ, Salzman E, eds. *Hemostasis and Thrombosis: Basic Principles and Clinical Practice*, 2d ed. Philadelphia: Lippincott; 1987;594–605.
13. Huang EM, Detwiler TC. Stimulus-response coupling mechanisms. In: Philips DR, Shuman MC, eds. *Biochemistry of Platelets*. New York: Academic Press; 1986;1–68.
14. Badimon L, Badimon JJ, Fuster V. Pathogenesis of thrombosis. In: Verstraete M, Fuster V, Topol E, eds. *Cardiovascular Thrombosis: Thrombocardiology*. Philadelphia: Lippincott-Raven; 1998:23–44.
15. Kieffer N, Phillips DR. Platelet membrane glycoproteins: Functions in cellular interactions. *Annu Rev Biol* 1990;6:329–357.
16. Kunicki TJ. Organization of glycoproteins within the platelet plasma membrane. In: George JN, Nurden AT, Philips DR, eds. *Platelet Membrane Glycoproteins*. New York: Plenum Press; 1985:87–101.
17. Fitzgerald LA, Phillips DR. Calcium regulation of the platelet membrane glycoprotein IIb-IIIa complex. *J Biol Chem* 1985;260:11366–11376.
18. Calvete JJ, Henschen A, Gonzalez-Rodriguez J. Complete localization of the intrachain disulphide bonds and the N-glycosylation points in the subunit of human platelet glycoprotein IIb. *Biochem J* 1989;261: 561–568.
19. Beer J, Coller BS. Evidence that platelet glycoprotein IIIa has a large disulfide bonded loop that is susceptible to proteolytic cleavage. *J Biol Chem* 1989;264:17564–17573.
20. Plow EF, Ginsberg MH, Marguerie GA. Expression and function of adhesive proteins on the platelet surface. In: Phillips DR, Shuman MA, eds. *Biochemistry of Platelets*. New York: Academic Press; 1986; 225–256.
21. Ruoslahti E, Pierschbacher MD. New perspectives in cell adhesion: RGD and integrins. *Science* 1987;238:491–497.
22. Doolittle RF, Watt KWK, Cottrell BA, et al. The amino acid sequence of the $\alpha$-chain of human fibrinogen. *Nature* 1979;280:464–467.
23. Kloczewiak M, Timmons S, Lukas TJ, et al. Platelet receptor recognition site on human fibrinogen. Synthesis and structure-function relationship of peptides corresponding to the carboxyterminal segment of the g chain. *Biochemistry* 1984;23:1767–1774.
24. Ginsberg MH, Xiaoping D, O'Toole TE, et al. Platelet integrins. *Thromb Haemost* 1993;70:87–93.
25. Shattil SJ. Regulation of platelet anchorage and signaling by integrin aIIbb3. *Thromb Haemost* 1993;70:224–228.
26. Vicente V, Houghten RA, Ruggeri ZM. Identification of a site in the $\alpha$-chain of platelet glycoprotein Ib that participates in von Willebrand factor binding. *J Biol Chem* 1990;265:274–280.
27. Fujimura Y, Titani K, Holland LZ, et al. Von Willebrand factor. A reduced and alkylated 52/48-kDa fragment beginning at amino acid residue 449 contains the domain interacting with platelet glycoprotein Ib. *J Biol Chem* 1986;261:381–385.
28. Fox JEB, Boyles JK, Berndt MC, et al. Identification of a membrane skeleton in platelets. *J Cell Biol* 1988;106:1525–1538.
29. Meyer D, Girma JP. Von Willebrand factor: Structure and function. *Thromb Haemost* 1993;70:99–104.

30. Vu TH, Hung DT, Wheaton VI, et al. Molecular cloning of a functional thrombin receptor reveals a novel proteolytic mechanism of receptor activation. *Cell* 1991;64:1057–1068.
31. Coughlin SR. Thrombin receptor structure and function. *Thromb Haemost* 1993;70:184–187.
32. Sakariassen KS, Nievelstein PF, Coller BS, et al. The role of platelet membrane glycoproteins Ib and IIb/IIIa in platelet adherence to human artery subendothelium. *Br J Haematol* 1986;63:681–691.
33. Sakariassen K, Bolhuis PA, Sixma J. Human blood platelet adhesion to artery subendothelium is mediated by factor VIII–von Willebrand factor bound to the subendothelium. *Nature* 1979;279:636–638.
34. Badimon L, Badimon JJ, Turitto VT, et al. Role of von Willebrand factor in mediating platelet–vessel wall interaction at low shear rate: The importance of perfusion conditions. *Blood* 1989;73:961–967.
35. Nemerson Y. Mechanism of coagulation. In: Williams WJ, Beutler E, Erslev AJ, Lichtman MA, ed. *Hematology*. New York: McGraw-Hill; 1990:1295–1304.
36. Rimon S, Melamed R, Savion N, et al. Identification of a factor IX/IXa binding protein on the endothelial cell surface. *J Biol Chem* 1987; 262:6023–6031.
37. Colman RW, Marder VJ, Salzman EW, et al. Overview of hemostasis. In: Colman RW, Hirsh J, Marder VJ, Salzman EW, eds. *Hemostasis and Thrombosis: Basic Principles and Clinical Practice*. Philadelphia: Lippincott; 1987:3–17.
38. Mann KG. Membrane-bound enzyme complexes in blood coagulation. In: Spaet TH, ed. *Progress in Hemostasis and Thrombosis*. New York: Grune & Stratton; 1984:1–23.
39. Mann KG, Nesheim ME, Church WR, et al. Surface dependent reactions of the vitamin K dependent enzyme complexes. *Blood* 1990; 76:1–16.
40. Rawala-Sheikh R, Ahmad SS, Ashby B, et al. Kinetics of coagulation factor X activation by platelet bound factor IXa. *Biochemistry* 1990; 29:2606–2611.
41. Rosing J, van Rijn JLML, Bevers EM, et al. The role of activated human platelets in prothrombin and factor X activation. *Blood* 1985;65: 319–332.
42. Nesheim ME, Furmaniak-Kazmierczak E, Henin C, et al. On the existence of platelet receptors for factor Va and factor VIIIa. *Thromb Haemost* 1993;70:80–86.
43. Ahmad SS, Rawala-Sheikh R, Monroe DM, et al. Comparative platelet binding and kinetic studies with normal and variant factor IXa molecules. *J Biol Chem* 1990;265:20907–20911.
44. Comp PC. Kinetics of plasma coagulation factors. In: Williams WJ, Beutler E, Erslev AJ, Lichtman MA, eds. *Hematology*. New York: McGraw-Hill, 1990:1285–1290.
45. Esmon NL, Owen WG, Esmon CT. Isolation of a membrane-bound cofactor for thrombin-catalyzed activation of protein C. *J Biol Chem* 1982;257:859–864.
46. Nemerson Y, Williams WJ. Biochemistry of plasma coagulation factors. In: Williams WJ, Beutler E, Erslev AJ, Lichtman MA, eds. *Hematology*. New York: McGraw-Hill; 1990:1267–1284.
47. Francis CW, Marder VJ. Physiologic regulation and pathologic disorders of fibrinolysis. In: Colman RW, Hirsh J, Marder VJ, Salzman EW, eds. *Hemostasis and Thrombosis: Basic Principles and Clinical Practice*. Philadelphia: Lippincott; 1987:358–379.
48. Collen D, Lijnen HR. Molecular and cellular basis of fibrinolysis. In: Hoffman R, Benz EJ Jr, Shattil SJ, et al, eds. *Hematology: Basic Principles and Practice*. New York: Churchill Livingstone; 1991: 1232–1242.
49. Badimon L, Badimon JJ, Turitto VT, et al. Platelet thrombus formation on collagen type I. Influence of blood rheology, von Willebrand factor and blood coagulation. *Circulation* 1988;78:1431–1442.
50. Badimon L, Badimon JJ, Galvez A, et al. Influence of arterial damage and wall shear rate on platelet deposition. Ex vivo study in swine model. *Arteriosclerosis* 1986;6:312–320.
51. Badimon L, Badimon JJ. Mechanism of arterial thrombosis in non-parallel streamlines: Platelet grow at the apex of stenotic severely injured vessel wall. Experimental study in the pig model. *J Clin Invest* 1989;84:1134–1144.
52. Lassila R, Badimon JJ, Vallbhajosula S, et al. Dynamic monitoring of platelet deposition on severely damaged vessel wall in flowing blood. Effects of different stenosis on thrombus growth. *Arteriosclerosis* 1990;10:306–315.
53. Drake TA, Morrissey JH, Edgington TS. Selective cellular expression of tissue factor in human tissues: Implication of hemostasis and thrombosis. *Am J Pathol* 1989;134:1087–1097.
54. Wilcox JN, Smith SM, Schwartz SM, et al. Localization of tissue factor in the normal vessel wall and atherosclerotic plaque. *Proc Natl Acad Sci USA* 1989;86(8):2839–2843.
55. Fuster V, Chesebro JH. Mechanisms of unstable angina. *N Engl J Med* 1986;315:1023–1025.
56. Fernández-Ortiz A, Badimon JJ, Falk E, et al. Characterization of the relative thrombogenicity of atherosclerotic plaque components: Implications for consequences of plaque rupture. *J Am Coll Cardiol* 1994;23:1562–1569.
57. Toschi V, Gallo R, Lettino M, et al. Tissue factor modulates the thrombogenicity of human atherosclerotic plaques. *Circulation* 1997; 95:594–599.
58. Badimon JJ, Lettino M, Toschi V, et al. Local inhibition of tissue factor reduces the thrombogenicity of disrupted human atherosclerotic plaques. Effects of TFPI on plaque thrombogenicity under flow conditions. *Circulation* 1999;99:1780–1787.
59. Sánchez-Gómez S, Casani L, Vilahur G, et al. FFR-rFVIIa inhibits thrombosis triggered by ruptured and eroded vessel wall. *Thromb Haemost* 2001;A:#OC999.
60. Libby P, Simon DI. Inflammation and thrombosis: The clot thickens. *Circulation* 2001;103:1718–1720.
61. Hani J, Corti R, Hutter R, et al. The interplay between inflammation and thrombosis in atherosclerosis. *Acute Coron Syndr* 2002;4:71–78.
62. Davies MJ. Stability and instability: Two faces of coronary atherosclerosis. The Paul Dudley White Lecture 1995. *Circulation* 1996;94:2013–2020.
63. Moreno PR, Falk E, Palacios IF, et al. Macrophage infiltration in acute coronary syndromes. Implications for plaque rupture. *Circulation* 1994; 90:775–778.
64. Galis ZS, Khatri JJ. Matrix metalloproteinases in vascular remodeling and atherogenesis: The good, the bad, and the ugly. *Circ Res* 2002;90: 251–262.
65. Libby P. Current concepts of the pathogenesis of the acute coronary syndromes. *Circulation* 2001;104:365–372.
66. Rodríguez C, Raposo B, Martínez-González J, et al. Low density lipoproteins downregulate lysyl oxidase in vascular endothelial cells and in the arterial wall. *Arterioscl Thromb Vasc Biol* 2002;22:1409–1414.
67. Mallat Z, Tedgui A. Current perspective on the role of apoptosis in atherothrombotic disease. *Circ Res* 2001;88:998–1003.
68. Mallat Z, Hugel B, Ohan J, et al. Shed membrane microparticles with procoagulant potential in human atherosclerotic plaques: A role for apoptosis in plaque thrombogenicity. *Circulation* 1999;99:348–353.
69. Badimon JJ, Fernández-Ortiz A, Meyer B, et al. Different response to balloon angioplasty of carotid and coronary arteries: Effects on acute platelet deposition and intimal thickening. *Atherosclerosis* 1998;140: 307–314.
70. Van de Werf F, Arnold AER, and the European Cooperative Study Group for Recombinant Tissue-Type Plasminogen Activator (rt-PA). Effect of intravenous tissue plasminogen activator on infarct size, left ventricular function and survival in patients with acute myocardial infarction. *BMJ* 1988;297:374–379.
71. Van Lierde, De Geest H, Verstraete M, et al. Angiographic assessment of the infarct-related residual coronary stenosis after spontaneous or therapeutic thrombolysis. *J Am Coll Cardiol* 1990;16:1545–1549.
72. Fuster V, Stein B, Badimon L, et al. Atherosclerotic plaque rupture and thrombosis: Evolving concepts. *Circulation* 1990;82(suppl II):47–59.
73. Davies SW, Marchant B, Lyon JP, et al. Coronary lesion morphology in acute myocardial infarction: Demonstration of early remodeling after streptokinase treatment. *J Am Coll Cardiol* 1990;16:1079–1086.
74. Badimon L, Badimon JJ, Lasilla R, et al. Thrombin inhibition by hirudin decreases platelet thrombus growth on areas of severe vessel wall injury. *J Am Coll Cardiol* 1989;13:145A.

75. Waller BF, Rothbaum DA, Pinkerton CA, et al. Status of the myocardium and infarct-related coronary artery in 19 necropsy patients with acute recanalization using pharmacologic (streptokinase, r-tissue plasminogen activator), mechanical (percutaneous transluminal coronary angioplasty) or combined types of reperfusion therapy. *J Am Coll Cardiol* 1987;9:785–801.
76. Meyer BJ, Badimon JJ, Mailhac A, et al. Inhibition of growth of thrombus on fresh mural thrombus: Targeting optimal therapy. *Circulation* 1994;90:2432–2438.
77. Meyer B, Badimon JJ, Chesebro JH, et al. Dissolution of mural thrombus by specific thrombin inhibition with r-hirudin: Comparison with heparin and aspirin. *Circulation* 1998;97;681–685.
78. Gosgnach W, Challah M, Coulet F, et al. Shear stress induces angiotensin converting enzyme expression in cultured smooth muscle cells: Possible involvement of bFGF. *Cardiovasc Res* 2000;279: C797–C805.
79. Burke AP, Kolodgie FD, Farb A, et al. Healed plaque ruptures and sudden coronary death: Evidence that subclinical rupture has a role in plaque progression. *Circulation* 2001;103:934–940.
80. Virmani R, Kolodgie FD, Burke AP, et al. Lessons from sudden coronary death: A comprehensive morphological classification scheme for atherosclerotic lesions. *Arterioscl Thromb Vasc Biol* 2000;20: 1262–1275.
81. Burke AP, Farb A, Pestaner J, et al. Traditional risk factors and the incidence of sudden coronary death with and without coronary thrombosis in blacks. *Circulation* 2002;105:419–424.
82. Kelleher CC. Plasma fibrinogen and factor VII as risk factors for cardiovascular disease. *Eur J Epidemiol* 1992;8:79–82.
83. Markovitz JH, Tolbert L, Winders SE. Increased serotonin receptor density and platelet GPIIb/IIIa activation among smokers. *Arterioscl Thromb Vasc Biol* 1999;19:762–766.
84. Badimon JJ, Badimon L, Turitto VT, et al. Platelet deposition at high shear rates is enhanced by high plasma cholesterol levels. In vivo study in the rabbit model. *Arterioscler Thromb Vasc Biol* 1991;11:395–402.
85. Osende JI, Badimon JJ, Fuster V, et al. Blood thrombogenicity in type 2 diabetes mellitus patients is associated with glycemic control. *J Am Coll Cardiol* 2001;38:1307–1312.
86. Rauch U, Crandall J, Osende JI, et al. Increased thrombus formation relates to ambient blood glucose and leukocyte count in diabetes mellitus type 2. *Am J Cardiol* 2000;86:246–249.
87. Corti R, Badimon JJ. Value or desirability of hemorheological-hemostatic parameter changes as endpoints in blood lipid-regulating trials. *Curr Opin Lipidol* 2001;12:629–637.
88. Erhardtsen E, Nilsson P, Johannessen M, et al. Pharmacokinetics and safety of FFR-rFVIIa after single doses in healthy subjects. *J Clin Pharmacol* 2001;41:880–885.
89. Eriksson BI, Bauer KA, Lassen MR, et al. Fondaparinux compared with enoxaparin for the prevention of venous thromboembolism after hip-fracture surgery. *N Engl J Med* 2001;345:1298–1304.
90. Turpie AG, Bauer KA, Eriksson BI, et al. Postoperative fondaparinux versus postoperative enoxaparin for prevention of venous thromboembolism after elective hip-replacement surgery: A randomised double-blind trial. *Lancet* 2002;359:1721–1726.
91. Coussement PK, Bassand JP, Convens C, et al. A synthetic factor-Xa inhibitor (ORG31540/SR9017A) as an adjunct to fibrinolysis in acute myocardial infarction. The PENTALYSE study. *Eur Heart J* 2001;22: 1716–1724.
92. Van de Werf F. New data in treatment of acute coronary syndromes. *Am Heart J* 2001;142:S16–S21.
93. Heit JA, Colwell CW, Francis CW, et al. Comparison of the oral direct thrombin inhibitor ximelagatran with enoxaparin as prophylaxis against venous thromboembolism after total knee replacement: A phase 2 dose-finding study. *Arch Intern Med* 2001;161:2215–2221.
94. Cauwenberghs N, Meiring M, Vauterin S, et al. Antithrombotic effect of platelet glycoprotein Ib-blocking monoclonal antibody Fab fragments in nonhuman primates. *Arterioscl Thromb Vasc Biol* 2000;20: 1347–1353.
95. Vilahur G, Juan O, Duran X, et al. Local blockade of the collagen binding domain to vWF-A3 with Saratin decreases thrombotic risk in human atherosclerotic lesions. *Thromb Haemost* 2003;A:#PO526.
96. Ingall AH, Dixon J, Bailey A, et al. Antagonists of the platelet P2T receptor: A novel approach to antithrombotic therapy. *J Med Chem* 1999;42:213–220.

CHAPTER 46

# CORONARY BLOOD FLOW AND MYOCARDIAL ISCHEMIA

Gaetano Antonio Lanza / Stefano Coli / Domenico Cianflone / Attilio Maseri



## REGULATION OF CORONARY BLOOD FLOW

The task of the coronary circulation is to supply the myocardium with oxygen and substrates and remove metabolic waste products. Contractile cardiac function relies on aerobic metabolism and, as basal oxygen extraction is more than 60 percent,[1] an adequate increase of coronary blood flow is required to meet the myocardium's increased need for oxygen consumption ($M\dot{V}O_2$).

During strenuous exercise, coronary blood flow can increase about five times.[2] The maximal increase in coronary flow above resting levels is defined as *coronary flow reserve* and is expressed as the ratio between the flow during maximal vasodilatation and basal flow.[3]

Vascular resistance in the coronary circulation is distributed into several functional compartments arranged in series. It is mainly determined by $M\dot{V}O_2$ and modulated by neural stimuli, local vasoactive autacoids, and circulating vasoactive substances. The transmural distribution of coronary resistance across the ventricular wall is largely determined by the compressive forces of extravascular tissue.

A brief description—as given below—of determinants of $M\dot{V}O_2$, the functional anatomy of the coronary circulation, and the distribution of coronary vascular resistance is useful for a better understanding of the regulation of myocardial blood flow.

### Determinants of Myocardial Oxygen Consumption

Mechanical work performed by the myocardium is the most important determinant of $M\dot{V}O_2$, as the latter decreases to only 15 to 20 percent in the nonbeating heart. Heart rate, myocardial wall tension, and myocardial inotropic state are the major determinants of metabolic activity and, therefore, of $M\dot{V}O_2$.[4]

In dogs, heart rate is by far the major determinant of $M\dot{V}O_2$: when heart rate doubles, myocardial oxygen uptake also approximately doubles. Myocardial tension developed during systole is directly proportional to aortic pressure (afterload), myocardial fiber length, and ventricular volume (preload).* Myocardial oxygen uptake approximately doubles as mean aortic pressure is increased from 75 to 175 mmHg at constant heart rate and stroke volume. Finally, myocardial inotropic state determines ventricular performance independent of both preload and afterload. $M\dot{V}O_2$ increases by about 30 percent when dP/dt† is doubled by extrasystolic potentiation or by norepinephrine at constant heart rate, aortic pressure, and cardiac output.

Direct measurement of $M\dot{V}O_2$ requires determination of coronary blood flow and the arteriovenous difference of blood oxygen content. In clinical practice, $M\dot{V}O_2$ can be estimated by the rate-pressure product (heart rate × systolic blood pressure), a simple parameter, which correlates with direct measures of $M\dot{V}O_2$ in a variety of physiologic and experimental conditions.

### Functional Compartments of the Coronary Circulation

About 75 percent of total vascular resistance occurs in the arterial system, which can be divided into three functional compartments arranged in series (Fig. 46-1).

1. The proximal compartment is represented by the large epicardial coronary arteries; these vessels have a conductive function and do not contribute significantly to vascular resistance. During systole, their blood content increases by about 25 percent as a result of anterograde flow from the aorta and retrograde flow from

*According to Laplace's law, wall tension = (pressure × radius / 2 × wall thickness.

†The expression dp/dt indicates the rate of pressure development in the left ventricle.

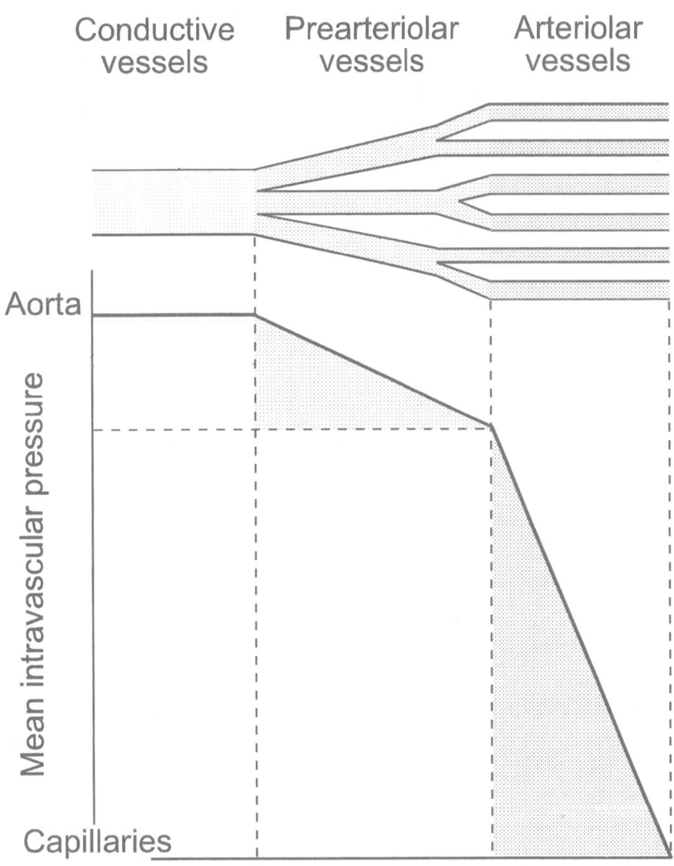


FIGURE 46-1 Schematic illustration of the subdivision of the coronary arterial system into conductive, prearteriolar, and arteriolar vessels. Resistance to flow is negligible in conductive vessels (epicardial arteries) and maximal in arterioles, which are under the control of myocardial metabolic activity. Prearteriolar vessels offer an appreciable resistance to flow, but, at variance with arterioles, are not under direct metabolic vasodilator control. Their specific function is to maintain pressure at the origin of arterioles within a narrow range when aortic pressure and coronary flow vary. The arterioles are the major site of metabolic regulation of flow. (From Maseri.[50] With permission.)

squeezed intramyocardial vessels. The elastic energy accumulated in the vessel wall during systole is transformed into blood kinetic energy at the beginning of diastole. About 60 percent of the wall thickness of conductive vessels is represented by the muscular media, which is responsible for myogenic autoregulation of the vascular lumen in response to changes in aortic pressure and for modulation of coronary tone in response to flow-mediated endothelium-dependent vasodilators, circulating vasoactive substances, and neural stimuli. Conversely, the large conduit arteries are unaffected by myocardial metabolites, due to their extramural position.

2. The intermediate compartment is represented by prearterioles, which are resistive vessels connecting epicardial conduit arteries to the arterioles. The proximal and distal ends of prearterioles cannot be defined anatomically, but their diameter is in the range of 100 to 500 $\mu$m and they contribute to about 30 percent of total coronary flow resistance. The main function of prearterioles is to maintain the driving pressure at the origin of arterioles within an optimal range. This regulatory function is mediated by myogenic autoregulation and flow-dependent vasodilatation in response to shear stress. Prearteriolar resistance is also modulated by neural stimuli and by local autacoids, whereas it is unaffected by myocardial metabolic vasodilators.
3. The distal arterial compartment is represented by the arterioles, which are the main site of metabolic regulation of coronary blood flow. Arterioles are smaller than 100 $\mu$m in diameter and are responsible for about 40 percent of coronary flow resistance. Also, their tone can be modulated by neural stimuli and local autacoids.

According to the integrated response model proposed by Kuo,[5] an increase in myocardial metabolic demand initially causes arteriolar vasodilatation (metabolic domain), followed by a transient decrease in pressure at their origin, with consequent myogenic regulation (myogenic domain), as well as by an increase in flow, leading to flow-mediated, endothelium-dependent vasodilatation in proximal vessels (flow-sensitive domain).

Arterioles branch into meta-arteriolar and capillary vessels, which provide a regional microdistribution of flow that, under physiologic conditions, exhibits spatial and temporal heterogeneity. Such physiologic heterogeneity may have pathophysiologic consequences, as coronary hypoperfusion severe enough to cause ischemia was shown to produce a nonuniform maximal dilation of microvessels and a variable response to adenosine in adjacent myocardial regions.[6]

Diffusion of oxygen and substrates to myocardial cells takes place at the capillary level. On average, there is one capillary for each myocardial fiber, but the density of these capillaries is about 20 percent higher in the subendocardial layers.

The venous side of the coronary circulation has so far received little attention, although it contributes a detectable fraction of total coronary flow resistance and can influence capillary recruitment and blood volume content in the ventricular wall, increasing diastolic fiber length and, therefore, myocardial oxygen consumption ("garden hose" effect).

## Physiologic Control of Myocardial Perfusion

The in-series distribution of resistance as well as total vascular resistance are largely determined by changes of coronary vasomotor tone, while the transmural distribution of perfusion is largely determined by extravascular compressive forces.

### EXTRAVASCULAR MECHANICAL FORCES

Unlike all other organs, the heart generates its own perfusion pressure.[7] During systole, intramyocardial left ventricular pressure is sufficiently high to prevent systolic flow across the whole wall (perhaps with the exception of the outermost layers). Furthermore, the high extravascular pressure squeezes intramyocardial blood forward out of the capillaries, venules, and veins toward the coronary sinus and backward from subendocardial and midwall layers toward epicardial arteries.[8] The extravascular compressive forces are highest in the subendocardium and decrease linearly toward the subepicardium.[9] Thus subendocardial vessels are squeezed more than subepicardial ones, so they take a longer time to refill and resume their caliber during diastole,[10] particularly when perfusion pressure is low (e.g., distal to flow-limiting coronary stenosis or in the presence of aortic stenosis) (Fig. 46-2). When poststenotic pressure is reduced, subendocardial perfusion is further impaired by tachycardia, which shortens the duration of diastole,[11] and by increased left ventricular diastolic pressure, which increases extravascular compressive forces in subendocardial layers. The higher extravascular resistance, together with a higher basal $M\dot{V}O_2$, determines a greater susceptibility to ischemia in subendocardial layers.

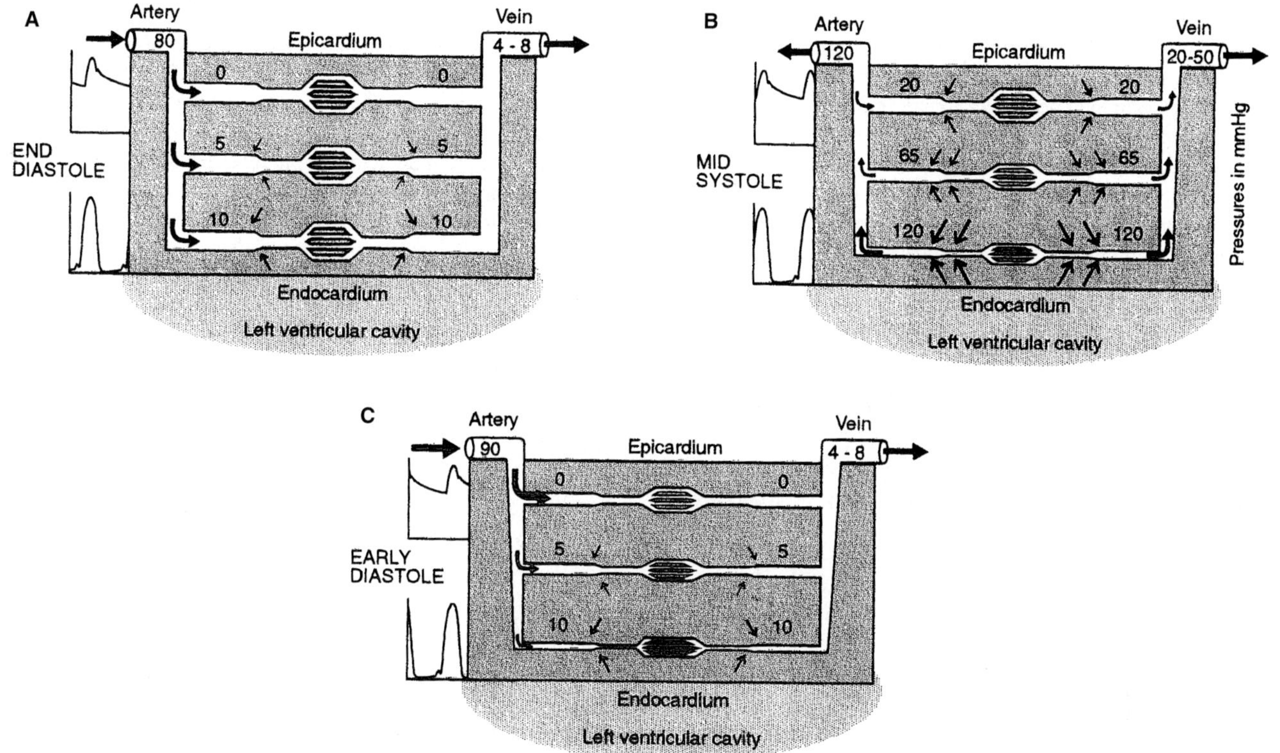


FIGURE 46-2 Changes in interstitial and intravascular pressure and vessel caliber across the left ventricular free wall during the cardiac cycle. During systole, the pressure of interstitial tissue is greater in subendocardial than in subepicardial layers, therefore subendocardial vessels are squeezed more than subepicardial ones at the end of systole and take longer to resume their full diastolic dimension. In the presence of a low perfusion pressure subendocardial flow is also impaired by reduced diastolic time, during tachycardia, and by elevated left ventricular diastolic pressure. (Modified from Hoffman et al.[10] With permission.)

## REGULATION OF CORONARY VASOMOTOR TONE

The mechanisms of contraction and relaxation of vascular smooth muscle cells are influenced by several factors and are not the same in the different compartments of the coronary circulation. Vasomotor tone is mainly determined by $M\dot{V}O_2$ in arteriolar vessels (metabolic vasodilatation) pressure, and flow-mediated vasodilatation in prearterioles and in large arteries (myogenic and endothelial control); it is influenced by neurogenic stimuli, local autacoids, and circulating vasoactive substances in all vascular compartments.

***Metabolic Regulation*** Arteriolar vasomotor tone is under metabolic control, as arterioles are directly exposed to the effects of the myocardial metabolites. When $M\dot{V}O_2$ increases, vasodilator metabolites released from myocardial cells diffuse into the arteriolar wall, causing smooth muscle cells to relax. The resulting arteriolar vasodilatation causes flow to increase, so that vasodilator metabolites are washed out and flow is reset at a higher level.

Adenosine has been considered a major component of myocardial metabolic regulation of flow.[12] According to a "microhypoxia" model, adenosine production reflects adenosine triphosphate (ATP) degradation resulting from a local myocardial imbalance between oxygen supply and demand. ATP dephosphorylation first results in the formation of adenosine monophosphate (AMP), and then, by 5′-nucleotidase action, in adenosine production. Adenosine stimulates $A_2$ receptors of smooth muscle cells, inducing adenylate-cyclase activation, cyclic-AMP synthesis, and consequent relaxation of smooth muscle cells. Adenosine may also favor vasodilation by inducing the opening of ATP-sensitive potassium channels on smooth muscle cells by means of the activation of both tyrosine and calcium-dependent protein kinases.

However, adenosine is unlikely to be the only component of metabolic vasodilatation.[13,14] Oxygen tension, pH, potassium, osmotic pressure,[15] and ATP-sensitive potassium channels[16] also contribute to metabolic regulation of flow. Moreover, adenosine probably plays a major role in pathologic conditions, such as myocardial ischemia, but does not seem to explain the increase in coronary blood flow observed during physiologic conditions, such as the exercise-induced increase in $M\dot{V}O_2$.[17]

***Myogenic Regulation*** When metabolic requirements do not vary, the heart, like other organs, exhibits an intrinsic tendency to maintain blood flow constant despite changes in arterial perfusion pressure. Pressure/flow curves in experimental models show that flow remains nearly constant over a range of perfusion pressure from 60 to 120 mmHg. This partly results from myogenic control of vasomotor tone, which tends to keep the vessel wall tension constant in response to changes in vascular distending pressure; myogenic tone increases when pressure increases and decreases when pressure decreases.

The role of myogenic control of vasomotor tone cannot be easily separated from the effects of stretch-induced release of endothelium-derived relaxing factor (EDRF, see below) and of metabolic regulation. However, myogenic activity has been demonstrated in coronary vessels 40 to 200 $\mu$m in diameter[18] and the responses of vascular tone to changes in transmural pressure are not affected by endothelial denudation, confirming that myogenic activity is an intrinsic property of vascular smooth muscle cells.

***Neural Regulation*** Coronary vessels are innervated by both sympathetic and parasympathetic efferents of the autonomic nervous system.[19] Nerve endings are located mainly at the adventitial-medial border of vessels and their density is greater in prearterioles and arterioles than in epicardial coronary arteries. Besides acetylcholine and norepinephrine, several "nonadrenergic noncholinergic" neurotransmitters identified in axonal varicosities may play a modulatory role in adrenergic and cholinergic output.[20] These substances include purines (ATP), amines (serotonin and dopamine), and peptides [neuropeptide Y (NPY), calcitonin gene–related peptide (CGRP), substance P, and vasoactive intestinal peptide (VIP)].

SYMPATHETIC CONTROL Both $\alpha_1$ and $\alpha_2$ and both $\beta_1$ and $\beta_2$ adrenergic receptors have been identified in coronary arteries. Electrical stimulation of sympathetic nerves and intracoronary infusion of norepinephrine cause an increase in coronary flow resistance mediated by $\alpha$-receptors, whereas pharmacologic stimulation of $\beta$ receptors results in a modest reduction (20 to 30 percent) in coronary flow resistance.[21] In humans, abolition of $\alpha$-adrenergic tone causes an approximately 10 percent increase in resting coronary blood flow, indicating the presence of a tonic basal, $\alpha$-mediated coronary vasoconstriction. Subepicardial $\alpha$-adrenergic–mediated coronary vasoconstriction may counterbalance the greater extravascular compressive forces in subendocardial layers.[22] Sympathetic innervation is particularly important during exercise. In exercising dogs, beta-adrenoceptor–mediated vasodilation can account for about 25 percent of the observed total increase in coronary blood flow.[23] Of note, an integrated response to sympathetic alpha and beta stimulation of coronary vessels likely contributes significantly to optimizing myocardial blood flow during exercise. Indeed, beta-receptor stimulation is involved in mediating the increase in coronary blood flow, whereas alpha vasoconstriction, which mainly concerns prearteriolar vessels (>100 $\mu$m), favors subendocardial flow by stiffening intramyocardial vessels—thus contrasting the myocardial compressive forces—and by improving transmural flow distribution.[23]

PARASYMPATHETIC CONTROL The role of the parasympathetic nervous system in the regulation of coronary blood flow is still unclear. Muscarinic receptors are present on smooth muscle cells, where they trigger contraction; on sympathetic nerve varicosities, where acetylcholine inhibits norepinephrine release; and on the endothelium, where their activation induces EDRF release.[24] However, the extent to which acetylcholine released at the site of vagal nerve endings in the adventitia reaches endothelial receptors is unknown. The variable effect of cholinergic stimulation may depend on the balance among its different sites of action. VIP coreleased with acetylcholine exerts a significant vasodilator effect.[25]

PURINERGIC CONTROL Two types of purinergic receptors have been identified: (1) $P_1$ (which includes $A_1$ and $A_2$ receptors), which is most sensitive to adenosine and mediates smooth muscle cell relaxation both directly and by endothelial release of EDRF, and (2) $P_2$, which is most sensitive to ATP and mediates endothelial release of EDRF but also direct vasoconstriction. ATP was found to be released from nerve terminals together with norepinephrine. However, the role of purine release by nerve endings in the regulation of coronary blood flow and coronary vasomotion is not well defined. Interestingly, ATP may be released by cardiomyocytes and circulating red blood cells during hypoxia to contribute to local vasodilation.[26]

PEPTIDES NPY is released with norepinephrine during sympathetic nerve stimulation[27]; its infusion was shown to cause severe myocardial ischemia by microvascular constriction in patients with normal coronary arteries (see below). Both CGRP and substance P are also found in cardiac nerves; their intracoronary infusion causes EDRF release and dose-dependent dilation of epicardial coronary arteries.

REFLEX CONTROL Afferent stimuli arising outside the heart (e.g., from chemoreceptors in the carotid bodies and from mechanoreceptors in the carotid sinus, aortic arch, and lungs) may produce efferent stimuli that influence coronary flow resistance. Hypotension at the level of carotid sinus baroceptors would tend to increase coronary flow resistance by $\alpha$-adrenergic stimulation, but this effect in vivo is obscured by metabolic vasodilatation in response to the increase in heart rate and contractility consequent to enhanced cardiac sympathetic drive.

## ENDOTHELIUM-MEDIATED REGULATION

Endothelial cells release several vasodilator autacoids that contribute to the physiologic regulation of coronary vasomotor tone—including endothelium-derived relaxing factor (EDRF), prostacyclin ($PGI_2$) and endothelium-derived hyperpolarizing factor (EDHF)—as well as vasoconstrictor autacoids, such as endothelin-1 (ET-1), angiotensin II, and endothelium-derived contracting factors (EDCFs), which may have a pathologic role in some conditions (Fig. 46-3).

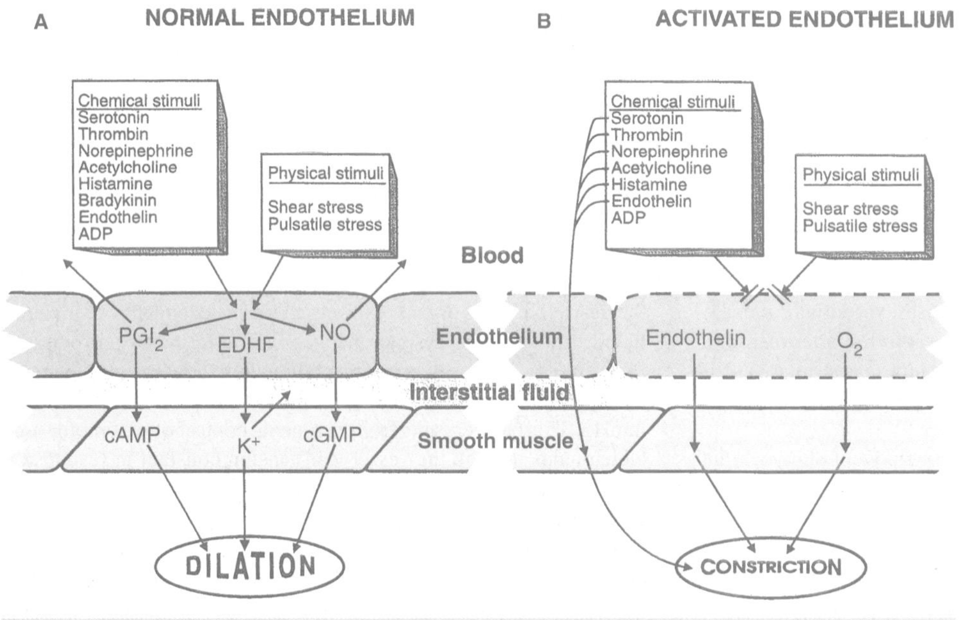

PHYSIOLOGIC VASODILATOR FUNCTION The maintenance of tonic basal vasodilatation and flow-mediated reg-

FIGURE 46-3 Vasoactive functions of the endothelium. *A*. Normal endothelium produces a variety of vasodilator substances. *B*. Activated endothelium causes loss of vasodilator functions and produces vasoconstrictor substances. ADP = adenosine diphosphate; $PGI_2$ = prostacyclin; EDHF = endothelium-derived hyperpolarizing factor; NO = nitric oxide; cAMP = cyclic adenosine monophosphate; $K^+$ = potassium ions; cGMP = cyclic guanosine monophosphate; $O_2^-$ = superoxide anion (From Maseri.[50] With permission.)

ulation of vascular tone are largely dependent on the release of EDRF, identified as nitric oxide (NO) or NO-carrier compound.[28] NO exerts its vasodilator action on vascular smooth muscle cells by activating the enzyme guanylate cyclase, which leads to the production of cyclic-GMP. EDRF is released in response to a large number of agonists acting on endothelial receptors, including neurotransmitters (acetylcholine and norepinephrine), substances released by platelets (serotonin, adenosine diphosphate) or formed during coagulation of the blood (thrombin), and autacoids formed in the vessel wall, such as histamine, bradykinin, and endothelin. Moreover, EDRF is also released in response to pulsatile stretch and flow shear stress; it is believed to be the major regulator of flow-mediated vasodilation in large arteries and in prearteriolar vessels.

EDRF has a 5-s half-life and is continuously released, tonically reducing basal vasomotor tone as the infusion of its inhibitor, NG-monomethyl-L-arginine (LNMMA), reduces forearm blood flow and coronary diameter in humans[29,30] and causes an increase in blood pressure in animals.[31]

The endothelium also modulates coronary vascular resistance by releasing $PGI_2$ and EDHF. $PGI_2$ is synthesized from arachidonic acid, has a 10-s half-life, and is released in response to pulsatile pressure, bradykinin, thrombin, serotonin, and platelet-derived growth factor (PDGF). It contributes to the tone of resting conduits and resistance vessels and to flow-mediated vasodilatation.[32] EDHF is most likely a short-lived metabolite of arachidonic acid,[33] thought to open ligand-gated potassium channels; it is released in response to several stimuli, including shear stress, pulsatile flow, acetylcholine, substance P, bradykinin, and CGRP.

Pathologic Vasoconstrictor Function Vasoconstrictor autacoids are released by endothelial cells in several pathologic conditions (hypertension, diabetes, atherosclerosis, acute inflammation), whereas their role in the physiologic control of the coronary circulation is uncertain.

Endothelin-1 (ET-1), a 21-aminoacid peptide released abluminally by endothelial cells, is the most powerful vasoconstrictor known.[34] Despite its short plasmatic half-life (about 5 min), it exerts a prolonged action, interacting with two major types of receptors ($ET_A$ and $ET_B$) and activating the membrane phospholipase C. Its release is reduced by NO and stimulated by thrombin, angiotensin II, catecholamines, interleukin-1$\beta$, and transforming growth factor $\beta$ as well as by hypoxia and ischemia.[35] ET-1 was shown to exert a potent vasoconstrictor effect on small coronary vessels; in dogs, intracoronary infusion of ET-1 causes a severe reduction in coronary flow without constricting angiographically detectable arteries (see below). Recent findings suggest that ET-1 may have some role in the physiologic control of coronary tone, as flow and resistance in apparently normal coronary arteries can be influenced by ET-1 antagonists.[36]

Other endothelial constrictor substances released from activated endothelium may include angiotensin II (produced through a local angiotensin-converting enzyme) and endothelium-derived contracting factors such as prostaglandin $H_2$ and oxygen-derived free radicals.[37]

## Blood/Vessel Wall Interface

In addition to its vasomotor function, the endothelium plays a major role in the homeostasis of the vessel wall and the control of the blood/vessel wall interface. The latter is of fundamental importance, as coronary thrombosis is a major pathogenetic mechanism of acute coronary syndromes.

### HOMEOSTASIS OF THE VESSEL WALL

Endothelial cells produce several constituents of the basement membrane and of the intercellular intimal matrix. They also synthesize growth factors for smooth muscle cells as well as inhibitors of cellular growth and migration, such as heparan sulfates and NO.[38,39] The integrity of the endothelium is essential for preventing the diffusion of atherogenic components into the arterial wall. The response of smooth muscle cells to trophic stimuli produced by the endothelium depends on their phenotype[40]: cells in the proliferative phenotype respond with increased protein synthesis and proliferation to growth factors and to constrictor stimuli, whereas cells in the mature contractile phenotype respond with contraction.

### CONTROL OF BLOOD/VESSEL WALL INTERFACE

The endothelium plays a key role in preserving blood fluidity and preventing thrombosis (Fig. 46-4*A*). This function is performed by different mechanisms. The glycocalyx of endothelial cells, represented by proteoglycans such as heparan sulfate, forms an electronegative barrier that prevents adhesion of platelets and circulating cells. The production of NO and $PGI_2$ also prevents platelet adhesion and aggregation.[41] Moreover, endothelial cells produce and bind anticoagulants such as heparan sulfate, which catalyze the inactivation of thrombin by plasma antithrombin III, and thrombomodulin, which binds thrombin and protein C, leading ultimately to the inactivation of factors V and VIII. Finally, endothelial cells are involved in fibrinolysis by the secretion of two plasminogen activators, a urokinase type (u-PA) and a tissue type (t-PA).

### ALTERATIONS OF ENDOTHELIAL FUNCTION

***Chronic Endothelial Dysfunction*** Patients with coronary atherosclerosis and also individuals with cardiovascular risk factors (such as hypertension, diabetes, hypercholesterolemia, hyperhomocysteinemia, and smoking) show a reduced or abolished vasodilator response to acetylcholine, suggesting an impairment of NO synthesis.[33] However, acetylcholine is also a direct, powerful constrictor of vascular smooth muscle cells; therefore it is impossible to establish whether an abnormal vasomotor response to acetylcholine is due to defective endothelial EDRF production or to an enhanced smooth muscle vasoconstrictor response. The latter possibility is suggested by the preserved dilator effect to substance P in atherosclerotic vessels.[42] It is also unknown to what extent an abnormal response to acetylcholine implies alterations of the endothelial antithrombotic properties.

***Acute Inflammatory Activation*** Increasing evidence suggests that inflammatory activation of the endothelium may play a role in the pathogenesis of some acute ischemic syndromes, determining a rapid switch of its functional properties from vasodilator to vasoconstrictor and from anticoagulant to procoagulant.[43,44] Also, in the absence of detectable histologic changes such as erosion or fissure, endothelial activation by inflammatory cytokines abolishes the release of EDRF and $PGI_2$ and stimulates ET-1 release, induces the expression of tissue factor and of adhesive receptors for platelets and leukocytes on the luminal surface, causes the production of plasminogen activator inhibitors (PAI-1), and inhibits that of plasminogen activators (u-PA, t-PA) and of heparan sulfate (Fig. 46-4*B*). In addition, cytokines may also activate metalloproteases, with consequent endothelial erosions and lysis of the plaque caps.[45,46] The causes of such an inflammatory process may be multiple, acute and chronic, infectious or noninfectious,[47] and variably modulated by the individual inflammatory and immune responses.[48,49]

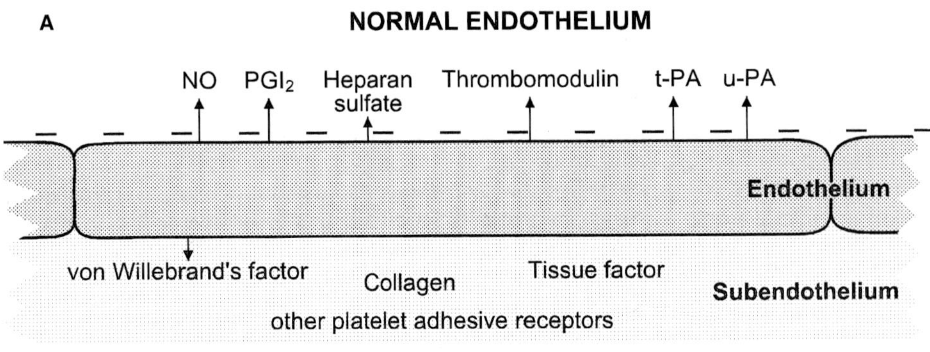


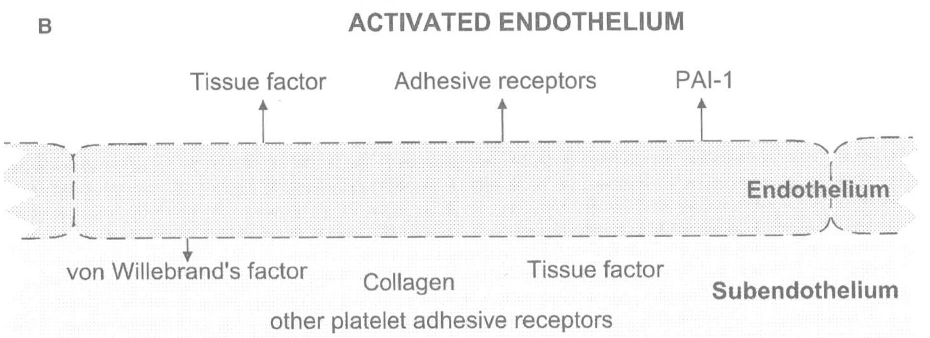


FIGURE 46-4 Anticoagulant role of normal endothelium (*A*) and procoagulant role of activated endothelium (*B*). The anticoagulant properties are due to electronegative charges, to the production of nitric oxide (NO) (which antagonizes platelet adhesion), prostacyclin ($PGI_2$) (which antagonizes platelet aggregation), heparan sulfate (which catalyzes binding of antithrombin III to thrombin), thrombomodulin (which activates protein C), and tissue and urokinase plasminogen activators (t-PA and u-PA) (which activate plasminogen). Activation of the endothelium causes the loss of anticoagulant functions, the expression of adhesive receptors for leukocytes and platelets, and the production of tissue factor and of plasminogen activator inhibitors (PAI-1). (From Maseri and Sanna.[46] With permission.)

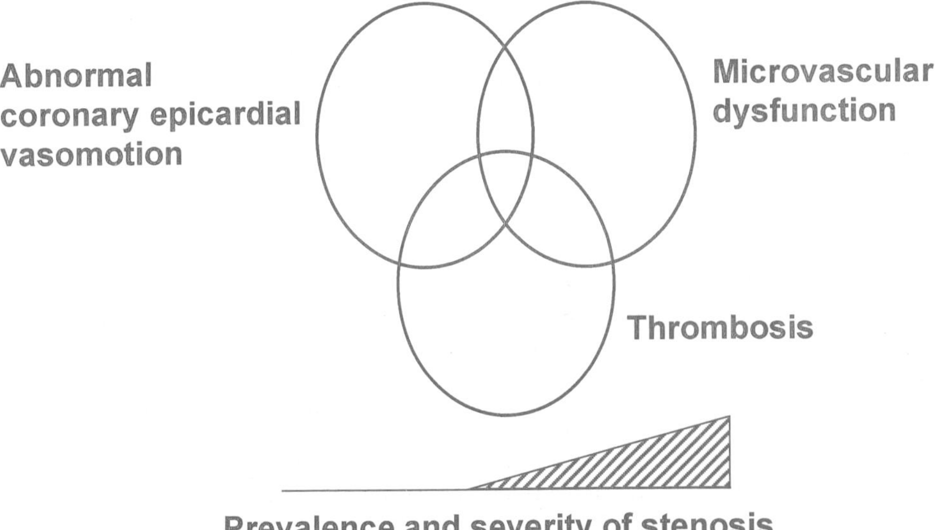


FIGURE 46-5 Pathophysiologic components of myocardial ischemia. The different clinical ischemic syndromes may result from fixed obstruction to coronary blood flow caused by atherosclerotic plaques, from coronary vasoconstriction of epicardial or of microvascular vessels, and from coronary thrombosis. (Modified from Maseri A, Crea F, Lanza GA: Coronary vasoconstriction: Where do we stand in 1999. An important, multifaceted but elusive role. *Cardiologia* 1999;44:115. With permission.)

Therefore, acute activation of the endothelium and of the vascular wall is one of the possible mechanisms that set the stage for local thrombosis and vasoconstriction in the presence of a very variable severity of the chronic atherosclerotic background.

## MECHANISMS OF MYOCARDIAL ISCHEMIA

Myocardial ischemia develops when coronary blood flow becomes inadequate to meet the requirements of the myocardium for oxygen and metabolic substrates to maintain adequate cardiac function. Myocardial ischemia can result from (1) an increase of myocardial workload, and hence oxygen demand, in the presence of a flow-limiting coronary artery stenosis or (2) a reduction of coronary blood flow caused by epicardial or microvascular coronary artery constriction or by acute thrombosis. These mechanisms may act in combination in some patients as well as in different ischemic episodes in a same patient (Fig. 46-5).[50]

In clinical practice, coronary stenoses are often considered the only or main cause of myocardial ischemia because they are the most obvious and readily plausible culprit. Acute thrombosis can be recognized only until thrombi are lysed or become incorporated into the atherosclerotic plaques. The detection of coronary spasm and of dynamic stenosis is even more elusive, because they are very transient and usually require repetition of angiography following nitrates or provocative tests. Finally, microvascular constriction may be inferred only indirectly by slow distal progression of the flow of dye at angiography or by special diagnostic studies.

The clinical presentation of anginal syndromes can provide useful clues as to the role of these distinct pathogenetic mechanisms in precipitating myocardial ischemia.

### Flow-Limiting Stenosis

#### EFFECTS OF FLOW-LIMITING STENOSIS ON BLOOD FLOW

The presence of epicardial coronary artery stenosis, caused by atherosclerotic plaques, is by far the most frequent angiographic finding in any cardiac ischemic syndrome. However, a stenosis becomes flow-limiting only when it determines a measurable transstenotic pressure gradient at rest. The transstenotic pressure gradient increases with increases in flow, more than doubling when blood flow doubles.

A basal gradient at rest may not cause myocardial ischemia, as flow is maintained by compensatory distal arteriolar dilatation. This, however results in a local reduction of coronary flow reserve. The greater the basal transstenotic pressure gradient, the greater the reduction of coronary flow reserve and the lower the level of cardiac work at which myocardial ischemia appears during effort (*ischemic threshold*). Experimental studies in dogs have shown that the acute reduction of coronary diameter by >50 percent causes a measurable basal transstenotic pressure gradient.[51] Further decreases in diameter cause an exponential increase of transstenotic pressure gradient and a reduction of maximal coronary blood flow (Fig. 46-6). A sudden 85 to 90 percent reduction in diameter of an epicardial coronary artery is required to cause myocardial ischemia at rest. The decrease in poststenotic pressure may be reduced by the gradual development of collateral blood flow (see below).

The general relationship between the severity of coronary stenosis, as assessed on coronary angiography, and impairment of coronary flow reserve has been confirmed in patients.[52,53] However, angiographic judgment of the hemodynamic consequences of coronary stenoses is difficult because (1) quantitative angiography does not permit an accurate three-dimensional measure of stenosis; (2) the luminal reduction is estimated with reference to the coronary segment proximal to the stenosis, which may be restricted by atheroma or, conversely, enlarged because of vascular remodeling; (3) the stenotic resistance is linearly related to the length of the stenosis and the flow turbulence caused by stenotic irregularities.

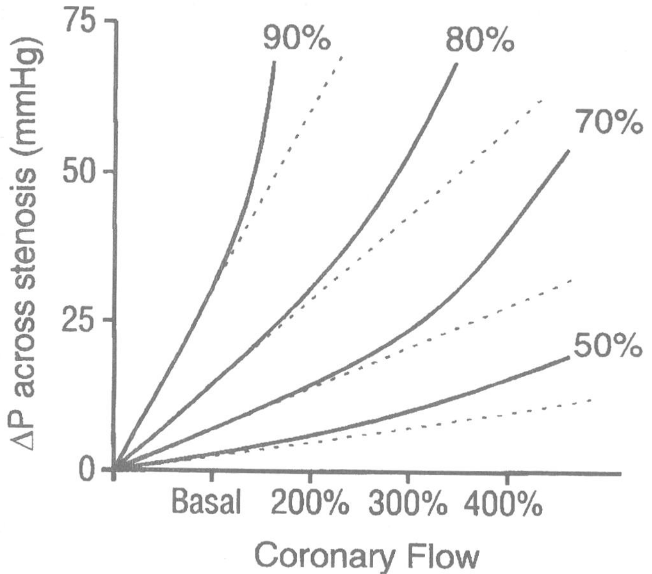


FIGURE 46-6 Schematic illustration of the relationship between coronary blood flow and the transstenotic pressure gradient. This relationship becomes curvilinear because of energy losses caused by blood flow turbulence across the stenosis (*solid lines*). Poststenotic pressure decreases progressively with the increase of stenosis severity and, for a given stenosis, it decreases markedly with increasing flow. In the absence of collateral flow, a stenosis 80 percent in diameter causes a drop in poststenotic pressure of about 12 mmHg, which would increase to about 30 mmHg when flow doubles. (Modified from Gallagher et al.[170] With permission.)

Several invasive and noninvasive methods have been proposed to assess the hemodynamic significance of coronary stenosis.[54] The measurement of fractional flow reserve (FFR) has been suggested as one of the most reliable of these.[55] FFR is calculated as the ratio between the mean pressures distal and proximal to the stenosis during maximal vasodilatation, usually obtained by intracoronary adenosine.* A FFR <0.75 is usually believed to indicate that the stenosis is capable of causing myocardial ischemia. However, the assessment of coronary stenoses can also more easily be done—after intracoronary nitrates have been administered to eliminate the possible vasomotor component of the stenosis—by direct measurement of the basal transstenotic pressure gradient. Indeed, in the absence of a measurable basal gradient, the development of ischemia, at rest or even during effort, should not be attributed to the hemodynamic effect of the stenosis.

## DYNAMIC MODULATION OF CORONARY STENOSES

Coronary flow-limiting stenoses are caused by concentric or eccentric atherosclerotic plaques with or without the potential for local vasomotor changes. Fixed flow-limiting stenoses present as smooth muscle cell atrophy and/or plaque rigidity and are associated with a predictable ischemic threshold during physical effort. Dynamic stenoses are usually eccentric, with compliant segments of the wall and preserved muscular media, and are associated with a variable ischemic threshold. The vasomotor potential of coronary stenoses can also be assessed directly at angiography by intracoronary infusion of vasodilator and/or vasoconstrictor substances.[56,57] Vasoconstriction at the site of stenosis may result from increased release of neural or local vasoconstrictor stimuli, impaired vasodilator mechanisms, abnormal response of dysfunctional vascular smooth muscle cells to vasoactive stimuli, or a variable combination of these mechanisms. For example, exercise and cold pressor testing cause vasodilatation in normal vessels but vasoconstriction at the site of stenosis.[58,59] Vasoconstrictor autacoids, produced locally by the endothelium (endothelin),[60,61] in the adventitia (histamine, leukotrienes), or released by activated platelets (thromboxane $A_2$, serotonin) are also powerful potential constrictor stimuli. Defective production and/or release of vasodilator substances (in particular EDRF) may increase basal coronary tone and prevent flow-mediated arterial vasodilatation during increased $M\dot{V}O_2$.[62–64] In animal models and possibly also in unstable patients, the severity of the stenosis may be modulated by the transient deposition of platelet aggregates.

## CORONARY COLLATERAL CIRCULATION

The drop in poststenotic pressure caused by flow-limiting stenoses stimulates the development of collateral circulation from other coronary artery beds. The blood flow from collateral vessels increases poststenotic pressure, thus improving coronary flow reserve.

Collateral vessels develop from the progressive enlargement of preexisting intercoronary arterial anastomoses. These vary greatly in number among mammalian species, being more numerous in guinea pigs and dogs, less so in pigs and rats, and practically absent in rabbits and sheep. Blood flow through these anastomoses begins, as a consequence of the flow-limiting stenosis, when a pressure gradient develops between their origin and termination.[50]

*Specifically, FFR is calculated by using the formula

$$(P_d - P_v)/(P_a - P_v)$$

where $P_d$ = intracoronary pressure distal to stenosis, $P_a$ = mean aortic pressure, and $P_v$ = central venous pressure (which, in normal conditions, can be considered equal to 0 mmHg).

Preexisting anastomoses are progressively transformed into mature collaterals over a period of 3 to 6 months by initial widening and remodeling, subsequent proliferation of endothelial and smooth muscle cells, and the development of a smooth muscle coat, leading to vessels with a final diameter of 20 to 200 $\mu$m. Collateral blood flow may also develop by the formation of new vessels, but in the dog this mechanism contributes less than 5 percent of total collateral flow.[50]

Blood flow through collaterals is determined by the driving pressure and the vessels' resistance, which is influenced by neural and humoral stimuli and by local vasoactive autacoids.[65–68]

In patients with flow-limiting stenoses, the number and size of collateral vessels is quite variable. At one extreme, some patients with an occluded coronary artery do not have signs of ischemia because the collateral circulation provides an adequate blood supply to the territory of the occluded coronary branch. At the other extreme, some patients with severe flow-limiting coronary stenosis do not show detectable improvement of their ischemic threshold over time; when the vessel occludes, they develop myocardial infarction. These individual differences in coronary collateral circulation are probably due to genetic factors.[69]

In experimental animals, no intervention was convincingly shown to improve the development of collateral vessels. In patients, heparin[70] and fibroblastic growth factor-1 (FGF-1)[71,72] have been suggested to promote collateral growth, but the data are not yet definitive. Recent observations have demonstrated a role for insulin in regulating the gene expression for VEGF and its receptors in microvascular and cardiac tissue.[73]

### CORONARY STEAL DISTAL TO FLOW-LIMITING STENOSIS

In the presence of flow-limiting stenosis, myocardial ischemia may develop as a result of a diversion of blood flow from a myocardial region with a very severe impairment of coronary flow reserve—determining an almost maximal arteriolar dilatation in basal conditions—to a myocardial region with sufficiently preserved coronary flow reserve.

Such a coronary diversion may occur (1) from the subendocardium, as a result of vasodilatation of subepicardial vessels, which increases subepicardial flow but causes a further critical decline in poststenotic pressure (*transmural coronary steal*),[50,74] or (2) from collateralized territories when the coronary artery supplying the collaterals also presents a flow-limiting stenosis proximal to their origin. In the latter case, arteriolar dilatation in the territory of the stenosed parent artery causes increased flow but a further drop in perfusion pressure at the origin of collaterals, which reduces collateral flow (*lateral coronary steal*).[75] In both instances the vasodilatation responsible for the steal can be induced by vasodilator drugs or an increase in $M\dot{V}O_2$.

## Coronary Artery Spasm

Coronary artery spasm is the pathogenetic mechanism of variant angina, but it can play a role in some patients who present with acute coronary syndromes.

### CORONARY SPASM IN VARIANT ANGINA

In patients who present with a variant form of angina (see below), myocardial ischemia is caused by an occlusive epicardial coronary spasm.[50] Spasm may develop at the site of subcritical or critical stenosis as well as in angiographically normal coronary arteries. Occlusive spasm usually causes transmural ischemia with ST-segment elevation. In some cases, however, spasm is subocclusive and causes subendocardial ischemia with ST-segment depression.[76]

In patients with variant angina, spasm tends to recur in the same arterial segment and can be precipitated by sympathetic and parasympathetic stimuli and by a variety of triggers—such as ergonovine, histamine, dopamine, acetylcholine, and serotonin—acting on different receptors as well as by an increase in arterial pH to 7.65 or 7.70.[77–82] Collectively, these findings suggest a hyperreactivity of local smooth muscle to a wide variety of constrictor stimuli. This may be caused by a variety of postreceptorial intracellular abnormalities.[50,65] Some cellular mechanisms potentially able to contribute to the induction of coronary spasm have recently been described; these include increased rho-kinase activity,[83] ATP-sensitive membrane potassium channels,[84] and membrane sodium-hydrogen countertransport.[85]

The postmortem findings at the site of coronary spasm are not specific, but fibromuscular hyperplasia was observed in some cases. The animal model of coronary spasm developed in minipigs,[86] on the other hand, is unlikely to adequately reflect the mechanisms of vasospastic angina occurring in patients.

### CORONARY SPASM IN ACUTE CORONARY SYNDROMES

Although occlusive spasm is typically observed in patients with variant angina, it may also represent a pathogenetic component of other, more common acute coronary syndromes, including unstable angina,[87] unheralded myocardial infarction,[88,89] resuscitated sudden cardiac death,[90] and post–coronary bypass graft angina.[91] In fact, there appears to be a higher prevalence of coronary spasm in patients with acute coronary syndromes (20 to 38 percent) than in those with stable angina (<6 percent).[50] Coronary spasm has been found to occur more frequently in Asian than in Caucasian patients with a recent acute myocardial infarction[89] (Fig. 46-7).

The differences in clinical presentation between variant angina and other ischemic syndromes suggest possible different underlying pathogenetic mechanisms. In the case of unstable plaques, the degree of constriction produced by thromboxane $A_2$, serotonin, and thrombin can be amplified at the site of fresh mural thrombi; in some patients, a local smooth muscle coronary hyperreactivity may contribute to the transition from a nonocclusive platelet-fibrin mural thrombus to an occlusive red thrombus.[50]

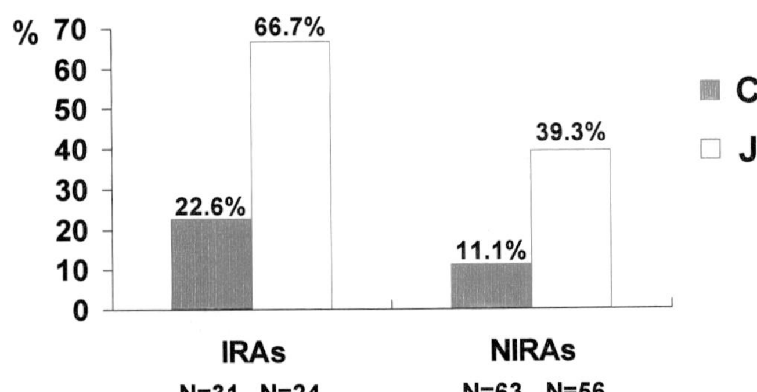


FIGURE 46-7 Induction of coronary spasm by intracoronary acetylcholine injection in infarct-related arteries (IRAs) and non-infarct-related arteries (NIRAs) of Japanese (J) and Italian (C) patients with recent acute myocardial infarctions. Japanese patients had about a threefold higher prevalence of spastic response in both IRAs and NIRAs. The spastic response was more frequent in IRAs than in NIRAs in Japanese but not in Italian Caucasian patients. (Modified from Pristipino et al.[89] With permission.)

## Small Coronary Vessel Dysfunction

The possibility that an impairment of coronary blood flow might occur at the level of distal rather than proximal coronary vessels has received little consideration until recently, as epicardial coronary artery stenoses, spasm, and thrombosis seemed to provide readily available, plausible mechanisms for ischemia. However, several animal and clinical studies have indicated that ischemia can also be caused by the constriction of small coronary vessels.[92,93]

### PHARMACOLOGIC STUDIES IN HUMANS

In patients with angiographically normal coronary arteries, the intracoronary infusion of neuropeptide Y and of high doses of acetylcholine were found to induce myocardial ischemia without any change in the large epicardial vessels but with extremely slow progression of dye or diffuse constriction of distal branches, respectively, indicating microvascular constriction.[50,94] Furthermore, in patients with coronary stenosis, the intracoronary infusion of serotonin caused myocardial ischemia with only small changes in the size of the stenotic lumen but with diffuse constriction of distal branches and reduced filling of collateral vessels.[50,94]

### CLINICAL CLUES TO MICROVASCULAR DYSFUNCTION

In some patients in whom myocardial ischemic episodes cannot be blamed on fixed or dynamic epicardial coronary stenosis, constriction of small coronary vessels may account for the development of myocardial ischemia. Patients with occlusion of a single epicardial coronary artery and no other stenosis may present very wide variations in the ischemic threshold during daily life and exercise testing, which cannot be attributed to dynamic modulation of the stenosis or spasm and are most likely caused by vasomotor changes in small, distal coronary vessels.[95]

*Patients with single-vessel disease following successful coronary angioplasty (PTCA) may* continue to present with angina, ST-segment depression on exercise testing, and perfusion defects on stress myocardial scintigraphy[96]; in such patients a dysfunction of small coronary vessels has been confirmed by intracoronary Doppler blood flow measurements and myocardial positron emission tomography (PET) following administration of vasodilator stimuli.[97,98] Microvascular dysfunction is most likely responsible for the reduced coronary dilator response of nonstenosed coronary arteries in patients with coronary disease[99,100] and also in those with risk factors but no flow-limiting coronary stenoses.[101,102]

*Patients with syndrome X,* who present angina pectoris, positive exercise testing, but angiographically normal coronary arteries and no evidence of epicardial spasm,[103] may suffer from some form of microvascular dysfunction. Such a possibility is suggested by stress-induced myocardial perfusion defects on radionuclide studies,[104,105] by transient ischemic ST-segment changes during effort testing, and by the reproduction of typical anginal pain, with or without ST-segment ischemic changes, on dipyridamole testing.

An ischemic origin of this syndrome is widely questioned because in the vast majority of studies, no myocardial lactate production or left ventricular dysfunction can be detected during angina and transient ischemic ST-segment changes.[106,107] This apparent paradox may be explained by a patchily distributed coronary microvascular dysfunction that is causing dispersed small foci of ischemia. A patchily distributed small vessel constriction may not cause detectable contractile abnormalities or lactate production but produce electrocardiographic (ECG) changes and myocardial perfusion defects when sufficiently confluent.[50,94] Observations in animal models, in which ischemia was caused by impairing coronary microcirculation with microspheres[50] or endothelin-1 infusion,[108] support this concept.

Recent data in syndrome X patients showing intracardiac production of lipid peroxidation products[109] following atrial pacing, stress-induced metabolic evidence of myocardial ischemia by phosphorous nuclear magnetic resonance, *and an abnormal flow response to adenosine on nuclear magnetic resonance strongly support the microvascular ischemic origin of this syndrome.*[110–113]

### SITE OF MICROVASCULAR DYSFUNCTION

Theoretically, myocardial ischemia caused by microvascular dysfunction may result from abnormal constriction or failure of adequate dilatation of arteriolar or prearteriolar vessels. Arteriolar constriction as a cause of myocardial ischemia would require constrictor stimuli sufficiently strong to overcome the dilator effect of ischemic metabolites on the arterioles themselves.[50,94] The constriction of prearteriolar vessels appears a more likely cause of the microvascular alterations responsible for myocardial ischemia. An increased patchy distribution of prearteriolar vasoconstriction has been proposed as a causal mechanism of syndrome X[50,94] (Fig. 46-8).

### MECHANISMS OF MICROVASCULAR DYSFUNCTION

In patients with coronary stenoses, small coronary vessel dysfunction is commonly attributed to atherosclerosis, although it may also be related to neurohumoral stimuli[114] or vascular abnormalities (e.g., perivascular fibrosis, medial hypertrophy) associated with systemic diseases, such as hypertension or diabetes.[115,116] Small vessel dysfunction in these patients is also frequently attributed to EDRF deficiency on the basis of an abnormal vasomotor response to acetylcholine, but a reduced vasodilator response or a vasoconstrictor response to acetylcholine[117,118] could also be caused by an increased constrictor effect of the drug on smooth muscle cells.

In patients with syndrome X, the mechanisms responsible for microvascular dysfunction can be multiple and not necessarily the same in all patients. They may include (1) structural abnormalities, such as fibrosis and medial hyperthrophy[50]; (2) impaired endothelial and nonendothelial vasodilator function[119]; (3) enhanced constrictor response of smooth muscle cells, possibly involving increased membrane $Na^+$-$H^+$ exchanger or intracellular rho-kinase activity[120–122]; (4) increased release of local vasoconstrictor autacoids (e.g., endothelin-1[123,124] or angiotensin[50]); and (5) abnormal neural stimuli. Evidence of abnormal cardiac sympathetic function was documented by $^{123}$I-metaiodobenzylguanidine (MIBG) scintigraphy, which showed total absence of cardiac MIBG uptake in 42 percent of patients and regional defects, matching thallium perfusion defects, in another 33 percent.[125] (Fig. 46-9).

## Acute Thrombosis

Intraluminal thrombi are the most common finding in patients with acute coronary syndromes. Most thrombi are composed of platelets and fibrin in variable proportions; they often develop at the site of non-flow-limiting coronary stenosis. Thrombosis may reduce or interrupt blood flow by itself or in combination with local or distal vasoconstriction (triggered by thromboxane, serotonin, and thrombin)[126] (Fig. 46-10). Fresh thrombi may have a different fate, as they may grow to occlude the artery, lyse completely, or become organized and contribute to plaque growth.

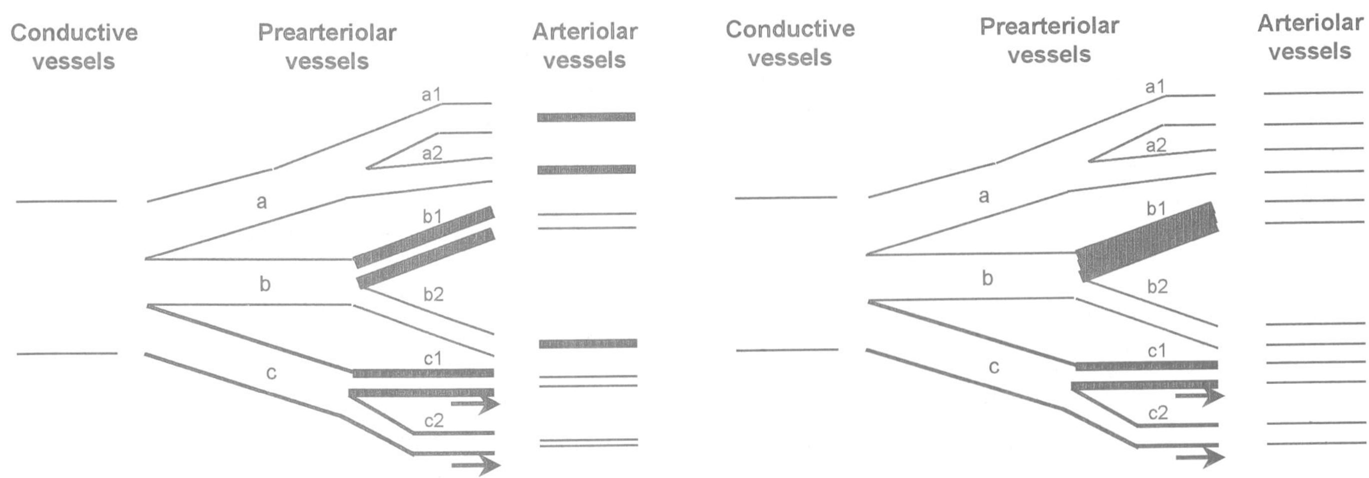


FIGURE 46-8 Model of patchily distributed prearteriolar vasoconstriction in syndrome X. Such a constriction may be present in basal conditions (b1,c1,c2) (*left panel*). As flow increases during metabolic or pharmacologic arteriolar dilation, the pressure drop through constricted prearterioles increases and perfusion pressure at the origin of distal arterioles decreases, thus resulting in small focal areas of myocardial ischemia (*right panel*). Blood flow steal may also occur from the territory supplied by the most constricted prearterioles toward regions supplied by less constricted prearteriolar vessels (c1,c2). At the ends of severely constricted prearterioles, distending pressure may become lower than the critical closing pressure, thus resulting in prearteriolar occlusion (b1). Compensatory myocardial release of adenosine in response to blood flow reduction distal to constricted prearterioles may be sufficient to maintain adequate flow, thus avoiding ischemia, but it may cause angina, particularly when it is associated with enhanced pain sensitivity. (Modified from Maseri A, Crea F, Kaski JC, et al. Mechanisms of angina pectoris in syndrome X. *J Am Coll Cardiol* 1991;17:499. With permission)

## MECHANISMS OF ACUTE THROMBOSIS

Intracoronary thrombosis may result from strong or weak thrombogenic stimuli.[126] *Strong thrombogenic stimuli* cause rapid thrombus growth with massive inclusion of red cells in the fibrin mesh (*red thrombi*), leading to persistent vessel occlusion within few minutes, as in the copper coil animal model. Strong thrombogenic stimuli may be represented by the mechanical rupture of a lipid-rich atherosclerotic plaque. *Weak thrombogenic stimuli* cause slow, progressive deposition of platelets and formation of platelet-fibrin thrombi (*white thrombi,* as in the electrical wire animal model). Weak thrombogenic stimuli may result from the fissure of plaques with low thrombogenic potential or from a local inflammatory activation of the vascular wall caused by infectious or noninfectious stimuli.[44,127–129] Thrombus growth is determined mainly by the intensity, duration, and recurrence of the weak inflammatory stimuli.

The hypothesis that thrombosis may occur at the site of identifiable "vulnerable" coronary plaques is attractive and is currently stimulating the development of new research tools for their clinical

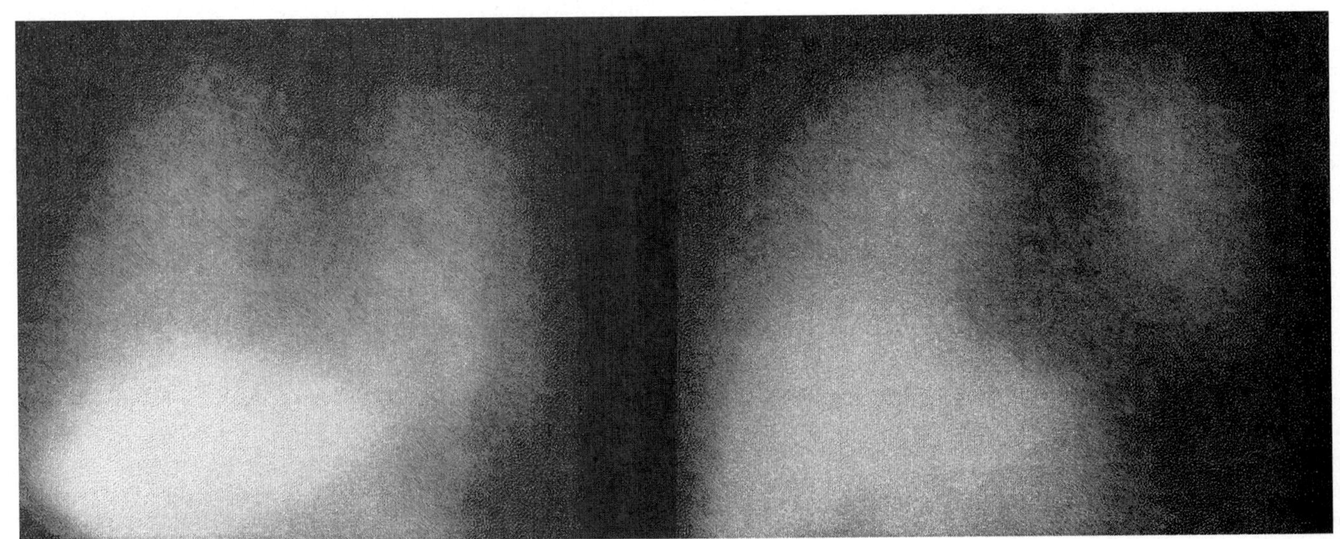

FIGURE 46-9 Typical cardiac scintigrams obtained 3 h after the injection of half a dose of $^{123}$I-metaiodobenzylguanidine (MIBG) in a healthy subject (*left panel*) and the other half in a patient with syndrome X (*right panel*). Cardiac MIBG uptake was normal in the control subject and totally absent in the patient with syndrome X, in contrast with his normal lung and liver MIBG uptake. The total absence of cardiac MIBG uptake was confirmed in follow-up studies at 1 and 12 months, consistent with a persistent impairment of cardiac sympathetic function. (From Ianza et al.[125] With permission.)

detection. However, morphologically or functionally vulnerable plaques may be potential sites of thrombosis because of mechanical rupture (as they have a large central lipid pool and a thin cap)[130] or because they are the site of acute inflammatory processes,[49] which cause endothelial activation and possibly also erosion and rupture. Plaque vulnerability may persist for days, weeks or months. Interestingly, in acute coronary syndromes, vascular inflammation[131] may be associated with multiple fissured and complicated plaques throughout the coronary bed,[132–134] and possibly also in remote vascular areas.[135]

The different mechanisms responsible for or contributing to coronary thrombosis and acute coronary occlusion may not have the same prevalence in different geographic, ethnic, age, and sex groups, yet they may influence the individual response to antiplatelet, antithrombotic, and acute reperfusion strategies.

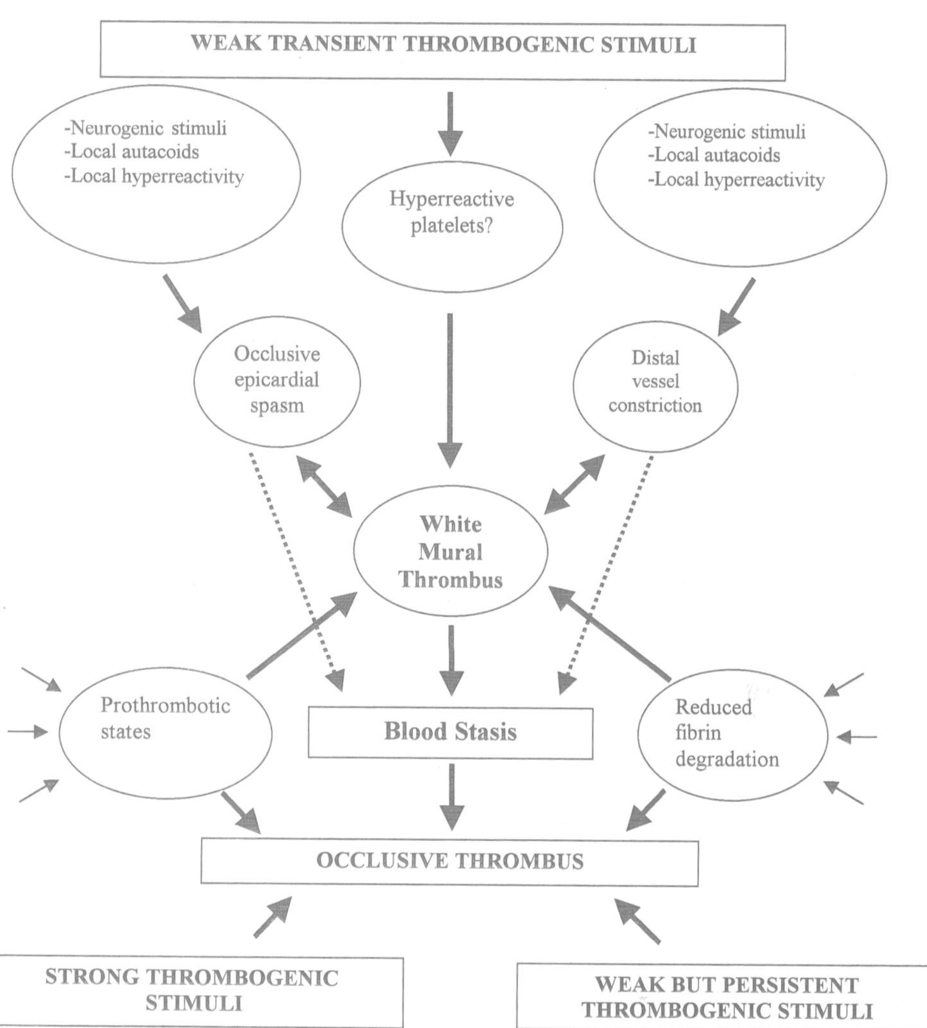


FIGURE 46-10. Vicious cycles leading to the formation and growth of an occlusive coronary thrombus. An occlusive red thrombus can form rapidly, within minutes, at the site of a highly thrombogenic injury (for example, the rupture of a strongly thrombogenic plaque). An occlusive platelet thrombus can form gradually at the site of weak but very persistent thrombogenic stimuli (for example, a persisting inflammatory process). A mural thrombus resulting from a weakly thrombogenic plaque fissure or from a transient local inflammatory process may evolve into occlusive thrombosis only in the presence of prothrombotic states or of blood flow stasis induced by local or distal coronary constriction. The components of these vicious cycles and their gain may have variable importance and prevalence in different groups of patients. Prothrombotic states may result from any acquired or genetic alteration that leads to enhanced platelet reactivity or thrombin activity or to reduced fibrinolysis. (From Virdis et al.[115] With permission.)

## CONSEQUENCES OF MYOCARDIAL ISCHEMIA

### Metabolic Consequences

During ischemia, several metabolic changes occur. Adenosine triphosphate (ATP) is degraded to adenosine, which, diffusing out of cardiomyocytes, causes arteriolar dilation and anginal pain. Free fatty acids and acyl-carnitine accumulate and protein synthesis and turnover are impaired in myocardial cells. Furthermore, myocardial ischemia/reperfusion produces free radicals, which contribute to postischemic myocardial cell dysfunction by reacting with proteins, lipids, and nucleic acids. Impaired $Ca^{2+}$ release from sarcolemma and sarcoplasmic reticulum, inhibition of crossbridge cycling,[136] and the competition of $H^+$ accumulating during ischemia for $Ca^{3+}$ binding sites on contractile proteins, also contribute to systolic dysfunction. Reduced ATP availability, decreasing $Ca^{2+}$ reuptake into sarcoplasmic reticulum, also prolongs interaction of $Ca^{2+}$ with myofilaments, causing diastolic dysfunction.

Impairment of ion pumps causes loss of intracellular $K^+$ and accumulation of intracellular $Na^+$, $Ca^{2+}$, and $H_2O$. Alterations of transsarcolemmal ion gradients may cause increased automaticity, triggered activity, and abnormalities of impulse conduction, which favor the development of reentry circuits.[137]

The consequences of ischemia and ischemia/reperfusion injury may not be limited to the myocytes but extend to endothelial cells, with inflammatory changes[138–140] resulting in vasoconstriction and a local thrombogenic tendency.

### Effects on Cardiac Function

The effects of myocardial ischemia have been studied in experimental animals by producing a sudden coronary occlusion, by gradually reducing coronary flow at rest, and by increasing $M\dot{V}O_2$ in the presence of a flow-limiting coronary stenosis. Such experimental models mimic, at least in part, the consequences of myocardial ischemia observed in variant angina, unstable angina, and effort angina, respectively (see below).

#### EFFECTS OF SUDDEN CORONARY OCCLUSION

Occlusion of a major coronary artery is followed within a few seconds by a typical sequence of events that includes a reduction in the velocity of ventricular relaxation and contraction, ST-segment elevation, increased end-diastolic pressure with dyssynchrony -

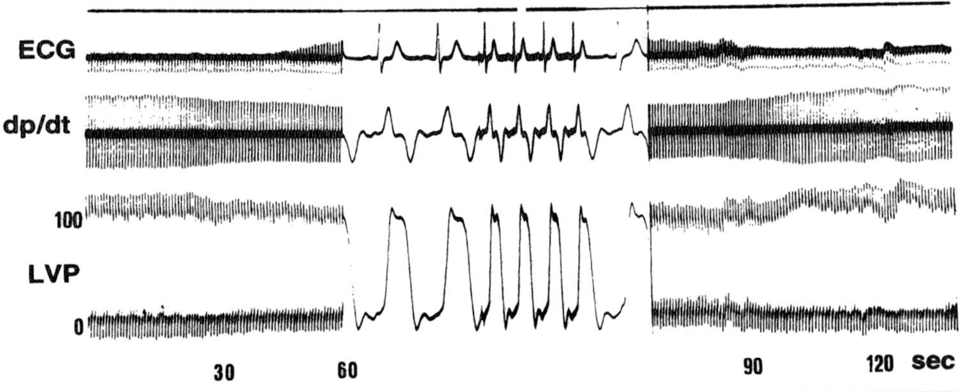


FIGURE 46-11 Sequence of alterations during an ischemic episode caused by left anterior descending coronary artery spasm. The playback at low and high speeds of a spontaneous episode of silent ischemia recorded in the coronary care unit shows a decrease in left ventricular peak relaxation and contraction dp/dt and in systolic pressure; an increase in proto- and end-diastolic pressure clearly precedes the onset of peaking of T waves on the ECG, which is followed by slight ST-segment elevation. The episode resolved spontaneously. This sequence of events is similar to that observed during coronary angioplasty and in the dog following sudden coronary artery ligation. LVP = left ventricular pressure; dp/dt = left ventricular dp/dt; ECG = electrocardiographic tracing. (From Maseri and Sanna.[46] With permission.)

(delayed onset of contraction in ischemic myocardial segments), hypokinesis (reduced contractility), akinesis (cessation of contraction), and dyskinesis (paradoxical expansion of the affected segment during systole). The sequence of hemodynamic and ECG events observed in experimental animals is similar to that observed in patients during episodes of occlusive epicardial coronary artery spasm (Fig. 46-11) or during coronary angioplasty balloon occlusion, typically characterized by the following sequence of events: a decrease in peak relaxation dp/dt, a decrease of peak contraction dp/dt, an increase in diastolic pressures, and a fall in systolic and in pulse pressure. In patients with transmural ischemia caused by occlusive coronary spasm, anginal pain, when it occurs, usually appears later, several seconds or minutes after the induction of ischemia.

## EFFECTS OF GRADED REDUCTION OF CORONARY FLOW AT REST

In anesthetized dogs, a 25 percent reduction of basal coronary blood flow through a major coronary branch is associated with increased myocardial extraction of oxygen and decreased oxygen consumption. Further reductions of flow are followed by a decrease in the rate of left ventricular relaxation and contraction, then by ST-segment depression, elevation of end-diastolic pressure, decreased stroke volume, and finally by elevation of the ST segment, which develops when flow reduction is about 70 percent and myocardial ischemia becomes transmural. Local contractile function in subendocardial layers begins to fall slightly when regional subendocardial flow is reduced by 10 to 20 percent and becomes marked as flow decreases by 50 to 80 percent. Segments with a flow reduction greater than 80 percent show paradoxical movement with bulging of the left ventricular wall (Fig. 46-12).

## EFFECT OF INCREASED WORKLOAD IN THE PRESENCE OF A FLOW-LIMITING STENOSIS

When exercise reduces mean transmural blood flow by 30 percent in chronically instrumented dogs with a coronary artery stenosis, a mild reduction of systolic thickening is observed, whereas in the normally perfused wall, thickening increases by 20 percent. During exercise, severe regional dysfunction develops when mean flow is about 80 percent lower than in nonischemic myocardial segments. Thus a severe reduction in coronary blood flow is necessary to produce detectable effects on global ventricular contractile function.

At variance with the late occurrence of pain following sudden coronary occlusion by spasm, anginal pain during effort induced ischemia may precede ECG changes in about one-third of the cases.

## PRECONDITIONING

The term *preconditioning* was originally used with reference to the ability of short periods of ischemia to limit infarct size after subsequent prolonged coronary occlusion in animals. However, it is now more broadly used also to indicate the improved tolerance of myocardium to ischemia after exposure to previous ischemic episodes. An early ischemic preconditioning after an ischemic episode was reported during the initial 2 h (early preconditioning), but a later protection was also reported beginning 24 h after the preconditioning stimulus and extending to 48 h (delayed preconditioning).[141] Findings compatible with early ischemic preconditioning were reported following balloon occlusion during coronary angioplasty, preinfarction angina, coronary artery bypass surgery, and exercise-induced ischemia (warmup phenomenon).[50] In experimental settings, ischemic preconditioning was also shown to reduce ventricular tachyarrhythmias appearing in the ischemic or reperfusion phase of ischemic episodes, and a reduction of ischemia-related ventricular arrhythmias following episodes of transmural myocardial ischemia was reported in patients with vasospastic angina.[142] Moreover, preconditioning anginal episodes

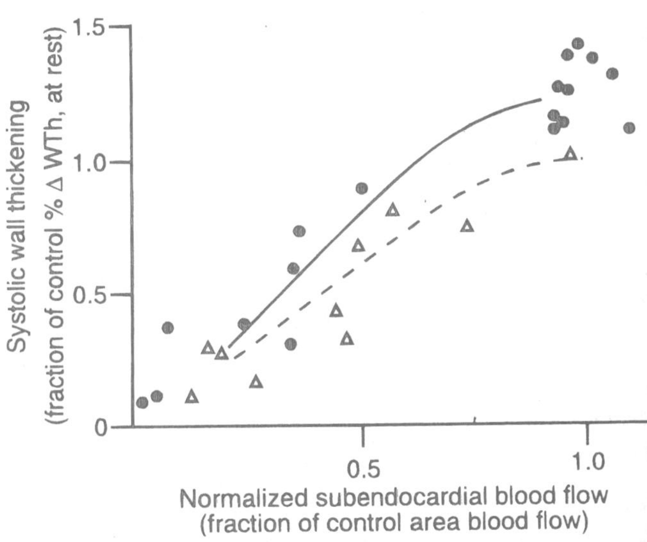


FIGURE 46-12 Effect of decrease of subendocardial blood flow on systolic segment shortening. In conscious dogs, the percentage decrease of subendocardial segment shortening is small until blood flow is reduced by 20 percent. Systolic bulging (segment lengthening) develops only when flow is reduced by more than 80 percent. (Modified from Maseri and Sanna[46] and Gallagher et al.[170] With permission.)

preceding acute myocardial infarction have recently been shown to decrease the occurrence of life-threatening tachyarrhythmias during the acute phase of infarction.[143] Preconditioning could partly explain the more favorable prognosis of patients in whom acute myocardial infarction is preceded by unstable angina.[144,145] The bases of preconditioning are not completely understood. Extrapolation of experimental results to patients should be done with caution. Various mediators released during ischemia, such as adenosine, but also bradykinin, catecholamines, endothelin, opioids and others, can activate G protein–coupled receptors to stimulate phospholipase C and generate diacylglycerol, which is responsible for the translocation and activation of protein kinase C. Other pathways, such as the generation of nitric oxide and intracellular reactive oxygen species, may also activate protein kinase C. Protein kinase C, in turn, activates mithochondrial $K^+_{ATP}$ channels, which appear to play a major role in ischemic preconditioning, probably acting both as mediators and effectors of the protective response.[146] Moreover, protein kinase C and other kinases (such as tyrosine kinase) activate a series of transcription factors to enhance the expression of various genes—including heat-shock proteins, manganese superoxide dismutase, and inducible nitric oxide synthase—that contribute to the resistant phenotype of delayed preconditioning[147] (see Table 46-1). Preconditioning in the human can be abolished by the administration of the oral hypoglycemic glibenclamide, which is a selective inhibitor of $K^+_{ATP}$ channels.[148]

TABLE 46-1 Features of Ischemia, Stunning, and Hibernation[a]

| | Coronary Blood Flow | Lactate Production | Contractile Function |
|---|---|---|---|
| Ischemia | Markedly reduced | Yes | Impaired<br>Recovers after relief of ischemia |
| Stunning | Preserved | No | Impaired<br>Transiently restored by inotropic stimulation<br>Recovers spontaneously over time |
| Hibernation | Reduced in the presence of typical histologic changes | No | Impaired<br>Recovers only after revascularization |

[a]Ischemia is characterized by inadequate perfusion, resulting in lactate production and impaired contractile function. Stunning develops after an ischemia/reperfusion sequence and is characterized by preserved regional blood flow and transient impairment of contractile function, which recovers spontaneously over time. Hibernation may develop after repeated episodes of ischemia/reperfusion and is characterized by myocardial histologic changes, absence of contraction, reduced $M\dot{V}O_2$, and reduced regional blood flow but no lactate production. Contractile function recovers following revascularization over a period of weeks and months.

## STUNNING

The term *stunning* defines a prolonged but reversible contractile dysfunction observed after an episode of transient myocardial ischemia. It has been observed in animals following sudden coronary occlusion lasting 10 to 15 min or after repeated shorter periods of occlusion as well as in patients after positive exercise test, in ischemic periinfarction regions, and following extracorporeal circulation. The spontaneous recovery of cardiac contractile function may take hours or days, depending on the severity and duration of ischemia, but contraction can be transiently restored by inotropic stimuli such as post-extrasystolic potentiation or beta-adrenergic drugs. In stunned myocardium, the delayed recovery of contractile function is associated with normal average myocardial perfusion in presence of reduced myocardial oxygen consumption. It is not clear to what extent stunning represents a gradual physiologic recovery from the ischemic insult or a consequence of a reperfusion-induced injury, which could delay or reduce the benefits of reperfusion.

Several components may contribute to stunning.[149] A decreased $Ca^{2+}$ sensitivity of myofilaments, troponin I degradation by $Ca^{2+}$-activated proteases, $Ca^{2+}$ overload and free radicals generation,[150] slow resynthesis of adenosine nucleotides, microvascular damage with leukocyte activation, myocyte electromechanical uncoupling,[151] and extracellular matrix alterations were all observed in experimental models (see also Table 46-1).

## HIBERNATION

Myocardial *hibernation* was originally defined as a condition of persistent impairment of contractile function at rest in the presence of both reduced $M\dot{V}O_2$ and coronary blood flow and in absence of metabolic evidence of ischemia, which partially or totally recovers when myocardial blood flow is restored. The time to functional recovery of hibernated myocardium after revascularization varies from 10 days to 6 months and is related to the severity of structural changes of cardiomyocytes and interstitium.

Hibernation is characterized[152] by progressive loss of sarcomeres, sarcoplasmic reticulum, and T tubules in cardiomyocytes with glycogen replacement. Mitochondria appear small and scattered and nuclei distorted, with uniformly dispersed heterochromatin. Hibernated myocardial cells have normal ATP, total adenine nucleotides, and phosphocreatine content and exhibit normal glucose uptake and no lactate production. Several of these characteristics suggest that hibernation may be the result of a dedifferentiation process related to changes in gene expression, as hibernated cardiomyocytes show many features of neonatal cardiomyocytes.[152,152a] Hibernation is caused by a severe reduction of coronary flow reserve, as a result of which any increase in $M\dot{V}O_2$ and any further reduction in coronary blood flow (e.g., by vasoconstriction or platelet aggregation) results in repeated episodes of myocardial ischemia/reperfusion (see also Table 46-1).

# Clinical Manifestations of Myocardial Ischemia

## CHEST PAIN

The most obvious clinical manifestation of myocardial ischemia, irrespective of its multiple causal mechanisms, is angina pectoris. However, myocardial ischemia may occur without angina and angina may occur without detectable signs of myocardial ischemia. Typically anginal pain is retrosternal in location, with a crushing, squeezing, or burning character. It may radiate to the throat, neck, ulnar side of the left and/or right arm, interscapular region, epigastrium, and the jaw and teeth. Headache may also be an unusual manifestation of myocardial ischemia.[153] The intensity of the discomfort can vary greatly, from a mild feeling of retrosternal fullness or tingling in only one dermatome to a diffuse, unbearable pain. These features are unrelated to the causes of ischemia and are not completely specific for ischemia, as they may also be due to nonischemic cardiac and extracardiac causes.

Myocardial ischemia with or without angina may occasionally present with other symptoms, including dyspnea (in the case of extensive ischemia with transient impairment of left ventricular function or ischemia of the papillary muscles with mitral regurgitation), palpitations, syncope, or cardiac arrest.

Anginal pain originates from the stimulation of polimodal receptors (more abundant around small coronary vessels) by chemical mediators produced during ischemia.[50] The best-studied of such mediators is adenosine. The algogenic effects of adenosine were studied by its intracoronary infusion and are mediated by $A_1$ receptors, while its vasodilator effects are mediated by $A_2$ receptors.[154] Comparison of pain location during selective intracoronary infusion of adenosine in the right and left coronary artery has shown that in nearly 70 percent of patients, afferent stimuli from different myocardial regions cannot be discriminated, thus suggesting that they converge on the same neurons of the dorsal roots of spinal cord.[155] However, in 30 percent of patients, anginal pain during the infusion of adenosine in the separate coronary beds caused a different location of pain. The possibility that a different location of pain in the same person reflects a different location of myocardial ischemia has been confirmed in patients undergoing PTCA or those with a second myocardial infarction.[156,157] Moreover, convergence of afferent painful stimuli from different visceral organs and somatic dermatomes on the same ascending neurons can cause noncardiac pain to have features indistinguishable from angina.

The central transmission of painful stimuli is modulated at the spinal cord level by a gating system regulated by descending and by afferent stimuli. From the dorsal horns of the spinal cord, afferent stimuli reach thalamic centers and are finally projected to the cortex, where their processing and decoding occur. The pain signal may also undergo modulation in supraspinal centers.

**PAINLESS ISCHEMIA**

Diagnostic techniques capable of detecting myocardial ischemia have shown that ischemic episodes in most cases occur without anginal pain; in some cases, silent ischemia may be the only manifestation of coronary artery disease. Continuous ECG recordings has revealed that about 70 percent of episodes of transient myocardial ischemia do not cause chest pain or any other symptom.[50] The percentage of episodes of silent ischemia is similar in chronic stable angina, unstable angina, variant angina and microvascular angina. Thus, the presence or absence of pain is totally unrelated to the actual cause of transient ischemia. Furthermore, also myocardial infarction may be totally silent in about 20 percent of the cases.

The reasons why myocardial ischemia does not elicit pain in the majority of cases are multiple.[155] Although angina is less likely to accompany myocardial ischemia when it is short lasting, there is no strict relationship between duration and extension of ischemia and development of chest pain also in the same patient.

The gating system at the spinal cord and possibly at the thalamic level, together with the cortical decoding of afferent stimuli, probably plays a major role in determining the perception of pain. Moreover, personality, emotional status, and previous experience of pain may modulate such perception (see also Chap. 57).

**ARRHYTHMIAS**

Arrhythmias are major potential consequences of acute ischemia, as they are responsible for the most part of deaths observed during the early phases of acute myocardial infarction as well as in variant angina, and thus for sudden death in the community.

During ischemia, increased automaticity, triggered activity, conduction delay and re-entry may all cause the development of ventricular tachycardia and fibrillation. Moreover, altered impulse formation and conduction defects may cause asystole and atrioventricular block.

Arrhythmic response to ischemic insult of individual patients is unpredictable, but is influenced by the cardiac anatomical background (left ventricular hypertrophy, previous infarction) and by nervous autonomic imbalance with predominance of sympathetic activity. It may also be related to the regulation of cardiac sodium channels ($Na_v1.5$) by growth factors (FGF12B) whose level of expression in adult heart may vary.[158]

Fatal ventricular arrhythmias are exceptional during mild subendocardial ischemia, but may develop during or soon after the termination of episodes of transmural ischemia, caused by occlusive spasm or thrombosis, or even of severe subendocardial ischemia. Reperfusion arrhythmias, although particularly common in anaesthetized animals, are less frequently observed both in patients with variant angina and during myocardial reperfusion in acute myocardial infarction.[50]

### Effects of Persistent Myocardial Ischemia: Myocardial Infarction

In dogs, focal cell necrosis begins about 20 minutes following coronary flow interruption. Such foci become confluent in subendocardial layers by 40 minutes, reaching subepicardial layers with a progressive wavefront at about 3–4 hours. By this time, necrosis has developed, on average, to about 90 percent of its final extension, which is reached after 6 hours. Apoptosis has also been shown to accompany necrosis as a mechanism of cell death during myocardial infarction.[159]

In patients, the extension of myocardial necrosis depends not only on the area perfused by the occluded vessel, the level of myocardial oxygen consumption and the presence of collaterals, but also on the intermittence of coronary occlusion. Actually, myocardial infarction is a dynamic process with intermittence of occlusion occurring in about 2/3 of the cases during the initial 6 hours[50]. Therefore, it is reasonable to undertake reperfusion strategies in all patients irrespective of actual delay from the onset of symptoms as long as ECG shows persistent massive ischemia without completed necrosis. The impairment of global myocardial function depends on the extension of myocardial necrosis. When infarction involves more than 15 percent of left ventricle, ejection fraction decreases. When it involves more than 25 percent of left ventricle, signs of heart failure develop, and when it involves more than 40 percent, cardiogenic shock occurs.

The development of primary ventricular fibrillation is independent of infarct size, but strongly influenced by high adrenergic tone.

## RELATIONSHIP BETWEEN MECHANISMS OF ISCHEMIA AND CLINICAL SYNDROMES

The mechanisms responsible for the development of ischemia do no influence the location and radiation of anginal pain but may deter mine specific clinical patterns of anginal episodes which, at least in typical cases, provide useful clues for personalized patient manage ment. Therefore a carefully collected clinical history is the fundamental first step in the assessment of the pathogenetic mechanisms of myocardial ischemia and for the selection of the appropriate sequence of diagnostic tests.

## Chronic Stable Angina

Among patients presenting with chronic stable angina, some report that anginal pain develops predictably only and every time they exceed a rather fixed level of exertion that they learn to recognize and avoid. Pain disappears within 1 to 2 min after the interruption of the effort or after the ingestion of sublingual nitrates. In these patients, the fixed anginal threshold suggests that myocardial ischemia is caused exclusively by an excessive increase in oxygen demand in the presence of a fixed coronary stenosis (*fixed threshold effort angina*).

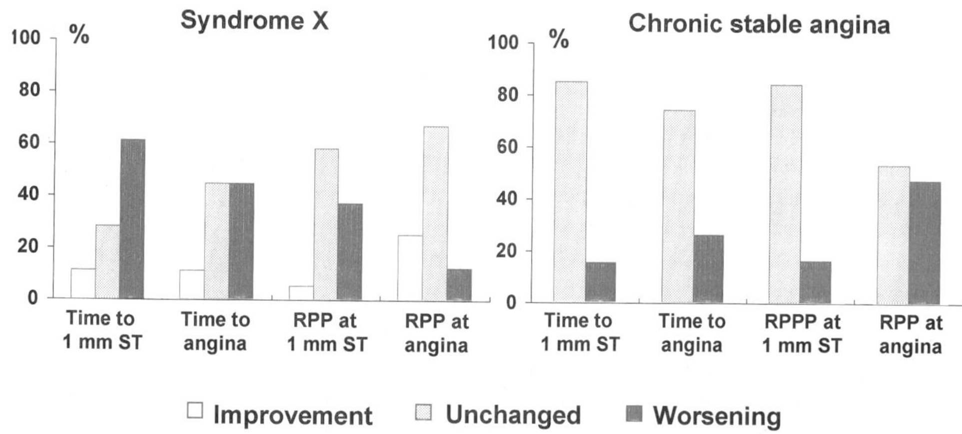


FIGURE 46-13 Acute effects of nitrates on exercise testing in syndrome X. The administration of isosorbide dinitrate (ISDN, 5 mg sublingual) significantly improved exercise test variables in patients with chronic stable angina and documented coronary artery disease (*right panel*). In contrast, ISDN caused a worsening of exercise variables in a significant number of patients with syndrome X (*left panel*). ST = ST segment; RPP = rate pressure product. (Modified from Lanza GA, Manzoli A, Bia E, et al. Acute effects of nitrates on exercise testing in patients with syndrome X. Clinical and pathophysiologic implications. *Circulation* 1994;90:2695. With permission.)

On careful questioning, however, the majority of patients with chronic stable angina report that they have a variable threshold for angina, which sometimes develops in the course of efforts that are usually well tolerated and occasionally also at rest (*mixed angina*). A variable ischemic threshold is suggestive of a strong modulation of residual flow reserve by changes in vasomotor tone at the level of a potential flow-limiting stenosis or in distal vessels and may represent an indication for vasodilator therapy.

## Syndrome X

Patients with a chronic stable pattern of effort or mixed angina, "ischemic" ST-segment depression, and/or myocardial perfusion defects during stress testing but with angiographically normal coronary arteries are classified as having syndrome X.[103] In these patients, angina also predominantly occurs on exertion, typically with a variable ischemic threshold, and occasionally at rest but very seldom at night. Although the location and radiation of pain are often indistinguishable from those of patients with flow-limiting stenosis, some distinct features raise the suspicion of syndrome X: (1) patients usually report persistence of angina for several minutes after the end of exertion, and many report attacks lasting over 30 min; (2) they often have a poor response to sublingual nitrates, which may also impair the results of exercise testing, in contrast to the established favorable effects of nitrates in patients with flow-limiting stenosis (Fig. 46-13); (3) they show a variable individual response to prophylactic long-acting nitrates, calcium antagonists, and beta blockers[160]; (4) they develop their typical pain (often with ischemic ECG changes) during dipyridamole testing but without developing left ventricular contractile abnormalities; (5) they often have an enhanced sensitivity to painful cardiac stimuli,[161] which helps to explain the paradox of severe angina in the absence of detectable myocardial contractile dysfunction (Fig. 46-14); (6) Holter monitoring demonstrates that some episodes of chest pain and ST segment depression in these patients are not associated with tachycardia, and it may show episodes of transient ST-segment depression in patients with a negative exercise test.[162]

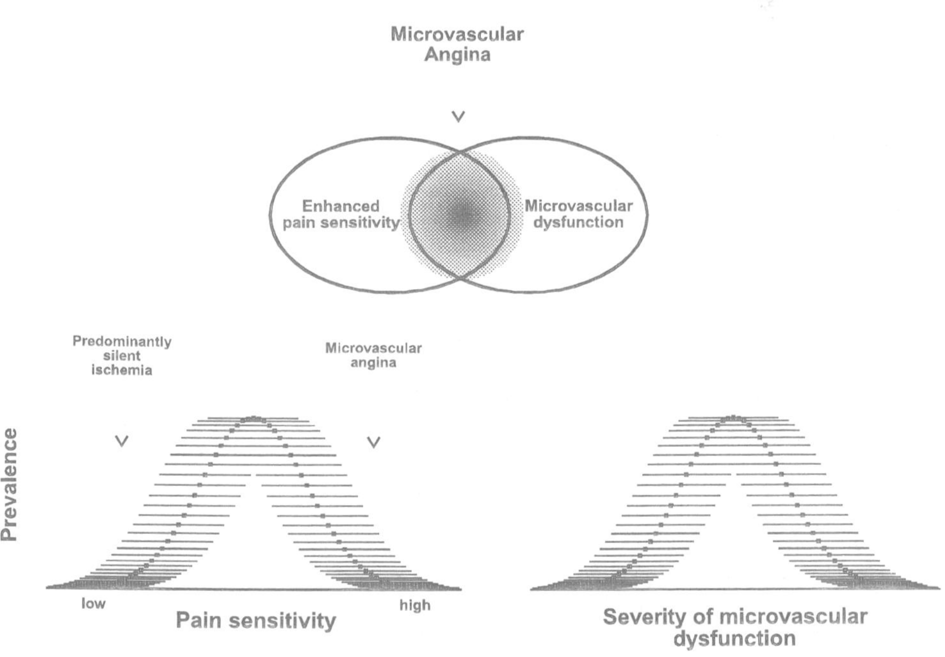


FIGURE 46-14 Main pathogenetic mechanisms of syndrome X, which probably results from a variable combination of two components: a coronary microvascular dysfunction and an increased pain sensitivity, the prevalence of both of which may follow a bell-shaped curve in the population. (From Maseri.[50] With permission.)

The diagnosis of syndrome X is confirmed by (1) evidence of a cardiac origin of pain because of its consistent association with transient ischemic ECG changes and/or myocardial perfusion defects during exercise testing or by diagnostic ECG changes on Holter monitoring[162]; (2) a normal coronary angiogram; (3) the exclusion of epicardial coronary spasm on the basis of distinct clinical history, absence of transient episodes of ST-segment elevation, and failure to induce coronary spasm by provocative tests.

## Unstable Angina

The characteristic clinical feature of unstable angina is the sudden appearance and/or worsening of angina, with more frequent and prolonged attacks occurring at rest or in association with efforts that were previously well tolerated. In patients with de novo angina and those with known ischemic heart disease and in the absence of secondary causes of instability (e.g., anemia, fever, hyperthyroidism, tachyarrhythmias), this pattern of presentation suggests a transient, recurring impairment of myocardial perfusion by thrombosis and vasoconstriction. A sudden reduction in the ischemic threshold on exertion, on the other hand, points to the rapid development or increased severity of a flow-limiting stenosis by organized thrombus. Many patients continue to present recurrent instability and/or develop myocardial infarction in the initial weeks and months following hospital discharge; unstable patients are also at an increased risk of restenosis following PTCA. The recurrence of instability and the higher rate of restenosis following PTCA may be predicted by elevated blood levels of systemic markers of inflammation (e.g., C-reactive protein[163] and interleukin-6[164]), consistent with the hypothesis that inflammatory cytokines may be an important component of instability (see also Chap. 51).

## Variant Angina

The clinical diagnosis of variant angina can be suspected only when sufficient time has elapsed from the onset of symptoms to allow the emergence of a distinctive pattern of angina. The following features suggest the clinical diagnosis of variant angina: (1) a report of pain occurring predominantly at rest, without apparent cause, more often at night, in the early morning hours, or at the same time each day, often with preserved effort tolerance; (2) the episodes are usually of short duration (2 to 5 min) and respond to sublingual nitrates within 1 to 2 min; (3) the episodes may occur in clusters of two or three in the early morning hours and be absent throughout the rest of the day; (4) they may be associated with syncope caused by either ventricular tachyarrhythmias[90] or atrioventricular block; (5) the exercise stress test is often negative, but in some patients it may cause ST-segment elevation, which can typically be prevented on repeating the test by the administration of nitrate sublingually.

The clinical suspicion elicited by these features is supported by the demonstration of ST-segment elevation during angina. This can be obtained by chance with a 12-lead ECG, by 24- or 48-h Holter monitoring, and during or soon after the exercise stress test. The diagnosis is confirmed by the angiographic demonstration of spasm occurring spontaneously or following provocative tests. Among these, ergonovine and hyperventilation have a 100 percent specificity but a lower sensitivity, compared to intracoronary acetylcholine which seems to have a greater sensitivity but a lower specificity. The occlusive spasm may occur either at the site of coronary stenosis or also in angiographically normal coronaries.[165] The diagnosis of variant angina is a mandatory indication for calcium antagonists and nitrates. In contrast, beta-blockers are usually contraindicated as they can facilitate spasm induction (see also Chap. 57).

## Myocardial Infarction

In some patients, myocardial infarction develops totally unheralded. In others, the final persistent episode of pain is preceded by a typical history of unstable angina. During the initial 6 h from the onset of symptoms in unselected patients with acute myocardial infarction, the infarct-related artery recanalizes spontaneously in 40 percent of the cases and exhibits occasional transient reperfusion in about 70 percent. Spontaneous early reperfusion seems to be more frequent in patients in whom myocardial infarction is preceded by unstable angina.[166] The presence of systemically detectable inflammatory markers in about 70 percent of patients with Braunwald class III B unstable angina and the much higher occurrence of cardiac events among the 50 percent of patients in whom the elevation persists at discharge[167] may represent an objective marker of inflammatory thrombogenic triggers. This possibility is supported by the elevation of such markers at the time of hospital admission in nearly all patients in whom myocardial infarction was preceded by unstable angina but in less than 50 percent of those in whom myocardial infarction was totally unheralded.[168] The presence of inflammatory markers also makes unlikely the diagnosis of variant angina, which sometimes has a clinical presentation indistinguishable from the more common form of unstable angina. Different pathogenetic components of coronary occlusion are also suggested by the earlier recanalization in response to t-PA observed in patients with preinfarction angina compared to those with a totally unheralded myocardial infarction.[144]

The prodromal symptoms of myocardial infarction also provide clues as to its pathogenetic mechanisms. In some patients, myocardial infarction occurs without any apparent cause; in others, a history of severe psychological distress[169] or a flu-like syndrome can be elicited on careful questioning. These prodromal symptoms may be associated with a different mode of presentation of acute myocardial infarction and can provide clues of distinct pathogenetic mechanisms that may not have the same prevalence in different age, sex, geographic, and ethnic groups.

An understanding of the precise mechanisms of acute coronary occlusion would allow more effective and complex coronary reperfusion strategies to be reserved for those patients who are unlikely to respond to simpler ones.

## References


1. Porenta G, Cherry S, Czernin J, et al. Noninvasive determination of myocardial blood flow, oxygen consumption and efficiency in normal humans by carbon-11 acetate positron emission tomography imaging. *Eur J Nucl Med* 1999;26:1465.
2. Pitkanen OP, Nuutila P, Raitakari OT, et al. Coronary flow reserve in young men with familial combined hyperlipidemia. *Circulation* 1999; 99:1678.
3. Vassalli G, Hess OM. Measurement of coronary flow reserve and its role in patient care. *Basic Res Cardiol* 1998;93:339.
4. Braunwald E. Myocardial oxygen consumption: The quest for its determinants and some clinical fallout. *J Am Coll Cardiol* 1999;34: 1365.
5. Kuo L, Davis MJ, Chilian WM. Longitudinal gradients for endothelium-dependent and independent vascular responses in the coronary microcirculation. *Circulation* 1995;92:518.
6. Coggins DL, Flynn AE, Austin RE, et al. Non uniform loss of regional flow reserve during myocardial ischemia in dogs. *Circ Res* 1990;67: 253.
7. Beyar R, Sideman S. Dynamic interaction between myocardial contraction and coronary flow. *Adv Exp Med Biol* 1997;430:123.
8. Spaan JAE. Mechanical determinants of myocardial perfusion. *Basic Res Cardiol* 1995;90:89.

9. Armour JA, Randall WC. Canine left ventricular intramyocardial pressures. *Am J Physiol* 1995;220:1833.
10. Hoffman JIE, Baer RW, Hanley FL, et al. Regulation of transmural myocardial blood flow. *J Biochem Eng* 1985;107:2.
11. Merkus D, Kajiya F, Vink H, et al. prolonged diastolic time fraction protects myocardial perfusion when coronary blood flow is reduced. *Circulation* 1999;100:75.
12. Berne RM. Cardiac nucleotides in hypoxia: Possible role in regulation of coronary blood flow. *Am J Physiol* 1963;204:317.
13. Yada T, Richmond KN, Van Bibber R, et al. Role of adenosine in local metabolic coronary vasodilation. *Am J Physiol* 1999;276:H1425.
14. DeFily DV, Chilian WM: Coronary microcirculation: Autoregulation and metabolic control. *Basic Res Cardiol* 1995;90:112.
15. Ishizaka H, Kuo L. Endothelial ATP-sensitive potassium channels mediate coronary microvascular dilation to hyperosmolarity. *Am J Physiol* 1997;273:H104.
16. Dellsperger KC. Potassium channels and the coronary circulation. *Clin Exp Pharmacol Physiol* 1996;23:1096.
17. Tune JD, Richmond KN, Gorman MW, et al. Control of coronary blood flow during exercise. *Exp Biol Med* 2002;227:238.
18. Miller FJ Jr, Dellsperger KC, Gutterman DD. Myogenic constriction of human coronary arterioles. *Am J Physiol* 1997;273:H257.
19. Feigl EO. Neural control of coronary blood flow. *J Vasc Res* 1998;35:85.
20. Saetrum Opgaard O, Gulbenkian S, Edvinsson L. Innervation and effects of vasoactive substances in the coronary circulation. *Eur Heart J* 1997;18:1556.
21. Saetrum Opgaard O, Edvinsson L. Mechanical properties and effects of sympathetic co-transmitters on human coronary arteries and veins. *Basic Res Cardiol* 1977;92:168.
22. Baumgart D, Heusch G. Neuronal control of coronary blood flow. *Basic Res Cardiol* 1995;90:142.
23. Gorman MW, Tune JD, Richmond KN, et al. Quantitative analysis of feedforward sympathetic coronary vasodilation in exercising dogs. *J Appl Physiol* 2000;89:1093.
24. Saetrum Opgaard O, Edvinsson L. Effect of parasympathetic and sensory transmitters on human epicardial coronary arteries and veins. *Pharmacol Toxicol* 1996;78:273.
25. Feliciano L, Henning RJ. Vagal nerve stimulation during muscarinic and beta-adrenergic blockade causes significant coronary artery dilation. *J Auton Nerv Syst* 1998;68:78.
26. Dietrich HH, Ellsworth ML, Sprague RS, et al. Red blood cell regulation of microvascular tone through adenosine triphosphate. *Am J Physiol Heart Circ Physiol* 2000;269:H1294.
27. Tanaka E, Mori H, Chujo M, et al. Coronary vasoconstrictive effects of neuropeptide Y and their modulation by the ATP-sensitive potassium channel in anesthetized dogs. *J Am Coll Cardiol* 1997;29:1380.
28. Fleming I, Busse R. NO: The primary EDRF. *J Mol Cell Cardiol* 1999;31:5.
29. Tousoulis D, Crake T, Tentolouris C, et al. Effects of inhibition of nitric oxide synthesis in proximal and distal segments in patients with normal arteries and in patients with coronary artery disease. *J Am Coll Cardiol* 1995;(suppl):117A.
30. Tousoulis D, Tentolouris C, Crake T, et al. Basal and flow-mediated nitric oxide production by atheromatous coronary arteries. *J Am Coll Cardiol* 1997;29:1256.
31. Bassenge E. Control of coronary blood flow by autacoids. *Basic Res Cardiol* 1995;90:112.
32. Duffy SJ, Castle SF, Harper RW, et al. Contribution of vasodilator prostanoids and nitric oxide to resting flow, metabolic vasodilation, and flow-mediated dilation in human coronary circulation. *Circulation* 1999;100:1951.
33. Campbell WB, Gebremedhin D, Pratt PF, et al. Identification of epoxyeicosatrienoic acids as endothelium-derived hyperpolarizing factors. *Circ Res* 1996;78:415.
34. Masaki T. Possible role of endothelin in endothelial regulation of vascular tone. *Annu Rev Pharmacol Toxicol* 1995;35:235.
35. Lüscher TF, Oemar BS, Boulanger CM, et al. Molecular and cellular biology of endothelin and its receptors. *Molecular Reviews.* London: Chapman & Hall: 1996:96.
36. McCarthy PA, Pegge NC, Prendergast BD, et al. The physiological role of endogenous endothelin in the regulation of human coronary vasomotor tone. *J Am Coll Cardiol* 2001;37:137.
37. Mombouli JV, Vanhoutte PM: Endothelial dysfunction: From physiology to therapy. *J Mol Cell Cardiol* 1999;31:61.
38. Ruschitzka FT, Noll G, Luscher TF. The endothelium in coronary artery disease. *Cardiology* 1997;88:3.
39. Luscher TF. Endothelial control of vascular tone and growth. *Clin Exp Hypertens A* 1990;12:897.
40. Li S, Sims S, Jiao Y, et al. Evidence from a novel human cell clone that adult vascular smooth muscle cells can convert reversibly between noncontractile and contractile phenotypes. *Circ Res* 1999;85:338.
41. Bombeli T, Mueller M, Haeberli A. Anticoagulant properties of the vascular endothelium. *Thromb Haemost* 1997;77:408.
42. Crossman DC, Larkin SW, Dashwood MR, et al. Responses of atherosclerotic human coronary arteries in vivo to the endothelium-dependent vasodilator substance P. *Circulation* 1991;84:2001.
43. Vallance P, Collier J, Bhagat K. Infection, inflammation, and infarction: Does acute endothelial dysfunction provide a link? *Lancet* 1997; 349:1391.
44. Kinlay S, Selwyn AP, Libby P, et al. Inflammation, the endothelium, and the acute coronary syndromes. *J Cardiovasc Pharmacol* 1998;32:S62.
45. Libby P: Molecular bases of the acute coronary syndromes. *Circulation* 1995;91:2844.
46. Maseri A, Sanna T. The role of plaque fissures in unstable angina: Fact or fiction? *Eur Heart J* 1998;19(suppl K):K2.
47. Maseri A. Anthibiotics for acute coronary syndromes: Are we ready for megatrials? *Eur Heart J* 1999;20:89.
48. Caligiuri G, Liuzzo G, Biasucci LM, et al. Immune system activation follows inflammation in unstable angina: pathogenetic implications. *J Am Coll Cardiol* 1998;32:1295.
49. Liuzzo G, Kopecky Sl, Frye RL, et al. Perturbation of the T-cell repertoire in patients with unstable angina. *Circulation* 1999;100: 2135.
50. Maseri A. *Ischemic Heart Disease.* New York: Churchill Livingstone; 1995
51. Klocke FJ. Measurements of coronary blood flow and degree of stenosis: Current clinical implications and continuing uncertainties. *J Am Coll Cardiol* 1983;1:31.
52. Di Carli M, Czernin J, Hoh CK, et al. Relation among stenosis severity, myocardial blood flow, and flow reserve in patients with coronary artery disease. *Circulation* 1995:91:1944.
53. Beanlands RSB, Muzik O, Melon P, et al. Noninvasive quantification of regional myocardial flow reserve in patients with coronary atherosclerosis using nitrogen-13 ammonia positron emission tomography. Determination of Extent of Altered Vascular Reactivity. *J Am Coll Cardiol* 1995;26:1465.
54. Rutishauser W. The Denolin Lecture 1998. Towards measurement of coronary blood flow in patients and its alteration by interventions. *Eur Heart J* 1999;20:1076.
55. De Bruyne B, Banohuin T, Melin J, et al. Coronary flow reserve calculated from pressure measurements in humans. *Circulation* 1994; 89:1013.
56. Tousoulis D, Davies GJ, Toutouzas PC. Vasomotion of coronary arteries: From nitrates to nitric oxide. *Cardiovasc Drugs Ther* 1999;13:295.
57. Tousoulis D, Crake T, Kaski JC, et al. Enhanced vasomotor responses of complex coronary stenoses to acetylcholine in stable angina pectoris. *Am J Cardiol* 1995;75:725.
58. Dubois-Rande JL, Dupouy P, Aptecar E, et al. Comparison of the effects of exercise and cold pressor test on the vasomotor response of normal and atherosclerotic coronary arteries and their relation to the flow-mediated mechanism. *Am J Cardiol* 1995;76:467.
59. Julius BK, Vassalli G, Mandinov L, et al. Alpha-adrenoceptor blockade prevents exercise-induced vasoconstriction of stenotic coronary arteries. *J Am Coll Cardiol* 1999;33:1499.
60. Petronio AS, Amoroso G, Limbruno U, et al. Endothelin-1 release from atherosclerotic plaque after percutaneous transluminal coronary angioplasty in stable angina pectoris and single-vessel coronary artery disease. *Am J Cardiol* 1999;84:1085.

61. Lerman A, Holmes DR Jr, Bell MR, et al. Endothelin in coronary endothelial dysfunction and early atherosclerosis in humans. *Circulation* 1995;92:2426.
62. Yokoyama I, Momomura S, Ohtake T, et al. Improvement of impaired myocardial vasodilatation due to diffuse coronary atherosclerosis in hypercholesterolemics after lipid-lowering therapy. *Circulation* 1999; 100:117.
63. Nishikawa Y, Ogawa S. Importance of nitric oxide in the coronary artery at rest and during pacing in humans. *J Am Coll Cardiol* 1997; 29:85–92.
64. Schachinger V, Zeiher AM. Quantitative assessment of coronary vasoreactivity in humans in vivo. Importance of baseline vasomotor tone in atherosclerosis. *Circulation* 1995;92:2087.
65. Traverse JH, Judd D, Bache RJ. Dose-dependent effect of endothelin-1 on blood flow to normal and collateral-dependent myocardium. *Circulation* 1996;93:558.
66. Lamping KG. Response of native and stimulated collateral vessels to serotonin. *Am J Physiol* 1997;272(5 Pt 2):H2409.
67. Klassen CL, Traverse JH, Bache RJ. Nitroglycerin dilates coronary collateral vessels during exercise after blockade of endogenous NO production. *Am J Physiol* 1999;277(3 Pt 2):H918–23.
68. Altman JD, Klassen CL, Bache RJ. Cyclooxygenase blockade limits blood flow to collateral-dependent myocardium during exercise. *Cardiovasc Res* 1995;30:697.
69. Schultz A, Lavie L, Hochberg I, et al. Interindividual heterogeneity in the hypoxic regulation of VEGF: Significance for the development of the coronary artery collateral circulation. *Circulation* 1999;100:547.
70. Fujita M, Kihara Y, Hasegawa K, et al. Heparin potentiates collateral growth but not growth of intramyocardial endarteries in dogs with repeated coronary occlusion. *Int J Cardiol* 1999;70:165.
71. Schumacher B, Pecher P, von Specht BU, et al. Induction of neoangiogenesis in ischemic myocardium by human growth factors: First clinical results of a new treatment of coronary heart disease. *Circulation* 1998;97:645.
72. Sellke FW, Laham RJ, Edelman ER, et al. Therapeutic angiogenesis with basic fibroblast growth factor: Technique and early results. *Ann Thorac Surg* 1998;65:1540.
73. Chou E, Suzuma I, Way JK, et al. Decreased cardiac expression of vascular endothelial growth factor and its receptors in insulin resistance and diabetic states. A possible explanation for impaired collateral formation in cardiac tissue. *Circulation* 2002;105:373.
74. Hamasaki S, Arima S, Fukumoto N, et al. Mechanisms of limited maximum coronary flow in severe single-vessel coronary artery disease in humans due to vertical steal. *Am J Cardiol* 1997;80:1597.
75. Holmvang G, Fry S, Skopicki HA, et al. Relation between coronary "steal" and contractile function at rest in collateral-dependent myocardium of humans with ischemic heart disease. *Circulation* 1999; 99:2510.
76. Lanza GA, Maseri A. Diagnosis and treatment of coronary artery spasm. *Cardiol Rev* 1996;1:1.
77. Lanza GA, Pedrotti P, Pasceri V, et al. Autonomic changes associated with spontaneous coronary spasm in patients with variant angina. *J Am Coll Cardiol* 1996;28:1249.
78. Yamakado T, Kasai A, Masuda T, et al. Exercise-induced coronary spasm: Comparison of treadmill and bicycle exercise in patients with vasospastic angina. *Coron Artery Dis* 1996;7:819.
79. Song JK, Lee SJ, Kang DH, et al. Ergonovine echocardiography as a screening test for diagnosis of vasospastic angina before coronary angiography. *J Am Coll Cardiol* 1996;27:1156.
80. Kugiyama K, Murohara T, Yasue H, et al. Increased constrictor response to acetylcholine of the isolated coronary arteries from patients with variant angina. *Int J Cardiol* 1995;52:223.
81. Ishida T, Hirata K, Sakoda T, et al. 5-HT1D beta receptor mediates the supersensitivity of isolated coronary artery to serotonin in variant angina. *Chest* 1998;113:243.
82. Nakao K, Ohgushi M, Yoshimura M, et al. Hyperventilation as a specific test for diagnosis of coronary artery spasm. *Am J Cardiol* 1997;80:545.
83. Masumoto A, Mohri M, Shimokawa H, et al. Suppression of coronary artery spasm by the rho-hinase inhibitor fasudil in patients with vasospastic angina. *Circulation* 2002;105:1545.
84. Chutkow WA, Pu J, Wheeler MT, et al. Episodic coronary artery vasospasm and hypertension develop in the absence of Sur2 K(ATP) channels. *J Clin Invest* 2002;110:203.
85. Lanza GA, De Candia E, Romagnoli E, et al. Increased platelet sodium-hydrogen exchanger activity in patients with variant angina. *Heart* 2003;89:935.
86. Katsumata N, Shimokawa H, Seto M, et al. Enhanced myosin light chain phosphorylations as a central mechanism for coronary artery spasm in a swine model with interleukin-1 beta. *Circulation* 1997; 96:4357.
87. Maseri A, Crea F, Lanza GA. Coronary vasoconstriction: Where do we stand in 1999. An important, multifaceted but elusive role. *Cardiologia* 1999;44:115.
88. Mongiardo R, Finocchiaro ML, Beltrame J, et al. Low incidence of serotonin-induced occlusive coronary artery spasm in patients with recent myocardial infarction. *Am J Cardiol* 1996;78:84.
89. Pristipino C, Beltrame JF, Finocchiaro ML, et al. Major racial differences in coronary constrictor response between Japanese and Caucasians with recent myocardial infarction. *Circulation* 2000;101:1102.
90. Chevalier P, Dacosta A, Defaye P, et al. Arrhythmic cardiac arrest due to isolated coronary artery spasm: Long-term outcome of seven resuscitated patients. *J Am Coll Cardiol* 1998;31:57.
91. Caputo M, Nicolini F, Franciosi G, et al. Coronary artery spasm after coronary artery bypass grafting. *Eur J Cardiothorac Surg* 1999; 15:545.
92. DeFily DV, Nishikawa Y, Chilian WM. Endothelin antagonists block $alpha_1$-adrenergic constriction of coronary arterioles. *Am J Physiol* 1999;276(3 Pt 2):H1028.
93. Miao L, Nunez BD, Susulic V, et al. Cocaine-induced microvascular vasoconstriction but differential systemic haemodynamic responses in Yucatan versus Yorkshire varieties of swine. *Br J Pharmacol* 1996; 117:559.
94. Cianflone D, Lanza GA, Maseri A. Microvascular angina in patients with normal coronary arteries and with other ischaemic syndromes. *Eur Heart J* 1995;16(suppl I):96.
95. Pupita G, Maseri A, Kaski JC, et al. Myocardial ischemia caused by distal coronary-artery constriction in stable angina pectoris. *N Engl J Med* 1990;323:514.
96. Versaci F, Tomai F, Nudi F, et al. Differences of regional coronary flow reserve assessed by adenosine thallium-201 scintigraphy early and six months after successful percutaneous transluminal coronary angioplasty or stent implantation. *Am J Cardiol* 1996;78:1097.
97. Kern MJ, Puri S, Bach RG, MJ, et al. Abnormal coronary flow velocity reserve after coronary artery stenting in patients: role of relative coronary reserve to assess potential mechanisms. *Circulation* 1999;100:2491.
98. Kosa I, Blasini R, Schneider-Eicke J, et al. Early recovery of coronary flow reserve after stent implantation as assessed by positron emission tomography. *J Am Coll Cardiol* 1999;34:1036.
99. Gregorini L, Marco J, Kozakova M, et al. Alpha-adrenergic blockade improves recovery of myocardial perfusion and function after coronary stenting in patients with acute myocardial infarction. *Circulation* 1999; 99:482.
100. Kramer CM, Rogers WJ, Theobald TM, et al. Remote Noninfarcted region dysfunction soon after first anterior myocardial infarction: A magnetic resonance tagging study. *Circulation* 1996;94:660.
101. Zeiher AM, Krause T, Schächinger V, et al. Impaired endothelium-dependent vasodilation of coronary resistance vessels is associated with exercise-induced myocardial ischemia. *Circulation* 1995;91: 2345.
102. Yokoyama I, Ohtake T, Momomura S, et al. Reduced coronary flow reserve in hypercholesterolemic patients without overt coronary stenosis. *Circulation* 1996;94:3232.
103. Kaski JC. Cardiac syndrome X and microvascular angina, in Kaski JC (ed). *Chest pain with Normal Coronary Angiograms.* Dordrecht: Kluwer; 1999:1.

104. Kao CH, Wang SJ, Ting CT, Chen YT. Tc-99m sestamibi myocardial SPECT in syndrome X. *Clin Nucl Med* 1996;21:280.
105. Rosano GM, Peters NS, Kaski JC, et al. Abnormal uptake and washout of thallium-201 in patients with syndrome X and normal-appearing scans. *Am J Cardiol* 1995;75:400.
106. Panza JA, Laurienzo JM, Curiel RV, et al. Investigation of the mechanism of chest pain in patients with angiographically normal coronary arteries using transesophageal dobutamine stress echocardiography. *J Am Coll Cardiol* 1997;29:293.
107. Rosano GMC, Kaski JC, Arie S, et al. Failure to demonstrate myocardial ischaemia in patients with angina and normal coronary arteries. Evaluation by continuous coronary sinus pH monitoring and lactate metabolism. *Eur Heart J* 1996;17:1175.
108. Watanabe S, Buffington CW, Moresea G. Comparison of myocardial ischemia induced by endothelin vs. mechanical stenosis in pigs. *Am J Physiol* 1995;268(3 Pt 2):H1276.
109. Rigattieri S, Buffon A, Ramazzotti V, et al. Oxidative stress in ischemia-reperfusion injury: assessment by three independent biochemical markers. *Ital Heart J* 2000;1:68.
110. Buffon A, Santini SA, Rigattieri S, et al. Transient intracardiac lipid peroxidation induced by atrial pacing in syndrome X: A definitive demonstration of an ischemic mechanism? *Circulation* 1997;96:I-270.
111. Crea F, Buffon A, Gaspardone A, et al. Alternative mechanisms for myocardial ischemia in syndrome X—New diagnostic markers, in Kaski JC (ed). *Chest Pain with Normal Coronary Angiograms. Pathogenesis, Diagnosis and Management.* Boston: Kluwer; 1999;123.
112. Panting JR, Gatehouse PD, Yang GZ, et al. Abnormal subendocardial perfusion in cardiac syndrome X detected by cardiovascular magnetic resonance imaging. *N Engl J Med* 2002;346:1948.
113. Buchthal SD, den Hollander JA, Merz NB, et al. Abnormal myocardial phosphorus-31 nuclear magnetic resonance spectroscopy in women with chest pain but normal coronary angiograms. *N Engl J Med* 2000; 342:829.
114. Baumgart D, Haude M, Gorge G, et al. Augmented alpha-adrenergic constriction of atherosclerotic human coronary arteries. *Circulation* 1999;99:2090.
115. Virdis A, Ghiadoni L, Lucarini A, et al. Presence of cardiovascular structural changes in essential hypertensive patients with coronary microvascular disease and effects of long-term treatment. *Am J Hypertens* 1996;9(4 Pt 1):361.
116. Kawaguchi M, Techigawara M, Ishihata T, et al. A comparison of ultrastructural changes on endomyocardial biopsy specimens obtained from patients with diabetes mellitus with and without hypertension. *Heart Vessels* 1997;12:267.
117. Zeiher AM, Krause T, Schachinger V, et al. Impaired endothelium-dependent vasodilation of coronary resistance vessels is associated with exercise-induced myocardial ischemia. *Circulation* 1995;91:2345.
118. Quyyumi AA, Dakak N, Andrews NP, et al. Contribution of nitric oxide to metabolic coronary vasodilation in the human heart. *Circulation* 1995;92:320.
119. Chauhan A, Mullins PA, Taylor G, et al. Both endothelium-dependent and endothelium-independent function is impaired in patients with angina pectoris and normal coronary angiograms. *Eur Heart J* 1997; 18:60.
120. Koren W, Koldanov R, Peleg E, et al. Enhanced red cell sodium-hydrogen exchange in microvascular angina. *Eur Heart J* 1997;18: 1296–1299.
121. Gaspardone A, Ferri C, Crea F, et al. Enhanced activity of sodium-litium countertransport in patients with cardiac syndrome X: A potential link between cardiac and metabolic syndrome X. *J Am Coll Cardiol* 1998;32:2031–2034.
122. Mohri M, Shimokawa H, Hirakawa Y, et al. Rho-kinase inhibition with intracoronary fasudil prevents myocardial ischemia in patients with coronary microvascular spasm. *J Am Coll Cardiol* 2003;41:15.
123. Kaski JC, Elliot PM, Salomone O, et al. Concentration of circulating plasma endothelin in patients with angina and normal coronary arteries. *Br Heart J* 1995;74:620.
124. Lanza GA, Luscher TF, Pasceri V, et al. Effects of atrial pacing on arterial and coronary sinus endothelin-1 levels in syndrome X. *Am J Cardiol* 1999;84:1187.
125. Lanza GA, Giordano A, Pristipino C, et al. Abnormal cardiac adrenergic nerve function in patients with syndrome X detected by [$^{123}$I]metaiodobenzylguanidine myocardial scintigraphy. *Circulation* 1997;96:821.
126. Maseri A. From syndromes to specific disease mechanisms. The search for the causes of myocardial infarction. *Ital Heart J* 2000;1:20.
127. Dechend R, Maass M, Gieffers J, et al. *Chlamydia pneumoniae* infection of vascular smooth muscle and endothelial cells activates NF-kappaB and induces tissue factor and PAI-1 expression: A potential link to accelerated arteriosclerosis. *Circulation* 1999;100: 1369.
128. Mayr M, Metzler B, Kiechl S, et al. Endothelial cytotoxicity mediated by serum antibodies to heat shock proteins of *Escherichia coli* and *Chlamydia pneumoniae:* Immune reactions to heat shock proteins as a possible link between infection and atherosclerosis. *Circulation* 1999; 99:1560.
129. Ikeda U, Takahashi M, Shimada K. Monocyte-endothelial cell interaction in atherogenesis and thrombosis. *Clin Cardiol* 1998;21:11.
130. Gutstein DE, Fuster V: Pathophysiology and clinical significance of atherosclerotic plaque rupture. *Cardiovasc Res* 1999;41:323.
131. Buffon A, Biasucci LM, Liuzzo G, et al. Widespread coronary inflammation in unstable angina. *N Engl J Med* 2002;347:5.
132. Goldstein JA, Demetriou D, Grines CL, et al. Multiple complex coronary plaques in patients with acute myocardial infarction. *N Engl J Med* 2000;343:915.
133. Rioufol G, Finet G, Ginon I, et al. Multiple atherosclerotic plaque rupture in acute coronary syndrome. A three-vessel intravascular ultrasound study. *Circulation* 2002;106:804.
134. Spagnoli LG, Bonanno E, Mauriello A, et al. Multicentric inflammation in epicardial coronary arteries of patients dying of acute myocardial infarction. *J Am Coll Cardiol* 2002;40:1579.
135. Rothwell PM, Villagra R, Donders RCJM, et al. Evidence of a chronic systemic cause of instability of atherosclerotic plaques. *Lancet* 2000; 355:19–24.
136. Shah AM, Mebazaa A, Yang ZK, et al. Inhibition of myocardial crossbridge cycling by hypoxic endothelial cells: A potential mechanism for matching oxygen supply and demand. *Circ Res* 1997;80: 688.
137. Ehlert FA, Goldberger JJ. Cellular and pathophysiological mechanisms of ventricular arrhythmias in acute ischemia and infarction. *PACE* 1997;20:967.
138. Niessen HW, Lagrand WK, Visser CA, et al. Upregulation of ICAM-1 on cardiomyocytes in jeopardized human myocardium during infarction. *Cardiovasc Res* 41:603,1999.
139. Kaikita K, Ogawa H, Yasue H, et al. Increased plasma soluble intercellular adhesion molecule-1 levels in patients with acute myocardial infarction. *Jpn Circ J* 1997;61:741.
140. Siminiak T, Dye JF, Egdell RM, et al. The release of soluble adhesion molecules ICAM-1 and E-selectin after acute myocardial infarction and following coronary angioplasty. *Int J Cardiol* 1997;61:113.
141. Tomai F, Crea F, Chiariello L, et al. Ischemic preconditioning in humans. Models, mediators and clinical relevance. *Circulation* 1999; 100:559.
142. Pasceri V, Lanza GA, Patti G, et al. Preconditioning by transient myocardial ischemia confers protection against ischemia-induced ventricular arrhythmias in variant angina. *Circulation* 1996;94:1850.
143. Gheeraert PJ, Henriques JP, De Buyzere ML, et al. Preinfarction angina protects against out-of-hospital ventricular fibrillation in patients with acute occlusion of the left coronary artery. *J Am Coll Cardiol* 2001;38:1369.
144. Andreotti F, Pasceri V, Hackett DR, et al. Preinfarction angina as a predictor of more rapid coronary thrombolysis in patients with acute myocardial infarction. *N Engl J Med* 334:7, 1996.
145. Braunwald E. Acute myocardial infarction—The value of being prepared. *N Engl J Med* 1996;334:51.

146. O' Rourke B. $K^+{}_{ATP}$ channels in myocardial preconditioning. *Circ Res* 2000;87:845.
147. Kloner RA, Jennings RB. Consequences of brief ischemia: Stunning, preconditioning and their clinical implications: Part 2. *Circulation* 2001;104:3158.
148. Tomai F, Crea F, Gaspardone A, et al. Ischemic preconditioning during coronary angioplasty is prevented by glibenclamide, a selective ATP-sensitive $K^+$ channel blocker. *Circulation* 1994;90:700–705.
149. Baker AJ. Cellular and extracellular mechanisms causing myocardial stunning. *J Am Coll Cardiol* 1999;34:603.
150. Bolli R. Causative role of oxyradicals in myocardial stunning: a proven hypothesis. A brief review of the evidence demonstrating a major role of reactive oxygen species in several forms of postischemic dysfunction. *Basic Res Cardiol* 93:156, 1998.
151. Murphy AM, Kogler H, Georgakapoulos D, et al. Transgenic mouse model of stunned myocardium. *Science* 2000;287:488.
152. Vanoverschelde J-L J, Wijns W, Borgers M, et al. Chronic myocardial hibernation in humans. From bedside to bench. *Circulation* 1997;95: 1961.
152a. Kudej RK, Vatner SF. Nitric oxide-dependent vasodilation maintains blood flow in true hibernating myocardium. *J Mol Cell Cardiol* 2003;35:931–935.
153. Lanza GA, Sciahbasi A, Sestito A, et al. Angina pectoris: A headache. *Lancet* 2000;356:998.
154. Crea F, Gaspardone A. New look to an old symptom: Angina pectoris. *Circulation.* 1997;96:3766.
155. Crea F, Gaspardone A, Kaski JC, et al. Relationship between stimulation site of cardiac afferent nerves by adenosine and location of cardiac pain: Results of a study in patients with stable angina. *J Am Coll Cardiol* 1992;20:1498.
156. Pasceri V, Patti G, Maseri A. Changing features of anginal pain after PTCA suggest a stenosis on a different artery rather than restenosis. *Circulation* 1997;96:3278.
157. Pasceri V, Cianflone D, Finocchiaro ML, et al. Relation between myocardial infarction site and pain location in acute Q-wave myocardial infarction. *Am J Cardiol* 1995;75:224.
158. Liu CJ, Sulayman D, Hajj D. Modulation of the cardiac sodium channel $Na_v1.5$ by fibroblast growth factor homologous factor 1B. *J Biol Chem* 2003;278:1029.
159. Kajstura J, Cheng W, Reiss K, et al. Apoptotic and necrotic myocyte cell deaths are independent contributing variables of infarct size in rats. *Lab Invest* 1996;74:86.
160. Lanza GA, Colonna G, Pasceri V, et al. Atenolol-vs-amlodipine-vs-isosorbide-5-mononitrate on anginal symptoms in syndrome X. *Am J Cardiol* 1999;84:854.
161. Pasceri V, Lanza GA, Buffon A, et al. Role of abnormal pain sensitivity and behavioral factors in determining chest pain in syndrome X. *J Am Coll Cardiol* 1998;31:62.
162. Lanza GA, Manzoli A, Pasceri V, et al. Ischemic-like ST-segment changes during holter monitoring in patients with angina pectoris and normal coronary arteries but negative exercise testing. *Am J Cardiol* 1997;79:1.
163. Liuzzo G, Biasucci LM, Gallimore R, et al. The prognostic value of C-reactive protein and serum amyloid a protein in severe unstable angina. *N Engl J Med* 1994;331:417.
164. Biasucci LM, Vitelli A, Liuzzo G, et al. Elevated levels of interleukin-6 in unstable angina. *Circulation.* 1996;94:874.
165. Beltrame JF, Sasayama S, Maseri A: Racial heterogeneity in coronary artery vasomotor reactivity: Differences between Japanese and Caucasian patients. *J Am Coll Cardiol* 1999;33:1442.
166. Masahatu I, Ikaru U, Hironobu T, et al. Implications of prodromal angina pectoris in anterior wall acute myocardial infarction: Acute angiographic findings and long-term prognosis. *J Am Coll Cardiol* 1997;30:970.
167. Biasucci LM, Liuzzo G, Grillo RL, et al. Elevated levels of C-reactive protein at discharge in patients with unstable angina predict recurrent instability. *Circulation* 1999;99:885.
168. Liuzzo G, Biasucci LM, Gallimore R, et al. Enhanced inflammatory response in patients with pre-infarction angina. *J Am Coll Cardiol* 1999;15:1696.
169. Pignalberi C, Patti G, Chimenti C, et al. Role of different determinants of psychological distress in acute coronary syndromes. *J Am Coll Cardiol* 1998;32:613.
170. Gallagher KP, Matsuzaki M, Osakada G, et al. Effect of exercise on the relationship between myocardial blood flow and systolic wall thickening in dogs with acute coronary stenosis. *Circ Res* 1983;52:716.

CHAPTER 47

# NONATHEROSCLEROTIC CORONARY HEART DISEASE

Bruce F. Waller



Atherosclerotic (atherothrombotic) disease of the coronary arteries is prevalent and by far the most common cause of luminal narrowing and critical coronary heart disease. However, there are also many nonatherosclerotic (congenital and acquired) causes of severe luminal narrowing and subsequent clinical coronary events (angina pectoris, acute myocardial infarction (MI), and sudden death; Table 47-1).

Various nonatherosclerotic coronary artery diseases can reduce or interrupt coronary blood flow by three predominate mechanisms: (1) fixed luminal obstructions (internal narrowing), (2) encroachment of the lumen by disease of the arterial wall or adjacent tissues (external narrowing), or (3) both.[1] Reduction in coronary arterial blood flow may also result from dynamic changes in the walls of an otherwise normal artery (spasm) or from a disproportion of myocardial oxygen supply and demand. In view of current trends toward rapid coronary artery reperfusion to salvage jeopardized myocardium during evolving acute coronary syndromes, the various nonatherosclerotic etiologies of coronary artery disease (CAD) must be kept in mind.

## FREQUENCY OF NONATHEROSCLEROTIC CORONARY NARROWING PRODUCING FATAL MYOCARDIAL INFARCTION

Approximately 4 to 7 percent of all patients with acute MI and nearly four times this percentage for patients under age 35 do not have atherosclerotic *CAD* as demonstrated by coronary arteriography, at necropsy, or both.[1–4] Since coronary angiography simply represents

TABLE 47-1 **Nonatherosclerotic Causes of Coronary Artery Disease** (Coronary Heart Disease)

| | |
|---|---|
| Congenital anomalies | Metabolic disorders |
| Anomalous origin from the aorta | Mucopolysaccharidoses (Hurler, Hunter) |
| Right-from-left sinus of Valsalva | Homocystinuria |
| Left-from-right sinus of Valsalva | Fabry's disease |
| Single coronary artery | Amyloid |
| Atresia of coronary ostium | Intimal proliferation |
| High-takeoff coronary ostium | Irradiation therapy |
| Ostial ridges | Cardiac transplantation |
| Anomalous origin from the pulmonary trunk | Fibromuscular hyperplasia (methysergide therapy) |
| Fistula | Ostial cannulation |
| Myocardial bridges (tunneled epicardial artery) | Transluminal balloon angioplasty |
| Embolus | Idiopathic infantile arterial calcification (juvenile internal sclerosis) |
| Natural | Cocaine |
| Thrombus | External compression |
| Tumor | Aortic aneurysm |
| Calcium | Tumor metastases |
| Vegetation (infective, noninfective) | Muscle bridges |
| Iatrogenic | Thrombosis without underlying atherosclerotic plaque |
| Cardiac surgery | Polycythemia |
| Cardiac catheterization | Thrombocytosis |
| Coronary angioplasty | Hypercoagulability |
| Prosthetic valves | Substance abuse |
| Paradoxical | Cocaine |
| Dissection | Amphetamines |
| Coronary artery | Myocardial oxygen demand-supply disproportion |
| Aortic | Aortic stenosis |
| Spasm | Systemic hypotension |
| Trauma | Carbon monoxide poisoning |
| Nonpenetrating | Increased myocardial function (thyrotoxicosis) |
| Penetrating | Intramural coronary artery disease (small vessel disease) |
| Surgery | Hypertrophic cardiomyopathy |
| Catheterization | Amyloid |
| Arteritis | Cardiac transplantation |
| Takayasu's disease | Neuromuscular |
| Polyarteritis nodosa | Diabetes mellitus |
| Systemic lupus erythematosus | Normal coronary arteries |
| Kawasaki's syndrome (mucocutaneous lymph node syndrome) | |
| Syphilis | |
| Other infections (infective endocarditis, *Salmonella*, parasites) | |
| Buerger's disease | |
| Giant-cell arteritis | |

SOURCES: Adapted from Waller,[1] Alpert and Braunwald,[2] Cheitlin et al.,[4] and Baim and Harrison.[5]

an image of one lumen, the specificity for etiology of the coronary *luminal* narrowing is extremely low. Review of necropsy studies[1–3] suggests that approximately 95 percent of patients with fatal acute MI have at least one major epicardial coronary artery with severe luminal narrowing or total occlusion Fig. 47-1. The remaining 5 percent of patients apparently have normal major epicardial coronary arteries. Of the 95 percent of patients with severe coronary luminal narrowing, 95 percent have typical atherosclerotic plaque with a superimposed thrombus in 85 percent of these.

The remaining 5 percent of the patients with severe coronary luminal narrowing have a host of etiologies (see Table 47-1), including coronary arteritis, trauma, systemic metabolic disorders, intimal fibrous proliferation, and coronary emboli. Medical centers with large populations of cardiac transplant patients will exceed this 5 percent nonatherosclerotic approximation due to the high frequency of intimal fibrous proliferation in the coronary arteries late after transplantation. Of the 5 percent of patients seen at necropsy after fatal acute MI with normal or nearly normal epicardial coronary arteries, perhaps 50 to 60 percent represent clinical coronary spasm, but the remaining 40 to 50 percent represent a combination of congenital coronary artery anomalies, spontaneous recanalization, and mismatches of coronary supply and myocardial demand (Chap. 37).

## CONGENITAL CORONARY ARTERY ANOMALIES

Variation in the origin, course, or distribution of the epicardial coronary arteries are found in 1 to 2 percent of the population (Table 47-2; Fig. 47-2).[1,5–13] Certain types of these anomalies—including

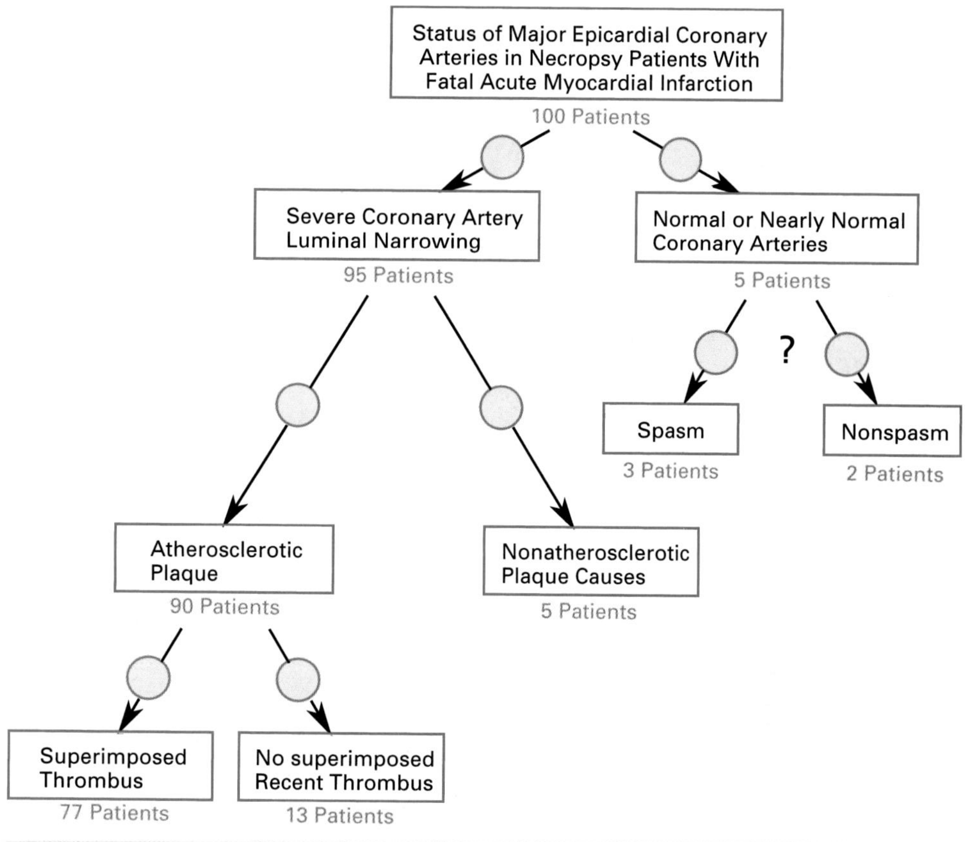


FIGURE 47-1 Diagram displaying the approximate breakdown of status of major epicardial coronary arteries in necropsy patients with fatal acute myocardial infarction. (From Waller.[9] Reproduced with permission from the publisher, editor, and author.)

TABLE 47-2 Certain Coronary Arterial Anomalies Associated with Clinical Coronary Events or Coronary Artery Narrowing

| | |
|---|---|
| Anomalous origin of one or more coronary arteries from the aorta | High-takeoff coronary ostia |
| Origin of both right (R) and left (L) from same sinus of Valsalva | Ostial narrowing |
| R + LM (left main) from right sinus | Syphilis |
| R + LM (left main) from left sinus | Takayasu's disease (pulseless disease) |
| Single coronary artery | Fibromuscular hyperplasia (druginduced) |
| Arising from right sinus | Aortic valve surgery |
| Arising from left sinus | Fibrous ridges |
| Arising from posterior sinus | Protruding masses |
| Anomalous origin of one or more coronary arteries from pulmonary trunk (PT) | Calcific nodules |
| Origin of R from PT | Supravalvular aortic stenosis |
| Origin of LM from PT | Aortic dissection |
| Origin of left anterior descending from PT | Adhesion of aortic cusp to sinus wall |
| Origin of left circumflex from PT | Embolism |
| Coronary artery atresia | Fibroelastosis |
| Atresia of R | Coronary artery fistula |
| Atresia of LM | Myocardial bridges |

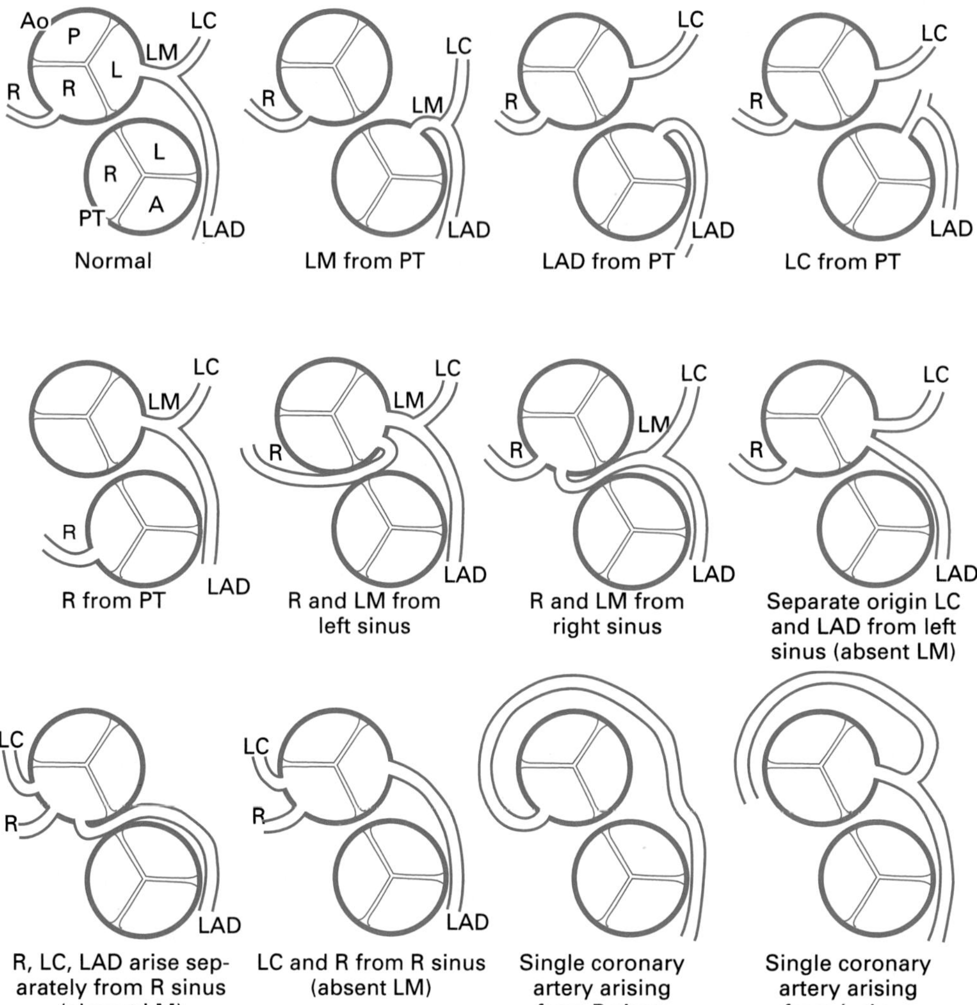


FIGURE 47-2 Diagram showing various congenital coronary artery anomalies that have been associated with clinical symptomatic heart disease. A = anterior cusp; Ao = aorta; L = left cusp; LAD = left anterior descending; LC = left circumflex; LM = left main; P = posterior cusp; PT = pulmonary trunk; R = right cusp or right coronary artery.

ostial lesions, passage of major artery between the walls of the pulmonary trunk, a major coronary artery originating from the pulmonary trunk, or perhaps myocardial "bridges"—may produce ischemia with subsequent MIs[8] (see Chap. 74).

## ORIGIN OF BOTH RIGHT AND LEFT CORONARY ARTERIES FROM THE SAME SINUS OF VALSALVA

When either the right or left coronary artery arises from the left or right sinus of Valsalva, respectively, the anomalous vessel transverses the base of the heart in a course anterior to the pulmonary trunk, posterior to the aorta, or between the aorta and pulmonary trunk (Figs. 47-3 and 47-4). At least 43 cases have been reported with necropsy where the origin of the left main coronary artery is from the right sinus with passage between the aorta and pulmonary trunk.[6] In 79 percent of these patients,[2,3] death was related to the anomaly by sudden death or an acute MI. At necropsy, 5 of 26 patients aged less than 20 years old had myocardial infarcts.[6] When the right coronary artery originates from the left sinus of Valsalva and passes between the aorta and pulmonary trunk, symptoms of myocardial ischemia, infarction, or sudden death may occur.[6] Of 12 patients with this anomaly,[6] 3 died suddenly and 2 had angina or syncope. At necropsy, transmural ventricular scars (healed infarction) were seen in two.

The mechanism of ischemia, infarction, and/or sudden death in this coronary anomaly appears related to the shape of the coronary ostium of the anomalous vessel (see Figs. 47-2 to 47-4). Normally, the coronary ostia are round to oval in shape, but in this anomaly, the coronary artery has an acute angle of takeoff that makes the ostium slitlike in shape. With increased cardiac output, the aorta dilates with stretching of the aortic wall, so that this slitlike ostium may become severely narrowed (Figs. 47-3 to 47-6). It is unlikely that there is "compression" of the anomalous coronary artery by the aorta and pulmonary trunk, in view of the marked differences in diastolic pressures. At best, there would be an anterior shift of the anomalous vessel rather than a viselike compression.

## SINGLE CORONARY ARTERY

Origin of the entire coronary circulation from a single aortic ostium has been termed *single coronary*. This anomaly is rare in the absence of other associated anomalies of the heart (see Fig. 47-1). One or more branches of the single artery may cross the base of the heart in a fashion described earlier and thus may be exposed to the risks of ischemia owing to acute angulation.[4] Angina pectoris and myocardial lactate production have been demonstrated in patients with single coronary arteries when coronary atherosclerosis or an anomalous coronary artery passage was absent.[12]

## CORONARY ARTERY ATRESIA

Atresia of one of the two main coronary ostia may be associated with myocardial ischemia and infarction in infancy or childhood.[4] The involved vessel becomes dependent on collateral coronary blood flow from the contralateral coronary artery.

## HIGH-TAKEOFF CORONARY OSTIA

Normally, the coronary ostia are located within the sinuses of Valsalva, which optimizes coronary artery blood flow in diastole. Location of the ostia in the tubular portion of the aorta (i.e., "high-

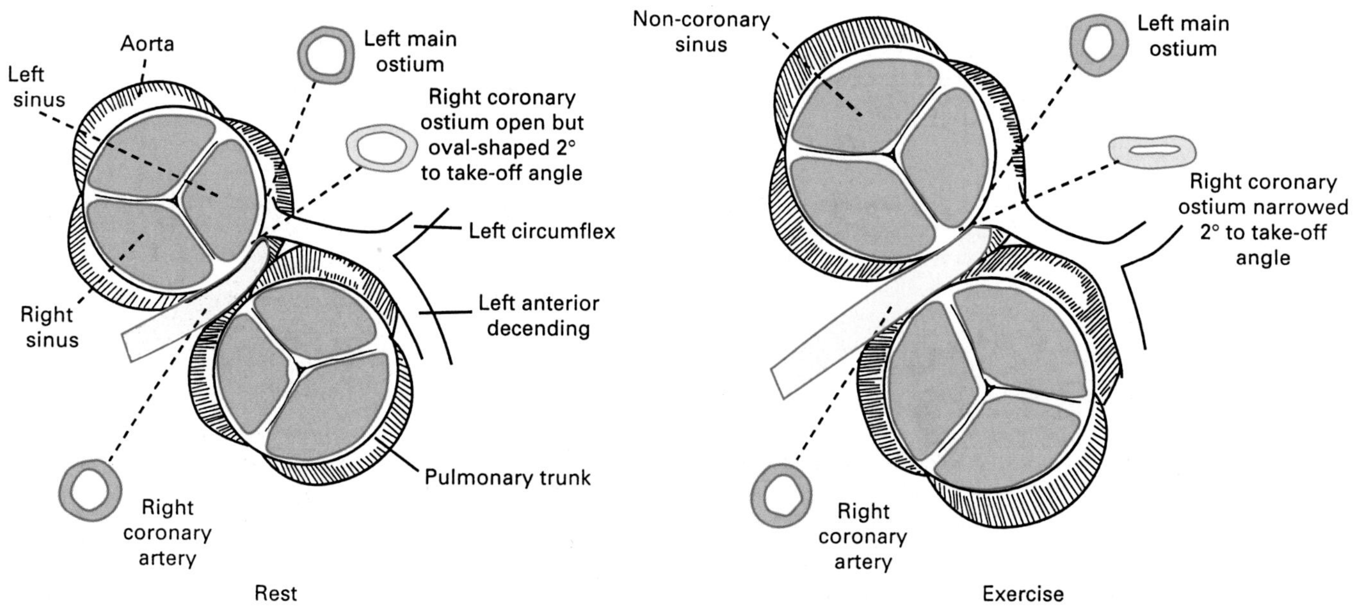


FIGURE 47-3 Diagram showing the proposed mechanism of myocardial ischemia produced by anomalous origin of the right coronary artery from the left sinus of Valsalva. With exercise, the aorta and pulmonary trunk dilate, thereby reducing the already narrowed coronary ostium of the anomalous right coronary. (From Waller.[9] Reproduced with permission from the publisher, editor, and author.)

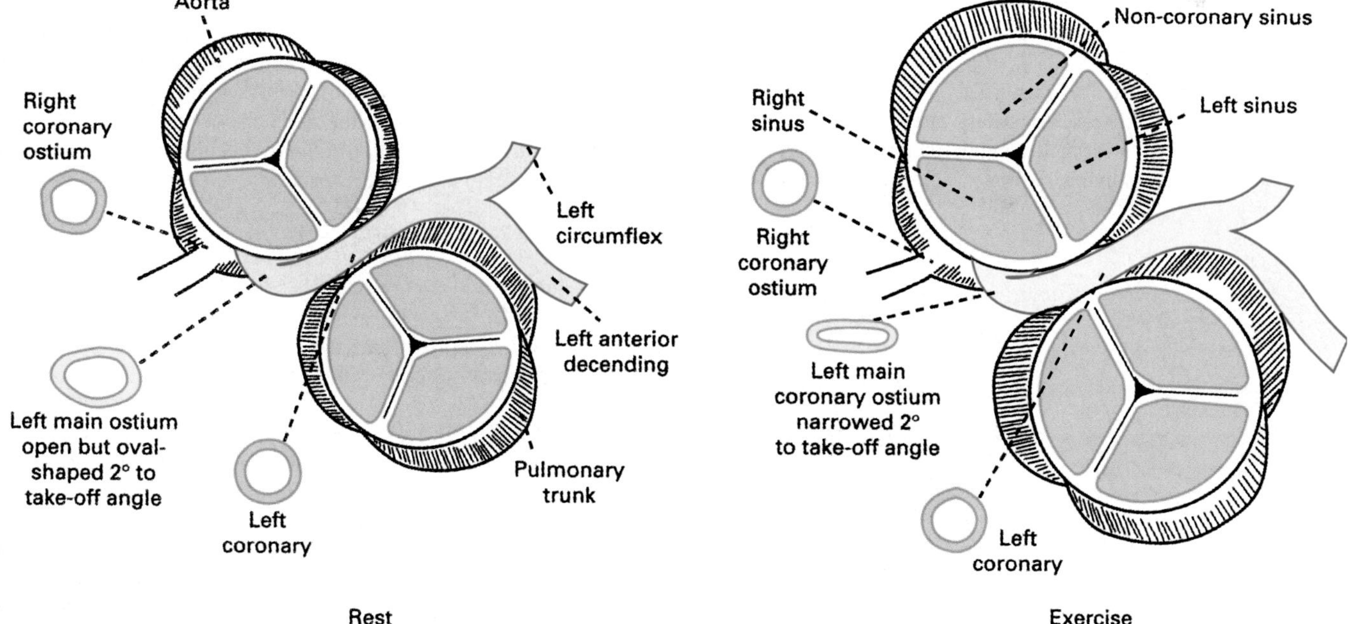


FIGURE 47-4 Diagram showing the proposed mechanism of myocardial ischemia produced by anomalous origin of the left coronary artery from the right sinus of Valsalva. With exercise, the aorta and pulmonary trunk dilate, thereby reducing the already narrowed coronary ostium of the anomalous left coronary. (From Waller.[9] Reproduced with permission from the publisher, editor, and author.)

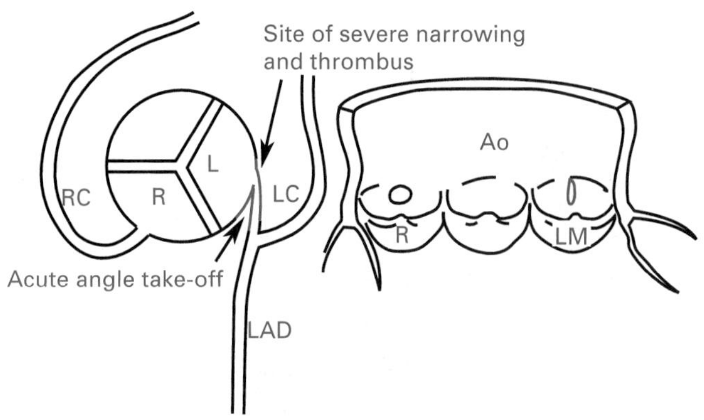


FIGURE 47-5 Diagram showing acute angle takeoff of the left main coronary artery with ostial ridge and slitlike orifice. The proximal left main is occluded by atherosclerotic plaque and thrombus, but the remaining vessels are normal. Accelerated coronary atherosclerosis may result from the acute angle takeoff malformation. Ao = aorta; L = left cusp; LM = left main; LC = left circumflex; LAD = left anterior descending; R = right cusp; RC = right coronary. (From Menke.[10] Reproduced with permission from the publisher and author.)

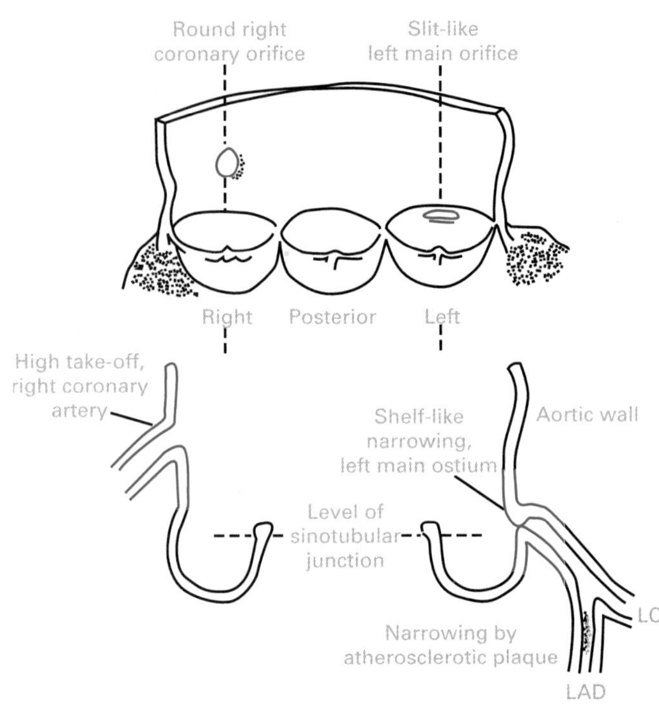


FIGURE 47-7 Diagram showing high-takeoff position of the right coronary artery and the nonatherosclerotic fibrous ridge occluding the left main coronary ostium. LAD = left anterior descending; LC = left circumflex. (From Foster et al.[13] Reproduced with permission from the publisher and author.)

takeoff" position) may be associated with decreased coronary perfusion (Figs. 47-7 and 47-8). Morphologic evidence of chronic ischemia has been reported in a patient with a high-takeoff right coronary artery who had right and left ventricular (LV) wall scarring.[13,14] High-takeoff position of the coronary ostium also has been postulated as a cause of sudden coronary death.[15] In a series of 54 major and minor coronary artery anomalies,[16] both coronary artery ostia arose above the sinotubular junction in two, the right coronary artery ostium arose high in five, and the left coronary artery ostium was in a high-takeoff position in three. In two cases of high origin of the right coronary artery ostium, ischemia and death were attributed to the ostial lesion in one.[17]

## Ostial Fibrous Ridges

Nonatherosclerotic causes of coronary ostial narrowing include syphilis,[18] Takayasu's disease (pulseless disease),[19] fibromuscular hyperplasia associated with methysergide therapy,[20,21] aortic valve surgery with or without coronary artery cannulation,[13,22] and ostial valvelike ridges (see Fig. 47-7). A nonatherosclerotic fibrous shelflike ridge can project from the wall of the aorta into the left main ostium.[13,14] It may have been responsible for chronic ischemia and myocardial necrosis. Other rare diseases that may narrow or occlude the coronary ostia have been summarized by Baroldi[23]: (1) a nonatheromatous, calcific protrusion from the sinotubular junction into the right or left ostium; (2) saccular aneurysm of the aorta; (3) aortic dissection extending into the coronary ostium; (4) supravalvular aortic stenosis with severe intimal thickening; (5) obliteration of the ostium due to adhesion of the free edge of an aortic cusp to the aortic wall above the coronary ostium; (6) occlusion by embolus (see later); and (7) occlusive fibroelastosis.

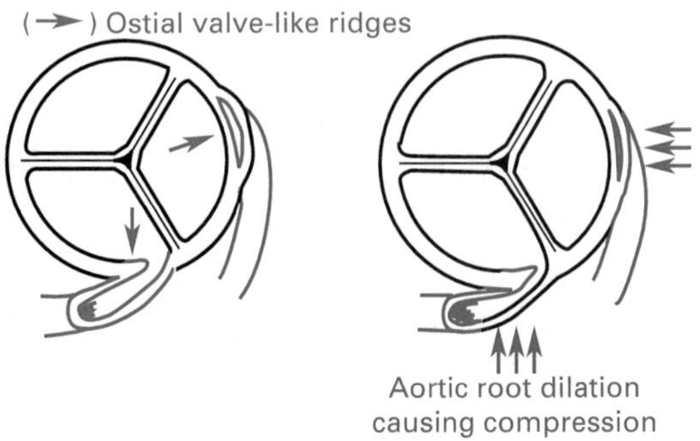


FIGURE 47-6 Diagram illustrating ostial valvelike ridges and the proposed mechanism of ostial compression with aortic root dilation. (From Virmani et al.[11] Reproduced with permission from the publisher and author.)

## ANOMALOUS ORIGIN OF ONE OR TWO CORONARY ARTERIES FROM THE PULMONARY TRUNK

Anomalous origin of a coronary artery from the pulmonary trunk (Figs. 47-9 and 47-10) may be responsible for myocardial ischemia and infarction in infants and children. In more than 90 percent of cases,[4,6] the left main artery is the anomalous artery; thus the anteroseptal and anterolateral left ventricular myocardium may be at jeopardy for injury. Asymptomatic older patients with this coronary anomaly are usually found when they present with an abnormal *electrocardiogram (ECG),* systolic murmur, or sudden death.[6] The murmur and abnormal *ECG* are the result of papillary muscle and/or anteroseptal myocardial wall damage (see Chap. 18).

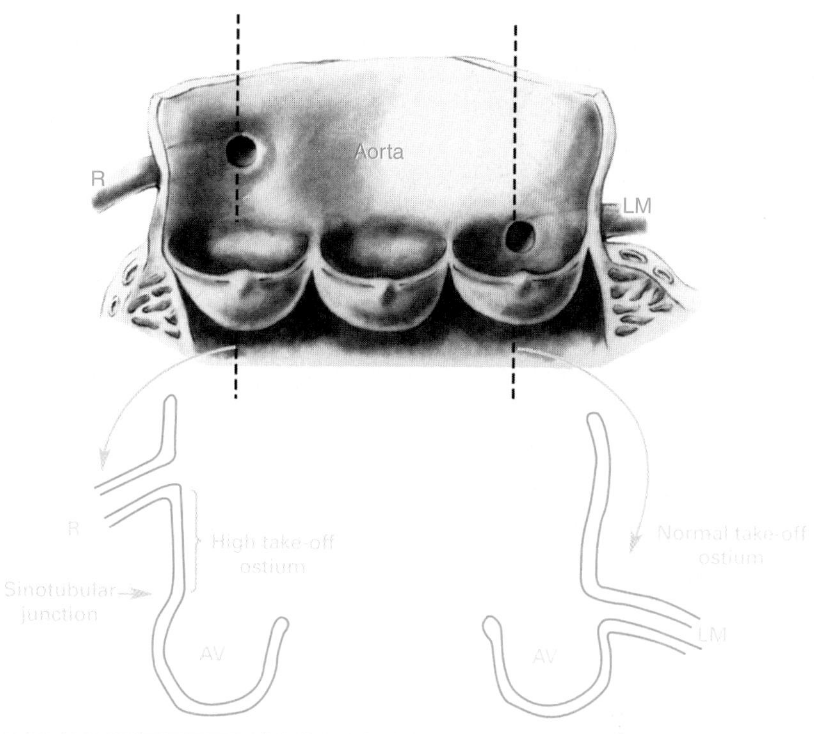


FIGURE 47-8 Diagram showing origin of right coronary ostium above the sinotubular junction—"high-takeoff position." AV = aortic valve; L = left cusp; LM = left main; R = right cusp or right coronary artery.

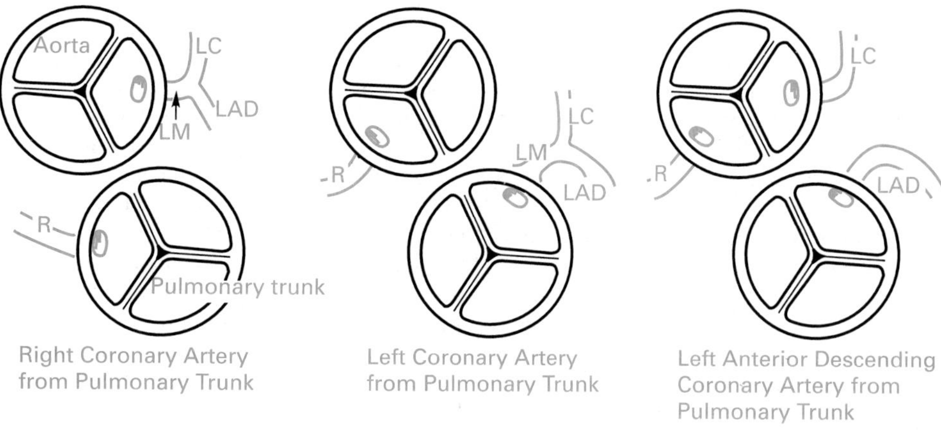


FIGURE 47-9 Anomalous origin of one or two major epicardial coronary arteries from the pulmonary trunk. (From Waller.[1] Reproduced with permission from the publisher, editor, and author.) For abbreviations, see Fig. 47-2.

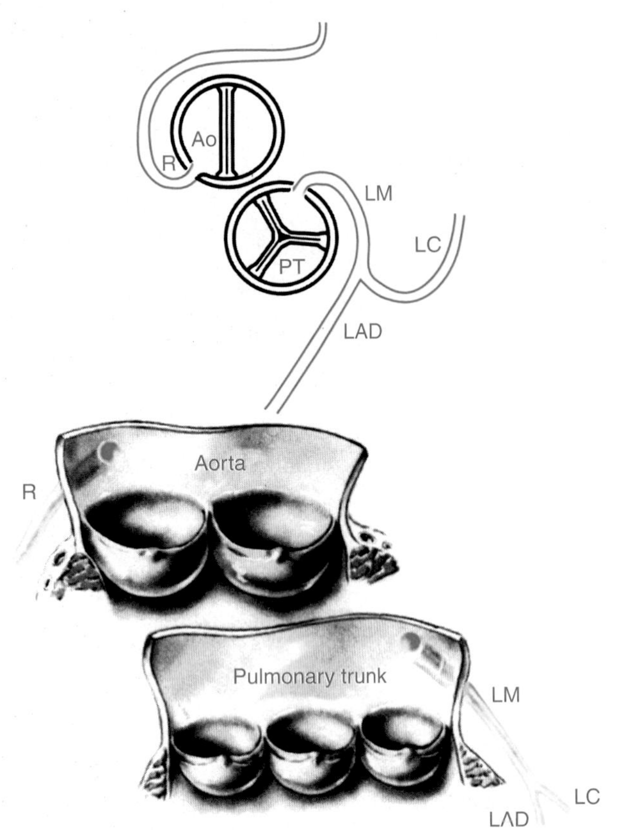


FIGURE 47-10 **Anomalous origin of the main (LM) coronary artery from the pulmonary trunk causing acute MI in an infant. Of interest is both the anomalous LM and normal right coronary arteries arise in high-takeoff positions from the pulmonary trunk and aorta (Ao) respectively. LAD = left anterior descending; LC = left circumflex.**

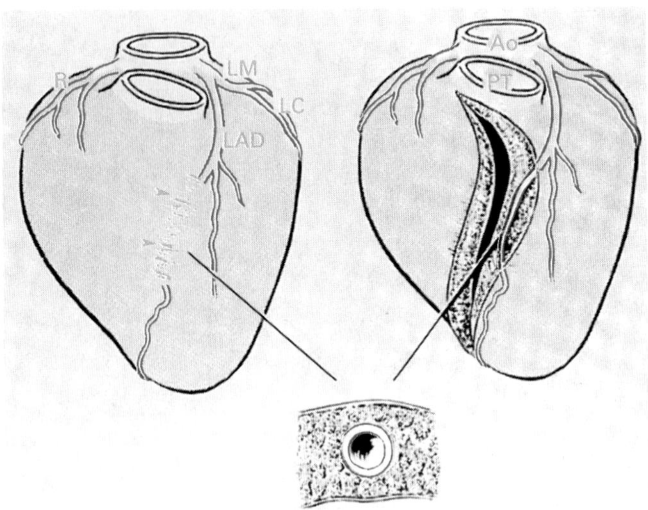


FIGURE 47-11 *Left:* Diagram showing tunneled left anterior descending coronary artery (LAD) (*arrowheads*). *Right:* Opened left ventricle showing intramyocardial segment. *Below:* Transverse section of left ventricular wall showing tunneled coronary artery surrounded by myocardium. (From Waller. [1] Reproduced with permission from the publisher, editor, and author.)

## MYOCARDIAL BRIDGES ("TUNNELED" EPICARDIAL CORONARY ARTERY)

**The coronary arteries may dip into the myocardium for varying lengths and then reappear on the heart's surface (Figs. 47-11 to 47-18). The muscle overlying the intramyocardial segment of the epicardial coronary artery is termed a *myocardial bridge,* and the artery coursing within the myocardium is called a *tunneled artery* (see Figs. 47-11 to 47-13).[24–35] Tunneled coronary arteries have long been recognized anatomically,[24] but suggested associations between myocardial ischemia and myocardial bridges have heightened their clinical relevance.[25,26]**

**Tunneled coronary arteries have been presumed congenital in origin.[27] At least three factors have been postulated to account for differences between the high frequency of tunneled major coronary arteries observed at necropsy (5[28] to 86 percent[29,32]) and the lower frequency of tunneled coronary arteries observed angiographically (0.5[25] to 12 percent[31,33,35]) or associated with symptoms of myocardial ischemia (18 percent[31]): (1) length of the tunneled coronary segment, (2) degree of systolic compression, and (3) heart rate. Longer tunneled segments of coronary arteries,[26] more severe systolic diameter narrowing of the tunneled segment,[26] and tachycardia[33] may contribute to the production of myocardial ischemia with myocardial bridging (see Figs. 47-17 and 47-18). The length of coronary tunneling may not always be an important factor in causing myocardial** ischemia, as three cases with left main intramyocardial tunneling of greater than 40 mm have been described without evidence of myocardial ischemia[35] (Fig. 47-19).

## CORONARY ARTERY FISTULA

A coronary artery fistula is an abnormal communication between an epicardial coronary artery and a cardiac chamber, major vessel (vena cava, subpulmonary veins, pulmonary artery), or other vascular structures (mediastinal vessels, coronary sinus) (Fig. 47-20).[4,36–77] This infrequent abnormality can affect any age and is the most important hemodynamically significant coronary artery anomaly.[4,36–78] Many are small and found incidentally during coronary arteriography, while others are identified as the cause of a continuous murmur, angina, acute MI, sudden death coronary steal, congestive heart failure, endocarditis, stroke, arrhythmias, coronary aneurysm formation (rupture, emboli), or superior vena cava syndrome.[36–48] Of over 33,000 patients undergoing coronary arteriography, coronary artery fistula occurred in 0.1 percent,[48] whether due to congenital[49–56] or acquired causes[48–77] (Table 47-3). Fistulas from the right coronary artery are more common than from the left[36–77] and over 90 percent of the fistulas drain into the venous circulation.[36–77] Most fistulas are single communications, but multiple fistulas have been identified.[71] The natural history of coronary artery fistulas is variable, with long periods of stability in some and sudden onset or gradual progression of symptoms in others. Spontaneous closure is uncommon.[71–73] Surgical repair of the fistula is recommended for symptomatic patients and for those asymptomatic patients at risk for future complications (coronary steals, aneurysms, large shunts).[74–77] Transcatheter embolization of fistulas has been reported.[78] Direct connection between a major epicardial coronary artery and a cardiac chamber or major vessel (vena cava, coronary sinus, pulmonary artery) is the most common hemodynamically significant coronary artery anomaly (see Fig. 47-19).[4] Fistulas from the right coronary artery are more common than they are from the left. Over 90 percent of the fistulas drain into the venous circulation.[4] Myocardial ischemia has been documented in some patients with coronary artery fistulas who have no evidence of coronary atherosclerosis.[4]

Treatment of symptomatic, clinically recognized myocardial bridges has included beta blockers and calcium channel blockers (control of tachycardia and antispasmodic effects) and surgery. Several cases have now been reported[79–81] in which "supraarterial myotomy" (release of myocardial bridge, excision of myocardial bridge) has resulted in relief of symptoms and improvement in previously abnormal nuclear imaging tests. High-frequency intraoperative echocardiography has been used to image the intramyocardial coronary artery before and after surgical release.[79]

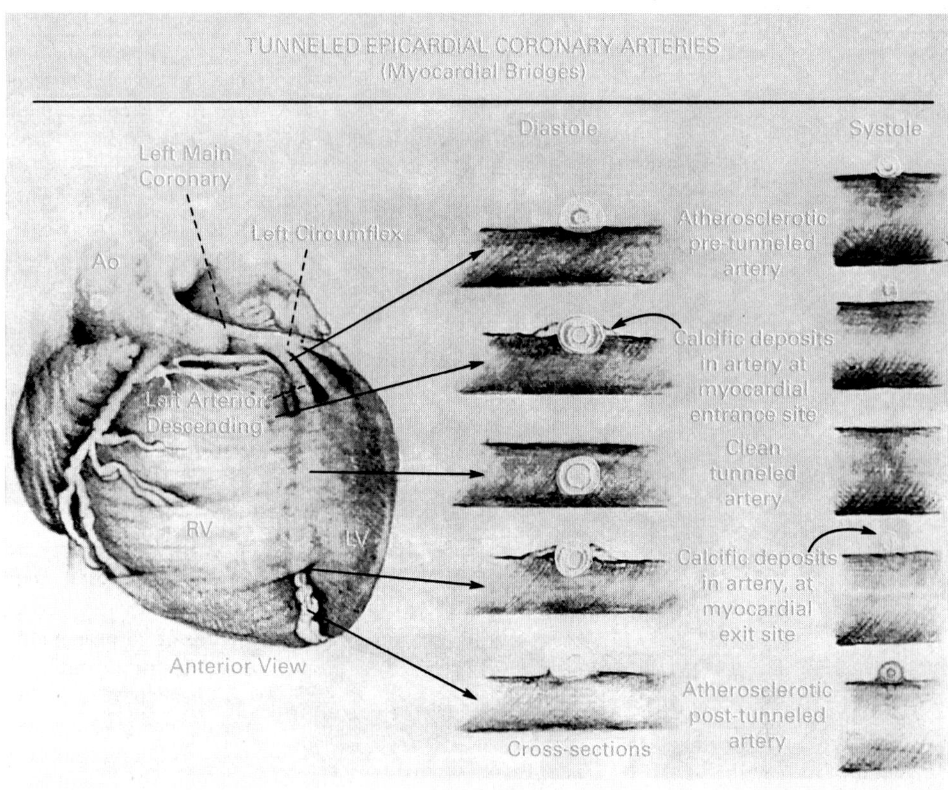


FIGURE 47-12 **Diagram showing segments of tunneled and nontunneled epicardial coronary artery with changes** during ventricular systole and diastole. Ao = aorta; LV = **left ventricle; RV = right ventricle. (From Waller.[9] Reproduced with permission from the publisher, editor, and author.)**

## CORONARY ANEURYSMS

Aneurysm formation of the coronary arteries may result from congenital or acquired conditions. Congenital coronary artery aneurysms are found most commonly in the right coronary artery.[82] Abnormal flow patterns within the aneurysm may lead to thrombus formation, with subsequent vessel occlusion, distal thromboembolization, and MI.[83] In general, angina pectoris or acute MI present in patients less than 20 years of age should prompt suspicion of a congenital coronary artery anomaly or a congenital coronary artery aneurysm.[82] Coronary artery aneurysms are found in about 1.5 percent of patients studied at necropsy or by coronary arteriography. Coronary artery aneurysms, which may be multiple, can be congenital or the result of atherosclerosis, trauma, angioplasty, atherectomy, laser procedures, arteritis (including syphilis), mycotic emboli, mucocutaneous lymph node syndrome (Kawasaki's disease), systemic lupus erythematosus,[84] or dissection (spontaneous or secondary; Table 47-4). Atherosclerosis-induced aneurysms are thought to result from primary thinning and/or destruction of the media and may represent up to 50 percent of the causes (see Table 47-4). Angioplasty, atherectomy, vasculitis, and arteritis may also damage the arterial wall (media) and lead to coronary aneurysms.

## CORONARY ARTERY EMBOLI

Coronary arterial emboli (Figs. 47-21 to 47-25) are clinically suspected in patients who develop severe chest pain with acute MI in the presence of a prosthetic left-sided valve, active infective endocarditis, native left-sided valve stenosis, atrial fibrillation, left ventricular aneurysm, dilated cardiomyopathy (see Fig. 47-22), known cardiac tumor, or during cardiac catheterization or cardiac surgery. Coronary emboli can be due to natural, iatrogenic, or "paradoxical" causes (Table 47-5; see Figs. 47-21 to 47-25).[85–97] Coronary embolism most often involves the left anterior descending coronary artery. Coronary artery embolism of tumor fragments or thrombus from the surface of tumors is an unusual cause of acute MI. Left-sided primary cardiac tumors (myxoma, angiosarcomas, rhabdomyosarcoma, rhabdomyoma, fibrosarcoma, or lipoma papillary fibrosarcoma) or metastatic cardiac tumors (primary or metastatic pulmonary tumors, osteogenic sarcoma, or renal cell carcinoma) can give rise to coronary emboli traveling from the left atrium or left ventricle to the coronary circulation. Right-sided cardiac primary or metastatic tumors can only produce coronary emboli in the presence of an intracardiac shunt.

Coronary embolism is suspected as the cause of acute MI when, at necropsy, the zone of necrosis is large but discrete (since there was little time to develop effective collaterals). Embolic coronary artery lesions can resolve completely and spontaneously and provide an explanation for angiographically normal coronary arteries several months following an acute MI.

The consequences of coronary embolism depend on two major factors (see Fig. 47-25): the size of the embolus and the size of the lumen of the artery in which it becomes impacted.[48, 99] The smaller the embolus, the greater the chance that it will travel distally to a small coronary arterial segment and the less likelihood of MI or fatal arrhythmia.[98] An embolus so small that it travels distally and impacts in a single intramural vessel is probably clinically silent and observed only at necropsy.[98, 99] The status of the coronary lumen before the embolus appears also determines the subsequent myocardial consequences. An embolus to a previously normal coronary artery is likely to migrate distally and result in localized MI because of absence of collaterals. An embolus traveling to a previously diseased

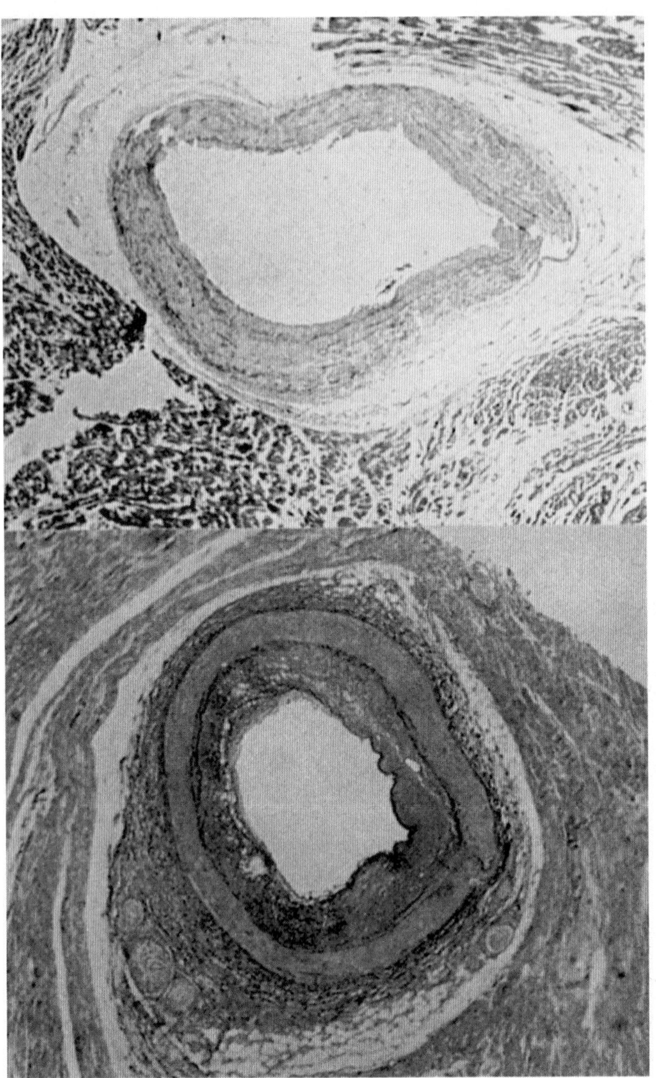

FIGURE 47-13 Tunneled epicardial coronary arteries. Two examples of tunneled left anterior descending coronary arteries. Each artery is surrounded by myocardium. (From Waller.[1] Reproduced with permission from the publisher, editor, and author.)

coronary artery is more likely to impact proximally. Emboli to the left main coronary arteries are rare but usually fatal (see Fig. 47-24).[99]

## CORONARY ARTERY DISSECTION

Separation of the media by hemorrhage with or without an associated intimal tear is termed *coronary artery dissection*. The medial separation forces the intimal-medial layer (wall of true channel) toward the true coronary lumen and produces distal myocardial ischemia and infarction (Figs. 47-26 and 47-27). Coronary artery dissections may be primary or secondary (Table 47-6).[100–110] Secondary coronary artery dissections are more frequent, especially those associated as an extension from aortic root dissection (8 percent).[4] Primary coronary artery dissections may occur spontaneously or as a consequence of coronary angioplasty or angiography, cardiac surgery, or chest trauma (0.3 percent).[106] Most spontaneous coronary artery dissections occur in women who are most commonly postpartum; they may be associated with coronary artery wall eosinophils.[100–110] The left anterior descending artery is the one most frequently involved. Systemic hypertension does not appear to provide a significant factor of risk.[82]

Spontaneous coronary artery dissection may result in sudden death or acute MI and subsequent death. Spontaneous coronary artery dissection, which becomes chronic (chronic dissection), may result in congestive heart failure. This circumstance is found primarily in postpartum women.[109] In a series reported by DeMaio and associates [109] 75 percent of cases were diagnosed only at autopsy and 75 percent of these patients were women (one half of the women were postpartum).[109] In a few patients with multivessel coronary artery dissection, systemic hypertension was the only association identified. Use of thrombolytic therapy in the acute phase may extend the dissection process or promotion rupture of the false channel due to "engorgement" tearing a thin medial-adventitial wall of the false channel. Recognition of the associated causes and conditions of spontaneous coronary artery dissection (including absence of classic coronary atherosclerotic disease risk factors) should alert clinicians to the possibility of coronary dissection producing acute MI and use of urgent coronary arteriography instead of automatic infusion of thrombolytic agents.

Localized and limited coronary artery dissection (i.e., intimal-media tear) appears necessary for a clinically successful coronary artery balloon angioplasty procedure[101,102] (see Chap. 55). Coronary angioplasty dissections viewed in short- or long-axis tomographic images help distinguish dissections that are *therapeutic* (mechanism) from those which are *complications of angioplasty* (complications).[110] In the short-axis image, dissection involving more than 50 percent of the coronary media circumference has been considered a complication. Similarly, in the long-axis image, dissections (antegrade, retrograde, or both) longer than 1 cm in length have also been defined as a complication of angioplasty (Fig. 47-28). A combination of dissection >50 percent of short-axis circumference and >1 cm antegrade or retrograde of long-axis length may result in "intussusception" of intimal-medial tissue. Spiral dissections ("the ugly") are among the most serious dissection injuries after balloon angioplasty (Fig. 47-29). The spiral dissection as reviewed angiographically appears to alternate from side to side, extending antegrade and retrograde (see Fig. 47-29*A*), or it has an unaltered dissection course but appears alternating from limited angiographic views (see Fig. 47-29*B*).

## CORONARY ARTERY SPASM

Coronary artery luminal narrowing produced by spasm has been associated with angina pectoris, acute MI, and sudden death[111–122] (see Chap. 51). Despite the extensive clinical information about coronary artery spasm, relatively few necropsy data are available.[111–152] Smooth muscle cells in the coronary artery wall may contract in response to various neurologic and pharmacologic stimuli and temporarily reduce the vessel lumen. Specific pathogenesis of this disorder is unknown[144] (see Chap. 51). Enhanced alpha-adrenergic tone[121] and various vasoactive substances—such as histamine, catecholamines, prostaglandins, thromboxane[119–121]—are presently thought to be relevant factors. Necropsy findings have been reviewed in 13 previously reported cases and in 3 new cases[114] (Figs. 47-30 and 47-31).

Most of the 13 previous patients with clinical evidence of spasm had significant fixed coronary luminal narrowing due to atherosclerotic plaque, although coronary angiograms during life did not recognize these lesions found at necropsy.[100] In one of the original patients described by Prinzmetal and colleagues,[111] both major epicardial coronary arteries were "markedly sclerotic," and the "posterior coronary artery" was 80 percent narrowed. Of the subsequent 12 necropsy patients, 10 had at least one major artery severely narrowed by atherosclerotic plaque at necropsy.[111–116] The three necropsy patients with clinical spasm[100,114] all had severe luminal coronary narrowing by atherosclerotic plaque at least in the artery in which spasm had been demonstrated during life (see Figs. 47-30 and 47-31). In general, histologic sections of the left anterior descending artery at the site of spasm disclosed luminal concentric plaque that had a predominance of smooth muscle cells, suggesting that the lesion may have been responsive to pharmacologic and neurologic stimuli compared with "garden-variety" fibrotic and calcified atherosclerotic plaque (see Fig. 47-31). In a patient with normal angiograms and documented MI, "intimal ridges" were observed on postmortem angiography; these were interpreted as evidence of spasm.[123] Similar ridges have been noted at necropsy in a patient with coronary artery spasm.[125] Histology of the ridges disclosed typical atherosclerotic plaque,[124] suggesting that varying degrees of dynamic muscular contraction may be superimposed upon fixed atherosclerotic lesions, presumably related to the amount of smooth muscle present.[100] Coronary artery smooth muscle depletion ("medial attenuation"), which accompanies advanced degrees of luminal narrowing by atherosclerotic plaque, suggests diminished potential for coronary wall spasm.[124] It has been suggested that medial "contraction" bands may represent a morphologic-histologic marker for arteries that have spasm during life[125] (see Chap. 51).

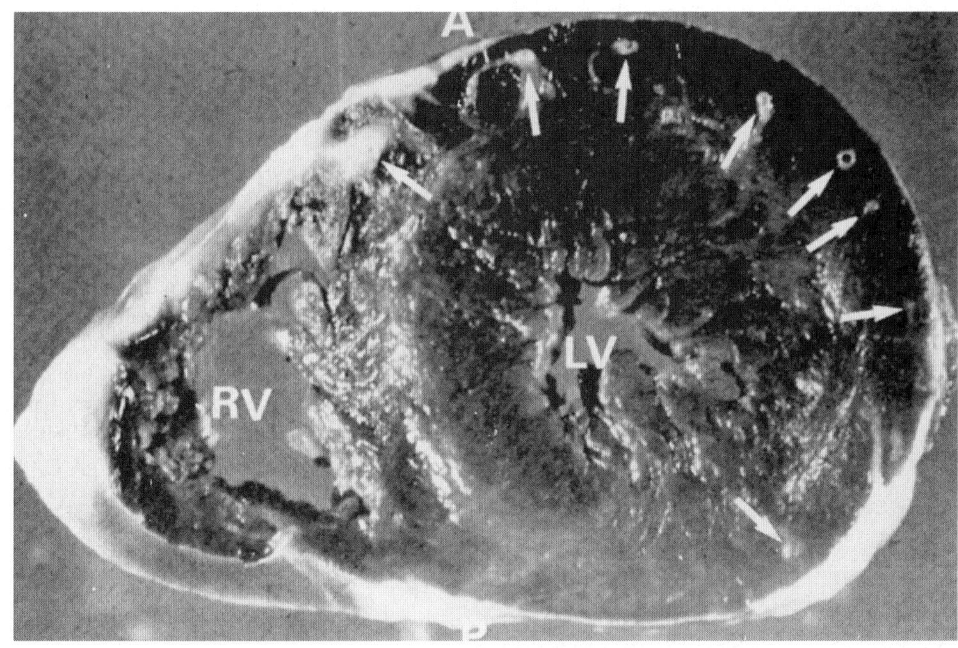

FIGURE 47-14 Transverse section of ventricular myocardium showing the "arcade" of tunneled epicardial coronary arteries (*arrows*). A = anterior; LV = left ventricle; RV = right ventricle; P = posterior. (From Waller.[1] Reproduced with permission from the publisher, editor, and author.)

Eccentric atherosclerotic plaques have a segment of disease-free wall with preserved media, which presumably has the potential for spasm[126] (see Chap. 51). In patients with clinical coronary spasm, unstable and stable angina pectoris, and episodes of silent myocardial ischemia, 448 segments were narrowed by more than 75 percent in cross-sectional area by plaques, 15 percent of these segments had a variable arc of disease-free wall with normal media. Other studies have found a similar 15 to 20 percent of the coronary wall normal in 70 percent of the cases studied.[127–128] This disease-free coronary segment represents a site of "vasospastic potential" and could convert a hemodynamically insignificant lesion of less than 50 percent cross-sectional area into a hemodynamically significant one of more than 75 percent narrowing.

Three newly recognized associations and/or causes of coronary spasm include general anesthesia,[116] "allergic angina" (histamine-induced), and postpartum bromocriptine usage. Acute ST-segment elevation has been noted following induction of general anesthesia in some patients with angiographically normal coronary arteries. In postpartum women receiving bromocriptine in the presence of pregnancy-induced hypertension acute MI has occurred.[117]

Coronary spasm also occurs with balloon angioplasty and coronary interventional procedures, catheter-related angiography, and neurofibromatosis.[118]

Endothelial cell dysfunction has been proposed to explain coronary vasospasm.[119] In response to increases in shear stress, platelet products, and other agonists, normal endothelial cells release endothelium-derived relaxing factor (nitric oxide), resulting in vasodilation.[119] When endothelium is damaged, as occurs with hypertension, elevated cholesterol, smoking, or use of cocaine, endothelial nitric oxide is reduced or lost. Thus, when platelets aggregate at such sites with release of vasospastic substances such as serotonin (5-HT) and thromboxane $A_2$, arterial smooth muscle cells contract, causing spasm.[120]

Pheochromocytomas result in excess catecholamine production. Coronary artery vasoconstriction has been reported with the excess catecholamine production resulting in decreased myocardial perfusion, myocardial inflammation, cell deaths, and fibrosis.[120]

## CORONARY ARTERY TRAUMA

Coronary artery trauma may produce myocardial ischemia and/or acute MI. Traumatic injury may result from a nonpenetrating blunt chest wall injury such as a steering-wheel injury; penetration trauma such as a laceration from a stab wound or bullet; coronary bypass surgery as from inadvertent ligation, laceration, or intimal dissection; or after coronary angiography or angioplasty resulting in dissection, rupture, or embolus. Nonpenetrating trauma may produce coronary injury and subsequent MI due to coronary dissection, contusion and thrombosis, fistula formation, and/or coronary artery aneurysm formation.[4] Extensive coronary artery dissections occur more commonly as the result of catheter or cannula injury in normal or nearly normal arteries as opposed to coronary arteries with severe atherosclerotic plaque (see Chap. 93).

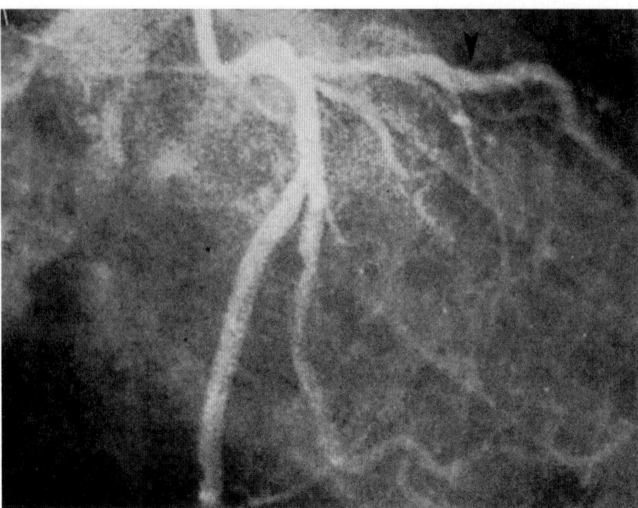

A

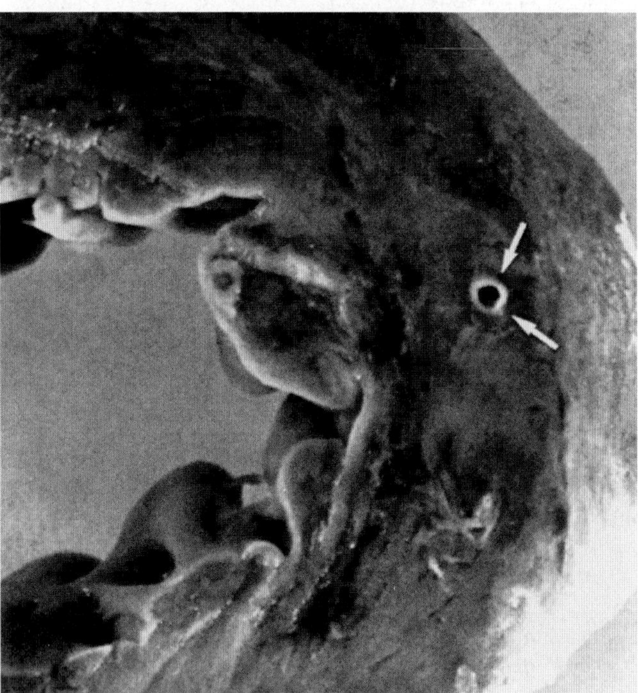

B

FIGURE 47-15 Tunneled epicardial coronary artery. *A*. Coronary angiogram showing tunneled segment of epicardial coronary artery. *B*. Corresponding segment of tunneled left circumflex coronary artery (*arrow*). (From Waller.[1] Reproduced with permission from the publisher, editor, and author.)

## CORONARY ARTERY ARTERITIS (VASCULITIS)

Epicardial coronary arteritis (vasculitis) is a rare event but has been reported in several conditions (Table 47-7). The resulting coronary injury may lead to myocardial ischemia or infarction with or without associated coronary artery thrombosis. This type of coronary artery damage has been classified by routes of entry[23]: *direct extension* from adjacent organ or tissue infections, e.g., epicardial or myocardial abscess from aortic valve endocarditis, pericardial infections such as tuberculosis; *hematogenous spread* through the coronary lumen or vasa vasorum; and *unknown* route of entry. In the direct extension route of entry, the adventitial layer of the artery is initially involved, whereas in the hematogenous route the coronary intimal layer is initially involved. Evidence of coronary arteritis has included[23] the following: (1) focal artery necrosis with or without calcification; (2) acute coronary artery thrombosis or recanalized thrombus associated with underlying atherosclerotic plaque; (3) rupture of the vessel wall unassociated with trauma or an interventional procedure; (4) coronary artery wall thickening with secondary luminal narrowing; or (5) wall thickening with aneurysm formation.[127] Specific coronary lesions may also be seen with systemic diseases such as tuberculosis or periarteritis.

A more recent classification of coronary vasculitides has been based upon known and unknown causes and involvement of size of vessel (medium-sized, small-sized; Table 47-8).[128] With the exception of infectious angiitis resulting from syphilitic, mycobacterial, or rickettsial infection, the causes and pathogenesis of most coronary vasculitides are either unknown or incompletely understood. Vasculitic syndromes may be caused by deposition of immune complex in the vessel walls.[129–133] The specific antigen has been identified in only a few cases, such as hepatitis B. Circulating immune complexes associated with hepatitis B infection may cause more than one type of vasculitic syndrome,[128] producing periarteritis nodosa in arteries of muscles and hypersensitivity angiitis in venules, while eliciting the production of anti-immunoglobulin antibodies, leading to cryoglobulinemia. Thus, a classification of vasculitides *based solely* on immunological studies is incomplete[128] (see Chap. 85).

## GENERAL CONCEPTS

The earliest vasculitic syndrome was named *periarteritis nodosa* because of the nodules along the course of small arteries.[128] Because the inflammatory changes are not only periarterial, *polyarteritis* may be a better term.[134] Periarteritis nodosa has become a "wastebasket designation" of any vasculitis whose cause was unknown.[128] The term *necrotizing angiitis* [135] has been used to designate arterial and venous lesions; there are 5 types[135,136]: (1) hypersensitivity angiitis, (2) allergic granulomatous angiitis, (3) rheumatoid arteritis, (4) periarteritis nodosa, and (5) temporal arteritis. The term *hypersensitivity angiitis* has been considered synonymous with small-vessel vasculitis and is used to imply that the angiitis is due to an allergic response to proteins, drugs, vaccines, or infections.[128] Allergic *granulomatous angiitis* (Churg-Strauss syndrome) is a variant of polyarteritis characterized by necrotizing vasculitis with extravascular granulomas and eosinophilia associated with asthma or allergic rhinitis.[128,137,138] *Rheumatic arteritis*[139] describes vascular lesions in rheumatic diseases with both rheumatic and necrotizing vascular lesions. *Temporal arteritis* (giant-cell arteritis) involves large and small extracranial arteries, including the coronary arteries, and blindness may be a serious complication.[128,140–143] Despite its limitations, this classification[134,135] remains a basis for the diagnosis of vasculitides. The classification of coronary vasculitis is closely tied to that of vasculitides in general[128] and relates to the predominant type and size of vessels affected (see Table 47-8; Chap. 85).[141,142]

## INFECTIOUS ANGIITIS

Various microorganisms may cause vasculitis in vessels of any size and involve the vessel by extension of the acute or chronic infective process from an adjacent tissue or organ[23] or from the lumen by hematogenous spread (see Table 47-8). The inflammatory response produces variable reactions including suppurative inflammation

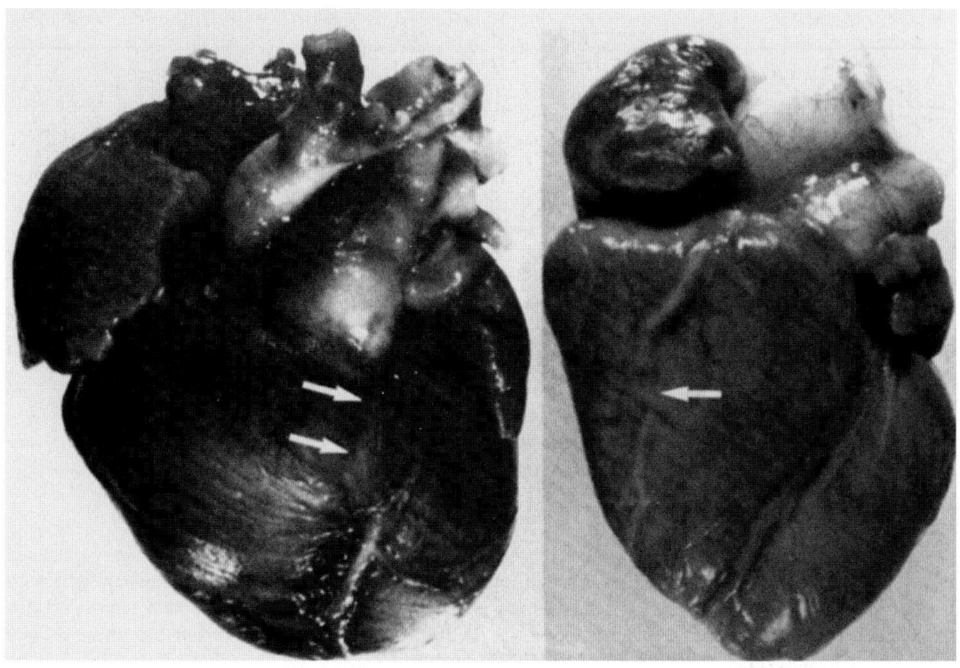

FIGURE 47-16 Tunneled left anterior epicardial coronary arteries from two newborn infants. *Left:* Tunneled left anterior descending. *Right:* Tunneled marginal branch of right coronary artery. (From Waller.[1] Reproduced with permission from the publisher, editor, and author.)

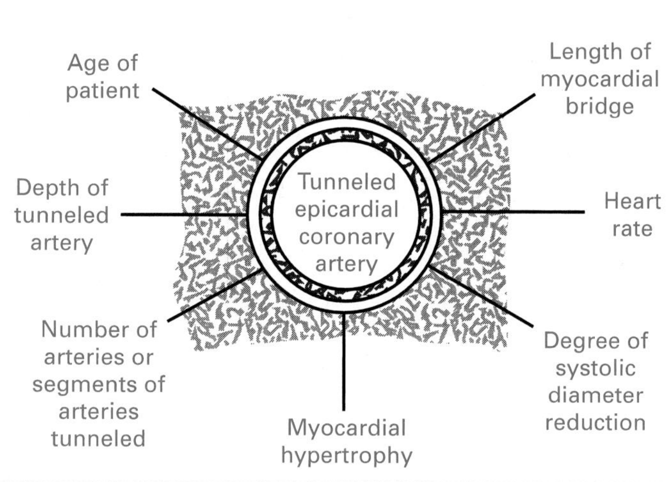


FIGURE 47-17 Diagram showing some of the clinical and anatomic factors in a tunneled epicardial coronary artery. (From Waller.[1] Reproduced with permission from the publisher, editor, and author.)

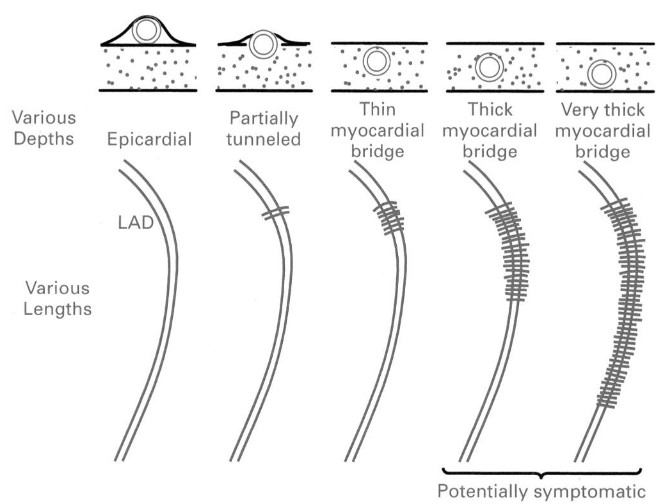


FIGURE 47-18 Diagram showing morphologic variations in tunneling (length of tunneled segment, depth of tunneled segment). (From Waller.[1] Reproduced with permission from the publisher, editor, and author.)

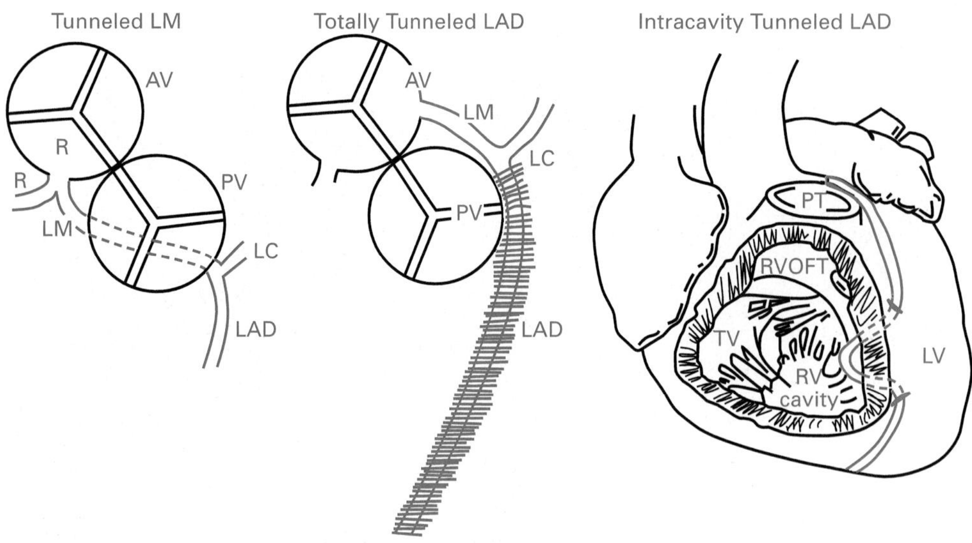


FIGURE 47-19 Diagram showing extremes of tunneled coronary arteries: left main (LM) tunneled through the ventricular septum, total length of the left anterior descending (LAD) located within the myocardium, tunneled segment of LAD becoming intracavitary. AV = aortic valve; LAD = left anterior descending; LC = left circumflex; LM = left main; LV = left ventricular; PT = pulmonary trunk; PV = pulmonary valve; RVOFT = right ventricular outflow tract; RV = right ventricle; TV = tricuspid valve. (From Waller.[1] Reproduced with permission from the publisher, editor, and author.)

bacteria, proliferative response (typhoid[146]), hemorrhagic (anthrax), and histiocytic and granulomatous response (leprosy, syphilis, tuberculosis).[128] The most important angiitic infections affecting the coronary arteries include syphilis, tuberculosis, and syphilitic arteritis. All three stages of syphilis show arteritic features. The most important vascular lesion of tertiary syphilis, coronary ostial stenosis, seen in up to 4 percent of patients with tertiary syphilis,[4,147,148] can occur independent of aortic involvement.[128,147] Syphilitic arteritis is characterized by a chronic inflammation with adventitial fibrosis and patchy destruction of media with a lymphoplasmacytic infiltrate. Gummas can be found in 20 percent of cases,[149] but spirochetes are rarely detected.[128] The first 3 to 4 mm of the left and right coronary arteries may be involved with an obliterative arteritis[82]; angina and acute MI may result from syphilitic involvement.[148]

## TUBERCULOUS ARTERITIS

Tuberculous coronary arteritis occurs mainly in patients with pericardial and myocardial tuberculosis.[150,151] Granuloma may involve the adventitia, intima, or the entire wall[23,151] and result from several infectious angiitic agents. Endocarditis and septicemia are the most common underlying causes of infectious angiitis and mycotic aneurysm formation.[128,152] Any type of gram-positive or gram-

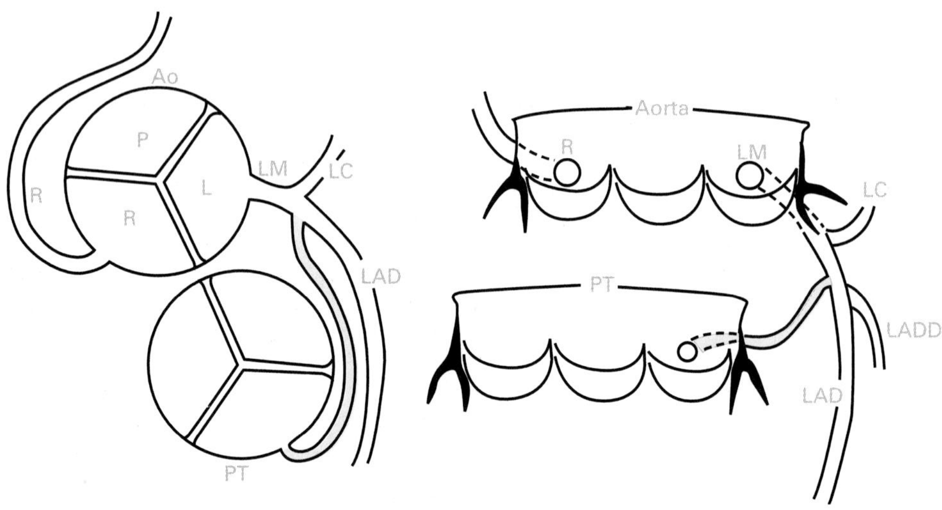


FIGURE 47-20 Diagram showing coronary artery fistula connecting pulmonary trunk and left anterior descending (LAD) artery. It originally was misdiagnosed as an anomalous coronary artery. LADD = diagonal branch of LAD: LC = left circumflex; LM = left main; R = right.

TABLE 47-3 Causes and Associations of Coronary Artery Fistula

I. Congenital[49–56]
  1. Embryonic
  2. Multiple; systemic hemangioma
II. Acquired
  1. Closed-chest ablation of accessory pathway[57]
  2. Percutaneous coronary balloon angioplasty[58–60]
  3. Hypertrophic cardiomyopathy[61]
  4. Right/left ventricular septal myectomy[66]
  5. Penetrating and nonpenetrating trauma[67–69]
  6. Acute myocardial infarction[62,64]
  7. Dilated cardiomyopathy[65]
  8. Mitral valve surgery[283]
  9. "Sign" of mural thrombus[284]
  10. Tumor[285]
  11. Permanent pacemaker placement[286]
  12. Cardiac transplant[63]
  13. Endomyocardial biopsy[287,298]
  14. Coronary artery bypass grafting[70]

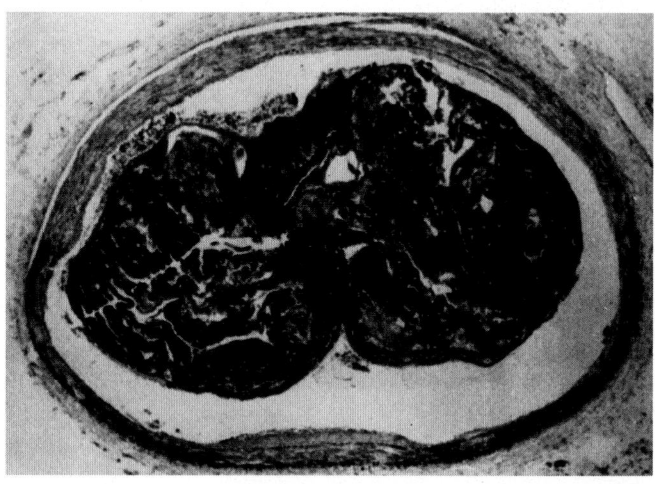

FIGURE 47-21 **Coronary artery embolus. Fibrin-platelet thrombus occluding the left anterior descending coronary artery. The source of the embolus was not established, but the patient recently underwent cardiac surgery. (From Waller.[1] Reproduced with permission from the publisher, editor, and author.)**

negative organism may be involved. Myocarditis with abscesses and pericarditis frequently accompany infectious coronary angiitis. Mucormycosis, aspergillosis, and *Candida* (Fig. 47-32) are examples of fungi and systemic yeast infections associated with coronary angiitis. Malarial parasites and parasitized red blood cells also may plug larger coronary arteries.[153] *Schistosoma haematobium* has been found in a major epicardial coronary artery associated with MI.[154] Rickettsial infections may produce angiitis in small vessels of the heart[128,155]; these infections consist of a lymphomononuclear infiltrate with or without thrombosis. A direct toxic effect from rickettsiae may produce angiitis.[156] Viruses have also been implicated in vasculitis by direct invasion of immunologic mechanisms.[128] Virus-induced vasculitides in humans are represented by polyarteritis associated with hepatitis-B antigenemia[128,157,158] and herpes zoster.[128]

## NONINFECTIOUS ANGIITIS

Various noninfectious causes of angiitis involve large- to medium-sized (predominately medium- and small-sized) blood vessels (see Table 47-8).[128]

TABLE 47-4 Causes of Coronary Arterial Aneurysms

Atherosclerosis (destruction of coronary media)
Trauma
Angioplasty
Atherectomy
Laser
Arteritis (including syphilis, lupus erythematosus)
Mycotic emboli
Mucocutaneous lymph node syndrome (Kawasaki's disease)
Congenital
Dissection
Neoplasm
Connective tissue disorders (Ehlers-Danlos, Marfan's)

### Takayasu's Arteritis

Takayasu's disease (pulseless disease) is one of the coronary vasculitides associated with aortitis; others are temporal arteritides and rheumatic disease. Takayasu's disease is a chronic, occlusive inflammatory disease of unknown etiology[128,159–165] with a worldwide distribution and greater incidence in young to middle-aged female Asians.[161] Involvement of the coronary arteries occurs 15 to 25 percent of cases and may be a lethal complication (Fig. 47-33),[160, 162–164] commonly involving the coronary ostium[160,166–170] with segmental involvement of distal coronary arteries.[163, 164, 171] Rarely, diffuse coronary arteritis is produced by Takayasu's disease.

Takayasu arteritis[172] should be considered in a patient without classic atherosclerotic risk factors under the age of 40 years presenting with acute MI. The average age at onset of symptoms is about 24 years and another coronary event occurs in 40 percent in the next 10 years.[172]

### Granulomatous Giant-Cell Arteritis (Temporal Arteritis)

Granulomatous giant-cell arteritis may occur independently or, more commonly, may be associated with temporal arteritis in 10 to 15 percent of patients.[128,142,143,173–180] Histologically proven giant-cell coronary arteritis is rare, and cases leading to fatal MI are even more rare (Fig. 47-34).[128,173–175,177] The arterial wall lesion is a granulomatous inflammation with giant cells found along degenerative internal elastic membrane.[177] The intima becomes greatly thickened, and ultimately the vessel is converted into a fibrous cord. Luminal thrombosis may also be present in 16 cases of temporal arteritis reported by Harrison[178]; only 1 case involved the epicardial coronary arteries. Giant-cell arteritis of the intramural (intramyocardial) coronary arteries (Fig. 47-35) may also occur in association with temporal arteritis and giant-cell arteritis[173] (see Chap. 85).

### Arteritis of Rheumatic Disease

Rheumatic diseases commonly affect the aorta and are morphologically indistinguishable from granulomatous aortitis.[128,179–188] Coronary arteritis at necropsy has been detected in up to 20 percent of

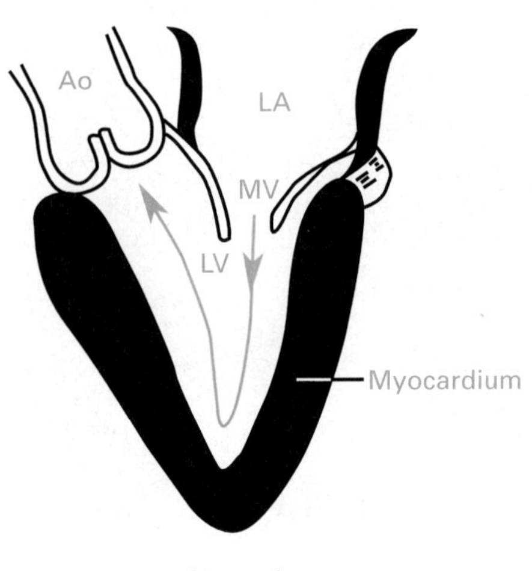


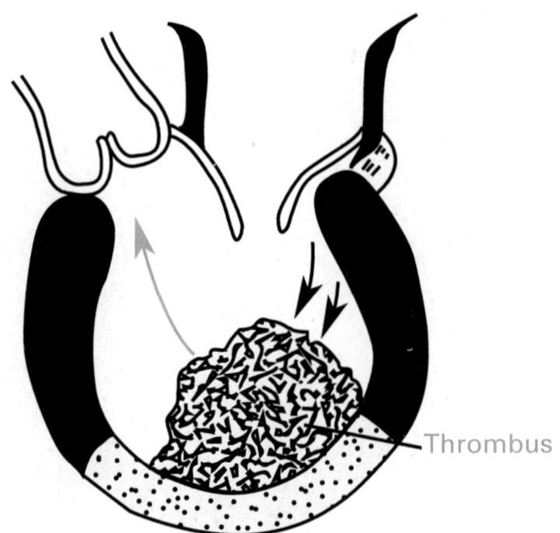


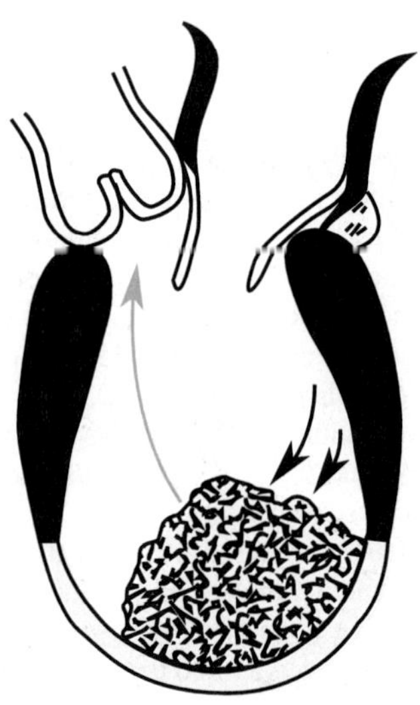


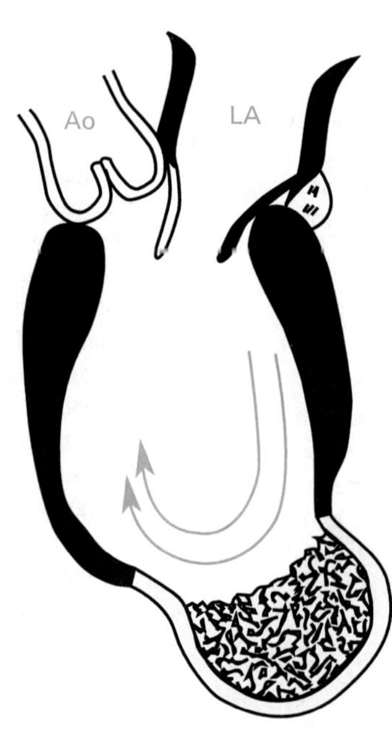


FIGURE 47-22 Diagram showing factors associated with emboli from left ventricular (LV) thrombus in three conditions: (1) idiopathic dilated cardiomyopathy (IDC); (2) coronary dilated cardiomyopathy (CDC); and (3) left ventricular aneurysm. Thrombus protruding into the LV cavity (IDC, CDC) is more likely to embolize than thrombus protected within the sac of an LV aneurysm. Underlying myocardial contraction is more likely to propel thrombus out the LV outflow tract than paradoxical motion of LV aneurysm. Ao = aorta; LA = left atrium; MV = mitral valve. (From Cabin HS, Roberts WC. Left ventricular aneurysm, intraaneurysmal thrombus and systemic embolus in coronary heart disease. *Chest 1980;77:586–590*. Reproduced with permission from the publisher, editor, and author.)

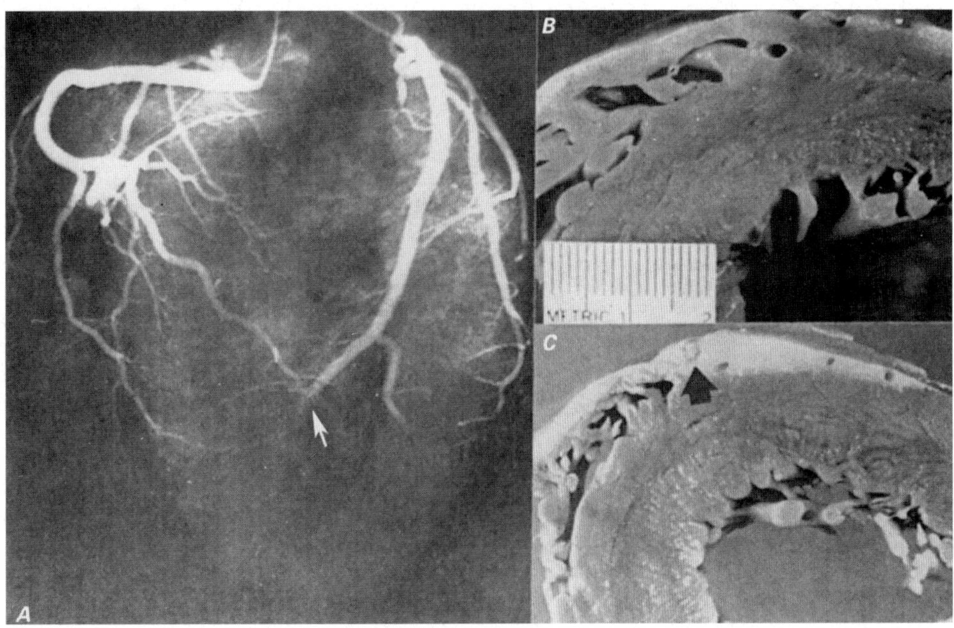


FIGURE 47-23 Coronary artery embolus. *A*. Postmortem coronary angiogram showing normal epicardial coronary arteries except for sudden cutoff of the distal third of the left anterior coronary artery (*arrow*). *B*. Portion of anterior left ventricle and proximal left anterior descending coronary artery showing normal artery. *C*. Site (*arrow*) of embolic occlusion of the left anterior descending coronary artery. The remaining distal left anterior descending, right, left circumflex, and left main coronary arteries were normal. (From Waller.[1] Reproduced with permission from the publisher, editor, and author.)

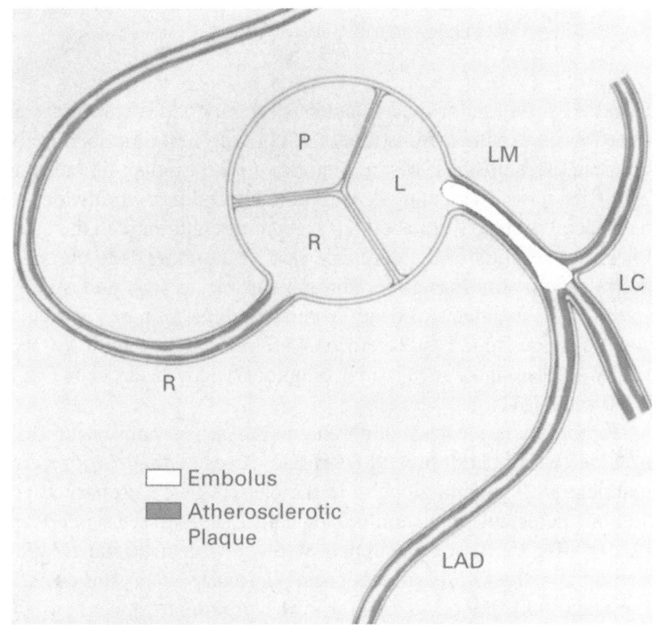


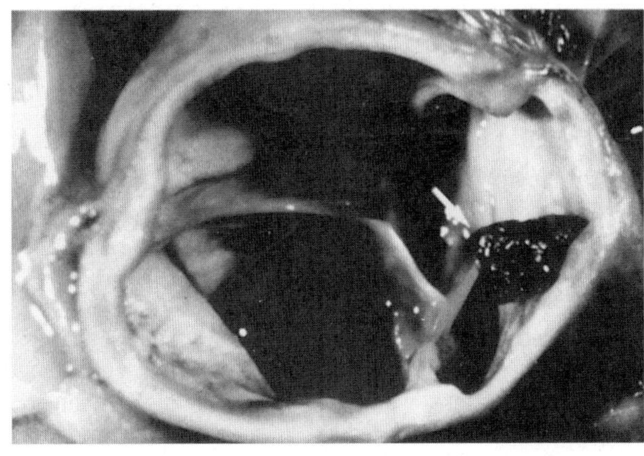


FIGURE 47-24 Coronary artery embolism. *A*. Diagram showing location and extent of occlusion of the left main (LM) coronary artery by an embolus. *B*. Photograph of aortic root showing embolus protruding from the LM coronary ostium (*arrow*). LAD = left anterior descending; LC = left circumflex; R = right. (From Waller et al.[99] Reproduced with permission from the publisher, editor, and author.)

CORONARY ARTERIAL EMBOLI

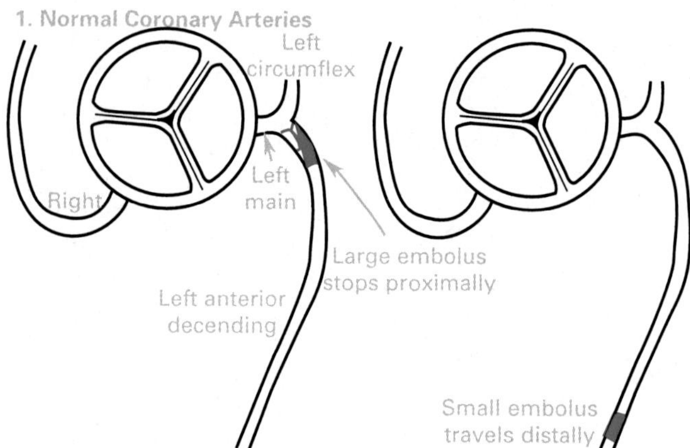


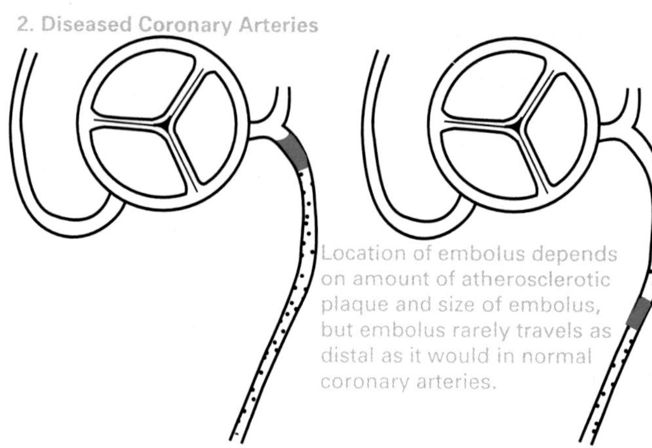

2. Diseased Coronary Arteries
Location of embolus depends on amount of atherosclerotic plaque and size of embolus, but embolus rarely travels as distal as it would in normal coronary arteries.


FIGURE 47-25 Coronary emboli in normal and diseased coronary arteries. (From Waller.[1] Reproduced with permission from the publisher, editor, and author.)

patients with rheumatoid arthritis, usually involving small intramural vessels.[179–191] The small-vessel arteritis may also involve conduction system vessels leading to various forms of heart block.[186–188] Rheumatoid coronary vasculitis producing MI is rare.[183–185,190,191] Histologically, extraaortic rheumatoid vasculitis (coronary artery vasculitis) is usually a polyarteritis type of necrotizing angiitis[128] and not a giant-cell arteritis (Fig. 47-36). Small myocardial vessels may also be severely narrowed in ankylosing spondylosis. Occlusion of the left main ostium has been described.[188]

### Thromboangiitis Obliterans (Buerger's Disease)

Thromboangiitis obliterans (Buerger's disease), which is rare (Fig. 47-37),[128,192–194] is a nonatherosclerotic, occlusive, inflammatory vascular disease of unknown cause occurring mainly in young males who are heavy smokers of cigarettes. In a few patients, the coronary arteries have shown focal polymorphonuclear infiltrates, histiocytes, and giant cells with or without coronary artery thrombosis.[192] Coronary involvement is rare, [192] although coronary thrombosis may be seen.[195] Buerger's disease involving a saphenous vein bypass graft has also been documented.

## POLYARTERITIS GROUP OF NECROTIZING ANGIITIS

### Classic Polyarteritis Nodosa

Classic polyarteritis nodosa is a chronic systemic disease manifest by infarction or hemorrhage in various target organs as the result of necrotizing vasculitis. Male patients are affected twice as often as female, with a mean age of 45 years.[128,196,197] It is probably the most common cause of coronary angiitis with both epicardial and intramural coronary arteries being affected (Fig. 47-38).[23,196–200] In a review of 66 necropsy cases,[198] 41 (62 percent) had involvement of the epicardial coronary arteries, including 25 cases (61 percent) with involvement of both the epicardial and intramural coronary arteries, while 16 cases (39 percent) had only involvement of the intramural arteries. Frequently, various stages of acute disease and healing are seen in the same arterial segment. The acute phase has an acute cellular reaction with destruction of the media and internal elastic membrane. The healing stage results in fibrous internal proliferation. Coronary arteries may dilate to form small berry-like aneurysms (becoming occluded by thrombus), rupture, or produce fatal MI, pericardial tamponade, or sudden death.[198–200]

### Infantile Polyarteritis

Polyarteritis nodosa occurring in infants under 2 years of age (infantile polyarteritis) differs from the clinical pathologic features of classical polyarteritis nodosa.[128,201–204] Infantile disease involves a higher frequency (79 percent) of coronary vasculitis and aneurysmal disease of the coronary arteries with sparing of vessels in other locations (Fig. 47-39).[126,201–204] Kawasaki's disease may involve children up to 8 or 10 years of age[128] rather than being confined to patients under 2 as in infantile polyarteritis.[129]

### Kawasaki's Disease (Mucocutaneous Lymph Node Syndrome)

Kawasaki's disease, or mucocutaneous lymph node syndrome, is an acute febrile exanthematous illness of children first described in the Japanese literature in 1967 and reported in the English literature in 1974.[206] It has subsequently been reported in children worldwide and in all racial groups.[207] In about 20 percent of children with the acute illness, a vasculitis of the coronary vasa vasorum leads to coronary arterial aneurysm formation, thrombosis, acute MI, and sudden death.[206–213] Estimates of death from acute infarction or ventricular analytic range from 1 to 2 percent. Late presentation with MI secondary to dislodged aneurysmal thrombosis may also occur (Figs. 47-40 and 47-41).[202–205]

Coronary artery ectasia or coronary artery aneurysms occur in 15 to 25 percent of children with Kawasaki disease who do *not* receive treatment with gamma globulin in the phase.[207,208] Coronary artery dilation (detectable echocardiographically) can be seen as early as 4 days after the first appearance of fever with maximal dilation peaking at 4 weeks after illness onset. Coronary aneurysms in early Kawasaki's disease occur mainly in the proximal segments of the major coronary arteries. The presence of distal coronary aneurysms is nearly always associated with proximal coronary aneurysms. Coronary aneurysms have resolved angiographically 1 to 2 years after disease onset in about half to two-thirds of vessels.[215] The likelihood of resolution of coronary artery aneurysms in Kawasaki's

TABLE 47-5 Etiology of Coronary Artery Emboli

| Natural | Iatrogenic |
|---|---|
| Vegetation | Cardiac surgery (ostial cannulization, prosthetic valve, patch repair) |
| Active infective endocarditis (native valve) | Cardiac catheterization and angiography (catheter thrombus, catheter fragments) |
| Active infective endocarditis (prosthetic valve) | Coronary angioplasty, other interventions, catheter balloon valvuloplasty and thrombolysis |
| Mural endocarditis | Prosthetic valves (thrombus, vegetation, occluders, leaflets, cloth covering, struts) |
| Noninfective (marantic) endocarditis | Cardioversion (left atrial thrombus, left ventricular thrombus) |
| Calcific deposit | Cardiac resuscitation (thrombus) |
| Aortic valve stenosis | Trauma—blunt penetrating, nonpenetrating, foreign body (bullet) |
| Mitral valve stenosis | "Paradoxical" |
| Intracardiac thrombus | Congenital heart disease (atrial septal defect, ventricular septal defect) |
| Left ventricle (myocardial infarction, cardiomyopathy, fibroelastosis with mural thrombus, ventricular aneurysm) | Probe patent foramen ovale defect (thrombophlebitis, right atrial catheters) |
| Left atrium—appendage (low-cardiac-output states) | Pulmonary hypertension (acquired atrial septal defect) |
| Left atrium—body (mitral stenosis, native or prosthetic) | Interatrial flap valve (fossa ovale aneurysm) |
| Pulmonary veins (mitral stenosis) | |
| Intracardiac tumor | |
| Primary (myxoma) | |
| Secondary (extension from pulmonary veins, lymphatic extension, direct extension) | |
| Coronary artery | |
| Plaque rupture (cholesterol) | |
| Thrombus dislodgment | |

SOURCE: Waller.[1] Reproduced with permission from the author, editor, and publisher.

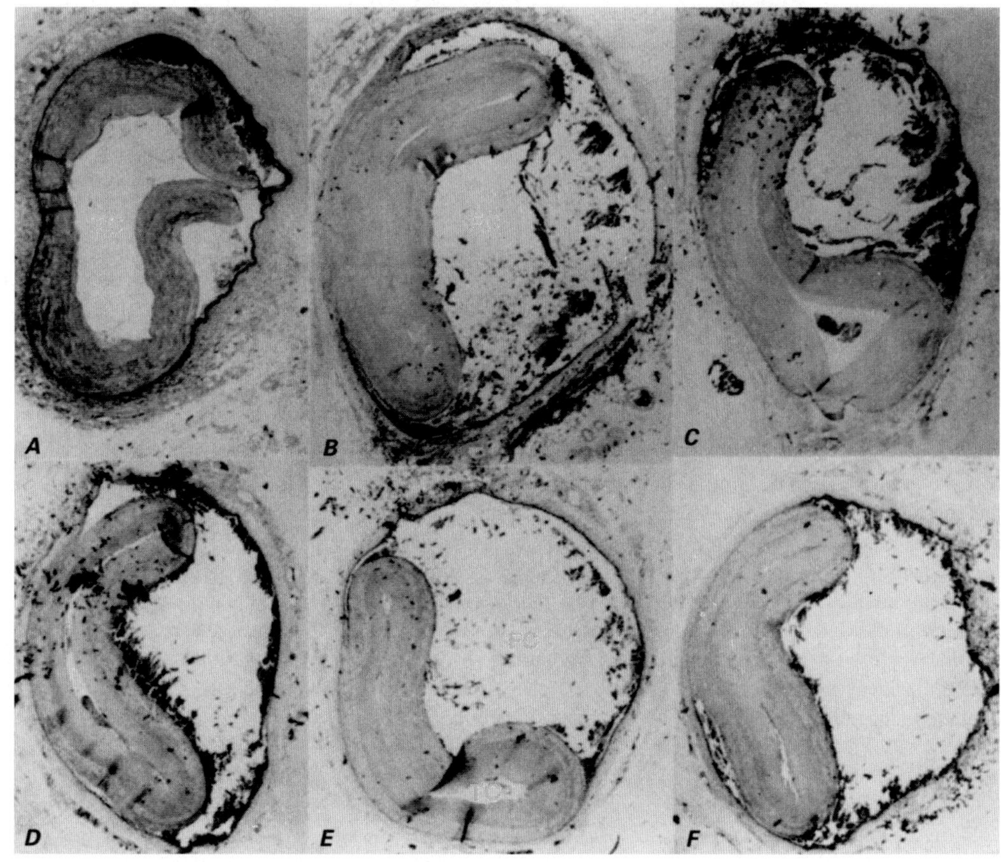


FIGURE 47-26 Coronary artery dissection. Serial cross-section (A-F) showing dissection of the left anterior descending coronary artery. The true channel (TL) is severely compromised by external compression from the false channel (FC; "dissection channel"). (From Waller.1 Reproduced with permission from the publisher, editor, and author.)

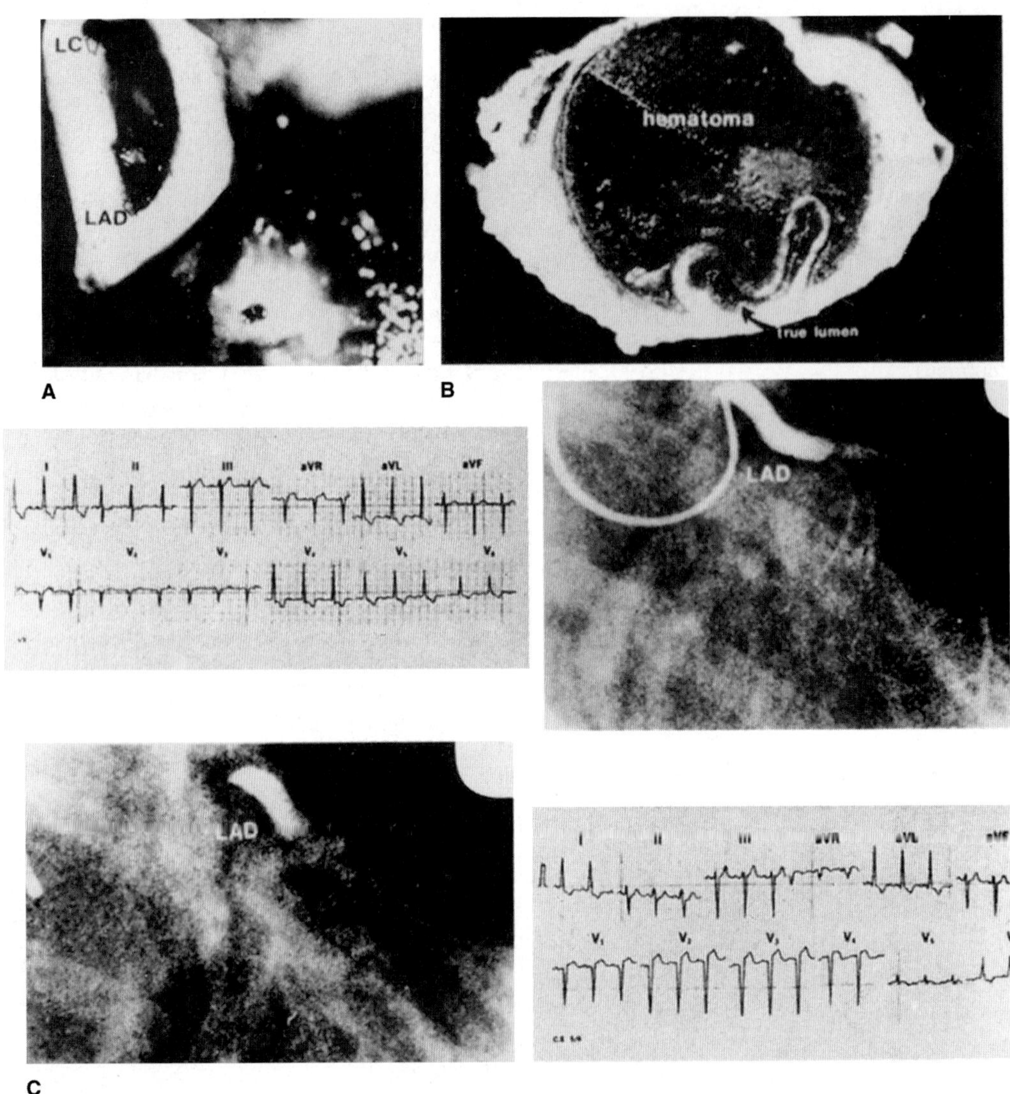


FIGURE 47-27 Coronary artery dissection. Occlusion of the left anterior descending (LAD) artery due to dissection. *A*. The LAD and left circumflex (LC) are seen through the left main artery. *B*. Cross-section shows hematoma in the false channel severely narrows native (true channel) unobstructed lumen. *C*. Sequential electrocardiographic and angiographic findings. (From Isner and Donaldson.[100] Reproduced with permission from the publisher, editor, and author.)

disease is determined largely by the initial size of the aneurysm. Takahashi and associates reported regression of coronary aneurysms also associated with *age* of the patient (regression more likely in children under age 1 year), aneurysm *morphology* (saccular more commonly than fusiform type), and *vessel location* of the aneurysm (regression more likely with distal coronary artery location). Angiographic regression of aneurysms occurs by intimal proliferation within the aneurysm or recanalization of a previously thrombotically occluded aneurysm. Necropsy "regressed coronary artery aneurysms" are historically abnormal and show reduced vascular reactivity.[216,217]

Pathologically, the acute phase shows a necrotizing angiitis involving media and adventitial layers. Some children have survived into adulthood, with coronary artery aneurysms identified later in life (see Figs. 47-40 and 47-41).[214] The differential diagnosis of coronary artery aneurysms in adults includes previously undiagnosed Kawasaki's disease presumably occurring during childhood. Coronary arteriography results in 1100 children ages 4 months to 13 years identified 262 (24 percent) patients with the disease. In these, coronary occlusion was present in 76 percent; segmental stenosis in 5.7 percent; localized stenosis in 23.7 percent; aneurysms in 35.5 percent; and dilatation in 27.5 percent.[212] The incidence of both occlusion and segmental stenosis was lowest in the group studied shortly after the onset of the illness, whereas the prevalence of coronary aneurysm was highest in this early group.

## Allergic Granulomatosis and Angiitis: Wegener's Granulomatosis and Churg-Strauss Syndrome

Wegener's granulomatosis is a necrotizing vasculitis of unknown cause classically involving the upper and lower respiratory tracts and the kidneys.[128,218–222] Cardiovascular involvement in Wegener's granulomatosis was described in one of three cases reported in 1936.[219] About 30 additional necropsy cases have been described

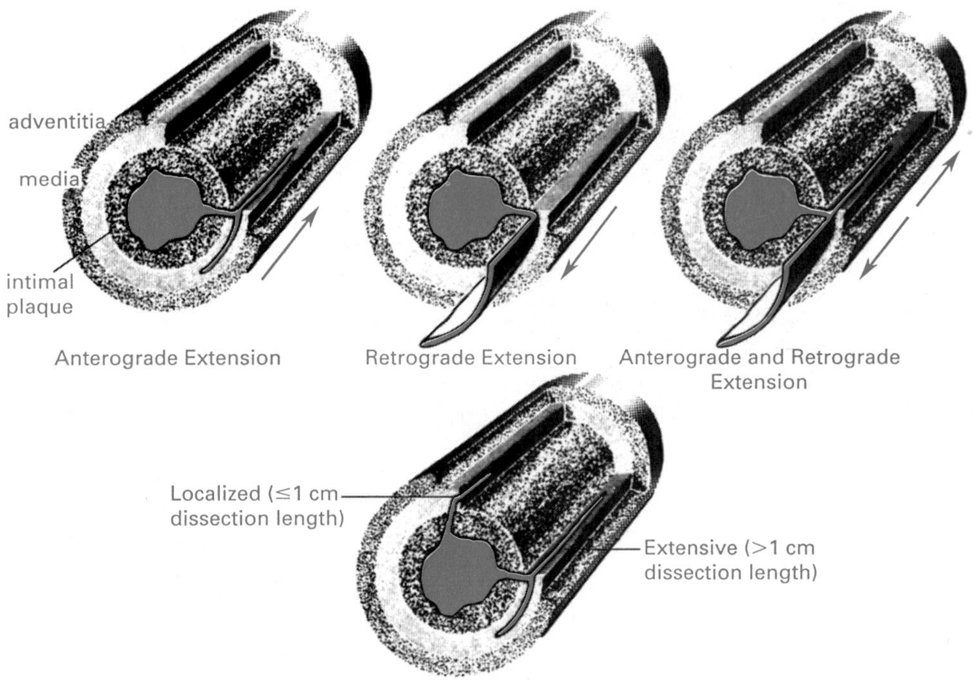


FIGURE 47-28 Diagram showing morphologic definition of coronary artery dissections in balloon angioplasty (long-axis plane): localized (mechanism) (1 cm in total dissection length) and extension (complications; ≥ 1 cm in total length). (From Waller et al.[110] Reproduced with permission from the author, editor, and publisher.)

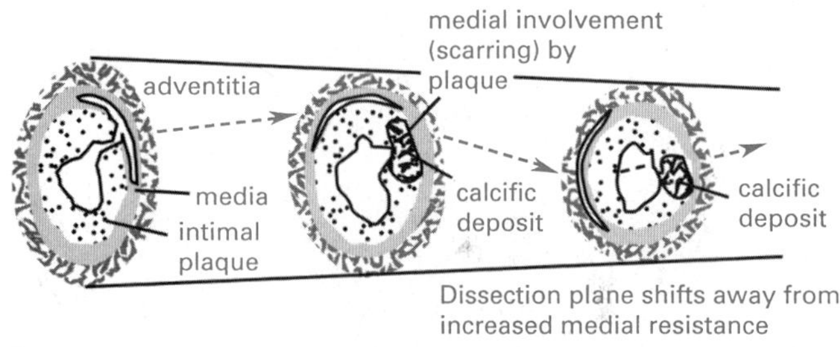


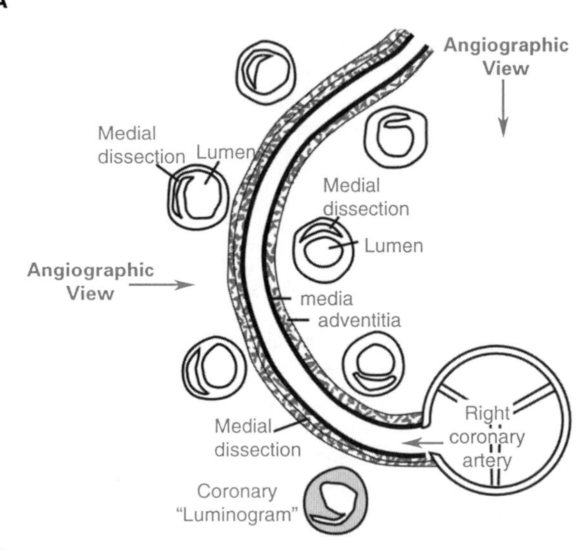


FIGURE 47-29 Diagram showing pathologic change accounting for angiographic appearance of coronary artery "spiral" dissection. *A*. Alteration in course of dissection. *B*. Angiographic appearance of unaltered course of dissection. (From Waller et al.[110] Reproduced with permission from the author, editor, and publisher.)

TABLE 47-6 Causes of Coronary Artery Dissections[100–110]

I. Spontaneous
   A. Post- or peripartum[103–105,107,108]
   B. With or without eosinophilia[105,107]
   C. Idiopathic[106,107]
   D. Systemic hypertension[107]
   E. Coronary spasm
   F. Aortic root dissection[107] (hypertension, medial degeneration)
   G. Arteritis
   H. Fibromuscular hyperplasia
II. Trauma
   A. Post- or peripartum[103,104,108]
   B. Blunt chest[304] (penetrating, nonpenetrating)
   C. Coronary angiography
   D. Coronary interventions[110] (angioplasty, atherectomy, laser, stenting, rotablade)
   E. Cardiac surgery (coronary bypass, coronary ostial cannulation, endarterectomy)
   F. Aortic root dissection (surgery, nonpenetrating, penetrating)

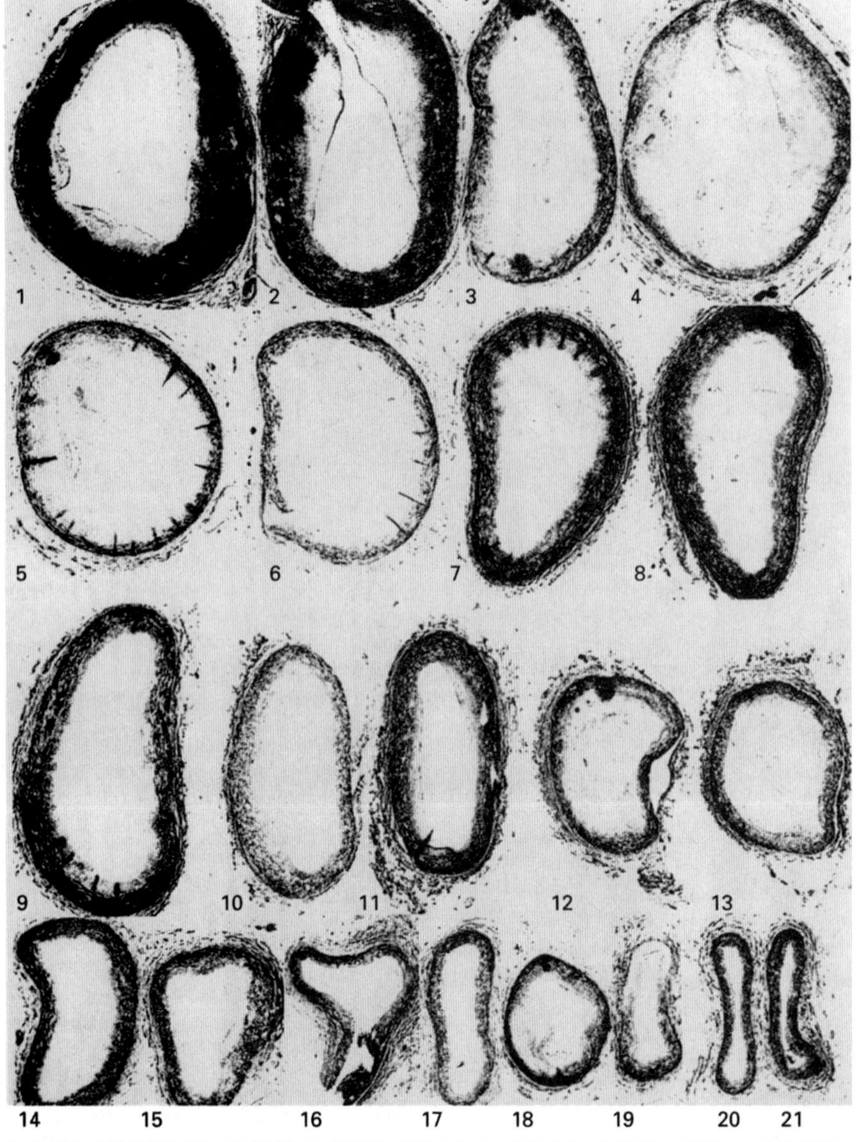


FIGURE 47-30 Coronary artery spasm. Composite of coronary artery cross-sections of a patient with coronary spasm during life. Clinical spasm involved segments 3 to 7. Severe atherosclerotic plaque is seen in 8 of the 21 segments. (From Roberts et al.[114] Reproduced with permission from the author, editor, and publisher.)

subsequently, 14 of these (47 percent) showed small-vessel necrotizing coronary vasculitis (Fig. 47-42).[128,220,221] Fibrinoid necrosis of the small- and medium-sized coronary arteries[218] and occlusion of large epicardial coronary arteries with MI[219] have been reported. In a large clinical series of patients with Wegener's granulomatosis, 12 percent had cardiac involvement largely manifest by pericarditis and coronary arteritis.[223] Some patients with this disease develop unusual cardiac complications such as pericardial tamponade and later constrictive pericarditis, high-grade atrioventricular block, and atrial tachycardia resistant to usual treatment measures. In this series,[223] all patients improved with cyclophosphamide therapy.

Churg-Strauss syndrome (allergic granulomatosis and angiitis) is a variant of polyarteritis nodosa[128,137] occurring in patients with asthma or an allergy history.[137,138,224] It is characterized by necrotizing angiitis with extravascular granulomas and eosinophilia. The heart is commonly involved with this disease, with granulomatous vasculitis of the coronary arteries (see Fig. 47-42). Granulomatous myocarditis may occur with or without coronary angiitis[225] (see Chap. 85).

## COLLAGEN VASCULAR DISEASE VASCULITIS

Collagen vascular diseases generally involve arthritis, myositis, carditis, dermatitis, and inflammatory vascular changes to varying degrees.[226] They include systemic lupus erythematosus, rheumatoid vasculitis, systemic sclerosis, and polymyositis. Rheumatoid vasculitis has been discussed earlier. One of the most common conditions with coronary vasculitis is systemic lupus erythematosus (Fig. 47-43). Several young patients with this disease and absent coronary atherosclerosis have suffered acute MI[227,228] (see Chap. 85). Grant coronary artery aneurysms also have been associated with systemic lupus erythematosus and acute MI.[229] At necropsy, the coronary arteries in these patients have shown internal fibrous proliferation, possibly representing healed arteritis. Necrotizing vasculitis frequently leads to fatal coronary thrombosis and MI,[128,228] rarely associated with thrombotic occlusion of all three major arteries.[228] Smaller intramural coronary arteries are also involved frequently with fibrinoid necrosis and subsequent fibrosis.[82] MI has been seen with a proximal right coronary artery aneurysm at necropsy. It was postulated that the coronary aneurysm represented a sequela of systemic lupus erythematosus arteritis similar to Kawasaki's disease. Necrotizing vasculitis occurs less commonly in other entities of collagen vascular disease such as dermatopolymyositis, systemic sclerosis,[230] Behçet's syndrome,[231] and Cogan's syndrome.[128,232] The antiphospholipid syndrome is characterized by arterial and venous thrombus in the *absence* of underlying coronary atherosclerosis in patients with lupus. The antiphospholipid antibiotics have been associated with unstable angina and acute MI.[233]

## HYPERSENSITIVITY ANGIITIS (ALLERGIC VASCULITIS)

*Hypersensitivity angiitis* describes a miscellaneous group of necrotizing vasculitides that involve both epicardial and intramural coronary arteries.[128] This includes drug-induced vasculitis,[234] which, when generalized, may involve the heart. Histologically, drug-induced vasculitis cannot be separated from primary vasculitis or from hypersensitivity angiitis associated with a known underlying disease or malignancy such as serum sickness, mixed cryoglobulinemia, or Schönlein-Henoch purpura (see Table 47-8).[128] Correct diagnosis cannot be made without clinical information about drug usage. Organ-transplantation arteritis[128] is also in this category representing a form of immune-mediated vascular injury (see Chap. 25).

## METABOLIC DISORDERS NARROWING CORONARY ARTERIES

Specific metabolic substances may accumulate in the walls of large and small coronary arteries as a result of inborn errors of metabolism. The deposition of this material may severely narrow the coronary artery lumen and produce acute MI.[4] Inherited inborn errors of metabolism that are known to affect major epicardial coronary arteries include Hunter's and Hurler's diseases (mucopolysaccharidoses).[188,235–237] The involvement of the coronary arteries in these disorders may be so severe as to occlude totally the vessel and to produce myocardial ischemia or infarction. Other disorders of metabolism such as primary oxalosis,[238] Fabry's disease,[82] Sandhoff's disease (gangliosidoses),[239] and homocystinuria may affect smaller coronary vessels by severe intimal proliferation[240] (see Chap. 72).

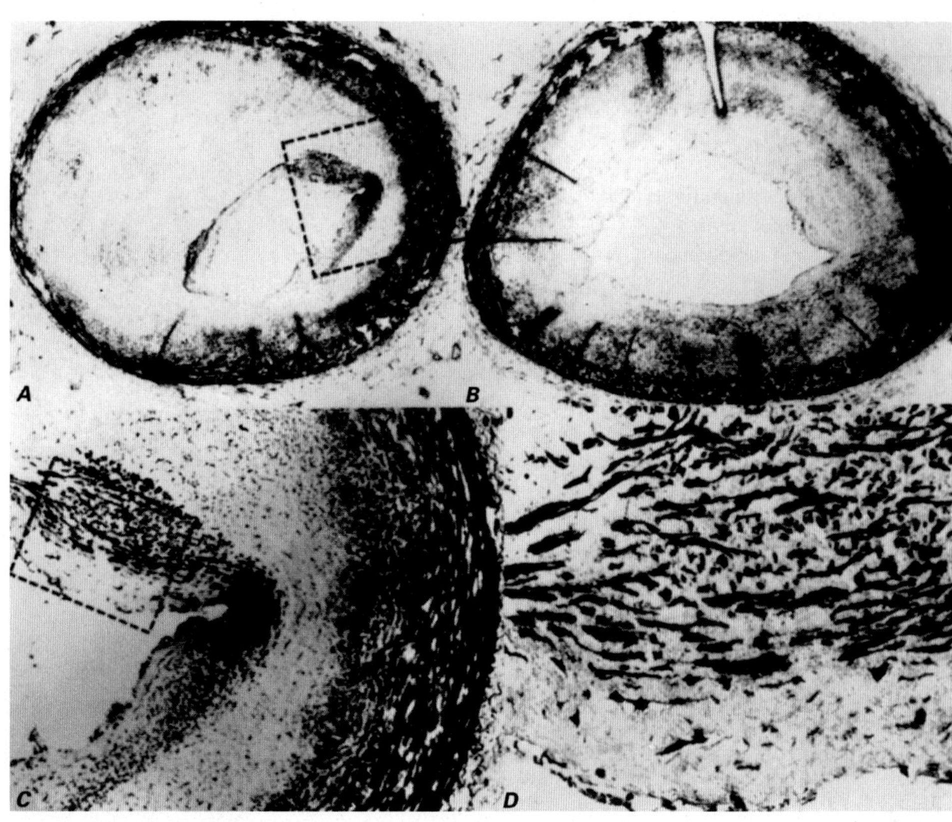


FIGURE 47-31 Coronary artery spasm. *A* and *B*. Histology sections of the left anterior descending coronary artery at the approximate site of spasm showing severe luminal narrowing. *C* and *D*. Higher magnifications of the internal plaque showing the predominance of smooth muscle cells. (From Roberts et al.[114] Reproduced with permission from the author, editor, and publisher.)

## INTIMAL PROLIFERATION

Fibrous hyperplasia and smooth muscle proliferation in the coronary arteries may severely narrow the lumen and produce myocardial ischemia or infarction. The process may be associated with mediastinal irradiation,[241] fibromuscular hyperplasia of the renal arteries,[4] the use of methysergide,[21,242] ostial cannulation during cardiac surgery, aortic valve replacement,[22] and unknown causes.[243–246] Up to 50 percent of patients undergoing cardiac transplantation develop significant narrowing of epicardial coronary arteries or total occlusion by intimal fibrous proliferation within 3 to 5 years after transplantation.[247] MI and sudden death may result from this "chronic rejection" process. Fibrosis of the intramural vessels may also occur. Intimal damage from immunologic rejection is believed to be the basis for the accelerated intimal fibrous hyperplasia involving the coronary arteries (see Chap. 25). A morphologic assessment of 61 human cardiac allografts of short- and long-term survival has been provided.[248] Allographs were divided into two groups: fibrous lesions confined to the proximal regional of epicardial arteries and those with diffuse necrotizing vasculitis of the entire system. Disease in the proximal region begins as concentric fibrous thickening. Diffuse disease (necrotizing vasculitis) was invariably associated with acute myocardial rejection with severe intimal lesions of large and small epicardial and intramural arteries.[248] These authors and others[249] have postulated that disease results from healing of a necrotizing vasculitis. Intravascular ultrasound[250] has shown intimal hyperplasia, which was easily detected; its severity predicted the development of cardiac events including MI, unstable angina, or sudden death, despite the presence of a normal coronary arteriogram.

A similar histologic picture of intimal fibrous proliferation is seen in epicardial coronary arteries late after undergoing percutaneous balloon angioplasty (Fig. 47-44).[101,102] Intimal fibrous proliferation

TABLE 47-7 Some Conditions Associated with Coronary Artery Arteritis (Vasculitis)

| |
|---|
| Tuberculosis[23,150,151] |
| Polyarteritis nodosa[23,128,196–204] |
| Giant-cell arteritis[128,142,143,173,180] |
| Systemic lupus erythematosus[128,226–228] |
| Buerger's disease (thromboangiitis obliterans)[128,192–194] |
| Wegener's granulomatosis[128,218–223] |
| *Salmonella*[4] |
| Leprosy[3] |
| Mucocutaneous lymph node syndrome[206–212] |
| Takayasu's disease[159–171] |
| Typhus[146] |
| Infective endocarditis |
| Rheumatic diseases[128,179–187] |
| Ankylosing spondylitis[188] |
| Syphilis[4,82,128,147–149] |
| Malaria[153] |
| Schistosoma haematobium[154] |
| Rickettsial infections[128,154–156] |
| Viruses[128,157,158] |

SOURCE: Waller.[1] Reproduced with permission from the author, editor, and publisher.

TABLE 47-8 Classification of Vasculitides

1. **Infectious angiitis**
   - Syphilitic
   - Mycobacterial
   - Pyogenic bacteria or fungal
   - Rickettsial
   - Viral
   - Whipple bacillus
2. **Noninfectious angiitis**
   - A. Involving large, medium-sized, and small blood vessels
     - Takayasu's arteritis
     - Granulomatous (giant-cell) arteritis
     - Cranial (temporal) arteritis and extracranial giant-cell arteritis
     - Disseminated visceral granulomatous angiitis
     - Granulomatous angiitis of the central nervous system
     - Arteritis of rheumatic-rheumatoid disease and sponduloarthropathies
   - B. Involving predominantly medium-sized and small blood yessels
     - Thromboangiitis obliterans (Buerger's disease)
     - Polyarteritis (periarteritis)
     - Polyarteritis nodosa
     - Infantile polyarteritis
     - Microscopic polyarteritis
     - Kawasaki's disease
     - Pathergic-allergic granulomatosis and angiitis
     - Wegener's granulomatosis
     - Churg-Strauss syndrome
     - Necrotizing sarcoid granulomatosis
     - Vasculitis of collagen vascular disease:
     - Rheumatic fever
     - Relapsing polychondritis
     - Rheumatoid arthritis
     - Systemic sclerosis
     - Seronegative arthropathies
     - Sjögren's syndrome
     - Systemic lupus erythematosus
     - Behçet's syndrome
     - Cogan's syndrome
     - Dermatomyositis/polymyositis
   - C. Involving predominantly small blood vessels
     - Hypersensitivity angiitis (synonym: leukocytoclastic or allergic vasculitis)
     - Serum sickness
     - Mixed cryoglobulinemia
     - Schönlein-Henoch purpura
     - Drug-induced angiitis
     - Hypocomplementemia
     - Inflammatory bowel disease
     - Malignancy-associated vasculitis
     - Primary biliary cirrhosis
     - Retroperitoneal fibrosis
     - Goodpasture's syndrome

SOURCE: Lie.[128] Reproduced with permission from the author, editor, and publisher.

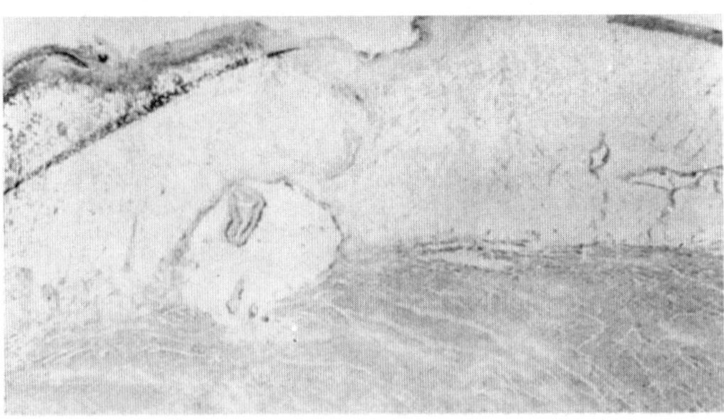

A

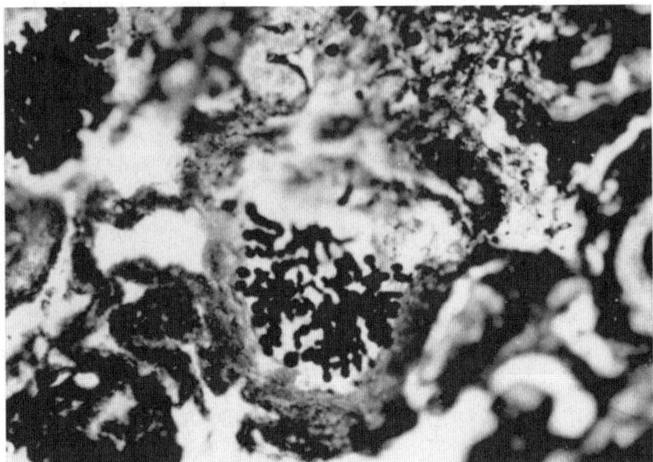

B

FIGURE 47-32 Coronary arteritis. *A.* Extensive yeast (*Candida*) percarditis, which involves the adventitial layer of a branch of a major subepicardial coronary artery. *B.* Closeup shows the budding yeast organisms (GMS stain). (From Waller.[1] Reproduced with permission from the author, editor, and publisher.)

of the left main coronary artery has been reported late after balloon angioplasty of a lesion in the proximal left anterior descending coronary artery.[251] This may be due to intimal reaction from balloon rubbing of the intimal surface and/or extension of the fibrous process from the angioplasty dilation site (see Chap. 48).

## EXTERNAL COMPRESSION

External compression of the epicardial coronary arteries may result in severe luminal narrowing and progressive myocardial ischemia. External compression of a major epicardial coronary artery has been reported in patients with sinus of Valsalva aneurysms, chronic aortic dissection,[252] and epicardial tumor metastases.[253,254] Myocardial bridging (external muscle compression during ventricular systole) has been reviewed earlier.

## METASTATIC IMPLANTS

Myocardial metastatic lesions from various tumors—including carcinomas, sarcomas, and lymphomas—may mimic a healed myocardial infarct at necropsy (Fig. 47-45). The discrete location or

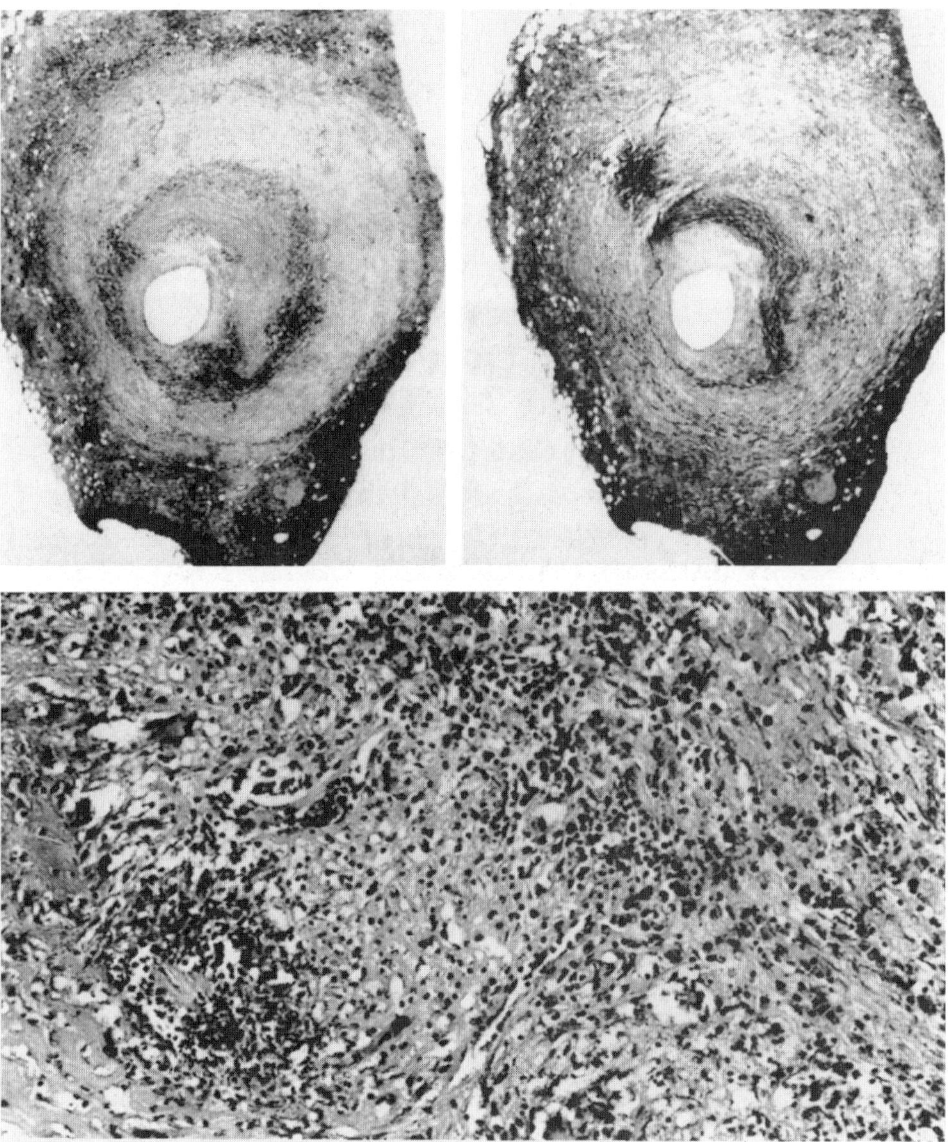

FIGURE 47-33 *Top:* Matching hematoxylin-eosin (*left*) and elastic stain (*right*) sections of coronary artery in Takayasu's arteritis. Note transmural fibrosis and inflammatory infiltrate in media of artery (×16). *Bottom:* Closeup view of lymphoplasmacytic infiltrate with giant cells in media of coronary artery (×160). (From Lie.[128] Reproduced with permission from the author, editor, and publisher.)

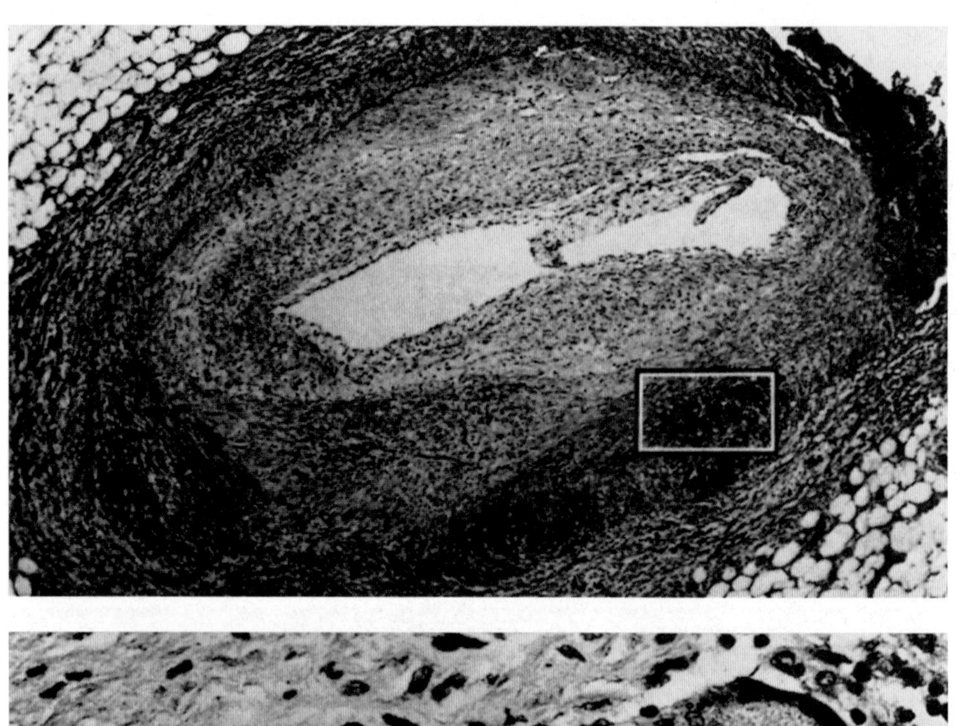

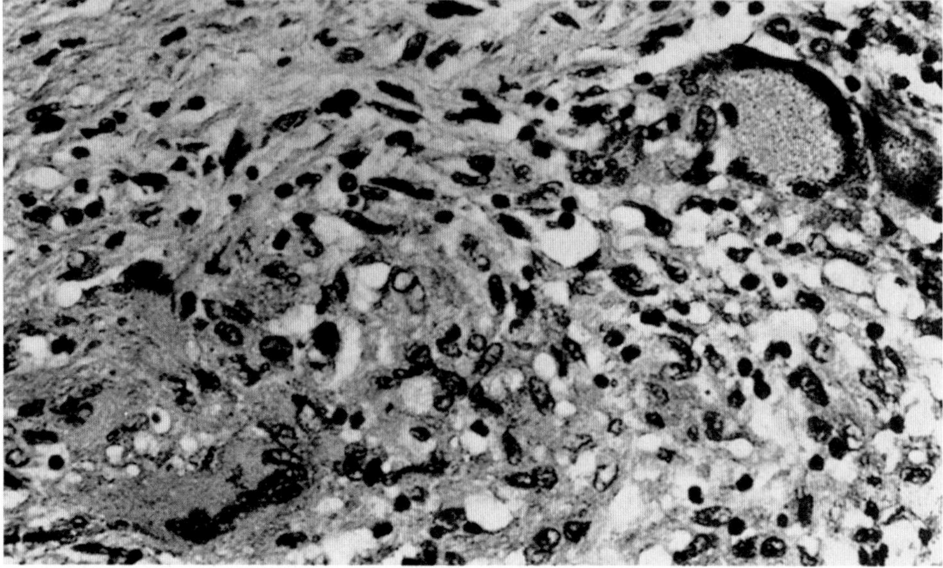

FIGURE 47-34 *Top:* Low-power view of granulomatous coronary arteritis associated with giant-cell aortitis (hematoxylin-eosin, ×40). *Bottom:* Closeup view of boxed area (hematoxylin-eosin ×400). (From Lie.[128] Reproduced with permission from the author, editor, and publisher.)

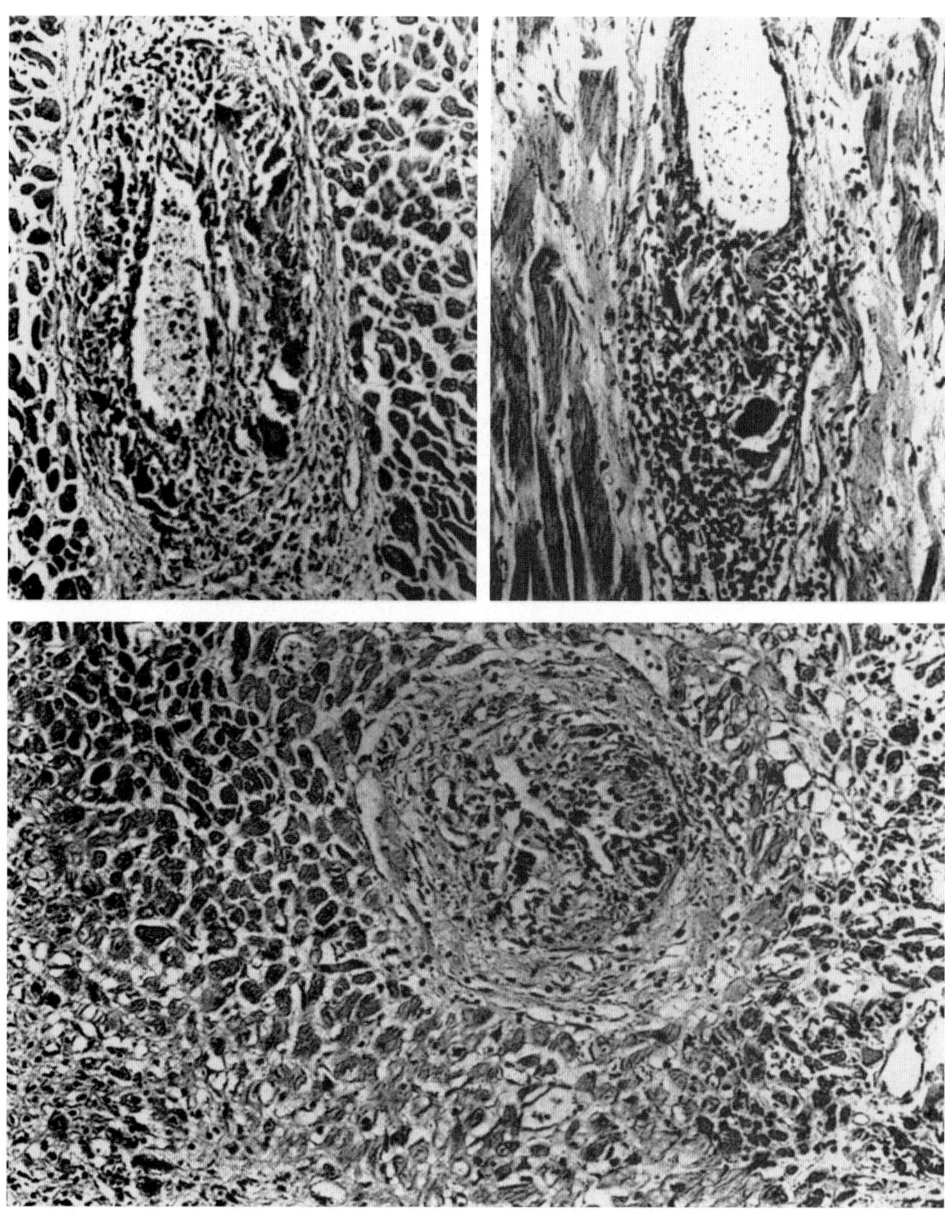

FIGURE 47-35 *Top left* and *right:* Giant-cell arteritis of intramural coronary arteries associated with temporal arteritis and giant-cell arteritis (hematoxylin-eosin, ×160). *Bottom:* Granulomatous coronary arteritis in disseminated visceral giant-cell angiitis (hematoxylin-eosin, ×160). (From Lie.[128] Reproduced with permission from the author, editor, and publisher.)

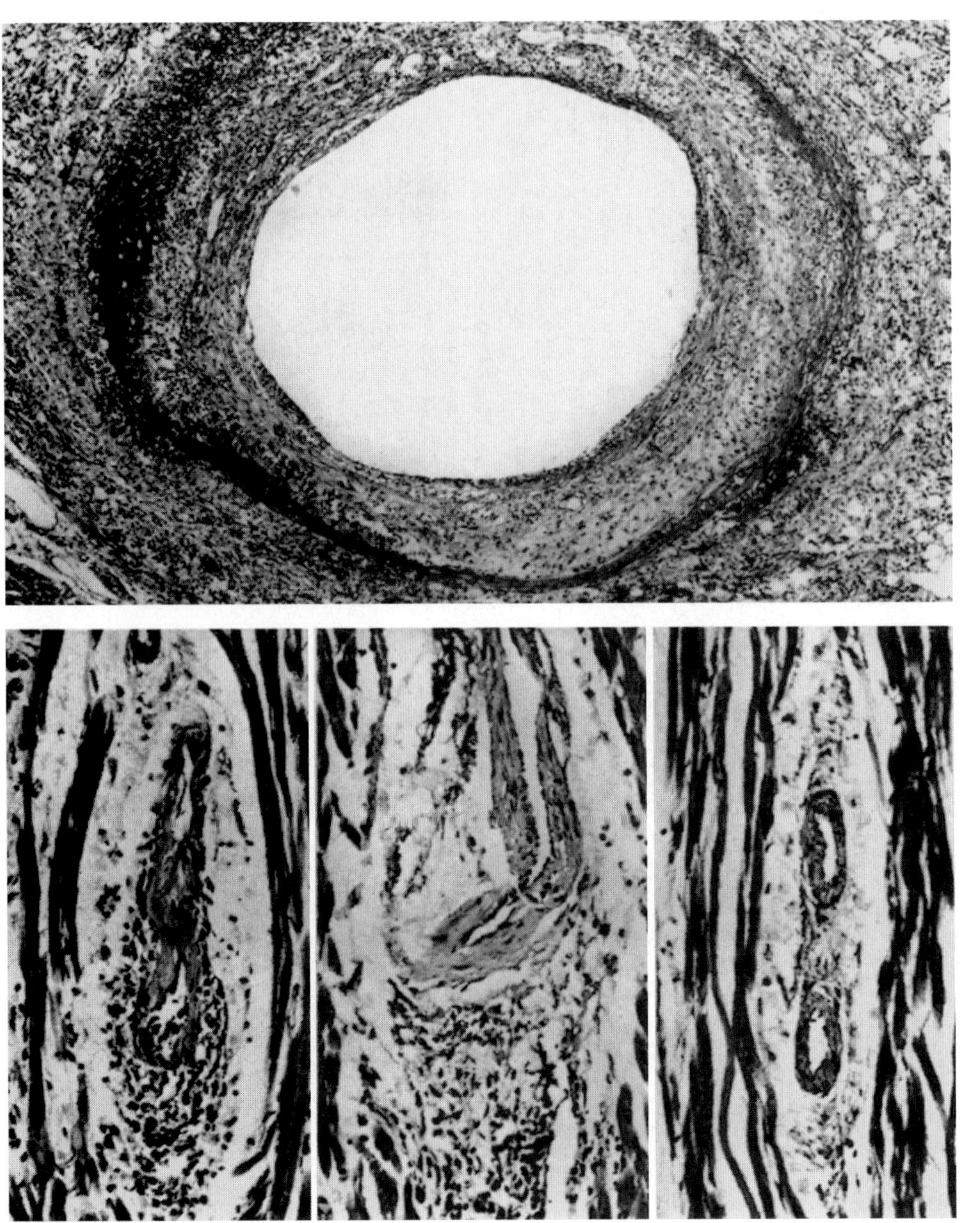

FIGURE 47-36 *Top:* Polyarteritis-type necrotizing angiitis of epicardial coronary artery in rheumatoid arthritis (hematoxylin-eosin, ×160). *Bottom:* Variations of small-vessel coronary arteritis in rheumatic fever (hematoxylin-eosin, ×160). (From Lie.[128] Reproduced with permission from the author, editor, and publisher.)

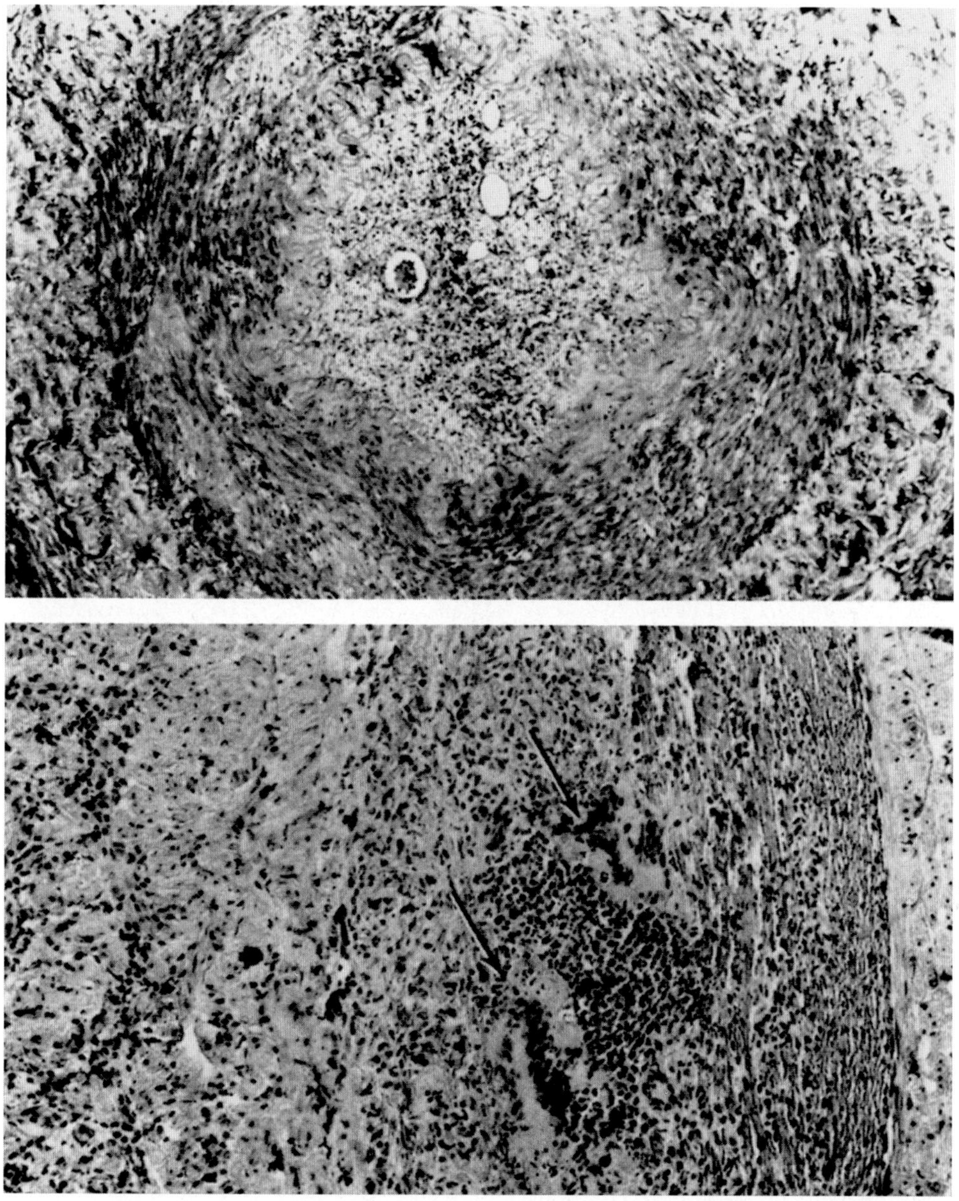

FIGURE 47-37 *Top:* Subacute stage of Buerger's disease of coronary artery with organizing thrombus (hematoxylin-eosin, ×160). *Bottom:* Involvement of the coronary vein in Buerger's disease with typical intraluminal microabscesses and giant cells (*arrows;* hematoxylin-eosin, ×160). (From Lie.[128] Reproduced with permission from the author, editor, and publisher.)

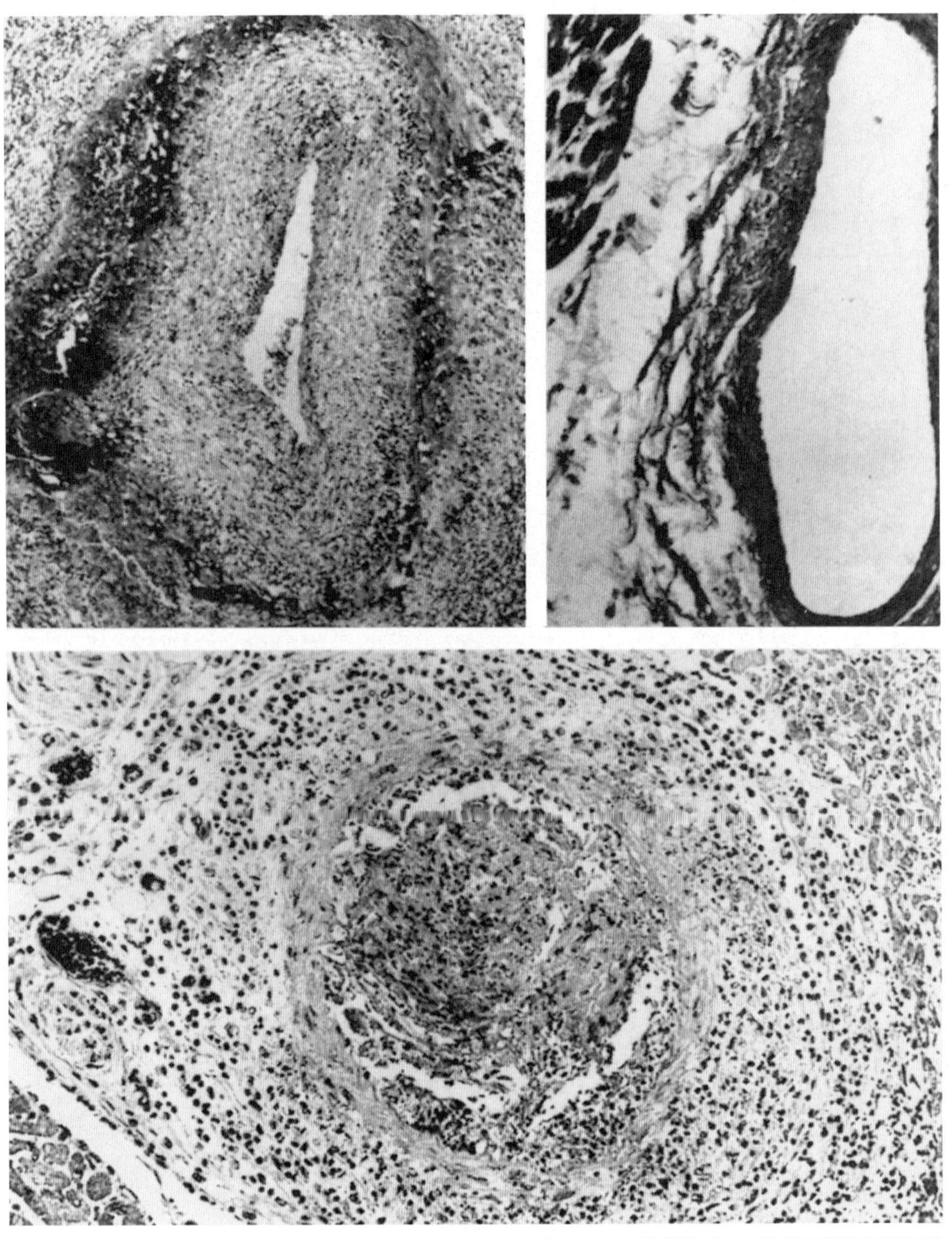

FIGURE 47-38 *Top:* Necrotizing angiitis (*left*) and histologically normal (*right*) segments of epicardial coronary arteries in classic polyarteritis nodosa (hematoxylin-eosin, ×16). *Bottom:* Necrotizing angiitis with fibrinoid necrosis of intramural coronary artery (hematoxylin-eosin, ×160). (From Lie.[128] Reproduced with permission from the author, editor, and publisher.)

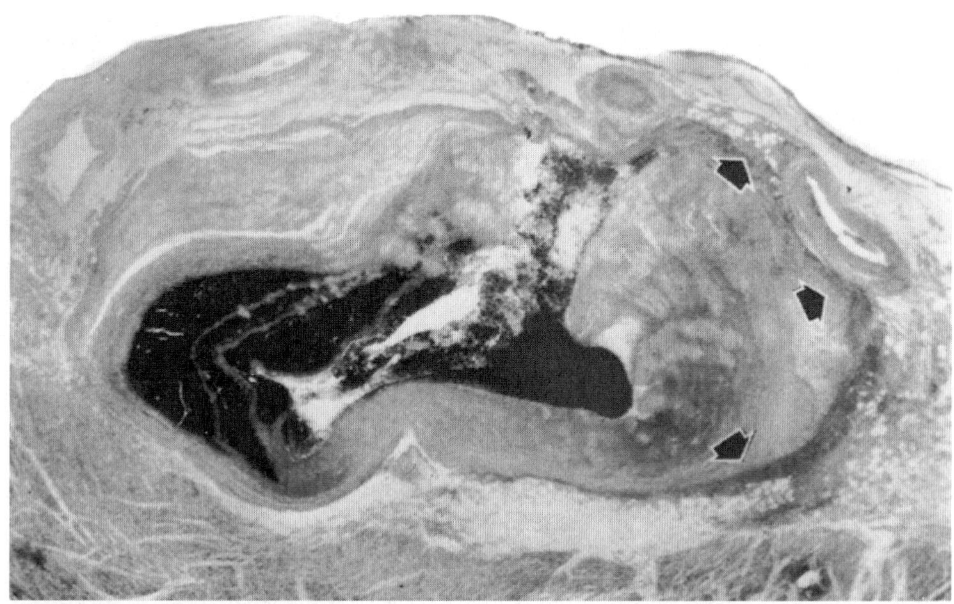

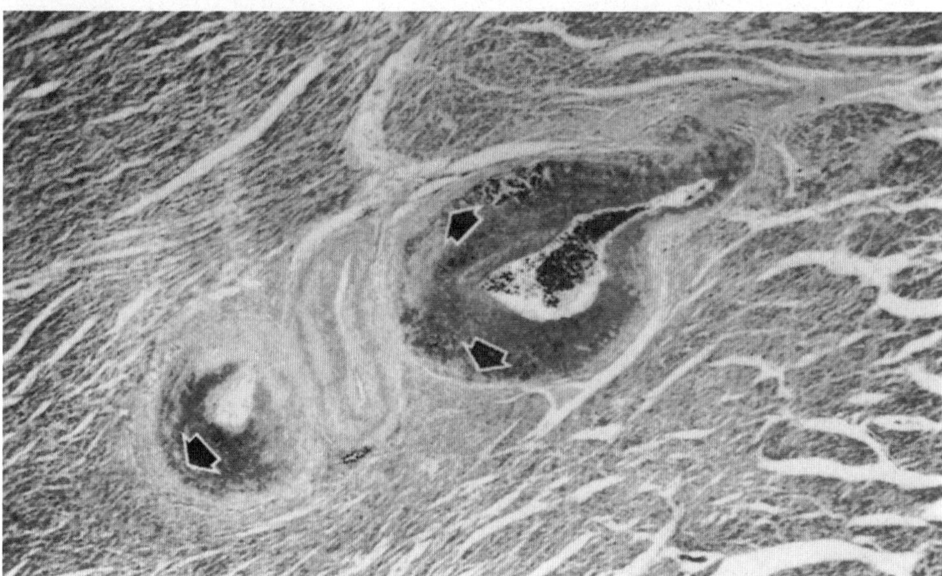

FIGURE 47-39 Necrotizing angiitis with aneurysmal disruption of epicardial (*arrows, top*) and intramural (*arrows, bottom*) coronary arteries in infantile polyarteritis nodosa (hematoxylin-eosin, ×160). (From Lie.[128] Reproduced with permission from the author, editor, and publisher.)

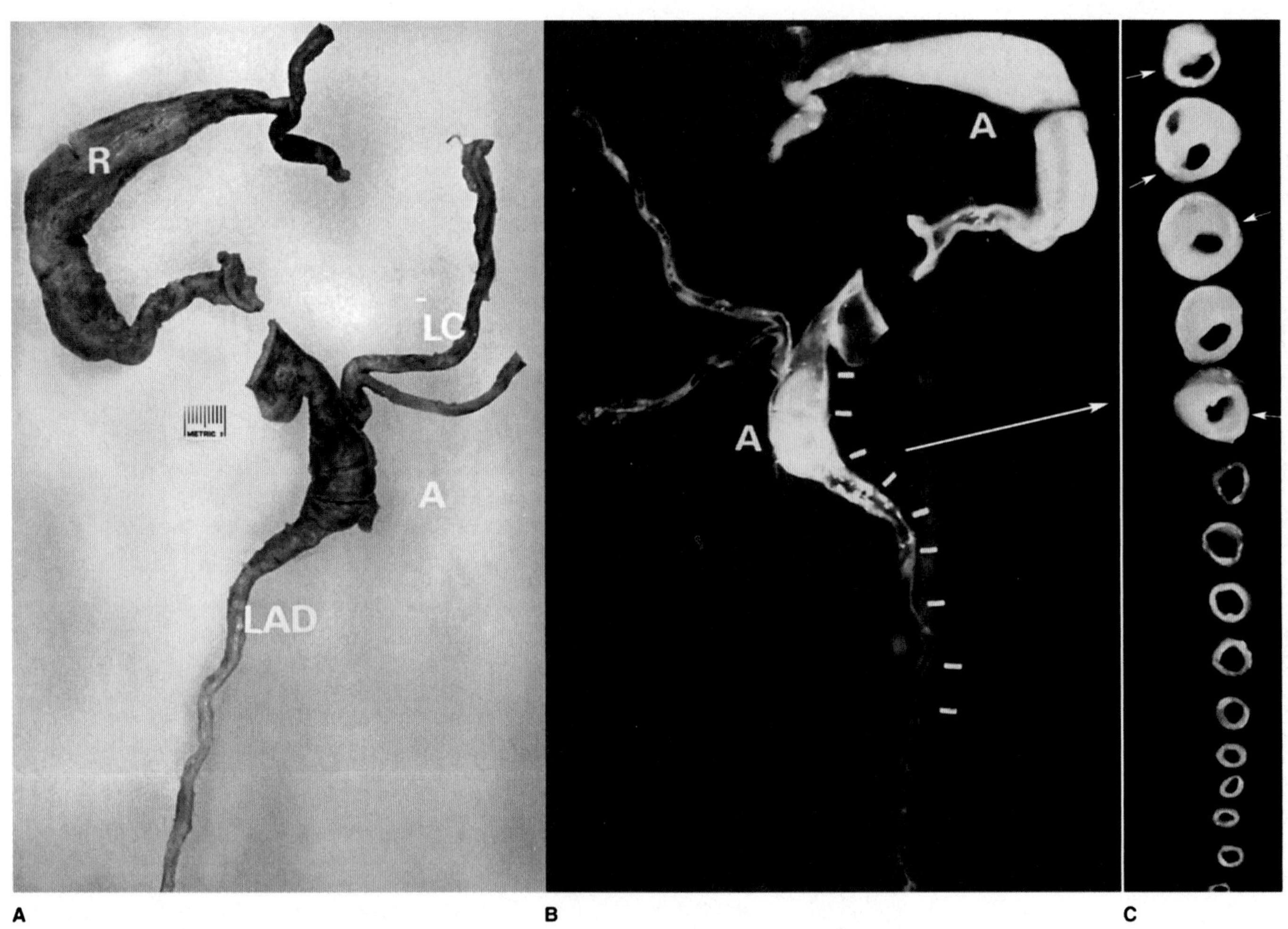


FIGURE 47-40 *A*. Epicardial coronary artery aneurysm involving the proximal left anterior descending (LAD) and right coronary artery (A) from an adult with probable Kawasaki's disease as a child. LC = left circumflex. *B*. Radiograph of coronary arterial tree in *A* showing calcific deposits. Cross-section of the aneurysm (*A*) is shown in (*C*). Arrows indicate calcific deposits.

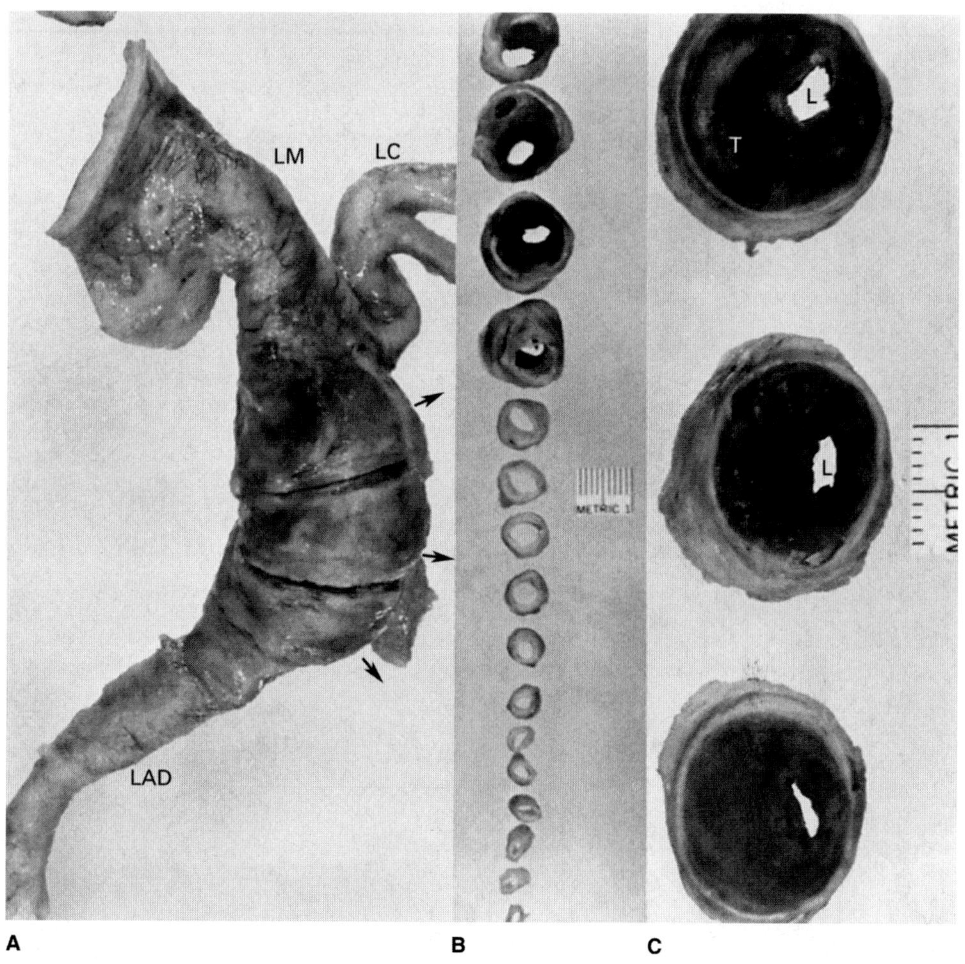


FIGURE 47-41 *A.* Close-up of left anterior descending (LAD) coronary aneurysm from Fig. 47-40 with cross-sections displayed in *B*. Note the intraaneurysmal thrombus. *C.* Close-up of three transverse sections of coronary aneurysm shown in *A* and *B*. LM = left main; LC = left circumflex.

locations of these metastatic deposits generally are unrelated to specific coronary arterial supply zones, and the lesions are usually surrounded by normal myocardium. These two gross observations suggest the lesions are metastatic tumor implants rather than healed myocardial infarcts (see Chap. 86).

## RADIATION-INDUCED CORONARY DISEASE

Intimal proliferation of epicardial coronary arteries involving the ostium, main segment, or both is well known and increasingly reported.[241,255–262] "Accelerated" or "premature" coronary atherosclerosis has been noted in young individuals undergoing previous mediastinal irradiation for various types of malignancies.[263] Internal proliferation following mediastinal radiation 5 to 10 years earlier is described as "intimal thickening *without* medial abnormalities." The intimal lesions (ostial or main segment of artery) consists of fibrous tissue *without* extracellular lipid deposits.[235,255] Coronary ostial stenosis has an incidence of 0.13 to 2.7 percent of patients undergoing mediastinal irradiation treatment.[241,262] A few patients have developed acute MI or unstable angina as a result of the radiation-induced lesions treated by myocardial revascularization or angioplasty (see Chap. 89).[255–263]

Because of their fibrous nature, many radiation-induced lesions do not provide the best substrate for dilation techniques.[101,102,251] Chemotherapy-induced MI in a young man without coronary disease has been reported.[264] Cardiac invasion by tumor, hypercoagulable states, and coronary artery spasm are possible etiologies.[264] Vascular toxicity, including MI, has been reported following antineoplastic regimens containing Vinca alkaloids.[264]

## CORONARY ARTERY THROMBOSIS WITHOUT UNDERLYING ATHEROSCLEROTIC PLAQUE (THROMBOSIS IN SITU)

Thrombotic occlusion of the coronary system unassociated with underlying atherosclerotic plaque may be seen with several hematologic diseases: thrombocytopenic purpura,[34] leukemia,[265] polycythemia vera,[266] sickle cell anemia,[82] and primary thrombocytosis.[267] Occasionally, acute MI may be the initial manifestation of these hematologic disorders. A main factor responsible for the myocardial ischemia in these conditions is blockage of small intramural coronary vessels by platelet aggregates.[268] These platelet aggregates initially may form in the major coronary arteries, then embolize distally.

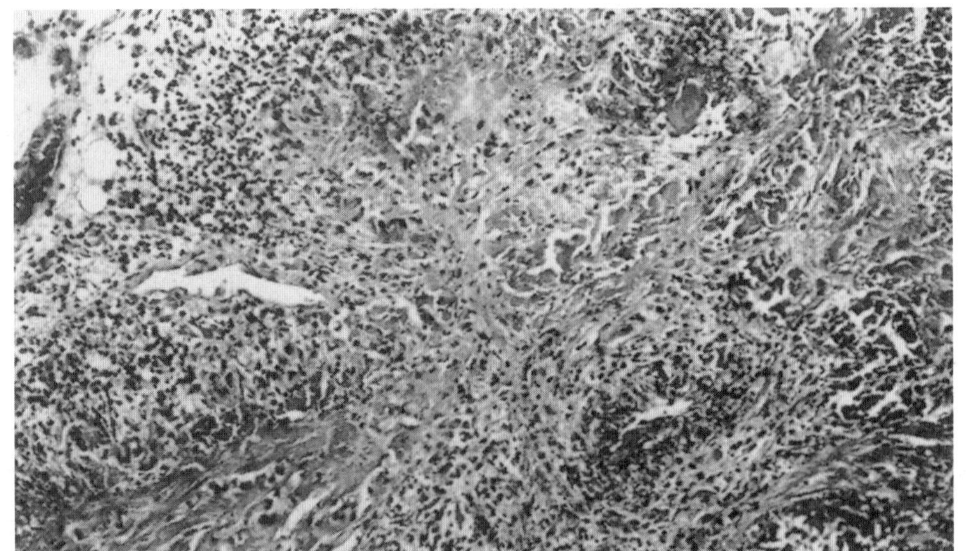

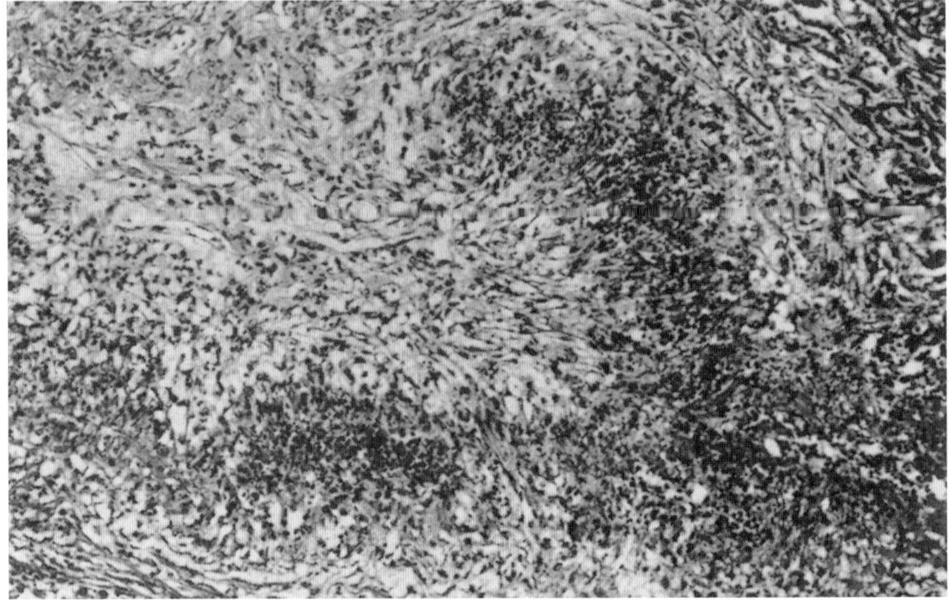

FIGURE 47-42 Granulomatous necrotizing angiitis of coronary arteries in Wegener's granulomatosis (*top*) and Churg-Strauss syndrome (*bottom*; hematoxylin-eosin, ×160). (From Lie.[128] Reproduced with permission from the author, editor, and publisher.)

## SUBSTANCE ABUSE (COCAINE)

Cocaine abuse is now a major health hazard; more than 22 million Americans have tried cocaine at least once, and 5 million are current users.[269] Reports have documented that cocaine abuse can result in myocardial ischemia and infarction in the absence of coronary artery disease,[269,270] and cocaine-induced coronary artery vasoconstriction has been reported in patients following the intranasal administration of cocaine[271] (see Chap. 89).

Several instances of coronary artery thrombosis and spasm have been reported in patients who abuse cocaine. Acute coronary thrombosis in association with cardiac events—including angina, acute MI, and sudden death—has been reported.[269,271] In some instances, there is underlying atherosclerotic plaque; in others, the coronary arteries are normal. Coronary thrombosis occurring in coronary arteries free of atherosclerotic plaque suggests the role of cocaine-induced spasm, massive norepinephrine release in the heart, or possible primary thrombogenicity of cocaine or its metabolites. Coronary spasm has been associated with cocaine usage and has been postulated as a mechanism of MI in cocaine users with clean coronary arteries.[269,272] In such cases, fibrointimal proliferation with coronary narrowing was attributed to underlying coronary artery spasm that caused focal vessel endothelial injury, platelet adherence, and aggregation. Platelets liberate *platelet-derived growth factor (PDGF),* which can induce intimal proliferative lesions. In patients with underlying coronary plaque, cocaine-induced spasm also may produce endothelial disruption at the surface of the plaque and promote platelet aggregation and further vasoconstriction from the release of platelet prostaglandins[273] (see Chap. 89).

Two drugs have been the center of debate over their potential for abuse versus use as psychotherapeutic agents and their complication in induction of arrhythmias.[274] Use of *MDMA ("Ecstasy") (3, 4-methylenedioxymethamphetamine)* and *MDEA ("Eve") (3,4-methylenedioxymethamphetamine)* have been associated with five sudden deaths.[268] In three of these, Eve and Ecstasy may have induced fatal arrhythmias.

## MYOCARDIAL OXYGEN DEMAND–SUPPLY DISPROPORTION

In this category are disease states in which there is failure to deliver adequate oxygen to the myocardium over a prolonged period or increased myocardial wall tension requiring increased oxygen supply. The classic example of the first situation is carbon monoxide poisoning,[3] which has been associated with extensive nontransmural infarction in the presence of normal epicardial coronary arteries. Prolonged shock from any cause can also result in extensive nontransmural necrosis and is frequently associated with transmural necrosis of the papillary muscles. One example of increased myocardial wall tension requiring increased coronary oxygen supply is aortic valve stenosis[4] (see Chap. 63). In the face of increased oxygen demand with increased muscle mass, coronary blood supply may be limited by poor perfusion resulting from the lower coronary arterial pressure. In addition, poor perfusion results from the high coronary resistance caused by increased wall pressure on the intramural coronary arteries and the high left ventricular end-diastolic pressure from a stiff ventricle, with further limitation of the time in diastole for coronary blood flow occasioned by tachycardia.[3] Excessive myocardial oxygen demand exceeding supply and resulting in myocardial ischemia or infarction may also be seen in thyrotoxicosis,[275] which reflects increased metabolic rates and the adverse affects of tachycardia.

Left ventricular hypertrophy (LVH) is an independent risk factor of cardiac mortality in renal failure patients. Arrhythmias, left ventricular dysfunction, and myocardial ischemia may result from the LVH from multiple factors such as small vessel smooth muscle hypertrophy vascular endothelial abnormalities microvascular calcification and alterations in oxygen demand and supply.[276]

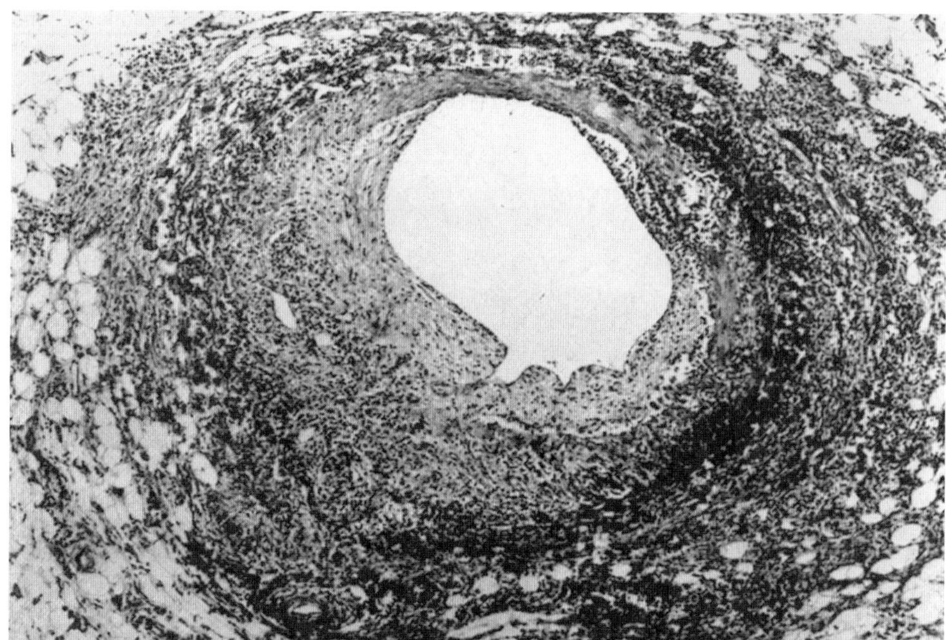

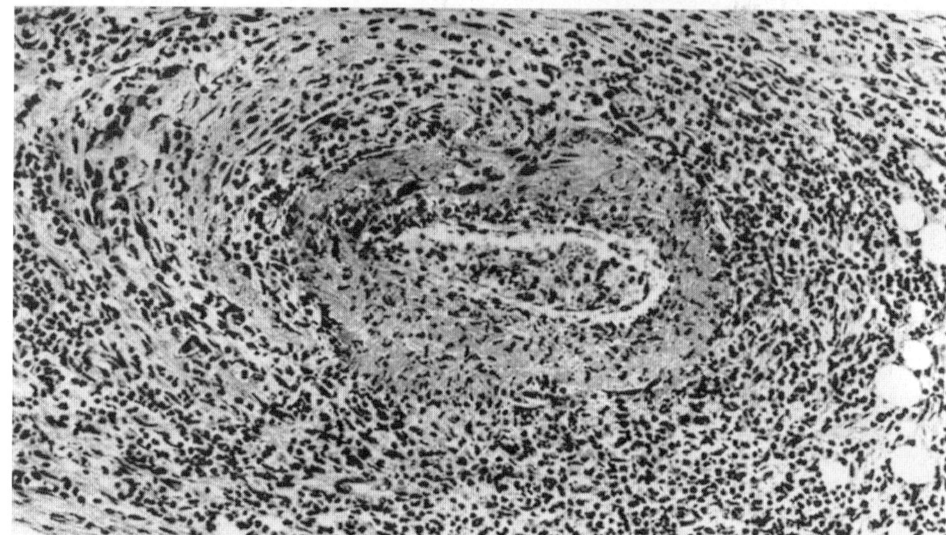

FIGURE 47-43 Necrotizing angiitis of epicardial (*top*) and intramural (*bottom*) coronary arteries in systemic lupus erythematosus (hematoxylin-eosin, ×160).

## INTRAMURAL CORONARY ARTERY DISEASE (SMALL-VESSEL DISEASE)

Acute MI may result from abnormally thickened or totally occluded intramural coronary arteries in the presence of normal extramural (epicardial) coronary arteries. A few of the conditions in this category include (1) hypertrophic cardiomyopathy, (2) diabetes mellitus, (3) amyloid heart disease,[274] (4) neuromuscular disorders (Friedreich's ataxia, progressive muscular dystrophy), (5) cardiac transplantation, (6) rheumatoid arthritis, (7) collagen- vascular disorders (scleroderma, systemic lupus erythematosus), (8) metabolism abnormalities (mucopolysaccharidoses, gangliosidoses), and (9) polyarteritis nodosa.

Histologic abnormalities of small-vessel coronary arteries have been reported in individuals who have died from toxic oil syndrome involving rapeseed oil adulterated with aniline.[277] Many of those who later died had scleroderma-like illnesses. Dense fibrosis of the sinus node, resembling scleroderma, was found with cystic degeneration of the sinus node (resembling lupus erythematosus) and fibromuscular dysplasia of small coronary vessels.

## NORMAL EPICARDIAL CORONARY ARTERIES

There have been relatively few necropsy reports of patients with acute MI who had angiographically normal coronary arteries and normal coronary arteries at necropsy.[2,3,275,278] Of 100 consecutive necropsy cases of *acute myocardial infarction (AMI)*,[2] 7 percent had infarcts without evidence of coronary luminal narrowing. In 10 patients with a typical picture of *AMI* who died within 25 days of onset of symptoms, the coronary arterial systems showed minimal or no luminal narrowing by atherosclerosis. No thrombotic material was observed in the coronary arteries despite the fact that the *AMI* was 2 days old in 5 patients and 3 to 4 days old in 3. Possible explanations for this have included coronary artery spasm, coronary artery disease in vessels too small to be visualized angiographically, or coronary artery thrombosis or embolus with subsequent clot lysis. MI in postpartum women with normal epicardial coronary arteries has included two additional causes for possible spasm in these patients: bromocriptine utilized for suppression of lactation[117,279] and antiphospholipid syndrome with elevated anticardiolipin antibody levels, false-positive syphilis serology, and a history of deep venous thrombosis.

## SYNDROME X

The syndrome of angina or angina-like pain with angiographically normal coronary arteries has been referred to as *syndrome X*.[280,281] The cause of symptoms in this syndrome is unclear, but true myocardial ischemia (lactate production during exercise[280]) may result from microvascular dysfunction, spasm (microvascular angina), or abnormal pain perception or sensitivity (sympathovagal imbalance)

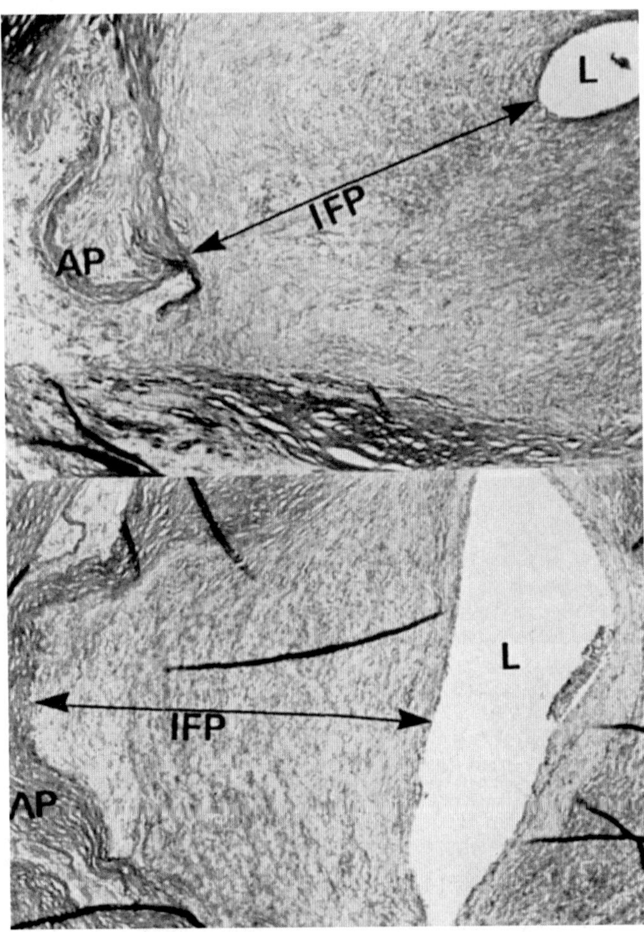


FIGURE 47-44 Intimal fibrous proliferation. Severe luminal narrowing of the left anterior descending coronary artery by intimal fibrous proliferation (IFP) several months after percutaneous balloon angioplasty. The IFP superimposes underlying atherosclerotic plaque (AP). L = lumen. (From Waller.[1] Reproduced with permission from the author, editor, and publisher.)

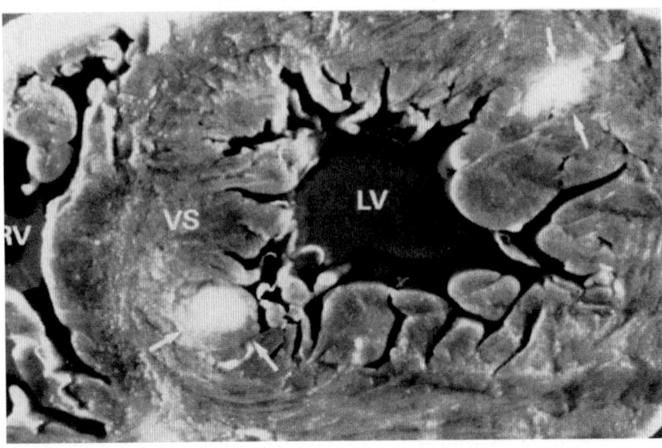


FIGURE 47-45 Metastatic deposits mimicking myocardial infarction. Transverse section of cardiac ventricle showing two discrete myocardial metastatic deposits of lymphoma. These whitish deposits may be mistakenly interpreted as healed myocardial infarctions in a patient with clean epicardial coronary arteries. LV = left ventricle; RV = right ventricle; VS = ventricular septum. (From Waller.[1] Reproduced with permission from the author, editor, and publisher.)

with sympathic predominance. In patients with evidence of myocardial ischemia, the incidence of coronary calcific deposits on computed tomography scanning is higher than with healthy controls (63 vs 22 percent) but lower than with patients who more coronary artery atherosclerosis (63 vs 96 percent).[281]

## References


1. Waller BF. Atherosclerotic and nonatherosclerotic coronary artery factors in acute myocardial infarction. In: Pepine CJ (ed). *Acute Myocardial Infarction*. Philadelphia: Davis, 1989:29–104.
2. Eliot RS, Baroldi G. Necropsy studies in myocardial infarction with minimal or no coronary luminal reduction due to atherosclerosis. *Circulation* 1974;49:1127–1131.
3. Cheitlin MD, McAllister HA, deCastro CM. Myocardial infarction without atherosclerosis. *JAMA* 1975;231:951–959.
4. Baim DS, Harrison DC. Nonatherosclerotic coronary heart disease (including coronary artery spasm). In: Hurst JW, et al (eds). *The Heart*, 5th ed. New York: McGraw-Hill, 1982:1158–1170.
5. Engel HJ, Torres C, Page HL. Major variations in anatomical origin of the coronary arteries: Angiographic observations in 4,250 patients without associated congenital heart disease. *Catheter Cardiovasc Diag* 1975;1:157–161.
6. Roberts WC. Major anomalies of coronary arterial origin seen in adulthood. *Am Heart J* 1986;111:941–963.
7. Levin DC, Fellows KE, Abrams HL. Hemodynamically significant primary anomalies of the coronary arteries. Angiographic aspects. *Circulation* 1978;58:25–34.
8. Roberts WC, Siegel RJ, Zipes DP. Origin of the right coronary artery from the left sinus of Valsalva and its functional consequences: Analysis of 10 necropsy patients. *Am J Cardiol* 1982;49:863–868.
9. Waller BF. Exercise related sudden death in young (age <30 years) and old (age >30 years) conditioned athletes. In: Wenger NK (ed). *Exercise and the Heart,* 2d ed. (Cardiovascular Clinics Series). Philadelphia; Davis, 1985:9–73.
10. Menke DM, Jordan MD, Sut CH, et al. Isolated and severe left main coronary atherosclerosis and thrombosis: A complication of acute angle takeoff of the left main coronary artery. *Am Heart J* 1986; 112:1319–1320.
11. Virmani R, Chun PKC, Goldstein RE, et al. Acute takeoffs of the coronary arteries along the aortic wall and congenital coronary ostial valve-like ridges: Association with sudden death. *J Am Coll Cardiol* 1984;3:766–771.
12. Joswig BF, Warren SE, Vieweg, WV, Hagan AD. Transmural myocardial infarction in the absence of coronary arterial luminal narrowing in a young man with single coronary arterial anomaly. *Catheter Cardiovasc Diag* 1978;4:297–301.
13. Foster L, Waller BF, Pless JE. Hypoplastic coronary arteries and high takeoff position of the right coronary artery. *Chest* 1985;88:299–301.
14. Foster L, Waller BF. Nonatherosclerotic fibrous ridges: A previously unrecognized cause of ostial left main stenosis. *J Indiana Med Assoc* 1983;76:682–683.
15. Vlodaver Z, Amplatz K, Burchell HB, Edwards JE. *Coronary Heart Disease: Clinical, Angiographic and Pathologic Profiles*. New York; Springer-Verlag, 1976.
16. Alexander RW, Griffith GC. Anomalies of the coronary arteries and their clinical significance. *Circulation* 1956;14:800–805.
17. Burth HC. Hoher und trichterformiger Ursprung der Herz Kanzarterien. *Beitr Pathol Anal* 1963;28:139–148.
18. Holt S. Syphilitic ostial occlusion. *Br Heart J* 1977;39:469–470.
19. Young JA, Sengupta A, Khaja FU. Coronary arterial stenosis, angina pectoris and atypical coarctation of the aorta due to nonspecific arteritis: Treatment, with aortocoronary bypass graft. *Am J Cardiol* 1973; 32:356–361.
20. Rozavi M. Unusual forms of coronary artery disease. In: D Vedt (ed). *Cleveland Clinic Cardiovascular Consultations*. Philadelphia: Davis, 1975:25.

21. Hudgson P, Foster JB, Walton JN. Methysergide and coronary artery disease. *Am Heart J* 1967;74:854–855.
22. Yates JD, Kirsh MM, Sodeman TM, et al. Coronary ostial stenosis: A complication of aortic valve replacement. *Circulation* 1974;49: 530–534.
23. Baroldi G. Diseases of the coronary arteries. In: Silver MD (ed). *Cardiovascular Pathology*. New York: Churchhill Livingstone, 1983:341.
24. Reyman HC. Disertatis de vasis cordis propiis. *Bibl Anat* 1737;2: 366–373.
25. Noble J, Bourassa MG, Petitclerc R, Dyrda I. Myocardial bridging and milking effect of the left anterior descending coronary artery: Normal variant or obstruction? *Am J Cardiol* 1976;37:993–999.
26. Faruqui AM, Maloy WC, Felner JM, et al. Symptomatic myocardial bridging of the coronary artery. *Am J Cardiol* 1978;41:1305–1310.
27. Visscher DW, Mildes BM, Waller BF. Tunneled ("bridged") left anterior descending coronary artery in a newborn without clinical or morphological evidence of myocardial ischemia. *Catheter Cardiovasc Diag* 1983;9:493–498.
28. Edwards JC, Burnsides C, Swarm RL, Lansing AJ. Arteriosclerosis and extramural portions of coronary arteries in the human heart. *Circulation* 1956;13:235–241.
29. Polacek P. Relation of myocardial bridges and loops in the coronary arteries to coronary occlusions. *Am Heart J* 1961;61:44–52.
30. Levin DC, Fellows KE, Abrams HL. Hemodynamically significant primary anomalies of the coronary arteries. Angiographic aspects. *Circulation* 1978;58:25–34.
31. Kramer JR, Kitazume H, Proudin WI, Sones IM. Clinical significance of isolated coronary bridges: Benign and frequent condition involving the left anterior descending artery. *Am Heart J* 1982;103:283–288.
32. Ferreira AG Jr, Trotter SE, Konig B Jr, et al. Myocardial bridges: Morphological and functional aspects. *Br Heart J* 1991;66:364–367.
33. Irvin RG. The angiographic prevalence of myocardial bridging in man. *Chest* 1982;81:198–202.
34. Channer KS, Bukis E, Hartnell G, Rees JR. Myocardial bridging of the coronary arteries. *Clin Radiol* 1989;40:355–359.
35. Wymore P, Yedlicka JW, Garcia-Medina V, et al. The incidence of myocardial bridges in heart transplants. *Cardiovasc Int Radiol* 1989; 12:202–206.
36. Gupta NC, Beauvais J. Physiologic assessment of coronary artery fistula. *Clin Nucl Med* 1991;16:40–42.
37. Theman TE, Crosby DR. Coronary artery steal secondary to coronary arteriovenous fistula. *Can J Surg* 1981;24:231–233, 236.
38. Nakashima M, Takashima S, Hashimoto K, Shiraishi M. Association of stroke and myocardial infarction in children. *Neuropediatrics* 1982; 13:47–49.
39. Macri R, Capulzini A, Fazzini L, et al. Congenital coronary artery fistula: Report of five patients, diagnostic problems and principles of management. *Thorac Cardiovasc Surg* 1982;30:167–171.
40. Sethia B, Pollock JC. Coronary artery fistula following rupture of aneurysm of the sinus node artery into the right atrium. *Thorac Cardiovasc Surg* 1985;33:191–192.
41. Zalman F, Andia AM, Wu KT, et al. Atherosclerotic coronary artery aneurysm progressing to coronary artery fistula: Presentation as myocardial infarction with continuous murmur. *Am Heart J* 1987;114: 427–429.
42. Fyfe DA, Edwards WD, Driscoll DJ. Myocardial ischemia in patients with pulmonary atresia and intact ventricular septum. *J Am Coll Cardiol* 1986;8:402–406.
43. Lau G. Sudden death arising from a congenital coronary artery fistula. *Forensic Sci Int* 1995;73:125–130.
44. Takahashi M, Sekiguchi H, Fujikawa H, et al. Multiple saccular aneurysm formation in a patient with bilateral coronary artery fistula: A case report and review of the literature. *Cardiology* 1995;86:174–176.
45. Takahashi M, Sekiguchi H, Fujikawa H, et al. Multicystic aneurysmal dilatation of bilateral coronary artery fistula. *Catheter Cardiol Diagn* 1994;31:290–292.
46. Cason BA, Gordon HJ. Coronary steal caused by a coronary artery fistula. *J Cardiothorac Vasc Anesth* 1992;6:65–67.
47. Rein AJ, Yatsiv I, Simcha A. Intracardiac causes of superior vena cava obstruction. *Eur J Pediatr* 1988;148:98–100.
48. Vavuranakis M, Bush CA, Boudoulas H. Coronary artery fistulas in adults: Incidence, angiographic characteristics, natural history. *Catheter Cardiovasc Diagn* 1995;35:116–120.
49. Aydogan U, Onursal E, Cantez T, et al. Giant congenital coronary artery fistula to left superior vena cava and right atrium with compression of left pulmonary vein simulating cor triatriatum—Diagnostic value of magnetic resonance imaging. *Eur J Cardiovasc Surg* 1994;8: 97–99.
50. Vigneswaran WT, Pollock JC. Pulmonary atresia with ventricular septal defect and coronary artery fistula: A late presentation. *Br Heart J* 1988;59:387–388.
51. Shizukuda Y, Yonekura S, Tsuchihashi K, et al. A case of a right coronary artery to left ventricle fistula observed over twenty years. *Jpn J Med* 1989;28:510–514.
52. Wilde P, Watt I. Congenital coronary artery fistulae: Six new cases with a collective review. *Clin Radiol* 1980;31:301–311.
53. Mori K, Onoe T, Ooka T. Three main coronary arteries to pulmonary artery fistula. *Jpn Circ J* 1981;45:209–212.
54. Adams P, Morris L, Ross I. Congenital left coronary artery-right ventricular fistula. *Austr Pediatr J* 1983;19:47–50.
55. Nakashima T, Tsuji T, Miyanaga H, et al. A case of blue rubber bleb nevus syndrome with coronary artery fistula to left ventricle. *Gastroenterol Jpn* 1983;18:255–259.
56. Liu PR, Leong KH, Lee PC, Chen YT. Congenital coronary artery-cardiac chamber fistulae: A study of fourteen cases. *Chung Hua i Hsueh Tsa Chih* 1994;54:160–165.
57. Mabo P, Le Breton H, De Place C, Daubert C. Asymptomatic pseudoaneurysm of the left ventricle and coronary artery fistula after closed-chest ablation of an accessory pathway. *Am Heart J* 1992; 124:1637–1639.
58. Bata IR, MacDonald RG, O'Neill BJ. Coronary artery fistula as a complication of percutaneous transluminal coronary angioplasty. *Can J Cardiol* 1993;9:331–335.
59. Iannone LA, Iannone DP. Iatrogenic left coronary artery fistula-to-left ventricle following PTCA: A previously unreported complication with nonsurgical management. *Am Heart J* 1990;120:1215–1217.
60. Cheng TO. Coronary artery fistula related to dilatation of totally occluded vessel. *Clin Cardiol* 1994;17:166.
61. Geist M, Rozenman Y, Hasin Y, Gotsman MS. Coronary artery-pulmonary artery fistula associated with hypertrophic cardiomyopathy. *Clin Cardiol* 1994;17:93–94.
62. Shirai K, Ogawa M, Kawaguchi H, et al. Acute myocardial infarction due to thrombus formation in congenital coronary artery fistula. *Eur Heart J* 1994;15:577–579.
63. Uchida N, Baudet E, Roques X, et al. Surgical experience of coronary artery-right ventricular fistula in a heart transplant patient. *Eur J Cardiothorac Surg* 1995;9:106–108.
64. Uy R, Sharma B, Franciosa JA. Acquired coronary artery fistula to the left ventricle after acute myocardial infarction. *Am J Cardiol* 1986; 58:557–558.
65. Doi YL, Takata J, Hamashige N, et al. Congenital coronary arteriovenous fistula associated with dilated cardiomyopathy. *Chest* 1987;91: 464–466.
66. Gildein HP, Kleinert S, Layangool T, Wilkinson JL. Acquired coronary artery fistula in children after ventricular septal myectomy of the right or left ventricular outflow tract. *Am Heart J* 1995;130:1124–1126.
67. Lowe JE, Adams DH, Cummings RG, et al. The natural history and recommended management of patients with traumatic coronary artery fistulas. *Ann Thorac Surg* 1983;36:295–305.
68. Haas GE, Parr GV, Trout RG, Hargrove WC III. Traumatic coronary artery fistula. *J Trauma* 1986;26:854–857.
69. Kwan T, Salciccioli L, Elsakr A, et al. Coronary artery fistula coexisting with a ventricular septal defect due to a penetrating gunshot wound. *Catheter Cardiovasc Diagn* 1995;34:235–239.
70. Tami LF. Coronary artery-right ventricular fistula after coronary artery bypass grafting. *Clin Cardiol* 1993;16:155–157.

71. Sapin P, Frantz E, Jain A, et al. Coronary artery fistula: An abnormality affecting all age groups. *Medicine* 1990;69:101–113.
72. Hackett D, Hallidie-Smith KA. Spontaneous closure of coronary artery fistula. *Br Heart J* 1984;52:477–479.
73. Griffiths SP, Ellis K, Hordof AJ, et al. Spontaneous complete closure of a congenital coronary artery fistula. *J Am Coll Cardiol* 1983; 2:1169–1173.
74. John S, Perianayagam WJ, Muralidharan S, et al. Surgical treatment of congenital coronary artery fistula. *Thorax* 1981;36:350–354.
75. Rim RS, Yang YJ, Chiu IS, et al. Surgical management of congenital coronary artery fistula. *J Formos Med Assoc* 1985;84:683–692.
76. Wellens F, Deuvaert F, Leclerc JL, Primo G. Coronary artery fistula: An absolute surgical indication. *Acta Chirurg Belg* 1984;84:339–344.
77. Kostis JB, Burns JJ, Moreyra AE, Pichard AD. Recurrent coronary artery fistula. *Clin Cardiol* 1984;7:307–313.
78. Reidy JF, Anjos RT, Qureshi SA, et al. Transcatheter embolization in the treatment of coronary artery fistulas. *J Am Coll Cardiol* 1991;18:187–192.
79. Watanabe G, Ohhira M, Takemura H, et al. Surgical treatment for myocardial bridge using intraoperative echocardiography. *J Cardiovasc Surg* 1989;30:1009–1012.
80. Betriu A, Tubau J, Sanz G, et al. Relief of angina by periarterial muscle resection of myocardial bridges. *Am Heart J* 1980;100:223–226.
81. Pey J, de Dios RM, Epeldegui A. Myocardial bridging and hypertrophic cardiomyopathy: Relief of ischemia by surgery. *Int J Cardiol* 1985;8:327–330.
82. Wenger NK. Nonatherosclerotic causes of myocardial ischemia and necrosis. In: Hurst JW, et al. (eds). *The Heart,* 4th ed. New York: McGraw-Hill, 1978:1345–1362.
83. Glickel SZ, Maggs PR, Ellis FH. Coronary artery aneurysm. *Ann Thorac Surg* 1978;25:372–376.
84. Sumino H, Kanda T, Sasaki T, et al. Myocardial infarction secondary to coronary aneurysm in systemic lupus erythematosus: An autopsy case. *Angiology* 1995;46:527–530.
85. Teja K, Crampton RS. Intramural coronary arteritis from cholesterol emboli: A rare case of unstable angina preceding sudden death. *Am Heart J* 1985;110:168–170.
86. Choy DS, Stertzer S, Loubeau JM, et al. Embolization and vessel wall perforation in argon laser recanalization. *Lasers Surg Med* 1985; 5:297–308.
87. Arvan S. Mural thrombi in coronary artery disease: Recent advances in pathogenesis, diagnosis, and approaches to treatment. *Arch Intern Med* 1984;144:113–116.
88. Charles RG, Epstein EJ. Diagnosis of coronary embolism: A review. *J R Soc Med* 1983;76:863–869.
89. Hartman RB, Harrison EE, Pupello DF, et al. Characteristics of left ventricular thrombus resulting in perioperative embolism: A complication of coronary artery bypass grafting. *J Thorac Cardiovasc Surg* 1983;86:706–709.
90. Rath S, Har-Zahav Y, Battler A, et al. Coronary arterial embolus from left atrial myxoma. *Am J Cardiol* 1984;54:1392–1393.
91. Charles RG, Epstein EJ, Holt S, Coulshed N. Coronary embolism in valvular heart disease. *Q J Med* 1982;51:147–161.
92. Wiegand V, Tebbe U, Helmchen U, Kreuzer H. Coronary arterial embolism due to valvular debris after percutaneous valvuloplasty of calcific mitral stenosis. *Clin Cardiol* 1988;11:793–796.
93. Saenz CB, Harrell RR, Sawyer JA, Hood WP. Acute percutaneous transluminal coronary angioplasty complicated by embolism to a coronary artery remote from the site of infarction. *Catheter Cardiovasc Diagn* 1987;13:266–268.
94. Lifschultz BD, Donoghue ER, Leestma JE, Boade WA. Embolization of cotton pledgets following insertion of porcine cardiac valve bioprostheses. *J Forensic Sci* 1987;32:1796–1800.
95. Johnson D, Gonzalez-Lavin L. Myocardial infarction secondary to calcific embolization: An unusual complication of bioprosthetic valve degeneration. *Ann Thorac Surg* 1986;42:102–103.
96. Cina SJ, Raso DS, Crymes LW, Upshur JK. Fatal suture embolism to the left anterior descending coronary artery: A case report and review of the literature. *Am J Forens Med Pathol* 1994;15:142–145.
97. Saber RS, Edwards WD, Bailey KR, et al. Coronary embolization after balloon angioplasty or thrombolytic therapy: An autopsy study of 32 cases. *J Am Coll Cardiol* 1993;22:1283–1288.
98. Roberts WC. Coronary embolism: A review of causes, consequences and diagnostic considerations. *Cardiovasc Med* 1978;3:699–709.
99. Waller BF, Dixon DS, Kem RW, Roberts WC. Embolus to the left main coronary artery. *Am J Cardiol* 1982;50:658–660.
100. Isner JM, Donaldson RF. Coronary angiographic and morphologic correlation. In: Waller BF (ed). *Cardiac Morphology.* (Cardiology Clinics Series). Philadelphia: Saunders; 1984:571–592.
101. Waller BR. Pathology of transluminal balloon angioplasty used in the treatment of coronary heart disease. *Hum Pathol* 1987;18:476–484.
102. Waller BF. Crackers, breakers, stretchers, drillers, scrapers, shavers, burners, welders and melters: The future of atherosclerotic coronary artery disease? A clinical-morphologic assessment. *J Am Coll Cardiol* 1989;13:969–987.
103. Mather PJ, Hansen CL, Goldman B, et al. Postpartum multivessel coronary dissection. *J Heart Lung Transpl* 1994;13:533–537.
104. Ehya H, Weitzner S. Postpartum dissecting aneurysm of coronary arteries in a patient with sarcoidosis. *South Med J* 1980;73:87–88.
105. Virmani R, Forman MB, Robinowitz M, McAllister HA. Coronary artery dissections. *Cardiol Clin* 1984;2:633–646.
106. Nishikawa H, Nakanishi S, Nishiyama S, et al. Primary coronary artery dissection: Its incidence, mode of the onset and prognostic evaluation. *J Cardiol* 1988;18:307–317.
107. Bateman AC, Gallagher PJ, Vincenti AC. Sudden death from coronary artery dissection. *J Clin Pathol* 1995;48:781–784.
108. Sage MD, Koelmeyer TD, Smeeton WM. Fatal postpartum coronary artery dissection: A light- and electron-microscope study. *Am J Forens Med Pathol* 1986;7:107–111.
109. DeMaio SJ Jr, Kinsella SH, Silverman ME. Clinical course and long-term prognosis of spontaneous coronary artery dissection. *Am J Cardiol* 1989;64:471–475.
110. Waller BF, Orr CM, Pinkerton CA, et al. Coronary balloon angioplasty dissections: The good, the bad, and the ugly. *J Am Coll Cardiol* 1992; 20:701–706.
111. Prinzmetal M, Kennamer R, Merliss R, Wada T. Angina pectoris: I. A variant form of angina pectoris. Preliminary report. *Am J Med* 1959; 27:375–388.
112. Silvermann ME, Flamm MD. Variant angina pectoris: Anatomic findings and prognostic implications. *Ann Intern Med* 1971;75:339–343.
113. Maseri A, L'Abbate A, Baroldi G, et al. Coronary vasospasm as a possible cause of myocardial infarction: A conclusion derived from the study of "preinfarction" angina. *N Engl J Med* 1978;299:1271–1277.
114. Roberts WC, Curry RC, Isner JM, et al. Sudden death in Prinzmetal's angina with coronary spasm documented by angiography: Analysis of 3 necropsy patients. *Am J Cardiol* 1982;50:203–210.
115. Conti CR. Large vessel coronary vasospasm: Diagnosis, natural history and treatment. *Am J Cardiol* 1985;55:41B–49B.
116. Kounis NG, Zavras GM. Histamin induced coronary artery spasm: The concept of allergic angina. *Br J Clin Prac* 1991;45:121–128.
117. Ruch A, Duhring JL. Postpartum myocardial infarction in a patient receiving bromocriptine. *Obstet Gynecol* 1989;74:448–451.
118. Halper J, Factor SM. Coronary lesions in neurofibromatosis associated with vasospasm and myocardial infarction. *Am Heart J* 1984;108: 420–422.
119. Shepherd JT, Katusic ZS, Vedernikov Y, Vanhoutte PM. Mechanisms of coronary vasospasm: Role of endothelium. *J Mol Cell Cardiol* 1991;23(suppl 1):125–131.
120. Simons M, Downing SE. Coronary vasoconstriction and catecholamine cardiomyopathy. *Am Heart J* 1985;109:297–300.
121. Hillis LD, Braunwald E. Coronary artery spasm. *N Engl J Med* 1978; 299:695–702.
122. Maseri A, Severi S, De Nes M, et al. "Variant" angina: One aspect of a continuous spectrum of vasospastic myocardial ischemia. *Am J Cardiol* 1978;42:1019–1035.
123. El-Maraghi NRH, Sealey BJ. Recurrent myocardial infarction in a young man with coronary arterial spasm, demonstrated at autopsy. *Circulation* 1980;61:199–207.

124. Isner JM, Fortin AH, Fortin RV. Depletion of smooth muscle from the media of atherosclerotic coronary arteries: A potential factor in the pathogenesis of myocardial ischemia and the variable response to antianginal therapy (abstr). *Clin Res* 1983;31:193A.
125. Factor SM, Cho S. Smooth muscle contraction bands in the media of coronary arteries: A postmortem marker of antemortem coronary spasm? *J Am Coll Cardiol* 1985;6:1329–1337.
126. Waller BF. The eccentric coronary atherosclerotic plaque: Morphologic observations and clinical relevance. *Clin Cardiol* 1988;12: 14–20.
127. Manion WC. Infectious angiitis. In: Orbison JL, Smith DE (eds): *The Peripheral Blood Vessels*. Baltimore: Williams & Wilkins; 1963:221.
128. Lie JT. Coronary vasculitis: A review in the current scheme of classification of vasculitis. *Arch Pathol Lab Med* 1987;111:224–233.
129. Paronetto F. Systemic nonsuppurative necrotizing angiitis. In: Miescher PA, Muller-Eberhard HJ, eds. *Textbook of Immunopathology*, 2d ed. New York: Grune & Stratton, 1976;1012–1024.
130. Christian CL, Sergent JS. Vasculitis syndromes: Clinical and experimental models. *Am J Med* 1976;61:385–392.
131. Fauci AS, Hayne BF, Katz P. The spectrum of vasculitis: Clinical, pathogenic, immunologic, and therapeutic considerations. *Ann Intern Med* 1978;89:660–676.
132. Soter NA, Austen KF. Pathogenetic mechanisms in necrotizing vasculitides. *Clin Rheum Dis* 1980;6:233–253.
133. McCluskey RT, Fienberg R. Vasculitis in primary vasculitides, granulomatoses, and connective tissue diseases. *Hum Pathol* 1983;14: 305–315.
134. Dickson WE. Polyarteritis acuta nodosa and periarterits nodosa. *J Pathol Bacteriol* 1908;12:31–57.
135. Zeek PM. Periarteritis nodosa: A critical review. *Am J Clin Pathol* 1952;22:777–790.
136. Zeek PM. Periarteritis and other forms of necrotizing angiitis. *N Engl J Med* 1953;248:764–772.
137. Churg J, Strauss L. Allergic granulomatosis, allergic angiitis, and periarteritis nodosa. *Am J Pathol* 1951;27:277–294.
138. Lanham JG, Elkon KB, Pusey CD, Hughes GF. Systemic vasculitis with asthma and eosinophilia: A clinical approach to the Churg-Strauss syndrome. *Medicine* 1984;63:65–81.
139. Von Glahn WC, Pappenheimer AM. Specific lesions of peripheral blood vessels in rheumatism. *Am J Pathol* 1926;2:235–250.
140. Huthinson J. Diseases of the arteries: On a peculiar form of thrombotic arteritis of the aged which is sometimes productive of gangrene. *Arch Surg London* 1890;1:323–329.
141. Huton BT, Magath TB, Brown GE. An underscribed form of arteritis of the temporal vessels. *Mayo Clin Proc* 1932;7:700–701.
142. Hamilton CR, Shelley WM, Tumulty PA. Giant cell arteritis: Including temporal arteritis and polymyalgia rheumatica. *Medicine* 1971;50: 1–27.
143. Ostberg G. On arteritis: With special reference to polymyalgia arteritica. *Acta Pathol Microbiol Immunol Scand A* 1973;237:1–59.
144. Somer T. Thrombo-embolic and vascular complications in vasculitis syndromes. *Eur Heart J* 1993;14(suppl K):24–29.
145. Kawai S, Fukuda Y, Okada R. Atherosclerosis of the coronary arteries in collagen disease and allied disorders with special reference to vasculitis as a preceding lesion of coronary atherosclerosis. *Jpn Circ J* 1982;46:1208–1221.
146. Allen AC, Spitz S. A comparative study of the pathology of scrub typhus (Tsutsugamushi disease) and other rickettsial diseases. *Am J Pathol* 1945;21:603–682.
147. Scharfman WB, Wallach JB, Angrist A. Myocardial infarction due to syphilitic coronary ostial stenosis. *Am Heart J* 1950;40:603–613.
148. Holt S. Syphilitic ostial occlusion. *Br Heart J* 1977;39:469–470.
149. Heggtveit HA. Syphilitic aortitis: A clinicopathologic study of 100 cases, 1950 to 1960. *Circulation* 1964;29:346–355.
150. Rose AG. Cardiac tuberculosis. A study of 19 patients. *Arch Pathol Lab Med* 1987;111:422–426.
151. Gouley BA, Bellet S, McMillan TM. Tuberculosis of the myocardium: Report of six cases with observations on involvement of coronary arteries. *Arch Intern Med* 1933;51:244–263.
152. Manion WC. Infectious angiitis. In: Orbison JL, Smith DE (eds). *The Peripheral Blood Vessels*. Baltimore: Williams & Wilkins, 1963;221–231.
153. Merkel WC. Plasmodium falciparum malaria: The coronary and myocardial lesions observed in autopsy in two cases of acute fulminating *P. falciparum* infection. *Arch Pathol* 1946;41:290–298.
154. Gazayerli M. Unusual site of a schistosome worm in the circumflex branch of the left coronary artery. *J Egypt Med Assoc* 1939;22:34–39.
155. Allen AC, Spitz S. A comparative study of the pathology of scrub typhus (Tsutsugamuschi's disease) and other rickettsial diseases. *Am J Pathol* 1945;21:603–681.
156. Moe JB, Mosher DF, Kenyon RH, et al. Functional and morphological changes during experimental Rocky Mountain spotted fever in guinea pigs. *Lab Invest* 1976;35:235–245.
157. Sergent JS. Vasculitides associated with viral infections. *Clin Rheum Dis* 1980;6:339–350.
158. Sergent JS, Lockshin MD, Christian CL, Gocke DJ. Vasculitis with hepatitis B antigenemia: Long-term observations in nine patients. *Medicine* 1976;55:1–18.
159. Heibel RH, O'Toole JD, Curtiss EI, et al. Coronary arteritis in systemic lupus erythematosus. *Chest* 1976;69:700–703.
160. Cipriano PR, Silverman JF, Perlroth MG, et al. Coronary arterial narrowing in Takayasu's aortitis. *Am J Cardiol* 1977;39:744–750.
161. Judge RD, Currier RD, Gracie WA, Figley MM. Takayasu's arteritis and the aortic arch syndrome. *Am J Med* 1962;32:379–392.
162. Ueda H. Clinical and pathological studies of aortitis syndrome: Committee report. *Jpn Heart J* 1968;9:76–87.
163. Lupi-Herrera E, Sanchez-Torres G, Marcus-Hamer J, et al. Takayasu's arteritis: Clinical study of 107 cases. *Am Heart J* 1977;93:94–103.
164. Rose AG, Sinclair-Smith CC. Takayasu's arteritis: A study of 16 cases. *Arch Pathol Lab Med* 1980;104:231–237.
165. Hall S, Barr W, Lie JT, et al. Takayasu arteritis: A study of 32 North American patients. *Medicine* 1985;64:89–99.
166. Hashimoto Y, Numano F, Maruyama Y, et al. Thallium 201 stress scintigraphy in Takayasu arteritis. *Am J Cardiol* 1991;67:879–882.
167. Takei M, Sasaki Y, Suyama K, et al. Surgically treated case of complete obstruction of the left main coronary artery caused by Takayasu's arteritis. *Am Heart J* 1993;126:458–459.
168. Tanaka M, Abe T, Takeuchi E, et al. Revascularization for coronary ostial stenosis in Takayasu's disease with calcified aorta. *Ann Thorac Surg* 1992;53:894–895.
169. Nakano S, Shimazaki Y, Keneko M, et al. Transaortic patch angioplasty for left coronary ostial stenosis in a patient with Takayasu's aortitis. *Ann Thorac Surg* 1992;53:694–696.
170. Aufderheide AC, Henke BW, Parker EH. Granulomatous coronary arteritis. *Arch Pathol Lab Med* 1981;105:647–649.
171. Rosen H, Gaton E. Takayasu's arteritis of coronary arteries. *Arch Pathol Lab Med* 1972;94:225–229.
172. Kihara M, Kimura K, Yakuwa H. Isolated left coronary ostial stenosis as the sole arterial involvement in Takayosu's disease. *J Intern Med* 1992;232:353–356.
173. Lie JT, Failoni DD, Davis DC. Temporal arteritis with giant cell aortitis, coronary arteritis, and myocardial infarction. *Arch Pathol Lab Med* 1986;110:857–860.
174. Morrison AN, Abitbol M. Granulomatous arteritis with myocardial infarction: A case report with autopsy findings. *Ann Intern Med* 1955; 42:691–700.
175. Save-Soderbergh J, Malmvall BE, Andersson R, Bengtsson RA. Giant cell arteritis as a cause of death: Report of nine cases. *JAMA* 1985; 255:493–496.
176. Lie JT. Disseminated visceral giant cell arteritis: Histopathologic description and differentiation from other granulomatous vasculitides. *Am J Clin Pathol* 1978;69:299–305.
177. Ainsworth RW, Gresham GA, Balmforth GV. Pathologic changes in temporal arteries removed from unselected cadavers. *J Clin Pathol* 1961;14:115–119.
178. Harrison CV. Giant-cell or temporal arteritis: A review. *J Clin Pathol* 1948;1:197–211.
179. Paulley JW. Coronary ischemia and occlusion in giant cell (temporal) arteritis. *Acta Medica Scand* 1980;208:257–263.

180. Zvaifler NJ, Weintraub AM. Aortitis and aortic insufficiency in chronic rheumatic disorders: A reappraisal. *Arthritis Rheum* 1963;6:241–245.
181. Heggtveit HA, Hennigar GR, Morrione TG. Panaortitis. *Am J Pathol* 1963;42:151–172.
182. Reimer KA, Rodgers RF, Oyasu R. Rheumatoid arthritis with rheumatoid heart disease and granulomatous aortitis. *JAMA* 1976;235: 2510–2512.
183. Swezey RL. Myocardial infarction due to rheumatoid arthritis. *JAMA* 1967;199:855–857.
184. Voyles WF, Searles RP, Bankhurst AD. Myocardial infarction caused by rheumatoid vasculitis. *Arthritis Rheum* 1980;23:860–883.
185. Morris PB, Imber MJ, Heinsimer JA, et al. Rheumatoid arthritis and coronary arteritis. *Am J Cardiol* 1986;57:689–690.
186. James TN. De Subitaneis Mortibus: XXIII. Rheumatoid arthritis and ankylosing spondylitis. *Circulation* 1977;55:669–677.
187. Hoffman FG, Leight L. Complete atrioventricular block associated with rheumatoid disease. *Am J Cardiol* 1965;16:585–592.
188. Grismer JT, Anderson WR, Weiss L. Chronic occlusive rheumatic coronary vasculitis and myocardial dysfunction. *Am J Cardiol* 1976; 20:739–745.
189. Kawai S, Okada R, Sugimoto H, et al. An autopsied case of a two month old infant with granulomatous pancarditis having severe vasculitis and valvulitis. *Jpn Circ J* 1983;47:1325–1330.
190. Voyles WF, Searles RP, Bankhurst AD. Myocardial infarction caused by rheumatoid vasculitis. *Arthritis Rheum* 1980;23:860–863.
191. Fujita M, Abe M, Itoh T, et al. Nonarthritic rheumatoid valvulitis with coronary arteritis causing myocardial infarction. *Virchows Arch* 1992; 420:109–112.
192. Saphir O. Thromboangiitis obliterans of the coronary arteries and its relation to arteriosclerosis. *Am Heart J* 1936;12:521–535.
193. Gore I, Burrows S. A reconsideration of the pathogenesis of Buerger's disease. *Am J Clin Pathol* 1958;29:319–330.
194. Ohno H, Matsuda Y, Takashiba K, et al. Acute myocardial infarction in Buerger's disease. *Am J Cardiol* 1986;57:690–691.
195. Averbuck SH, Silbert S. Thromboangiitis obliterans: Cause of death. *Arch Intern Med* 1934;54:436–465.
196. Fronert PP, Sheps SG. Long-term follow-up study of polyarteritis nodosa. *Am J Med* 1967;43:8–14.
197. Scott DG, Becon PA, Elliott PJ, et al. Systemic vasculitis in a district general hospital 1972–1980: Clinical and laboratory classification and prognosis in 80 cases. *Q J Med* 1982;51:292–311.
198. Holsinger DR, Osmondson PJ, Edwards JE. The heart in polyarteritis nodosa. *Circulation* 1962;25:610–617.
199. Swalwell CI, Reddy SK, Rao VJ. Sudden death due to unsuspected coronary vasculitis. *Am J Forensic Med Pathol* 1991;12: 306–312.
200. Sugihara N, Genda A, Shimizu M, et al. Intramural coronary angiitis of periarteritis nodosa proved by endomyocardial biopsy. *Am Heart J* 1990;119:1414–1416.
201. Ettinger RE, Nelson AM, Buske EC, Lie JT. Polyarteritis nodosa in childhood: A clinical pathologic study. *Arthritis Rheum* 1979;22:820–825.
202. Petty RE, Maligilavy DB, Cassidy JT, Sullivan DB. Polyarteritis in childhood: A clinical description of eight cases. *Arthritis Rheum* 1977; 20:392–394.
203. Roberts FB, Fetterman GH. Polyarteritis nodosa in infancy. *J Pediatr* 1963;63:519–529.
204. Munro-Faure H. Necrotizing arteritis of the coronary vessels in infancy: Case report and review of the literature. *Pediatrics* 1959;23: 914–926.
205. Tanaka N, Naoe S, Masuda H, Ueno T. Pathological study of sequelae of Kawasaki disease (MCLS): With special reference to the heart and coronary arterial lesions. *Acta Pathol Japon* 1986;36:1513–1527.
206. Kawasaki T, Kosaki F, Okawa S, et al. A new infantile acute febrile mucocutaneous lymph node syndrome (MLNS) prevailing in Japan. *Pediatrics* 1974;54:271–276.
207. Melish ME. Kawasaki syndrome (the mucocutaneous lymph node syndrome). *Annu Rev Med* 1982;33:569–585.
208. Langing BH, Larson EJ. Are infantile periarteritis nodosa with coronary artery involvement and fatal mucocutaneous lymph node syndrome the same? Comparison of 20 patients from North America with patients from Hawaii and Japan. *Pediatrics* 1977;59:651–662.
209. Kitamura S, Kawashima Y, Fujita T, et al. Aortocoronary bypass grafting in a child with coronary artery obstruction due to mucocutaneous lymph node syndrome: Report of a case. *Circulation* 1976;53: 1035–1040.
210. Kato H, Koike S, Yamamoto M, et al. Coronary aneurysms in infants and young children with acute febrile mucocutaneous lymph node syndrome. *J Pediatr* 1975;86:892–898.
211. Kitamura S, Kawachi K, Harima R, et al. Surgery for coronary heart disease due to mucocutaneous lymph node syndrome: Report of 6 patients. *Am J Cardiol* 1983;51:444–448.
212. Suzuki A, Kamiya T, Kuwahara N, et al. Coronary arterial lesions of Kawasaki disease: Cardiac catheterization findings of 1100 cases. *Pediatr Cardiol* 1986;7:3–9.
213. Kato H, Ichinose E, Kawasaki T. Myocardial infarction in Kawasaki disease: Clinical analyses in 195 cases. *J Pediatr* 1986;108:923–928
214. Suzuki A, Kamiya T, Kuwahara N. Coronary arterial lesions of Kawasaki disease: Cardiac catheterization findings in 1100 cases. *Pediatr Ca*rdiol 1986;7:3–11
215. Kato H, Sugimura T, Akagi T. Long form consequences of Kawasaki disease. A 10- to 21-year follow-up of 594 patients. *Circulation* 1996;94:1379–85.
216. Sugimura T, Kato H, Inoue O. Vasodilatory response of the coronary arteries after Kawasaki disease. Evaluation by intracoronary injection of isosorbide dinitrate. *J Pediatr* 1992;121:684–689.
217. Iemura M, Ishii M, Sugimura T. Long-term consequences of regressed coronary aneurysms after Kawasaki disease: Vascular wall morphology and function. *Heart* 2000;83:307–311.
218. Parrillo JE, Fauci AS. Necrotizing vasculitis, coronary angiitis and the cardiologist. *Am Heart J* 1980;99:547–554.
219. Gatenby PA, Lytton DG, Bulteau VG, et al. Myocardial infarction in Wegener's granulomatosis. *Aust NZ J Med* 1976; 6:336–340.
220. Wegener F. Uber generalisierte, septische Gefasserkrankugen. *Verh Dtsch Ges Pathol* 1936;29:202–210.
221. Forstot JZ, Overlie PA, Neufeld GK, et al. Cardiac complications of Wegener granulomatosis: A case report of complete heart block and review of the literature. *Semin Arthritis Rheum* 1980;10:148–154.
222. Allen DC, Doherty CC, O'Reilly DP. Pathology of the heart and the cardiac conduction system in Wegener's granulomatosis. *Br Heart J* 1964;52:674–678.
223. Schiavone WA, Ahmad M, Ockner SA. Unusual cardiac complications of Wegener's granulomatosis. *Chest* 1985;88:745–748.
224. Lie JT. Classification of vasculitis and a reappraisal of allergic granulomatosis and angiitis. *Mt Sinai J Med* 1986;53:429–439.
225. Cupps TR, Fauci AS. *The Vasculitides*. Philadelphia: Saunders, 1981:211.
226. Rich AR. Hypersensitivity in disease, with special reference to periarteritis nodosa, rheumatic fever, disseminated lupus erythematosus, and rheumatoid arthritis. *Harvey Lect* 1947;42:106–147.
227. Meller J, Conde CA, Deppisch LM, et al. Myocardial infarction due to coronary atherosclerosis in three young adults with systemic lupus erythematosus. *Am J Cardiol* 1975;35:309–314.
228. Bonfiglio TA, Botti RE, Hagstrom JWC. Coronary arteritis, occlusion and myocardial infarction due to lupus erythematosus. *Am Heart J* 1972;83:153–158.
229. Nobreg TP, Klodas E, Breen JF. Giant coronary artery aneurysms and myocardial infarction in a patient with systemic lupus erythematosus. *Catheter Cardiovasc Diagn* 1996;39:75–78.
230. Follansbee WP. The cardiovascular manifestations of systemic sclerosis. *Curr Probl Cardiol* 1986;11:245–297.
231. Schimizu T, Ehrlich GE, Inaba G, Hayashi K. Behçet disease. *Semin Arthritis Rheum* 1979;8:223–260.
232. Haynes BF, Kaiser-Kupfer MI, Mason P, Fauci AS. Cogan syndrome: Studies in 13 patients, long term follow-up and a review of the literature. *Medicine* 1980;59:426–441.
233. Vaarala O. Antiphospholipid antibiodies and myocrdial infarction. *Lupus* 1998;7(suppl 2):132–134.

234. Mullick FG, McAllister HA, Wagner BM, Fenoglio JJ Jr. Drug related vasculitis: Clinicopathologic correlation in 30 patients. *Hum Pathol* 1979;10:313–325.
235. Brosius FC, Roberts WC. Coronary artery disease in the Hurler syndrome. *Am J Cardiol* 1981;47:649–653.
236. Renteria VG, Ferrans VJ, Roberts WC. The heart in the Hurler syndrome: Gross histologic and ultrastructural observations in five necropsy cases. *Am J Cardiol* 1976;38:487–501.
237. Lindsay S. The cardiovascular system in gargoylism. *Br Heart J* 1950; 12:17–32.
238. Stauffer M. Oxalosis: Report of a case with a review of the literature and discussion on pathogenesis. *N Engl J Med* 1960;263:386–390.
239. Blieden LC, Desnick RJ, Carter JB, et al. Cardiac involvement in Sandhoff's disease: An inborn error of glycosphingolipid metabolism. *Am J Cardiol* 1974;34:83–88.
240. Blieden LC, Moller JH. Cardiac involvement in inherited disorders of metabolism. *Prog Cardiovasc Dis* 1974;16:615–631.
241. Brosius FC III, Waller BF, Roberts WC. Radiation heart disease: Analysis of 16 young (aged 15 to 33 years) necropsy patients who received over 3500 rads to the heart. *Am J Med* 1981;70:519–530.
242. Brill IC, Brodeur MTH, Oyama AA. Myocardial infarction in two sisters less than 20 years old. *JAMA* 1971;217:1345–1348.
243. Trimble AS, Bigelow WG, Wigle ED. Coronary ostial stenosis: A late complication of coronary perfusion in open-heart surgery. *J Thorac Cardiovasc Surg* 1969;57:792–795.
244. Lie JT, Berg KK. Isolated fibromuscular dysplasia of the coronary arteries with spontaneous dissection and myocardial infarction. *Hum Pathol* 1987;18:654–656.
245. Przybojewski JZ, Rossouw J. Severe isolated left mainstem coronary artery stenosis: A case report. *S Afr Med J* 1986;69:133–136.
246. Dominguez FE, Tate LG, Robinson MJ. Familial fibromuscular dysplasia presenting as sudden death. *Am J Cardiovasc Pathol* 1988;2: 269–272.
247. Billingham M. Personal communication. Stanford University, Stanford, CA, 1988.
248. Johnson DE, Gao SZ, Schroeder JS, et al. The spectrum of coronary artery pathologic findings in human cardiac allografts. *J Heart Transpl* 1989;8:349–359.
249. Gravanis MB. Allograft heart accelerated atherosclerosis: Evidence for cell mediated immunity in pathogenesis. *Mod Pathol* 1989;2: 495–505.
250. Mehra MR, Ventura HO, Stapleton DD, et al. Presence of severe intimal thickening by intravascular ultrasonography predicts cardiac events in cardiac allograft vasculopathy. *J Heart Lung Transpl* 1995; 14:632–639.
251. Waller BF, Pinkerton CA, Foster LN. Morphologic evidence of accelerated left main coronary artery stenosis: A late complication of percutaneous transluminal angioplasty of the proximal left anterior descending coronary artery. *J Am Coll Cardiol* 1987;9: 1019–1023.
252. Giritsky AS, Ricci MT, Reitz BA, Shumway NE. Extrinsic coronary artery obstruction by chronic aortic dissection. *Ann Thorac Surg* 1981; 32:289–293.
253. Gardia-Rinaldi R, Von Koch L, Howell JP. Aneurysm of the sinus of Valsalva producing obstruction of the left main coronary artery. *J Thorac Cardiovascular Surg* 1976;72:123–126.
254. Kopelson G, Herwig KJ. The etiologies of coronary artery disease in cancer patients. *Int J Radiat Oncol Biol Phys* 1978;4:895–906.
255. Applefeld MM, Wiernik PH. Cardiac disease after radiation therapy for Hodgkin's disease: Analysis of 48 patients. *Am J Cardiol* 1983; 51:1679–1681.
256. Sebag-Montefiore D, Hope Stone H. Radiation induced coronary heart disease. *Br Heart J* 1993;69:481–482.
257. Radwaner BA, Geringer R, Goldmann AM, et al. Left main coronary artery stenosis following mediastinal irradiation. *Am J Med* 1987; 82:1017–1020.
258. Schulman HE, Korr KS, Myers TJ. Left internal thoracic artery graft occlusion following mediastinal radiation therapy. *Chest* 1994;105: 1881–1882.
259. Benoff LJ, Schweitzer P. Radiation therapy induced cardiac injury. *Am Heart J* 1995;129:1193–1196.
260. Reber D, Birnbaum DE, Tollenaere P. Heart diseases following mediastinal irradiation: Surgical management. *Eur J Cardiothor Surg* 1995; 9:202–205.
261. Grollier G, Commeau P, Mercier V, et al. Post radiotherapeutic left main coronary ostial stenosis: Clinical and histological study. *Eur Heart J* 1988;9:567–570.
262. Tenet W, Missri J, Hager D. Radiation induced stenosis of the left main coronary artery. *Catheter Cardiovasc Diagn* 1986;12:169–171.
263. McEniery PT, Dorosti K, Schiavone WA, et al. Clinical and angiographic features of coronary artery disease after chest irradiation. *Am J Cardiol* 1987;60:1020–1024.
264. House KW, Simon SR, Pugh RP. Chemotherapy induced myocardial infarction in a young man with Hodgkin's disease. *Clin Cardiol* 1992; 15:122–125.
265. Fomina LG. A case of myocardial infarct in acute leukemia. *Sov Med* 1960;24:141–143.
266. Wirth L. Myocardial infarction as the initial manifestation of polycythemia vera. *Mil Med* 1960;125:544–548.
267. Spach MS, Howell DA, Harris JS. Myocardial infarction and multiple thrombosis in a child with primary thrombocytosis. *Pediatrics* 1963; 31:268–276.
268. James TN. Pathology of the small coronary arteries. *Am J Cardiol* 1963;20:679–691.
269. Isner JM, Estes NAM III, Thompson PD, et al. Acute cardiac events temporally related to cocaine abuse. *N Engl J Med* 1968;315: 1438–1443.
270. Virmani R, Robinowitz M, Smialek JE, Smyth DF. Cardiovascular effects of cocaine: An autopsy study of 40 patients. *Am Heart J* 1988; 115:1068–1076.
271. Hollander JE, Hoffman RS. Cocaine-induced myocardial infarction: An analysis and review of the literature. *J Emerg Med* 1992;10:169–177.
272. Miller GW. The cocaine habit. *Am Fam Physician* 1985;31:173–176.
273. Virmani R, Robinowitz M, Smialek JE, Smyth DF. Cardiovascular effects of cocaine: An autopsy study of 40 patients. *Am Heart J* 1988; 115:1068–1076.
274. Dowling GP, McDonough ET, Bost RO. Eve and ecstasy: A report of five deaths associated with the use of MDEA and MDMA. *J Am Coll Cardiol* 1987;257:1615–1617.
275. Masani ND, Northbridge DB, Hall RJ. Severe coronary vasospasm associated with hyperthyroidism causing myocardial infarction. *Br Heart Journal* 1995;74:700–701.
276. Silberberg JS, Barre PE, Prichard SS, Sniderman AD. Impact of left ventricular hypertrophy on survival in end-stag renal disease. *Kidney Int* 1989;36:286–290.
277. James TN, Posada de la Paz M, Abaitua Borda I, et al. Histologic abnormalities of large and small coronary arteries, neural structures, and the conduction system of the heart found in postmortem studies of individuals dying from the toxic oil syndrome. *Am Heart J* 1991; 121:803–815.
278. Friedberg CK, Horn H. Acute myocardial infarction not due to coronary artery occlusion. *JAMA* 1939;112:1675–1679.
279. Department of Health and Human Services, Food and Drug Administration Docket No. 94N-0304. Notice of Hearing on Proposal to Withdraw Approval of the Indication for Prevention of Physiological Lactation: Bromocriptine. Center for Drug Evaluation and Research, 7500 Standish Pl, Rockville MD pp 1–12.
280. Camici PG, Marraccini P, Lorenzoni R. Coronary hemodynamics and myocardial metabolism in patients with syndrome X. *Cardiol* 1991; 17:1461–1466.
281. Shenesh J, Fisman EZ, Tenenbaum A. coronary artery calcification in women with syndrome X: Usefulness of double-helical CT for detection. *Radiology* 1997;205:697–301.

CHAPTER 48

# DEFINITIONS OF ACUTE CORONARY SYNDROMES

Michael C. Kim / Annapoorna S. Kini / Valentin Fuster



Coronary artery disease (CAD) is a worldwide health epidemic. In the United States, for example, it is estimated that 12.2 million Americans have CAD, including 7.2 million individuals of whom already have had a myocardial infarction (MI).[1] In the United States, it is estimated that for those over 30 years of age, 213 per 100,000 individuals have ischemic heart disease.[1] Worldwide, it is estimated that 30 percent of all deaths can be attributed to cardiovascular disease, and the forecasts in the future estimate a growing number due to lifestyle changes in developing countries.[1] The Centers for Disease Control estimate that life expectancy might be increased by 7 years if CAD and its complications were eradicated.[2]

CAD represents a continuum of disease pathologies and its subsequent risks. CAD has been classified as chronic CAD, acute coronary syndromes, and sudden death from lowest to highest risk and may present clinically as an asymptomatic entity to unexpected cardiac collapse. Chronic CAD is almost always secondary to coronary atherosclerosis leading to an oxygen supply and demand mismatch and a stable pattern of coronary ischemia.[3] This chapter, however, will focus on the definitions of a more high-risk population, those with acute coronary syndromes (ACS) (see also Chap. 57).

## ACUTE CORONARY SYNDROMES

*ACS* is actually a unifying term representing a common end result, acute myocardial ischemia. Acute ischemia is usually, but not always, caused by atherosclerotic CAD and is associated with an increased risk of cardiac death and myonecrosis.[4] It encompasses acute MI (both resulting in ST elevation or non-ST elevation) and unstable angina. The importance of recognizing a cardiac patient with ACS concerns both triage and management. Those deemed to have an ACS in the emergency department should be triaged immediately to an area with continuous electrocardiogram (ECG) monitoring and defibrillation capability. An ECG should be able to be obtained and accurately interpreted within 10 min. Moreover, those with suspected ACS should be managed immediately with antiplatelet and anticoagulant therapies and considered for immediate revascularization mechanically or pharmacologically if new ST elevation is noted.[5]

Because of the life-threatening nature of an ACS, it is prudent to have a low threshold in suspecting a patient with acute chest pain as potentially having an ACS. Because the efficient diagnosis and optimal management of these patients are derived from information mostly only readily available from initial clinical presentation, there is overlap of those with true ACS and those that ultimately do not have CAD as a cause of their cardiac symptoms. In addition, it may not be possible to differentiate patients with MI (either ST elevation or non-ST elevation) from those with unstable angina in the initial hours.

Nonetheless, proper initial triage of patients suspected to have acute coronary ischemia should eventually identify patients as having (1) ACS; (2) a non-ACS cardiovascular condition such as pericarditis, aortic dissection, or pulmonary embolism; (3) a noncardiac cause of chest pain such as gastroesophageal reflux; and (4) a noncardiac condition that is yet undefined.[6] ACS patients with new evidence of ST-segment elevation on the presenting ECG are labeled as having an ST-segment elevation myocardial infarction (STEMI) and should be considered for immediate reperfusion therapy by thrombolytics or percutaneous coronary intervention (PCI). Those without ST-segment elevation but with evidence of myonecrosis are determined to have a non-ST-segment elevation myocardial infarction (NSTEMI); and those without any evidence of myonecrosis are diagnosed with unstable angina (Fig. 48-1).

### Definition of Unstable Angina

Unstable angina is usually secondary to reduced myocardial perfusion resulting from coronary artery atherothrombosis. In this event, however, the nonocclusive thrombus that developed on a disrupted atherosclerotic plaque does not result in any biochemical evidence of myocardial necrosis. Unstable angina and NSTEMI can be viewed as very closely related clinical conditions with similar presentations and pathogenesis but of differing severity.

Because of the lack of objective data associated with the condition, unstable angina (also known as preinfarction angina, intermediate coronary syndrome, or acute coronary insufficiency) must be diagnosed from careful history taking and is thus the most subjective of the ACS diagnoses. The Agency for Health Care Policy and Research (AHCPR) has published guidelines listing features that signify the likelihood of signs and symptoms suggestive of an ACS likely due to CAD (Table 48-1).[7] There are 3 principal presentations of unstable angina: (1) rest angina or angina with minimal exertion usually lasting at least 20 min, (2) new-onset severe angina usually defined as within the last month, and (3) crescendo angina defined as previously diagnosed angina that has become distinctly more frequent, longer in duration, or more severe in nature.[8]

Because of the heterogenous group of patients who fall under these loose definitions, many classification schemes have been

A.

Thrombosis
Mechanical obstruction
↑ $MVO_2$
Dynamic obstruction
Inflammation / infection

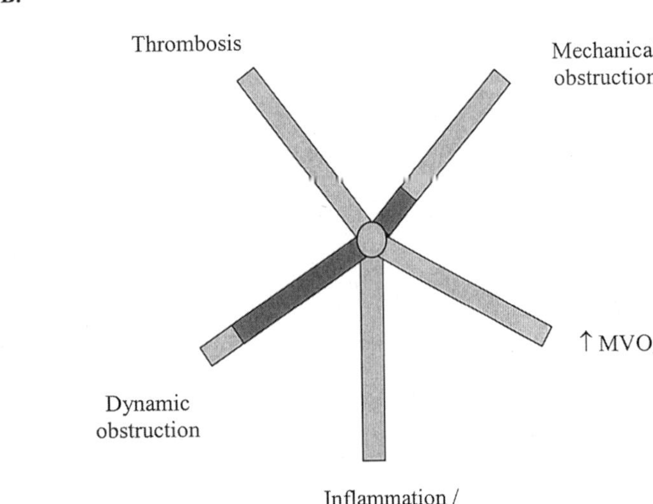


FIGURE 48-1 Schematic representation of the causes of unstable angina. Each of the five bars represents one of the etiologic mechanisms, and the dark portion of the bar represents the extent to which the mechanism is operative. *A.* Most common form of unstable angina in which atherosclerotic plaque causes moderate (60 percent diameter) obstruction, and acute thrombus overlying plaque causes very severe (90 percent diameter) narrowing. *B.* Mild coronary obstruction, adjacent to which there is intense (90 percent vasoconstriction). (From Braunwald E: Unstable angina: An etiologic approach to management. *Circulation* 1998;98:2219–2222.)

proposed for unstable angina. While not devised precisely to help define unstable angina, the Canadian Cardiovascular Society (CCS) has developed an easy classification system to grade anginal symptoms (Table 48-2; see also Chap. 12).[9] Class I angina is the least symptomatic and denotes that ordinary physical activity does not illicit anginal symptoms. Class II angina implies anginal symptoms that slightly impair ordinary activity such as walking and climbing stairs. For example, Class II angina would occur after walking more than 2 blocks on a level surface or climbing more than 1 flight of stairs. Class III angina is defined as symptoms that limit markedly ordinary physical activity. For example, symptoms that occur less than 1 block of walking on a level ground or less than 1 flight of stairs. Finally, Class IV angina is symptoms at rest or that cause an inability to carry on any physical activity without discomfort. The relevance of this classification system is exemplified in the definition of crescendo angina. Worsening angina can be defined as symptoms that result in at least 1 CCS Class increase or to at least CCS Class III severity.[10]

Braunwald has developed a useful classification of unstable angina assessing risk.[10] By differentiating the severity and clinical circumstances surrounding the presentation of unstable angina and considering also the presence or absence of ECG changes and the intensity of medical therapy, Braunwald has estimated the risk of death or MI at 1 year (Table 48-3). In terms of severity, Class I unstable angina is new onset or accelerated angina but with no rest pain. Class II presents with rest angina within the last month but not within the previous 48 h. Class III angina presents at rest and within the last 48 h or initial evaluation. In terms of clinical circumstances, Class A represents unstable angina in the setting of a secondary noncoronary cause of demand ischemia such as anemia, hypotension, or prolonged tachycardia. Class B is worsening primary CAD in the absence of extracardiac conditions. Class C is postinfarction unstable angina within 2 weeks of a documented MI. Furthermore, patients fared worse over the following 12 months if they presented with transient ST-T wave changes during pain and if they had angina despite maximal anti-ischemic therapy. In summary, patients with a 48-h pain-free interval and the absence of ECG changes were at decreased risk while those with postinfarction angina and the need for maximal medical therapy have the highest risk of death or MI over the next 1 year after presentation with UA. The AHCPR has also published guidelines assessing the short-term risk of death or nonfatal MI in patients with unstable angina using similar clinical features (Table 48-4). It should be noted that an elevated level of a cardiac marker such as a troponin places the patient at high risk. These patients would now be considered to have an NSTEMI instead of high risk unstable angina.[4]

As mentioned earlier while nonocclusive thrombus on a preexisting atherosclerotic plaque is the most common cause of unstable angina/NSTEMI, other causes may lead to acute coronary ischemia[6] (Table 48-5 and Fig. 48-2). A less common cause is dynamic obstruction of an epicardial artery leading to intense focal spasm (Prinzmetal's angina). It is thought that this spasm is caused by hypercontractility of vascular smooth muscle and/or endothelial dysfunction. Abnormal constriction of small intramural resistance vessels can also lead to dynamic obstruction and acute ischemia. A third cause of unstable angina is severe mechanical obstruction without spasm or thrombus. An example would be restenosis after percutaneous coronary intervention (PCI) or some patients with progressive atherosclerosis. A fourth cause is arterial inflammation and/or infection. It is thought that chronic inflammation perhaps related to infection leads to activation of macrophages and T-lymphocytes at the shoulder of a vulnerable plaque and increased expression of metalloproteins resulting in distruption and rupture of the plaque. Finally, a fifth cause of unstable angina is alluded to in Braunwald's classification as unstable angina from a secondary cause. These patients generally have chronic stable CAD, which worsens due to a noncoronary condition that increases myocardial oxygen demand such as fever or tachycardia, reduces coronary blood flow such as in hypotension, or reduces myocardial oxygen delivery such as hypoxemia or anemia. These causes are not mutually exclusive.

## Non-ST-Segment Elevation Myocardial Infarction

NSTEMI represents a clinical condition presenting very similarly to unstable angina but with evidence of myonecrosis by some form of

TABLE 48-1 Likelihood that Signs and Symptoms Represent an ACS Secondary to CAD

| Feature | High Likelihood *Any of the following:* | Intermediate Likelihood *Absence of high-likelihood features and presence of any of the following:* | Low Likelihood *Absence of high- or intermediate-likelihood features but may have:* |
|---|---|---|---|
| History | Chest or left arm pain or discomfort as chief symptom reproducing prior documented angina<br>Known history of CAD, including MI | Chest or left arm pain or discomfort as chief symptom<br>Age > 70 years<br>Male sex<br>Diabetes mellitus | Probable ischemic symptoms in absence of any of the intermediate-likelihood characteristics<br>Recent cocaine use |
| Examination | Transient MR, hypotension, diaphoresis, pulmonary edema, or rales | Extracardiac vascular disease | Chest discomfort reproduced by palpation |
| ECG | New, or presumably new, transient, ST-segment deviation ($\geq$ 0.05 mV) or T-wave inversion ($\geq$ 0.2 mV) with symptoms | Fixed Q waves<br>Abnormal ST segments or T waves not documented to be new | T-wave flattening or inversion in leads with dominant R waves<br>Normal ECG |
| Cardiac markers | Elevated cardiac TnI, TnT or CK-MB | Normal | Normal |

ABBREVIATIONS: ACS = acute coronary syndrome; CAD, coronary artery disease; CK-MB = creatine kinase-MB; ECG = electrocardiogram; MI = myocardial infarction; MR = mitral regurgitation; TnI = troponin I; TnT = troponin T.
SOURCE: Braunwald E, Mark DB, Jones RH, et al. Unstable angina: Diagnosis and management. Rockville, MD: Agency for Health Care Policy and Research and the National Heart, Lung, and Blood Institute, US Public Health Service, US Dept. of Health and Human Services; 1994:1. AHCPR Publication 94-0602.

cardiac markers without ST-segment elevation on ECG. Patients presenting with NSTEMI have an intermediate risk of acute complications when compared to unstable angina (lower risk) and STEMI-higher risk.[11] Because evidence of myonecrosis is required, the diagnosis of NSTEMI is less subject to error than is unstable angina and requires more careful monitoring and aggressive therapy. In fact, the most important reason to differentiate true unstable angina from NSTEMI is in determining the ideal management strategy in the early hospitalization period. It is becoming more and more evident from large, randomized multicenter clinical trials that early aggressive management with enhanced antiplatelet (clopidogrel and glycoprotein IIb/IIIa inhibitors) and earlier angiography/mechnical revascularization is superior to conservative traditional medical therapy and ischemia-guided revascularization[12–14] (see Figure 48-2).

Because the diagnosis of NSTEMI implies ischemia severe enough to cause sufficient myocardial damage to release detectable quantities of a maker of myocardial injury, it is important to discuss the different cardiac markers of injury. Biochemical markers such as troponins, creatinine kinase, and myoglobin are useful for both the diagnosis of myonecrosis and prognostically.[15] An ideal cardiac marker would be very specific to cardiac muscle and absent from nonmyocardial tissue. It would be released quickly into the peripheral blood after onset of injury and would measure quantitatively the magnitude of necrosis. Finally, the marker should be convenient and inexpensive to use.

Until recently creatine kinase (CK) activity has been the most widely used serum cardiac marker in the evaluation of ACS. Although this marker is very sensitive for detecting myocardial damage (average time to peak is 24 h and becomes initially elevated in 4 to 8 h after insult) and can accurately predict the magnitude of necrosis, several limitations do exist with this marker. CK levels are elevated in patients with muscle disease, alcohol intoxication, skeletal muscle trauma, seizures, vigorous exercise, thoracic outlet syndrome, and pulmonary embolism. Even the more cardiac muscle specific MB isoform may be present in the tongue, small intestine, uterus, and prostate.

Recent methods to improve specificity include measurement of CK-MB levels by specific enzyme immunoassays that use monoclonal

TABLE 48-2 Grading of Angina Pectoris According to CCS Classification (See also Chap. 12)

| Class | Description of Stage |
|---|---|
| I | "Ordinary physical activity does not cause . . . angina," such as walking or climbing stairs. Angina occurs with strenuous, rapid, or prolonged exertion at work or recreation. |
| II | "Slight limitation of ordinary activity." Angina occurs on walking or climbing stairs rapidly; walking uphill; walking or stair climbing after meals; in cold, in wind, or under emotional stress; or only during the few hours after awakening. Angina occurs on walking >2 level blocks and climbing >1 flight of ordinary stairs at normal pace and under normal conditions. |
| III | "Marked limitation of ordinary physical activity." Angina occurs on walking 1 to 2 level blocks and climbing 1 flight of stairs under normal conditions and at a normal pace. |
| IV | "Inability to carry on any physical activity" without discomfort—anginal symptoms may be present at rest. |

ABBREVIATION: CCS = Canadian Cardiovascular Society

TABLE 48-3 Braunwald Classification of Unstable Angina

| Severity | Clinical Circumstances: A. Develops in Presence of Extracardiac Condition that Intensifies Myocardial Ischemia (Secondary UA) | B. Develops in Absence of Extracardiac Condition (Primary Unstable UA) | C. Develops within 2 Weeks After Acute MI (Post-infarct UA) |
|---|---|---|---|
| I. New onset of severe angina or accelerated angina; no rest pain | IA | IB | IC |
| II. Angina at rest within last month, but not within preceding 48 h (angina at rest, subacute) | IIA | IIB | IIC |
| III. Angina at rest within 48 h (angina at rest, acute) | IIIA | IIIB | IIIC |

ABBREVIATIONS: MI = myocardial infarction; UA = unstable angina.

antibodies directed against CK-MB (mass method) and by measuring CK-MB isoforms. The mass method of CK-MB levels has proved to be more accurate than traditional radioimmunoassay or agarose gel electrophoresis methods, especially in patients presenting within 4 h of injury.[16] CK-MB isoforms exist in only 1 form in cardiac muscle ($CK\text{-}MB_2$) while they exist in different isoforms in the plasma ($CK\text{-}MB_1$). An absolute value of $CK\text{-}MB_2$ of greater than 1 U/L and a ratio of $CK\text{-}MB_2/CK\text{-}MB_1$ of greater than 2.5 has significantly improved the sensitivity of diagnosing myonecrosis at 6 h.[17] However, these isoform assays are not readily available and are still limited by

TABLE 48-4 Short-Term Risk of Death or Nonfatal MI in Patients with UA

| Feature | High Risk *At least 1 of the following features must be present:* | Intermediate Risk *No high-risk feature but must have 1 of the following:* | Low Risk *No high- or intermediate-risk feature but may have any of the following features:* |
|---|---|---|---|
| History | Accelerating tempo of ischemic symptoms in preceding 48 h | Prior MI, peripheral or cerebrovascular disease, or CABG, prior aspirin use | |
| Character of pain | Prolonged ongoing (> 20 min) rest pain | Prolonged (> 20 min) rest angina, now resolved, with moderate or high likelihood of CAD<br>Rest angina (< 20 min) or relieved with rest or sublingual NTG | New onset or progressive CCS Class III or IV angina the past 2 weeks without prolonged (> 20 min) rest pain but with moderate or high likelihood of CAD (see Table 48-1) |
| Clinical findings | Pulmonary edema, most likely due to ischemia<br>New or worsening MR murmur<br>$S_3$ or new/worsening rales<br>Hypotension, bradycardia, tachycardia<br>Age > 75 years | Age > 70 years | |
| ECG | Angina at rest with transient ST-segment changes > 0.05mV<br>Bundle branch block, new or presumed new<br>Sustained ventricular tachycardia | T-wave inversions > 0.2 mV<br>Pathologic Q waves | Normal or unchanged ECG during an episode of chest discomfort |
| Cardiac markers | Elevated (e.g., TnT or TnI > 0.1 ng/mL) | Slightly elevated (e.g., TnT > 0.01 but < 0.1 ng/mL) | Normal |

ABBREVIATIONS: CABG = coronary artery bypass graft; CAD = coronary artery disease; ECG = electrocardiogram; MI = myocardial infarction; MR = mitral regurgitation; NTG = nitroglycerin; TnI = troponin I; TnT = troponin T; UA = unstable angina.
SOURCE: Braunwald E, Mark DB, Jones RH, et al. Unstable angina: Diagnosis and management, Rockville, MD: Agency for Health Care Policy and Research and the National Heart, Lung and Blood Institute. US Public Health Service, US Dept. of Health and Human Services; 1994:1. AHCPR Publication 94-0602.

TABLE 48-5 Secondary Precipitants of Myocardial Ischemia

**Increased Myocardial Oxygen Demand**
1. Fever
2. Thyrotoxicosis
3. Tachycardia
4. Malignant hypertension
5. Pheochromocytoma
6. Aortic stenosis
7. High output state
8. Pregnancy
9. Drugs: cocaine, amphetamine

**Decreased Oxygen Supply**
1. Anemia
2. Hypoxemia
3. Carbon monoxide poisoning
4. Polycythemia vera
5. Hyperviscosity syndromes

specificity issues concerning CK-MB levels in the heart versus other tissues.

Cardiac troponins represent a major clinical shift in the diagnosis of NSTEMI.[18] The troponin complex consists of 3 subunits that regulate contraction of cardiac muscle: Troponin I (TnI), TnT, and TnC. Troponin C binds to calcium; TnI binds to actin and inhibits the actin-myosin interaction; TnT binds to tropomyosin, which attaches the troponin complex to the thin filament. Monoclonal antibody-based immunoassays have been developed to detect these cardiac-specific TnT and TnI. Because cardiac and smooth muscle share isoforms for TnC, no immunoassays of TnC have been developed to date. Because of the increased sensitivity and specificity of cardiac troponins relative to CK, it is estimated that up to 30 percent of patients who present with rest pain and normal CK-MB levels previously diagnosed with unstable angina actually can be reclassified as having NSTEMI when assessed with troponins.[19] There has been some controversy as to whether this subgroup of patients with negative CK-MB levels and minor elevations in troponins should be labeled as having high-risk unstable angina or NSTEMI. Some investigators have used the term *microinfarction,* or *minor myocardial damage,* to describe this situation.[20] Similarly, there is controversy in labeling a patient with no significant ECG changes and a minor troponin elevation as having unstable angina or NSTEMI.

There is no disagreement concerning the utility of elevated cardiac troponin levels in establishing prognosis.[21,22] Elevated levels indicate a high risk subgroup independent of ECG presentation and predischarge exercise testing.[23] There is an incremental risk of death or MI in patients with elevated troponins that can be seen in a quantitative fashion, even in patients with chronic renal insufficiency.[24] Even patients in whom CK-MB levels are within normal limits, troponin elevation signifies a higher risk of death than it does in those without elevation.[25] It should be emphasized that cardiac troponins should be used only as one tool in the initial evaluation along with the history, physical exam (heart failure, hypotension, tachycardia, mitral regurgitation all portend a poor prognosis), and baseline ECG in making a diagnosis of ACS. Most patients with high-risk clinical and ECG features will have elevated troponin levels. Still, it has been documented that decompensated heart failure can elevate troponin levels, indicating that myocardial damage from any etiology may lead to elevated levels.[26]

It is of interest that the intravenous infusion of a glycoprotein IIb/IIIa inhibitor in the acute medical management of coronary ischemia is mostly beneficial in patients with elevated troponin levels.[27,28] Furthermore, there are convincing data that early angiography and mechanical revascularization are superior to medical therapy in patients with NSTEMI and troponin elevation.[12–14]

Myoglobin is a low-molecular-weight heme protein found in both cardiac and skeletal muscle. While not specific for cardiac muscle, it is released rapidly (usually within 2 h) from necrotic myocardium after onset of injury. Levels are only elevated from 24 h limiting the period of use. Confirmation of myonecrosis should be made with a more specific marker such as cardiac troponins or CK-MB levels. Because of its high sensitivity, however, myoglobin measurements made within 4 to 8 h of symptom onset can be used to rule out an MI if normal levels are documented.[29]

The Diagnostic Marker Cooperative Study evaluated the role of these biochemical markers in the evaluation of ACS patients.[30] This large, multicenter, randomized, double-blind study of patients suspected of an MI in the emergency department compared the

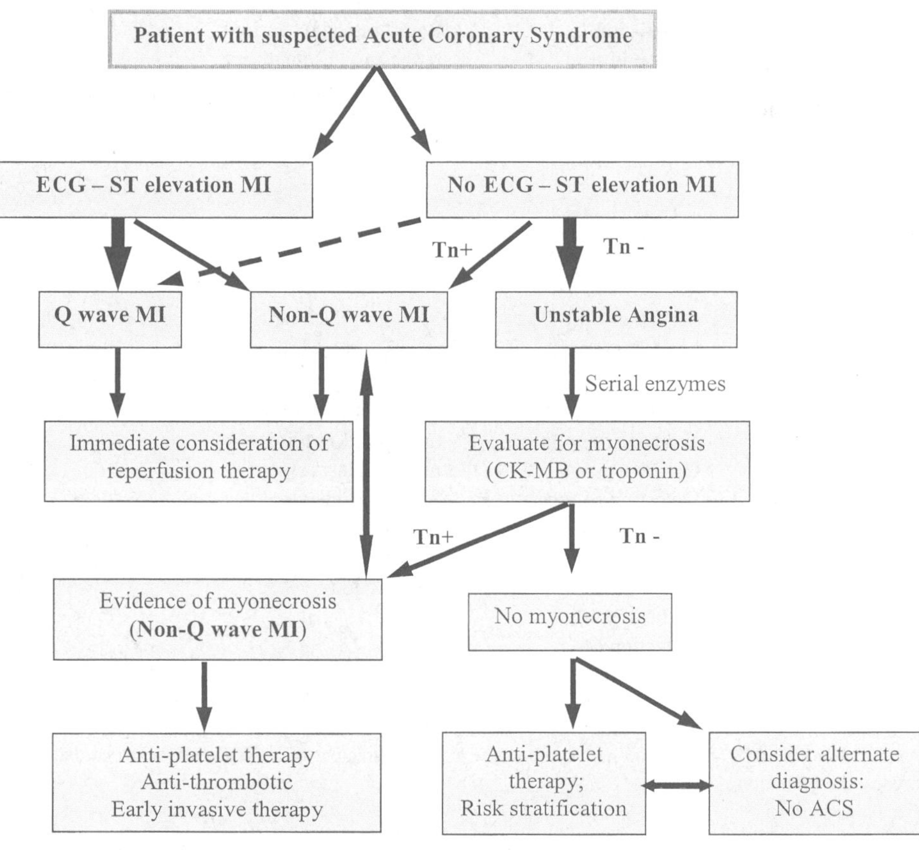


FIGURE 48-2 Approach to suspected acute coronary syndrome. Tn = troponin.

TABLE 48-6 Biochemical Cardiac Markers for the Evaluation and Management of Patients with Suspected ACS but Without ST-Segment Elevation of 12-Lead

| Marker | Advantages | Disadvantages | Point of Care Test Available? | Comment | Clinical Recommendation |
|---|---|---|---|---|---|
| CK-MB | 1. Rapid, cost-efficient, accurate assay<br>2. Ability to detect early reinfarction | 1. Loss of specificity in setting of skeletal muscle disease or injury, including surgery<br>2. Low sensitivity during very early MI (< 6 h after symptom onset) or later after symptom onset (> 36 h) and for minor myocardial damage (detectable with troponins) | Yes | Familiar to majority of clinicians | Prior standard and still acceptable diagnostic test in most clinical circumstances |
| CK-MB isoforms | 1. Early detection of MI | 1. Specificity profile similar to that of CK-MB<br>2. Current assays require special expertise | No | Experience to date predominantly in dedicated research centers | Used for extremely early (3–6 h after symptom onset) detection of MI in centers with demonstrated familiarity with assay technique |
| Myoglobin | 1. High sensitivity<br>2. Useful in early detection of MI<br>3. Detection of reperfusion<br>4. Most useful in ruling out MI | 1. Very low specificity in setting of skeletal muscle injury or disease<br>2. Rapid return to normal range limits sensitivity for later presentations | Yes | More convenient early marker than CK-MB isoforms because of greater availability of assays for myoglobin; Rapid-release kinetics make myoglobin useful for noninvasive monitoring of reperfusion in patients with established MI | |
| Cardiac troponins | 1. Powerful tool for risk stratification<br>2. Greater sensitivity and specificity than CK-MB<br>3. Detection of recent MI up to 2 weeks after onset<br>4. Useful for selection of therapy<br>5. Detection of reperfusion | 1. Low sensitivity in very early phase of MI (< 6 h after symptom onset) and requires repeat measurement at 8–12 h, if negative<br>2. Limited ability to detect late minor reinfarction | Yes | Data on diagnostic performance and potential therapeutic implications increasingly available from clinical trails | Useful as a single test to efficiently diagnose NSTEMI (including minor myocardial damage), with serial measurements. Clinicians should familiarize themselves with diagnostic "cutoffs" used in their local hospital laboratory |

ABBREVIATIONS: ACS = acute coronary syndrome; CK-MB = creative kinase-MB; MI = myocardial infarction; NSTEMI = non-ST-segment elevation myocardial infarction.

sensitivity and specificity of both cardiac troponin assays, CK-MB mass levels, CK-MB isoforms, and myoglobin for the diagnosis of myonecrosis. Within the first 6 h of symptom onset, CK-MB isoforms and myoglobin were the most efficient for diagnosis, whereas both cardiac troponins proved to be the most cardiac specific and were very useful for the late diagnosis of MI as their levels usually remain elevated for 7 to 14 days.

In summary, cardiac troponins have become the biochemical marker of choice in the evaluation of myonecrosis and the diagnosis of NSTEMI. Its superb sensitivity and specificity to cardiac muscle damage, in addition to its proven prognostic value, has established its current clinical position. CK-MB levels by mass method remains a reliable technique to diagnose more than minor myocardial damage. CK-MB isoforms are particularly useful in detecting early myocardial damage. Because of its high sensitivity to detect myonecrosis, myoglobin levels can be used in the early hours after symptom onset to rule out MI. Table 48-6 summarizes the strengths and weaknesses of each cardiac marker (see also Chaps. 51 and 52).

Research continues on new biochemical cardiac markers for injury. For example, there has been much interest in documenting levels of inflammatory markers such as C-reactive protein (CRP), serum amyloid A, and interleukin-6 in patients with unstable angina.[31–33] While there is hard evidence now that these inflammatory markers can help risk-stratify patients with unstable angina/NSTEMI on presentation, they are not valid for diagnosing myonecrosis at this time. Levels of circulating soluble adhesion molecules such as E-selectin and intercellular adhesion molecule-1 are under investigation.[34] Finally, markers of the coagulation cascade such as fibrinopeptide and fibrinogen levels appear to signify an increased risk of death in ACS patients.[35,36] To reiterate, however, none of these markers is currently accepted as a biochemical means of demonstrating MI.

## ST-Segment Elevation Myocardial Infarction

STEMI represents the most lethal form of ACS, one in which a completely occlusive thrombus results in total cessation of coronary blood flow in the territory of the occluded artery and the resultant ST-segment elevation on the ECG. Typically new Q waves evolve due to full or nearly full thickness necrosis of the ventricular wall supplied by the occluded artery. As this may only occur in up to 70 percent of patients and because a minority of patients without ST-segment elevation can eventually develop new Q waves, the nomenclature has changed from Q-wave MI to STEMI.[37]

The actual diagnosis of an STEMI does not completely rely on the ECG itself as the name might imply. The classic World Health Organization criteria for an acute MI requires that two of the following three elements be present: (1) a history suggestive of coronary ischemia for a prolonged period (>30 min), (2) evolutionary changes on serial ECGs suggestive of MI, and (3) a rise and fall in serum cardiac markers consistent with myonecrosis.[38] Only 2 out of 3 criteria are needed because of the wide variability in the pattern of patient presentation with acute MI. It has been estimated that up to one-third of patients with STEMI do not describe classic chest pain.[39] In contrast, due to the multitude of etiologies producing chest pain, objective evidence of myocardial necrosis is needed in order to confirm an MI. ST-segment elevation from noncoronary causes such as pericarditis, left ventricular hypertrophy, or J-point elevation must be differentiated from true myocardial ischemia

The accurate diagnosis of STEMI is of paramount importance for two reasons. First, the diagnosis mandates immediate consideration for reperfusion therapy, either by thrombolytic agents or by mechanical revascularization, most probably PCI. Mortality has been significantly decreased by reperfusion with 12 h of onset of symptoms in patients with STEMI.[40] However, both pharmacologic and mechanical means of reperfusion have potentially fatal side-effects or complications and should not be employed unless diagnosis is relatively certain. In order to prevent unnecessary dangers, thrombolytic agents are only recommended for at least 2-mm ST-segment elevation in at least two contiguous leads in the precordium or at least 1-mm ST-segment elevation in two contiguous limb leads in addition to biochemical marker data and clinical history.[41] It should be noted that a new left bundle branch block in the clinical setting of an acute MI also meets criteria for aggressive revascularization therapy with thrombolytic agents or by mechanical means.

# CONCLUSIONS

The definitions of ACSs have become more important as new therapies have been developed. Unstable angina, NSTEMI, and STEMI all share similar pathophysiologic characteristics, but the severity of its clinical presentation differs. Whereas patients with unstable angina with high-risk features and those with NSTEMI and biochemical evidence of myonecrosis should be treated in a similar fashion with additional antiplatelet agents and early revascularization, there are no convincing data to suggest that the large subgroup of unstable angina patients with no biochemical markers providing evidence of myonecrosis should be treated as aggressively.[42] Patients with STEMI appear to have evidence of a more fibrin-rich thrombus, which responds to thrombolytic therapy in addition to aggressive antiplatelet agents if urgent mechanical revascularization is not available.[43] As more attention to risk factor modification and secondary prevention of CAD with statins and antiplatelet agents such as aspirin and clopidogrel have become more widespread, the incidence of STEMI has declined while the incidence of NSTEMI appears to be increasing.[44]

As more large scale, randomized, multicenter, prospective trials are being conducted in patients with ACS evaluating more aggressive medical therapy along with the role of earlier and earlier revascularization, it has become more urgent for clinical researchers to identify and correctly define the subgroup of patients that will benefit from these potentially risky therapies. If the risk profile of the study population is not adequate, potentially beneficial therapies that would have been shown to be beneficial in high-risk patients will instead just appear as toxic if low-risk patients are only identified. In this sense, there should not be a cavalier attitude in diagnosing a patient with true ACS. The term *ACS* identifies a patient that must be monitored carefully and treated aggressively. These patients are at high risk of short- and long-term complications if not properly managed. To this end, cardiac troponins, accurate biochemical markers of myonecrosis, have become especially useful in diagnosing high-risk patients and now form the basis of differentiating those with unstable angina and NSTEMI.

## References


1. The American Heart Association. 1999 Heart and Stroke Statistical Update. Dallas: American Heart Association, 1999.
2. Anderson RN. US decennial life tables for 1989–91, Vol. 1 No. 4, United States life tables. Eliminating certain causes of death. Hyattsville, MD: National Center for Health Statistics; 1999.
3. Fuster V, Badimon L, Badimon JJ, Chesebro JH. The pathogenesis of coronary artery disease and the acute coronary syndromes. Part 1. *N Engl J Med* 1992:326;242–250.

4. Theroux P, Fuster V. Acute coronary syndromes: Unstable angina and non-Q-wave myocardial infarction. *Circulation* 1998;97:1195–1206.
5. Braunwald E, Mark DB, Jones RH, et al. Unstable angina: Diagnosis and management. Rockville, MD: Agency for Health Care Policy and Research and the National Heart, Lung, and Blood Institute, US Public Health Service, US Department of Health and Human Services; 1994:1. AHCPR Publication 94-0602.
6. Braunwald E, Antman EM, Beasley JW, et al. ACC/AHA Guideline for the management of patients with unstable angina and non-ST-segment elevation myocardial infarction: A report of the American College of Cardiology/American Heart Association Task Force on Practice Guidelines (Committee on the Management of Patients with Unstable Angina). *J Am Coll Cardiol* 2002;40:1366–1374.
7. Braunwald E. Unstable angina: An etiologic approach to management (editorial). *Circulation* 1998;98:2219–2222.
8. Betriu A, Heras M, Cohen M, Fuster V. Unstable angina: Outcome according to clinical presentation. *J Am Coll Cardiol* 1992;19:1659–1663.
9. Campeau L: Grading of angina pectoris (letter). *Circulation* 1976;54:522.
10. Braunwald E. Unstable angina: A classification. *Circulation* 1989;80: 410–414.
11. Fuster V, Badimon L, Badimon JJ, Chesebro JH. The pathogenesis of coronary artery disease and the acute coronary syndromes. Part 2. *N Engl J Med* 1992;326:310–318.
12. Cannon CP, Weintraub WS, Demopolous LA, et al. Comparison of early invasive and conservative strategies in patients with unstable coronary syndromes treated with the glycoprotein IIb/IIIa inhibitor tirofiban. *N Engl J Med* 2001;344:1879–1887.
13. The FRagmin and Fast Revascularization during InStability in Coronary artery disease Investigators, Invasive compared with non-invasive treatment in unstable coronary artery disease: FRISC II prospective randomized multicentre study. *Lancet* 1999;354:708–715.
14. Fox KAA, Poole-Wilson PA, Henderson RA, et al, for the Randomised Intervention Trial of unstable Angina (RITA) investigators. Interventional versus conservative treatment for patients with unstable angina or non-ST-elevation myocardial infarction: The British Heart Foundation RITA 3 randomised trial. *Lancet* 2002;360:743–751.
15. Roberts R, Fromm RE. Management of acute coronary syndromes based on risk stratification by biochemical markers: An idea whose time has come. *Circulation* 1998;98:1831–1833.
16. Mair J, Morandell D, Genser N, et al. Equivalent early sensitivities of myoglobin, creatinine kinase MB mass, creatinine kinase isoform ratios, and cardiac troponins I and T for acute myocardial infarction. *Clin Chem* 1995;41:1266–1272.
17. Puleo PR, Meyer D, Wathen C, et al. Use of a rapid assay of subforms of creatinine kinase-MB to diagnose or rule out acute myocardial infarction. *N Engl J Med* 1994;331:561–566.
18. Apple FS, Falahati A, Paulsen PR, et al. Improved detection of minor ischemic myocardial injury with measurement of serum cardiac troponin I. *Clin Chem* 1997;43:2047–2051.
19. Bertrand ME, Simoons ML, Fox KA, et al. Management of acute coronary syndromes: Acute coronary syndromes without ST-elevation: Recommendations of the Task Force of the European Society of Cardiology. *Eur Heart J* 2000;21:1406-1432.
20. Hamm CW, Goldmann BU, Heesschen C, et al. Emergency room triage of patients with acute chest pain by means of rapid testing for cardiac troponin T or troponin I. *N Engl J Med* 1997;337:1648–1653.
21. Ohman EM, Armstrong PW, Christenson RH, et al, for the GUSTO IIA Investigators. Cardiac troponin T levels for risk stratification in acute myocardial ischemia. *N Engl J Med* 1996;335:1333–1341.
22. Antman EM, Tanasijevic MJ, Thompson B, et al. Cardiac-specific troponin I levels to predict the risk of mortality in patients with acute coronary syndromes. *N Engl J Med* 1996;335:1342–1349.
23. Galvani M, Ottani F, Ferrini D, et al. Prognostic influence of elevated troponin I in patients with unstable angina. *Circulation* 1997;95: 2053–2059.
24. Aviles RJ, Askari AT, Lindahl B, et al. Troponin T levels in patients with acute coronary syndromes, with or without renal dysfunction. *N Engl J Med* 2002;346:2047–2052.
25. Stubbs P, Collinson P, Moseley D, et al. Prospective study of the role of cardiac troponin T in patients admitted with unstable angina. *BMJ* 1996;313:262–264.
26. Del Carlo CH, O'Connor CM. Cardiac troponins in congestive heart failure. *Am Heart J* 1999:138:646–653.
27. Hamm CW, Heeschen C, Goldmann B, et al, for the c7E3 Fab Antiplatelet Therapy in Unstable Refractory Angina (CAPTURE) Study Investigators. Benefit of abciximab in patients with refractory unstable angina in relation to serum troponin T levels. *N Engl J Med* 1999;340: 1623–1629.
28. Heeschen C, Hamm CW, Goldmann B, et al, for the PRISM Study Investigators: Platlet Receptor Inhibition in Ischemic Syndrome Management. Troponin concentrations for stratification of patients with acute coronary syndromes in relation to therapeutic efficacy of tirofiban. *Lancet* 1999;354:1757–1762.
29. Zaninotto M, Altinier S, Lachin M, et al. Strategies for the early diagnosis of acute myocardial infarction using biochemical markers. *Am J Clin Path* 1999;111:399–405.
30. Zimmerman J, Formm R, Meyer D, et al. Diagnostic Marker Cooperative Study for the diagnosis of myocardial infarction. *Circulation* 1999;99:1671–1677.
31. Morrow DA, Rifai N, Antman EM, et al. C-reactive protein is a potent predictor of mortality independently of and in combination with troponin T in acute coronary syndromes: A TIMI 11A substudy. Thrombolysis in myocardial infarction. *J Am Coll Cardiol* 1998;31: 1460–1465.
32. Morrow DA, Rifai N, Antman EM, et al. Serum amyloid A predicts early mortality in acute coronary syndromes. A TIMI 11A substudy. *J Am Coll Cardiol* 2000;35:358–362.
33. Biasucci LM, Vitelli A, Liuzzo G, et al. Elevated levels of interleukin-6 in unstable angina. *Circulation* 1996;94:874–877.
34. Ghasias NK, Shahi CN, Foley B, et al. Elevated levels of circulating soluble adhesion molecules in peripheral blood of patients with unstable angina. *Am J Cardiol* 1997;80:617-619.
35. Ardissino D, Merlini PA, Gamba G, et al. Thrombin activity and early outcome in unstable angina pectoris. *Circulation* 1996;93:1634–1639.
36. Becker RC, Cannon CP, Bovill EG, et al. Prognostic value of plasma fibrinogen concentration in patients with unstable angina and non-Q-wave myocardial infarction (TIMI IIIB Trial). *Am J Cardiol* 1996; 78:142–147.
37. Myocardial infarction redefined—A consensus document of the Joint European Society of Cardiology/American College of Cardiology Committee for the redefinition of myocardial infarction. *J Am Coll Cardiol* 2000;36:959–969.
38. Pedoe-Tunstall H, Kuulasmaa K, Amouyel P, et al. Myocardial infarction and coronary deaths in the World Health Organization MONICA Project. *Circulation* 1994;90:583–612.
39. Canto JG, Every NR, Magid DJ, et al. The volume of primary angioplasty procedures and survival after acute myocardial infarction. National Registry of Myocardial Infarction 2 Investigators. *N Engl J Med* 2000;342:1573-1580.
40. Califf RM. Ten years of benefit from a one-hour intervention. *Circulation* 1998;98:2649–2651.
41. Ryan TJ, Antman EM, Brooks NH, et al. 1999 update: ACC/AHA Guidelines for the Management of Patients With Acute Myocardial Infarction: Executive Summary and Recommendations: A report of the American College of Cardiology/American Heart Association Task Force on Practice Guidelines (Committee on Management of Acute Myocardial Infarction). *Circulation* 1999;100:1016–1030.
42. Fox KAA, Goodman SG, Klein W, et al. Management of acute coronary syndromes: Variations in practice and outcome. *Eur Heart J* 2002; 23:1177–1189.
43. Topol EJ. Toward a new frontier in myocardial reperfusion therapy: Emerging platelet preeminence. *Circulation* 1998;97:211–218.
44. Rogers WJ, Canto JG, Lambrew CT, et al. Temporal trends in the treatment of over 1.5 million patients with myocardial infarction in the US from 1990 through 1999: The National Registry of Myocardial Infarction 1, 2 and 3. *J Am Coll Cardiol* 2000;36:2056–2063.

CHAPTER 49

# PATHOLOGY OF MYOCARDIAL ISCHEMIA, INFARCTION, REPERFUSION, AND SUDDEN DEATH*

Renu Virmani / Allen P. Burke



## PATHOPHYSIOLOGY OF MYOCARDIAL ISCHEMIA

Despite recent declines in the incidence of acute myocardial infarction (MI), more than 1.5 million Americans still suffer from an acute infarct annually.[1] Mortality is highest in patients >65 years of age[2]; patients aged 65 to 74 years have a higher mortality than patients younger than 65 years, independent of infarct size.[3,4] Although men have a fivefold higher risk of MI than females between the ages of 45 to 54 years, this differential decreases to a twofold difference in the eighth decade, and women have a higher mortality than men after an MI at all age ranges. There has been a significant decrease in the death rate and case fatality rate for acute MI in persons 45 to 64 years of age in the United States from 1970 through 1995.[5,6] Deaths from MI due to coronary heart disease among 35- to 74-year-old residents of four communities in the United States have decreased. In-hospital mortality rates have fallen by 5.1 percent per year, whereas out-of-hospital mortality has declined by 3.6 percent per year, with the greatest decline seen in white men, followed by white women, black women, and black men.[7] The major cause of acute MI is coronary atherosclerosis with superimposed luminal thrombus, accounting for >80 percent of all infarcts. MIs resulting from nonatherosclerotic diseases of the coronary arteries are rare.

*The opinions or assertions contained herein are the private views of the authors and are not to be construed as official or reflecting the views of the Department of the Army, the Department of the Air Force, or the Department of Defense.

### Consequences of Reduction of Arterial Blood Flow

The normal function of the heart muscle is supported by high rates of myocardial blood flow, oxygen consumption, and combustion of fat and carbohydrates (glucose and lactate). Under normal aerobic conditions, cardiac energy is derived from fatty acids, supplying 60–90 percent of the energy for the synthesis of adenosine triphosphate (ATP) (Fig. 49-1). The rest of the energy (10 to 40 percent) comes from oxidation of pyruvate, formed from glycolysis and lactate oxidation. Almost all of the ATP formed comes from oxidative phosphorylation in the mitochondria; only a small amount of ATP (<2 percent) is synthesized by glycolysis. Approximately two-thirds of the ATP used by the heart goes to contractile shortening; the remaining one-third is used by sarcoplasmic reticulum $Ca^{2+}$ ATPase and other ion pumps.

Sudden occlusion of a major branch of a coronary artery is followed by a metabolic change that shifts from aerobic or mitochondrial metabolism to anaerobic glycolysis within seconds of reduced arterial flow. Myocardial ischemia primarily affects mitochondrial metabolism, resulting in decrease in ATP formation by shutting off oxidative phosphorylation. The reduced aerobic ATP formation stimulates glycolysis and an increase in myocardial glucose uptake and glycogen breakdown (Fig. 49-2). During ischemic conditions,

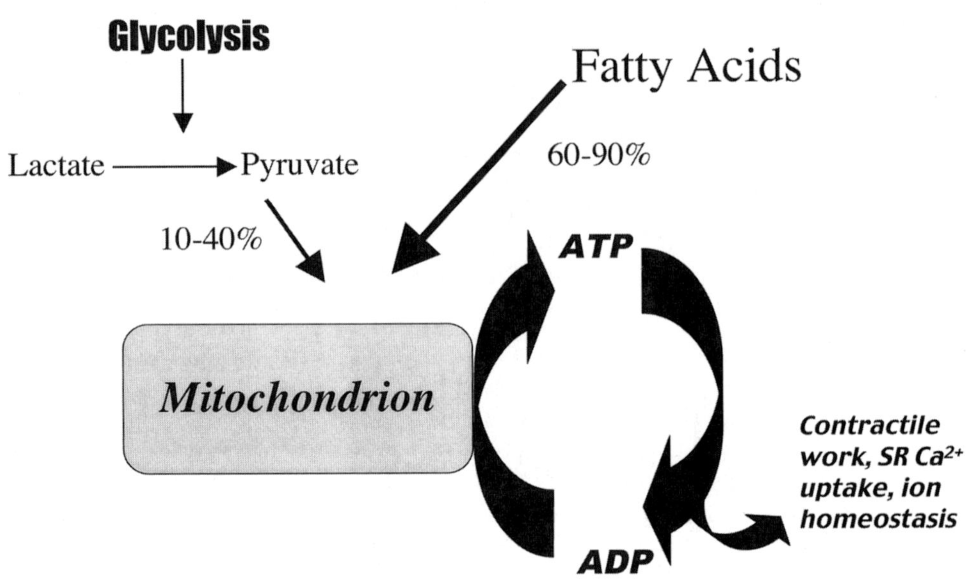


FIGURE 49-1 Cardiac energy metabolism under normal aerobic conditions. Fatty acids are the primary source of energy for the heart, supplying 60 to 90 percent of the energy for adenosine triphosphate (ATP) synthesis. The balance (10 to 40 percent) comes from the oxidation of pyruvate formed from glycolysis and lactate oxidation. Almost all of the ATP formation comes from oxidative phosphorylation in the mitochondria; only a trivial amount of ATP (<2 percent of the total) is synthesized by glycolysis. ADP = adenosine diphosphate; SR = sarcoplasmic reticulum. [From Stanley WC. Changes in cardiac metabolism: A critical step from stable angina to ischemic cardiomyopathy. *Eur Heart J* 2001;3(suppl):3. With permission.]

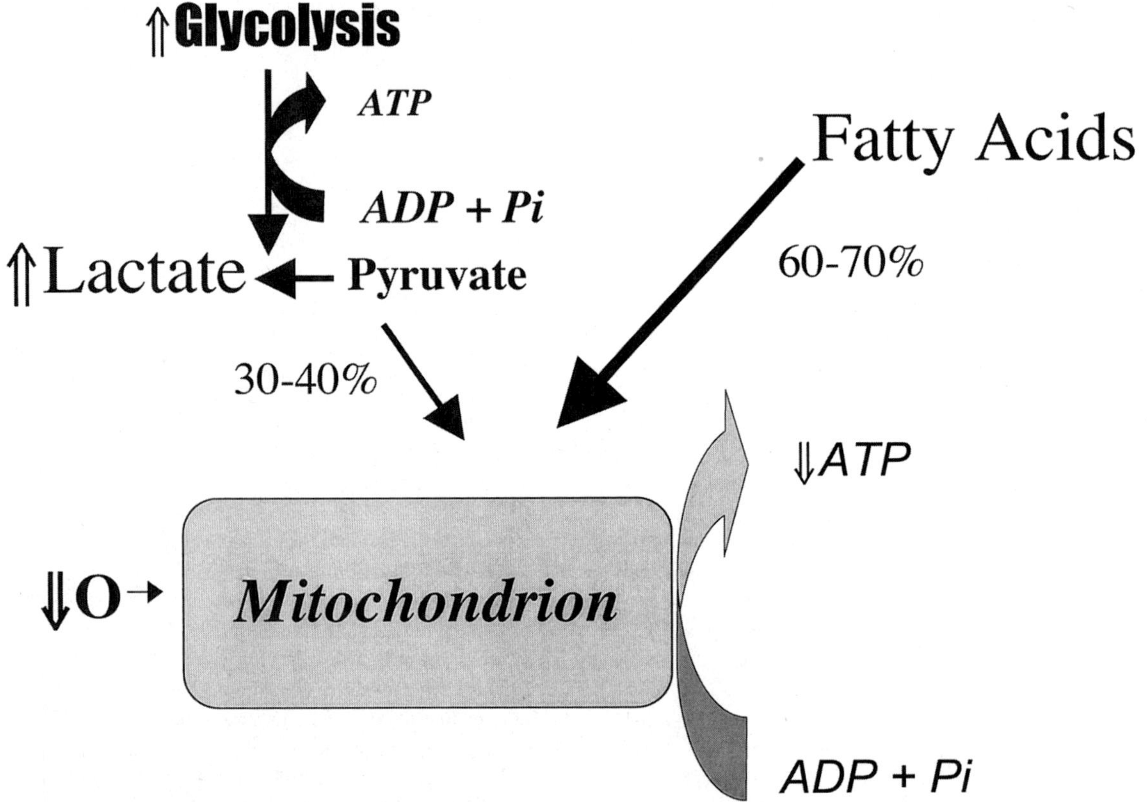


FIGURE 49-2 Cardiac energy metabolism during ischemia of moderate severity (approximately 40 percent of normal blood flow). The up and down arrows indicate the changes compared with normal conditions. Relative to aerobic conditions, ischemia results in an increase in glycolysis without an increase in the rate of pyruvate oxidation, thus causing lactate to accumulate in the cell. Despite accelerated glycolysis and lactate production, the relatively high rate of residual oxygen consumption is fueled primarily by the oxidation of fatty acids. ADP = adenosine diphosphate; ATP = adenosine triphosphate; $P_i$ = inorganic phosphate. [From Stanley WC. Changes in cardiac metabolism: A critical step from stable angina to ischemic cardiomyopathy. *Eur Heart J* 2001;3(suppl):5. With permission.]

pyruvate is not readily oxidized in the mitochondria; instead, there is greater production of lactate from pyruvate, which leads to a rise in tissue lactate and $H^+$, resulting in a fall in intracellular pH and a reduction in contractile function. Instead of normal uptake of lactate from blood, the ischemic myocardium switches to production of lactate. The fall in pH also leads to a greater ATP requirement in order to maintain $Ca^{2+}$ homeostasis.[8]

## Myocardial Ischemia

Myocardial ischemia occurs when the oxygen supply does not meet demand; necrosis or infarction occurs when ischemia is severe and prolonged. Although biochemical and functional abnormalities begin almost immediately at the onset of ischemia, severe loss of myocardial contractility occurs within 60 s, while other changes take a more protracted course—e.g., the loss of viability (irreversible injury) takes as least 20 to 40 min following total occlusion of blood flow.

For the clinical diagnosis of acute myocardial infarction, the World Health Organization requires that at least two of the following three criteria be present: (1) a history of chest pain or discomfort; (2) a rise and subsequent fall in serum cardiac enzymes; and (3) the development of electrocardiogram (ECG) abnormalities (new Q waves or ST-segment or T-wave changes) on serially obtained ECGs.[9] Since the ECG lacks sufficient sensitivity and specificity to detect myocardial necrosis, the presence of myocardial injury is often dependent upon the release of cardiac-specific serum markers such as troponin T, troponin I, and CK-MB.[10–13] It has been shown that infarct size generally correlates with the peak rise in serum CK-MB level.[14]

Two zones of myocardial damage are seen: a central zone with no or very low flow and a zone of collateral vessels in a surrounding marginal zone. The survival of the marginal zone is dependent on the level and duration of ischemia. The extent of coronary collateral flow is one of the principal determinants of infarct size. Indeed, at autopsy it is not uncommon to see chronic total coronary occlusion and an absence of MI in the distribution of that artery. Absence of myocardial ischemia (revealed by ECG changes or angina during transient coronary balloon occlusion) is associated with the presence of well-developed collateral vessels, suggesting that the patients with such vessels have a low risk of developing acute MI on abrupt closure of the culprit coronary artery.[15] Collaterals have been shown to be better developed in patients with angina and in younger individuals as compared to older patients with acute infarcts.[16] Since infarct size is an important determinant of survival as well as development of congestive heart failure, efforts have been directed toward limiting infarct size by early reperfusion, reduction of myocardial oxygen demand, and prevention of reperfusion injury. In 1971, Page et al. showed that infarcts ≥40 percent of left ventricle are predictors of cardiogenic shock and death.[17]

## The Wavefront Phenomenon

Reimer and Jennings, in a landmark paper in 1979, showed that if a canine coronary artery was occluded for 15 min, 40 min, 3 h, or uninterruptedly for 4 days, myocardial necrosis progressed as a "wavefront phenomenon" (Fig. 49-3*A*).[18] The extent of myocardial necrosis therefore depended on the duration of coronary occlusion. After only 15 min of occlusion, no infarct occurred. At 40 min, the infarct was subendocardial, involving only the papillary muscle, placing 28 percent of the myocardium at risk. At 3 h following coronary artery occlusion and reperfusion, the infarct was significantly smaller compared with nonreperfused permanently occluded infarct (62 percent of area at risk). The infarct size was greatest in permanent occlusion, becoming transmural and involving 75 percent of the area at risk[19] (Fig. 49-3*B*). In the dog model, it is impossible to achieve 100 percent infarction of area at risk because of species-related native collaterals.

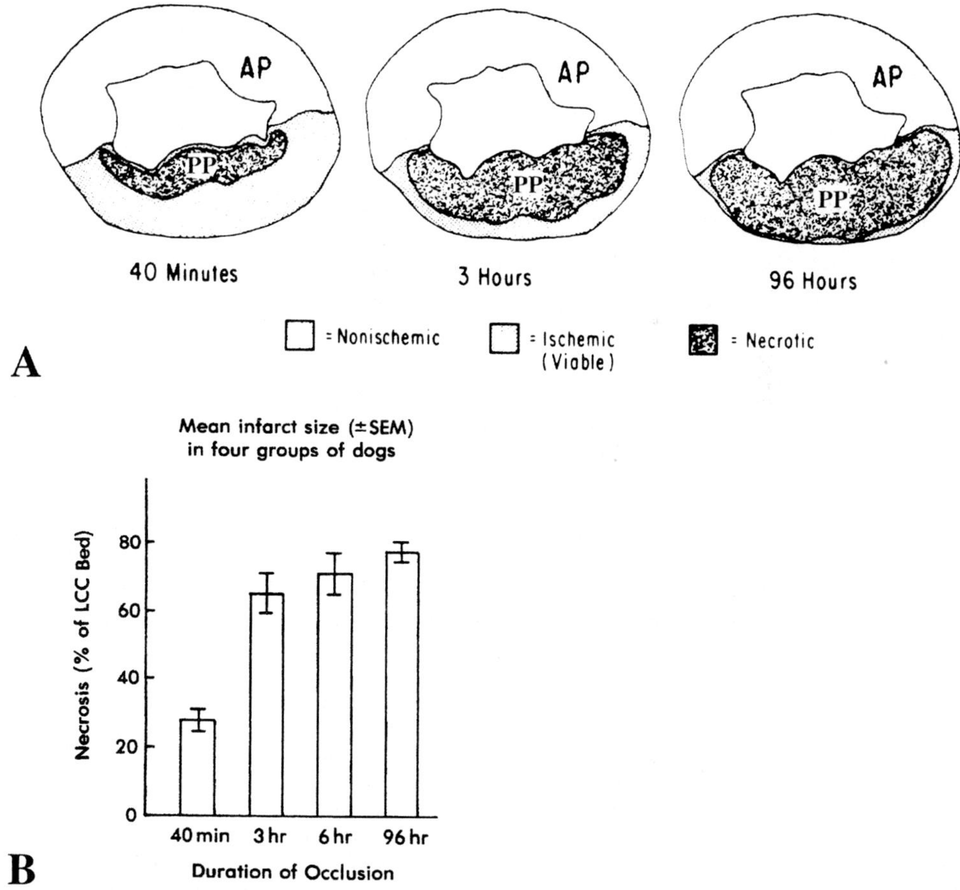


FIGURE 49-3 *A.* Progression of cell death versus time after experimental occlusion of the left circumflex coronary artery in the dog. Necrosis occurs first in the subendocardial region of the myocardium. With extension of the occlusion time, a wavefront of cell death moves from the subendocardial zone across the wall to involve progressively more of the transmural thickness of the ischemic zone. AP = anterior; PP = posterior. *B.* Infarct size variation with increasing duration of coronary occlusion. Infarct size dramatically increases from 40 min to 3 h; however, there is very little increase between 3 and 6 h and between 6 and 96 h of coronary artery occlusion. LCC = left circumflex coronary bed. [From Reimer KA, Jennings RB. The "wavefront phenomenon" of myocardial ischemic cell death: II. Transmural progression of necrosis with the framework of ischemic bed size (myocardium at risk) and collateral flow. *Lab Invest* 1979;40:633–644. With permission.]

In humans, it has been shown that approximately 40 percent of patients with acute MI have a well-developed collateral circulation.[16]

### Electron Microscopic Changes of Reversible and Irreversible Injury

Electron microscopic criteria for reversible versus irreversible myocardial ischemic injury are well established in various animal models, but the degree and the time to establish these changes varies from species to species.[20,21] Reversible injury is defined as injury that can be reversed to normal functioning state without any structural damage if the offending agent is removed.[22] An irreversible injury is said to set in if the cell can no longer perform its normal metabolic functions, even when the offending agent is removed.

Reversibly injured myocytes are edematous and swollen from the osmotic overload. The cell size is increased with a decrease in the glycogen content.[19,23] The myocyte fibrils are relaxed and thinned; I bands are prominent secondary to noncontracting ischemic myocytes.[19] The nuclei show mild condensation of chromatin at the nucleoplasm. The cell membrane (sarcolemma) is intact and no breaks can be identified. The mitochondria are swollen, with loss of normal dense mitochondrial granules and incomplete clearing of the mitochondrial matrix but without amorphous or granular flocculent densities (Fig. 49-4*A* and *B*).

Irreversibly injured myocytes contain shrunken nuclei with marked chromatin margination. The two hallmarks of irreversible injury are cell membrane breaks and mitochondrial presence of small osmiophilic amorphous densities.[19,20] These densities are composed of lipid, denatured proteins, and calcium.[20,24,25] The cell membrane breaks are small and are associated with subsarcolemmal blebs of edema fluid[19] (Fig. 49-4*B*).

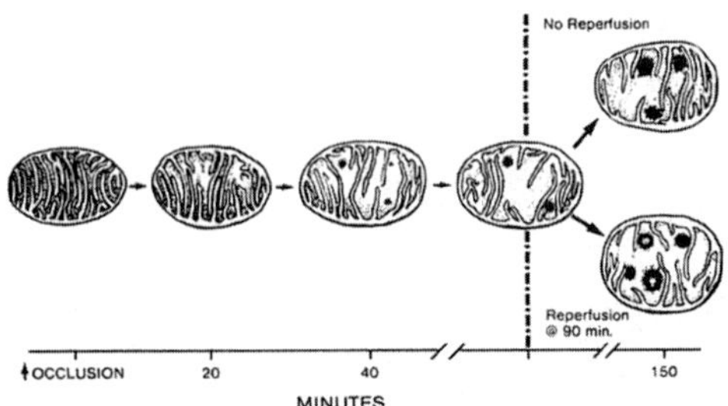


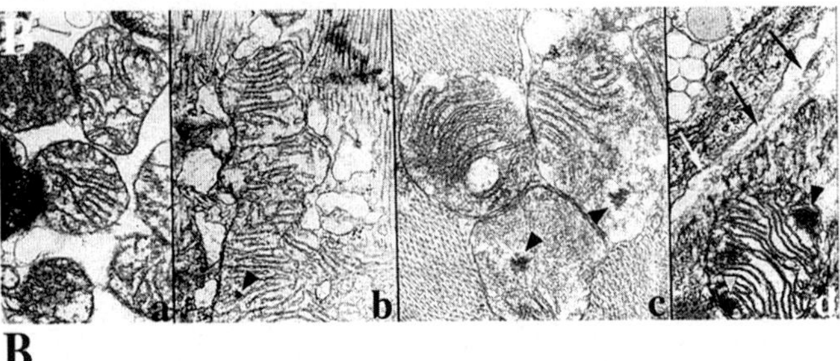


FIGURE 49-4 *A.* Sequential changes within mitochondria with varying time intervals of myocardial ischemia. At 20 min of ischemia, there is mild mitochondrial swelling. The matrix spaces between cristae show disorganization. At 40 min of ischemia, there is greater mitochondrial swelling; prominent amorphous matrix densities are present, indicating irreversible injury. With longer duration of coronary occlusion, mitochondria show larger amorphous matrix densities, and they also become more numerous. On reperfusion, both amorphous and granular densities are seen. Granular densities, however, seem larger and more fully developed. [Adapted from Jennings RB, Ganote CE. Structural changes in myocardium during acute ischemia. *Circ Res* 1974;35(suppl III):III-156–III-172. With permission from the American Heart Association.] *B.* Electron micrographs showing progressive changes in mitochondria as a result of ischemia in the canine model. *a.* Mitochondria showing reversible changes of ischemia after 10 min of coronary occlusion and reperfusion: mitochondria are swollen, there is clearing of mitochondrial matrix, and some cristae show disorganization. *b.* Similar changes as in *A* with only one of the mitochondria showing amorphous matrix densities (*arrowhead*) after 90 min of ischemia. *c.* Note the presence of large amorphous matrix densities (*arrowheads*) in two of the three mitochondria in a dog with 120 min of coronary occlusion. *d.* Ischemic myocyte with mitochondria containing multiple large amorphous matrix densities (*arrowheads*) after 3 days of permanent coronary occlusion. Note the break in the plasma lemma (*arrow*). [Adapted from Virmani R, Forman MB, Kolodgie FD. Myocardial reperfusion injury. Histopathologic effects of perfluorochemical. *Circulation* 1990;81(suppl IV): IV-57–IV-68. With permission from the American Heart Association.]

## PLAQUE MORPHOLOGY AND SITE OF THROMBUS IN ACUTE MYOCARDIAL INFARCTION

The vast majority of MIs occur in patients with coronary atherosclerosis; of these, over 90 percent are associated with superimposed luminal thrombus. We have shown, in sudden coronary death, that coronary thrombosis is most frequently the result of plaque rupture (65 percent) and less frequently due to plaque erosion (30 to 35 percent). Uncommonly it is the result of a calcified nodule (2 to 5 percent).[26,27] In contrast, Arbustini et al. found coronary thrombi in 98 percent of patients dying with clinically documented acute MI; of these, 75 percent were caused by plaque rupture and 25 percent by plaque erosion. There are gender differences in the causation of coronary thrombi leading to acute myocardial infarcts, as Arbustini showed that 37 percent of thrombi in women were due to erosion, as compared to only 18 percent in men.[28] Although an individual severe stenosis is more likely to become occluded by a thrombus than a lesion with less severe stenosis, the less severely narrowed plaques give rise to more occlusions, as there are many more sites that are mildly to moderately narrowed.[29] We have observed that 82 percent of fatal plaque erosions occur in coronary segments with relatively little stenosis (<79 percent narrowing of cross-sectional area) compared to only 57 percent, respectively, of plaque ruptures. The culprit coronary artery of infarction at autopsy is most frequently the left anterior descending artery (approximately one-half), followed by the right coronary artery (30 to 45 percent) and then the left circumflex (15 to 20 percent). No thrombi are found in fewer than 5 percent of acute MIs.

## PATHOPHSIOLOGY OF ACUTE MYOCARDIAL INFARCTION

### Gross Pathology of Acute Myocardial Infarction

The earliest change that can be grossly discerned in the evolution of acute MI—pallor of the myocardium—occurs 12 h or later after the onset of irreversible ischemia. The gross detection of infarction can be enhanced by the use of tetrazolium salt solutions, which form a colored precipitate on gross section of fresh heart tissue in the presence of dehydrogenase-mediated activity. The tetrazolium salts [nitroblue tetrazolium (NBT) and 2,3,5-triphenyltetrazolium chloride (TTC)] are dyes that are sensitive to the presence of tissue dehydrogenase enzyme activity, which is depleted in the infarcted myocardium. It has been shown that myocardial infarct can be detected

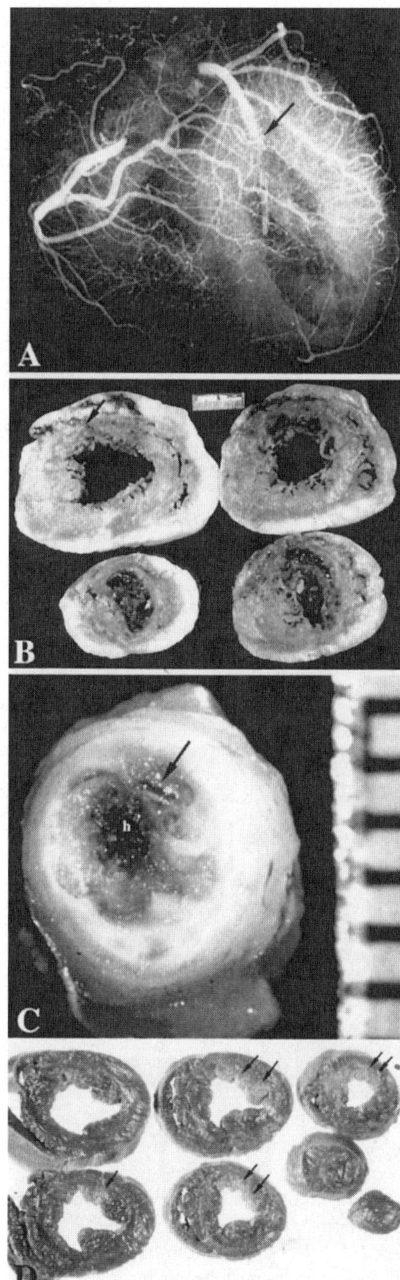

FIGURE 49-5 Regional distribution of vascular supply to the ventricles with right coronary artery dominance. *A.* Postmortem angiogram of the heart in a patient with acute myocardial infarction with total occlusion (*arrow*) of the proximal left anterior descending coronary artery in a 65-year-old female who presented with persistent chest pain of 6 h duration. *B.* At autopsy, she had a hemopericardium with a rupture site (*arrow*) identified on the anterior wall of the left ventricle. Note extensive hemorrhagic (h) transmural infarction involving the anterior wall of the left ventricle near the base of the heart (*upper slices*) and extending into the septum in the middle and apical slices (*lower slices*). *C.* Gross photograph of the left anterior descending coronary artery showing hemorrhage into the necrotic core and >90 percent luminal narrowing; barium is seen within the lumen (*arrow*). *D.* Slices of a dog heart following 15 min of incubation in 2% triphenyltetrazolium chloride (TTC) at 37°C. The animal had undergone 60 min of left anterior descending (LAD) coronary artery occlusion distal to the first diagonal branch, followed by reperfusion and sacrifice at 24 h. An injection of monastery dye following reocclusion of the LAD, just prior to sacrifice, identified the myocardium at risk of infarction. The heart was sliced and then immersed in TTC. The viable myocardium at risk stains red; the area not at risk is blue-red; whereas the infarcted region is creamy white (*arrows*). (From Virmani R, Burke AP, Farb A, Atkinson J, eds. *Cardiovascular Pathology,* 2d ed. Philadelphia: Saunders; 2001. With permission.)

by NBT as early as 2 to 3 h in the dog and a little less in the pig because of poor collaterals.[30] Red (TTC) or blue color (NBT) will form only in the normal noninfarcted myocardium, thus revealing the pale, unstained infarcted region (Fig. 49-5). In humans, the necrotic myocardium can be detected within 2 to 3 h after infarct by immersion of the fresh heart slices in a solution of TTC or NBT. TTC staining demonstrated a diagnostic sensitivity of 77 percent and a specificity of 93 percent compared with routine histology, with predictive values of positive and negative test of 81 and 91 percent, respectively.[31]

At approximately 24 h after the onset of irreversible ischemia, the pallor is enhanced (Fig. 49-6). However, in this era of thrombolytic therapy, most in-hospital patients will have received tissue plasminogen activator, streptokinase, or IIb/IIIa inhibitors, which lyse the thrombus and restore blood flow into the area of infarction. Therefore, in a reperfused infarct, the infarcted region will appear red from trapping of the red cells and hemorrhage due to the rupture of the necrotic capillaries (Fig. 49-7). However, if there has been no reperfusion, the area of the infarct is better defined at 2 to 3 days, with a central area of yellow discoloration surrounded by a thin rim of highly vascularized hyperemia (Fig. 49-6). At 5 to 7 days, the regions are much more distinct, with a central soft area and a depressed hyperemic border.[32–34] At 1 to 2 weeks, the infarct begins to heal, with infiltration by macrophages as well as early fibroblasts at the margins. At the same time, the infarct begins to be more depressed, especially at the margins, where organization takes place, and there is a white border (Table 49-1) (Fig. 49-6). Healing may be complete as early as 4 to 6 weeks in small infarcts or may take as long as 2 to 3 months when the area of infarction is large. Healed infarcts are white from the scarring, and the ventricular wall may or may not be thinned (aneurysmal). In general, infarcts that are transmural and confluent are likely to result in thinning, whereas subendocardial and nonconfluent infarcts are not.

## Light Microscopic Findings in Nonreperfused Infarction

The earliest morphologic characteristic of MI that can be discerned, between 12 to 24 h after onset of chest pain is the hypereosinophilic myocyte (Fig. 49-8). Despite the hypereosinophilia of the cytoplasm, which is seen best on routine hematoxylin-and-eosin staining, the myocyte striations appear normal and some chromatin condensation may be seen in the nucleus. The area of infarction may show interstitial edema; however, this change is difficult to appreciate in human autopsy hearts and better appreciated in animal experiments. It has been suggested in experimentally induced infarction that the appearance of "wavy fibers" may be the earliest change; this is thought to be the result of stretching of the ischemic noncontractile fibers by the adjoining viable contracting myocytes.[35] Wavy fiber change is, however, nonspecific and occurs in the absence of ischemia, especially in the right ventricle. Neutrophil infiltration is present by 24 h at the border areas. As the infarct progresses between 24 and 48 h, coagulation necrosis is established, with various degrees of nuclear pyknosis, early karyorrhexis, and karyolysis. The myocyte striations are preserved and the sarcomeres elongate. The border areas show prominent neutrophil infiltration by 48 h (Fig. 49-8).

At 3 to 5 days, the central portion of the infarct shows loss of myocyte nuclei and striations; in smaller infarcts, neutrophils invade

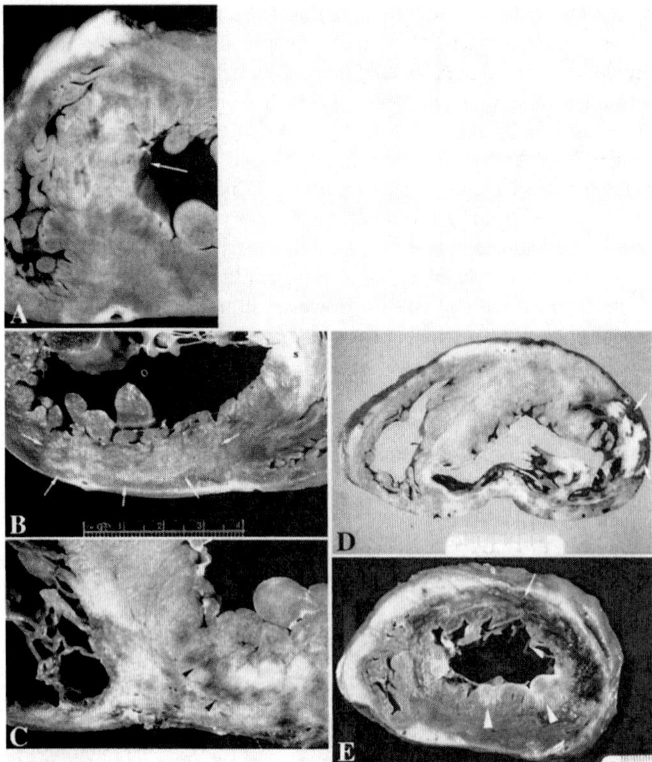

FIGURE 49-6 Gross photographs of the hearts with varying ages of acute myocardial infarction. *A.* 50-year-old hyperlipidemic and hypertensive male presented with unstable angina, underwent emergency percutaneous transluminal coronary angioplasty (PTCA) of the LAD, and died 20 h following onset of chest pain. At autopsy there was a pale ill-defined, slightly raised region in the anterior ventricular septum suggestive of an acute transmural infarct (*arrow*), which was confirmed by the presence of hypereosinophilic myocytes localized to the septum, with sparing of the subendocardial myocytes. The LAD at the PTCA site was totally occluded by a luminal thrombus and an underlying 60 percent atherosclerotic lesion. *B.* Another high-power view of a different acute transmural myocardial infarct involving the posterior wall of the heart showing a well-defined, pale, creamy tan and slightly raised infarct. Note absence of hyperemia in the border region. The infarct is 24 to 36 h old. An older infarct can be seen in the septa. *C.* An older infarct dated 36 to 72 h showing hyperemic areas (*arrowheads*) surrounding the subendocardial infarct (age 3 days), with a paler area in the outer half of the posterior wall of the left ventricle (infarct extension). The more recent infarct involves the posterior portion of the ventricular septum and the posterior wall of the right ventricle (36 to 48 h). *D.* Gross photograph of a heart slice close to the base of the heart shows a 1-week-old acute transmural myocardial infarct involving the posterolateral wall of the heart. Note the marked pale region in the inner two-thirds of the infarct with a surrounding prominent hyperemic zone (*arrows*). Also present is a healed transmural myocardial infarct involving the posterior wall and posteroseptal region of the heart. The patient died in severe congestive heart failure. *E.* Gross photograph of a transmural healing myocardial infarct involving the septum as well as the anterior and lateral walls of the left ventricle in an apical slice of the heart. Note the depressed, gelatinous appearance (*arrow*) of the infarct, which is 3 weeks old. Focal areas of scarring can be seen (*arrowheads*). (From Virmani R, Burke AP, Farb A, Atkinson J, eds. *Cardiovascular Pathology,* 2d ed. Philadelphia: Saunders; 2001. With permission.)

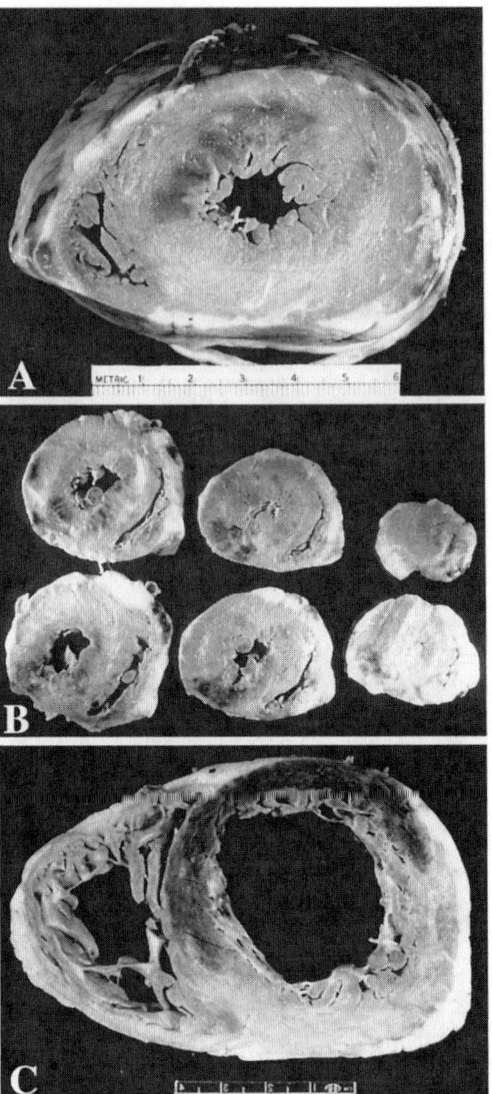

FIGURE 49-7 *A.* 47-year-old black male presented with unstable angina, evolved into a Q-wave infarct, on catheterization had a total occlusion of the left anterior descending coronary artery and had severe stenosis of the right and left circumflex coronary arteries, and underwent emergency bypass graft to all three vessels. He died secondary to refractory arrhythmias on the third hospital day. Note subendocardial hyperemic region in the anteroseptal wall of the left ventricle. *B.* Patient presented with acute myocardial infarction of 6 h duration, received streptokinase in the emergency room, and died 2 days following successful reperfusion of a cerebral bleed. Note a hemorrhagic transmural infarct involves the posteroseptal wall of the left ventricle, extending from the base to the apex of the heart with approximately 20 to 25 percent of the myocardium infarcted. *C.* A 60-year-old male admitted with onset of chest pain while mowing the lawn did not seek medical treatment until 8 h after onset of chest pain. He received streptokinase, developed arrhythmias, was treated with lidocaine, went into cardiogenic shock, and died 3 days following infarction. Note transmural confluent hemorrhagic infarct of the anteroseptal wall of the left ventricle involving at least 40 percent of the left ventricle. (Virmani R, Burke AP, Farb A, Atkinson J, eds. *Cardiovascular Pathology,* 2d ed., vol. 40 of *Major Problems in Pathology* series, Philadelphia: Saunders; 2001, Fig. 5-6. With permission.)

within the infarct and fragment, resulting in more severe karyorrhexis (nuclear dust). Loss of myocyte striations is best appreciated by Mallory's trichrome stain. Another stain that has been used to detect early areas of infarction is hematoxylin–basic fuchsin–picric acid; however this technique for the early detection of necrosis (6 to 8 h) in humans has not proven to be reliable.

Immunohistochemical staining has also been used to study early changes of necrosis, but these—including antibodies directed against creatine kinase, ceruloplasmin, myoglobin, C-reactive protein, complement complex (C5b-9), fibronectin, and others—have also not

TABLE 49-1 Gross and Microscopic Evolution of Reperfused and Nonreperfused Acute Myocardial Infarct

| Time of Occlusion | Permanent Occlusion/No Reperfusion | | Reperfusion following Occlusion | |
|---|---|---|---|---|
| | Gross | Histologic | Gross | Histologic |
| 12 h | No change/pallor | Wavy fibers | Mottled, prominent hemorrhage | CBN |
| 24–48 h | Pallor—yellow, soft | Hypereosinophilic fibers, PMNs at borders | Prominent hemorrhage | Hypereosinophilic fibers + CBN + PMNs + hemorrhage throughout |
| 3–5 days | Yellow center, hyperemic borders | Large number of PMNs at border, coagulation necrosis, loss of nuclei | Prominent hemorrhage | Aggressive phagocytosis profuse fibroblast infiltration + collagen77<None> |
| 6–10 days | Yellow, depressed central infarct, tan-red margins | Mummified fibers in center, macrophage phagocytosis + granulation tissue at borders | Depressed red-brown infarct with gray-white intermingled | Aggressive healing with greater collagen |
| 10–14 days | Gray red borders, infiltrating central tan-yellow infarct if large | Marked granulation tissue, collagen deposition, subendocardial myocyte sparing | Gray-white intermingled with brown | Aggressive healing with greater collagen |
| 2–8 weeks | Gelatinous to gray-white scar, greater healing at border zone | Collagen deposition with prominent large capillaries | White intermingled with groups of myocytes with red myocardium | Collagen intermingled with groups of myocytes |

Abbreviations: PMN = polymorphonuclear leukocyte; CBN = contraction band necrosis.
Source: Virmani R, Burke AP, Farb A, Atkinson J, eds. *Cardiovascular Pathology,* 2d ed. Philadelphia, Saunders; 2001.

been found to be useful.[30] Macrophages and fibroblasts begin to appear in the border areas. By 1 week, neutrophils decline and granulation tissue is established, with neocapillary invasion as well as lymphocytic and plasma cell infiltration. Although lymphocytes may be seen as early as 2 to 3 days, they are not prominent at any stage of infarct evolution. Eosinophils may be seen within the inflammatory infiltrate but are present in only 24 percent of infarcts.[36] There is phagocytic removal of the necrotic myocytes by macrophages, and pigment is seen within macrophages.

By the second week, fibroblasts are prominent, but their appearance may be seen as early as day 4 at the periphery of the infarct. There is continued removal of the necrotic myocytes, as the fibroblasts are actively producing collagen and angiogenesis occurs in the area of healing. The healing continues, and depending on the extent of necrosis, the healing may be complete as early as 4 weeks, or it may require 8 weeks or longer to complete (Fig. 49-8). The central area of infarction may remain unhealed, showing mummified myocytes for extended periods, despite the fact that the infarct borders are completely healed. For this reason, it is important to evaluate the age of the infarct by examining the border with noninfarcted muscle.

The magnitude of repair and healing is dependent not only on infarct size but also on local and systemic factors. If there is good collateral blood flow locally, healing will be relatively rapid, especially at the lateral borders, where viable myocardium interdigitates with necrotic myocardium. There may be various levels of healing within an infarct, because of differences in blood flow in adjoining vascular beds caused by variable extents of coronary narrowing. The border areas may show hemorrhage and contraction-band necrosis, depending on regional variations in blood flow. Systemic factors that influence repair of myocardium are the systemic blood pressure and cardiac output, which are severely decreased in heart of patients with multisystem failure.

## Light Microscopic Appearance of Reperfused Acute Myocardial Infarction

In dogs, the amount of myocardium that can be salvaged depends on the duration of total occlusion of the artery supplying the area of infarction. Maximal salvage is possible, in both dogs and humans, if the artery is opened within 6 h. The myocardium in the dog following 90 min of occlusion followed by reperfusion and sacrifice at 24 h shows a hemorrhagic infarct limited to the area of occlusion, which is subendocardial in extent. Hemorrhage occurs when the myocardial blood flow during the occlusion period is less than one-fifth of normal. The myocytes are thin, hypereosinophilic, devoid of nuclei or

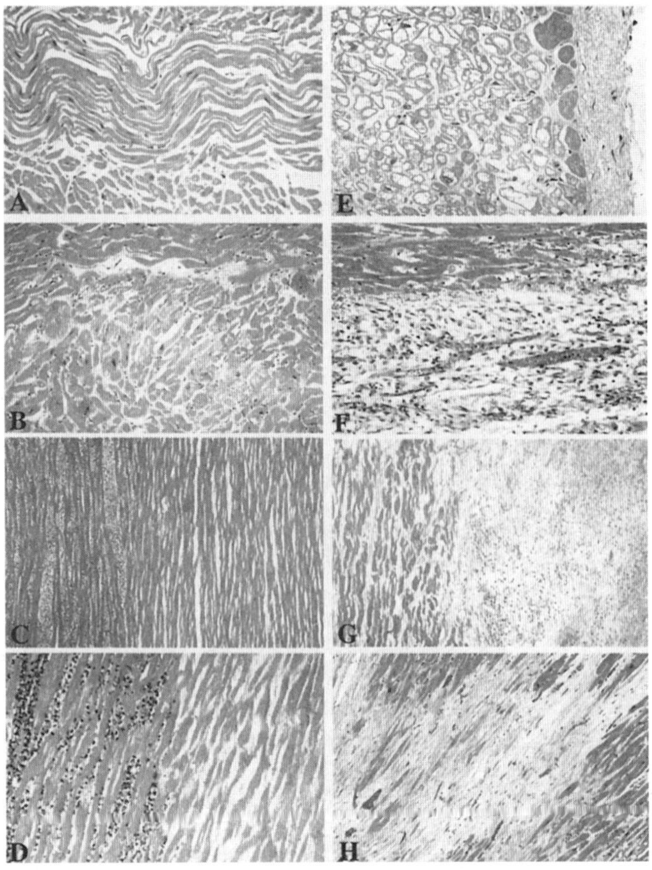

FIGURE 49-8 Histologic characteristics of myocardial infarction following total occlusion of a coronary artery. *A.* The earliest change seen is within 12 h after the onset of chest pain and has been described as wavy fibers with elongation of myocytes and narrowing of the myocyte diameter. *B.* Hypereosinophilic myocyte fibers representing early features of coagulation necrosis can be seen between 12 to 24 h after onset of chest pain; the nucleus is intact and the cross-striation are well seen. *C.* By 48 to 72 h the neutrophils are concentrated at the border of the infarcted and viable myocardium. The extent of neutrophil infiltration depends on the collateral flow as well as the extent of coronary perfusion of the adjacent bed. The central zone of infarction now shows all the features of coagulation necrosis with karyolysis and loss of cross-striations. *D.* Photomicrograph showing a high-power view of the border zone of a 5-day-old infarct, with marked neutrophil infiltration, that has undergone karyopyknosis and karyorrhexis. The adjoining infarcted myocardium shows coagulation necrosis with loss of nuclei and cross striations. *E.* A high-power view of the subendocardial region, which is usually ischemic but viable, showing myocyte vacuolization and loss of myofibrils. *F.* Almost complete removal of the necrotic myocardium. Note presence of neovascular channels and surrounding macrophages and a few lymphocytes (granulation tissue) at 7 to 10 days following acute myocardial infarction. *G.* The infarct is heavily infiltrated with fibroblasts, with early collagen deposition and interspersed neocapillaries and a few lymphocytes. The infarct is 3 to 4 weeks old. *H.* A fully healed infarct with dense collagen and few interspersed myocytes at the border region of the healed infarct. The infarct age may be 6 or more weeks. (From Virmani R, Burke AP, Farb A, Atkinson J, eds. *Cardiovascular Pathology,* 2d ed. Philadelphia: Saunders; 2001. With permission.)

showing karyorrhexis, with ill-defined borders and interspersed areas of interstitial hemorrhage. There is a diffuse but mild neutrophil infiltration. Within 2 to 3 days, macrophage infiltration is obvious and there is phagocytosis of necrotic myocytes and early stages of granulation tissue. Healing of the infarct in the dog is more rapid than that in the human, most likely due to nondiseased adjoining coronary arteries (collaterals) and a lack of underlying myocardial disease. In humans with acute MI, there is often chronic ischemia secondary to extensive atherosclerotic disease.

In humans, if reperfusion occurs within 4 to 6 h following the onset of chest pain or ECG changes; there is myocardial salvage and the infarct is likely to be subendocardial without transmural extension. There will be a nearly confluent area of hemorrhage within the infarcted myocardium, with extensive contraction-band necrosis. The extent of hemorrhage is dependent on the extent of reperfusion of the infarct as well as the extent of capillary necrosis. The larger the infarct and the longer the duration of the infarct, the greater the hemorrhage. The degree of hemorrhage may be variable and nonuniform, as blood flow is dependent upon the residual area of coronary narrowing and the amount of thrombolysis. Within a few hours of reperfusion, neutrophils are evident within the area of necrosis, but they are usually sparse (Fig. 49-9). In contrast to nonreperfused infarcts, neutrophils do not show concentration at the margins. However, reperfused infarcts often demonstrate areas of necrosis at the periphery, with interdigitation with noninfarcted myocardium. Macrophages begin to appear by day 2 to 3 and stromal cells show enlarged nuclei and nucleoli by days 3 and 4 (Fig. 49-9). Neutrophil debris, which may be concentrated at the border areas in cases of incomplete reperfusion, is seen by 3 to 5 days. By days 3 to 5, fibroblasts appear, with an accelerated rate of healing as compared to nonreperfused infarcts. By 1 week, there is collagen deposition, with disappearance of neutrophils; there is also prominence of macrophages containing pigment derived from ingested myocytes (Fig. 49-9). Angiogenesis is prominent and lymphocytes are often seen. Infarcts at 5 to 10 days are more cellular, and there is prominent myocytolysis (loss of myofibrils). As early as 2 to 3 weeks, subendocardial infarcts may be fully healed (Fig. 49-9). Some 5 to 10 layers of subendocardial myocytes are spared without necrosis. However, myofibrillar loss, which is a result of ischemia not severe enough to cause cell death, is prominent in this subendocardial zone. Larger infarcts and those reperfused after 6 h take longer to heal. Infarcts reperfused after 6 h show larger areas of hemorrhage as compared to occlusions with more immediate reperfusion (Fig. 49-7). However, myocytes maintain their striations, become stretched and elongated, and—as they do not respond to calcium influx—do not show significant contraction-band necrosis. Despite the fact that reperfusion should occur within 6 h of occlusion for maximal myocyte salvage, there appears to be some benefit in opening an artery regardless of the duration of coronary occlusion.

## THE NO-REFLOW PHENOMENON

The no-reflow phenomenon was originally described by Kloner and Jennings in 1974 in an experimental canine model of myocardial infarction.[37] They demonstrated homogenous distribution of thioflavin S dye after 40 min of ischemia and reperfusion; however, after 90 min of ischemia, areas of no reflow were identified mainly in the subendocardial regions as zones not staining with thioflavin S. By electron microscopy, they showed swollen endothelial protrusions and membrane-bound intraluminal bodies, which obstructed the capillary lumen and resulted in plugging of the capillaries by red cells, neutrophils, platelets, and fibrin thrombi. The areas not stained by thioflavin S were characterized by low regional myocardial blood flow. The term *reperfusion injury* was coined to describe reperfusion-related expansion or worsening of the ischemic cardiac injury as assessed by contractile performance, the arrhythmogenic threshold,

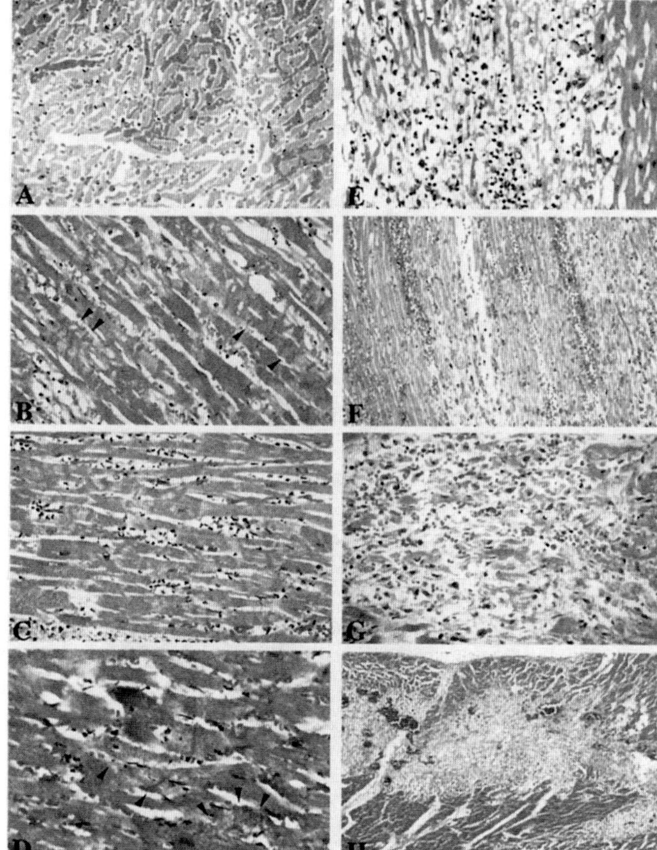


FIGURE 49-9 Histologic characteristics of a reperfused infarct following occlusion and reperfusion either with thrombolysis (tissue plasminogen activator, streptokinase, or IIb/IIIa) or balloon angioplasty with or without stenting or surgical revascularization. *A.* A cross section of myocytes shows necrosis with interstitial hemorrhage. Note pale myocyte nuclei and very early neutrophil infiltration. *B.* Myocytes cut longitudinally in a patient who was admitted with chest pain of 2 h duration, followed by infusion of streptokinase. The patient died within 6 h. Note the extensive contraction-band necrosis (dark bands alternating with lighter bands, *arrowheads*), a hallmark of reperfusion injury. There are interstitial red cells and a few neutrophils, which were scattered throughout the infarct. *C.* Note that the number of neutrophils is greater than in the previous example. There is mild red cell extravasation and contraction-band necrosis. The duration of chest pain was 3 h prior to reperfusion, and the patient died 24 h later. *D.* It is not uncommon to see one or a few necrotic myocytes with calcification (*arrowheads*) in patients with reperfused infarcts. *E.* Note the presence of macrophages and lymphocytes with early dissolution of the necrotic myocytes. These areas of necrosis are interdigitating with viable noninfarcted myocardium (4- to 5-day-old reperfused infarct). *F.* Note interstitial hemorrhage and infiltrating macrophages seen in the lower fifth and the right third of photomicrograph. *G.* High-power view of another infarct showing dissolution of the infarct and replacement with macrophages—also early angiogenesis. Hemorrhage is still present, but no neutrophils are seen. (5- to 7-day-old infarct) *H.* Low-power view of a healing infarct at 7 to 10 days. Note angiogenesis and early replacement fibrosis. (From Virmani R, Burke AP, Farb A, Atkinson J, eds. *Cardiovascular Pathology,* 2d ed. Philadelphia: Saunders; 2001. With permission.)

conversion of reversible to irreversible myocyte injury, and microvessel dysfunction. Recent studies have shown that the angiographic no-reflow phenomenon is a strong predictor of major cardiac events, such as congestive heart failure, malignant arrhythmias, and cardiac death after acute MI.

## COMPLICATIONS OF MYOCARDIAL INFARCTION

The in-hospital mortality of patients with acute MI has declined from 16 percent in the 1970s and early 1980s to 8 to 10 percent in the early 1990s. The reasons are multifactorial and include myocardial salvage from reperfusion, small infarction, and remodeling.[38] However, the incidence of cardiogenic shock in community studies has not declined.[39] The complications of MI infarction may manifest immediately or appear late and are dependent on the location and extent of infarction. The acute complications consist of arrhythmias and sudden death, cardiogenic shock, infarct extension, fibrinous pericarditis, cardiac rupture including papillary muscle rupture, and mural thrombus and embolization.

### Arrhythmias and Sudden Death

Before one can understand the arrhythmia patterns, it is essential to know the blood supply of the conduction system. The blood supply of the sinus node is from the right coronary artery in 60 percent of cases and from the left circumflex artery in 40 percent. The atrioventricular node is supplied from the right coronary artery in 90 percent of cases and from the left circumflex in 10 percent.[40] The bundle of His is supplied from the artrioventricular branch of the right coronary artery and a small contribution comes from the septal perforator of the left anterior descending artery. The His bundle divides into the right and left bundle branches; the right bundle branch receives most of its blood from the septal perforators of the left anterior descending artery, but there may be collaterals from the right and left circumflex arteries. The left bundle branch proximally divides into left anterior fascicle and the left posterior fascicle. The left anterior branch receives its blood supply from the septal perforators from the left anterior descending artery and is particularly susceptible to ischemia or infarction. The proximal portion of the left posterior fascicle receives its blood supply from the artrioventricular nodal artery (which is a branch of the right coronary artery) and from the septal perforators of the left anterior descending artery. The distal portion of posterior fascicle is supplied from two sources: the anterior and posterior septal perforating arteries.

Bradyarrhythmias during the first few hours of acute MI are triggered from inferior MI and are usually benign, while conduction disease beyond the first 24 h requires the most attention. Conduction disturbances (right bundle branch block and left anterior fascicular block) resulting from anterior MI are associated with higher mortality due to necrosis of the conduction system. Tachyarrhythmias that occur during acute MI often result form reperfusion, altered automatic tone, or hemodynamic instability.

Sudden death occurs in 25 percent of patients after MI, often before they reach the hospital. The proportion of deaths from ischemic heart disease that are sudden is almost 60 percent; therefore it is crucial to understand the causes and mechanisms of sudden death. Most arrhythmias responsible for out-of-hospital sudden coronary deaths are ventricular tachycardia and fibrillation, which may be monomorphic or polymorphic. In all patients, ventricular tachyarrhythmias are seen in 67 percent of cases within the first 12 h of acute myocardial infarction.[41] Nonsustained ventricular tachycardia is not associated with increased mortality, whereas sustained ventricular tachycardia seen during the first 48 h following acute myocardial infarction is associated with a 20 percent hospital mortality.[42] Arrhythmias most likely arise from the adjoining ischemic but noninfarcted myocardium. In this acidotic arrhythmogenic zone, there is the release of metabolites such as potassium, calcium, and catecholamines, with low levels of ATP and hypoxemia.[43,44] Later in the course of MI, arrhythmias may occur as a result of scar tissue surrounding viable myocytes.[45] The conduction system is relatively protected against ischemic injury, because conduction fibers are relatively inactive metabolically, as their function is not to provide contractility but to propagate the impulse.[46,47]

## Cardiogenic Shock

Cardiogenic shock is the most common cause of death in patients hospitalized with acute MI, and its incidence has remained high (approximately 10 percent). However, in-hospital death rates have recently fallen from 70 percent in 1975 to 1990 to 57 percent in 1997.[48] Cardiogenic shock is caused by decreased systemic cardiac output in the presence of adequate intravascular volume. Cardiogenic shock after MI usually occurs if there is loss of at least 40 percent of the left ventricular mass, either acutely or in combination with scarred myocardium from old healed infarcts.[17,49,50] In about 10 percent of patients who develop cardiogenic shock, shock occurs before hospitalization, immediately on presentation. Much more commonly, shock develops while the patient is in the hospital, presumably from infarct extension (Fig. 49-10*A*).[51,52] As a proportion of short-term deaths after MI, cardiogenic shock accounts for 44 percent. The remainder of deaths are the result of cardiac rupture (26 percent) and arrhythmias (16 percent).[45] Patients with extension of infarction (reinfarction) into subendocardial zones remote from the larger infarct may develop cardiogenic shock (Fig. 49-10*B*). In turn, cardiogenic shock renders the remaining viable myocardium prone to ischemic necrosis because of poor perfusion.[53]

Two related but distinct complications of MI are infarct extension and infarct expansion. Infarct extension results from an incremental increase in absolute necrotic myocardium and may be the result of infarction remote from the original infarct in either the right or left ventricle (Fig. 49-10). It has been suggested that the more general term *recurrent infarction* be used for *infarct extension*.[54] Infarct extension usually occurs between 2 and 10 days following infarction, at a time when ECG changes are evolving and the troponin I or T is still high. However, a rapidly falling serum creatine kinase (CK-MB) after the first 24 h may be useful for the detection of infarct extension along with a new Q wave on the ECG. The risk factors associated with infarct expansion are cardiogenic shock, subendocardial infarct, female gender, and previous infarcts.[55,56]

Infarct expansion is the thinning of the area of the infarcted region, not an increase in myocardial necrosis. In contrast, infarct expansion is caused by stretching of myocyte bundles, reducing the density of myocytes in the area of the infarcted wall and resulting in loss of tissue within the necrotic myocardium.[57] Infarct expansion typically results in dilatation and thinning of the infarct and is associated with heart failure, ventricular aneurysm, and high mortality. Risk factors for infarct expansion are anterior transmural infarcts and life-threatening arrhythmias.[58] Another term often applied to infarct expansion is *ventricular remodeling,* which involves remodeling of both the infarcted and the noninfarcted myocardium. As so defined, infarct expansion is a combination of changes in left ventricular dilation and hypertrophy of noninfarcted myocardium.[59,60]

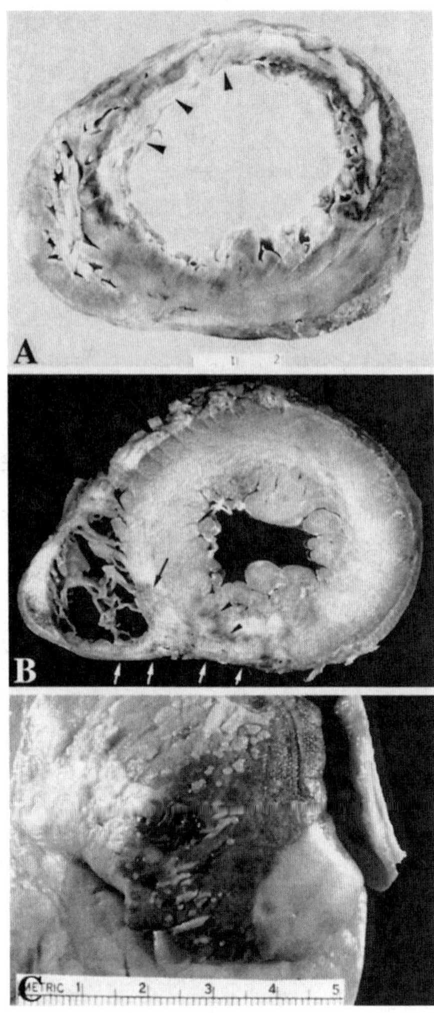


FIGURE 49-10 A 54-year-old man with a history of acute myocardial infarction had an anteroseptal transmural myocardial infarction. On day 3, the patient went into severe congestive heart failure; he died on the 10th day. Note markedly thinned transmural anteroseptal infarct (*arrowheads*) involving 60 percent of the basal slice of the heart. The anteroseptal region shows infarct expansion. *B.* A 47-year-old man presented with chest pain as well as elevated CK and CK-MB. On ECG, he was found to have a non-Q-wave myocardial infarction involving the posterior wall of the left ventricle. The patient had an uneventful hospital course with cardiac enzymes (CK-MB) falling close to baseline. On the third hospital day he developed another episode of chest pain with a rise in cardiac enzymes and new ECG changes of ST-segment elevation in the precordial leads and was diagnosed with infarct extension and right ventricular infarction. The ventricular slice shows an older subendocardial infarct with a hyperemic border (*arrowheads*) and a more recent infarction involving the full thickness of the posterior wall and a portion of the left ventricular septum with extension into the posterior wall of the right ventricle (*arrows*). *C.* A 51-year-old man presented with chest pain of $>$24 h duration; a diagnosis of acute myocardial infarction was made, involving the inferior wall of the left ventricle as well as the right atrium. Note the hemorrhagic right atrial border. Its the tip is pale and dusky, and there are fibrin deposits on the pericardial surface. (From Virmani R, Burke AP, Farb A, Atkinson J, eds. *Cardiovascular Pathology,* 2d ed. Philadelphia: Saunders; 2001. With permission.)

## Rupture of the Myocardial Free Wall

The incidence of rupture of the left ventricular free wall was higher (10 percent) than rupture of the ventricular septum (2 percent) in the prethrombolytic era among patients dying of transmural MI. Reperfusion therapy has reduced the incidence of cardiac rupture; however, late thrombolytic therapy may increase the risk of this occurrence (Fig. 49-11). Risk factors for cardiac rupture after MI include multivessel atherosclerotic disease, female gender and age above 60 years, hypertension, absence of hypertrophy and previous infarction, poor collateral flow, the presence of a transmural infarct involving at least 20 percent of the wall, and location of the infarct in the midanterior or lateral wall of the left ventricle.[61–66] Cardiac rupture usually occurs in the first few days (1 to 4 days) following the infarct, when coagulation necrosis and neutrophilic infiltration are at their peak and have weakened the left ventricular wall.[67,68] Left ventricular wall rupture is seven times more common than rupture of the right ventricle.[67,68] Infarcts with rupture contain more extensive inflammation and are more likely to demonstrate eosinophils (30 percent eosinophilic infiltration, as compared to 12 percent eosinophils in nonruptured infarcts[69]). However, at least 13 to 28 percent of ruptures occur within 24 h of onset of infarction, when inflammation and necrosis are not prominent.[70] Rupture most frequently occurs at the border between the infarcted region and the viable myocardium. Ruptures are usually not seen beyond 10 days after healing occurs. However, ruptures in infarcts with healing generally occur in the center of the infarct, unlike earlier ruptures (Fig. 49-11).[67,68] Nearly half the deaths from cardiac rupture occur as out-of-hospital sudden deaths and therefore are never seen by the clinician.[70] Clinical signs of cardiac rupture in patients who survive to the hospital include new murmur, a palpable thrill, and an echocardiographic finding of pericardial effusion.[71]

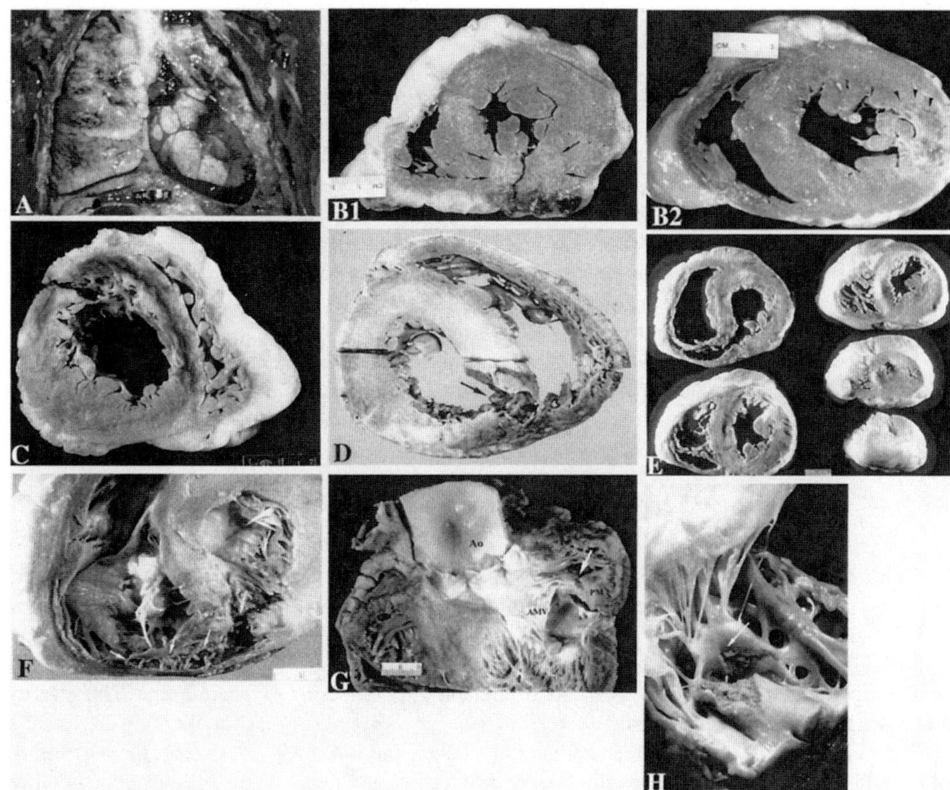


FIGURE 49-11 Ruptured acute myocardial infarction. *A.* Hemopericardium in a 70-year-old male with history of chest pain and diagnosis of acute transmural infarction who died suddenly while walking to the bathroom 24 h following admission. The pericardium contained 300 mL of blood, and a rupture site was identified on the posterior wall of the left ventricle (*B1*). Note an early transmural infarct (pale area on the posterior wall—*arrows*) with the rupture site close to the viable myocardium but within the infarct zone. A lateral wall rupture (*B2*). Note that the rupture site is close to the viable and infarcted myocardium (*arrowheads*). *C.* A 50-year-old man presented with chest pain of 7-h duration. He received streptokinase and underwent balloon angioplasty of the proximal left anterior descending coronary artery. At autopsy, the patient had hemopericardium and a transmural hemorrhagic reperfused infarct involving the anteroseptal wall of left ventricle. The rupture occurred close to the viable myocardium on the anterior wall. *D.* Rupture of the posterior ventricular septum (*arrow*) 2 weeks following an acute myocardial infarction. The patient died with severe congestive heart failure; the diagnosis of ventricular septal rupture had been missed clinically. (A four-chamber cut had been made prior to short-axis slicing). *E.* Ventricular septal rupture involving the inferobasal portion of the heart, which extends through the posterior septum and into the right ventricle, causing a dissection of the posterior wall of the right ventricle. *F.* A is a high-power view of the inferobasal portion of the heart showing the rupture through the septum extending into the right ventricle and piercing the right ventricular wall (*arrow along rupture tract*). *G.* A patient with transmural myocardial infarction of the posterior left ventricular wall with rupture of one of the two heads of posteromedial (PM) papillary muscle (*arrow*). The base of the heart has been opened along the left ventricular outflow tract. Ao = aorta, AMV = anterior mitral leaflet. High-power view shows total severance of one of the papillary heads (*arrow*) of the posteromedial papillary muscle. (From Virmani R, Burke AP, Farb A, Atkinson J, eds. *Cardiovascular Pathology*, 2d ed. Philadelphia: Saunders; 2001. With permission.)

Figuer as et al. reported an 18 percent incidence of cardiac rupture in patients admitted with a first MI. Ruptures of the left ventricular free wall and septum were equally frequent (8 percent), whereas rupture of the papillary muscle was less frequent (2 percent). Delayed hospitalization and undue in-hospital activity appeared to increase the risk of rupture.[72] Rupture of the free wall usually leads to hemopericardium and death from cardiac tamponade. Ruptures of the ventricular septum have been classified into simple or complex. Simple ruptures have a discrete defect and a direct through-and-through communication across the septum; they are usually associated with anterior MI and are located in the apex. Complex ruptures are characterized by extensive hemorrhage with irregular serpiginous borders of the necrotic muscle; they usually occur in inferior infarcts and involve the basal inferoposterior septum.[73] The mortality rate in the prethrombolitic era was extremely high, with a 50 percent mortality in surgically treated patients and 90 percent in those treated medically. The mortality rates have not declined significantly since the introduction of thrombolysis. Patients with septal rupture from inferior rather than anterior MI have the shortest survival.

Rupture of papillary muscle is less common than septal or free wall rupture and may occur as a complication of small subendocardial or larger transmural myocardial infarctions.[74,75] More than 80 percent of infarcts underlying papillary muscle rupture involve the posteromedial muscle, which has a single blood supply from the right coronary artery (Fig. 49-11). Because the anterolateral papillary muscle has a dual blood supply from the left anterior descending and the left circumflex coronary arteries, it rarely undergoes isolated ischemic rupture.[67,75,76] The patient with papillary muscle rupture presents with sudden mitral regurgitation of variable severity. Complete transection of a left ventricular papillary muscle is incompatible with life because of massive sudden mitral regurgitation.[68]

## Right-Sided Infarction

Right ventricular infarction is a common complication of inferior transmural MI (Fig. 49-10*B*). Necropsy studies have demonstrated right ventricular infarction in 14 to 60 percent of patients dying with inferior left ventricular MI. This is usually seen as a triad of findings consisting of contiguous inferoposterior wall, posterior septum, and posterior right ventricular wall necrosis; rarely, there may be anterolateral right ventricular wall extension.[77,78] We reported that 78 percent of right ventricular infarctions occurring in patients with inferior left ventricular infarcts had concomitant right ventricular hypertrophy.[79] Isolated right ventricular infarction may infrequently occur in the absence of coronary disease in patients with chronic lung disease and right ventricular hypertrophy.[80] Atrial infarction occurs in 10 percent of all left ventricular inferior wall infarcts and typically involves the right atrium.[81]

## Pericardial Effusion and Pericarditis

Pericardial effusion is reported in 25 percent of patients with acute MI and is more common in patients with anterior MI, large infarcts, and congestive heart failure.[82,83] Pericardial effusion secondary to acute MI may occur as a transudative effusion or as an exudate in association with acute pericarditis. Pericardial effusion after MI usually takes several months to reabsorb.

Pericarditis occurs less often than pericardial effusion and is seen only in transmural acute MI. Pericarditis, in contrast to postinfarction effusions, may be localized to the area of necrosis and is accompanied by chest pain. Pericarditis consists of fibrin deposition in addition to inflammation, and may be present from the first day after infarction to as late as 6 weeks later. Risk factors for the development of postinfarction pericarditis include heparinization and thrombolytic therapy.[84] Pericardial involvement is related to infarct size and associated with a poor prognosis. Postinfarction syndrome (Dressler's syndrome) consists of pleuropericardial chest pain, friction rub, fever, leukocytosis, and pulmonary infiltrates; it occurs weeks to months after MI and is often recurrent. It is reported to occur in 3 to 4 percent of all patients experiencing MI.[68] At autopsy, there is localized fibrinous pericarditis along with neutrophil infiltration. The cause of Dressler's syndrome is unknown, but antibodies to cardiac tissue have been reported, suggesting an immunologic process.[85] The incidence of postinfarction syndrome has markedly decreased since the institution of thrombolytic therapy; and the reasons for this are unclear.

## Chronic Congestive Heart Failure

Survival has improved from 28 to 56 percent after hospitalization for MI. Enhancements in medical care have primarily benefited the young as compared to diabetics and older patients.[86] Patients with large acute MIs and persistent ischemia are the most likely to develop heart failure. The severity of congestive heart failure is a predictor of mortality.[87] Congestive heart failure usually occurs in the presence of two- or three-vessel disease and may appear even in the presence of well-developed collaterals.[88] Grossly, the atria and the ventricles are dilated and the ventricle shows either a large healed infarct (Fig. 49-12) or multiple smaller infarcts with or without a transmural scar.[89] Scarring of the inferior wall of the left ventricle often involves the posteromedial papillary muscle, which gives rise to mitral regurgitation contributing to congestive heart failure (Fig. 49-12).[89] Microscopically, the subendocardial regions of ischemia will show myocytes with myofibrillar loss; they are rich in glycogen, suggesting a state of "hibernation" (see below).[90] Sometimes it is difficult to differentiate ischemic cardiomyopathy from idiopathic dilated cardiomyopathy when infarcts are few and small and only one-vessel disease is present; in such situations we tend to call these *idiopathic dilated cardiomyopathy with incidental coronary artery disease.*[91]

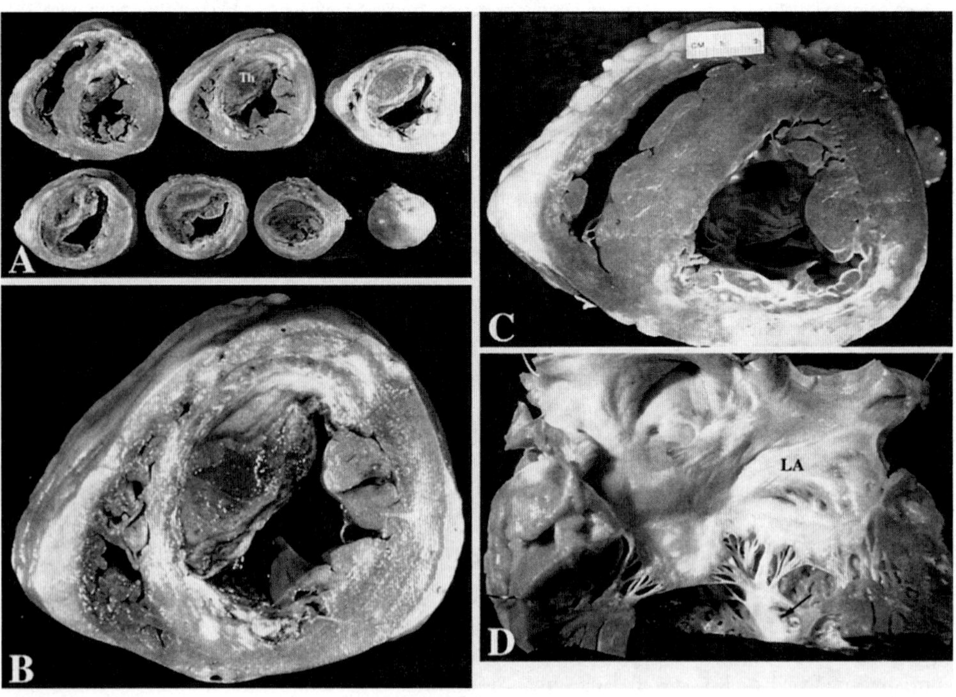


FIGURE 49-12 Thrombus of the left ventricle with healed myocardial infarct. *A*. Ventricular slices of a heart with healed myocardial infarction involving the anteroseptal wall of the left ventricle with extension from the base to the apex. Note dilatation of the left ventricular cavity and presence of an organizing thrombus (Th). *B*. Close-up of the basal ventricular slice (middle slice from top row in *A*). Note large transmural healed infarct with overlying organizing infarct. Patient at autopsy had multiple infarcts in the kidneys and one in the spleen. *C*. At autopsy, a 60-year-old man with congestive heart failure and mitral regurgitation had a healed myocardial infarction of the posterolateral left ventricular wall. *D*. Note scarred and thinned posteromedial papillary muscle (*arrow*), whereas the anterolateral papillary muscle is hypertrophied. Note dilated left atrium (LA). (From Virmani R, Burke AP, Farb A, Atkinson J, eds. *Cardiovascular Pathology,* 2d ed. Philadelphia: Saunders; 2001. With permission.)

## True and False Aneurysm

A large acute transmural myocardial infarct that has undergone expansion is the most likely infarct to result in a true aneurysm.[92,93] The pulsatile force from the blood in the cavity stretches and thins the necrotic muscle, which, when it heals, forms the wall of a true aneurysm.[94] An aneurysm is defined clinically as a discrete thinned segment of the left ventricle that protrudes during both systole and diastole and has a broad neck (Fig. 49-13). Morphologically, the wall of a true aneurysm develops after MI and consists of fibrous tissue with or without interspersed myocytes. In contrast, a false aneurysm has a small neck (from a prior rupture of the free wall of left ventricle due to infarct—it is contained by the adherent pericardium) and a wall of the aneurysm is formed by fibrous pericardium (not from the left ventricular MI and healing); the aneurysm is usually filled by a thrombus, which is organizing (Fig. 49-13). False aneurysms often require urgent surgical repair because of their propensity to rupture; they may also give rise to congestive heart failure. The cavity of the false aneurysm is usually filled with large blood clots, both old and new. The presence of hypertension and the use of steroids and nonsteroidal anti-inflammatory drugs may promote aneurysm formation.[95]

The incidence of true aneurysm following MI is 5 to 10 percent and is more frequent in transmural infarction than subendocardial infarction.[68] Aneurysms are usually associated with two-vessel or greater coronary disease with poorly developed collaterals.[96] Four of five aneurysms involve the anteroapical wall of the left ventricle[67]; they are four times more frequent in this wall than the inferior or posterior wall.[68] The pericardium is usually adherent to the aneurysm and may calcify. True aneurysm rarely rupture, whereas rupture is more common with a false aneurysm (Fig. 49-13).[97] The cavity of the aneurysm usually contains an organizing thrombus, and the patient may present with embolic complications. The mortality is six times higher in patients with aneurysm than in those without.[98]

Mills et al. have suggested that aneurysmectomy should be performed in patients having true aneurysms because of their poor prognosis. They reported a 27 percent 3-year survival in an autopsy series and a 70 percent survival in the Coronary Artery Surgery Study.[99] The survival of patients with pseudoaneurysm is also better following surgery. It has been said that over half of pseudoaneurysms are located in the posterior or inferior walls, whereas most true aneurysms involve the anterior wall. The reasons for these differences have been speculated to be because large inferoposterior infarcts that could lead to aneurysms are more often fatal, and therefore such patients would not survive, while posterior rupture is more often contained by the pericardium, allowing a pseudoaneurysm to develop.[100]

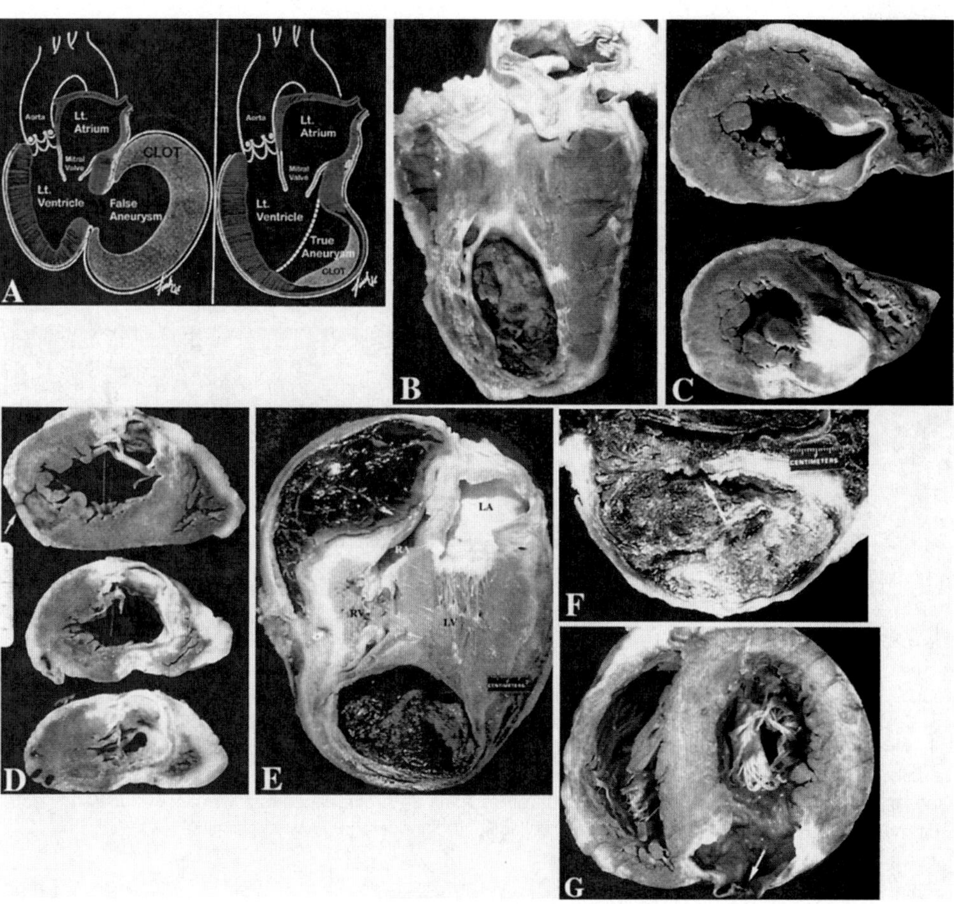


FIGURE 49-13 Diagram of a false (*left*) and a true (*right*) aneurysm. Note a rupture of the left ventricular wall, with the blood contained by the pericardial wall. The left ventricle does not form the wall of the aneurysm and the neck of the aneurysm is narrow. The wall of the true aneurysm is formed by the wall of the infarcted myocardium and the neck of the aneurysm is wide. (Courtesy of Dr. William C. Roberts.) *B.* A true aneurysm is seen at the apex of the heart, involving the anteroseptal apical two-thirds of the left ventricle. The aneurysm is filled with thrombus and there is endocardial thickening around the edges of the infarct. *C.* Healed transmural infarction of the posteroseptal wall of the left ventricle. Note the thinned and bulging aneurysm of the posterior and septal wall, with marked endocardial thickening. No thrombus was identified within the cavity of the aneurysm. *D.* A 54-year-old man without any significant medical history died suddenly. At autopsy there was cardiac tamponade with ventricular rupture of the posterolateral wall (*arrow*) secondary to a transmural acute infarction. Ventricular slices of the heart showing the presence of a localized small anterior aneurysm from a healed myocardial infarction involving the anterior and septal wall of the left ventricle. Note organizing thrombus in the aneurysmal cavity. *E.* False aneurysm. A 47-year-old male presented with sudden onset shortness of breath and died in the emergency room. At autopsy there was a loculated hemopericardium and a left ventricular anteroapical aneurysm secondary to a healed myocardial infarction with overlying thrombus. A four-chamber cut of the heart showed extensive adhesions between the visceral and the parietal pericardium, and loculated fresh blood was present in the pericardial space above the right atrium (RA) and right ventricle (RV) as well as organizing hemorrhage around the heart. LA = left atrium, LV = left ventricle *F.* A deeper posterior cut revealed the rupture site in the aneurysmal wall (*arrow*). Note the narrow communicating neck of the true aneurysm with the false aneurysm. A diagnosis of rupture of a true aneurysm with a secondary false aneurysm was made. *G.* Rupture of a healed inferior wall aneurysm (*arrow*) in a 56-year-old man who developed chest pain and died while undergoing a stress test. At autopsy, there was hemopericardium (500 mL). (From Virmani R, Burke AP, Farb A, Atkinson J, eds. *Cardiovascular Pathology*, 2d ed. Philadelphia: Saunders; 2001. With permission.)

## Mural Thrombus and Embolization

Mural thrombus forming on the endocardial surface over the area of the acute infarction occurs in 20 percent of all patients. However, the incidence is 40 percent for anterior infarcts and 60 percent for apical infarcts.[101–105] Patients with left ventricular thrombi have poorer global left ventricular function and a poorer prognosis as compared to those without thrombi.[101] The poor prognosis is secondary

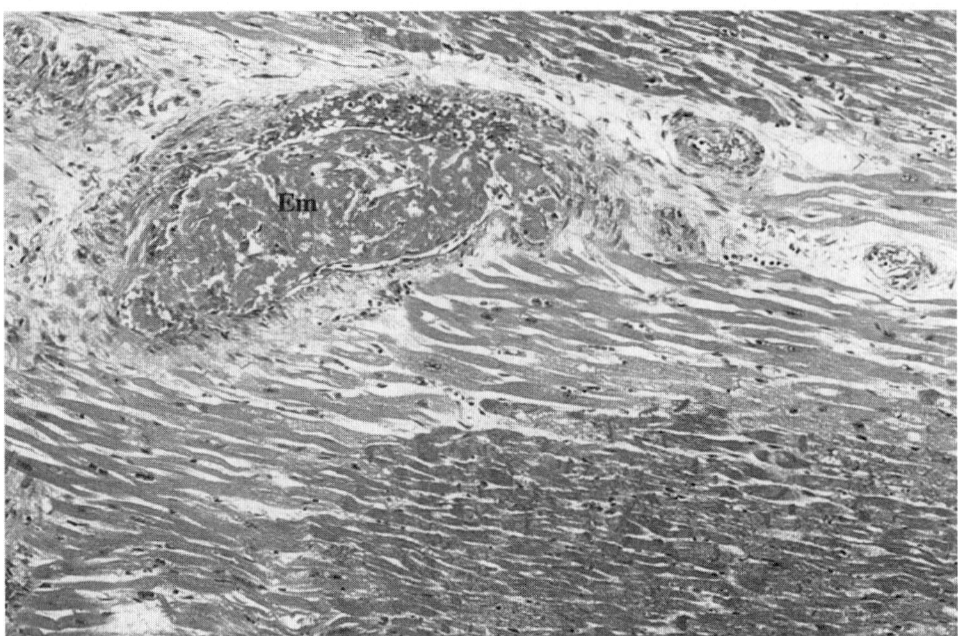


FIGURE 49-14 Intramyocardial thrombus with surrounding acute myocardial infarction in a patient with history of myocardial infarction 6 months prior to the current presentation with chest pain. On echocardiography, he had a thrombus in the left ventricular cavity overlying the healed infarct. No acute thrombus was seen in any of the epicardial coronary arteries at autopsy. However, the anterolateral wall of the left ventricle showed intramyocardial coronary emboli (Em) and surrounding infarction of less than 24 h duration. (From Virmani R, Burke AP, Farb A, Atkinson J, eds. *Cardiovascular Pathology*, 2d ed. Philadelphia: Saunders; 2001. With permission.)

to complications of a large infarct and not from emboli.[102] It has been reported that those that form thrombi have associated endocardial inflammation during the phase of acute infarction. The thrombi tend to organize, but the superficial portions may embolize in about 10 percent of cases (Fig. 49-14).[101] The usual sites of symptomatic embolization are the brain, eyes, kidney, spleen, bowel, legs, and coronary arteries. Symptomatic emboli are usually due to larger fragments, whereas small particles of thrombus that embolize generally do not cause symptoms.[103] The risk of embolization is greatest in the first few weeks after acute MI.[104] Anticoagulation has been show to reduce the incidence of left ventricular thrombus formation.[68]

## HIBERNATING MYOCARDIUM

In the early 1980s, Rahimtoola found a significant improvement in left ventricular function after coronary revascularization in a subset of patients with depressed ventricular performances.[106] He postulated that the mechanism of poor myocardial contractility was chronic ischemia, which could be improved by revascularization. The premise behind this rationale was dependent on the surviving myocardium being in a functional albeit in a depressed, "hibernating" state,[107,108] suggesting that the myocardium may adapt to chronic ischemia by decreasing its contractility but preserving viability. Subsequently, Sheiban et al.[109] have shown that 5 to 7 min of angioplasty balloon inflations in the coronary arteries of patients undergoing interventional procedures, followed by tracking of the resolution of the regional wall motion abnormalities over the next 5 days, showed persistence of regional wall motion abnormities up to 36 h. Similarly, return of left ventricular function has been studied following MI. Delayed recovery of wall motion was observed in the infarct region, with a positive change in wall motion from 0.2 at 3 days to 1.0 at 6 months in patients with reperfusion but not in those without reperfusion.[110]

Morphologically, hibernating myocytes show loss of contractile elements, especially in the perinuclear region and occasionally throughout the cytoplasm. The space left by the dissolution of myofibrils is occupied by glycogen, as evidenced by strong positivity for the periodic acid–Schiff reagent. Ultrastructurally, there is depletion of sarcomeres, most pronounced in the perinuclear region, with increased glycogen. The nuclei are enlarged, with a tortuous nuclear membrane and evenly distributed heterochromatin. The mitochondria are elongated, shrunken, and osmiophilic.[111]

## ISCHEMIC PRECONDITIONING

Ischemic preconditioning was first described by Murry et al. in 1986, when they observed that canine MI size was markedly reduced if it follows four 5-min episodes of occlusion followed by 5 min of reperfusion.[112] Infarct size in the absence of preconditioning has been shown to be related to collateral blood flow. However, this relationship is altered in the presence of preconditioning. Preconditioning has also been observed with only one episode of brief occlusion followed by reperfusion. If the duration between ischemic preconditioning and the long duration of occlusion is extended to 24 to 96 h, the protective effect is not equally marked.[113] The original description of preconditioning was applied only to the reduction of infarct size; this definition is now extended to cardiac function and arrhythmias, although the latter are not as consistent.[114]

The mechanisms of preconditioning are unclear, but it has been shown that preconditioning reduces the energy demand of the myocardium, both in animals and humans. Yellon and associates have shown that intermittent aortic cross-clamping can precondition the human left ventricle during coronary artery bypass surgery, resulting in the preservation of ATP levels.[115] Other observations that confirm the existence of preconditioning in patients have been observed in patients undergoing percutaneous transluminal coronary angioplasty (PTCA). Repeated balloon inflations of 60 to 90 s have been associated with decreasing chest pain, reduced ST-segment elevation, and a decrease in lactate production with subsequent inflations; these phenomenon are observed irrespective of the presence or absence of collaterals.[116] In TIMI-9, which studied the timing of angina in relation to MI, it was found that only patients with angina within 24 h of infarction showed a smaller infarct size and a better clinical outcome.[117]

The mediators of preconditioning are believed to involve the $K_{ATP}$ channel and specific isoforms of protein kinase C (PKC). The protective effect of temporary ischemia can be blocked by pretreatment of the myocardium with inhibitors of the $K_{ATP}$ channel, such as glibenclamide and 5-hydrocydeconate (5HD).[118,119] Similarly, inhibitors of PKC and tyrosine kinase, but not PKC alone, will prevent ischemic preconditioning. Also, agonists of adenosine ($A_1$ receptor) will pharmacologically precondition the heart against ischemia.[120] The benefits of preconditioning in humans cannot be applied to patients with acute MI, as the therapy must be instituted prior to coronary occlusion. However, it may be useful if administered before cardioplegia or to the heart prior to its removal for transplantation.[119]

## References


1. Tavazzi L. Clinical epidemiology of acute myocardial infarction. *Am Heart J* 1999;138:48–54.
2. Pashos CL, Newhouse JP, McNeil BJ. Temporal changes in the care and outcomes of elderly patients with acute myocardial infarction, 1987 through 1990. *JAMA* 1993;270:1832–1836.
3. Miller TD, Christian TF, Hodge DO, et al. Comparison of acute myocardial infarct size to two-year mortality in patients < 65 to those > or = 65 years of age. *Am J Cardiol* 1999;84:1170–1175.
4. Rosamond WD, Chambless LE, Folsom AR. Survival trends, coronary event rates, and the MONICA project. Monitoring trends and determinants in cardiovascular disease. *Lancet* 1999;354:864–865.
5. Levy D, Thorn TJ. Death rates from coronary disease—Progress and a puzzling paradox. *N Engl J Med* 1998;339:915–917.
6. Beller GA. Coronary heart disease in the first 30 years of the 21st century: Challenges and opportunities: The 33rd Annual James B. Herrick Lecture of the Council on Clinical Cardiology of the American Heart Association. *Circulation* 2001;103:2428–2435.
7. Rosamond WD, Chambless LE, Folsom AR, et al. Trends in the incidence of myocardial infarction and in mortality due to coronary heart disease, 1987 to 1994. *N Engl J Med* 1998;339:861–867.
8. Stanley WC. Cardiac energetics during ischaemia and the rationale for metabolic interventions. *Coron Artery Dis* 2001;12:S3–S7.
9. Tunstall-Pedoe H, Kuulasmaa K, Amouyel P, et al. Myocardial infarction and coronary deaths in the World Health Organization MONICA Project. Registration procedures, event rates, and case-fatality rates in 38 populations from 21 countries in four continents. *Circulation* 1994; 90:583–612.
10. Hedges JR, Young GP, Henkel GF, et al. Serial ECGs are less accurate than serial CK-MB results for emergency department diagnosis of myocardial infarction. *Ann Emerg Med* 1992;21:1445–1450.
11. Young GP, Gibler WB, Hedges JR, et al. Serial creatine kinase-MB results are a sensitive indicator of acute myocardial infarction in chest pain patients with nondiagnostic electrocardiograms: The second Emergency Medicine Cardiac Research Group Study. *Acad Emerg Med* 1997;4:869–877.
12. Morrow DA, Rifai N, Tanasijevic MJ, et al. Clinical efficacy of three assays for cardiac troponin I for risk stratification in acute coronary syndromes: A Thrombolysis In Myocardial Infarction (TIMI) 11B Substudy. *Clin Chem* 2000;46:453–460.
13. Antman EM, Grudzien C, Sacks DB. Evaluation of a rapid bedside assay for detection of serum cardiac troponin T. *JAMA* 1995;273: 1279–1282.
14. Hackel DB, Reimer KA, Ideker RE, et al. Comparison of enzymatic and anatomic estimates of myocardial infarct size in man. *Circulation* 1984;70:824–835.
15. Miwa K, Fujita M, Kameyama T, et al. Absence of myocardial ischemia during sudden controlled occlusion of coronary arteries in patients with well-developed collateral vessels. *Coron Artery Dis* 1999; 10:459–463.
16. Fujita M, Nakae I, Kihara Y, et al. Determinants of collateral development in patients with acute myocardial infarction. *Clin Cardiol* 1999; 22:595–599.
17. Page DL, Caulfield JB, Kastor JA, et al. Myocardial changes associated with cardiogenic shock. *N Engl J Med* 1971;285:133–137.
18. Reimer KA, Jennings RB. The "wavefront phenomenon" of myocardial ischemic cell death: II. Transmural progression of necrosis within the framework of ischemic bed size (myocardium at risk) and collateral flow. *Lab Invest* 1979;40:633–644.
19. Jennings RB, Steenbergen C Jr, Reimer KA. Myocardial ischemia and reperfusion. *Monogr Pathol* 1995;37:47–80.
20. Jennings RB, Ganote CE. Structural changes in myocardium during acute ischemia. *Circ Res* 1974;35(suppl 3):156–172.
21. Jennings RB, Ganote CE, Reimer KA. Ischemic tissue injury. *Am J Pathol* 1975;81:179–198.
22. Virmani R, Forman MB, Kolodgie FD. Myocardial reperfusion injury. Histopathological effects of perfluorochemical. *Circulation* 1990;81: IV57–IV68.
23. Jennings RB. Acute myocardial ischemic injury. Ultrastructural and biochemical studies of the early phase of lethal injury. *Arch Inst Cardiol Mex* 1980;50:365–371.
24. Buja LM, Fattor RA, Miller JC, et al. Effects of calcium loading and impaired energy production on metabolic and ultrastructural features of cell injury in cultured neonatal rat cardiac myocytes. *Lab Invest* 1990;63:320–331.
25. Buja LM, Burton KP, Chien KR, Willerson JT. Altered calcium homeostasis and membrane integrity in myocardial cell injury. *Adv Exp Med Biol* 1988;232:115–124.
26. Farb A, Burke AP, Tang AL, et al. Coronary plaque erosion without rupture into a lipid core. A frequent cause of coronary thrombosis in sudden coronary death. *Circulation* 1996;93:1354–1363.
27. Virmani R, Kolodgie FD, Burke AP, et al. Lessons from sudden coronary death: A comprehensive morphological classification scheme for atherosclerotic lesions. *Arterioscler Thromb Vasc Biol* 2000;20: 1262–1275.
28. Arbustini E, Dal Bello B, Morbini P, et al. Plaque erosion is a major substrate for coronary thrombosis in acute myocardial infarction. *Heart* 1999;82:269–272.
29. Falk E, Shah PK, Fuster V. Coronary plaque disruption. *Circulation* 1995;92:657–671.
30. Vargas SO, Sampson BA, Schoen FJ. Pathologic detection of early myocardial infarction: A critical review of the evolution and usefulness of modern techniques. *Mod Pathol* 1999;12:635–645.
31. Adegboyega PA, Adesokan A, Haque AK, Boor PJ. Sensitivity and specificity of triphenyl tetrazolium chloride in the gross diagnosis of acute myocardial infarcts. *Arch Pathol Lab Med* 1997;121:1063–1068.
32. Schoen FJ. *The Heart,* 6th ed. Philadelphia: Saunders; 1999.
33. Mallory GK, White PD, Salcedo-Salgar J. The speed of healing of myocardial infarction: A study of the pathologic anatomy in seventy-two cases. *Am Heart J* 1939;18:647–671.
34. Lodge-Patch I. The aging of cardiac infarcts and its influence on cardiac rupture. *Br Heart J* 1951;13:37–42.
35. Bouchardy B, Majno G. Histopathology of early myocardial infarcts. A new approach. *Am J Pathol* 1974;74:301–330.
36. Cowan MJ, Reichenbach D, Turner P, Thostenson C. Cellular response of the evolving myocardial infarction after therapeutic coronary artery reperfusion. *Hum Pathol* 1991;22:154–163.
37. Kloner RA, Ganote CE, Jennings RB. The "no-reflow" phenomenon after temporary coronary occlusion in the dog. *J Clin Invest* 1974;54: 1496–1508.
38. Hohnloser SH, Gersh BJ. Changing late prognosis of acute myocardial infarction: Impact on management of ventricular arrhythmias in the era of reperfusion and the implantable cardioverter-defibrillator. *Circulation* 2003;107:941–946.
39. Menon V, Hochman JS. Management of cardiogenic shock complicating acute myocardial infarction. *Heart* 2002;88:531–537.
40. Zimetbaum PJ, Josephson ME. Use of the electrocardiogram in acute myocardial infarction. *N Engl J Med* 2003;348:933–940.
41. Campbell RW, Murray A, Julian DG. Ventricular arrhythmias in first 12 hours of acute myocardial infarction. Natural history study. *Br Heart J* 1981;46:351–357.
42. Eldar M, Sievner Z, Goldbourt U, et al. Primary ventricular tachycardia in acute myocardial infarction: Clinical characteristics and mortality. The SPRINT Study Group. *Ann Intern Med* 1992;117: 31–36.
43. Corr PB, Gillis RA. Autonomic neural influences on the dysrhythmias resulting from myocardial infarction. *Circ Res* 1978;43:1–9.

44. Corr PB, Sobel BE. Mechanisms contributing to dysrhythmias induced by ischemia and their therapeutic implications. *Adv Cardiol* 1978: 110–129.
45. Stevenson WG, Linssen GC, Havenith MG, et al. The spectrum of death after myocardial infarction: A necropsy study. *Am Heart J* 1989; 118:1182–1188.
46. Bloor CM, White FC. Coronary artery reperfusion: Effects of occlusion duration on reactive hyperemia responses. *Basic Res Cardiol* 1975;70:148–158.
47. Bloor CM, Ehsani A, White FC, Sobel BE. Ventricular fibrillation threshold in acute myocardial infarction and its relation to myocardial infarct size. *Cardiovasc Res* 1975;9:468–472.
48. Hasdai D, Topol EJ, Califf RM, et al. Cardiogenic shock complicating acute coronary syndromes. *Lancet* 2000;356:749–756.
49. Mark DB, Naylor CD, Hlatky MA, et al. Use of medical resources and quality of life after acute myocardial infarction in Canada and the United States. *N Engl J Med* 1994;331:1130–1135.
50. Califf RM, Bengtson JR. Cardiogenic shock. *N Engl J Med* 1994;330: 1724–1730.
51. Holmes DR Jr, Califf RM, Topol EJ. Lessons we have learned from the GUSTO trial. Global Utilization of Streptokinase and Tissue Plasminogen Activator for Occluded Arteries. *J Am Coll Cardiol* 1995;25: 10S–17S.
52. Holmes DR Jr, Bates ER, Kleiman NS, et al. Contemporary reperfusion therapy for cardiogenic shock: The GUSTO-I trial experience. The GUSTO-I Investigators. Global Utilization of Streptokinase and Tissue Plasminogen Activator for Occluded Coronary Arteries. *J Am Coll Cardiol* 1995;26:668–674.
53. Gutovitz AL, Sobel BE, Roberts R. Progressive nature of myocardial injury in selected patients with cardiogenic shock. *Am J Cardiol* 1978; 41:469–475.
54. Califf RM. Myocardial reperfusion: Is it ever too late? *J Am Coll Cardiol* 1989;13:1130–1132.
55. Comparison of invasive and conservative strategies after treatment with intravenous tissue plasminogen activator in acute myocardial infarction. Results of the thrombolysis in myocardial infarction (TIMI) phase II trial. The TIMI Study Group. *N Engl J Med* 1989;320: 618–627.
56. Ellis SG, Topol EJ, George BS, et al. Recurrent ischemia without warning. Analysis of risk factors for in-hospital ischemic events following successful thrombolysis with intravenous tissue plasminogen activator. *Circulation* 1989;80:1159–1165.
57. Weisman HF, Bush DE, Mannisi JA, et al. Cellular mechanisms of myocardial infarct expansion. *Circulation* 1988;78:186–201.
58. Weisman HF, Healy B. Myocardial infarct expansion, infarct extension, and reinfarction: Pathophysiologic concepts. *Prog Cardiovasc Dis* 1987;30:73–110.
59. Gaudron P, Eilles C, Ertl G, Kochsiek K. Adaptation to cardiac dysfunction after myocardial infarction. *Circulation* 1993;87:IV83–IV89.
60. Gaudron P, Eilles C, Kugler I, Ertl G, Progressive left ventricular dysfunction and remodeling after myocardial infarction. Potential mechanisms and early predictors. *Circulation* 1993;87:755–763.
61. Mann JM, Roberts WC. Rupture of the left ventricular free wall during acute myocardial infarction: Analysis of 138 necropsy patients and comparison with 50 necropsy patients with acute myocardial infarction without rupture. *Am J Cardiol* 1988;62:847–859.
62. Reeder GS. Acute myocardial infarction: Enhancing the results of reperfusion therapy. *Mayo Clin Proc* 1995;70:1185–1190.
63. Pohjola-Sintonen S, Muller JE, Stone PH, et al. Ventricular septal and free wall rupture complicating acute myocardial infarction: Experience in the Multicenter Investigation of Limitation of Infarct Size. *Am Heart J* 1989;117:809–818.
64. Reddy SG, Roberts WC. Frequency of rupture of the left ventricular free wall or ventricular septum among necropsy cases of fatal acute myocardial infarction since introduction of coronary care units. *Am J Cardiol* 1989;63:906–911.
65. Shapira I, Isakov A, Burke M, Almog C. Cardiac rupture in patients with acute myocardial infarction. *Chest* 1987;92:219–223.
66. Oliva PB, Hammill SC, Edwards WD. Cardiac rupture, a clinically predictable complication of acute myocardial infarction: Report of 70 cases with clinicopathologic correlations. *J Am Coll Cardiol* 1993;22: 720–726.
67. Edwards WD. *Pathology of Myocardial Infarction and Reperfusion.* New York: Elsevier; 1991.
68. Antman EM, Braunwald E. *Acute Myocardial Infarction,* 5th ed. Philadelphia: Saunders; 1997.
69. Atkinson JB, Robinowitz M, McAllister HA, Virmani R. Association of eosinophils with cardiac rupture. *Hum Pathol* 1985;16:562–568.
70. Batts KP, Ackermann DM, Edwards WD. Postinfarction rupture of the left ventricular free wall: Clinicopathologic correlates in 100 consecutive autopsy cases. *Hum Pathol* 1990;21:530–535.
71. Reardon MJ, Carr CL, Diamond A, et al. Ischemic left ventricular free wall rupture: Prediction, diagnosis, and treatment. *Ann Thorac Surg* 1997;64:1509–1513.
72. Figueras J, Cortadellas J, Calvo F, Soler-Soler J. Relevance of delayed hospital admission on development of cardiac rupture during acute myocardial infarction: Study in 225 patients with free wall, septal or papillary muscle rupture. *J Am Coll Cardiol* 1998;32:135–139.
73. Birnbaum Y, Fishbein MC, Blanche C, Siegel RJ. Ventricular septal rupture after acute myocardial infarction. *N Engl J Med* 2002;347: 1426–1432.
74. Reeder GS. Identification and treatment of complications of myocardial infarction. *Mayo Clin Proc* 1995;70:880–884.
75. Barbour DJ, Roberts WC. Rupture of a left ventricular papillary muscle during acute myocardial infarction: Analysis of 22 necropsy patients. *J Am Coll Cardiol* 1986;8:558–565.
76. Wei JY, Hutchins GM. The pathogenesis of papillary muscle rupture complicating myocardial infarction: Hemorrhage accompanying contraction band necrosis. *Lab Invest* 1978;39:204–209.
77. Isner JM, Roberts WC. Right ventricular infarction complicating left ventricular infarction secondary to coronary heart disease. Frequency, location, associated findings and significance from analysis of 236 necropsy patients with acute or healed myocardial infarction. *Am J Cardiol* 1978;42:885–894.
78. Goldstein JA. Pathophysiology and management of right heart ischemia. *J Am Coll Cardiol* 2002;40:841–853.
79. Forman MB, Wilson BH, Sheller JR, et al. Right ventricular hypertrophy is an important determinant of right ventricular infarction complicating acute inferior left ventricular infarction. *J Am Coll Cardiol* 1987;10:1180–1187.
80. Kopelman HA, Forman MB, Wilson BH, et al. Right ventricular myocardial infarction in patients with chronic lung disease: Possible role of right ventricular hypertrophy. *J Am Coll Cardiol* 1985;5: 1302–1307.
81. Lazar EJ, Goldberger J, Peled H, et al. Atrial infarction: Diagnosis and management. *Am Heart J* 1988;116:1058–1063.
82. Galve E, Garcia-Del-Castillo H, Evangelista A, et al. Pericardial effusion in the course of myocardial infarction: Incidence, natural history, and clinical relevance. *Circulation* 1986;73:294–299.
83. Sugiura T, Iwasaka T, Takayama Y, et al. Factors associated with pericardial effusion in acute Q wave myocardial infarction. *Circulation* 1990;81:477–481.
84. Erhardt LR. Clinical and pathological observations in different types of acute myocardial infarction. *Acta Med Scand Suppl* 1974;560:1–78.
85. Uuskiula MM, Lamp KM, Martin SI. Relation between the clinical course of acute myocardial infarction and specific sensitization of lymphocytes and lymphotoxin production. *Kardiologiia* 1987;27:57–60.
86. Ali AS, Rybicki BA, Alam M, et al. Clinical predictors of heart failure in patients with first acute myocardial infarction. *Am Heart J* 1999; 138:1133–1139.
87. Pantely GA, Bristow JD. Ischemic cardiomyopathy. *Prog Cardiovasc Dis* 1984;27:95–114.
88. Schuster EH, Bulkley BH. Ischemic cardiomyopathy: A clinicopathologic study of fourteen patients. *Am Heart J* 1980;100:506–512.
89. Virmani R, Roberts WC. Quantification of coronary arterial narrowing and of left ventricular myocardial scarring in healed myocardial in-

farction with chronic, eventually fatal, congestive cardiac failure. *Am J Med* 1980;68:831–838.

90. Kloner RA, Bolli R, Marban E, et al. Medical and cellular implications of stunning, hibernation, and preconditioning: An NHLBI workshop. *Circulation* 1998;97:1848–1867.
91. Atkinson JB, Virmani R. Congestive heart failure due to coronary artery disease without myocardial infarction: Clinicopathologic description of an unusual cardiomyopathy. *Hum Pathol* 1989;20:1155–1162.
92. Erlebacher JA, Weiss JL, Weisfeldt ML, Bulkley BH. Early dilation of the infarcted segment in acute transmural myocardial infarction: Role of infarct expansion in acute left ventricular enlargement. *J Am Coll Cardiol* 1984;4:201–208.
93. Erlebacher JA, Richter RC, Alonso DR, et al. Early infarct expansion: Structural or functional? *J Am Coll Cardiol* 1985;6:839–844.
94. Hamer DH, Lindsay J Jr. Redefining true ventricular aneurysm. *Am J Cardiol* 1989;64:1192–1194.
95. Friedman BM, Dunn ML. Postinfarction ventricular aneurysms. *Clin Cardiol* 1995;18:505–511.
96. Forman MB, Collins HW, Kopelman HA, et al. Determinants of left ventricular aneurysm formation after anterior myocardial infarction: A clinical and angiographic study. *J Am Coll Cardiol* 1986;8:1256–1262.
97. Vlodaver Z, Coe JI, Edwards JE. True and false left ventricular aneurysms. Propensity for the latter to rupture. *Circulation* 1975;51: 567–572.
98. Meizlish JL, Berger HJ, Plankey M, et al. Functional left ventricular aneurysm formation after acute anterior transmural myocardial infarction. Incidence, natural history, and prognostic implications. *N Engl J Med* 1984;311:1001–1006.
99. Mills NL, Everson CT, Hockmuth DR. Technical advances in the treatment of left ventricular aneurysm. *Ann Thorac Surg* 1993;55:792–800.
100. Brown SL, Gropler RJ, Harris KM. Distinguishing left ventricular aneurysm from pseudoaneurysm. A review of the literature. *Chest* 1997;111:1403–1409.
101. Keeley EC, Hillis LD. Left ventricular mural thrombus after acute myocardial infarction. *Clin Cardiol* 1996;19:83–86.
102. Fuster V, Halperin JL. Left ventricular thrombi and cerebral embolism. *N Engl J Med* 1989;320:392–394.
103. Meltzer RS, Visser CA, Fuster V. Intracardiac thrombi and systemic embolization. *Ann Intern Med* 1986;104:689–698.
104. Kupper AJ, Verheugt FW, Peels CH, et al. Left ventricular thrombus incidence and behavior studied by serial two-dimensional echocardiography in acute anterior myocardial infarction: Left ventricular wall motion, systemic embolism and oral anticoagulation. *J Am Coll Cardiol* 1989;13:1514–1520.
105. Visser CA, Kan G, Meltzer RS, et al. Incidence, timing and prognostic value of left ventricular aneurysm formation after myocardial infarction: A prospective, serial echocardiographic study of 158 patients. *Am J Cardiol* 1986;57:729–732.
106. Rahimtoola SH, Grunkemeier GL, Teply JF et al. Changes in coronary bypass surgery leading to improved survival. *JAMA* 1981;246: 1912–1916.
107. Rahimtoola SH. The hibernating myocardium. *Am Heart J* 1989;117: 211–221.
108. Rahimtoola SH. Concept and evaluation of hibernating myocardium. *Annu Rev Med* 1999;50:75–86.
109. Sheiban I, Tonni S, Marini A, Trevi G. Clinical and therapeutic implications of chronic left ventricular dysfunction in coronary artery disease. *Am J Cardiol* 1995;75:23E–30E.
110. Schmidt WG, Sheehan FH, von Essen R, et al. Evolution of left ventricular function after intracoronary thrombolysis for acute myocardial infarction. *Am J Cardiol* 1989;63:497–502.
111. Vanoverschelde JL, Wijns W, Depre C, et al. Mechanisms of chronic regional postischemic dysfunction in humans. New insights from the study of noninfarcted collateral-dependent myocardium. *Circulation* 1993;87:1513–1523.
112. Murry CE, Jennings RB, Reimer KA. Preconditioning with ischemia: A delay of lethal cell injury in ischemic myocardium. *Circulation* 1986; 74:1124–1136.
113. Kuzuya T, Hoshida S, Yamashita N, et al. Delayed effects of sublethal ischemia on the acquisition of tolerance to ischemia. *Circ Res* 1993;72: 1293–1299.
114. Hagar JM, Hale SL, Kloner RA. Effect of preconditioning ischemia on reperfusion arrhythmias after coronary artery occlusion and reperfusion in the rat. *Circ Res* 1991;68:61–68.
115. Yellon DM, Alkhulaifi AM, Pugsley WB. Preconditioning the human myocardium. *Lancet* 1993;342:276–277.
116. Kloner RA, Yellon D. Does ischemic preconditioning occur in patients? *J Am Coll Cardiol* 1994;24:1133–1142.
117. Kloner RA, Shook T, Antman EM, et al. Prospective temporal analysis of the onset of preinfarction angina versus outcome: An ancillary study in TIMI-9B. *Circulation* 1998;97:1042–1045.
118. Critz SD, Liu GS, Chujo M, Downey JM. Pinacidil but not nicorandil opens ATP-sensitive K+ channels and protects against simulated ischemia in rabbit myocytes. *J Mol Cell Cardiol* 1997;29:1123–1130.
119. Kloner RA, Jennings RB. Consequences of brief ischemia: Stunning, preconditioning, and their clinical implications: Part 2. *Circulation* 2001;104:3158–3167.
120. Takano H, Bolli R, Black RG Jr. A(1) or A(3) adenosine receptors induce late preconditioning against infarction in conscious rabbits by different mechanisms. *Circ Res* 2001;88:520–528.

CHAPTER 50

# THE PATHOLOGIC AND BIOCHEMICAL BASIS FOR MYOCARDIAL ISCHEMIA AND REPERFUSION INJURY

Maksim A. Fedarau / Yoshifumi Naka / David J. Pinsky



The heart is a critical organ, which, like all other organs, is extremely dependent on a continual and adequate supply of oxygen and nutritive substances to perform its vital function. When this blood supply is interrupted, due to pathologic obstruction of the vascular lumen by clot or atheromatous debris, profound damage to the myocardium can ensue. This damage can be apparent at the micromolecular as well as the macroscopic level and certainly to the organism as a whole. The clinical condition is represented by patients experiencing angina or, more drastically, myocardial infarction. Although the basic interruption of blood flow results in clinically manifest pathology, homeostatic mechanisms are set into motion at the same time, trying to limit the resulting injury and rescue the damaged myocardium. These mechanisms may represent the body's own attempts to limit damage, but they may inadvertently exacerbate injury due to processes set in motion during reperfusion, which share many common features with the inflammatory response. These potential deleterious effects of reperfusion on the myocardium have been loosely called *reperfusion injury,* which can be brought about by the interaction of a number of different inflammatory cells as well as components of the coagulation and complement cascades. These interactions promote the formation of harmful substances, which may further contribute to myocardial cell damage. Our understanding of these basic pathophysiologic mechanisms that ultimately trigger myocyte death has led to new therapies designed to reduce the tissue injury accompanying myocardial ischemia and reperfusion.

## PATHOPHYSIOLOGY OF MYOCARDIAL ISCHEMIA/REPERFUSION INJURY

With the occlusion of the coronary artery, a number of electrical, mechanical, and chemical changes take place in the ischemic area of the myocardium. *Myocardial ischemia* refers to an imbalance between the supply and demand for arterial blood flow to the heart resulting in an inadequate supply of oxygen.[1] Ischemia of the myocardium develops whenever the flow of arterial blood through the obstructed vessels is inadequate to meet the metabolic needs of the myocardium to support its high metabolic demand. There is a characteristic sequence of events that occurs following interruption to the continual supply of arterial blood feeding the heart: the myocardium becomes cyanotic and tissue oxygen tension diminishes due to consumption of oxygen in its freely diffusible form as well as from stores of oxymyoglobin.[2] If the amount of oxygen is insufficient, intracellular respiration shifts from its aerobic to its anaerobic form. Adenosine triphosphate (ATP) stores are rapidly depleted,[3] causing adenosine diphosphate (ADP), and adenosine monophosphate (AMP) and adenosine to accumulate in the tissue. Shortly thereafter, the ischemic region of the myocardium loses its ability to maintain the negative resting membrane potential.[4] Depleted supplies of ATP or alteration in the availability of $Ca^{2+}$ causes the cessation of cardiac contraction.[4,5] This is followed by a distention of the ischemic myocardium, which perhaps occurs as the result of stretch due to tugging by adjacent nonischemic (and still contracting) myocytes.[6] Characteristic metabolic changes occur in the ischemic tissue, including an accumulation of tissue lactate,[3,7] $H^+$ ions,[8] phosphate,[7] and potassium.[9,10] There is also a rise in tissue tension of carbon dioxide ($P_{CO_2}$)[11] as an accumulated by-product of cellular metabolism without an egress mechanism during the stasis that characterizes ischemia. Mitochondrial calcium increases as well,[12] which may further contribute to ischemic contracture and perhaps even the ultimate death of the vulnerable myocyte. Arterioles exhibit a profound vasodilator response,[11] which might, under nonobstructing conditions, result in a restoration of nutritive flow; however, it is often futile. If complete obstruction to blood flow persists for as little as 20 min, myocardial necrosis may be observed.[13] Under circumstances in which myocardial reperfusion is reestablished with great rapidity, however, mechanical function can return to near baseline levels.[14]

When ischemic myocardial tissue is subjected to detailed histopathologic examination, there are characteristic structural changes, including, as one of the earliest changes, a decrease in the size and number of glycogen granules within the myocytes. The amount of glycogen decreases significantly following 30 min of ischemia and almost disappears during the subsequent $2\frac{1}{2}$ h.[15–17] Myofibrils appear to arrest in a relaxed state.[18] Ischemic tissue shows marked enlargement of interfibrillar and subsarcolemmal spaces with swelling of T tubules. Mitochondria also appear swollen and demonstrate decreased matrix density.[15–17] This swelling reflects changes in intracellular fluid distribution and increases in myocardial water content, which can represent nearly a 50 percent increase following an extended period of interrupted blood flow.[19,20] In addition to the contribution of intracellular fluid shifts, there is an expansion of the extracellular water content, presumably brought about by increases in the vascular permeability of vessels in the ischemic zone.[21–23]

There remains considerable controversy in the field as to exactly at which point the death of cardiac myocytes can be considered irreversible. Many pathologic mechanisms are triggered, which, if unchecked, would certainly lead to the inevitable death of the myocyte. However, other death-sparing pathways may be simultaneously activated, which can counterbalance the prodeath signals. The ultimate fate of the cardiac myocyte, therefore, depends on the prevailing balance of forces promoting or inhibiting their death. Clinically, it is often difficult to know where this balance lies or whether a given therapy will hasten or salvage myocyte death. An ischemic insult can be considered to cause irreversible myocyte death if it is of sufficient magnitude and duration, so that cells continue their march toward death even after restoration of blood supply.[24] Dead myocytes exhibit a characteristic histologic appearance, including the presence of contraction bands[25–27] and amorphous densities within swollen mitochondria.[25] Irreversible damage to mitochondria and cell membranes causes the release into blood of numerous plasma markers, which are used to quantify the degree of myocardial necrosis in patients. Markers of cardiac myocyte death appear in the plasma as plasma membrane integrity is compromised; these include enzymes such as lactate dehydrogenase (LDH), creatinine phosphokinase (CK), serum glutamic oxaloacetic transaminase (sGOT), and other intracellular proteins, such as myoglobin, troponin T and I, and cardiac-specific myosin light chains.[28] The other factor that contributes to rapid washout of these markers into blood is reperfusion of the myocardium following the period of ischemia. Integration of the area under the time-activity curves provides a rough estimate of the extent and degree of infarction,[29] although the presence of reperfusion causes early washout peaks, which can somewhat confound quantitative interpretation of this information.

## MYOCARDIAL REPERFUSION

Myocardial ischemia/reperfusion represents a clinically relevant problem associated with thrombolysis (brought about by the endogenous lytic system or by pharmacologic means), percutaneous coronary interventions, and coronary bypass surgery. Timely coronary reperfusion as a treatment for acute myocardial infarction has potential beneficial effects of reducing infarct size and improving the function of the myocardium as well as survival. Despite this, there has been concern that the reperfusion of a previously ischemic zone itself might have a deleterious effect on both the myocardium and the vasculature in the reperfused zone. This process of further tissue damage due to restoration of blood flow is called *reperfusion injury*. Reperfusion injury can be manifest as vascular compromise resulting in postischemic hypoperfusion or no reflow.[30] This flow compromise is brought about for several reasons, including frank vascular damage, thrombus formation, and neutrophil adhesion during reperfusion, which is accompanied by impairment of the coronary vasculature's ability to dilate in response to endogenous stimuli, such as adenosine release, which normally result in vasodilation. One important factor underlying impaired flow-mediated vasodilation is quenching of nitric oxide (NO), the available natural vasodilator, by reactive oxygen intermediates produced during reperfusion[31,32] When blood flow is insufficient to meet the demands of the tissue, myocardial contractility ceases and myocardial stunning is said to be present. *Stunned myocardium* refers to mechanical dysfunction that persists after reperfusion despite the restoration of coronary flow and absence of irreversible damage. Myocardial stunning is associated with the generation of oxygen-derived free radicals and by a loss of sensitivity of contractile filaments to calcium.[33–35]

Although, from a theoretical point of view, reperfusion injury is likely to be a real phenomenon, it must clearly be noted that rapid restoration of blood flow can arrest the progression of ischemic myocardial death.[36] Clinical trials of patients receiving thrombolytic agents for acute myocardial infarction have repeatedly shown that timely reperfusion is beneficial.[15] It is quite possible that the optimal therapy for acute myocardial infarction in the future will consist of a combination of rapid restoration of blood flow as well as an optimization of the reperfusion milieu.

The causes of reperfusion injury are multifold. Reperfusion injury is accompanied by the rapid generation of highly toxic reactive oxygen species (ROS),[37] with sites of production occurring in endothelial cells,[32] recruited/activated leukocytes, and even the myocytes themselves.[38–40] This ROS production can peak within minutes but may persist for many hours following restoration of blood flow.[41–43] Many species of ROS can be formed in the reperfusion milieu; examples include superoxide anion, hydroxyl radical, and hydrogen peroxide. The production of these ROS overwhelms the scavenging capacities of protective antioxidant enzymes, causing membrane phospholipid peroxidation, protein denaturation, and inactivation of key homeostatic enzymes.[44–46] Mitochondria, which are densely packed in cardiac myocytes, are likely to play the central role in free radical generation.[47,48] Superoxide production may also come from recruited neutrophils,[49] thus contributing to ROS formation, along with transition metal–catalyzed formation of hydroxyl radical by the Haber-Weiss pathway.[50] Xanthine oxidase represents another potential source of oxidative stress that generates superoxide as a by-product of purine metabolism—although controversy remains as to the importance of this particular oxidant-generating enzyme in the human heart.[51–53]

Evidence supporting the in vivo formation of ROS in the human heart comes from several studies that have detected by-products of membrane lipid peroxidation[54] such as malondialdehyde in coronary sinus effluent following percutaneous coronary intervention.[55] Similar evidence for the presence of lipid oxidation by-products comes from peripheral blood sampled following acute myocardial infarction.[56]

When cardiac myocytes are exposed to a period of ischemia followed by reperfusion, there is a characteristic increase in intracellular sodium and calcium,[57,58] which results in myofibrillar swelling.[59–61] Cardiac microvessels may exhibit similar swelling, and as prothrombotic and leukoadhesive mechanisms are triggered, there is a progressive decline in blood flow.[18,32,62] This may continue even if the head of pressure supporting blood flow increases, such as may occur with percutaneous coronary intervention (rescue angioplasty) or spontaneous or pharmacologic thrombolysis.

Taken together, these processes are termed the *no-reflow phenomenon*.[30,63] There is clinical evidence that this phenomenon is more than just an observation in laboratory animals; using perfusion scintigraphy, it has been shown that perfusion defects persist for several weeks after successful resolution of coronary artery occlusion in humans.[64]

The mechanical function of previously ischemic myocardium can remain depressed over a prolonged period of time, even in the absence of objective evidence of irreversible myocyte damage and despite restoration of normal or near-normal coronary blood flow. This postischemic dysfunction, called *myocardial stunning*,[65] is associated with depletion of ATP. The proposed mechanism(s) underlying this phenomenon include calcium overload and excitation contraction uncoupling secondary to dysfunction of the sarcoplasmic reticulum.[33,66] When the heart is examined by a technique permitting simultaneous assessment of both perfusion and wall motion, such as perfusion scintigraphy with a gated wall motion study, it can be apparent that there are regions which appear to have normal flow yet have depressed contractility. This is considered to be a flow/function mismatch,[67,68] which can be considered the hallmark of myocardial stunning in the setting of an ischemic cardiac event.

## MECHANISMS OF MYOCYTE DEATH AND APOPTOSIS

A number of theories have been advanced to explain the final common pathway by which myocardial and endothelial cells die during ischemia and reperfusion. Because of the unavailability of molecular oxygen during ischemia and the relatively inadequate degree of glycolysis, the myocyte—with its intrinsically high energy requirements—is unable to maintain the cell energy charge (i.e., ATP levels plummet). The shift from aerobic metabolism to anaerobic glycolysis leads to an increase in tissue lactate concentration.[11] As ATP demands outstrip ATP supply, cellular energy storages are depleted, resulting in the inability of ATP-dependent metabolic pumps to maintain a normal ionic gradient across cell membranes.[59] The generation of ROS upon restoration of blood flow to the previously ischemic myocardium results in oxidation of cell and mitochondrial membranes,[11] where enzymes of the oxidative phosphorylation chain are located; this leads to a further decrease in ATP production. Moreover, these free radicals may also inactivate glycolytic enzymes, thereby inhibiting the glycolytic production of $NADPH^+$.[69]

Cytosolic calcium overload is believed to be an important mechanism underlying the development of ischemic contracture[70] and cardiomyocyte death.[71] As a consequence of reduced cellular energy charge, stores of the general-purpose antioxidant reduced glutathione (GSH) decline, with a concomitant accumulation of the oxidized form of glutathione (GSSG). The function of an antioxidant protective enzyme, glutathione peroxidase[71,72]—which under normal conditions dissipates hydrogen peroxide[12,71,72]—is thereby impaired. Acid (protons)[7,73] and lactate accumulate, particularly in areas of ongoing stasis.

Current understanding of the pathophysiology of ischemic heart injury now incorporates a new elemental observation, whose importance was not recognized until recently: namely, cardiac myocytes die by a self-driven process of cellular suicide termed *apoptosis*.[74–76] Although apoptosis is not a unique feature of the cardiac myocyte, cells such as cardiac myocytes or neurons, which are terminally differentiated, can easily be driven into the apoptotic vortex. The executioners of this process are a family of cysteine proteases called *caspases*, which cleave proteins following aspartic acid residues.[77] Caspases are activated either by cell surface death receptors[78] or by the mitochondrial release of apoptotic activators such as cytochrome *c*.[79] Formation of ROS may be an important proximate cause of the release of cytochrome *c* from mitochondria.[80] Apoptosis is ultimately brought about when the activation of endogenous nucleases eventuate in the fragmentation of DNA.[74] Recent reports suggest that *LOX-1*, a newly recognized endothelial lectin-like receptor for oxidized low-density lipoproteins (such as oxidized LDL), plays a significant role in the induction of apoptosis and phagocytosis of dead cells.[81–84] Expression of the *LOX-1* gene is upregulated by different signals, including ox-LDL, inflammatory cytokines, and ROS[85–87] generated during the reperfusion of ischemic myocardium. It has been shown that blockage of the *LOX-1* pathway inhibits the apoptosis associated with reperfusion injury.[88]

## ROLE OF THE ENDOTHELIUM

Blood vessels within ischemic and reperfused tissue such as the myocardium are important structures whose proper functioning can determine the ultimate outcome for the organ or even the organism. Endothelial cells maintain vascular homeostasis by ensuring a proper balance between the nutrient supply and the dissipation of waste byproducts of metabolism. Furthermore, coagulation and leukocyte traffic are kept in tight check by quiescent endothelium. Endothelial cells have a central role in maintaining blood fluidity by preventing coagulation, modulating the vasomotor tone of the underlying vascular smooth muscle, thus regulating the blood vessel diameter. They also have an important function in regulating neutrophil adherence and egress into the underlying tissue. Disruption of any of these endothelial functions may be observed in the setting of myocardial ischemic/reperfusion injury; in fact, disruption of these generally occurs in concert. These changes lead to the characteristic highly permeable, thrombotic, proinflammatory phenotype of the endovascular wall. An important model system—which has been quite informative in simplifying the components of the ischemic vascular milieu for the study of specific cell functions—is a paradigm in which endothelial cells are exposed to hypoxia (to simulate ischemia/stasis) and subsequent reoxygenation (as a paradigm for reperfusion).

### Endothelium as a Barrier Permitting Restricted Diffusion

Cells of intact endothelium are typically tightly adherent to one another due to adherens junctions at their lateral margins and their discrete cytoskeletal architecture. In this way, they form a barrier to the passage of solutes and cells circulating within the bloodstream. Endothelial barrier function can be quantified in vitro by using measurements of electrical conductivity as well as by quantifying passage of radiolabeled molecules of various sizes across the endothelial layer. When exposed to a period of hypoxia of the same severity as that which accompanies cardiac ischemia ($Po_2$ of 12 to 16 Torr), endothelial cells develop changes in their actin cytoskeleton, which cause their margins to retract from each other.[89] New data also indicate that changes in the protein connections between cells (adherens and occluding junctions) may become altered, further facilitating large gap formation.[89,90] This results in the disruption of "restricted diffusion," in which molecules normally transit the endothelium as a function of their size; rather, unrestricted diffusion ensues, including mass transport of solutes by convective forces as well as by simple

Brownian motion. Ultimately, this allows large solutes and protein macromolecules to pass into underlying tissue.[89] Clinically, this becomes apparent as the interstitial space fills with solutes, proteins, and accompanying fluid along an oncotic gradient, resulting in interstitial edema.[91] The magnitude and duration of exposure of endothelial cells to hypoxia are key factors in determining the loss of endothelial barrier function.[89,90] As oxygen tension declines, certain important signaling cascades are disrupted, which may be the proximate cause of the disruption in endothelial barrier properties. There is a profound hypoxia-associated decrease in cyclic adenosine monophosphate (cAMP) levels within the endothelial cells, caused by a reduction in both basal and stimulated adenylate cyclase activity.[92] Experimentally, provision of the deficient second messenger in the form of a membrane-permeable cAMP analogue (dibutyryl-cAMP), can restore endothelial barrier function.[92] Other means of increasing cAMP, as by inhibiting the cAMP-specific phosphodiesterase or by stimulating the beta-adrenergic receptor cascade, are similarly effective for reducing capillary hyperpermeability.[93–96]

## Vascular Smooth Muscle Tone

The endothelium plays the key role in regulating vascular tone by releasing substances that modulate vascular smooth muscle contractility. cAMP itself has an important vasodilatory function, relaxing vascular smooth muscle[97] by either decreasing the concentration of intracellular calcium, required for actin-myosin bridging, or by inhibiting the myosin light-chain kinase, also an important participant in contractility. Perhaps the most important mediator of vascular smooth muscle relaxation is the formation by endothelium of NO, previously known as the endothelium-derived relaxation factor (EDRF),[98] from precursor L-arginine. NO causes relaxation of vascular smooth muscle by activating intracellular guanylate cyclase, causing an increase in cGMP levels.[99–101] Coronary ischemia/reperfusion dramatically suppresses the basal as well as stimulated generation of nitric oxide.[102–104] Although the synthesis of NO is ongoing during the ischemic phase, reoxygenation triggers a precipitous drop in NO—a decline caused by the quenching effect of ROS generated during reperfusion.[31,32] In addition to its vasodilatory function, NO subserves a number of other important vascular functions as well, such as inhibition of platelet adhesion and aggregation,[99,100,105,106] maintenance of restricted diffusion,[107] and inhibition of neutrophil adhesion.[102,108,109] In the heart, NO has other more organ-specific roles, such as its negative inotropic[110] and chronotropic[111] effects on the myocardium. NO may have two roles in terms of cardiac myocyte apoptosis—it may inhibit apoptotic myocyte death by nitrosylation of active sites of caspases[112] or, alternatively, it may directly contribute to apoptosis when levels are high.

The specific role of nitric oxide in damaging the myocardium and contributing to ischemia/reperfusion injury remains controversial. Several studies have demonstrated that the administration of NO donors[102,113,114] or induction/overexpression of the enzyme responsible for synthesis of NO[115,116] may potentially prevent myocardial ischemia/reperfusion injury. On the other hand, there is equally compelling evidence that pharmacologic inhibition of nitric oxide production may also reduce infarct size, probably by preventing peroxynitrite formation from NO and superoxide during reperfusion.[117–120]

## Contribution of Thrombosis to Myocardial Ischemia/Reperfusion Injury

The intact endothelium lining blood vessels has an anticoagulant phenotype that maintains blood fluidity. Normally the luminal surface of vascular endothelium repels platelets and coagulant events and prevents contact of the coagulation system with the subjacent and highly procoagulant endothelial matrix (which is rich in collagen and tissue factor).[121] The endothelial surface is rich in heparin-like proteoglycans that can function to accelerate the inactivation of coagulation proteases by antithrombin III. The other mechanism by which prevention of clot formation is achieved involves the membrane-spanning thrombin-binding protein thrombomodulin, which converts thrombin into a potent protein C activator.[122] In addition, local production of NO potently inhibits platelet aggregation.[105,123]

When oxygen availability is limited, as in myocardial ischemia, endothelium develops a procoagulant phenotype. Endothelial cell expression of thrombomodulin (both message and activity) is significantly reduced,[89] de novo synthesis of interleukin-1 in macrophages[124] or endothelial cells[125] can promote endothelial cell expression of tissue factor,[126] and the retraction of endothelial cell margins reveals subendothelial procoagulant matrix to circulating elements in the coagulation cascade. Additionally, hypoxia triggers the calcium-dependent exocytosis of Weibel-Palade bodies, leading to increased secretion of von Willebrand factor.[127] The rapid superoxide-mediated dissipation of NO also contributes to the local prothrombotic diathesis by potentiating platelet aggregation.

## Contribution of Inflammation to Myocardial Ischemia/Reperfusion Injury

A critical aspect of ischemia/reperfusion injury is the infiltration of polymorphonuclear leukocytes into the ischemic zone, which plays a central role in producing damage to myocardium.[128–132] Multiple chemotactic factors (components of complement activation C5a and C3a and leukotrienes) as well as cytokines, serve to activate the neutrophils and draw them into the area of ischemic injury. These proinflammatory cytokines include interleukin-1 (IL-1),[133,134] tumor necrosis factor (TNF),[135] and interleukin-8 (IL-8).[135,136] De novo synthesis of IL-1 occurred in endothelial cells exposed to hypoxia in cell culture as well as in in vivo experiments in which mice were subjected to hypoxic exposure. Similar studies have demonstrated that exposure to hypoxia leads to enhanced synthesis of IL-8 in endothelial cell culture and blood vessels.[137] As IL-8 is a potent neutrophil chemoattractant and activator, these studies are of great relevance to the pathogenesis of myocardial ischemia/reperfusion injury. Concurrent with formation of these cytokines is the upregulation of a number of adhesion molecules located both on endothelial cells and neutrophils. Ischemia/reperfusion drives expression of P-selectin, a member of the selectin family of glycoprotein adhesion receptors, which drives early neutrophil adhesion (via a rolling deceleration of circulating neutrophils). The importance of P-selectin as well as P-selectin glycoprotein adhesion ligand 1 (PSGL-1) has recently been verified in feline and other models of ischemic vascular injury.[138–141] Activation of endothelium with receptor agonists, such as thrombin and histamine,[142] as well as exposure of endothelial cells to ROS generated during reperfusion[38,39] promotes rapid surface expression of P-selectin,[143,144] with further rapid adhesion of neutrophils to the endothelial surface.[145] Other adhesion mechanisms act at later time points during the cascade of events, culminating in leukocyte adhesion and ultimately diapedesis. IL-1 and TNF are potent activators of adhesion molecule expression[124,126] as well as the further production of chemoattractive substances.[135] For instance, IL-1 significantly upregulates the endothelial cell expression of E-selectin[125] and intracellular adhesion molecule 1 (ICAM-1).[146] Recent observations have shown that oxidant injury to the endothelium also stimulates neutrophil adhesion through the rapid production of platelet activating factor (PAF), a lipid mediator of leukocyte adhesion.[147–149]

## ROLE OF ACTIVATED NEUTROPHILS

Neutrophils (polymorphonuclear leukocytes, or PMNs) have long been believed to participate in the pathogenesis of myocardial ischemia/reperfusion damage.[132,150–155] Infiltration of PMNs into the ischemic zone begins within 60 min of the onset of ischemia and increases significantly for up to 90 min after reperfusion. Activated neutrophils are able to elicit myocardial injury through different mechanisms. At sites of accumulation, activated PMNs release a veritable firestorm of caustic chemicals into the vicinity; these include hypochlorous acid, superoxide, hydrogen peroxide, singlet oxygen, and cytotoxic lysosomal enzymes (elastase, the metalloproteases collagenase and gelatinase, neutral proteases, and heparinase).[156] Chemotaxic factors such as C5a, PAF, and cytokines are also released in the vicinity and are capable of further activating neutrophils. Stimulation of PMNs by one or more of these factors elicits the respiratory burst characterized by sudden release of oxygen-derived free radicals, including superoxide anion, hypochlorous acid, hydroxyl radical, chloramine, and hydrogen peroxide.[156] This cytotoxic milieu damages endothelial cells and impairs physiologic vasodilatory and anticoagulant mechanisms. It promotes further increases in vascular permeability and stimulates neutrophil and platelet adhesion as well. Evidence for the role of leukocytes in ischemia/reperfusion injury comes from studies showing the protective effects of neutrophil depletion through administration of nonsteroidal anti-inflammatory drugs (such as ibuprofen) prior to ischemia/reperfusion[150] or by interfering with PMN adhesive mechanisms.[157,158]

A number of events must occur in order to recruit a sufficient number of neutrophils to elicit myocardial damage in the setting of ischemia/reperfusion. Neutrophils are first activated and attracted by specific chemotactic factors, such as fragments generated during complement activation (C3a and C5a)[156] as well as by IL-8.[159–161] PMNs are decelerated in their transit by initially engaging the activated endothelial surface by rolling, a process mediated by P-selectin on the endothelial cell and its carbohydrate ligand sialyl Lewis$^x$ on the PMN.[162] This interaction brings the neutrophils into close approximation with the vascular wall to engage other cognate receptors, such as L-selectin, PAF, ICAM-1 on the endothelial cells, and leukocyte beta$_2$ integrins (CD11/CD18 complex) on the PMNs.[156]

## ROLE OF THE COMPLEMENT SYSTEM

Recent studies have focused on the role of the complement cascade in ischemia/reperfusion injury.[111,112,163] Briefly, the complement system consists of three components, the classic pathway, the alternative pathway, and the mannose-binding pathway. These are activated by proteolytic cascades in a similar manner as the activation of the coagulation system. These pathways converge at the C3 component, the cleavage of which leads to the formation of anaphylatoxins (C3a and C5a) plus the amphiphilic membrane attack complex (MAC), consisting of complement components C5a to C9. This complex inserts itself into membranes and essentially "punctures" the cell, causing rapid dissipation of ionic gradients and extrusion of cytoplasmic contents.

Two primary mechanisms have been described to explain how complement activation elicits damage to myocardium. The first is brought about by the generation of chemotactic factors and anaphylatoxins (C3a, C4a, and C5a), which stimulate mast cells and basophils to release histamine, thus increasing vascular permeability as well as attracting neutrophils to the ischemic area. Activation of the complement system also causes direct myocardial damage through the formation of the MAC (C5b to C9), which has been detected using immunohistochemical techniques in areas of myocardial infarction, with relatively little deposition in adjacent nonischemic regions.[164] Even small amounts of C5b to C9, below the threshold levels required for cell lysis, may precipitate translocation of P-selectin to the endothelial surface, further contributing to neutrophil adhesion.[165]

A number of studies have demonstrated that the ROS generated upon reoxygenation has the ability to activate the complement cascade by converting C5 to a C5b active form. It is also an important observation that ischemia and reperfusion may metabolically impair the myocardial and endothelial cells, increasing their vulnerability to attack by complement. There is a plethora of evidence from experimental models indicating that local activation of the complement system is harmful to the heart.[154,164,166] In other studies, depletion of complement by the administration of cobra venom toxin significantly reduced ischemic injury.[154,167] Other strategies to eliminate the deleterious effect of complement cascade activation on myocardium that have been investigated have used a soluble complement inhibitor (sCR-1) or a C1 esterase inhibitor.[168–170]

## CONCLUSION

Despite considerable progress, the pathophysiology of cardiac ischemia/reperfusion has not been definitively deciphered. The entire process of myocardial injury due to ischemia/reperfusion can be thought of as a complex interaction between myocardial cells and surrounding tissue. A number of recruited cellular effector mechanisms (neutrophils, platelets), humoral factors (cytokines), components of coagulation and complement cascade and chemical species (ROS, lytic enzymes) are involved. Despite all of the recent advances, a burning question still remains: to what extent is the reperfusion after ischemia responsible for myocardial injury? Would therapeutic interventions designed to reduce endothelial dysfunction limit the consequences of leukocyte and complement activation and thereby be beneficial to the patient in the throes of a myocardial infarction? A detailed understanding of the mechanisms of myocardial ischemia and reperfusion will significantly guide the development of novel therapeutic strategies that could play an adjunctive role, along with thrombolytic therapy or percutaneous revascularization, in the treatment of acute myocardial infarction.

## References

1. Jennings RB. Myocardial ischemia observations, definitions, and speculations. *J Mol Cell Cardiol* 1970;1:345–349.
2. Sayen JJ, Sheldon WF, Pierce G, Kuo PT. Polarigraphic oxygen, the epicardial electrocardiogram and muscle contraction in experimental acute regional ischemia of the left ventricle. *Circ Res* 1958;6:779–798.
3. Braasch W, Gudbjarnason S, Puri PS, et al. Early changes in energy metabolism in the myocardium following acute coronary artery occlusion in anesthetized dogs. *Circ Res* 1968;23:429–438.
4. Jennings RB. Early phase of myocardial ischemic injury and infarction. *Am J Cardiol* 1969;24:753–765.
5. Katz AM, Hecht HH. The early "pump" failure of the ischemic heart. *Am J Med* 1969;47:497–501.
6. Kloner RA, Ellis SG, Lange R, Braunwald E. Studies of experimental coronary artery reperfusion. Effects on infarct size, myocardial

function, biochemistry, ultrastructure and microvascular damage. *Circulation* 1983;68:8–15.

7. Herdson PB, Kaltenbach JP, Jennings RB. Fine structural and biochemical changes in dog myocardium during autolysis. *Am J Pathol* 1969;57:539–557.
8. Krug A. Der Fruhnachweis des Herzinfarktes durch Bestimmung der Wasserstoffionenkonzentration im Herzmuskel mit Idicatorpapier. *Virchows Arch* 1965;338:339–341.
9. Berne RM, Rubio R. Acute coronary occlusion: Early changes that induce coronary dilatation and the development of collateral circulation. *Am J Cardiol* 1969;24:776–781.
10. Harris AS, Bisteni A, Russell RA, et al. Excitatory factors in ventricular tachycardia resulting from myocardial ischemia: Potassium is a major excitant. *Science* 1954;119:200–203.
11. Corr PB, Gross RW, Sobel BE. Arrhythmogenic amphiphilic lipids and the myocardial cell membrane. *J Mol Cell Cardiol* 1982;14:619–626.
12. Ferrari R, Ceconi C, Curello S, et al. Myocardial damage during ischaemia and reperfusion. *Eur Heart J* 1993;14(suppl G):25–30.
13. Jennings RB, Sommers HM, Smyth GA, et al. Myocardial necrosis induced by temporary occlusion of a coronary artery in the dog. *AMA Arch Pathol* 1960;70:68–78.
14. Tennant R, Wiggers CJ. The effect of coronary occlusion on myocardial contraction. *Am J Physiol* 1935;112:351–361.
15. Sobel RE. Acute myocardial infarction. In: Pasternak RC, Braunwald E, eds. *Heart Disease, A Textbook of Cardiovascular Medicine.* Philadelphia: Saunders; 1992:1200–1272.
16. Kloner RA, Rude RE, Carlson N, et al. Ultrastructural evidence of microvascular damage and myocardial cell injury after coronary artery occlusion: Which comes first? *Circulation* 1980;62:945–952.
17. Kloner RA, DeBoer LW, Carlson N, Braunwald E. The effect of verapamil on myocardial ultrastructure during and following release of coronary artery occlusion. *Exp Mol Pathol* 1982;36:277–286.
18. Jennings RB, Reimer KA. Salvage of ischemic myocardium. *Mod Concepts Cardiovasc Dis* 1974;43:125–130.
19. Garcia-Dorado D, Oliveras J. Myocardial oedema: A preventable cause of reperfusion injury? *Cardiovasc Res* 1993;27:1555–1563.
20. Garcia-Dorado D, Theroux P, Munoz R, et al. Favorable effects of hyperosmotic reperfusion on myocardial edema and infarct size. *Am J Physiol* 1992;262:H17–H22.
21. Steenbergen C, Hill ML, Jennings RB. Volume regulation and plasma membrane injury in aerobic, anaerobic, and ischemic myocardium in vitro. Effects of osmotic cell swelling on plasma membrane integrity. *Circ Res* 1985;57:864–875.
22. Dauber IM, Vanbenthuysen KM, McMurtry IF, et al. Functional coronary microvascular injury evident as increased permeability due to brief ischemia and reperfusion. *Circ Res* 1990;66:986–998.
23. Pilati CF. Macromolecular transport in canine coronary microvasculature. *Am J Physiol* 1990;258:H748–H753.
24. Jennings RB, Ganote CE, Reimer KA. Ischemic tissue injury. *Am J Pathol* 1975;81:179–198.
25. Jennings RB, Schaper J, Hill ML, et al. Effect of reperfusion late in the phase of reversible ischemic injury. Changes in cell volume, electrolytes, metabolites, and ultrastructure. *Circ Res* 1985;56:262–278.
26. Baroldi G. Different types of myocardial necrosis in coronary heart disease: A pathophysiologic review of their functional significance. *Am Heart J* 1975;89:742–752.
27. Hutchins GM, Bulkley BH. Correlation of myocardial contraction band necrosis and vascular patency. A study of coronary artery bypass graft anastomoses at branch points. *Lab Invest* 1977;36:642–648.
28. Adams JE, Abendschein DR, Jaffe AS. Biochemical markers of myocardial injury. Is MB creatine kinase the choice for the 1990s? *Circulation* 1993;88:750–763.
29. Devries SR, Jaffe AS, Geltman EM, Sobel BE, Abendschein DR. Enzymatic estimation of the extent of irreversible myocardial injury early after reperfusion. *Am Heart J* 1989;117:31–36.
30. Kloner RA. Does reperfusion injury exist in humans? *J Am Coll Cardiol* 1993;21:537–545.
31. Lefer AM, Tsao PS, Lefer DJ, Ma X-L. Role of endothelial dysfunction in the pathogenesis of reperfusion injury after myocardial ischemia. *FASEB Journal* 1991;5:2029–2034.
32. Pinsky DJ, Oz MC, Koga S, et al. Cardiac preservation is enhanced in a heterotopic rat transplant model by supplementing the nitric oxide pathway. *J Clin Invest* 1994;93:2291–2297.
33. Bolli R. Basic and clinical aspects of myocardial stunning. *Prog Cardiovasc Dis* 1998;40:477–516.
34. Appleyard RF, Cohn LH. Myocardial stunning and reperfusion injury in cardiac surgery. *J Card Surg* 1993;8:316–324.
35. Bolli RF, Marban E. Molecular and cellular mechanisms of myocardial stunning. *Physiol Rev* 1999;79:609–634.
36. Reimer KA, Vander Heide RS, Richard VJ. Reperfusion in acute myocardial infarction: Effect of timing and modulating factors in experimental models. *Am J Cardiol* 1993;72:13G–21G.
37. Zhang Y, Bissing JW, Xu L, et al. Nitric oxide synthase inhibitors decrease coronary sinus-free radical concentration and ameliorate myocardial stunning in an ischemia-reperfusion model. *J Am Coll Cardiol* 2003;38:546–554.
38. Zweier JL, Kuppusamy P, Lutty GA. Measurement of endothelial cell free radical generation: Evidence for a central mechanism of free radical injury in postischemic tissues. *Proceedings of the National Academy of Sciences of the United States of America* 1988;85:4046–4050.
39. Babbs CF, Cregor MD, Turek JJ, Badylak SF. Endothelial superoxide production in the isolated rat heart during early reperfusion after ischemia. A histochemical study. *Am J Pathol* 1991;139:1069–1080.
40. Kramer JH, Arroyo CM, Dickens BF, Weglicki WB. Spin-trapping evidence that graded myocardial ischemia alters post-ischemic superoxide production. *Free Radic Biol Med* 1987;3:153–159.
41. McCord JM, Roy RS, Schaffer SW. Free radicals and myocardial ischemia. The role of xanthine oxidase. *Adv Myocardiol* 1985;5:183–189.
42. Zweier JL, Rayburn BK, Flaherty JT, Weisfeldt ML. Recombinant superoxide dismutase reduces oxygen free radical concentrations in reperfused myocardium. *J Clin Invest* 1987;80:1728–1734.
43. Bolli R, Patel BS, Jeroudi MO, et al. Demonstration of free radical generation in "stunned" myocardium of intact dogs with the use of the spin trap alpha-phenyl N-tert-butyl nitrone. *J Clin Invest* 1988;82:476–485.
44. McCord JM. Oxygen-derived free radicals in postischemic tissue injury. [Review.] *N Engl J Med* 1985;312:159–163.
45. Lefer DJ, Scalia R, Nossuli T, et al. Peroxynitrite inhibits leukocyte-endothelial cell interactions and protects against ischemia-reperfusion injury in rats. *J Clin Invest* 1997;99:684–691.
46. Mehta JL, Nichols W, Donnelly W, et al. Protection by superoxide dismutase from myocardial dysfunction and attenuation of vasodilator reserve after coronary occlusion and reperfusion in dog. *Circ Res* 1989;65:1283–1295.
47. Ide T, Tsutsui H, Kinugawa S, et al. Mitochondrial electron transport complex I is a potential source of oxygen free radicals in the failing myocardium. *Circ Res* 1999;85:357–363.
48. Boveris A, Chance B. The mitochondrial generation of hydrogen peroxide. General properties and effect of hyperbaric oxygen. *Biochemical Journal* 1973;134:707–716.
49. Lucchesi BR, Werns SW, Fantone JC. The role of the neutrophil and free radicals in ischemic myocardial injury. *J Mol Cell Cardiol* 1989;21:1241–1251.
50. Halliwell B. Oxidants and human disease: Some new concepts. *FASEB J* 1987;1:358–364.
51. Eddy J, Stewart R, Jones H, et al. Xantine oxidase is detected in ischemic rat heart but not in human hearts. *Physiologist* 1986;29:166–170.
52. Eddy LJ, Stewart JR, Jones HP, et al. Free radical-producing enzyme, xanthine oxidase, is undetectable in human hearts. *Am J Physiol* 1987;253:H709–H711.
53. Muxfeldt M, Schaper W. The activity of xanthine oxidase in heart of pigs, guinea pigs, rabbits, rats, and humans. *Basic Res Cardiol* 1987;82:486–492.
54. Gutteridge JMC. Aspects to consider when detecting and measuring lipid peroxidation. *Free Radic Res Commun* 1986;1:173–184.

55. Roberts MJ, Young IS, Trouton TG, et al. Transient release of lipid peroxides after coronary artery balloon angioplasty. *Lancet* 1990;336: 143–145.
56. Davies SW, Ranjadayalan K, Wickens DG, et al. Lipid peroxidation associated with successful thrombolysis. *Lancet* 1990;335:741–743.
57. Hearse DJ. Stunning: A radical review. *Cardiovasc Drugs Ther* 1991; 5:853–876.
58. Heusch G. Myocardial stunning: A role for calcium antagonists during ischaemia? *Cardiovasc Res* 1992;26:14–19.
59. Whalen DA Jr, Hamilton DG, Ganote CE, Jennings RB. Effect of a transient period of ischemia on myocardial cells. I. Effects on cell volume regulation. *Am J Pathol* 1974;74:381–397.
60. Shen AC, Jennings RB. Kinetics of calcium accumulation in acute myocardial ischemic injury. *Am J Pathol* 1972;67:441–452.
61. Kloner RA, Ganote CE, Whalen DA Jr, Jennings RB. Effect of a transient period of ischemia on myocardial cells. II. Fine structure during the first few minutes of reflow. *Am J Pathol* 1974;74:399–422.
62. Pinsky D, Oz M, Liao H, et al. Restoration of the cAMP second messenger pathway enhances cardiac preservation for transplantation in a heterotopic rat model. *J Clin Invest* 1993;92:2994–3002.
63. Kloner RA. No reflow revisited. *J Am Coll Cardiol* 1989;14: 1814–1815.
64. Schofer J, Montz R, Mathey DG. Scintigraphic evidence of the "no reflow" phenomenon in human beings after coronary thrombolysis. *J Am Coll Cardiol* 1985;5:593–598.
65. Braunwald E, Kloner RA. The stunned myocardium: Prolonged, postischemic ventricular dysfunction. *Circulation* 1982;66:1146–1149.
66. Bolli R. Mechanism of myocardial "stunning." *Circulation* 1990;82: 723–738.
67. Takeishi Y, Tono-oka I, Kubota I, et al. Functional recovery of hibernating myocardium after coronary bypass surgery: Does it coincide with improvement in perfusion? *Am Heart J* 1991;122:665–670.
68. Stack RS, Phillips HR, Grierson DS, et al. Functional improvement of jeopardized myocardium following intracoronary streptokinase infusion in acute myocardial infarction. *J Clin Invest* 1983;72: 84–95.
69. Corretti MC, Koretsune Y, Kusuoka H, et al. Glycolytic inhibition and calcium overload as consequences of exogenously generated free radicals in rabbit hearts. *J Clin Invest* 1991;88:1014–1025.
70. Owen P, Dennis S, Opie LH. Glucose flux rate regulates onset of ischemic contracture in globally underperfused rat hearts. *Circ Res* 1990;66:344–354.
71. Opie LH. The mechanism of myocyte death in ischaemia. *Eur Heart J* 1993;14(suppl G):31–33.
72. Ferrari R, Alfieri O, Curello S, et al. Occurrence of oxidative stress during reperfusion of the human heart. *Circulation* 1990;81:201–211.
73. Dennis SC, Gevers W, Opie LH. Protons in ischemia: Where do they come from? Where do they go to? *J Mol Cell Cardiol* 1991;23: 1077–1086.
74. Gottlieb RA, Burleson KO, Kloner RA, et al. Reperfusion injury induces apoptosis in rabbit cardiomyocytes. *J Clin Invest* 1994;94: 1621–1628.
75. Stadler B, Phillips J, Toyoda Y, et al. Adenosine-enhanced ischemic preconditioning modulates necrosis and apoptosis: Effects of stunning and ischemia-reperfusion. *Ann Thorac Surg* 2003;72:555–563.
76. Xie YW, Wolin MS. Role of nitric oxide and its interaction with superoxide in the suppression of cardiac muscle mitochondrial respiration. Involvement in response to hypoxia/reoxygenation. *Circulation* 1996; 94:2580–2586.
77. Thornberry NA, Lazebnik Y. Caspases: Enemies within. *Science* 1998; 281:1312–1316.
78. Ashkenazi A, Dixit VM. Death receptors: Signaling and modulation. *Science* 1998;281:1305–1308.
79. Green DR, Reed JC. Mitochondria and apoptosis. *Science* 1998;281: 1309–1312.
80. Atlante A, Calissano P, Bobba A, et al. Cytochrome *c* is released from mitochondria in a reactive oxygen species (ROS)-dependent fashion and can operate as a ROS scavenger and as a respiratory substrate in cerebellar neurons undergoing excitotoxic death. *J Biol Chem* 2003; 275:3759–3766.
81. Sawamura T, Kume N, Aoyama T, et al. An endothelial receptor for oxidized low-density lipoprotein. *Nature* 1997;386:73–77.
82. Li DY, Chen HJ, Staples ED, et al. Oxidized low-density lipoprotein receptor LOX-1 and apoptosis in human atherosclerotic lesions. *J Cardiovasc Pharmacol Ther* 2002;7:147–153.
83. Kataoka H, Kume N, Miyamoto S, et al. Oxidized LDL modulates Bax/Bcl-2 through the lectinlike Ox-LDL receptor-1 in vascular smooth muscle cells. *Arterioscler Thromb Vasc Biol* 2001;21:955–960.
84. Iwai-Kanai E, Hasegawa K, Sawamura T, et al. Activation of lectin-like oxidized low-density lipoprotein receptor-1 induces apoptosis in cultured neonatal rat cardiac myocytes. *Circulation* 2001;104: 2948–2954.
85. Li DY, Zhang YC, Philips ME, et al. Upregulation of endothelial receptor for oxidized low-density lipoprotein (LOX-1) in cultured human coronary artery endothelial cells by angiotensin II type 1 receptor activation. *Circ Res* 1999;84:1043–1049.
86. Nagase M, Ando K, Nagase T, et al. Redox-sensitive regulation of LOX-1 gene expression in vascular endothelium. *Biochem Biophys Res Commun* 2003;281:720–725.
87. Kume N, Murase T, Moriwaki H, et al. Inducible expression of lectin-like oxidized LDL receptor-1 in vascular endothelial cells. *Circ Res* 1998;83:322–337.
88. Kataoka K, Hasegawa K, Sawamura T, et al. LOX-1 pathway affects the extent of myocardial ischemia-reperfusion injury. *Biochem Biophys Res Commun* 2003;300:656–660.
89. Ogawa S, Gerlach H, Esposito C, et al. Hypoxia modulates the barrier and coagulant function of cultured bovine endothelium. Increased monolayer permeability and induction of procoagulant properties. *J Clin Invest* 1990;85:1090–1098.
90. Ogawa S, Shreeniwas R, Brett J, et al. The effect of hypoxia on capillary endothelial cell function: Modulation of barrier and coagulant function. *Br J Haematol* 1990;75:517–524.
91. Stelzner TJ, O'Brien RF, Sato K, Weil JV. Hypoxia-induced increases in pulmonary transvascular protein escape in rats. Modulation by glucocorticoids. *J Clin Invest* 1988;82:1840–1847.
92. Ogawa S, Koga S, Kuwabara K, et al. Hypoxia-induced increased permeability of endothelial monolayers occurs through lowering of cellular cAMP levels. *Am J Physiol* 1992;262:C546–C554.
93. Minnear FL, Johnson A, Malik AB. Beta-adrenergic modulation of pulmonary transvascular fluid and protein exchange. *J Appl Physiol* 1986;60:266–274.
94. Minnear FL, DeMichele MA, Moon DG, et al. Isoproterenol reduces thrombin-induced pulmonary endothelial permeability in vitro. *Am J Physiol* 1989;257:H1613–H1623.
95. Farrukh IS, Gurtner GH, Michael JR. Pharmacological modification of pulmonary vascular injury: Possible role of cAMP. *J Appl Physiol* 1987;62:47–54.
96. Stelzner TJ, Weil JV, O'Brien RF. Role of cyclic adenosine monophosphate in the induction of endothelial barrier properties. *J Cell Physiol* 1989;139:157–166.
97. Haynes J Jr, Robinson J, Saunders L, et al. Role of cAMP-dependent protein kinase in cAMP-mediated vasodilation. *Am J Physiol* 1992; 262:H511–H516.
98. Feelisch M, te Poel M, Zamora R, et al. Understanding the controversy over the identity of EDRF. *Nature* 1994;368:62–65.
99. Lefer DJ, Nakanishi K, Johnston WE, Vinten-Johansen J. Antineutrophil and myocardial protecting actions of a novel nitric oxide donor after acute myocardial ischemia and reperfusion in dogs. *Circulation* 1993;88(Pt 1):2337–2350.
100. Sneddon JM, Vane JR. Endothelium-derived relaxing factor reduces platelet adhesion to bovine endothelial cells. *Proc Natl Acad Sci USA* 1988;85:2800–2804.
101. Moncada S, Palmer RM, Higgs EA. Nitric oxide: Physiology, pathophysiology, and pharmacology. *Pharmacol Rev* 1991;43:109–142.
102. Lefer DJ. Myocardial protective actions of nitric oxide donors after myocardial ischemia and reperfusion. *New Horiz* 1995;3:105–112.

103. Lefer DJ, Nakanishi K, Vinten-Johansen J. Endothelial and myocardial cell protection by a cysteine-containing nitric oxide donor after myocardial ischemia and reperfusion. *J Cardiovasc Pharmacol* 1993;22: S34–S43.
104. Weyrich AS, Ma X-L, Lefer AM. The role of L-arginine in ameliorating reperfusion injury after myocardial ischemia in the cat. *Circulation* 1992;86:279–288.
105. Radomski MW, Palmer RM, Moncada S. Endogenous nitric oxide inhibits human platelet adhesion to vascular endothelium. *Lancet* 1987; 2(8567):1057–1058.
106. Groves PH, Lewis MJ, Cheadle HA, Penny WJ. SIN-1 reduces platelet adhesion and platelet thrombus formation in a porcine model of balloon angioplasty. *Circulation* 1993;87:590–597.
107. Kubes P, Granger DN. Nitric oxide modulates microvascular permeability. *Am J Physiol* 1992;262:H611–H615.
108. Kubes P, Suzuki M, Granger DN. Nitric oxide: An endogenous modulator of leukocyte adhesion. *Proc Natl Acad Sci USA* 1991;88:4651–4655.
109. Jones SP, Giron WG, Palazzo AJ, et al. Myocardial ischemia-reperfusion injury is exacerbated in absence of endothelial cell nitric oxide synthase. *Am J Physiol* 1999;276:H1567–1573.
110. Finkel MS, Oddis CV, Jacob TD, et al. Negative inotropic effects of cytokines on the heart mediated by nitric oxide. *Science* 1992;257: 387–389.
111. Balligand JL, Kelly RA, Marsden PA, et al. Control of cardiac muscle cell function by an endogenous nitric oxide switches apoptosis to necrosis. *Exp Cell Res* 1993;249:396–403.
112. Leist M, Single B, Haumann H, et al. Inhibition of mitochondrial ATP generation by nitric oxide switches apoptosis to necrosis. *Exp Cell Res* 1999;249:396–403.
113. Mizuno T, Watanabe M, Sakamoto T, Sunamori M. L-arginine, a nitric oxide precursor, attenuates ischemia-reperfusion injury by inhibiting inositol-1, 4, 5-triphosphate. *J Thorac Cardiovasc Surg* 1998;115: 931–996.
114. Beresewicz A, Karwatowska-Prokopczuk E, Lewartowski B, et al. A protective role of nitric oxide in isolated ischaemic/reperfused rat heart. *Cardiovasc Res* 1995;30:1001–1008.
115. Kanno S, Lee PC, Zhang Y, et al. Attenuation of myocardial ischemia/reperfusion injury by superinduction of inducible nitric oxide synthase. *Circulation* 2000;101:2742–2748.
116. Brunner F, Maier R, Andrew P, et al. Attenuation of myocardial ischemia/reperfusion injury in mice with myocyte-specific overexpression of endothelial nitric oxide synthase. *Cardiovasc Res* 2003;57: 55–62.
117. Parrino PE, Laubach VE, Gaughen JR, et al. Inhibition of inducible nitric oxide synthase after myocardial ischemia increases coronary flow. *Ann Thorac Surg* 1998;66:733–779.
118. Flogel U, Decking UK, Godecke A, Schrader J. Contribution of NO to ischemia-reperfusion injury in the saline-perfused heart: A study in endothelial NO synthase knockout mice. *J Mol Cell Cardiol* 1999;31: 827–836.
119. Igarashi J, Nishida M, Hoshida S, et al. Inducible nitric oxide synthase augments injury elicited by oxidative stress in rat cardiac myocytes. *Am J Physiol* 1998;274:C245–C252.
120. Woolfson RG, Patel VC, Neild GH, Yellon DM. Inhibition of nitric oxide synthesis reduces infarct size by an adenosine-dependent mechanism. *Circulation* 1995;91:1545–1551.
121. Gerlach H, Clauss M, Ogawa S, Stern D. *Perturbation of Endothelial Barrier and Coagulant Properties by Environmental Factors: Endothelial Cell Dysfunction*. New York: Plenum Press; 1991:525–545.
122. Esmon C. The regulation of natural anticoagulant pathways. *Science* 1987;235(4794):1348–1352.
123. Broekman MJ, Eiroa A, Marcus A. Inhibition of human platelet reactivity by endothelium-derived relaxing factor from human umbilical vein endothelial cells in suspension: Blockade of aggregation and secretion by an aspirin-insensitive mechanism. *Blood* 1991;78(4):1033–1040.
124. Koga S, Ogawa S, Kuwabara K, et al. Synthesis and release of interleukin 1 by reoxygenated human mononuclear phagocytes. *J Clin Invest* 1992;90:1007–1015.
125. Shreeniwas R, Koga S, Karakurum M, et al. Hypoxia-mediated induction of endothelial cell interleukin-1$\alpha$. An autocrine mechanism promoting expression of leukocyte adhesion molecules on the vessel surface. *J Clin Invest* 1992;90:2333–2339.
126. Pober J. Cytokine-mediated activation of vascular endothelium. *Am J Pathol* 1988;133:416–422.
127. Oz M, Rose E, Michler R, et al. Coronary vascular endothelium may release contents of Weibel-Palade bodies but does not shed membrane proteins during cardiac surgery. *Circulation* 1993;88(suppl):I-247–I-250.
128. Horgan MJ, Wright SD, Malik AB. Antibody against leukocyte integrin (CD18) prevents reperfusion-induced lung vascular injury. *Am J Physiol* 1990;259:L315–L319.
129. Simpson PJ, Todd RF, Fantone JC, et al. Reduction of experimental canine myocardial reperfusion injury by a monoclonal antibody (anti-Mo1, anti-CD11b) that inhibits leukocyte adhesion. *J Clin Invest* 1988; 81:624–629.
130. Repine JE, Cheronis JC, Rodell TC, et al. Pulmonary oxygen toxicity and ischemia-reperfusion injury. A mechanism in common involving xanthine oxidase and neutrophils. *Am Rev Respir Dis* 1987;136: 483–485.
131. Colletti LM, Remick DG, Burtch GD, et al. Role of tumor necrosis factor-alpha in the pathophysiologic alterations after hepatic ischemia/reperfusion injury in the rat. *J Clin Invest* 1990;85:1936–1943.
132. Dreyer WJ, Michael LH, West M, et al. Neutrophil accumulation in ischemic canine myocardium. Insights into time course, distribution, and mechanism of localization during early reperfusion. *Circulation* 1991;84:400–411.
133. Dinarello CA. Interleukin-1 and its biologically related cytokines. *Adv Immunol* 1989;44:153–205.
134. Sherry B, Cerami A. Cachectin/tumor necrosis factor exerts endocrine, paracrine, and autocrine control of inflammatory responses. *J Cell Biol* 1988;107:1269–1277.
135. Strieter RM, Kunkel SL, Showell HJ, et al. Endothelial cell gene expression of a neutrophil chemotactic factor by TNF-alpha, LPS, and IL-1 beta. *Science* 1989;243:1467–1469.
136. Baggiolini M, Walz A, Kunkel SL. Neutrophil-activating peptide-1/interleukin 8, a novel cytokine that activates neutrophils. *J Clin Invest* 1989;84:1045–1049.
137. Karakurum M, Shreeniwas R, Chen J, et al. Hypoxic induction of interleukin-8 gene expression in human endothelial cells. *J Clin Invest* 1994;93:1564–1570.
138. Weyrich AS, Ma XY, Lefer DJ, et al. In vivo neutralization of P-selectin protects feline heart and endothelium in myocardial ischemia and reperfusion injury. *J Clin Invest* 1993;91:2620–2629.
139. Hattori R, Hamilton K, Fugate R, et al. Stimulated secretion of endothelial vWF is accompanied by rapid redistribution to cell surface of the intrecellular granule membrane protein GMP-140. *J Biol Chem* 1989;264:7768–7771.
140. McEver RP, Beckstead JH, Moore KL, et al. GMP-140, a platelet $\alpha$-granule membrane protein, is also synthesized by vascular endothelial cell and is localized in Weibel-Palade bodies. *J Clin Invest* 1989;84: 92–99.
141. Ewenstein BM, Warhol MJ, Handin RI, Pober JS. Composition of the von Willebrand factor storage organelle (Weibel-Palade body) isolated from cultured human umbilical vein endothelial cells. *J Cell Biol* 1987;104:1423–1433.
142. Birch KA, Pober JS, Zavoico GB, et al. Calcium/calmodulin transduces thrombin-stimulated secretion: Studies in intact and minimally permeabilized human umbilical vein endothelial cells. *J Cell Biol* 1992;118:1501–1510.
143. Lorant DE, Patel KD, McIntyre TM, et al. Coexpression of GMP-140 and PAF by endothelium stimulated by histamine or thrombin: A juxtacrine system for adhesion and activation of neutrophils. *J Cell Biol* 1991;115:223–234.
144. Patel KD, Zimmerman GA, Prescott SM, et al. Oxygen radicals induce human endothelial cells to express GMP-140 and bind neutrophils. *J Cell Biol* 1991;112:749–759.

145. Geng J-G, Bevilacqua MP, Moore KL, et al. Rapid neutrophil adhesion to activated endothelium mediated by GMP-140. *Nature* 1990;343: 757–760.
146. Vadas MA, Gamble JR. Regulation of the adhesion of neutrophils to endothelium. *Biochem Pharmacol* 1990;40:1683–1687.
147. Yoshida N, Granger DN, Anderson DC, et al. Anoxia/reoxygenation-induced neutrophil adherence to cultured endothelial cells. *Am J Physiol* 1992;262:H1891–H1898.
148. Arnould T, Michiels C, Remacle J. Increased PMN adherence on endothelial cells after hypoxia: Involvement of PAF, CD18/CD11b, and ICAM-1. *Am J Physiol* 1993;264:C1102–C1110.
149. Kubes P, Ibbotson G, Russell J, et al. Role of platelet-activating factor in ischemia/reperfusion-induced leukocyte adherence. *Am J Physiol* 1990;259:G300-G305.
150. Hoffmann G, Gobel B, Harbrecht U, et al. Platelet cAMP and cGMP in essential hypertension. *Am J Hypertens* 1992;5:847–850.
151. Mullane KM, Read N, Salmon JS, Moncada S. Role of leukocytes in acute myocardial infarction in anesthetized dogs: Relationship to myocardial salvage by anti-inflammatory drugs. *J Pharmacol Exp Ther* 1984;228:510–521.
152. Lucchesi B, Mullane K. Leukocytes and ischemia-induced myocardial injury. *Annu Rev Pharmacol Toxicol* 1986;26:201–224.
153. Entman M, Michael L, Rossen R, et al. Inflammation in the course of early myocardial ischemia. *FASEB J* 1991;5(11):2529–2537.
154. Crawford MH, Grover FL, Kolb WP, et al. Complement and neutrophil activation in the pathogenesis of ischemic myocardial injury. *Circulation* 1988;78:1449–1458.
155. Kurose I, Wolf R, Grisham MB, Granger N. Effects of an endogenous inhibitor of nitric oxide synthesis on postcapillary venules. *Am J Physiol* 1995;268:H2224–H2231.
156. Kilgore KS, Lucchesi BR. Reperfusion injury after myocardial infarction: The role of free radicals and the inflammatory response. *Clin Biochem* 1993;359:370.
157. Ma XL, Lefer DJ, Lefer AM, Rothlein R. Coronary endothelial and cardiac protective effects of a monoclonal antibody to intercellular adhesion molecule-1 in myocardial ischemia and reperfusion. *Circulation* 1992;86(3):937–946.
158. Ma XL, Tsao PS, Lefer AM. Antibody to CD-18 exerts endothelial and cardiac protective effects in myocardial ischemia and reperfusion. *J Clin Invest* 1991;88(4):1237–1243.
159. Rot A. Endothelial cell binding of NAP-1/IL-8: Role in neutrophil emigration. *Immunol Today* 1992;13:291–294.
160. Peveri P, Walz A, Dewald B, Baggiolini M. A novel neutrophil-activating factor produced by human mononuclear phagocytes. *J Exp Med* 1988;167:1547–1549.
161. Detmers PA, Lo SK, Olsen-Egbert E, et al. Neutrophil-activating protein 1/interleukin 8 stimulates the binding activity of the leukocyte adhesion receptor CD11b/CD18 on human neutrophils. *J Exp Med* 1990;171:1155–1562.
162. Mayadas TN, Johnson RC, Rayburn H, et al. Leukoctye rolling and extravasation are severely compromised in P selectin-deficient mice. *Cell* 1993;74:541–554.
163. Hill JH, Ward P. The physiologic role of C3 leukotactic fragments in myocardial infarcts of rats. *J Exp Med* 1971;133(4):885–900.
164. Homeister JW, Satoh P, Lucchesi BR. Effects of complement activation in the isolated heart. Role of the terminal complement components. *Circ Res* 1992;71:303–319.
165. Hattori R, Hamilton KK, McEver RP, Sims PJ. Complement proteins C5b-9 induce secretion of high molecular weight multimers of endothelial von Willebrand factor and translocation of granule membrane protein GMP-140 to the cell surface. *J Biol Chem* 1989;264:9053–9060.
166. Homeister JW, Satoh PS, Kilgore KS, Lucchesi BR. Soluble complement receptor type 1 prevents human complement-mediated damage of the rabbit isolated heart. *J Immunol* 1993;150:1055–1064.
167. Maroko PR, Carpenter CB, Chiariello M, et al. Reduction by cobra venom factor of myocardial necrosis after coronary artery occlusion. *J Clin Invest* 1978;61:661–670.
168. Weisman HF, Bartow T, Leppo MK, et al. Soluble human complement receptor type 1: In vivo inhibitor of complement suppression post-ischemic myocardial inflammation and necrosis. *Science* 1990;249: 146–151.
169. Homeister JW, Lucchesi BR. Complement activation and inhibition in myocardial ischemia and reperfusion injury. *Annu Rev Pharmacol Toxicol* 1994;34:17–40.
170. Pugsley MK, Abramova M, Cole T, et al. Inhibitors of the complement system currently in development for cardiovascular disease. *Cardiovasc Toxicol* 2003;3:43–70.

C H A P T E R 51

# UNSTABLE ANGINA AND NON-ST-SEGMENT ELEVATION MYOCARDIAL INFARCTION: CLINICAL PRESENTATION, DIAGNOSTIC EVALUATION, AND MEDICAL MANAGEMENT

Robert A. O'Rourke



## INTRODUCTION

As discussed in detail in Chap. 48, *acute coronary syndrome* (ACS) has become a useful operative term for referring to any pattern of clinical symptoms that is consistent with acute myocardial ischemia[1,2] (Fig. 51-1). This chapter is confined to two closely related forms of ACS, namely unstable angina (UA) and non-ST-segment elevation myocardial infarction (NSTEMI). The latter (Fig. 51-1) usually does not progress to a Q-wave MI (QWMI) but rather to a non-Q-wave MI (NQMI). The use of early revascularization therapy—thrombolysis or percutaneous coronary intervention (PCI)—may "convert" a potential ST-segment-elevation MI (STEMI) to a NQMI. Infrequently, an NSTEMI evolves to become a QWMI by electrocardiography (ECG).

UA and the closely related condition, NSTEMI are very common manifestations of coronary artery disease (CAD). In 1996 alone, the National Center for Health Statistics reported 1,433,000 hospitalizations for UA or NSTEMI.[3]

Previously, these two forms of ACS had been classified separately as unstable angina and NQMI. However, as described in detail in chapters 44, 45, and 48, the usual underlying pathophysiologic mechanism for both involves the rupture (most commonly) or erosion of an atherosclerotic (atherothrombotic) plaque with thrombus formation that severely obstructs the coronary artery lumen. There is a complex overlap between the two syndromes; their clinical presentations early in the course of ACS are difficult to distinguish with certainty. Accordingly, patients with either of these syndromes are frequently treated identically, with individual variations in management

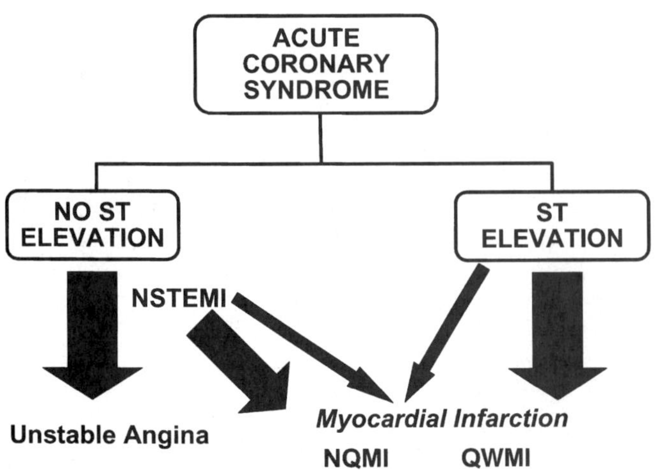


FIGURE 51-1 Nomenclature of ACSs. Patients with ischemic discomfort may present with or without ST-segment elevation on the ECG. The majority of patients with ST-segment elevation (*large arrows*) ultimately develop a Q-wave MI (QWMI), whereas a minority (*small arrow*) develop a non-Q-wave MI (NQMI). Patients who present without ST-segment elevation are experiencing either UA or an ST-segment-elevation MI (NSTEMI). (Adapted from Antman EM, Braunwald E. Acute myocardial infarction. In: Braunwald EB, ed. *Heart Disease: A Textbook of Cardiovascular Medicine*. Philadelphia: Saunders; 1997. With permission.)

depending on the classification of high, intermediate, or low risk.[1] They differ primarily in whether the ischemia is severe enough to cause sufficient myocardial damage to release detectable quantities of a marker of myocardial injury (troponin I, troponin T, or CK-MB)(see Chap. 52). In the past decade, considerable new information has come to light concerning the diagnosis and subsequent management of patients with either of these two types of ACS.[1,2]

Serum biochemical markers such as troponins I and T and C-reactive protein (CRP) enable more accurate risk stratification. New therapies, specifically low-molecular-weight heparin, platelet glycoprotein (GP) IIb/IIIa receptor antagonists and other antiplatelet drugs, particularly clopidogrel, have improved outcomes in high-risk patients, specifically when combined with the use of PCI employing coronary artery stents.[1] The aggressive medical and invasive treatment of these ACSs reduce the incidence of acute vessel closure. Also, restenosis has been markedly diminished in multiple randomized clinical research trials.[1]

Unfortunately, there has been considerable confusion among practicing physicians resulting from the many and often conflicting randomized clinical trials in patients with ACS; the reasons for this are listed in Table 51-1. This chapter discusses the current management of patients with these two presentations of ACS, which are very common manifestations of CAD. It also discusses another angina syndrome that is not "stable"—namely, *variant angina*.

TABLE 51-1 Sources of Inconsistency in Outcomes of Clinical Trials in Acute Coronary Syndromes

| |
|---|
| Criteria for diagnosis vary |
| Inclusion/exclusion criteria frequently differ |
| Heterogeneous group of patients enrolled |
| Primary endpoints are often composite in order to obtain significance |
| Duration of follow-up and medications frequently differ |
| In actuality, many do not practice what they preach |

SOURCE: From Freemantle et al.[208] With permission.

## DEFINITION AND CLASSIFICATION

UA/NSTEMI constitutes a clinical syndrome that is usually caused by CAD and is associated with an increased risk of subsequent cardiac death and QWMI. Angiographic and angioscopic studies indicate that UA/NSTEMI often results from the disruption of an atherothrombotic plaque with a subsequent cascade of pathologic processes that decrease coronary blood flow (Fig. 51-2).[2] Most patients who die during UA/NSTEMI do so because of sudden death or the development of a new or recurrent acute myocardial infarction (MI). Effective diagnosis and optimal management of these patients is based on information readily available at the time of the initial presentation.[1] The initial clinical features of patients with a life-threatening ACS often overlap with those of patients subsequently found not to have CAD.[1] Also, some forms of MI cannot be differentiated from unstable angina at the time of initial presentation. There are important differences in the initial management of patients with UA/NSTEMI compared to patients with QWMI, who usually respond to early revascularization therapy. Therefore, patients diagnosed as having acute MI (AMI) suitable for reperfusion with ST elevation are excluded from the specific treatment regimen benefiting NSTEMI (see Chap. 52).[2]

The National Heart Attack Alert Program (NHAAP) summarizes the clinical information necessary to make the diagnosis of possible ACS at the earliest phase of clinical assessment.[4] First, the patient should be placed in an environment with the capability for continuous electrocardiographic (ECG) recording and defibrillation and where a 12-lead ECG can be obtained expeditiously and interpreted accurately within 10 min. The most urgent priority is to identify patients with acute MI who should be considered for immediate reperfusion therapy, whether in the emergency department (ED) or during the initial hours of hospitalization. Each patient should have a

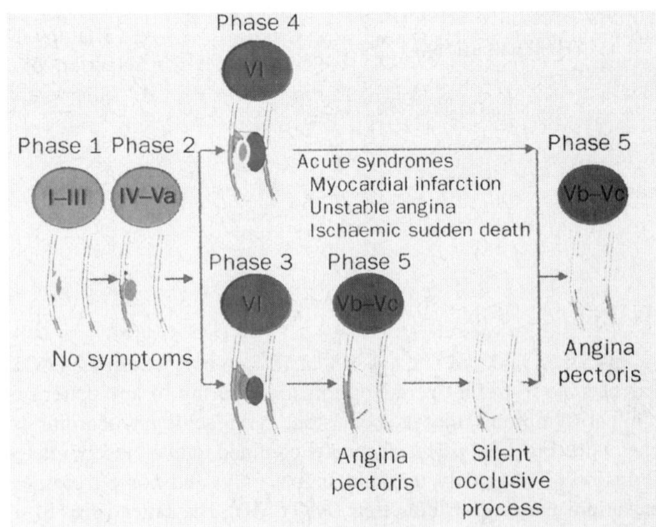


FIGURE 51-2 Phases of coronary lesion morphology and progression, with correlation to clinical syndromes. Unstable angina is caused by phase 2, type IV, and type Va—lesions that are disrupted and progress to phases 3 and 4, or type VI. (From Fuster V, Fayal ZA, Badimon JJ. Acute coronary syndromes: Biology. *Lancet* 1999; 353(suppl II):5–9. With permission.)

provisional diagnosis, ruled in or ruled out, of (1) ACS, which, in turn, is classified as STEMI, NSTEMI, or UA; (2) a non-ACS cardiovascular condition; (3) another specific noncardiac disease (e.g., esophageal spasm), or (4) a noncardiac condition that is undefined. Also, the initial assessment should include risk determination and treatment of life-threatening events.[1]

Updated American College of Cardiology/American Heart Association (ACC/AHA) clinical practice guidelines for the treatment of patients with NSTEMI/UA have recently been published.[1]

## CAUSES

UA and NSTEMI are characterized by an imbalance between myocardial oxygen supply and demand. A schematic representation of their causes is depicted in Fig. 51-3.

The most common cause of UA/NSTEMI is reduced myocardial perfusion due to coronary artery luminal narrowing caused by a nonocclusive thrombus that developed following rupture or erosion of an atherothrombotic plaque (Fig. 51-3). The thrombus is usually not occlusive and microembolization of platelet aggregates and components of the disruptive plaque are likely responsible for the release of myocardial biochemical markers in many patients. A second but much less common cause (Fig. 51-3) is dynamic obstruction, which may be due to intense focal spasm of a segment of an epicardial coronary artery (Prinzmetal's or variant angina, as discussed specifically in the final section of this chapter). A third cause of UA/NSTEMI is severe narrowing without spasm or thrombosis. This occurs in some patients with progressive atherothrombosis or with restenosis after PCI. The fourth cause is arterial inflammation perhaps caused by or related to infection, which may result in arterial narrowing, plaque destabilization, rupture, and thrombogenesis. Activated macrophages and T lymphocytes located at the shoulder of a plaque increase the expression of enzymes that may cause thinning and disruption of the fibrous cap. Multiple recent reports[5–11] implicate inflammation as an important related or causal factor for acute coronary events. The fifth cause is "secondary UA/NSTEMI" (Fig. 51-3), in which the precipitating condition is extrinsic to the coronary arterial bed. Such patients have underlying coronary atherosclerotic narrowing that limits myocardial perfusion; they also often have prior chronic stable angina. UA/NSTEMI occurs with sudden increases in myocardial oxygen demands (e.g., fever, tachycardia), reductions in coronary blood flow, (e.g., hypotension), or diminution in myocardial oxygen delivery (e.g., severe anemia).

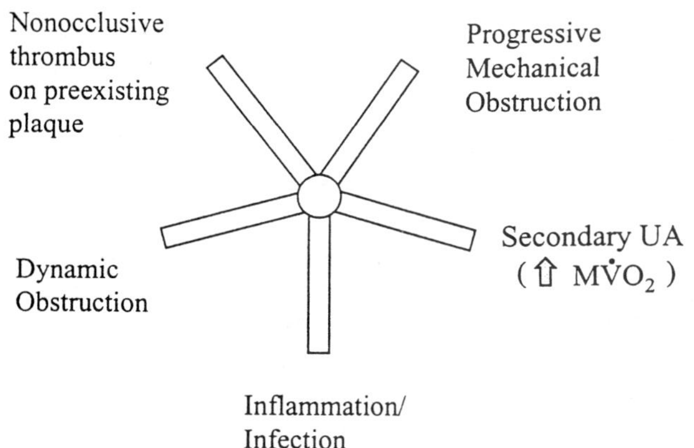


FIGURE 51-3 Framework for considering the pathophysiologic components that contribute to unstable angina in a specific patient. Varying contributions are possible from each of the five arms. Some patients will have predominantly one cause, while in others two or more mechanisms will contribute significantly. (From Braunwald E. Unstable angina: An etiologic approach to managment. *Circulation* 1998; 98: 2219–2222. With permission.)

## INITIAL PRESENTATION

There are three principal manifestations of UA/NSTEMI: (1) rest angina; (2) new-onset severe angina; and (3) increasing angina.[1] Criteria for diagnosis of UA/NSTEMI are based on duration and intensity of angina as graded according to the Canadian Cardiovascular Society Classifications (Chap. 12).

The designation of three specific forms of UA/NSTEMI is useful because the pathophysiology, prognosis, and management of these forms are different. The de novo form resulting from the development of an unstable coronary plaque was described above. Other settings include UA/NSTEMI within 6 months after PCI, which is almost invariably caused by restenosis. Intravenous nitroglycerin provides effective therapy. Repeat PCI is usually performed. UA/NSTEMI in a patient with previous coronary bypass surgery often involves advanced atherothrombosis of venous bypass grafts and a lower likelihood of long-term symptomatic relief compared with other patients with UA.[12,13]

## PATHOPHYSIOLOGY

Progression of a coronary atherothrombotic plaque can be divided into five phases and different lesions (Fig. 51-2).[7] Disruption of a type IV or Va lesion exposes the underlying thrombogenic substrate, leading to the formation of a thrombus. This acute type VI lesion can be healed without producing symptoms. However, when the thrombus totally or subtotally occludes the lumen, an ACS may result. The factors that contribute to the development of an ACS also represent potential targets for therapy (Table 51-2).

### Plaque Disruption or Erosion

As described in Chaps. 44 and 48, mechanical factors contribute to plaque disruption; a thin fibrous cap is more prone to rupture than is

TABLE 51-2 Factors That Modulate the Development of Acute Coronary Syndromes

| |
|---|
| Location of the culprit coronary lesion |
| Stenosis length, contour, and severity |
| Extent of plaque rupture or erosion |
| Inflammatory substrate |
| Endothelial function |
| Degree of coronary vasoconstriction |
| Extent of collaterals |
| Thrombotic factors |
| Platelet aggregability and reactivity |
| Leukocyte activation |
| Intrinsic clotting factor |
| Plaque tissue factor levels |
| Level of fibrinolytic activity |
| Blood viscosity |
| Systemic factors |
| Heart rate and blood pressure |
| Catecholamine levels (smoking, cocaine, stress) |
| Cholesterol levels, including Lp(a) |

a thick one. *Plaque rupture* commonly occurs at the shoulders, where the plaque joins the adjacent vessel wall.[14,15] A lipid pool within a plaque influences the biomechanical properties of the plaque and increases the likelihood of rupture ("high risk" or "vulnerable"). Conversely, fibrosis and *calcification* appear to decrease the risk of rupture.[15,16]

*Erosion* usually occurs centrally through a thinning cap rather than at the plaque shoulders.[17] Erosion appears to be more common among women smokers and plaque rupture occurs more frequently in hyperlipidemic men.[18,19]

## Inflammation

Inflammation appears to play a major role in plaque disruption and ACS (Fig. 51-4). Macrophages and T lymphocytes accumulate in atherothrombotic plaques because of the expression of adhesion molecules on monocytes, endothelial cells, and leukocytes.[20,21] These cells are active in the local oxidation of low-density-lipoprotein (LDL) cholesterol and other products.

The matrix metalloproteinases—which include collagenases and gelatinases—are released from foam cells and degrade the collagen that provides strength to the fibrous cap.[22] Tissue inhibitors of metalloproteinases (TIMPS) are normally expressed by vascular smooth muscle cells (VSMC). Unfortunately, in the critical areas of the fibrous cap, foam cells predominate and smooth muscle cells are sparse.[2]

Elevated peripheral blood levels of specific matrix metalloproteinases have been reported in patients with ACS.[23] Also, atherectomy specimens from patients with unstable angina exhibit active synthesis of a specific gelatinase.[24] Nuclear factor-$\kappa$B (a transcription factor that is a marker of inflammation) has been found to be increased in the peripheral blood of patients with unstable angina but not of patients with stable angina (Fig. 51-4).[25]

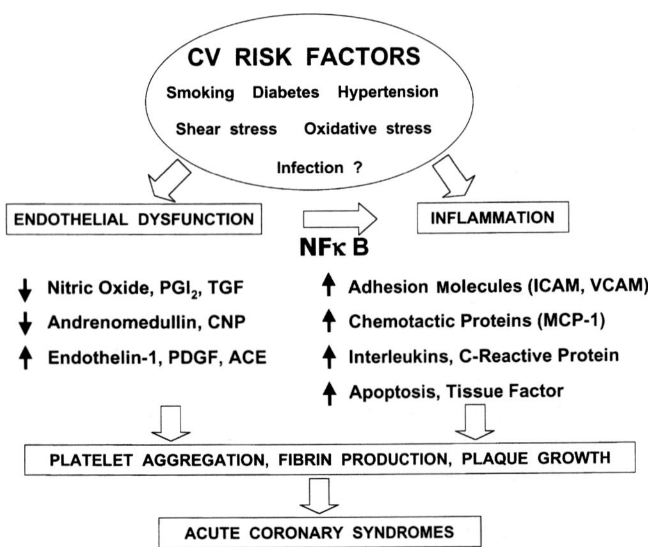


FIGURE 51-4 Link between cardiovascular risk factors, endothelial dysfunction, inflammation, and acute coronary syndromes. Endothelial dysfunction can be caused by many proinflammatory atherogenic factors. Endothelial cells thereafter increase expression of adhesion molecules. ACE = angiotensin converting enzyme; CNP = c-type natriuretic peptide; ICAM = intercellular adhesion molecule; MCP-1 = monocyte chemoattractant protein-1; NF$\kappa$ = nuclear factor kappa; PDGF = platelet-derived growth factor; $PGI_2$ = prostaglandin; TGF = transforming growth factor; VCAM = vascular cell adhesion molecule.

In a detailed study of 20 culprit plaques, macrophages and T lymphocytes were found to be clustered at the intermediate site of plaque rupture.[26] These cells and nearby vascular smooth muscle cells (VSMCs) expressed high levels of the same human leukocyte antigen, indicating both activation and "cross talk" among the cells. Mast cells have also been found in culprit lesions of UA patients only.[27] Together, these findings indicate that an inflammatory stimulus causes a "biochemical storm" within the high-risk plaque, leading to rupture of its fibrous cap.

High-sensitivity (hs) C-reactive protein (CRP) is a nonspecific acute-phase reactant. Increased serum levels have been reported in most patients with UA and MI but not in those with stable angina.[28] The short-term prognosis is worse in unstable angina patients with elevated levels of CRP.[29,30] It is currently being assessed as an "emerging" risk factor for subsequent coronary events (Chap. 43).

Recently Brennan and colleagues[30a] demonstrated increased myeloperoxidase (secreted by activated leukocytes) as a marker of acute coronary events as well as an indicator of a poor six-month cardiac prognosis in patients presenting with chest pain. Further validation of this "diagnostic test" is indicated.

## Infection

The stimulus initiating the acute inflammatory process in UA has *not* been clearly delineated. Atherothrombosis itself, as defined by the "response to injury" hypothesis, is a chronic, low-grade inflammatory condition.[31] Controversy persists as to whether infectious agents play a primary role either in atherothrombosis or in the transformation of stable to unstable CAD.[32,33]

*Chlamydia pneumoniae,* cytomegalovirus, and *Helicobacter pylori* have been identified within human atherosclerotic lesions.[32] Furthermore, antibodies against *Chlamydia* heat-shock proteins can cross-react against heat-shock proteins produced by endothelium, resulting in endothelial damage and accelerated atherosclerosis.[34,35]

Although antibodies to *Chlamydia,* cytomegalovirus, and *H. pylori* are found more often in patients with atherothrombosis than in controls,[32,33] these associations do not indicate causality. Antibodies to these agents due to prior infection are found in a high proportion of the population, particularly the elderly.

In a small study of post-MI patients, more adverse cardiovascular events occurred during follow-up in those with increasing antibody titers to *Chlamydia.*[36] Patients with high chlamydia blood titers were randomized to azithromycin or placebo; events were reduced significantly in the antibiotic-treated group.[37] The results in similar patients have been variable and contradictory in several other small group trials.[38,39]

## Platelets and Leukocytes

Platelet deposition onto the exposed thrombogenic surface of a ruptured plaque is an important event in the pathogenesis of UA/NSTEMI. Postmortem studies in accident victims with coronary atherothrombosis suggest that plaque ruptures are common.[40] In patients with UA, the production of nitric oxide by the platelets themselves is impaired and its release by the endothelium is attenuated[41,42] (Fig. 51-4).

In UA/NSTEMI, activated platelets generate thromboxane and prostaglandin metabolites.[43] Severe or persistent UA is associated with the highest thromboxane output; stabilization of ACS is accompanied by a return to normal levels.[44,45] Importantly, activated platelets and activated leukocytes interact in the acute phase of UA/NSTEMI to facilitate platelet-thrombus deposition.[46–48]

### Thrombosis and Fibrinolysis

The interplay of activated platelets and leukocytes stimulates the coagulation system. Monocytes release tissue factor, a small glycoprotein that initiates the extrinsic clotting cascade, resulting in an augmentation in thrombin generation.[49,50] Intermittent thrombus deposition causes reductions in transient coronary flow and thus symptoms due to myocardial ischemia at rest.

Tissue factor is also present in the lipid-rich core of atherothrombotic plaques and is likely one of the major determinants of the thrombogenicity of ruptured plaques.[51] Thus, tissue factor content plays a major role in the evolution of the "high risk" plaque.[52]

### Vasoconstriction

Culprit lesions in UA/NSTEMI demonstrate an increased response to vasoconstrictor stimuli,[53] but other coronary artery segments or culprit lesions of patients with stable angina are unaffected. Vasoconstriction or the lack of appropriate vasodilation probably contributes significantly to the development of ischemic episodes in patients with UA and is a potential target for therapy.[2] In the author's experience, vasodilators (e.g., nitroglycerin, chronic calcium blockers) are underutilized in the treatment of most patients with ACS or chronic stable angina (Chap. 57).

### Evolution of the Culprit Lesion

The angiographic characteristics of the culprit lesion have been defined before, during, and after an episode of unstable angina.[2] If a patient with UA has had a prior coronary angiogram, the culprit lesion has usually progressed markedly since the time of the prior angiogram.[54] At the time of UA/NSTEMI, the culprit lesion is likely to be asymmetric or eccentric, with a narrow base or neck, compared with control lesions.[55] Lesions with irregular borders, overhanging edges, or obvious thrombus at angiography are more likely to initiate another cardiac event in the ensuing months. Preliminary data suggests that more aggressive treatment with antiplatelet or antithrombotic drugs can modify the course of such complex lesions.[56]

## DIAGNOSIS

Patients with suspected ACS must be evaluated expeditiously. Decisions based on the early evaluation have important clinical and economic consequences. A prompt and accurate diagnosis permits the timely initiation of appropriate therapy which is paramount; complications are clustered in the early phases of ACS and appropriate treatment reduces the rate of their occurrence. This may result from plaque stabilization or passivation.

Patients with chest pain lasting for longer than 20 min, hemodynamic instability, recent syncope or presyncope should be referred to a hospital ED.[1] Other individuals with suspected UA/NSTEMI may be seen initially in an outpatient facility where a 12-lead ECG can be obtained quickly.

### Initial Evaluation

In a patient with known CAD, typical symptoms are highly likely to be caused by myocardial ischemia, especially if the patient reports that the current symptoms, including shortness of breath and/or chest discomfort, are identical to previous episodes when CAD was objectively documented as the cause. The evaluation of a patient with UA/NSTEMI requires not only the establishment of the diagnosis but also an assessment of the short-term risk, which determines the intensity of initial and often subsequent treatment.

### History

When unstable angina is suspected in a patient younger than age 50, it is particularly important to consider cocaine use.[1] Cocaine can cause coronary vasospasm and thrombosis in addition to its direct effect on heart rate and arterial blood pressure; it has been implicated as a cause of ACS[1,2] (Chap. 84).

The characteristic association between stable angina and physical exertion or other activities is often lacking in UA/NSTEMI. Also, chest discomfort due to UA/NSTEMI is less likely than stable angina to be relieved by nitroglycerin. The duration of chest discomfort is usually longer and more variable in UA/NSTEMI. Patients with ACS often experience discomfort typical of angina but the episodes are more severe and prolonged; they often occur at rest and commonly are precipitated by less exertion than previously. Some patients may have no chest discomfort but present solely with jaw, neck, ear, arm, and epigastric discomfort. These should be considered as "angina equivalents."

Evaluation of patients with suspected UA/NSTEMI should include the physician's opinion of whether the chest discomfort's *likelihood* of being due to myocardial ischemia is in one of three categories: high, intermediate, or low (Table 51-3).

TABLE 51-3 Likelihood That Unstable Angina Symptoms Are Caused by Myocardial Ischemia

HIGH LIKELIHOOD
- Any of the following features:
- Known coronary disease
- Definite angina in men age ≥60 years or women age ≥70 years
- Hemodynamic or ECG changes during pain
- Variant angina
- ST-segment elevation or depression of at least 1 mm
- Marked symmetric T-wave inversion in multiple precordial leads

INTERMEDIATE LIKELIHOOD
Absence of high-likelihood features and any of the following:
- Definite angina in men age <60 years or women age <70 years
- Probable angina in men age ≥60 years or women age ≥70 years
- Probably not angina in diabetics or in nondiabetics with two or more other risk factors
- Extracardiac vascular disease
- ST-segment depression of 0.05 to 1 mm
- T-wave inversion of at least 1 mm in leads with dominant R waves

LOW LIKELIHOOD
Absence of high- or intermediate-likelihood features but may have:
- Chest pain, probably not angina
- One risk factor but not diabetes
- T waves flat or inverted <1 mm in leads with dominant R waves
- Normal ECG

Nausea, sweating, or shortness of breath may accompany episodes of chest discomfort. In elderly or diabetic patients, these symptoms may be the only indication that myocardial ischemia is present. Both groups of patients have an increased incidence of multivessel disease. Women are less likely than are men to be smokers, and more men are likely to have had a previous myocardial infarction.[57] At coronary angiography, women are less likely to have significant coronary heart disease.[57]

## The Electrocardiogram

An ECG is an integral part of the initial evaluation of a patient with a suspected ACS. The diagnostic yield is enhanced greatly if an ECG can be recorded during an episode of chest discomfort. While a normal ECG during chest pain does not rule out ACS, it is a relatively favorable prognostic sign.

Transient ST-segment depression of at least 1 mm (Fig. 51-5) that appears during chest discomfort and disappears after relief provides objective evidence of transient myocardial ischemia. When it is a constant finding with or without chest pain, it is less specific. A common ECG pattern in patients with unstable angina is a persistent negative T wave over the involved area (Fig. 51-6). Deeply negative T waves across all the precordial leads suggest a proximal, severe left anterior descending (LAD) coronary artery stenosis as the culprit lesion.[58]

In UA/NSTEMI patients, the ECG may show Q waves from an old infarction or a left bundle branch block resulting from extensive prior LV damage. Patients with such findings are at increased risk.[59,60]

ECG abnormalities may appear or progress in the absence of new symptoms or signs in patients with ACS. Accordingly, it is appropriate to obtain serial ECGs during the first 48 h as well as during episodes of chest pain.

## Biochemical Cardiac Markers

Biochemical cardiac markers are useful for both the diagnosis of myocardial necrosis and the estimation of prognosis (Chap. 52). The loss of membrane integrity of necrotic myocytes causes intracellular macromolecules to diffuse into the cardiac interstitium, endolymphatics, and cardiac microvasculature. Eventually, these biochemical markers are detectable in the peripheral circulation. Traditionally, elevated serum levels of cardiac enzymes or the MB isoenzyme of creatine kinase (CK) were used to distinguish between UA and acute MI. The diagnosis of UA *without* MI was made when minor elevations in CK or CK-MB were detected by serial sampling because it was recognized that this was a negative prognostic sign.[61]

The widespread availability of other, more sensitive biochemical cardiac markers, particularly troponins, has improved the ability to diagnose lesser degrees of myocardial necrosis.[62] As many as 25 to 33 percent of patients with UA will have elevated levels of troponin T or I on admission or soon thereafter.[1,2] Many of these will have normal levels of CK-MB.[2] Several large studies have demonstrated that elevations of either troponin T or troponin I are independent predictors of adverse events in populations with either UA alone or UA and NQMI.[62–65] The elevated troponin T or I levels may be only slightly above the upper limits of the assay for a normal healthy population (Chap. 52). Accordingly, some investigators use the term *minor my-*

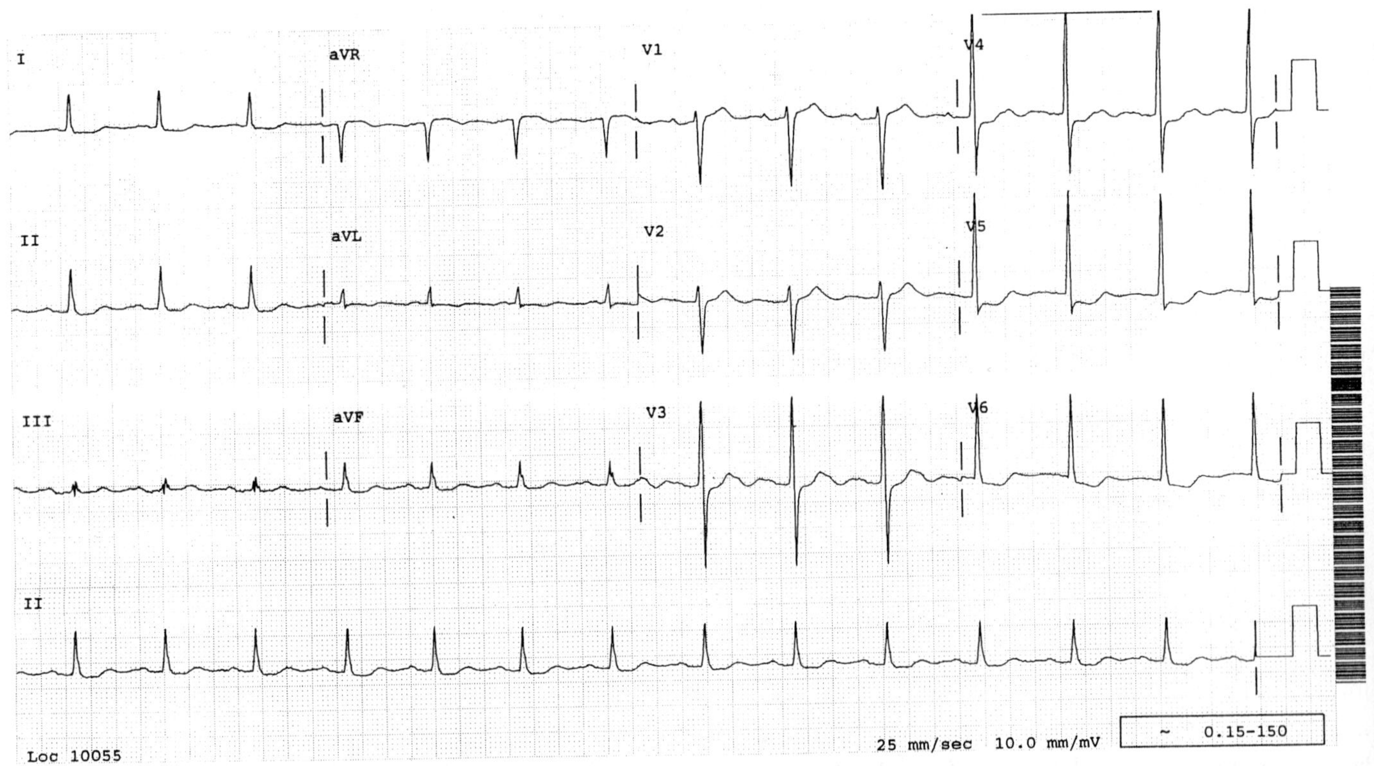


FIGURE 51-5 Electrocardiogram recorded during an episode of chest pain at rest in a patient with unstable angina. ST-segment depression >1 mm is present in leads $V_4$ to $V_6$. This abnormality was not present on the baseline tracing. The chest pain and ST-segment depression disappeared promptly after the administration of sublingual nitroglycerin.

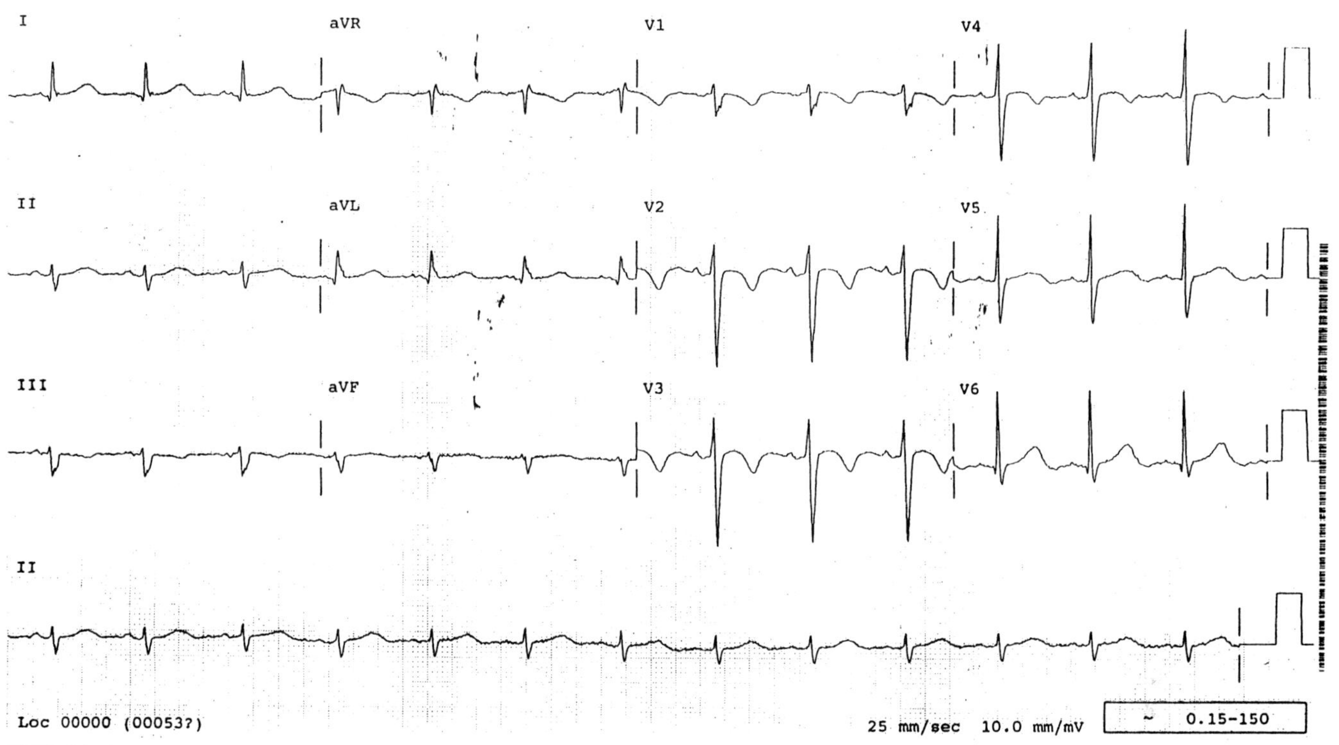


FIGURE 51-6 Electrocardiogram recorded during a pain-free interval from a patient hospitalized with unstable angina. The negative T waves in $V_1$ to $V_4$ had been upright on a previous tracing. The culprit lesion was located in the left anterior descending coronary artery.

*ocardial damage* or *mild myocardial infarction* for patients with detectable troponin but no CK-MB in the blood. Approximately 30 percent of patients who present with rest pain without ST-segment elevation and who would otherwise be diagnosed as having UA because of a lack of CK-MB elevation actually have NSTEMI when assessed with cardiac-specific troponin monoclonal antibody–based immunoassays.[1] Troponins are accurate also in identifying myocardial necrosis that is not due to atherosclerotic CAD. Therefore, in making a diagnosis of NSTEMI, cardiac troponins *should be used in conjunction* with appropriate signs or symptoms and/or ECG changes.[1]

Troponin T or I measurements may be normal early after the onset of ACS and become positive later. As alluded to, patients with elevation of troponins should be treated as being at *high risk* compared with UA patients with normal troponin levels. These high-risk patients should be classified as having NSTEMI even in the presence of normal CK-MB levels.

Only a minority of UA/NSTEMI patients assessed in a good ED or chest pain unit will have elevated troponin levels on admission, so the diagnosis is usually made by other means. However, an elevated troponin level may be the only objective evidence of the presence of an ACS in many patients.[1,2]

## Acute Myocardial Perfusion Imaging

Intermittent reductions in coronary blood flow distal to the responsible coronary stenosis can occur in UA without either ECG changes or release of biochemical cardiac markers. Acute rest myocardial perfusion imaging with either thallium or sestamibi is a relatively sensitive and specific diagnostic test for ACS. In practice, sestamibi is more useful than thallium for this purpose because imaging can be delayed for up to several hours after injection as a result of the minimal redistribution of this imaging agent.[2] ECG-gated images provide an assessment of wall motion in addition to perfusion (Chap. 19).

The sensitivity and specificity of acute rest imaging are very high if sestamibi is injected during an episode of chest pain, but sensitivity decreases if the injection is done within the ensuing hours.[66] The negative predictive value of a normal perfusion study is *extremely high* when the isotope is injected during symptoms. However, acute rest imaging will miss a few patients with ACS (less than 5 percent); therefore patient management decisions should not be made solely on the basis of one test result.

Another potential method for diagnosing ACS early is the use of magnetic resonance imaging (MRI), which can assess cardiac function, LV motion, and myocardial perfusion in the ED.[67] (See Chap. 21.)

## Chest Pain Units

The evaluation of patients with chest pain who may have UA or MI is often difficult and uncertain. Hospitalizing all such patients for an extensive workup is neither cost-effective nor necessary. However, missing the diagnosis of UA/NSTEMI may result in unnecessary QWMI and death. The chest pain unit was developed as a solution to this problem.[1] (See Chap. 52.)

Most chest pain units are in or adjacent to the ED and utilize a set of criteria designed to select *low-risk* patients.[68–70] Criteria usually include chest pain that may indicate myocardial ischemia but with a normal or unchanged ECG and a normal initial set of cardiac enzymes.[70] The likelihood of a major cardiovascular event declines over time, with 41 percent of cardiac events occurring within 12 h and 62 percent within 24 h.[71] Events can be predicted by a set of simple clinical measures available at baseline and updated at 12 h.[64] (See Chap. 52.)

In most units, CK-MB is measured every 3 to 4 h for 12 h duration, sometimes with other serum markers. Patients receive an aspirin, an intravenous line, ECG monitoring, and a 12-lead ECG during chest pain at specific intervals. If no evidence of active CAD is detected, a stress test may be performed for diagnostic and prognostic purposes or the patient may be discharged and sent home.[1,2]

Chest pain units have been reported to reduce the rate of missed MIs from approximately 5 percent to 0.5 percent, as estimated from return visits within 72 h.[70–72] (See Chap. 52.)

## RISK STRATIFICATION

The evaluation of a patient with UA/NSTEMI requires both establishing the diagnosis and determining the short-term risk. This risk assessment dictates the appropriate intensity of therapy. At the low end of the risk scale, a patient may be discharged home with aspirin and beta blockers, to be followed as an outpatient, often with a subsequent test for exercise inducible myocardial ischemia. At the high end of the scale, patients may be hospitalized in a coronary care unit, treated with multiple drugs, and undergo coronary arteriography urgently as a prelude to revascularization if feasible.

### Clinical Features

The ACC/AHA 2002 Guideline Update for the Management of Patients with UA and Non-ST Segment Elevation Myocardial Infarction categorizes patients with UA into low-, intermediate-, and high-risk groups[1] (Table 51-4). High-risk patients have ongoing chest pain that lasts longer than 20 min, reversible ST-segment changes of at

TABLE 51-4 Short-Term Risk of Death or Nonfatal Myocardial Infarction in Patients with Unstable Angina[a]

| Feature | High Risk<br>At least one of the following features must be present: | Intermediate Risk<br>No high-risk feature but must have one of the following features: | Low Risk<br>No high- or intermediate-risk feature but may have any of the following features: |
|---|---|---|---|
| History | Accelerating tempo of ischemic symptoms in preceding 48 h | Prior MI, peripheral or disease, or CABG, prior aspirin use | New-onset or progressive CCS Class III or IV angina the past 2 weeks without prolonged (>20 min) rest pain but with moderate or high likelihood of CAD |
| Character of pain | Prolonged ongoing (>20 min) rest pain | Prolonged (>20 min) rest angina, now resolved, with moderate or high likelihood of CAD<br>Rest angina (<20 min) or relieved with rest or sublingual NTG | |
| Clinical findings | Pulmonary edema, most likely due to ischemia<br>New or worsening MR murmur<br>$S_3$ or new/worsening rales<br>Hypotension, bradycardia, tachycardia<br>Age >75 years | Age >70 years | |
| ECG | Angina at rest with transient ST-segment changes >0.05 mV<br>Bundle branch block, new or presumed new<br>Sustained ventricular tachycardia | T-wave inversions >0.2 mV<br>Pathologic Q waves | Normal or unchanged ECG during an episode of chest discomfort |
| Cardiac markers | Elevated (e.g., TnT or TnI > 0.1 ng/mL) | Slightly elevated (e.g., TnT > 0.01 but < 0.1 ng/mL) | Normal |

[a]Estimation of the short-term risk of death and nonfatal cardiac ischemic events in UA is a complex multivariable problem that cannot be fully specified in a table such as this; therefore, this table is meant to offer general guidance and illustration rather than rigid algorithms.

ABBREVIATIONS: MR = mitral regurgitation; TnT = troponin T; TnI = troponin I; MI = myocardial infarction; CABG = coronary artery bypass graft; CAD = coronary artery disease; NTG = nitroglyerin; CCC = Canadian cardiovascular class; ECG = electrocardiogram.

SOURCE: Adapted from AHCPR Clinical Practice Guideline No. 10, Unstable Angina: Diagnosis and Management, May 1994. Braunwald E, Mark CB, Jones RH, et al. Unstable angina: Diagnosis and management. Rockville, MD: Agency for Health Care Policy and Research and the National Heart, Lung, and Blood Institute, US Public Health Service, US Department of Health and Human Services; 1994; AHCPR Publication No. 94-0602.

least 1 mm, or signs of serious LV dysfunction. Low-risk patients have worsening angina without rest pain, are age 65 or younger, and have a normal or unchanged ECG without evidence of previous infarction.

The risk assessment should be updated during hospitalization because patients frequently change categories. Continuing angina with ST changes despite medical therapy is an ominous sign of "high risk" that should initiate urgent coronary arteriography with probable revascularization. Episodes of silent ST-segment depression detected by ambulatory ECG recordings predict an unfavorable outcome.[73]

## Serum Biochemical Markers

Troponin measurements should be used in the risk stratification of patients with UA/NSTEMI to supplement the assessment from clinical features and the results of the ECG. Elevated troponin levels strongly predict coronary events over the short term, as noted. (See Chap. 52.) The combination of troponin T or I elevation and ST-segment depression identifies a group at particularly high risk.[74–76] Measuring troponin not just at baseline but also at 8, 12 and 16 h after admission has been shown to add useful prognostic information.[74]

High levels of the inflammatory markers such as CRP, serum amyloid A, and interleukin-6 are associated with a poorer prognosis in UA/NSTEMI.[77] Markers of activation of the coagulation system have also been reported to predict risk, including fibrinopeptide A[78] and fibrinogen.[79] The early rise in von Willebrand factor was an independent predictor of events within 30 days in one study.[80] However, *in practice,* the only serum marker that *should be measured routinely* for *risk stratification* in UA is troponin I or T.[1,2]

## Stress Testing

Stress testing is often used for risk assessment in patients with UA/NSTEMI.[2] Low-risk and some intermediate-risk patients whose symptoms stabilize with medical therapy undergo stress testing for advanced risk stratification.[2] Those with high-risk findings, such as large reversible perfusion defects or ST-segment depression at low exercise levels, should undergo coronary arteriography; those with negative or low-risk results can be treated medically (Chap. 19). This approach has been validated in patients with UA/NSTEMI, demonstrating that high-risk abnormalities correlate with a higher event rate during follow-up.[81–84] Patients with low exercise tolerance, exercise-induced ST-segment depression, and large myocardial perfusion defects on imaging studies are more likely to have three-vessel disease than patients without these high-risk findings[85] (Chaps. 16 and 19).

Patients who complete a stay in a chest pain unit without objective evidence of myocardial ischemia can safely undergo stress testing for diagnosis and prognostic purposes either immediately or within the next 24 to 48 h.[86]

In patients who are unable to exercise, pharmacologic testing with dipyridamole, adenosine, or dobutamine can be used as the stress and sestamibi imaging or echocardiography can be used as a method of assessment (Chaps. 15, 16, and 19). Stress testing is not needed in patients whose clinical features already put them at high risk; they should proceed directly to coronary arteriography.

## Coronary Angiography

Risk in coronary patients traditionally has been assessed according to the number of vessels with ≥50 percent diameter stenosis and the presence and severity of LV dysfunction. However, the relative prognostic impact is probably less with ACS, since the risk of short-term events in UA/NSTEMI patients is dominated by features of the *culprit lesion,* such as whether it induces ST-segment depression or troponin release. Culprit lesions for UA/NSTEMI are far more likely to progress and initiate other coronary events, including MI and death, than are other coronary lesions in the same patients.[87–89]

Among patients with UA/NSTEMI who undergo arteriography, approximately 25 percent will have one-vessel disease, 25 percent two-vessel disease, and 25 percent three-vessel disease. Ten percent will have significant main coronary stenosis; and the other 15 percent will have coronary luminal narrowings of less than 50 percent or normal vessels on arteriography.[90,91]

Patients with left main stenosis of at least 50 percent or three-vessel disease with LV dysfunction will obtain a survival benefit from coronary artery bypass graft (CABG) surgery.[91,92] Importantly, patients with *no* significant lesions at angiography benefit from a reorientation of their management.[2] Noncardiac causes of chest pain should be considered, as well as "syndrome X" and variant angina. Antithrombotic and antiplatelet drugs can often be discontinued, and the need for antianginal medication can be reassessed. The UA/NSTEMI patients who are most likely to have no significant lesions at angiography tend to be women with no ST-segment depression on ECG.[92] Nevertheless, the finding of no significant lesions at angiography is usually unanticipated. As a note of caution, symptomatic patients with "normal" coronary artery contrast luminography may have severe coronary atherosclerosis on intravascular ultrasound, with coronary artery remodeling (Chap. 18).

## Risk Stratification with Combinations of Predictors

The combination of ST-segment abnormalities and elevated troponin levels is useful for prognostication. In one study using these two indicators, the risk of death or infarction within 30 days was 25.8, 3.1, and 1.7 percent in high-, intermediate-, and low-risk groups, respectively.[2] In a Thrombin Inhibition in Myocardial Ischemia (TRIM) substudy,[93] the composite endpoint of death, MI, or refractory angina within 30 days was predicted by ST-segment depression, inverted T waves in at least five leads, elevated troponin or myoglobin levels, female sex, and age of 65 years or older. Death or infarction occurred in 14, 6, and 3 percent of high-, intermediate-, and low-risk groups, respectively.[93]

In summary, the short-term outcome of UA/NSTEMI can be predicted by a variety of methods (Table 51-4).[1,2] The most important predictors are the clinical presentation, ST-segment depression during attacks, elevated troponin levels, and continuing episodes of pain in spite of medical therapy.

# PROGNOSIS

Prognosis in patients with UA or UA/NSTEMI depends on the combination of the morbidity or mortality expected from the extent of coronary stenosis and left ventricular (LV) function and the unstable short-term risk associated with the culprit lesion and the unstable state of ACS.[93,94] The short-term risk is related entirely to MI and its complications and to the recurrences of ACS. Risk is highest early after the onset of symptoms.[2]

Published reports concerning the survival of patients with UA are influenced by patient selection and treatment and can be quite misleading (Table 51-1). The inclusion and exclusion criteria for the clinical trials bias the prognosis by often eliminating low- or high-risk patients. Aspirin was not routinely used in the treatment of UA until the early 1980s. Results from that era are therefore far below current expectations.[2]

In a collation of 10 representative series with nearly 2000 UA patients, excluding those with new-onset or postinfarction angina, the mortality was 4 percent in the hospital and 10 percent at 1 year.[95] Survival without infarction was 89 percent at 1 month and 79 percent at 1 year.[95] Among 4488 UA patients in GUSTO-IIb, the mortality rate was 2.4 percent at 30 days, 5 percent at 6 months, and 7 percent at 1 year.[96] The MI rate was 4.8 percent at 30 days and 6.2 percent at 6 months. Recurrent ischemia had a major impact on these rates. Outcomes are representative of the results of modern therapy in the late 1990s and have even improved further by the year 2004.

## TREATMENT

The aims of therapy for UA/NSTEMI patients are to control symptoms and prevent further episodes of myocardial ischemia and/or necrosis. Nitroglycerin, beta blockers, and, to a lesser extent, calcium channel blockers reduce the risk of recurrent ischemic attacks. Revascularization eliminates ischemia in many patients. The risk of MI is diminished by antiplatelet and antithrombotic drugs.

### In-Hospital Treatment

The initial care for the patient who presents to an ED or a chest pain clinic has been detailed above.

Hospitalized moderate- to high-risk ACS patients should be treated with aspirin (ASA), a beta blocker, antithrombin therapy, and a glycoprotein (GP) IIb/IIIa inhibitor.[1] Also, oral statin therapy is usually started or continued. Furthermore, critical decisions are required regarding the angiographic strategy. One option is a *routine* angiographic approach in which coronary angiography and revascularization are performed unless a contraindication exists. Within this strategy, the most common approach has included an initial period of medical stabilization. More recently, many physicians are taking an earlier aggressive approach, with coronary angiography and revascularization performed within 24 h of admission when possible. Their rationale is the demonstrated protective effect of careful, early administration of antithrombin and antiplatelet therapy on procedural outcome. The alternative approach, commonly referred to as the *initially conservative strategy,* is guided by myocardial ischemia, with angiography reserved for patients with recurrent ischemia or a "high-risk" noninvasive imaging test at rest or with stress despite medical therapy. Regardless of the angiographic strategy, an assessment of LV function should be strongly considered in patients with documented ischemia because it is imperative to treat patients who have impaired LV systolic function with both angiotensin-converting enzyme (ACE) inhibitors and beta blockers unless contraindicated and, when the coronary anatomy is appropriate (e.g., severe three-vessel coronary disease), with CABG surgery. When the coronary angiogram is performed, a left ventriculogram should be obtained at the same time. When coronary angiography is not scheduled, the patient is evaluated at rest and/or with stress for inducible myocardial ischemia or LV systolic dysfunction.

The optimal management of UA/NSTEMI has the dual goals of the immediate relief of ischemia and the prevention of serious adverse outcomes (i.e., death or MI/reinfarction). Table 51-5 lists the recommendations of the ACC/AHA class I guidelines for anti-ischemic therapy in the presence or absence of continuing ischemia or high-risk features.[1]

#### USE OF ANTI-ISCHEMIC DRUGS

***Nitrates*** Nitroglycerin (NTG) reduces myocardial oxygen demand while enhancing myocardial oxygen delivery (Chap. 57). NTG, an endothelium-independent vasodilator, has both peripheral and coronary vascular effects. By dilating the capacitance vessels, it increases venous pooling, which diminishes myocardial preload, thereby reducing LV wall tension, a determinant of myocardial oxygen consumption ($M\dot{V}O_2$). NTG promotes the dilation of large coronary arteries as well as collateral flow and redistribution of coronary blood flow to ischemic regions.

Patients whose symptoms are not relieved with three 0.4-mg sublingual NTG tablets or spray taken 5 min apart may benefit from intravenous NTG, and such therapy is recommended in the absence of contraindications. The use of sildenafil (Viagra) within the previous 24 h and the presence of hypotension are important contraindications.[96]

Intravenous NTG may be initiated at a rate of 10 μg/min through continuous infusion with nonabsorbing tubing and increased by 10 μg/min every 3 to 5 min until some symptom or blood pressure response is noted. Caution should be exercised when systolic blood pressure declines to less than 110 mmHg in previously normotensive patients or to greater than 25 percent below the starting mean arterial blood pressure if hypertension was present.[1] An upper limit of 200 μg/min is commonly used.

The rationale for NTG use in UA/NSTEMI is extrapolated from pathophysiologic principles and extensive, although uncontrolled, clinical observations.

TABLE 51-5 ACC/AHA Class I Recommendations for Anti-ischemic Therapy in the Presence or Absence of Continuing Ischemia or High-Risk Features[a]

| Present | Absent |
|---|---|
| Bed rest with continuous ECG monitoring | |
| Supplemental $O_2$ to maintain $Sa_{O_2}$ >90% | |
| NTG IV | |
| Beta blockers, oral or IV | Beta blockers, oral |
| Morphine IV for pain, anxiety, pulmonary congestion | |
| IABP if ischemia or hemodynamic instability persists | |
| ACE inhibitor for control of hypertension or LV dysfunction after MI | ACE inhibitor for control of hypertension or LV dysfunction after MI |

[a]Recurrent angina and/or ischemia-related ECG changes (greater than or equal to 0.05-mV ST-segment depression or bundle branch block) at rest or low-level activities; or ischemia associated with CHF symptoms, $S_3$ gallop, or new or worsening mitral regurgitation; or hemodynamic instability or depressed LV function (EF <0.40 on noninvasive study); or malignant ventricular arrhythmia.

ABBREVIATIONS: ACC/AHA = American College of Cardiology/American Heart Association; ECG = electrocardiogram; NTG = nitroglycerin; IABP = intraaortic balloon pump; ACE = angiotensin-converting enzyme; LV = left ventricular; MI = myocardial infarction; EF = ejection fraction.

***Morphine Sulfate*** Morphine sulfate (1 to 5 IV) is recommended for patients whose symptoms are not relieved after three serial sublingual NTG tablets or whose symptoms recur despite adequate anti-ischemic therapy. Unless contraindicated by hypotension or intolerance, morphine may be administered along with intravenous NTG, with careful blood pressure monitoring, and may be repeated every 5 to 30 min as needed to relieve symptoms and maintain patient comfort (Chap. 52).

***Beta-Adrenergic Blockers*** Beta blockers competitively block the effects of catecholamines on cell membrane beta receptors. Thus they blunt the heart rate and contractility responses to chest pain, exertion, and other stimuli. They also decrease systolic blood pressure. All of these effects reduce $M\dot{V}O_2$. In UA/NSTEMI, the primary benefits of beta blockers are due to effects on $beta_1$-adrenergic receptors that decrease cardiac work and myocardial oxygen demand. Slowing of the heart rate also has a very desirable effect, not only by reducing $M\dot{V}O_2$ but also by increasing the duration of diastole and diastolic pressure-time, a determinant of coronary flow and collateral flow (Chap. 57).

Beta blockers should be started early in the absence of contraindications. These agents should be administered *intravenously,* followed by oral administration in high-risk patients as well as in patients with ongoing rest pain, or orally for intermediate- and low-risk patients.[1]

The choice of beta blocker for an individual patient is based primarily on pharmacokinetic and side-effect criteria. The initial choice of agents includes metoprolol, propranolol, or atenolol. Esmolol can be used if an ultra-short-acting agent is required.[1]

The contraindications to the use of beta blockers on an acute basis are detailed elsewhere (Chap. 57 specifically).[96] Patients with significant sinus bradycardia (heart rate less than 50 beats per minute) or hypotension (systolic blood pressure less than 90 mmHg) generally should not receive beta blockers until these conditions have resolved. If there are concerns about possible intolerance to beta blockers, initial selection should favor a short-acting $beta_1$-specific drug such as metoprolol. Mild wheezing or a history of chronic obstructive pulmonary disease (COPD) mandates a short-acting cardioselective agent at a reduced dose (e.g., 2.5 mg metoprolol IV or 12.5 mg metoprolol orally or 25 $\mu g \cdot kg^{-1} \cdot min^{-1}$ esmolol IV as initial doses) rather than the complete avoidance of a beta blocker.[1]

Metoprolol may be given in 5-mg increments by slow intravenous administration (5 mg over 1 to 2 min), repeated every 5 min for a total initial dose of 15 mg. In patients who tolerate the total 15 mg IV dose, oral therapy should be initiated 15 min after the last intravenous dose at 25 to 50 mg every 6 h for 48 h. Thereafter, patients should receive a maintenance dose of 100 mg twice daily.[1] Intravenous esmolol is administered as a starting dose of 0.1 $mg \cdot kg^{-1} \cdot min^{-1}$, with titration in increments of 0.05 $mg \cdot kg^{-1} \cdot min^{-1}$ every 10 to 15 min as tolerated by the patient's blood pressure until the desired therapeutic response has been obtained, limiting symptoms develop, or a dosage of 0.3 $mg \cdot kg^{-1} \cdot min^{-1}$ is reached. A loading dose of 0.5 mg/kg may be given by slow intravenous administration (2 to 5 min) for a more rapid onset of action. In patients suitable to receive a longer-acting agent, intravenous atenolol can be initiated with a 5-mg IV dose followed 5 min later by a second 5-mg IV dose and then 50 to 100 mg/day orally initiated 1 to 2 h after the intravenous dose.[1] Monitoring during intravenous beta-blocker therapy should include frequent checks of heart rate and blood pressure and continuous ECG monitoring as well as auscultation for rales and bronchospasm (Chaps. 57 and 90).

Evidence for the beneficial effects of beta blockers in patients with UA/NSTEMI is based on limited randomized clinical trials along with pathophysiologic considerations and extrapolation from experience with CAD patients who have other types of ischemic syndromes (Chap. 57).

***Calcium Antagonists*** These agents reduce cell transmembrane inward calcium flux, which inhibits both myocardial and vascular smooth muscle contraction; some also slow atrioventricular (AV) conduction and depress sinus node impulse formation. Agents in this class vary in the degree to which they produce vasodilation, decrease myocardial contractility, cause AV block, and sinus node slowing (Chaps. 57 and 90). Nifedipine and amlodipine have the most peripheral arterial dilatory effect but little or no AV or sinus node effects, whereas verapamil and diltiazem have prominent AV and sinus node effects and some peripheral arterial dilatory effects as well.[1,2]

Calcium antagonists may be used to control ongoing or recurring ischemia-related symptoms in patients who are already receiving adequate doses of nitrates and beta blockers, in patients who are unable to tolerate adequate doses of one or both of these agents, or in those with variant angina.

Rapid-release short-acting dihydropyridines (e.g., nifedipine) *must be avoided* in the absence of adequate concurrent beta blockade in ACS because controlled trials suggest increased adverse outcomes.[96,97]

Several randomized trials assessing the use of calcium antagonists in ACS generally confirm that these agents relieve or prevent symptoms and related ischemia to a degree similar to that of beta blockers[98,99] (Chap. 57).

***Angiotensin-Converting Enzyme Inhibitors*** ACE inhibitors have been shown to reduce mortality rates in patients with AMI or who recently had an MI and have LV systolic dysfunction.[100–102] They are also effective in diabetic patients with LV dysfunction[103] and in a broad spectrum of patients with high-risk chronic CAD, including those with normal LV function.[104] Accordingly, ACE inhibitors should be used in such patients as well as in those with hypertension that is not controlled with beta blockers and nitrates (Chaps. 61 and 86).

Other, less extensively studied techniques for the relief of ischemia—such as spinal cord stimulation, prolonged external counterpulsation, and laser transmyocardial revascularization—are under evaluation for patients with refractory angina and particularly for those who are no longer candidates for PCI or CABG surgery.[1]

## ANTIPLATELET THERAPY

Antithrombotic therapy is essential to modify the active disease process and prevent its progression to death, MI, or recurrent MI. A combination of ASA, unfractionated heparin (UFH), and a platelet GP IIb/IIIa receptor antagonist represents the most effective therapy. The intensity of treatment is tailored to individual risk; triple antithrombotic treatment is used in patients with continuing ischemia or with other high-risk features and in those requiring early invasive strategy.[1] A low-molecular-weight heparin (LMWH) can be advantageously substituted for UFH, although experience with the former in PCI, in patients referred for urgent CABG, and in combination with both a GP IIb/IIIa antagonist and with a thrombolytic agent is somewhat limited.[1,2] A recent preliminary report (A to Z Trial) showed that enoxaparin was not inferior to UFH in the treatment of ACS (ACC Scientific Session 2003).

***Aspirin*** By irreversibly inhibiting cyclooxygenase-1 within platelets, ASA prevents the formation of thromboxane $A_2$, thereby diminishing platelet aggregation promoted by this pathway but not by others. This platelet inhibition is the likely mechanism for the clinical benefits of ASA in ACS because it is fully present with low doses of ASA (80 to 325 mg/day) and because platelets represent one of the principal participants in thrombus formation after plaque disruption.[104–106]

ASA clinical trials in patients with UA/NSTEMI have consistently documented a marked benefit of the drug in decreasing cardiac events independent of differences in study design, such as time of entry after the acute phase, duration of follow-up, and doses used[107–110] (Fig. 51-7).

It appears reasonable to initiate ASA treatment in patients with UA/NSTEMI at a dose of 160 or 325 mg.[1] Patients who present with suspected ACS who are not already receiving ASA may chew the first dose to rapidly establish a high blood level. Subsequent doses may be swallowed. Thereafter, daily doses of 75 to 325 mg are prescribed.

The prompt action of ASA and its ability to reduce mortality rates in patients with suspected AMI enrolled in the ISIS-2 trial (Chap. 50) led to the recommendation that ASA be initiated immediately in the ED as soon as the diagnosis of ACS is made or suspected. In patients who are already receiving ASA, it should be continued.

***Adenosine Diphosphate Receptor Antagonists and Other Antiplatelet Agents*** Two thienopyridines—ticlopidine and clopidogrel—are adenosine diphosphate (ADP) antagonists that are currently approved for antiplatelet therapy.[1] The platelet effects of ticlopidine and clopidogrel are reversible but take several days to become completely manifest. Because the mechanisms of the antiplatelet effects of ASA and ADP antagonists differ, a potential exists for additive benefit with the combination.[1]

Ticlopidine has been used successfully for the secondary prevention of stroke and MI and for the prevention of stent closure and graft occlusion.[1]

The adverse effects of ticlopidine limit its usefulness: gastrointestinal problems (diarrhea, abdominal pain, nausea, vomiting), neutropenia in approximately 2.4 percent of patients, severe neutropenia in 0.8 percent of patients, and, rarely, thrombotic thrombocytopenia purpura (TTP).[111]

Most clinical experience with clopidogrel is derived from the Clopidogrel versus Aspirin in Patients at Risk of Ischaemic Events (CAPRIE) trial.[112] A total of 19,185 patients were randomized to receive 325 mg/day of ASA or 75 mg/day clopidogrel. Entry criteria consisted of atherosclerotic vascular disease manifest as recent ischemic stroke, recent MI, or symptomatic peripheral arterial disease. Follow-up extended for 1 to 3 years. The endpoint composite risk ratio (RR) of ischemic stroke, MI, or vascular death was reduced by 8.7 percent in favor of clopidogrel from 5.83 to 5.32 percent ($p = 0.043$). However, *no* differences in the frequency of death and/or MI occurred between ASA and clopidogrel.

The **C**lopidogrel in **U**nstable Angina to Prevent **R**ecurrent Ischemic **E**vents (CURE) trial randomized 12,562 patients with UA and NSTEMI presenting within 24 h to placebo or clopidogrel (loading dose of 300 mg followed by 75 mg/day) followed for 3 to 12 months.[113] All patients received ASA. The composite endpoint of cardiovascular death, MI, or stroke occurred in 11.5 percent of patients assigned to placebo and 9.3 percent assigned to clopidogrel (RR = 0.80, $p < 0.011$). In addition, clopidogrel was associated with significant reductions in the rate of in hospital severe myocardial ischemia and revascularization as well as the need for thrombolytic therapy or intravenous GP IIb/IIIa receptor antagonists.

There was an excess of major bleeding (2.7 in the placebo group vs. 3.7 percent in the clopidogrel group, $p = 0.003$) as well as of minor, not of life-threatening bleeding. The risk of bleeding was increased in patients undergoing CABG surgery within the first 5 days of stopping clopidogrel. CURE was conducted at centers with no routine policy of early invasive procedures; revascularization was performed during the initial admission in only 23 percent of the patients. Additional information on the safety of the addition of heparin (LMWH or UFH) and a GP IIb/IIIa inhibitor in patients already receiving ASA and clopidogrel is being assessed in clinical trials. Also, it is not yet clear whether clopidogrel improves the outcome in patients who receive GP IIb/IIIa antagonists.

The CURE trial provides strong but not definitive evidence for the addition of clopidogrel to ASA on admission in the management of patients with UA/NSTEMI in whom a noninterventional approach is intended. This is an especially useful approach in hospitals that do not have a routine policy of early invasive procedures. The optimal dura-

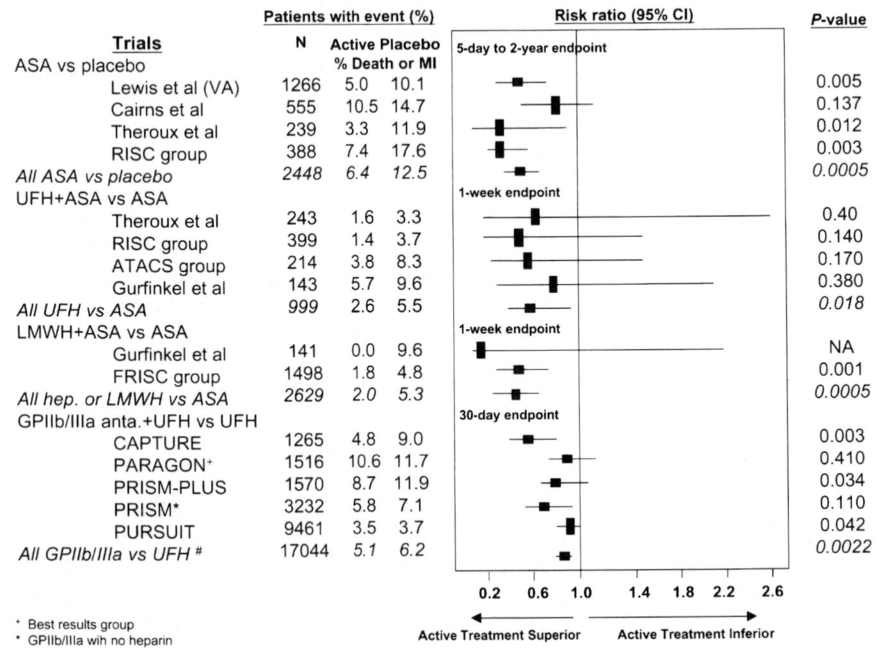

Patients with event (%)
Risk ratio (95% CI)
P-value
Trials
N
Active Placebo
% Death or MI
5-day to 2-year endpoint
ASA vs placebo
Lewis et al (VA) 1266 5.0 10.1 0.005
Cairns et al 555 10.5 14.7 0.137
Theroux et al 239 3.3 11.9 0.012
RISC group 388 7.4 17.6 0.003
All ASA vs placebo 2448 6.4 12.5 0.0005
1-week endpoint
UFH+ASA vs ASA
Theroux et al 243 1.6 3.3 0.40
RISC group 399 1.4 3.7 0.140
ATACS group 214 3.8 8.3 0.170
Gurfinkel et al 143 5.7 9.6 0.380
All UFH vs ASA 999 2.6 5.5 0.018
1-week endpoint
LMWH+ASA vs ASA
Gurfinkel et al 141 0.0 9.6 NA
FRISC group 1498 1.8 4.8 0.001
All hep. or LMWH vs ASA 2629 2.0 5.3 0.0005
30-day endpoint
GPIIb/IIIa anta.+UFH vs UFH
CAPTURE 1265 4.8 9.0 0.003
PARAGON+ 1516 10.6 11.7 0.410
PRISM-PLUS 1570 8.7 11.9 0.034
PRISM* 3232 5.8 7.1 0.110
PURSUIT 9461 3.5 3.7 0.042
All GPIIb/IIIa vs UFH # 17044 5.1 6.2 0.0022
0.2 0.6 1.0 1.4 1.8 2.2 2.6
Active Treatment Superior
Active Treatment Inferior
* Best results group
+ GPIIb/IIIa wih no heparin
# All trials except PRISM compared BP IIb-IIIa with UFH vs UFH


FIGURE 51-7 Summary of trials of antithrombotic therapy in unstable angina. Metanalysis of randomized trials in unstable angina/non-ST-segment-elevation myocardial infarction that have compared aspirin (ASA) with placebo, the combination of unfractionated heparin (UFH) and ASA with ASA alone, the combination of a low-molecular-weight heparin (LMWH) and ASA with ASA alone, and the combination of a platelet glycoprotein (GP) IIb/IIIa antagonist (anta.), UFH (hep.), and ASA with UFH plus ASA. The RR values, 95 percent CIs, and probability value for each trial are shown. The timing of the endpoint (death or MI) varied. Results with the platelet GP IIb/IIIa antagonists are reported at the 30-day time point. Incremental gain is observed from single therapy with ASA to double therapy with ASA and UFH and to triple antithrombotic therapy with ASA, UFH, and a platelet GP IIb/IIIa antagonist. In the CAPTURE trial, nearly all patients underwent percutaneous coronary intervention after 20 to 24 h per study design.

tion of therapy with clopidogrel has not been determined, but the favorable results in CURE were observed over a period averaging 9 months.[113]

In the PCI-CURE study, 2658 patients undergoing PCI had been randomly assigned double-blind treatment with clopidogrel ($n = 1313$) or placebo ($n = 1345$).[114] Patients were pretreated with ASA and the study drug for a median of 10 days. After PCI, most patients received open-label thienopyridine for about 4 weeks, after which the study drug was restarted for a mean of 8 months. Overall (including events before and after PCI), there was a 31 percent reduction in cardiovascular death or MI ($p = 0.002$). Thus, in patients with UA and NSTEMI receiving ASA and undergoing PCI, a strategy of clopidogrel pretreatment followed by at least 1 month and probably longer-term therapy appeared beneficial in reducing major cardiovascular events. Therefore the ACC/AHA Guideline ACS Update Committee recommended that clopidogrel should be used routinely in patients who undergo PCI.[1]

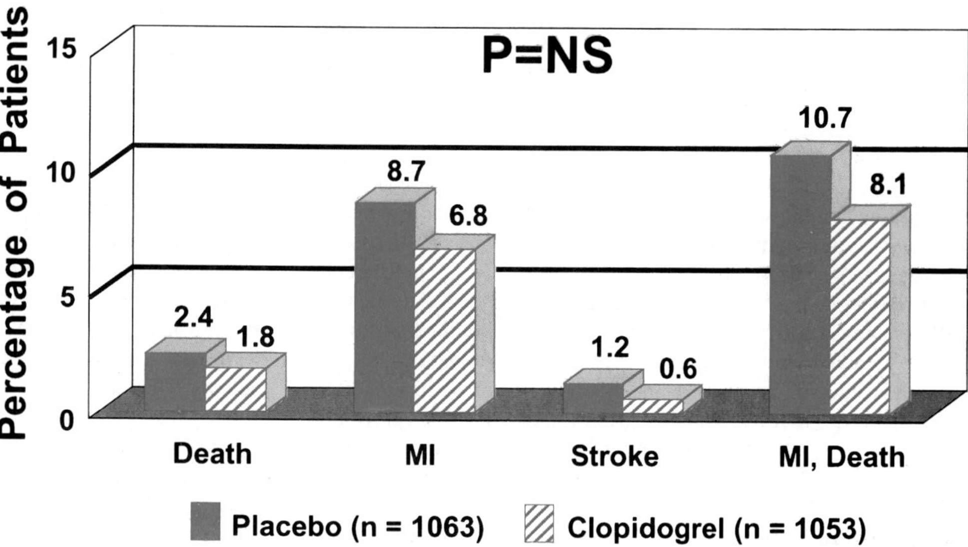


FIGURE 51-8 The differences in the endpoints of death, myocardial infarction (MI), stroke, or a combination of MI and death did not significantly change between patients who were randomized to clopidogrel and those who were not.

In a more recent trial, Clopidogrel for the Reduction of Events During Observation (CREDO),[115] a statistically significant reduction of thrombotic outcomes was reported in patients treated with combination clopidogrel and ASA for 1 year compared to aspirin alone[115] (Fig. 51-8). Over 2000 patients who were expected to undergo PCI were randomized to clopidogrel versus placebo. The clopidogrel group received a 300-mg loading dose. Both groups received clopidogrel 75 mg and ASA for the following 28 days.

Investigators found a *nonsignificant* trend toward a reduction in the primary composite endpoint of cardiovascular death, MI, and stroke at 28 days (19.7 percent relative risk reduction CI: 13.3 to 43.1). These patients were then followed for another 11 months using two different treatment strategies. The group that had received the initial clopidogrel bolus was given clopidogrel plus ASA, whereas the placebo group was given ASA alone. At 1 year there was a statistically significant 26.9 percent risk reduction in the *composite primary endpoint* in the combination-therapy group versus the ASA-only group (8.5 vs. 11.5 percent, $p = 0.02$, CI: 3.9 to 44.4). The results were similar across the various subgroups studied: men, women, those with and without ACS or with and without diabetes, and those who had received and not received GP IIb/IIIa inhibitors at the time of intervention. Importantly, there was *no difference* in death and/or MI alone (Fig. 51-8).

While these findings were positive, some questions still remain.[116,117] As with CURE, there was an increased risk of major bleeding in the combination-therapy group (8.8 vs. 6.7 percent, $p = 0.07$), but this was almost entirely in the group that underwent CABG. Thus, it may be difficult to modify this bleeding risk without delaying a patient's surgery beyond the currently recommended 5 days after having received a dose of clopidogrel.

Recent clinical data suggesting that atorvastatin attenuates the antiplatelet effects of clopidogrel have generated considerable debate and unrest in the pharmaceutical community. Since clopidogrel is being prescribed for an ever-increasing portion of patients with CAD, most of whom are receiving statins for secondary prevention, any negative interaction between these two classes of drugs could have profound detrimental effects.

In a series of sophisticated in vitro studies, Clarke and Waskell[118] have demonstrated that cytochrome P450 3A4 metabolized clopidogrel. When clopidogrel and atorvastatin are present at equimolar concentration, clopidogrel metabolism is inhibited by greater than 90 percent. Lau and colleagues[119] have demonstrated that the concomitant use of atorvastatin, which is metabolized by the same P450 enzyme system in the liver, reduces the antiplatelet effect of clopidogrel.

The clinical importance of this interaction will be difficult to prove without a randomized clinical trial comparing patients on clopidogrel with and without concomitant therapy with CYP3A4 inhibitors. Patient variation has recently been described.[119a]

In many hospitals in which patients with UA/NSTEMI undergo diagnostic catheterization within 24 to 36 h of admission, clopidogrel is not started until it is clear that CABG surgery will not be scheduled within the next several days. A loading dose of clopidogrel can be given to a patient on the catheterization table if a PCI is to be carried out immediately. If PCI is not carried out, the clopidogrel can be begun after the catheterization. Despite the strong recommendation by the ACC/AHA Guidelines Committee, many clinicians oppose this routine use of clopidogrel because of associated bleeding effects and no differences in the death rate.[116,117]

## ANTICOAGULANT THERAPY

Anticoagulants available for parenteral use include UFH, various LMWHs, and hirudin; for oral use, the anti–vitamin K drugs are available (Chap. 54).[1] Synthetic pentasaccharides and synthetic direct thrombin inhibitors (argatroban, bivaluridine) as well as oral direct and indirect thrombin inhibitors are under clinical investigation.

UFH is a heterogenous mixture of polysaccharides of various molecular weights, which accelerate the action of circulating antithrombin, a proteolytic enzyme that inactivates factor IIa (thrombin), factor

IXa, and factor Xa. It prevents thrombus propagation but does not lyse existing thrombi.[120] LMWHs are relatively more potent in catalyzing the inhibition of factor Xa by antithrombin than in the inactivation of thrombin (Chap. 54). Relative to UFH, LMWH has decreased nonspecific binding, a longer half-life, and predictable anticoagulation, permitting once- or twice-daily subcutaneous administration. Use of LMWHs does not usually require laboratory monitoring. Their ratios of anti-Xa factor to anti-IIa factor vary, ranging from 1.9 to 3.8.[121]

By contrast, direct thrombin inhibitors act by binding directly to the anion binding and catalytic sites of thrombin to produce potent, predictable anticoagulation.[121,122] (See Chap. 54.) Several large trials have compared hirudin with UFH in UA/NSTEMI, with a modest short-term reduction in the composite endpoint of death or nonfatal MI and a modest increase in the risk of bleeding. Hirudin is approved for use in patients with heparin-induced thrombocytopenia.[1]

Bivalurudin (Hirulog) is a synthetic analogue of hirudin that binds reversibly to thrombin. It has been compared with UFH in several small trials in UA/NSTEMI and in PCI, with some evidence of a reduction in death or MI and less bleeding than with UFH.[123,124]

***Unfractionated Heparin*** Seven randomized, placebo-controlled trials with UFH have been reported[1] (Chap. 54).

The results of the studies that have compared the combination of ASA and heparin with ASA alone are shown in Fig. 51-7. With UFH, the reduction in the rate of death or MI during the first week was 54 percent ($p = 0.016$); in the trials that used either UFH or LMWH, the reduction was 63 percent. Two published metanalyses have included different studies.[1] In one metanalysis, which involved three randomized trials and an early endpoint (less than 5 days), the risk of death or MI with the combination of ASA and heparin was reduced by 56 percent ($p = 0.03$). In the second metanalysis of 6 trials, the endpoints ranged from 2 to 12 weeks, and the RR was reduced by 33 percent ($p = 0.06$).[1] Most of the benefits of the various anticoagulants are short-term, however, and not maintained on a long-term basis (Chap. 54). Reactivation of the disease process after the discontinuation of anticoagulants may contribute to this loss of early gain, which has been described with UFH, dalteparin, and hirudin. The combination of UFH and ASA and continuation of ASA appears to mitigate this reactivation in part.[125]

Pharmacokinetic limitations of UFH translate into poor bioavailability, especially at low doses, and marked variability in anticoagulant response[126] The effects of heparin requires monitoring with the activated partial thromboplastin time (aPTT) (Chap. 54). A weight-adjusted regimen is recommended, with an initial bolus of 60 to 70 U/kg (maximum 5000 U) and an initial infusion of 12 to 15 U $\cdot$ kg$^{-1}$ $\cdot$ h$^{-1}$ (maximum 1000 U/h). The American College of Chest Physicians consensus conference[126] has recommended dosage adjustments of the nomograms to correspond to a therapeutic range equivalent to heparin levels of 0.3 to 0.7 U/mL by anti–factor Xa determinations, which correlates with aPTT values between 60 and 80 s.[1]

Even though weight-based UFH dosing regimens are used, the aPTT should be monitored for adjustment of UFH dosing (Chap. 54). Because of variation in the control aPTT values, nomograms should be established at each institution to achieve target aPTT values. Measurements should be made 6 h after any dosage change to adjust UFH infusion to an appropriate aPTT. When two consecutive aPTT values are therapeutic, the measurements may be made every 24 h and, if necessary, the dose adjusted. Also, a significant change in the patient's clinical condition should prompt a similar response[1] (Chap. 54).

Serial platelet counts are necessary to monitor for heparin-induced thrombocytopenia. Severe thrombocytopenia (platelet count less than 100,000) occurs in 1 to 2 percent of patients and typically appears after 4 to 14 days of therapy. A rare but dangerous complication (less than 0.2 percent incidence) is autoimmune UFH-induced thrombocytopenia with thrombosis.[126]

***Low-Molecular-Weight Heparin*** In a pilot open-label study, 219 patients with UA were randomized to receive ASA (200 mg/day), ASA plus UFH, or ASA plus nadroparin, an LMWH. The combination of ASA and LMWH significantly reduced the total ischemic event rate, the incidence of recurrent angina, and the number of patients requiring interventional procedures.[127]

Because the level of anticoagulant activity cannot easily be measured in patients receiving LMWH, interventional cardiologists have expressed concern about the substitution of LMWH for UFH in patients scheduled for catheterization with possible PCI. However, Collet et al.[128] found, in a study of 293 patients with UA/NSTEMI undergoing PCI, that these patients received the usual dose of enoxaparin with complete safety.

In the National Investigators Collaborating on Enoxaparin Trial (NICE-1), an observational study, intravenous enoxaparin (1.0 mg/kg) was used in 828 patients undergoing elective PCI without an intravenous GP IIb/IIIa inhibitor. The rate of bleeding (1.1 percent for major bleeding and 6.2 percent for minor bleeding in 30 days) was comparable to historical controls with UFH.[1]

An alternative approach is to use LMWH during the period of initial stabilization.[1] The dose can be withheld on the morning of the procedure, and if an intervention is required and more than 8 h has elapsed since the last dose of LMWH, UFH can be used for PCI according to usual practice patterns. Because the anticoagulant effect of UFH can be more readily reversed than that of LMWH, UFH is preferred in patients likely to undergo CABG within 24 h.

***LMWH versus UFH*** Four large randomized trials have directly compared an LMWH with UFH (Fig. 51-9) (Chap. 54). In the FRagmin In unstable Coronary artery disease (FRIC) study,[129] 1482

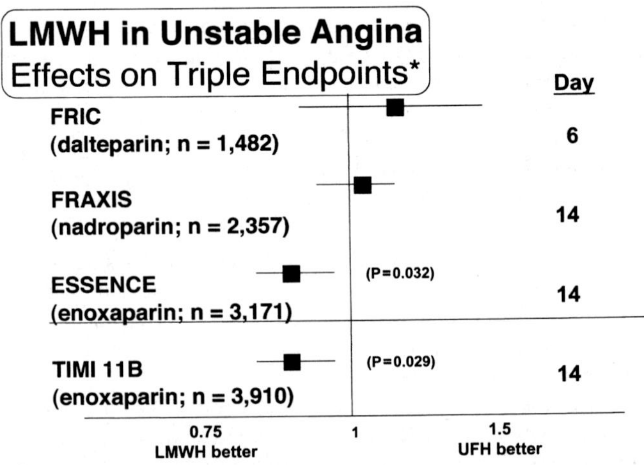


FIGURE 51-9 The use of low-molecular-weight heparin (LMWH) in unstable angina showing effects on the triple endpoints of death, myocardial infarction, and recurrent ischemia with or without revascularization. Early (6-day) and intermediate outcomes of the four trials that compared LMWH and unfractionated heparin: ESSENCE, TIMI 11B, FRIC, and FRAXIS. Nadroparin in FRAXIS was given for 14 days.

patients with UA/NSTEMI received open-label dalteparin or UFH for 6 days.[130] At day 6 and until day 45, patients were randomized a second time to double-blind administration of dalteparin or placebo. During the first part of the study, the composite risk of death, MI, or recurrent angina was not significantly increased with dalteparin (9.3 vs. 7.65 percent, $p = 0.33$), and the risk of death or MI was unaffected (3.9 vs. 3.6 percent, $p = 0.8$). Between days 6 and 45, the rates of death, MI, and recurrence of angina were comparable between the active treatment and placebo groups.

The ESSENCE trial[131] compared enoxaparin, with standard UFH, in 3171 patients, followed by an infusion titrated to an aPTT of 55 to 86 s, administered for 48 h to 8 days (median duration in both groups of 2.6 days).[132] With UFH, only 46 percent of patients reached the target aPTT within 12 to 24 h. The composite outcome of death, MI, or recurrent angina was reduced by 16.2 percent at 14 days with enoxaparin (19.8 UFH vs. 16.6 percent enoxaparin, $p = 0.019$) and by 19 percent at 30 days (23.3 vs. 19.8 percent, $p = 0.017$). The rates of death were unaffected, whereas there were trends to reductions in the rates of death and MI by 29 percent ($p = 0.06$) at 14 days and by 26 percent ($p = 0.08$) at 30 days.

The TIMI 11B trial[133] randomized 3910 patients with UA/NSTEMI to enoxaparin or UFH. The acute-phase therapy was followed by an outpatient phase, during which enoxaparin or placebo for patients who were initially randomized to UFH was administered in a double-blind manner twice a day. Enoxaparin was administered for a median of 4.6 days and UFH was administered for a median of 3.0 days. The composite endpoint of death, MI, or need for an urgent revascularization was reduced at 8 days from 14.5 to 12.4 percent ($p = 0.048$) and at 43 days from 19.6 to 17.3 percent ($p = 0.048$). The rates of death or MI were reduced from 6.9 to 5.7 percent ($p = 0.114$) at 14 days and from 8.9 to 7.9 percent ($p = 0.276$) at 43 days (Chap. 54).

The FRAXiparine in Ischaemic Syndrome (FRAXIS)[134] trial had three parallel arms and compared the LMWH nadroparin administered for 6 or 14 days with control treatment with UFH. A total of 3468 patients with UA or NSTEMI were enrolled. The composite outcome of death, MI, or refractory angina occurred at 14 days in 18.1 percent of patients in the UFH group, 17.8 percent of patients treated with nadroparin for 6 days, and 20.0 percent of patients treated with nadroparin for 14 days; the values at 3 months were 22.2, 22.3, and 26.2 percent of patients, respectively ($p < 0.03$ for the comparison of 14-day nadroparin therapy with UFH therapy). Trends to *more frequent* death and to death or MI were observed at all time points in nadroparin-treated patients (Chap. 54).

Thus, two trials with enoxaparin have shown a moderate benefit over UFH, and two trials (one with dalteparin and one with nadroparin) showed neutral or unfavorable trends (Fig. 51-9). Whether these heterogeneous results are explained by different populations, study designs, various heparin dose regimens, properties of the various LMWHs (e.g., specifically different molecular weights and anti–factor Xa/anti–factor IIa ratios), or other unrecognized influences is speculative.

For patients who are receiving subcutaneous LMWH and for whom CABG is planned, it is recommended that LMWH be discontinued and UFH be used during the operation. Additional experience with regard to the safety and efficacy of the concomitant administration of LMWHs with GP IIb/IIIa antagonists and thrombolytic agents may modify this approach (Chap. 54).

***Hirudin and Other Direct Thrombin Inhibitors*** Hirudin, the prototype of the direct thrombin inhibitors, has been extensively studied.[135–137] The GUSTO-IIb trial randomized 12,142 patients to 72 h of therapy with either intravenous hirudin or UFH.[138] No differences in drug efficacy were seen between patients with and without ST-segment elevation early or by 30 days.

A metanalysis of the GUSTO-IIB,[135] TIMI 9B,[136] OASIS 1, and OASIS 2 trials[137] showed risks of death or MI at 35 days relative to heparin after randomization of 0.90 ($p = 0.015$) with hirudin compared with UFH.[132] At 72 h, the RR values of death or MI were 0.78, 0.89, and 0.72, respectively. Additional trials of direct antithrombins in UA/NSTEMI appear warranted[1] (Chap. 54).

Hirudin (lepirudin) is presently indicated only for anticoagulation in patients with heparin-induced thrombocytopenia[138] and for the prophylaxis of deep veinous thrombosis in patients undergoing hip replacement surgery.[1]

***Long-Term Anticoagulation*** The long-term administration of warfarin has been evaluated in a few pilot studies,[139] and it is not recommended for patients presenting only with UA/NSTEMI.[1]

Warfarin should be prescribed, however, for UA/NSTEMI patients who also have other well-proven indications for warfarin, such as atrial fibrillation and mechanical prosthetic heart valves.

## Antiplatelet and Anticoagulant Therapy

The GP IIb/IIIa receptor is present on the platelet surface (Chap. 54). When activated, this receptor improves its binding affinity for fibrinogen. The binding of fibrinogen to receptors on different platelets results in aggregation.[140] The platelet GP IIb/IIIa receptor antagonists act by occupying the receptors sites, thus opposing fibrinogen binding.[1] The occupancy of ≥ 80 percent of the receptor sites and inhibition of platelet aggregation to ADP by ≥ to 80 percent results in potent antithrombotic effects.[140] The various GP IIb/IIIa antagonists, however, possess significantly different pharmacokinetic and pharmacodynamic properties[141] (Chap. 54).

The efficacy of GP IIb/IIIa antagonists in prevention of the complications associated with PCI has been documented in numerous trials, many of them composed totally or largely of patients with UA (Fig. 51-10). Two trials with tirofiban and one trial with eptifibatide have also documented their efficacy in UA/NSTEMI patients, only some of whom underwent interventions.[142–144]

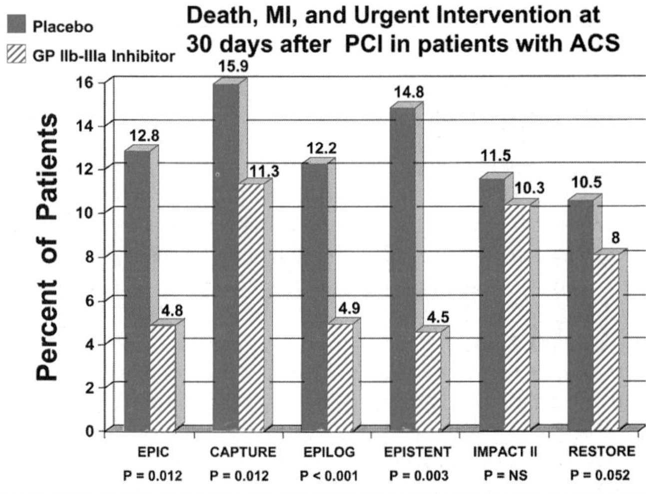


FIGURE 51-10 A comparison of death, myocardial infarction, and urgent intervention at 30 days after percutaneous coronary intervention in patients with acute coronary syndrome. Note that in all cases but one, fewer coronary events occur in the group randomized to GP IIb/IIIa inhibitors.

Abciximab has been studied primarily in PCI trials, and its administration prior to PCI consistently showed a significant reduction in the rate of MI and the need for urgent revascularization.[1] The CAPTURE trial assessing abciximab enrolled patients with refractory UA.[145]

The GUSTO IV-ACS trial[146] enrolled 7800 patients with UA/NSTEMI who were admitted to the hospital with more than 5 min of chest pain and either ST-segment depression and/or elevated troponin T or troponin I concentration. All received ASA and either UFH or LMWH. Revascularization was not intended. Abciximab in the dosing regimen used in GUSTO IV-ACS is not indicated in the management of patients with UA or NSTEMI in whom an early invasive management strategy is *not planned*.[1]

Tirofiban was studied in the Platelet Receptor Inhibition in Ischemic Syndrome Management (PRISM) Study[142] and Platelet Receptor Inhibition in Ischemic Syndrome Management in Patients Limited by Unstable Signs and Symptoms (PRISM-PLUS)[143] trials. The primary composite outcome (death, MI, or refractory ischemia at the end of a 48-h infusion period) was reduced from 5.6 percent with UFH to 3.8 percent with tirofiban (RR 0.67, $p = 0.01$).

Eptifibatide was studied in the PURSUIT trial, which enrolled 10,948 patients who had chest pain at rest within the previous 24 h and ST-T changes or CK-MB elevation.[144]

In the PRISM-PLUS trial, 1069 patients did not undergo early PCI.[143] Even though tirofiban treatment was associated with a lower incidence of death, MI or death, or of MI or refractory ischemia at 30 days, these reductions were not statistically significant. In a high-risk subgroup of these patients not undergoing PCI (TIMI risk score ≥4), tirofiban appeared to be beneficial whether they underwent PCI or not. However, no benefit was observed in patients at lower risk. In the PURSUIT trial, eptifibatide given for at least 72 h reduced the incidence of death or MI at 30 days from 15.7 to 14.2 percent (RR 0.91, 95 percent CI = 0.79 to 1.00, $p = 0.032$).[144]

Boersma et al. performed a metanalysis of GP IIb/IIIa antagonists of all six large randomized placebo-controlled trials (including GUSTO IV[146]) involving 31,402 patients with UA/NSTEMI not routinely scheduled to undergo coronary revascularization. Reductions in the endpoints of death or nonfatal MI considered individually did not achieve statistical significance.

Although the data are not definitive, it appears that GP IIb/IIIa inhibitors can be used with LMWH.[1] In the Antithrombotic Combination Using Tirofiban and Enoxaparin (ACUTE II) study,[1] UFH and enoxaparin were compared in patients with UA/NSTEMI receiving tirofiban.

In general, aspirin and UFH or LMWH are administered to all patients with UA/NSTMI. Clopidogrel is usually given (300 mg loading dose) to patients at moderate to severe risk prior to or at the time of a percutaneous coronary intervention. In many centers it is not given until the patient has been ruled out for coronary bypass surgery. The IIb/IIIa glyco protein inhibitors are usually reserved for those patients likely to undergo early PCI.

## THROMBOLYSIS

Thrombolytic agents in UA/NSTEMI have had no significant beneficial effect and actually increased the risk of MI in TIMI IIIB.[147]

## RISK STRATIFICATION

The management of ACS patients requires continuous risk stratification. Important prognostic information is derived from careful initial assessment, the patient's course during the first few days of management, and the patient's response to anti-ischemic and antithrombotic therapy. Angina at rest within 48 h in the absence of an extracardiac condition and UA in the early postinfarction period—along with age, male sex, hypertension, and maximal intravenous antianginal/anti-ischemic therapy—were independent predictors of death or nonfatal MI.[1] The baseline ECG on presentation has also been found to be extremely useful for risk stratification in the TIMI III registry.[148] Patients with ST-segment depression of ≥0.1 mV had an 11 percent rate of death or nonfatal MI at 1 year. Those with left bundle branch block (LBBB) had rates of 22.9 percent. The majority of patients had no ECG change or only isolated T-wave changes, with 6.8 to 8.2 percent rates of death or MI, respectively, at 1 year. In one study, the rates of death or MI associated with these initial ECG findings in ACS patients were even higher[148] (Fig. 51-11).

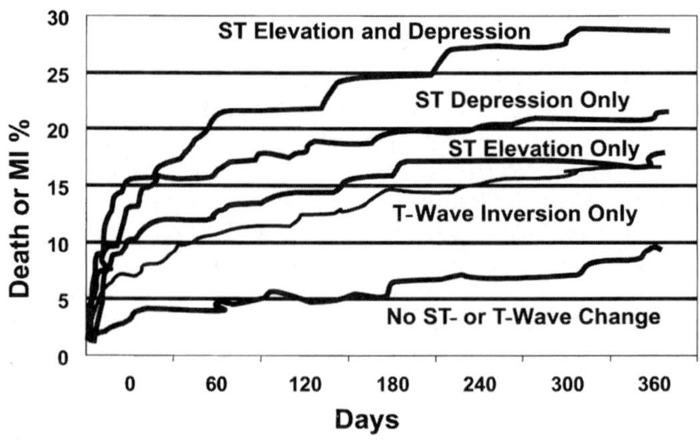


FIGURE 51-11 Adverse outcomes in acute coronary syndrome (ACS) patients stratified by initial electrocardiogram. (Adapted from Nyman I, Areskog M, Areskog NH, et al. Very early risk stratification by electrocardiogram at rest in men with suspected unstable coronary heart disease. (From the RISC Study Group. *J Intern Med* 1993;234:293-301. With permission.)

## NONINVASIVE TEST SELECTION

A detailed discussion of noninvasive stress testing in CAD is presented in the ACC/AHA Guidelines for Exercise Testing, ACC/AHA Guidelines for the Clinical Use of Cardiac Radionuclide Imaging, and ACC/AHA Guidelines for the Clinical Application of Echocardiography.[149–153] Ischemia that develops at greater than 6.5 metabolic equivalents (METs) may be associated with severe coronary artery obstruction, but unless other high-risk markers are present [greater than 0.2-mV ST-segment depression or elevation, fall in blood pressure, ST-segment shifts in multiple leads reflecting multiple coronary regions, or prolonged (greater than 6 min of ST-segment shifts) during recovery], these patients may also be *safely* managed *conservatively.*

The Veterans Affairs Non-Q-Wave Infarction Strategies in Hospital (VANQWISH) trial used symptom-limited thallium exercise treadmill testing at 3 to 5 days to direct the need for angiography in 442 NQMI patients randomized to an early conservative strategy.[154] This strategy included an effort to detect ischemia with noninvasive testing that would be associated with a high risk for adverse outcome. Cumulative death rates in the 238 conservative strategy patients directed to angiography on the basis of recurrent ischemia or high-risk stress test results were 3, 10, and 13 percent at 1, 6, and 12 months, respectively, whereas the rates were 1, 3, and 6 percent in the patients who were not directed to angiography (no recurrent ischemia or high-risk test). These findings support the concept that noninvasive stress testing can be used successfully to identify a high-risk subset of patients who could be directed to coronary angiography. It is unlikely that any an-

TABLE 51-6 ACC/AHA Recommendations for Noninvasive Risk Stratification

High risk (>3% annual mortality rate)
1. Severe resting LV dysfunction (LVEF <0.35)
2. High-risk treadmill (score ≤ −11)
3. Severe exercise LV dysfunction (exercise LVEF <0.35)
4. Stress-induced large perfusion defect (particularly if anterior)
5. Stress-induced multiple perfusion defects of moderate size
6. Large, fixed perfusion defect with LV dilation or increased lung uptake (thallium 201)
7. Stress-induced moderate perfusion defect with LV dilation or increased lung uptake (thallium 201)
8. Echocardiographic wall motion abnormality (involving more than two segments) developing at a low dose of dobutamine (≤10 mg/kg/min) or at a low heart rate (≤120 beats per minute)
9. Stress echocardiographic evidence of extensive ischemia

Intermediate risk (1–3% annual mortality rate)
1. Mild/moderate resting LV dysfunction (LVEF 0.35–0.49)
2. Intermediate-risk treadmill score (score −11 to +5)
3. Stress-induced moderate perfusion defect without LV dilation or increased lung intake (thallium 201)
4. Limited stress echocardiographic ischemia with a wall motion abnormality only at higher doses or dobutamine involving ≤2 segments

Low risk (<1% annual mortality rate)
1. Low-risk treadmill (score ≥ +5)
2. Normal or small myocardial perfusion defect at rest or with stress
3. Normal stress echocardiographic wall motion or no change of limited resting wall motion abnormalities during stress

ABBREVIATIONS: ACC/AHA = American College of Cardiology/American Heart Association; LV = left ventricular; LVEF = left ventricular ejection fraction.

giographically directed early revascularization strategy could alter the very low early event rates observed in patients without a high-risk stress test. The ACC/AHA Guidelines for Noninvasive Risk Stratification are presented in Table 51-6.

## Selection of Coronary Angiography

In contrast to the noninvasive tests, coronary angiography provides detailed structural information for assessing prognosis and to provide direction for appropriate management (Chap. 15). When combined with LV angiography, it also allows an assessment of global and regional LV function. Indications for coronary angiography are interwoven with indications for possible therapeutic plans such as PCI or CABG surgery.[155]

Coronary angiography is usually indicated in patients with UA/NSTEMI who either have recurrent symptoms of ischemia despite adequate medical therapy or who are at high risk as categorized by clinical signs (CHF, malignant ventricular arrhythmias) or noninvasive test findings [significant LV dysfunction: ejection fraction (EF) less than 0.35, large anterior or multiple perfusion defects].

### EARLY CONSERVATIVE VERSUS INVASIVE STRATEGIES

When the early conservative strategy is chosen, a plan for noninvasive evaluation is required to detect severe ischemia that occurs spontaneously or at a low threshold of stress and to promptly refer these patients for coronary angiography and revascularization if feasible. The ACC/AHA Guidelines for guiding strategies for early conservative versus invasive approaches in ACS are presented in Table 51-7.

In patients with UA/NSTEMI without recurrent ischemia in the first 24 h, the use of early angiography provides an invasive approach to risk stratification. It can identify the 10 to 15 percent of patients with no significant coronary stenoses and the approximately 20 percent with three-vessel disease with LV dysfunction or left main CAD.

Most patients with UA/NSTEMI do not benefit from *routine,* early invasive management and a conservative, *ischemia-guided* initial approach was both safe and effective even in the predominantly high-risk male population of the VANQWISH trial.

It may be concluded from FRISC II[156] that patients with UA/NSTEMI who are not at very high risk for revascularization and who first receive an average of 6 days of treatment with LMWH, ASA, nitrates, and beta blockers have a better outcome at 6 months with a *(delayed)* routine invasive approach than with a routine conservative approach.

In the TACTICS-TIMI 18 trial,[157] 2220 patients with UA or NSTEMI were treated with ASA, heparin, and the GP IIb/IIIa

TABLE 51-7 ACC/AHA Class I Recommendations for Early Conservative versus Invasive Strategies

An early invasive strategy in patients with unstable angina/non-ST-segment-elevation myocardial infarction and any of the following high-risk indicators:
- Recurrent angina/ischemia at rest or with low-level activities despite intensive anti-ischemic therapy
- Elevated TnT or TnI
- New or presumably new ST-segment depression
- Recurrent angina/ischemia with CHF symptoms, an $S_3$ gallop, pulmonary edema, worsening rales, or new or worsening MR
- High-risk findings on noninvasive stress testing
- Depressed LV systolic function (e.g., EF <0.40 on noninvasive study)
- Hemodynamic instability
- Sustained ventricular tachycardia
- PCI within 6 months
- Prior CABG

In the absence of these findings, either an early conservative or an early invasive strategy in hospitalized patients without contraindications for revascularization.

ABBREVIATIONS: ACC/AHA = American College of Cardiology/American Heart Association; TnT = troponin T; TnI = troponin I; CHF = congestive heart failure; MR = mitral regurgitation; LV = left ventricular; EF = ejection fraction; PCI = percutaneous coronary intervention; CABG = coronary artery bypass graft.

inhibitor tirofiban. They were randomized to an early invasive strategy with routine coronary angiography within 48 h followed by revascularization if the coronary anatomy was deemed suitable or to a more conservative strategy. In the latter, catheterization was performed only if the patient had recurrent ischemia or a positive stress test. Death, MI, or rehospitalization for ACS at 6 months occurred in 15.9 percent of patients assigned to the invasive strategy versus. 19.4 percent assigned to the more conservative strategy ($p = 0.025$).

Thus, both the FRISC II[156] and TACTICS-TIMI 18[157] trials, the two most recent trials comparing invasive versus conservative strategies in patients with UA/NSTEMI, showed a benefit in patients assigned to the invasive strategy. In contrast to earlier trials, a large majority of patients undergoing PCI in these two trials received coronary stenting as opposed to balloon angioplasty alone. Therefore an invasive strategy is associated with a better outcome in UA/NSTEMI patients *at high risk,* as defined in Table 51-7 and in TACTICS-TIMI 18[157] and who receive a GP IIb/IIIa inhibitor.[156]

## CORONARY REVASCULARIZATION

Coronary angiography is useful for defining the coronary artery anatomy in patients with UA/NSTEMI and for identifying subsets of high-risk patients who may benefit from early revascularization.[1] Coronary revascularization (PCI or CABG) is carried out to improve prognosis, relieve symptoms, prevent ischemic complications, and improve functional capacity. The decision to proceed from diagnostic angiography to revascularization is influenced not only by the coronary anatomy but also by a number of additional factors, including anticipated life expectancy, LV function, comorbidity, functional capacity, severity of symptoms, and quantity of viable myocardium at risk.

### Percutaneous Coronary Intervention

In recent years, technological advances, coupled with high acute success rates and low evidence of complications, have increased the use of PCI in patients with UA/NSTEMI (Chap. 55).

In the absence of active thrombus, rotational atherectomy is useful to debulk arteries that contain large atheromatous burdens and to modify plaques in preparation for more definitive treatment with adjunctive balloon angioplasty or stenting (Chap. 55).

Data from both retrospective observations and randomized clinical trials indicate that PCI can lead to angiographic success in most patients with UA/NSTEMI (Fig. 51-10). The safety of these procedures in these patients is enhanced by the addition of intravenous platelet GP IIb/IIIa receptor inhibitors to the standard regimen of ASA, heparin, and anti-ischemic medications.

### Surgical Revascularization

Two randomized trials conducted in the early years of CABG compared medical and surgical therapy in UA. The National Cooperative Study Group randomized 288 patients at nine centers between 1972 and 1976.[159] The Veterans Administration (VA) Cooperative Study randomized 468 patients between 1976 and 1982 at 12 hospitals.[160] Both trials included patients with progressive or rest angina accompanied by ST-T-wave changes. Patients greater than 70 years old or with a recent MI were excluded; the VA study included only men. In the National Cooperative Study, the hospital mortality rate was 3 percent for patients undergoing medical therapy and 5 percent after CABG ($p$ = NS). Follow-up to 30 months showed no differences in survival rates between the treatment groups.

A metanalysis was performed on the results of six trials conducted between 1972 and 1978 to compare long-term survival in CAD patients treated medically or with CABG.[1] A clear survival advantage was documented only for CABG in patients with left main and three-vessel coronary disease that was independent of LV function.

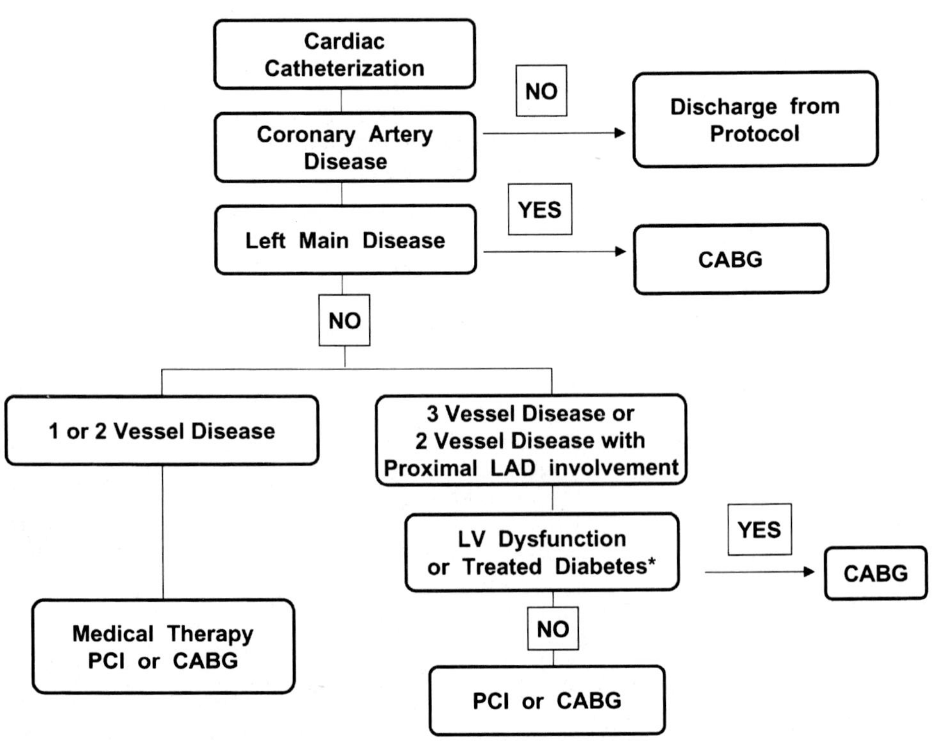


FIGURE 51-12 Revascularization strategy in unstable angina/non-ST-segment-elevation myocardial infarction (UA/NSTEMI). There is conflicting information about these patients. Most authors consider CABG to be preferable to PCI.

### Conclusions

In general, the indications for PCI and CABG in UA/NSTEMI are similar to those for stable angina.[1] High-risk patients with LV systolic dysfunction, patients with diabetes mellitus, and those with two-vessel disease with severe proximal involvement of the left anterior descending (LAD) artery or severe three-vessel or left main disease should be considered for CABG (Fig. 51-12). Many other patients will have less severe CAD that does not put them at high risk for cardiac death. However, even less severe disease can have a substantial negative impact on quality of life. Low-risk patients will receive negligible or very modest increases in long-term survival with CABG. Therefore, quality of life and patient preferences are given more weight than are strict clinical outcomes in the selection of a treatment strategy. Low-risk patients whose symptoms do not respond well to maximal medical therapy and who experience a significantly reduced quality of life and functional status should be considered for revascularization. Patients who are unwilling to accept the increased short-term procedural risks to gain long-term benefits or who are satisfied with their existing capabilities should be managed medically at first and followed carefully as outpatients.

## POST-HOSPITAL DISCHARGE AND CARE

The acute phase of UA/NSTEMI is usually over within 2 months. The risk of progression to MI or the development of recurrent MI or death is highest during that period. At 1 to 3 months after the acute phase, most patients resume a clinical course similar to that in patients with chronic stable coronary disease (Chap. 57).

The broad goals during the hospital discharge phase are twofold: (1) to prepare the patient for normal activities to the extent possible and (2) to use the acute event as an opportunity to reevaluate long-term care, particularly lifestyle and risk-factor modification. *Aggressive risk-factor modification* is the mainstay of the long-term management of stable CAD (Chap. 57). Patients who have undergone successful PCI with an uncomplicated course are usually discharged the next day, and patients who undergo uncomplicated CABG are generally discharged 4 to 7 days after CABG. Medical management of low-risk patients after noninvasive stress testing and coronary arteriography can typically be accomplished rapidly with discharge on the day of testing or the day after. Medical management of a high-risk group of patients who are unsuitable for or unwilling to undergo revascularization may require prolonged hospitalization.

### Medical Regimen

The goals for continued medical therapy after discharge relate to potential prognostic benefits (primarily shown for ASA, beta blockers, cholesterol-lowering agents, and ACE inhibitors, especially for LVEF less than 0.40), control of ischemic symptoms (nitrates, beta blockers, and calcium antagonists), and treatment of major risk factors such as hypertension, smoking, hyperlipidemia, and diabetes mellitus (Chap. 86). Thus, the selection of a medical regimen is individualized to the specific needs of each patient based on the in-hospital findings and events, the risk factors for CAD, drug tolerability, or the type of recent procedure. The mnemonic *ABCDE* (aspirin and antianginals; beta blockers and blood pressure; cholesterol and cigarettes; diet and diabetes; education and exercise) has been found to be useful in guiding treatment[153] (Chap. 51).

### Long-Term Medical Therapy

Many patients with UA/NSTEMI have chronic stable angina at hospital discharge. The management of the patient with stable CAD is detailed in the ACC/AHA/ACP-ASIM Guidelines for the Management of Patients With Chronic Stable Angina[153] and in Chap. 57.

The health care team should work with patients and their families to educate them regarding specific targets for LDL cholesterol, blood pressure, weight, and exercise. The family may be able to further support the patient by making changes in risk behavior.

The National Cholesterol Education Program III has raised the target for high-density-lipoprotein (HDL) cholesterol to 40 mg/dL.[161] In the Myocardial Ischemia Reduction with Aggressive Cholesterol Lowering (MIRACL) study, 3086 patients were randomized to treatment with an aggressive lipid-lowering regimen of atorvastatin 80 mg/day or placebo 24 to 96 h after an ACS.[162] At 16 weeks of follow-up, the primary endpoint of death, nonfatal MI, resuscitated cardiac arrest, or recurrent severe myocardial ischemia was reduced from 17.4 percent in the placebo group to 14.8 percent in the atorvastatin group ($p = 0.048$). There were no significant differences in the risk of death or nonfatal MI in the two groups, but there were fewer strokes and a lower risk of severe recurrent ischemia. The Lipid-Coronary Artery Disease (L-CAD) study was a small trial that randomized 126 patients with an ACS to early treatment with pravastatin, alone or in combination with cholestyramine or niacin, or to usual care. At 24 months, the patients who received early aggressive treatment had a lower incidence of clinical events (23 percent) than the usual-care group (52 percent; $p = 0.005$).

## VARIANT (PRINZMETAL'S) ANGINA

In 1959, Prinzmetal and associates described a syndrome characterized by angina at rest with transient marked ST-segment elevation.[163] Exercise tolerance usually was well preserved, and the attacks were cyclic in nature, often occurring in the early morning hours (Chap. 57). The episodes lasted no longer than ordinary anginal episodes, and the ST-segment elevation disappeared rapidly as the chest pain receded. Ventricular arrhythmias and AV block sometimes occurred at the peak of an attack, and both MI and sudden death were common consequences (Chap. 50).

With the use of coronary angiography, it soon became evident that the syndrome was caused by coronary spasm, usually focal and often at the site of a coronary artery stenosis.[164] The underlying coronary lesion varies from subtotal occlusion to a very mild stenosis; in some cases the coronary arteries are angiographically normal. Coronary spasm occurs in more than one artery in some patients,[165] and the site of spasm can fluctuate from one coronary artery to another.[166]

### Pathophysiology

Many etiologic explanations for variant angina have been proposed or rejected. Evidence of parasympathetic nervous system overactivity[167] and reduced sympathetic activity[168] has been presented, but coronary spasm has also been demonstrated in the transplanted, denervated heart,[169] thus making a central neural mechanism unlikely. The frequency of episodes of variant angina is not diminished by alpha-adrenergic blockade,[170] blockade of serotonin receptors,[171] inhibition of thromboxane $A_2$ production,[172] or the administration of prostacyclin.[173] Magnesium deficiency,[174] hyperinsulinemia,[175] and vitamin E deficiency[176] have each been reported to be present in patients with variant angina. Vitamin C attenuates the abnormal coronary vasoconstriction in patients with variant angina, purportedly by inhibiting oxygen free radical generation[177] (Chap. 43).

Whether nitric oxide activity at sites of coronary spasm is normal or abnormal remains debatable.[178] A mutation of the endothelial nitric oxide synthetase (eNOS) gene is reportedly more common in patients with coronary spasm than in controls.[179] Decreased endothelial nitric oxide production could predispose patients with this defect to coronary spasm.

Coronary spasm usually is localized to the site of an atherosclerotic lesion. Even variant angina patients with no angiographic evidence of luminal narrowing (Chap. 43) invariably will have atherosclerosis demonstrable by intracoronary ultrasound (IVUS) at the site of focal spasm.[180] Asian patients with variant angina more commonly have generalized coronary artery hyperactivity, whereas in Caucasian patients the abnormality is more focal.[181]

The pathophysiologic sequelae of coronary spasm are well known. Severe spasm rapidly induces transmural ischemia, resulting in segmental myocardial dyskinesis and ST-segment elevation. If the ischemic zone is large, cardiac output and systemic arterial pressure decrease. The risk of serious ventricular arrhythmias increases in proportion to the severity and extent of ischemia. Prolonged spasm can cause intracoronary thrombosis, which results in MI.[182]

## Clinical Features

Variant angina is uncommon, and the presenting symptoms are usually not severe enough to be distinguished immediately from those of UA. Angina at rest occurs with a cyclic pattern, and episodes are more common in the early morning hours. Exertional angina coexists in more than half of these patients, but with a greater variability in ischemic threshold.[183] Variant angina can occur during the recovery phase of MI[184] or in the early hours after coronary bypass surgery[185] or PCI.[186]

Variant angina is more common in heavy cigarette smokers, but their age, sex, and risk-factor profiles are otherwise similar to those of other coronary patients.[187] Patients with normal coronary arteries tend to be younger and more often are women. One-quarter of patients with variant angina have a history of migraine headaches, and about 25 percent have symptoms of Raynaud's phenomenon.[188] Thus, in some cases variant angina may be part of a more generalized vasospastic diathesis. Syncope, likely due to ischemia-induced ventricular arrhythmia or AV block, during rest angina is a clue to the diagnosis. Rare cases of life-threatening ventricular arrhythmias caused by silent myocardial ischemia during coronary spasm have been reported.[189]

Cocaine causes coronary vasoconstriction and can precipitate coronary spasm, sometimes with myocardial infarction. This topic is discussed in Chaps. 46, 52, and 53.

Physical examination of variant angina patients between attacks usually reveals no abnormalities. Routine laboratory tests, including cardiac enzymes, are normal.

## Diagnostic Procedures

Variant angina can be diagnosed most easily by an ECG recording during an episode of rest angina. The ST-segment elevation that occurs during an attack disappears promptly after the administration of nitroglycerin. Coronary spasm can induce ST elevation, ST depression, or pseudonormalization of abnormally negative T waves (Fig. 51-13). When variant angina is a consideration, ambulatory ECG monitoring or an event monitor sometimes can be useful to confirm the diagnosis. Exercise testing will provoke angina with ST-segment elevation in approximately one-third of patients with variant angina during an active phase of the disease. Provocative testing has been used to confirm the diagnosis of variant angina when a spontaneous attack cannot be documented. The cold pressor response, exercise, and hyperventilation are physiologic stimuli for coronary spasm, but each has a sensitivity that is too low to be reliable clinically.[190] Pharmacologic agents ergonovine and acetylcholine provoke coronary spasm with a sensitivity of approximately 90 percent in patients with variant angina.[191,192] Intracoronary acetylcholine is probably the preferred method, but a temporary pacemaker must be placed before right coronary (or dominant left coronary) injections are done because of the high incidence of bradyarrhythmias and conduction disturbances from cholinergic effects in the AV node. All attempts to induce coronary spasm should be performed in the catheterization laboratory, since intracoronary nitroglycerin may be necessary to treat arterial hypotension due to a positive test.

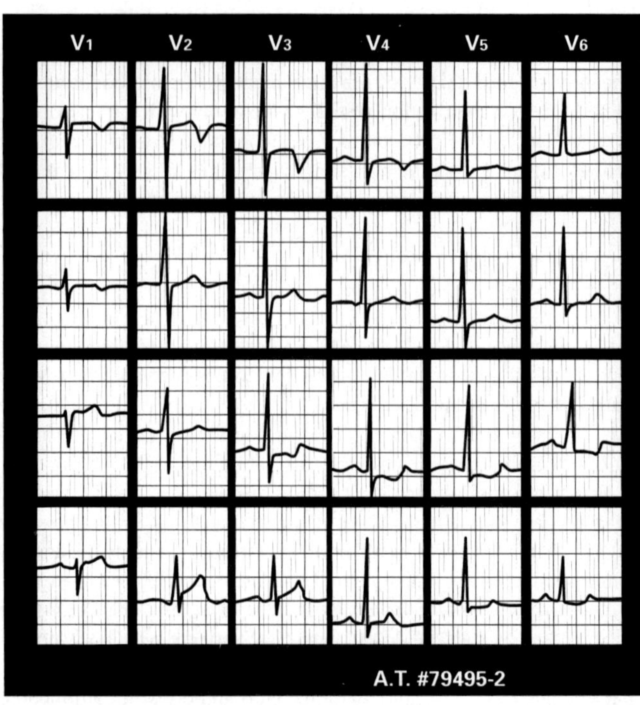


FIGURE 51-13 Electrocardiogram (leads $V_1$ to $V_6$) from a patient with active variant angina. Negative T waves are present in the control tracing (*top*). The other three tracings were recorded during separate episodes of rest angina and show pseudonormalization of T waves, ST depression, and ST elevation, respectively.

All patients with variant angina should undergo coronary angiography unless an absolute contraindication is present. Coronary angiography is the only certain method to distinguish between patients who have severe organic multivessel disease and those who have only mild luminal narrowings or angiographically normal arteries. An IVUS study (Chap. 18) may reveal more disease than indicated by angiography.

## Treatment

Variant angina is often difficult to treat because attacks are unpredictable and often occur without an obvious precipitating factor. The aim of therapy, therefore, should be the elimination of all attacks. Spontaneous remission is a common outcome,[193] but MI is a frequent consequence within the first 3 months after diagnosis, particularly in those with underlying multivessel disease.[194] Nitroglycerin relieves variant angina attacks within minutes and should be used promptly. Long-acting nitrates initially are effective in preventing variant angina attacks, but the development of nitrate tolerance often limits their utility. Beta-adrenergic blockers should not be used in variant angina because of their propensity to increase the frequency and duration of attacks.[195,196]

Calcium channel blockers are very effective in preventing attacks of variant angina.[197–199] More than 50 percent of patients treated with one of these drugs become completely asymptomatic, but higher doses are frequently required. For example, long-acting nifedipine 80 mg/day, diltiazem 360 mg/day, verapamil 480 mg/day, or amlodipine 20 mg/day are commonly used doses. The efficacy of these drugs in preventing variant angina is about equal. Patients with an incomplete response to one drug often become angina-free on a combination of nifedipine (or amlodipine) and either diltiazem or verapamil. Evidence from uncontrolled studies suggests that treatment with calcium channel blockers reduces the risk of MI.[200,201]

Approximately 20 percent of variant angina patients will not respond to treatment with two calcium channel blockers plus a long-acting nitrate. Although not approved by the U.S. Food and Drug Administration (FDA) for this indication, amiodarone,[202] guanethidine,[203] and clonidine[204] are reportedly effective in some of these refractory patients. Treatment for ventricular arrhythmias and conduction disturbances that complicate attacks should be directed toward the elimination of all episodes of spasm.[205] Patients with variant angina should also be treated with low-dose aspirin to reduce the risk of MI, even though very high doses of aspirin have been reported to aggravate coronary spasm.[206]

CABG surgery should be considered in most patients with variant angina and multivessel atherosclerotic disease even though operative mortality and the perioperative MI rate are higher than in comparable patients without variant angina.[207,208] Nevertheless, surgery almost invariably eliminates variant angina, and the long-term outcome is excellent. Bypass surgery will be successful when the anastomosis can be placed distal to the site of focal spasm but not when diffuse spasm involves the entire artery. Bypass surgery is *not* indicated for variant angina when there are no significant organic stenoses present.

Many patients with variant angina have coronary lesions that are ideal for PCI. When such patients are pretreated with calcium channel blockers and are given intracoronary nitroglycerin during the procedure, the primary success rate is high. Coronary spasm may persist or recur after successful angioplasty, however, and calcium channel blockers should therefore be continued. The restenosis rate in variant angina patients is substantially higher than usual. Whether coronary stenting improves outcomes for variant angina patients is yet unknown. PCI, like CABG, is not indicated for patients with coronary spasm who have normal or nearly normal arteries on coronary angiography.

## Prognosis

The long-term prognosis of variant angina has been reported for several large series of patients from different countries. The extent and severity of the underlying coronary disease appear to be the most important factors influencing the outcome. One-year survival without infarction in a consecutive series of 217 patients was 93 percent for those without stenoses of 70 percent or more, 86 percent for patients with single-vessel disease, and 65 percent for those with multivessel disease. At 5 years, the corresponding figures were 83 percent, 74 percent, and 44 percent, respectively. Other factors correlating with a poor outcome include the presence of depressed LV function, ventricular arrhythmias during attacks, multivessel spasm, and the absence of treatment with calcium channel blockers. Fortunately, the majority of these patients will become angina-free within months or years. Variant angina will recur in rare cases after a long asymptomatic interval. More commonly, patients will develop further manifestations of coronary atherothrombosis. It is likely that recurrent coronary spasm accelerates the progression of coronary atherosclerosis, with a histologic pattern of neointimal hyperplasia that resembles restenosis.

## References


1. Braunwald E, Antman EM, Beasley JW, et al. ACC/AHA 2002 guideline updates for the management of patients with UA and non-ST-segment elevation myocardial infarction. A report of the American College of Cardiology/American Heart Association Task Force on Practice Guidelines (Committee on the Management of Patients With UA). *J Am Coll Cardiol* 2002;40:1366–1374.
2. Waters DD. Diagnosis and management of patients with unstable angina. In: Fuster V, Alexander RW, O'Rourke, RA, et al, eds. Hurst's the Heart, 10th ed. New York: McGraw-Hill; 2001:1237–1274.
3. National Center for Health Statistics. Detailed diagnoses and procedures: National Hospital Discharge Survey, 1996. Hyattsville, MD: National Center for Health Statistics; 1998:13. Data from Vital and Health Statistics.
4. Nourjah P. et al. National Hospital Ambulatory Medical Care Survey: 1997 emergency department summary. Hyattsville, MD: National Center for Health Statistics; 1999:304. Advance data from Vital and Health Statistics.
5. Blake GJ, Ridker PM. Novel clinical markers of vascular wall inflammation. *Circ Res* 2001;89:763–771.
6. Ridker PM, Stampfer MJ, Rifai N. Novel risk factors for systemic atherosclerosis: A comparison of C-reactive protein, fibrinogen, homocysteine, lipoprotein(a), and standard cholesterol screening as predictors of peripheral arterial disease. *JAMA* 2001;2835:2481–2485.
7. Lowe GD, Yarnell JW, Rumley A, et al. C-reactive protein, fibrin D-dimer, and incident ischemic heart disease in the Speedwell study: Are inflammation and fibrin turnover linked in pathogenesis? *Arterioscler Thromb Vasc Biol* 2001;21:603–610.
8. Mueller C, Buettner JH, Hodgson JM, et al. Inflammation and long-term mortality after non-ST-elevation acute coronary syndrome treated with a very early invasive strategy in 1042 consecutive patients. *Circulation* 2002;105:1412–1415.
9. Vorchheimer DA, Fuster V. Inflammatory markers in coronary artery disease: Let prevention douse the flames. *JAMA* 2001;286:2154–2156.
10. Ridker PM, Glynn RJ, Hennekens CH. C-reactive protein adds to the predictive value of total and HDL cholesterol in determining risk of first myocardial infarction. *Circulation* 1998;97:2007–2011.
11. Blake GJ, Ridker PM. C-reactive protein and other inflammatory markers in acute coronary syndromes. *J Am Coll Cardiol* 2003;141: L23–L305.
12. Chen L, Théroux P, Lespérance J, et al. Angiographic features of vein grafts versus ungrafted coronary arteries in patients with unstable angina and previous bypass surgery. *J Am Coll Cardiol* 1996;28: 1493–1499.
13. Braunwald E, Jones RH, Mark DB, et al. Diagnosing and managing unstable angina. *Circulation* 1994;90:613–622.
14. Fuster V, Fayal ZA, Badimon JJ. Acute coronary syndromes: Biology. *Lancet* 1999;353(suppl II):5–9.
15. Davies MJ, Richardson PD, Woolf N, et al. Risk of thrombosis in human atherosclerotic plaques: Role of extracellular lipid, macrophages, and smooth muscle content. *Br Heart J* 1993;69:377–381.
16. Davies MJ. Stability and instability: Two faces of coronary atherosclerosis. *Circulation* 1996;94:2013–2020.
17. Farb A, Burke AP, Tang AL, et al. Coronary plaque erosion without rupture into a lipid core: A frequent cause or coronary thrombosis in sudden coronary death. *Circulation* 1996;93:1354–1363.
18. Burke AP, Farb A, Malcom GT, et al. Coronary risk factors and plaque morphology in men with coronary disease who die suddenly. *N Engl J Med* 1997;336:1276–1282.
19. Burke AP, Farb A, Malcom GT, et al. Effect of risk factors on the mechanism of acute thrombosis and sudden coronary death in women. *Circulation* 1998;97:2110–2116.
20. Sato T, Takebayashi S, Kohehi K. Increased subendothelial infiltration of the coronary arteries with monocytes/macrophages in patients with unstable angina. *Atherosclerosis* 1995;68:191–197.
21. Mazzone A, De Servi S, Ricevuti G, et al. Increased expression of neutrophil and monocyte adhesion molecules in unstable coronary artery disease. *Circulation* 1993;88:358–363.
22. Libby P. Molecular basis of acute coronary syndromes. *Circulation* 1995;91:2844–2850.
23. Kai H, Ikeda H, Yasukawa H, et al. Peripheral blood levels of matrix metalloproteinases-2 and -9 are elevated in patients with acute coronary syndromes. *J Am Coll Cardiol* 1998;32:368–372.
24. Brown DL, Hibbs MS, Kearney M, et al. Identification of 92-kD gelatinase in human coronary atherosclerotic lesions: Association of active enzyme synthesis with unstable angina. *Circulation* 1995;91:2125–2131.

25. Ritchie ME. Nuclear factor-$\kappa$B is selectively and markedly activated in humans with unstable angina pectoris. *Circulation* 1998;98:1707–1713.
26. van der Wall AC, Becer AE, van der Loos CM, Das PK. Site of intimal rupture or erosion of thrombosed coronary atherosclerotic plaques is characterized by an inflammatory process irrespective of dominant plaque morphology. *Circulation* 1994;89:36–44.
27. Kaartinen M, van der Wal AC, van der Loos CM, et al. Mast cell infiltration in acute coronary syndromes: Implications for plaque rupture. *J Am Coll Cardiol* 1998;32:606–612.
28. Berk BC, Weintraub WS, Alexander RW. Elevation of C-reactive protein in "active" coronary artery disease. *Am J Cardiol* 1990;65:168–172.
29. Liuzzo G, Biasucci LM, Gallimore JR, et al. The prognostic value of C-reactive protein and serum amyloid A protein in severe unstable angina. *N Engl J Med* 1994;331:417–424.
30. Ross R. Atherosclerosis—An inflammatory disease. *N Engl J Med* 1999;340:115–126.
30a. Brennan ML, Penn MS, VanLente F, et al. Prognostic value of myeloperoxidase in patients with chest pain. *N Engl J Med* 2003; 349:1595–1604.
31. Libby P, Egan D, Skarlatos S. Roles of infectious agents in atherosclerosis and restenosis: An assessment of the evidence and need for future research. *Circulation* 1997;96:4095–4103.
32. Ridker PM. Inflammation, infection and cardiovascular risk: How good is the evidence? *Circulation* 1998;97:1671–1674.
33. Kol A, Sukhova GK, Lichtman AH, Libby P. Chlamydial heat shock protein 60 localizes in human atheroma and regulates macrophage tumor necrosis factor-$\alpha$ and matrix metalloproteinase expression. *Circulation* 1998;98:300–307.
34. Mayr M, Metzler B, Kiechl S, et al. Endothelial cytotoxicity mediated by serum antibodies to heat shock proteins of *Escherichia coli* and *Chlamydia pneumoniae:* Immune reactions to heat shock proteins as a possible link between infection and atherosclerosis. *Circulation* 1999; 99:1560–1566.
35. Strachan DP, Mendall MA, Carrington D, et al. Relation of *Helicobacter pylori* infection to 13-year mortality and incident ischemic heart disease in the Caerphilly Prospective Heart Disease Study. *Circulation* 1998;98:1286–1290.
36. Gupta S, Leatham EW, Carrington D, et al. Elevated *Chlamydia pneumoniae* antibodies, cardiovascular events, and azithromycin in male survivors of myocardial infarction. *Circulation* 1997;96:404–407.
37. Gupta S, Leatham EW, Carrington D, et al. Elevated *Chlamydia pneumoniae* antibodies, cardiovascular events, and azithromycin in male survivors of myocardial infarction. *Circulation* 1997;96: 404–407.
38. Andersen JL, Muhlestein JB, Carlquist J, et al. Randomized secondary prevention trial of azithromycin in patients with coronary artery disease and serological evidence for *Chlamydia pneumoniae* infection: The Azithromycin in Coronary Artery Disease: Elimination of Myocardial Infection with Chlamydia (ACADEMIC) Study. *Circulation* 1999;99:1540–1547.
39. Gurfinkel E, Bozovich G, Daroca A, et al for the ROXIS Study Group. Randomized trial of roxithromycin in non-Q-wave coronary syndromes: ROXIS pilot study. *Lancet* 1997;350:404–407.
40. Davies M, Bland J, Hangartner J, et al. Factors influencing the presence or absence of acute coronary artery thrombi in sudden ischemic death. *Eur Heart J* 1989;10:203–208.
41. Furman MI, Benoit SE, Barnard MR, et al. Increased platelet reactivity and circulating monocyte-platelet aggregates in patients with stable coronary artery disease. *J Am Coll Cardiol* 1998;31:352–358.
42. Davi G, Gresele P, Violi F, et al. Diabetes mellitus, hypercholesterolemia, and hypertension but not vascular disease per se are associated with persistent platelet activation in vivo: Evidence derived from the study of peripheral arterial disease. *Circulation* 1997;96:69–75.
43. Fitzgerald DJ, Roy L, Catella F, Fitzgerald A. Platelet activation in unstable coronary disease. *N Engl J Med* 1986;315:983–989.
44. Grande P, Grauholt AM, Madsen JK. Unstable angina pectoris: Platelet behavior and prognosis in progressive angina and intermediate coronary syndrome. *Circulation* 1990;81(suppl I):I-16–I-19.
45. Hamm CW, Lorenz RL, Bleifeld W, et al. Biochemical evidence of platelet activation in patients with persistent unstable angina. *J Am Coll Cardiol* 1987;10:998–1004.
46. Ikeda H, Takajo Y, Ichiki K, et al. Increased soluble form of P-selectin in patients with unstable angina. *Circulation* 1995;92:1693–1696.
47. Ott I, Neumann FJ, Gawaz M, et al. Increased neutrophil-platelet adhesion in patients with unstable angina. *Circulation* 1996;94:1239–1246.
48. De Servi S, Mazzone A, Ricevuti G, et al. Clinical and angiographic correlates of leukocyte activation in unstable angina. *J Am Coll Cardiol* 1995;26:1146–1150.
49. Fitzgerald DJ, Roy L, Catella F, Fitzgerald A. Platelet activation in unstable coronary disease. *N Engl J Med* 1986;315:983–989.
50. Grande P, Grauholt AM, Madsen JK. Unstable angina pectoris: Platelet behavior and prognosis in progressive angina and intermediate coronary syndrome. *Circulation* 1990;81(suppl I):I-16–I-19.
51. Hamm CW, Lorenz RL, Bleifeld W, et al. Biochemical evidence of platelet activation in patients with persistent unstable angina. *J Am Coll Cardiol* 1987;10:998–1004.
52. Toschi V, Gallo R, Lettino M, et al. Tissue factor modulates the thrombogenicity of human atherosclerotic plaques. *Circulation* 1997;95: 594–599.
53. Bogaty P, Hackett D, Davies G, Maseri A. Vasoreactivity of the culprit lesion in unstable angina. *Circulation* 1994;90:5–11.
54. Moise A, Théroux P, Taeymans Y, et al. Unstable angina and progression of coronary atherosclerosis. *N Engl J Med* 1983;309:685–689.
55. Ambrose JA, Winters SL, Stern A, et al. Angiographic morphology and the pathogenesis of unstable angina pectoris. *J Am Coll Cardiol* 1985; 5:609–616.
56. De Feyter PJ, Ozaki Y, Baptista J, et al. Ischemia-related lesion characteristics in patients with stable or unstable angina: A study with intracoronary angioscopy and ultrasound. *Circulation* 1995;92: 1408–1413.
57. Hochman J, Tamis JE, Thompson D, et al., for the Global Use of Strategies to Open Occluded Coronary Arteries in Acute Coronary Syndromes IIb investigators. Sex, clinical presentation and outcomes in patients with acute coronary syndromes. *N Engl J Med* 1999;341:226–232.
58. De Zwaan C, Bär FW, Janssen JHA, et al. Angiographic and clinical characteristics of patients with unstable angina showing an ECG pattern indicating critical narrowing of the proximal LAD coronary artery. *Am Heart J* 1989;117:657–664.
59. Cannon CP, McCabe CH, Stone PH, et al., for the TIMI III Registry ECG Ancillary Study investigators. The electrocardiogram predicts one-year outcome of patients with unstable angina and non-Q wave myocardial infarction: Results of the TIMI III Registry ECG Ancillary Study. *J Am Coll Cardiol* 1997;30:133–140.
60. Ohman EM, Armstrong PW, Christenson RH, et al., for the GUSTO-IIa investigators. Cardiac troponin T levels for risk stratification in acute myocardial ischemia. *N Engl J Med* 1996;335:1333–1341.
61. Armstrong PW, Chiong MA, Parker JO. The spectrum of unstable angina: Prognostic role of serum creatine kinase determination. *Am J Cardiol* 1982;49:1849–1852.
62. Antman EM, Tanasijevic MJ, Thompson B, et al. Cardiac specific troponin I levels to predict the risk of mortality in patients with acute coronary syndromes. *N Engl J Med* 1996;335:1342–1349.
63. Lüscher MS, Thygesen K, Ravkilde J, Heickendorff L, for the TRIM Study Group. Applicability of cardiac troponin T and I for early risk stratification in unstable coronary artery disease. *Circulation* 1997;96: 2578–2585.
64. Galvani M, Ottani F, Ferrini D, et al. Prognostic influence of elevated values of cardiac troponin I in patients with unstable angina. *Circulation* 1997;95:2053–2059.
65. Olatidoye AG, Wu AHB, Feng YJ, Waters D. Prognostic role of troponin T versus troponin I in unstable angina pectoris for cardiac events with meta-analysis comparing published studies. *Am J Cardiol* 1998; 81:1405–1410.
66. Azar RR, Fram DB, Fossati AT, et al. How long do Tc-99m-sestamibi myocardial perfusion defects last after resolution of acute ischemia? An angioplasty model (abstr). *Circulation* 1997;96:(suppl I):I-309.

67. Kwong RY, Schussheim AE, Rekhraj S, et al. Detecting acute coronary syndrome in the emergency department with cardiac magnetic resonance imaging. *Circulation* 2003;107:531–537.
68. Gaspoz J, Lee TH, Weinstein MC, et al. Cost effectiveness of a new short-stay unit to "rule out" acute myocardial infarction in low risk patients. *J Am Coll Cardiol* 1994;24:1249–1259.
69. Gomez MA, Anderson JL, Karagounis LA, et al., for the ROMIO Study Group. An emergency department-based protocol for rapidly ruling out myocardial ischemia reduces hospital time and expense: Results of a randomized study (ROMIO). *J Am Coll Cardiol* 1996;28: 25–33.
70. Graff LG, Dallara J, Ross MA, et al. Impact on the care of the emergency department chest pain patient from the Chest Pain Evaluation Registry (CHEPER) Study. *Am J Cardiol* 1997;80:563–568.
71. Goldman L, Cook EF, Johnson PA, et al. Prediction of the need for intensive care in patients who come to emergency departments with acute chest pain. *N Engl J Med* 1996;334:1498–1504.
72. Farkouh ME, Smars PA, Reeder GS, et al. for the Chest Pain Evaluation in the Emergency Room (CHEER) Investigators. A clinical trial of a chest-pain observation unit for patients with unstable angina. *N Engl J Med* 1998;339:1882–1888.
73. Bugiardini R, Borghi A, Pozzati A, et al. Relation of severity of symptoms to transient myocardial ischemia and prognosis in unstable angina. *J Am Coll Cardiol* 1995;25:597–604.
74. Newby LK, Christenson RH, Ohman EM, et al, for the GUSTO-IIa Investigators. Value of serial troponin T measures for early and late risk stratification in patients with acute coronary syndromes. *Circulation* 1998;98:1853–1859.
75. Polanczyk CA, Lee TH, Cook EF, et al. Cardiac troponin I as a predictor of major cardiac events in emergency department patients with acute chest pain. *J Am Coll Cardiol* 1998;32:8–14.
76. Lindahl B, Venge P, Wallentin L, for the Fragmin in Unstable Coronary Artery Disease (FRISC) Study Group. Troponin T identifies patients with unstable coronary artery disease who benefit from long-term antithrombotic protection. *J Am Coll Cardiol* 1997;29:43–48.
77. Morrow DA, Rifai N, Antman EM, et al. C-reactive protein is a potent predictor of mortality independently of and in combination with troponin T in acute coronary syndromes: A TIMI 11A substudy: Thrombolysis in Myocardial Infarction. *J Am Coll Cardiol* 1998;31: 1460–1465.
78. Ardissino D, Merlini PA, Gamba G, et al. Thrombin activity and early outcome in unstable angina pectoris. *Circulation* 1996;93:1634–1639.
79. Becker RC, Cannon CP, Bovill EG, et al., for the TIMI III investigators. Prognostic value of plasma fibrinogen concentration in patients with unstable angina and NQWMI (TIMI IIIB Trial). *Am J Cardiol* 1996;78:142–147.
80. Montalescot G, Philippe F, Ankri A, et al., for the French investigators in the ESSENCE trial. Early increase of von Willebrand factor predicts adverse outcome in unstable coronary artery disease: Beneficial effects of enoxaparin. *Circulation* 1998;98:294–299.
81. Swahn E, Areskog M, Berglund U, et al. Predictive importance of clinical findings and a predischarge exercise test in patients with suspected unstable coronary artery disease. *Am J Cardiol* 1987;59:208–214.
82. Wilcox I, Freedman SB, Allman KC, et al. Prognostic significance of a predischarge exercise test in risk stratification after unstable angina pectoris. *J Am Coll Cardiol* 1991;18:677–683.
83. Brown KA. Prognostic value of thallium-201 myocardial perfusion imaging in patients with unstable angina who respond to medical treatment. *J Am Coll Cardiol* 1991;17:1053–1057.
84. Stratmann HG, Younis LT, Wittry MD, et al. Exercise technetium-99m myocardial tomography for risk stratification of men with medically treated unstable angina pectoris. *Am J Cardiol* 1995;76:236–240.
85. Freeman MR, Chisholm RJ, Armstrong PW. Usefulness of exercise electrocardiography and thallium scintigraphy in unstable angina pectoris in predicting the extent and severity of coronary artery disease. *Am J Cardiol* 1988;62:1164–1170.
86. Polanczyk CA, Johnson PA, Hartley LH, et al. Clinical correlates and prognostic significance of early negative exercise tolerance test in patients with acute chest pain seen in the hospital emergency department. *Am J Cardiol* 1998;81:288–292.
87. Alison HW, Russell RO, Mantle JA, et al. Coronary anatomy and arteriography in patients with unstable angina pectoris. *Am J Cardiol* 1978;41:204–209.
88. Ouyang P, Brinker JA, Mellits ED, et al. Variables predictive of successful medical therapy in patients with unstable angina: Selection by multivariate analysis from clinical, electrocardiographic, and angiographic evaluations. *Circulation* 1984;70:367–376.
89. Russell RO, Moraski RE, Kouchoukos N, et al. Unstable angina pectoris: National cooperative study group to compare medical and surgical therapy: II. In-hospital experience and initial follow-up results in patients with one, two and three vessel disease. *Am J Cardiol* 1978;42:839–848.
90. Luchi RJ, Scott SM, Dupree RH, and the principal investigators and their associates of Veterans Administration Cooperative Study No. 28. Comparison of medical and surgical therapy for unstable angina pectoris. *N Engl J Med* 1987;316:977–984.
91. Yusuf S, Zucker D, Peduzzi P, et al. Effect of coronary artery bypass graft surgery on survival: Overview of 10-year results from randomised trials by the Coronary Artery Bypass Graft Surgery Trialists Collaboration. *Lancet* 1994;344:563–570.
92. Diver DJ, Bier JD, Ferreira PE, et al., for the TIMI-IIIA Investigators. Clinical and arteriographic characterization of patients with unstable angina without critical coronary arterial narrowing (from the TIMI-IIIA Trial). *Am J Cardiol* 1994;74:531–537.
93. Holmvang L, Lüscher MS, Clemmensen P, et al., and the TRIM study group. Very early risk stratification using combined ECG and biochemical assessment in patients with unstable coronary artery disease (a Thrombin Inhibition in Myocardial Ischemia [TRIM] substudy). *Circulation* 1998;98:2004–2009.
94. Yusuf S, Wittes J, Friedman L. Overview of results of randomized clinical trials in heart disease: II. unstable angina, heart failure, primary prevention with aspirin, and risk factor modification. *JAMA* 1988;260: 2259–2263.
95. Betriu A, Heras M, Cohen M, Fuster V. Unstable angina: Outcome according to clinical presentation. *J Am Coll Cardiol* 1992;19: 1659–1663.
96. Van Domburg RT, van Miltenburg-van Zihl AJ, Veerhoek RJ, Simoons ML. Unstable angina: Good long-term outcome after complicated early course. *J Am Coll Cardiol* 1988;31:1534–1539.
97. Furberg CD, Psaty BM, Meyer JV. Nifedipine dose-related increase in mortality in patients with coronary heart disease. *Circulation* 1995; 92:1326–1331.
98. Gibson RS, Boden WE, Theroux P, et al. Diltiazem and reinfarction in patients with non-Q-wave myocardial infarction: Results of a double-blind, randomized, multicenter trial. *N Engl J Med* 1986;315:423–429.
99. Lubsen J, Tijssen JG. Efficacy of nifedipine and metoprolol in the early treatment of unstable angina in the coronary care unit: Findings from the Holland Interuniversity Nifedipine/metoprolol Trial (HINT). *Am J Cardiol* 1987;60:18A–25A.
100. Yusuf S, Pepine CJ, Garces C, et al. Effect of enalapril on myocardial infarction and unstable angina in patients with low ejection fractions. *Lancet* 1992;340:1173–1178.
101. ACE Inhibitor Myocardial Infarction Collaborative Group. Indications for ACE inhibitors in the early treatment of acute myocardial infarction: Systematic overview of individual data from 100,000 patients in randomized trials. *Circulation* 1998;97:2202–2212.
102. Flather M, Yusuf S, Kober L, et al. Long-term ACE-inhibitor therapy in patients with heart failure or left ventricular dysfunction: A systematic overview of data from individual patients. *Lancet* 2000;355:1575–1581.
103. Gustafsson I, Torp-Pedersen C, Kober L, et al. Effect of the angiotensin-converting enzyme inhibitor trandolapril on mortality and morbidity in diabetic patients with left ventricular dysfunction after acute myocardial infarction. Trace Study Group. *J Am Coll Cardiol* 1999;34:83–89.
104. Yusuf S, Sleight P, Pogue J, et al. for the Heart Outcomes Prevention Evaluation Study Investigators. Effects of an angiotensin-converting-enzyme inhibitor, ramipril, on cardiovascular events in high-risk patients. *N Engl J Med* 2000;342:145–153.

105. Antiplatelet Trialists' Collaboration. Collaborative overview of randomised trials of antiplatelet therapy: I. prevention of death, myocardial infarction, and stroke by prolonged antiplatelet therapy in various categories of patients [erratum appears in *Br Med J* 1994;308:1540]. *Br Med J* 1994;308:81–106.
106. Ridker PM, Cushman M, Stampfer MJ, et al. Inflammation, aspirin, and the risk of cardiovascular disease in apparently healthy men [erratum appears in *N Engl J Med* 1997;337:356]. *N Engl J Med* 1997;336:973–979.
107. Lewis HDJ, Davis JW, Archibald DG., et al. Protective effects of aspirin against acute myocardial infarction and death in men with unstable angina: Results of a Veterans Administration Cooperative Study. *N Engl J Med* 1983;309:396–403.
108. Cairns JA, Gent M, Singer J, et al. Aspirin, sulfinpyrazone, or both in unstable angina: Results of a Canadian multicenter trial. *N Engl J Med* 1985;313:1369–1375.
109. Theroux P, Ouimet H, McCans J, et al. Aspirin, heparin, or both to treat acute unstable angina. *N Engl J Med* 1988;319:1105–1111.
110. RISC Group. Risk of myocardial infarction and death during treatment with low dose aspirin and intravenous heparin in men with unstable coronary artery disease. *Lancet* 1990;336:827–830.
111. Love BB, Biller J, Gent M. Adverse haematological effects of ticlopidine: Prevention, recognition and management. *Drug Saf* 1998;19:89–98.
112. CAPRIE Steering Committee. A randomised, blinded, trial of Clopidogrel versus Aspirin in Patients at Risk of Ischaemic Events (CAPRIE). 1996;348:1329–1339.
113. Yusuf S, Zhao F, Mehta SR, et al. Effects of clopidogrel in addition to aspirin in patients with acute coronary syndromes without ST-segment-elevation. *N Engl J Med* 2001;345(7):494–502.
114. Mehta SR, Yusuf S, Peters RJ, et al. Effects of pretreatment with clopidogrel and aspirin followed by long-term therapy in patients undergoing percutaneous coronary intervention: The PCI-CURE study. *Lancet* 2001;358:527–533.
115. The CREDO Investigators. Clopidogrel for the Reduction of Events During Observation. *JAMA* 2002;288:2411–2420.
116. Hongo RH, Ley J, Dick ED, Yee RR. The effect of clopidogrel in combination with aspirin when given coronary artery bypass grafting. *J Am Coll Cardiol* 40(2):231–237.
117. Khot UN, Nissen SE. Is CURE a cure for acute coronary syndromes? Statistical versus clinical significance. *J Am Coll Cardiol* 2002;40(2):218–219.
118. Clarke TA, Waskell LA: The metabolism of clopidogrel is catalyzed by human cytochrome P450 3A and is inhibited by atorvastatin. *Drug Metab Dispos* 2003;31:53–59.
119. Lau WC, Waskell LA, Watkins PB, et al: Atorvastatin reduces the ability of clopidogrel to inhibit platelet aggregation. A new drug-drug interaction. *Circulation* 2003;107:32–37.
119a. Lau WC, Gurbel PA, Watkins PB, et al. Contribution of hepatic cytochrome P450 3A4 metabolic activity to the phenomenon of clopidogrel resistance. *Circulation* 2004;109:166–171.
120. Hirsh J. Heparin. *N Engl J Med* 1991;324:1565–1574.
121. Weitz JI. Low-molecular-weight heparins [erratum appears in *N Engl J Med* 1997;337:1567] *N Engl J Med* 1997;337:688–698.
122. Stone SR, Hofsteenge J. Kinetics of the inhibition of thrombin by hirudin. *Biochemistry* 1986;25:4622–4628.
123. Bittl JA, Strony J, Brinker JA, et al for the Hirulog Angioplasty Study Investigators. Treatment with bivalirudin (Hirulog) as compared with heparin during coronary angioplasty for unstable or postinfarction angina. *N Engl J Med* 1995;333:764–769.
124. Kong DF, Topol EJ, Bittl JA, et al. Clinical outcomes of bivalirudin for ischemic heart disease. *N Engl J Med* 1999;100:2049–2053.
125. Theroux P, Waters D, Lam J, et al. Reactivation of unstable angina after the discontinuation of heparin. *N Engl J Med* 1992;327:141–145.
126. Hirsh J, Warkentin TE, Raschke R, et al. Heparin and low-molecular-weight heparin: Mechanisms of action, pharmacokinetics, dosing considerations, monitoring, efficacy, and safety. *Chest* 1998;114:489S–510S.
127. Gurfinkel EP, Manos EJ, Mejail RI, et al. Low molecular weight heparin versus regular heparin or aspirin in the treatment of unstable angina and silent ischemia. *J Am Coll Cardiol* 1995;26:313–318.
128. Collet JP, Montalescot G, Lison L, et al. Percutaneous coronary intervention after subcutaneous enoxaparin pretreatment in patients with unstable angina pectoris. *Circulation* 2001;103:658–663.
129. Klein W, Buchwald A, Hillis SE, et al. Comparison of low-molecular-weight heparin with unfractionated heparin acutely and with placebo for 6 weeks in the management of unstable coronary artery disease. FRagmin In unstable Coronary artery disease study (FRIC) [erratum appears in *Circulation* 1998;97:413]. *Circulation* 1997;96:61–68.
130. FRagmin during InStability in Coronary Artery Disease (FRISC) study group. Low-molecular weight heparin during instability in coronary artery disease. *Lancet* 1996,347:561–568.
131. Cohen M, Demers C, Gurfinkel EP et al, for the Efficacy and Safety of Subcutaneous Enoxaparin in Non-Q-wave Coronary Events Study Group. A comparison of low-molecular-weight heparin in unfractionated heparin for unstable coronary artery disease. *N Engl J Med* 1997;337:447–452.
132. Organization to Assess Strategies for Ischemic Syndromes (OASIS) Investigators. Comparison of the effects of two doses of recombinant hirudin compared with heparin in patients with acute myocardial ischemia without ST elevation: A pilot study. *Circulation* 1997;96:769–777.
133. Antman E, McCabe CH, Gurfinkel EP, et al. Enoxaparin prevents death and cardiac ischemic events in unstable angina/non-Q-wave myocardial infarction: Results of the Thrombolysis in Myocardial Infarction (TIMI) 11B study. *Circulation* 1999;100:1593–1601.
134. FRAXIS study group. Comparison of two treatment durations (6 days and 14 days) of a low molecular weight heparin with a 6-day treatment of unfractionated heparin in the initial management of unstable angina or non-Q wave myocardial infarction. FRAXIS (FRAXiparine in Ischaemic Syndrome). *Eur Heart J* 1999;20:1553–1562.
135. The Global Use of Strategies to Open Occluded Coronary Arteries (GUSTO) IIb Investigators. A comparison of recombinant hirudin with heparin for the treatment of acute coronary syndromes. *N Engl J Med* 1991;335:775–778.
136. Antman EM. Hirudin in acute myocardial infarction. Thrombolysis and Thrombin Inhibition in Myocardial Infarction (TIMI) 9B trial. *Circulation* 1996;94:911–921.
137. Organisation to Assess Strategies for Ischemic Syndromes (OASIS-2) Investigators. Effects of recombinant hirudin (lepirudin) compared with heparin on death, myocardial infarction, refractory angina, and revascularisation procedures in patients with acute myocardial ischaemia without ST elevation: A randomised trial. *Lancet* 1999;353:429–438.
138. Warkentin TE, Levine MN, Hirsh J, et al. Heparin-induced thrombocytopenia in patients treated with low-molecular-weight heparin or unfractionated heparin. *N Engl J Med* 1995;332:1330–1335.
139. Coumadin Aspirin Reinfarction Study (CARS) Investigators. Randomised double-blind trial of fixed low-dose warfarin with aspirin after myocardial infarction. *Lancet* 1997;350:389–396.
140. Lefkovits J, Plow EF, Topol EJ. Platelet glycoprotein IIb/IIIa receptors in cardiovascular medicine. *N Engl J Med* 1995;332:1553–1559.
141. Theroux P. Tirofiban. *Drugs Today* 1999;35:59–73.
142. The Platelet Receptor Inhibition in Ischemic Syndrome Management (PRISM) Study Investigators. A comparison of aspirin plus tirofiban with aspirin plus heparin for unstable angina. *N Engl J Med* 1998;339:436–443.
143. The Platelet Receptor Inhibition in Ischemic Syndrome Management in Patients Limited by Unstable Signs and Symptoms (PRISM-PLUS) Study investigators. Inhibition of the platelet glycoprotein IIb/IIIa receptor with tirofiban in unstable angina and non-Q-wave myocardial infarction. *N Engl J Med* 1998;338:1488–1497.
144. Greenbaum AB, Harrington RA, Hudson MP, et al for the PURSUIT Investigators. Therapeutic value of eptifibatide at community hospitals transferring patients to tertiary referral centers early after admission for acute coronary syndromes. *J Am Coll Cardiol* 2001;37:492–498.

145. Hamm CW, Heeschen C, Goldmann B, et al for the c7E3 Fab Antiplatelet Therapy in Unstable Refractory Angina (CAPTURE) Study Investigators. Benefit of abciximab in patients with refractory unstable angina in relation to serum troponin T levels. *N Engl J Med* 1999;340: 1623–1629.
146. Simoons ML. Effect of glycoprotein IIb/IIIa receptor blocker abciximab on in patients with acute coronary syndromes without early coronary revascularization: The GUSTO IV-ACS randomized trial. *Lancet* 2001;357:1915–1924.
147. The TIMI IIIB investigators. Effects of tissue plasminogen activator and a comparison of early invasive and conservative strategies in unstable angina and non-Q wave infarction: Results of the TIMI IIIB Trial. *Circulation* 1994;89:1545–1556.
148. Nyman I, Areskog M, Areskog NH, et al for the RISC Study Group. Very early risk stratification by electrocardiogram at rest in men with suspected unstable coronary heart disease. *J Intern Med* 1993;234: 293–301.
149. Gibbons RJ, Balady GJ, Beasley JW, et al. ACC/AHA guidelines for exercise testing: A report of the American College of Cardiology/American Heart Association Task Force on Practice Guidelines (Committee on Exercise Testing). *J Am Coll Cardiol* 1997;30:260–311.
150. Eagle KA, Guyton RA, Davidoff R, et al. ACC/AHA guidelines for coronary artery bypass graft surgery: A report of the American College of Cardiology/American Heart Association Task Force on Practice Guidelines (Committee on Coronary Artery Bypass Graft Surgery). *J Am Coll Cardiol* 1999;34:1262–1347.
151. Cheitlin MD, Alpert JS, Armstrong WR, et al. ACC/AHA guidelines for the clinical application of echocardiography: A report of the American College of Cardiology/American Heart Association Task Force on Practice Guidelines (Committee on Clinical Application of Echocardiography). Developed in collaboration with the American Society of Echocardiography. *Circulation* 1997;95:1686–1744.
152. Ritchie JL, Bateman TM, Bonow RO, et al. Guidelines for the clinical use of cardiac radionuclide imaging: Report of the ACC/AHA Task Force on Assessment of Diagnostic and Therapeutic Cardiovascular Procedures (Committee of Radionuclide Imaging). Developed in collaboration with the American Society of Nuclear Cardiology. *J Am Coll Cardiol* 1995;25:521–547.
153. Gibbons RJ, Chatterjee K, Daley J, et al. ACC/AHA ACP-ASIM guidelines on the management of patients with chronic stable angina. *J Am Coll Cardiol* 1999;33:2092–2197.
154. Boden WE, O'Rourke RA, Crawford MH, et al, for the Veterans Affairs Non-Q-Wave Infarction Strategies in Hospital (VANQWISH) trial investigators. Outcomes in patients with acute non-Q-wave myocardial infarction randomly assigned to an invasive as compared with a conservative management strategy. *N Engl J Med* 1998;338:1785–1792.
155. Scanlon PJ, Faxon DP, Audet A, et al. ACC/AHA guidelines for coronary angiography a report of the American College of Cardiology/American Heart Association Task Force on Practice Guidelines (Committee on Coronary Angiography). *J Am Coll Cardiol* 1999;33:1756–1824.
156. Cannon CP, Weintraub WS, Demopoulos LA, et al. Comparison of early invasive and conservative strategies in patients with unstable coronary syndromes treated with the glycoprotein IIb/IIIa inhibitor tirofiban. *N Engl J Med* 2001;344:1879–1887.
157. FRagmin and Fast Revascularization during InStability in Coronary artery disease (FRISC II) investigators. Invasive compared with noninvasive treatment in unstable coronary-artery disease: FRISC II prospective randomized multicentre study. *Lancet* 1999;354:708–715.
158. FRagmin and Fast Revascularisation during InStability in Coronary artery disease investigators. Long-term low-molecular-mass heparin in unstable coronary-artery disease: FRISC II prospective randomised multicentre study. *Lancet* 1999;354:701–707.
159. National Cooperative Study Group to Compare Surgical and Medical Therapy. Unstable angina pectoris. *Am J Cardiol* 1978;42:839–848.
160. Veterans Administration Coronary Artery Bypass Surgery Cooperative Study Group. Eleven-year survival in the Veterans Administration randomized trial of coronary bypass surgery for stable angina. *N Engl J Med* 1984;311:1333–1339.
161. The Third Report of the Expert Panel on Detection, Evaluation and Treatment of High Blood Cholesterol in Adults (Adult Treatment Panel III, or ATPIII). *Circulation* 2002;107:3157–3421.
162. Schwartz GG, Olsson AG, Ezekowitz MD, et al. Effects of atorvastatin on early recurrent ischemic events in acute coronary syndromes: The MIRACL study: A randomized controlled trial. *JAMA* 2001;285: 1711–1718.
163. Prinzmetal M, Kennemer R, Merliss R, et al. Angina pectoris: I. A variant form of angina pectoris. *Am J Med* 1959;27:375–388.
164. MacAlpin RN, Kattus AA, Alvaro AB. Angina pectoris at rest with preservation of exercise capacity: Prinzmetal's variant angina. *Circulation* 1973;47:946–958.
165. Onaka H, Hirota Y, Shimada S, et al. Clinical observations of spontaneous angina attacks and multivessel spasm in variant angina pectoris with normal coronary arteries: Evaluation by 24-hour 12-lead electrocardiography with computer analysis. *J Am Coll Cardiol* 1996;27:38–44.
166. Ozaki Y, Keane D, Serruys PW. Fluctuation of spastic location in patients with vasospastic angina: A quantitative angiographic study. *J Am Coll Cardiol* 1995;26:1606–1614.
167. Yasue H, Horio Y, Nakamura N, et al. Induction of coronary artery spasm with acetylcholine in patients with variant angina: Possible role of the parasympathetic nervous system in the pathogenesis of coronary artery spasm. *Circulation* 1986;74:955–963.
168. Sakata K, Yoshida H, Hoshino T, Kurata C. Sympathetic nerve activity in the spasm-induced coronary artery region is associated with disease activity of vasospastic angina. *J Am Coll Cardiol* 1996;28:460–464.
169. Kushwaha S, Mitchell AG, Yacoub MH. Coronary artery spasm after cardiac transplantation. *Am J Cardiol* 1990;65:1515–1518.
170. Chierchia S, Davies G, Berkenboom G, et al. $\alpha$-Adrenergic receptors and coronary spasm: An elusive link. *Circulation* 1984;69:8–14.
171. Freedman SB, Chierchia S, Rodriguez-Plaza L, et al. Ergonovine-induced myocardial ischemia: No role for serotonergic receptors? *Circulation* 1984;70:178–183.
172. Robertson RM, Robertson D, Roberts LJ, et al. Thromboxane $A_2$ in vasotonic angina pectoris: Evidence from direct measurement and inhibitor trials. *N Engl J Med* 1981;304:998–1003.
173. Chierchia S, Patrono C, Crea F, et al. Effect of intravenous prostacyclin in variant angina. *Circulation* 1982;65:470–477.
174. Satake K, Lee JD, Shimizu H, et al. Relation between severity of magnesium deficiency and frequency of anginal attacks in men with variant angina. *J Am Coll Cardiol* 1996;28:897–902.
175. Shimabukuro M, Shinzato T, Higa S, et al. Enhanced insulin response relates to acetylcholine-induced vasoconstriction in vasospastic angina. *J Am Coll Cardiol* 1995;25:356–361.
176. Miwa K, Miyagi Y, Igawa A, et al. Vitamin E deficiency in variant angina. *Circulation* 1996;94:14–18.
177. Kugiyama K, Motoyama T, Hirashima O, et al. Vitamin C attenuates abnormal vasomotor reactivity in spasm coronary arteries in patients with coronary spastic angina. *J Am Coll Cardiol* 1998;32:103–109.
178. Kugiyama K, Yasue H, Okumura K, et al. Nitric oxide activity is deficient in spasm arteries of patients with coronary spastic angina. *Circulation* 1996;94:266–272.
179. Egashira K, Katsuda Y, Mohri M, et al. Basal release of endothelium-derived nitric oxide at site of spasm in patients with variant angina. *J Am Coll Cardiol* 1996;27:1444–1449.
180. Nakayama M, Yasue H, Yoshimura M, et al. $T^{-786}\rightarrow C$ mutation in the 5′-flanking region of the endothelial nitric oxide synthase gene is associated with coronary spasm. *Circulation* 1999;99:2864–2870.
181. Yamagishi M, Miyatake K, Tamai J, et al. Intravascular ultrasound detection of atherosclerosis at the site of focal vasospasm in angiographically normal or minimally narrowed coronary segments. *J Am Coll Cardiol* 1994;23:352–357.
182. Beltrame JF, Sasayama S, Maseri A. Racial heterogeneity in coronary artery vasomotor reactivity: Differences between Japanese and Caucasian patients. *J Am Coll Cardiol* 1999;33:1442–1452.
183. Maseri A, Severi S, De Nes M, et al. "Variant" angina: One aspect of a continuous spectrum of vasospastic myocardial ischemia. *Am J Cardiol* 1978;42:1019–1035.

184. Waters DD, Szlachcic J, Bourassa MG, et al. Exercise testing in patients with variant angina: Results, correlation with clinical and angiographic features and prognostic significance. *Circulation* 1982;65:265–274.
185. Koiwaya Y, Torii S, Takeshita A, et al. Postinfarction angina caused by coronary arterial spasm. *Circulation* 1982;65:275–280.
186. Waters D, Théroux P, Crittin J, et al. Previously undiagnosed variant angina as a cause of chest pain after coronary artery bypass surgery. *Circulation* 1980;61:1159–1164.
187. David PR, Waters DD, Scholl JM, et al. Percutaneous transluminal coronary angioplasty in patients with variant angina. *Circulation* 1982; 66:695–702
188. Scholl JM, Benacerraf A, Ducimetiere P, et al. Comparison of risk factors in vasospastic angina without significant fixed coronary narrowing and no vasospastic angina. *Am J Cardiol* 1986;57:199–202.
189. Miller D, Waters DD, Warnica W, et al. Is variant angina the coronary manifestation of a generalized vasospastic disorder? *N Engl J Med* 1981;304:763–766.
190. Myerburg RJ, Kessler KM, Mallon SM, et al. Life-threatening ventricular arrhythmias in patients with silent myocardial ischemia due to coronary artery spasm. *N Engl J Med* 1992;326:1451–1455.
191. Chevalier P, Dacosta A, Defaye P, et al. Arrhythmic cardiac arrest due to isolated coronary artery spasm: Long-term outcome of seven resuscitated patients. *J Am Coll Cardiol* 1998;31:57–61.
192. Waters DD, Szlachcic J, Bonan R, et al. Comparative sensitivity of exercise, cold pressor and ergonovine testing in provoking attacks of variant angina in patients with active disease. *Circulation* 1983;67: 310–315.
193. Okumura K, Yasue H, Matsuyama K, et al. Sensitivity and specificity of intracoronary injection of acetylcholine for the induction of coronary artery spasm. *J Am Coll Cardiol* 1988;12:883–888.
194. Waters DD, Bouchard A, Théroux P. Spontaneous remission is a frequent outcome of variant angina. *J Am Coll Cardiol* 1983;2:195–199.
195. Walling A, Waters DD, Miller DD, et al. Long-term prognosis of patients with variant angina. *Circulation* 1987;76:990–997.
196. Tilmant PY, Lablanche JM, Thieuleux FA, et al. Detrimental effect of propranolol in patients with coronary arterial spasm countered by combination with diltiazem. *Am J Cardiol* 1983;52:230–233
197. Morikami Y, Yasue H. Efficacy of slow-release nifedipine on myocardial ischemia episodes in variant angina pectoris. *Am J Cardiol* 1991; 68:580–584.
198. Pepine CJ, Feldman RL, Whittle J, et al. Effect of diltiazem in patients with variant angina: A randomized double-blind trial. *Am Heart J* 1981;101:719–725.
199. Johnson SM, Mauritson DR, Willerson JT, Hillis LD. A controlled clinical trial of verapamil for Prinzmetal's variant angina. *N Engl J Med* 1981;304:862–866.
200. Chahine RA, Feldman RL, Giles TD, et al. Randomized placebo-controlled trial of amlodipine in vasospastic angina. *J Am Coll Cardiol* 1993;21:1365–1370.
201. Yasue H, Takizawa A, Nagao M, et al. Long-term prognosis for patients with variant angina and influential factors. *Circulation* 1988; 78:1–9.
202. Rutitzky B, Girotti AL, Rosenbaum MB. Efficacy of chronic amiodarone therapy in patients with variant angina pectoris and inhibition of ergonovine coronary constriction. *Am Heart J* 1982;103:38–43.
203. Frenneaux M, Kaski JC, Brown M, Maseri A. Refractory variant angina relieved by guanethidine and clonidine. *Am J Cardiol* 1988;62: 832–833.
204. Miwa K, Kambara H, Kawai C. Exercise-induced angina provoked by aspirin administration in patients with variant angina. *Am J Cardiol* 1981;47:1210–1214.
205. Mark DB, Califf RM, Morris KG, et al. Clinical characteristics and long-term survival of patients with variant angina. *Circulation* 1984; 69:880–888.
206. Shubrooks SJ Jr, Bete JM, Hutter AM Jr, et al. Variant angina pectoris: Clinical and anatomic spectrum and results of coronary bypass surgery. *Am J Cardiol* 1975;36:142–147.
207. Bertrand ME, Lablanche JM, Thieuleux FA, et al. Comparative results of percutaneous transluminal coronary angioplasty in patients with dynamic versus fixed coronary stenosis. *J Am Coll Cardiol* 1986;8: 504–508.
208. Freemantle N, Calvert M, Wood J, et al. Composite outcomes in randomized trials. *JAMA* 2003;289:2554–2559.

CHAPTER 52

# ST-SEGMENT-ELEVATION MYOCARDIAL INFARCTION: CLINICAL PRESENTATION, DIAGNOSTIC EVALUATION, AND MEDICAL MANAGEMENT*

R. Wayne Alexander / Craig M. Pratt / Thomas J. Ryan / Robert Roberts



## BACKGROUND AND INTRODUCTION*

Progress in elucidating the pathogenesis of acute myocardial infarction (AMI) and of its treatment epitomizes scientific, evidence-based medicine at its best. Although myocardial infarction has long been a clinically recognized entity resulting from coronary artery atherosclerosis, its relative importance is a modern phenomenon. Its appearance as a modern epidemic reflects increasing longevity, permitting manifestation of chronic "degenerative" diseases, such as atherosclerosis, to appear; the adoption of high-fat diets based on meats, permitted by increasing affluence; and decreased exercise, made possible by the increased mechanization of society. Osler devoted only a few pages in his textbook, published in 1892, to the discussion of AMI.[3]

*The new American College of Cardiology/American Heart Association (ACC/AHA) Guidelines for the Management of Patients with ST-Elevation Myocardial Infarction have been published.[1] These guidelines represent a major revision of the 1999 ACC/AHA Guidelines for the Management of Patients with Acute Myocardial Infarction, which also included consideration of patients with unstable angina/non–ST-elevation myocardial infarction (UA/NSTEMI).[2] Guidelines for and management of patients with UA/STEMI are discussed in Chap. 51.

The modern era can be said to have begun with the autopsy studies of Herrick, who concluded in 1912 that the clinical syndrome of myocardial infarction results from acute thrombotic occlusion of a coronary artery, with resulting downstream necrosis.[4] This conclusion was generally accepted for 60 years, and the term *coronary thrombosis* was not uncommonly used as the equivalent of *heart attack* or, more formally, *acute myocardial infarction.* The conventional wisdom was challenged in 1972, when it was suggested that coronary artery thrombus may be the result rather than the cause of acute infarction, since autopsy studies—which were frequently performed several days after the acute event—did not uniformly show thrombus.[5] In retrospect, these findings can be explained by spontaneous lysis of a thrombus that had been occlusive for a sufficient amount of time to cause tissue necrosis. Definitive proof of the central role of thrombus formation in the pathogenesis of myocardial infarction came from angiographic studies performed during the first hours of the acute event,[6,7] a diagnostic strategy that had previously been thought to be contraindicated.[8]

The unequivocal demonstration of the role of the thrombus in AMI quickly led to the systematic testing of thrombolytic strategies to abort myocardial infarctions.[9–11] Analysis of data from several small trials of thrombolytic therapy with streptokinase suggested improved mortality in treated patients as early as 1982.[12] These early efforts were followed by a large number of major multicenter clinical trials on the treatment of AMI; these demonstrated in a rigorous fashion the efficacy of beta-adrenergic receptor blockers,[13] streptokinase versus no thrombolytic therapy,[14] and recombinant tissue plasminogen activator versus streptokinase[15] in reducing mortality. These and other major trials are discussed in detail further on. The major point to be made here is that large, adequately powered, randomized studies in the treatment of myocardial infarction have helped set a new standard and approach to the goal of enhancing the evidence-based practice of medicine while moving away from one based on previous practice patterns and intuitive extrapolations from pathophysiologic principles. Key to the success of these very large trials has been the generalizability achieved mostly by the use of broad-entry criteria that facilitated the rapid enrollment of suitable patients and gave the studies robust statistical power.

The availability of data from well-designed clinical trials has permitted the development, by panels of experts, of evidence-based practice guidelines for the treatment of myocardial infarction.[1,16] Furthermore, the confidence with which recommendations can be made for any particular diagnostic or therapeutic approach can be graded on the basis of judgments as to the strength of the supporting evidence. Thus, a committee convened by the American College of Cardiology/American Heart Association (ACC/AHA) Task Force on Practice Guidelines was charged with revising the ACC/AHA statement "Guidelines for the Early Management of Patients with Acute Myocardial Infarction," published in 1990.[16] The results of the deliberations of this committee, "Guidelines for the Management of Patients with Acute Myocardial Infarction," were published in 1996 and were updated in 1999.[2] As noted, these guidelines were recently revised to deal specifically with ST-elevation myocardial infarction (STEMI) and guidelines for UA/NSTEMI were developed separately as discussed in Chap. 51. The evidence and expert opinion supporting use of a therapy, intervention, or diagnostic procedure were weighed and expressed in ACC/AHA format as follows:

*Class I:* Conditions for which there is evidence and/or general agreement that a given procedure or treatment is beneficial, useful, and effective.

*Class II:* Conditions for which there is conflicting evidence and/or a divergence of opinion about the usefulness/efficacy of a procedure or treatment.

*Class IIa:* Weight of evidence/opinion is in favor of usefulness/efficacy.

*Class IIb:* Usefulness/efficacy is less well established by evidence/opinion.

*Class III:* Conditions for which there is evidence and/or general agreement that a procedure/treatment is not useful/effective and in some cases may be harmful.[2]

The new guidelines also add a "level of evidence" designation as follows:

*Level of evidence A:* Data derived from multiple randomized controlled trials or metanalyses.

*Level of evidence B:* Data derived from a single randomized control trial or nonrandomized studies.

*Level of evidence C:* Only consensus opinion by experts, case studies, or standards of care.

In general, recommendations in this chapter are associated with a class I, II, or III designation so as to guide the reader in weighing diagnostic and therapeutic options.

The pathophysiologic bases and consequences of coronary artery disease and myocardial infarction are discussed elsewhere: natural history and prognosis (Chap. 2); pathogenesis of atherosclerosis (Chap. 44); pathology of coronary atherosclerosis (Chap. 44); risk factors and prevention (Chap. 43); nonatherosclerotic causes of coronary heart disease (spontaneous coronary artery dissection, aortic dissection, thrombosis associated with the use of birth-control pills, emboli, congenital coronary anomalies, metabolic abnormalities, blunt chest trauma, vasculitis, and drug abuse, especially cocaine) (Chap. 47); pathophysiology of myocardial ischemia (Chap. 46); pathophysiology of coronary artery disease as related to myocardial ischemic syndromes (Chaps. 46 and 50); and thrombogenesis and antithrombotic therapy (Chap. 54).

The following are important general facts about myocardial infarction:

1. Approximately 800,000 people in the United States experience AMI annually; of these, about 213,000 die. Of those who die, approximately half do so within 1 h of the onset of symptoms, before reaching a hospital.[2,17,18]
2. The majority of early deaths are the result of ventricular arrhythmias that can be readily aborted by defibrillation, either during prehospital care or in the hospital's coronary care unit (CCU).
3. The major cause of myocardial infarction is atherosclerotic disease of the epicardial coronary arteries, as noted. Although luminal narrowing resulting in hemodynamically significant obstruction of blood flow is the major cause of symptoms of coronary ischemia (Chap. 57), the majority of myocardial infarctions occur as a result of the disruption of arterial lesions that are not hemodynamically significant (<60 percent). This breakdown of the structural integrity of the arterial intima occurs because of weakening induced by proteolytic degradation of matrix proteins by products released from inflammatory leukocytes[19] and results in the exposure of blood to thrombogenic intimal material, causing obstructive clot formation. Local vasospasm may contribute to the obstruction. *These observations have led to the concept that the biological state of atherosclerotic lesions and not the extent of stenosis is the major determinant of whether or not plaque rupture and myocardial infarction occur.*
4. Myocardial infarction, or ischemia, is a segmental process limited to the distribution of the affected artery. Impaired contractility usually occurs within seconds of the cessation of blood flow. The process usually begins in the endocardium and spreads toward the epicardium. If flow is restored before cell death occurs, prolonged contractile impairment (stunning) may occur.
5. Episodes of ischemia preceding coronary occlusion enhance the survivability of myocardial cells (*ischemic preconditioning*).
6. Irreversible cardiac injury occurs if occlusion is complete for at least 15 to 20 min. Irreversible injury occurs maximally in the area at risk when occlusion is sustained for 4 to 6 h, but most of the damage occurs in the first 2 to 3 h. Thus, restoration of flow within the first 4 to 6 h is associated with salvage of the myocardium, but the salvage is exponentially greater if restoration occurs in 1 to 2 h.
7. Restoration of blood flow by thrombolysis results in myocardial salvage and improved mortality. The extent of the benefit depends on restoration of near-normal blood flow *(open-artery hypothesis)* and is inversely related to the time between the onset of occlusion (symptoms) and the restoration of blood flow.

8. The percentage of tissue at risk that undergoes necrosis (infarct size) depends on existing collateral flow, which is highly variable and difficult to predict.
9. The major predictor of long-term outcome is infarct size, which is inversely related to the ejection fraction.
10. Q-wave infarction (usually presenting as ST-segment elevation) is a distinct clinical entity as compared with non-Q-wave infarction (usually presenting with ST-segment depression). There are differential features in their clinical courses. [Q-wave infarction, untreated, has a relatively high in-hospital mortality rate that is favorably influenced by thrombolysis, whereas non-Q-wave infarction (see Chap. 51) has a lower in-hospital mortality and complication rate with a prolonged vulnerability to reinfarction. Thrombolysis may worsen the clinical outcome.] Although there is no close anatomic correlation between the presence and absence of Q waves and transmural and nontransmural myocardial infarction, the distinct clinical outcomes of patients presenting with ST-segment elevation and ST-segment depression have made this electrocardiographic feature a major initial decision point in assigning therapeutic strategies to patients presenting with symptoms compatible with AMI.
11. Because of their salutary effects on thrombus formation and ventricular arrhythmias, aspirin and beta-adrenergic blockers, respectively, have proved to be effective for secondary prevention in patients who have had a myocardial infarction. Aspirin has also been shown to be modestly effective for primary prevention in middle-aged males.
12. Lipid lowering and smoking cessation have both been shown to be effective in the primary and secondary prevention of myocardial infarction. The enormous progress that has been made in understanding the pathogenesis and treatment of myocardial infarction has resulted in substantial improvements in outcomes in recent years. Indeed, the "natural history" of treated patients has improved dramatically. The mortality rate in the pre-CCU era has been estimated to have been about 30 percent.[20] The mortality rate then dropped dramatically, to about 15 percent, in the CCU era, which embraced the use of hemodynamic monitoring, defibrillation, and the use of beta blockers. The increased use of thrombolytics, coronary interventions, aspirin, and angiotensin-converting enzyme inhibitors has decreased the mortality of patients treated for the conventional ST-segment-elevated AMI to 6 to 7 percent.[15,18] The major challenge, however, is to bring the principles and lessons learned from the efforts of the past decade to everyday clinical practice.

## CLINICAL ASPECTS

### Predisposing Characteristics and Circumstances

The standard risk factors for the development of coronary artery disease (dyslipidemia, family history, age, male gender, cigarette smoking, diabetes mellitus, and hypertension) are well established and are discussed in Chap. 43. *Careful consideration of the probabilities of the presence of coronary artery disease is centrally important in the initial assessment and evaluation of testing results of any patient with chest pain.* The experienced clinician will calibrate his or her responses even within the context of algorithmic approaches to the evaluation of chest pain. For example, the 35-year-old male with atypical chest pain whose father died of coronary disease at less than age 50 and whose mother had a coronary bypass at age 55 would be viewed with a higher index of suspicion than if both his parents and grandparents were alive and well. This higher level of concern might translate into ordering diagnostic modalities with a higher level of sensitivity and specificity for detecting coronary artery disease in the former as opposed to the latter case.

As discussed in Chaps. 44 and 50, atherosclerosis generally, including the disease in the coronary arteries, is a chronic inflammation representing the response of the arterial wall to the stress imposed by various risk factors. AMI has commonly been shown to occur as a result of the disruption of a coronary artery plaque at a site of a high density of inflammatory cells.[21] Thus, AMI can be thought of as resulting from the acute exacerbation of a chronic inflammatory response. There is increasing clinical evidence supporting this view. Thus, unstable angina, a frequent antecedent of myocardial infarction,[22] has been shown to be associated with elevated plasma levels of the acute-phase reactant C-reactive protein.[23,24] Observations from the Physicians' Health Study, which showed that subjects with the highest levels of C-reactive protein have an increased long-term risk of cardiac events, are also supportive of the concept that inflammatory responses are important in the pathogenesis of AMI.[25] *Thus, events precipitating myocardial infarctions can be viewed as exacerbating the arterial inflammatory response and/or increasing the physical forces (rheological-platelet-arterial wall interactions) impinging on a coronary artery lesion weakened by inflammation, which leads to rupture.*

### Precipitating Events

There is little direct but intriguing indirect evidence that external factors might exacerbate the arterial inflammatory response. An association has been noted between AMI and antecedent mild respiratory syndromes.[26] It is possible that an infection, by activating systemic responses, could stimulate or activate previously quiescent atherosclerotic lesions. A more specific relation between AMI and an infectious agent has been posited in the case of *Chlamydia pneumoniae.*[27,28] Increased antibody titers to *C. pneumoniae* in subsets of patients have been associated with an increased risk of acute infarction, and acute infarction–associated increases in circulating immune complexes, followed by a subsequent increase in antibody titers, have been observed.[29] Evidence exists for the presence of chlamydiae in atherosclerotic coronary artery lesions.[30] Thus, it is possible that *C. pneumoniae* infection contributes to the inflammatory responses in atherosclerosis and that acute reinfection activates the inflammatory response, leading to myocardial infarction. This area requires further investigation.

There is considerable evidence associating AMI with emotional or environmental stresses. It is likely that the majority of these stresses involve activation of the sympathetic nervous system, with increases in locally released and circulating catecholamines. Increased sympathetic drive increases cardiac oxygen consumption by increasing contractility and rate. Sympathetic stimulation will also increase shear forces and stress on vascular atherosclerotic lesions by augmenting contraction and torque and elevating blood pressure. Superimposition of these forces on a vessel weakened by inflammation can lead to plaque rupture. Enhanced circulating catecholamine levels can increase the propensity for thrombus formation by activating platelets. Such a scenario likely explains the association (in about 4 to 7 percent of patients) between acute increases in physical exertion and the development of myocardial infarction, especially among those who do not exercise regularly.[31,32] Similarly, episodes of anger increase the risk of precipitating myocardial infarction in susceptible persons.[33] Distressing or changing life events reportedly occur with increased frequency in the months preceding a myocardial infarction.[34–36] Another well-controlled study, however, found no correlation between the occurrence of acute infarction and the presence of unusual life events for up to 4 weeks prior to the AMI.[31]

It is apparent that any acute stressful event or intervention can precipitate AMI in a patient with "active," susceptible coronary atherosclerotic lesions. Anesthesia and surgery are well known to enhance the risk of myocardial infarction, and cardiac events are the leading cause of perioperative morbidity.[37] Perioperatively, stress can be induced by tachycardia and hypotension,[38] anemia,[39] and hypothermia.[40] A study of patients with coronary disease undergoing noncardiac surgery has shown that the usual perioperative hypothermia was associated with a relative risk of cardiac events of 2.2, as contrasted to a similar group in whom normothermia was maintained.[41] The salutary effects of maintaining normothermia were thought to be due to the prevention of cardiac stress imposed by activation of the sympathetic nervous system. By extension, many of the stressful events—such as pulmonary emboli, stroke, hypoxia, allergic responses, blood loss, etc.—that have been associated with the precipitation of AMI can likely be related to the effects of adrenergic stimulation by an excess of catecholamines.

Myocardial infarction can occur because of low perfusion pressure in shock of any etiology and can arise in severe aortic stenosis even in the absence of coronary artery disease because of excessive oxygen demands in a very hypertrophic ventricle with, for example, marked tachycardia. Other nonatherosclerotic causes of myocardial infarction, including trauma, embolism, and dissection, are discussed in Chap. 47. Vasospasm in the absence of angiographically demonstrable coronary artery disease has been reported to have caused AMI in several patients during general anesthesia.[42] Also, it is likely that vasospasm plays a central role in cocaine-induced myocardial infarction.[43]

## Personality Types

It has been claimed that so-called coronary-prone individuals exhibit certain personality traits, such as being compulsively hard workers, being deadline-driven, and being excessively competitive. The categorization of people with such traits as "type A" and thus as being at increased risk for myocardial infarction was formerly widely discussed.[44] This concept is not widely accepted now,[45] as the psychological contributions to heart disease are generally considered to be more complex (see Chap. 91).

## Circadian and Seasonal Variation

Results of the Multicenter Investigation of Limitation of Infarct Size (MILIS) study showed a marked circadian periodicity in the occurrence of myocardial infarction, with a peak prevalence between 6 A.M. and noon. The circadian rhythm was present whether the onset of the infarction was marked subjectively by the appearance of pain or objectively by plasma MB-CK (creatine kinase) levels. There was a threefold increase in the frequency of infarction at peak (9 A.M.) periods as compared with trough (11 P.M.) periods.[46] As a corollary, sudden death attributed to ischemic heart disease has a similar circadian periodicity. Available data suggest that the rhythms both for the occurrence of myocardial infarction and for deaths from ischemic events are actually bimodal. These rhythms are characterized not only by the morning peak but also by a secondary, less pronounced late-afternoon or early-evening peak (6 to 8 P.M.).[47] The mechanisms underlying this temporal distribution of ischemic events are not completely understood but are probably related to diurnal variations in thrombotic tendencies and to sympathetic nervous system activity. There is both an enhanced platelet aggregation[48] and a trough in intrinsic fibrinolytic activity during the morning hours.[49] A similar circadian variation is observed for cerebral infarction,[50] which further implicates an increased propensity for thrombosis in the morning hours. The blunting of the morning peak of myocardial infarction by both aspirin and beta-adrenergic blockers emphasizes the contributions of both the sympathetic nervous system and the coagulation pathways to the circadian rhythm of cardiovascular events.[51]

Other endogenous daily rhythms may be causally related. Ambulatory ST-segment changes in patients with coronary artery disease have demonstrated a close correlation between basal heart rate (which is higher in the morning) and the frequency of ischemic ST-segment changes.[52] These observations may be mechanistically related to the morning increase in tone noted in coronary artery segments with dysfunctional endothelium-dependent dilation in patients with chronic stable angina (see Chaps. 7 and 50).[53] Circadian variations in blood pressure[54] and plasma catecholamine levels[55] that parallel those of ischemic events have been observed. The morning increase in sympathetic activity not only augments the metabolic demand but may also cause coronary vasoconstriction that is unopposed by normal endothelial vasodilator mechanisms, as implied earlier.

There also appear to be exogenous rhythms that influence the development of AMI. In a working population, there is an increased risk for infarction on Mondays.[56] Seasonal variations have also been commented on, with increases in the winter months of January through March.[57]

## Symptoms

Prodromal symptoms antedating AMI are common and occur in at least 60 percent of patients.[58] Since at least 8 to 10 percent of AMIs are painless (not necessarily silent) and many ischemic episodes are silent,[59] it is apparent that the great majority of patients capable of sensing cardiac pain during periods of unstable angina do so in the hours, days, or sometimes weeks prior to the acute event. Most of these symptoms are anginal or angina-like, especially when assessed retrospectively in the context of the character of the pain of the acute infarct. The antecedent symptoms may also be anginal equivalents, such as paroxysmal dyspnea (see Chap. 50). The clinical features of unstable angina are discussed in Chap. 51. If one considers the general feeling of malaise and fatigue that many patients report having experienced prior to acute infarction, it is apparent that it is relatively unusual for the episode to be totally unheralded—a conclusion that is consistent with general clinical experience.

The classic symptoms of AMI involve chest discomfort that is commonly retrosternal or precordial in location and is described as pressure, aching, burning, crushing, squeezing, heavy, swelling, or bursting in quality.[60,61] Typically it has all the features of prolonged angina pectoris, which was so eloquently described by William Heberden in his original report to the assembly of the Royal College of Physicians in 1772:

> There is a disorder of the breast marked with strong and peculiar symptoms considerable for the kind of danger belonging to it, and not extremely rare, which deserves to be mentioned more at length. The seed of it, and sense of strangling, and anxiety with which it is attended, may make it not improperly be called angina pectoris. They who are afflicted with it, are

> seized while they are walking (more especially if it be uphill, and soon after eating) with a painful and most disagreeable sensation in the breast, which seems as if it would extinguish life, if it were to increase or to continue; but the moment they stand still, all this uneasiness vanishes.

The location is usually of little help in differentiating ischemia/infarction from other causes of chest pain,[62] but severe chest pain (as opposed to vague discomfort) and the presence of associated symptoms (dyspnea, nausea, diaphoresis, etc.) are more commonly associated with AMI.[63] The discomfort often radiates over the anterior chest and frequently into the left arm or both arms (particularly the medial aspect) and/or into the neck or jaw. In unusual instances, the pain may be in the back, particularly between the scapulae. There may be skip areas with retrosternal pain—associated with jaw, antecubital fossa, or wrist pain—or no pain between the two sites. Moreover, the pain may appear only in the referral area. The duration of the pain of infarction is prolonged, lasting conventionally longer than 15 min. While the intensity of the pain is usually steady following an initial crescendo, there is occasionally some waxing and waning. Sudden relief of pain may accompany reperfusion. Associated symptoms may include dyspnea, diaphoresis, nausea, and vomiting. Marked apprehension is common. Occasionally, presenting symptoms include syncope, acute confusion, agitation, stroke, or palpitations.

Approximately 23 percent of myocardial infarctions go unrecognized by patients because of the absence of symptoms or the lack of recognition of the significance of symptoms.[64] The common symptoms in this latter instance are nonclassic or atypical pain, dyspnea, nausea, vomiting, and/or epigastric pain. A myocardial infarction may also masquerade as the development or worsening of congestive heart failure, the appearance of an arrhythmia, an overwhelming sense of apprehension, profound weakness, acute indigestion, pericarditis, embolic stroke, or peripheral embolus.[65] On the other hand, acute aortic dissection, acute myocarditis, pericarditis, and pneumothorax are conditions that can mimic AMI and must be excluded before initiating therapy in patients with presumed MI. Presentation with painless myocardial infarction is more common in the elderly (age >65 years) than it is in the nonelderly, and this subgroup has an increased frequency of congestive heart failure as the initial presenting symptom.[66]

## Physical Findings

### GENERAL EXAMINATION

Features of the physical examination during AMI have been the subject of several reviews.[67,68] The patient is frequently sitting up because of a sense of suffocation or a feeling of shortness of breath. Most patients with cardiac pain or myocardial infarction have some sense of impending doom that is reflected in their facial expression. They may have a grayish appearance or one of panic or exhaustion. Diaphoresis is frequent. In severe cases, patients may be quite anxious, with an ashen or pale face beaded with perspiration. The patient should be examined in both the supine and left lateral decubitus positions. The major findings pertaining to the heart appear on palpation of the precordium in the left lateral position. It is important to rapidly ascertain the vital signs and the nature, character, and rhythm of the arterial pulse; to observe the jugular venous pulse; to check the peripheral pulses; to palpate the precordium; and to auscultate the chest and precordium. Examination of the extremities should include subjective assessment of the temperature and color of the feet. The presence of very cool feet, especially with acrocyanosis in the setting of tachycardia, suggests low cardiac output.

The heart rate and rhythm are important indicators of cardiac function in the initial hours of myocardial infarction. *A normal rate usually indicates that the patient is not experiencing significant hemodynamic compromise.* In patients with inferior myocardial infarction, heart rates in the fifties and sixties are common in the initial hours. Up to 60 percent of these patients initially have bradycardia, but the rate gradually increases over the next few hours. The bradycardia, which may be associated with secondary hypotension, results from the stimulation of myocardial receptors with vagal afferents. *Persistent sinus tachycardia beyond the initial 12 to 24 h is predictive of a high mortality rate.* The pulse may be low in volume, reflecting decreased stroke volume. The blood pressure is usually normal but may be increased secondary to anxiety, or it may be decreased from cardiac failure. Blood pressure frequently normalizes temporarily with AMI in patients with hypertension. All peripheral pulses should be examined to observe their presence, and their status should be noted both to exclude current occlusion and provide a baseline in case of future embolic events. The carotid pulse is most useful in assessing systolic upstroke time and stroke volume, which are decreased in the patient with a low output state.

The rhythm of the pulse is important because of the frequency of ectopic atrial and, in particular, ventricular beats in AMI. Observation of the jugular venous pulse is useful in determining whether ectopic beats are atrial or ventricular. A large A wave, indicating that the right atrium is contracting against a closed atrioventricular (AV) valve, suggests that the ectopic beat is ventricular. The respiratory rate is usually within the normal range. However, patients who are extremely anxious often exhibit hyperventilation, and those with pulmonary edema and cardiac failure have an increased respiratory rate associated with shallow inspirations. Abnormal breathing patterns, such as Cheyne-Stokes respirations, are rare unless the patient is in cardiogenic shock.

Examination of the jugular venous pulse is important with AMI, especially in patients with an inferior infarction, because insights can be gained into possible involvement of the right ventricle. The right ventricle is commonly involved with inferior infarction, but right-sided failure is seen only with major right ventricular involvement. It may be manifest by an elevated jugular venous pressure. In addition, in many patients with right ventricular infarction or ischemia, there is also a prominent A wave because of the decreased compliance of the right ventricle.[69] Kussmaul's venous sign, or an inspiratory increase in the amplitude and pressure of the internal jugular vein, may also be seen in right ventricular infarction/ischemia because of decreased right ventricular compliance.[69a] Generally, right ventricular failure commonly reflects left ventricular failure, with a secondary elevation in pulmonary and right ventricular pressures. This circumstance usually occurs with large anterior or anterolateral infarction.

### EXAMINATION OF THE LUNGS

Basilar rales are frequently detected in AMI. Cardiac failure diagnosed on the basis of mild signs of pulmonary congestion occurs in 30 to 40 percent of patients with otherwise uncomplicated myocardial infarction. A clinical classification proposed by Killip provides some uniformity in terms of describing cardiac failure and pulmonary congestion.[70] Class I patients do not have any pulmonary rales or a third heart sound. Class II patients have crackles/rales of a mild-to-moderate degree, involving less than 50 percent of the lung fields, and may or may not have an $S_3$ gallop. Class III patients have crackles/rales more than halfway up the lung fields and an $S_3$ gallop. Class IV patients are those in cardiogenic shock.

### CARDIAC EXAMINATION

Palpation of the precordium may reveal evidence of regional wall motion abnormalities. Palpation should be performed with the patient initially lying in the supine position; this is often adequate to ascertain whether there is a localized normal apical impulse and also permits assessment for dyskinetic impulses (see Chap. 12). Frequently, one may not feel any precordial impulse with the patient in the supine position because of the decreased intensity of contraction and/or due to body habitus. With the patient in the left lateral decubitus position, one may palpate a diffuse rather than a localized apical impulse, akinesis, or a paradoxical bulging during late systole often located in the third left intercostal space in the midclavicular space; in some patients, there is a palpable atrial contraction corresponding to an audible $S_4$ gallop due to the decreased compliance of the left ventricle. One or more of these features of decreased contractility or lusitrophy and dyssynergy are frequently present in the early hours of AMI, particularly with extensive damage.

The first and second heart sounds are often very soft because of decreased contractility. The first heart sound may also be diminished because of a prolonged PR interval. If there is tachycardia, a shortened PR interval may result in a somewhat accentuated first heart sound. The second heart sound is usually normal; however, with extensive damage, there may be a single second sound. Rarely, paradoxical splitting may reflect severe left ventricular dysfunction. A fourth heart sound is often audible in patients with AMI. A third heart sound is heard in probably only about 15 to 20 percent of AMI patients. A pericardial friction rub can be heard anytime between 24 to 72 h after the onset of myocardial infarction; since its presence is often transient, frequently repeated auscultation is the best means of detection. The murmur of papillary muscle dysfunction is relatively common early in the course of infarction. This crescendo-decrescendo midsystolic murmur often reflects ischemia of the papillary muscles or the myocardial attachment rather than irreversible injury to these structures. This murmur usually disappears after the first 12 to 24 h if it is soft; however, if the murmur is moderate to loud in intensity, it may persist much longer, possibly throughout the patient's life. Mitral regurgitation is most commonly due to ischemia of the posteromedial papillary muscle (see also Chap. 12). Other findings on physical examination, such as the murmur of papillary muscle rupture or a ruptured ventricular septum, are described in appropriate sections under "Complications."

## Diagnosis of Acute Myocardial Infarction

### DIFFERENTIAL DIAGNOSIS

Myocardial infarction has typically been diagnosed on the basis of the triad of chest pain, electrocardiographic changes, and elevated plasma enzyme activity. Although AMI can occur without chest pain (20 to 25 percent of cases), chest pain remains the most common symptom and is usually responsible for the patient's seeking medical help. The differential diagnosis of prolonged chest pain is presented in Table 52-1. Chest pain, however, is not specific to cardiac disease, and it is often impossible, on the basis of history alone, to distinguish ischemia or infarction from other causes of chest pain. The differential diagnosis of chest pain is discussed in Chap. 57. Of patients presenting to the emergency department with chest pain, only about 14 percent are subsequently documented to have AMI.[71–74] Most patients at risk for myocardial infarction will be admitted to evaluate their chest pain unless definite noncardiac causes of chest pain—such as chest wall pain, hyperventilation, pleurisy, gastrointestinal (GI) pain, and so on, which are not imminently dangerous—can be identified. In the CCU, only about 20 percent of patients admitted with chest pain have AMI.

TABLE 52-1 Differential Diagnosis of Prolonged Chest Pain

- Acute myocardial infarction
- Aortic dissection
- Pericarditis
- Atypical anginal pain associated with hypertrophic cardiomyopathy
- Esophageal, other upper gastrointestinal, or biliary tract disease
- Pulmonary disease
  - Pleurisy: infectious, malignant, or immune disease–related
  - Embolus with or without infarction
  - Pneumothorax
- Hyperventilation syndrome
- Chest wall
  - Skeletal
  - Neuropathic
- Psychogenic

### ELECTROCARDIOGRAPHIC DIAGNOSIS

The electrocardiogram (ECG) is sensitive for detecting myocardial ischemia and infarction but frequently cannot differentiate between ischemia and necrosis (see Chap. 53).[71,72,75] Serial ECGs during AMI will show some evolutionary changes in the majority of patients.[76] An ECG obtained during cardiac ischemic pain frequently but not always exhibits changes in repolarization. The absence of ECG changes during pain provides evidence but not proof that the pain is not ischemic in nature. The early ECG changes of T-wave inversion or ST-segment depression may reflect ischemia or infarction. ST-segment elevation is more specific for AMI and reflects the epicardial injury–associated total occlusion of an epicardial coronary artery. In this case the event is classified as ST-elevation MI or STEMI. The hallmark of AMI is the development of abnormal Q waves,[77,78] which appear on average 8 to 12 h from the onset of symptoms but may not develop for 24 to 48 h. Abnormal Q waves usually reflect tissue death and the development of an electrical dead zone. Since abnormal Q waves do not develop immediately, they are not very helpful for initial diagnostic management and therapeutic triage except to signify the presence or absence of prior myocardial infarction. The diagnostic serial ECG changes consist of ST-segment elevation with the development of T-wave inversion and the evolution of abnormal Q waves.[79] The appearance of abnormal Q waves is very specific to AMI; however, they are present in less than 50 percent of patients with documented AMI.[80] Most of the other patients who have AMI will have ECG changes restricted to T-wave inversion or ST-segment depression or no change at all. These patients represent the group with non-Q-wave myocardial infarction,[81] also referred to as non-ST-segment-elevation infarction see Chap. 51. It is becoming conventional to refer to this entity or NQWMI.

The traditional concept that myocardial infarctions can be classified as transmural or nontransmural on the basis of the presence or absence of Q waves is misleading, since autopsy studies have demonstrated convincingly that pathologic Q waves may be associated with nontransmural infarction and may be absent with transmural infarction.[82–84] These misnomers have been replaced by the terms *Q-wave infarction* and *non-Q-wave infarction, for transmural and nontransmural infarction,* respectively.[85] The evolution of a NQWMI is characterized by a lack of development of an abnormal Q wave and by the appearance of reversible ST-T-wave changes with ST-segment depression that usually returns to normal over a few days but is occasionally permanent. Differentiation between these two types of infarctions has become entrenched, since there are major differences in their pathogenesis, clinical manifestations, treatment, and prognosis. The initiating events in the pathogenesis of Q-wave and NQWMI are thought to be identical—namely, coronary occlusion induced by a thrombus superimposed on a plaque together with vasoconstriction. NQWMI or non-ST-segment-elevation infarction is discussed in Chap. 51.

Traditional teaching has held that AMI could not be diagnosed electrocardiographically in the presence of a left bundle branch block (LBBB) because of the unpredictability of the depolarization and repolarization patterns. It has been suggested that marked ST-segment deviation, beyond what could be anticipated from the conduction abnormality, could be useful in the diagnosis of AMI in the setting of a left bundle branch block.[86]

The resting ECG is insensitive for detecting the presence of atherosclerotic coronary heart disease; it is normal in 50 percent of patients with angiographically significant coronary obstruction.[87] Nevertheless, an abnormally wide Q wave on a resting ECG has been the standard criterion for the diagnosis of a myocardial infarction for over 60 years.[88]

The ECG criteria for the diagnosis of STEMI as outlined in the MILIS study are the presence of any one of the following in the setting of chest pain: (1) new or presumably new Q waves (at least 30 ms wide and 0.20 mV deep) in at least two leads from any of the following: (a) leads II, III, or $aV_F$; (b) leads $V_1$ through $V_6$; or (c) leads I and $aV_L$; (2) new or presumably new ST-T-segment elevation or depression ($\geq$0.10 mV measured 0.02 s after the J point in two contiguous leads of the previously mentioned lead combination); or (3) a complete left bundle branch block in the appropriate clinical setting. An evaluation of these criteria in 1809 enzyme-confirmed infarctions found that 21 percent of the patients with an infarction had none of these changes.[89] Conversely, over 90 percent of patients who had ST-segment elevation of 0.1 mV, as described previously, were confirmed to have AMI. If the patients also had ST-segment depression in the so-called reciprocal leads, the infarction rate was 3 percent higher. Patients with a left branch bundle block or ST-segment depression without other abnormalities had a lower rate of infarction (46 and 52 to 56 percent, respectively) than those with ST-segment elevation. Furthermore, the presence of abnormal Q waves on the resting ECG accurately predicts the presence and location of left ventricular contraction abnormalities. In a study of 64 patients with abnormal Q waves on the ECG, all patients with abnormal Q waves in the anterior leads and 30 of 33 with abnormal Q waves in the inferior leads demonstrated contraction abnormalities in the corresponding left ventricular segments.[90] The evolution of a Q-wave myocardial infarction can be separated electrocardiographically into four phases: (1) hyperacute, (2) acute, (3) subacute, and (4) chronic stabilized (see Chap. 53).

In the hyperacute phase, the earliest ECG manifestation of an acute infarction is usually a straightening of the normal upward concavity of the ST-T segment.[91] With further evolution, the straightened ST-T segment becomes elevated. The ST-T segment usually slopes upward, since the portion of the ST-T segment nearest the T wave is more elevated than the proximal portion. Also, the amplitude of the T wave is usually increased. Occasionally, the ST-T segment may be markedly elevated and yet retain its upward concavity. ST-T depressions in leads oriented toward the presumably noninfarcted myocardium were traditionally termed *reciprocal changes*. Studies have indicated that such ST-T depressions usually reflect more extensive infarction. In the subacute phase, the abnormal Q wave representing myocardial necrosis begins to appear, but the T-wave vector still points toward the infarct zone. In the fully evolved phase, the ST-T segment begins to diminish in amplitude and becomes coved or convex upward. It blends into the now symmetrically inverted T waves. The abnormal Q waves (>0.03 s in duration and more than 25 percent of the R-wave amplitude) appear during this stage. During the chronic phase, there is generally resolution of the ST- and T-wave changes, with the only residual change being an abnormal Q wave. Although the ST-T segments again become isoelectric, they are frequently horizontal, with a sharp-angled ST-T junction, rather than exhibiting the normal concavity. Occasionally, in small inferior infarctions, even the abnormal Q waves resolve.

Posterior myocardial infarction occurs in the posterior left ventricular wall. An isolated true posterior infarction is quite uncommon, since such an infarction is usually associated with an inferior or lateral infarction. Since there are no ECG leads oriented toward the posterior left ventricular wall, the ECG changes of a true posterior infarction are seen as mirror-image representations in leads $V_1$ to $V_3$. Schamroth described the criteria for a true posterior infarction as follows: R waves of 0.04 s in lead $V_1$ and in contiguous right precordial leads with upright T waves, and, in the acute phase, ST-segment depression and an R/S ratio $\geq$1 in leads $V_1$ and $V_2$.[91] Usually, there are associated changes of an inferior or lateral infarction. As the infarction evolves, the ST-segment depression decreases and the upright T-wave amplitude increases. It is helpful to turn the ECG upside down and look at it from the back while holding it to a strong light. The changes in leads $V_1$ and $V_2$, which might be overlooked on a direct glance, are seen as abnormal Q waves, ST-segment elevation, and T-wave inversion when viewed from this perspective.

Similarly, ECG diagnosis of right ventricular infarction offers special challenges. Since right ventricular infarction generally occurs in the presence of inferior left ventricular infarction, the resulting ST-segment elevation is usually overwhelmed in the conventional precordial leads overlying the right ventricle ($V_2$ and $V_3$) by the ST-segment elevation in the opposing left ventricular myocardium on the inferior surface. The right ventricular electrical forces might be manifest in this setting as a diminution of the usual reciprocal ST-segment depression seen in the right precordial leads in inferior infarction. If the injury to the inferior wall is minimal, ST-segment elevation will occasionally be seen in $V_2$ through $V_4$ in the presence of right ventricular infarction.[92] Otherwise, ST-segment elevation must be sought in the right chest leads, $V_1$, and $V_{3R}$ through $V_{6R}$. ST-segment elevation in these leads provides reasonably strong evidence for the presence of right ventricular infarction.[93] It is well to note that ST-segment elevation in these leads in this situation often disappears within ten hours, and one postmortem study has shown that a 25 percent or greater involvement of the right ventricle was necessary to produce ST-T-segment elevation.[94] The diagnosis of acute right ventricular infarction by ECG has relatively good specificity but rather poor sensitivity.[95] Atrial infarction is usually reflected in PR-segment elevation or depression and P-wave abnormalities and is frequently associated with supraventricular arrhythmias, as discussed further on.[96]

The phenomenon of "ischemia at a distance" reflects the occurrence, in AMI with ST-segment elevation, of ST-segment depression in other, frequently reciprocal leads. It remains uncertain whether these changes represent true reciprocal changes or subendocardial ischemia in the area, but the presence of the finding is associated with a less favorable prognosis than its absence.[97,98]

Criteria for ECG diagnosis of AMI in various areas of the heart are discussed more fully in Chap. 53. In view of a lack of sensitivity and specificity of the chest pain history or of the ECG, confirmation of the diagnosis of AMI is based on elevated plasma levels of cardiac-specific markers.

## PLASMA DIAGNOSTIC MARKERS

***Tissue Distribution of MB-CK, Troponin T, Troponin I, and Myoglobin*** Myocardial necrosis is associated with the release of a variety of macromolecules, including enzymes, myoglobin, and contractile proteins that have been evaluated as potential diagnostic markers for AMI. The use of CK and MB-CK was shown to be highly sensitive, specific, and cost-effective for diagnosing myocardial infarction[99] and remained the standard over the past three decades. Release of CK into the circulation has been shown to reflect necrosis and does not occur with reversible ischemia.[100] However, cardiac troponins T and I are more specific and may in the future replace MB-CK.[101] The use of total CK alone without MB-CK yields a similar sensitivity, but specificity is markedly lower, in the range of 70 percent.[99] The use of total CK as a diagnostic marker for myocardial infarction is not ideal. Nevertheless, total CK as a diagnostic marker is used almost exclusively in large international trials because of its ease of measurement and the widespread availability of a universal standard assay. The proposed criterion is a twofold increase in plasma total CK.

CK consists of two monomers, each having a molecular weight of 43,000. The isoenzymes of CK are formed by the association of two M monomers (MM-CK), which predominate in muscle (hence the name) or of two B monomers (BB-CK), which predominate in the brain and internal visceral organs. A hybrid form (MB-CK), found in the heart, is composed of one M subunit and one B subunit. The isoenzymes MM, MB, and BB are located in the cytoplasm of the cell. There are separate genes for each of the monomers, which have been isolated, cloned, and sequenced.[102,103] About 5 percent of cellular MM-CK activity is associated with the M line of the sarcomere in both heart and skeletal muscle and a significant amount is in the Z line in heart muscle.

In the normal adult myocardium, 15 percent of the CK is in the form of MB-CK, with the remainder being MM-CK. Several investigators have found small amounts of MB-CK in normal adult skeletal muscle.[104,105] MB-CK is alleged to increase (1 to 5 percent) in skeletal muscle following injury, chronic exercise,[106] inflammation,[107] trauma,[108] and electrical injury.[109] In Duchenne muscular dystrophy (DMD), MB-CK in skeletal muscle is in the range of 1 to 5 percent. Myoglobin, with a molecular weight of 17,000, is ubiquitously distributed throughout cardiac and skeletal muscles and, while sensitive as an indicator of muscle injury, is very nonspecific and does not differentiate between skeletal and cardiac muscle.[110]

The recently introduced diagnostic markers cardiac troponins T and I[111] are part of the sarcomere complex. Troponin T has a molecular weight of 38,000, and troponin I, 23,000. There are three genes for each of the troponins, which encode for slow and fast skeletal and cardiac muscle.[112] Cardiac troponin I has 31 amino acids, which are not present in the skeletal forms. The recognition site of the antibody used in the assay is in the cardiac-specific region, which makes the test very specific as a marker for myocardial injury[113]; since normal plasma levels of troponin I are near 0, it is also very sensitive. Furthermore, studies indicate that cardiac troponin I is not upregulated in skeletal muscle with hypertrophy or injury and the skeletal form is not upregulated in the heart with hypertrophy or injury.[114] Cardiac troponin T has 11 amino acids not present in the skeletal forms, which has permitted the development of a specific diagnostic test.[117] Troponin T has sensitivity similar to that of troponin I, but the first-generation assay had less specificity, while the second-generation assay appears to have similar specificity to that of troponin I.[112]

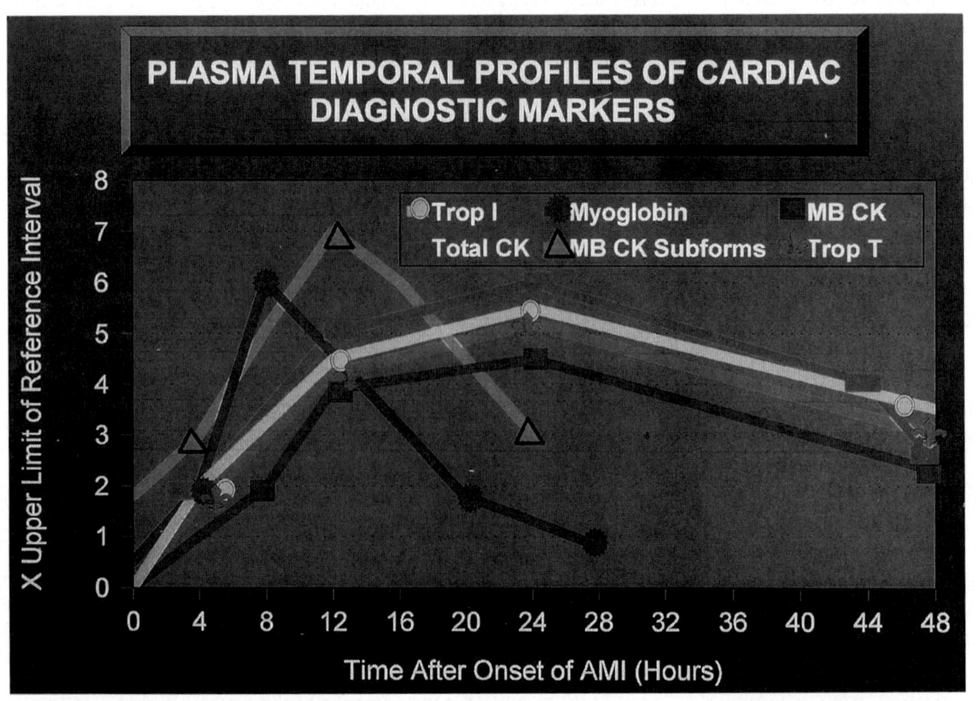


FIGURE 52-1 (Plate 84) Shown here is the temporal profile of the diagnostic biomarkers used for detecting myocardial infarction. The plasma temporal profile for early detection is illustrated for myoglobin and MB-CK subforms. The markers MB-CK, total CK, and cardiac troponins I and T are all released with a similar initial time profile. However, troponins I and T remain elevated for 10 to 14 days and thus are better markers for late diagnosis than that of MB-CK.

***Temporal Profiles of MB-CK, Myoglobin, Troponin I, and Troponin T Released into Plasma*** Plasma MB-CK activity following myocardial infarction is significantly elevated, such that reliable diagnostic sensitivity (>90 percent) is reached within 12 to 16 h of the onset of symptoms. Maximal levels[101] of MB-CK are reached between 14 and 36 h, with a return to normal levels occurring after 48 to 72 h (Fig. 52-1, Plate 84). In patients with minimal cardiac injury, as occurs in non-Q-wave infarction or following effective early reperfusion, plasma MB-CK reaches its maximal activity at about 12 to 15 h. In contrast, after Q-wave infarction with reperfusion, it reaches maximal activity at an average of 28 h. The plasma temporal profiles of troponins I and T are very similar to those of total CK and MB-CK. Troponins I and T are released into the plasma so that reliable diagnostic sensitivity (>90 percent) is reached by 12 to 16 h and maximal activity is reached by 24 to 36 h. However, the levels do not return to normal for 10 to 12 days.[101] Plasma myoglobin is increased within 2 h of the onset of symptoms and remains increased for at least 7 to 12 h.[110]

TABLE 52-2 Diagnostic Sensitivity and Specificity of Markers for Myocardial Infarction Based on Time from Onset of Chest Pain

| | Early Diagnosis | | | Late Diagnosis | | | |
|---|---|---|---|---|---|---|---|
| Time, hours | 2 | 4 | 6 | 10 | 14 | 18 | 22 |
| MARKER | | | | | | | |
| MB-CK subforms | | | | | | | |
| Sensitivity (%) | 21.1 | 46.4 | 91.5 | 96.2 | 90.6 | 80.9 | 53.1 |
| Specificity (%) | 90.5 | 88.9 | 89.0 | 90.2 | 90.0 | 89.9 | 92.2 |
| Myoglobin | | | | | | | |
| Sensitivity (%) | 26.3 | 42.9 | 78.7 | 86.5 | 62.3 | 57.5 | 42.9 |
| Specificity (%) | 87.3 | 89.4 | 89.4 | 90.2 | 88.3 | 88.8 | 91.3 |
| Troponin T | | | | | | | |
| Sensitivity (%) | 10.5 | 35.7 | 61.7 | 86.5 | 84.9 | 78.7 | 85.7 |
| Specificity (%) | 98.4 | 98.3 | 96.1 | 96.4 | 96.1 | 95.7 | 94.6 |
| Troponin I | | | | | | | |
| Sensitivity (%) | 15.8 | 35.7 | 57.5 | 92.3 | 90.6 | 95.7 | 89.8 |
| Specificity (%) | 96.8 | 94.2 | 94.3 | 94.6 | 92.2 | 93.4 | 94.2 |
| Total MB-CK activity | | | | | | | |
| Sensitivity (%) | 21.1 | 40.7 | 74.5 | 96.2 | 98.1 | 97.9 | 89.8 |
| Specificity (%) | 100.0 | 98.8 | 97.5 | 97.5 | 96.1 | 96.9 | 96.2 |
| Total MB-CK mass | | | | | | | |
| Sensitivity (%) | 15.8 | 39.3 | 66.0 | 90.4 | 90.5 | 95.7 | 95.7 |
| Specificity (%) | 99.2 | 98.8 | 100.0 | 99.6 | 98.9 | 99.6 | 99.1 |

***Comparison of the Markers for Diagnosis of Early- and Late-Onset Infarction*** MB-CK SUBFORMS AND MYOGLOBIN In the United States, over 5 million patients with chest pain go to the emergency department annually, but only about 10 percent of those with chest pain will subsequently be shown to have myocardial infarction.[101] About 50 percent of patients will have cardiac ischemia, 10 percent will have nonischemic cardiac pain, and about 30 percent will have pain of noncardiac origin.[101] It is important to have an early diagnosis to determine the initial therapeutic regimen and whether hospital admission is needed. In the United States, it is estimated that over $12 billion per year[115] is spent unnecessarily to exclude myocardial infarction in patients admitted to the hospital with chest pain without infarction. Thus, early, rapid diagnosis is required to triage patients, reduce costs, and select appropriate therapy in spite of the difficulty in distinguishing cardiac ischemia from infarction based on the patient's history, physical examination, and the ECG, as noted. This difficulty is emphasized by the observation that over 50 percent of AMI patients in the United States[116] have nonspecific ST-segment changes (non-Q-wave infarction) rather than ST-segment elevation (Q-wave infarction)(see Chap. 51). The only specific ECG finding on admission for myocardial infarction is the recent development of ST-segment elevation or new left bundle branch block. It is estimated that less than 50 percent of patients with AMI will have a diagnostic ECG, which represents only 5 percent of the total patients presenting with chest pain; thus, there is a need for an early objective marker (within 6 h of onset).[72] The ideal diagnostic test should have an assay performance time that is brief, and the marker must have a highly reliable negative predictive value, since only 10 percent of patients will have infarction, as noted. While a false-positive range of 5 to 10 percent is acceptable, a desirable false-negative range is 1 to 2 percent. Assessment of the plasma profile of the markers shows only two plausible candidates, namely, MB-CK subforms and myoglobin.

MB-CK upon release into plasma is converted from MB-2 into MB-1, due to the proteolytic activity of carboxypeptidase-N.[117,118] In the plasma, the MB-CK subforms are in equilibrium, with a ratio of MB-2 to MB-1 of 1 to 1. Normally, the baseline plasma MB-CK activity is in the range of 2 to 4 IU/L, or a protein concentration of 3 to 5 ng/L. Thus, for a reliable diagnosis of myocardial infarction based on total MB-CK activity, one requires an increase above 9 IU/L, or, for protein, above 7 ng/L. When infarction occurs, MB-2, the tissue form, is initially released into the circulation in minute amounts so that total plasma MB-CK activity remains within the normal range, but the ratio of MB-2 to MB-1 changes markedly and provides the basis for an early diagnosis of myocardial infarction. The current assay for MB-CK subforms is completely automated and requires about 25 min. In a large, blinded, prospective study involving 1110 patients presenting consecutively with chest pain, it was shown that MB-CK subforms reliably diagnosed myocardial infarction within 6 h of onset of symptoms.[119]

A large multicenter, prospective, double-blind study, the Diagnostic Marker Cooperative Study (DMCS), comprised 1004 patients admitted consecutively with chest pain.[101] A serial analysis of all markers (MB-CK activity, MB-CK mass, MB-CK subforms, myoglobin, and cardiac troponins T and I) was performed on a sample taken on admission, at 1 h, every 2 h for up to 6 h from onset, and subsequently every 4 h for up to 24 h (Table 52-2). In keeping with previous observations, only 11 percent of the patients with chest pain were subsequently documented to have infarction ($n$ = 118), of whom less than 47 percent had a diagnostic ECG (43 percent had ST-segment elevation and 4 percent had a left bundle branch block), with the remainder having nonspecific ST-T changes (NQWMI). Cardiac ischemia accounted for 51 percent and nonischemic cardiac pain for another 9 percent, while in 29 percent the pain was of noncardiac origin. MB-CK subforms afforded a sensitivity and specificity of 91 percent for the diagnosis of infarction within 6 h of the onset of symptoms. Myoglobin had a sensitivity of 83 percent during the same interval. The negative predictive value of MB-CK subforms within the initial 6 h of onset was 97 percent and that of myoglobin 95 percent. Thus, if a patient has a negative MB-CK subform test at 6 h after the onset of symptoms, one can reliably conclude that the patient does not have infarction. During the same interval of 6 h from onset, the total MB-CK (activity or mass assay) and troponins T and I afforded a sensitivity of only 65 percent. MB-CK subforms correctly diagnosed 92 percent of the patients with myocardial infarction within 60 min of arriving in the emergency department. For patients presenting after 6 to 10 h, troponin I or T or MB-CK has high sensitivity and specificity for the diagnosis of myocardial infarction (Table 52-2). It is noteworthy that the sensitivity of myoglobin decreases after about 7 or 8 h because of rapid renal clearance and thus may not be reliable after 10 to 12 h, particularly in patients with minimal injury.

***Sampling Intervals and the Diagnosis of Infarction*** In patients presenting within the first 6 to 10 h of the onset of myocardial infarction, the marker with most sensitivity is either MB-CK subforms or myoglobin. It is recommended that a blood sample be taken immediately on admission, 1 h later, then every 2 h until 6 h from the onset of symptoms, and then, if positive, every 6 h for 24 to 48 h. The MB-CK subform assay provides a diagnosis based on the first two samples (initial and 1 h) in more than 90 percent of the patients with infarction. Once a sample is positive, one can sample every 6 h for 24 to 48 h. If the sample shows normal values for the MB-CK subforms, one must sample until 6 h from the onset of symptoms to reliably exclude infarction, at which time sampling can be discontinued. Sampling for 24 to 48 h in patients with positive MB-CK subforms is optional, but it is recommended for the following reasons: to obtain maximal total plasma MB-CK activity as a rough index of the extent of damage; to follow the decline in MB-CK subform activity as a baseline for subsequent procedures often performed, such as cardiac catheterization or percutaneous transluminal coronary angioplasty (PTCA); and to facilitate detection of early reinfarction, which accounts for 30 to 40 percent of in-hospital deaths in patients recovering from AMI. If the myoglobin is analyzed, a similar sampling algorithm is followed except that the interval required to exclude or include infarction with myoglobin may be longer, since with MB-CK subforms, 90 percent of patients with AMI are diagnosed within 60 min (two samples), whereas only [illegible] percent over the same interval will be diagnosed with myoglobin. Patients presenting 10 to 12 h or later after the onset of symptoms should have a sample taken on admission; if this is positive, it should be repeated every 6 h for 24 to 48 h. Troponin I or T or MB-CK will provide the desired diagnostic sensitivity and specificity. Normal total plasma MB-CK activity or protein concentrations at 12 to 16 h from the onset of symptoms excludes infarction with 95 to 100 percent reliability, as does a normal troponin T or I. Plasma myoglobin is not a reliable marker 8 to 10 h after the onset of symptoms. The upper level of normal for MB-2 is $\geq$2.6 IU/L, with a ratio of MB-2 to MB-1 of $\geq$1.7. The upper limit of normal for myoglobin is 85 ng/mL. The upper limit of total MB-CK activity is 9 IU/L, and for protein (mass) assays, 7 ng/mL. The upper limit of normal for troponin T is 0.1 ng/mL and for troponin I 1.5 ng/mL. The following guidelines are suggested:

1. Preferably, the diagnosis is made on the basis of no fewer than two samples in a 24-h period, separated by at least 4 h.
2. If only a single sample is present, the diagnosis must be made on the basis of an elevation above normal by at least twofold.
3. In patients admitted beyond 72 h from the onset of infarction, troponin T or I is preferred, since MB-CK levels may have returned to normal.

***Limitations of Myoglobin, MB-CK, and Troponins I and T in the Diagnosis of AMI*** Elevated plasma MB-CK as a diagnostic marker for myocardial infarction is associated with a very low incidence of false-negative results when samples are collected frequently and appropriately within 48 to 72 h of the onset of symptoms. However, false-positive results do occur, since trace amounts of MB-CK can be released from tissues other than the heart. Skeletal muscle injury, as noted, may induce the synthesis of MB-CK and has been documented after crush injury,[108] electrical injury,[109] dermatomyositis and polymyositis,[107] and Duchenne muscular dystrophy[120] as well as in professional athletes and marathon runners.[106]

Troponin I has not been found to be elevated in patients with normal skeletal muscle despite severe exercise or injury[113] or in the blood of marathon runners.[121,122] Furthermore, in a study involving 100 patients undergoing noncardiac surgery with extensive skeletal muscle injury, only 1 patient had a slight elevation of cardiac troponin I.[123] Troponin I is not elevated in chronic renal failure.[113] An increase in troponin T has been reported in patients with polymyositis/dermatomyositis without cardiac involvement.[124]

***Rationale for Selecting a Diagnostic Marker*** In selecting a marker for *early diagnosis* upon admission to the emergency department, there is essentially a choice between MB-CK subforms and myoglobin. As compared with myoglobin, MB-CK subforms provide greater sensitivity as well as greater specificity overall for the early diagnosis of AMI. Both assays are automated and simple to perform, requiring only about 25 min, and are identical in cost. For the diagnosis of patients presenting 10 h or later after the onset of symptoms, cardiac troponin I or T is preferred over CK-MB because of increased sensitivity, since troponins are not normally present in the blood. The time required to assay each of these latter three markers is about 25 min, with identical costs. A single assay for both early and late diagnosis is the MB-CK subforms, which provide an early diagnosis and from which total MB-CK can be derived for the late diagnosis. Another is MB-CK subforms for early diagnosis plus either troponin I or T for late diagnosis. Myoglobin provides an early diagnosis but is less specific. Nevertheless, the combination of a troponin marker and myoglobin is rapidly becoming routine. In clinical situations where there is concommitant skeletal muscle involvement, MB-CK, if elevated, is less than 5 percent of total CK activity and is usually not a diagnostic problem. However, troponin I or T is more appropriate in those clinical conditions. The data from the DMCS indicate no advantage to analyzing myoglobin if one is assaying for MB-CK subforms; similarly, for late diagnosis, there is no advantage to analyzing multiple markers unless one is interested in diagnosing early reinfarction, in which case MB-CK is the choice.

***Diagnosis of Acute Myocardial Infarction in Patients 48 H or More from the Onset of Symptoms*** In patients admitted 48 to 72 h after the onset of symptoms, particularly when associated with minimal myocardial damage, plasma MB-CK may have returned to normal levels. In this situation, it has been traditional to utilize LDH isoenzymes, since LDH-1 activity peaks between 48 and 72 h and remains elevated for 10 to 14 days; but the preferred diagnostic marker is now troponin I or T. It is recommended that LDH, LDH isoenzymes, and SGOT (AST) be discontinued as diagnostic markers for AMI.

***Diagnostic Assessment of Patients Undergoing Fibrinolytic Therapy or Angioplasty*** Patients who receive fibrinolytic therapy or early angioplasty (within 4 to 6 h) for treatment of infarction should be assessed hourly for plasma MB-CK activity or one of the troponins for the first 4 to 6 h, then every 6 to 8 h for 36 h, with sampling reinitiated if chest pain or other features occur to suggest reinfarction. Following successful reperfusion, MB-CK is usually elevated within 30 to 60 min of the reperfusion, and plasma activity reaches maximum levels within 10 to 15 h. Studies have shown that 15 to 20 percent of patients undergoing elective PTCA have elevated plasma MB-CK,[125] and that these individuals have a worse prognosis over the subsequent 6 months.[126] It remains controversial whether routine sampling for MB-CK should be performed after elective PTCA, since changes in treatment based on increased MB-CK have not been assessed. In patients with triple-vessel disease or where complications are more likely, routine sampling with MB-CK subforms is recommended for 6 h; it should be discontinued if the results are normal. If they are positive, sampling should continue for at least 24 h, and the patient should be treated as having had myocardial damage. It is now recognized that increased plasma levels of MB-CK reflect cardiac cell death, and it is likely though not proven that cardiac troponin I and T do so also.

***Diagnosis of Early Reinfarction*** Diagnosis of early reinfarction (within 24 to 48 h) is difficult, since it represents an elevation superimposed on an already elevated plasma marker.[127,128] However, if MB-CK has returned to normal, the diagnosis is relatively easy, since one sees a secondary increase in plasma MB-CK activity. Detection of early reinfarction by measuring a secondary elevation in plasma MB-CK in patients who undergo successful thrombolysis is appropriate, since MB-CK activity usually peaks within the first 10 to 15 h and returns to normal by 36 to 48 h. A secondary elevation of MB-CK activity 36 to 48 h after the onset of symptoms provides for a sensitive and specific diagnosis of reinfarction. In the latter situation, reinfarction is defined as an increase of 50 percent or more in the plasma MB-CK activity above the preceding baseline (mean of the two preceding samples) in at least two samples separated by a minimum of 4 h within a 24-h interval, with an absolute value of ±9 IU/L or 7 ng/L in at least one sample.[129] If the MB-CK activity is on the downslope from the antecedent infarction, a 25 percent increase is considered diagnostic; however, this is always less reliable than a secondary elevation after the return of MB-CK activity to baseline. These criteria were found to be reliable in three large clinical trials.[81,130,131] Confirmation of reinfarction occurring early, however, is more appropriately diagnosed using the MB-CK subforms. The MB-2 is near normal by 18 to 24 h and usually peaks at 10 to 12 h, so a well-defined downslope is apparent after 12 to 16 h. The other markers, cardiac troponins T and I, since they remain elevated for 10 to 14 days, lack the necessary sensitivity. Myoglobin, since it returns to normal early after onset, is also a sensitive marker, but because of venipuncture or other minor skeletal muscle trauma commonly occurring in the hospital setting, it can be less specific.

***Prognostic Role for Biochemical Markers in the Assessment of Unstable Angina*** Several studies have shown that patients presenting with the clinical diagnosis of unstable angina and minor elevations in MB-CK, troponin T, or troponin I have a more adverse outcome with respect to clinical events such as death, myocardial infarction, or the need for revascularization. In the Global Use of Strategies to Open Occluded Coronary Arteries (GUSTO) IIA trial,[132] of 835 patients with unstable angina, 36 percent had elevated troponin T and experienced increased mortality and other clinical events. Similarly, in the Thrombolysis in Myocardial Infarction (TIMI) III trial,[133] of 1404 patients with NQWMI infarction and unstable angina, 41 percent had elevated troponin I and experienced increased mortality and other clinical events. In a study involving 593 patients with unstable angina, those with elevated MB-CK had increased mortality and other clinical events.[134]

It is now recommended that patients with unstable angina be assessed with one or more of these markers; preferably a troponin (see also Chap. 51). The new consensus is that an elevation of cardiac troponin I, troponin T, or CK-MB reflects myocardial injury and should be diagnosed as myocardial infarction.[134] Data[100] conclusively indicate release of CK reflects irreversible injury. This finding coupled with the observation that patients with proven obstructive coronary disease during exercise-induced ischemia, as documented by thallium scintigraphy, exhibited no increase in plasma MB-CK or MB-CK subforms provides the basis for interpreting elevated plasma MB-CK levels as reflective of irreversible injury.[135] Studies have not been performed to determine whether increased troponin I or troponin T reflects cell death, although, since they are structural sarcomeric proteins, it is highly likely that their release does reflect cell necrosis. Since the molecular weight of troponin I is 23,000, however, and that of troponin T is 39,000, both of which are significantly less than that of MB-CK (82,000), leakage with myocardial ischemia will have to be excluded by appropriate studies.

***Diagnosis of Myocardial Infarction after Surgery*** Myocardial infarction after noncardiac surgery is also reliably determined from serial analysis of plasma MB-CK, MB-CK subforms, troponin T, or troponin I every 4 to 6 h.[136] There is a marked elevation of other enzymes due to tissue trauma, including total CK, but MB-CK, troponin T, and troponin I are highly specific to the myocardium. There is at least one study[123] showing that troponin I is more reliable than either total MB-CK or troponin T for the diagnosis of AMI in this setting. In the setting of cardiac surgery, however, MB-CK, like other cardiac markers, is almost always elevated due to manipulation and involvement of the myocardium and thus is not a reliable diagnostic index.[137] Nevertheless a severalfold elevation of MB-CK postoperatively is highly suggestive of periprocedural infarction, even in the absence of Q-waves, although it lacks specificity as a sole criterion. Multifold elevations of troponin T or troponin I probably have the same implications postoperatively.

***Other Biochemical Alterations*** The stress of myocardial infarction elicits numerous hormonal and metabolic responses. For example, both catecholamines and growth hormones are elevated. It is noteworthy, however, that serum cholesterol and lipoprotein fractions are relatively unchanged in the initial 1 to 2 days but decrease significantly over subsequent days and weeks. In establishing the baseline levels of these values for guiding future therapeutic interventions, measurements should be performed on admission or should be delayed for 6 to 8 weeks.[138] It should also be recognized that if myocardial infarction is occurring in individuals who have hypertension or who for any reason are on medications such as diuretics, there may be significant electrolyte abnormalities that need to be treated, particularly in view of the increased propensity for arrhythmias, as with hypokalemia or alkalosis. The other abnormality seen on occasion is that of an increase in blood glucose following myocardial infarction, which in some cases, particularly in patients with mild or moderate diabetes, may be associated with the development of significant ketoacidosis.[139] Not infrequently, it has also been shown that in the early days following myocardial infarction, the glucose tolerance curve is abnormal. It returns to normal after a few weeks. The white blood cell count is usually mildly to moderately elevated in 3 to 5 days.

## NONINVASIVE IMAGING IN ACUTE MYOCARDIAL INFARCTION

***Chest Roentgenography*** The chest roentgenogram (x-ray) provides important information in the evaluation of chest pain and contributes to an integrative assessment of the clinical situation. The chest film may help to exclude causes of chest pain such as pneumothorax, pulmonary infarction with effusion, aortic dissection, skeletal fractures, and so on. In the patient with acute infarction, the chest film can be useful in establishing the presence of pulmonary edema, assessing heart size to assist in determining whether or not cardiomegaly is present, and deciding whether heart failure or myocardial or valvular disease is acute or chronic. It must be emphasized that severe left ventricular failure can be present without manifesting pulmonary edema on the chest x-ray and that, conversely, improvement in the x-ray appearance can lag behind hemodynamic resolution of pulmonary congestion (see Chap. 14).

***Echocardiography*** Because of the quality of the images provided, their wide availability, and the portability of these modalities, two-dimensional and Doppler echocardiography have become very useful tools in the assessment of the patient with suspected AMI[140] (see also Chap. 15). Echocardiography is particularly valuable in assessing the patient with a nondiagnostic ECG. The presence of a regional wall motion abnormality provides strong supportive evidence of acute coronary ischemia and is generally present in transmural or Q-wave myocardial infarction.[141] Wall motion abnormalities are less common in NQWMI but are still present in the majority of cases. Nonetheless, small infarctions can be missed, and a wall motion abnormality may not necessarily be acute.[142] Echocardiography also provides an assessment of ventricular function; it is useful in predicting the prognosis[143] and in diagnosing right ventricular infarction.[144] It can also provide information concerning alternative diagnoses such as aortic dissection and, coupled with Doppler, information on such complications as ruptured chordae tendineae with mitral regurgitation and ventricular septal defect[145] (see Chap. 15). It is useful in detecting ventricular thrombus and pericardial fluid. Thus, echocardiography is extremely useful in the initial assessment of AMI. General guidelines on its clinical use, including those for myocardial infarction, have been published.[146]

***Magnetic Resonance Imaging*** Magnetic resonance imaging (MRI) offers great promise in assessing AMI (see Chap. 21). Its major limitation is logistic, in that patients must be transported to the imaging facility, and this is a major concern in those who are acutely ill. It is potentially useful in the assessment of infarct size and viable myocardium and the extent of the ischemic insult as well as in estimating perfusion to ischemic and nonischemic areas.[147,148] Currently, MRI does not have a defined role in the routine management of AMI.

***Computed Tomography*** Computed tomography (CT) is a powerful tool for cardiac imaging that provides high-resolution structural information (see Chap. 20). Ventricular thickness and dimensions can be assessed.[149] Also, CT is highly sensitive for detecting a left ventricular thrombus.[150] It has the same logistic limitations as MRI in the management of AMI. It does not have a routine role in the management of infarction. Whether electron-beam CT, with its very rapid acquisition times, can have a role in routine management requires further investigation (see Chap. 20).

***Radionuclide Scintigraphy*** The radionuclide techniques available for the diagnosis of AMI are discussed in detail in Chap. 19 and summarized in Table 52-3. Guidelines for the use of cardiac radionuclide scanning have been published and suggest that the indications for its use in the diagnosis of acute infarction are limited to the unusual case in which history, ECG changes, and plasma markers are unreliable or unavailable.[151] There is no class I indication in the acute setting, and routine diagnostic use is not indicated (class III).[1,151] Radionuclide scintigraphy may have a diagnostic role in certain patients with right ventricular infarction by showing localized contractile abnormalities[152] or uptake of technetium-99m ($^{99m}$Tc) pyrophosphate (class IIa).[151]

***Assessment of Infarct Size by Imaging*** Infarct size can be assessed by echocardiography (see Chap. 15), CT (see Chap. 20), MRI (see Chap. 21), positron emission tomography (see Chap. 23), or radionuclide scintigraphy (Table 52-3) (see Chap. 19). $^{99m}$Tc sestamibi with tomographic imaging has been used to quantitate infarct size[153,154] and shown to be inversely related to the patient's outcome.[155,156] Thallium 201 can also be used to measure infarct size.[151]

TABLE 52-3 Uses of Radionuclide Testing in Acute Myocardial Infarction

| Diagnosis | | | Risk Assessment | | |
|---|---|---|---|---|---|
| Indication | Test | Class | Indication | Test | Class |
| 1. Right ventricular infarction | Rest RNA | IIa | 1. Residual ischemia | Stress (exercise/pharmacologic) thallium with redistribution | I |
| | $^{99m}$Tc pyrophosphate | IIa | | Stress (exercise/pharmacologic) sestamibi with redistribution | |
| 2. Infarction not diagnosed by standard means—early presentation with successful reperfusion | Rest myocardial perfusion imaging | IIb | 2. Myocardial infarct size | Tomographic thallium | IIa |
| | $^{99m}$Tc pyrophosphate | IIb | | Tomographic sestamibi | IIa |
| 3. Infarction not diagnosed by standard means—late presentation | $^{99m}$Tc pyrophosphate | IIa | 3. Hibernating myocardium | Early, late thallium | IIa |
| 4. Routine diagnosis | Any technique | III | 4. Ventricular function | RNA | I |

Abbreviations: RNA = radionuclide angiography; $^{99m}$Tc = technetium 99m.
Source: The ACC/AHA task force[151] With permission.

## PREHOSPITAL CARE

### Out-of-Hospital Cardiac Arrest

ACC/AHA recommendations are as follows[1]:

Class I

1. All communities should create and maintain a strong "chain of survival" for out-of-hospital cardiac arrest that includes early access [recognition of the problem and activation of the Emergency Medical Services (EMS) system by a bystander], early CPR, early defibrillation for patients who need it, and early advanced cardiac life support (ACLS) (*level of evidence C*).
2. Family members of victims of STEMI should be advised to take CPR training (*level of evidence C*).

As mentioned previously, modern in-hospital care of the AMI patient has resulted in a substantial reduction in mortality. Some 40 to 65 percent of deaths from AMI, however, occur within an hour of the onset of symptoms and prior to arrival at a hospital.[157,158] Most of these deaths are attributable to ventricular fibrillation (VF).[159] To achieve a further substantial decrease in the mortality rate, it will be necessary to reduce the incidence of deaths outside the hospital.[160] Since, as noted, the earlier thrombolytic therapy can be initiated in eligible patients, the better the outcome, it is also essential to bring patients with chest pain into the medical care system as soon as possible because of the need to shorten the time between the onset of symptoms and the initiation of thrombolytic therapy or primary coronary intervention (see Chap. 56). To that end, in the United States, the National Heart, Lung and Blood Institute of the National Institutes of Health has instituted the National Heart Attack Alert Program as a coordinated plan to extend the ACC/AHA guidelines promoting rapid identification and treatment of patients with AMI.[161,162]

### Recognition and Management

A further reduction in the mortality rate will require the combined efforts of the patient, bystanders, minimally trained "first responders" who are capable of applying defibrillation therapy, and/or paramedics as well as the patient's physician. It has been established that a prolonged delay time in responding to a patient's symptoms is the rate-limiting step in defining the prehospital phase of myocardial infarction. Mean delay time in such response is almost 3 h.[163] Most of this time is consumed in decision making while failing to recognize or acknowledge the seriousness of the problem.[164] Additional components of the delay between the onset of symptoms and the initiation of definitive therapy involve prehospital evaluation, treatment, and transport time and the time involved with the diagnosis and initiation of treatment in the hospital. The National Registry of Myocardial Infarction found, in a review of 48, 128 patients with confirmed AMI, that the average duration of the prehospital phase, defined as onset of chest pain to hospital presentation, was 5.1 h.

#### STRATEGIES TO REDUCE DELAY

Patient-specific issues for decreasing the delay in seeking assistance primarily involve education. The patient must perceive the symptoms, recognize their possible significance, and conclude that medical help is appropriate. For some patients, the decision time is prolonged because of a lack of knowledge. It is interesting, however, that the length of time patients take to get help is not dependent on educational level, occupation, socioeconomic class, or past history of cardiac disease. In fact, patients with a past history of myocardial infarction or angina have an unexpectedly long decision time,[165] a situation that must be viewed, at least in part, as a failure by physicians to educate patients with established coronary artery disease as to the appropriate response to a change in or reappearance of their symptoms. In other cases, the decision time is prolonged by denial or by "diagnostic trials" with household remedies, patent medications, or previously prescribed drugs. It has been noted that only 10 percent of patients arriving at the hospital within 1 h of the onset of pain utilized nonprescription medications, while 41 percent of those arriving after 12 h did so.[157] The remainder of the delay time is consumed by "human factors," including the time a patient takes to modify existing social obligations and to prepare for going to the hospital. There is evidence that public education can reduce the time required for decision making.[164] It follows that effective efforts by the physician and his or her staff in educating patients with coronary artery disease will have similar effects in inducing appropriate responses to ischemic coronary symptoms. Prodromal symptoms occur in about two-thirds of patients with AMI, as discussed previously, and patients must be taught to recognize them.[160] Patients and their families must be given a specific plan of action after the recognition of symptoms that includes medications to be taken (nitroglycerin and possibly aspirin), mode of transportation to the hospital, and the location of the nearest hospital that offers emergency cardiac care. It is desirable that coronary patients have a copy of their resting ECG with them. They should be instructed not to delay by attempting to contact their physician and should be shown how to use the EMS system and how to contact it (911 in the United States). As opposed to personal transportation, utilizing EMS is desirable because it permits the earliest possible access to expertise in defibrillation and resuscitation and facilitates evaluation in the field to prepare the hospital to receive the patient, as discussed further on. The use of the EMS usually decreases the delay in initiating definitive care.[161] Since the capabilities of the EMS vary by locale, the physician must be familiar with the system in the patient's home area.

Instructions concerning medications to be taken at the onset of symptoms should be individualized. In general, patients are instructed to take nitroglycerin immediately at the onset of angina or a recognized anginal equivalent. If pain is not relieved, another nitroglycerin dose is taken at 5 min and a third at 10 min. If there is no relief by the third dose of nitroglycerin, the patient should be transported to the appropriate emergency facility. The physician should decide whether to incorporate the chewing of an aspirin tablet into this regimen when the decision is made to proceed to the hospital.

Bystanders and family members can play an important role in both shortening patient delay time and responding to an arrest. It has been shown that a spouse's presence accelerated the hospital arrival time.[159] Furthermore, if basic life support is initiated by a bystander within 4 min of cardiac arrest and defibrillation is accomplished within 8 min, 40 percent of patients will survive and be discharged from the hospital.[166]

#### EMERGENCY MEDICAL SERVICES

ACC/AHA recommendations are as follows[1]:

Class I

1. All EMS first responders to patients with chest pain and/or suspected cardiac arrest should be trained and equipped to provide early defibrillation (*level of evidence A*).
2. All public safety first responders to patients with chest pain and/or suspected cardiac arrest should be trained and equipped to provide early defibrillation with automatic external defibrillators (AEDs) (provision of early defibrillation with AED by nonpublic safety

first responders is a promising new strategy, but further study is needed to determine its safety and efficacy) (*level of evidence B*).

3. EMS health care workers should advocate for enhanced cell telephone technology to identify call location on 911 systems (*level of evidence C*).
4. Dispatchers staffing 911 center emergency medical calls should have medical training, should use nationally developed and maintained protocols, and should have a quality improvement system in place to assure compliance with protocols.

Many communities in the United States are served by a two-tier ambulance service consisting of basic and advanced life support units. Since these are usually more basic support units, their response time is shorter and should ideally be less than 5 min.[1,167] The first responders may be any of a variety of public service employees who are trained in cardiopulmonary resuscitation (CPR) and defibrillation and have been taught to have a sense of urgency in order to identify and treat the AMI patient rapidly. Automatic external defibrillators are safe and effective and can be used by even minimally trained first responders to analyze rhythms and deliver defibrillatory shocks to convert VF.[1,168–172] The incorporation of automatic external defibrillators into emergency medical systems is highly desirable.[1] Minimally, it has been recommended that every ambulance transporting victims of cardiac arrest be equipped with a conventional defibrillator.[170]

## PREHOSPITAL CHEST PAIN EVALUATION AND TREATMENT

ACC/AHA recommendations are as follows[1]:

Class I

1. Prehospital EMS providers should administer 160–325 mg aspirin (chewed) to chest pain patients suspected of having STEMI unless contraindicated or already taken (*level of evidence C*).

Class IIa

1. It is reasonable for all 911 dispatchers to advise patients without a history of aspirin allergy who have symptoms of STEMI to chew aspirin (160–325 mg) while awaiting arrival of prehospital EMS providers (*level of evidence C*).
2. All prehospital advanced life support (ALS) providers should be trained and equipped to perform 12-lead ECGs routinely on chest pain patients suspected of STEMI (*level of evidence B*).
3. If the ECG shows evidence of STEMI, prehospital ALS providers should perform a fibrinolytic "checklist" and relay the ECG and checklist findings to the nearest appropriate receiving hospital facility (*level of evidence C*).

The goal of any emergency medical system should be to include individuals who are trained in advanced life support techniques—including the use of antiarrhythmics as well as the administration of intravenous fluids and analgesics—and who can reach the patient as soon as possible in a vehicle equipped as a CCU. Undirected EMS technicians can spend excessive amounts of time evaluating a patient with chest pain and actually delay the ultimate initiation of appropriate therapy.[1] The time elapsed between receiving a 911 call and the actual arrival in the hospital has been assessed, and, at over 46 min, was substantially longer than estimates (under 26 min) taken from the paramedics involved.[164] Most of this field time was consumed by the paramedic on-scene time, which was not prolonged by acquisition of a 12-lead ECG. It has been demonstrated that, by the use of a standardized protocol (Table 52-4), evaluation of the patient with chest pain by experienced EMS technicians, acquisition of a 12-lead ECG, and initiation of therapy can be accomplished within 20 min.[1] The protocol should facilitate de-

TABLE 52-4 Chest Pain Checklist for Use by EMT/Paramedic for Diagnosis of Acute Myocardial Infarction and Thrombolytic Therapy Screening

Check each finding below. If all "yes" boxes are checked and ECG indicates ST-segment elevation or new BBB, reperfusion therapy with thrombolysis or primary PTCA may be indicated. Thrombolysis is generally not indicated unless all "no" boxes are checked and BP $\leq$180/110 mmHg.

| | *Yes* | *No* |
|---|---|---|
| Ongoing chest discomfort (≥20 min and <12 h) | ☐ | — |
| Oriented, can cooperate | ☐ | — |
| Age >35 years (>40 if female) | ☐ | — |
| History of stroke or TIA | — | ☐ |
| Known bleeding disorder | — | ☐ |
| Active internal bleeding in past 2 weeks | — | ☐ |
| Surgery or trauma in past 2 weeks | — | ☐ |
| Terminal illness | — | ☐ |
| Jaundice, hepatitis, kidney failure | — | ☐ |
| Use of anticoagulants | — | ☐ |
| Systolic/diastolic blood pressure | | |
| Right arm: —/— | | |
| Left arm: —/— | | |
| | *Yes* | *No* |
| ECG done | ☐ | — |
| *High-risk profile*[a] | *Yes* | *No* |
| Heart rate ≥100 bpm | ☐ | — |
| BP ≤100 mmHg | ☐ | — |
| Pulmonary edema (rales greater than halfway up) | ☐ | — |
| Shock | ☐ | — |
| Pain began | — | AM/PM |
| Arrival time | — | AM/PM |
| Begin transport | — | AM/PM |
| Hospital arrival | — | AM/PM |

[a]Transport to hospital capable of angiography and revascularization if needed.

ABBREVIATIONS: EMT = emergency medical technician; ECG = electrocardiogram; BBB = bundle branch block; PTCA = percutaneous transluminal coronary angioplasty; BP = blood pressure; TIA = transient ischemic attack. Adapted from the Seattle/King County EMS Medical Record.

SOURCE: Ryan et al.[2] With permission.

termination of the likelihood of AMI and the presence of comorbid conditions in which thrombolytic therapy would be dangerous. It should also identify those suspected AMI patients who are at high risk. Patients in this category include those with sinus tachycardia, hypotension, or pulmonary edema or those with signs of shock. It is ideal to be able to record 12-lead ECGs in the field to be transmitted to the hospital physician. The availability of these data facilitates establishing the diagnosis and allows for accelerating preparations to administer thrombolytic therapy[173–175] or planning for acute cardiac catherization and coronary intervention[176] (see also Chap. 56).

### PREHOSPITAL THROMBOLYSIS

ACC/AHA recommendations are as follows[1]:

Class IIa

1. Prehospital fibrinolysis is reasonable in (1) settings in which physicians are present in the ambulance; or (2) well-organized EMS systems with full-time paramedics who have 12-lead ECGs in the field with transmission capability, paramedic initial and on-going training in ECG interpretation and MI treatment, online medical command, and a medical director with training/experience in STEMI management. Prehospital fibrinolysis should be especially considered in high-volume (more than 25,000 runs per year) EMS systems in which the prehospital transport times are greater than 60 min (*level of evidence B*).

As mentioned previously, there is unequivocal evidence that the earlier thrombolysis is administered to the AMI patient with ST-segment elevation, the more efficacious the outcome[14,177,178]; in particular, the most favorable results are achieved when therapy is initiated within the first 1 to 2 h after the symptoms appear. It seems logical, therefore, that if thrombolysis could be initiated in appropriate patients during the prehospital phase by general practitioners or by EMS technicians guided by protocol, the 12-lead ECG, and communication with the emergency department physician, outcomes would be improved. Prehospital thrombolysis has been evaluated in several trials.[173,179–181] A metanalysis of all of the trials showed a modest (17 percent) improvement in outcome, although none of the trials demonstrated significant improvement individually.[179] Prehospital thrombolysis, however, is fraught with a number of difficulties, beginning with the fact that only a small portion of chest pain patients (5 to 10 percent) have an AMI and are eligible to be treated with thrombolytics.[173,175,182,183] Thus, correctly selecting patients for thrombolytic therapy and avoiding its administration when not indicated or when contraindicated is difficult and has significant legal, medical, and economic implications. Because of these difficulties, prehospital thrombolysis should be emphasized primarily in those circumstances in which it can be administered 60 to 90 min before reaching the hospital (because of a long transport time) or when a physician is in the ambulance.[1] Generally, emphasis should be placed on rapid screening and diagnosis in the field to facilitate hospital triage and thrombolytic administration or coronary intervention within 30 min of the patient's arrival.

### PREHOSPITAL DESTINATION PROTOCOLS

ACC/AHA Recommendations are as follows[1]:

Class I

1. Patients with STEMI who have severe left ventricular (LV) dysfunction with shock should be brought immediately or secondarily transferred promptly to facilities capable of cardiac catheterization and rapid revascularization (PCI or CABG) (*level of evidence B*).
2. Every community should have a written protocol that guides EMS system personnel in determining where to take patients with suspected or confirmed STEMI (*level of evidence C*).

Class IIa

1. Patients with STEMI who have contraindications to fibrinolytic therapy should be brought immediately or secondarily transferred promptly (i.e., primary receiving hospital door-to-departure time less than 30 min) to facilities capable of cardiac catheterization and rapid revascularization (PCI or CABG) (*level of evidence B*).
2. Patients with STEMI and shock other than those more than 75 years of age who have severe LV dysfunction should be brought immediately or secondarily transferred promptly (i.e., primary receiving hospital door-to-departure time less than 30 min) to facilities capable of cardiac catheterization and rapid revascularization (PCI or CABG) (*level of evidence B*).

Every community should have a written protocol that guides EMS system personnel in determining where to take patients with suspected or confirmed STEMI. Active involvement of local health care providers, particularly cardiologists and emergency physicians, is needed to formulate local EMS destination protocols for these patients. In general, patients with suspected STEMI should be taken to the nearest appropriate hospital. However, patients with STEMI and shock are an exception to this general rule.[1]

## Optimal Strategies for Emergency Department Triage

ACC/AHA recommendations are as follows[1]:

Class I

1. Hospitals should establish multidisciplinary teams (including primary care physicians, emergency physicians, cardiologists, nurses, and laboratorians) to develop guideline-based written protocols for triaging and managing patients who present to the ED with symptoms suggesting STEMI.

### BACKGROUND

In general, the goals of the emergency department with respect to patients with chest pain are to rapidly identify those patients with AMI with both typical and atypical presentations so that appropriate therapy can be initiated; to recognize those patients with acute coronary syndromes (unstable angina) but without myocardial infarction and who, thus, are at high risk; and to assess accurately those patients at low risk who are candidates for noninvasive evaluation and early discharge.[184]

As mentioned previously, the earlier reperfusion therapy is initiated in the subset of patients with diagnostic ST-segment elevation, the more favorable the clinical results (Fig. 52-2).[177]

An important objective, obviously, should be a triage system that minimizes the number of patients at high risk (AMI or unstable angina) who are inadvertently discharged from the emergency department while also minimizing the admission to high-intensity CCUs of low-risk patients without myocardial infarction—a goal of increasing urgency in this era of intense pressures for cost containment. Of patients admitted to a CCU, for example, less than 20 percent will have AMI, as noted.[185,186] In contrast, even in the current era of an enhanced appreciation for atypical presentations, an increased potential for litigation, and a decreased threshold for admission to exclude myocardial infarction, the missed diagnosis rate has still been about 4 percent,[119] a percentage that appears not to have changed substantially since the 1980s.[187–189]

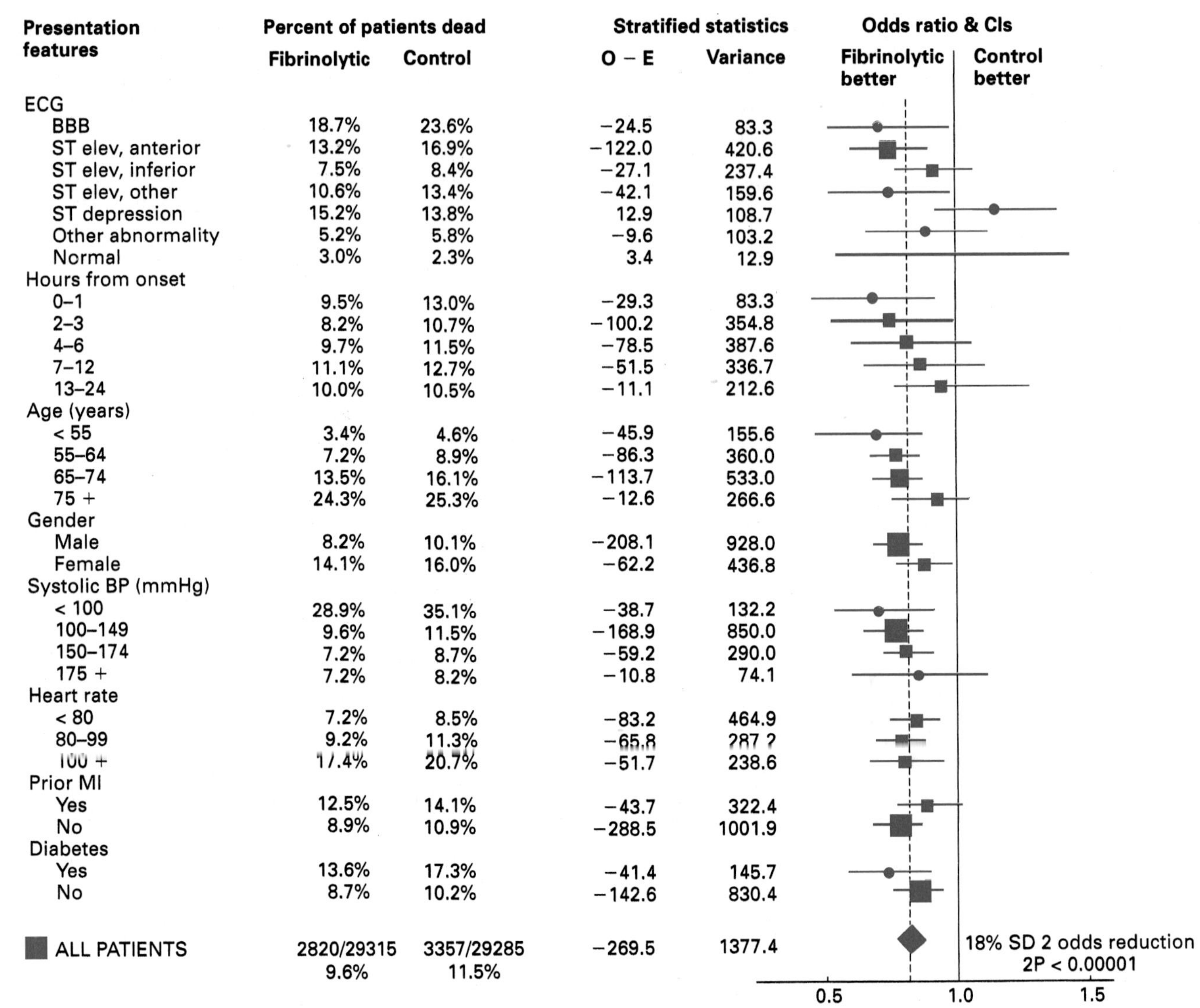

| Presentation features | Percent of patients dead: Fibrinolytic | Control | Stratified statistics: O − E | Variance |
|---|---|---|---|---|
| **ECG** | | | | |
| BBB | 18.7% | 23.6% | −24.5 | 83.3 |
| ST elev, anterior | 13.2% | 16.9% | −122.0 | 420.6 |
| ST elev, inferior | 7.5% | 8.4% | −27.1 | 237.4 |
| ST elev, other | 10.6% | 13.4% | −42.1 | 159.6 |
| ST depression | 15.2% | 13.8% | 12.9 | 108.7 |
| Other abnormality | 5.2% | 5.8% | −9.6 | 103.2 |
| Normal | 3.0% | 2.3% | 3.4 | 12.9 |
| **Hours from onset** | | | | |
| 0–1 | 9.5% | 13.0% | −29.3 | 83.3 |
| 2–3 | 8.2% | 10.7% | −100.2 | 354.8 |
| 4–6 | 9.7% | 11.5% | −78.5 | 387.6 |
| 7–12 | 11.1% | 12.7% | −51.5 | 336.7 |
| 13–24 | 10.0% | 10.5% | −11.1 | 212.6 |
| **Age (years)** | | | | |
| < 55 | 3.4% | 4.6% | −45.9 | 155.6 |
| 55–64 | 7.2% | 8.9% | −86.3 | 360.0 |
| 65–74 | 13.5% | 16.1% | −113.7 | 533.0 |
| 75 + | 24.3% | 25.3% | −12.6 | 266.6 |
| **Gender** | | | | |
| Male | 8.2% | 10.1% | −208.1 | 928.0 |
| Female | 14.1% | 16.0% | −62.2 | 436.8 |
| **Systolic BP (mmHg)** | | | | |
| < 100 | 28.9% | 35.1% | −38.7 | 132.2 |
| 100–149 | 9.6% | 11.5% | −168.9 | 850.0 |
| 150–174 | 7.2% | 8.7% | −59.2 | 290.0 |
| 175 + | 7.2% | 8.2% | −10.8 | 74.1 |
| **Heart rate** | | | | |
| < 80 | 7.2% | 8.5% | −83.2 | 464.9 |
| 80–99 | 9.2% | 11.3% | −65.8 | 287.2 |
| 100 + | 17.4% | 20.7% | −51.7 | 238.6 |
| **Prior MI** | | | | |
| Yes | 12.5% | 14.1% | −43.7 | 322.4 |
| No | 8.9% | 10.9% | −288.5 | 1001.9 |
| **Diabetes** | | | | |
| Yes | 13.6% | 17.3% | −41.4 | 145.7 |
| No | 8.7% | 10.2% | −142.6 | 830.4 |
| **ALL PATIENTS** | 2820/29315 9.6% | 3357/29285 11.5% | −269.5 | 1377.4 |



FIGURE 52-2 Proportional effects of fibrinolytic therapy on mortality during days 0 to 35 subdivided by presentation features. "Observed minus expected" (O − E) number of events among fibrinolytic-allocated patients (and its variance) is given for subdivisions of presentation features stratified by trial. This is used to calculate odds ratios (ORs) of death among patients allocated to fibrinolytic therapy to that among those allocated control. The ORs (squares with areas proportional to the amount of "statistical information" contributed by the trials) are plotted with their 99 percent confidence intervals (CIs) (*horizontal lines*). Squares to the left of the solid vertical line indicate benefit (significant at $2p < 0.01$ only where the entire CI is to left of vertical line). Overall result and 95 percent CI represented by diamond, with overall proportion reduction in the odds of death and statistical significance given alongside. (From Fibrinolytic Therapy Trialists' Collaborative Group.[177] With permission.)

The reasons for misdiagnosis of acute coronary syndromes in the emergency department have been studied extensively and have been reviewed.[184] The misinterpretation of ECGs has been reported to occur in approximately 20 to 40 percent of missed AMIs.[189–191] Equally disturbing are the reports, which are indictments of training or focus, that patients are discharged even though the physician has recognized ischemic symptoms or ECG changes.[188,190,191] A major contributing problem is that even experienced clinicians are imprecise in their clinical judgment as to the presence or absence of myocardial infarction in a given patient. Sensitivities of 80 to 90 percent and specificities of approximately 70 to 80 percent in diagnostic precision in determining the presence or absence of AMI based on clinical impressions have been reported.[71,189,192] The diagnostic problem, however, is not limited to the diagnosis of myocardial infarction but also applies to whether unstable angina is present (see also Chap. 51). Patients who are admitted to the hospital with chest pain and only transient ST-segment changes and without aggressive therapy have a 22 percent incidence of death and myocardial infarction after a 28-month follow-up,[193] a figure not dissimilar to that for patients with an initial confirmed infarction. These similarities in outcome of unstable angina and myocardial infarction are not surprising, since the fundamental underlying pathophysiologic mechanisms—disruption of the atherosclerotic plaque and thrombus formation, with or without vasospasm—are likely to be identical, the major difference being the extent of luminal compromise by the thrombus. Thus, the clinical focus should not be simply to "rule out" AMI but, taking a proactive approach, to "rule in" either acute infarction or unstable angina in an expeditious manner.[184] Once these urgent conditions have been excluded or ascertained to be of low probability, the next level of concern is determining the presence of other acute cardiovascular or cardiopulmonary conditions, such as aortic dissection, pulmonary embolus, and pericarditis. The focus, subsequently, in a hierarchical fashion, is to establish whether or not stable coronary artery disease is present, to identify cardiovascular risk factors, and to consider noncardiac diagnoses, which, in nonurgent cases, can be evaluated further on an outpatient basis.

It has been suggested[184] that management of chest pain in the emergency department can be optimized by having the appropriate clinical focus, developing effective risk-stratification approaches, and implementing systematic algorithmic protocols. There has been a great deal of interest in the development of actual or virtual chest pain units to facilitate the expeditious triage and management of patients with chest pain, as discussed further on.

## INITIAL APPROACH, DETECTION, AND ASSESSMENT OF RISK

ACC/AHA recommendations are as follows[1]:

Class I

1. An ECG should be performed and shown to an experienced ED physician within 10 min of ED arrival on all patients with chest discomfort or other symptoms suggestive of STEMI (*level of evidence C*).
2. Since patient delay time is variable and not under direct control of the health care provider, the delay from patient contact with the health care system (arrival at the ED, or contact with paramedics if prehospital fibrinolytic therapy is available in the EMS system) and initiation of fibrinolytic therapy should be less than 30 min. Alternatively, if PCI is chosen, the delay from patient contact with the health care system (typically, arrival at the ED, or contact with paramedics) should be less than 90 min (*level of evidence B*).
3. If the initial ECG is not diagnostic of STEMI, but the patient remains symptomatic and there is a high clinical suspicion for MI or ACS, serial ECGs should be performed at 5–10 min intervals to detect potential development of ST elevation (*level of evidence C*).

Class IIa

1. The choice of initial STEMI treatment should be made by the ED physician on duty based on a predetermined, institution-specific, written protocol that is a collaborative effort of cardiologists (both those involved in coronary care unit management and interventionalists), emergency physicians, primary care physicians, nurses, and other appropriate personnel. For cases in which the initial diagnosis and treatment plan is unclear to the emergency physician or is not covered directly by the agreed-upon protocol, immediate cardiology consultation is advisable (*level of evidence C*).

A major goal of the emergency department in dealing with patients with chest pain is the establishment of a routine approach that leads to a rapid (10 min) preliminary evaluation, acquisition of a 12-lead ECG, and establishment of intravenous access and continuous ECG monitoring. The initial physical examination and assessment of the history are guided by the differential diagnosis of chest pain, with the goal of establishing whether or not myocardial ischemia is a likely or possible diagnosis. Blood is drawn for baseline cardiac marker levels, and if coronary ischemia is suspected and there are no contraindications, the patient is given aspirin of 160 to 325 mg to chew and swallow. Also, the patient with suspected coronary ischemia is given sublingual nitroglycerin unless the systolic blood pressure is less than 90 mmHg. This should be avoided with severe bradycardia or tachycardia. Because of the potentially catastrophic implications, the history of chest pain alone usually dictates entry into the system for evaluation. In general, the only patients with chest pain who are not systematically evaluated for myocardial ischemia would be those in whom a clear noncardiac cause, such as chest wall tenderness, can be demonstrated unequivocally to be the etiology of the presenting symptoms. Continuous ECG monitoring is essential because of the propensity for the development of sudden and potentially lethal ventricular arrhythmias in any patient with an acute coronary ischemic syndrome. Intravenous access is essential for therapeutic interventions under such circumstances as well as for more general purposes. Additionally, paroxysmal changes in the ST segment may be recognizable on the monitor. The differential diagnosis of chest pain and the clinical recognition of AMI were discussed previously. The causes of chest pain that are not the result of acute pathologic changes compromising the structural integrity of the large coronary arteries are listed in Table 52-5 (see also Chap. 12).

As a general rule, and as previously mentioned, one should begin the evaluation of the patient with chest pain with the assumption that one is dealing with myocardial ischemia until proven otherwise. As noted previously, the three most serious and urgent alternative diagnoses that need to be considered specifically during the initial evaluation are aortic dissection, acute pulmonary embolus, and acute pneumothorax. Acute pericarditis and myopericarditis must be considered as well.

Although relatively uncommon, aortic dissection must be considered and ruled in or out during the initial evaluation of the patient with chest pain, since specific intervention can decrease its high mortality. Furthermore, and not unexpectedly, administration of thrombolytic agents in the presence of aortic dissection is associated with high mortality.[194–196] Suspicion of dissection should be heightened especially in hypertensive patients or in those with marfanoid habitus

TABLE 52-5 Causes of Chest Pain Other Than Acute Coronary Artery Syndromes

- Cardiovascular
  - Aortic dissection
  - Aortic stenosis
- Pericarditis
  - Mitral valve prolapse
  - Microvascular angina
    - Hypertrophic cardiomyopathy
    - Syndrome X
  - Pulmonary embolus
  - Arrhythmia/palpitations
- Noncardiovascular
  - Pleurisy
  - Pneumonia
  - Pneumothorax
  - Costochondritis
  - Gastrointestinal
    - Esophageal spasm/reflux
    - Acid peptic disease
    - Cholecystitis
    - Gastritis
- Psychiatric
  - Panic attack
  - Cardiac neurosis
  - Depression
  - Malingering

(see also Chaps. 72 and 98). Most patients with aortic dissection who have mistakenly received thrombolytic therapy did not meet the ECG criteria of ST-segment elevation that is usually required.[195] Aortic dissection is usually associated with sudden onset of a severe, tearing pain that may migrate and is frequently felt in the back at some point. Differential blood pressures in the arms may be noted, and pulse differences in the carotids or arms may be observed. An echocardiogram and, in particular, transesophageal echocardiography can be very efficacious in the diagnosis of aortic dissection (see Chaps. 15 and 98).

Pulmonary embolus can be life-threatening and should be suspected in anyone with a sudden onset of shortness of breath and chest pressure or pain, especially if there is a history of being sedentary or immobilized and/or of deep venous thrombosis. There may be a pleural rub, and the chest roentgenogram is usually normal, although arterial hypoxia may be present (see Chap. 63). Similarly, pneumothorax may be associated with persistent chest pain, hypoxemia, and evidence of hypoventilation on physical examination.

Acute pericarditis may mimic AMI in that the pain can be substernal and persistent. Frequently, however, there will be a positional component as well as characteristics of pleurisy, with accentuation by deep breathing. Furthermore, the diffuse ST-segment elevation may lead to a misdiagnosis of myocardial infarction. The key differentiating features in pericarditis include PR depression, the diffuse nature of ST-segment elevation in most leads, and the absence of reciprocal changes (see Chaps. 13 and 80). The presence of a pericardial rub is a key diagnostic finding. Echocardiography, by demonstrating a pericardial effusion in the case of pericarditis or a wall motion abnormality in acute ischemia, can be helpful in making the appropriate diagnosis. Hemorrhagic pericardial effusions have been reported in patients given thrombolytic therapy in the setting of acute pericarditis.[194,196]

Although usually not urgent, it should be kept in mind that esophageal disorders, as assessed retrospectively by motility studies, are very common in patients presenting with chest pain in whom cardiac ischemia is ruled out[197–200] (see also Chap. 57). In fact, among all patients presenting with chest pain, gastroesophageal disease has been observed to be the most common etiology (42 percent), whereas ischemic heart disease was present in 31 percent and chest wall syndromes were responsible in 28 percent.[201] Because of the high frequency of GI disease in patients with chest pain, "GI cocktails" or antacids have been used as a diagnostic tool to guide triage and disposition. Only 25 percent of patients with esophageal pain, however, have been reported to obtain pain relief with antacids.[202] Furthermore, coincidental, spontaneous relief of ischemic chest pain at the time of administration of the GI cocktail could be misleading. Similarly, administration of nitroglycerin as a diagnostic strategy for ischemic disease could be misleading because it can relieve esophageal spasm. Moreover, it has been found that pain relief after nitroglycerin did not predict unstable angina or AMI in the chest pain patient.[203] The use of these "response-to-treatment" strategies as major decision points in the evaluation of chest pain has been discouraged.[184] This reservation, however, applies primarily to those patients without diagnostic ECG changes and does not preclude giving sublingual nitroglycerin to patients with chest pain and ST-segment elevation as a test of vasospasm or Prinzmetal's angina.

***Detection*** THE 12-LEAD ELECTROCARDIOGRAM AS A GUIDE TO MANAGEMENT STRATEGY The results of the 12-lead ECG guide the next level of decision making for the patient with chest pain thought to be compatible with myocardial ischemia. The ECG interpretation is assigned to one of three categories: (1) ST-segment elevation in two or more leads or a presumptively new bundle branch block implicating acute coronary occlusion, usually thrombotic; (2) ST-segment depression and/or T-wave inversion implying subtotal occlusion or non-Q infarction; and (3) normal or nondiagnostic. The group with ST-segment elevation or a left bundle branch block is particularly important to define, as it is this group that has been shown to benefit from thrombolytic therapy. ST-segment elevation has a 46 percent sensitivity and a 91 percent specificity for the diagnosis of AMI.[89] Non-ST-segment elevation myocardial infarction and the acute coronary syndromes are discussed in Chap. 51.

As discussed previously, the initial ECG is diagnostic in less than 50 percent of patients with AMI,[204,205] and the measurement of serum markers of myocardial damage plays a major role in diagnosis. Measurement of MB-CK is the benchmark laboratory test, and the specificity and sensitivity of samples taken 2 h apart during serial sampling have been reported to be 91 and 94 percent, respectively.[206] The limitations of conventional MB-CK measurements and the role of myoglobin and the troponins have been discussed. The rapid high-voltage method to separate MB-CK-1 and MB-CK-2 and to determine the ratio of the isoforms was described and may be particularly relevant to the initial evaluation in the emergency department, since it quickly provides information that not only facilitates establishing the appropriate diagnosis but also contributes to assigning a risk category to a patient.

***Risk Stratification*** Stratifying risk in the patient with AMI is an essential part of the management strategy during all phases of care. It permits not only the more precise calibration of treatment and diagnostic approaches with the level of risk but also, increasingly, facilitates the appropriate utilization of hospital resources. Traditional approaches to initial risk assessment have involved combinations of ECG changes and clinical manifestations. The ECG serves as a basis for initial risk assessment. ST-segment elevation or a new left bundle branch block in the patient with chest pain defines a high-risk group, and in those with elevated ST segments, the mortality correlates positively with the number of leads with the ST changes.[207] The presence of ST-segment depression or T-wave inversion also defines a high-risk group. In patients with unstable angina or non-Q-wave myocardial infarction, ST-segment depression on the initial ECG of at least 1 mm in two leads during pain predicted major clinical events in the subsequent 3 months[208] (see also Chap. 51). A nondiagnostic or normal ECG is associated with low risk. For example, the incidence of myocardial infarction has been reported to be 10, 8, and 41 percent in patients who, at admission, had a normal, a nonspecific, or an abnormal ECG, respectively.[209] The incidence of complications paralleled the infarction rate—a predictable conclusion corroborated by other studies.[210,211] *High risk has been associated with age, ST-segment elevation or depression, T-wave inversions, and Q waves as well as prolonged chest pain, especially if it radiates to cardiac referral areas.*[71,189,212–214]

Quantitative assessments of risk have been developed to guide the management of patients with chest pain in the emergency department.[211] *Predictors of an increased risk of complications included ECG evidence of ST-segment elevation or Q waves in two or more leads that are not known to have been present previously; ST-segment depression or T-wave inversions consistent with myocardial ischemia and not known to be present previously; pain worse than prior angina or the same as that experienced with prior myocardial infarction; systolic blood pressure of less than 100 mmHg; or rales bilaterally above the bases.* On the basis of these predictors, patients could be divided into four risk groups.[211] Furthermore, the risk could be updated if a complication occurred. This general approach can guide decisions concerning the level of intensity of the unit to which a patient is admitted and the length of observation required.

Blood levels of cardiac markers are prognostically important, as noted. In particular, increased levels of any of the markers—CK-MB or the subforms or troponins (I and T) but not myoglobin—at presentation appear to be strong predictors of risk in patients with acute ischemic syndromes[132,133] (see Chap. 51).

## INITIAL MANAGEMENT

As discussed, one frequently does not have a definitive diagnosis of AMI in the patient with chest pain in the emergency department, although this situation may ultimately be improved by the wider availability of the very rapid assays of blood cardiac markers, as discussed earlier. Nevertheless, the initial general treatment of the acute coronary syndromes is the same.

***Routine General Measures*** OXYGEN ADMINISTRATION The recommendations are as follows[2]:

Class I

1. Overt pulmonary congestion
2. Arterial oxygen desaturation ($Sa_{O_2}$ less than 90 percent)

Class IIa

1. Routine administration of oxygen to all patients with uncomplicated myocardial infarction during the first 2 to 3 h

Class IIb

1. Routine administration of supplemental oxygen to patients with uncomplicated myocardial infarction beyond 3 to 6 h

Hypoxemia is not uncommon in patients with AMI, even with an uncomplicated course, and presumably because of ventilation/perfusion mismatch.[215] Oxygen administration has been reported to decrease ST-segment elevation in anterior myocardial infarction.[216] Thus, oxygen administration for up to several days has previously been routine. There is concern with this practice, however, since oxygen may increase vascular resistance, and there may not necessarily be increased delivery to tissues. Because of these concerns and because of the expense of prolonged oxygen administration, there appears to be little justification for extending its use in uncomplicated myocardial infarction with an ($Sa_{O_2}$ of greater than 90 percent beyond 2 to 3 h.[1] Justification of its use in uncomplicated infarction can be based on its potential for limiting ischemic injury and on the fact that nitroglycerin can induce ventilation/perfusion abnormalities due to its pulmonary vasodilator activity, thus contributing to hypoxia.

Oxygen administration should be continued in patients with pulmonary congestion and desaturation. In patients with complicated myocardial infarction, nasal oxygen or oxygen by face mask may be insufficient to maintain saturation, and positive-pressure breathing or intubation and mechanical ventilation may have to be considered. If necessary, they should be initiated promptly.

ANALGESIA ACC/AHA recommendations are as follows[1]:

Class IIA

1. Morphine sulfate (4–8 mg IV with 2–8 mg repeated at 5–15 min intervals) is the analgesic of choice for the treatment of patients with STEMI.

The alleviation of pain and anxiety remains an essential element in the care of the patient with AMI. The pain and accompanying anxiety contribute to excessive activity of the autonomic nervous system and to restlessness. These factors, in turn, increase the metabolic demands of the myocardium. Physician reassurance from the beginning is an essential part of treatment and should be provided with compassion, patience, and confidence. Optimal care of the patient with AMI requires a team of experienced individuals who can help alleviate anxiety by their air of competence and caring.

It is a common clinical observation that reperfusion in AMI is associated with rapid relief of pain, suggesting that the pain is due to ongoing ischemia of the viable myocardium rather than to the effects of tissue necrosis. Thus, the approach to pain consists of the dual strategy of relieving ischemia and attacking the pain directly. Anti-ischemic therapy consists of reperfusion, beta blockers (if appropriate), nitrates, and oxygen administration, as discussed. Narcotics not only relieve pain directly but also indirectly by diminishing the sympathetic nervous system's drive and catecholamine secretion, which will increase blood pressure and drive cardiac chronotrophic and inotrophic responses to increase oxygen consumption and ischemia. The increased sympathetic drive will also enhance the propensity for serious ventricular arrhythmias. Morphine, in most instances, is the drug of choice, since it is well tolerated and offers analgesia without significant cardiac depression.[217] It also relieves anxiety and the feeling of doom commonly described. Morphine sulfate can be given at doses of 2 to 4 mg every 15 min until adequate relief has been obtained, which, in some patients, may require 25 to 30 mg.[218] The peak effect of intravenous morphine occurs within 15 to 20 min, thus requiring titration. Morphine has frequently been given in inadequate doses because of fear of respiratory depression or hypotension. Respiratory depression is less common in patients with myocardial infarction than it is in patients generally, because of the anxiety and respiratory drive from hypoxia, and can be treated with intravenous naloxone should it occur.[1] Hypotension related to morphine is usually orthostatic and volume-dependent and is less common in supine patients.[219] In patients with severe ongoing pain, it may be prudent to avoid concomitant administration of substantial doses of morphine and vasodilators, such as nitroglycerin. In patients with an acute inferior myocardial infarction with bradycardia with or without hypotension, the vagolytic narcotic meperidine may be substituted for the parasympathomimetic morphine. If the patient's anxiety is not controlled by the administration of narcotics, mild sedation with a benzodiazepine is appropriate. Diazepam in doses of 5 mg orally every 8 to 12 h or alprazolam in doses of 0.25 mg every 8 h are most often used.

NITROGLYCERIN ACC/AHA recommendations are as follows[1]:

Class I

1. Patients with ongoing ischemic discomfort should receive sublingual nitroglycerin (0.4 mg).
2. IV nitroglycerin is indicated for relief of ongoing ischemic discomfort, control of hypertension, or management of pulmonary congestion (*level of evidence C*).

Class III

1. Nitrates should not be administered to patients with systolic pressure less than 90 mm Hg or right ventricular infarction.
2. Nitrates should not be administered to patients who have received sildenafil within the last 24 h (*level of evidence B*).

Nitroglycerin has become very widely used in the treatment of AMI. It is an antiischemic agent not only by virtue of its actions to decrease preload and afterload, and thus to decrease oxygen demand, but also because of its vasodilator actions on epicardial coronary arteries and coronary collaterals. Consequently, and especially in patients with good collaterals, nitroglycerin is likely to increase flow into the ischemic regions.[220,221] Apart from relieving ischemia and pain, intravenous nitroglycerin, in early studies, appeared to reduce the likelihood of developing cardiac failure, infarct extension, or cardiac death. Both clinical data[222,223] and animal studies suggest that the early administration of nitroglycerin limits the extent of myocardial damage and favorably affects survival.[224] Long-term nitrates after reperfusion in animals favorably affect ventricular remodeling.[225]

Small, early trials before the widespread use of reperfusion suggested that the early administration of intravenous nitroglycerin was associated with improved morbidity and mortality. A metanalysis of these trials suggested that the use of nitrates reduced the odds of mortality after AMI by greater than 30 percent.[226] The efficacy of nitrates in improving short-term mortality after AMI was tested prospectively in the GISSI-3 trial.[227] At 6 weeks, there was no significant difference between the nitrate and control groups. The power to distinguish between the two, however, was diminished, because about half of the control group received nitrates during the first 2 days at the discretion of the attending physician. The angiotensin-converting enzyme (ACE) inhibitor lisinopril was tested in a similar fashion in GISSI-3. Mortality was decreased slightly at 6 weeks. The combined use of nitrates and lisinopril was associated with decreased mortality at both 6 weeks and 6 months compared with the no-nitrate group or with the group that received lisinopril alone. There was no significant difference noted at 35 days in comparison with the control group in another large trial, International Study of Infarct Survival (ISIS)-4, which evaluated the effects of nitrates on mortality after myocardial infarction.[228] This trial was also compromised by the high frequency of discretionary nitrate use in the control group. A metanalysis of all randomized, controlled trials involving the use of nitrates in AMI show a small, statistically significant reduction in mortality (about 5 percent).

The weight of the evidence does not justify the routine, long-term use of nitrates in uncomplicated AMI. The use of intravenous nitroglycerin early after acute infarction is justified because of its ease of titration, rapid onset, and ability to be quickly withdrawn in case of complications. Long-term use of nitrates is appropriate in the case of recurrent ischemia, large infarction, congestive heart failure, or hypertension.

COMPLICATIONS AND LIMITATIONS The most serious complication of nitroglycerin is hypotension. The fall in blood pressure may cause reflex tachycardia, and, together with decreased perfusion pressure, may cause or worsen angina. Thus, nitroglycerin should be avoided with a systolic pressure of less than 90 mmHg. Caution should be exercised in the case of inferior wall infarction because of the possibility of right ventricular involvement. Nitroglycerin should be used only with extreme caution if at all in right ventricular infarction, because the right ventricle in this circumstance becomes extremely dependent on preload, which can be diminished by the venodilating properties of the drug.[229] Similarly, nitroglycerin should be avoided in patients with severe bradycardia (heart rate less than 50 beats per minute), as hypotension may result.[230] If hypotension and bradycardia develop, nitroglycerin should be stopped, legs elevated, fluid administered, and atropine given if needed. Headache is a common side effect of nitrate administration.

Nitrate tolerance is common (see Chap. 90). With intravenous nitroglycerin, this may be recognized only as a diminution of clinical effect after 24 to 48 h. An increase in dose may be required.

DOSAGE OF NITROGLYCERIN Long-acting nitrates should generally not be used as initial therapy in AMI. Intravenous nitroglycerin is preferable, as noted, because of its rapidity of onset, ease of titration, and ease of removal in case of complications. Dose titration can be assessed by frequent determinations of blood pressure and heart rate. Invasive monitoring is not essential but is probably prudent if high doses are required or if there is hemodynamic instability or uncertainty about the adequacy of ventricular preload.

Treatment should be initiated with a bolus injection of 12.5 to 25 $\mu$g and should be followed by infusion by pump of 10 to 20 $\mu$g/min, with increases of 5 to 10 $\mu$g every 5 to 10 min while assessing hemodynamic and clinical responses.[1] Control of symptoms is a major endpoint; in the case of high left ventricular filling pressure, a decrease of 10 to 30 percent in pulmonary artery wedge pressure is the objective. Limitations of nitroglycerin dosing are a decrease in mean arterial pressure of 10 percent in normotensive patients or a decrease of 30 percent in hypertensive patients, but not below a systolic pressure of 90 mmHg or an increase in heart rate of 10 beats per minute, not to exceed 110 beats per minute.

Doses of nitroglycerin greater than 200 $\mu$g/min are associated with an increased risk of hypotension. The development of such high requirements may indicate tolerance, and alternative drugs such as ACE inhibitors or nitroprusside should be considered. If tolerance is the issue, responsiveness should return after a 12- to 18-h period off of nitroglycerin.

ASPIRIN ACC/AHA recommendations are as follows[1]:

Class I

1. Nonenteric aspirin should be chewed by patients who have not taken aspirin prior to presentation with STEMI (*level of evidence A*).
2. The dose should be 162 mg (*level of evidence A*) to 325 mg (*level of evidence C*).

Class IIa

1. Other antiplatelet agents such as clopidogrel (loading dose of 300 mg, maintenance dose 75 mg), which is preferred, or ticlopidine (250 mg bid) may be substituted if true aspirin allergy is present (*level of evidence C*).

Aspirin has become a standard part of the armamentarium for treating not only AMI but also atherosclerotic vascular disease generally. A 23 percent reduction in mortality at 35 days in patients treated with aspirin during the early stages of AMI was observed in the Second International Study of Infarct Survival (ISIS-2).[178] The reduction in mortality due to aspirin in combination with streptokinase was 42 percent. In a summary of a large number of clinical trials, aspirin has been shown to reduce the incidence of vascular events in patients with AMI at 1 month, a prior history of MI (2 years), a history of transient cerebral ischemia or stroke, and/or unstable angina.[231]

Aspirin irreversibly inhibits platelet cyclooxygenase, an enzyme that causes formation of thromboxane $A_2$, a mediator of platelet aggregation.[232] Its antithrombotic and side effects are discussed in detail in Chap. 54. Aspirin should be avoided in cases of true hypersensitivity. In the case of a history of bleeding from acid peptic disease, aspirin rectal suppositories can be used. Ticlopidine or clopidogrel, which are antiplatelet drugs acting as adenosine diphosphate receptor antagonists, can be used in acute infarction in patients in whom aspirin is contraindicated. Their actions do not develop immediately. They are discussed in Chap. 54. Clopidogrel is safer than ticlopidine and was shown to be more effective than aspirin in the CAPRIE (Clopidogrel versus Aspirin in Patients at Risk of Ischemic Events) trial.[233]

Aspirin is an effective antithrombotic at doses as low as 80 mg, but the rapid, acute effect probably requires 162 mg, which is absorbed and is thus clinically effective more quickly if the tablet is chewed rather than swallowed whole. *Thus the patient suspected of having a coronary ischemic syndrome should receive, early in the course, 162 to 325 mg of non-enteric-coated aspirin, which is chewed.*

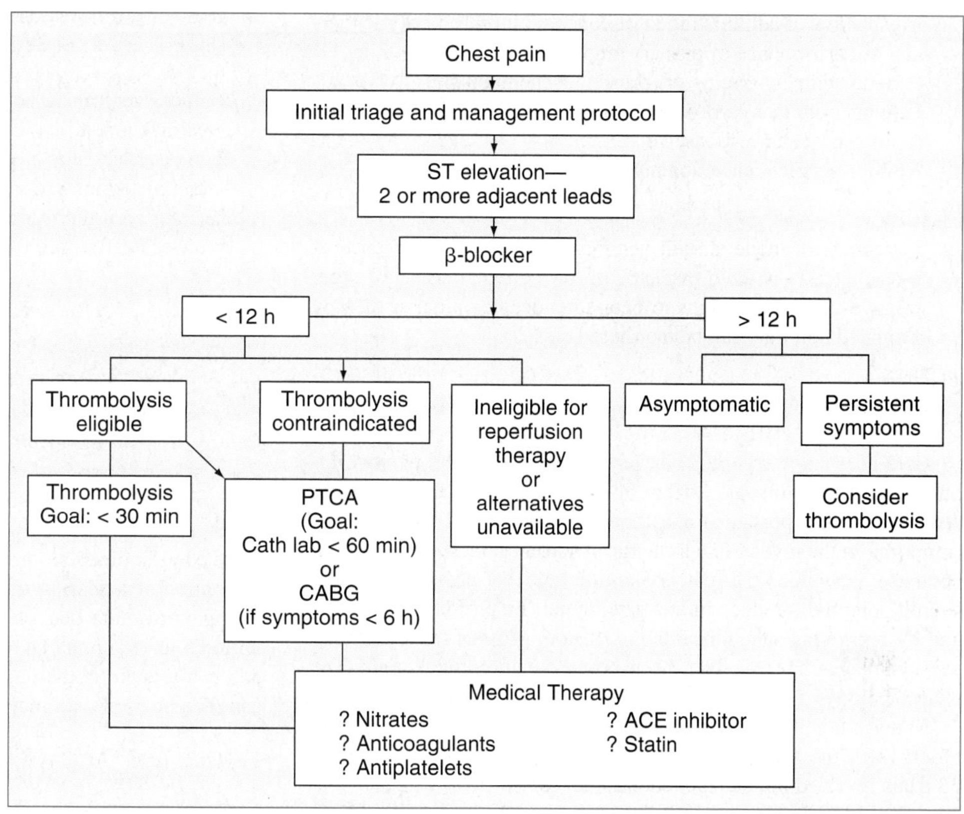


FIGURE 52-3 Evaluation of patients with ST-segment elevation. Algorithm for initial decision making in regard to reperfusion therapy in patients with suspected AMI and ST-segment elevation. Whether or not to administer thrombolytics or to perform primary PTCA is determined by the time from onset of symptoms. For patients in whom more than 12 h have elapsed since the onset of symptoms, reperfusion should be considered only if there are persistent or recurrent symptoms associated with ST-segment elevation. For patients with ST-segment elevation and duration of symptoms between 7 and 12 h, the decision to proceed with a reperfusion strategy requires careful clinical judgment in weighing the risk/benefit issues, as discussed in the text. (Modified from Ryan et al.[1] With permission.)

## Management after Triage into Electrocardiographic Subgroups

As discussed earlier, the initial ECG, as a first approximation, permits the assignment of patients with chest pain into subgroups that are distinguishable in terms of therapeutic responsiveness and risk. Thus, those with either ST-segment elevation and presumptively new bundle branch block or those with ST-segment depression and/or T-wave inversion are in high-risk groups, whereas those with either normal ECGs or nonspecific changes are in a low-risk category. Furthermore, the high-risk groups can be subdivided into those (ST-segment elevation or new bundle branch block) who have a favorable therapeutic response to thrombolytics and those who do not (ST-segment depression and/or T-wave inversion). *It must be kept in mind that these initial categorizations do not necessarily define ultimate outcome. Thus, patients with no ST-segment elevation at presentation may, in fact, have unstable angina and ultimately have no infarction or may progress to have either a Q-wave or a non-Q-wave infarction. Similarly, those presenting with ST-segment elevation may have a non-Q-wave infarction, although the majority of these will develop Q waves.* This potential for variable outcomes provides the underlying rationale for close monitoring and continuous reassessment of clinical course, risk, and therapeutic strategies during the period of observation and for monitoring both in the emergency department and subsequently in other hospital units.

## APPROACH TO THE PATIENT WITH ST-SEGMENT ELEVATION

The approach to the patient with chest pain and ST-segment elevation is guided heavily by the evidence that this subgroup has a high frequency of epicardial coronary artery occlusion by a thrombus that can be halted by prompt reperfusion.[234,235] Furthermore, multiple clinical trials of thrombolytic therapy have shown clinical benefit, but only in those with ST-segment elevation (Fig. 52-2).[177] This efficacy, moreover, has been shown in men, women, and diabetics and is manifest regardless of any history of previous myocardial infarction, existing heart rate, or recorded blood pressure (if less than 175 mmHg).[177] The greatest benefit is seen in patients with anterior myocardial infarction (and inferior infarction with right ventricular involvement), those with signs of a large infarction (systolic blood pressure less 100 mmHg or heart rate greater than 100 beats per minute), and in those with diabetes. Thus, the evaluation and management of the patient with ischemic chest pain and ST-segment elevation is focused on the rapid assessment of suitability for and delivery of reperfusion therapy. The approach to these patients is summarized in Fig. 52-3.[2]

During the initial evaluation, the patient will have had aspirin given, blood drawn, intravenous access established, a 12-lead ECG showing ST-segment elevation in at least two adjacent leads, nasal oxygen administered, appropriate analgesia, and continuous ECG monitoring initiated. The appropriate next steps are to administer a beta-adrenergic blocker, if not contraindicated and to initiate evaluation for reperfusion therapy. Based on the data from nine major clinical trials of thrombolytic therapy summarized by the Fibrinolytic Therapy Trialists Collaborative Group, thrombolytic therapy is efficacious in AMI (although linearly decreasing with the passage of time) for up to 12 h after the onset of symptoms.[177] There was a statistically uncertain benefit from 13 to 18 h. Thus, the 12-h point was chosen as defining the time frame in which the risk-benefit ratio is clearly favorable for administering thrombolytic therapy (Fig. 52-2).

***Beta-Adrenergic Receptor Blockers*** The recommendations are as follows[2]:

Class I

1. Patients without a contraindication to beta-adrenoceptor blocker therapy who can be treated within 12 h of onset of infarction,

irrespective of administration of concomitant thrombolytic therapy or performance of primary angioplasty

2. Patients with continuing or recurrent ischemic pain
3. Patients with tachyarrhythmias, such as atrial fibrillation with a rapid ventricular response
4. Non-ST-segment elevation myocardial infarction

Class IIa

1. Patients with moderate left ventricular failure (the presence of bibasilar rales without evidence of low cardiac output) or other relative contraindications to beta-adrenoceptor blocker therapy provided that they can be monitored closely

Class III

1. Patients with severe left ventricular failure

Beta-adrenergic receptor blockers interfere with the positive inotropic and chronotropic effects of catecholamines, thus reducing afterload (blood pressure) and therefore myocardial oxygen consumption. In the myocardial ischemic syndromes, these drugs should decrease ischemia and catecholamine-induced arrhythmias and should potentially reduce infarct size, in part by prolonging diastole and by improving subendocardial perfusion. Most of these theoretical advantages have, in fact, been borne out in clinical trials. The pharmacology of beta-adrenergic blockers is discussed in Chap. 90.

Many studies have demonstrated the clinical efficacy of beta blockers in the treatment of AMI. Analysis of pooled data from 28 trials revealed an average reduction of mortality of 28 percent at 1 week, and the majority of the benefit was seen in the first 48 h.[236] The Beta-Blocker Heart Attack Trial demonstrated that the benefits on mortality persisted and were about 20 percent after 2.5 years.[13] In the First International Study of Infarct Survival, patients were enrolled within the first 12 h from the onset of symptoms and atenolol, 5 to 10 mg, was immediately given intravenously and followed by oral atenolol, 100 mg daily.[13] Seven-day mortality was reduced by 14 percent. In the Metoprolol in Acute Myocardial Infarction (MIAMI) trial, metoprolol 15 mg was given intravenously in three divided doses early in the course and followed by 50 mg orally every 6 h for 48 h and then by 100 mg twice daily.[237] Mortality relative to placebo was reduced 12 percent at 15 days. In both of these trials, benefit was seen after 1 day and was sustained. Beta blockers have also enhanced therapeutic efficacy when given adjunctively with thrombolytic therapy. In the Thrombolysis in Myocardial Infarction phase II (TIMI-II) trial of conservative versus invasive strategies after treatment with recombinant tissue-type plasminogen activator (rt-PA), a subgroup was selected to receive either early intravenous followed by daily oral metoprolol or to begin oral metoprolol on day 6 after AMI.[238] The beta-blocker regimen was metoprolol 15 mg intravenously, followed by 50 mg orally twice daily for 1 day and 100 mg twice daily subsequently. The alternative protocol involved beginning the oral metoprolol regimen on day 6. The immediate intravenous metoprolol regimen was associated with a 45 percent reduction in nonfatal reinfarction and a 27 percent reduction in recurrent ischemic events in comparison with the group beginning beta-blocker therapy on day 6. *Thus, available data strongly support the use of beta blockers early in the course of acute STEMI in the absence of contraindications.* The data supporting the use of beta blockers in non-Q-wave myocardial infarction are less compelling, but these drugs are generally utilized (see Chap. 51). The effects of beta blockers in Q-wave MI are summarized in Table 52-6. While metoprolol and atenolol are the only beta blockers approved for use by the U.S. Food and Drug Administration (FDA) in the United States in AMI, it is generally thought that therapeutic efficacy is a class effect of beta blockers lacking intrinsic sympathomimetic activity.

TABLE 52-6 Effects of Beta Blockade in STEMI

| |
|---|
| Reduces ventricular ectopy, atrial fibrillation, and nonfatal cardiac arrest |
| Reduces frequency of progression of threatened infarction to completed infarction |
| Reduces recurrent ischemia and infarction during first 6 weeks after initial event |

*The relative contraindications to beta-blocker therapy are as follows*[2]*: (1) heart rate less than 60 beats per minute, (2) systolic blood pressure less than 100 mmHg, (3) moderate or severe left ventricular failure, (4) signs of peripheral hypoperfusion, (5) PR interval greater than 240 ms, (6) second- or third-degree AV block, (7) severe chronic pulmonary disease, (8) history of asthma, (9) severe peripheral vascular disease, and (10) insulin-dependent diabetes mellitus.* Since these contraindications are relative and not absolute, the clinician has the option of assessing the effects of beta blockade with the short-acting intravenous beta blocker esmolol, which has an onset of action within 5 to 10 min and a half-life of about 30 min. If the beta blockade is tolerated by the patient, long-acting oral beta-blocking drugs can then be used with increased confidence.

***Thrombolysis*** ACC/AHA recommendations are as follows[1]:

Class I

1. In the absence of absolute contraindications: fibrinolytic therapy should be administered to patients with symptoms of STEMI within the prior 12 h and ST-segment elevation greater than 0.1 mV in at least two contiguous precordial leads or at least two adjacent limb leads (*level of evidence A*).
2. In the absence of absolute contraindications: fibrinolytic therapy should be administered to patients with symptoms of STEMI within the prior 12 h and new or presumably new left bundle branch block (*level of evidence A*).

Class IIa

1. In the absence of absolute contraindications: fibrinolytic therapy should be administered to patients with symptoms of STEMI within the prior 12 h and 12-lead ECG findings consistent with a true posterior MI (*level of evidence C*).

Class III

1. Fibrinolytic therapy should not be administered to asymptomatic patients whose initial symptoms of STEMI began more than 24 h earlier (*level of evidence C*).
2. Fibrinolytic therapy should not be administered to patients whose 12-lead ECG shows only ST-segment depression except if a true posterior MI is suspected.

*Comment: In the absence of ST-segment elevation, there is no evidence for benefit in patients with normal ECG or nonspecific changes. Using current thrombolytic regimens, there is some suggestion of harm (including increased bleeding risk) for patients with ST-segment depression only.*[177] *When marked ST-segment depression is confined to leads $V_1$ through $V_4$, there is a likelihood that this reflects a posterior current of injury; it suggests a circumflex artery occlusion, for which thrombolytic therapy would be considered appropriate.*

INDICATIONS FOR THROMBOLYTIC THERAPY Reperfusion therapy should be given immediate consideration in all patients presenting with AMI. Patients with ST-segment elevation in two or more contiguous leads or a bundle branch block masking ST-segment changes occurring within 12 h of symptoms are candidates for thrombolytic therapy.[177,239] In the ISIS-2 trial,[240] patients with bundle branch block had a mortality of 28 percent when treated with a placebo versus 19.8 percent when treated with streptokinase and aspirin. A similar beneficial effect was noted in ISIS-3.[241] Patients of unknown age with bundle branch block and with the clinical features of AMI are candidates for thrombolytic therapy.[239] *Patients with ongoing symptoms suggestive of myocardial ischemia should be repeatedly evaluated by 12-lead ECGs as frequently as every 10 to 15 min in order to identify ST-segment elevation as soon as possible.* Conversely, ST-segment elevation in the absence of suggestive symptoms should raise such possibilities as early repolarization, pericarditis, and previous infarction with aneurysm formation. Elderly patients should not be excluded from thrombolytic therapy primarily because of their age or because of the increased risk of bleeding.

Large, placebo-controlled clinical trials have consistently demonstrated reduced mortality in patients receiving thrombolytic therapy within 6 h of the onset of an STEMI.[242] In comparison with conventional medical therapy, thrombolytic therapy reduces the 35-day mortality by 21 percent. It is estimated that 34 lives per 1000 patients treated are saved when thrombolysis is used within the first hour of symptom onset, compared to 16 lives saved per 1000 treated when thrombolytics are given 7 to 12 h after the onset of symptoms.[1] The true benefit of thrombolytic therapy between 6 and 12 h has been somewhat unresolved; however, the ACC/AHA guidelines[1] have indicated acceptance that there may be a definite benefit between 6 and 12 h and have, therefore, recommended that the time limit for therapy be up to 12 h from the onset of symptoms. The benefit of thrombolytics given between 6 and 12 h postinfarction is greater in patients classified with high-risk infarction, such as those with severe heart failure. In patients with anterior infarction, left bundle branch block, or severe hypotension, thrombolytic therapy should be given even if the precise time of onset of symptoms is unknown. Conversely, the young patient with inferior infarction having ST-T-segment elevation might not benefit greatly from thrombolytic therapy after 6 h from the onset of symptoms.

In contrast, patients with ST-segment depression, T-wave inversion, or no ECG changes have not been shown to benefit from thrombolytic therapy, as noted earlier[243] (see Chap. 51). A major problem in patients with nonspecific ST-segment depression or T-wave inversion is that less than 20 percent will have infarction. Patients with unstable angina receiving rt-PA experienced an increased incidence of reinfarction and death compared with conventional therapy, and the trial had to be discontinued.[244] However, the mean time of initiating thrombolytic therapy in patients with NQWMI was 9 h from the onset of symptoms, which was probably too late to have a significant beneficial effect. An appropriate trial in which NQWMI is diagnosed upon presentation to the emergency department within 20 to 30 min, as with MB-CK subforms or myoglobin, and is followed by thrombolytic therapy or PTCA is yet to be performed. This would be an important trial, since about 50 percent of infarctions in the United States are now NQWMI.[116]

Contraindications to Thrombolytic Therapy ACC/AHA recommendations are as follows[1]:

Class I

1. Neurologic absolute contraindications to fibrinolytic therapy include any history of intracranial hemorrhage (ICH), significant closed head trauma within the past three months, ischemic stroke within the past three months (*level of evidence A*).
2. It is preferable to treat STEMI patients at substantial (greater than or equal to four percent) ICH risk with percutaneous coronary intervention rather than with fibrinolytic therapy (*level of evidence A*).

Class IIa

1. Neurologic relative contraindications to fibrinolytic therapy include history of transient ischemic attack/ischemic stroke within the past three to six months and a history of dementia (*level of evidence A*).

The major contraindication to thrombolytic therapy is a cerebrovascular accident (CVA) within the preceding 3 months. A hemorrhagic CVA in the past is an absolute contraindication, whereas a nonhemorrhagic CVA in the more distant past with complete or nearly complete recovery is only a relative contraindication. Patients who have undergone recent (within 2 weeks) major surgery or vaginal delivery are not candidates for thrombolytic therapy; neither are those with active internal bleeding or bleeding from a peptic ulcer. Puncture of a noncompressible vessel within the previous 10 days makes thrombolytic therapy inadvisable. Other absolute contraindications to thrombolytic therapy include suspected aortic dissection, recent head trauma or known intracranial neoplasm, and pregnancy. Previous exposure to streptokinase or anistreplase (APSAC) requires the use of alteplase (rt-PA), tenecteplase (TNK-PA), or reteplase (r-PA) in subsequent attempts at thrombolysis. Systemic arterial hypertension and cardiopulmonary resuscitation should no longer be regarded as absolute contraindications to thrombolytic therapy. The ISIS-2 trial found that, among patients with a systolic blood pressure greater than 175 mmHg, the mortality rate was lower in those receiving streptokinase than it was in control subjects (5.7 vs. 8.7 percent). Some practitioners consider a recorded blood pressure greater than 200/120 mmHg to be an absolute contraindication. A history of severe chronic hypertension with diastolic blood pressure greater than 100 mmHg, with or without drug therapy, is a relative contraindication. Most clinicians either perform PTCA or proceed with thrombolytic therapy in a high-risk patient if elevated blood pressure normalizes promptly, with the easing of pain and anxiety through the use of narcotics and more direct therapy, including nitroglycerin and beta blockers. Califf et al. noted that patients who had brief (<10 min), nontraumatic cardiopulmonary resuscitation had no evidence of tamponade or hemothorax with thrombolytic therapy.[245] Prior administration of cardiopulmonary resuscitation should be considered a relative contraindication, since the risk of further bleeding in the chest may not outweigh the benefit. Other relative contraindications include trauma or surgery less than 2 weeks previously, active peptic ulcer disease, and bleeding diathesis or current use of anticoagulants. The absolute and relative contraindications for thrombolytic therapy are summarized in Table 52-7.

Choice of Thrombolytic Agent Several thrombolytic agents have been approved in the United States: streptokinase (SK), urokinase, APSAC, alteplase (rt-PA), tenecteplase (TNK-PA), and reteplase (r-PA). Each has been shown to limit infarct size, preserve ventricular function, and improve survival rates. These drugs and their pharmacologic properties are discussed in detail in Chap. 54.

In angiographic studies,[246,247] rt-PA, r-PA, and TNK-PA recanalized the coronary artery at 90 min in about 70 to 75 percent of patients, compared with 55 to 60 percent of those receiving SK, urokinase, or APSAC. Patency determined at 24 to 36 h is essentially the same for all agents. The time course for this "catch-up" phenomenon in vessel patency, as defined by the GUSTO angiographic substudy, occurs within the first 3 h after administration of the lytic

TABLE 52-7 Absolute and Relative Contraindications to Thrombolytic Therapy

| Absolute Contraindications | Relative Contraindications |
|---|---|
| Active internal bleeding | History of nonhemorrhagic cerebrovascular accident in distant past with complete recovery |
| Intracranial neoplasm or recent head trauma | Prolonged, traumatic CPR |
| Suspected aortic dissection | Recent trauma or surgery >2 weeks previously |
| Pregnancy | Active peptic ulcer disease |
| History of hemorrhagic cerebrovascular accident or recent nonhemorrhagic cerebrovascular accident | History of severe hypertension with diastolic blood pressure >100 |
| Recorded blood pressure >200/120 | Bleeding diathesis or concurrent use of anticoagulants |
| Trauma or surgery that is a potential bleeding source within previous 2 weeks | Previous treatment with SK or APSAC if being considered (does not apply to rt-PA) |
| Allergy to SK or APSAC if being considered | |

ABBREVIATIONS: CPR = cardiopulmonary resuscitation; SK = streptokinase; APSAC = anistreplase; rt-PA = recombinant tissue plasminogen activator.

agent.[15] Conversely, the GUSTO trial found a 30-day mortality rate of 6.3 percent for the accelerated rt-PA regimen, which was significantly less than the 7.2 percent mortality with SK and subcutaneous heparin and less than the 7.4 percent mortality with SK and intravenous heparin.[248] This absolute reduction of 1 percent reflects a 14 percent reduction in the risk of death, compared with that of SK or APSAC. A major reason why GUSTO I demonstrated an advantage for rt-PA and GISSI-2 as well as ISIS-3 did not was the adjunctive effect of heparin. The 1-year follow-up on the GUSTO-I patients[249] showed that the 1 percent lower mortality rate compared with SK was maintained, which provided further evidence that rt-PA is more effective than SK.

r-PA is a modified recombinant form of rt-PA with a longer half-life (15 min) and can be given as 2 boluses 30 min apart (see Chap. 54). In the International Joint Efficacy Comparison of Thrombolytics (INJECT) trial of 6000 patients, r-PA was compared with SK.[250] The mortality and the incidence of complications for r-PA were identical to those of SK. This was followed by the GUSTO-III trial,[251] which compared r-PA with rt-PA and showed that mortality and bleeding complications were similar. At 30 days, the mortality rate in the r-PA group was 7.43 percent; with rt-PA, it was 7.22 percent. The rate of hemorrhagic strokes was very similar: 0.91 percent for r-PA versus 0.88 percent for rt-PA. The overall stroke rate was 1.67 for r-PA versus 1.83 for rt-PA. The rate of bleeding events was virtually identical between the two treatments. The generally accepted conclusion is that the two drugs have similar efficacy and safety.

Tenecteplase (TNK-PA) is a variant of the original rt-PA molecule but with a longer half life, and it can be given as a single bolus injection. TNK-PA, in comparison to rt-PA, has a longer half-life[252] is more fibrin specific,[252] and has increased resistance to PAI-1.[253] In early trials, a dose of 40 mg of TNK-PA was determined to be as effective and safe rt-PA, but a weight-adjusted dose appeared appropriate. In ASSENT-2,[253] a large trial of 16,950 patients with STEMI, TNK-PA was compared to rt-PA. The dose of TNK-PA was weight-adjusted to 0.53 mg/kg and given in 5-mg increments with total doses ranging from 30 to 50 mg. Overall mortality was the same for TNK-PA and rt-PA (6.17 vs. 6.15), as was intracerebral hemorrhage (ICH) (0.93 vs. 0.95 percent) and total stroke was similar at 1.78 percent for TNK-PA versus 1.66 percent for rt-PA. However, there were two differences within subgroups. Patients treated more than 4 h from onset had higher patency rates with TNK-PA than with rt-PA, and this was confirmed in angiographic trials.[15] This is opposite to results with streptokinase, which is less effective if the time from onset is greater than 4 h. This is believed to be due to the increased fibrin-specificity, which provides continued activity despite increasing resistance of the clot with time. Another benefit of TNK-PA over rt-PA was found in the elderly (>75 years). The ICH rate was lower (1.7 vs. 2.6 percent) with TNK-PA over rt-PA in such patients. Total bleeding was also less with TNK-PA: 4.77 versus 5.9 percent.

The selection of a thrombolytic agent must be based on its adverse effects as well as upon its efficacy. The major risk with any thrombolytic agent is its propensity for causing bleeding, with the most devastating bleeding being a hemorrhagic stroke. The combined endpoint of death or nonfatal hemorrhagic stroke was, however, significantly reduced in the rt-PA group compared with the SK groups (6.6 vs. 7.5 percent; $p = 0.004$).[254] One reason to choose rt-PA, TNK-PA, or r-PA over SK is the 14 percent decreased risk of mortality. Nevertheless, the 10-fold greater cost of the tPA therapies must be considered. TNK-PA has a half-life of about 17 min and can be given as a single bolus. TNK-PA is preferred over accelerated rt-PA since it can be given as a single dose over a few minutes rather than as an intravenous infusion. This assures that the complete dose is given. Second, TNK-PA, as indicated previously, is more effective than rt-PA in patients presenting 4 h or more from onset and is associated with less bleeding, particularly in the elderly. One may choose TNK-PA over r-PA since the latter requires the injection of two boluses separated by 30 min. In the United States, the two preferred preparations are TNK-PA and r-PA. Streptokinase and rt-PA are being used less and less frequently.

DOSE AND ADMINISTRATION OF THROMBOLYTIC AGENTS Streptokinase is given in a dose of 1.5 million U intravenously over 30 to 60 min. Since antibodies develop and may persist for several years, a subsequent need for thrombolytic therapy, as for early or late reocclusion, would require the use of a rt-PA derivative. If the patient has had a streptococcal infection within 3 to 6 months, the use of an rt-PA derivative is preferable. Although APSAC is identical to SK as a thrombolytic agent, it can be given as a rapid infusion of 30 U over 5 to 10 min. Its therapeutic half-life is similar to that of SK, which is about 90 min. In contrast, the half-life of rt-PA is about 5 min. The FDA-approved dose of rt-PA is an initial bolus of 15 mg, followed by an infusion of 50 or 0.75 mg/kg body weight over the next 30 min and an infusion of 35 or 0.50 mg/kg over the subsequent 60 min for a total of up to 100 mg given over 90 min. Reteplase is given as an initial bolus of 15 megaunits (MU), followed by a second bolus of 15 MU in 30 min. TNK-PA is given 0.53 mg/kg in 5-mg increments for a full dose not exceeding 50 mg.

***Combination Therapy with GPIIb-IIIa Inhibitors*** ACC/AHA recommendations are as follows[1]:

Class IIb

1. Combination pharmacologic reperfusion with abciximab and half-dose reteplase or tenecteplase may be considered for pre-

vention of reinfarction (*level of evidence A*) and other complications of STEMI (without proven mortality benefit) in selected patients: anterior location of MI, age less than 75 and low risk for bleeding (*level of evidence B*).
2. Combination pharmacologic reperfusion with abciximab and half-dose reteplase or tenecteplase may be considered for prevention of reinfarction and other complications of STEMI in selected patients: anterior location of MI, age less than 75 and no risk factors for bleeding in whom an early referral for angiography and percutaneous coronary intervention (PCI) (i.e., facilitated PCI) is planned.

Class III
1. Combination pharmacologic reperfusion with abciximab and half-dose reteplase or tenecteplase may be harmful to patients greater than 75 years of age due to an increased risk of intracranial hemorrhage.

## OVERALL STRATEGY FOR REPERFUSION OF PATIENTS WITH ACUTE MYOCARDIAL INFARCTION

The criteria for initiating thrombolytic therapy are as follows (Table 52-8):

1. Patients presenting with chest pain suggestive of myocardial ischemia having ST-T-segment elevation greater than 1 mm in two contiguous limb leads or greater than 2 mm in two contiguous precordial leads or new left bundle branch block and who are within 6 h of the onset of symptoms should receive thrombolytic therapy if there are no contraindications. In patients presenting between 6 and 12 h of the onset of symptoms, one must weigh more heavily the risk versus the benefit. Patients presenting after 12 h are no longer routinely considered for thrombolytic therapy.
2. Contraindications for thrombolytic therapy are absolute or relative, as discussed earlier (Table 52-7).
3. In patients receiving rt-PA, r-PA, or TNK-PA it is recommended that heparin be given as a bolus at the initiation of infusion (60 U/kg) and then an additional maintenance dose of 12 U/kg/h (with a maximum of 4000 U bolus and a 1000 U/h infusion for patients weighing >70 kg), adjusted to maintain a partial thromboplastin time (PTT) at 1.5 to 2.0 times control (50 to 70 s) for 48 h. Continuation of heparin infusion beyond 48 h should be considered in patients at high risk for systemic or venous thromboembolism. In patients treated with nonselective thrombolytic agents (streptokinase, anistreplase, or urokinase), heparin should be given intravenously to those who are at high risk for systemic emboli (large or anterior myocardial infarction, atrial fibrillation, previous embolus, or known left ventricular thrombus). It is recommended that heparin be withheld for 6 h and that an activated partial thromboplastin time (aPTT) testing begin at that time. Heparin should be started when the aPTT returns to two times control (approximately 70 s) and then infused to keep the aPTT at 1.5 to 2.0 times control (initial infusion rate approximately 1000 U/h). After 48 h, a change to subcutaneous heparin or warfarin or aspirin alone should be considered.
4. Patients allergic to SK or APSAC who require thrombolytic therapy should receive an rt-PA derivative. Patients who received SK or APSAC and who again require thrombolytic therapy should also receive an rt-PA derivative.
5. Patients presenting with ST-T-segment depression and chest pain are not candidates for thrombolytic therapy. These patients must be triaged as to whether their pain is of cardiac or noncardiac origin. If the former, those with either unstable angina (see Chap. 51) or non-ST-elevated infarction should be treated with intravenous unfractionated heparin or low-molecular-weight heparin subcutaneously. In all patients not treated with thrombolytic therapy who do not have a contraindication to heparin, subcutaneous unfractionated heparin (e.g., 7500 U bid) or low-molecular-weight heparin (e.g., enoxoparin) 1 mg/kg bid should be used. In patients who are at high risk for systemic emboli, intravenous heparin is preferred.
6. As discussed further on and in detail in Chap. 56, PTCA as a primary procedure is an alternative to thrombolytic therapy and must be performed in a timely fashion by individuals skilled in the procedure and supported by experienced personnel in high-volume centers (class I). The individual must perform 75 such PTCA procedures per year and the center a minimum of 200 PTCAs per year. PTCA is indicated in patients with a contraindication to thrombolytic therapy, such as severe bleeding diathesis or cardiogenic shock (class IIa).
7. Elective angioplasty should be given to patients who develop ischemia or reinfarction or in whom thrombolytic therapy appears ineffective. In patients in whom angioplasty cannot be performed and who develop recurrent ischemia with possible infarction, the possibility of readministering a thrombolytic agent should be considered.

TABLE 52-8 Criteria for Initiating Thrombolytic Therapy

Chest pain consistent with angina
ECG changes
  ST ↑ ≥ 1 mm, ≥ 2 contiguous limb leads
  ST ↑ ≥ 2 mm, ≥ 2 contiguous precordial leads
  New left bundle branch block
Absence of contraindications

## PERCUTANEOUS TRANSLUMINAL CORONARY ANGIOPLASTY AS A PRIMARY THERAPY FOR ACUTE MYOCARDIAL INFARCTION

Percutaneous coronary intervention is a very effective method for reestablishing coronary perfusion and is suitable for at least 90 percent of patients with STEMI. Considerable data support the use of PCI for patients with acute STEMI. Reported rates of achieving TIMI III flow, the goal of reperfusion therapy, range from 70 to 90 percent.[273,274] Late follow-up angiography demonstrates that at least 87 percent of infarct arteries remain patent. Although most evaluations of PCI have been on patients who are eligible to receive fibrinolytic therapy, considerable experience supports the value of PCI for patients who may not be suitable for fibrinolytic therapy due to an increased risk of bleeding (see Chap. 56 for detailed discussion).

***Coronary Angiography*** ACC/AHA recommendations are as follows[1]:

Class I
1. Acute diagnostic coronary angiography should be performed:
   in candidates for primary or rescue PCI,
   in patients with cardiogenic shock who are candidates for revascularization,
   in candidates for CABG, and candidates for surgical repair of ventricular septal rupture and MR,
   in patients with persistent hemodynamic instability.

2. Diagnostic coronary angiography should be performed for:
recurrent ischemia/angina at rest or with low-level activities,
evidence of moderate or severe ischemia at a low level of noninvasive stress testing,
sustained ventricular tachycardia.

Class IIa
1. It is reasonable to perform coronary angiography in STEMI patients with diabetes.
2. It is reasonable to perform coronary angiography in STEMI patients with a left ventricular ejection fraction less than 40 percent or CHF.
3. It is reasonable to perform coronary angiography in STEMI patients with prior coronary revascularization.
4. It is reasonable to perform coronary angiography when STEMI is suspected to have occurred by a mechanism other than thrombotic occlusion at an atherosclerotic plaque. This would include coronary embolism, arthritis, certain metabolic or hematological diseases, or coronary artery spasm.

Class IIb
1. It is debatable whether to perform routine coronary angiography as part of an invasive strategy after STEMI.

Class III
1. Coronary angiography should not be performed in patients with extensive co-morbidities (e.g., liver or pulmonary failure, cancer), in whom the risks of revascularization are likely to outweigh the benefits.

Acute cardiac catheterization has been proposed as an anatomic risk stratification strategy. A subset of patients will have severe three vessel or left main artery disease, or anatomic features unfavorable for PCI, and would be candidates for urgent or emergency CABG. Another subset of patients will have spontaneously reperfused and have minimal evidence for atherosclerotic disease. They can be treated medically, avoiding the risks of fibrinolytic therapy or PCI. Additionally, identifying high-risk patients may facilitate additional strategies that will improve outcome, whereas low-risk patients may be eligible for early hospital discharge.

***Primary Percutaneous Coronary Intervention*** ACC/AHA recommendations are as follows[1]:

Class I
1. If immediately available, primary PCI should be performed in patients with STEMI or MI with new or presumably new LBBB who could undergo PCI of the infarcted artery within 12 h of onset of symptoms (or more than 12 h if ischemic symptoms persist), if performed in a timely fashion (balloon inflation within 90 min of admission) by persons skilled in the procedure (individuals who perform more than 75 PCI procedures per year). The procedure should be supported by experienced personnel in an appropriate laboratory environment (a center that performs more than 200 PCI procedures per year, of which at least 36 are primary PCI for STEMI, and has cardiac surgery capability).
2. Primary PCI should be performed with the goal of a door-to-balloon time as short as possible and with a target of less than 90 min (*level of evidence B*).
3. Fibrinolytic therapy is generally preferred if symptom duration is less than or equal to 3 h and the expected door-to-balloon time minus the expected door-to-needle time is greater than one h (*level of evidence B*).
4. Primary PCI is generally preferred if symptom duration is less than or equal to 3 h and the expected door-to-balloon time minus the expected door-to-needle time is less than 1 h.
5. If the symptom duration is greater than 3 h, primary PCI is generally preferred with the goal of a door-to-balloon time as short as possible and with a target of less than 90 min.
6. Primary PCI is recommended for patients less than 75 years of age with ST-elevation or LBBB or posterior MI who develop shock within 36 h of MI and are suitable for revascularization that can be performed within 18 h of shock unless further support is futile based on patient's wishes or contraindications/unsuitability for further invasive care (*level of evidence A*).
7. Primary PCI should be performed in patients with severe congestive heart failure and/or pulmonary edema.

Class III
1. Primary PCI should not be performed in patients eligible for fibrinolysis by an operator who performs fewer than 75 PCI procedures per year in a laboratory without surgical capability.
2. Primary PCI should not be performed in a noninfarct-related artery at the time primary PCI of infarct-related artery.
3. Primary PCI should not be performed in asymptomatic patients more than 12 h after onset of STEMI, who are hemodynamically and electrically stable.

*Comment: There is serious concern that a routine policy of primary PTCA for patients with AMI will result in unacceptable delays in achieving reperfusion in a substantial number of cases and less than optimal outcomes if performed by less experienced operators. Strict performance criteria must be mandated for primary angioplasty programs so that such delay in revascularization and performance by low-volume operators and centers do not occur. Interventional cardiologists and centers must operate within a specified "corridor of outcomes" to include (1) balloon dilatation within 90 (±30) min of admission and diagnosis of AMI; (2) a documented clinical success rate with TIMI-2 through 3 flow attained in >90 percent of patients without emergency coronary artery bypass graft, stroke, or death; (3) emergency coronary artery bypass graft rate <5 percent among all patients undergoing the procedure; (4) actual performance of angioplasty in a high percentage of patients (85 percent) brought to the laboratory; and (5) mortality rate <10 percent. Otherwise, the focus of treatment should be the early use of thrombolytic therapy.*

## Angioplasty as Primary or Adjunctive Therapy to Thrombolysis

Detailed discussions of PTCA and its indications appear in Chap. 55. Comprehensive discussions of PTCA in the treatment of AMI are presented in Chap. 56. Direct angioplasty has been compared with thrombolytic therapy in a metanalysis of 10 randomized trials involving 2606 patients.[255] In 1290 patients treated with primary PTCA, the mortality rate at 30 days was 4.4 percent, compared to 6.5 percent in 1316 patients treated with thrombolytic therapy. Pooled rates of nonfatal reinfarction or death were also lower in the PTCA as opposed to the thrombolysis groups. The incidence of stroke was also lower with PTCA than it was with thrombolysis. These authors concluded that "primary PTCA appears to be superior to thrombolytic therapy for treatment of patients with AMI, with the proviso that success rates for PTCA are as good as those achieved in these trials. Data evaluating longer-term outcome, operator expertise, and time delays before treatment are needed before primary PTCA can be recommended universally as the preferred treatment."[255] Registry data (Second National Registry of Myocardial Infarction) of 4939 patients with acute AMI (ST-segment elevation) who received primary PTCA and 24,705 who received alteplase showed similar in-hospital mortality (5.2 and 5.4 percent, respectively) in the absence of shock.[256] These results also add some caution against the general adoption of primary PTCA over thrombolysis in the treatment of ST-segment-elevation myocardial infarction.

In the case of cardiogenic shock in AMI (ST-segment elevation/new left bundle branch block), primary angioplasty, if rapidly available, offers benefit over thrombolysis as part of a strategy of emergency revascularization.[257] In the Should We Emergently Revascularize Occluded Coronaries for Cardiogenic Shock (SHOCK) Trial, a strategy of emergency revascularization was compared with initial medical stabilization and delayed revascularization based on clinical indicators. The 30-day mortality showed a favorable but not significant ($p = 0.11$) trend for emergency revascularization over initial medical restabilization in the case of mortality at 30 days (46.7 vs. 56.0 percent, respectively). The mortality at 6 months, however, was significantly lower ($p = 0.027$) for the emergently revascularized group (53.5 percent) compared to the initially medically stabilized group (65.7 percent). Patients <75 years old had a more favorable outcome with emergency revascularization than did older patients (>75), with a 15.4 percent reduction in 30-day mortality (56.8 vs. 41.4 percent, $p < 0.01$). Patients in the emergency revascularization group who were >75 years old fared worse than similar patients did in the medical stabilization group. PTCA was the revascularization procedure in 60 percent and coronary artery bypass grafting was used in 40 percent of patients, with similar outcomes.

Thus, there is increasing evidence of the efficacy of PTCA as an alternative to thrombolysis in the treatment of ST-segment elevation/new left bundle branch block myocardial infarction. It is the method of choice in cardiogenic shock and in the presence of contraindications for thrombolytic therapy. There is increasing consensus that, in high-volume centers with skilled, experienced operators, PTCA is the procedure of choice if it can be performed in a timely manner (generally within the first 2 h). Indeed, a report showed a 53 percent reduction in 30-day mortality in patients having PTCA within the first 2 h of pain in comparison to those more than 2 h into their pain.[1,258] Because of the logistic issues involved (including transfer from a community hospital to an interventional center) in obtaining PTCA within an appropriate time frame, the approach of combining a low-dose thrombolytic (to obtain early patency) with PTCA outside of the 2-h time is being explored.[1] These and other issues including the use of stents are discussed in detail in Chap. 55.

*Several caveats must be considered before embracing PTCA as the therapy of choice for AMI generally. Only about 20 percent of hospitals in the United States have cardiac catheterization laboratories and relatively few can perform PTCA on an emergency basis. In many cases the time delay involved in transferring a patient to a hospital capable of performing emergency PTCA may outweigh any benefit.*[1] *The excellent results for emergency PTCA described earlier were achieved by highly experienced and enthusiastic investigators in hospitals that have devoted extraordinary support and personnel to achieving opening of the coronary artery within 60 to 90 min of the patient's arrival.*[1,259,260] Available data suggesting that emergency PTCA may be comparable to thrombolysis in many community settings were alluded to previously.

## HEPARIN AS CONJUNCTIVE OR ADJUNCTIVE THERAPY

Class I

1. Patients undergoing percutaneous surgical revascularization should receive unfractionated heparin.
2. Unfractionated heparin should be given intravenously to patients undergoing reperfusion therapy with alteplase, reteplase, or tenecteplase with dosing as follows: 60 U/kg (maximum 4000 U) as a bolus, 12 U/kg per hour (maximum 1000 U) adjusted to maintain aPTT at 1.5 to 2.0 times control.
3. Unfractionated heparin should be given intravenously to patients treated with nonselective fibrinolytic agents (streptokinase, anistreplase, urokinase) who are at high risk for systemic emboli (large or anterior MI, AF, previous embolus or known LV thrombus).
4. Platelets should be monitored daily in patients on heparin.

It is recommended that heparin not be started immediately but that an aPTT be obtained at 4 h and that heparin be started when the aPTT returns to less than twice control (about 70 s).

The necessity of heparin for maintaining coronary patency induced by rt-PA was established in the Heparin-Aspirin Reinfarction Trial (HART) trial.[246] Coronary angiographic studies performed at 18 to 81 h showed a patency of 82 percent in the group receiving heparin and 52 percent in the group receiving aspirin. The findings of HART were confirmed by Bleich et al.,[261] who showed that rt-PA given with heparin had a patency of >90 percent; without heparin, the patency rate was 44 percent. Heparin appears to act by preventing early reocclusion, at least after rt-PA.[262] A subcutaneous heparin dose of 12,500 U twice a day used in the megatrials failed to provide therapeutic anticoagulation for at least 24 h in various cohort analytic studies.[263,264] The administration of SK without adjunctive heparin has not been properly tested. At present, heparin is recommended in a bolus of 5000 U intravenously followed by an infusion of 1000 to 1200 U/h to keep the PTT at 1.5 to 2.0 times normal. It is recommended that the PTT not be measured until 4 h after heparin therapy is initiated because otherwise it will not yet have reached a steady state. If the PTT has increased more than twofold over normal, the same dose of heparin should be continued; if PTT exhibits less than a twofold increase, the infusion rate of heparin should be increased. Initiation of heparin is recommended either during or following completion of thrombolytic therapy, as discussed earlier, and it should be maintained in uncomplicated cases for 24 to 48 h.

Low-molecular-weight heparins are cleavage products of heparin with a mean molecular weight of ≈5000 that have higher anti-Xa activity and less antithrombin activity. Low-molecular-weight heparin preparations are widely used in non-ST-segment elevation acute coronary syndromes (unstable angina, non-Q-wave myocardial infarction), as discussed in Chap. 51. Low-molecular-weight heparins are being evaluated as adjunctive therapy for thrombolysis.[2] Their use has a class IIa recommendation in all patients with ST-segment elevation AMI who have not been treated with thrombolytics and who do not have a contraindication to heparin.[2] High-risk patients for systemic embolization should be treated with heparin, as noted.

## EVOLUTION OF CONCEPTS CONCERNING ACUTE INTERVENTION IN STEMI

Routine immediate or delayed angioplasty was not traditionally recommended as a standard mode of therapy following thrombolysis. The TIMI-IIA and TIMI-IIB trials,[265] the TAMI study,[266] The European Cooperative Study Group trial,[267] and the SWIFT trial[268] all showed no reduction in the incidence of coronary reocclusion or hospital mortality rates and no evidence of improved ventricular function with routine immediate or delayed angioplasty compared with elective angioplasty in the case of manifest ischemia following thrombolytic therapy. The TIMI-II trial found that angioplasty either performed routinely at 18 to 48 h when anatomically appropriate or in response to induced or spontaneous ischemia did not improve survival or reduce the reinfarction rate at either 6 weeks or 1 year[269]; neither did it reduce the need for surgery (Fig. 52-4). The most

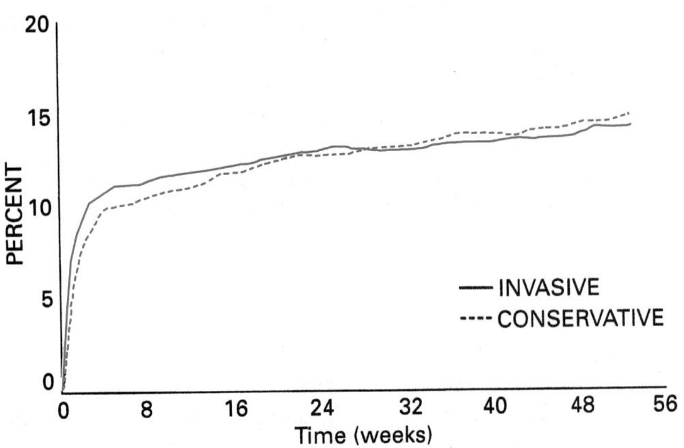


FIGURE 52-4 Kaplan-Meier curves for death and infarction in patients assigned to the invasive or conservative strategies in TIMI-2. Routine cardiac catheterization after thrombolytic therapy and revascularization with PTCA or bypass grafting (when anatomically appropriate) was not a superior strategy to catheterization and revascularization when there is development of spontaneous ischemia or ischemia induced by exercise testing. (Reproduced with permission from Williams DO, Braunwald E, Knatterud G, et al. One-year results of the thrombolysis in myocardial infarction investigation (TIMI) phase II trial. *Circulation* 1992;85:533–542.[269] Copyright 1992 American Heart Association.)

widely accepted recommendation traditionally has been to perform cardiac catheterization for possible angioplasty or bypass surgery in patients who develop angina or manifest evidence of myocardial ischemia during submaximal exercise testing or who develop hemodynamic or ischemic instability. Views about this issue are evolving rapidly. In general, a consensus is developing that favors early intervention for STEMI when it can be delivered expeditiously and experted as discussed subsequently and in detail in Chap. 56.

Rescue angioplasty to open occluded arteries after presumptive failed thrombolysis has been advocated and, in fact, studies indicate that TIMI grade 3 flow can be achieved in a high percentage of these patients.[270] In the reported TIMI-IV trial, however, it was found that although a strategy of rescue angioplasty could restore flow that is superior to that from thrombolysis alone, the incidence of adverse events for the strategy as a whole was the same as for not undertaking PTCA (35 percent adverse event rate whether or not PTCA was performed for an occluded artery). Both rates tended to be higher than the incidence in patients with patent arteries (23 percent, $p = 0.07$).[271] A major concern is that the patency status of the infarct-related artery is often uncertain and requires acute angiography to define the issue. Complete resolution of ST-segment elevation predicts patency of the infarct-related artery with good specificity (>70 percent) but this occurs in less than a majority of patients.[272] Rescue angioplasty previously has not been recommended as a routine strategy for failed or presumptively failed thrombolysis. Acute angiography and rescue angioplasty should be considered in patients with large and especially anterior myocardial infarctions who are thought to have failed thrombolysis, as reflected by persistent chest pain and ST elevation or hemodynamic compromise lasting more than 90 min after treatment (see Chap. 56). The potential impact of coronary stenting and especially the evolving strategy of facilitated coronary intervention in which a lower-than-usual dose of a thrombolytic agent is administered prior to a planned intracoronary procedure in AMI are discussed in Chap. 56. As alluded to above, the efficacy of primary PCI in acute STEMI is leading to recommendations for expanding use of early coronary arteriography if it can be associated with PCI as defined.[273,274]

Patients with cardiogenic shock have a very high mortality (>70 percent) with or without thrombolysis. As noted previously, the results of the reported SHOCK Trial now provide data to suggest that emergency revascularization results in a 41.4 percent survival rate at 30 days.[275] All of these patients received intraaortic balloon assist whether they received revascularization urgently or whether they had initial medical stabilization. These data suggest that other means of metabolically manipulating the myocardial cell may be required for further advances in the management of this lethal complication of AMI.

## PRIMARY PCI AND FIBRINOLYTIC INELIGIBLE PATIENTS

ACC/AHA recommendations are as follows[1]:

Class I

1. Primary PCI should be performed in fibrinolytic ineligible patients who present with STEMI within 12 h of symptoms onset or arrival of ongoing or recurrent symptoms after 12 h.

   Randomized clinical trials evaluating the outcome of PCI for patients who present with ST-segment elevation but who are ineligible for fibrinolytic therapy have not been performed. Few data are available to characterize the value of primary PCI for this subset of acute STEMI patients. Nevertheless, these patients are at increased risk for mortality and there is a general consensus that PCI is an appropriate means for achieving reperfusion in those who cannot receive fibrinolytics because of increased risk of hemorrhage. Other reasons also exclude acute STEMI patients from fibrinolytic therapy and criteria for undertaking PCI in these patients may differ from those eligible for fibrinolytic therapy.

## RESCUE PERCUTANEOUS CORONARY INTERVENTION

Class I

1. Rescue PCI should be performed in patients with cardiogenic shock.

Class IIa

2. Rescue PCI is reasonable to perform in patients with anterior STEMI with continuing or recurrent myocardial ischemia after fibrinolytic therapy.
3. Rescue PCI is reasonable to perform in patients with nonanterior STEMI with continuing or recurrent ischemia associated with hemodynamic or electrical instability.

Class IIb

1. It is debatable whether to perform rescue PCI in patients with nonanterior STEMI with continuing or recurrent ischemia not associated with hemodynamic or electrical instability. It is debatable whether to perform elective PCI in occluded arteries after unsuccessful fibrinolysis.

Great improvements in equipment, operator experience, and adjunctive pharmacotherapy have increased PCI success rates and decreased complications. More recently, the invasive strategy for NSTEMI patients has been given a Class I recommendation by the ACC/AHA Guidelines Committee.[276] STEMI patients are increasingly being treated similarly as an extension of this approach. One study supports the policy of performing catheterization and subsequent revascularization for patients who do have spontaneous or inducible angina after STEMI. The Danish Acute Myocardial Infarction (DANAMI) Trial[277] randomly assigned 1008 survivors of a first acute MI treated with fibrinolytic therapy within 12 h of onset of symptoms to catheterization and subsequent revascularization or standard medical therapy if they showed evidence of spontaneous or inducible angina. Those who underwent revascularization had less unstable angina and fewer nonfatal MIs during a 21/2 year period of follow-up compared with those patients randomly assigned to medical treatment only (18 percent and 5.6 percent versus 30 percent and 10.5 percent, respectively).

## EMERGENCY OR URGENT CORONARY ARTERY BYPASS SURGERY

ACC/AHA recommendations are as follows:[1]

Class I

1. Failed angioplasty with persistent pain or hemodynamic instability in patients with coronary anatomy suitable for surgery (*level of evidence B*).
2. Persistent or recurrent ischemia refractory to medical therapy in patients who have coronary anatomy suitable for surgery, have a significant area of myocardium at risk, and who are not candidates for PCI (*level of evidence B*).
3. At the time of surgical repair of postinfarction ventricular septal rupture (VSR) or mitral valve insufficiency (*level of evidence B*).
4. Cardiogenic shock in patients less than 75 years of age with ST-segment elevation or LBBB or posterior MI who develop shock within 36 h of MI and are suitable for revascularization that can be performed within 18 h of shock unless further support is futile based on patient's wishes or contraindications/unsuitability for further invasive care (*level of evidence A*).
5. Life-threatening ventricular arrhythmias in the presence of greater than or equal to 50 percent left main stenosis and/or triple vessel disease (*level of evidence B*).

Class IIa

1. Emergency CABG can be performed as primary reperfusion in the early hours (6–12 h) of an evolving STEMI (*level of evidence B*).

Class III

1. Emergency CABG should not be performed in patients with persistent angina and a small area of risk who are hemodynamically stable (*level of evidence C*).
2. Emergency CABG should not be performed in patients with successful epicardial reperfusion with unsuccessful microvascular reperfusion (*level of evidence C*).

## ARRHYTHMIAS EARLY IN THE COURSE OF ACUTE MYOCARDIAL INFARCTION

***Bradycardia*** Bradyarrhythmias are relatively common (30 to 40 percent) early in the course of AMI, especially in inferior infarction or after reperfusion of the right coronary artery, because of the activation of vagal afferents that ultimately result in enhanced parasympathetic tone.[2] Atropine, because of its anticholinergic effects, can be very useful in this situation, since it enhances the discharge rate of the sinus node and facilitates AV conduction[278] as well as reversing the peripheral effects of excessive cholinergic activity, such as vasodilation with associated hypotension. Parasympathomimetic effects with bradycardia, hypotension, and nausea and vomiting are also produced by morphine and can be reversed by atropine. Atropine should be used sparingly and appropriately in AMI, however, because of the protective effect of vagal stimulation against VF.[279]

THE USE OF ATROPINE The recommendations are as follows[2]:

Class I

1. Sinus bradycardia with evidence of low cardiac output and hypoperfusion peripherally or frequent ventricular premature complexes at the onset of symptoms of AMI
2. Acute inferior infarction with type I second- or third-degree AV block associated with symptoms of hypotension, ischemic discomfort, or ventricular arrhythmias
3. Sustained bradycardia and hypotension after administration of nitroglycerin
4. Morphine-induced nausea and vomiting
5. Ventricular asystole

Class IIa

1. In patients with inferior infarction and type I second- or third-degree block at the AV-nodal level (narrow QRS complex or known preexisting bundle branch block) who are symptomatic from the low output and/or vagal predominance

Class IIb

1. Vagal symptoms and sinus bradycardia associated with the administration of morphine
2. Patients with inferior infarction who are asymptomatic with type I second-degree heart block or third-degree block at the AV node
3. Second- or third-degree AV block of uncertain mechanism and unavailability of pacing

Class III

1. Asymptomatic sinus bradycardia and a rate of greater than 40 beats per minute with no signs of hypoperfusion or frequent ventricular premature contractions
2. Type II and third-degree AV block and third-degree AV block with new, wide QRS complex (i.e., block below the AV junction)

***Sinus Bradycardia, Atrioventricular Block, or Ventricular Asystole*** Atropine is indicated for the treatment of type I second-degree AV block, especially with complicating inferior myocardial infarction, and is useful at times in third-degree AV block at the AV node in restoring AV conduction or for increasing the junctional response rate.[2] By increasing the sinus node rate or improving AV conduction, atropine may improve signs or symptoms of congestive heart failure, hypotension, or frequent, complex ventricular arrhythmias associated with AV block or sinus bradycardia; thus, pacemaker insertion may be avoided.[1] Treatment of sinus bradycardia or first- or second-degree AV block is generally not indicated in the absence of hemodynamic compromise,[1] and atropine should seldom be used in the treatment of type II AV block (location of block below the AV node). Symptomatic bradycardia that is unresponsive to atropine should be treated with pacing.

Atropine should be administered intravenously at a dosage of 0.5 to 1.0 mg and repeated as necessary to achieve an adequate heart rate every 3 to 5 min, up to a total maximum dose of 2.5 mg, which provides complete vagal blockade.[1] Atropine may also be efficacious in ventricular asystole and should be given intravenously at a dosage of 1.0 mg every 3 to 5 min during cardiopulmonary resuscitation up to a maximum of 2.5 mg if asystole persists.[280]

At doses of 0.5 mg or less, atropine may produce, paradoxically, bradycardia and suppression of AV nodal conduction due to a central or peripheral parasympathomimetic effect.[281] Atropine dosage should be titrated carefully, because tachycardia can be induced and ischemia can be worsened. Thus, atropine should be given in 0.5-mg increments, as noted, to achieve an adequate heart rate of 50 to 60 beats per minute.

***Heart Block*** Heart block develops in about 10 percent of patients with AMI and is associated with an increased mortality during hospitalization, but it does not predict long-term mortality in those who survive to be discharged.[281,282] Intraventricular conduction delay or bundle branch block is also associated with increased in-hospital mortality.[177] The increase in mortality associated with heart block reflects the extent of myocardial damage, not heart block per se. Thus, heart block in the setting of anterior myocardial infarction reflects extensive infarction and concomitant destruction of the conduction system and is associated with relatively high mortality. In contrast, heart block with inferior myocardial infarction may primarily reflect ischemia of the AV node rather than extensive tissue damage and is associated with a more favorable prognosis. Because of the overwhelming effect of the extent of myocardial damage on prognosis, pacing has not been shown to lessen mortality associated with AV block or bundle branch block.[283] It is likely, however, that pacing will benefit subgroups of these patients with severe slowing of ventricular rates but without extensive myocardial damage[283,284] by preventing hypotension, ischemia, and ventricular escape arrhythmias associated with the appearance of a heart block. In AMI, the risk of developing heart block is augmented by the presence of any evidence of conduction system abnormality including first-degree AV block, Mobitz type I or II AV block, left anterior or posterior hemiblock, or a left or right bundle branch block.[1]

TEMPORARY PACING EARLY IN THE COURSE OF ACUTE MYOCARDIAL INFARCTION The "Guidelines for the Management of Patients with Acute Myocardial Infarction"[2] placed increased emphasis on transcutaneous pacing in view of the availability of new systems that provide standby status for pacing in AMI patients who do not require immediate pacing and are at intermediate risk for developing heart block. These systems use a single pair of multifunctional electrodes, permitting ECG monitoring, transcutaneous pacing, and defibrillation.[285] Transcutaneous pacing does not entail the risk and complications of transvenous pacing and, because invasive procedures may thus be avoided or delayed, is well suited for use in the patient who has undergone thrombolysis. Percutaneous pacing is painful; if prolonged pacing is required, the patient should be switched to transvenous systems.

PLACEMENT* OF TRANSCUTANEOUS PATCHES AND ACTIVE (DEMAND)† TRANSCUTANEOUS PACING The recommendations are as follows[2,286]:

Class I
1. Sinus bradycardia (rate less than 50 beats per minute) with symptoms of hypotension (systolic blood pressure less than 80 mmHg) unresponsive to drug therapy†
2. Mobitz type II second-degree AV block†
3. Third-degree heart block†
4. Bilateral bundle branch block (alternating left and right bundle branch block (RBBB) or RBBB with alternating left anterior and posterior fascicular block—irrespective of time of onset)*
5. Newly acquired or age-indeterminant left bundle branch block, right bundle branch block, and anterior or posterior fascicular block*
6. Right bundle branch block or LBBB and first-degree AV block*

Class IIa
1. Stable bradycardia (systolic blood pressure greater than 90 mmHg, no hemodynamic compromise, or compromise responsive to initial drug therapy)*
2. Newly acquired or age-indeterminant right bundle branch block*

Class IIb
1. Newly acquired or age-indeterminant first-degree AV block*

Class III
1. Uncomplicated AMI without evidence of conduction system disease

*Put pacing system in place.
†Activate system.

As noted, transcutaneous pacing is intended to be temporary; if prolonged pacing is required, transvenous pacing should be instituted (discussed further on). In addition, patients with a high probability of requiring pacing should have it instituted early on.[2] Technical aspects of transcutaneous pacing have been reviewed.[287]

***Ventricular Ectopy, Tachycardia, and Fibrillation*** SUMMARY RECOMMENDATIONS FOR ATRIOVENTRICULAR AND INTRAVENTRICULAR CONDUCTION DISTURBANCES The new recommendations for treatment of atrioventricular and intraventricular conduction disturbances during acute STEMI have been summarized in the following Table 52-9 from the latest revision of ACC/AHA Guidelines for the Management of Patients with ST-Segment Elevation Myocardial Infarction

VENTRICULAR FIBRILLATION The use of lidocaine to treat VF refractory to electrical shock or pulseless VT followed by unsynchronized electric shock has not been demonstrated to be beneficial in this setting and has been labeled "Class Indeterminant" by the Guidelines 2000 For Cardiopulmonary Resuscitation and Emergency Cardiovascular Care.[287a]

ACC/AHA recommendations are as follows[1]:

Class I
1. VF or pulseless VT should be treated with unsynchronized electric shock with an initial energy of 200 J; if unsuccessful, a second shock of 200–300 J should be given, and, if necessary, a third shock of 360 J (*level of evidence B*).
2. Recurrent intractable ventricular arrhythmia with hemodynamic instability must be treated immediately (*level of evidence C*).

Class IIa
1. VF or pulseless VT that is refractory to electrical shock should be treated with amiodarone 300 mg IV bolus, followed by a repeat unsynchronized electric shock (*level of evidence B*).
2. Electrolyte and acid-based disturbances should be corrected (K greater than 4.0 and Mg greater than 2.0) to prevent recurrent episodes of VF when an initial episode of VF has been treated.

Class IIb
1. Procainamide bolus and infusion to treat VT or shock refractory VF has limited value due to the length of time required for administration.

Class III
1. Prophylactic administration of antiarrhythmic therapy is not recommended when using fibrinolytic agents.

Ventricular rhythm abnormalities are common during the early phases of AMI, with an incidence of VF within the first 4 h, so-called primary VF, of 3 to 5 percent, which declines rapidly thereafter.[288] Primary VF is thought to be the result of microreentry mechanisms in the infarct zone.[1] Postulated triggering mechanisms include hypokalemia, hypomagnesemia, enhanced adrenergic tone, acidosis, increased intracellular calcium, increased free fatty acids, and reperfusion-induced production of free radicals.[289,290] Although the relative contribution of each of these factors to early ventricular tachycardia/fibrillation (VT/VF) and the effects of their specific treatment are not known, epidemiologic evidence suggests that there has been a decrease in the incidence of primary VF,[291] which may be related generally to more aggressive treatment strategies, including the use of beta blockers. Primary VF is associated with increased in-hospital mortality but not with increased long-term mortality for patients who survive and are discharged.[292]

TABLE 52-9 Recommendations for Treatment of Atrioventricular and Intraventricular Conduction Disturbances during Acute STEMI

| | Atrioventricular Conduction | | | | | | | |
|---|---|---|---|---|---|---|---|---|
| Intraventricular Conduction | Normal | | First degree AV block | | Mobitz I second degree AV block | | Mobitz II second degree AV block | |
| | | | STEMI | | STEMI | | STEMI | |
| Normal | Action | Class | Action | Class | Action | Class | Action | Class |
| | Observe | I | Observe | I | Observe | IIa | Observe | III |
| | A | III | A | III | A* | III | A | III |
| | TC | IIb | TC | IIb | TC | I | TC | I |
| | TV | III | TV | III | TV | III | TV | IIa |
| Left anterior fascicular block | Observe | I | Observe | IIb | Observe | IIb | Observe | III |
| | A | III | A | III | A* | III | A | III |
| | TC | IIb | TC | IIa | TC | I | TC | I |
| | TV | III | TV | III | TV | III | TV | IIa |
| Left posterior fascicular block | Observe | I | Observe | IIb | Observe | IIb | Observe | III |
| | A | III | A | III | A* | IIb | A | III |
| | TC | IIb | TC | I | TC | I | TC | IIa |
| | TV | III | TV | IIa | TV | III | TV | IIa |
| Old right bundle branch block | Observe | I | Observe | III | Observe | III | Observe | III |
| | A | III | A | III | A* | III | A | III |
| | TC | IIa | TC | I | TC | I | TC | I |
| | TV | III | TV | IIb | TV | IIb | TV | I |
| Old left bundle branch block | Observe | I | Observe | III | Observe | III | Observe | III |
| | A | III | A | III | A* | III | A | III |
| | TC | IIa | TC | I | TC | I | TC | I |
| | TV | III | TV | IIb | TV | IIb | TV | IIa |
| New bundle branch block | Observe | III | Observe | III | Observe | III | Observe | III |
| | A | III | A | III | A* | III | A | III |
| | TC | I | TC | I | TC | I | TC | I |
| | TV | IIb | TV | IIa | TV | IIa | TV | I |
| Fascicular block + right bundle branch block | Observe | III | Observe | III | Observe | III | Observe | III |
| | A | III | A | III | A* | III | A | III |
| | TC | I | TC | I | TC | I | TC | I |
| | TV | IIb | TV | IIa | TV | IIa | TV | I |
| Alternating left and right bundle branch block | Observe | III | Observe | III | Observe | III | Observe | III |
| | A | III | A | III | A* | III | A | III |
| | TC | I | TC | I | TC | I | TC | I |
| | TV | I | TV | I | TV | I | TV | I |

SOURCE: Antman et al.[1] With permission.

Post-AMI VT occurs in about 15 percent of patients and is also most commonly manifest during the relatively early period.[288] Ventricular tachycardia is classified according to its ECG morphology (monomorphic or polymorphic) and by its duration and consequences: sustained (lasting more than 30 s and/or causing hemodynamic compromise earlier, which requires intervention) and nonsustained (not resulting in hemodynamic compromise and lasting less than 30 s).[1] Short runs (5 beats or less) of nonsustained VT are common in the early postmyocardial infarction period and do not require specific treatment.

Because primary VF is one of the major contributors to mortality in the first 24 to 48 h after AMI, a great deal of attention has been paid to attempting to define characteristics of ventricular premature beats that predict VT/VF in order to provide prophylaxis. The hierarchical classification of ventricular arrhythmias according to propensity to cause VT/VF—for example, early coupled R-on-T premature beats as opposed to late-cycle, coupled beats—has fallen out of favor because of the realization that the late-cycle premature beats were equally likely to induce VT/VF.[293]

Accelerated idioventricular rhythm normally occurs frequently during the first hours of AMI[1] and after thrombolysis as a reperfusion arrhythmia. In neither case is it a premonitory rhythm for VT/VF.[294–296] *Accelerated idioventricular rhythm should ordinarily be observed and not treated specifically.*[1] It has been suggested, however, that if accelerated idioventricular rhythm speeds up to a rate of about 120 beats per minute, it should be considered an automatic rhythm for which suppression with lidocaine should be considered.[293]

Formerly, it was common practice, in order to prevent VT/VF, to treat prophylactically with lidocaine either all patients with AMI or, selectively, those with patterns of premature ventricular contractions thought to predict VT/VF. This approach is no longer common practice, because metanalysis of trials of lidocaine prophylaxis, although confirming a substantial reduction in primary VF, showed evidence of increased mortality, probably because of episodes of profound bradycardia and asystole.[297] Thus, *routine use of prophylactic lidocaine in AMI in the presence or absence of thrombolysis is not recommended.*

Two prophylactic approaches to the prevention of VT/VF, however, are recommended.[1] Routine administration of beta blockers, as described previously, has been shown to reduce the incidence of VT/VF. Also, since evidence suggests that hypokalemia is a risk factor for VT/VF,[290] it is recommended that serum potassium levels be kept above 4.0 meq/L by supplementation as necessary. Although the supporting evidence is less compelling, it is also considered to be good clinical practice to maintain serum magnesium levels above 2.0 meq/L in AMI patients.[1]

TREATMENT OF VENTRICULAR TACHYCARDIA/FIBRILLATION Electrical cardioversion of VT that is hemodynamically compromising should be performed immediately.[288] Rapid polymorphic VT should be considered the equivalent of VF and cardioverted with an unsynchronized shock of 200 J; monomorphic VT at a rate of greater than 150 beats per minute can be treated initially with a synchronized discharge of 100 J.[2,286] Urgent cardioversion for VT with rates of under 150 beats per minute is usually not needed. Ventricular tachycardia that is tolerated hemodynamically can be approached initially with trials of lidocaine, procainamide, or amiodarone, as outlined earlier, with attention being paid to need for dose modifications based on age and renal and hepatic function.

VF should initially be treated with an unsynchronized shock of 200 J, then incrementally with 200 to 300 J, and finally with 360 J as needed.[286] There are no definitive data concerning appropriate adjunctive therapy for fibrillation that is difficult to cardiovert.[1] The Advanced Cardiac Life Support (ACLS) protocol recommends the following hierarchical approach, as needed, to adjunctive therapy of resistant VF:[298,299] (1) epinephrine (1 mg IV, repeat every 3 to 5 min, or, alternatively, 40 U of vasopressin IV, single dose, one time only (level IIb); (2) amiodarone (150 mg IV bolus) (IIb for persistent or recurrent ventricular fibrillation/pulseless ventricular tachycardia); or (3) lidocaine (1.5 mg/kg IV)(recommendation level: indeterminate). In the case of resistant or recurrent VT/VF, electrolyte imbalances should be sought and corrected and ongoing ischemia suspected. Beta-adrenergic blockers should be used in recurrent VT or primary VF to decrease both sympathetic input to the heart and ischemia.[1] Intravenous amiodarone should be used in these life-threatening ventricular tachyarrhythmias.[300] *If ongoing ischemia is involved, intraaortic balloon pumping or emergency revascularization should be considered.*

## PROTOCOLS, CLINICAL PATHWAYS, AND CHEST PAIN EVALUATION UNITS

There are increasing pressures, driven by both economic and clinical imperatives, to improve the management of patients with chest pain. The goal of controlling costs has contributed to the need to triage patients with chest pain accurately to levels of care that are appropriate to need and to facilitate evaluation and treatment in the shortest time that is commensurate with good medical care. For example, low-risk patients with normal ECGs frequently do not have to be admitted to the hospital, much less to the intensive care unit (ICU), and can have a total time in the health care facility of hours rather than of days. The medical necessity of achieving rapid, accurate diagnoses has been discussed earlier. These two driving forces have led to the development of predictive algorithms to guide triage decisions.[71,192] For example, one analysis provided evidence that patients with chest pain with ECG changes of ischemia or infarction were, depending on age, the only subgroup with a probability of AMI high enough (21 percent or moderate) to justify admission to the CCU as opposed to an intermediate care unit of reduced intensity.[301] While these algorithms have been shown to be effective in, for instance, reducing ICU admissions without compromising clinical care,[192,212] they have not been widely adopted for a variety of reasons, including the fact that most experienced clinicians are comfortable with their decision making in triaging patients with chest pain.[184]

The continuing need to improve the process of chest pain management has led to the development of clinical pathways, protocols, and practice guidelines that differ from predictive instruments in that they provide structure to the decision-making process rather than driving decision making.[184,302] A chest pain evaluation unit, which may either be a defined area, frequently near the emergency department, or a virtual entity embracing a team approach to chest pain evaluation and management, is frequently central to the strategy to systematize the approach.

In general, the approach is to triage the patient to evaluation and management pathways according to risk based on ECG findings, history, and symptoms. For example, and at the opposite ends of the clinical spectrum, the patient with ST-segment elevation would receive thrombolytic therapy within 30 min of arrival and be rapidly admitted to the CCU, whereas the low-risk patient with a normal ECG would be evaluated in a unit of low intensity and acuity and would be discharged within a matter of hours. There is a great deal of interest in the use of imaging modalities such as nuclear scanning with sestamibi or stress echocardiography to guide decision making in cases of intermediate or low probability for AMI during the initial evaluation period.[184] While the results using the systematized approach of a chest pain evaluation unit appear promising, further assessment is needed in large-scale trials to test both clinical value and cost-effectiveness before a specific strategy can be recommended. The general strategy of systematizing the approach to the patient with chest pain, however, is strongly encouraged.

## MANAGEMENT AFTER HOSPITAL ADMISSION

### General Approach

The recommendations are as follows[2]:

Class I

1. Selection of ECG monitoring leads based on infarct location and rhythm to maximize diagnostic utility
2. Bed rest with bedside commode privileges for initial 12 h in hemodynamically stable patients who are free of ischemic-type chest discomfort
3. Avoidance of the Valsalva maneuver and straining
4. Optimization of pain relief

Class IIb

1. Routine use of anxiolytics

Class III

1. Prolonged bed rest (more than 12 to 24 h) in stable patients without complications

The general issues involved in the management of the patient with suspected or manifest AMI in the intensive or moderate care unit are to provide for adequate monitoring for the detection of arrhythmia, ischemia, and hemodynamic instability; to provide the patient with a calm, supportive, and reassuring environment; to control the level of activity; to begin the education process for a lifetime of living with coronary heart disease; to control pain and inappropriate anxiety; and to treat adverse events promptly. It is assumed, as previously discussed, that oxygen therapy, beta-adrenergic blockers, aspirin, thrombolytics, unfractionated heparin, low-molecular-weight heparin, and nitroglycerin have been begun or given as appropriate in the emergency department. Also, it is assumed that a decision has been made about the appropriateness of adding glycoprotein IIb/IIIa inhibitors.

## Patient Care Environment

### CORONARY CARE UNIT (CCU)

ACC/AHA recommendations for CCU environment are as follows[1]:

Class I

1. STEMI patients should be admitted to an environment that provides for continuing monitoring of ECG and pulse oximetry and has ready access to facilities for hemodynamic monitoring and defibrillation.
2. The patient's medications orders should be reviewed to confirm the administration of aspirin, and beta blockers in an adequate dosage to control heart rate and to assess the need for intravenous nitroglycerin for control of angina, hypertension, or heart failure (*level of evidence A*).
3. The ongoing need for supplemental oxygen should be assessed by monitoring arterial oxygen saturation. Supplemental oxygen should be discontinued after the first 2 to 3 h in patients who consistently maintain an arterial oxygen saturation greater than or equal to 90 percent of room air.
4. Nursing care should be provided by individuals certified in critical care with the appropriate nurse:patient ratio (minimum 1:2) to address evolving patient acuity.
5. Care of STEMI patients in the CCU should be structured around protocols derived from practice guidelines.

Class III

1. It is not an effective use of the CCU environment to admit terminally ill "do not resuscitate" patients with STEMI unless their clinical and comfort needs require a critical care environment.

### STEP-DOWN UNIT

Class I

1. It is an effective use of clinical resources to admit low-risk STEMI patients who have undergone successful PCI directly to the step-down unit.
2. STEMI patients originally admitted to the CCU who demonstrate 12 to 24 h of clinical stability (absence of recurrent ischemia, heart failure, or hemodynamically compromising dysrhythmias) should be transferred to the step-down unit.

Class IIa

1. Patients recovering from STEMI who have clinically symptomatic heart failure can be cared for in the step-down unit provided facilities for continuous monitoring of pulse oximetry and appropriately skilled nurses are available.
2. Patients recovering from STEMI who have dysrhythmias that are hemodynamically well tolerated (e.g., atrial fibrillation with a controlled ventricular response; paroxysms of nonsustained ventricular tachycardia (lasting <30 s) can be cared for in the step-down unit provided facilities for continuous monitoring of the ECG, defibrillators, and appropriately skilled nurses are available.

Class IIb

1. Patients recovering from STEMI who have clinically significant pulmonary disease requiring high flow supplemental oxygen or noninvasive mask and ventilatory bilevel positive airway pressure (BIPAP)/continuous positive airway pressure (CPAP) can be considered for care in a step-down unit provided facilities for continuous monitoring of pulse oximetry and appropriately skilled nurses with a sufficient nurse:patient ratio are available.

Class III

1. It is not an effective use of the step-down unit to admit terminally ill STEMI patients for whom "do not resuscitate" orders are written unless their clinical and comfort needs require the level of nursing care in a step-down unit.

***Monitoring*** The patient must have continuous ECG monitoring and frequent hemodynamic evaluation by the assessment of blood pressure and heart rate. ECG monitoring leads should be selected to maximize the ability of the CCU staff to detect and diagnose arrhythmias and recurrent ischemic ST-segment changes. Thus, the lead selected should ideally permit identification of the P wave as well as providing a QRS complex of adequate size. Furthermore, the lead should be selected to interrogate the area of known infarction or ischemia.[2] Blood pressure and pulse rate should be monitored with a frequency to be determined by the perceived level of acuity, but generally every half hour until stable and then every 4 h. Pulse oximetry has become standard. Precise orders should be given to notify the physician of, for example, systolic pressures >150 and <90 mmHg, heart rates >110 or <60 beats per minute, respiratory rate of >22 or <8 per minute, or significant decreases in blood oxygen saturation.[2]

***Activity*** Minimizing physical exertion is an important approach, in addition to minimizing sympathetic nervous system drive by administering beta-adrenergic blockers and by controlling pain and excessive anxiety, so as to decrease myocardial oxygen demand and thus decrease myocardial ischemia and necrosis. *Prolonged bed rest and a severe limitation of activities such as self-feeding are no longer recommended except in the case of continuing ischemic pain and/or hemodynamic instability because of evidence that cardiovascular deconditioning and unfavorable shifts in intravascular volume develop very rapidly in immmobilized patients in the supine position.*[303] Losses of plasma volume occur that decrease preload and stimulate compensatory reflexes, enhancing sympathetic activity. These fluid shifts may be the major cause of cardiovascular dysfunction with prolonged bed rest.[304] It is prudent to prescribe about 12 h of bed rest and a bedside commode for the patient with uncomplicated AMI.[1]

Subsequently, low-level activities such as routine self-care, assisted bathing, and brief ambulation should be permitted to prevent deconditioning.

The major coronary precaution that should be strictly adhered to is the avoidance of the Valsalva maneuver, which increases cardiac wall stress because of increases in systolic blood pressure and heart rate.[2] These changes in wall stress may cause localized repolarization abnormalities in the infarct zone that may precipitate ventricular arrhythmias.[305,306] Constipation should be avoided and stool softeners routinely prescribed. A bedside commode is preferable to a bedpan in all but the most unstable patients.

***Analgesics and Anxiolytics*** The importance of controlling chest pain and excessive anxiety and the use of morphine and diazepam were discussed previously (see "Evaluation and Management of the Patient with Chest Pain in the Emergency Department"). Morphine is sometimes used in inadequate doses because of fear of side effects, and anxiolytics may be overused. Ischemic chest pain, heart rate, blood pressure, and perceived anxiety level have not been found to be different in patients treated with diazepam or with a placebo.[307] Conversely, strong psychological support in hospitals has prolonged effects to prevent anxiety and depression after AMI.[308] Anxiolytics may be useful in treating symptoms of nicotine withdrawal in smokers during hospitalization. Psychosis manifesting as delirium and agitation is not uncommon, particularly in the elderly, during prolonged stays in the ICU ("ICU psychosis"). Intravenous haloperidol can be useful and safe in this setting. Drug-induced psychosis or delirium caused by lidocaine, for example, should be considered.

***Education*** Education of the AMI patient by both the CCU staff and the physician are essential components of medical management and should be begun early during hospitalization. Presenting the patient with information about the management of symptoms and prevention of a recurrence gives a sense of empowerment associated with changes in behavior[309] and decreased anxiety.[310] Information should be presented in a direct fashion at a relatively simple level and should emphasize issues relevant to patient behavior, such as control of chest pain, diet, smoking, and exercise, rather than the pathophysiology of the disease. Family members, in particular the spouse, should participate in the education process. Because of the substantial risk of cardiac arrest in the 18 months after AMI, family members should be taught cardiopulmonary resuscitation.[311,312] Ideally, educational materials can be presented in a permanent printed form so that the self-education process can continue after discharge and can supplement that given by health care professionals during cardiac rehabilitation and physician visits.

## Adjunctive Therapy during the Early In-Hospital Period

### ANGIOTENSIN-CONVERTING ENZYME INHIBITORS

ACC/AHA recommendations are as follows[1]:

Class I

1. ACE inhibitors should be administered orally within the first 24 h of STEMI to all patients in the absence of hypotension (systolic blood pressure less than 100 mmHg or more than 30 mmHg below baseline systolic pressure) or known contraindications to the use of ACE inhibitors (*level of evidence A*).
2. ACE inhibitors should be administered orally long-term during and after convalescence from STEMI in patients who have left ventricular ejection fraction less than 40 percent or clinical heart failure arising from systolic pump dysfunction (*level of evidence A*).

Class IIa

1. Asymptomatic STEMI patients with diabetes or age 55 or older, with a history of vascular disease, or another cardiovascular risk factor should stay on ACE inhibitor therapy long term (*level of evidence A*).

Class IIb

1. It is debatable whether to administer ACE inhibitors long term to patients who have recently recovered from STEMI but have normal or mildly abnormal global LV function and no other high-risk vascular features and who are younger than 55 years of age (*level of evidence B*).

Class III

1. Intravenous ACE inhibitors should not be given to patients within the first 24 h of STEMI because of the risk of hypotension, unless these drugs are needed to manage hypertension (*level of evidence B*).

A number of clinical trials have shown that ACE inhibitors reduce left ventricular dysfunction and dilatation and slow the progression to congestive heart failure in patients with left ventricular dysfunction after AMI.[313–315]

The ACE inhibitors have also been shown, with few exceptions, to reduce mortality after AMI. Metanalysis of 4 major and 11 minor trials involving, collectively, more than 100,000 patients showed an odds reduction in the ACE-inhibitor group of 6.5 percent ($2p = 0.006$).[316] Originally, there was some doubt about the timing of initiation of the ACE inhibitor after AMI because of the results of the Cooperative New Scandinavian Enalapril Survival Study (CONSENSUS) II.[317] In this randomized study, patients were assigned to intravenous placebo or enalapril during the first day of AMI and were subsequently given an oral placebo or enalapril. The trial was stopped in its early stages by the Safety Monitoring Committee because it was unlikely to show a positive effect and because of hypotension in elderly patients. The issue of timing of the initiation of ACE inhibitor therapy has subsequently been clarified. In GISSI-3, patients with either ST-segment elevation or depression were given oral lisinopril or assigned to an open control group starting on the first day of AMI.[227] There was a significant reduction in mortality at 6 weeks (odds ratio 0.88), and the majority (60 percent) of lives saved were in the first 5 days. In ISIS-4, patients were assigned to an oral placebo or to captopril within the first 24 h, and a 7 percent mortality reduction was seen at 5 weeks in the captopril group.[228] The majority of the decrease in deaths was seen in the first 2 days. There was no increase in adverse events in the elderly in ISIS-4 or in GISSI-3. Thus, the hypotension in CONSENSUS II may be attributed to the use of intravenous enalapril.

Initiation of ACE-inhibitor therapy within the first few days after AMI in patients with left ventricular dysfunction and continuation of therapy over the long term was associated with a decrease in mortality and in fatal and severe nonfatal cardiovascular events in three other trials: Survival and Ventricular Enlargement (SAVE), captopril[314]; Acute Infarction Ramipril Efficacy (AIRE2), ramipril[318]; and Trandolapril Cardiac Evaluation (TRACE), trandolapril.[319]

Thus, trials of ACE inhibitors have shown clear evidence of benefit in AMI from their use early in the course of AMI. Efficacy may be greatest in those at highest risk—that is, patients with prior MI, anterior MI, tachycardia, or congestive heart failure (CHF). Therapy should begin within the first 24 h after hemodynamic stabilization whether or not thrombolytic therapy has been administered. Intravenous forms should be avoided, and therapy should be started with low doses. The ACE inhibitors should not be given if systolic blood pressure is below 100 mmHg or if there are contraindications—that is, bilateral renal artery stenosis, renal failure, history of severe cough, or angioedema with previous treatment.[1] In the presence of significant left ventricular dysfunction, therapy should probably be continued indefinitely. Evidence from the Heart Outcomes Prevention Evaluation (HOPE) trial using the ACE inhibitor ramipril has shown significant decreases in cardiovascular events in high-risk individuals, including but not limited to those with prior AMI.[320] These data, which will be discussed in more detail subsequently, provide support for the strategy of using ACE inhibitors in most patients indefinitely after AMI.

**MAGNESIUM**

ACC/AHA recommendations are as follows[1]:

Class IIa

1. Documented magnesium deficits should be corrected, especially in patients receiving diuretics before onset of STEMI.
2. Episodes of torsades de pointes-type VT associated with a prolonged QT interval should be treated with 1–2 g of magnesium administered as an IV bolus over 5 min.

Class III

1. In the absence of documented electrolyte deficits or torsades de pointes-type VT, there is no indication for the routine administration of intravenous magnesium to STEMI patients at any level of risk.

There has been conflicting evidence concerning the clinical efficacy of magnesium administration in ST-segment-elevation AMI. Several studies in the 1980s indicated a salutary effect on mortality.[321,322] Furthermore, the Leicester Intravenous Magnesium Intervention Trial (LIMIT-2) reported that treatment with magnesium was associated with significant reductions in overall mortality and in the incidence of CHF in the CCU.[323] On the other hand, the results of the large ISIS-4 trial, which was published in 1995, showed no benefit and even raised the possibility of some harm.[228] The uncertainty resulting from conflicting data led to the performance of the Magnesium in Coronaries (MAGIC) trial.[324] MAGIC was a large (6213 patients), randomized, double-blind trial of the effects of intravenous magnesium sulfate in the setting of acute ST-segment-elevation myocardial infarction. The primary endpoint was 30-day all-cause mortality. The patients were at high risk, with a median age of 70, and were stratified at randomization into categories of age greater than 65 years and eligible for reperfusion therapy and of any age who were not eligible for reperfusion therapy. No benefit or harm of magnesium was seen in any of multiple prespecified or exploratory subgroups. Overall, the available evidence suggests that the routine use of intravenous magnesium in ST-segment-elevation AMI has no place in current practice. Magnesium should continue to be used, of course, in the setting of known or suspected hypomagnesemic states and especially when these are associated with severe ventricular arrhythmias or QT prolongation, as recommended above.

## Management of the Low-Risk Patient

As discussed previously, there are increasing pressures to minimize resource utilization while not compromising safety in the patient with ischemic-type chest discomfort. As a practical matter, this means matching patient acuity and risk appropriately with the hospital facilities required to deal with their situation and appropriately controlling the time spent in these units. For example, the patient who is at low risk for AMI may be evaluated in the emergency department or in a chest pain evaluation unit, and if AMI or unstable angina are excluded, he or she may be discharged within a matter of hours without having been formally admitted to the hospital. The patient with AMI who has an uncomplicated initial course and is at low risk for the development of complications is a candidate for transfer out of the CCU within 24 to 36 h.[325–328] *Such a low-risk patient does not have a history of prior AMI and has not had recurrent ischemic pain, hypotension, CHF, persistent sinus tachycardia, heart block, or sustained VT. This patient may be a candidate for early discharge at 3 to 4 days.*

Patients who have been treated with thrombolytics are frequently candidates for early discharge from the CCU.[329–332] In this setting, the *absence* of early sustained VT or VF as well as the absence of early sustained hypotension or shock and the *presence* of a left ventricular ejection fraction (LVEF) > 40 percent and of only one- or two-vessel coronary artery disease are independent predictors of freedom from late complications.[331]

Approaches to risk stratification and noninvasive testing to guide management decisions in the post-AMI patient are discussed further on (see "Noninvasive Risk Stratification in Patients Surviving Acute Myocardial Infarction"). Excessive diagnostic testing in all post-AMI patients, especially those at low risk, should be discouraged. The variability in practice in this regard, without demonstrable correlative changes in outcomes, suggests the need for more rigorous adherence to guidelines and protocols.[2]

As discussed previously, AMI can be diagnosed rapidly using serum cardiac markers. If AMI is effectively ruled out and the patient is at low risk (i.e., normal ECG and absence of the characteristics noted earlier, especially the absence of prolonged initial pain or the recurrence of pain), noninvasive testing can establish the safety of early discharge (3 to 12 h) from the emergency department, chest pain evaluation unit, or CCU and further evaluation as an outpatient.[184] In general, such patients do not necessarily need to be admitted to the CCU unless noninvasive testing is positive for ischemic heart disease. Patients with ischemic-type chest discomfort and intermediate probabilities of AMI—that is, duration of chest pain >20 to 30 min and nondiagnostic ECG changes (without significant ST-segment elevation or depression, T-wave inversion, or bundle branch block) without known coronary artery disease—should be admitted to an observation unit or to the CCU if an intermediate unit is unavailable. They should be placed on a fast track to rule in AMI or unstable angina, as previously outlined. If the clinical course is unrevealing and early imaging negative, stress testing and further evaluation can be planned. Clinical decisions can usually be made within 12 h in this setting.[184]

## Management of the High-Risk Patient with STEMI

The STEMI patient at low risk is defined in the previous section by the absence of certain characteristics. By contrast, the *high-risk AMI patient is defined by the presence of one or more of the following clinical features, including recurrent chest pain; CHF and low cardiac output; arrhythmias and, in particular, recurrent or sustained VT or VF; mechanical cardiac complications of AMI such as ruptured papillary muscle or intraventricular septum; and/or inducible ischemia and extensive coronary artery disease.*

**RECURRENT CHEST PAIN**

The most common causes of recurrent chest pain after AMI are coronary ischemia and pericarditis. ACC/AHA recommendations for the diagnosis and treatment of recurrent ischemia/infarction are as follows[1]:

***Recurrent Ischemia***

Class I

1. Patients with recurrent ischemic-type chest discomfort after initial reperfusion therapy for STEMI should undergo escalation of medical therapy with nitrates and beta blockers to decrease myocardial oxygen demand and reduce ischemia. Intravenous anticoagulation should be initiated if not already accomplished (*level of evidence B*).
2. In addition to escalation of medical therapy, patients with recurrent ischemic-type chest discomfort and signs of hemodynamic instability, poor LV function, or large areas of myocardium at risk should have an intraaortic balloon pump inserted and referred for cardiac catheterization.

Class IIa

1. Patients with recurrent ST-segment elevation and ischemic-type chest discomfort who are not considered candidates for revascularization or for whom coronary angiography and PCI cannot be rapidly implemented (ideally less than 60 min) should undergo readministeration of fibrinolytic therapy.

Recurrence of chest pain in the patient who has had an AMI is a serious development and requires immediate attention to establish the correct diagnosis and initiate treatment, especially if the pain represents recurrent ischemia, which is a more serious development than if the pain is a manifestation of pericarditis. Early postinfarction angina is an important predictor of the severity of coronary artery disease and has an overall incidence of about 18 percent.[333] Postinfarction angina is defined as chest pain that is frequently similar to the original discomfort, occurring at rest or with limited activity during hospitalization 24 h or more after onset of the AMI. The pain may or may not be associated with ST-segment elevation or depression or with pseudonormalization of inverted T waves on the post–myocardial ischemia ECG.[334] The pain is usually a result of ischemia in the territory of the myocardium supplied by the vessel that precipitated the initial myocardial ischemia. At least three categories of patients are at high risk for postinfarction angina: (1) patients with non-Q-wave myocardial infarction (NQWMI) (see Chap. 51); (2) patients who have received thrombolysis; and (3) patients with multiple risk factors.[335–337] The incidence of postinfarction angina is almost twice as high after NQWMI (25 to 35 percent) than after Q-wave myocardial infarction. Thrombolytic therapy for AMI created a new high-risk group for postinfarction angina (35 to 45 percent incidence), with a 12 to 15 percent incidence of reinfarction during the early experience with lytic therapy for reperfusion.[338] Regardless of whether postinfarction angina occurs after Q-wave myocardial infarction, NQWMI, or thrombolytic therapy, it is more likely to occur in patients with two- or three-vessel disease than in patients with single-vessel disease.[333] Postinfarction angina is important because it is associated with a twofold increase in the incidence of reinfarction. The 1-year mortality rate and acute risk of reinfarction is two- to fourfold greater in patients with postinfarction angina associated with ECG changes than in patients without chest pain or in those with chest pain but without associated ST-T changes.[339,340]

The incidence of reinfarction following thrombolytic therapy has been reduced from 12 to 15 percent to 5 to 7 percent with the use of adjunctive therapy, including heparin, aspirin, nitroglycerin, and beta blockers, as discussed previously. Nevertheless, reinfarction, despite the use of heparin and aspirin, still accounts for one-quarter of all deaths that occur following thrombolytic therapy and thus remains a major concern.[341] Patients with Q-wave myocardial infarction who do not receive thrombolytic therapy were previously likely to have an incidence of postinfarction angina of only about 12 to 15 percent and a reinfarction rate of about 5 to 7 percent, although these absolute rates have probably decreased with the more widespread use of adjunctive therapy with beta blockers, aspirin, and ACE inhibitors. Death, ventricular arrhythmias, and severe CHF are early sequelae of reinfarction, and there is an increased rate of sudden death and cardiogenic shock.[107,342]

Diagnosis of reinfarction within 18 h after thrombolytic therapy is based on the recurrence of ischemic-type chest pain, as noted, lasting at least 30 min, which may be associated with ST-T-wave changes. There is a reelevation of MB-CK, and the diagnostic criteria were discussed previously. Adequate beta-adrenergic blockade should be achieved. Sublingual nitroglycerin should be administered, and restarting of intravenous infusion should be considered. Pain should be controlled. Coronary arteriography generally should be performed early after the redevelopment of ischemic chest pain, and a high-grade stenosis is commonly found. If the lesion is suitable, PTCA should be performed, or additional thrombolysis should be administered if mechanical reperfusion is not feasible or available. With appropriate ECG changes—that is, ST-segment elevation—thrombolysis should be considered if cardiac catheterization and PTCA are not immediately available. If either APSAC or SK was used originally, it should not be readministered and rt-PA or r-PA should be utilized. These latter agents can be readministered. If multiple high-grade stenoses are found, coronary artery bypass grafting should be considered.

***Pericarditis*** ACC/AHA recommendations for treatment of post-STEMI pericarditis are as follows[1]:

Class I

1. Aspirin is recommended for treatment of pericarditis after STEMI, but doses as high as 650 mg orally every 4 to 6 hours may be needed (*level of evidence B*).

Class IIb

1. Ibuprofen (300 to 600 mg every 6 to 8 h) may be considered for pericarditis that is not controlled by aspirin. However, ibuprofen is associated with an increased risk of infarct expansion.
2. Corticosteroids although effective for pain relief should only be used as a last resort in patients with pericarditis refractory to aspirin or nonsteroidals because their use is associated with an increased risk of scar thinning and myocardial rupture.
3. Colchicine 0.6 mg orally every 12 h may be considered for recurrent or persistent pericarditis.

Class III

1. Indomethacin should not be used to treat pericarditis because of an increased risk of reduction of coronary blood flow and increased risk of myocardial scar thinning and infarct expansion.

Pericardial involvement associated with AMI assumes one of two forms. By far the most common type is pericardial inflammation overlying the necrotic segment of a transmural myocardial infarction. This particular pericarditis is usually an incidental finding in the course of a more significant illness. The less frequent form of postinfarction pericarditis is generally a delayed complication, which may represent an immunologic or autoimmune reaction. This pericarditis, a component of Dressler's syndrome, generally represents a major complication that often outlasts the basic illness (see also Chap. 80)

Early Postinfarction Pericarditis The prevalence of early postinfarction pericarditis, as reflected by the presence of typical symptoms and a friction rub, is 6 to 11 percent.[343,344] However, the general consensus among cardiologists is that this entity occurs fa more frequently than is clinically recognized. This suspicion is supported by postmortem studies finding evidence of postinfarction pericarditis when it was not recognized clinically.[345] The pericarditis usually becomes evident between the second and fourth days following the AMI, but it may occur up to several weeks later. In comparison to post-AMI patients without pericarditis, those who develop the condition have larger infarcts, a lower ejection fraction, and a higher incidence of CHF.[346,347]

The most common manifestation of pericarditis other than the chest pain is a scratchy two- or three-component friction rub along the left sternal border. The friction rub may have only a single component and may be dismissed erroneously as a systolic murmur. The rub is evanescent, generally lasting 1 to 6 days. The pain of pericarditis is generally perceived by the patient to be different from that of the AMI. The location of the pain may be the same, but any radiation is usually to the neck, shoulder, or scapula rather than to the arms or jaw. Characteristically, the pain is aggravated by inspiration, swallowing, coughing, or recumbency. Fever, usually less than 39°C, frequently accompanies the pericardial inflammation and typically lasts longer than 3 days, unlike the fever in an uncomplicated myocardial infarction.[348] The ECG is frequently not helpful in these patients, partially because it is usually distorted by the infarction and perhaps because of the localized nature of the inflammation. The cardiac rhythm is generally sinus, but there is an increased prevalence of atrial fibrillation.[349] Since significant effusion is unusual with this form of pericarditis, the echocardiogram is of limited diagnostic value.

*The treatment of choice is aspirin (160 to 325 mg daily), although higher doses (650 mg every 4 to 6 h) may be required.*[1,350,351] Indomethacin is effective in relieving symptoms[1] but experimentally causes thinning of scar formation.[352] Corticosteroids and ibuprofen provide pain relief but have also been associated with thinning of scar formation as well as with cardiac rupture.[353,354] The use of anticoagulants is relatively contraindicated in AMI complicated by pericarditis. Situations ordinarily calling for anticoagulation, such as mural thrombosis seen on echocardiography, require excellent clinical judgment in assessing the risk-benefit ratio if pericarditis is also present.

POSTMYOCARDIAL INFARCTION SYNDROME (DRESSLER'S SYNDROME) The clinical features of this syndrome are fever, chest pain, evidence of polyserositis, and a tendency to recur.[350] The reported frequency is 1 to 3 percent of AMIs.[349,350] The incidence, however, has appeared to diminish dramatically in the reperfusion era.[355] While there is usually a latency period of at least 1 week before its appearance, the pleuropericarditis may develop within the first week following the AMI.[356] The syndrome can occur in association with NQWMI, and it is usually associated with fever in the range of 38 to 39°C and occasionally up to 40°C. The chest pain is the most sensitive index of this syndrome and often precedes the fever. Aggravation of the pain by deep inspiration and turning is its most distinctive feature. The pericarditis is manifest by a friction rub, usually occurring between the second and eleventh week after the infarction and lasting from 3 days to 3 weeks. Pericardial effusion is common. While pericarditis is the dominant feature, as many as two-thirds of patients have pleural effusions. These effusions are usually small and are frequently bilateral but may be large and hemorrhagic. About one-quarter of patients have linear or patchy infiltrates in the lung bases.

The clinical features, pathologic findings, and prompt response to steroids all suggest an immunologic or autoimmune reaction. The presence of antimyocardial antibodies has been demonstrated in the majority of patients tested with the syndrome.

Treatment is similar to that of early postinfarction pericarditis but is more likely to require a course of oral corticosteroids. Recurrences are common for several months and require the reinstitution of corticosteroids with a more gradual tapering. Anticoagulants should generally be discontinued in the presence of postmyocardial infarction syndrome.[357]

## HEART FAILURE IN ACUTE MYOCARDIAL INFARCTION

***Pathophysiology and Hemodynamics*** The immediate hemodynamic consequences of myocardial infarction include both systolic and diastolic dysfunction. Systolic dysfunction is secondary to a loss of contractile function of the infarcted and ischemic myocardium.[358] Experimentally, over a period of 1 to 3 min, the regional disturbance of contraction progresses from dyssynchrony (disturbed temporal sequence of contraction) through hypokinesis (diminished motion) and akinesis (total lack of motion) to dyskinesia (paradoxical systolic expansion).[359] This loss of contractile function results in a decreased systolic ejection, increased end-systolic volume, increased end-diastolic volume, and a secondary increase in diastolic filling pressure caused by the increase in ventricular volume. The diastolic impairment often precedes the systolic dysfunction, which is characterized immediately by a transient increase in left ventricular diastolic distensibility,[360,361] followed by decreased distensibility due in part to adenosine triphosphate depletion and restraint by the pericardium and perhaps ultimately by the infiltration of inflammatory fluid and cells. The hemodynamic consequence of the reduced distensibility is increased diastolic pressure. The systolic stress on the ischemic segment, which contributes to "cell stretch" and "cell slippage," results in expansion of the infarcted segment[362] and provides the stimulus for volume overload hypertrophy, characterized by sarcomere replication, fiber elongation, and chamber enlargement. The chamber enlargement accommodates the increased volume and allows the diastolic pressure to return toward normal.[359]

Cardiac failure develops when left ventricular function is reduced to 30 percent or more of normal and usually occurs within minutes or hours of the onset of a large infarction. Since even with sustained coronary occlusion only 60 to 70 percent of the ischemic region undergoes necrosis, compromise of cardiac function associated with AMI is transient (24 to 72 h) in perhaps more than two-thirds of the cases. *Unlike the situation with chronic heart failure, the circulatory volume is normal or decreased in acute ventricular dysfunction associated with myocardial infarction.* The usual clinical scenario is one of left ventricular dysfunction with pulmonary congestion and without hypoperfusion. There is sometimes biventricular failure, and in about 5 to 10 percent of cases there is predominantly right ventricular failure, as discussed later. The severity of the failure, its duration, and whether or not it is reversible are predominantly dependent on infarct size.[363,364] If more than 40 percent of the myocardium is destroyed, decompensation occurs, resulting in shock.[365–367] In a few patients, failure develops later as a consequence of expansion of the infarcted segment, reinfarction, or ischemia.[360] Less commonly, failure is precipitated by papillary muscle dysfunction or ventricular septal rupture. The compromised heart will also be negatively affected by supraventricular or ventricular arrhythmias, conduction disturbances, drugs with negative inotropic effects, fever, and hypovolemia.

Left ventricular dysfunction with the clinical signs of failure is said to occur in 30 to 40 percent of patients and usually develops when the abnormally contracting segment exceeds 30 percent of the left ventricular circumference.[368] Another factor contributing to cardiac failure is residual scarring from previous episodes of infarction, which limits the extent of compensation. After myocardial infarction, adjacent normal myocardium increases its contractility because of increased stimulation by catecholamines; it also utilizes the Starling mechanism in an attempt to maintain cardiac output. The pathophysiology of heart failure is discussed in Chap. 24. That intravascular volume may be normal or decreased in acute heart failure in AMI is important in considering the therapeutic approach to low cardiac output and pulmonary congestion in acute infarction.

## RIGHT VENTRICULAR INFARCTION

Until about 15 to 20 years ago, right ventricular infarction was recognized infrequently and was usually thought not to be of great consequence. Subsequently, it was shown that the majority of patients with acute inferior infarction had abnormal regional function of the right ventricle,[369–371] although typical hemodynamic abnormalities are seen in only 10 to 15 percent of patients.[372,373] Right ventricular function returns to normal in most of these patients, suggesting that substantial stunning, rather than massive infarction, has occurred[1] (see also Chap. 46).

Inferior myocardial infarction associated with right ventricular infarction defines a high-risk subset with a mortality rate of 25 to 30 percent, as opposed to an overall mortality of about 6 percent in inferior myocardial infarction.[372] This group should be approached aggressively with consideration for reperfusion therapy. *Right ventricular involvement should always be considered and should be specifically sought out in inferior myocardial infarction with clinical evidence of low cardiac output, because the therapeutic approaches are quite different in the presence of right ventricular involvement from those for predominantly left ventricular failure.*

***Pathophysiology of Right Ventricular Infarction*** Right ventricular infarction is unusual in the absence of inferior infarction because occlusion of the right coronary artery proximal to the right ventricular branches usually also causes infarction in the inferior left ventricle, which is supplied by the distal distribution of the vessel.[374] The infarction usually involves the posterior septum and posterior wall rather than the right ventricular free wall. The relative sparing of the free wall results from the high degree of collateralization of the right ventricular arterial blood supply, from the blood flow derived from thebesian vessels, and from diffusion of oxygen from the ventricular cavity as well as from the fact that the free wall is thin and has comparatively low oxygen demands because of its mass and low workload.[375–378]

The hemodynamic consequences of right ventricular ischemia or infarction share features previously described for the left ventricle. Thus, there is impairment of contractility and diastolic dysfunction related to dilatation and pericardial restraint. In a low-pressure volume pump, such as the right ventricle, this combination has even more deleterious effects than in the left ventricle and causes substantial increases in diastolic pressure and decreases in systolic pressure. If the right ventricular afterload is also increased because of left ventricular dysfunction, then right-sided output can decrease dramatically and the driving force becomes essentially the right atrial pressure. Under these circumstances, right atrial transport essentially becomes critical, and anything decreasing it, such as diminished volume and filling pressure or loss of AV synchrony, may cause severe decreases of right and, secondarily, left ventricular output.[337,379,380]

***Diagnosis of Right Ventricular Infarction*** As noted, right ventricular infarction should be considered in all cases of acute inferior myocardial infarction, especially in the setting of low cardiac output. A typical presentation would include inferior myocardial infarction, clear lung fields, and jugular venous distention. Jugular venous distention that is enhanced by inspiration (Kussmaul's sign) in the setting of inferior myocardial infarction is highly suggestive of right ventricular involvement but may not be manifest with volume depletion and might become apparent only with repletion.[381] A right atrial pressure >10 mmHg that is >80 percent of the pulmonary wedge pressure is a sensitive and specific sign of right ventricular infarction.[382]

TABLE 52-10 Differential Diagnosis of Congestive Heart Failure in Inferior STEMI

| |
|---|
| Arrhythmia: high-degree AV block, atrial fibrillation, or sustained ventricular tachycardia |
| Ischemia at a distance, with the occluded artery to the inferior wall supplying the anterior wall via collaterals |
| Previous infarction at another location |
| Mechanical complication, such as papillary muscle dysfunction |
| Right ventricular infarction |

The differential diagnosis of heart failure or low cardiac output in inferior infarction includes (1) arrhythmia, such as atrial fibrillation, sustained ventricular arrhythmia, or high-degree AV block; (2) ongoing ischemia, such as ischemia at a distance if the occluded artery to the inferior wall was also supplying, through collaterals, the anterior wall; (3) previous infarction at another location; (4) a mechanical complication such as papillary muscle dysfunction or, less commonly, a ventricular septal defect; or (5) right ventricular infarction.[383] This differential diagnosis of causes of CHF in inferior STEMI is summarized in Table 52-10.

*ST-segment elevation in lead $V_{4R}$ is the single most powerful predictor of right ventricular involvement in inferior infarction and identifies a patient subset with a markedly increased in-hospital mortality.*[372] All patients with inferior infarction should be screened by recording ECG lead $V_{4R}$. Echocardiography can also be useful as an adjunctive diagnostic approach[146] and can be particularly valuable in detecting right-to-left shunting of blood through the foramen ovale, which can occur because of the high right atrial pressures in right ventricular ischemia. Such shunting can be a cause of hypoxemia unresponsive to oxygen administration in this setting.[384]

***Treatment of Right Ventricular Ischemia and Infarction*** ACC/AHA recommendations are as follows[1]:

Class I

1. Patients with inferior STEMI and hemodynamic compromise should be assessed with echocardiography and a right precordial V4R lead to detect ST-segment elevation.
2. The following principles apply to therapy of patients with STEMI and RV ischemia:
   - Early reperfusion should be achieved if possible.
   - AV synchrony should be achieved and bradycardia should be corrected.
   - RV preload should be optimized, usually requiring initial volume challenge in patients with hemodynamic instability.
   - RV afterload should be optimized, usually requiring therapy for concomitant LV dysfunction.
   - Inotropic support should be used for hemodynamic instability not responsive to volume challenge.

The major objectives in treating right ventricular infarction are to maintain right ventricular preload, provide inotropic support, reduce afterload of the right ventricle, and achieve early reperfusion.[229] The

TABLE 52-11 Treatment Strategy for Right Ventricular Ischemia/ Infarction

Maintain right ventricular preload
  Volume loading (IV normal saline)
  Avoid use of nitrates and diuretics
  Maintain AV synchrony
    AV sequential pacing for symptomatic high-degree heart block unresponsive to atropine
  Prompt cardioversion for hemodynamically significant SVT
Inotropic support
  Dobutamine (if cardiac output fails to increase after volume loading)
Reduce right ventricular afterload with left ventricular dysfunction
  Intraaortic balloon pump
  Arterial vasodilators (sodium nitroprusside, hydralazine)
  ACE inhibitors
Reperfusion
  Thrombolytic agents
  Primary PTCA
  CABG (in selected patients with multivessel disease)

ABBREVIATIONS: IV = intravenous; AV = atrioventricular; SVT = supraventricular tachycardia; ACE = angiotensin-converting enzyme; PTCA = percutaneous transluminal coronary angioplasty; CABG = coronary artery bypass graft.
SOURCE: Ryan et al.[2] With permission.

recommendations are summarized in Table 52-11.[2] Venodilators such as nitrates should be avoided and diuretics should be used with caution. Volume loading with 1 to 2 L of saline will frequently restore cardiac output and correct hypotension; this should be the initial step. Excessive volume loading, however, may dilate the ventricle and decrease output. Inotropic support should be initiated if saline administration does not restore output and correct hypotension.[1] Dobutamine is an ideal initial choice.[69a]

The critical role of atrial transport in maintaining output in right ventricular infarction and the need to maintain AV synchrony have been discussed. High-degree AV block occurs in about 50 percent of patients in this setting, and AV sequential pacing can restore cardiac output.[385,386] Atrial fibrillation occurs in up to one-third of these patients, in whom prompt cardioversion should be considered if there is any evidence of hemodynamic compromise.[387] If there is significant left ventricular dysfunction—which may further compromise right ventricular function, as noted—afterload reduction by nitroprusside infusion or intraaortic balloon pumping is indicated.[1]

Reperfusion with thrombolytic therapy or primary PTCA improves right ventricular ejection fraction and hemodynamic status[388] and decreases the incidence of complete heart block.[388–390] Coronary artery bypass grafting should be considered if multivessel disease is found.

***Management of Congestive Heart Failure in Acute Myocardial Infarction: General Issues*** HEMODYNAMIC MONITORING Recommendations for monitoring via balloon-flotation right-heart catheterization[1]:

Class I
1. Severe or progressive CHF or pulmonary edema
2. Cardiogenic shock or progressive hypotension
3. Suspected mechanical complications of acute infarction, i.e., ventricular septal defect, papillary muscle rupture, or pericardial tamponade

Class IIa
1. Hypotension that does not respond promptly to fluid administration in a patient without pulmonary congestion
2. Persistent signs of hypoperfusion without hypotension or pulmonary congestion

Class III
1. Patients with acute infarction without evidence of cardiac or pulmonary complications

The balloon flotation (Swan-Ganz) catheter fundamentally permits one, in the setting of low cardiac output, to distinguish between inadequate ventricular filling pressures and inadequate systolic function. The former is treated with volume expansion and the latter with inotropic support and frequently afterload reduction. The catheter, even when used correctly, is not totally benign; during manipulation, it may precipitate VT and pulmonary hemorrhage or infarction. To minimize the risk of infection, the catheter should not be left in place longer than 5 days.[1]

INTRAARTERIAL PRESSURE MONITORING The recommendations are as follows[1]:

Class I
1. Patients with severe hypotension (systolic arterial pressure less than 80 mmHg) and/or cardiogenic shock
2. Patients receiving vasopressor agents

Class IIa
1. Patients receiving intravenous sodium nitroprusside or other potent vasodilators

Class IIb
1. Hemodynamically stable patients receiving intravenous nitroglycerin for myocardial ischemia
2. Patients receiving intravenous inotropic agents

Class III
1. Patients with acute infarction who are hemodynamically stable. Arterial monitoring in AMI is useful in all hypotensive patients but especially in those who are in shock. The radial artery is the preferred site, although the brachial and femoral arteries can be used. Intraarterial catheters should not be left in place longer than 72 h because of the risk of thrombosis and infection.[1]

INTRAORTIC BALLOON COUNTERPULSATION The recommendations are as follows[1]:

Class I
1. Cardiogenic shock not quickly reversed with pharmacologic therapy as a stabilizing measure for angiography and prompt revascularization
2. Acute mitral regurgitation or ventricular septal defect complicating myocardial infarction as a stabilizing therapy for angiography and repair and revascularization
3. Recurrent intractable ventricular arrhythmias with hemodynamic instability
4. Refractory postmyocardial infarction angina as a bridge to angiography and revascularization

Class IIa
1. Signs of hemodynamic instability, poor left ventricular function, or persistent ischemia in patients with large areas of the myocardium at risk

Class IIb

1. In patients with successful PTCA after failed thrombolysis or those with three-vessel coronary disease, to prevent reocclusion
2. In patients known to have large areas of myocardium at risk, with or without active ischemia

By inflating in the aorta during diastole and by deflating during systole, the intraaortic balloon pump reduces afterload during ventricular systole and increases coronary perfusion during diastole. The decrease in afterload and increased coronary perfusion account for its efficacy in cardiogenic shock and ischemia. It is particularly useful as a stabilizing bridge to facilitate diagnostic angiography and revascularization and repair of mechanical complications of AMI.[1] The use of the intraaortic balloon pump after thrombolysis for AMI or after PTCA has not been uniformly successful in improving clinical outcome, including reocclusion rate or global or regional left ventricular function.[391] Thus, the routine use of the intraaortic balloon pump after either drug or mechanical reperfusion cannot be recommended.[1]

DIURETICS AND POSITIVE INOTROPIC AGENTS DIURETICS AND CARDIAC FAILURE IN ACUTE MYOCARDIAL INFARCTION As previously mentioned, patients with failure due to AMI have normal total body water, and the transudation of fluid into the lungs may induce hypovolemia. As ventricular compliance is decreased, an increased left ventricular end-diastolic pressure is necessary to maintain cardiac output, since the heart operates on the steep portion of the ascending limb of Starling's curve.[392,393] The administration of a diuretic in this setting may be associated with a decrease in cardiac output.[394–396] Thus, diuretics should not be the drugs used initially in the treatment of pulmonary congestion in AMI. Their use early in the course should usually be guided by hemodynamic measurements from a Swan-Ganz catheter. Diuretic therapy may become appropriate later if salt and water retention occur and left ventricular filling pressures become excessively high, → up to 18 to 20 mmHg, for example.

INOTROPIC AGENTS IN CONGESTIVE HEART FAILURE ASSOCIATED WITH ACUTE MYOCARDIAL INFARCTION Digoxin is a relatively weak inotropic agent and is not the drug of choice in acute heart failure in myocardial infarction. In a direct comparison, dobutamine was shown to increase cardiac output by 40 percent and to decrease left ventricular filling pressure, whereas digoxin increased cardiac output by only 10 percent and did not decrease filling pressure.[397] Since endogenous catecholamine levels can be quite elevated, digoxin may contribute little. The primary use of digoxin in AMI is to control heart rate in atrial fibrillation.

Dobutamine has favorable pharmacologic properties for use in heart failure in myocardial infarction (see Chap. 25). It has a rapid onset of action and increases cardiac output because of its positive inotropic properties. It is a vasodilator and increases coronary flow. It decreases filling pressure, as noted. Dopamine has a tendency to increase heart rate more than dobutamine. With higher doses, dopamine may increase peripheral resistance and filling pressures, offsetting some of the positive inotropic effects. There is concern that positive inotropic agents may increase infarct size. Evaluation of dobutamine in AMI showed that, as long as heart rate was not increased more than 10 percent above baseline, there was no increase in infarct size or in the incidence of reinfarction or arrhythmia.[398]

***Management of Uncomplicated Cardiac Failure after Acute Myocardial Infarction*** The major determinant of left ventricular dysfunction is the extent of myocardial injury.[363,364,399] The loss of contractile function in the initial minutes or hours (1 to 4) is potentially reversible and accounts in part for the transient nature of cardiac failure in the setting of uncomplicated AMI, as noted above. The presence of cardiac failure and its severity depend not only on the extent of damage but also upon the extent of injury from previous episodes.

Since the introduction of the Swan-Ganz catheter, considerable data have accumulated correlating hemodynamics with clinical features. In 1967, prior to invasive monitoring, Killip and Kimball[70] devised a clinical classification based on physical findings present on admission that provided a prognostic guide. That guide was followed by the classification of Forrester and colleagues,[400,401] based on extensive data obtained from invasive monitoring of patients with acute MI (Table 52-12). The latter classification combined the presence or absence of pulmonary congestion with the presence or absence of systemic hypoperfusion. They added the underlying hemodynamics to this classification based on the pulmonary arterial occlusive (wedge) pressure and the cardiac

TABLE 52-12 Clinical and Hemodynamic Subsets in Acute Myocardial Infarction

| Subset | Clinical Features | Approximate % of Patients with AMI | Hospital Mortality, % |
|---|---|---|---|
| | **KILLIP CLASS** | | |
| 1 | No signs of congestive heart failure | 40–50 | 6 |
| 2 | $S_3$ gallop and bibasilar rales | 30–40 | 17 |
| 3 | Acute pulmonary edema | 10–15 | 38 |
| 4 | Cardiogenic shock | 5–10 | 81 |
| | **CEDARS-SINAI CLINICAL SUBSETS** | | |
| 1 | No pulmonary congestion or tissue hypoperfusion | 25 | 1 |
| 2 | Pulmonary congestion only | 25 | 11 |
| 3 | Tissue hypoperfusion only | 15 | 18 |
| 4 | Pulmonary congestion and tissue hypoperfusion | 35 | 60 |
| | **CEDAR-SINAI HEMODYNAMIC SUBSETS** | | |
| | Hemodynamic features | | |
| 1 | PCW $\leq$ 18; CI $>$ 2.2 | 25 | 3 |
| 2 | PCW $>$ 18; CI $>$ 2.2 | 25 | 9 |
| 3 | PCW $\leq$ 18; CI $\leq$ 2.2 | 15 | 23 |
| 4 | PCW $>$ 18; CI $\leq$ 2.2 | 35 | 51 |

ABBREVIATIONS: AMI = acute myocardial infarction; CI = cardiac index (L/min/m$^2$); PCW = pulmonary capillary wedge pressure (mmHg).

index. These classifications also provide important diagnostic and therapeutic guidelines, despite the observation that patients frequently cross over from one class to the other and are seldom restricted to one particular hemodynamic subset. Each classification illustrated that with increasing severity of ventricular dysfunction, there is an increased risk of mortality. Nevertheless, there is imprecision in predicting mortality rates from hemodynamics. Rackley and coworkers[402] observed that patients with a ventricular filling pressure >29 mmHg had a 100 percent mortality rate; those with a filling pressure >15 mmHg and a cardiac index <2 L/min per square meter of body surface had a mortality rate of 93 percent; while those with a ventricular filling pressure <15 and a cardiac index <2 L/min per square meter of body surface had a mortality rate of 63 percent.

*In patients with uncomplicated AMI, there is no need to perform invasive monitoring if careful clinical observations are made.* There should be repeated assessment of the heart and lungs; examination of the skin and mucous membranes; monitoring of the systemic arterial pressure, cardiac rhythm, and heart rate; and routine laboratory examinations, including chest x-ray and determinations of urine output and arterial blood-gas values. If there are clinical indications of pulmonary congestion and/or decreased peripheral perfusion, invasive monitoring includes the insertion of a Swan-Ganz catheter in order to monitor right ventricular hemodynamics and pulmonary artery occlusive pressure (which will reflect ventricular end-diastolic pressure) and to obtain serial determinations of the cardiac output. Occasionally, it may be necessary to insert an arterial catheter to measure the arterial pressure; however, one can usually follow the pressure adequately with the use of a sphygmomanometer or an automatic blood pressure monitoring device. Frequently, it is also essential to insert a Foley catheter to follow the urine output, particularly in patients with sustained hypotension or cardiogenic shock.

In most patients in whom cardiac failure is not complicated by mechanical factors—such as mitral valve rupture, ventricular septal rupture, pulmonary embolus, or tamponade—the failure is transient and of mild-to-moderate severity. If the cardiac output is normal, aggressive treatment is often not recommended.[129] In patients with rales at the base of the lungs with only a minimal increase in heart rate and no other signs of hypoxemia (Killip class III), conventional therapy with morphine; nasal oxygen; intravenous, oral, or transdermal nitrates; and bed rest is adequate without any specific therapy for failure. In patients with extensive pulmonary edema who are normotensive and exhibit hypoxia and dyspnea (Forrester class II), the treatment of choice is nitroglycerin given intravenously at 0.1 $\mu$g/kg per minute and increased in increments of 5 to 10 $\mu$g/min, stopping at a dose that does not decrease the systolic blood pressure below 100 mmHg. On the average, nitroglycerin in a dose of 0.5 $\mu$g/kg per minute is required in patients with evolving acute infarction and failure. Another vasodilator that has been used extensively in the past in AMI is sodium nitroprusside, which is initiated at 0.5 $\mu$g/kg per minute and increased by 10- to 20-$\mu$g/min increments every 10 to 15 min until the desired therapeutic point or a maximum of 10 $\mu$g/kg per minute is reached. Nevertheless, nitroglycerin is the preferred agent, since it has been shown to offer some cardioprotection when given in the early phase of myocardial infarction and to be both reliable and safe. In contrast, in experimental infarction in the dog, it has been shown that nitroprusside is more likely to redirect coronary flow away from the ischemic area to normal areas and to induce coronary steal.[220] The effect of nitroprusside on cardioprotection has been inconsistent and in one large study was shown to be detrimental.[403] In view of the data showing ACE inhibitors to be effective in cardiac failure, these agents are being used more generally in this setting. It is preferable that hemodynamics be monitored invasively (by Swan-Ganz catheter) when one gives a vasodilator to reduce the ventricular filling pressure to 15 to 17 mmHg while maintaining adequate cardiac output and coronary perfusion. Whether or not one monitors hemodynamics invasively will depend in part on the confidence that clinical features reflect the volume status. Mitral valve regurgitation due to papillary muscle dysfunction is commonly an aggravating factor even in mild-to-moderate cardiac failure and responds well to a vasodilator, as does systemic hypertension. Usually a vasodilator is not adequate, in which case an intravenous inotropic agent should be added. The inotropic agents are generally those of sympathomimetic drugs, including dobutamine, dopamine, and norepinephrine (see Chap. 25). Dobutamine, a synthetic direct-acting agent, is preferred, as noted, and has actions that include vasodilatation, increased cardiac output, decreased ventricular filling pressure, and increased coronary flow.[398] The infusion should be initiated at 2 to 5 $\mu$g/kg per minute and should be increased such that adequate systemic pressure is maintained and the heart rate does not increase by more than 10 to 15 percent. Dobutamine is preferably titrated to cardiac output and ventricular filling pressure. The ventricular filling pressure should be decreased to a range of 14 to 18 mmHg while maintaining adequate cardiac output and blood pressure. In general, the objective is to maintain adequate cardiac output and blood pressure without inducing tachycardia while maintaining a filling pressure that is normal or minimally increased.

In patients with inferior infarction and low cardiac output, right ventricular infarction should be suspected, as discussed. If it is present, a Swan-Ganz catheter should be inserted to determine the filling pressure. Therapy with a positive inotropic agent, such as dobutamine, should be used after assuring that there is appropriate intravascular volume to facilitate right ventricular filling.[404,405]

In patients with borderline blood pressure and evidence of peripheral hypoperfusion, therapy should be initiated with an inotropic agent and not a vasodilator. Similarly, in patients with left ventricular failure and frank hypotension (<95 mmHg), a vasodilator must be avoided and initial therapy should be with a positive inotropic agent. Dopamine would frequently be the choice under these circumstances, since it exerts cardiovascular effects similar to those of dobutamine, but it also possesses an alpha$_1$-adrenergic activity and releases endogenous norepinephrine from sympathetic nerve endings. Low doses of dopamine (2 to 7 $\mu$g/kg per minute) are associated with increased stroke volume, cardiac output, and renal blood flow and moderate effects to increase peripheral resistance. High doses of dopamine induce significant vasoconstriction and may increase the left ventricular filling pressure due to increased afterload, which further exacerbates pulmonary congestion. Dopamine also has a more positive chronotropic effect than does dobutamine, which can be a disadvantage in AMI. Norepinephrine, which produces potent arteriolar and venous constriction, is used for hypotension in other settings but is otherwise relatively contraindicated in AMI. It is seldom used unless patients are hypotensive and do not respond to dopamine, the phosphodiesterase inhibitor milrinone, or dobutamine. It is used in cardiogenic shock after dopamine has failed, since it is the major alternative that can be used for maintaining adequate perfusion pressure.

As indicated earlier, diuretics should be used with more caution in acute heart failure associated with AMI than in chronic heart failure, since volume expansion is usually not the primary problem. If high filling pressure (>18 to 20 mmHg) persists after adequate output is achieved with positive inotropic agents and/or vasodilators, diuretics may be added. However, this effect can be achieved by vasodilator therapy, which avoids the hypovolemia and hypotension that may occur secondary to the subsequent diuresis (1 to 2 h). The preferred diuretics are intravenous furosemide or ethacrynic acid.[406] These drugs also provide some acute venodilation.

***Complicated Heart Failure after Myocardial Infarction*** Some AMI patients present with acute, fulminating pulmonary edema (with severe respiratory distress; generalized inspiratory crackles and wheezing; expectoration of pink, frothy sputum; cool, clammy, diaphoretic skin; and cyanosis) and require much more aggressive therapy than do patients with uncomplicated AMI. The condition is usually associated with a pulmonary artery wedge pressure exceeding 25 mmHg and an in-hospital mortality rate of at least 15 to 20 percent.[407] The systolic blood pressure is usually either low normal or borderline normal (95 to 105 mmHg). The maintenance of adequate oxygenation must be the primary concern. Administration of high concentrations (60 to 100 percent) of oxygen via a face mask is essential. If the patient appears moribund, endotracheal intubation should be performed. While an assessment of arterial blood gases is appropriate, the speed with which clinical events change in these emergent situations may demand that decisions be made without benefit of these values. After the institution of mechanical ventilation, positive end-expiratory pressure may be needed to maintain adequate oxygenation while keeping the inspired oxygen concentration within safe levels ($FIO_2 < 60$ percent). Positive end-expiratory pressure should be applied only with an awareness of its risks of pneumothorax and reduction in cardiac output secondary to decreased left ventricular preload.[407] Invasive hemodynamic monitoring is particularly useful in these patients. Therapeutic interventions, however, should not be delayed until the monitoring is established. The therapy for severe pulmonary edema should include intravenous morphine unless the patient is known to have chronic $CO_2$ retention. From 5 to 10 mg of morphine sulfate should be given slowly, with careful observation for evidence of respiratory depression. If the systolic blood pressure is adequate (>100 mmHg), nitroglycerin is administered intravenously. In the patient with severe pulmonary edema, the improvement in left ventricular pump performance afforded by the prompt reduction in systemic vascular resistance by nitroprusside[408] may be essential for the rapid reversal of this life-threatening situation (particularly if systemic hypertension had been present). Either nitroglycerin or nitroprusside will provide a reduction in preload. If the systolic blood pressure is 100 mmHg or less, treatment with a positive inotropic agent should probably be initiated, with the subsequent addition of a vasodilator or an agent to improve cardiac output. The adjunctive use of intravenous diuretics is the same as outlined for mild degrees of heart failure.

PERIPHERAL HYPOPERFUSION WITHOUT PULMONARY CONGESTION Patients with clinical hypoperfusion without pulmonary congestion (with cool, cyanotic extremities, somnolence or confusion, and decreased urine flow) usually have a cardiac index <2.2 L/min. The mortality rate in these patients is four times greater than that in patients without hypoperfusion.[408] Invasive hemodynamic monitoring of the pulmonary capillary wedge pressure is essential. Volume augmentation is the initial therapeutic step in patients with a pulmonary capillary wedge pressure <15 mmHg. If possible, this pressure should be maintained below the level of pulmonary congestion (>20 mmHg). Vasodilators are usually not indicated, at least until adequate filling pressures have been achieved and cardiac output is augmented with positive inotropic agents. This situation is commonly seen with severe biventricular infarction and thus should be suspected with inferior and right ventricular infarction. In this case, bradycardia should be treated with atropine if it is thought to be contributing to the systemic hypoperfusion. Excessive treatment with nitroglycerin and volume contraction from previous diuretic therapy can also contribute to systemic hypotension.

HYPOTENSION AND CARDIOGENIC SHOCK Cardiogenic shock may occur when 40 percent or more of the left ventricle is destroyed.[365,366,409] It is the most common cause of in-hospital death with myocardial infarction. The incidence of cardiogenic shock was about 15 percent in the early 1970s, but it has now decreased to approximately 5 to 7 percent.[407] The mortality rate is frequently over 80 percent.[410] The most effective therapy in the treatment of cardiogenic shock is prevention, since its major determinant is infarct size.[364,411] Cardiogenic shock usually occurs within hours of the onset of infarction due to massive ischemia and necrosis.[412] In other cases, a relatively small infarction that is superimposed on extensive previous damage may precipitate cardiogenic shock. Less commonly, cardiogenic shock may develop days after the initial event. This occurrence is almost always due to development of new necrosis (extension or early reinfarction) in the area of the preceding infarction. The decrease in the incidence of cardiogenic shock is believed to be in part due to better treatment of angina and ischemia, together with the widespread use of thrombolytic therapy and other cardioprotective agents. Cardiogenic shock by definition represents a more severe form of cardiac failure, resulting in decreased organ perfusion in addition to the conventional features of pulmonary congestion and left ventricular dysfunction. Cardiac failure with hypoperfusion and that regarded as cardiogenic shock may differ only in the severity of decreased perfusion. Clearly, every effort must be made to treat hypoperfusion whether or not it satisfies the strict criteria of cardiogenic shock. Characteristics of cardiogenic shock are (Table 52-13) (1) evidence of organ hypoperfusion with cold, clammy skin, especially on the feet and hands, that may be associated with peripheral cyanosis of the nail beds; (2) oliguria, disordered mentation, and systolic blood pressure <80 to 90 mmHg; (3) left ventricular end-diastolic pressure or, more commonly, pulmonary capillary wedge pressure >18 mmHg; (4) evidence of a primary cardiac abnormality; and (5) a cardiac index *not* >1.8 L/min per square meter of body surface. Hypotension or shock due to a primary abnormality of cardiac rhythm or conduction is not considered cardiogenic shock.

The advantage of early revascularization in reducing mortality in the acute setting (SHOCK trial)[257] was discussed earlier. Since the prognosis is extremely poor for patients with cardiogenic shock due primarily to loss of muscle mass, reversible causes associated with a better prognosis must be excluded. Potentially reversible causes include mitral valve rupture, ventricular septal rupture, right ventricular infarction, pulmonary embolus, and cardiac tamponade. While the mortality associated with surgical correction of infarct-associated mitral rupture or ventricular septal defect is still high, it is far less

TABLE 52-13 Characteristics of Cardiogenic Shock

Evidence of hypoperfusion: cold, clammy skin, especially of feet and hands; impaired mentation; oliguria
Systolic blood pressure <80–90 mmHg
LVED pressure (or PCW pressure) ≥18 mmHg
Evidence of primary cardiac abnormality
Cardiac index ≤1.8 $L/min/m^2$

ABBREVIATIONS: LVED = left ventricular end-diastolic; PCW = pulmonary capillary wedge.

than that associated with cardiogenic shock due solely to myocardial injury. The details of management of these mechanical causes of shock are discussed further on. Hypotension may be due to inadequate fluid administration, to vasodilatation induced by such drugs as morphine and vasodilators, and occasionally to depressed contractility due to antiarrhythmic therapy. Inadequate filling pressure is a very important cause of hypotension and should be corrected immediately. It is particularly common in patients with inferior infarction, as noted. A Swan-Ganz catheter should be inserted to determine the circulatory status and assess the response to therapy.

Therapeutic objectives are to establish and maintain a systemic arterial pressure adequate for perfusing the vital organs and for reducing pulmonary congestion. The approaches to pulmonary congestion include the judicious use of morphine and the maintenance of adequate oxygenation together with endotracheal intubation and mechanical ventilation if necessary. In addition to instituting hemodynamic monitoring, one should assess urinary output using an indwelling catheter. If the pulmonary artery wedge pressure is <15 mmHg, prompt volume expansion to raise the capillary pressure to 18 to 20 mmHg should be initiated. The cornerstones of therapy are inotropic and vasopressor agents. If the systemic arterial pressure is below 80 to 90 mmHg, a pressor agent such as dopamine should be infused.[412] At relatively low doses of 2 to 5 μg/kg per minute, increases in stroke volume and cardiac output are mediated by beta-adrenergic stimulation and increases in renal blood flow by the dopaminergic-specific receptors. The alpha-adrenergic vasoconstrictor effects are manifest progressively at doses above 5 μg/kg per minute. The use of intravenous dopamine requires careful titration, beginning with a low dose and gradually increasing until an adequate (90 to 100 mmHg) systemic pressure is achieved. If high doses of dopamine are necessary to maintain adequate perfusion, a change to norepinephrine infusion should be considered. This drug is a potent arteriolar and venous constrictor that is mediated through alpha-adrenergic stimulation. It demonstrates relatively modest beta-adrenergic stimulation. It is, therefore, a very potent pressor agent with less chronotropic or arrhythmogenic effects than dopamine.[234] The drug should be started at low doses of 1 to 4 μg/min. Extravasation should be avoided, since it will produce tissue sloughing.

When the systemic blood pressure is 90 mmHg or more, dobutamine is frequently the preferred agent. By increasing cardiac output, dobutamine may produce a rise in systemic blood pressure, but this increase would not be expected to be >10 to 15 mmHg.[413,414] Dobutamine will not support arterial pressure except by its effect on cardiac output. As the cardiac output rises, the left ventricular filling pressure should decline. Dobutamine therapy should begin with a dose of 2 to 5 μg/kg per minute with increases every 5 to 10 min. Inappropriate increases in heart rate are unlikely to occur with doses <15 to 20 μg/kg per minute.[398]

On occasion, the severity of cardiac pump dysfunction will require the use of two divergent therapeutic modalities in order to facilitate left ventricular emptying.[415] The most commonly utilized of these combined therapies is nitroprusside and dopamine. The principal advantage offered by nitroprusside in this combination is a reduction in left ventricular preload. The cardiac output is not appreciably increased by the addition of nitroprusside to dopamine therapy. The advantage offered by dopamine in this combination is an augmentation of cardiac output and the maintenance of systemic arterial pressure.[416] A less frequently used combination, dobutamine and nitroprusside, has been shown to result in higher cardiac output and lower pulmonary capillary wedge pressures than has resulted with either drug alone.[415] Stabilization of the patient with cardiogenic shock may be achieved by mechanical circulatory assist devices, such as the intraaortic balloon as demonstrated in the SHOCK trial.[257] Aortic balloon counterpulsation reduces afterload while simultaneously improving coronary perfusion by increasing diastolic aortic pressure, as discussed. It is the only intervention that will increase diastolic aortic pressure without increasing myocardial oxygen demand. Aortic counterpulsation is often helpful for patients in cardiogenic shock due to a potentially reversible condition or in whom cardiac transplantation is being considered. Such conditions include an acute but still evolving MI or AMI with a severe mechanical complication (e.g., mitral regurgitation or ventricular septal defect). In such cases, aortic counterpulsation should be used to stabilize the patient's condition in preparation for salvage of the jeopardized but still viable myocardium or correction of the mechanical defect.[234] Intraaortic counterpulsation in patients without a reversible defect is now being used with greater frequency, especially in patients <75 years of age based on the compelling data emerging from the long-term follow-up of the SHOCK trial patients.[257]

Restoration of coronary blood flow is the most effective therapy in salvaging patients with cardiogenic shock who are unresponsive to fluid and pharmacologic management in the early hours after a myocardial infarction. If angioplasty and/or coronary artery bypass grafting are not readily available, thrombolytic therapy should be tried if it has not already been utilized—although it has not been shown to improve survival in this setting.[417,418] These patients should be transferred quickly to a tertiary care center. Blood pressure should be stabilized with an intraaortic balloon pump, and cardiac catheterization should be performed as soon as possible. Assessment of correctable mechanical lesions, such as ruptured papillary muscles, can be made together with evaluation of coronary anatomy. Depending upon this anatomy, a judgment can be made as to whether to attempt PTCA or to proceed to coronary artery bypass surgery. Mechanical revascularization appears to improve survival in cardiogenic shock complicating AMI.[257,419]

### Mechanical Dysfunction Contributing to Cardiac Failure

**Papillary muscle rupture** ACC/AHA recommendations are as follows[1]:

Class I

1. Patients with acute papillary muscle rupture should be considered for urgent cardiac surgical repair, unless further support is considered futile based on patient's wishes or contraindications/unsuitability for further invasive care.
2. Coronary artery bypass surgery should undertaken at the same time as mitral valve repair surgery.

Rupture of the left ventricular papillary muscle occurs in approximately 1 percent of myocardial infarctions and accounts for 0.4 to 5.0 percent of infarct-related deaths.[420] It occurs slightly less frequently than ventricular septal rupture. The posteromedial papillary muscle is involved 6 to 12 times more frequently than is the anterolateral muscle.[421] Thus, papillary muscle rupture with an acute anterior myocardial infarction is uncommon. The rupture may occur distally and may involve one or several of the smaller heads of the muscle or, less commonly, may occur proximally and produce complete dehiscence of the papillary muscle.

Papillary muscle rupture is manifest by the sudden appearance of pulmonary edema, usually 2 to 7 days after the infarction. The abruptness of onset and severity of pulmonary edema are usually greater than seen with ventricular septal rupture. A mid- or holosystolic murmur with wide radiation is usually audible. Although the murmur is generally loud, a thrill is rarely present, and the murmur may seem inconsequential. The diagnosis can be established by Doppler echocardiographic studies (see Chap. 15). The two-dimensional echocardiogram will generally show a flail mitral leaflet and may reveal a portion of the papillary muscle visualized as a mass attached to the chordae. Even when the flail leaflet is not observed, documentation of relatively intact ventricular systolic function in the postinfarction patient with pulmonary edema should suggest the diagnosis. The Doppler study will establish the presence and severity of the mitral regurgitation. Bedside right-heart catheterization can be used to exclude an oxygen step-up from the right atrium to the right ventricle, indicative of ventricular septal rupture, and to confirm elevated pulmonary capillary wedge pressures with tall V (regurgitant) waves characteristic of acute mitral regurgitation.

Studies in the presurgical era demonstrated a poor prognosis for these patients, with a 50 percent mortality rate in the first 24 h and a 6 percent survival rate for longer than 2 months.[357] Thus, immediate recognition and treatment are essential. Intraaortic counterpulsation alone or with vasodilator and inotropic therapy may frequently be required for temporary stabilization. During this period, the patient should undergo cardiac catheterization to define coronary anatomy and should be transferred to surgery for mitral valve replacement or repair.

PAPILLARY MUSCLE DYSFUNCTION The sudden development of an apical systolic murmur after a myocardial infarction is much more often secondary to papillary muscle dysfunction than it is to rupture. Twenty percent of patients who die from infarction have histologic evidence of papillary muscle necrosis, usually without rupture.[422] Papillary muscle dysfunction is frequently compatible with long-term survival.

The posteromedial papillary muscle is involved with ischemia or infarction more commonly than the anterolateral muscle because the latter receives blood from two arteries (left anterior descending and circumflex), whereas the posteromedial muscle is supplied predominantly from the circumflex.[423] Dysfunction may be transient during ischemia. Papillary muscle ischemia is usually accompanied by ischemia of the contiguous ventricular wall.[424] Involvement of the contiguous ventricular wall is a key factor in the development of significant mitral regurgitation, since isolated papillary muscle ischemia or even infarction is usually not sufficient to cause important mitral regurgitation.[425]

Papillary muscle dysfunction typically presents with an apical systolic murmur. The murmur may be holosystolic, late systolic, or even early systolic. Echocardiography coupled with Doppler flow studies will confirm the presence of mitral regurgitation, grade its severity, and permit assessment of left ventricular function. There is generally no hemodynamic deterioration associated with the appearance of the murmur. It is the unusual patient who develops pulmonary edema, and these patients usually have concomitant significant left ventricular dysfunction. The ordinary patient with papillary muscle dysfunction will require no specific therapy for the regurgitation, while the unusual patient with severe regurgitation should be treated as in the case of papillary muscle rupture. In intermediate cases with moderate to moderately severe regurgitation where cardiac surgery is not contemplated, afterload reduction with ACE inhibitors should be considered.

VENTRICULAR SEPTAL RUPTURE (VSR) ACC/AHA recommendations are as follows[1]:

Class I

1. Patients with STEMI complicated by the development of VSR should be considered for urgent cardiac surgical repair, unless further support is considered futile based on patient's wishes or contraindications/unsuitability for further invasive care (*level of evidence B*).
2. CABG should be undertaken at the same time as repair of the VSD.

Rupture of the interventricular septum is estimated to occur in 1 to 3 percent of AMIs and accounts for approximately 5 percent of all infarct-related deaths.[426] Ventricular septal rupture occurs with an approximately equal frequency between anterior and inferior infarctions. There is a higher prevalence in first infarctions and the majority occur within the first week. Some 20 to 30 percent may develop as early as the first 24 h after the infarction.[427,428] Septal rupture rarely occurs after 2 weeks. Ventricular septal rupture is usually manifest by the appearance of a new harsh, holosystolic murmur along the left sternal border (often associated with a thrill) and sudden clinical deterioration with hypotension and pulmonary congestion. Right ventricular volume overload secondary to the shunt may produce signs of systemic venous congestion out of proportion to those of pulmonary venous congestion. Often the event is heralded by a recurrence of chest pain.

The diagnosis can be established by two-dimensional and Doppler echocardiographic studies that will demonstrate the site and approximate size of the rupture as well as the left-to-right shunt. Right-heart catheterization is useful in confirming the diagnosis (an increase in $O_2$ saturation of >5 percent from right atrium to right ventricle) and is an aid in managing the patient. The primary diagnostic concern is to exclude rupture of the papillary muscle. The presence of a thrill or an anterior infarction would be unusual with papillary muscle rupture, and results of the Doppler echocardiographic studies and/or the oxygen step-up on right side of the heart catheterization would confirm the presence of septal rupture.

When medical therapy alone is used, most patients with ventricular septal rupture deteriorate rapidly and virtually all patients die, many within 24 h after rupture. Except for the rare case in which there is no clinical or hemodynamic deterioration, medical therapy can be expected to be ineffective. *It is now axiomatic, that upon discovery of rupture of the ventricular septum, prompt surgical repair should take place, even for those patients who are clinically stable.* Inotropic and vasopressor agents may be required to sustain arterial blood pressure but can increase the left-to-right shunt. Prompt but temporary stabilization can be achieved with intraaortic balloon counterpulsation alone or in conjunction with vasodilator and inotropic drug therapy. Cardiac catheterization should be performed in an expeditious manner to define cardiac anatomy, left ventricular function, and mitral valve competence. An aggressive approach of immediate operative repair of these patients results in a short-term survival rate of 42 to 75 percent.[429–431] The 5-year actuarial survival rate for the operative survivors has been reported to be as high as 88 percent.[432] Surgical results are worse when ventricular septal rupture complicates inferior infarction and when there is combined right ventricular and septal dysfunction.[431]

CARDIAC RUPTURE ACC/AHA recommendations are as follows[1]:

Class I

1. Patients with free wall rupture should be considered for urgent cardiac surgical repair, unless further support is considered futile based on patient's wishes or contraindications/unsuitability for further invasive care.
2. CABG should be undertaken at the same time as repair of the LV free wall rupture (*level of evidence B*).

Cardiorrhexis, or rupture of the heart, occurs in up to 24 percent of fatal AMIs. After cardiogenic shock and arrhythmias, it is the most common cause of death. The free wall of the ventricle is the most common site of rupture.[433]

Rupture of the free wall generally occurs within the first 2 weeks of the infarction and may occur within the first 24 h.[427,428] Rupture occurring after this interval usually represents extension of the infarction or rupture through a false aneurysm.[434]

The rupture occurs primarily in the left ventricle, with a fairly even distribution between the anterior, inferior, and lateral walls. Given the relatively smaller number of lateral infarctions, the incidence of rupture with lateral wall infarctions would presumably be relatively smaller than at other sites.[435] Free wall rupture is more likely to occur with the initial myocardial infarction, in women, in the sixth decade of life or later, and in patients with systemic arterial hypertension, particularly if there is no associated ventricular hypertrophy.[427] The prolonged use of corticosteroids might predispose a patient to cardiac rupture.

Cardiac rupture generally presents as sudden, unanticipated death. Symptoms such as pain, agitation, sinus tachycardia, or vagally mediated bradycardia seldom precede death by more than minutes. Occasionally, intermittent chest pain and/or transient hypotension may precede and portend the final catastrophic event. Cardiac rupture is diagnosed terminally by the development of electromechanical disassociation in the setting of recurrent chest pain. Few cases, and only those with immediate recognition, can be salvaged. Even these few cases require heroic measures, such as immediate pericardiocentesis, emergency thoracotomy, and surgical repair.

## OTHER COMPLICATIONS OF ACUTE MYOCARDIAL INFARCTION

***Pulmonary Embolism*** ACC/AHA recommendations are as follows[1]:

Class I

1. Deep venous thrombosis (DVT) or pulmonary embolism (PE) after STEMI should be treated with full-dose low-molecular-weight heparin (LMWH) for a minimum of 5 days and until the patient is adequately anticoagulated with warfarin. Start warfarin concurrently with LMWH and titrate to an INR of 2 to 3 (*level of evidence A*).
2. Patients with CHF post-STEMI, hospitalized for prolonged periods, unable to ambulate, or considered at high risk with DVT and not otherwise anticoagulated should receive low-dose heparin prophylacticly, preferably with low molecular weight heparin (*level of evidence A*).

The prevalence of deep venous thrombosis in AMI is reported to be between 12 and 38 percent. Patients with large infarctions in any location, anterior infarctions, evidence of CHF, and complicated infarctions have a greater frequency of deep venous thrombosis.[436,437] Reduced cardiac output and immobilization are additional predisposing factors for deep venous thrombosis (see Chap. 101).

Venous thrombosis is usually a minor and frequently unrecognized complication of infarction but is potentially life-threatening. A prevalence of pulmonary embolism of 10 to 15 percent and a prevalence of fatal embolism in 3 to 6 percent of cases has been reported in the past.[438] More recently, pulmonary embolism has been reported to account for less than 1 percent of deaths in myocardial infarction, probably because of earlier ambulation and better therapy of low output.[434]

Early mobilization combined with therapy directed toward improving cardiac output, when appropriate, is probably the most effective means of preventing pulmonary emboli. Prophylactic anticoagulant therapy is not routinely recommended for all patients after a myocardial infarction but is advisable for patients with increased risk factors for deep venous thrombosis and pulmonary embolism.

***Systemic Emboli*** Emboli to the cerebrovascular, renal, mesenteric, iliofemoral, or other arterial systems may complicate the AMI. The reported prevalence of clinically apparent systemic emboli in patients with myocardial infarction varies from 0.6 to 6.4 percent.[439,440] These emboli result from dislodgement of left ventricular thrombi, which are found in 20 to 40 percent of anterior myocardial infarctions. A ventricular thrombus is unusual in patients with an inferior infarction.[440,441] The predilection of the apical wall for thrombus development appears to be related to a combination of stagnant blood flow and poor wall contractility. Severe depression of left ventricular function is not a prerequisite for thrombus formation. The development of a mural thrombus in a small infarction (CK $<$ 1000 U), however, is unusual.[442,443] Thrombus morphology and mobility would seem to correlate with systemic embolization.[439,444,445] Pedunculated and freely mobile thrombi have been thought to have a greater chance of embolization. At least two studies, however, could not correlate risk of embolization to any particular thrombus morphology.[440,443]

Left ventricular thrombosis usually occurs within the first 3 days after a myocardial infarction,[443,446] but it may occur at any time during the hospital course. Early mural thrombosis occurs in large infarctions that have an unfavorable prognosis.[443] Systemic embolization occurs an average of 14 days after AMI and is unlikely to occur after more than 4 to 6 weeks.[447] Anticoagulation appears to reduce the incidence of mural thrombus formation[448] and the prevalence of systemic embolization.[439,441,442] All patients with an anterior myocardial infarction should have two-dimensional echocardiography performed within 24 to 72 h following the infarction, with particular emphasis on the two- and four-chamber apical views. Those with a severe apical wall contraction abnormality (akinesis or dyskinesis) should receive heparin for several days, followed by warfarin (INR 2 to 3) for 1 to 3 months. In patients with a left ventricular thrombus demonstrated by echocardiographic studies, chronic warfarin therapy (Chap. 54) is continued for approximately 3 months. Warfarin administration should be maintained indefinitely for atrial fibrillation.

Two-dimensional echocardiography has a sensitivity of 83 to 95 percent and a specificity of 86 to 90 percent in diagnosing a mural thrombus.[440,442,443,449] Angiography has a sensitivity of 20 to 63 percent and a specificity of 67 to 75 percent.[439,450] Occasionally, a technically unsatisfactory echocardiogram may require the use of alternative noninvasive imaging modalities. Both computed tomography and magnetic resonance imaging offer a similar sensitivity and perhaps superior specificity to echocardiography in this setting.[450]

***Ventricular Aneurysm*** The true prevalence of ventricular aneurysm after myocardial infarction is not well defined. Probably the best approximation comes from postmortem studies estimating a 3 to 15 percent prevalence.[446,451] The Coronary Artery Surgery Study (CASS) registry documented angiographically defined left ventricular aneurysms in 7.6 percent of patients with coronary artery disease. The location of the aneurysm is usually anterior, anteroapical, or apical. True posterior ventricular aneurysms located in the diaphragmatic wall between the septum and insertion of the posterior papillary muscle have been observed but are quite uncommon.[452]

Pathologically, the aneurysmal area is characterized by a thinned-out transmural scar that has completely lost its trabecular pattern. The scar, which may eventually calcify, is clearly delineated from surrounding ventricular muscle. Aneurysms characteristically have a wide base (the diameter of the mouth is equal to or larger than its greatest internal diameter), and half are lined by a laminated thrombus.[453]

As many as 80 percent of chronic ventricular aneurysms can be diagnosed clinically by the presence of an abnormal precordial impulse, most often located in the third left intercostal space at the midclavicular line; a typical bulge on the left ventricular border on chest x-ray, frequently with calcification around the apex; and ECG evidence of a large anterior infarction with ST-segment elevation persisting beyond 2 weeks following the infarction. Two-dimensional echocardiographic studies can confirm the diagnosis.[440] Left ventricular aneurysms are associated with a reduced survival rate. The prognosis for these patients, however, is primarily related to the left ventricular dysfunction and not to the presence of the aneurysm. True ventricular aneurysms rarely rupture. In fact, the survival rate for patients with an aneurysm is no different than that for patients without an aneurysm but with a similar degree of left ventricular dysfunction. Moreover, the incidence of sudden death is no different. Whether or not clinical recognition of the presence of a ventricular aneurysm is important in the management of the patient after STEMI remains to be answered.[449]

Most patients with ventricular aneurysms should be treated the same as any other postinfarction patient with a similar degree of left ventricular dysfunction. Vasodilators, digoxin, anticoagulants, and antiarrhythmics should be used, based not on the presence of the aneurysm but as dictated by presence of heart failure, mural thrombi, and life-threatening arrhythmias. Occasionally, surgical resection of the aneurysm is justified in order to correct refractory heart failure, recurrent life-threatening arrhythmias, or multiple systemic emboli. The aneurysm resection should usually be combined with coronary bypass grafting and, in cases of ventricular arrhythmias, should be guided by electrophysiologic mapping.

***Pseudoaneurysm*** A pseudoaneurysm is a rare complication of myocardial infarction; its prevalence is not known. The probable sequence of events in the development of a pseudoaneurysm is as follows: occurrence of a transmural infarction with localized pericarditis arising at the site of infarction; development of adhesions between the visceral and parietal pericardium; rupture of the infarcted myocardium, with the extravasated blood confined by the adherent pericardium; progressive enlargement of the aneurysmal sac; and development of thrombus within the sac.[434]

Unlike a true ventricular aneurysm, a pseudoaneurysm has a narrow base (site of rupture). The wall is composed only of a thrombus and pericardium, and the risk of rupture is high.[454] While the neck is small (its diameter is $<50$ percent of the diameter of the fundus), the pseudoaneurysm may progressively enlarge to become larger than the left ventricle. The pseudoaneurysm may be clinically silent or may present as progressively worsening heart failure, an abnormal bulge on the cardiac border, persistent ST-segment elevation in the area overlying the infarction, or systolic murmurs.[455]

The diagnosis can be established by two-dimensional echocardiographic studies, ventriculographic radionuclide studies, magnetic resonance imaging (MRI), or left ventriculographic contrast studies.[454] Surgical resection is always indicated.

***Arrhythmias and Conduction Disturbances Complicating Acute Myocardial Infarction*** Arrhythmias and conduction disturbances that are likely to be significant problems during the early phases of AMI and their management have been discussed earlier, under "Evaluation and Management of the Patients with Chest Pain in the Emergency Department." The arrhythmias and conduction abnormalities discussed include sinus bradycardia, AV block, idioventricular rhythm, VT, and VF. In general, the acute management of these rhythm disturbances is the same in the early and in the late phases of AMI. Sustained VT and VF are exceptions, however, in that their occurrence after the first 24 h has more ominous implications for long-term electrical instability and sudden cardiac death. Other rhythm and conduction abnormalities that may be manifest throughout the course of AMI and are not characteristically associated with the early phases are discussed here.

VENTRICULAR ECTOPY, VENTRICULAR TACHYCARDIA, AND VENTRICULAR FIBRILLATION The management of VT and VF after the first 24 h of hospitalization for AMI is similar to that discussed for the early phase. The occurrence of symptomatic, sustained VT or VF in the later phases of the hospital course, however, suggests that a chronic arrhythmogenic focus may be developing in the damaged ventricle. These ventricular arrhythmias are classified as secondary and indicate increased risk for subsequent sudden cardiac death. These clinical developments are usually an indication for electrophysiologic evaluation and consideration for implantation of an automatic intracardiac defibrillator (AICD) (see Chaps. 31, 34, and 38).

***Intracardiac Defibrillator (ICD) Implantation in Patients after STEMI*** ACC/AHA recommendations are as follows[1]:

Class I

1. An ICD is indicated for patients with VF or hemodynamically significant sustained VT greater than three days post-STEMI, provided the arrhythmia is not judged to be due to transient or reversible ischemia or reinfarction (*level of evidence A*).

Class IIa

1. If there is a reduced ejection fraction (EF) (40 percent or less), nonsustained VT 4 to 30 days post-STEMI, an inducible VT on EPS, an ICD may be indicated (*level of evidence B*).
2. If there is a reduced EF (30 percent or less), at least one month post-STEMI, an ICD may be indicated (*level of evidence B*).
3. If there is a reduced EF (31 to 40 percent) more than 30 days post-STEMI, nonsustained VT, and inducible VT on EPS, an ICD may be indicated.

Class IIb

1. If there is a reduced EF (30 percent or less) within 30 days of MI and no sustained VT that needs to be monitored, the benefit of an ICD is uncertain and the EF should be repeated more than 30 days after STEMI.

Class III

1. If there is an EF greater than 40 percent without VF or sustained VT, ICD is not indicated.

***Sinus Tachycardia or Atrial Premature Beats*** Sinus tachycardia following AMI is common and is frequently an unfavorable prognostic sign. The increased heart rate enhances myocardial oxygen demand, while the decreased diastolic time decreases diastolic coronary flow. Patients with a large area of infarcted myocardium may have sinus tachycardia on the basis of left ventricular dysfunction, which causes reflex sympathetic nervous system activation. Other obvious causes of sinus tachycardia—such as fever, anxiety, pain, pulmonary embolism, anemia, hypovolemia, or hypoxemia—must be evaluated and treated. Sinus tachycardia may occur as a result of the effects of drugs such as dobutamine, dopamine, theophylline, and atropine.[456] In the absence of precipitating causes, a persistent sinus tachycardia most likely reflects progressive left ventricular dysfunction, which should be evaluated and managed accordingly.

Frequent atrial premature complexes are relatively common in AMI and are caused by atrial ischemia or infarction and pericarditis.[456–460] No specific therapy is indicated; rather, attention should be given to the underlying disease process.

PAROXYSMAL SUPRAVENTRICULAR TACHYCARDIA Episodes of paroxysmal supraventricular tachycardia occur rather commonly in AMI and are usually transient.[457] Underlying causes are similar to those of atrial premature complexes. For reasons discussed, the tachycardia may worsen ischemia. Rate control is essential, and the therapeutic approaches—which may include carotid sinus massage, adenosine, digoxin, verapamil, or diltiazem—are discussed in Chaps. 29 and 30.

ATRIAL FLUTTER AND ATRIAL FIBRILLATION Atrial flutter is relatively uncommon in AMI, whereas atrial fibrillation has an incidence of 10 to 15 percent.[457,458] Atrial fibrillation is associated with an increased in-hospital mortality rate, probably because it is associated with large infarcts and is seen relatively more commonly in older patients and those with cardiac failure, complex ventricular arrhythmias, advanced AV block, atrial infarction, and pericarditis.[461] The pathophysiologic implications are similar to those for paroxysmal supraventricular tachycardia in that a rapid ventricular response can worsen ischemia and infarction by increasing oxygen consumption. Furthermore, the loss of atrial transport can worsen cardiac output and lead to hemodynamic instability.

Atrial fibrillation increases in incidence with age; it occurs in less than 5 percent of patients with AMI under the age of 60 and in about 16 percent of those over age 70.[1] The incidence of atrial fibrillation has been reported to be lower in patients receiving thrombolytic therapy than in control patients.[462]

Systemic embolization occurs more commonly in AMI in the presence of atrial fibrillation (1.7 percent) than in its absence (0.6 percent). Fifty percent of these emboli occur during the first hospital day and 90 percent have occurred by the fourth day.[463] Thus, heparin therapy is indicated in patients not already receiving it, despite the fact that the rhythm is usually transient.

If the patient experiences new or worsening pain, ischemic ST-segment changes, or hemodynamic instability during atrial fibrillation with a rapid ventricular response rate, immediate electrical cardioversion is indicated. In the conscious patient, brief anesthesia is indicated (see Chaps. 28 and 29).

If the clinical situation is less urgent, the ventricular rate can be reduced with drugs. Rapid digitalization with intravenous digoxin is effective but will not result in an immediate response, which may take 1 to 2 h. In the absence of contraindications such as CHF or bronchospastic pulmonary disease, intravenously administered beta-blocking drugs are highly effective in slowing the ventricular rate. Intravenous administration of the calcium channel blockers, verapamil or diltiazem, can also be effective in slowing the ventricular response, but these are not considered to be first-line drugs.

Firm recommendations have not been made about the use of class I and III antiarrhythmics to prevent the recurrence of atrial fibrillation in AMI.[1] Since recurrence is associated with a worse prognosis, however, it seems prudent to consider amiodarone or sotalol or, alternatively, quinidine or procainamide. Neither anticoagulation nor antiarrhythmic therapy should be continued for the long term. With stable sinus rhythm, either or both, as the case may be, should be stopped after 6 weeks.

JUNCTIONAL RHYTHM An escape AV junctional rhythm at a rate of 40 to 60 beats per minute in patients with inferior myocardial infarction and high-degree heart block is not uncommon.[457] Therapy usually is not required. Accelerated junctional rhythms are occasionally seen in AMI, more likely at rates of 70 to 130 beats per minute,[464] but are rarely seen at considerably higher rates. Treatment generally focuses on the underlying conditions, such as ischemia or digitalis toxicity.

HEART BLOCK First-, second-, and third-degree AV blocks have been discussed briefly. First-degree block is frequently seen in AMI, especially in inferior myocardial infarction. This is attributable to ischemia or enhanced vagal activity. It can be worsened by drugs such as beta blockers. Treatment is seldom required.

Second-degree AV block is also relatively common, especially Mobitz type I or Wenckebach block. This block, characterized by progressive lengthening of the PR interval before the atrial beat, is not conducted and may occur in as many as 10 percent of AMI patients.[465] It is associated with a narrow QRS and frequently is the result of AV node ischemia in inferior myocardial infarction. It is usually transient, and its presence does not affect the prognosis. Mobitz type II block is uncommon but is associated with more serious complications and a worse prognosis. It usually occurs with anterior myocardial infarction and reflects trifascicular block. It is characterized by a wide QRS and a nonvarying PR interval before a nonconducted atrial beat. Heart block may develop suddenly and is an ominous sign, with a mortality of about 80 percent. It is usually permanent.

Third-degree AV block, or complete heart block, occurs in about 5 percent of patients with AMI and is most commonly seen with inferior infarction, usually with block at the AV node. As indicated, complete heart block in inferior myocardial infarction is usually transient and may occur early or late in the hospital course with the same implications for prognosis. There is some increase in in-hospital mortality rates in this setting, but complete heart block in inferior myocardial infarction is not an independent predictor of poor long-term prognosis.[280] In contrast, patients with anterior infarction who develop third-degree AV block have a mortality rate of 80 percent.[466] Implications for temporary and permanent pacing are discussed further on.

INTRAVENTRICULAR CONDUCTION DISTURBANCES The development of bundle branch block during AMI usually signifies an extensive infarct. In one multicenter trial, the presence of bundle branch block was associated with a twofold increase in the in-hospital mortality rate (28 vs. 14 percent), compared with the absence of bundle branch block.[283,467] Data indicate that the presence of bundle branch block identifies patients who (1) are more likely to develop CHF, (2) are more likely to develop high-degree heart block, (3) are more likely to have an episode of ventricular fibrillation, and (4) have a higher mortality rate.[467]

INDICATIONS FOR TEMPORARY TRANSVENOUS PACING The recommendations are as follows[2]:

Class I

1. Asystole
2. Symptomatic bradycardia (including sinus bradycardia with hypotension and type I second-degree AV block with hypotension not responsive to atropine)
3. Bilateral bundle branch block (alternating or right bundle branch block with alternating left anterior fascicular/posterior fascicular block; any age)
4. New or indeterminate-age bifascicular block (right bundle branch block with left anterior or posterior fascicular block) with first-degree AV block
5. Mobitz type II second-degree AV block

Class IIa
1. Right bundle branch block and left anterior or left posterior fascicular block (new or indeterminate)
2. Right bundle branch block with first-degree AV block
3. Left bundle branch block, new or indeterminate
4. Incessant VT, for atrial or ventricular overdrive pacing
5. Recurrent sinus pauses (greater than 3 s) not responsive to atropine

Class IIb
1. Bifascicular block of indeterminate age
2. New or age-indeterminate isolated right bundle branch block

Class III
1. First-degree heart block
2. Type I second-degree AV block with normal hemodynamics
3. Accelerated idioventricular rhythm
4. Bundle branch block or fascicular block known to exist before AMI

Cardiac pacing is discussed in Chap. 32. The indications generally agreed on for temporary pacemaker insertion in AMI include asystole, complete heart block in the setting of anterior myocardial infarction, new onset of right or left bundle branch block with persistent Mobitz II second-degree AV block in the setting of anterior myocardial infarction, or other symptomatic bradycardias unresponsive to atropine.[166]

Bundle branch block in the setting of AMI, as noted, identifies a population at risk for both electrical and mechanical complications. Such patients must be monitored for evidence of transient high-degree heart block. Prolonged intermediate care with telemetry monitoring and repeat assessments of heart failure status are important.

***Permanent Pacing*** The recommendations are as follows[2]:

Class I
1. Persistent second-degree AV block in the His-Purkinje system with bilateral bundle branch block or complete heart block after AMI
2. Transient advanced (second- or third-degree) AV block and associated bundle branch block
3. Symptomatic AV block at any level

Class IIb
1. Persistent advanced (second- or third-degree) block at the level of the AV node

Class III
1. Transient AV conduction disturbances in the absence of intraventricular conduction defects
2. Transient AV block in the presence of isolated left anterior fascicular block
3. Acquired left anterior fascicular block in the absence of AV block
4. Persistent first-degree AV block in the presence of bundle branch block that is old or age-indeterminate

The use of permanent pacemakers is discussed in detail in Chap. 32. The subject is reviewed extensively in the ACC/AHA guidelines for pacemaker implantation.[468] That temporary pacing may have been required in the course of AMI does not necessarily indicate a need for permanent pacing. Patients who have had permanent pacemakers inserted after AMI usually have a relatively unfavorable prognosis primarily related to the extensiveness of the underlying disease and myocardial damage.[2] Thus, these patients are at increased risk for death from progressive CHF and VTs. The generally accepted indications for insertion of a permanent pacemaker after AMI are summarized in the previous recommendations.

## DISCHARGE FROM THE CORONARY CARE UNIT

The length of stay in the CCU should be based on the risk of developing VT and VF. The risk of developing primary VF after AMI decreases exponentially, with the majority of arrhythmic deaths occurring within the first 24 h. After the third day, the episodes of life-threatening arrhythmias are fairly evenly distributed over the remainder of the hospitalization.[469] Thus, a patient with an uncomplicated infarction can be transferred from the CCU on the third day. Since 31 to 34 percent of in-hospital deaths from AMI occur after discharge from the CCU and half of them are sudden and unexpected, certain patients need more prolonged cardiac monitoring.[470,471] Those patients who are prime candidates for late-hospital sudden deaths manifest, while in the CCU, one or more of the following: (1) the arrhythmias of pump failure (sinus tachycardia, atrial flutter, or atrial fibrillation); (2) the arrhythmias of electrical instability (VT or VF); (3) acute interventricular conduction disturbances; (4) evidence of circulatory failure (CHF, pulmonary edema, or significant hypotension); or (5) large anterior infarction. The effectiveness of prolonged monitoring of this select group of patients in an intermediate care unit following CCU discharge is evident in a doubling of the rate of successful resuscitations.[472,473] Patients who do not fit into these high-risk subgroups can be discharged from the CCU to a medical unit without continuous monitoring. The wide availability of continuous monitoring in many hospitals in nonacute care units, however, permits easy further monitoring even on lower-risk patients and is preferable if available.

The activity permitted the patient with uncomplicated infarction has changed immensely during the last two decades. In an uncomplicated myocardial infarction, the patient does not need to be confined to bed for longer than 24 h. In fact, the patient may use a bedside commode from the time of admission. The safety and benefits of chair rest were initially promoted by Samuel Levine and Bernard Lown in 1951.[474] Upon transfer from a CCU, the patient should be started on a program of progressive ambulation. The speed with which the patient progresses from one stage to the next depends on the severity of the infarction, the presence or absence of complications, the patient's age, and the presence of comorbid conditions. The length of hospitalization following an AMI should likewise depend on these same factors. If the patient has not manifested the arrhythmias of pump failure or electrical instability, evidence of circulatory failure, or advanced AV block during the first 4 days of hospitalization, he or she is very unlikely to do so at any later time.[475] This patient could probably be discharged after 7 or fewer days in the hospital.[476] The last 2 to 3 days of the hospitalization are generally necessary to resolve the questions pertaining to residual ventricular function, the presence or absence of ventricular ectopy, and the adequacy of the remainder of the coronary circulation. In addition, time is needed for instruction in risk-factor modification (see Chap. 43 and 60). As discussed previously, time in the hospital is being shortened, especially after successful thrombolysis.

### Noninvasive Risk Stratification in Patients Surviving Acute Myocardial Infarction

The purpose of risk stratification of patients surviving AMI assumes that the information provided will enhance decision making, resulting in improved long-term outcome. While numerous tests provide prognostic information, only some have resulted in a treatment strategy that improves outcome. No single noninvasive cardiac test better exemplifies this potential "benefit gap" than ventricular premature beats after AMI, which are associated with an increased risk of death; however, no antiarrhythmic intervention has been demonstrated to reduce mortality; some have even paradoxically increased the mortality rate.[477]

Survivors of AMI have a substantial risk of incurring subsequent cardiovascular events. Noninvasive risk assessment provides useful information to individualize the extent of further workup and therapy by (1) targeting specific long-term therapies that are established to alter mortality and morbidity; (2) identifying high-risk patients requiring aggressive diagnostic tests and therapies; (3) identifying low-risk groups as targets for a conservative approach emphasizing early discharge and established long-term prophylactic therapies; (4) providing information that facilitates counseling the patient on prognosis; (5) providing data to recommend an exercise program; and (6) providing information used in planning and prioritizing modifications of lifestyle.

Three interrelated prognostic factors are the focus of predischarge assessment: (1) assessment of left ventricular function, (2) detection of myocardial ischemia (jeopardized myocardium), and (3) assessment of the risk of arrhythmic (sudden cardiac) death. Most proposed algorithms of noninvasive test selection focus on these three important clinical areas.[478,479] High-risk patients can be clinically identified, as previously discussed, without such noninvasive assessments because of evidence of one or more of the following: decompensated CHF, angina associated with ECG changes, in-hospital cardiac arrest, spontaneous sustained VT, or the development of a high-degree heart block.[480–483] In contrast to these high-risk groups, the majority of postinfarct patients have a relatively benign hospital course. In these patients, noninvasive testing can accurately identify a group at very low risk whose annual mortality is 1 to 3 percent.[331,332,484,485] The practical consequences of identifying a low-risk group is that emphasis is focused on early discharge, lifestyle modification, and targeted prophylactic medical therapy rather than expensive, invasive diagnostic testing.

Since there is general agreement that early coronary angiography and aggressive interventional therapy are indicated in patients with recurrent episodes of spontaneous angina or ischemia or with evidence of persistent decompensated CHF or cardiogenic shock, the emphasis will be on the noninvasive evaluation of asymptomatic patients.

## ASSESSMENT OF LEFT VENTRICULAR FUNCTION AND LEFT VENTRICULAR EJECTION FRACTION

Many clinical features are associated with an increased risk for the development of CHF, including anterior and anterolateral infarction, papillary muscle dysfunction and associated mitral regurgitation, as well as recurrent AMI and the development of transient episodes of high-degree heart block. CHF in the setting of inferior AMI associated with right ventricular infarction is also a prognostically important category necessitating an aggressive management strategy, as discussed. Measurement of LVEF is mandatory in such patients but also useful in patients without such obvious left ventricular dysfunction. Left ventricular ejection fraction can be assessed by either echocardiographic, radionuclide, or angiographic techniques.[486,487] Left ventricular ejection fraction is an important determinant of survival after AMI regardless of reperfusion status. In-hospital mortality is directly related to the severity of left ventricular dysfunction. In the absence of significant ischemia or ventricular arrhythmias, patients with a LVEF >40 percent have mortality rates in the range of 5 percent over 1 to 2 years, whereas a LVEF of 30 to 39 percent or <30 percent have mortality rates that increase to 10 to 15 percent and 20 to 25 percent, respectively.[478,486,487] Although measured much less frequently, the end-systolic volume index is also an accurate predictor of survival following AMI.[487,488]

In the prethrombolytic era, the Multicenter Postinfarction Research Group (MPRG) reported long-term follow-up in 799 patients. The majority of deaths occurred with patients with a LVEF <40 percent, with a 1-year mortality rate of 47 percent in patients with an LVEF <20 percent.[489]

In more recent trials utilizing thrombolytic therapy, survival at any increment of LVEF is better with patients receiving thrombolytic therapy than patients with identical LVEF without thrombolytic therapy. This may be due to the improvement in arterial patency and prevention of long-term remodeling.[490–492] Although LVEF is routinely measured within the first week of AMI, LVEF may be underestimated in patients with significant myocardial infarction; this can be clarified by a repeat measurement of LVEF within the first 1 to 2 months. Postinfarction measurement of a normal LVEF (e.g., LVEF >50 percent) identifies a very low risk group (1-year mortality = 1.2 percent), as noted in multiple large thrombolysis trials.[491,492]

Clinical reflections of the degree of left ventricular systolic dysfunction include the patient's exercise capacity as judged by exercise testing and/or the New York Heart Association clinical classification, which is an independent predictor of outcome. Patients with good exercise capacity, even in the presence of a reduced ejection fraction, have a superior long-term outcome in comparison with those who cannot perform mild-to-moderate exercise.[493]

## ASSESSMENT OF MYOCARDIAL ISCHEMIA

***Role of Exercise Testing*** ACC/AHA recommendations for exercise testing for myocardial ischemia after STEMI are as follows[1]:

Class I

1. Exercise testing should be performed in STEMI patients not selected for cardiac catheterization and without high-risk features to assess the presence and extent of inducible ischemia, either in-hospital or early postdischarge (*level of evidence B*).
2. In patients with baseline abnormalities which compromise ECG interpretation, echocardiography or myocardial perfusion imaging should be added to standard exercise testing (*level of evidence B*).

Class IIb

1. It is debatable whether to perform exercise testing prior to discharge of patients recovering from STEMI to guide postdischarge exercise prescription (*level of evidence B*).

Class III

1. Stress testing should not be performed within two to three days of STEMI in patients who have not undergone successful reperfusion.
2. Stress testing should not be performed to evaluate patients with STEMI who have unstable postinfarction angina, decompensated CHF, life-threatening cardiac arrhythmias, or noncardiac conditions that severely limit the ability to exercise.
3. Stress testing should not be used for risk stratification in patients with STEMI who have already been selected for cardiac catheterization. In this situation an exercise test may be useful after catheterization to evaluate function or identify ischemia in the distribution of a coronary lesion of borderline severity.

Exercise testing provides useful information for risk stratification, determining the need for coronary angiography, and prognosis. During the hospitalization of patients recovering from AMI, a practical and safe approach to exercise testing has been to utilize a submaximal treadmill exercise protocol (modified Naughton or modified Bruce protocol) rather than the standard Bruce protocol.[494] The target for completing the test is often symptom-limited exercise to a specific heart rate goal (e.g., 70 to 75 percent age-predicted) or to a peak work level (e.g., 5 metabolic equivalents, or METs) unless other factors (>2 mm ST-segment depression, chest pain, ventricular arrhythmia, or hypotension) arise first (see Chap. 16). The exercise ECG more accurately reflects the risk of subsequent ischemic events when baseline ECG is normal.

Exercise testing is also useful in planning the exercise prescription for a cardiac rehabilitation program (see Chap. 60). For safety, patients should be angina-free and free of cardiac failure before exercise testing. Patients selected in this fashion under the supervision of a physician are at minimal risk for complications.[484,485,495,496] A third category in which exercise testing is useful is the assessment of adequacy of antischemic therapy or indication of need for further treatment options.

***Clinical Significance of Predischarge Submaximal Exercise Testing*** Predischarge exercise testing for prognostic assessment is a class I AHA/ACC indication.[497] Numerous studies have analyzed the predictive value of predischarge exercise testing during a 6- to 12-month follow-up after AMI.[484,485] Exercise variables indicating increased risk of cardiac events include (1) exercise-induced ST-segment depression; (2) ST-segment elevation; (3) development of angina during exercise; (4) inadequate blood pressure response to exercise; or (5) exercise of short duration. From the practical standpoint, it is important to consider all of these exercise variables rather than to focus solely on the presence or absence of ST-segment depression. Done appropriately, submaximal exercise testing consistently identifies a high risk for recurrent cardiac events (AMI, unstable angina) or mortality in the first year after the AMI. The ACC/AHA guidelines support the use of submaximal exercise testing in uncomplicated patients with interpretable 12-lead ECGs before discharge.[1]

For patients with a normal exercise test before discharge, symptom-limited maximal exercise testing can be repeated 2 to 6 weeks after AMI. The maximal exercise test can be used to identify additional high-risk patients.[498,499] Since many cardiovascular events can occur in the first 4 to 6 weeks, predischarge assessment of ischemia risk is preferable. Evidence of exercise-induced ischemia generally mandates cardiac catheterization to define the coronary anatomy and the consideration of revascularization (see algorithm in Fig. 52-5[497]). The consensus opinion of the ACC/AHA guidelines management group is that exercise testing is still useful in the risk stratification of STEMI patients who have received thrombolytic therapy and who have not been selected for cardiac catheterization, and it retains a class I indication in uncomplicated patients postinfarction.[1,500,501]

The clinical inference is that the detection of ischemia should lead to coronary arteriography. A randomized trial supports the performance of coronary arteriography in post–myocardial infarction patients with evidence of inducible ischemia before hospital discharge. In the DANAMI trials of 503 patients who survived AMI who were randomized to receive thrombolytic therapy, those patients with evidence of inducible ischemia prior to discharge had a nearly twofold higher cardiac event rate than did a group receiving early invasive intervention.[502] These study results are supportive of the recommendation for performing coronary arteriography in asymptomatic STEMI patients with evidence of inducible ischemia.

***Ambulatory Electrocardiographic Detection of Myocardial Ischemia*** As with other modalities to measure ischemia, the detection of ambulatory ECG ischemia has been predictive of a poor outcome in long-term follow-up trials in patients surviving AMI. The correlations among exercise testing, ambulatory ECGs, and ischemia detected by thallium have some overlap but are not identical.[503] No studies show that a treatment strategy to reduce episodes of silent ischemia result in an improved outcome. Thus, routine ambulatory ECG assessment of ischemia is not recommended.[1,504]

***Detection of Myocardial Ischemia by Imaging*** Adenosine stress perfusion nuclear scintigraphy or dobutamine two-dimensional echocardiography or comparable exercise studies continue to have a class IIa indication. These evaluations become a class I indication when baseline 12-lead ECG abnormalities (e.g. left bundle branch block or significant ST and T wave changes) compromise interpretation.[1]

THALLIUM-201 OR TECHNETIUM-99M SESTAMIBI There are several alternatives to standard exercise testing. One well-studied technique is exercise thallium-201 ($^{201}$Tl) scintigraphy, as discussed previously (see Chap. 19). Exercise $^{201}$Tl scintigraphy has a number of potential advantages over routine exercise testing: (1) it can be used when the 12-lead ECG is uninterpretable for ischemic ST-segment shifts because of baseline changes, such as a left bundle branch block, where it has a class I indication; (2) it allows assessment of reversible and irreversible perfusion defects, both within and outside the vascular region involved in the AMI; (3) the technique of single photon emission computed tomography (SPECT) $^{201}$Tl scintigraphy provides a semiquantitative evaluation of ischemia; (4) exercise $^{201}$Tl scintigraphy offers superior sensitivity and specificity for the detection of multivessel disease when compared with standard exercise testing; and (5) if pharmacologic adenosine stress is used, it can be safely performed on day 3 or 4 after myocardial infarction.[506,507]

High-risk patients are identified if (1) perfusion defects exist in more than one discrete vascular zone; (2) there is distinct evidence of redistribution; or (3) there was evidence of increased lung uptake. Low-risk patients are defined by $^{201}$Tl scintigraphy showing involvement of a single vascular region without redistribution, with no evidence of increased lung uptake. A high-risk $^{201}$Tl scintigram is correlated with multivessel coronary disease. $^{201}$Tl scintigraphy has been shown to be excellent at identifying high-grade stenoses of 90 percent or greater, especially high-grade lesions of the left anterior descending coronary artery.[506]

As in routine exercise testing, a limited number of studies have evaluated the value of pharmacologic stress $^{201}$Tl tomography in patients with thrombolytic therapy, with some conflicting results. Provocative pharmacologic studies using $^{201}$Tl tomography also predicted risk of subsequent ischemic events after AMI.[505] Adenosine pharmacologic stress tomography offers the advantage of allowing the safe assessment of ischemia as early as 2 to 4 days following AMI. In the era of cost containment and pressure for early hospital discharge, this approach, although not proven, may be beneficial in identifying patients who can safely be discharged early.[506,508]

Since adenosine SPECT can safely be performed early in asymptomatic post–myocardial infarction patients,[508] it may gain more general acceptance as the preferred test for post–myocardial infarction ischemia. At present ACC/AHA guidelines give a class I indication to performing this test only when the 12-lead ECG is abnormal (uninterpretable). Adenosine SPECT imaging can identify high-risk patients and also track the relation between therapeutic changes and subsequent changes in risk of cardiac events by tracking changes in perfusion defect size. In a preliminary trial, cardiac event-free sur-

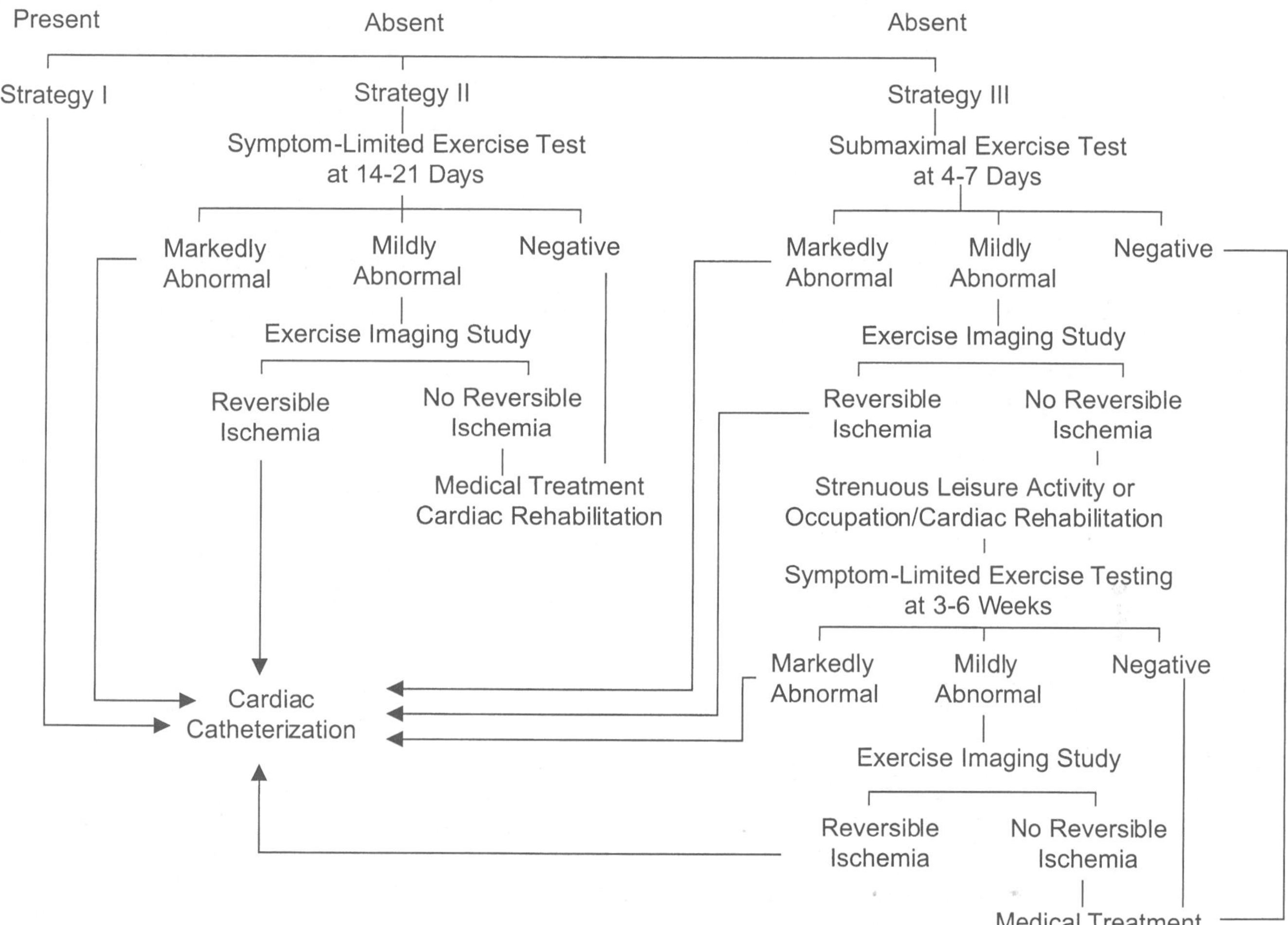


FIGURE 52-5 Strategies for exercise test evaluations soon after myocardial infarction. If patients are at high risk for ischemic events based on clinical criteria, they should undergo invasive evaluation to determine whether they are candidates for coronary revascularization procedures (strategy I). For patients initially deemed to be at low risk at time of discharge after myocardial infarction, two strategies for performing exercise testing can be used. One is a symptom-limited exercise test at 14 to 21 days (strategy II). If the patient is on digoxin or if the baseline ECG precludes accurate interpretation of ST-segment changes (e.g., baseline left bundle branch block or left ventricular hypertrophy), then an initial exercise imaging study can be performed. Results of exercise testing should be stratified to determine need for additional invasive or exercise perfusion studies. Another strategy (strategy III) is to perform a submaximal exercise test at 4 to 7 days after myocardial infarction or just before hospital discharge. The exercise test results may be stratified using the guidelines in strategy I. If exercise test studies are negative, a second symptom-limited exercise test can be repeated at 3 to 6 weeks for patients undergoing vigorous activity during leisure time activities, at work, or exercise training as part of cardiac rehabilitation. A small area contiguous to the infarct zone may not necessarily require catheterization. Modified from ACC/AHA guidelines. (From Gibbons, et al.[498] With permission.)

vival was 96 percent at 1 year for patients in whom the ischemic burden could be reduced to ≤9 percent by pharmacologic and/or invasive therapy.[508] The Adenosine Sestamibi Post-Infarction Evaluation (INSPIRE) trial is a prospective, multicenter, randomized study of 728 patients with recent AMI. Stratification of risk is based on adenosine $^{99m}$Tc sestamibi gated SPECT performed within the first several days postinfarction. High-risk patients (total defect size ≥20 percent and ischemic defect size >10 percent) randomized to coronary intervention or optimal anti-ischemic therapy following scintigraphy at 6 to 8 weeks and clinical followup for 1 year will be used to assess this modality to stratify and track prognosis. Results of this pilot study will be available soon.[507]

Other radionuclide techniques are useful in the evaluation of patients after AMI. These techniques include the use of radionuclide angiography for the assessment of ventricular function, including the evaluation of right ventricular infarction, and the use of technetium pyrophosphate to estimate myocardial infarct size and hibernating myocardium. These are summarized in Table 52-3.[151] The choice between nuclear imaging, stress echocardiography, and standard exercise testing depends on ECG interpretability, test availability, cost, and clinical experience.[508]

ROLE OF ECHOCARDIOGRAPHY ACC/AHA recommendations are as follows[1]:

Class I

1. Echocardiography should be used in patients with STEMI not undergoing left ventricular angiography to assess baseline LV

function, especially if the patient is hemodynamically unstable (*level of evidence C*).

2. Echocardiography should be used to evaluate patients with inferior STEMI, clinical instability, and clinical suspicion of RV infarction (*level of evidence C*).
3. Echocardiography should be used in patients with STEMI to evaluate suspected complications including acute mitral regurgitation, VSR, cardiogenic shock, infarct expansion, ventricular septal rupture, intracardiac thrombus, and pericardial fusion (*level of evidence C*).
4. Stress echocardiography (or myocardial infusion imaging) should be used in patients with STEMI for in-hospital or early post–discharge assessment for inducible ischemia when baseline abnormalities are expected to compromise electrocardiographic interpretation.
5. Dobutamine echocardiography is indicated in hemodynamically and electrically stable patients 4 to 10 days after STEMI to assess myocardial viability when required to define the potential efficacy of revascularization.

Class IIa

1. Echocardiography (or myocardial perfusion imaging) should be used in patients with STEMI for in-hospital or early post-discharge for assessment for inducible ischemia in the absence of baseline abnormalities are expected to compromise ECG abnormalities.
2. Echocardiography should be used in patients with STEMI to reevaluate ventricular function during recovery when results are used to guide therapy.
3. In STEMI patients who have not undergone contrast ventriculorography, echocardiography should be used in patients with STEMI to assess ventricular function after revascularization.

Class III

1. Echocardiography should not be used in patients with STEMI for routine reevaluation in the absence of any change in clinical status or revascularization procedure.

Exercise two-dimensional echocardiography is an alternative technique for identifying postinfarction ischemia. A reversible segmental wall motion defect is felt to represent an area of significant ischemia. Studies from specialized centers with expertise in echocardiography have shown that exercise or pharmacologic stress echocardiographic studies have a high sensitivity and specificity in identifying patients with multivessel coronary disease (see Chap. 15).[509–511]

The definition of high risk on dobutamine stress echocardiograms includes (1) the presence of four or more akinetic or dyskinetic segments in the infarct territory during low-dose dobutamine (an index of infarct size); (2) the presence of two or more coronary artery territories demonstrating abnormal wall motion at rest or during peak-dose dobutamine; and (3) a lack of improvement in wall thickening (i.e., lack of viability) within the infarct region during low-dose dobutamine infusion.[509,510] Like those of $^{201}$Tl scintigraphy, the findings of dobutamine stress echocardiography may provide comparable or superior risk stratification to that of coronary angiography. The procedure is predictive of cardiac events in patients treated with thrombolytic agents as well as in those who did not receive thrombolytic therapy.[512] In general, negative tests with exercise, dipyridamole, or dobutamine echocardiography are associated with a low rate of cardiac events.[509–512] Variation among institutions in expertise in the quality of echocardiographic study and interpretation are limitations to a widespread recommendation for the preferred use of echocardiography.

A multinational study provides long-term validation for the use of pharmacologic stress echocardiography in post–myocardial infarction patients with single-vessel coronary artery disease.[513] Either persantine or dobutamine stress resulted in useful long-term prognostic information, with stress echocardiographic "ischemia" detection associated with high 4-year rates of myocardial infarction. The investigators emphasized that stress echocardiography provided effective risk stratification at a relatively low cost.[513]

***Metanalysis of Various Methodologies of Exercise Testing*** POST–MYOCARDIAL INFARCTION In the comprehensive metanalysis of alternative methodologies of post–myocardial infarction exercise testing by Peterson and colleagues, a few general patterns are apparent (Table 52-14). All exercise testing modalities share a high negative predictive value. However, all testing modalities have a suboptimal positive predictive value. None of the more sophisticated technologies appear to have a positive predictive value for subsequent cardiac events that substantially exceeds that of simple stress echocardiography. The prognostic value of the testing modalities appears equally valid in patients receiving thrombolytic therapy.[514]

## SUGGESTED ALGORITHM FOR THE EVALUATION OF MYOCARDIAL ISCHEMIA AFTER MYOCARDIAL INFARCTION

Based on all of the evaluable data, the task force on practice guidelines for the management of AMI created a strategy for the evaluation of myocardial ischemia after AMI in low-risk patients; this is presented in Fig. 52-5. If there are clinical indications of high risk in given patients, such patients are considered for early cardiac catheterization and coronary angiography, as detailed earlier (strategy I).[1] The evaluation of myocardial ischemia in low-risk patients is alternatively presented for strategies II and III. Strategy III favors using a submaximal exercise test or alternative imaging study prior to hospital discharge. Strategy II alternatively suggests that a symptom-limited exercise test be performed soon after hospital discharge. Regardless of whether exercise testing or a more sophisticated exercise imaging study is ordered in the hospital, a negative test does not preclude the repeat evaluation for myocardial ischemia once the patient is fully ambulatory, after 3 to 6 weeks. Because of the "front-loaded" nature of cardiac events postinfarction, predischarge detection of ischemia seems preferable for guiding both additional diagnostic and therapeutic intervention.

## ASSESSMENT OF THE RISK OF ARRHYTHMIC (SUDDEN CARDIAC) DEATH: OVERVIEW

Although the technology to assess the risk of arrhythmic death in patients after AMI has improved in sophistication, antiarrhythmic therapies to reduce risk have thus far proved disappointing. For comparison, there is consensus that the identification of postinfarction patients with a LVEF of ≤40 percent mandates the use of ACE inhibitors.[314,315,515] Likewise, the identification of asymptomatic postinfarction patients with ischemia indicates the need for early performance of coronary angiography to assess the potential for PTCA or coronary artery bypass surgery.[1] Unfortunately, the identification of asymptomatic but high-risk patients for arrhythmic death after AMI is not similarly associated with a successful treatment strategy. This section addresses AMI patients who are asymptomatic and have not had sustained VT or VF—identifiers that all agree require aggressive management, most commonly the placement of an implantable cardioverter defibrillator (ICD) as discussed.

The preponderance of evidence is that the majority of asymptomatic AMI patients who experienced arrhythmic (sudden cardiac)

TABLE 52-14 Predischarge Risk Stratification Done Using Noninvasive Testing[a]

| Test Result | Sensitivity | | Specificity | | Positive Predictive Value | | Negative Predictive Value | |
|---|---|---|---|---|---|---|---|---|
| | Cardiac Death | Cardiac Death or MI | Cardiac Death | Cardiac Death or MI | Cardiac Death | Cardiac Death or MI | Cardiac Death | Cardiac Death or MI |
| Exercise electrocardiography[b] | | | | | | | | |
| ST-segment depression | 0.42 | 0.44 | 0.75 | 0.70 | 0.04 | 0.16 | 0.98 | 0.91 |
| Impaired systolic blood pressure | 0.44 | 0.23 | 0.79 | 0.87 | 0.11 | 0.21 | 0.96 | 0.88 |
| Limited exercise duration | 0.56 | 0.53 | 0.62 | 0.65 | 0.10 | 0.18 | 0.95 | 0.91 |
| Chest pain on exercise | 0.23 | 0.29 | 0.83 | 0.82 | 0.08 | 0.19 | 0.94 | 0.89 |
| Exercise myocardial perfusion imaging[c] | | | | | | | | |
| Reversible perfusion defect | 0.89 | 0.80 | 0.38 | 0.48 | 0.07 | 0.16 | 0.98 | 0.95 |
| Multiple perfusion defects | 0.64 | 0.75 | 0.71 | 0.76 | 0.07 | 0.17 | 0.98 | 0.97 |
| Exercise ventricular function imaging | | | | | | | | |
| Exercise radionuclide angiography[d] | | | | | | | | |
| Peak EF <40% | 0.63 | 0.60 | 0.77 | 0.75 | 0.27 | 0.31 | 0.94 | 0.91 |
| Change in EF <5% | 0.80 | 0.55 | 0.67 | 0.74 | 0.15 | 0.18 | 0.98 | 0.94 |
| New dyssynergy | — | 0.78 | — | 0.50 | — | 0.17 | — | 0.94 |
| Exercise echocardiography[e] | | | | | | | | |
| Change in EF <5% | — | 0.56 | — | 0.60 | — | 0.14 | — | 0.92 |
| New dyssynergy | 1.00 | 0.62 | 0.62 | 0.79 | 0.18 | 0.48 | 1.00 | 0.86 |
| Pharmacologic stress imaging | | | | | | | | |
| Myocardial perfusion imaging[f] | | | | | | | | |
| Reversible perfusion defect | 0.56 | 0.71 | 0.46 | 0.49 | 0.10 | 0.19 | 0.90 | 0.91 |
| Multiple perfusion defects | — | 0.50 | — | 0.64 | — | 0.17 | — | 0.90 |
| Echocardiography[g] | | | | | | | | |
| New dyssynergy | 0.67 | 0.55 | 0.56 | 0.54 | 0.05 | 0.08 | 0.98 | 0.94 |

[a]All event rates are for 1 year after infarction. EF = ejection fraction; MI = myocardial infarction.
[b]Rate of cardiac death, 3.3%; rate of cardiac death or MI, 7.8%.
[c]Rate of cardiac death, 4.6%; rate of cardiac death or MI, 13.1%.
[d]Rate of cardiac death, 9.3%; rate of cardiac death or MI, 13.2%.
[e]Rate of cardiac death, 5.6%; rate of cardiac death or MI, 15.9%.
[f]Rate of cardiac death, 6.6%; rate of cardiac death or MI, 15.0%.
[g]Rate of cardiac death, 2.5%; rate of cardiac death or MI, 5.0%.
SOURCE: Peterson et al.[515] With permission.

death have had sustained VT and/or VF.[516] A review of selected clinical trials of antiarrhythmic therapy focusing on patients after AMI is presented in Table 52-15[517] for the purpose of demonstrating the total deaths attributable to arrhythmic or sudden cardiac death, which vary widely in the placebo groups of these trials. The Cardiac Arrhythmia Suppression (CAST) trials[477,518] and the Canadian Amiodarone Myocardial Infarction Arrhythmia Trial (CAMIAT)[519] identified high-risk patients after AMI using the criteria of ventricular arrhythmia on ambulatory ECGs. In the placebo groups, the range of death attributable to arrhythmia varied from 48 to 66 percent. The Survival and Ventricular Enlargement (SAVE) trial,[314] the European Myocardial Infarction Amiodarone Trial (EMIAT),[520] and the Survival With Oral d-sotalol (SWORD)[521] trial identified patients after AMI using an ejection fraction cutoff. The range of deaths attributable to arrhythmia in the placebo group was 45 to 67 percent. Patients in trials with a mixture of etiologies of left ventricular dysfunction including old AMI, such as the Studies of Left Ventricular Dysfunction (SOLVD) prevention and SOLVD treatment trials, have a lower percentage of deaths attributable to arrhythmia.[315,515] The wide variation in arrhythmic death rates and the variety of screening tests used to identify high-risk patients highlight the lack of precision of current arrhythmic death classifications.[517]

The changing proportion of deaths over time attributable to arrhythmia and other causes after AMI is conceptually depicted in Fig. 52-6. Sustained VT and VF occur most frequently in the first year following AMI.[478] As ischemic cardiomyopathy develops over many years, deaths attributable to VT/VF decrease and proportionately more "sudden deaths" are attributable to asystole, electromechanical dissociation, or a high-degree heart block.[522] Also, noncardiac conditions emulate the circumstances of VT or VF (for instance, massive pulmonary embolism, ruptured abdominal or thoracic aortic aneurysm, or massive stroke).[517] Thus, the temporal influence on cause-specific mortality after AMI is an important consideration. Risk stratification for arrhythmic death seems most relevant immediately following myocardial infarction (Fig. 52-6).

This discussion is limited to tests available for evaluating asymptomatic patients. The preponderance of evidence does not support a class I or even a class IIa indication for any of the testing modalities

TABLE 52-15 Review of Representative Clinical Trials: Placebo Cause-Specific Mortality

| Trial (No. of Placebo Patients), Entrance Criteria | Mean Follow-up (months) | Annualized Mortality, % | Arrhythmia/SCD, % |
|---|---|---|---|
| CAST I[519] (743), VPC ≥6/VT/AMI | 10 | 4.2 | 62 |
| CAST II[478] (574), VPC ≥6/VT/AMI/EF ≤40% | 18 | 6.4 | 66 |
| SAVE[315] (1116), EF ≤40%/AMI 3–16 d | 42 | 7.1 | 45 |
| SOLVD PREV[516] (2117), No CHF/EF ≤35% | 37 | 5.3 | 31 |
| SOLVD Rx[316] (1294), CHF (II/III) + EF ≤35% | 41 | 11.7 | 22 |
| SWORD[522] (1572), MI, EF ≤40% | 5 | 1.5 | 67 |
| EMIAT[521] (743), MI + <40% | 21 | 7.8 | 49 |
| CAMIAT[520] (596), MI + VPC ≥10 or VT | 20 | 4.7 | 48 |

ABBREVIATIONS: SCD = sudden cardiac death; CAST = Cardiac Arrhythmia Suppression Trial; VPC = ventricular premature complexes; VT = ventricular tachycardia; AMI = acute myocardial infarction; EF = ejection fraction; SAVE = Survival and Ventricular Enlargement; SOLVD = Studies of Left Ventricular Dysfunction; PREV = prevention; CHF = congestive heart failure; Rx = treatment; SWORD = Survival With Oral d-Sotalol; EMIAT = European Myocardial Infarction Amiodarone Trial; CAMIAT = Canadian Amiodarone Myocardial Infarction Arrhythmia Trial.
SOURCE: Adapted from Pratt et al.[518] With permission.

to be discussed. What is lacking in each is the absence of compelling data that the identification of "arrhythmic death risk" is coupled with a strategy to improve outcome.[1]

***Ambulatory Electrocardiographic Recordings: Ventricular Arrhythmias*** Asymptomatic spontaneous ventricular arrhythmias detected on ambulatory ECGs are predictive of an increased risk of arrhythmic (sudden) death in the first 1 to 2 years following AMI.[478,523] The mechanism responsible for the majority of arrhythmic deaths in post–myocardial infarction patients is, as noted, sustained VT or VF.[516] Vulnerability for arrhythmic death appears to be highest in the first year after AMI, probably accounting for half of the first-year mortality.[478,523] Thus, it appears that arrhythmic death risk should be assessed prior to hospital discharge. The use of ambulatory ECG recording to identify a high-risk group, however, has a poor positive predictive value.[518,524] Postinfarction patients with no baseline ventricular arrhythmia on ambulatory ECG recording uniformly have a low risk for arrhythmic death.[478,524] Frequent premature ventricular complexes and nonsustained VT are generally associated with a two- and threefold increased risk, respectively.[13,478,523,524] Because of poor positive predictive value, a fair view from these studies is that for every 100 patients identified with "warning arrhythmias," only 4 to 7 will have arrhythmic death in the 1 to 2 years following infarction. Thus, a treatment strategy that would include routine prophylactic administration of an antiarrhythmic drug would necessitate a superb safety profile, since approximately 95 percent of the patients cannot benefit but all patients would be exposed to potentially lethal proarrhythmic risk. Such potential hazards have been documented to be real in prophylactic antiarrhythmic drug trials.[477,518,521] Thus, ambulatory ECG has an adequate negative predictive value but a poor positive predictive value, consistent with its class IIb rating. The Multicenter Unsustained Tachycardia Trial (MUSTT) trial required unsustained ventricular tachycardia and low LVEF ≤40 percent; it demonstrated an improvement survival with ICD implantation.[525] Because approximately 50 percent of patients had the index myocardial infarction at least 3 years previously, the relevance to AMI risk stratification is very limited.

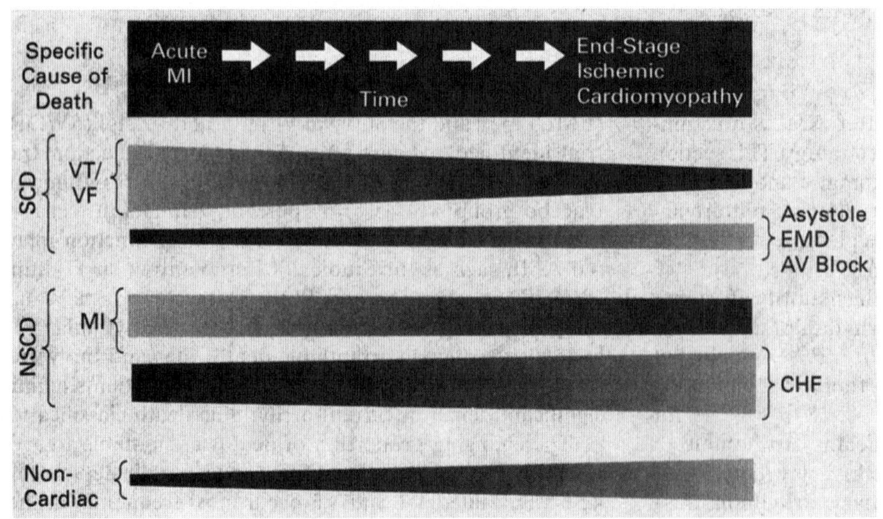


FIGURE 52-6 A theoretical view of approaches to identify a post–myocardial infarction population dying of ventricular tachycardia/fibrillation. This concept is presented in a qualitative fashion and represents estimates based on the literature (see text). SCD = sudden cardiac death; NSCD = non–sudden cardiac death; VT = ventricular tachycardia; VF = ventricular fibrillation; MI = myocardial infarction; EMD = electromechanical dissociation; CHF = congestive heart failure.

***Ambulatory Electrocardiogram Recordings: Heart Rate Variability*** Heart rate variability, measured by the standard deviation of the RR interval on monitored ECG leads, is an indirect assessment of proportional autonomic tone. Extensive variability in the heart rate connotes a preponderance of parasympathetic activity, whereas less variability in the heart rate is consistent with proportionately more sympathetic activity.[526–528] In animal models, enhanced sympathetic activity increases the vulnerability of the ischemic myocardium to the development of VF.[529]

Clinical trials have assessed the relation of heart rate variability to mortality rate in patients surviving AMI. Depressed heart rate variability is associated with an increased risk of death. Multivariate analysis has identified reduced heart rate variability as an independent predictor of arrhythmic death.[526–528,530] In one study, patients selected for depressed heart rate variability and ventricular arrhythmias, excluding patients with the lowest ejection fractions, identified a patient population in whom 75 percent of the deaths were presumed to have been arrhythmic.[531] Heart rate variability measured after thrombolytic therapy still has clinical relevance, and an improvement in heart rate variability correlated with TIMI grade 3 flow.[532]

Practical approaches to minimizing cost while focusing noninvasive testing on a targeted group are under evaluation. In a study of 729 survivors of AMI prior to hospital discharge from St. George's Hospital in London, a 24-h heart rate variability index was compared to a 5-min analysis of an ectopic-free segment of the Holter recording, measuring the standard deviation of normal-to-normal RR intervals (SDNN).[533] The 5-min analysis of SDNN measurement was a useful and inexpensive tool to select patients for more extensive 24-h heart rate variability index evaluation.[534]

The Azimilide Post-Infarct Survival Evaluation (ALIVE) was the first trial to incorporate low heart rate variability as well as low LVEF (15 to 35 percent) to prospectively stratify risk.[534] While azimilide therapy was not associated with a mortality reduction, low heart rate variability did independently identify a high-risk population. The trial did not result in a better clinical outcome based on a strategy using stratification by heart rate variability. Thus, heart rate variability assessment, like other noninvasive "arrhythmic markers," has a class IIb indication.

At present, while heart rate variability is a very promising method of evaluating parasympathetic and sympathetic effects in the heart, it cannot be recommended as a standard clinical test in AMI patients unless and until trials demonstrate an improved outcome to a treatment strategy based upon risk assessment by heart rate variability.[1,535]

***Baroreflex Sensitivity*** Baroreflex sensitivity is another autonomic marker that is a measure of the change in heart rate (anticipated reduction) to an increase in blood pressure. In this respect, it provides an index of the ability to reflexly increase cardiac vagal activity. Heart rate variability, in contrast, is a marker of vagal tone.[536]

The importance of these two autonomic markers is demonstrated by the results of the Autonomic Tone and Reflexes After Myocardial Infarction (ATRAMI) trial, a study of 1284 patients with a recent ( ≤28 days) myocardial infarction.[537] One-year mortality was increased in patients with a reduced baroreflex sensitivity as well as a low heart rate variability (see Table 52-16).[536] There was an additive value to the measurement of the two markers: If both are low there is a 15-fold increased risk of death than if both markers are normal (15 versus 1 percent; $p < 0.0001$). The interaction of LVEF and these autonomic markers is also apparent from Table 52-16, each being associated with a twofold greater risk of death in patients with LVEF <35 percent than it is in those with better preserved left ventricular systolic function. It is reasonable to conclude that both baroreflex sensitivity and heart rate variability have independent prognostic value for stratifying the risk of death after myocardial infarction.[75]

TABLE 52-16 Multivariate Analysis of Influence of Baroreceptor Sensitivity and Heart Rate Variability on Relative One-Year Mortality Risk after Acute Myocardial Infarction

| Variable Examined | Variable in Analysis | Groups | RR | 95% CI | *p* Value |
|---|---|---|---|---|---|
| Baroreflex sensitivity | LVEF | 35–50% | 2.1 | 0.90–4.69 | 0.08 |
| | | <35% | 4.7 | 2.04–10.9 | 0.0003 |
| | BRS (ms/mmHg) | 3.0–6.1 | 1.7 | 0.81–3.69 | 0.15 |
| | | <3.0 | 2.8 | 1.24–6.16 | 0.01 |
| | VPCs per h | ≥10 | 1.8 | 0.94–3.46 | 0.07 |
| Heart rate variability | LVEF (%) | 35–50% | 1.9 | 0.87–4.49 | 0.10 |
| | | <35% | 3.9 | 1.69–9.25 | 0.001 |
| | SDNN | 70–105 | 1.9 | 0.86–4.04 | 0.11 |
| | | <70 | 3.2 | 1.42–7.36 | 0.005 |
| | VPCs per h | ≥10 | 1.8 | 0.97–3.50 | 0.06 |

ABBREVIATIONS: RR = relative rate; CI = confidence interval; LVEF = left ventricular ejection fraction; BRS = baroreflex sensitivity; VPC = ventricular premature complex; SDNN = standard deviation of all normal beats.

SOURCE: Schwartz.[536] With permission.

***Signal-Averaged Electrocardiogram*** Time-domain analysis of the signal-averaged ECG can be used to detect low-amplitude, high-frequency potentials at the end of the QRS complex, termed *ventricular late potentials*. The presence of late potentials identifies patients likely to have inducible sustained monomorphic VT during programmed electrical stimulation and is associated with an increased risk of subsequent arrhythmic events.[526,538,539] The predictive value of late potentials is best established in patients with AMI and is of less established value in other patient populations.

In some studies, an abnormal signal-averaged ECG, frequent ventricular premature complexes on the ambulatory ECG recording, and left ventricular aneurysm were independent predictors of VT, regardless of whether or not a patient had received thrombolytic therapy.[539] If results of the signal-averaged ECG are negative—that is, there are no after depolarizations—the negative predictive value in this population is good and the likelihood of subsequent arrhythmic death low. As with the evaluation of heart rate variability, the interpretation of the signal-averaged ECG can be improved by combining it with other variables, especially the LVEF. Even when multiple tests are combined for assessing the risk of sudden cardiac death, the strength is in their negative rather than their positive predictive value, which usually falls below 50 percent.[538,539] There is an adverse prognostic consequence of a positive signal-averaged ECG and an occluded infarct-related artery.[540] The routine use of signal-averaged ECGs in AMI is not at present recommended.[1]

***T-Wave Alternans*** T wave alternans (TWA) consists of ECG changes in the amplitude, polarity, or contour of the T wave occurring with some regular rhythmic pattern (e.g., every other beat). TWA has been predictive of both spontaneous and inducible ventricular arrhythmias. In some trials, T-wave alternans has been a predictor for cardiac death postinfarction. Variables across studies include the timing of assessment of TWA postinfarction as well as adequacy of pharmacologic therapy at the time of TWA measurement. A number of trials have concluded that TWA is a marker for arrhythmic death, including patients who have had infarctions.[541–545] A number of investigators have assessed the additive power of TWA to proven risk stratifiers like LVEF and nonsustained ventricular tachycardia. While such combined studies appear to be additive in their predictive value, it is not clear if there is improved risk assessment for arrhythmic death or total mortality.

TWA is a heart rate–dependent measure of vulnerability to arrhythmia, with improved accuracy at heart rates in the range of 100 to 120, usually achieved by atrial pacing or low-level exercise testing.[546] Such an approach in postinfarction patients can allow assessment of ischemia as well as potential arrhythmia risk. As with other arrhythmia markers, no trial has used this risk marker to achieve a better clinical outcome in a postinfarction population.

***Invasive Electrophysiologic Testing (Programmed Electrical Stimulation)*** Invasive electrophysiologic assessment has been evaluated in two distinct populations who survived AMI. The first and relatively small group had a cardiac arrest or an episode of sustained VT following an AMI. In such patients, the risk of recurrent cardiac arrest or arrhythmic events is high, and electrophysiologic studies are an alternative for assisting in therapy selection.[547]

The much larger patient populations are those with an increased risk of arrhythmic death based on the results of one or more noninvasive tests, as discussed previously. Performing electrophysiologic studies on all asymptomatic high-risk patients is not justified.[1] Reports on the utility of electrophysiologic studies have been inconsistent in predicting total mortality and are only slightly more consistent in identifying patients likely to have subsequent arrhythmic events.[548,549]

Both Multicenter Automatic Defibrillator Implantation Trials (MADIT) I and II used postinfarction risk markers and had favorable mortality outcomes of implantable defibrillation devices.[550,551] Both used LVEF cutoffs (LVEF 35 and 30 percent respectively for MADIT I and II, respectively), and the former required inducible, nonsuppressible ventricular tachycardia. However, Q-wave infarction was not recent; in fact, recent acute MI was an exclusion in both trials (3 weeks and 1 month, respectively). Thus, the relevance of the MADIT I and II populations to postinfarction risk stratification is tenuous.

The recently published Multicenter Unsustained Tachycardia Trial Investigators (MUSTT) trial enrolled patients with coronary artery disease (90 percent with a previous myocardial infarction), LVEF ≤40 percent, and unsustained ventricular tachycardia.[525] Inducible ventricular tachycardia identified a patient group with a favorable mortality reduction by ICD implantation.

These three trials all show favorable mortality results from ICD using three separate risk stratification strategies. The majority of infarcts in all three trials were old. Relevance to acute infarction risk stratification algorithms is reduced.

***Assessing Arrhythmic Death: Conclusion*** In the ACC/AHA guidelines, none of the noninvasive techniques is generally agreed upon to be beneficial, useful, and effective, either unequivocally (class I) or based on the weight of evidence or opinion (class IIa) for predicting arrhythmic death. These techniques have class IIb indications, meaning that their usefulness and efficacy are not well established by either scientific evidence and/or general opinion.[1] In addition to their poor positive predictive value, no clinical trial has demonstrated that the use of any one or a combination of these modalities of testing identifies a high-risk population in whom an interventional strategy results in clinical benefit.

Unless and until studies are carried out to show that targeting a high-risk population and using the data to direct subsequent prophylactic therapy result in patient benefit, these modalities of risk assessment remain interesting tools for investigational studies and for use on selected individual patients. Other assessments of risk for sudden death, such as QT dispersion, are being investigated and at present there is little supporting evidence that its use improve the management and outcome of AMI patients.[1,552]

## Coronary Angiography and Percutaneous Transluminal Coronary Angioplasty

ACC/AHA recommendations are as follows[1]:

Class I

1. Cardiac catheterization should be performed in patients with spontaneous episodes of myocardial ischemia or episodes of myocardial ischemia provoked by minimal exertion during recovery from STEMI (*level of evidence B*).
2. Cardiac catheterization should be performed for provocable myocardial ischemia on an exercise stress test (*level of evidence B*).
3. Cardiac catheterization should be performed before definitive therapy of a mechanical complication of STEMI such as acute MR, VSR, pseudo-aneurysm or LV aneurysm (*level of evidence B*).
4. Cardiac catheterization should be performed in patients with persistent hemodynamic instability (*level of evidence B*).
5. It is reasonable to perform cardiac catheterization in survivors of STEMI with LVEF less than 40 percent, CHF, prior revascularization, or malignant ventricular arrhythmias (*level of evidence B*).

Class IIa

1. It is reasonable to perform cardiac catheterization when STEMI is suspected to have occurred by a mechanism other than thrombotic occlusion of an atherosclerotic plaque. This would include coronary embolism, certain metabolic or hematologic diseases, or coronary artery spasm.
2. It is reasonable to perform cardiac catheterization in survivors of acute STEMI who had clinical heart failure during the acute episode but subsequently demonstrated well-preserved LV function.
3. It is reasonable to perform cardiac catheterization for recurrent VT or VF or both, despite antiarrhythmic therapy, in patients without evidence of ongoing myocardial ischemia to identify a possible ischemic cause of the tachyarrhythmia.

Class IIb

1. It is debatable whether to perform PCI as part of an invasive strategy after fibrinolytic therapy.

Class III

1. Cardiac catheterization should not be performed in survivors of STEMI who are thought not to be candidates for coronary revascularization.

The selection of patients for cardiac catheterization and coronary angiographic studies prior to hospital discharge should be based on identifying patients at risk for ischemic events and on whether the information provided by cardiac catheterization and coronary angiography will change patient management.

Studies analyzing the prognostic utility of cardiac catheterization prior to hospital discharge are from the prethrombolytic era and demonstrate that the angiographic extent of coronary artery disease was related to survival.[553,554] Other trials have addressed the utility of routine coronary angiographic studies in patients who have received thrombolytic therapy.[555–558] The timing of cardiac catheterization during hospitalization has been addressed in several studies. In general, studies that have compared acute or early cardiac catheterization to a more conservative approach of performing cardiac catheterization and coronary angiographic studies only for patients with spontaneous recurrent angina or exercise-induced ischemia have demonstrated no benefit to the strategy of routine catheterization.[1,238] As discussed previously, opinion on the issue of early angiography and PCI in STEMI is evolving rapidly.[1]

Figure 52-5 presents a strategy for identifying symptomatic and asymptomatic high-risk patients who should have cardiac catheterization and coronary angiographic studies before discharge. Patients who have a complicated clinical course characterized by refractory cardiac failure, unstable angina, an episode of sustained VT, or cardiac arrest should be studied, as discussed previously. An aggressive approach to these patients is justified because of the observed 1-year mortality rate, ranging from 10 to 25 percent.[489] In the case of patients with symptomatic cardiac failure, right heart catheterization should be included.

The recommended algorithm for selecting asymptomatic, uncomplicated post-AMI patients for cardiac catheterization is also presented in Fig. 52-5. Decision making focuses on the presence or absence of myocardial ischemia. Because of the high incidence of residual ischemia in patients with a NQWMI, the task force for guidelines for coronary angiographic studies after myocardial infarction originally recommended such studies in all NQWMIs.[559] The more conservative recommendation here emphasizes evidence of objective ischemia. Where patients have received thrombolytic therapy, it seems reasonable that those who have evidence of residual ischemia are still at increased risk of future ischemic events and should undergo coronary angiography prior to discharge. Consideration of PTCA following coronary angiographic studies should be based on established clinical and anatomic guidelines[1,560] as discussed (see Chap. 55). Coronary artery bypass surgery should be considered in those groups in whom it has been shown to be of proven benefit: patients with triple-vessel disease, patients with ischemia, and those with significant left ventricular dysfunction (see also Chap. 58).[561]

## SECONDARY PREVENTION AND CARDIAC REHABILITATION DURING AND AFTER HOSPITAL DISCHARGE

### Risk-Factor Reduction

The relation between the level of activity of the inflammatory response in the arterial wall (which is the characteristic feature of atherosclerosis) and the tendency of the structural integrity of the artery to break down, with the resultant exposure of thrombogenic material and clot formation, is discussed in Chap. 44. The inflammatory response is caused by and/or exacerbated by the presence of the classic risk factors. It follows that favorably modifying the risk factors would, intuitively, reduce coronary events. There is now abundant evidence that this is the case. Thus, since those who have had AMI are among those at highest risk for recurrence, management strategies to mitigate this risk are very important in patient management.[562]

#### SMOKING

Smoking has multiple cardiovascular effects that can promote AMI, including enhanced platelet aggregation, coronary vasospasm, and vascular inflammation. Smoking cessation is an essential goal after AMI, since the recurrence rate and death rate after AMI are doubled by the continuation of smoking (see also Chap. 43).[563] After AMI, however, in those who break the habit the risk associated with smoking declines rapidly to that of the nonsmoking cohort survivors within 3 years.[564] The psychological and physiologic aspects of smoking should be addressed, and a number of programs have been developed to deal with these needs. Most smokers who have quit, however, have done so without an organized program.[565] The role of the physician in motivating the patient to quit smoking is extremely important and the likelihood of success appears to be directly related to the extent of his or her involvement. Transdermal nicotine patches and oral preparations can be used to aid withdrawal but are not risk-free and should be used temporarily and adjunctively with physician counseling and/or a formal program in behavior modification.[566] The transdermal patches or oral nicotine preparations should not be used during the period just after AMI and should not be used concurrently with smoking. Difficult cases are probably handled best by referral to a formal smoking cessation program. Clonidine hydrochloride has also been used to ameliorate symptoms of smoking withdrawal as well as in conjunction with behavioral intervention.[562]

***Dyslipidemia*** ACC/AHA recommendations for lipid management are as follows[1]:

Class I

1. Dietary therapy that is low in saturated fat and cholesterol (less than 7 percent of total calories as saturated fat and less than 200 mg/d cholesterol) should be started upon discharge after recovery from STEMI. Increased consumption of the following should be encouraged: omega-3 fatty acids, fruits, vegetables, and grains (*level of evidence B*).
2. Patients with LDL cholesterol levels greater than 100 mg/dL should be discharged on drug therapy with the goal of reducing LDL to less than 100 mg/dL (*level of evidence B*).
3. Patients with normal plasma cholesterol levels who have a high-density lipoprotein (HDL) cholesterol level less than 40 mg/dL should receive nonpharmacologic therapy (e.g., exercise, weight loss, smoking cessation) to increase HDL (*level of evidence B*).

Class IIa

1. Patients with normal total cholesterol levels but HDL cholesterol less than 40 mg/dL despite dietary and other nonpharmacologic therapy may be started on drugs such as niacin to raise HDL levels (*level of evidence A*).
2. It is reasonable to add drug therapy using either niacin or a fibrate to diet regardless of low-density lipoprotein (LDL) and HDL levels when triglyceride levels are greater than 200 mg/dL (*level of evidence B*).
3. It is reasonable to discharge patients with low-density lipoprotein cholesterol (LDL-C) less than 100 mg/dL or unknown LDL-C on statin therapy (*level of evidence B*).

*The β-hydroxy-β-methylglutaryl-CoA (HMG-CoA) reductase inhibitors are the most effective drugs in lowering LDL cholesterol. Niacin is effective in raising HDL and, in combination with resins, is also effective in lowering LDL. Triple therapy with a reductase inhibitor, niacin, and resin can be useful in resistant cases. Drug therapy of dyslipidemias is discussed in Chap. 43.*

As mentioned earlier, patients who have had an AMI are generally at high risk for recurrence. Furthermore, an abnormally elevated serum cholesterol level is a powerful risk factor for death in this group.[567,568] Early primary prevention studies and relatively small angiographic trials showed decreases in cardiovascular event rates with cholesterol-lowering therapy (see Chap. 43). Large secondary prevention trials have provided compelling evidence that in patients who have had an AMI, therapy with HMG-CoA reductase inhibitors to lower serum cholesterol levels that were either initially elevated—as in the Scandinavian Simvastatin Survival Study (4S),[569] or within "average" range, as in the Cholesterol and Recurrent Events (CARE) trial[570]—was effective in reducing both cardiovascular and total mortality as well as cardiovascular events. In CARE, a treatment effect was not observed in the group with baseline LDL values <125 mg/dL. The guidelines of the expert panel of the National Cholesterol Education Program provide target goals for patients with manifest coronary artery disease. These goals are as follows: LDL cholesterol, <100 mg/dL (2.59 mmol/L); HDL cholesterol, >35 mg/dL (0.91 mmol/L).[571]

Serum lipid levels are decreased within several hours after AMI, presumably by the inflammatory response to tissue necrosis.[572] Evaluation of serum lipid levels should be made within the first 6 to 8 h from onset of symptoms or after recovery at 6 to 8 weeks. All AMI patients should have serum lipids evaluated and treated intensively in order to achieve target goals. Treatment should start in the hospital with initiation of the AHA step II diet. With established very high lipid levels (for example, LDL-C >200 mg/dL), many clinicians would have a low threshold for initiating drug therapy early on, anticipating that diet therapy alone might not be sufficient for achieving target LDL goals. Initiating lipid-lowering therapy before hospital discharge in STEMI patients with LDL-C levels >100 mg/dL is a Class I recommendation as noted. Low HDL is a powerful risk factor for AMI. It is prudent (Class I) to attempt to raise HDL levels by prescribing a regimen of diet, weight loss, and exercise.[1] Niacin is also efficacious in raising HDL levels; it may be used, especially if indicated as adjunctive therapy with HMG-CoA reductase inhibitors or with resins, to lower LDL. Recommendations have changed for treating elevated (>200 mg/dL) triglycerides in STEMI patients. Adding to the hygienic regimen drug therapy using niacin or a fibrate in these patients is regarded as reasonable to consider (Class IIa) (see Chap. 43).

***Inactivity*** There have been numerous studies of post-AMI patients documenting the beneficial effects of aerobic exercise on functional capacity and myocardial oxygen demand at a given submaximal workload.[573] Such exercise can decrease angina pectoris and ischemia. Conversely, a sedentary lifestyle is a risk factor for coronary artery disease. Metanalysis of cardiac rehabilitation studies has shown a reduction in mortality in the exercise group as opposed to a control group.[573] These analyses have not permitted separating the effects of exercise per se from the other beneficial aspects of the programs. The greatest benefits of exercise are those observed with moderate, regular exercise as contrasted with the nonexercise group. The benefit can be obtained by exercising about 4200 kJ a week, which can be achieved by walking about 1.5 miles (2.4 km) per day. Long-term, regular exercise training can best be sustained by participating in a supervised exercise program beginning several weeks after discharge from the hospital.[562,573] A standard exercise program might involve three 20- to 30-min sessions three to four times per week at 60 to 75 percent of maximal aerobic capacity. This target activity level should be achieved progressively over several weeks, and progress should be monitored by the physician at regular intervals. The exercise regimen should be initiated and guided by monitored exercise testing.

Regular aerobic exercise should be prescribed for post-AMI patients in stable condition at an intensity, duration, and frequency as determined by formal testing and clinical judgment. Optimum benefit is achieved in a supervised program, although asymptomatic, stable patients can exercise without direct supervision but should receive regular monitoring by a physician (see also Chap. 50).

***Low-Estrogen States (Women)*** The recommendations are as follows[1]:

Class IIa

1. Hormone replacement therapy (HRT) with estrogen plus progestin for secondary prevention of coronary events should not be given de novo to postmenopausal women after myocardial infarction.
2. Postmenopausal women who are already taking HRT with estrogen plus progestin at the time of an AMI can continue this therapy.

Estrogen replacement therapy and the primary or secondary prevention of cardiovascular disease continues to be a somewhat contentious and emotional issue that involves weighing the potential efficacy of ERT in reducing cardiovascular risk against the possible increases in breast cancer rates.[574,575] Clinical trials have demonstrated that estrogen with or without progestins lowers both LDL-C and fibrinogen,[576] an effect that would be expected to reduce cardiovascular risk. Contrary to conventional wisdom and expectations, the first large double-blind, placebo-controlled trial to assess the effects of estrogen and progestin treatment on the secondary prevention of coronary heart disease in postmenopausal women showed no reduction in any cardiovascular outcome after 4.1 years of follow-up.[577] Furthermore, the Heart and Estrogen-Progestin Replacement Study (HERS) Research Group reported a significant trend for more primary cardiac events in the treatment group than it did in the placebo group in year 1, although there were fewer events in years 4 and 5 in the treatment group than there were in the placebo group.[577] These observations led to the recommendation that, post-AMI, women on hormone replacement therapy at the time of the event should continue but that initiation of therapy could not be recommended.[1]

## DRUG THERAPY

***Beta-Adrenergic Blockers*** ACC/AHA recommendations for long term therapy with β-blockers in STEMI patients are as follows[1]:

Class I

1. All patients after STEMI except those at low risk and those with contraindications should receive beta-blocker therapy. Treatment should begin within a few days of the event (if not initiated acutely) and continue indefinitely. (*level of evidence: A*).
2. Patients with moderate or severe LV failure should receive beta-blocker therapy with a gradual titration scheme. Patients should have no or minimal evidence of fluid retention and should not have had required treatment recently with an intravenous positive inotropic agent.

Class IIa

1. It is reasonable to prescribe beta-blockers to low-risk patients after STEMI without a clear contraindication. (after deleting a section continue with existing paragraph: "The benefits of beta-blocker therapy given. . . .")

The benefits of beta-blocker therapy given early in the course of AMI were previously discussed. Multiple clinical trials have also demonstrated the benefits of long-term treatment of post-AMI patients with beta blockers.[578] Long-term efficacy has been demonstrated for propranolol,[13] timolol,[579] and metoprolol.[580] Mortality has been shown to be reduced by about 25 to 35 percent. The beneficial effect is highest in high-risk patients with large (usually anterior) myocardial infarction, and compensated left ventricular dysfunction. The beneficial effects in low-risk patients are less clear, but the consensus is that these patients should probably be treated because of the relatively favorable side-effect profile.[1] This recommendation extends to the patient with NQWMI although, as discussed, the data are less compelling. Beta blockers with intrinsic sympathomimetic activity should not be used in this context.

***Aspirin*** ACC/AHA recommendations are as follows[1]:

Class I

1. A daily dose of aspirin 75 to 160 mg should be given indefinitely to patients recovering from STEMI (*level of evidence A*).

Class IIa

1. If true aspirin allergy is present, preferably clopidogrel 75 mg daily or alternatively ticlopidine 250 mg twice daily should be substituted (*level of evidence B*).
2. If true aspirin allergy is present, warfarin therapy with a target INR of greater than or equal to 2.5 is an alternative to clopidogrel in patients less than 75 years of age who are at low risk for bleeding and can be adequately monitored for dose adjustment to maintain a target INR range.

The role of aspirin during the early phases of STEMI was discussed earlier. Aspirin use over the long term after STEMI is also associated with a reduction in mortality. Metanalysis of six major trials of aspirin treatment showed an overall reduction in vascular mortality in the treated group of 13 percent, with 31 and 42 percent reductions in nonfatal infarction and nonfatal stroke, respectively.[581] These trials used relatively large aspirin doses (300 to 1500 mg/day), but one trial showed efficacy at only 75 mg/day,[582] suggesting that long-term use of more modest doses would be effective. Thus, aspirin at relatively low doses is recommended for all patients with AMI in the absence of contraindications (see also Chap. 54).

***Anticoagulation*** WARFARIN THERAPY ACC/AHA recommendations for warfarin therapy are as follows[1]:

Class I

1. Warfarin is useful for secondary prevention of MI in STEMI patients unable to take daily aspirin (*level of evidence A*).
2. Warfarin should be prescribed for post-STEMI patients in persistent AF (*level of evidence A*).
3. Warfarin should be prescribed for at least three months in post-STEMI patients with LV thrombus noted on an imaging study (*level of evidence B*).

Class IIa

1. It is reasonable to prescribe warfarin to post-STEMI patients with extensive wall motion abnormalities (*level of evidence B*).
2. It is reasonable to prescribe warfarin to post-STEMI patients with paroxysmal AF (*level of evidence B*).
3. It is reasonable to prescribe warfarin to post-STEMI patients with LV systolic dysfunction with or without CHF (*level of evidence A*).
4. It is reasonable to prescribe warfarin alone to post-STEMI patients without contraindications who are less than 75 years old (target INR 2.5–3.5) or in combination with low-dose ASA (75 or 81 mg) (target INR 2–3) in post-STEMI patients who are at high risk for thromboembolic events or reinfarction and who can be monitored carefully.

Anticoagulation can reduce mortality, recurrent myocardial infarction, and stroke after STEMI, as indicated by an analysis of multiple trials.[578] Because of relatively high rates of bleeding with warfarin, the need for monitoring, and, in particular, the efficacy and low risk of aspirin, the role of warfarin is rather limited to those at increased risk for developing mural thrombi[562] with demonstrable left ventricular thrombus or atrial fibrillation. The duration of anticoagulation should be limited to 3 months in the case of left ventricular thrombus (see also Chap. 54).

***Angiotensin-Converting Enzyme Inhibitors*** The ACE inhibitors and recommendations for their use early in the course of AMI were previously discussed. Studies have documented their efficacy in secondary prevention. The reduction in late morbidity and mortality was most obvious in those with large infarctions with reduced ejection fraction and in those with anterior myocardial infarction. In these patients, left ventricular remodeling and progression to heart failure were reduced.[314,318,583] The beneficial effects of ACE inhibitors have been less obvious when low-risk patients were included.[584] The decrease in ischemic events in the SAVE trial[314] and in other ACE-inhibitor trials suggests that the threshold for use of ACE inhibitors for long-term therapy may be lowered by many clinicians to include those with only modest left ventricular dysfunction. Thus, ACE inhibitors have been recommended for chronic use after AMI in those patients with significant left ventricular dysfunction, and their use should be considered in those with only mild-to-moderate left ventricular dysfunction (ejection fraction <45 percent).

The publication of the Heart Outcomes Prevention Evaluation (HOPE) trial in patients with significant risk factors for cardiovascular events showed significant reduction in new events and new-onset diabetes mellitus in those treated with the ACE inhibitor ramipril.[320] It is likely that the recommendations for use of ACE inhibitors will be extended to all patients at high risk for cardiovascular events regardless of blood pressure or left ventricular function (see Chap. 43).

## Modification of Lifestyle and Cardiac Rehabilitation after Acute Myocardial Infarction

Because of the relatively high risk of recurrence and the need for lifelong modification of lifestyles and risk factors, most post-AMI patients should be enrolled in a cardiac rehabilitation program that emphasizes dietary modification, risk-factor reduction, and exercise. The low-risk patient does not require prolonged supervised exercise, as previously discussed. All patients, however, can benefit from a structured environment to launch a lifetime of healthy living. Cardiac rehabilitation is discussed in Chap. 60 and risk factors and the prevention of coronary artery disease are discussed in Chap. 43.

There has been considerable reinvigoration of interest in the potential of dietary interventions in secondary prevention after AMI since the publication of the results of the Lyon Diet Study[585] and of the GISSI-Prevention Study.[586] Both of these studies showed a dramatic (>30 percent) reduction in recurrence of cardiovascular events in patients in whom a diet and supplements rich in omega-3 fatty acids was added to adequate conventional therapy. Thus, in view of the minimal or absent risk, it seems prudent to recommend that patients incorporate into their dietary regimens sources of omega-3 fatty acids (fish, especially tuna, salmon, and sardines; nuts, such as walnuts; and probably fish oil supplements).

## References


1. Antman EM, Anbe DT, Armstrong PW, et al. ACC/AHA Guidelines for the management of patients with ST-elevation myocardial infarction. *Circulation.* In press (2004).
2. Ryan TJ, Antman EM, Brooks NH, et al. 1999 update: ACC/AHA guidelines for the management of patients with acute myocardial infarction: A report of the American College of Cardiology/American Heart Association Task Force on Practice Guidelines (Committee on Management of Acute Myocardial Infarction). *J Am Coll Cardiol* 1999;34:890–911.
3. Osler W. *The Principles and Practice of Medicine.* New York: Appleton & Co; 1892.
4. Herrick JB. Clinical features of sudden obstruction of the coronary arteries. *JAMA* 1912;59:2015.
5. Roberts WC, Buja LM. The frequency and significance of coronary arterial thrombi and other observations in fatal acute myocardial infarction. *Am J Med* 1972;52:425–443.
6. Rentrop KP, Blanke H, Karsch KR, et al. Coronary angiographic findings and left ventricular pump function in acute infarction and changes in chronic stage infarction. *Z Kardiol* 1979;68:335–350.
7. DeWood MA, Spores J, Notske R, et al. Prevalence of total coronary occlusion during the early hours of transmural myocardial infarction. *N Engl J Med* 1980;303:897–902.
8. Bristow JD, Burchell HB, Campbell RW, et al. Report of the ad hoc committee on the indications for coronary arteriography. *Circulation* 1977;55:969A–974A.
9. Rentrop KP, Blanke H, Karsch KR, et al. Acute myocardial infarction: Intracoronary application of nitroglycerine and streptokinase. *Clin Cardiol* 1979;2:354–363.
10. European Cooperative Study Group for Streptokinase Treatment in Acute Myocardial Infarction. Streptokinase in acute myocardial infarction. *N Engl J Med* 1979;301:797–802.
11. Mathey DG, Kuck K-H, Tilsner V, et al. Nonsurgical coronary artery recanalization in acute transmural myocardial infarction. *Circulation* 1981;63:489–497.
12. Stampfer MJ, Goldhaber SZ, Yusuf S, et al. Effect of intravenous streptokinase on acute myocardial infarction: Pooled results from randomized trials. *N Engl J Med* 1982;307:1180–1182.
13. Beta-Blocker Heart Attack Study Group. The beta-blocker heart attack trial. *JAMA* 1981;246:2073–2084.
14. GISSI: Gruppo Italiano per lo Studio della Streptochinasi nell'Infarto Miocardio. Effectiveness of intravenous thrombolytic treatment in acute myocardial infarction. *Lancet* 1986;1:397–402.
15. GUSTO Investigators. An international randomized trial comparing four thrombolytic strategies for acute myocardial infarction. *N Engl J Med* 1993;329:673–682.
16. Gunnar (ACC/AHA) RM, Passamani ER, Bourdillon PD, et al. Guidelines for the early management of patients with acute myocardial infarction. *J Am Coll Cardiol* 1990;16:249–292.
17. Herlitz J, Blohm M, Hartford M, et al. Delay time in suspected acute myocardial infarction and the importance of its modification. *Clin Cardiol* 1989;12:370–374.
18. National Heart Lung and Blood Institute. Morbidity and Mortality: Chartbook on cardiovascular, lung, and blood diseases. 1992.
19. Galis ZS, Sukhova GK, Lark MW, et al. Increased expression of matrix metalloproteinases and matrix degrading activity in vulnerable regions of human atherosclerotic plaques. *J Clin Invest* 1994;94: 2493–2503.
20. Friesinger GC. The natural history of atherosclerotic coronary heart disease, in Schlant RC, Alexander RW (eds). *The Heart,* 8th ed. New York: McGraw-Hill; 1994;1185–1204.
21. van der Wal AC, Becker AE, van der Loos CM, et al. Site of intimal rupture or erosion of thrombosed coronary atherosclerotic plaques is characterized by an inflammatory process irrespective of the dominant plaque morphology. *Circulation* 1994;89:36–44.
22. Mounsey P. Prodromal symptoms in myocardial infarction. *Br Heart J* 1951;13:215–226.
23. Berk BC, Weintraub WS, Alexander RW. Elevaton of C-reactive protein in "active" coronary artery disease. *Am J Cardiol* 1990;65:168–172.
24. Liuzzo G, Biasucci LM, Gallimore JR, et al. The prognostic value of C-reactive protein and serum amyloid a protein in severe unstable angina. *N Engl J Med* 1994;331:417–424.
25. Ridker PM, Cushman M, Stampfer MJ, et al. Inflammation, aspirin, and the risk of cardiovascular disease in apparently healthy men. *N Engl J Med* 1997;336:973–979.
26. Spodick DH, Flessas AP, Johnson MM. Association of acute respiratory symptoms with onset of acute myocardial infarction: Prospective investigation of 150 consecutive patients and matched controls. *Am J Cardiol* 1984;53:481–482.
27. Saikku P. *Chlamydia pneumoniae* infection as a risk factor in acute myocardial infarction. *Eur Heart J* 1993;14:62–65.
28. Miettinen H, Lehto S, Saikku P, et al. Association of *Chlamydia pneumoniae* and acute coronary heart disease events in non-insulin dependent diabetic and non-diabetic subjects in Finland. *Eur Heart J* 1996;17:682–688.
29. Patel P, Mendall MA, Carrington D, et al. Association of *Helicobacter pylori* and *Chlamydia pneumoniae* infections with coronary heart disease and cardiovascular risk factors. *BMJ* 1995;311:711–714.
30. Campbell LA, Kuo C-C. *Chlamydia pneumoniae* and atherosclerosis. *Semin Respir Infect* 2003;18:48–54.
31. Willich SN, Lewis M, Lowel H, et al. Physical exertion as a trigger of acute myocardial infarction. Triggers and mechanisms of myocardial infarction study group. *N Engl J Med* 1993;329:1684–1690.
32. Mittleman MA, Maclure M, Tofler GH, et al. Triggering of acute myocardial infarction by heavy physical exertion. Protection against triggering by regular exertion. Determinants of Myocardial Infarction Onset Study Investigators. *N Engl J Med* 1993;329:1677–1683.
33. Mittleman MA, Maclure M, Sherwood JB, et al. Triggering of acute myocardial infarction onset by episodes of anger. Determinants of Myocardial Infarction Onset Study Investigators. *Circulation* 1995; 92:1720–1725.
34. Rahe RH, Romo M, Siltanen P. Recent life changes, myocardial infarction, and abrupt coronary death. *Arch Intern Med* 1974; 133:221–228.
35. Lundberg U, Theorell T, Lind E. Life changes and myocardial infarction: Individual differences in life changes scaling. *J Psychosom Res* 1975;37:27–32.
36. Jenkins CD. Recent evidence supporting psychologic and social risk factors for coronary disease. *N Engl J Med* 1976;294:1033–1038.
37. Mangano DT. Perioperative cardiac morbidity. *Anesthesiology* 1990; 72:153–184.
38. Leiberman RW, Orkin KF, Jobes DR, et al. Hemodynamic predictors of myocardial ischemia during halothane anesthesia for coronary artery revascularization. *Anesthesiology* 1983;59:36–41.
39. Nelson AH, Fleisher LA, Rosenbaum SH. Relationship between postoperative anemia and cardiac morbidity in high risk vascular patients in the intensive care unit. *Crit Care Med* 1993;21:860–866.
40. Frank SM, Beattie C, Christopherson R, et al. Unintentional hypothermia is associated with post-operative myocardial ischemia. *Anesthesiology* 1993;78:468–476.
41. Frank SM, Fleisher LA, Breslow MD, et al. Perioperative maintenance of normothermia reduces the incidence of morbid cardiac events. *JAMA* 1997;277:1127–1134.
42. Zainea M, Duvernoy WF, Chauhan A, et al. Acute myocardial infarction in angiographically normal coronary arteries following induction of general anesthesia. *Arch Intern Med* 1994;154:2495–2498.
43. Moliterno DJ, Willard JE, Lange RA, et al. Coronary-artery vasoconstriction induced by cocaine, cigarette smoking, or both. *N Engl J Med* 1994;330:454–459.
44. Friedman M, Rosenman RH. Type A behavior pattern: Its association with coronary heart disease. *Ann Clin Res* 1971;3:300–312.
45. Dimsdale JE. A perspective on type A behavior and coronary disease. *N Engl J Med* 1988;318:110–112.
46. Muller JE, Stone PH, Turzi ZG, et al. Circadian variation in the frequency of onset of acute myocardial infarction. *N Engl J Med* 1985; 313:1315–1322.

47. Mitler MM, Kripke DF. Circadian variation in myocardial infarction. *N Engl J Med* 1986;314:1187–1188.
48. Petralito A, Mangiafico RA, Giblino S, et al. Daily modifications of plasma fibrinogen, platelet aggregation, Howell's time, PTT, PT, and antithrombin III in normal subjects and in patients with vascular disease. *Chronobiologia* 1982;9:195–201.
49. Rosing DR, Brakma P, Redwood DR, et al. Blood fibrinolytic activity in man: Diurnal variation and the response to varying intensities of exercise. *Circ Res* 1970;27:171–184.
50. Marshall J. Diurnal variation in occurrence of strokes. *Stroke* 1977;8: 230–231.
51. Sayer JW, Wilkinson P, Ranjadayalan K, et al. Attenuation or absence of circadian and seasonal rhythms of acute myocardial infarction. *Heart* 1977;77:325–329.
52. Quyyumi AA, Mockus L, Wright C, et al. Morphology of ambulatory ST segment changes in patients with varying severity of coronary artery disease: Investigation of the frequency of nocturnal ischemia and coronary spasm. *Br Heart J* 1985;53:186–193.
53. el-Tamimi H, Mansour M, Pepine CJ, et al. Circadian variation in coronary tone in patients with stable angina. Protective role of the endothelium. *Circulation* 1995;92:3201–3205.
54. Millar-Craig MW, Bishop CN, Raftery EB. Circadian variation of blood pressure. *Lancet* 1978;1:795–797.
55. Turton MB, Deegan T. Circadian variations of plasma catecholamine, cortisol, and immunoreactive insulin concentrations in supine subjects. *Clin Chim Acta* 1974;55:389–397.
56. Willich SN, Lowel H, Lewis M, et al. Weekly variation of acute myocardial infarction. Increased Monday risk in the working population. *Circulation* 1994;90:87–93.
57. Spielberg C, Falkenhahn D, Willich SN, et al. Circadian, day-of-week, and seasonal variability in myocardial infarction: Comparison between working and retired patients. *Am Heart J* 1996;132: 579–585.
58. Hofgren C, Karlson BW, Herlitz J. Prodromal symptoms in subsets of patients hospitalized for suspected acute myocardial infarction. *Heart Lung* 1995;24:3–10.
59. Gill JB, Cairns JA, Roberts RS, et al. Prognostic importance of myocardial ischemia detected by ambulatory monitoring early after acute myocardial infarction. *N Engl J Med* 1996;334:65–70.
60. Maseri A, Crea F, Kaski JC, et al. Mechanisms and significance of cardiac ischemic pain. *Prog Cardiovas Dis* 1992;35:1–18.
61. Maseri A. The changing face of angina pectoris: Practical implications. *Lancet* 1983;1:746–749.
62. Everts B, Karlson BW, Wahrborg P, et al. Localization of pain in suspected acute myocardial infarction in relation to final diagnosis, age and sex, and site and type of infarction. *Heart Lung* 1996;25:430–437.
63. Herlitz J, Bang A, Isaksson L, et al. Ambulance dispatchers' estimation of intensity of pain and presence of associated symptoms in relation to outcome in patients who call for an ambulance because of acute chest pain. *Eur Heart J* 1995;16:1789–1794.
64. Margolis JR, Kannel WB, Feinleich M, et al. Clinical features of unrecognized myocardial infarction—silent and symptomatic. *Am J Cardiol* 1973;32:1–7.
65. Bean WB. Masquerades of myocardial infarction. *Lancet* 1977;1: 1044–1045.
66. Madias JE, Chintalapaly G, Choudry M, et al. Correlates and in-hospital outcome of painless presentation of acute myocardial infarction: A prospective study of a consecutive series of patients admitted to the coronary care unit. *J Invest Med* 1995;43:567–574.
67. Jaffe AS, Roberts R. Precordial inspection and palpation in patients with acute myocardial infarction. *Prac Cardiol* 1981;7:46–50.
68. Fowler NO. Physical signs in acute myocardial infarction and its complications. *Prog Cardiovasc Dis* 1968;10:287–297.
69. Harvey WP. Some pertinent physical findings in the clinical evaluation of acute myocardial infarction. *Circulation* 1969;40 (suppl 4): 175–181.
69a. O'Rourke RA, Dell'Italia LJ. Diagnosis and management of right ventricular myocardial infarction. *Curr Probl Cardiol* 2004;29:1–48.
70. Killip T III, Kimball JT. Treatment of myocardial infarction in a coronary care unit: A two year experience with 250 patients. *Am J Cardiol* 1967;20:457–464.
71. Goldman L, Cook EF, Brand DA, et al. A computer protocol to predict myocardial infarction in emergency department patients with chest pain. *N Engl J Med* 1988;318:797–803.
72. Lee TH, Rouan GW, Weisberg MC, et al. Sensitivity of routine clinical criteria for diagnosing myocardial infarction within 24 hours of hospitalization. *Ann Intern Med* 1987;106:181–186.
73. Lee TH, Juarez G, Cook EF, et al. Ruling out acute myocardial infarction. *N Engl J Med* 1991;324:1239–1246.
74. Lee TH, Weisberg MC, Brand DA, et al. Candidates for thrombolysis among emergency room patients with acute chest pain. *Ann Intern Med* 1989;110:957–962.
75. Roberts R. The two out of three criteria for the diagnosis of infarction—Is it passe? *Chest* 1984;86:511–513.
76. Parker ABI, Waller BF, Gering LE. Usefulness of the 12-lead electrocardiogram in detection of myocardial infarction: Electrocardiographic-anatomic correlations. Part I. *Clin Cardiol* 1996;19:55–61.
77. Cook RW, Edwards JE, Pruitt RD. Electrocardiographic changes in acute subendocardial infarction. I. Large subendocardial and large transmural infarcts. *Circulation* 1958;18:603–612.
78. Gunnar RM, Pietras RJ, Blackaller J, et al. Correlation of vectocardiographic criteria for myocardial infarction with autopsy findings. *Circulation* 1967;35:158–171.
79. Wagner NB, White RD, Wagner GS. The 12-lead ECG and the extent of myocardium at risk of acute infarction: Cardiac anatomy and lead locations, and the phases of serial changes during acute occlusion. In: Califf RM, Mark DB, Wagner GS, eds. *Acute Coronary Care in the Thrombolytic Era.* Chicago: Year Book; 1988;31–45.
80. Ambos HD, Moore P, Roberts R. A database for analysis of patient diagnostic data. In: *Computers in Cardiology.* Long Beach, CA: IEEE Computer Society; 1978.
81. Gibson RS, Boden WE, Theroux P, et al. Diltiazem and reinfarction in patients with non-Q-wave myocardial infarction. Results of a double-blind, randomized, multicenter trial. *N Engl J Med* 1986;315: 423–429.
82. Bodenheimer MM, Banka VS, Trout RG, et al. Relationship between myocardial fibrosis and epicardial and surface electrocardiographic Q-waves in man. *J Electrocardiol* 1979;12:205–210.
83. Pratt CM, Roberts R. Non-Q-wave myocardial infarction: Recognition, pathogenesis, prognosis and management, in McIntosh HD, ed. *Baylor Cardiology Series,* 8th ed. Houston: Baylor College of Medicine; 1985;5–19.
84. Wilson FN, Johnston FD, Hill IGW. The form of the electrocardiogram in experimental myocardial infarction: IV. Additional observations with later effects produced by ligation of the anterior descending branch on the left coronary artery. *Am Heart J* 1935;10:1025–1035.
85. Spodick DH. Q-wave infarction versus S-T infarction: Nonspecificity of electrocardiographic criteria for differentiating transmural and nontransmural lesions. *Am J Cardiol* 1983;51:913–915.
86. Sgarbossa EB, Pinski SL, Barbagelata A, et al. Electrocardiographic diagnosis of evolving acute myocardial infarction in the presence of left bundle branch block. GUSTO-1 (Global Utilization of Streptokinase and Tissue Plasminogen Activator for Occluded Coronary Arteries) Investigators. *N Engl J Med* 1996;334:481–487.
87. Helfant RH, Banka VS. *A Clinical and Angiographic Approach to Coronary Heart Disease,* Philadelphia: Davis; 1978.
88. Fenichel NM, Kugell VH. The large Q wave of the electrocardiogram. A correlation with pathologic observations. *Am Heart J* 1931;7:235.
89. Rude RE, Poole WK, Muller JE, et al. Electrocardiographic and clinical criteria for recognition of acute myocardial infarction based on analysis of 3,697 patients. *Am J Cardiol* 1983;52:936–942.
90. Bodenheimer MM, Banka VS, Helfant RH. Q-waves and ventricular asynergy: Predictive value and hemodynamic significance of anatomic localization. *Am J Cardiol* 1975;35:615–618.
91. Schamroth L. Posterior wall myocardial infarction. In: *The 12-lead Electrocardiogram,* Book 1 (of 2). Boston: Blackwell;1989:176–180.

92. Geft IL, Shah PK, Rodriguez L, et al. ST elevations in leads $V_1$ to $V_5$ may be caused by right coronary artery occlusion and acute right ventricular infarction. *Am J Cardiol* 1984;53:991–996.
93. Lopez-Sendon J, Coma-Canella I, Alcasena S, et al. Electrocardiographic findings in acute right ventricular infarction: Sensitivity and specificity of electrocardiographic alterations in right precordial leads V4R, V3R, V1, V2, and V3. *J Am Coll Cardiol* 1985;6:1273–1279.
94. Erhardt L, Sjogren A, Wahlberg I. Single right-sided precordial lead in the diagnosis of right ventricular involvement in inferior myocardial infarction. *Am Heart J* 1976;91:571–576.
95. Kabakci G, Yildirir A, Yildiran L, et al. The diagnostic value of 12-lead electrocardiogram in predicting infarct-related artery and right ventricular involvement in acute inferior myocardial infarction. *Ann Noninvas Electrocardiol* 2001;6:229–239.
96. Sivertssen E, Hoel B, Bay G, et al. Electrocardiographic atrial complex and acute atrial myocardial infarction. *Am J Cardiol* 1973;31: 450–456.
97. Mirvis DM. Physiologic bases for anterior ST segment depression in patients with acute inferior wall myocardial infarction. *Am Heart J* 1988;116:1308–1322.
98. Muller DW, Topol EJ, Califf RM, et al. Relationship between antecedent angina pectoris and short-term prognosis after thrombolytic therapy for acute myocardial infarction. Thrombolysis and Angioplasty in Myocardial Infarction (TAMI) Study Group. *Am Heart J* 1990;119 (2 Pt 1):224–231.
99. Roberts R, Gowda KS, Ludbrook PA, et al. Specificity of elevated serum MB CPK activity in the diagnosis of acute myocardial infarction. *Am J Cardiol* 1975;36:433–437.
100. Ishikawa Y, Saffitz JE, Mealman JE, et al. Reversible myocardial ischemic injury is not associated with increased creatine kinase activities in plasma. *Clin Chem* 1997;43:467–475.
101. Zimmerman J, Fromm R, Meyer D, et al. Diagnostic marker cooperative study (DMCS) for the diagnosis of myocardial infarction. *Circulation* 1999;99:1671–1677.
102. Perryman MB, Kerner SA, Bohlmeyer TJ, et al. Isolation and sequence analysis of a full-length cDNA for human M creatine kinase. *Biochem Biophys Res Commun* 1986;140:981–989.
103. Villarreal-Levy G, Ma TS, Kerner SA, et al. Human creatine kinase: Isolation and sequence analysis of cDNA closes for the B subunit, development of subunit specific probes and determination of gene copy number. *Biochem Biophys Res Commun* 1987;144:1116–1127.
104. Tsung JS, Tsung SS. Creatine kinase isoenzymes in extracts of various human skeletal muscles. *Clin Chem* 1986;32:1568–1570.
105. Wilhelm AH, Albers KM, Todd JK. Creatine phosphokinase isoenzyme distribution in human skeletal and heart muscles. *IRCS Med Sci* 1976;4:418.
106. Apple FS, Rogers MA, Sherman WM, et al. Profile of creatine kinase isoenzymes in skeletal muscles of marathon runners. *Clin Chem* 1984;30:413–416.
107. Keshgegian AA, Feiberg NW. Serum creatine kinase MB isoenzyme in chronic muscle disease. *Clin Chem* 1984;30:575–578.
108. Shahangian S, Ash KO, Wahlstrom NO Jr, et al. Creatine kinase and lactate dehydrogenase isoenzymes in serum of patients suffering burns, blunt trauma, or myocardial infarction. *Clin Chem* 1984;30: 1332–1338.
109. McBride JW, Labrosse KR, McCoy HG, et al. Is serum creatine kinase MB in electrically injured patients predictive of myocardial injury? *JAMA* 1986;255:764–768.
110. Plebani M, Zaninotto M. Diagnostic strategies in myocardial infarction using myoglobin measurement. *Eur Heart J* 1998;19:N12–N15.
111. Hartmann F, Kampmann MF, Frey N, et al. Biochemical markers in the diagnosis of coronary artery disease. *Eur Heart J* 1998;19:N2–N7.
112. Apple FS, Ricchiuti V, Voss EM, et al. Expression of cardiac troponin T isoforms in skeletal muscle of renal disease patients will not cause false-positive serum results by the second generation cardiac troponin T assay. *Eur Heart J* 1998;19:N31–N33.
113. Adams JE, Bodor GS, Davila-Roman VG, et al. Cardiac troponin I: A marker with high specificity for cardiac injury. *Circulation* 1993;88: 101–106.
114. Bodor GS, Porterfield D, Voss EM, et al. Cardiac troponin I is not expressed in fetal and healthy or diseased adult human skeletal muscle tissue. *Clin Chem* 1995;41:1710–1715.
115. HCIA. *Diagnostic Regional Groupings Handbook.* Washington, DC: 1993.
116. Guadagnoli E, Hauptman PJ, Ayanian JZ, et al. Variation in the use of cardiac procedures after acute myocardial infarction. *N Engl J Med* 1995;333:573–578.
117. George S, Ishikawa Y, Perryman MB, et al. Purification and characterization of naturally occurring and in vitro induced multiple forms of MM creatine kinase. *J Biol Chem* 1984;259:2667–2674.
118. Perryman MB, Knell JD, Roberts R. Carboxypeptidase-catalyzed hydrolysis of C-terminal lysine: Mechanism for in vivo production of multiple forms of creatine kinase in plasma. *Clin Chem* 1984;30: 662–664.
119. Puleo PR, Meyer D, Wathen C, et al. Use of rapid assay of subforms of creatine kinase MB to diagnose or rule out acute myocardial infarction. *N Engl J Med* 1994;331:561–566.
120. Somer H, Dubowitz V, Donner M. Creatine kinase isoenzymes in neuromuscular diseases. *J Neurol Sci* 1976;29:129–136.
121. Cummins B, Auckland M, Cummins P. Cardiac-specific troponin I radioimmunoassay in the diagnosis of acute myocardial infarction. *Am Heart J* 1987;113:1333–1344.
122. Cummings P, Young A, Auckland ML, et al. Comparison of serum cardiac specific troponin I with creatine kinase, creatine kinase-MB isoenzyme, tropomyosin, myoglobin and C-reactive protein release in marathon runners: Cardiac or skeletal muscle trauma? *Eur J Clin Invest* 1987;17:317–324.
123. Adams JE, Sicard GA, Allen BT, et al. Diagnosis of perioperative myocardial infarction with measurement of cardiac troponin I. *N Engl J Med* 1994;330:670–674.
124. Kobayashi S, Tanaka M, Tamura N, et al. Serum cardiac troponin T in polymyositis/dermatomyositis. *Lancet* 1992;340:726.
125. Abdelmeguid AE, Topol EJ, Whitlow PL, et al. Significance of mild transient release of creatine kinase MB fraction after percutaneous interventions. *Circulation* 1996;94:1528–1536.
126. Abdelmeguid AE, Topol EJ. The myth of the myocardial "infarctlet" during percutaneous coronary revascularization procedures. *Circulation* 1996;94:3369–3375.
127. Roberts R. Recognition, diagnosis, and prognosis of early reinfarction: The role of calcium channel blockers. *Circulation* 1987;75: V139–V147.
128. Turi ZG, Rutherford JD, Roberts R, et al. Electrocardiographic, enzymatic and scintigraphic criteria of acute myocardial infarction as determined from study of 726 patients (a MILIS Study). *Am J Cardiol* 1985;55:1463–1469.
129. Roberts R. Enzymatic diagnosis of acute myocardial infarction. *Chest* 1988;93:3S–6S.
130. Muller JE, Morrison J, Stone PH, et al. Nifedipine therapy for patients with threatened and acute myocaridal infarction: A randomized, double-blind, placebo-controlled comparison. *Circulation* 1984;69: 740–747.
131. MILIS Study Group, ed. National Heart, Lung, and Blood Institute Multicenter Investigation of the Limitation of Infarct Size (MILIS): Design and methods of the clinical trial. an investigation of beta-blockade and hyaluronidase for treatment of acute myocardial infarction (monograph 100). Dallas: American Heart Association; 1984.
132. Ohman EM, Armstrong PW, Christenson RH, et al. Cardiac troponin T levels for risk stratification in acute myocardial ischemia. GUSTO IIA Investigators. *N Engl J Med* 1996;335:1333–1341.
133. Antman EM, Tanasijevic MJ, Thompson B, et al. Cardiac-specific troponin I levels to predict the risk of mortality in patients with acute coronary syndromes. *N Engl J Med* 1996;335:1342–1349.
134. Lindahl B, Venge P, Wallentin L, et al. Relation between troponin T and the risk of subsequent cardiac events in unstable coronary artery disease. For the FRISC Study Group. *Circulation* 1996;93: 1651–1657.
135. Hamburg RJ, Verani MS, Mahmarian JJ, et al. Absence of trace MB creatine kinase release following stress-induced myocardial ischemia (Abstr). *J Am Coll Cardiol* 1993;21:161A.

136. Roberts R, Sobel BE. Elevated plasma MB creatine phosphokinase activity. A specific marker for myocardial infarction in perioperative patients. *Arch Intern Med* 1976;136:421–424.
137. Righetti A, O'Rourke RA, Schelbert H, et al. Usefulness of preoperative and postoperative Tc-99m (Sn)-pyrophosphate scans in patients with ischemic and valvular heart disease. *Am J Cardiol* 1977;39:43–49.
138. Gore JM, Goldberg RJ, Matsumoto AS, et al. Validity of serum total cholesterol level obtained within 24 hours of acute myocardial infarction. *Am J Cardiol* 1984;54:722–725.
139. Ceremuzynski L. Hormonal and metabolic reactions evoked by acute myocardial infarction. *Circ Res* 1981;48:767–776.
140. Katz AS, Harrigan P, Parisi AF. The value and promise of echocardiography in acute myocardial infarction and coronary artery disease. *Clin Cardiol* 1992;15:401–410.
141. Horowitz RS, Morganroth J, Parrotto C, et al. Immediate diagnosis of acute myocardial infarction by two-dimensional echocardiograpy. *Am Heart J* 1982;103:814–822
142. Sabia P, Afrookteh A, Touchstone DA, et al. Value of regional wall motion abnormality in the emergency room diagnosis of acute myocardial infarction: A prospective study using two-dimensional echocardiography. *Circulation* 1991;84(suppl I):I-85–I-92.
143. Kuhn MB, Egeblad H, Hojberg S, et al. Prognostic value of echocardiography compared to other clinical findings: Multivariate analysis based on long-term survival in 456 patients. *Cardiology* 1995;86: 157–162.
144. D'Arcy B, Nanda NC. Two-dimensional echocardiographic features of right ventricular ejection fraction in patients with coronary artery disease. *J Am Coll Cardiol* 1983;2:911–918.
145. Tice FD, Kisslo J. Echocardiographic assessment and monitoring of the patient with acute myocardial infarction. Prospects for the Thrombolytic Era, in Califf RM, Mark DB, Wagner GS, eds. *Acute Coronary Care.* St Louis: Mosby–Year Book; 1994:49.
146. Cheitlin MD, Alpert JS, Armstrong WF, et al. ACC/AHA Guidelines for the Clinical Application of Echocardiography. A report of the American College of Cardiology/American Heart Association Task Force on Practice Guidelines (Committee on Clinical Application of Echocardiography). Developed in collaboration with the American Society of Echocardiography. *Circulation* 1997;95:1686–1744.
147. Johnston DL, Gupta VK, Wendt RE, et al. Detection of viable myocardium in segments with fixed defects on thallium-201 scintigraphy: Usefulness of magnetic resonance imaging early after acute myocardial infarction. *Magn Reson Imaging* 1993;11:949–956.
148. Cherryman GR, Pirovano G, Kirchin MA. Gadobenate dimeglumine in MRI of acute myocardial infarction: Results of a phase III study comparing dynamic and delayed contrast enhanced magnetic resonance imaging with EKG, $^{201}$TI SPECT, and echocardiography. *Invest Radiol* 2002;37:135–145.
149. Hirose K, Reed JE, Rumberger JA. Serial changes in regional right ventricular free wall and left ventricular septal wall lengths during the first 4 to 5 years after index anterior wall myocardial infarction. *J Am Coll Cardiol* 1995;26:394–400.
150. Foster CJ, Sekiya T, Love HG, et al. Identification of intracardiac thrombus: Comparison of computed tomography and cross-sectional echocardiography. *Br J Radiol* 1987;60:327–331.
151. Ritchie JL, Bateman TM, Bonow RO, et al. Guidelines for clinical use of cardiac radionuclide imaging: Report of the American College of Cardiology/American Heart Association Task Force on Assessment of Diagnostic and Therapeutic Cardiovascular Procedures (Committee on Radionuclide Imaging), developed in collaboration with The American Society of Nuclear Cardiology. *J Am Coll Cardiol* 1995;25: 521–547.
152. Reduto LA, Berger HJ, Cohen LS, et al. Sequential radionuclide assessment of left and right ventricular performance after acute transmural myocardial infarction. *Ann Intern Med* 1978;89: 441–447.
153. Gibson WS, Christian TF, Pellikka PA, et al. Serial tomographic imaging with technetium-99m-sestamibi for the assessment of infarct-related arterial patency following reperfusion therapy. *J Nucl Med* 1992;33:2080–2085.
154. Christian TF, Schwartz RS, Gibbons RJ. Determinants of infarct size in reperfusion therapy for acute myocardial infarction. *Circulation* 1992;86:81–90.
155. McCallister BD Jr, Christian TF, Gersh BJ, et al. Prognosis of myocardial infarctions involving more than 40% of the left ventricle after acute reperfusion therapy. *Circulation* 1993;88:1470–1475.
156. Miller TD, Christian TF, Hopfenspirger MR, et al. Infarct size after acute myocardial infarction measured by quantitative tomographic 99mTc sestamibi imaging predicts subsequent mortality. *Circulation* 1995;92:334–341.
157. Fulton M, Julian DG, Oliver MF. Sudden death and myocardial infarction. *Circulation* 1969;40:182–191.
158. Kuller L. Sudden death in arteriosclerotic heart disease: The case for preventive medicine. *Am J Cardiol* 1969;24:617–628.
159. Adgey AAJ, Allen JD, Geddes JS, et al. Acute phase of myocardial infarction. *Lancet* 1971;2:501–504.
160. Simon AB, Feinleib M, Thompson HK Jr. Components of delay in the prehospital phase of acute myocardial infarction. *Am J Cardiol* 1972; 30:476–482.
161. National Heart Lung and Blood Institute. *Rapid Identification and Treatment of Acute Myocardial Infarction.* NHLBI;1994.
162. National Heart Attack Alert Program Coordinating Committee. *Patients/Bystander Recognition and Action: Rapid Identification and Treatment of Acute Myocardial Infarction.* IN National Heart Attack Alert Program (NHAAP). 1993.
163. Pressley JC, Severance HW, Jr, Raney MP, et al. A comparison of paramedic versus basic emergency medical care of patients at high and low risk during acute myocardial infarction. *J Am Coll Cardiol* 1988;12:1555–1561.
164. Kareiakes DJ, Weaver WD, Anderson JL, et al. Time delays in the diagnosis and treatment of acute myocardial infarction: A tale of eight cities. Report from the Prehospital Study Group and the Cincinnati Heart Project. *Am Heart J* 1990;120:773–780.
165. Goldstein S, Moss AJ, Greene W. Sudden death in acute myocardial infarction: Relationship to factors affecting delay in hospitalization. *Arch Intern Med* 1972;129:720–724.
166. ACC/AHA Task Force, Gunnar RM, et al. ACC/AHA Guidelines for the early management of patients with acute myocardial infarction. *Circulation* 1990;82:664–707.
167. Lewis RP, Lanese RR, Stang JM, et al. Reduction of mortality from prehospital myocardial infarction by prudent patient activation of mobile coronary care system. *Am Heart J* 1982;103:123–130.
168. Eisenberg MS, Horwood BT, Cummins RO, et al. Cardiac arrest and resuscitation: A tale of 29 cities. *Ann Emerg Med* 1990;19:179–186.
169. Cummins RO, Eisenberg MS, Litwin PE, et al. Automatic external defibrillators used by emergency medical technicians: A controlled clinical trial. *JAMA* 1987;257:1605–1610.
170. Cummins RO, Ornato JP, Thies WH, et al. Improving survival from sudden cardiac arrest: The "chain of survival" concept. A statement for health professionals from the Advanced Cardiac Life Support Subcommittee and the Emergency Cardiac Care Committee, American Heart Association. *Circulation.* 1991;83:1832–1847.
171. Weaver WD, Hill D, Fahrenbruch CE, et al. Use of the automatic external defibrillator in the management of out-of-hospital cardiac arrest. *N Engl J Med* 1988;319:661–666.
172. Stults KR, Brown DD, Schug VL, et al. Prehospital defibrillation performed by emergency medical technicians in rural communities. *N Engl J Med* 1984;310:219–223.
173. Weaver WD, Cerqueira M, Hallstrom AP, et al. Prehospital-initiated vs. hospital-initiated thrombolytic therapy: The Myocardial Infarction Triage and Intervention Trial. *JAMA* 1993;270:1211–1216.
174. Weaver WD, Litwin PE, Martin JS, et al. Effect of age on use of thrombolytic therapy and mortality in acute myocardial infarction: The MITI Project Group. *J Am Coll Cardiol* 1991;18:657–662.
175. Karagounis L, Ipsen SK, Jessop MR, et al. Impact of field-transmitted electrocardiography on time to in-hospital thrombolytic therapy in acute myocardial infarction. *Am J Cardiol* 1990;66:786–791.
176. Grines C, Westerhausen DJ, Grines L, et al. A randomized trial of transfer for primary angioplasty versus on-site thrombolysis in patients

with high-risk myocardial infarction: The Air Primary Angioplasty in Myocardial Infarction Study. *J Am Coll Cardiol* 2002;29:1713–1719.

177. Fibrinolytic Therapy Trialists' (FTT) Collaborative Group. Indications for fibrinolytic therapy in suspected acute myocardial infarction: Collaborative overview of early mortality and major morbidity results from all randomized trials of more than one thousand patients. *Lancet* 1994;343:311–322.
178. ISIS-2 (Second International Study of Infarct Survival) Collaborative Group. Randomised trial of intravenous streptokinase, oral aspirin, both, or neither among 17,187 cases of suspected acute myocardial infarction: ISIS-2. *Lancet* 1988;2:349–360.
179. GREAT Group. Feasibility, safety, and efficacy of domiciliary thrombolysis by general practitioners: Grampian Region Early Anistreplase Trial. *Br Med J* 1992;305:548–553.
180. Castaigne AD, Herve C, Duval-Moulin AM, et al. Prehospital use of APSAC: Results of a placebo-controlled study. *Am J Cardiol* 1989;64 (suppl 2):30A–33A.
181. Schofer J, Buttner J, Geng G, et al. Prehospital thrombolysis in acute myocardial infarction. *Am J Cardiol* 1990;66:1429–1433.
182. European Myocardial Infarction Project Group. Prehospital thrombolytic therapy in patients with suspected acute myocardial infarction. *N Engl J Med* 1993;329:383–389.
183. Gibler WB, Kereiakes DJ, Dean EN, et al. Prehospital diagnosis and treatment of acute myocardial infarction: A North-South perspective. The Cincinnati Heart Project and the Nashville Prehospital TPA Trial. *Am Heart J* 1991;121:1–11.
184. Jesse RL, Kontos MC. Evaluation of chest pain in the emergency department. *Curr Probl Cardiol* 1997;22:149–236.
185. Stark ME, Vacek JL. The initial electrocardiogram during admission for myocardial infarction. *Arch Intern Med* 1987;147:843–846.
186. Karlson BW, Herlitz J, Wiklund O, et al. Early prediction of acute myocardial infarction from clinical history, examination and electrocardiogram in the emergency room. *Am J Cardiol* 1991;68:171–175.
187. Lee TH, Rouan GW, Weisberg MC, et al. Clinical characteristics natural history of patients with acute myocardial infarction sent home from the emergency room. *Am J Cardiol* 1987;60:219–224.
188. Rouan GW, Hedges JR, Tolzis R, et al. A chest pain clinic to improve the follow-up of patients released from an urban university teaching hospital emergency department. *Ann Emerg Med* 1987;16:1145–1150.
189. Tierney WM, Roth BJ, Psaty B, et al. Predictors of myocardial infarction in emergency room patients. *Crit Care Med* 1985;13:526–531.
190. McCarthy BD, Beshansky JR, D'Agostino RB, et al. Missed diagnoses of acute myocardial infarction in the emergency department: Results from a multicenter study. *Ann Emerg Med* 1993;22:579–582.
191. Rusnak RA, Stair TO, Hansen K, et al. Litigation against the emergency physician: Common features in cases of missed myocardial infarction. *Ann Emerg Med* 1989;18:1029–1034.
192. Goldman L, Weinberg M, Weisberg M, et al. A computer-derived protocol to aid in the diagnosis of emergency room patients with acute chest pain. *N Engl J Med* 1982;307:588–596.
193. Schroeder JS, Lamb IH, Hu M. Do patients in whom myocardial infarction has been ruled out have a better prognosis after hospitalization than those surviving infarction? *N Engl J Med* 1980;303:1–5.
194. Kahn JK. Inadvertent thrombolytic therapy for cardiovascular diseases masquerading as acute coronary thrombosis. *Clin Cardiol* 1993;16:67–71.
195. Butler J, Davies AH, Westaby S. Streptokinase in acute aortic dissection. *BMJ* 1990;300:517–519.
196. Eriksen UH, Molgaard H, Ingerslev J, et al. Fatal haemostatic complications due to thrombolytic therapy in patients falsely diagnosed as acute myocardial infarction. *Eur Heart J* 1992;13:840–843.
197. Katz PO, Dalton CB, Richter JE, et al. Esophageal testing of patients with noncardiac chest pain or dysphagia. *Ann Intern Med* 1987;106: 593–597.
198. Goyal RK. Changing focus on unexplained esophageal chest pain. *Ann Intern Med* 1996;124:1008–1011.
199. Nevens F, Janssens J, Piessens J, et al. Prospective study on prevalence of esophageal chest pain in patients referred on an elective basis to a cardiac unit for suspected myocardial ischemia. *Dig Dis Sci* 1991;36:229–235.
200. Hewson EG, Sinclair JW, Dalton CB, et al. Twenty-four-hour esophageal pH monitoring: The most useful test for evaluating noncardiac chest pain. *Am J Med* 1991;90:576–583.
201. Fruergaard P, Launbjerg J, Hesse B, et al. The diagnoses of patients admitted with acute myocardial infarction: A comparison between patients with and without confirmed myocardial infarction. *Eur Heart J* 1996;17:1028–1034.
202. Levene DL. Chest pain: Prophet of doom or nagging neurosis? *Acta Med Scand Suppl* 1981;644:11–13.
203. Ornato JP, Jesse RL, Tatum JL, et al. Lack of correlation between relief of chest pain after sublingual nitroglycerin and reversible radionuclide perfusion defects or presence of significant coronary atherosclerosis on coronary angiography (abstr). *J Am Coll Cardiol* 1995;25:12A.
204. Gibler W, Lewis L, Erb R, et al. Early detection of acute myocardial infarction in patients presenting with chest pain and non-diagnostic ECGs: Serial CK-MB sampling in the emergency department [published erratum appears in *Ann Emerg Med* 1991 Apr;20(4):420]. *Ann Emerg Med* 1990;19:1359–1366.
205. Goldberg R, Gore J, Alpert J, et al. Incidence and case fatality rates of acute myocardial infarction (1975–1984): The Worcester Heart Attack Study. *Am Heart J* 1988;115:761–767.
206. Marin MM, Teichman SL. Use of rapid serial sampling of creatine kinase MB for very early detection of myocardial infarction in patients with acute chest pain. *Am Heart J* 1992;123:354–361.
207. Mauri F, Gasparini M, Barbonaglia L, et al. Prognostic significance of the extent of myocardial injury in acute myocardial infarction treated by streptokinase (the GISSI Trial). *Am J Cardiol* 1989;63: 1291–1295.
208. Cohen M, Hawkins L, Greenberg S, et al. Usefulness of ST segment changes in greater than or equal to 2 leads on the emergency room electrocardiogram in either unstable angina pectoris or non-Q-wave myocardial infarction in predicting outcome. *Am J Cardiol* 1991;67: 1368–1373.
209. Slater DK, Hlatky MA, Mark DB, et al. Outcome in suspected acute myocardial infarction with normal or minimally abnormal admission electrocardiographic findings. *Am J Cardiol* 1987;60:766–770.
210. Brush JE Jr, Brand DA, Acampora D, et al. Use of the initial electrocardiogram to predict in-hospital complications of acute myocardial infarction. *N Engl J Med* 1985;312:1137–1141.
211. Goldman L, Cook EF, Johnson PA, et al. Prediction of the need for intensive care in patients who come to emergency departments with acute chest pain. *N Engl J Med* 1996;334:1498–1504.
212. Pozen MW, D'Agostino RB, Selker HP, et al. A predictive instrument to improve coronary-care-unit admission practices in acute ischemic heart disease. *N Engl J Med* 1984;310:1273–1278.
213. Selker HP, Griffith JL, D'Agostino RB. A tool for judging coronary care unit admission appropriateness, valid for both real-time and retrospective use. *Med Care* 1991;29:610–627.
214. Grijseels EWM, Deckers JW, Hoes AW, et al. Pre-hospital triage of patients with suspected myocardial infarction. *Eur Heart J* 1995;16: 325–332.
215. Fillmore SJ, Shapiro M, Killip T. Arterial oxygen tension in acute myocardial infarction: Serial analysis of clinical state and blood gas changes. *Am Heart J* 1970;79:620–629.
216. Madias JE, Hood WB Jr. Reduction of precordial ST-segment elevation in patients with anterior myocardial infarction by oxygen breathing. *Circulation* 1976;53(suppl I):I-198–I-200.
217. Lowenstein E. Morphine "anesthesia"—A perspective. *Anesthesiology* 1971;35:563–565.
218. Herlitz J. Analgesia in myocardial infarction. *Drugs* 1989;37:939–944.
219. Antman EM. General hospital management, in Julian DG, Braunwald E, eds. *Management of Acute Myocardial Infarction.* London:, Saunders; 1994:42–44.
220. Chiariello M, Gold HK, Leinbach RC, et al. Comparison between the effects of nitroprusside and nitroglycerin on ischemic injury during acute myocardial infarction. *Circulation* 1976;54:766–773.

221. Mann T, Cohn PF, Holman L, et al. Effect of nitroprusside on regional myocardial blood flow in coronary artery disease: Results in 25 patients in comparison with nitroglycerin. *Circulation* 1978;57: 732–738.
222. Bussmann WD, Passek D, Seidel W, et al. Reduction of CK and CK-MB indexes of infarct size by intravenous nitroglycerin. *Circulation* 1981;63:615–622.
223. Flaherty JT, Becker LC, Bulkley BH, et al. A randomized prospective trial of intravenous nitroglycerin in patients with acute myocardial infarction. *Circulation* 1983;68:576–588.
224. Jugdutt BI, Becker LC, Hutchins GM, et al. Effect of intravenous nitroglycerin on collateral blood flow and infarct size in the conscious dog. *Circulation* 1981;63:17–28.
225. Jugdutt BI, Khan MI, Jugdutt SJ, et al. Impact of left ventricular unloading after late reperfusion of canine anterior myocardial infarction on remodeling and function using isosorbide-5-mononitrate. *Circulation* 1995;92:926–934.
226. Yusuf S, Collins R, MacMahon S, et al. Effect of intravenous nitrates on mortality in acute myocardial infarction: An overview of the randomized trials. *Lancet* 1989;1:1088–1092.
227. GISSI-3, Gruppo Italiano per lo Studio della Streptochinasi nell'Infarto Miocardico. Effects of lisinopril and transdermal glycerol trinitrate singly and together on 6-week mortality and ventricular function after acute myocardial infarction. *Lancet* 1994;343:1115–1122.
228. ISIS-4 Collaborative Group. ISIS-4: A randomized factorial trial assessing early oral captopril, oral mononitrate, and intravenous magnesium sulphate in 58,050 patients with suspected acute myocardial infarction. *Lancet* 1995;345:669–685.
229. Kinch JW, Ryan TJ. Right ventricular infarction. *N Engl J Med* 1994; 330:1211–1217.
230. Come PC, Pitt B. Nitroglycerin-induced severe hypotension and bradycardia in patients with acute myocardial infarction. *Circulation* 1976;54:624–628.
231. Fourth American College of Chest Physicians Consensus Conference on Antithrombiotic Therapy. Consensus Conference on Antithrombotic Therapy. *Chest* 1995;108 (suppl):225S–522S.
232. Monocada S, Vane JR. The role of prostacyclin in vascular tissue. *Fed Proc* 1979;38:66–71.
233. CAPRIE Steering Committee. A randomised, blinded trial of clopidogrel versus aspirin in patients at risk of ischaemic events (CAPRIE). *Lancet* 1996;348:1329–1339.
234. Reimer KA, Lowe JE, Rasmussen MM, et al. The wavefront phenomenon of ischemic cell death. I. Myocardial infarc size vs duration of coronary occlusion in dog. *Circulation* 1977;56:786–794.
235. Reimer KA, Jennings RB. The "wave front phenomenon" of myocardial ischemia cell death. II. Transmural progression of necrosis within the framework of ischemic bed size (myocardium at risk) and collateral flow. *Lab Invest* 1979;40:633–644.
236. Lau J, Antman EN, Jimenez-Silva J, et al. Cumulative meta-analysis of therapeutic trials for myocardial infarction. *N Engl J Med* 1992; 327:248–254.
237. MIAMI Trial Research Group. Metoprolol in acute myocardial infarction: Patient population. *Am J Cardiol* 1985;56:1G–57G.
238. TIMI Study Group. Comparison of invasive and conservative strategies after treatment with intravenous tissue plasminogen activator in acute myocardial infarction. Results of thrombolysis in myocardial infarction (TIMI) phase II trial. *N Engl J Med* 1989;320:618–627.
239. Collins R, Peto R, Baigent C, et al. Aspirin, heparin, and fibrinolytic therapy in suspected acute myocardial infarction. *Drug Ther* 1997;36: 847–860.
240. ISIS-2 (Second International Study of Infarct Survival) Collaborative Group. Randomized trial of intravenous streptokinase, oral aspirin, both, or neither among 17,187 cases of suspected acute myocardial infarction: ISIS-2. *J Am Coll Cardiol* 1988;12:3A–13A.
241. ISIS-3 Collaborative Group. A randomized comparison of streptokinase vs tissue plasminogen activator vs anistreplase and of aspirin plus heparin vs aspirin alone among 41,299 cases of suspected acute myocardial infarction. *Lancet* 1992;339:753–770.
242. Kennedy JW. Thrombolytic therapy for acute myocardial infarction: A brief review. *Heart Lung* 1987;16(6 Pt 2):740–745.
243. TIMI IIIB Investigators. Effects of tissue plasminogen activator and a comparison of early invasive and conservative strategies in unstable angina and non-Q-wave myocardial infarction: Results of the TIMI IIIB Trial. Thrombolysis in Myocardial Ischemia. *Circulation* 1994; 89:1545–1556.
244. Cannon CP, Thompson B, McCabe CH, et al. Predictors of non-Q-wave acute myocardial infarction in patients with acute ischemic xsyndromes: An analysis from the Thrombolysis in Myocardial Ischemia (TIMI) III trials. *Am J Cardiol* 1995;75:977–981.
245. Califf RM, Topol EJ, Kereiakes DJ, et al. Cardiac resuscitation should not be a contraindication to thrombolytic therapy for myocardial infarction (abstr). *Circulation* 1988;78:II-127.
246. Hsia J, Hamilton WP, et al for HART Investigators. A comparison between heparin and low-dose aspirin as adjunctive therapy with tissue plasminogen activator for acute myocardial infarction. Heparin-Aspirin Reperfusion Trial (HART) Investigators. *N Engl J Med* 1990;323:1433–1437.
247. Roberts R, Kleiman NS. *The Open Artery: Perspectives on Coronary Reperfusion in Acute Myocardial Infarction.* Hamilton, Ontario, Canada: Decker Periodicals; 1992.
248. Granger CG, Califf RM, Hirsch J, et al. APTTs after thrombolysis and standard intravenous heparin are often low and correlate with body weight, age and sex: Experience from the GUSTO Trial (abstr). *Circulation* 1992;86:I-258.
249. Roberts R. La difference: Long-term benefit of one thrombolytic over another. *Circulation* 1996;94:1203–1205.
250. Hampton JR, Schroder R, Wilcox RG, et al. Randomised, double-blind comparison of reteplase double-bolus administration with streptokinase in acute myocardial infarction (INJECT): Trial to investigate equivalence. *Lancet* 1995;346:329–336.
251. Cody RJ. Results from late breaking clinical trials sessions at ACC '97. *J Am Coll Cardiol* 1997;30:1–7.
252. Cannon CP, Gibson CM, McCabe C, et al. TNK-tissue plasminogen activator compared with front-loaded alteplase in acute myocardial infarction. Results of the TIMI 10B Trial. *Circulation* 1998;98:2805–2814.
253. Single-bolus tenecteplase compared with front-loaded alteplase in acute myocardial infarction: the ASSENT-2 double-blind randomised trial. Assessment of the Safety and Efficacy of a New Thrombolytic Investigators. *Lancet* 1999;354:716–722.
254. Ryan TJ, Bauman WB, Kennedy JW, et al. ACC/AHA guidelines for percutaneous transluminal coronary angioplasty: A report of the American College of Cardiology/American Heart Association Task Force on Assessment of Diagnostic and Therapeutic Cardiovascular Procedures (Committee on Percutaneous Transluminal Coronary Angioplasty). *J Am Coll Cardiol* 1993;22:2033–2054.
255. Weaver WD, Simes RJ, Betriu A, et al. Comparison of primary coronary angioplasty and intravenous thrombolytic therapy for acute myocardial infarction: A quantitative review [published erratum appears in *JAMA* 279:1876, 1998]. *JAMA* 1997;278:2093.
256. Tiefenbrunn AJ, Chandra NC, French WJ, et al. Clinical experience with primary percutaneous transluminal coronary angioplasty compared with alteplase (recombinant tissue-type plasminogen activator) in patients with acute myocardial infarction: A report from the Second National Registry of Myocardial Infarction (NRMI-2). *J Am Coll Cardiol* 1998;31:1240–1245.
257. Hochman JS, Sleeper LA, Webb JG, et al. Early revascularization in acute myocardial infarction complicated by cardiogenic shock. *N Engl J Med* 1999;341:625–634.
258. Brodie BR, Stuckey TD, Wall TC, et al. Importance of time to reperfusion for 30-day and late survival and recovery of left ventricular function after primary angioplasty for acute myocardial infarction. *J Am Coll Cardiol* 1998;32:1312–1319.
259. Grines CL, Browne KF, Marco J, et al. A comparison of immediate angioplasty with thrombolytic therapy for acute myocardial infarction: The Primary Angioplasty in Myocardial Infarction Study Group. *N Engl J Med* 1993;328:673–679.

260. Zijlstra F, deBoer MJ, Hoorntje JC, et al. A comparison of immediate coronary angioplasty with intravenous streptokinase in acute myocardial infarction. *N Engl J Med* 1993;328:680–684.
261. Bleich SD, Nochols TC, Schumacher RR, et al. Effect of heparin on coronary arterial patency after thrombolysis with tissue plasminogen activator in acute myocardial infarction. *Am J Cardiol* 1990;66: 1412–1417.
262. Kander NH, Holland KJ, Pitt B, et al. A randomized pilot trial of brief versus prolonged heparin after successful reperfusion in acute myocardial infarction. *Am J Cardiol* 1990;65:139–142.
263. Hull RD, Raskob GE, Hirsch J, et al. Continuous intravenous heparin compared with intermittent subcutaneous heparin in the initial treatment of proximal vein thrombosis. *N Engl J Med* 1986;315: 1109–1114.
264. Prins MH, Hirsch J. Heparin as an adjunctive treatment after thrombolytic therapy for acute myocardial infarction. *Am J Cardiol* 1991; 67:3A–11A.
265. Simoons MS, Arnold AER, Betriu A, et al. Thrombolysis with tissue plasminogen activator in acute myocardial infarction. No additional benefit from immediate percutaneous coronary angioplasty. *Lancet* 1988;1:197–203.
266. Topol EJ, George BS, Kereiakes DJ, et al. A randomized controlled trial of intravenous tissue plasminogen activator and early intravenous heparin in acute myocardial infarction. *Circulation* 1989;79: 281–286.
267. Verstraete M, Bory M, Collen D, et al. Randomized trial of intravenous recombinant tissue-type plasminogen activity versus intravenous streptokinase in active myocardial infarction. Report from the European Cooperative Study Group for Recombinant Tissue-Type Plasminogen Activator. *Lancet* 1985;1:842–847.
268. SWIFT Trial Study Group. SWIFT Trial of delayed elective intervention versus conservative treatment after thrombolysis with anistreplase in acute myocardial infarction. *BMJ* 1991;302:555–560.
269. Williams DO, Braunwald E, Knatterud G, et al. One-year results of the Thrombolysis in Myocardial Infarction (TIMI) phase II trial. *Circulation* 1992;85:533–542.
270. Juliard JM, Himbert D, Golmard JL, et al. Can we provide reperfusion therapy to all unselected patients admitted with acute myocardial infarction? *J Am Coll Cardiol* 1997;30:157–164.
271. Gibson CM, Cannon CP, Greene RM, et al. Rescue angioplasty in the Thrombolysis In Myocardial Infarction (TIMI) 4 trial. *Am J Cardiol* 1997;80:21–26.
272. Zeymer U, Schroder R, Tebbe U, et al. Non-invasive detection of early infarct vessel patency by resolution of ST-segment elevation in patients with thrombolysis for acute myocardial infarction: Results of the angiographic substudy of the Hirudin for Improvement of Thrombolysis (HIT)-4 trial. *Eur Heart J* 2001;22:769–775.
273. Jacobs AK. Primary angioplasty for acute myocardial infarction—Is it worth the wait? *N Engl J Med* 2003;349:798–800.
274. Keeley EC, Boura JA, Grines CL. Primary angioplasty versus intravenous thrombolytic therapy for acute myocardial infarction: A quantitative review of 23 randomised trials. *Lancet* 2003;361:13–20.
275. Hochman JS, Boland J, Sleeper LA, et al. Current spectrum of cardiogenic shock and effect of early revascularization on mortality: results of an International Registry. SHOCK Registry Investigators. *Circulation* 1995;91:873–881.
276. Braunwald E, Antman E, Beasley J, et al. ACC/AHA 2002 Guideline update for the management of patients with unstable angina and non-ST-segment elevation myocardial infarction—Summary article. Committee on the Management of Patients with Unstable Angina. *J Am Coll Cardiol* 2002;40:1366–1374.
277. Madsen JK, Grande P, Saunamaki K, et al. Danish multicenter randomized study of invasive versus conservative treatment in patients with inducible ischemia after thrombolysis in acute myocardial infarction (DANAMI). *Circulation* 1997;96:748–755.
278. Das G, Talmers FN, Weissler AM. New observations on the effects of atropine on the sinoatrial and atrioventricular noeds in man. *Am J Cardiol* 1975;36:281–285.
279. Kent KM, Smith ER, Redwood DR, et al. Electrical stability of acutely ischemic myocardium: Influences of heart rate and vagal stimulation. *Circulation* 1973;47:291–298.
280. Kottmeier CA, Gravenstein JS. The parasympathomimetic activity of atropine and atropine methylbromide. *Anesthesiology* 1968;29: 1125–1133.
281. Berger PB, Ruocco NA, Jr, Ryan TJ, et al. Incidence and prognostic implications of heart block complicating inferior myocardial infarction treated with thrombolytic therapy: Results from TIMI-II. *J Am Coll Cardiol* 1992;20:533–540.
282. McDonald K, O'Sullivan JJ, Conroy M, et al. Heart block as predictor of in-hospital death in both acute inferior and acute anterior myocardial infarction. *Am J Med* 1990;74:277–282.
283. Fisch GR, Zipes DP, Fisch C. Bundle branch block in sudden death. *Prog Cardiovasc Dis* 1980;23:187–224.
284. Hindman MC, Wagner GS, JaRo M, et al. The clinical significance of bundle branch block complicating acute myocardial infarction: Part I: Clinical characteristics, hospital mortality, and one-year follow-up. *Circulation* 1978;58:679–688.
285. Zoll PM, Zoll RH, Falk RH, et al. External noninvasive temporary cardiac pacing: Clinical trials. *Circulation* 1985;71:937–944.
286. Emergency Cardiac Care Committee and Subcommittees, American Heart Association. Guidelines for cardiopulmonary resuscitation and emergency cardiac care. Part III: Adult advanced cardiac life support. *JAMA* 1992;268:2199–2241.
287. Wood MA. Temporary transvenous pacing. In: Ellenbogen KA, Kay GN, Wilkoff BL, eds. *Clinical Cardiac Pacing.* Philadelphia: Saunders; 1995;687–700.
287a. Guidelines 2000 for cardiopulmonary resuscitation and emergency cardiovascular care. Part 6: Advanced cardiovascular life support section 6. Pharmacology II. Agents to optimize cardiac output and blood pressure. The American Heart Association in Collaboration with the International Liaison Committee on Resuscitation. *Circulation* 2000; 102:II29–II35.
288. Campbell RW, Murray A, Julian DG. Ventricular arrhythmias in first 12 hours of acute myocardial infarction: Natural history study. *Br Heart J* 1981;46:351–357.
289. Campbell RWF. Arrhythmias. In: Julian DG, Braunwald E, eds. *Management of Acute Myocardial Infarction,* London: Saunders; 1994;223–240.
290. Higham PD, Adams PC, Murray A, et al. Plasma potassium, serum magnesium and ventricular fibrillation: A prospective study. *Q J Med* 1993;86:609–617.
291. Antman EM, Berlin JA. Declining incidence of ventricular fibrillation in myocardial infarction: Implications for the prophylactic use of lidocaine. *Circulation* 1992;86:764–773.
292. Behar S, Goldbourt U, Reicher-Reiss H, et al. Prognosis of acute myocardial infarction complicated by primary ventricular fibrillation: Principal investigators of the SPRINT Study. *Am J Cardiol* 1990;66: 1208–1211.
293. Reeder GS, Gersh BJ. Modern management of acute myocardial infarction. *Curr Probl Cardiol* 1996;21:591–667.
294. Dhurandhar RW, MacMillan RL, Brown KW. Primary ventricular fibrillation complicating acute myocardial infarction. *Am J Cardiol* 1990;66:1208–1211.
295. Lie KI, Wellens HJ, Durrer D. Characteristics and predictability of primary ventricular fibrillation. *Eur J Cardiol* 1974;1:379–384.
296. Solomon SD, Ridker PM, Antman EM. Ventricular arrhythmias in trials of thrombolytic therapy for acute myocardial infarction: A meta-analysis. *Circulation* 1993;88:2575–2581.
297. MacMahon S, Collins R, Peto R, et al. Effects of prophylactic lidocaine in suspected acute myocardial infarction: An overview of results from the randomized controlled trials. *JAMA* 1992;260:1910–1916.
298. American Heart Association. Guidelines 2000 for cardiopulmonary resuscitation and emergency cardiovascular care. *Circulation* 2000; 102(suppl):I1–I384.
299. Kern KB, Halperin HR, Field J. New guidelines for cardiopulmonary resuscitation and emergency cardiac care: Changes in the management of cardiac arrest. *JAMA* 2001;285:1267–1269.

300. Scheinman MM, Levine JH, Cannom DS, et al. Dose-ranging study of intravenous amiodarone in patients with life-threatening ventricular tachyarrhythmias. The Intravenous Amiodarone Multicenter Investigators Group. *Circulation* 1995;92:3264–3272.
301. Tosteson ANA, Goldman L, Udvarhelyi IS, et al. Cost-effectiveness of a coronary care unit versus an intermediate care unit for emergency department patients with chest pain. *Circulation* 1996;94:143–150.
302. Tatum JL, Jesse RL, Kontos MC, et al. Comprehensive strategy for the evaluation and triage of the chest pain patient. *Ann Emerg Med* 1997;29:116–125.
303. Chobanian AV, Lille RD, Tercyak A, et al. The metabolic and hemodynamic effects of prolonged bed rest in normal subjects. *Circulation* 1974;49:551–559.
304. Winslow EH. Cardiovascular consequences of bed rest. *Heart Lung* 1985;14:236–246.
305. Metzger BL, Therrien B. Effect of position on cardiovascular response during the Valsalva maneuver. *Nurs Res* 1990;39:198–202.
306. Taggart P, Sutton P, John R, et al. Monophasic action potential recordings during acute changes in ventricular loading induced by the Valsalva manoeuvre. *Br Heart J* 1992;67:221–229.
307. Dixon RA, Edwards IR, Pilcher J. Diazepam in immediate post–myocardial infarct period: A double blind trial. *Br Heart J* 1980;43: 535–540.
308. Thompson DR, Meddis R. A prospective evaluation of in-hospital counselling for first time myocardial infarction in men. *J Psychosom Res* 1990;34:237–248.
309. Duryee R. The efficacy of inpatient education after myocardial infarction. *Heart Lung* 1992;21:217–225.
310. Fletcher V. An individualized teaching programme following primary uncomplicated myocardial infarction. *J Adv Nurs* 1987;12:195–200.
311. Dracup K, Moser DK, Guzy PM, et al. Is cardiopulmonary resuscitation training deleterious for family members of cardiac patients? *Am J Public Health* 1994;84:116–118.
312. Myerburg RJ, Kessler KM, Castellanos A. Sudden cardiac death: Epidemiology, transient risk, and intervention assessment. *Ann Intern Med* 1993;119:1187–1197.
313. Pfeffer MA, Lamas GA, Vaughan DE, et al. Effect of captopril on progressive ventricular dilatation after anterior myocardial infarction. *N Engl J Med* 1988;319:80–86.
314. SAVE Investigators, Pfeffer MA, Braunwald E, et al. Effect of captopril on morbidity and mortality in patients with left ventricular dysfunction after myocardial infarction: Results of the Survival and Ventricular Enlargement Trial. *N Engl J Med* 1992;327:669–677.
315. SOLVD Investigators. Effect of enalapril on survival in patients with reduced left ventricular ejection fractions and congestive heart failure. *N Engl J Med* 1991;325:293–302.
316. Latini R, Maggioni AP, Flather M, et al. Ace-inhibitor use in patients with myocardial infarction: Summary of evidence from clinical trials. *Circulation* 1995;92:3132–3137.
317. Sigurdsson A, Swedberg K. Left ventricular remodelling, neurohormonal activation and early treatment with enalapril (CONSENSUS II) following myocardial infarction. *Eur Heart J* 1994;15(suppl B):14–19.
318. Acute Infarction Ramipril Efficacy (AIRE) Study Investigators. Effect of ramipril on mortality and morbidity of survivors of acute myocardial infarction with clinical evidence of heart failure. *Lancet* 1993;342:821–828.
319. Kober L, Torp-Pedersen C, Carlsen JE, et al. A clinical trial of the angiotensin-converting-enzyme inhibitor trandolapril in patients with left ventricular dysfunction after myocardial infarction. Trandolapril Cardiac Evaluation (TRACE) Study Group. *N Engl J Med* 1995;333: 1670–1676.
320. HOPE Investigators. Effects of an angiotensin-converting-enzyme inhibitor, ramipril, on cardiovascular events in high-risk patients. The Heart Outcomes Prevention Evaluation Study Investigators. *N Engl J Med* 2000;342:145–153.
321. Teo KK, Yusuf S, Collins R, et al. Effects of intravenous magnesium in suspected acute myocardial infarction: Overview of randomised trials. *BMJ* 1991;303:1499–1503.
322. Woods K, Abrams K. The importance of effect mechanism in the design and interpretation of clinical trials: The role of magnesium in acute myocardial infarction. *Prog Cardiovasc Dis* 2002;44:267–274.
323. Woods KL, Fletcher S, Roffe C, et al. Intravenous magnesium sulphate in suspected acute myocardial infarction: Results of the second Leicester Intravenous Magnesium Intervention Trial (LIMIT-2). *Lancet* 1992;339:1553–1558.
324. MAGIC Trial Investigators. Early administration of intravenous magnesium to high-risk patients with acute myocardial infarction in the Magnesium in Coronaries (MAGIC) Trial: A randomised controlled trial. *Lancet* 2002;360:1189–1196.
325. Gheorghiade M, Anderson J, Rosman H, et al. Risk identification at the time of admission to coronary care unit in patients with suspected myocardial infarction. *Am Heart J* 1988;116:1212–1217.
326. Pozen MW, Stechmiller JK, Voigt GC. Prognosis efficacy of early clinical categorization of myocardial infarction patients. *Circulation* 1977;56:816–819.
327. Krone RJ. The role of risk stratification in the early management of a myocardial infarction. *Ann Intern Med* 1992;116:223–237.
328. Kloner RA, Parisi AF. Acute myocardial infarction: Diagnostic and prognostic applications of two-dimensional echocardiography. *Circulation* 1987;75:521–524.
329. Hopkins LE, Crabbe SJ, Chase SL. Use of a proprietary database to examine lengths of hospital stay of patients who received drug therapy for acute myocardial infarction. *Am J Hosp Pharm* 1989;46: 957–961.
330. Topol EJ, Burek K, O'Neill WW, et al. A randomized controlled trial of hospital discharge three days after myocardial infarction in the era of reperfusion. *N Engl J Med* 1988;318:1083–1088.
331. Mark DB, Sigmon K, Topol EJ, et al. Identification of acute myocardial infarction patients suitable for early hospital discharge after aggressive interventional therapy: Results from the Thrombolysis and Angioplasty in Acute Myocardial Infarction Registry. *Circulation* 1991;83:1186–1193.
332. Newby LK, Califf RM, Guerci A, et al. Early discharge in the thrombolytic era: An analysis of criteria for uncomplicated infarction from the Global Utilization of Streptokinase and t-PA for Occluded Coronary Arteries (GUSTO) Trial. *J Am Coll Cardiol* 1996;27:625–632.
333. Bosch X, Theroux P, Waters DD, et al. Early postinfarction ischemia: Clinical, angiographic, and prognostic significance. *Circulation* 1987;5:988–995.
334. Oliva PB, Hammill SC. The clinical distinction between regional postinfarction pericarditis and other causes of postinfarction chest pain: Ancillary observations regarding the effect of lytic therapy upon the frequency of postinfarction pericarditis, postinfarction angina, and reinfarction. *Clin Cardiol* 1994;17:471–478.
335. Kudenchuk PJ, Ho MT, Weaver WD, et al. Accuracy of computer-interpreted electrocardiography in selecting patients for thrombolytic therapy: MITI Project Investigators. *J Am Coll Cardiol* 1991;17: 1486–1491.
336. Rothbaum DA, Linnemeier TJ, Landin RJ, et al. Emergency percutaneous transluminal coronary angioplasty in acute myocardial infarction: A 3-year experience. *J Am Coll Cardiol* 1987;10:264–272.
337. Ferguson JJ, Diver DJ, Boldt M, et al. Significance of nitroglycerin-induced hypotension with inferior wall acute myocardial infarction. *Am J Cardiol* 1989;64:311–314.
338. Cragg DR, Friedman HZ, Bonema JD, et al. Outcome of patients with acute myocardial infarction who are ineligible for thrombolytic therapy. *Ann Intern Med* 1991;115:173–177.
339. Gibson RS, Young PM, Boden WE, et al. Prognostic significance and beneficial effect of diltiazem on the incidence of early recurrent ischemia after non-Q-wave myocardial infarction: Results of the Diltiazem Reinfarction Study. *Am J Cardiol* 1987;60:203–209.
340. Schechtman KB, Capone RJ, Kleiger RE, et al. Differential risk patterns associated with 3 month as compared with 3 to 12 month mortality and reinfarction after non-Q-wave myocardial infarction. The Diltiazem Reinfarction Study Group. *J Am Coll Cardiol* 1990;15: 940–947.

341. Loop FD, Lytle BW, Cosgrove DM, et al. Reoperation for coronary atherosclerosis: Changing practice in 2509 consecutive patients. *Ann Surg* 1990;212:378–385.
342. Yasmineh WG, Ibrahim GA, Abbasnezhad MA, et al. Isoenzyme distribution of creatine kinase and lactate dehydrogenase in serum and skeletal muscle in Duchenne muscular dystrophy, collagen disease, and other muscular disorders. *Clin Chem* 1978;24:1985–1989.
343. Krainin FM, Flessas AP, Spodick DH. Infarction-associated pericarditis: Rarity of diagnostic electrocardiogram. *N Engl J Med* 1984;311:1211–1214.
344. Thadani U, Chopra MP, Aber CP. Pericarditis after acute myocardial infarction. *BMJ* 1971;2:135–137.
345. Erhardt LR. Clinical and pathological observations in different types of acute myocardial infarction: A study of 84 patients deceased after treatment in a coronary care unit. *Acta Med Scand* 1974;560:1–78.
346. Tofler GH, Muller JE, Stone PH, et al. Pericarditis in acute myocardial infarction: Characterization and clinical significance. *Am Heart J* 1989;117:86–92.
347. Wall TC, Califf RM, Harrelson-Woodlief L, et al. Usefulness of a pericardial friction rub after thrombolytic therapy during acute myocardial infarction in predicting amount of myocardial damage: The TAMI Study Group. *Am J Cardiol* 1990;66:1418–1421.
348. Barman PC, Krishnaswami V, Geraci AR. Pericarditis in acute myocardial infarction. *NYS J Med* 1973;73:645–648.
349. Guillevin L, Valere PE. Pericarditis in acute myocardial infarction (letter). *Lancet* 1976;1:429.
350. Berman J, Haffajee CI, Alpert JS. Therapy of symptomatic pericarditis after myocardial infarction: Retrospective and prospective studies of aspirin, indomethacin, prednisone, and spontaneous resolution. *Am Heart J* 1981;101:750–753.
351. Lavie CJ, Gersh BJ. Mechanical and electrical complication of acute myocardial infarction. *Mayo Clin Proc* 1990;65:709–730.
352. Hammerman H, Schoen FJ, Braunwald E, et al. Drug-induced expansion of infarct: Morphological and functional correlations. *Circulation* 1984;69:611–617.
353. Bulkley BH, Roberts WC. Steroid therapy during acute myocardial infarction: A cause of delayed healing of ventricular aneurysm. *Am J Med* 1974;56:244–250.
354. Kloner RA, Fishbein MC, Lew H, et al. Mummification of the infarcted myocardium by high dose corticosteroids. *Circulation* 1978;57:56–63.
355. Shahar A, Hod H, Barabash GM, et al. Disappearance of a syndrome: Dressler's syndrome in the era of thrombolysis. *Cardiology* 1994;85:255–258.
356. Dressler W. The post-myocardial-infarction syndrome. *Arch Intern Med* 1959;103:28–42.
357. Kossowsky WA, Epstein PJ, Levine RS. Post myocardial infarction syndrome: An early complication of acute myocardial infarction. *Chest* 1973;63:35–39.
358. McKay RG, Pfeffer MA, Pasternak RC, et al. Left ventricular remodeling after myocardial infarction: A corollary to infarct expansion. *Circulation* 1986;74:693–702.
359. Forrester JS, Wyatt HL, da Luz PL, et al. Functional significance of regional ischemic contraction abnormalities. *Circulation* 1976;54:64–70.
360. Aroesty JM, McKay RG, Heller GV, et al. Simultaneous assessment of left ventricular systolic and diastolic dysfunction during pacing-induced ischemia. *Circulation* 1985;71:889–900.
361. Tyberg JV, Forrester JS, Wyatt HL, et al. An analysis of segmental ischemic dysfunction utilizing the pressure-length loop. *Circulation* 1974;49:748–754.
362. Weisman HF, Healey B. Myocardial infarct expansion, infarct extension, and reinfarction: Pathophysiologic concepts. *Prog Cardiovasc Dis* 1987;30:73–110.
363. Sobel BE, Bresnahan GF, Shell WE, et al. Estimation of infarct size in man and its relation to prognosis. *Circulation* 1972;46:640–648.
364. Roberts R, Henry PD, Sobel BE. An improved basis for enzymatic estimation of infarct size. *Circulation* 1975;52:743–754.
365. Page DL, Caulfield JB, Kastor JA, et al. Myocardial changes associated with cardiogenic shock. *N Engl J Med* 1971;285:133–137.
366. Alonso DR, Scheidt S, Post M, et al. Pathophysiology of cardiogenic shock: Quantification of myocardial necrosis, clinical, pathologic and electrocardiographic correlations. *Circulation* 1973;48:588–596.
367. Harnarayan C, Bennett MA, Pentecost BL, et al. Quantitative study of infarcted myocardium in cardiogenic shock. *Br Heart J* 1970;32:728–732.
368. Rigaud M, Rocha P, Boschat J, et al. Regional left ventricular function assessed by contrast angiography in acute myocardial infarction. *Circulation* 1979;60:130–139.
369. Marmor A, Geltman EM, Biello DR, et al. Functional response of the right ventricle to myocardial infarction: Dependence on the site of left ventricular infarction. *Circulation* 1981;64:1005–1011.
370. Wackers FJT, Lie KI, Sokole EB, et al. Prevalence of right ventricular involvement in inferior wall infarction assessed with thallium 201 and technetium-99m pyrophosphate. *Am J Cardiol* 1978;42:358–362.
371. Rigo P, Murray M, Taylor DR, et al. Right ventricular dysfunction detected by gated scintiphotography in patients with acute inferior myocardial infarction. *Circulation* 1975;52:268–274.
372. Zehender M, Kasper W, Kauder E, et al. Right ventricular infarction as an independent predictor of prognosis after acute inferior myocardial infarction. *N Engl J Med* 1993;328:981–988.
373. Berger PB, Ryan TJ. Inferior myocardial infarction: High-risk subgroups. *Circulation* 1990;81:401–411.
374. Andersen HR, Falk E, Nielsen D. Right ventricular infarction: Frequency, size and topography in coronary heart disease: A prospective study comprising 107 consecutive autopsies from a coronary care unit. *J Am Coll Cardiol* 1987;10:1223–1232.
375. Lee FA. Hemodynamics of the right ventricle in normal and diseased states. *Cardiol Clin* 1992;10:59–67.
376. Cross CE. Right ventricular pressure and coronary flow. *Am J Physiol* 1962;202:12–16.
377. Haupt HM, Hutchins GM, Moore GW. Right ventricular infarction: Role of the moderator band artery in determining infarct size. *Circulation* 1983;67:1268–1272.
378. Setaro JF, Cabin HS. Right ventricular infarction. *Cardiol Clin* 1992;10:69–90.
379. Goldstein JA, Barzilai B, Rosamond TL, et al. Determinants of hemodynamic compromise with severe right ventricular infarction. *Circulation* 1990;82:359–368.
380. Goldstein JA, Tweddell JS, Barzilai B, et al. Importance of left ventricular function and systolic ventricular interaction to right ventricular perfomance during acute right heart ischemia. *J Am Coll Cardiol* 1992;19:704–711.
381. Dell'Italia LJ, Starling MR, Crawford MH, et al. Right ventricular infarction: Identification by hemodynamic measurements before and after volume loading and correlation with noninvasive techniques. *J Am Coll Cardiol* 1984;4:931–939.
382. Cohn JN, Guiha NH, Broder MI, et al. Right ventricular infarction: Clinical and hemodynamic features. *Am J Cardiol* 1974;33:209–214.
383. Wellens H. Right ventricular infarction (editorial). *N Engl J Med* 1993;328:1036–1038.
384. Manno BV, Bemis CE, Carver J, et al. Right ventricular infarction complicated by right to left shunt. *J Am Coll Cardiol* 1983;1:554–557.
385. Braat SH, DeZwaan C, Brugada P, et al. Right ventricular involvement with acute inferior wall myocardial infarction identifies high risk of developing atrioventricular nodal conduction disturbances. *Am Heart J* 1984;107:1183–1187.
386. Love JC, Haffajee CI, Gore JM, et al. Reversibility of hypotension and shock by atrial or atrioventricular sequential pacing in patients with right ventricular infarction. *Am Heart J* 1984;108:5–13.
387. Sugiura T, Iwasaka T, Takahashi N, et al. Atrial fibrillation in inferior wall Q-wave acute myocardial infarction. *Am J Cardiol* 1991;67:1135–1136.
388. Braat SH, Ramentol M, Halders S, et al. Reperfusion with streptokinase of an occluded right coronary artery: Effects on early and late right and left ventricular ejection fraction. *Am Heart J* 1987;113:257–260.

389. Schuler G, Hofmann M, Schwarz F, et al. Effect of successful thrombolytic therapy on right ventricular function in acute inferior wall myocardial infarction. *Am J Cardiol* 1984;54:951–957.
390. Moreyra AE, Suh C, Porway MN, et al. Rapid hemodynamic improvement in right ventricular infarction after coronary angioplasty. *Chest* 1988;94:197–199.
391. Griffin J, Grines CL, Marsalese D, et al. A prospective, randomized trial evaluating the prophylactic use of balloon pumping in high risk myocardial infarction patients: PAMI-2 (Abstr #715-2). *J Am Coll Cardiol* 1995;25:86A.
392. Parmley WW, Chuck L, Chatterjee K, et al. Acute changes in the diastolic pressure-volume relationship of the left ventricle. *Eur J Cardiol* 1976;4:105–120.
393. Smiseth OA, Rufsum H, Junemann J, et al. Ventricular diastolic pressure-volume shifts during acute ischemic left ventricular failure in dogs. *J Am Coll Cardiol* 1984;3:966–977.
394. Dikshit K, Vyden JK, Forrester JS, et al. Renal and extrarenal hemodynamic effects of furosemide in congestive heart failure after acute myocardial infarction. *N Engl J Med* 1973;288:1087–1099.
395. Biddle TL, Yu PN. Effect of furosemide on hemodynamics and lung water in acute pulmonary edema secondary to myocardial infarction. *Am J Cardiol* 1979;43:86–90.
396. Kiely J, Kelly DT, Taylor DR, et al. The role of furosemide in the treatment of left ventricular dysfunction associated with acute myocardial infarction. *Circulation* 1973;48:581–587.
397. Goldstein RA, Passamani ER, Roberts R. A comparison of digoxin and dobutamine in patients with acute infarction and failure. *N Engl J Med* 1980;303:846–850.
398. Gillespie TA, Ambos HD, Sobel BE, et al. Effects of dobutamine in patients with acute myocardial infarction. *Am J Cardiol* 1977;39: 588–594.
399. Kahn JC, Gueret P, Menier R, et al. Prognostic value of enzymatic (CPK) estimation of infarct size. *J Mol Med* 1977;2:223–231.
400. Forrester JS, Diamond GA, Chatterjee K, et al. Medical therapy of acute myocardial infarction by appliaction of hemodynamic subsets (first of two parts). *N Engl J Med* 1976;295:1356–1362.
401. Forrester JS, Diamond GA, Chatterjee K, et al. Medical therapy of adult myocardial infarction by application of hemodynamic subsets (second of two parts). *N Engl J Med* 1976;295:1404–1413.
402. Rackley CE, Satler LF, Pearle DL, et al. Use of hemodynamics measurements for management of acute myocardial infarction. *Cardiovasc Clin* 1976;16:3–15.
403. Cohn JN, Franciosa JA, Francis GS, et al. Effect of short-term infusion of sodium nitroprusside on mortality rate in acute myocardial infarction complicated by left ventricular failure. *N Engl J Med* 1982;306:1129–1135.
404. Clark G, Strauss HD, Roberts R. Dobutamine versus furosemide in the treatment of cardiac failure due to right ventricular function. *Chest* 1980;77:220–223.
405. Roberts R. Inotropic therapy for cardiac failure associated with acute myocardial infarction. *Chest* 1988;93:22S–24S.
406. Young JB, Roberts R. Heart failure. In: Dirks JH, Sutton RAI, eds. *Diuretics: Physiology, Pharmacology and Clincial Use.* Philadelphia: Saunders; 1986:51–167.
407. Schreiber TL, Miller DH, Zola B. Management of myocardial infarction shock: Current status. *Am Heart J* 1989;117:435–443.
408. Hill NS, Antman EM, Green LH, et al. Intravenous nitroglycerin: A review of pharmacology, indications, therapeutic effects and complications. *Chest* 1981;79:69–76.
409. Wackers FJ, Lie KI, Becker AE, et al. Coronary artery disease in patients dying from cardiogenic shock or congestive heart failure in the setting of acute myocardial infarction. *Br Heart J* 1976;38:906–910.
410. Cercek B, Shah PK. Complicated acute myocardial infarction: Heart failure, shock, mechanical complications. *Cardiol Clin* 1991;9: 569–593.
411. Gutovitz AL, Sobel BE, Roberts R. The progressive nautre of myocardial injury in selected patients with cardiogenic shock. *Am J Cardiol* 1978;41:469–475.
412. Goldberg LI. Cardiovascular and renal actions of dopamine: Potential clinical application. *Pharmacol Rev* 1972;21:1–29.
413. Gunnar R, Loeb HS. Shock in acute myocardial infarction: Evolution of physiologic therapy. *J Am Coll Cardiol* 1983;1:154–163.
414. Mikulic E, Cohn JN, Franciosa JA. Comparative hemodynamic effects of inotropic and vasodilator drugs in severe heart failure. *Circulation* 1977;56:528–533.
415. Miller RR, Awan NA, Joyce JA, et al. Combined dopamine and nitroprusside therapy in congestive heart failure. *Circulation* 1977;5: 881–884.
416. Richard C, Ricome JL, Rimailho A, et al. Combined hemodynamic effects of dopamine and dobutamine in cardiogenic shock. *Circulation* 1983;67:620–626.
417. Lee L, Erbel R, Brown TM, et al. Multicenter registry of angioplasty therapy of cardiogenic shock: Initial and longterm survival. *J Am Coll Cardiol* 1991;17:599–603.
418. Waller BF, Rothbaum DA, Pinkerton CA, et al. States of the myocardium and infarct-related coronary artery in 19 necropsy patients with acute recanalization using pharmacologic (streptokinase, recombinant tissue plasminogen activator), mechanical (percutaneous transluminal coronary angioplasty) or combined types of reperfusion therapy. *J Am Coll Cardiol* 1987;9:785–801.
419. Brodie BR, Weintraub RA, Stuckey TD, et al. Outcomes of direct coronary angioplasty for acute myocardial infarction in candidates and noncandidates for thrombolytic therapy. *Am J Cardiol* 1991;67:7–12.
420. Wei JY, Hutchins GM, Buckley BH. Papillary muscle rupture in fatal acute myocardial infarction: A potentially treatable form of cardiogenic shock. *Ann Intern Med* 1979;90:149–152.
421. Nishimura RA, Schoff HV, Shub C, et al. Papillary muscle rupture complicating acute myocardial infarction: Analysis of 17 patients. *Am J Cardiol* 1983;51:373–377.
422. Lie JT, Wright KE, Jr, Titus JL. Sudden appearance of a systolic murmur after acute myocardial infarction. *Am Heart J* 1975;90:507–512.
423. Shelburne JC, Rubinstein D, Gorlin R. A reappraisal of papillary muscle dysfunction: Correlative clinical and angiographic study. *Am J Med* 1969;46:862–871.
424. DeBusk RF, Harrison DC. The clinical spectrum of papillary-muscle disease. *N Engl J Med* 1969;281:1458–1467.
425. Burch GE, DePasquale NP, Phillips JH. The syndrome of papillary muscle dysfunction. *Am Heart J* 1968;75:399–414.
426. Radford MJ, Johnson RA, Daggett WM, et al. Ventricular septal rupture: A review of clinical and physiologic features and an analysis of survival. *Circulation* 1981;64:545–553.
427. Rasmussen S, Leth A, Kjoller E, et al. Cardiac rupture in acute myocardial infarction: A review of 72 consecutive cases. *Acta Med Scand* 1979;205:11–16.
428. Maker JF, Mallory GK, Laurenz GA. Rupture of the heart after myocardial infarction. *N Engl J Med* 1956;255:1–10.
429. Held AC, Cole PL, Lipton B, et al. Rupture of the interventricular septum complicating acute myocardial infarction: A multicenter analysis of clinical findings and outcome. *Am Heart J* 1988;116:1330–1336.
430. Gaudiani VA, Miller DG, Stinson EB, et al. Postinfarction ventricular septal defect: An argument for early operation. *Surgery* 1981;89: 48–54.
431. Gray RJ, Sethna D, Matloff JM. The role of cardiac surgery in acute myocardial infarction. I. With mechanical complications. *Am Heart J* 1983;106:723–728.
432. Moore CA, Nygard TW, Kaiser DS, et al. Postinfarction ventricular septal rupture: The importance of location of infarction and right ventricular function in determining survival. *Circulation* 1986;74:45–55.
433. Bates RJ, Beutler S, Resnekor L, et al. Cardiac rupture—Challenge in diagnosis and management. *Am J Cardiol* 1970;40:429–437.
434. Roberts WG, Morrow AG. Pseudoaneurysm of the left ventricle: An unusual sequel of myocardial infarction and rupture of the heart. *Am J Med* 1967;43:639–644.
435. Cabin HS, Roberts WC. Left ventricular aneurysm, intraaneurysmal thrombus and systemic embolus in coronary heart disease. *Chest* 1980;77:586–589.

436. Hayes MJ, Morris GK, Hampton JR. Lack of effect of bed rest and cigarette smoking on development of deep venous thrombus after myocardial infarction. *Br Heart J* 1976;38:981–983.
437. Miller RR, Lies JE, Carretta RF, et al. Prevention of lower extremity venous thrombus by early mobilization. *Ann Intern Med* 1976;84: 700–703.
438. Emerson PA, Marks P. Preventing thromboembolism after myocardial infarction: Effect of low-dose heparin or smoking. *BMJ* 1977;1: 18–20.
439. Weinreich DJ, Burke JF, Pauletto FJ. Left ventricular mural thrombi complicating acute myocardial infarction. *Ann Intern Med* 1984;100: 789–794.
440. Visser CA, Kan G, Meltzer RS, et al. Embolic potential of left ventricular thrombus after myocardial infarction: A two-dimensional echocardiographic study of 119 patients. *J Am Coll Cardiol* 1985;5: 1276–1280.
441. Kouvaras G, Chronopoulas G, Soufras G, et al. The effects of long term antithrombotic treatment of left ventribular thrombi in patients after an acute myocardial infarction. *Am Heart J* 1990;119:73–78.
442. Keating EC, Gross SA, Schlamowitz RA, et al. Mural thrombi in myocardial infarctions: Prospective evaluation by two dimensional echocardiography. *Am J Med* 1983;74:989–995.
443. Spirito P, Bellotti P, Chiarella F. Prognostic significance and natural history of left ventricular thrombi in patients with acute anterior myocardial infarction: A two-dimensional echocardiographic study. *Circulation* 1985;72:774–780.
444. Jugdutt BI, Sivaram CA. Prospective two-dimensional echocardiographic evaluation of left ventricular thrombus and embolism after acute myocardial infarction. *J Am Coll Cardiol* 1989;13:554–564.
445. Johannssen KA, Nordrehoug JE, Vonder Lippe G, et al. Risk factors for embolization in patients with left ventricular thrombi and acute myocardial infarction. *Br Heart J* 1988;60:104–110.
446. Davis MJE, Ireland MA. Effect of early anticoagulation on the frequency of left ventricular thrombi after anterior wall acute myocardial infarction. *Am J Cardiol* 1986;57:1244–1247.
447. Lapeyre AC, III, Steele PM, Kazmier FJ, et al. Systemic embolism in chronic left ventricular aneurysm: Incidence and the role of anticoagulation. *J Am Coll Cardiol* 1985;6:534–538.
448. Turpie ACG, Robinson JG, Doyle DJ, et al. Comparison of high-dose with low-dose subcutaneous heparin to prevent left ventricular mural thrombosis in patients with acute transmural anterior myocardial infarction. *N Engl J Med* 1989;320:352–357.
449. Takamoto T, Kim D, Urie PM, et al. Comparative recognition of left ventricular thrombi by echocardiography and cineangiography. *Br Heart J* 1985;53:36–42.
450. Sechtem U, Theissen P, Heindel W, et al. Diagnosis of left ventricular thrombi by magnetic resonance imaging and comparison with angiocardiography, computed tomography and echocardiography. *Am J Cardiol* 1989;64:1195–1199.
451. Faxon DP, Ryan TJ, Davis KB, et al. Prognostic significance of angiographically documented left ventricular aneurysm from the Coronary Artery Surgery Study (CASS). *Am J Cardiol* 1982;50:157–164.
452. Loop FD, Effler DB, Webster JS, et al. Posterior ventricular aneurysms. Etiologic factors and surgical treatment. *N Engl J Med* 1973;288:237–239.
453. Loop FD, Effler DB, Navia JA, et al. Aneurysms of the left ventricle: Survival and results of a ten-year surgical experience. *Ann Surg* 1973; 178:399–405.
454. Catherwood E, Mintz GS, Kotler MN, et al. Two-dimensional echocardiographic recognition of left ventricular pseudo-aneurysm. *Circulation* 1980;62:294–303.
455. Martin RH, Almond CH, Saab S, et al. True and false aneurysms of the left ventricle following myocardial infarction. *Am J Med* 1977;62: 418–424.
456. Liberthson RR, Salisbury KW, Hutter AM, et al. Atrial tachyarrhythmias in acute myocardial infarction. *Am J Med* 1976;60:956–960.
457. Zoni-Berisso M, Carratino L, Ferroni A, et al. Frequency, characteristics and significance of supraventricular tachyarrhythmias detected by 24-hour electrocardiographic recording in the late hospital phase of acute myocardial infarction. *Am J Cardiol* 1990;65:1064–1070.
458. Gordon S, Finck DR, Perera RD, et al. Atrial infarction complicating an acute inferior myocardial infarction. *Arch Intern Med* 1984;144:193.
459. Nielsen FE, Andersen HH, Gram-Hansen P, et al. The relationship between ECG signs of atrial infarction and the development of supraventricular arrhythmias in patients with acute myocardial infarction. *Am Heart J* 1992;123:69–72.
460. James TN. Myocardial infarction and atrial arrhythmias. *Circulation* 1961;24:761–776.
461. Goldberg RJ, Seeley D, Becker RC, et al. Impact of atrial fibrillation on the in-hospital and long-term survival of patients with acute myocardial infarction: A community-wide perspective. *Am Heart J* 1990;119:996–1001.
462. Nielsen FE, Sorensen HT, Christensen JH, et al. Reduced occurrence of atrial fibrillation in acute myocardial infarction treated with streptokinase. *Eur Heart J* 1991;12:1081–1083.
463. Behar S, Zahavi Z, Goldbourt U, et al. Long-term prognosis of patients with paroxysmal atrial fibrillation complicating acute myocardial infarction: SPRINT Study Group. *Eur Heart J* 1992;13:45–50.
464. Konecke LL, Knoebel SB. Nonparoxysmal junctional tachycardia complicating acute myocardial infarction. *Circulation* 1972;45: 367–374.
465. Meltzer LE, Cohen HE. The incidence of arrhythmias associated with acute myocardial infarction., In: Meltzer LE, Dunning AJ, eds. *Textbook of Coronary Care.* Philadelphia: Charles Press; 1972.
466. Kostuk WJ, Beanlands DS. Complete heart block associated with acute myocardial infarction. *Am J Cardiol* 1970;26:380–384.
467. Hindman MC, Wagner GS, JaRo M, et al. The clinical significance of bundle branch block complicating acute myocardial infarction: Part II Indications for temporary and permanent pacemaker insertion. *Circulation* 1978;58:689–699.
468. Dreifus LS, Fisch C, Griffin JC, et al. Guidelines for implantation of cardiac pacemakers and antiarrhythmia devices: A report of the American College of Cardiology/American Heart Association Task Force on Assessment of Diagnostic and Therapeutic Cardiovascular Procedures (Committee on Pacemaker Implantation). *J Am Coll Cardiol* 1991;18:1–13.
469. Goble AJ, Sloman G, Robinson JS. Mortality reduction in a coronary care unit. *BMJ* 1966;1:1005–1009.
470. Graboys TB. In-hospital sudden death after coronary care unit discharge: A high risk profile. *Arch Intern Med* 1975;135:512–514.
471. Grace WJ, Yarvote PM. Acute myocardial infarction: The course of the illness following discharge from the coronary care unit. A description of the intermediate coronary care unit. *Chest* 1971;59:15–17.
472. Christensen D, Ford M, Reading J, et al. Sudden death in the late hospital phase of acute myocardial infarction. *Arch Intern Med* 1977; 137:1675–1679.
473. Frieden J, Cooper JA. The role of the intermediate cardiac care unit. *JAMA* 1976;235:816–819.
474. Levine A, Lown B. The "chair" treatment of coronary thrombosis. *Trans Assoc Am Phys* 1951;64:316.
475. McNeer JF, Wagner GS, Ginsburg PB, et al. Hospital discharge one week after acute myocardial infarction. *N Engl J Med* 1978;298: 229–232.
476. Madsen EB, Hougaard P, Gilpin E, et al. The length of hospitalization after acute myocardial infarction determined by risk calculation. *Circulation* 1983;68:9–16.
477. Cardiac Arrhythmia Suppression Trial II (CAST) Investigators. Effect of the antiarrhythmic agent moricizine on survival after myocardial infarction. *N Engl J Med* 1992;327:227–233.
478. Bigger JT, Fleiss JL, Kleiger R, et al. The relationships among ventricular arrhythmias, left ventricular dysfunction, and mortality in the 2 years after myocardial infarction. The Multicenter Post-Infarction Research Group. *Circulation* 1984;69:250–258.
479. Epstein SE, Palmeri ST, Patterson RE. Evaluation of patients after acute myocardial infarction: Indications for cardiac catheterization and surgical intervention. *N Engl J Med* 1982;307:1487–1492.

480. Hillis LD, Forman S, Braunwald E. Risk stratification before thrombolytic therapy in patients with acute myocardial infarction: the Thrombolysis in Myocardial Infarction (TIMI) Phase II co-investigators. *J Am Coll Cardiol* 1990;16:313–315.
481. Schuster EH, Bulkley BH. Early post-infarction angina: Ischemia at a distance and ischemia in the infarct zone. *N Engl J Med* 1981;305: 1101–1105.
482. Normand SL, Glickman ME, Sharma RG, et al. Using admission characteristics to predict short-term mortality from myocardial infarction in elderly patients: Results from the Cooperative Cardiovascular Project. *JAMA* 1996;275:1322–1328.
483. Lee KL, Woodleif LH, Topol EJ, et al. Predictors of 30-day mortality in the era of reperfusion for acute myocardial infarction: Results from an international trial of 41,021 patients. *Circulation* 1995;91: 1659–1668.
484. Krone RJ, Miller JP, Gillespie JA, et al. Usefulness of low-level exercise testing early after acute myocardial infarction in patients taking beta-blocking agents. *Am J Cardiol* 1987;60:23–27.
485. Krone RJ, Gillespie JA, Weld FM, et al. Low-level exercise testing after myocardial infarction: Usefulness in enhancing clinical risk stratification. *Circulation* 1984;71:80–89.
486. Van Reet RE, Quinones MA, Poliner LR, et al. Comparison of two-dimensional echocardiography with gated radionuclide ventriculography in the evaluation of global and regional left ventricular function in acute myocardial infarction. *J Am Coll Cardiol* 1984;3:243–252.
487. White HD, Norris RM, Brown MA, et al. Left ventricular end-systolic volume as the major determinant of survival after recovery from myocardial infarction. *Circulation* 1987;76:44–51.
488. Mahmarian JJ, Moye L, Verani MS, et al. Criteria for the accurate interpretation of changes in left ventricular ejection fraction and cardiac volumes as assessed by rest and exercise gated radionuclide angiography. *J Am Coll Cardiol* 1991;18:112–119.
489. Multicenter Postinfarction Research Group. Risk stratification and survival after myocardial infarction. *N Engl J Med* 1983;309: 331–336.
490. Simoons ML, Vos J, Tijssen JG, et al. Long-term benefit of early thrombolytic therapy in patients with acute myocardial infarction. 5-year follow-up of a trial conducted by the Interuniversity Cardiology Institute of The Netherlands. *J Am Coll Cardiol* 1989;14: 1609–1615.
491. Zaret B, Wackers F, et al. for the TIMI Study Group. Value of radionuclide rest and exercise left ventricular ejection fraction in assessing survival of patients after thrombolytic therapy for acute myocardial infarction: Results of the Thrombolysis in Myocardial Infarction (TIMI) Phase II Study. *J Am Coll Cardiol* 1995;26:73–79.
492. Volpi A, DeVita C, Franzosi MG, et al. Determinants of 6-month mortality in survivors of myocardial infarction after thrombolysis. Results of the GISSI-2 data base. *Circulation* 1993;88:416–429.
493. Pilote L, Silberberg J, Lisbona R, et al. Prognosis in patients with low left ventricular ejection fraction after myocardial infarction. Importance of exercise capacity. *Circulation* 1989;80:1636–1641.
494. Fletcher GF, Balady G, Froelicher VF, et al. Exercise standards: A statement for healthcare professionals from the American Heart Association. *Circulation* 1995;91:580–615.
495. Starling MR, Crawford MH, Kennedy GT, et al. Exercise testing early after myocardial infarction: Predictive value for subsequent unstable angina and death. *Am J Cardiol* 1980;46:909–914.
496. Weld FM, Chu KL, Bigger JT, et al. Risk stratification with low-level exercise testing 2 weeks after acute myocardial infarction. *Circulation* 1981;64:306–314.
497. Gibbons R, Balady G, Bricker J, et al. ACC/AHA 2002 Guideline Update for Exercise Testing. A report of the American College of Cardiology/American Heart Association Task Force on Practice Guidelines (Committee on Exercise Testing). American College of Cardiology website: www.acc.org/clinical/guidelines/exercise/dirIndex.htm 2002.
498. Senaratne MPJ, Hsu L, Rossall RE, et al. Exercise testing after myocardial infarction: Relative values of the low level predischarge and the postdischarge exercise test. *J Am Coll Cardiol* 1988;12:1416–1422.
499. Starling MR, Crawford MH, Kennedy GT, et al. Treadmill exercise tests predischarge and six weeks post-myocardial infarction to detect abnormalities of known prognostic value. *Ann Intern Med* 1981;94: 721–727.
500. Villella A, Maggioni AP, Villella M, et al. Prognostic significance of maximal exercise testing after myocardial infarction treated with thrombolytic agents: The GISSI-2 data base. Gruppo Italiano per lo Studio della Sopravvivenza Nell'Infarto. *Lancet* 1995;346:523–529.
501. Chaitman BR, McMahon RP, Terrin M, et al. Impact of treatment strategy on predischarge exercise test in the Thrombolysis in Myocardial Infarction (TIMI) II Trial. *Am J Cardol* 1993;71:131–138.
502. Madsen JK, Grande P, Saunamaki K, et al. Danish multicenter randomized study of invasive versus conservative treatment in patients with inducible ischemia after thrombolysis in acute myocardial infarction (DANAMI). *Circulation* 1997;96:748–755.
503. Mahmarian JJ, Steingart RM, Forman S, et al. Relationship between ambulatory electrocardiographic monitoring and myocardial perfusion imaging to detect coronary artery disease and myocardial ischemia. An ACIP ancillary study. *J Am Coll Cardiol* 1997;29:764–769.
504. Knatterud G, Bourassa M, Pepine C, et al. Effects of treatment strategies to suppress ischemia in patients with coronary artery disease: 12-week results of the Asymptomatic Cardiac Ischemia Pilot (ACIP) Study. *J Am Coll Cardiol* 1994;24:11–20.
505. Mahmarian JJ, Mahmarian AC, Marks GF, et al. The role of adenosine thallium-201 tomography for precisely defining long-term risk in patients following acute myocardial infarction. *J Am Coll Cardiol* 1995;25:1333–1340.
506. Mahmarian JJ. Prediction of myocardium at risk. Clinical significance during acute infarction and in evaluating subsequent prognosis. *Cardiol Clin* 1995;13:355–378.
507. Mahmarian J. Risk assessment in acute coronary syndromes. In: Iskandrian A, Verani M, eds. *Nuclear Cardiac Imaging: Principles and Applications,* 3rd ed. New York: Oxford University Press; 2003: 207–243.
508. Dakik HA, Kleiman NS, Farmer JA, et al. Intensive medical therapy versus coronary angioplasty for suppression of myocardial ischemia in survivors of acute myocardial infarction. *Circulation* 1998;98: 2017–2023.
509. Carlos ME, Smart SC, Wynsen JC, et al. Dobutamine stress echocardiography for risk stratification after myocardial infarction. *Circulation* 1997;95:1402–1410.
510. Geleijnse ML, Elhendy A, VanDomburg RT, et al. Cardiac imaging for risk stratification with dobutamine-atropine stress testing in patients with chest pain: echocardiography, perfusion scintigraphy, or both? *Circulation* 1997;96:137–147.
511. Quinones MA. Risk stratification after myocardial infarction: Clinical science versus practice behavior. *Circulation* 1997;95:1352–1354.
512. Minardi G, Disegni M, Manzara C, et al. Diagnostic and prognostic value of dipyridamole and dobutamine stress echocardiography in patients with acute myocardial infarction. *Am J Cardiol* 1997;80:847–851.
513. Cortigiani L, Picano E, Landi P, et al. Value of pharmacologic stress echocardiography in risk stratification of patients with single-vessel disease: A report from the echo-persantine and echo-dobutamine international cooperative studies. *J Am Coll Cardiol* 1998;32:69–74.
514. Peterson ED, Shaw LJ, Califf RM. Risk stratification after myocardial infarction. *Ann Intern Med* 1997;126:561–582.
515. SOLVD Investigators. Effect of enalapril on mortality and the development of heart failure in asymptomatic patients with reduced left ventricular ejection fraction. *N Engl J Med* 1992;327:685–691.
516. Pratt CM, Francis MJ, Luck JC, et al. Analysis of ambulatory electrocardiograms in 15 patients during spontaneous ventricular fibrillation with special reference to preceding arrhythmic events. *J Am Coll Cardiol* 1983;2:789–797.
517. Pratt CM, Greenway PS, Schoenfeld MH, et al. An exploration of the precision of classifying sudden cardiac death: Implications for the interpretation of clinical trials. *Circulation* 1996;93:519–524.
518. Cardiac Arrhythmia Suppression Trial (CAST) Investigators. Preliminary report: Effect of encainide and flecainide on mortality in a

randomized trial of arrhythmia suppression after myocardial infarction. *N Engl J Med* 1989;321:406–412.

519. Cairns JA, Connolly SJ, Robert R, et al. Randomized trial of outcome after myocardial infarction in patients with frequent or repetitive ventricular premature depolarisations: CAMIAT. *Lancet* 1997;349: 675–682.
520. Julian DG, Camm AJ, Fragin G, et al. Randomised trial of effect of amiodarone on mortality in patients with left-ventricular dysfunction after recent myocardial infarction: EMIAT. *Lancet* 1997;349:667–674.
521. Waldo AL, Camm AJ, deRuyter H, et al. Effect of d-sotalol on mortality in patients with left ventricular dysfunction after recent and remote myocardial infarction. The SWORD Investigators. Survival With Oral d-Sotalol. *Lancet* 1996;348:7–12.
522. Luu M, Stevenson WG, Stevenson LW, et al. Diverse mechanisms of unexpected cardiac arrest in advanced heart failure. *Circulation* 1989; 80:1675–1680.
523. Moss AJ, DeCamilla J, Davis H. Cardiac death in the first 6 months after myocardial infarction: Potential for mortality reduction in the early posthospital period. *Am J Cardiol* 1977;39:816–820.
524. Cardiac Arrhythmia Pilot Study (CAPS) Investigators. Effects of encainide, flecainide, imipramine, and moricizine on ventricular arrhythmias during the year after acute myocardial infarction: The CAPS. *Am J Cardiol* 1988;61:501–509.
525. Buxton A, Lee K, et al for the Multicenter Unsustained Tachycardia Trial Investigators. A randomized study of the prevention of sudden death in patients with coronary artery disease. *N Engl J Med* 1999; 341:1882–1890.
526. Farrell TG, Bashir Y, Cripps T, et al. Risk stratification for arrhythmic events in postinfarction patients based on heart rate variability, ambulatory electrocardiographic variables and the signal-averaged electrocardiogram. *J Am Coll Cardiol* 1991;18:687–697.
527. Bigger JT Jr, LaRovere MT, Steinman RC, et al. Comparison of baroreflex sensitivity and heart period variability after myocardial infarction. *J Am Coll Cardiol* 1989;14:1511–1518.
528. Odemuyiwa O, Malik M, Farrell T, et al. Comparison of the predictive characteristics of heart rate variability index and left ventricular ejection fraction for all-cause mortality, arrhythmic events and sudden death after acute myocardial infarction. *Am J Cardiol* 1991;68:434–439.
529. Schwartz PJ, Vanol E, Stramba-Badiale M, et al. Autonomic mechanisms and sudden death: New insights from analysis of baroreceptor reflexes in conscious dogs with and without a myocardial infarction. *Circulation* 1988;78:669–679.
530. Makikallio TH, Hoiber S, Kober L, et al. Fractal analysis of heart rate dynamics as a predictor of mortality in patients with depressed left ventricular function after acute myocardial infarction. *Am J Cardiol* 1999;83:836–839.
531. Copie X, Hnatkova K, Staunton A, et al. Predictive power of increased heart rate versus depressed left ventricular ejection fraction and heart rate variability for risk stratification after myocardial infarction. Results of a two-year follow-up study. *J Am Coll Cardiol* 1996;27:270–276.
532. Singh N, Mironov D, Armstrong PW, et al. Heart rate variability assessment early after acute myocardial infarction. Pathophysiological and prognostic correlates. GUSTO ECG substudy investigators. Global Utilization of Streptokinase and TPA for Occluded Arteries. *Circulation* 1996;93:1388–1399.
533. Faber TS, Staunton A, Hnatkova K, et al. Stepwise strategy of using short- and long-term heart rate variability for risk stratification after myocardial infarction. *Pacing Clin Electrophysiol* 1996;19:1845–1851.
534. Camm A, Karam R, Pratt CM. The azimilide post-infarct survival evaluation (ALIVE) trial. *Am J Cardiol* 1998;81:35D–46D.
535. American College of Cardiology Cardiovascular Technology Assessment Committee. Heart rate variabiity for risk stratification of life-threatening arrhythmias. *J Am Coll Cardiol* 1993;22:948–950.
536. Schwartz PJ. The neural control of heart rate and risk stratification after myocardial infarction. *Eur Heart J* 1999;1(suppl H):H33–H44.
537. LaRovere MT, Bigger JT Jr, Marcus FI, et al. Baro-reflex sensitivity and heart-rate variability in prediction of total cardiac mortality after myocardial infarction. *Lancet* 1998;351:478–484.
538. Gomes JA, Winters SL, Martinson M, et al. The prognostic significance of quantitative signal-averaged variables relative to clinical variables, site of myocardial infarction, ejection fraction and ventricular premature beats: A prospective study. *J Am Coll Cardiol* 1989;13:377–384.
539. Hohnloser SH, Franck P, Klingenheben T, et al. Open infarct artery, late potentials, and other prognostic factors in patients after acute myocardial infarction in the thrombolytic era: A prospective trial. *Circulation* 1994;90:1747–1756.
540. Vatterott PJ, Hammill SC, Bailey KR, et al. Late potentials on signal-averaged electrocardiograms and patency of the infarct-related in survivors of acute myocardial infarction. *J Am Coll Cardiol* 1991;17: 330–337.
541. Tapanainen J, Still A-M, Airaksinen K, et al. Prognostic significance of risk stratifiers of mortality, including T wave alternans, after acute myocardial infarction: Results of a prospective follow-up study. *J Cardiovasc Electrophysiol* 2001;12:645–652.
542. Rosenbaum D, Jackson L, Smith J, et al. Electrical alternans and vulnerability to ventricular arrhythmias. *N Engl J Med* 1994;330: 235–241.
543. Armoundas A, Rosenbaum D, Ruskin J, et al. Prognostic significance of electrical alternans versus signal averaged electrocardiography in predicting the outcome of electrophysiological testing and arrhythmia-free survival. *Heart* 1998;80:251–256.
544. Hohnloser S, Klingenheben T, Li Y, et al. T wave alternans as a predictor of recurrent ventricular tachyarrhythmias in ICD recipients: Prospective comparison with conventional risk markers. *J Cardiovasc Electrophysiol* 1998;9:1258–1268.
545. Ikeda T, Sakata T, Takami M, et al. Combined assessment of T-wave alternans and late potentials used to predict arrhythmic events after myocardial infarction. A prospective study. *J Am Coll Cardiol* 2000;35:722–730.
546. Gold M, Spencer W. T wave alternans for ventricular arrhythmia risk stratification. *Curr Opin Cardiol* 2003;18:1–5.
547. Zipes DP, Akhtar M, Denes P, et al. Guidelines for clinical intracardiac electrophysiologic studies: A report of the American College of Cardiology/American Heart Association Task Force on assessment of diagnostic and therapeutic cardiovascular procedures. *J Am Coll Cardiol* 1989;14:1827–1842.
548. Bourke JP, Richards DAB, Ross DL, et al. Routine programmed electrical stimulation in survivors of actue myocardial infarction for prediction of spontaneous ventricular tachyarrhythmias during follow-up: Results, optimal stimulation protocol and cost-effective screening. *J Am Coll Cardiol* 1991;18:780–788.
549. Richards DA, Byth K, Ross DL, et al. What is the best predictor of spontaneous ventricular tachycardia and sudden death after myocardial infarction? *Circulation* 1991;83:756–763.
550. Moss AJ, Hall J, Cannom DS, et al. Improved survival with an implanted defibrillator in patients with coronary disease at high risk for ventricular arrhythmia. *N Engl J Med* 1996;335:1933–1940.
551. Moss A, Zareba W, et al for the Multicenter Automatic Defibrillator Implantation Trial II Investigators. Prophylactic implantation of a defibrillator in patients with myocardial infarction and reduced ejection fraction. *N Engl J Med* 2002;346:877–883.
552. Glancy JM, Garratt CJ, Woods KL, et al. QT dispersion and mortality after myocardial infarction. *Lancet* 1995;345:945–948.
553. Gibson RS, Watson DD, Craddock GB, et al. Prediction of cardiac events after uncomplicated myocardial infarction: A prospective study comparing predischarge exercise thallium-201 scintigraphy and coronary angiography. *Circulation* 1983;68:321–336.
554. De Feyter PJ, van Eenige MJ, Dighton DH, et al. Prognostic value of exercise testing, coronary angiography and left ventriculography 6–8 weeks after myocardial infarction. *Circulation* 1982;66:527–536.
555. Grines CL, Topol EJ, Bates ER, et al. Infarct vessel status after intravenous tissue plasminogen activator and acute coronary angioplasty: Prediction of clinical outcome. *Am Heart J* 1988;115:1–7.
556. Topol EJ, Califf RM, George BS, et al. A randomized trial of immediate versus delayed elective angioplasty after intranveous tissue plas-

minogen activator in acute myocardial infarction. *N Engl J Med* 1987;317:581–588.

557. Muller DW, Topol EJ, Ellis EG, et al. Multivessel coronary artery disease: A key predictor of short-term prognosis after reperfusion therapy for acute myocardial infarction. *Am Heart J* 1991;121:1042–1049.
558. Aguirre FV, Kern MJ, Hsia J, et al. Importance of myocardial infarction artery patency on the prevalence of ventricular arrhythmia and late potentials after thrombolysis in acute myocardial infarction. *Am J Cardiol* 1991;68:1410–1416.
559. Ross J, Jr, Brandenburg RO, Dinsmore RE, et al. Guidelines for coronary angiography: A report of the American College of Cardiology/American Heart Association Task Force on assessment of diagnostic and therapeutic cardiovascular procedures. *J Am Coll Cardiol* 1987; 10:935–950.
560. Ryan TJ, Faxon DP, Gunnar RM, et al. Guidelines for percutaneous transluminal coronary angioplasty: A report of the American College of Cardiology/American Heart Association Task Force on the assessment of diagnostic and therapeutic cardiovascular procedures. *J Am Coll Cardiol* 1988;1:889–893.
561. European Coronary Surgery Study Group. Prospective randomized study of coronary artery bypass surgery in stable angina pectoris: A progress report on survival. *Circulation* 1982;65:67–71.
562. Deedwania PC, Amsterdam EA, Vagelos RH. Evidence-based, cost-effective risk stratification and management after myocardial infarction. *Arch Intern Med* 1997;157:273–280.
563. Ronnevik PK, Gundersen T, Abrahamsen AM. Effect of smoking habits and timolol treatment on mortality and reinfarction in patients surviving acute myocardial infarction. *Br Heart J* 1985;54:134–139.
564. Rosenberg L, Kaufman DW, Helmrich SP, et al. The risk of myocardial infarction after quitting smoking in men under 55 years of age. *N Engl J Med* 1985;313:1511–1514.
565. Ockene JK. Smoking intervention: A behavioral, educational, and pharmacologic perspective. In: Okene IS, Ockene JK, eds. *Prevention of Coronary Heart Disease.* Boston: Little, Brown; 1992:201–230.
566. Henningfield JE. Nicotine medications for smoking cessation. *N Engl J Med* 1995;333:1196–1203.
567. Pekkanen J, Linn S, Heiss G, et al. Ten-year mortality from cardiovascular disease in relation to cholesterol level among men with and without preexisting cardiovascular disease. *N Engl J Med* 1990;322: 1700–1707.
568. Stampfer MJ, Sacks FM, Salvini S, et al. A prospective study of cholesterol, apolipoproteins, and the risk of myocardial infarction. *N Engl J Med* 1991;325:373–381.
569. Scandinavian Simvastatin Survival Study Group. Randomised trial of cholesterol lowering in 4444 patients with coronary heart disease: The Scandinavian Simvastatin Survival Study (4S). *Lancet* 1994;344: 1383–1389.
570. Sacks FM, Pfeffer MA, Moye LA, et al. The effect of pravastatin on coronary events after myocardial infarction in patients with average cholesterol levels. Cholesterol and Recurrent Events (CARE) Trial. *N Engl J Med* 1996;335:1001–1009.
571. Expert Panel on Detection and Treatment of High Blood Cholesterol in Adults. Summary of the second report of the National Cholesterol Education Program (NCEP) Expert Panel on Detection, Evaluation, and Treatment of High Blood Cholesterol in Adults (Adult Treatment Panel II). *JAMA* 1993;22:933–940.
572. Rosenson RS. Myocardial injury: The acute phase response and lipoprotein metabolism. *J Am Coll Cardiol* 1993;22:933–940.
573. Haskell WL. Sedentary lifestyle is a risk factor for coronary artery disease. In: Pearson TA, Criqui MH, Leupker RV, et al, eds. *Primer in Preventive Cardiology.* Dallas: American Heart Association; 1994; 173–187.
574. Stanford JL, Weiss NS, Voight LF, et al. Combined estrogen and progestin hormone replacement therapy in relation to risk of breast cancer in middle-aged women. *JAMA* 1995;274:137–142.
575. Colditz GA, Hankinson SE, Hunter DJ, et al. The use of estrogens and progestins and the risk of breast cancer in postmenopausal women. *N Engl J Med* 1995;332:1589–1593.
576. Healy B. Effects of estrogen or estrogen/progestin regimes on heart disease risk factors in postmenopausal women: The Postmenopausal Estrogen/Progestin Interventions (PEPI) Trial. *JAMA* 1995;273: 199–208.
577. Hulley S, Grady D, Bush T, et al. Randomized trial of estrogen plus progestin for secondary prevention of coronary heart disease in postmenopausal women. Heart and Estrogen/Progestin Replacement Study (HERS) Research Group. *JAMA* 1998;280:605–613.
578. Yusuf S, Lessem J, Jha P, et al. Primary and secondary prevention of myocardial infarction and strokes: An update of randomly allocated, controlled trials. *J Hypertens* 1993;11(suppl 4):S61–S73.
579. Norwegian Multicenter Study Group. Timolol-induced reduction in mortality and reinfarction in patients surviving acute myocardial infarction. *N Engl J Med* 1981;304:801–807.
580. Hjalmarson A, Elmfeldt D, Herlitz J, et al. Effect on mortality of metoprolol in acute myocardial infarction: A double-blind randomised trial. *Lancet* 1981;2:823–827.
581. Becker RC. Antiplatelet therapy in coronary heart disease: Emerging strategies for the treatment and prevention of acute myocardial infarction. *Arch Pathol Lab Med* 1993;117:89–96.
582. Juul-Moller S, Edvardsson N, Jahnmatz B, et al. Double-blind trial of aspirin in primary prevention of myocardial infarction in patients with stable chronic angina pectoris: The Swedish Angina Pectoris Aspirin Trial (SAPAT) Group. *Lancet* 1992;340:1421–1425.
583. Ambrosioni E, Borghi C, Magnani B, et al. The effect of the angiotensin-converting enzyme inhibitor zofenopril on mortality and morbidity after anterior myocardial infarction. For the Survival of Myocardial Infarction Long-Term Evaluation (SMILE) Study Investigators. *N Engl J Med* 1995;332:80–85.
584. Ball SG, Hall AS. What to expect from ACE inhibitors after myocardial infarction. *Br Heart J* 1994;72(suppl 3):S70–S74.
585. deLorgeril M, Salen P, Martin J-L, et al. Mediterranean diet, traditional risk factors, and the rate of cardiovascular complications after myocardial infarction. Final report of the Lyon Diet Heart Study. *Circulation* 1999;99:779–785.
586. GISSI Prevention Trial. Dietary supplementation with n-3 polyunsaturated fatty acids and vitamin E after myocardial infarction: Results of the GISSI-Prevention Trial. *Lancet* 1999;354:447–455.

CHAPTER 53

# THE ELECTROCARDIOGRAM IN ACUTE MYOCARDIAL INFARCTION

Anton P. Gorgels / Domien J. Engelen / Hein J. J. Wellens



The possibility of treating an acute coronary occlusion by thrombolytic therapy or percutaneous intracoronary interventions makes it necessary to determine which coronary artery is involved and the size of the area at risk.

This chapter discusses the value of the electrocardiogram (ECG) in dealing with this problem; it is therefore placed in the section on coronary heart disease. Chapter 13 provides a general discussion of the ECG in the diagnosis of cardiac disease (see also Chaps. 51 and 52).

## CLINICAL PRESENTATION OF ACUTE MYOCARDIAL INFARCTION IN RELATION TO THE INFARCT VESSEL

The presentation of acute myocardial infarction (MI) varies depending on the coronary artery involved. The left anterior descending branch (LAD) supplies the anterior, lateral, septal, and frequently the inferoapical segments of the left ventricle, including the proximal part of the bundle branches, leading to large MIs. The right coronary artery (RCA) perfuses the sinus node (in 55 percent of patients), the right ventricle, the atrioventricular (AV) node, the posteromedial papillary muscle, the inferior part of the left ventricle, and variably also the posterior and lateral segments. The clinical picture may be impressive due to (1) activation of the vagal nervous system and/or (2) ischemia of the sinus and AV node, leading to sinus bradycardia and delay or block in the AV node, (3) right ventricular involvement with cardiogenic shock, and (4) ischemia of the papillary muscle, leading to mitral regurgitation.

The circumflex (CX) branch perfuses the posterior wall and variably the inferior and lateral segments. In case of posterior wall involvement following occlusion, abnormalities in ventricular activation occur in the second half of the QRS complex and are therefore difficult to pick up on the 12-lead ECG, frequently causing underestimation of the area at risk and undertreatment of the patient.[1]

## THE ELECTROCARDIOGRAM IN ANTERIOR WALL INFARCTION

The ECG signs of an anterior MI are ST-segment elevation in precordial leads $V_2$, $V_3$, and $V_4$. The behavior of the ST segments in the other precordial and frontal leads depends on the presence of ischemia in three vectorially opposite areas[2]: (1) the basoseptal area, perfused by the proximal septal branch; (2) the basolateral area, perfused by the first diagonal (anterolateral or intermediate) branch; and (3) the inferoapical area, when the distal LAD wraps around the apex. This leads schematically to occlusion either (1) proximally to the septal and first diagonal branch (40 percent of cases), or (2) distally to these two branches (40 percent), or (3) proximally to the first diagonal but distally to the septal branch (10 percent), or (4) proximally to the septal but distal to the first diagonal (or intermediate) branch (10 percent).

### DOMINANCE OF BASAL AREA: PROXIMAL LAD OCCLUSION

Typical features include ST elevation in aVR and ST elevation of ≥2.5 mm in $V_1$, ST depression in the inferior leads and in $V_5$,[3,4] and an abnormal Q in aVL (Fig. 53-1). Figure 53-2, Plate 85, depicts the likely mechanism of these findings: all areas are ischemic and contribute to the ST-segment vector. Because of the larger mass of the basal parts, the ST-segment vector will point in a superior direction

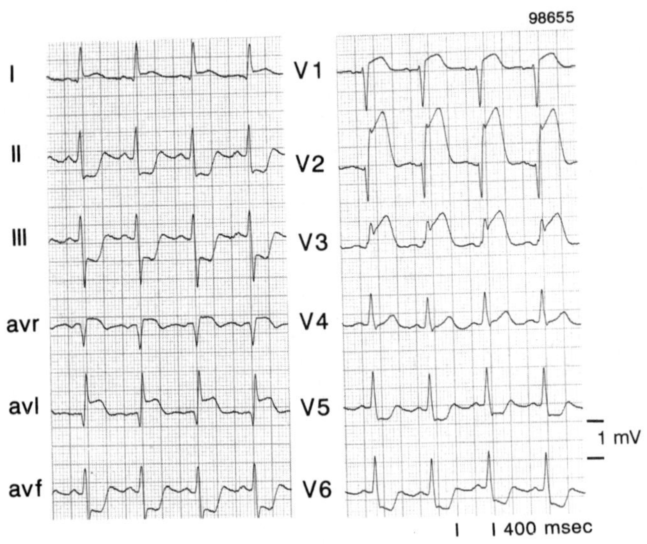


FIGURE 53-1 Acute anterior MI in proximal LAD occlusion. Anterior MI is present, as indicated by ST-segment elevation in leads $V_2$ and $V_3$. In addition, the precordial leads show marked ST-segment elevation in lead $V_1$ and ST-segment depression in leads $V_5$ and $V_6$. The extremity leads show ST-segment elevation in lead $aV_R$ and ST-segment depression in inferior leads II, III, and aVF.

(Fig. 53-2, left panel). In the frontal plane, this results in ST elevation in leads aVR, aVL, and $V_1$ (Fig. 53-2, right panel). This upward orientation of the ST vector causes reciprocal ST depression in the inferior leads and sometimes in leads $V_5$ and $V_6$. Local conduction delay in the lateral area will lead to widening of the Q wave in lead aVL.

## DOMINANCE OF INFEROAPICAL AREA: DISTAL LAD OCCLUSION

Typical is the absence of ST-segment depression in the inferior leads (Fig. 53-3).[5] Sometimes also, wide Q waves are recorded in $V_4$ through $V_6$. The inferoapical part is the dominant ischemic area, with the ST vector pointing inferiorly (Fig. 53-4, left panel; Plate 86) leading to positive or isoelectric inferior leads (Fig. 53-4, right panel, Plate 86, and Table 53-1). The Q waves in the left precordial leads are likely caused by the combination of local conduction delay in that area combined with the regular septal q wave in these leads.

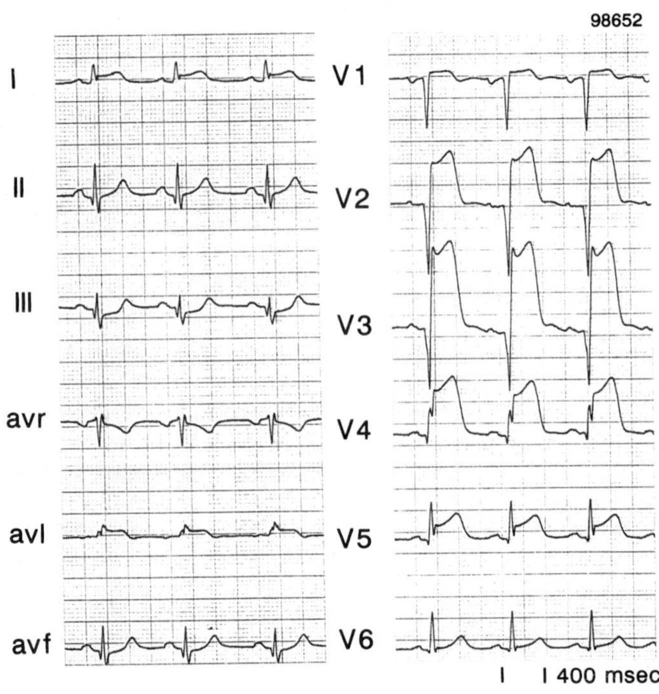


FIGURE 53-3 Acute anterior MI in distal LAD occlusion. Signs of acute anterior MI are seen, but ST-segment elevation is present in the inferior leads. Note also ST-segment depression in lead aVR.

## DOMINANCE OF SEPTAL AREA: FIRST DIAGONAL NOT INCLUDED

The anterobasal-lateral area is not involved (Fig.53-5). First septal branch occlusion leads to ST-segment elevation in aVR and ≥2.5 mm in $V_1$, and ST-segment depression in $V_5$. The right precordial lead $V_{3R}$ may also show ST-segment elevation.[6] Lead aVL now

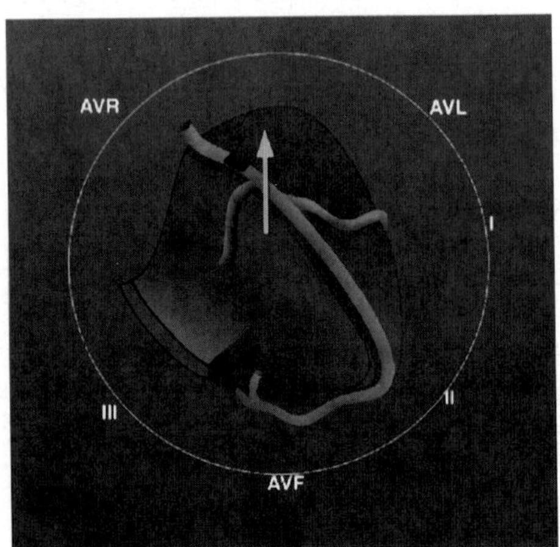


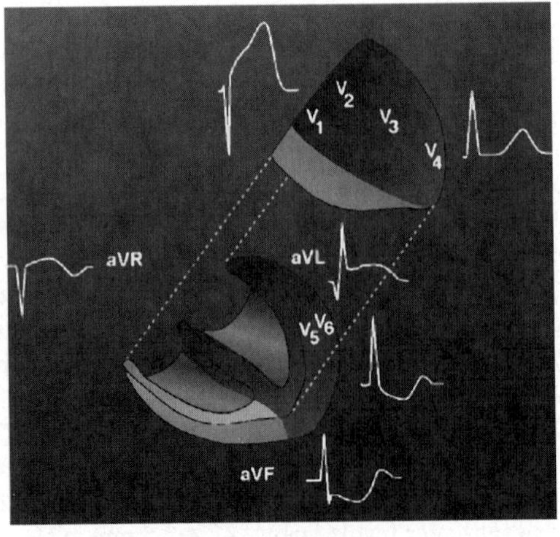


FIGURE 53-2 (Plate 85) Areas of left ventricular ischemia in LAD occlusion proximal to the first septal and first diagonal branch. *Left panel:* There is ischemia of the left ventricle. The ST-segment vector points in a superior direction because ischemia predominates in the basal areas. *Right panel:* The superiorly oriented ST vector leads to ST-segment elevation in lead aVR and lead $V_1$ and ST-segment depression in the inferior leads and in $V_5$ and $V_6$.

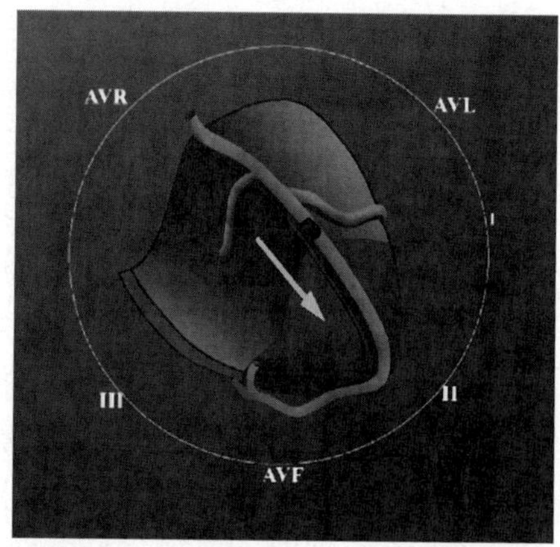


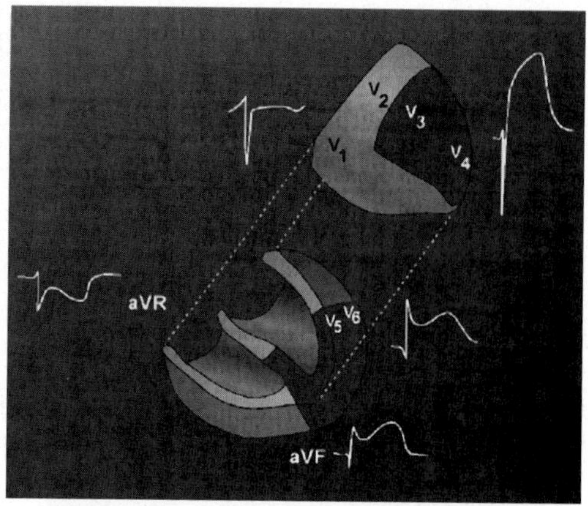


FIGURE 53-4 (Plate 86) Ischemic areas in distal LAD occlusion. *Left panel:* The ST vector points inferiorly due to ischemia of the inferoapical area. *Right panel:* The inferiorly directed ST vector leads to ST-segment depression in lead aVR and ST-segment elevation in the inferior leads.

TABLE 53-1 ECG Criteria to Identify Site of Occlusion in the LAD

| Criterion | Occlusion site | Sens | Spec | PPA | NPA |
|---|---|---|---|---|---|
| CRBBB | Proximal to S1 | 14 | 100 | 100 | 62 |
| ST ↑ V1 >2.5 mm | Proximal to S1 | 12 | 100 | 100 | 61 |
| ST ↑ avR | Proximal to S1 | 43 | 95 | 86 | 70 |
| ST ↓ V5 | Proximal to S1 | 17 | 98 | 88 | 62 |
| Q avL | Proximal to D1 | 44 | 85 | 67 | 69 |
| ST ↓ II ≥1.0 mm | Proximal to S1/D1 | 34 | 98 | 93 | 68 |
| Q V5 | Distal to S1 | 24 | 93 | 71 | 53 |
| ST ↓ avL | Distal to D1 | 22 | 95 | 87 | 46 |
| No ST ↓ III | Distal to S1/D1 | 41 | 95 | 92 | 53 |

ABBREVIATIONS: NPA = negative predictive accuracy; PPA = positive predictive accuracy; RBBB = right bundle branch block.

shows ST-segment depression, being a very specific finding (Table 53-1), and the inferior leads positive ST segments. Figure 53-6, Plate 87, is a diagrammatic presentation of this situation.

## DOMINANCE OF THE LATERAL AREA, FIRST SEPTAL BRANCH NOT INCLUDED

Typical features are Q waves in the left lateral leads, ST-segment depression in lead III, and the absence of this finding in lead II (Fig. 53-7). Figure 53-8, Plate 88, shows the distribution of ischemia in that situation, the ischemia vector pointing in the lateral direction. Local conduction delay in the lateral area with persistence of the septal Q wave results in widening of the Q wave in leads aVL and $V_5$ (right panel).

## ECG Criteria to Identify the Site of Occlusion in Anterior MI2

Right bundle branch block is a very specific marker of an occlusion before the first septal branch[7,8] as well as ST-segment elevation in $V_1 \geq$ 2.5 mm, any ST-segment elevation in aVR, and ST-segment depression in $V_5$. Lead aVL is useful in detecting occlusion proximally (Q wave) or distally (negative ST segment) to the first diagonal branch. The specificity of these criteria is high, implying that their presence, but not their absence, predicts the occlusion site (Table 53-1).

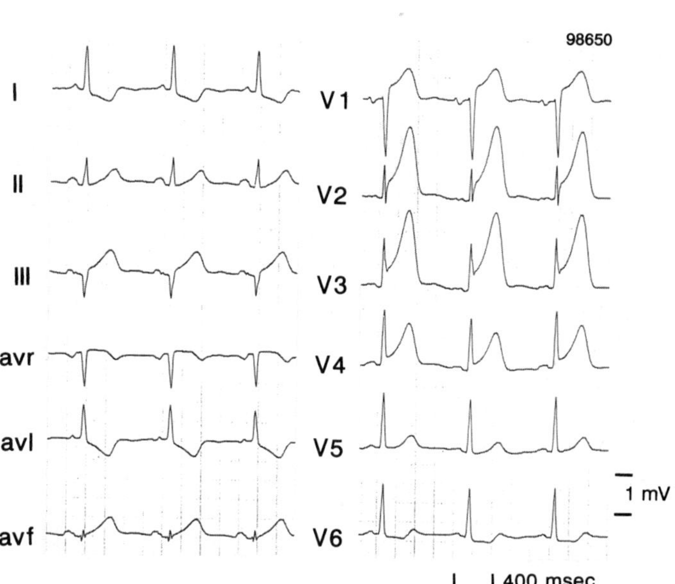


FIGURE 53-5 Acute anterior MI due to LAD occlusion distal to the first diagonal but proximal to the first septal branch. The precordial leads show evidence of acute anterior MI, but lead aVL shows ST-segment depression.

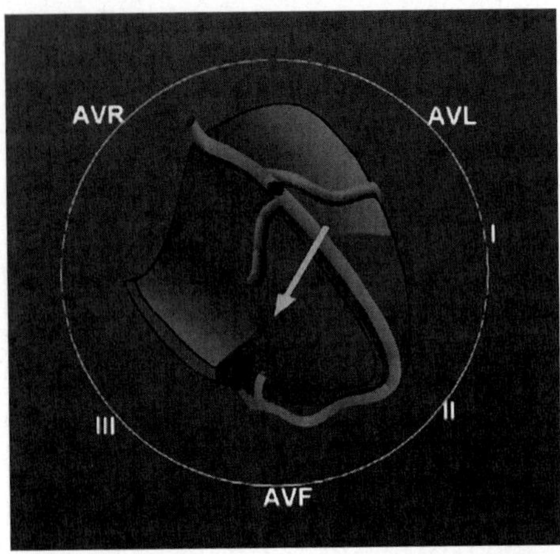


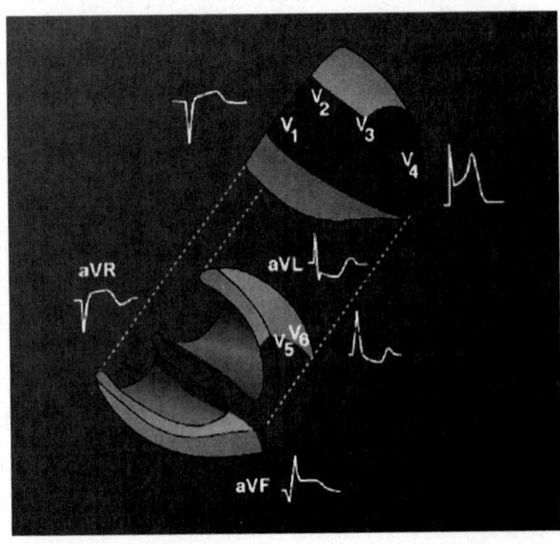


FIGURE 53-6 (Plate 87) Ischemic areas in LAD occlusion between the first diagonal (or intermediate) and first septal branch. *Left panel:* Predominance of ischemia in the septal-apical area leads to an ST-segment vector pointing in a rightward direction. *Right panel:* Apart from ST-segment elevation in the precordial leads, ST-segment elevation is also seen in leads III and aVR. Negativity of the ST segment is seen in lead aVL.

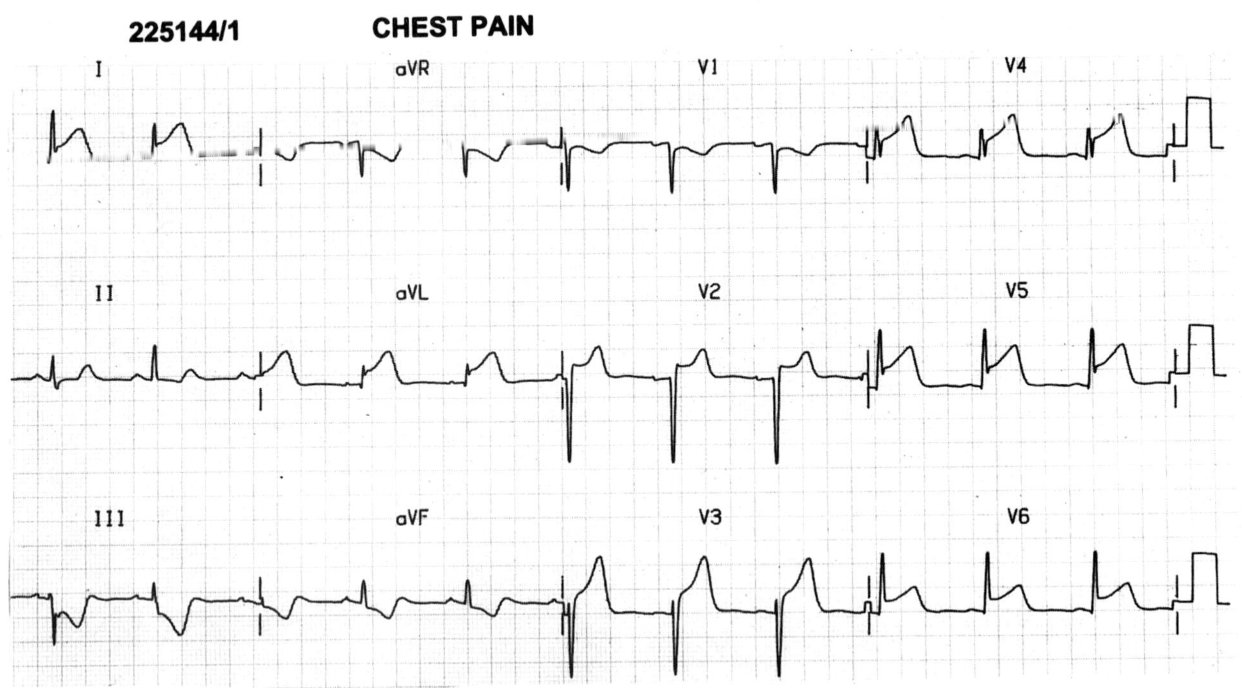


FIGURE 53-7 12-lead ECG with acute anterior MI due to an occlusion site distal to the first septal branch. ST-segment elevation is present in the precordial leads and lead aVL, whereas leads III and aVR clearly show ST-segment depression.

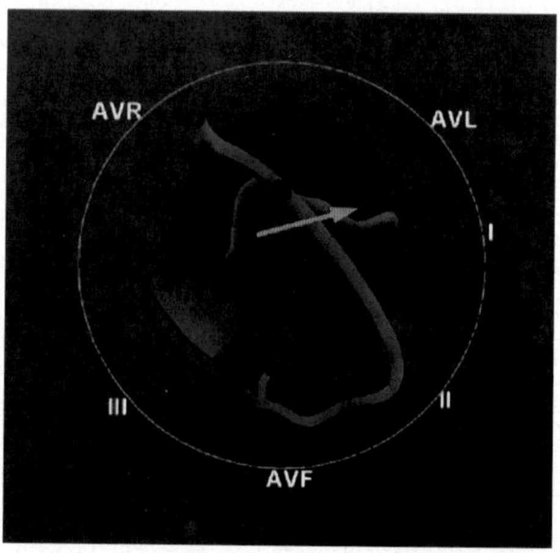


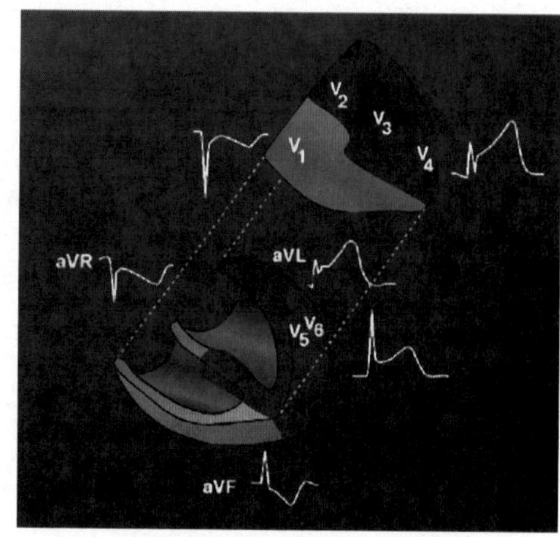


FIGURE 53-8 (Plate 88) Ischemic areas in LAD occlusion distal to the septal and proximal to the first diagonal branch. *Left panel:* Predominance of ischemia in the lateral area leading to an ST vector pointing in that direction. *Right panel:* The lateral orientation of the ST vector leads to ST-segment negativity of leads III and aVR. Lead II is isoelectric due to the perpendicular orientation of the ST vector in that lead. The lateral leads I and aVL show ST-segment elevation.

## INFEROPOSTERIOR WALL INFARCTION

The ECG in inferoposterior MI is able to assess the culprit coronary artery and involvement of the right ventricle.

### The Distinction between a Right Coronary Artery and a Circumflex Coronary Artery Occlusion

Because RCA occlusion results in inferoseptal ischemia, the ST-segment vector is directed toward lead III; in CX occlusion, there is inferoposterolateral ischemia with a vector pointing toward lead II. Therefore, in RCA occlusion, ST-segment elevation is greater in lead III than lead II (resulting in ST-segment depression more in aVL than in lead I).[9] In CX occlusion, lead II will show more ST-segment elevation than lead III (with lead I showing an isoelectric or elevated ST-segment (Figs 53-9 and 53-10).

The amount of ST-segment depression and number of leads with ST-segment depression in the precordial leads depend on the extent of posterior ischemia. The leads $V_5$ and $V_6$ are of little value in differentiating between an RCA or CX occlusion. ST-segment elevation in these leads implies a larger area at risk.[10]

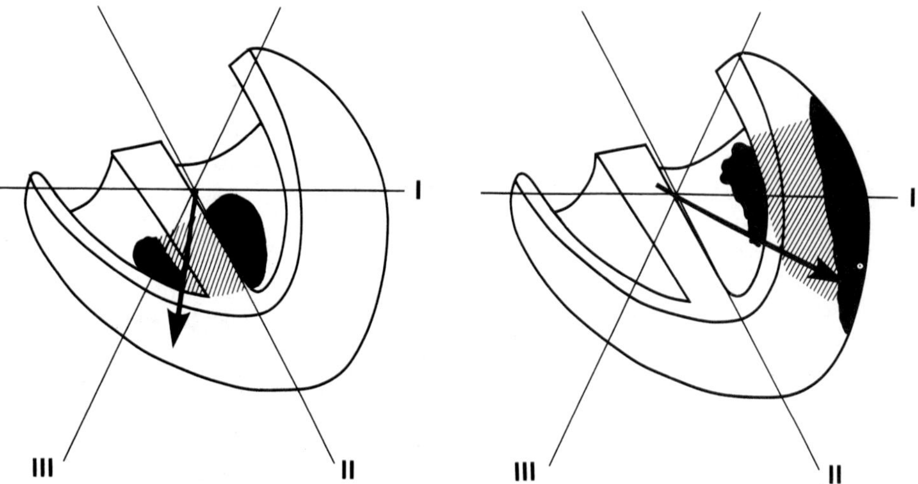


FIGURE 53-9 Schematic presentation of the ST-segment vector with inferoposterior MI caused by a right coronary artery (RCA) or circumflex coronary artery (CX). As shown, RCA occlusion leads to predominant ischemia in the inferoseptal area with an ST-segment vector pointing toward lead III. In CX occlusion, the ischemic area is located posterolaterally, resulting in an ST-segment vector directed toward lead II.

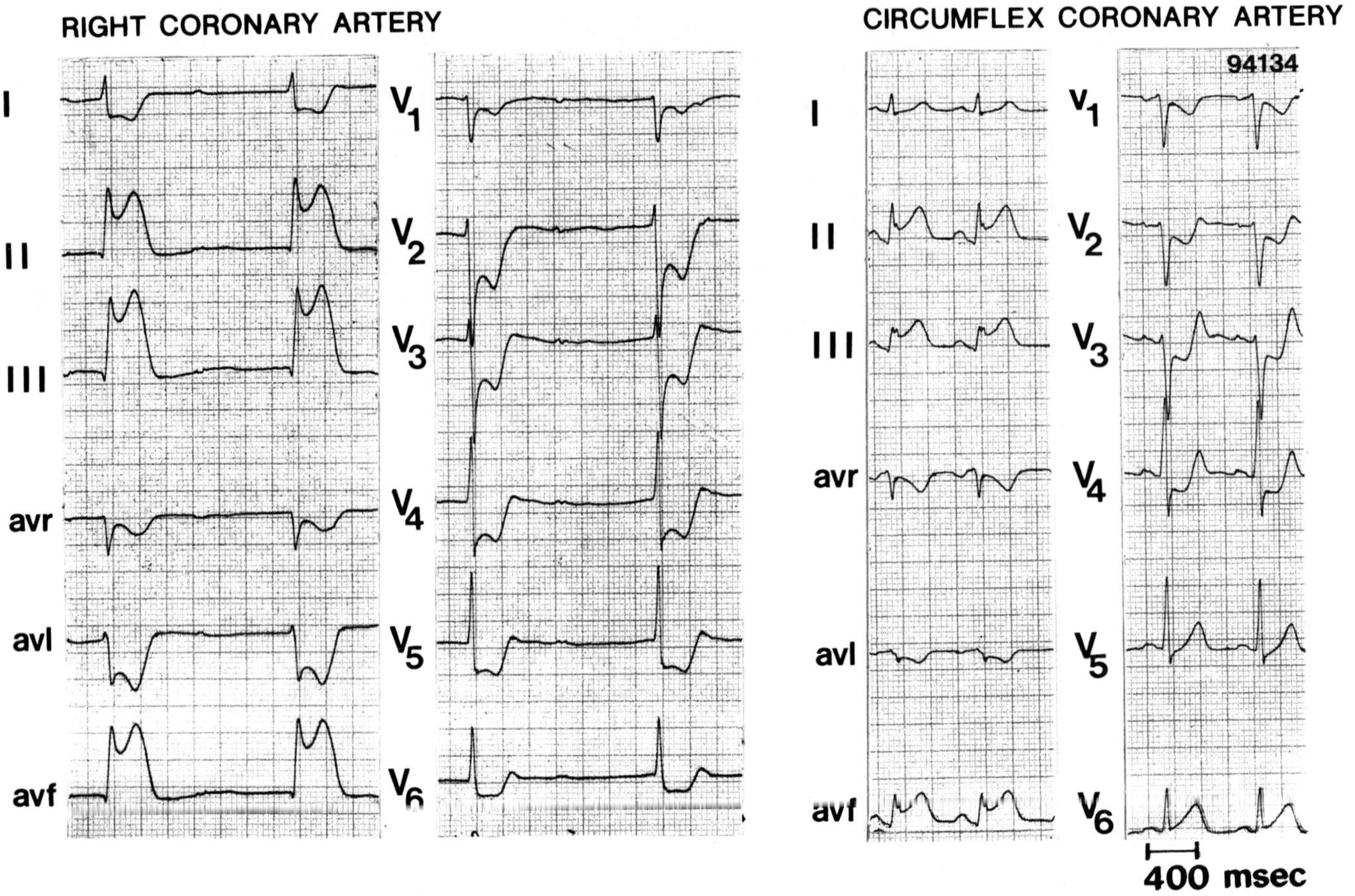

RIGHT CORONARY ARTERY

CIRCUMFLEX CORONARY ARTERY

94134

I II III avr avl avf V1 V2 V3 V4 V5 V6

400 msec

FIGURE 53-10 *Left panel:* The typical picture of an RCA occlusion. ST-segment elevation in lead III is higher than in lead II, resulting in ST-segment depression in lead I. In this patient with a dominant RCA complete AV block, right atrial and posterior MI is also present. *Right panel:* An example of a CX occlusion. ST-segment elevation is more marked in lead II than in lead III, leading to a positive T wave in lead I.

## Diagnosing Right Ventricular Infarction

The right ventricle (RV) is supplied by branches of the RCA. Occlusions are classified as proximal or distal to the RV branch(es). RV involvement may lead to cardiogenic shock in the acute and to ventricular tachycardia in the chronic phase. A proximal RCA occlusion shows ST-segment elevation with a positive T wave in lead $V_{4R}$, a distal occlusion an isoelectric ST-segment with a positive T wave, and a negative T wave indicates an occlusion of the CX.[11] Sufficient ST-segment elevation in the inferior leads is needed to use lead $V_{4R}$ reliably (Figs. 53-11 through 53-13).

## ST-Segment Depression in the Anterior Leads in Inferior MI

ST-segment depression implies posterior wall involvement; it may extend from $V_1$ through $V_6$ (Fig. 53-10) and indicate a larger MI.[12] Maximal ST-segment depression in leads $V_4$ through $V_6$ is more frequently seen in three-vessel disease and lower LV ejection fractions.[13] Precordial ST-segment depression occurs both in RCA or CX

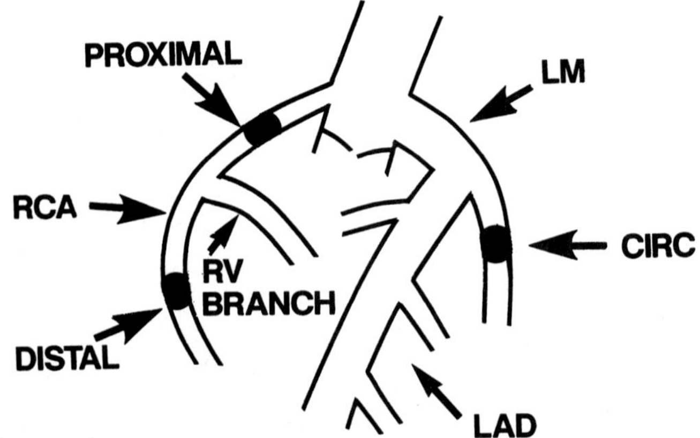


FIGURE 53-11 Diagram showing the coronary arteries and the possible sites of coronary artery occlusion leading to inferoposterior MI. In the right coronary artery (RCA), the occlusion may be before (proximal) the right ventricular (RV) branch or after it (distal). As shown in proximal RCA occlusion, the RV is involved in the MI.

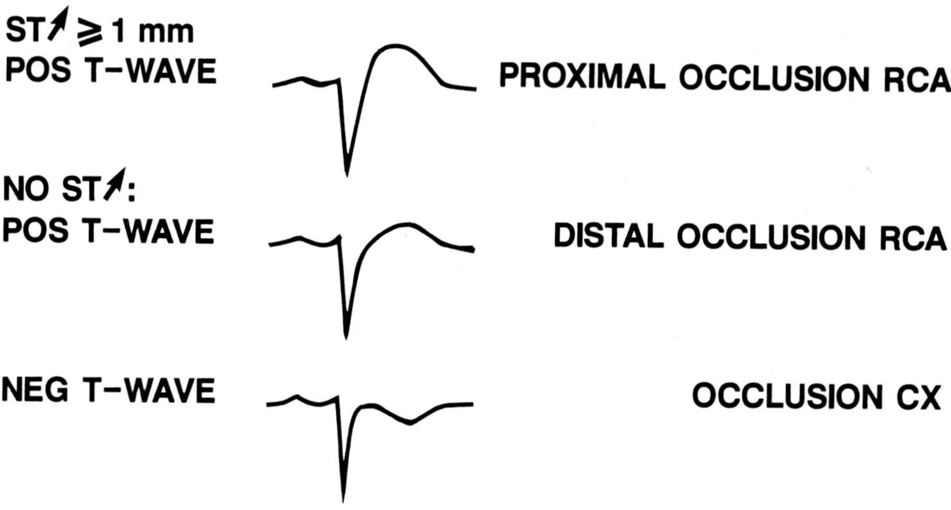


FIGURE 53-12 Characteristic ST-T-segment changes in lead $V_{4R}$ in cases of proximal RCA, a distal RCA occlusion, or a CX occlusion (see text).

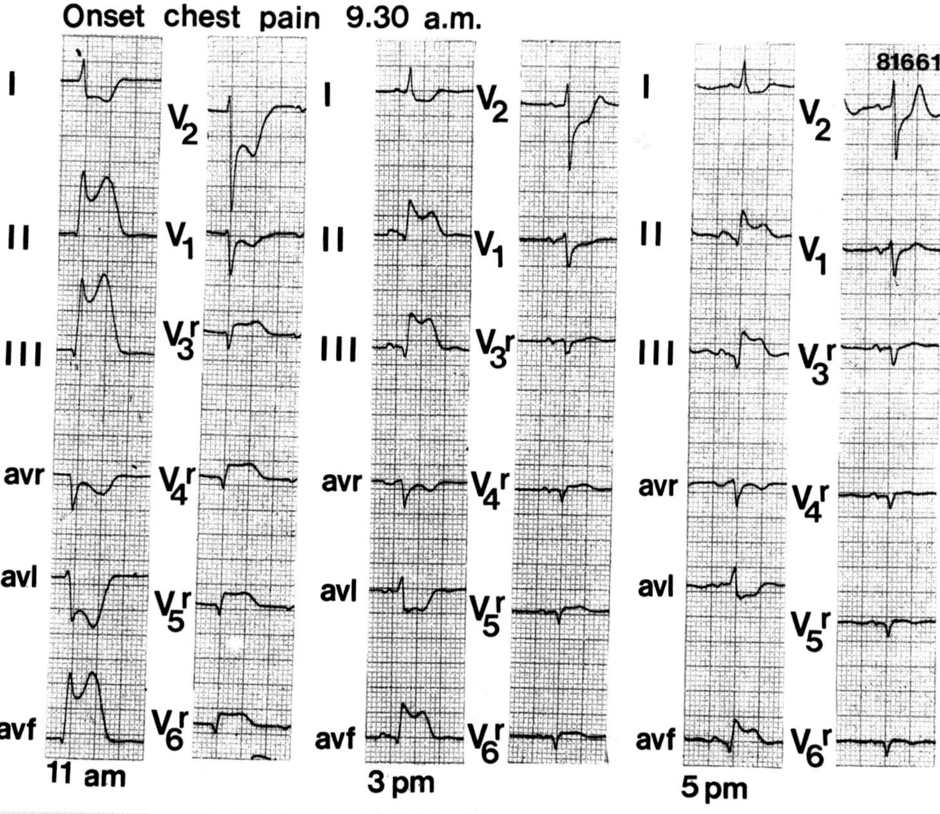


FIGURE 53-13 The relation between ST-segment elevation in leads II, III, and aVF and in the right precordial leads in proximal RCA. Note that changes diagnostic for RV involvement in lead $V_{4R}$ have disappeared $7\frac{1}{2}$ h after the onset of chest pain. As shown, there is a relation between the amount of ST-segment elevation in the inferior leads and lead $V_{4R}$.

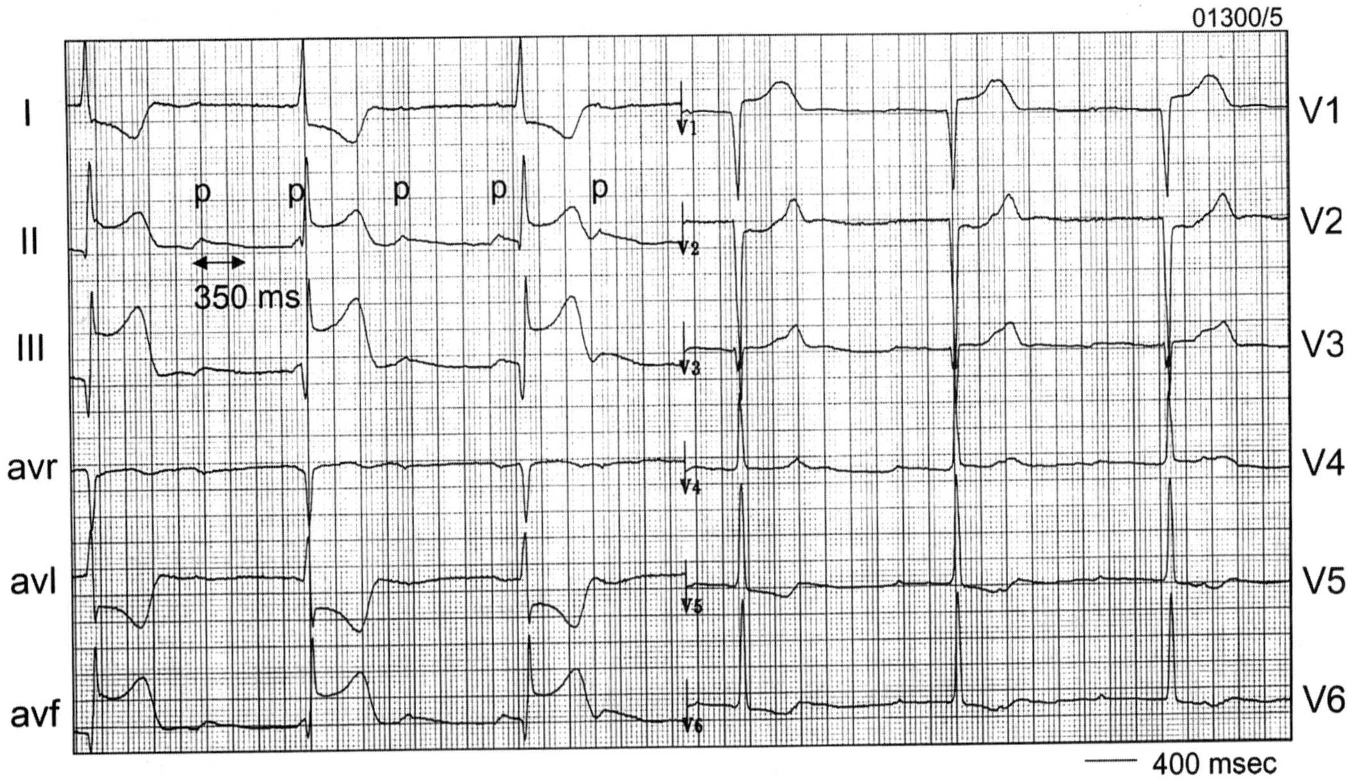


FIGURE 53-14 Sinus rhythm of 75 beats per minute with complete AV block, AV junctional escape rhythm of 35 beats per minute, increase of ST-segment elevations in III > II, and ST-segment depressions in I and aVL. Note the marked Ta elevation with markedly prolonged atrial conduction time (350 ms) (*arrow*). (Published with permission from the *J Cardiovasc Electrophysiol*.)

involvement (Fig. 53-10), but its absence points to the RCA.[14] In isolated ST-segment depression, CX occlusion with a true posterior MI or nonocclusive myocardial ischemia is possible. Localization of maximal ST-segment depression in $V_2$ and $V_3$ is predictive of acute CX occlusion.[15] Also, leads $V_7$ to $V_9$ have been recommended for that purpose.[16]

## Isolated Right Ventricular Infarction

Sometimes only minor changes are seen in the inferior leads, but ST-segment elevation is prominent in leads $V_1$ and $V_2$ and the right precordial leads.[17] This reflects a RV MI and is found in either a small or collaterally filled RCA or an occlusion of an RV branch only.

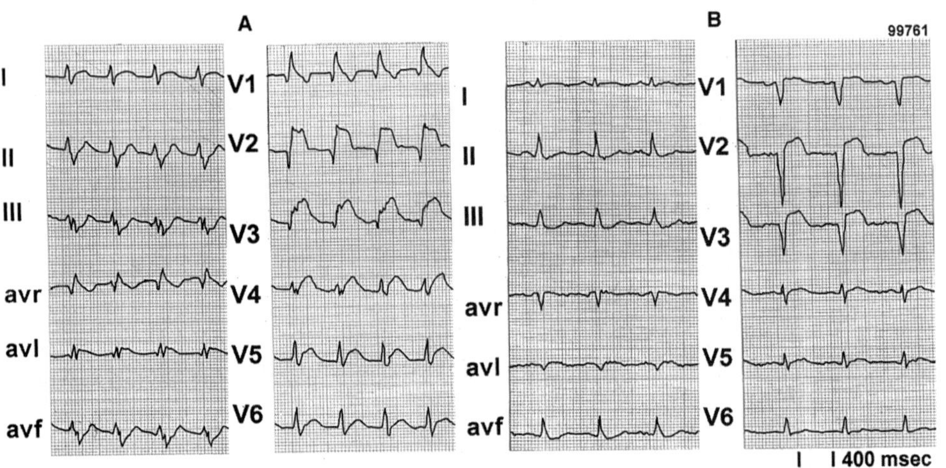


FIGURE 53-15 *Left panel:* Sinus tachycardia with a prolonged PR interval and right bundle branch block (RBBB) in a patient with an acute anterior MI. These findings point to an LAD occlusion proximal to the first septal branch. *Right panel:* Same patient after primary PTCA of the proximal LAD occlusion. Note disappearance of PR prolongation and RBBB. The precordial QRS picture indicates a small anterior MI.

## Atrioventricular Conduction Disturbances

### ATRIOVENTRICULAR NODAL BLOCK

AV nodal conduction delay and block occurs in inferior MI with proximal RCA occlusion, frequently with RV involvement (Fig. 53-14),[18] and is accompanied by a higher in-hospital morbidity and mortality.[19]

### SUBATRIOVENTRICULAR NODAL BLOCK

Right bundle-branch block with or without hemiblock during acute anterior MI indicates proximal LAD occlusion.[7] Bundle branch block or complete AV block indicates a poor prognosis.[20–22] Left anterior fascicular block in acute inferior MI suggests additional LAD disease (Fig. 53-15).[23]

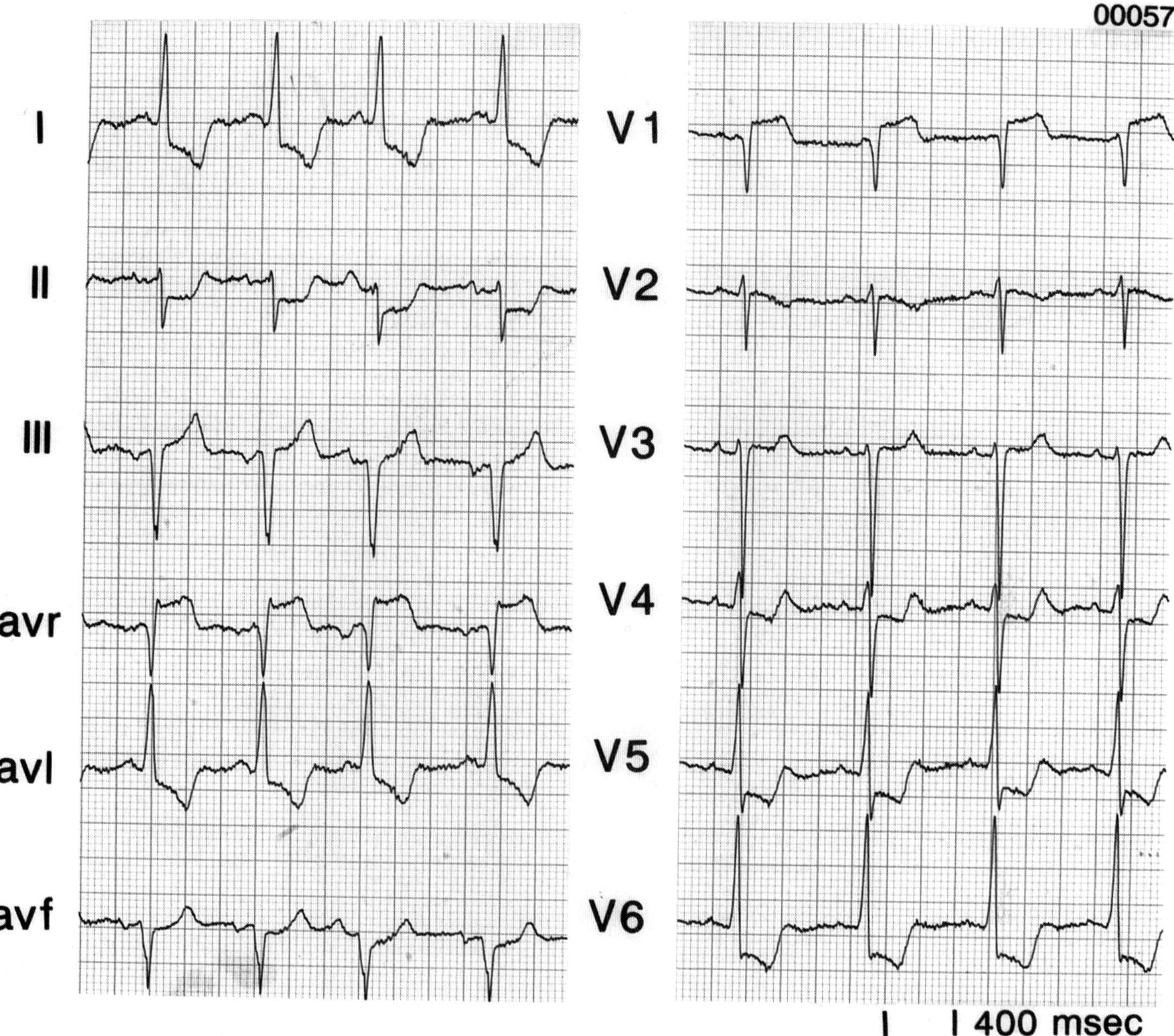


FIGURE 53-16 Left main coronary artery obstruction. Sinus rhythm of 75 beats per minute and slight widening of the QRS complexes, with absence of the initial septal q wave. Note the extensive downsloping ST-segment depressions, especially in leads I, II, and $V_4$ to $V_6$. Moreover, marked ST-segment elevation is present in leads aVR and $V_1$, typically being more pronounced in lead aVR.

## LEFT MAIN STEM STENOSIS OR THREE-VESSEL DISEASE

Acute complete obstruction of the left main coronary artery (LMCA) is rare but causes severe hemodynamic deterioration. More frequently, subtotal stenosis is seen or with collateral filling from the RCA, presenting as unstable angina. The ECG in the latter situation is similar to that of severe proximal three-vessel disease[24]: marked, downsloping ST-segment depression in leads I, II, and $V_4$ through $V_6$ and ST-segment elevation in lead aVR. The negative predictive and positive accuracy of this pattern was 78 and 62 percent, but when the total amount of ST-segment change was $\geq$ 12 mm, the chance for three-vessel or left main stem coronary artery disease (CAD) rose to 86 percent.

In total LMCA obstruction[25] (Fig. 53-16), lead aVR ST-segment elevation ($\geq$0.05 mV) occurred more often (88 percent) than in LAD (43 percent) or RCA (8 percent) occlusion and was higher (0.16 mV) than in LAD occlusion (0.04 mV). Lead $V_1$ ST-segment elevation was lower in the LMCA group (0.00 mV) than in the LAD group (0.14 mV). This finding had an 81 percent sensitivity, 80 percent specificity, and 81 percent accuracy to distinguish both conditions. Death occurred more frequently in those with higher ST segment elevation in lead aVR.

## ATRIAL INFARCTION

The signs of atrial MI are seen during the repolarization phase of the atria, the Ta segment. Elevation of the Ta segment occurs in leads I,

II, III, $V_5$, or $V_6$ or a depression is observed in the precordial leads (Fig. 53-14)[26,27] Atrial MI may be seen in 10 percent of acute inferoposterior MI. It occurs in the setting of ventricular MI; isolated occurrence is rare,[28] Atrial MI indicates proximal occlusion of the RCA or CX. Complications are atrial fibrillation or flutter, chaotic atrial rhythm, sinus standstill, and, less frequently, thromboembolic events or rupture of the atrial wall.

## LIMITATIONS

Assessment of the site of occlusion of a coronary vessel by the ECG is most reliable in case of a first MI and is impaired by multivessel disease, an old MI, collateral circulation, and when ventricular activation is altered, as in preexistent left bundle branch block, preexcitation, and paced rhythms.

## CONCLUSION

In acute cardiac ischemia, the aggressiveness of therapy should be determined by the occlusion site and the related size of the area at risk. The ECG can be of great help in providing that information.

## ACKNOWLEDGMENT

The art work of Ms. Adri van den Dool and of Ms. Mary Anne Williams is gratefully acknowledged.

## References

1. O'Keefe JH, Sayed-Taha K, Gibson W, et al. Do patients with left circumflex coronary artery-related acute myocardial infarction without ST-segment elevation benefit from reperfusion therapy? *Am J Cardiol* 1995;75:718–720.
2. Engelen DJ, Gorgels AP, Cheriex EC, et al. Value of the electrocardiogram in localizing the occlusion site in the left coronary artery in acute anterior myocardial infarction. *J Am Coll Cardiol* 1999;34:389–395.
3. Tamura A, Kataoka H, Mikuriya Y, Nasu M. Inferior ST-segment depression as a useful marker for identifying proximal left anterior descending artery occlusion during acute anterior wall myocardial infarction. *Eur Heart J* 1995;16:1795–1799.
4. Porter A, Sclarovsky S, Ben-Gal T, et al. Value of T wave direction with lead III ST-segment depression in acute anterior myocardial infarction: Electrocardiographic prediction of a wrapped left anterior descending coronary artery. *Clin Cardiol* 1998;21:562–566.
5. Tamura A, Kataoka H, Nagase K, et al. Clinical significance of inferior ST elevation during acute myocardial infarction. *Br Heart J* 1995; 74:611–614.
6. Kataoka H, Tamura A, Yano S, et al. ST elevation in the right chest leads in anterior wall ventricular acute myocardial infarction. *J Am Coll Cardiol* 1990;66:1146–1147.
7. Lie KJ, Wellens HJJ, Schuilenburg RM, Durrer D. Factors influencing prognosis of bundle branch block complicating acute antero-septal infarction. *Circulation* 1974;50:935–941.
8. Melgarejo-Moreno A, Galcera-Tomas J, Garcia-Alberola A, et al. Incidence, clinical characteristics, and prognostic significance of right bundle-branch block in acute myocardial infarction: A study in the thrombolytic era. *Circulation* 1997;96:1139–1144.
9. Herz I, Assali AR, Adler Y, et al. New electrocardiographic criteria for predicting either the right or left circumflex artery as the culprit coronary artery in inferior wall acute myocardial infarction. *Am J Cardiol* 1997;80:1343–1345.
10. Assali A, Sclarovsky S, Herz I, et al. Comparison of patients with inferior wall acute myocardial infarction with versus without ST-segment elevation in leads V5 and V6. *Am J Cardiol* 1998;81:81–83.
11. Braat SH, Gorgels APM, Bär FWHM. Value of the ST-T segment in lead $V_{4R}$ in inferior wall acute myocardial infarction to predict the site of coronary artery occlusion. *Am J Cardiol* 1988;62:140–142.
12. Peterson ED, Hathaway WR, Zabel M, et al. Prognostic significance of precordial ST segment depression during inferior myocardial infarction in the thrombolytic era: Results in 16521 patients. *J Am Coll Cardiol* 1996;28:305–312.
13. Birnbaum Y, Wagner GS, Barbash GI, et al. Correlation of angiographic findings and right (V1-V3) versus left (V4-V6) precordial ST-segment depression in inferior wall acute myocardial infarction. *Am J Cardiol* 1999;83:143–148.
14. Kontos M, Desai PV, Jesse RL, Ornato JP. Usefulness of the admission electrocardiogram for identifying the infarct related artery in inferior wall acute myocardial infarction. *Am J Cardiol* 1997;79:182–184.
15. Shah A, Wagner GS, Green CL, et al. Electrocardiographic differentiation of the ST-segment depression of acute myocardial injury due to the left circumflex artery occlusion from that of myocardial ischemia of nonocclusive etiologies. *Am J Cardiol* 1997;79:512–513.
16. Matetzky S, Freimark D, Chouraqui P, et al. Significance of ST segment elevations in posterior chest leads ($V_7$ to $V_9$) in patients with acute inferior myocardial infarction: Application for thrombolytic therapy. *J Am Coll Cardiol* 1998;31:506–511.
17. Mittal SR. Isolated right ventricular infarction. *Int J Cardiol* 1994;46: 53–60.
18. Braat S, de Zwaan C, Brugada P, et al. Right ventricular involvement with acute myocardial infarction identifies high risk of developing atrioventricular nodal conduction disturbances. *Am Heart J* 1984;107: 1103–1107.
19. Berger P, Ruocco N, Ryan T, et al. Incidence and prognostic implications of heart block complicating acute inferior myocardial infarction treated with thrombolytic therapy: Results from TIMI II. *J Am Coll Cardiol* 1992;20:533–540.
20. Newby KH, Pisano E, Krucoff MW, et al. Incidence and clinical relevance of the occurrence of bundle branch block in patients treated with thrombolytic therapy. *Circulation* 1996;94:2424–2428.
21. Barron HV, Bowlby LJ, Breen T, et al. Use of reperfusion therapy for acute myocardial infarction in the United States: Data from the national registry of myocardial infarction. *Circulation* 1998;97:1150–1156.
22. Harpaz D, Behar S, Gotlieb S, et al. Complete atrioventricular block complicating acute myocardial infarction in the thrombolytic era. *J Am Coll Cardiol* 1999;34:1721–1728.
23. Assali A, Sclarovsky S, Herz I, et al. Importance of left anterior hemiblock development in inferior wall acute infarction. *Am J Cardiol* 1997;79:672–674.
24. Gorgels AP, Vos MA, Mulleneers R, et al. Value of the electrocardiogram in diagnosing the number of severely narrowed coronary arteries in rest angina pectoris. *Am J Cardiol* 1993;72:999–1003.
25. Yamaji H, Iwasaki K, Kusachi S, et al. Prediction of acute left main coronary artery obstruction by 12-lead electrocardiography. ST segment elevation in lead aVR with less ST segment elevation in lead V(1). *J Am Coll Cardiol* 2001;38:1348–1354.
26. Nielsen FE, Andersen HH, Gram-Hansen P, et al. The relationship between ECG signs of atrial infarction and the development of supraventricular arrhythmias in patients with acute myocardial infarction. *Am Heart J* 1992;123:69–72.
27. Neven K, Crijns H, Gorgels A. Atrial infarction: A neglected ECG sign with important clinical implications. J Cardiovasc Electrophysiol 2003; 14:306–308.
28. Ventura T, Colantonio D, Leocata P, et al. Isolated atrial myocardial infarction: Pathological and clinical features in 10 cases. *Cardiologia* 1991;36:345–350.

# INDEX

NOTE: Boldface page numbers indicate main discussions; page numbers followed by *f* indicate figures and those followed by *t* indicate tables.

B

## D

G

I